SKILLS

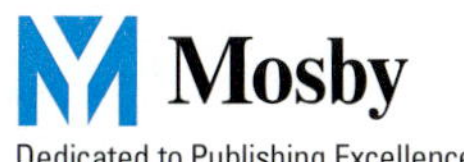

Publisher: Nancy L. Coon
Editor: Susan R. Epstein
Associate Developmental Editor: Laurie K. Muench
Project Manager: Carol Sullivan Weis
Senior Production Editor: Pat Joiner
Design Manager: Betty Schulz, Sheilah Barrett
Designer: Elizabeth Rohne Rudder
Manufacturing Manager: Theresa Fuchs
Illustrator: Lydia V. Kibiuk

Printed in the United States of America

Composition by The Clarinda Company
Printing/binding by Von Hoffman Press

Mosby–Year Book, Inc.
11830 Westline Industrial Drive
St. Louis, Missouri 63146

Library of Congress Cataloging in Publication Data

Foundations of nursing / edited by Barbara Lauritsen Christensen,
Elaine Oden Kockrow.—2nd ed.
p. cm.
Includes bibliographical references and index.
ISBN 0-8016-7784-X
1. Practical nursing. I. Christensen, Barbara Lauritsen.
II. Kockrow, Elaine Oden.
[DNLM: 1. Nursing. WY 100 F771 1994]
RT62.F68 1994
610.73—dc20
DNLM/DLC
for Library of Congress 94-20168
CIP

94 95 96 97 98 / 9 8 7 6 5 4 3 2 1

FOUNDATIONS OF NURSING

SECOND EDITION

Edited by

Barbara Lauritsen Christensen, RN, MS
Nurse Educator
Mid-Plains Community College
North Platte, Nebraska

Elaine Oden Kockrow, RN, MS
Nurse Educator
Mid-Plains Community College
North Platte, Nebraska

With 614 illustrations, with 346 in color

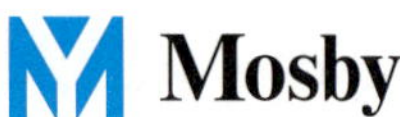

St. Louis Baltimore Berlin Boston Carlsbad Chicago London Madrid
Naples New York Philadelphia Sydney Tokyo Toronto

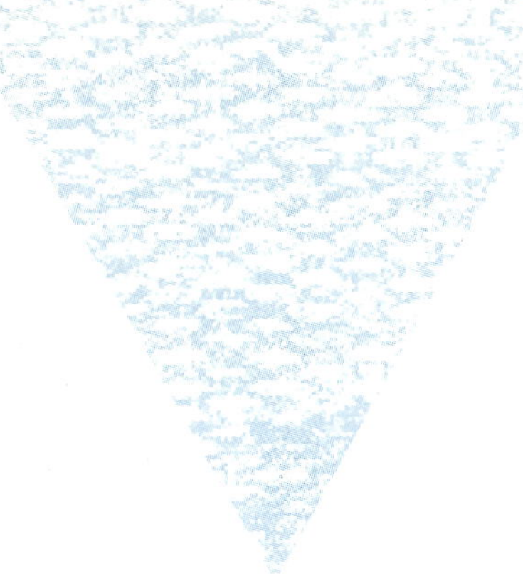

CONTRIBUTORS

First Edition

M. LYNNE ACHESON, RN, BSN
Staff Education Coordinator
Great Plains Regional Medical Center
North Platte, Nebraska

PERSEPHONE C. AGRAFIOTIS, RN, PhD
Management Consultant
Manchester, New Hampshire

JENANN ALLEN, RN, BS
Vocational Nursing Instructor
Grayson County College
Denison, Texas

LORA JEAN ALLEY, RN
Medical Assistant Instructor
Draughons Junior College
Bristol, Tennessee;
LPN Instructor, Jacksboro Vocational Technical School
Jacksboro, Tennessee

DONNA M. BABAO, RN, MA, MSN
Nursing Instructor, Yuba College
Marysville, California

SYLVIA LONG BALDWIN, RN, BSN
Instructor, Howard College Vocational Nursing Program
San Angelo Campus, San Angelo, Texas

SALLY L. PERSONS BECK, RN, MS, CPC
Rehabilitation Supervisor
Centennial Rehabilitation Associates, Inc.
Lincoln, Nebraska

BOBBIE BLOCH, RN, MSN
Doctoral Student
Department of Educational Technology
University of Toledo, Toledo, Ohio

LINDA CUTCHEN-CLARK, RN, MSN
Chair, Nursing Department
Butte College, Oroville, California

GLORIA DePOLE COSCHIGANO, RN, MSN
Assistant Professor of Nursing
Iona College, Elizabeth Seton School
Yonkers, New York

CYNTHIA M. DAVIS, MEd
Associate Professor of Nursing
Bainbridge College
Bainbridge, Georgia

CAROLYN DEAN, RN, BSN
Coordinator, Practical Nursing Program
North Central Missouri College
Trenton, Missouri

CAROLYN S. EDWARDS, RN, MEd
Coordinator, Wood County Vocational School of Practical Nursing
Parkersburg, West Virginia

JOSEPHINE M. ESTRADA, RN. BSN
Patient Care Coordinator for Home Health/Hospice
Great Plains Regional Medical Center
North Platte, Nebraska

JEANETTE M. JEFFERS, RN, C, PhD
Assistant Professor, Department of Nursing, The Wichita State University
Wichita, Kansas

FRANCES JEAN KELLEY, RN, PhD
Instructor, The University of Texas Health Science Center
Houston, Texas

SANDRA KLOCKE, RN, MS
Administrator
Statewide Home Health Program and Horizon Home Health Care Subunit
Nebraska State Health Department
Division of Community Health Nursing, North Platte, Nebraska

GRETCHEN H. LeGAULT, RN, MSN
Instructor, Fundamentals of Nursing, Psychiatric, Mental Health Nursing
Pima Community College, Tucson

KRISTEN KARTCHNER MAUGHAN, BS, RD
Nutrition Instructor, Mid-Plains Community College
North Platte, Nebraska

MARY MILLER-WERLINGER, RN, MSN, ANP
Staff Development Coordinator
Goodall-Witcher Hospital Foundation
Clifton, Texas

IVA L. MUELLER, RN, BSN
Assistant Director, Home Health Aides
Visiting Nurses' Association of Omaha; Graduate Student,
Creighton University—Pastoral Ministry, Omaha, Nebraska

RUTH BECKMANN MURRAY, RN, EdD
Professor and Coordinator
Psychiatric/Mental Health Nursing Graduate Major
St. Louis University School of Nursing, St. Louis, Missouri

JOYCE ELIZABETH MYERS, RN, MSN
Nursing Professor, Florida Community College at Jacksonville
Jacksonville, Florida

CHRISTINE NEFF, RN, BSN
Nursing Instructor, Mid-East Ohio Vocational School
Zanesville, Ohio

LINDA NORTH, RN, MSN
LPN Coordiantor and Instructor
Reid State Technical College, Evergreen, Alabama

PATRICIA HELMER OLES, RN, MSN
Assistant Professor of Nursing
Pasco-Hernando Community College
New Port Richey, Florida

KAREN H. RICHARDSON, RN, MA
Assistant Professor of Nursing
Pasco-Hernando Community College
New Port Richey, Florida

LINDA RICKEL, RNP, MSN
University of Arkansas at Pine Bluff;
John L. McClellan Veterans Hospital
Little Rock, Arkansas

ELIZABETH SCHENK, RN, MSN
Vice President of Nursing, Heather Hill, Inc.
Chardon, Ohio;
Clinical Faculty Member
Frances Payne Bolton School of Nursing
Case Western Reserve University, Cleveland, Ohio

GLADYS M. SCIPIEN, RN, MS
Assistant Professor, University of Massachusetts Boston, Harbor Campus
Boston, Massachusetts

ALITA SELLERS, RN, MDEd, PhD
Course Coordinator and Instructor
Western Pennsylvania Hospital, School of Nursing
Pittsburgh, Pennsylvania

ANNABELLE SITLER, RN, BSN
Instructor, Hannah E. Mullins School of Practical Nursing, Salem, Ohio

GEORGEANNA TEMRES SMITH, RN, MEd
Nursing Program Director
Northern Nevada Community College, Elko, Nevada

MARTHA E. SPRAY, RN, BSN
Adult Practical Nursing Instructor
Mid-East Ohio Vocational School District
Zanesville, Ohio

AUDREY WADMAN SZCZESIUL, RN, MS
Instructor, Practical Nurse Education Program
A.I. Prince Regional Vocational School
Hartford, Connecticut

PHYLLIS J. TURNER, RN. MS
Coordinator of Health Occupations Education
Jefferson Technical Institute, Metairie, Louisiana

HAZEL WALKER, RN. MNEd
Formerly Administrative Director, Division of Nursing
St. Francis Regional Medical Center
Wichita, Kansas

CONNIE M. WALLACE, RN, MSN
Nurse Educator, Jennie Edmundson Memorial Hospital
School of Nursing
Council Bluffs, Iowa

LOIS WHITE, RN, PhD
Director, Vocational Nursing
Del Mar College, Corpus Christi, Texas

GLORIA E. WOLD, RN, MS
Instructor, Laboratory Manager
Milwaukee Area Technical College
Milwaukee, Wisconsin

FOUNDATIONS OF NURSING

Second Edition

MARY LYNNE TODD ACHESON, RN, MSN
Staff Training and Development Coordinator
Great Plains Regional Medical Center
North Platte, Nebraska

PERSEPHONE C. AGRAFIOTIS, RN, PhD
Management Consultant
Manchester, New Hampshire

LORA MILLER ALLEY, RN
Formerly Practical Nurse Instructor/Medical Assistant Instructor
Abingdon, Virginia

DONNA M. BABAO, RN, BSN, MA, MSN
Nursing Instructor
Yuba College
Marysville, California

SYLVIA LONG BALDWIN, RN, BSN
Instructor, Vocational Nursing
Howard County Junior College
San Angelo, Texas

BOBBIE BLOCH, RN, BSN, MSN, PhD
Director of Education and Training
Calvert Memorial Hospital
Prince Frederick, Maryland

GERALD R. CHRISTENSEN, RP
Chief Pharmacist
Omaha Tribe of Nebraska
Macy, Nebraska

GLORIA DePOLE COSCHIGANO, RN, MSN, CS
Assistant Professor of Nursing
Iona College
New Rochelle, New York

CYNTHIA M. DAVIS, RN, BA, BSN, MEd
Associate Professor of Nursing
Bainbridge College
Bainbridge, Georgia

CAROLYN DEAN, RN, BSN
Coordinator, LPN Nursing Program
North Central Missouri College
Trenton, Missouri

SUSAN DE RIENZO DE VIVIO, RN, MPH
Pediatric Nurse Practitioner
Nassau County Medical Center
East Meadow, New York

CAROLYN EDWARDS, RN, BSN, MEd
Coordinator
Wood County Vocational School of Nursing
Parkersburg, West Virginia

JANICE BRIDGES FLYNN, BSN, MN
Assistant Professor of Nursing
Kennesaw State College
Marietta, Georgia

JOHN G. GUZALLIS, RP
Assistant Director of Pharmacy
Great Plains Regional Medical Center
North Platte, Nebraska

FRANCES JEAN KELLEY, RN, PhD
Assistant Professor of Clinical Nursing
The University of Texas Houston Health Science Center
Houston, Texas

SANDRA TROXEL KLOCKE, RN, BSN, MSEd
Administrator, Home Health Program
Nebraska Department of Health
Division of Community Health Nursing
North Platte, Nebraska

JAMES L. MANNING, RP
Director of Pharmacy
Great Plains Regional Medical Center
North Platte, Nebraska

MARIE ANN MARINO, RN, EdD, PNP
Pediatric Nurse Practitioner, Nassau County Medical Center
East Meadow, New York
Clinical Associate Professor, State University of New York at Stony Brook
Stony Brook, New York

KRISTEN KARTCHNER MAUGHAN, BS, RD
Adult Educator/Staff Dietitian, Great Plains Regional Medical Center
Nutrition Instructor, Mid-Plains Community College
Consultant, West Central Nebraska Area Agency on Aging
North Platte, Nebraska

JOYCE E. MYERS, RN, BSN, MN
Associate Professor of Nursing
DeKalb College
Clarkston, Georgia

M. CHRISTINE NEFF, RN, BSN
LPN Nursing Instructor
Mid-East Ohio Vocational School District
Zanesville, Ohio

LINDA NORTH, RN, MSN
LPN Coordinator/Instructor
Reid State Technical College
Evergreen, Alabama

PATRICIA HELMER OLES, RN, MSN, CS
Assistant Professor of Nursing
Pasco-Hernando Community College
New Port Richey, Florida

SALLY L. PERSONS-BECK, RN, BS, MSEd, CPC
Branch Manager
GENEX Rehabilitation Services
Des Moines, Iowa

ELAINE U. POLAN, RNC, BSN, MS
Assistant Nursing Supervisor
Vocational Education and Extension School of Practical Nursing
Uniondale, New York

CLAIRE RAYMOND, PHARM D
Medical Services Manager
Bristol-Myers Squibb
Cincinnati, Ohio

KAREN H. RICHARDSON, BSN, MA
Assistant Professor of Nursing
Pasco-Hernando Community College
New Port Richey, Florida

JUDY HOLT ROLLINS, RN, MS
Consultant, Rollins and Associates, Inc.
Instructor, Georgetown University School of Medicine
Coordinator, Studio G, Georgetown University Medical Center
Washington, DC

ELIZABETH SCHENK, RN, MSN
Vice President of Nursing, Heather Hill, Inc.
Clinical Faculty Member, Frances Payne Bolton School of Nursing
Case Western Reserve University
Cleveland, Ohio

ALITA K. SELLERS, RN, BSN, MNEd, PhD
Chairperson, Nursing
West Virginia University at Parkersburg
Parkersburg, West Virginia

ANNABELLE SITLER, RN, BSN
Instructor
Hannah E. Mullins School of Practical Nursing
Salem, Ohio

GEORGEANNA TEMRES SMITH, BSN, MEd, MSN
Nursing Program Director
Northern Nevada Community College
Elko, Nevada

SUE SMITH, RN, MHSc, MA
Counsellor/Consultant in Private Practice
Victoria, British Columbia

MARTHA E. SPRAY, RN, MS
Adult Practical Nursing Instructor
Mid-East Ohio Vocational School District
Zanesville, Ohio

PAULA L. STOBBS, RP
Staff Pharmacist
Great Plains Regional Medical Center
North Platte, Nebraska

AUDREY WADMAN SZCZESIUL, RN, BSN, MSEd
Instructor
A.I. Prince Regional Vocational Technical School
Hartford, Connecticut

MARY MILLER WERLINGER, RN, MS, CS, FNP-C
Family Nurse Practitioner, Community Internal Medicine Clinic
Scott and White Hospital
Temple, Texas

VIRGINIA F. WILKINSON, BSN
Program Administrator
HIV/AIDS Program
Nebraska Department of Health
Lincoln, Nebraska

GLORIA E. WOLD, RN, MS
Instructor/Nursing Laboratory Manager
Milwaukee Area Technical College
Milwaukee, Wisconsin

TONI C. WORTHAM, RNC, BSN, MSN
Associate Professor
Madisonville Community College
Madisonville, Kentucky

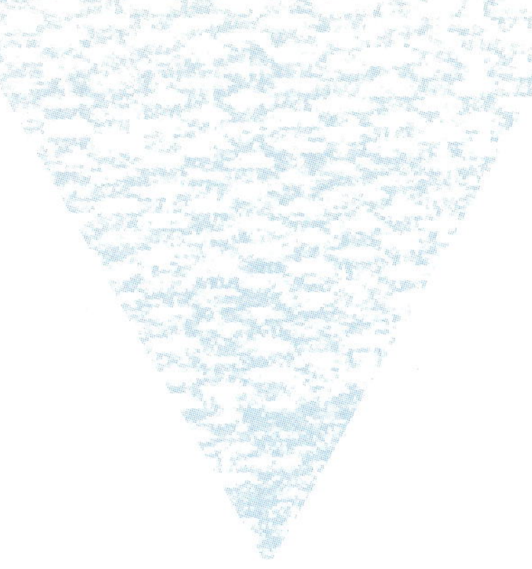

CONSULTANTS

JUDY ARMBRUSTER, BSN
Instructor, Practical Nursing
Northeast Community College
Norfolk, Nebraska

PEGGY BOHANNON, BS, MSN
Lead Instructor, LVN Program
Lee College
Baytown, Texas

CATHERINE BURKE, RN, MS
Nursing Instructor
Kankakee Community College
Kankakee, Illinois

DORIS BUSH, RN, MSN
Chair, Nursing and Allied Health
Bishop State Community College
Mobile, Alabama

DARLENE CHILES, RN, BSN
Practical Nursing Coordinator
Ohio Hi-Point JVSD School of Practical Nursing
Bellefontaine, Ohio

VIRGINIA CLEVENGER, RN, MA
Coordinator, Health Occupations
Mercer County Vocational School
Trenton, New Jersey

DOROTHY CREWS, RN, AS, BSN, MA, PhN
Nursing Instructor, LDN/ADN Program
Modesto Junior College
Modesto, California

FAITH DARILEK, RN, BSN
Director/Instructor
The Victoria College School of Vocational Nursing
Gonzales, Texas

PATRICIA DeVRIES, RN, MSN
Nursing Faculty
Muskegon Community College
Muskegon, Michigan

JUDITH DIEHL, RN, MS
Registered Nursing Instructor
Jefferson Davis Community College
Brewton, Alabama

MARIA DIXON, RN, MSN
Practical Nursing Instructor
Center for Arts and Technology–Brandywine Campus
Coatesville, Pennsylvania

JODY ECKLER, RN, BSN
Public Health Nurse
Huron County Health Department
Norwalk, Ohio

LINDA ELLSWORTH, RN, BSN
Practical Nursing Instructor
W. Howard Nicol School of Practical Nursing
Greensburg, Ohio

SANDRA L. EWUSIAK, RN, BSN
Assistant Professor
Jefferson Technical College
Steubenville, Ohio

ELIZABETH FAYRAM, BSN, MSN
Associate Professor
Edgewood College
Madison, Wisconsin

SHEILA FEENEY, RNC, NP, BSN
Staff Nurse, Emergency Room
Great Plains Regional Medical Center
North Platte, Nebraska

MARY K. FIET, RN, BSN
Hospice Coordinator
Beatrice Community Hospice
Beatrice, Nebraska

CAROL GREEN-NIGRO, RN, MSN, PhD CANDIDATE
Instructor
Johnson County Community College
Overland Park, Kansas

BETTY HAMLIN, RN, BA
Administrative Instructor, Placement and Follow-Up
Dalton School of Health Occupations
Dalton, Georgia

SALLY HOLLAND, RN, BSE, MEd
Coordinator, Health Occupations
James L. Walker Vocational Technical Center
Naples, Florida

BARBARA HUTCHINSON, BSN, MS, MSN
Professor
Mt. San Antonio College
Walnut, California

GARNET LAURITSEN JOHNSTON, RN
Staff Nurse, CCU
Mercy Hospital-Anderson
Cincinnati, Ohio

NANCY JO KASTOR, RN, BSN
Instructor
Portage Lakes Career Center
W. Howard Nicol School of Practical Nursing
Greensburg, Ohio

JOYCE KEENAN, RN, BSN, MSN
Assistant Professor
Thiel College
Greenville, Pennsylvania

LINDA KERBY, BA, BSN, MA
Hospice Nurse
Leawood, Kansas

SANDRA KIRKLAND, BS, MSN, CETN
Instructor
University of South Alabama
Mobile, Alabama

PATTY KNECHT, ADN, BSN
Practical Nursing Instructor
Center for Arts and Technology-Brandywine Campus
Coatesville, Pennsylvania

ELAINE MASEBERG, RN, BSN, MSN
Instructor
Mid-Plains Community College
North Platte, Nebraska

SHARON NEANOVER, RNC
Instructor
Butler County Practical Nurse Program
Fort Hamilton Hughes Memorial Hospital
Hamilton, Ohio

MURIEL OWEN, RN, BSN, MN
Director, Education and Vocational Nursing
Concorde Career Institute
San Diego, California

BARBARA D. POWE, RN, PhD, CCRN
Nursing Faculty
Florence Darlington Technical College
Florence, South Carolina

SUZANNA SALMON, RN, BSN
Practical Nursing Instructor
W. Howard Nicol School of Practical Nursing
Greensburg, Ohio

JOANNA SCALABRINI, RNC, BSN, MSN, MA
Chair, Practical Nursing
Westchester Community College
Valhalla, New York

ELAINE SCHMIDT, RN, MSN
Nursing Instructor, IVY Tech State College
Evansville, Indiana

MARY ANN SHEA, JD, RN, BS
Attorney at Law/Registered Nurse
St. Louis, Missouri

ANITA KAY SWARTZWELDER, BSN, CNOR
Practical Nursing Instructor
Kentucky Tech-Ashland Campus
Ashland, Kentucky

JULIE THELAN, RN
Director, Home & Community Health Agency
Great Plains Regional Medical Center
North Platte, Nebraska

KAREN TINDALL, ADN, BSN, MA
Coordinator/Associate Professor, Practical Nursing
Central Florida Community College
Ocala, Florida

CAPTAIN CANDACE TULL, RNC, BSN, CCE, CBE
Perinatal Education Case Manager
USAF Nurse Corps, Wilford Hall Medical Center
San Antonio, Texas

JUDY WHITE, RN, BS
Lead Instructor, Practical Nursing
Ivy Tech State College
Richmond, Indiana

BEVERLY POST YESHION, RN, BSN, ACCE
Instructor/Nurse Consultant
Hillsborough Community College
Tampa, Florida

To My Three Children
Jennifer Holly, MD
Jessica Heather, BA
Jason Heath, BA
Who have so lovingly enhanced
my exciting voyage through life.

To My Siblings
Shirlee, Ann, Lowell Chris, and Garnet
Whose friendship and interest have
lasted a lifetime. Our parents
would be so pleased.

BARBARA CHRISTENSEN

To My Beloved Father
Charles T. Oden
Whose pride and dignity in life
provide a role model.

To My Dear Husband
Donald
Whose patience, support, sense of humor,
and attentiveness have given me strength
and the freedom to complete this labor of love.

ELAINE KOCKROW

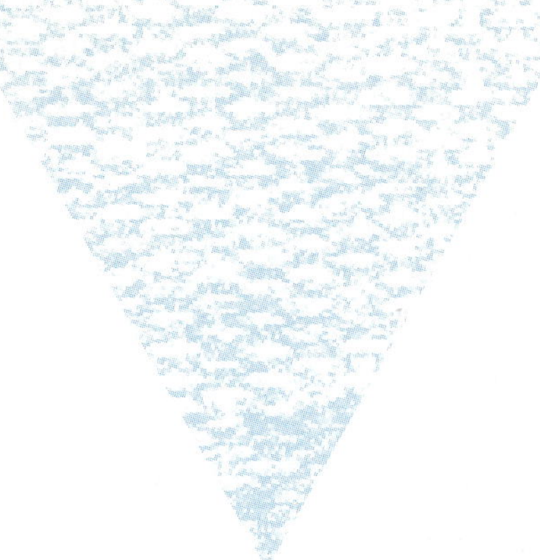

PREFACE

Foundations of Nursing was developed to provide practical and vocational nursing students (RNA students in Canada) with the knowledge required to competently and safely care for a wide variety of patients in numerous settings. Unique to this text is its comprehensive coverage of all areas of the practical/vocational nursing curriculum. Coverage includes the historical, legal, and ethical aspects of nursing, as well as communications, life span development, anatomy and physiology, medical-surgical nursing, cultural aspects of nursing, basic nursing skills, care of the surgical patient, mathematics review, and medication administration. The text also includes maternal and neonatal, pediatric, gerontological, mental health, community health, and emergency nursing, as well as dying and death, and the world of the graduate. The text may stand alone or be used with a few supplemental titles.

The future of nursing promises dynamic change and continual challenge. The role of the nurse as caregiver and teacher will continue to broaden in scope, reflecting the changing needs of society and the evolution of innovative health care delivery. Regardless of the technological advances or reforms to the health care system that lie ahead, the heart of nursing practice will, and must, remain the same—people caring for other people with sensitivity, knowledge, skill, and compassion. This philosophy is echoed by the students whose personal reasons for pursuing a career in nursing begin each unit.

As nursing education addresses changes in practice, so must nursing textbooks. This edition has been revised and expanded to reflect current practice and anticipated developments through the end of the century. We are indebted to the educators and students who have shared their thoughts and ideas with us, and credit each of them as valuable collaborators for this revision.

FEATURES

The numerous features of *Foundations of Nursing* are designed to enhance learning, promote understanding, and emphasize essential aspects of today's practice. These features include:

- A readable writing style engages the student and ensures comprehension.
- An attractive, logical design provides bold headings and large, clear type to make the text easy to read and follow.
- Numerous boxes and tables highlight and summarize important content.
- Hundreds of large, clear illustrations, many in full color, reinforce and clarify key concepts and techniques.
- Detailed, full-color anatomical drawings help students visualize the intricacies of the body.
- Nursing process provides a consistent format for presenting care that reflects the focus of current practice, as well as the test plan for the licensure examination.
- Dozens of skills are presented in a logical, step-by-step format with rationales for nursing actions to help students understand how and why procedures are performed. Sample documentation is included to illustrate what information to record and provide examples of proper phrasing and accurate descriptions. Special concerns highlight gerontological considerations that may require modifying technique or ob-

serving for potential problems. Patient teaching regarding variations for the home or long-term care facility is provided to address the growing trend of community-based care.

- Therapeutic dialogues provide examples of effective communication techniques to reduce students' anxiety and promote positive nurse-patient interaction.
- Sample care plans are based on realistic case studies to help students learn to plan individualized care. Based on tenth conference NANDA nursing diagnoses, care plans focus on patient-centered goals and expected outcomes.
- Learning aids in each chapter are designed to help students identify and review important content. Objectives, key terms, and related topics of interest begin each chapter; the objectives and key terms for anatomy and physiology are listed separately for clarity. Key terms are boldfaced and defined in the chapter. Chapters conclude with Chapter Challenges that feature key concepts and clinically based study questions that reflect the new NCLEX format.
- A glossary of terms allows students quick access to nursing and medical terminology.

Many new features address the expanding roles and responsibilities of the practical/vocational nurse in the nineties and include:

- Critical thinking questions conclude each nursing care plan to help students learn to better evaluate care and address patient needs.
- Patient teaching content helps students identify topics and develop teaching techniques.
- Gerontological considerations boxes alert students to the normal changes of aging as well as the special needs of the older adult.
- Medication tables provide essential information on the action, dosage, side effects, and nursing considerations for commonly used drugs.

NEW AND EXPANDED CONTENT

All content in this second edition has been thoroughly reviewed and revised to incorporate the most accurate, current, and clinically relevant information available. To reflect changes in practice and in response to suggestions from students and educators, a number of areas have been substantially rewritten and expanded, and new content has been developed. Throughout the text, prognosis statements have been added for each disease condition. Other changes include the following:

- Legal aspects have been revised and expanded based on reviews by a nurse attorney.
- Chapters on communication and nursing process were completely rewritten to enhance student comprehension.
- Normal growth and development is now presented in one logical, comprehensive chapter to provide a clear overview.
- The unit on pediatric nursing has been revised and expanded by pediatric nurse practitioners to provide complete coverage of health maintenance and care of the child with physical or emotional problems.
- Nursing skills, including sterile technique, nasogastric tube insertion, and application of heat and cold therapy, have been added.
- The chapter on care of the surgical patient has been revised and expanded to better prepare students to care for these patients and ready them for early discharge.
- Separate chapters provide expanded coverage of patients with cardiovascular conditions and blood or lymphatic disorders.
- The chapter on AIDS, updated and rewritten by Nebraska's program administrator for HIV and AIDS, now includes the most current information and therapies.
- The chapter on care of the older adult has been revised by Gloria Wold, author of *Basic Geriatric Nursing,* to thoroughly prepare students to deal with the physiological and psychological needs of this important population.
- The final chapter includes a discussion of the computerized NCLEX-PN CAT examination.

TEACHING-LEARNING PACKAGE

We recognize that educators today have limited time in which to prepare classroom and clinical activities. We have therefore provided an expanded *Instructor's Resource Manual* that includes numerous suggested activities as well as a totally revised *Test Bank* that follows the new NCLEX format. In addition, we have added a set of full-color transparency acetates designed to supplement and enhance lectures.

To help students make maximum use of their study time and reinforce learning, we again offer a comprehensive study guide (prepared by Brenda Goodner). This guide is keyed chapter by chapter to the text and includes a wide variety of questions and activities to promote understanding and retention of key content. Performance checklists for skills in the text are also provided.

We are pleased to note the growing number of men currently involved in the practice of nursing and acknowledge their dedication, skill, and professionalism. We have therefore made every effort to eliminate any gender-specific pronouns. In a very few instances, we have used "she" to refer to the nurse and "he" to refer to the patient to clearly communicate to the reader.

ACKNOWLEDGMENTS

This edition has been achieved through research, attention to detail, and response to the many educators and students throughout the nation. We are grateful for the success of the first edition and are honored to contribute to the continuing education of student nurses.

For the completion of this text, one must have the contribution of knowledgeable and creative individuals. We wish to recognize those persons who have assisted us with this text.

We would first like to acknowledge the editorial staff at Mosby: our Editor, Suzi Epstein, for her confidence in our nursing expertise and her outstanding creativeness; Kathy Sartori, our Developmental Editor, for her kindness and organizational skills; Laurie Muench, our Associate Developmental Editor for her sincerity, promptness, and interest; Pat Joiner, our Senior Production Editor, for her punctuality and attention to detail; Liz Rudder, our Book Designer, and Betty Schulz and Sheilah Barrett, our Design Managers, for their ability to add brightness and interest to the textbook.

We are indebted to Lydia Kibiuk, Medical Illustrator, for her infectious enthusiasm and multiple talents and to James Helie of the Camera and Lab Shop for the use of his talents on the photo shoot. We also wish to thank all of the authors from Mosby for the use of their artwork.

We are grateful for the knowledge and skills of our authors, contributors, and reviewers. Without the broad demographic representation, the completion of the most current nursing knowledge could not have been achieved. We extend a heartfelt "thank you" to Brenda Goodner for her efforts to expand the Study Guide.

The staff of Great Plains Regional Medical Center have contributed in numerous ways to enhance this textbook. Our special thanks to Cindy Bradley, Nancy Hudson, Dr. Dorothy Wycoff, Dr. Richard Byrne, Bonnie Reynolds, Karen Exon, Janelle Hawks, and Sheila Feeney.

Mid-Plains Community College has enthusiastically supported our efforts to complete this second edition. Pauline Shahan, Director of Health Occupations, has quietly encouraged the undertaking of this edition. We wish to give special acknowledgment to Debbie Beebout, our typist, whose outstanding secretarial skills assisted us in the many revisions and numerous additions.

Special thanks to Gloria Wold, who not only revised the chapter on care of the older adult, but also provided the gerontological considerations boxes that appear throughout the text. Our thanks to Claire Raymond, RP; Gerald R. Christensen, RP; John G. Guzallis, RP; James L. Manning, RP; and Paula L. Stobbs for their expertise in preparing the excellent medication tables and helpful pharmacology consultation.

We wish to thank our families for their love, kindness, and interest that provided us with strength and encouragement to complete this laborious task. Last, we wish to express to each other our gratitude for the gift of friendship that is sterling and has provided us with courage, enthusiasm, energy, and purpose.

Barbara Lauritsen Christensen
Elaine Oden Kockrow

CONTENTS

14 COMMUNITY HEALTH NURSING

15 EMERGENCY NURSING

1

INTRODUCTION TO NURSING

I hold within my mind a dream. A dream I've carried for 36 years—to become a nurse. A dream which almost became reality 30 years ago. However, like Florence Nightingale's lamp, it flickered with the winds of time. A dream dampened down, put on hold. Yet flickering under the surface of marriage, a family, and discontent. Too far away for educational opportunities, that tiny flame continued to be fed by work at a hospital. Nudging my mind frequently with "Someday it will become reality." Just waiting for the fuel of a short phrase heard with a small corner of a busy mind, "LPN program starting soon." Wait! Wait! Tell me, tell me, tell me more! With encouragement from a loving husband, "Go for it, if that's what you want. I'll get by." A weekend wife, longing for home, studing with all my might. With Practical Nursing a big step toward that continual need to help others. A stepping stone on the way up. . .

Sue Lucht
Student Nurse

1

THE EVOLUTION OF NURSING

Persephone C. Agrafiotis

KEY TERMS

accreditation
approved program
health
health care system
holistic
holistic health care
illness
licensure
medicine
patient
wellness

LEARNING OBJECTIVES

After reading this chapter, the student should be able to do the following:

- Define the key terms.
- Describe the evolution of nursing and nursing education from early civilization to the twentieth century.
- Define the four purposes of NAPNES and NFLPN.
- List the major developments of practical/vocational nursing.
- Identify the components of the health care system.
- Identify the participants of the health care system.
- Describe the complex factors involved in the delivery of patient care.
- Define practical/vocational nursing.
- Describe the purpose, role, and responsibilities of the practical/vocational nurse.

RELATED TOPICS OF INTEREST

- Legal aspects of nursing (Chapter 2)
- Ethical aspects of nursing (Chapter 3)
- Communication (Chapter 4)
- The nursing process (Chapter 5)
- Documentation (Chapter 6)

THE HISTORY OF NURSING AND NURSING EDUCATION

Nursing has evolved over many years, influenced by the means by which the sick were cared for. Changes in the way people live, the interrelationship of people with their environment, the search for knowledge and truth through education, and technological advances have made nursing and nursing education what they are and what they will be. Nursing evolves as society and health care needs and policies change. Nursing responds and adapts to these changes, meeting new challenges as they arise.

Care of the Sick During Early Civilization

In 5000 BC there was little reference to nursing, per se. **Illness** (an abnormal process in which aspects of the social, emotional, or intellectual condition and function of a person are diminished or impaired) was considered to be directly related to disfavor with God. Primitive people believed that a person became sick when an evil spirit entered the body and that the presence of a good spirit kept disease away.

Medicine men performed witchcraft on the affected part of the body to induce the bad spirits to leave the body. Some of the techniques involved the use of frightening masks, noises, incantations, vile odors, charms, spells, and even sacrifices.

Men assisted the medicine men in treating illnesses. They used purgatives, emetics, application of hot and cold substances, cauterization, cupping, blistering, and massage. Few women assisted the medicine men. They assisted mostly women in childbirth.

The Babylonians were intellectually, socially, and scientifically well developed. Many wars brought misery, suffering, illness, and injury to their people. There is evidence that some form of medical service existed and that laypersons provided this service. It is believed that these caregivers were usually men. If they were women, they were probably of low status because the actions of Babylonian women were dominated by men.

The ancient Hebrews, according to the Talmud and the Old Testament, attributed their misfortunes and illnesses to God's wrath. They depended on Him to restore them to **health** (a condition of physical, mental, and social well-being and the absence of disease or other abnormal conditions) when they were sick. They combined their religious beliefs with the hygienic practices that they acquired from Babylonia, where they had been in captivity. These practices included the inspection of all meats and the careful selection and preparation of all foods. They prevented the spread of communicable disease by burning infected garments and scrubbing the homes of those infected with the disease. Nurses were mentioned occasionally in the Talmud as persons caring for the sick in their homes. This appears to have been a demonstration of the first public health/home care movement.

Ancient records of early Egyptian civilization described nursing procedures, such as feeding a **patient** (a recipient of a health care service) with tetanus and dressing wounds.

Records of pre-Christian India reported the establishment of hospitals where the sick were cared for. The reports described a body of attendants, probably male, who were of good behavior, who were distinguished for purity and cleanliness of habits, and who were clever, skillful, and endowed with kindness. They bathed patients, made beds, and were always willing to do whatever they could to assist the sick.

By 500 BC the Hellenic civilization showed keen intellect, independent thinking, democratic action, and a thirst for knowledge and truth. **Medicine** (the art and science of the diagnosis, treatment, and prevention of disease and the maintenance of good health) progressed from the belief that demons and spirits caused human ills to the founding of temples suitable for rest and restoration of health. These temples, often referred to as hospitals, resembled our health centers of today: they had spas, mineral springs, bath gymnasiums, and treatment and consultation rooms. The religious influence was still present in the form of prayer, thanks offerings, and rituals. Priestesses served as attendants and cared for the sick. Pregnant women and people with incurable diseases were not admitted.

Hippocrates, born in 460 BC on the island of Cos in the Mediterranean, was a brilliant, progressive physician and teacher. He rejected the belief in the supernatural origin of disease and adopted a system of physical assessment, observation, and record keeping as an integral part of patient care. As his patient-centered care approach and medical ethics were adopted, Hippocrates was named the "Father of Medicine" and is credited with the Hippocratic Oath, which is still taken by physicians today. The work of Hippocrates is the basis for the **holistic** (of or pertaining to the whole; considering all factors, as *holistic medicine*) approach to patient care.

The Greek influence on the care of the sick changed the approach from one of mysticism to that of public health and safety. The religious influence was still prevalent, but with an emphasis on the poor, the sick, the widowed, and the children. Deacons and deaconesses were designated by the Roman bishops to assist the church by providing services, such as visiting sick women in their homes, visiting and tending to the needs of prisoners, and watching over the sick in the hospitals. One of the first deaconesses, Phoebe, performed nursing functions about AD 60. She was known as a visiting nurse, attending the sick and poor in their homes. Another Roman woman, Fabiola, spent her wealth and time nursing the sick and poor. She is credited with providing the first free hospital in Rome in AD 390.

Monastic and military orders were charged with caring for the sick over the next 1000 years, but the rise and fall of feudalism in Central Europe hindered the progress made in Greece and Rome. Famine, disease, war, and the emphasis on survival resulted in an increased need to care for the sick and poor, but the ongoing battles between the church and state hindered the development of any one approach to patient care. Care of the sick was performed by both men and women. Female religious orders were concerned with the care of the sick and needy, but the concern for religious problems took priority. Male military personnel served the medical needs of soldiers on the battlefield.

Organized Nursing Education in the Nineteenth Century

In the early nineteenth century, hospitals were overcrowded, and there was a lack of trained and qualified people who were interested in caring for the sick and the infirm. Hospitals were a place to contract diseases rather than be cured of them, because of patients with open wounds and unchecked infection and the dirty physical conditions of the plant itself. Women of "proper upbringing" did not work outside of the home during this time. As a result, nursing attracted inferior and undesirable lower-class women who drank heavily and engaged in prostitution. The best sources of nurses were the religious nursing orders, but these orders could not begin to meet the ever-increasing need for nursing services.

The Lutheran Order of Deaconesses established the first real school of nursing under the guidance of Theodor Fliedner, a German pastor in Kaiserswerth, Germany. The reputation of the school spread throughout Europe. It reached a young woman in England whose interest in nursing overshadowed the opposition of her family, her friends, and the social class to which she belonged. Florence Nightingale (Fig. 1-1), a strong-minded, intelligent, and determined young woman, joined the Kaiserswerth program in 1851 at the age of 31.

Armed with the education and training she received at Kaiserswerth and with her administrative and organizational skills, Florence Nightingale became the superintendent of a charity hospital for ill governesses in 1853. The governing board of the hospital was not always pleased with the changes and innovations she made and the guidance she gave her uneducated nurses, even though the quality of patient care improved.

In the following year, when she was preparing to become Superintendent of King's College Hospital in London, news of the atrocious conditions befalling the wounded soldiers in the Crimean War reached England. People were greatly concerned over the number of casualties and deaths that were reported. The Secretary of War, a long-standing friend of Miss Nightingale, asked her to lead a group of nurses to Scutari, Turkey, to care for the wounded. Ironically she had sent him a letter offering her services at about the same time. Within a week of receiving the Secretary's letter, she and 38 nurses left England for Turkey.

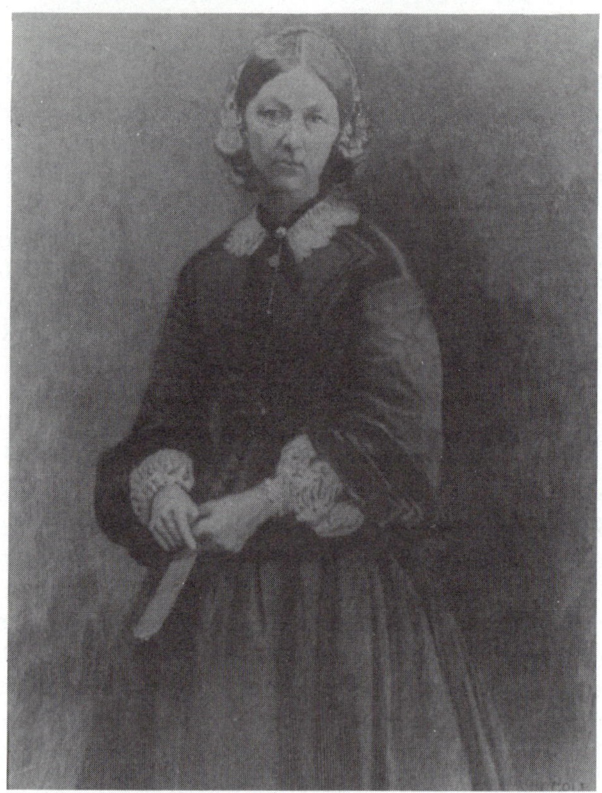

FIG. 1-1 Florence Nightingale. (From Cole T: Florence Nightingale, Wood engraving, National Library of Medicine, Bethesda, Md.)

Once again Florence Nightingale applied the principles of nursing she had learned at Kaiserswerth. These concepts, coupled with her dedication and leadership, turned the tide. The hospital units were cleaned, clothes were washed regularly, and sanitary conditions, which were nonexistent before her arrival, were established. The mortality among the casualties dropped significantly. Not only had the physical environment of the hospital been changed by Florence Nightingale's actions, but through her patience, dedication, and empathetic treatment of the soldiers, a psychological change took place as well. The soldiers grew to respect her and looked forward to her presence on the wards. They looked for her smile and took strength from her self-fulfilled personality. When she made her rounds through the wards late at night, she carried a lamp to light her way through the rows of beds of the injured and sick. This practice became a ritual, and soon she was known as "The Lady with the Lamp." The small lamp she carried became her trademark and continues to be the symbol of the nursing profession around the world.

The standards of nursing care established by Florence Nightingale gained the respect of the medical community and led to improved care for the sick and a much improved image of nursing in general. The need for educated and trained nurses became painfully evident, and the time was right for a shift in the approach to nursing education.

In 1860 Florence Nightingale began the reformation of nursing from occupation to profession by establishing the nursing school at Saint Thomas Hospital in London. She chose this hospital for the location of the school because of its reputation as a progressive medical facility, and therefore it was the ideal place to promote the new standards of nursing in which she so strongly believed.

The nursing program operated separately from the hospital and was financially independent to ensure that the major emphasis of its activity was directed exclusively toward educating nursing students. A nurses' residence was provided for the students, who had to pass strict admission procedures. The length of nurses' training was 1 year and included both formal instruction and practical experience. Complete records were kept on each student's progress while at the school. This practice became known as the "Nightingale Plan," which was to become the model for nursing education in the twentieth century. After the students graduated, records were also kept on where they were employed. This eventually became a "register," which was the beginning of a movement to exercise control over the nursing graduate and to establish a standard for the practicing nurse.

Students admitted into the nursing program at Saint Thomas had to provide excellent character references, show a strong commitment to a career in nursing, and demonstrate that they were intellectually capable of passing the course of study before them. The resultant demand for "Nightingale nurses" was overwhelming. The improved patient care provided by this new breed of nurse included such measures as good hygiene, sanitation, patient observation, accurate record keeping, nutritional improvements, and the introduction and use of certain new medical equipment.

During the time that Florence Nightingale was active in Europe, the same kinds of patient care problems were occurring in America. Both the American Revolution and the Civil War were characterized by severe casualties, disease, infected wounds, and archaic medical care. As in the Crimean War, nurses were scarce and those who were available were poorly trained to handle the horrors of war. Women such as Dorothy Dix, Superintendent of Female Nurses of the Union Army in 1861, and Clara Barton, the founder of the Red Cross in 1881, tried to meet the needs of both the battlefield casualties and civilian casualties.

By the end of the nineteenth century, three schools of nursing had been established in the United States. All three of these schools were modeled after the Nightingale Plan. In May 1873 the Bellevue Hospital School of Nursing in New York established itself as the foremost proponent of the Nightingale Plan in America. In October of that same year the Connecticut Training School was opened in New Haven. In November the Boston Training School at the Massachusetts General Hospital began operating.

In the interest of establishing standards for the new nursing schools, dedicated women such as Isabelle Hampton Robb and Lavinia Dock organized The American Society of Superintendents of Training Schools of Nursing in 1894. The major goal of this organization was to set educational standards for nurses. The structure of the organization was modeled after that of the American Medical Association. A code of ethics for nurses was adopted by the Society, and this code, known as the Nightingale Pledge, is subscribed to by the nursing profession of today.

Changes in Nursing Practice and Education in the Twentieth Century

While the superintendents of the nurses' training schools organized at the national level, the graduates of those training schools organized in their own fashion at the local levels. They established the Alumnae Association in an attempt to establish standards for the actual practice of nursing.

However, change in nursing education and practice could not come about in a vacuum. Any change had to be affected by the social issues of the times. This resulted in the need for rigid standards and laws, which were bound to affect the supply of well-trained nurses. In 1903 the first nursing **licensure** (the granting of permission by a competent authority [usually a government agency] to an organization or individual to engage in a practice or activity that would otherwise be illegal) laws to protect the public, were passed in North Carolina, New Jersey, New York, and Virginia. As a result, the nursing organizations recognized the need to amend their purpose and redirect their focus. As part of the reorganization that followed, The American Society of Superintendents of Training Schools became the Education Committee of the National League for Nursing Education in 1903. The Alumnae Association became the American Nurses Association in 1911.

Concurrent with these changes, Isabelle Hampton Robb and Mary Adelaide Nutting developed a program at Columbia University to train and develop teachers of nursing. They were convinced that nurses needed not only a college education and clinical practice, but also specific training in theoretical knowledge. The belief that nurses needed such a balance of liberal arts education and nursing practice skills brought a new, balanced perspective to the profession of nursing.

World War I brought an increased demand for nurses. The newly formed Army and Navy Nurse Corps sought nurses whom school superintendents certified as having "good moral character and professional qualifications." The available supply of nurses could not meet the demand, so once again untrained women volunteered their services to their country. Nursing leaders, concerned that these untrained personnel would be caring directly for wounded and ailing soldiers without adequate training, quickly established the Army School of Nursing.

After the war the women who had served as military nurses returned to their homes and their previous jobs and careers. They had no desire to remain in nursing as civilians. The image attached to professional nurses still posed a problem for most women. Furthermore, they were disenchanted because nurses' training still focused heavily on "service to the patient" rather than on a comprehensive professional education. This was far removed from what the Nightingale Plan had proposed for aspiring nurses.

Twenty-five years later, the demand for trained nurses was once again escalated almost overnight because of World War II. Although medicine had advanced, so had the art of war, and the casualties were high and severe. Early in the war, the Cadet Nurse Corps was established to provide nursing education and training. The Corps provided an abbreviated training program designed to meet the needs of the war effort. Additionally, federally subsidized programs in nursing were developed and implemented to offer women and, for the first time, men an education and career in nursing while serving their country in the war. After the war, many of the nurses trained by these programs remained in military service. Prestige, pay, and the opportunity for advancement were much greater in the military service than for civilian nurses. Civilian nurses received low pay and worked long shifts under atrocious conditions in the major hospitals, particularly in urban areas. These conditions in no way could attract those who became nurses as a result of the war and who, ironically, enjoyed a certain life-style that war invariably provides. As a result, the shortage of nurses in the United States and other countries worsened.

The effects of World War I, the Great Depression, and World War II strongly influenced this deficit. Pressure was exerted on the state boards of nursing, which had licensure responsibility, to mandate requirements for nurses. State-administered licensing examinations were no longer considered adequate for the country's needs. The parochial state examinations were in no way standardized and allowed a wide spectrum of competence to enter nursing. National norms of competence were needed and quickly established.

The characteristics of health care changed rapidly as health care became an industry. Growth and diversity became the major emphasis as the industry of health care became increasingly lucrative. The need for nurses, particularly well-educated nurses, increased at a rate much greater than could be provided.

The nursing organizations continued to deliberate on the future of nursing as a profession. In 1965 the American Nurses Association (ANA) took the position that nursing education should take place in institutions of learning within the general system of education, much as Robb and Nutting had proposed in 1903. Their position paper further delineated that the minimum preparation for the beginning professional nurse should be a baccalaureate degree in nursing and that the minimum education for technical nursing practice should be an associate degree in nursing. Assistants to nurses, they said, should have preservice programs in vocational education rather than just on-the-job training. This position has had a profound effect. Since 1965 many hospital-based nursing programs have been disbanded and an increasing number of baccalaureate and associate degree nursing programs have been established in the colleges and universities. The intent is obviously to change the trend from "training" nurses to "educating" nurses.

DEVELOPMENT OF PRACTICAL/ VOCATIONAL NURSING IN THE UNITED STATES

The first school for training the practical nurse started in Brooklyn, New York, in 1892 and was conducted under the auspices of the Young Women's Christian Association (YWCA). The Ballard School, as it was known, was approximately 3 months in duration and trained its students to care for the chronically ill, the invalid, children, and the elderly. The main emphasis was on home care and included cooking, nutrition, basic science, and basic nursing procedures. Graduates of this program were referred to as *attendant nurses.*

Two other programs were started, and they were patterned after the Ballard School. In 1907 the Thompson Practical Nursing School opened in Brattleboro, Vermont, and in 1918 the Household Nursing Association School of Attendant Nursing (later changed to the Shepard-Gill School of Practical Nursing) opened in Boston. The focus of these programs continued to be on home nursing care and light housekeeping duties. Hospital experience was not a part of the training in the early programs. The Thompson School is still in operation and continues to be accredited by the National League for Nursing (NLN). Practical nursing programs developed slowly during the first half of the twentieth century. A total of 36 schools opened during this period.

There were few controls, little educational planning, and minimal supervision of practical nursing schools before 1940. The increased demand for nursing services brought on by World War II and the postwar years and the excellent bedside nursing care evidenced by the practical nurse resulted in the opening of 260 practical/vocational nursing programs between 1948 and 1954. These programs varied in administrative design. Some were affiliated with hospitals or chronic care institutions, whereas others aligned themselves with private agencies or private schools. Their commitment was meeting the needs of the sick. Students in these programs provided nursing services while they were obtaining their education and training. This apprentice training emphasized vocational/technical education. The allocation of federal funds for training practical/vocational nurses helped recruit men and women.

Practical nursing programs were increasing rapidly. The need to establish standards again became a major issue. The Association of Practical Nurse Schools was founded in 1941 and was dedicated exclusively to practical nursing. Its membership was multidisciplinary and included licensed practical nurses, registered nurses, physicians, hospital and nursing home administrators, students, and public figures. Together they planned the first standard curriculum for practical nursing. By 1942 they saw the need to change the name to the National Association of Practical Nurse Education (NAPNE). They broadened their focus to include education and practice and established an accrediting service for schools of practical/vocational nursing in 1945. The association changed its name in 1959 to the National Association for Practical Nurse Education and Service (NAPNES).

In 1949 the National Federation of Licensed Practical Nurses (NFLPN) was founded by Lillian Kuster. This association is the official membership organization for licensed practical and vocational nurses, and membership is limited to LVNs and LPNs.

These two organizations, the NAPNES and the NFLPN, set standards for practical/vocational nursing practice, promote and protect the interests of practical/vocational nurses, and educate and inform the general public about practical/vocational nursing.

In 1961 the NLN broadened its scope of service because of the growth of practical/vocational nursing programs. The NLN established a Department of Practical Nursing Programs and developed an accreditation service for these programs, which is now called the *Council of Practical Nursing Programs.*

For 20 years both the NLN and NAPNES provided accreditation services. Nursing programs had the option of selecting either organization from which to seek accreditation. In recent years, however, the NAPNES has discontinued this service.

Accreditation of a program differs from program approval. An **approved program** is one that meets minimum standards set by the respective state agency responsible for overseeing educational programs. The state seeks to ensure that a given program, for example, meets the needs of the student, has adequate course content and qualified faculty, is of sufficient length, has adequate facilities, and provides clinical experience. All these elements are needed for licensure. The state also ensures that the welfare of the public is protected by maintaining minimum standards. Approval is required for the program to operate. **Accreditation** involves the administration of a program voluntarily seeking a review by a given organization to determine whether the program meets the preestablished criteria of that organization. Many times the standards established by professional organizations that accredit are far higher than those established by the state. Although graduates of nonaccredited programs can take the licensure examination required in most states, accreditation is extremely important when programs seek federal funding.

Practical/vocational nursing programs continued to proliferate, and by the 1990-91 school year, 1125 practical/vocational nursing programs in the United States produced 38,100 graduates. Nursing programs are still offered by various organizations, such as high schools, trade or technical schools, hospitals, junior and community colleges, colleges and universities, and private education agencies. Health care corporations such as the Galen Health Institutes, Inc. (formerly, Humana Health Institute, Inc.) also offer practical/vocational programs. However, they must all meet minimum state standards. The length of the programs is usually 12 to 18 months, with a focus on nursing skills and theory that is correlated with clinical practice. On completing the program, the graduate is eligible to take the National Council Licensing Examination for Practical Nursing (NCLEX-PN).

Creative educational programs in nursing today offer various approaches to educating student practical/vocational nurses. The combination of practical/vocational nurse education with associate degree programs in 2-year colleges is available. At the successful completion of the first academic year, the student can either exit and take the licensure examination for practical/vocational nursing or continue for another year and earn an associate degree in nursing, becoming eligible to take the licensure examination for registered nursing. Many other programs offering other combinations of education and degrees are available throughout the United States. Twenty-four states have some type of articulation plan.

Events That Changed Practical/Vocational Nursing (Box 1-1)

Before 1860 nursing care in the United States was provided generally by persons who were self-taught and who gained what experience they could as they practiced their nursing skills. Registration, licensing, and title differentiation were not clear or were nonexistent. Clearly defined duties and responsibilities were absent.

Box 1-1 IMPORTANT DATES OF MAJOR EVENTS IN THE UNITED STATES

1892	The Ballard School at the YWCA in Brooklyn, New York, established the first school to train practical nurses.
1907	The Thompson Practical Nursing School in Brattleboro, Vermont, was the second practical nursing school to be established.
1914	The Mississippi State Legislature was the first political body to pass license laws controlling practical nurses.
1917	The Smith-Hughes Act was passed. It provided federal funding for vocationally oriented practical nursing programs.
1918	The Household Nursing Association School of Attendant Nursing in Boston, Massachusetts, later called the Shepard-Gill School of Practical Nursing, was the third practical nursing school established.
1941	The association of Practical Nursing Schools was founded. It set standards for practical nursing education.
1942	The Association of Practical Nursing Schools became the National Association of Practical Nurse Education (NAPNE).
1944	The U.S. Department of Vocational Education commissioned an intensive study to differentiate tasks of the practical nurse.
1945	New York became the only state to have mandatory licensure laws for practical nurses.
1949	The National Federation of Licensed Practical Nurses (NFLPN) was founded by Lillian Kuster. This association is the official membership organization for licensed practical and vocational nurses, and membership is limited to LVNs and LPNs.
1955	All the states passed licensure laws affecting practical/vocational nursing.
1959	The National Association of Practical Nurse Education (NAPNE) changed its name to the National Association for Practical Nurse Education and Service (NAPNES).
1961	The National League for Nursing established a Department of Practical Nursing. Through this department, schools of practical nursing could be accredited by the NLN.
1990	Galen Health Institutes, Inc., opened practical/vocational nursing programs in Louisville, Kentucky, St. Petersburg, Florida, and San Antonio, Texas.

The term *nurse* was used only in the broadest sense as "a person who takes care of the sick."

The early creation and development of practical nursing in the United States evolved from the need for a caregiver who could be trained and ready for service in a short time. The cost of the services provided by these caregivers was expected to be reasonable and easily affordable by the patient. There was also the need at that time to provide a vocation for the many unskilled women who were migrating to the larger cities to seek better lives. This need prompted the YWCA in New York City to start the first practical nursing program in the late 1800s. During this time women generally were not skilled or trained for jobs other than manual labor. Practical/vocational nursing education enabled women to secure a vocation, and at the same time it expanded the availability of health care nursing.

World War I escalated the need for trained nurses abroad, while in the United States, the Spanish influenza epidemic strained the resources of the nursing community. The Smith-Hughes Act was passed in 1917 to provide vocational and public education. Federal funding then provided the means for vocational-based practical/vocational nursing programs throughout the country. Even with these resources, the demand for nurses caused by the war and the epidemic could not be met.

By 1940 thousands of self-taught "practical nurses" were working to meet the needs of the country. However, they lacked the education and experience that can be obtained only under supervision in an established program. They could not really be called practical/vocational nurses nor could they be licensed by the states. In fact, few states had even established minimal standards for the practice of practical/vocational nursing. Only 19 states and one territory had considered or passed legislation dealing with practical/vocational nursing. Licensure of the practical/vocational nurse was mandatory in only one state by the end of 1945. Many job descriptions and titles were used in referring to the work done by the practical/vocational nurse. There was no agreement on the duties, the role, or the responsibilities of these people. These facts and the absence of standards and licensing practices created difficulties.

Even before the United States entered World War II, the Depression caused a great demand for nurses. The Cadet Navy Corps and the American Red Cross provided expedient training in nursing. Practical nursing programs flourished throughout the United States. The need for skilled medical care personnel, although important, was upstaged by the need to prepare people for nursing in the shortest time. A 1-year program provided the minimal amount of training for practical/vocational nursing. As the shortage of nurses in the hospitals and other health care facilities became critical, the practical/vocational nurse, practicing in the home environment, was hired to work in those institutions.

In 1944 the U.S. Department of Vocational Education commissioned an intensive study of practical/vocational nursing tasks. The outcome of this study differentiated the tasks performed by the practical/vocational nurse in relation to those tasks performed by the registered nurse. As a result of this study, individual state boards of nursing began to specify the duties and responsibilities that could be accomplished by both groups of nurses.

Another event that influenced change in attitude about practical/vocational nursing was the 1965 position paper of the American Nurses Association. This position paper clearly defined two levels of nursing practice: that of the registered nurses and that of the technical nurse. The term *practical nurse* was not included in this position paper. However, even with the exclusion of the practical/vocational nurse in the position paper, the practical/vocational nurse has certainly proved her worth and provides excellent bedside nursing skills in many areas of service. The practical nurse provides valuable nursing interventions under the supervision of a registered nurse or physician.

Licensure for Practical/ Vocational Nursing

Licensing laws have been passed throughout the states to protect the public from unqualified persons practicing in almost any field or profession. Every state and the District of Columbia, American Samoa, the Northern Mariana Islands, and the Virgin Islands have licensing laws that apply to the practical/vocational nurse. These laws are put into effect through various state agencies, usually the state boards of nursing and the Nurse Practice Acts of the respective states.

Licensing for practical nurses in the United States began in 1914 when the state legislature in Mississippi passed the first laws pertaining to that group. This followed the passage of laws on licensing registered nurses by 11 years. The passage of such laws governing practical/vocational nursing in other states was slow in coming. Only six states passed such laws between 1920 and 1940. This may have been because there were not many practical nurses' training programs initiated during that period. After the outbreak of World War II and the opening of a large number of practical/vocational nurses' training programs, all the states were forced to pass legislation concerning the licensing of practical/vocational nurses. By 1955 all states had passed laws in this area in consonance with the standards set by NAPNE. The State Board Test Pool of the NLN Education Committee established a testing mechanism for all states and administered the examination several times a year throughout the United States. Graduates of a state-approved practical/vocational nursing education program were eligible to take the examination and, if they passed, became licensed practical nurses (LPNs) or licensed vocational nurses (LVNs), as they are called in Texas and California. Each state established its own required passing score on the examination.

Currently graduates of a state-approved LPN/LVN education program are eligible to take the NCLEX-PN. On completing the examination with a "pass" score (numerical scores are no longer given), the graduate is issued a license to practice as an LPN or an LVN.

Licensing laws for nursing are now established in all states. It is the individual's responsibility to be informed regarding licensure in the state in which she resides or intends to practice. Interstate endorsement (reciprocity between states) exists, and licensing for practice in other states can be obtained without repeating the NCLEX-PN if resident state requirements are met (see Chapter 54).

HEALTH CARE DELIVERY SYSTEMS

LPNs/LVNs practice within the established health care delivery system. For them to practice to their fullest, they must recognize the complexity of this system and their vital role in its functioning.

Identification of the Health Care System

The **health care system** is the complete network of agencies, facilities, and all providers of health care in a specified geographical area. This system depends on a variety of health care professionals who interact with their external environment. This environment includes the patient, the patient's family, the community in which the system is operating, the current technology, governmental agencies, the medical profession in the community, third-party participants, such as insurance companies, and many other forces that affect the patient's care. The major goal of the system is to achieve optimal levels of health care for a defined population through adequate and appropriate health care services. The LPN/ LVN is an integral member of the team of health care professionals within the overall system who will provide her services within the scope of practice as defined by the state's Nurse Practice Act.

Wellness/Illness Continuum. Health care services provided by the LPN/LVN depend on the wellness/illness continuum of the consumer, as well as on the environment where the services are provided.

The wellness/illness continuum is defined as the range of a person's total health. This continuum is ever changing and is influenced by the individual's physical condition, mental condition, and social well-being. **Wellness** (a dynamic state of health in which an individual progresses toward a higher level of functioning, achieving an optimal balance between internal and external environment), at one end of the spectrum, represents the highest level of optimal health. Illness, at the opposite end of the spectrum, represents a diminished or impaired state of health (Fig. 1-2).

Maintaining one's health requires constant effort to achieve a balance of all aspects of life. For the individual to achieve this equilibrium, a number of interrelated factors must be considered when health care is provided to the consumer. Such factors include age, sex, family relationships, cultural influences, and economic status. This comprehensive approach to health care is known as **holistic health care** (a system of comprehensive or total patient care that considers the physical, emotional, social, economic, and spiritual needs of a person).

Health Promotion and Illness Prevention. From the earliest recorded civilizations to the twentieth century, the primary focus of health care has been on the care of the sick. As time passed, the focus broadened to include the determination of the cause of illness and the prevention of its spread.

Hospitals, which were historically dirty, unsanitary, and ill-kept institutions where unsuspecting patients acquired diseases, slowly became clean, sterile, well-kept places where patients were fairly well assured that their disease or illness would be attended to and, it was hoped, cured, without risking the exposure to additional medical problems. The phenomenal death rates in the hospitals during the Crimean War decreased dramatically when the hospital units were cleaned and strict sanitary requirements were imposed.

As more and more standards were established and adhered to, health statistics gathered by the U.S. Department of Public Health began to identify what types of diseases were most prevalent, which age groups seemed to be affected by certain illnesses, and which illnesses were predominant in various parts of the country. These statistics identified problem areas for researchers and health care providers, whose efforts were then directed at developing treatment for the illness, establishing methods to decrease its spread, and isolating its cause. Childbirth without prenatal care increased the mortality of infant and mother; lack of milk in an infant's diet affected bone development and contributed to crippling deformities; coal miners' constant exposure to coal dust and contaminated air in the mines deteriorated their lungs.

Once causes for these and other problems were found, the focus shifted from curing the problem to preventing it. With the focus on decreasing the risk factors for a given illness or disease and thereby preventing it, the quality of life and life expectancy in general were enhanced in the United States. General medical research and specific research for the cause and cure of cancer, cystic fibrosis, heart disease, and many other life-threatening conditions continue to be integral parts of the health care system in this country.

Continuity of Care. The patient is the most important person in the health care system. However, he is not the only factor in the total scheme of the holistic health care system that has evolved. The number of health care providers and health care agencies involved in the care and treatment of a single patient is extensive. Increased specialization by health care providers and health care institutions, reimbursement procedures by third-party payers (such as insurance companies), cumbersome federal regulatory organizations, and state health care regulatory agencies all affect the consumer (the patient) and the type and quality of care provided.

Maintaining one's autonomy and ensuring that continuity of care is received within the maze of the present health care delivery system is an ongoing challenge for the medical care consumer. Understanding what procedures are done, why, and by whom is a discouraging and often impossible task for patients already bewildered and frightened by medical conditions that threaten their well-being. The right to choose which method of care will be provided or who will provide that care becomes a terrifying dilemma, which many times cannot be resolved by the patient.

Delivery of Patient Care

The delivery of patient care is an extremely humanistic activity. It is the delivery of services by human beings to human beings. It involves not only the treatment of disease and injury but the prevention of disease, the restoration of optimal wellness through rehabilitation, the maintenance of a desirable level of wellness through such procedures as kidney dialysis, the care of the chronically ill, the provision of assistance to the patient

Wellness – – – – – – – – – – – – – – – – Illness

Highest level of optimum health	Diminished or impaired state of health

FIG. 1-2 Wellness/illness continuum.

in the arduous process of self-care, and patient education.

The development of an individualized care plan is needed to identify individual needs of the patient and to plan a systematic approach to meet those needs. The nursing process (discussed in Chapter 5) provides the means by which a patient's individual needs are identified, and a plan of health care is developed to meet those expressed needs. The care plan involves all health care providers who, through a coordinated and cooperative effort, work toward meeting the patient's total needs in a holistic, caring manner.

Participants in the Health Care System. The patient, the recipient of health care services, is the central focus of those activities performed by more than 200 types of health providers identified in the health care system in the United States. Physicians, dentists, osteopathic physicians, surgeons, psychiatrists, and other professional health care specialists must pass examinations in their specialty to become *board certified* and be permitted to practice in their area of specialization. In many cases physicians employ persons who have specialized training to function in cooperation with the physician. These people may be physician assistants or nurse practitioners.

The registered nurse (RN), a direct health caregiver, has completed one of three types of nursing education programs: a 4-year baccalaureate degree program, a 2-year associate degree program, or a 3-year diploma program. On satisfactory completion of one of these programs, the graduate nurse is eligible to take the National Council Licensing Examination for Registered Nurses (NCLEX-RN). The RN practices in a variety of settings, performing skills within the parameters of the education received and the scope of nursing practice as outlined in the state's Nurse Practice Act.

The LPN/LVN practices under the supervision of the RN, medical physician, osteopathic physician, or dentist. Working together, they are the direct patient caregivers in most institutions. Nursing recognizes the benefit of having this bedside caregiver on the health care team. The activity of the LPN/LVN is based on the scope of practice outlined in a given state's Nurse Practice Act.

Other caregivers are required to be registered and to have the specialized education and training dictated by their professional organizations. For example, the social worker is trained to counsel patients who have social, emotional, or environmental problems. The patient may be referred to other agencies or professionals for specific care and treatment. The physical therapist, on the other hand, uses precise methods of massage, exercise, and hydrotherapy to help restore physical muscular functioning of the body. The dietician is trained to provide the intake of foods that will meet the nutritional requirements of the patient. The respiratory therapist assists the patient by administering oxygen, monitoring and maintaining ventilators, drawing blood for blood gas analysis, and performing other pulmonary function tests.

Technologists and medical technicians are among the group of laboratory, radiology and other diagnostic personnel who are prepared to assist the medical professional staff in their attempt to diagnose and treat disease and injury. The term *technologist* refers to those who have a baccalaureate degree, whereas the term *technician* refers to those who have an associate degree or less. Paraprofessionals are those persons educated to assist the professional in providing care for the patient. The nursing assistant is educated in basic nursing techniques and performs under the supervision of the RN. The ward clerk is mainly a secretary, preparing and maintaining patients' records, ordering supplies, scheduling diagnostic tests, performing receptionist duties, and directing the flow of traffic in the patient care unit. These are only a sampling of the health care participants in the health care system. Each participant makes a valuable contribution in ensuring the safety and well-being of the patient.

Environmental Factors Affecting Health and Illness. Social and physical environmental factors do not necessarily cause illness, but they do influence the development or progression of an illness. Personal financial hardship, life-style, social pressures, and major societal issues, such as AIDS, abortion, and drug abuse, are some of the more obvious social factors. Stress, conflict, smoking, excessive weight, alcoholism, and the impact of high technology are among the physical factors.

Reactions to these factors vary from patient to patient. Fear of illness and dehumanization, loss of identity, and loss of control can affect one's mental state, whereas an imbalance in body functions can affect one's physical condition. Although we tend to separate social factors from physical factors, it must be emphasized that one group affects the other and vice versa.

Early recognition of the effect of environmental factors on a patient and prompt intervention by family, health care providers, or the patient himself can decrease or minimize any negative impact.

Expectations of the Patient and Health Care Team. Each patient is special, possessing a unique personality, background, life-style, and level of education. His needs, expectations, and response to health care are influenced by all these factors.

The belief held by most people in the United States is that everyone has a right to health care, regardless of race, color, creed, or economic status. This health care includes the treatment of disease, as well as preventive medicine. The acute awareness of preventive medicine

Box 1-2 THE PATIENT'S BILL OF RIGHTS

- The patient has the right to considerate and respectful care.
- The patient has the right to obtain from his physician complete current information concerning his diagnosis, treatment, and prognosis in terms the patient can be reasonably expected to understand. When it is not medically advisable to give such information to the patient, the information should be made available to an appropriate person in his behalf. He has the right to know, by name, the physician responsible for coordinating his care.
- The patient has the right to receive from his physician information necessary to give informed consent prior to the start of any procedure and/or treatment. Except in emergencies, such information for informed consent should include, but not necessarily be limited to, the specific procedure and/or treatment, the medically significant risks involved, and the probable duration of incapacity. Where medically significant, alternatives for care or treatment exist, or when the patient requests information concerning medical alternatives, the patient has the right to such information. The patient also has the right to know the name of the person responsible for the procedures and/or treatment.
- The patient has the right to refuse treatment to the extent permitted by law, and to be informed of the medical consequences of his action.
- The patient has the right to every consideration of his privacy concerning his own medical care program. Case discussion, consultation, examination, and treatment are confidential and should be conducted discreetly. Those not directly involved in his care must have permission of the patient to be present.
- The patient has the right to expect that all communications and records pertaining to his care should be treated as confidential.
- The patient has the right to expect that within its capacity a hospital must make reasonable response to the request of a patient for services. The hospital must provide evaluation, service, and/or referral indicated by the urgency of the case. When medically permissible the patient may be transferred to another facility only after he has received complete information and explanation concerning the needs for and alternatives to such a transfer. The institution to which the patient is to be transferred must first have accepted the patient for transfer.
- The patient has the right to obtain information as to any relationship of his hospital to other health care and educational institutions insofar as his care is concerned. The patient has the right to obtain information as to the existence of any professional relationships among individuals, by name, who are treating him.
- The patient has the right to be advised if the hospital proposes to engage in or perform human experimentation affecting his care or treatment. The patient has the right to refuse to participate in such research projects.
- The patient has the right to expect reasonable continuity of care. He has the right to know in advance what appointment times and physicians are available and where. The patient has the right to expect that the hospital will provide a mechanism whereby he is informed by his physician or a delegate of the physician of the patient's continuing health care requirements following discharge.
- The patient has the right to examine and receive an explanation of his bill regardless of source of payment.
- The patient has the right to know what hospital rules and regulations apply to his conduct as a patient.

today has resulted in an emphasis on the wellness continuum through education about issues such as smoking, heart disease, drug and alcohol abuse, weight control, stress syndrome, and social diseases.

Ironically, there is less emphasis on the treatment of illness than on its prevention in the minds of most people. They believe that once they become ill, they are no longer in control of their health. Therefore, when a person does become ill and seeks medical attention, there is an expectation that it will be provided in a knowledgeable, safe, expeditious manner that will lead to a cure. It is expected that health care providers will work in a cooperative manner for the benefit of the patient and that the cost of the care will be reasonable and, most important, paid for by somebody else (an insurance company or the government). It is presumed that the service will be highly satisfactory, and it is hoped that a cure will follow.

There is one more vital expectation that must be recognized and practiced by all health care workers. Patients expect to be treated with dignity and compassion and to have their rights respected. In 1972 the American Hospital Association issued a "Patient's Bill of Rights" (Box 1-2) in an effort to ensure that this expectation be realized. This document assured patients that they have the right to high-quality care, the right to respect and dignity, the right of access to information about the illness and/or treatment, the right to be involved in decisions about the care being provided, the right of informed consent, the right to express concerns about the care being provided, and the right to refuse care.

The delivery of health care needs to be a process of mutual exchange between patients and health care givers. Whereas patients expect the "rights" as outlined, health care workers expect something as well. Health care professionals expect that patients will actively participate in their care as much as possible by taking an active role in the planning process, by having an understanding of the care and the treatment given, by asking questions, by following the treatment plan prescribed, by acting responsibly with respect to their own conditions, and by giving health care workers the same respect that patients are entitled to.

Interdisciplinary Approach to Health Care. The primary goal of the health care team is the optimal physical, mental, and social well-being of the patient. This goal is achieved by promoting and restoring health within the wellness/illness continuum. It is imperative that health care personnel, when working to meet the needs of the patient, work together as a health care team. Each member of the team must coordinate his activity with every other member of the team by developing a comprehensive care plan, by effectively communicating, and by keeping accurate records. A care plan is a document that outlines the individual needs of the patient and the approach to meeting these needs. It further identifies who will assist in treating the patient. The document guides and directs the activities surrounding the patient's care and ensures that continuity and consistency of care will be provided.

Good communication is essential for the exchange of information among the members of the health care team. This communication ensures that either the care plan is meeting the needs of the patient or, if it is not, there is opportunity to make appropriate changes. (See Chapter 4 for a further discussion of communication.)

Documentation in any form is the permanent record of the patient's progress and treatment. It constitutes the formal and legal record of care received by the patient and the patient's response to that care. The information recorded during the entire course of treatment serves many purposes. It provides a progress record of treatment so that all the involved health care members are aware of what treatment the patient is receiving. It also provides a history of events, which may be valuable in the future treatment of the same condition. (See Chapter 6 for a further discussion of documentation.)

Following this interdisciplinary approach to treatment prevents the fragmentation of patient care. Just as the plan of care for patients is developed in a holistic manner, so is the actual delivery of health care. Health care providers must never forget that the central focus of all their activity is the patient.

PRACTICAL/VOCATIONAL NURSING

The role of the practical/vocational nurse is not new within the health care delivery system. The role and responsibilities have expanded from bathing patients and light housekeeping to performing skilled tasks needed to provide health care to people within the wellness/illness continuum.

The role of the LPN/LVN continues to evolve. This evolution is influenced by the various states' Nurse Practice Acts, individual changes within the health care agencies, the availability of health care workers, and the needs of patients. The practical/vocational nurse is finding a career in hospitals, clinics, outpatient agencies, home health agencies, long-term care facilities, insurance companies, physician offices, and the military services.

The blend of nursing history and today's health care delivery system sets the foundation for the career of an LPN/LVN.

Definition

Practical/vocational nursing is defined as the activity of providing specific services to patients under the direct supervision of a licensed physician or dentist and/or RN. The services are provided in a structured setting surrounding the caring for the sick, the rehabilitation of the sick and injured, and the prevention of sickness and injury. This definition is adapted from the NAPNES and several states' Nurse Practice Acts.

The unique function of the nurse is to assist individuals, sick or well, in the performance of those activities contributing to health, to their recovery, or to a peaceful death—activities that patients would perform unaided if they had the necessary strength, will, or knowledge—and if feasible to do this in such a way as to help patients gain independence as rapidly as possible. The practical/vocational nurse is educated to be a responsible member of a health care team, performing basic therapeutic, rehabilitative, and preventive care for anyone who needs it.

Objectives, Components, and Characteristics of Practice

The stated objectives for practical/vocational nursing practice are the following:

- To acquire the specialized knowledge and skills needed to meet the health care needs of patients in a variety of settings
- To be a graduate of a state-approved practical/vocational nursing program
- To take and pass the NCLEX-PN examination
- To acquire a state license to practice

To accomplish these objectives, students must assume responsibility for their own education, intensive

Box 1-3

CHARACTERISTICS, ROLES, AND RESPONSIBILITIES OF THE PRACTICAL/VOCATIONAL NURSE

- Being a responsible and accountable member of the health care team
- Maintaining a current license
- Practicing within the scope of the Nurse Practice Act
- Practicing under the supervision of a medical physician, RN, osteopathic physician, or dentist
- Participating in continuing education activities
- Being an effective member of the health care team
- Using the nursing process to meet patients' needs
- Promoting and maintaining health, preventing disease, and encouraging and assisting in rehabilitation
- Maintaining a professional appearance
- Subscribing to recognized ethical practices
- Performing within legal parameters
- Participating in activities of professional organizations
- Assisting in developing the role of the licensed practical/vocational nurse of tomorrow

study, and dedication to duty. Organizing one's time effectively helps accomplish these objectives and ultimately assures the patient of safe and competent care.

Distinguishing characteristics for practice by the LPN/LVN are shown in Box 1-3.

Roles and Responsibilities

In 1981 NAPNES issued the following statement of responsibilities required for practice as a practical/vocational nurse:

- Recognizes the LPN/LVN's role in the health care delivery system and articulates that role with those of other health care team members
- Maintains accountability for one's own nursing practice within the ethical and legal framework
- Serves as a patient advocate
- Accepts their role in maintaining developing standards of practice in providing health care
- Seeks further growth through educational opportunities

Practical/vocational nursing is an exciting, challenging career that provides an opportunity to care for others while receiving personal satisfaction. The focus is on bedside/personal care of patients in a variety of settingsthat require knowledge, skill, and expertise to perform in a responsible, accountable manner.

REFERENCES AND SUGGESTED READINGS

1. Apple RD: Sentimental women need not apply: a history of American nursing, *J Am Hist* 78(3):1170, 1991.
2. Becker BG, Fendler DJ: *Vocational and personal adjustments in practical nursing,* ed 6, St Louis, 1993, Mosby.
3. Bunning S, Campbell JC: Feminism and nursing: historical perspectives, *Adv Nurs Sci* 12(4):11, 1990.
4. Cooke H: An introduction to the social history of nursing, *Br J Sociol* 41:593, 1990.
5. Dietz LD, Lehozky AR: *History and modern nursing,* ed 2, Philadelphia, 1993, FA Davis.
6. Dolan J: *History of nursing,* ed 12, Philadelphia, 1970, WB Saunders.
7. Donahue MP: *Nursing: the finest art—an illustrated history,* St Louis, 1986, Mosby.
8. Fairman JA: Sources and references for research in nursing history, *Nurs Res* 36(1):56, 1987.
9. Griffin GJ, Griffin JK: *Jensen's history and trends of professional nursing,* ed 6, St Louis, 1969, Mosby.
10. Harrion L: *Professional issues in practical/vocational nursing,* Albany, NY, 1992, Delmar.
11. Hood G, Dincher JR: *Total patient care: foundations and practice,* ed 8, St Louis, 1992, Mosby.
12. Humana revamps its staffing and opens three LPN schools, *Am J Nurs* 90(2):106, 1990.
13. Jameson EM et al: *Trends in nursing history,* ed 6, Philadelphia, 1968, Saunders.
14. Kelly, LY: *Dimensions of professional nursing,* ed 4, New York, 1981, Macmillan.
15. Kenny E: An LPN looks at the developing LPN role, *Issues* 7(2):6, 1986.
16. Kippinbrock TA: I wish I had been there: a sense of nursing history, *Nurs Health Care* 12(4):208, 1991.
17. Kuczin CR: *Contemporary practical/vocational nursing,* ed 2, Philadelphia, 1993, Lippincott.
18. McClosky JC, Grace HK: *Current issues in nursing,* ed 3, St Louis, 1990, Mosby.
19. McMahon, M: Nursing histories: reviving life in abandoned selves, *Feminist Review* 37:23, Spring 1991.
20. Minkowski WL: Women healers of the middle ages, *Am J Public Health* 82(2):288, 1992.
21. Mitchell PR, Grippando GM: *Nursing perspectives and issues,* ed 5, New York, 1993, Delmar.
22. *Mosby's medical, nursing and allied health dictionary,* ed 4, St Louis, 1994, Mosby.
23. Nightingale F: *Notes on nursing: what it is and what it is not,* London, 1859, Harrison and Sons.
24. Pokorney ME: An historical perspective of confederate nursing during the Civil War, 1861-1865, *Nurs Res* 41(1):28, 1992.
25. Steward IM, Austin AL: *A history of nursing,* ed 5, New York, 1962, Putnam's.
26. Walters S: And why I choose to remain an LPN, *J Pract Nurs* 39(1):44, 1989.
27. Woodham SG: *Florence Nightingale,* New York, 1981, McGraw-Hill.

CHAPTER CHALLENGE

KEY POINTS

- The evolution of nursing was greatly influenced by the way the sick and injured were cared for.
- The influence of Florence Nightingale on nursing practice and nursing education was highly significant in the nineteenth century.
- Nursing practice and education in the United States were significantly influenced by activities of Florence Nightingale.
- The Association of Practical Nurse Schools was organized in Chicago in 1941, to address the needs of practical nursing education. Its name was changed to the National Association of Practical Nurse Education (NAPNE) in 1942.
- NAPNE changed its name in 1959 to the National Association for Practical Nurse Education and Service (NAPNES).
- In 1949 the National Federation of Licensed Practical Nurses (NFLPN) was founded by Lillian Kuster.
- Mandatory licensure laws were established for practical/vocational nursing education and practice.
- The wellness/illness continuum is the range of a person's total health situation.
- Prevention of illness and injury and continuity of patient care are integral components of holistic health care.
- The practical/vocational nurse is one of many of the large groups of health care workers who provide health care services.
- The role and responsibilities of the practical/vocational nursing community function in accordance with the several states' Nurse Practice Acts.

STUDY QUESTIONS

1. Miss Dregis is interested in attending an accredited school for practical nursing. She is aware that an accredited program:
   1. voluntarily seeks a review by a given organization to determine if the program meets preestablished criteria of that organization
   2. is one that meets the minimal standards set by the respective state agencies responsible for overseeing educational programs
   3. is necessary before the graduate is eligible to take the National Council Licensing Examination for Practical Nursing (NCLEX-PN)
   4. is a federally funded health care program that educates practical nurse students
2. The acute awareness by the health care consumer of preventive medicine has resulted in an increase in:
   1. anxiety over diagnostic workups such as colonoscopies or gynecological exams
   2. the number of admissions for inpatient services
   3. the length of a hospitalization stay
   4. knowledge and services to promote health and prevent illness (wellness continuum)
3. The factor that best advanced the practice of nursing in the first century was the:
   1. growth of cities
   2. better education of nurses
   3. teachings of Christianity
   4. improved conditions for women
4. Nursing education programs may seek voluntary accreditation by the appropriate council of the:
   1. American Nurses Association
   2. International Council of Nurses
   3. Congress for Nursing Practice
   4. National League for Nursing
5. When developing a definition of "health," a person should consider that health is:
   1. a condition of physical, mental, and social well-being and absence of disease
   2. the ability to pursue activities of daily living
   3. a function of the physiological state
   4. a static condition; the absence of pathology
6. Mr. Morton, practical student nurse, is educated to understand the concepts of a system of comprehensive or total patient care that considers the physical, emotional, social, economic, and spiritual needs of the person; the person's response to the illness; and the impact of the illness on the person's ability to meet self-care needs. The modern nursing practice that expresses this philosophy of care is called:
   1. wellness/illness continuum
   2. Patient's Bill of Rights
   3. holistic nursing
   4. health care delivery system

2

LEGAL ASPECTS OF NURSING

Persephone C. Agrafiotis

KEY TERMS

answer
appeal
complaint
damages
defendant
deposition
discovery
informed consent
interrogatories
judgment
law
liability
litigation
malpractice
negligence
plaintiff
standards of care
statute
standard operating procedure
summons

LEARNING OBJECTIVES

After reading this chapter, the student should be able to do the following:

- Define the key terms.
- Outline the development of the legal influence on health care.
- Describe the parts of the legal process.
- Define the legal relationship between the patient and the practical/vocational nurse.
- Describe standards of care.
- Discuss the terms *negligence* and *malpractice.*
- Discuss the three Ds of nursing malpractice defense.
- Describe the legal protection system and controls available for both the patient and practical/vocational nurse.

RELATED TOPICS OF INTEREST

- The evolution of nursing (Chapter 1)
- Ethical aspects of nursing (Chapter 3)
- Communication (Chapter 4)
- Documentation (Chapter 6)
- Principles and practice of medication administration (Chapter 21)
- The surgical patient (Chapter 22)
- The world of the graduate (Chapter 54)

No system operates in a vacuum, and the health care delivery system is no exception. As the health care providers within the system deliver numerous services to the consumer, they must practice within the limits established by federal and state legislation. Court-rendered definitions of health care and court decisions that establish precedents have operational implications that affect how, when, where, and to whom health care will be provided.

The law requires that a minimum standard of care should be met. Ethical standards may require a higher standard and are set by the requirements and/or needs of a particular situation.

HISTORICAL PERSPECTIVE

In early times laws were developed by a monarch, the church, the ruling class, or other persons whom the people accepted as having the "right" to make decisions for them. Either these persons were given the right to make these decisions because of their knowledge, expertise, and position or they assumed the right based on power they were able to exert over the people.

Laws were developed from **judgments** (the decision of the law given by a court as a result of court proceedings) that came forth when those having the right or the power to make decisions did so on a case-by-case basis. Future laws and rules continued to be developed on such decisions and contributed to the establishment of a system of rules by which the people lived. This form of case law established by a given society's rulers, and later by judges, became known as "common law" or "judge-made law."

With societal development, governing rules for the people became more formal and legislative bodies were added to the common law approach. The formation of the legislative bodies followed the creation of Parliament in England and Congress in the United States.

Law became known as the reference to a rule, principle, or regulation established and made known by a government to protect or to restrict the people affected.

As we have seen from the historical perspective of nursing, clearly defined laws for health care were nonexistent well into the nineteenth century. Until then, laws that were passed emphasized human freedom, personal liberty, and property rights.

In the health care field, the fundamental principles that governed behavior came from people such as Hippocrates, Florence Nightingale, Dorothea Dix, and Clara Barton. Their efforts to assist the poor, the sick, and the infirm brought about significant changes in the delivery of health care that became the foundation for the standards of practice and eventually the passage of laws for the protection of the consumer.

LEGAL PROCESS

The legal process enables a person to look at societal issues and to respond to problems with a broad background of experience based on laws established by and for the people whom they affect. The laws provide fundamental rights and establish relationships between governmental bodies and the citizenry. The validity of the legislation passed and the regulations established is measured against federal or state constitutional standards, or both, depending on the issue in question.

Legal System in the United States and Its Influence on the Health Care System

Law refers to man-made rules and regulations that derive their authority from various sources. In the United States there are three levels of government involved with establishing law: federal, state, and local. These governmental bodies produce statutory law. These laws are passed by the legislative bodies created by the United States Congress, state legislative bodies, and city councils. **Statutes** (legislative acts declaring, commanding, or prohibiting something) are officially acted on or voted on by the legislative bodies and are compiled into codes, collections of statutes, or city ordinances.

To enact these laws, administrative agencies are established with the power to implement the rules and regulations that enforce statutory law. These rules and regulations are known as administrative laws.

Judicial or case laws are made by courts of law that interpret legal issues that are being disputed. The interpretation of statutes and regulations decides which of two conflicting approaches applies to a given situation. Once decided, a precedent is established for future interpretation of the law in question.

Legal health care issues began to surface in the courts as early as 1852 when a case before the North Carolina Supreme Court asked that court to define the health status of a slave suffering with myopia (nearsightedness). The court noted that healthy meant "free from disease or bodily ailments." The court extended the definition by adding the word "sound," which in its opinion meant "whole, right, nothing the matter, and free from any defect." The court's interpretation and subsequent decision supported the claim that the slave was unfit to work because of his condition.

Five years later the North Carolina Supreme Court was again asked to determine the level of health of a slave who had a contracted finger. In a lengthy opinion, the court interpreted health, healthy, and soundness with regard to the contracted finger. It decided that the condition was somewhat less than healthy but not totally unhealthy and that therefore the slave could perform the work required of him.

Such questions surrounding health care continue to be debated in the courts today. However, the complexity of the cases and the adequacy of the treatment or care of the patient have increased dramatically as evidenced by some of the malpractice suit judgments and awards made by the courts. The outcome of these court debates, from the seemingly insignificant to the more serious, continue to influence the health care delivery system and the individual behavior of everyone working in that system, including the practical/vocational nurse. An example of a court case is presented as follows:

> *Eyoma v. Falco* (NJ 1991). Nurse Falco, a recovery room nurse at the Hackensack Medical Center in New Jersey, failed to adequately monitor a patient, which later resulted in the patient's death. The patient's family sued Nurse Falco and Dr. Brotherton, who had operated on the patient, for wrongful death. The Superior Court of Bergen County held Nurse Falco 100% liable and exonerated Dr. Brotherton. Nurse Falco appealed the decision but lost.

Components and Characteristics of the Legal Process

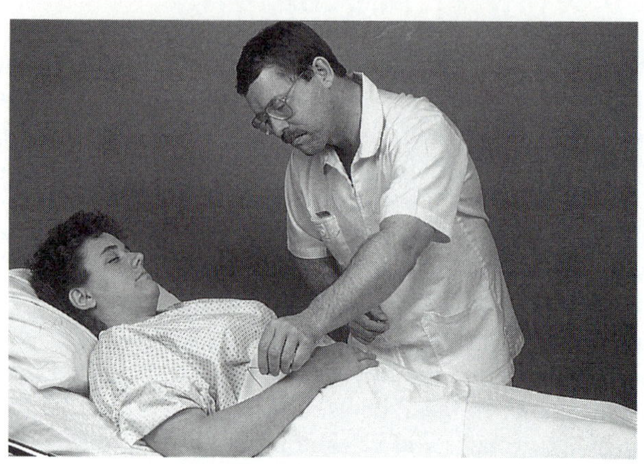

Judicial or case law involving the health care delivery system is increasing because of issues being litigated between the consumer and the health care provider.

Litigation (a lawsuit) begins when a complaining party (the **plaintiff**) files a document known as a **complaint** (pleading by a plaintiff made under oath to initiate a lawsuit) with the court. This document states the basis for the complaint and outlines the **damages** (money asked for by the plaintiff as compensation for any loss, detriment, or injury to the plaintiff's person, property, or rights caused by the wrongdoing or negligence of the defendant). The person at whom the complaint is directed is known as the **defendant.** The filing of a complaint is followed by the issue of a **summons,** which is a court order advising the defendant that a lawsuit against him is pending. It further notifies the defendant what he must do with respect to the lawsuit and the time constraints involved.

If the defendant, once served, chooses to do nothing in response to the summons, such as hire an attorney or file a countercomplaint, the court may enter a default judgment against the defendant, which is based on the uncontested testimony of the plaintiff.

A defendant presented with a summons normally retains an attorney, who then files a document called an appearance, which prevents the court from entering a default judgment. The defendant, through his attorney, then files a response **(answer)** to the allegations made in the complaint. This response either admits or denies the allegations made. If the response by the defendant includes significant information not referred to in the original complaint, the plaintiff, through his attorney, has the option to file a reply.

When all the allegations by both parties have been addressed, the case is ready to move forward and the parties are said to be "at issue." **Discovery** (pretrial procedures allowing one party to examine vital witnesses and/or documents held exclusively by the adverse party) procedures are then initiated, whereby relevant information is gathered by both sides. **Depositions** (out-of-court, under-oath statements of a witness) and **interrogatories** (written questions) are taken from or asked of witnesses before the scheduled trial. During this pretrial period, efforts may be made by either side to influence the outcome of the lawsuit. Such efforts include, but are not limited to, motions to dismiss the complaint, requests to change the trial date, and offers of a settlement out of court.

If motions to dismiss the lawsuit are denied and all other motions have been resolved by the court, the case then goes to trial. The court hears the evidence, comes to certain conclusions, and decides on a verdict. Once the judge or jury reaches a decision and a verdict is declared, either party may **appeal** (request review and/or retrial of legal issues) that verdict to an appellate court. If an appeal is granted, the testimony and the procedures of the trial are reviewed by the appellate court. That court may choose to uphold or reverse the decision of the lower court. The right to an appeal is a constitutional right and serves as part of the system of checks and balances on the court system of the United States.

The time period for the process of litigation and the outcome of that litigation vary, depending on many factors that are peculiar to each case. Predominant factors are (1) the severity of the complaint, (2) whether an injury or a death is involved, and (3) the backlog of cases pending before the court.

Legal Relationship of the Patient and Practical/Vocational Nurse

The licensed practical/vocational nurse must practice within the confines of the scope of practical nursing. Yet the reality of the current status of nursing is that there is a shortage of registered nurses. Because of this, the role of the licensed practical/vocational nurse has expanded to include more responsibility for patient care and sometimes patient care management, a role formerly designated only to registered nurses. When faced with a trend toward expansion of practice, the nurse must be cognizant of the practice limitations imposed by law. Just because a patient has a need, the licensed practical/vocational nurse cannot necessarily fulfill the need within legal guidelines, if doing so requires that the licensed practical/vocational nurse must operate outside the scope of practical/vocational nursing licensure restrictions. The prudent licensed practical/vocational nurse knows the limits of practice and operates within them at all times.

Knowledge of the law, rules and regulations, and even existing institutional policy is essential to (1) make informed decisions concerning patient care, (2) become a responsive and responsible employee in the health care system, (3) achieve personal and professional satisfac-

Box 2-1 COMMON LEGAL TERMS

abandonment of care Wrongful cessation of the provision of care to a patient.

affidavit Written or printed statement of facts that is sworn to before a notary public or an officer of the court.

assault Any willful attempt or threat to harm another, coupled with the ability to actually harm the other person; injury is not a requirement.

battery Any intentional touching of another's body or anything the person is touching or holding without consent.

civil law Concerned with relationships among people and the protection of a person's rights. Although violations of civil law might cause harm to an individual or property, no grave threat to society as a whole usually exists.

competency Legal presumption that, when one attains the age of majority, a person is able to make legally enforceable acts.

criminal law Concerned with relationships between individuals and governments and with acts that threaten society and its order. Misuse of controlled substances is an example of criminal conduct for nurses.

deposition An out-of-court, under-oath statement of a witness.

informed consent A person of legal competency voluntarily agrees to allow something to happen (for example, surgery) based on a full disclosure of facts needed to make an intelligent decision (that is, knowledge of risks involved, benefits, alternatives, or consequences of refusal).

legal procedure Rules governing how a lawsuit will proceed.

liability Legal concept that one is responsible and will be held accountable for one's actions (personal liability), that a corporation is responsible and answerable for its own decisions (corporate liability), or that an employer is responsible for an employee's acts done within the scope of employment.

libel Defamation in the form of written words.

malpractice In law, professional negligence that is the proximate cause of injury or harm to a patient; resulting from a lack of professional knowledge, experience, or skill that can be expected in others in the profession or from a failure to exercise reasonable care of judgment in the application of professional knowledge, experience, or skill. Malpractice is the failure to meet a professional standard of care.

negligence The commission of an act that a prudent person would not have done or the omission of a duty that a prudent person would have fulfilled, resulting in injury or harm to another person. Failure to meet the ordinary standards of care, one not involving special knowledge or skill, which leads to harm.

slander Defamation in the form of spoken words.

standards of care Acts permitted to be performed or prohibited from being performed by a prudent person working within the parameters of his or her training, license, and experience and the conditions existing at the time; the nurse's duty to a patient with whom there is an established nurse-patient relationship to provide reasonable, prudent care required by the circumstances.

tort Category of law involving civil wrongs against another's person or property; torts include negligence, false imprisonment, assault, battery, defamation, invasion of privacy, and fraud.

tion, and (4) protect oneself from lawsuits and legal charges.

LEGAL ISSUES

Legal precedents over the years have well established the right of both patient and nurse to be protected when involved in receiving or giving health care services.

The patient has the right to expect that the practical/vocational nurse will act in the patient's best interest by providing proper care based on existing standards, the Patient's Bill of Rights, and the principle of informed consent. See Box 2-1 for a list of common legal terms.

Nurses, on the other hand, must rely on the rights that are granted in their respective states' Nurse Practice Acts. These rights vary from state to state, but they generally are intended to provide basic legal protection for nurses, provided that the nurses are operating professionally, prudently, and within the scope of their authority.

Controls for the Protection of the Patient

Devotion to duty by the health care professional is an expectation that every patient depends on when suffering from an illness or injury and under medical care. However, the legal system requires more stringent and tangible controls that can be recorded, observed, and measured against a standard. These standards provide the key control for patient protection.

Standards of Care. Standards of care are determined in a variety of ways. They are devised by professional organizations, the Nurse Practice Acts of each state, guidelines established by accrediting bodies for hospitals, nursing homes, educational programs, and other health care agencies, and finally by the people who are charged with providing that care.

One of the functions of law, applied to nursing practice, is to define the standard of care that nurses must provide. All U.S. state legislatures and Canadian provincial parliaments have passed nursing practice acts that define the scope of nursing practice in their particular state or providence. The nursing practice acts set educational requirements for nurses, distinguish between nursing and medical practice, and generally define nursing practice. All nurses are responsible for knowing the provisions of the act for the state or providence in which they work.

These **standards of care** define those acts that are permitted to be performed or prohibited from being performed by a prudent person working within the parameters of her training, license, and experience and the conditions existing at the time. A standard of care is the nurse's duty to a patient with whom there is an established nurse-patient relationship to provide reasonable, prudent care required by the circumstances. These standards are the ruler against which the practical/vocational nurse's performance is measured with respect to providing patient care. Standards of care concern nurses' accountability or obligations to account for their actions. All nurses should know the standards of care they are expected to meet.

Standards of care are very important. They are the guidelines by which nurses should practice. If nurses do not perform duties within accepted standards of care, they may place themselves in jeopardy of legal action. In a malpractice lawsuit, these standards are used to determine whether the nurse has acted as any reasonably prudent nurse with the same level of education and experience would act. Standards of care are thus guidelines for determining whether nurses performed duties in an appropriate manner. If nurses are named as defendants in malpractice lawsuits and it is shown that neither the accepted standards of care outlined by the state or province nursing practice act nor the policies of the employing institution were followed, the nurse's legal liability is clear (Box 2-2).

Patients' Rights. Today's consumers of health care services are very knowledgeable about their own medical and health care needs. They are also extremely knowledgeable about what they can and cannot expect in health care services.

Over the years, a number of documents regarding patients' rights have been published. The National League for Nursing (NLN) in 1959 published a document titled "What People Can Expect of Modern Nursing Practice." In 1972 the American Hospital Association (AHA) issued the "Statement on a Patient's Bill of Rights" (see Box 1-2). In that same year the Pennsylvania Insurance Department issued a document called the "Citizen's Bill of Hospital Rights."

In 1973 Minnesota became the first state to incorporate patients' rights into a law and the Congress of the United States passed the Rehabilitation Act, which granted services to handicapped persons. In 1980 the Mental Health Patient's Bill of Rights and the Pregnant Patient's Bill of Rights became law.

Box 2-2 EVIDENCE OF NURSING STANDARDS

- Practice protocols, contracts, collaborative practice agreements, employment agreements, personnel manuals
- Agency policy and procedure manuals
- State nurse practice acts and regulations and standards incorporated by reference
- American Nurses' Association's Code for Nurses (1985)
- American Nurses' Association's Standards of Practice (1991)
- Accreditation criteria of the Joint Commission on Accreditation of Healthcare Organizations
- Other accreditation standards, depending on the practice setting (e.g., National League for Nursing, National Association of Home Care)
- State and federal licensing laws and regulations governing health care agencies; state, professional, and occupational legislation and regulations
- Nursing specialty standards of care and certification
- Nursing literature, textbooks, journals
- Education, continuing education, staff development, orientation
- Experience
- Expert nurse witnesses, other experts and peers, material witnesses
- Customary and usual practices of nurses

The Joint Commission on Accreditation of Healthcare Organizations (JCAHO) includes an entire section on the "Rights and Responsibilities of Patients" in its accreditation manual. Among the rights that hospitals must provide to patients to be accredited are access to health care, the right to respect and dignity, the right to privacy and confidentiality, the right to personal safety, the right to their identity, the right to information about their treatment and hospital rules and regulations, the right to communication with the health care staff, the right to give or not give consent, the right to consultation, the right to refuse treatment, the right to know what the charges for the treatment or care will be, and the right to transfer and continuity of care.

On the other hand, patients also have responsibilities, such as providing information about themselves and their condition, complying with instructions given them in conjunction with their care and treatment, and behaving within the rules and regulations of the institution.

Informed Consent. One important aspect of the Patient's Bill of Rights is the matter of informed consent (Fig. 2-1). **Informed consent** is a person's agreement to allow something to happen (for example, surgery) based on a full exclosure of facts needed to make an intelligent decision (that is, knowledge of risks involved, benefits, alternatives, or consequences of refusal). The law has long recognized that individuals have the right to be free from bodily intrusion. Before any invasive treatments or procedures can be performed, the patients must consent to treatment. Not only must they give their consent, they must also be allowed to make an informed choice as to whether an alternative method of treatment and/or care will be provided or whether the proposed treatment is necessary.

Procedures must be followed that provide in nontechnical terms an explanation to patients of the preferred treatment, the risks involved, alternative courses of treatment, and who will be performing the treatment or procedure. A method to ensure that patients understand what they are told should be included in these procedures.

Following such procedures not only helps to avoid unnecessary lawsuits but establishes a relationship of trust between the patient and the health care providers. One who performs a procedure on a patient without informed consent may be found civilly liable for committing battery.

Controls for the Protection of the Practical/Vocational Nurse

Standards of care not only assure patients that practical/vocational nurses will perform their duties based on the criteria established by the profession, they also protect the nurses.

The standards of care that a reasonable person would use in a particular circumstance are made known through the Nurse Practice Acts of each state, the rules and regulations established by administrative law, standing operating procedures of the various health care agencies, and employee policies of the health care institutions.

Deviations from the standards of care provide grounds for charges of **negligence** (the commission of an act that a prudent person would not have done or the omission of a duty that a prudent person would have fulfilled, resulting in injury or harm to another person; the failure to meet the ordinary standards of care, one not involving special knowledge or skill, which leads to harm) or **malpractice** (professional negligence that is the proximate cause of injury or harm to a patient, resulting from a lack of professional knowledge, experience, or skill that can be expected in others in the profession or from a failure to exercise reasonable care or judgment in the application of professional knowledge, experience, or skill). The nurse has a responsibility to behave in a reasonable and prudent manner within the parameters of the accepted standards of care. The best protection that nurses have against potential lawsuits is that they act within the scope of the standards of care that are expected in a given circumstance.

Nurse Practice Acts. One aspect of the nurse-society relationship is spelled out in the state nursing practice act (NPA). To practice nursing, one must be licensed. This is one way to protect the public from incompetent, unscrupulous, and illegal behavior.

Every state has laws governing professions or occupations, with general provisions for all professionals and specific provisions for each profession, including nursing. The latter is generally known as the state's *nursing practice act.* This law defines nursing practice, identifies the scope of practice, outlines professional and unprofessional conduct, and creates a board of nursing empowered to make decisions about nursing to protect the public. Board of nursing activities include the following:

1. Approving schools, curriculum, and programs in nursing
2. Defining the scope of nursing and the entry requirements into nursing practice, such as licensure examination
3. Participating in disciplinary actions involving nurses
4. Identifying standards of care

Specific nursing practice act provisions allow graduates of nursing programs who are waiting to take the licensing examination to practice nursing for a limited time between the time of graduation and receiving the results of the licensing examination. With the CAT examination, the waiting period will be very short. The licensed practical/vocational nurse is required by law to practice under the supervision of a registered nurse, li-

Great Plains Regional Medical Center
601 West Leota - P.O. Box 1167
North Platte, Nebraska 69103-1167
308-534-9310

AUTHORIZATION FOR AND CONSENT TO OPERATION, ADMINISTRATION OF ANESTHETICS, SPECIAL DIAGNOSTIC OR THERAPEUTIC PROCEDURES AND THE RENDERING OF OTHER MEDICAL SERVICES

Addressograph

Patient Barbara McVey Date January 9, 1995 Time 0800

1. **Operation or Procedure and Alternatives**
   a. I hereby authorize Dr. Jennifer H. Christensen and whomever he may designate as his assistants to perform the following procedure and/or alternative procedure necessary to treat my condition: (state nature of procedure(s) to be performed).

   Right total hip replacement
   OK for blood transfusion
   (LIST PROCEDURE(S))

   b. I understand the reason for the procedure is: to replace my right hip joint and the head of my right hip bone. OK to receive blood transfusion

   c. For the purpose of advancing medical education and care, I consent to the admittance of observers to the Operating Room.
   d. It has been explained to me that conditions may arise during this procedure whereby a different procedure or an additional procedure may need to be performed and I authorize my physician and his assistants to do what they feel is needed and necessary.
   e. I understand that no guarantee or assurance has been made as to the results of the procedure and that it may not cure the condition.
   f. I consent to the examination and disposal by hospital authorities of any tissues or body parts which may be removed.
2. **Risks:** This authorization is given with the understanding that any operation or procedure involves some risks and hazards. The more common risks include: infection, bleeding nerve injury, blood clots, heart attack, allergic reactions, and pneumonia. These risks can be serious and possibly fatal. Specific risks for this procedure have been explained to me by my physician.
3. **Anesthesia:** The administration of anesthesia also involves risks, most importantly a rare risk of reaction to medications causing severe injury or death. I consent to the use of such anesthetics as may be considered necessary by the person responsible for these services.
4. **Photography:** I consent to the photographing of operations to be performed, including appropriate portions of my body for medical, scientific, or educational purposes, providing my identity is not revealed by the pictures or by the descriptive texts accompanying them.
5. **Patient's Consent:** I have read and fully understand this consent form, and I understand I should not sign this form if all items, including all my questions, have not been explained or answered to my satisfaction or if I do not understand any of the terms or words contained in this consent form.

   IF YOU HAVE ANY QUESTIONS AS TO THE RISKS OR HAZARDS OF THE PROPOSED SURGERY OR TREATMENT, OR ANY QUESTIONS CONCERNING THE PROPOSED SURGERY OR TREATMENT ASK YOUR SURGEON NOW!
   BEFORE SIGNING THIS CONSENT FORM.

   DO NOT SIGN UNLESS YOU HAVE READ AND THOROUGHLY UNDERSTAND THIS FORM!
6. I certify that I have read and fully understand the above consent after adequate explanations were made to me, and after all blanks were filled in or crossed out before I signed.

Dr. J.H. Christensen
(Doctor Signature)

Signed Barbara McVey
(Patient, Parent, or Legal Guardian's Signature)
or

Jessica H. DeBoom LPN
(Witness to Signature only)

(Second Witness Signature if needed)
(i.e. Telephone Consent)

FIG. 2-1 Sample consent form for a special procedure. (Courtesy Great Plains Regional Medical Center, North Platte, Neb.)

censed medical physician, osteopathic physician, or dentist. Specific provisions describe the scope of student nurse practice while in training.

Rules and Regulations. Administrative rules and regulations are written within the scope of the authority granted by the legislative body of the respective state.

Administrative agencies, such as the board of nursing in each state, develop the rules and regulations that ensure that the Nurse Practice Act can be effectively implemented. These rules and regulations detail how the act will be implemented and describe procedures that are measureable and enforceable.

Standard Operating Procedures. Each health care agency has established standard operating procedures that have been approved by its administrative body.

Standard operating procedures are written documents that contain rules, policies, procedures, regulations, and orders for the conduct of patient care in various stipulated circumstances that are unique to the agency making them known. In such procedures, conditions are usually specified under which a prescribed action is to be taken. Health care providers are guided as they provide care in their institution or agency. The standard operating procedures of an organization are the means of establishing and maintaining the standards for the organization.

Employee Policies. Employee policies, often described in a handbook that is distributed to all newly hired employees, should provide personnel with key information about the operation of the organization. These policy statements should include such information as the organization's philosophy, goals, rules, regulations, procedures, and behavioral expectations. It is important for all employees to understand the operation and responsibility of the organization as it relates to their positions in that organization.

Good Samaritan Acts. Good Samaritan Acts provide rules that govern how a citizen within a state can, by law, act in lending assistance to another citizen. Such an act is especially written to encourage health care providers to render assistance to people in distress or at the scene of an accident.

These acts protect health care providers from civil liability while rendering help to people in need. Because of these acts, health care providers are immune from any liability from suit that might be brought against them as long as they are acting within the level of skill and training and act reasonably.

Liability Protection. The ever-changing environment of health care and the complexity of the legal system contribute to a higher incidence of medical malpractice lawsuits in the United States than ever before. Whereas in the past, the physician and the health care institution were usually the targets of lawsuits, health care providers at every level are now equally vulnerable.

Health care agencies and institutions usually provide an adequate level of malpractice insurance to cover their employees under normally adverse situations. However, this coverage does not always provide the full range of protection that is sometimes needed under unusual or unforeseen circumstances. This kind of protective insurance can be found only in a personal, professional **liability** (legal concept that one is responsible and will be held accountable for one's actions [personal liability], that a corporation is responsible and answerable for its own decisions [corporate liability], or that an employer is responsible for an employee's acts done within the

Box 2-3 DO'S AND DO NOT'S

Do:

- Document all unusual incidences.
- Report all unusual incidences.
- Know your job description.
- Follow policies and procedures as established by your employing agency.
- Keep current your license to practice.
- Perform procedures that you have been taught and that are within the standard scope of your practice.
- Protect patients from injuring themselves.
- Remain alert and focused.
- Establish and maintain rapport with patients and family.
- Question and clarify orders when the patient's medical condition changes.
- Practice safety with verbal physician's orders.

Do not:

- Remove side rails on patients' beds unless there is an order or hospital policy to do so.
- Allow patients to leave the hospital or nursing home unless there is an order or signed release. (However, current rules prevent holding patients against their will. This can lead to a charge of false imprisonment. The nurse should attempt to have the patient sign a form, "Against Medical Advice," if they insist on leaving without a physician's dismissal.)
- Accept money or gifts from patients.
- Give advice that is contrary to physician orders or the nursing care plan.
- Give medical advice to friends and neighbors.
- Attempt to "practice medicine."
- Witness a patient's will.
- Take medications that belong to patients.
- Work as a licensed practical/vocational nurse in a state in which you are not licensed.

scope of employment) insurance policy. Carrying malpractice insurance, once the burden only of a physician, now is a consideration for the nurse as well. Malpractice insurance provides personal protection by paying damages, when warranted, against the nurse. It also pays for legal fees, bonds, and lost wages under certain circumstances. The nurse may obtain liability insurance through various professional organizations or through advertisements in professional journals. The premium ranges from \$50 to \$100 per year for \$1,000,000 to \$1,500,000 policies.

Although this is neither an endorsement of malpractice insurance for the nurse nor an indictment of society's view of the medical and health care profession's behavior, it is a fact that every nurse must accept. Box 2-3 on p. 23 lists *do's* and *do not's* as guidelines for safe practice.

DEFENSES: HOW TO AVOID LAWSUITS

Prevention is the best defense to a lawsuit. If the lawsuit cannot be prevented, a well-written medical record provides the second-best defense. The nurse who wants to stay out of court should always remember the following three Ds of nursing malpractice defense: dedication, demeanor, and documentation.

Dedication to competency is of primary importance in avoiding lawsuits. The licensed practical/vocational nurse must know and do what is expected by virtue of licensure and must always abide by the appropriate standards of care. The licensed practical/vocational nurse must maintain the highest level of competency at all times, including maintaining skills through continuing education. A dedicated nurse always gives the best quality care.

The nurse's *demeanor* is often the determining factor in whether the patient sues the nurse. A warm and caring demeanor may prevent a lawsuit. The nurse must never underestimate the significance of demeanor and rapport in malpractice prevention.

Documentation in the medical record provides the only credible proof in court that the appropriate care was given and the standards of care were met. The nurse should always remember that if it was not charted, it was not done.

The nurse who is conscientious about the three Ds of defense significantly minimizes the risk of ending up in court.[5]

SUMMARY

There are many legal issues confronting practicing nurses today, but nurses should view the law, not with apprehension, but as a helpful partner in defining nursing practice. Nurses aware of legal rights and obligations are better prepared to care for patients.

Nursing standards of care outline and define appropriate nursing interventions. Some standards are stated in general terms such as those enacted in nursing practice acts and those provided by professional nursing organizations. More specific standards are defined by the employing institutions. If nurses act within the accepted standard of care, their chances of being involved in a malpractice lawsuit are reduced.

Some legal issues, such as the necessity for informed consent and avoiding negligence, are involved in almost every branch of nursing. Nurses are responsible for knowing the laws that apply to their areas of nursing practice.

REFERENCES AND SUGGESTED READINGS

1. American Nurses Association: *Standards of continuing education in nursing,* Washington, DC, 1991, The Association.
2. Anderson BJ et al: Serving justice: how to give a deposition, *Am J Nurs* 91(3):32, 1991.
3. Badzek LA: What you need to know about advance directives, *Nursing* 22(6):58, 1992.
4. Beare PG, Myers JL: *Adult health nursing,* ed 2, St Louis, 1994, Mosby.
5. Becker BG, Fendlerd T: *Vocational and personal adjustments in practical nursing,* ed 6, St Louis, 1991, Mosby.
6. Calfee BE: Protecting yourself from allegations of nursing negligence, *Nursing* 21(12):34, 1991.
7. Calfee BE: *Staying out of court: a self assessment guide for nurses,* Beachwood, Ohio, 1991, Calfee & Associates.
8. Calfee JD et al: A question of informed consent, *Nursing* 21(4):66, 1991.
9. Donavan NM: Confidentiality vs. duty to warn—whose life is it anyway? *Nurs Health Care* 12(8):432, 1991.
10. Feutz SA: Do you need professional liability insurance? *Nursing* 21(1):56, 1991.
11. Hall JK: Understanding the fine line between law and ethics, *Nursing* 29(10):34, 1990.
12. Harrion L: *Professional issues in practical/vocational nursing,* Albany, NY, 1992, Delmar.
13. Johnson LG: Preparing for a deposition, *Nursing '90* 29(7):44, 1990.
14. Lacombe DC: Avoiding a malpractice nightmare, *Nursing '90* 29(6):42, 1990.
15. Lagerquist SL: Myths and facts . . . about legal issues, *Nursing* 20(2):30, 1990.
16. LPNs widen their role: disagreement grows, *Am J Nurs* 90(2):16, 1990.
17. Mason DJ: Nursing and politics: a professional comes of age, *Orthop Nurs* 9(5):11, 1990.
18. McCluree ML: Nursing and hospital cost containment, *J Prof Nurs* 7(1):4, 1991.
19. Mendall M: Practical ways to survive a lawsuit, *Nursing* 22(8):56, 1992.
20. Mitchell PR, Grippand GM: *Nursing perspectives and issues,* ed 5, Albany, NY, 1993, Delmar.
21. Moore G: Surviving a malpractice lawsuit, *Nursing* 23(10)54, 1993.
22. *Mosby's medical, nursing, and allied health dictionary,* ed 3, St Louis, 1994, Mosby.
23. Northrop CE: How good samaritan laws do and don't protect you, *Nursing* 20(2):50, 1990.
24. Pesto, MM: If you're asked to be an expert witness, *RN* 54(12):65, 1991.
25. Potter PA, Perry AG: *Fundamentals of nursing concepts, process and practice,* ed 3, St Louis, 1993, Mosby.

CHAPTER CHALLENGE

KEY POINTS

- Laws were developed on a case-by-case basis and were known as common law.
- The interpretation of statutes and regulations decides which of two conflicting approaches applies to a given situation, thus establishing precedent.
- Laws control the practice of the practical/vocational nurse.
- The patient has the right to expect care that is based on established standards of care.
- The legal process is becoming more and more prevalent in today's health care delivery system.
- The Nurse Practice Act of each state contains a legal definition of nursing practice and delineates the area of practice that the law seeks to regulate.
- Prevention is the best defense to a lawsuit. The nurse should always remember the three Ds of nursing malpractice defense: dedication, demeanor, and documentation.
- Standards of care are acts permitted to be performed or prohibited from being performed by a prudent person working within the parameters of training, license, and experience and the conditions existing at the time; the nurse's duty to a patient with whom there is an established nurse-patient relationship to provide reasonable, prudent care required by the circumstances.
- The Patient's Bill of Rights outlines what the patient can expect from the health care delivery system.
- Liability protection for the practical/vocational nurse provides personal protection in a society where increasing numbers of malpractice lawsuits are filed.
- Malpractice is professional negligence that is the proximate cause of injury or harm to a patient, resulting from a lack of professional knowledge, experience, or skill that can be expected in others in the profession or from a failure to exercise reasonable care or judgment in the application of professional knowledge, experience, or skill. Malpractice is the failure to meet a professional standard of care.

STUDY QUESTIONS

1. Ms. Grayston is a new LPN who is going to begin working in home health nursing. She carefully reads the Nurse Practice Act of the state in which she will practice. The primary purpose of the Nurse Practice Act is to:
   1. set standards of nursing practice
   2. define areas of activity for nursing practice
   3. set standards of education for nursing practice
   4. determine quality of nursing care
2. Mr. Borden is a staff LVN working on an orthopedics floor. He realizes nurses' roles are interrelated. The role prominently expressed when protecting the patient's human rights is that of:
   1. caregiver
   2. manager
   3. patient advocate
   4. rehabilitator
3. Mr. Bradinski is a 56-year-old patient with a CVA. He is unable to reposition himself in bed. To win a malpractice lawsuit against the nursing staff, Mr. Bradinski would need to establish that:
   1. his decubitus ulcer resulted from lack of care
   2. a felony has been committed against him
   3. empathetic rapport was not maintained
   4. the nurses intended to cause bodily harm
4. Miss Solos and Mr. Krion were discussing the incompetency of a patient's physician. The patient overheard the two nurses' discussion. The nurses could be held liable for:
   1. assault
   2. invasion of privacy
   3. slander
   4. malpractice
5. Mr. Rodrine has signed a consent for an abdominoperineal surgical procedure. Which of the following responses would indicate the patient had given consent?
   1. "My wife wants me to go through with this."
   2. "I understand, but what exactly will be done?"
   3. "I'm in so much pain that I'll sign anything."
   4. "I realize the stoma will be permanent."
6. Nurses must rely on the rights granted in their respective states to provide them basic legal protection; they must operate professionally, prudently, and within the scope of their authority. This provision is in the document called:
   1. Nurse Practice Act
   2. Standards of Care
   3. informed consent
   4. Patient's Bill of Rights
7. Administrative law is written within the scope of the authority granted by:
   1. the hospital
   2. the legislative body
   3. the nursing home
   4. the school of nursing

3

ETHICAL ASPECTS OF NURSING

Persephone C. Agrafiotis

KEY TERMS

advocate
accountability
autonomy
customs
dilemma
ethics
morals
mores
responsibility
value system

LEARNING OBJECTIVES

After reading this chapter, the student should be able to do the following:

- Define the key terms.
- Describe the evolution of ethical codes involved in the delivery of health care.
- Identify the importance of value clarification in the delivery of patient care.
- Outline the ethical issues of health care.
- List ethical dilemmas faced in practicing as a practical/vocational nurse.
- Discuss the nurse's role in responsibility and accountability for nursing interventions.
- Discuss the proper guidelines for reporting unethical behavior of a fellow nurse.

RELATED TOPICS OF INTEREST

- The evolution of nursing (Chapter 1)
- Legal aspects of nursing (Chapter 2)
- Care of the HIV-positive or AIDS patient (Chapter 37)
- Care of the patient with cancer (Chapter 38)
- Care of the mother and newborn at risk (Chapter 42)
- Hospice care (Chapter 53)
- The world of the graduate (Chapter 54)

EVOLUTION OF ETHICAL CODES AND CONSIDERATIONS

Shifting of today's attitudes and values is an obvious consequence of the tremendous change in society as a whole. Advances in medical knowledge and technology, combined with these societal changes, have greatly influenced ethical considerations of the health care delivery system.

Nursing **ethics** (science or study of moral values or principles, including ideals of self-determination, kindness, and justice), the study of principles of right and wrong conduct for nurses, provide the standards for professional behavior. Nursing ethics state the duties and obligations of nurses to their patients, other health professionals, the profession, and the community. The nurse is accountable to act under a code of ethical conduct and with belief in the dignity and worth of her patients. Nurses are constantly refining the nursing profession's guidelines to meet the daily challenges of an ever-changing and increasingly complex society. Respect for persons is the fundamental principle of professional behavior. Nurses are obligated to respect human existence and the individuality of persons to whom they provide nursing interventions. This respect is essential if meaningful, individual, and holistic patient care is to be provided. Nurses must take all responsible means to protect and sustain human life where there is hope of recovery or when patients can benefit from life-prolonging treatment. The nurse must meet the demands of a dynamic and pluralistic society by providing effective, responsible, and ethical health care.

Nurses should explore, assess, and determine their own personal values and should recognize their own priorities in the decision-making process. Nurses must be nonjudgmental in making decisions about their patients. This process must consider the patient's value system and needs.

Historical Perspective

Early history defines man as a member of a well-defined group known as the family. This family group was organized to provide solidarity and a means of survival against the hardships and adversities of the environment.

The primary means of perpetuating the family, or tribe as it was called early on, was to hand down the customs and mores that represented the way all members of the family were expected to behave. These **customs** (habitual practice; the usual way of acting under given circumstances) and **mores** (folkways of central importance, accepted without question and embodying the fundamental moral views of a group) became the law of the land, and strict enforcement by the family leaders strongly influenced family members to obey them. Noncompliance with these customs and mores meant banishment from the group or even death.

The health care needs of the family were provided by the members themselves, usually the women. As the need for care of the sick and infirm increased and became more complex, the need evolved for a designated "expert" to provide health care. This person was the family or tribal "medicine man." The medicine man learned how to care for the sick and to keep people well. The primary method used was to ward off evil spirits, which were believed to be the cause of all illness.

The medicine man was the primary caregiver until approximately 525 BC, when the Egyptians established the position of priest physician. The priest physician was responsible for performing both the religious and medical tasks required in Egyptian society. These combined practices assured the people that not only would they be cared for while they were alive, their status in life would be preserved after death.

Hippocrates, the Father of Medicine, did not accept this combination of medical and religious practice. He sought to dispel the mystical approach to a healthy body. His approach saw man as having three faculties: the mind, the body, and the spirit. These faculties, he believed, existed in unison, and for an individual to attain the ideal virtuous state, these faculties must be in perfect balance. He further proposed that physician and patient share a common set of values that would allow them to agree on what is considered beneficial or harmful to one's health. This was the basis for the Hippocratic Oath.

Over the years, the affiliation between the physician and the nurse was not always equitable. The ethical standards and practices of the physician did not include the nurse. As a result, the nursing profession sought to establish its own code of ethics as the ethical issues involved with medicine and health care increased.

The work of Florence Nightingale, Lavinia Dock, and Isabel Hampton Robb persuaded the members of the American Society of Superintendents of Training Schools of Nursing to include the development of a code of ethics as one of the objectives of that organization. In 1893 Lystra E. Gretter, of the Farrand School of Nursing in Detroit, Michigan, developed an oath resembling the Hippocratic Oath, called the Nightingale Pledge. The Code for Licensed Practical/Vocational Nurses was adopted by the National Federation of Licensed Practicel Nurses in 1961.

Ethics has always been an integral part of nursing. Throughout history one can find codes of ethics, statements of **moral** (generally accepted customs of conduct and right living in a society) principles, treatises on maintaining high ideals, and recorded discussions of moral and ethical issues. Caring for and comforting the sick and protecting the suffering are human activities of nurses.

These human activities and how society views them directly affect the mores, customs, and beliefs of humankind.

Values Associated with Health Care

A person's **value system** is the accepted mode of conduct and set of norms, goals, and values that the person has developed over many years, beginning in childhood. This system serves as a guide for the individual to determine what is right and what is wrong, what is good and what is bad, and what is desirable and what is undesirable. A person uses his value system in making decisions and achieving a meaningful life.

A person holds many values simultaneously and without conflict until faced with a severe state of stress or serious illness. when these situations occur, some values become more prominent and take precedence over all others. Most evident are the values of self-determination, well-being, and equity.

The principle of self-determination recognizes that people define their values and assume responsibility for particular life-styles and certain health practices. They are entitled to accept or reject health care interventions on the basis of these values and their personal goals.

The principle of well-being preserves and improves one's state of health by avoiding harm and seeking good physical and mental health care practices. The person's own best interest becomes the first priority and allows the choice of many options in health care.

The principle of equality causes the person to expect fair and equal treatment by sharing in the health care decision-making process as it relates to him. Common areas where shared decision making is needed include: the question of when life begins, abortion, contraception, sterilization, surrogate motherhood, organ transplant, AIDS, and drug testing.

In all cases, the right of free choice is an important value and must be respected by all who work in the health care delivery system.

Patient Advocacy

An **advocate** is a person who works on behalf of another person who is in a vulnerable or underprivileged position. Patients often are vulnerable when in the high-technology environment of a health care facility. Such an environment tends to threaten their **autonomy** (ability or tendency to function independently, personal liberty of action) because they do not always have the knowledge or the control to make meaningful decisions about their care. When this occurs, the patient advocate, acting on the patients' behalf, provides information to patients about their situation, helps patients understand their situation, assists health care providers in understanding patients and patients' perceptions of what is happening, and helps patients negotiate therapeutic relationships as these relationships pertain to their care and well-being.

Patient advocates provide relief and remedies against wrongdoing by members of the health care system. The advocates' activities, if accomplished within the scope of their charter, safeguard patients against possible abuse and violation of their basic rights.

Code of Ethics

Within any given profession, a code of ethics serves as a means of self-regulation and a source of guidelines for individual behavior and responsibility. Ideally, codes of ethics are a response to a society's needs for trustworthy, competent, and accountable practitioners. Professional codes of ethics are a system of rules and principles by which that profession is expected to regulate its members and demonstrate its responsibility to society. They provide an enforceable standard of minimal conduct and indicate the ethical considerations of professional conduct.

A code of ethics provides a standard of behavior that serves as a guide for (1) education and practice of nurses, (2) legislation affecting nurses, (3) licensing of nurses, and (4) public participation of nurses.

The Nightingale Pledge (Box 3-1), prepared by Gretter, included the basic principles governing ethical practices.

The pledge that was prepared for the practical nurses addressed similar aspects of the Nightingale Pledge (Box 3-2).

As ethical decision making became prevalent with the advancement of medical technology, the need for a code of ethics became apparent. In 1965 the Interna-

Box 3-1 THE NIGHTINGALE PLEDGE

I solemnly pledge myself before God and in the presence of this assembly:

To pass my life in purity and to practice my profession faithfully;

I will abstain from whatever is deleterious and mischievous and will not take or knowingly administer any harmful drug;

I will do all in my power to maintain and elevate the standard of my profession, and will hold in confidence all personal matters committed to my keeping and all family affairs coming to my knowledge in the practice of my calling;

With loyalty will I endeavor to aid the physician in his work, and devote myself to the welfare of those committed to my care.

tional Council of Nurses, which met in Geneva, Switzerland, decided that these pledges did not meet the needs of nurses in some countries, so they adopted an International Code of Ethics. In 1973 the Code was revised to reflect the changes of the health care delivery system (Box 3-3).

VALUE CLARIFICATION

Value clarification is the expression of a person's preferences, likes, and dislikes about those things affecting life and living that are important to her.

Issues such as life and death, belief or disbelief in God, what is good and what is bad, the concept of truth, and the concept of love are only a few of the values that must be considered when the health care provider must make a health care decision.

Patient's Values

Each patient's character is defined by the value choices he makes and then incorporates into his value system. These values are statements (nonverbal) that a patient makes through behavior, expression of need, or actions. They define what is important to the patient at a time when health care decisions must be made.

These value choices (1) contribute to the development of health care goals, attitudes, and feelings experienced when people are patients and (2) grow from people's experiences as patients to become a permanent part of their value systems.

Box 3-2 THE PRACTICAL NURSE'S PLEDGE

Before God and those assembled here, I solemnly pledge:

To adhere to the code of ethics of the nursing profession;

To cooperate faithfully with the other members of the nursing team and to carry out faithfully and to the best of my ability the instructions of the physician or the nurse who may be assigned to supervise my work;

I will not do anything evil or malicious and I will not knowingly give any harmful drug or assist in malpractice;

I will not reveal any confidential information that may come to my knowledge in the course of my work;

And I pledge myself to do all in my power to raise the standards and the prestige of practical nursing.

May my life be devoted to service, and to the high ideals of the nursing profession.

Box 3-3 ETHICAL CONCEPTS AND NURSING

The fundamental responsibility of the nurse is fourfold: to promote health, to prevent illness, to restore health, and to alleviate suffering.

The need for nursing is universal. Inherent in nursing is respect for life, dignity, and rights of man. It is unrestricted by considerations of nationality, race, creed, colour, age, sex, politics, or social status.

Nurses render health services to the individual, the family, and the community and coordinate their services with those of related groups.

NURSES AND PEOPLE

The nurse's primary responsibility is to those people who require nursing care.

The nurse, in providing care, promotes an environment in which the values, customs, and beliefs of individuals are respected.

The nurse holds in confidence personal information and uses judgment in sharing this information.

NURSES AND PRACTICE

The nurse carries personal responsibility for nursing practice and for maintaining competence by continual learning.

The nurse maintains the highest standards of nursing care possible within the reality of a specific situation.

The nurse uses judgment in relation to individual competence when accepting and delegating responsibilities.

The nurse when acting in a professional capacity should at all times maintain standards of personal conduct which reflect credit upon the profession.

NURSES AND SOCIETY

The nurse shares with other citizens the responsibility for initiating and supporting action to meet the health and social needs of the public.

NURSES AND CO-WORKERS

The nurse sustains a cooperative relationship with co-workers in nursing and other fields.

The nurse takes appropriate action to safeguard the individual when his care is endangered by a co-worker or any other person.

NURSES AND THE PROFESSION

The nurse plays the major role in determining and implementing desirable standards of nursing practice and nursing education.

The nurse is active in developing a core of professional knowledge.

The nurse, acting through the professional organization, participates in establishing and maintaining equitable social and economic working conditions in nursing.

From The International Council of Nurses, 3, place Jean Marteau CH-1201, Geneva. Reaffirmed by the Council of National Representatives, 1989.

Choices made by patients, then, are based on what is perceived as important to them at the time they are confronted with a traumatic situation.

Practical/Vocational Nurse's Practice Values

The practical/vocational nurse is a vital and active member in decision making about patient care. This is accomplished in an ever-changing environment of health care technology. Such developments include human experimentation, euthanasia, right to life, abortion, living wills, informed consent, Do Not Resuscitate orders, drug and alcohol abuse and testing, sterilization, use of blood, care of the elderly, and organ transplant.

The ultimate goals in health care are to achieve maximum health potential, to maintain good health, to prevent disease, and to provide rehabilitative care.

The practical/vocational nurse is responsible for assisting the patient to achieve these goals by adhering to the standards of ethical practice and conduct set for in the Code for Licensed Practical/Vocational Nurses adopted by the National Federation of Licensed Practical/Vocational Nurses (NFLPN), revised in 1991 (Box 3-4).

Box 3-4 THE CODE FOR LICENSED PRACTICAL/VOCATIONAL NURSES

1. Know the scope of maximum utilization of the LP/VN as specified by the nursing practice act and function within this scope.
2. Safeguard the confidential information acquired from any source about the patient.
3. Provide health care to all patients regardless of race, creed, cultural background, disease, or lifestyle.
4. Refuse to give endorsement to the sale and promotion of commercial products or services.
5. Uphold the highest standards in personal appearance, language, dress, and demeanor.
6. Stay informed about issues affecting the practice of nursing and delivery of health care and, where appropriate, participate in government and policy decisions.
7. Accept the responsibility for safe nursing by keeping oneself mentally and physically fit and educationally prepared to practice.
8. Accept responsibility for membership in NFLPN and participate in its efforts to maintain the established standards of nursing practice and employment policies which lead to quality patient care.

From National Federation of Licenced Practical Nurses, Inc, 1991.

ETHICAL ISSUES

Nursing has a commitment to keep the well-being of a patient the primary focus in the delivery of health care. Ethical codes of practice emphasize the obligation to fulfill this commitment. Making difficult, complex ethical decisions is an inherent part of the practical/vocational nurse's role.

Ethical decisions are not made in a vacuum. Many factors influence the process as one searches for the right decision. It is important to understand all the factors involved in the decision-making process and to appreciate that these factors are not independent or mutually exclusive but act and react with one another.

Right to Know

In response to patients' demands and as an outcome of court decisions regarding the methods by which health care is delivered, the "right to know movement" has had a significant effect on the health care system. This movement prompted the American Hospital Association to issue its "Patient's Bill of Rights" in 1973 (see Chapter 1).

Patients who receive health care in the context of organized institutions, such as hospitals, nursing homes, and ambulatory care centers, depend on health care providers for all aspects of care. Patients should not be treated as persons incapable of learning, and they should not be manipulated and coerced into making decisions about their care that suit the health care provider. Rather, the health care provider should assist the patient in making intelligent decisions based on adequate information regarding her condition and within the scope of the patient's values.

Confidentiality

Confidentiality is the cornerstone of the nurse-patient relationship. Because it instills trust, promotes autonomy, enables human relationships, and ensures fidelity, it is an inherent and respected ethical duty.[6] Confidentiality allows patients to seek assistance without fear of public disclosure, preserves the patient's right to self-determination, and facilitates free disclosure of information.[1] A nurse who discloses privileged information violates the patient's rights to privacy and autonomy and jeopardizes the nurse-patient relationship, threatening the quality and effectiveness of further nursing care.[20]

The development of a trusting relationship contributes positively to the total environment of patient care. The practical/vocational nurse has an obligation to preserve patients' privacy by holding information regarding their care in strict confidence.

All information about a patient and his care belongs to that patient. The nurse safeguards the patient's right to privacy by prudently protecting information of a confidential nature. Nurses avoid discussing the condition of

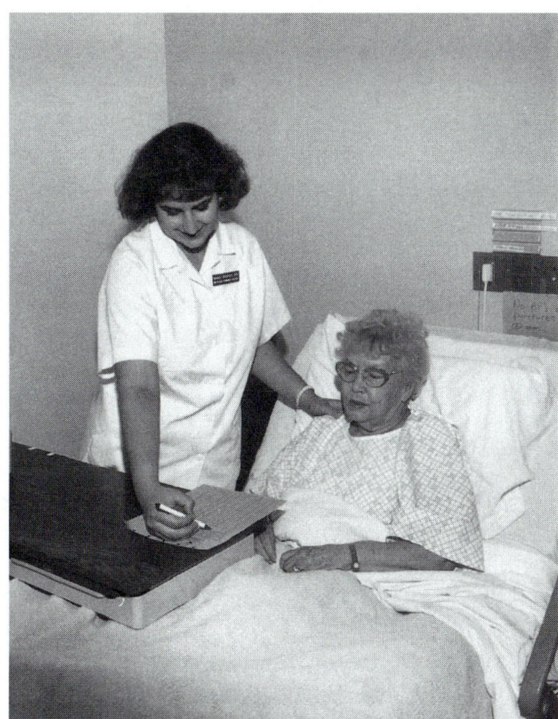

a patient with anyone who is not involved in the patient's care. The ANA's Code for Nurses (1987) maintains that the nurse safeguards the patient's right to privacy by protecting confidential information.

Maintaining patient confidentiality is a valuable tool because by creating an atmosphere of trust, the health care provider makes it possible for patients to feel comfortable about telling the truth about their condition. Furthermore, there may be serious legal ramifications when the privacy of a patient is invaded, misused, or otherwise compromised.

Policies have been adopted within health care agencies that provide specific guidelines about what information must be revealed according to existing freedom-of-information laws. In most cases this information does not violate patient confidentiality.

Accountability and Responsibility

A nurse assumes responsibility and accountability for nursing interventions provided. **Responsibility** refers to the execution of duties associated with the nurse's particular role. When administering medications, the nurse is responsible for assessing the patient's need for the drugs, giving them safely and correctly, and evaluating the responses. A nurse who acts in a responsible manner gains the trust of patients and co-workers. A responsible nurse maintains competence in knowledge and skills and demonstrates a willingness to perform within the ethical guidelines of the profession.

Box 3-5 MAINTAINING PROFESSIONAL ACCOUNTABILITY

SELF

- Report any personal conduct that endangers patients
- Stay informed of current nursing practice theory and issues
- Make judgments based on facts

PATIENT

- Provide patients with accurate information about care
- Conduct nursing care in a manner that ensures patient safety and well-being

PROFESSION

- Maintain ethical standards in practice
- Encourage peers to follow the same
- Report a colleague's unethical behavior

EMPLOYING INSTITUTION

- Follow policy and procedures defined by the institution

SOCIETY

- Maintain ethical conduct in the care of all patients in all settings

Accountability means being answerable for one's own actions. A nurse is accountable to self, the patient, the profession, the employer, and society (Box 3-5). If an incorrect dose of medication is given, the nurse is accountable to the patient who received it, the physician who ordered it, the nursing service that set standards of expected performance, and society, which demands professional excellence. To be accountable, the nurse acts according to the professional code of ethics. Thus, when an error is made, the nurse reports it and initiates care to prevent further injury. Accountability calls for an evaluation of a nurse's effectiveness in practice. Professional accountability serves the following purposes:

1. Allows evaluation of new professional practices and reassessment of existing ones.
2. Maintains standards of health care.
3. Facilitates personal reflection, ethical thought, and personal growth on the part of health care professionals.
4. Provides a basis for ethical decision making.

To be accountable, the nurse practices within the code of the profession. Accountability requires an evaluation of the nurse's performance in providing nursing interventions. The Joint Commission on Accreditation of Healthcare Organizations (JCAHO) has recommended the establishment of standards for the delivery of nursing interventions. The standards are developed by clinical experts within the department of nursing. These standards provide a basic structure against which nursing interventions are objectively measured. These standards do not eliminate the need for individualized care plans. Instead, the nurse incorporates the standards into care plans. Accountability is better ensured because the quality of care can be measured.

Reporting Unethical Behavior

Reporting a fellow nurse is never an easy decision to make, but it is an ethical responsibility to patients and the nursing profession as well as to one's own conduct. Some of the factors to consider are the following:

1. Has the behavior caused harm to a patient?
2. Is the behavior against the ethical code of nursing practice?

It is important to remember that the nurse's primary commitment is to the health, welfare, and safety of the patient. If these areas are being adversely affected by the unethical behavior, it must be documented and reported.

The following guidelines should be followed for reporting unethical behavior:

1. Always follow the proper channels.
2. Be clear and specific. Document carefully the conduct and the issues.
3. Be absolutely accurate. Describe only those areas that you know to be true.
4. Be consistent and honest.
5. Document all actions taken. Be certain to include names, dates, times, place, and actions taken.
6. Continue to follow the proper channels and procedures.

Before beginning any actions against a fellow nurse, it is advisable to discuss the problem with the nurse directly. If the outcome of the discussion is not satisfactory, a consultation with a trusted professional and an appropriate course of action must be pursued.

Box 3-6 ETHICAL DILEMMAS: WHAT WOULD YOU DO IF . . .

You are a nurse caring for Mr. Jones, a patient who is critically ill with *Pneumocystis carinii* pneumonia. Mr. Jones has just been diagnosed with acquired immunodeficiency syndrome (AIDS). He is comatose, and the physician doesn't expect him to survive. The patient lived with a woman, Ms. Jinkins, and her three young children. Ms. Jinkins doesn't know Mr. Jones is infected with the human immunodeficiency virus (HIV). Mr. Jones's doctor believes that only the patient's next of kin—in this case, his mother—are entitled to this confidential information. The mother and Ms. Jinkins have a hostile relationship, so you doubt that Ms. Jinkins will learn the truth about his condition from her. What would you do?[27]

You have just received confirmation that you are 10 weeks pregnant. Your obstetrician cautions you to avoid exposure to infectious diseases because of the effects it may have on the fetus. You are assigned to take care of a newly admitted patient with AIDS. What would you do?

You are assigned to the operating room as an assistant scrub nurse. You are scheduled to assist with an abortion. Abortion is contrary to your religious belief. What would you do?

You attended a party with a nurse with whom you work. She was drinking heavily and began to disclose that she was addicted to drugs such as morphine, Librium, Valium, and codeine. She showed you a handful of the drugs that she was taking. The next day you are assigned to work on the same unit with her. At the end of the shift, the narcotic count is incorrect. What would you do?

You are assigned to care for a 75-year-old female patient who has a cerebral vascular accident, has brain damage, and is on a respirator. You overheard family members discussing whether they should give approval for a "Do Not Resuscitate" order to be written by their physician. The respirator alarm has just gone off. What would you do?

ETHICAL DILEMMAS

A **dilemma** is defined as a situation requiring a choice between two equally desirable or undesirable alternatives. In an ethical dilemma, each alternative course of action can be justified by the way in which a person views the course of action based on her value system.

Issues in health care delivery practices present different alternatives based on whether the issue or course of action is viewed by the patient, the health care agency, the legal system, or the practical/vocational nurse.

The dilemma occurs when opposing views are seen for the solution of an issue and a decision must be made. There are no set procedures or easy answers for how an ethical dilemma should be resolved. A list of challenging ethical dilemmas is presented in Box 3-6.

Box 3-7 PRIMARY FUNCTIONS OF ETHICS COMMITTEES

- To direct educational programs that provide knowledge regarding ethical principles and issues for the medical and professional community
- To assist the hospital nursing and medical staff in the development and review of policies related to ethical responsibilities. Examples include the "Do Not Resuscitate" policy and the advance directives policy
- To serve in an advisory capacity and/or as a resource for persons involved with a specific patient to resolve ethical situations or make decisions related to the patient's care
- To evaluate institutional experiences related to reviewing decisions having ethical implications

ETHICS COMMITTEES

The patient's rights movement, in conjunction with the complexity and rising costs of health care, has accelerated the consumer movement in today's society. Consumers are demanding greater participation in the decision-making process as it affects them in the delivery of health care. At the same time, health care workers are recognizing that scientific and technological advances and increased public awareness have raised complex ethical, legal, and social questions about patients and the medical and nursing care provided to them. These changes led to the formation of ethics committees.

Ethics committees include physicians, administrators, nurses, social workers, spiritual advisors, attorneys, public policy makers, and consumers. Any member of the health care team can bring issues to an ethics committee for formal review. Nurses have the responsibility to be knowledgeable about the existence of an ethics committee within the health care environment and about ways to access committee members for assistance in ethical situations (Box 3-7).

REFERENCES AND SUGGESTED READINGS

1. Brown ML: AIDS and ethics: concerns and considerations, *Oncol Nurs Forum* 14:69, 1987.
2. Davis AJ, Aroska MA: *Ethical dilemmas and nursing practice,* ed 3, Norwalk, Conn, 1991, Appleton & Lange.
3. Flarey DL: Advanced directive: in search of self-determination, *JONA* 21(11):16, 1991.
4. Grant AB: Exploring an ethical dilemma, *Nursing* 22(12):52, 1992.
5. Greve J, Paul A: Keep quiet or speak up? Issues in patient confidentiality, *RN* 53(12):53, 1990.
6. Haddad A: The dilemma of keeping confidences, *AORN* 50(159):162, 1989.
7. Hall JK: Understanding the fine line between law and ethics, *Nursing* 20(10):34, 1990.
8. Harrion L: *Professional issues in practical/vocational nursing,* Albany, NY, 1992, Delmar.
9. Joint Commission on the Accreditation of Healthcare Organizations: *Accreditation manual for health care organizations,* Oakbrook Terrace, IL, 1991, The Commission.
10. Kurzen CR: *Contemporary practical/vocational nursing,* ed 2, New York, 1993, Lippincott.
11. Lund M et al: Speaking out on ethics, *Geriatr Nurs* 11(5):223, 1990.
12. Melia K: Everyday ethics for nurses, *Nurs Times* 83:28, 1987.
13. Miedema F: A practical approach to ethical decisions, *Am J Nurs* 91(12):20, 1991.
14. Mitchell PR, Grippando GM: *Nursing perspective and issues,* ed 5, Albany, NY, 1993, Delmar.
15. Mitty EL: The nurse as an advocate: issues in long term care, *Nurs Health Care* 12(10):520, 1991.
16. *Mosby medical, nursing, and allied health dictionary,* ed 4, St Louis, 1994, Mosby.
17. Murphy P: Helping Jeanne die with dignity: a nursing profile in courage, *Nursing* 20(9):44, 1990.
18. Pauly OS: Dilemmas in practice: questioning the use of invasive technology, *Am J Nurs* 91(1):19, 1991.
19. Potter PA, Perry AG: *Fundamentals of nursing concepts, process, and practice,* ed 3, St Louis, 1993, Mosby.
20. Reisman EC: Ethical issues confronting nurses, *Nurs Clin North Am* 23(4):789, 1988.
21. Salladay SA, McDonnel MM: Facing ethical conflicts, *Nursing* 22(2):44, 1992.
22. Saloman Cohen S: Health care policy and abortion: a comparison, *Nurs Outlook* 38(1):20, 1990.
23. Saylor DC: The LP/VN's role in bioethical decision-making, *J Pract Nurs Clin North Am* 23(4):789, 1988.
24. Scanlon C et al: Confronting ethical issues: a nursing survey, *Nurs Manage* 2(5):63, 1990.
25. Smith S: When ethics and orders conflict, *RN* 54(9):61, 1991.
26. Stark L: Health care under siege: the challenge for change, *Nurs Health Care* 12(1):26, 1991.
27. Stewer K: Dilemmas in practice: AIDS, the way it is, *Am J Nurs* 90(12):16, 1990.
28. The ethics of HIV disclosure: to tell or not to tell, *Nursing* 23(3):50, 1993.
29. Winslow BJ, Winslow GR: Integrity and compromise in nursing ethics, *J Med Philos* 16(3):307, 1991.
30. Young-Mason J: The secret sharer as a guide to compassion, *Nurs Outlook* 39(2):62, 1991.

CHAPTER CHALLENGE

KEY POINTS

- Early civilization contributed to the development of humans' value systems as they exist in today's pluralistic society.
- A person's value system influences the ethical decisions made regarding health care.
- Codes of ethics are systems of rules and principles that guide the members of a profession in meeting the ethical standards of that profession.
- Value clarification is the process whereby personal values of the practical/vocational nurse and the patient are considered when providing holistic health care.
- Early ethical principles for nurses were outlined in the Nightingale Pledge.
- The quality of a practical/vocational nurse's practice is performed within the scope of the standards of practice established by the profession, the Nurse Practice Acts, and the policies, rules, and regulations of the health care agency.
- Health care workers recognize that scientific and technological advances have raised complex ethical, legal, and social questions about patients and the medical and nursing care provided to them.
- Nurses have a responsibility to be knowledgeable about the existence of an ethics committee within the health care environment and about how to access committee members for assistance in ethical situations.

STUDY QUESTIONS

1. Ms. Serrotus is a nurse who is assigned to work on a medical floor. Ms. Serrotus is aware in her practice of nursing that a nurse's use of ethical responsibility can best be seen in which of the following ways:
   1. delivery of competent patient care
   2. formation of interpersonal relationships
   3. application of the nursing process
   4. evaluation of medical technologies
2. Miss Islom, a student nurse, realizes that she has administered the wrong dose of medication to a patient. She immediately informs her nurse educator. This student nurse is described ethically as:
   1. honest
   2. trustworthy
   3. sorry
   4. accountable
3. Nurses have a professional code of ethics. The purpose of such a code is to:
   1. state the specific decision-making steps in an ethical dilemma
   2. provide standards of conduct for the practice of nursing
   3. clearly govern nurse practice
   4. provide a tool for interpretation of individual expectations
4. Mr. Karto, general duty nurse, has been asked by the patient to increase the dosage of a tranquilizer above the prescribed order. Mr. Karto did not comply because he adheres to the accepted code of conduct and set of norms and goals that he has developed over many years. This is referred to as his:
   1. patient advocacy
   2. ethical dilemma
   3. principles of beneficence
   4. value system
5. Mrs. Justin, LPN, is working as a staff member in a nursing home. One of the patients, Mrs. Laurens, an 89-year-old with Alzheimer's disease is restless, wanders, and has slept poorly for several nights. Mrs. Justin is told in report by Miss Tremal, a fellow nurse, that she borrowed a Halcion (hypnotic) and Darvocet N 100 (analgesic) from another patient and gave them unprescribed to Mrs. Laurens to "calm her down." After Mrs. Justin discusses the problem with Miss Tremal and reports the error to the physician, the next appropriate action would be to:
   1. do nothing because an oral reprimand was given
   2. report the problem to the State Department of Health
   3. bring the issue to the organization's ethics committee
   4. call her attorney to file a complaint
6. Mrs. Langson, 83 years old, is a patient in the hospital with congestive heart failure. She is alert, but forgetful and unsteady on her feet. In the past she has fallen, and the nurses are concerned for her safety. The nurse explains the need for Mrs. Langson to wear a safety reminder device when the nurse cannot be in attendance. This necessary action for the protection of the patient must, of necessity, interfere with Mrs. Langson's ability or tendency to function independently and thus has threatened her:
   1. beneficence
   2. autonomy
   3. value clarification
   4. informed consent

2

COMMUNICATING IN HEALTH CARE

There is a great satisfaction in being a student nurse. You can spend extra time with patients and are given the chance to make a difference and provide some comfort in an ill patient's life or death. Nursing can be frustrating and emotional, but the reward is much greater than the burden. Nursing gives a sense of worthiness, importance, and pride in yourself. I feel if you can leave a patient's bedside with the feeling that if you were in that bed and received the care you had given and felt as though someone does care and wants to help, then it's been a job well done. Nursing is a wonderful gift; giving it is even better.

Ginger Carole Snapp Medley
Student Nurse

4

COMMUNICATION

Sue Smith

KEY TERMS

aggression
aggressive communication
assertive communication
assertiveness
comfort
commiseration
communication
compassion
confrontation
consolation
empathy
feedback
first-level patient-focused response
humanistic nursing approach
nonverbal communication
ordinariness
pity
second-level patient-focused response
self-disclosure
sympathy
unassertive communication
verbal communication

LEARNING OBJECTIVES

After reading this chapter students should be able to do the following:

- Define the key terms.
- Discuss the meaning of effective communication.
- Discuss the importance of nurses communicating effectively with their patients.
- Explain the purpose of communication between patients and nurses.
- Discuss the importance of communicating assertively with patients as opposed to communicating unassertively or aggressively.
- Discuss the four categories of requests patients make of nurses: understanding, information, action, and comfort.
- Relate several ways to use effective communication to provide patients with understanding, information, and comfort.
- Describe the six steps of the systematic nursing process for communicating effectively with your patients.
- State effective ways of asking questions.
- Relate the ways in which nurses' communication can help patients feel important and valued or insignificant and unworthy.
- Discuss how nurses can improve their interpersonal communication with patients.

RELATED TOPICS OF INTEREST

- The nursing process (Chapter 5)
- Documentation (Chapter 6)
- Cultural aspects of nursing care (Chapter 8)
- Comfort, rest, and sleep (Chapter 15)
- Mental health concepts (Chapter 46)

As a practical/vocational nurse you perform a wide range of nursing functions for patients with a variety of physical and emotional health problems. The safety and proficiency with which you carry out your nursing care activities are of utmost importance. You must call upon a sound knowledge of physical sciences and technical skills to provide good nursing interventions for your patients, but technical competence is only part of the essential requirements for being a caring nurse. Equally significant are the interpersonal style and interpersonal communication skills you employ when communicating with your patients.

To demonstrate caring for your patients you must be a competent humanitarian as well as a competent practitioner. Using a **humanistic nursing approach** you will consider interactions with your patients as human-to-human interventions, not simply nurse-to-patient communication. "To humanistically 'care' requires the presence and the use of the nurse 'self' and the sharing of the 'self' with another."[2] Effective communication is a fundamental and essential part of every nurse's skill repertoire. When the nurse's communication is ineffective, patients complain that they are not heard or understood and that they are treated disrespectfully.[12]

The intent of this chapter is to increase your knowledge about communicating effectively with your patients. "A nurse with good communications skills is one who is able to assess patients' problems, gives patients the information they require, supports them in their distress [and] has the ability to determine when patients' problems require specialist intervention."[30]

Stuart and Sundeen's[24] definition of communication underlines the importance of interpersonal communication in the nurse-patient relationship. Included in their definition is that **communication** is the vehicle for establishing a therapeutic relationship since it involves conveying information and exchanging thoughts and feelings and that communication is also the means by which people influence the behavior of another.[24] Take some time to consider the impact of this definition and you will agree that communication is one of the strongest aspects of your nursing practice. To create a strong communication foundation for your nursing practice you must know essential ways to communicate effectively in a variety of circumstances with different patients.

Being an effective nurse-communicator is a challenge that requires a commitment to practice communicating effectively, a willingness to receive feedback from others, and the capacity for self-evaluation. Reading may improve your knowledge about communication but "you can only transform yourself through practice."[21] You have entered nursing with the knowledge and skills for being an effective interpersonal communicator. This chapter outlines ways you can add to this knowledge to build confidence and competence in your abilities to communicate effectively as a nurse.

PURPOSE OF COMMUNICATION BETWEEN NURSES AND PATIENTS

Every interpersonal interaction is an opportunity for you to make a positive difference in your patient's healing process. When nurses use good interpersonal communication skills, it increases patients' satisfaction with their health care services and compliance with their treatment. Patients make judgments about nurses' competence based on the effectiveness of nurses' interpersonal communication. It is, therefore, imperative for you, as a nurse, to become a sensitive and effective communicator with your patients.

Importance of Communication Skills

Everything you do as a nurse has communicative value.[10] The way you take in and make sense of information through your senses (hearing, sight, taste, smell, touch) and the way you send messages (verbal, nonverbal, written) are aspects of the way you communicate as a nurse (Box 4-1).

Function of Communication

A critical function of communication between you and your patients is the transmission of messages from one to the other in order to create understanding of each other's meaning. The real purpose of creating understanding between you and your patients is to effect some change. One such change is to influence another to respond to a request. Gerrard, Boniface, and Love[7] outlined four categories of requests your patients might make of you as a nurse: requests for understanding, information, comfort, and action.

Request for Understanding. Patients request that nurses comprehend their feelings and concerns. Patients want to hear in your own words that you understand

Box 4-1 WHY COMMUNICATION SKILLS ARE IMPORTANT FOR NURSES

- Communication is the vehicle nurses use to provide assistance to patients.
- Communication allows a person to establish, maintain, and improve contacts with others.
- Communication enables nurses to establish a working relationship with patients and eventually to help them meet their health care needs.
- Communication establishes relationships among the health care team and promotes continuity of care.
- Communication creates ways to effect change.[6]

exactly what they are feeling and experiencing. Whatever your patients experience—whether they are hurting, disoriented, excited, anxious, relieved, alienated, hopeful, terrified, or reassured—they want you as their nurse to demonstrate that you understand how they are feeling and the reasons they are reacting a particular way. For example, your patient tells you that he is scared *(feeling)* to have anesthesia because his mother died during an operation 4 years ago *(reason for feeling),* or your patient tells you that she feels frustrated *(feeling)* and trapped *(feeling)* in the hospital and longs *(feeling)* to get back home because her 4-year-old cries all night and won't go to preschool since she's been admitted *(reason for feelings).*

The request for understanding is met when nurses show patients that they comprehend what patients are feeling or experiencing and why they are reacting that way.

Request for Information. The request for information is the factual need for knowledge that patients require to understand and make decisions about their health care. Feedback, confrontation, and expressing opinions are some of the ways nurses provide patients with information.

Being hospitalized is an unusual and sometimes fearful experience for most people, and the unfamiliar surroundings and routines raise many questions. Patients often ask nurses to provide the information they require to understand and make decisions about their health care. Patients may request information about hospital routines, nursing interventions for their illness, pain control methods, and expected outcomes. For example, as you are changing his dressing, your patient asks you why you do things in a certain order and what is the purpose of the liquid you are applying to his open wound *(request for information about routines and treatment),* or your patient wants to know how long he will have his cast and when he can return to work *(request for information about his healing process and outcome).*

Request for Comfort. The request for comfort is the patients' requests to nurses for strength, cheer, or the easing of grief or trouble. Comfort is a demonstration that nurses care for their patients as people and evidence that they have personal interest in meeting patients' needs. Requests for comfort may be emotional or physical.

Patients need to know that nurses care about them as people, not simply as patients. Patients find it comforting when nurses show personal interest in meeting their health care needs. Requests for comfort may be emotional (e.g., requests for hope, cheer, or reassurance) or physical (e.g., requests for a blanket, warmer water for bathing, or an extra cup of coffee) (Fig. 4-1). For example, your patient wants to know if his reactions to treatment are "normal" and if his progress is going "as expected" *(request for emotional comfort in the form of reassurance),* or your patient tells you that he will start a course of radiation recommended by his physician for cancer, which has spread to his lymph nodes *(request for emotional comfort in the form of hope).*

Request for Action. The request for action is the patients' request for physical activities or treatments nurses carry out, such as providing physical comfort measures or ensuring a safe and convenient environ-

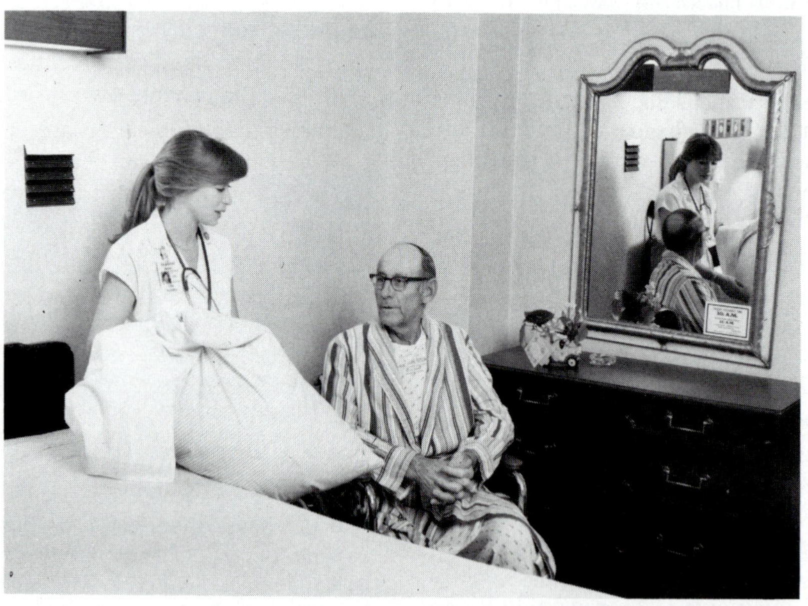

FIG. 4-1 The nurse integrates therapeutic communication skills into all aspects of care.

ment. It might be as simple as getting a glass of water, or performing a more complex nursing function such as assisting a patient with a total hip replacement to reposition in bed. For example, your patient asks you to limit *(request for action)* the number of visitors his roommate has during visiting hours because when seven relatives gather round the bed next to him, the noise of their talking and laughing sets off a migraine headache, or your patient tells you he has vomited and soiled his gown and asks you to change his sheets *(request for action).*

Direct and Indirect Requests

Your patients may make requests in clear and direct ways, or you may have to "read between the lines" to fully understand requests that are made in unclear or indirect ways. Illness is often accompanied by worry, anxiety, and fear, and the turmoil of these emotions might affect the clarity of your patients' communication. Since your patients' requests may be masked, you must listen carefully to pick out the request your patient is making.

Example One:

One of your postoperative patients asks you, "How long have I been in this position? When am I supposed to be turned next?" He touches his hip-to-toe cast on his left side and then rubs his lower back while grimacing.

Your patient's direct request is for information about the length of time he has been lying in his present position, and for information about when he can be assisted to turn to a more comfortable position. Some of his requests are unspoken. One unverbalized request is for your understanding that he is uncomfortable. As well, he is indirectly asking that you comfort him with the reassurance that you will not forget to turn him (action) as soon as it is time to rotate to a new position.

Example Two:

Your patient has been prepared for surgery and is awaiting her preoperative medications. She is scheduled for the surgical removal of a malignant growth from her left breast. She has been told that if the surgeon discovers metastases to the lymph nodes, her surgery will take longer and she will not return to the unit until much later. You are making your last checks to ensure that she is comfortable and warm when she says, "I wonder when I'll be back to the unit—for afternoon or evening visiting hours?"

It might sound as if she is requesting information about the length of surgery, but it is her indirect requests that are most important here. She wants you to show her you understand her fear about the surgery, which might reveal that her malignant growth has spread further than her breast tissue. Although you cannot reassure her about the surgical outcome, you may provide **comfort** that she is in capable surgical hands and that you (or one of your competent colleagues) will be present to care for her when she returns to the unit.

Example Three:

One of your patients is a 14-year-old boy whose malleolus has been severely crushed in a motor vehicle accident. It is unlikely that he will enjoy competitive athletics again. He had demonstrated remarkable potential in hockey, rising to the top of his league to receive the All-Star award for 2 consecutive years. It is time for him to go to the physiotherapy department for his daily therapy. When you pass his room, you notice that he has not dressed and is lying on top of his bed watching television. In response to your reminder about his physiotherapy appointment, he states, "I'm not going. What's the point anyway? It's just a stupid waste of time."

The most important request this patient is making is for understanding of what he is going through—coming to grips with a future of dashed hopes and dreams. He may be looking for comfort in the form of encouragement and hopefulness to continue with his physiotherapy treatments.

To be an effective nurse-communicator you must show initiative to discover the real requests your patients are making. Answering the following questions will help you determine your patients' requests: What does my patient want me to understand? What information does my patient require? What kind of action would be helpful to my patient? What kind of comfort is my patient requesting? Doing this mental check will help you to respond effectively to your patients.

TYPES OF COMMUNICATION: VERBAL AND NONVERBAL

Any message has two parts: the verbal expression of the sender's thoughts and feelings and the nonverbal expression of the sender's thoughts and feelings. **Verbal communications** are sent through words, voice inflection, and rate of speech. **Nonverbal communications** are conveyed by eye movements, facial expressions, and body posturing. When the verbal and nonverbal aspects of nurses' communication are congruent (harmonious) or matched, nurses are demonstrating genuineness. For example, you may wish to convey to your patient that you enjoy working with him and that you are pleased to have been assigned to his care. When you verbally tell him, "I am pleased to see you," and nonverbally you smile, and you make eye contact with him, your communication is genuine and congruent. If you were to verbally tell him, "I am pleased to see you" and nonverbally refrain from smiling, and avoid eye contact, your patient would get a different message from the one you gave verbally. In this example, the verbal communication does not match the nonverbal communication and is noncongruent. Your patient would get an unclear and confusing message and likely doubt the sincerity of your words.

Interpersonal communication is complex. There are many factors that influence it other than verbal and non-

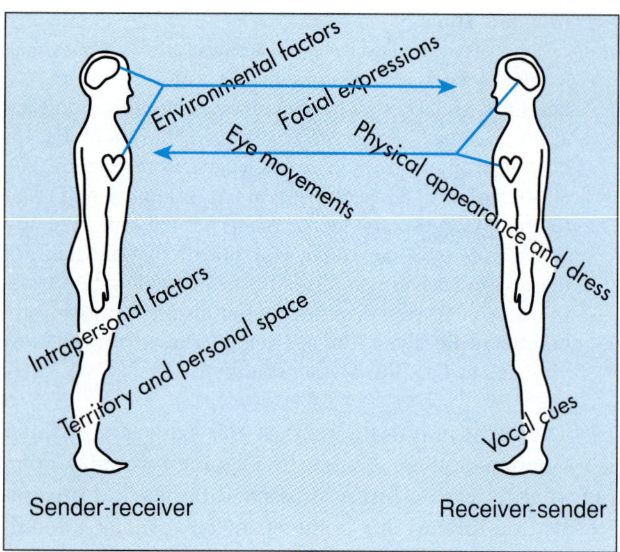

FIG. 4-2 Factors influencing interpersonal communication.

Box 4-2 ASSERTIVE COMMUNICATION FOR NURSES

Communicating assertively means:

- Being skilled in a variety of communication strategies for expressing your thoughts and feelings in a way that simultaneously protects your rights and those of your patients
- Having a positive attitude about communicating in a forthright and fair way
- Feeling comfortable and in control of negative feelings such as anxiety, tenseness, shyness, or fear
- Feeling comfortable that you can conduct yourself in a self-respecting manner
- Keeping your rights and those of your patients equally paramount

verbal messages. Here is a partial list of factors that affect your communication.[22]

- Environmental factors: formality, warmth, privacy, physical distance between people, climate, arrangement of furniture
- Territory and personal space: crowding, seating arrangements, roles and status (e.g., employer and employee), soundproofing, privacy
- Physical appearance and dress: body shape, body color, body odor, gender, body movements, posture, touch, height
- Intrapersonal factors: development stage, language mastery, values, self-concept

The above factors have the potential to enhance or detract from the effectiveness of communication (Fig. 4-2).

ASSERTIVE STYLE AS A RESPECTFUL APPROACH FOR NURSE-PATIENT COMMUNICATION

Assertiveness is the nurse's ability to confidently and comfortably express her thoughts and feelings while still respecting the legitimate rights of patients. Interpersonal communication that takes into account the feelings and requests of your patients yet honors your rights as a nurse in the relationship is the most effective approach. This style of communication is call **assertive communication.** Deep values of respect for self and other are the basis of assertive communication (Box 4-2).

Assertion is not continual confrontation; it is a conscious choice about verbal and nonverbal communication. Assertion involves choosing what to say, when and how to say it, and with whom to communicate. One intent of this chapter is to help you foster an assertive style in your communication with your patients by providing you with the communication skills to feel confident about the choices you make to solidify an attitude of mutual respect with your patients.

Every time you interact with your patients you exert an influence. The words you choose (verbal communication) and the posture or stance you assume (nonverbal communication) are merely two of the obvious factors that can make the difference between your patients feeling important and valued or feeling insignificant and unworthy. Here is an illustration of the power you have as a nurse to make a difference to your patients. Picture yourself as the nurse in the scene described below.

> It is mid-morning, and you are engaged in morning care activities with your patients on the orthopedic unit. One of your patients is scheduled for surgery immediately after lunch, and your assignment is to complete the surgical skin preparation. Time dictates that you complete this assignment soon. You are just about to collect your equipment when one of your patients asks if you will transfer her from her wheelchair back to bed. Time pressure makes you feel torn between starting your preoperative preparations and responding to Mrs. Jones' request for action and comfort (reassurance) that you will help. There are three ways you can respond, and each intervention has the power to affect your patient and you.

Aggression is interpersonal behavior that dominates, humiliates, or violates the rights of others. **Aggressive communication** is an overpowering, bold, forceful way of trying to get what we need at the expense of others. When communicating aggressively, we respond to our own rights at the expense of the rights of patients.

Aggressive communication results in hurting patients and likely embarrassing ourselves. Aggressive communication is not assertive.

Unassertive communication is failing to stand up for our legitimate rights as nurses. **Unassertive communication** is uncertain and unconfident, and fails to show patients our respect for ourselves as nurses. Communicating unassertively diminishes our self-esteem.

Assertive communication has positive benefits for nurses and patients because it solidifies an attitude of mutual respect and helps build trust between nurses and patients.

The following examples illustrate aggressive, unassertive, and assertive ways nurses can communicate with patients and the powerful influence each style has on both patients and nurses.

The Aggressive Way

> "I just got you up, Mrs. Jones *(exasperated tone)*. Please don't bother me now. I've got an important treatment to do. Ask me later."

This response would hurt Mrs. Jones and make her feel less important than your other patients. Your rejection of both her request for action and comfort belittles her needs, making her feel unworthy. You would likely feel badly that you responded so harshly and disrespectfully. Neither you nor Mrs. Jones benefits from this reply: this is a "lose-lose" situation.

The Unassertive Way

> "Well . . . *(looking at your watch)*, I don't have too much time just now. Could you . . . well, I guess . . . OK. I'll be there soon."

Although you have agreed to Mrs. Jones' request for action, it is abundantly clear that your reluctance denies her request for comfort. Your nonverbal hesitancy outweighs your verbal agreement. Mrs. Jones "wins" because she will get your assistance to transfer, but at the cost of feeling as though she is imposing. You "lose" because you are now further behind in your schedule; you know you have not been able to say "no" assertively; and you probably feel somewhat ashamed that you have hurt Mrs. Jones' feelings by indirectly conveying that she is "a nuisance." This is a "lose-win" response.

The Assertive Way

> "I regret I'm not available to help you transfer just now, Mrs. Jones *(calm voice)*. I could find one of the other nurses to help you, or if you can wait about 20 minutes, I could help you then. Which would work better for you?"

This is a "win-win" response. Mrs. Jones feels secure that she will be taken care of (requests for comfort and action met) because you have taken her request seriously. You feel that you have managed your time well by offering some alternatives to Mrs. Jones yet still reserving sufficient time for completing your preoperative preparation. Your interpersonal communication makes both your patient and you feel respected.

Assertive communication is effective communication. The literature reports that poor communication can lead to more patient suffering than many of the symptoms of terminal illness.[6] Knowledge of your potential impact should motivate you to plan your communication so that it will meet your patient's requests and honor your needs in the situation as well.

SYSTEMATIC COMMUNICATION IS EFFECTIVE COMMUNICATION

Effective communication also means communicating in a logical, systematic way, demonstrating accurate problem-solving behavior for the situation. See Box 4-3 for the problem-solving steps of the nursing process to improve communication.

Box 4-3 STEPS TO COMMUNICATING EFFECTIVELY WITH YOUR PATIENTS

1. **Collection of data:** Collect the essential verbal and nonverbal data about your patient's thoughts and feelings. Listen to what your patient is requesting of you both directly and indirectly: understanding, information, action, and/or comfort.
2. **Assessment of the data:** Analyze the information you secure from your patient. Determine what request your patient is making.
3. **Establish expected outcomes (objectives):** Determine how you would like your patient to respond to your communication. For example, you may want your patient to feel respected, appreciated, relieved, informed, relaxed, reassured, etc. At this point you decide what you hope to achieve by your communication.
4. **Plan how you will communicate:** Select a communication strategy that will likely help your patient achieve the expected or desired outcome(s).
5. **Implement your plan:** Communicate assertively, respecting your patient's request and your rights as a nurse in the situation.
6. **Evaluate your communication:** Assess the effect of your communication on your patient. Did your communication help your patient achieve the desired outcome(s)? Evaluate how assertive your strategy was in respecting both your patient's request and your requirements in the situation.

COMMUNICATING WHEN YOUR PATIENT'S REQUEST IS FOR UNDERSTANDING

All human beings have a need to be understood, and that requirement intensifies under the stressfulness of illness and hospitalization. When you can convince your patients that you fully understand them, without judging them for how they are feeling, questioning why they are reacting in a particular way, or advising them to feel differently, it provides them with a wonderful feeling of acceptance.[22] A nonjudgmental reception is reassuring and opens up feelings of relief and freedom. When patients are assured that nurses understand them, they no longer have to struggle to get their point across nor do they have to justify their reactions. Your understanding as a nurse is reassuring acknowledgment to patients that they have a right to be and feel themselves. The "ability to understand and to demonstrate understanding must always matter in a caring profession, especially at a time when strenuous attempts are being made to introduce primary nursing. Primary nursing is a system in which nurse and patient are obliged to interact more closely than ever before, for the duration of the patient's hospital stay."[8]

Nurses can use first-level and second-level patient-focused communication responses to convey understanding to patients.[13] **First-level patient-focused responses** are reflexive and spontaneous responses, the ones with which the nurse identifies with the patients' suffering. To communicate using a first-level response, nurses must be willing to experience or share the patient's suffering in order to respond meaningfully and appropriately. The engagement through identification makes first-level responses comforting for patients. First-level patient-focused communication strategies include the following:

- Ordinariness
- Sympathy
- Pity
- Compassion
- Commiseration
- Consolation

Second-level patient-focused responses are learned professional communication responses, and therefore the nurse's amount of personal investment in the patient's suffering is controlled. When using second-level responses, nurses imagine what it is like for patients rather than becoming involved in patients' suffering. Second-level responses require less of the nurse's energy than first-level responses. Second-level communication strategies include the following:

- Empathy
- Self-disclosure

First-Level Patient-Focused Responses

Taylor's[27] study of nurses as persons instead of exclusively as helpers showed that when nurses and patients shared a common humanity, patients felt connected with the nurses because of this bond. When nurses showed their humanness to their patients, it provided a shared sense of **ordinariness,** making them as one in their humaness. Ordinariness is comforting to patients in the unfamiliar and sometimes threatening environment of a health care setting. This bond creates a special place in which the relative strangeness of being in a health care setting can be made familiar and manageable. Patients in Taylor's study perceived nurses as being ordinary people who were extraordinarily effective by the very ways in which their humanness shone through their knowledge and skills to make their whole interaction with patients something more than just professional helping.

For students learning to become professionals in nursing, Taylor's work may provide a word of wisdom: maintain comfort in being yourself with your patients, for it will provide the patient with a link of being understood as a fellow human.

Reflexive, Patient-Focused, Connected Responses.

First-level patient-focused responses are triggered by the emotional insight of the nurse. Nurses see the patient's suffering, become engaged with the suffering, and experience the suffering themselves. Thus, the patient's suffering becomes a shared experience. To use first-level responses nurses must be willing to engage in the sufferer's experience, that is, to be able to identify with what the patient is experiencing. First-level responses are reflexive rather than learned. First-level patient-focused responses of sympathy, pity, compassion, commiseration, and consolation demonstrate understanding, develop connectedness between nurses and patients, and are naturally comforting to patients.

Sympathy is the expression of the nurse's own sorrow or regret at the patient's plight. Sympathy is a first-level patient-focused communication response to the patient's request for understanding. Sympathy has an "I" focus, expressing "I'm sorry" rather than "poor you." It is the nurse's verbal and nonverbal expression of dismay for patients' suffering.[13] Given appropriately, sympathy legitimizes and justifies patients' feelings of suffering, making it "all right" for them to feel that way. Nurses' acceptance of patients' suffering is comforting. For example, you could express sympathy to a teen athlete whose sprained ankle prevents her from competing in the track and field finals in her event:

> "I feel so sorry *(expression of own sorrow)* that you were injured just at this crucial time—the finals *(appropriate verbal expression of sorrow)!*"

This example demonstrates how sympathy conveys understanding in a human-to-human way.

Pity is an expression of regret or sorrow for patients who are suffering, distressed, or unhappy. Pity is a first-level patient-focused communication response to meet patients' request for understanding. When nurses feel deep sorrow for situations experienced by patients or their families, pity can be used to confirm patients' state. Pity may be required for only a short time, and is especially useful during episodes of extreme suffering. Nurses' pity can facilitate sufferers' acceptance of reality and hastens their adjustment to difficult events. For example, you could express pity to a diabetic patient who is traumatized from the news that her toes will have to be amputed:

> "I'm so sorry *(expression of pity)* that your toes can't be saved. You've worked so hard over the years to prevent amputation. . . . It's terribly disappointing."

For this patient, who is likely in shock after receiving news of a pending amputation, expression of pity shows understanding of her plight.

Compassion is a strong emotion or sentiment stimulated by the presence of suffering that evokes recognition and mutual sharing of the despair or pain of patients. Compassion is a first-level patient-focused communication response to meet patients' request for understanding. Compassion echoes the patient's sentiments and in this way differs from sympathy, which is an expression of the nurse's sorrow. Nurses' expression of compassion strengthens and comforts patients. Being compassionate means nurses come in touch with their own suffering; therefore, it is not possible to avoid pain and still be compassionate. For example, you could enjoin a patient's grief and express compassion by echoing your patient's suffering after a house fire has severely burned him and his 10-year-old son and asphyxiated their dog, a family pet for many years.

> "It's so horrible *(shared reaction)* what you and your family are going through . . . having a fire is something we all fear *(shared reaction)* and pray doesn't happen . . . . I feel deeply for you and your son *(expression of compassion).*"

Receiving this compassion would reassure the patient that you understand the shock and horror of this tragedy.

Commiseration is the sharing of mutual predicaments. Commiseration is appropriate when nurses have experienced patients' circumstances firsthand in their lives. Commiseration is a first-level patient-focused communication response to meet patients' request for understanding. Commiseration involves reflecting on a mutual response to a common experience. While commiserating, nurses and patients share feelings of identity, enabling nurses to listen and communicate sincere expressions of agreement and understanding. For example, you could commiserate with a patient who has a full-length cast on her right leg and will be unable to drive her car for 6 weeks. Her situation brings back memories of your own situation when you were temporarily disabled after tearing your Achilles tendon.

> "Isn't it frustrating! Your car is your passport to freedom and you can't even drive it! The thing I found so frustrating was having to wait to be chauffeured places *(commiseration).* It takes away your independence."

Commiserating from your own experience demonstrates that you understand how hindered your patient feels without access to her vehicle.

Consolation is soothing and encouraging expressions used to ease discomfort or pain. Consolation is a first-level patient-focused communication response to meet the patient's request for understanding. Consolation is initiated by nurses to, at least temporarily, reduce patients' distress, discomfort, and pain. Hope is induced by consolation without being unrealistic. For example, you could console a patient with the fact that his post-trauma healing is progressing quickly because he was physically fit at the time of the accident.

> "Your rehabilitation is progressing so well, and so quickly, probably because you are in such good shape. All that physical exertion in the gym is paying off to help you heal quickly after your accident *(expression of consolation).*"

This expression of consolation conveys the understanding that you are aware of how difficult the rehabilitation process is and how important it is to receive encouragement.

In summary, first-level patient-focused responses involve nurses' engagement and identification with patients' suffering. Nurses' instantaneous recognition of a patient's plights, called emotional insight, induces reflexive feelings of helping, triggering expressions of first-level patient-focused responses. It is the nurse's engagement and involvement that are the essence of the nurse-patient relationship.[13]

The critical factor in eliciting any one of the first-level patient-focused responses is that the nurse become emotionally involved and able to identify with the patient's suffering. Nurses must be willing and able to experience and share with patients' suffering in order to respond meaningfully and appropriately. It is this process of engagement between nurses and patients that makes first-level patient-focused responses comforting for patients. Paradoxically, it is nurses' immersion in patients' pain that enlarges their own experience of pain or suffering.

Second-Level Patient-Focused Responses

Nurses' sharing of suffering experiences requires strength and consumes emotional energy.[13] In the clinical area there are limits to how much shared suffering nurses can tolerate or may find desirable. Nurses are exposed to much patient suffering, are constantly bombarded with emotional stresses, and frequently are required to carry out nursing procedures that inflict more pain. Nurses learn to redirect, alter, or squelch the spontaneous arousal of first-level responses by using second-level patient-focused responses.[13] Empathy and self-disclosure are two such second-level communication strategies you can use to meet your patients' requests for understanding.

Empathy. **Empathy** is a communication skill for demonstrating understanding of what patients feel and the reasons for their emotions. When using empathy you still have the energy to care for other patients and can avoid becoming emotionally drained and exhausted. Empathy is a second-level patient-focused communication response to meet patients' request for understanding.

Empathy is best described as *trying to imagine* what the suffering is like for your patient rather than becoming genuinely involved in your patient's experience, as in first-level patient-focused responses. Empathy is an alternative skill you can employ to reflect accurately and specifically in words what your patients are experiencing. When you convey empathy to your patients, it increases their feelings of being connected with another person, enhances self-esteem, and creates assurance of being accepted. Empathy helps your patients relax with the knowledge that you have understood them.

Empathy is a reflection of your understanding of patients' feelings and the reasons for their emotional reactions. Your empathic response must be accurate, with no exaggerating or minimizing of what your patients express to you. The feeling words you choose must match what your patients intended; the exact meaning of the patients' feelings needs to be expressed. For example, a patient may tell you he is "looking forward" to his discharge from the hospital. Many feeling words may come to mind to reflect this intended meaning, such as "eager," "hopeful," "excited," "relieved," and "expectant." When communicating your understanding, you should select the feeling word that most closely matches your patient's meaning.

Being empathic does not mean repeating verbatim what patients tell you. Parroting can be inappropriate at times and can imply that you have not processed or understood your patient's situation and reactions to it. It is this act of processing that makes empathy a second-level patient-focused response.

When using empathy with your patients, ask yourself, "What does my patient want me to hear?" Attempt to pick out the most important message and verbally reflect your patient's feelings and the reason for specific reactions. Here are some examples of empathic responses:

> Example One:
>
> Your patient, who is scheduled for coronary angioplasty, states, "I hope they know what they're doing tomorrow. I've only got one heart, and I'd hate to have anything else happen to it. I hope I'll be OK."

Your patient wants you to understand his fear and his need for reassurance.

Your empathic reply: "It's a natural response to be worried *(feeling reflection)* about having an important procedure like an angioplasty *(content reflection)*. I noticed that Dr. May will be doing your procedure and she's done hundreds successfully over the 5 years I've been working on the unit. Most patients feel well by the time they return to the unit and grateful that they are pain-free. Can I do anything to help you feel less anxious?"

> Example Two:
>
> When you bring the bed bath supplies to the bedside, your patient says, "I'm so tired. I didn't get any sleep last night. My roommate snored all night long. I'm already stressed enough being in here without being kept up at night."
>
> You reply empathically: "It must have been totally frustrating *(feeling reflection)* to be kept awake in an unfamiliar bed. You already have enough concerns without losing your sleep on top of everything else *(content reflection)*. Today we'll have to figure out some way to solve this problem so that you can get the sleep you need tonight."

Empathy leaves no doubt that you understand your patients' feelings and what is responsible for their reactions. The accuracy and specificity of empathy make it an excellent communication strategy for responding to your patients' requests for understanding.

Self-Disclosure. Another type of second-level patient-focused response to convey understanding to your patients is self-disclosure. **Self-disclosure** is the nurse's revelations of personal information for the purpose of demonstrating deep understanding of patients' situations. Because the nurse-patient relationship is established for the benefit of your patients, anything you self-disclose in the helping relationship should be revealed for the benefit of your patients. Anything you reveal about yourself—your thoughts, feelings, and experiences—should be revealed for the purpose of demonstrating to your patients that you understand their experiences.

When you have had similar experiences, thoughts, feelings, and reactions to those of your patient, and you deem it would benefit your patient to hear your responses, then self-disclosure is a strategy you can employ. Before disclosing you must be sure that your revelation will demonstrate understanding and that you feel comfortable providing your patients with this information about yourself.

A complete self-disclosure begins with an empathic reflection to your patient. Then add your self-disclosure, and close by checking with your patient to see whether you have been accurate in your understanding:

Example One:

Your postpartum patient, mother of a newborn baby girl, tells you she is disappointed that her daughter isn't able to suckle and that she won't be able to breastfeed. "It's just not fair. I looked forward to nursing her for so long. All my friends have told me what a wonderful experience breastfeeding is. I feel like a failure."

Your patient wants you to understand her disappointment and feelings of inadequacy.

Your empathic reply followed by a self-disclosure might go something like this: "Naturally you are disappointed *(empathic feeling reflection)* to miss out on the special experience of breastfeeding your daughter *(content reflection)*. I was unable to breastfeed my first child, and, like you, at first I felt cheated and a bit inferior *(self-disclosure feeling reflection to show understanding)* because I couldn't breastfeed my son. What turned things around for me was when I saw how much it meant to my husband to be able to bottlefeed our son, and help me out by taking turns getting up for night feedings (*self-disclosure* to provide hope). Maybe there will be something that helps compensate for your disappointment."

Summary

When your patients request understanding, you can meet their request with the first-level patient-focused responses of ordinariness, sympathy, pity, compassion, commiseration, or consolation. Employment of first-level patient-focused responses depends on identification with patients' suffering. This requires the nurse's emotional energy and strength, which can be emotionally draining for nurses to employ constantly. To help decrease the amount of emotional fatigue nurses experience, the options of empathy and self-disclosure, two second-level patient-focused responses, can be implemented to meet patients' requests for understanding.

COMMUNICATING WHEN YOUR PATIENT'S REQUEST IS FOR INFORMATION

Patients today are more informed about health and illness and more assertive about getting the essential information needed to make knowledgeable decisions about their health care. As nursing personnel you will be asked for information frequently. Three strategies that you can employ to provide information your patients require are feedback, confrontation, and expressing opinions.

Feedback

Feedback is giving patients the benefit of your reactions—your thoughts and feelings about their behavior. Feedback is a communication response that nurses can use to meet patients' request for information. Your feedback is information patients can use to assess how they are progressing. Patients can use nurses' feedback to help them decide whether to make changes in their health behaviors.

Feedback is information to be accepted or rejected by patients, depending on their personal preferences, values, and priorities. When giving feedback you must deliver it in ways that are receivable and inviting for patients to consider. Here are some steps to take when giving feedback:

1. **Gain permission to give feedback to your patients.** Usually you can simply ask, "You look like you'd like my thoughts about your progress with the training program. May I tell you what I've noticed?"
2. **Be specific when giving feedback to your patients:** "Lately I've noticed that when you require a nurse, you shout my name hoping I'll hear. Sometimes I don't hear you because I might be in another patient's room, but your shouting can be distressing to the other patients in your room."

   This feedback tells your patient specifically how you are reacting to a behavior and, without exaggeration, describes why that behavior is problematic.
3. **Convey your perspective in a respectful way.** When you give feedback, remember that you are reporting your view of things. Although your reactions are important to your patients, there is nothing objectively right or wrong about your perspective; it is simply how you see things. To ensure that your feedback is delivered respectfully, you can deliver it with such phrases as the following: "From my perspective," "The way I see it," and "I felt *(describe your feelings)* when you *(specifically indicate what your patient did)*."
4. **Invite comments from your patients.** Check out your patient's reactions to your feedback so that you maintain a mutual relationship. One never knows how patients will respond to feedback, and you must allow time for patients to grasp what you are saying, think it over, ask for more information, and express their feelings and thoughts about what you have said.
5. **Be genuine.** When you are sincere in giving feedback, it builds trust. If what you are saying is different from the expression on your face or the tone of your voice, your patients will pick up this incongruency and get a mixed or confusing message.

Confrontation

Confrontation is the interpersonal skill you can use to give your patients information about how their behavior is destructive to themselves or others. Confrontation also includes asking others to change their behavior. This request for a change in behavior is the difference between feedback (which is simply a reflection of your thoughts and feelings) and confrontation. The request for change is information that must be delivered in a clear, direct way so that patients understand exactly what is expected. Here is an example of confrontation used when a patient's behavior is unproductive or self-destructive.

Example One:

You are preparing your preoperative patient for his postoperative care. He is doing a return demonstration of deep breathing and coughing. You confront him with: "Your hands were just lying lightly on your abdomen that time, Mr. Wright *(feedback)*. For this to be effective, you need to splint your abdomen firmly with your hands *(request for change)*, so that you support your incision. After your surgery, you'll find it provides comfort to hold your abdomen firmly, and doing so will prevent pressure on your incision *(positive consequences for making the change)*."

Here is an example of confrontation used when a patient's behavior invades your rights or the rights of others:

Example Two:

One of your male patients has made several unprofessional comments to you. You confront him with: "When you make inappropriate statements to me, it is embarrassing *(feedback)*. I would like you to treat me more respectfully by stopping your inappropriate remarks *(specific request for change)*. If you can do that, I can continue to be your nurse *(positive consequence for changing)*; but if you won't stop, I will ask to be reassigned *(negative consequence for not changing)*. Will you change your behavior *(checking out)*?"

Notice that both examples include consequences to encourage the patient to change. Consequences can emphasize the positive implications if change occurs or the negative outcomes if no change occurs.

Expressing Opinions

Expressing opinions refers to disclosing what you think or believe about health care situations or options affecting your patients. Expressing opinions is a communication response that nurses can use to meet patients' request for information.

Your opinions are additional information your patients can use for problem solving and decision making. In contrast, giving advice is more unilateral, and has the risk of sending the message that you think patients are incapable of self-direction. The opinions you express can provide your patients with a fuller picture to make choices about their health and treatment plans. Here are some suggestions for expressing opinions in a mutually respectful way.

Suggestions for Expressing Opinions in an Assertive Way

- **Get the consent of your patient before expressing your opinions.** Ask your patient if he is interested in hearing your viewpoint. There are several natural phrases you can use to complete this courteous step that will flow naturally into your conversation:

"A patient who was recently discharged told me a good idea for handling a problem like yours. Would you like to hear his suggestion?"

"I recently read an article that had some excellent pointers for solving a problem like yours. Would you like to have a copy of it?"

"Many patients on our unit have had a problem similar to yours. The nursing staff has compiled some recommendations. Would you like to hear them?"

Your patients will confirm that they would like to receive your input or let you know that they are not interested. More assertive patients will tell you directly, and those who are less direct will send you nonverbal signals indicating that you can proceed or that you should refrain from sharing your opinions. Looking away, changing the subject, or arguing that this situation is unique are warning signs to you to refrain and keep your opinions to yourself. Such gestures are clues that patients are not ready to hear your opinions. If you receive nonverbal gestures that show signs of interest, it is your signal to continue.

- **Make allowances for the uniqueness of your patient.** It is impossible to know all the circumstances and personal factors that might account for the appropriateness or acceptance of your opinions with a particular patient. Therefore, when you offer your persuasions to your patients, do it tentatively and show consideration of your patient's circumstances.

"Mrs. Smith, do you think this idea will help in your situation?"

"Mr. Jones, what do you think about these recommendations?"

"Mr. Garcia, how do you think this suggestion will fit your life-style?"

"Ms. Lorin, how does my viewpoint strike you?"

- **Include your rationale for your viewpoint.** Giving your rationale for your opinions is a responsible way to defend your position. It provides information for patients to make their final decision. "In response to your question. I think doing it this way would be the most helpful to get the results you want. What do you think?"
  "It will be difficult to ambulate with your cast when you are discharged. Since you are new in town and haven't yet built a support network, I would like to recommend some of our home care agencies to help you manage at home."

COMMUNICATING WHEN YOUR PATIENT'S REQUEST IS FOR COMFORT

One of the greatest challenges for nurses is to provide comfort to patients. To **comfort** means to give strength and hope, to cheer, and to ease the grief or trouble of another. Promoting physical and psychological comfort is a vital part of the role of a nurse.[13] One of the nursing interventions you can use to comfort your patients is support. Support is anything nurses communicate or provide to patients that helps them function more effectively or makes them feel better about how they are functioning. Here are some of the kinds of support you can provide your patients so as to comfort them.

Inspiration is access to knowledge or skills that show patients how to improve their situation. For example, your 18-year-old patient with a torn cartilage may be inspired by meeting another patient with the same knee injury who is now walking smoothly and without pain, because he adhered faithfully to the prescribed rehabilitation program. The hope inspired by this introduction would be comforting.

Recognition is acknowledgment of the skills patients possess and encouragement of their independence in decision making. For example, asking a patient who is a teacher by profession for feedback on improving your unit's preoperative classes or your diabetic teaching pamphlets is a way of providing the comfort of acknowledgment of his talents.

Praise is expressed admiration for your patients' progress. For example, you might compliment a patient for keeping his chest clear through his strict adherence to the deep breathing and coughing exercises. Or, you might praise a patient's progress in losing weight through his dedication to following the diabetic meal preparation plan. Your praise is a source of comfort when patients are making difficult adjustments to the imposed changes of illness.

Reassurance is providing acceptance and encouragement to patients. One example of reassurance is forgiveness for imperfections of omission or commission. For example, you might tell one of your patients who has strained her muscles from overdoing her exercise program that after rest she will likely be able to continue with her program. This intervention would be comforting because it eases her disappointment.

Adequate physical facilities that are conducive for the activities in which your patients engage for healing are supportive. For example, you might invite a grieving family to use the private family room on the unit to talk quietly together and console one another. Provision of privacy acknowledges the family's grief and shock and would be comforting.

Sharing relates to the exchange of information (thoughts, feelings, experiences) between patients with similar concerns or health problems. For example, you might suggest that the two teenage girls on the unit be placed in the same room so that they can share their mutual interests. This move would cheer the two patients and be a comfort measure to offset hospitalization. Another example would be arranging for three patients who have been recently diagnosed with diabetes to join a discussion group with the nutritionist about dietary management after they have viewed a video tape on the same topic. Access to sharing similar reactions is supportive and comforting and adds to patient confidence.

Adequate supplies refers to materials that patients might use in their recovery. For example, you might ask the unit secretary to order more brochures describing the out-patient services available in your community for patients being discharged. Having adequate materials makes patients feel cared for and comforted.

This list of ways of providing the comfort of support is just a beginning. As you progress through your education program and gain experience as a practical/vocational nurse, you will add to this list of comfort measures to provide your patients.

COMMUNICATING WHEN YOUR PATIENT'S REQUEST IS FOR ACTION

The skills required for taking action to provide physical comfort, ensure hygiene, secure safety, complete treatments, and perform the various nursing interventions are covered in the chapters of this comprehensive textbook. One important skill to practice when meeting patients' requests for action is to treat all nurse-patient interactions as human-to-human encounters (Fig. 4-3).

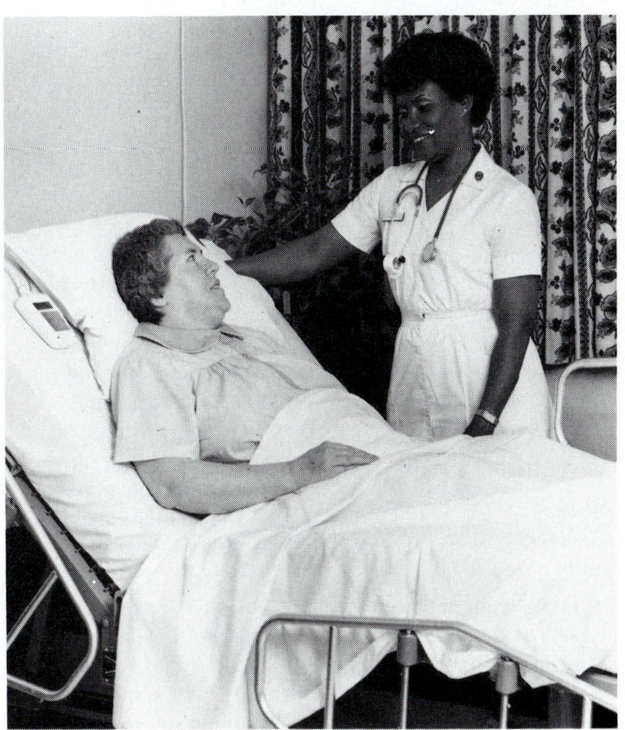

FIG. 4-3 Gently touching the patient's hand conveys encouragement and support.

One way to ensure that you bring such a humanistic perspective to your patient is to be genuine in your communication. As discussed earlier, a basic feature of genuineness is congruency of verbal and nonverbal communication. Another ingredient of genuineness is nurses presenting their honest thoughts and feelings verbally and nonverbally to patients. Nurse genuineness has positive benefits for patients, and incongruence has negative consequences. Table 4-1 presents an overview of the benefits of nurse genuineness; the negative effects of incongruence are shown in Table 4-2.

TABLE 4-1 Benefits of Nurse Genuineness for Patients

Nurse Genuineness	Benefits for Patients
■ Speaks deep from within without apology	■ Feel free to express their true thoughts and emotions ■ Develop a feeling of trust for the nurse
■ Expresses what she is thinking, feeling, and experiencing in the here and now	■ Are provided with information they can use in the relationship here and now
■ Shows spontaneity	■ Unwind in a relaxed atmosphere
■ Conveys openness	■ Enjoy a climate of realness

TABLE 4-2 Negative Effects of Nurse Incongruence for Patients

Nurse Incongruence	Negative Effects for Patients
■ Puts up facade or pretense	■ Distrust for nurse ■ Suspicion of nurse
■ Withholds how she is thinking or what she is experiencing	■ Strained, tense relationship ■ Valuable information missing from the interchange
■ Mismatch between verbal and nonverbal messages	■ Decode the message as two distinct and dissimilar ones ■ Confusion ■ May believe only the nonverbal message ■ Question the credibility of the nurse ■ Find it difficult to maintain meaningful dialogue in the presence of mixed messages
■ Is rigid and contrived; acts as though scripted or how she thinks she should act	■ Don't feel as though they are talking to a real person ■ Feel that the nurse is trying to impress, rather than reach or connect with them

Being genuine sets the tone that you are human, that you have human reactions, and that you are willing to share your reaction to show that you understand some of the reactions your patients are experiencing. Despite the many varied ways you meet patients' requests for action, you can always carry out your nursing functions with a manner of genuineness.

The preceding framework provides ways of assessing and meeting requests for understanding, information, comfort, and action. The next section provides an overview of the important skill of asking questions.

ASKING QUESTIONS EFFECTIVELY

A communication skill that you will use repeatedly for collecting information, verifying your assessments, and evaluating the effectiveness of your nursing interventions is that of *asking questions.* The more effective you are at asking questions, the more pertinent and useful information you will collect, the more time you will save yourself and others, and the more streamlined your interviewing experience will be.[22] "Nurses need to be able to relate quickly and easily with patients of all ages and from widely different backgrounds. Assessment of patient data is therefore a highly complex skill."[14] Here are a few key reminders about effective ways to ask questions:

- The *why* of asking questions: Consider why you require the information from your patients. When patients understand your purpose in asking questions, they are more likely to be open and provide you with what you need to know.
- The *what* and *how* of asking questions: You must plan what to ask your patients and how to phrase your questions in ways that invite them to respond. Closed questions are focused and posed to elicit a specific, brief response from patients. Open questions invite patients to elaborate in whatever direction they choose. If you want to know about your patient's pain in a general way, it would be appropriate to ask an open-ended question such as the following:
  - "Where is your pain?" Your patient will tell you. This question is more effective than a guessing game with closed questions such as: "Is it in the front of your head or the back?"
  - "What is your pain like?" This question will provide you with a full description and is more effective than closed questions that try to guess the nature of the pain: "Is it a squeezing pain?" "Does it come and go?"

Closed questions are effective when a specific response is required. For example, if you want to know if ice helps relieve your patient's pain, the appropriate closed question would be: "Does the pain ease up when you apply ice?" You require a "yes" or a "no" response and therefore a closed question works best.

- The *who* of asking questions: It is important to consider who is the most significant person from whom to get information. There are times when patients cannot answer questions, and as the nurse, you will have to find the essential people from whom to secure the information you require.
- The *when* and *where* of asking questions: Timing of questioning is important to consider for a number of reasons. It might be embarrassing to question patients about private matters at your first meeting. Because privacy and confidentiality are important to all your patients, the soundproofing and visibility of the place in which you choose to ask questions must take patients' needs into account. A patient might be in too much pain, be too grief-stricken, or be too fatigued to answer questions.

BARRIERS TO COMMUNICATING EFFECTIVELY IN NURSING

The following list summarizes some of the common blocks and barriers to effective nurse-patient communication.[6]

- Asking patients "why?" can put them on the defensive and cause insecurity and resentment. Rather than intimidating a patient through "why" questioning, phrase the question to mutually explore the problem or issue.
- Changing the subject inappropriately leaves patients feeling ignored and possibly worried that you are avoiding discussing something important about their treatment.
- Excessive questioning can be upsetting to patients. Instead of getting the message that you care, excessive questioning can make patients feel interrogated.
- Labeling patients with negative or positive categories is destructive and prevents acceptance of the patient as an individual.
- False reassurance makes patients feel that nurses do not care, or that they do not comprehend the gravity or importance of the situation. Do not attempt to put a bandage over a severed artery.
- Giving advice, especially unsolicited, takes control away from patients. To ensure that patients have an investment in the outcome, it is best that they be involved at all stages of the nursing process.
- Language barriers and physical changes, including deafness or blindness, are potential barriers to communication.

Despite emphasis on the importance of effective communication with patients and communication skills training courses for nurses, there are situations in which nurses have been reported to be ineffective, unengaged, and seemingly uncaring communicators. Nurses cite pressure of time, inadequate knowledge, feeling unprepared for emotional involvement with patients, and fear of being overwhelmed by patients' feelings or their own responses as some of the reasons for communicating ineffectively.[12] Others claim that anxiety, authoritarian attitudes, and trying too hard to be professional prevent nurses from showing patients understanding.[27] By practicing the communication strategies described in this chapter and receiving supportive feedback, you can overcome these potential barriers to the effectiveness of your interpersonal communication with patients.

Research findings suggest that the extent to which nurses can develop therapeutic relationships with patients depends a great deal on support and resources in the workplace, including the environment created by nurse managers.[19,31] When selecting a workplace after graduation, give consideration to factors that might enhance or detract from effective communication with patients so that you select a working environment where effective communication is prized and encouraged (Box 4-4).

YOUR COMMITMENT TO IMPROVING YOUR NURSE-PATIENT COMMUNICATION

This chapter outlines several ways to communicate effectively with your patients. Continued improvement in your communication effectiveness requires self-monitoring. Effective nurse communicators habitually think before communicating, and evaluate and reflect after speaking. This monitoring may sound like a lot of effort, but it is well worth the investment. As a nurse you play a significant role in your patients' assessment, treatment, and recovery process. Awareness that your interpersonal communication makes a major impact on patients' healing and recovery is an invitation to communicate humanistically—offering your therapeutic self in a caring way to your patients (Fig. 4-4).

Tatano Beck[26] writes that nurses who know what caring is, what it is reflected in practice, and how it is transacted interpersonally will be better able to provide caring to their patients. You can grow in insight about yourself as a caring communicator by practicing effective interpersonal communication with your student colleagues. ". . . To nurture caring, nursing students need to be surrounded in a caring environment. Caring can

Box 4-4 MAINTAINING EFFECTIVE COMMUNICATION

PROMOTING EFFECTIVE COMMUNICATION

Maintaining silence. Silence can help the nurse and patient to organize their thoughts. It also enables the nurse to observe the patient more closely. A nurse's silence acknowledges patients' needs for a few moments of privacy. Silence shows that the nurse is interested and will accept any response patients can express.

Listening attentively. Attentive listening allows one to understand an entire message conveyed, verbally and nonverbally. It also facilitates trust.

Conveying acceptance. Acceptance means that one is nonjudgmental. Acceptance is not synonymous with agreement; rather, it is a willingness to hear the person's message. One conveys acceptance through positive feedback and making certain verbal and nonverbal cues are congruent.

Asking related questions. Questioning is a direct method of communicating. Asking related questions allows the patient to give information logically. Open-ended questions are useful for eliciting more information from the patient about a subject.

Paraphrasing. Paraphrasing sends feedback to the patient that information has been accurately received.

Clarifying. Clarifying helps retain important information. Using examples can clarify abstract ideas. All clarification should be specific.

Focusing. When a discussion becomes vague or ill defined, focusing directs conversation to a specific topic or issue. It limits the area of discussion to which the patient can respond. The nurse seeks meaning in the patient's message.

Stating observations. Describing a patient's observed behavior can provide feedback as to whether an intended message was received. It can clarify conflicts between verbal and nonverbal cues.

Offering information. Offering information provides a patient with relevant data and prevents one-sided conversations. It is useful for health teaching and helps in decision making. If the nurse avoids sharing information or gives only partial information, patients may lose trust in the nurse.

Summarizing. Summarizing is a concise review of main ideas from a discussion. It sets the tone for further interactions. By reviewing a conversation the participants can focus on key issues and any relevant information previously deleted.

BLOCKS TO EFFECTIVE COMMUNICATION

Offering false reassurance. Offering false reassurance can do more harm than good. False reassurance may allow the nurse to promise something that will not occur or is unrealistic.

Being defensive. Defensiveness in the face of criticism implies that the patient has no right to an opinion. The patient's concerns often become ignored. Attentive listening helps the patient open up but does not imply agreement.

Showing approval or disapproval. Showing approval or disapproval is judgmental and may halt a conversation. It inhibits the patient's ability to share ideas and make decisions independently. Disapproval can indicate rejection.

Asking why. Asking why may imply an accusation. It can cause resentment, insecurity, and mistrust. If additional information is needed, the nurse can phrase a question to avoid use of "why."

Changing the subject inappropriately. Changing the subject inappropriately is rude and shows a lack of empathy. It stalls communication. The patient may then give incomplete or inadequate information.

Forming communication barriers. Forming communication barriers by saying something inadvertently that blocks a patient's communication can break down communication. By acknowledging the mistake, the nurse can start the communication process anew.

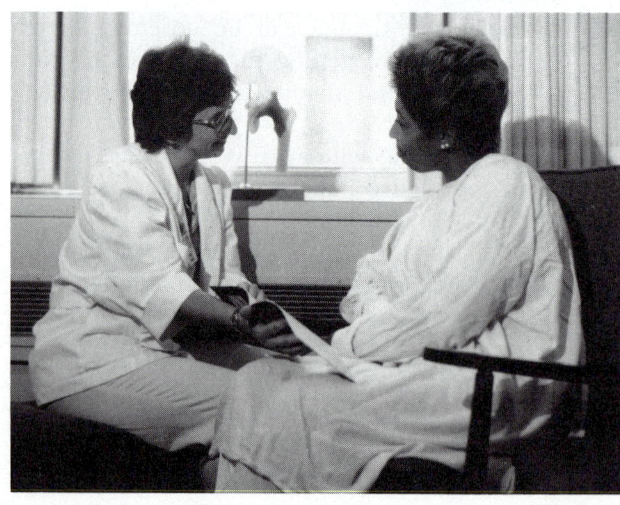

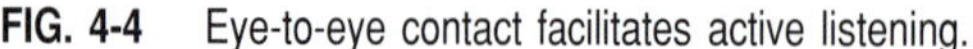

FIG. 4-4 Eye-to-eye contact facilitates active listening.

be integrated throughout schools of nursing by fostering not only faculty but also student role models of caring. Caring is contagious."[26]

You have a choice. The option this chapter invites you to embrace is to enhance your communication through active self-monitoring. Effective nurse communicators are not born, they are made through their sensitive evaluation of their competence to respond to patients' requests for understanding, information, comfort, and action.

REFERENCES AND SUGGESTED READINGS

1. Bradley J, Edingerg MA: *Communication in the nursing context,* ed 3, Norwalk, Conn, 1990, Appleton & Lange.
2. Chipman Y: Caring: its meaning and place in the practice of nursing, *J Nurs Educ* 30(4):171, 1991.
3. Christensen BL: *Comfort, rest, and sleep.* In Christensen BL, Kockrow EO, editors: *Foundations of nursing,* St Louis, 1991, Mosby.
4. Egan G: *The skilled helper: a systematic approach to effective helping,* ed 4, Pacific Grove, Calif, 1990, Brooks/Cole.
5. Farrell GA: How accurately do nurses perceive patients' needs? A comparison of general and psychiatric settings, *J Adv Nurs* 16:1062, 1991.
6. Gerrard BA, Boniface WJ, Love BH: *Interpersonal skills for health professionals,* Reston, Va, 1980, Reston.
7. Gooch J: Dying in the ward, *Nurs Times* 84(21):38, 1988.
8. Gould D: Empathy: a review of the literature with suggestions for an alternative research strategy, *J Adv Nurs* 15:1167, 1990.
9. Lalli-Ascosi S: Polishing your self image, *Health Trends Transition* 1(2):15, 1990.
10. LeGault GH: Communication. In Christensen BL, Kockrow EO, editors: *Foundations of nursing,* St Louis, 1991, Mosby.
11. Lindberg JB et al: *Introduction to nursing concepts, issues and opportunities,* Philadelphia, 1990, Lippincott.
12. Macleod Clark J, Hopper L, Jesson A: Progression to counseling, *Nurs Times* 87(8):41, 1991.
13. Morse JM et al: Beyond empathy: expanding expressions of caring, *J Adv Nurs* 17:809, 1992.
14. Pike AW: On the nature and place of empathy in clinical nursing practice, *J Prof Nurs* 6:235, 1990.
15. Perry AG, Potter PA: *Clinical nursing skills and techniques,* ed 3, St Louis, 1994, Mosby.
16. Potter PA, Perry G: *Fundamentals of nursing: concepts, process and practice,* ed 3, St Louis, 1993, Mosby.
17. Purtilo R: *Health professional and patient interaction,* ed 4, Philadelphia, 1990, Saunders.
18. Raudseff E: 7 ways to cure communication breakdowns, *Nurs 90* 20(4):132, 1990.
19. Savage J: Keeping in touch, *Nurs Times* 88(49):30, 1992.
20. Severtsen BM: Therapeutic communication demystified, *J Nurs Educ* 29(4):190, 1990.
21. Slade M: Are you sitting comfortably? *Nurs Times* 88(39):32, 1992.
22. Smith SP: *Communication in nursing: communicating assertively and responsibly in nursing: a guidebook,* ed 2, St Louis, 1992, Mosby.
23. Stanhope M, Lancaster J: *Community health nursing: process and practice for promoting health,* ed 3, St Louis, 1993, Mosby.
24. Stuart GW, Sundeen SJ: *Principles and practice of psychiatric nursing,* ed 4, St Louis, 1991, Mosby.
25. Tannen D: *You just don't understand: women and men in conversation,* New York, 1990, Morrow.
26. Tatano Beck C: Caring among nursing students, *Nurse Educator* 17(6):22, 1992.
27. Taylor BJ: From helper to human: a reconceptualization of the nurse as person, *J Adv Nurs* 17:1042, 1992.
28. Timby BK, Lewis LW: *Fundamental skills and concepts in patients care,* ed 5, Philadelphia, 1992, Lippincott.
29. Vortherms RC: Clinically improving communication through touch, *J Gerontol Nurs* 17(5):6, 1991.
30. Wilkinson S: Confusions and challenges: communication skills among nurses: a research review, *Nurs Times* 88(35):24, 1992.
31. Wilkinson S: Factors which influence how nurses communicate with cancer patients, *J Adv Nurs* 16:677, 1991.

CHAPTER CHALLENGE

KEY POINTS

- Effective communication with patients is the means of establishing a therapeutic relationship with patients.
- Effective interpersonal communication allows the exchange of information, thoughts, and feelings.
- Effective communication is the means by which nurses and patients influence each other's behavior.
- Assertive communication that takes into account the feelings and requests of patients yet honors nurses' rights in the relationship is the most effective communication.
- Effective nurse communicators are perceptive at assessing direct and indirect requests from patients.
- Effective nurse communicators can employ several communication strategies in order to meet patients' requests for understanding, information, comfort, and action.
- Effective nurse communicators follow the steps of the systematic nursing process for communicating with patients.
- Effective nurse communicators demonstrate efficiency and sensitivity when asking patients questions.
- Effective nurse communicators demonstrate genuineness by maintaining congruency between their verbal and nonverbal communication.
- Effective nurse communicators know how to avoid or overcome the common barriers to effective communication with patients.
- Effective nurse communicators believe that they can make patients feel important and valued and are consequently committed to improving their interpersonal communication through practice, feedback, and self-evaluation.

STUDY QUESTIONS

1. The real purpose of creating understanding between you and your patients is to effect some change. One such change is to influence another to respond to a request. Four categories of requests patients might make of nurses are for:
   1. Understanding, empathy, caring, and action
   2. Understanding, action, information, and support
   3. Understanding, information, action, and comfort
   4. Understanding, information, knowledge, and reassurance
2. The most effective interpersonal communication takes into account the feelings and requests of your patients yet honors nurses' rights in the relationship. This style of communication is called:
   1. Assertiveness
   2. Confidence
   3. Caring
   4. Actualizing
3. Mr. Brown, the husband of an obstetrical patient who has just delivered a healthy baby boy, says to the nurse: "This is our third child, and even though I've been here for each delivery, I feel so useless. It's my wife who has all the pain and I'm just on the sidelines." The nurse's most appropriate response would be:
   1. "Yes, it must be hard for husbands to watch their wives going through the agony of labor and delivery."
   2. "Sounds like you wish you could have done more—maybe even taken some of your wife's pain yourself."
   3. "From what I saw, you were right there soothing and coaching your wife and doing all kinds of things to comfort her. It looked like a team effort."
   4. "You attended the prenatal classes, so you must know that just being present is helpful. Lots of husbands aren't as good as you in delivery—believe me, I've seen lots."
4. There are several ways nurses can demonstrate to their patients that they understand them. They are:
   1. Ordinariness, empathy, reflexive-connected responses, self-disclosure
   2. Communicated understanding, reality checking, empathy
   3. Sympathy, nonverbal facilitators, warmth, respect
   4. Listening, empathy, ordinariness, closeness
5. The mother of your pediatric patient comes to the nursing station and says: "I just got reprimanded by Jimmy's doctor. He told me I shouldn't be feeding Jimmy cookies because you are doing a series of allergy tests. Why didn't one of you tell me so that I know what's going on? Now I've ruined the tests." The nurse's most appropriate response would be:
   1. "Well, I did put a sign above his bed to ask any visitors not to feed him. I guess you didn't see it."
   2. "I can see you feel bad because you fed Jimmy something that may interfere with his allergy tests. Somehow we missed out on informing you about this plan. We can restart it tomorrow, and I can explain it to you now."
   3. "No one told you? That's hard to believe . . . (checking the Kardex); it says right here that you were notified. Somebody's at fault here. I'm going to check this out."
   4. "Dr. Jones' bark is worse than his bite. Don't let him get to you. He yelled at our head nurse this morning, too."
6. Confrontation is the interpersonal skill that you can use to give patients information about how their behavior is destructive to themselves or others. The way in which confrontation differs from the interpersonal communication skill of feedback is:
   1. Confrontation is more threatening and difficult
   2. Confrontation includes asking patients to make a change
   3. Feedback requires asking permission first
   4. Feedback can be delivered nonverbally and is less complex
7. There are several factors nurses need to remember when expressing opinions to their patients. It is important to:
   1. Get the consent of patients before expressing opinions and be straightforward, because nurses have information that will likely benefit their patients.
   2. Get the patient's consent, make allowances for the uniqueness of each patient and include a rationale for one's viewpoint
   3. Make allowances for the uniqueness of each patient and remember to protect other patients' confidentiality
   4. Proceed with caution and include a rationale for one's viewpoint if a patient is not direct about whether he wants feedback

5

THE NURSING PROCESS

Toni C. Wortham

KEY TERMS

actual nursing diagnosis
assessment
biographical data
collaborative problem
data base
defining characteristics/cues
diagnose
evaluation
goal
high-risk nursing diagnosis
implementation
medical diagnosis
NANDA
nursing diagnosis
nursing interventions
nursing process
objective data
planning
possible nursing diagnosis
problem
subjective data
wellness nursing diagnosis

LEARNING OBJECTIVES

After reading this chapter, the student should be able to do the following:

- Define the key terms.
- Discuss the role of the licensed practical nurse in the nursing process.
- Discuss the five phases of the nursing process.
- Describe methods of collecting data.
- Discuss the steps used to develop a nursing diagnosis.
- Differentiate among types of nursing diagnoses.
- Describe the development of patient-centered goals.
- Discuss the creation of nursing orders.
- Explain the evaluation of a nursing care plan.
- Demonstrate the nursing process by writing a nursing care plan.

RELATED TOPICS OF INTEREST

- Communication (Chapter 4)
- Documentation (Chapter 6)
- Signs, symptoms, and physical assessment (Chapter 9)

Nursing is "the diagnosis and treatment of human response to actual or potential health problems."[2] The nursing process serves as the organizational framework for the practice of nursing. The **nursing process** is a systematic method by which nurses plan and provide care for patients. This involves a problem-solving approach that enables the nurse to identify patient problems and to plan, deliver, and evaluate nursing care in an orderly, scientific manner. The nursing process consists of five dynamic phases: assessment, diagnosis, planning, implementation, and evaluation (Fig. 5-1).

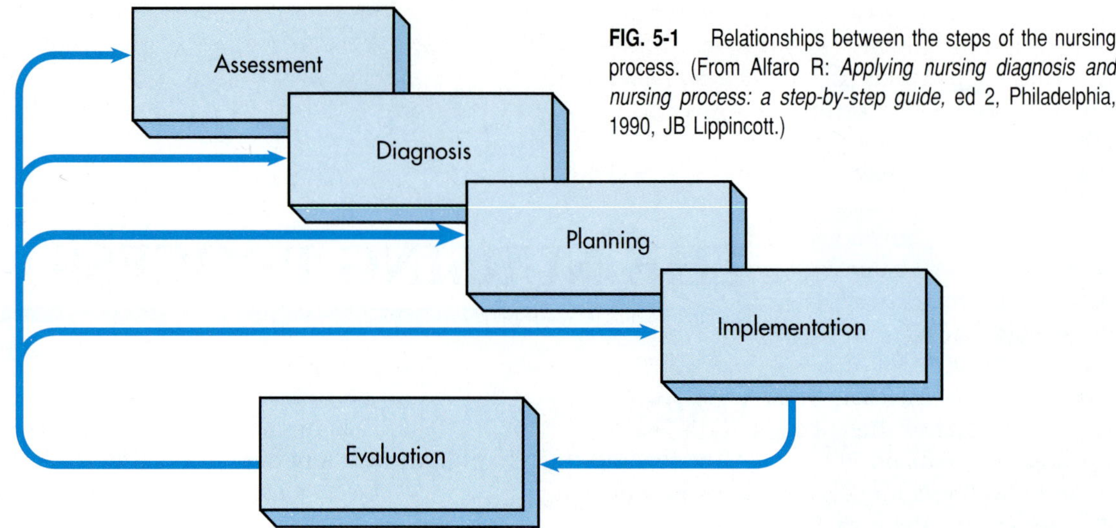

FIG. 5-1 Relationships between the steps of the nursing process. (From Alfaro R: *Applying nursing diagnosis and nursing process: a step-by-step guide,* ed 2, Philadelphia, 1990, JB Lippincott.)

ASSESSING

Assessment means the evaluation or appraisal of a condition. The nurse gathers information to identify the health status of the patient. Assessments are made initially and continuously throughout patient care. The remaining phases of the nursing process are dependent upon the accurateness and completeness of this initial data collection.

When the patient enters the health care system, the nurse begins the data collection. The nurse uses judgment about the appropriateness of performing a complete assessment. If the patient is critically ill, disoriented, or unable to respond, it is better to postpone a complete assessment. A focus assessment is performed instead of a complete assessment.

A focus assessment differs from a complete head-to-toe assessment because a focus assessment gathers information about a specific health problem of the patient. When the nurse must gather specific data to confirm or eliminate a problem, a focus assessment is performed.

Focus assessments can be performed during the establishment of the initial data base. For example, if the patient reports right upper abdominal pain, the nurse who suspects gallbladder disease will ask further questions about nausea and vomiting, pain referred to the scapular area, and the relationship of signs and symptoms to dietary fat intake.

Focus assessments are also performed continuously. The nurse who monitors intake and output, skin turgor, and oral mucous membranes is performing a focus assessment for Fluid Volume Deficit.[1,4,25]

TABLE 5-1 Comparison of Subjective and Objective Data

Subjective Data	Objective Data
"I feel nauseated."	50 cc green-tinged vomitus.
"My chest hurts."	BP 150/100, pulse 110, respirations 32, holding fist over sternum.
"I'm nervous."	Wringing hands, pacing in hall, pulse 112, respirations 28, BP 152/98.
"I'm tired."	Dark circles under eyes, yawning, catnaps during the day.
"My foot hurts."	1″ × 2″ open lesion on left heel.

Types of Data

When performing an assessment the nurse gathers subjective and objective data. **Subjective data** are the verbal statements provided by the patient. Statements about nausea and descriptions of pain, fatigue, and anxiety are examples of subjective data. Other terms for subjective data are symptoms and cues. Subjective data are secret until *s*hared by the *s*ubject, the patient.

Objective data are observable and measurable signs. Objective data can be recorded. A camera can record a rash, a skin lesion, or puffy eyes. A tape recorder can give evidence of crying or slurred speech. A thermometer can record a temperature elevation. Other terms for objective data are signs and cues. (See Table 5-1 for comparison of subjective and objective data.)

Sources of Data

Data can be obtained from primary or secondary sources. The primary source of data is the patient. In most instances, the patient is considered the most accurate reporter. The alert and oriented patient can provide information about past illnesses and surgeries and present signs, symptoms, and life-style.

When the patient is unable to supply information because of deterioration of mental status, age, or seriousness of illness, secondary sources are used. Secondary sources include family, significant others, additional health care professionals, medical records, diagnostic procedures, and nursing literature. Members of the patient's support system may be able to furnish information about the patient's health status, current illness, allergies, and current medications.

Other health team professionals are also helpful secondary sources. Physicians, other nurses, dietitians, respiratory and physical therapists, and others can provide data about the patient.

Past and present medical records can supply important information about the health status of the patient. Diagnostic and laboratory test results are also information sources.

The nurse reviews nursing literature to determine what information may be needed. Knowing the etiology, pathophysiology, clinical manifestations, assessment, diagnostic tests, medical management, nursing interventions, patient teaching needs, and prognosis can provide important information that can guide further data collection.

Methods of Data Collection

There are two basic methods used to collect data. In the first method the nurse conducts an interview to obtain information about the patient's health history. The second method is the performance of a physical examination to gather objective data. A review of systems is a common format used to ensure completeness of the health history (see Chapter 9). The health history provides a collection of information from the patient and from other sources. The history provides a **data base** (a large store or bank of information) from which a plan for nursing diagnosis, medical management, nursing interventions, and discharge planning for the patient may be made. When the nurse has completed the assessment form, the data base has been established.

There are several common components assessed in a nursing health history. The nurse inquires about **biographical data** that provide information about the facts or events in a person's life. Other information sought includes the reason for seeking health care, a history of the present illness, the past health history, and the family history. Because it is important to determine substances, forces, and conditions in and about a community that affect health, an environmental history is obtained. A psychosocial history obtains information about a combination of psychological and social factors. A review of systems follows, during which the nurse gathers information about the function of each body system.

The physical examination is guided by subjective data provided by the patient. To avoid omitting any area, the physical examination is also done using a systematic approach. A head-to-toe or systems format may be used.

During the physical examination, vital signs are taken and the entire body is assessed. Inspection, percussion, palpation, and auscultation are used (see Chapter 9).

Data Clustering

Data clustering is the grouping of related information from the patient's health history, physical examination, and laboratory results as part of the process of making a diagnosis. After collecting and validating the subjective and objective data, the nurse organizes the information into meaningful clusters.

During data clustering, the nurse organizes data and focuses attention on functions needing support and assistance for recovery. Examples of appropriate data clustering are as follows:

> Intact, flushed skin, which is hot and dry to touch; dry oral mucosa, coated tongue and cracked lips
>
> or
>
> Complaining of intermittent abdominal cramping, with periods of diarrhea and constipation; denies vomiting, states, "I haven't eaten for the past 24 hours," hyperactive bowel sounds in all 4 quadrants.

DIAGNOSING

To **diagnose** is to identify the type and cause of a health condition. The licensed practical nurse and the registered nurse may both observe and collect data. Once the initial assessment has been completed, the data must be analyzed. It is usually the responsibility of the registered nurse to analyze and interpret that data to identify health problems.

A **problem** is any health care condition that requires diagnostic, therapeutic, or educational actions. When the patient has a problem or a potential problem, cues are usually present that will help the nurse identify the area of concern.

There are three basic guidelines that help the nurse identify the cues that are significant for nursing interventions. The nurse considers any of the following to be important: (1) any change in the patient's usual pattern; (2) any difference from the normal functioning of any body system; (3) any difference from the normal pattern of growth and development[9] (see Table 5-2).

Nursing Diagnosis

One of the types of health problems that can be identified is a nursing diagnosis. In 1990 the North American Nursing Diagnosis Association **(NANDA)** approved an

TABLE 5-2 Determination of Significant Cues

Patient Values	Norm	Conclusion*
42-year-old male: BP 165/92	Average: 120/80	Hypertension
18-year-old: respirations 32	16-22	Tachypnea
Small-frame, 5′2″ female, weight 178 lb	106-118	Weight above accepted normal standard
22-month-old: not walking	12 months	Walking delayed
Adult male: hemoglobin 8 g/dl	14-18 g/dl	Below normal limits
Adult female: hemoglobin 12 g/dl	12-16 g/dl	Within normal limits
25-year-old: pulse 120 bpm	60-100 bpm	Tachycardia
Newborn: pulse 132	130-150	Within normal limits
Adult: thrombocytes 20,000	150,000-400,000/mm^3	Thrombocytopenia

*The conclusion is based on appropriate norm for age and sex.

official definition of a nursing diagnosis. A **nursing diagnosis** is "a clinical judgment about individual, family, or community responses to actual or high risk (potential) health problems/life processes. Nursing diagnosis provides the basis for selection of nursing interventions to achieve outcomes for which the nurse is accountable."[5] Nurses can legally identify and prescribe the primary interventions to treat or prevent the problem that is identified as a nursing diagnosis. The nurse should be aware of this important point. By definition, if the nurse cannot prescribe the primary treatment, the problem is not a nursing diagnosis.

Components of a Nursing Diagnosis

Nursing research is ongoing in its identification of nursing diagnoses. Every 2 years the members of NANDA receive research from nurses. When nurses submit nursing diagnoses for approval, the following four components are addressed: (1) nursing diagnosis title/label; (2) definition; (3) contributing/etiological/related factors; and (4) defining characteristics/cues (which can be objective or subjective data). The selection of an accurate nursing diagnosis is dependent upon closely matching the elements in the patient situation with all four components of the nursing diagnosis. These four components are found in numerous nursing diagnoses handbooks and are defined and explained in the following discussion.

Nursing Diagnosis Title/Label. The cluster of signs and symptoms or cues that define the problem is given a title or label. Frequently this diagnosis title/label is simply called the nursing diagnosis. *Nursing diagnosis* is the term that will be used to describe this component in this chapter. The nursing diagnosis provides a concise name for the identified health problem. Lists of nursing diagnoses are presented in alphabetical order. Constipation, diarrhea, fatigue, hopelessness, and pain are examples of nursing diagnoses.

Adjectives add meaning by describing the nursing diagnosis. Examples of adjectives are ineffective, impaired, altered, and anticipatory. When writing the nursing diagnosis the nurse may place the adjective in front of the noun modified. This provides a more natural word order. For example: Impaired physical mobility follows a more natural word order than does Mobility, impaired physical; however, either order is correct and acceptable.

Definition. The definition gives a clear, precise description of the problem. This description helps to identify the difference between similar nursing diagnoses. For example, if the nurse needed to select either colonic constipation or perceived constipation, the following definitions would be helpful. Colonic constipation is defined as "The state in which an individual's pattern of elimination is characterized by hard, dry stool which results from a delay in passage of food residue."[25] Perceived constipation is defined as "The state in which an individual makes a self-diagnosis of constipation and ensures a daily bowel movement through abuse of laxatives, enemas, and suppositories."[25]

Contributing/Etiological/Related Factors. Contributing/etiological/related factors are conditions that may be involved in the development of a problem. This factor may become the focus for nursing interventions. Some authors also speak about contributing factors as the "related to's." A contributing factor for the nursing diagnosis of anxiety is hospitalization.

Risk factors are those circumstances that increase the susceptibility of a patient to a problem. Prolonged immobility increases the risk of skin impairment and is the risk factor for the nursing diagnosis of impaired skin integrity. The risk factors are then written as "related to" in the nursing diagnosis statement.

Defining Characteristics/Cues. The defining characteristics or cues tell how the diagnosis is manifested. **Defining characteristics/cues** are the clinical signs and symptoms that furnish evidence that the problem exists. These cues or defining characteristics are written as "manifested by" in the nursing diagnosis statement. Examples will be presented in the discussion of writing nursing diagnosis statements.

Writing Nursing Diagnosis Statements

There are four types of nursing diagnoses: actual, high risk, possible, and wellness. The following discussion provides descriptions of each type and furnishes guidelines for writing each type of nursing diagnosis statement.

Actual Nursing Diagnosis. An **actual nursing diagnosis** represents a condition that is currently present. Cues indicate the presence of a problem. An actual nursing diagnosis statement is usually represented by a three-part statement. The three parts are written in the following order: (1) the nursing diagnosis from the NANDA list; (2) the contributing/related factor; and (3) the specific cues from the patient's assessment that indicated the presence of the problem. Connecting phrases are used to join the three parts of the statement. "Related to (R/T)" links the first and second parts of the statement. "Manifested by (M/B)" joins the second and third parts of the diagnostic statement. A sample three-part actual nursing diagnosis statement is given below.

> Colonic constipation related to decreased fluid intake manifested by abdominal distention, lack of bowel movement for 5 days, and straining at stool.

High-Risk Nursing Diagnosis. A **high-risk nursing diagnosis** is a "clinical judgment that an individual, family, or community is more vulnerable to develop the problem than others in the same or similar situation."[5] The assessment indicates that risk factors are present that are known to contribute to the development of the problem. High-risk nursing diagnoses are written as two-part statements. The two parts are: (1) the nursing diagnosis from the NANDA list and (2) the risk factor(s). As in an actual nursing diagnosis, the two parts are connected by the words "related to." An example of a high-risk nursing diagnosis statement is given below.

> High risk for impaired skin integrity related to prolonged immobility.

There is no third part ("manifested by") in the nursing diagnostic statement because there are no signs or symptoms.

Possible Nursing Diagnosis. A **possible nursing diagnosis** is used when a problem is considered feasible. Additional data must be gathered to confirm or eliminate the problem. Possible nursing diagnoses are written as two-part statements. The two parts are: (1) the nursing diagnosis from the NANDA list and (2) the contributing or related factor(s). An example of a possible nursing diagnosis follows:

> Possible colonic constipation related to the effects of anesthesia on smooth muscle tone.

Wellness Nursing Diagnosis. A **wellness nursing diagnosis** is defined as a "clinical judgment about an individual, group, or community in transition from a specific level of wellness to a higher level of wellness."[5] A wellness nursing diagnosis is written as a one-part statement. The words "Opportunities for Enhanced . . ." are used to precede the desired health change. Opportunities for Enhanced Nutrition is an example of a wellness nursing diagnosis statement.

Other Types of Health Problems

Collaborative problems and medical diagnoses must be *distinguished* from nursing diagnoses. These two types of problems will be defined and discussed separately.

Collaborative Problems. A **collaborative problem** is "an actual or potential health problem (complication) that focuses on the pathophysiologic response of the body (to trauma, disease, diagnostic studies, or treatment modalities), and that nurses are responsible and accountable to identify and treat in collaboration with the physician."[1,4] An example for a diabetic patient on insulin would be Potential Complication of Hypoglycemia.

Medical Diagnoses. A **medical diagnosis** is the identification of a disease or condition by a scientific evaluation of physical signs, symptoms, history, laboratory tests, and procedures. The physician is licensed to make medical diagnoses. Examples of medical diagnoses are congestive heart failure, pneumonia, diabetes mellitus, and hepatitis B.

PLANNING

During the **planning** phase of the nursing process, the nurse establishes priorities of care, writes desired patient outcomes, selects and converts nursing interventions into nursing orders, and communicates the plan of care. The nurse must decide what can be done to lessen or solve an actual problem or to prevent a high-risk problem from becoming an actual problem. The decision about what interventions will be effective is made during the planning phase.

Priority Setting

The nurse in today's busy health care facility is caring for many patients with complex problems and is challenged daily to use time and effort wisely. Priorities must be established to provide care for each patient.

Once a list of nursing diagnoses has been developed, the problems can be ranked. A useful framework to guide the prioritization is Maslow's hierarchy. The basis of this structure is that lower-level needs must be met before higher-level needs can be satisfied. The physiological needs are more vital than the safety and security needs, and the safety and security needs are more critical than the love and belonging needs. (Review Maslow's hierarchy in Fig. 5-2.) Life-threatening and health-threatening problems are ranked before other types of problems. Actual problems may be ranked before high-risk problems unless the high-risk problem, if it were to develop, would be life threatening. For example, High Risk for Ineffective Airway Clearance might be prioritized higher than an actual problem of Colonic Constipation.

Patients should be consulted about their prioritization of problems. Mutually established plans are more effective because of the active involvement of the patient.

Time factors and severity of illness are important in determining which problems are addressed. The patient who is admitted to the emergency department with a possible myocardial infarction is not ready to hear dietary instructions to reduce cholesterol.

Priorities change as the patient progresses through hospitalization. As problems are resolved, other problems may be approached. The following example illustrates how the nursing diagnoses change during hospitalization.

> A 28-year-old woman admitted for an abdominal hysterectomy may have the preoperative diagnosis of Fear/Anxiety. Pain is an important nursing diagnosis in the first few days after surgery. As the pain is controlled, nutrition and elimination concerns are managed. When the patient approaches dismissal, teaching about wound care and activity restrictions must be done. Because of the loss of reproductive ability, self-esteem problems should be confirmed or eliminated as a nursing diagnosis for this patient.

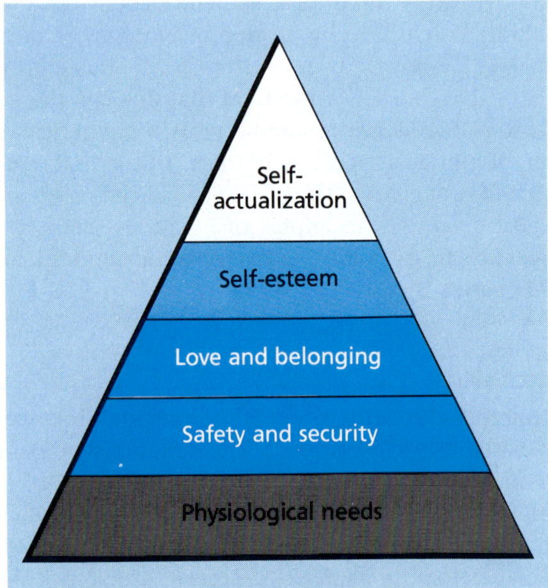

FIG. 5-2 Maslow's hierarchy of needs. Physical needs include physiological (personal hygiene, activity, sexuality) and homeostatic (vital functions [oxygenation], eating and drinking, sleep and rest, elimination). Safety and security needs include safety and accident prevention, religion and philosophy, and feelings of well-being. Love and belonging needs are communication, affection, identity, modesty, companionship, and dependence. The self-esteem need is recognition, and the self-actualization need is a desire for self-fulfillment.

Establishing Desired Patient Outcomes

During the planning phase, the nurse predicts the condition of the patient following nursing interventions. This prediction is expressed in a statement that indicates the degree of wellness desired, expected, or possible for the patient to achieve. This statement may be referred to as a patient goal, a patient-centered goal, an objective, a behavioral objective, or a patient outcome. A patient outcome statement provides a description of the specific, measurable behavior (outcome criteria) that the patient will be able to exhibit following the nursing interventions.

A **goal** is defined as the purpose to which an effort is directed. Incorrectly written goal statements indicate the nursing action rather than a patient behavioral change. For example, "prevent constipation or promote activity" are goals for nursing interventions, but do not describe the desired behavior that the patient will exhibit after the nurse has intervened. To avoid this problem the student should use the terms *patient-centered goal* or *desired patient outcome* when referring to this part of the nursing care plan. Patient-centered goals or desired patient outcomes are written as follows:

> Patient will have one soft, formed bowel movement every other day during hospitalization.
>
> Patient will ambulate 200 feet by the third day after surgery.

The patient-centered goals or desired patient outcomes state the behaviors that the patient will be able to perform rather than what the nurse will do. Patient-centered goal/outcome statements serve two functions. First, they guide the selection of nursing interventions. Nursing interventions are selected to achieve the desired outcomes. Second, the outcome statement establishes the measuring standard that is used to evaluate the effectiveness of the nursing interventions. Therefore the outcome statement must provide the specific details that can be used as the yardstick to judge progress and/or problem solution.

A well-written patient-centered goal/outcome statement does the following:

1. Uses the word patient or a part of the patient as the subject of the statement.
2. Uses a measurable verb.
3. Is specific for the patient and the problem.
4. Is realistic for the patient and the problem.
5. Includes a time frame for patient reevaluation.[1]

The subject of a patient-centered goal/outcome statement should be the patient or a part of the patient.[1] Therefore the outcome statement should begin with the words, "The patient will . . ."

Measurable verbs indicate the precise behavior that the nurse anticipates hearing or seeing. Define, describe, list, walk, and verbalize are examples of measurable verbs.

The patient-centered goal/outcome statement should be specific to the patient and the problem. A patient who is in traction because of a bone fracture has mobility restrictions. An outcome statement indicating that all joints will be moved through full range of motion is not a safe patient-centered goal/outcome statement for this patient's problem.

The patient-centered goal/outcome statement should also be realistic for the patient and the problem. It would not be realistic to expect an 88-year-old to learn to jog.

A time frame is written into the patient-centered goal or outcome statement to provide a deadline for evaluation of the patient's progress. Nursing experience will increase the student's ability to predict realistic time frames.

Patient-centered goal/outcome statements indicate a reversal of the problem identified by the NANDA nursing diagnosis label, as is shown by the following example:

NURSING DIAGNOSIS	GOAL/OUTCOME STATEMENT
Impaired skin integrity related to prolonged immobility manifested by 2″ diameter ulcer on coccyx.	Patient will have intact skin within 3 weeks.

Selecting Nursing Interventions

Nursing interventions are those activities that should promote the achievement of the desired patient outcome. Interventions may include activities that the nurse selects to resolve a nursing diagnosis, to monitor for the development of a high-risk problem, or to carry out physician orders.

Nursing interventions are classified as independent, dependent, and interdependent. Independent interventions are those actions that the nurse can perform without direction from others. Providing a back massage and turning a patient every 2 hours are examples of independent nursing interventions.

Interdependent interventions are those actions that the nurse and other health care personnel perform together. For example, the physical or occupational therapist may be using special splints for a patient's extremities. The nurse will continue with the application and monitoring of these devices.

Dependent nursing interventions are prescribed by the physician or dentist and are carried out by the nurse. The nurse follows orders when administering medications, performing wound care, and ordering diagnostic tests. Nursing judgment is used in regard to dependent nursing activities. Assessing, teaching, and validating the safety of physician orders remain within the realm of nursing practice.

When determining appropriate nursing interventions, the nurse should consider the contributing/etiological/related factor, the patient-centered goal/outcome, and the nursing diagnosis label itself. Nursing interventions often are aimed at reducing or eliminating the causative factor.

Example: Anxiety related to lack of knowledge of hospital procedures.

Nursing interventions would direct the nurse to teach the patient about typical routines and procedures. Providing information should help reduce the fear of the unknown and thus reduce anxiety.

The patient-centered goal/outcome statement is also considered when selecting nursing interventions.

Example: The patient will plan a week's menu for an 1800-calorie diabetic diet by 2/14/95.

Interventions would be selected to increase the patient's knowledge of diabetic diets. The nursing diagnosis label may also direct the interventions.

Example: Acute pain related to tissue trauma secondary to appendectomy incision.

The nurse can direct interventions to relieve the nursing diagnosis label of acute pain.

A variety of sources list nursing interventions. Nursing textbooks, periodicals, and special "care plan" books are available in bookstores and libraries. Co-workers can suggest ideas for intervention that have worked previously. Nursing conferences held to plan patient care often provide an environment for the development of creative approaches to patient care. The patient also may provide suggestions for interventions. If the patient states that a hot cup of coffee first thing in the morning stimulates a bowel movement, the wise nurse will include that intervention on the care plan unless it is contraindicated.

Writing Nursing Orders

Interventions offered in textbooks and care planning manuals are broad, general statements that indicate the activity to be performed. For example, a text might suggest the following interventions for constipation.

1. Increase dietary bulk.
2. Increase activity.
3. Encourage fluids.

This information is helpful because it does prescribe a direction for care, but the information provided is incomplete. How will the nurse carry out those interventions? The nurse must translate the broad intervention statements into nursing orders. This is necessary because the nurse who initiates the plan of care is providing instructions for all care givers. Instructions must therefore be extremely clear and concise. Nursing orders must be written to reduce the likelihood of misinterpretation. Details are provided to convey the intended meaning. Nursing orders should include the following:

1. Date/signature
2. Subject
3. Action verb
4. Qualifying details

In most cases the subject of the nursing order is understood to be the nurse. When the nurse is not the subject, identify the person responsible for the action.

Example: Physical therapy will ambulate patient tid at 0900, 1400, 1900.

The nursing order should begin with an action verb. Action verbs tell what the care giver should do. Examples of action verbs are: offer, assist, encourage, demonstrate, turn, and assess.

Clarity is increased by adding qualifying details to the instruction. Explanations about how, when, where, how often, and how much are vital parts of the nursing order.

The nursing order should be written within the field of nursing, be realistic for the patient, correlate with the medical plan of care, and be based on scientific principles. The examples below illustrate appropriate translation of the nursing interventions into nursing orders.

1. Add four servings of fruits and vegetables to daily menu.
2. Ambulate patient with the assistance of two personnel 200 feet at 1000, 1500, and 2100.
3. Offer water and juices up to 2000 ml per day according to the following schedule
   7-3 shift 1200 ml
   3-11 shift 600 ml
   11-7 shift 200 ml

Communicating the Nursing Care Plan

After completing the initial assessment, analyzing the data, writing the nursing diagnoses, and selecting the appropriate nursing interventions, the nurse must communicate the detailed plan of care for the patient. The written nursing care plan is the product of the previous phases of the nursing process (Table 5-3).

Because the nursing staff is constantly changing, it is important to have written guidelines to promote continuity of patient care. Continuity increases patient trust in the nursing staff and promotes outcome achievement.

TABLE 5-3 Nursing Care Plan Form

Nursing Diagnosis	Nursing Order	Scientific Principle	Evaluation
Acute pain R/T tissue trauma from fractured fibula and tibia M/B grimaces, statements that right leg hurts, and elevated BP 140/100. **Desired goal/outcome** Patient will demonstrate improved comfort level as evidenced by relaxed facial expression, statements of pain relief, and return of vital signs to patient's normal range within 30 min of nursing interventions.	1. Assess verbal and nonverbal indications of pain. 2. Monitor BP and pulse for increase over baseline value every 4 hr. 3. Elevate right leg on 2 pillows at all times except meals. 4. Offer back rub and position change with statements of pain.	1. Fractures cause edema and pressure on nerves. Patient pain report establishes need for intervention. 2. Pain increases heart rate and BP. 3. Gravity helps reduce edema, which reduces pain. 4. Sensory nerve impulses from the skin "close the gate" and prevent pain transmission.	Outcome achieved. Focus: Pain. D (data)—States pain in lower right leg. BP 140/100. A (action)—Right leg elevated on 2 pillows. Back rub given for 10 min. R (response)—States pain relieved. BP 132/88.

Formats for the written nursing care plan vary from institution to institution according to individual needs. Nursing diagnoses, patient-centered goals/outcomes, and nursing orders are components common to nursing care planning systems.

Nursing faculty frequently require the student to provide scientific principles to explain "why" the intervention is needed and "how" the intervention will work. The student usually provides reference page numbers to show the source of the scientific principle.

Nursing care plans may be individually prepared, standardized, or computerized. Individually prepared care plans are time consuming but often provide the most individualized care.

Standardized nursing care plans are appropriate for routine, expected care requirements. Many standardized care plans have blank spaces that are filled in by the nurse to increase the individualization.

Some computerized systems print an updated nursing care plan for each shift. The nurse reads the printed interventions, intervenes for the patient, and documents the nursing interventions on the computerized care plan.

IMPLEMENTING

During the implementation phase of the nursing process the established plan is put into action to promote outcome achievement. This is the fourth phase of the nursing process. The **implementation** phase includes ongoing activities of data collection, prioritization, performance of nursing intervention, and documentation.[1]

In emergency situations the nurse proceeds directly from assessment of the problem to intervention. For example, the nurse initiates cardiopulmonary resuscitation for a patient whose respiratory or cardiac function has failed.

Daily contact with the patient and patient's family provides opportunities for additional data collection. Increasing pain, fatigue, or changes from the patient's initial health status may be noted.

As a result of this ongoing assessment, priorities of care may need to be altered. Activities may need to be delayed or canceled if the patient's condition warrants.

Interventions that the nurse may perform include the following:

- Performing an activity for a patient.
- Assisting the patient to perform an activity.
- Teaching the patient or family about health maintenance.
- Counseling the patient and family.
- Monitoring for problems or complications.
- Administering medications and monitoring for therapeutic and nontherapeutic effects.
- Referring the patient for care and follow-up activities.[1,20]

Nursing interventions include both nurse-prescribed and physician-prescribed activities. (If this is not clear, this is a good time to review the previous discussion of independent, dependent, and interdependent interventions.)

Documentation is a vital component of the implementation phase. The written documentation of the nursing process is a legal record of what has transpired while the patient was in the health care facility. "If it was not charted, it was not done," remains a constant principle of nursing. (See Chapter 6 for further content on documentation.)

EVALUATING

Evaluation is the determination made about the extent to which the established outcomes have been achieved in the nursing care plan. There are several steps the nurse takes to complete the evaluating phase. First, the nurse reviews the patient-centered goals/outcomes established in the planning phase of the nursing process. These outcome statements present criteria that are observable and measurable. Second, the nurse reassesses the patient to gather data indicating the patient's actual response. Third, the nurse compares the actual outcome with the desired outcome and makes a critical judgment about whether or not the patient-centered goal/outcome was achieved.

The nurse should make one of three judgments or decisions: the outcome was achieved, the outcome was partially achieved, or the outcome was not achieved. The nurse should document the basis for that decision. For example:

GOAL/OUTCOME STATEMENT	EVALUATION AND DOCUMENTATION
The patient will demonstrate self-administration of insulin by using sterile technique and selecting correct site by 1/14/95.	1/14/95—Outcome achieved. Pt correctly administered 4 units of regular insulin into upper thigh using sterile technique.

The plan of care is changed during this phase of the nursing process. Modification would occur if the outcome has been achieved, partially achieved, or not achieved. If the problem has been resolved, the nurse removes that problem from the nursing care plan.

When the outcome has been partially achieved or not achieved, further analysis is needed. At this point the nurse reviews all phases of the nursing process. The following are examples of questions the nurse might ask to ensure the accuracy of the nursing process. Was the assessment complete and accurate? Was the problem identified correctly? Was the patient-centered goal/outcome realistic and specific? Were the interventions realistic and were they implemented consistently by all personnel? Did new problems develop? Was adequate time allowed?

Once these questions have been answered, the nursing care plan can be changed. The nurse will intervene appropriately to correct the errors and will then refine the nursing care plan as needed.

ROLE OF THE LICENSED/ VOCATIONAL PRACTICAL NURSE

The role of the licensed practical nurse (LPN)/licensed vocational nurse (LVN) with the nursing process may vary from state to state and with different institutions. Student practical/vocational nurses should review their state's nurse practice acts for guidance in determining the LPN's/LVN's responsibility in their state.

Box 5-1 ROLE OF THE LPN/LVN IN THE NURSING PROCESS

ASSESSING

Observe and report significant cues (signs, symptoms), defining characteristics to nurse in charge or to the physician.

DIAGNOSING

Assist with the determination of accurate nursing diagnoses.
Gather further data to confirm or eliminate problems.

PLANNING

Assist with priority setting.
Suggest interventions.
Assist with the development of realistic patient-centered goals/outcomes.

IMPLEMENTING

Assist with establishment of priorities.
Carry out physician and nursing orders.
Evaluate the effectiveness of nursing activities.

EVALUATING

Assist with reevaluation of patient's health state after nursing intervention.
Suggest alternative nursing interventions when necessary.

The LPN/LVN is in the unique position of providing direct bedside nursing care. This direct care position allows the LPN/LVN to closely assess, prioritize, intervene, and evaluate the care provided to and for the patient. See Box 5-1 for a summary of the LPN's/LVN's role in the nursing process.

REFERENCES AND SUGGESTED READINGS

1. Alfaro R: *Applying nursing diagnosis and nursing process: a step-by-step guide,* ed 2, Philadelphia, 1990, Lippincott.
2. American Nurses' Association: *Standards of nursing practice,* Kansas City, Mo, 1973, The Association.
3. Carpenito LJ: *Nursing diagnosis: application to clinical practice,* ed 4, Philadelphia, 1992, Lippincott.
4. Carroll-Johnson RM, editor: *Classification of nursing diagnoses: proceedings from the ninth NANDA National Conference,* Philadelphia, 1991, Lippincott.
5. Carton G, Langton D, Robinson D: Teaching the nursing process, *Nurs Stand* 5(8):23, 1990.
6. Craven RF, Hirnle CJ: *Fundamentals of nursing: human health and function,* Philadelphia, 1992, Lippincott.
7. Doenges ME, Moorhouse MF: *Application of nursing process and nursing diagnosis: an interactive text,* Philadelphia, 1992, FA Davis.
8. Gettrust KV, Brabec PD: *Nursing diagnosis in clinical practice: guides for care planning,* Albany, NY, 1992, Delmar.
9. Hickey PW: *Nursing process handbook,* St Louis, 1990, Mosby.
10. Iyer P, Taptich BJ, Bernocchi-Losey D: *Nursing process and nursing diagnosis,* ed 2, Philadelphia, 1991, Saunders.
11. Kim MJ, McFarland GK, McLane AM: *Pocket guide to nursing diagnoses,* ed 4, St Louis, 1991, Mosby.
12. Kozier B, Erb G, Olivieri R: *Fundamentals of nursing: concepts, process, and process,* ed 4, Redwood City, Calif, 1991, Addison-Wesley.
13. Lederer JR et al: *Care planning pocket guide: a nursing diagnosis approach,* ed 4, Redwood City, Calif, 1991, Addison-Wesley.
14. Long BC, Phipps WJ, Cassmeyer VL: *Medical-surgical nursing: a nursing process approach,* ed 3, St Louis, 1993, Mosby.
15. Mills WC: Nursing diagnosis: the importance of a definition, *Nurs Diagn* 2(1):3, 1991.
16. *Mosby's dictionary of medicine, nursing, and allied health,* ed 4, St Louis, 1994, Mosby.
17. Pesut DJ, Herman J: Metacognitive skills in diagnostic reasoning: making the implicit explicit, *Nurs Diagn* 3(4):1489, 1992.
18. Potter PA, Perry AG: *Fundamentals of nursing: concepts, process, and practice,* ed 3, St Louis, 1993, Mosby.
19. Seidel H et al: *Mosby's guide to physical examination,* ed 2, St Louis, 1991, Mosby.
20. Sparks SM, Taylor CM: *Nursing diagnosis reference manual,* ed 2, Springhouse, Pa, 1993, Springhouse Corporation.
21. Swearingen PL: *Manual of nursing therapeutics: applying nursing diagnoses to medical disorders,* ed 2, St Louis, 1990, Mosby.
22. Taylor C, Lillis C, LeMone P: *Fundamentals of nursing: the art and science of nursing care,* Philadelphia, 1993, Lippincott.
23. Tucker SM et al: *Patient care standards: nursing process, diagnosis, and outcome,* ed 5, St Louis, 1992, Mosby.
24. Whaley LF, Wong DL: *Nursing care of infants and children,* ed 4, St Louis, 1991, Mosby.
25. Wilkinson JM: *Nursing process in action: a critical thinking approach,* Redwood City, Calif, 1992, Addison-Wesley.
26. Wright K: An overview of nursing process, *Gastroenterol Nurs* 15(1):14, 1992.

CHAPTER CHALLENGE

KEY POINTS

- The nursing process consists of five interconnected phases: assessment, diagnosis, planning, implementation, and evaluation.
- A complete and valid assessment influences the remaining phases of the nursing process.
- The patient is the primary source of data; all others are secondary sources.
- The nurse identifies four types of nursing diagnoses: actual, high risk, possible, and wellness.
- The nurse prescribes the primary interventions to treat a nursing diagnosis.
- During the planning phase of the nursing process, the nurse establishes priorities of care, writes desired patient outcomes, and communicates the plan of care.
- A patient-centered goal/outcome statement describes measurable, observable behavior that the patient should demonstrate after nursing interventions.
- Nursing interventions are planned activities to promote outcome achievement.
- Evaluation is ongoing for each phase of the nursing process.
- During evaluation the actual patient response is compared with the patient-centered goal/outcome and a judgment is made about outcome achievement.
- The plan of care is changed according to need.
- The licensed practical/vocational nurse has a significant role in the nursing process.

STUDY QUESTIONS

1. Ms. Robin, 49 years of age, has just been admitted to the medical floor. She is accompanied by several family members. When gathering information for an assessment, the nurse realizes the best source of data is usually the:
   1. patient.
   2. family.
   3. physician.
   4. old chart.
2. Mr. Laird states, "My right calf muscle aches when I walk." This is an example of:
   1. objective data
   2. subjective data
   3. personal data
   4. overt data
3. Mr. Reade states that he takes his medication regularly. His wife states that her husband takes his medicine only when reminded. Which step would the nurse take next?
   1. Validate the data.
   2. Cluster the data.
   3. Interpret the data.
   4. Identify the problem.
4. Which of the following data would be considered abnormal when compared with usual standards for a 44-year-old man?
   1. Temperature 100.2° F.
   2. Pulse 78.
   3. Respirations 18.
   4. BP 132/84.
5. Which of the following is the best example of an appropriate data cluster?
   1. Nonproductive cough, no bowel movement in 3 days, and incision pain.
   2. Pulse 100, difficulty voiding, and weight 161 pounds for 5′4″ height.
   3. Drags right foot when walking, respiration 32, states lack of appetite.
   4. Productive cough, respirations 24, and adventitious breath sounds.
6. Which of the following nursing diagnostic title/labels would be ranked first in priority?
   1. Constipation.
   2. Altered nutrition: less than body requirements.
   3. Social isolation.
   4. Ineffective airway clearance.
7. "Potential for Fetal Distress related to umbilical cord compression" is an example of a(n):
   1. actual nursing diagnosis.
   2. "high risk for . . ." nursing diagnosis.
   3. wellness nursing diagnosis.
   4. collaboration problem.
8. The phrases used to connect the parts of a nursing diagnosis are:
   1. related to and due to.
   2. due to and manifest by.
   3. related to and manifested by.
   4. due to and as evidenced by.

6

DOCUMENTATION

Donna M. Babao

KEY TERMS

auditors
chart (health care record)
charting
charting by exception
computer terminals
diagnosis related groups (DRGs)
documenting
focus charting
Kardex/Rand
narrative charting
nursing care plan
nursing notes
peer review
problem list
problem-oriented medical record (POMR)
quality assurance/ assessment/ improvement
recording
SOAPE
SOAPIER
traditional or block chart

LEARNING OBJECTIVES

After reading this chapter, the student should be able to do the following:

- Define the key terms.
- List the five purposes for written patient records.
- Describe the differences between traditional and problem-oriented medical records.
- State important legal aspects of chart ownership, access, confidentiality, and patient care documentation.
- Describe the purpose of and relationship between the Kardex and the nursing care plan.
- Explain the relationship of the nursing care plan to care documentation and patient care reimbursement.
- Describe the basic guidelines for and mechanics of charting.
- Describe the differences in documenting care using activity of daily living and physical assessment forms, narrative, SOAPE, and focus formats.
- Discuss the use of computers for record keeping and documentation in health care facilities.

RELATED TOPICS OF INTEREST

- The evolution of nursing (Chapter 1)
- Legal aspects of nursing (Chapter 2)
- Communication (Chapter 4)
- The nursing process (Chapter 5)
- Principles and practice of medication administration (Chapter 21)

A medical record should furnish all health care providers with a concise, accurate, written picture of a patient's medical and nursing problems, care planned and given, and the patient's response to treatments. The **chart (health care record)** has never been more important in the health care system than it is today; it is a legal record that is used to meet the many demands of the health, accreditation, medical insurance, and legal systems.

A nurse must understand how to use these records effectively and efficiently. This chapter will cover the purposes for written records, common types of records, basic guidelines and rules for documentation, and legal concerns. The knowledge of these guidelines and the ability to chart completely, accurately, and legibly are a requirement for licensure and employment as a nurse.

The process of adding written information to the chart is called **charting, recording,** or **documenting.** Although there are many details to remember when documenting in the chart, the process is not difficult but can be time consuming. Documentation is part of the implementation phase of the nursing process (see Chapter 5) and is necessary for the evaluation of patient care as well as for care cost reimbursement.

PURPOSES OF PATIENT RECORDS

There are five basic purposes for written patient records: (1) written communication, (2) permanent record for accountability, (3) legal record of care, (4) teaching, and (5) research and data collection.

The patient's chart provides a permanent written record of past and current medical and nursing problems, plans for care, care given, and the patient's responses to various treatments. The record facilitates accurate communication and continuity of care among all members of the health care team. Written information is not as easily lost or altered as the spoken word.

This permanent written record may also be used by various government and other agencies to evaluate the institution's patient care and to prove that care was given for cost reimbursement. Current regulations require chart audits (review of specific chart components for completion and appropriateness) by officially appointed **auditors** (persons appointed to examine patients' charts and health records to assess quality of care). Institutions have medical and **peer review** systems (an appraisal by professional co-workers of equal status). Peer review appraises the manner in which an individual nurse conducts practice, education, or research. Institutions also have specific procedures to provide for **quality assurance/assessment/improvement.** An audit in health care is any evaluation of services provided and the results achieved compared with accepted standards. Accurate and legible records are the only means institutions have to prove that they are providing care to meet the patient's needs and established standards.

Cost reimbursement rates by the government plans (Medicare, Medicaid) are based on **diagnosis related groups (DRGs)** (a system that classifies patients by age, diagnosis, and surgical procedure, producing 300 different categories used in predicting the use of hospital resources, including length of stay). Many private insurance companies now use similar illness categories when setting hospital payment rates. The **nursing notes** (the form on the patient's chart on which nurses record their observations, care given, and the patient's responses) are carefully reviewed when deciding whether the necessary and ordered care is being or was given. Institutions are reimbursed by insurance companies or government programs only for the patient care documented.

The patient chart or health record is a legal document and can be called into court. Although the physician or institution owns the original record, lawyers and courts can gain access to it, so it is important to chart in a very detailed, defensive manner. Most states now also grant patient access through channels established by the individual facility. Patients usually do not have immediate access to their full records (see Chapter 2).

Patient health records are also used for teaching. Students in the health care professions can learn more quickly and easily if examples of good charting are shared. Individuals can also learn from their mistakes and the mistakes of others.

Individuals involved in research and data collection in the health field have many uses for patient records. For example, the government periodically publishes data on certain diseases and the effectiveness of new treatments. The usual length of hospitalization and the cost of treatment for specific illnesses or surgeries have become very important to the government and other health insurance providers because of the pressure to contain or limit health care costs.

COMMON MEDICAL ABBREVIATIONS AND TERMINOLOGY

A nurse cannot effectively and efficiently use a health record until some understanding and knowledge of common abbreviations and medical terms have been developed. This information is also required for concise and accurate documentation of care. Most facilities have a published list of generally accepted medical abbreviations and terms approved for use in charting. The use of ambiguous abbreviations and terms should be avoided because may lead to misinterpretations and errors. (Consult the inside back cover of this text.)

TYPES OF PATIENT RECORDS

There are basically two types of forms for patient health records: the traditional or block chart and the problem-oriented medical record (POMR). Both formats, while different in style, contain the same information.

Traditional Chart

The **traditional** or **block chart** is divided into specific sections or blocks. Emphasis is placed on specific sheets

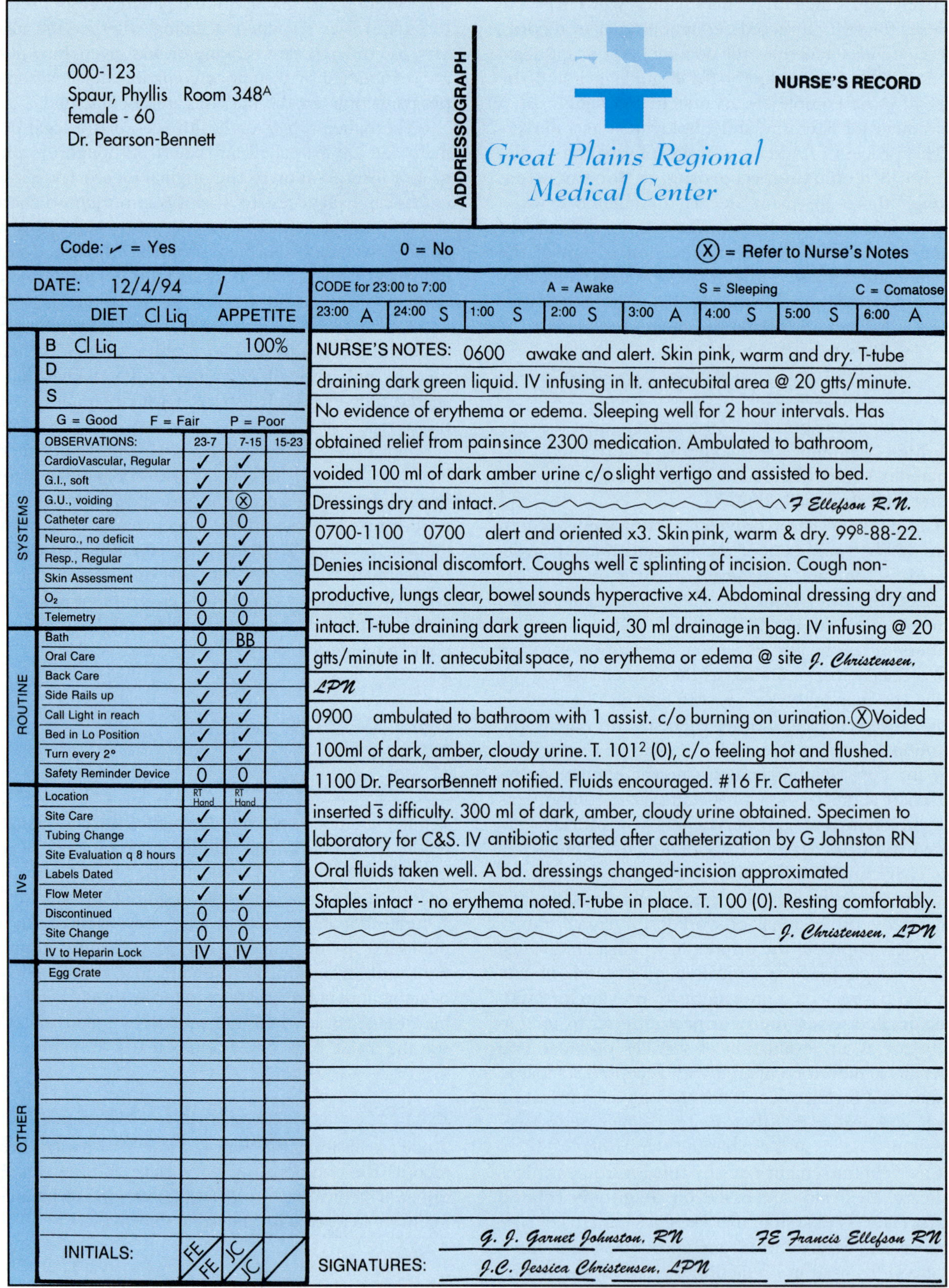

000-123
Spaur, Phyllis Room 348A
female - 60
Dr. Pearson-Bennett

ADDRESSOGRAPH

Great Plains Regional Medical Center

NURSE'S RECORD

Code: ✓ = Yes 0 = No ⓧ = Refer to Nurse's Notes

DATE: 12/4/94 /

DIET Cl Liq APPETITE

B	Cl Liq	100%
D		
S		

G = Good F = Fair P = Poor

	OBSERVATIONS:	23-7	7-15	15-23
SYSTEMS	CardioVascular, Regular	✓	✓	
	G.I., soft	✓	✓	
	G.U., voiding	✓	ⓧ	
	Catheter care	0	0	
	Neuro., no deficit	✓	✓	
	Resp., Regular	✓	✓	
	Skin Assessment	✓	✓	
	O_2	0	0	
	Telemetry	0	0	
ROUTINE	Bath	0	BB	
	Oral Care	✓	✓	
	Back Care	✓	✓	
	Side Rails up	✓	✓	
	Call Light in reach	✓	✓	
	Bed in Lo Position	✓	✓	
	Turn every 2°	✓	✓	
	Safety Reminder Device	0	0	
IVs	Location	RT Hand	RT Hand	
	Site Care	✓	✓	
	Tubing Change	✓	✓	
	Site Evaluation q 8 hours	✓	✓	
	Labels Dated	✓	✓	
	Flow Meter	✓	✓	
	Discontinued	0	0	
	Site Change	0	0	
	IV to Heparin Lock	IV	IV	
OTHER	Egg Crate			
	INITIALS:	FE/FE	JC/JC	

CODE for 23:00 to 7:00 A = Awake S = Sleeping C = Comatose

23:00	24:00	1:00	2:00	3:00	4:00	5:00	6:00
A	S	S	S	A	S	S	A

NURSE'S NOTES: 0600 awake and alert. Skin pink, warm and dry. T-tube draining dark green liquid. IV infusing in lt. antecubital area @ 20 gtts/minute. No evidence of erythema or edema. Sleeping well for 2 hour intervals. Has obtained relief from painsince 2300 medication. Ambulated to bathroom, voided 100 ml of dark amber urine c/o slight vertigo and assisted to bed. Dressings dry and intact. F Ellefson R.N.

0700-1100 0700 alert and oriented x3. Skin pink, warm & dry. 99⁸-88-22. Denies incisional discomfort. Coughs well c̄ splinting of incision. Cough non-productive, lungs clear, bowel sounds hyperactive x4. Abdominal dressing dry and intact. T-tube draining dark green liquid, 30 ml drainage in bag. IV infusing @ 20 gtts/minute in lt. antecubital space, no erythema or edema @ site J. Christensen, LPN

0900 ambulated to bathroom with 1 assist. c/o burning on urination.ⓧVoided 100ml of dark, amber, cloudy urine. T. 101² (0), c/o feeling hot and flushed. 1100 Dr. PearsonBennett notified. Fluids encouraged. #16 Fr. Catheter inserted s̄ difficulty. 300 ml of dark, amber, cloudy urine obtained. Specimen to laboratory for C&S. IV antibiotic started after catheterization by G Johnston RN Oral fluids taken well. A bd. dressings changed-incision approximated Staples intact - no erythema noted. T-tube in place. T. 100 (0). Resting comfortably. J. Christensen, LPN

SIGNATURES: G. J. Garnet Johnston, RN FE Francis Ellefson RN J.C. Jessica Christensen, LPN

FIG. 6-1 Narrative charting. (Courtesy Great Plains Regional Medical Center, North Platte, Neb.)

of information. Typical blocks are admission sheet, physician's orders, progress notes, history and physical examination data, nurse's admission information, care plan, and nursing notes, graphics, and laboratory and x-ray reports. The order, content, and number of the sections vary among institutions. Nurses use flow sheets, graphics, and **narrative charting** (recording of patient care in descriptive form) to chart observations, care, and responses (Fig. 6-1).

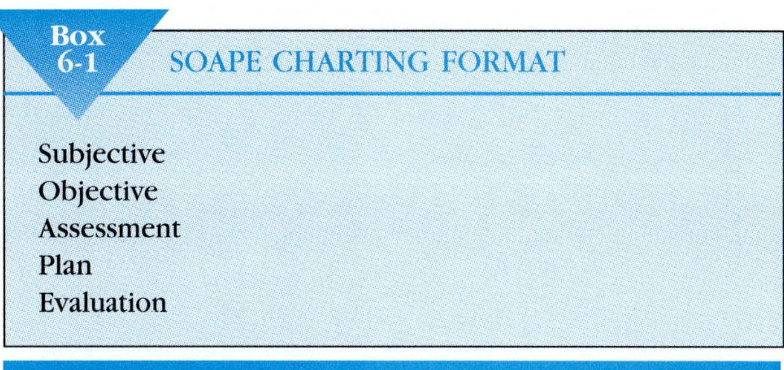

Box 6-1 SOAPE CHARTING FORMAT

Subjective
Objective
Assessment
Plan
Evaluation

Problem-Oriented Medical Record

The organization of the **problem-oriented medical record (POMR)** is based on the scientific problem-solving system or method. The principal sections are data base, problem list, initial plan, and progress notes. The accumulated data or data base from the history, physical examination, and diagnostic tests are used to identify and prioritize the health problems on the master medical and other problem list.

This **problem list** of active, inactive, potential, and resolved problems serves as the index for chart documentation. All health care providers—physicians, nurses, social workers, and therapists—chart on the same progress notes. This is done to facilitate and enhance communication between care providers. The charting format used is called SOAPIER or SOAPE.

SOAPIER is an acronym for seven different aspects of charting. For notes on specific patient problems, only the necessary parts needed for completeness are used.

- **S** *Subjective* information is what the patient states or feels; *only* the patient can provide this information.
- **O** *Objective* information is what the nurse can measure or factually describe.
- **A** *Assessment* refers to an analysis or potential diagnosis of the cause of the patient's problem or need.
- **P** *Plan* is the general statement of the plan of care to be given or action to be taken.
- **I** *Implementation* is the specific care given or action taken.
- **E** *Evaluation* is an appraisal of the response and effectiveness of the plan.
- **R** *Revision* includes the changes that may be made to the original plan of care.

SOAPE (Box 6-1) is the briefer adaptation of the charting format for the problem-oriented record. In this more compact form, the care given or action taken (implementation) *(I)* is included in the plan notations. The needed plan revisions *(R)* are noted after the evaluation of the response to treatment in the evaluation section. The commonly used charting forms in the progress notes in medical records are shown in Figs. 6-2 through 6-4.

Focus Charting Format

One other charting form used in some institutions has similarities to the problem list for the POMR. This focus charting format (Box 6-2), developed by nurses, could be used with both traditional and POMR charting. In **focus charting,** instead of problem lists, a modified list of nursing diagnoses is used as an index for nursing documentation. This form of charting uses the nursing process and the more positive concept of the patient's needs rather than medical diagnoses and problems.

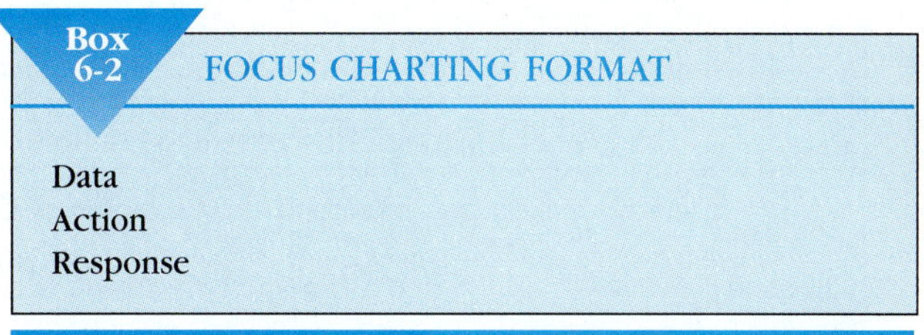

Box 6-2 FOCUS CHARTING FORMAT

Data
Action
Response

The focus can be a current patient concern or behavior, significant change in patient status or behavior, or significant event in the patient's therapy. A focus is not a medical diagnosis.

Data *(D)* is equivalent to the assessment step of the nursing process. Action *(A)* is a combination of planning and implementation. Response *(R)* is the same as evaluation. Not all the DAR steps need to be used each time notes are made on a particular focus (Fig. 6-5).

BASIC GUIDELINES FOR DOCUMENTATION

The quality and accuracy of the nurse's notes are very important. The words used can clearly and concisely convey the intended message or can cause confusion and errors in communication and patient care. Correct spelling, grammar, and punctuation, as well as good penmanship and other writing skills, are important in documentation.

The information recorded in the chart should be clear, concise, complete, and accurate. The forms used to make these notes vary, but each institution's policy should be followed. Each facility uses a combination of graphics, care flow sheets, and narrative or SOAPE notes to document observations, care, and responses. The

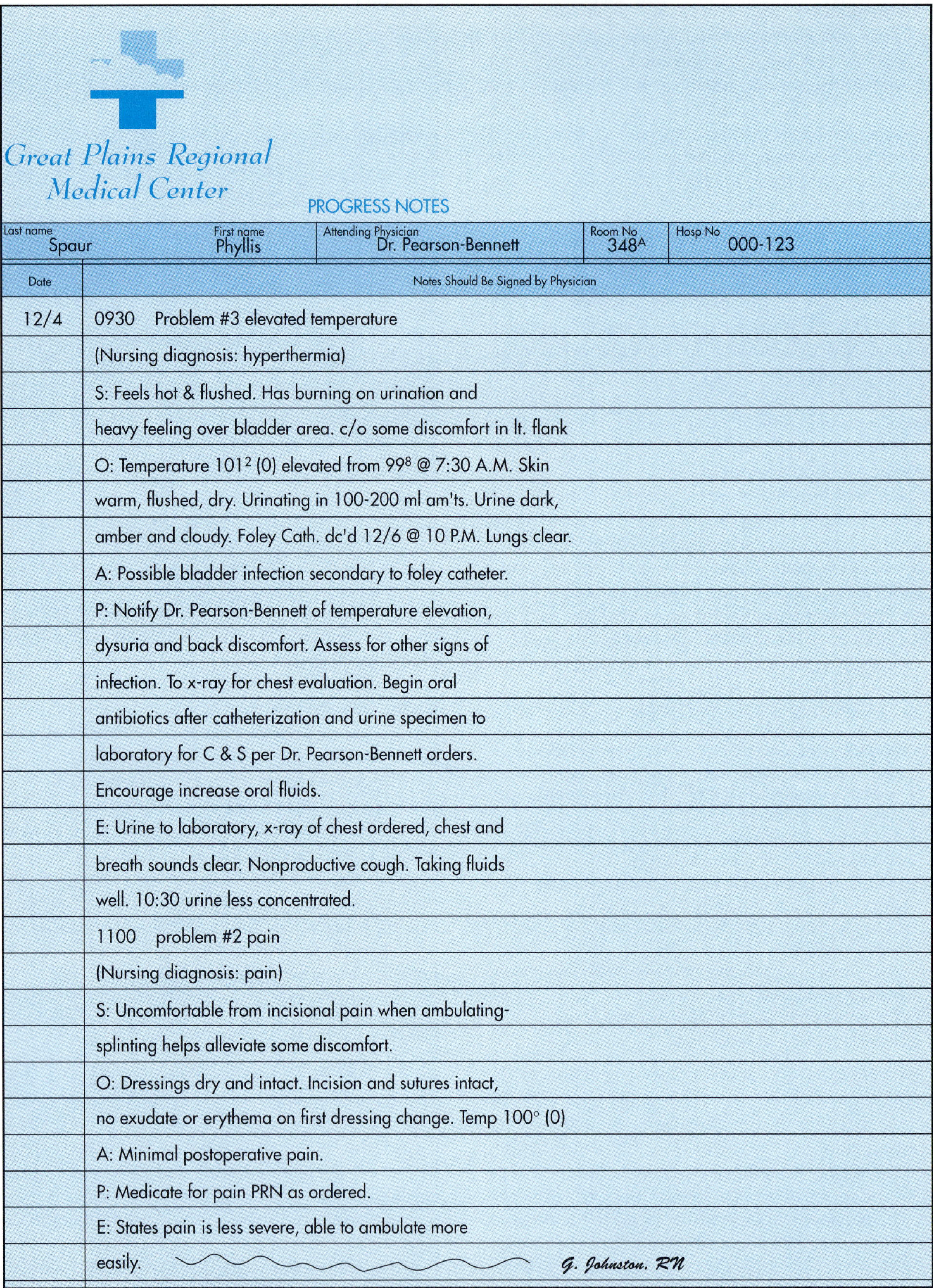

Great Plains Regional Medical Center

PROGRESS NOTES

Last name	First name	Attending Physician	Room No	Hosp No
Spaur	Phyllis	Dr. Pearson-Bennett	348A	000-123

Date	Notes Should Be Signed by Physician
12/4	0930 Problem #3 elevated temperature
	(Nursing diagnosis: hyperthermia)
	S: Feels hot & flushed. Has burning on urination and
	heavy feeling over bladder area. c/o some discomfort in lt. flank
	O: Temperature 101^2 (0) elevated from 99^8 @ 7:30 A.M. Skin
	warm, flushed, dry. Urinating in 100-200 ml am'ts. Urine dark,
	amber and cloudy. Foley Cath. dc'd 12/6 @ 10 P.M. Lungs clear.
	A: Possible bladder infection secondary to foley catheter.
	P: Notify Dr. Pearson-Bennett of temperature elevation,
	dysuria and back discomfort. Assess for other signs of
	infection. To x-ray for chest evaluation. Begin oral
	antibiotics after catheterization and urine specimen to
	laboratory for C & S per Dr. Pearson-Bennett orders.
	Encourage increase oral fluids.
	E: Urine to laboratory, x-ray of chest ordered, chest and
	breath sounds clear. Nonproductive cough. Taking fluids
	well. 10:30 urine less concentrated.
	1100 problem #2 pain
	(Nursing diagnosis: pain)
	S: Uncomfortable from incisional pain when ambulating-
	splinting helps alleviate some discomfort.
	O: Dressings dry and intact. Incision and sutures intact,
	no exudate or erythema on first dressing change. Temp 100° (0)
	A: Minimal postoperative pain.
	P: Medicate for pain PRN as ordered.
	E: States pain is less severe, able to ambulate more
	easily. G. Johnston, RN

FIG. 6-2 SOAPE charting progress notes. (Courtesy Great Plains Regional Medical Center, North Platte, Neb.)

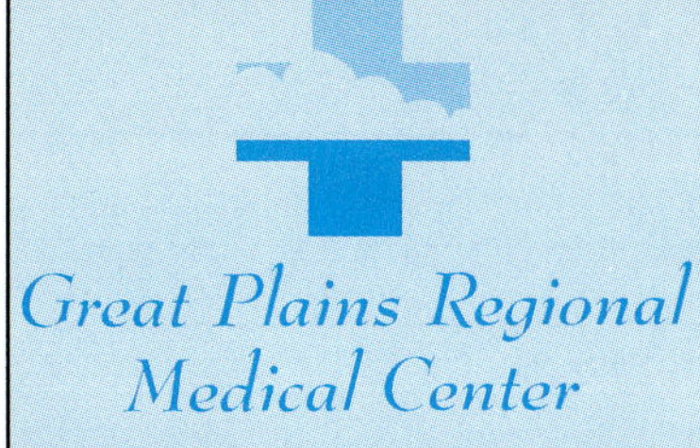

Great Plains Regional Medical Center

000-123
Spaur, Phyllis - Room 348A
Female - 60
Dr. Pearson-Bennett

Page 1 of 2

PATIENT CARE PLAN

Admitting Diagnosis: Cholelithiasis/Cholecystitis | Operation: Cholecystectomy | Surgery Date: 12/5/94

Additional Diagnosis: | Surgeon: Dr. Pearson-Bennett | Adm. Date: 12/4 | Dism. Date:

Nursing Diagnosis with outcome	Start Date	Nursing Interventions	Date D/Cd	Init	Reassessment	Date D/Cd	Init
#1 Knowledge deficit	12/5	Explain preoperative routine NPO	12/6	JC	Has learned to		JC
Preoperative and		laboratory blood work. Demonstrate			cough, deep breath		
postoperative care		postoperative deep breathing coughing			and do leg exercise		
R/T Scheduled surgery		and leg exercises. Explain about I.V.,					
Goal: will verbalize		tubes, vital signs, pain control c̄					
routines and demonstrate		medication.					
postop. deep breathing coughing							
and leg exercise							
#2 Pain R/T incision	12/6	Review incisional splinting. Assist c̄	12/6	JC	Is moving more		JC
and muscle spasms		splinting by using pillow or bath			easily, resting well		
M/B verbalization		blanket. Encourage requesting			for several hours. Is		
of pain, guarded		medication for pain before complaints			splinting incision		
movements.		are too severe. Teach relaxation			well and able to		
Goal: Relate that		exercises. Administer analgesics			cough and deep		
she feels more		PRN. Assess response to medication			breath.		
comfortable, moves		within 1/2 hour					
more easily, rests							
and sleeps well							
@ intervals							

INITIALS AND SIGNATURE JC J. Christensen LPN

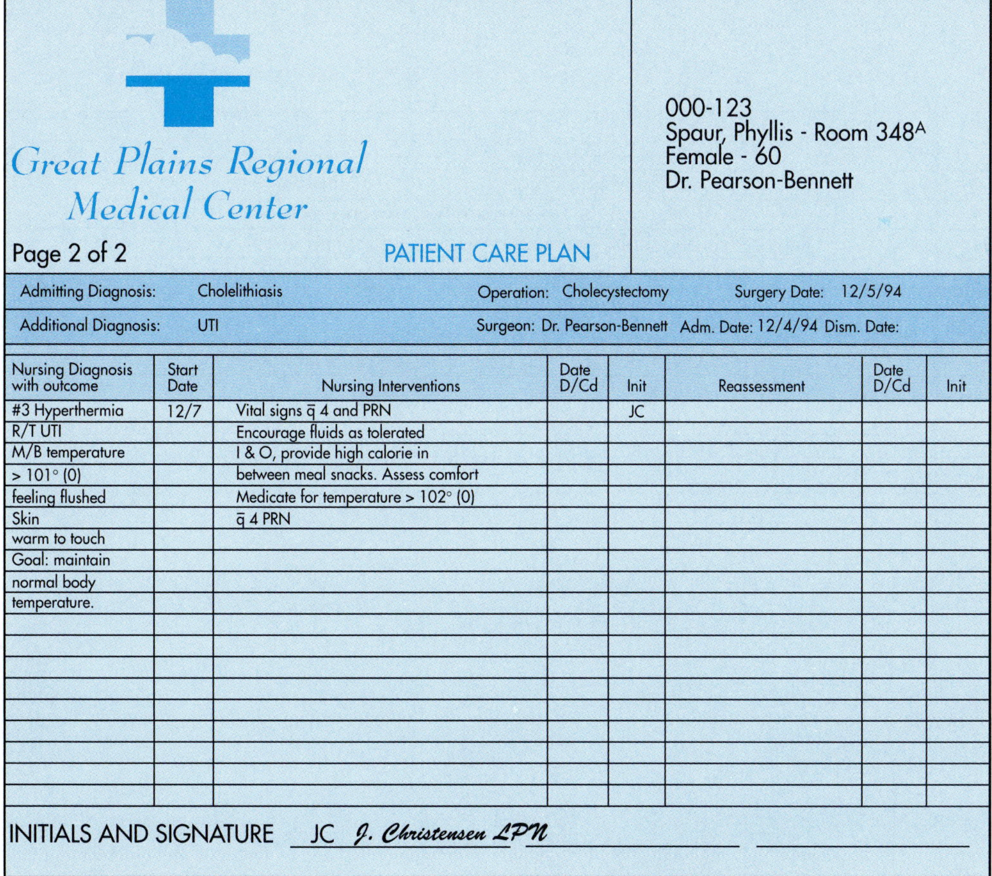

Great Plains Regional Medical Center

000-123
Spaur, Phyllis - Room 348A
Female - 60
Dr. Pearson-Bennett

Page 2 of 2

PATIENT CARE PLAN

Admitting Diagnosis: Cholelithiasis | Operation: Cholecystectomy | Surgery Date: 12/5/94

Additional Diagnosis: UTI | Surgeon: Dr. Pearson-Bennett | Adm. Date: 12/4/94 | Dism. Date:

Nursing Diagnosis with outcome	Start Date	Nursing Interventions	Date D/Cd	Init	Reassessment	Date D/Cd	Init
#3 Hyperthermia	12/7	Vital signs q̄ 4 and PRN		JC			
R/T UTI		Encourage fluids as tolerated					
M/B temperature		I & O, provide high calorie in					
> 101° (0)		between meal snacks. Assess comfort					
feeling flushed		Medicate for temperature > 102° (0)					
Skin		q̄ 4 PRN					
warm to touch							
Goal: maintain							
normal body							
temperature.							

INITIALS AND SIGNATURE JC J. Christensen LPN

FIG. 6-3 Patient care plan with nursing diagnosis. (Courtesy Great Plains Regional Medical Center, North Platte, Neb.)

MASTER PROBLEM LIST				
Date	Problem	Resolved	Reviewed	Reactivate
12/5/94	#1 Knowledge deficit R/T Preoperative and postoperative procedures.	12/6/94		
12/6/94	#2 Pain R/T incision.	12/7		
12/7/94	#3 Temperature elevation 2° to bladder infection.			

Addressograph

000-123
Spaur, Phyllis - Room 348A
Female - 60
Dr. Pearson-Bennett

FIG. 6-4 Master problem list.

DATE	12/7	
TIME	FOCUS	NURSES NOTES
1400	post-op pain	Ambulating in hall c̄ moderate assist. I.V. infusing
		@ 20 gtts/min. Still feels warm, main concern is
		incisional pain, splinting is helpful. Positioned in
		bed c̄ pillows for support. Medicated for pain.
		Practiced relaxation breathing exercises. J. Christensen LPN
1400	pain/fever	States, "I am more comfortable and relaxed now." Skin warm
		and dry. T. 99^6 (0). c/o some burning on urination,
		less than in a.m. Taking fluids well. Urine light
		yellow and less cloudy. ——— J. Christensen LPN

FIG. 6-5 Focus charting nurse's notes.

nurse's notes should always correlate with the medical orders, Kardex information, and nursing care plan.

The registered nurse has primary responsibility for each patient's initial admission nursing history, physical assessment, and development of the care plan based on the nursing diagnoses identified. Contributions by all team members during this initial process and during later updating sessions are very important.

Some facilities want a minimum of three entries per shift made on the narrative notes, as well as all care given or not given charted on a flow sheet. This is a policy that fulfills the charting concept that care was not given if it was not charted. Although all care should be charted, this is a time-consuming and detailed manner of defensive charting.

Many hospitals now have a policy called **charting by exception.** Complete physical assessments, observations, vital signs, IV site and rate, and other pertinent data are charted at the beginning of each shift. During the shift only additional treatments done or withheld, changes in patient condition, and new concerns are charted. All active nursing diagnoses on the nursing care plan should have notations reflecting progress or revisions. More detailed flow sheets, which reduces the time needed to chart, are used with this method of documentation.

Auditors will check to see whether all ordered care was charted as given and whether responses to specific care plan items and treatments are noted. Accuracy and completeness of documentation are important for communication, continuity of patient care, legal matters, accreditation and quality assurance/assessment/improvement audits, and cost reimbursement purposes. Charting should cover all areas of patient needs and concerns: physical, emotional, psychological, social, and spiritual.

NARRATIVE CHARTING

The idea of writing narrative charting is often intimidating to students. This form of nurse's notes is easier to complete if the writer remembers that the steps of the nursing process are followed and that the notes should include the same information as a SOAPE note. Narrative charting should include the basic patient need or problem data (subjective and/or objective), whether someone was contacted, care and treatments provided (implementation), and the patient's response to treatment (evaluation). This type of charting is written in an abbreviated story form instead of in the outline style of the POMR note format (see Fig. 6-1).

CHARTING RULES

Generally accepted charting rules were developed to provide consistency in documentation between health care providers and facilities (Box 6-3). These rules also meet the standards expected by the individuals and agencies using the charts.

Box 6-3 BASIC RULES FOR CHARTING

- All sheets should have the correct patient name, date, and time if appropriate.
- Use only approved abbreviations and medical terms.
- Be timely, specific, accurate, and complete.
- Write legibly (print if handwriting is not legible).
- Follow rules of grammar and punctuation.
- Fill all spaces; leave no empty lines.
- Chart after care, not before.
- Chart as soon and as often as possible.
- Chart only your own care, observations, and teaching; *never* chart for anyone else.
- Use direct quotes when appropriate.
- Describe each item as you see it—"white metal ring with clear stone."
- Be objective in charting—only what you hear, see, feel, smell.
- Chart facts; avoid judgmental terms and placing blame.
- Sign each block of charting or entry with full legal name and title.
- When a patient leaves a unit (e.g., to go to x-ray, lab, or office), chart the time and method of transportation on departure and return.
- Chart all ordered care as given or explain the deviation (NPO for lab, off unit, refused, etc.).
- Note patient response to treatments and response to analgesics or other special medications.
- Use only hard-pointed, permanent black ink pens; no erasures or correcting fluids are allowed on charts.
- If a charting error is made, draw one line through the faulty information, mark error, initial if required, and make the correct entry (~~simple~~ error sample).
- When making a late entry, note it as a late entry and then proceed with your notation: for example, Late entry___ ___ ___ ___ ___ .
- Follow each institution's policies and procedures for charting.

OTHER DOCUMENTATION FORMS AND EXAMPLES

The nursing **Kardex/Rand** is a card system used to consolidate patient orders and care needs in a centralized, concise way. The cumulative care file or Rand is kept at the nursing station for quick reference. Card forms vary between institutions based on information required for care (Fig. 6-6).

The **nursing care plan** is developed to meet the nursing care needs of a patient. A standard care plan for a certain condition or surgery may be used and special

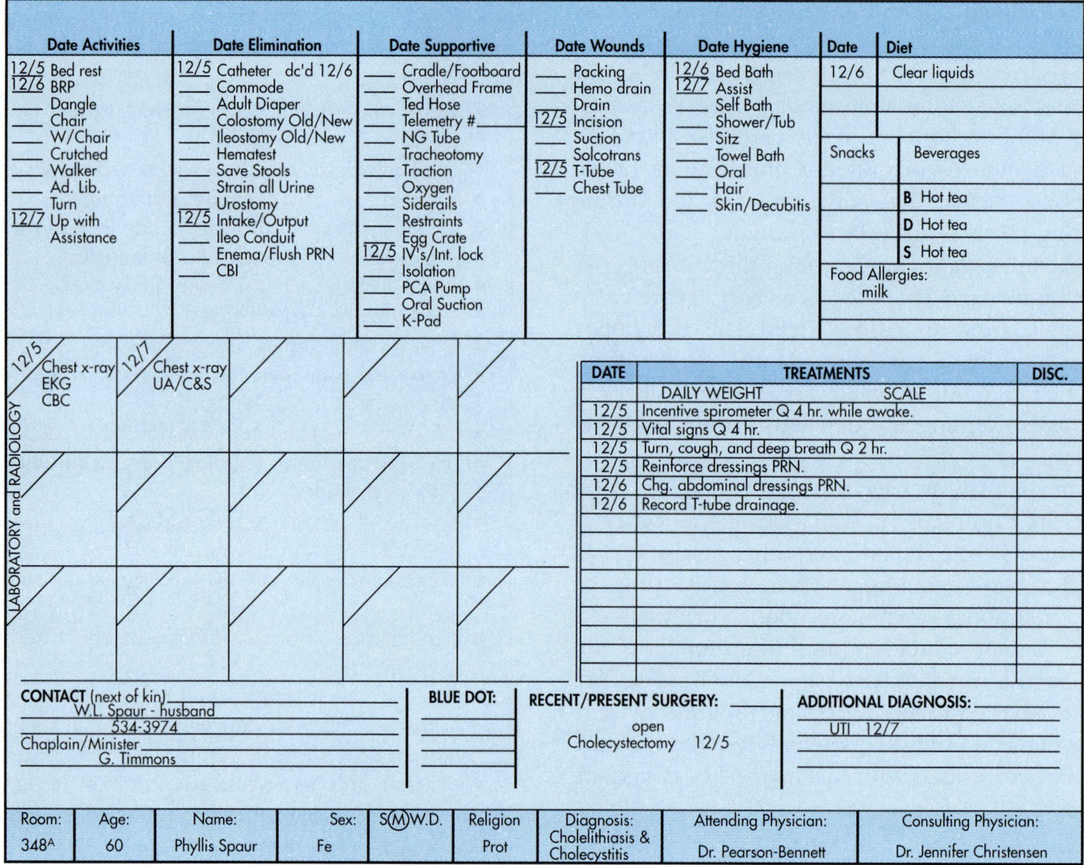

Date Activities	Date Elimination	Date Supportive	Date Wounds	Date Hygiene
12/5 Bed rest	12/5 Catheter dc'd 12/6	___ Cradle/Footboard	___ Packing	12/6 Bed Bath
12/6 BRP	___ Commode	___ Overhead Frame	___ Hemo drain	12/7 Assist
___ Dangle	___ Adult Diaper	___ Ted Hose	___ Drain	___ Self Bath
___ Chair	___ Colostomy Old/New	___ Telemetry #___	12/5 Incision	___ Shower/Tub
___ W/Chair	___ Ileostomy Old/New	___ NG Tube	___ Suction	___ Sitz
___ Crutched	___ Hematest	___ Tracheotomy	___ Solcotrans	___ Towel Bath
___ Walker	___ Save Stools	___ Traction	12/5 T-Tube	___ Oral
___ Ad. Lib.	___ Strain all Urine	___ Oxygen	___ Chest Tube	___ Hair
___ Turn	___ Urostomy	___ Siderails		___ Skin/Decubitis
12/7 Up with Assistance	12/5 Intake/Output	___ Restraints		
	___ Ileo Conduit	___ Egg Crate		
	___ Enema/Flush PRN	12/5 IV's/Int. lock		
	___ CBI	___ Isolation		
		___ PCA Pump		
		___ Oral Suction		
		___ K-Pad		

Date	Diet
12/6	Clear liquids

Snacks	Beverages
	B Hot tea
	D Hot tea
	S Hot tea

Food Allergies: milk

LABORATORY and RADIOLOGY
12/5 Chest x-ray, EKG, CBC
12/7 Chest x-ray, UA/C&S

DATE	TREATMENTS	DISC.
	DAILY WEIGHT SCALE	
12/5	Incentive spirometer Q 4 hr. while awake.	
12/5	Vital signs Q 4 hr.	
12/5	Turn, cough, and deep breath Q 2 hr.	
12/5	Reinforce dressings PRN.	
12/6	Chg. abdominal dressings PRN.	
12/6	Record T-tube drainage.	

CONTACT (next of kin) W.L. Spaur - husband 534-3974
Chaplain/Minister G. Timmons

BLUE DOT:

RECENT/PRESENT SURGERY: open Cholecystectomy 12/5

ADDITIONAL DIAGNOSIS: UTI 12/7

Room:	Age:	Name:	Sex:	S(M)W.D.	Religion	Diagnosis:	Attending Physician:	Consulting Physician:
348A	60	Phyllis Spaur	Fe		Prot	Cholelithiasis & Cholecystitis	Dr. Pearson-Bennett	Dr. Jennifer Christensen

FIG. 6-6 Nursing Kardex or Rand card.

needs added for individualized care. This plan is based on nursing assessment and nursing diagnosis; it is developed by nurses for nurses. Nursing care plans include the pertinent nursing diagnoses, goals, and plans for care, and specific actions for care implementation and evaluation (Fig. 6-3).

An *incident report* (Fig. 6-7) or other hospital notification form is filled out when patient care was not consistent with facility or national standards of expected care. For example, a medication or treatment was forgotten or an incorrect dose of a drug was given; either of these events could or may have caused injury. Incident reports are also filled out for any unusual event in a hospital (e.g., patient, visitor, or hospital personnel injuries). Many staff members are reluctant to fill out these forms, but this information helps the facility risk manager and unit managers prevent future problems through education and other corrective measures.

When filling out an incident report, give only objective, observed information. Do not admit liability or give unnecessary details. Do list date, time, care given the patient, and the name of the physician notified. When charting the incident in the patient's nurse's notes, do not mention the incident report because this makes it easier for an attorney to request that document for a court case.

SPECIAL ISSUES IN DOCUMENTATION

Record Ownership and Access

As mentioned earlier, the original health care record or chart is the property of the institution or physician. On admission to the health care facility the patient is usually asked to sign a form granting permission for appropriate persons to have access to the record as necessary.

Patients have gained access rights to their records in most states, but only if they follow the established policy of each facility. Usually a written request for chart access must be submitted, and institutions state an allowed period of time for the physician and the facility to review the record and give a response. The institution may require that a staff member or physician be present while the individual looks through the chart to answer questions and to protect the integrity of the record.

If no addressograph, write in name, age, sex, and chart number. For a visitor, please include address and telephone number.

Addressograph

GREAT PLAINS REGIONAL MEDICAL CENTER

Report of Medication, (Patient), Visitor Safety Variance

To be completed by the person most closely involved or the person discovering the incident/occurrence.

PATIENT NAME: John Jordan AGE: 76 SEX: male

ADDRESS: 506 South Ash Street North Platte, Ne 69101

TYPE OF PATIENT: (check one)
X Inpatient ___ Outpatient ___ Emergency
___ Visitor ___ Employee

Social Security #: 405-38-2948

Date and Time of Variance: 4-9-95 0900

Exact Location of Variance: 230A

Description of Variance: Found patient lying on floor at foot of bed sts "I was having a liquid bowel movement and I couldn't push the nurse's call light." Noted a large liquid stool on floor near patient. Side rails up x 2.

What was the nature of the injury to the (patient)/visitor, etc.: 4 cm. abrasion to left trochanteric area.

Equipment or supplies involved: none

ID # & Present Location: 3001

Why did variance occur? patient too weak to push nurse's call light and an unsteady gait.

Physician Notified? yes X no ___ when? 0915

Signature *Cheryl Nichols RN* Physician: *Dr. J.H. Christensen*

Witness *Lois Gallman RN*

If the incident is related to patient care, this sheet must remain on inpatient medical record for 24 hours, after which it shall be taken to the Risk Management Department.

CONFIDENTIAL - NOT PART OF THE MEDICAL RECORD

FIG. 6-7 Incident report. (Courtesy Great Plains Regional Medical Center, North Platte, Neb.)

A lawyer can gain access to a chart with the patient's written permission. Courts can legally obtain records for their review and use.

Confidentiality

Health care personnel must respect the confidentiality of the patient's record. The Patient's Bill of Rights and the law guarantee that the patient's medical information will be kept private, except if the information is needed in providing care or the patient gives permission for others to see it. The nurse should not read a record unless there is a clinical reason and should hold the information regarding the patient in confidence. Ethical codes of practice emphasize the nurse's obligation to preserve patients' privacy by holding patient information in highest confidentiality. Trust is necessary for good nurse-patient relationships, and breaking confidences is a way to lose patient trust. If laws concerning record confidentiality are broken, a nurse can also face a lawsuit. (See Chapter 2.)

Use of Computers

Many institutions have mainframe computers for data processing tasks. Most billing information is now stored and processed on this type of computer. Individuals enter data through desktop **computer terminals** that include a screen, keyboard, and printer. It is a very efficient means of retrieving individual records to change or add information.

Some progressive hospitals have installed computer systems that can handle physician orders, pharmacy, laboratory, and diagnostic imaging orders, central supply requests, care planning, documentation, and billing. All departments are interconnected in the system. Information is relayed quickly and efficiently, and use of the computer avoids duplication of efforts. Time is not wasted recording data in several places and relying on runners or a tube system to deliver messages.

A computerized system is very expensive to install, and nurses must be willing to attend classes to learn how to use it. Computers are becoming easier to understand and use; they are an effective tool to save nurses documentation time and energy so that they can use that time caring for patients.

The most efficient computer systems have bedside or handheld terminals for data entry by nurses and other staff. Many hospitals currently use these systems. To protect patient confidentiality, all users of the computer system are assigned entry passwords; these passwords should not be shared with others. The password is the individual's legal signature when using a computer.

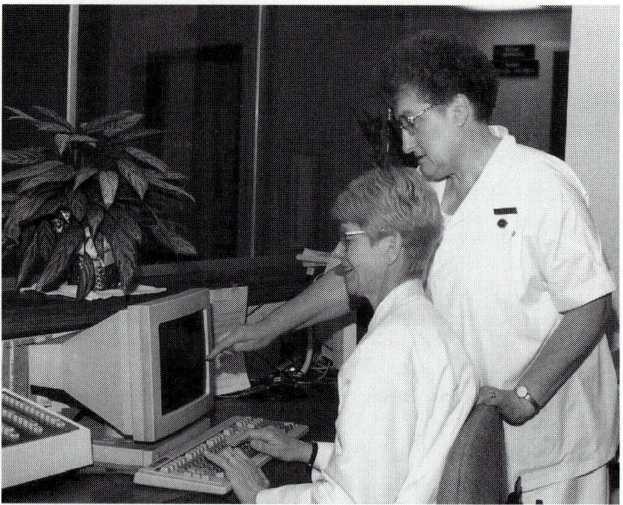

Whenever a nurse finishes charting, she should store the information and log off the computer so that no one else can access or enter data under her password. Students and other temporary users of the system may have to sign confidentiality statements before being issued a password for system entry.

Computer use for nursing documentation and care plan development is expected to increase. All nurses need to become familiar with basic computer use skills. See Chapter 54 for use of computers for the National Council Licensure examination (NCLEX) for RN and LPN candidates.

Use of Facsimile Machines

Facsimile (fax) machines are being used to quickly transmit patient data between offices, hospitals, and other facilities. Any written document can be sent over telephone lines between fax machines. This advance in information communication has radically improved the ability to receive written documentation immediately. Fax machines are a vital channel for rapid information transmission and are becoming as important as computers for documentation and data handling.

REFERENCES AND SUGGESTED READINGS

1. Badzek L: What you need to know about Advance Directives, *Nursing* 22:58, 1992.
2. Brider P: The move to patient focused care, *Am J Nurs* 92(9):26, 1992.
3. Brider P: Who killed the nursing care plan? *Am J Nurs* 91(5):35, 1991.
4. Calfee B: Protecting yourself: nursing negligence, *Nursing* 21:34, 1991.
5. Collins H: Legal risks of computer charting, *RN* 81(53):5, 1990.
6. Darland N: Called to testify, *Am J Nurs* 91(7):22, 1991.

7. Doenges M, Moorhouse M: *Nurse's pocket guide: nursing diagnoses with interventions,* ed 3, Philadelphia, 1991, FA Davis.
8. Fralic M, Kowalski P, Llewellyn F: The staff nurse as quality monitor, *Am J Nurs* 91(4):40, 1991.
9. Gordon M: *Manual of nursing diagnosis, 1991-1992,* St Louis, 1991, Mosby.
10. Green E, Katz J: Make your bulletin board a QA tool, *RN* 53(1):38, 1990.
11. Hurley M: What do the new JCAHO standards mean for you? *RN* 54(6):42, 1991.
12. Iyer P: Filling out an incident report, *Nursing* 22(10):17, 1992.
13. Iyer P: New trends in charting, *Nursing* 21(1):48, 1991.
14. Iyer P: Six more charting rules to keep you legally safe, *Nursing* 21(7):34, 1991.
15. Iyer P: Thirteen charting rules to keep you legally safe, *Nursing* 21(6):40, 1991.
16. Lacombe D: Avoiding a malpractice nightmare, *Nurs 90* 20(6):42, 1990.
17. Mandell M: Practical ways to survive a lawsuit, *Nursing* 22(8):56, 1992.
18. Marrelli T: *Nursing documentation handbook,* St Louis, 1992, Mosby.
19. Mehne C: On tract with bedside terminals, *For The Record* 4(4):4, 1992.
20. *Mosby's medical and nursing dictionary,* ed 3, St Louis, 1990, Mosby.
21. Murphy J, Burke L: Charting by exception, *Nurs 90* 20(5):65, 1990.
22. Potter P, Perry A: *Basic nursing: theory and practice,* ed 2, St. Louis, 1991, Mosby.
23. Rutkowski B: How D.R.G.'s are changing your charting, *Nurs 85* 15:49, 1985.
24. Tribulski J: Why aren't more nurses using this valuable tool? (point of care terminals), *RN* 55(7), 53, 1989.

CHAPTER CHALLENGE

KEY POINTS

- Documentation is part of the implementation phase of the nursing process and is used in evaluation.
- Only approved abbreviations and medical terms should be used when charting in a patient's record. Knowledge of the common abbreviations and terms is required.
- There are five purposes for written patient records. Records are (a) a means of written communication to facilitate continuity of care, (b) a permanent record for accountability (audits, accreditation, and cost reimbursement), (c) a legal record, (d) used in teaching, and (e) used for research and data collection.
- Two common types of medical records or charts are the traditional or block chart and the problem-oriented medical record (POMR).
- The POMR uses a master patient problem list as an index to the chart. These listed problems are usually medical diagnoses.
- SOAPIER is one format for charting in the POMR. The letters stand for subjective *(S),* objective *(O),* assessment *(A),* plan *(P),* implementation *(I),* evaluation *(E),* and revision *(R).*
- Two other common formats for charting nurse's notes are narrative and focus. Focus charting has a data *(D),* action *(A),* and response *(R)* format.
- Charting needs to be legible, clear, concise, accurate, and complete. These guidelines serve as a national standard for licensed nurses.
- Each institution or unit may have specific forms and charting formats, but the general guidelines and rules for charting should be followed.
- Medical records are legal documents. The physician or institution owns the original record.
- Lawyers, courts, and patients can gain access to the record but must follow specified access procedures.
- The contents of a health record are confidential information protected by the law and the Patient's Bill of Rights.
- The nursing Kardex or Rand is a card-filing system used by nurses to condense all the orders and other care information needed quickly for each patient. It is kept at the nursing station for quick reference and is updated frequently.
- The nursing care plan is a plan of care for a patient and a part of the health record. The nurse uses the assessment data to make nursing diagnoses of the patient's responses to illness and problems. This plan includes the nursing diagnosis, treatment goals, specific directions for care implementation, and evaluation guidelines. The care plan should serve as a guide for individualized nursing care delivery and recording.
- Nursing access to computer terminals and care documentation systems has the potential to save time and energy needed for patient care services. These systems are expensive but are a great benefit to the nurses able to use them.
- Fax machines are now in use in sending written documents over telephone lines to quickly transmit data between hospitals and other facilities.

STUDY QUESTIONS

1. Documentation is part of what phase of the nursing process:
   1. assessment
   2. planning
   3. implementation
   4. evaluation
2. When documenting care and observations in a patient record,
   1. approved medical terms and abbreviations can be used.
   2. any locally used abbreviations can be used.
   3. to prevent errors no abbreviations should be used.
   4. a nurse does not worry about the use of abbreviations.
3. Patient health care records are:
   1. confidential information and cannot be taken to court.
   2. owned by the patient, who has a right to see the data.
   3. not used by anyone else but the direct care providers.
   4. concise, legal records of all care given and responses.
4. There are basically two types of medical records:
   1. the traditional and block chart records
   2. the traditional and problem-oriented medical records
   3. the focus and problem-oriented medical records
   4. the problem-oriented medical and SOAPE records
5. When the POMR method is used for documentation:
   1. the problem list has only active and resolved problems.
   2. only the physician charts on the progress notes.
   3. the charting format is SOAPE or SOAPIER.
   4. focus or the DAR charting format is never used.
6. The nurse is using the SOAPE method to chart. In this method the *S* stands for:
   1. signs and symptoms that were measured by the nurse.
   2. subjective information the patient states or feels.
   3. subjective information the nurse can measure.
   4. solutions to problems identified by the nurse.
7. When charting the nurse should:
   1. chart as soon and as often as possible.
   2. remember to chart only basic care information.
   3. leave blank lines for others if asked.
   4. chart facts using judgmental terms if needed.
8. Understanding that health care personnel must respect the confidentiality of patients' records, the nurse
   1. ethically can look at a friend's chart to see the diagnosis.
   2. knows that only the Patient's Bill of Rights advocates confidentiality.
   3. reads charts only for a professional reason.
   4. shares information from a chart to protect a friend.
9. The use of computers in the hospital by nurses:
   1. can save on charting time once nurses are computer comfortable.
   2. is not considered important or efficient.
   3. can be done only on a shared terminal at the desk.
   4. lacks security measures to protect confidentiality.

3

DEVELOPMENTAL, SOCIOCULTURAL, AND FAMILY INFLUENCES

It isn't so much that I chose nursing as it is that nursing chose me. I think that it should be a calling rather than a job. There is a nurse inside me that my continued education will free. Nursing for me is just as much who I am as what I want to be.

Lori Meyer-Lee
Student Nurse

7

LIFE SPAN DEVELOPMENT

Elaine U. Polan

KEY TERMS

adoptive family
ageism
autocratic family pattern
blended/reconstructed family
chromosomes
conception (fertilization)
concrete operational phase
democratic family pattern
development
disengagement stage
engagement/ commitment stage
establishment stage
expectant stage
extended family
formal operational thought phase
foster family
growth
homosexual family
matriarchal family pattern
nuclear family
parenthood stage
patriarchal family pattern
preoperational thought stage
presbycusis
presbyopia
schema
senescence stage
sensorimotor
single parent family
social contract family/cohabitation
teratogen
zygote

LEARNING OBJECTIVES

After reading this chapter, the student should be able to do the following:

- Define the key terms.
- Differentiate between the types of family patterns and their functions in society.
- Describe different types of stresses that commonly impact on today's families.
- Describe the physical characteristics at each stage of the life cycle.
- List the psychosocial changes at the different stages of development.
- Discuss Erikson's stages of psychosocial development.
- Describe Piaget's four stages of cognitive development.
- Describe the cognitive changes occurring in the early childhood period.
- Discuss the developmental tasks of the adolescent period.
- List the developmental tasks for early adulthood.
- Describe the developmental tasks for middle adulthood.
- Define *aging.*
- Discuss the theories of aging.
- Describe the normal age-related changes affecting the major body systems.
- Discuss the effect of the aging process on personality, intelligence, learning, and memory.

RELATED TOPICS OF INTEREST

- Cultural aspects of nursing care (Chapter 8)
- Basic nutrition (Chapter 18)
- Diet therapy (Chapter 19)
- Care of the patient with a reproductive disorder (Chapter 33)
- Care of the Patient with an immune disorder (Chapter 36)
- Care of the patient with cancer (Chapter 38)
- Care of the mother and newborn (Chapter 41)
- Basic pediatric nursing care (Chapter 43)
- Care of the older adult (Chapter 45)

Development is considered a lifelong process that begins at **conception (fertilization),** the beginning of pregnancy, and ends with death. Only recently has the impact of middle adulthood and late adulthood been recognized as having equal importance as the earlier stages of development. There is a continuity of development throughout the life span. Experiences at one time of life affect future development. People are influenced by their genes, their families, and the world in which they live. The study of life-span development is the study of how and why people change over time as well as of how and why they remain the same. There are eight stages of life-span development. These stages and their approximate ages are as follows:

1. Infancy	Birth-1 year
2. Toddler	1-3 years
3. Preschool	3-5 years
4. School age	6-12 years
5. Adolescence	13-19 years
6. Early adulthood	20-40 years
7. Middle adulthood	40-65 years
8. Late adulthood	65 years and over

Each stage of the life span is unique and has certain distinguishable features. The goal of studying the life span is to enable the student to better understand and relate to individuals at various stages of development. Finally, with the increasing older population, we must become more aware of the unique characteristics, needs, and problems of the older adult.

GROWTH AND DEVELOPMENT

An individual undergoes continuous changes throughout life in order to exist and function. These changes include the continuous replacement of cells, tissues, and fluids. Some changes are not physical in nature; they are changes in emotions, behavior, and feelings.

Growth (an increase in the size of an organism or in any of its parts) is a term that refers to a change or increase in size. The term **development** makes reference to the gradual process of change and differentiation from a simple to a more advanced level of complexity. It is an orderly sequential series of changes in function. Growth and development are continuous and interdependent. The principles of growth and development may be summarized as follows:

- Growth and development proceed at a highly individualized rate that varies from person to person. No two persons should be expected to react in the same manner to the same stimuli.
- Growth and development are a continuous process characterized by spurts of growth and periods of rest.
- Growth and development proceed from the simple to the complex in a predictable sequence.
- Growth and development vary for specific structures at specific times. In other words, not all organs grow and develop at the same rate; for example, the ovaries in the female and the testes in the male do not mature until puberty.
- Last, growth and development are a total process that involves the whole person. The person grows physically, socially, mentally, and emotionally. Each type of growth is interrelated.

Patterns of Growth

Growth patterns appear to be genetically controlled. Nutrition, heredity, and environment play an important role in the patterns. The blueprint for all inherited traits is contained in the **chromosomes** (any one of the threadlike structures in the nucleus of a cell that functions in the transmission of genetic information). At conception (fertilization), the individual is endowed with a complex set of biological potentials involving characteristics such as height, skin, hair and eye color, and talents and interests, to name a few. Only identical twins have the same combinations of chromosomes (karyotype). The process of division, transmission, and mixing of chromosomes accounts for either the variations in or the continuity of distinctive family traits. This is discussed further in Chapter 39.

The Beginnings. Development begins with conception (fertilization) or the union of the sperm and ovum. This merger combines the genetic material of both parents. The role environment plays is difficult to determine. Heredity and environment are interrelated, and their interaction results in the creation of a unique individual.

After fertilization the **zygote** (the developing ovum from the time it is fertilized until, as a blastocyst, it is implanted in the uterus) contains 23 pairs of chromosomes or a total of 46 chromosomes. One of each pair has been contributed by the mother and one by the father. A question immediately asked by prospective parents following the birth of their baby is, Is it a boy or girl? One of the pairs of chromosomes determines the sex of the baby (Fig. 7-1 on p. 80). The ovum always carries an X chromosome, while the sperm may carry either an X or a Y chromosome.

X ovum + Y sperm = XY male
X ovum + X sperm = XX female

In addition to these gender characteristics there are many other potential traits that may be inherited. Certain abnormalities may be genetically transmitted. Examples of such inherited disorders include Tay-Sachs disease, sickle cell disease, phenylketonuria, and spina bifida.

In some instances environmental factors may also play a role in contributing to certain diseases or defects in the unborn. Any substance, agent, or process that in-

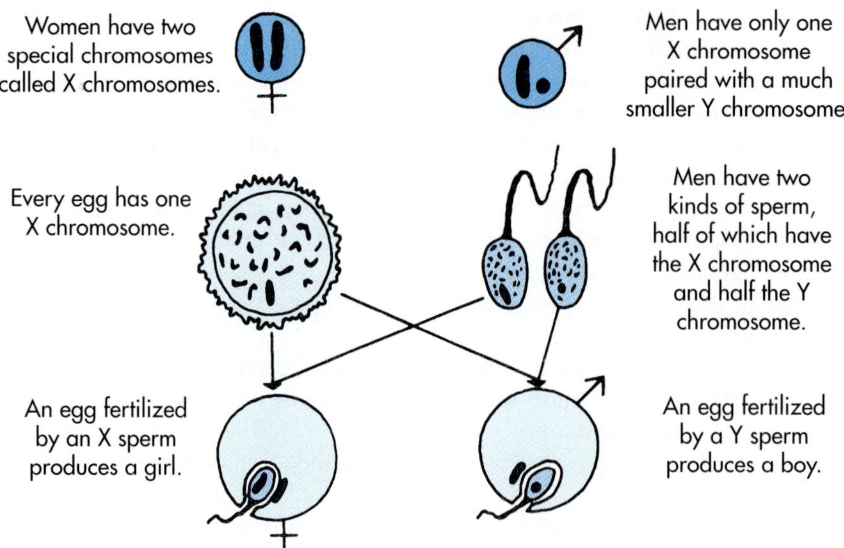

FIG. 7-1 Sex determination. (From Morgan C: *Introduction to psychology,* ed 2, New York, 1961, McGraw-Hill.)

terferes with normal prenatal development, causing the formation of one or more developmental abnormalities in the fetus, is called a **teratogen.** Drugs, alcohol, and cigarette smoke are just a few of the known harmful substances that need to be avoided during pregnancy. Research data indicate that 5% to 25% of unfavorable outcomes in all pregnancies may be attributed to smoking. Other studies have supported the finding that smoking increases the incidence of low-birth-weight babies.

THE FAMILY

The family is the basic unit of society. Families are composed of two or more individuals united by marriage, blood, adoption, emotional bonds, and social roles. The individuals of the family share emotional ties that usually last a lifetime.

Several significant changes in American families are visible today. The factors that have contributed to the changed family are given in Box 7-1. As a result of these influences, family roles and life-styles have changed to meet society's needs.

Box 7-1 CHANGES AFFECTING MODERN FAMILIES

- Economic changes—resulting in an increase in the number of women in the work force
- The feminist movement
- More effective birth control
- Legalization of abortion
- Postponement of marriage, childbearing
- Increase in divorce rate

Types of Families

Nuclear Family. The **nuclear family** is a family unit consisting of the biological parents and their offspring. For a number of years the nuclear family was been thought of as the traditional family. This family type has sex-based roles assigned to its members. The nuclear family usually consists of a husband and wife and their children living in an independent household setting. In the past, one parent, usually the male, was the breadwinner. Today these roles have been redefined in their structure and function. In many families both parents work and share equally in the financial support, roles, and responsibilities of the family unit.

Extended Family. The **extended family** is a family group consisting of the biological parents, their children, the grandparents, grandchildren, aunts, uncles, and other family members. This family type consists of the nuclear or traditional family and some additional family members all living in the same household. A sharing of support, roles, and responsibilities is common to this family structure. This family structure is the basic family group in many societies.

Single Parent Family. The **single parent family** exists today as a family style of choice or as the result of death, divorce, separation, or abandonment. Over 40% of single parent families are the result of divorce. The head of the household may be either female or male. This type of family unit may also result from an unwed parent living alone or from the decision of a single person to adopt a child. The single parent family has the unique responsibility of carrying out the functions that are typically shared by two members.

Blended or Reconstructed Family. The **blended or reconstructed family** (also called the stepfamily) includes all the relatives from four adults (the married pair, plus both former spouses, if each has previously been married, and any children from either adult). This type of family can present many stresses. Because of losses resulting from death or divorce, both children and adults may be afraid to trust or to love. A child's loyalties to an absent or dead parent may interfere with forming ties to a stepparent, especially when the child goes back and forth between two households. This family arises when one or both adults remarry or agree to cohabit and bring together their children from a previous marriage.

Social Contract and Cohabitation. The **social contract family** style is also referred to as **cohabitation.** It involves an unmarried couple living together and sharing roles and responsibilities similar to those of the nuclear family structure.

Homosexual Family. The **homosexual family** is a family group made up of a same sex couple. In recent years homosexual adults have formed family units. Their members share bonds of emotional commitment and roles of childrearing. Many of these family structures consist of either natural children (from a heterosexual relationship) or adopted or foster children. Regardless of the family structure each family type has common parenting concerns and responsibilities.

Adoptive Family. The **adoptive family** is a family unit with adopted children. Each year millions of couples increase their family size through adoption. Childless or infertile couples often are lonely and lack fulfillment of the joys of parenthood. The ordeal of adoption may be time consuming and anxiety provoking. The role of parenting can be both exciting and fulfilling for natural and adoptive families alike.

Foster Family. **Foster families** allow for the care, supervision, and nurturing of children whose parents are unable to care for them. The length of stay in the foster home may be temporary and depends on the individual circumstances.

Refer to Box 7-2 for a summary of family types.

• • •

Regardless of the type of family, there are certain basic functions inherent to the family unit. These basic functions include protection, nurturance, education, sustenance, and socialization. Usually unconditional affection, acceptance, and companionship are guaranteed to each family member. The family attempts to meet the individual's needs for growth and development, and in doing so it helps support personal fulfillment and strengthen each individual's self-esteem.

The family is the first socializing agent for teaching children society's expectations and limitations. As a part of that socialization, the family is responsible for ensuring that the child receives a formal education. The fam-

Box 7-2 SUMMARY OF FAMILY TYPES

NUCLEAR

- Consists of married man and woman and their children
- Lives in independent household

EXTENDED

- Consists of nuclear plus additional family members living in same household
- Provides a sharing of responsibilities

SINGLE PARENT

- Occurs by divorce, death, separation, abandonment, or choice
- More common in recent years
- Typically adult must perform roles of two persons

BLENDED OR RECONSTRUCTED

- Occurs when adults from previous marriage remarry and combine children within new household

SOCIAL CONTRACT AND COHABITATION

- Made up of man and woman living together without legal commitment but sharing roles and responsibilities similar to those of nuclear structure

HOMOSEXUAL

- Involves homosexual partners living together with shared responsibilities

ADOPTIVE

- Consists of usually traditional members, husband, wife, and adoptive child

FOSTER

- Responsible for care, supervision, and nuturing of children in their charge

ily is also responsible for instilling morals, values, and ideals[16] into the children. These roles and functions of families are not constant and may change at any time. The birth of a baby and the death of a family member are happenings that create the need to rearrange family roles and structures.

Family Patterns

Family patterns refer to the way in which family members relate to each other. Examples of family patterns include autocratic, patriarchal, matriarchal, and democratic patterns.

Autocratic Family Pattern. In the **autocratic family pattern,** the relationships are unequal. The parents attempt to control the children with strict rigid rules and expectations. This family pattern is least open to outside influence.

Patriarchal Family Pattern. In the **patriarchal family pattern** the male usually assumes the dominant role. The male member functions in the work role and is responsible for control of finances and makes most decisions.

Matriarchal Family Pattern. In the **matriarchal family pattern** (also known as the matrifocal family) the female assumes primary dominance in areas of child care and homemaking as well as financial decision making. In some families of this type an older female relative provides child care so that the mother of the children is free to work outside of the home.

Democratic Family Pattern. In the **democratic family pattern** the adult members function as equals. Children are treated with respect and recognized as individuals. This style encourages joint decision making, and it recognizes and supports the uniqueness of each individual member. This family pattern favors negotiation, compromise, and growth.

• • •

Several researchers have identified 12 qualities of strong families. These qualities are listed in Box 7-3.

Box 7-3 QUALITIES OF STRONG FAMILIES

1. A sense of commitment toward promoting the member's well-being
2. A sense of appreciation and encouragement for tasks accomplished
3. Directed effort toward spending quality time with individual members
4. A sense of purpose that encourages progress during good or difficult times
5. A sense of harmony between members of the family
6. Effective communications between individuals
7. Established values, rules, and beliefs
8. A variety of different coping techniques to enhance functioning
9. The use of effective problem-solving measures and the use of a variety of options
10. Positive outlook
11. The ability to be flexible and adapt to changes
12. The use of varied resources to facilitate coping skills

Stages of Family Development

Engagement/Commitment Stage. The **engagement/commitment stage** begins when the couple acknowledges to themselves and others that they are considering marriage. At this time, opposition or support will be evident from friends and/or parents. Wedding plans must be arranged. Housing, work, and furnishings are some of the items discussed and explored.

Establishment Stage. The **establishment stage** extends from the wedding up until the birth of the first child. During this phase, one of the important tasks is the adjustment from the single independent to the married interdependent state. The challenges facing the newly married couple include learning to live with another person, decision making, conflict resolution, and communication. The relationship established with the couple's parents and family can enhance or lessen the cohesiveness and strengthen or weaken the couple's ties. To the average young adult, marriage is an important serious change that requires major adjustments. A good marriage doesn't just happen. It is something both parties must work at and contribute to for success. Equal energy must be aimed at commitment, goals, and respect for each other. Success at marriage satisfies Erikson's task of intimacy and helps fulfill the individual's need for love and belonging.

Expectant Stage. The **expectant stage** begins when conception occurs and continues through the pregnancy. The most important decision of one's life is that of starting a family. Becoming parents may be described as one of the most challenging as well as rewarding roles. Pregnancy requires both physiological and psychological adjustments. Important decisions must be considered during pregnancy, including continuation of employment, child care, feeding, and childbirth methods. The desired outcome of pregnancy is that a bond or attachment will be established between the parents and the new baby.

Parenthood Stage. The **parenthood stage** begins at the birth or adoption of the first child. The transition to parenthood is seen as a major event. Even couples with good preparation express a great deal of anxiety associated with the onset of this new role. One of the most frequently described problems is the lack of time. There appears to be less free time, less sleep time, less time together, and less intimate sexual time. Compounding the lack of time is the stress of parenting and the self-doubt in one's ability and competency in this new role.

Disengagement Stage of Parenthood. The **disengagement stage** of parenthood is that period of family life when the grown children depart from the home. The role of parenting changes during this phase of the life cycle. The departure of children does not end the role of parenting. Even though grown children may not be living with their parents, they usually continue to need emotional guidance and some financial support. Many grown children return to living at home for financial reasons. Regardless, during the disengagement stage couples or the single parent needs to redefine personal roles and structure time so that there is a sense of usefulness, accomplishment, and self-fulfillment.

Senescence Stage. The **senescence stage** is the last stage of the life cycle, which requires the individual to cope with a large range of changes. For the older adult the family unit continues to be a major source of satisfaction and pleasure. Most older adults prefer to live independently. The greater life expectancy for women means that it is not uncommon that many older women outlive their spouses and continue life alone. Most older adults have regular contact with other family members. The grandparenting role requires new adaptations. This role requires a change in one's identity and changing roles. In the past, grandparents often lived with their extended families because they had to, not necessarily because they wanted to. Grandparents of today are an independent breed. Grandparents want close, stable, emotionally satisfying family ties. Simultaneously, they want an independent life, away from kin. They want to see and love their grandchildren, but not be responsible for them. They want to see and love their grown children, but not live with them.

Causes of Family Stress

Various stressors may impact on the family unit. Chronic illness, abuse, and divorce are some of the factors that affect the family.

Chronic Illness. Chronic physical or emotional illness of the parent or child affects all family members. Factors, such as financial resources, family stability, and an adequate support system, determines an individual's ability to cope with a family member's chronic illness.

Abuse. Abuse refers to physical, emotional, financial, verbal, or sexual assault and/or neglect. Each year 6 million women, children, and men are victims of physical abuse inflicted by parents, spouses, siblings, children, and other relatives. Abuse is common in many families. Certain visible factors have been identified as related to family violence. They include financial strain, social isolation, low self-esteem, and previous history of abuse. The presence of several of these risk factors may indicate that the individual is more prone to abuse and may possess ineffective coping skills that would prevent maintaining family wellness and safety. Following are some characteristics of parents who abuse their children: they were often abused themselves as children; they are often loners; they are harsh, strict, and punitive; they have unreasonable expectations; and they are immature and lack self-control and have low self-esteem.

Early recognition, prompt reporting, and preventive measures must be employed to help detect and end all forms of abuse and neglect.

Divorce. Divorce is widespread. It continues to affect more than 1 million children annually. The effects of divorce on children are varied and complex. One of the factors is the age of the child at the time of the divorce. Younger children often feel abandoned and feel they are no longer loved by both parents. Other factors that may affect the child are the bitterness surrounding the conflicts, the child's prior relationship with the absent parent, the effects of the divorce on the custodial parent, and the postdivorce relationship of the parents. Many children have reconciliation fantasies for extended periods after the divorce is finalized. Changes in one parent's status will create changes in emotional milieu, family role, finances, life-style, and often neighborhood.

STAGES OF GROWTH AND DEVELOPMENT

Infancy: 1 to 12 Months

Physical Characteristics. An infant's physical development happens so rapidly that size, shape, and skills seem to change daily. (See Chapter 41 for discussion of the newborn.) Growth is very rapid during the first 6 months of life. The infant is expected to gain about 1.5 lb a month until 5 months. The infant usually will double the birth weight by 4 months. By the time the baby is 1 year of age, the birth weight has tripled (average weight

21.5 lb). Most of the weight gain in the first months of life is fat, providing insulation and a source of nourishment that can be drawn on if teething or other problems decrease food intake for a few days. After 8 months, weight gain includes more bone and muscle.

Height increases by about 1 inch a month for the first 6 months. By 12 months of age, the infant's birth length has increased about 50%; the typical length is 30 inches (75 cm).

Vital Signs. Infants are subject to wide variation in temperature related to activity levels and state of health. Apical rates slow down in infancy. At 2 months, the average apical rate is about 120 beats/min.

The apical pulse should be counted for a full minute, noting variations in rate, volume, and rhythm. Respiratory rates also decrease during infancy; these rates are related to activity level. Average resting respiratory rate for the 12-month-old is about 30 breaths/min. Blood pressure reading will gradually increase to 90/60 at 12-months.

Motor Development. At 2 months the infant is able to hold the head up while in the prone position. By 4 months of age the infant can hold the head up steadily to a 90-degree angle while in the prone position. At 6 months most infants can balance the head quite well.

Locomotion. Crawling, an early means of movement, is a motion made with the infant's abdomen touching the floor (Fig. 7-2, *F*). A more advanced form of locomotion is creeping. This is accomplished by the infant's resting the weight on the hands and knees. Infants may crawl at 7 months and creep at about 9 months. Creeping appears after the age of 9 months in most children (see Fig. 7-2, *G*).

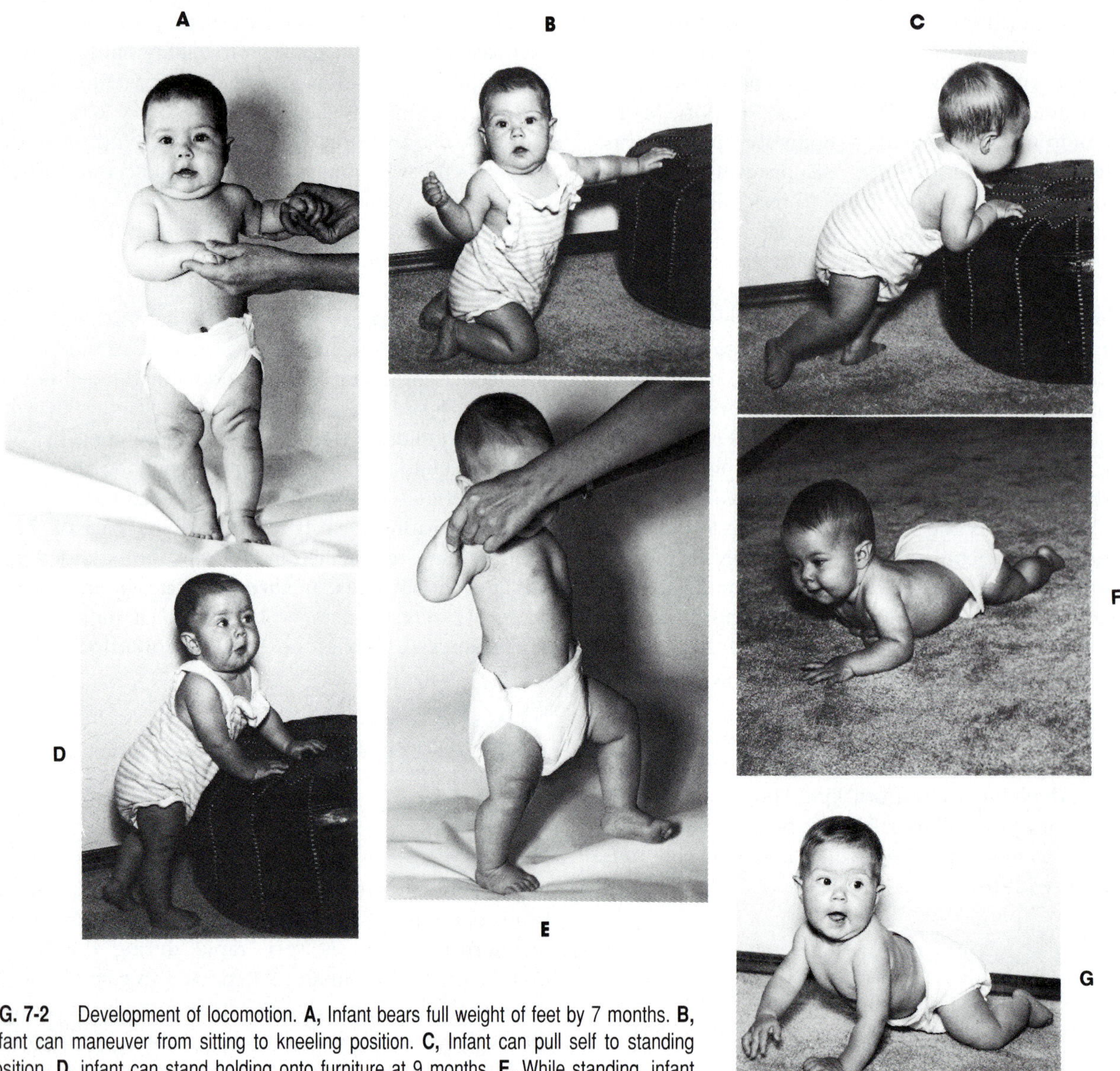

FIG. 7-2 Development of locomotion. **A,** Infant bears full weight of feet by 7 months. **B,** Infant can maneuver from sitting to kneeling position. **C,** Infant can pull self to standing position. **D,** infant can stand holding onto furniture at 9 months. **E,** While standing, infant takes deliberate step at 10 months. **F,** Infant crawls with abdomen on floor and pulls self forward with hands at 10 months. **G,** Infant creeps on hands and knees at 11 months.

Standing with support and walking follow at about 8 months to 15 months (Fig. 7-2, *D*).

Dentition. Teething begins at about 5 to 6 months of age. Signs of teething—irritability, edematous red gums, excessive drooling, and change in stooling—begin 3 to 4 weeks before the appearance of the tooth. See Box 7-4 for the schedule of eruption of primary teeth. Dental decay can begin at any time after tooth development. Oral hygiene for the young infant consists of offering sips of clear water and wiping and massaging the infant's gums.

Toothbrushing should begin after the first teeth appear and continue throughout the life span. The use of fluoride toothpaste is recommended in areas without added fluoride in the water. To prevent bottle-mouth syndrome, care givers are instructed to avoid putting anything but water in the infant's night bottle. Sugar in milk, formula, or juice has been shown to severely decay and destroy the tooth enamel. In addition, all care givers should be instructed not to prop up the bottle as this can lead to aspiration. Holding the infant during feeding provides warmth, comfort, and bonding, all vital factors in providing a feeling of love and security.

Psychosocial Development. Basic trust involves order and security. Erikson describes the task of the infant as basic trust vs. mistrust. The responsiveness of others to the needs of the infant helps establish the basis of trust. When the infant's emotional and physical needs are met, the foun-dation for later optimism and responsiveness to others is developed. Infants learn to trust their world significantly more if they are well fed, warm, and dry than if they are constantly hungry, cold, and wet. Infants begin to develop a secure sense of self when their primary care giver (usually the mother or father) provides a "consistency, continuity, and sameness of experience," so they know that their needs will be met predictably and benevolently. The infant whose needs are not met develops a sense of dissatisfaction or mistrust. Feelings of sus-

Box 7-4 PRIMARY DENTITION SCHEDULE

- **6 months:** teething begins with eruption of two lower central incisors
- **7 months:** eruption of upper central incisors
- **9 months:** eruption of upper lateral incisors
- **11 months:** eruption of lower lateral incisors
- **12 months:** approximately 6-8 teeth present
- **24 months:** approximately 16 teeth present
- **30 months:** completion of primary dentition—20 teeth

TABLE 7-1 Erikson's Stages of Psychosocial Development

Stage	Approximate Age, Years	Developmental Task	Outcomes
1. Infant	Birth-1	Basic trust vs. mistrust	Infants learn either to trust or to mistrust that significant others will properly care for their basic needs, including nourishment, sucking, warmth, cleanliness, and physical contact
2. Toddler	1-3	Autonomy vs. shame and doubt	Children learn either to be self-sufficient in many activities, including toileting, feeding, walking, and talking, or to doubt their own abilities
3. Preschool	4-6	Initiative vs. guilt	Children want to undertake many adultlike activities, sometimes going beyond the limits set by parents and feeling guilty because of it
4. School age	7-11	Industry vs. inferiority	Children eagerly learn to be competent and productive or feel inferior and unable to do any task well
5. Adolescence	12-19	Identity vs. role confusion	Adolescents try to figure out "Who am I?" They establish sexual, ethnic, and career identities or are confused about what future roles to play
6. Young adult	20-44	Intimacy vs. isolation	Young adults seek companionship and love with another person or become isolated from others
7. Middle adulthood	45-65	Generativity vs. stagnation	Middle-aged adults are productive, performing meaningful work and raising a family, or become stagnant and inactive
8. Late adulthood	65+	Ego, integrity vs. despair	Older adults try to make sense out of their lives, either seeing life as meaningful and whole or despairing at goals never reached and questions never answered

Box 7-5 PIAGET'S STAGES OF COGNITIVE DEVELOPMENT

SENSORIMOTOR: BIRTH-2 YEARS

- Uses senses and motor abilities to understand the world; this period begins with reflexes and coordinates sensorimotor skills
- Develops schema
- Begins to interact with environment
- Learns that an object still exists when it is out of sight (object permanence) and begins to remember and imagine experiences (mental representation)
- Develops thinking and goal-directed behavior

PREOPERATIONAL THOUGHT: 2-6 YEARS

- Develops egocentric thinking (understands the world from only one perspective, that of the self)
- Uses trial and error to discover new traits and characteristics
- Conceptualizes time as being limited to present
- Uses symbols to represent objects
- Develops more logical, intuitive thinking
- Centers or focuses on a single aspect of an object, producing some distortion of reality
- Gains in imaginative ability
- Gradually begins to "de-center" (becomes less egocentric and understands other points of view)

CONCRETE OPERATIONAL THOUGHT: 7-11 YEARS

- Understands and applies logical operations or principles to help interpret specific experiences or perceptions
- Has more realistic views; better understands other viewpoints
- Improves use of memory
- Focuses on more than one task; develops logical, socialized thoughts
- Recognizes cause-and-effect relationships
- Learns to identify behavior outcome
- Understands basic ideas of conversation, number classification, and other concrete ideas

FORMAL OPERATIONAL THOUGHT: 12+ YEARS

- Uses a systematic, scientific problem-solving approach
- Recognizes past, present, and future
- Is able to think about abstractions and hypothetical concepts and is able to move in thought "from the real to the possible"
- Becomes more interested in ethics, politics, and all social and moral issues as ability to take a broader and more theoretical approach to experience increases

picion and fear and general difficulties with relating to people may develop.

Refer to Table 7-1 on p. 85 for an overview of Erikson's stages of psychosocial development.

Cognitive and Intellectual Development. During this stage the infant uses the senses to learn about self and the environment. The infant learns by exploration of objects and events and by interaction. Piaget describes the infant as in the sensorimotor stage of cognitive development. (Box 7-5).

In the **sensorimotor** stage an infant's knowledge comes about primarily through sensory impressions and motor activities. Behavior is completely reflective. The infant develops images or **schema** (an innate knowledge structure that allows a child to mentally organize ways to behave in the immediate environment) and assimilates and interprets the information. Infants learn by actively encountering stimulation from the environment. As the infant interacts with the environment, there are changes in mental structure and in development of thinking ability. During the first 1 to 4 months, the infant follows objects visually with the eyes and auditorily with the ears. By 4 months of age, infants become notably better at using both eyes together. This makes them more astute observers. By the age of 4 months, many infants can identify the voices of the most familiar people in their lives. Smiling occurs in response to different people and events. From 4 to 8 months of age the infant can recognize and imitate. Reaching and grasping are improved skills. From 8 to 12 months of age anxiety is shown when separated from the primary care giver. There is shyness and a fear of strangers. The infant may cling and protest any separation from the primary care giver(s).

By the age of 3 months most infants are responding differently to the parents or primary care giver than they do to other people. At the sight of the parents or primary care giver, the infant will smile and begin to vocalize. By the age of 9 months, most children will show alarm at the presence of a stranger. Parents and child develop a form of synchrony (happening at the same time; moving or operating at the same rate). It is thought that infants who develop a secure early attachment will later have the confidence to seek out future relationships. Studies on children ages 15 to 30 months who had good attachment relationships showed that they experienced a predictable behavior following separation, known as *separation anxiety.* The behaviors recognized during separation are listed in Box 7-6.

Communication and Language. Humans have an innate capacity to learn language. They are born with the mechanism and capacity to develop speech and language skills. During infancy, the unique ability of the brain to sort out basic sounds and to extract from sentences the most meaningful elements becomes apparent. During early childhood the brain's language acquisition ability becomes even more sophisticated. Parents and other care givers can have an enormous influence on the infant's intellectual and language development. However, infants will not speak spontaneously. The environment must provide a means for them to acquire these skills. Speech requires intact physiological functioning of (1) the respiratory system, (2) speech control centers in the cerebral cortex, and (3) articulation and resonance structures of the mouth and nasal cavities. In addition, acquisition of language requires (1) an intact and discriminating auditory apparatus, (2) intelligence, (3) a need to communicate, and (4) stimulation. The rate of speech development varies from child to child and is directly related to neurological competence and intellectual development. All children go through the same sequence of stages in language and speech development in early childhood unless there are abnormal conditions present (Table 7-2).

The basic sequence of language is as follows:

- **3 months**—babbling. When infants babble, they typically explore all the possible sounds they can make by enhancing the force of the air stream as it passes their vocal cords and by varying the positions of their tongue and mouth.
- **1 year**—recognizes words. Between ages 1 and 2 infants generally acquire the ability to produce

Box 7-6 SEPARATION ANXIETY

Protest: In the first phase the behavior is expressed by loud crying, restlessness, and rejection of surrogate adult figures.

Despair: In the second phase the behavior demonstrates hopelessness, quiet crying, inactivity, and withdrawal.

Detachment: The last phase is characterized by apathy even when the mother returns. The infant shows renewed interest in the environment.

TABLE 7-2 Normal Language and Speech Development During Early Childhood

Age (years)	Normal Language Development	Normal Speech Development	Intelligibility
1	Says two or three words with meaning Imitates sounds of animals	Omission of most final and some initial consonants Substitution of consonants "m," "w," "p," "b," "k," "g," "n," "t," "d," and "h" for more difficult sounds Height of unintelligible jargon at age 18 months	Usually no more than 25% intelligible to unfamiliar listener
2	Uses two- to three-word phrases Has vocabulary of about 300 words and uses "I," "me," and "you"	Use of above consonants with vowels but inconsistently and with much substitution Omission of final consonants Articulation lags behind vocabulary	At age 2, 65% intelligible in context
3	Says four- to five-word sentences Has vocabulary of about 900 words Uses "who," "what," and "where" in asking questions Uses plurals, pronouns, and prepositions	Mastery of "b," "t," "d," "k," and "g"; "r" and "l" may still be unclear; omission or substitution for "w" Repetitions and hesitations common	At age 3, 70%-80% intelligible
4-5	Has vocabulary of 1500-2100 words Able to use most grammatical forms correctly, such as past tense of verb with "yesterday" Uses complete sentences with nouns, verbs, prepositions, adjectives, adverbs, and conjunctions	Mastery of "f" and "v"; possible distortion of "r," "l," "s," "z," "sh," "ch," "y," and "th" Little or no omission of initial or last consonant	Speech is totatlly intelligible, although some sounds are still imperfect
5-6	Has vocabulary of 3000 words, comprehends "if," "because," and "why"	Mastery of "r," "l," and "th"; possible continuing distortion of "s," "z," "sh," "ch," and "j" (usually mastered by 7½-8 years of age)	Speech is totally intelligible

holo phrases (one-word sentences that convey a complete message ["up"]. Infants learn to expand their holo phrases by attaching them back-to-back to other nouns or verbs. They thus form two-word sentences ("mommy milk," "daddy come"). Early speech is often referred to as telegraphic speech because, as in telegram messages, the articles, pronouns, prepositions, and conjunctions are omitted. In organizing and coding language infants acquire an understanding of the most meaningful units of speech. No one teaches infants to use nouns and verbs first. They learn this sequence on their own.

- **Preschool**—acquiring structure of native language. The language explosion that occurs during the preschool years is most obvious in the growth of vocabulary, from 50 words at 18 months to 200 words at age 2 to between 8000 and 14,000 words at age 6. From age 2 to age 6, the average child learns between 6 and 10 words a day. Preschoolers have an outstanding ability to learn language. Most researchers regard early childhood as a crucial period for language learning.
- **6 years**—able to speak and understand new words and sentences. Although the preschool years are the time of a language explosion, language development from 6 years on is also remarkable, albeit much more subtle, as children consciously come to understand more about the many ways language can be used. This understanding gives them greater control in their comprehension and use of language, and in turn, enhances the range of their cognitive powers generally.

A common rule of thumb helpful in evolution of early speech acquisition is that the number of words in an average response should correspond to the chronological age of the child. For example, a 2-year-old child might say, "me do"; a 3-year-old might add a word, "me do it"; and a 4-year-old child might say, "let me do it."

Girls advance more rapidly in language development than do boys. First-born children develop language earlier than do later-born children, and children of multiple births (twins, triplets) develop language later than children of single births.

Health Maintenance.

Nutrition. Both human breast milk and commercially prepared formula are available to meet the nutritional needs of the infant. Even though today's excellent infant formulas approximate human milk, breast milk is still almost always the best food for newborns. It has been called the "ultimate health food," because it offers so many benefits. However, infants who are fed with properly prepared formula and raised with love also grow up healthy and well-adjusted. Breast milk or formula is the only food most babies need until they are about 4 to 6 months of age. Full-term infants have enough stored iron to last for at least the first 5 to 6 months of age. After this time iron supplements or food sources can be given to replenish the diminishing supply. It is generally accepted that certain foods be avoided in the first 6 months of life. Those foods include citrus fruits, egg whites, and wheat flour, all frequently identified as allergy-producing substances.

Much controversy exists regarding when solid foods should best be introduced into the infant diet. Many physicians believe that very early introduction of solids can lead to many problems. Rather than deciding on when to introduce solid food, it is simpler to describe how to first introduce these foods into the infant diet. The rules for solid foods include the following:

- Introduce only one new food at a time, allowing several days between new foods.
- Introduce cereals first, then fruits and vegetables, and lastly meats.
- Avoid mixing foods to allow the infant to develop interest in different foods and tastes. In warmer weather, febrile conditions, prolonged vomiting, and diarrhea may place infants at higher risk for dehydration because of their small fluid volume. At these times extra care is needed to ensure that the infant receives 100 to 150 ml of water per kg of body weight per day.

By the age of 8 to 9 months most babies can master eating mashed or junior foods. Self-feeding of finger foods allows the infant further exploration. By 9 months of age a training cup can be introduced and the process of weaning begins. This is usually a gradual process with the cup substituted for one bottle at a time, usually at lunch.

Immunization.

Routine childhood immunization has never been as complex a process as it is today. New recommendations for the hepatitis B (HBV) vaccine, a new vaccine for pneumococcal infections, and the welcome addition of a single vaccine combining two old ones—DTP and *Haemophilus influenzae* type b (Hib)—make for important changes in what was once a relatively simple vaccination schedule.

Understanding the current immunization guidelines for both the traditional and new vaccines will become increasingly important for all nurses as the need for preventive care takes on national importance. In fact, the Standards for Pediatric Immunization Practices released in January 1993 by the CDC's National Vaccine Advisory Committee, recommends that health-care providers screen immunization status whenever a child presents for care—whether it's in an office, clinic, ED, or on your unit.*

*From National Vaccine Advisory Committee: Standards for pediatric immunization practices, *Morb Mortal Wkly Rep* 42(RR-5):5, 1993. Quoted in Vessey JA, Ritchie SR: The who, what, and when of pediatric immunization, *RN* 56(4):42, 1993.

The American Academy of Pediatrics recommends that immunization against hepatitis B be initiated in the neonatal period. The recommended schedule for immunization is given in Table 7-3.

Sleep, play, and safety. Newborn and infants sleep 18 hours out of 24. These sleep periods usually consist of short naplike periods. The infant may be restless and make noises during these periods. Toward the end of the first 3 months definite sleep patterns emerge, with nap periods and wake periods clearly established. By the end of the first year the infant will usually sleep 12 hours at night and take one nap during the day. Persistent crying during usual sleep or nap periods may signal discomfort or illness and should be investigated.

TABLE 7-3 Vaccinations: Who, What, and When

Patients can be protected from a wide variety of infectious diseases. This table covers routine childhood vaccines, which now include the HBV vaccine and one intended for patients at risk for pneumococcal infections—a serious public health concern.

Vaccine	Schedule	Contraindications	Side Effects
Diphtheria Toxoid derived from *Corynebacterium diphtheriae* exotoxin	Primary: 2, 4, 6, and 18 months Boosters: 4 to 6 years, then every 10 years with reduced dose	Previous anaphylactic or encephalopathic reaction to the vaccine Moderate to severe illness with or without fever	Slight fever, malaise, local irritation, and sterile abscess 1 to 2 weeks after injection
Tetanus Toxoid derived from *Clostridium tetani* exotoxin	Primary: 2, 4, 6, and 18 months Boosters: 4 to 6 years, then every 10 years	Previous anaphylactic or encephalopathic reaction to the vaccine Moderate to severe illness with or without fever	Local redness and swelling and, rarely, anaphylaxis
Pertussis Inactivated whole-cell bacterial suspension of *Bordetella pertussis*	Primary: 2, 4, 6, and 18 months Booster: 4 to 6 years Never give after 6 years of age.	Previous anaphylactic or encephalopathic reaction to the vaccine Moderate to severe illness with or without fever	Fever, irritability, local redness and swelling, sterile abscess 1 to 2 weeks after injection More rare are seizures, anaphylaxis, very high fever, and high-pitched, persistent crying
Haemophilus influenzae type b (Hib) Purified capsular polysaccharide antigens conjugated to diphtheria protein, meningococcal protein, or tetanus protein	Primary: 2 and 4 months, and 6 months depending on type of vaccine Booster: 15 months If child is over 60 months, vaccinate only if at high risk.	Anaphylactic reaction to previous Hib vaccine Moderate to severe illness with or without fever	Local tenderness, fever, and rarely, anaphylaxis
DTP and Hib combination (Tetramune)	Primary: 2, 4, 6, and 15 to 18 months; optional at 6 months	Previous anaphylactic or encephalopathic reaction to DTP vaccine Moderate to severe illness with or without fever	Fever, malaise, irritability, local redness and swelling, and sterile abscess 1 to 2 weeks after injection More rare are seizures, anaphylaxis, very high fever, and high-pitched, persistent crying
Polio Live poliovirus types 1, 2, and 3	Primary: 2, 4, 6, and 18 months; optional at 6 months Booster: 4 to 6 years	Anaphylactic reaction to previous polio vaccine Moderate to severe illness with or without fever HIV infection or household contact with same Altered immune status or household contact with same Give with caution during pregnancy	Rarely, paralysis

Continued.

TABLE 7-3 Vaccinations: Who, What, and When—cont'd

Vaccine	Schedule	Contraindications	Side Effects
Rubeola Live attenuated measles virus	Primary: 15 months, 12 months if there is an epidemic Booster: 4 to 6 years or 11 to 12 years	Anaphylactic reaction to previous rubeola vaccine, eggs, or neomycin Moderate to severe illness with or without fever Pregnancy Altered immune status (does not include HIV infection) Give with caution if immunoglobulin was administered within 3 months.	Adverse effects may occur about 1 week after immunization and include fever of 103° F (39.4° C) or higher, transient rash, and, rarely, encephalitis
Mumps Live attenuated mumps virus	Primary: 15 months Booster: 4 to 6 years or 11 to 12 years	Anaphylactic reaction to previous mumps vaccine, eggs, or neomycin Moderate to severe illness with or without fever Pregnancy Altered immune status (doesn't include HIV infection) Give with caution if immunoglobulin was administered within 3 months	Rarely, unilateral orchitis Neurological complications also suspected
Rubella Live attenuated rubella virus	Primary: 15 months Booster: 4 to 6 years or 11 to 12 years	Anaphylactic reaction to previous rubella vaccine, eggs, or neomycin Moderate to severe illness with or without fever Pregnancy Altered immune status (doesn't include HIV infection) Give with caution if immunoglobulin was administered within 3 months.	Rash, fever, lymphadenopathy, joint pain, and, rarely, arthritis in adults
Hepatitis B Inactivated viral surface antigen derived by means of recombinant DNA technology	Primary when mother is not infected: At 0 to 2 days, then at 1 to 2 and 6 to 18 months; alternative: 1 to 2, 2 to 4, and 6 to 18 months Primary when mother is infected: On the day of birth, then at 1 and 6 months Also give to adolescents and high-risk individuals, e.g., health-care workers and household and sexual contacts of HBV carriers	Anaphylactic reaction to previous HBV vaccine Moderate to severe illness with or without fever Pregnant women should only receive the vaccine if it is clearly needed.	Local soreness and redness, headache, fever, malaise, upper respiratory infection, and gastrointestinal distress Rarely, joint pain and neurological reactions such as vertigo and paresthesia
Pneumococcus Purified capsular polysaccharide antigens with conjugate carrier	Single dose given to high-risk children over 2 years, high-risk adults, and senior citizens	Pregnancy and previous pneumococcal vaccination	Local redness and pain, fever, myalgia, and, rarely, anaphylaxis

From Vessey JA, Ritchie SR: The who, what and when of pediatric immunizations, *RN* 56(4):42, 1993.

Play is important for learning. Play that captures the pleasures of using the senses and motor abilities is called *sensorimotor play*. Early play items include turning mobiles, mirrors, colorful shapes, and toys of different textures. As hand coordination improves, other items, such as rattles and shapes, become useful play objects. Toward the end of the first year, stacking items, blocks, and puzzles encourage developing motor skills. Music can be used to soothe or stimulate awareness of sounds and rhythms. Play style during infancy is described as solitary play. This means that the infant plays alone, not needing other children with whom to play.

Accidents are the leading cause of injury and death of infants and young children. Safety precautions must be instituted immediately at birth of the child. Box 7-7 contains a list of safety rules for infants and young children. Infancy is also a time of daily changes. Goals for the developmental tasks of infancy are shown in Box 7-8 on p. 92.

The Toddler: 1 to 3 Years

Physical Characteristics. Rate of growth in the toddler years is slower than in infancy but follows the same general principles. It is orderly. It proceeds from head to foot, from the center outward, and from general to specific movements.

One of the most striking changes from infancy is the upright stance of the toddler. The chubby look of infancy is gone by 12 to 15 months. In the beginning of this stage the toddler's body proportions result in a top-heavy appearance, but by the end of this period rapid growth of the extremities and slowed growth in the trunk produce a more proportionate body appearance. Noticeable in the toddler is the exaggerated lumbar lordosis (convex lumbar curve) and protruding abdomen. This potbelly appearance disappears as the abdominal muscles strengthen. By age 2½ years all 20 deciduous teeth are present. Routine dental examinations and toothbrushing should begin during this period.

Box 7-7 SAFETY RULES FOR INFANTS and YOUNG CHILDREN

- Never leave an unsupervised infant on an elevated surface.
- Never leave an infant unattended in a highchair, stroller, walker, or any other device.
- Secure stairways and exits.
- Keep crib sides up and set mattress at lowest setting.
- Never leave infants or young children unattended in a bath for even a few seconds.
- Windows should be kept locked and secured with child guards.
- Never use plastic bags or coverings on mattresses or near infant's playthings.
- Avoid the use of pillows with small infants.
- Infant cribs must meet U.S. Consumer Product Safety regulations to prevent strangulation between crib bars.
- Remove wires and dangling electric cords from the crawling child's reach. Cover outlets with protective caps.
- Inspect all toys carefully for long strings and small removable parts.
- Use pacifiers that have one-piece construction.
- Do not allow a child to play with balloons.
- Avoid giving infants and young children hard candies, nuts, popcorn, and other foods that may easily be aspirated.
- Lock all poisons and medicines out of infants' and young children's reach (Fig. 7-3 on p. 92).
- Avoid holding an infant while drinking hot fluids.
- Check temperature of foods and formula before feeding.
- Turn pot handles toward back of stove and remove burner knobs if within child's reach.
- Avoid smoking near infants and children to prevent burns and smoke inhalation.
- Keep infants and children away from hot surfaces, stoves, fireplaces, barbecues.
- Use flame-retardant sleepwear.
- Never administer medication and say that it is candy.
- Keep poison control phone number accessible.
- Remove plants from child's reach.
- Use plastic rather than glass eating and drinking utensils.
- Inspect toys and household items for sharp points.
- Inspect for chipped lead-based paint on surfaces painted before 1978 (production of lead paint for consumer use was banned in 1978).
- Keep knives and forks away from young children.
- Supervise infants and children playing around animals and pets.
- Teach children early about street dangers and supervise their play.
- Instruct children to never go anywhere with strangers.
- Teach young children the use of the telephone for emergencies.
- Instruct children that others should not touch their "private" body parts and to report happenings if they occur. Accept the child's story unless you can prove otherwise.

Box 7-8 DEVELOPMENTAL TASKS OF INFANCY

- Establish a trusting, meaningful relationship; recognizes primary care giver, develops attachment behavior
- Learns to orient to objects, develop exploration skills, predict responses to environment
- Develops communication skills by beginning vocalization, developing nonverbal communication system, and imitating simple vocalizations
- Develops muscular control, eye/hand coordination, and object manipulation
- Develops mobility; crawling, creeping, cruising, walking
- Establishes patterns of living: eating, sleeping, and elimination habits
- Begins to develop independent living skills, including self-feeding, walking, undressing, and communication of needs

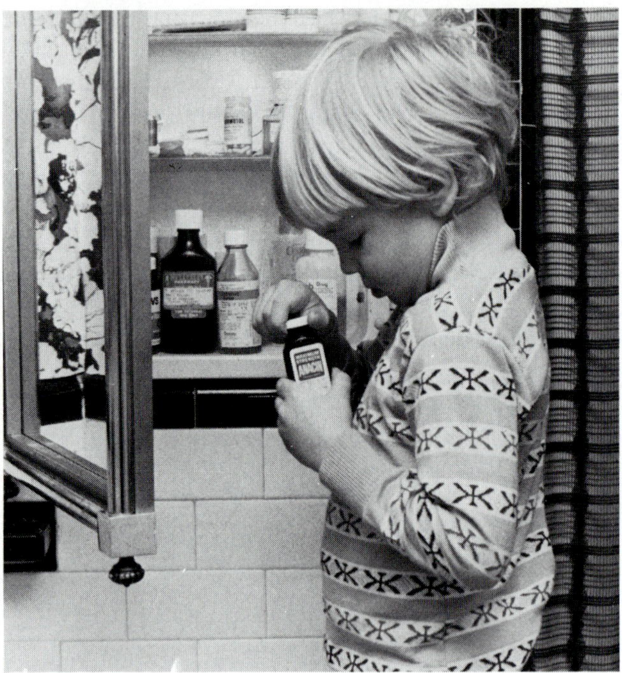

FIG. 7-3 Preschoolers are still impulsive and curious and cannot be expected to avoid all dangers. (Photograph by Douglas Bloomquist.)

Vital Signs. During the toddler period the pulse ranges between 90 to 120 beats per minute. Blood pressure averages 80 to 100 systolic and 64 diastolic. Body temperature ranges between 98° and 99° F (36.6 and 37.2° C). Respiration slows to 20 to 30 breaths/minute.

Neuromuscular Development. The emergence of gross motor skills includes walking, climbing stairs (2 years), and hopping (3 years). The toddler develops running, pulling, and holding on tight skills, exploring the world in ways theretofore impossible. Fine motor skills, such as beginning to scribble (2 years) and copying a circle (3 years), are acquired.

Toilet Training. Children do not reach physiological or psychological maturity necessary to begin toilet training until 18 to 24 months of age. Children need to reach maturity so they have neuromuscular control, the cognitive ability to understand what is expected of them, and the language skills to express their needs. Bowel control is achieved first. Bladder control begins at the same time but takes longer to achieve. Nighttime control may be achieved after daytime control is established. Parents and care givers should expect setbacks and accidents, particularly during times of stress or illness. Accidents should be deemphasized; the child should never be made to feel inadequate. That is, success should be praised and accidents should be ignored. If praise is given for toileting successes and accidents are cleaned up without negativism, the toddler will gain a sense of self-control, inner goodness, and pride. However, if the toddler is punished and made to feel foolish, a sense of shame will develop. If the toddler is kept in diapers and given no opportunities to control the urges, a sense of doubt will be fostered. Feeling of shame and doubt are not healthy personality attributes.

Psychosocial Development. The toddler is an uninhibited, energetic little person, always seeking attention, approval, and personal goals (Fig. 7-4). Sometimes the toddler is cuddly and loving; at other times, biting, hitting, or pinching prevails. The toddler only slowly realizes that everything desired cannot be had and that some behavior annoys others. The toddler tries to be independent, yet becomes easily frightened and runs to the care giver for protection, security, reassurance, and approval.

Erikson sees the toddler struggling with autonomy versus shame and doubt. With newfound skills of independence, walking, talking, self-feeding, and beginning toilet training, the toddler is struggling to be independent. Characteristics of this search for autonomy is the toddler's use of the word "no," which gives a sense of control. The toddler possesses endless energy, yet often falls asleep almost in motion. As toddlers struggle for independence, one frequently sees possessiveness and a desire to have things go their way. Ritualistic behavior is common at this stage. Toddlers enjoy the same story, the same routine, the same foods at each meal. Rituals decrease their anxiety by helping them know what to expect. When health care providers follow a hospitalized child's usual rituals, the toddler will feel safer and more secure in the strange environment.

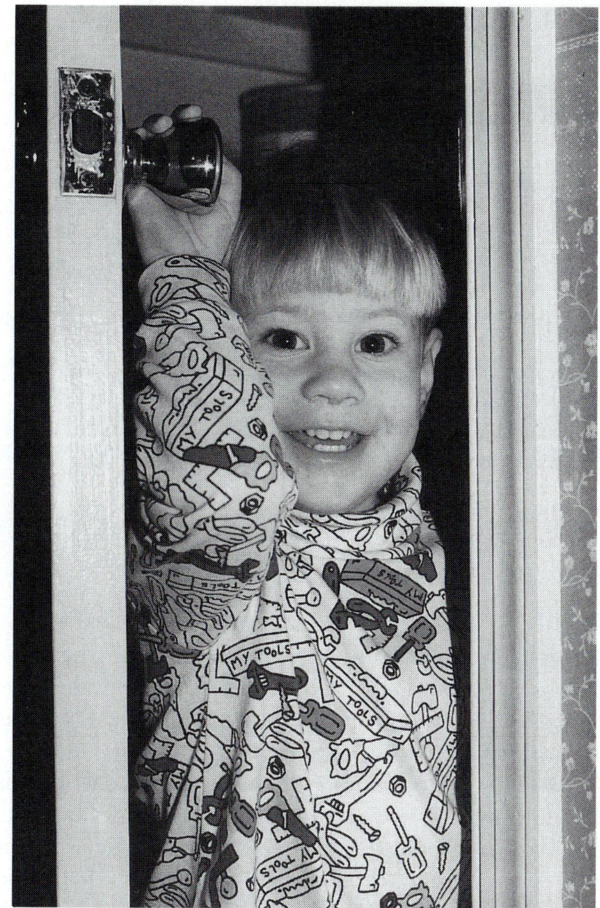

FIG. 7-4 Uninhibited, energetic little toddler.

> **Box 7-9** BASIC PRINCIPLES OF DISCIPLINE
>
> - **Consistency:** Apply rules uniformly
> - **Follow-through:** Say and do what you mean
> - **Positive modeling:** Practice role model–approved behavior
> - **Promptness:** Administer punishment in a nonhostile manner immediately after incident occurs
> - **Trust:** Express trust in the child
> - **Avoidance:** Remove temptation
> - **Reinforcement:** Offer positive reinforcement for acceptable behavior

Temper tantrums are common and are the result of frustration. A combination of wanting things "my way," the inability to communicate feelings, and the lack of impulse control may produce outbursts of temper. This type of negativism is best ignored unless the child or others are in danger of harm.

Toddlers need many experiences of being able to choose among alternatives (to play inside or outside, to wear the green pants or red pants). However, care givers should phrase questions for children to allow situations in which either choice will be acceptable. When a particular behavior is necessary (such as going to bed, holding hands to cross a street, letting go of another child's hair), care givers should not give a choice. Erikson stressed that young children do not have the wisdom to know what behaviors are acceptable or unacceptable, healthy or unhealthy.

Discipline is a necessary means of teaching limit setting, and impulse control. Basic principles of discipline are given in Box 7-9.

Cognitive and Intellectual Development. The period from 12 to 24 months of age is the last phase of sensorimotor development, in which the toddler's knowledge of the world comes about primarily through sensory impression and motor activities. The period of early childhood is the **preoperational thought stage.** (When the child focuses on the use of language as a tool to meet needs, the child has the emerging ability to think mentally.) The child uses trial and error to discover new traits and characteristics. Piaget states that this stage extends from 2 to 7 years of age.

Toddlers are constantly absorbing new ideas, widening the cognitive world, and expanding memory. Activities can be connected to past events or memories. The toddler's concept of time is limited to the present. The child's thinking is egocentric at this stage. He may be demanding, wanting things to go his way.

Communication and Language. Cognitive and language development make it possible for toddlers to think about their actions and make their wills known to their care givers. "No!" and "Me!" (meaning "Let me do it myself") are oft-repeated holo phrases of 2- and 3-year-olds.

During the toddler period the child identifies objects by use. At age 2½ the toddler's vocabulary consists of about 450 words and two-word sentences consisting of a noun and verb, for example, "my toy." By 3½ years of age the child can answer questions, can use brief sentences, and may recite TV commercials. The 3-year-old's vocabulary is approximately 900 words. Parents are strongly encouraged to read to their toddlers. Being read to not only increases the child's vocabulary but provides a pleasant environment that enhances child/care giver bonding.

Health Maintenance.

Nutrition. Good nutrition requires that the toddler's daily diet consist of one serving from the meat group, two or more servings of vegetables, and at least two servings of fruit, cereal, or breads. The Food Pyramid guidelines should be followed. The child needs

Box 7-10 GUIDELINES FOR BEDTIME PREPARATION

- Reduce activity level before bedtime.
- Establish a simple ritual, i.e., bathroom, story time, goodnight song, etc.
- Make bedtime a pleasurable experience.
- Familiarize child with routine nightly.
- Reassure child that he is not alone.
- Use a night light.
- Expect disruptions or setbacks during and after illness and stress or after stimulating activities.

Box 7-11 DEVELOPMENTAL TASKS OF THE TODDLER

- Recognizes self as a separate person; tolerates separation from primary care giver; expresses own ideas and needs.
- Develops increased attention span.
- Begins to develop communication skills.
- Begins to develop self-control skills.
- Masters toilet-training basics.
- Achieves independent mobility.
- Develops independent skills of daily living, feeding, dressing, toileting, managing simple tasks.

about 1 quart of milk a day. Most children are more likely to eat foods with which they are familiar. Therefore gradual introduction of new foods is advisable. Bite-size pieces, finger foods, and smaller portions are generally more acceptable. Idiosyncratic eating patterns are common at this stage. Toddles need less food per unit of body weight than they did during infancy. A general guideline for serving size is 1 tablespoon of each solid food for each year of age.

Parents need to be informed that during illness, brief periods of anorexia are usually not serious.

Immunizations. Refer to Table 7-3 for recommended immunization schedule.

Sleep, play, and safety. Toddlers expend a high level of energy in daily growing, playing, and exploring. Adequate rest and sleep are essential for maintaining optimal wellness. The toddler requires 12 hours of sleep each night plus a daytime nap. Suggestions helpful in assisting health sleeping patterns include limiting stimulation prior to sleep time, using of quiet-time activities before sleep, allowing a favorite bedtime toy, telling a specified number of stories, and establishing and maintaining bedtime rituals. See Box 7-10 for guidelines for bedtime preparation.

Play improves muscle coordination, balance, and muscle strength. Play style for the toddler is described as parallel play. This play style refers to the need that toddlers have to play alongside of, but not with, peer mates. Toddlers play with similar toys in similar ways, but they do not interact with others. They are unable to share and interact with their peers at this stage.

More than half of all childhood deaths are caused by accidents, many of which are motor vehicle accidents. About 90% of the accidents that occur in the home are believed to be preventable. Prevention methods must include both supervision and education. A list of safety rules is found in Box 7-7. Toddlers seek attention, approval, and love as they struggle for independence.

The developmental tasks of toddlers are summarized in Box 7-11.

Preschool: 3 to 5 Years

Physical Characteristics. Physical development during early childhood occurs on many fronts, with the most important—maturation of the nervous system and mastery of skills—being the least obvious; the most obvious are the striking changes in size and shape.

Growth during the preschool period is described as slow and steady. The preschooler looks taller and thinner. Average weight gain is less than 5 lb a year. Linear growth is about 2 to 2½ inches a year. The 4-year-old has usually doubled the birth length. The preschooler's body contour changes in a loss of the lordosis and protuberant abdomen (as the abdominal muscles strengthen, the child loses the potbelly appearance). The gait of the preschooler becomes more steady. The preschooler is more capable of focusing and refining activities, and the body grows slimmer, stronger, and less top heavy. Because of these developments, gross motor skills (large body movements such as running, climbing, jumping, and throwing) improve dramatically. Fine motor skills (skills that involve small body movements) are much harder for preschoolers to master than gross motor skills. Such things as tying shoelaces, cutting food with a knife and fork, and putting together a puzzle prove difficult because of their undeveloped fine motor skills. It is important to encourage development of fine motor skills. The scribbling of the young child can be compared to the babbling of the infant. Both are ways to master certain raw materials that at some later date will lead to communication. Providing pencils, crayons, markers, and paper is as important as providing things to climb, things to throw, and places to run.

Vision in the preschooler is described as farsighted. Vision improves and most children achieve 20/20 visual accuracy by age 5. By age 6, the child begins to lose the deciduous teeth.

Vital Signs. Heart rate for the preschooler ranges between 70 and 110 beats/minute. Respiratory rate slows

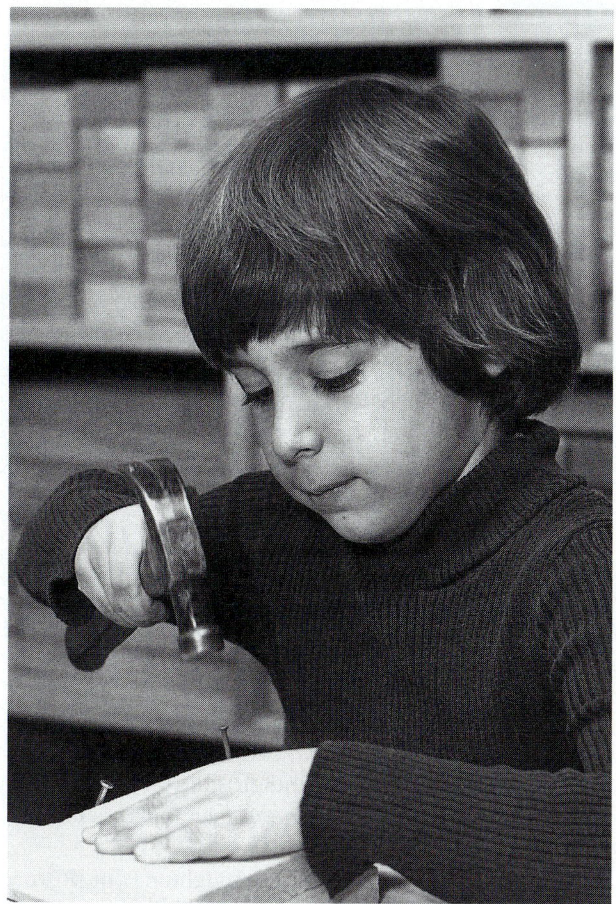

FIG. 7-5 Trying out new roles.

down to about 23 breaths/minute at rest. BP averages 110/60. Temperature ranges from 97° to 99° F (36.1° to 37.2° C), depending upon method used.

Psychosocial Development. First the child learns to function independently, and then he begins to use imagination to creatively explore new experiences (Fig. 7-5). Erikson describes the task of the preschooler as initiative versus guilt. Preschoolers search for and create fantasies about the different kinds of people they would like to become. They pretend to be grown up and try a variety of roles. During the preschool period the child's superego (conscience) functions as a censor of behavior. The crisis, according to Erikson, is to test one's initiative without creating an overwhelming sense of guilt. Typical development of the preschooler includes gender identification. It is common at this time for the child to stereotype roles and to show marked interest in sexual differences.

Cognitive and Intellectual Development. According to Piaget the preschool child is at the preoperational stage of cognitive development. Preschoolers use symbols to represent objects. They use trial and error to discover new traits and characteristics. Between the ages of 4 and 7 years intuitive thinking develops and the child begins to think logically. Preoperational children see the world from their own viewpoint. They see things as being black or white or as absolutes. All things to the preschool child are seen as either good or bad.

During the preschool stage, time is associated with weekly and seasonal events. Magical thoughts are typical of the child of this age, who believes that wishes can make things happen. As a result the preschool child may feel powerful and responsible for events. Sometimes the preschooler feels guilty over the belief that a wish has caused serious harm or death to a loved one. White lies or untruths may express some of the child's fantasies. During this stage of development the child needs trust and guidance to distinguish truth from fantasy. At this stage, the child is more vulnerable to certain fears, probably stemming from a vivid imagination. Excessive exposure to undesirable television and other media may further distort reality testing. Common fears manifesting at this stage include fear of thunder, lightning, the dark, pain, abandonment, and monsters.

Communication and Language. By the age of 3 years children can carry on a conversation. Pronunciation problems continue into the school years. Language becomes more adultlike. By the age of 3 years if the child is not talking, evaluation by a physician for possible hearing loss or other speech pathologies is necessary. Parents should continue to read to their child because this helps to expand the language ability and comprehension and continues to foster positive child/care giver relationships.

Health Maintenance

Nutrition. Since body systems and muscles are still growing steadily, the preschool child continues to need high levels of protein. Calcium and phosphorus are important to both toddlers and preschool children because of the increased mineralization of their teeth and bones. Food habits, likes, dislikes, and appetites vary greatly from child to child. Supplementary vitamins are recommended by some physicians. Vitamins, like any other medication, should not take the place of good eating habits (see Chapter 18).

Immunization. See immunization schedule in Table 7-3.

Sleep, play, and safety. Preschoolers may resist nap periods but still need 11 to 12 hours of sleep at night. Rest periods offered during the day enable children to reenergize and carry out the rest of their daily activities.

Play for the preschool child becomes a cooperative style of play. The child begins to share, take turns, and interact with playmates. Preschoolers enjoy pretend play such as cooking, shopping, and driving. Through dramatic play the child tries on different roles and identi-

Box 7-12 STEPS FOR DISCIPLINE AND LIMIT SETTING

1. Define acceptable vs. unacceptable behaviors.
2. Set limits: "I will not let you hurt anyone."
3. Be consistent; keep the same rules.
4. Recognize escalating emotions and intervene: "I can see you're upset—let's go over there and sit down."
5. Suggest "time out" or call for help.
6. Choose punishment to "fit" wrongdoing and enact in a timely manner (given in a nonhostile manner).
7. Praise and reinforce positive behavior: "I like the way you. . . ."
8. Always start with a clean slate.
9. Stay calm; avoid arguing.
10. Avoid putdowns: "You're acting like a bad boy."
11. Remember to listen to your child.

Box 7-13 DEVELOPMENTAL TASKS OF PRESCHOOLERS

- Develops stronger sense of self; can express own needs, ideas, and feelings; can postpone immediate gratification
- Learns greater attention span, listens more attentively
- Develops and refines gross motor skills and fine motor skills
- Recognizes sex identification
- Begins to work and play more cooperatively with others
- Improves communication skills
- Develops self-control skills; learns socially acceptable ways of expressing anger, frustration, and disappointment; obeys simple rules; develops self-awareness and sense of self-protection
- Seeks information, asks questions, learns values and beliefs of the family

fies with adult models. Dramatic play encourages social development when two or more children cooperate in creating their own drama. Not only is dramatic play fun for the preschooler, but it also helps children try out social roles, express their fears and fantasies, and learn to cooperate. Experiences with imaginary playmates are not uncommon in this age group. Children often feel in control of what happens in their "imaginary world" and slowly learn to deal with reality through practice and experimentation.

All the safety precautions described earlier apply to the preschool child as well as the infant and toddler (Box 7-7). Preschool children should be taught their full names, addresses, and telephone numbers. They should know how to use the phone in case of an emergency.

Discipline and limit setting are needed and are as important to the child as are love and security. Guidance must include offering alternative ways of expressing feelings and meeting needs (Box 7-12).

The preschool period is a time of learning to function independently and exploring the imagination. See Box 7-13 for the preschool developmental tasks.

School-Age Child: 6 to 12 Years

Physical Characteristics. During the school-age period the growth pattern is usually gradual and subtle. The most obvious growth is in the long bones of the extremities and in the development of the facial bones. As a result of this bone growth some children complain of "growing pains," particularly at night. Persistent pains should be evaluated by a physician to rule out any underlying pathology. Height and weight increase by about 2 inches and 2 lb a year for both boys and girls from age 6 to 12. Motor skills in boys and girls develop with some differences; boys may become stronger and girls may become more graceful and accurate.

The child's posture becomes straighter. Poor posture may be due to fatigue or minor skeletal defects. School-age children should be routinely screened for scoliosis (abnormal lateral curvature of the spine). Muscle mass and strength gradually increase, and the body loses its "baby fat" appearance of earlier childhood. Both gross and fine motor development continues to be refined during the school-age years.

Vital Signs. Heart and respiratory rate steadily decrease, while blood pressure increases. Normal pulse rate is between 55 and 90, respiratory rate is 22 to 24, and blood pressure is 110/65.

Vision improves, and most children achieve 20/20 vision at this stage. Regular vision testing should be performed throughout the school years.

Psychosocial Development. Entrance into school challenges the child and creates demands for new social and cognitive skills (Fig. 7-6). The child becomes more independent and participates in a broader world of peers and new experiences. School-age children are becoming increasingly aware of rules and socialization skills and expectations. The beginning skills of compromise and competition are the challenges facing this age group.

Erikson identified the task of the school-age years as industry versus inferiority. During these years the child learns to work and master skills that produce satisfaction as the result of that work. After the child realizes that "there is no workable future within the womb of his family," says Erikson, the school-age child "becomes ready to apply himself to given skills and tasks." Children develop their own goals and direct their efforts toward mastery of these goals. As children discover their talents and accomplishments, they gain self-confidence and a sense of purpose. Successful mastery of learning in school leads to strengthening and stabilizing the child's sense of self. According to Erikson, as children busily try to master whatever skills are valued in their culture, they develop views of themselves as either competent or incompetent, as either industrious and productive or inferior and inadequate.

If the environment inadequately supports a child's pursuits, the stage may be set for the development of feelings of inferiority and the lack of self-confidence. The school setting should be a pleasant, comfortable environment. Teachers and care givers need to use praise, encouragement, and rewards to positively reinforce the school-age child's efforts. Teachers need to be positive role models. School helps the child learn new routines and establish important social relationships.

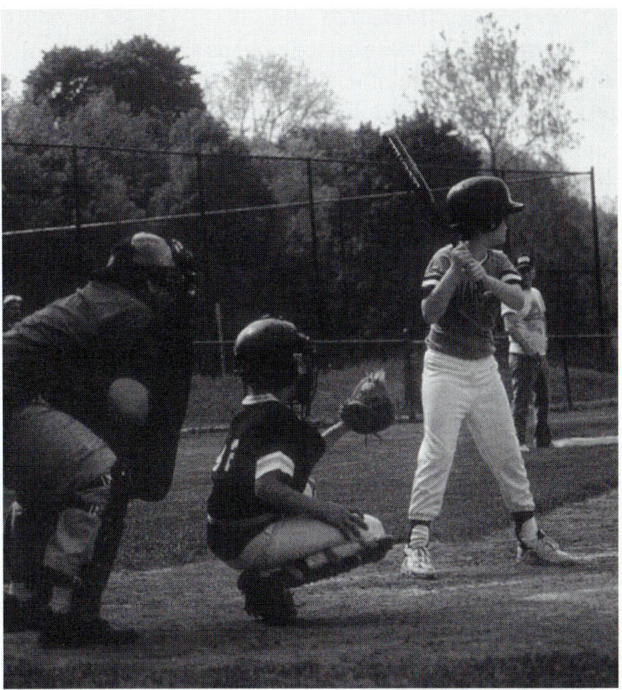

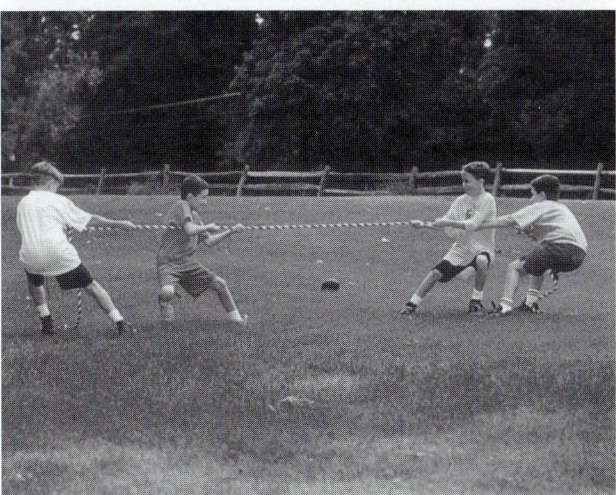

FIG. 7-6 Playground interaction

Cognitive and Intellectual Development. According to Piaget, children in the school years move into the **concrete operational phase.** During this phase, thoughts become increasingly logical and coherent, so that the child is able to classify, sort, and organize facts while still being incapable of generalizing or dealing with abstractions. Children can reason about almost anything specific they perceive. Between the ages of 7 and 11, children usually come to understand logical principles, as long as the principles can be applied to concrete, specific cases. They view the world more realistically, and they are capable of understanding the views of others. They can distinguish purpose from behavior and outcome. This age group can focus on more than one aspect of a task. The child has begun to develop logical socialized thought. There is a movement away from fantasy as the child realizes that a physical cause is behind an event. The child's developing cognitive skills serve as a motivator for learning how to work. A supportive learning environment can enhance the child's approach to problem solving and can help lead to success.

Communication and Language. Most 6-year-olds have a good command of sentence structure. The child's vocabulary has become more extensive and includes slang and swear words, which may be used to create an effect. By age 7 the hands of the child have become more steady. Printing becomes clearer and smaller. Between the ages of 8 and 10 years, the hand becomes more efficient, which enables the child to write rather than print. The 10- to 12-year-old child can accomplish complex, intricate, fine-quality handcrafts or may begin piano, violin, or guitar lessons.

Health Maintenance

Nutrition. Total metabolic needs are affected by the energy expenditure of each individual child. The sedentary quiet child who prefers fine motor activities requires fewer calories than the child who is more oriented to athletics or is more physically active. The recommended daily intake of food is listed in the Food Guide Pyramid (see Chapter 18).

Dietary habits and food preferences are strongly established during the school-age period. Cultural influences, family habits, and peer pressure are all critical factors in a child's developing food habits. Childhood obesity is closely correlated with obesity in adult years and therefore it is necessary to maintain the child's weight within normal limits. In middle childhood, obese children are teased, picked on, and rejected. They know they are overweight and they often hate themselves for it. Obese children usually have fewer friends than other children. The best way to get children to lose weight is to increase their physical activity. Indeed inactivity may be as much a cause of childhood obesity as overeating. Studies have shown that diets high in saturated fat increase a child's risk for high blood cholesterol and heart disease, unless steps are taken to lower these levels.

Immunization. See Table 7-3 for the immunization schedule. Health and dental checkups should be done regularly to identify minor problems early, before they become serious.

Sleep, play, and safety. Fatigue, irritability, inattention, and poor learning are often signs of inadequate sleep. The 6-year-old needs about 12 hours of sleep at night. By 12 years of age the child usually needs about 10 hours of sleep. Some children have frequent nightmares, which disrupt their sleep. Stress, violence on television, or overtiredness may contribute to a child's nightmares. Relaxation techniques such as quiet music, story time, and bathing may help the child relax before sleep.

School-age children need adequate exercise to enhance muscle development, coordination, balance, and strength. In addition, music, craft projects, board games, appropriate television, and video games are all enjoyed by the school-age child. Privacy and a place for their belongings are important at this age. The school-age child is often a willing worker and enjoys being paid for small jobs. The collection and hoarding of "treasures" as their belongings are a part of this stage of development.

Many children during the school years become involved with competitive or team sports. Children of this age show interest and loyalty to peers of the same sex. They learn to follow the rules of the game. Some are able to benefit from team competitiveness and use it to motivate them to practice in order to excel. Others shy away from the competition and become disinterested or develop feelings of inadequacy and disappointment.

Accidents are still the leading cause of death in this age group. Impulsiveness, poor judgment, curiosity, and incomplete control over motor coordination are some of the factors that may increase the school-age child's incidence of accidents.

Dentition. Permanent teeth develop rapidly. Regular dental checkups are recommended every 6 months throughout childhood.

The school-age child experiences gradual and subtle growth changes while learning new social and cognitive skills. Box 7-14 contains a list of the developmental tasks of the school-age child.

Adolescent: 12 to 19 Years

Physical Characteristics. The term *adolescence* covers the transition period from childhood to adulthood. Adolescence begins at puberty (the period of life at which the ability to reproduce begins), and accompanying the pubertal changes are corresponding changes in the personality.

Puberty refers to the maturation of the reproductive system, including all the primary and secondary sexual developmental changes. Primary changes occur in the organs related to reproduction (ovaries, breasts, uterus, testes, and penis). Secondary sexual changes occur in other parts of the body (development of pubic and facial hair, voice changes, and fat deposits). Adolescence literally means "to grow into maturity" and is generally regarded as the psychological, social, and maturational process initiated by pubertal changes.

Adolescence is characterized as the second major period of rapid growth. Females grow 2 to 8 inches (5 to 20 cm) while males grow 4 to 12 inches (10 to 30 cm). During this adolescent period weight gains for females are 15 to 55 lb (7 to 25 kg), and males gain 15 to 65 lb (7 to 30 kg). While females develop more body fat, males develop more muscle tissue. Males average 50% muscle and 10% fat, while females average 40% muscle and 25% fat after puberty. Muscle strength and muscle mass increase in the male, causing the average male to

Box 7-14 DEVELOPMENTAL TASKS OF THE SCHOOL-AGE CHILD

- Develops a sense of belonging with family, peers
- Develops work habits; learns to organize, set and reach goals, evaluate work, accept criticism
- Learns competence in reading, writing, calculation, grammar, and communication
- Refines fine and gross motor coordination.

have more muscle strength. Exercise facilitates the size, strength, and endurance of each adolescent.

In the female, menarche (the first menstrual period) is the identification point used to signify the onset of the postpuberty period. In the male, sperm production signals the beginning of adolescence.

Body shapes are sex differentiated after puberty. Boys have broader shoulders, narrower hips, and larger limbs. Girls have larger breasts, narrower waists, wider hips, and lower centers of gravity.

Both boys and girls experience voice changes. Girls' voices become fuller and richer because the lengthening of their vocal cords. Boys' voices become lower and louder. The deeper male voice results from enlargement of the larynx (the Adam's apple) lengthening of the vocal cords.

Sexual interests increase markedly in vigor and intensity and are usually focused on members of the opposite sex. New problems arise as adolescents find social disapproval and prohibitors of their own consciences conflicting with intense sexual drives.

Vital Signs. Average pulse rate is 70 beats/minute. Respiratory rate averages 20 breaths/minute. Blood pressure increases to 120/70 mm Hg.

Psychosocial Development. The period of adolescence is frequently described as a difficult period or a stormy search for oneself (Fig. 7-7). Confronting every adolescent are a changing body, sexual demands, responsibilities, expectations, and questions about values and beliefs. The search for one's identity amid a world of social pressures creates a painful struggle. Erikson described the developmental task of adolescence as establishing a sense of identity. He proposed the conflict of identity versus role confusion as characteristic of adolescence. The search for a sense of identity, he believed, reaches crisis proportions at this time. Not only does the adolescent need to adjust to a sexually mature body, but all previous conflicts (trust versus mistrust, autonomy versus doubt, initiative versus guilt, and industry versus inferiority) must be re-resolved in light of the newly sensuous self. The period of adolescence requires major reorganization of the personality, resolution of childhood insecurities, and acceptance of adult responsibilities. The value of peers is usually significant to the adolescent (Fig. 7-8). Peers influence preferences, dress, speech, and leisure activities. The peer group is often the place to learn and test developing interpersonal skills. Conforming behavior may be exhibited to win praise and acceptance by peers.

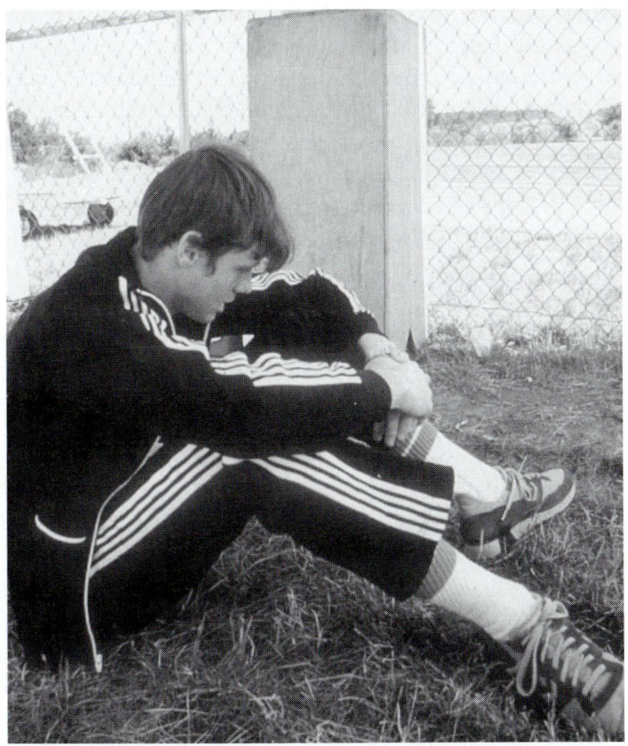

FIG. 7-7 Many adolescents become very introspective. (Photograph by David S. Strickland.)

Cognitive Development. According to Piaget, an individual's cognitive function reaches maturity during adolescence. Piaget describes this stage as the **formal operational thought phase.** This is a higher process that permits abstract reasoning and systematic scientific problem solving. The adolescent thinks beyond the present. At this time thoughts can be influenced more by logical principles than by personal perceptions and experiences. Adolescents become capable of scientific reasoning and formal logic. Without having to center attention on the immediate situation, they can imagine the possible—a sequence of events that might occur, such

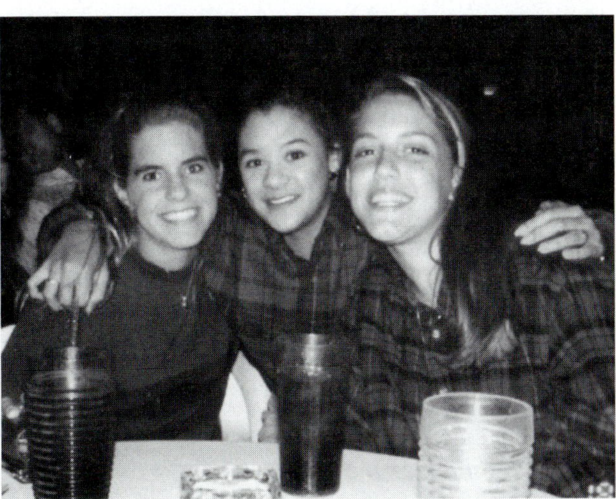

FIG. 7-8 Adolescence is a time when best friends share their most intimate ideas and concerns. (Photograph by David S. Strickland.)

as college and occupational possibilities; how things might change in the future, such as relationships with parents; and the consequences of their actions, such as dropping out of school.

Moral Development. As children move through the stages of cognitive and logical thought, they also progress through stages of moral development. As with other developmental processes, moral development approaches or achieves adult levels during a person's adolescence.

When old principles are challenged but new and independent values have not yet emerged, young people search for a moral code that preserves their personal integrity and guides their behavior, especially in the face of strong pressure to violate the old values. Their decisions involving moral dilemmas must be based on an internalized set of principles that provide them with resources to evaluate the demands of the situation and to plan a course of action consistent with their ideals.

Health Maintenance.

Nutrition. The rate of body growth and the adolescent's increased basal metabolic rate require an increase in the individual's caloric needs. At peak growth females may need as much as 2600 calories a day, males as much as 3600 calories a day. Many factors affect the individual's dietary habits, including cultural influence, family habits, work schedules, school, concerns about weight gain, peer influence, and lack of knowledge concerning correct food choices. Protein needs are increased, related to the rapid growth of this period. Protein should comprise 12% to 16% of the total daily food intake.

The adolescent diet is most likely to be deficient in calcium, iron, and zinc. There is a substantial increase in the need for these minerals during the period of rapid growth—calcium for skeletal growth; iron for expansion of muscle mass and blood volume, soft tissue growth, and the rapid growth demands of the expanding red cell mass; and zinc for the generation of both skeletal and muscle tissue. Adolescent boys have greater muscle mass, but adolescent girls have an additional iron loss from menstruation. Consequently, the need is probably equivalent in both sexes.

Increased amounts of milk are usually required to supplement an average diet to ensure an adequate calcium intake during this time.

The adolescent should follow the guidelines of the Food Pyramid (see Chapter 18).

Immunization. Refer to Table 7-3 for the immunization schedule.

Sleep and safety. The adolescent needs to pace activities to allow for adequate rest. The adolescent often has the need for increased hours of sleep to restore energy levels.

Box 7-15 GUIDELINES FOR PRACTICE OF SAFE SEX

- The safest sexual practice is abstinence.
- Be familiar with your sexual partners. Ask about their sexual life-style before you engage in sexual relations.
- Avoid engaging in sexual relations with IV drug users or with individuals who have had multiple sex partners.
- Use a latex *condom* as the best type of protection from infection.
- Condoms should be inspected for tears prior to use. Avoid lengthy storage and exposure to excessive heat.
- Fit the condom over the erect penis, leaving a small space at the end for the collection of semen.
- Hold the upper end of the condom when withdrawing from the vagina to prevent slippage.
- Avoid sexual relations with individuals who have genital lesions or unusual drainage.
- Be aware that there is an increased risk of HIV infection with oral sexual practices. Anal intercourse requires additional education for safe practice.

Accident prevention is vitally important to this age group. The greatest number of deaths in this age group are due to accidents. Driver's education, water safety training, education about safe sexual practices, and drug education are necessary to inform adolescents of the risks and dangers inherent in these activities. Box 7-15 lists safe sex practices that need to be emphasized early in adolescence with emphasis on abstinence.

Adolescence is a period of maturation, covering the transition from childhood to adulthood. The developmental tasks of adolescence are given in Box 7-16.

Early Adulthood: 20 to 40 Years

The transition to adulthood in the United States is marked by several events such as taking on financial responsibilities, making career choices, beginning social relationships, entering marriage, and becoming a parent. All the challenges and accomplishments of the earlier developmental stages have assisted in the preparation of the individual for the responsibilities of adult maturity. The unrealistic impressions of adulthood are usually replaced with realistic expectations and anticipation.

Physical Characteristics. The body during early adult years is at its optimal level of functioning. The typical young adult is a fine physical specimen. Strength, energy, and endurance are now at their peak. From the middle 20s most body functions are fully developed, and the peak of muscular strength occurs. At about age 50, de-

Box 7-16

DEVELOPMENTAL TASKS OF ADOLESCENCE

- Recognizes individuality
- Accepts strengths and weaknesses
- Develops own value system
- Assumes responsibility for one's own behavior
- Develops philosophy of life
- Adapts to somatic changes (changes affecting the body)
- Acquires skills necessary for adult living
- Defines social skills
- Develops independent living skills

Box 7-17

RECOMMENDATIONS FOR A HEALTHY LIFE-STYLE

- Follow the guidelines of the Food Pyramid
- Drink adequate fluids
- Avoid smoking and drugs
- Consume little or no alcohol
- Maintain optimum weight
- Participate in a scheduled program of daily exercise
- Receive adequate restorative sleep
- Practice stress reduction
- Enjoy leisure activities

clines in physical capabilities occur but are usually so gradual that they are hardly noticed.

Physical appearance is always influenced by one's heredity, environment, and general state of wellness. Females usually reach their maximum height at about 16 to 17 years of age. Males may continue to grow until 18 to 20 years of age. Between the ages of 30 and 45, height is stable, then it begins to decline because of a settling of spinal disks. There is often an increase in fatty tissue, causing weight gain; a decrease in muscle strength; and a stabilization of reaction time. The senses are also at their sharpest during young adulthood. Visual acuity is keenest at about age 20 and does not begin to decline until about age 40. Both vision and hearing diminish slightly in middle adulthood. Cardiac output, vital capacities, and organ reserves gradually decrease in middle adulthood.

Diet plays an important role throughout the developmental stages. Both heart disease and cancer are major concerns for the adult years. Heart disease caused by increased cholesterol deposits occluding the walls of blood vessels may be controllable by proper diet and exercise. Likewise low-fat, increased fiber, and decreased cholesterol diets are recommended as preventive measures against cancer of the breast, stomach, and intestine (see Chapter 19). Other life-style habits such as the use of tobacco, drugs, and alcohol will also affect the adult's health status. See Box 7-17 for a list of recommendations for good health.

In the past 15 years physical fitness has increased in popularity. Regular, paced exercise increases heart and lung capacity, lowers blood pressure, helps control weight, enhances body function, and improves emotional health.

By adulthood, both male and females have reached their sexual maturity. Research shows that sexual drive continues for both males and females throughout adulthood.

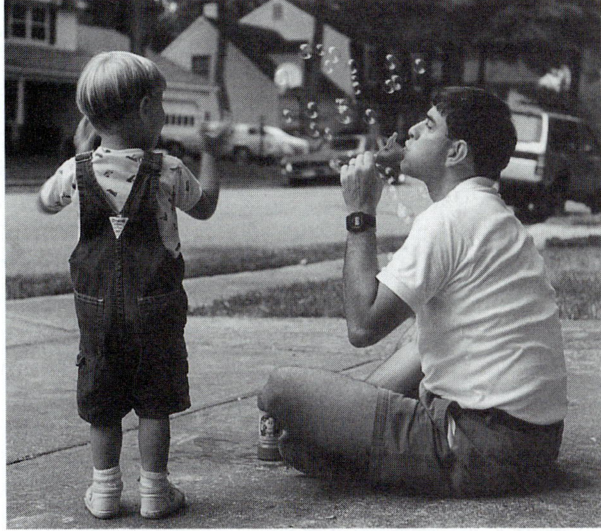

FIG. 7-9 Father and child at play.

Psychosocial Development. About 95% of Americans marry at some point in their lives. Dual-career families have grown out of economic realities as well as the woman's interest in pursuing a career. The feminist movement has resulted in many positive social changes. The dual-career life-style has affected both the home and workplace.

Another important choice of this age group is the decision to start a family (Fig. 7-9). If procreation is the choice, a subsequent issue is the number and training of children. Additional thought must be given to considerations such as money, safety, family support, housing, the relationship to members of the extended family, and the roles and responsibilities of the nuclear family unit. Today it is important for young adults establishing a family to have open communication about self-development, which includes issues of dual careers, childbearing practices, and domestic duties within the home.

Family development and harmony are major goals for many young adults, both male and female. Although family size and structure have undergone dramatic changes in the past several years, concerns about individual members' health and safety continue as a prime focus within the family as a unit. Family life is influenced by the qualities of individual family members. Typically, the age of the individuals, job security, place in the community, and healthy patterns of living (good nutrition, personal cleanliness, physical fitness) are associated with healthy family adjustment. Therefore the physical and mental health of one family member affects all family members.

Erikson identified intimacy vs. isolation as the developmental task of adulthood. Intimacy is the ability to relate one's deepest hopes and concerns to another person. Part of intimacy is the capacity of the person to accept the closeness of another person. Intimacy leads to commitment, sharing, and compromise. The "virtue" that develops in young adulthood is the virtue of love, or mutuality of devotion between partners who have chosen to share their lives. As young adults resolve conflicting demands of intimacy, competitiveness, and distance, they develop an ethical sense, which Erikson considers the mark of the adult. The opposite of intimacy or the negative resolution leads to isolation and self-absorption or the distancing of one self from intimate relationships.

Box 7-18 DEVELOPMENTAL TASKS OF EARLY ADULTHOOD

- Achieves independence, both financial and social
- Maximizes personal worth and identity
- Develops meaningful and satisfying social relationships
- Assumes responsibilities and independent decision making
- Learns to balance personal needs and societal expectations
- Accepts self and others
- Distinguishes physical attraction from love and permanent commitment
- Decides on a marriage, career, and children

Cognitive Development. Piaget saw adulthood as actively developing the formal operational approach to learning and problem solving. He felt that the same cognitive operations apply throughout adulthood to a larger, more expansive list of experiences. Adults tend to think in an integrative way.

Health Maintenance.

Nutrition. Fewer total numbers of calories are needed than during adolescence, since the adult has completed biophysical growth. Enough calories are needed to maintain body functioning for cell replacement and repair and for provision of energy. Calorie needs vary based on age, gender, size, physical activity, metabolism, and stress.

Rest and sleep. Most adults function with 7 to 9 hours of restorative sleep. Planning for rest during the day to avoid fatigue is not commonly done by adults; however, they can increase their productivity with adequate rest periods during the day. Adequate rest is essential for the pregnant woman to ensure the health of both herself and her unborn baby.

Physical health. Annual physical and dental examinations are recommended. For the male a routine testicular exam and for the female annual Papanicolaou (Pap) smears are essential for early detection of cancer. Monthly breast self-examinations for women over age 20 and a baseline mammogram between ages 35 and 40 are recommended. Beginning at age 40 males' yearly physical examination should include a digital examination and PSA to screen for prostate cancer (see Chapter 38).

Adults who have completed their primary immunizations should have booster immunization against diphtheria and tetanus every 10 years. Repeats of other immunizations are based on an individual's previous history and exposure risks.

Recently the hepatitis B vaccine has been recommended for adults who are at increased risk of exposure to blood and body fluids, those with multiple sexual partners, or those with a history of shared needle usage (see Box 7-15).

Routine dental examinations should be scheduled for adults every 6 months. Eye examinations are necessary every 2 years unless otherwise indicated.

Safety. Accidents are the leading cause of disability and death in this age group. Injuries commonly result from work, vehicle, and sports accidents as well as from violence.

Early adulthood, the period of optimal physical condition, is marked by momentous changes in life-style. Box 7-18 contains a list of the developmental tasks of early adulthood.

Middle Adulthood: 40 to 65 Years

Most individuals during the middle adult years enjoy a healthy body. This period is arbitrarily the period of life between 40 and 65 years of age. There are some changes that result in a gradual shift of balance away from peak performance. The extent of these changes is directly related to diet, heredity, exercise, rest, mental outlook, stress, and disease.

The middle adulthood period is characterized by shifts in responsibilities and physical adjustments. Box 7-19 contains a list of the developmental tasks for middle adulthood.

Box 7-19

DEVELOPMENTAL TASKS FOR MIDDLE ADULTHOOD

- Balances goals and realities and redirects energies as necessary
- Extends caring and concern beyond immediate family (to neighborhood, community, society)
- Develops career/job satisfaction
- Adapts to physical changes
- Establishes new roles and relationships with spouse, children, grandchildren, and parents

Physical Characteristics. Bone mass decreases one's skeletal growth cells. Females lose calcium from bone tissue after menopause. This bone loss leads to an increased risk of osteoporosis. Males lose calcium from bones but at a more gradual rate than females. Slight changes in height occur as a result of compression of the spinal vertebrae and hardening of collagen fibers. A decrease in muscle fibers results in a reduction of muscle mass. Heredity, nutrition, and exercise patterns may account for variation in different individuals. Changes in muscle strength may be more related to level of activity than to age. Body shape and contour changes are related to a redistribution of body weight. A decrease in basal metabolism and less activity may necessitate calorie reductions to prevent weight gain.

Basic neurological functioning remains at a high level during this age period.

Changes in vision are noticeable because of **presbyopia** (defect in vision in advancing age involving loss of accommodation or the recession of near vision caused by loss of elasticity of crystalline lens).

Other sensory changes may include **presbycusis** (a normal loss of hearing acuity, speech intelligibility, auditory threshold, and pitch associated with aging), a progressive loss of hearing in advancing age. These changes usually begin around age 40, and occur more commonly in males than in females.

One of the most noticeable changes is in the appearance of the individual's skin. There is a decrease in the elastic fibers and a slight loss of subcutaneous tissue, giving a looser, more wrinkled appearance to the skin. Hair color may change with age, the onset of graying. Graying usually begins at the temples. Hair growth and distribution may change during the middle adult years. Scalp hair may become thinner.

There is a higher incidence of periodontal (gum) disease in the middle adult years. Preventive treatment programs should include fluoride usage, regular flossing, and dental cleaning.

Hormonal changes include the female's inability to produce estrogen and progesterone. Menopause (female climacteric) is a gradual process that takes about 5 years to complete. A female's perception of menopause is likely to be affected by her perceptions of her general health. During this process the functions of the ovaries will diminish and eventually cease. Noticeable signs and symptoms of menopause may include irregular menstrual periods, flow changes, excess fluid retention, breast tenderness, hot flashes, flushes, palpitations, night sweats, and irritability or mood swings. Some women have very few signs or symptoms related to menopause. Women may be given small doses of estrogen to relieve the complications of decreased estrogen levels. It is suggested that hormone replacement therapy (HRT) can reduce osteoporosis and the risk of atherosclerosis and heart disease; however, HRT may increase the risk of endometrial cancer and breast disease as well as elevate the blood pressure. Therefore, the risks versus the benefits must be evaluated on an individual basis. The female can continue to have positive, satisfying sexual experiences and responses throughout the middle adult years. Many females, without the fear of pregnancy, enjoy an enhanced sexual period.

The male climacteric may consist of decreased libido (sex drive), loss of body hair, and delayed erection. Men do not lose the ability to reproduce during the middle adult years. Changes in body appearance, including weight gain, hair loss, and decreased muscle strength, may affect the male's perception and mental outlook rather than his actual capacity to function. The changes seen in the male are often more related to psychological than physiological occurrences. As a result of these changes some males go through what is described as a "midlife crisis." During this time the midlife male may engage in extramarital affairs and divorce.

Many males are unaffected by the physiological and psychological occurrences of the climacteric.

Psychosocial Development. According to Erikson the developmental task of middle age is generativity vs. stagnation. This means accepting responsibility for and offering guidance to the next generation. Generativity encourages productivity, continuity, and creativity. If this developmental task is not met, people become stagnant—inactive or lifeless. The impulse to foster development of the young is not limited to guiding one's own children. It can be expressed through activities such as teaching and mentorship, a mutually fulfilling relationship that satisfies a younger protegé's need for guidance as well as an older person's need for generativity. The middle adult years are a time for vocational, interpersonal, and personal fulfillment. Resumption of education, career growth or changes, reentry into the work force, and involvement with community activities create a multitude of possibilities for personal growth and satisfaction during the middle adult years.

The past two decades have probably been the best time ever to be an American grandparent and to enjoy grandparenting as a joyful experience. Grandparents now have the longest, healthiest life spans ever, the best social services, and the most independence. Although many still hover just above the poverty line, and some are below it, as a group grandparents are more prosperous than ever. As the parents of the baby-boom generation, grandparents have lots of grandchildren to enjoy. Many American grandparents are not involved in the upbringing and disciplining of their grandchildren, preferring a "norm of noninterference." Grandparents often refrain from telling their grown children how to raise the grandchildren, even when they do not like something they see. Most contemporary grandparents value their independence; many would be unwilling to give up their life-styles for the hard, often frustrating work of raising children again.

Family roles change during this stage. Children may or may not be present in the home. For caregivers, the end of the daily active responsibility for children is usually a significant change in their lives. Relationships between spouses change, and couple may have to refamiliarize themselves with each other. For many this may be a time for new or renewed companionship. Survival of the marriage after children leave home may depend on the growth, maturity, and commitment of each partner. Research shows that the majority of empty-nest females actually look forward to the emancipation from parenting duties, seeing it as an opportunity to further develop their personal and social roles.

The role of grandparenting often begins at this developmental stage. Because it often does not have the constraints and responsibilities of childrearing, grandparenting becomes a rich and rewarding experience for many middle-aged adults.

On the other hand, most adults are not prepared for the increased responsibility of caring for aging parents. Economic stress and emotional pressure are both associated with the role reversals sometimes known as "parenting the parent." Studies have indicated that a midlife daughter is most likely to be involved in elder care with her parents and her husband's parents.

Health Maintenance.

Nutrition. Many adults slow down in their middle adult years; therefore, they need fewer calories than they did in their teens and twenties. About 34 million adult Americans, or 25% of the population, are overweight. This is defined as being 20% over the desirable weight for one's sex, height, and body build. Inadequate calorie intake, or undernutrition, is also becoming more common. In some cases, this is due to poverty; however, in many cases it is due to self-inflicted dieting.

Average adults without special dietary restrictions will be healthier if they choose plenty of dark-green leafy vegetables, fresh fruits, and whole grain breads, rice, pasta, and cereal products to make up a large proportion of their total daily caloric intake, as per the recommendations of the Food Pyramid guidelines. A reduced intake of fat is recommended; most of it should come from unsaturated fats such as soy, sunflower, corn, or safflower oil. High blood levels of saturated fats and cholesterol contribute to atherosclerosis, coronary heart disease, and cancer.

Physical and dental examinations. The person in middle adulthood should have regular physical and dental examinations. Preventive American Cancer Society guidelines should be followed (see Chapter 38).

Sleep and rest. The adult in this age group sleeps less and has more awakenings than younger adults. The need for additional daytime rest may lessen the number of nighttime hours of sleep required.

Late Adulthood: 65 and Older

The experience of growing old can be examined from many different approaches. Aging is a normal condition of human existence, and has been studied from sociological, physiological, and psychological perspectives. All these views are interrelated throughout the life span. Gerontologists, who study the older adult and the aging process, note that many 70-year-olds today act and think as 50-year-olds did 10 or 20 years ago.

The fact remains that everyone must age. The physiological changes are not universal or necessarily inevitable, and the changes are often compatible with many interventions and treatments.

How an individual responds to the age-related changes visible in the mirror is related to the person's self-esteem. Successful aging depends on the individual's capacity to cope and ability to change. The process of aging affects the individual, the family, and society at large (see gerontological box).

The sociological issues of aging are concerned with work, retirement, social security, and health care. As more and more people reach late adulthood, society needs to recognize and value these individuals' knowledge, skills, and contributions. Preparation and planning for the future need to be addressed and encouraged in the early adult years because this helps to prepare, support, and enhance future adjustments. Flexible services and financial assistance programs need to be implemented to help people fulfill their goals.

The response to getting older can also be related to one's lifelong health habits, diet, and exercise patterns. Family, love, friendships, and intimate relationships are additional factors important to survival and well-being (Fig. 7-10). Regardless of one's age, these relationships are crucial to the individual's happiness. Love relationships vary in intensity and meaning in adulthood. Early on, these relationships usually have an intense physical basis, which leads to intimacy, respect, and commitment; although intense sexual drive decreases with age, sexual

GERONTOLOGICAL CONSIDERATIONS

- Each generation has its own central life tasks to complete. As more generations coexist, the needs of one age group can conflict with that of others. This increases intergenerational stress and can lead to altered family dynamics.
- Changes in roles and relationships present major developmental challenges to older adults.
- Currently 12% of the population is older than 65. By the year 2030, this will increase to 20%.
- With increased emphasis on wellness and preventive care, today's older adults are living longer, healthier lives. However, longer lifespans result in an increased presence of chronic and degenerative disorders.
- Health care needs of the aging population will place increased demands of the health care delivery system.
- The cost of providing care for the increasing large older adult population is a major societal concern. It is likely to have a significant impact on the amount and type of health care coverage provided by insurance companies and the government.
- Older Adults are a politically active group, and as their numbers increase, they are having an impact on all aspects of the society, including the entertainment, travel, and housing industries.
- Although some are poor older adults as a group they generally have more discretionary income than younger individuals and therefore have a significant impact on the economy.

behavior remains an important part of many adult relationships.

Ageism. **Ageism**—a form of discrimination and prejudice against the older adult—definitely exists. Like racism and sexism, ageism works to prevent people from being as happy and productive as they can be. It is passed on from generation to generation by the process of socialization. Society today must relinquish old stereotypes about the older adult. The purpose of this section is to refute the negative stereotypes, to present a more realistic positive view of aging, and to help the reader identify the normal physical patterns of aging so that deviations from the norm may be recognized. Aging should not be seen only as a decline; it involves growth as well as decline.

Before reading this portion of the chapter, it is important for the reader to examine personal beliefs about aging. Box 7-20 on p. 106 has a brief list of true-false statements that will help you clarify your beliefs.

The number of older persons has grown steadily over the past century. Between 1900 and 1985 there was a 10-fold increase in the number of older persons. By 2020 we can expect 20% of the population to be over 65 years of age.

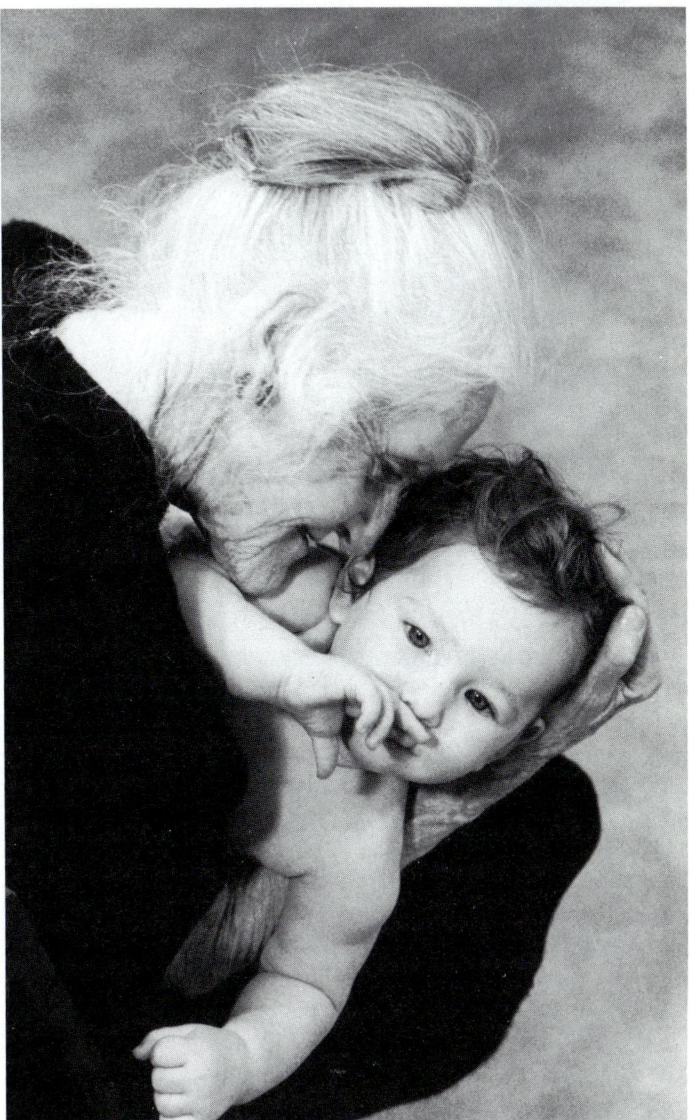

FIG. 7-10 Beauty throughout the life span.

Every year another group of adults reaches late adulthood. Who are these people? What are they like? In order to understand our older population, we must first consider what we mean by late adulthood. For our purposes, late adulthood will be defined as age 65 or older. We can further subdivide this state into: "young older adult" (ages 65 to 74), "middle older adult" (ages 75 to 84), and "older older adult" (over age 85). This population is constantly changing as new individuals enter the group and others leave through death. Each person has a uniquely personal history, reflecting many influences. Box 7-21 on p. 106 lists keys to successful aging.

Theories of Aging. For centuries, humanity has been fascinated with the concept of aging. Many theories have

Box 7-20 YOUR BELIEFS ON AGING

_____ 1. All old people become senile.
_____ 2. Most older people live in a nursing home or other institutional setting.
_____ 3. Most older persons are isolated from their families.
_____ 4. Most older persons have no interest in or capacity for sexual relationships.
_____ 5. Older workers are less productive than younger people.
_____ 6. Intelligence declines in old age.
_____ 7. Older persons should cease exercising and just rest.
_____ 8. Marked personality changes occur in the older person.
_____ 9. Older persons naturally become inflexible and demanding.
_____ 10. Older persons have less satisfaction from life.

All the answers to these 10 statements should be false.

Box 7-21 KEYS TO SUCCESSFUL AGING

- Practice pleasurable activities.
- View life as meaningful.
- Maintain a positive self-image.
- Accept responsibility for the past.
- Be optimistic.
- Remain motivated to maintain or expand intellectual capacity.
- Participate in a planned exercise program.

attempted to define the causes of and to develop measures to halt or postpone the aging process. One of the earliest theories of aging, generated by Hippocrates, speculated that aging was an irreversible natural event caused by a decrease in body heat. Later, Galen supported this concept and postulated (to make claim for as real or true) that aging was a lifelong process rather than an event occurring at the end of the life span. Leonardo DaVinci, among the first to attempt to identify the physical changes associated with aging, performed comparison autopsies on old men and young children. After 1900, only a few scientists focused on aging as their main interest. Finally, in the past 25 years, we have begun to see a renewed interest in researching the causes of the aging process. Recent theories now include autoimmunity, free radicals (a compound with an extra electron or protein), wear and tear, and biological programming, among others.

Autoimmunity theory. The autoimmunity theory holds that with aging the body becomes less able to recognize or tolerate the "self." As a result, the immune system produces antibodies that act against the "self." This theory is supported by the increased accumulation of lymphocytes, plasma cells found in the tissues of normal, healthy, older persons.

The primary organs of the immune system (thymus and bone marrow) are believed to be affected by the aging process. As one ages, the thymus decreases in size and weight and becomes less able to produce T cells. The bone marrow stem cells also show reduced efficiency in performing certain functions. As the ability of the immune system decreases, there is an increased risk of developing infection and cancer (see Chapter 36).

Free radical theory. Free radicals are highly reactive cellular components derived from unstable atoms or molecules. Free radicals have a reduced cellular efficiency and cause an accumulation of cellular waste. Some free radicals are produced by radiation, heat, or oxidation. The presence of free radicals may accelerate aging and result in the death of an organism. Lipofuscin is a pigmented material that accumulates in many organs as a part of aging. This accumulation interferes with the diffusion and transportation of essential metabolites and may also contribute to the aging process.

Wear-and-tear theory. According to the wear-and-tear theory, age is not based on one's chronological age, but is determined by the amount of wear and tear that one experiences. Many believe that structural and functional changes associated with growing old are accelerated by abuse of the body.

Biological programming theory. Some theorists claim that there is a hereditary basis for aging, evidenced by the similarities in life expectancies in a particular family. Further evidence supporting the theory of biological programming comes from "in vitro" cell studies. One early theory suggested that aging was a programmed genetic occurrence that was due to specific aging genes. Another theory cited aging as the result of progressive environmental damage to cells, interfering with normal cell functions. Aging has been attributed to the accumulation of lipofuscin, lipids, and fat. Changes in collagen structure and degenerative changes in elastin make tissues more stiff, less pliable, and less elastic and efficient.

All that is conclusive at this time is that aging is a slow, continuous, complex process that probably involves both intrinsic and extrinsic factors.

Psychological theories

Disengagement theory. According to supporters of the disengagement theory of aging, there should be a natural withdrawal or disengagement between the individual and society. This withdrawal can be initiated either by the individual or by others in society. Believers suggest that such withdrawal prevents older adults from experiencing frustration when they can no longer function adequately, while allowing a younger member of society to fulfill the now-empty role. This process is characterized as a normal, inevitable, universal process. The major criticisms of this disengagement theory include:

1. It does not allow for the many active, functional older adult.
2. The process is not seen in all cultural groups and it is, therefore, not universal.

Activity theory. According to this theory, the older person who is more active socially will more likely adjust well to aging. Various studies have shown that those with more social involvement have higher morale and better life satisfaction and personal adjustment. The number and quality of the activities are important. If activities or roles are given up, replacements should be found. Meaningful activities involving close, personal contact are extremely important. Activities of this nature reinforce one's self-concept, which in turn is associated with a higher life satisfaction.

Continuity theory. Supporters of this theory suggest that the critical factors in one's adjustment to old age are previously developed coping abilities and the ability to maintain previous roles and activities. Knowledge of and an understanding of a person's personality type can be useful in predicting the response to the aging process. Persons who were never highly involved will likely maintain the same level of involvement in old age. On the other hand, individuals who were highly involved and actively engaged with society need to remain active and involved with similar intensity. Supporters of the continuity theory contend that a person's adjustment to the aging process will be eased by maintaining similar roles and interests as developed earlier in life.

Physical Characteristics. Aging is a complex process that affects cells, tissues, and organs. Like growth and development, aging occurs at a highly individualized rate. There is a gradual reduction in the number and a change in the composition of aging cells. There is usually a slow increase in body weight until 45 to 50 years of age and then a gradual decline begins. Body fat content and distribution differ in men and women. The accumulation of adipose tissue in females can be found over the chest, waist, hips, and thighs. Adipose tissue in the male is deposited mostly in the waist, chest, and lower abdomen.

Loss of height begins after the age of 50. Most of the noticeable decrease in the trunk length is a result of the increase in spinal curvature caused by a slight thinning of the intervertebral disks. In addition to the shortening of the spine, certain abnormal postures and contours are noted. Kyphosis, an exaggeration of the thoracic curvature, may increase with aging. This can lead to a barrel-chest appearance, which may affect the position of the diaphragm and reduce the effectiveness of inspiration. These and other postural changes may affect body posture, mobility, gait, and respiratory efficiency.

Common age-related changes specific to each body system are listed in Table 7-4 on pp. 108-109, along with suggested nursing interventions to minimize the effect of these changes.

Psychosocial Development. Years of living, successes, failures, strengths, weaknesses, and all the early experiences influence the emotional stability of the older individual. Despite the physiological changes associated with the aging process, the older years should be viewed as a time of satisfaction and pleasure. Older adults must recognize their physical limitations and begin a process of adjustment and acclimation to their new needs.

Erikson described the challenge of late adulthood as ego integrity versus a sense of despair. The task here is to evaluate one's life and accomplishments and find satisfaction and meaning to life (Fig. 7-11). The process of

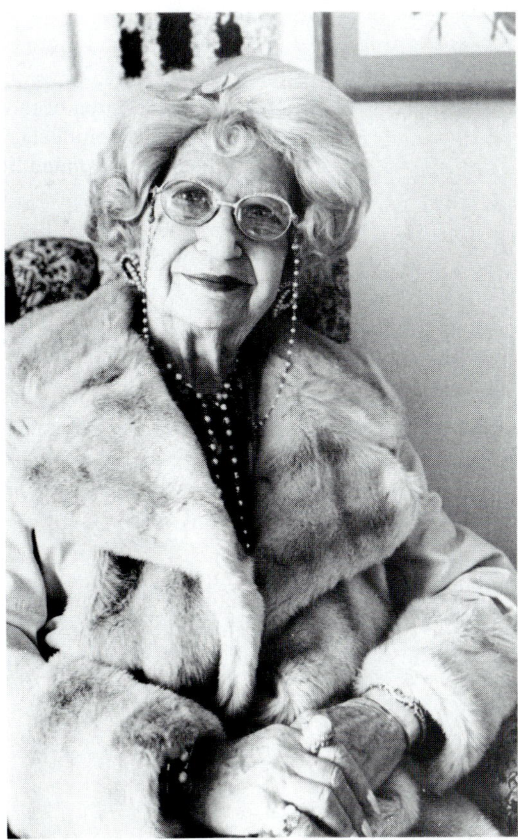

FIG. 7-11 Tranquility. (Photograph by Christine Becker.)

TABLE 7-4 Common Age-Related Changes

System	Normal Changes	Suggested Nursing Interventions
Musculoskeletal system		
Bones, muscles, joints, and connective tissue	Mineral salts move from bones to blood, making bones more porous; tendons, ligaments less elastic; increase in joint stiffness with less range of motion; varying degrees of increase of flexion at wrists, hips, knees, producing less joint mobility, agility, and endurance; thinning of vertebral disks	Maintain mobility. Encourage passive and active exercises. Avoid fatigue. Use assistive aids when indicated.
Nervous system	Fewer, smaller neurons (nerve cells), slowed reaction time, decrease in tactile sensitivity, decrease in pain perception, altered motor coordination	Allow adequate time to complete activities. Avoid burning and chilling related to diminished sensitivity. Encourage position changes; inspect skin daily.
Special senses		
Taste and smell	Decline in taste and smell perception.	Use smoke detectors. Serve attractive, colorful food.
Vision	Decreased tear production, increase in lens density; presbyopia (farsightedness; loss of elasticity of lens); yellowing of lens; slowing of accommodation (reaction to changes in light and distance); narrowing of visual field; decrease in depth perception	Encourage annual eye exams. Use more diffuse lighting. Use bright colors (red, yellow). Place articles within visual field. Use night lights.
Hearing	Presbycusis (increased difficulty hearing high-pitched sounds); increase in degenerative changes within ear structure; increase in buildup of wax production	Speak slowly, clearly. Face individual. Do not shout. Speak in lower tones. Decrease background noises. Encourage use of aids if available.
Respiratory system		
Ribcage	Increase in calcification of thorax; respiratory muscles weaken, producing diminished respiratory efficiency; maximum breathing capacity reduced; more susceptible to respiratory infection; easily fatigued	Allow for rest periods. Encourage coughing and deep breathing.
Lungs	Alveoli (air sacs) thinner, smaller, with decreased alveolar surface for gaseous exchange; decreased cough reflex action; decreased ciliary action, reduced maximum breathing capacity	Maintain adequate exercise and nutrition. Avoid high-fat diets. Encourage regular physical examinations. Avoid overexertion and allow for rest between activities.
Cardiovascular system	Fewer blood cells produced; loss of elasticity and narrowing of blood vessels, with an increase in blood pressure, valves thicker, more rigid; heart requires more time to return to resting state; decreased cardiac output	Encourage regular, paced exercise with adequate rest periods. Maintain low-fat diet.
Integumentary system		
Skin	Paler, thinner, irregularly pigmented; decrease in moisture; decrease in sweat and sebaceous gland activity; less elastic, more wrinkling; loss of subcutaneous fat; skin more fragile and prone to injury	Inspect skin for impairment or signs of pressure. Change position frequently. Wash with water and mild soap as needed. Rinse thoroughly and pat dry skin. Use lotions to replenish moisture. To maintain body warmth, provide adequate clothing.
Reproductive system		
Female	Fallopian tubes atrophy and shorten; ovaries smaller, thinner; uterus, cervix smaller in size; vagina less elastic, more alkaline, drier; reproduction ceases	Suggest use of vaginal lubricants if indicated.

TABLE 7-4 Common Age-Related Changes—cont'd

System	Normal Changes	Suggested Nursing Interventions
Male	Increased size of prostate; decreased testosterone levels; decreased circulation and decreased rate and force of ejaculation	Instruct person to have annual prostate examinations and prostatic specific antigen (PSA) level test.
Endocrine	Slowing of thyroid gland activity; BMR decreases; decreased hormone production, affecting other systems	Recommend annual physical examination with thyroid function testing.
Urinary system	Fewer cells in kidney, decreased renal blood flow; less effective filtration; decreased bladder elasticity and capacity; need to void more frequently	Observe for signs of urinary tract infections. Observe closely for adverse drug reactions.
Hair	Increase in graying; balding changes occur; changes in distribution of body hair	
Nails	More fragile, brittle; appear dull opaque yellow or gray in color; toenails thicken	Have toenails trimmed by podiatrist as indicated.
Gastrointestinal system	Decrease in saliva produced; chewing efficiency decreases; decreased esophageal motility; total capacity of stomach reduced; decrease in gastric enzyme secretions; liver smaller in size; less absorption of nutrients; slowing of peristalsis	Ensure adequate fluid intake. Encourage annual dental checkups. Offer 5-6 small meals, rather than 3 large ones. Assess for indigestion. Encourage regular toileting habits.

reminiscing with others can further validate the meaning and importance of the individual's life. Those who can feel that their lives have been well spent and are satisfied with their decisions and achievements have mastered this task of integrity. This allows the person to continue life with a sense of dignity and peacefulness. Adults who are dissatisfied with their accomplishments often experience conflict and despair. Dissatisfaction contributes to a feeling of restlessness and a sense of panic that time is "running out." Often the individual feels the need for more time and a chance to do things over again differently.

There are many other factors that will also affect the older adult's adjustment to this stage of life. Retirement is a major adjustment for the older adult. Health and financial resources are critical elements in determining one's life satisfaction after retirement. Generally speaking, our society is relatively unprepared for the phenomenon known as retirement. Retirement creates many changes—some welcome, some not. Examples are changes in roles, self-esteem, support systems, life patterns, and leisure time. Retirement brings more time to spend as one wishes. Individuals, therefore, need to plan and discuss their hopes and expectations for the retirement period. Planning for retirement helps persons identify activities that will be meaningful and promote self-esteem and a sense of usefulness to both the person and society.

Family Roles Change with Time. For many individuals, the older years become a time to explore their feelings about parenting and grandparenting. Grandparenting today is often very different from the role of grandparenting three to four decades ago. Today's grandparent may be working and very active. During this stage, couples may need to adjust to increased time together, companionship, and closeness. Maintaining old friendships and exploring ways to form new ones along with continuing strong family ties can help soften the losses that might be experienced during this period.

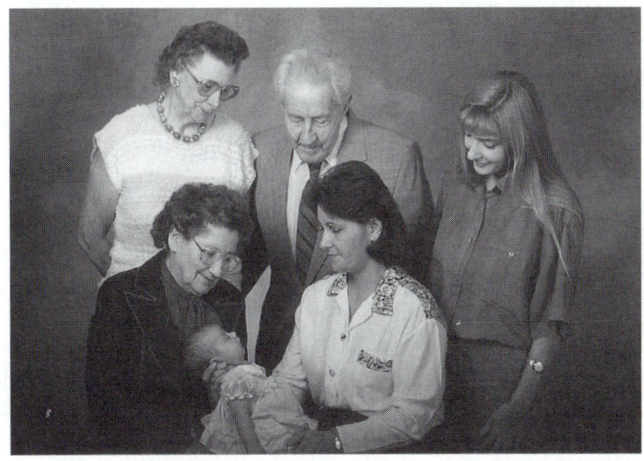

FIG. 7-12 Life span of five generations.

The impact of the death of a spouse is traumatic at any age. In the older years, being widowed is more common for women than men. Children and a strong social network may play important roles in supporting the surviving person. The experience of being widowed goes beyond ending a partnership. Role changes, changes in life-style, and access to fewer financial resources are just some of the adjustments created by the death of a spouse. Some older persons seeking companionship, love, and security find remarriage as a solution to the challenge of being widowed.

Cognitive and Intellectual Development. It is strongly suggested that older adults in good health and nurturing environments will have the capacity to maintain or increase their level of functioning, particularly in their areas of interest or specialization. Several factors have been identified as being important to continued cognitive functioning: level of education, work roles, personality, health, life-style, and the relevancy of the tasks. It is possible that some "practical" abilities may decline with age, while others may be stable or improve with age.

Memory. Some older adults notice some changes in memory. This benign forgetfulness is far more common than the forgetfulness associated with Alzheimer's disease. As adults advance in years, there appears to be a greater loss of recent memory over remote memory. An older individual may forget what was served for breakfast 2 hours earlier and yet may remember in great detail the events of a wedding many decades ago. Older persons are slower than younger people, but often are more accurate. Many people believe that the older person is more willing to sacrifice speed for accuracy.

Health Maintenance. Health promotion rests on the belief that individuals can have a strong influence on their health status. Environment, social patterns, diet, exercise, and personal habits are all factors that determine a person's state of health. It is imperative that health care workers clarify the common misconceptions about health and aging. It needs to be emphasized that persons of all ages can benefit from a change in life-style, even in the later years (see Box 7-17).

Nutrition. Considerable evidence has been documented supporting the relationship between dietary habits and health. Older adults should have a diet of foods that are higher in quality and lower in quantity while maintaining the basic nutrient content. Although caloric needs are highly individualized, generally speaking, older adults are less active with more adipose tissue and less body mass, and therefore, may need less daily calorie intake. Most frequently recommended are diets that are lower in saturated fats and carbohydrates and high in fiber. Common threats to the older adult's adequate diet are such things as poor oral health, lack of appetite, food intolerances, and constipation. Proper nutritional assessment and counseling can identify problems and offer interventions. To ensure dietary compliance, long-standing habits and cultural influences must be taken into consideration when introducing any dietary changes. Various psychosocial factors may also affect the older person's diet. Economic factors may determine what foods are purchased and included in the diet. Loneliness can also contribute to an inadequate diet. Often the inability to shop for and prepare meals may result in less than desirable diets. Another crucial component in the older person's diet is adequate fluid intake. Older adults should maintain a minimum daily intake of 1500 ml/day. Avoidance of fluids is commonly attributed to the person's fear of incontinence and a lack of thirst.

Activity. Throughout the life span, evenly paced, satisfying exercise is crucial to general well-being. Exercise has been related to improving cardiovascular functioning, lowering blood pressure while enhancing oxygen utilization, and maintaining joint mobility. Exercise should never be to the point of exhaustion and always should be followed by rest periods to recuperate and restore the body to its maximum level of functioning.

Sleep. Older individuals require more rest, but need less actual sleep. More accidents occur on awakening at night, and safety concerns need to be considered. Using night lights and reducing excess furniture or clutter may decrease the risk of night-time injury. Sleep for the older person may be affected by medications, alcohol, caffeine, stress, and environmental noise and temperature.

Immunization. In addition to annual physical examinations, the older adult is best protected by being immunized yearly against influenza and pneumonia.

Safety. Most accidents are preventable. The key to prevention is the knowledge and the recognition of the contributory factors that place the person at greater risk for accident or injury. Diminished sight along with changes in posture or balance can dispose the older person to the risk of falls. A single fall may produce an injury requiring a long period of immobilization and diminishing the person's independence and self-esteem. For a summary of safety tips for the older adult, see Box 7-22.

Since older adults represent a rapidly growing segment of the population, it is important for individuals to prepare for and understand the aging process. An individual's adjustment to aging is a uniquely complex process. Aging can be viewed from many different approaches: sociological, physiological, and psychosocial.

Box 7-22

SAFETY TIPS FOR THE OLDER ADULT

- Minimize clutter or excess furniture in rooms and hallways.
- Remove scatter rugs.
- Use hand rails on stairs.
- Install grab bars in showers and bathroom.
- Use night lights.
- Get up slowly from a lying flat position.
- Use caution in going from well-lighted areas to darkened areas or vice versa.
- If self-medicating, use dispensing aids to decrease the risk of error.
- Wear properly fitting shoes and clothing.
- Allow enough time—do not rush or hurry.

Box 7-23

DEVELOPMENTAL TASKS OF LATE ADULTHOOD

- Accepts one's life
- Recognizes accomplishments
- Finds satisfaction with new roles, relationships, and leisure time
- Maximizes independence and maintains high level of involvement
- Accepts one's own mortality and prepares for death (see Fig. 7-12).

Health promotion is the belief that people can have an influence on their own health. Measures to maintain good health relate to nutrition, exercise, and life-style practices.

The major tasks of late adulthood are listed in Box 7-23.

REFERENCES AND SUGGESTED READINGS

1. Adlersberg M, Thorne S: Emerging from the chrysalis: older widows in transition, *J Gerontol Nurs* 16(1):4, 1990.
2. Ali N, Bennett S: Postmenopausal women: factors in osteoporosis preventive behaviors, *J Gerontol Nurs,* 18(12):23, 1992.
3. Aligood K: Caring for victims of child abuse, *Imprint,* 39(2):63, 1992.
4. Bender P: Deceptive distress in the elderly, *Am J Nurs,* 92(10):29, 1992.
5. Biester D: Childhood immunization: Nursing's role and responsibility, *J Pediatr Nurs* 7(1):65, 1992.
6. Bowlby J: *Attachment and loss,* New York, 1982, Basic Books.
7. Brazelton T: *On becoming a family: the growth of attachment,* New York, 1992, A Merlbyd Lawrence Book.
8. Burke M, Walsh M: *Gerontologic nursing: care of the frail elderly,* St Louis, 1992, Mosby.
9. Caplan F: *The first twelve months of life,* New York, 1985, Bantam Books.
10. Cavanagh JC: *Adult development and aging,* Belmont, Calif, 1990, Wadsworth.
11. Christensen B, Kockrow E: *Foundations of nursing,* St Louis, 1991, Mosby.
12. Christiansen J, Grzybowski J: *Biology of aging,* St Louis, 1993, Mosby.
13. Clawson J, Sears J: A stepmother in the family, *Pediatr Nurs,* 15(3):249, 1989. May/June 1990.
14. Coffman S: Parent and infant attachment: review of nursing research, 1981-1990, *Pediatr Nurs* 18(4):421, 1992.
15. Coppens N: Parental responses to children in unsafe situations, *Pediatr Nurs* 16(6):571, 1990.
16. Dickson E, Schulte M, Silverman B: *Maternal-infant nursing care,* ed 2, St Louis, 1994, Mosby.
17. Eliopoulos C: *Gerontological nursing,* Philadelphia, 1993, Lippincott.
18. Erikson E: *The life cycle completed,* New York, 1985, Norton.
19. Fraiberg S: *The magic years,* New York, 1981, Scribners.
20. Gorby R: Assessing child abuse in community health nursing, *Imprint,* 39(2):77, 1992.
21. Green C: Clinical considerations: midlife daughters and their aging parents, *J Gerontol Nurs* 17(11):6, 1991.
22. Hartford S: Overview of child maltreatment, *Imprint* 39(2):56, 1992.
23. Hauck M: Cognitive abilities of preschool children: implications for nurses working with young children, *J Pediatr Nurs* 6(4):230, 1991.
24. Hiatt S, Bross D: Nursing, child abuse and child protection teams, *Imprint* 39(2):69, 1992.
25. Igoe J: Health promotion, health, protection, and disease prevention in childhood, *Pediatr Nurs* 12(3):291, 1992.
26. Igoe J, Goodwin L: Meeting the challenge of immunizing the nation's children, *Pediatr Nurs* 17(6):583, 1991.
27. Jacobson J: Nursing's response to the aging population, *Home Health Nurse* 8(3):24, 1990.
28. Jordan P: Laboring for relevance: expectant and new fatherhood, *Nurs Res* 39(1):11, 1990.
29. Kelly S: Methodological issues in child sexual abuse research, *J Pediatr Nurs,* 6(1):21, 1991.
30. Koepke J et al: Becoming parents: feelings of adoptive mothers, *Pediatr Nurs,* 17(4):333, 1991.
31. Logsdon D: Conceptions of health and health behaviors of preschool children, *J Pediatr Nurs* 6(6):396, 1991.
32. Loranger N: Play intervention: strategies for the Hispanic toddler with separation anxiety, *Pediatr Nurs* 18(6):571, 1992.
33. Masters W, Johnson V: *Human sexual response,* Boston, 1966, Little, Brown.
34. Mays R: Response to "maternal role satisfaction: a new approach to assessing parenting," *Scholar Inq Nurs Pract* 6(2):151, 1992.
35. Melnyk B: Changes in parent-child relationship following divorce, *Pediatr Nurs,* 17(4):337, 1991.
36. Mercer R, Ferketich S: Predictors of parental attachment during early parenthood, *J Adv Nurs* 15:268, 1990.
37. *Mosby's dictionary of Medicine, nursing, and allied health,* ed 4, St Louis, 1994, Mosby.
38. Ohashi J: Maternal role satisfaction: a new approach to assessing parenting, *Scholar Inq Nurs Pract* 6(2):135, 1992.

39. Palkovitz R: Changes in father-infant bonding beliefs across couples' first transition to parenthood, *Matern Child Nurs J* 20(3):141, 1992.
40. Palmieri D: Clearing up the confusion: adverse effects of medications in the elderly, *J Gerontol Nurs* 17(10):32, 1991
41. Phipps W et al: *Medical-surgical nursing: concepts and clinical practice,* St Louis, 1991, Mosby.
42. Preston D, Dellasegas C: Elderly women and stress: does marriage make a difference? *J Gerontol Nurs* 16(4):27, 1990.
43. Summers K: Providing for play in the care of children, *Pediatr Nurs,* 17(3):266, 1991.
44. Thomas D: Caring for the perimenopausal woman at home, *Home Health C Nurse,* 8(4):9, 1990.
45. Tucker S: Adolescent patterns of communication about the menstrual cycle, sex and contraception, *J Pediatr Nurs* 5(6):393, 1990.
46. Vessey J, Mahon M: Therapeutic play and the hospitalized child, *J Pediatr Nurs* 5(5):308, 1990.
47. Vessey JA, Ritchie SR: The who, what, and when of pediatric immunization, *RN* 56(9):42, 1993.
48. Whaley L, Wong D: *Nursing care of infants and children,* St Louis, 1991, Mosby.
49. Williams M: Creating a positive impact on the health & well-being of children & families through education, *J Pediatr Nurs* 6(1):72, 1991.
50. Wilson J: What do we owe our aging parents? *Home Healthc Nurse* 8(6):42, 1990.

CHAPTER CHALLENGE

KEY POINTS

- Development is a lifelong process that begins at conception and ends at death.
- All types of families serve similar basic functions: protection, nurturance, education, sustenance, and socialization of its members.
- Growth patterns suggest rapid growth during infancy, continued growth during toddler and preschool years, slowed steady growth during the school years, followed by a rapid surge of growth during puberty and adolescence.
- Erikson identified a central task that needed resolution at each stage of the life span: infancy, toddler, preschool, school age, adolescence, early adulthood, middle adulthood, and late adulthood.
- Piaget focused on the concept of cognitive development beginning in infancy and continuing throughout the childhood years.
- Immunization follows an age-based schedule.
- Accidental injuries are a major cause of death during infancy, childhood, and adolescence.
- Consistent discipline and supervision are needed throughout childhood.
- Peer relationships become significant at school age.
- Adolescence is the transitional period between childhood and adulthood.
- Adulthood is marked by significant events: career decisions, marriage, new social relationships, and financial concerns.
- Certain physical changes become evident during middle age, including graying of hair and vision changes.
- Menopause and hormonal changes characterize the reproductive changes of the middle-aged female.
- Role changes emerge during middle adulthood, including change in family roles, relationships with grown children, grandparenting, and possible career changes.
- Late adulthood is marked by a gradual slowing of the body's functioning.
- Several significant physical changes become evident in the older adult.
- Family changes and an increased awareness of one's mortality are common adjustments of the aging process.
- Life review and acceptance of one's strengths and weaknesses are a necessary part of the aging process.
- Several theories attempt to explain aging; however, no one theory is universally accepted.
- Aging, like growth, is a highly individualized process.

STUDY QUESTIONS

1. Bob and Sally are parents of an infant girl. The pediatric nurse advises them that regular brushing of a baby's teeth should begin:
   1. When the baby is able to hold the toothbrush
   2. When the baby's first tooth appears
   3. When the first four teeth erupt
   4. When the child begins preschool
2. Alice, a 5-month-old, has been brought to well-child clinic. Alice's vital signs are measured. Which of the following sets of readings would be considered normal for Alice?

1.	T: 96	Ht. rate: 100	R: 20	BP: 100/70
2.	T: 97	Ht. rate: 80	R: 30	BP: 120/70
3.	T: 98	Ht. rate: 120	R: 30	BP: 90/50
4.	T: 99.6	Ht. rate: 160	R: 60	BP: 80/40

3. Steve is 10 months of age. He is a very active and healthy infant. Since falls are a common cause of injury to infants, parents should be advised to:
   1. Place the infant in an infant seat on the table top
   2. Use blankets around the infant on a bed or couch
   3. Place gates at top and bottom of stairs
   4. Use pillows to secure infant when he is left on the bed

4. Joey, age 2, is seen in the physician's office for a regular checkup. His parents state that "he must be sick because he doesn't eat as much as he used to." After assessing Joey the nurse might explain that:
   1. Toddlers should have an increase in their appetite
   2. Toddlers need less food per unit of weight than infants
   3. Appetite lags may indicate discipline problems in the toddler
   4. The toddler should be encouraged to eat more at each meal
5. At approximately how many months of age does the child's vocabulary increase to include two-word sentences:
   1. 12 months
   2. 24 months
   3. 36 months
   4. 48 months
6. Sarah and Joey are 4 years of age. They are busily engaged in a play activity in preschool. Observing preschoolers at play in preschool reveals typical play as:
   1. Imitative
   2. Competitive
   3. Parallel
   4. Solitary
7. The correct order of Piaget's four stages of cognitive development is:
   1. Preoperational, sensorimotor, concrete operational, formal operational
   2. Sensorimotor, preoperational, concrete operational, formal operational
   3. Preoperational, concrete operational, sensorimotor, formal operational
   4. Sensorimotor, concrete operational, preoperational, formal operational
8. Sammy is a 9-year-old school-age child. Peer relationships are important to the school-age child. Which of the following is characteristic of 9-year-old Sammy:
   1. Boys and girls play together.
   2. Activities are noncompetitive.
   3. Loyalties and peer attachments are with peers of the same sex.
   4. He has difficulty sharing and taking turns.
9. Erikson identified the psychosocial task for the adolescent period as the task of identity. Which of the following would be a positive sign of identity in a young adolescent:
   1. Continuous dieting
   2. Getting pregnant
   3. Obtaining a job and saving money
   4. Focusing on peer relationships
10. According to the text the onset of puberty refers to:
    1. Cognitive development
    2. Psychosocial development
    3. Production of eggs and sperm
    4. Spiritual development

8

CULTURAL ASPECTS OF NURSING CARE

Bobbie Bloch

KEY TERMS

cultural healing beliefs
culture
dominant group
ethnic stereotype
ethnicity
ethnocentrism
minority group
racism
subculture
values

LEARNING OBJECTIVES

After reading this chapter, the student should be able to do the following:

- Define the key terms.
- Describe ways in which culture influences an individual.
- Explain how ethnocentrism can cause cultural conflicts in the nurse/patient relationship.
- Discuss how cultural variables may influence health behavior.
- Use cultural data to bring about change in health behavior of a patient.
- Evaluate the effects of nurses' values, beliefs, and practices on the patient related to ethnicity.

RELATED TOPICS OF INTEREST

- Communication (Chapter 4)
- Life span development (Chapter 7)

Cultural beliefs and personal characteristics determine health behavior in individuals and families. More than half of all health problems are the result of behavior and life-style. If nursing's goal is to promote health while respecting individual value systems and life-styles, culture-based health behavior must be understood.

Nurses as a group reflect society's cultural mix. In North America, the majority of nurses hold values, beliefs, and attitudes typical of the dominant middle class. In addition, nurses belong to a separate culture as members of the health care team. When two people of differing cultural backgrounds interact, significant communication barriers may arise unless at least one of the persons is willing and able to recognize and adapt to other's values. To care for others, nurses must be able to accept a wide diversity of beliefs, practices, and ideas about health and illness, including many that differ from their own.

Acceptance of alternative beliefs about health and illness can be more difficult for nurses than might initially be assumed. As health care professionals educated in and exposed to the established health care system, nurses share certain values, attitudes, and beliefs about health and illness about which they may not consciously think. These ways of thinking have been shaped by more than 2000 years of Western thought broadly known as *Hippocratic medicine.* Modern health care is based on rational, scientific, and biomedical principles directed at solving human health problems. As part of the dominant culture, the health care culture is interwoven with established social, religious, political, and economic systems. Certain aspects of the health care culture, such as nurse-physician relationships and provider-patient relationships, are governed by a broadly shared set of customs and protocols.

The cultural beliefs of some patients may conflict with the cultural beliefs many nurses share. Nurses cannot hope to plan meaningful health care for their patients without at least understanding their own health beliefs.

Thousands of subcultures exist within a culture, and everyone is a member of several. Although subcultures have an identity uniquely their own, they are also related to the overall culture in certain ways. Major subcultural groups in the United States include African Americans (12.1%), Hispanic Americans (9%), Asian Americans (2.9%), and Native Americans (0.8%). In Canada, major subcultures include French Canadians (27%) and Natives (2%).

WAYS TO DEVELOP CULTURAL SENSITIVITY

- Recognize that cultural diversity exists.
- Demonstrate respect for people as unique individuals, with culture as one factor that contributes to their uniqueness.
- Respect the unfamiliar.
- Identify and examine your own cultural beliefs.
- Recognize that some cultural groups have definitions of *health* and *illness* as well as practices that attempt to promote health and cure illness, which may differ from the nurse's own.
- Be willing to modify health care delivery in keeping with the patient's cultural background.
- Do not expect all members of one cultural group to behave in exactly the same way.
- Appreciate that each person's cultural values are ingrained and therefore very difficult to change.

This chapter will give some examples of cultural characteristics of several ethnic minority groups, but it is beyond the scope of this discussion to present in greater detail every group known.

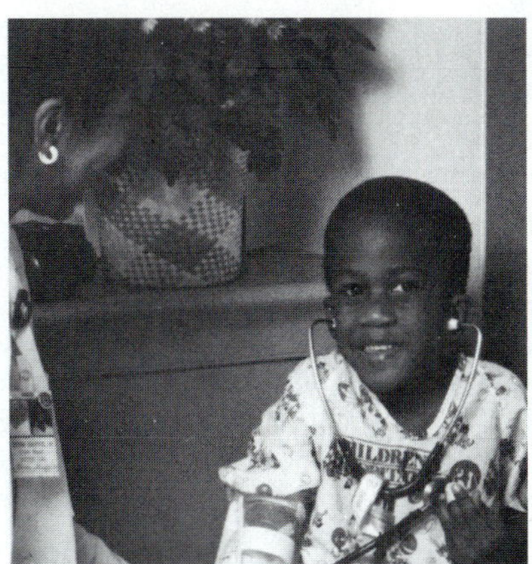

CULTURE

Definition of Culture

Culture may be defined as the learned ways of acting and thinking which are transmitted by group members and which provide for each individual ready-made and tested solutions for vital problems. Culture includes such areas as diet, language and communication process, religion, art and history, family life processes, social groups' interactive patterns, value orientations, and healing beliefs and practices. How persons resolve problems related to basic human needs is strongly influenced by these cultural elements. Because culture is devised by people to solve human problems, it is universal.

Characteristics of Culture

Murray and Zentner[16] have identified three major characteristics of culture as follows:

1. Culture is learned. A person learns behaviors, values, attitudes, and beliefs within his cultural family system. This learning is influenced mainly by the person's social status within a society and adaptation to his environment.
2. Culture is capable of change but remains stable. Language, traditions, and norms or customs may act as stabilizers for a culture.
3. Components or patterns are present in every culture. These include communication systems, means of economic and physical survival, transportation systems, family systems, social customs and mores, and religious systems.

Influences of Culture

Nurses providing care should consider all patients as individuals, because each person is unique. How a person is influenced, as well as the extent of the influence, depends on the individual. How a person is influenced by

GERONTOLOGICAL CONSIDERATIONS

- Cultural background has an impact on family dynamics and plays an important role in determining the role and status of the older person
- Older adults form a unique cultural group based on shared historical experiences. There may be fewer differences between two older individuals of diverse cultural backgrounds than between two persons of the same culture but from different age groups because of shifts in value systems that occurred over time.
- Some older adults may be less tolerant of other cultures as a result of influences or experiences early in their lives. This may result in misunderstandings and distrust when the care giver is of a cultural group different from the older person.
- Older persons experiencing disturbed cognitive function such as Alzheimer's disease often speak without regard for the cultural sensitivity of others. This can result in harmful comments being made to care givers and other persons.
- Many of older adults value "home remedies" and cultural practices regarding health care and may resist the attempts of care givers to change their practices even when they are harmful.
- Many older persons persist in religious practices of their yourth such as fasting or the use of religious symbols even though they are not currently promoted by their church. If these practices are not harmful, the older person's wishes should be respected.

his culture depends on the unique life experiences of the individual (e.g., family factors, "critical events," age, and socioeconomic level). Culture influences behavior patterns, communications process, and health and illness beliefs and practices. The nurse and the patient each have their own cultural life-styles. Because of these differences in cultural life-styles, nurses may find it diffi cult to accept diseases categorized as "hot" or "cold" or as the result of "God's will." Nurses may also question the use of herbal medicines such as ginseng as used for treatment by cultural healers. It is not that a nurse should change her beliefs, values, and practices related to health and illness to fit those of her patients, but she needs to gain an understanding of her patient's characteristics to provide effective care. If a nurse is not aware of a patient's cultural background, she may (1) misjudge the culture's effect on health care, (2) make culturally incorrect and improper nursing care judgments, and (3) provide poor and even unsafe interventions.[9]

To provide individualized nursing care, it is important for nurses to develop a positive approach in interacting with patients who are culturally and racially different. We all have a cultural background, and each person will decide which cultural characteristics are important. Even if a person considers herself to be mainstream American, she also has a cultural life-style. Trends or similarities that exist among persons belonging to a distinct cultural or racial group can be seen in their behavior and communication in the clinical or community setting. Gerontological considerations are listed in the box.

Box 8-1 FACTORS RELATED TO CULTURAL VARIATIONS AMONG ETHNIC/MINORITY GROUPS

Age
Religion
Dialect/language spoken
Gender identity and roles
Socioeconomic background
Geographical location in country of origin or current residence
Amount and type of interaction between younger and older generations
Degree of adoption of values in current country

The cultural variables described in this chapter are group characteristics of ethnic minorities. Again, these characteristics may not be shown by every member of a cultural group. A person never acquires a culture as a complete and absolute pattern; instead, he merely learns the main components of a **subculture** (an ethnic, regional, economic, or social group with characteristic patterns of behavior and ideals that distinguish it from the rest of a culture or society). Variations within a cultural group usually occur because of individual differences.[1] Examples of these differences are displayed in Box 8-1.

Because culture influences different individuals' values, attitudes, and behaviors in various ways, the nurse must not stereotype members of any cultural group. Porter[19] defined stereotype as "attitudinal sets in which we assign characteristics to another person solely on the basis of the class or category to which that person belongs." An **ethnic stereotype** is a fixed concept of how all members of an ethnic group act or think. Stereotypes may or may not bear any relationship to reality. For example, stereotypes based on racism are unrelated to reality.[23] An example of a stereotype is the belief that all patients of Japanese ancestry are uncomplaining and cooperative.

ETHNOCENTRISM AND CULTURAL CONFLICTS

Definition of Ethnocentrism

Ethnocentrism is the tendency to view members of other cultural or ethnic groups in terms of the standards of behavior and values of a person's own group.[19] Ethnocentrism restricts a person from accepting another culture favorably. For instance, an ethnocentric nurse might view all healing methods that differ from her own as primitive and unscientific. Both ethnocentrism and stereotyping can affect the quality of patient care.

When ethnocentrism increases, cultural racism can result. **Racism** is any ethnocentric activity—cultural, individual, or institutional, deliberate or not—that is based on the belief of the superiority of one racial group over other racial groups.

Racial/Cultural Conflicts

Cultural conflict between health professionals and their patients occurs when health care is perceived as unequal. For example, if a minority group has been stereotyped as dirty, a patient from the minority group may receive a nurse's emphasis on cleanliness and bathing as prejudice.

Aggression occurs when **minority group** (a racial, religious, or political group smaller than and differing from the larger, controlling group in a community or nation) members strike out against their subordinate status by engaging in hostile acts against members of the **dominant group** (a group exercising authority or influence; ruling or prevailing). The patient from a minority group may react to prejudice and discrimination with overt (direct) or covert (indirect) aggression. One form in which hostility may find expression is in humor—the joke. For example, a Puerto Rican patient says to a nurse: "Hey, Mr. Jones changed his room. Is he afraid of catching something from me? He acted like I was a strange thing from outer space or something (laughing)." The "joke" illustrates the patient's underlying feeling or belief that his roommate left because of his racial or ethnic minority status, and that it is safer to express that belief using humor rather than anger or hostility. It is in reality not meant to be funny, but to mask the patient's true feelings in a clinical environment. The astute nurse can often pick up significant clues concerning the patient's real sentiments and attitudes from such jokes. In contrast, sullenness or stubbornness and verbal hostility might be used by patients of a minority group to express more direct forms of frustration. Nurses should interact by showing sympathy and understanding to break down the wall of resistance.[10]

Sometimes it is impossible to change a patient's ideas, but if a nurse has dealt with her own feelings of racial prejudice, this is a step in the right direction and offers an example for others. Piero said, "Think through beliefs about people of other races. Most of us harbor prejudices. To be fair with ourselves, fellow workers, and patients, we must find them and overcome them."[6] Nurses also need to expand their knowledge of culture and analyze nurse/patient interactions in an attempt to resolve cultural conflicts.

Box 8-2 CULTURAL VARIABLES

1. Ethnic and racial identity
2. Value orientations
3. Language and communication process
4. Family system
5. Healing beliefs and practices
6. Religious beliefs and practices
7. Nutritional behavior and cultural influences

CULTURAL VARIABLES

Cultural variables (differences) are those characteristics generally identified with a particular cultural group. These variables may or may not be exhibited by every person from a cultural group. An understanding of the underlying development of the cultural variables is essential for carrying out an appropriate and effective cultural assessment. Box 8-2 highlights those variables that form the basis for cultural assessment.

Ethnic and Racial Identity

Werner[26] defines **ethnicity** as a group's "affiliation as a result of shared linguistic, racial, religious, and/or cultural background." For example, Africans and Puerto Ricans are members of ethnic groups, whereas the terms *Black* and *Oriental* describe membership in racial groups.

Value Orientations

Values are intrinsic beliefs about the worth of an entity or concept. They provide the basis for attitudes and behaviors, and they help a person establish a hierarchy of needs and goals. For example, different cultures place different values on privacy, courtesy, respect for elders, and the work ethic. Value orientations are defined as principles that assist in the solution of common human problems.

Language and Communication Process

The most difficult area for nurses and ethnic/cultural patients is in the communication process, since so much of the nursing process depends on communication. One example of communication variations is in the Filipino communication process. The patient who is Filipino is likely to view the nurse as an authority figure who should be treated with formality; thus a patient who is Filipino may appear aloof and reserved, even in an anxiety-provoking clinical situation. Another example is the different traditional communication patterns of Caucasians and African-Americans: the White tradition relies on a relatively rigid pattern of expression characterized by heavy dependence on the written word, whereas the African-American tradition is more memory-oriented and favors oral communication. Thus the nurse might find that visual aids could be used to address this communication style among African-American patients.

Family System

The extended family, including relatives beyond the basic family unit, is highly valued among many ethnic minority groups. Usually the entire family is involved when a person becomes ill. Older adults play a significant role in family functions in ethnic families. For example, the "issei" (first generation) Japanese expect their children, the "nisei" (second generation), to practice "oya koko," meaning caring for parents in old age. McGoldrick, Pearce, and Giordano[15] state that "individual behavior cannot be understood in isolation from the family context and that family behavior makes sense only in the larger framework of culture." Known characteristics of groups may assist in formulating initial thoughts and concerns about health and illness behavior of ethnic families.

For example, strong kinship bonds are highly prevalent among African-Americans as a means of survival, regardless of social class. If a family member cannot take care of a young child, often the child is informally adopted by another family member.[4] La Fargue[11] states that nurses are often not aware of this survival strategy among African-Americans "to immerse themselves in a domestic circle of kinfolk who will help them."

Four points to remember when assessing the ethnic/cultural importance of a patient's family system are described in Box 8-3.

Box 8-3 FACTORS TO CONSIDER IN ASSESSING FAMILY SYSTEM

1. Consider the family as a unit when planning a patient's care.
2. Consider how the family structure influences the patient's response to health/illness.
3. Consider the family's participation in the patient's care.
4. Consider the family's role in health promotion or illness causation.

Healing Beliefs and Practices

Cultural healing beliefs reflect a specific cultural group's orientation to health and illness. Alternative healing beliefs and practices may be the most difficult factors for the nurse to assess, because they differ greatly from the traditional scientific medical theories about health and illness with which nurses are familiar. Much research has been done to show these beliefs and practices are prevalent among ethnic/cultural groups.

For example, the Hmong from Southeast Asia believe in the idea of a "bad fate" person. Any child or adult who is disfigured or disabled is viewed as having become this way because the ancestor spirits and other spirits in nature have produced the malady.

Healing practices among ethnic minority groups commonly involve using herbs, potions, oils, powders, tokens, rituals, ceremonies, candles, and incense. The nurse on occasion may ask patients who are from an ethnic minority group if they are using cultural healing practices or employing cultural healers (spiritualist, voodoo priest, curandero, or Asian herbalist) that may impact on Western orthodox medicine. Nurses must understand that these beliefs often have great psychological impact on whether the patient gets well.

Religious Beliefs and Practices

Religious beliefs and practices often overlap with the cultural beliefs about the cause of illness and methods of cure. For example, pledges, prayers, and the wearing of clothing identified with saints are still practiced by some Hispanics during illnesses. Many Hispanics also believe that wellness or illness is the will of God. Religion is a major psychological support system for many ethnic minority patients. Patients should be encouraged to use this support system, and they should be allowed to keep or use talismans, tokens, or religious ceremonies that may help them combat the anxiety and stress associated with their illness and/or its treatment.

Nutritional Behavior and Cultural Influences

The nurse should assess food preferences and restrictions, meaning of foods, style of food preparation and consumption, frequency of eating, time of eating, and eating utensils that are culturally determined. Chinese believe that conditions such as dry mouth, constipation, or poor digestion are caused by eating too many hot foods (fried/spicy) and that hot foods must be balanced with cold foods (leafy vegetables). Finally, some American Indians use corn in many religious ceremonies, because corn is thought to possess medicinal qualities and may be sprinkled around an ill person to protect him.

Understanding the cultural basis of a patient's behavior will help the nurse appreciate differences in custom or practice that might otherwise be viewed as harmful to the patient's health. To provide effective care to patients from diverse cultural backgrounds, nurses must develop an understanding of ethnic/cultural data for those populations in their communities.

REFERENCES AND SUGGESTED READINGS

1. Anderson JM: Health care across cultures, *Nurs Outlook* 38:136, 1990.
2. Barkauskas V, et al: *Health and physical assessment,* St Louis, 1994, Mosby.
3. Bobak IM, Jensen MD: *Essentials of maternity nursing,* ed 3, St Louis, 1991, Mosby.
4. Bloch B: *The black family: rules and modes of communication.* In Wang F, Nath CL, Simoni PS, editors: *Living with change and choice in health,* Morgantown, W Va, 1986, Sigma Theta Tau, Alpha Rho Chapter.
5. Daniel JL, Smitherman G: *How I got over: communication dynamics in the black community.* In Carbaugh D, editor: *Cultural communication and intercultural contact,* Hillsdale, NJ, 1990, Lawrence Erlbaum Associates.
6. DeSantio L, Thomas J: The immigrant Haitan mother: transcultural nursing perspective on preventive health care for children, *J Transcult Nurs* 2(2), 1990.
7. Dossey B: Awakening the inner healer, *Am J Nurs* 91(8)30, 1991.
8. Giger JN, Davidhizar RE: Transcultural nursing assessment and intervention, St Louis, 1991, Mosby.
9. Henkle JO et al: Cultural diversity: a resource in planning and implementing nursing care, *Pub Health Nurs* 7:145, 1990.
10. Kuhni CQ: When cultures clash at the bedside, *RN* 53(1):23, 1990.
11. La Fargue JP: A survival strategy: kinship networks, *Am J Nurs* 80:1636, 1980.
12. Leininger M: Issues, questions, and concerns related to nursing diagnosis cultural movement from a transcultural nursing perspective, *J Transcult Nurs* 2(23), 1990
13. Leininger M: The significance of cultural concepts in nursing, *J Transcult Nurs* 2(52), 1990.
14. Long BC, Phipps WJ, Cassmeyer VL: *Medical-surgical nursing: a nursing process approach,* ed 3, St Louis, 1993, Mosby.
15. McGoldrick M, Pearce JK, Giordano J, editors: *Ethnicity and family therapy,* New York, 1982, Guilford Press.
16. Murray RB, Zentner JP: *Nursing concepts for health promotion,* ed 2, Englewood Cliffs, NJ, 1979, Prentice-Hall.
17. Phipps W, Long B, Woods N: *Medical-surgical nursing: concepts and clinical practice,* St Louis, 1991, Mosby.
18. Piero P: Black-White crisis, *Am J Nurs* 74:281, 1974.
19. Porter RE: An overview of intercultural communication. In Samovar LA, Porter RE, editors: *Intercultural communication: a reader,* Belmont, Calif, 1972, Wadsworth.
20. Potter PA, Perry AG: *Basic nursing: theory and practice,* ed 3, 1995, Mosby.
21. Potter PA, Perry AG: *Fundamentals of nursing: concepts, process, and practice,* ed 3, 1993, Mosby.
22. Rosenbaum JN: A cultural assessment guide: learning cultural sensitivity, *Can Nurse* 87(4):32, 1991.
23. Spector RE: *Cultural diversity in health and illness,* ed 3, Norwalk, Conn, 1991, Appleton & Lange.
24. Stone L: Cultural influences in community participation in health, *Soc Sci Med* 35(4):409, 1992.
25. Swaby-Ellis D: Why worry about cultural differences? *J Christ Nurs* 7:31, 1990.
26. Werner EE: *Cross-cultural child development: a view from the planet Earth,* Monterey, Calif, 1979, Brooks/Cole.

CHAPTER CHALLENGE

KEY POINTS

- Cultural background affects a person's health in all dimensions, and therefore the nurse should consider the patient's cultural background when planning care.
- The impact of culture on behaviors, attitudes, and values depends on individual factors and varies among members of a specific cultural group.
- How a person seeks to meet basic human needs is influenced by culture.
- Ethnocentrism can impede the delivery of care to ethnic minority patients and when pervasive can become cultural racism.
- Stereotyping ethnic group members can lead to mistaken assumptions about an individual ethnic minority patient.
- Cultural groups vary widely in value orientations, use of language, family systems, healing beliefs and practices, religious beliefs and practices, and food and eating habits.

STUDY QUESTIONS

1. Nurses who care for persons in predominantly ethnic minority communities should learn about their life-styles. The best way nurses might obtain firsthand information from ethnic minority communities in their local area is by:
   1. Eating ethnic foods at a vendor in a shopping mall.
   2. Scheduling a home visit to a family of a different racial group.
   3. Conducting a library study of a cultural group.
   4. Observing cultural behaviors in a movie shown at a theater in the community.
2. Mrs. Garcia was admitted to the hospital exhibiting symptoms of listlessness, loss of appetite, and withdrawal characteristic of the cultural condition called "susto" (fright). Which one of the following nursing interventions would be appropriate for this patient whose cultural beliefs may differ from the nurse's beliefs about physical illness?
   1. Adhering to the philosophy, "I treat all my patients the same."
   2. Encouraging patients to describe their symptoms by using only the English language.
   3. Including the services of the "curandero" on the health care team for Hispanic patients.
   4. Using the magic of the "evil eye" to cure physical conditions of patients.
3. To provide effective nursing care to ethnic minority patients the nurse will need to gain an understanding of cultural variables (differences) as part of the cultural assessment process. This process includes which one of the following?
   1. Using stereotypic terms such as "issei" to describe health behaviors of Japanese-Americans.
   2. Describing skin color as a basis for dealing with feelings of loss of dignity and respect.
   3. Assuming the role of cultural healer when curing the symptoms of "bad fate."
   4. Clarification of a patient's perception of his values and customs based on his ethnic/cultural background.
4. A sacred talisman was removed from Mr. Grayhorse, an American Indian, before surgery; the patient and family members became highly upset. What would be an appropriate intervention by the nurse in this situation?
   1. Explain to Mr. Grayhorse and his family that hospital policy does not allow him to keep his sacred talisman.
   2. Discuss with the patient and family the significance of the sacred talisman and attempt an acceptable solution that considers hospital policy.
   3. Give the sacred talisman back to Mr. Grayhorse to calm both him and his family.
   4. Consult with the medicine man and have him wear the sacred talisman for Mr. Grayhorse during surgery.
5. Miss Johnson is a 25-year-old Caucasian nurse who was born and raised in the Midwest. She is typical of most Americans who believe that illness is generally attribut to:
   1. fate and God's will.
   2. socioeconomic class.
   3. getting what you deserve.
   4. physiological changes.
6. The student nurse states to her nurse educator that she doesn't understand why the Japanese-American family members are not grieving for their dying father. The educator's response is based on the knowledge that the student nurse is:
   1. subculture oriented.
   2. stereotyping.
   3. ethnocentric.
   4. culturally racist.
7. The nurse should know that the concept of culture is best defined as:
   1. learned ways of acting and thinking.
   2. fixed concept of how the older adults of that culture act or think.
   3. tendency to view members of other cultural or ethnic groups as inferior.
   4. intrinsic beliefs about the work of an entity or concept.

4

VITAL SIGNS AND PHYSICAL ASSESSMENT

I chose to become a nurse because I wanted a challenging, rewarding career, and this profession gives me the opportunity to fulfill my desire. It also provides me with unlimited opportunities to advance my education and specialize my skills in many different fields of the profession. In addition to this, I have the satisfaction of knowing I can and will make a difference in people's lives.

Joan Sunnzfranz
Student Nurse

9

SIGNS, SYMPTOMS, AND PHYSICAL ASSESSMENT

Audrey Wadman Szczesiul

KEY TERMS

acute
anomaly
assessment
auscultation
bruit
crackles
crepitus
chronic
drainage
dullness
edema
erythema
etiology
exudate
flatness
focused assessment
inspection
leukoplakia
LOC
neoplastic
nursing health history
objective data
palpation
percussion
pruritus
purulent
sign
subjective data
symptom
turgor
tympany
wheeze

LEARNING OBJECTIVES

After reading this chapter, the student should be able to do the following:

- Define the key terms.
- Discuss the difference between a sign and a symptom.
- List the origins of disease.
- Discuss the four major risk categories for development of disease.
- Discuss frequently noted signs and symptoms of disease conditions.
- List the universal signs of inflammation/infection.
- Describe the nursing responsibilities when assisting a physician with the physical examination.
- Discuss equipment and supplies necessary for the physical examination/assessment.
- Explain the necessary skills for the physical examination/nursing assessment.
- Discuss the nurse-patient interview.
- List the basic essentials for a patient's health history.
- Discuss the sequence of steps when performing a nursing assessment.
- Discuss normal assessment findings in the head-to-toe assessment.
- Describe documentation of the physical examination/nursing assessment.

RELATED TOPICS OF INTEREST

- Communication (Chapter 4)
- The nursing process (Chapter 5)
- Documentation (Chapter 6)
- Vital signs (Chapter 10)
- Medical asepsis and infection control (Chapter 12)
- Hygiene and care of the patient's environment (Chapter 16)
- Specimen collection and diagnostic examinations (Chapter 17)

SIGNS AND SYMPTOMS

Signs are **objective data,** as perceived by the examiner, in this case the nurse. A sign can be seen, heard, measured, or felt by the examiner. Examples of signs are rashes, altered vital signs, and visible drainage or exudate. **Drainage** refers to the removal of fluids from a body cavity, wound, or other source of discharge by one or more methods. Examples are the closed urinary drainage system or an open drainage system, such as from a Penrose drain. **Exudate** refers to fluid, cells, or other substances that have been slowly exuded, or discharged, from cells or blood vessels through small pores or breaks in cell membrane, usually as a result of inflammation or injury. Perspiration, pus, and serum are sometimes identified as exudates.)

The nurse uses the senses of sight, hearing, touch, and smell to gather these objective data or signs. In addition, laboratory findings as well as diagnostic imaging and other diagnostic studies are included in the objective data.

Symptoms are subjective indications of illness that are perceived by the patient. Examples of symptoms are pain, nausea, vertigo, and anxiety. The nurse is unaware of symptoms unless the patient describes the sensation. Symptoms are referred to as **subjective data.**

In subjective data collection the interviewer encourages a full description by the patient of the onset, the course, and the character of the problem and any factors that aggravate or ameliorate (improve) it. Many signs accompany symptoms; for example, erythema and a rash are often seen when a patient complains of **pruritus** (itching). Some symptoms may be objectively confirmed; for example, patient complaints of numbness of a body part may be confirmed by absence of response to a pin prick.

Disease and Diagnosis

A disease is a specific illness characterized by a recognizable set of signs and symptoms. These signs and symptoms are clustered into a group that allows the physician to make a medical diagnosis. The nurse also relies on assessment of signs and symptoms to formulate a nursing diagnosis. Unlike a medical diagnosis, which deals with pathophysiological factors and the cure of a disease, the nursing diagnosis recognizes holistic needs of the patient that can be treated with independent and dependent nursing interventions. These needs are patient problems, either real or high risk.

Origins of Disease. Disease or illness originates from many causes, including hereditary, congenital, infectious, metabolic, deficiency, neoplastic, traumatic, and environmental. There are other diseases for which no apparent cause is known. These illnesses have an unknown **etiology** (cause of a disease).

Hereditary diseases are transmitted genetically from parent to offspring. An example of a genetically transmitted disease is cystic fibrosis. The offspring has a 25% chance of acquiring cystic fibrosis if both the parents have the recessive trait. The child with cystic fibrosis develops lifelong respiratory and digestive difficulties.

Congenital diseases are present at birth. The disease results from a condition during the pregnancy that interferes with the normal development of the fetus, such as the mother's having rubella (German measles) during early gestation (pregnancy). Congenital conditions include **anomalies** (structural defects) and defects in the functioning of a body organ. An example of an anomaly is the absence of a limb or the presence of an extra finger. Defects in the body's functioning include Down's syndrome, which results in a physical and/or cognitive impairment (mentally delayed).

Infectious diseases result from the invasion of bacteria or viruses into the body. Examples of infectious diseases include acquired immunodeficiency syndrome (AIDS), tuberculosis, and measles.

Deficiency disease result from the lack of a specific nutrient. Nutrients are minerals, vitamins, proteins, fats, and carbohydrates. Scurvy is a deficiency disease resulting from a lack of vitamin C. Kwashiorkor results from a severe deficiency of protein in the diet.

Metabolic disease is caused by a dysfunction that results in a loss of metabolic control of homeostasis in the body. The dysfunction usually involves endocrine glands, which secrete hormones to regulate body processes. Diabetes mellitus results from the dysfunction of the pancreas. Other examples of metabolic disease are hypothyroidism and acromegaly, which involve the thyroid and pituitary glands (see Chapter 32).

Neoplastic disease is described as an abnormal growth of new tissues. The new growth may be benign or malignant (cancerous). Malignant neoplasms are a serious threat to health, because the rapid growth of the cells robs nutrients from the body's normal cells.

Traumatic conditions result from both physical and emotional trauma. Physical trauma, such as a motor vehicle accident, can result in traumatic brain injury (TBI). TBI may leave the individual mentally and physically impaired. Emotional trauma, such as the loss of a loved one, can result in the individual being unable to manage the activities of daily living (ADLs) participated in before the trauma.

Environmental diseases are a group of conditions that develop from exposure to a harmful substance in the environment. The "tight building syndrome" is an example of an environmental illness. The individual complains of headache, vertigo (dizziness), and respiratory infections. These signs and symptoms result from the fact that the well-built buildings of today do not allow circulation of fresh air and instead recycle air containing fumes and microorganisms. Radon gas and asbestos are also substances in the environment that can lead to disease.

Although many disease conditions have an unknown cause, many conditions are now thought to result from autoimmune responses. In an autoimmune response, the body develops immunoglobulins (antibodies) against its own tissues or body substances. Rheumatoid arthritis and ulcerative colitis are being researched as possible autoimmune diseases (see Chapter 36).

Risk Factors for Development of Disease. A risk factor is any situation, habit, environmental condition, physiological condition, or other variable that increases the vulnerability of an individual or group to illness or accident. Risk factors do not necessarily mean that a person will develop a disease condition but that the chances of disease are increased. For example, risk factors for the development of coronary artery disease include heredity, cigarette smoking, high blood levels of cholesterol, and stressful work conditions. The nurse assesses the patient's risk factors, because nursing diagnoses are made for high risk as well as actual patient problems.

Risk factors are placed into four major categories: genetic and physiological, age, environment, and life-style (Box 9-1).

Terms Used to Describe Disease. Diseases are described in terms of duration. **Chronic** disease develops slowly and persists over a long period, often for a person's lifetime. Diabetes mellitus (inability of the body to use glucose) is an example of a chronic disease. Chronic disease can be further described as early, late, or terminal. Chronic disease can also be described as being in remission. Remission means there has been a partial or complete disappearance of clinical and subjective characteristics of the disease. Remission may be spontaneous or a result of therapy.

In comparison, a disease described as **acute** begins abruptly with marked intensity of severe signs and symptoms and then often subsides after a period of treatment. An episode of appendicitis would be considered acute.

Disease can also be described as functional or organic. Organic disease results from changes in an organ that interfere with its functioning. Cerebrovascular accident (CVA, stroke) is an organic disease of the brain. A functional disease may be manifested as an organic disease, but careful examination fails to reveal evidence of structural or physiological abnormalities. A headache can be an organic or a functional disorder.

Box 9-1 RISK FACTORS FOR DISEASE

GENETIC, PHYSIOLOGICAL

- A family history of cancer increases the risk that an individual will develop cancer (genetic).
- Malnourishment predisposes an individual to illness (physiological).

AGE

- Thinning skin in the elderly makes this group more susceptible to skin trauma.

ENVIRONMENT

- Radon gas seeping from the earth into a basement can increase the risk of cancer development.
- Air, water, and noise pollution increases the risk of illness.
- High crime rates or overcrowding can also lead to stresses that make individuals more susceptible to disease.
- Within the family, conflicts or other problems may create stressors that put individual members or the family as a whole at increased risk of illness.

LIFE-STYLE

- Smoking increases the risk of lung cancer.
- Overeating or poor nutrition, insufficient rest and sleep, and poor personal hygiene also add to increased risk for illness for the individual.
- Other habits that place a person at risk for illness include alcohol or drug abuse.
- Sunbathing increases the risk of skin cancer.
- Any emotional stress can be a risk factor if severe or prolonged or if the person is unable to adequately cope. In such a case, emotional stress may increase the chance of illness. Events such as death, divorce, or pregnancy, as well as job-related stressors, are known to place the individual at risk.

Frequently Noted Signs and Symptoms of Disease Conditions (Table 9-1)

Signs and symptoms: inflammation and infection. Inflammation differs from infection. Infection is caused by invasion of a microorganism, such as a bacterium or a parasite. Inflammation does have signs and symptoms similar to those of infection but is not necessarily the result of an invading organism. The universal signs of inflammation/infection are pain, **erythema** (redness), **edema** (swelling), heat, purulent drainage (pus), and loss of function. The purulent drainage may also have a foul (fetid) odor.

The inflammatory process is actually a body defense against the causative agent. The erythema and edema are the result of increased blood flow to the area. Pain occurs because of increased pressure on pain sensors in the area. Heat occurs as blood flow and metabolism in the area are increased. Loss of function is the body's

TABLE 9-1 Frequently Noted Signs and Symptoms of Disease Conditions

Term	Definition
Anorexia	Lack of appetite resulting in the inability to eat. This symptom can occur in many disease conditions.
Constipation	Difficulty in passing stools or an incomplete or infrequent passage of hard stools. There are many causes, both organic and functional.
Coughing	A sudden audible expulsion of air from the lungs. Coughing is an essential protective response that serves to clear the lungs, bronchi, or trachea of irritants and secretions or to prevent aspiration of foreign material into the lungs. It is a common sign of diseases of the chest and larynx.
Cyanosis	Bluish discoloration of the skin and mucous membranes caused by an excess of deoxygenated hemoglobin in the blood.
Diarrhea	Frequent passage of loose liquid stools; generally results from increased motility in the colon. This is usually a sign of an underlying disorder. The characteristics of the diarrhea give evidence as to the source. Dark black tarry stools can mean there is bleeding in the intestines. Bright red blood in the feces indicates active bleeding from the lower portion of the intestinal tract.
Dyspnea	A shortness of breath or difficulty in breathing that may be caused by certain heart and lung conditions, strenuous exercise, or anxiety.
Edema	An abnormal accumulation of fluid in interstitial spaces. It may be caused by overhydration, excess sodium intake, or a loss of serum albumin (a protein), which causes fluid to leave the vessels and collect in the interstitial space. Skin that is edematous will be taut and shiny. Pitting may occur when the skin is pressed; a small indentation will remain after the finger is removed.
Erythema	Redness or inflammation of the skin or mucous membranes that is the result of dilation and congestion of superficial capillaries; erythema is seen in a mild sunburn.
Febrile (fever, pyrexia)	An abnormal elevation of the temperature of the body above 98.6° F (37° C) because of disease. It results from an imbalance between the elimination and production of heat. Infection and many different diseases may lead to elevated temperature.
Jaundice	Yellow tinge to the skin and may indicate obstruction in the flow of bile from the liver.
Orthopnea	An abnormal condition in which a person must sit or stand to breathe deeply or comfortably. Occurs in many disorders of the respiratory and cardiac system.
Nausea	A sensation often leading to the urge to vomit. Common causes include intense pain, gallbladder disease, inflammation of the stomach, and food poisoning.
Pain	An unpleasant sensation caused by noxious (extremely destructive or harmful) stimulation of the sensory nerve endings. It is a cardinal symptom of inflammation and is valuable in the diagnosis of many disorders and conditions. Pain may be mild or severe, chronic, acute, burning, dull or sharp, precisely or poorly localized, or referred.
Pallor	An unnatural paleness or absence of color in the skin; it may result from a decrease in hemoglobin and erythrocytes (red blood cells).
Pruritus	A symptom of itching and an uncomfortable sensation leading to an urge to scratch. Some causes are allergy, infection, jaundice, and skin irritation.
Sallow	An unhealthy, yellow color: usually said of a complexion or skin.
Tachycardia	An abnormal condition in which the heart contracts regularly but at a rate greater than 100 beats per minute. The heart rate accelerates in response to fever, exercise, or nervous excitement.
Tachypnea	An abnormally rapid rate of breathing seen in many diseased conditions.
Vomiting	To expel the contents of the stomach through the esophagus and out of the mouth. The quality of the vomitus can give a clue to the underlying cause. "Coffee ground" vomitus indicates bleeding in the stomach. The blood takes on a coffee ground appearance because of the effect of the digestive juices. Vomiting of bright red blood could be a sign of gastric hemorrhage.

method of resting the injured part. Purulent exudate is the accumulation of the white blood cells, dead cells, bacteria, and other debris from an infectious process. An infectious process differs from an inflammatory process in that infection is caused by pathogenic microorganisms and inflammation can be caused by nonpathogenic irritation of local tissue, as in the case of tissue injury. The heat felt when fever is present during an illness is a body defense, since many bacteria will be destroyed by the higher temperature.

ASSESSMENT

Assessment is an evaluation or appraisal of a condition. It includes gathering, verifying, and communicating information about the patient.

Medical Assessment

When the physician conducts a physical examination, the nurse is often requested to assist the examiner. There are certain functions the nurse will be expected to carry out. Preparing the examining room, assisting with equipment, preparing the patient, and collecting specimens are a few examples of tasks the nurse should be familiar with to facilitate the physical exam. There are preexamination responsibilities as well as postexamination responsibilities. For specific interventions for special examinations, see Table 17-1.

As the nurse prepares the patient for the physical examination, certain questions need to be answered. They are as follows:

- Is an informed consent necessary? Has it been signed by the patient or next of kin? Has it been witnessed? Has it been dated?
- Have all test prerequisites been completed? Have vital signs been obtained? Have the patient's height and weight been determined? (See Chapter 10.) Is a skin prep required? Has a urinalysis been ordered? A CBC? Chest x-ray? (See Box 9-3.) Has the patient voided? Is the patient wearing a hospital gown?
- Has the patient been adequately advised concerning the examination? Time? Place? Examiner? Sequence of events? Does the patient have any unanswered questions? (See Box 9-2 for psychological preparation for a physical examination.)
- Will the physical exam be performed in the patient's room? Is the working area cleared of unnecessary articles? Have the curtains been pulled? Have visitors been asked to leave and shown where to wait? Has the door been closed? (Privacy is essential.)
- If an examination room is provided, how should the patient be transferred to the room? By gurney? By wheelchair? Ambulation? Has the examining room been prepared? Are all necessary supplies and equipment arranged for easy access? (See Fig. 9-1 and Box 9-3.)
- How much assistance will the patient need to safely recline on the examining table? What position will the patient be required to assume during procedures? (See Table 9-2.) For perineal ex-

Box 9-2 PSYCHOLOGICAL PREPARATION FOR A PHYSICAL EXAMINATION

Psychological preparation may be the nurse's highest priority before the examination. Patients become embarrassed when required to answer sensitive questions about body functions or when certain body parts are exposed and examined. The possibility that the examiner may find something abnormal also creates anxiety. The nurse first tells the patient about the examination in general terms. Then as each body system is examined, a more detailed explanation is given. The examiner will use simple terms when describing steps of the examination as complicated terminology will perplex some patients and may add to their fears.

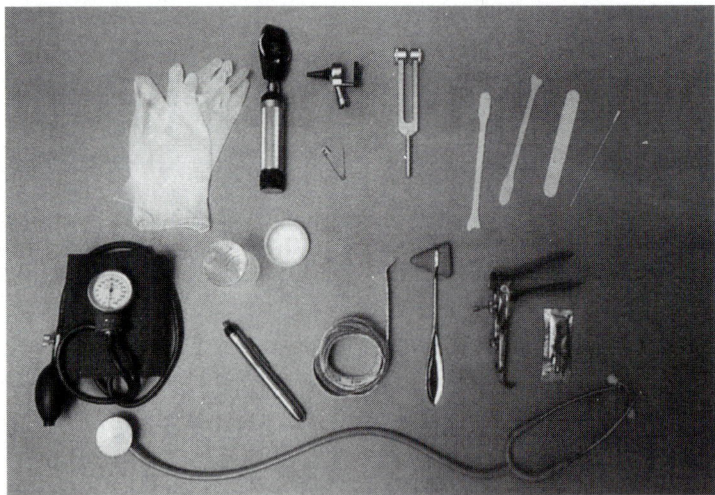

FIG. 9-1 Equipment used during a physical examination *(clockwise from upper left):* disposable gloves, ophthalmoscope, otoscope attachment, sterile safety pin, tuning fork, cervical spatulas, tongue depressor, cotton-tip swab, lubricant, vaginal speculum, reflex hammer, tape measure, penlight, specimen cup, sphygmomanometer, and stethoscope *(bottom).*

Box 9-3 EQUIPMENT AND SUPPLIES FOR PHYSICAL EXAMINATION AND ASSESSMENT

- Cotton applicators
- Cytobrush
- Disposable pad
- Drapes
- Eye chart (e.g., Snellen chart)
- Flashlight and spotlight
- Forms (e.g., physical, laboratory)
- Gloves (sterile and clean)
- Gown for patient
- Lubricant
- Ophthalmoscope
- Otoscope
- Papanicolaou smear slides
- Paper towels
- Percussion hammer
- Safety pins
- Scale with height measurement rod
- Spatula
- Specimen containers and microscope slides
- Sphygmomanometer and cuff
- Stethoscope
- Swabs or sponge forceps
- Tape measure
- Thermometer
- Tissues
- Tongue depressor
- Tuning fork
- Vaginal speculum
- Wristwatch with second hand

TABLE 9-2 Positions for Examination

Position	Areas Assessed	Rationale	Limitations
Sitting 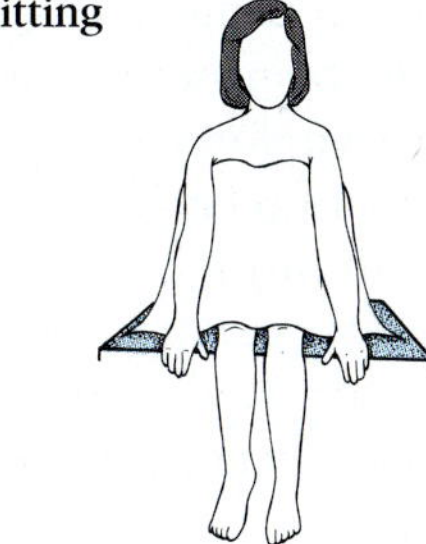	Head and neck, back, posterior thorax and lungs, anterior thorax and lungs, breasts, axillae, heart, vital signs, and upper extremities	Sitting upright provides full expansion of lungs and provides better visualization of symmetry of upper body parts.	A physically weakened patient may be unable to sit. Use supine position with head of bed elevated instead.
Supine	Head and neck, anterior thorax and lungs, breasts, axillae, heart, abdomen, extremities, pulses	This is the most normally relaxed position. It prevents contracture of abdominal muscles and provides easy access to pulse sites.	If patient becomes short of breath easily, examiner may need to raise head of bed.
Dorsal recumbent	Head and neck, anterior thorax and lungs, breasts, axillae, heart	Certain patients with painful disorders are more comfortable with knees flexed.	Position is not used for abdominal assessment, because it promotes contracture of abdominal muscles.
Lithotomy 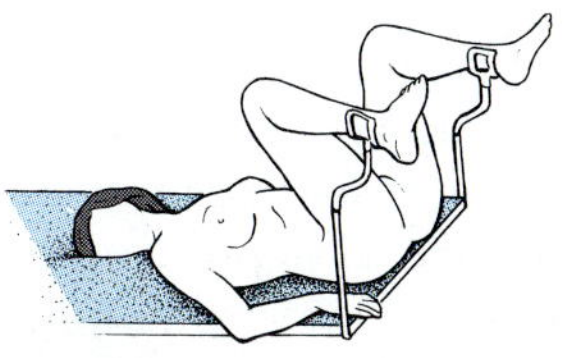	Female genitalia and genital tract	This position provides maximal exposure of genitalia and facilitates insertion of vaginal speculum.	This is an embarrassing and uncomfortable position, so minimize time the patient spends in this position. Keep patient well draped. A patient with severe arthritis or other joint deformity may be unable to assume this position.
Sims'	Rectum	Flexion of hip and knee improves exposure of rectal area.	Joint deformities may hinder the patient's ability to bend hip and knee.
Prone 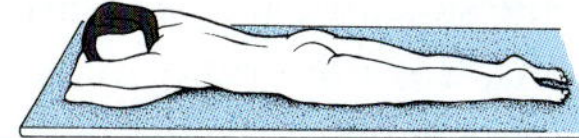	Musculoskeletal	This position is used only to assess extension of the hip joint.	This position is intolerable for a patient with respiratory difficulties.

amination, has the patient been draped adequately to expose only the area being examined?

- Will the nurse be required to remain in the examining room? Do not leave the patient alone. Most examiners appreciate a nurse in attendance; however, on occasion this may not be necessary.
- Is the patient acquainted with the examiner? Are introductions necessary?
- Does the lighting need adjustment? Does the examiner expect the nurse to provide instruments, supplies, and equipment as they are needed?
- Will specimens be obtained? How should they be labeled? Where should they be sent? How? (See Chapter 17.)
- How much attention and encouragement will the patient need during the examination?
- How much assistance will the patient need to assume a comfortable position following the examination? To cleanse herself? To get dressed? To return to the room? To call for further assistance if needed?
- What signs and symptoms related to the procedure should the nurse note? (Assessment should be made at frequent intervals.)
- What information needs to be included in documenting the procedure? (Vital signs, pertinent signs and symptoms, complaints of pain, anxiety level, and specimens obtained should all be noted.)
- What other members of the health care team need to be informed of the procedure? (Usually those who are directly responsible for the patient's care.)
- Does the examination room need attention? Was order maintained? Does equipment need to be disposed of or cleaned and returned to its proper location? (Special examining rooms and equipment should always be kept in readiness for the next patient.)

The nurse can perform an assessment to determine the actual or potential (high risk for) patient problems that will require nursing interventions for the safety and well-being of the patient. For example, if during the assessment the nurse observes that the patient has a need for oxygen (a basic human need), positioning, deep breathing, and coughing can be instituted to meet this need.

It is imperative that the nurse perform accurate assessments because the nurse is the care giver who is in constant contact with the patient. The nurse can monitor the patient to discover developing complications as well as to evaluate medical treatments.

Nursing Assessment

Nursing assessment is the process of gathering, verifying, and communicating data about a patient. The purpose of the assessment is to establish a data base about the patient's level of wellness, health practices, past illnesses, related experiences, and health care goals. The information contained in the data base is the basis for an individualized plan of nursing care developed throughout the nursing process (see Chapter 5).

Collection of data includes the nursing health history, physical examination, results of laboratory and diagnostic tests, and information from health care team members and the patient's family or significant other. Data gathered during the health history are obtained when the nurse interviews the patient. To collect data from an interview, the nurse initiates the nurse-patient relationship (see Chapter 4), uses various interview techniques, and progresses through the interview.

The skills of inspection, palpation, percussion, and auscultation permit the nurse to collect data from the physical examination/assessment (Box 9-4). Laboratory and diagnostic tests validate the findings of the history and examination and can lead to identification of problems not previously noted (Box 9-5 on p. 130).

Initiating the Nurse-Patient Relationship. Perhaps the most difficult patient interview for a nurse to conduct is the first one. For some patients, being interviewed by a nurse is a new experience. Therefore the nurse must establish an effective nurse-patient relationship before proceeding to the nursing health history.

The first step in initiating the relationship is for the nurse to introduce herself, stating her name, position, and the purposes of the interview (see example below).

THERAPEUTIC DIALOGUE

Nurse: Good morning, Mr. Carney. I am Mrs. Auen, a student nurse. I will be caring for you today. A portion of my nursing care is to conduct an assessment of you. Your temperature, pulse, blood pressure, heart rate, breath sounds, abdominal sounds, and skin color will be included in my assessment. It will take me about 30 minutes. Do you have any questions? *(pause)* My assessment will help me plan your nursing care. May I begin now? *(pause)* I will start with your vital signs.

In the above example the nurse introduced herself as the nurse, gave an estimate of the time needed for the assessment, and told Mr. Carney the reason for the assessment. Indicating the length of time is important because it helps ensure cooperation. A patient, even one in a hospital, should not be considered a captive audience, and the nurse should take steps to ensure that a patient's time is not used inappropriately. Stating the length of time demonstrates that the time will not be abused. In the example, the nurse also gave Mr. Carney an opportunity to ask questions. It is important to determine whether the patient has any pressing questions be-

Box 9-4

NECESSARY SKILLS FOR PHYSICAL EXAMINATION AND NURSING ASSESSMENT

INSPECTION

The nurse inspects the patient's body and observes moods, including all responses and nonverbal behaviors. This **inspection** (purposeful observation of the patient) begins with the nurse's first contact with the patient and continues throughout the gathering of the nursing history. Inspection is used to systematically collect data about significant behaviors or physical features. It is important to be accurate and thorough, using a systematic approach such as head-to-toe assessment.

PALPATION

With **palpation,** the examiner uses the hands and sense of touch to gather data. Hands are very sensitive to texture, temperature, and moisture and thus help to determine the quality of an area. Palpation is used to detect tenderness, temperature, texture, vibration, pulsations, masses, and other changes in structural integrity. Each body part is palpated, usually after a systematic assessment pattern. Palpation rules out or confirms suspicions raised during interview and inspection. Because touching may elicit fear, embarrassment, pain, or other strong emotions, the nurse should explain the actions and the reasons for them. In addition, the patient should be instructed to let the nurse know whether palpation produces tenderness, pressure, or pain. The two palpation techniques, light and deep, are illustrated in Fig. 9-2 on p. 130.

When using palpation, the nurse should warm the hands before touching the patient. Social conversation during palpation is appropriate at times to distract the patient and help him relax. Pads of the fingers should be used and placed flat against the skin with slight pressure and gentle rotation of the area under examination. The thumb and forefinger can be used to palpate muscle mass on arms and legs. Pulses are palpated with the pads of the fingers.

When doing palpation the nurse should also observe the patient's facial expressions; a grimace may indicate pain, which the patient can be asked to describe.

PERCUSSION

Percussion is use of the fingertips to tap the body's surface to produce vibration and sound. The sounds indicate the density of the underlying tissue and thus detect the location of body organs and structures. For example, percussion over a hollow organ such as the stomach produces a high-pitched, drumlike sound called **tympany.** Percussion over a dense organ such as the liver produces a low-pitched, thudlike sound called **dullness.** Percussion over a muscle produces a soft, high-pitched, flat sound called **flatness.** Percussion requires the examiner to place the palmar surface of one hand against the patient's body while tapping with the fingers of the other hand. Percussion should not be painful for the patient, but if it does cause discomfort, it should be discontinued and the results documented. Each area should be tapped two or three times.

AUSCULTATION

Auscultation is the process of listening to sounds produced by the body. Three systems produce sounds for the examiner to auscultate: the cardiovascular system, the respiratory system, and the gastrointestinal system. For auscultation of these systems the nurse uses a stethoscope, an instrument that amplifies sounds produced by internal organs. The technique of auscultation is also used to detect the fetal heart sound (see Chapter 39).

Mastering auscultation technique requires practice; when auscultating, the nurse realizes that the body produces many sounds that are normal and must be able to ignore those normal sounds and concentrate on abnormal sounds. Adventitious (abnormal) breath sounds may be superimposed over normal sounds. The environment must be quiet for accurate assessment. Television, sounds from nasogastric suction, movement of bed linen, and conversation can all interfere with accurate auscultation. Auscultation should not be rushed: time is taken to assess each area properly.

The diaphragm of the stethoscope is placed gently over the patient's skin. If the area is hairy, the area can be dampened to decrease the sound made by the hair against the diaphragm.

fore beginning the interview. By answering these questions, the nurse can meet some of the patient's immediate needs, and the patient may feel more comfortable about answering questions. For example, a patient who is unsure about how the hospital bed operates may be thinking about the bed instead of the nurse's questions and therefore may not provide complete information for the data base. Finally, the nurse asked whether it was acceptable to conduct the interview at that time, thereby giving the patient a choice.

The next step in initiating the nurse-patient relationship is to communicate trust and confidentiality to patients. Illnesses that cause people to seek help are often accompanied by anxiety, powerlessness, altered family processes, economic concerns, and changes in self-image. Frequently, patients are asked to provide very personal information about themselves and their families. Generally, people share such information only with family members or close friends. The patient must be comfortable that this information will be shared only with

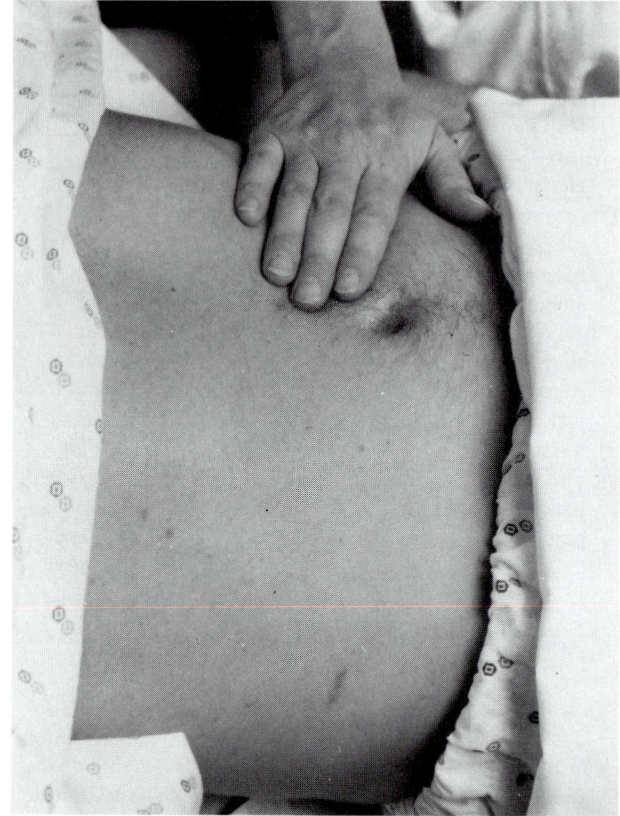

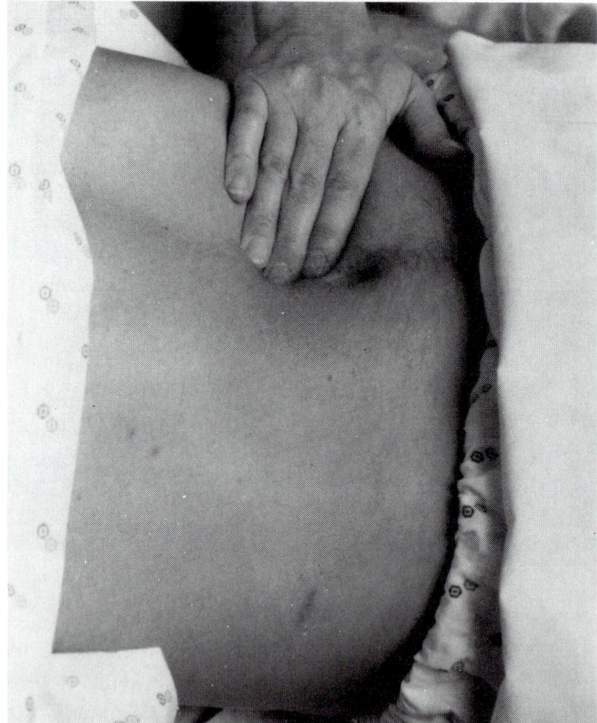

FIG. 9-2 **A,** To perform light palpation, the examiner presses gently on the patient's skin, indenting approximately ½ to 1 inch. The hand is moved in a circular motion. **B,** To perform deep palpation, fingertip pressure is increased, indenting about 2 inches.

Box 9-5

COMMON LABORATORY AND DIAGNOSTIC TESTS

BLOOD ANALYSIS

- Complete blood count (CBC), includes RBC, Hgb, hematocrit, platelets, WBC with differential
- Electrolyte tests: sequential multiple analysis—6 (SMA_6), SMA_{12}
- Arterial blood gas (ABG) analysis
- Fasting blood sugar (FBS) test
- Blood chemistry profile

URINE ANALYSIS

- Urinalysis (UA)
- Urine culture and sensitivity test

DIAGNOSTIC IMAGING EXAMINATIONS

- Chest roentgenogram (CXR)
- Upper gastrointestinal (UGI) examination
- Barium enema (BE) examination
- Intravenous pyelogram (IVP)
- Scans of the body, head, chest, and bones

STOOL ANALYSIS

- Guaiac tests
- Ova and parasite tests
- Culture and sensitivity
- *Clostridium difficile*

SPUTUM ANALYSIS

- Culture and sensitivity test
- Acid-fast bacilli (AFB) test
- Cytology tests

OTHER

- Electrocardiogram (ECG)
- Stress test
- Tuberculosis (TB) skin test

care givers who need this knowledge to provide proper care. The nurse assures patients that information concerning past or present levels of wellness or family relationships is strictly confidential.

Finally, the nurse-patient relationship is enhanced by the professionalism and competence conveyed by the nurse. The nurse's attitude of professionalism and professional manner and appearance encourage a supportive therapeutic relationship with the patient so that the nurse and patient can communicate freely, thereby allowing identification of health care needs and objectives. The nurse establishes a rapport with the patient and family and becomes an advocate for the patient. The nurse as a patient advocate intercedes for the patient and encourages others to put the patient's needs high on their list of priorities.

The Interview. The nurse conducts the interview in a relaxed, unhurried manner in a quiet, private, well-lighted setting. The nurse must convey feelings of compassion and concern while remaining objective. The patient must feel that the information being given is important to the nurse; the nurse must demonstrate an interest in the patient's state of wellness.

The nurse should determine by what name the patient wishes to be addressed and then use that name during the interview. An accepting posture, in which the nurse is sitting in a relaxed manner at eye level with the patient, will definitely enhance the interview. A pleasant facial expression will promote communication, and eye contact assists the patient in believing she has the nurse's full attention.

The nurse can enhance communication by using nonjudgmental language. Statements by the nurse such as, "Yes I see," or "What happened next?" can encourage the patient to clarify without feeling threatened. Reflecting what the patient has said in her own words clarifies statements, as does summarizing and restating what the patient has said. The nurse's approving nods and gestures facilitate the exchange of information (Box 4-4).

Nursing Health History. The **nursing health history** is data collected about the patient's level of wellness, changes in life patterns, sociocultural role, and mental and emotional reactions to illness. The nursing history obtained during the interview is the first step in assessment. The objective is to identify patterns of health and illness, risk factors for physical and behavioral health problems, deviations from normal, and available resources for adaptation to life's changes (Box 9-6).

Biographical data. In most facilities the biographical data are obtained in the admitting department, and the nurse may refer to this information to begin the interview.

Reasons for seeking health care. The nurse asks why the patient sought health care, because the information contained on the admission form may differ greatly from the subjective reason for seeking health care. This may also be referred to as the *chief complaint.* The nurse may simply ask, "What is the reason for your admission?" This allows the patient not only to describe the reason for admission, but also to make his expectations known to the nurse. To get the most information from the patient about health concerns, the nurse can use the PQRST method (Box 9-7 on p. 132).

Box 9-6 BASIC ESSENTIALS FOR HEALTH HISTORY

- **Biographical data:** date of birth, sex, address, family members' names and addresses, marital status, religious preference and practices, occupation, source of health care, and insurance
- **Reasons for seeking health care:** goals of care, expectations of the health care system, and expectation of services and care delivered
- **Present illness or health concern:** onset, signs and symptoms, nature of signs and symptoms (e.g., sudden or gradual), duration, precipitating factors, relief measures, and weight loss or gain
- **Past health history:** prior illnesses throughout development, injuries and hospitalizations, surgeries, blood transfusions, allergies, immunizations, habits (e.g., smoking, caffeine intake, alcohol or drug abuse), prescribed and self-prescribed medications, work habits, relaxation activities, and sleep, exercise, and eating or nutritional patterns
- **Family history:** health status of the immediate family and living relatives, cause of death of relatives, and risk factors for cancer, heart disease, diabetes mellitus, kidney disease, hypertension, or mental disorders
- **Environmental history:** hazards, pollutants, and physical safety
- **Psychosocial and cultural history:** primary language, cultural group, educational background, community resources, mood, attention span, and developmental stage
- **Review of systems (ROS):** head-to-toe review of all major body systems, as well as the patient's knowledge of and compliance with health care (e.g., frequency of breast or testicular self-examination or last visual acuity examination)

It is also appropriate to elicit the patient's expectations of the health care providers. The nurse determines whether patients expect to be "cured," "free of pain," or "able to care for themselves." This information assists in establishing the goals of nursing interventions, as well as in determining whether patients' expectations of themselves and the health care providers are realistic. In addition, such expectations provide the nurse with information on patient perceptions about patterns of illness or changes in life-style.

Past health history. The information collected about past health history provides data on the patient's health care experiences. The nurse determines whether the patient has ever been hospitalized or has undergone surgery. Also essential in planning nursing interventions are descriptions of allergies, including allergic reactions to food, drugs, or pollutants. If an allergy is present, the

Box 9-7 HISTORY OF PRESENT ILLNESS

When discussing the history of present illness with your patient, make sure she describes her problems fully. To do this, ask the patient the following questions about each complaint:

Time of onset. When was the first date (the problem) happened? What time did it begin?

Type of onset. How did (the problem) start: suddenly? gradually?

Original source. What were you doing when you first experienced or noticed (the problem)? What seems to trigger it: stress? position? certain activities? arguments? If describing a discharge: thick? runny? clear? colored? If describing a psychological problem: Do the voices drown out other sounds? Whose voice does it sound like?

Severity. How bad is (the problem) when it's at its worst? Does it interfere with your normal activities? Does it force you to lie down, sit down, slow down?

Radiation. In the case of pain, does it travel down your back or arms, up your neck, or down your legs?

Time relationship. How often do you experience (the problem): hourly? daily? weekly? monthly? When do you usually experience it: daytime? at night? in the early morning? Are you ever awakened by it? Does it ever occur before, during, or after meals? Does it occur seasonally?

Duration. How long does an episode last?

Course. Does (the problem) seem to be getting better, to be getting worse, or does it remain the same?

Associations. Does (the problem) lead to anything else? Is it accompanied by other signs and symptoms?

Source of relief. What relieves it: changing diet? changing position? taking medications? being active?

Source of aggravation. What makes it worse?

You can remember all these questions using the letters *PQRST:*

- **P** Provocative/palliative
  What causes it? What makes it better?
  What makes it worse?
- **Q** Quality/quantity
  How does it feel, look, or sound, and how much of it is there?
- **R** Region/radiation
  Where is it? Does it spread?
- **S** Severity scale
  Does it interfere with activities?
  How does it rate on a severity scale of 1 to 10?
- **T** Timing
  When did it begin? How often does it occur? Is it sudden or gradual?

specific reaction and treatment are noted on the assessment form.

The nurse also identifies habits and life-style patterns. Use of alcohol, tobacco, caffeine, or drugs or routinely taken medications can place the patient at risk for diseases involving the liver, lungs, heart, nervous system, or thought processes. Noting the type of habit, as well as the frequency and duration of use, provides essential data. This may be an uncomfortable area for both the patient and the nurse, but a more accurate response may be obtained if the question is asked, "How much do you drink?" rather than asking the patient if he drinks.

The patient's ability to perform ADLs should be assessed. Assessing patterns of sleep, exercise, and nutrition is important when planning nursing interventions. The nursing care plan within a health care setting should be correlated with a patient's life-style patterns. If possible, variations in sleep, activity, and nutritional patterns should be accommodated.

Family history. The purpose of the family history is to obtain data about immediate and blood relatives. The objectives are to determine whether the patient is at risk for illnesses of a genetic or familial nature and to identify areas of health promotion and illness prevention. The family history also provides information about family structure, interaction, and function that may be useful in planning care. For example, a cohesive, supportive family can be a resource in assisting a patient to adjust to an illness or disability and should be incorporated into the plan of care. Conversely, if the patient's family is not supportive, it may be more therapeutic to refrain from involving them in care, particularly if the family history reveals that the patient is experiencing stress related to familial relationships.

Environmental history. The environmental history provides data about patients' home environments. The environmental history, for example, identifies exposure to pollutants that can affect health, high crime rates that prevent patients from walking around their neighborhoods, and resources that can assist patients in the return to the community.

Psychosocial history. The psychosocial history includes information about ways that the patient and family cope with stressors and any support systems that the patient or family members may need to use. The nurse asks about resolved stressors to determine the types of stressors encountered and available coping resources.

Review of Systems. The review of systems (ROS) is a systematic method for collecting data on all body systems (Box 9-8). During the ROS, the nurse asks the patient about normal functioning of each system and any noted changes. Such changes are usually subjective data because they are described as perceived by the patient.

As the nurse proceeds through the nursing health history, the data obtained are recorded in a clear, con-

Box 9-8

REVIEW OF SYSTEMS

It is probable that all the questions in each system will not be included every time a nursing health history is taken. Nevertheless, some questions regarding each system should be included in every history. These essential areas are listed in bold type in the outline that follows. More comprehensive and detailed areas for questions relating to each system are listed afterward and should be included whenever the patient gives positive responses to the first group of questions for that system. Keep in mind that these lists do not represent an exhaustive enumeration of questions that might be appropriate within an organ system. Even more detailed questions may be required, depending on the patient's problem.

A. **General constitutional symptoms:** fever, chills, malaise, fatigability, night sweats; weight (average, preferred, present, change, appetite)

B. **Skin:** rash or eruption, pruritus, pigmentation or texture change; diaphoresis (excessive sweating), abnormal nail or hair growth

C. **Skeletal:** joint stiffness, pain, restriction of motion, edema, erythema, heat, bone deformity

D. **Head**

1. General: frequent or unusual headaches, vertigo (dizziness), syncope (fainting), severe head injuries
2. Eyes: visual acuity, blurring, diplopia (double vision), photophobia (abnormal sensitivity to light), pain, recent change in appearance or vision; glaucoma, use of eye drops or other eye medications; history of trauma or familial eye disease
3. Ears: hearing loss, pain, discharge, tinnitus, vertigo
4. Nose: sense of smell, frequency of colds, obstruction, epistaxis (nosebleed), postnasal discharge, sinus pain
5. Throat and mouth: hoarseness or change in voice; frequent sore throats, bleeding or edema of gums; recent tooth abscesses or extractions; soreness of tongue or buccal mucosa, ulcers; disturbance of taste

E. **Endocrine:** thyroid enlargement or tenderness, heat or cold intolerance, unexplained weight change, diabetes mellitus, polydipsia (excessive thirst), polyuria, changes in facial or body hair, increased hat and glove size, skin striae

F. **Reproduction**

1. Males: onset of puberty, erections, emissions, testicular pain, libido, infertility
2. Females:
   a. Menses: onset, regularity, duration of flow, dysmenorrhea (pain in association with menstruation), last period, intermenstrual discharge or bleeding, pruritus, date of last Pap smear, age at menopause, libido, frequency of intercourse, sexual difficulties
   b. Pregnancies: number, miscarriages, abortions, duration of pregnancy in each and any complication during any pregnancy or postpartum period; use of oral or other contraceptives
   c. Breasts: pain, tenderness, discharge, lumps, mammograms; family history of breast cancer

G. **Respiratory:** pain relating to respiration, dyspnea, cyanosis, wheezing, cough, sputum (character and quantity), hemoptysis (expectorating blood from respiratory tract), night sweats, exposure to TB; date and result of last chest x-ray examination

H. **Cardiac:** chest pain or distress, precipitating causes, timing and duration, relieving factors, palpitations, dyspnea, orthopnea (number of pillows needed), edema, claudication (weakness of legs accompanied by cramplike pain), hypertension, previous myocardial infarction, CHF, estimate of excerise tolerance, past ECG or other cardiac tests; history of coronary artery bypass surgery, percutaneous transluminal coronary angioplasty, or percutaneous balloon valvuloplasty

I. **Hematological:** anemia, tendency to bruise or bleed easily, thromboses, thrombophlebitis, any known abnormality of blood cells, transfusions

J. **Lymph nodes:** enlargement, tenderness, suppuration (to produce purulent [pus] material)

K. **Gastrointestinal:** appetite, digestion, intolerance for any type of foods, dysphagia (difficulty swallowing), heartburn, nausea, vomiting, hematemesis, regularity of bowels, constipation, diarrhea, change in stool color or contents (clay-colored, tarry, fresh blood, mucus, undigested food), flatulence, hemorrhoids, hepatitis, jaundice, dark urine; history of ulcer, gallstones, polyps, tumor; previous x-ray examinations (where, when, findings)

L. **Genitourinary:** dysuria, flank or suprapubic pain, urgency, frequency, nocturia, hematuria, polyuria, hesitancy, dribbling, loss in force of stream, passage of stone; edema of face, stress incontinence, hernias, sexually transmitted disease (inquire what kind and signs and symptoms, and list results of serological test for syphilis [STS], if known)

M. **Neurological:** syncope (brief lapse in consciousness caused by transient cerebral hypoxia), history of CVA, seizures, weakness or paralysis, abnormalities of sensation or coordination, tremors, loss of memory; unusual frequency, distribution, or severity of headaches, serious head injury in past

N. **Psychiatric:** depression, mood changes, difficulty concentrating, nervousness, tension, suicidal thoughts, irritability, sleep disturbances

cise manner using appropriate terminology. A clear, concise record is necessary because other health care professionals may use the nursing health history when delivering health care. Fig. 9-14 on p. 135 illustrates the correct way to record such information.

When the nurse is determining the status of each body system, the patient is asked specific questions relating to the functioning of the organ. For example, assessment of the respiratory system might begin with the question, "Do you have any difficulty with your breathing?" If the answer is yes, then the questioning may continue with, "Please explain," or more specific questions, such as "Do you have shortness of breath?" An ROS guide can be used to guarantee a complete interview.

THERAPEUTIC DIALOGUE

Mr. Jones is admitted to the hospital with a diagnosis of possible peptic ulcer.

Nurse: Mr. Jones, can you tell me about your pain? What brings it on?

Mr. Jones: I get the pain several times a day after I eat. *(provocative) (timing)*

Nurse: What does it feel like?

Mr. Jones: It feels like burning. *(quality)*

Nurse: Where does the pain occur?

Mr. Jones: In my stomach. *(region)*

Nurse: How does the pain rate on a scale of 1 to 10?

Mr. Jones: About an 8. *(severity)*

Nurse: How long have you had this pain?

Mr. Jones: It began about 6 months ago. *(timing)*

GERONTOLOGICAL CONSIDERATIONS

- All systems will manifest changes to a greater or lesser extent with aging. All older adults do not show the physical signs of aging at the same rate.
- It is essential to allow adequate time for a thorough assessment. Several shorter sessions are likely to be better tolerated than one long session.
- During the assessment, the nurse monitors for signs of fatigue such as slumping, sighing, or irritability.
- For comfort during the assessment, the nurse should:
  - Ensure privacy. If the older person has cognitive difficulty or wishes family members' assistance, allow it. Be careful that the family member does not dominate the conversation.
  - Encorage the older person to void before the assessment.
  - Conduct the assessment in a room where bathroom facilities are readily available.
  - Verify that the temperature of the room is warm enough for the older person and free from drafts.
- The nurse should explain what she is doing in terms the older person can understand and should avoid the use of medical jargon.
- The nurse should be patient and listen. The older person may take longer to reply, but it is important to allow him to complete ideas in his own words without interruption.
- The nurse should watch for objective and subjective data during the assessment.

The patient interview at the beginning of the physical assessment gives the nurse much more information about the patient than what is actually spoken. The therapeutic dialogue above is an example of an interview using the PQRST technique. The nurse observes patient mobility and gains insight about the patient's intellect, level of orientation, and emotional and psychological state.

The nurse should assess the appropriateness of the patient's answers. By asking questions such as "Who are you?" "Why are you here?" and "Where are you?" the nurse determines the level of consciousness **(LOC)** and orientation of the patient is made.

Once the interview has been completed, the nurse can proceed to the physical assessment. When assessing the patient, the nurse should pay special attention to areas about which the patient has expressed concern.

NURSING PHYSICAL ASSESSMENT

The physical examination as performed by the nurse may be referred to as the nursing assessment. The purpose of the nursing assessment is to determine the patient's state of health or illness. The data collected are completed as the first step of the nursing process. The nursing assesment is the initial step in forming the nursing care plan, just as the physician performs a physical examination to determine the medical diagnosis. Many of the questions raised by the nurse in preparation to assist the physician are also a necessary part of the nursing physical assessment. Special considerations for assessing older adults are listed in the geronological box.

When to Perform a Nursing Physical Assessment

The best time to assess the patient is as soon after admission as possible. In some facilities, policy dictates that the assessment be done within 24 hours of admission. The initial nursing assessment is performed by a registered nurse; however, the ongoing assessment is the responsibility of both the registered nurse and the licensed practical/vocational nurse.

Obtaining an accurate, comprehensive history requires skill in communicating with individuals who are ill and who may feel that giving a history of their illness is not what they need at that time. The skilled nurse will be able to obtain the essential information despite resistance.

The formal head-to-toe assessment (which will be described in detail) is initially done when the patient is admitted; however, portions of the assessment can be performed when the nurse observes a change in the patient's condition. This is also referred to as a **focused assessment** (concentrated attention on that part of the body where the signs and symptoms are localized or most active in order to determine their significance). The nurse can make a nursing assessment part of daily nursing care. A complete physical assessment performed initially on the patient will help establish a data base (a large store or bank of information) from which the nursing care plan is developed.

Where to Perform a Nursing Assessment

Regardless of the type of nursing interventions performed, whether it be home care, hospital care, or nursing in an extended care facility (ECF), the area in which the nursing assessment is performed should be comfortable for the patient, with a table or bed to allow for the positioning of the patient. It should provide for the patient's privacy and be free of distracting sights and sounds. In most cases the patient's own room works very well and is convenient for both patient and nurse.

Methods of Nursing Physical Assessment

The assessment may be organized as head-to-toe or system-by-system. In either case, the nurse must proceed sys-tematically. If special concerns are expressed by the patient or noted by the nurse, it may be best to perform assessment of the system involved (focused assessment). For example, if the patient complains of abdominal pain, the nurse can then concentrate on assessment of the abdomen, employing percussion, palpation, and auscultation.

The head-to-toe method of assessment is best when performing a complete examination. The nurse begins with the head and neck, including the eyes, ears, nose, and mouth. The chest, back, arms, abdomen, perineal area, legs, and feet are examined in that order.

Performing the Nursing Physical Assessment

Items essential to the nurse's assessment are a penlight or flashlight, stethoscope, blood pressure cuff, thermometer, gloves, and a tongue blade (see Box 9-3). The nurse also makes use of the senses of touch, smell, sight, and hearing. The nurse should always wash the hands before beginning the physical assessment.

The patient should be provided the opportunity to empty the bladder before the examination. This makes the patient more comfortable and allows easier assessment of the bladder.

The patient's vital signs are obtained, including temperature, pulse, respirations, and blood pressure. The patient's height and weight can also be measured at the outset of the examination. Height and weight should be measured by the nurse for accuracy rather than taking the patient's stated height and weight. Vital sign data gathered at the beginning of the assessment may give the nurse a clue as to areas that will warrant more critical evaluation.

Head-to-Toe Assessment.

Head and neck. Assessment of the head includes the eyes, ears, nose, and mouth. The neck involves assessment of arteries, veins, lymph nodes, and the thyroid gland. Examination of the face begins with the assessment of the skin, including the hair.

The nurse should note the symmetry of the face; facial movements should also be symmetrical and appropriate. The facial expression can give clues to the emotional state of the patient. The hair should be of smooth texture and not oily or dry. The scalp should be free of dandruff, lesions, or parasites. The nurse may wish to wear gloves for the inspection of the hair and scalp. The skin's color, texture, temperature, and moisture can be noted. Normal skin tones vary with race, heredity, and exposure to the sun. Color should be observed in the sclera (tough, white, fibrous tissue that covers the white of the eye), conjunctiva (mucous membrane that lines eyelids), buccal mucosa (mucous membranes of the mouth), tongue, lips, nail beds, palms, and soles.

Normally, the skin should be dry and smooth, with good turgor. **Turgor** is the normal resiliency of the skin caused by the outward pressure of the cells and interstitial fluid. Dehydration results in decreased skin turgor, manifested by lax skin that when grasped and raised between two fingers, slowly returns to a position level with the adjacent tissue (Fig. 9-3). Marked edema results in in-

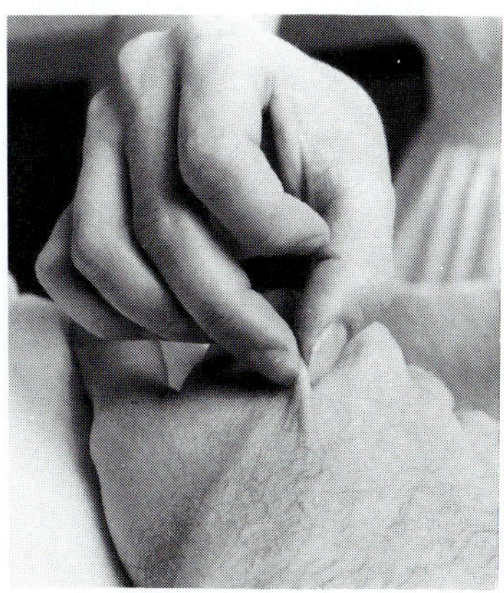

FIG. 9-3 Assess skin turgor by first grasping fold of skin on back of patient's hand, sternum, forearm, or abdomen. Note ease and speed with which skin returns to place.

creased turgor manifested by smooth, taut, shiny skin that cannot be grasped and raised. The nurse should note whether the patient has a normal pattern of hair growth.

Gross assessment of range of motion (ROM) can be done by having the patient move the head from side to side and in a nodding motion. The patient is asked to touch the chin to the chest; the patient should be able to move the head comfortably through these motions. The temporomandibular joint (TMJ) is palpated and the patient is directed to open and close the jaw. There should be no clicking or **crepitus** felt, crepitus being a "crackly" sensation beneath the skin. Using the pads of the fingers, the nurse palpates beneath the jaw and down each side of the neck to feel for enlarged lymph nodes. Although it is not abnormal for a person to have an enlarged node, it should not be tender. The nurse palpates the carotid pulses gently and one at a time (Fig. 9-4). The pulses should be even and palpable without a thrill (vibrating sensation).

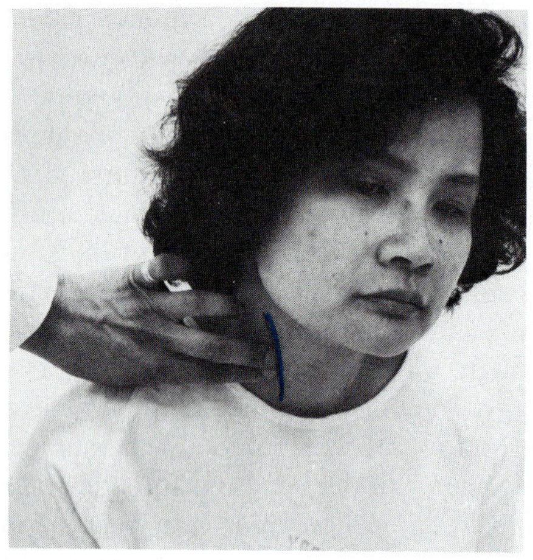

FIG. 9-4 Palpation of carotid artery.

The nurse next inspects for jugular vein distention (JVD). Normally, the veins will not be observable.

The thyroid gland can be palpated for enlargement. This is best done standing behind the patient. The pads of the fingers are placed on either side of the trachea below the Adam's apple, and the patient is asked to tilt the head back slightly and swallow. The nurse should be able to feel the gland sliding up beneath the fingers. The gland should not be noticeably enlarged, nor should it be tender or uneven. Palpation of the thyroid gland takes practice (Fig. 9-5).

Auscultation of the carotid artery can be performed at this point. The artery should be heard just below the mandible (lower jaw) with the bell of the stethoscope. There should be no bruits heard. **Bruits** are abnormal "swishing" sounds heard over organs, glands, and arteries.

Mouth and throat. Inspection of the lips and mucous membranes of the mouth is done with a tongue blade and penlight to assess all surfaces of the oral cavity. The mucous membrane should be pink and free of lesions. The lips should be smooth, moist, and free of cracking. The teeth and gums can be inspected for periodontal disease and dental caries. Assessment of the teeth can give the nurse insight into the health habits of the patient. To examine the throat, the patient is asked to say "ah." The movement of the tongue is noted, and the light is directed to the back surface of the throat to inspect the tonsils and throat for erythema, **leukoplakia** (thickened white patches), edema, or **purulent** discharge (pus). Tonsils may be enlarged, but this is consid-

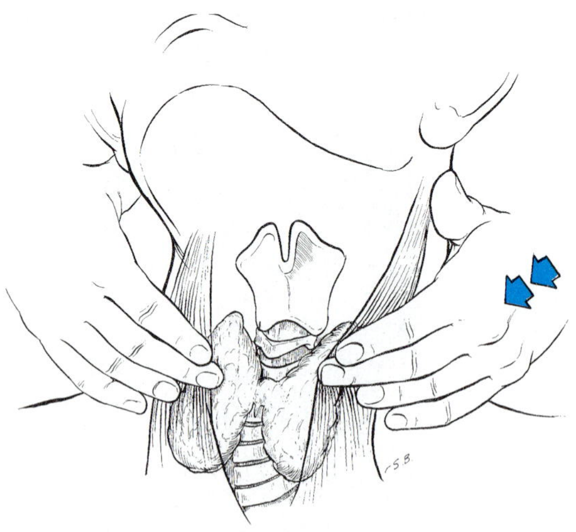

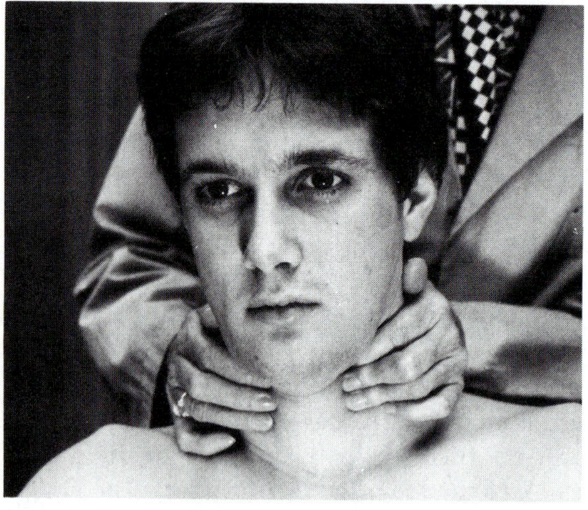

FIG. 9-5 Posterior approach to thyroid examination. To examine the right lobe of the thyroid gland, the examiner displaces the trachea slightly to the right with the fingers of the left hand and palpates for the right thyroid lobe with the fingers of the right hand.

ered normal if other findings are negative. Breath odors can indicate disease; the breath should not be foul, fruity, or musty.

Eyes. The nurse should first note whether the eyes are symmetrical. There should be no exudate from the eyes, and the lids should be open. The sclera of the eye should be white and the conjunctiva pink. There should be no signs of icterus (yellowing of the sclera) or ptosis (drooping of the eyelid). The conjunctiva is observed by gently depressing the lower lid. Periorbital edema (edema around the eyes) is abnormal.

Both eyes should be assessed individually. The nurse also observes the eyes for pupillary reflex. This is done easily by darkening the room, using the penlight to shine the light into the pupil. The light should come from the side of the eye with the patient looking straight ahead at a focal point. The normal eye will show the pupil constricting when the light is applied. The rate and size of constriction should be equal. This finding can be recalled by using the acronym PERRLA, which stands for pupils equal, round, and reactive to light and accommodation.

Eye movement can be assessed by having the patient hold the head still and follow the tip of the nurse's finger with the eyes. The patient should be able to follow the examiner's finger without difficulty. The hand is moved in a star pattern to check all possible movements. The patient should have no extraocular movements. Visual acuity (clearness of perception) can be simply assessed by having the patient read newsprint. If the patient uses glasses or contact lenses, she should wear them. Examination with the ophthalmoscope (a device for examining the interior of the eye) is an advanced procedure, and the ophthalmoscope may not be available to the nurse in a particular setting. The screening mentioned above can give adequate information for the nurse to make a nursing diagnosis.

Ears. The nurse first notes that the ears are symmetrical and the level at which they are attached to the head. There should not be any discharge from the ears. The ear canal can be examined by using the penlight and pulling gently back and up on the external ear with the fingers. Moving the ear in this manner will straighten the canal and allow the nurse to look further into it. With a child under the age of 3, the ear is pulled back and down. There should not be any pain associated with this movement. The ear canal should be free of excess cerumen (earwax), blood, or any purulent discharge.

During this assessment, the nurse should note whether the patient is appropriately following commands, indicating ability to hear. A simple hearing test can be conducted by standing behind the patient and having him repeat whispered words; another test involves rubbing the patient's hair between the fingers near the ear and asking the patient if the sound can be heard. Examination with an otoscope (an instrument used to examine the ear) is an advanced procedure, and the otoscope may not be available to the nurse in a particular setting. The above screening procedure can give adequate information for the nurse to make a nursing diagnosis.

Nose. The nose should be symmetrical, although variations in size are considered normal. To test for patency (condition of being opened or unblocked), the nurse presses against one nostril and asks the patient to breathe. Air should flow through the nose. Both nostrils are assessed, observing for bleeding or drainage. The nurse palpates on either side of the nose beneath the eyes with the fingertips to assess for sinus tenderness. Sinuses should not be tender. The functioning of the first cranial nerve is checked by having the patient smell and name a common odor. The first cranial nerve is the olfactory nerve for the sense of smell. An alcohol wipe or lemon glycerine swab can be used.

Chest, lungs, and heart. Assessment of the chest, lungs, and heart is performed with the patient in a sitting position. The nurse inspects the chest for bilateral chest expansion, which should be symmetrical. The respiratory rate and depth of respirations are noted. Audible congestion is noted and can later be auscultated to determine the quality. The normal respiratory rate for an adult is 12 to 20 breaths per minute. Breathing should be quiet. Posture can indicate pulmonary status: the patient who is unable to lie supine or who must lean forward to breathe may have respiratory difficulty. A large, rounded "barrel chest" may be a sign of increased respiratory effort such as in emphysema.

Breasts. The breasts should be examined once a month on a regular basis. (See Chapter 38 for the breast self-examination [BSE] and the assessment of the breasts.)

Lung sounds. Auscultation of breath sounds is a major method of assessing the lungs' status. When beginning to assess breath sounds, it is sufficient for the nurse to recognize the sound of normal respirations; this later allows recognition of abnormal sounds. Both the bell and diaphragm of the stethoscope should be used. Labeling the sounds will come with practice. Lung sounds are best heard by placing the stethoscope on the patient's back. The diaphragm of the stethoscope is used to pick up the lung sounds. The nurse should listen for one full inspiratory/expiratory cycle at each point. Adventitious breath sounds that are not normally heard are superimposed over normal sounds. The nurse's eyes should be closed and the breath held when listening so that she can concentrate on the sounds (Figs. 9-6 and 9-7 on p. 138). Breath sounds are classified as either crackles (rales) or wheezes (rhonchi). **Crackles** can be fine, medium, or coarse. Fine crackles sound like hair being rubbed between the fingers and are heard at the end of the inspiratory phase. They are high pitched and discrete. Medium crackles have a deeper tone and a more moist sound and

FIG. 9-6 Thoracic landmarks. **A,** Anterior thorax. **B,** Posterior thorax.

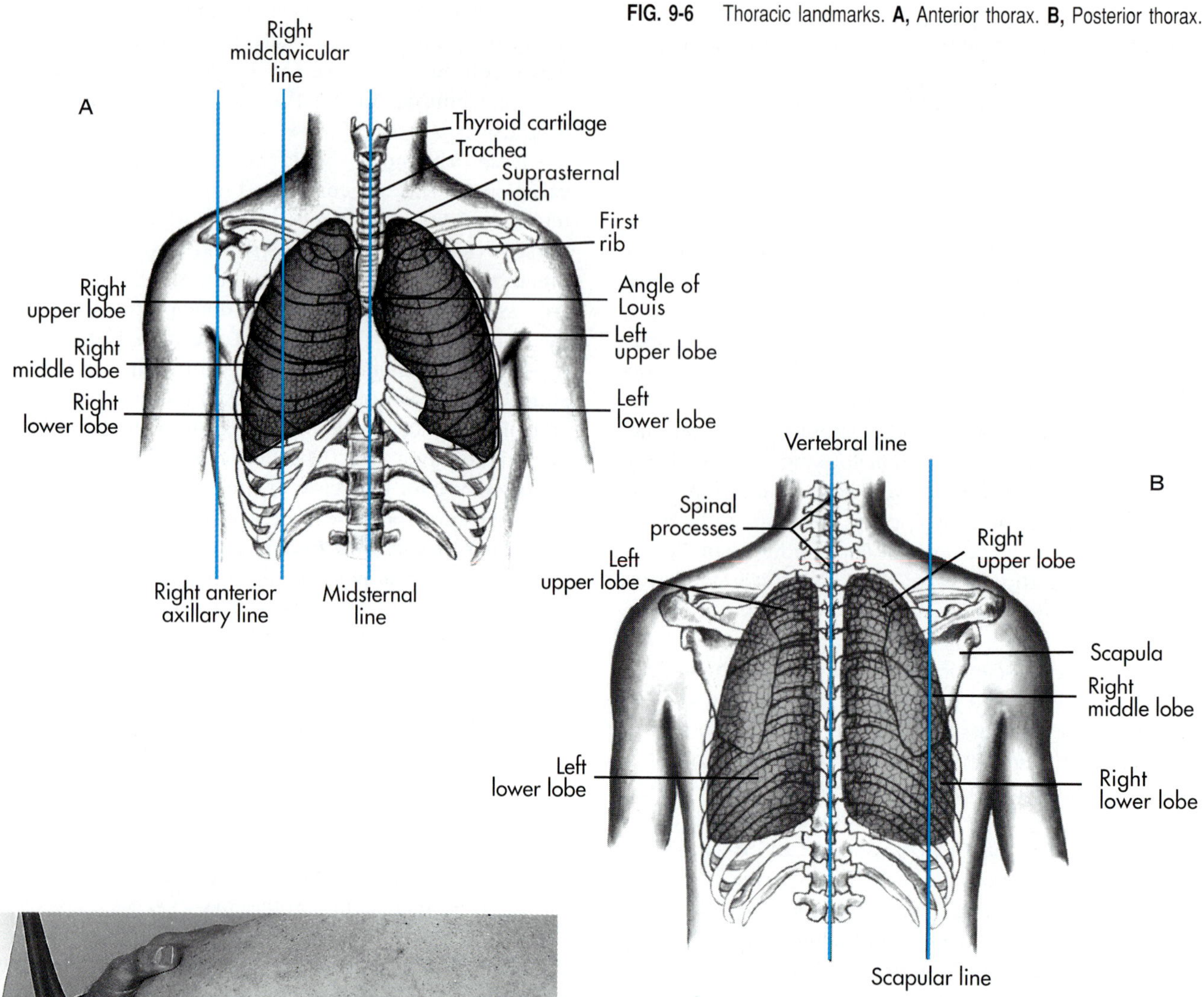

A
Right midclavicular line
Thyroid cartilage
Trachea
Suprasternal notch
First rib
Angle of Louis
Right upper lobe
Right middle lobe
Right lower lobe
Left upper lobe
Left lower lobe
Right anterior axillary line
Midsternal line

B
Vertebral line
Spinal processes
Left upper lobe
Right upper lobe
Scapula
Right middle lobe
Left lower lobe
Right lower lobe
Scapular line

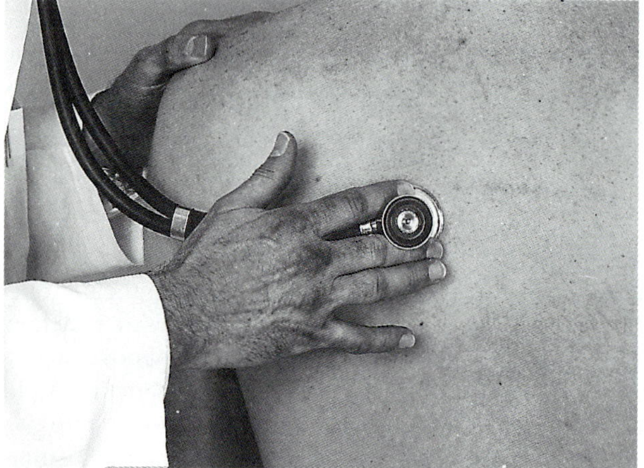

FIG. 9-7 In an adult the nurse uses the diaphragm of the stethoscope to auscultate breath sounds.

are usually heard in the middle of the inspiration. Medium crackles sound like the "fizzing" of a carbonated beverage. Coarse crackles make a loud, bubbling sound and are heard at the beginning of inspiration. Coarse crackles are sometimes referred to as the "death rattle." **Wheezes** are classified as sibilant or sonorous. Sibilant wheezes may be heard on both inspiration and expiration and sound like high-pitched crowing. Sonorous wheezes are lower-pitched sounds. Wheezes characteristically clear when the patient coughs, whereas crackles do not. As a rule, crackles indicate congestion in the smaller alveoli, and wheezes indicate narrowing or congestion in the larger airways of the bronchial tree and trachea (Fig. 9-8). Pleural friction rubs can also be heard and sound like "pieces of leather being rubbed together." This sound indicates inflammation of the pleura (refer to Table 31-1).

Spine. With the patient in a sitting position, the curvature of the spine is noted. The nurse should also assess the posture when the patient is standing. The nurse can run the fingers down the patient's spine. The spine should be straight. There should be a normal lumbosacral curve. The skin of the back should be of normal color, temperature, and moisture (see Chapter 26).

Heart sounds. Heart sounds are auscultated with the stethoscope. The nurse places the stethoscope at four

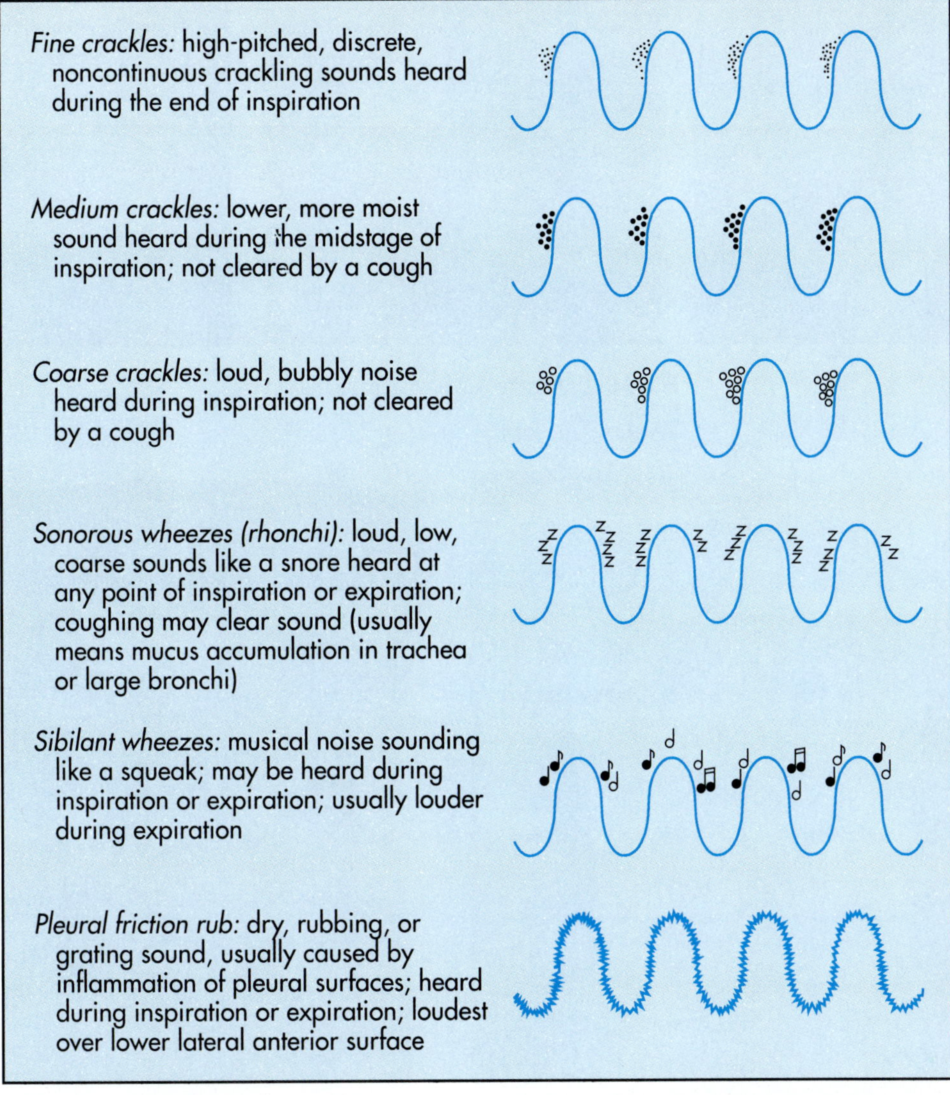

FIG. 9-8 Adventitious breath sounds. (Modified from Stiesmeyer JK: Pulmonary assessment: A four step approach, *Am J Nurs* 93(8):22, 1993.)

points on the patient's chest and listens for several cardiac cycles at each point. The normal "lub-dub" sound of the heart occurs because of the contraction of the atria and ventricles, respectively. When listening, the nurse uses both the bell and the diaphragm of the stethoscope to hear low- and high-pitched sounds (Fig. 9-9 on p. 140; see Chapter 28).

Abdomen. During the remaining portion of the examination the patient can remain in the supine position. The nurse then examines the abdomen. During this portion of the assessment, the patient should be properly draped to decrease exposure of the pubic area. The nurse first inspects the abdomen for shape, contour, lesions, scars, lumps, or rashes. The abdomen's contour should be even, and skin color should be the same as that of the thorax. Before palpating, the nurse auscultates for bowel sounds by placing the diaphragm of the stethoscope over the divisions of the abdomen and listening for the peristaltic sounds produced by the intestines (Fig. 9-10 on p. 140). Because peristalsis (wavelike movements of the intestines) is continuous, sound should be present in all quadrants. Bowel sounds occur every 15 to 60 seconds and are classified as hyperactive, hypoactive, or absent. If the patient is on a nasogastric suction machine or if a radio or television is on, it should be turned off. The nurse listens to bowel sounds for 1 minute in all quadrants. However, if the patient does not have abdominal complaints, it is not necessary to listen to each quadrant for 1 minute. The normal rate of bowel sounds is 4 to 32 per minute.

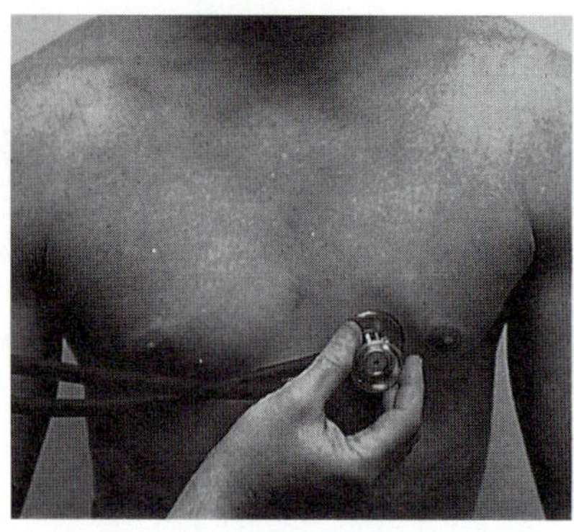
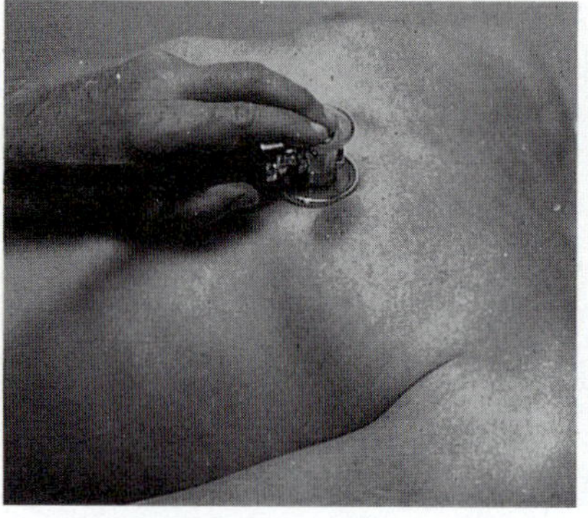
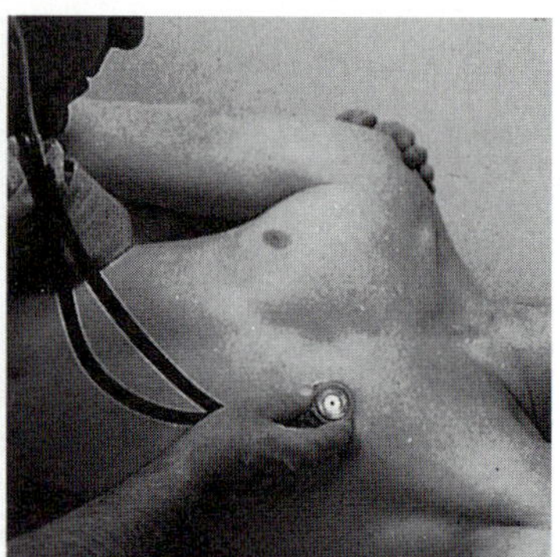

FIG. 9-9 Areas for auscultation of the heart.

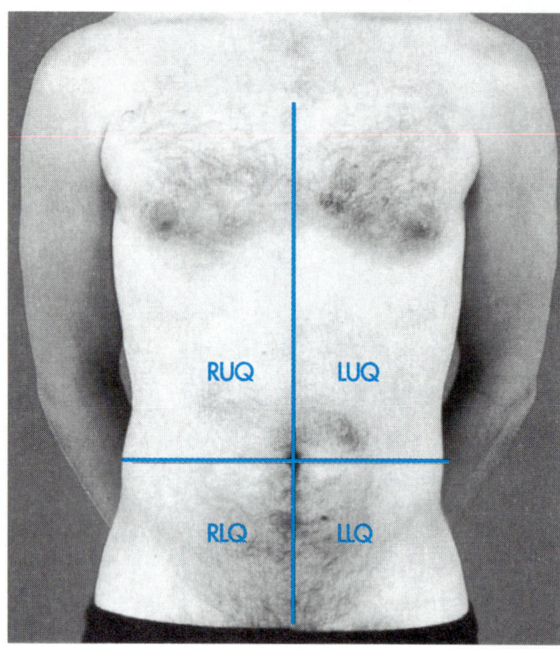

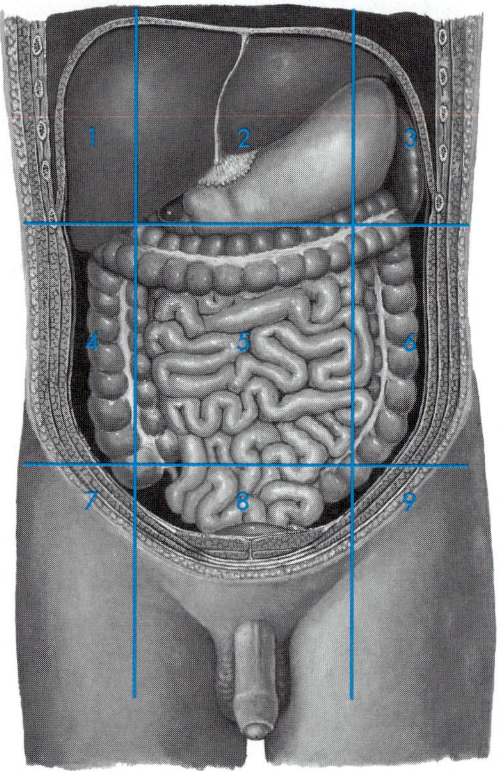

FIG. 9-10 Anatomical divisions of the abdomen.

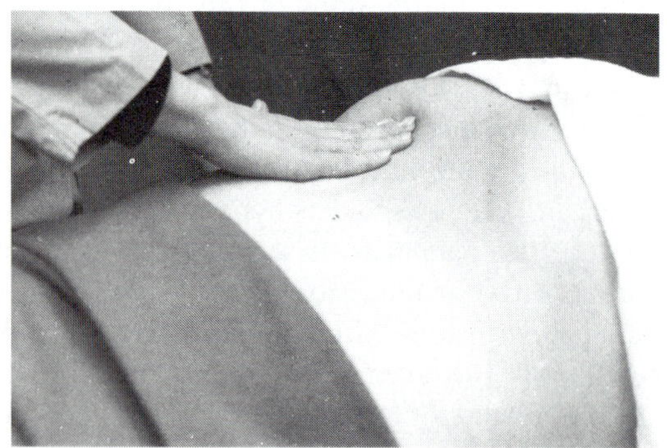
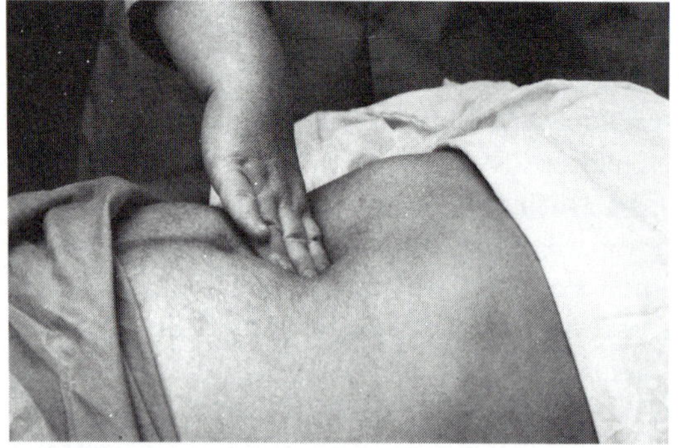

FIG. 9-11 Palpation of the abdomen to assess organs such as the liver and spleen.

After auscultating for bowel sounds, the nurse can then palpate the underlying structures. Both light and deep palpation is used. Beginning with light palpation, the nurse notes the texture, temperature, and moisture of the skin in all regions. To ensure that the patient is relaxed during the palpation, the hands should be warmed, and conversation can be used to distract the patient. Light palpation can detect superficial lesions just below the skin. The skin of the abdomen should be smooth, dry, and warm. Deep palpation is used to detect tenderness or masses of the abdomen. In the upper right quadrant just below the rib cage, the liver may be palpated. If the liver can be felt, this may mean that it is enlarged. The patient's liver should be smooth and nontender. The abdomen itself should be free of masses, and palpation should not be uncomfortable for the patient (Fig. 9-11).

The nurse notes the patient's face when palpating and looks for grimacing. The patient may also guard a tender area, which means he will tighten up abdominal muscles when the area is touched.

Percussion is used on the abdomen to note the density of underlying tissue. It is also used to locate the margins of internal organs. The abdomen has a tympanic (drumlike) sound, with dullness noted over the liver. A hollow sound heard over the stomach or intestines indicates flatus.

Genitourinary system. Nurses do not perform the vaginal examination with a speculum unless they have had advanced training. Assessment of the urinary system is performed using observation and palpation. It is most convenient for the nurse to perform this inspection during the perineal care of the patient. Gloves should be worn when inspecting the labia for lesions. The pubic hair is inspected for lice, and any vaginal discharge is noted. Normal labia are pink, moist, and free of lesions. A normal white vaginal discharge known as leukorrhea can be present in the female.

The male genitalia are inspected for lesions and lice; the nurse looks for discharge from the penis. The scrotum is palpated for lumps or hernias. If the male is uncircumcised, the foreskin should be retracted to inspect for lesions on the glans penis.

While inspecting the genitalia on both the male and female, the nurse can palpate the femoral artery in that area (Fig. 9-12). Palpation of the suprapubic area can also be performed to determine bladder distention. Tenderness at the costovertebral angle (CVA) could indicate kidney disease.

Rectum. The rectal area is best examined with the patient in a Sims' position. The buttocks can be spread to look for hemorrhoids or lesions. Normal skin around the anus is darker than surrounding skin. To further assess the intestinal system, the nurse can explain the procedure for obtaining a stool specimen to the patient and leave a Hemoccult slide with the patient. The results of the test may indicate whether gastrointestinal bleeding is present.

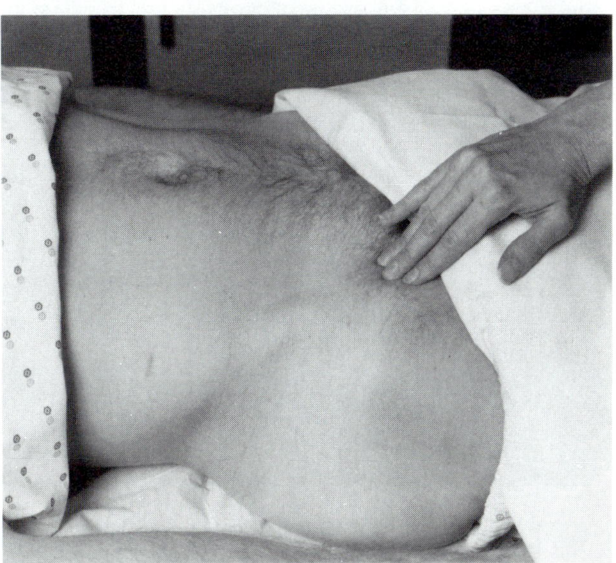

FIG. 9-12 Palpation of the femoral artery.

Legs and feet. The legs and feet are the final area of assessment. Femoral, popliteal, posterior tibial, and pedal pulses should be palpated (Fig. 9-13 on p. 141). The legs and feet should be observed and palpated for edema. Edema is a sign of interstitial fluid. To check for edema, press the bony prominence over the tibia or medial malleolus (a rounded bony process on the midline of the ankle) for several seconds and lift the finger. If the depression does not fill almost immediately, pitting edema is present (see Table 28-3 and Fig. 28-22). The nurse directs the patient to flex knees and ankles to test for ROM, although a better assessment of this is made by observing the patient's gait. Skin color on the legs should be similar to the rest of the body. Varicosities (enlarged veins) should not be present.

Check the CMS (color, motion, and sensation) of both feet. The nurse can test for sensation by touching the toes and asking the patient whether she feels it. The patient's feet should be equally warm. Pedal pulses should be present (see Table 10-2). Corns or bunions may interfere with the patient's mobility.

Neurological assessment. The neurological assessment can be integrated with the head-to-toe assessment. For instance, after taking a radial pulse the nurse can have the patient grasp the nurse's hands to test for equal grip. Gross motor and coordination skills can be assessed by having the patient touch the tip of the nose with the finger and then touch the tip of the nurse's finger as it is moved to different positions. The patient should be able to follow the movement of the nurse's finger. (See Chapter 35 for further assessment of the nervous system.)

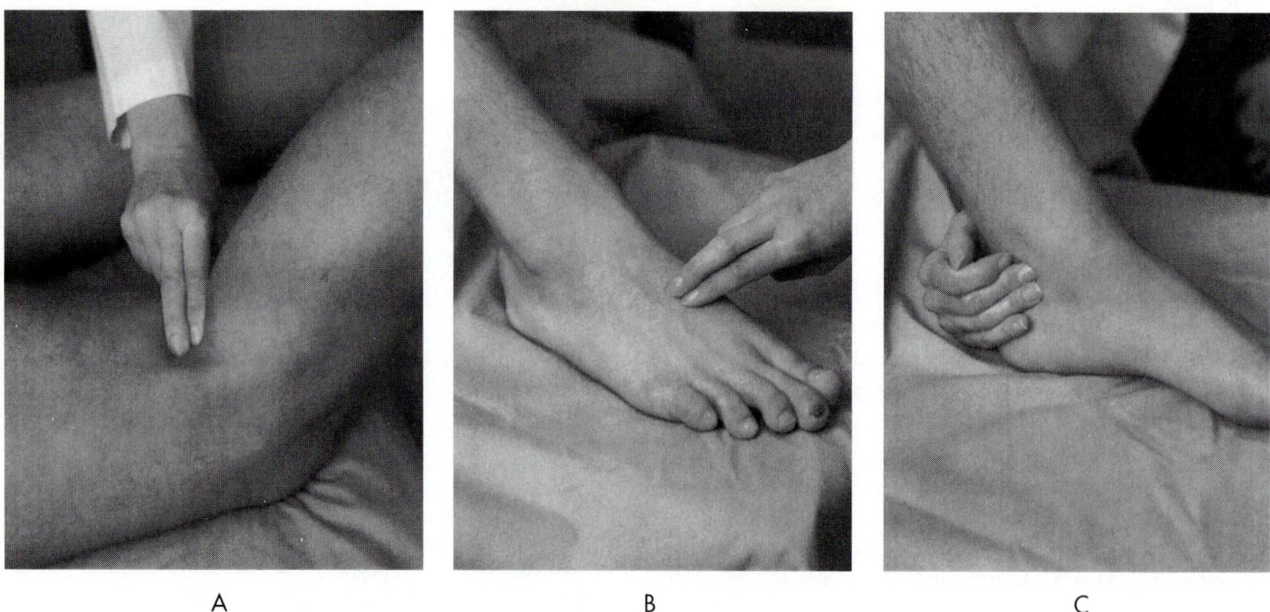

FIG. 9-13 **A,** The patient lies with knee flexed to give the nurse access to the popliteal pulse. **B,** The dorsalis pedis pulse is palpated at a point along a line with the groove between the extensor tendons of the great and first toes. **C,** Palpation of posterior tibial pulse below the medial malleolus.

Great Plains Regional Medical Center

NURSING ADMISSION ASSESSMENT

Admitted: Ambulatory, Cart, Wheelchair, Arms, Ambulance

From: Office, ER, Surgery, Radiology, Recovery Room Transferred From: physician's office

Oriented to Room: Call Light, Siderails, TV, Phone, Safety/Smoking Policy: Yes ✓ No ____

Vital Signs: T 101² P 92 P 24 BP 160/92 HT 5'4" WT 190 Dentures upper/lower

Diet at home: 2 gm sodium

Allergies: Drug penicillin Reaction hives

Other none Organ Donor: Yes ____ No X

Reason for Admission Elevated temperature & fluid retention Signature E. Fletcher, LPN

Date: 12/20/94 **Time:** 2000

EYES Impaired Vision, Blind, Cataract, Glaucoma, Contacts, Glasses, Prosthesis R. L.
Comments: cataract surgery (rt eye) 1993 OD

EARS, NOSE, THROAT: Hard of hearing, Deaf, Lesions, Hearing Aid, R L., Tracheotomy
Comments:

RESPIRATORY: Pain, Dyspnea, Wheeze, Asthma, Sinusitis, COPD, Cough,
Productive ____ Non Productive X
Oxygen needed, Smoker
Comments: c/o shortness of breath upon exertion crackles right base

CIRCULATION: Apical, Radial, Strong, Weak, Thready, Bounding, Regular, Palpitations, Chest pain, Numbness, Bruising, Edema, Hypertension, Hx MI, CHF, Pacer, Bypass Surgery
Comments: st " 4 pound weight gain in the last 3 days 3t pitting edema bilaterally

ENDOCRINE: Thyroid, Diabetes
Comments: no problems

GI TRACT: Heartburn, ulcers, Pain, Hernia, Dysphagia, Nausea, Vomiting, Loss of Appetite, Distention, Diverticulities
Comments:

ELIMINATION: Last BM 2 days ago Normal, Constipated, Diarrhea, Tarry, Bright red, Clay colored, Hemorrhoids, Involuntary, Use of laxatives, Yes/No
Enema, Yes/No Ileostomy, Colostomy
Comments:

URINARY: Incontinence, Nocturia, Hematuris, Dysuria, Burning, Frequency, Urgency, Dribbling, Infections,
Cath: Yes/No
comments:

NEUROLOGICAL: Convulsions, Paralysis, Syncope, Paresthesia, Dizziness, Coordination, Weakness, Headaches,
Comments:

SKIN: Color pale Turgor poor Temp warm
Describe any rashes, Lesions, Exxhymosis, Petechiae, Scars, Diabetic sores,
Comments: central abdominal scar

MUSCULOSKELETAL: Pain, Stiffness, Contractures, Deformities, Tremors, Backaches, Weight bearing, Amputation
Comments:

FEMALE REPRODUCTION: LMP EDC
Menopause, Breast pain, Breast tenderness, Vaginal discharge,
Comments: post

PREVIOUS SURGERIES: hemiorrhaphy ventral 1990
Rt eye Cataract surgery 1993

MEDS TAKEN AT HOME:

Med:	Dose:	Last Taken:
Lanoxin	25 mgm qam	AM
Lasix	40 mgm qam	AM
K-Lor	10 mEq BID	AM
Halcion	25 mgm HS	Last pm

DISPOSAL OF MEDS:
Did no bring ✓
Pt. has ____ Family took home ____
Retained/taken to Pharmacy ____
Other:

Signature: Carolyn Oden RN
Time:

FIG. 9-14 Nursing admission assessment. (Courtesy Great Plains Regional Medical Center, North Platte, Neb.)

Recording the Interview

Most institutions have a form to follow when conducting the patient interview and review of systems (Fig. 9-14). The nurse should state the patient's complaints in the patient's own words. It is acceptable to record information as it is obtained; therefore a pad and pencil may be helpful during the assessment.

REFERENCES AND SUGGESTED READINGS

1. American Nurses Association: *Standards of clinical nursing practice,* Kansas City, Mo, 1991, The Association.
2. Anonymous: Assessing the lungs, *Nursing* 21:32, 1991.
3. Brigdon P, Todd M: In search of the perfect assessment, *Prof Nurse* 5(4):181, 1990.
4. Bright LD, Georgi S: Peripheral vascular disease: is it arterial or venous? *Am J Nurs* 92(9):34, 1992.
5. Brown M: How do you spell assessment? . . . Simple mnemonic device to organize your work, *Am J Nurs* 7:55, 1991.
6. Collier JAH: Developmental and systems perspectives on chronic illness, *Holistic Nurs Pract* 5(1):31, 1990.
7. Cooper KM: Measuring blood pressure the right way, *Nursing* 22:75, 1992.
8. Dykes PC: Mending the Five P's of neurovascular assessment, *Am J Nurs* 93(6):38, 1993.
9. Edelman CL, Mandle CL: *Health promotion throughout the life span,* ed 2, St Louis, 1990, Mosby.
10. Erickson R, Kirklin S: Comparison of methods for core temperature measurement, *Heart Lung* 55(2):297, 1992.
11. Finesilver C: Respiratory assessment, *RN* 55(2):22, 1992.
12. Gehring PE: Physical assessment begins with a history, *RN* 54:26, 1991.
13. Gehring PE: Vascular assessment, *RN* 55:40, 1992.
14. Holmgren C: Abdominal assessment, *RN* 55:28, 1992.
15. Hood GH, Dincher JR: *Total patient care,* ed 8, St Louis, 1992, Mosby.
16. Joint Commission on Accreditation of Healthcare Organizations: *Manual of hospital accreditations: 1992 standards,* Chicago, 1992, The Commission.
17. Lower J: Rapid neuro assessment, *Am J Nurs* 92:38, 1992.
18. Malasanos L et al: *Health assessment,* ed 4, St Louis, 1990, Mosby.
19. McConnell EA: Clinical do's and don'ts: assessing the skin, *Nursing* 22:86, 1992.
20. Morley CJ: Measuring infants' temperatures, *Midwives Chronicle,* Feb 1992, p 26.
21. *Mosby's medical and nursing dictionary,* ed 3, St Louis, 1990, Mosby.
22. Perry A, Potter P: *Clinical nursing skills and technique,* ed 3, St Louis, 1994, Mosby.
23. Phipps W et al: *Medical-surgical nursing: concepts and clinical practice,* ed 5, St Louis, 1995, Mosby.
24. Potter P, Perry A: *Basic nursing: theory and practice,* ed 3, St Louis, 1995, Mosby.
25. Potter P, Perry A: *Fundamentals of nursing concepts, process, and practice,* ed 3, St Louis, 1993, Mosby.
26. Seidel HM et al: *Mosby's guide to physical examination,* ed 2, St Louis, 1991, Mosby.
27. Selby TL: RNs work to keep America healthy, *Am Nurse* 22(2):3, 1990.
28. Stiesmeyer JK: Pulmonary assessment: a four-step approach, *Am J Nurs* 93(8):22, 1993.
29. The Staff: *Nursing procedures,* Springhouse, Penn, 1992, Springhouse.
30. Thomas CL: *Taber's cyclopedic medical dictionary,* ed 17, Philadelphia, 1993, FA Davis.
31. Timby BK, Lewis LW: *Fundamental skills and concepts in patient care,* ed 5, Philadelphia, 1991, Lippincott.

CHAPTER CHALLENGE

KEY POINTS

- A sign is perceived by the nurse using the senses of sight, touch, smell, and hearing.
- A symptom is a sensation felt only by the patient, such as pruritus (itching), pain, or dizziness.
- Diseases originate from several different causes, and may be hereditary, congenital, traumatic, neoplastic, infectious, deficiency, or environmental in nature.
- Risk factors for acquiring a disease include age, genetics, environment, and life-style variables.
- The universal signs of infection are erythema, edema, pain, heat, loss of function, and purulent, malodorous drainage.
- Some frequently noted signs and symptoms of disease are cyanosis, pallor, erythema, edema, nausea, vomiting, diarrhea, dyspnea, tachycardia, and fever.
- When a physician conducts a physical exam, the nurse is often requested to assist the examiner. There are certain responsibilities for the nurse, such as preparing the examining room, assisting with equipment, and preparing the patient.
- Becoming cognizant of results of laboratory evaluation of specimens such as urine and stool can add to the information about the patient.
- The nurse can perform an assessment to determine the actual or high risk for patient problems that will require nursing interventions to promote the safety and well-being of the patient.
- A complete nursing physical assessment should be performed as soon after admission as possible.
- Interviewing the patient initially determines signs, symptoms, and areas of patient concern that can be clarified by the examination.
- The physical assessment should proceed in an orderly fashion: head-to-toe or system-by-system.
- Assessment should be performed with specific skills of observation, palpation, percussion, and auscultation.
- The practical/vocational nurse should be familiar with normal assessments and thus be able to identify abnormalities.

STUDY QUESTIONS

1. Mr. Jones, age 31, has been admitted with a diagnosis of pneumonia. He has many signs of the disease. One sign of the disease would be:
   1. Fatigue
   2. Anorexia
   3. Pain
   4. Fever
2. John Manns, age 9, has a congenital condition, cystic fibrosis, which affects his ability to breathe effectively. This condition is an example of a disease originating from:
   1. Exercise
   2. Heredity
   3. Dieting
   4. Environment
3. Lisa Ann, age 13, has an infection in her finger resulting from a cat scratch. Her hand is painful and reddened. This redness of the skin would be documented as:
   1. Jaundice
   2. Erythema
   3. Edema
   4. Bruising
4. Mr. Baurer, age 90, has chronic obstructive pulmonary disease. He sleeps sitting in a chair leaning over a table in order to breathe more easily. This condition would be called:
   1. Orthopnea
   2. Tachypnea
   3. Apnea
   4. Bradypnea
5. Mr. Brown, 80 years of age, lives alone in his apartment. The visiting nurse is contacted to assess Mr. Brown's ability to care for himself. During the interview, Mr. Brown acts suspicious and reluctant to talk. Communication with Mr. Brown can be enhanced by the nurse's:
   1. Asking questions requiring "yes" or "no" responses
   2. Sitting down during the interview process
   3. Avoiding eye contact with Mr. Brown
   4. Using prolonged periods of silence
6. While obtaining a history of 36-year-old Mr. Parrot's present illness, colitis, the nurse uses the PQRST method to elicit more details of his condition. A question that might be asked during the "P" portion of the interview would be:
   1. How does it feel?
   2. What causes the diarrhea?
   3. When does the pain occur?
   4. When did the diarrhea begin?
7. During the review of systems, the nurse questions Mrs. Smith, age 40, regarding the functioning of her lungs. An appropriate question to ask of Mrs. Smith would be, Do you have:
   1. Any wheezing
   2. Any vertigo
   3. Any syncope
   4. Any palpitations

10

VITAL SIGNS

Audrey Wadman Szczesiul

KEY TERMS

apical pulse
apnea
auscultate
auscultatory gap
axillary
blood pressure
bradycardia
bradypnea
Cheyne-Stokes respirations
diastolic
dyspnea
dysrhythmia
expiration
febrile
hypertension
hyperthermia
hyperventilation
hypotension
hypothermia
hypoventilation
inspiration
Korotkoff sounds
orthostatic hypotension
pulse
pulse deficit
pulse pressure
pyrexia
radial pulse
respirations
sphygmomanometer
stethoscope
systolic
tachycardia
tachypnea
temperature
tympanic
vital signs

LEARNING OBJECTIVES

After reading this chapter, the student should be able to do the following:

- Define the key terms.
- Discuss guidelines for vital sign measurement.
- Discuss the procedures for obtaining oral, rectal, axillary, and tympanic temperatures.
- List various sites for the pulse measurement.
- Describe the procedure for obtaining an apical pulse, a radial pulse, and a pulse deficit.
- Describe the procedure for determining the respiratory rate.
- List the steps in obtaining the blood pressure.
- State the normal limits of each vital sign.
- List the factors that affect vital sign readings.
- Describe the procedure for obtaining accurate height and weight measurements.
- Discuss frequency of vital signs measurement.
- Discuss methods by which the nurse can ensure accurate measurement of vital signs.
- Describe the benefits of and precautions to follow for self-measurement of blood pressure.

RELATED TOPICS OF INTEREST

- Documentation (Chapter 6)
- Signs, symptoms, and physical assessment (Chapter 9)
- Medical asepsis and infection control (Chapter 12)
- Care of the patient with a cardiovascular disorder (Chapter 28)
- Care of the patient with a respiratory disorder (Chapter 31)

Vital signs include temperature, pulse, respirations, and blood pressure. It is necessary for the nurse to be able to obtain accurate measurements of these. Because vital signs are an indication of basic body functioning, it is appropriate to begin the physical assessment by obtaining these data.

Box 10-1

GUIDELINES FOR VITAL SIGN MEASUREMENT

- The nurse who cares for the patient is ideally the one to assess vital signs, interpret their significance, and participate in decisions about care.
- Equipment used to measure vital signs (e.g., thermometer, stethoscope, sphygmomanometer) must be in proper working condition to ensure accurate findings.
- The nurse should be aware of the normal range for all vital signs. This knowledge will help the nurse detect abnormalities.
- The nurse must be aware of the patient's normal range of vital signs. The patient's normal range may differ from the standard range. These values serve as a baseline for comparison with findings obtained later.
- It is wise for the nurse to know the patient's medical history, therapies, and medications prescribed. Some illnesses or treatments cause predictable vital signs changes.
- The nurse will know to control or minimize environmental factors that may affect vital signs. Assessing the patient's pulse after ambulation or an emotional trauma and obtaining a temperature reading in a warm, humid room may yield values that are not true indicators of the patient's condition.
- The nurse uses an organized, systematic approach when obtaining vital signs. When using a glass thermometer, measure temperature while assessing the pulse, respirations, and blood pressure.
- The nurse and physician decide the frequency of vital sign measurement on the basis of the patient's condition. Most acute care facilities have a policy of assessing patient's vital signs at least every shift. However, certain conditions dictate more frequent measurement of vital signs, such as after a patient has had surgery or a major diagnostic procedure: frequent measurements are taken until vital signs stabilize to the patient's baseline prior to the procedure. If a patient's physical condition begins to worsen, the nurse takes vital signs more frequently, perhaps every 5 to 10 minutes.
- The nurse studies the results of vital sign measurement. Vital signs are only one measurement of the patient's condition. The nurse must also assess other signs and symptoms and be aware of the patient's ongoing health status. Vital signs are only a part of the assessment of the patient's physical and psychological condition.
- The nurse verifies and communicates significant changes in vital signs. The baseline measurement allows the nurse to identify changes in vital signs; the nurse reports abnormal vital signs to the physician. The nurse must also record and report any changes to the nurses working the oncoming shift.

The skills required to measure vital signs are simple but should never become routine. Vital signs and other physiological measurements can be the bases for problem solving. Careful technique ensures accurate findings.

GUIDELINES FOR OBTAINING VITAL SIGNS

Vital signs are a part of the data base that a nurse obtains during assessment. The procedure for assessing vital signs is not routine but is individualized to a patient's needs and condition. The nurse must be able to:

- Measure vital signs correctly
- Understand and interpret the values
- Communicate findings appropriately
- Begin interventions as needed

The nurse's judgment determines the need for and frequency of vital signs measurement (Box 10-1).

TEMPERATURE

The body strives to maintain a **temperature** (a relative measure of sensible heat or cold) of 98.6° F (37° C) (Box 10-2), which is considered normal. However, variations of from 97° F to 99.6° F (36.1° C to 37.5° C) are considered to be within normal range. Many factors can cause body temperature variances, including the environment, the time of day, the patient's state of health, activity levels, and stage of monthly menstrual cycle (Box 10-3).

Body temperature is regulated by the hypothalamus, which is located in the brain, forming the floor and part of the lateral wall of the third ventricle. The hypothalamus helps maintain a balance between heat lost and heat produced by the body.

Box 10-2

NORMAL BODY TEMPERATURES ACCORDING TO SITES

	Oral	Rectal	Axillary	Tympanic
Fahrenheit (F)	98.6°	99.5°	97.6°	98.6°
Centigrade (C)	37.0°	37.5°	36.4°	37.0°

When it is necessary to convert temperature readings, formulas can be used. To convert Fahrenheit to centigrade, the nurse subtracts 32° from the Fahrenheit reading and multiplies the results by 5/9:

$$C = (F - 32° \times 5/9)$$

To convert centigrade to Fahrenheit, the nurse multiplies the centigrade reading by 9/5 and adds 32° to the reading:

$$F = (9/5 \times C) + 32°$$

The body produces heat by metabolism. The amount of heat produced can be increased by increasing metabolism, as with exercise and digestion. Constriction of peripheral vessels helps conserve heat by preventing loss of heat through the skin surface.

Temperature measurements are obtained by several methods. Glass and electronic thermometers are used to obtain oral, rectal, and **axillary** (armpit) temperatures. Heat-sensitive patches are used also. The patches are placed on an area of skin, such as the forehead. Color changes on the patch indicate temperature readings. **Tympanic** (membranous "eardrum") temperature measurement is becoming more popular today (see Skill 10-5 and Fig. 10-1).

Box 10-3 FACTORS AFFECTING BODY TEMPERATURE

Age. The neonate's temperature normally ranges from 35.5° to 37.5° C (96° to 99.5° F). Temperature regulation is labile during infancy because of immature physiological mechanisms. This can continue until puberty. In older adults the normal range commonly lowers, with 35° C (95° F) not being unusual for some older patients in cold weather. With aging, sensitivity to temperature extremes develops because of deteriorating control mechanisms.

Exercise. Any form of exercise can increase body temperature. Prolonged strenuous exercise can temporarily raise body temperatures to as high as 31° to 41° C (103.2° to 105.8° F).

Hormonal influences. Women generally have greater variations in body temperature than men. Hormone changes during ovulation and menopause cause body temperature fluctuations.

Diurnal variations (happening daily). Body temperatures normally change throughout the day, with the lowest reading occurring between 1 AM and 4 AM (36.5° C [97.7° F] on average). The temperature usually peaks around 4 to 6 PM.

Stress. Physical or emotional stress, such as anxiety, may raise body temperature.

Environment. Environmental temperature extremes can raise or lower the body temperature. The changes depend on the extent of exposure, air humidity, and the presence of convection currents.

Ingestion of hot and cold liquids. Drinking hot or cold liquids can cause slight variations in actual oral temperature readings (−0.2° to −1.6° F after drinking iced water).

Smoking. Smoking cigarettes or cigars may alter body temperature measurement (−0.2° F to 0.2° F).

The sensor probe on the tympanic thermometer is placed in the external ear and infrared heat is measured. The benefits of this method are that the results are fast (2 seconds) and accurate, since measurement is from an enclosed cavity unaffected by the environmental temperature. Probe covers decrease spread of infection, and neither the exposure of the patient nor active participation is needed as with rectal/oral measurement. A switch on the thermometer provides oral and rectal equivalents (Fig. 10-1 on p. 148).

Glass thermometers have been widely replaced by the electronic thermometer, since the electronic method is fast and accurate (Fig. 10-2 on p. 148). Determining body core temperature rectally is most accurate, since the thermometer is placed in a closed cavity (Skill 10-1 on p. 149). There are two basic styles of glass thermometers for oral and rectal temperature measure. They are color coded: red tipped for rectal, and blue or clear tipped for oral. The mercury bulb of the rectal thermometer is short and rounded; of the oral thermometer, long and narrow (Fig. 10-3, *A* to *C* on p. 150). Because glass thermometers contain mercury (a hazardous material), the nurse should not clean up a broken thermometer without a mercury spill kit. This is a kit that includes a bulb syringe and sealed container. The mercury is aspirated with the syringe and transferred into a labeled container for safe disposal by the facility.

Temperature readings are documented in either centigrade (Celsius; C) degrees or Fahrenheit (F) degrees (Fig. 10-3, *D* to *E*). Glass thermometers are calibrated in either F or C scales. The type of scale used is determined by facility policy.

Because glass thermometers are not disposable, several policies have been adopted by health facilities to prevent cross-contamination among patients. In some cases, each patient is issued a thermometer, which is kept at the bedside. Also, disposable plastic sheaths are used to cover both glass and electronic thermometers when these thermometers are used for more than one patient. The nurse may be responsible for cleaning and disinfecting glass thermometers. A common method of cleaning/disinfecting is to first cleanse the thermometer from fingertips to bulb after the patient use. The thermometer is then washed with detergent and rinsed with cool water to avoid breakage. The next step is to soak glass thermometers in a disinfectant, for example, alcohol, for a length of time specified by policy. The last step is to rinse thermometers in tepid water, dry, and store in a dry place.

Temperature elevations may be the first sign of illness. When body temperature is above normal, the patient's condition is said to be **pyrexia, febrile,** or **hyperthermia.** Fever is actually a body defense. Elevated body temperature will destroy invading bacteria. Unfortunately, if temperature exceeds 105° F (40.5° C), normal body cells can be damaged (Box 10-4 on p. 148).

Text continued on p. 152.

Tympanic Temperature Instructions

1. Remove probe from base unit by lifting firmly near RELEASE button.

2. Note equivalence setting on display: CORE, REC, ORAL, CAL.

3. Select TYMPANIC by pressing MODE button (if TYMPANIC not already displayed).

4. Place disposable cover on probe tip.

5. Place probe in ear canal and seal opening. In infants, seal outer opening of ear canal.

6. Press and release SCAN button.

7. Remove probe from ear as soon as triple beep is heard and display flashes DONE.

98.6 °F
TYMPANIC
DONE

8. Read temperature in display window.

9. Press blue RELEASE button to discard probe cover.

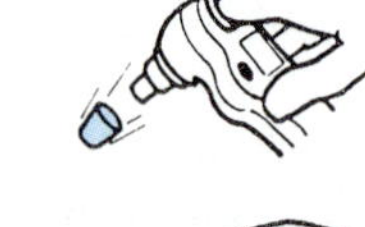

10. Return probe to base unit for storage.

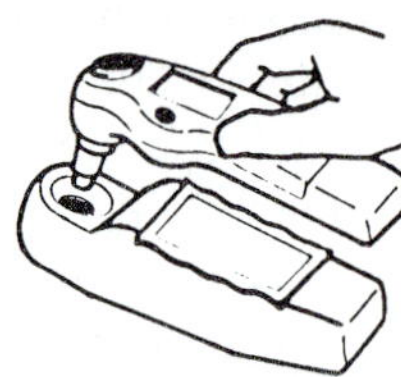

Tips On Technique

Although the technique for using the Genius is not as critical as with oral or rectal thermometry, the following guidelines will improve the consistency and accuracy of measurement:

1. If necessary, gently restrain the patient's head movements while taking temperature.
2. Insert probe tip into ear canal just far enough to SEAL opening. No additional pressure or tugging on the ear is required.
3. In infants, where the probe tip cannot enter the outer ear canal, SEAL OUTER OPENING with probe tip, then gently press SCAN button.
4. Remove probe as soon as triple beep is heard and display blinks DONE. Removal of the thermometer from the ear before DONE is displayed may result in a low temperature.

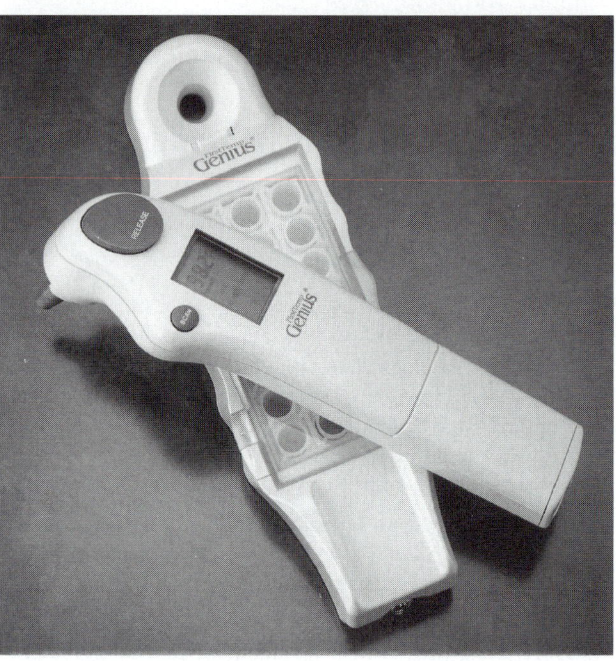

FIG. 10-1 Tympanic membrane thermometer and instructions and technique. (Courtesy Sherwood Medical Instruments, Inc, St Louis, Mo.)

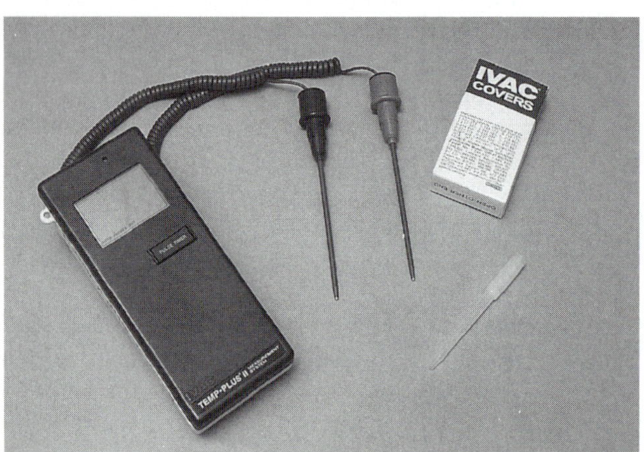

FIG. 10-2 Electronic thermometer.

Box 10-4 SIGNS AND SYMPTOMS OF ELEVATED BODY TEMPERATURE

- Thirst
- Anorexia
- Flushed, warm skin
- Irritability
- Glassy eyes/photophobia (sensitivity to light)
- Headache
- Elevated pulse and respiratory rates
- Restlessness or excessive sleepiness
- Increased perspiration
- Disorientation
- Convulsions in infants and children

OBTAINING A TEMPERATURE READING USING AN ELECTRONIC THERMOMETER

SKILL 10-1

Nursing action/*Rationale*

1. Wash hands *to inhibit spread of microorganisms.*
2. Introduce self *to patient to decrease anxiety.*
3. Identify patient by identification band *to ensure correct patient for procedure.*
4. Explain procedure to patient *to seek cooperation and assistance and to decrease anxiety level.*
5. Prepare for procedure by:
   a. Collecting all necessary supplies *to organize procedure efficiently:* electronic thermometer, probe covers, lubricant if rectal reading is to be taken.
   b. Providing for patient privacy if necessary *to decrease anxiety level.*
6. Implement procedure:
   a. Insert probe snugly into probe cover: red probe for rectal readings; blue probe for oral, axillary, and groin readings.
   b. Inspect digital display *to ensure that unit is ready to take reading.*
   c. Place probe on correct body surface: Oral — sublingual pocket; axillary—axilla; rectal — 1½ inches into rectum with lubricated tip (wear gloves).
   d. Wait for audible signal *to indicate temperature reading is complete.*
   e. Remove probe cover by pressing button on top of probe; direct into trash container.
   f. Provide for patient's comfort.
7. Read and write down reading from digital display (before reinserting probe into holder) *for documentation later.*
8. Wash hands *to inhibit spread of microorganisms.*
9. Document reading on graphic sheet. (e.g., 101° F) (see illustration).
10. Follow up by reporting any abnormal readings.

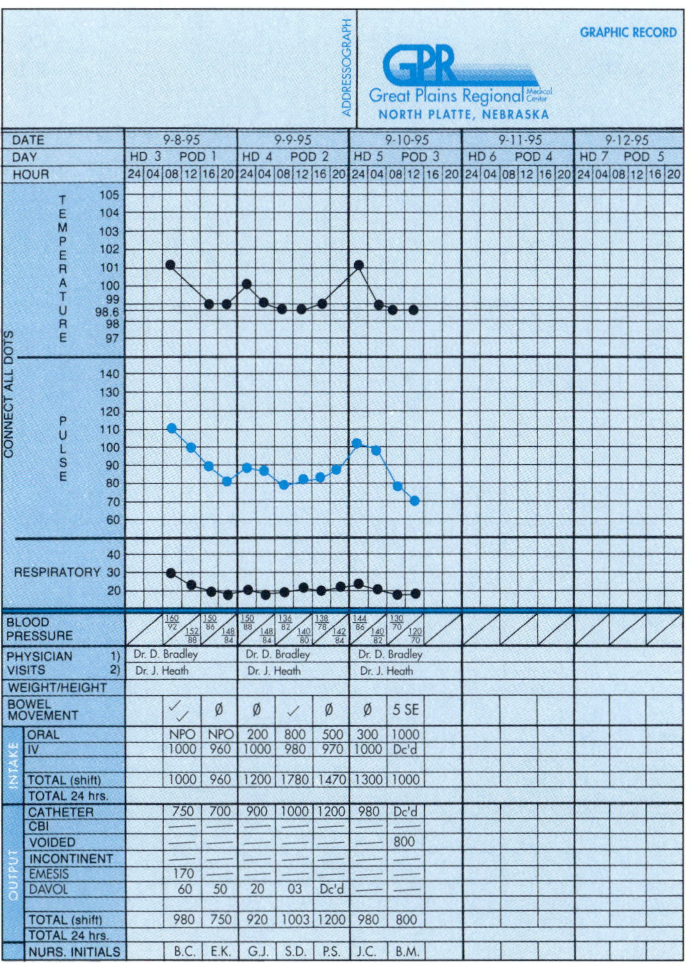

DATE	9-8-95						9-9-95						9-10-95						9-11-95						9-12-95					
DAY	HD 3 POD 1						HD 4 POD 2						HD 5 POD 3						HD 6 POD 4						HD 7 POD 5					
HOUR	24	04	08	12	16	20	24	04	08	12	16	20	24	04	08	12	16	20	24	04	08	12	16	20	24	04	08	12	16	20

	9-8-95			9-9-95			9-10-95			9-11-95			9-12-95		
BLOOD PRESSURE		160/92, 152/88	150/86, 148/84	150/88, 148/84	136/82, 140/80	138/78, 142/84	144/86, 140/82	130/70, 120/70							
PHYSICIAN VISITS 1)	Dr. D. Bradley			Dr. D. Bradley			Dr. D. Bradley								
2)	Dr. J. Heath			Dr. J. Heath			Dr. J. Heath								
WEIGHT/HEIGHT															
BOWEL MOVEMENT		✓✓	Ø	Ø	✓	Ø	Ø	5 SE							
INTAKE ORAL		NPO	NPO	200	800	500	300	1000							
IV		1000	960	1000	980	970	1000	Dc'd							
TOTAL (shift)		1000	960	1200	1780	1470	1300	1000							
TOTAL 24 hrs.															
OUTPUT CATHETER		750	700	900	1000	1200	980	Dc'd							
CBI		—	—	—	—	—	—	—							
VOIDED		—	—	—	—	—	—	800							
INCONTINENT		—	—	—	—	—	—	—							
EMESIS		170	—	—	—	—	—	—							
DAVOL		60	50	20	03	Dc'd	—	—							
TOTAL (shift)		980	750	920	1003	1200	980	800							
TOTAL 24 hrs.															
NURS. INITIALS		B.C.	E.K.	G.J.	S.D.	P.S.	J.C.	B.M.							

STEP 8

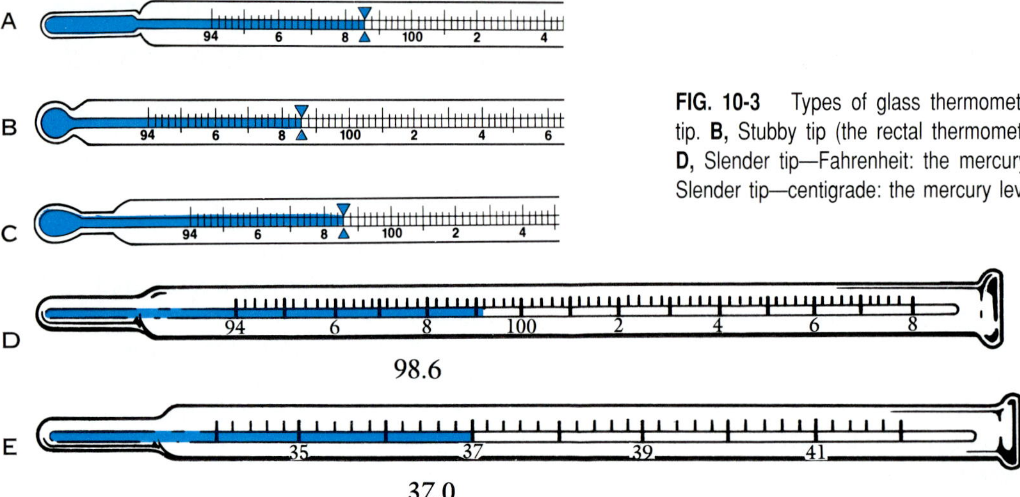

FIG. 10-3 Types of glass thermometers. **A,** Long or slender tip. **B,** Stubby tip (the rectal thermometer). **C,** Pear-shaped tip. **D,** Slender tip—Fahrenheit: the mercury level is at 99.2° F. **E,** Slender tip—centigrade: the mercury level is at 37° C.

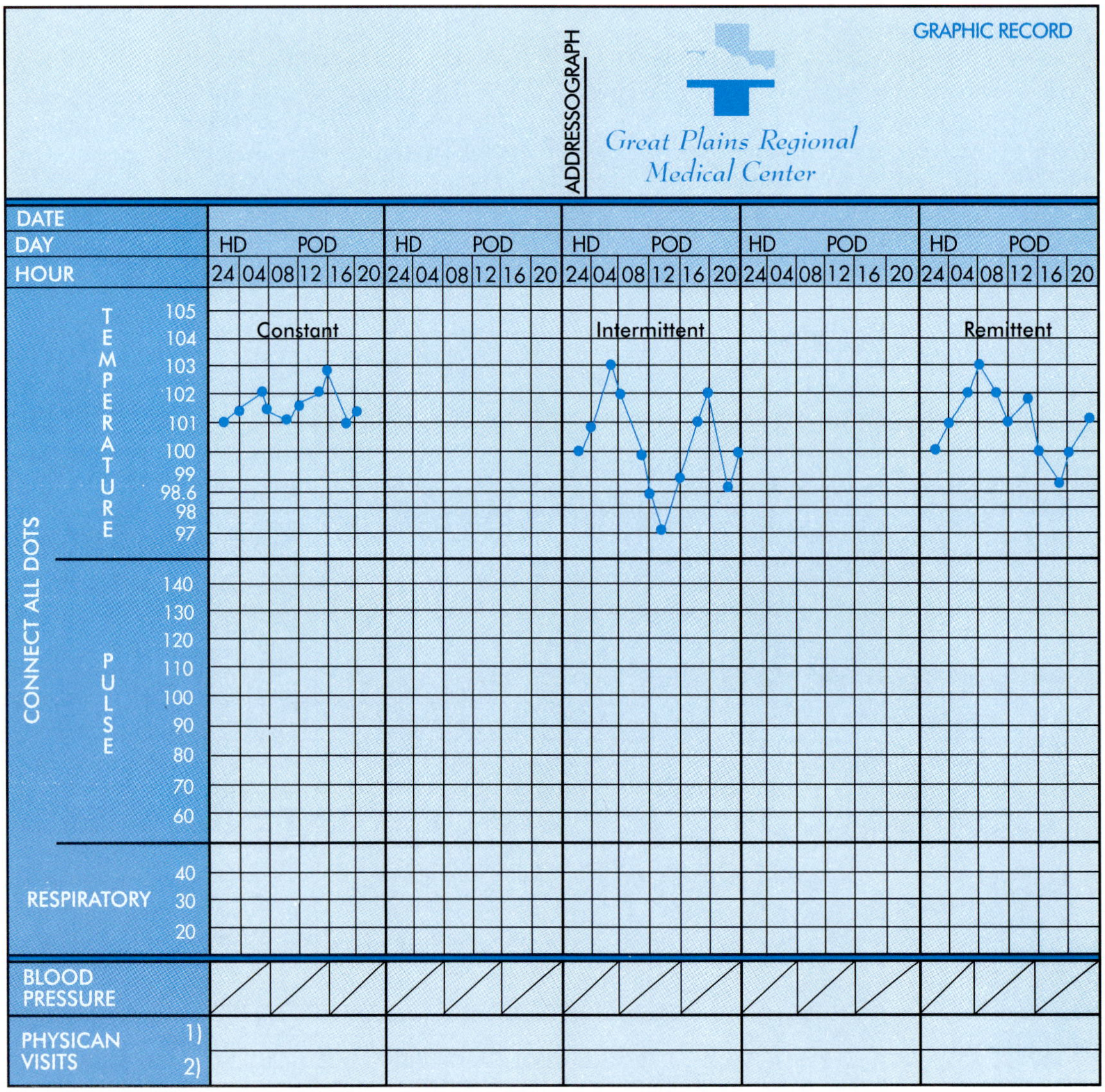

GRAPHIC RECORD

ADDRESSOGRAPH

Great Plains Regional Medical Center

DATE					
DAY	HD POD	HD POD	HD POD	HD POD	HD POD
HOUR	24 04 08 12 16 20	24 04 08 12 16 20	24 04 08 12 16 20	24 04 08 12 16 20	24 04 08 12 16 20
TEMPERATURE 105 104 103 102 101 100 99 98.6 98 97	Constant		Intermittent		Remittent
PULSE 140 130 120 110 100 90 80 70 60					
RESPIRATORY 40 30 20					
BLOOD PRESSURE					
PHYSICAN VISITS 1) 2)					

CONNECT ALL DOTS

FIG. 10-4 Form for recording vital signs. Note temperature graphic showing types of fevers. (Courtesy Great Plains Regional Medical Center, North Platte, Neb.)

SKILL 10-2

OBTAINING AN ORAL TEMPERATURE READING

Nursing action/*Rationale*

1. Wash hands *to inhibit spread of microorganisms.*
2. Introduce self *to patient to decrease anxiety level.*
3. Identify patient by identification band *to ensure correct patient for procedure.*
4. Explain procedure *to seek cooperation and assistance from patient and to decrease anxiety level.*
5. Prepare for procedure by:
   a. Collecting all necessary supplies *to organize procedure efficiently:* oral thermometer, alcohol pledgets, disposable sheaths, if used.
   b. Providing for patient privacy if necessary *to decrease anxiety level.*
   c. Determine if the patient has consumed hot or cold beverage or has been smoking. If so, wait 15 minutes *to ensure accuracy.*
6. Implement procedure:
   a. Cleanse thermometer from bulb to fingertips with pledget cleaning from clean to less clean area of thermometer.
   b. Inspect thermometer for defects and mercury level. Shake down mercury with snaps of the wrist to a level of 96 degrees. Cover with sheath if used or rinse with cool water.
   c. Place bulb end of thermometer in sublingual pocket (see illustration).
   d. Wait 5 minutes for accurate reading.
   e. Remove thermometer and wipe with pledget from fingertips to bulb. Remove sheath if used.
   f. Read thermometer, holding at eye level and rotating until mercury line can be read.
7. Write down reading *for documentation later* (e.g., 98.6° O).
8. Wash hands to inhibit spread of microorganisms.
9. Document reading on graphic sheet (see illustration, p. 149).
10. Follow up by reporting any abnormal temperature readings.

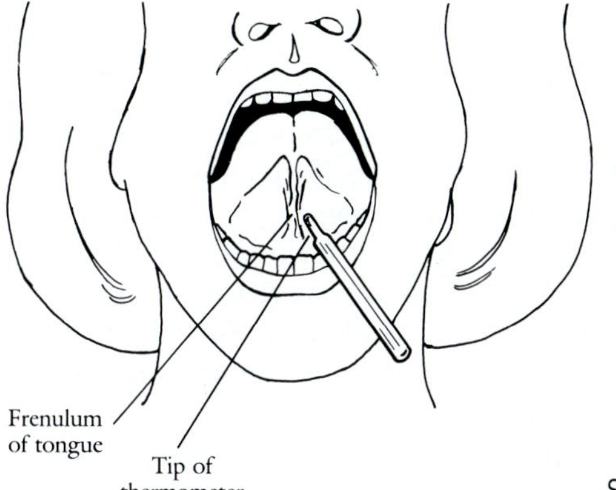

STEP 6c

TABLE 10-1 Selection of Sites for Temperature Measurement

Advantages	Disadvantages
Oral	
Most accessible site; comfortable for patient	It should not be used for patients who could be injured by thermometer, who are unable to hold thermometer properly, or who might bite down on thermometer; infants or small children; disoriented or unconscious patients; patients who have had oral surgery; patients with trauma to face or mouth; patients experiencing oral pain; patients who breathe only with mouth open; patients with history of convulsions; patients experiencing a shaking chill.
Rectal	
Thought to provide most reliable measurement	It should not be used for patients after rectal surgery, patients who have a rectal disorder such as tumor or hemorrhoids, or patients who cannot be positioned for proper thermometer placement, such as those in traction.
Axilla	
Safe method because noninvasive	Least accurate
Tympanic	
Noninvasive, accurate, safe	Excessive cerumen (earwax) may interfere with accurate reading.

SKILL 10-3

OBTAINING A RECTAL TEMPERATURE READING

Nursing action/*Rationale*

1. Wash hands *to inhibit spread of microorganisms.*
2. Introduce self to patient *to decrease anxiety level.*
3. Identify patient by identification band *to ensure correct patient for procedure.*
4. Explain procedure *to seek cooperation and assistance from patient and to reduce anxiety level.*
5. Prepare for procedure by:
   a. Collecting all necessary supplies *to organize procedure efficiently:* gloves, rectal thermometer, lubricant, alcohol pledgets, disposable sheaths, if used.
   b. Provide for patient privacy *to decrease anxiety level.*
6. Implement procedure:
   a. Don gloves.
   b. Cleanse thermometer from bulb to fingertips with pledget cleaning from clean to less clean area on thermometer.
   c. Inspect thermometer for defects and mercury line. Shake down mercury with snaps of the wrist to a reading of 96 degrees.
   d. Lubricate tip of thermometer 1½ inches *to ease insertion.*
   e. With patient in Sims' position, gently spread buttocks and insert thermometer 1½ inches (see illustration). Hold thermometer throughout procedure for safety purposes.
   f. Wait 2 minutes.
   g. Remove thermometer, cleanse from fingertips to bulb or discard sheath, if used.
   h. Read thermometer, holding at eye level and rotating until mercury line can be read.
   i. Provide for patient comfort by repositioning and removing excess lubricant from rectal area.
7. Write down reading *for documenting later.*
8. Remove gloves and wash hands *to inhibit spread of microorganisms.*
9. Document reading on graphic sheet. (e.g., 99.6° R) (see illustration, p. 149).
10. Follow up by reporting any abnormal temperature readings.

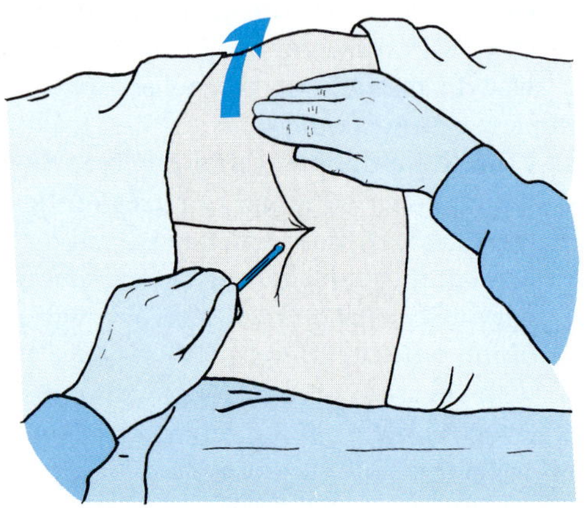

STEP 6e

Fevers are classified as constant, intermittent, or remittent. Constant fevers remain elevated consistently and fluctuate very little. Intermittent fevers rise and fall, for example, normal or subnormal in the morning and "spiking" (elevated) in the afternoon. Remittent fevers are similar to intermittent fevers except the temperature never returns to normal until the patient becomes well (Fig. 10-4 on p. 150).

The condition of an abnormally low body temperature is **hypothermia.** Death can occur if the body temperature falls below 93.2° F (34° C). There have been documented cases of persons surviving with much lower temperatures. The patient may intentionally be placed in hypothermia for a surgical procedure. Certain conditions, such as hypothyroidism, produce a subnormal temperature.

The method to measure the temperature is determined by the nurse's assessment of the patient (Table 10-1 on p. 151). Oral temperature is not obtained in the comatose or disoriented patient or in small infants, since this method requires patient cooperation (Skill 10-2 on p. 151). Rectal temperatures are contraindicated for patients with recent rectal surgery or certain conditions of the perineum (Skill 10-3). Axillary temperature (Skill 10-4) is considered the least accurate method and is used less frequently since the advent of the tympanic membrane thermometer (Skill 10-5). The nurse should be aware that rectal readings are normally 1 degree higher than oral, and axillary readings are 1 degree lower than oral. When an oral reading or a tympanic reading is obtained, it is not usually necessary to provide privacy for the patient.

SKILL 10-4

OBTAINING AN AXILLARY TEMPERATURE READING

Nursing action/*Rationale*

1. Wash hands *to inhibit spread of microorganisms.*
2. Introduce self *to patient to decrease anxiety.*
3. Identify patient by identification band *to ensure correct patient for procedure.*
4. Explain procedure *to seek cooperation and assistance from patient and to decrease anxiety.*
5. Prepare for procedure by:
   a. Collecting all necessary supplies *to organize procedure efficiently:* oral thermometer, alcohol pledgets, disposable sheath, if used.
   b. Providing for patient privacy if necessary *to decrease anxiety.*
6. Implement procedure:
   a. Cleanse thermometer from bulb to fingertips with pledget cleaning from clean to less clean area of thermometer.
   b. Inspect thermometer for defects and mercury line. Shake down mercury with snaps of the wrist until reading is at 96 degrees. Cover with sheath, if used.
   c. Place bulb of thermometer against axilla. If skin is wet, dry *to ensure accurate reading.* Hold arm snugly along side of body with forearm resting across chest (see illustration).
   d. Wait 5 to 10 minutes *to ensure accuracy.*
   e. Remove thermometer and wipe with a pledget from fingertips to bulb, or if the electronic thermometer is used, discard disposable sheath.
   f. Read thermometer, holding at eye level and rotating until mercury line can be read; if electronic thermometer is used, read digital display.
   g. Provide for patient comfort by assisting to redress exposed arm.
7. Write down reading *for documenting later.*
8. Wash hands *to inhibit spread of microorganisms.*
9. Document reading on graphic sheet (e.g., 97.6° ax) (see illustration, p. 149).
10. Follow up by reporting any abnormal temperature readings.

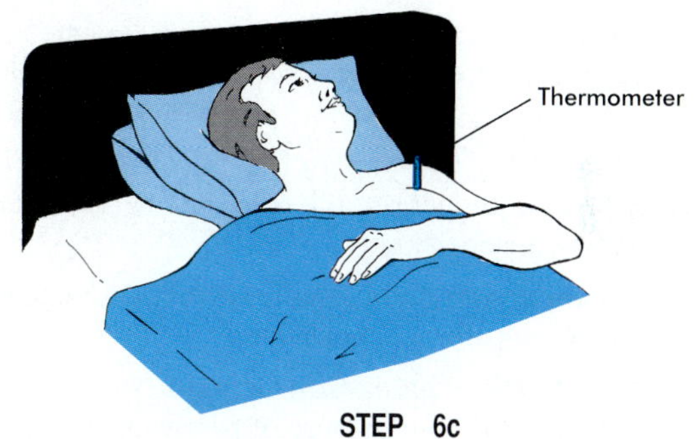

STEP 6c

SKILL 10-5

OBTAINING A TYMPANIC MEMBRANE TEMPERATURE

Nursing action/*Rationale*

1. Wash hands *to inhibit spread of microorganisms.*
2. Introduce self *to patient to decrease anxiety.*
3. Identify patient by identification band *to ensure correct patient for procedure.*
4. Explain procedure *to seek cooperation and assistance from patient and to decrease anxiety.*
5. Prepare for procedure by:
   a. Collecting all necessary supplies *to organize procedure efficiently:* tympanic membrane thermometer and probe cover.
   b. Providing for patient privacy if necessary *to decrease anxiety level.*
6. Implement procedure:
   a. Attach probe cover to thermometer unit *to inhibit spread of microorganisms.*
   b. Insert probe cover into ear canal, applying a gentle but firm pressure *to ensure accurate reading* (see Fig. 10-1).
   c. Remove thermometer after reading has been displayed on digital unit, about 2 seconds *because tympanic core temperatures are rapid and extremely accurate.*
   d. Remove probe cover and place in proper receptacle *to inhibit spread of microorganisms.*
   e. Return thermometer to storage unit *to recharge battery.*
7. Write down reading for documentation later (e.g., 99.2°).
8. Wash hands to inhibit spread of microorganisms.
9. Document reading on graphic sheet (see p. 149).
10. Follow up by reporting any abnormal temperature reading.

PULSE

A **pulse** is a rhythmic beating or vibrating movement. It is the regular, recurrent expansion and contraction of an artery produced by waves of pressure caused by the ejection of blood from the left ventricle of the heart as it contracts. It corresponds to each beat of the heart. When taking the pulse, the nurse notes the rate, rhythm, and volume of the pulse. The adult pulse rate is normally between 60 and 100 beats per minute with the approximate average being 80.

The patient's age, sex, emotional state, size, temperature, condition of the heart, and amount of physical activity can influence the pulse rate. If the pulse is faster than 100 beats per minute, the patient has **tachycardia;** if it is slower than 60 beats per minute, the patient has **bradycardia.** Tachycardia can result from shock, hemorrhage leading to hypovolemia (an abnormally low circulating blood volume), exercise, fever, and acute pain. Drugs such as epinephrine can also increase the pulse rate. Bradycardia can result from unrelieved, severe pain, because it stimulates the parasympathetic nervous system, which slows the heart rate. Drugs such as digitalis may lower the heart rate. Resting in a supine position

Box 10-5 FACTORS INFLUENCING PULSE RATES

Age. The pulse rate decreases as the aging process progresses from infancy through adulthood. Pulse rate in the older adult may be greater than 80 beats per minute because of weakened heart muscle or because of medication.

Exercise. Short-term exercise increases pulse rate. Long-term exercise strengthens heart muscle, resulting in lower than normal rate at rest and a quicker return to resting rate after exercise.

Fever, heat. Both increase the pulse rate because of increased metabolic rate.

Acute pain, anxiety. These increase the pulse rate because of sympathetic stimulation.

Unrelieved severe pain, chronic pain. These decrease the pulse rate because of parasympathetic stimulation.

Medications. Various medications alter pulse rate. For example, digitalis decreases the pulse rate; atropine and epinephrine increase the pulse rate.

Hemorrhage. Loss of blood increases the pulse rate because of the sympathetic stimulation.

Postural changes. Lying down initially decreases the pulse rate. On the other hand, standing or sitting increases the pulse rate.

Metabolism. Certain diseases such as hyperthyroidism can cause a chronic elevated pulse rate. Hypothyroidism can cause a slowing of the pulse.

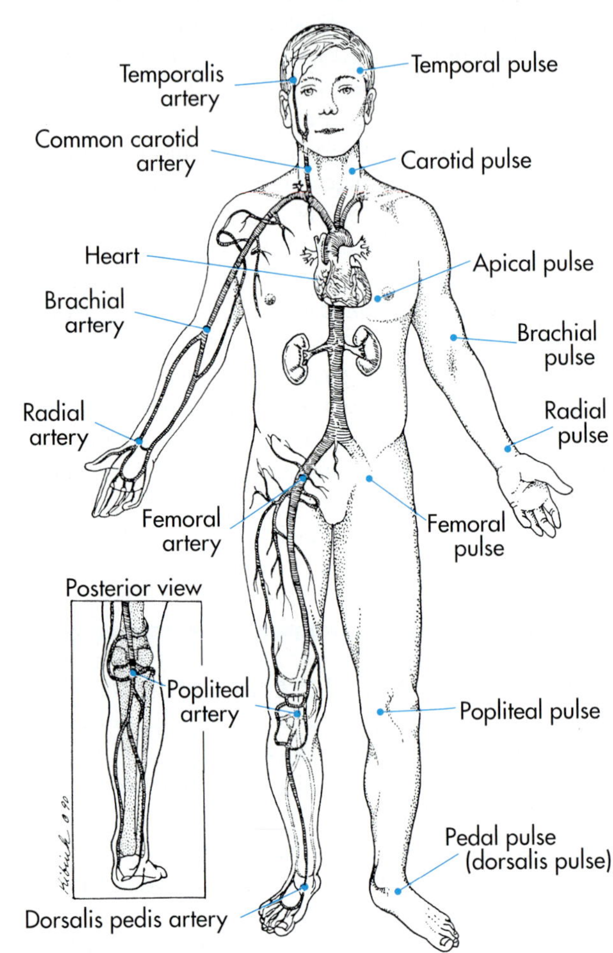

FIG. 10-5 The pulse sites.

TABLE 10-2 Pulse Volume Variations

Number	Type	Description
0	Absent pulse	None felt
1+	Thready pulse	Difficult to feel; not palpable when only slight pressure applied.
2+	Weak pulse	Somewhat stronger than a thready pulse but not palpable when light pressure applied.
3+	Normal pulse	Easily felt but not palpable when moderate pressure applied.
4+	Bounding pulse	Feels full and springlike even under moderate pressure.

may decrease the heart rate, as will the cardiac condition heart block (Box 10-5). If the amount of time between beats varies, there will be an irregular pulse or **dysrhythmia** (any disturbance or abnormality in a normal rhythmic pattern, specifically irregularity in the normal rhythm of the heart).

The normal pulse reflects an equal amount of time between beats. The volume of the pulse refers to the amount of blood pushing against the artery wall with each beat. A weak pulse is difficult to palpate; a bounding pulse is easily felt with light palpation. A pulse that cannot be felt at all is imperceptible. Another means to communicate the volume of the pulse is by the use of numbers. The numbering system and descriptions can be seen in Table 10-2. Follow agency policy when describing the pulse.

The pulse rate is usually obtained at the radial artery, which is located on the thumb side of the inner wrist **(radial pulse)**. When assessing the patient, the nurse should palpate all major pulses and **auscultate** (act of listening for sounds within the body to evaluate the condition of the heart, lungs, pleura, intestines, or other organs or to detect fetal heart tones) the apical rate. For example, a pulse palpated at the dorsalis pedis indicates blood flow to the foot. Major pulses include the temporal, facial, carotid, brachial, radial, femoral, popliteal, and posterior tibial and dorsalis pedis (Fig. 10-5).

Pulses are palpated using the pads of the index and middle fingers. Only slight pressure is applied over the artery to avoid obliterating the pulse (by occluding blood flow) (Fig. 10-6). See Skill 10-6 for obtaining a radial pulse rate.

The apical rate is auscultated when the radial pulse is irregular or is difficult to palpate or when certain medications such as digoxin (Lanoxin) require it. Apical refers to apex of the heart. The **apical pulse** represents the actual beating of the heart. When the apical rate is auscultated, the "lub dub" heard by the nurse represents one cardiac cycle, or heartbeat. See Skill 10-7 on p. 156 for obtaining apical pulse rate and Fig. 10-7 on p. 156 for the anatomical position of the apical pulse.

The nurse may note a difference between the radial and apical rates. This is called a **pulse deficit.** To confirm a pulse deficit, the nurse listens to the apical rate, and a second nurse palpates the radial pulse at the same time, using the same watch. A deficit results when the radial rate is less than the apical rate. For example, an apical rate of 92 and a radial rate of 88 result in a pulse deficit of 4. A pulse deficit signifies that the pumping action of the heart is faulty. This can be seen in atrial fibrillation.

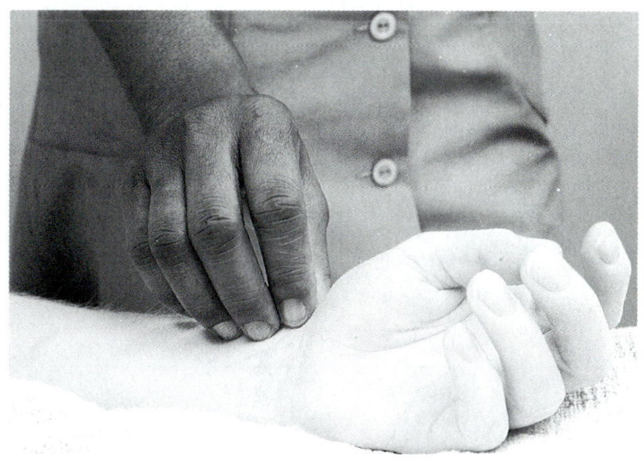

FIG. 10-6 Finger placement for a radial pulse measurement.

SKILL 10-6

OBTAINING A RADIAL PULSE RATE

Nursing action/*Rationale*

1. Wash hands *to inhibit spread of microorganisms.*
2. Introduce self to patient *to decrease anxiety level.*
3. Identify patient by identification band *to ensure correct patient for procedure.*
4. Explain procedure *to seek cooperation and assistance from the patient and to decrease anxiety level.*
5. Prepare for procedure by:
   a. Collecting all necessary supplies *to organize procedure efficiently:* wristwatch with second hand.
   b. Providing privacy for the patient if necessary *to decrease anxiety.*
6. Implement procedure:
   a. Palpate the radial pulse with index and middle finger by placing them on thumb side of patient's wrist using gentle pressure *so that pulse is not obliterated.*
   b. Count pulse for 60 seconds *to ensure accuracy.*
7. Write down radial rate *for documentation later.*
8. Wash hands *to inhibit spread of microorganisms.*
9. Document rate on graphic sheet (e.g., P-60) (see illustration, p. 149).
10. Follow up by reporting any abnormal pulse rates.

SKILL 10-7

OBTAINING AN APICAL PULSE RATE

Nursing action/*Rationale*

1. Wash hands *to inhibit spread of microorganisms.*
2. Introduce self to patient *to decrease anxiety level.*
3. Identify patient by identification band *to ensure correct patient for procedure.*
4. Explain procedure *to seek cooperation or assistance from patient and to decrease anxiety.*
5. Prepare for procedure by:
   a. Collecting all necessary supplies *to organize procedure efficiently:* stethoscope and watch with second hand.
   b. Providing privacy for patient if necessary *to decrease anxiety.*
6. Implement procedure:
   a. Expose patient's chest as necessary.
   b. Place stethoscope against patient's chest (see illustration).
   c. Count pulse rate for 60 seconds *to ensure accuracy.*
   d. Provide for patient's comfort by assisting to redress.
7. Write down pulse rate *for later documentation.*
8. Wash hands *to inhibit spread of microorganisms.*
9. Document pulse rate on graphic sheet (e.g., P-64 ap) (see illustration, p. 149).
10. Follow up by reporting an abnormal pulse rate.

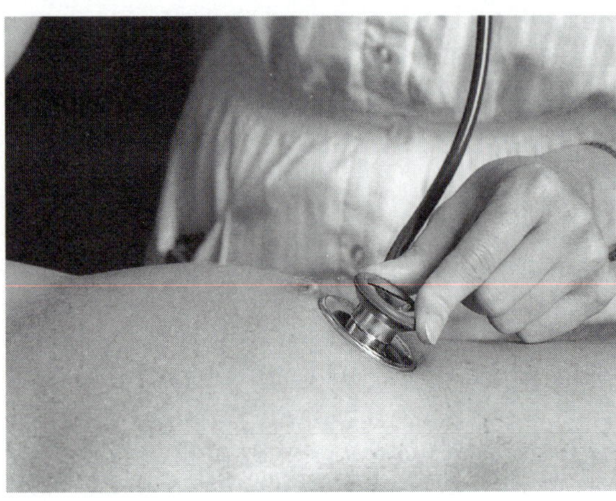

STEP 6b

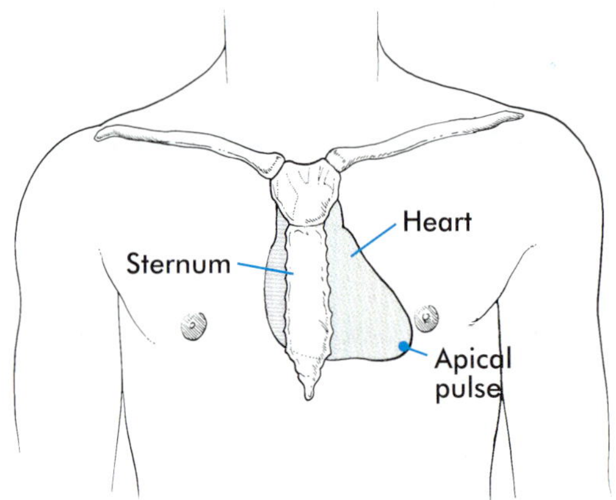

FIG. 10-7 Anatomical positioning of an apical pulse.

RESPIRATIONS

Respirations (the taking in of oxygen, its utilization in the tissues, and the giving off of carbon dioxide; the act of breathing, i.e., inhaling and exhaling) can be internal or external. Internal respiration refers to the exchange of gas at the alveolar level. There is a molecule exchange of oxygen and carbon dioxide with the body's tissues, from the lungs to cellular oxidation (any process in which the oxygen content of a compound is increased) processes. The breathing movements of the patient that can be observed by the nurse are called external respirations. External respirations have two parts in the cycle: inspiration and expiration. **Inspiration** is inhaling air with oxygen into the lungs, and **expiration** is exhaling air with carbon dioxide out of the lungs. The rate of respiration is controlled by the medulla oblongata in the brain.

Any activity that increases metabolism (the aggregate of all chemical processes that take place in living organisms resulting in growth, generation of energy, elimination of wastes, and other bodily functions as they relate to the destruction of nutrients in the body after digestion) will increase the need for oxygen by the body and will increase respiratory rate. In assessing respirations, the nurse notes the rate, depth, rhythm, and quality. The normal rate for an adult is between 12 to 20 respirations per minute (Box 10-6 and Skill 10-8).

The patient with a rapid respiratory rate has **tachypnea.** Exercise and fever increase respiratory rate. A slow respiratory rate, below 12, is known as **bradypnea.** The depth of respiration is determined by the amount of

Box 10-6

FACTORS INFLUENCING RESPIRATION

- **Disease or illness.** Chronic lung disease (e.g., emphysema or bronchitis) alters the normal stimulus for ventilation. Lung tissue disease, reduced red blood cell levels, chest pain, kidney diseases, febrile disease, and diseases of the heart are a few of the conditions that alter the rate and depth of respiration.
- **Stress.** An anxious or fearful patient will likely have increases in the rate and depth of respiration, and as a result, hyperventilation occurs.
- **Fever.** Hyperpyrexia (greatly elevated temperature) results in an abnormally rapid rate of breathing.
- **Age.** With growth from infancy to adulthood, the lungs' capacity increases and respiratory rate gradually declines. With older adults, lung capacity and depth of respiration decrease, and respiratory rate increases.
- **Gender.** Men have a greater lung capacity than women.
- **Body position.** In slumped or stooped position, ventilation is often impaired, with a reduced depth of respiration.
- **Medications.** Narcotic analgesics depress the patient's ability to increase the volume of air inspired, and the rate of respiration is decreased. Other medications may increase or decrease the rate and depth of respiration and may affect the rhythm.
- **Exercise.** Exercise increases the rate and depth of respirations.
- **Acute pain.** Pain increases rate and depth of respirations as a result of sympathetic stimulation.
- **Smoking.** Long-term smoking changes the lungs' airways, resulting in an increased respiratory rate.
- **Brain stem injury.** Injury to the brain stem impairs the respiratory center and inhibits respiratory rate and rhythm.

SKILL 10-8

OBTAINING A RESPIRATORY RATE

Nursing action/*Rationale*

1. Wash hands *to inhibit spread of microorganisms.*
2. Introduce self to patient *to decrease anxiety.*
3. Identify patient by identification band *to ensure correct patient for procedure.*
4. Explain procedure *to seek cooperation or assistance from the patient and to decrease anxiety.*
5. Prepare for procedure by:
   a. Collecting all necessary supplies *to organize procedure efficiently:* wristwatch with second hand.
   b. Provide privacy for patient if necessary *to decrease anxiety.*
6. Implement procedure:
   a. Place fingertip as if to obtain a radial pulse. *Since the patient may unconsciously alter the respiratory rate when being observed, it is best to obtain the respiratory rate at the same time as the radial pulse reading.*
   b. Observe respiratory rate for 60 seconds *to ensure accuracy.* Count each rise of the chest wall. One inhalation/exhalation = one respiration.
   c. Provide for patient comfort if necessary
7. Write down rate *for documentation later.*
8. Wash hands *to inhibit spread of microorganisms.*
9. Document the rate on the graphic sheet (e.g., R-20) (see illustration, p. 149).
10. Follow up by reporting any abnormal respiratory rates.

air taken in with inhalation. Normally 500 ml of air is inspired. Movement by the diaphragm (a dome-shaped musculofibrous partition that separates the thoracic and abdominal cavities; the diaphragm aids respirations by moving down during inspiration and moving up during expiration) and intercostal muscles allows the nurse to judge the depth of respirations. Shallow respirations make ventilation difficult to observe and only a small amount of air is exchanged in the lungs. The rhythm of respiration should be regular and uninterrupted. Occasional sighing is normal and allows all alveoli (plural for *alveolus,* an air cell of the lungs where gases are exchanged in respirations) to be aerated. Respirations should not be audible except with the aid of a **stethoscope** (an instrument used in auscultation, consisting of two earpieces connected by flexible tubing to a diaphragm that is placed against the patient's chest or back to hear heart and lung sounds).

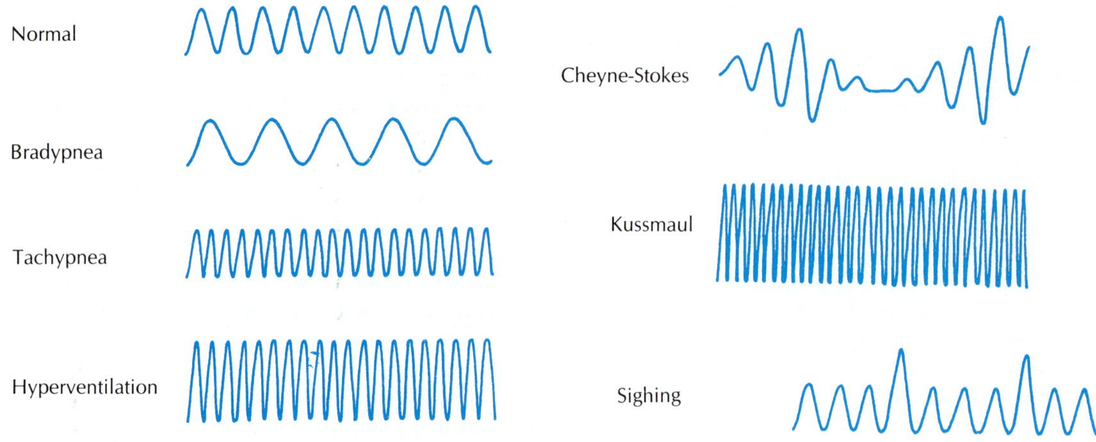

FIG. 10-8 Patterns of respirations.

Patterns of breathing should be assessed (Fig. 10-8). **Dyspnea** is breathing with difficulty. The patient may be laboring to get enough oxygen, with pursed lips, flared nostrils, and clavicular and costal retractions (the visible sinking-in of the soft tissues of the chest between and around the firmer tissues of the cartilaginous and body ribs, as occurs with increased inspiratory effort). **Apnea** is a lack of spontaneous respirations. **Cheyne-Stokes respirations** are an abnormal pattern of respiration characterized by alternating periods of apnea and deep, rapid breathing. The periods of apnea increase as time goes on. Cheyne-Stokes respirations are noted in the critically or terminally ill patient. **Hyperventilation** is when the rate of ventilation exceeds normal metabolic requirements for exchange of respiratory gases, such as during emotional trauma. Rate and depth of respirations increase. **Hypoventilation** occurs when the rate of ventilation entering the lungs is insufficient for metabolic needs. Respiratory rate is below normal and depth of ventilation is depressed. Postoperative open cholecystectomy in which deep breathing would result in discomfort is an example of hypoventilation.

The best time to assess respirations is when counting a radial or apical pulse. The patient is unaware and unable to alter respirations.

BLOOD PRESSURE

The **blood pressure** is the pressure exerted by the circulating volume of blood on the arterial walls, veins, and chambers of the heart. Blood pressure is measured in millimeters of mercury (mm Hg). There are actually two pressures that make up blood pressure. The **systolic** pressure is the higher number and represents the ventricles contracting, forcing blood into the aorta and pulmonary arteries. This occurrence of systole is indicated by the first sound heard on auscultation. The second number is the **diastolic** pressure and represents the pressure within the artery between beats. It is the period between contractions of the atria or the ventricles during which blood enters the relaxed chambers from the systemic circulation and the lungs. Diastole represents the initial absence of sound. The difference between the two readings is called the **pulse pressure.** A reading of 120/80 mm Hg reveals a pulse pressure of 40.

Blood pressure reflects cardiac output (the amount of blood discharged from the left or right ventricle per minute), the quality of the arteries, the blood volume, and blood viscosity.

When blood is pumped by the heart into the arteries, the pressure within the arteries rises. Therefore the greater the amount of blood pumped by the heart, the greater the pressure. Likewise, if the blood volume is increased, the pressure within the artery will increase.

When the arteries' lumens (channels within the arteries) narrow and become less flexible, blood pressure rises because there is less space for the blood to enter. Increased viscosity (thickness) of the blood causes a slower flow of blood in the capillaries, which causes backup pressure in the larger vessels (Box 10-7).

Normal blood pressure in the adult is 120/80 mm Hg. **Hypertension** occurs when the sustained elevated pressure is above 140/90 mm Hg. Primary or essential hypertension is the most common form. The cause is unknown but is believed to be related to aging. Risk factors also have a contributing significance and should be considered when doing patient teaching. These risk factors include family history of hypertension, obesity, smoking, heavy alcohol consumption, elevated blood cholesterol level, and continued exposure to stress.

A blood pressure below normal is **hypotension.** It is considered healthy to have a low blood pressure providing there are no ill effects, such as vertigo (dizziness) or syncope (fainting). **Orthostatic hypotension** (a drop of 25 mm Hg in systolic pressure and a drop of 10 mm Hg in diastolic pressure when moving from a lying

Box 10-7

FACTORS INFLUENCING BLOOD PRESSURE

Age. Normal blood pressure levels vary throughout life.

AGE	ARTERIAL PRESSURE*
Newborn (3000 g [6.6 lb])	Systolic 50-52 Diastolic 25-30 Mean 35-40
4 years	85/60
6 years	95/62
10 years	100/65
12 years	108/67
16 years	118/75
Middle adult	120/80
Older adult	140-160/90-100

Anxiety, fear, pain, and emotional stress. May increase blood pressure because of increased heart rate and increased peripheral vascular resistance.

Medications. Can either lower or increase blood pressure depending on their pharmacological action.

Hormones. Variations in blood pressure may be manifested as a person ages, because of hormonal alterations. Pregnancy may cause mild to severe elevations in blood pressure.

Diurnal (happening daily). Variations may include a lower blood pressure in the morning, rising throughout the day, peaking in late afternoon or evening, and lowering at night; individual variations are significant.

Race. The rate of hypertension is higher in urban African-Americans than in European-Americans. Hypertension-related deaths are also higher among African-Americans. The tendency for this population to have hypertension is believed to be genetically and environmentally related.

*In mm Hg.

TABLE 10-3 Conditions Causing Alterations in Blood Pressure

Conditions	Effect	Cause
Hemorrhage	Lowers pressure	Decreased blood volume
Increased intracranial pressure	Raises pressure	Disturbance of cardiovascular control mechanisms in brain stem resulting from pressure exerted on the medulla oblongata
Acute pain	Raises pressure	Increased vasomotor tone and peripheral vascular resistance as a result of sympathetic stimulation
End stage renal disease	Raises pressure	Increased blood volume resulting from increased retention of sodium and water; release of renin, a vasopressor that increases peripheral vascular resistance
Primary essential hypertension	Raises pressure	Increased peripheral vascular resistance resulting from progressive thickening of arterial walls
General anesthesia	Lowers pressure	Decreased vasomotor tone resulting from depression of vasomotor center in brain stem
Exercise	Raises pressure	Increased cardiac output
Postural change	Lowers pressure	Decreased blood volume as person moves from lying to sitting or standing position; normally, variations are minimal
Smoking	Raises pressure	Increased vasoconstriction

to sitting or sitting to standing position) occurs when a person rises too quickly from a supine position. The patient may feel light-headed and unstable. This patient should be advised to rise slowly from lying to sitting to standing, thus preventing blood volume from shifting suddenly. Hypotension resulting from shock or massive hemorrhage is very serious and requires immediate medical intervention (Table 10-3).

The patient is assessed for hypertension and hypotension. The diagnosis of hypertension is not made with only one random elevated reading. The diagnosis of hypertension in adults is made when an average of two or more diastolic readings on at least two subsequent visits is 90 mm Hg or higher or when an average of two or more systolic readings on at least two visits is higher than 140 mm Hg.

Blood pressure readings are taken with a sphygmomanometer and a stethoscope. A **sphygmomanometer** (a device for measuring the arterial blood pressure) consists of an inflatable cuff and a gauge. The gauge can be

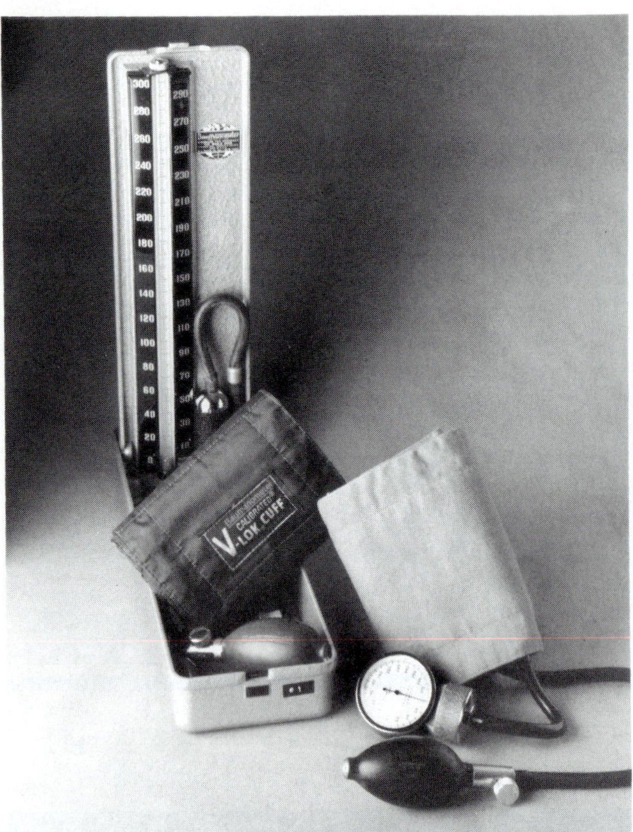

FIG. 10-9 Sphygmonmanometer is composed of pressure manometer, cloth cuff with rubber bladder and pressure bulb. Mercury manometer is at left; aneroid manometer at right.

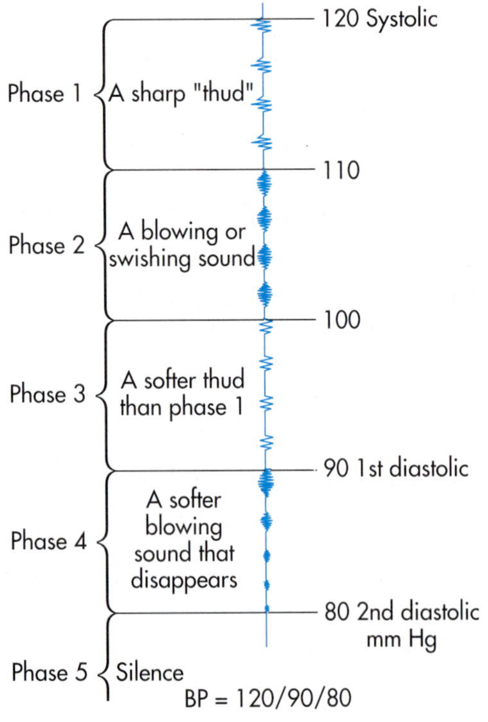

FIG. 10-10 Phases of the Korotkoff sounds.

aneroid or mercury (Fig. 10-9). The cuff is inflated around the patient's arm to compress the artery, which will occlude blood flow; then it is slowly deflated, which will allow blood flow to resume. While performing this, the nurse listens at the brachial artery with the stethoscope and hears pulsating sounds. These are called **Korotkoff sounds.** The sounds go through five phases (Fig. 10-10). When the first sound is heard, the nurse makes a mental note of that point on the sphygmomanometer gauge and again notes when the sound disappears. The point when the first sound is heard is the systolic pressure. The point at which the last sound is heard is the diastolic pressure. At times the sounds are heard to zero. In this case the nurse must listen for a subtle change in the quality of the sound as it approaches the diastolic reading. This then is the diastolic pressure, and the blood pressure is written using the three readings, for example, 120/80/0 mm Hg.

In patients with hypertension, the sounds usually heard over the brachial artery disappear as pressure is reduced and then reappear at a lower level. This temporary disappearance of sound is the **auscultatory gap.** It typically occurs between the first and second Korotkoff sounds. The gap in sound may cover a range of 40 mm Hg and thus may cause an underestimation of systolic pressure or overstimulation of diastolic pressure. The examiner must be certain to inflate the cuff enough to hear the true systolic pressure before the auscultatory gap. Palpation of the radial artery helps determine how high to inflate the cuff. The nurse inflates the cuff 30 mm Hg above the pressure at which the radial pulse was palpated. The range of pressures in which the auscultatory gap occurs is recorded (for example, "BP 190/94, with an auscultatory gap from 190 to 160").

If a nurse is unable to auscultate sounds because of a weakened arterial pulse, a Doppler ultrasonic stethoscope can be used. This stethoscope allows the nurse to hear low-frequency sounds and is commonly used with adults who have very weak blood pressures and with infants and children (Fig. 10-11 on p. 163).

To ensure an accurate blood pressure reading, the environment must be quiet. The equipment must be in good working order, and the cuff should fit correctly. The gauge should be read at eye level; that is, the level of the meniscus (curved portion at the top of the mercury column) should be at eye level. Reading above the meniscus will give a false low reading. Reading below the meniscus will give a false high reading. The patient should be lying down or sitting up with both feet flat on the floor (legs should not be crossed) (Skill 10-9).

Assessment of Blood Pressure in the Lower Extremities

Occasionally, dressings, casts, intravenous catheters, or other devices make the upper extremities inaccessible,

PALPATORY-AUSCULTATORY METHOD OF OBTAINING A BLOOD PRESSURE READING

Nursing action/*Rationale*

1. Wash hands *to inhibit spread of microorganisms.*
2. Introduce self *to decrease anxiety level.*
3. Identify patient by identification band *to ensure correct patient for procedure.*
4. Explain procedure *to seek cooperation and assistance from patient and to decrease anxiety.*
5. Prepare for procedure by:
   a. Collecting all necessary supplies *to organize procedure efficiently:* sphygmomanometer and stethoscope. Determine the correct cuff size. *An improper size will give an inaccurate reading.* The length of the cuff should be 80% of the upper arm circumference and be two thirds the width of the upper arm. *A higher inaccurate reading will be obtained if too small a cuff is used. Conversely a lower inaccurate reading will be obtained if too large a cuff is used.*
   b. Provide privacy for patient if necessary *to decrease anxiety.*
   c. Determine site for blood pressure measurement. Avoid applying cuff to arm when: (1) catheter is in antecubital fossa and if fluids are infusing; (2) arteriovenous shunt is in place; (3) breast or axillary surgery has been performed on that side; (4) an arm or hand has been traumatized or is diseased; (5) a lower arm cast or bulky bandage is in place.
6. Implement procedure:
   a. Apply cuff to bare arm with patient's palm facing upward. The cuff is applied 1 to 2 inches above the antecubital space (see illustrations). The cuff is centered over the brachial artery. The patient's upper arm is held at the level of the heart and the lower arm is rested on a firm surface *to ensure accuracy.*
   b. Palpate radial artery (see illustrations).
   c. Inflate cuff. Note the point on the manometer gauge when the radial pulse is obliterated. This is the approximate systolic pressure.

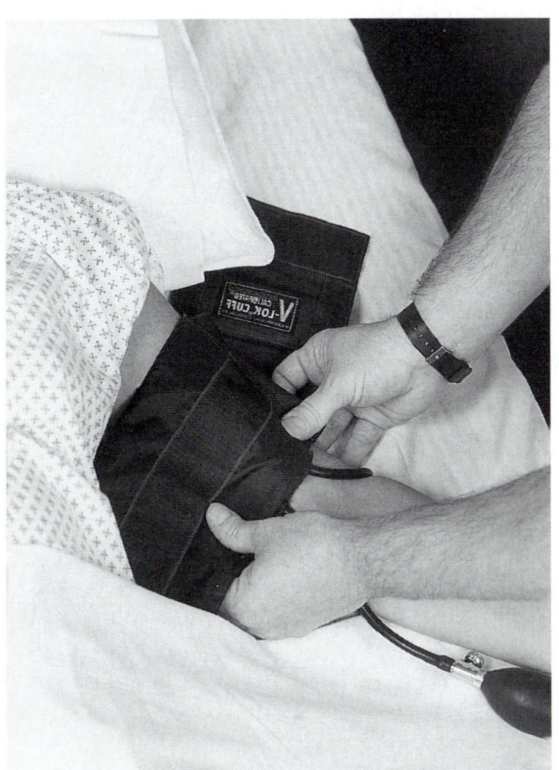

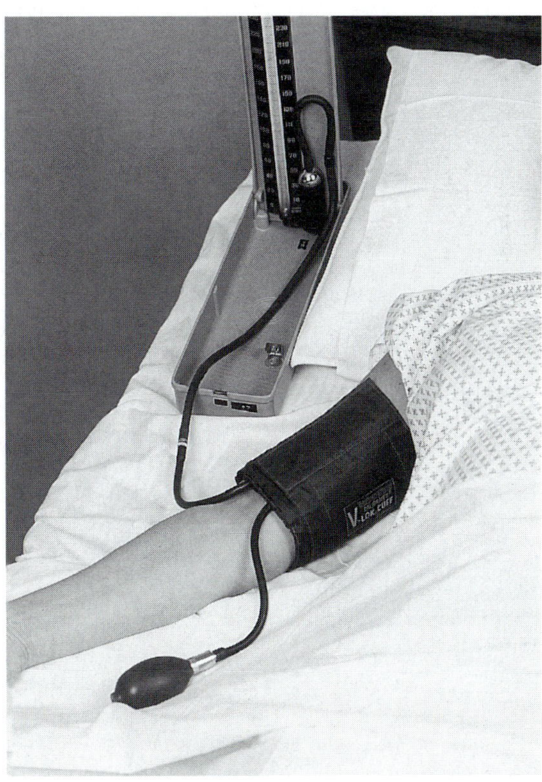

STEP 6a

Continued.

PALPATORY-AUSCULTATORY METHOD OF OBTAINING A BLOOD PRESSURE READING—cont'd

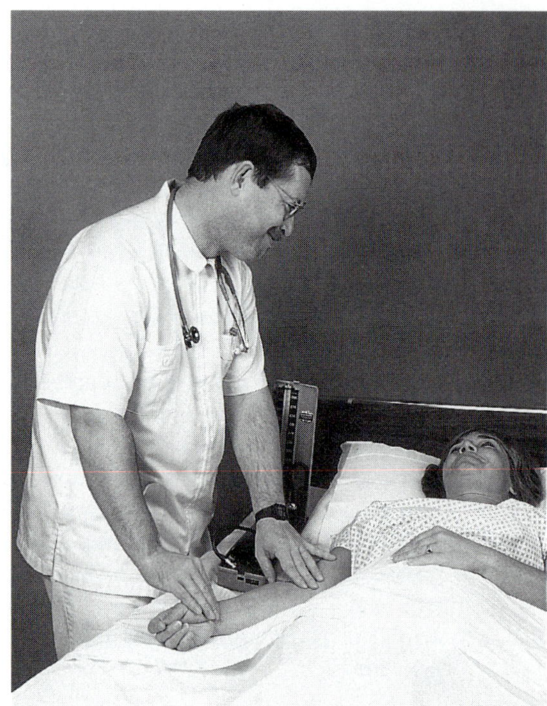

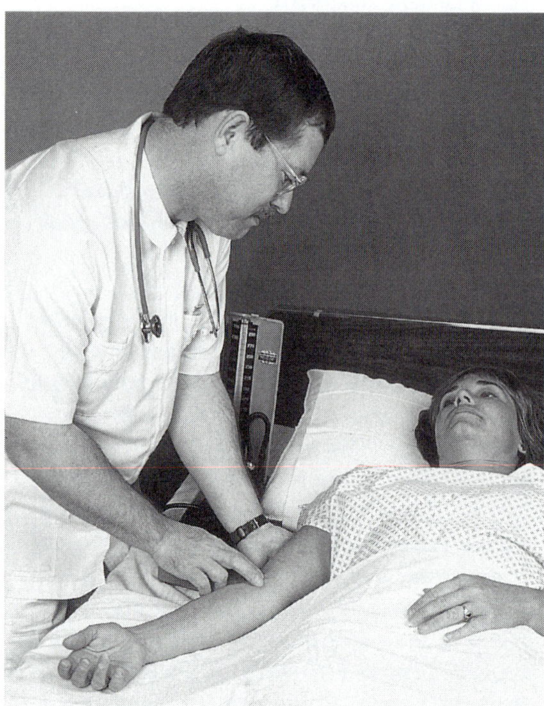

STEP 6b

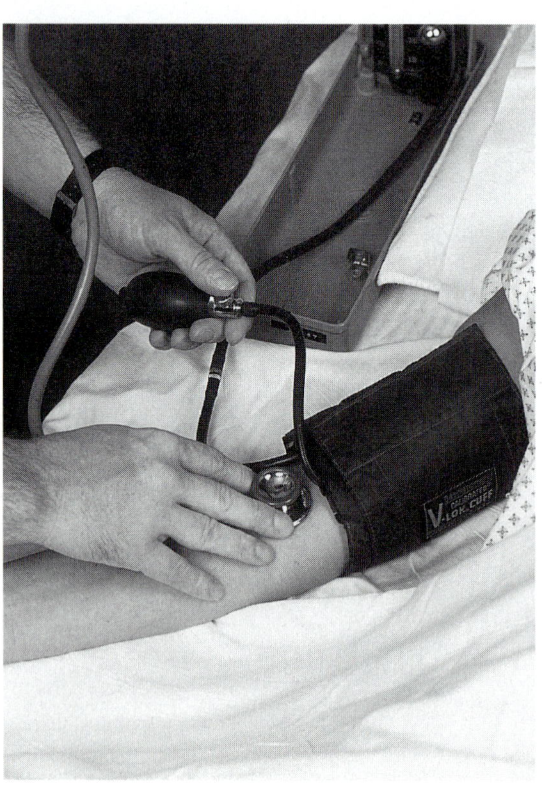

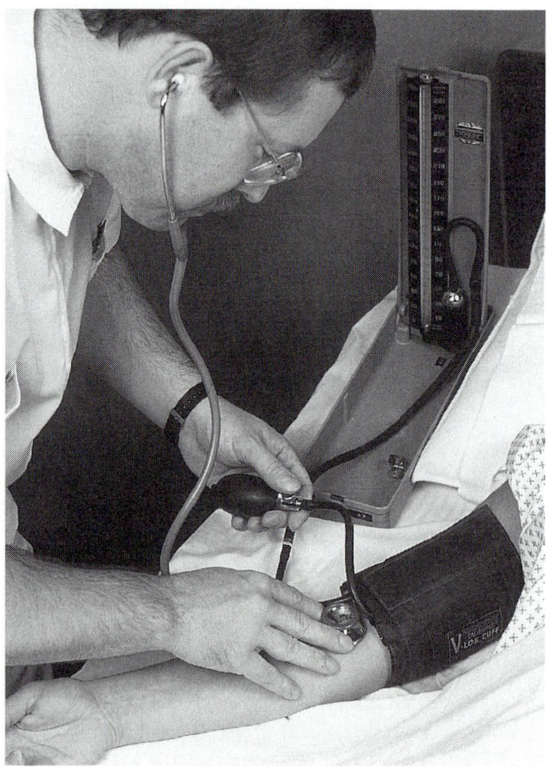

STEP 6e

SKILL 10-9

PALPATORY-AUSCULTATORY METHOD OF OBTAINING A BLOOD PRESSURE READING—cont'd

d. Deflate the cuff. *Deflating the cuff allows congestion to leave the arm, preventing a false high reading. Rest arm for 1 minute.*
e. Palpate the brachial artery and place the bell/diaphram of the stethoscope over it (see illustrations).
f. Reinflate cuff 20 to 30 mm Hg above point at which radial artery was obliterated to *avoid the auscultatory gap.*
g. Slowly deflate cuff. Cuff is deflated at a rate of 2 mm Hg per second. Note the point at which the pulse is heard. This is the systolic pressure. Note the point at which no pulse is heard. This is the diastolic pressure.
h. Completely deflate and remove the cuff.
i. Provide for patient comfort by replacing clothing.

7. Write down reading *for documentation later.*
8. Wash hands *to inhibit spread of microorganisms.*
9. Document reading on graph sheet (e.g., BP 120/80) (see illustration, p. 149).
10. Follow up by reporting abnormal readings immediately.

See Box 10-8. For accurate assessment of blood pressure, initially measure BP in both arms.

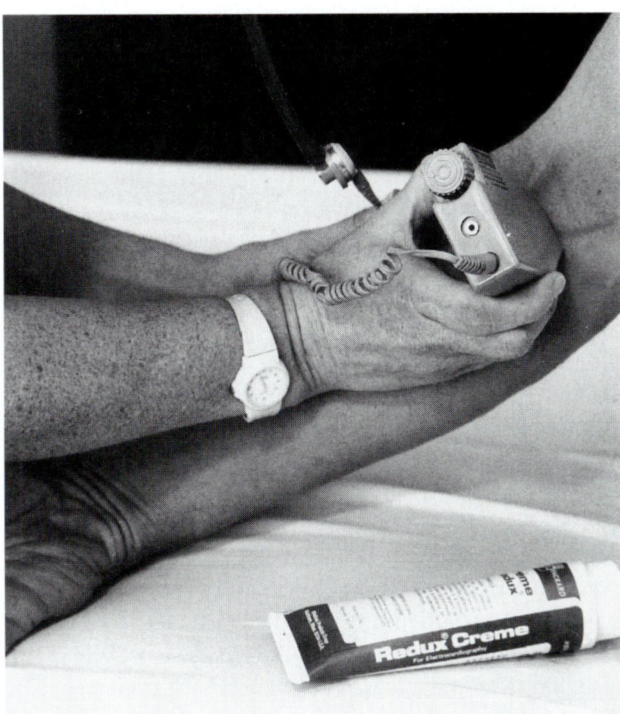

FIG. 10-11 Ultrasound stethoscope in position on brachial artery.

Box 10-8 ASSESSING BLOOD PRESSURE IN BOTH ARMS

- The nurse should initially measure blood pressure in both arms, especially if the patient has heart disease or if the reading in the first arm is abnormal.
- Normally a difference of 5 to 10 mm Hg exists between the arms. In subsequent assessments the blood pressure should be measured in the arm with the higher pressure.
- Pressure differences higher than 10 mm Hg indicate conditions such as aortic stenosis or an arterial occlusion in the arm with the lower pressure.

so blood pressure must be measured in the lower extremities. Also, in patients with certain circulatory abnormalities, it helps to compare blood pressure in the upper extremities with that in the legs. The popliteal artery, located behind the knee in the popliteal space, is the site for auscultation. The cuff must be wide and long enough to allow for the larger girth of the thigh and is positioned with the bladder over the posterior aspect of the midthigh. Placing the patient in a prone position is best. If such a position is impossible, the patient should be asked to flex the knee slightly for easier access to the artery. The procedure is the same as that for brachial artery auscultation. Systolic pressure in the lower extremities is usually higher by 10 to 40 mm Hg than that in the brachial artery, but the diastolic pressure is essentially the same (Fig. 10-12 on p. 164).

Self-Measurement of Blood Pressure

More people measure their own blood pressures because of improved technology in home monitoring devices and a greater interest in health promotion. Two of the more common devices used by the general public are portable home devices and stationary automated machines.

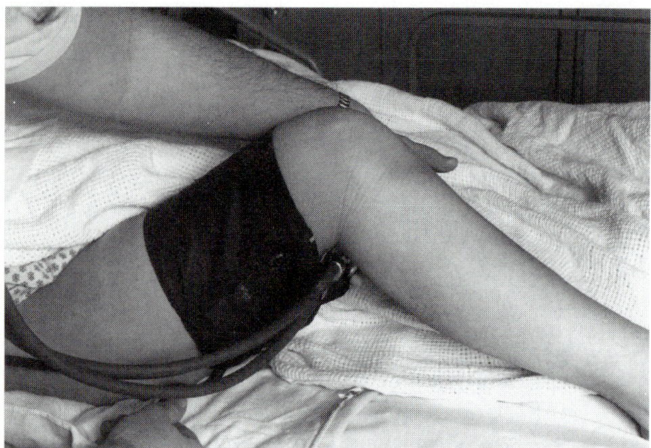

FIG. 10-12 Assessment of blood pressure in the lower extremity.

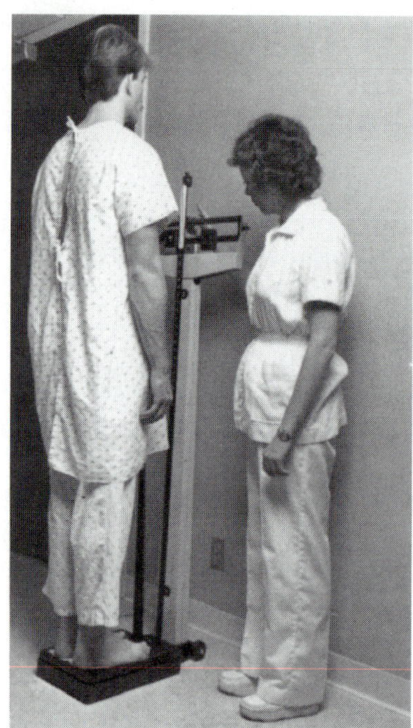

FIG. 10-13 Measuring weight.

The portable home devices include the mercury and aneroid sphygmomanometers and electronic digital readout devices that do not require use of a stethoscope. The electronic devices inflate and deflate cuffs with the push of a button. The electronic devices may be easier to manipulate but can easily become inaccurate and require recalibration more than once a year. Because of their sensitivity, improper cuff placement or movement of the arm can cause electronic devices to give incorrect readings.

Stationary automated machines can be found in public places such as grocery stores, fitness clubs, banks, airports, or work sites. Users simply rest the arm within the machine's inflatable cuff, which contains a pressure sensor. The cuff fits over the clothing. A visual display tells users their blood pressure within 60 to 90 seconds. The reliability of the stationary machines is limited. Blood pressure values may vary by 5 to 10 mm Hg or more (for both the systolic and diastolic values) compared with the pressures taken with a manual sphygmomanometer.

Consumers can learn to use self-measurement devices if they have the information that they need to perform the procedure correctly and if they know when to seek medical attention. The nurse can advise patients of possible inaccuracies in the machines, help patients understand the meaning and implications of readings, and teach patients proper measurement techniques.

HEIGHT AND WEIGHT

With the initial measurement of vital signs, the nurse measures the patient's height (the vertical measurement of a structure, organ, or other object from bottom to top, when it is placed or projected in an upright position) and weight (the force exerted on a body by the gravity of the earth; normal weight depends upon the frame of the individual). Height and weight determination is important because it helps to assess normal growth and development, aids in proper drug dosage calculation, and may be used to assess the effectiveness of drug therapy, such as diuretics. A significant loss of weight may be a sign of an underlying disease.

Patients should be weighed at the same time of day, on the same scale, and in the same clothes to allow an objective comparison of subsequent weighings. Patients are weighed to give the physician information for prescribing medication dosages and to determine nutritional status and water balance. Because 1 liter (L) of fluid equals 1 kilogram (kg) (2.2 pounds [lb]), a weight change of 1 kg (2.2 lb) will reflect a loss or gain of 1 L of body fluids. An ideal time to weigh patients is at 6 AM, after voiding and before breakfast is served. Patients capable of bearing their own weight use a standing scale (Skill 10-10). The nurse calibrates the scale by setting the weight at zero and noting whether the balance beam registers in the middle of the mark (Fig. 10-13). Scales with a digital display should read zero before each use. The patient stands on the scale platform and remains still. The nurse slowly adjusts the scale weight on the balance beam until the tip of the beam registers in the middle of the mark. Digital scale readouts display weight in a matter of seconds.

Stretcher and chair scales are available for patients unable to bear weight. After being transferred to the scale, the patient is lifted above the bed by a hydraulic device, and the weight is measured on a balance beam or digital display. Caution must be used to promote patient safety when transferring patients to and from the scales.

SKILL 10-10

MEASURING HEIGHT AND WEIGHT

Nursing action/*Rationale*

1. Wash hands *to inhibit spread of microorganisms.*
2. Introduce self to patient *to decrease anxiety level.*
3. Identify patient by identification band *to ensure correct patient for procedure.*
4. Explain procedure to patient *to gain cooperation and assistance and to decrease anxiety.*
5. Prepare for procedure by:
   a. Collecting supplies *to organize procedure efficiently:* scale—standing, chair, or bed type.
   b. Providing privacy, if necessary, *to decrease anxiety.*
6. Implement procedure:
   a. Balance scale at zero *to ensure accurate reading.*
   b. Have patient step on to scale. Patient should be weighed in same amount of clothing each time—preferably gown and slippers.
   c. Measure height with patient standing upright, if patient can tolerate.
   d. Measure weight.
   e. Assist patient off scale. Have patient step to side, *which is safer than stepping backward.*
   f. Provide for patient comfort by assisting to bed or chair as needed.
7. Write down measurement *for documentation later.*
8. Wash hands *to inhibit spread of microorganisms.*
9. Document measurements (e.g., Ht. 64 inches, Wt. 136 lb).
10. Follow up by reporting measurement if required.

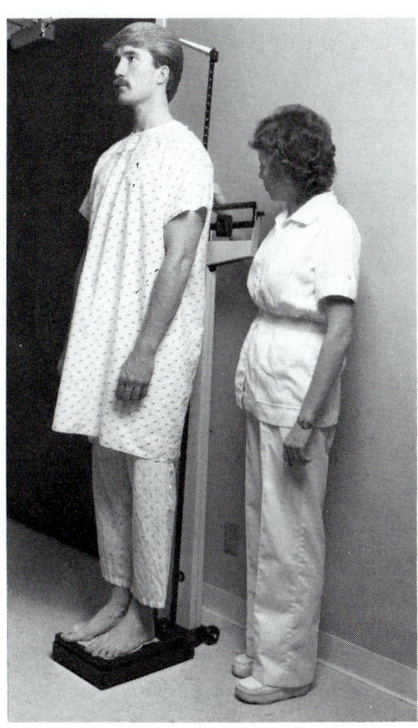

FIG. 10-14 Measuring height.

To facilitate weighing very ill patients portable bed scales are available in some agencies. The scale is positioned next to the bed. The patient is carefully transferred to and from the scale platform.

Different techniques exist for measuring the height of weight-bearing and non-weight-bearing patients. Patients who are able to stand should remove their shoes. Paper towels are placed on the scale platform or floor so that the patient's feet remain clean. A measuring stick or tape is attached vertically to the weight scales or wall. The nurse asks the patient to stand erect, exercising good posture. On the standing scale, a metal rod, which is attached to the back of the scale, swings out and over the top of the head (Fig. 10-14).

The nurse should never accept a stated height and weight. Only in cases of extreme illness should the nurse delay obtaining these valuable assessments.

The nurse weighs malnourished patients, patients who are undergoing diuretic therapy, and patients who have diseases that increase fluid retention, such as heart, liver, and kidney disease (see Skill 10-9).

WHEN VITAL SIGNS ARE ASSESSED

Although temperature, pulse, respiration, and blood pressure are presented as separate procedures, all of them are usually assessed at the same time at set intervals. A set of vital signs is taken when a patient is admitted to a facility, and then as prescribed by the physician or as policy dictates, for example, every 4 hours, once a shift, or even weekly in some extended-care facilities (Box 10-9). The more ill the patient, the more frequently vital signs are taken. The nurse uses her judgment in cases where the patient's condition worsens, at which times

TABLE 10-4 Age-Related Vital Signs

Age Group	Heart Rate (per minute)	Respiratory Rate (per minute)	Blood Pressure (mm Hg)
Neonate	130-150	36-60	Systolic 20-60
Infant	125-135	40-46	Systolic 70-80
Toddler	90-120	20-30	Systolic 80-100
School-age (6-10)	65-105	22-24	Systolic 90-100 Diastolic 60-64
Adolescent (10-18)	65-100	16-22	Systolic 100-120 Diastolic 70-80
Adult	60-100	12-20	Systolic 100-120 Diastoli 70-80
Older adult	60-100	12-18	Systolic 130-140 Diastolic 90-95

Box 10-9 WHEN TO OBTAIN VITAL SIGNS

- During admission to a health care facility
- On a routine schedule as determined by physician's order or hospital policy
- Before and after surgical procedure
- Before and after invasive diagnostic procedures
- Before and after administering certain medications
- When the patient's general condition changes (loss of consciousness, hemorrhage, cardiac dysrhythmias, or the onset of intense pain)
- Before and after certain nursing interventions (when a patient ambulates for the first time or after tracheal suctioning)
- When the patient reports nonspecific symptoms of physical distress (complaints of "feeling funny" or "different")
- Routinely as part of a procedure (blood transfusion, liver biopsy, paracentesis, thoracentesis)

vital signs should always be obtained. Vital sign readings are interrelated. A rise in temperature of 1 degree may cause an increase in pulse rate of 4 beats per minute. Respiratory rate and blood pressure readings likewise increase with a rise in temperature; however, when blood pressure falls because of hemorrhage, the pulse and respirations increase and the temperature usually decreases. It is also important to recognize the age-related differences in vital signs (Table 10-4 and gerontological box).

If there is a possibility of contact with body secretions, the nurse wears gloves while obtaining vital signs.

Before measurement of vital signs, the patient should be given an explanation of the procedure to elicit cooperation and decrease anxiety, which could alter measurements.

GERONTOLOGICAL CONSIDERATIONS

- An active older adult generally maintains a core body temperature within the accepted norms for younger adults. After age 75, core temperature averages 97.2° F (36° C).
- Environmental temperature plays a more significant role in the older than in younger adults and is more likely to contribute to hypothermia and hyperthermia.
- Pulse irregularities are more commonly seen in older adults. Apical pulses should be auscultated as part of a thorough assessment.
- Pulses can be easily occluded in older adults; therefore gentle pressure should be applied.
- With aging, there is typically a decrease in depth of respirations. Respiratory rate may increase to compensate.
- Often a standard adult cuff is too large for an older individual who has lost upper arm mass. Incorrect cuff sizing can result in significant errors.
- Accurate measurement of blood pressure is essential for older adults receiving antihypertensive medication.
- Orthostatic hypotension, a sudden drop in blood pressure with positional change, is commonly observed in inactive older adults, particularly when rising after a period of bed rest.
- Older persons receiving antihypertenives and vasodilators should be monitored closely for orthostatic hypotension. A systolic pressure of less than 100 mm Hg or a drop of 20 mm Hg or more in the systolic blood pressure should be promptly reported.

RECORDING VITAL SIGNS

Most facilities have graphic flow sheets for charting vital signs. In some facilities a rectal temperature would be indicated with a small circled R, and axillary with a small circled A next to the reading. Blood pressures are always written with the systolic first and the diastolic beneath: 120/80. When charting the pulse on a graphic sheet, note that the pulse was an apical measurement by writing "ap" next to the number: 78 ap. An example of graphic flow sheet is shown in the illustration on p. 149. Any abnormal findings are reported to the nurse-manager or physician immediately. In addition to any actual vital sign values, the nurse records in the nurses' notes any accompanying or precipitating signs and symptoms such as chest pain, vertigo, shortness of breath, flushing, and diaphoresis. The nurse documents any interventions initiated as a result of vital sign measurement, such as tepid sponging.

REFERENCES AND SUGGESTED READINGS

1. American Heart Association: *Techniques for blood pressure measurement palpatory and auscultory method,* 1988, The Association.
2. Anderson MH: Evaluation of an infrared tympanic membrane thermometer in pediatric patients, *Pediatrics* 85(5):854, 1990.
3. Baird SC, White NE, Basinger M: Can you rely on tympanic thermometers? *RN* 55(8):48, 1992.
4. Brown S: Temperature taking: getting it right, *Nurs Stand Suppl* 4, 1990.
5. Camberlain JM et al: Comparison of a tympanic thermometer to rectal and oral thermometers in a pediatric emergency department, *Clin Pediatr Suppl* 24, Apr 1991.
6. Erickson R, Yount S: Comparison of tympanic and oral temperature in surgical patients, *Nurs Res* 40(2):90, 1991.
7. Giuffre M et al: The relationship between axillary and core body temperatures, *Appl Nurs Res* 3(2):52, 1990.
8. Hill MN, Grim CM: How to take a precise blood pressure, *Am J Nurs* 91:38, 1991.
9. Huston CJ: Hyperthermia, *Nursing* 20(12):33, 1990.
10. *Illustrated manual of nursing practice,* Springhouse, Penn, 1991, Springhouse.
11. Intelligent Medical Systems: Tympanic thermometry: a first temp clinical monography, Calsbad, Calif, 1991, The Publisher.
12. Jolly A: Taking a blood pressure, *Nurs Times* 87:40, 1991.
13. Kenney RD et al: Evaluation of an infrared tympanic membrane thermometer in pediatric patients, *Pediatrics* 85(5):856, 1990.
14. Malasanos L et al: *Health assessment,* ed 4, St Louis, 1990, Mosby.
15. Margolius FR: Accuracy of apical pulse rate measurement in young children, *Nurs Res* 39:378, 1991.
16. McCaffery M: How vital are vital signs? *Nursing* 22:42, 1992.
17. *Mosby's medical, nursing, and allied health dictionary,* ed 4, St Louis, 1994, Mosby.
18. Oregon JM: The inaccuracy of axillary temperatures measured with an electronic thermometer, *Am J Dis Child* 144(1):109, 1990.
19. Perry AG, Potter PA: *Clinical nursing skills and techniques,* ed 3, St Louis, 1994, Mosby.
20. Potter PA, Perry AG: *Basic nursing:* theory and practice, ed 3, St Louis, 1995, Mosby.
21. Potter PA, Perry AG: *Fundamentals of nursing: concepts, process, and practice,* ed 3, St Louis, 1993, Mosby.
22. Scharff K: Vital signs revisited: what you may be missing, *Nurs 91,* 21:59, 1991.
23. Seidel H et al: *Mosby's guide to physical examination,* ed 3, St Louis, 1995, Mosby.
24. Sheehan MM: Blood pressure monitoring: completing the picture-ambulatory blood pressure monitor, *Nurs '90* 20(4):79, 1990.
25. The Staff: *Nursing procedures,* Springhouse, Penn, 1992, Springhouse.
26. Thibodeau GA, Patton K: *Anatomy and physiology,* ed 2, St Louis, 1993, Mosby.
27. Timby BK, Lewis LW, *Fundamental skills and concepts in patient care,* ed 5, Philadelphia, 1992, Lippincott.

CHAPTER CHALLENGE

KEY POINTS

- Vital signs include the physiological measurement of temperature, pulse, respiration, and blood pressure.
- Vital signs may be measured as part of a complete physical examination or more commonly in a review of the patient's condition.
- Vital signs should be obtained whenever the patient's condition changes adversely.
- Knowledge of the factors influencing vital signs assists the nurse in interpreting abnormal values.
- Vital sign measurements provide a basis for evaluating the patient's response to medical and nursing interventions.
- The nurse assesses the presence and character of peripheral pulses to determine the adequacy of peripheral blood flow.
- Temperatures can be obtained by oral, rectal, axillary, and tympanic routes.
- When assessing blood pressure, having the proper equipment is as important as using the correct technique.
- Temperature, pulse, respiration, and blood pressure are interrelated; a change in one may alter other vital signs.
- Height and weight is a ratio. Knowing the weight or height alone usually does not supply useful information.
- Self-measurement of blood pressure can be useful in detecting an elevated blood pressure in persons previously unaware of a problem or in monitoring blood pressure in persons already diagnosed with hypertension.

STUDY QUESTIONS

1. Mr. Jones, age 44, is undergoing antibiotic therapy for pneumonia. His oral temperature reading is 100.6° F. His rectal temperature would be:
   1. 101.6° F
   2. 100.6° F
   3. 99.6° F
   4. 97.6° F
2. Mrs. Kurgak, age 30, develops a postpartum temperature that is elevated in the evening but returns to a normal reading in the morning. This has occurred for several days. This pattern of fever would be classified as:
   1. Constant
   2. Intermittent
   3. Remittent
   4. Crisis
3. Mr. Smith, age 66, has a 10-year history of coronary artery disease. He is presently recovery from a myocardial infarction. The most accurate assessment of pulse rate would be to obtain a(n):
   1. Carotid pulse
   2. Radial pulse
   3. Apical pulse
   4. Brachial pulse
4. Ms. Beideck, age 16, enters the emergency room with an exacerbation of asthma. Her respirations are 40 per minute. After treatment, her rate returns to normal limits. Normal limits for Ms. Beideck's respirations would be:
   1. 30-60
   2. 16-22
   3. 8-12
   4. 24-30
5. Mrs. Adams is 48 years old. During a routine physical her blood pressure is noted at 180/90. She fears she is hypertensive. The nurse would explain that the diagnosis of hypertension is made when there is a sustained elevated blood pressure of over:
   1. 160/100
   2. 140/90
   3. 130/70
   4. 120/80
6. Mr. Pauly, age 65, has a history of emphysema resulting from a 30-year history of cigarette smoking. He frequently complains of dyspnea. Dyspnea is defined as:
   1. Pallor
   2. Absence of retractions
   3. Cyanosis
   4. Difficult respirations
7. Mrs. Gerring, age 52, complains of palpitations resulting from anxiety over her impending surgery. Her pulse rate is found to be 110 per minute. Mrs. Gerring's heart rate could be described as:
   1. Bradycardia
   2. Tachycardia
   3. Tachypnea
   4. Hypertensive
8. Mrs. Pace, age 66, suddenly develops rectal hemorrhaging. Her radial pulse is difficult to palpate even with slight pressure. This type of pulse would be described as:
   1. Absent
   2. Nonpalpable
   3. Thready
   4. Bounding

5

BASIC NURSING SKILLS

Nursing is a career in which I can give care not only by professional techniques but also by giving a part of myself that has matured during my lifetime. There is more to good nursing care than knowing all the correct procedures. You must be able to extend yourself into understanding not only yourself but your patient as well. This may consist of only holding a hand to comfort or being available to listen when a prognosis is not so good.

Marquitta Crabtree
Student Nurse

11

ADMISSION, TRANSFER, AND DISCHARGE

Lois White
Elaine Kockrow
Barbara Christensen

KEY TERMS

admission
against medical advice (AMA)
continuity of care
discharge
discharge planning
disorientation
empathy
health care facility
home health agency
separation anxiety
third party payers
transfer

LEARNING OBJECTIVES

After reading this chapter, the student should be able to do the following:

- Define the key terms.
- Identify guidelines for admission, transfer, and discharge of a patient.
- Describe common patient reactions to hospitalization.
- Identify nursing interventions for common patient reactions to hospitalization.
- Discuss the nurse's responsibilities in performing an admission.
- Describe how the nurse prepares a patient for transfer to another unit or facility.
- Discuss discharge planning.
- Describe how the nurse prepares a patient for discharge.
- Identify the nurse's role when a patient chooses to leave the hospital against medical advice.

RELATED TOPICS OF INTEREST

- Communication (Chapter 4)
- Documentation (Chapter 6)
- Life span cycle (Chapter 7)
- Signs, symptoms, and physical assessment (Chapter 9)
- Safety (Chapter 13)
- Basic pediatric nursing care (Chapter 43)
- Home health nursing (Chapter 48)
- Hospice care (Chapter 53)

COMMON PATIENT REACTIONS TO HOSPITALIZATION

Admission (entry of a patient into the health care facility) to a hospital or other **health care facility** (any agency that provides health care) is an anxious time for patients and their families. The patient is usually very concerned about health problems, or potential health problems, and the potential outcome of treatment. Often the patient is having pain or some other discomfort. The first contact with nurses and other health care workers is important; anxiety and fears can be lessened and a positive attitude regarding the care to be received can be initiated.

The environment of a health care facility differs from a patient's home and has new sights, sounds, and smells that may interfere with the patient's comfort. It is the nurse's responsibility to assist the patient in maintaining dignity and a sense of control and to become comfortable in this new environment.

Each person's reaction to hospitalization is unique; however, there are some common reactions the nurse can anticipate, such as fear of the unknown, loss of identity, **disorientation** (mental confusion characterized by inadequate or incorrect perception of place, time, and identity), **separation anxiety** (fears and apprehension caused by separation from familiar surroundings and significant persons), and loneliness. These reactions are related to some of the needs described by Maslow.[9]

Fear of the unknown, which causes insecurity, may be the most common reaction. This relates to the need Maslow calls safety. Such questions as these can cause anxiety and insecurity if unanswered: How do I work the bed? how do I call the nurse? how or when do I get some food? when can my family visit? and what are they going to do to me next? A caring nurse can relieve some of the anxiety by orienting the patient and family to the room and explaining how the equipment works. Explanations about hospital policies, information about medical orders and procedures, and simple direct answers to questions the patient or family may ask help the person feel more comfortable and in control.

During the admission process to a health care facility, a patient may feel a loss of identity that reflects a need for esteem, including recognition, as described by Maslow. When an identification band is put on the patient's wrist, the patient may feel recognized only as the number and name on the identification band rather than as a person. Thus, it is important to explain that this is a necessary procedure to provide a positive means of identification, because medications, anesthesia, discomfort, and emotional reactions may cause the patient to be disoriented or unresponsive.

The nurse must learn new patients' names quickly and use Mr., Mrs., Ms., or Miss with the last name. First names are used only at the patient's request. Using "honey, dear, gramps, or grandma" is *never* appropriate.

GERONTOLOGICAL CONSIDERATIONS

- The older person admitted to the hospital today is likely to be seriously ill.
- In a normally alert and oriented older adult, medical conditions that necessitate hospitalization often result in some level of disorientation.
- Older adults, who often have some limitation of vision or hearing, are more likely to become agitated or fearful during hospitalization. Many experience relocation stress.
- Transfers, even within the hospital, tend to be confusing and upsetting to them.
- Hospitalized older adults frequently are concerned that they will be unable to return to their homes and will need institutional placement.
- Appropriate referrals for home nursing, therapy, homemaking, Meals on Wheels, or other services are essential for older adults.

The reactions of separation anxiety and loneliness reflect a need for belongingness and love that Maslow identified. Separation anxiety is widely recognized in young children, but adults and the elderly often have this reaction as well. It generally is expressed in children by crying; adults may be either very quiet or very talkative; the older adult may exhibit disorientation or depression.

Liberal visiting hours in health care facilities encourage family and friends to visit. Many hospitals now allow small children to visit relatives, especially their mother with a new baby. Parents are encouraged to stay with their hospitalized child to prevent the anxiety of separation from the parents. This also gives the child a feeling of security. In some facilities pets are allowed to visit; pets may even live in some nursing homes.

The nurse may help reduce the severity of these common reactions to hospitalization with a warm, caring attitude and with courtesy and **empathy** (ability to recognize and to some extent share the emotions and state of mind of another and to understand the meaning and significance of that person's behavior). Treating patients with respect, maintaining their dignity, involving them in the plan of care, and, whenever possible, adjusting hospital routine to meet their desires will help them adapt. Special considerations for the older adult are listed in the gerontological box.

SKILL 11-1: ADMITTING A PATIENT

Guidelines

The admission procedure generally begins in the admitting department. Here the admissions staff gathers information to start the patient's record. This information usually includes name, address, telephone number, age, birth date, Social Security number, next of kin, insurance company and policy number, place of employment, physician's name, and reason for this admission and for previous admissions. This information is primarily used in the business office for billing purposes. The identification band is prepared with the patient's name, age, ID number, physician's name, and the room number. The admitting clerk usually puts the band on the patient's wrist. The unit where the patient is assigned for care is notified, and the patient is escorted to the room.

Some hospitals have telephone admitting. The day before a planned admission, a clerk from the admitting office calls the patient at home and gathers all the information needed to begin the records. Instructions are given regarding time to arrive at the hospital, items to bring to the hospital, and things that should not be brought to the hospital (e.g., jewelry and large sums of money). When the patient arrives the next day, the records and identification band need only the room number put on them.

Persons brought to the emergency room may be admitted directly to a patient care room or a special care unit such as an intensive care unit (ICU), coronary care unit (CCU), or burn unit. In these situations a family member, usually the next of kin, goes to the admitting office to provide the necessary information.

When the unit staff are notified that a new patient is being escorted to a room, the room should be made ready. A room that is neat and clean, with lighting and temperature appropriate, and personal care items in place, makes the patient feel expected and welcome. A room that is not prepared may make the patient feel unexpected or that the arrival is inconvenient to the nurse. This makes a poor first impression and impedes the development of a therapeutic nurse-patient relationship.

If special equipment will be required by the new patient, such as oxygen or traction, it should be in place and ready when the patient arrives. A patient arriving on a stretcher will need the bed in the high position; the low bed position is best for a patient arriving by wheelchair or walking.

Greeting the patient by name and making him feel welcome is one of the most important aspects of the admission procedure. Be careful to call the patient by his surname if the patient is an adult, unless otherwise directed. The nurse should introduce herself by name and title (e.g., Miss Rodriquez, SPN [or SVN], or Mr. Smith, LPN [or LVN]). A person who is warmly welcomed will be more at ease in this new environment.

It is important for the nurse to remember that patients do not get ill and require hospitalization at the nurse's convenience. Regardless of the time or activity occurring on the nursing unit, the nurse should be courteous, interested in, and receptive of the new patient. The new patient should be given an orientation to the unit and the room. The orientation should include the following:

1. The relationship of the room to the nurses' station
2. The location of lounge areas
3. The location of shower and bathroom facilities
4. How to call the nurse from the bed and the bathroom
5. How to use the intercom system
6. How to adjust the bed and lights
7. How to operate the television
8. How to operate the telephone and the radio
9. Explanation of policies that are applicable to the patient

The hospital routine should also be explained. Knowing when meals are served, when family and friends may visit, when laboratory tests or diagnostic imaging evaluations are scheduled, when the physician usually makes rounds, and the policy on side rails will give the patient a sense of security and lessen anxiety. Many hospitals have booklets for the patient explaining these routine activities; these serve as reminders of what the nurse explains. Some booklets include information about the availability of various social services, religious services, and facilities such as cafeteria, library, and gift shop.

The admitting procedure on the patient care unit is much more extensive than that in the admitting department. The nurse should check the identification band and verify the information with the patient. Assessment of immediate needs such as pain, shortness of breath, or severe anxiety should be made and reported. If there is another patient in the room, the roommate should be introduced.

Jewelry, money, and medication should be given to the family to take home. If no family member is present, the valuables may be put in the hospital safe. The nurse must carefully follow the hospital policy for patient valuables. Losing a patient's valuables can have serious legal implications for both the hospital and the nurse. Disposition of valuables must be documented on the medical record.

The patient is usually asked to put on pajamas or a hospital gown. Sometimes the nurse must help the patient change clothes. If this help is not needed, provide the patient a few minutes of privacy to change. Clothing should be inventoried along with other personal items the patient uses, such as glasses, contacts, dentures, prostheses, crutches, hearing aids, wigs, or Bible. Jewelry and money kept in the patient's room must also be recorded. Fig. 11-1 is a sample clothing and valuable inventory check.

Once the patient is established in his room, the nurse should take the health history and do the initial nursing assessment. The health history generally includes the reason for admission, signs and symptoms the patient is experiencing, past illnesses or surgical procedures or hospitalizations, medications (both prescription and nonprescription), allergies (food, medications,

SPOHN HOSPITAL

VALUABLES FORM

VAUABLES BROUGHT WITH PATIENT TO HOSPITAL DATE ______

Clocks ______ Hearing Aids ______

Dentures: no. of plates______ Jewelry ______

Bridgework: no. of pieces______ Money (billfold) ______

Eyeglasses ______ Money (purse) ______

Contact lens ______ Radio ______

Watches ______ T.V. ______

Electric toothbrush______ Electric razor ______

Prosthesis (any type)______ Others ______

I take entire responsibility for retaining in my possesion the articles listed above. I am holding nothing in my possession which I have not declared here. I understand and agree that Spohn Hospital is not liable or responsible for any of patient's property left in the care, custody and control of the Hospital at patient's or patient representative's request if items are not secured in the Valuables Storage Envelope or in the Hospital safe.

SIGNATURE OF PATIENT ______

I have fully explained to this patient that Spohn Hospital takes no responsibility for articles retained by the patient.

SIGNATURE OF EMPLOYEE RECORDING ARTICLES ______

VALUABLES STORAGE ENVELOPE

When Valuables Storage Envelope is used, record the following information:

Envelope Number ______

Date property received ______

Employee taking envelope to Cashier ______

T 278 902830 Revised 7-88

FIG. 11-1 Clothing and valuables inventory check form. (Courtesy Spohn Hospital, Corpus Christi, Tex.)

other), eating habits, urinary and bowel patterns, sleep routine, and activity/exercise. Other information to be included in a history is the language spoken and understood, family members or significant others, home situation, interests, abilities, activities of daily living, and occupation.

The initial assessment should include level of consciousness, vital signs, height, weight, breath sounds, bowel sounds, range of motion, condition of skin, vision, and hearing. Fig. 11-2 on pp. 174-175 is an example of a record used to collect this information. The health history and initial nursing assessment may be performed by the RN in some hospitals. In others, either an RN or an LPN/LVN may collect this information.

The physician is notified when the patient has been admitted. If no orders have been previously received, the physician will give the nurse orders at this time.

Skill 11-1 identifies the general steps to follow in admitting a patient. Specific hospital policies and the patient's condition may alter these steps.

SPOHN HOSPITAL
DEPARTMENT OF NURSING
PATIENT DATA BASE/ASSESSMENT

ARRIVED: DATE: 11-9-94 1445
BY: AMB ___ W/C X ARMS ___
STRETCHER ___
AMULANCE ___

HEIGHT: STATED 5'6" ACTUAL 5'6"
WEIGHT: STATED 140 ACTUAL 145
TEMP 98^6 PULSE 82 RESP 20 BP 118/76

LANGUAGE SPOKEN: ENG ___
SPANISH X OTHER ___

STATED ALLERGIES: (NONE)
DRUG: ___
FOOD: ___
OTHER: ___

REASON FOR HOSPITALIZATION AND DESCRIPTION FOR SYMPTOMS:
(use Patient's or Significant Other's own words)
To have knee surgery in AM

ONSET OF SYMPTOMS: Twisted knee in basketball practice last week

HEALTH HISTORY: PAST SURGERIES/DATES: NONE

PREVIOUS DIET Regular

PREVIOUS ILLNESSES:			COMMENTS
GLAUCOMA	YES ___	NO X	
DIABETES	YES ___	NO X	
CANCER	YES ___	NO X	
LUNG DISEASE	YES ___	NO X	
ASTHMA	YES ___	NO X	
HEART DISEASE	YES ___	NO X	
TUBE FEEDING	YES ___	NO X	
HYPERTENSION	YES ___	NO X	
PACEMAKER	YES ___	NO X	
G.I. DISEASE	YES ___	NO X	
ARTHRITIS	YES ___	NO X	
JAUNDICE	YES ___	NO X	
NERVE DIS/PARALYSIS	YES ___	NO X	
OTHER			

MEDICATIONS NAME	DOSE	FREQ.	REASON FOR TAKING	LAST DOSE
NONE				

ASSISTANCE NEEDED WITH:

AMBULATION	YES X	NO ___
FEEDING	YES ___	NO X
HYGIENE	YES ___	NO X
ELIMINATION	YES ___	NO X

EQUIPMENT BROUGHT:

EYEGLASSES	YES X	NO ___
CONTACTS	YES ___	NO X
HEARING AID	YES ___	NO X
CRUTCHES	YES X	NO ___
CANE	YES ___	NO X
WALKER	YES ___	NO X
DENTURES/UPPER ___	LOWER ___	
BRIDGE		
OTHER		

PROSTHESIS:

EYE	RT ___	LT ___
BREAST	RT ___	LT ___
ARM/LEG	RT ___	LT ___

PATIENT INSTRUCTIONS:

SIGNAL LIGHT	✓
BED CONTROLS	✓
LIGHT CONTROLS	✓
BATHROOM	✓
SHOWER	✓
T.V.	✓
TELEPHONE	✓
UNIT INTRODUCTORY/ WELCOME LETTER	✓
VISITING PRIVILEGES	✓
HIGH RISK PRECAUTIONS	
I.D. BAND ON	✓
ALLERGY BAND ON	
URINALYSIS: OBTAINED	✓
INSTRUCTED	

HIGH RISK FALL CHECKLIST

___ (2) AGE GREATER THAN 70
___ (5) HISTORY OF PREVIOUS FALLS
___ (3) FROM NURSING HOME
___ (3) HAS HAD SITTER/COMPANION AT HOME

STATUS: MENTAL/PHYSICAL

___ (5) CONFUSED/DISORIENTED
___ (5) SENSORY IMPAIRMENT
___ (5) SEDATED
___ (5) NONCOMPLIANCE/ UNCOOPERATIVENESS
X (3) MOBILITY IMPAIRMENT/AMPUTEE (circled)
___ (3) WEAKNESS/DEBILITATION
___ (5) URGENT ELIMINATION NEEDS

MEDICATIONS

___ (3) DIURETICS
___ (3) LAXATIVES/G.I. PREPS
___ (3) ANTIHYPERTENSIVES
___ (3) ANTISEIZURES
___ (3) SEDATIVE/HYPNOTICS
___ (3) ANALGESICS
___ (3) CHEMOTHERAPY

3 TOTAL

IF SCORE IS 15 OR GREATER, INITIATE HIGH RISK MEASURES.

SKIN IMPAIRMENT HIGH RISK FOR CHECKLIST

GENERAL PHYSICAL CONDITION:
___ (1) FAIR (MAJOR BUT STABLE)
___ (2) POOR (CHRONIC/SERIOUS, NOT STABLE)

LEVEL OF CONSCIOUSNESS: (RESPONSE TO STIMULI)
___ (1) LETHARGIC (SLOW)
___ (2) SEMI-COMATOSE: (VERBAL/PAINFUL STIMULI)
___ (3) COMATOSE (NO RESPONSE)

ACTIVITY:
X (2) AMBULATORY WITH ASSISTANCE
___ (4) CHAIRFAST
___ (6) BEDFAST

MOBILITY:
___ (2) RESTRICTED MOVEMENT
___ (4) MOVES ONLY WITH ASSISTANCE
___ (6) IMMOBILE

INCONTINENCE:
___ (2) OCCASIONAL (<2 per 24 HRS.)
___ (4) USUALLY (>2 per 24 HRS.)
___ (6) TOTAL (NO CONTROL)

NUTRITION:
___ (1) FAIR (EATS/DRINKS 50% OR LESS)
___ (2) POOR (UNABLE/REFUSES DIET)
2 TOTAL

PTS. WITH A SCORE OF 8 OR ABOVE ARE HIGH RISK: INITIATE INTERVENTION PROTOCOL.

SIGNATURE & TITLE OF ADMITTING NURSE: Cory Sommer LPN DATE: 11-9-94 TIME: 1500

PATIENT DATA BASE/ASSESSMENT

FIG. 11-2 Patient data base assessment form, first page. (Courtesy Spohn Hospital, Corpus Christi, Tex.)

SPOHN HOSPITAL
DEPARTMENT OF NURSING
PATIENT DATA BASE/ASSESSMENT

DISCHARGE PLANNING ADMISSION SCREEN

	YES	NO
Do you live in a nursing home?		X
Do you have a visiting nurse?		X
Do you have help at home with your daily care or needs?	X	
Do you have a dependent person at home with no one to care for him/her?		X

A yes answer to any of the above questions require a referral to Social Services

ADDITIONAL COMMENTS: ______

SYSTEMS	YES	NO	COMMENTS
CNS			
L.O.C.			
- alert	✓		
- drowsy		✓	
- comatose		✓	
- disoriented		✓	
EYES			
- PEARLS			
- vision normal	✓		
- prosthesis		✓	
EARS			
- responds to normal voice tone	✓		
- drainage		✓	
SPEECH			
- clear	✓		
- slurred			
- hoarse/raspy			
- aphasic			
INTEGUMENTARY SKIN - color normal	✓		
- warm, dry	✓		
- turgor good	✓		
- bruises, abrasions, lacerations		✓	
- rash, lesions		✓	
- scars		✓	
- decubitus		✓	
- dressing		✓	

SYSTEMS	YES	NO	COMMENTS
CARDIOVASCULAR			
PULSES			
- radial			82
- carotid		✓	
- pedal			80
APICAL RATE ______			
CHEST PAIN		✓	
RESPIRATORY			
RESPIRATIONS			
- rapid		✓	
- slow		✓	
- deep		✓	
- shallow		✓	
- labored		✓	
BREATH SOUNDS			
- clear	✓		
- wheezes		✓	
- rales		✓	
COUGH			
- present		✓	
- productive		✓	
GASTROINTESTINAL			
ABDOMEN			
- soft	✓		
- distended		✓	
- tenderness		✓	
ELIMINATION			
- bowel sounds	✓		
- diarrhea		✓	
- constipation		✓	
- incontinence		✓	
- ostomy		✓	
LAST B.M. this AM			

SYSTEMS	YES	NO	COMMENTS
MUSCLE/SKELETAL EXTREMITIES			
- moves all on command	✓		
- WEAKNESS (SPECIFY) RA ____ LA ____			pain from injury
RA ____ LA ____	✓		
- edema		✓	
- normal ambulation			c̄ crutches
- prosthesis (SPECIFY)			
GENITOURINARY			
VOIDING			
- normal	✓		
- frequency		✓	
- burning		✓	
- incontinence		✓	
- catheter		✓	
CATHETER INSERTION DATE ____			
DATE OF LAST MENSTRUAL PERIOD:			
PSYCHO-SOCIAL			
- cooperative	✓		
- agitated		✓	
- depressed		✓	
- frightened		✓	anxious about surgery
- combative		✓	
HABITS			
- smoking		✓	
- alcohol		✓	
- drugs		✓	

After assessing this patient's physical condition, psycho-social needs, the Data Base and the Discharge Planning Admission screen, is Discharge Planning indicated at this time? ____ YES ____ NO

Referred to Social Services ____ YES X NO

Reviewed for Discharge Planning:
High Risk ____ YES X NO

Paula Sokol RN — Signature of Registered Nurse — 11/9/94 Date

Mary Pendleton — Signature of Social Worker — 11/9/94 Date

PATIENT DATA BASE/ASSESSMENT

FIG. 11-2—cont'd Patient data base assessment form, second page.

SKILL 11-1

ADMITTING A PATIENT

Nursing action/*Rationale*

1. Wash hands thoroughly *to inhibit the spread of microoganisms.*
2. Prepare the room before the patient arrives: care items in place; bed at proper height and open; light on *to make the patient feel expected and welcome.*
3. Courteously greet the patient and family. Introduce yourself. Project interest and concern. Introduce roommate(s) if any because *the patient and family are more at ease when they know the people around them.*
4. Check the identification band and verify accuracy *to ensure identification before tests or surgery is performed or medication is given.*
5. Assess immediate needs *to establish trust as needs are recognized and met.*
6. Orient the patient to the unit, lounge, and nurses' station *to promote safety.*
7. Orient the patient to the room. Explain the use of equipment, call system, bed, telephone, and television *to allow the patient some control over the environment* and *promote safety.*
8. Explain hospital routines, such as visiting hours, meal times, and morning wake-up *to decrease fear of unknown and give a feeling of security.*
9. Provide privacy if the patient desires. Family may be asked to leave the room. Assist the patient to undress if needed *to help maintain dignity and show respect for the patient.* Helping the patient undress prevents fatigue and falls. Range of motion and the skin may be assessed.
10. Follow hospital policy for care of valuables, clothing, and medications *to avoid loss of valuables, clothing, or medications, which is disturbing to the patient and family and could result in legal problems.*
11. Obtain the patient's health history, and do the initial nursing assessment *to provide a basis for individualized care.*
12. Provide for safety: bed low, side rails up *to help promote safety.*
13. Begin care as ordered by the physician *because the patient and family will develop a positive attitude about the institution when care is started immediately.*
14. Invite the family back into the room if they left earlier *to decrease family anxiety when they observe the patient is settled.*
15. Wash hands thoroughly *to inhibit the spread of microorganisms.*
16. Record the information on the patient's chart according to hospital policy *to provide information that can also be used by other health professionals. It is the beginning of the permanent record.*

Sample charting

Date	Time	Notes
11/9/94	1445	17-year-old white male admitted per wheelchair accompanied by parents. T—96^{6}, P—78, R—18, BP 128/74. C/O pain in R knee. Limps when walking. Edema noted in R knee. To have right knee surgery in AM. Wallet given to mother. No known allergies. Health history taken and initial assessment completed. Reported to G. Fullor, RN.

(nurse's signature)

SPECIAL CONCERNS

When a patient is admitted in critical condition, only the most pertinent information need be collected immediately. The remaining information may be obtained at a later time.

Children. Admission of an infant or small child requires emotional support for both child and parents. Parents are generally encouraged to stay with their child to prevent separation anxiety The most reliable source of admission information is the parents (see Chapter 43).

Young children are very curious about what is happening to them and the environment around them. Encouraging the child to use equipment on dolls helps reduce anxieties. Children should be encouraged to express how they feel. It is generally best to perform invasive procedures (e.g., obtaining

ADMITTING A PATIENT—CONT'D

blood specimens, starting intravenous lines) in a treatment room so the child can perceive the association that his room is a safe area.

Older children and adolescents are often self-conscious about the changes in their bodies. Be aware of their reservations and provide them with privacy. Trust can be established by asking them the health questions instead of the parents.

Older adults. Older adult patients should be conversed with slowly and clearly, because hearing may be less acute with age. The nurse should face the patient to make lip-reading possible. Older patients should not be rushed; the nurse should wait for the patient to answer rather than letting family members answer. The change in environment and daily routine may cause disorientation, loss of appetite, or reversal of sleeping-waking patterns. Anxiety about hospitalization may interfere with memory.

HOME HEALTH VARIATIONS

A patient requiring care at home may be referred to a **home health agency** (an organization that provides health care in the home). The services may include skilled nursing care or simply assistance with activities of daily living. There must be a physician's order for these services to be reimbursable from insurance or Medicare/Medicaid. A health history and initial assessment are performed, just as in the hospital (see Chapter 48).

NURSING HOME VARIATIONS

Admission to a nursing home may be a transfer from the hospital (see Skill 11-2) or a direct admission. A health history and initial nursing assessment are done to determine the patient's condition. The patient is encouraged to bring clothing and other personal items such as pictures; even personal furniture may be brought to place in the room to give a feeling of familiarity.

Purposes

The nurse performs the accepted procedure for admitting a patient for the following reasons:

- to assist in orienting the patient to the hospital environment
- to obtain information about the patient that will serve as a basis for care *(data base)*
- to begin to establish a therapeutic nurse/patient relationship

SKILL 11-2: TRANSFERRING A PATIENT

Guidelines

The changing condition of a patient, whether improved or more critical, may require **transfer** (moving a patient from one unit to another *[intraagency transfer]* or moving a patient from one health care facility to another *[interagency transfer]*) either to another unit in the hospital or to another health care institution, such as a nursing home or rehabilitation hospital. (See Fig. 11-3 on p. 179 for an example of a patient transfer form for home health.) A patient whose condition becomes critical may be moved to special care areas, such as the ICU or CCU. A patient whose condition improves may be moved from a special care area to a general care area. Other patients may be transferred to a nursing home for continued care at a lower cost. Transfers may also be done at the patient's request; for example, a patient may wish to have a private room or a quieter room.

Transfer combines admission and discharge. The patient is discharged from one unit and received on the new unit, much like an admission. A physician's order may be needed to begin the transfer process. The patient's family should be notified of the transfer. Skill 11-2 gives general steps to follow when transferring a patient.

Purposes

The nurse performs the accepted procedure for transferring a patient for the following reasons:

- to adjust the type and intensity of nursing interventions to the patient's needs
- to situate the patient in the facility best able to provide the care needed
- to accommodate the patient's request for a specific type of room when possible

SKILL 11-2

TRANSFERRING A PATIENT

Nursing action/*Rationale*

1. Wash hands thoroughly *to inhibit the spread of microorganisms.*
2. Check physician's order for transfer *to verify if and when a patient is to be transferred.*
3. Inform the patient and family of the transfer *to reduce the fear of the unknown and strengthen the nurse/patient relationship.*
4. Notify the receiving unit that the patient is being transferred and when to be expected *to allow time to prepare to welcome the new patient and begin care in a courteous, thoughtful, and unhurried manner.*
5. Gather *all* the patient's belongings and necessary care items to accompany the patient *to build trust and prevent loss of items.*
6. Assist in transferring the patient, usually by stretcher or wheelchair, *to ensure patient safety. Condition will determine mode of transportation.*
7. Introduce patient and family to nurses on new unit and to roommate *to establish the beginning of new therapeutic nurse/patient relationship and give a sense of belonging.*
8. Provide a brief summary of medical diagnosis, treatment care plan, and medications. Review medical orders with nurse assuming care. If transfer is to another facility, complete an interagency transfer form *to give personnel on the receiving unit pertinent information for continuing care. Reviewing records together to prevents errors.*
9. Explain equipment, policies, and procedures that are different on the new unit *to give the patient some control and reduce anxiety.*
10. Wash hands thoroughly *to inhibit the spread of microorganisms.*
11. Record condition of patient and means of transfer. The nurse on the new unit should also record an assessment of the patient's condition on arrival because *the chart should reflect all care given and the patient's response to that care while in the hospital.*
12. Notify other hospital departments, such as diagnostic imaging, laboratory, switchboard, dietary, and business offices, of the transfer *to keep records current and avoid errors.*

Sample charting

Date	Time	Notes
1/15/95	1230	Transferred by private care with personal belongings to *(name)* nursing home. Accompanied by son and daughter-in-law. Alert and smiling. Physician's orders and nursing care plan sent.

____

(nurse's signature)

SPECIAL CONCERNS

An interagency transfer may be made by air or ground ambulance or private car. The patient must be dressed or covered appropriately for environmental comfort. If oxygen is required, a small transport tank may be used. A nurse generally accompanies a critically ill patient who is being transferred.

Children. Infants are generally transported in an Isolette that is returned to the sending health care facility. Parents usually accompany their child during transfer unless the transfer is by air ambulance. The parents generally would then follow in family transportation.

HOME HEALTH AND NURSING HOME VARIATIONS

Following agency policies and requirements of **third party payers** (entities [persons or elements] other than the giver or receiver of service responsible for payment, e.g., Medicare or insurance company) is important so that benefits will not be lost.

Home care patients may be either transferred for a few hours to a clinic or outpatient services for diagnostic tests or treatments, or transferred for admission to the hospital or nursing home. (See Fig. 11-3 for an example of a home health transfer form.)

Patient Transfer Form

Patient Transfer Form	Date: 1-31-95	Medical Record No.: 432-612-1111
Patient's Name: Nels Lauritsen — Phone #: 262-1349	Diet on Transfer: Low sodium	Date of Transfer: 1-31-95
Address: 28 West Park, Spenser, Ia	Attending Physician at Time of Transfer: Dr. Fieselman	

Diagnosis:
Primary: myocardial infarction
Secondary: congestive heart failure
All Other Conditions: ______ Allergies: penicillin

Current Medications: (Date andTime Last Dose)

Bumex 1 mgm '0' daily
Lanoxin .25 mgm '0' daily
Colace tabs '0' H.S.
Slow K 10 mEq '0' B.I.D.
Procardia XL 30 mgm '0' B.I.D.
Nitrostat 6.5 mgm '0' daily

Nursing Evaluation

a. Speech	☒ Normal	☐ Impaired	☐ Unable to Speak	
b. Hearing	☐ Normal	☒ Impaired	☐ Deaf	
c. Sight	☐ Normal	☒ Impaired	☐ Blind	
d. Mental Status	☒ Always Alert	☐ Occasionally Confused	☐ Always Confused	
e. Feeding	☒ Independent	☐ Help with Feeding	☐ Cannot Feed Self	
f. Dressing	☒ Independent	☐ Help with Dressing	☐ Cannot Dress Self	
g. Elimination	☐ Independent	☒ Help to Bathroom	☐ Bedpan or Urinal Required	☐ Incontinent
h. Bathing	☐ Independent	☒ Help with Bathing	☐ Bed Bath with Help	☐ Bed Bath
i. Ambulatory Status	☐ Independent	☒ Walks with Assistance	☐ Help from Bed to Chair	☐ Bed Bound

Appliances or Support: walker
up c̄ assistance

Physical Activity: ______

Nursing assessment and Other Pertinent Information: grieving the loss of wife 2 months ago
alert and oriented x3
crackles in right apex
last BM this am - brown semi-formal stool
last set of vitals = 97^8-80-22 $^{100}/_{60}$
Abdomen soft and non distended
pedal pulse +2 bilaterally

Nurse's Signature: Barbara J. Christensen Title: RN MS Date: 1-31-95

FIG. 11-3 Example of home health patient transfer form. (Courtesy Great Plains Regional Medical Center, North Platte, Neb.)

SKILL 11-3: DISCHARGING A PATIENT

Guidelines

As soon as a patient is admitted to a hospital, all members of the health care team begin preparations for **discharge** (release of a patient from a health care facility). Successful **discharge planning** (a set of decisions and activities involved in providing continuity and coordination of nursing care when a patient is discharged from a health care agency) is a centralized, coordinated, multidisciplinary/multidepartmental process that ensures the patient has continuing care after leaving the hospital (Box 11-1). Discharge planning facilitates the transition of the patient from one environment to another. The following goals (levels of outcomes) must be ensured for a patient's successful discharge plan:

1. Patient and family understand the diagnosis, anticipated level of functioning, discharge medications (Fig. 11-4), and anticipated medical follow-up.
2. Specialized instruction or training is provided to the patient and family to ensure **continuity of care** (continuing patient care from one setting to another).
3. Community support systems are coordinated to enable the patient to return home.
4. The relocation of the patient and the coordination of support systems or transfer to another health care facility are performed.

Every patient in a hospital requires discharge planning. There are conditions, however, that place a patient at greater risk for being unable to meet continuing health care needs after discharge (Box 11-2). When a patient has one of these conditions, it is especially important to coordinate referrals to appropriate outside agencies such as a home health care agency or a rehabilitation center.

All care givers who care for a patient with a specific health problem must participate in discharge planning. Development of a plan with mutually accepted goals (outcomes) and ongoing communication about its progress are essential. For example, a patient admitted to the hospital for a major surgical procedure involving the lung will probably require the collaboration of the physician, nurses, respiratory therapists, physical therapists, social workers, and home health care staff. The patient will need pain control, early physical ambulation, aggressive pulmonary therapy, and training for improved exercise tolerance. The patient's smooth transition from hospital to home may not be accomplished if, for example, the nurse's pain control measures are not used before physical therapy, the physician chooses to prescribe bed rest an extra day, or the social worker is not informed of the lack of family support. All care givers

Box 11-1 HEALTH DISCIPLINES USED AS REFERRALS IN DISCHARGE PLANNING

DIETITIAN

- Provides proper nutrient and food source requirements in patients' diets.
- Instructs patients on meal planning and diet restrictions.

SOCIAL WORKER

- Provides counseling for major life crises such as terminal illness and family problems.
- Assists in finding community resources such as equipment for home health care or an agency that will accept patients after discharge from a hospital.
- Assists in finding financial resources to cover medical costs.

PHYSICAL THERAPIST

- Assists in the examination and treatment of physically disabled or handicapped persons.
- Assists in rehabilitating patients and restoring musculoskeletal function to the patients' greatest potential.

OCCUPATIONAL THERAPIST

- Teaches patients to adapt to physical handicaps by learning new vocational skills or activities of daily living.

SPEECH THERAPIST

- Assists patients with disorders affecting normal oral communication.

CLINICAL NURSE SPECIALIST

- Consults with nursing staff on appropriate nursing interventions for complex nursing diagnoses.
- Provides instruction to patients and family members who will assume patient self-care.

HOME HEALTH CARE NURSE

- Provides follow-up discharge visits to a patient's home for the delivery of nursing services.

must work together for a discharge plan to be successful.

At the time of discharge, a review of the medications, diet, activity, and treatments to be continued at home should be conducted with the patient and family. If they cannot manage this care, arrangements should be made for home health care or nursing home care.

Many hospitals have a form with written instructions and teaching documentation for the patient to sign acknowledging understanding of the instructions. These instructions serve as a guide for the patient to use at home (Fig. 11-5 on p. 182).

Sometimes a patient will insist on leaving the hospital without the physician's consent, that is, **against medical advice (AMA).** A special form must be signed

Box 11-2

PATIENT RISK FACTORS FOR DISCHARGE PLANNING

- Lack of knowledge of treatment plan
- Newly diagnosed chronic disease
- Major surgery
- Radical surgery
- Prolonged recuperation from major surgery or illness
- Social isolation
- Emotional or mental instability
- Complex home care regimen
- Lack of financial resources
- Lack of available or approximate referral sources
- Terminal illness

MEDICAL INFORMATION

Medical Conditions: CHF and Hypertension

My Doctor(s): Dr. J. Bernard-Stevens

Allergies: Darvon

Pharmacy or Pharmacist: James Manning

GPR
Great Plains Regional Medical Center
Box 1167-601 West Leota
North Platte, Nebraska 69101
308-534-9310

MEDICATION RECORD

Mable Lauritsen
Name

28 West Park
Address (street)

Spencer,	Iowa	59101
City	State	Zip

8-28-1904
My Birth Date

262 lbs	5' - 4"
My Weight	My Height

	MEDICATION (Prescription & Over-the-Counter)	FOR WHAT CONDITION	DOSAGE	WHEN & HOW TO TAKE
1)	Lasix	CHF	40 mgm	by mouth every AM
2)	Lanoxin	CHF	.125 mgm	by mouth every AM
3)	Micro K	CHF	8 mEq.	by mouth twice a day
4)	Metamucil	constipation	ī Tbs.	at bed time
5)	Mycalog	leg ulcers	topical	apply to lesions daily
6)				
7)				
8)				
9)				
10)				
11)				
12)				

FIG. 11-4 Example of a medical record. (Courtesy Great Plains Regional Center, North Platte, Neb.)

GPR
Great Plains Regional Medical Center
Box 1167-601 West Leota
North Platte, Nebraska 69101
308-534-9310

Name Marjorie Oden Allergies no known allergies

1. Diet: Regular ____ Soft X Liquid ____ Special Instructions: ____

2. Activity: Walking X Rest X Lifting 10 lbs Driving No
Work ____ Other ____

3. Bowels: Laxative of choice

4. Bathing: Shower X Tub No Sponge —

5. Wound Care: Incision care ____
Dressing change ____
Special instructions leave steri strips in place on abdomen until physicians' visit

6. Tubes, drains, heplock, appliances: Special instructions ____

Heparin lock patient instruction sheet given: yes ____
Physician's instruction sheet given: yes ____

7. Medications:

Drug	Dose	Frequency	Route	Special Instructions
Keflex	250 mgm	three times daily	by mouth	take with food or milk
Darvocet N100	tabs 1	every 4 hours	by mouth	as needed for pain control
Colace	caps 2	daily	by mouth	hours of sleep
Halcion	.125 mgm	daily	by mouth	as needed for sleep

8. Other instructions: Call physician if any reddness of incision or temperature greater than 100°

9. Office visit: Call for an appointment on 12-6-94 @ 2 pm (date)
Doctor A. Yocum Address 1402 Iowa Avenue Phone number 308-2890

Instructions received and understood,
Patient or Responsible party Marjorie Oden
Signature Relationship

Nurse Signature Elaine Kockrow, RN MS Date 12-6-94

DISMISSAL INSTRUCTION SHEET

FIG. 11-5 Example of discharge instructions. (Courtesy Great Plains Regional Medical Center, North Platte, Neb.)

DISCHARGING A PATIENT

Nursing action/*Rationale*

1. Wash hands thoroughly *to inhibit the spread of microoganisms.*
2. Make certain there is a written discharge order *to verify physician's decision regarding time for the patient to be discharged.*
3. If no discharge order has been written, have patient sign AMA form *because generally patients cannot be held against their wishes.* The patient's signature acknowledges full responsibility for what happens after leaving.
4. Notify the family or person who will be transporting the patient home *to avoid delay in discharge.*
5. Verify that the patient and family understand the instructions for care—medications, special diet, exercise—*to help ensure appropriate home care.*
6. Gather equipment, supplies, and prescriptions that the patient is to take home *to provide service patient is unable to do.*
7. Check to see that business office has given a release *to prevent undue waiting for the patient when leaving.*
8. Assist the patient in dressing and packing items to go home *to conserve patient's strength.*
9. Check clothing and valuables list made on admission according to policy *to avoid patient leaving personal items at facility.*
10. Transfer the patient and belongings via wheelchair to the vehicle. Assist patient into the vehicle if needed *to provide patient safety and comply with policy of most hospitals.*
11. Wash hands thoroughly *to inhibit spread of microorganisms.*
12. Chart entire discharge procedure *to document teaching, patient's condition, and method of discharge so as to complete the record. Legally this is important and may prevent problems in the future.*

Sample charting

Date	Time	Notes
11/14/94	1300	Diet and activity instructions reviewed. Copy of instructions and prescription for Tylenol #3 given to mother. Mother can state name, dosage, frequency to give, desired and unexpected effects of Tylenol #3. Given appointment card to see Dr. Smith. Dismissed by wheelchair to parent's car.

____
(nurse's signiature)

SPECIAL CONCERNS

Children. The parents must be included in all aspects of teaching and the entire discharge procedure for children. Some hospitals have a special form to be signed by the person legally responsible for taking the child away from the facility.

AMA. If the patient is leaving without a physician's discharge order, the appropriate forms must be signed and the physician notified (Fig. 11-6 on p. 184)

HOME HEALTH VARIATIONS

Discharge from a home health agency involves the same kind of teaching as from the hospital. The nurse must be sure the patient or family can provide any care still needed. Since the patient is al ready home, it is the nurse who must gather any equipment and supplies to be returned to the agency.

NURSING HOME VARIATIONS

Discharge from a nursing home is essentially the same as from a hospital. There will be more personal belongings to gather and pack.

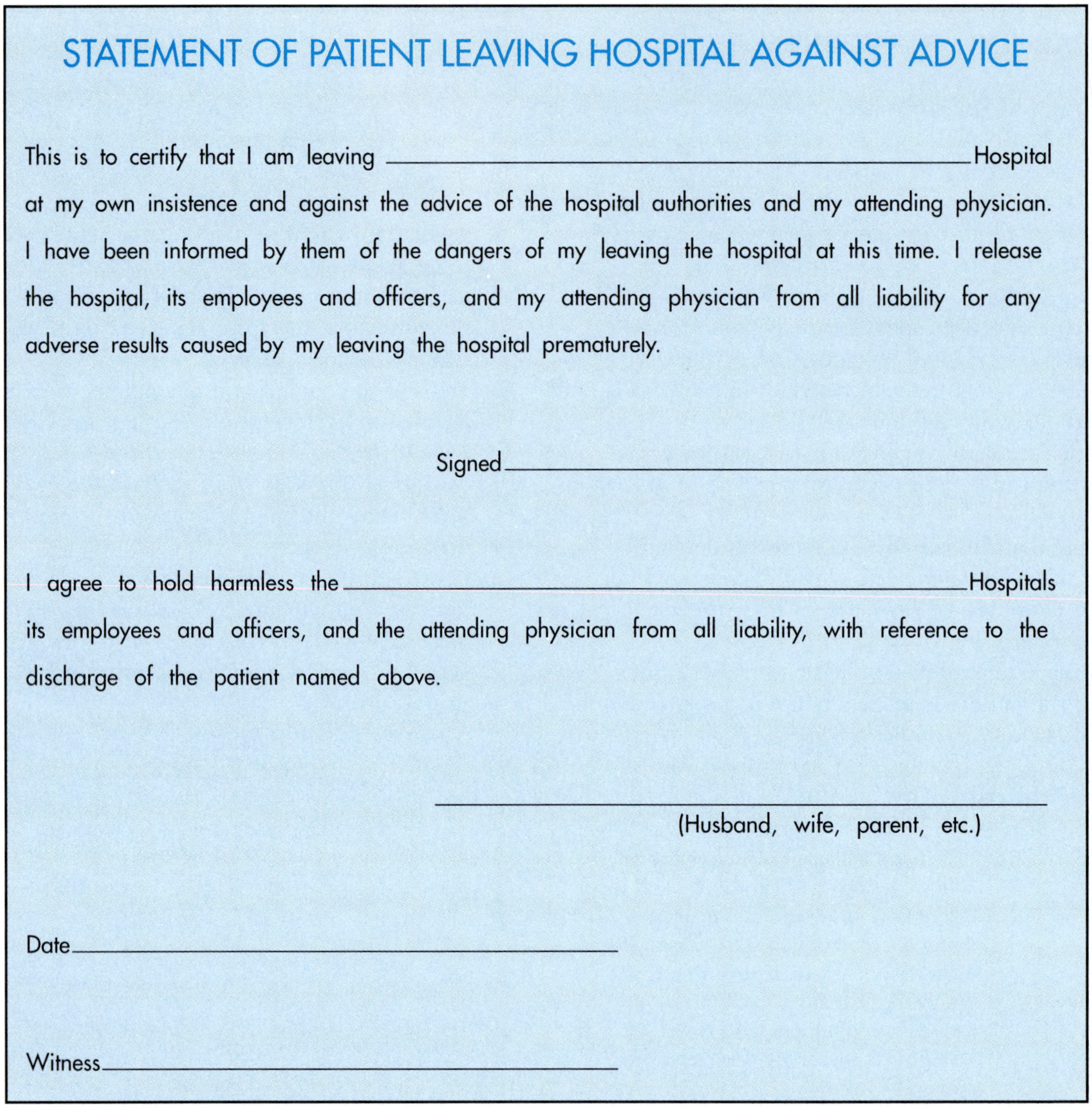

STATEMENT OF PATIENT LEAVING HOSPITAL AGAINST ADVICE

This is to certify that I am leaving ______________________________ Hospital at my own insistence and against the advice of the hospital authorities and my attending physician. I have been informed by them of the dangers of my leaving the hospital at this time. I release the hospital, its employees and officers, and my attending physician from all liability for any adverse results caused by my leaving the hospital prematurely.

Signed ______________________________

I agree to hold harmless the ______________________________ Hospitals its employees and officers, and the attending physician from all liability, with reference to the discharge of the patient named above.

____
(Husband, wife, parent, etc.)

Date ______________________________

Witness ______________________________

FIG. 11-6 Example of form used when patient leaves hospital against physician's advice. (Courtesy Great Plains Regional Center, North Platte, Neb.)

by the patient in which the patient acknowledges leaving without the physician's discharge order and that the physician, hospital, and hospital personnel will not be responsible for any problems that might occur because of this action.

A rational adult patient who will not sign the form cannot be forcibly detained. Only if a court order was issued for the admission, as in some cases of mental illness, can a patient be detained forcibly. A lawsuit for false imprisonment could be filed against the hospital and/or personnel for keeping patients against personal wishes. Documentation of the refusal to sign the form and the information given about the risks of leaving should be made in the patient's chart.

Skill 11-3 outlines the steps for discharging a patient.

Nurse's Role in Discharge Planning

The nursing process (see Chapter 5) is a systematic, purposeful method of helping patients regain, maintain, or promote health. Often the first health care provider to encounter a patient, the nurse must ensure that an organized approach to care begins immediately. Application of the nursing process ensures effective discharge planning. *Assessment* of patient's health care problems and responses to those problems, identification of specific problems *(nursing diagnoses [ndxs])* requiring intervention, development of a *plan* to eliminate or modify problems, provision of appropriate interventions *(implementation),* and *evaluation* of interventions are the nursing process. If any step is incorrectly performed, discharge will not go smoothly.

Nurses in different health care facilities conduct the discharge planning process differently. When the delivery-of-care system is primary nursing, a single nurse is responsible for coordinating care from admission to discharge. This primary nurse would then make a follow-up telephone call a day or two after discharge to discuss progress and/or problems.

Many hospitals also have discharge planning rounds on nursing divisions. During rounds, various members of the health care team discuss the status of each patient with respect to potential discharge. Rounds allow members of all disciplines (departments) to interact and discuss the best treatment options for each patient.

In some hospitals, nurses assume the role of case manager. The role builds on the accountability practiced in primary nursing. The case manager is responsible for specific patient goals/expected outcomes. Care expected to be delivered by various disciplines (departments) throughout a hospital is planned and managed through formal case management plans.

Referrals for Health Care Services

Often a patient will require the services of various disciplines (departments) within a hospital, such as dietary, social work, or physical therapy. The nurse is often the first to recognize the patient's needs. For example, a patient may have had a poor appetite for several days and reveals to the nurse a dislike for many of the food choices on the menu. A referral to a dietitian could result in identifying food preferences appropriate to the patient's diet. It is important to remember that other health professionals specialize in skills and knowledge that give a patient services that the nurse cannot offer. Referrals should be made as soon as possible after the patient's need is identified.

In many agencies a physician's order is needed for a referral, especially when specific therapies are planned (for example, physical therapy). It is ideal to have patients participate in referral processes so that they are involved in decision making. If patients fail to understand the purpose of referrals, they may refuse proposed treatment measures. Box 11-1 summarizes the role that various disciplines (departments) can play in a treatment plan.

When multiple referrals are made for a patient's plan of care, the nurse coordinates referral activities. Often it is necessary to have different therapists work together so that a patient's care is uninterrupted. For example, there may be certain times in the day when a patient can better tolerate physical therapy or is most receptive to instruction. The nurse attempts to plan referral activities at these times.

Purposes

The nurse performs the accepted procedure for discharging a patient for the following reasons:

- to assist the patient in making the change from the hospital environment to the home environment
- to provide for continuity of care at home so that the patient can return to the best state of wellness possible

REFERENCES AND SUGGESTED READINGS

1. Anderson BW, Ross JM: Smoothing the transition home, *Clin Manage* 12(5):46, 1992.
2. Dellasega C, Shellenbarger T: Discharge planning for cognitively impaired, *Nurs Health Care* 13(10):526, 1992.
3. Frederick C, Holter AN: Discharge planning for the head injured patient, *Crit Care Nurse* 11(6):42, 1991.
4. Herking Kruse D: Interhospital transfers: how to prepare your patient, *Nursing* 21(2):41, 1991.
5. Hood GH, Dincher JR: *Total patient care,* ed 8, St Louis, 1992, Mosby.
6. Joint Commission on Accreditation of Healthcare Organizations: *Manual of hospital accreditation: 1992 standards,* Chicago, 1992, The Commission.
7. Long BC, Phipps WJ, Cassmeyer VL: *Medical-surgical nursing: a nursing process approach,* ed 3, St Louis, 1993, Mosby.
8. Maslow AH: *Motivation and personality,* New York, 1954, Harper & Row.
9. *Mosby's medical, nursing, and allied health dictionary,* ed 4, St Louis, 1994, Mosby.
10. Naylor MD: Comprehensive discharge planning for hospitalized elderly: a pilot study, *Nurs Res* 39(3):156, 1990.
11. Perry A, Potter P: *Clinical nursing skills,* ed 3, St Louis, 1994, Mosby.
12. Phipps WJ, Long BC, Woods FN et al: *Medical-surgical nursing concepts and clinical practice,* ed 4, St Louis, 1991, Mosby.
13. Portnoff Geer M: Top 25 discharge drugs, *Nursing* 21(6):53, 1991.
14. Potter P, Perry A: *Fundamentals in nursing: concepts process and practice,* ed 3, St Louis, 1993, Mosby.
15. Prescott T: We get an early start on AM admits, *RN* 53(8):21, 1990.
16. Rarden JW, Taft ED: *Discharge planning guide for nurses,* Philadelphia, 1990, Saunders.
17. Timby BK, Lewis LW: *Fundamental skills and concepts in patient care,* ed 5, Philadelphia, 1992, Lippincott.
18. Tisk JE: Determining discharge priorities: how to prepare your patient for early discharge and on-going care at home, *Nursing* 22(7):55, 1992.

CHAPTER CHALLENGE

KEY POINTS

- Admission into a hospital begins with making certain that the patient is knowledgeable about routine procedures and activities that will occur during the hospital stay.
- The patient has the right to be treated with dignity, courtesy, and respect.
- The nurse's attitude often influences the patient's feelings about the care received.
- Common reactions to hospitalization are fear of the unknown, loss of identity, disorientation, separation anxiety, and loneliness.
- An adult patient should always be addressed as Miss, Ms., Mrs., or Mr. (last name), unless the patient grants permission to do otherwise.
- Transfers may be intraagency (patient is discharged from one unit and received on the new unit, much like an admission).
- Transfers may also be interagency (patient leaving one health care facility to enter another health care facility).
- Coordination is the key to the efficient and safe transfer of a patient.
- Discharge planning begins when a patient is admitted to a hospital.
- A medical condition may place a patient at risk for needing thorough discharge planning.
- Nurses may find it necessary to involve other health care providers in discharge planning when it becomes apparent that the expertise of those providers is needed.
- Every patient in the hospital requires discharge planning.
- Successful discharge planning is a centralized, coordinated, multidisciplinary process that ensures the patient has a plan for continuing care after leaving the hospital.
- The ultimate goal of discharge planning is to give patients/families the knowledge, skills, and resources needed to assume self-care/patient care after discharge.
- When the patient is leaving without a physician's discharge order, the appropriate forms must be signed and the physician notified.
- Generally, a person may not be kept in a health care facility against his will.

STUDY QUESTIONS

1. Mr. Aspinal, a 65-year-old rancher, is being admitted to the surgical unit in preparation for a bowel resection the following morning. As his nurse you remember that an admission to a health care facility may cause a person to feel a loss of identity. This reflects which of Maslow's needs?
   1. safety
   2. esteem
   3. self-actualization
   4. belongingness and love
2. Mrs. Burke, a 36-year-old schoolteacher, is being admitted for observation and various diagnostic tests. As her nurse you remember the initial action in her admission process is to:
   1. introduce self and roommates
   2. measure vital signs
   3. help her get undressed and into bed
   4. notify the physician
3. Mr. Nelson, a 90-year-old great-grandfather, has been hospitalized with pneumonia. You find it necessary to reorient him to his surroundings periodically throughout your 8-hour shift. As the nurse assisting him with his AM care, you remember that to call an older male patient "Gramps" is:
   1. just fine if he has grandchildren
   2. acceptable if you cannot remember his name
   3. acceptable if you feel comfortable calling him Gramps
   4. Never appropriate
4. Mrs. Kucera has been transferred out of the ICU to a medical unit. You have been assigned to complete the transfer. This type of transfer is called a(n):
   1. patient-initiated transfer
   2. interagency transfer
   3. business office transfer
   4. intraagency transfer
5. Mr. Dowhower, 52 years old, is being transferred to the surgical unit from the recovery room following extensive surgery as the result of trauma from an automobile accident. As the nurse assigned to complete his care you are knowledgeable that an important principle to remember when admitting, transferring, or discharging a patient is that:
   1. the patient is a human being deserving dignity, courtesy, and respect
   2. the patient is ill and unable to make decisions or give accurate information
   3. the nurse knows best and should tell the patient what to do
   4. families get in the way and should be encouraged not to get involved in the patient's care

6. Mrs. Beal, 45 years old, has been recently diagnosed and hospitalized for type I diabetes mellitus. The multidisciplinary health care team has been preparing her for dismissal. The nurse knows the purpose of discharge planning is to:
   1. make certain she takes her medication as prescribed
   2. provide medical treatment
   3. provide on going patient education
   4. ensure continuity of care
7. Mr. Peterson, 84 years old, has been hospitalized for six days with a diagnosis of a cerebral vascular accident (stroke). The nurse knows planning for Mr. Peterson's dismissal should begin:
   1. when his condition has stabilized
   2. upon his admission to the hospital
   3. when he begins to ask questions
   4. when his family asks for information
8. Mr. Yoshida is determined to leave the hospital. His physician is not aware of his intent to leave nor is it within his best interest to be dismissed at this time. The nurse recalls when a patient chooses to leave a health care facility without a physician's written order, she should:
   1. call the family so they can expect the patient at home
   2. allow the patient to leave because no one can be held against her will
   3. call security because there must be a physician's order before a patient may leave
   4. explain the risks of leaving and have the patient sign a paper accepting responsibility for problems that may occur

12

MEDICAL ASEPSIS AND INFECTION CONTROL

Annabelle Sitler
Elaine Kockrow

KEY TERMS

asepsis
body substance isolation (BSI)
carrier
Centers for Disease Control and Prevention (CDC)
contamination
disinfection
double bagging
endogenous
exogenous
fomite
host
isolation precautions
medical asepsis
microorganism
nosocomial infection
reservoir
spore
sterilization
surgical asepsis
universal precautions
vehicle
virulent

LEARNING OBJECTIVES

After reading this chapter, the student should be able to do the following:

- Define the key terms.
- Explain the difference between medical and surgical asepsis.
- Explain how each element of the chain of infection contributes to infection.
- List five major classifications of pathogens.
- Differentiate between *Staphylococcus aureus* and *Staphylococcus epidermidis* regarding virulence.
- Discuss nursing interventions used to interrupt the sequence in the infection process.
- Explain conditions that promote the onset of nosocomial infections.
- Discuss examples for preventing infection for each element in the chain of infection.
- Demonstrate the appropriate procedure for 2-minute handwashing.
- Discuss universal precautions.
- Discuss body substance isolation.
- Discuss category-specific isolation practices.
- Demonstrate appropriate gowning and gloving techniques.
- Demonstrate the appropriate method for double bagging contaminated articles.
- Describe the accepted techniques of preparation for disinfection and sterilization.
- Discuss patient teaching for infection control.

RELATED TOPICS OF INTEREST

- Communication (Chapter 4)
- Signs, symptoms, and physical assessment (Chapter 9)
- Hygiene and care of the patient's environment (Chapter 16)
- Specimen collection and diagnostic examination (Chapter 17)
- Care of the patient with an immune disorder (Chapter 36)

With research and the discovery that microorganisms cause infection came the realization that somehow their growth and reproduction must be inhibited or stopped to prevent infection. Although many scientists, researchers, and doctors contributed to the progress made in aseptic technique, Joseph Lister (1827-1912) is known as the father of aseptic technique.

Lister's method of aseptic technique helped reduce morbidity and mortality from surgery and wound care. These methods are still used in asepsis today.

ASEPSIS

There is a great societal concern regarding the increase of transmissible infections, not only in health care institutions but also in the home. **Microorganisms** (any tiny, usually microscopic, entity capable of carrying on living processes) are naturally present on and in the human body, as well as in the environment. Many of these microorganisms are harmless (nonpathogenic) and do not produce disease in most individuals; some are even helpful. However, if an individual is highly susceptible to infection, the nonpathogenic microorganisms could be dangerous. There are also known microorganisms (pathogens) that do cause specific diseases or infections.

Infection control is routine in whatever action a nurse performs. Any patient entering a health care facility because of lowered resistance, increased exposure to numbers and types of disease-causing organisms, or the need for an invasive procedure is at a greater risk of developing an infection. The nurse's knowledge of infection, application of infection control principles, and use of common sense help protect patients from infection. Control of infection is an important part of every action the nurse performs. In many situations nurses are exposed to pathogenic microorganisms and should use both specialized and routine practices of cleanliness and disinfection to prevent the spread of infection. These techniques aid in accomplishing **asepsis,** or freedom from pathogenic microorganisms. Asepsis is divided into the following two categories:

1. **Medical asepsis** consists of techniques that inhibit the growth and spread of pathogenic microorganisms. Medical asepsis is also known as *clean technique* and is used in many daily activities, such as handwashing and changing the patients' bed linen daily. Principles of medical asepsis are commonly followed in the home, as in the case of washing hands before preparing food.
2. **Surgical asepsis** destroys all microorganisms and their **spores** (the reproductive cell of some microorganisms (for example, fungi or protozoa). Surgical asepsis is known as *sterile technique* and is used in specialized areas or skills, such as care of surgical wounds, urinary catheter insertion, invasive procedures, and surgery.

INFECTION PROCESS

For a microorganism to be transported and be effective in continuing contamination, it follows a definite cycle or chain and must have the following six elements (Fig. 12-1 on p. 190):

1. The infectious agent—a pathogen
2. Reservoir—where the pathogen can grow
3. Exit from reservoir
4. Method of transportation, such as exudate, feces, air droplets, hands, and needles
5. Entrance through skin, mucous lining, or mouth
6. Host—another person or animal

For the prevention of the spread of a microorganism, the cycle must be interrupted. This is accomplished through daily practices of medical asepsis. These practices help to inhibit (to stop or slow a process) the growth and reduce the number of microorganisms, especially pathogens.

Infectious Agent

Bacteria. The study of bacteria has shown that they have many different characteristics. In addition to the three basic shapes—round, oblong, and spiral—there are many variations of these shapes. Some may be elongated or have pointed ends, or they may be flattened on one side. Some are shaped like a comma, and others may appear square. Spirilla may be tightly coiled like a corkscrew. During cell division some bacteria remain together to form pairs, whereas others may form long chains. All these modifications are important in identifying specific kinds of bacteria.

Bacteria may also have different chemical compositions, require different nutrients, and form different waste products. Aerobic bacteria grow only in the presence of oxygen, whereas anaerobic bacteria grow only in the absence of oxygen. Some bacteria are capable of movement. Their motility is possible because of fine, hairlike projections—flagella—that arise from the bacterial cell. These projections cause a wavelike motion that moves the cell. A bacterium may have only one flagellum attached to one end of the cell, or there may be many flagella surrounding the cell. Locomotion of the spirochete is achieved by a wiggling motion involving the entire cell body.

Some bacteria form a specialized structure called a spore. Spore formation appears to occur when conditions are unfavorable for growth of the bacterium. The spore is a round body that is formed by the bacterium in the presence or absence of oxygen. The spore enlarges until it is as large as the bacterial cell and is surrounded by a capsule. Eventually the portion of the cell surrounding the spore disintegrates. The spore remains dormant until environmental conditions become favorable for growth. At that time the spore will germinate and begin reproducing in a normal manner. Characteris-

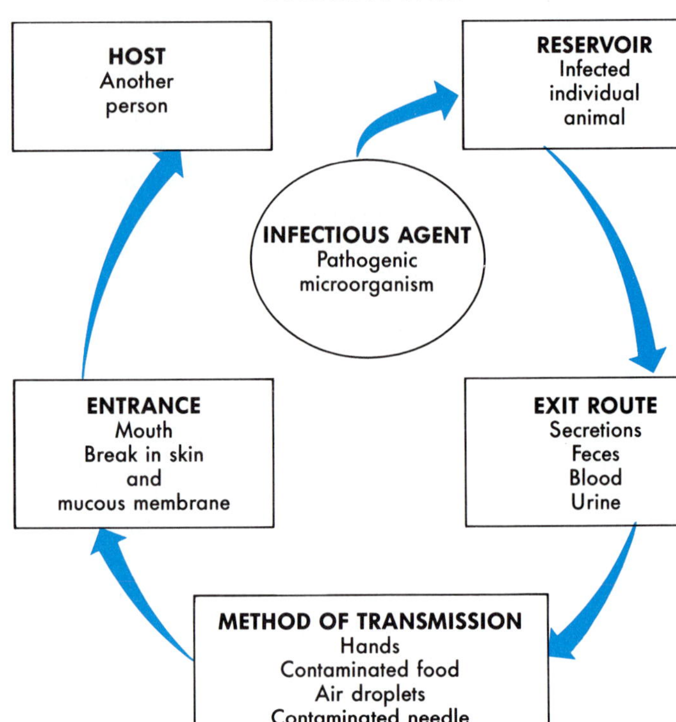

FIG. 12-1 The chain of infection.

tically, spores have a high degree of resistance to heat and disinfectants. They cannot be stained by the usual laboratory methods but require special staining techniques.

Some bacteria have the ability to form capsules about the cell wall. These mucilaginous (thick, sticky, slimy substance) envelopes seem to form when the bacterial environment is unfavorable; it is also believed that the formation may be defensive to protect the bacteria. The composition of the capsules varies with the species of bacteria. However, they may be composed of protein or fat substances, and some may contain nitrogen and phosphorus. As with spores, staining in the laboratory may require special procedures. When capsules are present, antibiotic therapy may be ineffective because the capsule may prevent the drug from reaching the bacteria within the capsule.

Many diseases cannot be diagnosed and properly treated until the specific microorganism causing the illness has been identified. Identification of microorganisms is made by specially trained laboratory personnel. Most bacteria cannot be seen until a special staining process has been done. In some instances examination may be done before staining, but this is usually less satisfactory. Staining is accomplished by the use of a dye applied to a specially prepared glass slide containing a small amount of the material to be examined. Most bacteria can be identified by this simple process; however, other bacteria require additional staining. Depending on whether a color can be removed by a solvent or is retained after the use of the solvent, the organism is identified as being gram positive or gram negative. This identification is important in the treatment of the patient. This is a simple laboratory test that will assist in the selection of effective antibiotics. Different antibiotics may be required for their destruction. Some bacteria are known as acid-fast bacteria, depending on the staining process. Special staining is required for bacteria having flagella, spores, or capsules (Fig. 12-2).

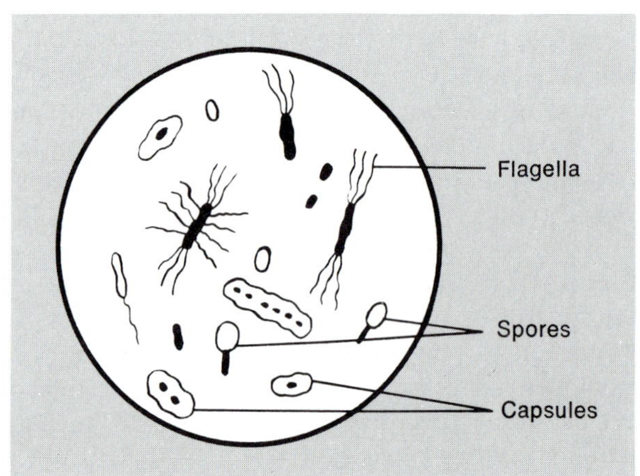

FIG. 12-2 Flagella, spores, and capsules.

Body fluids and secretions suspected of containing pathogenic organisms can be collected in sterile containers and sent to the laboratory for culture and sensitivity tests. In the laboratory the collected specimens are transferred to a special culture medium that promotes growth. The culture is then studied, and the pathogens are identified. Sensitivity tests are carried out to deter-

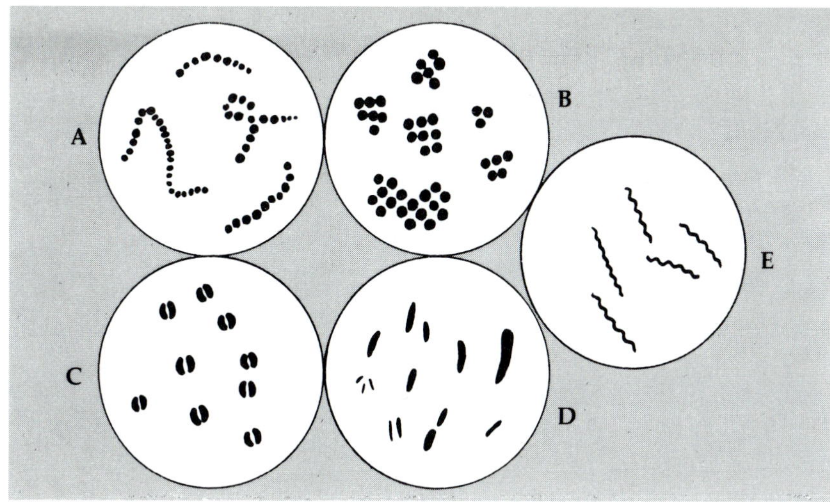

FIG. 12-3 Some common disease-producing bacteria: **A,** Streptococci; **B,** Staphylococci; **C,** Diplococci; **D,** Bacilli; **E,** Spirilla.

mine which antibiotics will effectively inhibit the pathogens' growth. Appropriate antibiotics are ordered on the basis of these tests.

Bacterial infections are transmitted from person to person by direct contact, by inhaling droplet nuclei, and by indirect contact with articles contaminated with the pathogen. Some are also transmitted through the ingestion of contaminated food and drink.

Bacteria have been divided into three major groups: (1) cocci, (2) bacilli, and (3) spirilla. In addition, the Rickettsiae are now classified as bacteria (Fig. 12-3).

Streptococci, staphylococci, and diplococci. The streptococcus bacterium is responsible for more diseases than is any other organism. Some strains produce serious or even fatal diseases; other strains produce disease only under special conditions; and other strains are nonpathogenic. Disease-producing strains include β-hemolytic streptococci and the viridans groups, also called α-hemolytic streptococci.

The β-hemolytic group of streptococci is responsible for about 90% of streptococcal infections. Some of the diseases caused by this group are extremely serious and may be fatal. They include osteomyelitis, septicemia, scarlet fever, rheumatic fever, and pneumonia, as well as relatively common diseases like tonsillitis and impetigo. The organisms may also invade surgical wounds or malignant lesions. Wound infection may occur as the result of improper handwashing before changing dressings. The organisms live in the upper respiratory tract and may be spread from one person to another by direct or indirect contact.

Viridans streptococci may cause subacute bacterial endocarditis, in which the valves of the heart may be affected. Viridans streptococci may also be found in the nose and throat of well persons.

There are two primary species of *Staphylococcus* bacteria: *Staphylococcus aureus* and *Staphylococcus epidermidis. S. aureus* belongs to the pyogenic (pus-producing) group. Staphylococci may be found on the skin at all times and cause boils, abscesses, and carbuncles. Sometimes they get into the bloodstream and cause serious complications (see Chapter 25).

S. epidermidis is a nonpathogenic species of the *Staphylococcus* organism that inhabits the human skin. Although this species may cause minor infections, the incidence of such infections is low.

There are several kinds of diplococcus bacteria. One type causes pneumonia and was previously called the *pneumococcus;* it is now called *Streptococcus pneumoniae.* One characteristic of this organism is that it is encased in a capsule, or gelatinous envelope. Two other forms of diplococci cause gonorrhea (gonococcus) and meningitis (meningococcus).

Bacilli. The name *bacillius* means "little rod"; however, its rodlike shape is extremely variable. Certain forms of the bacillus produce spores. These forms are present in the intestinal tract of humans and animals and are discharged onto the soil. These spore-forming bacilli produce tetanus, gas gangrene, and anthrax. Numerous other diseases are caused by these organisms, including tuberculosis, diphtheria, pertussis, typhoid fever, and bacillary dysentery.

Spirilla. Spirilla organisms are spiral shaped, like a corkscrew. Some forms of spirilla are rigid, whereas others are flexible. One form, which resembles a comma, is the cause of Asiatic cholera. Most of the diseases caused by the spirilla bacteria are uncommon. The spirochetes that cause syphilis are spiral shaped, but they have been separated and classed in a different order of bacteria.

Rickettsiae. Rickettsiae are microorganisms now classified as bacteria. They are parasites (an organism living in or on and obtaining nourishment from another organism) that flourish only within living susceptible cells. The cells provide a suitable environment and the nutrients needed for parasite growth. The most serious diseases caused by rickettsiae are typhus fever and Rocky Mountain spotted fever. Typhus fever is spread from person to person through bites from infected body lice or fleas from rats. Epidemic typhus is an acute, severe disease associated with overcrowding, famine, and filth. It has caused devastating epidemics, responsible for the deaths of millions of persons over the past centuries. Although it is rare, cases can be found in the southern United States bordering Mexico.

Rocky Mountain spotted fever has been found in almost every area of the United States, and its prevalence seems to be increasing. It is transmitted to humans through the bite of an infected tick. Several varieties of ticks carry the disease. The ticks live on many different kinds of animals found in rural and wooded areas. They may also live on common house pets, such as cats and dogs. Persons working in areas where ticks are known to be abundant are more likely to become infected. The tick attaches itself to the skin, and the longer it remains attached to the skin, the more likely the person is to become infected. In removing the tick from the skin, great care should be taken not to crush or squeeze it.

Signs and symptoms of Rocky Mountain spotted fever and typhus fever are similar; in both diseases patients are usually extremely ill. Preventive vaccines are available for both diseases, and persons going into areas where the diseases are known to exist should avail themselves of the preventive vaccines.

Viruses. Viruses are the smallest known agents that cause disease. They are not complete cells, but consist of a protein coat around a nucleic acid core and depend on the metabolic processes of the cell they enter. Before 1900, scientists discovered that certain agents, unlike bacteria, would pass through a laboratory filter. In addition, they were unable to observe these tiny bodies with the ordinary microscope. In 1898 Martinus W. Beijerinck called these small bodies viruses, and they became known as filterable viruses.

For years scientists knew little about viruses, even though they were able to observe their effect on humans and animals. In 1941 the electron microscope became available, and a whole new era in the study of human disease was opened. With this advancement the science of virology was born. In addition the use of certain dyes that become luminous when exposed to ultraviolet light (fluorescent microscopy), tissue culture methods, ultracentrifuge, cytochemistry, and the development of other technical laboratory aids have resulted in rapid advances in the study of viruses.

A virus may gain entrance to the body through the respiratory tract, the gastrointestinal tract, or the broken skin resulting from an animal bite, or it may be injected by a mosquito or hypodermic needle. Viruses are selective in the type of body cells they attack, but once they have found cells showing affinity, they enter the cell and reproduce rapidly. As they multiply, they interrupt the cell activities and use the cell material to produce new virus material.

Viral infections are usually self-limiting. They run a given course, and recovery usually occurs. One exception is rabies, which is almost always fatal. Another exception is acquired immunodeficiency syndrome (AIDS), which is the most severe disease state observed to date of a continuum of illnesses related to infection by the human immunodeficiency virus (HIV) (see Chapter 37). Other viral diseases may be fatal if complications occur or if they attack extremely weak, elderly, or debilitated persons. The common cold is caused by a virus, and the aching feeling, fever, and chilling sensations may be relieved by staying in bed and taking certain medicines. No medicine will cure the cold; medicine only relieves the discomfort. In nearly all viral diseases, antibiotics and sulfonamide agents do not alter the course of the disease.

Viruses are classified in various ways. They can be classified according to the human diseases they cause or by the characteristics of a specific group. In the latter classification system, each subgroup may have many types or strains.

Fungi. The fungal (mycotic) infections are among the most common diseases found in humans. Fungi belong to the plant kingdom, and although many of them are harmless, some are responsible for infections. Types of fungi that are familiar to everyone include the fuzzy, black, green, or white growth on stale bread, decayed fruit, or damp clothing. Fungi are among the most plentiful forms of life. Mycotic infections are diseases caused by yeasts and molds. They may be superficial, involving the skin and mucous membranes. The most frequently involved areas include the external layers of the skin, hair, and nails. These infections are commonly referred to as ringworm (dermatomycosis). The most frequent site in children is the scalp. The condition is considered infectious, and the child may not be permitted to attend school until the infection has been cured. Other sites include men's beards (barber's itch) and the feet (athlete's foot). The infection may also occur on other parts of the body, frequently about the nails. Domestic pets may also have ringworm infection and are frequently the source of infection for humans (see Chapter 25).

Fungi also invade the deeper tissues of the body. Most of these infections produce no signs or symptoms; however, some become serious and may be fatal. Those most common in the United States are coccidioidomycosis (valley fever) and histoplasmosis.

1. *Coccidioidomycosis* was discovered in southern California, although the disease is found in other areas of the Southwest where the climate is hot and dry. The disease affects the lungs and is believed to be contracted by inhaling the spores in soil, which are blown about in the wind.

2. *Histoplasmosis* also affects the lungs. This disease is widespread throughout the world; in some areas 80% of the population may be infected. The disease occurs as the result of inhaling spores present in the soil, and there is also a possibility that ingestion of the spores may cause the disease. Histoplasmosis has often been associated with various kinds of birds; however, it is now believed that the only relationship is that bird droppings enrich the soil, providing fertile media in which the fungi may proliferate.
3. *Candida albicans* may cause superficial or systemic infections. This fungus is a normal inhabitant of the gastrointestinal tract, the mouth, and the vagina. An infection develops when something, such as change in pH, interferes with the balance of the normal flora, allowing the organism to grow. This change in balance can occur as a result of antibiotic therapy.

Protozoa. The protozoa are single-celled animals existing everywhere in nature in some form. Some of the parasitic forms of protozoa are found in the intestinal tract, genitourinary tract, respiratory tract, and circulatory system of humans and animals. The disease-producing protozoa are responsible for malaria, amebic dysentery, and African sleeping sickness. In 1981 pneumonia caused by *Pneumocystis carinii,* which is a protozoan, was the first opportunistic infection reported in AIDS. It remains a serious, life-threatening infection in AIDS. Another form of protozoa causes vaginal trichomoniasis in women, often as a complication of pregnancy. It may also live in the male urethra and may be acquired or transmitted through coitus. Of the diseases caused by protozoa, the three of importance in the United States are *P. carinii* pneumonia, malaria, and amebic dysentery. The last is more prevalent where sanitation is poor and personal hygiene neglected. The source of infection can be the excreta of convalescent patients or carriers, and the disease is transmitted by food handlers, contaminated food, or contaminated water supplies. The common housefly may be an intermediary vector by transmitting the organism to food.

The malaria protozoan is transmitted to humans through the bite of the female *Anopheles* mosquito. Malaria is a worldwide health problem and is one of the most serious handicaps to the development of many countries.

Pathogenic microorganisms are infectious agents. These pathogens could be bacteria, viruses, yeasts, fungi, or protozoa. All these microorganisms require food for growth and the proper environment in which to live. Areas such as unwashed hands, wound dressings, soiled linen, or oral cavities are ideal for pathogenic growth. The strength of the microorganism, the number of microorganisms present, the effectiveness of a person's immune system, and the length of exposure to the microorganisms determine a pathogen's ability to produce disease. It is important for the nurse to provide a safe environment for a patient. This can be accomplished by handwashing, donning gloves, use of disinfectants, and sterilization techniques.

Reservoir

Any natural habitat of a microorganism that promotes growth and reproduction is a **reservoir.** There are different microorganisms found in many areas of the body, but the presence of these microorganisms does not always cause illness.

Examples of a reservoir are soiled or wet dressings; hospital equipment, such as a bedside stand, overbed table, suction equipment, or urinary drainage bags; and a carrier. A **carrier** is a person or animal who harbors and spreads an organism causing disease in others but who does not become ill.

To thrive, organisms require food and a proper atmosphere. Characteristics of an environment that supports organism growth include food, oxygen, water, temperature, pH, and light.

The nurse prevents known carriers from coming into contact with the patient, appropriately change wet or soiled dressings, clean hospital equipment, change suction bottles routinely, and use medical asepsis when handling urinary drainage bags (Box 12-1, p. 194).

Exit Route

A microorganism cannot cause disease in another host unless it finds a point of escape from the reservoir. Human exit routes are gastrointestinal, respiratory, genitourinary, tissue, and blood.

By handwashing, the nurse can prevent the spread of microorganisms or cross-contamination. The nurse can also teach the patient to cover the nose when coughing or sneezing.

Method of Transmission

Once the microorganism has exited a reservoir, there are many **vehicles** (the means by which organisms are carried about) on or by which it can travel to the next host. These vehicles are then considered contaminated. **Contamination** means a condition of being soiled, stained, touched by, or otherwise exposed to harmful agents, such as by the entry of infectious or toxic materials into a previously clean or sterile environment, making an object potentially unsafe for use. If the vehicle is an inanimate (nonliving) object, it is called a **fomite,** which may be a stethoscope, thermometer, bandage scissors, tissue, drinking glass, needles, or one of many other objects. This is known as the indirect method of transmission.

The microorganism can be transmitted through direct contact, such as when the nurse turns or bathes a patient or uses inappropriate handwashing technique.

Box 12-1 INFECTION CONTROL TO REDUCE RESERVOIRS OF INFECTION

BATHING

- Use soap and water to remove drainage, dried secretions, excess perspiration, or sediment from disinfectants.

DRESSING CHANGES

- Change wet or soiled dressings (see Chapter 22).

CONTAMINATED ARTICLES

- Place tissues, soiled dressings, or soiled linen in moisture-resistant bags for proper disposal.

CONTAMINATED NEEDLES

- Place syringes and uncapped hypodermic needles and intravenous needles in moisture-resistant, puncture-proof containers, which should be located in patients' rooms or treatment areas so that exposed, contaminated equipment need not be carried any distance.
- Do not recap needles or attempt to break them.

BEDSIDE UNIT

- Keep table surfaces clean and dry.

BOTTLED SOLUTIONS

- Do not leave bottled solutions open for prolonged periods.
- Keep solutions tightly capped.
- Date bottles when opened.

SURGICAL WOUNDS

- Keep drainage tubes and collection bags patent to prevent accumulation of serous fluid under the skin surface.

DRAINAGE BOTTLES AND BAGS

- Empty and dispose of drainage suction bottles according to agency policy.
- Empty all drainage systems on each shift unless otherwise ordered by a physician.*
- Never raise a drainage system (e.g., urinary drainage bag) above the level of the site being drained unless it is clamped off.

*Closed water-sealed chest drainage system's receptacles are *never* emptied.

Air currents can carry microorganisms easily. Therefore when beds are made, the linens should not be shaken. A dampened or treated cloth should be used when dusting to prevent circulation of dust particles.

The floor is the dirtiest area in any building. Anything dropped, such as soiled linens and other supplies, should be discarded. Feet and furniture are the only items that belong on the floor.

All hospital personnel providing direct care (physical therapists and physicians as well as nurses) and those performing diagnostic and support services (laboratory technicians, respiratory therapists, dietary workers) must follow practices to minimize the spread of infection. Because so many factors can promote the spread of infection to a patient, all health care workers must be conscientious in using infection control practices.

Entrance of Microorganisms

Once the microorganism has exited one host and been transmitted, it must find a way to enter the susceptible host. Often the route or method of entrance is the same as the method of exit. When the host's defense mechanisms are reduced, the microorganism has a greater chance to enter. If the patient's skin is punctured with a contaminated needle, microorganisms may enter and be absorbed into the bloodstream. Incorrect handling of a wound dressing allows microorganisms to enter the open wound and cause an infection.

The methods used to prevent entrance of microorganisms are similar to the ones used in controlling the exit of microorganisms. The skin is the first line of defense and should be kept intact, lubricated, and clean. Areas of possible skin impairment should be closely observed, and treated accordingly.

Accidental needle sticks are a hazard for all health personnel and should be reported immediately so that prophylactic measures can be started. There should be appropriate waste containers for safe disposal of sharp instruments. Needles should never be recapped.

Inappropriate care of Foley catheter or other drainage apparatus can provide an entrance for microorganisms and allow the infectious process to continue. Tubes should remain connected and intact. Care should be taken when turning, positioning, or transferring a patient to prevent tubes from becoming tangled or pulling apart.

Appropriate cleansing of wounds will prevent the entrance of microorganisms. This is accomplished by cleaning away from the wound, wearing sterile gloves, and using an antiseptic agent. Gloves should be worn when handling soiled dressings, and the dressings should be placed in a container for infectious waste.

Host

A **host** is an organism in which another, usually parasitic organism is nourished and harbored.

How susceptible a person is to an infection is determined by the amount of resistance shown to the pathogen. Microorganisms are constantly in contact with people, but an infection will not develop unless a person is susceptible to the strength and numbers of the microorganism. As the pathogen's strength and numbers increase, the person becomes more susceptible. Factors that affect a person's immunological defense mechanisms are described in Box 12-2. The microorganism must accept the host for it to continue to exist.

Immunizations have proven effective in providing additional protection against infectious disease. These may be given before a person has been exposed to a dis-

Box 12-2 FACTORS AFFECTING IMMUNOLOGICAL DEFENSE MECHANISMS

- Increasing age and being very young
- Stress
- Nutritional status
- Hereditary factors
- Disease processes
- Environmental factors
- Medical therapy
- Chemotherapy
- Radiation

TABLE 12-1 Normal Defense Mechanisms Against Infection

Defense Mechanisms	Action	Factors That May Alter Defense
Skin		
Intact multilayered surface (body's first line of defense against infection)	Provides barrier to microorganisms	Cuts, abrasions, puncture wounds, areas of maceration
Shedding of outer layer of skin cells	Removes organisms that adhere to skin's outer layers	Failure to bathe regularly
Sebum	Contains fatty acid that kills some bacteria	Excessive bathing
Mouth		
Intact multilayered mucosa	Provides mechanical barrier to microorganisms	Lacerations, trauma, extracted teeth
Saliva	Washes away particles containing microorganisms Contains microbial inhibitors (e.g., lysozyme)	Poor oral hygiene, dehydration
Respiratory tract		
Cilia lining upper airway coated by mucus	Trap inhaled microbes and sweep them outward in mucus to be expectorated or swallowed	Smoking, high concentration of oxygen and carbon dioxide, decreased humidity, cold air
	Engulf and destroy microorganisms that reach lungs' alveoli	Smoking
Urinary tract		
Flushing action of urine flow	Washes away microorganisms on lining of bladder and urethra	Obstruction to normal flow by urinary catheter placement, obstruction from growth or tumor, delayed micturition Introduction of urinary catheter, continual movement of catheter in urethra
Gastrointestinal tract		
Acidity of gastric secretions	Chemically destroys microorganisms incapable of surviving low pH	Antacids
	Prevents retention of bacterial contents	Delayed motility resulting from impaction of fecal contents in large bowel or mechanical obstruction by masses
Vagina		
At puberty, normal flora cause vaginal secretions to achieve low pH	Inhibit growth of many microorganisms	Antibiotics, excessive douching, and oral contraceptives disrupting normal flora

ease (to provide protection before contact) or after exposure (if the person's history indicates possible contact with an infectious microorganism). See Table 12-1 on p. 195 for normal defense mechanisms against infection.

NOSOCOMIAL INFECTIONS

The term *nosocomial* is taken from the Greek word *nosocomium* meaning health care facility. A **nosocomial infection** is one that is acquired while in a hospital or other health agency, an infection acquired at least 12 hours after admission. This is a far-reaching and serious problem. More than 40 million people are admitted to hospitals each year, and, while there, as many as 10% of these people acquire infections. A hospital harbors microorganisms that may be highly **virulent** (of or pertaining to a very pathogenic or rapidly progressive condition), making it a more likely place to acquire an infection. The patient's immune system may already be weakened from disease or therapy, which makes the patient more susceptible to pathogens. Nosocomial infections not only extend hospital care for the patient but increase costs for both patient and hospital.

An **exogenous** (growing outside the body) infection is an infection caused by microorganisms from another person. An **endogenous** (growing within the body) infection is an infection caused by the patient's own normal microorganisms becoming altered and overgrowing or being transferred from one body site to another (e.g., microorganisms found in fecal material can be transferred to skin by hands and infect a wound).

Nosocomial infections are most commonly transmitted by direct contact between health personnel and patients or from patient to patient. For this reason a very strong emphasis is placed on sanitary procedures, such as handwashing.

To decrease the occurrence or continuation of nosocomial infections, many agencies have an infection control department, which investigates and establishes policies to develop sanitary procedures. These procedures include clean technique, which is used in all areas, and sterile technique, which is used in specialized areas.

The nurse is responsible for providing the patient with a clean and safe environment. The conscientiousness and accuracy of the nurse in performing clean and aseptic procedures increase the effectiveness of infection control.

Nosocomial infections significantly increase costs of health care. Extended lengths of stay in health care institutions increase disability, and prolonged recovery times add to the expenses of the patient as well as those of the health care institution and funding bodies (Medicare and Medicaid). Often, costs for nosocomial infections are not reimbursed; as a result, prevention has a beneficial financial impact.

Role of the Infection Control Nurse

Many hospitals employ nurses who are specially trained in infection control. These nurses are responsible for advising hospital personnel on safe aseptic practices and for monitoring infection outbreaks within the hospital. Duties of an infection control nurse include the following:

- Providing staff education on infection control
- Reviewing infection control policies and procedures
- Reviewing patients' medical records and laboratory reports to recommend appropriate isolation procedures
- Screening patient records for community-acquired infections
- Consulting with employee health departments concerning recommendations to prevent and control the spread of infection among personnel, such as tuberculosis testing
- Gathering statistics regarding the epidemiology of nosocomial infections
- Notifying the public health department of incidences of communicable diseases
- Conferring with all hospital departments to investigate unusual events or clusters of infection
- Educating patients and families
- Identifying infection control problems with equipment
- Checking microorganism sensitivity to antibiotics in use and reminding medical staff of resistance on sensitivity examination

An infection control nurse can be a valuable resource for controlling nosocomial infections.

UNIVERSAL PRECAUTIONS AND BODY SUBSTANCE ISOLATION

With the increased awareness of contamination from blood-borne pathogens—for example, the hepatitis B virus (HBV) and the human immunodeficiency virus (HIV) that causes AIDS—came the realization that definite precautions should be taken to prevent infections.

The Centers for Disease Control and Prevention (CDC) is part of the U.S. Department of Health and Human Services, providing facilities and services for investigation, prevention, and control of disease. The CDC has conducted studies on health care workers with documented skin or mucous membrane exposure to blood or body fluids of infected patients. The studies show infection when health care workers did not use protective measures.

It is difficult to accurately identify all patients infected with blood-borne pathogens. The CDC recommends that "universal blood and body fluid precautions" or "universal precautions" be used by health care workers when caring for all patients.

With the increase in the incidence of tuberculosis (TB), the importance of wearing correct protective masks against air borne pathogens has also been stressed along with universal precautions.

Universal precautions is an approach to infection control designed to prevent transmission of blood-borne diseases such as AIDS and hepatitis B in health care settings. Instituted in 1987 by the CDC and in 1989 by the Bureau of Communicable Disease Epidemiology in Canada, universal precautions are the minimum standard of practice recommended in the Occupational Safety and Health Act of 1991 for all health care agencies (Box 12-3).

Both universal precautions and body substance isolation involve the use of the same barrier precautions. Specifically, the recommendations for glove use differ. Body substance isolation requires that clean gloves be worn before contact with body fluids, mucous membranes, nonintact skin, and insertion sites. **Body substance isolation (BSI)** emphasizes the potential infectiousness of all moist body substances. For universal precautions, gloves are used only for anticipated contact with blood or body secretions containing blood. Health care workers use protective apparel based on the type of patient care anticipated (Box 12-4 on p. 198). The precautions for BSI are adequate for all patients except for those with diseases spread by the respiratory tract (for example, TB).

Hepatitis B, or serum hepatitis, is the infection most commonly transmitted by contaminated needles. A needlestick should be reported immediately. Health care agencies require workers who have had a needlestick to complete an injury report and seek appropriate treatment (Box 12-5 on p. 198).

Hospital Infection Control Update

As of January 1994, the Isolation System under discussion by Hospital Infection Control Practices Committee (HICPC) essentially calls for incorporating elements of universal precautions and body substance isolation (BSI) system into a new "standard precautions" component.

Universal precautions essentially emphasize barrier precautions to protect health care workers from HIV and other blood-borne pathogens, while BSI is designed to protect both workers and patients from pathogens in any body substance. The use of standard precautions would eliminate the need for existing auxiliary isolation measures such as enteric precautions.

The standard precautions will include recommendations on handwashing, use of gloves, and other barriers. There will also be an occupational health section that will address exposure control and work restrictions. The

Box 12-3 UNIVERSAL PRECAUTIONS TO MINIMIZE TRANSMISSION OF INFECTIOUS DISEASES

- Gloves are worn for touching body fluids, mucous membranes, or nonintact skin of all patients.
- Gloves are worn for handling items or surfaces soiled with blood or body fluids
- Gloves are worn when a health care staff member has a break in the skin.
- Gloves are *not* worn when 1, 2, or 3 above is neither present nor likely (e.g., when transporting patients)
- Gloves are worn for performing venipuncture and other vascular access procedures.
- Gloves should be changed after contact with each patient.
- Hands are washed immediately after gloves are removed.
- Hands or other skin surfaces are washed immediately and thoroughly if contaminated with blood or other body fluids.
- Used sharps, such as needles or scalpels, are placed in a biohazard needle box.
- Needles are *not* purposely bent, broken, or recapped.
- The needle container is not overfilled.
- Disposable wastes and articles contaminated with blood or large amounts of body fluids are placed in impervious (no holes present) containers for a trash pickup.
- Spills of blood or body fluids are cleaned up with a 1:10 solution (prepared daily) of Clorox and water.
- Masks, protective eyewear, or face shields are worn during procedures that are likely to generate droplets of blood or body fluid (e.g., nasotracheal suctioning) and airborne pathogens to prevent exposure of mucous membrane.
- Gowns are worn during procedures that are likely to generate splashes of blood or other body fluids (e.g., wound irrigation, cleansing a patient with bowel or bladder incontinence).
- Reusable items (e.g., suction bottles and oxygen setups) are emptied with care to avoid splashing.
- *All* soiled linen is placed in a laundry bag, and the bag is *not* overfilled.
- For patients with diarrhea—there is no change in practice by a staff member, whether a patient has been diagnosed as having AIDS or not.
- For patients who are coughing—there is no change in practice by a staff member, whether a patient has been diagnosed as having AIDS or not.
- To reduce the need for mouth-to-mouth resuscitation, mouth pieces, resuscitator bags, or other ventilation devices should be used.
- Health care workers with exudative (draining) lesions should refrain from all direct patient care and from handling patient care equipment.

Box 12-4 BODY SUBSTANCE ISOLATION GUIDELINES

- Personnel wear clean, disposable gloves before contact with mucous membranes, nonintact skin, or moist body substances.
- Personnel change gloves between patients and between activities with the same patient when gloves become excessively soiled.
- Personnel wash hands for at least 30 seconds when the hands are soiled, before each new patient contact, and after gloves are removed. (Wearing gloves does not eliminate the need to wash hands.)
- Additional barriers such as gowns or plastic aprons, masks, goggles or glasses, hair covers, and shoe covers are used as needed to keep moist body substances off clothing, skin, and mucous membranes of the wearer. For example, the nurse wears a mask and goggles when performing a procedure in which the face can be sprayed with mucus, blood, or any body fluid.
- All sharp instruments and needles are discarded uncapped in a rigid, puncture-proof container located at the point of use, such as a patient's room or treatment area.
- Laboratory specimens from all patients are handled as if they are infectious.
- Handling and reprocessing practices are uniform for all articles and equipment used on all patients. For example, soiled reusable articles are transported in plastic bags or rigid containers.
- Soiled linen is bagged securely before transport.
- Private rooms are used for patients with communicable diseases transmitted via the air or patients who soil their environment uncontrollably with body substances. A large red sign reading STOP is placed at the door of this patient's room; it also instructs all persons, "Check with the nurse before entering." For certain diseases (e.g., meningococcal meningitis), masks are worn when personnel or family enter the patient's room. Roommates who are immune to the patient's disease or who are currently infected with the same disease may share rooms (institutional policy may vary on this specific procedure).

standard precautions will be increased by three "transmission" categories that have thus far been designated as airborne (tuberculosis), contact (streptococcus) and droplet (pertussis).

Throughout the Committee's deliberations there has been discussion of the distinction between relative merits of BSI—which advocates precautions with all body substances—vs the transmission-driven approaches. The Committee's position, however, is that BSI does not address all the potential transmission of airborne droplet, dry skin, environment, and fomite contacts.[11]

Box 12-5 HEPATITIS B VACCINATION AND FOLLOW-UP AFTER EXPOSURE

- Health care employers shall make available the hepatitis B vaccine and vaccination series to all employees who have occupational exposure. Evaluation and follow-up care will be available to all employees who have been exposed.
- All medical evaluations and procedures, including the vaccine and vaccination series and evaluation after exposure (prophylaxis), are made available at no cost to employees.
- A confidential written medical evaluation will be available to employees with exposure incidents.
- Hepatitis B vaccinations will be made available to employees within 10 working days of assignment.

From Occupational Safety and Health Act of 1991, *Federal Register,* 1991.

Box 12-6 HANDWASHING IS ESSENTIAL

- Before and after caring for a patient
- After contact with organic material, such as feces, wound drainage, and mucus
- In preparation for an invasive procedure, such as suctioning, catheterization, or injections
- Before changing a dressing or contact with open wounds
- Before preparing and administering medications
- After removing disposable gloves or handling contaminated equipment

SKILL 12-1: PERFORMING A 2-MINUTE HANDWASHING

Guidelines

Handwashing is the most important and basic preventive technique for interrupting the infectious process. Box 12-6 indicates when it is essential to initiate handwashing.

A 2-minute handwashing will provide appropriate protection before the nurse cares for a patient. A 30-second handwashing before caring for another patient should be sufficient to ensure minimal transmission of microorganisms between patients. If a nurse has handled organic material or a contaminated article, a 1-minute handwashing would be appropriate.

Teaching patients and visitors about appropriate times for handwashing is an important role for the nurse. This enables the patient and family to inhibit the spread

PERFORMING A 2-MINUTE HANDWASHING

Nursing action/*Rationale*

1. Inspect hands, observing for visible soiling, breaks, or cuts in the skin and cuticles *because poor personal hygiene and an open area of the skin provide areas in which microorganisms can grow.*
2. Determine contaminant of hands *because this helps determine the need for a 2-minute handwash.*
3. Assess areas around the skin that are contaminated or clean *to prevent contamination of hands during and after handwashing procedure.*
4. Explain to the patient the importance of handwashing, *which helps the patient understand that handwashing slows down the spread of infection.*
5. Remove jewelry (except plain wedding band), and push watch and long sleeves above wrist *because microorganisms can collect in jewelry and watch bands. Also, removing jewelry makes it easier to wash all areas of hands and wrists.*
6. Adjust the water to appropriate temperature and force *because water that is too hot can chap skin, and too much force will cause splashing and spread microorganisms to other areas.*
7. Wet hands and wrists under the running water, always keeping hands lower than elbows *because hands are the most contaminated part of the arm, water should flow from the wrists (least contaminated area), over the hands, and then down the drain (see illustration).*
8. Lather hands with liquid soap (about 1 teaspoon) *because soap lather emulsifies fat and aids in cleansing.*
9. Wash hands thoroughly using a firm, circular motion and friction on back of hands, palms, and wrists. Wash each finger individually, paying special attention to areas between fingers and knuckles by interlacing fingers and thumbs and moving hands back and forth *causing friction which helps to loosen dirt and microorganisms—both resident (normally present) and transient (acquired from contamination) (see illustration).*
10. Wash 1 minute, rinse thoroughly, relather, and wash another minute, using a continuous amount of friction *because the rinsing removes the loosened microorganisms, and relathering ensures more thorough cleaning. The greater the contamination, the more need for longer washing.*
11. Rinse wrists and hands completely, keeping hands lower than elbows *because water should run from cleaner area (the wrists) over the hands, and then down the drain, rinsing the dirt and microorganisms away (see illustration).*
12. Clean fingernails carefully under running water using fingernails of other hand or blunt end of an orange stick—*this reduces chance of microorganisms remaining under nails.*
13. Dry hands thoroughly with paper towels. Start by patting at fingertips, hands, and then wrists and forearms *to prevent chapping. The cleanest areas are now the fingers and hands, so drying should progress from clean to less clean.*
14. Turn off faucets with a dry paper towel *to keep clean hands from touching contaminated handles (see illustration).*
15. Use hand lotion if desired *to keep skin soft and lubricated so skin will not crack easily.*

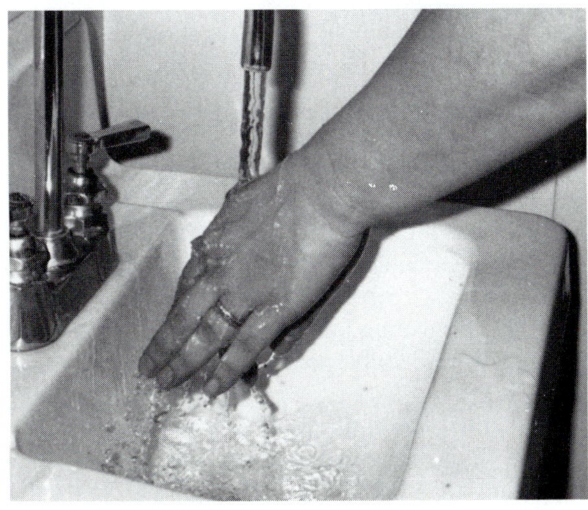

STEP 7

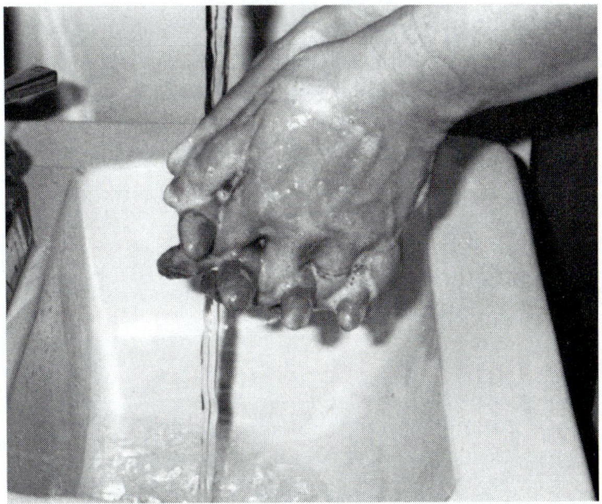

STEP 9

Continued.

PERFORMING A 2-MINUTE HANDWASHING—cont'd

16. Inspect hands and nails for cleanliness. *which ensures cleanliness of hands and nails.*

17. Record procedure to provide documentation of performance of 2-minute handwashing before administering patient care.

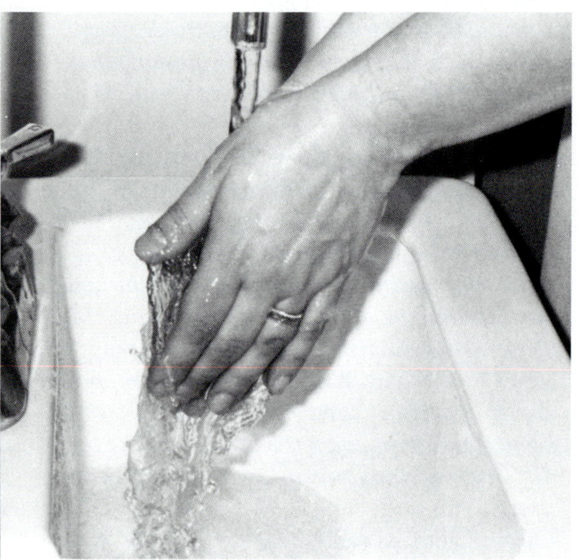

STEP 11

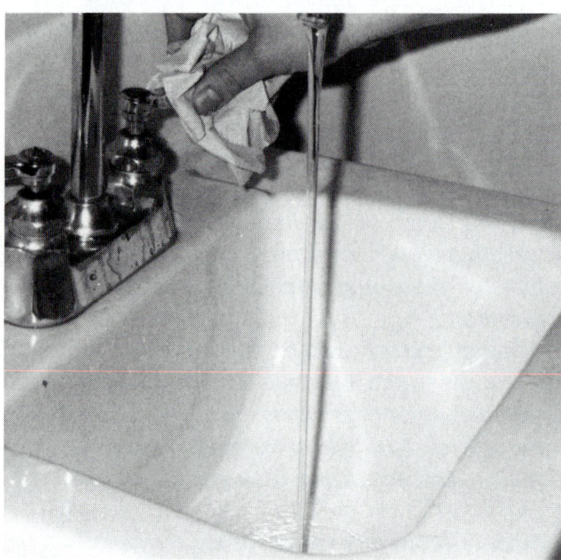

STEP 14

Sample charting

DATE	TIME	NOTES
1/12/95	0745	Two-minute handwashing procedure performed by the nurse.

____

(nurse's signature)

FOLLOW-UP

1. Two-minute handwashing should be performed each morning before beginning patient care, *because initial handwashing aids in removing surface soil from outside influences encountered on the way to work.*
2. Perform handwashing between care of patients *because additional handwashing prevents cross-contamination.*

SPECIAL CONCERNS

- If hands touch sink during handwashing, repeat procedure because inside of sink is contaminated.
- Avoid splashing water against uniform as microorganisms travel and grow in moisture.
- Avoid using water that is too hot or too cold when washing hands because breaks in the skin may occur and cause the hands to become contaminated when performing patient care.
- The very young patient and the older adult are highly susceptible to infection.

PATIENT TEACHING

- Demonstrate handwashing in view of the patient whenever possible to emphasize the importance of effective handwashing technique.
- Ask the patient questions and answer patient's questions regarding medical asepsis when appropriate.

of microorganisms when health care is continued at home. The importance of handwashing before and after handling food, after handling contaminated articles, and before and after elimination should be stressed in the teaching process.

In addition to handwashing, other actions can be taken to reduce the chance of transmitting microorganisms. A patient should receive her own set of personal care articles, such as a bedpan, urinal, bath basin, thermometer, water pitcher, and drinking glass, to prevent cross-contamination.

Microorganisms are transmitted by indirect contact with contaminated equipment and soiled linen. These articles should be placed in special waste containers or laundry bags and kept away from the nurse's uniform.

By following these recommendations the health care worker will be protected from infection and will prevent the patient acquiring a nosocomial infection.

Purposes

The nurse performs routine handwashing for the following reasons:

- To prevent nosocomial infection
- To maintain a safe, clean environment for the patient
- To provide safety for the nurse and prevent cross-contamination of patients or the spread of microorganisms

Supplies/equipment

Warm running water	Orange stick
Paper towels	Hand lotion
Liquid soap	

The risk of transmitting nosocomial infections or infectious disease among patients is high. When a patient has a known source of infection, health care workers are alerted and follow infection-control practices.

Isolation precautions are practices of infection control. They control the transmission of pathogens. These precautions may consist of wearing protective gowns and gloves, masks, and eyewear and the use of private rooms to keep the pathogens confined to an area. Care givers follow procedures to prevent organisms from leaving the rooms of patients or to prohibit organisms from entering the rooms of susceptible patients (Skills 12-2, through 12-5).

SKILL 12-2: DONNING GLOVES

Guidelines

Nurses or health care personnel don gloves if there is any possibility of contact with infectious material. Advice from the CDC on wearing gloves follow:

1. Gloves are worn only once and then placed into infectious-waste containers for safe disposal.
2. If the nurse has not completed the patient's care but has come into contact with infectious material, the gloves should be changed before continuing the patient's care.
3. There is a chance that gloves could be perforated during use, so hands should be washed after gloves are removed.

Family members should understand the importance of appropriate use of gloves. It is necessary for the nurse to explain that gloves will become contaminated if they have touched infected material or a contaminated object.

Purposes

The nurse wears gloves for many types of patient care for the following reasons:

- To protect the nurse and the nurse's family from disease
- To protect the patient from the nurse, who may be considered a contaminator to the patient
- To comply with 1987 CDC recommended use in order to (1) protect personnel from contact with infectious microorganisms, (2) reduce the possibility of patient contact with the health care worker's endogenous flora or normal bacteria, and (3) lessen the chance of personnel becoming infected with pathogenic microorganisms, which then could be carried to other patients

Supplies/equipment

Pair of gloves

SKILL 12-3: GOWNING FOR ISOLATION

Guidelines

The use of gowns in isolation is important primarily to protect clothing from being soiled while patient care is being administered. The gown also is protection against infectious microorganisms that could have exited from the patient. It is recommended that gowns not be reused but be discarded when leaving the patient's room. This aids in preventing the spread of pathogens to other patients or personnel. This procedure also applies to visitors.

Another rationale for use is protection of a patient whose immune system is inadequate. In this situation, a sterile gown is worn to prevent the transfer of pathogens from health care personnel and visitors to the patient.

There are many types of isolation, and some require wearing a gown, whereas others do not.

Donning an isolation gown is indicated when caring for patients with diseases characterized by heavy drainage and/or exudate, infectious and acute diarrhea,

SKILL 12-2

DONNING GLOVES

Nursing action/*Rationale*

1. Remove gloves from dispenser *in order to have gloves readily available for use.*
2. Don gloves when ready to begin patient care, *which provides protection for the patient and nurse (see illustrations).*
3. Inspect gloves for possibility of perforation *because perforated gloves can allow entry of pathogenic microorganisms.*
4. Change gloves after direct handling of infectious drainage, *which prevents contamination of patient.*
5. Remove one glove by grasping at cuff edge and turning glove inside out over hand. With ungloved hand, tuck finger inside cuff of remaining glove and pull it off, inside out and discard into waste container (see illustration), *which prevents nurse from touching outside area of gloves, which is considered contaminated.*
6. Wash hands thoroughly *to remove microorganisms that could be on nurse's hands.*
7. Record use of gloves during patient care, if agency's policy, *which provides documentation of wearing gloves for protection of patient and nurse.*

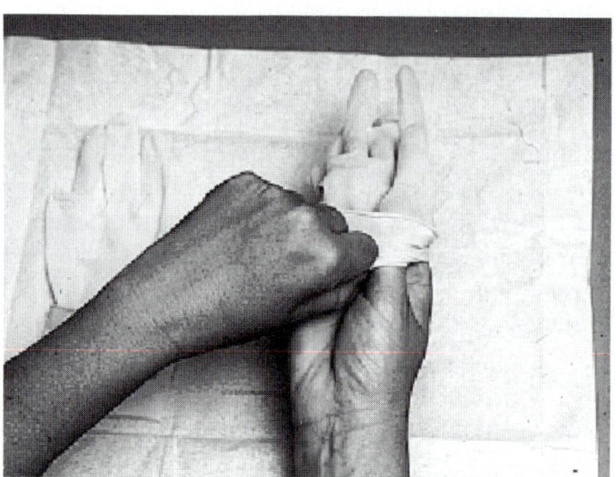

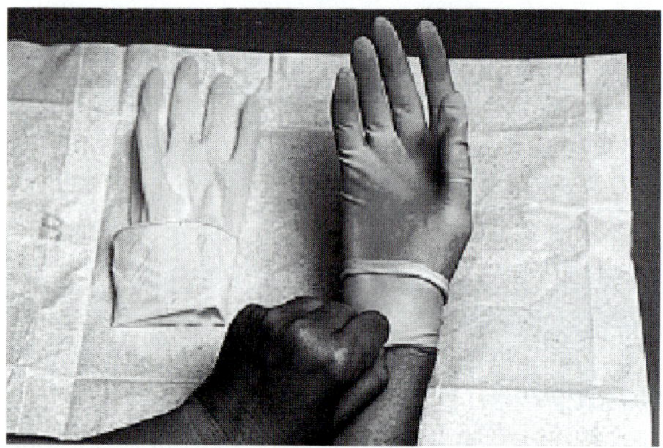

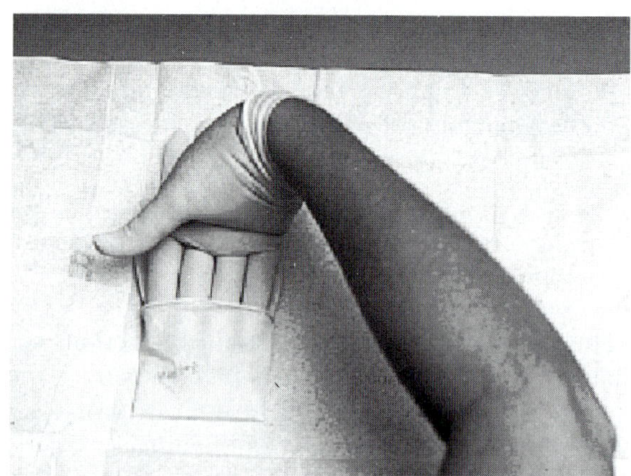

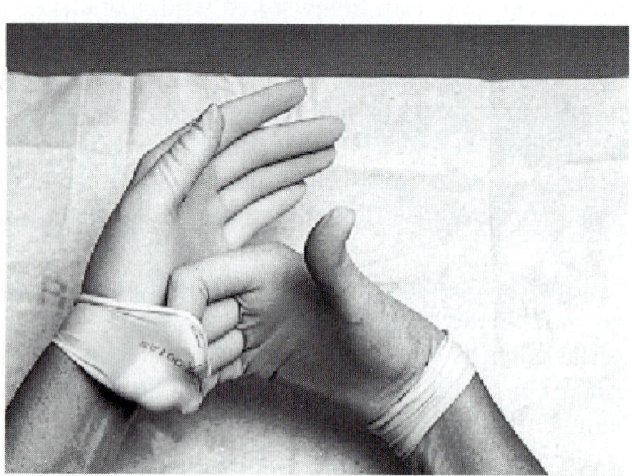

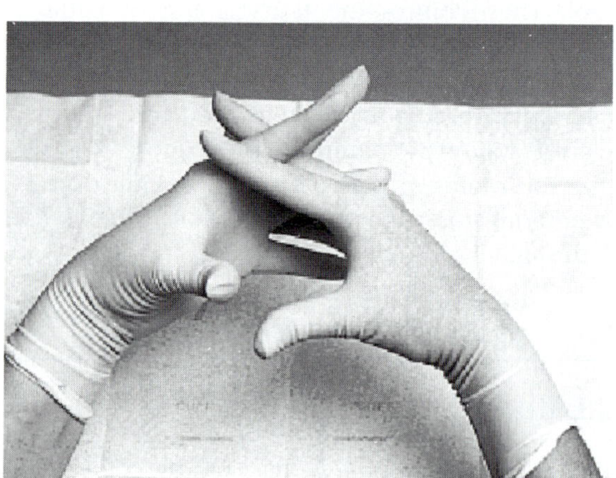

STEP 2

SKILL 12-2

DONNING GLOVES—cont'd

Sample charting

DATE	TIME	NOTES
1/12/95	0800	Gloves worn by nurse during administration of bed bath and AM care. Patient asked why gloves were worn. Explained reason for use of gloves. Patient voiced satisfisfaction with explanation.

____
(nurse's signature)

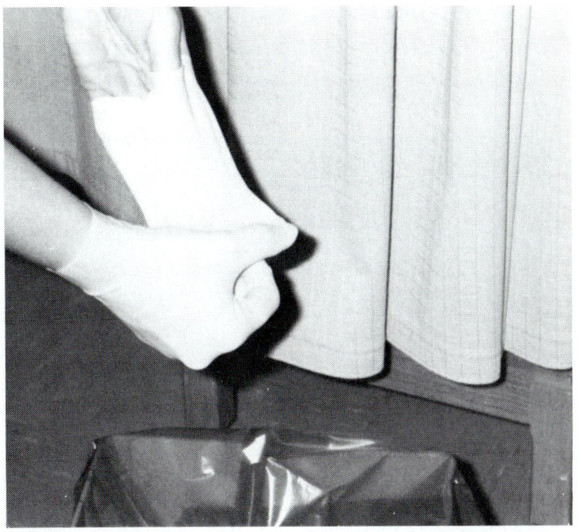

STEP 5

FOLLOW-UP

1. Make certain patient knows nurse is isolating the microorganism and not the patient *because this assists in patient's well-being and does not offend patient.*

SPECIAL CONCERNS

- If contamination continues, nurse must have technique reassessed.

PATIENT TEACHING

- Patient may need special assistance in understanding the precautions.
- The nurse should demonstrate donning gloves to patient.
- The nurse should allow time for a question and answer session for the patient.

SKILL 12-3

GOWNING FOR ISOLATION

Nursing action/***Rationale***

1. Remove watch and push up long sleeves *to ensure that uniform sleeve is under gown sleeve for protection.*
2. Place watch on a paper towel or see-through baggie before taking vital signs *to prevent cross-contamination of the watch.*
3. Wash hands *to inhibit spread of microorganisms.*
4. Don gown by securely tying gown at neck and waist *to provide protective covering of the entire uniform (see illustration).*
5. Remove gown, *which has protected the nurse.*
6. Wash hands *to prevent spread of microorganisms.*

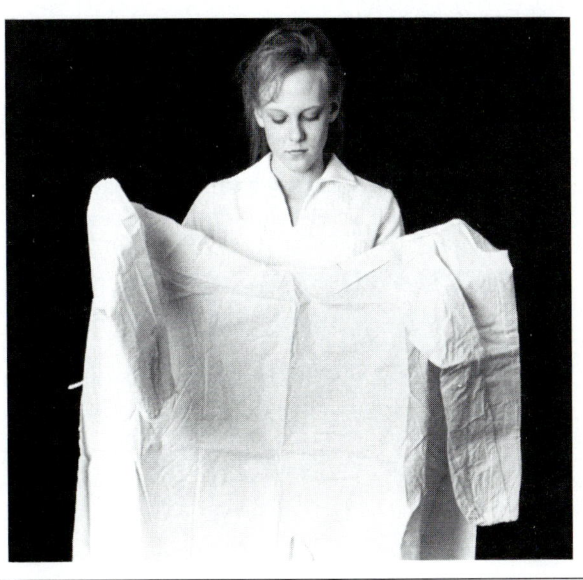

STEP 4

Continued.

SKILL 12-3

GOWNING FOR ISOLATION—cont'd

7. Record use of gown in isolation procedure if agency's policy, *to provide proof that appropriate procedure was followed.* Some agencies charge a daily rate for isolation precautions. This is noted on a daily basis in the patient's record. Therefore repeated notations throughout the 24 hours are not necessary.

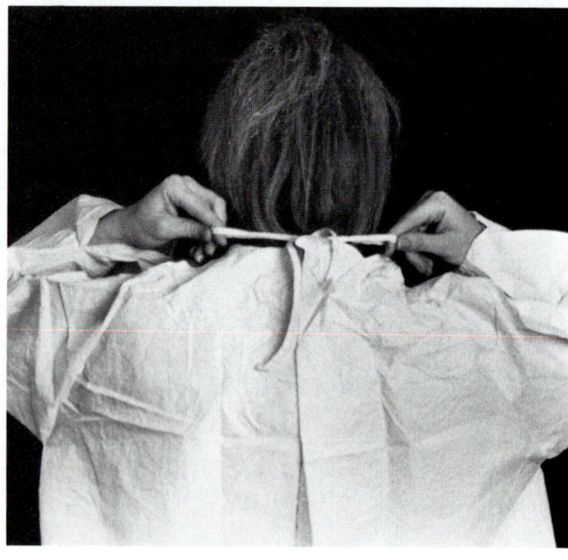

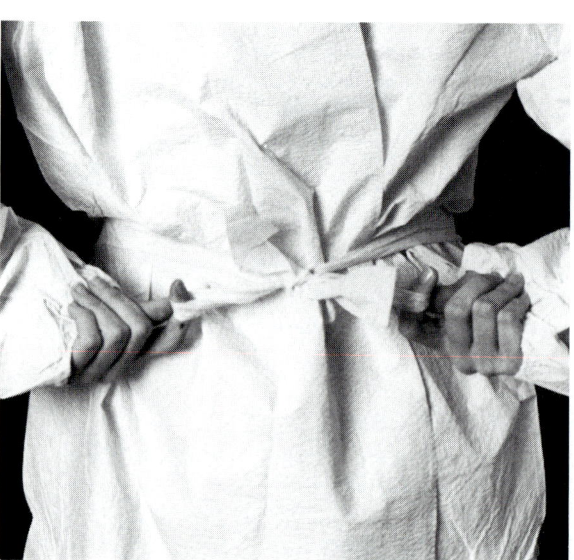

STEP 4, cont'd

Sample charting

DATE	TIME	NOTES
1/23/95	0930	Followed strict isolation procedure for heavy drainage from wound. Explained purpose for carrying out isolation technique.

____

(nurse's signature)

FOLLOW-UP

1. Discard soiled gown appropriately to prevent contamination.

SPECIAL CONCERNS

- Gown must be disposed of appropriately.
- Patient should feel comfortable and accepted.

PATIENT TEACHING

- Teach precautions appropriate to patient and significant others.
- Explain risks of inappropriate isolation technique.

other gastrointestinal disorders, respiratory disorders, skin wounds or burns, and urinary disorders.

Isolation gowns open at the back with ties at the neck and the waist. This keeps the gown securely closed, protecting the back of the uniform, as well as the front. The gown should be long enough to cover the nurse's uniform and have long sleeves with cuffs for added protection.

To don gowns correctly, follow the procedures listed in Skill 12-3.

Purposes

The nurse dons a gown for isolation for the following reasons:

- to protect the nurse from contracting an infection from the patient
- to prevent medical personnel from exposing an immunocompromised patient

Supplies/equipment
Isolation gown

SKILL 12-4: DONNING A MASK/PROTECTIVE EYEWEAR

Guidelines

When a mask is appropriately applied, it will fit snugly and securely over the nose and the mouth and the top edge will fit below eyeglasses, if worn. (This prevents fogging of the glasses.) Masks with eyeshields are designed to cover the eyes (glasses). The device should be changed at least every 20 to 30 minutes or if it becomes moist. Masks should not be reused or dangled around the neck and then reused. The patient and significant others should be instructed on appropriate use of the mask.

Purposes

A mask should be worn for the following reasons:

- to protect the wearer from inhaling microorganisms that travel on airborne droplets for short distances or that remain suspended in the air for longer periods or if slashing should occur
- to prevent inhaling pathogens if resistance is reduced or if being transported to another area (patient use)
- to discourage the wearer from touching the mouth, nose, or eyes and from transmitting infectious material

Supplies/equipment
Isolation mask

SKILL 12-5: DOUBLE BAGGING

Guidelines

A single bag is adequate if the contaminated articles can be placed in the bag without contamination of the outside of the bag. **Double bagging** (an infection control practice that involves placing a bag of contaminated items into another, clean bag that is held outside an isolation room by other personnel) is recommended by the CDC when it is impossible to keep the outer surface of a single bag free from contamination. The second bag should be labeled or color-coded to alert nursing personnel and to prevent contamination of housekeeping personnel when handling contaminated material. Double bagging can be used for safe removal of any article from the room.

The CDC recommends the following guidelines for handling isolation linen:

- Soiled linen should be placed in a laundry bag in the patient's room.
- The laundry bag should be labeled or it should be a special color (for example, red or yellow) designated for such linen so it is easily recognized.
- Linen requires less handling if the bag is soluble in hot water; however, such a bag may need to be double bagged because it punctures or tears easily.

Purposes

The nurse uses special bagging technique to remove contaminated articles from the patient's environment for the following reasons:

- to prevent the spread of microorganisms to the surrounding environment if it is impossible to prevent contamination of the bag's outer surface
- to prevent potential accidental exposure of personnel to contaminated articles

Supplies/equipment
Single isolation bag
Special color-coded double bag
Holder for isolation bag
Isolation gown
Isolation mask
Clean gloves
Holder for laundry bag

SKILL 12-6: ISOLATION TECHNIQUE

Guidelines

The type of isolation techniques followed will depend on how transmissible the pathogen is. The use of environmental barriers will keep pathogens in a confined

SKILL 12-4

DONNING A MASK

Nursing action/***Rationale***

1. Remove mask from container *so that the mask is readily available for use.*
2. Don mask when ready to begin patient care by covering the nose, mouth, and eyes (glasses) with the device. Mask with protective eye shield is worn when the risk of splashing is imminent. Secure mask in place with elastic band or by tying the strings behind the head, *which provides protection from microorganisms (see illustrations).*
3. Wear mask until it becomes moist but no longer than 20 to 30 minutes *because moisture renders a mask ineffective.*
4. Remove mask by untying the strings or moving the elastic. Make certain not to touch contaminated area *so that nurse will not come into contact with contaminated mask.*
5. Dispose of soiled mask *to protect other health care workers.*
6. Wash hands thoroughly *to remove microorganisms*
7. Record use of mask during patient care *to provide proof of wearing mask for protection of patient and nurse.*

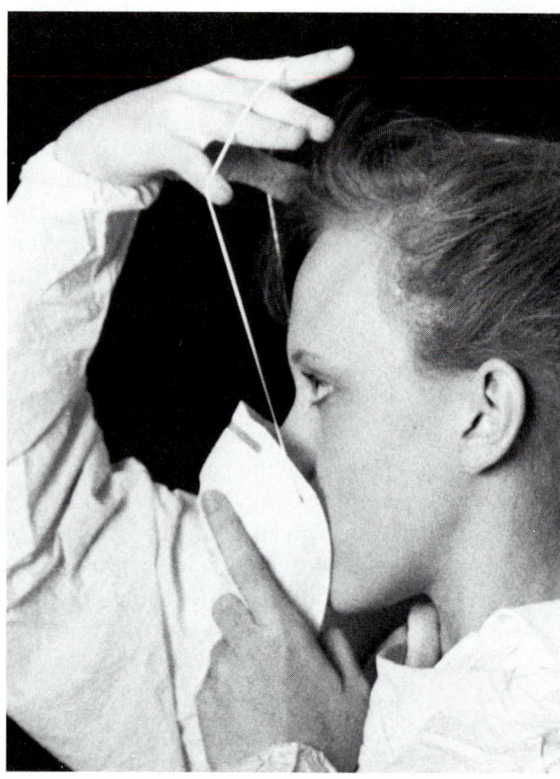

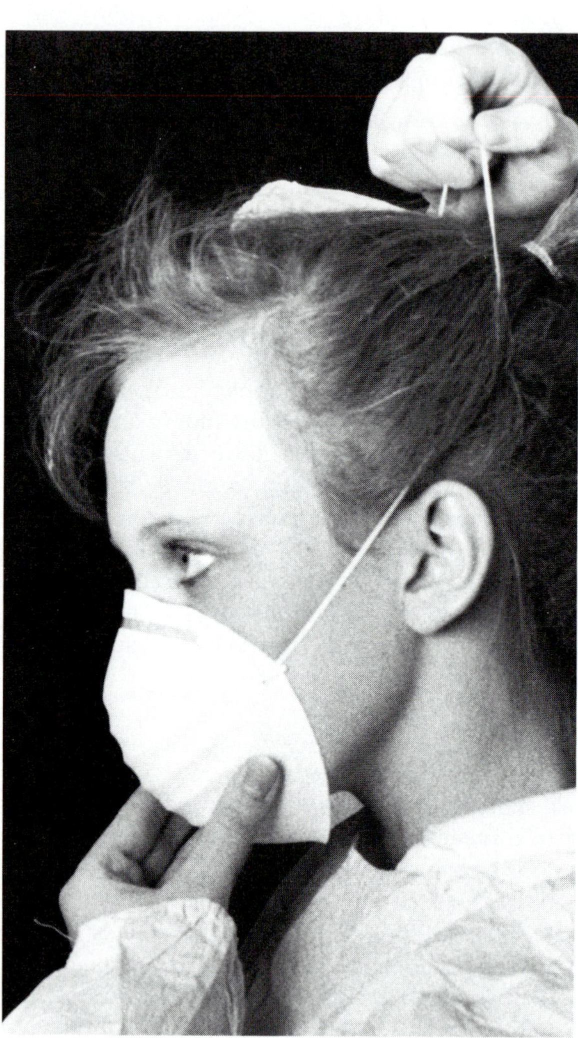

STEP 2

Sample charting

DATE	TIME	NOTES
1/30/95	0800	Mask worn by nurse during patient care.

____

(nurse's signature)

FOLLOW-UP

1. Make certain patient feels comfortable and accepted *because this assists in patient's well-being and prevents patient's being offended.*

SPECIAL CONCERNS

- If contamination of patient continues, technique must be reassessed.

PATIENT TEACHING

- Patient may need special assistance in understanding the precautions.
- Allow a question and answer session for the patient.

SKILL 12-5

DOUBLE BAGGING

Nursing action/***Rationale***

1. Don gown, mask, and gloves before entering patient's room *to prevent contact with contaminated articles.*
2. Collect all contaminated disposable articles in isolation bag *to prepare for double bagging.*
3. Summon second health care worker to remain outside patient area *because this prevents risk of contamination of personnel.*
4. Second person holds double bag with the top edge of bag covering hands *to prevent risk of contamination of personnel (see illustration).*
5. First person drops contaminated bag in double bag without touching edges of bag *so that the outside of the double bag remains clean.*
6. Bags are sealed or tied and labeled, *which prevents spread of infectious microorganisms.*
7. First person places new bags in holders *to keep articles ready for use.*
8. Remove gloves, gown, and mask without contamination, *which prevents spread of pathogens.*
9. Wash hands thorougly *to prevent contamination of nurse and others.*
10. Record double bagging procedure, *which provides proof of use of appropriate technique.*
11. Document patient's response to isolation, *which could indicate need for patient teaching.*

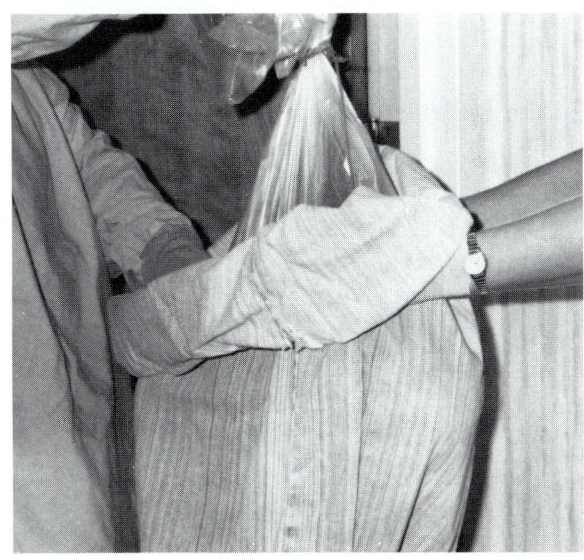

STEP 4

Sample charting

DATE	TIME	NOTES
1/31/95	0940	All disposable, contaminated articles double bagged and placed outside rooms for pickup. Patient understands and cooperates with isolation procedures.

____

(nurse's signature)

FOLLOW-UP

1. Ensure positive feelings of patient toward being in isolation *in order to prevent the patient from feeling rejected.*

SPECIAL CONCERNS

- If contamination continues, the technique must be reassessed.

PATIENT TEACHING

- Patient may need special assistance in understanding the precautions.
- Allow a question and answer session for the patient.

area. Examples of such barriers are a private room, isolation room, closed door, protective gown, mask, goggles, gloves, and shoe covers.

There are specific guidelines issued by the CDC for isolation technique in a controlled environment. There are two systems for implementing these guidelines: the disease-specific system, where certain procedures are performed for each type of infectious disease, and the category-specific system. The category-specific system recognizes eight ways a microorganism is transmitted (Box 12-7 on p. 210). In this category similar isolation precautions are used for different diseases because the microorganisms are transmitted in the same manner. Although the disease-specific system has proven to be less time consuming and less costly because some diseases need only minimum precautions, the category-specific system is most commonly used in health care agencies.

SKILL 12-6

ISOLATION TECHNIQUE

Nursing action/***Rationale***

1. Determine causative microorganism or effectiveness of patient's immune system *to help nurse know virulence of causative pathogen.*
2. Recognize mode of transmission and how microorganism exits the body *to determine the category or type of isolation to use.*
3. Follow agency policy for specific type of isolation used, *which increases awareness of isolation categories available in the agency.*
4. Provide an environment with adequate equipment and supplies:
   a. Private room or isolation with anteroom *to reduce possibility of transmission of pathogens.*
   b. Sign stating isolation category *because it alerts personnel, patient, family, and visitors about special precautions to be followed.*
   c. Adequate handwashing facilities *so handwashing can easily be performed on entering and leaving the area.*
   d. Special containers for trash, soiled linen, and sharp instruments, such as needles, *which ensures safe disposal of contaminated articles.*
5. Plan time to explain isolation technique to patient, family, and visitors *because this relieves apprehension and promotes cooperation of those involved.*
6. Post card on door of patient's room or wall outside room stating the protective measures in use for patient care *so it informs those entering room of precautions to be followed and encourages cooperation.*
7. Supply the room with designated lined containers for soiled linens and for trash, *which prevents transmission of pathogens from seepage through container.*
8. Assess vital signs, administer medications, administer hygiene, and collect specimens (see Table 12-2).
9. Report changes in patient's health status, whether positive or negative, *to ensure continued care and help determine progress of patient.*
10. Record assessments and performance of protective asepsis *to provide proof of appropriate patient care.*

Sample charting

DATE	TIME	NOTES
2/1/95	0745	Isolation procedure carried out. Patient answered questions clearly and demonstrated understanding of procedures performed

____
(nurse's signature)

FOLLOW-UP

1. Determine patient's understanding of activities in room *because it increases patient's comfort and feeling of well-being.*

SPECIAL CONCERNS

- Make certain that patient does not feel alone and isolated from loved ones.
- Ensure patient safety.

PATIENT TEACHING

- Teach patient how to carry out handwashing precautions.

There are some basic principles to be followed no matter what protective system is used. They follow:

1. Thorough handwashing should be performed before entering and after leaving a patient's room when using protective asepsis.
2. An understanding of the disease process and method of transmission of the infectious microorganism helps determine the use of protective barriers.
3. Contaminated equipment and articles are to be disposed of in a safe and effective manner to prevent transmission of pathogens to other individuals.
4. If the patient is to be transported to other areas in the agency (away from the isolation room), necessary measures should be taken to protect those who may be exposed. This is accomplished by having the patient wear a gown and mask.

The patient with an infectious disease should be placed in a private or isolation room equipped with the appropriate handwashing and toilet facilities. Private rooms used for isolation have negative-pressure airflow

TABLE 12-2 Specimen Collection Techniques for the Patient in Isolation

Amount Needed*	Collection Device*	Specimen Collection and Transfer
Wound culture		
As much as possible (after cleaning skin to remove flora)	Cotton-tipped swab or syringe	Don gloves and place clean test tube or culturette tube on clean paper towel. After swabbing center of wound site, grasp collection tube by holding it with paper towel. Carefully insert swab without touching outside of tube. After removing gloves, washing hands, and securing tube's top, transfer labeled tube into bag for transport to laboratory.
Blood culture		
10 ml per culture bottle, from two different venipuncture sites (volume may differ based on collection containers)	Syringes and culture media bottles	Don gloves and perform venipuncture at two different sites to decrease likelihood of both specimens being contaminated by skin flora. Inject 10 ml of blood into each bottle. Remove gloves and wash hands. Secure tops of bottles, label specimens, and send to laboratory.
Stool culture		
Small amount, approximately size of a walnut	Clean cup with seal top (not necessary to be sterile) and tongue blade	Don gloves and place cup on clean paper towel in patient's bathroom. Using tongue blade, collect needed amount of feces from bedpan. Transfer feces to cup without touching cup's outside surface. Remove gloves, wash hands, and place seal on cup. Repeat handwashing. Transfer specimen cup into clean bag for transport to laboratory.
Urine culture		
1-5 ml	Syringe and sterile cup	Don gloves and place cup or tube on clean towel in patient's bathroom. Use alcohol swab pad, syringe, and needle to collect specimen if patient has Foley catheter. Otherwise, have patient follow procedure to obtain clean-voided specimen (see Chapter 17). Transfer urine into sterile container by injecting urine from syringe or pouring it from container. Remove gloves, wash hands, and secure top of labeled container. Transfer labeled specimen into clean bag for transport to laboratory.

*Agency policies may differ on type of container, amount of specimen material required, and bagging.

to prevent infectious particulates from flowing out of the closed environment. There are also special rooms with positive-pressure airflow that are used for highly susceptible patients such as transplant recipients. In this case, no organisms are able to enter the room. The routine care of a patient in isolation is the same hygienic care given to all patients. The health care worker should remember that all articles that come into contact with the patient are contaminated and should be handled in the correct manner to maintain protective asepsis. Equipment for assessing vital signs remains in the room if possible. Otherwise, the equipment must be disinfected safely when removed from the room. The nurse's watch may be placed on a clean paper towel or sealed in a plastic bag and placed on the bedside unit stand before the nurse touches any article in the room.

It is important in the care of this patient to consider the psychological/or emotional deprivation created by

Box 12-7 CATEGORY-SPECIFIC ISOLATION PRECAUTIONS

1. Strict isolation—Diseases transmitted by air or contact require full-isolation technique. Disease examples: diphtheria or varicella (chicken pox).
2. Contact precautions—The nurse should wear gown, mask, and gloves only when coming into contact with the infectious substance. Disease examples: impetigo, herpes simplex, and acute respiratory infections in infants and small children.
3. Respiratory isolation—Health care personnel must wear a mask whenever in the room with the patient, because the pathogen is transmitted by airborne droplets over short distances. Disease examples: pneumonia, measles, tuberculosis, or bacterial meningitis.
4. Enteric precautions—Disease spread through fecal material. The nurse should wear gown and gloves for protection against feces. Disease examples: viral hepatitis or infectious diarrhea.
5. Tuberculosis isolation (acid-fast bacillus [AFB]—Pathogen transmitted by air droplet and sputum. The nurse may need to wear gown and a mask if the patient is coughing without covering the mouth, but gloves are not indicated. A specially designed mask is available to be worn when caring for patients with tuberculosis; this mask prevents inhalation of fine respiratory particulates (Particulate Respirator).
6. Drainage/secretion precautions—The pathogen is transmitted by direct or indirect contact with drainage from an infected body site. The nurse should wear gown and gloves to prevent contact with the infectious material. A mask is not needed unless there is a high risk of exposure to splash. Disease example: infected burns or wounds.
7. Universal blood/body fluid precautions—Direct or indirect contact with infected body fluids or blood requires the use of gown and/or gloves. Caring for a patient with AIDS requires blood/body fluid precautions.
8. Care of immunosuppressed patient—This was previously known as reverse or protective isolation. Health care personnel caring for an immunosuppressed patient should wear a gown, mask, and gloves to prevent transmission of pathogens by contact or air droplet. Disease examples: leukemia, burns, or patients with organ transplants.

isolation. The patient is forced into solitude and deprived of normal social contacts. The patient should feel wanted and cared for like all other patients. Extra time should be spent with the patient, the room should be kept clean and pleasant, and the patient should be taught the rationale for use of this technique. The emotional state of the patient can interfere with recovery unless the nurse minimizes the feeling of psychological and physical isolation. The patient and significant others should have an understanding of the patient's disease and know the importance of following isolation precautions. Family and visitors should be taught how to wear isolation apparel, and the nurse should ensure that the procedure is followed.

Purpose

The nurse follows isolation procedure for the following reason:

- to prevent the transmission of infectious microorganisms by preventing pathogens from leaving the room of the infected patient or from entering the room of a highly susceptible patient

Supplies/equipment

Outside Patient's Room or in Anteroom:
Isolation gowns
Isolation masks
Isolation gloves
Clean linens
Single isolation bags
Double isolation bags
Paper towels
Running water
Soap with dispenser

Inside the Patient's Room or in Anteroom:
Holder for isolation bag
Holder for laundry bag

SKILL 12-7: PREPARING FOR DISINFECTION AND STERILIZATION

Guidelines

Pathogenic microorganisms are believed to be present on most articles in the home and public areas, including health agencies. **Disinfection** (a process by which pathogens, but not necessarily their spores, are destroyed) and **sterilization** (a process by which all microorganisms, including their spores, are destroyed) are two processes used to prevent spread of pathogens and disease.

Most health agencies have a central supply department, which sterilizes some supplies and disinfects reusable equipment and supplies. Although most supplies used today for patient care are disposable, there are situations that still require the use of sterilization and disinfection techniques. The patient and significant others can also be taught cleansing and disinfecting principles for the home environment (see patient teaching box on p. 212).

There are two accepted methods of sterilization and disinfection (see Box 12-8). One is a physical process that uses heat or radiation; the second process uses chemicals. Both methods destroy microorganisms. The method used depends on the following factors: (1) the type of mi-

SKILL 12-7

PREPARING FOR DISINFECTION AND STERILIZATION

Nursing action/***Rationale***

1. Prepare equipment and supplies *to ensure organization of task.*
   a. Disinfectant to use for cleansing, *which aids in appropriate care of equipment and reusable supplies.*
   b. Method of sterilization *to ensure that appropriate method is used.*
   c. Gloves *to protect the nurse from contamination.*
   d. Running water, *because it aids in cleansing and rinsing of articles.*
   e. Scrub brush *is used to aid in cleansing grooves.*
   f. Cloth wrapper *to provide the means for wrapping articles requiring sterilization.*
2. Don gloves *because they protect the nurse from contamination.*
3. Rinse article under cool running water, *which emulsifies or softens dirt for removal.*
4. Wash article with detergent, *which emulsifies or softens dirt for easy removal.*
5. Use scrub brush to remove material in grooves *because friction loosens material in corners and grooves.*
6. Dry article thoroughly *to prevent the growth of microorganisms.*
7. Prepare article for sterilization by wrapping it in cloth wrapper, *which ensures appropriate sterilization of the article.*
8. Clean work area and put in order *to prevent the growth of microorganisms.*

SPECIAL CONCERNS

- In the home an oven or a pressure cooker may be used for sterilization. Microwaves are widely used now.
- Exposure to sunlight is helpful.
- Boiling of contaminated articles destroys microorganisms.

PATIENT TEACHING

- Teach patient to recognize possible sources of infection to perform the necessary protective measures.
- Set a personal example of cleanliness.
- Teach patient and significant others to understand the steps performed in protective asepsis to help prevent transmission of pathogens.
- Teach and assist patient and significant others to control infection in the home by improvising or using available materials to maintain hygienic techniques.
- Inform patient about nature of infections and techniques to control and prevent the spread of disease. Topics that can be discussed in teaching sessions are presented in the patient teaching box.

croorganisms present, since spore-forming bacteria are resistant to destruction; (2) how many microorganisms are present, since it takes longer to kill a large number; and (3) the type of article in need of cleansing, since some materials are so sensitive that heat or certain chemicals can destroy the article. Other determinants of the sterilization method used are (1) the intended use for the article (e.g., surgery requires that all organisms be destroyed, whereas medical asepsis requires only removal of pathogens) and (2) the methods of sterilization available.

Effective chemicals used in disinfection and sterilization are iodine, alcohol, and chlorine compounds. Chlorine is useful for household disinfecting and in disinfection of water but should never be mixed with ammonia because of the resulting emission of toxic fumes. Chlorine has a tendency to corrode some metals. Iodine is a good bactericidal agent (i.e., it kills the bacteria but not spores). Iodine stains articles and is not used as widely as it once was.

Purpose

The nurse follows basic clean or aseptic technique for the following reason:

- to interrupt the infection process in order to prevent and control the spread of infection

Supplies/equipment
Disinfection
Gloves
Running water
Scrub brush
Sterilization
Cloth wrappers

PATIENT TEACHING FOR INFECTION CONTROL

- The nurse should teach the patient about the infection process, especially how an infection is transmitted, and stress the importance of interrupting the process. A simple diagram can be used to illustrate this (see Fig. 12-1). The nurse should use an example for each step that is familiar to the patient.
- Although handwashing is a basic aseptic technique, the nurse should stress when and how the procedure should be performed to be effective in preventing infection.
- The nurse should emphasize the importance of adequate exercise, a well-balanced diet, and current immunizations. This is good preventive health care for patients to follow.
- The nurse should discuss the susceptibility of the patient to infection.
- The patient should be taught correct and safe methods of storing and preparing food.
- The patient should practice good methods of hygiene to minimize microorganism growth and spread. The nurse may suggest a list of disinfectants that could be used in daily cleaning.
- The patient should be aware of family members/significant others who are susceptible to infections.
- Instruct patient about signs and symptoms of wound infection.
- For patients who receive tube feedings at home, explain the importance of preparing enough formula for only 8 hours (commercially prepared) or 4 hours (home prepared). Tell patient that contaminated enteral feeding can cause salmonellal or staphylococcal infections. Rinse feeding bag and tubing with mild soap and water daily.
- Instruct patient to place contaminated dressings and other disposable items containing infectious body fluids in impervious (incapable of being penetrated) plastic bags. Place needles in metal containers such as soda cans and tape the openings shut.
- Clean noticeably soiled linen separate from other laundry. Wash in water that is as hot as the fabric will tolerate. Add 1 cup of bleach or Lysol to detergent.

Box 12-8 PRINCIPLES OF STERILIZATION OR DISINFECTION

PHYSICAL METHOD

1. **Steam under pressure,** or moist heat, is the most practical and dependable method for destruction of all microorganisms. This technique is called *sterilization.* Examples of sterilization equipment are the autoclave, which is used in hospitals and other agencies, and the pressure cooker, which is used in a home environment.
2. **Boiling water** is the best method for home use and is the least expensive. However, this technique will not destroy bacterial spores and some viruses. The article should be boiled for a minimum of 15-20 minutes for disinfection. (e.g., glass baby bottle).
3. **Radiation** sterilizes pharmaceutical goods, foods, and heat-sensitive items. It is extremely effective on articles that are difficult to sterilize.
4. **Dry heat** is a method used for disinfecting articles that are destroyed by moisture. Health agencies seldom use this method, but in the home an article can be disinfected by being placed in the oven for 2 hours at 320° F or for 45 minutes at 350° F.

CHEMICAL PROCESS

1. **Gas** (ethylene oxide) is used for sterilization. It destroys spores formed by bacteria.
2. **Chemical solutions** are often used to disinfect instruments because they are effective in destroying microorganisms. Clinical thermometers can be stored in a chemical solution, and some articles are soaked in a solution to prepare them for another method of disinfection or sterilization.

REFERENCES AND SUGGESTED READINGS

1. Banick B: Light at the end of a decade, *Am J Nurs* 90:37, 1990.
2. Brigham CJ, Foster SL, Hodson KE: Asepsis and universal precautions: a participatory learning module, *Nurse Educ* 16(22), 1991.
3. Boutotte J: Protecting yourself against T.B., *Nursing* 23(10):64, 1993.
4. Burtis RE, Evangelisti J: Will universal precautions protect me? *Nurs Outlook* 40(3):133, 1992.
5. Centers for Disease Control Update: Universal precautions for prevention of transmission of human immunodeficiency virus, hepatitis B virus, and other blood-borne pathogens in health care settings, *MMWR* 37(24):337, 1988.
6. Centers for Disease Control and Prevention: Nosocomial enterococci resistant to vancomycin, United States, 1989-1993, *MMWR* 42:597, 1993.
7. Controversies in care: new OSHA rules under fire from all angles, *Am J Nurs* 90(1):18, 1990.
8. Craft K: Do you really know how to handle sharps? *RN* 58(8):33, 1990.
9. Crow S: Common sense asepsis. Adapted from Asepsis—the right touch, *Nursing* 24(3):32C, 1994.
10. Czurylo KT et al: M-R-S-A: methicillin-resistant *Staphylococcus aureus, Nursing* 21(12):68, 1991.
11. DeWit S: *Keane's essentials of medical-surgical nursing,* ed 3, Philadelphia, 1992, Saunders.
12. Editor: HICPAC warns of resistant bugs, hammers out new guidelines, *Hosp Infect Control* 21(1):1, 1994.
13. Editors: Infection control update, *Nursing* 23(10):61, 1993.
14. Editor: New CDC guidelines unveiled as ICPs take APIC "global view," *Hosp Infect Control* 20(9):89, 1993.
15. Eggleston B: Infection control update. I. *Nursing* 24(3):70, 1994.
16. English JFP: Reported hospital needle stick injuries in relation to knowledge/skill, design, and management problems, *Infect Control Hosp Epidemiol* 13(5):259, 1992.
17. Gregory E: Use of gloves in infection control, *Nurs Res* 39(2):5, 1990.
18. *Illustrated manual of nursing practice,* Springhouse, Penn, 1991, Springhouse.
19. Jackson M, Lynch P: In search of a rational approach, *Am J Nurs* 90(10):65, 1990.
20. Joint Commission on Accreditation of Healthcare Organizations: *Accreditation manual for hospitals,* Oakbrook Terrace, Ill, 1992, The Commission.
21. Kiyosawa K et al: Hepatitis C in hospital employees with needlestick injuries, *Ann Intern Med* 115(5):367, 1991.
22. Long BC, Phipps WJ, Cassmeyer VL: *Medical-surgical nursing: a nursing process approach,* ed 3, 1993, St Louis, Mosby.
23. Lynch P et al: Implementing and evaluating a system of generic infection precautions: body substance isolation, *Am J Infect Control* 18(1):1, 1990.
24. *Mosby's medical, nursing, and allied health dictionary,* ed 4, St Louis, 1994, Mosby.
25. Much JK, Colleta T: Stress of occupational exposure to blood or body fluids: managing the response, *Med Surg Nurs* 2(1):49, 1993.
26. Parker L: From pestilence to asepsis, *Nurs Times* 86(63):1990.
27. Perry AG, Potter PA: *Clinical nursing skills and techniques,* ed 3, St Louis, 1994, Mosby.
28. Phipps WJ et al: *Medical-surgical nursing: concepts and clinical practice,* ed 4, St Louis, 1991, Mosby.
29. Potter PA, Perry AG: *Basic nursing: theory and practice,* ed 3, St Louis, 1995, Mosby.
30. Potter PA, Perry AG: *Fundamentals of nursing: concepts, process, and practice,* ed 3, St Louis, 1993, Mosby.
31. Pritchard V, Sanders N: Universal precautions: how effective are they against methicillin-resistant *Staphylococcus aureus? J Gerontol Nurs* 17(1):7, 1991.
32. Rodts MF, Benson DR: HIV: precautions for prevention in the workplace, *Orthop Nurs* 11(5):51, 1992.
33. Rogers B, Travers P: Overview of work-related hazards in nursing: health and safety issues, *Heart Lung* 20:486, 1991.
34. Statka JL et al: An analysis of blood and body fluid exposures sustained by house officers, medical students and nursing personnel on acute care general medical wards: a prospective study, *Infect Control Hosp Epidemiol* 12(10):583, 1991.
35. Tattam A: Unhygienic practices, *Nurs Times* 87(20):1991.
36. The Staff: *Fundamental nursing skills,* Springhouse, Penn, 1994, Springhouse.
37. The Staff: *Nursing procedures: student version,* Springhouse, Penn, 1993, Springhouse.
38. Thompson JM et al: *Mosby's clinical nursing,* ed 3, St Louis, 1993, Mosby.
39. Timby BK, Lewis LW: *Fundamental skills and concepts in patient care,* ed 5, Philadelphia, 1992, Lippincott.
40. Weber D et al: Management of the health care worker infected with human immunodeficiency virus: lessons from nosocomial transmission of hepatitis B virus, *Infect Control Hosp Epidemiol* 12(10): 625, 1991.

CHAPTER CHALLENGE

KEY POINTS

- An infection can develop as long as the six elements composing the infectious chain are uninterrupted.
- A microorganism's virulence depends on its ability to resist attack by the body's normal defenses.
- Age, poor nutrition, stress, inherited conditions, chronic disease, and treatments or conditions that compromise the immune system increase susceptibility to infection.
- Surgical asepsis requires more stringent techniques than medical asepsis and is directed toward eliminating microorganisms.
- The CDC recommends that health care workers consider all patients as potentially infected with HIV and other blood-borne pathogens and reduce risk of exposure to blood and body fluids.
- Body substance isolation (BSI) involves taking precautions before waiting for a patient to be diagnosed with an infection.
- Following aseptic principles is the key to a nurse's success in preventing patients from acquiring infection.
- The nurse does not take an article (e.g., sphygmomanometer/blood pressure cuff) into an isolation room if the article is to be used by another patient.

- Lack of handwashing is the main cause of infections.
- An infection-control nurse monitors the incidence of infections within an institution and provides educational and consultative services to maintain aseptic practices.
- Isolation practices prevent personnel and patients from acquiring infections and prevent transmission of microorganisms to other persons.
- A patient in isolation is subject to psychological and emotional deprivation because of the restricted environment.

STUDY QUESTIONS

1. Mr. Jones, age 24, has been admitted to a medical unit with the diagnosis of hepatitis A and placed in enteric isolation. The purpose of this is to:
   1. Prevent transmission of infectious microorganisms
   2. Control the environment of the patient
   3. Protect the patient from infectious microorganisms
   4. Protect only the family
2. Mr. Smith, LPN, is working on a clinical medical area with a census of 15. Each patient has somewhat different illnesses. The most important method Mr. Jones can use to protect each patient from microorganisms is:
   1. Wearing a gown
   2. Placing each patient in isolation
   3. Handwashing
   4. Wearing gloves
3. Mrs. Brown, age 40, has an immunocompromised condition as a result of chemotherapy. A room is being prepared to put her in reverse isolation. The main goal while preparing this room is to:
   1. Prevent transmission of microorganisms from patients' rooms to other areas
   2. Keep all articles sterile
   3. Prevent only visitors from coming into contact with microorganisms
   4. Protect only the patient from the invasion of microorganisms
4. Mr. Brown, age 42, has been admitted to the clinical area with a diagnosis of infectious diarrhea. A private room, equipped with appropriate handwashing and toilet facilities, has been prepared because:
   1. It facilitates prevention of the spread of disease
   2. A "No Visitors" rule can be better controlled
   3. There is more room
   4. The patient will be kept isolated from others
5. Mr. Voss, age 47, recently returned to the United States from traveling abroad. He came into the emergency room complaining of diarrhea and abdominal pain and was admitted to the clinical area. The diagnosis was possible salmonella gastroenteritis, and Mr. Voss was placed on enteric precautions, which would include:
   1. Mask only
   2. Gloves and mask if the nurse is in contact with secretions
   3. Gowns only
   4. Gowns and gloves if the nurse is in contact with feces
6. Mrs. Cook, age 63, admitted with a diagnosis of bacterial meningitis, has been placed in respiratory isolation. A visitor or nurse entering the room to visit or care for Mrs. Cook must:
   1. Wear gloves
   2. Wear a mask
   3. Wear mask, gown, and gloves
   4. Wear gown and gloves
7. Mrs. Pauly, age 54, has been admitted to the burn unit and placed in isolation for protection against pathogenic microorganisms. This type of isolation indicates health care personnel should wear:
   1. Gown, gloves, and mask
   2. Mask only
   3. Gloves and gown
   4. Gloves and mask
8. At Great Plains Regional Medical Center Mr. McGee, age 36, diagnosed with hepatitis A, has been placed on enteric precautions. Mr. McGee has a perineal wound that is being treated with normal saline irrigations bid. Which of the following is the correct way to dispose of the contaminated articles?
   1. Place with soiled linens in a clear plastic bag
   2. Double bag and appropriately discard
   3. Single bag and place in utility room
   4. Leave in the patient's room
9. Ms. Myers, LVN, is caring for several patients in different category-specific isolation situations. Which of the following would require gloves to be worn?
   1. Direct contact with blood or body fluids
   2. When infection is spread through fecal matter
   3. When in contact with wound drainage
   4. All the above
10. Mr. Peeks, age 45, was admitted to the hospital with cellulitis of the right foot. Three days later he developed bacterial pneumonia. This type of an infection is classified as:
    1. Acute primary
    2. Nosocomial
    3. Interstitial
    4. Mycoplasmic

13

SAFETY

Frances Jean Kelley

KEY TERMS

Centers for Disease Control (CDC)
code
disaster manual
disaster situation
Hazard Communication Act
Omnibus Budget Reconciliation Act (OBRA)
poisoning
RACE
safety reminder device (SRD)
toxicological analysis

LEARNING OBJECTIVES

After reading this chapter, the student should be able to do the following:

- Define the key terms.
- Discuss necessary modifications of the hospital environment for the left-handed patient.
- Summarize safety precautions that can be implemented to prevent falls.
- Relate specific safety considerations to the development level and needs of individuals across the lifespan.
- Identify nursing interventions that are appropriate for individuals across the lifespan to help ensure a safe environment.
- Discuss safety concerns specific to the health care environment.
- Describe safe and appropriate methods for the application of safety reminder devices.
- Discuss nursing interventions that are specific to the patient requiring safety reminder device.
- List the steps to be followed in the event of a fire.
- Discuss the role of the nurse in disaster planning.
- Describe nursing interventions in the event of accidental poisoning.

RELATED TOPICS OF INTEREST

- Documentation (Chapter 6)
- Signs, symptoms, and physical assessment (Chapter 9)
- Comfort, rest, and sleep (Chapter 15)
- Hygiene and care of the patient's environment (Chapter 16)
- Care of the patient with a musculoskeletal disorder (Chapter 26)
- Care of the patient with a neurological disorder (Chapter 35)
- Care of the older adult (Chapter 45)

SAFE ENVIRONMENT

The need for a safe environment is ever present. Concerns range from a focus on the immediate environment of a patient to local and national concerns about the environment in which one lives and works. Such issues as water and air pollution, disposal of waste and toxic materials, safety on the highways, protection of endangered species, and the preservation of forests illustrate general environmental concerns about safety. The hospital environment in terms of overall safety for the patient has traditionally been a primary concern of nursing. Today the focus on a safe hospital environment has expanded with the recognition and identification of potential hazards and threats faced by hospital personnel.

A safe environment implies freedom from injury with focus on helping to prevent falls, electrical injuries, fires, burns, and poisoning. The nurse must be aware of potential safety problems and must know how to report and respond when safety is threatened.

The responsibility for providing and maintaining a safe environment involves the patient, visitors, and members of the health care team. Both protection and education are primary nursing responsibilities, with nurses directly and actively involved in ensuring a safe health care environment. Checking to see that the call light or signal system is working and accessible is an example of how the nurse helps maintain a safe environment.

Left-Handed Patient

The left-handed patient presents a unique challenge to the health care team, especially to the nurse. The typical hospital room environment is set up to accommodate the right-handed patient (see Fig. 16-1). Seldom, if ever, is the patient asked, "Which is your dominant hand?" Patients will struggle and strain to cope by contorting (twisting) the body, which creates a "high risk for injury" situation.

The nurse is able to gather baseline data as to the handedness of a patient by asking, "Which hand do you write with?" The nurse would then adjust the patient's environment by placing the bed stand and table to the patient's left. This would allow the water pitcher and glass, tissues, telephone, and wastebasket to be at the patient's left. The call light is also placed near the left hand. The discerning nurse will document in the patient's record the fact that the patient is left handed.

Additional safety features are listed in Box 13-1.

Box 13-1 SAFETY FOR THE LEFT-HANDED PATIENT.

- During personal hygiene, place all bathing articles at the patient's left.
- As back care is performed, allow patient to turn to the right side as the left arm and hand will be stronger to assist in turning over.
- Place the drainage receptacle for the indwelling catheter to patient's left.
- Arrange meal trays by placing all liquids on the left side of the trays.
- When ambulating the left-handed patient, the nurse should walk to the patient's left side.
- Use the patient's right hand and arm for intravenous therapy and injections whenever possible.
- Allow more time for the patient to master skills during patient teaching if the nurse is right handed. The left-handed patient must translate the hand movements to the opposite hand.
- Left-handed nurses need to consider the problems that right-handed patients have with their instructions. Unlike left handers, right handers are not accustomed to making modifications.

Falls

Falls are a common problem, and nurses should be aware of patients who may fall. The very young and older adults are not the only individuals at risk in the health care environment. Individuals who become ill or who are injured are at risk for falls. An unfamiliar environment and the various symptoms and signs associated with the patient's diagnosis may also place the individual at risk. The use of anesthesia, sedatives, or narcotics increases the risk of falling, as does an unstable gait or problems with balance. Various safety precautions can be taken to prevent falls (Box 13-2). Gait belts are an added safety feature in ambulating patients. See Box 13-3 for correct technique in the use of the gait belt.

Infants and Children

Ensuring the safety of the environment of infants and children requires protection of the child and education of the parents. Anticipating injuries assists nurses in individualizing care and teaching. Growth and the acquisition of new motor skills place the child at great risk for injury (see Chapter 43).

For example, most children younger than 6 years of age cannot read labels on cleaning materials or medication containers. All household cleaning items are potentially poisonous when ingested and should be kept out of the reach of children. Young infants in the oral stage of development put almost anything into their mouths, and as infants learn to crawl, electric sockets and cords become a danger. Toddlers and young children should be protected from burns: handles of pots on a stove should be turned away from the child's reach, and bathwater temperature should be carefully monitored. No infant, toddler, or preschool child should be left unattended in a bathtub or pool of water, not even for a moment. Infants and toddlers should be protected from falling out of bed. Side rails must be up at all times. The nurse should always place her hand on the infant or toddler if she must turn to obtain supplies, for example.

Older Adults

Changes associated with aging significantly affect the ability of older adults to protect themselves from injury (see gerontological box on p.218). For example, unsteadiness in gait causes falls. Age-related eye changes may affect the ability to see the height of stairs. Vertigo (dizziness) is often related to a side effect of some medications and to chronic disease conditions (see Chapter 45). Eyeglasses, hearing aids, and assistive devices such as canes should be used by patients with deficits. The nurse should be certain that frail or disoriented older patients are assisted when drinking hot liquids, such as soups, coffee, or tea. These persons are vulnerable to burns from spilled hot liquids. Long, loose clothing and straps from SRDs that might cause tripping should be changed or correctly positioned for safety.

Using the nursing process, nurses can reduce the risk of injury to patients.Patients at risk for injury should be identified. Specific interventions can help ensure a safe environment by removing threats to safety. If safety is threatened, guidelines should be followed to resolve the situation (Table 13-1).

Hospital Environment

The hospital environment itself is a source of potential safety hazards to health care workers. Various biological, chemical, and physical hazards have been identified. The increased use of lasers in the health care setting requires specific precautions in order to keep the environment safe. Laser precautions are necessary as a laser can cause skin and eye injury as well as start a fire if used improperly. As a result, the eyes of the patient and the staff working with the laser must be protected. Specially designed eyewear is worn by personnel when working with laser-based procedures. Because a laser beam generates an enormous amount of energy, dry combustibles in the surgical field could accidentally ignite, posing a threat to the patient and staff. Water and a halon fire extinguisher should be readily available.

Hospital workers are also exposed to blood and body fluids, contaminated needles, radiation, and vaccine-preventable diseases such as rubella and hepatitis B. Immunization programs help protect hospital personnel and, in turn, patients at risk of being infected by hospital personnel. For example, health care facilities require the hepatitis B vaccine for employees who work in high-risk areas. Some schools of nursing also require that students have the hepatitis B vaccine prior to beginning their clinical experiences. Newer IV tubing and accessories are now available that do not require "needles," thus reducing the risks associated with needle

Box 13-2 SAFETY PRECAUTIONS TO PREVENT FALLS

1. Orient patient to the environment to provide familiarity.
2. Place bedside table and overbed table within reach. Ensure that frequently used items, such as the telephone, eyeglasses, or other personal belongings, are easily accessible.
3. Assist patients who have had surgery, who have received narcotics for analgesia, or who have been in bed for an extended period when they get out of bed.
4. Keep environment free of litter because such items as books, magazines, and shoes can cause the patient to trip and fall.
5. Follow facility policies regarding the use of side rails.
6. Keep adjustable beds in the low position except when care is given.
7. If bed is equipped with an alarm, turn on for the restless, disoriented patient.
8. Encourage patients to wear slippers or shoes with low heels when ambulating. Terrycloth slippers with rubber, skid-resistant soles are recommended; loose, poor-fitting soft shoes should be avoided.
9. Wipe or mop up spilled liquids promptly. Personnel and patients should be alert to signs warning of wet or slippery floors.
10. Encourage the use of handrails in the bathrooms and halls.
11. Provide adequate lighting.
12. Demonstrate the proper use of emergency call buttons or cords.
13. Instruct patient to use the call bell for assistance.

Box 13-3 TECHNIQUE FOR USE OF GAIT BELTS

1. Apply gait belt securely around patient's waist.
2. Walk to the side of patient, one arm around waist, hand on belt (walk on strong or unaffected side).
3. Patient can support himself by leaning or holding onto nurse's arm.
4. The nurse should walk with her closest leg just behind the patient's knee.
5. Walk with knees and hips flexed (see Chapter 13, nurse ambulating patient using the gait belt).
6. If patient is weak:
   A. Walk beside bed or heavy furniture.
   B. Use handrail in hallway, if available.
   C. Encourage patient to use furniture or rails.
7. Following ambulation, the gait belt is loosened or removed.
8. Document procedure.

TABLE 13-1 Safety Nursing Diagnosis, Goals, Expected Outcomes, and Interventions

Nursing Diagnosis	Patient Goals/Expected Outcomes	Nursing Interventions
Injury, high risk for r/t disease process, weakness, lack of mental acuity, medications or age.	Patient will demonstrate knowledge and understanding of potential hazards and practice preventative measures or will be protected from injury as necessary during hospitalization.	Assess patient's mental, visual, and auditory acuity (fall assessment). Assess patient's level of consciousness. Assess patient's ability to perform ADLs, exercise, and ambulation. Maintain safe environment; avoid clutter. Orient patient to surroundings. Assess effectiveness of reality orientation. Maintain siderails and bed alarm. Maintain bed in low position. Assist with ADLs as needed. Obtain medication history and administer medications according to agency policy. Document nursing interventions for medications and monitor side effects. Use SRDs as per protocol. Assess respiratory status every 2 hours if the chest SRD is used. Offer fluids every 2 hours while awake unless contraindicated. Offer use of commode, bed pan, or urinal every 2 hours while awake. Release SRDs and exercise extremities every 2 hours. Assess extremities for alteration in peripheral tissue perfusion by: testing capillary refill (blanch response); palpating radial and pedal pulses; assessing for edema, pallor, cyanosis, and coldness of extremities; and eliciting description of extremity sensations from patient (paresthesia) suggesting that nerve compression has disrupted nerve function. Document type of SRD used, including patient response and patient and family teaching about need for SRD. Review use of SRD every 24 hours or when reapplied if temporarily discontinued.

GERONTOLOGICAL CONSIDERATIONS

- Physiological changes in aging increase the need for safety precautions:
  - Changes in vision, including alteration in depth perception, increased sensitivity to glare and decreased visual acuity in dim light, increase the risk of falls because of misperception of visual cues.
  - Changes in hearing, including varying degrees of deafness and tinnitus, increase the risk of injury from hazards in the environment, such as motor vehicle horns, alarms, or even spoken warnings, that are commonly detected by auditory cues.
  - Changes in muscle strength and joint function resulting in slowed reaction time, alteration in gait, and altered sense of balance increase the risk of falls resulting from stumbling.
  - Changes in the cardiovascular system such as anemia, orthostatic hypotension, and heart block increase the risk of falls because of syncope.
  - Changes in the peripheral vascular system can result in loss of sensitivity to heat, cold, or foreign objects, which increases the risk of tissue damage resulting from burns, frostbite, and pressure.
- Older adults take many medications that increase the need for safety precautions. For example, sedatives, hypnotics, and tranquilizers affect the reaction time and increase the risk of injury. Antihypertensives, diuretics and antihistamines increase the risk of orthostatic hypotension, which increases the risk of falls.
- Use of safety reminder devices should be kept to a minimum with older adults and when necessary, the minimal amount of restraint possible should be used. Safety reminder devices reduce mobility and result in a loss of strength that can increase the risk of falls or injury.
- Accidental poisoning is a significant problem in older adults. Visual changes can lead to misreading of labels on medication or other package labels, resulting in overdosage or other complications. In addition, many older adults do not consider over-the-counter medications to be real medicine, so they take them freely and fail to mention them when questioned regarding drug use. Many over-the-counter medications can increase the risk of injury to the older adult by potentiating or interfering with the effects of prescription drugs.

sticks. Needle sticks can be dramatically reduced when the "Do Not Recap" procedure is followed and needles are properly disposed of after use.

The National Institute for Occupational Safety and Health (NIOSH) focuses on safety and issues related to health. Identifying risks associated with the preparation of certain drugs and looking at ways to control exposure during preparation and administration represent efforts by this group to ensure a safe health care environment. The Occupational Safety and Health Administration's (OSHA) **Hazard Communication Act** requires hospitals to inform employees about the presence of or potential for harmful exposures and how to reduce the risk of exposure. The **Centers for Disease Control (CDC)** (a federal agency that provides facilities and services for the investigation, identification, prevention, and control of disease) also provides guidelines for working with infected patients (e.g., universal precautions). The nurse should request information and follow recommended guidelines for reducing exposure to hazards in the hospital environment.

SKILL 13-1: APPLYING SAFETY REMINDER DEVICES

Guidelines

A **safety reminder device (SRD)** is defined as any one of numerous devices used to immobilize a patient. The most common type of SRD is the soft restraint. This is often referred to as a *Posey* restraint after the company that manufactures this type of restraint.

SRDs are used for various reasons. Patient safety is the primary consideration. These devices are used to maintain treatment (e.g., the wrist SRD prevents patients from removing intravenous lines, feeding tubes, or drainage tubes). SRDs also prevent the disoriented patient from wandering and prevent or reduce the risk of the patient falling from a bed, chair, or wheelchair. Movement of an aggressive patient may also be restricted to protect other patients and staff from harm.

The use of SRDs is widespread in North America: they are used on 7% to 10% of the hospital population. Certain patient populations, such as the older adult and the disoriented, are more likely to need SRDs. Today ethical and legal issues surround their use. There is a focus on using alternative strategies before SRDs are applied. Individual patient needs, characteristics of the environment, and organizational changes should be assessed when interventions are planned to decrease SRD use. Patient safety or the safety of others should be the priority reason an SRD is applied.

The use of SRDs can also result in increased restlessness, disorientation, agitation, anxiety, and a feeling of powerlessness. It also contributes to patient immobility and the problems associated with immobility such as dehydration, nosocomial infection, and incontinence. The disuse of body parts can increase disability and lead to further patient weakness and unsteadiness. Patients often pull against the SRDs, causing skin and circulation problems.

Documentation about the need for the SRDs, the type of device used, and patient response is crucial. A comprehensive assessment focusing on the patient's behavior, activity, and skin condition is necessary. All nursing interventions, including patient and family teaching about the SRDs, must be noted.

Recent legislation has greatly affected the use of SRDs in the long-term facility. Under the **Omnibus Budget Reconciliation Act (OBRA)** of 1987, residents' rights are specifically addressed in terms of SRDs. This act, effective October 1, 1990, mandates specific guidelines and prohibits routine use of SRDs in nursing homes. The act regulates the use of extremity SRDs, hand mitts, safety vests, and wheelchair safety bars. SRDs may be used only to ensure the physical safety of the resident or other residents. There must be a written order by the physician detailing the duration and circumstances under which the SRDs are to be used.

Most health care facilities have specific policies and procedures related to the use of SRDs. Most facilities require a specific order from a physician. The nurse should be familiar with the policies regarding the application of SRDs. They should be used judiciously and with kindness. The nurse should explain to the patient the need for the devices even if the patient does not seem to understand the explanation. Family members should also be informed about the need for SRDs. Information about the specific device used and the approximate period for use should be shared. If the nurse has any questions, the supervisor should be consulted.

Purposes

The nurse, usually in response to a physician's order or facility unit policy, may apply SRDs for the following reasons:

- to promote safety when the patient is in bed or up in a chair or wheelchair
- to prevent injury to the patient and/or others caring for the patient
- to prevent injury or interruption of therapeutic interventions (e.g., dislodging tubes, pulling out IV needle or catheter, or removing a dressing)

Related Knowledge and Skills

Before applying SRDs, the nurse should know the health care facility's policy concerning SRD use and documentation and should understand the following:

- assisting with the collection of subjective and objective data with a focus on assessment of the skin (see Chapters 9 and 25).

Text continued on p. 225.

SKILL 13-1

APPLYING SAFETY REMINDER DEVICES

Nursing action/*rationale*

1. Wash hands *to inhibit spread of microorganisms.*

2. Introduce self *to decrease anxiety level.*

3. Identify patient by identification band *to identify correct patient for procedure.*

4a. Explain procedure *to seek cooperation or assistance from patient and family and to decrease anxiety.*

b. Prepare for procedure by providing privacy and collecting necessary supplies *to organize procedure and decrease anxiety.*

5. Apply appropriate type of SRD:

a. **Wrist** or **ankle** (extremity) SRD designed *to immobilize one or more extremities.*

1) If using Kerlix gauze, make a clove hitch by forming a figure eight and picking up the loops *as the clove hitch does not tighten when pulled.*

2) Place gauze or padding around the extremity *to decrease injury to underlying skin.*

3) Slip the wrist(s) or ankle(s) through loops directly over the padding—if using a commercially made SRD, wrap the padded portion of the device around affected extremity, thread tie through slit in restraint, and fasten to second tie with a secure knot (see illustration).

4) Secure ends of ties to bed frame, NOT SIDE RAILS. *If side rails are lowered with the SRD attached, injury could result* (see illustration).

5) Leave as much slack as possible (1-2 inches) *to provide for movement.*

6) Palpate pulses below the safety reminder device *to ensure that the device is not too tight, thus occluding circulation.*

b. **Elbow SRD**

1) Place SRD (a piece of fabric with slots for the insertion of tongue blades to keep the elbow straight) over the elbow or elbows. *Elbow SRDs are often used with children to prevent elbow flexion so they cannot disturb tubes, catheters, and dressings* (see illustrations).

2) Wrap SRD (s) snugly, tying the SRDs at the top. For small infants, tie or pin SRDs to their shirts *to secure them* (see illustration).

c. **Vest** (may be referred to as wrap jacket or chest SRDs)

1) Apply device over the patient's gown *to protect the skin.*

2) Put vest on patient with V-shaped opening in the front. *If vest is on backward and patient becomes restless, choking could result.*

3) Pull tie at end of vest flap across the chest and slip tie through slit on opposite side of vest.

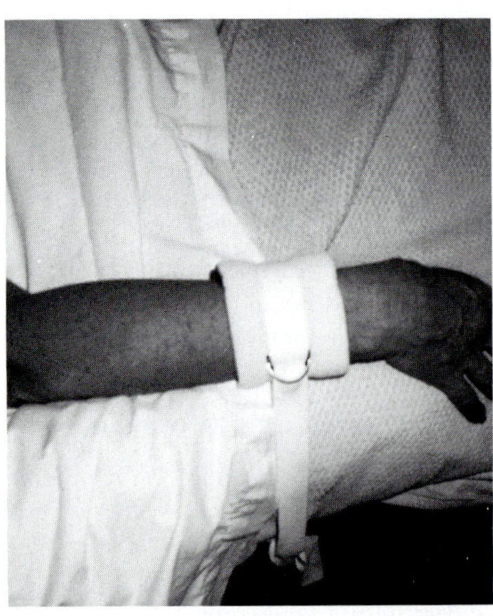

STEP 5a(3)

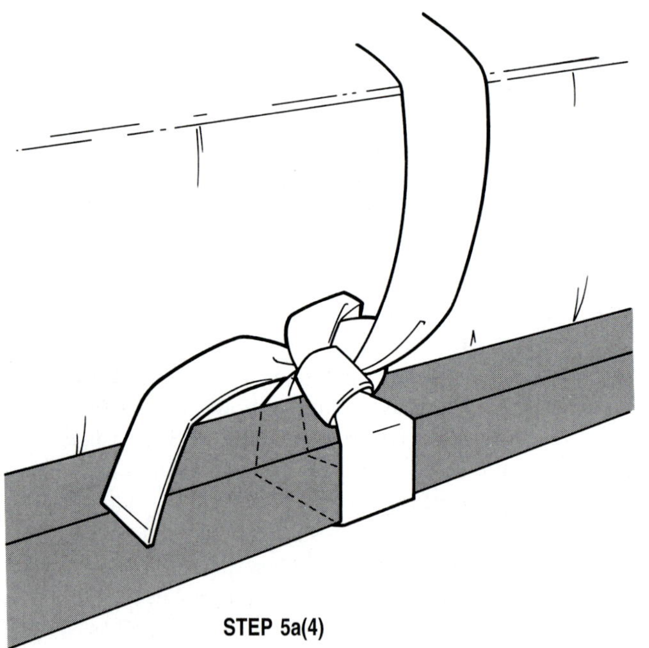

STEP 5a(4)

APPLYING SAFETY REMINDER DEVICES—cont'd

4) Wrap the other end of the flap across patient and tie the straps to frame of bed or behind wheelchair *to help secure vest SRD to the patient* (see illustration).
5) There should be room for a fist in the space between the vest and the patient. *This determines the vest is not too tight.*

d. **Gait or safety reminder belts**
1) Apply belt over the patient's gown *to protect the skin* (see illustration).
2) If patient is ambulating, place belt around the patient's waist. The belt usually has a buckle to secure the belt in place *to provide a snug fit and to prevent slipping.*
3) If the belt does not have a buckle, use a slip knot *to allow for quick removal in case of emergency.*

6. A square knot rather than a regular knot should be used to secure the safety reminder devices to bed frame. *A square knot can be released quickly in an emergency* (see illustration).
7. SRDs should be secured so that the patient cannot untie them *so that injury is prevented.*
8. Apply SRD with gentleness and compassion.
9. Wash hands *to inhibit spread of microorganisms.*

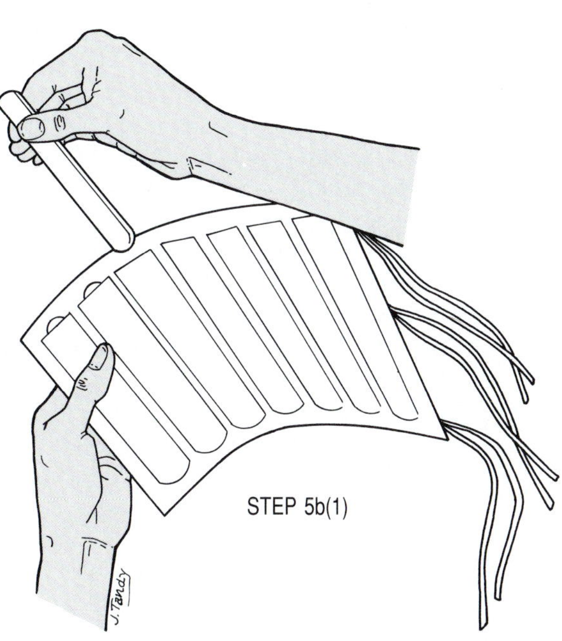

STEP 5b(1)

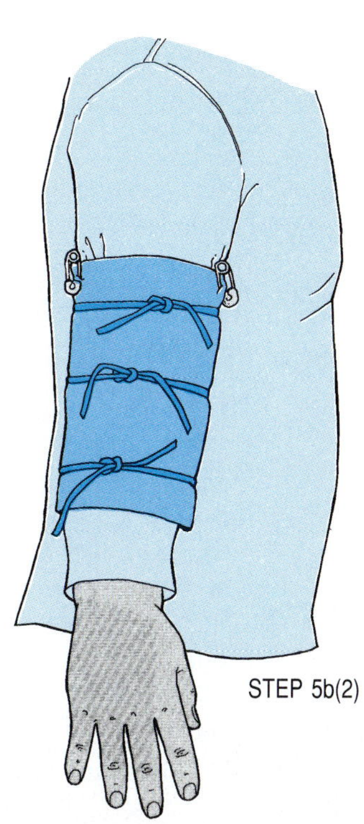

STEP 5b(2)

STEP 5c(4)

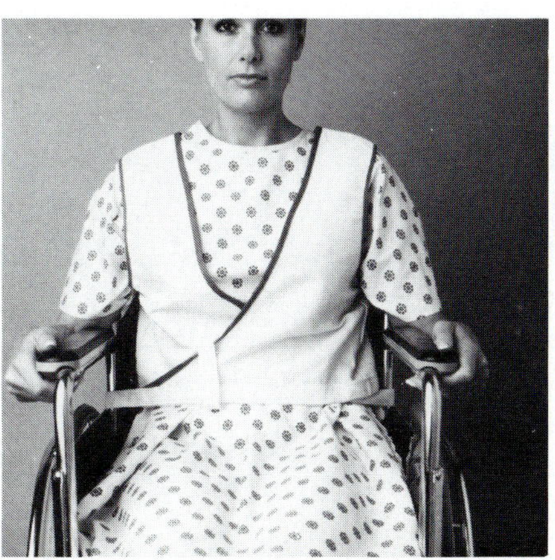

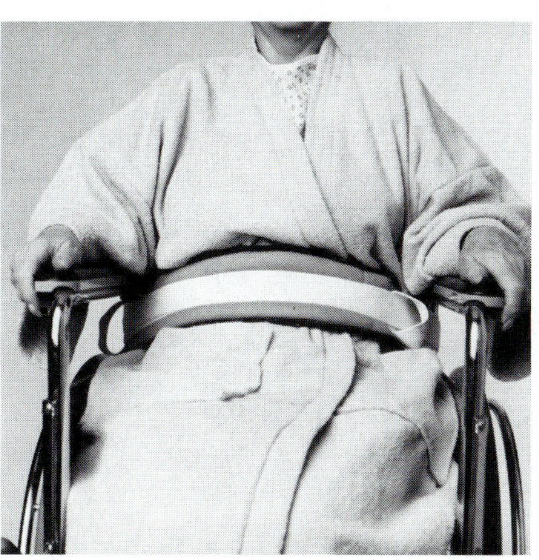

STEP 5d(1)

Continued.

SKILL 13-1

APPLYING SAFETY REMINDER DEVICES—cont'd

10. Document procedure *to note procedure and patient's response.*

11. Documentation should include:
- reason(s) SRD was needed
- if appropriate, the notification of the physician and time order was obtained
- the time and type of SRD applied
- the ongoing assessment and monitoring of the patient's skin, extremity circulation, and mental status
- the responses of the patient
- the periodic removal of the SRD and any skin care performed
- if SRD removed, note time and follow-up assessments
- if reapplication needed, note reasons, time, and patient assessment

Sample charting

Date	Time	Notes
1/4/95	22:30	Restless. Thrashing about in bed. Attempting to get out of bed. Explained to patient danger of falling. Attempts to quiet patient unsuccessful.
	22:45	Dr. D. Bradley notified. Orders to use wrap jacket SRD on patient noted.
	22:55	Wrap jacket applied. Fastened to underside of bed frame. Patient offered no resistance.
	23:15	Quiet. Color pink. Pulse, 82. Fluids offered.
	23:45	Remains quiet. Respirations even and unlabored.

(nurse's signature)

12. Follow-up
a. Monitor for skin impairment *as excessive pressure may lead to loss of skin integrity.*
b. With the use of extremity SRD, assess extremity distal to SRD at least every 2 hours *to identify any problems or need to remove or adjust SRD.*
   1) Remove SRD on one extremity at a time at least every 2 hours (see agency policy) for 5 minutes *to allow supervised movement of extremity, enhance circulation, and reduce apprehension.*
c. Monitor position of SRD, circulation, and skin condition frequently *to ensure patient safety.*
d. With the use of vest SRD, monitor respiratory status *as respiratory distress may occur if there is restriction from the vest.*
e. SRD should be removed at least every 2 hours; patient should NOT be left unattended during this time. *Patient's position can be changed and skin inspected. An unattended patient may be injured.*
f. Massage skin beneath SRD—lotion or powder may be applied. *Massage of the skin increases circulation to area.*
g. SRD should be changed when soiled or wet *to reduce risk of skin impairment and infection.*
h. Check frequently for tangled ties or pressure points from knots; adjust SRD device(s) as needed. *Excess pressure leads to loss of skin integrity and impaired circulation.*

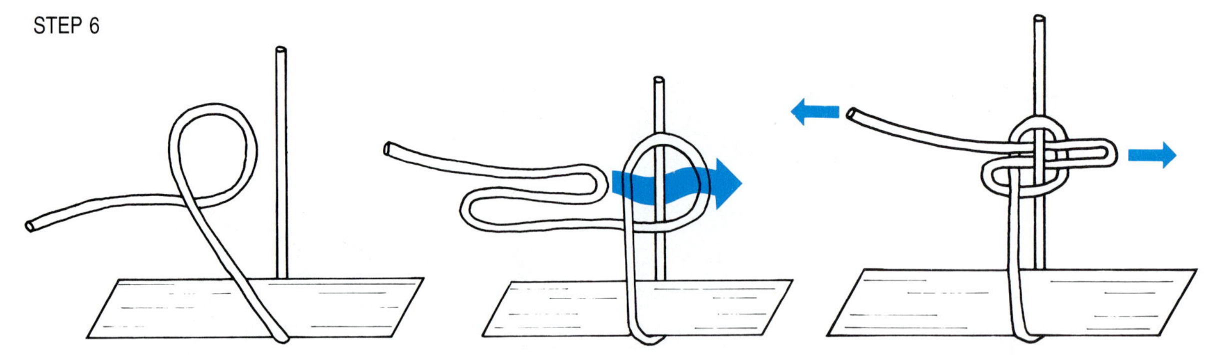

APPLYING SAFETY REMINDER DEVICES—cont'd

i. Monitor and document physical and mental status, circulation, and need for SRD. *SRDs should be removed when they are no longer required.*

j. If SRD use is necessary because of changes in the patient's condition, document the changes and efforts to calm or safeguard the patient without SRD use.

k. Assess for any related problems, i.e., to the skin or to the musculoskeletal system. *Complications can be prevented with timely intervention.*

13. Evaluation

a. The SRD is adequate and appropriate for the individual patient's condition *to prevent interruption of treatment or therapy and/or prevent patient from falling from bed, chair, or wheelchair.*

b. SRDs are correctly applied *as correct application prevents injury to the patient.*

c. Tied knots are easily released *to ensure quick access to the patient.*

d. Related problems, i.e., to the skin or to the musculoskeletal system, are identified *so complications can be prevented with timely interventions.*

SPECIAL CONCERNS

The nurse should know agency policy and procedures for the use and monitoring of SRD.

Select the least restrictive device that will keep the patient *safe.*

- A physician's order is usually required before SRDs are applied.
- Some facilities may have specific requirements for SRD use in certain situations (e.g., the presence of an endotracheal tube).
- Older adults' skin is frequently very thin and fragile. Skin impairment can result also because of a decreased sensitivity to pressure. The older adult should be restrained loosely with soft SRDs. The skin should be assessed more frequently, at least every hour.
- A comprehensive nursing assessment of the patient's potential for injury and/or treatment-related need for SRDs is critical before SRDs are supplied.
- The use of SRDs increases the need for observation and ongoing assessment.
- While SRDs are in use, the patient will need assistance with activities of daily living.
- Restraining a patient without a physician's order or without a reasonable cause could result in being charged with false imprisonment.

PATIENT TEACHING

- Explain to the patient and members of the family why SRDs are necessary.
- Provide information about the type of SRD to be used and approximate time frame for use.
- Inform patient and family that patient will still receive comfort measures such as repositioning and limb exercises.

NURSING HOME VARIATIONS

Recent legislation has greatly affected the use of SRDs in the long-term facility. Under the Omnibus Budget Reconciliation Act (OBRA) of 1987, resident rights are specifically addressed in terms of restraint use. SRDs may be used only to ensure the physical safety of the resident or other residents. There must be a written order by the physician detailing the duration and circumstances under which the SRDs are to be used.

SKILL 13-2

FIRE SAFETY

Nursing action/*rationale*

1. Wash hands *to inhibit spread of microorganisms.*
2. Introduce self *to decrease anxiety level.*
3. Identify patient by identification band *to identify correct patient for procedure.*
4. Explain procedure *to seek cooperation or assistance from patient and family and to decrease anxiety.*
5. Follow facility fire plan in the event of a fire. *Fire plan outlines procedures to follow.*
   a. Identify patient's age, sensory impairments, level of mobility, ability to comprehend instructions, and overall need for protection *to protect and assist patient in interpreting environmental stimuli relevant to safety.*
   b. Identify type of fire extinguisher needed. *The appropriate fire extinguisher must be used for each type of fire.*
   c. If indicated, assess patients for type of evacuation assistance needed. *Individuals at risk for injury must be moved to a safer area.*
   d. Provide clear explanations to patients and visitors in a calm manner. *Anxiety hinders understanding of situation and ability to follow instructions.*
   e. Assist with evacuations if needed:
      1) Usually patients are moved horizontally, i.e., out of rooms, across halls, and through next set of fire doors. *The fire and its potential for spreading may necessitate movement to a safer area.*
      2) If smoke or fire prevents the nurse from moving patients across the floor, proceed vertically down to a lower level. *Never use elevators to escape.*
      3) If a patient cannot walk or be moved by bed, stretcher, or wheelchair from the fire area, the patient may need to be carried. *Use the carrying method that is safe for both the nurse and the patient; fire department personnel can help with the evacuation.*
6. Follow-up
   a. Listen to the all-clear announcement after a drill or follow specific instructions from the fire department and/or supervisor regarding the return of patients. *The area is safe for patients and staff.*
   b. Reduce the potential for fire-related injuries by:
      1) Knowing the location of fire alarm boxes and fire extinguishers.
      2) Knowing the location of the fire exits.
      3) Being familiar with the hospital fire safety program and protocols for evacuation.
      4) Keeping hallways free of unnecessary supplies, furniture, and other obstacles.
      5) Checking to see that electrical equipment is operating safely. *Planning saves valuable time and improves overall performance.*
   c. Participate, when possible, in fire drills. *Drills are helpful in evaluating the overall fire safety program and are required by accrediting agencies.*
7. Evaluation
   a. The immediate environment of the patient is safe from potential fire hazards. *Fire safety practices can help prevent fires.*
   b. In the event of a fire, established protocols are followed. *The emergency can be handled rapidly and appropriately.*

SPECIAL CONCERNS

- Certain areas of the health care facility require additional fire safety programs and precautions. For example, fires and smoke inhalation are potential problems associated with the use of lasers in surgery and with oxygen therapy.
- Other common ignition sources in the operating area are electric cautery equipment and high-intensity light cords.
- In the event of a fire, patients on life support systems may need manual respiratory support with an Ambu bag.
- Fire safety education programs are necessary to meet the requirements of accrediting agencies, such as the Joint Commission on Accreditation of Healthcare Organizations.
- Learning experiences are provided through participation in fire drills and formal critiques of the activity.
- Many facilities are adopting a *No Smoking* policy to promote a smoke-free environment for patients and employees.

FIRE SAFETY—cont'd

PATIENT TEACHING

- The nurse should use the fire drill procedure as an opportunity to talk about fire safety.

HOME HEALTH VARIATIONS

Today, as more patients are discharged with follow-up care in the home, the nurse has an excellent opportunity to evaluate fire safety practices in the home environment. Patients who are elderly or patients with mobility limitations may require the assistance of the nurse to help achieve an environment that is free of potential fire hazards. Instructions should be given about the proper use of monitoring or therapy equipment used. Several electrical circuits should be used to prevent overloading. Electrical appliances and equipment should not be used near sinks, bathtubs, or showers.

Smoking practices should be reviewed, with instructions to not smoke in bed or when sleepy. Smoking by the patient, family, or visitors should not be permitted in areas where oxygen is used. The installation of fire alarms and detectors should be encouraged, as well as the purchase of a portable fire extinguisher. The family should be involved in planning fire escape routes from each room and should practice exit drills.

SKILL 13-2: ENSURING FIRE SAFETY

Guidelines

Both the home and the health care facility are at risk for fires. Fires in the health care facility are often related to smoking in bed or faulty electrical equipment. Approximately 8100 hospital fires and 4300 nursing home fires are reported each year.

An established fire safety program is mandatory for all health care facilities. Most facilities have a safety committee that is actively involved in establishing and monitoring prevention and fire education programs. Fire prevention includes good housekeeping, maintenance, and employee discipline.

The housekeeping responsibilities include the elimination of all unnecessary combustible material; maintenance responsibilities include ensuring the proper functioning of fire protection devices, such as alarms, extinguishers, and sprinklers. Cooking and laundry equipment, filters, and ducts should be kept free of lint and grease. All mechanical and electrical equipment must be regularly inspected and maintained to minimize fire hazards.

All employees should know the telephone number and procedure for reporting a fire, as well as the location of the nearest alarms and firefighting equipment. Additionally, health care workers must know their roles in the overall hospital evacuation plan. Checking for fire hazards should be ongoing.

An important element in any fire safety program is knowing what type of fire extinguisher to use on different types of fires.

Paper, wood, and cloth fires require a type A fire extinguisher.

Flammable liquid fires, such as those caused by grease and anesthetics, require a type B fire extinguisher.

Electrical fires require a type C fire extinguisher.

Fire extinguishers marked ABC can be used on any type of fire. Knowing which type of extinguisher is on the unit *before* a fire occurs is vital. Most fire safety programs afford health care workers the opportunity to handle the different types of fire extinguishers.

In the event of fire, patients in *immediate* danger should be rescued and then the facility's procedure should be followed for activating the fire alarm and reporting the location and extent of the fire. Measures should then be taken to contain or extinguish the fire if there is no immediate threat to safety. Measures to contain or extinguish the fire include closing doors and windows, turning off oxygen and electrical equipment, and using the appropriate fire extinguisher. By remembering the formula **RACE** (**R**escue patients, sound the **A**larm, **C**onfine the fire, and **E**xtinguish or **E**vacuate), nurses can be prepared when safety is threatened by fire.

Enforcing the facility's smoking policy and monitoring for potential electrical hazards help *prevent* fires. For example, frayed or broken electrical cords or a faulty piece of equipment should not be used. The maintenance department should be notified of any defects in the equipment. Any shocks felt while using equipment must be reported. *No Smoking* rules must be monitored carefully, especially with patients receiving oxygen. The safety of patients and staff depends on the staff's knowledge of fire prevention guidelines and fire procedures.

SKILL 13-3 DISASTER PLANNING

Nursing action/*rationale*

1. Wash hands *to inhibit spread of microorganisms.*
2. Introduce self *to decrease anxiety level.*
3. Identify patient by identification band *to identify correct patient for procedure.*
4. Explain procedure *to seek cooperation or assistance from patient and family and to decrease anxiety.*
5. Follow facility disaster plan in the event of a disaster. *Disaster plan outlines procedures to follow and is most effective when personnel respond appropriately.*
   a. Identify the type of disaster emergency by recognizing the code that is used to announce the specified disaster. *Unfamiliarity with the codes could result in loss of valuable time and cause injury to patients and/or personnel.*
   b. Identify patient's age, sensory impairments, level of mobility, ability to comprehend instructions, and overall need for protection *to protect and assist patient in interpreting environmental stimuli relevant to safety.*
   c. If indicated, assess patients for possible discharge and/or transfer. *Space may be needed for disaster victims.*
   d. Provide clear explanations to patients and visitors in a calm manner. *Anxiety hinders understanding of situation and ability to follow instructions.*
   e. If an actual disaster occurs when off duty, health care personnel should report to the facility. *Additional personnel, e.g., student nurses and clinical faculty, could assist with inpatient care to free staff for more critical disaster victims.*
   f. Assist with "early" discharges and transfers as indicated. *Space may be needed for disaster victims.*
   g. If an internal disaster occurs, assist with planned evacuations as needed. *The disaster may necessitate movement to a safer area.*
6. Follow-up
   a. Listen to the all-clear announcement after a disaster drill. *The drill is over.*
   b. Review facility disaster plan frequently to update knowledge. *Information helps health care workers anticipate role in the event of a disaster.*
   c. Know own particular responsibilities in a disaster emergency. *Valuable time is saved and overall performance improved.*
   d. Participate, when possible, in disaster drills. *Drills are helpful in evaluating the overall safety program and are required by accrediting agencies.*
   e. Participation in a crisis support group is desirable if directly involved in a disaster or a disaster response. Individuals may experience some level of emotional or critical incident stress. *Crisis support teams or groups encourage staff to share thoughts and feelings related to the experience (debriefing).*
7. Evaluation
   a. Compare actual outcomes and performances with disaster-preparedness plan (usually a critique session is held). *Evaluation allows facility to examine whether plan accomplished goals and objectives; necessary changes can be made.*

SPECIAL CONCERNS

- Protection of inpatients, as well as casualties from a disaster, is a top priority.
- The development of the disaster-preparedness plan is an evolving and ongoing process.
- The disaster-preparedness plan must prepare the facility and health care workers for both external and internal disasters.
- Learning experiences are provided through disaster drills and formal critiques of the responses.
- Community agencies and resources are incorporated into the overall plan.

PATIENT TEACHING

The amount of information the patient and family has about the situation (drill, disaster event) will affect their ability to cooperate and participate in any planned or unplanned activity.

DISASTER PLANNING—cont'd

NURSING HOME VARIATIONS

Nursing home residents may also require evacuation and relocation because of an internal disaster situation. The successful nursing home disaster-preparedness plan, like those for hospitals, outlines the sequence of events to be followed. Residents will require some type of identification card. At the designated triage site, nurses will decide where residents will go. Residents may require admission to a hospital or other building, such as a school or church, for temporary shelter and care. The disaster plan must include instructions and guidelines for what is to be done after the relocation is completed. Families and physicians must be notified. A log is usually kept to document events and transfers as they occur.

Purposes

The nurse is knowledgeable of fire safety practices and fire procedures for the following reasons:

- to prevent or decrease the likelihood of fires
- to provide safety and protection for patients, visitors, and health care workers
- to be prepared to respond to a simulated (fire drill) or actual fire

Related Knowledge and Skills

To be prepared to function effectively in preventing fires and in a fire emergency, the nurse should fulfill the following responsibilities:

- periodically review the facility's overall and unit fire emergency procedures, including patient evacuation procedures
- know the location of fire exits
- know the location of fire alarms and fire extinguishers and how to appropriately use them
- participate, when possible, in fire drills to become familiar with the protocols

SKILL 13-3 DISASTER PLANNING

Guidelines

Disaster planning or emergency preparedness enables rescuers to respond effectively and efficiently when confronted with a disaster situation. A **disaster situation** is an uncontrollable, unexpected, psychologically shocking event. The disaster situation is unique and directly affects health care facilities. Examples of natural threats to safety are earthquakes, hurricanes, floods, and tornados. Bombings, arson, riots, and hostage taking represent acts of violence carried out by people.

Factors that affect disaster response include the time of the day; the scope and duration of the triggering event; readiness of the health care facility, personnel, equipment, and procedures; and the extent to which the various community agencies and institutions collaborate with one another. Health care facilities are expected to receive victims and survivors and to assist rescuers.

Disasters are also referred to as *external* or *internal*. The external disaster originates outside the health care facility and results in an influx of casualties brought to the facility. The emergency department is the main focus of activity. There is no immediate safety threat to staff, patients, or hospital property.

The internal disaster represents an extraordinary situation that is brought about by events within the health care facility. The organization's ability to function normally is threatened. The internal disaster often threatens the safety of patients, visitors, staff, and facility property.

Disaster planning represents the means by which health care facilities and personnel meet the responsibilities associated with managing the disaster. The conduction of disaster drills on a routine basis helps ensure that health care personnel respond effectively. Personnel should be familiar with the location and contents of the facility's **disaster manual.** This manual specifies departmental responsibilities, chain of command, callback procedures, assignment procedure, patient evacuation procedure and routes, procedures for the receipt and management of casualties, and policies related to the overall management of supplies and equipment.

Purposes

The nurse is knowledgeable of the health care facility's overall disaster plan for the following reasons:

- to recognize the various **codes** (a system of notification that allows information to be transmitted rapidly) used by the health care facility to alert physicians and hospital personnel to the various emergencies affecting the facility
- to be prepared to respond to a simulated (drill) or actual disaster emergency

SKILL 13-4

ACCIDENTAL POISONING

Nursing action/rationale

1. Wash hands *to inhibit spread of microorganisms.*
2. Introduce self *to decrease anxiety level.*
3. Identify patient by identification band *to identify correct patient for procedure.*
4. Explain procedure *to seek cooperation or assistance from patient and family and to decrease anxiety.*
5. If a poisoning occurs
   a. Obtain an accurate history *to identify possible antidote(s) and method of treatment needed.*
      1) Identify the route (e.g., injected, ingested, inhaled), type, and amount of poisonous substance(s) received.
      2) Determine how long ago it happened.
      3) Obtain a history of allergies, prescribed medications, medical problems, and general state of physical and mental health.

   b. Assess for changes in mental status and the presence of motor and sensory deficits *as incomplete data may result in incorrect identification of patient's health needs.*
   c. Notify the poison control center and/or follow facility protocols. *Treatment guidelines will be furnished.* If instructed to use ipecac syrup to induce vomiting, follow dose instructions (see Chapter 51).
      1) Make sure gag reflex is intact *to reduce risk of aspiration.*
      2) Ipecac syrup should be administered with adequate amounts of fluids. *Ipecac syrup is considered the safest and most effective way to induce emesis.*
      3) If instructed, save emesis; note the presence or absence of such material as pill particles *for* **toxicological analysis** (scientific study of poisons, their detection, and their effect).
      4) Place individual with head turned to side to reduce risk of aspiration.

   d. Do not induce vomiting if poisoning is related to the following substances: household cleaners, lye, furniture polish, grease, or petroleum products *as vomiting can increase risk of internal burns.*
   e. Do not induce vomiting in an unconscious individual *as vomiting increases danger of aspiration.*
6. Wash hands *to inhibit spread of microorganisms.*
7. Document procedure *to note procedure and patient's response.*
8. Follow-up
   a. Continue to monitor vital signs and response to treatment *as ongoing assessment is a part of the treatment.*
   b. Reduce the potential for accidental poisoning by
      (1) being aware of potentially poisonous substances (e.g., drugs, plants, and cleaning solutions)
      (2) informing patients and families about how to handle a poisoning emergency
      (3) ensuring that poisonous substances are labeled, locked, and out of the reach of children. *The risk of accidental poisoning can be greatly reduced. Quick and appropriate action can decrease the effects of the poisoning.*

   c. Know where emergency instructions are located. *The procedures and guidelines for handling the emergency are outlined.*
   d. Know the number of the poison control center and be prepared to provide information about the poison. *The poison control center will provide information needed to treat the patient or offer referral assistance.*

Evaluation

1. The immediate environment is safe from potential poisoning hazards (e.g., poisonous substances are labeled, locked, and properly stored). *Safety practices can reduce the risk of accidental poisoning.*
2. In the event of an accidental poisoning, established protocols are followed. *The emergency is handled rapidly and appropriately.*

SPECIAL CONCERNS

- Drug administration policies and procedures should always be followed. Nurses should have their dosage calculations checked, especially if a mixed or prepared drug is to be infused.
- Nurses should keep informed of new medications and recommended dosages.
- Cleaning solutions and disinfectants should be properly labeled and stored.
- Substances from unmarked containers should never be used.

ACCIDENTAL POISONING—cont'd

- Inform patients and parents about potential sources of poisoning found in the home and appropriate safety precautions (see Box 13-4).
- Inform patients and parents about poison control centers.
- Teach basic interventions to follow in the case of a poisoning.
- Inform that safety items, such as ipecac syrup or stickers with poison center information, should be available for use.
- Teach that to decrease problems associated with taking medication, label medications in print large enough to be seen, write instructions in a clear manner, or use a color-coded calendar or chart and pill holders to assist in proper administration of medications. Instruct to not give medications to others or take medication from others.
- Instruct to keep all medications, both prescribed and over-the-counter, out of the reach of children, to discard medications that do not have labels or medications no longer taken, and to check expiration dates.

Box 13-4 COMMON POISONOUS HOUSEHOLD CHEMICALS

- Alcoholic beverages
- Ammonia
- Antifreeze
- Ant syrup or paste
- Automotive products
- Bathroom bowl cleaner
- Bleach
- Boric acid
- Campho-Phenique
- Charcoal lighter
- Cleaning fluid
- Clinitest tablets
- Cologne
- Copper and brass cleaners
- Corn and wart remover
- Detergents
- Dishwasher detergents
- Disinfectants
- Drain cleaners
- Epoxy glue kit
- Furniture polish
- Garden sprays
- Gasoline
- Gun cleaners
- Hair dyes
- Insecticides
- Iodine
- Iron medications
- Kerosene
- Lighter fluid
- Model cement
- Muriatic acid
- Mushrooms
- Nail polish
- Nail polish remover
- Oven cleaner
- Paint
- Paint remover
- Paint thinner
- Perfume
- Permanent wave solutions
- Pesticides
- Pine oil
- Plants
- Prescription and nonprescription medicines
- Rat poisons
- Rubbing alcohol
- Shaving lotion
- Silver polish
- Snail bait
- Spot removers
- Strychnine
- Sulfuric acid
- Super glue
- Turpentine
- Veterinary products
- Weed killers
- Window wash solvent

From Regional Poison Center Network: *Poisonous household chemicals,* St Louis, 1983, Cardinal Glennon Children's Hospital.

Related Knowledge and Skills

To function effectively in the event of a disaster, the nurse should do the following:

- periodically review the established facility's protocols related to disaster preparedness
- participate, when possible, in disaster drills to become familiar with the protocols

SKILL 13-4: ACCIDENTAL POISONING

Guidelines

Childhood **poisoning** (the condition or physical state produced by the ingestion, injection, inhalation, or exposure of a poisonous [toxic] substance) is one of the major causes of death in children under 5 years of age.

Whaley and Wong[23] note that there are more than 500 toxic substances in the average home. Although legislation passed in the early 1970s required the use of child safety packaging for certain substances, a significant number of accidental poisonings continue to occur. Specific antidotes and treatments are not available for all types of poisons.

The older adult is also at risk. Changes associated with aging interfere with the individual's ability to absorb or excrete drugs. Older adults may "share" drugs with friends or limit their medications because of the expense. Changes in eyesight may lead to an accidental ingestion. If there is any memory impairment, elderly patients may forget when they last took either prescribed or over-the-counter medication.

Hospitalized patients can be at risk for accidental poisoning because there are many poisonous substances in the environment (e.g., cleaning solutions). Drugs, of course, are potentially hazardous if prepared or administered inappropriately. Human carelessness can cause errors. Drug administration procedures should always be followed (see Chapter 21). Staff-development inservice programs that present new drugs or provide updated information on frequently used drugs should be attended when scheduled.

To prevent poisoning, toxic agents should be removed from areas where accidental poisoning could occur. Toxic or poisonous substances should not be removed from their original containers because substances may be incorrectly identified. Poisonous substances should be labeled conspicuously and after use should immediately be stored appropriately.

Poison control centers are valuable sources of information when poisoning is suspected or does occur. Information received from the center can aid in both treatment and referral if needed. Most health care facilities also have posted instructions about how to handle poisoning cases. The nurse should know where these are located. (See Chapter 51.)

Purposes

The nurse is aware of substances and practices that may contribute to accidental poisoning and is knowledgeable of procedures to be followed for the following reasons:

- to prevent or decrease the likelihood of accidental poisoning
- to take appropriate measures in the event of a poisoning

Related Knowledge and Skills

In the event of a poisoning, the nurse should know the following:

- the location of the emergency instructions for handling victims of poisonings

REFERENCES AND SUGGESTED READINGS

1. Bailes BK, Fasano N: The left handed patient: is there a difference? *J Pract Nurs* 9:28, 1986.
2. Ball KA: The basics of laser technology, *Nurs Clin North Am* 25(3):619, 1990.
3. Blakeslee JA, Goldman BD, Papougenis D et al: Making the transition to restraint-free care, *J Gerontol Nurs* 17(2):4, 1991.
4. Brower HT: The alternatives to restraints, *J Gerontol Nurs* 17(2):18, 1991.
5. Cassidy DJ: Involving the staff in fire safety, *Nurs Homes Sen Cit Care* 40(15):15, 1991.
6. Collins HL: Who'd survive a fire on your unit? *RN* 51(7):32, 1988.
7. Cutchins CH: Blueprint for restraint-free care, *Am J Nurs* 91(7):36, 1991.
8. Dinerman N: Disaster preparedness: observations and perspectives, *J Emerg Nurs* 16(4):252, 1990.
9. Eliopoulos C: *Gerontological nursing,* ed 3, Philadelphia, 1992, Lippincott.
10. Farrell J: *Nursing care of the older person,* Philadelphia, 1990, Lippincott.
11. Hayes G, Goodwin T, Miars B: After disaster, *Am J Nurs* 90(2):61, 1990.
12. Jacobson E: New hospital hazards, *Am J Nurs* 90(2):36, 1990.
13. Michelson SA: A laser primer for orthopaedic nurses, *Orthop Nurs* 9(5):57, 1990.
14. Miller DM: Care for the caregivers, *RN* 55(9):58, 1992.
15. Mion LC, Mercurio AT: Methods to reduce restraints: process, outcomes, and future directions, *J Gerontol Nurs* 18(11):5, 1992.
16. *Mosby's medical, nursing, and allied health dictionary,* St Louis, 1994, Mosby.
17. Norris J: Fire safety in the operating room, *Today's OR Nurse* 14(3):8, 1992.
18. Potter PA, Perry AG: *Basic nursing: theory and practice,* ed 2, St Louis, 1991, Mosby.
19. Rader J, Donius M: Leveling off restraints, *Geriatr Nurs* 12(2):71, 1991.
20. Rubin JG: Critical incident stress debriefing: helping the helpers, *J Emerg Nurs* (16)4:255, 1990.
21. Tamamelleo AD: Restraints: a legal catch-22? *RN* 55(4):71, 1992.
22. Timby BK, Lewis LW: *Fundamental skills and concepts in patient care,* ed 5, Philadelphia, 1992, Lippincott.
23. Whaley LF, Wong DL: *Nursing care of infants and children,* ed 4, St Louis, 1991, Mosby.

CHAPTER CHALLENGE

KEY POINTS

- Preventing falls, electrical injuries, fires, burns, and accidental poisoning are key components in maintaining a safe environment.
- Left-handed patients need special considerations to cope in a right-handed hospital environment.
- Infants, young children, older adults, and the ill or injured patient are at risk for falling.
- Patient orientation should include information about the use of the call light and bed controls. Frequently used items should be placed within reach of patients.
- Adjustable beds should be kept in the low position except when care is given.
- Gait belts are an added safety feature for ambulating patients.
- Patient safety or the safety of others should be the priority reason an SRD is applied.
- SRD use can result in increased restlessness, disorientation, agitation, anxiety, and feelings of powerlessness.
- Once physical SRDs are applied to a patient, the position of the device, circulation, physical and mental status, and ongoing need for the device should be documented.
- When extremity SRDs are applied, gauze or padding should be placed around the extremity and the ends of the ties secured to the bed frame, *not* to the side rails.
- SRDs should be removed at least every 2 hours and the skin assessed. During this time the patient should not be left unattended.
- The nurse should be knowledgeable of agency policy and procedures regarding SRDs use and documentation.
- Electrical accidents can be prevented by reporting frayed or broken electrical cords or any shocks felt while using equipment.
- Fire-related injuries can be reduced by knowing the location of exits, fire alarm boxes, and fire extinguishers.
- By remembering the formula *RACE* (Rescue patients, sound the Alarm, Confine the fire, and Extinguish or Evacuate), nurses can be prepared when safety is threatened by a fire.
- Participation in fire and disaster drills helps staff become familiar with established protocols.
- Poison control centers are valuable sources of information when poisoning is suspected or has occurred.
- Several national organizations, such as the Occupational Safety and Health Administration (OSHA), the National Institute for Occupational Safety and Health (NIOSH), and the Centers for Disease Control (CDC), provide guidelines that help reduce safety hazards in the workplace.

STUDY QUESTIONS

1. SRDs are frequently used in the hospital setting to prevent patient injury. Which of the following statements is correct:
   1. SRDs often decrease anxiety because the patient feels safer.
   2. All elderly patients should have some type of SRDs at night.
   3. As much freedom of movement as possible should be allowed when the SRDs are applied.
   4. When used to prevent injury from falling out of bed, the soft SRDs should be tied to the side rail.
2. The initial step taken to protect the patient in the event of a fire is to:
   1. Notify the fire department
   2. Disconnect the oxygen supply
   3. Use any extinguisher on the fire
   4. Remove the patient from the area
3. The nurse is working 7 AM to 3 PM on the adult surgical unit and hears the code announced for an external disaster emergency. Which event best represents this type of situation:
   1. A school bus accident
   2. A bomb threat in the mail room
   3. A hostage-taking event in the emergency room
   4. An electrical fire in the maintenance department
4. Which factor MOST places a child at risk for specific types of injuries:
   1. Sex of the child
   2. Overall health
   3. Educational level
   4. Developmental level
5. An appropriate nursing intervention when caring for a patient requiring the use of safety reminder devices is to:

1. Monitor the skin for signs of impairment
2. Remove the safety reminder devices once every 24 hours
3. Secure the ends of the ties to the side rails
4. Ensure that the safety reminder devices are in place at all times

6. The nurse's assessment of the patient who requires the use of an extremity safety reminder device reveals an edematous extremity. The MOST appropriate nursing action is to:
   1. Elevate the involved extremity
   2. Increase the padding around the extremity
   3. Notify the physician for a different type of safety reminder device
   4. Remove the safety reminder device and watch the patient more closely
7. Type **C** fire extinguishers are required for the following type of fire:
   1. Paper
   2. Cloth
   3. Grease
   4. Electrical
8. Which action indicates the need for further fire safety instruction:
   1. Fire exits and corridors are kept clear
   2. A *No Smoking* sign is posted when oxygen is in use
   3. A heating pad cord is taped when a frayed area is noted
   4. Facility smoking policies are a part of the admission procedure
9. Vomiting would MOST likely be induced if poisoning is related to the ingestion of the following substance(s):
   1. Lye
   2. Petroleum products
   3. Household cleaners
   4. Salicylates, such as aspirin
10. Mr. Gonzales, age 63, is brought to the emergency department for treatment of an accidental poisoning. The first step in the treatment is to:
    1. Induce vomiting
    2. Assess the patient
    3. Place the patient in an upright position
    4. Notify the poison control center

14

BODY MECHANICS

Lora Miller Alley

KEY TERMS

abduct
adduct
alignment
base of support
body mechanics
contracture
dorsal (supine)
dorsal recumbent
dorsiflexion
extension
genupectoral
hyperextension
joint
lithotomy
orthopneic
pronate
prone
ROM
semi-Fowler's
Sims'
supinate
Trendelenburg

LEARNING OBJECTIVES

After reading this chapter, the student should be able to do the following:

- Define the key terms.
- State the principles of body mechanics.
- Explain rationale for using appropriate body mechanics.
- Describe the purposes for properly positioning the patient.
- Demonstrate positioning in Fowler's, supine (dorsal), Sims', side-lying, prone, dorsal recumbent, and lithotomy
- Explain range-of-motion exercises.
- Identify complications caused by inactivity.
- Explain appropriate technique for turning, moving, lifting, and carrying the patient.

RELATED TOPICS OF INTEREST

- Documentation (Chapter 6)
- Signs, symptoms, and physical assessment (Chapter 9)
- Comfort, rest, and sleep (Chapter 15)
- Hygiene and care of the patient's environment (Chapter 16)
- Principles and practice of medication administration (Chapter 21)
- Care of the patient with a musculoskeletal disorder (Chapter 26)
- Care of the patient with a neurological disorder (Chapter 35)
- Care of the older adult (Chapter 45)

GERONTOLOGICAL CONSIDERATIONS

- The skin of older adults is more fragile and susceptible to injury. When moving or transferring older adults, it is essential to avoid pulling them across bed linens because this may cause shearing or tearing of the skin.
- Always support older adults under the joints when moving them in bed. Lifting in any other manner increases the stress on the joint and causes increased pain, particularly if there is some degenerative joint disease.
- Aging can result in loss of flexibility and joint mobility. This may interfere with normal transfer techniques and require modifications to protect patient and nurse.
- Weakness and hypotension are common signs and symptoms noted in an older adult on bed rest. The nurse should proceed slowly and cautiously when ambulating a patient for the first time. The nurse should provide adequate help to ensure patient safety.
- Older adults, particularly those with altered sensory perception, may become fearful when hydraulic lifts are used for transfers.

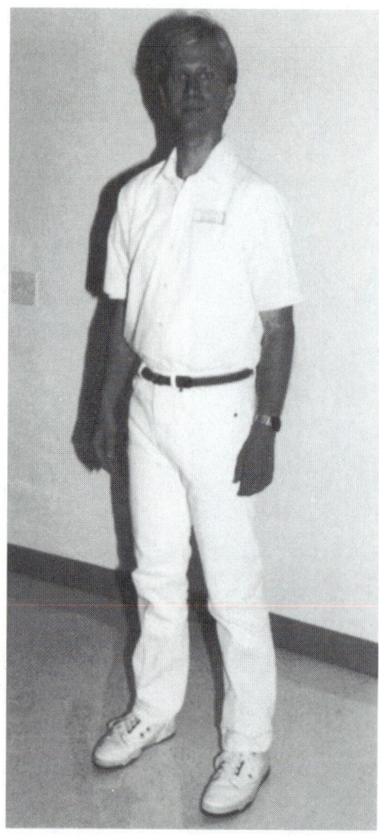

FIG. 14-1 Good position for body mechanics: Chin is high, abdomen is tight, buttocks are tucked in, and feet are spread apart.

Using appropriate body mechanics or movements protects the nurse's large muscle groups from injury and provides safety for patients when they are ambulating. Also the patient must be taught appropriate positioning for home care, and a family member must learn to assist the patient at home. The nurse uses body mechanics daily in making beds, assisting the patient to walk, carrying supplies and equipment, lifting, providing patient care, and carrying out other procedures. Special care should be taken with older adults (see gerontological box).

SKILL 14-1: USING APPROPRIATE BODY MECHANICS

Understanding **body mechanics** (the field of physiology that studies muscular actions and the functions of muscles in maintaining the posture of the body) includes understanding how certain muscle groups are used. The musculoskeletal system must be protected to prevent injury to the patient and nurse. The nurse must learn self-protection and teach the patient to protect himself.

Guidelines

The nurse must maintain a wide **base of support** (a stance with foot slightly apart) when standing. Keeping the feet slightly apart helps provide better stability (Fig. 14-1). This stability prevents becoming overbalanced while carrying out an activity such as assisting the patient in and out of bed or ambulating in the room.

Equilibrium, or balance, is maintained by skeletal muscles and the nervous system and aids appropriate body alignment when lifting, bending, moving, and doing other activities. The back can be well protected when the nurse bends the knees before attempting these activities. If the base of support is widened in the direction of movement, less effort is required to carry out an activity. Standing in front of the object helps avoid twisting the spine.

When stooping, the nurse flexes or bends the hips and knees and maintains appropriate body alignment. The nurse should avoid bending from the waist, since this will, in time, strain the lower back (Fig. 14-2).

Using large muscle groups helps in performing a bigger workload more safely. The more muscle groups used, the more evenly the workload is distributed. The nurse's back is vulnerable to stress and potential injury because of the physical work required in nursing.

Adjusting the working level to one of comfort and ease for the nurse helps prevent undue stress and strain of the back muscles. This can be accomplished by adjusting the height of the bed appropriate to the height of the nurse.

Carrying objects close to the midline of the body (Fig. 14-3), avoiding reaching too far, avoiding lifting

SKILL 14-1

USING APPROPRIATE BODY MECHANICS

Nursing action/*Rationale*

1. Position feet 6 to 8 inches apart *to provide adequate base of support.*
2. Align and balance weight on both feet; *this distributes weight evenly.*
3. Flex knees slightly *to prevent* ***hyperextension*** *(extreme or abnormal stretching).*
4. Tilt pelvis forward by pulling buttocks inward, *which helps straighten the lumbar curve of the spine.*
5. Hold abdomen in and up *to provide support and reduce muscle strain.*
6. Hold chest up *to allow better lung expansion.*
7. Keep head erect *to help maintain appropriate alignment of the spine.*
8. Use appropriate body mechanics in all activities:
   a. standing *to demonstrate appropriate body movement*
   b. sitting *to demonstrate appropriate body movement*
   c. bending *to demonstrate appropriate body movement*
   d. lifting *to demonstrate appropriate body movement*

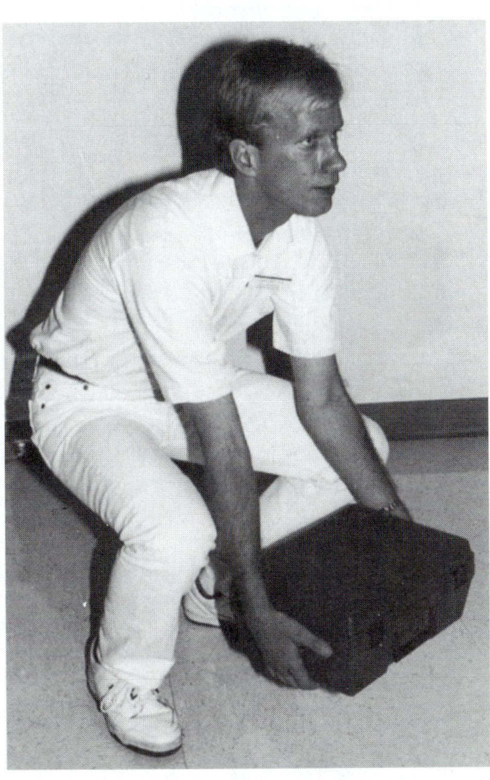

FIG. 14-2 Lifting heavy objects from the floor. Bend at the hips and knees, with the feet apart.

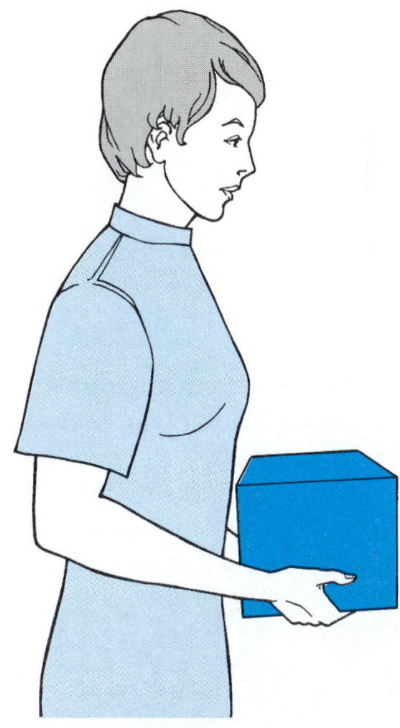

FIG. 14-3 Box carried close to the nurse's body and base of support.

when other means of movement are available, and using alternating periods of rest and activity are ways in which the patient and the nurse can be protected from any injury.

The appropriate use of body mechanics should be practiced daily and used in personal life. Maintaining appropriate body alignment is the key factor in proper body mechanics. The term **alignment** refers to the relationship of various body parts to each other. Alignment helps balance and helps coordinate movements smoothly and effectively.

Purposes

Nurses use appropriate body mechanics for the following reasons:

- to prevent strain and injury to patients
- to prevent strain and injury to nurses
- to use appropriate technique when moving patients
- to provide safety for patients

Supplies/equipment
Chair

POSITIONING PATIENTS

Nursing action/*Rationale*

1. Wash hands *to inhibit spread of microorganisms.*
2. Introduce self *to decrease anxiety level.*
3. Identify patient by identification band *to identify correct patient for procedure.*
4. a. Explain procedure *to seek cooperation from patient and to decrease anxiety.*
   b. Prepare for procedure by providing privacy and collecting necessary supplies *to organize procedure and decrease anxiety.*
5. Position patient:
   a. **Dorsal (supine** [lying horizontally on the back]) (see illustration)
      1) Slide patient and mattress to head of bed, and remove pillow *to ensure appropriate body alignment.*
      2) Lower head of bed unless contraindicated *to provide patient safety.*
      3) Turn patient onto back *to position patient.*
      4) Replace pillow to provide patient comfort
      5) Wash hands to inhibit spread of microorganisms.
      6) Document procedure to note procedure and patient's response.

   b. **Dorsal recumbent** (supine position with patient lying on back, head, and shoulder with extremities moderately flexed, legs may be extended) (see illustration)
      1) Slide patient and mattress to head of bed, to ensure appropriate body alignment and remove pillow.
      2) Lower head of bed unless contraindicated to provide patient safety.
      3) Turn patient onto back to appropriately position patient.
      4) Assist patient to raise legs, bend knees, and allow legs to relax *to position patient in dorsal recumbent.*
      5) *Replace pillow to provide comfort.*
      6) Wash hands *to inhibit spread of microorganisms.*
      7) Document. procedure *to note procedure and patient's response.*

   c. Fowler's (posture assumed by patient when head of bed is raised 45 to 60 degrees) (see illustration)
      1) Slide patient and mattress to head of bed, and remove pillow *to ensure appropriate body alignment.*
      2) Raise head of bed to 45 to 60 degrees *to position appropriately.*
      3) Replace pillow *to provide comfort.*
      4) Raise foot of bed *to help prevent patient from slipping down in bed.*
      5) Wash hands *to inhibit spread of microorganisms.*
      6) Document procedure *to note procedure and patient's response.*

   d. **Semi-Fowler's** (posture assumed by patient when head of bed is raised approximately 30 degrees) (see illustration)
      1) Slide patient and mattress to head of bed and remove pillow *to help ensure appropriate body alignment.*
      2) Raise head of bed to about 30 degrees *to position appropriately.*

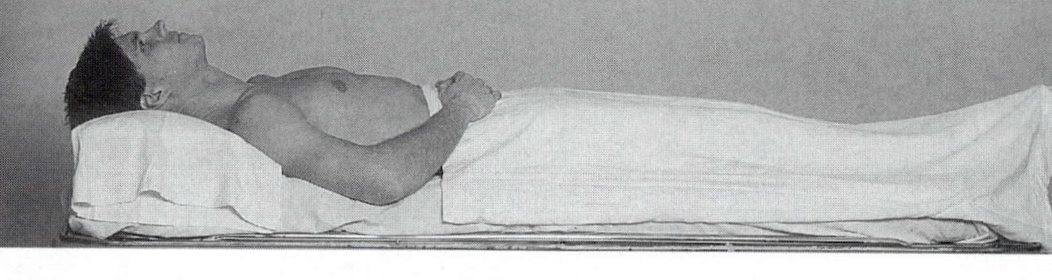

Step 5a

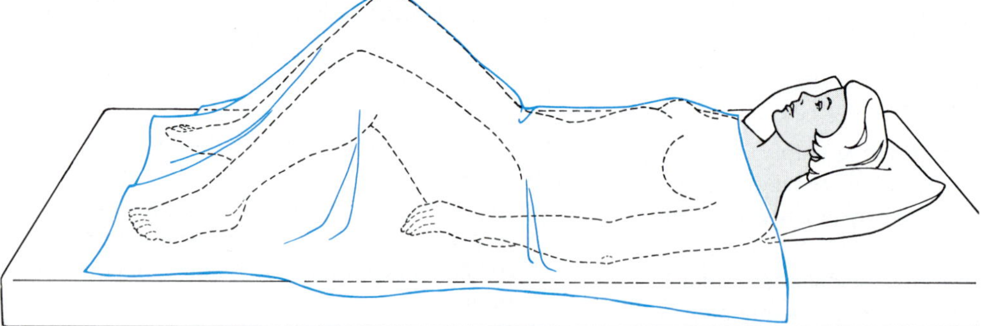

Step 5b

POSITIONING PATIENTS—cont'd

3) Replace pillow *to provide patient comfort.*
4) Slightly raise foot of bed *to prevent patient from slipping in bed.*
5) Wash hands *to inhibit spread of microorganisms.*
6) Document procedure *to note procedure and patient's response.*

e. **Orthopneic** (the posture assumed by the patient sitting up in bed at 90-degree angle, sometimes resting forward supported by pillow on overbed table) (see illustration)
   1) Elevate head of bed to 90 degrees *to facilitate positioning.*
   2) Place pillow between patient's back and mattress *to provide back support.*
   3) Place pillow on over-bed table and assist patient to lean over, placing head on pillow *to facilitate ease of breathing.*
   4) Wash hands *to inhibit spread of microorganisms.*
   5) Document procedure *to note procedure and patient's response.*

f. **Sims'** (position in which patient lies on left side with right knee and thigh drawn upward toward chest) (see illustration)
   1) Turn patient on left side *to initiate position placement.*

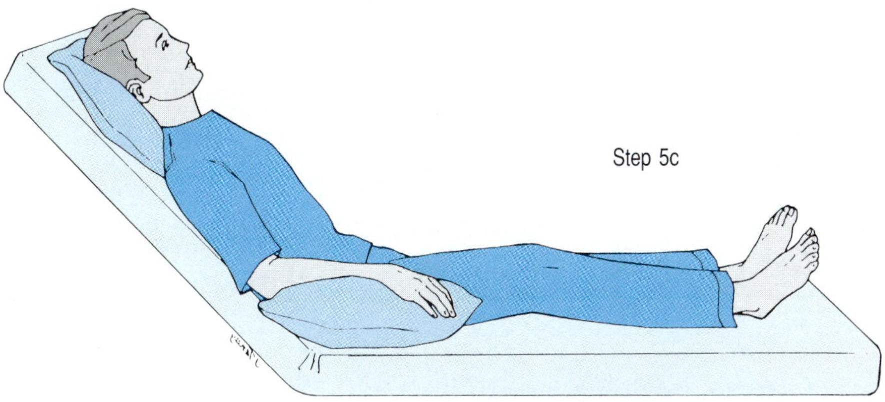

Step 5c

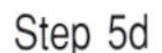

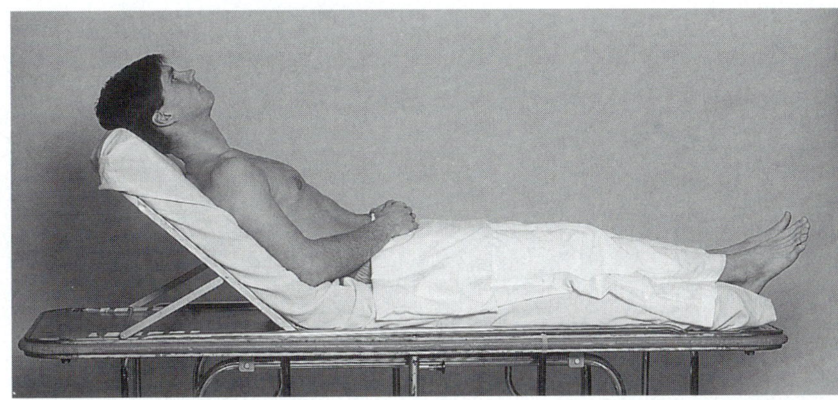

Step 5d

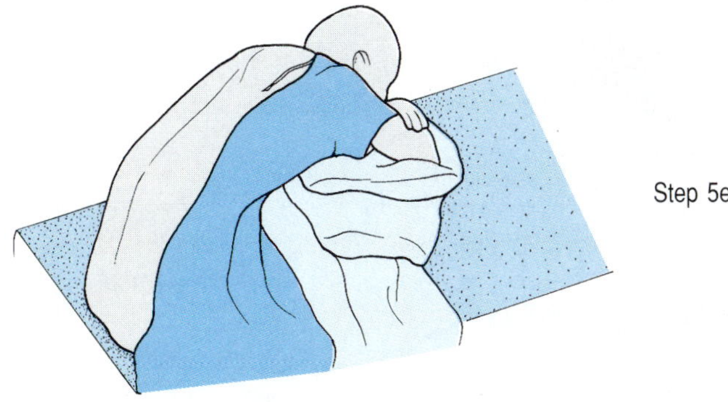

Step 5e

Continued.

POSITIONING PATIENTS—cont'd

2) Draw right knee and thigh up near abdomen *to provide appropriate position for administering enema.*
3) Place patient's left arm along the back *to provide appropriate body alignment.*
4) Bring right arm up and flex elbow and support with pillow *to provide comfort and decrease strain on joints.*
5) Allow patient to lean forward to rest on chest *to provide comfort.*
6) Wash hands *to inhibit spread of microorganisms.*
7) Document procedure *to note procedure and patient's response.*

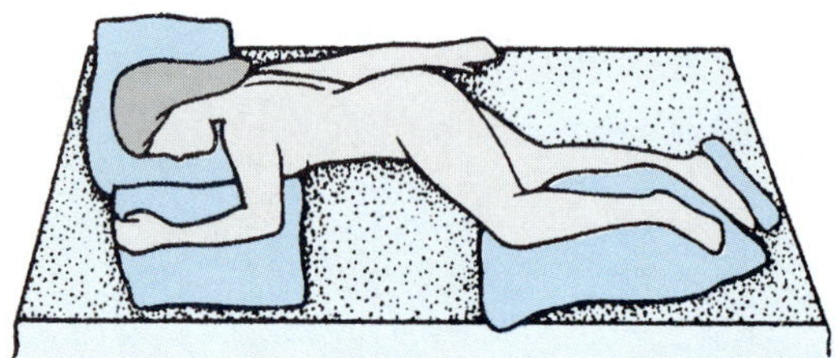

Step 5f

g. **Prone** (being in horizontal position when lying face down) (see illustration)
   1) Assist patient onto abdomen with face to one side *to position patient.*
   2) Flex arms toward the head *to provide appropriate body alignment.*
   3) Wash hands *to inhibit spread of microorganisms.*
   4) Document procedure *to note procedure and patient's response.*

h. Knee-chest **(genupectoral** [patient kneels so that weight of body is supported by knees and chest, with abdomen raised, head turned to one side, and arms flexed) (see illustration)
   1) Turn patient onto abdomen *to facilitate positioning.*
   2) Assist patient to kneeling position; arms and head should rest on pillow while upper chest rests on bed *to complete knee-chest position.*
   3) Wash hands *to inhibit spread of microorganisms.*
   4) Document procedure *to note procedure and patient's response.*

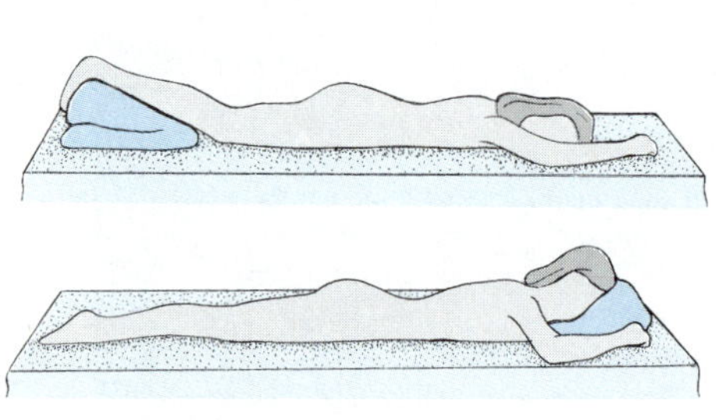

Step 5g

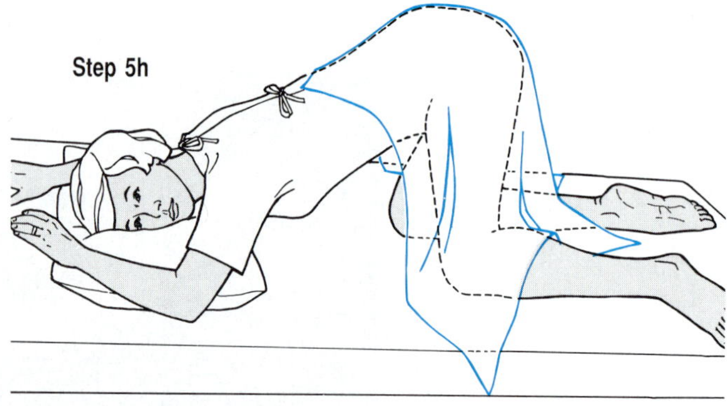

Step 5h

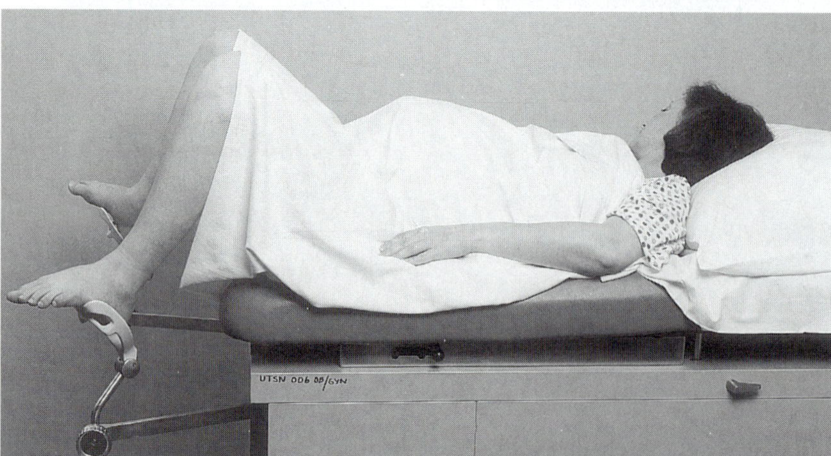

Step 5i

POSITIONING PATIENT'S—cont'd

i. **Lithotomy** (lying supine with hips and knees flexed and thighs abducted and rotated externally) (see illustration)
   1) Request patient to slide buttocks to edge of examinating table *to facilitate positioning.*
   2) Lift both legs, have patient bend knees, and place feet in stirrups *to position patient appropriately.*
   3) Drape patient *to provide privacy and prevent exposure.*
   4) Wash hands *to inhibit spread of microorganisms.*
   5) Document procedure *to note procedure and patient's response.*

6. Record appropriate alignment and position of patient *to provide documentation of patient's safety and response.*

Sample charting

DATE	TIME	NOTES
1/30/95	0900	Placed in semi-Fowler's position in appropriate body alignment. States feels comfortable.

____
(nurse's signature)

Follow-up

1. Make certain patient remains as appropriately positioned to follow-up and provide appropriate patient care.

Evaluation

1. Assess for appropriate body alignment and positioning of patient *to evaluate and determine safety and welfare of patient.*

SPECIAL CONCERNS

- Performing a back massage after turning from one position to another helps prevent impaired skin integrity.
- Appropriate body alignment should be assessed after every change of position.
- Skin of the elderly is often thin and nonelastic and needs special care to prevent tearing and further impaired skin integrity.
- Small children must often be propped with pillows to help them maintain a position.

j. **Trendelenburg** (position in which head is low and body and legs are on inclined plane) (see illustration)
   1) Place patient's head lower than body with body and legs elevated and on an incline (bed may be elevated on blocks) *for performing ainal surgery (not used if patient has a head injury).* Trendelenburg position is not usually used to treat shock because of pressure it causes on diaphragm by organs in the abdomen.
   2) Wash hands *to inhibit spread of microorganisms.*
   3) Document procedure *to note procedure and patient's response.*

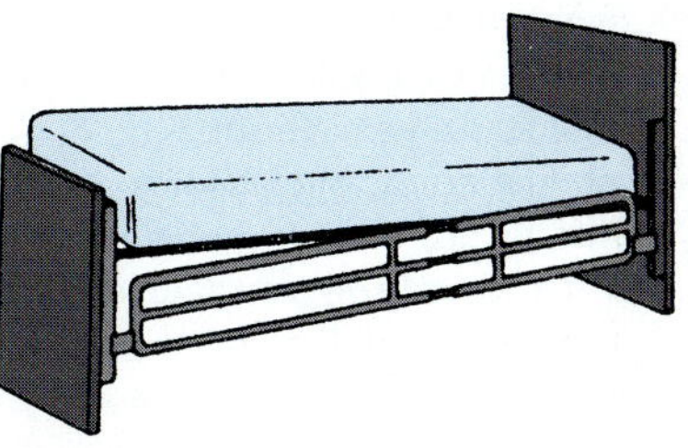

Step 5j

HOME HEALTH VARIATIONS

- Teach family members how to position and maintain body alignment.

PATIENT TEACHING

- Explain the importance of maintaining skin integrity.
- Explain the importance of appropriate body alignment.

SKILL 14-2: POSITIONING PATIENTS

Guidelines

Positioning patients is performed daily by nurses. There are many positions a nurse must learn to prevent patients from developing complications. Permanent disability can occur from inappropriate positioning.

Purposes

Nurses position patients for the following reasons:

- to provide movement for patients
- to prepare a patient for a procedure
- to provide patient comfort

Supplies/equipment

Chair Hospital bed Pillow

TABLE 14-1 Normal ROM

Body Part	Motion	Measurement
Jaw	Open and close jaw.	Able to insert three fingers
	Move jaw side to side.	Bottom side teeth overlapping top side teeth
	Move jaw forward.	Top teeth behind lower teeth
Neck	Touch chin to sternum.	Flexion 70 degrees to 90 degrees
	Extend neck with chin pointing toward ceiling.	Hyperextension 55 degrees
	Bend neck laterally with ear toward shoulder.	Lateral bending 35 degrees
	Rotate neck with ear toward chest.	Rotation 70 degrees to left and right
Spine	Bend forward at the waist.	Flexion 75 degrees
	Bend backward.	Extension 30 degrees
	Bend to each side.	Lateral bending 35 degrees
Shoulder	Abduct arm straight up.	Abduction 180 degrees
	Abduct arm toward midline of trunk.	Adduction 45 degrees
	Abduct arm straight horizontally to floor; bring arm backward toward spine and forward across chest.	Horizontal extension 45 degrees Horizontal flexion 130 degrees
	Flex or elevate forward with arm straight.	Flexion 180 degrees
	Extend backward with arm straight.	Extension 60 degrees
Elbow	Extend lower arm to normal extreme.	Extension 150 degrees
	Flex lower arm toward biceps.	Flexion 150 degrees
	Hyperextend arm beyond normal resting point.	Hyperextension up to 10 degrees
	Supinate lower arm (palm of hand turned up).	Supination 90 degrees
	Pronate lower arm (palm of the hand facing downward and backward).	Pronation 90 degrees
Wrist	Flex wrist toward lower arm.	Flexion 80 degrees to 90 degrees
	Extend wrist backward.	Extension 70 degrees
	Deviate wrist laterally toward radius.	Radial deviation 20 degrees
	Deviate wrist laterally toward ulna.	Ulnar deviation 30 degrees to 50 degrees
Fingers	Flex fingers into fist and then extend them flat.	Flexion 80 degrees to 100 degrees (varies with joint)
	Spread fingers apart.	Extension up to 45 degrees
	Cross fingers together.	Abduction 20 degrees (between fingers)
	Oppose fingers: touch each fingertip with thumb.	Adduction (fingers will touch) Includes abduction and flexion
Hip	Raise leg with knee straight.	Flexion 90 degrees
	Raise leg with knee flexed.	Flexion 110 degrees to 120 degrees
	Lying prone, extend leg straight back.	Extension 30 degrees
	Abduct partially flexed leg outward.	Abduction 45 degrees to 50 degrees
	Adduct partially flexed leg inward.	Adduction 20 degrees to 30 degrees
	Flex knee and swing foot away from midline.	Internal rotation 35 degrees to 40 degrees
	Flex knee and swing foot toward midline.	External rotation 45 degrees
Knee	Flex knee with calf touching thigh.	Flexion 130 degrees
	Extend knee beyond normal point of extension.	Hyperextension 15 degrees
	Rotate knee and lower leg toward midline.	Internal rotation 10 degrees
Ankle	Dorsiflex foot with toes pointing toward head.	Dorsiflexion 20 degrees
	Plantar flex foot with toes pointing down.	Plantar flexion 45 degrees
	Turn foot away from midline.	Eversion 20 degrees
	Turn foot toward midline.	Inversion 30 degrees
Toes	Curl toes under foot.	Flexion 35 degrees to 60 degrees (varies with joints)
	Raise toes to point upward.	Extension up to 90 degrees (varies with joints)
	Spread toes apart.	Varies

PERFORMING RANGE-OF-MOTION EXERCISES

Nursing action/*Rationale*

1. Wash hands *to inhibit spread of microorganisms.*
2. Introduce self *to decrease anxiety level.*
3. Identify patient by identification band *to identify correct patient for procedure.*

4a. Explain procedure *to seek cooperation or assistance from patient and to decrease anxiety.*

b. Prepare for procedure by providing privacy and collecting necessary supplies *to organize procedure and decrease anxiety.*

5. Assist patient in putting each joint through full ROM. (Begin with the head and progress toward the feet, appropriately supporting the body part being exercised [see Table 14-1].)
6. *Neck*—Place palm of each hand against side of patient's face or place one hand under patient's head and one hand on patient's chin.
   a. Bring head forward until chin touches sternum *to flex neck.*
   b. Return head to straight position and have patient look straight ahead *to extend neck.*
   c. Bend head backward with chin pointing toward ceiling *to hyperextend (position of maximum extension) neck.*
   d. Return head to **extension** (movement allowed by certain joints of the skeleton that increases angle between two adjoining bones) position and assist patient to rotate head until ear is toward chest. Turn head

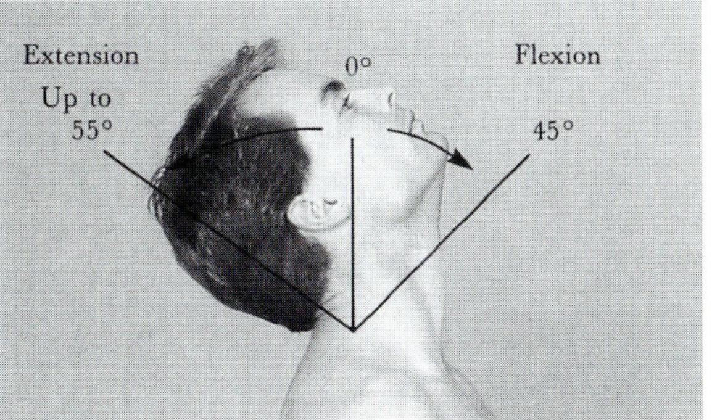

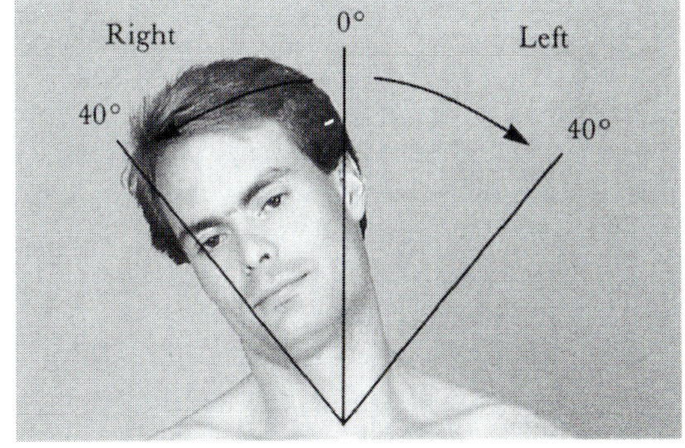

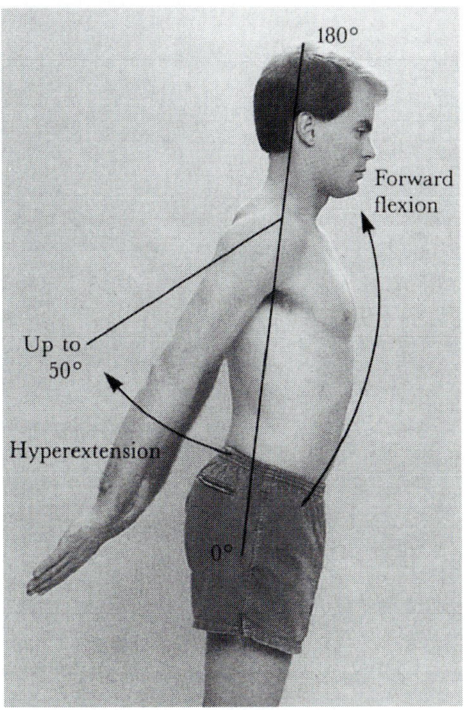

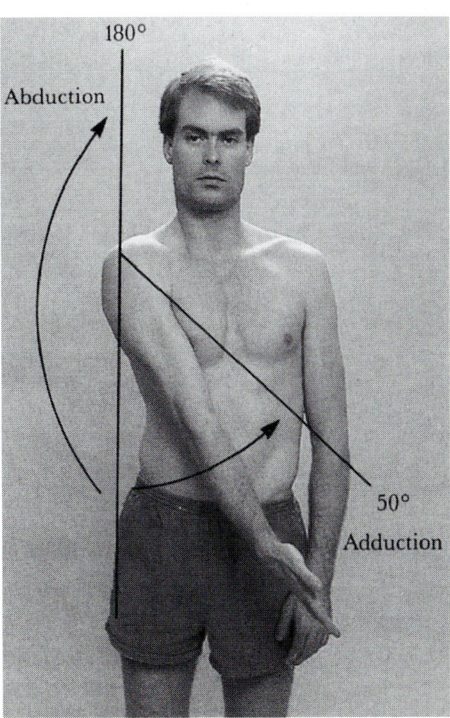

Continued.

PERFORMING RANGE-OF-MOTION EXERCISES—cont'd

until right ear and then left ear are toward chest *to rotate neck.*

e. Return head to extension and bend head laterally with ear toward shoulder, first toward right ear and then left *to laterally flex neck.*

7. Shoulder—Cup one hand beneath elbow and grasp wrist with other hand.

a. Bring arm away from body so that it is level with shoulder *to abduct arm.*

b. Return arm toward side of body *to* ***adduct*** *(movement of limb toward axis of body) arm.*

c. **Abduct** (movement of limb away from body) the arm; continue movement until patient's hand is toward head of bed. *(Bending elbow will avoid striking head of the bed with patient's hand.)*

d. Abduct arm to shoulder level; flex elbow; bring forearm down until palm of hand touches the bed; and swing forearm up until back of hand touches bed *to rotate shoulder.*

8. *Elbow:* Support patient's arm by grasping center of forearm with one hand and just above elbow with other hand. (These exercises may be combined with shoulder exercises.)

a. Bend lower arm toward biceps *to flex elbow.*

b. Straighten lower arm *to extend elbow.*

c. Hold patient's hand as if to shake hands and turn palm upward *to* ***supinate*** *(kind of rotation allowed by certain skeletal joints that allows palm of hand to turn upward).*

d. Continue holding patient's hand and turn palm of hand downward *to* ***pronate.***

9. *Wrist:* Hold wrist joint with one hand and hold palm of patient's hand with other hand.

a. Bend wrist toward lower arm with fingers pointing downward *to flex wrist.*

b. Return wrist to a straight position (in alignment with forearm) *to extend wrist.*

c. Bend wrist with fingers pointing upward toward ceiling *to hyperextend wrist.*

d. Extend wrist and bend it laterally toward radial (thumb) side *to radially deviate.*

e. Extend wrist and bend it laterally toward ulna (little finger) side *to deviate outwardly on side of ulna bone of lower arm.*

10. *Fingers:* Place palm and fingers of one hand directly against back of patient's hand and fingers *to exercise all fingers at one time.*

a. Curve fingers with nurse's fingers to resemble a fist *to flex fingers.*

b. Straighten all fingers *to extend fingers.*

c. Using thumb and index finger of one hand, spread fingers apart by moving each one away from nearest finger *to abduct.*

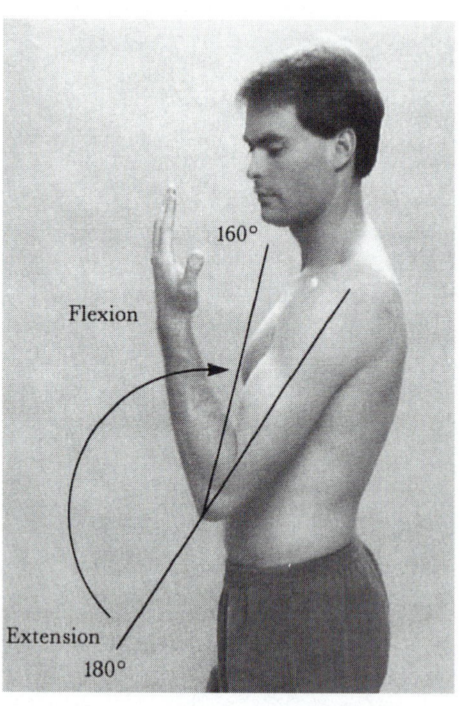

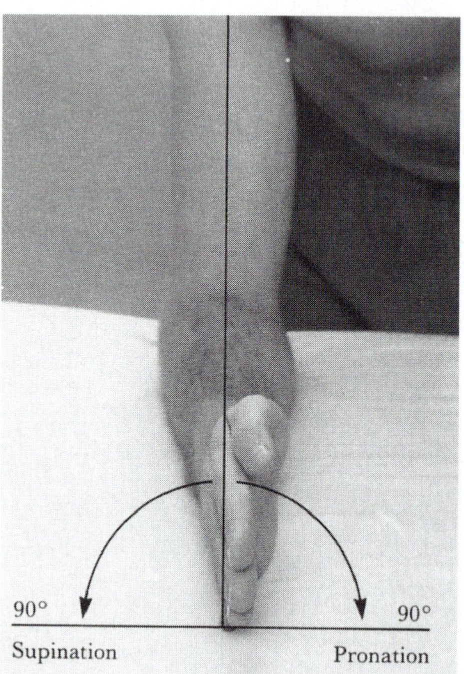

SKILL 14-3

PERFORMING RANGE-OF-MOTION EXERCISES—cont'd

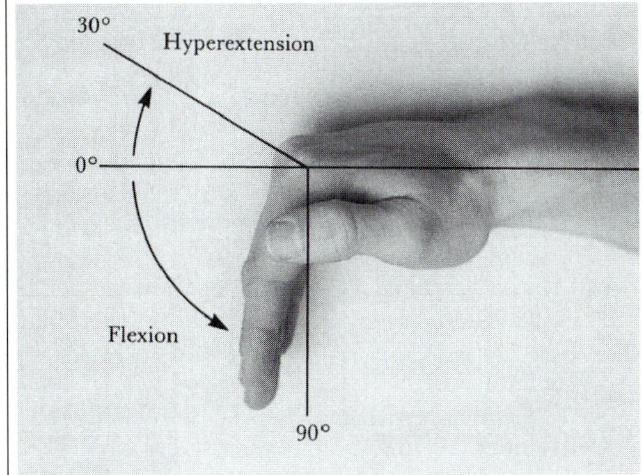

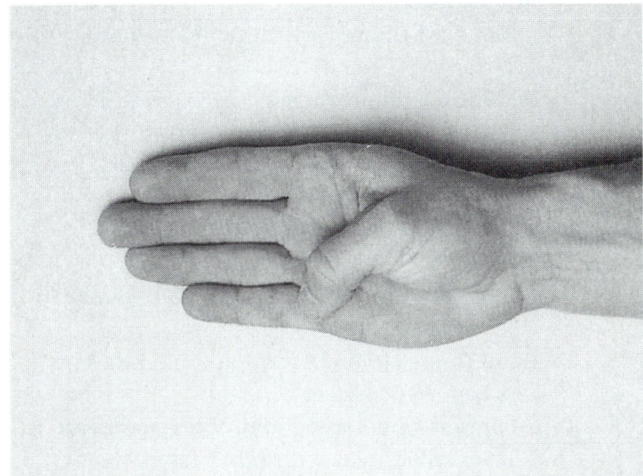

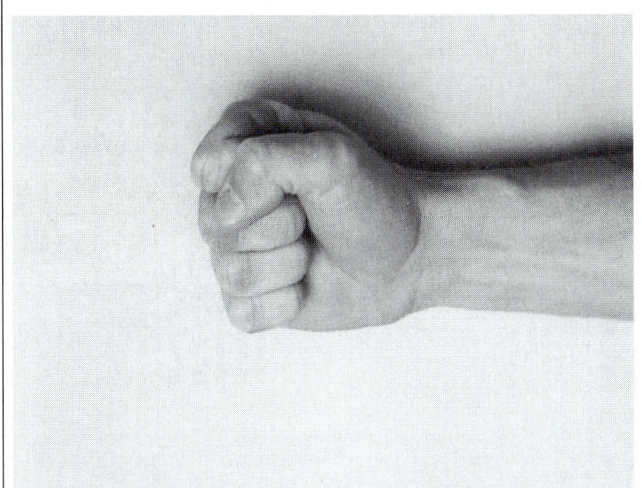

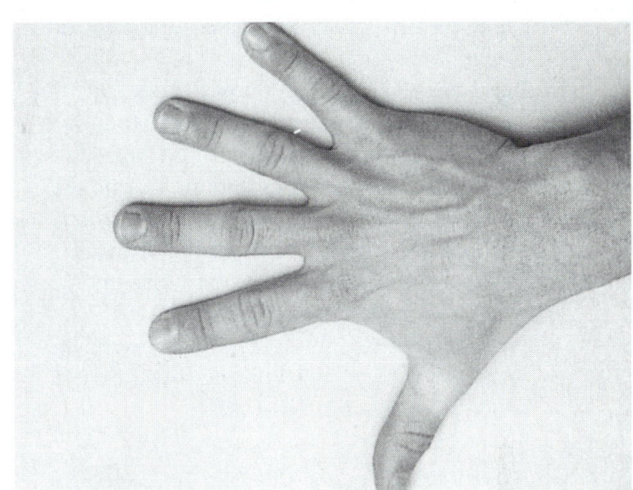

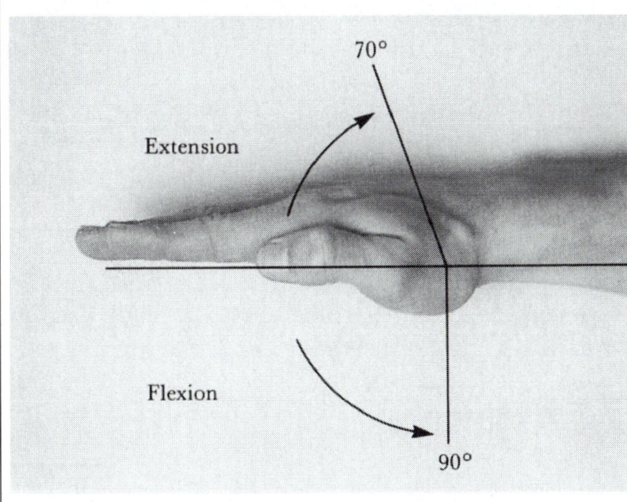

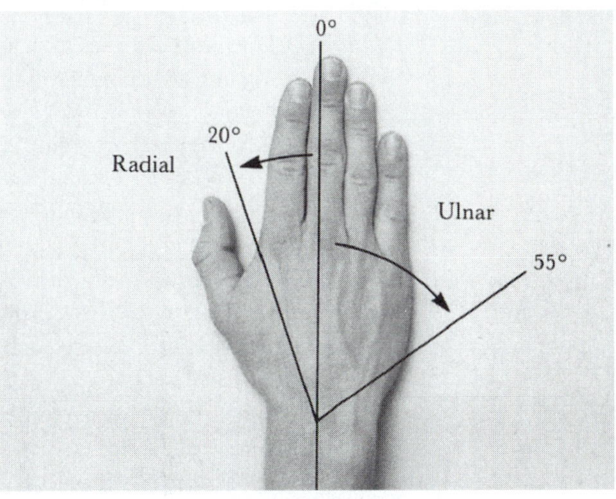

Continued.

SKILL 14-3

PERFORMING RANGE-OF-MOTION EXERCISES—cont'd

   d. Return fingers together until touching each other *to adduct.*

11. *Thumb:* Hold thumb with thumb and index finger.
    a. Manipulate thumb across the palm of hand to touch tip of each finger to tip of thumb *to place thumb in normal functioning position called opposition.*
    b. Move thumb away from index finger *to abduct.*
    c. Return thumb toward index finger *to adduct.*
    d. Bend thumb joint forward and backward *to flex and hyperextend joint.*
12. *Hip:* Support under knee joint with one hand and grasp ankle joint with other hand.
    a. Raise leg with knee straight *to flex 90 degrees.* Return leg to bed in straight position *to extend hip.*
    b. Raise leg and bend knee toward chest to flex to 110 to 120 degrees *to flex hip;* straighten knee and return to bed *to extend hip.*
    c. Move leg out away from midline *to abduct.*
    d. Bring leg back toward other leg *to adduct.*
    e. Position legs straight and roll leg outward (away from other leg), toes pointing outward, *to rotate hip externally.*
    f. Position legs straight and roll leg inward (toward other leg), toes pointing toward each other, *to rotate hip internally.*
13. Knee: Support under knee joint with one hand and grasp ankle joint with other hand. (These exercises may be easily combined with hip exercises.)
    a. Bend knee with calf touching thigh *to flex.*
    b. Straighten knee *to extend joint.*
    c. Extend knee beyond the normal point of extension *to hyperextend knee joint.*
    d. Rotate knee and lower leg toward midline *to internally rotate the knee joint.*
14. Ankle: Grasp heel in the palm of one hand, touching inner aspect of the forearm to sole of foot. Support top of foot just above ankle with other hand.
    a. Gently press against the sole of the foot with inner arm, toes pointing upward *to stretch the Achilles tendon (*__dorsiflexion__ [to bend or flex backward, as in the upward bending of the toes]).
    b. Press on top of foot to point toes downward *to relax Achilles tendon.*
    c. Turn foot away from midline (away from other foot) *to evert (move outward).*
    d. Turn foot inward (toward other foot) *to invert (move inward).*

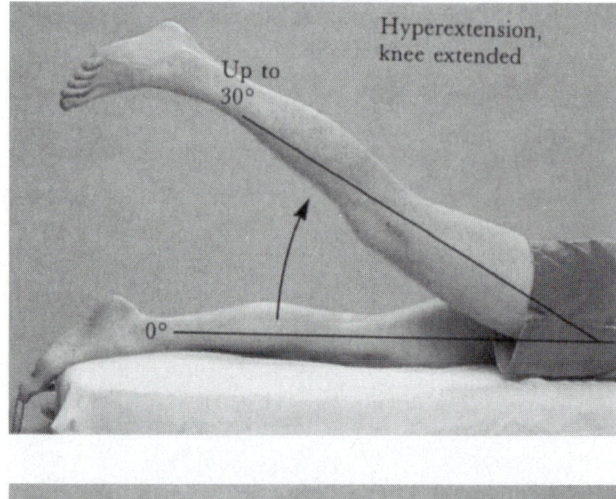

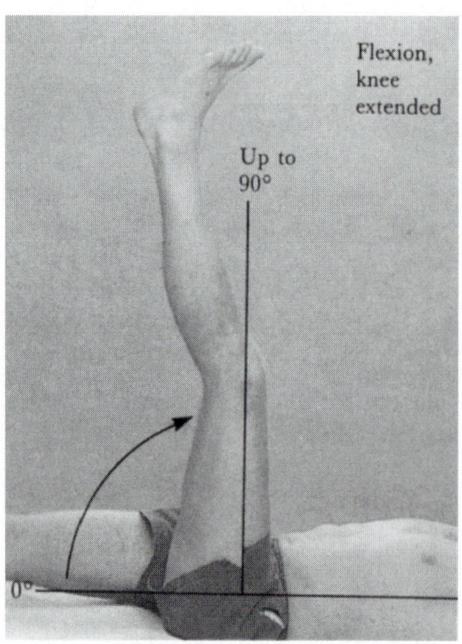

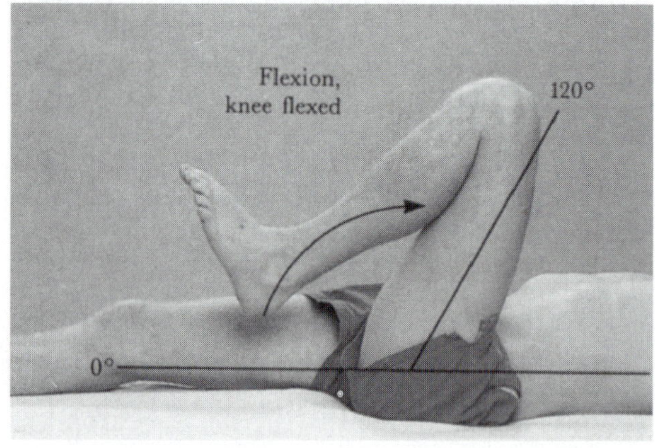

SKILL 14-3

PERFORMING RANGE-OF-MOTION EXERCISES—cont'd

15. Toes: Place fingers over toes *to exercise all appendages at one time.* Support bottom of foot with hand and bottom of toes with other hand.

a. Curl toes downward toward bottom of foot *to flex.*

b. Raise toes to point upward *to extend.*

c. Spread toes apart (away from each other) *to abduct.*

d. Return toes toward each other *to adduct.*

16. Documentation

a. Report and record any abnormal findings *to provide information for patient care.*

b. Report and record normal findings *to provide information of normal patient assessment.*

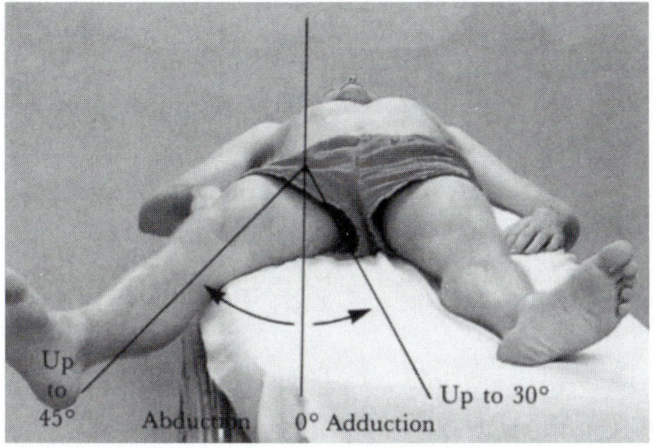

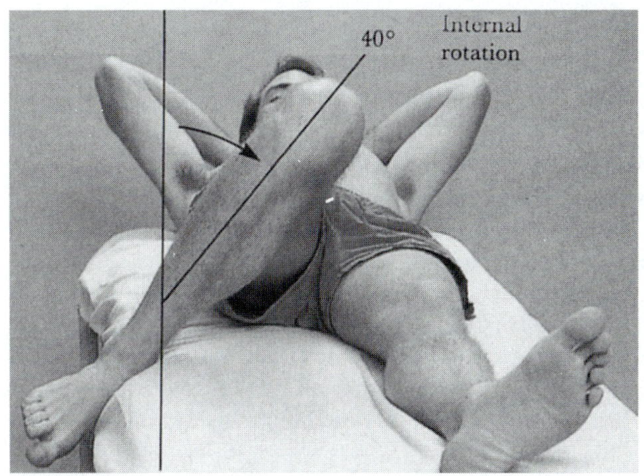

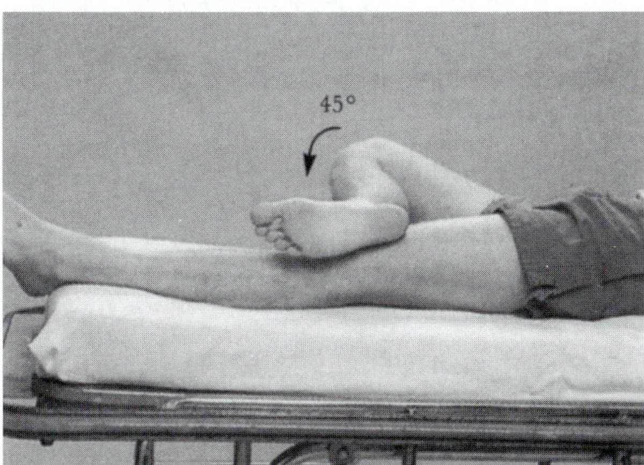

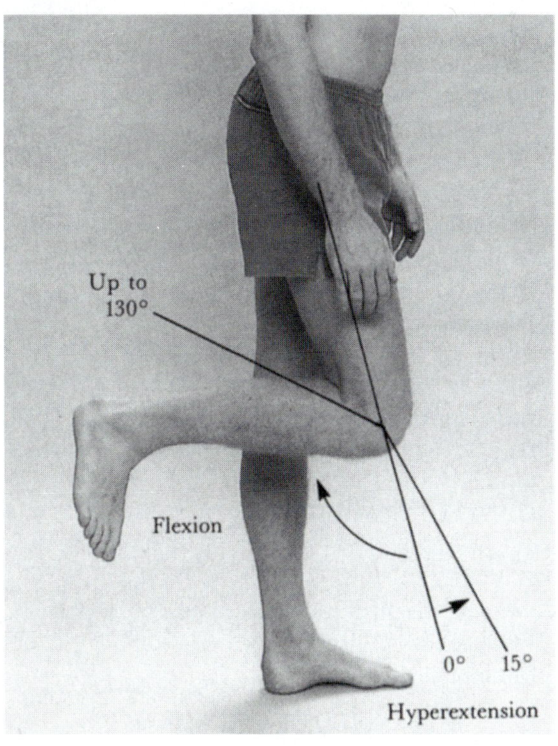

Continued.

PERFORMING RANGE-OF-MOTION EXERCISES—cont'd

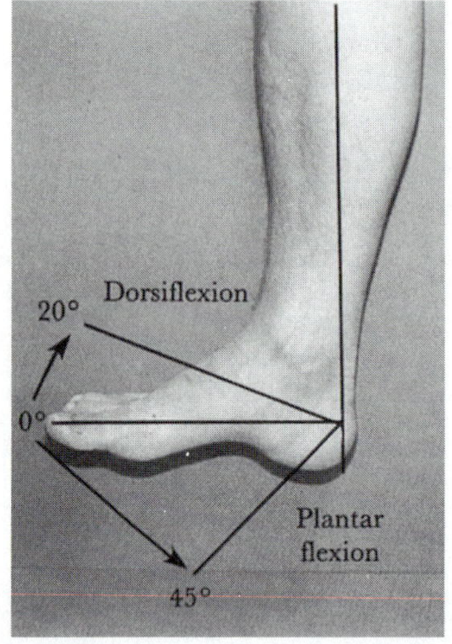

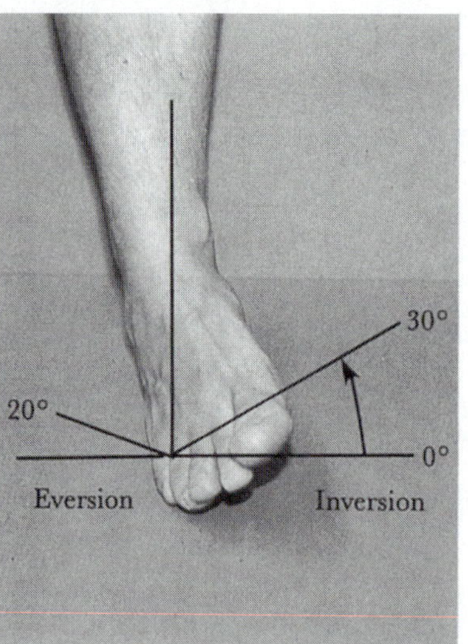

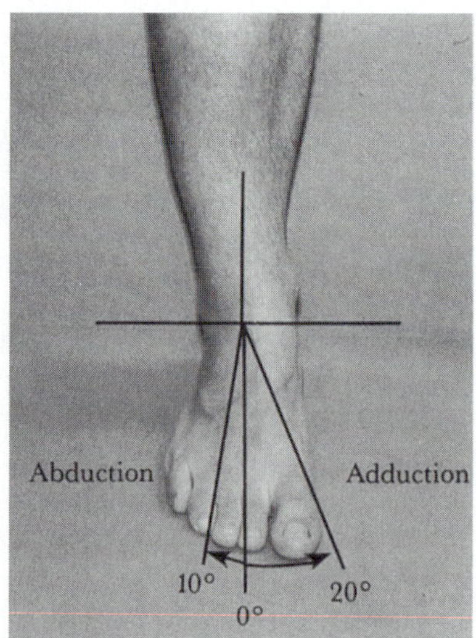

Evaluation

Compare information found with normal joint assessment *to determine abnormal findings.*

Sample charting

DATE	TIME	NOTES
1/27/95	0800	Carried out full ROM to all joints. Stated felt pain in wrist joint left hand (patient is left-handed). Reported joint pain to M. McHarness, RN.

(nurse's signature)

Follow-up

1. Turn patient *to prevent acquired deformities.*
2. Maintain appropriate body alignment *to prevent joint immobility.*

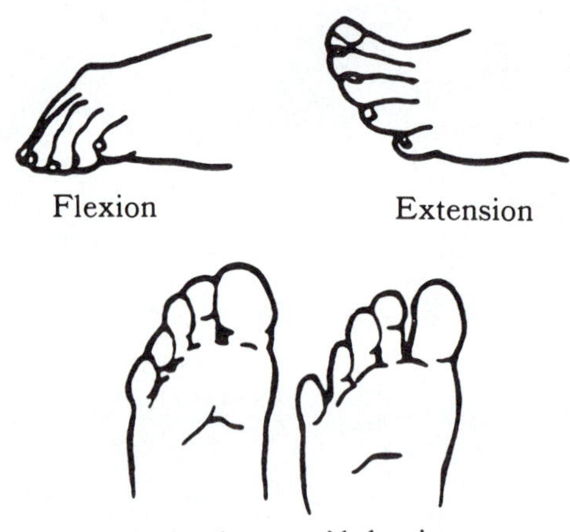

SPECIAL CONCERNS

- To prevent contractures, the nurse should not allow patients with joint pain to remain continuously in position of comfort; joints must be exercised routinely.
- The nurse should periodically provide back massage for patient comfort.

PATIENT TEACHING

- Emphasize importance of patient performing active ROM exercises when possible.

HOME HEALTH VARIATIONS

- Nurse must teach patient and family member ROM exercises.
- Full ROM exercises must be carried out on geriatric bedfast patients to prevent further complications of immobility.
- Avoid injury to joints in children because of more rapid metabolism.

SKILL 14-3: PERFORMING RANGE-OF-MOTION EXERCISES

Guidelines

Range-of-motion (**ROM,** any body action involving the muscles, joints, and natural directional movements) exercises may be performed by the physical therapy department or by the nurse. The exercises are ordered for patients confined to bed for long periods. ROM may be performed passively by the nurses or actively by patients. Designated body **joints** (connections between bones) are moved to the point of resistance, using care to avoid injury. The nurses or therapists gradually increase the ROM with subsequent exercises as tolerated.

Purposes

Nurses perform ROM exercises for the following reasons:

- to increase circulation
- to prevent **contractures** (abnormal, usually permanent conditions of joints)
- to provide joint motion and flexibility

SKILL 14-4: MOVING THE PATIENT

Guidelines

The nurse often is required to assist in moving the patient. Moving includes lifting the patient up in bed, turning, dangling, and assisting the patient in and out of the bed for ambulation. Other techniques include using mechanical equipment for lifting patients, such as the hydraulic lift, roller board, and gurney lift. Nurses must remember to lift twice—once mentally and then physically—to be certain that they have sufficient assistance from other health care personnel. Patients are reluctant to move if moving will cause more pain for them. The nurse should administer medication to the patient before any such activity.

Purposes

Nurses move (e.g., left, turn, dangle, assist for ambulation) patients for the following reasons:

- to move patient up toward head of bed
- to move patient for appropriate positioning
- to assist patient into bed
- to assist patient out of bed
- to turn patient

Supplies/Equipment
Hospital bed
Chair
Siderails
Patient slippers
Cotton blanket
Pillows
Extra personnel

SKILL 14-4

MOVING THE PATIENT

Nursing action/*Rationale*

1. Wash hands *to inhibit spread of microorganisms.*
2. Introduce self *to decrease anxiety level.*
3. Identify patient by identification band *to identify correct patient for procedure.*
4. a. Explain procedure *to seek cooperation or assistance from patient and to decrease anxiety.*
   b. Prepare for procedure by providing privacy and collecting necessary supplies *to organize procedure and decrease anxiety.*
5. Lifting and moving patient up in bed (This may require one or more nurses.)
   a. Place patient supine with head flat *to provide less resistance on flat surface.*
   b. Face side of bed and provide base of support *to protect nurse's back.*
   c. Place one arm under axilla and opposite arm under shoulder and neck *to support patient.*
   d. Ask patient to flex knees and push up with feet on count of 3 while assisting *to protect nurse's back and promote patient mobility.*
   e. Nurses position selves on both sides of patient and support patient's back with one arm, with the second arm under shoulder and neck *to protect nurses and provide patient safety.*
   f. On count of 3, each nurse pulls patient up *to head of bed to move patient in unison.*
6. Turning the patient:
   a. Stand with feet slightly apart, and flex knees *to provide base of support for nurse.*
   b. Place one arm under patient's neck and shoulders and other arm under waist *to provide patient safety and support.*

Continued.

MOVING THE PATIENT—cont'd

c. Pull patient toward nurse *to reduce strain on nurse.*
d. Turn patient on side facing raised siderail *to prevent falling out of bed.*
e. Flex one leg over the other *to reduce pressure on lower leg.*
f. Align shoulders *to ensure appropriate body alignment.*
g. Support back with pillows if necessary *to help keep patient in position.*
h. Assess appropriate body alignment *to provide patient safety and comfort.*

7. Dangling patient:

a. Assess pulse and respirations *to provide baseline for assessing patient's reaction to dangling.*
b. Move patient to side of bed toward nurse *to make it easier for patient to sit up* (see illustration).
c. Lower bed to lowest position *to provide patient safety when getting up.* (see illustration).
d. Raise head of bed *to make it easier for patient to swing around to sitting position.*
e. Support patient's shoulders and help to swing legs around and off bed; do this all in one motion; feet must touch floor *to prevent strain on patient, especially if patient has an incision.*
f. Help patient don slippers; cover legs *to protect from chilling.*
g. Assess patient's pulse and respiration *to determine patient's response to dangling.*

8. Logrolling the patient:

a. Three nurses (if possible) stand by side of bed *because the use of three nurses provides safety for the patient.*
b. One nurse places arms under patient's legs; second nurse places arms under patient's buttocks; third nurse places arms under patient's chest, shoulders, and neck *to ensure that patient is turned like log is rolled (as a unit)* (see illustration).
c. The nurse nearest head of patient gives prearranged signal to turn patient simultaneously *to ensure appropriate logrolling by one designated person* (see illustration).
d. Make patient comfortable *to provide comfort and relaxation for the patient.*

9. Transferring the patient from bed to straight chair and wheelchair:

a. Lower bed to lowest position *to provide patient safety when getting up.*
b. Raise head of bed *to make it easier for patient to swing around to sitting position.*
c. Support patient's shoulder and help to swing legs around and off bed; perform all in one motion *to prevent strain on patient, especially if patient has incision.*
d. Help patient don robe and slippers *to prevent chilling.*
e. Have chair placed beside bed with seat facing foot of bed *to provide easy access to chair.*
   1) Lock wheels of wheelchair *to provide safety.*
   2) Place straight chair against wall *to provide safety.*
f. Stand in front of patient, and place hands under patient's axillae *to prepare patient for movement to chair.*

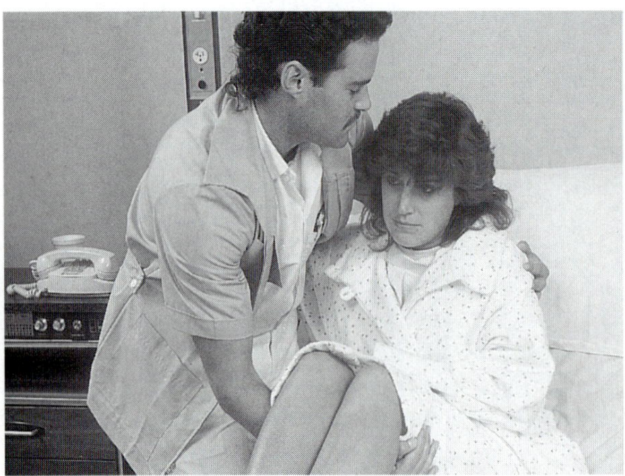

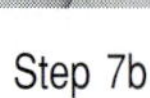

Step 7b

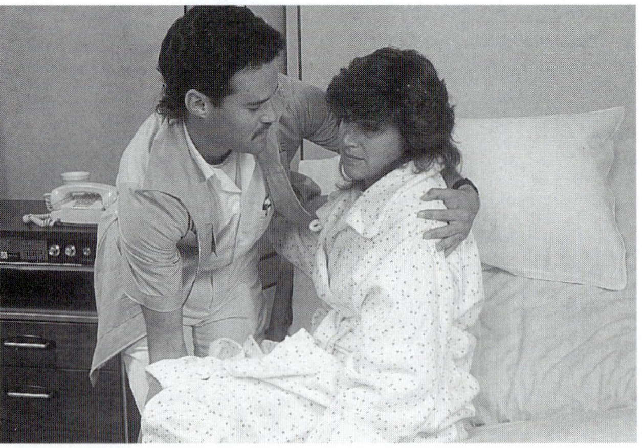

Step 7c

MOVING THE PATIENT—cont'd

g. Assist patient to stand and swing around with back toward seat of chair *to provide patient safety.*
h. Help patient to sit down as nurse bends knees to assist process *to prevent patient from slipping and falling.*
i. Apply blanket to legs *to provide extra warmth.*

10. Wash hands *to inhibit spread of microorganisms.*
11. Document procedure *to note procedure and patient's response.*
12. Assess for appropriate body alignment after patient movement *to evaluate and determine safety and comfort.*

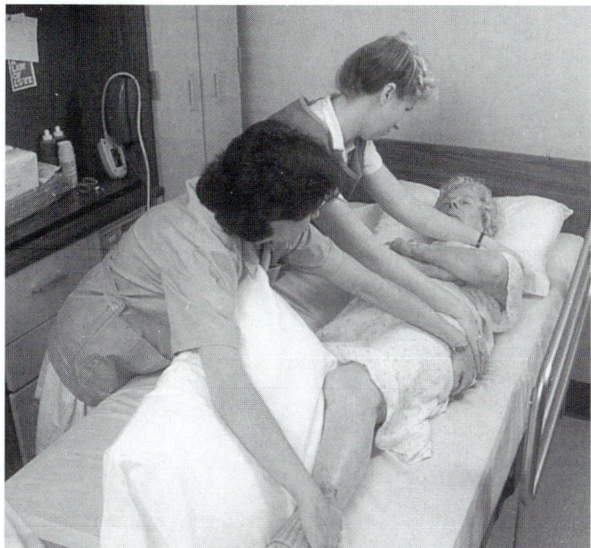

Step 8b

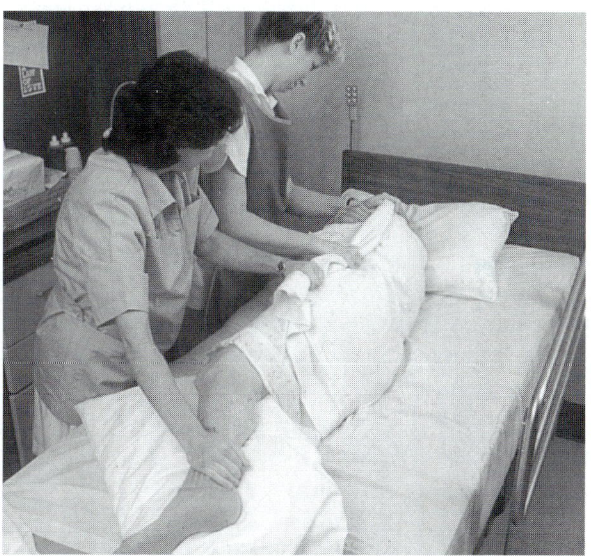

Step 8c

Sample charting

DATE	TIME	NOTES
1/5/95	1000	Moved up to head of bed. Placed in appropriate body alignment.
		_______________ *(nurse's signature)*
1/5/95	1100	Repositioned to lt. Sims'
		_______________ *(nurse's signature)*
1/5/95	0800	Dangled at side of bed 10 minutes. Tolerated well. P 74, with regular rate and rhythm. Respirations 18 and regular.
		_______________ *(nurse's signature)*

Follow-up

13. Follow up and assess that wheelchair locks are in working order *to provide patient safety.*

SPECIAL CONCERNS

- Do not overtire patient during ambulation.
- Give patient time to talk about ambulation needs.
- Children on bed rest may be irritable because of restrained activity.
- Older patients on bed rest are at risk for impairment.
- If patient begins to fall, protect by holding patient and allow patient to sit down on floor to prevent patient injury.

PATIENT TEACHING

Explain the importance of proper physical movement

USING LIFTS FOR MOVING PATIENTS

Nursing action/*Rationale*

1. Wash hands *to inhibit spread of microorganisms.*
2. Introduce self *to decrease anxiety level.*
3. Identify patient by identification band *to identify correct patient for procedure.*
4. Explain procedure *to seek cooperation or assistance from patient and to decrease anxiety.*
   a. Prepare for procedure by providing privacy and collecting necessary supplies *to organize procedure and decrease anxiety.*
5. Secure appropriate number of personnel *to assist and provide patient safety.*
6. Place chair near bed *to prepare seat for patient.*
7. Raise bed to maximum height *to ensure appropriate body mechanics.*
8. Appropriately place canvas seat under patient *to help in lifting safely.*
9. Slide horseshoe-shaped bar under bed on one side *to place lift close to bed.*
10. Lower horizontal bar to level of sling by releasing hydraulic valve and lock valve *to place lift close to patient.*
11. Fasten hooks on chain to openings in sling *to place lift to sling seat.*
12. Raise head of bed *to place patient in sitting position.*
13. Fold patient's arms over chest *to prevent patient injury.*
14. Pump lift handle until patient is raised off bed *to ensure patient safety during lifting.*
15. With steering handle, pull lift off bed and down to chair *to place patient safely in chair provided.*
16. Release valve slowly to left and lower patient toward chair *to appropriately place patient in chair.*
17. Close off valve, and release straps *to prevent patient injury from boom.*
18. Remove straps and hydraulic lift *to provide safety and comfort.*
19. Wash hands *to inhibit spread of microorganisms.*
20. Document procedure *to note procedure and patient's response.*
21. a. Evaluate body alignment to help prevent skin impairment.
    b. Evaluate patient's response to movement to help determine patient's mobility potential.

Follow-up

1. Follow up by assessing for skin impairment and effects of procedure to ensure comfort and safety of the patient.

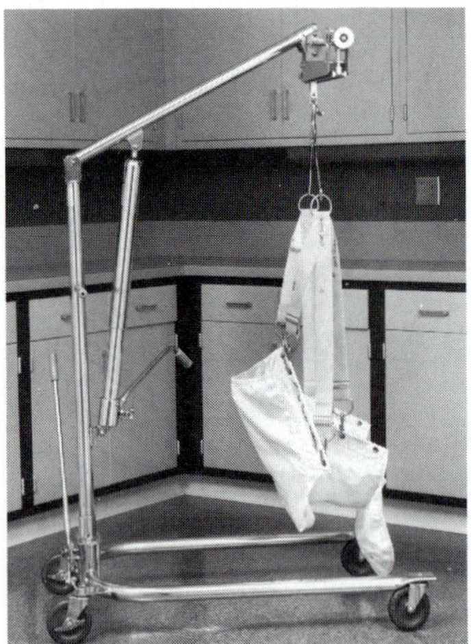

FIG. 14-4 Hydraulic lift with a Hoyer sling.

SKILL 14-5: USING THE LIFT FOR MOVING PATIENTS

Guidelines

Mechanical devices, such as the hydraulic lift used with a Hoyer sling (Fig. 14-4) are used for moving patients safely, protecting the nurse's back, and full-weight lifting of patients who cannot assist. Agency policy is followed for use of the lift.

Purposes

Nurses use lifts for moving patients for the following reasons:

- to place patient in chair
- to place patient on gurney
- to place patient in tub

Supplies/equipment
2 cotton blankets
Sling hydraulic lift, such as the Hoyer

REFERENCES AND SUGGESTED READINGS

1. Ellis JR, Nowlis EA, Bentz PM: *Modules for basic nursing skills,* ed 5, vol 1, Philadelphia, 1992, Lippincott.
2. Lederer JR et al: *Care planning pocket guide,* ed 3, Redwood City, Calif, 1990, Addison-Wesley.
3. Long BC, Phipps WJ, Cassmeyer VL: *Medical-surgical nursing: a nursing-process approach,* ed 3, 1993, St Louis, Mosby.
4. Kottke F, Stillwell G, Lehmann J: *Krusen's handbook of physical medicine and rehabilitation,* ed 4, Philadelphia, 1990, Saunders.
5. Kozier B, Erb G, Olivieri R: *Fundamentals of nursing: concepts, process, and practice,* ed 4, Redwood City, Calif, 1991, Addison-Wesley.
6. McCauley M: The effect of body mechanics instruction on work performance among young workers, *Am J Occup Ther* 44(4):402, 1990.
7. McConnell EA: Placing your patient in the lateral position, *Nursing 90* 20:65, 1990.
8. *Mosby's medical, nursing, and allied health dictionary,* ed 4, St Louis, 1994, Mosby.
9. Olson EV, Johnson BJ, Thompson LF: The hazards of immobility, *Am J Nurs* 90:43, 1990.
10. Owen BD, Garg A: Reducing risk for back pain in nursing personnel, *AAOHN J* 39(1):24, 1991.
11. Perry AG, Potter PA: *Clinical nursing skills and techniques,* ed 3, St Louis, 1995, Mosby.
12. Potter PA, Perry AG: *Fundamentals of nursing: concepts, process, and practice,* ed 3, St Louis, 1993, Mosby.
13. Suddarth DS: *The Lippincott manual of nursing practice,* ed 5, Philadelphia, 1991, Lippincott.
14. Tucker SM et al: *Patient care standards: nursing process, diagnosis, and outcome,* ed 5, St Louis, 1992, Mosby.
15. United States Department of Health and Human Services, Public Health Service: *Healthy people 2000: health promotion and disease preventions objectives,* Washington, DC, 1990, Government Printing Office.

CHAPTER CHALLENGE

KEY POINTS

- The musculoskeletal system must be protected to prevent injury to both patient and nurse.
- Less effort is required to carry out an activity if the base of support is widened in the direction of movement.
- Appropriate body mechanics should be practiced daily.
- Maintaining correct body alignment is the key to proper body mechanics.
- Correct body alignment promotes balance and helps coordinate movements.
- Permanent disability can occur from inappropriate positioning.
- Proper positioning provides activity to enhance comfort and prepares patients for procedures.
- The nurse performs range-of-motion exercises to promote circulation, prevent contractures, and provide joint mobility.
- When turning, moving, lifting, or carrying a patient, the nurse secures enough assistance to reduce strain and prevent injury to both nurse and patient.
- Mechanical devices such as hydraulic lift, roller board, and gurney lift are used for moving patients safely.

STUDY QUESTIONS

1. The nurse is assigned to care for Mr. Horten, an 82-year-old patient who weighs 252 lb and is a bilateral below-the-knee amputee. The safest method to transfer Mr. Horten from bed to chair would be:
   1. log rolling
   2. using two nurses to lift
   3. hydraulic lift with Hoyer sling
   4. gurney lift
2. The nurse is ambulating Ms. Draden, an 84-year-old patient who has peripheral vascular disease causing severe stasis ulcer. Ms. Draden becomes very weak, complains of feeling faint, and begins to fall. The most appropriate action to prevent injury to Ms. Draden would be:
   1. support Ms. Draden and allow her to sit on the floor
   2. carefully attempt to return Ms. Draden to her room
   3. tell Ms. Draden to hold onto the wall and that you will get more assistance
   4. ask Ms. Draden to take deep breaths and look straight ahead
3. Mr. Gordon is a 56-year-old patient who had an open cholecystectomy. The nurse is going to dangle Mr. Gordon before ambulation. After sitting him on the edge of the bed, what nursing intervention should be performed before proceeding with the ambulation:
   1. assess his temperature
   2. assess his pulse and respiration
   3. perform an oximetry check
   4. remove antiembolism stockings
4. The nurse is placing the overhead table over the bed of 65-year-old Mr. Noonan, who is on bed rest for pulmonary embolism. He accidentally knocks the emesis basin to the floor. When picking up the emesis basin, the proper body mechanics for the nurse would be:
   1. lower the body by flexing the knees and bending the hips
   2. bend from the waist and hips
   3. flex the knees and bend at the waist
   4. keeping the legs straight and flex the waist
5. Mrs. Tomlinson is a 72-year-old patient with a cerebrovascular accident who has slid to the foot of the bed. To use appropriate body mechanics, the nurse maintains a wide base of support and faces the patient in the direction of movement, thus allowing her to:
   1. use her back muscles
   2. use her large muscles across the scapula
   3. exert less physical effort
   4. use her gluteal muscles
6. Ms. Graysen is an 82-year-old patient who has had a right total hip replacement. On the first postoperative day, the nurse repositions Ms. Graysen to her left side, placing a pillow between her legs and another to her back. The nurse assesses the proper placement of Ms. Graysen's body to evaluate:
   1. base support
   2. body alignment
   3. head, chin tilt
   4. gluteal pressure
7. It is the first night after an abdominal hysterectomy for Mrs. Bauck. She has not voided for 9 hours, and the nurse is to insert a #16 Foley catheter into her bladder. The preferred position to place Mrs. Bauck for the procedure is:
   1. dorsal recumbent
   2. lithotomy
   3. Sims'
   4. prone
8. The nurse is assigned to care for 64-year-old Mr. Fullerton who was admitted for exacerbation of chronic obstructive pulmonary disease and pneumonia. He has dyspnea (shortness of breath) and is unable to rest in a supine position. The nurse elevates the head of the bed to 90 degrees, places a pillow on the overbed table, and assists Mr. Fullerton to lean forward, placing his head on the pillow. This position is called:
   1. semi-Fowler's
   2. dorsal
   3. Sims'
   4. orthopneic
9. Mr. Kildon is a 45-year-old patient who has had a spinal fusion. He is to be logrolled every 3 hours. The number of nurses required to perform this nursing intervention is:
   1. one
   2. two
   3. three
   4. four
10. Mr. Jurgon is a 45-year-old patient with rheumatoid arthritis. To prevent contractures, the nurse should not allow Mr. Jurgon to:
    1. remain continuously in position of comfort
    2. carry out full ROM to all joints
    3. rotate his knees and lower legs toward the midline
    4. supinate his lower arms and abduct his legs

15

COMFORT, REST, AND SLEEP

Barbara Lauritsen Christensen

KEY TERMS

acute pain
chronic pain
endorphin
gate control theory
nonrapid eye movement (NREM)
noxious
patient-controlled analgesia (PCA)
placebo
rapid eye movement (REM)
referred pain
synergistic
transcutaneous electrical nerve stimulation (TENS)
visual analogue scale

LEARNING OBJECTIVES

After reading this chapter, the student should be able to do the following:

- Define the key terms.
- List 10 possible causes of discomfort.
- Explain McCaffery's description of pain.
- Explain the relationship of the gate control theory to selecting nursing interventions for pain relief.
- Identify subjective and objective data in pain assessment.
- Discuss the synergistic relationship of fatigue, sleep disturbance, and depression to one's perception of pain.
- Explain three recently developed tools to identify intensity of pain.
- Discuss the responsibilities of the nurse in pain control.
- List six methods for pain control.
- Identify nursing interventions to control painful stimuli in the patient's environment.
- Describe the difference and similarities between sleep and rest.
- Outline nursing interventions that promote rest and sleep.
- Discuss the sleep cycle, differentiating between NREM and REM sleep.
- List six signs and symptoms of sleep deprivation.
- Identify two nursing diagnoses related to sleep problems.

RELATED TOPICS OF INTEREST

- Signs, symptoms, and physical assessment (Chapter 9)
- Hygiene and care of the patient's environment (Chapter 16)
- Principles and practice of medication administration (Chapter 21)
- The surgical patient (Chapter 22)
- Care of the patient with a neurological disorder (Chapter 35)

THE MEANING OF COMFORT

One of the greatest challenges of the nurse is to provide comfort to the patient. *To comfort* means to give strength and hope, to cheer, and to ease the grief or trouble of another. Promoting physical and psychological comfort is a vital part of the role of a nurse.

For the patient, the lack of comfort can be the result of many factors and can take many forms, including the following:

- anxiety
- constricting edema
- depression
- diaphoresis
- distention
- dry mouth
- dyspnea
- fatigue
- fear
- flatus
- headache
- hopelessness
- hyperthermia
- hypothermia
- incontinence
- muscle cramping
- nausea
- pain
- powerlessness
- pruritus
- retention
- sadness
- singultus
- thirst
- vomiting

The nurse should pursue methods to assist the patient in achieving relief from discomfort.

It is important to explore the patient's concept of what constitutes comfort. By actively listening to the patient, the nurse will be better prepared to plan nursing interventions. The nurse who knows what might constitute patient discomfort will recognize discomfort signals even when the patient cannot verbalize, as in the case of a patient who is aphasic or one who is semicomatose.

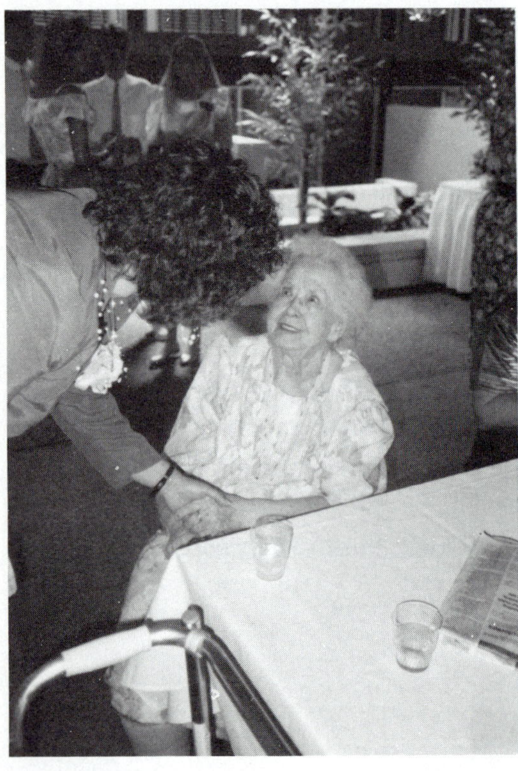

FIG. 15-1 Comfort and well-being can be promoted with eye contact and gentle touch.

The nurse must be diligent in her efforts to relieve patients' discomfort. If interventions are not successful, alternative interventions should be pursued.

Regardless of age, patients receive comfort and a sense of well-being from gentle touch and eye contact (Fig. 15-1). The following depicts the nurse's role in bringing physical and psychological comfort to the patient.

Case study: discomfort to comfort

Mr. Donavon is a 91-year-old patient hospitalized for pneumonia and exacerbation of COPD. The night nurse reported that he had been belligerent and occasionally combative.

Upon entering Mr. Donavon's room, the nurse sees a pale, thin, and slightly dyspneic patient. He appears fragile and vulnerable. Mr. Donavon complains of pain and tenderness on his lower left gum line. He also states, "I can't hear without my hearing aids, and I am cold."

The nurse acknowledges Mr. Donavon's complaints of oral discomfort, inability to hear, and being cold. Immediate nursing interventions are to place a warm bath blanket over him, put his hearing aids in place, encourage him to cough, and assist in repositioning. The nurse assesses his oral cavity, using a flashlight for better visualization; an erythematous area is noted. She gently cleanses the area with a soothing mouthwash applied with toothettes to sooth his erythematous and tender mouth. She offers him a glass of apple juice. These interventions are followed with a warm towel bath to enhance his feeling of well-being.

The nurse speaks slowly and distinctly while facing Mr. Donavon to improve his ability to hear. Gentle touch, eye contact, and a projection of concern are employed during the interventions.

Mr. Donavon verbalizes that he is more comfortable. He then makes a significant comment: "I have very little jaw bone left, and I drool; the nurses have to wipe it off my face and that makes me feel like a bum." The nurse listens to this revealing statement and acknowledges his feelings of powerlessness over his ability to contain his saliva. After providing opportunity for Mr. Donavon to verbalize his feelings of powerlessness, the nurse places facial tissues within his reach to assist him in wiping secretions from his face. Mr. Donavon has a comfortable morning and does not display belligerent or combative behavior.

The interventions addressed the patient's discomfort, physically as well as psychologically, and comfort was established.

NATURE OF PAIN

Pain is a complex, abstract, personal experience. It is an unpleasant sensation caused by **noxious** (injurious to physical health) stimulation of the sensory nerve endings. Pain cannot be seen. It serves as a warning to the body because it often occurs where there is actual or potential tissue damage. Pain can also occur when there is no tissue damage. Examples of this are the pain of grief at the death of a loved one or the pain of migraine headaches, in which there is no tissue damage.

Pain is subjective; the interpretation and significance of pain depend on the individual's learned experiences and involve psychosocial and cultural factors. Only the person who is bearing the pain is an expert about that pain. McCaffery has a realistic description of pain: "Pain is whatever the experiencing person says it is, existing whenever he says it does." According to McCaffery's definition of pain, the nurse must believe every patient who says he has pain. The nurse should remember also that some patients may deny pain for a variety of reasons and that this situation must be explored as well.

Because so many health care providers have difficulty with the concept of pain, it must be emphasized that *there is no test for pain.* Even though some nurses with years of experience think they can identify all patients in pain, it is not always possible. Lack of pain expression does not mean lack of pain.

Function and Types of Pain

Pain may be a cardinal symptom of inflammation and is valuable in the diagnosis of many disorders and conditions. There are many types of pain: mild or severe, chronic or acute, intermittent or intractable (constant), burning, dull, or sharp, precisely or poorly localized, or referred. **Referred pain** is felt at a site other than the injured or diseased organ or part of the body. An example of referred pain is angina: the pain of coronary artery insufficiency may be felt in the left shoulder, arm, or jaw.

Acute and chronic pain. **Acute pain** is intense and of short duration; the pain lasts less than 6 months. Generally acute pain provides a warning to the individual of actual or potential tissue damage. It creates an autonomic response commonly referred to as the *fight-or-flight* response. When healing occurs, the pain also resolves. There is usually anxiety associated with the pain. Because the pain is of short duration, physicians are more likely to prescribe narcotics and analgesics.

Chronic pain is generally characterized by pain lasting longer than 6 months. The pain can be continuous or intermittent and can be as intense as acute pain. The fight-or-flight response is no longer present. Chronic pain does not serve as a warning of tissue damage. In rheumatoid arthritis, for example, joint pain may continue when the disease process is no longer active, because of the structural damage that has already occurred in the joint. The reason for some forms of chronic pain may not be known. Because of the prolonged time involved in chronic pain, the patient often develops chronic low self-esteem, change in social identity, changes in role and social interaction, fatigue, sleep disturbance, and depression.

It is possible that fatigue, sleep disturbance, and depression act in a type of **synergistic** (the action of two or more substances or organs to achieve an effect of which each is individually incapable) relationship, which can markedly change one's perception of pain. Depression is associated with sleep disturbance, usually lack of sleep, which in turn increases the intensity of the fatigue. In addition, a decrease in activity increases fatigue. The patient's world becomes smaller and smaller, which is, in the worse case, limited to just his own body and mind. As one's attention draws inward like this, it entraps the individual in a vicious cycle, making the pain difficult to treat.

Because of the general differences between acute and chronic pain, some aspects of nursing interventions for these conditions may differ. The nurse must remember the realness of the pain, whether acute or chronic, and use appropriate measures to relieve that pain.

Behavioral Characteristics of Pain

The defining characteristic of pain is the verbal or nonverbal communication by the patient of the presence of pain. Behavioral characteristics are noted in Box 15-1.

Box 15-1 BEHAVIORAL CHARACTERISTICS OF PAIN

1. Is self-protective; guards the painful area—places hands over the area
2. Has narrowed focus: cannot think of anything but the pain, has reduced attention span
3. Withdraws from social contact, avoids conversation or social contacts
4. Has impaired thought processes
5. Demonstrates distraction behavior, which includes moaning, rocking, crying, pacing, restlessness, or seeking out other people or activities
6. Presents facial mask of pain, recognized by eyes that appear dull or lusterless, fixed or scattered facial movements, grimace, clenching of teeth, biting of lips, or tightening of jaw
7. Experiences alterations in muscle tone, ranging from lassitude to rigidity
8. Exhibits diaphoresis, changes in blood pressure and pulse rate, pupillary dilation, and increased or decreased rate of respiration
9. May demonstrate no outward expressions of pain. However, the nurse must remember that lack of pain expression does not mean lack of pain. There is no specific "picture" of a patient in pain

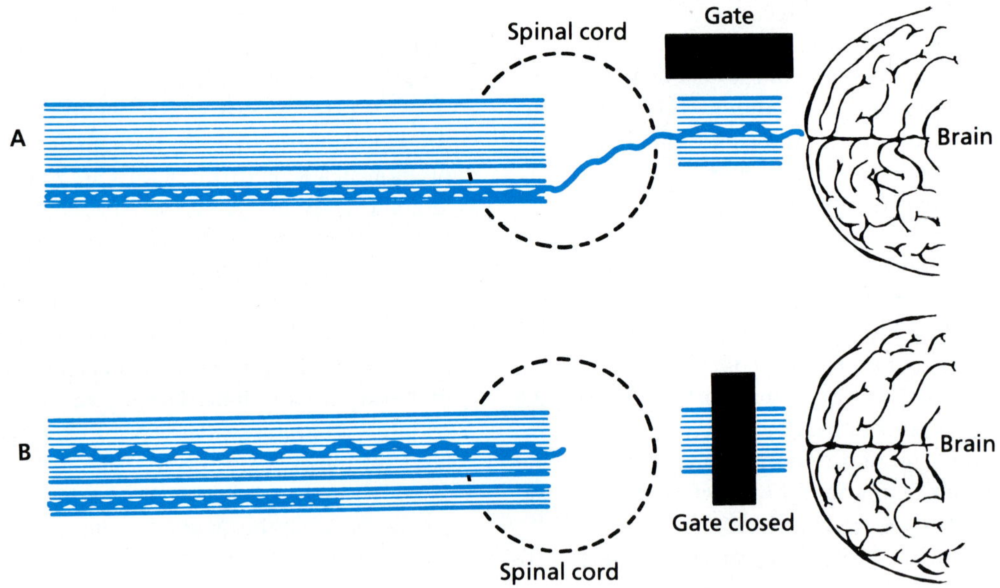

FIG. 15-2 Diagrammatic sketch of gate control theory.

Theories of Pain Transmission

The **gate control theory** of pain, proposed by Melzack,[18] suggests that pain impulses can be regulated or even blocked by gating mechanisms located along the central nervous system. The proposed location of the gates is in the dorsal horn of the spinal cord. Pain and other sensations of the skin and muscles travel the same pathways through the large nerves in the spinal cord. If other cutaneous stimuli besides pain are transmitted, the "gate" through which the pain impulse must travel is temporarily blocked by the stimuli. The brain cannot acknowledge the pain while it is interpreting the other stimuli. When gates are open, pain impulses flow freely. When gates are closed, pain impulses become blocked. Partial openings may occur. A bombardment of sensory impulses, such as those from the pressure of a backrub, the heat of a warm compress, or the cold from ice applications, will close the gates to painful stimuli. Some patients can be distracted from pain by removing the sensation of pain from their center of attention. Auditory or visual stimuli can distract patients and help make pain more tolerable (Fig. 15-2).

Gating mechanisms can also be altered by thoughts, feelings, and memories. The cerebral cortex and thalamus can influence whether pain impulses reach a person's conscious awareness. There is conscious control over how pain is perceived, and this helps explain the various ways people react and adjust to pain.

Endorphins. The body contains a natural supply of morphine-like substances called **endorphins** (potent polypeptides composed of many amino acids found in the pituitary gland and other areas of the CNS). Stress and pain activate endorphins. Analgesia results when certain endorphins attach to opiate receptors in the brain. People who have less pain than others from a similar injury have higher endorphin levels. Pain relief measures, such as transcutaneous electrical nerve stimulation (TENS), acupuncture, and placebos, are believed to cause the release of endorphins.

NURSING ASSESSMENT OF PAIN

Collection of Subjective Data

Because pain is a subjective experience, it is vital that the nurse become a well-versed and competent practitioner of the art of pain assessment. It is important for the nurse to obtain accurate information from the patient concerning the pain, including characteristics and description of the pain. The characteristics may include the site, severity, duration, and location of pain. When documenting the presence of pain, the nurse should describe the specific location and intensity. Charting "patient complains of pain" provides no useful information. It is necessary to ask the patient what relieves the pain and what does not relieve the pain. Sociocultural information includes identifying usual coping mechanisms and the patient's, family's, and friends' expectations of appropriate behavior when in pain. If medications are taken for pain, the name, dose, frequency, and effect of the drugs must be determined.

The nurse must be sensitive to the patient's condition. Obviously, patients who are critically ill or in excruciating pain should be asked only a few key questions at any given time rather than be subjected to a long list

Box 15-2 PAIN INTENSITY SCALES

CATEGORICAL SCALE

0-No pain
1-Mild pain
2-Discomforting pain
3-Distressing pain
4-Horrible pain
5-Excruciating pain

NUMERICAL SCALE

0—1—2—3—4—5—6—7—8—9—10

No Pain **Worst Pain Imaginable**

VISUAL ANALOGUE SCALE (VAS)

No Pain **Worst Pain**

____

Box 15-3 OBJECTIVE SIGNS OF PAIN

PHYSIOLOGICAL SIGNS

Pulse: increased rate
Respirations: increased depth and frequency
Blood pressure: increased systolic and diastolic
Diaphoresis, pallor
Dilated pupils
Muscle tension (face, body)
Nausea and vomiting (if pain is severe)

BEHAVIORAL SIGNS

Rigid body position
Restlessness
Frowning
Clenched teeth
Clenched fists
Crying
Moaning

of questions. The nurse must project an interest and concern for the patient so he will openly discuss his pain.

There has been interest recently in developing tools specifically for assessment of pain. Nurses are frequently faced with difficulties in assessing pain. A pain scale will help with this assessment; it allows the patient to rate the pain so that the nurse can measure its intensity.

Categorical scales, numerical scales, and visual analogue scales (VAS) are commonly used to qualify the intensity of the pain experience[28] (Box 15-2). With the **visual analogue scale,** the patient marks a spot on a horizontal line to indicate pain intensity (intensity increases as the line moves from left to right), or the patient may use a number scale by choosing a number from 0 to 5 or 0 to 10, with 0 being no pain and 5 or 10 being the worst pain imaginable. For clinical assessment, any of these scales is adequate and appropriate. It is important that the same scale always be used with the same patient. If one nurse uses a 0 to 10 scale and the next nurse uses a 0 to 5 scale, a patient's rating of 4 will mean something different to both patient and nurse.

Collection of Objective Data

The nurse must carefully observe the patient. Some objective signs may be tachycardia, increased rate and depth of respirations, diaphoresis, increased systolic or diastolic blood pressure, pallor, dilated pupils, and increased muscle tension. The patient may complain of nausea or weakness (Box 15-3).

If the pain is chronic or less severe, the physiological changes may be less prominent. The nurse may notice changes in facial expressions, such as frowning or gritting of teeth. Some persons clench their fists and withdraw when in pain. Others may complain bitterly, cry, moan, toss about in bed, assume a fetal position, or clutch at the affected body part. Still others will pace if they have energy to do so. Some patients in pain want someone in constant attendance, whereas others want to be left alone.

Nurses must be nonbiased and nonjudgmental when gathering objective data: the patient is doing the best possible at the given moment. The immediate intervention by the nurse is to relieve or decrease the pain. It should be remembered that pain is what the patient says it is. The nurse should not expect the patient to behave in any set manner when in pain.

NURSING DIAGNOSES FOR PAIN

The following nursing diagnoses are directly associated with the care of patients with pain:

- Pain, acute
- Pain, chronic

Possible other nursing diagnoses that may be appropriate because of the effects of pain on other aspects of a patient's life include the following:

- Anxiety
- Body image disturbance
- Caregiver role strain
- Colonic constipation
- Coping, ineffective individual
- Family coping, disabling

NURSING CARE PLAN: THE PATIENT WITH CHRONIC PAIN

Mr. Johns is a 45-year-old patient with a 15-year history of severe, crippling rheumatoid arthritis. He has had numerous joint replacements, has had a weight loss of 40 pounds in the past year, and has developed corneal ulcers from the presence of Sjögren's syndrome. He is in constant chronic pain and has limited mobility. He states he has difficulty accomplishing activities of daily living (ADLs).

Nursing diagnoses	Patient goals/expected outcomes	Nursing interventions
Pain, chronic, related to joint/muscle inflammation and degeneration manifested by complaints of pain, narrow focus of interest, guarded movement, and social withdrawal	Patient and/or family will verbalize a reduction in anxiety and pain when using relaxation, massage, cutaneous stimulation, and analgesics.	Teach relaxation exercises. Perform massage to relieve pain and to enhance communication. Administer analgesics and apply cold/heat applications as ordered. Maintain TENS as ordered.
Physical mobility, impaired, related to musculoskeletal degeneration, pain, and edema manifested by slow, painful movement, decreased range of motion, and loss of muscle strength	Patient will demonstrate increase in mobility of joints.	Place patient in position of comfort, support joints with pillows or pads, and change position hourly. Assist with ROM exercise. Avoid restrictive clothing. Assist to ambulate as tolerated. Maintain safety: handrails in shower, tub, and toilet; raised toilet seat; and rubber-tipped cane or walker.
Self-care deficit, dressing/grooming, related to pain, decreased vision, lack of range of motion, and weakness manifested by difficulty performing ADLs	Patient's independence in self-care activities will increase within parameters of disability.	Teach self-care activities. Establish and teach plan for ADLs. Set with patient short-term, easily accomplished goals. Discuss use of snaps on clothing and slip-on shoes.
Low self-esteem, chronic, related to inability to work, and body image change manifested by preoccupation with body changes and verbalization of powerlessness	Patient will verbalize understanding of changes in body image caused by disease process and will begin to exhibit increased confidence in dealing with self-esteem.	Encourage verbalization about fears and anxiety; listen attentively. Deal with behavioral changes, denial, powerlessness, anxiety, and dependence. Be supportive in setting goals. Encourage independence, and give praise for tasks accomplished. Modify environment, and allow time for patient to accomplish goals.
Knowledge deficit, related to home care management manifested by statements of concern/misconceptions about medication regimen, exercise program, and diet	Patient and/or significant others will demonstrate understanding of home care follow-up instructions through interactive discussion and actual demonstration.	Stress importance of maintaining prescribed exercise, activities, rest, diet, and medication regimen. Reinforce physician explanation of disease, expectations, and limitations. Discuss diet management; stress importance of balanced diet.

Sleep pattern disturbance, related to chronic pain manifested by social withdrawal and fatigue	Patient will sleep uninterrupted for 4 to 6 hours.	Determine the patient's usual rest and sleep patterns, decide if they are sufficient, and note why the patient is not getting sufficient rest. Wash patient's back, gently massage it, and freshen the linens. Have the patient void. Reduce environmental stimuli by dimming lights and decreasing noise. Do not awaken for vitals or procedure unless absolutely necessary. Administer an analgesic or hypnotic as prescribed.

CRITICAL THINKING QUESTIONS

1. During the morning ADLs, Mr. Johns states, "I feel so useless. I can't even place the urinal for myself." What would be the most therapeutic responce by the nurse?
2. For Mr. Johns to have reduced pain during assisted ambulation, what would be the most useful nursing intervention to achieve this goal?
3. Which comfort measures could the nurse perform to ensure Mr. Johns several hours of restorative sleep?
4. Mr. Johns complains of his eyes burning and feeling dry and the lights annoying him. What measures would be useful to relieve his symptoms?

- Family processes, altered
- Fatigue
- Fear
- Grieving, anticipatory
- Hopelessness
- Knowledge deficit (specify)
- Mobility, impaired physical
- Nutrition, altered: less/more than body requirements
- Powerlessness
- Role performance, altered
- Self-care deficit, dressing/grooming
- Self-care deficit, toileting
- Sexual dysfunction
- Sleep pattern disturbance
- Social isolation
- Thought processes, altered

The extensiveness of the list alerts the nurse to the numerous problems that may develop because of pain.

RESPONSIBILITY OF THE NURSE IN PAIN CONTROL

The nurse can assist the patient in pain relief by telling the patient, "I believe that you are in pain, and I will assist you in whatever way I can to relieve your pain." This reduces the patient's anxiety level. A patient should not be required to expend energy convincing the nurse that the pain is real. The nurse should begin pain intervention as soon as the patient states he is in pain.

Pain management is a challenge that every nurse must face, regardless of the practice setting. In fact, the nurse's role in pain management is probably more important than that of any other member of the health care team (see nursing care plan).

Probably no other area of nursing involves patient advocacy as much as pain control. In all nursing fields, the nurse should advocate for the patient by clarifying concerns, answering questions, supplying all the information the patient needs to make decisions about care, and supporting the patient's decisions. Effective patient advocacy requires time, patience, and courage. Good listening skills are essential. A nurse should ask a patient how he is and attentively wait to hear the answer.

At times the nurse may be the only person who "advocates" or believes that the patient has pain. This can be a very disconcerting experience for the nurse, one that requires patience and energy. Advocacy is critical if the nurse is to be effective in pain management.

The founding principle of effective pain management is Meinhart and McCaffery's statement that "the failure to treat pain is inhumane and constitutes professional negligence."[17] Every patient has the right to be free of pain; it is the nurse's responsibility to do everything possible to alleviate the patient's pain.

GUIDELINES FOR INDIVIDUALIZING PAIN THERAPY

In providing pain relief measures it is important for the nurse to choose therapies suited to the patient's unique pain experience. McCaffery suggests patient's unique guidelines for individualizing pain therapy.

1. **Use different types of pain relief measures**—using more than one therapy has an additive effect in reducing pain. In addition, the character of pain may change throughout the day, requiring several different therapies. Combining physical and psychological approaches (e.g., analgesics and relaxation) controls all components of the pain experience.
2. **Provide pain relief measures before pain becomes severe**—an ounce of prevention is worth a pound of cure (it is easier to prevent severe pain than to relieve it). Giving an analgesic 30 minutes before a patient must walk or perform an activity is an example of controlling pain early.
3. **Use measures the patient believes are effective**—the patient is the expert on the pain. He may have ideas about what measures to use (e.g., rubbing lotion on an edematous finger) and when to use them that will make pain therapy successful.
4. **Consider the patient's ability or willingness to participate in pain relief measures**—some patients cannot actively assist with pain therapy because of fatigue, sedation, or altered levels of consciousness. However, there are variations of pain relief measures that require little effort, such as relaxation exercises in bed or listening to music as a distraction. The nurse will not relieve pain by forcing an unwilling patient to participate in therapy. The depressed patient with chronic pain has little motivation to participate.
5. **Choose pain relief measures appropriate to the severity of the pain as reflected by the patient's behavior**—it would be poor judgment to administer a potent narcotic to a patient who is displaying only mild pain. The nurse carefully assesses what the patient says and behaves before choosing pain therapy. Some patients acquire relief from severe pain after using only mild analgesics. Only the patient can determine the degree of effectiveness of a therapy.
6. **If a therapy is ineffective at first, encourage the patient to try it again before abandoning it**—often anxiety or doubt prevents patient from gaining relief from therapy. Some approaches, such as distraction, require practice. Some measures that seem ineffective may merely require adjustment to become effective. For example, the dosage of an analgesic may be increased if severe pain is initially unrelieved. The nurse should be persistent and understanding in helping the patient learn to use measures that do not afford immediate relief.
7. **Keep an open mind about what may relieve pain**—new ways are found to control pain. There is much to be learned about the pain experience. Rejecting a patient's nonconventional therapies will lead to mistrust. It is, however, the nurse's responsibility to monitor therapies to ensure the patient's safety and well-being.
8. **Keep trying**—the nurse can easily become frustrated when efforts at pain relief fail. It is important not to abandon the patient when pain persists. The patient in severe chronic pain who is ignored may choose suicide as an alternative. If the patient gains no relief, the nurse should reassess the situation and consider whether alternative therapies are needed.
9. **Protect the patient**—pain therapy should not cause more distress than the pain itself. The nurse always observes the response to therapy. Any pain relief measure may cause side effects, such as fatigue, anxiety, or additional pain. The nurse's aim is to relieve pain without disabling the patient mentally, emotionally, or physically.

NURSING INTERVENTIONS TO CONTROL PAINFUL STIMULI IN PATIENTS' ENVIRONMENT

The following measures can be performed by the nurse to assist in pain control:

- Tighten wrinkled bed linens
- Reposition drainage tubes or other objects on which patient is lying
- Place warm bath blankets for coldness
- Loosen constricting bandages
- Change wet dressings
- Check tape to prevent pulling on skin
- Position patient in anatomical alignment
- Check temperature of hot and cold applications, including bath water
- Lift, not pull, patient up in bed; handle gently
- Position patient correctly on bedpan
- Avoid exposing skin or mucous membranes to irritants (e.g., diarrheal stool or wound drainage)
- Prevent urinary retention by ensuring patency of Foley catheter
- Prevent constipation by encouraging appropriate fluid intake, diet, and exercise

Noninvasive Pain Relief Techniques

Noninvasive pain relief measures can be helpful alone or in conjunction with other methods of management of pain. These approaches include cutaneous stimulation (heat, cold, massage, and TENS), distraction, relaxation, imagery, hypnosis, and biofeedback.

Whether these techniques work because of the gate control theory or because they decrease anxiety, they undoubtedly have many advantages for pain control; most are inexpensive and easy to perform, have low risk and few side effects, and may not require a physician's order. Probably the greatest advantage of these techniques is the patient's ability to have some control over the treatment of his pain. Although not everyone will react successfully to these pain relief measures, it is worthwhile to attempt any of them before advancing to more invasive techniques. It also enables the nurse to offer options for pain relief to patients.

Transcutaneous Electrical Nerve Stimulation (TENS). A special pain relief system, **transcutaneous electrical nerve stimulation (TENS),** pocket-sized, battery-operated device provides a continuous, mild electrical current to the skin via electrodes (see Chapter 22). Generally the electrodes are placed on or near the painful site. As with other forms of cutaneous stimulation, it is thought that TENS works by stimulating large nerve fibers to "close the gate" in the spinal cord. In addition, TENS may stimulate endorphin production.

Invasive Approach to Pain Management

Invasive means anything that enters the body. Examples of invasive techniques are nerve blocks, neurosurgical procedures, and acupuncture. Certain invasive techniques can be helpful for the patient with pain. However, careful patient selection and proper technique are essential, because the costs and risks are high.

Medication Approach to Pain Management

Analgesics can provide patients effective pain relief. Nurses and physicians frequently have misconceptions about the dangers and effects of analgesics. They often undertreat patients because of (1) incorrect pharmacological information, (2) concerns about contributing to addiction, (3) anxiety over errors in judgment while using a narcotic analgesic, and (4) administering less medication than is ordered. Often because of a nurse's uncertainty about the correct administration of analgesics, pain is only reduced, not relieved.

Nurses must understand the medications available for pain relief and their effects. A drug may act at the peripheral receptor level or at the central nervous system level. The most common peripheral analgesics include acetylsalicylic acid (aspirin), acetaminophen (Tylenol), and the nonsteroidal antiinflammatory drugs, ibuprofen (Motrin) and naproxen (Naprosyn) PO and ketorolac tromethamine (Toradol) IM and PO. These drugs act primarily as peripheral receptors to diminish reception of pain stimuli.

Narcotic analgesics, such as morphine, meperidine (Demerol), and codeine, act on higher centers of the brain to modify perception and reaction to pain. The danger of morphine and other narcotic analgesics is the potential for depression of vital nervous system functions. Opiates cause respiratory depression by depressing the respiratory center within the brainstem.

The nurse must learn what is the most effective analgesic and means of administration for the patient's specific need. It takes skill to determine if the medication should be given orally, IM, or IV (see Chapter 21).

Because nurses sometimes fear overtreating patients' pain, a helpful rule is that severe pain requires a greater amount of analgesic for relief. Dosages at the upper end of normally prescribed ranges are usually safe. If a nurse administers a low dose that proves ineffective, the patient may suffer until the required time interval has passed before a drug can again be given.

The patient should be an active participant by telling the nurse when pain perception occurs. The nurse also assesses the patient for nonverbal expressions of pain. If any pain-producing procedure, such as ambulating, coughing, or a dressing change, is scheduled, the nurse should give an analgesic before the activity. The drug should be administered so that its peak effect is reached during the patient's most active time.

Patient-Controlled Analgesia. A drug delivery system called **patient-controlled analgesia (PCA)** allows patients to administer pain medications when they need them. The PCA is a portable, computerized pump with a chamber for a syringe. The pump intravenously delivers a small, preset dose of medication, usually morphine or meperidine (Demerol). To receive a dose, the patient pushes a button on a cord attached to the pump (Fig. 15-3 on p. 262). A timer prevents the system from delivering more than a specified number of doses every hour, to avoid overdoses. Each dose may be as small as 1 ml or 1 mg of morphine every 6 to 12 minutes. It has a locked safety system that prevents tampering.

Epidural Analgesia. Another method of delivery for pain control is the insertion of an epidural catheter and the infusion of opiates into the epidural space. The epidural medication diffuses slowly from the epidural space across the dura and arachnoid membranes into the cerebrospinal fluid (Fig. 15-4 on p. 262). The epidural space, which is filled with fatty tissue and an extensive venous system, is separated from the spinal cord by the dura mater. Thus a higher dose of opiate is needed when the epidural route is used. An epidural dose may be 10 times as much as a dose that would be injected directly into the cerebral spinal fluid.

Drugs used for epidural analgesia are morphine, fentanyl, hydromorphone, and meperidine. The epidural opioids also have side effects: urinary retention, postural hypotension, pruritus, nausea, vomiting, and respiratory depression. Respiratory rate is monitored carefully every 2 hours during infusion.[3]

The insertion and maintenance of the epidural catheter for the infusion are invasive techniques that are the responsibility of the anesthetist or anesthesiologist. Nursing staff members are responsible for monitoring the patient's level of consciousness, pain intensity, respiratory rate, and infusion rate/volume on the pump. The dressing site is examined for signs of infection or leakage of medication around the catheter.[29]

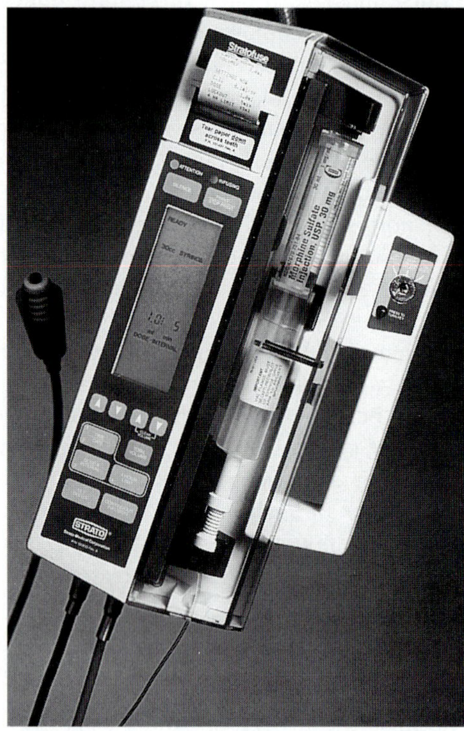

FIG. 15-3 Patient-controlled analgesic device.

Placebos. A **placebo** is an inactive substance or procedure that is given to a patient for its suggestive effect. A placebo is any treatment that produces an effect because of its intent and not its physical or chemical properties, according to McCaffery.[13] An inactive substance, such as injectable normal saline or an oral preparation of sugar, is often prescribed as if it were medication. Some researchers believe that placebos increase endorphin levels. Others believe they create a psychological sense of pain relief, lowering a patient's pain perception. The patient's belief that a placebo is a real form of therapy may be the necessary factor in relieving pain.

SLEEP AND REST

A patient at rest feels mentally relaxed, free from worry, and physically calm. A patient at rest is free from physical or mental exertion. All persons have their own method of obtaining rest and can usually adjust to new environments or conditions affecting the ability to rest.

Nurses frequently care for patients for whom bed rest has been prescribed. This treatment confines patients to bed to decrease physical or psychological demands on the body. Bed rest does not necessarily mean a patient is resting. Emotional or metabolic stressors may cause the patient to be restless.

Sleep is a state of rest that occurs for a sustained period. The reduced consciousness during sleep pro

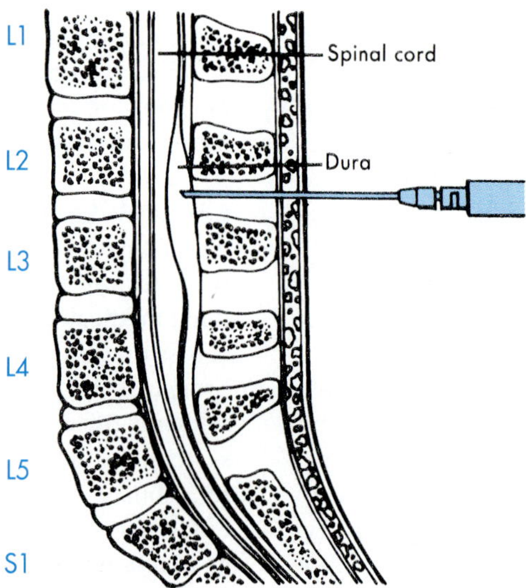

FIG. 15-4 Epidural analgesia. (Courtesy Ross Laboratories, Columbus, Ohio.)

vides time for repair and recovery of body systems for the next period of wakefulness. Sleep restores a person's energy and feeling of well-being.

When the patient enters the hospital or other health care facility, rest and sleep habits can easily be disrupted by hospital routines. The extent of the change depends on the gravity of the illness, as well as the environment in which the patient is placed. The nurse must remain aware of the patient's need for rest. Without rest, the patient becomes fatigued and irritable and has a decreased ability to cope with stressors. Special considerations for the older adult are listed in the gerontological box.

Sleep Cycle

Sleep involves two phases: **rapid eye movement (REM)** and **nonrapid eye movement (NREM).** NREM sleep is further divided into four stages, through which a sleeper progresses during a typical sleeping cycle. The sleeping states are highly individualized (Fig. 15-5 and Box 15-4 on p. 264).

Normally in an adult the routine sleep pattern begins with a presleep period during which the person is aware only of a gradually developing drowsiness. This period normally lasts 10 to 30 minutes, but if a person has difficulty falling asleep, it may last an hour or longer.

As adults fall asleep, they progress through the four stages of NREM sleep. At the end of the fourth stage, they come out of a deep sleep, go back to stage 2, and then enter a period of REM. A person reaches REM sleep in about 90 minutes (average). Each person differs, but a typical night's sleep consists of four to six such cycles. People on the average awaken five times and are twice as likely to awaken from REM sleep as any other stage.

Dreams occur during both the NREM and REM stages. The dream of REM sleep is believed to be functionally important, more vivid, and elaborate. Dreaming allows a person to clarify emotions and prepare the mind for events of the next day. Most medications used to promote sleep, relieve anxiety, and overcome depression interfere with REM sleep. The person may sleep but not feel rested.

Sleep Deprivation

Sleep deprivation is a problem many patients experience as a result of hospitalization. Sleep deprivation involves decreases in the amount, quality, and consistency of sleep. When sleep is interrupted or fragmented, changes in the normal sequence of sleep stages occur, and cycles cannot be completed. Gradually a cumulative deprivation develops.

Patients may experience a variety of physiological and psychological signs and symptoms. Physiological signs and symptoms include hand tremors, decreased reflexes, slowed response time, reduction in word memory, decreased reasoning and judgment, and cardiac dysrhythmias. Psychological signs and symptoms include mood swings, disorientation, irritability, decreased motivation, fatigue, sleepiness, and hyperexcitability.

GERONTOLOGICAL CONSIDERATIONS

- Older adults require about the same amount of sleep as younger persons but are more likely to achieve it in separated episodes; they take more naps and get less sleep at night.
- The sleep of an older adult is less deep. This increases the risk of early awakening and complaint of sleep disturbance.
- Sleep is likely to be disturbed in older adults with chronic health problems such as arthritis, congestive heart failure, and chronic obstructive pulmonary disease. Adequate pain control and positioning facilitates breathing and helps promote rest and sleep.
- Older adults often take medications such as diuretics and theophylline that are likely to disturb sleep. Time of administration and the affect on sleep should be carefully assessed and modified when possible.
- Insufficient sleep may lead to memory and personality changes in older adults.
- Initial nursing interventions to promote rest and sleep should include nonpharmacological comfort measures.

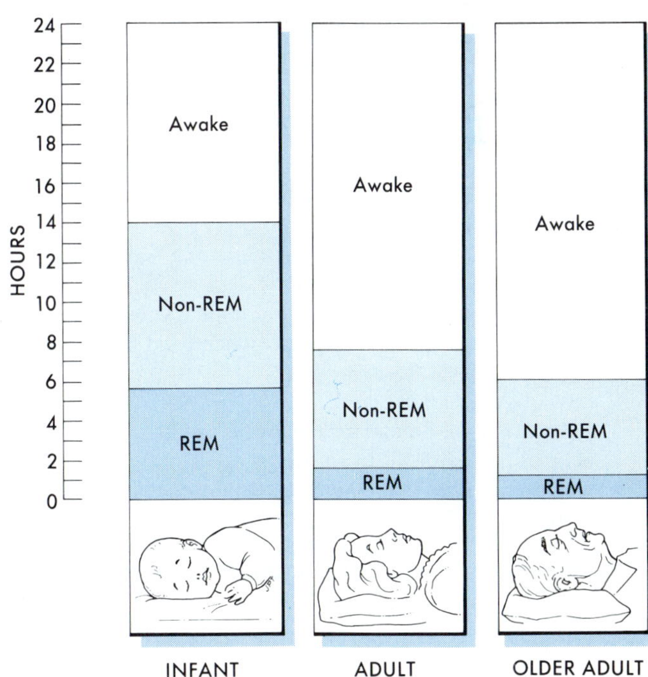

FIG. 15-5 Sleep-wake cycles across the lifespan. *Infants:* approximately 40% of total sleep time is REM. *Adults:* 20% of total sleep time is REM. *Older adults:* total sleep time is slightly reduced, REM remains 20% of total.

Box 15-4 STAGES OF SLEEP

STAGE 1: NREM

- Lightest level of sleep
- Lasts a few minutes
- Decreased physiological activity begins with gradual fall in vital signs and metabolism
- Person easily aroused by sensory stimuli, such as noise
- If person awakes, feels as though daydreaming

STAGE 2: NREM

- Period of sound sleep
- Relaxation progresses
- Arousal is still easy
- Lasts 10 to 20 minutes
- Body functions continue to slow

STAGE 3: NREM

- Initial stages of deep sleep
- Sleeper is difficult to arouse and rarely moves
- Muscles completely relax
- Vital signs decline but remain regular
- Lasts 15 to 30 minutes

STAGE 4: NREM

- Deepest stage of sleep
- Very difficult to arouse sleeper
- If sleep loss has occurred, sleeper will spend considerable portion of sleep in this stage
- Stage responsible for restoring and resting body
- Vital signs significantly lower than during waking hours
- Lasts approximately 15 to 30 minutes
- Sleepwalking and enuresis may occur

REM SLEEP

- Stage of vivid, full-color dreaming (less vivid dreaming may occur in other stages)
- Usually begins every 50 to 90 minutes after sleep has begun
- Typified by autonomic response of rapidly moving eyes, fluctuating heart and respiratory rates, and blood pressure
- Loss of skeletal muscle tone
- Responsible for mental restoration
- Sleeper most difficult to arouse
- Duration of REM sleep increases with each cycle and averages 20 minutes

Promoting Rest and Sleep

The nurse should determine the patient's usual rest and sleep patterns, decide if they are sufficient, and note why the patient is not getting sufficient rest. A plan should be developed with the patient and family to provide for more rest. The plan might include limiting interruptions during the night for vital sign checks and other procedures, providing a quiet environment with a comfortable room temperature, limiting the number of visitors and the duration of visits, and carrying out all procedures within a given time frame.

In preparing the patient for sleep, the nurse should wash the patient's back if the patient is on bed rest, gently massage it, freshen the linens, make certain the patient is warm enough, offer a noncaffeine beverage, such as milk, change soiled dressings, and have the patient void.

Environmental stimuli should be decreased by dimming the lights and decreasing the noise level. The nurse should direct the patient to assume a comfortable position and assist if needed. The patient should be instructed to concentrate on each extremity, one at a time, to focus on how light and relaxed each extremity is, and to begin to breathe slowly, but carefully, allowing no other thoughts to enter the mind. With practice, this approach can be used by the patient when going to sleep. A sleeping medication or analgesic may be administered if the patient cannot sleep.

Nursing diagnoses and interventions for the patient with sleep disturbance include but are not limited to the following:

NURSING DIAGNOSES	NURSING INTERVENTIONS
Sleep pattern disturbance, related to illness and psychological stress manifested by change in behavior performance and increased irritability and listlessness	Encourage patient to ambulate 15 min if able, 1 to 2 hr before bedtime. Provide glass of milk 30 min before bedtime unless contraindicated. Perform all necessary procedures before 9 PM to ensure uninterrupted sleep. Massage back, freshen linens, reduce noise, and dim lights. Administer hypnotic as ordered.
Thought processes altered related to sleep deprivation manifested by slower reaction time, altered attention span, and disorientation	Maintain periods of uninterrupted rest. Provide safe environment. Close door to patient room. Orient to reality. Administer analgesic and/or sedative about 30 min before bedtime, if ordered.

REFERENCES AND SUGGESTED READINGS

1. American Pain Society: *Principles of analgesic use in the treatment of acute and chronic cancer pain: a concise guide to medical practice,* ed 2, Skokie, Ill, The Society.
2. Beare PG, Meyers JL: *Principles and practices of adult health nursing,* ed 2, St Louis, 1994, Mosby.
3. Cahill Wright C: Managing postoperative pain, *Nursing* 21(12):42, 1991.
4. Coylen N: The last four weeks of life, *Am J Nurs* 90(12):75, 1990.
5. Donovan MI, Dillon P, McGuire L: Incidence and characteristics of pain in a sample of medical-surgical inpatients, *Pain* 30:69, 1987.
6. Ferrell BA: Pain management in elderly people, *J Am Geriatr Soc* 39:64, 1991.
7. Fulton JS: Using high-dose morphine to relieve cancer pain, *Nursing* 23(2):34, 1993.
8. Grainger RD: How to manage your own fatigue, *Am J Nurs* 90(3):13, 1990.
9. Harkness-Hood G, Dincher JR: *Total patient care: foundations and practice of adult health nursing,* ed 8, St Louis, 1992, Mosby.
10. Jacox A et al: *Managing acute pain: guidelines for the nation,* Am J Nurs 92(5):49, 1992.
11. Kim MJ, McFarland GK, McLane AM: *Pocket guide to nursing diagnoses,* ed 5, St Louis, 1993, Mosby.
12. Long BC, Phipps WJ, Cassmeyer VL: *Medical-surgical nursing,* ed 3, St Louis, 1993, Mosby.
13. McCaffery M: *Nursing management of the patient with pain,* ed 2, Philadelphia, 1979, Lippincott.
14. McCaffery M, Beebe A: *Pain: clinical manual for nursing practice,* St Louis, 1989, Mosby.
15. McCaffery M, Ferrell B: How vital are vital signs? *Nursing* 22(1):43, 1992.
16. McCaffery M, Ferrell B: Patient age: does it affect your pain control decisions? *Nursing* 21(9):44, 1991.
17. Meinhort NT, McCaffery M: *Pain: a nursing approach to assessment and analysis,* New York, 1983, Appleton-Century-Crofts.
18. Melzack R: *Pain measurement and assessment,* New York, 1983, Raven Press.
19. Metzler D, Finesilver C: When to worry if your patient can't sleep . . . sleep apnea, *RN* 53(3):52, 1990.
20. Miaskowski C: Current concepts in the assessment and management of acute pain, *Med-Surg Nurs* 2(1):28, 1993.
21. Morton P: *Health assessment in nursing,* ed 2, Springhouse, Pa, 1993, Springhouse Corporation.
22. *Mosby's medical, nursing, and allied health dictionary,* St Louis, 1994, Mosby.
23. Phipps WJ, Long BC, Woods NF: *Medical-surgical nursing: concepts and clinical practice,* ed 4, St Louis, 1991, Mosby.
24. Potter PA, Perry AG: *Basic nursing: theory and practice,* ed 3, St Louis, 1995, Mosby.
25. Potter PA, Perry AG: *Fundamentals of nursing: concepts, process, and practice,* ed 3, St Louis, 1993, Mosby.
26. Timby BK, Lewis LW: *Fundamental skills and concepts in patient care,* ed 5, Philadelphia, 1992, Lippincott.
27. Tucker S et al: *Patient care standards: nursing process, diagnosis, and outcome,* ed 5, St Louis, 1992, Mosby.
28. Watt-Watson JH, Ivers Donovan M: *Pain management: nursing perspective,* St Louis, 1992, Mosby.
29. Wild L, Coyne C: The basics and beyond: epidural analgesia, *Am J Nurs* 92(4):26, 1992.

CHAPTER CHALLENGE

KEY POINTS

- McCaffery has a realistic description of pain: "Pain is whatever the experiencing person says it is, existing whenever he says it does."
- Pain is largely a subjective experience.
- Pain is often a protective mechanism that warns of tissue injury.
- A nurse's bias and misconception of pain may result in ineffective control of the patient's pain.
- Pain scales are used to objectively evaluate pain intensity and the effectiveness of pain therapies.
- The nurse individualizes pain therapy by working closely with the patient, using assessment findings, and trying a variety of therapies.
- Patient-controlled analgesic devices and epidural analgesia give pain control with low risk of overdose.
- Nursing implications for administering epidural analgesia include closely monitoring for respiratory depression.
- Fatigue, sleep disturbance, and depression act in a type of synergistic relationship that can markedly change one's perception of pain.

STUDY QUESTIONS

1. Following surgery for a total knee replacement, Mrs. DeBoom was given an epidural catheter for epidural analgesia. An important nursing intervention for the nurse caring for Mrs. DeBoom would be to:
   1. administer additional analgesic medications prn
   2. change epidural dressing every shift
   3. assess respiratory rate carefully
   4. encourage unassisted ambulation
2. Mr. Nichols is a 52-year-old patient admitted for deep vein thrombosis of the left internal iliac vein. He complains of excruciating pain in his left leg. The most appropriate response the nurse could give Mr. Nichols to assure him of her belief in his pain and its control is:
   1. "Pain is what you say it is; I will assist you in whatever way I can."
   2. "Your pain is an unpleasant sensation caused by inflammation of the vein and difficult to control."
   3. "Your pain is one of the cardinal signs of inflammation."
   4. "I know you are in pain, but it is important that we guard against possible addiction to narcotics."
3. Ms. Johnson, age 63, is a first day postoperative patient who has undergone a lower anterior bowel resection. A common central nervous system analgesic often prescribed for control of her pain is:
   1. aspirin
   2. Tylenol
   3. morphine
   4. Motrin
4. A drug delivery system that would allow Mr. Long, a 62-year-old, second day postoperative patient with a below-the-knee amputation, to control his pain via a portable computerized pump with a chamber for a syringe is called:
   1. patient-controlled analgesia
   2. transcutaneous electrical nerve stimulation
   3. a venous access device
   4. a placebo
5. The gate control theory of pain suggests that:
   1. the body contains a natural supply of a morphine-like substance called endorphins
   2. pain is a specific modality and there are specific nerve fibers that transmit pain impulses to the brain
   3. pain impulses can be regulated or even blocked by mechanisms located along the central nervous system
   4. pain is a manifestation of an intricate chain of electrochemical events
6. Mrs. Smith is admitted with severe cellulitis of the left breast. She states, "I have a severe burning pain, and it feels like my breast is on fire." This collection of data by the nurse in assessing Mrs. Smith's pain would be:
   1. deductive
   2. speculative
   3. objective
   4. subjective
7. The nurse listens attentively while Ms. Thompson describes her angina pectoris pain as radiating down her left inner arm to the little finger and upward to the jaw and shoulder. This type of pain is called:
   1. precisely localized
   2. referred
   3. intermittent
   4. chronic
8. The most frequently quoted authority on pain is:
   1. Wiese
   2. Champagne
   3. Hood
   4. McCaffery
9. The nurse is assessing Mr. Torkins' description of his back pain. He states it is "immobilizing, intense and on a scale of 0 to 10, it is a 6." The intensity of pain scale Mr. Torkin is using is called:
   1. visual analogue
   2. categorical
   3. functional
   4. numerical
10. A visual analogue scale may be helpful for:
    1. comparison of a person's concept of pain intensity over time
    2. rating the pain on a scale of 0 to 5
    3. determining the proposed location of pain in the dorsal horn of the spinal cord
    4. use by a critical ill patient
11. People who have less pain than others from a similar injury have a:
    1. higher level of endorphins
    2. lower level of endorphins
12. Research shows nurses treating pain have a tendency to:
    1. overtreat
    2. undertreat
13. Ms. Jones was admitted to the orthopedic section for acute back pain. The physician chose to use cutaneous stimulation management, in which the analgesic effects are achieved by closing the gate to pain impulses and release of endorphins. An example of this pain control method is:
    1. epidural analgesia
    2. transcutaneous electrical nerve stimulation
    3. NSAIDS
    4. patient-controlled analgesia
14. Most medications used to promote sleep, relieve anxiety, and overcome depression:
    1. enhance REM sleep
    2. interfere with REM sleep

16

HYGIENE AND CARE OF THE PATIENT'S ENVIRONMENT

Elaine Oden Kockrow

KEY TERMS

axilla
bedpan
canthus
cerumen
Chux
circumorbital
denture
erythematous
flatus
hygiene
labia majora
labia minora
medical asepsis
microorganisms
oral hygiene
pathogenic
perineal care
personal hygiene
prone
range of motion
sanguineous
Sims'
supine
syncope
umbilicus
urinal
vertigo

LEARNING OBJECTIVES

After reading this chapter, the student should be able to do the following:

- Define the key terms.
- Discuss a therapeutic hospital room environment.
- Describe factors that influence personal hygienic practices.
- Discuss variations of the bath procedure determined by the patient's condition and physician's orders.
- Demonstrate the correct procedure for administering the bed bath.
- Identify nursing interventions for the prevention and treatment of decubitus ulcers.
- Describe components of the bath procedure: oral hygiene, shaving, hair care, nail care, eye, ear, and nose care.
- Demonstrate the correct procedure for administering the back rub.
- Demonstrate the correct procedure for administering perineal care to the male and female.
- Demonstrate the correct procedure for administering skin care.
- Demonstrate the correct procedure for making the unoccupied bed: open, closed, and surgical.
- Demonstrate the correct procedure for making the occupied bed.
- Discuss measures to assist the patient in the use of the bedpan, urinal, and bedside commode.

RELATED TOPICS OF INTEREST

- Communication (Chapter 4)
- Documentation (Chapter 6)
- Signs, symptoms, and physical assessment (Chapter 9)
- Medical asepsis and infection control (Chapter 12)
- Safety (Chapter 13)
- Body mechanics (Chapter 14)
- Comfort, rest, and sleep (Chapter 15)
- Care of the patient with an integumentary disorder (Chapter 25)
- Care of the patient with a urinary disorder (Chapter 30)
- Care of the patient with an eye or ear disorder (Chapter 34)

When providing the patient's hygiene needs, the nurse has an opportunity to observe the patient's ability to perform self-care.

During the bath the nurse notes the patient's physical and emotional state. All body systems can be assessed during the patient's bath. Because the bath, especially the bed bath, involves close contact with the patient, the nurse uses communication skills to enhance the therapeutic relationship, thereby learning about the emotional needs of the patient.

Patients are often placed in a dependent role, dependent on the nurse to assist them in carrying out **personal hygiene** (the self-care measures people use to maintain their health). The nurse should preserve the patient's well-being, encourage as much of the patient's independence as possible, and respect the patient's privacy.

At times the nurse will need to teach health promotion practices, and hygiene care provides an excellent opportunity for this. The nurse must project an attitude of acceptance when caring for a patient whose hygiene is obviously poor. Many factors influence the practice of an individual's personal hygiene: (1) physical condition, (2) personal preferences, (3) cultural variables, (4) knowledge, (5) socioeconomic status, (6) social practices, and (7) body image (see Box 16-1). The prudent nurse will consider all of these factors when assisting the patient with personal hygiene.

Hygiene (the science of health) includes care of not only the skin but also the hair, hands, feet, eyes, ears, nose, mouth, back, and perineum. This chapter will include the bath, components of the bath, bed making, and assisting the patient in the use of the bedpan, urinal, and bedside commode.

Conscientious personal hygienic practices are essential for the nurse. Nurses are role models because teaching can be done by example (Box 16-2). These practices promote **medical asepsis,** also known as *clean technique.* This is a technique that inhibits the growth and spread of **pathogenic** (disease-producing) microorganisms. **Microorganisms** are tiny living plants or animals that can be seen only through a microscope.

Box 16-1 FACTORS INFLUENCING THE PATIENT'S HYGIENIC PRACTICES

SOCIAL PRACTICES

Social groups, family customs, age, friends, and work groups all influence practices of personal hygiene.

BODY IMAGE

Body image is a person's subjective concept of physical appearance. This body image affects the manner in which hygiene is maintained. The nurse will need to provide education to the unclean patient about the importance of hygiene. However, the nurse must not convey feelings of disapproval when caring for the patient whose hygienic practices differ from the nurse's.

SOCIOECONOMIC STATUS

The patient's economic resources may influence the type or extent of hygienic practices used.

KNOWLEDGE

Knowledge alone is not enough. The patient must also be encouraged to maintain self-care. Often, learning about an illness or condition encourages patients to improve hygienic practices. For example, teaching the patient with diabetes the importance of foot care helps to prevent infections. It is important that the nurse maintain a nonjudgmental attitude while providing hygiene for the patient.

PERSONAL PREFERENCE

Individual patients will have individual desires and choices as when to bath, shave, and shampoo. Patients choose different shampoos, deodorants, and toothpastes, according to personal needs or selections. Nurses do not try to change the patient's preferences unless the patient's health is affected.

PHYSICAL CONDITION

Patients in the late stages of terminal illness or those who have undergone surgery often lack the physical energy or dexterity to perform personal hygiene. Some disease conditions may exhaust or incapacitate patients, thereby requiring the nurse to perform total hygiene. Other disease conditions, such as serious cardiac or pulmonary problems, may cause severe activity intolerance.

CULTURAL VARIABLES

Patients from diverse cultural backgrounds follow different self-care practices. For example, in North America, people take daily baths (tub or shower), but in many European countries, it is not unusual to bathe completely only once a week. The nurse will avoid being judgmental when caring for patients with different hygienic practices.

Patient's Room Environment

Patients with severe illnesses may be restricted to prolonged bed rest. Patients with limitations such as traction, casts, or monitoring equipment may not be allowed to leave their rooms. Patients with chronic disabilities and patients in long-term care facilities are often confined to their rooms for long periods. Rooms should be comfortable and safe. The nurse's control of factors such as room temperature, ventilation, noise, and odors can create a more therapeutic environment. Keeping the room clean, neat, and orderly helps to contribute to a sense of well-being (Fig. 16-1 on p. 270).

Box 16-2 PRACTICES OF PERSONAL HYGIENE FOR NURSES

1. Take a daily bath, tub or shower.
2. Use a strong, odorless, and effective deodorant every day.
3. Wear clean undergarments every day.
4. Wear a clean uniform every day.
5. Shampoo hair as often as necessary to maintain cleanliness.
6. Keep hair off the collar or at least pulled back away from the face and in a contained hairstyle. Barrettes and bows should blend in with the hair.
7. Wear hose that are nylon, white, and free from defects; launder following each wearing. Male nurses wear white cotton socks.
8. Wear white, comfortable shoes; keep clean and polished. Shoestrings should be laundered on a regular basis.
9. Keep fingernails short, clean, and well manicured. If polish is worn, it should be clear or pale pink (never have chipped polish).
10. Wear make-up only in moderation.
11. Wear only an engagement ring and/or wedding ring.*
12. Wear only small, unobtrusive earrings; wear only one pair.*
13. Use only a very light cologne, perfume, or after-shave (strong odors are objectionable to patients).
14. Male nurses should wear white only t-shirts under uniform tops.
15. Wear the standard departmental uniform. Jeans, sport slacks, blouses, and shirts are not recommended.
16. Keep beards and mustaches clean, short, and well trimmed.
17. Use breath mints; the smell of coffee or nicotine can be offensive to patients.

*Large and/or dangling earrings are not recommended , nor are numerous rings. These are considered hazardous in departments such as pediatrics and some mental health areas. In departments such as the operating and delivery rooms, rings are not worn at all (surgical asepsis).

Maintaining Comfort

The nurse will want to consider the patient's age, severity of illness, and activity tolerance when maintaining the patient's comfort.

The recommended room temperature should be 68° to 74° F (20° to 23° C). Infants, older adults (see gerontological box), and the acutely ill may need warmer temperatures. Physically active patients may be more comfortable in a cooler environment.

Good ventilation is necessary to keep stale air and odors from lingering in the room. The nurse must be aware of protecting the patient from drafts.

Nurses must be conscientious about emptying and rinsing bedpans and urinals promptly after use. Visitors should not be allowed to smoke in patients' rooms. (Many health care facilities have instituted a no-smoking policy throughout the facility.)

Noise is an unpleasant sound. Ill patients are more sensitive to the noises commonly heard within the hospital environment. All hospital personnel should moni-

GERONTOLOGICAL CONSIDERATIONS

- Older individuals are more likely to become chilled during bathing or when left uncovered. The room temperature should be warmer than for younger persons, and drafts should be minimized.
- Older adults should be properly draped during care to prevent chilling and provide for modesty.
- Impaired circulation or neurological changes may decrease the older person's ability to sense temperature changes in water, so caution should be used to prevent burns during tub or shower bathing.
- Too frequent bathing and use of detergent soaps can have harmful effects on the skin of older adults. Type and frequency of bath's and choice of soap should be based on individual needs.
- Immobility, incontinence, and poor nutrition increase the risk of skin impairment in older adults. Adequate diet, frequent change of position, use of pressure-reducing devices, regular toileting, and prompt cleansing of the skin after incontinence reduce the risks.
- Decreased production of saliva in aging necessitates more frequent oral hygiene. Good cleaning of the oral cavity and teeth or dentures helps reduce the alteration in taste common with aging.
- Older adults should be treated with respect. Grooming, including hair care and use of cosmetics, should be age appropriate.
- Because of normal changes in the nails and an increased incidence of circulatory problems or diabetes mellitus, older individuals are more likely to require special foot care.

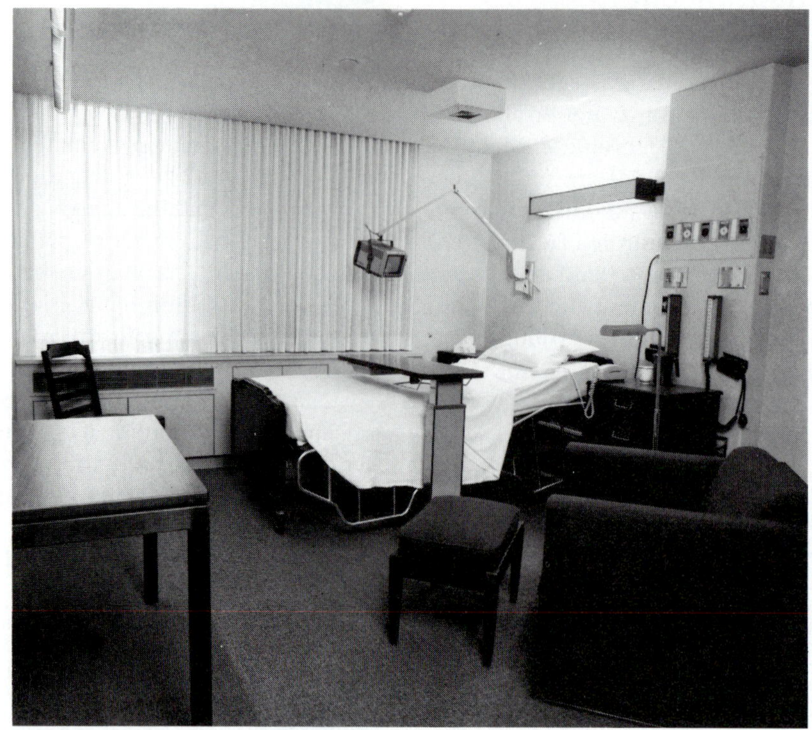

FIG. 16-1 A typical hospital room.

tor the noise level that results from the moving of metal equipment on and off the elevator, TVs and radios, telephones ringing, loud talking, and laughter at the nurses' station. The nurse will want to manage equipment properly, answer phones immediately, and control voice volume. Patients should be asked to keep TVs and radios turned down.

Proper lighting is necessary for the safety of the nurse as well as that of the patient. The nurse will reduce lighting levels to encourage sleep or will brighten the room for stimulation. The nurse may adjust the lighting by closing or opening the drapes, adjusting overbed and floor lights, as well as by opening or closing room doors.

All of the patient's energy must be directed toward recovery. The nurse must do everything possible to control stimuli within the patient's personal environment. This will promote a sense of security and enhance the ability to gain needed rest and sleep (see Chapter 15).

Room Equipment

The usual hospital room (see Fig. 16-1) contains certain basic furniture: bedside stand, bed, overbed table, chairs, and lights. In addition, the standard hospital room will have either a closet or drawer space.

The bedside stand is used to store the patient's personal articles and hygienic equipment such as towels, the emesis and the bath basin, toothpaste and toothbrush, and comb and brush. The telephone, drinking glass, and water pitcher are ordinarily kept on the patient's bedside stand.

The overbed table is on wheels and is adjustable to various heights over the bed or a chair. Usually there is a storage area under the table top. This table top is ideal as a working space for the nurse performing procedures. It also serves as a surface for meal trays, toileting items during hygienic care, and other objects frequently used by the patient.

Chairs are a necessity in the hospital room. Both straight chairs and lounge chairs can be found in the patient's room. The lounge chair can be used by both the patient and visitor. Straight chairs are more convenient because they are more maneuverable than lounge chairs. They are also more convenient when temporarily transferring the patient from the bed as, for example, during bedmaking. Recliner chairs may be used by relatives when sitting with the patient for several hours at a time or all night.

Lights in each patient's room provide comfort, safety, and ease. A call light is available at each bedside. The call light signal indicates that a patient needs assistance. Many facilities are designed so that the call light from a patient's bathroom will blink off and on, perhaps many times, denoting a call of a more serious nature, whereas the bedside call light does not blink. The nurse should respond as soon as possible when a patient indicates a need for assistance.

Beds are designed for comfort, safety, and adaptability to position changes. The standard hospital bed will have a firm mattress on a metal frame that may be raised and lowered horizontally. Most beds are powered by electricity, but some are operated manually. The bed is also constructed so that the head and the foot can be raised and lowered independently.

Most beds will have a firm, water-repellent mattress. The mattress should have an even surface for comfort. Most mattresses will have handles on the sides to use when removing or turning the mattress over.

The controls are conveniently situated on the side of the bed. However, some beds are designed with the controls in the side rail, at the foot of the bed, or as part of the bedside stand. The nurse will teach the patient the proper use of the controls, and will caution the patient to leave the bed at its lowest level to prevent injuries from falls. These Hi-Low beds are convenient to raise while the nurse is working at the bedside and then lower when the patient is being transferred or when the nurse leaves the patient's room.

Hospital beds have a number of safety features. Locks on the wheels can be used to prevent movement. Side rails (adjustable metal frames that raise and lower by pushing or pulling a knob) are located on both sides of the bed. These side rails protect patients from falling, aid patients in positioning themselves, and provide upper extremity support as the patient gets out of bed. The nurse will never leave the bedside when the side rail is lowered with the patient in bed. Each bed will probably have a special removable headboard. This is important when the medical team must have easy access to the patient's head during cardiopulmonary resuscitation.

Throughout the day, the nurse provides a variety of hygienic measures and often schedules other care measures at the same time as hygienic care.

Box 16-3 describes the types of hygienic care that are usually performed at certain times of the day. These times may change due to other factors influencing the nurse's organization and scheduling of care. These factors may include the patient's preferences and habits or the patient's need for further attention, such as when soiling occurs from urine or bowel incontinency (inability to control urine or feces). Other factors influencing care might be scheduled activities or procedures, the nurse-patient staffing ratio, and the nurse's other assignments (for example, administering medications or accompanying the physicians on patient rounds).

Box 16-3 HYGIENIC CARE SCHEDULE

EARLY MORNING CARE

Nursing personnel on the night shift provide basic hygiene to patients getting ready for breakfast, scheduled tests, or early morning surgery. "AM care" includes offering a bedpan or urinal if the patient is not ambulatory, washing the patient's hands and face, and assisting with oral care.

MORNING OR AFTER-BREAKFAST CARE

This care is performed after breakfast. The nurse assists by offering a bedpan or urinal to patients confined to bed; providing a bath or shower; providing oral, foot, nail, and hair care; giving a backrub; changing the patient's gown or pajamas; changing the bed linens; and straightening the patient's bedside unit and room. This is often referred to as *complete AM care.*

AFTERNOON CARE

Because hospitalized patients often undergo many exhausting diagnostic tests or procedures in the morning, afternoon care is greatly appreciated. Afternoon hygiene care includes washing the hands and face, assisting with oral care, offering a bedpan or urinal, and straightening bed linen.

EVENING OR HOUR-BEFORE-SLEEP CARE

Before bedtime the nurse offers personal hygiene care that helps a patient relax to promote sleep. "PM care" may include changing soiled bed linens, gowns, or pajamas; assisting the patient in washing the face, hands, and back; providing oral hygiene; giving a back massage; and offering the bedpan or urinal to nonambulatory patients.

BATHING

The extent of the patient's bath and methods used for bathing depend on the patient's capabilities, the degree of hygiene required, and the physician's order, as in the case of therapeutic baths (Box 16-4 on p. 272).

A complete bed bath is for patients who are totally dependent and require total hygiene (Skill 16-1on pp. 273-275).

The seriously or critically ill patient may need a towel bath (Skill 16-2 on pp. 276-277).

As the patient improves, only partial assistance may be required. The nurse assists the patient to bathe those body parts that are inaccessible to the patient.

If the patient's condition warrants and ambulation has been ordered, the patient may be allowed to take a tub bath or shower (Skill 16-3 on p. 278).

Box 16-4 THERAPEUTIC BATHS

SITZ BATH

This bath cleanses and aids in reducing inflammation of the perineal and anal areas of the patient who has undergone rectal or vaginal surgery or childbirth. Discomfort from hemorrhoids or fissures is relieved by a sitz bath also.

Appliances for the sitz bath are shown in Fig. 16-2. Depending on the patient's diagnosis and the physician's order, the desired results could be obtained from a tub bath. However, the tub is the least desirable method because heat is also applied to the legs, thus reducing the effects on the pelvic region.

The nurse maintains a water temperature of 110° F (about 43° C) if the purpose is to apply heat to the affected area. If the purpose is to promote healing or to produce relaxation, a water temperature of about 98° to 102° F (34° to 39° C) is used. The nurse also should remember to prevent chilling by covering the patient's legs with a bath blanket and his shoulders with a towel. A towel may be placed behind the patient's back for comfort.

The sitz bath should last from 20 to 30 minutes. If the patient has reading material, the time will seem to pass more quickly.

The patient should be observed for signs and symptoms of weakness, such as rapid, weak pulse, tachypnea, and dizziness **(vertigo)** or fainting **(syncope).** The patient should never be left alone unless the nurse is sure the patient is safe; then a call signal should be placed within easy reach.

The patient should be instructed to stay out of drafts and to rest after a sitz bath.

COOL WATER TUB BATH

This bath may be given to relieve tension or lower body temperature. The nurse must institute measures to prevent the patient from chilling. The water temperature is tepid, not cold—98.6° F (37° C).

WARM WATER TUB BATH

This bath is given chiefly to reduce muscle tension. The recommended water temperature is 109.4° F (43° C).

HOT WATER TUB BATH

This bath is given to assist in relieving muscle soreness and muscle spasms. This procedure is not recommended for children. The water temperature for adults should be 113 to 115° F (45° to 46° C). The nurse should remember that danger of burns exists and should take precautions to avoid this.*

*Not used for patients with neurological disorders or circulatory impairment because of the danger of burning.

A sitz bath may be ordered for the patient who has undergone rectal or vaginal surgery. This bath promotes healing and pain relief (see Box 16-4).

A tepid sponge bath is administered to reduce an elevated temperature. This procedure is commonly used for patients who are febrile (elevated body temperature) (Skill 16-4 on p. 279).

A medicated bath may be ordered. This bath may include agents such as oatmeal, cornstarch, Burow's solution, and soda bicarbonate (alkaline bath). The medicated bath is ordered to reduce tension and relax the patient and to relieve pruritus caused by certain skin disorders (Skill 16-5 on p. 280).

Purposes

The nurse provides or facilitates a patient's bath for the following reasons:

- to cleanse the skin
- to apply medication
- to stimulate circulation
- to improve self-image
- to reduce body odors
- to promote range of motion
- to demonstrate caring—an important aspect of the nurse/patient relationship

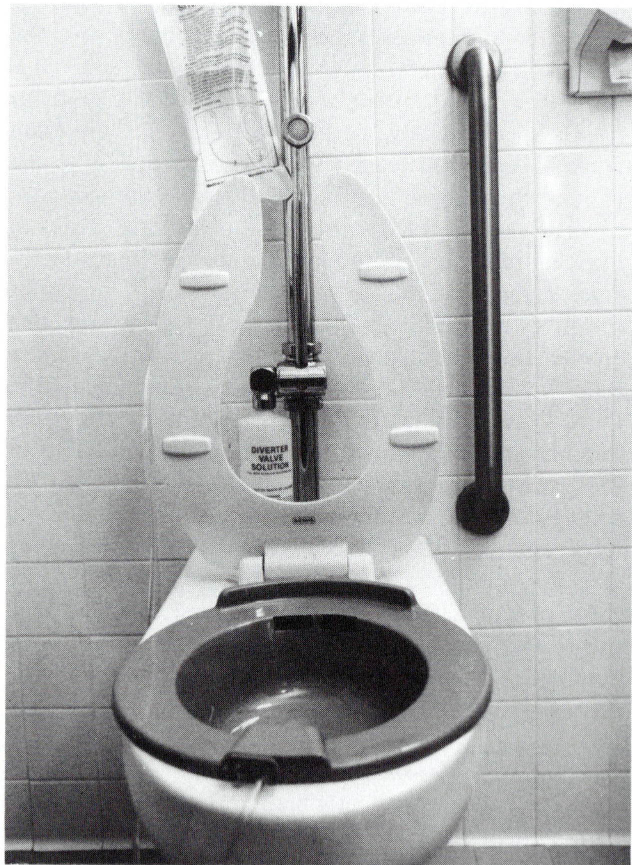

FIG. 16-2 The disposable sitz bath.

ADMINISTERING A BED BATH/PARTIAL BATH

Nursing action/*rationale*

1. Check physician's orders *to provide a basis for care.*
2. Introduce self, and explain procedure *to promote cooperation.*
3. Adjust room temperature, and provide privacy *to prevent chilling and encourage relaxation.*
4. Prepare the following supplies *to promote organization.*
   - bath towels (2)
   - wash cloths (2)
   - wash basin
   - soap and soap dish
   - bath blanket
   - gown
   - hygiene articles, such as lotion, powder, and deodorant
   - laundry bag or hamper
   - disposable gloves

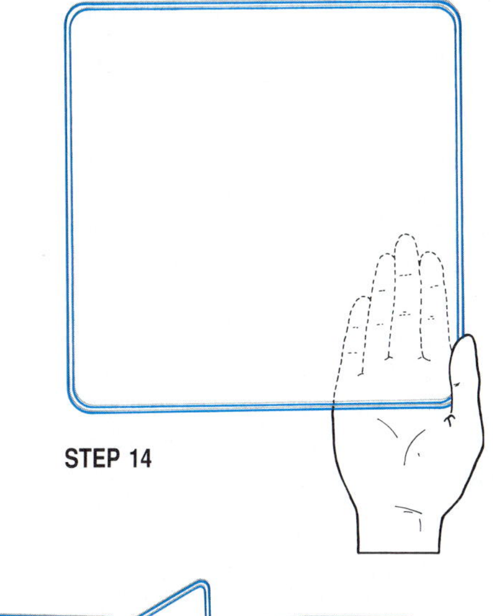

STEP 14

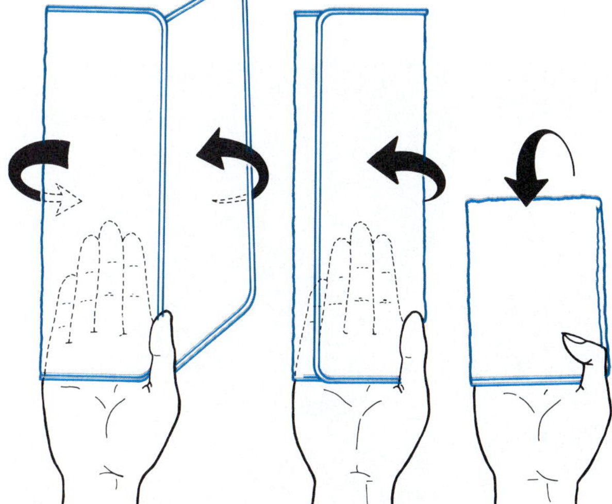

5. Suggest use of bedpan/urinal/bathroom *to prevent interruptions during procedure and provide for patient comfort.*
6. Wash hands *to prevent spread of microorganisms.*
7. Lower side rail, position patient on side of bed closest to nurse, and raise bed to working level *to ensure good body mechanics.*
8. Loosen top linens from the foot of the bed; place bath blanket over the top linens. Ask patient to hold bath blanket while nurse removes top linens. If patient is unable, nurse will need to hold bath blanket in place while removing linens *to provide warmth and privacy.*
9. Place soiled laundry in laundry bag—do not touch uniform with soiled laundry *to prevent spread of microorganisms.*
10. Assist patient with oral hygiene *to prevent mouth diseases, improve self-image, and improve appetite.* If patient is unable, the nurse performs procedure (see Skills 16-6 and 16-7).
11. Remove patient's gown, all undergarments, and jewelry *to facilitate a more effective bed bath.*
12. Raise side rail, and fill water basin two-thirds full with water at 110° to 115° F (43° to 46° C) *to maintain patient's safety.*
13. Remove pillow, and raise head of bed to semiFowler's position if patient can tolerate it *to make the patient's face, ears, and neck more accessible for cleansing.*
14. Form mitt with bath cloth around your hand (see illustration); dip mitt and hand into bath water. Squeeze out excess water *to facilitate handling of bath cloth and prevent corners from brushing against patient.*
15. Wash around patient's eyes using a different portion of wash cloth for each eye. Cleanse from inner to outer **canthus** (corner of eye) (see illustration). Dry gently *to prevent irritation, spread of infection, and injury.*

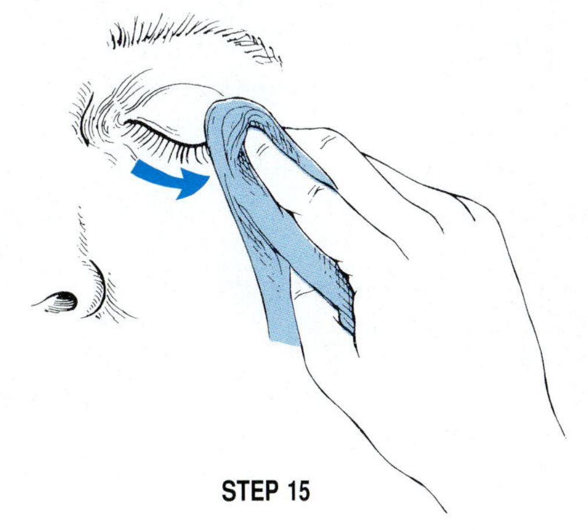

STEP 15

Continued.

ADMINISTERING A BED BATH/PARTIAL BATH—cont'd

16. Rinse bath cloth (continue to use as mitt), and finish washing face. (Ask patient about using soap on face, since some patients, especially female patients, do not use soap on face.) Ears and neck are washed at this time. Cleanse pinna (the projection part of the external ear) with cotton-tipped applicators.
17. Expose arm farthest from nurse. Place towel lengthwise under patient's arm. Place wash basin on towel, and place patient's hand in basin of water. Bathe arms using long, firm strokes. Supporting arm, raise it above patient's head to bathe the **axilla** (the underarm area or armpit). Rinse and dry well. Nail care is done at this time (see Skill 16-10). Deodorant may be applied. Beginning on far side *prevents reaching over clean area;* long, firm strokes *stimulate circulation.* Raising arm *promotes* ***range of motion*** (normal movement that any given joint is capable of making), *as well as exposes axilla.* (Axilla should be bathed last because it is considered less clean than arm.)
18. When doing nail care, allow hand to soak for 3 to 5 min; push back cuticles gently with wash cloth. Clean under nails, and file smoothly as needed. Dry thoroughly *to enhance feeling of self-worth and to decrease spread of infection. Soaking softens cuticles and loosens debris under nails.*
19. Bathe arm closest to nurse. Follow steps 17-18.
20. Cover patient's chest with bath towel; fold bath blanket down to waist, and wash chest with circular motion. Be certain to cleanse and dry well in skin folds and under breasts. Using circular motion while bathing chest *prevents injury to delicate breast tissue.* Covering chest with towel *prevents unnecessary exposure.* Cleansing well in skin folds and under breasts *maintains skin integrity.*
21. Fold bath blanket down to pubic area, keeping chest covered with dry towel. Wash abdomen including **umbilicus** (the depressed point in the middle of the abdomen) (using cotton-tipped applicators) and skin folds. Dry thoroughly *to maintain patient's privacy, to prevent unnecessary exposure, and to prevent skin impairment.*
22. Raise side rail; empty basin into hopper or stool. Rinse basin and wash cloth. Refill basin two thirds full with water at 110° to 115° F (43° to 46° C) *to promotes patient safety and comfort.*
23. Expose leg farthest away from nurse, keeping perineum (the genital area) covered. Place bath towel lengthwise on bed under patient's leg. Place wash basin on towel, and place foot in basin (see illustration). (Make certain to support patient's leg properly; flex knee and grasp heel.) (If patient is unable to place foot in wash basin, wash leg and foot with mitted wash cloth.)
24. Using long, firm strokes to promote circulation, bathe leg. After soaking, do nail care (see Skill 16-10). If skin is dry, lotion may be applied. Do not massage legs. Lower extremities are never massaged, *to prevent possible embolus (a moving blood clot).*
25. Bathe other leg and foot as in steps 23 and 24.
26. Raise side rail. Make sure patient is covered with bath blanket. Change water (see step 22) to maintain patient's safety and privacy.
27. Lower side rail. If patient tolerates, position in **prone** (on abdomen) or in **Sims'** (side-lying)

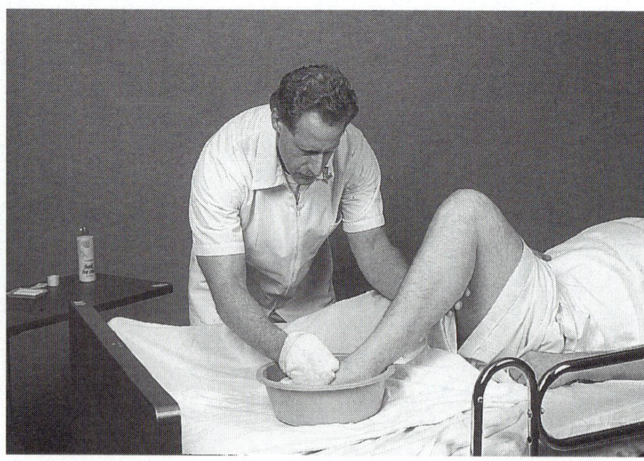

STEP 23

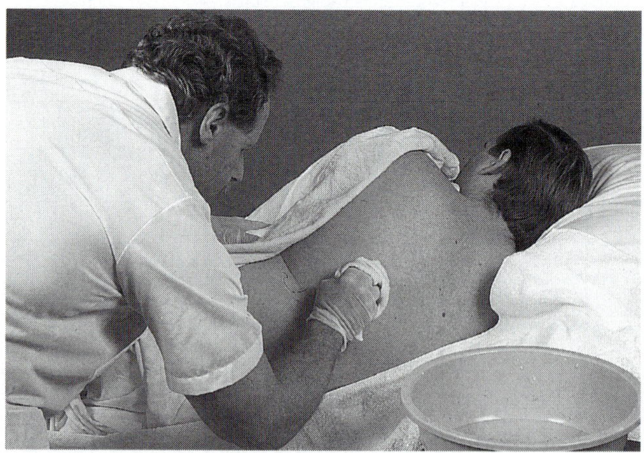

STEP 27

Nursing action/*rationale*

position. Place towel lengthwise on bed along back. Wash and dry back from neckline down to buttocks (see illustration). If patient can tolerate a massage action, do so while washing back *to promote circulation, thus preventing skin impairment.*

28. Reposition patient in **supine** (face up) position. Provide basin of water, soap, wash cloth, and towel, and instruct patient to cleanse perineal area. (Give patient privacy while this is done.) If patient is unable to finish bath, nurse will don gloves and complete this aspect of patient care (see Skill 16-11).
29. Make certain patient is covered with blanket to prevent chilling. Raise side rail to promote safety. Empty basin, and wash and rinse basin. Replace basin in bedside stand. Place wash cloth in laundry bag for soiled linen to maintain medical asepsis.
30. Position patient in Sims' or prone position close to nurse. Place towel lengthwise along patient's back. Give back rub (see Skill 16-13). to facilitate back care. Back care provides comfort and promotes skin integrity.
31. Assist patient into clean gown. If ordered, ambulate patient to chair, place towel over shoulders, and comb hair to promote positive self-image. Women may wish to apply makeup at this time.
32. While patient is in chair, make unoccupied bed (see Skill 16-15). If patient is not ambulatory, nurse must make occupied bed (see Skill 16-14) to maintain clean environment.
33. Place all soiled linen into laundry bag. Make certain all bath equipment is clean and replaced as necessary. Place call light, overbed table, night stand, and telephone within easy reach. Prevents the spread of microorganisms. Promotes safety.
34. Wash hands to *prevent spread of microorganisms.*

The partial bed bath differs from the bed bath only in that the patient does not need assistance bathing various anatomical regions. The nurse then assists to bathe those areas that the patient cannot reach. All steps of the bath are followed, and the same considerations prevail. Supplies are placed within easy reach. Water is changed as noted in the bed bath skill, and back care, skin care, nail care, and hair care are given.

DOCUMENTATION

1. Record procedure *to prove performance.*

Sample charting

DATE	TIME	NOTES
1/30/95	0830	Awake but lethargic. Complains of "muscle soreness." Cast to right forearm clean and dry. Slight digital edema noted. Fingers pale but mobile. Bed bath given. Noted small-intact, erythematous (reddened) area over coccyx. Massage given. States "that felt good." Positioned for comfort. Reported to P. Shahan, RN.

____

(nurse's signature)

DATE	TIME	NOTES
1/30/95	0830	Awake. Denies discomfort. Left leg cast clean and dry. Left toes pink, warm, and mobile. Capillary refill is prompt. States "I hope to go home this evening." Partial bed bath given. This nurse assisted with back, legs, feet, and nail care. Color pink, and skin warm and dry. Respirations unlabored. Very talkative this AM. Reported to E. Maseberg, RN.

____

(nurse's signature)

SPECIAL CONCERNS

- Do not place soap in bath water—too much suds will prevent adequate rinsing.
- The nurse observes the condition of the patient's skin, degree of mobility, and behavior. She encourages the patient to verbalize concerns.
- Patients with diabetes mellitus require special foot care.
- Be certain to expose only those body parts being bathed.
- If danger of contact with body fluids exists, don gloves.
- A firm stroke rather than a light stroke prevents a tickling sensation.
- Maintain a neat, clean work area.

PATIENT TEACHING

- When appropriate, the nurse should take the opportunity to instruct the patient in personal hygiene and skin care.

SKILL 16-2

ADMINISTERING A TOWEL BATH

Nursing action/*rationale*

1. Check physician's order. Confer with charge nurse to determine need for towel bath *to ensure accuracy of procedure.*
2. Explain procedure *to reduce anxiety.*
3. Adjust room temperature, and provide privacy *to prevent chilling, and to encourage relaxation.*
4. Obtain the following supplies *to promote orderly procedure.*
   - concentrate/solution (e.g., Septi-Soft)
   - measuring device, such as plastic medication cup or liter-calibrated container
   - towel-bath towel (3 ft × 7½ ft)
   - large plastic bag
   - bath towel
   - wash cloths (2)
   - bath blankets (2 or 3)
   - disposable gloves
   - linens for bedmaking
   - articles for personal hygiene—comb, toothbrush, lotion, toothpaste, and mouthwash
5. Prepare patient *to ensure bath towel will be warm enough for patient's comfort, as well as for effective towel bath.*
   a. Remove patient's clothing and excess bedding (top linens, bedspread). Place patient on bath blanket, and cover patient with bath blanket.
   b. Cover with plastic any surgical dressings, casts, or areas that should not be wet *to prevent contamination of dressing or cast.*
   c. Fan fold a clean bath blanket at foot of the bed.
   d. Position patient supine (lying on back with legs partially separated and arms loosely at sides).
6. Prepare towel *to prevent unnecessary cleanups and to promote effective procedure.*
   a. Fold towel in half, top to bottom; fold in half again, top to bottom; now half again, side to side. Then roll towel-bath towel, with bath towel and wash cloth inside, beginning with folded edge (see illustration).
   b. Place rolled-up towel-bath towel (with bath towel and wash cloths inside) in plastic bag with selvage edges toward open end of bag.
   c. Draw 2000 ml of water at 115° to 120° F (46° to 49° C) into plastic pitcher. Measure 30 ml of concentrate or 90 ml of solution. (If using dispenser with a pump, a single stroke measures 30 ml.) Mix 2000 ml of water and Septi-Soft.
   d. Pour mixture over towel in plastic bag.

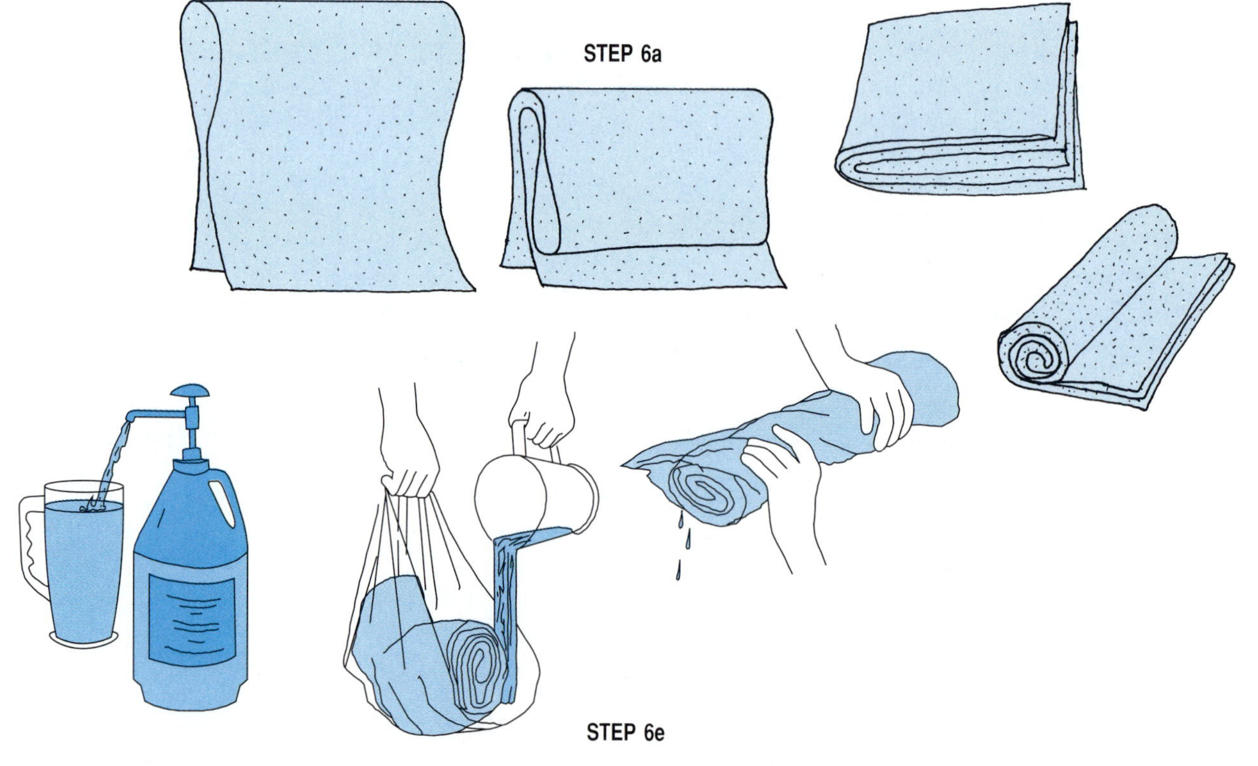

ADMINISTERING A TOWEL BATH—cont'd

e. Knead the solution quickly into towel, position plastic bag with open end in sink, and squeeze out excess water, giving added wringing twist to selvage edges of towel.

7. Bathe patient using the following procedure *to promote effective towel bath, provide warmth, and keep bed dry, avoiding causing the patient to chill.*

a. Fold bath blanket down to waist. Remove warm, moist towel from plastic bag and place on patient's right or left chest with open edges up and outward. (Unroll towel across chest.)

b. Open towel to cover entire body while removing top bath blanket. Tuck towel-bath towel in and around body (leave bath towel and wash cloths in plastic bag to keep warm) (see illustration).

c. Begin bathing at feet, using gentle, massaging motion. Employ clean section of towel for each part of body as nurse moves toward patient's head.

d. Fold lower part of towel upward away from feet as bathing continues.

e. Put clean bath blanket up over patient as nurse moves upward. Leave 3 in of exposed skin between towel and bath blanket. Skin will dry in 2 or 3 sec.

f. Wash face, neck, and ears with one of prepared wash cloths.

g. Turn patient onto side.

h. Use prepared bath towel for back care.

i. Use second wash cloth for perineal care (don disposable gloves).

j. When bath is completed, remove towel and place with soiled linens in plastic laundry bag.

k. If top bath blanket is not soiled, fold for reuse later.

8. Make occupied bed (see Skill 16-14) *to provide comfort and to promote practices of medical asepsis.*

9. Document procedure and any abnormal findings, such as skin impairment *to record patient care in a timely fashion.*

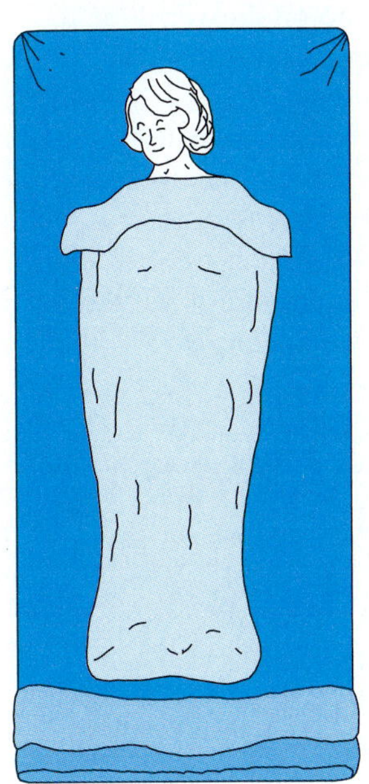

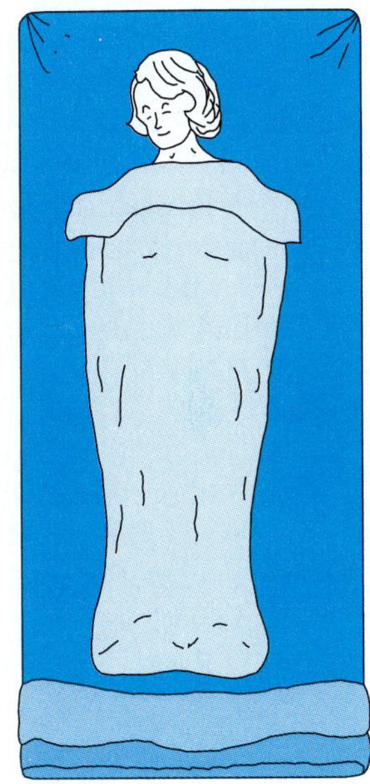

STEP 7b

DOCUMENTATION

Many agencies have flow sheets for recording the type of bath; if the facility requires narrative charting, see example. Record procedure *to prove performance.*

Sample charting

DATE	TIME	NOTES
12/4/94	0900	Color pale. Respirations 30 and labored. Complains of weakness. Towel bath given. A harsh, nonproductive cough noted at infrequent intervals. Positioned for comfort. Sleeping. Reported to Linda Miles, RN.

____

(nurse's signature)

SPECIAL CONCERNS

- The patient must be readied before the bath towel is prepared—the temperature cools down quickly.
- If the towel is not warm, saunalike effect will not be produced and the patient will chill.
- A basin of warm water, soap, wash cloth, towel, and gloves may be necessary to perform perineal care.
- If the towel bath is given properly, the patient will be refreshed and relaxed.
- If the nurse has an assistant, the bath is given more efficiently.

SKILL 16-3

ASSISTING THE PATIENT TO TAKE A TUB BATH OR SHOWER

Nursing action/*rationale*

1. Determine if activity is allowed: consult with RN in charge, and check physician's order, *to provide a basis for patient care.*
2. Make certain tub or shower appliance is clean. See agency's policy. Place nonskid mat on tub or shower floor and disposable mat outside of tub or shower *to promote patient safety.*
3. Gather all items necessary for bathing, including the following, *to prevent unnecessary interruptions.*
   - towel
   - washcloth
   - soap
   - deodorant
   - lotion
   - clean gown
4. Assist patient to tub or shower. Be certain patient wears robe and slippers *to promote patient safety and to prevent patient from chilling.*
5. Instruct patient on how to use call signal and place "in use" sign on tub or shower door if private bath is not being used *to provide for patient safety and privacy.*
6. If tub is used, fill with warm water: 109° F (43° C). Have patient test water, and adjust temperature. Instruct patient on use of faucets—which is hot and which is cold. If shower is used, turn water on and adjust temperature *to prevent accidental burns and promote safety.*
7. Caution patient to use safety bars, and discourage use of bath oil in water. Check on patient q 5 min. Do not allow patient to remain in tub more than 20 min *to maintain patient safety and to prevent vertigo and syncope.*
8. Return to room when patient signals, to assist from tub. Knock before entering *to provide privacy.*
9. Assist patient out of tub and with drying. If patient complains of weakness, vertigo, or syncope, drain tub before patient gets out and place towel over patient's shoulder *to prevent falls and to promote comfort.*
10. Assist patient into clean gown, robe, and slippers. Accompany to room, and position for comfort, in either chair or bed *to maintain warmth and safety.*
11. Make unoccupied bed if patient can tolerate sitting in chair. Perform back, hair, nail, and skin care *to maintain clean environment, to promote positive self-image and medical asepsis.*
12. Return to shower or tub. Clean according to agency policy. Place all soiled linens in laundry bag and return all articles to patient's bedside *to promote orderly environment.*
13. Wash hands *to reduce spread of microorganisms.*

DOCUMENTATION

1. If hospital policy requires, record procedure to prove performance.

Sample charting

DATE	TIME	NOTES
12/4/94	1000	Color pink. Skin warm and dry. NPO for upper GI series. Denies discomfort. Up to shower assisted by this nurse. Respirations even and unlabored. Ambulated down to end of west hall and returned to bed assisted by this nurse. Denies abdominal pain. Reported to Betty Berg, RN.

____

(nurse's signature)

SPECIAL CONCERNS

- Safety must be maintained at all times.
- An unoccupied bed may be made while the patient bathes unless patient condition is such that the nurse should remain with the patient.
- Return to the tub or shower room, and offer to wash the patient's back.
- Observe the patient for signs and symptoms of weakness, which are rapid pulse, pale color, diaphoresis, unsteady gait, tachypnea, vertigo, and syncope.
- Shower chairs are available in most facilities. The patient may be transported from the bedside to the shower, bathed, dried, and returned to bed.

PATIENT TEACHING

- The nurse should emphasize to the patient the importance of safety.

ADMINISTERING A TEPID SPONGE BATH FOR TEMPERATURE REDUCTION

Nursing action/*rationale*

1. Observe patient for elevated temperature. Review physician's orders *to provide basis for care.*
2. Explain to patient: outline steps of the procedure *to reduce anxiety.*
3. Prepare the following equipment *to promote organization.*
   - bath basin
   - tepid water (37° C or 98.6° F)
   - wash cloths (4)
   - bath thermometer
   - bath blanket
   - patient thermometer
4. Provide privacy, and wash hands *to promote relaxation and to prevent spread of microorganisms.*
5. Cover patient with bath blanket, remove gown, and close widows and doors *to prevent chilling.*
6. Test water temperature. Place wash cloths in water, and then apply wet cloths to each axilla and groin (the depressed area between the thigh and trunk). If patient is in tub, allow to stay in water for 20 to 30 min *to promote cooler temperature and to allow for more effective heat loss because blood vessels are close to the surface of the body in the axilla and groin.*
7. Gently sponge an extremity for about 5 min. If patient in tub, gently sponge water over upper torso, chest, and back *to prevent sudden drop in body temperature.*
8. Continue sponge bath to other extremities, back, and buttocks for 3 to 5 min each. Determine temperature q 15 min *to minimize risk of patient chilling.*
9. Change water, and reapply freshly moistened wash cloths to axilla and groin as necessary *to maintain tepid water temperature.*
10. Continue with sponge bath until body temperature falls to slightly above normal. Discontinue procedure according to agency's policy *to prevent body temperature from falling below normal.*
11. Dry patient thoroughly, and cover with light blanket or sheet *to prevent chilling.*
12. Return equipment to storage, clean area, and change bed linens as necessary. Wash hands *to prevent spread of microorganisms.*
13. Record time procedure was started, when ended, vital signs, and patient's response *to indicate patient's response to treatment.*

DOCUMENTATION

1. Record procedure *to prove performance.*

Sample charting

DATE	TIME	NOTES
12/4/94	0230	Color flushed. Skin very warm and moist. C/o headache. Temperature 102.2° F, pulse 100, respirations 28, BP 160/92. Sponge bath for temperature reduction performed for 15 min. Temperature 101.6° F. Reported to N. Hudson, RN.

____

(nurse's signature)

DATE	TIME	NOTES
12/4/94	0250	Sponge bath continued for 15 min. Temperature 100.8° F.
	0310	Sponge bath continued for 15 min. Temperature 99.6° F. States "I'm feeling better." Sponge bath continued for 15 mins. Temperature 99° F, pulse 88, respirations 20, BP 138/82. Denies headache. Skin cool; color pink. Reported to N. Hudson, RN.

____

(nurse's signature)

DATE	TIME	NOTES
12/4/94	0315	Sponge bath discontinued. Complete bed change done. Fluids encouraged. Reported to N. Hudson, RN.

____

(nurse's signature)

SPECIAL CONCERNS

- Measure temperature and pulse every 15 minutes.
- Keep body parts covered that are not being sponged.
- Observe patient's response to therapy and document accurately.
- Avoid rubbing the skin too vigorously, because this may cause an increase in heat production.

PATIENT TEACHING

- Remind patient to call for assistance when getting up; the combination of the elevated temperature and sponge bath could weaken the patient.

SKILL 16-5

ADMINISTERING A MEDICATED BATH

Nursing action/*rationale*

1. Prepare tub bath (see Skill 16-3) *to promote an orderly procedure.*
2. Add appropriate agent as ordered by physician *to follow physician's orders.*
3. Assist patient to tub *to maintain patient safety.*
4. Allow patient to remain in tub for required time *to promote effective procedure.*
5. Assist patient out of tub *to maintain patient's safety.*
6. Gently pat dry *to allow medication to remain on patient's skin.*
7. Assist patient into gown or pajamas *to prevent patient from chilling.*
8. Assist patient to return to bed, and position for comfort *to allow patient to rest and relax.*
9. Wash hands *to prevent spread of microorganisms.*

DOCUMENTATION

1. Record procedure *to prove performance and communicate patient care.*

Sample charting

DATE	TIME	NOTES
1/4/95	0830	Alkaline bath with soda bicarbonate 1:5 solution administered as tub bath for 30 min. Patted dry gently. Assisted to bed and positioned for comfort. States "the itching is not quite as bad." Edematous, erythematous patches over lower extremities are not as prominent as yesterday. Reported to D. Hoffmann, RN.

(nurse's signature)

PATIENT TEACHING

- Teach patient not to scratch the lesions to avoid further irritation and to prevent infection.

COMPONENTS OF THE PATIENT'S HYGIENE

Care of the Skin

When a person's physical condition changes, the skin often reflects this by alterations in color, thickness, texture, turgor, temperature, and hydration (see Chapter 25). As long as the skin remains intact and healthy, its physiological function remains optimal.

Collection of Data. The nurse will determine the condition of the patient's skin by observing its color, texture, thickness, turgor, temperature, and hydration (Box 16-5).

The nursing diagnosis of impairment of skin integrity, either actual or high risk for, applies to every patient with whom the nurse has contact. Prevention and treatment of skin impairment are often responsibilities of the nurse. Prevention is the ultimate goal, but when this is not possible, good nursing interventions can result in (1) optimal healing of the impaired skin without complications, (2) a decrease in the patient's discomfort, (3) a decrease in length of hospitalization, and (4) a decrease in the cost of ongoing care.

A major manifestation of impairment of skin integrity is decubitus ulcers (pressure sores). A patient who

Box 16-5 NORMAL SKIN CHARACTERISTICS

Intact, without abrasions
Warm
Localized changes in texture across surface
Good turgor (elastic and firm) and generally smooth and soft
Skin color variations from body part to body part

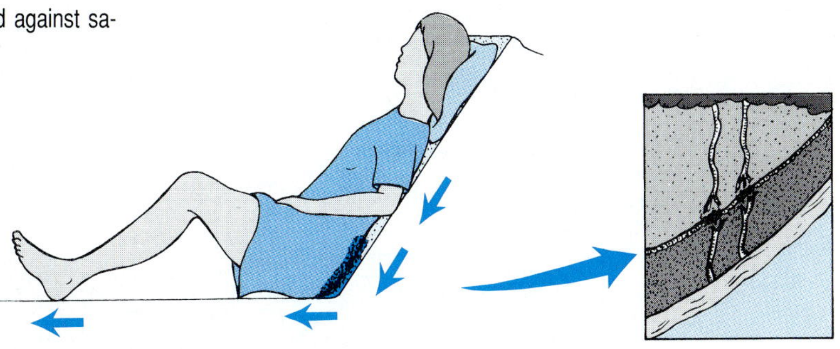

FIG. 16-3 Diagrammatic sketch of shearing force exerted against sacral area.

stays in one position without relief of pressure, especially over bony prominences, can develop a decubitus ulcer. Patients especially at risk are chronically ill, debilitated, older, or disabled or have spinal cord injuries.

Decubitus ulcers occur when there is sufficient pressure on the skin to cause the blood vessels in an area to collapse. The flow of blood and fluid to the cells is impaired, resulting in ischemia, or lack of oxygen and nutrients, to the cells. When the external pressure against the skin is greater than the pressure in the capillary bed (network of capillaries), blood flow decreases to the adjacent tissue. If the pressure continues without relief for more than 2 hours, cell necrosis (death of tissue) may occur in the layers of skin involved. Pressure is usually most severe over bony prominences (e.g., the sacrum, ischial tuberosities, trochanteric areas of the hips, heels, and malleoli of the ankles).

In addition to unrelieved pressure, two mechanical factors can result in decubitus ulcers. The first is *shearing force.* This occurs when the tissue layers of skin slide on each other, resulting in kinking or stretching of subcutaneous blood vessels, which results in an interruption of blood flow to the skin (Fig. 16-3).

The second mechanical factor is *friction.* The rubbing of skin over a surface produces friction, which may remove layers of tissue. Examples of when this might occur are (1) moving the patient in bed by sliding over the linen, (2) improperly lifting the patient, and (3) improperly placing the bedpan.

The first goal in the care of the patient's skin is to prevent skin impairment. A critical factor in achieving this goal is careful observation of each patient to determine who is at increased risk for impaired skin integrity. The six areas to include in data collection follow:

1. General physical condition
2. Level of consciousness
3. Level of activity
4. Degree of mobility
5. Presence of continence or incontinence
6. Nutritional state

The patients at highest risk are those who are confined to a bed or chair, who have limited mobility, who are incontinent, and who have poor overall nutrition. Those who are incontinent are at risk because continual contact of the skin with urine and feces may cause chemical irritation, resulting in skin impairment. Nutritional factors are pertinent for those who are overweight and those who are underweight. Obesity increases the risk because fat tissue has decreased vascularity and resilience and increases weight and pressure on bony prominences. Underweight increases the risk because of a lack of cushion over the bones and muscles. In addition, any condition that results in a decrease in oxygen and nutrients to the cells, such as anemia, atherosclerosis, or edema (swelling), increases the risk of skin impairment because the cells are not adequately nourished.

Patients who are at increased risk for any reason will need careful, ongoing observation and a plan of care aimed at the prevention of skin impairment.

Nursing diagnoses and interventions for the patient with risk for impaired skin integrity include, but are not limited to, the following:

NURSING DIAGNOSIS	NURSING INTERVENTIONS
Skin integrity, impaired, high risk for, related to immobilization	Inspect skin for presence of pressure points at least tid. Provide daily baths. Provide perineal care after each voiding and defecation. Apply skin lotion to areas of skin that become easily **erythematous** (a redness), such as coccyx, heels, scapulae, and greater trochanteric regions. Keep bed linen clean, dry, neat, and as wrinkle-free as possible. Encourage a nutritious diet. Encourage adequate fluid intake. Perform range-of-motion exercises. Use mechanical means, such as sheepskin pads, eggcrate mattress, heel and elbow protectors, and foam- or water-filled chair cushions, but pressure-reducing devices are preferred. Turn q 2 hr.

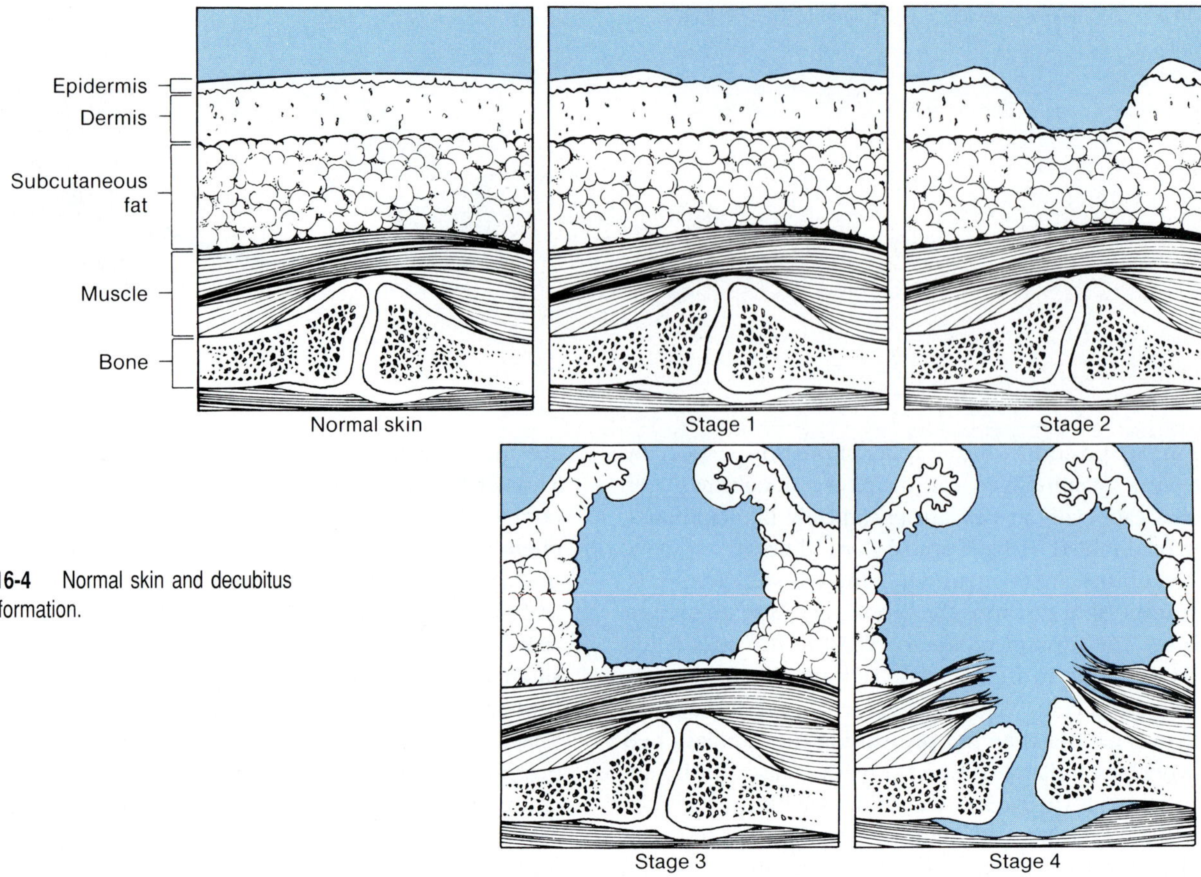

Epidermis
Dermis
Subcutaneous fat
Muscle
Bone
Normal skin
Stage 1
Stage 2
Stage 3
Stage 4

FIG. 16-4 Normal skin and decubitus ulcer formation.

Box 16-6 FOUR STAGES OF DECUBITUS ULCERS AND BEYOND

STAGE I

Transient circulatory disturbance: erythema and/or blanching (to whiten or make pale, as with digital pressure) that disappears when pressure is removed.

The signs are the result of a compensatory mechanism. When pressure is released, circulation is restored to the area. With prolonged pressure, estimated to be more than 2 hr, this compensatory mechanism may not be able to respond and the skin at the site suffers ischemia (lack of blood supply) and necrosis.

STAGE II

Erythematous and/or blanched area with no impairment of skin integrity. patient may complain of pain at the site.

STAGE III

Erythema and edema with vesicle (partial-thickness lesion) and/or impairment of skin integrity.

STAGE IV

Full-thickness lesion extending to subcutaneous fat with or without serosanguineous exudate. (Beyond stage IV, full-thickness lesion extending to deep fascia, muscle, and bone.)

Nursing diagnoses are formulated, goals are determined by stage of the decubitus ulcer (Fig. 16-4), and interventions are implemented. If the patient already has a skin impairment, it is necessary to assess its severity. A commonly accepted classification system divides ulcers into four stages (Box 16-6).

Nursing interventions for these patients include ongoing assessment for evaluating whether improvement is occurring. Assessment data include the size and depth of the ulcer, the amount and color of any exudate, the presence of pain or odor, and the color of the exposed tissue. Healing is a long-term process; therefore the plan of care should be consistent over time and evaluated for effectiveness.

Nursing interventions are aimed at preventing, as well as healing, the ulcers. Specific interventions are determined by the stage of the ulcer.

The nurse will practice surgical asepsis when caring for the decubitus ulcer to prevent a secondary infection. Sterile (free of all living microorganisms) asepsis includes the use of sterile dressings, sterile gloves, and sterile irrigating solution.

The nurse will remember to gently massage the skin over a bony prominence. A vigorous massage could impair skin integrity.

Nutritional support, which promotes healthy tissue repair, may be as important as local wound care for the patient.

Also observe the patient's hydration. If it is inadequate or if signs of dehydration (decreased skin tugor and recessed eyes) are present, carefully observe the patient's intake and output (I&O) and monitor fluid replacement therapy as ordered.

The nurse must be mindful of the primary medical or nursing problem for the patient's hospitalization. Patients are rarely admitted solely because they have a decubitus ulcer that has not healed. The multidisciplinary team of health care professionals—nurses, doctors, physical therapists, and social workers, to name just a few—are available to deliver comprehensive care to the patient.

Patients who are on complete bed rest should be turned every 2 hours. It is important to avoid the full lateral position, which results in direct pressure on the trochanteric region. It is preferable to use the 30-degree lateral-incline position.

Reposition chairbound patients every hour. If the chairbound patient can shift his weight, he should be taught to do so every 15 minutes.

Place patients who are at risk for skin impairment on a pressure-reducing mattress or chair cushion.* Doughnut-type cushions are not advisable because they may cause a congestion of blood to the area, resulting in edema and decrease blood flow to the area.

Other pressure-reducing devices could be therapeutic beds and mattresses. Examples of pressure-relieving beds are the low air-loss bed, (Kin Aire) and the oscillating support surface bed, (Rotorest), both produced by Kinetic Concepts, and the Clinitron bed produced by Support Systems International. Examples of the therapeutic mattress are the Roho, produced by Roho, and the First Step, produced by Kinetic Concepts. In addition, there are the alternating air mattress and the water mattress.

Many kinds of topical agents are available for application to the wound and edges of the wound to facilitate healing. Care should be used to evaluate the effectiveness of any product used on the ulcer. Products that might damage fragile skin and prevent epithelialization (formation of new cells), such as hydrogen peroxide or alcohol, should be used with caution.

Nursing diagnoses and interventions for the patient with decubitus ulcer include, but are not limited to, the following:

NURSING DIAGNOSES	NURSING INTERVENTIONS
Skin integrity, impaired, related to decubitus ulcer (stages I, II, and III)	Assess skin, and identify stage of ulcer development. Eliminate causative factors, and initiate appropriate ulcer care. Cleanse area at least q 4 hr with mild soap and water, and pat dry. Massage area *gently* to increase circulation; avoid vigorous rubbing. If possible, expose area to sunlight and air q 2 to 4 hr or to heat lamp every day for 15 min; observe area frequently to prevent burning. Position patient on unaffected areas. Protect skin surface and affected area with one or combination of the following: ■ Apply karaya powder lightly; dust off excess. ■ Apply skin prep or skin gel. ■ Cover area with moisture-permeable adhesive or wafer barrier. ■ Apply Granulex spray q 8 hr or commercial fat pad, according to manufacturer's directions. ■ Continue one type of application or combination for 48 to 72 hr; if improvement is apparent, continue applications; if no improvement is noted, begin another type of treatment for the patient. ■ Continue use of various mechanical devices.
Skin integrity, impaired, related to decubitus ulcer (stages IV and beyond)	Assess ulcer for size, color, odor, and amount and type of exudate. Monitor temperature for elevation. Culture ulcer as needed. Continue applications to promote healing. If healing is not evident, prepare for débridement as ordered. After débridement, change dressings as ordered. Administer antibiotics as ordered. If available, consult enterostomal therapist. Evaluate various mechanical devices and continue use accordingly.

*These pressure-reducing devices are preferred over the use of sheepskin heel protectors. Placing a rolled bath blanket under the distal extremity to raise the heel off the bed is a much preferred method as this device would totally relieve pressure on the heel.

SKILL 16-6

ADMINISTERING ORAL HYGIENE

Nursing action/*rationale*

1. Position patient's head to side toward nurse (dependent side if possible) as close to nurse as possible *to prevent aspiration.*
2. Explain procedure, even to unconscious patient *because unconscious patients may be able to hear.*
3. Prepare the following equipment *to organize procedure.*
   - cleansing solution, such as diluted hydrogen peroxide, toothpaste, normal saline, soda solution, or mouthwash
   - Toothette, toothbrush, or tongue blade wrapped with gauze
   - towel
   - emesis basin
   - disposable wash cloths
   - water glass filled with cool water
   - water-soluble lubricant
   - disposable gloves
   - flashlight
4. Wash hands, and don gloves *to prevent spread of microorganisms.*
5. Provide privacy, and arrange equipment *to promote an orderly procedure.*
6. Raise bed to working level, and lower side rail *to enable good body mechanics.*
7. Place towel under patient's face and emesis basin under patient's chin *to facilitate procedure and prevent soiling of bed.*
8. Carefully separate patient's jaws *to protect nurse's fingers.*
9. Cleanse mouth using brush, tongue blade, or Toothette moistened with cleansing agent (see illustration). Clean inner and outer teeth surfaces. Swab roof of mouth and inside cheeks. Use flashlight for better visualization of oral cavity. Gently swab tongue. Rinse and repeat. Rinse several times *to remove food particles, secretions, and dried exudate; to moisten mucosa; to leave mouth fresh.*
10. Apply lubricant to lips *to provide moisture to prevent drying and cracking.*
11. Remove gloves and dispose of properly *to prevent spread of microorganisms.*
12. Position patient for comfort, raise side rail, and lower bed *to promote comfort and safety.*
13. Clean and return equipment to storage. Place soiled linen in laundry bag *to maintain clean environment.*
14. Wash hands *to prevent spread of microorganisms.*
15. Record procedure. Include any pertinent observations, such as gum bleeding or ulcerations *to document patient response—any unusual findings may indicate more serious problems.*

SPECIAL CONCERNS

- Complete oral hygiene requires preventive and therapeutic measures. Proper care will prevent oral disease and tooth destruction.
- Patients in hospitals or long-term care facilities often do not receive the aggressive care they need.
- Oral care must be provided on a regular basis; frequency of hygiene measures will depend on the condition of the patient's mouth.
- The beneficial outcomes of oral hygiene may not be seen for several days.
- Repeated cleansing is often needed to remove tenacious, dried exudate of the tongue and to restore the mucosa's hydration to normal.

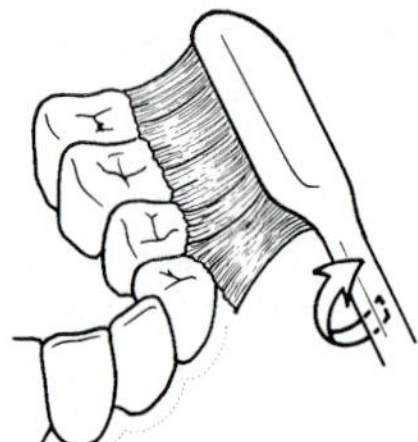
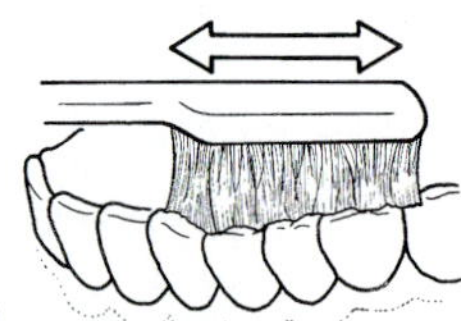
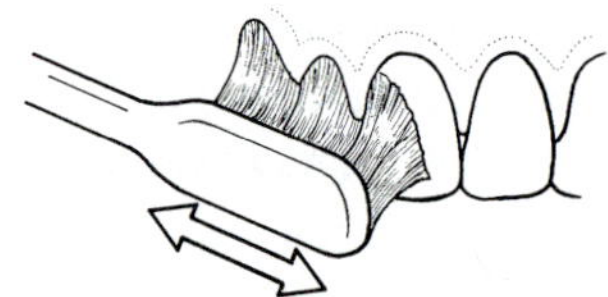

STEP 9

Oral Hygiene

Oral hygiene (care of the oral cavity) helps maintain a healthy state of the mouth, teeth, gums, and lips. Brushing the teeth removes food particles, plaque, and bacteria; massages the gums; and relieves discomfort resulting from unpleasant odors and tastes. Complete oral hygiene gives a sense of well-being and thus can stimulate appetite.

Certain patients are at risk for oral disorders because of (1) a lack of knowledge about oral hygiene, (2) an inability to perform oral care, or (3) an alteration in the integrity of teeth and mucosa resulting from disease or treatments.

Patients who are particularly at risk are those who (1) are paralyzed, (2) are seriously ill, (3) have upper extremity activity limitations, (4) are unconscious, (5) are disoriented, (6) are diabetic, or (7) are NPO status. Patients undergoing radiation therapy, receiving chemotherapeutic drugs, or undergoing oral surgery also are at risk.

Patients should brush their own teeth when possible. When the patient is unable to do so, the nurse will need to perform this procedure (Skill 16-6 and Skill 16-7 [pp. 286-287]).

Shaving the Patient

Many patients prefer to shave at the time of bathing. The nurse should remember that those patients who have a bleeding disorder or are taking anticoagulants (medications that increase the tendency to bleed) should use electric razors. The nurse will not allow a disoriented or depressed patient to use a razor with a blade, to prevent accidental or self-inflicted injury. A patient's beard, mustache, or sideburns are never removed without written consent, except for emergency purposes.

The nurse will need to shave the patient when he is unable to, e.g., because he is too ill or an arm is immobilized in traction or a cast (Skill 16-8 on p. 287).

Hair Care

Proper hair care is important to the patient's self-image. Combing, brushing, and shampooing are basic hygiene measures for all patients. Illness or disability may prevent patients from performing their own daily hair care. A bedfast patient's hair may soon become tangled. It is important for the nurse to remember that most patients are aware of their appearance at all times. Therefore good hair care must be performed routinely, at least daily, to meet the hygiene needs of the patient. If the patient cannot carry out this part of self-care, the nurse will be required to give assistance. If the patient can take a shower or tub bath, the hair can be shampooed easily. A portable chair may be used in the shower, or a chair may be placed in front of a sink.

For the helpless, bedfast patient, the shampoo must be performed in bed. A physician's order may or may not be necessary. Most facilities have portable blow dryers and curling irons available, as well as shampoo boards (Skill 16-9 on pp. 288-289).

Hands and Feet Care

Hands and feet often require special attention to prevent infection, odors, and injury. Problems arise from abuse or poor care of the hands and feet, for example, biting the nails or wearing ill-fitting shoes.

Assessment of the feet involves a thorough examination of all skin surfaces. The area between the toes should be carefully checked. Patients with diabetes mellitus or peripheral vascular disease should be observed for adequate circulation to the feet. The elderly also are at risk for foot disorders, because of poor vision or decreased mobility.

Care of the hands and feet can be administered during the morning bath or at another time (Skill 16-10 on pp. 290-291).

Eye, Ear, and Nose Care

Special attention is given to the cleansing of the eyes, ears, and nose during the patient's bath. The nurse often has the responsibility of assisting patients in the care of eye glasses, contact lenses, or artificial eyes. For patients who wear eye glasses, contact lenses, artificial eyes, or hearing aids, the nurse will assess the patient's knowledge and methods used to care for the aids, as well as any problems caused by the aids. Patients who cannot grasp small objects, have limited mobility in the upper extremities, have reduced vision, or are seriously fatigued will require assistance from the nurse.

The eyes, ears, and nose are sensitive, and therefore extra care should be taken to avoid injury to these tissues (see Chapter 34).

Care of the Eyes. Cleansing of the **circumorbital** (circular area around the eye) area of the eyes is usually performed during the bath and involves washing with a clean wash cloth moistened with clear water. The use of soap is generally omitted because it may cause burning and irritation. The eye is cleansed from the inner to outer canthus. A separate section of the wash cloth is used each time to prevent spread of infection. If the patient has dried exudate that is not removed easily with gentle cleansing, the nurse may first place a damp cotton ball or gauze on the lid margins to loosen secretions. Never apply direct pressure over the eyeball, because this may cause serious injury. Exudate from the eyes should be removed carefully and as often as necessary to keep the eye clean.

CLEANING DENTURES

Nursing action/*rationale*

1. Explain procedure to patient *to promote cooperation.*
2. Prepare the following equipment *to promote orderly procedure:*
   - soft-bristled toothbrush
   - denture brush
   - emesis basin or sink
   - cleansing agent
   - water glass
   - wash cloth
   - 4 × 4 gauze
   - denture cup
   - disposable gloves
3. Wash hands *to prevent spread of microorganisms.*
4. Arrange supplies close by *to promote organized procedure.*
5. Fill emesis basin half full of tepid water *to act as a cushion for the dentures if accidentally dropped, preventing damage to dentures.*
6. Don gloves *to prevent spread of microorganisms.*
7. Ask patient to remove dentures and place in emesis basin. If patient is unable to remove own dentures, break suction that holds upper denture in place by using thumb and finger. With gauze apply gentle downward tug and carefully remove from patient's mouth. Next remove lower denture by carefully lifting up and turning sideways. Remove and place in emesis basin *to prevent slipping while handling dentures.*
8. Cleanse biting surfaces. Cleanse outer and inner teeth surfaces (see illustration). Be certain to cleanse under surface of dentures *to prevent food, bacteria, odor, and stain formation.*
9. Rinse dentures thoroughly with tepid water *because warm water is more effective than cold water.*
10. Replace dentures either in patient's mouth or in container of solution placed in safe place *because dentures may become brittle and warped if not kept moist.*
11. Before replacing dentures in patient's mouth or after storing dentures properly, gently brush patient's gums, tongue, and inside of cheek, and rinse thoroughly *because the oral cavity needs cleansing also to promote healthy gums and mucosa.*
12. Remove gloves, and discard appropriately. Clean and store equipment. Wash hands *to prevent spread of microorganisms.*

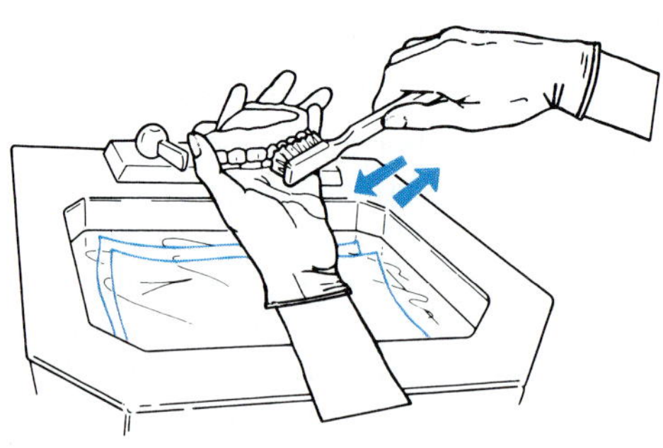

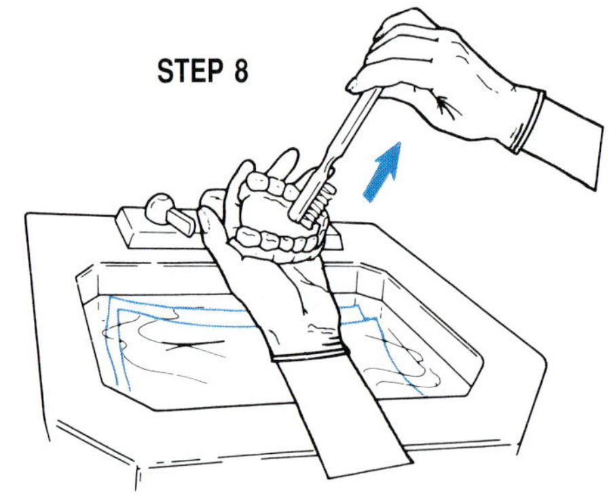

STEP 8

DOCUMENTATION

1. Record procedure *to prove performance and communicate patient care.*

Sample charting

DATE	TIME	NOTES
1/4/95	0935	Oral care given. Dentures cleaned. Tongue, gums, and mucosa cleaned. Slight **sanguineous** (bloody) exudate noted. Dentures replaced in patient's mouth. Lubricant applied to lips. States, "Oh, that feels better." Reported to L. Stebbins, RN.

____

(nurse's signature)

SPECIAL CONCERNS

- Dentures are expensive, are the patient's personal property, and are easily broken; Care must be taken to prevent breakage or loss. Hold over a basin or sink of water or over a soft cloth while cleaning.
- When reinserting the dentures, replace the upper denture first if patient has both dentures. Apply gentle pressure to reestablish the suction. Moisten dentures for easier insertion. Make certain dentures are comfortably situated in patient's mouth before leaving the bedside.

SKILL 16-7

CLEANING DENTURES—cont'd

- Observe dentures for a loose fit. Observe the gums and mucous membrane for tenderness and irritation. These areas may need special care.
- Report any unusual findings.
- Patients should be encouraged to care for their own **dentures** (a set of artificial teeth not permanently fixed or implanted) as often as for natural teeth to prevent infection and irritation.
- If the patient becomes disabled, incapacitated, or disoriented, the nurse must assist with denture care.
- Dentures should be stored in an enclosed and labeled cup during soaking or when not worn; patients should be discouraged from wrapping them in tissue or placing them on meal trays, since the dentures may be accidentally discarded.

PATIENT TEACHING

- Teach patient proper method of caring for dentures, including storage and avoiding damage to dentures.

SKILL 16-8

SHAVING THE PATIENT

Nursing action/*rationale*

1. Determine patient's usual shaving method. Explain procedure *to follow patient's pattern as much as possible.*
2. Wash hands *to prevent spread of microorganisms.*
3. Assemble the following equipment *to organize procedure. Choose equipment with safety in mind.*
   - razor with sharp blade
   - shaving cream/soap/brush
   - bath towel
   - face towel
   - wash cloth
   - bath blanket
   - basin with hot water, 115° F (46° C) or as patient prefers
   - after-shave lotion/powder
   - mirror
4. Assist patient to sitting position if patient is able. Provide privacy. Drape patient with bath blanket *to simulate the normal position. Some patients prefer privacy. Keeps patient warm.*
5. Observe face and neck for lesions, moles, or birthmarks *because cutting could cause infection, bleeding, or irritation.*
6. Use shaving cream or soap *because lathering will soften beard and facilitate shave.*
7. Shave in direction hair grows. Use short strokes. Start with upper face and lip, and then extend to neck. If patient is able, it will help if he will hyperextend (tilt backward) his head to help shave curved areas *to provide for closer shave without irritation.*
8. Pull skin taut with nondominant hand below the area being shaved *to promote uniform shaving* (see illustration).
9. Rinse razor after each stroke *to keep cutting edge clean.*
10. Rinse and dry face *to remove remnants of lather and shaved hair.*
11. If patient desires, apply lotion or cologne *to cause cooling sensation that feels refreshing.*
12. Clean and store equipment. Dispose of used blades in safety container *to protect others from accidental injury.*
13. Wash hands *to prevent spread of microorganisms.*

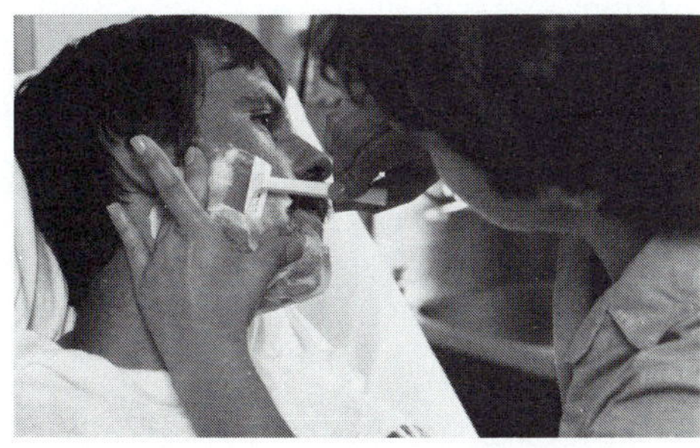

STEP 8

ADMINISTERING A BED SHAMPOO

Nursing action/*rationale*

1. Review physician's order *because special shampoos may be ordered.*
2. Explain procedure *as patient may be anxious.*
3. Prepare the following equipment *to promote an orderly procedure:*
   - bath towels (2):
   - wash cloth or hand towel
   - water pitcher
   - shampoo
   - shampoo board
   - wash basin
   - bath blanket
   - comb and brush
   - hair dryer and curling iron if needed
4. Wash hands *to prevent spread of microorganisms.*
5. Arrange equipment conveniently *to prevent interruptions during procedure.*
6. Position patient close to one side of bed. Place shampoo board under patient's head and wash basin at end of spout (see illustration). Make sure spout extends over edge of mattress *to prevent wetting of bed linens.*
7. Position rolled-up bath towel under patient's neck *to minimize discomfort.*
8. Brush and comb patient's hair *to remove tangles and loosen dried secretions.*
9. Obtain water in pitcher about 110° F (43° C) *to prevent burns.*
10. If patient is able, instruct patient to hold wash cloth over eyes. Completely wet hair, and apply small amount of shampoo *to prevent water and shampoo from getting into eyes.*
11. Massage scalp with fingertips, not nails. Shampoo hairline, back of neck (lift head slightly), and sides of hair *to ensure thorough cleansing and increase scalp circulation.*
12. Rinse thoroughly and apply more shampoo, repeating steps 10 and 11. Rinse, and repeat rinsing until hair is free of shampoo *to prevent scalp irritation.*
13. Wrap dry towel around patient's head. Dry patient's face, neck, and shoulders. Dry hair and scalp using second towel if necessary *to prevent patient from chilling.*
14. Comb hair and/or dry with blow dryer as quickly as possible *to keep patient from chilling* (see illustration).
15. Complete styling hair, and position patient for comfort *to promote sense of well-being.*
16. Place soiled linens in hamper. Clean and store equipment. Wash hands *to prevent spread of microorganisms.*

DOCUMENTATION

Record procedure *to prove performance.*

Sample charting

DATE	TIME	NOTES
1/9/95	0920	Bed shampoo given. Scalp pink and intact. Denies discomfort. Dried hair immediately with hair dryer and styled. States "I'm so glad to have that done." Reported to H. Tufts, RN.

____

(nurse's signature)

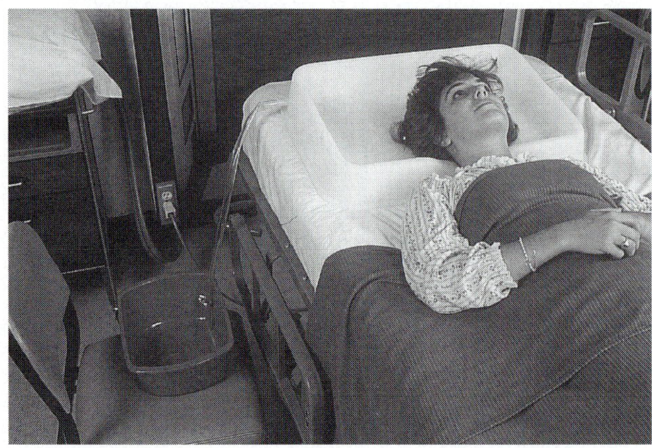

STEP 6

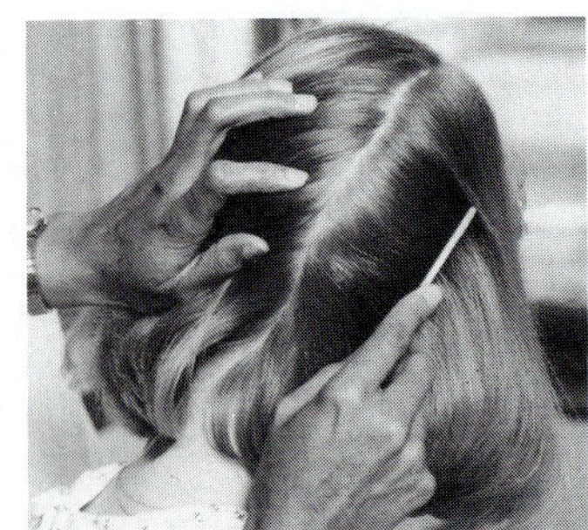

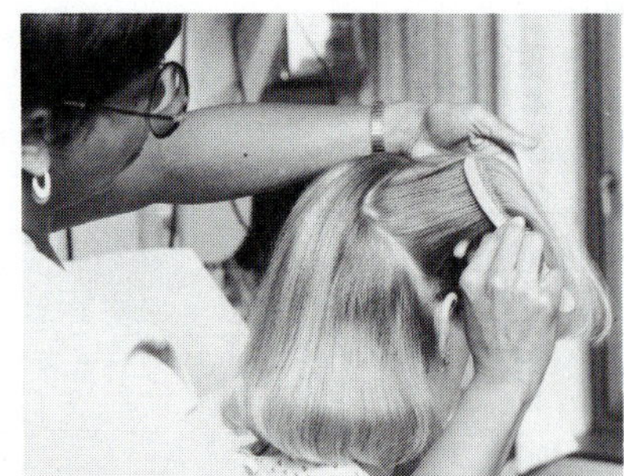

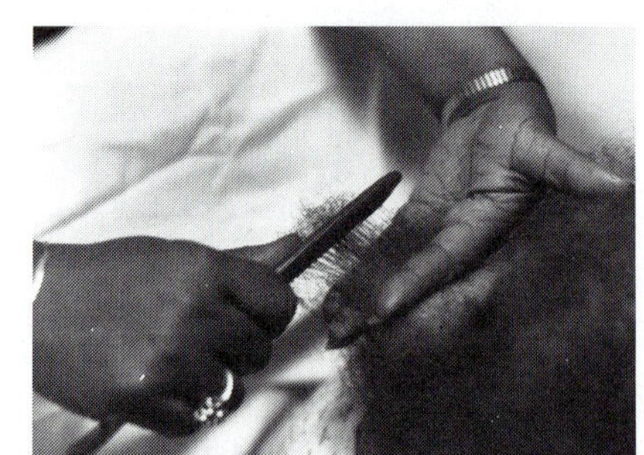

STEP 14

ADMINISTERING A BED SHAMPOO—cont'd

SPECIAL CONCERNS

- Certain conditions, such as cervical neck injuries, open incisions, or a tracheostomy, may place the patient at risk for injury.
- In extreme cases a physician's order may be necessary.
- If hair is matted with blood, hydrogen peroxide is effective as a cleansing agent.
- Inspect condition of scalp; report any unusual findings.
- Make every effort to prevent the patient from chilling.
- Document procedure according to agency policy.

PATIENT TEACHING

- It may be necessary to teach a significant other shampooing techniques.

The eyes are well protected with eyelashes, tearing, and a split-second blink reflex and usually do not require special care. However, the unconscious patient may need frequent special eye care. Secretions may collect along the margins of the lid and inner canthus when the blink reflex is absent or when the eyes do not completely close. Lubricating eye drops may be ordered by the physician. Sometimes the eyes may be medicated and covered to prevent corneal drying and irritation.

Many patients wear eye glasses. This represents a large financial investment for them. Therefore the nurse will use care when cleaning glasses and should protect them from breakage or other damage when not worn.

Eye glasses should be stored in the case and placed in the drawer of the bedside stand when not in use to avoid accidental damage. Glasses are made of hardened glass or plastic that is impact resistant to prevent shattering but can be easily scratched. Plastic lenses require special cleansing solutions and drying tissues. Warm water is adequate to clean glass lenses, and the use of a soft cloth to dry is best to prevent scratching of the lenses.

Most patients prefer caring for their own contact lenses. A contact lens is a small, round, sometimes colored disk that fits on the cornea of the eye over the pupil. If the patient's condition does not permit self removal of the lenses, the nurse should seek assistance from someone who is familiar with the procedure. The lenses need not be reinserted until the patient is more capable of caring for the lenses. It is important that the nurse protect those patients who are unable to care for their lenses properly, because prolonged wearing of contact lenses may cause serious damage to the cornea. There is a large variety of products available for lens care. Each type of lens (hard, soft, or rigid gas-permeable) requires a different cleansing technique. Each set of lenses is stored in a case with solution according to manufacturer's directions.

Care of the Ears. The ears are cleansed by the nurse during the bed bath. A clean corner of a moistened wash cloth rotated gently into the ear canal works best for cleaning. Also, a cotton-tipped applicator is useful for cleansing the pinna. The nurse should teach patients never to use bobby pins, toothpicks, or cotton-tipped applicators to clean the internal auditory canal. These objects may damage the tympanic membrane (eardrum) or cause **cerumen** (wax) to become impacted in the canal.

Hearing aids. Hearing loss is a common health problem. The ability to hear enables patients to communicate and react appropriately within their environment. There are several types of hearing aids available (see Chapter 34). The care of the hearing aid involves routine cleanings, battery care, and proper insertion technique. The nurse will assess the patient's knowledge of and routines for cleaning and caring for the hearing aid. The nurse will determine whether the patient can hear clearly with the use of the aid by talking slowly and clearly in a normal voice tone. The nurse should have the patient suggest any additional tips for care of the hearing aid. When not in use, the hearing aid should be stored where it will not become damaged. The hearing aid should be turned off when not in use to prolong the life of the battery. The outside of the hearing aid should be cleaned with a dry, soft cloth.

Care of the Nose. The patient can usually remove secretions from the nose by gently blowing into a soft tissue. This could be the only daily hygiene necessary. The nurse should teach the patient that harsh blowing causes pressure capable of injuring the tympanic membrane

CARING FOR THE HANDS AND FEET

Nursing action/*rationale*

1. Obtain physician's order if necessary *because the patient's physical condition may place him at risk for infection.*
2. Explain procedure *because patient may be anxious or fatigued.*
3. Prepare the following equipment *to prevent interruptions during procedure.*
   - wash basin
   - emesis basin
   - wash cloth
   - hand towel
   - nail clippers, emery board, and orangewood stick
   - lotion
   - disposable bath mat
   - disposable gloves (optional)
4. Wash hands. Arrange supplies within easy reach *to prevent spread of microorganisms.*
5. Provide privacy. Position patient in chair. If possible place disposable mat under patient's feet *to protect patient's bare feet from floor.*
6. Fill basin with water at 100° to 110° F (43° to 44° C). Place basin on disposable mat, and assist patient to place feet into basin. Allow to soak 10 to 20 min (see illustration). Rewarm water as necessary *because soaking in warm water will soften nails and ensures easy manipulation of cuticles.*
7. Place overbed table in low position in front of patient. Fill emesis basin with water at 100° to 110° F (43° to 44° C). Place basin on table, and place patient's fingers in basin. Allow fingernails to soak 10 to 20 min (see illustration). Rewarm water as necessary *because soaking loosens foreign particles under nails and ensures easy manipulation of cuticles.*
8. Using orange stick, gently clean under fingernails. With clippers, trim nails straight across and even with tip of fingers (see illustration). With emery board shape fingernails. Push cuticles back gently with wash cloth or orangewood stick *to prevent injury to delicate nail beds.*
9. Don gloves, and with wash cloth scrub areas of feet that are callused *to prevent spread of microorganisms.*
10. Trim and clean toenails following step 8.
11. Apply lotion or cream to hands and feet. Return patient to bed, and position for comfort. *Creams and lotions lubricate dry skin.*
12. Remove and dispose of gloves in proper container. Clean and store equipment. Place soiled linen in laundry bag. Wash hands *to prevent spread of microorganisms.*

STEP 6

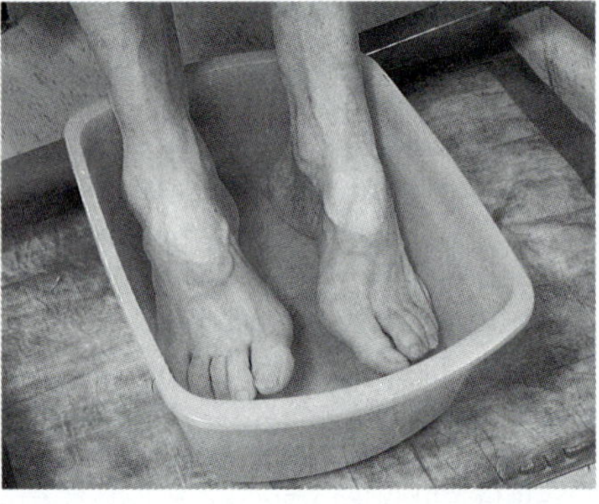

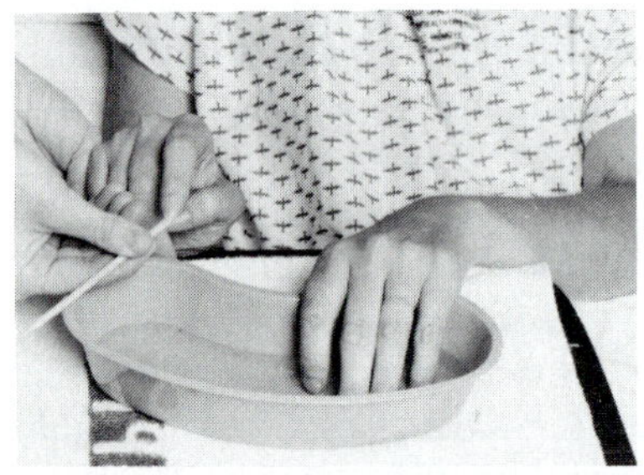

STEP 8

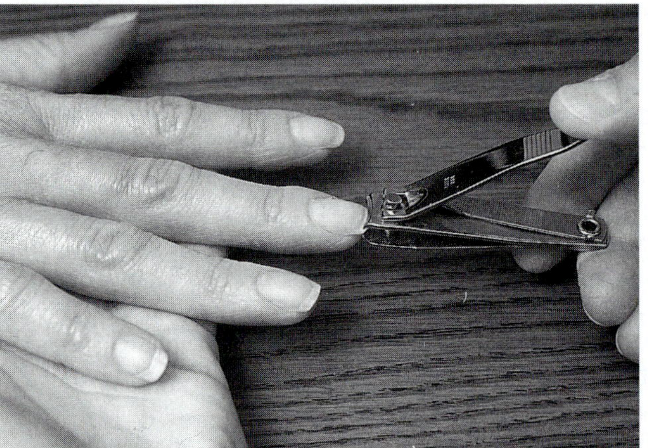

STEP 8

DOCUMENTATION

1. Record procedure *to prove performance and to communicate patient care.*

Sample charting

DATE	TIME	NOTES
12/4/94	1015	Hands and feet soaked for 15 minutes. Nails trimmed straight across. Hands and feet dried thoroughly. Skin areas dry and intact. Lotion applied. Reported to J. Peterson, RN.

____

(nurse's signature)

CARING FOR THE HANDS AND FEET—cont'd

SPECIAL CONCERNS

- Care of the feet and nails may be accomplished during the bath procedure, especially the bed bath. However, for those patients who have special problems, such as the elderly patient or the patient with diabetes mellitus, special attention must be given to this important part of the patient's hygiene.
- Other health disorders that put the patient at risk for foot and/or nail problems are heart failure, renal disease, cerebral vascular accident (CVA), and peripheral vascular conditions.
- On completion of procedure, observe the nails and surrounding tissue for condition of skin and any remaining rough edges.
- If a patient's nails are extremely hard or if a patient is unable to perform personal nail care, a podiatrist (a person trained in the treatment of nail and foot problems) can provide nail care.

PATIENT TEACHING

- The nurse must take time during the procedure to teach the patient the appropriate techniques for cleaning and trimming the nails.

(eardrum), nasal mucosa, and even sensitive eye structures. If the patient is not able to clean the nose, the nurse will assist, using a saline-moistened wash cloth or cotton-tipped applicator. The applicator should not be inserted beyond the cotton tip. If nasal secretions are excessive, suctioning may be necessary. When patients receive oxygen per nasal cannula or have a nasogastric tube, the nurse should cleanse the nares every 8 hours with a cotton-tipped applicator moistened with saline. Because secretions are more likely to collect and dry around the tube, the nurse will also need to gently cleanse the tube with soap and water.

Perineal Care

Perineal care (pericare or care of the genitalia) is part of the complete bed bath. Those patients most in need of scrupulous pericare are those at risk for acquiring an infection, for example, patients with indwelling catheters, patients recovering from rectal or genital surgery, or postpartum patients. If patients are able to do their own pericare, they should be allowed to do so. Embarrassment should never cause the nurse to overlook this nursing intervention. A professional, dignified attitude can diminish embarrassment and put patients at ease (Skill 16-11 on pp. 292-293).

The nurse should be alert for signs of vaginal or urethral exudate (discharge), skin impairment, unpleasant odors, complaints of burning during urination, or localized tenderness or pain of the perineum. The nurse should also observe for skin impairment in the perineal area in those patients with urinary or fecal incontinence, rectal and perineal surgical dressings, and indwelling urinary catheters (Skill 16-12 on p. 294).

Perineal Care for the Patient with an Indwelling Catheter. Catheter care is to be performed twice daily on all patients with indwelling catheters unless otherwise ordered by the physician. Daily catheter care should include cleansing of the meatal-catheter junction with soap and water and application of a water-soluble microbicidal ointment (Betadine or Neosporin, unless another ointment or cream is ordered by physician).

Indwelling urinary catheters should never be used solely as a matter of convenience and should be discontinued promptly when they are no longer necessary. Insertion of an indwelling urinary catheter should be done only by trained personnel using sterile technique, including gloves, catheter, microbicidal antiseptic solution (Betadine) and a water-soluble microbicidal ointment (Betadine), or as ordered.

A sterile, closed-drainage system with disposable, clear plastic bag and connecting tubes should be used. The system should provide for removal of urine without break in sterile continuity and should be changed if sterility is compromised by a break in tubing or technique. Drainage bags should never be inverted or elevated to or above the level of the patient's bladder.

Back Care/Backrub

The backrub is usually administered after the patient's bath. It should be offered to the patient because it promotes relaxation, relieves muscular tension, and stimu-

SKILL 16-11

ADMINISTERING PERINEAL CARE FOR MALE AND FEMALE PATIENTS

Nursing action/*rationale*

1. Explain procedure *to minimize anxiety.*
2. Prepare the following equipment *to promote organization:*
   - soap dish/soap
   - wash basin
   - wash cloths (2)
   - bath towel
   - bath blanket
   - bedpan
   - toilet tissue
   - disposable gloves

When perineal care is given other than routinely during the bath, the nurse will need perineal bottle (peribottle) filled with cleansing solution.

3. Provide privacy. Arrange supplies within easy reach *to reduce anxiety and to ensure orderliness.*
4. Raise bed to working height, and lower the side rail. Assist patient to the dorsal recumbent position for females or supine position for males *to enable good body mechanics.*
5. Female perineal care
   a. Drape patient with bath blanket *to prevent unnecessary exposure.*
   b. Raise side rail, and fill basin two-thirds full with water at 105° to 109° F (41° to 43° C) *to promote patient safety.*
   c. Wash hands, and don gloves *to prevent spread of microorganisms.*
   d. Wash and dry patient's upper thighs *because surrounding skin surfaces need cleansing also.*
   e. Wash both **labia majora** (larger fold or lip) and **labia minora** (smaller fold or lip). Wash carefully in skin folds. Cleanse in direction anterior to posterior *remember to use separate corner of wash cloth for each skin fold to prevent spread of microorganisms.*
   f. Separate labia to expose the urinary meatus (opening) and vaginal orifice. Wash *downward* toward rectum with smooth strokes (see illustration). Use separate corner of wash cloth for each smooth stroke, *to prevent spread of microorganisms.*
   g. Cleanse, rinse, and dry thoroughly *because retained moisture harbors microorganisms.* (If patient is on bedpan and peribottle is used, direct flow of cleansing solution *down* over perineal area and dry thoroughly.)
   h. Assist patient to side-lying position, and cleanse rectal area with toilet tissue, if necessary. Wash area by cleansing from perineal area *toward* anus (see illustration). (Several wash cloths may be needed.) Wash, rinse, and dry thoroughly *to prevent spread of microorganisms and to prevent skin impairment.*
   i. Remove and discard gloves properly *to prevent spread of microorganisms.*
   j. Position patient for comfort, and provide warmth *to promote patient's comfort.*
   k. Clean and store equipment. Place soiled linen in laundry bag *to promote an orderly environment.*
   l. Wash hands *to prevent spread of microorganisms.*
6. Male perineal care
   a. Position patient *to facilitate procedure.*
   b. Raise bed to working height *to enable good body mechanics.*
   c. Drape patient *to provide privacy.*
   d. Raise side rail, Fill basin two-thirds full with water 105° to 110° F (41° to 43° C) *to provide for patient safety.*
   e. Wash hands, and don gloves *to prevent spread of microorganisms.*
   f. Gently grasp shaft of penis. Retract foreskin of uncircumcised patient *because secretions collect under foreskin.*
   g. Wash tip of penis with circular motion. Cleanse from meatus outward *to prevent microorganisms from entering urethra* (see illustration). Two wash cloths may be necessary. Wash, rinse, and dry gently. .
   h. Replace foreskin, and wash shaft of penis with a firm but gentle downward stroke.

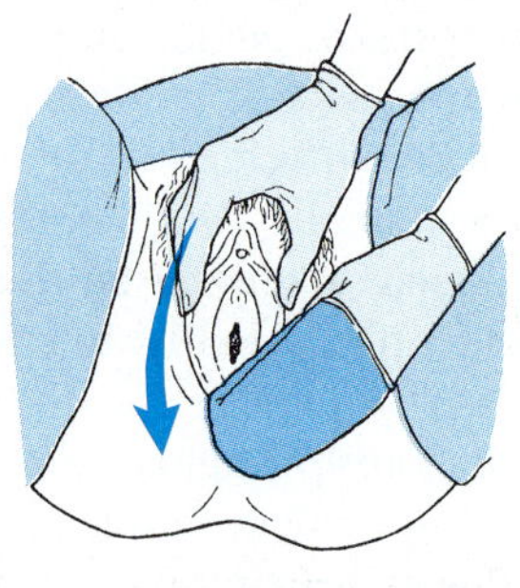

STEP 5f

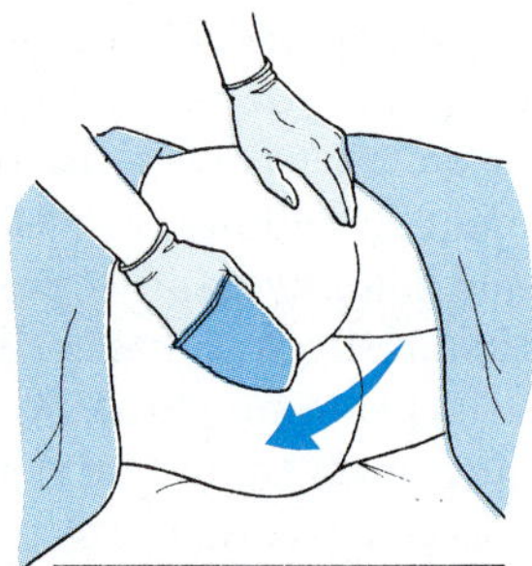

STEP 5h

SKILL 16-11

ADMINISTERING PERINEAL CARE FOR MALE AND FEMALE PATIENTS—cont'd

Rinse and dry thoroughly *because retained moisture harbors microorganisms.*

i. Cleanse stcrotum gently. Cleanse carefully in underlying skin folds. Rinse and dry gently *because pressure on scrotal tissue can be very painful.*

j. Assist patient to a side-lying position *to facilitate procedure.* Cleanse anal area following step a of female perineal care.

k. Follow steps [.] of female perineal care.

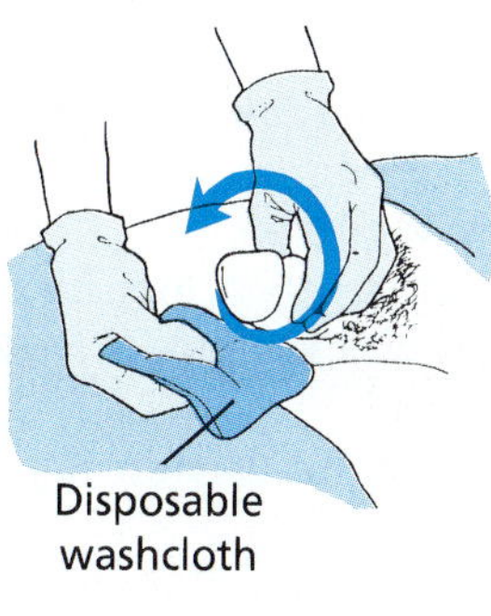

STEP 6g

DOCUMENTATION

1. Record procedure and any abnormal findings *to prove performance and to communicate patient care.*

Sample charting

DATE	TIME	NOTES
12/4/94	1000	Noted moderate amount of tenacious, white, oderless vaginal exudate. Perineal care given. Vulva area crythematous and edematous. Complaints of burning on urination. Fluids encouraged. Reported to K. Williams, RN. __________ *(nurse's signature)*

SPECIAL CONCERNS

- The foreskin of the uncircumcised male patient *must* be replaced after thorough cleansing to prevent edema and discomfort.
- If the patient has an indwelling catheter, the nurse should make certain the catheter is cleansed thoroughly and should apply antibacterial ointment if ordered (see Skill 16-12)
- Patients with indwelling catheters or surgical incisions and patients with fecal or urinary incontinence are at risk for developing infection of the urinary or reproductive tract. Perineal care twice daily decreases this risk.
- Careful observation can assist in determining the need for additional therapy (treatment).

lates circulation. During the backrub the nurse observes the skin. To give an effective backrub, the nurse massages for 3 to 5 minutes (Skill 16-13 on p. 295).

Bedmaking

The patient's bed is usually made in the morning after the bath. When possible the bed is made while not occupied. The patient may be in the tub, showering, or out of the room for a diagnostic examination or procedure. When the patient is unable to be out of bed, the nurse will make an occupied bed.

The patient's safety is always foremost in the nurse's mind. Comfort and privacy are also important. The nurse remembers to use side rails, to keep the call light within easy reach, and to maintain the bed in the proper position: high position while working at the bedside, and low position when work is completed, to protect the patient from accidental falls.

It is the nurse's responsibility to keep the bed as clean and comfortable as possible. This may require frequent inspections to make certain bedding is clean, dry, and wrinkle-free. The nurse will check the linens for food particles after meals and for urine incontinence or involuntary stool. If linens are soiled with urine, feces, blood, or emesis, they should be changed.

The nurse will follow basic principles of medical asepsis. These principles are the following:

1. Keep soiled linens away from uniform.
2. Place soiled linens in hamper or plastic bag.

SKILL 16-12

ADMINISTERING PERINEAL CARE FOR THE PATIENT WITH AN INDWELLING CATHETER

Nursing action/*rationale*

1. Check physician's orders *to provide basis for care.*
2. Introduce self, and explain procedure *to promote cooperation.*
3. Provide privacy *to encourage relaxation.*
4. Obtain the following supplies *to promote orderly procedure.*
   - Betadine (or ointment of physician's choice)
   - soft wash cloth
   - soap and water
   - sterile cotton-tipped applicator and gloves
5. Wash hands, and don gloves *to prevent cross-contamination.*
6. Position patient for comfort *to promote ease of procedure.*
7. Cleanse around urethral meatus and adjacent catheter. Cleanse entire catheter with soap and water *to prevent urinary tract infections.*
8. Repeat cleansing to remove all exudate from meatus and catheter *because exudates can be irritating and serve as good medium for infectious organisms.*
9. Open package of sterile cotton-tipped applicators. Do not touch cotton tip. Apply Betadine ointment to applicator. Do not touch wrapper to cotton tip *to maintain sterility.*
10. Apply ointment to junction of catheter and urethral meatus *to reduce irritation and to prevent spread of microorganisms.*
11. Remove gloves. Clean and store equipment. Dispose of contaminated supplies in proper receptacle *to prevent spread of microorganisms.*
12. Wash hands *to prevent spread of microorganisms.*
13. Position patient for comfort *to promote relaxation.*

DOCUMENTATION

Record any unusual findings *to communicate patient care in timely fashion.*

Sample charting

DATE	TIME	NOTES
1/4/95	1015	Perineal care with catheter care performed. Genitalia pink and moist. Betadine ointment applied. Catheter draining clear, amber urine. Fluids encouraged. Reported to C. Oden, RN.

____

(nurse's signature)

SPECIAL CONCERNS

- Catheter care is to be done 2 times daily on all patients with indwelling catheters unless ordered otherwise by the physician.

PATIENT TEACHING

- Teach patient importance of washing hands before and after performing catheter care.

3. Never fan linens in the air. (This causes air currents, which spread microorganisms.)
4. Never place soiled linens on the floor. If clean linens touch the floor, place in laundry hamper immediately.

The nurse must use proper body mechanics while making the bed, such as raising the bed to a working level to avoid bending down or stretching. Also, the principles of body mechanics should be applied while turning and repositioning the patient.

An occupied bed is made with the patient in it (Skill 16-14 on pp. 296-298). An unoccupied bed may be made open or closed. In the open bed the top linens are fan folded toward the foot of the bed to allow the patient to return to bed more easily. A closed bed is prepared after the patient is dismissed, transferred, or dies, before another patient is admitted (Skill 16-15 on pp. 299-300).

Text continued on p. 300.

ADMINISTERING THE BACKRUB

Nursing action/*rationale*

1. Explain procedure *to promote relaxation.*
2. Prepare the following equipment *because lotion lubricates skin, whereas alcohol has drying effect:*
   - bath blanket (optional)
   - bath towel
   - skin lotion, alcohol, or powder
3. Adjust bed height to working level *to ensure proper body mechanics.*
4. Provide privacy and quiet environment *to promote relaxation.*
5. Lower side rail. Position patient with back toward nurse. Cover patient so that only parts to massage are exposed *to prevent unnecessary exposure.*
6. Wash hands, and warm if necessary. Warm lotion by holding some in hands. Explain that lotion may feel cool *to enhance relaxation.*
7. Begin massage by starting in sacral area using circular motions. Stroke upwards to shoulders. Use firm, smooth strokes to massage over scapulae. Continue to upper arms with one smooth stroke and down along side of back to iliac crests (see illustration). Do not break contact with patient's skin. Complete massage in 3 to 5 min *because a firm, gentle pressure provides relaxation.* Using firm pressure *prevents tickling sensation.* Continuous contact with skin surface is *soothing and stimulates circulation.*
8. Gently but firmly knead skin by grasping area between thumb and fingers. Work across each shoulder and around nape of neck (see illustration). Continue downward along each side to sacrum to increase circulation.
9. With long, smooth strokes because they are relaxing and the most soothing of all massage movements end massage. Remove excess lubricant from patient's back with towel, and retie gown. Position for comfort. Lower bed and raise side rail as needed *to promote patient safety.*
10. Place soiled laundry in proper receptacle. Wash hands *to prevent spread of microorganisms.*

STEP 7

STEP 8

DOCUMENTATION

1. Record procedure, condition of skin, and patient's response *to prove performance and to communicate patient care and condition.*

Sample charting

DATE	TIME	NOTES
1/4/95	2250	Complaining of generalized fatigue. Restless. Expressing concerns over financial matters. Back rub given with lotion. Noted several small erythematous areas over both scapulae. Special massage given to these areas. Denies discomfort. Positioned for comfort.
1/4/95	2330	Asleep. Reported to L. Reid, RN.

____

(nurse's signature)

SPECIAL CONCERNS

- The backrub is contraindicated if the patient has such conditions as fractures of the ribs or vertebral column, burns, pulmonary embolism, or open wounds.
- Monitor pulse and blood pressure of those patients with a history of hypertension or dysrhythmias.

PATIENT TEACHING

- Perhaps a significant other can be taught how to perform the backrub. A backrub could become part of the patient's sleep routine.

SKILL 16-14

MAKING THE OCCUPIED BED

Nursing action/*rationale*

1. Explain procedure *because the patient could be feeling anxious if uncomfortable or fatigued.*
2. Prepare the following supplies *to organize procedure:*
   - laundry bag
   - mattress pad (optional)
   - bottom sheet—many facilities use the contour/fitted sheet
   - protective draw sheet (optional)
   - linen draw sheet
   - top sheet, flat
   - blanket
   - spread
   - **Chux** (waterproof disposable underpad) and/or bath blanket (2)
   - pillow case(s)
   - bedside chair or table
3. Wash hands *to prevent spread of microorganisms.*
4. Assemble equipment, and arrange conveniently *to provide for smooth procedure.*
5. Provide privacy, lower side rail, remove call light, and adjust bed height *to ensure proper body mechanics.*
6. Remove spread and blanket separately, and if soiled, place in laundry bag. If linens will be reused, fold neatly and place over back of chair. (Keep linens away from uniform.) Do not fan or shake linens *to prevent spread of microorganisms.*
7. Place bath blanket over patient on top of sheet. Request patient to hold onto bath blanket while nurse removes top sheet by drawing sheet out from under bath blanket at foot of bed. If patient is unable to assist, nurse will need to hold bath blanket in place while removing sheet. Place soiled sheet in laundry bag *to prevent unnecessary exposure.*
8. With assistance from coworker, slide mattress to top of bed *because if mattress has shifted to foot of bed, it will be difficult to tuck in linens.*
9. Position patient to far side of bed with the back toward nurse. Adjust pillow for comfort. Be sure side rail is up *to provide patient safety.*
10. Beginning at head and moving toward foot, loosen bottom linens. Fan fold linen draw sheet, protective draw sheet, and bottom sheet, tucking edges of linens under patient *to provide maximum work space.*
11. Apply clean linens to bed by first placing mattress pad (if used). Fold lengthwise, making sure crease is in center of bed. Likewise, unfold bottom sheet and place over mattress pad. Hem of bottom sheet should be placed with rough edge down and just even with bottom edge of mattress *to minimize energy and time needed by nurse for bedmaking.*
12. Miter corners (if flat sheet) at head of bed (see illustrations). Continue to tuck in sheet along side toward front, keeping linens smooth *to prevent linens from becoming easily loosened.*
13. Reach under patient to pull out protective draw sheet (if used), and smooth out over clean bottom sheet. Tuck in. Unfold linen draw sheet, and place center fold along middle of bed, smooth out over protective draw sheet, and tuck in. Tuck in folded linens in center of bed so they are under patient's buttocks and torso. Keep palms down as linens are tucked under mattress *to provide for patient's comfort* (see illustrations).
14. Raise side rail, and assist patient to roll slowly toward nurse over folds of linen. Go to opposite side of bed and lower side rail *to maintain patient's safety.*
15. Loosen edges of all soiled linens. Remove by folding into a bundle (see illustration), and place in laundry bag *to prevent spread of microorganisms.*
16. Spread clean linens including protective draw sheet out over mattress, and smooth out wrinkles. Assist patient to supine position, and

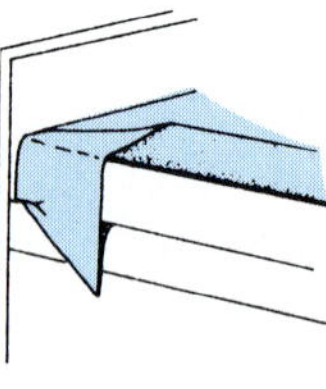

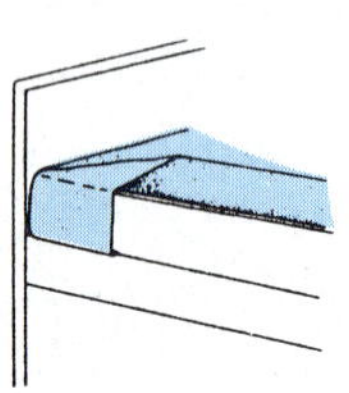

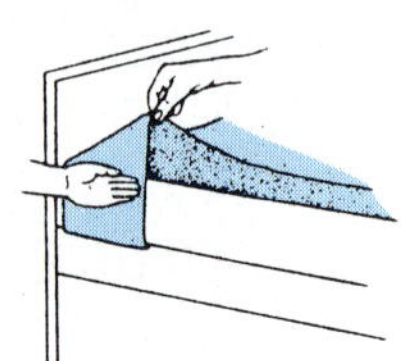

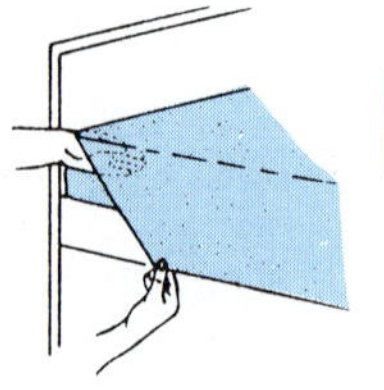

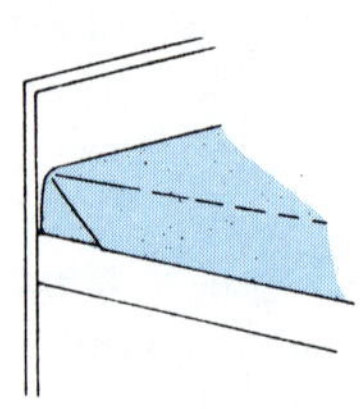

STEP 12

MAKING THE OCCUPIED BED—cont'd

position pillow for comfort *to maintain patient's comfort.*

17. Miter top corner of bottom sheet, pulling sheet taut (see illustrations of step 12). Tuck bottom sheet under mattress all the way to foot of bed *to maintain smooth linens.* Avoid lifting mattress too fat, *to ensure tight fit.*
18. Smooth out draw sheets. Pulling sheet taut, tuck in protective draw sheet and then tuck in linen draw sheet, first in center, then top, and last, bottom *to ensure tight fit.*
19. Place top sheet over bath blanket that is over patient. Request patient to hold top sheet while nurse removes bath blanket. Place blanket in laundry bag. (Make sure center fold of sheet is in center of bed.) If blanket is used, place over sheet and place spread over blanket. Form cuff with top linens under patient's chin *to provide for patient comfort and warmth* (see illustration).
20. Tuck in all linens at foot of bed, making modified miter corner (see illustration). Raise side rail and make opposite side of bed. Remember to allow for toe pleat. Make toe pleat by placing fold either lengthwise down center of bed or across foot of bed *to prevent unnecessary pressure on patient's feet, possibly causing footdrop.*
21. Change pillow case. Remove case by grasping pillow through opened end, and draw pillow

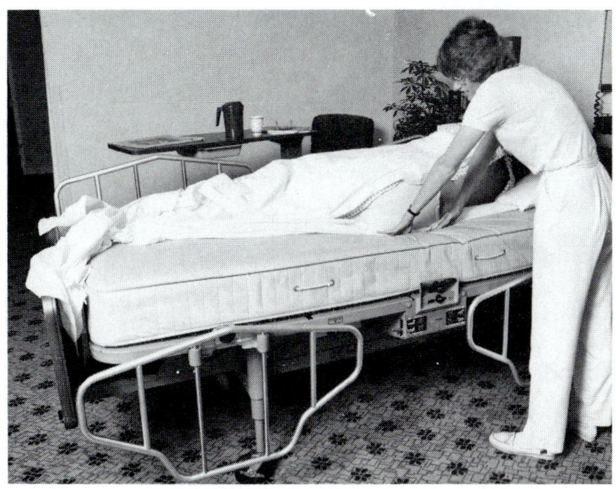

STEP 13

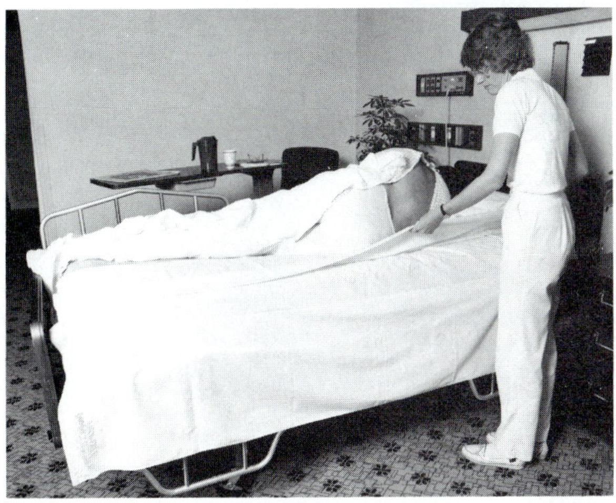

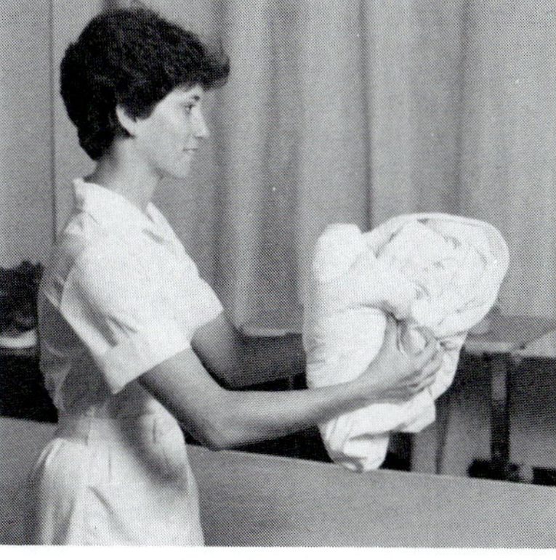

STEP 15

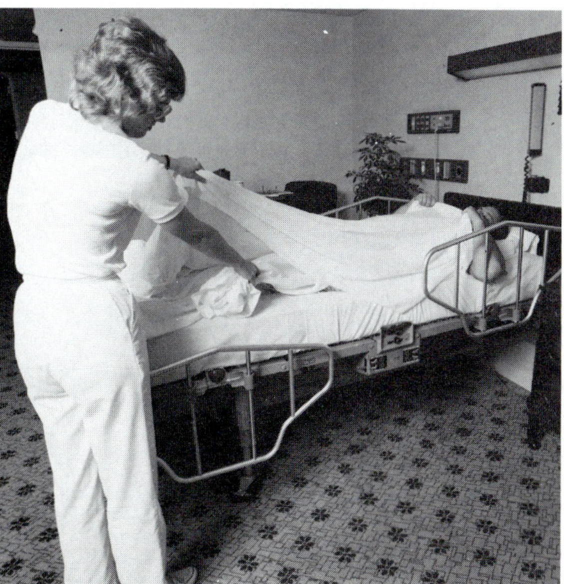

Continued.

MAKING THE OCCUPIED BED—cont'd

out through case. Grasp closed end of pillow case, turning case inside out over hand. Now grasp one end of pillow with hand in the case. With other hand pull pillow case over pillow and smooth out wrinkles, making sure pillow corners fit into pillow case corners (see illustration below). As pillow is removed from under patient, support neck muscles *to prevent injury.* Nurses should never hold pillow under their chin to prevent the spread of microorganisms.

22. Place call light within easy reach, and lower bed. Place personal items within easy reach on bedside stand or table *to provide safety and comfort.*
23. Remove all soiled linens, and place in proper receptacle. Wash hands *to prevent spread of microorganisms.*

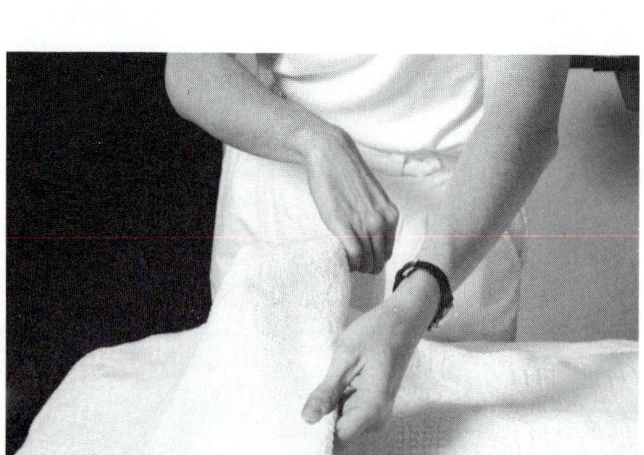

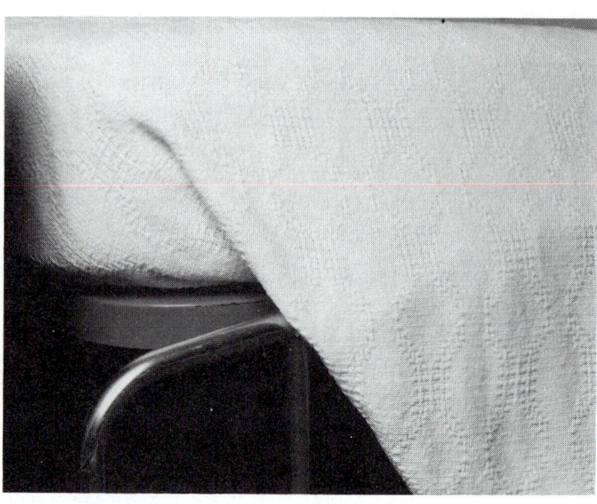

STEP 20

SPECIAL CONCERNS

- If patient is incontinent or if there is excessive drainage, waterproof pads or an extra bath blanket may be necessary.
- Check physician's order for any precautions in moving or positioning the patient.
- Remove all unnecessary equipment, and maintain a neat work area.
- Rough hem edges should be away from the patient to prevent skin impairment.
- All linens should be smooth and wrinkle free to promote patient's comfort.
- Assure patient that he will not fall out of bed.
- Patients with certain conditions, such as a respiratory disorder, may not be able to tolerate lying flat.

PATIENT TEACHING

- Explain steps of procedure in which patient will be participating.

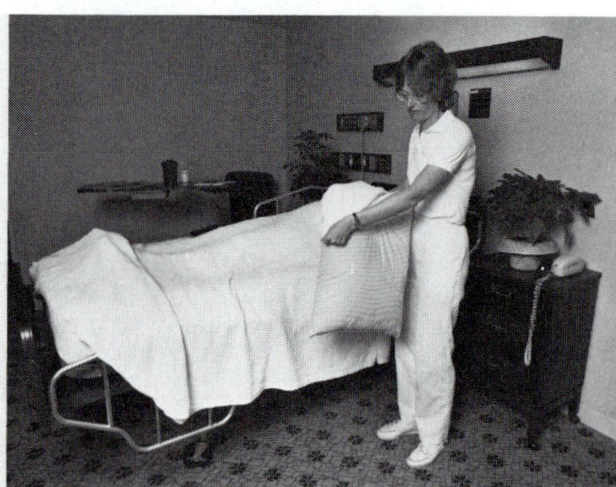

STEP 20

MAKING THE UNOCCUPIED BED

Nursing action/*rationale*

1. Prepare supplies *to ensure orderly procedure.*
   - laundry bag
   - mattress pad (optional)
   - bottom sheet (may be contoured)
   - protective draw sheet (optional)
   - linen draw sheet
   - top sheet (flat)
   - blanket
   - spread
   - Chux and/or bath blanket (optional)
   - pillow case(s)
   - bedside chair or table
2. Wash hands *to prevent spread of microorganisms.*
3. Assemble equipment, and arrange conveniently *to provide for a smooth procedure.*
4. Lower side rail. Adjust bed level, and remove call light *to ensure good body mechanics.*
5. Starting at head of bed, loosen linens all the way to foot. Go to opposite side of bed, loosen linens, roll all linens up in ball, and place in soiled laundry bag. Do not permit linens to come in contact with uniform. Do not shake or fan linens because linen is easier to remove and *to prevent spread of microorganisms.*
6. If blanket and spread are to be reused, fold neatly and place over back of chair. Remove soiled pillow case as in Skill 16-14, step 21 *to facilitate replacement, and to prevent wrinkles.*
7. Slide mattress to head of bed because it is easier to tuck in linens.
8. If necessary, cleanse mattress with moistened cloth with antiseptic solution and dry thoroughly *to prevent spread of microorganisms.*
9. Begin to make bed standing on side where linens are placed. Unfold bottom sheet, placing fold lengthwise down center of bed. Make certain rough edge of hem lies down away from patient's heels and even with edge of mattress (see illustration). Smooth out sheet over top edge of mattress, and miter corner. (See Skill 16-14 and step 12.) Tuck remaining sheet under mattress all the way to foot. Keep linens smooth. Time is saved if one side of bed is made at a time. Fan folding all linen lengthwise down bed *promotes neatness and prevents wrinkling.*
10. Place draw sheet on bed so that center fold lies down middle of bed. If protective draw sheet is to be used, place it on first. Smooth out over mattress, and tuck in *to prevent loosening and wrinkling.* Keep palms down.
11. Place top sheet over bed, and smooth out. Place blanket over top sheet. Smooth out. Place spread over blanket, and smooth out. Make cuff with top linens (see illustration) *to provide for patient's comfort.*

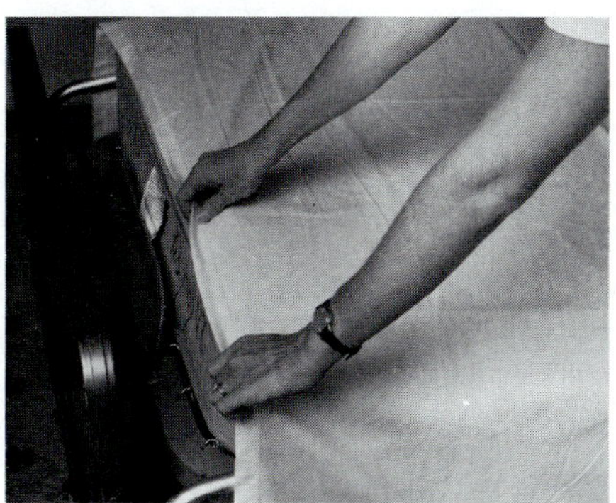

STEP 9

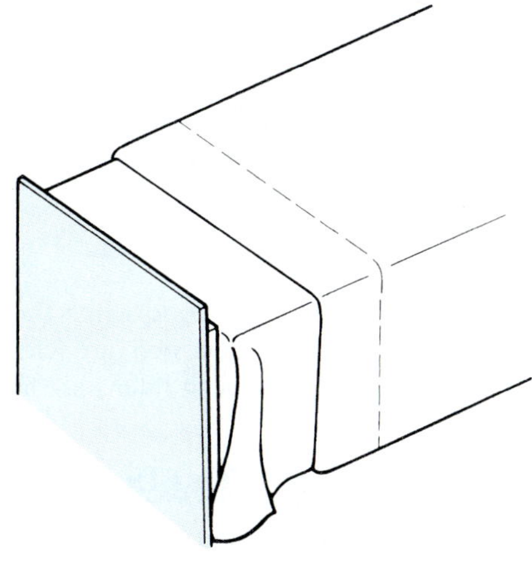

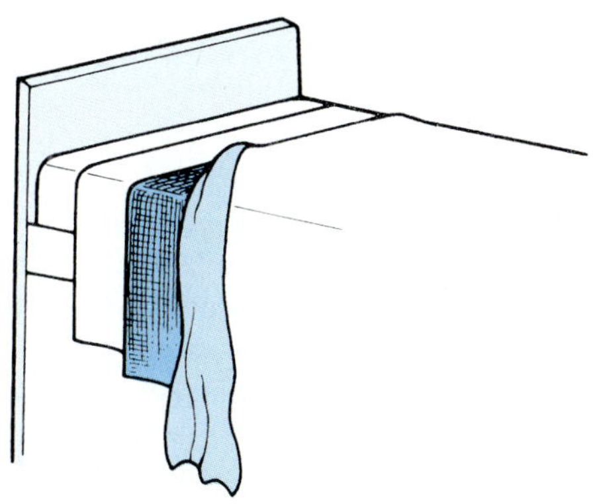

STEP 11

Continued.

SKILL 16-15

MAKING THE UNOCCUPIED BED—cont'd

12. Allow for toe pleat. Make modified mitered corner by not tucking tip of triangle under mattress (see Skill 16-14, step 20) *to provide for patient comfort.*
13. Move to opposite side of bed, and complete making bed as described in steps 9 to 12 *to save nurse's time and energy.* Pull linens tight, and keep taut as linens are tucked in (see illustration).
14. Put on clean pillow case (see Skill 16-14, step 21). Position pillow at head of bed *to make it easy to slide case over pillow.* Place call light within easy reach, and lower bed level.
15. If patient is to return to bed, fan fold top linens down to foot of bed. Make sure cuff at top of linens is easily accessible to patient *to make it easier for patient to return to bed.*
16. Arrange personal items on bed table or bedside stand, and place within patient's easy reach. Leave area neat and clean *to promote sense of well-being.*
17. Place all soiled linens in proper receptacle. Wash hands *to prevent spread of microorganisms.*
18. Assist patient to bed, and position for comfort *to provide safety and patient's comfort.*

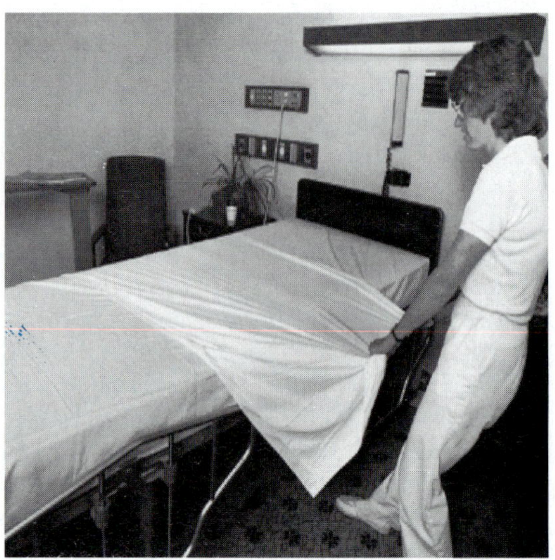

STEP 8

Box 16-7 CHARACTERISTICS OF NORMAL URINE

1. Ranges from a pale, straw color to amber (depends on the concentration)
2. Is transparent at the time of voiding
3. Has a characteristic odor: faintly aromatic
4. Is negative for protein, glucose, ketone bodies, red blood cells, white blood cells, and bacteria

Box 16-8 CHARACTERISTICS OF NORMAL STOOL

1. Is brown in color
2. Odor is affected by food types
3. Has soft, formed consistency
4. Frequency ranges from once a day to two or three a week
5. Resembles the shape of the rectum
6. Contains undigested food, dead bacteria, fat, bile pigment, living cells, intestinal mucosa, and water

The postoperative bed is a form of the open bed. The top sheet and the spread are not mitered or tucked in at the corners of the patient's bed. The top linens may be fan folded lengthwise or crosswise at the foot of the patient's bed. The top bed linens should be arranged in such a way that they allow easy transfer of the surgical patient from the gurney to the bed. A complete linen change is done if the patient is returning from surgery.

A complete linen change is done when the patient is discharged. The mattress and bed are cleaned by housekeeping personnel, and fresh linens are applied.

Assisting the Patient with Elimination

The **bedpan** (device for receiving feces or urine from either male or female patients confined to bed) or **uri-**

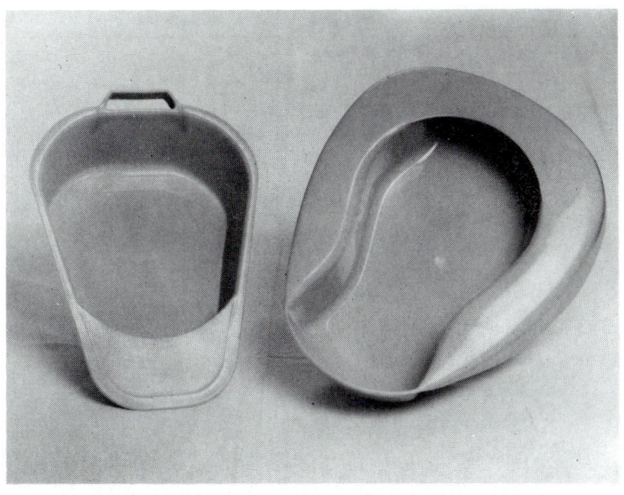

FIG. 16-5 Types of bedpans. *Left,* Fracture bedpan; *right,* regular bedpan.

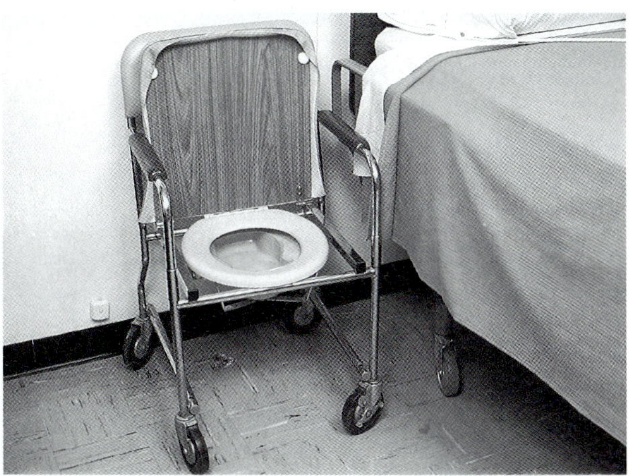

FIG. 16-7 The bedside commode has a toilet seat with a container underneath. The container slides out from under the toilet seat for emptying.

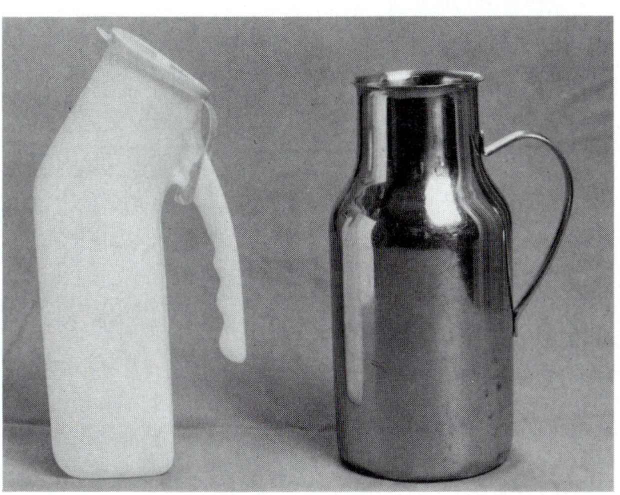

FIG. 16-6 Male urinals.

nal (a device for collecting urine from male patients) is used when a patient is unable to get up to the bathroom for the purpose of urination (the act of emptying the urinary bladder) or of defecation (the act of eliminating feces [BM]). This procedure is personal, and the patient should be afforded as much privacy as the condition allows.

The nurse should offer the bedpan or urinal frequently, because patients may accidentally soil bedclothes if their elimination needs are not met. It is not unusual for a patient to procrastinate using a bedpan because it is uncomfortable and embarrassing. Patients may try to get to the bathroom unassisted even if their condition prohibits ambulation. The nurse should remind patients of the possibility of accidents or falls. See Box 16-7 for the characteristics of normal urine. The nurse should note any abnormalities (see Chapter 33). See Box 16-8 for the characteristics of normal stool. Again, the nurse should note any abnormalities (see Chapter 27).

The bedpan is made of metal or plastic. There are two types of bedpans. One type has a high back. The second type is flat and smaller and is called a *fracture pan* (Fig. 16-5).

A urinal is made of metal or plastic. There are two types of urinals. One type is used by the male for voiding (Fig. 16-6). The other type is called a *female urinal* and has a different shape than the male urinal. The metal urinal may be warmed by running warm water over its surface.

If the patient is unable to place the urinal for himself, the nurse will need to assist him:

1. Request the patient to abduct his legs a slight distance.
2. Holding the urinal by the handle and directing the urinal at an angle, place the urinal between the patient's legs, making certain the long, flat side, which is opposite the handle of the urinal, is resting on the bed.
3. Gently raising the penis, place it fully within the urinal.

The bedpan and urinal should be emptied immediately after use, cleansed, and stored properly. If the patient's intake and output are being monitored, urine should be measured and recorded. Liquid stool is estimated on the appropriate form according to the agency's policy. The nurse will remember to wear gloves. (Skill 16-16 on pp. 302-303 and Fig. 16-7). Positioning the bedpan.

SKILL 16-16

POSITIONING THE BEDPAN

Nursing action/*rationale*

1. Assess patient's needs *to allow nurse to note any potential problems in elimination.*
2. Check physician's order *to provide basis for care.*
3. Wash hands *to prevent cross contamination.*
4. Gather supplies *to organize procedure.*
5. Introduce self *to decrease anxiety level.*
6. Explain procedure to patient *to encourage cooperation.*
7. Provide privacy *to promote relaxation.*
8. Don gloves *to protect the nurse from patient's body fluids.*
9. Place protector under patient if necessary *to provide protection for bed.*
10. Warm metal bedpan under running warm water *to provide for patient comfort.*
11. When patient is able to assist self onto bedpan, nurse will position patient in supine position with knees flexed and bottom of feet flat on bed surface. As patient raises hips, nurse supports patient's lower back with her arm and slides bedpan under patient. When patient has finished with elimination, nurse removes bedpan in same manner *to allow for some measure of independence.*
12. For patient unable to assist self on bedpan:
    - Turn patient away from nurse toward opposite side rail, moving linens out of way *to provide for patient safety.*
    - Fit bedpan to patient's buttocks *to prevent injury to patient's skin (see illustration).*
    - Assist patient to turn over onto bedpan while nurse secures bedpan *to allow nurse to use appropriate body mechanics.*
    - Raise head of bed 30 degrees *to promote patient comfort.*
    - Place toilet tissue and call light within easy reach *for patient convenience and to promote certain measure of independence.*

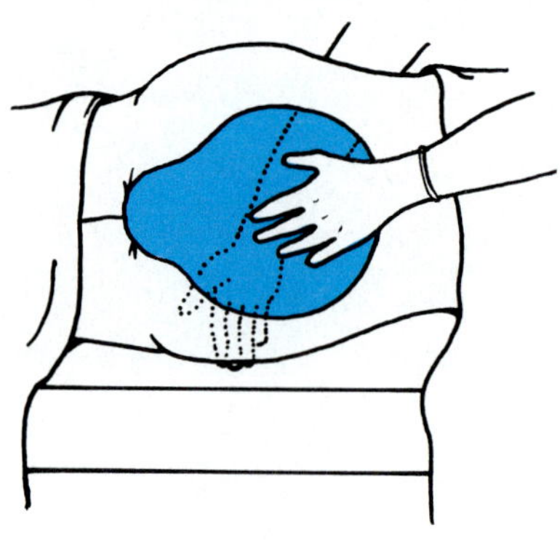

STEP 12

DOCUMENTATION

1. Record amount, color, and consistency of urine and feces *to record patient's pattern of elimination.*

Sample charting

DATE	TIME	NOTES
12/4/95	0920	Voided 300 ml in bedpan. Urine clear amber. Denies discomfort. Perineal care given. Fluids encouraged. ______________________ *(nurse's signature)*
12/4/95	0920	Voided 500 ml in urinal. Urine red with moderate amount of sediment. Complains of urgency and frequency. Fluids encouraged. Reported to B. Anderson, RN. ______________________ *(nurse's signature)*
12/4/95	1045	Up to bathroom with assistance. Large, soft, brown stool with moderate amount **flatus** (gas in digestive tract) expelled. Perineal care given. Returned to bed and positioned for comfort. ______________________ *(nurse's signature)*

POSITIONING THE BEDPAN—cont'd

12/4/95 1045 Assisted onto bedpan. Moderate amount of green, liquid stool and much flatus expelled. Complains of abdominal cramping. Bowel sounds hyperactive. Reported to J. Gutschenritter, RN.

____
(nurse's signature)

SPECIAL CONCERNS

- Allow the patient enough time for elimination. Ignoring the urge to defecate or urinate or not taking time to eliminate completely is a common cause of constipation or urine retention.
- The nurse must be prompt to assist the patient to the bathroom or onto the bedpan or bedside commode.
- When the patient shares a room with another patient, be certain to curtain off the patient's area. This enables the patient to relax, knowing that interruptions will not occur.
- Bathroom doors must be closed. If necessary to remain nearby, stand outside door or curtains.
- For those patients unable to assume the normal squatting position, there are stool risers, which require less effort to sit or stand.
- For those patients who can be out of bed but are unable to ambulate far, there is the bedside commode (see Fig. 16-7). Some are equipped with wheels, which allow the patient to be moved to the bathroom for more privacy.
- When transferring a patient to the commode, assist the patient in the same manner as if assisting to a chair.

PATIENT TEACHING

- Teach patients who have trapeze bars on their beds how to lift themselves on and off the bedpan.

REFERENCES AND SUGGESTED READINGS

1. Bryant RA et al: *Pressure ulcer.* In Bryant RA, editor: *Acute and chronic wounds: nursing management,* St Louis, 1992, Mosby.
2. Collins L: Preventing pressure ulcers: how to recognize and care for patients at risk, *Nurs '90,* 20(12):60, 1990.
3. Cooper DM: Wound assessment and evaluation of healing. In Bryant RA, editor: *Acute and chronic wounds: nursing management,* St Louis, 1992, Mosby.
4. Ellis JR, Nowlis EA, Bentz PM: *Basic nursing skills,* ed 4, vol 2, Boston, 1988, Houghton Mifflin.
5. Flynn JM, Hackel R: *Technological foundations in nursing,* East Norwalk, Conn, 1990, Appleton & Lange.
6. Greifzu S, Radjesk D, Winnick B: Oral care is part of cancer care, *RN* 53(6):43, 1990.
7. Kim MJ, McFarland GK, McLane AM: *Pocket guide to nursing diagnosis,* ed 5, St Louis, 1993, Mosby.
8. Krasner D: Resolving the dressing dilemma: selecting wound dressings by category, *Ostomy Wound Management,* pp 35, 64, July/August 1991.
9. Krasner D: The 12 commandments of wound care, *Nursing* 22(12):34, 1992.
10. Long BC, Phipps WJ, Cassmeyer VL: *Medical-surgical nursing: a nursing process approach,* ed 3, St Louis, 1993, Mosby.
11. Makebust J, Suggreen M: *Pressure ulcers: guidelines for prevention and nursing management,* West Dundee, Ill, 1991, S-N Publications.
12. Malasanos L, Barkauskas V, Stoltenberg-Allen K: *Health assessment,* ed 4, St Louis, 1990, Mosby.
13. *Mosby's medical, nursing, and allied health dictionary,* ed 3, St Louis, 1994, Mosby.
14. Osterman HM, Stuck RM: The aging foot, *Orthop Nurs* 9:43, 1990.
15. Panel for the Prediction and Prevention of Pressure Ulcers in Adults: *Pressure ulcers in adults: prediction and prevention,* Rockville, Md, 1992, Agency for Health Care Policy and Research.
16. Perry AG, Potter PA: *Clinical nursing skills and techniques,* ed 3, St Louis, 1994, Mosby.
17. Potter PA, Perry AG: *Fundamentals of nursing: concepts, process, and practice,* ed 3, St Louis, 1992, Mosby.
18. Powers I, William D: Urinary incontinence, *Nursing* 22(12):46, 1992.
19. Pues M, Mueller A: Detection and management of early tissue pressure indication: a pictorial essay, *Progressions* 3(3):3, 1991.
20. Timby BK, Lewis LW: *Fundamental skills and concepts in patient care,* ed 5, Philadelphia, 1992, Lippincott.
21. Tucker SM et al: *Patient care standards: nursing process, diagnosis, and outcome,* ed 5, St Louis, 1992, Mosby.

CHAPTER CHALLENGE

KEY POINTS

- Hygiene is a personal matter, and the nurse considers all factors influencing personal hygiene routine.
- The nurse assumes responsibility for providing the daily hygienic needs of patients if they are unable to care for themselves adequately.
- Providing hygienic care gives the nurse the opportunity to assess all external body surfaces and the patient's emotional state.
- Assisting or providing the patient with daily hygienic needs allows the nurse to use teaching and communication skills to develop a meaningful relationship with the patient.
- The patient's personal preferences should be considered as the nurse plans the daily hygienic care.
- The nurse must maintain the patient's privacy and comfort when providing daily care.
- During assessment of the skin, the nurse observes characteristics most influenced by hygienic measures.
- Patients who are immobilized, who are poorly nourished, and who have reduced sensation are at risk for impaired skin integrity.
- External pressure, shearing force, moisture, impaired peripheral circulation, edema, and obesity contribute to the development of decubitus ulcers.
- When the external pressure against the skin is greater than the pressure in the capillary bed, blood flow decreases to the adjacent tissues.
- There are four stages of pressure ulcer development.
- Meticulous assessment of the skin and underlying tissue and identification of risk factors are important in decreasing the opportunity for decubitus ulcer development.
- Preventive skin care is aimed at controlling external pressure on bony prominences and keeping the skin clean, well lubricated, and hydrated and free of excess moisture.
- Proper positioning reduces the effects of pressure and guards against the shearing force.
- Cleansing and topical agents used to treat decubitus ulcers vary according to the stage of the ulcer.
- Assessment of the ulcer enables the nurse to select proper skin care agents.
- Gloves should be worn by nurses during hygienic care when the risk of contacting body fluids is high.
- Techniques used during tepid sponging are designed to minimize the risk of a patient becoming chilled.
- Patients with diabetes mellitus require special consideration when a nurse provides nail and foot care.
- When administering oral care to unconscious patients, the nurse takes measures to prevent aspiration.
- The evaluation of hygienic care is based on the patient's expression of a sense of relaxation and well-being and an understanding of personal hygienic techniques.

STUDY QUESTIONS

1. The student nurse is knowledgeable that microorganisms are spread by:
   1. fresh air and sunshine
   2. carrying linens away from one's uniform
   3. placing soiled linens on the floor
   4. using a common handwashing station
2. During the bed bath the nurse covers the patient with a bath blanket:
   1. to prevent skin impairment
   2. for cosmetic purposes
   3. to prevent the spread of microorganisms
   4. to prevent chilling
3. Mr. James has severe crippling rheumatoid arthritis. He is confined to bed for extended periods of time. An erythematous and edematous area over the coccyx that could become an open lesion is noted in Mr. James. This is referred to as:
   1. an inflammatory ulcer
   2. a decubitus ulcer
   3. a stasis ulcer
   4. the inner canthus
4. The nurse educator instructs the student nurse that Ms. Ontego, a 64-year-old patient with terminal cancer, is too weak to perform her own perineal care. The student nurse knows she will include bathing which of the following areas for perineal care:
   1. back and buttocks
   2. eyes, ears, and nose
   3. upper torso and thighs
   4. upper thighs, genitalia, and anal area
5. Which of the following patients assigned to the nurse for AM cares would be at greatest risk for skin impairment:
   1. child on bed rest
   2. infant with cool skin temperature
   3. young man with diarrhea
   4. elderly patient in a body cast
6. Mrs. Johnson 52 years old, is in her second postoperative day after an abdominal hysterectomy. The nurse plans to give Mrs. Johnson a bed bath. When caring for Mrs. Johnson's face, the nurse should:

1. use only water
2. ask the patient her preference
3. use soap in all areas except the eyes
4. use a cleansing cream

7. Tammy Jones is a 12-year-old patient with a leg cast placed to correct a fracture of her femur. The nurse bathing Tammy is aware that proper eye care would be:
   1. to wash from outer canthus to inner canthus
   2. to cleanse dried exudate with hot water
   3. to avoid drying circumorbital area after washing
   4. to use a different section of wash cloth for each eye

8. Mr. Rodriquez is stabilizing well with congestive heart failure. He states he would enjoy a tub bath. The nurse assists Mr. Rodriquez in filling the bathtub. The correct water temperature is:
   1. 105° to 110° F
   2. 110° to 115° F
   3. 98° to 100° F
   4. 85° to 98° C

9. Sarah Cregas is an 11-month-old infant who is admitted with a temperature of 105° F (tympanic) of unknown origin. The physician orders a tepid sponge bath. The nurse is cognizant that the purpose of the tepid sponge bath is to:
   1. reduce temperature in febrile patients
   2. cleanse patient's groin and axillary areas
   3. stimulate circulation to the skin
   4. calm and relax the patient

10. Mr. Curtis is an 80-year-old uncircumcised male who is in the first postoperative day after a TURP. When administering perineal care to this uncircumcised male patient, the nurse should:
    1. retract the foreskin, cleanse the penis, and allow the foreskin to return to former position
    2. sprinkle powder under the foreskin to facilitate retraction of the foreskin
    3. leave the foreskin slightly damp to allow retraction to its former state
    4. retract the foreskin, cleanse the penis, and return the foreskin with a gentle forward motion

11. Mrs. Gonzas is a 50-year-old patient who had a percutaneous plication of a prolapsed urethra. She was discharged home with a Foley catheter. The student nurse instructed Mrs. Gonzas in the proper procedure for cleansing the female perineal area by instructing her to:
    1. cleanse the area in circular motions around the rectum
    2. cleanse from the rectum toward the pubis
    3. cleanse from the pubis toward the rectum
    4. cleanse in circular motions around the vaginal area

12. The nurse is knowledgeable that the following patient is most at risk for complications of the feet:
    1. young man in a career that requires standing
    2. disoriented, elderly man
    3. 60-year-old person with diabetes mellitus
    4. 62-year-old patient with total hip replacement

13. Mr. Johnson is an 82-year-old who is in the terminal stage of lung cancer. He is unconscious and requires meticulous oral hygiene. The optimal position for providing oral hygiene to this patient is:
    1. high Fowler's position
    2. high Fowler's position with head hyperextended
    3. supine with the head lowered
    4. side-lying with head lowered

14. Mrs. Smith is a 72-year-old patient with diffuse pancreatitis that developed after a perforated diverticulum with temporary colostomy. The nurse in giving her a soothing bed bath will cleanse her ears. Which of the following interventions for cleansing her ears is correct:
    1. cleansing the outer ear with the wash cloth during the bath
    2. retracting the outer ear downward to loosen visible cerumen
    3. irrigating to remove tenacious cerumen
    4. using cotton-tipped applicators to remove cerumen

15. The student nurse has completed her educational instructions on the correct procedures for bedmaking. She understands that the following intervention is correct for the bedmaking process:
    1. preparing a closed bed for receiving postoperative patients
    2. shaking soiled linen before placement in the hamper
    3. mitering the corners of the bottom fitted sheet
    4. washing hands thoroughly after handling soiled linen

16. Mr. Hoover, a retired dentist, has been admitted to the hospital for a thrombophlebitis of his left leg. The nurse is giving Mr. Hoover a relaxing backrub. Which of the following strokes should the nurse use when finishing his backrub:
    1. long firm strokes across the width of the back
    2. light strokes while moving up the back in a circular motion
    3. long, smooth strokes along the length of the back
    4. circular motion upward from buttocks to shoulder

17. Mr. Koldesk is a 92-year-old patient who is in his first postoperative day after a lypsis of adhesions to correct a small bowel obstruction. As part of his morning care, the nurse will remove and cleanse his dentures. Which of the following techniques is correct:
    1. working over an open sink convenient to the water faucet
    2. rinsing dentures thoroughly with hot water
    3. brushing dentures with a soft toothbrush
    4. holding dentures securely in the palm of the hand

17

SPECIMEN COLLECTION AND DIAGNOSTIC EXAMINATION

Elaine Kockrow
Barbara Christensen
Jenann Allen

KEY TERMS

coffee ground vomitus/emesis
culture
cytology
expectorate
fixative
hemoccult test
midstream urine specimen
occult
residual urine
sensitivity
specimen

LEARNING OBJECTIVES

After reading this chapter the student should be able to do the following:

- Define key terms.
- Discuss guidelines for specimen collection.
- Identify the role of the nurse when performing a procedure for specimen collection.
- Discuss patient teaching for a specimen collection.
- State appropriate labeling for a collected specimen.
- List the proper steps for teaching self-blood glucose monitoring.
- Demonstrate the correct procedure for the glucose/acetone determination using Keto-diastix, Reagent tablet, Tes-Tape, and Acetest tablet.
- Discuss the procedure for obtaining stool specimens.
- State the correct procedure for collecting a sputum specimen.
- List the proper steps when obtaining urine specimens.
- List the nursing responsibilities for the glucose tolerance test.
- Discuss the nursing interventions necessary for proper preparations for a patient having diagnostic examinations.
- List the diagnostic tests for which the nurse should determine whether the patient is allergic to iodine.

RELATED TOPICS OF INTEREST

- Communication (Chapter 4)
- Documentation (Chapter 6)
- Signs, symptoms, and physical assessment (Chapter 9)
- Medical asepsis and infection control (Chapter 12)
- Care of the patient with a gastrointestinal or accessory organ disorder (Chapter 27)
- Care of the patient with a urinary disorder (Chapter 30)
- Care of the patient with a respiratory disorder (Chapter 31)

SPECIMEN COLLECTION

Nurses are often responsible for the collection of specimens of body secretions and excretions. Laboratory examination of specimens of urine, stool, sputum, blood, and wound drainage provides important information about body functioning and contributes to the assessment of health status. Laboratory test results can facilitate the diagnosis of health care problems, provide information about the stage and activity of a disease process, and measure the response to therapy.

Patients often experience embarrassment or discomfort when giving a sample of body excretions or secretions. Most persons believe excretions should be handled discreetly; therefore it is important to provide the patient with as much comfort and privacy as possible. Anxiety is also provoked by the invasive nature of some collection procedures or by the fear of unknown test results. Patients given a clear explanation about the purpose of the specimen and how it is to be obtained will be more cooperative in its collection. With proper instruction, many patients are able to obtain their own specimens of urine, stool, and sputum, thus avoiding embarrassment. Often the success of specimen collection depends on cooperation.

Laboratory tests are often expensive. The nurse can prevent unnecessary costs by using the correct procedure for obtaining and processing specimens. When there are questions about laboratory tests, the nurse should consult the agency's procedure manual or call the laboratory.

Normal values for laboratory tests can be found in reference books, but the nurse should know that each laboratory establishes its own values for each test. These values are usually readily available on the laboratory slips of the agency. Any major deviations should be immediately discussed with the physician. See Box 17-1 for guidelines for specimen collection.

Box 17-1 GUIDELINES FOR SPECIMEN COLLECTION

- Consider the patient's need and ability to participate in specimen collection procedures.
- Recognize that collection of a specimen may provoke anxiety, embarrassment, or discomfort.
- Provide support for patients who are fearful about the results of a specimen examination.
- Recognize that children require a clear explanation of procedures and may benefit from support of parents or family members.
- Obtain specimens in accordance with specific prerequisite conditions (e.g., fasting, NPO) as required.
- Wear gloves when collecting specimens of blood or other body fluids because it is not possible to identify all persons infected with HIV or other pathogens such as hepatitis B. (These universal precautions are advocated by the CDC.)
- Wash hands and other skin surfaces immediately and thoroughly if contaminated with blood or body fluids; wash hands immediately after removing gloves.
- Collect specimens in appropriate containers, at the correct time, in the appropriate amount.
- Properly label all specimens with the patient's identification; complete laboratory requisition form as necessary.
- Deliver specimens to the laboratory within the recommended time or ensure that they are stored properly for later transport.
- Use aseptic technique in all collections to prevent contamination, which can cause inaccurate test results.
- Transport specimens under special conditions (e.g., iced specimens or special containers with preservatives) as required.

DIAGNOSTIC EXAMINATION

Diagnostic examinations may be performed by a physician at the patient's bedside or in a specially equipped room for therapeutic or diagnostic purposes. The nurse is responsible for assessing the patient's knowledge of and preparing the patient for the procedure, assisting the physician with the procedure, and caring for the patient

GERONTOLOGICAL CONSIDERATIONS

- Because of a decrease in the agility required to collect a midstream urinalysis, catheterization of the older person may be necessary. It is important to explain the purpose of the procedure and provide privacy during specimen collection.
- Decreased peripheral circulation can cause difficulty when collecting a specimen for blood glucose determination. Wrapping the hand in a warm, moist washcloth for a few minutes may facilitate the procedure.
- Changes in blood vessels can make venipuncture more difficult in older adults. The need to perform repeated sticks to obtain blood samples can lead to mental and physical trauma in the older adult.
- Stool specimens can be collected from older adults by use of a bedpan or specimen pan in the toilet or commode. At home, stool can be collected by supporting a large piece of waxed paper under the toilet seat.
- Collection of sputum is often difficult because of poor cough in older adults. Respiratory-induced sputum collection may be needed to obtain a specimen.
- Collection of wound drainage may increase pain. Older persons should receive adequate analgesics before this is performed.

after tests are completed. The nurse's knowledge and organization of the diagnostic procedure can be the key to success.

The nurse anticipates the needs of the physician and has the proper supplies ready, but most important, the nurse keeps the patient adequately informed of procedural details that could cause discomfort.

The nurse must be aware of legal considerations when dealing with diagnostic procedures. Most invasive diagnostic tests require a signed, informed consent. Usually the physician is responsible for getting consent, but the nurse must be aware of institutional policies regarding consent forms and ensure that informed consent is obtained before the procedure. The nurse must also record and report the patient's status before and after the procedure.

The nurse assists the patient through a procedure. Many procedures cause moderate discomfort. The patient may tolerate the procedure better if a well-informed nurse stays at the bedside and describes each step and possible reactions. See Box 17-2 for guidelines for diagnostic examinations.

Special care should be taken with older adults during specimen collection and diagnostic examination (see gerontological box on p. 307).

SKILL 17-1: PREPARING THE PATIENT FOR DIAGNOSTIC EXAMINATIONS

Guidelines

The nurse must inform the patient that a test is to be performed and answer questions for which the patient may need clarification. The patient needs to know if nothing can be taken by mouth (NPO) after 12 midnight or if breakfast will be held until the examination is completed. The patient needs to know if a special room or equipment is required for the test, as well as special medications needed before or during the test. An informed patient will be more cooperative during any test (see Box 17-2).

Text continued on p. 315.

Box 17-2 GUIDELINES FOR DIAGNOSTIC EXAMINATION

- Know the patient's baseline vital signs. Some diagnostic tests are invasive procedures and have associated complications. Changes from baseline vital signs can provide early physiological data about potential complications.
- Know the patient's level of education. Diagnostic tests require the nurse to teach the patient about the test. Knowing the patient's educational background enables the nurse to develop an individualized teaching plan.
- Determine the patient's awareness of actual or potential medical diagnoses. This determination provides the nurse with data about the patient's knowledge and perception of medical diagnoses.
- Through nursing assessment, determine abnormal findings, which can indicate or contraindicate a diagnostic test.
- Determine the patient's previous experience with diagnostic testing. Patients who have had smooth, uncomplicated diagnostic tests are usually less anxious about a test. If a patient has had a complication from a diagnostic test, the patient may require more preprocedure education and support.

For a more comprehensive look at diagnostic examinations, refer to Table 17-1.

SKILL 17-1

PREPARING THE PATIENT FOR DIAGNOSTIC EXAMINATIONS

Nursing action/*Rationale*

1. Read physician's order *because this will provide a basis for care.*
2. Collect supplies *to organize procedure.*
3. Introduce self *to decrease anxiety level.*
4. Identify patient by identification band *to identify correct patient for procedure.*
5. Explain procedure to patient *to seek cooperation and decrease anxiety.*
6. Wash hands, and don clean gloves, *which helps prevent cross-contamination.*
7. Assist physician with procedure *to provide help to physician while providing support to patient.*
8. Answer questions from patient; *this provides security and emotional support to patient.*
9. Ensure delivery of specimen to laboratory when applicable. Using correct protocol; be certain specimen is accurately labeled with patient's name, age, room number, physician, date, and type of specimen. *This is important to ensure accuracy of appropriate specimen.*
10. Document *to communicate performance of procedure and patient's response.*

TABLE 17-1 Nurses' Role in Diagnostic Examinations

Nursing Interventions Before Examination	Nursing Interventions After Examination
Abdominal scan	
Prepare requisition form. Explain procedure. Instruct patient to be NPO for 4 hours before examination.	No specific follow-up care.
Amniocentesis (see Chapter 39)	
Explain procedure. Encourage verbalization. Obtain written consent. Monitor fetal heart tones.	Monitor fetal heart tones. If patient complains of vertigo, allow her to rest on her left side for several minutes before leaving examination room. If patient has any fluid loss or temperature elevation, instruct her to notify her physician. Inform patient to contact her physician to obtain results.
Arteriogram (see Chapter 28)	
Explain procedure.	Keep patient at bed rest for 8 hours. Monitor vital signs and observe for bleeding.
Barium enema (see Chapter 27)	
Prepare requisition form. Explain procedure. Provide needed emotional support. Assist with required preparations—monitor effects of cathartics and/or enemas. Instruct patient to be NPO after midnight (some facilities allow liquids for breakfast).	Allow patient to resume regular diet as soon as exam is completed. Monitor stools—barium may cause constipation. A local anesthetic ointment may be applied after examination to relieve anal discomfort as per physician order. Instruct patient that a warm bath may be soothing. Administer milk of magnesia, 2 oz, after examination as per hospital protocol. Allow time for rest.
Blood chemistries	
Prepare requisition form. Instruct patient to be NPO. Explain procedure. Smoking prohibited, as per agency policy.	Observe site for bleeding. Be certain patient's meal is served after test is completed. Report results.
Brain scan (see Chapter 35)	
Explain procedure. Keep patient NPO for 4 hours before examination. Instruct patient not to wear wig, hairpins, or clips. Observe patient for iodine allergies. If ordered, give sedation.	No special care required after procedure. Encourage fluid intake.
Bone marrow aspiration (Fig. 17-1) (see Chapter 29)	
Prepare requisition form. Explain procedure. Obtain written consent. Assist in obtaining specimens. Provide needed emotional support.	Observe the puncture site for bleeding. Monitor patient for signs and symptoms of shock. Allow patient to resume normal activity 30-60 min after examination. Mild analgesics may be needed for complaints of tenderness at the puncture site.

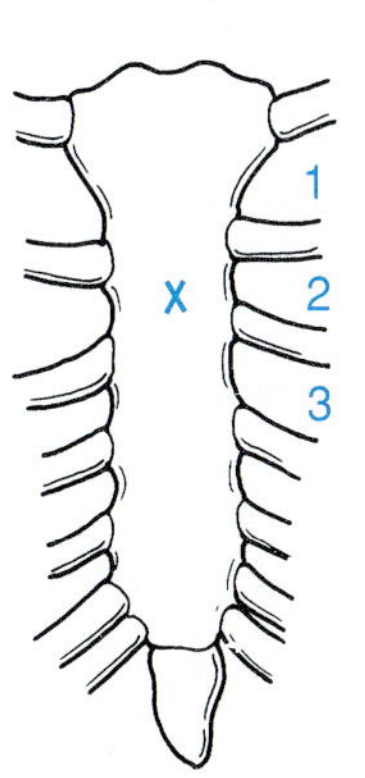

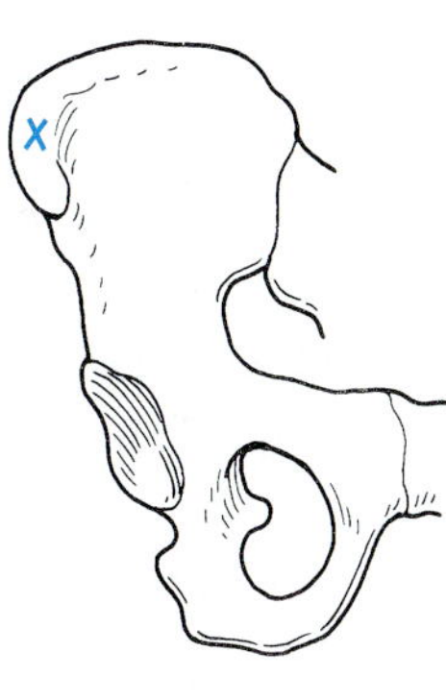

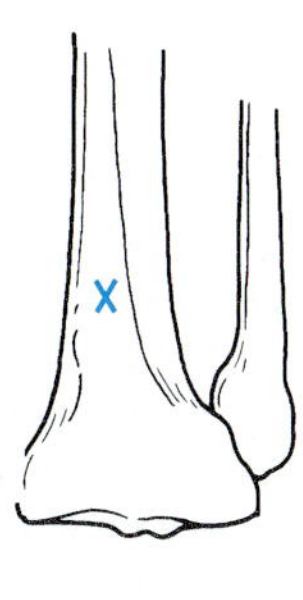

FIG. 17-1 Bone marrow is located in spongy bone. The iliac crest is the most common area used for bone marrow aspirations.

Continued.

TABLE 17-1 Nurses' Role in Diagnostic Examinations—cont'd

Nursing Interventions Before Examination	Nursing Interventions After Examination
Body scan	
Prepare requisition form. Explain procedure. No specific preparation.	No specific follow-up care.
Bone scan (see Chapter 38)	
Prepare requisition form. Explain procedure. Instruct patient to remove jewelry or any metal objects. Encourage patient to drink several glasses of water. Have patient void before examination.	Observe injection site for erythema or edema; if hematoma forms, apply warm soaks to the area to relieve pain.
Bronchoscopy (Fig. 17-2) (see Chapter 31)	
Prepare requisition form. Explain procedure. Obtain an informed consent before patient is premedicated. Instruct patient to be NPO after midnight. Administer preoperative medication as ordered. Remove and safely store contact lenses, dentures, glasses. Reassure patient.	Do not allow patient to eat or drink after procedure until the effect of anesthesia no longer exists and gag reflex has returned—usually about 2 hr. Observe any sputum for blood. Monitor vital signs frequently: fever is normal within the first 24 hr after bronchoscopy. Observe for impaired respirations. Observe closely until effects of anesthesia no longer exist. If patient complains of sore throat, warm saline gargles and lozenges may be provided.

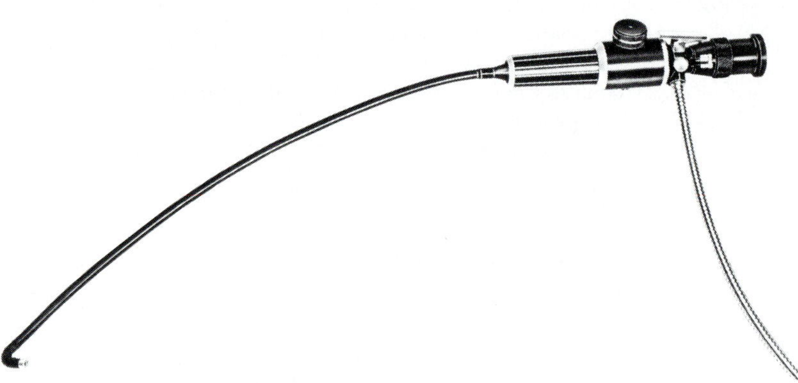

FIG. 17-2 Flexible fiberoptic bronchoscope. (Courtesy American Cystoscope Makers, Inc, Pelham, NY.)

Nursing Interventions Before Examination	Nursing Interventions After Examination
Cardiac catheterization (see Chapter 28)	
Explain procedure. Obtain written consent. Provide needed emotional support. Instruct patient to be NPO for 6-8 hr. Determine if patient has any dye allergies. Administer preexamination medications as ordered.	Monitor vital signs. Observe catheter site for bleeding. Monitor pedal pulses for adequate circulation. Encourage rest. Encourage fluids.
CBC (see Chapter 29)	
Prepare requisition form. Explain procedure.	Observe site for bleeding. Report results.
Chest x-ray (see Chapter 31)	
Prepare requisition form. Explain procedure. Be certain there are no snaps or pins on gown.	Report results.
Colonoscopy (see Chapter 27)	
Prepare requisition form. Explain procedure. Obtain written consent. Assist with the bowel prep. Record the results from the cathartics and enemas.	Observe for abdominal pain, tenderness, and bleeding. Examine stools for gross blood. Encourage fluids. Offer normal diet. Suggest a warm bath for relaxation. Allow time for rest. Take precautions until the medication effects no longer exist.

TABLE 17-1 Nurses' Role in Diagnostic Examinations—cont'd

Nursing Intervention Before Examination	Nursing Intervention After Examination
Computed tomography (Fig. 17-3) (see Chapter 35)	
Explain the procedure. Obtain informed consent if required. Assess for allergies to iodine. Inform patient that wigs, hair pins or clips, and partial denture plates must be removed if scan will include head. Maintain NPO status 4 hours before oral contrast is administered, except in emergencies.	Encourage patient to drink fluids to avoid renal complications and to promote excretion of dye.

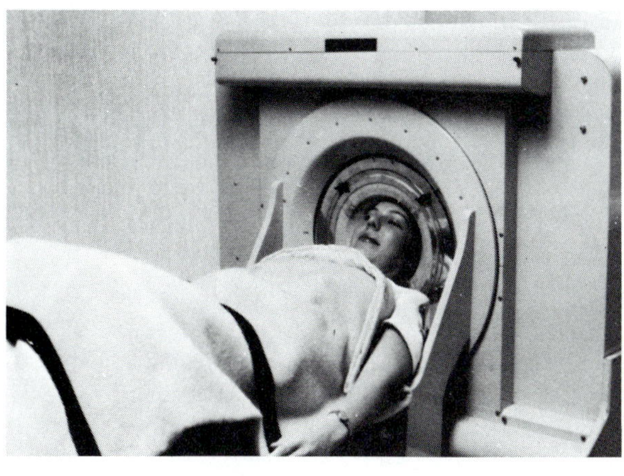

FIG. 17-3 Person undergoing CT scanning.

Nursing Intervention Before Examination	Nursing Intervention After Examination
Cystoscopy (see Chapter 30)	
Explain procedure. Obtain written consent. Administer enemas as ordered, and record results. If patient will be under local anesthesia, a liquid breakfast may be allowed. If patient will be under general anesthesia, keep patient NPO. Administer preprocedure medications as ordered.	Assess patient's ability to void for at least 24 hr after procedure. Record urine color—if bright red, report to physician. Suggest warm sitz baths for relaxation. Encourage fluid intake. Observe vital signs. Observe for hemorrhage and for sepsis. Administer antibiotic as ordered.
Echocardiogram (see Chapter 28)	
Prepare requisition form. Explain procedure. Answer questions.	Remove the gel from the patient's chest with a tissue.
Endoscopy and gastroscopy (Fig. 17-4) (see Chapter 27)	
Prepare requisition form. Administer preexamination medication if ordered. Explain procedure. Obtain written consent. Keep patient NPO after midnight. Provide emotional support. Remove patient's dentures and eye glasses. Perform oral hygiene measures.	Perform oral hygiene measures. Do not allow food or drink until the gag reflex returns (2-4 hr). Explain that drinking cool fluids and gargling will help relieve some soreness. Observe the patient for bleeding, fever, abdominal pain, dysphagia, and dyspnea. Monitor vital signs. Observe safety precautions until the effects of the sedatives no longer exist.

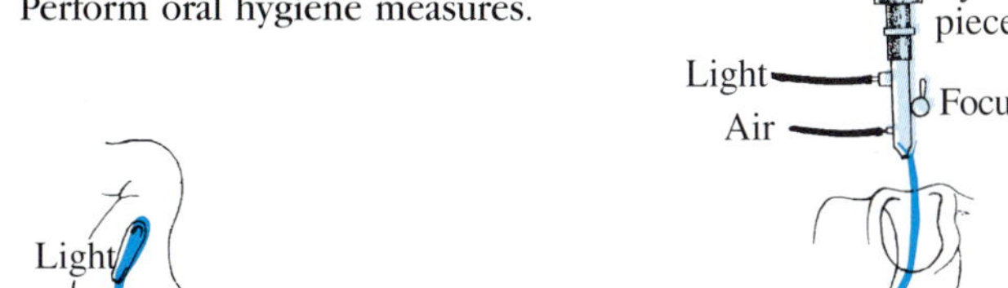

FIG. 17-4 Fiberoptic endoscope.

Continued.

TABLE 17-1 Nurses' Role in Diagnostic Examinations—cont'd

Nursing Intervention Before Examination	Nursing Intervention After Examination
Electrocardiogram (see Chapter 28)	
Prepare requisition form. Explain procedure.	Remove gel from patient's skin with a tissue.
Electroencephalogram (see Chapter 35)	
Prepare requisition form. Explain procedure. Hair should be clean; administer shampoo as necessary. Confer with physician if any medications should be discontinued before examination. Administer sedatives or hypnotics as ordered. Encourage food intake but eliminate coffee, tea, and colas.	Assist the patient to remove the electrode paste. Shampoo hair. Ensure safety precautions until effects of the sedatives no longer exist.
Exercise tolerance test (see Chapter 28)	
Explain procedure. Keep patient NPO until after the test except for water. Hold medications. Instruct patient not to smoke. Instruct patient to wear suitable clothing.	Diet as usual. Resume medication regime. Have patient rest for several hours after examination and instruct not to shower immediately after examination.
Femoral angiogram (see Chapter 28)	
Provide emotional support. Observe patient for allergies to iodine dye. Obtain written consent. Keep patient NPO after midnight.	Observe catheter insertion site for inflammation, hemorrhage, hematoma at the site, or absence of peripheral pulses. Observe the involved extremity for numbness, tingling, pain, or loss of function. Monitor vital signs. Apply cold compresses to the puncture site as needed to reduce discomfort and edema. If patient complains of continuous, severe pain, notify physician.
Glucose tolerance (see Chapter 32)	
Prepare requisition slip. Explain procedure. Keep NPO—encourage H_2O intake so patient can provide urine samples. Obtain urine samples at designated times. Collect blood and urine specimen at the same time. The procedure will be as follows: 1. Make certain the patient empties the bladder; 30 min later obtain a fasting UA. 2. Laboratory will administer 75 g of dextrose orally. 3. The nurse will collect urine specimen ½ hr, 1 hr, 1½ hr, 2½ hr, 3½ hr, up to 5 hr after dextrose, depending on the physician's orders.	Observe venipuncture site for bleeding. Make certain patient receives meal when test is completed. Report results: An elevated blood glucose level at the 2-hr point usually indicates some disorder of carbohydrate metabolism; depending on the elevation of the blood glucose, there may be glucose present in the urine.
Gallbladder series/cholecystogram (see Chapter 27)	
Prepare requisition form. Explain procedure. Allow a fat-free meal the evening before examination. Assess patient for allergy to iodine. Administer the iopanoic acid tablets (Telepaque) as ordered the day before the examination—usually early evening (a number of tablets are ordered; the tablets should not be crushed and should be taken one at a time, waiting 15 min after each tablet).	Monitor patient for side effects to the tablets. Usual diet may be resumed as soon as series is completed.

TABLE 17-1 Nurses' Role in Diagnostic Examinations—cont'd

Nursing Intervention Before Examination	Nursing Intervention After Examination
Hematest of stools (see Chapter 27)	
Explain procedure. Assist patient in obtaining specimens. Document specimens as sent to laboratory.	No specific follow-up care. Read results.
Intravenous pyelogram (see Chapter 30)	
Prepare requisition form. Be certain IVP is done before barium x-rays are performed. Explain procedure. Check for allergies to iodine (the intravenous dye usually contains iodine). Administer cathartics or laxatives as ordered (children and infants are not given cathartics or laxatives). Keep patient NPO after midnight (if an intravenous solution is infusing, ask physician if he wishes to decrease IV to a keep-open-rate to prevent hydration: in an IVP the patient needs to have fluid restricted for the dye to be taken up by the kidney).	Observe for anaphylaxis (respiratory distress, shock, and drop in blood pressure). Allow patient normal diet. Encourage fluid intake to help eliminate any dye left in body. Assess for weakness. Encourage to ambulate with assistance unless contraindicated.
Liver biopsy (see Chapter 27)	
Explain procedure. Obtain written consent. Assess blood coagulation profile. Keep patient NPO before examination. Assist physician. Send specimens to laboratory promptly. Have specimen placed in proper **fixative** (any substance used to preserve gross or histologic specimens of tissue for later examination); usually 10% formalin is used, but the nurse must consult with the laboratory or pathologist. If the liver specimen is for detection of lymphoma, saline solution is used.	Keep patient at bed rest for 24 hours. Observe for hemorrhage. Monitor vital signs. Observe biopsy site.
Lumbar puncture (see Chapter 35)	
Explain before procedure and after procedure routine. Obtain written consent. Have patient empty bladder and bowel if possible. Provide necessary equipment. Assist patient to assume appropriate position. Hold manometer straight, if requested. Label and number specimens.	Keep patient flat after procedure. Observe patient for mobility of extremities, pain, drainage, and ability to void. Notify physician if any unusual occurrences. Report results.
Lung scan (see Chapter 31)	
Prepare requisition form. Explain procedure. Instruct patient to be NPO for 4 hr before examination. Observe the patient for allergies to iodine.	No specific follow-up care. Encourage fluid intake.
Magnetic resonance imaging (see Chapter 35)	
Prepare requisition form. Explain procedure. Obtain informed consent. Assess the patient for any contraindications for testing (aneurysm clips, plates). Instruct patient to remove all metal objects: dentures, partials, jewelry, hair clips, belts. Inform patient of the need to remain motionless. Have patient empty bladder for comfort.	Inform patient that no postprocedural care is necessary. Report results.

Continued.

TABLE 17-1 Nurses' Role in Diagnostic Examinations—cont'd

Nursing Intervention Before Examination	Nursing Intervention After Examination
Mammography (see Chapter 33)	
Prepare requisition form. Explain procedure. If patient is embarrassed by the procedure, ask patient to verbalize her feelings. Provide emotional support. Instruct patient not to wear deodorant, powder, or lotion.	Explain how test results can be obtained.
Myelogram (see Chapter 35)	
Instruct patient to be NPO for 4 hr before examination. Explain procedure. Obtain written consent.	If necessary, assist with proper positioning, as prescribed by the physician. Observe the patient for fever, stiff neck, occipital headache, or photophobia. Monitor vital signs. Monitor ability to void. Encourage fluids so patient does not get dehydrated; this will result in a severe headache.
Paracentesis (see Chapter 27)	
Explain procedure. Obtain written consent. Provide emotional support. Obtain equipment. Assist physician.	Observe puncture site. Observe for syncope. Monitor vital signs. Encourage a period of rest after examination. Send specimen to laboratory for examination if requested.
Positron emission tomography (PET) (see Chapter 35)	
Prepare requisition form. Explain procedure. Obtain informed consent. Instruct patient not to have alcohol, caffeine, or tobacco for 24 hr before examination. Instruct patient not to take sedatives or tranquilizers before examination. Have patient empty bladder before exam.	Instruct patient to change position slowly from lying to standing to avoid postural hypotension. Encourage patient to drink fluids and urinate frequently to aid in removal of the radioisotope from the bladder. Report results.
Proctoscopy and sigmoidoscopy (Fig. 17-5) (see Chapter 27)	
Prepare requisition form. Explain procedure. Provide emotional support. Obtain written consent. Allow patient a light breakfast on day of exam. Administer enemas as ordered, and record results.	Observe the patient for fever, bleeding, abdominal distention, and unusual complaints of pain.
Renal angiography (see Chapter 30)	
Explain procedure. Answer questions. Obtain written consent. Assess patient for allergy to iodine dye. Keep patient NPO after midnight. Administer cathartics as ordered. Administer preprocedure medications.	Observe arterial puncture site frequently. Monitor the extremity for adequate circulation. Monitor pedal pulses and vital signs frequently. Keep patient on bed rest for 12-24 hr. Inform patient that cold compresses to puncture site will help reduce discomfort and edema. Encourage fluids.

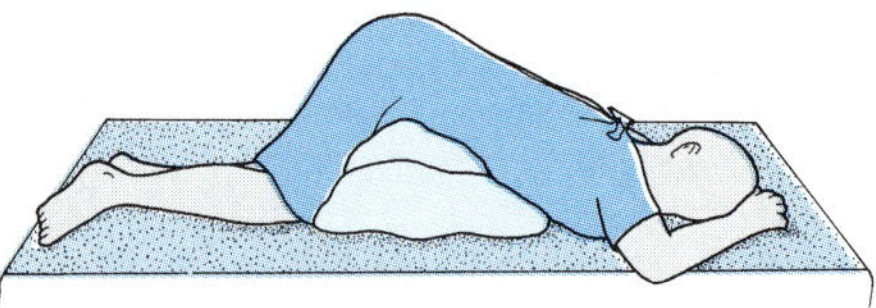

FIG. 17-5 Position for proctoscopy.

TABLE 17-1 Nurses' Role in Diagnostic Examinations—cont'd

Nursing Intervention Before Examination	Nursing Intervention After Examination
Thoracentesis (Fig. 17-6) (see Chapter 31)	
Explain procedure. Obtain written consent. Obtain equipment. Assist patient to assume the appropriate position (usually sitting). Offer emotional support.	Monitor vital signs. Monitor patient for coughing or for hemoptysis. Monitor patient for complications; notify physician if any unusual signs and symptoms occur. Monitor patient's lung sounds. If no complaints of dyspnea, normal activity can be resumed in an hour. Send specimen to laboratory for examination if requested.
Ultrasound/sonogram (see Chapters 27 and 33)	
Prepare requisition form. Explain procedure. If a pelvic sonogram is ordered, the patient needs a full bladder. If a gallbladder sonogram is ordered, keep patient NPO. Obtain signed consent form, if required.	Because this procedure is noninvasive, no specific follow-up care is needed. Usual diet may be resumed after examination.
Upper gastrointestinal series (see Chapter 27)	
Prepare requisition form. Explain procedure. Answer questions. Offer emotional support. Keep patient NPO after midnight.	Patient may eat as soon as series is completed unless contraindicated. Encourage fluids. Monitor stools. Administer milk of magnesia, 2 oz, or per hospital protocol.
Urinalysis (see Chapter 30)	
Prepare requisition form. Explain purpose and specific method of urine collection. Wash perineal area, if soiled. If patient is menstruating, note this on requisition form.	Report results.

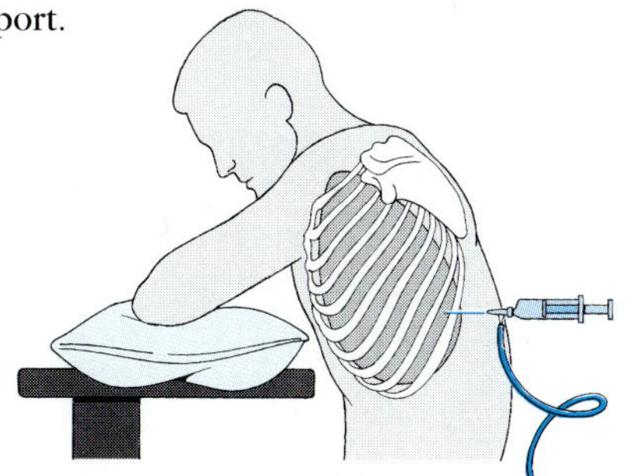

FIG. 17-6 Position for thoracentesis.

Purposes

The nurse prepares the patient for tests for the following reasons:

- to ensure the patient is ready for the test to be performed
- to avoid prolonging hospital stay because of inadequate test preparation

SKILL 17-2: COLLECTING A MIDSTREAM URINE SPECIMEN

Guidelines

There are several methods for collecting a urine **specimen** (a small sample of something, intended to show the nature of the whole) for urinalysis, one of the most commonly ordered diagnostic tests. Several tests can be ordered on one sample of urine, including pH, protein, glucose, ketones, blood, and specific gravity. The responsibilities of the nurse are to collect and label the urine sample, to ensure its safe delivery to the laboratory, and to assess the results. The nurse also explains test collection to the patient. If appropriate, notify the physician of the results.

The patient must be aware of the upcoming test and told to contact the nurse before the next voiding. The nurse should instruct the patient to drink extra water to assist voiding, to not put toilet tissue in container, and to not allow fecal matter to come in contact with the urine specimen. A **midstream urine specimen** is urine

SKILL 17-2

COLLECTING A MIDSTREAM URINE SPECIMEN

Nursing action/*Rationale*

1. Read physician's order *to provide basis for care.*
2. Collect supplies: sterile cotton balls, antiseptic, and sterile specimen container *to organize procedure* (see illustration).
3. Introduce self. *This decreases the patient's anxiety level.*
4. Identify patient by identification band *to identify correct patient for procedure.*
5. Explain procedure to patient. Make certain patient understands how to perform procedure. *This ensures patient's cooperation, decreases anxiety, and ensures accuracy.*
6. Wash hands, and don clean gloves *to prevent cross-contamination.*
7. If patient is able, allow patient to cleanse perineum from anterior to posterior with antiseptic solution. Separate the labia well on a female patient. Retract foreskin of an uncircumcised male. Use each cotton ball that is saturated with antiseptic solution one time only. If patient is unable to cleanse area, the nurse will don gloves and assist with procedure. *All this provides a cleaner specimen and prevents organisms at or near the meatus from being washed into the specimen.*
8. Request that patient (1) begin to void into container about 30 ml; then place the sterile specimen container so the sides of the labia of the female do not touch; (2) without stopping flow, void a small amount into specimen cup; and (3) without stopping flow, finish voiding into toilet seat collector. *This procedure collects midstream urine specimen appropriately. The first 30 ml is discarded so that the organisms at the meatus will be washed away.*
9. Secure lid on container *to prevent spillage.*
10. Cleanse and return toilet seat collector, if applicable, *which will ready it for the next use.*
11. Label specimen appropriately *to provide accuracy.*
12. Ensure that specimen is taken to laboratory with requisition *to ensure fresh specimen for testing.*
13. Document procedure performed *to provide communication of procedure and patient's response.*

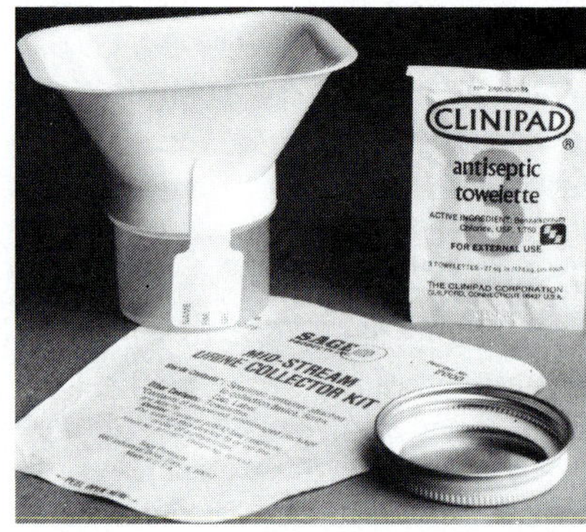

STEP 2

Sample charting

DATE	TIME	NOTES
1/28/95	1110	Voided 300 ml of clear amber urine. Collected midstream urine specimen. Specimen sent to laboratory.

____
(nurse's signature)

FOLLOW-UP

1. Allow patient to wash hands after procedure *to prevent cross-contamination.*

SPECIAL CONCERNS

- Have all supplies ready for patient to perform procedure.
- Make certain patient understands the proper procedure for collecting the urine specimen.
- Be certain specimen is labeled correctly: patient's name, room number, date, physician, and type of specimen.
- Varying degrees of assistance will be required by patients who are seriously ill, have difficulty standing, or are disoriented. Some patients may need assistance in the bathroom, whereas others require bedpan or urinal in bed. Older patients have difficulty in maintaining balance and raising or lowering toilet seats.

PATIENT TEACHING

- Teach patient the importance of appropriate collection of urine specimen.

PEDIATRIC CONSIDERATIONS

- Young children are often unable to void on request. Offer fluids they enjoy (juice, popsicles) and allow them to suggest when they are ready to void.
- Children may prefer assistance of parent in cleansing genitalia and collecting urine.

COLLECTING A STERILE URINE SPECIMEN VIA CATHETER PORT

Nursing action/*Rationale*

1. Read physician's order *to provide basis for care.*
2. Collect supplies *to organize procedure.*
3. Introduce self, *which helps to decrease patient's anxiety level.*
4. Identify patient by identification band *to identify correct patient for procedure.*
5. Explain procedure to patient, *as this will ensure patient cooperation and decrease anxiety.*
6. Wash hands, and don clean gloves *to help prevent cross-contamination.*
7. Catheter port collection:
   a. Clamp just below catheter port for about 30 min *to allow urine to collect for removal* (see illustration).
   b. Return in 30 min; clean port with alcohol prep *to cleanse port for needle puncture.*
   c. Insert needle into port at 30-degree angle, and withdraw 5 to 10 ml of urine for a specimen *to provide urine for testing* (see illustration).
   d. Place urine in sterile specimen cup *to keep specimen sterile.*
   e. Unclamp catheter *to allow continuous urine flow.*
   f. Label specimen, and send to laboratory with requisition *to provide accuracy of specimen.*
8. Remove gloves and wash hands.
9. Document procedure and observations *to communicate with others the patient care administered.*

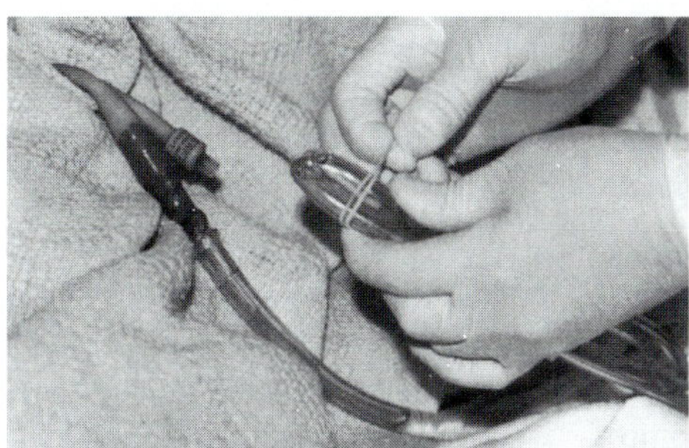

STEP 7a

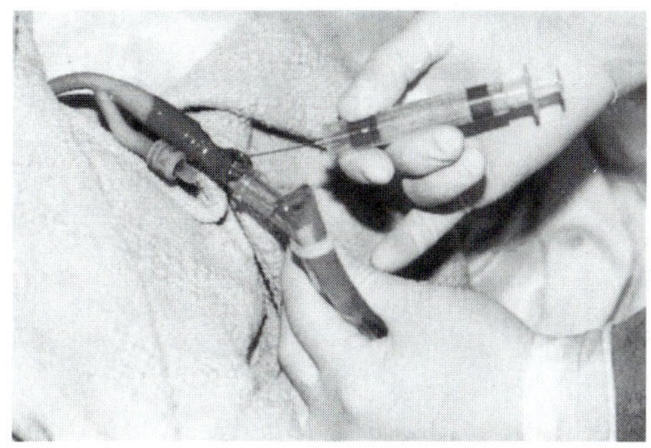

STEP 7c

Sample charting

DATE	TIME	NOTES
1/28/95	1030	10 ml sterile urine specimen collected from catheter port and sent to laboratory.

____

(nurse's signature)

FOLLOW-UP

1. Make patient comfortable, and position appropriately *to provide safe patient environment.*

SPECIAL CONCERNS

- Use strict sterile technique to prevent infection in urinary system.

PATIENT TEACHING

- Answer patient questions about the procedure.

collected after voiding is initiated (midstream) and before voiding is completed. This is the cleanest part of the voided specimen.

Purposes

The nurse collects a urine specimen and ensures its delivery to the laboratory for the following reasons:

- to help the physician make a diagnosis
- to evaluate the effectiveness of treatment

Supplies/equipment

Gloves	Label
Sterile midstream collection kit	Laboratory requisition

SKILL 17-3: COLLECTING A STERILE URINE SPECIMEN

Guidelines

A sterile urine specimen can be obtained either by inserting a straight catheter into the urinary bladder and removing urine or by obtaining a specimen from the port of an indwelling catheter using sterile technique. Urine from a dependent drainage bag should not be used for a specimen, since it is not fresh and would not reflect accurate test results. **Residual urine,** urine left in the bladder after voiding, can be measured at the time of catheterization. The patient voids, and catheterization is performed within 10 minutes. Residual urine is more than 50 ml of urine remaining in the bladder; the patient may need to have an indwelling catheter inserted.

The nurse must prepare the patient by explaining which type of urine specimen will be collected. It is important to relieve any anxiety by assuring the patient that there should be no discomfort if the patient remains relaxed; the patient should experience only mild pressure as the catheter is inserted and will feel nothing when urine is collected from the catheter port. See Chapter 30 for insertion of sterile urinary catheter.

If a urinary catheter is already in place, then the nurse may take steps to obtain a sterile urine specimen from the port of the urinary drainage system. When this approach is carried out, the sterility of the urinary drainage system is not compromised.

Purposes

The nurse collects a sterile urine specimen for the following reasons:

- to prevent risk of infection to the patient
- to obtain uncontaminated urine for diagnostic testing
- to obtain uncontaminated urine to ascertain effectiveness of treatment

Supplies/equipment

Port collection
Sterile specimen cup with lid
20-ml syringe
21- or 22½-inch needle
Tube clamp
Alcohol prep
Label
Requisition slip

Straight catheter collection
Straight catheter tray
Label
Requisition

SKILL 17-4: COLLECTING A 24-HOUR URINE SPECIMEN

Guidelines

Tests of renal function and urine composition, such as measurements of levels of adrenocortical steroids, hormones, protein, and creatinine clearance, require a 24-hour collection of urine. The procedure for ensuring that the test can be performed accurately should be followed carefully.

Purposes

Some tests require that the entire volume of urine from a 24-hour period be collected.

Supplies/equipment
Urinal/bedpan/specimen hat
Specimen container with added preservative of agency's choice

SKILL 17-5: PERFORMING A URINE GLUCOSE/ACETONE, DETERMINATION

Guidelines

A glucose/acetone determination test is performed to measure the amount of sugar (glucose) and acetone in a sample of urine from a diabetic patient. Several types of products, such as Clinitest tablets, Tes-Tape, Dipstick, Acetest tablets, and Keto-diastix, are used for the test.

The patient is taught to perform the test at certain times during the day, such as before meals and at bedtime. The specimen should be a double-voided one to ensure accurate test results. This test is done far less often now for glucose determination in the urine because of availability of self-blood glucose monitoring or blood glucose monitoring by the laboratory personnel or the nurse. Blood glucose monitoring provides more current and accurate information on glucose levels in the body.

The patient should be informed of the times during the day the test will be performed in order to give a urine sample as needed. Test results are usually charted on a flow sheet and are reported to the medication nurse when a sliding scale for insulin is ordered. In this case, insulin is administered according to the test results. This test is easy to perform but must be done accurately, since the amount of insulin may be determined by results.

Purposes

The nurse performs the urine glucose/acetone determination test for the following reasons:

- to aid the physician in deciding the amount of insulin to order
- to assist in controlling diabetes
- to detect elevated glucose levels before the patient is given more glucose
- to help adjust food intake, exercise, and insulin requirements

Supplies/equipment

For reagent tablet testing
Bedpan or urinal
Specimen container
10-ml test tube
Test tube holder
Medicine dropper
Clean container for water
Clinitest tablets
Acetest tablets
Color charts
Tissues or paper towel

For reagent strip testing
Specimen container
Glucose/ketone test strip
Test strip color chart

SKILL 17-4

COLLECTING A 24-HOUR URINE SPECIMEN

Nursing action/*Rationale*

1. Read physician's order *to verify procedure.*
2. Wash hands *to promote medical asepsis.*
3. Identify patient *to ensure accuracy.*
4. Post signs on patient's door, bathroom door, and near patient's bed. *This will alert the staff and reminds the patient to save all urine.*
5. Explain procedure *to ensure patient's cooperation.*
6. Instruct patient about the importance of collecting *all* urine for a period of 24 hours, *which ensures a valid test of 24-hour kidney function can be obtained.*
7. Instruct patient not to place toilet tissue or fecal material in urine. *This will prevent contamination of specimen and alterations of results.*
8. Have patient void when the 24-hour specimen collection is to begin; discard this voiding *as this voiding has been formed in urinary system before the study began.*
9. Place labeled container on ice if required. (Some agencies require refrigeration of all specimens. Others advocate that the urine container be placed on ice. For some collection procedures, such as the creatinine clearance test, refrigeration may not be necessary.) *This keeps the specimen cool, which decreases decomposition and odor.*
10. Save all urine for the 24-hour period; place each voided specimen into the larger container with preservative. *All urine must be saved or results will be altered.*
11. Instruct patient to void a few minutes before end of 24 hours; this urine is part of the 24-hour specimen. *This will empty bladder before the end of testing.*
12. Send specimen to lab promptly; be certain label includes date and time specimen started, patient's name, room number, and test ordered. If more than one container is necessary, make certain both are labeled and numbered *to ensure proper identification of specimen.*
13. Document procedure and observations *to communicate with others the patient care administered.*

Sample charting

DATE	TIME	NOTES
1/6/95	0700	Voided 300 ml light amber urine. Urine discarded; 24-hour urine specimen collection begun. According to verbal response, patient demonstrates understanding of procedure.

____

(nurse's signature)

SPECIAL CONCERNS

- Wash hands and don gloves each time a specimen is collected and transferred to the large collection container to prevent spread of microorganisms.
- If more than one collection container is necessary, be certain to label containers as #1, #2, etc. In this manner the lab personnel will know another container will follow. This will ensure the accuracy of results.
- If patient is menstruating, be certain to note this on requisition form to ensure accuracy of results.

PATIENT TEACHING

- Encourage and teach appropriate handwashing.

SKILL 17-5

PERFORMING A URINE GLUCOSE/ACETONE DETERMINATION

Nursing action/*Rationale*

1. Read physician's order *to provide basis for care.*
2. Collect supplies *to organize procedure.*
3. Introduce self *to decrease anxiety level.*
4. Identify patient by identification band *to identify correct patient for procedure.*
5. Explain procedure to patient, *as this will ensure patient's cooperation and decrease anxiety.*
6. Wash hands, and don clean gloves *to help prevent cross-contamination.*
7. Obtain double-voided specimens ½ hour apart *to provide most accurate results from freshest urine.*
8. Perform glucose reagent tablet test:
   a. Drop 5 drops of urine from medicine dropper into test tube, and rinse dropper *to provide accuracy of test results.*
   b. Add 10 drops water to urine in test tube *to provide accuracy of test results.*
   c. Add reagent tablet to test tube *to provide chemical reaction for test.*
   d. Hold test tube near top or place tube in holder *to prevent nurse from receiving burn from chemical reaction.*
   e. *Shake test tube gently 15 seconds after boiling action stops, and compare color of solution with color chart to give results of test.*
   f. Cleanse test tube and rinse; *this prepares equipment for the next use.*
   g. There is also a 2-drop method; it follows the same procedure except 2 drops of urine is used and this method has a different color chart.
9. Perform glucose reagent tape test:
   a. Tear 1½ inches Tes-Tape from holder, and immerse end of strip in and immediately out of urine *to help determine accuracy of test.*
   b. Tap gently on side of container; *this removes excess urine that can dilute reagent.*
   c. After appropriate amount of time, compare with color chart *to provide test results.*
10. Perform acetone reagent tablet test:
    a. Place Acetest tablet on dry paper towel; do not touch with bare hands *because moisture can cause inaccurate results.*
    b. Place 1 drop of urine from medicine dropper onto tablet *to provide chemical reaction.*
    c. After appropriate amount of time, compare with color chart *to provide test results.*
11. Wash hands *to reduce number of microorganisms.*
12. Record glucose/acetone determination *to verify performance of procedure, patient's test response, and test results.*

Sample charting

DATE	TIME	NOTES
1/26/95	1040	Voided 300 cc of clear amber urine.
	1110	Voided 100 ml clear, yellow urine. Glucose/acetone test performed. Clinitest negative and Acetest negative. Reported to medication nurse. Both urine samples discarded.

____

(nurse's signature)

FOLLOW-UP

1. Clean and replace supplies and equipment *because this prepares for next procedure to be performed and keeps environment clean.*
2. Make sure bottle cap is replaced tightly *because the tablets may react to moisture in the air, which renders the tablets chemically inactive.*

SPECIAL CONCERNS

- Patient must be given enough time to give a double-voided specimen. Save first specimen.
- Offer extra water to drink to increase renal perfusion.
- Read instructions carefully on all glucose/acetone testing materials before performing tests.
- Chart glucose/acetone results on flow sheet.
- Test first specimen of urine if patient cannot give double-voided specimen, and report and record even though not considered accurate.

PATIENT TEACHING

- Teach patient to perform glucose/acetone urine tests.
- Explain results of tests where applicable.
- Teach skin puncture for blood glucose if applicable; this test is replacing urine glucose testing and gives more accurate information.
- Teach patient importance of washing hands before and after performing procedure.

SKILL 17-6: MEASURING BLOOD GLUCOSE LEVELS

Guidelines

The use of a meter to measure blood glucose is a more meaningful test for use by diabetics than testing urine for the presence of glucose. A skin puncture can be easily performed by the patient at home and provides more accurate information than does the urine glucose/acetone determination test.

Purposes

The nurse measures blood glucose for the following reasons:

- to monitor blood glucose levels, especially for the patient who is diabetic and the patient who is receiving IV hyperalimentation
- to formulate a nursing diagnosis
- to teach the diabetic patient how to control blood glucose levels
- to teach the diabetic patient to measure blood glucose levels to perform procedure at home

Supplies/equipment
Lancet
Automatic lancing device
Cotton balls
Vial of test strips
Meter to measure glucose

SKILL 17-7: COLLECTING A STOOL SPECIMEN

Guidelines

Stool specimens are collected and examined for a variety of reasons, including to determine the presence of infection, bleeding, or hemorrhage; to observe the amount, color, consistency, and presence of fats; and to identify parasites, ova, and bacteria. The nurse collects the feces, labels the specimen appropriately, and sends the specimen and laboratory request to the laboratory. Stool to be examined for parasites must be taken immediately to the laboratory in order for parasites to be examined under the microscope while alive. A stool specimen may also be collected from a colostomy or ileostomy.

The patient must be informed that a stool specimen is needed, but collection must be carried out in such a manner that will not cause stress or make the patient feel hurried or embarrassed. Arrange supplies if patient will collect the stool. When a stool specimen is to be obtained, the speciman hat is placed toward the back of the stool. When a urine specimen is to be obtained, the speciman hat is placed toward the front of the stool. The nurse must understand why the stool specimen is being collected to use the appropriate supplies. If stool specimen is for ova and parasite (0 & P), an appropriate container with special solution is obtained.

Purposes

The nurse collects stool specimens for the following reasons:

- to test for abnormal elements in the stool
- to determine malabsorption problems

Supplies/equipment
Stool specimen cup/container
Tongue depressor
Bedpan, specimen device, or commode
Gloves
Label
Laboratory requisition

SKILL 17-8: DETERMINING THE PRESENCE OF OCCULT BLOOD IN STOOL

Guidelines

The presence of blood in body waste is abnormal. Blood in the stool may be bright red, which indicates that the blood is fresh and that the site of bleeding is in the lower GI tract. On the other hand, black tarry feces means the presence of old blood and that the site of bleeding is higher in the gastrointestinal tract. When blood is present in the stool but cannot be seen without the use of a microscope, it is referred to as **occult** (hidden). A **hemoccult test** detects occult blood in feces.

The nurse must instruct the patient on how many stool specimens are ordered by the physician and how to collect a stool specimen. The Hemoccult card is then labeled appropriately and sent to the laboratory.

Purposes

The nurse collects a stool specimen and sends it to the laboratory for the following reasons:

- to detect the presence of blood in the stool
- to aid the physician in making a diagnosis

Supplies/equipment
Hemoccult card
Wooden applicator
Clean bedpan or specimen device for commode
Clean gloves

Text continued on p. 326.

SKILL 17-6

MEASURING BLOOD GLUCOSE LEVELS

Nursing action/*Rationale*

1. Read physician's order *to provide basis for care.*
2. Collect supplies *to organize procedure.*
3. Introduce self *to decrease anxiety level.*
4. Identify patient by identification band *to identify correct patient for procedure.*
5. Explain procedure to patient *to seek cooperation and decrease anxiety.*
6. Wash hands, and don clean gloves *to help prevent cross-contamination and protect nurse from blood and body fluids.*
7. Remove cap from lancet using sterile technique *to maintain sterility of point.*
8. Place lancet into automatic lancing device according to instructions in operating manual; *this allows proper puncture of skin.*
9. Select site on side of any fingertip (heel used for infant) *because the side of finger is less responsive to pain from puncture.*
10. Wipe selected site with alcohol swab, and discard *to prepare site.*
11. Ask patient to hold arm at side 30 seconds, *as this increases blood flow to site and allows site to dry.*
12. Gently squeeze fingertip with thumb of same hand *to increase blood supply to site.*
13. Hold lancing device *to provide easy access to device.*
14. Place trigger platform of lancing device on side of finger, and press (see illustration). *This activates lancing mechanism.*
15. Squeeze finger in downward motion (wipe off first drop of blood) *to obtain enough blood to cover test pad on test strip and to remove surface contaminant.*
16. While holding strip level, touch drop of blood to test pad; *this enables covering of test pad without smearing.*
17. Begin recommended timing. After 60 seconds blot blood off test strip (A), place reagent strip into appropriate site on meter (B), and wait for numeric readout (C) *to ensure test accuracy* (see illustration).
18. Remove lancet from device, and discard *to prevent needle puncture of nurse.*
19. Remove gloves, discard, and wash hands *to prevent cross-contamination.*
20. Document procedure and observations, *as this communicates with others the patient care administered.*

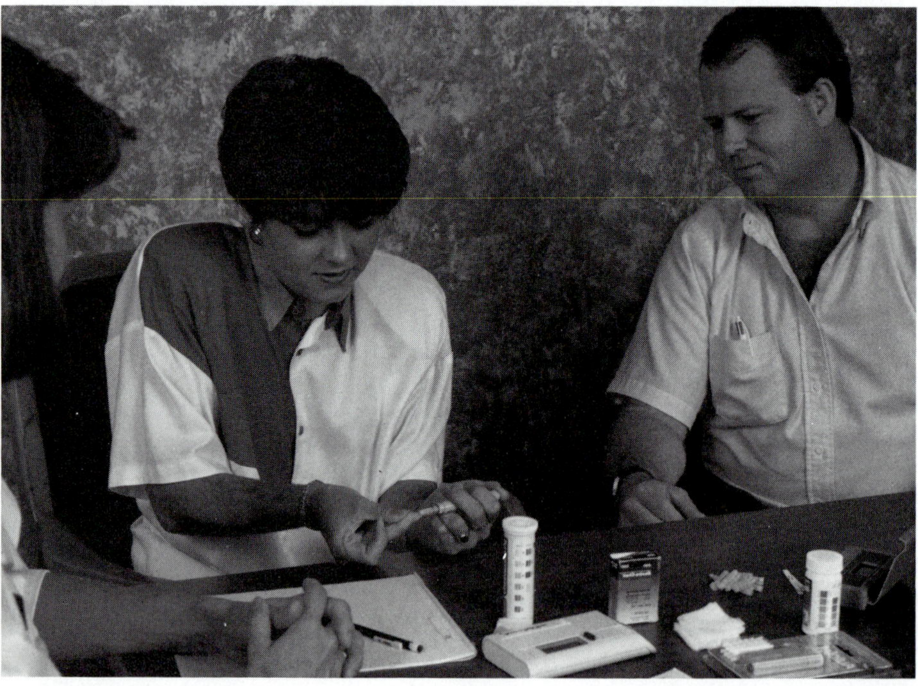

STEP 14

MEASURING BLOOD GLUCOSE LEVELS—cont'd

Sample charting

DATE	TIME	NOTES
2/20/95	1730	Skin puncture performed on left index finger for blood glucose. Results: 84 per glucometer. Tolerated well. Verbalizes understanding of blood glucose level. Dr. Smith notified per phone of test results.

____

(nurse's signature)

SPECIAL CONCERNS

- Make certain staff is aware of what tests are scheduled for each day.
- Have all supplies available if patient is to perform procedure (see *illustrations*).
- Carry out sterile technique during procedure.
- Wear clean gloves when in contact with body fluids.
- Make certain patient understands how to perform procedure to ensure patient safety and accurate test results.

PATIENT TEACHING

- Teach patient to perform a skin puncture when appropriate.
- Have patient return demonstration for a skin puncture.
- Explain normal blood glucose levels to the patient.
- Explain to patient which blood glucose levels should be reported to the physician.
- Teach patient importance of handwashing before and after procedure.

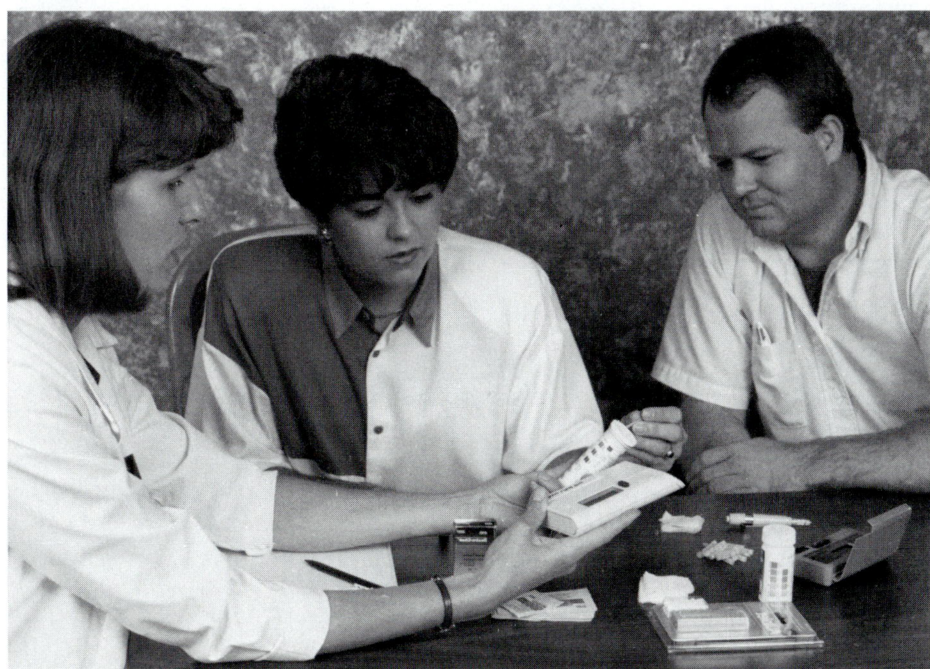

STEP 17

SKILL 17-7

COLLECTING A STOOL SPECIMEN

Nursing action/*Rationale*

1. Read physician's order *to provide basis for care.*
2. Collect supplies *to organize procedure.*
3. Introduce self *to decrease anxiety level.*
4. Identify patient by identification band *to identify correct patient for procedure.*
5. Explain procedure to patient; make certain patient understands what is expected *to seek cooperation and decrease anxiety.*
6. Wash hands and don gloves *to help prevent cross-contamination.*
7. Assist to bathroom when necessary *to provide patient safety.*
8. Request patient to defecate into commode, specimen device, or bedpan, and to prevent urine from entering specimen *to prevent contamination of specimen* (see illustration).
9. Transfer stool to specimen cup with use of a tongue blade, and close lid *to protect specimen* (see illustration).
10. Remove gloves, and wash hands *to protect nurse from contamination.*
11. Attach lab slip and send specimen to laboratory *to identify specimen for laboratory.*
12. Assist patient to bed *to provide patient safety.*
13. Document procedure and observations *to communicate with others the care administered.*

Sample charting

DATE	TIME	NOTES
12/4/95	1040	Specimen of soft, brown stool collected and taken with requisition form to laboratory.

____
(nurse's signature)

PATIENT TEACHING

- Explain how to collect a stool specimen appropriately.
- Teach purpose for collecting a stool specimen.
- Encourage and teach appropriate handwashing.

SPECIAL CONCERNS

- Nurse must know what type of stool specimen is ordered and how to collect the specimen.
- Make certain patient understands what is expected, to provide patient safety.
- Specimen to be examined for ova and parasites must be taken to the laboratory immediately.
- Other stool specimens may be kept at room temperature.

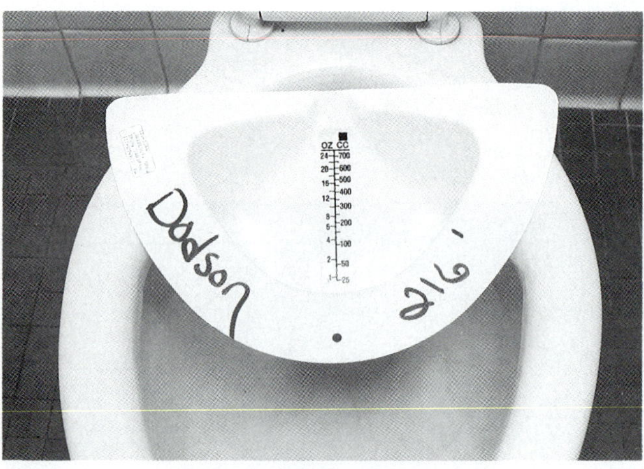

STEP 8

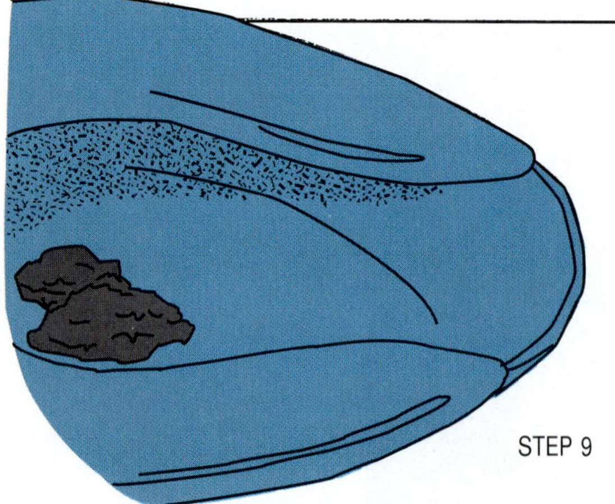

STEP 9

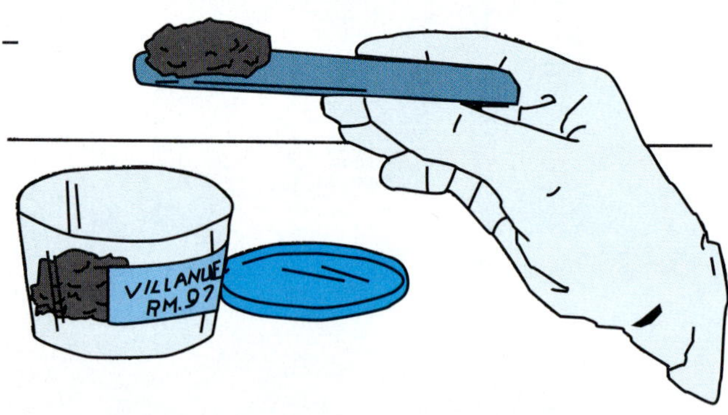

DETERMINING THE PRESENCE OF OCCULT BLOOD IN STOOL

Nursing action/*Rationale*

1. Read physician's order *to provide basis for care.*
2. Collect supplies *to organize procedure.*
3. Introduce self *to decrease anxiety level.*
4. Identify patient by identification band *to identify correct patient for procedure.*
5. Explain procedure to patient *to ensure cooperation and decrease anxiety.*
6. Wash hands, and don gloves *to prevent cross-contamination.*
7. Collect stool specimen *to provide stool for Hemoccult.*
8. Follow steps on Hemoccult slide test:
   a. Open flap *to begin test* (see illustration).
   b. Smear very small amount with tongue blade in first box (A) *to prepare slide.*
   c. Smear very small amount with tongue blade from another part of stool, and transfer to box B *to prepare second slide* (see illustration).
   d. Close card, and label *to ensure accurate identification of specimen.*
   e. Send specimen to lab *to provide fresh specimen for testing.*
9. Remove gloves and wash hands *to help prevent cross-contamination.*
10. Document procedure and observations *to communicate with others collection of stool specimen.*

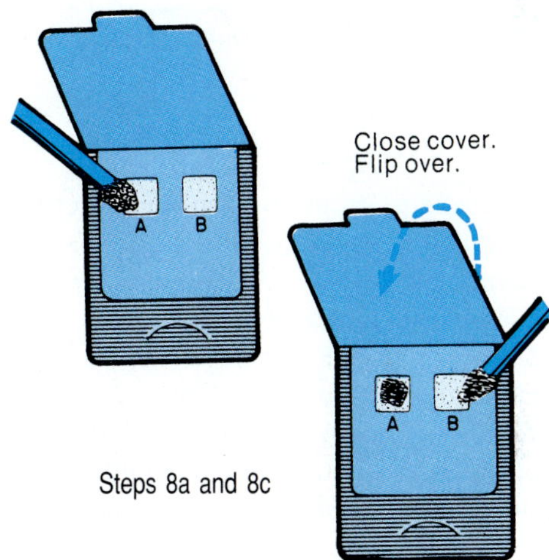

Steps 8a and 8c

Sample charting

DATE	TIME	NOTES
1/28/95	1310	Expelled large amount soft, brown stool. First specimen for occult blood collected and sent to laboratory. Instructed regarding need for total of three specimens.

____

(nurse's signature)

According to verbal response, patient demonstrates understanding of procedure.

FOLLOW-UP

1. Read physician's orders for changes in regimen after test completion *as results of tests can lead to further nursing interventions.*

SPECIAL CONCERNS

- Do not confuse hemorrhoidal bleeding with upper gastrointestinal bleeding, such as in **coffee ground vomitus/emesis** (dark brown vomitus the color and consistency of coffee grounds and composed of gastric juices and old blood and indicative of slow upper GI bleeding.)
- Meat-free diet may be ordered 3 days before test.

PATIENT TEACHING

- Make certain patient understands test and why it is being performed.
- Teach patient how to perform procedure if discharged before three specimens are collected.
- Encourage and teach appropriate handwashing.

SKILL 17-9

COLLECTING SPUTUM

Nursing action/*Rationale*

1. Read physician's order *to provide basis for care.*
2. Collect supplies *to organize procedure.*
3. Introduce self *to decrease anxiety level.*
4. Identify patient by identification band *to identify correct patient for procedure.*
5. Explain procedure to patient *to seek cooperation and decrease anxiety.*
6. Wash hands and don gloves *to help prevent cross-contamination.*
7. Position patient in Fowler's position *to assist coughing.*
8. Instruct patient to take three breaths and force cough into sterile container *to help patient expectorate mucus* (see illustration).
9. Label specimen container *to ensure appropriate specimen reaches laboratory.*
10. Attach laboratory requisition, and immediately send specimen to laboratory *to ensure specimen is sent to the laboratory.*
11. Remove gloves, and wash hands *to help prevent cross-contamination.*
12. Document procedure and observations *to communicate the care administered.*

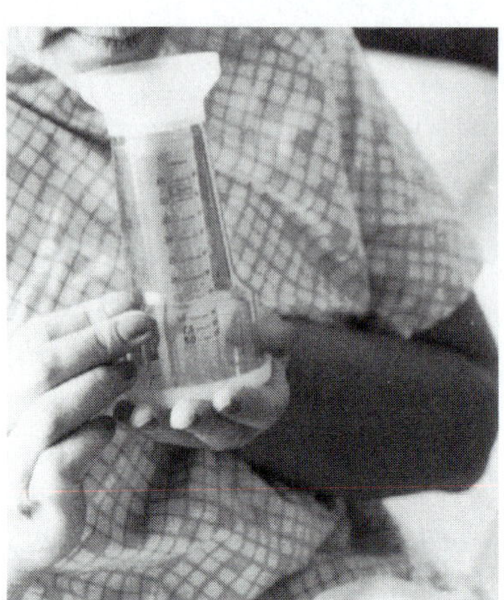

STEP 8

Sample charting

DATE	TIME	NOTES
12/4/95	0630	Sputum specimen collected and sent to lab for culture and sensitivity. Obtained moderate amount of light green, tenacious sputum. Some dyspnea noted but subsided with rest. Respirations 22 and regular.

____

(nurse's signature)

SPECIAL CONCERNS

- Oral hygiene should be provided after the procedure for patient comfort.
- Accuracy of test decreases if delivery of specimen to laboratory is delayed.
- Make certain patient knows how to perform sputum collection.
- The nurse must be prepared to obtain the specimen by suctioning if the patient cannot cough. (See Chapter 31 for suctioning procedure).

PATIENT TEACHING

- Instruct patient regarding the importance of drinking fluids to decrease thickness of mucus.
- Stress to patient the importance of coughing from deep in the bronchial tree.
- Encourage and teach patient appropriate handwashing.

SKILL 17-9: COLLECTING A SPUTUM SPECIMEN

Guidelines

Sputum is secretions from the lung. It contains mucus, cellular debris, or microorganisms, and it may contain blood or pus. A sputum specimen must come from deep in the bronchial tree. Expectoration from throat and mouth secretions cannot be used as a sputum specimen. Early morning is the best time to collect a sputum specimen because the patient has not yet cleared the respiratory passages. Many tests can be performed on sputum, such as **culture** (a laboratory test involving cultivation of microorganisms or cells in a special growth medium) and **sensitivity** (a laboratory method of determining the effectiveness of antibiotics, usually performed in conjunction with culture), **cytological** (the study of cells, including their formation, origin, structure, function, biochemical activities, and pathology) examination, and test for acid-fast bacillus. Some patients cannot **expectorate** (the ejection of mucus, sputum, or fluids from the trachea and lungs by coughing or spitting) a specimen and must have tracheal suctioning to obtain sputum (see Chapter 31 for the suctioning procedure). Closed-method collection containers protect the nurse from contamination from body fluids. The nurse explains the procedure and prepares the patient for the test.

The nurse instructs the patient the night before the test to drink extra fluids, since this will assist loosening secretions to more easily expectorate for the specimen. Saliva cannot be used as a specimen, and the patient must be so instructed. Saliva will be clear whereas sputum is thick, colored, and tenacious (sticky).

Purposes

The nurse collects a sputum specimen for the following reasons:

- to determine (1) if pathogenic microorganisms are present in the sputum, (2) the type of microorganism present, and (3) to what drugs it is sensitive (by doing a culture and sensitivity)
- to determine if cancer cells are present (cytological examination)
- to determine the presence of an organism called the *tubercle bacillus,* which causes tuberculosis (acid-fast bacillus)

Supplies/equipment
Sterile sputum collector
Tissues
Label for specimen
Laboratory requisition
Gloves

REFERENCES AND SELECTED READINGS

1. Brown SJ: Behind the numbers on the CBC, *RN* 52(2):46, 1990.
2. Buffington S: How much do you know about laboratory studies? *Nursing* 21(12):46, 1991.
3. Cheny AM, MaQuindang ML: Patient teaching for x-ray and other diagnostics, *RN* 56(4):54, 1993.
4. Eyles MY: *Mosby's comprehensive review of practical nursing,* ed 11, St Louis, 1994, Mosby.
5. Flyn JM, Hackel R: *Technological foundations in nursing,* East Norwalk, Conn, 1990, Appleton & Lange.
6. Hood GH, Dincher JR: *Total patient care: foundations and practice,* ed 8, St Louis, 1992, Mosby.
7. Kestel F: Using blood glucose meters: what you and your patient need to know. I. *Nursing* 23(3):34, 1993.
8. Kestel F: Using blood glucose meters: what you and your patient need to know. II. *Nursing* 23(4):50, 1993.
9. Kestel F: Using blood glucose meters: what you and your patient need to know. III. *Nursing* 23(5):51, 1993.
10. McConnell EA: Understanding diagnostic tests, *Nursing* 24(3):39, 1994.
11. McDonagh A: Getting your patient ready for a nuclear medicine scan, *Nurs '91* 21(2):53, 1991.
12. Monroe D: Patient teaching for x-ray and other diagnostics, *RN* 53(4):52, 1990.
13. Monroe D: Patient teaching for x-ray and other diagnostics, *RN* 53(9):42, 1990.
14. *Mosby's medical, nursing, and allied health dictionary,* ed 4, St Louis, 1994, Mosby.
15. Pagana KD, Pagana TJ: *Mosby's diagnostic and laboratory reference,* St Louis, 1992, Mosby.
16. Peragalo-Ditko V: Buyers' guide to blood glucose meters, *Diabetes Self Management* 8(3):34, 1991.
17. Perry AG, Potter PA: *Clinical nursing skills and techniques,* ed 3, St Louis, 1994, Mosby.
18. Potter PA, Perry AG: *Basic nursing: theory and practice,* ed 3, St Louis, 1995, Mosby.
19. Potter PA, Perry AG: *Fundamentals of nursing: concepts, process, and practice,* ed 3, St Louis, 1993, Mosby.
20. Renkes J: GI endoscopy: managing the full scope of care, *Nursing* 23(6):50, 1993.
21. The Staff: *Fundamental nursing skills,* Springhouse, Penn, 1993, Springhouse.
22. The Staff: *Nursing procedures: student version,* Springhouse, Penn, 1993, Springhouse.
23. Tietz N: *Clinical guide to laboratory tests,* ed 2, Philadelphia, 1994, Saunders.
24. Timby BK, Lewis LW: *Fundamental skills and concepts in patient care,* ed 5, Philadelphia, 1992, Lippincott.
25. Whaley LF, Wong DL: *Nursing care of infants and children* ed 4, St Louis, 1991, Mosby.
26. Wilkinson MM: Your role in needle biopsy of the liver, *RN* 53(8):62, 1990.

CHAPTER CHALLENGE

KEY POINTS

- Laboratory examinations of specimens of urine, stool, sputum, blood, and wound drainage provide important information about body functioning and contributes to the assessment of health status.
- Patients given a clear explanation about the purpose of the specimen and how it is obtained will be more cooperative in its collection.
- The nurse properly prepares to ensure that the patient is ready for the test and to avoid prolonging hospital stay because of inadequate test preparations.
- Most persons believe that excretions should be handled discreetly; therefore it is important to provide the patient with as much comfort and privacy as possible.
- The nurse wears gloves when collecting specimens of blood or other body fluids to prevent spread of HIV, hepatitis B, and other pathogens.
- The nurse collects specimens in appropriate containers at the correct time and in the appropriate amount.
- The nurse properly labels all specimens with the patient's identification and completes laboratory requisition as necessary.
- Most invasive diagnostic tests require a signed informed consent.

STUDY QUESTIONS

1. Mrs.George, age 64, newly diagnosed with diabetes mellitus, has been learning how to perform her own blood glucose monitoring. The nurse is aware that having Mrs. George hold her arm at her side for 30 seconds before obtaining a blood sample to measure glucose will:
   1. Increase blood to the site
   2. Provide easy access to device
   3. Prepare the site
   4. Prevent needle puncture of the nurse
2. Several residents in a long-term care facility have a urine glucose/acetone determination test ordered. A second voided specimen is advised. The purpose of a double-voided specimen is to:
   1. Provide a chemical reaction
   2. Determine insulin requirements for the patient
   3. Ensure accurate test results
   4. Obtain a pooled urine specimen
3. A sputum specimen has been ordered for Mr. Burke, a 75-year-old admitted with possible pneumonia of the right lower lobe. Mr. Burke is not able to cough. The nurse is aware that for patients who cannot expectorate sputum from deep in the bronchial tree, the specimen must be collected by:
   1. Pharyngeal suctioning
   2. Endotracheal suctioning
   3. Oropharyngeal suctioning
   4. Percussion and vibration
4. The physician has ordered a stool specimen for blood that cannot be seen by the naked eye. This examination is for:
   1. Hemoccult blood
   2. Gross blood
   3. Melena
   4. Occult blood
5. Mr. Lander, age 46, is seen by the physician for recurrent symptoms of cystitis. He is to have a urine culture and sensitivity determination and a 24-hour urine collection for laboratory analysis. Mr. Lander should be informed that a urine culture study is required to:
   1. Identify the causative organisms
   2. Determine the presence of malignant cells
   3. Analyze the elements present in the urine
   4. Localize the site of the inflammatory process
6. To obtain a 24-hour urine specimen, a patient should be given which of the following instructions:
   1. Collect each voiding in separate containers for the next 24 hours
   2. Discard the first voided specimen and then collect the total volume of each voiding for 24 hours
   3. For the next 24 hours, retain a 30-ml specimen of each voiding after recording the amount voided
   4. Keep a record of the time and amount of each voiding for 24 hours
7. Mrs. Clough, age 72, has an indwelling urinary catheter. A sterile urine specimen has been ordered for a culture and sensitivity. The sterile specimen should be obtained by:
   1. Obtaining 60 ml of urine from the collection bag
   2. Removing the present catheter, having the patient void, and then recatheterizing
   3. Disconnecting the tubing from the catheter and draining 2 cc of urine
   4. Aspirating 10 cc of urine with a sterile syringe from the tubing port
8. A patient performing a finger stick for blood glucose determination asks why the side of the fingertip is advised as the preferred site. The nurse is aware that it is because:
   1. The blood supply is greater in this area
   2. It is easier for the self-determination method
   3. The side of the finger is less responsive to pain
   4. It leaves more room for other site selection
9. An important preexamination nursing intervention for the patient undergoing an invasive diagnostic examination is:
   1. A cleansing bath with Hebiclens
   2. Obtaining the informed consent
   3. Encouraging patient to drink several glasses of water
   4. Instructing patient not to wear deodorant, powder, or lotion
10. A patient is scheduled for an upper GI series and a barium enema. The nurse explains that because of the procedure for an upper gastrointestinal study and barium enema, the patient can expect to:
    1. Be NPO after midnight and have enemas until clear
    2. Have coffee and toast the morning of the test
    3. Take radiographic dye tablets
    4. Have a needle inserted into the liver area

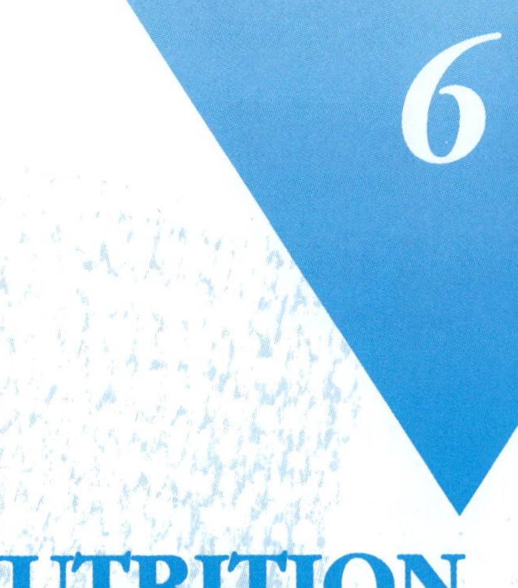

6 NUTRITION

I have always been a person of few but often poignant words! I narrowed my thoughts to just a few!

N-Nurturing
U-Unique
R-Responsibility
S-Satisfaction
E-Enthusiasm!

These are the qualities I feel reflect my feelings regarding nursing. This pretty will spells it out for me!

Patricia S. McConnell
Student Nurse

18

BASIC NUTRITION

Kristen Kartchner Maughan

KEY TERMS

adipose tissue
amino acid
anabolism
antioxidant
carbohydrate
catabolism
dietary cholesterol
dietary fiber
electrolyte
enzyme
essential nutrient
fat
glycogen
iron deficiency anemia
kilocalorie
kwashiorkor
lipid
lipoprotein
marasmus
metabolism
mineral
nitrogen balance
nutrient
nutrient dense
nutrition
pellagra
pernicious anemia
satiety
scurvy
serum cholesterol
vegan
vitamin

LEARNING OBJECTIVES

After reading this chapter, the student should be able to do the following:

- Define the key terms.
- Discuss the role of the nurse in promoting good nutrition.
- Explain how to use the Food Guide Pyramid, the Dietary Guidelines for Americans, and the Recommended Dietary Allowances (RDAs) in diet planning and assessment.
- List the six classes of essential nutrients and identify those that provide energy.
- Identify the three basic functions of nutrients in the body.
- List food sources and possible health benefits of dietary fiber.
- List the functions and food sources of protein, carbohydrates, and fats.
- Discuss the difference between saturated and unsaturated fats, and explain the effect of excess fat intake on health.
- Discuss the effects of deficiencies and toxicities of vitamins and minerals.
- List food sources of each of the vitamins and minerals.
- Discuss the benefits of receiving nutrients from food rather than from dietary supplements.
- Discuss the changes in nutrient needs throughout the life cycle.
- Suggest ideas for developing sound dietary habits in children.
- Identify factors that may lead to poor nutrition in the elderly.
- Discuss ways nutrients and drugs may interact.

RELATED TOPICS OF INTEREST

- Life span development (Chapter 7)
- Diet therapy (Chapter 19)
- The surgical patient (Chapter 22)
- Care of the patient with a gastrointestinal or accessory organ disorder (Chapter 27)
- Mental health concepts (Chapter 46)
- The patient with an addictive personality (Chapter 47)

Prevention—perhaps this word best describes why nutrition is becoming increasingly important in health care. **Nutrition** is the total of all processes involved in the taking in and utilization of food substances for proper growth, functioning, and maintenance of health. More and more evidence points to the fact that nutrition plays a role in many disease states and that, in many cases, proper nutrition may help prevent or delay the onset of certain diseases. It has long been known that optimal nutrition ensures proper growth in children, teens, and pregnant women. But nutrition is important at every age, not only for growth, but for quality of life. Nutrition is vital for the proper functioning of the cardiovascular, renal, pulmonary, nervous, digestive, and immune systems, among others. In short, nutrition plays a role directly or indirectly in all body processes. Its importance must not be overlooked.

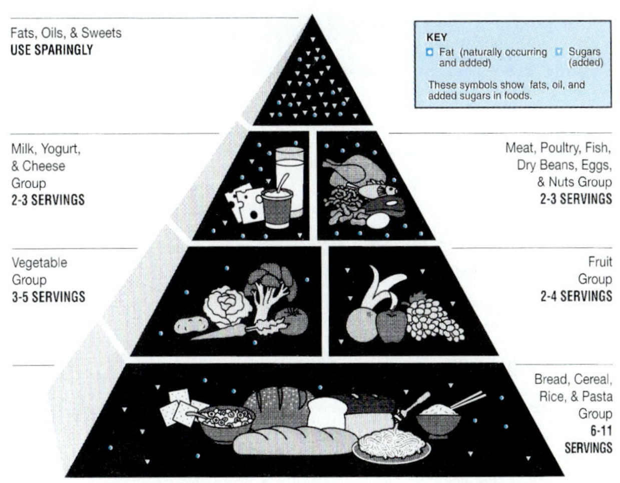

ROLE OF THE NURSE IN PROMOTING NUTRITION

Because the nurse is most directly involved with the patient, the patient looks to the nurse as a source of health information. Therefore nurses should have a basic knowledge of nutrition. Although the dietitian is the nutrition expert, the nurse will have opportunities to apply nutrition knowledge in a number of ways by:

- Helping the patient understand the importance of the diet
- Assisting some patients with the eating process
- Taking and recording patient weights
- Recording patient intakes
- Observing clinical signs of poor nutrition and reporting them
- Serving as a communication link among the patient, dietitian, physician, or other members of the health care team

Nurses can also apply nutrition knowledge in their personal lives. What better reason for understanding nutrition?

DIET PLANNING GUIDES

Food Guide Pyramid

A number of guidelines have been established in the United States to help in planning for optimal nutrition. The most recent of these is the US Department of Agriculture's Food Guide Pyramid (Fig. 18-1). This food guide was developed to replace the four food groups pie chart in use since the 1950s. The pyramid's intent is to illustrate which foods should be included in a healthful diet and in what proportion.

Foods are divided into six groups. The Bread, Cereal, Rice, and Pasta group (Table 18-1 on p. 332) is at the base of the pyramid to indicate that these grain-based foods should make up the bulk of the diet. A recommended 6 to 11 servings should be consumed each day.

In contrast to the old four food groups, which included fruits and vegetables in the same category, the pyramid separates these groups, placing them side by side atop the grain-based group. This change indicates the importance of including both vegetables and fruits in the diet each day. The guide suggests at least three servings of vegetables and two servings of fruit daily.

Two to three servings of the Milk, Yogurt, and Cheese group will provide most of the daily calcium needs, along with protein and many other nutrients necessary for health. For most people, low-fat and nonfat milk products are recommended to keep the diet low in fat and cholesterol. In the past, some have included other dietary products in this group. Items such as butter and cream are high in fat; however, these foods are now included in the Fats, Oils, and Sweets group.

The Meat, Poultry, Fish, Dry Beans, Eggs, and Nuts group supplies protein and other nutrients such as iron. Two to three servings daily supply adequate amounts of protein when consumed with a balance of the other food groups. Again, to control the amount of fat in the diet, lean meats and low-fat cooking methods are suggested.

Fats, Oils, and Sweets occupy the very tip of the pyramid, indicating the need for moderation in the use of these foods. Fats, oils, and sweets may be included as an accompaniment or an enhancement to an already healthful diet. They should never replace adequate servings of foods from the other groups.

The *Basic Four* has probably been the most widely recognized food guide in the past. With the development of the Food Guide Pyramid, it is preferable to discontinue use of the four food groups and begin using the six groups outlined in the pyramid.

TABLE 18-1 HOW MANY SERVINGS DO YOU NEED EACH DAY?

	Women and Some Older Adults	Children, Teenage Girls, Active Women, Most Men	Teenage Boys and Active Men
Calorie Level*	About 1600	About 2200	About 2800
Bread group	6	9	11
Vegetable group	3	4	5
Fruit group	2	3	4
Milk group	2-3†	2-3†	2-3†
Meat group	2 (for a total of 5 oz)	2 (for a total of 6 oz)	3 (for a total of 7 oz)

What Counts as 1 Serving?

Bread, Cereal, Rice, and Pasta Group	***Vegetable Group***	***Fruit Group***
1 slice bread ½ c cooked rice or pasta ½ c cooked cereal 1 oz ready-to-eat cereal	½ c chopped raw or cooked vegetables 1 c leafy raw vegetables	1 piece fruit or melon wedge ¾ c juice ½ c canned fruit ¼ c dried fruit
Milk, Yogurt, and Cheese Group	***Meat, Poultry, Fish, Dry Beans, Eggs, and Nuts Group***	***Fats, Oils, and Sweets***
1 c milk or yogurt 1½ oz natural cheese 2 oz process cheese	2½ to 3 oz cooked lean meat, poultry, or fish Count ½ c cooked beans, 1 egg, or 2 tbsp of peanut butter as 1 oz of lean meat	*Limit calories from these,* especially if you need to lose weight

*These are the calorie levels if you choose low-fat lean foods from the five major food groups and use foods from the fats, oils, and sweets group sparingly.

†Women who are pregnant or breastfeeding, teenagers, and young adults to age 24 need three servings.

Box 18-1 DIETARY GUIDELINES FOR AMERICANS AND SUGGESTIONS FOR THEIR USE

1. EAT A VARIETY OF FOODS. The Food Guide Pyamid (see Fig. 18-1) can provide a guide for eating a variety of foods. Remember to include a variety of foods from each group. For example, eat different types of vegetables rather than the same ones each day. No one food can provide all dietary needs.
2. MAINTAIN HEALTHY WEIGHT. Use moderation in the use of high-calorie, nutrient-poor foods such as fatty foods, sweets, and alcohol. Use more nutrient-dense foods (those high in nutrients relative to calories). Include physical activity regularly.
3. CHOOSE A DIET LOW IN FAT, SATURATED FAT, AND CHOLESTEROL. Choose low-fat dairy products, lean meats, poultry, and fish. Limit the use of eggs and organ meats, and add less fat to foods. Bake, broil, or poach rather than fry. Limit rich desserts.
4. CHOOSE A DIET WITH PLENTY OF VEGETABLES, FRUITS, AND GRAIN PRODUCTS. The bulk of the diet should be provided by these foods. Try to select whole-grain products, beans, peas, nuts, and seeds. Use a wide variety of fruits and vegetables. These foods are the best source of dietary fiber and many of the vitamins and minerals.
5. USE SUGARS ONLY IN MODERATION. Limit intake of sugar, honey, syrup, molasses, candy, cakes, sweetened beverages, and gelatins. Use fresh fruits or fruits canned in light syrup or their own juices.
6. USE SALT AND SODIUM ONLY IN MODERATION. Use less salt in cooking and at the table. Limit the use of processed foods, snack foods, canned soups, and cured and pickled products. Generally, the more processed a food, the more sodium it will contain. Read labels for sodium content.
7. IF YOU DRINK ALCOHOLIC BEVERAGES, DO SO IN MODERATION. Those who drink should consume no more than two alcoholic beverages per day. One alcoholic beverage is equivalent to 12 oz of beer, 4 oz of wine, or 1 oz of hard liquor. Pregnant women should refrain from drinking.

From US Department of Agriculture and US Department of Health and Human Services: Home and Garden Bull No 232, 1990.

GERONTOLOGICAL CONSIDERATIONS

- Older adults experience changes in digestive secretions, stomach mucosa, and enzyme production that affect how food is digested, absorbed, and excreted. The decreased glomerular filtration rate affects the removal of the waste products of protein metabolism.
- Because of a decrease in muscle, the basal metabolic rate decreases with aging.
- Calorie needs decrease with aging: 5% for each decade between 55 and 75, 7% for each decade after age 75.
- Protein, carbohydrate, and fat needs do not change significantly with age.
- Vitamin needs do not change significantly in healthy older adults. Supplements may be required if the dietary intake is inadequate.
- Water and dietary fiber play an important role in preventing constipation in older adults.
- Age-related changes in taste, medication use, loss of teeth, loneliness, forgetfulness, and apathy can affect the eating habits of older adults.
- Many food-medication interactions are possible. Because older adults generally take several medications, the nurse should explain needed diet modifications.
- Because of restricted mobility and financial limitations, older adults may have difficulty obtaining and preparing nutritious food.

Dietary Guidelines for Americans

In 1980 the first *Dietary Guidelines for Americans* was published, with subsequent revisions in 1985 and 1990. These guidelines, developed specifically for the United States population, address the prevention of overnutrition and disease. Overnutrition is evident in the typical American diet, which is rich in fat, high in sodium, and sometimes filled with excess calories and other nutrients. Since the development of the Dietary Guidelines for Americans, other reports, such as the *Surgeon General's Report on Nutrition and Health,* have issued similar guidelines. Box 18-1 lists the Dietary Guidelines for Americans with suggestions for their use.

Recommended Dietary Allowances (RDAs)

The RDAs are the "levels of intake of essential nutrients that . . . are judged . . . to be adequate to meet the known nutrient needs of practically all healthy persons." These guidelines are determined by a group of distinguished scientists chosen by the National Academy of Sciences. Recommendations are given for various age groups of both sexes (Table 18-2 on p. 334). RDAs are not absolute requirements but are recommendations. Each person's nutrient needs are individual, so to say that everyone needs exactly what the list is unrealistic. Rather, RDAs are better used as a guide to evaluate average intakes of groups of people. Special considerations for older adults are listed in the gerontological box.

Using Diet Planning Guides Simultaneously

There are disadvantages to using just one guide in diet planning. The Food Guide Pyramid may not provide adequate nutrients if one uses no variety, and it can also be high in calories if calorie-rich foods are selected. The Dietary Guidelines for Americans focus on prevention of overnutrition but do not present a specific guide of food selection. The RDAs may be too complex for the lay public. Used as a whole, however, these guides can aid in proper food selection. By including the suggested number of servings from each group in the Food Guide Pyramid, using *variety* in food selection, and exercising *moderation* in the intake of fat, sugar, sodium, alcohol, and calories, one can eat both well and nutritiously. Variety and moderation are the key principles in diet planning. The RDAs can further help in label reading and assessment of various nutrient intakes in the diet.

ESSENTIAL NUTRIENTS

Basic Functions

A **nutrient** is a chemical compound or element found in food that is necessary for good health. **Essential nutrients** are those that our bodies cannot make in amounts necessary for good health, and therefore we must obtain them through diet or other sources. There are six classes of essential nutrients: carbohydrates, fats, proteins, vitamins, minerals, and water. Each is necessary for life.

Nutrients may perform any or all of these basic functions: (1) provide energy, (2) build and repair tissue, and (3) regulate body processes.

Provide Energy. A **kilocalorie** (kcal) is a measurement of energy, much as pound is a measurement of weight. When we say a certain food has so many kilocalories, we are actually saying it will provide energy. The more kilocalories in a food, the greater its energy-giving potential. Of the six essential nutrients, three provide energy—carbohydrate, fat, and protein. Alcohol, although not a nutrient, provides energy as well. Carbohydrate and protein provide approximately 4 kcal/g, whereas fat provides 9 kcal/g. Alcohol supplies 7 kcal/g. Most authorities recommend that about 55% to 60% of daily kilocalories be supplied by carbohydrate, 25% to 30% of kilocalories from fat, and 15% to 20% of daily kilocalories from protein. This distribution is called the *caloric distribution* of the diet.

Vitamins, minerals, and water do not provide energy. They have no energy or kilocalorie value.

TABLE 18-2 Food and Nutrition Board, National Academy of Sciences–National Research Council Recommended Dietary Allowances,[a] Revised 1989

Category	Age (Years) or Condition	Weight[b] (kg)	Weight[b] (lb)	Height[b] (cm)	Height[b] (in)	Protein (g)	Fat-Soluble Vitamins: Vitamin A (μg RE)[c]	Vitamin D (μd[d]	Vitamin E (mg α-TE)[e]	Vitamin K (μg)
Infants	0.0-0.5	6	13	60	24	13	375	7.5	3	5
	0.5-1.0	9	20	71	28	14	375	10	4	10
Children	1-3	13	29	90	35	16	400	10	6	15
	4-6	20	44	112	44	24	500	10	7	20
	7-10	28	62	132	52	28	700	10	7	30
Males	11-14	45	99	157	62	45	1000	10	10	45
	15-18	66	145	176	69	59	1000	10	10	65
	19-24	72	160	177	70	58	1000	10	10	70
	25-50	79	174	176	70	63	1000	5	10	80
	51+	77	170	173	68	63	1000	5	10	80
Females	11-14	46	101	157	62	46	800	10	8	45
	15-18	55	120	163	64	44	800	10	8	55
	19-24	58	128	164	65	46	800	10	8	60
	25-50	63	138	163	64	50	800	5	8	65
	51+	65	143	160	63	50	800	5	8	65
	Pregnant					60	800	10	10	65
	Lactating									
	1st 6 months					65	1300	10	12	65
	2nd 6 months					62	1200	10	11	65

[a]The allowances, expressed as average daily intakes over time, are intended to provide for individual variations among most normal persons as they live in the United States under usual environmental stress. Diets should be based on a variety of common foods in order to provide other nutrients for which human requirements have been less well defined. See text for detailed discussion of allowances and of nutrients not tabulated.
[b]Weights and heights of Reference Adults are actual medians for the United States population of the designated age, as reported by National Health and Nutrition Survey II. The use of these figures does not imply that the height-to-weight ratios are ideal.

Build and Repair Tissue. Protein is a nutrient necessary for building and repairing tissue. Examples of other nutrients that perform this function include calcium and phosphorus, necessary nutrients in bone structure; iron, a major constituent of hemoglobin in the red blood cells; and fat, a component found in all cell walls.

Regulate Body Processes. **Metabolism** is the combination of all chemical processes that take place in living organisms. Nutrients play various roles in metabolism and thereby help to regulate certain body processes. For example, carbohydrate must be present in order for fat to be utilized correctly and completely. The B vitamins are necessary for the body to derive energy from foods. Water is an integral part of almost all chemical reactions in the body.

Carbohydrates

Carbohydrates are any of a group of organic compounds, the most important being sugar, starch, cellulose, and gum. The main function of carbohydrates is to provide energy. Carbohydrates should provide the bulk of the kilocalories in the diet—55% to 60%. Carbohydrates are also important in adequate amounts to spare protein from being used as an energy source. Carbohydrates may be classified as either simple or complex. Table 18-3 summarizes the classification of carbohydrates.

Simple Carbohydrates. From a chemical view carbohydrates are made of molecular units called saccharides. The simple carbohydrates include the monosaccharides and disaccharides. Monosaccharides are single carbohydrate units. They include glucose, fructose, and galactose. Glucose is the main monosaccharide found in the body. It circulates in the blood stream and is used by the cells for energy. The brain derives almost all its energy from glucose. Fructose, the sweetest of all the carbohydrates, is found most commonly in fruits and honey. Galactose is not found singularly in nature; rather, it is chemically bonded to glucose in the disaccharide lactose. All other carbohydrates are made of combinations of these monosaccharides or sugar units.

Disaccharides, as indicated by the name, are sugars made from two bonded saccharide units. These include sucrose, lactose, and maltose. Sucrose is a combination of glucose and fructose. It is the common table sugar. Lactose is made of glucose and galactose and is only found in milk products. Maltose is made from two glucose units and is not as common as the other disaccha-

Water-Soluble Vitamins							Minerals						
Vitamin C (mg)	Thiamin (mg)	Riboflavin (mg)	Niacin (mg NE)	Vitamin B_6 (mg)	Folate (μg)	Vitamin B_{12} (μg)	Calcium (mg)	Phosphorus (mg)	Magnesium (mg)	Iron (mg)	Zinc (mg)	Iodine (μg)	Selenium (μg)
30	0.3	0.4	5	0.3	25	0.3	400	300	40	6	5	40	10
35	0.4	0.5	6	0.6	35	0.5	600	500	60	10	5	50	15
40	0.7	0.8	9	1.0	50	0.7	800	800	80	10	10	70	20
45	0.9	1.1	12	1.1	75	1.0	800	800	120	10	10	90	20
45	1.0	1.2	13	1.4	100	1.4	800	800	170	10	10	120	30
50	1.3	1.5	17	1.7	150	2.0	1200	1200	270	12	15	150	40
60	1.5	1.8	20	2.0	200	2.0	1200	1200	400	12	15	150	50
60	1.5	1.7	19	2.0	200	2.0	1200	1200	350	10	15	150	70
60	1.5	1.7	19	2.0	200	2.0	800	800	350	10	15	150	70
60	1.2	1.4	15	2.0	200	2.0	800	800	350	10	15	150	70
50	1.1	1.3	15	1.4	150	2.0	1200	1200	280	15	12	150	45
60	1.1	1.3	15	1.5	180	2.0	1200	1200	300	15	12	150	50
60	1.1	1.3	15	1.6	180	2.0	1200	1200	280	15	12	150	55
60	1.1	1.3	15	1.6	180	2.0	800	800	280	15	12	150	55
60	1.0	1.2	13	1.6	180	2.0	800	800	280	10	12	150	55
70	1.5	1.6	17	2.2	400	2.2	1200	1200	320	30	15	175	65
95	1.6	1.8	20	2.1	280	2.6	1200	1200	355	15	19	200	75
90	1.6	1.7	20	2.1	260	2.6	1200	1200	340	15	16	200	75

[c]Retinol equivalents. 1 retinol equivalent = 1 μg retinol or 6 μg β-carotene.
[d]As cholecalciferol, 10 μg cholecalciferol = 400 IU of vitamin D.
[e]α-Tocopherol equivalents. 1 mg d-α tocopherol = 1 α-TE.
[f]1 NE (niacin equivalent) = 1 mg of niacin or 60 mg of dietary tryptophan.
Recommended Dietary Allowances by the National Academy of Sciences, Washington, DC, 1989, National Academy Press.

TABLE 18-3 Summary of Carbohydrate Classification

Chemical Class	Class Members	Dietary Sources
Simple carbohydrate		
Monosaccharides	Glucose	Dextrose, corn syrup
	Fructose	Fruit, honey
	Galactose	Milk (only found in lactose)
Disaccharides	Sucrose	Table sugar, sugar cane, beet sugar, powdered and brown sugar
	Lactose	Milk
	Maltose	Malted grain products
Complex carbohydrate		
Polysaccharides	Starch	Grains and grain products, i.e., cereals, breads, crackers, pasta, rice, legumes, corn, potatoes, vegetables
	Glycogen	No significant dietary source (storage form of carbohydrate in animal tissue)
	Dietary fiber	Whole grains, legumes, fruits, vegetables, nuts, seeds

rides. It may be found in products containing malted barley or other grains.

Complex Carbohydrates. Complex carbohydrates are termed polysaccharides because they are made from many bonded glucose units. They include starch, glycogen, and dietary fiber. Starch is found in many plant foods such as grains, legumes, and vegetables, particularly starchy vegetables like corn and potatoes. **Glycogen,** a polysaccharide, is not generally consumed in the diet but is the body's storage form of carbohydrate. It is found mainly in the liver, with some storage in the muscles.

Digestion and Metabolism of Carbohydrate. All carbohydrates are broken down in the digestive tract into monosaccharides. They are then absorbed and may be converted to glucose for energy. If energy needs are met, carbohydrate will be stored as glycogen, with any excess carbohydrate being converted to fat and stored as adipose tissue (body fat).

Dietary Fiber. **Dietary fiber** is a generic term for nondigestible chemical substances found in plants. Fiber is a complex carbohydrate made of long chains of bonded glucose units; however, fiber is bonded in such a way that the body cannot digest it. Therefore most of the fiber we consume is eventually excreted in the feces. Fiber has received much attention recently, focusing on its relationship to health and disease. There are a number of fiber types having varying effects on the body. Fiber may be categorized as either water-soluble or water-insoluble.

Insoluble fibers include cellulose and many hemicelluloses. They are found most abundantly in vegetables, wheat, and most whole grains. Insoluble fiber appears to be effective in softening stools, speeding transit of foods through the digestive tract, and reducing pressure in the colon. Thus it may help relieve constipation and reduce the risk of certain gastrointestinal disorders such as diverticulosis or hemorrhoids.

Water-soluble fibers include pectins, gums, mucilages, and some hemicelluloses. This type of fiber is found in fruits, oats, barley, and legumes. Oat bran and beans are particularly good sources of soluble fiber. Soluble fiber binds with the bile acids and cholesterol in the digestive tract, preventing their absorption and thereby helping to lower blood cholesterol. It also helps delay gastric emptying and provides a feeling of fullness, which may be beneficial in the treatment of obesity.

Both types of fiber may enhance weight reduction efforts if fiber-rich foods are included in the diet in place of high-fat and high-kilocalorie foods. Soluble and insoluble fibers seem to delay glucose absorption. This is particularly beneficial for control of blood glucose levels in diabetes and may help reduce the need for insulin. Many medical professionals now recommend a high-fiber diet for patients with diabetes.

Colon cancer incidence is lower in populations consuming a high-fiber diet. Fiber may reduce colon cancer by reducing concentration and bacterial synthesis of carcinogens (cancer-causing substances) in the bowel. It also reduces the amount of time the carcinogens are in contact with the lining of the colon. Both types of fiber appear beneficial in reducing colon cancer risk.

Carbohydrates and Wellness. Carbohydrate is often overlooked as an important nutrient for wellness. When carbohydrates are emphasized in the diet, both fat and sodium intakes tend to decrease. This may be particularly important in reducing the risk of heart disease and certain cancers. In addition, diets high in complex carbohydrates and fiber are useful in achieving top athletic performance, controlling weight, regulating diabetes, and reducing the risk for gastrointestinal disorders.

Carbohydrates should make up 55% to 60% of the calories in the diet. Encourage patients to consume at least five servings of fruits and vegetables and six or more servings of grains, cereals, pasta, or rice each day. Most carbohydrates should come from complex sources and natural sugars. Refined sugar consumption is high in the United States. Table sugar and sweeteners such as honey and corn syrup are high in kilocalories, are virtually void of nutrients, and contribute to dental caries (cavities). Recommendations have been made to reduce sugar consumption to less than 10% of total kilocalories. Sugar and sweets can be used to complement a healthy diet, but should never be used in place of nutritious foods.

For an adequate dietary fiber intake, choose fiber-rich carbohydrate sources. Box 18-2 lists the fiber content of some foods. Use foods as close to their "whole" state as possible; for example, use whole wheat bread rather than white, a fresh apple (with the skin) rather than apple juice, or a baked potato (skin included) instead of dehydrated mashed potato flakes. Generally, the more processing a food has undergone, the less fiber it contains. Because fiber research is relatively new, precise recommendations for levels of intake have not been made; however, tentative recommendations range from 25 to 50 g of dietary fiber a day. If the diet is well-planned, most individuals can receive adequate fiber in the diet without using supplements. There may be hazards to consuming too much fiber, including poor mineral absorption. Moderation should be used with fiber consumption as with any dietary component.

Fats (Lipids)

Lipids are a group of organic substances of a fatty nature that are insoluble in water and that are necessary in the body for good health. Fats and cholesterol are both lipids.

With all the attention recently given to fat and cholesterol and their relationship to disease, many erroneously believe that fat should be totally eliminated from the diet. This is incorrect. Fat performs a number of functions in the body. **Fat** (a substance composed of lipids or fatty acids and occurring in various forms or consistencies ranging from oil to tallow) provides the most concentrated source of energy of all the nutrients (9 kcal/g). Both the fat in foods and that stored as adipose tissue can be used for energy. **Adipose tissue** is the body's storage form of fat and helps to insulate the body from temperature extremes. It serves as a cushion to protect organs and other tissues from being bumped or

Box 18-2

FIBER CONTENT OF SELECTED FOODS

FOOD/SERVING SIZE	FIBER (g)
Beans, Peas, Legumes (½ cup cooked)	
Pinto beans	9.5
Kidney beans	9.2
Pork and beans, Campbell's	8.7
Black-eyed peas	8.2
Navy beans	6.0
Lima beans	5.0
Lentils	3.7
Split peas	2.7
Breads	
Whole wheat (1 slice)	2.0
White (1 slice)	<1.0
Part wheat (1 slice)	1.0
Bran muffin (1)	3.0
Bagel, plain (1)	<1.0
Cereals	
Servings in parentheses are equal to 1 oz. Hot cereal servings apply to prepared cereal.	
Fiber One (½ c)	13.0
Wheat bran (⅓ c)	12.6
All Bran (⅓ c)	10.0
100% Bran (½ c)	10.0
Bran buds (⅓ c)	8.0
Bran Chex (⅔ c)	6.1
Rice bran (⅓ c)	6.1
Fruitful Bran (⅔ c)	5.0
Raisin Bran (¾ c)	5.0
Fruit & Fibre (½ c)	5.0
Wheatena (½ c)	4.0
Oat bran, hot cereal (⅔ c)	4.0
Wheat germ (¼ c)	3.3
Grape Nuts (¼ c)	3.0
Total or Wheaties (1 c)	3.0
Shredded wheat (1)	3.0
Oatmeal, quick cooking (⅔ c)	4.0
Oatmeal, instant (⅔ c)	2.7
Corn flakes (1 c)	1.0
Cream of wheat (⅔ c)	1.0
Oat Granola (⅓ c)	1.0
Rice Krispies (1 c)	<1.0
Special K (1 c)	<1.0
Sugar Smacks (1 c)	<1.0

FOOD/SERVING SIZE	FIBER (g)
Snack Foods	
Wheat 'n Bran Triscuits (3)	2.0
Oat Thins (8)	1.0
Triscuits (3)	<1.0
Saltines (4)	<1.0
Popcorn (3 c)	3.9
Snickers bar (1)	1.4
Fig bars (2)	1.3
Graham crackers (4)	1.0
Potato chips (14)	1.0
Nature Valley Granola Bar	0.8
Almonds (¼ c)	3.8
Peanuts (¼ c)	2.9
Cashews (¼ c)	2.0
Peanut butter (2 tbsp)	2.0
Fruits and Vegetables	
Figs, dried (3)	5.3
Apple, large w/skin (1)	4.7
Pear (1)	4.3
Baked potato w/skin (1 med)	4.2
Orange (1)	3.5
Brussels sprouts (½ c)	3.3
Strawberries (½ c)	3.1
Corn (½ c)	3.1
Peas or winter squash (½ c)	2.9
Carrot, raw (1)	2.3
Broccoli or spinach (½ c)	2.0
Raisins (¼ c)	2.0
Banana (1 med)	1.8
Tomato (1)	1.6
Cauliflower (½ c)	1.4
Peach (1)	1.4
Green pepper, raw (1)	1.2
Cantaloupe (¼)	1.1
Grapefruit (½)	0.7
Lettuce, iceberg (1 c)	0.6
Mushrooms or cucumbers (½ c)	0.5
Orange juice (6 oz)	0.4
Grapes (10)	0.4
Pasta and Rice	
Whole wheat spaghetti (1 c)	5.9
Brown rice (1 c)	3.3
Macaroni or spaghetti (1 c)	2.1
White rice (1 c)	1.0

From Center for Science in the Public Interest (CSPI): New fiber scorecard, *Nutrition Action Newsletter* 17(2):8, 1990.

jarred. Likewise, fat is a component in all cell membranes.

Dietary fat provides **satiety** or a feeling of fullness and satisfaction from food. It adds flavor and aroma to foods. Fat provides the body with the three essential fatty acids—linoleic acid, linolenic acid, and arachidonic acid. It also carries the fat-soluble vitamins, A, D, E, and K. Most dietary fat is found in the form of triglycerides. Triglycerides are composed of glycerol, a three-carbon chain with three fatty acids attached to it, hence the name *triglyceride.* Fatty acids can be classified as either saturated or unsaturated.

Saturated Fatty Acids. A saturated fatty acid is one whose chemical bonds are completely filled or saturated with hydrogen. Saturated fats share similar characteristics. They are generally of animal origin and solid at room temperature. Oils that have undergone hydrogenation, the process of adding hydrogen to a fatty acid, are also saturated. Those fats in which the majority of fatty acids are saturated are listed in Table 18-4. Saturated fats tend to increase blood cholesterol levels, thus increasing the risk of atherosclerosis (the buildup of fatty deposits on the artery walls).

Unsaturated Fatty Acids. An unsaturated fatty acid has one or more places on its chemical chain where hydrogen is missing. These are called points of unsaturation. A fatty acid with only one point of unsaturation is called a monounsaturated fatty acid. Fatty acids with two or more points of unsaturation are termed polyunsaturated.

TABLE 18-4 Summary of Fatty Acid Classification

Fatty Acid Class	Food Sources
Saturated	Coconut, palm, and palm kernel oils
	Beef tallow
	Fat in and on meats
	Skin on poultry
	Egg yolk
	Butter, cream, milkfat
	Hydrogenated oils
Monounsaturated	Olive oil, olives
	Canola oil
	Peanuts and peanut oil
	Most other nuts
	Avocados
Polyunsaturated	Safflower oil
	Sunflower oil
	Cottonseed oil
	Soybean oil
	Corn oil
	Most fish oils

From *USDA Handbook 8-4.*

Unsaturated fats are usually from plant sources and are liquid at room temperature. Sources of monounsaturated fats and polyunsaturated fats are seen in Table 18-3. Unsaturated fats seem to have a blood cholesterol lowering effect at moderate levels of intake and in combination with lowered saturated fat intake.

Cholesterol. Cholesterol is a lipid belonging to a class of chemical substances called *sterols.* Cholesterol performs specific functions in the body; however, it provides no energy (kcals). It is synthesized in the liver and, therefore, does not need to be consumed in the diet. Since cholesterol is produced in the liver, it is found only in foods of animal origin. Plant foods and oils do not contain cholesterol. **Dietary cholesterol** (a fat-soluble sterol found in animal fats and oils) is highest in organ meats and egg yolks. It is also found in smaller amounts in seafood, meats, poultry, and dairy products. Low-fat dairy products and lean meats have less cholesterol than their higher-fat counterparts. By decreasing intake of animal fats, dietary cholesterol intake will similarly be lowered. Dietary cholesterol seems to increase blood cholesterol levels but not as greatly as saturated fats.

Digestion and Metabolism of Fat. For fat to be digested, it must be emulsified, or pulled into suspension with digestive juices. Bile, a secretion of the liver, is necessary to emulsify fat. Bile is stored in the gallbladder and dispensed into the duodenum when fat is present. Once emulsified, fats can be broken down and absorbed. Fat may be used for various functions mentioned previously or may be used for energy. Excess dietary fat will be stored as adipose tissue.

After absorption, fats are carried in the blood stream in packages called lipoproteins. Simply stated, **lipoproteins** (a protein and lipid molecule that facilitates transport of lipids in the blood stream) are lipids wrapped in protein. Types of lipoproteins include chylomicrons, high-density lipoproteins (HDLs), low-density lipoproteins (LDLs), and very low-density lipoproteins (VLDLs). Of particular interest in cardiovascular disease are the LDLs and HDLs. Both lipoproteins carry cholesterol in the blood stream; however, it appears that the cholesterol found in the LDLs increases the risk of atherosclerosis by contributing to plaque buildup on the artery walls. On the other hand, HDL cholesterol seems to have the opposite effect. It appears that HDLs carry cholesterol *from* the blood stream to the liver to be degraded and excreted. LDLs are sometimes referred to as carrying the "bad" cholesterol, whereas HDLs carry the "good" cholesterol.

Dietary goals for the American population stress reducing total **serum** (blood) **cholesterol** (a fat-soluble sterol found circulating in the blood stream; it is continuously synthesized in the body, primarily in the liver) levels, particularly LDL cholesterol. Table 18-5 lists serum cholesterol values used to determine risk of atherosclerosis. LDL cholesterol may be reduced by implementing a fat-controlled diet with emphasis on reduced saturated fat and dietary cholesterol intake. Regular aerobic exercise appears to lower LDL cholesterol and increase HDL cholesterol, both beneficial effects.

Fats, Cholesterol, and Wellness. For all healthy individuals over the age of 2 years, a dietary pattern has been advocated that includes an average of no more than 30% of total kilocalories from fat, less than 10% of kilocalories from saturated fat, and less than 300 mg dietary cholesterol a day. These recommendations are consistent with guidelines given by numerous health organizations ([such as the American Heart Association AHA]) as well as the federal government.

To reduce dietary fat and cholesterol, use low-fat or nonfat dairy products; choose lean meats and use skinless poultry; limit meat, fish, and poultry to no more than 6 ounces (cooked) per day; use low-fat cooking methods such as baking and broiling rather than frying; use no more than four whole eggs per week; use no more than 5 to 8 teaspoons of fats and oils (i.e., margarine, butter, vegetable oils, and shortening) per day; and be sure to include plenty of fruits, vegetables, and grains in the diet.

Medical professionals can better enable a patient to control dietary fat by giving specific recommendations for fat intake rather than simply prescribing a "low-fat diet." For example, a 65-year-old woman who consumes 1400 kcal/day should keep her fat intake below 47 g of fat a day. Table 18-6 lists total fat and saturated fat allowances for men and women based upon their size and caloric intake. Patients should make it a point to read labels and printed nutrition information at restaurants to become familiar with amounts of fat and cholesterol in various products. For more information on reducing fat and cholesterol in the diet, see Chapter 19, Table 19-8.

TABLE 18-5 Screening and Monitoring for Elevated Blood Cholesterol Levels*

	Total Cholesterol†	LDL Cholesterol†
Adults		
Acceptable level	<200	<130
Borderline high level	200-239	130-159
High level	≥240	≥160
Children and adolescents		
Acceptable level	<170	<110
Borderline high level	170-199	110-129
High level	≥200	≥130

*An HDL cholesterol of <35 mg/dl in adults is considered low.
†In mg/dl.

Protein

The human body contains thousands of different proteins. Proteins make up the bulk of the body's lean tissues and organs. In comparison with either carbohydrate or fat, protein has numerous functions in the body. Carbohydrates, fat, and protein all contain carbon, hydrogen, and oxygen, but protein is unique in that it also contains nitrogen. Nitrogen is a necessary element in the formation of any type of protein. Proteins are necessary for tissue growth, repair, and wound healing. Collagen, a vital connective tissue, is made of protein. Some hormones, including thyroxine and insulin are protein. All **enzymes** (proteins produced by living cells that catalyze chemical reactions without being changed in the process) are necessary for digestion (the conversion of food into absorbable substances in the gastrointestinal tract) and metabolism. The plasma proteins aid in fluid balance within the body. Albumin, a plasma protein, attracts water and can pull fluid from one body compartment to another to attain balance. Immunoglobulins (an-

TABLE 18-6 Suggested Daily Fat Allowances

	Height	Calories per Day for Adults With Moderate Activity	Total Fat (g)	Saturated Fat (g)
Women	4′10″-5′2″	1400-2000	47-67	16-22
	5′3″-5′6″	1600-2200	53-73	18-24
	5′7″-5′10″	1800-2500	60-83	20-28
Men	5′1″-5′5″	1600-2000	53-73	18-24
	5′6″-5′10″	1800-2600	60-87	20-29
	5′11″-6′4″	2100-3000	70-100	23-33

*Calories are for maintaining weight in a moderately active 25-year-old. Older persons should subtract 100 calories and 3.5 g of fat for every 10 years of age over 25. Less active individuals should use the numbers at the lower end of the range.

tibodies) are also made of proteins, emphasizing the role protein plays in immune function. If necessary, protein may be used for energy. It supplies 4 kcal/g; however, if the body uses protein as an energy source, it is rendered useless for any other function.

Proteins are made of smaller units called **amino acids** (the building blocks of protein). There are 22 common amino acids, and they can be bonded in a variety of ways to form different proteins. The body uses all 22 amino acids, but only nine of them are considered essential amino acids. In other words, the body does not make them in sufficient quantity to sustain health. The nine essential amino acids must be obtained from the diet. The body can manufacture adequate amounts of the other amino acids from those that are essential.

Complete Proteins. Food proteins can be classified as either complete or incomplete. A complete protein is one that contains all nine essential amino acids in sufficient quantity and ratio for the body's needs. Complete proteins are generally of animal origin and are found in foods such as meat, poultry and fish, milk, cheese, and eggs.

Incomplete Proteins. Incomplete proteins are those that are lacking in one or more of the essential amino acids. Incomplete proteins are of plant origin. This includes the protein in grains, legumes, nuts, and seeds. For the body to use protein for functions other than energy, all nine essential amino acids must be present at the same time. When different incomplete proteins are consumed at the same time, the body can use those incomplete proteins together to obtain a balance of the essential amino acids. Incomplete proteins consumed together are called *complementary* proteins.

Vegetarian Diets. Some people choose not to consume any animal products in their diets and are called **vegans** (strict vegetarians). Others omit animal flesh but consume products such as milk and cheese (lacto-vegetarians) and eggs (lacto-ovo-vegetarians). Whatever the type of vegetarian diet, protein needs can be met. A vegan can receive adequate protein by eating a wide variety of protein-rich plant foods. Different plant foods eaten together will generally supply all nine essential amino acids. Lacto-vegetarians and lacto-ovo-vegetarians can receive adequate proteins from milk and eggs in combination with plant proteins.

Digestion and Metabolism of Protein. Proteins must be broken down to smaller amino acid units or individual amino acids before absorption.

Once absorbed, amino acids can be disassembled and used for energy or they may be reassembled into new proteins to be used for the various needs at hand. Protein metabolism—how the protein is used by the body—is determined by what type of nitrogen balance the body has. **Nitrogen balance** can be defined as the amount of nitrogen that is consumed compared with the amount of nitrogen excreted in a given period of time.

Nitrogen is obtained from eating foods and drinking beverages that contain protein. Nitrogen is excreted in urine, feces, and sweat. Other losses of nitrogen occur with the sloughing off of dead skin and intestinal cells and in hair and fingernails.

If kilocalorie intake is adequate, the body uses the nitrogen in protein to perform the functions listed earlier. If, however, inadequate kilocalories are being consumed, the body is forced to use dietary protein for energy. When protein is used for energy, the nitrogen is wasted and cannot be used to build or maintain tissues. Similarly, during times of increased kilocalorie and protein needs such as during illness or after surgery or trauma, the body may have to use its protein (lean tissue) stores for energy. When lean body tissue is broken down for energy, the nitrogen is excreted. If the body loses more nitrogen than it is consuming, it is in negative nitrogen balance. This may also be defined as **catabolism** (the breaking-down or destructive phase of metabolism).

On the other hand, during periods of growth, such as during infancy, childhood, and adolescence, during pregnancy, or in recovery periods, the nitrogen (protein) consumed is used to build tissues and therefore is retained by the body. In this case nitrogen consumed is greater than nitrogen excreted. This is called positive nitrogen balance or **anabolism** (the build up or constructive phase of metabolism). Zero nitrogen balance or nitrogen equilibrium occurs when nitrogen consumed is equal to nitrogen excreted. A healthy adult who is maintaining his weight might be at zero nitrogen balance.

Protein-Kilocalorie Malnutrition (PCM). When individuals suffer from a lack of kilocalories or protein, the body breaks down its own protein stores for energy. When this occurs for extended periods of time, the person may suffer from PCM (sometimes referred to as protein-energy malnutrition). Two types of PCM exist. **Kwashiokor** is malnutrition caused by severe protein deficiency. It may occur in the presence of adequate kilocalories. It generally occurs in infancy or childhood, and onset is usually at the time of weaning from the breast. Symptoms may include retarded growth, changes in skin and hair pigmentation, diarrhea, loss of appetite, irritability, edema, dermatoses, and fatty liver (causing distended abdomen) (Fig. 18-2). Multiple vitamin and mineral deficiencies may also occur. **Marasmus** is a condition of extreme malnutrition and emaciation from inadequate kilocalories and protein. It is most often seen in failure-to-thrive children and in starvation. A child with marasmus will be very thin with wasted muscles and

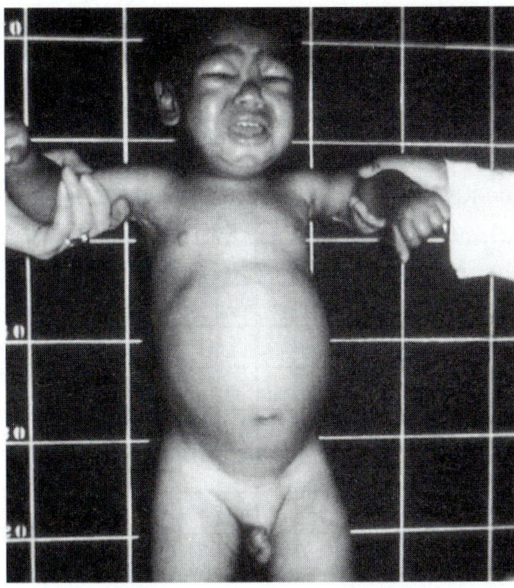

FIG. 18-2 Child with kwashiorkor.

Box 18-3 METHODS OF PRESERVING THE VITAMIN CONTENT OF FOODS

1. Expose food to as little water as possible; steam, microwave, stir-fry, or bake rather than boil.
2. Expose food to as little air as possible; keep prepared vegetables, fruits, and juices covered and airtight; cut and manipulate food as little as possible; keep lids on pans while cooking.
3. Avoid very high temperatures, long cooking times, and holding hot foods for an extended time as in a buffet line.
4. Keep and use the cooking water.
5. Store fruits and vegetables cold.
6. Keep milk in opaque containers.
7. Use foods in the whole form whenever possible.

little, if any, subcutaneous fat. If marasmus occurs during the first years of life, brain development may be impaired.

Protein and Wellness. Only 15% to 20% of total daily calories need come from protein. This is more than adequate to meet the needs of most healthy individuals. Despite popular opinion, athletes and body builders do not need large amounts of protein to build or maintain muscles. Protein and amino acid supplements are expensive and do not provide an edge over proteins found in foods. When protein is consumed in amounts greater than body needs, the amino acids will be chemically changed, converted to fat, and stored as adipose tissue. Therefore, more dietary protein does not necessarily make more muscle.

Research points to the fact that excess dietary protein may be unhealthy. Those consuming high-protein diets tend to excrete more calcium. This may put them at increased risk for osteoporosis. Too much dietary protein may also place an excessive burden on the kidneys, possibly leading to health problems.

Vitamins

Vitamins are organic compounds that are essential in small quantities for normal physiological and metabolic functioning of the body. The American population is very interested in vitamins. Claims have been made that vitamins can help reduce stress, prevent colds, increase sexuality, increase energy, and improve physical performance. Sometimes it is difficult for a consumer to divide fact from fiction. The simple truth is that for most people vitamins are best received from a balanced, varied diet, not from pills.

Nonetheless, vitamins are essential. They are noncaloric and needed in only small amounts. Vitamins are sometimes destroyed by heat, light, and exposure to air. They can also be lost when foods are cooked in water. Thus methods of preparation and storage can affect the final vitamin content of foods. Tips to preserve vitamin content of foods are found in Box 18-3. Vitamins are classified by whether they are soluble in fat or soluble in water.

The Fat-Soluble Vitamins. Vitamins A, D, E, and K are the fat-soluble vitamins. They are usually carried in the fatty portions of food. Fat-soluble vitamins can be stored by the body. It is possible for an excess of these to reach toxic levels in the body, so good dietary sources may be needed only every other day.

Toxicity is a condition that results from exposure to excess amounts of a substance that does not cause adverse effects in small amounts. Toxicity of a vitamin or mineral may occur when too much is consumed or stored by the body. When this occurs, it causes adverse, possibly harmful effects. It is rare for toxicity to occur from eating nutrient-rich foods; it is seen most often in those using excess vitamin and mineral supplements.

Vitamin A. Vitamin A is necessary for vision, tissue strength, and bone and soft tissue growth. A mild deficiency of vitamin A will produce night blindness. A severe deficiency can lead to drying and hardening of the cornea. This condition is called xerophthalmia. If allowed to progress, it may lead to irreversible blindness. Vitamin A is essential for healthy skin and mucous membranes. Deficiencies may lead to dry tissues and decreased resistance to infection. A deficiency of vitamin A may also lead to cessation of bone growth or changes in bone shape.

Foods that supply vitamin A include the dark leafy greens, such as spinach, collards, and kale, or the dark yellow or deep orange vegetables such as carrots, winter squash, and sweet potatoes. Other sources include liver, eggs, milk, and dairy products. Toxic or harmful effects from vitamin A can occur in adults with intakes of 5 to 10 times the RDA. Children may be affected by smaller dosages. Toxicity symptoms may include fatigue, irritability, headache, dry mucous membranes and skin, vomiting, double vision, hair loss, bone pain, and growth retardation. Toxicity generally occurs secondary to supplementation, and therefore, it is best to get vitamin A from food sources.

Vitamin D. The main function of vitamin D in the body is to aid in the mineralization of bones and teeth. Vitamin D stimulates calcium and phosphorus absorption from the intestine and regulates their action on bone tissue. Deficiency of vitamin D leads to weakening and softening of bones. In children this is called rickets (Fig. 18-3). In adults it is termed osteomalacia. Children with rickets often have bowed legs because their bones become malformed under their own weight.

Vitamin D can be obtained in two ways. It is found in small amounts in liver, eggs, and some fish, but the most common dietary sources include fortified milk and milk products. Nonfortified milk is a poor source of vitamin D. The body can also make vitamin D from exposure to sunlight, but the amount produced varies depending on skin pigmentation, age, and length of exposure. Dietary vitamin D sources are particularly important for those who are confined indoors, such as nursing home residents.

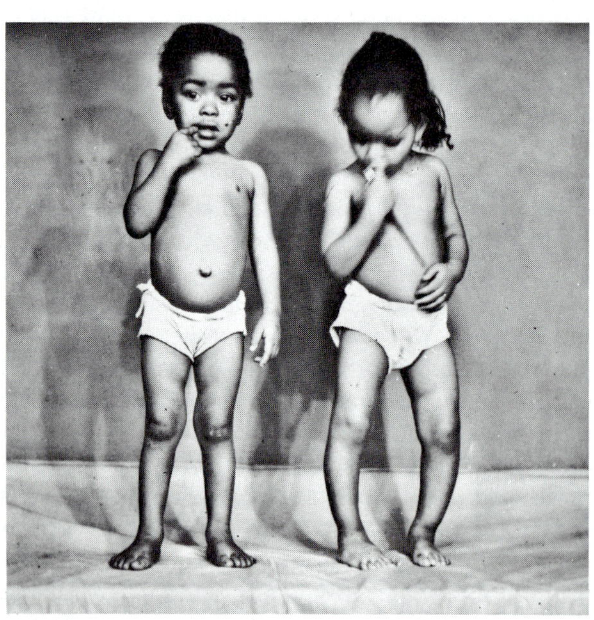

FIG. 18-3 Children with rickets.

Vitamin D may be toxic with intakes of only five times the RDA. Toxicity can lead to calcification of the body's soft tissues, leading to renal and cardiovascular damage. Dietary supplements of vitamin D may be detrimental to children and adults who regularly consume fortified milk.

Vitamin E. Vitamin E functions as an **antioxidant;** that is, it helps protect cell membranes from being oxidized (being altered or destroyed in the presence of oxygen). The vitamin E will be oxidized itself to spare the cell membrane. Vitamin E exerts its protective effect on the lung tissues, body lipids, and both white and red blood cells. Deficiency is rarely seen except in premature infants or individuals with fat malabsorption. Deficiency is often exhibited by excessive destruction of red blood cells (erythrocyte hemolysis).

Vitamin E is found in vegetable oils and products made with them, leafy green vegetables, wheat germ, and nuts. Large amounts of vitamin E may enhance anticoagulant effects of drugs used to prevent clotting. Patients on anticoagulant therapy should not take vitamin E supplements.

Vitamin K. Vitamin K is essential to the blood clotting process. It is necessary for the formation of various blood clotting factors. Deficiency is uncommon but may occur in fat malabsorption, during prolonged antibiotic treatments, and in infants not given vitamin K injections at birth. Deficiency results in hemorrhaging (excessive bleeding).

Vitamin K is synthesized by bacteria in the intestine, and much of the daily needs can be met by bacterial synthesis. Dietarily, vitamin K is found abundantly in green leafy vegetables. It is also present in milk, meat, eggs, cereals, fruits, and other vegetables.

The Water-Soluble Vitamins. The water-soluble vitamins include the B vitamins and vitamin C. Since they are water soluble, these vitamins are not readily stored in the body. Excesses are generally excreted in the urine. Daily intake of these vitamins is necessary, since body reserves are minimal.

Thiamin (Vitamin B_1). Thiamin is necessary for the metabolism of carbohydrates and the consequent release of energy. In the United States deficiency of thiamin is most commonly seen in those with alcoholism, because of both poor dietary intakes and an increased need for thiamin in alcohol metabolism. Beriberi is the name given the thiamin deficiency disease. Its signs and symptoms include mental confusion, peripheral paralysis, anorexia, muscle weakness and wasting, enlarged heart, and edema.

Since thiamin is needed for energy production, needs are based on energy expenditure. Requirements can easily be met by eating a varied diet. Sources include whole, unrefined grains, enriched and fortified grain products, liver, pork, legumes, and nuts.

Riboflavin (Vitamin B_2). Riboflavin is also necessary for energy production as well as functioning in protein metabolism. Deficiency symptoms often involve tissue impairment. Signs of riboflavin deficiency (ariboflavinosis) include cracked lips and mouth corners (cheilosis), dermatitis, and sensitivity to light.

Riboflavin is found in milk and milk products, meats, poultry and fish, enriched or fortified cereal products, and some green vegetables. The vitamin riboflavin is destroyed in ultraviolet light. This is why milk distributors package milk in opaque containers.

Niacin. Sometimes called vitamin B_3, niacin is another vitamin that is necessary for energy production. Deficiency is not common in the United States. It results in **pellagra,** a disease characterized by dermatitis, diarrhea, and dementia (deteriorating mental state).

Niacin is found abundantly in meats and poultry. Smaller amounts are found in milk, fish, and green leafy vegetables. Niacin is added to enriched and fortified cereal products. Niacin can be made in the body from tryptophan, one of the essential amino acids. Therefore, foods with complete proteins can contribute to the niacin needs of the body.

Niacin (nicotinic acid) is sometimes used in pharmacological doses to lower blood lipids. Large doses of niacin may produce vascular dilation, or "flushing," with a feeling of burning or stinging of the hands and face. Other body systems may also be affected. Caution should be used in taking large doses.

Vitamin B_6 (Pyridoxine). Vitamin B_6 functions in amino acid metabolism. It also plays a role in both carbohydrate and fat metabolism. Because of its role in protein metabolism, vitamin B_6 requirements are roughly based on protein intake. Deficiency of vitamin B_6 is rare and, if seen, is usually accompanied by other B complex deficiencies. It may result in anemia, dermatitis, smooth tongue (glossitis), irritability, and convulsions.

Vitamin B_6 is widely distributed in animal and plant foods. It is most highly concentrated in meats, poultry, fish, and eggs. Other sources include brown rice, wheat, oats, soybeans, some nuts, and seeds.

Toxicity of vitamin B_6 may occur if megadoses (very large doses) are taken over a long time. Symptoms include changes in peripheral nerve sensations and muscle coordination.

Folic Acid. Folic acid and folate or folacin all refer to this B vitamin. Folic acid is necessary for the production of deoxyribonucleic acid (DNA), the nucleic acid that carries genetic information and is the basis of heredity. Deficiency of folic acid affects rapidly growing tissues. It is manifested by a type of anemia called megaloblastic anemia (large-cell type). Folic acid is found in liver, green leafy vegetables, legumes, and some fruits.

Folic acid may be particularly important in pregnancy. Recent evidence indicates that adequate folic acid before conception and during the first few weeks of pregnancy may reduce the risk of bearing an infant with neural tube defects such as spina bifida. Folic acid may also improve the overall outcome of the pregnancy. The US Public Health Service recommends that women of childbearing age consume 400 μg of folic acid per day. This is twice the current RDA for nonpregnant women. Women who are planning to become pregnant may benefit from a multivitamin/mineral supplement containing 400 μg of folic acid.

Vitamin B_{12}. Vitamin B_{12} is also called cyanocobalamin. A deficiency of vitamin B_{12} appears similar to and is related to a folic acid deficiency. These two vitamins work together in the manufacture of red blood cells. Deficiency causes macrocytic megaloblastic anemia (large, immature red blood cells). Vitamin B_{12} deficiency over time may also result in paralysis and nerve damage.

Vitamin B_{12} requires a special *intrinsic factor* produced in the lower portion of the stomach for absorption. When the intrinsic factor is missing, for example, after stomach excision, **pernicious anemia** (a progressive macrocytic megaloblastic anemia, affecting mainly older people) develops. Pernicious anemia results because B_{12} is not absorbed. It manifests itself as a B_{12} deficiency. Treatment of pernicious anemia requires B_{12} injections for a lifetime.

Vitamin B_{12} is found in animal tissues and animal products. Dietary deficiency is uncommon and takes many years to manifest itself. Vegans (strict vegetarians) may be at risk of deficiency if they consume no animal foods over an extended time.

Biotin and Panotothenic Acid. Biotin and panotothenic acid are both B vitamins with specific functions in the body. Their importance cannot be discounted; however, both are widely distributed in the food supply and deficiencies are not seen in humans consuming a normal diet.

Vitamin C (Ascorbic Acid). The functions of vitamin C are not completely understood, and much controversy surrounds the issue of vitamin C requirements. Vitamin C functions in the formation of collagen, the strong matrix (framework) that is necessary for wound healing and bone formation. It is also an antioxidant, similar to vitamin E. When ingested in the same meal, vitamin C enhances the absorption of iron from the gastrointestinal (GI) tract. Vitamin C can also affect the immune response. A severe deficiency of vitamin C results in a condition called **scurvy.** Early signs of vitamin C deficiency include bleeding gums, pinpoint hemorrhages, and easy bruising. Further deficiency results in rough, scaly skin, mood changes, muscle atrophy, poor wound healing, increased infections, painful joints, and fractures.

Vitamin C is found almost exclusively in the fruits and vegetables food group. The other food groups are poor sources of vitamin C. Particularly rich sources of vitamin C include citrus fruits and juices, green and red peppers, cantaloupe, strawberries, kiwi fruit, and broc-

TABLE 18-7 Vitamin C Content of Selected Foods*

Food and Portion Size	Vitamin C (mg)
Orange juice, fresh squeezed (1 c)	124
Cantaloupe (½ melon)	112
Orange juice, from concentrate (1 c)	97
Strawberries, whole (1 c)	85
Grapefruit juice, from concentrate (1 c)	83
Kiwi (1 medium)	75
Green pepper (1)	70
Orange (1 medium)	70
Broccoli, cooked (½ c)	60
Brussels sprouts, cooked (½ c)	48
Grapefruit, pink (½ medium)	47
Watermelon (1 inch round)	47
Tomato juice (1 c)	45
Cauliflower, cooked (½ c)	34
Potato, baked (1)	26
Tomato (1)	22
Spinach, cooked (½ c)	20

*The adult RDA for vitamin C = 60 mg/day.
From *USDA Handbooks 4, 5, 6,* and *8.*

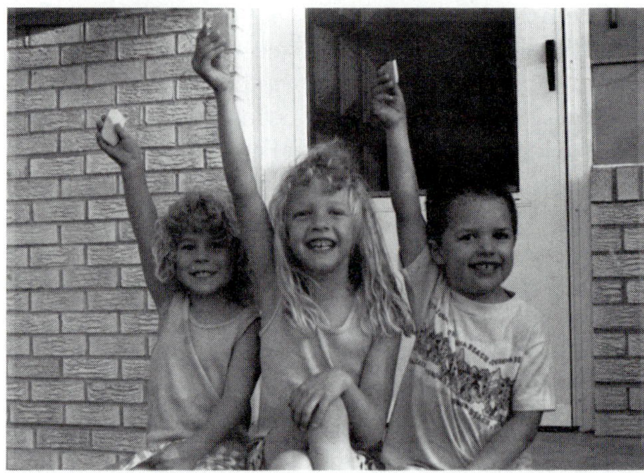

FIG. 18-4 Say cheese! a fun snack and a healthy way to help children meet their requirements.

coli. Table 18-7 lists the vitamin C content of some common foods.

The most recent RDA for vitamin C is 60 mg/day for the adult. Regular cigarette smokers need more vitamin C because of increased metabolic turnover of the vitamin. The RDAs suggest 100 mg/day for smokers. Vitamin C requirements can easily be obtained through diet without supplement usage.

Still, vitamin C supplementation has become a common practice of many. Claims have been made that megadoses of vitamin C may prevent colds and reduce or cure cancer. Although it is true that adequate vitamin C is necessary for proper immune function and may also be beneficial in reducing cancer risk, large doses of the vitamin have not been consistently and conclusively shown to be of greater value than that which can be obtained solely through diet. And whereas moderate doses of vitamin C do not seem to be harmful, larger doses may cause cramps and diarrhea. Routine supplementation with large amounts of vitamin C (1000 mg or more) is not recommended. Table 18-8 summarizes vitamins, their food sources, their functions, and their deficiency and toxicity signs and symptoms.

Minerals

Minerals differ from vitamins in that they are inorganic and they are single elements rather than compounds. Because they are elements, minerals cannot be destroyed as vitamins can. They can, however, be lost in cooking water. Similar to vitamins, minerals are needed in only small amounts in the body. Many minerals are stored in body tissues; thus excess may lead to toxicity. The major minerals are those needed in amounts greater than 100 mg/day. The trace minerals are needed in much smaller amounts.

The Major Minerals. The major minerals include calcium, phosphorus, magnesium, sulfur, sodium, potassium, and chloride.

Calcium. Of the calcium in the body 99% is found in the bones and teeth. Calcium is necessary for both the formation and the maintenance of bones and teeth. It is also essential in nerve conduction, muscle contraction, and blood clotting. Calcium is found in the blood stream as well as in the bones. Generally, blood calcium levels remain constant regardless of dietary calcium intake. If diet is inadequate, calcium may be pulled from the bones to maintain blood calcium levels. Thus a low intake of calcium over a long period may contribute to osteoporosis, an abnormal reduction in bone density leading to bone pain, fractures, loss of stature, and deformities.

The causes of osteoporosis are multiple. Growth and mineralization of bone occur from birth until approximately 25 years of age. Peak bone mass is determined not only by calcium intake, but by genetic influences, sex hormones, physical activity, and dietary intake of vitamin D, fluoride, and other trace minerals. During the fifth decade of life, bone mass begins to decline. In women menopause greatly accelerates the rate of bone loss. This results in weakened bones and a greater risk of fractures. If peak bone mass reached in young adulthood is higher, the risk of bone fractures at a given age will be reduced. Therefore calcium intake in childhood, adolescence, and young adulthood is very important (Fig. 18-4). Calcium is also necessary in adulthood for bone maintenance and to prevent excessive bone loss.

TABLE 18-8 Vitamins

Name	Food Sources	Function	Deficiency Signs and Symptoms	Toxicity Signs and Symptoms
Vitamin A (beta-carotene is a previtamin; it is converted to vitamin A in the body)	Egg yolk, liver, milk Carrots, winter squash, sweet potato, spinach, collards, kale, broccoli, apricots, cantaloupe	Vision, formation and maintenance of bone and epithelial tissue	Night blindness, xerophthalmia, dry skin, increased infections, bone growth abnormalities	Fatigue, headache, vomiting, double vision, dry mucous membranes, bone abnormalities, liver damage
Vitamin D (calciferol)	Fortified milk, fortified margarine, egg yolk, liver, fish oils Sunlight on skin	Formation and maintenance of bones and teeth	Rickets (children): abnormal shape and structure of bones Osteomalacia (adults): weakening and softening of the bones	Calcification of soft tissues
Vitamin E (α tocopherol)	Vegetable oils, dark-green leafy vegetables, wheat germ, nuts	Antioxidant; protection of cell membranes	Erythrocyte hemolysis: breakdown of red blood cells and release of hemoglobin (rare)	None exhibited
Vitamin K	Green leafy vegetables, milk, dairy products, liver, meat, egg yolks, green tea (synthesis by intestinal bacteria)	Formation of blood clotting factors	Hemorrhaging	Excess vitamin K_3 (menadione) administration in newborns may cause hemolytic anemia
Thiamin (vitamin B_1)	Unrefined whole grains, enriched and fortified grains and cereals, liver, pork, legumes, nuts	Carbohydrate metabolism	Beriberi: mental confusion, anorexia, muscle weakness and wasting, enlarged heart, edema, and peripheral paralysis	None exhibited
Riboflavin (vitamin B_2)	Milk, meats, poultry, fish, enriched and fortified grains and cereals	General metabolism	Ariboflavinosis: cheilosis (a disorder of the lips and mouth characterized by scales and fissures), dermatitis, and light sensitivity	None exhibited
Niacin	Meat, poultry, enriched and fortified grains and cereals (high-protein foods that contain tryptophan)	General metabolism	Pellegra: dermatitis, diarrhea, and dementia	Burning, pruritus (itching) of the skin, abnormal liver function
Vitamin B_6 (pyridoxine)	Meat, poultry, fish, eggs, brown rice, wheat, oats, soybeans	Amino acid metabolism, general metabolism	Anemia, convulsions, dermatitis, and glossitis	Peripheral neuropathy, irregular muscle coordination
Folic acid	Liver, green leafy vegetables, legumes, fruit	Nucleic acid synthesis, amino acid metabolism	Megaloblastic (large-cell) anemia	May mask vitamin B_{12} deficiency; interferes with the anti-convulsant drug phenytoin (Dilantin)
Vitamin B_{12} (cyanocobalamin)	Animal products, i.e., meat, fish, poultry, milk, dairy products, eggs	New cell synthesis, maintenance of nerve cells	Pernicious anemia: macrocytic megaloblastic anemia Nerve damage	None exhibited
Biotin	Liver, egg yolk, soy flour cereals, yeast (synthesis by intestinal bacteria)	General metabolism	Anorexia, nausea, vomiting, glossitis, depression, hair loss, and dermatitis (rare)	None exhibited

Continued.

TABLE 18-8 Vitamins—cont'd

Name	Food Sources	Function	Deficiency Signs and Symptoms	Toxicity Signs and Symptoms
Pantothenic acid	Widespread in foods; abundant in animal tissue, whole grains, and legumes	General metabolism	Listlessness and fatigue (rare)	Diarrhea and water retention
Vitamin C (ascorbic acid)	Citrus fruits and juices, strawberries, kiwi fruit, melons, broccoli, peppers, tomatoes, potatoes, fortified beverages	Antioxidant; wound healing, tissue growth and maintenance, proper immune function, absorption of iron	Scurvy: bleeding gums, easy bruising, increased infections, poor wound healing, rough skin, joint pain, muscle atrophy	Abdominal cramps and diarrhea

Box 18-4 CALCIUM CONTENT OF FOODS IN EQUIVALENT AMOUNTS OF MILK

The following examples have the same amount of calcium as 1 cup of milk (300 mg):

- 1 c yogurt
- 8 oz milkshake
- 1 c pudding or custard
- ¼ c nonfat dry milk
- 1¼ c ice milk or frozen yogurt
- 1¾ c ice cream
- 1½ oz cheese
- 1 c macaroni and cheese (home recipe)
- 2 c cottage cheese
- 2½ c cooked soybeans
- 3 oz tofu (soybean curd)
- 1 c cooked greens (kale, collards)
- 2 c broccoli
- 6-7 medium sardines
- 5 oz canned salmon

From *USDA Handbooks 4, 5, 6,* and *8*.

The RDA for calcium for adults is 800 mg/dl. For those 11 to 25 years of age, the RDA is 1200 mg/dl. The best sources of calcium come from the milk group. One cup of milk, 1½ oz of cheese, or 1 cup of yogurt provides about 300 mg of calcium. Three servings of milk would easily meet the RDA for calcium for the adult. Other sources of calcium include green leafy vegetables, such as collards or kale, broccoli, tofu (soybean curd), and fish with bones, such as sardines and salmon. Box 18-4 lists the calcium content of foods in equivalent amounts of milk.

Calcium absorption from the gastrointestinal (GI) tract varies depending on the circumstances surrounding its consumption. It appears that calcium in milk products is absorbed best. Calcium supplements are absorbed better when taken with milk or with a meal. Absorption is increased when body needs are great, such as during childhood, pregnancy, or lactation, and absorption decreases in old age.

Phosphorus. Phosphorus works together with calcium in bone and tooth formation. Phosphorus has many other roles in the body as well. It is part of DNA and ribonucleic acid (RNA), the genetic code material in each cell. Phosphorus is necessary for the release of energy in many chemical reactions, and phosphorus also assists in maintaining the acid-base balance of the patient's body fluids.

Phosphorus is present in nearly all foods. It is particularly abundant in protein-rich foods, such as meat and milk, and in cereal grains. Natural dietary deficiencies are not known.

Magnesium. Many body processes require magnesium. It is necessary for the release of energy, protein synthesis, transmission of genetic code, muscle contraction and relaxation, and activation of more than 300 enzymes. Magnesium deficiency has not been reported in people consuming typical diets. When it does occur, it is usually associated with other disease states such as alcoholism, protein malnutrition, excessive vomiting or diarrhea, renal dysfunction, or long-term intravenous feedings. A severe deficiency may lead to tetany, a severe and prolonged contraction of the muscles.

Magnesium is found in nuts, legumes, and unmilled grains. Green vegetables contain magnesium, which is found in the green pigment chlorophyll.

Sulfur. Sulfur is an essential nutrient, functioning in tissue structure and some metabolic reactions; however, no dietary requirements have been set. Sulfur is found in all proteins, and dietary deficiency of sulfur by itself has never been reported. Deficiency may be seen in severe protein malnutrition.

Box 18-5

SODIUM CONTENT OF FOODS**

1 tsp salt = 2100 mg sodium

800-1000+ mg/SERVING

Baking soda, 1 tsp
Cheeseburger, ¼ lb
Chili, canned, 1 c
Condensed canned soup, prepared, 1 c
Crab, canned, 3 oz
Dill pickle, 1 large
Ham, 3 oz
Soy sauce, 1 tbsp
Tomato juice, 6 oz

500-799 mg/SERVING

Frankfurter, 1
Gravy, from mix, ½ c
Nuts, roasted, salted, 1 c
Parmesan cheese, 1 oz
Sardines, 3 oz
Sauerkraut, ½ c
Tomato sauce, ½ c

300-499 mg/SERVING

Baking powder, 1 tsp
Bologna, 1 oz slice
Bran flakes, 1 c
Corn flakes, 1 oz
Cottage cheese, ½ c
Instant chocolate pudding, ½ c
Processed cheese, 1 oz
Tuna, canned, 3 oz

100-299 mg/SERVING

Bacon, 2 slices
Bread, 1 slice
Canned vegetables (corn, green beans, peas), ½ c
Catsup, 1 tbsp
Corn chips, 1 oz
French fries, 1 small bag
Lobster, 3 ozSaltines, 4
Margarine, 1 tbsp
Milk, 1 c
Milkshake, 1 medium
Natural cheeses, 1 oz
Potato chips, 1 oz
Sweet pickle, 1

LESS THAN 100 mg/SERVING

Beef, round, 3 oz
Carrot, 1 raw*
Celery, 1 stalk*
Chicken breast, 3 oz
Cola, 12 oz*
Diet cola, 12 oz*
Fresh cooked vegetables, ½ c
Fruit juices, 1 c*
Rice, cooked, ½ c*
Trout, 3 oz

From *USDA Handbooks 4, 5, 6, and 8.*
*Indicates less than 50 mg/serving.
**The National Research Council recommends consuming less than 2400 mg sodium/day.

The Electrolytes. Sodium, potassium, and chloride are all major minerals. They are also the principal **electrolytes** (compounds that when dissolved in water or another solvent dissociate into ions and are able to conduct an electrical current) found in the body. Other minerals such as calcium and magnesium may also serve as electrolytes in lesser capacities. A solution that contains electrolytes conducts electricity. Electrolytes function in regulating an individual's fluid and acid-base balance and in conducting electrical impulses such as those necessary for nerve conduction and muscle contraction.

Sodium. Sodium is the principal positively charged ion (cation) in the extracellular fluid. It functions as an electrolyte as previously discussed. Sodium deficiency is uncommon, possibly being seen in chronic diarrhea or renal failure or in prolonged diaphoresis (extreme perspiration).

Of more concern is the possibility that excess sodium may be detrimental to health. Excess sodium intake may be related to hypertension (high blood pressure) in sensitive individuals. Sodium reduction in some people helps to reduce blood pressure. Sodium attracts water; because of this, a high-sodium diet consumed by individuals who suffer with edema (fluid retention) may exacerbate the problem.

Sodium is found naturally in practically all foods. Most processed foods contain additional sodium in the form of salt and other additives. This, combined with the salt that many people add during cooking and at the table, adds up to an abundance of dietary sodium. The AHA recommends that individuals consume less than 3000 mg of sodium per day. The National Research Council recommends intake of less than 2400 mg per day. Although most people are concerned about using too much sodium, it is important to remember that sodium is an essential nutrient and that small amounts are necessary for good health. A minimum daily requirement for sodium is estimated at only 500 mg per day. Almost any diet of natural foods from all of the food groups with no added salt whatsoever would easily provide 500 mg of sodium. Box 18-5 lists the sodium content of some foods.

Potassium. Potassium is the major intracellular cation. It also performs the functions of an electrolyte. Potassium is particularly important in maintaining the

Box 18-6 POTASSIUM CONTENT OF FOODS*

(Serving size equals ½ cup unless otherwise indicated.)

601-800 mg/SERVING

Avocado, ½ fruit
Baked potato, 1 medium
Cantaloupe, ½ melon

401-600 mg/SERVING

Banana, 1 medium
Peaches, dried, 4 halves
Winter squash

301-400 mg/SERVING

Artichoke, 1 medium
Apricots, dried, 6 halves
Kidney beans, cooked
Lima beans, cooked
Milk, 1 cup
Spinach, cooked

201-300 mg/SERVING

Asparagus, cooked
Broccoli, cooked
Brussels sprouts, cooked
Chocolate pudding
Carrot, 1 whole
Meat, poultry, or fish, 3 oz
Orange, 1 medium
Orange juice
Parsnips, cooked
Peach, 1 medium
Pumpkin, mashed
Sweet potato, mashed
Tomato, 1 whole
Tomato juice

From *USDA Handbooks 4, 5, 6,* and *8.*
*The National Research Council suggests a minimum intake of 2000 mg potassium/day for healthy individuals.

heartbeat. Potassium deficiency may occur with use of potassium-wasting diuretics and in cases of chronic vomiting, diarrhea, or laxative use. Although dietary deficiency is uncommon, more and more evidence points to the fact that dietary potassium exerts a beneficial effect on hypertension, and recommendations have been made to increase potassium intake from foods. Potassium supplementation is not recommended except when prescribed by a physician. Toxicity may lead to cardiac arrest. The National Research Council has suggested 2000 mg potassium/day as a *minimum* requirement for adults. Box 18-6 lists potassium content of some foods.

Chloride. Chloride is a negatively charged ion or anion. It functions as an electrolyte and is also a principal component in gastric juice. Dietary deficiency of chloride does not occur; however, prolonged gastric secretion loss through nasogastric drainage may cause a decrease in serum chloride. The most common source of chloride is table salt.

The Trace Minerals. Trace minerals include iron, zinc, iodine, selenium, copper, manganese, fluoride, chromium, and molybdenum. Other trace minerals thought to be essential, but of which less is known, include arsenic, boron, nickel, and silicon.

Iron. Iron is a part of hemoglobin, myoglobin, and a number of enzymes. Hemoglobin is part of the red blood cell and carries oxygen to the cells. Myoglobin is a similar compound in the muscle tissue.

Iron deficiency anemia manifests itself as a microcytic (small cell size), hypochromic (less cell color) anemia. Not all anemia is caused by a marginal intake or excess loss of iron, but iron deficiency anemia is a major health problem around the world. Symptoms include fatigue, weakness, headaches, apathy, and pale skin and mucous membranes. Immune function may also be decreased. It is difficult to measure the effects of anemia, but work capacity and job performance may be greatly diminished. In children iron deficiency has been associated with a short attention span, irritability, and a reduced ability to learn.

Children 6 months to 4 years, adolescents, menstruating women, and pregnant women are at greatest risk for iron deficiency anemia. Dietary requirements for adult women are 50% higher than for men because of the monthly blood loss of menstruation. Iron RDAs are set at 15 mg/day for adolescent girls and premenopausal adult women. Postmenopausal women, adult men, and children have an RDA of 10 mg of iron per day. Male adolescents' RDA for iron is 12 mg/day. Pregnant women have an iron requirement set at twice that for nonpregnant women—30 mg/day.

Iron is found in liver, meat, poultry, fish, legumes, whole grains, enriched grain products, green leafy vegetables, and dried fruits (Table 18-9). Dietary iron is found in two forms—heme and nonheme. Heme iron is well absorbed. About 40% of the iron in animal tissues (meats, poultry, and fish) is heme iron, with the remaining 60% being nonheme iron. Nonheme iron is not well absorbed from the GI tract. The iron in plant products is nonheme. Supplemental iron also seems to be poorly absorbed. Iron absorption from the GI tract may be enhanced or inhibited by certain dietary factors. They are listed in Box 18-7. The use of vitamin C-rich foods and meat, fish, or poultry with meals may increase iron absorption by as much as fourfold.

Iron can be toxic and even fatal. Iron poisoning is seen each year in children who overdose on iron-containing vitamin/mineral supplements. Medical attention should be immediate if a child ingests large amounts of iron-containing supplements.

Zinc. Zinc functions in a number of metabolic pathways in the body and is necessary for the functioning of over 70 enzymes. Signs of zinc deficiency include loss of appetite, decreased taste perception, growth retardation, skin changes, and immune system dysfunction. Severe dietary deficiencies in the Middle East have resulted in dwarfism and retarded sexual maturation. In persons with low blood zinc levels, increased zinc intake seems to improve wound healing and taste acuity.

TABLE 18-9 Iron Content of Selected Foods

Heme Sources		Nonheme Sources*	
Food (Cooked Servings, 3 oz)	Total Iron (mg)	Food	Total Iron (mg)
Beef liver	5.3	Raisin bran (fortified), ½ c	4.5
Sirloin	2.6	Oatmeal, cooked, ½ c	0.8
Ground beef, lean	1.8	Whole wheat bread, 1 slice	1.0
Pork tenderloin	1.3	White bread, 1 slice	0.7
Boneless ham	1.2	Dried apricots, 7 halves	1.2
Pork loin chop	0.8	Dried prunes, 3 medium	0.8
Chicken liver	7.2	Raisins, 2 tbsp	0.4
Chicken leg	1.1	Potato, baked, with skin, 1 medium	2.8
Chicken breast	0.9	Peas, cooked, ½ c	1.3
Turkey leg	2.3	Spinach, raw, ½ c	0.8
Turkey breast	1.0	Broccoli, raw, ½ c	0.4
Tuna:		Kidney beans, boiled, ½ c	2.6
Light meat, canned	2.7	canned, ½ c	1.6
White meat, canned	0.5	Tofu (soybean curd), 2½″ × 2¾″ × 1″	2.3
Halibut	0.9	Egg, whole	1.0
Oysters, 6 medium, raw	5.6	Blackstrap molasses, 1 tbsp	5.1
Shrimp	2.6		

Adapted from National Livestock and Meat Board: *Iron in human nutrition,* Chicago, 1990, Education Department.
*Note: Nonheme sources of iron are poorly absorbed.

The best sources of zinc include meat, liver, eggs, and seafood. Cereals, grains, and legumes also contain zinc, but in a less absorbable form. Massive doses of zinc result in gastrointestinal upset, vomiting, and diarrhea. Even moderately elevated intakes of zinc may adversely affect the immune system and impair the body's use of copper. Zinc supplementation is not recommended without medical supervision.

Iodine. Iodine is part of the thyroid hormones that regulate the basal metabolic rate. Iodine deficiency is manifest by an enlarged thyroid gland, or goiter. If the thyroid gland is unable to function, the metabolic rate is reduced, causing sluggishness, weight gain, skin and hair changes, and intolerance to cold. Iodine deficiency in pregnancy results in severe mental and physical retardation of the newborn infant. This condition is called cretinism. Iodine deficiency is a worldwide problem, especially in underdeveloped countries.

Iodine content varies widely depending on geographical area. Soils in coastal regions contain iodine, and thus the plants grown on these soils will provide iodine. Seafood is also a source. The most reliable source of iodine in the United States is iodized salt, which has almost abolished goiter. Most North Americans receive sufficient amounts of iodine each day.

Selenium. Selenium functions as an antioxidant in conjunction with vitamin E. Deficiency may be manifest by muscular discomfort, weakness, and cardiomyopathy (disease of the myocardium).

Box 18-7 FACTORS AFFECTING IRON ABSORPTION FROM THE GI TRACT

Factors that enhance iron absorption

1. Meat, fish, and poultry (MFP). Animal tissues seem to have a factor, sometimes called the MFP factor, which enhances iron absorption.
2. Vitamin C (ascorbic acid), when eaten in the same meal with iron-containing foods.
3. Physiological need. Generally when needs are greater, such as in pregnancy, more iron is absorbed.

Factors that inhibit iron absorption

1. Bran and some fibers. Phytates in some fibers bind iron in the GI tract so that it is not absorbed.
2. Tea and coffee. The tannins present inhibit absorption of iron.
3. Some medications, such as antacids.
4. Soybeans and other legumes.*

From Monsen ER: Iron nutrition and absorption: dietary factors which impact iron bioavailability, *J Am Diet Assoc* 88:786, 1988.
*Further research is needed for conclusive evidence.

The major contributors of selenium in the diet include beef, pork, chicken and turkey, tuna fish, and bread. Grains and seeds contain selenium in varying amounts depending on soil content. Toxicity of selenium was seen in the United States in individuals who

TABLE 18-10 Minerals

Name	Food Source	Function	Deficiency Signs and Symptoms	Toxicity Signs and Symptoms
Calcium	Milk, cheese, milk products, green leafy vegetables, broccoli, legumes	Formation and maintenance of bones and teeth, blood clotting, nerve conduction, muscle contraction	Osteoporosis (adults): weak, more porous bones Stunted growth in children	Constipation, increased risk in males for urinary stone formation, reduced absorption of iron and zinc
Phosphorus	Milk, meat, poultry, fish, grains, food additives	Essential component of bone, general metabolism, acid-base balance	Bone loss, weakness, loss of appetite (rare, but may occur in patients using aluminum hydroxide antacids)	None exhibited
Magnesium	Nuts, legumes, whole grains, green leafy vegetables	Bone mineralization, muscle contraction and relaxation, general metabolism	Nausea, muscle weakness, confusion, tetany (rare, usually caused by other disease states)	None exhibited
Sulfur	All foods containing protein	Essential constituent of proteins, metabolism	None exhibited except in severe protein deficiency	None exhibited
Sodium	Salt, processed food, small amounts in whole unprocessed foods	Fluid and acid-base balance, nerve conduction, muscle contraction	Cramps, mental confusion, apathy, appetite loss (usually secondary to diarrhea or disease)	Hypertension in susceptible individuals
Potassium	Fruits, vegetables, fresh meat, legumes, milk	Nerve conduction; muscle contraction, including the heart; fluid and acid-base balance	Weakness, anorexia, nausea, listlessness, drowsiness, irrational behavior, cardiac dysrhythmias	Cardiac arrest
Chloride	Salt, processed foods, water supply	Fluid and acid-base balance	Metabolic alkalosis	None exhibited
Iron	Liver, meat, poultry, fish, legumes, whole and enriched grains	Part of hemoglobin and myoglobin; necessary for oxygen transport and use in the body; part of some enzymes; energy metabolism	Microcytic, hypochromic anemia: fatigue, weakness, headache, apathy, pale skin, decreased immune function In children: reduced attention span, decreased ability to learn	Tissue damage, increased infection Accidental poisoning in children: nausea, vomiting, diarrhea, rapid heartbeat, weak pulse, dizziness, shock, and disorientation
Zinc	Meat, liver, eggs, seafood, cereal grains, legumes	Part of many enzymes involved in metabolism	Loss of appetite, growth retardation, skin changes, immune system dysfunction	Vomiting, diarrhea, impaired immune response, and impaired copper status
Iodine	Iodized salt, seafood, plants grown in iodine-rich soil	Part of thyroxin, which helps regulate metabolism, growth, and development	Goiter: enlarged thyroid gland, weight gain, skin and hair changes Cretinism: mental and physical retardation of fetus	Enlarged thyroid gland
Selenium	Meat, poultry, fish, bread, grains, seeds	Antioxidant	Muscular discomfort, weakness, cardiomyopathy	Nail and hair changes, nausea, diarrhea, peripheral neuropathy, and fatigue

TABLE 18-10 Minerals—cont'd

Name	Food Source	Function	Deficiency Signs and Symptoms	Toxicity Signs and Symptoms
Copper	Organ meats, seafood, nuts, seeds, whole grains	Necessary for utilization of iron	Anemia, bone demineralization (rare)	Nausea, vomiting
Fluoride	Water supply, plants grown in fluoride-rich soil	Increases tooth resistance to decay	Increased susceptibility to tooth decay	Fluorosis: mottled tooth enamel, altered bone health, kidney function, and muscle and nerve function
Chromium	Brewer's yeast, whole grains, meats	Maintenance of normal glucose metabolism	Impaired glucose tolerance, diabetes-like symptoms	None exhibited
Manganese	Widely distributed in food; richest in whole grains, cereals, fruits, vegetables	General metabolism	None exhibited	Dietary toxicity not exhibited

consumed an improperly manufactured supplement containing excessive selenium. Symptoms included nausea, diarrhea, nail and hair changes, peripheral neuropathy, and fatigue.

Other trace minerals. Copper is essential for blood formation. Deficiencies are rare and result in anemia and bone changes.

Fluoride plays a role in increasing the strength of teeth and increasing resistance to tooth decay. It may also increase bone strength and help delay osteoporosis. Fluorine is found naturally in many water supplies and is added in small amounts to others. In areas where water is not fluoridated, fluoride supplements for children may be of benefit for dental health.

Chromium is necessary for glucose metabolism and seems to work with insulin in the regulation of blood glucose. Studies are now focusing on its relationship to diabetes mellitus. Deficiencies, although rare, produce a diabetes-like condition.

Manganese is an essential element, but deficiencies are rare. It is found abundantly in plant foods. Toxicities have been seen in miners, who inhale manganese dust on the job. See Table 18-10 for mineral food sources, function, and deficiency and toxicity signs and symptoms.

Nutrient Supplementation

The evidence regarding toxicity of some vitamins and minerals points to the fact that more is not necessarily better. Our food supply can provide adequate amounts of nutrients for health if the diet is well planned. Except in cases where nutritional needs are increased, such as during pregnancy and lactation and in certain disease states or medical/surgical conditions, supplementation is not necessary. For those who like to use a supplement as "insurance" against an imperfect diet, a simple multivitamin and mineral supplement providing about 100% of the US RDA should suffice. Large doses or megadoses of nutrients and the taking of numerous types of supplements should be avoided.

Water

Water is the nutrient most vital to life. Lack of this nutrient will bring detrimental effects faster than any other. Body weight is 55% to 60% water. Water performs many functions. It provides form and structure to body tissues. It acts as a solvent and is necessary for most of the body's chemical processes to occur. Water transports nutrients and other substances throughout the body by way of the blood, body secretions, and tissue fluids. It lubricates and protects moving parts of the body such as joints. It also lubricates food and aids in digestion. Water is necessary to regulate body temperature. If fluid needs are not met, dehydration will result. This can become life-threatening when more than 10% of body weight is lost. Signs of dehydration include poor skin turgor, flushed dry skin, dry mouth, decreased urine output, irritability, and disorientation.

Needs for water vary depending on factors such as activity level, metabolic needs, temperature, water losses, and age, so it is impossible to give a specific requirement. For most adults, 2 to 3 L (8 to 12 cups) of water per day is adequate. Pregnant and lactating women have increased water needs. Infants may be at a greater risk of dehydration because they have a higher percentage of water as body weight and are more susceptible to greater skin losses of water. In the young infant breast milk and formula normally provide adequate fluid, but extra fluids may be needed in warmer weather. The elderly have a decreased sensitivity to thirst and are at greater risk for dehydration. Special attention should be given to this population to make certain fluid needs are met.

LIFE CYCLE NUTRITION

Pregnancy and Lactation

Nutrient needs during periods of intensive growth, such as during pregnancy and in infancy, are greater than at any other time during the life cycle.

Evidence has always pointed to the fact that optimal nutrition during pregnancy reduces the risk of complications, premature deliveries, and low-birth-weight infants. Even before conception nutrition may play a role in the final outcome of a pregnancy. All women of childbearing age should be encouraged to consume a healthy diet and use care in the consumption of alcohol and caffeine. The focus of maternal care should be broadened to include preconceptional as well as prenatal nutrition care. Many women are unaware of their pregnancy during the first weeks after conception. Similarly, most women do not attend prenatal information classes until the later months of their pregnancy. Although any prenatal education is positive, it would be ideal to provide information before conception or within the first few weeks of pregnancy. During these early weeks of pregnancy, adequate folic acid may greatly reduce the risk of neural tube defects, such as spina bifida, in the infant. For this reason, some experts now advocate routine folic acid supplements for all women of childbearing age.

Diet during pregnancy should reflect changes in nutrient needs. During pregnancy a woman's need for protein, calcium, phosphorus, magnesium, and folic acid increases greatly. Other nutrients are also needed in greater amounts. Protein is necessary for tissue growth. Calcium, phosphorus, and magnesium contribute to skeletal development, whereas folic acid, iron, and vitamin B_{12} are necessary for the increase in blood volume.

The RDAs suggest that pregnant women consume an additional 300 kcal/dl. This is only a modest increase, and since kilocalorie needs increase less than nutrient needs, a woman should try to select **nutrient-dense** foods (that is, foods that contain large amounts of nutrients relative to kilocalories). Some nutrient-dense food choices might include skim or low-fat milk and yogurt, cottage cheese, lean meats, poultry, fish, whole grains, and fresh fruits and vegetables.

Pregnant women should use the Food Guide Pyramid as a basis for diet planning (see Figure 18-1, Box 18-1). The diet should include at least 3 servings from the milk group, 2 to 3 servings from the meat group (to equal 5 to 7 oz), 2 to 4 servings from the fruit group, 3 to 5 servings from the vegetable group, and 6 to 11 servings from the grain group. Table 18-11 gives some sample menus for the pregnant woman.

A varied, balanced diet can adequately meet the added nutrient needs brought on by pregnancy, with the exception of iron and possibly folic acid requirements. Supplementation with 30 mg iron/day is recommended. With the recent information on folic acid and birth defects, it would seem prudent to recommend a 400 μg (0.4 mg) supplement of folic acid a day. Other vitamin/mineral supplementation during pregnancy should be assessment-based rather than routine.

Concerns in Pregnancy.

Weight gain. Weight gain in pregnancy is important. Recommended weight gains vary based upon a woman's pre-pregnancy weight. Normal weight women should gain 25 to 35 lb. Underweight women should gain between 28 and 40 lb, while overweight women should gain 15 to 25 lb. Young adolescents and black women are encouraged to strive for gains at the upper end of the recommended range. Short women should strive for gains at the lower end of the range.

Under no condition should weight loss be attempted in pregnancy. Mothers who do not gain adequate weight in pregnancy may give birth to a low-birth-weight (LBW) infant. LBW infants have a birth weight of less than 2500 g (5½ lb). These babies have a greater risk of complications during and after birth. Mortality rates are higher for LBW infants.

Discomforts and complications. Many women experience discomforts during pregnancy. Some of these may be alleviated with dietary alterations. A few suggested nutritional aids to help relieve discomfort are listed in Box 18-8.

Occasionally, pregnancy will bring about medical conditions that may pose dangers for both the mother and the fetus. Pregnancy-induced hypertension (PIH), formerly called toxemia or preeclampsia, is a condition that may occur after about the fifth month of pregnancy. If occurs more frequently in the malnourished. Signs include hypertension, edema, and proteinuria. Proper nutrition is vital throughout pregnancy and may help to avert this condition. Once PIH has begun, adequate nutrition should be a part of therapy. Contrary to old practices, salt should not be restricted in most cases of PIH.

Gestational diabetes is a type of diabetes mellitus that occurs only in pregnancy. It usually develops in the latter part of pregnancy. Women should be screened for diabetes in about the sixth month of pregnancy. If gestational diabetes occurs, diet is a major part of therapy. Chapters 19 and 32 discusses diabetes in more detail.

Anemia is also a common nutritional problem in pregnancy. Both iron deficiency and folacin deficiency anemia may occur. Adequate diet including meats, poultry and fish, green leafy vegetables, and a variety of fruits

TABLE 18-11 Sample Menus for Diet During Pregnancy

Meal	Menu 1	Menu 2	Menu 3
Breakfast	1 c ready-to-eat cereal 1 slice wheat toast 1 tsp margarine 1 cup orange juice 1 c 1% milk	1 cup oatmeal with 2 tbsp raisins and 2 tsp cinnamon and sugar 1 cup 1% milk	2-egg omelet with 1 oz mozzarella ¼ cup green pepper 1 onion bagel with 2 tbsp cream cheese ½ pink grapefruit 1 c 1% milk
Snack	1 apple 2 tbsp peanut butter	1 cup strawberries 1 English muffin with 2 tsp margarine	1 c nonfat yogurt with ½ c granola
Lunch	2 oz turkey on 2 slices wheat bread 1 tsp mayonnaise 1 c spinach salad 6 crackers 1 c 1% milk	2 slices ham and cheese pizza 1 slice French bread 2 c iceberg lettuce with shredded carrots 2 tbsp low-cal ranch dressing Water	2 oz water-pack tuna with 1 c pasta spirals 1 stalk celery, chopped 2 tbsp low-cal Italian dressing 1 tomato 1 pumpernickel roll 1 c 1% milk
Snack	½ cantaloupe with ½ c low-fat cottage cheese	1 c tomato soup 6 crackers	½ cup skim milk pudding 6 vanilla wafers
Dinner	3 oz lean pork chop ½ sweet potato with 1 tsp margarine 1 c steamed broccoli Dinner roll with 1 tsp jelly Water	4 oz roast chicken ½ cup rice pilaf ½ cup asparagus 1 cup 1% milk	2 oz grilled hamburger on a bun ½ c baked beans 1 c steamed summer squash 1 kiwifruit mixed with ½ c mandarin oranges Water
Snack	2 oatmeal cookies 1 c 1% milk	½ c ice-milk ½ c fruit cocktail	3 c popcorn 1 c apricot nectar

Total Number of Servings Provided:			
Bread group	8	9	8
Fruit group	3	3	4
Vegetable group	4	4	4
Milk group	3½	3½	4
Meat group	6 oz	6 oz	7 oz
Fats, oils, and sweets	5	5	4

and other vegetables should be consumed along with a prenatal supplement containing iron and folic acid.

Practices to avoid. Some dietary practices should be avoided during pregnancy, especially alcohol consumption. Alcohol contributes to an increased risk of mental and physical retardation of the fetus. Fetal alcohol syndrome (FAS) is the name given to the cluster of signs and symptoms seen in an infant whose mother consumed excess alcohol during her pregnancy. It includes not only physical and mental retardation, but characteristic facial and body deformities. There has been no determination of a safe level of alcohol consumption during pregnancy, and most nutrition experts seem to favor total abstinence. The American Medical Association goes one step further in recommending that women of childbearing age abstain from drinking alcohol as soon as they plan to become pregnant.

Box 18-8 NUTRITIONAL AIDS FOR DISCOMFORTS IN PREGNANCY

Nausea and vomiting

Eat soda crackers before getting out of bed.
Eat smaller meals more often.
Drink liquids before or after meals, rather than with them.
Avoid high-fat or fried foods in excess.

Constipation

Drink plenty of fluids.
Include fiber-rich foods in each meal.
Include daily exercise or physical activity.

Gastric distress

Eat smaller, more frequent meals.
Avoid high-fat and fried foods.
Do not lie down after eating, and do not eat immediately before going to bed.

Caffeine consumption may affect fetal growth. Several studies indicate that maternal consumption of caffeine in excess of 300 mg/day (approximately 3 servings of coffee, or 300 mg from colas, teas, etc.) increases the risk of LBW infants. For more information on caffeine, see the section on nutrient-drug interactions in this chapter.

Smoking, although not dietary, should be discouraged. Low birth weight occurs more frequently in infants of mothers who smoke. Drugs of any kind should be avoided, except under the advice of a physician. Also, dieting for weight reduction is contraindicated during pregnancy.

Lactation. During lactation a woman would do well to follow a diet similar to that followed during pregnancy. Nutrient needs are similar, and kilocalorie needs are actually higher than during pregnancy. An increase of 500 kcal extra per day is recommended. Fluid needs are increased in lactation and can be obtained through the consumption of water, milk, juices, and other beverages. Coffee, tea, and alcohol, if consumed, should be used in moderation since caffeine and alcohol can enter the breast milk.

During lactation adequate nutrition is vital. Studies show that during lactation a poor kilocalorie and nutrient intake will decrease the quantity of milk produced. Nutritional quality of the milk remains fairly constant except in cases of severe nutrient deficiency. Therefore, it is essential for the lactating mother to be properly nourished to ensure lactation continues and milk supply is adequate. If a lactating mother complains that she is unable to produce "enough" milk for the infant, a nurse would do well to ask about her dietary intake.

Box 18-9 ADVANTAGES OF BREAST-FEEDING

ANTIINFECTIVE PROPERTIES

Immunoglobulins, lymphocytes, and other immune components are present in breast milk and provide protection against infection in the infant. The bifidus factor in breast milk is a substance that encourages growth of normal bacterial flora in the infant GI tract.

NUTRITION

Breast milk is specifically made for the human infant. Its protein, carbohydrate, and fat ratio is thought to be ideal for growth and development. It is well digested and readily absorbed.

GROWTH AND DEVELOPMENT

Breast-feeding promotes better tooth and jaw alignment. It may be less likely to produce obesity in the child, and it may favor optimum bonding between mother and infant.

ALLERGY

Breast-feeding may reduce the incidence of allergies in infants at high risk for allergic conditions.

MATERNAL BENEFITS

Hormones produced in breast-feeding help contract and shrink the uterus. Breast-feeding requires no formula preparation or bottle sterilization and is more economical than formula feeding.

Infancy

The time from birth to 1 year of age is one of rapid growth and development. The average infant's birth weight triples by the first birthday. Obviously, nutrition is important for proper growth and development.

Breast milk or iron-fortified infant formula is generally recommended in the first year of life. Breast-feeding has several advantages for the infant and mother. It should be encouraged whenever possible; however, if a woman prefers to formula feed her infant, she should be supported in that decision. Box 18-9 lists benefits of breast-feeding.

Regular cow's milk (whole, low-fat, or skim) is inappropriate during the first year of life. Unlike adults, infants need a high percentage of kilocalories from fat. Skim or low-fat milk provides inadequate fat, is more difficult to digest, and places undue physiological stress on the kidneys. Infants fed whole cow's milk have low intakes of iron, essential fatty acids, and vitamin E and excess intakes of sodium, potassium, and protein. Iron is the nutrient most greatly affected by the use of regular cow's milk. Recent evidence shows that iron status is impaired even in infants who did not receive whole cow's milk until 6 months of age. During the first year, the only acceptable alternative to breast milk is iron-fortified infant formula. Whole milk is acceptable after the first year, but skim and low-fat milk should not be used until the child is 2 years of age.

Sometime between 4 and 6 months of age, an infant begins to need more iron in the diet. This is a good time to introduce solids into the diet. Solids generally need not be given before 4 months of age. The tendency to develop allergies is greater, and most infants are not developmentally or physiologically ready to handle solid foods.

There is no absolute guideline for the introduction of solid foods to the infant; however, a few principles should be followed. Foods should be introduced singly at weekly intervals. This will allow sufficient time to de-

TABLE 18-12 A Guide for the Introduction of Foods to the Infant

Age	Foods Added to the Diet
4-6 months	Iron-fortified cereals for infants (rice, oats, barley)
5-7 months	Strained fruits, vegetables, and juices (from a cup)
6-8 months	Strained or ground meats, cheese, yogurt, egg yolks, cooked legumes
8-12 months	Finger foods, chopped meats, soft table foods, whole eggs, wheat cereal

- Introduce individual foods one at a time at weekly intervals. Watch for adverse affects to detect allergies. Of the cereals, introduce wheat last.
- Use a cup to introduce juices.
- Use a spoon. Do not put semisolid foods into a bottle or syringe. This may lead to overfeeding or choking and does not encourage proper development of eating skills.
- Do not use honey until after 1 year of age because of the risk of botulism.

tect any food-related allergies. Solid food should always be introduced by spoon feeding rather than in bottles or syringes, and juice should be given in a cup. This allows the infant to develop proper eating skills and may prevent overfeeding. No particular foods should be introduced first or last; however, rice cereal is usually recommended first because it is the least allergenic of any cereal. Fruits need not be given before vegetables. In fact, many mothers prefer to introduce vegetables before fruits so that the infant may enjoy their flavor before becoming accustomed to the naturally sweet taste of fruits. There is no need to introduce all of one food group before going on to another. If the family has a history of food allergies, wheat cereal, wheat products, and egg whites may need to be withheld until 1 year of age. Table 18-12 gives a general guide for the introduction of solid foods. By about age 1, most children can eat many of the same foods as the rest of the family and should be consuming a wide variety of solid foods (Fig. 18-5).

Most commercially prepared baby foods in the United States are nutritious, safe, and of high quality. However, it is important to read labels and use foods without added salt and sugar. Plain, simple foods are often better choices than the mixed dinner type of baby foods. The simple foods can be mixed to make a more nutritious meal having fewer fillers. If baby foods are prepared at home, care should be taken to reduce the risk of food poisoning by having a sanitary preparation area and proper storage conditions. Honey should not be given to infants until after the age of 1 year because it may carry botulism spores and cause food poisoning in the small body of the infant.

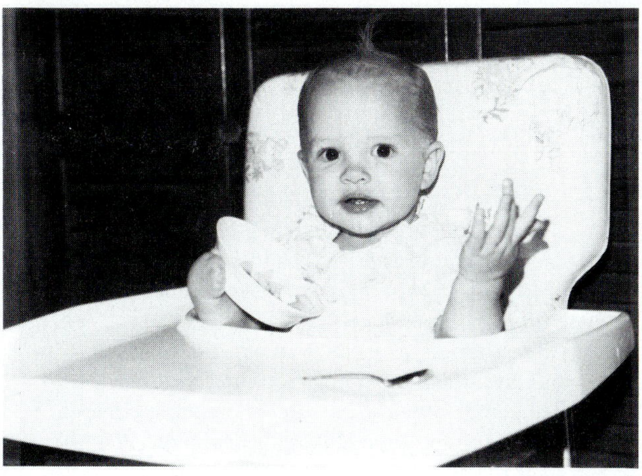

FIG. 18-5 The 1-year old child can eat a variety of solid foods, including many of the same foods the rest of the family eats.

Childhood

At approximately age 1, appetite generally tapers off, and the growth rate slows from that of infancy. Children still need adequate nutrition, although nutrient needs relative to weight are generally less than in infancy. The Food Guide Pyramid (see Fig. 18-1) recommends that children receive three servings of milk, two of meat, four of vegetables, three of fruits, and nine of grain each day. Obviously, the younger child may need smaller serving sizes than adults, and as the child grows, serving sizes will increase.

Childhood is a critical time for instilling good dietary habits. It is also a time for children to test their independence. Food is often a source of contention at mealtime, with the parents resorting to coaxing to get the child to eat or arguing with the child to gain compliance. Often, the more pressure that is placed on the child at mealtime, the more negative the experience will become, and the child may then be more resistant to developing sound eating habits. In general if children are offered nutritious foods in pleasant surroundings and in nonthreatening ways, they will most likely be adequately nourished. Ways to help make mealtimes more pleasant and food habits more appropriate are found in Box 18-10 on p. 356. A good rule to keep in mind is that parents and caregivers should decide which foods to serve and at what time. The child should be able to decide what and how much to eat. The development of good nutritional habits in childhood will provide a sound nutritional base with which to enter the adolescent years.

Adolescence

The adolescent years are years of both physical and emotional growth. In making food choices teenagers are influenced greatly by peer pressure and social acceptance.

Box 18-10 WAYS TO ENCOURAGE SOUND DIETARY HABITS IN CHILDREN

1. Children should be encouraged to eat meals and snacks at regular times and usually at the table. By having set eating times, children will learn that they cannot eat continually all day.
2. Try to make meals relaxed and enjoyable. Children need time to eat correctly, and mealtimes should be a positive experience.
3. Offer a variety of foods from all six food groups, and give children a choice of what they may eat.
4. Remember, physical growth and appetite come in spurts. Do not force children to eat more than they want to eat.
5. Give small servings, or teach children how to serve themselves small servings. Then let them have seconds if still hungry.
6. Offer new foods, but do not force children to eat foods they dislike. If the child will not eat a new food, quietly remove the food and offer it again at another time.
7. Encourage children to help with food selection and preparation.
8. Keep nutritious snacks available, such as fruit, cheese, crackers, raw vegetables, and bread. Most children need to snack.
9. Limit sweets, and do not use sweets and foods as rewards or bribes.
10. Encourage children to be physically active.
11. As adults, set a good example by practicing sound dietary and exercise habits.

Their diets are often filled with kilocalorie-rich and nutrient-poor snack foods. Fast foods make up a large portion of the diet, and although these foods do not lack nutrients, the fast food diet is often void of fruits and vegetables and, sometimes, milk. Common dietary inadequacies in adolescence include iron and calcium (particularly in girls) and vitamins A and C and folic acid. Iron needs increase with the onset of menstruation in girls, and anemia is a common problem. Boys' nutritional intakes are generally better than girls. During adolescence many teenagers experiment with alcohol and drugs, and these substances are not without detrimental effects on nutritional status.

Eating Disorders. Puberty brings with it hormonal changes and the emergence of sexual characteristics. In response to these changes as well as multiple other factors—physical, emotional, and psychological—some teenagers, particularly young women, turn to inappropriate dieting and eating behaviors.

Two eating disorders, anorexia nervosa and bulimia, may occur in adolescents and young adults. Eating disorders are discussed in Chapter 19.

Obesity in Childhood and Adolescence

Obesity in the young is a frequent problem in our society. As previously mentioned, these years are a time of growth, and although obesity is not ideal, restrictive diets can be harmful, may suppress development, and may lead to eating disorders. Attention should be focused on good eating habits rather than restrictions and should emphasize adequate physical activity. Limiting television viewing may help to increase the amount of energy expended by increasing physical activity. Weight reduction diets should be attempted only under the advice of a physician and with the guidance of a dietitian.

Adulthood

During adulthood, nutrient needs change very little in comparison to the adjustments during the years of growth and development. Energy needs, however, decrease with age. At the same time, many adults decrease activity levels. The combined effects of decreased energy needs and reduced physical activity often result in weight gain. As adults advance in years, it is important to use nutrient-dense foods and thereby receive adequate nutrition with fewer kilocalories. Emphasis should also be placed on maintaining an active life-style.

With age comes the increasing likelihood of age-related illness. Because many older Americans suffer from heart disease, arthritis, osteoporosis, diabetes, kidney disease, and other disorders, nutrient needs vary greatly from individual to individual.

Late adulthood also brings with it physical changes such as loss of eyesight, hearing, and teeth. Digestive function diminishes and physical stamina decreases. Psychological changes may take place, such as forgetfulness, depression, or apathy. Also, financial burdens often increase, whereas income is less. Social, psychological, physical, and financial factors can all contribute to malnutrition in the elderly. Malnutrition can then increase the likelihood of some diseases. The result is a vicious cycle. Older Americans must be encouraged to value good nutrition. They may sometimes need assistance with shopping or food preparation. Food assistance programs such as food stamps and Senior Citizen's Congregate Meals can help facilitate better nutrition.

Older Americans are particularly vulnerable to health fraud. They should be wary of products promoting quick and painless cures, "secret" formulas, or "scientific breakthroughs." Suspicious products and treatments should be discussed with a doctor, dietitian, nurse, or other health professional.

Nutrient-Drug Interactions. Medical conditions and disease states often require medication. Many elderly people take a number of prescription medications daily. Added to these medications are over-the-counter drugs, which are purchased and used without a prescription. Many medications can affect a person's nutritional status adversely.

Drugs may alter food intake by either increasing or decreasing appetite or the ability to eat. They may also affect the absorption, metabolism, and excretion of certain nutrients. On the other hand, food intake and vitamin/mineral supplementation may affect the absorption, distribution, metabolism, and action of some medications (Box 18-11). Some common medications used by the elderly and their nutritional implications are discussed in Table 18-13.

Box 18-11 NUTRIENT-DRUG INTERACTIONS

HOW DRUGS AFFECT NUTRITION

I. Drugs may alter food intake by:
*decreasing or increasing appetite
*interfering with taste perceptions and taste sensitivity
*causing mouth irritations, or sensitive gums, or dry mouth
*causing nausea and/or vomiting

II. Drugs may increase or decrease nutrient absorption by:
*causing diarrhea or constipation
*changing the acidity (pH) of the GI tract
*binding with nutrients so they cannot be absorbed
*damaging or altering the GI lining
*altering digestive juices and enzymes

III. Drugs may alter nutrient metabolism by:
*counteracting the effect of the nutrient
*interfering with enzymes necessary in nutrient metabolism
*affecting the function of the liver and other organs

IV. Drugs may increase or decrease nutrient excretion by:
*altering kidney function
*causing diuresis
*displacing nutrients in the body, causing nutrients to be excreted

HOW DIET AFFECTS DRUG UTILIZATION

I. Food and vitamin/mineral supplements in the GI tract may increase or decrease drug absorption by:
*changing the acidity (pH) of the GI tract
*binding with a drug so it is not absorbed
*slowing down the rate of drug absorption

II. Chemicals in food and vitamin/mineral supplements may alter drug metabolism by:
*increasing or decreasing the rate at which a drug is metabolized
*interfering with or potentiating the action of the drug
*interacting with the drug to cause different and adverse reactions

III. Food in the stomach may lessen gastric irritation caused by some drugs.

TABLE 18-13 Common Medications and Their Effect on Nutrition

Drug Type	Possible Dietary Significance
Antacids	Reduced phosphorus, vitamin A, and iron absorption; increased destruction of thiamin.
Antibiotics	Nausea, vomiting and diarrhea leading to reduced absorption from vomiting and in diarrhea increased excretion of multiple nutrients.
Aspirin	In long-term therapy: increased excretion of and decreased serum levels of ascorbic acid (vitamin C); possible GI bleeding leading to loss of iron; vitamin K depletion. *Encourage diet rich in vitamin C.*
Antihypertensives (hydralazine)	Vitamin B_6 depletion. *Vitamin B_6 supplementation encouraged for those with marginal diets.*
Diuretics (furosemide, chlorothiazide, hydrochlorothiazide)	Increased electrolyte excretion leading to potassium, magnesium, and calcium depletion. *Potassium-rich diet encouraged. May require potassium supplements. Avoid licorice—leads to lower potassium levels.*
Diuretics (spironolactone)	Decreased potassium excretion—avoid supplements.
Laxatives	Decreased absorption of calcium, potassium, fat-soluble vitamins especially vitamin D. *Encourage fiber- and fluid-rich diets. Encourage physical activity. This may reduce the need for laxatives.*

TABLE 18-14 Caffeine Content of Selected Beverages and Foods

Item	Average Caffeine/mg
Coffee (5 oz c)	
Brewed, drip	115
Brewed, percolated	80
Instant	60
Decaffeinated	3
Tea (5 oz cup)	
Brewed 5 min	50
Instant	30
Iced tea (12 oz glass)	70
Soft drinks (12 oz glass)	
Coca Cola, regular and diet	45
Dr. Pepper, regular and diet	40
Mountain Dew	54
Pepsi, regular and diet	37
Lemon-lime, orange, root beer	0
Hot cocoa (5 oz c)	4
Chocolate milk (8 oz glass)	5
Milk chocolate (1 oz)	6
Dark chocolate, semisweet (1 oz)	20

Adapted from Lecos C: Caffeine jitters: some safety questions remain, *FDA Consumer,* reprinted January 1993; and American Dietetic Association: *Manual of clinical dietetics,* Chicago, 1988, The Association.

Caffeine. Caffeine is a drug. It is a central nervous system stimulant and a diuretic. It can cause nervousness, irritability, anxiety, insomnia, and heart dysrhythmias and palpitations. It may also affect blood pressure, circulation, and gastric acid secretion. Often older people cannot tolerate caffeine as well as when they were younger. The effects of caffeine vary from individual to individual. One person may consume large amounts of caffeine with no apparent side effects, while another may be very sensitive to it. Older Americans should use moderation in their intake of caffeine. They should be aware of the possible effects of caffeine, which may resemble an anxiety attack in some people. In those who complain of these symptoms, caffeine consumption should be assessed. Reduction of caffeine intake may alleviate these negative effects and possibly avert the use of yet another drug to relieve anxiety. The caffeine content of selected foods and beverages is given in Table 18-14.

REFERENCES AND SUGGESTED READINGS

1. American Academy of Pediatrics, Committee on Nutrition: The use of whole cow's milk in infancy, *Pediatrics* 89(6):1105, 1992.
2. American Dietetic Association: Response to FDA's request for comments on dietary supplements, *J Am Diet Assoc* 91:1220, 1991.
3. Center for Science in the Public Interest: New fiber scorecard, *Nutrition Action Newsletter* 17(2):8, 1990.
4. Council on Scientific Affairs: Dietary fiber and health, *JAMA* 262(4):542, 1989.
5. Donatelle EP: Constipation: pathophysiology and treatment, *Am Fam Physician* 42(5):1335, 1990.
6. Fenster L et al: Caffeine consumption during pregnancy and fetal growth, *Am J Public Health* 81(4):458, 1991.
7. Food and Nutrition Board: *Nutrition during pregnancy,* Washington, DC, 1990, National Academy Press.
8. Glanze WD, editor: *Mosby's medical, nursing, and allied health dictionary,* ed 4, St Louis, 1994, Mosby.
9. Herbert V: Everyone should be tested for iron disorders, *J Am Diet Assoc* 92(12):1502, 1992.
10. Levander OA: Scientific rationale for the 1989 Recommended Dietary Allowance for selenium, *J Am Diet Assoc* 91(12):1572, 1991.
11. McDonald AD, Armstrong BG, Sloan M: Cigarette, alcohol, and coffee consumption and prematurity, *Am J Public Health* 82(1):85, 1992.
12. National Research Council: *Recommended dietary allowances,* ed 10, Washington, DC, 1989, National Academy Press.
13. Oliveria SA et al: Parent-child relationships in nutrient intake: the Framingham Children's Study, *Am J Clin Nutr* 56(3):593, 1992.
14. Position of the American Dietetic Association: health implications of dietary fiber, *J Am Diet Assoc* 88(2):216, 1988; reaffirmed, 1992.
15. Position of the American Dietetic Association: promotion of breast feeding, *J Am Diet Assoc* 86(11):1580, 1986; reaffirmed 1991.
16. Ryan AS, Craig LD, Finn SC: Nutrient intakes and dietary patterns of older Americans: a national study, *J Gerontol* 47(9):M145, 1992.
17. Shannon B, Peacock J, Brown MJ: Body fatness, television viewing and calorie intake of a sample of Pennsylvania sixth grade children, *J Nutr Ed* 23(6):262, 1991.
18. Siegenberg D et al: Ascorbic acid prevents the dose-dependent inhibitory effects of polyphenols and phytates on non-heme-iron absorption, *Am J Clin Nutr* 53(2):537, 1991.
19. Splett PL, Story M: Child nutrition: objectives for the decade, *J Am Diet Assoc* 91(6):665, 1991.
20. Tamura T et al: Maternal serum folate and zinc concentrations and their relationships to pregnancy outcome, *Am J Clin Nutr* 56(2):365, 1992.
21. Thacker SB, Millar JD: The epidemiology of neural tube defects: a review of dietary intake and related factors as etiologic agents, *Am J Epidemiol* 133(5):526, 1991.
22. USDA, Human Nutrition Information Service: The Food Guide Pyramid, *Home & Garden Bulletin No. 252,* 1992.
23. USDA and US Department of Health and Human Services: Dietary guidelines for Americans, ed 3, *Home and Garden Bull. No. 232,* 1990.
24. US Department of Health and Human Services: The National Cholesterol Education Program: report of the expert panel on Blood Cholesterol Levels in Children and Adolescents, *NIH Pub. No. 91-2732,* 1991.
25. US Department of Health and Human Services: The Surgeon General's Report on Nutrition and Health, *DHHS (PHS) Pub No 88-50211,* Washington, DC, 1989, National Academy Press.
26. US Department of Health and Human Services: The National Cholesterol Education Program: report of the Expert Panel on Population Strategies for Blood Cholesterol Reduction, *NIH Pub. No. 90-3046,* 1990.
27. Whitney EN, Hamilton EN, Rolfes SR: Understanding nutrition, ed 5, St Paul, 1990, West Publishing.
28. Williams SR: *Essentials of nutrition and diet therapy,* ed 6, St Louis, 1993, Mosby.

CHAPTER CHALLENGE

KEY POINTS

- Nutrients are necessary for the proper functioning of all life processes in the body.
- Nurses play an important role in promoting good nutrition.
- Food planning guides such as the Food Guide Pyramid, the Dietary Guidelines for Americans, and the Recommended Dietary Allowances (RDAs) have been developed to plan and assess diets for nutritional adequacy.
- The six classes of essential nutrients include carbohydrates, proteins, fats, vitamins, minerals, and water.
- Kilocalories are a measure of energy. Carbohydrates, proteins, and fats provide energy.
- Dietary fiber, found abundantly in whole grains, legumes, and fruits and vegetables, may exert a protective effect against certain diseases such as diverticulosis, constipation, cancer, and heart disease. It may also help in the control of diabetes mellitus and obesity.
- Fat and cholesterol are carried in the blood stream in the form of lipoproteins. Elevated levels of low-density lipoproteins (LDL) combined with lower levels of high-density lipoproteins (HDL) may lead to heart disease. Reduced consumption of saturated fats and cholesterol may help lower LDL levels.
- The essential nutrients perform specific functions in the body. Marginal intakes and deficiencies lead to dysfunction of various body systems.
- Excesses of nutrients may lead to system dysfunction as well. Overnutrition may be related to heart disease, hypertension, cancer, obesity, and dental caries.
- For normal, healthy Americans, well-planned diets can provide adequate nutrition without supplementation.
- Nutrient needs change during pregnancy and lactation to facilitate fetal and maternal growth and milk production. Nutrient-dense foods should provide the bulk of kilocalories. Iron and folic acid supplements are generally recommended.
- Infancy and childhood are years of rapid growth and change. Good nutrition is vital for proper development. During these years dietary habits are being formed.
- Adolescents' nutritional status may be affected by high consumption of fast foods and kilocalorie-rich snacks, the stress of puberty, alcohol and drug use, and peer pressure. The eating disorders anorexia nervosa and bulimia may appear at this age. Emphasis should be placed on promoting good health and individuality.
- Lower activity levels combined with a constant kilocaloric intake in adults often leads to obesity. Nutrient-dense foods and active life-styles should be encouraged.
- Social, physical, psychological, and financial factors can affect nutritional status of the elderly. Diet planning should be individualized, keeping these various factors in mind.
- The elderly often take many medications at one time. Drugs may affect nutritional status, and diet may alter drug utilization. The elderly should be aware of drug-nutrient interactions.

STUDY QUESTIONS

1. Rebecca, a 9-month-old infant, falls above the 90th percentile for her age group in weight measures. Her parents tell you they are thinking of starting her on a low-fat diet using skim milk. Your best response would be:
   1. "That's a good idea. Using skim milk is one of the best ways to decrease fat intake."
   2. "That's probably the best way to prevent obesity. Try to feed her foods with less than 30% of calories from fat."
   3. "Right now you may want to try increasing the amount of fiber in her diet, but wait until she is 12 months old to use skim milk."
   4. "Infants, unlike adults, need more calories from fat. I would suggest you wait until she is 2 years old to use skim and low-fat milk."
2. Mr. Adams has been complaining of constipation. The doctor has asked him to increase fiber in his diet. What dietary practice would best increase fiber?
   1. Drinking fruit juices every day.
   2. Including more lean meats and poultry in the diet.
   3. Including a cooked cereal such as Cream of Wheat each morning.
   4. Including at least two servings of fruit and three servings of vegetables each day.
3. Sharon is a single mother. She is in for her prenatal checkup. When asked if she will breastfeed or bottle-feed her newborn infant, she responds, "Well, I don't know. It probably doesn't make much difference. Aren't formula and breast milk about the same anyway?" The most appropriate response would be:

1. "Both are adequate to meet the baby's nutritional needs, but breast milk offers other advantages such as protection against infection for the baby and a lower cost for you."
2. "No, breast milk is by far the best choice. Formula feeding can increase the risk of allergies and obesity. It's too bad so many women choose to bottle-feed their babies."
3. "Yes, both are nutritionally adequate to meet the baby's needs. It really doesn't matter which method of feeding you choose."
4. "Breast milk has some advantages over formula, but I chose to formula-feed my children and they have all been healthy."

4. Mrs. Sullivan has osteoporosis and wants to include more foods in her diet to prevent its progression, but she dislikes dairy products. Which of the following foods would contribute the most calcium to her diet?
   1. Whole grain breads, cereals, and bran.
   2. Dark-green leafy vegetables and broccoli.
   3. Citrus fruits and fruit juices.
   4. Liver and organ meats.
5. Mrs. Abbot is concerned that her 8-year-old daughter is gaining too much weight. She asks for your recommendation on how to prevent obesity in her daughter. The most appropriate response would be:
   1. "Restrict all sweets, desserts, pastries, and sugary drinks in your daughter's diet. Enroll her in a sports program or dance class."
   2. "Together, you and your daughter could follow a low-calorie diet for weight loss."
   3. "Prepare balanced meals and snacks for your whole family. Limit how much television your family watches."
   4. "Weigh your daughter and record her weight each week so that she becomes more aware of her weight gain."
6. After experiencing chronic fatigue, headaches, and weakness, Susan is diagnosed with iron-deficiency anemia. Which dietary recommendations would best help improve iron status?
   1. Include more legumes such as soybeans, lentils, and split peas in the diet.
   2. Include more dried fruits such as raisins, prunes, and apricots in the diet.
   3. Drink at least 2 cups of milk per day and include other dairy products such as cheese and yogurt.
   4. Consume adequate amounts of meat, fish, and poultry and include good vitamin C sources at each meal.
7. An elderly patient is found to be taking laxatives on a daily basis. In what way could laxatives affect her nutritional status?
   1. By decreasing absorption of vitamins and minerals.
   2. By causing taste bud changes, thus leading to loss of appetite.
   3. By affecting vitamin metabolism in the liver.
   4. By increasing urinary potassium loss.
8. Mr. Simpson has a high incidence of heart disease in his family. He has his blood cholesterol tested. A desirable total blood cholesterol measure would be:
   1. 50-75 mg/dl.
   2. $<$200 mg/dl.
   3. 200-239 mg/dl.
   4. $<$240 mg/dl.
9. Mrs. Lau is recovering from surgery and needs extra protein for wound healing. Which of the following is a source of *complete* protein?
   1. Peanut butter.
   2. Legumes.
   3. Eggs.
   4. Whole wheat.
10. Mr. Anderson has been hospitalized for several days. A nitrogen balance study is conducted and shows that he is in negative nitrogen balance. This means he is:
    1. in an anabolic state and will probably gain weight.
    2. in a catabolic state and will probably lose weight.
    3. not getting enough nitrogen in his diet and should take a vitamin/mineral supplement.
    4. consuming too much protein and the excess nitrogen is being excreted in the urine.

19

DIET THERAPY

Kristen Kartchner Maughan

KEY TERMS

anorexia
anorexia nervosa
anuria
atherosclerosis
basal metabolic rate (BMR)
bulimia
diet therapy
diverticulitis
diverticulosis
dumping syndrome
enteral nutrition
exacerbation
hyperglycemia
hyperlipidemia
hypoglycemia
inflammatory bowel disease
ketoacidosis
mechanical soft diet
myocardial infarction (MI)
obesity
oliguria
parenteral nutrition
peptic ulcer
peripheral parenteral nutrition (PPN)
postprandial
residue
therapeutic diet
total parenteral nutrition (TPN)
tube feeding

LEARNING OBJECTIVES

After reading this chapter, the student should be able to do the following:

- Define the key terms.
- Discuss the nurse's role in diet therapy.
- Identify standard hospital diets and modifications for texture, consistency, and meal frequency.
- List medical or surgical conditions that require a high-kilocalorie diet, and discuss ways to increase kilocalories in the diet.
- Define obesity. List the three necessary components of an effective weight management program.
- Compare the diets in the treatment of insulin-dependent diabetes mellitus (IDDM) and non-insulin-dependent diabetes mellitus (NIDDM).
- Distinguish between anorexia nervosa and bulimia and discuss the dietary treatment of these disorders.
- List conditions that require a fat-modified diet, and compare fat-controlled and low-fat diets.
- Identify high-fat foods and food preparation methods that should be limited in fat-controlled and low-fat diets.
- Discuss medical or surgical conditions requiring modifications in sodium, potassium, and/or fluid.
- Identify food items to avoid or limit on sodium-restricted diets.
- Discuss rationale for protein restriction in renal and liver disease.
- Identify tube feeding routes of administration, and list medical or surgical conditions that may require a tube feeding.
- Define parenteral nutrition, and describe the two methods of administration. List medical or surgical conditions where parenteral nutrition may be indicated.
- Describe the responsibilities of the nurse in monitoring the patient on nutritional support.

RELATED TOPICS OF INTEREST

- Basic nutrition (Chapter 18)
- The surgical patient (Chapter 22)
- Fluids and electrolytes (Chapter 24)

- Care of the patient with an integumentary disorder (Chapter 25)
- Care of the patient with a gastrointestinal or accessory organ disorder (Chapter 27)
- Care of the patient with a cardiovascular disorder (Chapter 28)
- Care of the patient with a blood or lymphatic disorder (Chapter 29)
- Care of the patient with a urinary disorder (Chapter 30)
- Care of the patient with an endocrine disorder (Chapter 32)

Diet therapy is the treatment of disease through diet. It involves modifying diets in such a way as to meet the requirements created by disease or injury. A diet used as a medical treatment is called a **therapeutic diet.** If a patient needs a special diet, the physician should prescribe the diet and write the diet order in the medical record. The therapeutic diet is planned by the dietitian and usually served and monitored by the nurse. Nurses and other health professionals should consult with the physician when conditions may necessitate a change in diet order.

THE NURSE AND DIET THERAPY

Hospital food service must accommodate a wide range of patients from varying backgrounds. Many different therapeutic diets must be planned, and the number and type of meals to be served change daily. It is no wonder hospital food does not always measure up to "home cookin'." Nevertheless, hospital menus are planned to be nutritionally adequate and well balanced. Efforts are made to accommodate each individual patient. Patients sometimes have a negative perception of hospital food. If they are on a restricted diet, they may have even less of a desire to eat.

The nurse can make an impact on the patient's nutritional therapy in a number of ways. First, it is imperative for the nursing and dietary department to have a working communication link. For example, if a patient who has a food allergy is admitted, the nurse should inform the dietary department promptly so as to avoid having that particular food sent to the patient. Or, if a diagnostic test is being performed that requires that the patient omit breakfast, the nurse could alert dietary the night before and ask them to withhold breakfast but send a snack at the time the patient will be back from the test. Also, the nurse works closely with the patient on a daily basis and may notice whether inappropriate foods are served or whether the patient has an inadequate intake or manifests clinical signs of malnutrition. It is essential for the nurse to report these findings to the dietitian and physician so proper nutritional intervention can occur.

Second, meal trays should be served in a positive manner. Nurses should avoid making negative statements about the food. Meal trays should be served promptly while foods are at the correct temperature. Some patients may need assistance opening milk cartons, cutting meats, or sitting up to eat. The nurse must be sensitive to these needs, for many patients will leave the food uneaten rather than ask for help.

Third, the nurse can help reinforce and encourage adherence to therapeutic diets. Many therapeutic diets are difficult to learn and comply with. The patient may not see immediate benefits from following the diet or may not comprehend the effect noncompliance may have on disease progression and future health. A patient may feel deprived of certain preferred foods or beverages. The patient may also have to partake of unfamiliar or disliked food items. For these and other reasons, many patients abandon therapeutic diets. Encouragement and concern from the nurse may help stimulate the patient to continue with the diet and seek further help in diet adherence. A registered dietitian should instruct the patient with a therapeutic diet. Nurses do not give dietary instruction; however, it is important for nurses to be familiar with therapeutic diets not only to reinforce them, but also to be able to answer questions knowledgeably and avoid giving misinformation about the diet. Gerontological considerations are listed in the box.

GERONTOLOGICAL CONSIDERATIONS

- Increased incidence of acute and chronic medical conditions necessitates some form of diet therapy in a large number of older adults. The most common conditions include diabetes mellitus, cardiovascular disease, renal insufficiency, diverticulosis, anemia, osteoporosis, and lactose intolerance.
- Changes in dentition commonly seen with aging, decreased saliva production, and alterations in swallowing are likely to necessitate modification in the consistency of foods. Chopped, ground, pureed, and liquid diets may be less appealing to the older person and should be served in as palatable a manner as possible.
- Diet modification may be resisted by the older person who has long-standing dietary perferences and habits.
- Dietary fiber and adequate fluid intake play an important role in the prevention of constipation in older adults.
- The aroma and taste of food is affected by normal changes of aging. Sweet and salty foods are often preferred by older adults despite dietary restrictions.
- Many medications taken by the older adult have dietary considerations. Medications can interact with food, deplete the body of important nutrients, and alter the taste of food. The nurse should assess the dietary effects of medications.

THERAPEUTIC DIETS

Consistency, Texture, and Frequency Modifications

Often when we think of therapeutic. diets we think of nutrient-modified diets, such as low-fat or low-sodium diets. But modifications in textures, consistencies, and meal frequency may also be therapeutic. Most hospitals have standard diets based on consistency, specifically liquid, soft, and regular diets.

Liquid Diets. The two types of liquid diets are clear liquid and full liquid. The clear liquid diet is a nonirritating diet consisting of liquids that are easily digested and absorbed and leave little residue in the gastrointestinal (GI) tract. **Residue** is food, fiber, and other substances that remain in the colon after digestion is completed. The clear liquid diet may be used before diagnostic tests, particularly tests on the GI tract, or before surgery. It is commonly used postoperatively until the bowel resumes activity and may also be used during times of vomiting or diarrhea. The clear liquid diet is low in kilocalories, protein, and most nutrients. It should be used temporarily, preferably for 3 days or less.

The full liquid diet is used as a transition diet after a clear liquid diet. It may be used until the patient is ready for solid foods. A full liquid diet is more nutritionally complete than a clear liquid one but is still lacking in some nutrients, such as iron, zinc, and fiber. This diet too, should only be used temporarily. Box 19-1 lists foods included in both of the liquid diets.

Soft Diets. Soft diets can be used as an intermediate diet when the patient is progressing from a liquid to a regular diet. Soft diets may also be used on a long-term basis for those with conditions affecting the GI tract. A soft diet is sometimes called a low-fiber diet. It can include foods from all five food groups including meats, fish, poultry, eggs, milk, grains, fruits, and vegetables. Foods excluded are whole grains and cereals; nuts; seeds; bran; fried meats, fish, or poultry; fried eggs; fried breads and pastries; legumes, peas, corn, and gas-producing vegetables such as cabbage; raw fruits (except bananas); and raw vegetables. Foods with strong spices may also be limited.

Box 19-1 FOODS INCLUDED IN LIQUID DIETS

CLEAR LIQUID	FULL LIQUID
Bouillon	All clear liquids
Fat-free broth	Strained cereals
Grape,* apple, cranberry juice	Strained soups
Fruit drinks	Fruit and vegetable juices
Popsicles	Milk, milkshakes
Gelatin	Ice cream, sherbet
Tea,* coffee*	Custard
Ginger ale, lemon-lime soda	Puddings

*Some facilities restrict the use of these items.

Low-residue diet. The low-residue diet is a variation of the soft diet. Its restrictions are similar to the soft or low-fiber diet, but the diet may also exclude milk and milk products because they leave more residue in the colon. If milk is omitted, care should be taken that the patient receives adequate calcium from other sources.

Both soft and low-residue diets are used in the treatment of **diverticulitis,** a condition involving inflammation of diverticula (pouchlike herniations through the colon). Patients with inflammatory bowel disease may also follow soft or low-residue diets. **Inflammatory bowel disease** refers to both ulcerative colitis and Crohn's disease. Both involve inflammation and tissue changes in the intestinal walls. Patients with diverticulitis or inflammatory bowel disease often do not need to follow a low-residue diet except during periods of **exacerbation,** an increase in the seriousness and symptoms of the disease. Other GI conditions for which these diets are prescribed include gastritis, and periods of diarrhea or indigestion. See Chapter 27 for more information on GI disorders.

Mechanical soft diet. The **mechanical soft diet** is specifically for those with chewing or swallowing difficulties. The diet eliminates foods that are difficult to chew or swallow. Other foods may be chopped, pureed, or liquified. This diet must be individualized depending on the extent of the patient's chewing or swallowing difficulties.

Bland Diets. The bland diet of the past was a restrictive diet prescribed for patients with GI disorders. Spices and fiber were avoided, and milk and cream were consumed in excess. As long ago as 1971 the American Dietetic Association published a position paper stating that the rationale for the typical bland diet was not supported by scientific evidence.

The bland diet of today is much more liberal. It does not restrict dietary fiber and allows almost all spices except a select few that stimulate gastric acid secretion. Food choices for a bland diet are shown in Table 19-1 on p. 364. For patients with Crohn's disease (a type of inflammatory bowel disease affecting the small intestine), the bland diet is used with a low-residue diet during periods of exacerbation. The bland diet is also prescribed for patients with reflux esophagitis. Reflux esophagitis is an acute or chronic inflammation of the esophageal wall caused by reflux of gastric contents into the esophagus. The bland diet helps reduce secretion of

TABLE 19-1 Bland Diet

Food Type	Foods Allowed	Foods to Avoid
Beverages	Cereal beverages, caffeine-free carbonated beverages, and fruit-flavored drinks	Coffee, tea, carbonated beverages with caffeine, cocoa, alcohol
Milk and milk products	Use as desired; milk, yogurt, cheese (low-fat or nonfat recommended)	Chocolate milk
Breads and cereals	Use as desired; enriched and whole grain breads, cereals, crackers, pasta, rice	None
Fats and sweets	Use in moderation; butter, margarine, cream, sour cream, salad dressings, cooking oils, desserts, pastries, candies	Spicy salad dressings **only** if not tolerated; desserts using chocolate or cocoa
Fruits and vegetables	Use as desired; fresh, frozen, canned, dried (including juices)	Avoid citrus fruits or gas-forming vegetables such as cabbage, onion, broccoli, brussels sprout, and cauliflower **only** if not tolerated
Meats, fish, poultry, eggs, and legumes	Use in moderation; beef, veal, ham, lamb, poultry, liver, fish, eggs, peanut butter, legumes (as tolerated)	Highly seasoned meats such as bratwurst, sausage, and some lunch meats **only** if not tolerated; fried and high-fat meats and poultry should be avoided if they cause discomfort
Miscellaneous	Soups, spices, condiments	Gravies, bouillon, black pepper, chili powder, mustard seed, and nutmeg **only** if not tolerated

Box 19-2 DIETARY RECOMMENDATIONS FOR PEPTIC ULCER DISEASE

1. Eat regular, balanced meals each day. During the acute stages, provide six to eight small, frequent meals rather than three large meals. Optimal nutrition is important for healing.
2. Avoid known gastric acid stimulants:

Coffee (including decaffeinated)	Cocoa
Tea	Chocolate
Alcohol	Black pepper*
Caffeinated soft drinks	Chili powder*
Aspirin	Mustard seed*
	Nutmeg*

3. Individualize the diet according to patient tolerance, eliminating any specific food or spice that causes discomfort.

*These spices stimulate gastric acid secretion in some, but not all, individuals.

gastric acids that erode the esophageal walls. A low-fat diet and small, frequent meals may also be prescribed. Fat remains in the stomach longer than protein or carbohydrate. Therefore it may cause prolonged reflux. Patients who suffer from hiatal hernia, epigastric distress (heartburn), or gallbladder disease may also benefit from a bland, low-fat diet; however, dietary treatment should be individualized.

A **peptic ulcer** is an erosion of the stomach lining, the duodenum, or any portion of the GI tract exposed to gastric juices. Peptic ulcers may develop secondary to excess gastric acid secretion, or they may occur due to a decreased resistance of the stomach or duodenal lining. Cigarette smoking increases the risk of developing an ulcer, slows the healing process, and increases the likelihood of recurrence of the ulcer. Treatment of peptic ulcers includes a combination of diet, medication, and rest. Rather than being put on a strict bland diet, patients with peptic ulcers are instructed to individualize their diet, omitting foods that tend to bother them. In addition, all patients are to (1) eat smaller meals more often and eat in a relaxed environment, (2) avoid caffeinated beverages, such as coffee, tea, and colas (decaffeinated coffee is also restricted), (3) avoid pepper, chili powder, and cocoa, and (4) avoid alcohol. Adequate protein and kilocalories are necessary for the ulcer to heal. Box 19-2 lists dietary recommendations for peptic ulcer disease.

High-Fiber Diets. The high-fiber diet is a variation of the regular diet and may be used therapeutically. It may be used as a treatment for some GI disorders and may induce a preventive effect against some disease (see Chapter 18). High-fiber diets are used in the treatment of constipation. With adequate fluids, fiber can reduce constipation in the young, as well as the elderly, which may help reduce to eliminate the need for laxatives. A high-fiber diet is recommended for patients with **diverticulosis,** the presence of pouchlike herniations through the muscular walls of the colon. A high-fiber diet may help lessen the severity of symptoms and inflammation (diverticulitis). If diverticulitis occurs, the patient may need to follow a low-residue diet for a short time until symptoms subside and then gradually return to eating a high-fiber diet. Data also suggest that a high-fiber diet is protective against the development of diverticulosis.

High-fiber diets are used with other dietary controls in the treatment of diabetes mellitus. Complex carbohydrates and fiber seem to moderate the rise in **postprandial** (after a meal) blood glucose levels, thus ensuring better blood glucose regulation. Fiber may also help increase tissue sensitivity to insulin and thus help reduce the need for insulin. High-fiber diets may also be used in the treatment of **atherosclerosis,** a disorder characterized by buildup of cholesterol and lipids on the artery walls.

For most persons, doubling the intake of dietary fiber is a reasonable goal to achieve a high-fiber diet. A dietitian can assess a patient's current intake and help plan a diet that will gradually increase fiber intake twofold. The high-fiber diet uses foods with high-fiber content in place of similar foods with little, if any, fiber. For example, whole grain products, rather than refined, are used. Fresh cooked or raw fruits and vegetables, including peel where possible, should be used, rather than canned or processed fruits and vegetables. Nurses should advise patients who are just beginning a high-fiber diet to increase intake gradually so the body can become accustomed to larger amounts of fiber. Box 18-3 lists some high-fiber foods.

Meal Frequency Modifications. Often, especially in GI-related disorders, small, frequent meals will be used rather than three larger meals. Perhaps as many as six to eight small meals or snacks may be consumed daily. The workload placed on the GI tract and cardiovascular system by smaller meals is less than that with a large meal.

Small, frequent meals may be used for GI disorders, such as hiatal hernia and epigastric distress, during periods of nausea or indigestion, for reflux esophagitis or peptic ulcer, and in pancreatitis. They may also be prescribed after **myocardial infarction (MI;** an occlusion of a coronary artery caused by atherosclerosis or an embolus resulting from a necrotic area in the myocardium) and in congestive heart failure.

Kilocalorie Modifications

The body requires a specific amount of energy each day to carry out its tasks. Energy intake includes foods and beverages consumed daily. Energy output includes energy used for (1) **basal metabolic rate (BMR),** the amount of energy used by the body at rest to maintain vital functions; (2) physical activity; and (3) digestion of food. Energy balance may be better understood by imagining a balance scale with energy intake on one side and energy output on the other (Fig. 19-1). When intake equals output, the body is in zero energy balance, or equilibrium. During zero energy balance, weight should remain constant. If energy intake exceeds energy output, positive energy balance occurs. Positive energy balance results in weight gain. On the other hand, if intake is less than output, negative energy balance occurs, leading to weight loss.

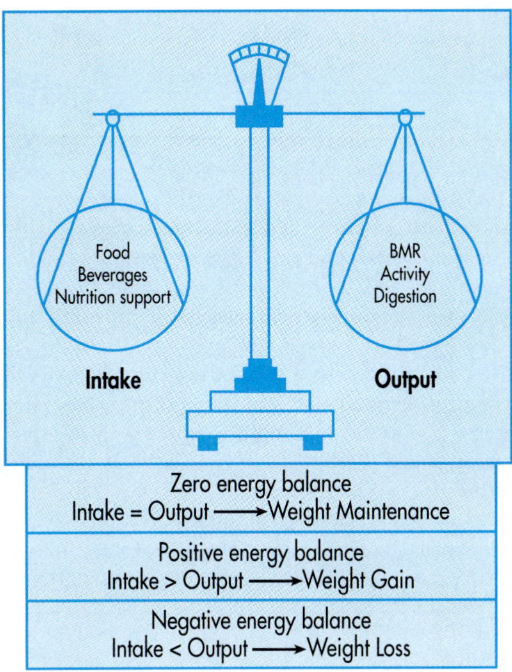

FIG. 19-1 Energy balance.

High-Kilocalorie and High-Protein Diets. During times of physiological stress, such as after surgery, bone fractures, sepsis, burns, cancer, and some other disease states, the body's energy and protein needs are increased. Medical trauma can greatly increase the BMR, so that if energy needs are not met by diet, negative energy balance and negative nitrogen balance will result. The patient will lose protein stores and weight.

Many trauma and cancer patients suffer from **anorexia,** or lack of appetite, and may also have difficulty with the eating process. This further complicates the problem of nutritional inadequacies. Dietary treatment should aim at restoring energy and nitrogen balance in the normal weight patient or creating a positive energy and nitrogen balance in the underweight patient. High-kilocalorie and high-protein diets should provide increased amounts of kilocalories and protein in a small volume. Commercially prepared liquid supplements may be used. They should be chilled and served in an attractive container to encourage intake. Other suggestions to

Box 19-3 SUGGESTIONS TO INCREASE KILOCALORIES AND PROTEIN

- Add extra powdered milk to milkshakes, beverages, soups, puddings, and cooked cereals
- Spread peanut butter on crackers, fruit, or celery
- Add cheese to casseroles, soups, and sauces
- Use extra meat, chicken, or fish in casseroles and soups
- Add sugar to foods where reasonable (this only adds kilocalories)
- Use generous amounts of kilocalorie-dense foods such as butter, margarine, mayonnaise, cream cheese, sour cream, and cream in recipes, as spreads, or as dips
- Add nuts and dried fruits to cereals, breads, or desserts
- Have snacks available at all times
- Encourage the patient to eat high-kilocalorie foods first and eat the lower-kilocalorie foods if still hungry

help increase kilocalories and protein are listed in Box 19-3.

Of course, the diet should still provide a balance of foods from all the food groups. It should be kept in mind that the appearance of the food and how it is served may determine whether or not it is eaten. Those serving foods should do so with a positive attitude and encouragement. The meals should be as attractive as possible. Beverages, especially liquid supplements, should be served in glasses, not cans. Foods should be served at the correct temperature: meals should be served promptly, and snacks and supplements should be refrigerated if necessary.

If a patient is not able to consume adequate kilocalories or refuses to eat, nutritional support in the form of tube feedings or intravenous (IV) feedings may be considered. This is discussed later in the chapter.

Kilocalorie-Controlled and Low-Kilocalorie Diets.

Kilocalorie-controlled and low-kilocalorie diets are used in the treatment of obesity and in the prevention of excess weight gain.

Obesity. **Obesity** is defined strictly as an excess of adipose tissue or body fat. In the simplest terms, it is overfatness. Occurrence of obesity in the United States is estimated at 15% to 50% of adults, 20% to 30% of adolescents, and 6% to 15% of children.

Assessment of obesity. A common method of assessing obesity is with height and weight tables. Using this method, *overweight* may be defined as body weight 10% above a desirable weight, whereas obesity is a body weight 20% or more above desirable standards. These norms are roughly based on life insurance weight tables (Table 19-2) and are simple to use, but are not always accurate. Weighing more than the norm does not necessarily mean obesity. Ideally, obesity should be determined using measures of body composition.

Treatment of obesity. Obesity is resistant to treatment. Some studies have shown that if the "cure" from obesity is defined as a reduction to the ideal weight and maintenance of that weight for 5 years, a person is more likely to recover from many forms of cancer than from obesity. Still, studies show that moderate weight loss de-

TABLE 19-2 Metropolitan Life Insurance Company Height and Weight Tables

	Weight in Pounds		
Height	Small Frame	Medium Frame	Large Frame
Men*			
5′ 2″	128-134	131-141	138-150
5′ 3″	130-136	133-143	140-153
5′ 4″	132-138	135-145	142-156
5′ 5″	134-140	137-148	144-160
5′ 6″	136-142	139-151	146-164
5′ 7″	138-145	142-154	149-168
5′ 8″	140-148	145-157	152-172
5′ 9″	142-151	148-160	155-176
5′ 10″	144-154	151-163	158-180
5′ 11″	146-157	154-166	161-184
6′ 0″	149-160	157-170	164-188
6′ 1″	152-164	160-174	168-192
6′ 2″	155-168	164-178	172-197
6′ 3″	158-172	167-182	176-202
6′ 4″	162-176	171-187	181-207
Women†			
4′ 10″	102-111	109-121	118-131
4′ 11″	103-113	11-123	120-134
5′ 0″	104-115	113-126	122-137
5′ 1″	106-118	115-129	125-140
5′ 2″	108-121	118-132	128-143
5′ 3″	111-124	121-135	131-147
5′ 4″	114-127	124-138	134-151
5′ 5″	117-130	127-141	137-155
5′ 6″	120-133	130-144	140-159
5′ 7″	123-136	133-147	143-163
5′ 8″	126-139	136-150	146-167
5′ 9″	129-142	139-153	149-170
5′ 10″	132-145	142-156	152-173
5′ 11″	135-148	145-159	155-176
6′ 0″	138-151	148-162	158-179

*Weights at ages 25 to 59 based on lowest mortality. Weight in pounds according to frame (in indoor clothing weighing 5 lb, shoes with 1″ heels).

†Weights at ages 25 to 59 based on lowest mortality. Weight in pounds according to frame (in indoor clothing weighing 3 lb, shoes with 1″ heels).

Courtesy Metropolitan Life Insurance Company.

creases health risks and medical problems in the majority of obese patients. Many people have improved the quality of their lives by losing weight and keeping it off. Treatment of obesity has ranged from diets, medications, and psychotherapy to surgery. The initial goal of any treatment is to cause a negative energy balance resulting in weight loss. It takes a deficit of 3500 kilocalories (Kcal) to lose 1 pound of body fat.

Ultimately, the goal of any obesity treatment should be improved health, a higher quality of life, and permanent weight control. Weight goals should be set to encourage health, not to attain an "ideal weight," which may be neither realistic nor healthy for the obese individual. A successful weight-control program should incorporate three major components: (1) a lower-kilocalorie and low-fat diet, (2) exercise and physical activity, and (3) behavior modification and other life-style changes. Treatment should focus on improving the quality of dietary intake. Severe restriction of kilocalories and the classification of certain foods as "good" or "bad" should be discouraged. Rather, patients should be taught to include a wide variety of foods from all the food groups. They can learn to include some of their favorite foods and still enjoy them in moderation. The major focus of diet should be a gradual reduction of dietary fat. Limiting fat intake is associated with reduced risk of disease and may be the most effective method of preventing the regain of body fat after weight loss.

Body composition analysis measures lean tissue and body fat mass. It provides information on the composition or quality of an individual's weight. Table 19-3 lists standards of body composition.

The cause of obesity is at best difficult to explain. Many factors may contribute to the positive energy balance that leads to obesity. Most experts agree that both heredity and life-style contribute to obesity. Regardless of cause, obesity is a major health problem, particularly in well-developed countries. Obese people have a higher incidence of non-insulin-dependent diabetes mellitus (NIDDM), high blood lipid levels, hypertension, coronary heart disease, postsurgical complications, gynecological irregularities, pregnancy-induced hypertension, and gout. Excess weight exacerbates arthritis and some respiratory problems. It can lead to varicose veins and abdominal hernias. Along with physical risks, obesity also has psychological and social consequences such as depression, poor self-esteem, and discrimination.

We all need some body fat for proper health. Essential fat is the fat present in bone marrow, nerve tissue, and body organs. Essential fat is estimated at 3% to 5% in men and 11% to 13% in women. Females have more essential fat because of their childbearing and hormonal functions. Storage fat is an energy reserve that accumulates mainly as adipose tissue under the skin. Some storage fat is normal and healthy. Excess storage fat leads to obesity. It is possible to be overweight, yet not be overfat. Take, for example, a 6 foot, 235 lb football player. According to the height/weight tables, this athlete would be obese; however, his fat percentage of only 11% means that his weight is mostly lean, muscular weight, not fat. On the other hand, an office worker who has a sedentary life-style may have a weight well within the normal of the height/weight tables, yet her body fat of 29% shows that she is overfat and therefore at an increased risk for health problems (see Table 19-3).

TABLE 19-3 Standards of Body Fat for Adults

Classification	% Fat	
	Males	Females
Essential fat	3-5%	11-13
Very low fat	7-10	14-17
Low fat	10-13	17-20
Average fat	13-17	20-27
Above normal fat	17-25	27-31
Very high fat	25 +	31 +

Adapted from Clark N: *Sports nutrition guidebook: fueling your active lifestyle,* 1990.

Methods of measuring body composition include hydrostatic weighing (submerging the body in a tank of water and measuring displacement), fatfold thickness measures (measuring a pinch of skin using skinfold calipers), and electrical impedance tests (a small electrical current is transmitted through the body and its resistance measured). These methods measure percentage of body fat and are better suited for determining obesity; however, they are not always available nor are they as simple as using a weight scale.

The body mass index (BMI) is another method of assessing obesity and health risk. The BMI is derived by taking the patient's weight in kilograms (kg) and dividing by the patient's height in meters squared (m^2): BMI $= kg/m^2$. Obesity is generally defined as a BMI of 28 to 30 or higher. Because of the ease of measuring height and weight, the BMI is the most widely used measure of obesity. The BMI correlates highly with body fat percentage and is more accurate than height and weight tables. Low-fat diets are discussed later in this chapter.

Many weight-control diets are based on the exchange lists for meal planning, discussed in the section of this chapter on diabetes mellitus (see Box 19-6 and Table 19-5). The program should help prepare patients to control weight throughout life and not just on a temporary basis. Diet should be no less than 1200 kcal/day, and weight loss should occur at an average rate of no more than 1 to 2 lb/week. Diets that require the purchase of specially prepared foods, supplements, or "magic" diet aids should be avoided. Persons trying to lose weight must learn to take charge of their own life and not rely on expensive products for weight control. Individuals consuming less than 1500 kcal/day may need to take a multivitamin/mineral supplement providing approximately 100% of the U.S. Recommended Dietary Allowance (RDA).

Exercise is an integral part of any weight-control program. Physical activity improves health, helps prevent the loss of lean body tissues during weight reduction, elevates basal metabolic rate, and promotes long-term weight maintenance. Aerobic (oxygen-using) exercise appears to be the best suited for weight control and loss of body fat. Aerobic exercise elevates the heart rate, uses large muscle groups (legs, buttocks, arms), and is sustained continuously for 20 to 30 minutes. Examples of aerobic exercise include brisk walking, jogging, cycling, cross-country skiing, rowing, swimming, and aerobic dance or stepping exercises. Aerobic exercise should be included at least 3 to 5 days a week for 30 minutes or more each session. Many obese individuals need to build up to this level slowly, beginning with as little as 5 minutes a day. Strength training, flexibility, and muscle toning exercises do not necessarily aid in weight loss but can help with maintenance of lean tissue and improved physical appearance. Weight-control participants must be committed to a regular program of exercise that should become a permanent part of their lives. Weight-control programs that claim weight may be lost permanently with no exercise should be avoided.

Behavior modification involves analyzing behaviors that lead to poor dietary control and health choices and then taking steps to change these behaviors. Patients often keep food records or diaries, listing what they have eaten, how much, when, and how they were feeling at the time. Food records can help the participant become more aware of eating behaviors. Psychological, social, and emotional factors may create powerful barriers to change. These factors must be identified and dealt with for weight loss to be successful in some individuals. A program that focuses only on weight loss and diet may overlook these psychological factors.

Very-Low-Calorie Diets (VLCD). VLCD programs, sometimes called liquid fasts, are being used increasingly in many hospital outpatient clinics and doctors' offices. These diets consist of a low-kilocalorie, nutritionally balanced, liquid diet providing 300 to 500 kcal/day. Throughout the liquid fast, patients are monitored by their physician and other health professionals. They should receive dietary and behavioral counseling and should be involved in an exercise program. The patient continues on the liquid fast for a given period, eating no other foods, and then begins a gradual refeeding program and is instructed on a diet for weight maintenance. In 1990 the American Dietetic Association issued the following statement on VLCDs:

> It is the position of the American Dietetic Association that while very-low-calorie diets promote rapid weight loss and may be beneficial for certain individuals, such diets may have health risks and should be undertaken only with the supervision of a multidisciplinary health team with monitoring by a physician and nutrition counseling by a registered dietitian.

Long-term results of VLCDs prove disappointing, showing a higher percentage of dieters regaining over half of the weight lost on the program. With VLCDs, as with any weight reduction regimen, the principles of weight management still apply. Unless exercise continues, food intake is controlled, and dietary habits are changed, weight loss will be only temporary.

It is estimated that almost half of American women and a quarter of American men are dieting to lose weight at any given time. In one survey, approximately 44% of teenagers in grades 9 to 12 reported that they were trying to lose weight. Another study showed that 63% of high school girls reported they were dieting. The majority of these girls were dieting in spite of the fact that they were at or below normal weight. It appears that the number of people dieting in this country exceeds the number of people who are obese. Therefore some are dieting unnecessarily. There are possible risks associated with unnecessary dieting, repeated dieting, and weight cycling (repeated weight loss followed by weight gain). These risks might include psychological consequences, slowing of the basal metabolic rate, and an increased risk for disease. Further research is needed to clarify these risks. Health professionals must realize that the ultimate goal of weight loss is better health. Unnecessary dieting should be discouraged.

Eating Disorders. Anorexia nervosa and bulimia are eating disorders that are complex psychiatric disorders thought to be caused by a number of factors, including individual mental and emotional processes, family relationships, cultural values, and genetic predisposition. These disorders manifest themselves in physical symptoms. Compulsive eating and obesity, when connected to underlying psychological and emotional issues, may also be considered eating disorders.

Anorexia nervosa. **Anorexia nervosa** is an eating disorder characterized by self-imposed starvation. Certain features are common in individuals with this disorder. They are generally women in their midteens, although young adult women and men sometimes develop the disorder. Often, they are high achievers from educated, middle-class families. The young person with anorexia nervosa is frequently a perfectionist and uses food and exercise as a means of controlling the body. These people become obsessed with weight loss and soon develop a distorted body image, seeing themselves as "fat" even when their weight is much less than the average for their height and age (Fig. 19-2). They become preoc-

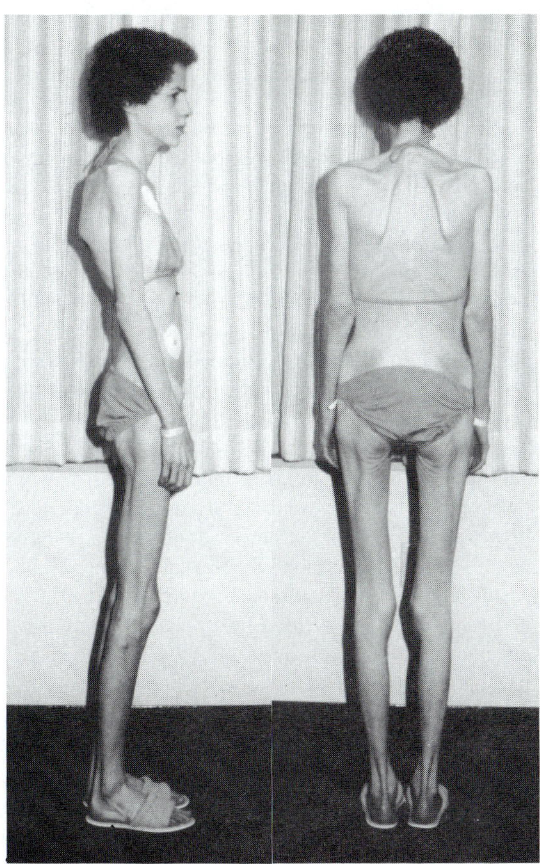

FIG. 19-2 Patient with anorexia nervosa.

cupied with food and exercise. Rigid and ritualistic eating behaviors develop, such as cutting food into very small pieces, hiding food so that it appears it has been eaten, or measuring foods meticulously before consuming unusually small amounts. The brain's electrical activity is affected, leading to altered thinking patterns, disturbed sleep, and bad dreams. Personality changes, depression, and apathy may occur. As weight loss continues, other physical symptoms occur such as cold intolerance, heart irregularities, and hypotension. GI function is affected, causing slowed peristalsis and feelings of distention. The lining of the digestive tract deteriorates so that on eating the person may experience malabsorption and diarrhea. This further compounds the negative perception of food. Amenorrhea occurs in women, whereas men experience loss of sexual interest. Loss of scalp hair may occur, and finally, a fine, downy hair (lanugo) may grow on the body and face. Death may occur in as many as 20% of those with anorexia nervosa.

Treatment requires a multidisciplinary approach involving nutritional therapy and counseling along with psychological and family counseling. Nutritional goals include increasing and improving dietary intake to reverse nutrient deficiencies, achieving a healthy weight for height, and reestablishing "normal" eating patterns. Box 19-4 lists some nutritional guidelines for treatment in anorexia nervosa.

Box 19-4

NUTRITIONAL GUIDELINES FOR INTERVENTION IN ANOREXIA NERVOSA

- Increase kilocalories slowly.
- Provide balanced meals, including adequate fiber to ease elimination.
- Use small, frequent meals to reduce sensations of fullness and distention.
- Use finger foods (snacks) and cold or room temperature foods to reduce feelings of satiety.
- Give multivitamin and mineral supplements at RDA levels.
- Add liquid supplements when desired intake cannot be achieved with solid foods.
- Limit caffeine intake.
- Monitor food intake and in behavioral programs, link rewards to kilocalorie intake, not to weight gain.
- Provide ongoing nutritional counseling.
- Use intravenous nutrition support or tube feedings only in severe states of malnutrition or ill health.

Modified from Rock CL, Yager J: Nutrition and eating disorders: a primer for clinicians, *Int J Eating Disorders* 6:276, 1987.

Bulimia. **Bulimia** is an eating disorder characterized by periods of binge eating followed by purging. A binge is the compulsive eating of what an individual considers to be too much. This may range from one unplanned cookie to a 20,000-kcal binge. Foods consumed during a binge are usually easily ingested, soft, high-kilocalorie foods such as ice cream, chocolate, soft candies, cakes, breads, and pastries. After a binge, the person with bulimia purges using one or more of the following methods: self-induced vomiting, laxative abuse or enemas, diuretic use, fasting, and/or excessive exercise.

Bulimia occurs more frequently than anorexia nervosa and is seen most often in young women. It is thought to be prevalent among college students. Those with bulimia are often of normal weight or even overweight. Most are aware that their eating patterns are abnormal. They often experience fear of not being able to stop eating and experience depression, guilt, and remorse after a binge. Clinical symptoms of bulimia may include tooth erosion, callused knuckles, a puffy, splotched face, broken blood vessels in the eyes or face, stomach lacerations, and esophageal and sinus infections from excessive vomiting. Electrolyte imbalances may occur, leading to muscle weakness and cramps, abnormal heart rhythms, and injury to the kidneys. Repeated infections of the bladder and kidney may lead to renal failure.

Treatment for bulimia, like that for anorexia nervosa, must be multidisciplinary. Psychological counseling and therapy are necessary. Nutritional goals include improvement of dietary intake to correct nutritional deficiencies and electrolyte imbalances and cessation of binge-purge behavior with reestablishment of normal eating. If the patient is overweight, weight loss should be delayed until after eating is normalized. Nutrition intervention differs somewhat from that for anorexia nervosa, and guidelines are listed in Box 19-5.

Eating disorders are relatively new in medical science, and their prevalence seems to be increasing. Bulimia was first medically defined as an eating disorder in 1980. Both disorders occur almost exclusively in developed nations, and it appears obvious that our society with its focus on thinness has helped bring about their occurrence. In young adolescence, women are already concerned that they are "too fat"; many are on diets. They see magazine pictures, models, and television images of beautiful and extremely thin women. For some the quest for unrealistic thinness, beauty, and happiness leads to eating disorders.

Recognizing and treating eating disorders early may lessen their effects. Table 19-4 lists some danger signs of these disorders. Above all, the greatest focus should be placed on prevention. As a society our focus should be on good health rather than on thinness. Each individual must learn to respect and value his own personal uniqueness.

Box 19-5 GUIDELINES FOR DIETARY TREATMENT OF BULIMIA

- Use structured, nonflexible eating plans during the initial stages of treatment. As treatment continues, add more flexibility on an individual basis.
- Follow a well-balanced diet. For variety and to help prolong the meal, include adequate amounts of vegetables, fruits, salads, and whole-grain and high-fiber breads and cereals. Include some fat in each meal to promote satiety and to help slow gastric emptying and enhance the feeling of fullness.
- To increase satiety, include warm foods rather than cold or room-temperature foods.
- Avoid labeling foods as "good" or "bad." Allow consumption of favorite foods in moderation as part of a balanced diet. The patient should not feel deprived; however, "trigger" foods (certain foods that usually lead to a binge) may need to be avoided initially.
- Avoid finger foods; plan meals requiring utensils.
- Use foods naturally divided into portions, such as precut meats and chicken parts; individual serving size packages of yogurt, ice cream, or cottage cheese; frozen dinners and entrees; and baked potatoes (as opposed to rice, pasta, or mashed potatoes).
- Avoid "all-you-can-eat" restaurants and stores with loose bins of bulk foods. Do not shop for food when hungry. Avoid shopping for food alone.
- Require that foods be eaten while sitting down.
- Identify vulnerable times when binge eating is likely and then substitute other activities for eating at these times.
- Keep a food diary requiring that food be planned and recorded before eating.

Carbohydrate-Modified Diets

Diabetes Mellitus. Probably the most common type of carbohydrate-modified diet is the diabetic diet used for those with diabetes mellitus. In diabetes mellitus beta cells in the pancreas do not produce enough insulin or cannot use it properly. Insulin is the hormone necessary to move glucose from the blood stream into the cells where it is used for energy. Without insulin, glucose builds up in the blood stream, leading to **hyperglycemia** (elevated blood glucose). Diabetes also may affect fat metabolism and increase levels of blood lipids (cholesterol and triglycerides). Over time, elevated blood glucose and lipid levels may cause serious long-term complications. See Chapter 32 for a discussion on diabetes mellitus.

Perhaps not enough emphasis has been placed on the role of diet in the management of diabetes. Proper diet is essential for blood glucose control and may help reduce insulin needs if strictly followed. By keeping blood glucose levels relatively constant and in an appropriate range, the risk of diabetic complications may be lessened. Persons with diabetes should continually be encouraged to follow their individualized meal plan. Dietary goals differ somewhat depending on the type of diabetes being treated (Table 19-5).

Insulin-dependent diabetes mellitus (IDDM). IDDM occurs most often in children and adolescents. Those with IDDM do not produce insulin. The body cannot use glucose for energy and begins to burn fat. When fat is burned for energy in the absence of glucose, acid wastes called *ketones* are formed. Ketones build up in the blood and lead to a life-threatening condition called **ketoacidosis** (acidosis accompanied by an accumulation of ketones in the body resulting from faulty carbohydrate metabolism). People with IDDM must take insulin to avoid this condition.

The most important principle for those with IDDM is consistency. Meals and snacks should be eaten at about the same time each day. The types and amounts of foods eaten should be similar from day to day. This is neces-

TABLE 19-4 Danger Signs of Eating Disorders

Diagnostic Category	Signs and Symptom or Behavior
Eating behaviors	Caloric restriction; preoccupation with dieting and calorie counting Binge eating; secretive eating Extreme preoccupation with food—reading cookbooks, recipes, shopping and preparing food for others Exhibition of peculiar eating rituals
Purging behaviors	Evidence of forced vomiting Abuse of laxatives, diuretics, enemas, or diet pills Fasting Excessive amounts of exercise Excessive time spent in the bathroom
Physiological changes	Insomnia, hair loss, dry skin, weak and brittle nails Bouts of constipation, diarrhea, and cramps Loss of sexual drive Amenorrhea in women Cold intolerance Edematous glands in the neck beneath the jaw Erosion of tooth enamel, cavities, tooth loss Weight loss
Psychological changes	Depression and/or apathy Irritability Withdrawal from friends, family, and social activities Inability to concentrate Distorted body image (feeling fat when actually being very thin)

TABLE 19-5 Nutrition Guidelines for Persons with IDDM and NIDDM

Dietary Component	IDDM	NIDDM
Kilocalories	Sufficient for growth in children, teens, and in pregnancy (kilocalorie intake should be evaluated every 3 months) Sufficient for maintenance of a healthy, reasonable weight in adults	Sufficient for maintenance of a healthy, reasonable weight Weight reduction encouraged for obese individuals
Carbohydrate	50%-60% of total kilocalories Emphasis on complex carbohydrates (unrefined grains, cereals, vegetables, and fruits)	55%-60% of total kilocalories Same
Sucrose	5%-10% of carbohydrate energy allowed, contingent upon metabolic control and adherence to meal plan	Modest amounts allowed on an individual basis contingent upon metabolic control and body weight
Fiber	High-fiber diet with emphasis on soluble fiber	Up to 40 g/day with emphasis on soluble fiber
Protein	12%-20% of total kilocalories High intakes may lead to deterioration of kidney function (diabetic nephropathy)	12%-20% of total kilocalories or 0.8 g/kg body weight
Fat	< 30% total kilocalories	Same
Saturated fat	< 10% total kilocalories	Same
Cholesterol	< 300 mg/day	Same
Sodium	Moderate consumption acceptable If hypertensive, limit to 3000-4000 mg/day	< 3000 mg/day
Vitamins/minerals	No evidence that diabetes causes increased need	Same

Continued.

TABLE 19-5 Nutrition Guidelines for Persons with IDDM and NIDDM—cont'd

Dietary Component	IDDM	NIDDM
Alcohol	No use recommended. If consumed: ■ Limit to no more than 1 to 2 alcohol equivalents (1½ oz liquor, 4 oz wine, or 12 oz beer) in 4-hour period. ■ Never get drunk. ■ Always eat a source of carbohydrate when drinking alcohol. ■ Do not substitute alcohol for food. ■ Do not increase insulin dose, since the overall effect of alcohol is to lower blood glucose levels. ■ Always eat a bedtime snack. ■ Wear a diabetes identification tag.	Occasional or no use; limit to 1 to 2 alcohol equivalents once or twice a week.
Alternative sweeteners	Use of a variety of types in moderation	Use is acceptable
Meals and snacks	Should be eaten at about the same time each day Amounts and types of food eaten at each meal and snack should be consistent day to day Bedtime snack should consist of a minimum of one protein source and one starch source	Should be planned on an individual basis If on insulin, meals and snacks should be coordinated with insulin schedule

From Connell JE, Thomas-Doberson D: Nutritional management of children and adolescents with insulin-dependent diabetes mellitus: a review by the Diabetes Care and Education Dietetic Practice Group, *J Am Diet Assoc* 91:1556, 1991; and Beebe CA et al: Nutrition management for individuals with noninsulin-dependent diabetes mellitus in the 1990s: a review by the Diabetes Care and Education Dietetic Practice Group, *J Am Diet Assoc* 91:106, 1991.

TABLE 19-6 1500-Kilocalorie Meal Plan* and Menu Examples Using the Exchange Lists for Meal Planning

Meal	Exchange List	Servings	Menu 1	Menu 2
Breakfast	Starch/bread	2	1 slice wheat toast ½ c oatmeal	1 whole wheat bagel (2 halves)
	Fruit	1	½ c orange juice	1 fresh peach
	Milk	1	1 c skim milk	1 c plain yogurt
	Fat	1	1 tsp margarine	1 tbsp cream cheese 1 c coffee, black (free)
Lunch	Starch/bread	3	2 slices wheat bread 3 gingersnaps	1 hamburger bun ½ c potato salad
	Meat	2	½ c tuna (water)	2 oz ground beef, lean
	Vegetable	1	1 c carrot & celery sticks, raw Iceberg lettuce (free)	½ c tomato juice Cucumber slices (free)
	Fruit	1	1 small apple	15 grapes
	Fat	1	2 tsp salad dressing	2 tsp dressing in potato salad
Supper	Starch/bread	2	⅔ c seasoned brown rice	½ c mashed potatoes ½ c stuffing
	Meat	2	2 oz top round steak	2 oz roast turkey
	Vegetable	2	1 c stir-fried vegetables	1 c steamed asparagus
	Fruit	1	¾ c fresh pineapple	1¼ c whole strawberries
	Fat	2	1 tsp oil for stir-frying 1 Tbls slivered almonds in stir-fry	2 tbsp whipped cream (for strawberries)
Snack	Starch/bread	1	3 c salted popcorn	3 squares graham crackers
	Milk	1	1 c sugar-free fruit-flavored yogurt	1 c skim milk

*This meal plan provides 204 g carbohydrate (54% of kilocalories); 74 g protein (19% of kilocalories); 45 g fat (27% of kilocalories).

Box 19-6 EXCHANGE LISTS FOR MEAL PLANNING

LIST 1: STARCH/BREAD LIST

Each serving contains:	15 g carbohydrate, 3 g protein, trace of fat 80 kcal
Representative servings:	½ c cooked cereal, pasta, or starchy vegetables; 1 oz of a bread product (1 slice bread); ¾ c ready-to-eat cereal; ⅓ c cooked rice

LIST 2: MEAT LIST

Each serving contains:	7 g protein, 5 g fat, no carbohydrate 75 kcal
Representative servings:	1 oz lean meat, fish, or poultry; 1 oz low-fat cheese or ¼ c cottage cheese; 1 egg *Note:* Some meats may be lower in fat or higher in fat.

LIST 3: VEGETABLE LIST

Each serving contains:	5 g carbohydrate, 2 g protein, no fat 25 kcal
Representative servings:	½ c cooked vegetables or vegetable juice; 1 c raw vegetables

LIST 4: FRUIT LIST

Each serving contains:	15 g carbohydrate, no protein or fat 60 kcal
Representative servings:	1 medium-sized piece fresh fruit; ½ c canned fruit or fruit juice; ½ c dried fruit; 1 c cubed melon or berries

LIST 5: MILK LIST

Each serving contains	12 g carbohydrate, 8 g protein, trace of fat 90 kcal
Representative servings:	1 c skim milk, 1% milk, or buttermilk; 1 c plain low-fat yogurt *Note:* Whole and 2% milk contribute more fat.

LIST 6: FAT LIST

Each serving contains:	5 g fat, very little protein or carbohydrate
Representative servings:	1 tsp butter, margarine, or oil; 1 tbsp cream or salad dressings; 1 tbsp chopped nuts; 1 tsp mayonnaise; 1 slice bacon; 2 tbsp coconut

From American Diabetes Association and American Dietetic Association: *Exchange lists for meal planning,* Alexandria, Va, and Chicago, 1986, The Associations.

sary because the carbohydrate eaten must balance the insulin administered each day. Carbohydrate intake should be distributed evenly throughout the day to provide adequate amounts of glucose for the available insulin to move from the blood stream to the cells. This is called carbohydrate distribution.

Those with IDDM should follow a diet that limits the use of simple sugars, emphasizes adequate fiber intake, and limits dietary fat and cholesterol. The Exchange Lists for Meal Planning were developed by the American Diabetes Association and the American Dietetic Association for use in diabetic meal planning. Because of the flexibility and variation allowed in the exchange lists, they are often used in weight reduction programs as well. Foods are divided into six food groups called *exchange lists.* The foods in each group are similar in protein, carbohydrate, fat, and caloric values. Thus a serving of any food from one exchange list should have approximately the same nutrient and caloric value as another food in the same list. The six exchange lists, their nutrient values, and representative foods are found in Box 19-6.

The patient should be given a meal plan to follow that specifies the number of food choices (exchanges) to be consumed at each meal and snack. Carbohydrate is distributed among the meals to correspond with insulin dosage. Table 19-6 shows an example of a 1500-kcal meal plan. Although the meal plan should be followed each day, the individual can vary food choices for variety. Menu 1 and menu 2 in Table 19-6 are examples of menus that fit into the same 1500-kcal meal plan.

If a person taking insulin fails to consume adequate carbohydrate, blood glucose levels may drop, causing **hy-**

poglycemia (low blood glucose). Symptoms of hypoglycemia may include headache, disorientation, weakness, perspiration, shallow breathing, nervousness, visual disturbances, and vertigo and may lead to unconsciousness. Sometimes the person experiencing hypoglycemia may be mistakenly judged to be intoxicated. Proper medical identification should be worn to prevent such a mistake. Hypoglycemia should be treated with immediate administration of glucose in a readily available form, such as orange juice, followed by food containing both carbohydrate and protein. If juice is not available, sugar or hard candy may be eaten. In the event unconsciousness has occurred, glucose should be administered intravenously.

In times of illness, the patient with diabetes may not want to eat the usual foods on the meal plan. In such cases, it is essential to provide carbohydrate in the diet to correspond with insulin dosage. Carbohydrate-containing beverages, such as juices and punch, should be offered. Popsicles, flavored gelatin, crackers, puddings, and ice milk provide carbohydrate and may be better accepted during illness.

Non-insulin-dependent diabetes mellitus (NIDDM). NIDDM usually occurs in adults, many of whom are overweight. People with NIDDM produce insulin, but either there is not enough insulin or the body is unable to use it properly. This type of diabetes often may be controlled by diet and exercise. Some people with NIDDM use oral hypoglycemic agents, medications that stimulate insulin production and use. In some instances insulin injections may be needed to help regulate blood glucose levels. Whenever insulin is administered, the dietary principles for IDDM should be used.

Many people with NIDDM are overweight, and one of the major dietary goals with this type of diabetes is weight control. For the obese person with NIDDM, weight reduction can help control blood glucose and reduce the need for medication. Kilocalorie control is more important than carbohydrate distribution in this type of diabetes. A diet using the exchange lists is an ideal method of weight control. As with IDDM, simple sugar should be limited and adequate fiber intake emphasized.

Exercise reduces blood glucose levels. This is helpful in the control of blood glucose and is also important for weight control. People with either type of diabetes may be able to reduce insulin or medication needs with regular exercise. Diet can also be adjusted to compensate for exercise. If a patient with IDDM is to be involved in unaccustomed physical activity, some carbohydrate-containing food (milk, fruits, vegetables, or starches) may be added to the meal just before engaging in the activity. In this way the extra carbohydrate will provide more glucose to satisfy the demands of exercise.

Dumping Syndrome. **Dumping syndrome** (the combination of profuse perspiration, nausea, vertigo, and weakness) may occur after surgery where a portion or all of the stomach is removed (partial or total gastrectomy). After partial or total gastrectomy, the stomach contents may empty too rapidly into the jejunum. The body reacts by sending water to the intestinal tract, thus reducing blood pressure. The load in the intestinal tract increases peristalsis (contractions that move food through the GI tract), leading to diarrhea. Signs and symptoms occur 15 to 30 minutes after meals and include cramping, weakness, diaphoresis, vertigo, nausea, and possibly vomiting.

Diet therapy involves giving small, frequent meals that are higher in protein and fat and lower in carbohydrates. Concentrated sweets should be avoided, and fluids should be taken 30 to 60 minutes before or after a meal. The dumping syndrome diet may be needed only temporarily until the body adjusts to the changes caused by surgery.

Lactose Intolerance. Lactose intolerance occurs as a result of a lack of the digestive enzyme *lactase.* Because of this, the GI tract is unable to break down lactose, the milk sugar. Symptoms occur after ingestion of milk products and include nausea, cramps, a bloated feeling, flatulence, and diarrhea.

Diet for lactose intolerance excludes milk and milk products, such as ice cream, puddings, cheese, and powdered milk. Foods with milk added, such as biscuit or muffin mixes, some soups, and other prepared foods, may need to be avoided.

Some individuals have a deficiency rather than a total absence of lactase. These individuals may be able to tolerate small amounts of milk products. Yogurt and cheese are often well tolerated. Lactase enzyme–containing preparations are available and can be added to milk before drinking.

Fat-Modified Diets

As mentioned in Chapter 18, fat- and cholesterol-controlled diets may be beneficial in reducing the risk of atherosclerosis and certain cancers. Dietary fat intake may also be modified in the treatment of disease.

Fat-Controlled Diets. A fat-controlled diet is desirable for the prevention and treatment of atherosclerosis, heart disease, and **hyperlipidemias** (elevated levels of blood lipids such as cholesterol and triglycerides). Diabetic diets also incorporate fat control. A fat-controlled diet limits both total fat and saturated fat intake.

The National Cholesterol Education Program (NCEP) and the American Heart Association (AHA) have developed Step One and Step Two diets for reducing blood cholesterol levels (see Table 19-7). The Step One diet is the less restrictive. It calls for an average saturated fat intake of less than 10% of kilocalories, a total fat intake of no more than 30% of kilocalories, and a dietary cho-

TABLE 19-7 Characteristics of Step-One and Step-Two Diets for Lowering Blood Cholesterol

Nutrient	Recommended Intake	
	Step-One Diet	Step-Two Diet
Total fat	Average of no more than 30% of total calories	Same
Saturated fatty acids	Less than 10% of total calories	Less than 7% of total calories
Polyunsaturated fatty acids	Up to 10% of total calories	Same
Monounsaturated fatty acids	Remaining total fat calories	Same
Cholesterol	Less than 300 mg/day	Less than 200 mg/day
Carbohydrates	About 55% of total calories	Same
Protein	About 15%-20% of total calories	Same
Calories	To promote normal growth and development and to reach or maintain desirable body weight	Same

From US Department of Health and Human Services: The National Cholesterol Education Program: *Report of the Expert Panel on Blood Cholesterol Levels in Children and Adolescents,* NIH Pub No 91-2732, 1991.

lesterol intake of less than 300 mg/day. These recommendations are the same as for the general population. The medical climate in which this diet is prescribed and the follow-up that should take place make this diet therapeutic. If, after 3 months of this diet, the minimal goals of therapy are not achieved, the patient should progress to the Step Two diet. This diet calls for further reduction of saturated fat to less than 7% of total kilocalories and a dietary cholesterol intake of less than 200 mg/day. Usually when saturated fat intake is reduced, cholesterol intake also drops, since it is often found in foods containing saturated fat. The individual who is reducing saturated fat in the diet may choose low-fat dairy products, lean meats, skinless poultry, and fish. Eggs should be limited to four or less per week and organ meats, such as liver, limited to one serving per week or less. Visible fats, such as butter, margarine, mayonnaise, cream, sour cream, nuts, and rich desserts, should be limited. Cooking methods may need to be altered as well. Patients should be encouraged to bake, broil, or poach food, rather than to fry. Sauces, gravies, salad dressings, and dips are often high in fat. Patients should use these in moderation or try low-fat varieties. When fat is necessary in food preparation, unsaturated fats (monounsaturated and polyunsaturated) should be used in place of saturated fats. Table 19-8 on p. 376 shows dietary guidelines for implementing a fat-controlled diet.

Fat is a nutrient. It performs essential functions in the body. It also enhances the flavor, aroma, and texture of food and the overall satiety of a meal. As medical professionals we must not forget the qualities fat possesses and the pleasure it can bring to eating. Many Americans believe that to have a low-fat diet they must completely eliminate all high-fat foods. This is not so. Choosing a low-fat and low-cholesterol diet does not mean "never eat cheese because it contains fat" or "never eat egg yolks because they contain cholesterol." It is the *total* amount of fat, saturated fat, and cholesterol that matters. Besides, foods such as cheese and egg yolks contribute important nutrients to the diet. Sometimes, eliminating all high-fat foods compromises the overall nutritional value of the diet. For example, an older woman has been prescribed a low-fat, low-cholesterol diet. In an effort to reduce fat and cholesterol, she decides to purchase a nondairy milk substitute instead of regular low-fat milk. Although she is consuming less saturated fat and cholesterol, she is also receiving less protein, calcium, riboflavin, and vitamin B_{12}. She may have reduced her risk for heart disease, but she has increased her risk for osteoporosis.

Rather than totally eliminating high-fat foods, encourage moderation. Balance high-fat foods with other foods that contain less fat and cholesterol. For example, if a patient desires a hot fudge sundae, which is high in fat, after dinner, he should choose a low-fat entree such as broiled fish or chicken. Patients can be educated to read nutrition labels and nutrition information materials to become familiar with the amounts of fat in various food items. They can then "budget" their fat intake to be less than or equal to their daily fat allowance (see Table 18-5). By adhering to balance, variety, and moderation, patients can still enjoy some of their favorite foods while following a healthy, fat-controlled diet. Tables 18-10 and 19-6 show meal plans that provide no more than 30% of kilocalories from fat.

Low-Fat Diets. Other medical conditions warrant the use of a low-fat diet. Low-fat diets differ from fat-controlled diets in that all fats are limited, regardless of saturation. Any time fat malabsorption occurs, dietary fat should be limited. GI diseases that involve malabsorption of fat include cystic fibrosis, inflammatory bowel disease, pancreatitis, and short-bowel syndrome (secondary to

TABLE 19-8 Guidelines for Lowering Fat, Saturated Fat, and Cholesterol

Food Groups	Choose . . .	Go Easy On. . .
Fish, chicken, turkey, and lean meats (up to 6 oz per day)	Fish, poultry without skin, lean cuts of beef, lamb, pork, or veal, shellfish	Fatty cuts of beef, lamb, pork, spare ribs, organ meats, regular cold cuts, sausages, hot dogs, bacon, sardines, roe
Skim and low-fat milk, cheese, yogurt, and dairy substitutes (2-3 servings per day)	Skim or 1%-fat milk (liquid, powdered, evaporated), buttermilk	Whole milk: (4% fat) regular, evaporated, condensed; cream, half and half; 2% milk, imitation milk products, most nondairy creamers, whipped toppings
	Nonfat (0% fat) or low-fat yogurt	Whole-milk yogurt
	Low-fat cottage cheese (1% or 2% fat)	Whole-milk cottage cheese (4% fat)
	Low-fat cheeses, farmer or pot cheeses (all of these should be labeled "no more than 2 to 6 g fat per oz")	All-natural cheeses (e.g., bleu, Roquefort, Camembert, cheddar, Swiss)
	Ice milk, frozen yogurt	Cream cheeses, sour cream
	Sherbet, sorbet	Ice cream
Eggs (up to 4 egg yolks per week)	Egg whites (2 whites = 1 whole egg in recipes), cholesterol-free egg substitutes	Egg yolks
Fruits and vegetables (2-4 servings of fruit per day; 3-5 servings of vegetables per day)	Fresh, frozen, canned, or dried fruits and vegetables	Vegetables prepared with butter, cream, or other sauces
Breads and cereals (6-11 servings per day)	Homemade baked goods using unsaturated oils sparingly, angel food cake, low-fat crackers, low-fat cookies	Commercially baked goods; pies, cakes, doughnuts, croissants, pastries, muffins, biscuits, high-fat crackers, high-fat cookies
	Rice, pasta	Egg noodles
	Whole-grain breads and cereals (e.g., oatmeal, whole wheat, rye, bran, multigrain)	Breads in which eggs are major ingredient
Fats and oils (up to 6 tsp per day)	Baking cocoa	Chocolate
	Unsaturated vegetable oils: corn, olive, rapeseed, safflower, sesame, soybean, sunflower	Butter, coconut oil, palm oil, palm kernel oil, lard, bacon fat
	Margarine or shortenings made from one of the unsaturated oils listed above	
	Diet margarine	
	Reduced-calorie mayonnaise, salad dressings made with unsaturated oils listed above	Dressings made with egg yolk
	Low-fat dressings	
	Seeds and nuts	Coconut

bowel resection). Gallbladder disease often requires a low-fat diet. The gallbladder stores bile and contracts whenever fat is present in the intestinal tract. If gallstones are present or inflammation of the gallbladder exists, contraction may be painful. A low-fat diet may alleviate some discomfort. After the gallbladder is removed (cholecystectomy), a low-fat diet is no longer required. Some patients with gallbladder disease may be overweight or obese. Weight reduction is indicated for these individuals and may reduce symptoms of disease.

Low-fat diets may restrict fat to as little as 25 g/day. In this severe fat restriction, no visible fats are allowed (i.e., butter, cream, oil). Only nonfat dairy products and lean meat, fish, and poultry (no more than 5 oz per day) are allowed. Adequate grains, cereals, fruits, and vegetables are emphasized.

Some patients may be unable to digest regular fats (long-chain triglycerides). Occasionally, the use of medium-chain triglycerides (MCT) is necessary. This type of fat is absorbed readily, requiring minimal digestion. MCTs are expensive and generally only available in special supplemental formulas.

Protein-, Electrolyte-, and Fluid-Modified Diets

Protein-Restricted Diets. In disease states, increased protein needs are often considered to facilitate healing. However, in the presence of defects in protein metabolism or excretion, protein intake should be reduced or controlled (Box 19-7). One such case is during renal failure. Renal failure can occur rapidly (acute renal failure) or may progress slowly (end-stage renal disease). Acute renal failure is often temporary, whereas end-stage renal disease is irreversible.

The kidney normally functions to excrete wastes, concentrate urine, and conserve needed electrolytes. During renal failure the nephrons (working units of the kidney) fail to maintain normal function. **Oliguria** (less than 500 ml in 24 hours) or **anuria** (no urine output or less than 100 ml in 24 hours) may result. Urea and other nitrogenous wastes, the end products of protein metabolism, build up in the blood stream, leading to a condition known as *azotemia.* Many electrolytes, particularly potassium, sodium, and phosphorus, are retained, and increased blood levels of these nutrients may occur.

Because of the buildup of protein waste products, dietary protein should be restricted. A therapeutic diet for renal failure limits the amount of protein consumed; the degree of limitation depends on the extent of renal failure. Patients are encouraged to consume moderate amounts of only high-quality, or complete, proteins found in milk, meat, fish, poultry, and eggs. Incomplete proteins, those found in plant products, contribute to azotemia and should be restricted. Other dietary modifications include the restriction of potassium, sodium, phosphorus, and fluids. Vitamin/mineral supplements are generally prescribed. Chapter 30 discusses urinary disorders.

Cirrhosis is a chronic, degenerative disease of the liver. It is most often seen secondary to alcoholism but may also be seen as a result of hepatitis A and B or other infection. Scar tissue develops in the liver, hampering its effectiveness in removing waste products from the blood stream. In this case ammonia, a waste product of protein metabolism, builds up in the blood stream. If not controlled, high ammonia levels may contribute to hepatic coma (coma secondary to liver disease), brain damage, and death. Ascites, a condition characterized by accumulation of fluid in the abdominal cavity, may occur. If the liver is unable to produce bile, fat malabsorption also may take place.

In the presence of cirrhosis, protein intake should initially be at or above the RDA to facilitate healing and tissue regeneration. However, if blood ammonia levels become elevated and signs of impending coma are present, such as disorientation, apathy, and drowsiness, a strict low-protein diet should be followed. The low-protein diets for cirrhosis restrict milk and milk products, meats, fish, poultry, cheese, eggs, legumes, and nuts. Box 19-7 on p. 378 shows examples of various levels of protein restriction. Special nutritional support formulas with modified protein content have also been developed for hepatic coma.

The veins at the lower end of the esophagus may become enlarged and tortuous during cirrhosis, a condition called *esophageal varices.* Esophageal varices are painful, and the use of a soft or liquid diet may be beneficial in this case. Other dietary modifications for cirrhosis include total abstinence from alcohol and may require restriction of sodium and fluid if ascites occurs and fat restriction if malabsorption is present. Vitamin/mineral supplements are also given. Chapter 27 discusses gastrointestinal and assessory organ disorders.

Sodium-Restricted Diets. Sodium restrictions may be used to treat a number of medical conditions. Hypertension is often responsive to a lowered sodium intake. It is estimated that 20% of the population is "sodium sensitive"; that is, they have a genetic sensitivity to sodium that leads to hypertension. In such individuals sodium reduction appears beneficial in controlling blood pressure.

Sodium is also restricted when water retention or edema is present. In the presence of congestive heart failure, sodium intake should be decreased to alleviate pulmonary and peripheral edema. Directly after a myocardial infarction, sodium, fluid, kilocalorie, and fat restrictions may be implemented. These restrictions are to minimize the work load on the heart. As recovery progresses, the diet will be liberalized as the individual's condition permits. If cirrhosis is accompanied by ascites, sodium intake should be reduced, and in renal failure, if anuria or oliguria exists, sodium should be restricted.

Sodium-restricted diets vary in degree of restriction. The no-added-salt (NAS) diet is the least restrictive, allowing 2000 to 3000 mg of sodium/day. This diet allows the use of most foods with the exception of highly salted snack foods and prepared foods. Patients following this diet should read nutrition labels to assess the sodium content of food products and determine which would be appropriate for their diet. Very little or no salt should be added in cooking or at the table. Other sodium-restricted diets range from 2000 mg (2 g) sodium to as little as 250 mg of sodium/day. Box 19-8 on p. 378 lists foods restricted on low-sodium diets. See Box 18-6 for sodium content of foods.

In the presence of cystic fibrosis, the sweat glands produce excessive amounts of sodium and chloride. In

Box 19-7 LOW-PROTEIN DIETS: 15 g, 30 g, 40 g, and 50 g PROTEIN

GENERAL DESCRIPTION

- The following diets are used when dietary protein is to be restricted.
- The patterns limit foods containing a large percentage of protein, such as milk, eggs, cheese, meat, fish, fowl, and legumes.
- Meat extractives, soups, broth, bouillon, gravies, and gelatin desserts should also be avoided.

BASIC MEAL PATTERNS (contain approximately 15 g of protein)

Breakfast	Lunch	Dinner
½ c fruit or fruit juice	1 small potato	1 small potato
½ c cereal	½ c vegetable	½ c vegetable
1 slice toast	Salad (vegetable or fruit)	Salad (vegetable or fruit)
Butter	1 slice bread	1 slice bread
Jelly	Butter	Butter
Sugar	1 serving fruit	1 serving fruit
1 tbsp cream	Sugar	Sugar
Coffee	Coffee or tea	Coffee or tea

	EXAMPLES OF MEAT PORTIONS
FOR 30 g PROTEIN	
Add: 1 c milk 28 g (1 oz) meat, 1 egg, or equivalent	28 g (1 oz) meat = 1 thin slice roast, 4 × 5 cm 1(½ × 2 in) 1 rounded tbsp cottage cheese 1 slice American cheese
FOR 40 g PROTEIN	
Add: 1 c milk 70 g (2½ oz) meat, or 1 egg and 42 g (1½ oz) meat	70 g (2½ oz) meat = Ground beef patty (5 from 448 g [1 lb]) 1 slice roast
FOR 50 g PROTEIN	
Add: 1 c milk 112 g (4 oz) meat, or 2 eggs and 56 g (2 oz) meat	112 g (4 oz) meat = 2 lamb chops 1 average steak

Box 19-8 FOODS TO LIMIT IN SODIUM RESTRICTION* (250 MG TO 2000 MG)

1. Salt in cooking or at the table
2. Salty snack foods, i.e., chips, nuts, crackers, pretzels, salted popcorn
3. Regular canned soups
4. Salty condiments, such as soy sauce, barbeque sauce, Worcestershire and steak sauces, bouillon, prepared mustard, meat tenderizers, monosodium glutamate (MSG), spice salts, and regular salad dressings
5. Regular cheese and peanut butter, smoked or cured meats, luncheon meats, canned meats, corned beef, shellfish
6. Canned vegetables with salt, pickled foods, sauerkraut, and olives
7. Leavening agents, such as baking soda and baking powder
8. Commercially prepared foods and mixes, such as pudding, instant breakfast cereals, beverage mixes, biscuit and muffin mixes, cake and pastry mixes
9. Most ready-to-eat cereals
10. Commercially prepared milk mixes, such as ice milk and milkshakes
11. Salted butter and margarine

*The diet becomes more flexible the higher the sodium limit. Very strict low-sodium diets (250-500 mg) also incorporate the use of special dietetic products, such as low-sodium milk and breads.

TABLE 19-9 Summary of Diet Modifications

Condition	Possible Diet Modifications
Acquired immune deficiency syndrome (AIDS)	High kilocalorie and protein; increased fluid intake; mechanical soft; possible tube feeding or TPN
Atherosclerosis	Fat controlled; high fiber; when necessary, kilocalorie- and/or sodium-restricted diet
Burns	High kilocalorie and protein; increased fluid intake; vitamin/mineral therapy
Cancer	High kilocalorie and protein; dietary adjustments made based on symptoms; possible tube feeding or TPN
Cirrhosis/hepatic coma	Protein restricted; possible sodium, fat, and fluid restriction; no alcohol; vitamin/mineral supplementation
Congestive heart failure	Sodium-restricted; fluid-restricted; small, frequent feedings; soft diet; possible kilocalorie restriction
Constipation	High fiber; increased fluid intake
Cystic fibrosis	High kilocalorie and protein; low fat; generous sodium; vitamin and mineral supplementation
Diabetes mellitus	
IDDM	Carbohydrate controlled; no concentrated sweets; fat controlled; high fiber
NIDDM	Kilocalorie restricted; no concentrated sweets; fat controlled; high fiber
Diverticulitis	Soft, low residue
Diverticulosis	High fiber
Dumping syndrome	Carbohydrate restricted; no concentrated sweets; small, frequent feedings; fluids before or after meals; when necessary, fluid and electrolyte replacement
Gallbladder disease	Low fat; when necessary kilocalorie restricted; bland
Gastritis	Low residue, bland
Hepatitis	High kilocalorie and protein
Hiatal hernia	Small, frequent feedings; low fat; bland; when necessary, kilocalorie restricted
Hyperlipidemia	Fat controlled; when necessary, kilocalorie restricted; carbohydrate controlled
Hypertension	Sodium restricted; high potassium; fat controlled; when necessary, kilocalorie restricted
Hypoglycemia	No concentrated sweets; small, frequent feedings
Inflammatory bowel disease	Low residue; low fat; high kilocalories and protein; fluid and electrolyte replacement; vitamin/mineral supplementation; possible lactose restriction, possible bland diet; tube feeding or TPN
Lactose intolerance	Lactose restricted
Malabsorption	Low fat; high kilocalorie and protein; fluid and electrolyte replacement
Mouth, conditions affecting	
Broken jaw/oral surgery	Mechanical soft; possible tube feeding
Dental caries/periodontal disease/ill-fitting dentures/missing teeth	Mechanical soft
Dry mouth	Mechanical soft; increased fluid intake
Dysphagia (difficulty swallowing)	Mechanical soft; possible tube feeding
Ulcers of mouth or gums	Mechanical soft; bland
Myocardial infarction	Low sodium; kilocalorie restricted; soft; bland; small, frequent feedings; fat controlled; fluid restricted (temporary); moderate temperature foods
Nausea	Soft; bland; small, frequent feedings
Obesity	Kilocalorie restricted; fat controlled; high fiber
Pancreatitis	Low fat; small, frequent feedings; possible tube feedings or TPN
Peptic ulcer	Individualized bland diet
Reflux esophagitis	Small frequent feedings; low fat; bland
Renal calculi (kidney stones)	Increased fluid intake; possible calcium controlled
Renal failure	
Acute	Protein restricted; high kilocalorie; fluid, sodium, and potassium controlled
Chronic	Protein restricted; low sodium; potassium, fluid, and phosphorus restricted; vitamin/mineral supplement
Underweight	High kilocalorie and protein
Vomiting	Fluid and electrolyte replacement

Modified from Cataldo CB, Nyenhuis JR, Whitney EN: *Nutrition and diet therapy: principles and practice,* ed 2, St Paul, 1989, West Publishing.

this special condition sodium intake is not restricted; indeed, generous amounts of sodium and salt are encouraged to compensate for the large losses of sodium.

Potassium-Modified Diets. Potassium is considered to play a role in blood pressure control. Evidence indicates that populations with higher potassium intakes have less incidence of hypertension. Increased potassium intake from foods may be beneficial for blood pressure control. Many patients with hypertension or other conditions that cause water retention may take potassium-wasting diuretics. An increased intake of potassium is needed to counteract the loss of potassium caused by the diuretic. Potassium-rich foods are listed in Box 18-7.

In end-stage renal disease and other kidney disease, potassium intake may need to be restricted to as little as 1500 to 2000 mg/day. During renal failure, potassium is retained, leading to a buildup of potassium in the blood stream. If dietary intake is not controlled, blood potassium levels could increase to the point of causing dysrythmias and sudden cardiac arrest. In a potassium-controlled diet, the foods listed in Box 18-7 should be restricted.

Fluid-Modified Diets. Fluid is found in the diet in a number of forms. Of course, all beverages—milk, juices, coffee, and tea—add fluid to the diet. Other dietary fluid sources include gelatins, ice cream, sherbet, puddings, popsicles, fruit ices, and soups.

During end-stage renal disease and other kidney disease with oliguria or anuria, fluid is restricted to 400 to 500 ml/day (approximately 2 cups) plus an amount equal to daily urine output, if any. Fluid restrictions may also be implemented during congestive heart failure, directly after an MI, or in hepatic coma or ascites.

In the hospital, fluid restrictions are often divided between the nursing and dietary departments. For example, if a patient is on a 1000-ml fluid restriction, the dietary department may be allowed to provide the patient with 600 ml, whereas the nursing department may give 400 ml per day. The amount of fluid allowed for nursing depends on the patient's IV and medication needs.

During fluid restrictions, patients may experience excessive thirst. Some suggestions to help alleviate thirst include rinsing the mouth with cold mouthwash, putting lemon into cold water to make it more refreshing, freezing fluid so it takes longer to consume, eating cold fruits and raw vegetables, chewing gum, sucking on breath mints or hard candies (in moderation), and brushing teeth often.

Increased fluid intake is a common dietary treatment for renal calculi (kidney stones) and urinary tract infection. Additional fluid helps to dilute the urine and increase urinary output. Fluid needs are also increased during periods of diarrhea, vomiting, or malabsorption, such as in inflammatory bowel disease. Care should be taken by the patient to replace fluids that are lost to prevent dehydration.

The burn victim loses a large volume of fluids from the wounds. Immediately after a severe burn, fluids, electrolytes, and protein are given intravenously rather than orally, because burn patients experience a temporary loss of bowel function. Once bowel activity resumes, adequate fluids should be a part of dietary treatment. Burn victims also require enormous amounts of protein, kilocalories, and certain vitamins and minerals. Chapter 25 discusses treatment of the burn patient.

Most conditions requiring diet therapy involve combinations of therapeutic diets. As a summary, Table 19-9 on p. 379 lists different medical conditions and their commonly prescribed diets.

NUTRITION SUPPORT

Occasionally a patient may not be able to consume an oral diet. For whatever reason, alternative feeding methods are available in the form of tube feedings or intravenous feedings.

Tube Feedings

A **tube feeding** (the administration of nutritionally balanced liquefied foods or formula through a tube inserted into the stomach, duodenum, or jejunum by way of a nasoenteric tube or a feeding ostomy) is often referred to as **enteral nutrition** (administration of nutrients into the GI tract) support. Tube feedings may be indicated when a patient is unable to chew or swallow, such as after oral surgery or facial trauma; when a person has no appetite or refuses to eat; in times of great nutritional need, such as in the burn or trauma patient; in the comatose patient; or during periods of moderate malabsorption or diarrhea. Box 19-9 lists conditions that may require a tube feeding.

Tube feedings should be used only when all or at least part of the GI tract is functioning. Tube feedings are most commonly administered by way of a nasogastric tube, that is, a tube that is passed through the nose and into the stomach (Fig. 19-3). If regurgitation is common or gastric residual is high, a nasojejunal or nasoduodenal tube (a tube that is passed through the nose and into the jejunum or duodenum) may be used to reduce the risk of aspiration.

In cases where long-term tube feedings are necessary, such as in a patient with a gastrectomy or intestinal resection, or in a patient with an upper GI obstruction, feeding ostomies may be employed. Ostomies are surgical openings through which a feeding tube may pass. Ostomies may be made into the esophagus (esophagostomy), stomach (gastrostomy), or jejunum (jejunostomy) (see Fig. 19-3). Ostomy feeding need not be con-

Box 19-9 INDICATIONS FOR THE USE OF ENTERAL NUTRITION SUPPORT (TUBE FEEDING)

- Protein kilocalorie malnutrition with inadequate intake for past 5 days
- Hospitalized patient consuming less than 50% of nutritional needs for past 7 to 10 days
- Severe dysphagia (difficulty swallowing)
- Major burns
- Sustained major trauma wounds
- Liver failure
- Renal dysfunction
- Radiation therapy
- Mild chemotherapy
- As adjunctive therapy with TPN for small bowel regeneration
- Low-output enterocutaneous fistulas (abnormal passage from the intestine to the body surface) that can be successfully bypassed with a tube

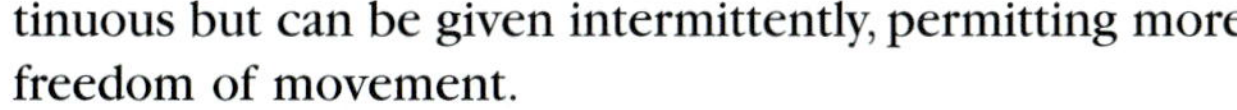

Modified from ASPEN Board of Directors: Guidelines for the use of enteral nutrition in the adult patient, *J Parenter Enteral Nutr* 11(5):435, 1987.

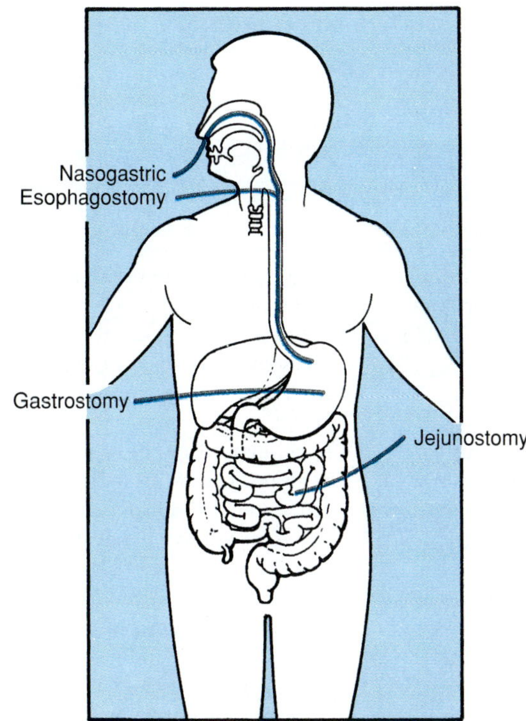

FIG. 19-3 Tube feeding sites.

tinuous but can be given intermittently, permitting more freedom of movement.

Formulas vary in composition. If the tube feeding is the sole source of nutrition, a complete formula that provides adequate kilocalories, protein, carbohydrate, fat, vitamins, and minerals to meet RDAs should be used. Intact formulas are formulas containing proteins, carbohydrates, and fats in whole forms, as found in foods. These formulas are available with or without fiber. Elemental or hydrolyzed formulas are available for individuals experiencing malabsorption, such as in inflammatory bowel disease and diarrhea. Elemental formulas are predigested; that is, the nutrients are already broken down into smaller units. Therefore they require little digestive action before being absorbed.

In the hospital, tube feedings can be done on a continuous basis, using a continuous drip pump that administers the formula slowly over 16 to 24 hours. Feedings may also be given intermittently. This involves giving a specific volume of formula over a short time, about 20 to 30 minutes. This may be done four to six times daily. Intermittent feeding is preferred by many long-term tube-fed patients. Bolus feedings (giving a 4- to 6-hour volume of formula in a matter of minutes) may also be given but are poorly tolerated in most patients.

Tube feedings should always be started slowly, and most formulas should be diluted to one third to one half of regular strength. The strength and the amount of formula can then be increased at different intervals until the full prescription is given. Distention, diarrhea, and nausea may indicate that the formula strength and/or volume is too great. Dumping syndrome may also occur with rapid and concentrated formula delivery.

Tube feeding is considered to be aggressive nutritional therapy. Complications may arise, including diarrhea; contamination of formula; infection; aspiration; overhydration or dehydration; abnormalities of blood concentrations of electrolytes, glucose, and other nutrients; and development of liver abnormalities. The patient should be monitored closely. A monitoring checklist for the tube-fed patient is found in Table 19-10 on p. 382. Guidelines for administering tube feedings are given in Box 19-10 on p. 382.

Parenteral Nutrition Support

Parenteral nutrition is the term used to describe intravenous feedings. Parenteral nutrition may be administered through peripheral veins, such as those in the arms or legs. This administration route is called **peripheral parenteral nutrition (PPN).**

Total parenteral nutrition (TPN) refers to the administration of a hypertonic solution into a large central vein. *TPN* is also sometimes referred to as *hyperalimentation.* The terms *total parenteral nutrition* and *hyperalimentation* are interchangeable. In TPN the solution is usually infused into the superior vena cava via a catheter threaded through either the subclavian or internal jugular vein (Fig. 19-4 on p. 382). TPN and PPN

TABLE 19-10 Guidelines for Monitoring the Tube-Fed Patient

Frequency	Procedure	Frequency	Procedure
Before starting a new or intermittent feeding	Review nutritional assessment; check tube placement; check residual formula in stomach (if 100 ml, consider reasons for delayed gastric emptying)	Every 8 hr	Check and record intake and output Chart patient's acceptance of an tolerance to tube feeding
Every ½ hr	Check gravity drip rate when applicable	Every day	Weigh patient; change feeding bag and tubing (except portion of tube in GI tract); monitor electrolytes, blood urea nitrogen, and blood glucose until stabilized
Every hour	Check pump drip rate when applicable		
Every 2 to 4 hr of continuous feeding	Check residual by aspirating through the tube. If residual is one half or more of hourly volume, hold feeding for 1 hour and reassess.	Every 7 to 10 days	Check all laboratory findings; review current nutritional assessment and dietary goals
Every 4 hr	Check vital signs, including blood pressure, temperature, pulse, and respiration; monitor blood glucose (may be discontinued after 48 hr if glucose is consistently normal in the nondiabetic patient)	As needed	Observe patient for any undesirable responses to tube feeding, for example, nausea, vomiting, or diarrhea; document and describe stools; check tube placement (nasogastric only); administer nasal and oral hygiene; chart significant details

Modified from Cataldo CB, Nyenhuis JR, Whitney EN: *Nutrition and diet therapy: principles and practice,* ed 2, St Paul, 1989, West Publishing.

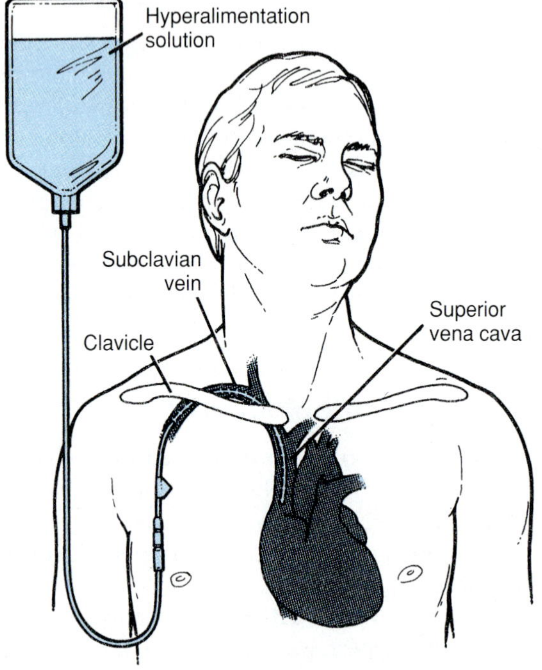

FIG 19-4 Administration of total parenteral nutrition.

Box 19-9 GUIDELINES FOR ADMINISTERING TUBE FEEDINGS

- Thoroughly wash hands with soap and water.
- Use the least manipulation possible when preparing and administering the formula.
- Avoid touching anything that will come in contact with the formula.
- Limit formula hang time to 8 hours.
- Discard any open, unused product within 24 hours.
- Never add new formula to a partially used reservoir of formula.
- Elevate the head of the bed 30 degrees while feeding is being infused (and for at least ½ hour after an intermittent or bolus feeding).

From DiLima SN, editor: *Dietitian's patient education manual,* vol 2, Gaithersburg, Md, 1991, Aspen.

Box 19-11 POSSIBLE INDICATIONS FOR THE USE OF TOTAL PARENTERAL NUTRITION

- Bone marrow transplantation
- Chronic intractable vomiting (such as hyperemesis gravidarum, the severe nausea and vomiting of pregnancy)
- Severe malabsorption and diarrhea
- Inflammatory bowel disease
- Enterocutaneous fistulas (abnormal passage from the intestine to the body surface)
- Small bowel obstruction or surgical resection
- Moderate to acute pancreatitis
- High-dose chemotherapy
- High-dose radiation therapy affecting the GI tract
- Preoperative therapy when intensive medical or surgical intervention is used in the malnourished
- Severe malnutrition in the face of a nonfunctioning GI tract
- Hospitalization, when adequate enteral nutrition cannot be established in 7 to 10 days

In any condition, TPN should not be used for those patients whose dependence on parenteral nutritional support is expected to be shorter than 5 days.

Modified from ASPEN Board of Directors: Guidelines for use of total parenteral nutrition in the hospitalized adult patient, *J Parenter Enteral Nutr* 10(5):441, 1986.

formulas are composed of glucose, amino acids, vitamins, minerals, and electrolytes. Fat, in the form of triglycerides, is also given as a supplement to the main formula. It is administered separately through a Y-connector tube.

Parenteral nutrition support is indicated for the patient with a nonfunctioning or dysfunctioning GI tract. Many patients with nonfunctioning GI tracts can be maintained on glucose and saline solutions for 5 to 7 days, but if the digestive tract is still nonfunctioning after that time, PPN or TPN should be initiated.

When IV nutrition is necessary, PPN should be the first choice of administration where possible. PPN carries less risk of complications, requires less monitoring, and costs less than the central venous route. Candidates for PPN are those needing 3000 or fewer kilocalories/day, those needing supplementation to oral diet, or those requiring short-term therapy (less than 3 weeks).

TPN is indicated for patients needing a highly concentrated formula, such as those who need more kilocalories than can be administered peripherally or those requiring fluid restriction—a concentrated formula delivers more kilocalories and nutrients in a smaller volume. Other candidates for TPN include those who must be on IV feedings for more than 3 weeks and those with unsuitable or unavailable peripheral veins. Box 19-11 identifies conditions requiring TPN.

TPN requires constant medical care. Central venous administration requires surgical placement of a catheter in one of the central veins. This imposes significant risks to the patient, including sepsis (major infection), pneumothorax (air in the pleural cavity), hemothorax (blood in the pleural cavity), phlebitis (inflammation of the vein), or thrombosis (blood clots). The catheter site must be kept aseptic, and feeding solutions must be sterile. Biochemical and clinical status of the patient must be constantly monitored.

The patient receiving TPN may experience fluid and electrolyte imbalances, hyperglycemia or hypoglycemia, metabolic disturbances, and bone disorders, such as osteomalacia (softening of the bones). For this reason blood chemistries should be monitored frequently. Blood glucose should be checked several times each day. Regular insulin may be administered on a sliding scale to maintain blood glucose levels below 200 mg/dl.

REFERENCES AND SUGGESTED READINGS

1. American Dietetic Association: Position of the American Dietetic Association: very low calorie weight loss diets, *J Am Diet Assoc* 90(5):722, 1990.
2. Beebe CA et al: Nutrition management for individuals with noninsulin-dependent diabetes mellitus in the 1990s: a review by the Diabetes Care and Education Dietetic Practice Group, *J Am Diet Assoc* 91(2):196, 1991.
3. Connell JE, Thomas-Dobersen D: Nutritional management of children and adolescents with insulin-dependent diabetes mellitus: a review by the Diabetes Care and Education Dietetic Practice Group, *J Am Diet Assoc* 91(12):1556, 1991.
4. Di Lima SN, editor: *Dietitian's patient education manual,* vol 1, Gaithersburg, Md, 1991, Aspen Publishers.
5. Di Lima SN, editor: *Dietitian's patient education manual,* vol 2, Gaithersburg, Md, 1991, Aspen Publishers.
6. Glanze WD, editor: *Mosby's medical, nursing, and allied health dictionary,* ed 4, St Louis, 1994, Mosby.
7. Hudnall M, Wellman NS: Missing the nutrition message of balance, variety and moderation, *J Nutr Ed* 24(6):3210, 1992.
8. National Research Council: *Recommended dietary allowances,* ed 10, Washington, DC, 1989, National Academy Press.
9. Position of the American Dietetic Association: Nutrition intervention in the treatment of anorexia nervosa and bulimia, *J Am Diet Assoc* 88(1):68, 1988; reaffirmed, 1992.
10. Robison JI et al: Obesity, weight loss, and health, *J Am Diet Assoc* 93(4):445, 1993.
11. Skipper A, editor: *Dietitian's handbook of enteral and parenteral nutrition,* Gaithersburg, Md, 1989, Aspen Publishers.
12. US Department of Health and Human Services: The National Cholesterol Education Program: *Report of the Expert Panel on Blood Cholesterol Levels in Children and Adolescents,* NIH Pub No 91-2732, 1991.
13. US Department of Health and Human Services: The National Cholesterol Education Program: *Report of the Expert Panel on Population Strategies for Blood Cholesterol Reduction,* NIH Pub No 90-3046, 1990.
14. Williams SR: *Basic nutrition and diet therapy,* ed 9, St Louis, 1992, Mosby.
15. Williams SR: *Essentials of nutrition and diet therapy,* ed 5, St Louis, 1990, Mosby.

CHAPTER CHALLENGE

KEY POINTS

- Diet therapy involves using the diet as medical treatment for disease or injury.
- Diets may be altered in consistency when GI function prohibits the use of a regular diet. Liquid diets are not nutritionally adequate and should be used only temporarily.
- In some GI disorders, in hypoglycemia, after MI, or in congestive heart failure, small frequent feedings are used as diet therapy.
- High-kilocalorie and high-protein diets are used when patients need to gain weight or maintain present weight in the face of increased metabolic needs.
- Low-kilocalorie and low-fat diets are used in conjunction with exercise and life-style changes in the treatment of obesity.
- The eating disorders anorexia nervosa and bulimia require multidisciplinary therapy, including nutritional, family, and psychological counseling. Nutritional goals include increasing and/or improving dietary intake, achieving a healthy weight, and establishing "normal" eating patterns. Emphasis should be placed on prevention of these disorders.
- Carbohydrate-controlled diets are used in diabetes, hypoglycemia, and lactose intolerance.
- Fat-controlled diets are prescribed in atherosclerosis, heart disease, hyperlipidemias, and diabetes. Attention should focus on reducing both total fat and saturated fat intake.
- Low-fat diets restrict all fats and are used to treat malabsorption syndromes and gallbladder disease.
- Reduced dietary sodium and increased dietary potassium seem to help lower blood pressure in susceptible individuals.
- Electrolyte and protein restrictions apply in many forms of renal disease including end-stage renal disease. They often apply in cirrhosis of the liver.
- Fluid restrictions may be necessary during heart failure, edema, and reduced urine output. Kidney stones and urinary tract infections necessitate the use of high fluid intakes.
- Nutritional support (tube feedings or total parenteral nutrition) may be necessary when oral intake is impossible or inadequate to meet needs. GI function usually indicates which type of feeding is to be used.

STUDY QUESTIONS

1. Mr. Hopkins is obese and desires to lose weight. He wants to lose 20 lb in the next month before his class reunion. A safe rate of weight loss would be:
    1. No more than ½ lb per week
    2. An average of no more than 1 to 2 lb per week
    3. An average of 3 to 5 lb per week
    4. Up to 10 lb per week as long as exercise is included
2. Sam Leland, a 40-year-old businessman, is admitted to the hospital with a bleeding ulcer. Mr. Leland's diet history reveals that he usually skips breakfast and drinks 8 to 10 cups of coffee over the course of the day. He usually eats fast food for lunch and especially enjoys Mexican and Italian foods. He snacks on fresh fruit and crackers in the afternoon, eats a large supper, and often drinks a beer or two before bed. Which of the following dietary changes would be most beneficial for Mr. Leland:
    1. Avoiding all spicy and high-fiber foods; eating smaller, more frequent meals, including breakfast
    2. Eating regular, balanced meals, including breakfast; avoiding coffee and alcohol
    3. Eliminating fast foods and bringing a sack lunch to work; altering the afternoon snack to be low in fiber
    4. Including milk or cream at all meals and snacks; avoiding high-fiber foods and alcohol
3. Mr. Taylor has hypertension and a family history of heart disease. He is prescribed a 2000-mg sodium diet. Which of the following meals would be most appropriate for this diet:
    1. Canned chili, baking powder biscuits with honey butter, tossed salad with bacon bits, milkshake
    2. Grilled chicken breast, baked potato with cottage cheese, steamed asparagus, dinner roll with low-fat spread, strawberry pie.
    3. Chicken chow mein, fried rice, won ton soup, egg roll, fresh pineapple, tea
    4. Tuna salad sandwich, cottage cheese with fruit, tomato juice, chocolate chip cookies
4. Mrs. Ivans is admitted to the hospital with congestive heart failure. She complains about receiving six small meals per day rather than the three regular-sized meals she is accustomed to. The purpose of small, frequent feedings is to:

1. Alleviate the strain placed upon abdominal and rectal muscles during constipation
2. Help regulate blood pressure and body fluids
3. Decrease the amount of stress placed on the GI tract and circulatory system at a given time
4. Prevent the patient from sleeping for long periods of time

5. Mr. Evans is suffering from acute renal failure and anuria. He is placed on a severe fluid restriction of 500 ml/day. He has received his full fluid allotment for the day, but is experiencing excessive thirst. You could recommend:
   1. Eating ice, since it does not count as fluid
   2. Chewing gum or brushing teeth often
   3. Drinking iced tea, since it is low in kilocalories
   4. Eating low-sodium bread

6. Mr. Slater is a cancer patient suffering from anorexia and weight loss. Which of the following suggestions may help Mr. Slater consume a higher kilocalorie diet?
   1. Eliminate between-meal snacks
   2. Eat high-kilocalorie foods first in each meal
   3. Eat larger portions at each meal
   4. Drink liquid nutritional supplements at room temperature

7. Jonathan Young has diabetes mellitus (IDDM). He is following a diet plan using the exchange lists for meal planning. For a bedtime snack Jonathan is allowed 1 milk serving, 1 starch serving, and 1 fruit serving. Which of the following snacks fits this pattern:
   1. 1 cup yogurt, ½ cup canned peaches, 3 graham cracker squares
   2. ½ cup cottage cheese, 1 cup orange juice, 1 glazed doughnut
   3. 1 grilled cheese sandwich, 1 apple
   4. ½ cup ice cream, 1 cup strawberries, 1 whole toasted bagel with jelly

8. Mrs. Wang is an obese, 50-year-old woman recently diagnosed with NIDDM. She is taking oral hypoglycemic agents daily and has been prescribed a 1500-kcal diabetic diet. The most important dietary factor for Mrs. Wang should be to:
   1. Avoid all sweets and concentrated carbohydrate sources
   2. Distribute carbohydrate evenly throughout the day to balance with medication
   3. Consume adequate protein during the bedtime snack to help prevent hypoglycemia during the night
   4. Control dietary intake of kilocalories and fat to help with the attainment of a healthy weight

9. During a visit to the doctor's office, Mrs. Oswald discusses her concerns that her 14-year-old daughter, Mary, may have an eating disorder. Which of the following statements by Mrs. Oswald might indicate the presence of an eating disorder:
   1. Does Mary look thinner to you? I'm afraid she is losing some weight. She seems more concerned about her appearance lately. I'm worried she may have an eating disorder.
   2. Mary is so irritable and withdrawn lately. She spends a lot of time alone in the bathroom and when she's not there, it seems she's always exercising. In fact, she'd rather exercise than go out with her friends!
   3. Mary eats so much junk food and then she will never eat the healthy food I make for dinner. She always wants to go to fast food restaurants and instead of eating school lunch, she'd rather buy a candy bar.
   4. Mary doesn't eat as much as she used to. She says she wants to lose some weight. Some of her friends are on diets and she wants to go on a diet with them.

10. A continuous-drip tube feeding has just been initiated on Janet Miller, a 20-year-old trauma patient. She is receiving an intact enteral formula through a nasogastric tube. One hour after initiation of the feeding she experiences nausea, cramps, and diaphoresis. These symptoms most likely indicate that:
    1. Janet is unable to tolerate an intact formula and should be placed on an elemental formula.
    2. Janet's GI tract is not functioning. The tube feeding should be discontinued and parenteral nutrition initiated.
    3. The formula strength and/or volume is too great. The formula should be diluted and administered at a slower rate.
    4. Janet is not able to tolerate the continuous drip mode of administration. Intermittent or bolus feedings would be more appropriate.

7

MEDICATION ADMINISTRATION

I want to be a nurse because I love caring for people. I don't like to see people hurting, so if I can do just one thing to make them feel better, I feel better. A diagnosis is a diagnosis, used many times, but every patient is a person, a person that needs individualized care. The older adult who tells me of his past, the smile when a patient goes home, the look of relief when the baby is here and everything is fine—every contact I make affects me. I hope my patients feel the same way about me as I feel about them.

Larisa Arnold
Student Nurse

20

MATHEMATICS REVIEW

Cynthia M. Davis

KEY TERMS

body surface area
denominator
extremes
means
milliequivalent
numerator
percent
proportion
ratio

LEARNING OBJECTIVES

After reading this chapter, the student should be able to do the following:

- Define key terms.
- Confidently use basic mathematical skills to solve dosage problems accurately.
- Set up and work problems using the formula:

$$\frac{\text{Desired dose}}{\text{Available dose}} \times \text{Amount}$$

- Set up and work problems using the proportion method.
- Use "key" equivalents of metric and apothecary measurement systems in dosage problems.
- Convert measurement units within the metric system.
- Convert between measurement units of the metric system and the apothecary system.
- Determine the appropriateness of dosage orders for children by the use of Young's, Clark's, and Fried's rule and the body surface area nomogram.

RELATED TOPICS OF INTEREST

- Documentation (Chapter 6)
- Medical asepsis and infection control (Chapter 12)
- Principles and practice of medication administration (Chapter 21)
- Basic pediatric nursing care (Chapter 43)

The nurse must accurately calculate drug dosages to provide safe medication administration to each patient. The review of basic mathematics section of this chapter will provide the LPN/LVN with a review of basic math, three measurement systems, two methods of solving dosage problems, and methods of determining the appropriateness of children's drug orders.

FRACTIONS

Are you afraid of fractions? Many students are. What *is* a fraction? A fraction is a "part" of a whole number. For example:

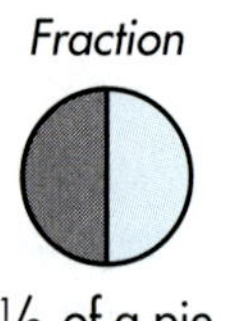

Definitions

numerator the "top" number of a fraction.
denominator the "bottom" number of a fraction.

Types of Fractions.

Proper fractions—the numerator is less than the denominator.

EXAMPLE: $\frac{1 \text{ Numerator}}{2 \text{ Denominator}}$

Improper fractions—the numerator is larger than the denominator.

EXAMPLE: $\frac{2 \text{ Numerator}}{1 \text{ Denominator}}$

Mixed fractions—consist of a whole number plus a fraction.

EXAMPLE: $1\frac{1}{2}$ 1 is the whole number; $\frac{1}{2}$ is the fraction

Changing an Improper Fraction to a Whole or Mixed Number.

RULE 1: Divide the denominator (bottom number) into the numerator (top number).

EXAMPLE: Change $\frac{10}{5}$ to a *whole* number.

$10 \div 5 = 2$ (a WHOLE number)

Change $\frac{40}{5}$ to a *whole* number.

$40 \div 5 = 8$ (a WHOLE number)

EXAMPLE: Change $\frac{20}{7}$ (an improper fraction) to a *mixed* number.

$$20 \div 7 = 7\overline{)20} = 2\frac{6}{7} \text{ (a MIXED number)}$$

$$\begin{array}{r} 2 \\ 7\overline{)20} \\ \underline{14} \\ 6 \\ \hline 7 \end{array}$$

Change $\frac{54}{5}$ to a *mixed* number.

$$54 \div 5 = 5\overline{)54}$$

$$\begin{array}{r} 10 \\ 5\overline{)54} \\ \underline{5} \\ \frac{4}{5} \end{array} = 10\frac{4}{5} \text{ (a MIXED number)}$$

Changing a Mixed Number to an Improper Fraction.

RULE 1: Multiply the denominator (bottom number) by the whole number.

RULE 2: Add numerator to the product; the sum is now the new number.

EXAMPLE: Change $2\frac{6}{7}$ (a mixed number) to an improper fraction.

Multiply the denominator 7 by the whole number 2.

$7 \times 2 = 14$ (The answer from numbers multiplied is called the *product.*)

Add the numerator to the product.

$6 + 14 = 20$ (The answer from numbers added is called the *sum.*)

Place the sum, 20, over the original denominator, 7, to have an improper fraction.

$$\frac{20}{7}$$

The mixed number $2\frac{6}{7}$ is now the improper fraction $\frac{20}{7}$.

Reducing Fractions to the Lowest Term.

Fractions are commonly reduced to the lowest term in which they can be expressed, because it is easier to work with smaller numbers. For example, $\frac{20}{80}$ or $\frac{25}{100}$, which can both be reduced to $\frac{1}{4}$, become more convenient to use in calculation.

RULE 1: Find a number that will evenly divide into the numerator *and* the denominator.

EXAMPLE: $\frac{2}{10}$

What number will divide into the numerator, 2?
2 will divide evenly into the numerator, 2, one time.
2 will divide into the denominator, 10, five times.

$\frac{2}{10} = \frac{1}{5}$ (Reduce all fractions to their lowest terms.)

EXAMPLE: $\frac{16}{60} = \frac{4}{15}$ (The number, 4, divides evenly into both the numerator and the denominator.)

Determining Which Fraction is Larger.

RULE 1: If the denominators are the *same,* the fraction with the *larger numerator* is the larger fraction.

PROBLEM: Which is larger? $\frac{4}{6}$ or $\frac{2}{6}$

$\frac{4}{6}$ is larger

RULE 2: If the denominators are *different,* such as $\frac{2}{5}$ and $\frac{1}{3}$, you must find a "common denominator." (Finding a common denominator means to find a number into which both denominators can be divided.) A common, or equivalent, will also be found.

PROBLEM: Find a common denominator for $\frac{2}{5}$ and $\frac{1}{3}$.

(Try multiplying the denominators to get a common denominator.)

EXAMPLE: $\frac{2}{5} = \frac{\ }{15}$ $\frac{1}{3} = \frac{\ }{15}$

PROBLEM: Which is larger? $\frac{2}{3}$ or $\frac{6}{8}$

$\frac{2}{3} = \frac{16}{24}$ $\frac{6}{8} = \frac{18}{24}$

$\frac{6}{8}$ is larger

RULE 3: After the common denominator is found, an equivalent numerator for each fraction must be found.

$\frac{2}{5} = \frac{?}{15}$ $\frac{1}{3} = \frac{?}{15}$

Find an equivalent numerator by dividing the first denominator into the equivalent denominator; multiply the answer by the first numerator.

EXAMPLE: $\frac{2}{5} = \frac{6}{15}$ $(15 \div 5 = 3; 3 \times 2 = 6)$

$\frac{1}{3} = \frac{5}{15}$ $(15 \div 3 = 5; 5 \times 1 = 5)$

RULE 4: Compare the two fractions.

PROBLEM: Which is larger? $\frac{6}{15}$ or $\frac{5}{15}$

$\frac{6}{15}$ is larger

Adding Fractions That Have the Same Denominator.

RULE 1: *Add* the numerators and place the sum of the numerators over the denominator.

EXAMPLE:

$$\frac{1}{6} + \frac{1}{6} = \frac{2}{6} = \frac{1}{3}$$

Adding Fractions That Have Different Denominators.

RULE 1: Find common denominators for all fractions in the problem.

EXAMPLE: $\frac{1}{3} = \frac{\ }{12}$ (3 and 4 will divide into 12; 12 is the common denominator.)

$+\frac{2}{4} = \frac{\ }{12}$

RULE 2: Find the equivalent numerators.

$\frac{1}{3} = \frac{4}{12}$ $(12 \div 3 = 4; 4 \times 1 = 4)$

$+\frac{2}{4} = \frac{6}{12}$ $(12 \div 4 = 3; 3 \times 2 = 6)$

$\frac{10}{12} = \frac{5}{6}$

$\frac{6}{20} = \frac{6}{20}$

$+\frac{12}{20} = \frac{12}{20}$

$\frac{18}{20} = \frac{9}{10}$

Adding Mixed Numbers.

RULE 1: Add the fractions of the mixed number. Then, add the sum of the fractions to the whole numbers.

EXAMPLE:

$$1\frac{2}{3} + 2\frac{1}{3} = 3\frac{3}{3} = 4$$

$1\frac{3}{5} = 1\frac{6}{10}$

$+4\frac{5}{10} = 4\frac{5}{10}$

$5\frac{11}{10} = 5 + 1 \text{ whole} + \frac{1}{10}$,

which $= 6\frac{1}{10}$

Subtracting Fractions with the Same Denominator.

RULE 1: Subtract the numerator and place it over the denominator in the answer.

EXAMPLE:

$$\frac{3}{5} - \frac{1}{5} = \frac{2}{5} \qquad \frac{4}{7} - \frac{2}{7} = \frac{2}{7}$$

Subtracting Fractions With Different Denominators.

RULE 1: Find a common denominator, then subtract. Hint: Try multiplying the two denominators as a way to find a common denominator.

EXAMPLE:

$$\begin{array}{r} \frac{3}{4} = \frac{9}{12} \\ -\frac{1}{3} = \frac{4}{12} \\ \hline \frac{5}{12} \end{array} \qquad \begin{array}{r} \frac{2}{3} = \frac{4}{6} \\ -\frac{1}{2} = \frac{3}{6} \\ \hline \frac{1}{6} \end{array}$$

Subtracting Mixed Numbers.

RULE 1: When the numerator of the top fraction is smaller than the bottom fraction, borrow one whole number from the whole number of the mixed fraction and express it as a fraction.

PROBLEM:

$$\begin{array}{r} 3\frac{9}{15} \\ -2\frac{10}{15} \\ \hline \end{array}$$

EXAMPLE: $3 = 2\frac{15}{15}$

RULE 2: Add the fraction of the original mixed number to the new fraction.

$$3\frac{9}{15} = 2\frac{15}{15} + \frac{9}{15} = 2\frac{24}{15}$$

RULE 3: Subtract fractions and whole numbers, if any.

$$\begin{array}{r} 2\frac{24}{15} - 2\frac{10}{15} \\ \hline \frac{14}{15} \end{array}$$

EXAMPLE:

$$\begin{array}{rl} 5\frac{6}{10} = 4\frac{10}{10} + \frac{6}{10} = & 4\frac{16}{10} \\ -3\frac{8}{10} = 3\frac{8}{10} & -3\frac{8}{10} \\ \hline & 1\frac{2}{10} \text{ or } 1\frac{1}{5} \end{array}$$

Multiplying Fractions.

RULE 1: Multiply the numerators; multiply the denominators.

EXAMPLE:

$$\frac{1}{2} \times \frac{3}{4} = \frac{1 \times 3}{2 \times 4} = \frac{3}{8}$$

$$\frac{4}{8} \times \frac{1}{3} = \frac{4 \times 1}{8 \times 3} = \frac{4}{24} = \frac{1}{6}$$

Multiplying Fractions and Mixed Numbers.

RULE 1: Change the mixed number to an improper fraction. (See the section on changing mixed numbers to improper fractions, p. 388.)

RULE 2: Multiply.

PROBLEM: Multiply $3\frac{1}{2}$ by $1\frac{2}{3}$

EXAMPLE: a. Change $3\frac{1}{2}$ and $1\frac{2}{3}$ to improper fractions.

$$3\frac{1}{2} = \frac{7}{2} \qquad 1\frac{2}{3} = \frac{5}{3}$$

b. Multiply.

$$\frac{7 \times 5}{2 \times 3} = \frac{35}{6} = 6\overline{)35} = 5\frac{5}{6}$$

(Long division: 35 ÷ 6 = 5, 30, remainder $\frac{5}{6}$)

PROBLEM: Multiply $1\frac{2}{3}$ by $2\frac{3}{4}$

EXAMPLE: $1\frac{2}{3} = \frac{5}{3} = 2\frac{3}{4} = \frac{11}{4}$

$$\frac{5}{3} \times \frac{11}{4} = \frac{55}{12} = 4\frac{7}{12}$$

Dividing Fractions.

RULE 1: Write the problem down *correctly;* invert the second fraction.

RULE 2: Multiply.

PROBLEM: Divide $\frac{1}{2}$ by $\frac{3}{4}$

EXAMPLE: a. Write the problem down *correctly.*

$$\frac{1}{2} \div \frac{3}{4}$$

b. Invert the second fraction; change the division sign to a multiplication sign; multiply.

$$\frac{1}{2} \times \frac{4}{3} = \frac{4}{6}$$

c. Reduce to the lowest terms.

$$\frac{4}{6} = \frac{2}{3}$$

Dividing Fraction and Whole Numbers.

RULE 1: Change the whole number to a fraction.

RULE 2: Divide.

PROBLEM: Divide 4 by $\frac{3}{5}$.

EXAMPLE: a. Change 4 to a fraction. Make 4 the numerator and use 1 as the denominator.

$$\frac{4}{1}$$

b. Invert second fraction; multiply.

$$\frac{4 \times 5}{1 \times 3} = \frac{20}{3}$$

c. Reduce to lowest terms.

$$\frac{20}{3} = 6\frac{2}{3} \qquad 3\overline{)20}\ \text{quotient } 6,\ \frac{18}{2},\ \frac{2}{3}$$

DECIMAL FRACTIONS

The decimal fraction is a type of fraction that uses a decimal to indicate the denominator of the fraction. The placement or position of the decimal point determines whether the denominator is 10, multiples of 10, or divisions of 10.

Names of Decimal Places

.00001	One-hundred thousandths
.0001	Ten thousandths
.001	Thousandths
.01	Hundredths
.1	Tenths
1.	Unit (whole numbers)
10	Tens
100	Hundreds
1,000	Thousands
10,000	Ten thousands
100,000	One-hundred thousands

RULE 1: A decimal point found left of a whole number means that the number is a *fraction* of a whole number.

EXAMPLE: 0.1 "Point one" is $\frac{1}{10}$ of the whole number, 1.

Hint: Place a zero left of the decimal point to avoid mistaking .1 with 1.
Correct placement of decimal points in drug dosages is *critical.*

RULE 2: A decimal point found *after* a number means that it is a whole number.

EXAMPLE: 5. = 5

RULE 3: A number *without* a decimal point is understood to have an "invisible" decimal point behind it.

EXAMPLE: 1 = 1.0

Adding Decimals.

RULE 1: Align the decimal point of each decimal fraction in a column.

RULE 2: Add.

PROBLEM: Add 3.34 and 0.6

EXAMPLE:

```
 3.34  Add decimal point in column; add.
+0.6
 3.94
 ↑ Make sure that the decimal point is
   aligned properly in the answer.
```

Hint: Zeroes may be added to the right of the decimal point if needed to help align the column. The value of the number is *not* changed by adding zeroes.

EXAMPLE: 1.00 = 1   5.0 = 5

Subtracting decimals.

RULE 1: Align the decimal points of each decimal fraction in a column.

RULE 2: Subtract.

PROBLEM: Subtract 7.45 from 15.

EXAMPLE: a. Align decimal points in column; subtract.

```
  15.00   (Note zeroes used to align the
 − 7.45    two columns.)
   7.55
```

Rounding a Number.

RULE 1: Numbers found after the decimal point that are 5 or larger can increase the number before it by one whole number.

EXAMPLE: 7.55 = 7.6 or 8

Hint: There are times when it is practical to round a volume of medication.

PROBLEM: How can 7.55 minims easily be given?

EXAMPLE: Round 7.55 to 8; give 8 minims.

Note: Minims are very small units of measurement. Milliliters/cubic centimeters are not rounded in this manner, since drug dosage would be altered.

Multiplying Decimals.

RULE 1: Multiply. Decimal points in the problem *do not* have to be aligned.

RULE 2: The decimal place in the answer is determined by how many numbers are found right of the decimal points in the numbers multiplied.

EXAMPLE:

```
     5.50
 ×   2.15   (There are 4 numbers found
     2750    after the decimal points; 2 on
     550     the top and 2 on the bottom.)
    1100
  11.8250x
   ↑____|  x = 11.8250 or 12 (rounded)
```

Note: A small "x" hereafter indicates the unexpressed decimal after a whole number or a decimal point that has been moved from one place to another.

Dividing Decimals.

RULE 1: Change a decimal fraction in the divisor to a whole number by moving the decimal point *all* the way to the right.

PROBLEM: Divide 2.5 by 1.5.

EXAMPLE: a. (divisor) 1.5⟌2.5 (dividend)
b. 1.5x⟌2.5 (15⟌2.5)

RULE 2: Move the decimal point in the dividend the *same number of places moved in the divisor.*

EXAMPLE: 1.5x⟌2.5x   The decimal point in the divisor is unexpressed after it is moved.

RULE 3: Place the decimal point in the answer directly over the decimal point in the dividend after moving the decimal point in the dividend.

EXAMPLE: $15\overline{)25.}$

RULE 4: If a decimal point is in the divisor, but not in the dividend (such as $.5\overline{)15}$), move it the same number of places as the divisor. Remember there is an unexpressed decimal point at the right of all whole numbers. Add zeroes after the decimal point in the dividend as needed.

EXAMPLE: $.5x\overline{)15.0x}$ $5\overline{)150.0}$

RULE 5: If the dividend contains a decimal fraction and the divisor does not, leave the divisor as it is.

EXAMPLE: $5\overline{)2.5}$ would remain unchanged.

Changing Fractions to Decimals.

RULE 1: Divide the numerator (the top number) by the denominator (the bottom number).

PROBLEM: Change $\frac{3}{4}$ to a decimal fraction.

EXAMPLE: $\frac{3}{4} = 4\overline{)3.00}$ = .75; 28; 20; 20

Changing a Decimal Fraction to a Common Fraction.

Decimal fractions are based on 10's, multiples of 10, and divisions of 10. The position or place of the decimal point indicates the denominator.

RULE 1: To change a decimal fraction to a common fraction, give the decimal fraction a denominator according to the position of the decimal point in the decimal fraction.

PROBLEM: Change .1 to a common fraction.

EXAMPLE: a. .1 (The decimal point is in the "tens" place; 10 is the denominator.)

$$\overline{10}$$

b. Now that the denominator is 10, place the 1 over it to make a common fraction.

$$\frac{1}{10}$$

PERCENTS

The word **percent** and its symbol, %, mean "hundredths." A hundredth is a fraction of a whole number; therefore a number followed by % is a *fraction*. The denominator of the fraction is understood to be 100.

EXAMPLE: 25% is the same as $\frac{25}{100}$

$\frac{25}{100}$ can be reduced to $\frac{1}{4}$

Changing a Percent to a Decimal Fraction.

RULE 1: Remove %; move the decimal point two places to the left to indicate "hundredths."

PROBLEM: Change 25% to a decimal fraction.

EXAMPLE: .25

Changing a Fraction to a Percent.

RULE 1: Change a fraction to a percent by dividing the numerator by the denominator.

RULE 2: Multiply the answer by 100.

RULE 3: Label the answer with the percent symbol.

EXAMPLE: $\frac{3}{4} = 4\overline{)3.00}$ = .75; 28; 20; 20

```
   100
×  .75
   500
  700
 75.00x
```

(There are two decimal places in this problem; move the decimal point in the answer two places to the left.)

75% Therefore $\frac{3}{4}$ = 75%

Multiplying by Percent.

RULE 1: Change percent to a decimal (move decimal point two places to the left).

RULE 2: Multiply.

PROBLEM: Multiply 80 by 7.5%.

EXAMPLE: 7.5% is .075

```
    80
× .075
   400
  560
  00
 6.000x
```

(Move decimal point three places to the left = 6)

RATIOS

Ratio shows the relationship of one number or quantity to another number or quantity. Numbers of a ratio are separated by a colon. A ratio is also a fraction. The value of a ratio is not changed if both terms are multiplied or divided by the same number.

EXAMPLE: 2:4 is the same as 1:2 or 4:8

When numbers are written in ratio, they must all be expressed in the same units.

EXAMPLE: 1 liter, 2 ounces, and 30 milliliters (ml) must all be expressed in the same way, as:

1000 ml:60 ml:30 ml

A fraction may be written as a ratio.

EXAMPLE: $\frac{1}{25} = 1:25 \quad \frac{3}{4} = 3:4$

Ratio is an important concept that is used in the following methods of calculating dosages.

PROPORTIONS

Proportion shows that the relationship between two ratios has equal value.

EXAMPLE: 1 is to 2 as 4 is to 8 or 1:2 :: 4: 8

Definitions

means the inner terms of the proportion.
extremes the outer terms of the proportion.

EXAMPLE: 1:2 :: 4:8 (means) 1:2 :: 4:8 (extremes)

Set up the left side of the proportion as the "known" side using information that is known or given. The known information will be:

EXAMPLE: a. An equivalent such as 60 milligrams = 1 grain (60 mg:1 gr)

or

b. A doctor's medication or IV order, such as "give 1000 ml in 8 hr" (1000 ml:8 hr)

or

c. A drug dosage you have on hand or available, such as information on a drug label that reads "50 mg/ml (50 mg:1 ml)"

PROBLEM: The doctor orders Demerol 25 mg q 3-4 hr prn for pain. On hand is a vial labeled "50 mg/1 ml."

RULE 1: Set up the known side.

EXAMPLE: 50 mg:1 (given on the label)

RULE 2: Set up the unknown side. Use x for what you are trying to find, such as "How many milliliters are needed to give 25 mg?"

	Known		**Unknown**
EXAMPLE:	50 mg:1 ml	::	25 mg:x ml

RULE 3: Set up the units, such as milligrams and milliliters, in the *same position on each side* of the problem.

EXAMPLE: ____ mg: ____ ml :: ____ mg: ____ ml

RULE 4: Multiply the means.
RULE 5: Multiply the extremes.

PROBLEM: 50 mg:1 ml::25 mg:x ml
EXAMPLE: Multiply the means.

50 mg:1 ml::25 mg:x ml
= 25

Multiply the extremes.

50 mg:1 ml::25 mg:x ml
50x = 25

RULE 6: Solve for x (divide the number with the x into the number on the opposite side of the problem).

EXAMPLE: 50 mg:1 ml::25 mg:x ml
50x = 25 = $50\overline{)25.0}$ = .5
x = .5

RULE 7: Label the answer with the unit of measurement that accompanies the x in the problem.

EXAMPLE: 50 mg:1 ml::25 mg:x ml
50x = 25
x = .5 ml

Review of Proportion Method.

1. Set up problems in the *same order* on both sides.
2. Multiply the means; multiply the extremes.
3. The number multiplied with the x is always that number with the x to the right of it.

   EXAMPLE: 2 mg: 1 ml: 5 mg:x ml

4. Divide the number with the x into the number on the other side of the problem.
5. Label the problem by looking to see what unit of measurement the x is with the proportion.

$$\frac{\textit{Desired dosage}}{\textit{Available dosage}} \times \textit{Amount method}$$

Many nurses use the following method of solving dosage problems.

RULE 1: Place the dose that the physician wants given over the dose that the nurse has available (on-hand).

PROBLEM: The physician orders 40 mg of furosemide (Lasix). The nurse has an ampule of furosemide labeled Lasix 20 mg/ml.

EXAMPLE: $\frac{\text{(Desired dosage) } 40 \text{ mg}}{\text{(Available dose) } 20 \text{ mg}} \times \frac{1 \text{ ml}}{1} = \frac{40}{20} =$
40 ÷ 20 = 2 ml

PROBLEM: The physician orders 15 mg of diazepam (Valium). The nurse has Valium tablets that contain 5 mg/tablet.

EXAMPLE:

$\frac{\text{(Desired dosage) } 15 \text{ mg}}{\text{(Available dose) } 5 \text{ mg}} \times \frac{1 \text{ tab}}{x \text{ tab}} = \frac{15}{5x} = x =$
15 ÷ 5 = 3 tablets

Box 20-1 NURSE ALERT

- There is no room for error in calculating dosages.
- Check math work with another nurse.
- Work problems systematically and carefully *on paper.*
- Reduce distractions while working problems.
- Recheck calculations.
- Is the answer reasonable?

See Box 20-1 on p. 393 for the nurse's responsibilities in solving dosage problems accurately.

THE METRIC SYSTEM

The metric system is the preferred system of weights and measures. It is more accurate and easier to use in calculating dosage problems.

Similar to the U.S. monetary system, which is based on the dollar, the metric system is also based on the decimal system. The decimal system uses the divisions and multiples of a unit, which is always in ratios of tens.

EXAMPLE:

1 dollar	=	10 dimes
10 dimes	=	20 nickles
20 nickles	=	100 pennies

All these units are multiples or divisions of tens.

The metric system uses the following basic units of volume, weight, and length:

liter (L) volume (amount) of fluids.
gram (g) weight of solids.
meter (m) measure of length.

Smaller units of the system are designated by the following prefixes:

deci 0.1 of the unit; tens (liter, gram, meter)
centi 0.01 of the units; hundredths
milli 0.001 of the unit; thousandths

Larger units of the system are designated with the following prefixes:

deka 10 times the unit (liter, gram, meter)
hecto 100 times the unit
kilo 1000 times the unit

Units of weight

1 gram (g)	= 1000 milligrams (mg)
0.001 gram (g)	= 1 milligram (mg)
1 kilogram (kg)	= 1000 grams (g)
0.001 kilogram (kg)	= 1 gram (g)

Units of volume

1 liter (L)	= 1000 milliliters (ml)
0.001 liter (L)	= 1 milliliter (ml)
1 milliliter (ml)	= 1 cubic centimeter (cc)

In addition to the preceding units of measurement, the nurse often encounters the term **milliequivalents,** abbreviated mEq. Milliequivalent refers to the concentration of electrolytes in a certain volume of solution, expressed as milliequivalents per liter (mEq/L). Potassium chloride (KCl) is an electrolyte that is sometimes ordered as an intravenous additive to a liter (1000 ml) of fluid. For example, the doctor orders:

Add 40 mEq KCl to 1 L D_5W to run at 125 ml/hr.

Approximate Equivalents of the Metric System and the Apothecary System

The apothecary system is a system of measurement that is still used by some physicians and hospitals. It is being replaced slowly by the metric system. Since it continues to be used, the following equivalents are needed to convert dosages from one system to another. The conversions are approximations only but are acceptable equivalents with which to work.

Volume.

Metric	**Apothecary**
1 milliliters (ml)	= 15 or 16 minims (♏ XV/XVI)
4 or 5 milliliters (ml)	= 1 fluid dram (f ʒ i̇)
30 milliliters (ml)	= 1 fluid ounce (f ℥ i̇)
500 milliliters (ml)	= pint (O i̇ or 1 pt)
1000 milliliters (ml) or 1 liter (L)	= 1 quart (1 Qt)

The symbols for the above apothecary units are:

Minim = ♏
Fluid dram = ʒ
Fluid ounce = ℥
Pint = O or pt
Quart = Qt

The symbols appear in front of the number (which is written in Roman numerals).

EXAMPLE: 16 minims is written ♏ XVI

Weight.

Metric	**Apothecary**
60 milligrams (mg)	= 1 grain (the symbol is gr. for grain)
1000 milligrams (mg)	= 15 grains (gr. XV)
4 grams (g or Gm)	= 1 dram (ʒ i̇)
30 grams (g)	= 1 ounce (℥ i̇)
0.45 kilogram (kg)	= 1 pound (lb)
1 kilogram (kg)	= 2.2 pounds (lb)

Convert from one system to another to work dosage problems in the same measurement units.

Metric Measurements of Length

The basic unit of length in the metric system is the meter. The meter is equal to 39.37 inches, about $3\frac{1}{2}$ inches longer than 1 yard (36 inches). Some of the tasks that the nurse will perform using the metric measurements of length will be to:

Measure area size for topical applications.
Measure results of intradermal skin tests (size of drug or allergen reaction on the skin).
Measure wound size.
Measure decubiti.
Measure height, length, and head circumference (such as is common in obstetrics and pediatrics).
Measure abdominal girth (obstetrics and patients with ascites and congestive heart failure).

Length.

0.001 meter	= 1 millimeter (mm)
0.01 meter	= 1 centimeter (cm)
0.1 meter	= 1 decimeter (dm)
10 meters	= 1 dekameter (dam)
100 meters	= 1 hectometer (hm)
1000 meters	= 1 kilometer (km)

Most frequently used equivalents are:

1 meter (m)	= 1000 millimeters (mm)
0.001 meter (m)	= 1 millimeter (mm)
1 meter (m)	= 100 centimeters (cm)
1 centimeter (cm)	= 10 millimeters (mm)
1 millimeter (mm)	= 0.1 centimeter (cm)

BIG TO SMALL RULE

Whatever method is used to solve dosage problems, the units of measurement in the problem must *always* be converted to the same unit of measurement.

Some students find it difficult to convert dosages that contain decimal fractions. Discussed here is a quick, easy method called the "big to small" rule. It is useful in converting dosages *within the same* system (the metric system).

Because there are 1000 ml in 1 L (and 1000 mg in 1 g), milliliters can be converted to liters (and milligrams to grams) by this method. Likewise, liters can be converted to milliliters (and grams to milligrams) by this method.

Converting Larger Units of Measurement to Smaller Units of Measurement (Grams to Milligrams; Liters to Milliliters).

RULE 1: Write down BIG → SMALL.

RULE 2: Place the large unit under the word BIG and the small unit under the word SMALL.

EXAMPLE: BIG ⟶ SMALL
2.5 g = — mg

RULE 3: Move the decimal point three places in the direction of the arrow; add zeroes.

EXAMPLE: BIG ⟶ SMALL
2.500 = 2500 mg

Converting Smaller Units of Measurement to Larger Units of Measurement (Milligrams to Grams; Milliliters to Liters).

RULE 1: Write down the big to small rule formula.

EXAMPLE: BIG → SMALL

RULE 2: Reverse the direction of the arrow.

EXAMPLE: BIG ← SMALL

RULE 3: Place the large unit under the word BIG and the small unit under the word SMALL.

EXAMPLE: BIG ← SMALL
x g = 2500 mg

RULE 4: Move the decimal point three places in the direction that the arrow points.

EXAMPLE: BIG ← SMALL
2.5 g = 2.500.

PEDIATRIC CONSIDERATIONS

Pediatric dosage refers to the determination of the correct amount, frequency, and total number of doses of a medication to be administered to a child or infant.

Age, weight, body surface area, and the ability of the child to absorb, metabolize, and excrete medication must be considered when administering medication to a child.

It is the physician's responsibility to determine medication orders and dosage for a pediatric patient, but the nurse must be able to recognize appropriate and inappropriate drug dosages and orders.

The nurse must be knowledgeable about the four standard formulas for calculating children's dosages. These are Young's rule, Clark's rule, Fried's rule, and the body surface area method.

Young's Rule

Young's rule is as follows:

$$\frac{\text{Age of child}}{\text{Age of child} + 12} \times \text{Average adult dose} = \text{Child's dose}$$

This rule applies to children up to the age of 12.

PROBLEM: The average adult dose of a particular medication is 50 mg. What is an appropriate dose of this medication for an 8-year-old child?

EXAMPLE:

$$\frac{8\text{ yr}}{8+12} \times 50\text{ mg} = \frac{8}{20} \times \frac{50}{1} = \frac{400}{20} = 20\overline{)400} = 20\text{ mg}$$

(long division: 400 ÷ 20 = 20; 40, 0, 0)

ANSWER: 20 mg is an appropriate dose.

Clark's Rule

Clark's rule is as follows:

$$\frac{\text{Weight of child}}{150} \text{ in pounds} \times \text{Average adult dose} = \text{Child's dose}$$

This rule uses the child's weight to determine dosage.

PROBLEM: The average adult dose of a particular medication is 25 mg. What is an appropriate dose of this medication for a child who weighs 40 pounds?

EXAMPLE:

$$\frac{40\text{ lb}}{150} \times 25\text{ mg} = \frac{40}{150} \times \frac{25}{1} = \frac{1000}{150} = 150\overline{)1000.00} = 6.66 = 6.7\text{ mg or } 7\text{ mg}$$

(long division: 1000.00 ÷ 150 = 6.66; 900, 1000, 900, 1000)

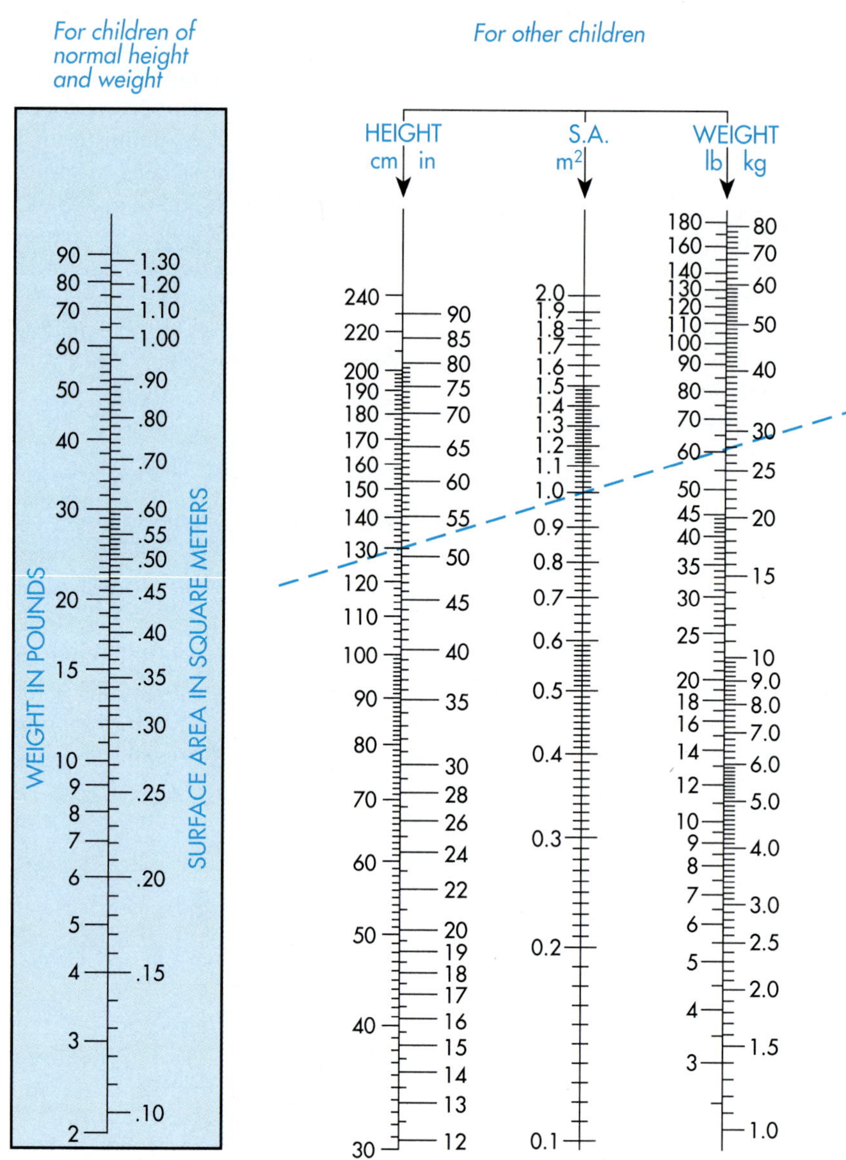

FIG. 20-1 Estimating body surface area in children. (From Behrman RE, Kliegman RM: *Nelson's Textbook of pediatrics,* ed 14, Philadelphia, 1992, Saunders.)

ANSWER: 6.7 or 7 mg is an appropriate dose.

Fried's Rule

Fried's rule is as follows:

$$\frac{\text{Age in months}}{150} \times \text{Average adult dose} = \text{Child's dose}$$

This rule is used for infants less than 2 years of age.

PROBLEM: The average adult dose of a particular medication is 25 mg. What is an appropriate dose of this medication for a child who is 22 months of age?

EXAMPLE:

$$\frac{22\text{ mo}}{150} \times 25\text{ mg} = \frac{550}{150} = 150\overline{)550.00} = 3.7 \text{ or } 4\text{ mg}$$

```
      3.66
150 ) 550.00
      450
      1000
       900
      1000
```

ANSWER: 3.7 or 4 mg is an appropriate dose.

Estimating Body Surface Area in Children

Body surface area is defined as the total area exposed to the outside environment. For pediatric patients of average size, body surface area may be estimated with the scale shown in Fig. 20-1. Match weight to the corresponding surface area. For other pediatric patients, use the other scale. Lay a straight edge on the correct height and weight points for your patient, and observe the point where it intersects on the surface area scale at center.[1]

PROBLEM: Trey, an 8-year-old, weighs 60 pounds and is 51 inches tall. His body surface area (as determined by using the nomogram, Fig. 20-1) is 1.0. If an adult dose is 50 mg, how many milligrams should Trey receive?

EXAMPLE: Use the formula:

$$\frac{SA(m^2)}{1.73\text{ m}^2} \times \text{Adult dose} = \text{Child's dose}$$

(Trey's surface area expressed in square meters = 1.0)

$$\frac{1.0}{1.73} \times 50\text{ mg} = \frac{1.0}{1.73} \times \frac{50}{1} = \frac{50}{1.73} = 1.73\overline{)50.00.00} = 29\text{ mg}$$

```
        28.9
1.73 ) 50.00.00
       356
       1440
       1384
         560
         557
           3
         173
```

ANSWER: 29 mg is appropriate for a child of Trey's height and weight.

Body surface area is used for determining pediatric dosages for burn patients in particular and also for determining radiation dosages.

REFERENCES AND SUGGESTED READINGS

1. Deglin JH, Russin MM, Vallerand AH: *Davis's drug guide for nurses,* ed 3, Philadelphia, 1993, FA Davis.
2. Dison N: *Simplified drugs and solutions for nurses,* ed 10, St Louis, 1992, Mosby.
3. LaRocca JC, Otto SE: *Pocket guide to intravenous therapy,* ed 2, St Louis, 1992, Mosby.
4. *Mosby's medical, nursing, and allied health dictionary,* ed 4, St Louis, 1994, Mosby.
5. Thomas CL: *Taber's cyclopedic medical dictionary,* ed 17, Philadelphia, 1993, FA Davis.
6. Tood CM, Erickson B: *Dosage calculations manual,* ed 2, Springhouse, Penn, 1992, Springhouse.

CHAPTER CHALLENGE

KEY POINTS

- The nurse must accurately calculate drug dosages to provide safe medication administration to each patient.
- A ratio shows the relationship of one number or quantity to another number or quantity.
- A proportion shows that the relationship between two ratios has equal value; extremes are the outer terms of the proportion, whereas means are the inner terms of the proportion.
- There is no room for error in calculating dosages; the nurse should check math work with another nurse, reduce distractions while working problems, and recheck calculations.
- The metric system is the preferred system of weights and measures; it is more accurate and easier to use in calculating dosage problems.
- Whatever method is used to solve dosage problems, the unit of measurement in the problem must always be converted to the same unit of measurement.
- Age, weight, body surface area, and the ability of the body to absorb, metabolize, and excrete medication must be considered when administering medication to a child.
- The nurse must be knowledgeable about the four standard formulas for calculating children's dosages; Young's rule, Clark's rule, Fried's rule, and body surface area method.

STUDY QUESTIONS

Work the following problems. Use the *proportion method* or *desired dose/available dose* formula, *key equivalents,* and the *big to small rule.*

1. The physician has ordered 0.5 g of ampicillin. You have available a vial labeled 250 mg/ml. How many milliliters will you give your patient:
   1. 2 ml
   2. 0.2 ml
   3. 0.05 ml
   4. 0.5 ml
2. Digoxin (Lanoxin) 0.125 mg is ordered. On hand is Lanoxin 0.5 mg/ml. How many milliliters will be given:
   1. 3 ml
   2. 0.25 ml
   3. 2.5 ml
   4. 0.025 ml
3. Mrs. Brown is to give her child 6 ml of a liquid medication. Her only measuring tool in her new apartment is a teaspoon. How many teaspoons of the medication should she give:
   1. 1 t
   2. 2 t
   3. 3 t
   4. ½ t
4. The pediatrician has requested Tim's weight in kilograms. Your scales say that Tim weighs 30 lb. How many kilograms will be reported to the physician:
   1. 20.6 kg
   2. 15 kg
   3. 13.6 kg
   4. 22 kg

Work these problems using the *proportion method.* Multiply milliliters by the drip factor to convert milliliters to drops.

1. Ordered is 1 L of D_5W to run over 8 hours. The drip factor stated on the IV tubing is 15 gtt/ml. How many milliliters will be infused every hour:
   1. 100/hr
   2. 125/hr
   3. 150/hr
   4. 175/hr
2. An IV of 1 L D_5 1/2 NS is to run at 150 ml/hr. How many hours will this IV run:
   1. 6 hr
   2. 6.6 hr
   3. 7.5 hr
   4. 8 hr
3. At 3 PM an 8-hour bag of 1 L D_5LR, which was started at 9 AM, has 100 ml left in the bag. Does this infusion need to run slower or faster or is it running at the correct rate:
   1. Needs to infuse slower
   2. Needs to infuse faster
   3. Is at the correct rate
   4. Needs to be discontinued

Insulin may be given in a tuberculin syringe if there are no insulin syringes available or if the dose to be given is extremely small. All insulin is now 100 units per milliliter. Use the *proportion method* to work these problems. (Hint: 100 U : 1 ml is the "known" in every problem.)

1. The physician orders 30 U of insulin. Using a tuberculin syringe, you will give how much of a milliliter:
   1. 0.03 ml
   2. 3.0 ml
   3. 0.3 ml
   4. 0.003 ml
2. The physician orders 50 U of insulin given. What part of a milliliter will be given:
   1. 5/100 of 1 ml
   2. 5/1000 of 1 ml
   3. 5/10,000 of 1 ml
   4. 5/10 of 1 ml
3. How many minims will be given in problem 2:
   1. 6 ♍
   2. 5 ♍
   3. 8 ♍
   4. 16 ♍
4. The nurse calculates that 8 ♍ is the correct amount that the physician has ordered. Cathy asks another LPN, "What part of a milliliter is 8 minims?" The correct answer given by the LPN was:
   1. 0.5 ml
   2. More than 0.5 ml
   3. 1 ml
   4. More than 1 ml
5. Dr. Wertz wants 15 U of insulin given. What part of a milliliter is this:
   1. 0.015 ml
   2. 0.15 ml
   3. 1.5 ml
   d. 15 ml

Are the following doses appropriate for these children?

1. Dr. Green orders 50 mg of meperidine HCl (Demerol) for Andrea, an 8-year-old. Is 50 mg appropriate for her age (the average adult dose of Demerol is 75 mg):
   1. 10 mg is appropriate
   2. 20 mg is appropriate
   3. 30 mg is appropriate
   4. 50 mg is appropriate
2. Dr. Jones ordered 125 mg of acetaminophen (Tylenol) for a 2-month-old infant who weighs 10 lb. Is this appropriate (the average adult dose of Tylenol is 500 mg):
   1. It is appropriate
   2. It is a little too much
   3. It is an extreme overdose
   4. It is not enough
3. The average dose of a medication is 0.4 mg (gr 1/150) for an adult. What is the dosage for a 12-year-old:
   1. 2 mg
   2. 0.002 mg
   3. 0.02 mg
   4. 0.2 mg
4. An adult dose of diazepam (Valium) is 5 mg. John weights 27 kilograms. How many milligrams is appropriate for John:
   1. 2 mg
   2. 1.5 mg
   3. 3 mg
   4. 2.5 mg

21

PRINCIPLES AND PRACTICE OF MEDICATION ADMINISTRATION

Cynthia M. Davis

KEY TERMS

adverse drug reaction
agonist
anaphylactic shock
antagonist
buccal
compatibility
cumulative
drip factor
drug interaction
enteral
enteric-coated
graduated
gauge
idiosyncratic
intermittent peripheral infusion device
lumen
metabolite
meniscus
parenteral
patient-controlled analgesia
percutaneous
pharmacology
potentiation
pulverized
souffle cup
sublingual
therapeutic
tolerance
topical application

LEARNING OBJECTIVES

After reading this chapter, the student should be able to do the following:

- Define the key terms.
- Explain each phase of drug action.
- Explain the importance of decreased hepatic and renal functioning.
- Discuss drug dosage.
- Discuss minimal dosage.
- Discuss maximal dosage.
- Discuss toxic dosage.
- Discuss lethal dosage.
- Discuss potentiation.
- Explain the importance of an antagonist counteracting an agonist.
- Describe factors to consider in choosing routes of administration.
- List the "five rights" of drug administration.
- Describe five factors that affect drug action in patients.
- Describe the importance of the accurate transcription of medication orders.
- Give the order of priority in the following terms: stat, ASAP, SOS, now, and prn.
- Explain what is meant by a controlled substance.
- List three ways medication orders are given.

RELATED TOPICS OF INTEREST

- Legal aspects of nursing (Chapter 2)
- Documentation (Chapter 6)
- Life span development (Chapter 7)
- Medical asepsis and infection control (Chapter 12)
- Comfort, rest, and sleep (Chapter 15)
- Mathematics review (Chapter 20)

PRINCIPLES OF PHARMACOLOGY

Pharmacology is the study of drugs and their action on the living body. Substances derived from plants and animals, from vitamins and minerals, and from synthetic (artificial) sources can be used as drugs in the treatment and prevention of disease; in the restoration and maintenance of the healthy functioning of body tissues, organs, and systems; and in diagnostic procedures.

The action of any drug on the body is a complicated process. This process begins with the pharmaceutical phase—the making of the drug until absorption of the drug takes place in the patient's body. Absorption occurs when the active ingredient of the drug enters the body fluids.

The pharmacokinetic phase involves the movement or distribution of the drug's active ingredients from the body fluids to the site where the intended action of the drug takes place.

In the pharmacodynamic phase the drug's active ingredient interacts with the intended body tissues. The body's cells respond to the action of the drug and change as the drug is metabolized.

The liver is the main organ that inactivates and metabolizes drugs; the kidneys are the principal organs that eliminate the metabolites of drugs from the body. **Metabolites** are substances produced by metabolic action.

The nurse must understand the process of drug action and elimination from the body, because each patient will be affected differently by the medications prescribed. Each patient's hepatic (liver) and renal (kidney) functions must be assessed and considered, because decreased hepatic and/or renal function may prolong the length of time a drug stays in the body.

Drugs that are not excreted in the urine, feces, sweat, tears, breast milk (in lactating mothers), and expired air may build up in the body. A drug that builds up in the body is said to have a **cumulative** effect, which can lead to *toxic* (harmful) or even lethal (deadly) effects.

Drug Dosage

Dosage is the amount of a drug prescribed for the patient by the physician (e.g., "Give 300 mg Dilantin po tid").

Three hundred milligrams is the dosage ordered in the example. The nurse will give three doses of Dilantin po three times a day. Each dose contains 100 mg per capsule. A *dose* of medicine refers to a single prescribed amount of drug given at one time. Nurses must become familiar with **therapeutic** (beneficial) dosages of frequently used drugs to confidently administer doses of medication to each patient (Box 21-1).

Box 21-1 DOSAGE TERMS

Minimal dose: The smallest amount of a drug that produces a therapeutic effect

Maximal dose: The largest amount of a drug that can be given safely

Toxic dose: The amount of a drug that produces signs and symptoms of poisoning

Lethal dose: The amount of a drug that will cause death

From Asperheim M: *Pharmacology: an introductory text,* ed 6, Philadelphia, 1987, Saunders.

Drug Actions and Interactions

There are two general types of drug action—local and systemic. Drugs that produce a local action affect only the area where the drug is placed. Systemic drug action affects the entire body, because the drug enters the systemic circulation.

When one drug alters the action of another drug, it is called a *drug interaction*. When two or more drugs are given together, the combined actions of the drugs may produce a totally different effect than the expected effect of either drug. These effects can be beneficial or harmful. When one drug increases the action or the effect of another drug, it is called **potentiation** or synergism. This is often done purposely to "boost" the action of one or the other of the drugs administered.

Some drugs *do not* combine chemically with other drugs. This is called drug *incompatibility*. For example, when two drugs are mixed and the solution changes color, becomes cloudy, or forms a precipitate (solid mass), incompatibility is suspected. **Compatibility** (the quality or state of existing together in harmony) charts allow quick reference to determine whether one drug may be given along with another drug in the same syringe or intravenous infusion.

Knowledge of agonistic and antagonistic drug action is helpful to the nurse and physician. A drug that produces a predictable response at the intended site of action is called an **agonist.** An **antagonist** is a drug that will block the action of another drug. Antagonistic drugs are used to counteract the effects of a previously given drug. For example, naloxone HCl (Narcan) works against the central nervous system depressant effects of meperidine HCl (Demerol) or other central nervous system depressants by blocking the action of the depressants.

Because each patient responds differently to medications, the nurse must be alert to the possibility of idiosyncratic drug reactions. An **idiosyncratic** response to a drug is an individual's unique hypersensitivity to a particular drug. It is an unexpected response to a medication. Idiosyncratic reactions are thought to have a genetic basis. An idiosyncratic reaction to a sedative that was given to produce calmness may unexpectedly cause the patient to become agitated and restless. For this reason, it is important to observe and assess patients for signs of overdose, toxicity, and unexpected drug reactions even though they are receiving the correct therapeutic dose.

A patient may be hypersensitive or allergic to a drug. The nurse should assess the patient's drug history *before* giving a drug. Has the patient taken the drug before? Does the patient have any known allergies to medications? If so, the drug should be withheld and this information reported to the charge nurse. When in doubt, "Don't."

A reduced response to a drug is called drug **tolerance.** The patient who has developed tolerance to a drug requires a larger dose of the drug to achieve the same effect that a smaller therapeutic dose once gave. Drug tolerance may either be acquired from taking increasing dosages of the drug over a period of time or result from genetic factors unique to the individual.

Drug administration is a tremendous nursing responsibility. The nurse must not give any unfamiliar medication and should look up the medication in a drug reference book *before* giving it to the patient.

Each patient's reaction to drug therapy must be observed, particularly when the patient is given a drug for the first time. The patient's mental and physical status must be assessed before a new medication is started to establish a baseline reference. Changes in mental or physical status should be reported to the RN. The change may be caused by an **adverse drug reaction** (a harmful, unintended reaction to a drug administered at a normal dosage), drug hypersensitivity, or drug intolerance.

The *Physicians' Desk Reference (PDR)* is a book usually found in the nurses' station. It can be used to find therapeutic dosage, indications for use of the drug, contraindications (conditions in which the drug should *not* be used), side effects, routes, generic and trade names, a list of poison control centers, and information for managing overdosages.

Drug interactions (a modification of the effect of a drug when administered with another drug) are more likely to occur with drugs that are especially potent (strong), such as digitalis. The cardiotonics (drugs that slow and strengthen the heart), antihypertensives (drugs that lower blood pressure), hypoglycemic agents (oral medications that lower blood glucose [sugar]), insulin (injectable medication that lowers blood glucose), and heparin (medication that decreases the clotting of blood) are all powerful agents that the nurse must be familiar with *before* giving. In drug interactions, the effect may be an increase or a decrease in the action of either substance, or it may be an adverse effect that is not normally associated with either drug. The particular interaction may be the result of a chemical-physical incompatibility of the two drugs or of a change in the rate of absorption or the quantity absorbed in the body.

Clayton and Stock[4] state that drug interactions are a frequent cause of adverse effects, decreased patient compliance, and prolonged hospitalizations. Continual awareness of the possibility of interactions and observation for these complications are the responsibility of all health professionals. The nurse should watch for changes in level of consciousness such as slurred speech or ataxia (unsteady gait) and for changes in vital signs. The nurse should *listen* to what the patient says about the medication's effects. The LPN/LVN reports observations to the RN and documents these observations objectively in the nurse's notes. Physicians depend on the ongoing nursing assessment of each patient's response to drug therapy.

The following factors affect how patients respond to medication and must be considered in patient assessment:

- *Age:* Very young and very old people generally react more acutely to drugs than others. Older persons tend to have a higher ratio of fat tissue to muscle tissue, and the higher fat percentage may affect the distribution and accumulation of fat-soluble drugs. Prolonged drug action is likely to occur in older adults, because renal and hepatic function may be decreased (Table 21-1 on p. 402). The very young do not have fully developed renal and hepatic functions; therefore drugs are inefficiently metabolized and excreted.
- *Weight:* Overweight persons may require higher drug dosages than those of average weight. Underweight individuals usually require lower drug dosages. Body surface area, height, and weight are important factors in determining drug dosages in children (see Chapter 43).
- *Physical health:* Persons in poor physical health do not tolerate average dosages as well as those in good health. Disease processes alter dosage requirements, particularly in patients with renal, hepatic, cardiovascular, and gastrointestinal (GI) dysfunctions.
- *Psychological status:* Stress, emotional conflict, anxiety, and fear may alter response to drug therapy. If the patient has faith in the drug, the hospital, the physician, and the nurse, he is more likely to adhere to the medication therapy. The nurse's actions, attitudes, and skills also affect the patient's response to drug therapy.
- *Environmental temperature:* Heat may increase the metabolism of a drug; cold may decrease the metabolic rate.
- *Gender:* Women tend to have a higher percentage of body fat than men, whereas men have a higher percentage of body fluid. Since some drugs are fat soluble, females with high body fat percentage may accumulate fat-soluble drugs in their body. Pregnant and lactating women must be advised that the substances taken during pregnancy may pass through the placenta and adversely affect the fetus. Drugs may also be passed to infants through breast milk.

TABLE 21-1 Influence of Drug Actions in Older Adults

Physiological Change	Drug Action/Patient Response	Nursing Interventions
Gastrointestinal tract		
Oral cavity		
Loss of elasticity in oral mucosa, which becomes dry and easily abraded	Difficulty in swallowing tablets or capsules; sensitivity to drugs that cause dryness of mouth; susceptibility to gum disease and dental caries	Have patient rinse oral cavity frequently with tepid clear water, floss daily, and brush teeth and gums gently. Recommend substitute saliva.
Esophagus		
Delayed esophageal clearance because of weakened contractions and failure of lower esophageal sphincter to relax	Difficulty in swallowing large tablets or capsules; tissue erosion caused by drugs such as aspirin and uncoated potassium chloride	Position patient upright. Administer full glass of liquid with drug. Crush tablets and mix with food (if gastric pH does not affect absorption).
Stomach		
Decrease in gastric acidity and peristalsis	Potentiation of irritating effects of highly acidic drugs (e.g., aspirin)	Have patient drink full glass of water and take medication with nonfat snack to reduce gastric distress.
Large intestine		
Reduced colon muscle tone; loss of defecation reflex; decreased intestinal blood flow	Slowing of drug excretion; overuse and abuse of laxatives by patient; delayed drug absorption	Provide normal fluid intake. Instruct patient to eat bulk-forming foods and avoid use of constipating drugs
Skin and vascular system		
Reduced SQ skinfold thickness in extremities (less body fat); reduced elasticity in skin and vascular system	Fragile blood vessels; patient prone to bleeding after injection	Avoid using veins in hand for IV injections. Apply pressure to injection sites after administration. Observe injection sites for bleeding
Liver		
Reduced liver size; decline in hepatic blood flow	Longer biotransformation time; longer-than-normal duration of drug action; greater risk for drug sensitivity and toxicity	Monitor for signs and symptoms of liver impairment (jaundice, pruritus, dark urine).
Kidneys		
Reduced glomerular filtration; decreased tubular function and renal blood flow	Risk of drug accumulation and toxicity	Prevent urinary retention (keep catheters free flowing and observe frequency of urination). Monitor for signs and symptoms of renal impairment (reduced output and difficulty in urinating).

- *Amount of food in the stomach:* Drugs taken on an empty stomach reach the bloodstream faster than those taken on a full stomach. Irritating drugs are given after or with meals so that they will not irritate the gastrointestinal tract.
- *Dosage forms:* Dosage forms influence the onset, intensity, and duration of a drug. Intravenous and intramuscular drugs react more quickly than drugs taken orally.

It is important to continually assess and evaluate drug action in each individual patient. The nurse must use judgment before giving medications, because any drug can be harmful.

The nurse must be knowledgeable about the basics of drug action, how drug orders are written, how to interpret them, and how they are transcribed. The basic practices and principles of safe medication administration must *always* be followed. High personal and professional standards protect the patient and prevent the nurse from making medication errors.

Medication Orders

The nurse is ethically and legally responsible for ensuring that the patient receives the correct medication ordered by the physician. Physicians write medication orders during patient admissions, during morning and evening rounds, after surgery, and any other time throughout the day or night as needed. As soon as possible after a physician writes an order, the nurse should read and interpret the order. The nurse then transcribes the drug order to the Medex (or Kardex, depending on the facility) *exactly* the same way that the order appears on the order sheet. If the handwriting is illegible, another nurse should be asked to help or the physician called for clarification.

The medication request for the patient's medications is sent to the pharmacy. The pharmacist will prepare and send the medications to the patient's unit.

Some drugs come in multidose vials or bottles; others come in unit dose (one dose per vial or package). The unit dose system was instituted to reduce medication errors and to make it easier to keep accurate records of medications used and not used. For example, if a patient goes home or dies, the unused unit dose medications are returned to the pharmacy for credit to the patient's account.

Whether unit dose or multidose is used, it is the nurse's responsibility to properly store medications on the ward. The storage instructions of each drug must be followed; some must be refrigerated, whereas others must be kept in a dark or cool area. Narcotics, barbiturates, and other controlled drugs that have a high potential for abuse must be safely and securely stored.

Frequently the drug received on the ward has a different name than that ordered by the physician. Each drug has several names; the two most commonly used are the trade name and the generic name. The trade name is the brand name given to it by the manufacturer. It is followed by the symbol ®. The trade name is short and easy to spell and to pronounce, such as "Demerol." It is capitalized. The generic name, frequently used, is usually longer, is not capitalized, and is used by the manufacturer. The generic name for Demerol is meperidine.

The nurse must make certain that the drug received is the same drug that was ordered. The pharmacist should be consulted if there is a question about the identity of a drug. Once assured that the medication is the correct one, the nurse clearly and accurately transcribes the medication name, dosage, times, and stop date on the Medex. In many facilities unit clerks transcribe drug orders. The RN or LPN/LVN who transcribes or verifies the order writes her signature and title and the time and date immediately after the last order on the order sheet. The nurse draws a line after the last order to indicate the end of that physician's particular order.

Medication orders should include the following:

1. Patient's name (on physician's order sheet)
2. Date and time of the order (usually on the left side of the order sheet); written by the physician
3. Name of drug
4. Dosage of the drug (e.g., give ASA grains [gr] X prn q 3-4 hr)
5. Route of administration (if none is given, it is understood to be by mouth)
6. Time or frequency drug is given (e.g., give bid [two times a day])
7. Signature of the physician
8. Any special instructions regarding any aspect of administering the drug (e.g., give ASA grains [gr] X q 3-4 hr if temp >101° F)

See Box 21-2 for common terms used with medication orders.

One-time-only orders, such as stat, now, ASAP, or SOS, are signed off on the physician's order sheet by the RN as soon as possible after the medication has been given. Doing so prevents another nurse from "double-dosing" the patient as a result of poor communication between nurses. If the order is written on the Medex (Fig. 21-1 on p. 404), the nurse must properly transcribe the order and discontinue the order immediately after giving the medication (see Medex examples).

Controlled Substances. Narcotics, barbiturates, and other controlled drugs that have a high possibility for abuse or addiction are double-locked. The "narcotic

Box 21-2 COMMON TERMS USED WITH MEDICATION ORDERS

STAT: Immediately; number one priority; give before any other type of order. Be careful to document that the medication was given to avoid mistakes. A "Stat" order is a one-time only dose.

Now: Give now; number two priority; give before orders of lower priority. Cancel order after giving.

ASAP: As soon as possible; number three priority; give before orders of lower priority. Cancel order after giving.

SOS: One time only, if needed; may be given *only* one time, *and if* it is needed according to the patient's wishes or according to the nurse's assessment of the patient's need. Cancel order after giving.

PRN: Give as necessary; the patient may request prn medication, or the nurse may offer a prn medication; prn medications should have a definite time interval within which the medication is to be given.

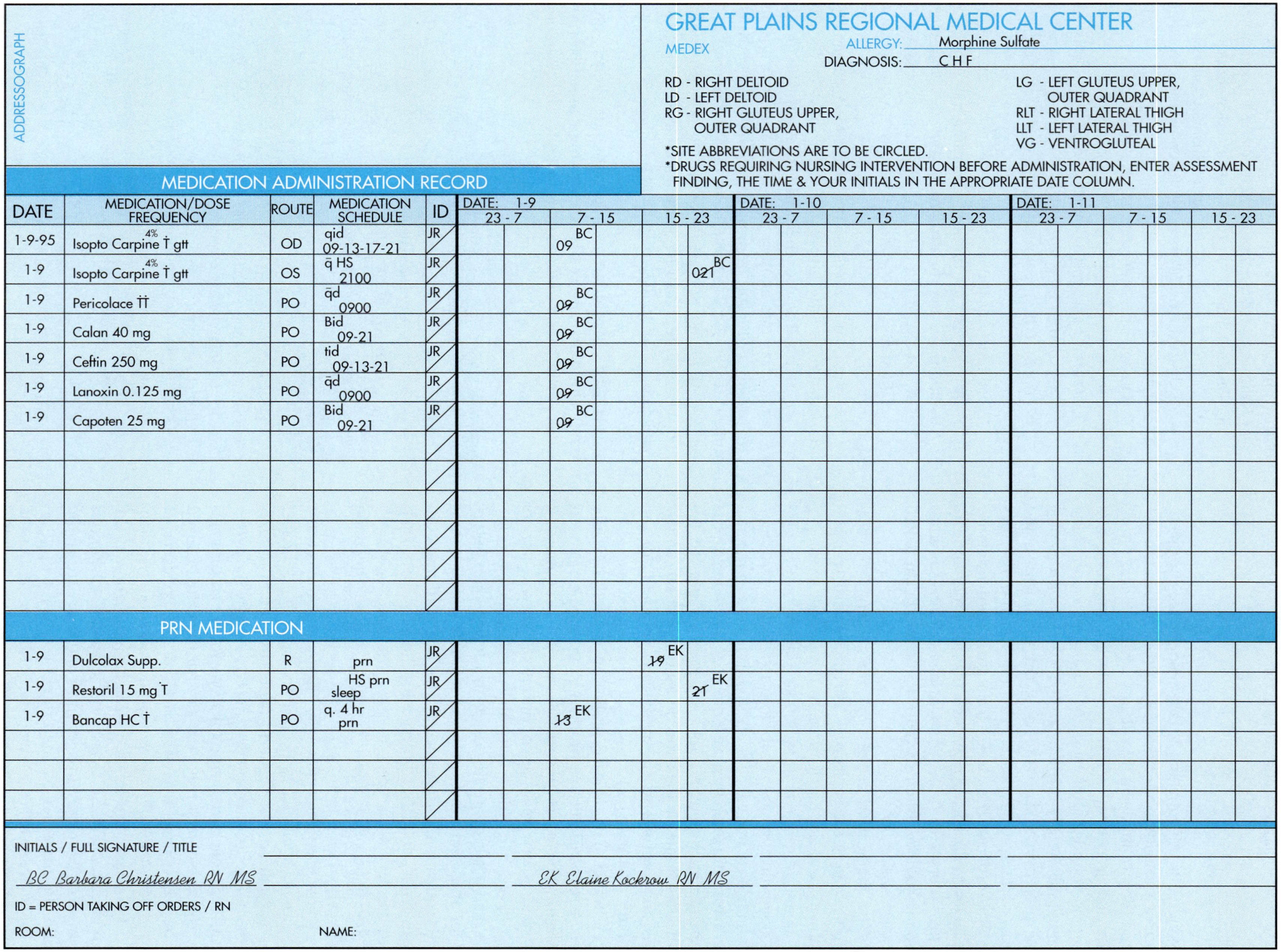

ADDRESSOGRAPH

GREAT PLAINS REGIONAL MEDICAL CENTER

MEDEX

ALLERGY: Morphine Sulfate

DIAGNOSIS: C H F

RD - RIGHT DELTOID
LD - LEFT DELTOID
RG - RIGHT GLUTEUS UPPER, OUTER QUADRANT
LG - LEFT GLUTEUS UPPER, OUTER QUADRANT
RLT - RIGHT LATERAL THIGH
LLT - LEFT LATERAL THIGH
VG - VENTROGLUTEAL

*SITE ABBREVIATIONS ARE TO BE CIRCLED.
*DRUGS REQUIRING NURSING INTERVENTION BEFORE ADMINISTRATION, ENTER ASSESSMENT FINDING, THE TIME & YOUR INITIALS IN THE APPROPRIATE DATE COLUMN.

MEDICATION ADMINISTRATION RECORD

DATE	MEDICATION/DOSE FREQUENCY	ROUTE	MEDICATION SCHEDULE	ID	DATE: 1-9			DATE: 1-10			DATE: 1-11		
					23 - 7	7 - 15	15 - 23	23 - 7	7 - 15	15 - 23	23 - 7	7 - 15	15 - 23
1-9-95	Isopto Carpine 4% ↑ gtt	OD	qid 09-13-17-21	JR		09 BC							
1-9	Isopto Carpine 4% ↑ gtt	OS	q̄ HS 2100	JR			021 BC						
1-9	Pericolace ↑↑	PO	q̄d 0900	JR		09 BC							
1-9	Calan 40 mg	PO	Bid 09-21	JR		09 BC							
1-9	Ceftin 250 mg	PO	tid 09-13-21	JR		09 BC							
1-9	Lanoxin 0.125 mg	PO	q̄d 0900	JR		09 BC							
1-9	Capoten 25 mg	PO	Bid 09-21	JR		09 BC							
PRN MEDICATION													
1-9	Dulcolax Supp.	R	prn	JR			19 EK						
1-9	Restoril 15 mg ↑	PO	HS prn sleep	JR			21 EK						
1-9	Bancap HC ↑	PO	q. 4 hr prn	JR		13 EK							

INITIALS / FULL SIGNATURE / TITLE

BC Barbara Christensen RN MS

EK Elaine Kockrow RN MS

ID = PERSON TAKING OFF ORDERS / RN

ROOM: NAME:

FIG. 21-1 Medication record.

keys" are kept by one designated nurse per shift. It is that nurse's responsibility to see that each controlled drug used that shift is logged in the narcotic log book. At the end of each shift controlled drugs in the locker are carefully counted by the key-holding nurse of the outgoing shift and the nurse of the incoming shift. The number of drugs given, according to the log book, and the actual number of medications contained in the locker *must* be exactly the same. The staff are *not* dismissed until the narcotic count is done. If the count is incorrect, the error or the missing drug must be found before anyone is dismissed. The nurse *must not* take the keys home.

The nurse should always have a witness to the "wasting" (disposal) of part of a controlled medication. The witness and the person wasting the medication must sign the log book to indicate that the medication was wasted. Controlled substances are handled only by people with licenses, such as an RN, an LPN/LVN or a student nurse under the supervision of the nurse educator (Box 21-3).

Types of Orders

Standing Orders. Standing orders are already written by a physician for all patients on a particular unit or area. They are carried out without having to call the physician and without the presence of the physician. A copy of the orders is kept on the unit. The nurse should know where the orders are located, be knowledgeable about standing orders, and use assessment and judgment skills in implementing these orders. A patient may be unnecessarily stressed or uncomfortable if the nurse is unaware that the physician has left standing orders. If there is *any* question about a standing order, the nurse should get verification or clarification from the physician who wrote them. Each physician leaves different standing orders; the nurse *must know* the physicians' orders.

There are two types of standing orders:

Standing order with expiration: The order is written and kept in a folder at the nurses' station. The order must be discontinued or reordered on the expiration date.

Standing order without expiration: The order is written and kept in a folder at the nurses' station, but no expiration date is given.

Box 21-3 GUIDELINES FOR SAFE NARCOTIC ADMINISTRATION AND CONTROL

- Store all narcotics in a locked, secure cabinet or container. (Computerized, locked cabinets are now available.)
- Nurses in charge carry a set of keys (or a special computer entry code) for the narcotics cabinet.
- During an institution's change-of-shift, the nurse going off duty counts all narcotics with the nurse coming on duty. Both nurses sign the narcotic record to indicate that the count is correct.
- Discrepancies in narcotic counts are reported immediately.
- A special inventory record is used each time a narcotic is dispensed.
- The record is used to document the patient's name, date, time of drug administration, name of drug, dosage, and signature of nurse dispensing the drug.
- The form provides an accurate ongoing count of narcotics used and remaining.
- If only one part of a premeasured dosage of a controlled substance is given, a second nurse witnesses disposal of the unused portion and documents such on the record form.

Verbal Orders. A verbal order from a physician may be given in the presence of an LPN/LVN or an RN directly or over the telephone. Hospital policy for LPNs/LVNs taking verbal and telephone orders should be observed. Verbal orders are written on the physicians' order sheet exactly as the physician gave them. The physician should sign the order as soon as possible. The nurse should be alert and careful when taking verbal orders. If the order is unclear or confusing, the nurse should not hesitate to ask the physician about the order. The nurse should always repeat the order to the physician to make sure that what was heard is what the physician actually said.

GENERAL PRINCIPLES AND PRACTICES OF MEDICATION ADMINISTRATION

The nurse uses each step of the nursing process in carrying out the responsibilities of drug administration.

Drugs are administered in a variety of ways. Regardless of the route by which a drug enters the body, the same practices and principles of medication administration apply.

Following the "five rights," performing the "three label checks," using universal precautions, and practicing good handwashing and aseptic technique ensure excellent drug administration practice.

The "five rights" are followed every time a drug is given (Box 21-4 on p. 406).

The Right Medication

The nurse must make sure the drug to be given is the correct drug, checking the label on its container three times (Box 21-5 on p. 406).

The nurse should *never* give a medication that has been prepared by another person and *never* prepare or

Box 21-4 THE FIVE RIGHTS OF MEDICATION ADMINISTRATION

1. Give the *right medication* in the
2. *Right dose* to the
3. *Right patient* at the
4. *Right time* by the
5. *Right route*

Box 21-5 THE THREE LABEL CHECKS OF MEDICATION ADMINISTRATION

1. Check the label when taking the medication from its storage area.
2. Check the label when removing the medication from its container.
3. Check the label when discarding or replacing the medication container.

use a medication that is not labeled. In both cases it is impossible to know for sure what medication was prepared or what medication was in the unlabeled container.

The nurse should check the physician's order to verify the Medex if there is a question about a medication. The nurse must become familiar with generic and trade names of frequently used medications. Consult the *PDR* or the pharmacist if necessary.

The Right Dose

The nurse should check the Medex to verify the dosage of a drug. If there is a question, then the physician's order should be checked. The nurse always checks the label on the container for the dose per milliliter or dose per tablet and consults with another nurse to check calculations or clarify a dosage.

The appropriateness of the dose must be assessed: Is the dose consistent with the age of the patient, the diagnosis of the patient, the gender of the patient? The nurse looks at the number of tablets that constitute the dose or the number of milliliters that make the dose. Does the number of tablets or the number of milliliters in the syringe "look" or "sound" reasonable? The decimal place in the dosage ordered and the nurse's calculations must be checked; a decimal in the wrong place can cause a serious drug error.

The Right Time

The nurse is responsible for placing the drug order on the right time schedule. A standardized schedule is generally specified by the hospital. A medication should be worked into the standardized schedule as soon as possible. Table 21-2 lists commonly used abbreviations.

Medications should be given on time. If it is impossible to give a medication exactly at the scheduled time, the nurse should give it at least within 30 minutes of the scheduled time. Antibiotics in particular should be given on time to maintain therapeutic blood levels.

Medications to be administered prn should not be given before the time specified by the physician's order. The nurse should check the date that the drug order was written to be sure that the drug, intravenous infusion, or blood product is started and given on the right day and at the right time. The order sheet and/or the Medex should be checked for dates and times to be sure that the medication has not been discontinued (d/c).

The Right Route

The route chosen for administering a drug depends on its properties and desired effect and the patient's physical and mental condition. The nurse frequently is involved in judging the best route for a medicine.

The drug order should indicate the preferred route of administration. If no route is given, it is understood that the route is po (per os; by mouth). If there is doubt, the nurse should verify the order with the physician.

If the medication is parenteral (intramuscular, IM; subcutaneous, SQ; intradermal, ID; and intravenous, IV), the nurse must be certain to inject the drug into the tissue specified.

The Right Patient

The nurse makes sure the medication is given to the right patient by systematically identifying the patient in every situation by checking the name, room number, and bed number of the patient against the drug order. Once in the patient's room, the nurse asks the patient to state his full name. The patient may also be asked to spell his name as the nurse checks the identification band.

An unconscious patient cannot identify himself; his safety depends on the nurse. A family member or visitor may be at the bedside, but do not rely on others to identify the patient. The nurse should *always* check the identification band on conscious or unconscious patients and *never* give medications or perform procedures on a patient who does not have an ID band.

After the five rights have been observed and the three label checks have been done, the nurse uses universal precautions (see Chapter 12).

TABLE 21-2 Commonly Used Abbreviations

Abbreviation	Meaning	Example
bid	Two times a day	0900-2100
tid	Three times a day	0900-1300-1700
qid	Four times a day	0800-1200-1600-2000
qd	Every day	0900
ac	Before eating	Varies with hospital or unit
pc	After eating	Varies with hospital or unit
hs	Hours of sleep	Varies with hospital or unit

Important Considerations of Medication Administration

While handling equipment during medication administration, the nurse must always think, "sterile to sterile and clean to clean." Hands must be washed after each patient. Work spaces and equipment must be kept clean and orderly, and practices should be established that will keep staff members and patients safe. Short cuts should not be taken, and staff should never deviate from principles that are effective. The following rules should be applied:

1. If you did not pour it, do not give it.
2. If you gave it, chart it.
3. Do not chart for someone else or have someone chart for you.
4. Do not transport or accept a container that is not labeled.
5. Do not put down an unlabeled syringe; keep it in your hand or label it before you put it down.
6. If given a verbal order, repeat the order to the physician.
7. If you make an error, report it *immediately* to the charge nurse or supervisor, or if you are in charge notify the physician.
8. *Never* leave a medication tray or cart unattended or unlocked.
9. *Do not* leave a medication with a patient or family member. *Watch* the patient take and swallow the medication.
10. *Always return* to assess the patient's response to the medication.
11. Chart as soon as possible after giving medication.
12. If a patient refuses medication, do not force it; chart "Refused medication because of . . . ."
13. If you elect to omit a dose based on your nursing judgment, let another nurse help make the decision. If medication is not given, document "Dose omitted because of . . . ." Be objective and exact in charting. Report your decision to the physician.

ROUTES OF ADMINISTRATION

Drugs enter the body through three general routes—enteral, percutaneous, and parenteral. The drugs that enter the body by these routes come in various forms.

Enteral

Drugs that enter through the **enteral** (by the GI tract) routes are given in these forms:

1. Powders: Often mixed with a liquid (diluent) before administration
2. Pills: Round, solid drug form that must be broken down into solution form (dissolution) in the stomach
3. Tablets: Round, spherical, or oddly shaped forms that dissolve in the stomach
   Types of tablets
   a. Scored: Indented to allow tablet to be broken in half
   b. **Enteric-coated:** Candylike coated shell encases tablet to keep tablet from being absorbed in the stomach; absorption takes place in the intestine. Enteric pertains to the small intestine.
   c. Capsule: Powders or pellets enclosed in a gelatin-like, elongated, spherical form; encapsulated because (1) substance may be bad tasting or (2) substance may be a spansule with time-released pellets to delay the action of the drug
   d. Lozenge/troche: A sweet mucilage-type tablet that dissolves in the mouth to release medication
4. Suspensions: Solid particles and liquid that must be *shaken to disperse* solid particles throughout the liquid portion *before* absorption by the body can occur
5. Suppositories: Drugs mixed with lubricated substance molded to insert into body cavities such as the rectum; *must melt* at body temperature to be absorbed

The above dosage forms are given by the enteral routes. The enteral routes are as follows:

1. po: by mouth
2. Tubal: by nasogastric tube (Levin tube) into the stomach
3. Suppository: by rectum, vagina, or urethra
4. Enema: by rectum

Percutaneous

Dosage forms used by the **percutaneous** route (through the skin or mucous membranes) include lotions, ointments, creams, and powders.

The percutaneous routes are as follows:

1. Topical: Applied to the skin
2. Instillation: To the mucous membranes of the mouth:
   a. **Sublingual** (under the tongue)
   b. **Buccal** (in the cheek)
   c. To the mucous membranes of the eye, ear, nose, and vagina
3. Inhalation: Aerosolized liquids, gases

Parenteral

The **parenteral** routes are methods other than the digestive system route. They are usually thought of as the "needle" route. Dosage forms are liquids that are contained in the following:

- *Ampules.* Ampules are glass containers that are opened by snapping off the top part of the ampule. They are intended for unit dose use.
- *Vials.* Vials are glass containers that are sealed with a metal cap with a rubber diaphragm in the middle of the cap. The rubber diaphragm permits a needle to enter the vial for either unit dose or multidose use (depending on the contents of the vial).

Large volumes of fluids are contained in plastic or glass containers, such as intravenous fluid bags. IV fluid bags or bottles range in amounts from 50 ml to 1000 ml.

The parenteral routes are as follows:

IM: Intramuscular (within the muscle)
SC, SQ, or Subq: subcutaneous (under the dermis; fatty tissue)
ID: Intradermal (within the dermis)
IV: Intravenous (within the vein)

ADMINISTERING VIA THE ENTERAL ROUTES

Preparation of Tablets, Pills, and Capsules

Tablets, pills, and capsules that enter the GI tract are absorbed more slowly into the bloodstream than by any other route. The slow absorption rate makes the po (by mouth; oral) route relatively safe.

SKILL 21-1

ADMINISTERING TABLETS, PILLS, AND CAPSULES

1. Follow the five rights (Box 21-4).
2. Perform the three label checks (Box 21-5).
3. Follow universal precautions (Box 12-3).
4. Wash hands.
5. If using unit dose package (see illustration), place unopened package in medicine cup.
6. If using a multidose bottle, pour tablet, without touching it, into cap of bottle.
7. Pour tablet from cap into medicine cup.
8. If using medicine tray (for several patients), set it up from left to right, front to back.
9. If pouring from multidose bottle and patient is to receive several tablets, use separate cup for medications such as digitalis. If the patient's pulse is less than 60/min, withhold the medication and report this to the RN. By placing digitalis in a separate cup marked with a red heart it will be identified easily.
10. Do not replace pills, tablets, or capsules that come from multidose bottles if they have been handled or dropped on the floor.
11. Take medication to the room.
12. Follow procedure for room, bed, and patient identification (p. 404).
13. Explain procedure to patient.
14. Document administration of medication on the Medex with time, date, and initials.
15. Return to assess patient's response to medication.
16. Document assessment in nursing notes.

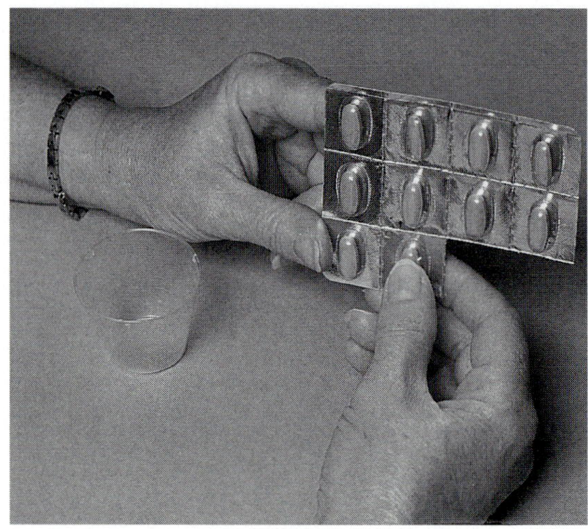

STEP 5

If an error is made, report it immediately to the RN. An incident report should be done to document the error. The nurse should not hesitate to report an error, because prompt intervention may prevent adverse effects on the patient.

Nurses must also be aware that some po medications are irritating to the patient's GI tract and that larger tablets may be difficult for some patients to swallow (Skill 21-1).

Preparation of Liquid Medications

Liquid medication is often given to children, to patients who cannot swallow tablets, pills, or capsules, and to geriatric patients. Liquids may be given po or via a nasogastric tube or gastrostomy tube.

Liquids must *not* be given to unconscious patients because of the possibility of aspirating (inhaling) the medication into the respiratory tract.

The nurse must be aware that some liquid medications are *not* to be followed with water and that some medications, such as iron, may stain the teeth. The nurse should look for and follow any instructions on the label (Skill 21-2).

Tubal Medications

Nasogastric (NG) tubes are used to administer liquid medications to unconscious patients, dysphagic patients (who have difficulty in swallowing), and those who are too ill to eat. A gastrostomy tube (placed through the abdominal wall and into the stomach) is also used in the same manner as the NG tube.

Many medicines come in liquid form. If they do not, solid tablets may be **pulverized** (crushed to a powder) in a mortar and pestle. Mix the crushed tablet with 30 ml of water and give through the tube. Capsules can also be opened, mixed with 30 ml of water, and administered (Skill 21-3 on p. 410).

Suppositories

A suppository is a cone-shaped, egg-shaped, or spindle-shaped medication made for insertion into the rectum,

SKILL 21-2

ADMINISTERING LIQUID MEDICATIONS

1. Follow the five rights (Box 21-4).
2. Perform the three label checks (Box 21-5).
3. Follow universal precautions (Box 12-3).
4. Wash hands.
5. Remove liquid preparation from patient's drug box/bin (or from medication cabinet).
6. Check dosage per milliliter and total volume of medication in container.
7. Calculate dosage; if the dosage ordered is different from the dosage per milliliter stated on the label, calculate correct dose; if ordered medication is labeled in a different measurement system, convert by using appropriate equivalent. Work problem on paper.
8. Check calculations with another nurse.
9. Obtain **graduated** (has markings indicating marked amount) medicine cup (total volume of cup is 30 ml or 1 oz).
10. Face label of bottle toward palm of hand to avoid soiling label; if label becomes soiled, return the bottle to the pharmacy; do not give medication if label is unreadable.
11. Place medicine cup on flat surface or hold at eye level while pouring.
12. Place cap of bottle with inner rim up to avoid contaminating inside of cap (which would contaminate remaining contents of bottle).
13. Read dosage amount at lower level of **meniscus** (curve formed by liquid's upper surface); see illustration.
14. Transport medication to patient's room.
15. Follow procedure for room, bed, and patient identification (p. 404).
16. Explain procedure to patient.
17. Document administration on Medex with time, date, and initials.
18. Return to assess patient's response to medication.
19. Document assessment in nursing notes.

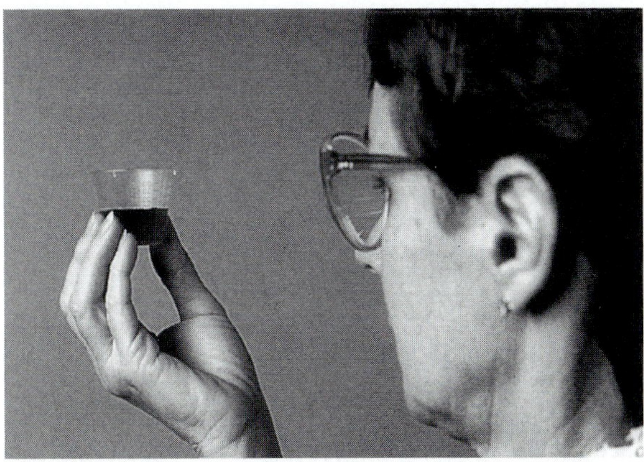

STEP 13

SKILL 21-3

ADMINISTERING TUBAL MEDICATIONS

1. Follow the five rights (Box 21-4).
2. Perform the three label checks (Box 21-5).
3. Follow universal precautions (Box 12-3).
4. Wash hands.
5. Prepare medication using the same procedure as for liquid medications.
6. Gather equipment: 10 ml syringe, towel, stethoscope, bulb or Asepto syringe, tap water.
7. Take equipment and medication to patient's room.
8. Follow procedure of room, bed, patient identification (see p. 404).
9. Explain procedure; answer questions patient may have about the procedure.
10. Place patient in high Fowler's position.
11. Put towel over patient's chest (to protect clothing and bed linen).
12. Don disposable, unsterile gloves.
13. Check and recheck placement and patency of tube with at least two methods to ensure that tube is in the stomach and *not* in the respiratory tract.
    Method A: Attach bulb or Asepto syringe to end of NG tube. Pull plunger back or release suction of bulb syringe to aspirate stomach contents. If stomach contents are seen, proceed with medication. Because of the difficulty in withdrawing fluid from small-bore feeding tubes, nurses incorrectly rely on the auscultatory method to confirm NG feeding tube placement.
    Currently used bedside methods to test placement of small-bore feeding tubes are frequently ineffective. At present, the most reliable method is radiographic verification. This method is cost prohibitive. Therefore new methods to test tube placement must be explored. In the meantime, the nurse must have a high index of suspicion for tube displacement in patients at risk and use meticulous assessment skills.
    Method B: Place stethoscope over stomach. Push 10 ml of air through NG tube with syringe. The rush of air is heard in stomach with stethoscope if tube is in stomach. Proceed with medication.
    Method C: Many authorities are now recommending the Litmus test instead of the auscultatory (air-instillation) method. Measure pH of aspirate with color-coded pH paper with range of whole numbers from 1 to 11. Gastric aspirates have decidedly acidic pH values, preferably value of 4 or less.
14. Clamp tube with rubber-tipped hemostats or other clamping device.
15. Attach syringe to end of tube (with plunger out of syringe).
16. Pour medication into syringe.
17. Unclamp tubing to allow medication to slowly flow by gravity.
18. Follow medication with 30 to 50 ml of water to flush the medication into stomach. Water is essential to enhance absorption of medication and is also used to clean and maintain patency of NG tube.
19. Clamp tubing; secure tube after medication is given.
20. If NG tube is attached to suction, do *not* reconnect suction for 30 minutes. The medication will then have time to absorb, since medication will not be aspirated through tube.
21. Remove towel from patient.
22. Remove gloves.
23. Leave patient in comfortable position.
24. Gather equipment; clean up patient and area.
25. Wash hands.
26. Document administration of NG medication in Medex with time, date, and initials.
27. Return to assess patient's response to medication.
28. Document assessment in nursing notes.

SKILL 21-4

ADMINISTERING RECTAL SUPPOSITORIES

1. Follow the five rights (Box 21-4).
2. Perform the three label checks (Box 21-5).
3. Follow universal precautions (Box 12-3).
4. Wash hands.
5. Obtain suppository from refrigerator or from patient's medication bin.
6. Place unopened suppository into medicine cup or **souffle cup** (ungraduated disposable paper cup).
7. Take disposable, unsterile gloves or finger cot (single-digit plastic finger cover) to room.
8. Follow procedure of room, bed, and patient identification (p. 404).
9. Explain procedure to patient.
10. Gain patient's cooperation.
11. Provide privacy.
12. Position patient in Sims' position (on left side with upper leg flexed at knee).
13. Unwrap suppository.
14. Maintain privacy; expose buttocks.
15. Don gloves.
16. Apply lubricant, such as KY jelly, to tapered end of suppository.
17. Ask patient to take deep breath; insert beyond internal anal sphincter. Insert suppository as patient exhales to relax anal sphincter.
18. Ask patient to retain suppository as long as possible to allow the medication to completely dissolve and absorb through mucous membranes of rectum into capillaries of systemic circulatory system. Hold the buttocks together to help patient to retain suppository.
19. Discard gloves.
20. Help patient assume comfortable position.
21. Wash hands.
22. Document administration of suppository in Medex with time and initials.
23. Return to assess patient's response to medication.
24. Document assessment in nurse's notes.

urethra, or vagina. Suppositories dissolve at body temperature and are absorbed directly into the bloodstream. Suppositories are useful for babies, patients who cannot take oral preparations, and patients with nausea and vomiting (Skill 21-4).

Suppositories should be stored in a cool place so that they do not melt; they may be placed in the refrigerator.

ADMINISTERING VIA THE PERCUTANEOUS ROUTES

The percutaneous routes are those routes by which medications are absorbed through the skin or the mucous membranes. Most percutaneous medications produce a local action, but there are some that produce a systemic action.

The percutaneous routes include **topical applications** (applied to the skin), instillations, and inhalations. Absorption is rapid, but of short duration.

Topical medications include ointments, creams, powders, and lotions.

Ointments

An ointment is an oil-based semisolid medication; it may be applied to the skin or a mucous membrane. Nitroglycerin (NTG) is a commonly used ointment that produces an effect of longer duration than the sublingual form. NTG ointment is applied topically by using applicator paper and is placed on the skin with the ointment side on the skin. The topical disk is a transdermal patch that provides controlled release of NTG through the semipermeable membrane of the disk. The adhesive side of the system is placed on a selected body site where there is little hair, and the disk is pressed into the site. The nurse should not touch the NTG side of the applicator paper or the NTG side of the disk.

Sites commonly used for NTG applications are the chest, flank, and upper arm. Ointments are removed with cottonseed oil and gauze.

Creams

Creams are semisolid, nongreasy emulsions that contain medication for external application. Creams are gently rubbed into the area and are easily removed with water and gauze.

Lotions

Lotions are generally aqueous preparations that are used as soothing agents that relieve pruritus, protect the skin, cleanse the skin, or act as astringents. Lotions contain suspended particles that must be brought into solution by shaking before application. Lotions are gently patted (not rubbed) onto the skin, and they may be removed with soap and water (Skill 21-5 on p. 412).

SKILL 21-5

APPLYING TOPICAL AGENTS

1. Follow the five rights (Box 21-4).
2. Perform the three label checks (Box 21-5).
3. Follow universal precautions (Box 12-3).
4. Wash hands.
5. Transport medication to room.
6. Identify room, bed, and patient (p. 404).
7. Introduce yourself; explain procedure to patient.
8. Provide privacy; place patient in comfortable position that allows exposure of selected site.
9. Cleanse site with appropriate materials (according to whether application is oil or water based).
10. Don gloves.
11. Prepare medicinal agent (ointments, creams, and lotions may have to be squeezed or removed with a tongue blade, depending on preparation used).
12. Apply paper applicator, disk, lotion, ointment, or cream.
13. Remove gloves.
14. Leave patient properly draped or clothed in comfortable position.
15. Answer patient's questions, and teach patient to perform self-applications if appropriate.
16. Clean work area.
17. Wash hands.
18. Record administration in Medex with initials, date, and time.
19. Return to assess patient's response to medication.
20. Document assessment in nursing notes.

Eyedrops and Eye Ointments

Eyedrops and ointments are sterile. Care should be taken to keep all ophthalmic (eye) preparations sterile by not touching the dropper or the tube of ointment to the eye. The container should be checked to ensure that the medication is marked "for ophthalmic use." Ophthalmic medications are used for only one patient and are not shared (Skill 21-6).

Eardrops

Containers of solutions to be used as eardrops will be labeled "otic." They must be at room temperature when applied. Individual bottles are used for each patient (Skill 21-7 on p. 414).

Nosedrops

Nosedrops are for individual use *only* (Skill 21-8 on p. 415).

Nasal Sprays

Because nasal sprays are absorbed quickly, less medication is used and wasted when administered in this manner. Nasal sprays are for individual use *only* (Skill 21-9 on p. 415).

Administering Medications by Inhalation

Drugs may be absorbed through the mucous membranes of the respiratory tract. They may produce a relatively limited effect or a systemic effect. The inhalation route is accessible to the bloodstream for vapors such as ammonia, anesthetic gases (such as chloroform, nitrous oxide, and halothane), and for respiratory therapy agents (such as acetylcysteine [Mucomyst] and Alevaire).

Respiratory therapy departments actively use the inhalation route, as do anesthesiologists and nurse anesthetists.

The nurse's participation in inhalation therapy may be limited to helping patients use metered-dose inhalers that contain bronchodilators or corticosteroids. Directions for use of these inhalers should be read and followed thoroughly, because methods of use may vary among manufacturers.

Sublingual Administration

Sublingual administration of a drug (usually in tablet form) is achieved by placing the tablet beneath the tongue until the tablet dissolves. After dissolution, the active ingredient, such as NTG, is rapidly absorbed into the bloodstream. Drugs given by sublingual routes bypass the liver, which reduces the time it takes for the drug to produce its desired action.

SKILL 21-6

ADMINISTERING EYE DROPS AND EYE OINTMENTS

1. Follow the five rights (Box 21-4).
2. Perform the three label checks (Box 21-5).
3. Follow universal precautions (Box 12-3).
4. Wash hands.
5. Transport medications to room.
6. Identify room, bed, and patient (p. 404).
7. Introduce yourself; explain procedure.
8. Provide privacy; position back of patient's head on pillow; direct patient's face upward toward ceiling.
9. Don gloves.
10. Remove exudate; clean eye as needed using sterile solution of saline; use cotton balls to wipe away exudate; use one cotton ball per stroke, wiping from inner canthus outward.
11. *To apply drops,* expose lower conjunctival sac by having patient look upward while gentle traction is applied to lower eyelid (see illustration).
12. Put prescribed number of drops into conjunctival sac, *not* onto eyeball.
13. Using a cotton ball or tissue, apply gentle pressure above bone at inner corner of eyelid for 1 to 2 minutes (see illustration).
14. Apply sterile dressing, if ordered.
15. *To apply ointment,* expose lower conjunctival sac by having patient look upward while gentle traction is applied to lower eyelid (see illustration).
16. Squeeze ointment into lower conjunctival sac.
17. Ask patient to close eye; and move it around in circular motion to spread medication.
18. Apply sterile dressing, if ordered.
19. After applying drops or ointment to an eye, leave patient in comfortable position; clean up the work area.
20. Remove gloves and wash hands.
21. Answer patient's questions and if appropriate, teach patient to perform self-care.
22. Record administration of medications in Medex with initials, date, and time.
23. Return to assess patient's response to medication.
24. Document assessment in nursing notes.

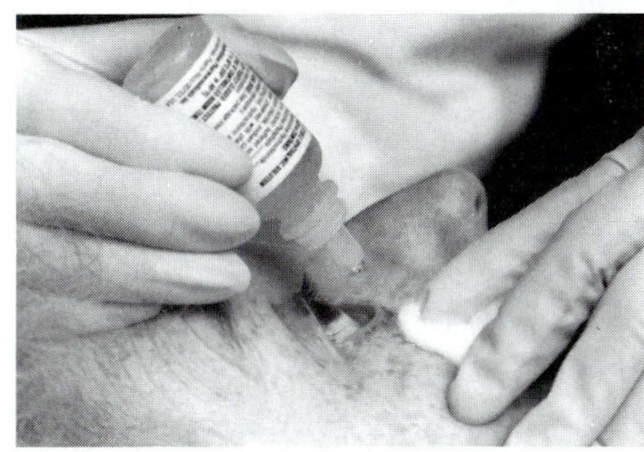

STEP 11

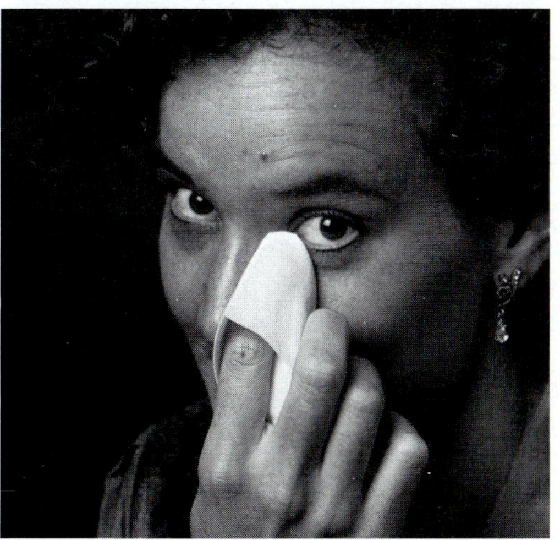

STEP 13

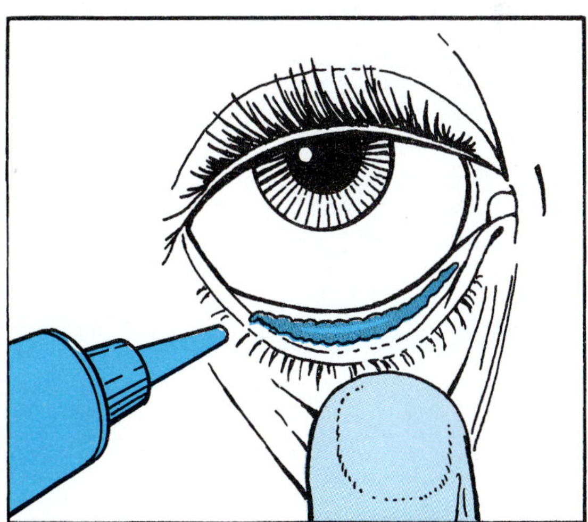

STEP 15

SKILL 21-7

ADMINISTERING EARDROPS

1. Follow the five rights (Box 21-4).
2. Perform the three label checks (Box 21-5).
3. Follow universal precautions (Box 12-3).
4. Wash hands.
5. Transport medication to room.
6. Identify room, bed, and patient (p. 404)
7. Introduce yourself; explain procedure.
8. Provide privacy; position patient with affected ear upward.
9. Don gloves.
10. Remove external exudate from ear; an order must be obtained before irrigating the ear.
11. Draw medication into dropper.
12. For adults and for children over 3 years old, turn head with affected side up; pull ear lobe *upward* and *back* to straighten external auditory canal; give drops without touching ear with dropper (see illustration).
13. For children under 3 years old, turn head with affected side up; pull earlobe *downward* and *back;* instill drops without touching ear with dropper (see illustration).
14. Tell patient to remain in same position for a few minutes to allow medication to drain into ear by gravity.
15. A cotton ball may be placed loosely into ear as needed.
16. Remove gloves.
17. Leave patient in comfortable position; clean work area.
18. Answer patient's questions and if appropriate, teach patient self-care.
19. Wash hands.
20. Record administration in Medex with initials, date, and time.
21. Return to assess patient's response to medication.
22. Document assessment in nursing notes.

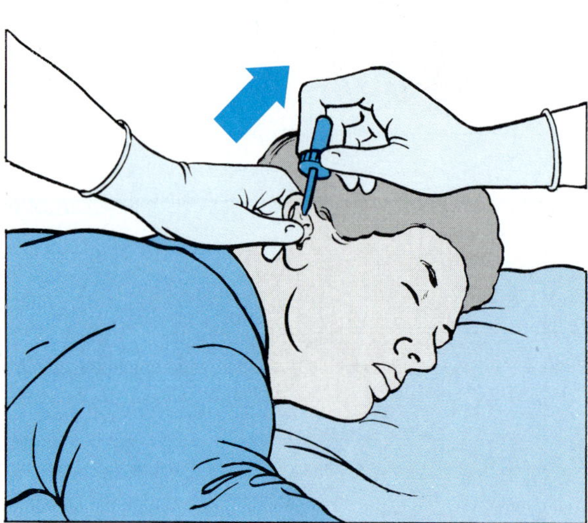

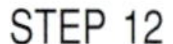
STEP 12

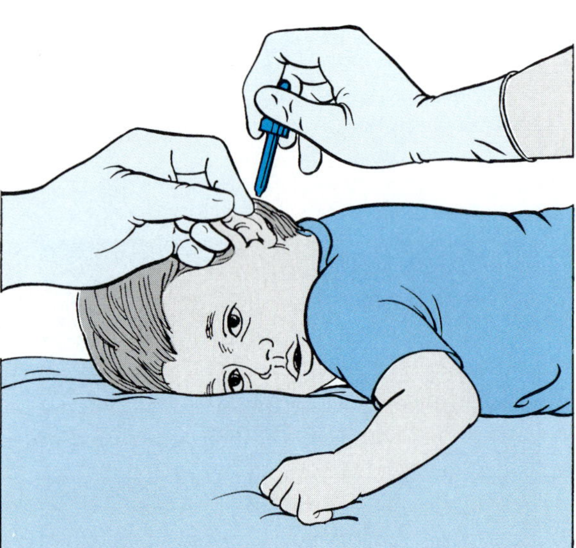

STEP 13

SKILL 21-8

ADMINISTERING NOSEDROPS

1. Follow the five rights (Box 21-4).
2. Perform the three label checks (Box 21-5).
3. Follow universal precautions (Box 12-3).
4. Wash hands.
5. Transport medication to room.
6. Identify room, bed, and patient (p. 404).
7. Introduce yourself; explain procedure.
8. Provide privacy.
9. Don gloves.
10. Ask adult or older child to clear nose of accumulations by blowing gently into tissue.
11. Have patient lie down, hanging head backward over edge of bed or with pillow under shoulders to hyperextend the neck if patient can tolerate it.
12. After drawing medication into dropper, instill medication while holding dropper above nostril being treated (see illustration).
13. If ordered, repeat procedure to instill drops in other nostril.
14. Tell patient to hold position for a few minutes to allow medication to remain in place.
15. Administer nosedrops to a younger child after positioning him on bed with head backward and downward, or to an infant while holding his with head backward and downward.
16. Administer drops in same way as to an adult.
17. Remove gloves.
18. Tell patient to refrain from blowing nose immediately after instillation.
19. Offer tissues for later use.
20. Leave patient in comfortable position; clean work area.
21. Answer patient's questions and if appropriate, teach patient self-care.
22. Wash hands.
23. Record administration in Medex with initials, date, and time.
24. Return to assess patient's response to medication.
25. Document assessment in nursing notes.

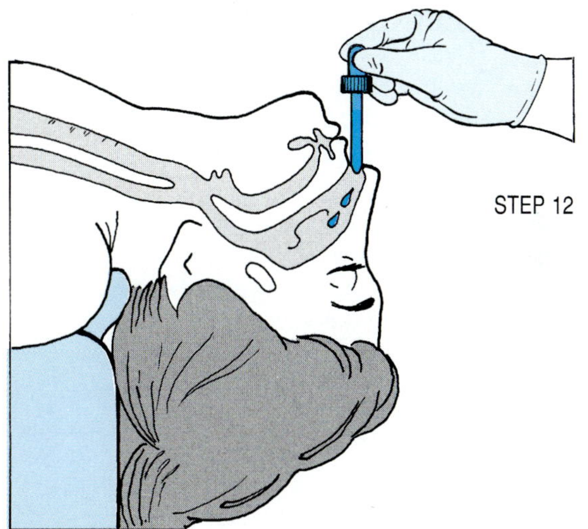

STEP 12

SKILL 21-9

ADMINISTERING NASAL SPRAYS

1. Follow the five rights (Box 21-4).
2. Perform the three label checks (Box 21-5).
3. Follow universal precautions (Box 12-3).
4. Wash hands.
5. Transport medication to patient.
6. Identify room, bed, and patient (p. 404).
7. Introduce yourself; explain procedure.
8. Provide privacy; position patient upright.
9. Don gloves.
10. Have patient gently blow nose to clear nasal passages of accumulations.
11. Compress one nostril.
12. Shake bottle while holding it upright.
13. Insert tip of spray bottle into patient's patent nostril.
14. Instruct patient to inhale; while he inhales, squeeze bottle.
15. If ordered, repeat procedure for other nostril.
16. Tell patient to refrain from blowing nose for a few minutes; offer tissues for later use.
17. Answer patient's questions and if appropriate, teach self-administration.
18. Remove gloves and wash hands.
19. Record administration in Medex with initials, date, and time.
20. Return to assess patient's response to medication.
21. Document assessment in nursing notes.

SKILL 21-10

ADMINISTERING SUBLINGUAL MEDICATIONS

1. Follow the five rights (Box 21-4).
2. Perform the three label checks (Box 21-5).
3. Follow universal precautions (Box 12-3).
4. Wash hands.
5. Follow procedure for room, bed, and patient identification (p. 404).
6. Wear gloves to place tablet under patient's tongue.
7. *Do not* follow with water.
8. Instruct patient *not* to swallow tablet.
9. Explain to patient how to place medication under tongue. Instruct patient to let it dissolve.
10. Remove gloves and wash hands.
11. Document sublingual administration in Medex with time, date, and initials.
12. Return to assess patient's response to medication.
13. Document assessment in nursing notes.

SKILL 21-11

ADMINISTERING BUCCAL MEDICATIONS

1. Follow the five rights (Box 21-4).
2. Perform the three label checks (Box 21-5).
3. Follow universal precautions (Box 12-3).
4. Wash hands.
5. Follow procedure for room, bed, and patient identification (p. 404).
6. Wear gloves to place medication between patient's cheek and gum.
7. *Do not* follow with water.
8. Instruct patient *not to swallow* tablet; let it dissolve.
9. Explain to patient how to place medication between gum and cheek.
10. Remove gloves and wash hands.
11. Document buccal administration in Medex with time, date, and initials.
12. Return to assess patient's response to medication.
13. Document assessment in nurse's notes.

Nitroglycerin is a common sublingual medication. It is usually ordered to be left at the bedside so the patient may take it ad lib (as desired). The patient is allowed to take the NTG tablets to the diagnostic imaging department or to any other diagnostic testing area in case a tablet is needed for anginal pain.

The administration of sublingual tablets follows the same procedure as the preparation of solid oral medication, with the exceptions noted in Skill 21-10.

Buccal Administration

Buccal administration is achieved by placing a tablet between the cheek and the teeth, or between the cheek and the gums. It is left there until it dissolves. Absorption into the capillaries of the mucous membranes of the cheek gives rapid onset of the drug's active ingredient because of its direct entry into the systemic circulation.

Buccal administration is accomplished by the same procedure as solid tablet administration or sublingual administration (Skill 21-11).

ADMINISTERING VIA THE PARENTERAL ROUTES

The intramuscular, subcutaneous, intradermal, and intravenous routes are called the *parenteral routes; parenteral* actually refers to all routes other than the GI, orenteral, routes. Parenteral routes are used for the following reasons:

1. Some medications, such as insulin, are altered by the secretions of the GI tract.
2. Some patients cannot take medications by mouth, such as those who are intubated, are severely dysphagic (unable to eat), or have full-thickness burns, shock, nausea, and/or vomiting.
3. The parenteral route gives a more rapid onset of action than the oral route.
4. The *duration* of the effects of parenteral administration is shorter than that of oral administration.
5. Smaller doses of parenteral drugs may be used, because active drug ingredients are not changed or lost in the GI tract and liver.

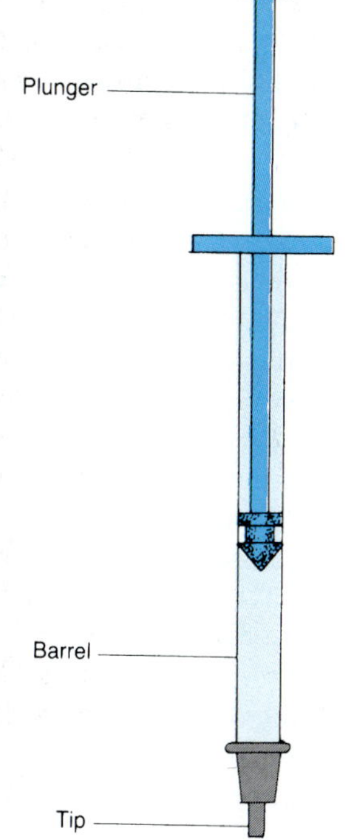

FIG. 21-2 Parts of a syringe.

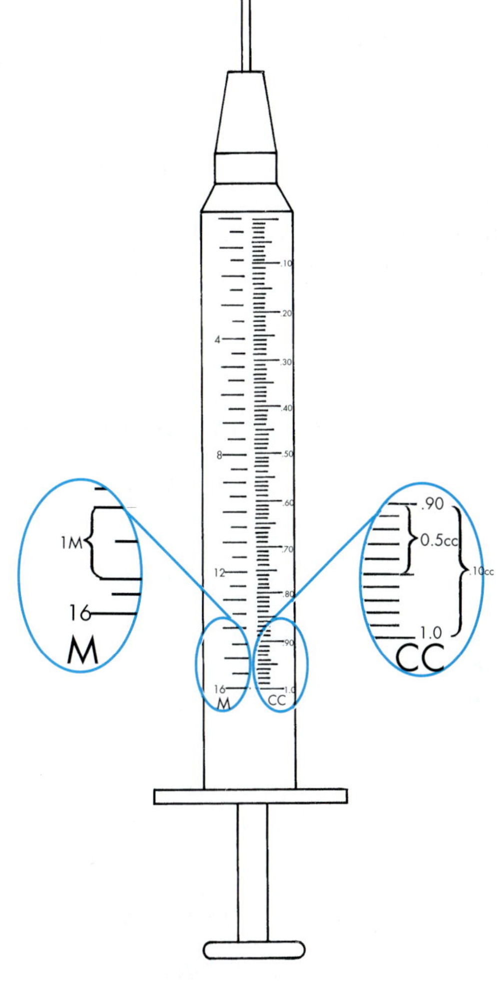

FIG. 21-3 Tuberculin syringe calibration.

6. Intravenous administration of a drug can be carefully regulated. Immediate entry into the bloodstream gives immediate onset of the drug's action.

Hands should be thoroughly washed before selecting and handling syringes, needles, and other equipment. Aseptic technique is used, because the skin is penetrated (which makes a portal of entry into the body for pathogenic organisms).

Parenteral medication administration must be performed skillfully and accurately. Dosages must be exact, and the proper site must be selected for the injection.

Equipment

Syringes. A syringe consists of a barrel, a plunger, and a tip (Fig. 21-2). The outside part of the barrel is calibrated in milliliters, minims, insulin units, or heparin units.

Barrels range in size from 1 ml to 50 ml. The outside of the barrel is not sterile, but the inside is. The tip of the barrel may be the plain or Luer-Lok. The needle slips directly onto the plain barrel tip, whereas the Luer-Lok needle must be turned to the right as it is placed onto the barrel tip.

The plunger inside of the barrel is also sterile; the nurse should avoid touching the plunger anywhere except the tip. The plunger is used to draw up and inject medication from the syringe. The plunger has a rubber stopper on the end that is inside the barrel. The volume of a medication is read at the point of the rubber stopper nearest the needle.

The most commonly used syringes are the 1 ml (tuberculin syringe), 3 ml, and 5 ml.

Tuberculin syringe. The tuberculin syringe (Fig. 21-3) holds a total of 1 ml or 16 minims (♍) (1 ml = 16 ♍). It is used to give volumes of medication of 1 ml volume or less. It is used for giving small doses of epinephrine, intradermal skin tests, insulin (U100, when no insulin syringe is available), and subcutaneous medication.

One side of the tuberculin syringe is measured in minims. The long line of the minim scale represents 1 ♍; the shorter lines represent 0.5 (5/10 or ½ ♍).

The other side is measured in milliliters (ml). The long lines represent 0.1 (1/10) ml, the shorter lines represent 0.05 (5/100) ml, and the shortest lines represent 0.01 (1/100) ml.

Insulin syringe. The insulin syringe is used only for insulin, because it is calibrated in units (Fig. 21-4 on p.

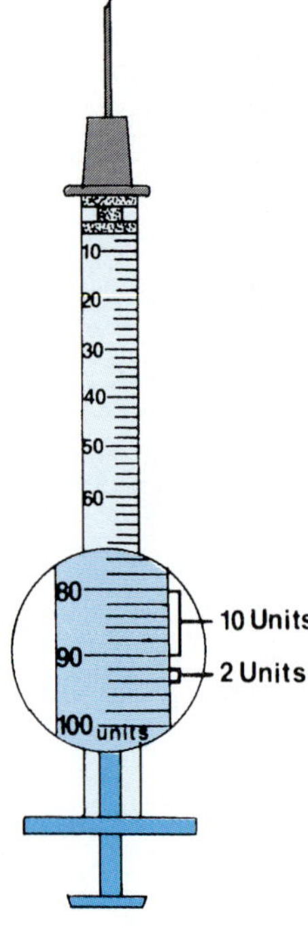

FIG. 21-4 Calibration of U100 insulin syringe.

418). Most insulin is made in the concentration of U100. The U100 syringe holds 100 units of insulin per 1 ml. All insulin dosages should be checked with another nurse before being administered to the patient.

Three-milliliter syringe. The most frequently used syringe is the 3-ml syringe (Fig. 21-5). The 3-ml syringe is chosen for giving volumes of medication of 1 ml to 3 ml. It is used for most intramuscular injections. The 3-ml syringe is calibrated in milliliters (ml) or cubic centimeters (cc), which are equivalent units. The short lines represent 0.1 ml; the longer lines represent 0.5 ml.

Syringe selection is based on the volume of medication that is to be given (see Fig. 21-6).

Safety-lok syringes. Safety-Lok syringes to prevent needle sticks from occurring are now on the market. See Fig. 21-7.

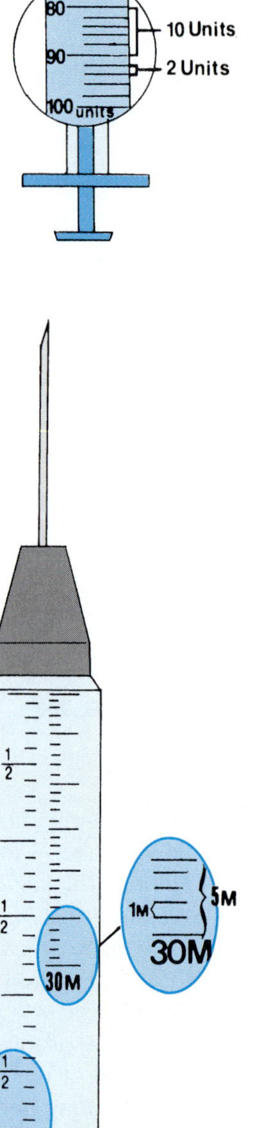

FIG. 21-5 Reading the calibrations of a 3-ml syringe.

Needles. The parts of a needle are the hub, shaft, and beveled tip (Fig. 21-8). The opening at the needle's beveled tip is the **lumen.** The size of the diameter of the inside of the needle's shaft determines the **gauge** (a standard or scale of measurement) of the needle (Fig. 21-9). The smaller the gauge, the larger the diameter of the needle. Needle gauge selection is based on the viscosity (thickness) of the medication. The thicker the medication, the smaller the gauge required. A 20- to 22-gauge needle is usually adequate for most nonviscous intramuscular injections. A 16- to 18-gauge intravenous needle is appropriate for blood administration, emergency IV

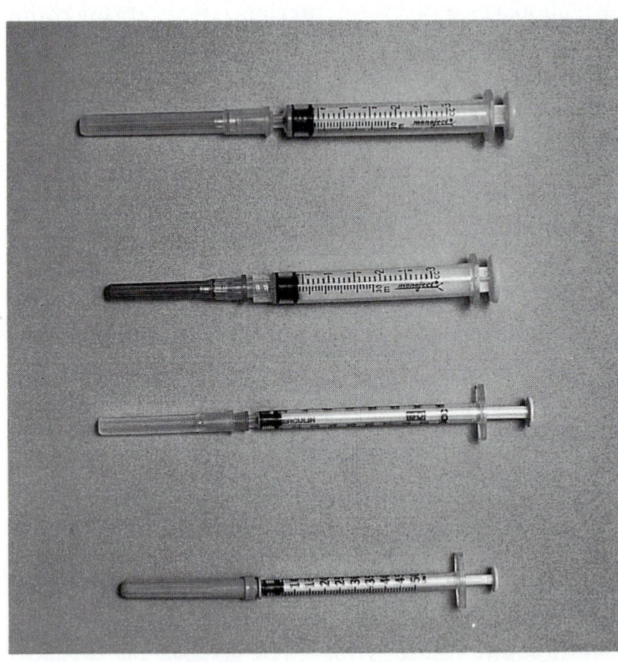

FIG. 21-6 Type of syringes. From *top* to *bottom:* disposable 3-ml hypodermic syringe (intramuscular), 3-ml hypodermic syringe (subcutaneous), insulin syringe, and tuberculin syringe.

routes, and surgical cases. A 23- to 26-gauge is frequently used for infants and children and for intradermal injections.

Needle length. Needle length is selected based on the depth of the tissue into which the medication is to be injected. Intradermal injections require only ⅜ to ½ inch needle length, whereas an intramuscular injection may require ½ to 1¼ inch needle length, depending on the amount of muscle tissue the patient has. Needle length for subcutaneous injections is based on depth of appropriate tissue (Fig. 21-9).

Intravenous needles. Two types of needles made especially for intravenous (IV) use are the butterfly and the over-the-needle catheter.

The butterfly (also called a scalp needle or a wing-tipped needle) is useful in administering intravenous fluids on a short-term basis. They are used in pediatric cases in which veins are sometimes hard to find except in the scalp. Butterflies are easy to put in, but some health care providers prefer over-the-needle catheters.

Over-the-needle catheters (Fig. 21-10) are called Angiocaths, Jelcos, Abbocaths, or Insytes, according to the manufacturer of the needle.

Over-the-needle catheters are preferred for emergency situations, surgery cases, blood and blood product transfusion, intensive care cases, transporting situations such as in helicopters or ambulances, and thick, intravenous infusions or hyperalimentation.

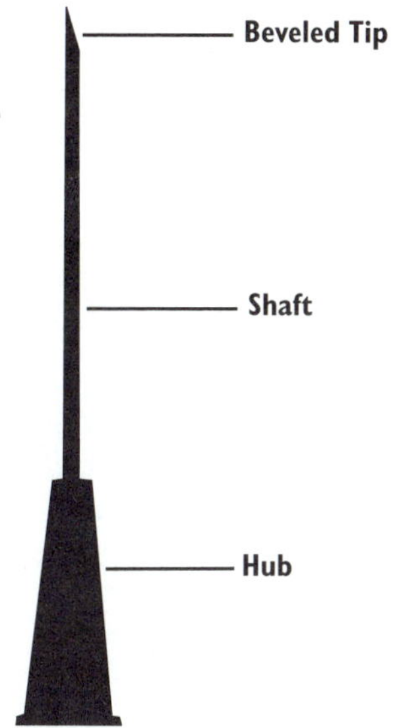

FIG. 21-8 Parts of a needle.

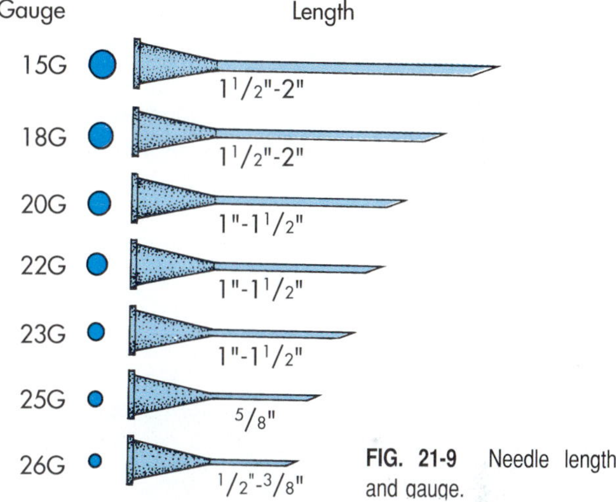

FIG. 21-9 Needle length and gauge.

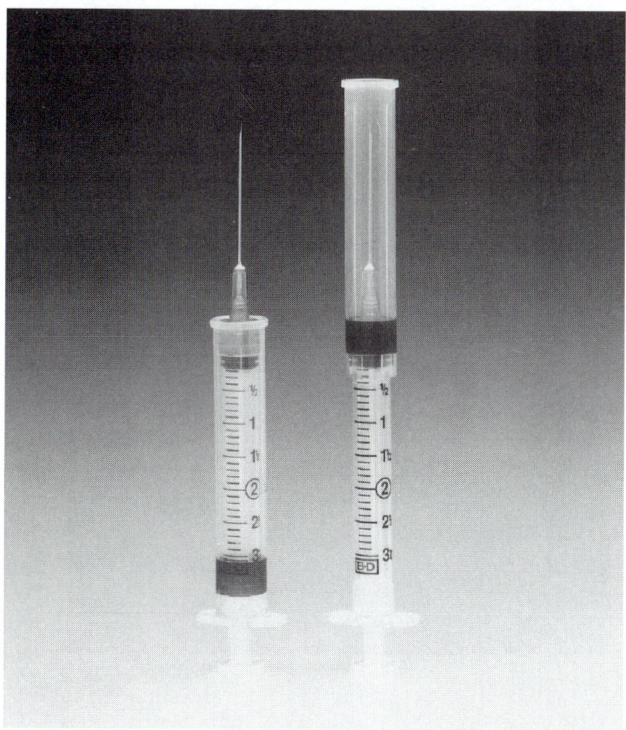

FIG. 21-7 Safety-Lok Syringe. (Courtesy Becton Dickinson and Co, Franklin Lakes, NJ.)

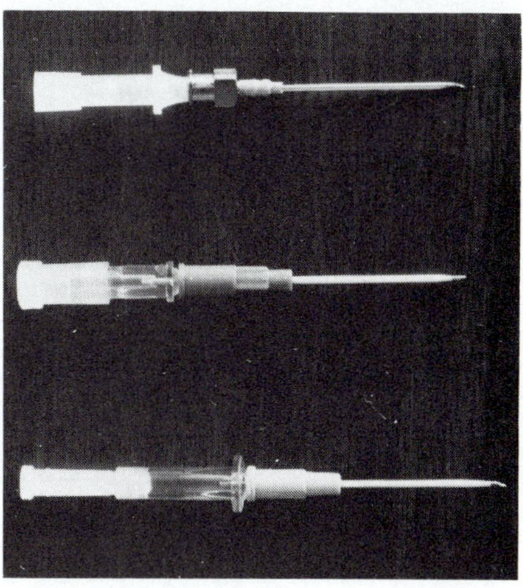

FIG. 21-10 Over-the-needle cannulae. (Courtesy Alton Ochsner Medical Foundation, New Orleans.)

SKILL 21-12

PREPARING PARENTERAL MEDICATIONS

1. Follow the five rights procedure (Box 21-4).
2. Perform the three label checks (Box 21-5).
3. Follow universal precautions (Box 12-3).
4. Wash hands before handling equipment; prepare medication in clean area; reduce distractions.
5. Keep sterile parts of syringe and needle sterile. Use aseptic technique throughout preparation.
6. Compare drug and dosage ordered with drug and dosage on hand; check expiration date, dosage per milliliter, total volume of solution in vial/ampule. Look for contaminants or defects in vial or ampule.
7. Calculate drug dosage and check calculations with another nurse.
8. Check compatibility chart or consult pharmacy if mixing two medications.

Withdrawing medication from a vial

9. Remove metal cap from top of vial; wipe rubber diaphragm briskly with alcohol sponge.
10. Pull plunger of syringe back to aspirate air into syringe equal to amount of drug to be withdrawn.
11. Insert needle into inverted vial; inject air and withdraw volume of solution to be given. Keep needle under solution to prevent aspiration of air into syringe.
12. Push plunger gently to disperse solution to tip of needle. Remove air bubbles by gently tapping syringe.

Withdrawing medication from an ampule

13. Tap the top of ampule to move solution from top of ampule to bottom of ampule (see illustration).
14. Cover neck of ampule with an alcohol sponge; break off top of ampule; deposit top of glass ampule in "sharps" container (see illustration).
15. Use a filter needle to aspirate medication from ampule. Filter or aspiration needles catch particles of glass that may be in the solution from the broken ampule.
16. Insert filter needle into open neck of ampule; invert ampule to withdraw correct dose.
17. Replace filter needle with needle appropriate for purpose of and viscosity of solution
18. Push plunger gently until the medication is at tip of needle.

Reconstituting a powdered dosage form

19. Follow instructions on manufacturer's box and drug insert. The instructions will specify the type and amount of diluent to use (e.g., add 10 ml bacteriostatic saline to prepare a ratio of 500 mg/ml).
20. Remove the protective cap from diluent; withdraw diluent using sterile technique.

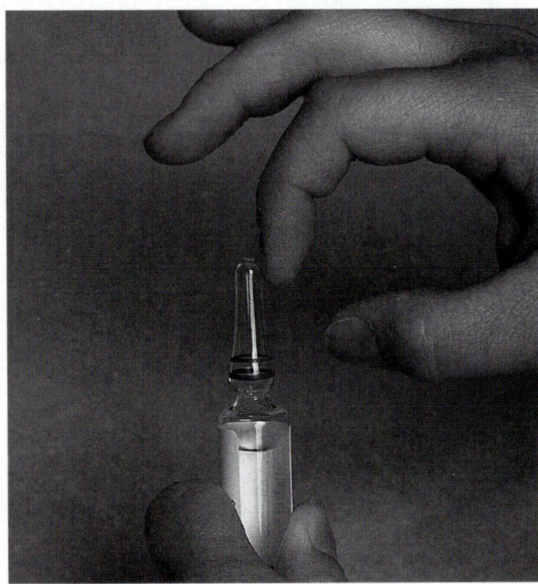

STEP 13

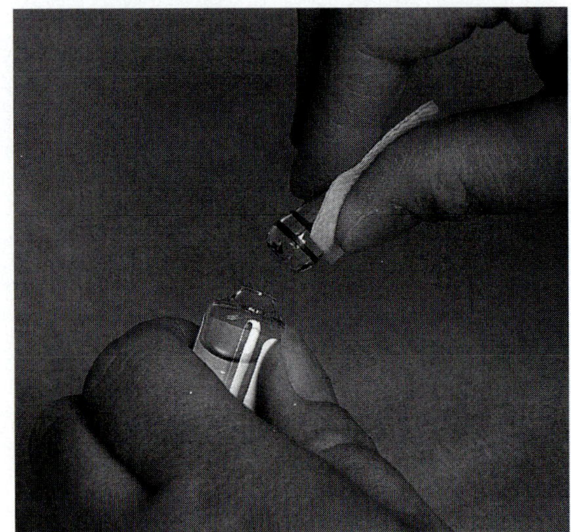

STEP 14

PREPARING PARENTERAL MEDICATIONS—cont'd

21. Withdraw needle from diluent vial (see illustration).
22. Inject diluent into vial of powdered drug; gently shake and tap vial to dissolve powder into solution (see illustration).
23. Label solution with:
    a. Date and time mixed
    b. Name of person who mixed drug and diluent
    c. Dosage per milliliter obtained (concentration)
    d. Amount and type of diluent used
24. Withdraw correct dose; select appropriate needle gauge and length for patient.

Placing two medications into one syringe (insulin example used)

25. Check compatibility of two drugs with a compatibility chart or call pharmacy.
26. Check and compare label of each drug ordered with label of each drug on hand.
27. Compare each label with medication order.
28. Roll long- and intermediate-acting insulin between the palms; do not shake any insulin.
29. Briskly wipe tops of both vials with separate alcohol swab.
30. Pull back plunger of syringe to amount equal to volume of longer-acting insulin to be given.
31. Insert needle and inject air into vial of longer-acting insulin.
32. Withdraw needle from vial; *do not* remove insulin.
33. Pull back plunger of syringe to amount equal to volume of shorter-acting (regular) insulin to be given.
34. Insert needle through rubber stopper of second vial; inject air into vial.
35. Invert vial; withdraw volume of shorter-acting (regular) insulin.
36. Check dosage in syringe against medication order.
37. Wipe rubber stopper of longer-acting insulin; insert needle of the syringe containing shorter-acting insulin and withdraw ordered dose of longer-acting insulin.
38. Remove needle/syringe from vial.
39. Check labels of both vials against medication order; check order/dosage with another nurse.
40. Pull plunger back enough to allow space in barrel of syringe for insulin to be gently mixed. Mix by tilting syringe back and forth; remove air.
41. Change needles; inject subcutaneously.

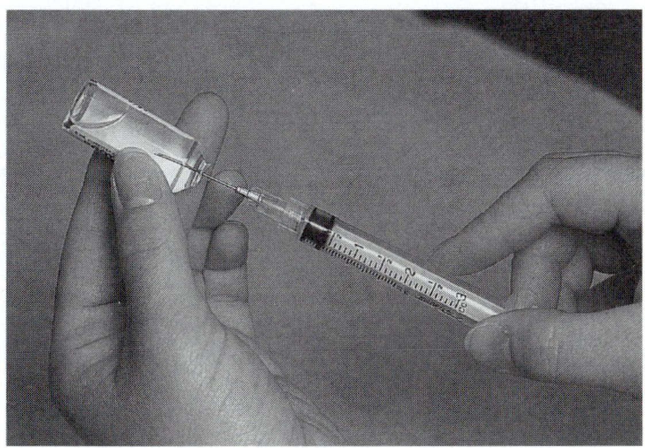

STEP 21

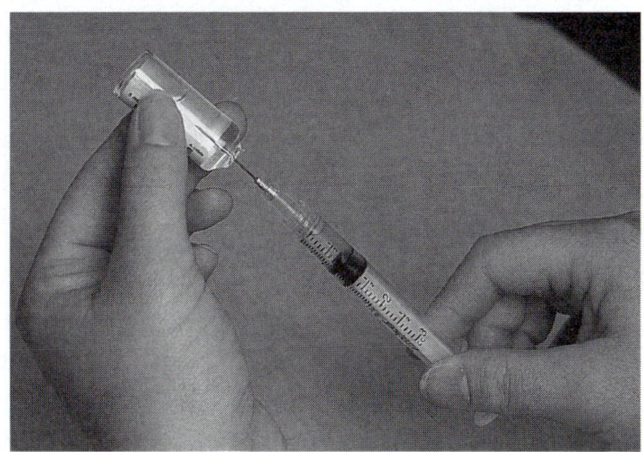

STEP 22

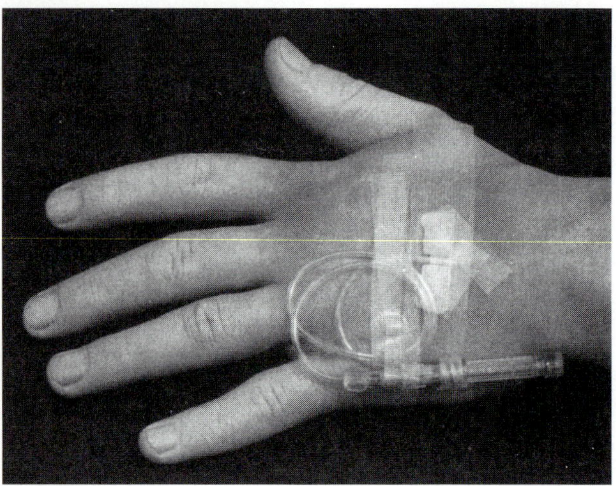

FIG. 21-11 Butterfly, scalp, or wing-tipped needle in place as a heparin lock.

Angiocaths are plastic catheters over a stainless steel needle stylet. A stylet is a sharp, bevel-tipped metal guide that is used to pierce the skin and vein. Once the catheter is in the vein, blood return is seen and the stylet is removed. The plastic catheter is left in the vein. The catheter is preferred for long-term IV use, because it is more flexible and can withstand patient movement.

Butterflies (Fig. 21-11) and Angiocaths cannot be used for an indefinite length of time and should be assessed for patency (openness) and intactness or complications every shift.

Intracaths are similar to Angiocaths, except that they are much longer. Physicians insert Intracaths for long-term intravenous administration or for intravenous nutritional feedings (hyperalimentation). See Skill 21-12 on pp. 420-421 for preparation of parenteral medications.

Box 21-6 CHARACTERISTICS OF INTRAMUSCULAR SITES

VASTUS LATERALIS MUSCLE

- This large, developed muscle lacks major nerves and blood vessels and is the most fully developed muscle in the newborn.
- Rapid drug absorption occurs.

VENTROGLUTEAL MUSCLE

- A deep site, the ventrogluteal muscle is situated away from major nerves and blood vessels. There is less chance of contamination in incontinent patients or infants because it is away from the rectum.
- It is easily identified by a prominent bony landmark.

DORSOGLUTEAL MUSCLE

- The nurse runs the risk of striking the underlying sciatic nerve, greater trochanter, or major blood vessels.
- This site is not used with infants or children under 3 years of age due to underdeveloped muscle.
- This site must be clean to avoid contamination.

DELTOID MUSCLE

- This site is easily accessible, but the muscle is not well developed in most patients.
- Nurses use this site for small amounts of medications.
- The nurse avoids using the deltoid muscle in infants or children with underdeveloped muscles.
- There is potential for injury to radial and ulnar nerves.
- Less discomfort is felt in the deltoid, and this site is less likely to impair circulation.

Intramuscular Injections

An intramuscular (IM) injection involves inserting a needle into the muscle tissue to administer medication. Since muscle tissue has a large blood supply, absorption of an IM medication is faster than a subcutaneous injection. The most commonly used sites are the upper, outer quadrant of the gluteal area, the ventrogluteal area, the vastus lateralis of the thigh, and the deltoid muscle of the arm.

Site selection is based on the amount and type of medication to be injected, the size of the individual's muscle mass, and the integrity of the individual's tissue. Damage to nerves or blood vessels may result from improper site selection (see Box 21-6 for characteristics of IM sites).

Site Selection.

Gluteal sites. The gluteal sites are the ventrogluteal and the dorsogluteal. The ventrogluteal site (Fig. 21-12) is located by using three landmarks—the greater trochanter, the anterior iliac spine, and the iliac crest (the hip bone).

With the palm of the hand on the lateral portion of the greater trochanter and the index (pointer) finger on the anterior superior iliac spine, the nurse extends the middle finger to the iliac crest. Medication is injected into the V formed by the index and middle fingers. The best position for the patient is prone. Muscle relaxation is promoted by turning the patient's toes inward. A side-lying position may also be used, with muscle relaxation promoted by flexing the upper leg.

The dorsogluteal site (Fig. 21-13) is located by using the posterior superior iliac spine and the greater trochanter. An imaginary line is drawn between these two landmarks, and medication is injected at any point along the imaginary line and below the curve of the iliac crest.

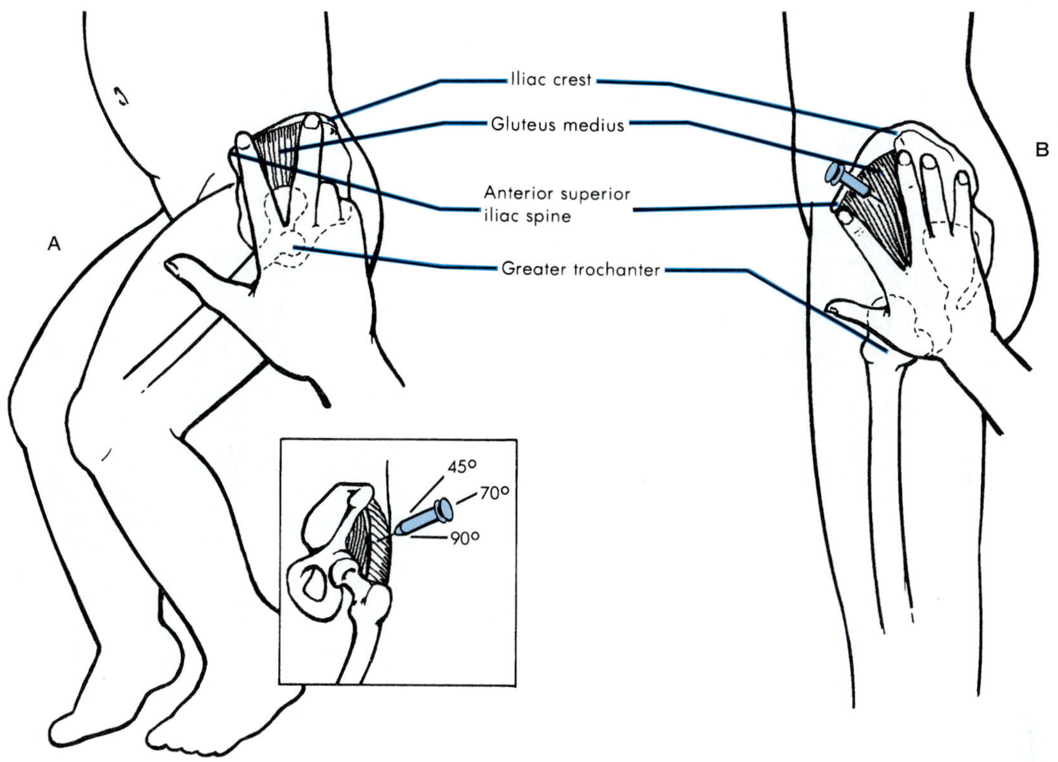

FIG. 21-12 Ventrogluteal site. **A,** Child/infant. **B,** Adult.

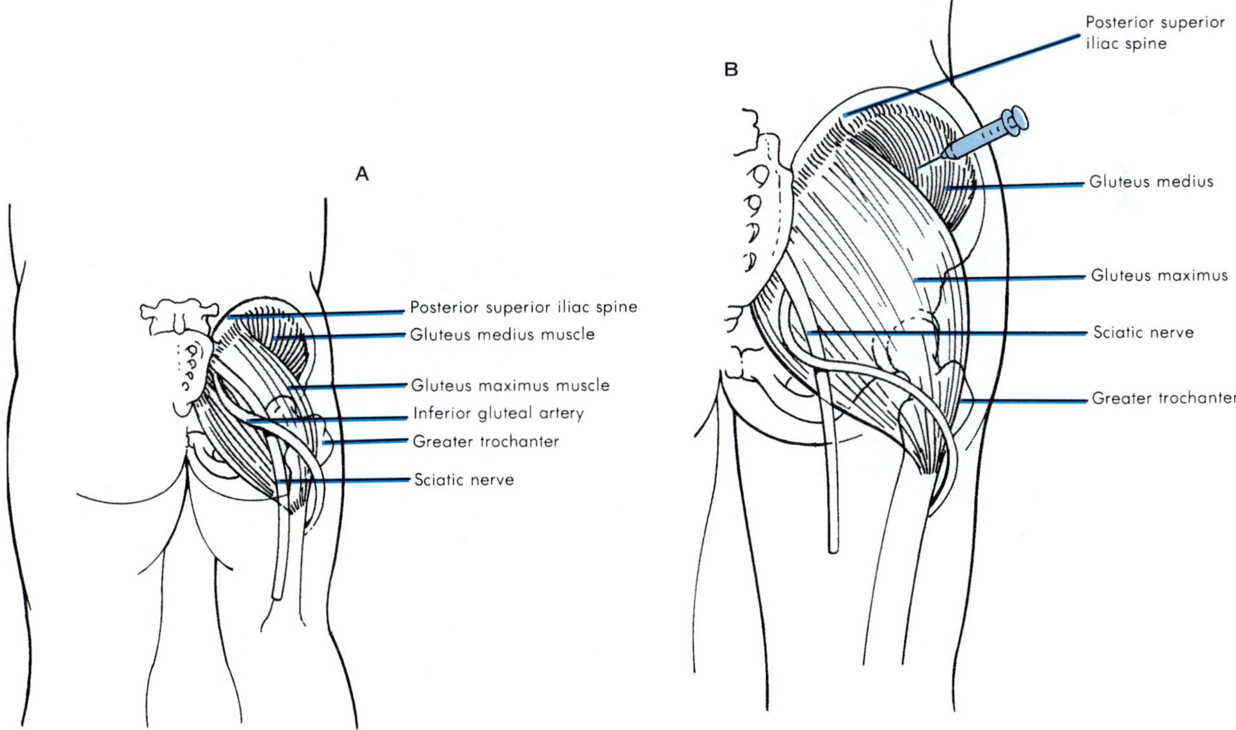

FIG. 21-13 Dorsogluteal site. **A,** Child/infant. **B,** Adult.

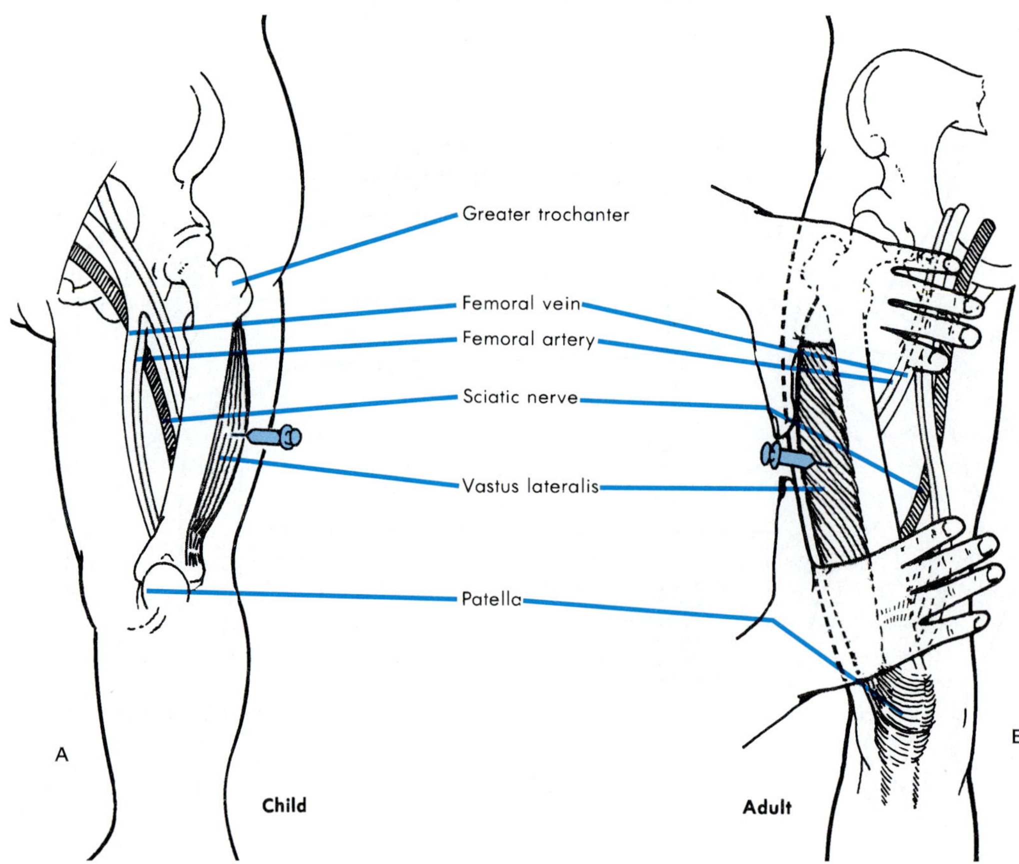

FIG. 21-14 Vastus lateralis muscle. **A,** Child/infant. **B,** Adult.

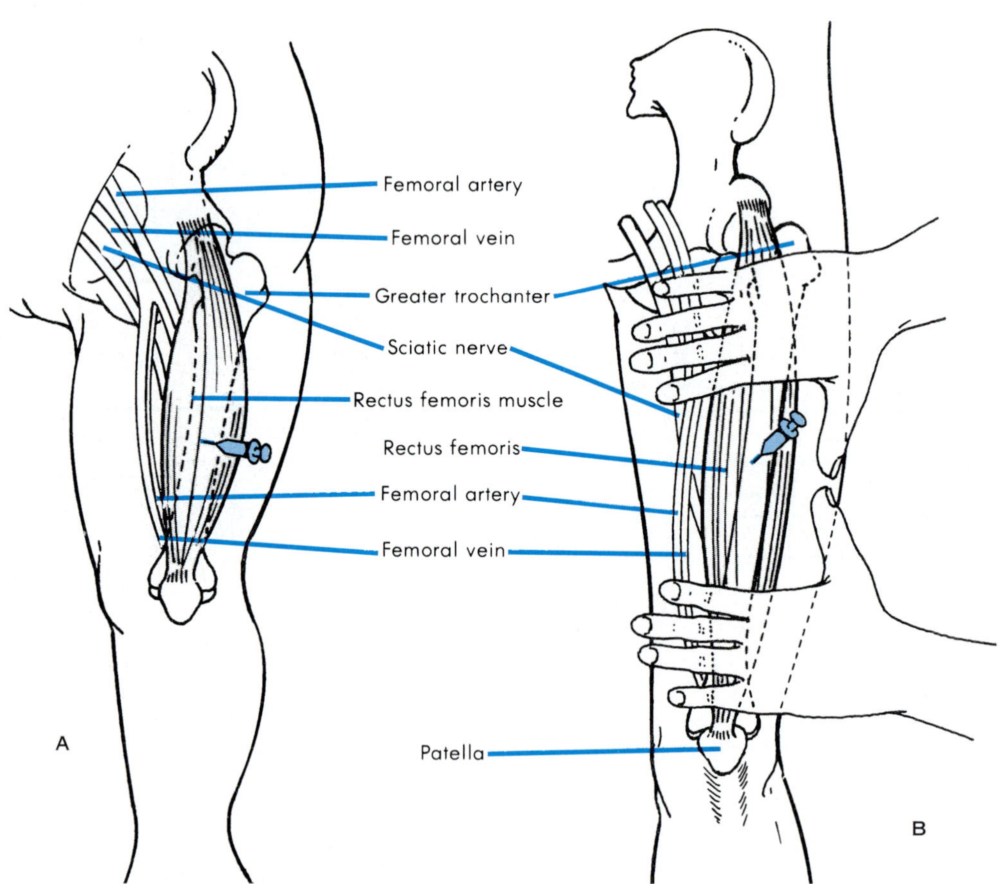

FIG. 21-15 Rectus femoris muscle. **A,** Child/infant. **B,** Adult.

The patient should be in a prone position with the toes turned inward to promote muscle relaxation. A side-lying position may be used, with muscle relaxation promoted by flexing the upper leg.

The gluteal sites are used commonly for IM preoperative medications or analgesic, because the gluteal muscles are large enough in most patients to inject up to 3 ml in one site. The gluteal muscles should not be used in children under 3 years of age, because their gluteal muscles are not developed from walking.

The sciatic nerve and superior gluteal artery are bypassed when proper site selection is carried out.

A second method is to visualize imaginary lines that divide the buttocks into a square box with four equal quadrants. The top of the square begins at the iliac crest; the bottom of the square is the gluteal fold where the buttocks join the thigh. The upper outer quadrant is the site for injection.

The vastus lateralis muscle (Fig. 21-14) is the preferred site for children under 3 years of age, because it is free of nerves and blood vessels. It is also used in adults when other sites are not accessible. The vastus is located on the anterior lateral thigh. The patient should be in a supine or sitting position. One hand is placed above the patient's knee and one hand below the greater trochanter. The IM injection is made in the area between the two hands. Depending on development of this muscle, up to 3 ml of medication may be injected.

The rectus femoris muscle (Fig. 21-15) is located by the same manner as the vastus lateralis. The rectus femoris is *medial* to the vastus lateralis. It is the common site for self-administration of medication. The sciatic nerve lies close to this muscle, and major blood vessels are also present, making the site potentially dangerous to use.

The deltoid muscle (Fig. 21-16) of the upper arm is a relatively small area. No more than 2 ml should be injected into this muscle. The patient may be positioned in a sitting, standing, prone, or supine position. The patient is asked to relax his arm during the injection to decrease discomfort.

The landmarks for locating the proper area for injection are the acromion process of the scapula and the axillary fold. An imaginary line can be drawn that extends from the axillary fold across the lateral aspect of the arm; the center of this area is the thicker midportion of the muscle, where the injection is given.

Generally, the deltoid is too small in children and older adults. Also the brachial vein and artery and the radial nerve are in this area. See Skill 21-13 and Fig. 21-17 on p. 426.

Z-track method. Z-track is used for injecting medications that are irritating to the tissues. Z-track IM administration seals medication deep within muscle tissue. Z-track does not allow staining or tracking of the medication into the tissue as the needle is withdrawn. This method is used when giving Imferon (iron) (Skill 21-14 on p. 427).

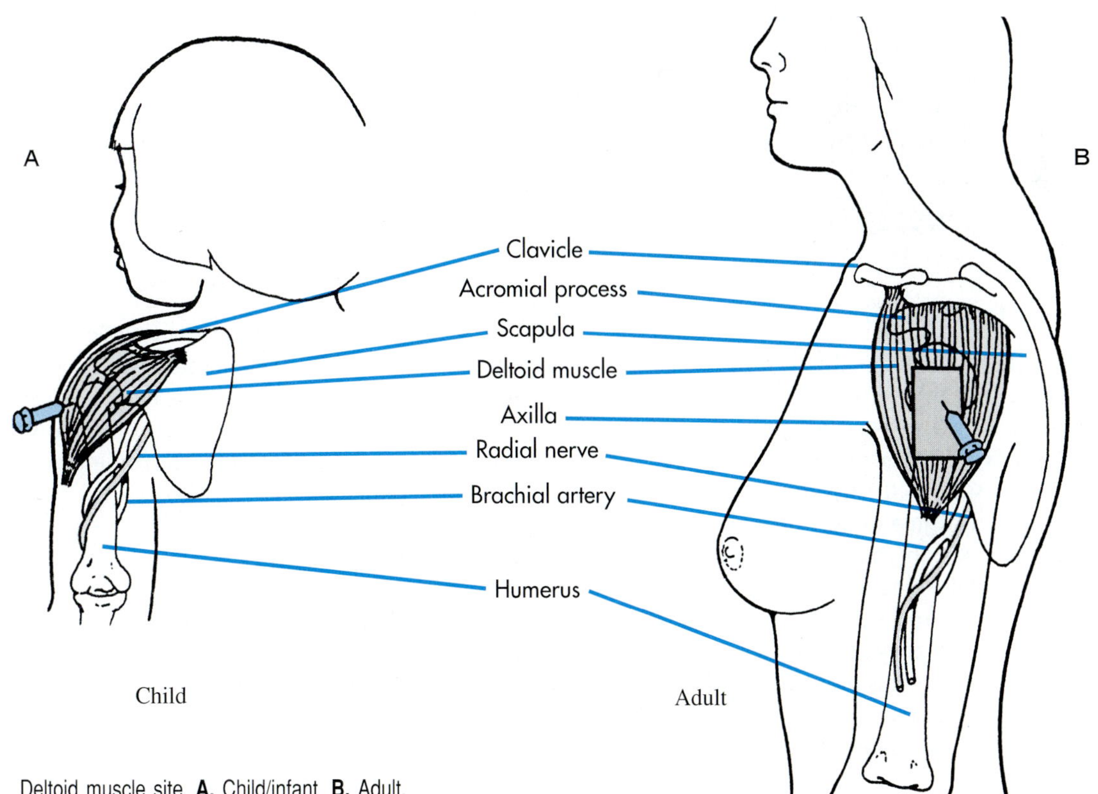

FIG. 21-16 Deltoid muscle site. **A,** Child/infant. **B,** Adult.

SKILL 21-13

GIVING AN INTRAMUSCULAR INJECTION

1. Follow the five rights procedure (Box 21-4).
2. Perform the three label checks (Box 21-5).
3. Follow universal precautions (Box 12-3).
4. Wash hands.
5. Prepare medication according to standard procedure for injectables.
6. Don gloves.
7. Identify patient and explain the procedure.
8. Select and expose site (according to IM site selection procedure); provide privacy.
9. Clean skin with alcohol swab (from center outward), spread skin tight with thumb and index finger; let dry.
10. Ask patient to take a deep breath and exhale slowly to relax muscle as needle is inserted (lessens pain from injection).
11. Insert needle at a 90-degree angle quickly in a dartlike motion (see illustration). Quickness reduces discomfort.
12. Maintain needle in muscle; gently aspirate (pull back plunger) to be certain needle is in muscle (and not in a vein or an artery).
13. If blood is seen, needle is in a vein or artery; withdraw needle; prepare new medication. Select another site.
14. Slowly inject medication into muscle to lessen discomfort.
15. Withdraw needle quickly without bending or twisting it.
16. Use pressure and gauze (2 × 2) to stop any bleeding.
17. *Do not* recap needle; dispose directly into sharps container.
18. Remove gloves and wash hands.
19. Chart site used and amount and type of medication (e.g., Demerol 50 mg given IM left ventrogluteal). Remember a quick, dartlike insertion followed by slow injection of the medication is much less painful to the patient.

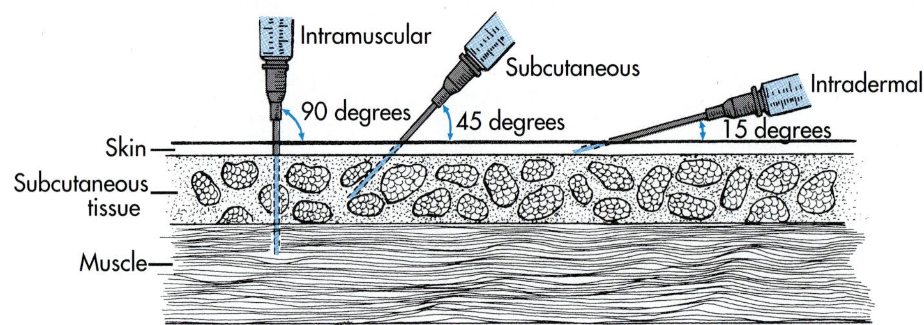

FIG. 21-17 Angles of insertion for intramuscular (90 degrees), subcutaneous (45 degrees), and intradermal (15 degrees) injections.

Intradermal Injections

An intradermal (ID) injection is the introduction of a hypodermic needle into the dermis for the purpose of instilling a substance such as a serum, vaccine, or skin test agent. Intradermals are not aspirated.

Small volumes such as 0.1 ml are injected to form a small bubblelike wheal just under the skin. Absorption is slow, which makes it the best route for allergy sensitivity tests, tuberculin screening, desensitization injections, local anesthetics, and vaccinations. Because these medications are potent, they are injected into the dermis, where the blood supply is reduced and drug absorption occurs slowly. A patient may have a severe anaphylactic reaction if the medications enter the circulation too rapidly.

A tuberculin syringe is used to give intradermals because the tuberculin syringe holds only a maximum of 1 ml or 16 ♍. A 25-gauge, ⅝ inch needle is used.

The upper chest, inner aspect of the lower arm, and scapular area are used for intradermal injections (see Fig. 21-17 and Skill 21-15 on p. 428).

Subcutaneous Injections

Insulin and heparin are given by the subcutaneous route. Injections are made into the loose, connective tissue between the dermis and the muscle layer. Because subcutaneous tissue is not as richly supplied with blood as the muscles, drug absorption is somewhat slower than with IM injections. The outer aspect of the upper arms, the

GIVING A Z-TRACK INJECTION

1. Follow the five rights procedure (Box 21-4).
2. Perform the three label checks (Box 21-5).
3. Follow universal precautions (Box 12-3).
4. Wash hands.
5. Prepare medication according to standard procedure for injectables.
6. Don gloves.
7. Use one needle to withdraw dose from container. Use another needle (1½ to 2 inches) to inject medication so that no solution remains on the outside needle shaft.
8. The nurse draws up 0.2 ml of air to create an air lock.
9. Expose and locate dorsogluteal or ventrogluteal site according to IM site selection procedure (see illustration); provide privacy.
10. Clean site with an alcohol swab.
11. Ask the patient to take a deep breath and to slowly exhale (to relax the muscle). Pull skin

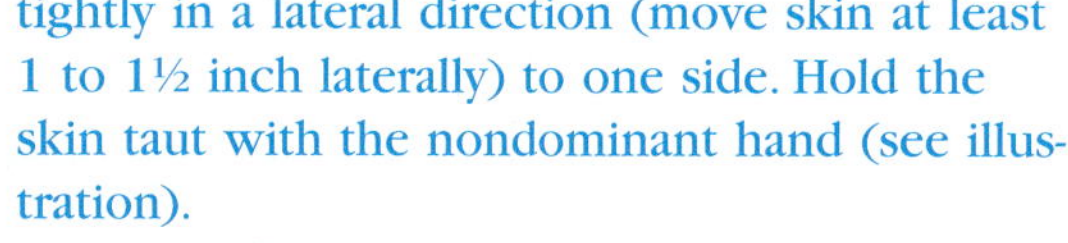

tightly in a lateral direction (move skin at least 1 to 1½ inch laterally) to one side. Hold the skin taut with the nondominant hand (see illustration).
12. Insert needle at a 90-degree angle; aspirate; if no blood is seen, inject medication and air slowly; wait 10 seconds to allow the medication to disperse slowly (see illustration).
13. Withdraw needle quickly; allow skin to return to its normal position, which leaves a zigzag path that seals the needle track wherever tissue planes slide across each other. The drug cannot escape from the muscle tissue (see illustration).
14. Use a 2 × 2 gauze pad or Band-Aid as needed.
15. *Do not* massage site.
16. *Do not* recap needle; dispose directly into sharps container.
17. Remove gloves and wash hands.
18. Chart site used, Z-track method used, and amount and type of medication given.

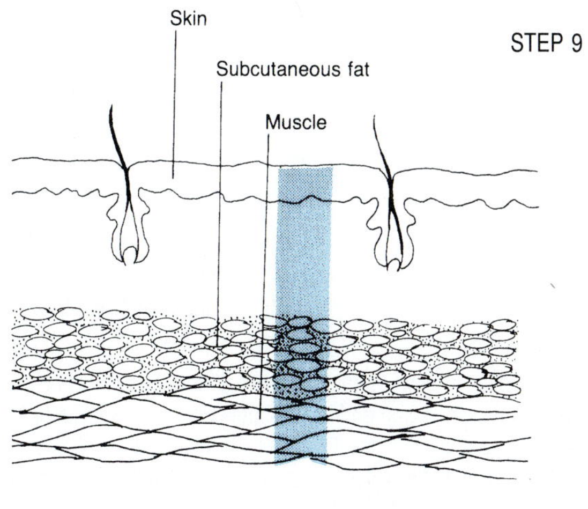

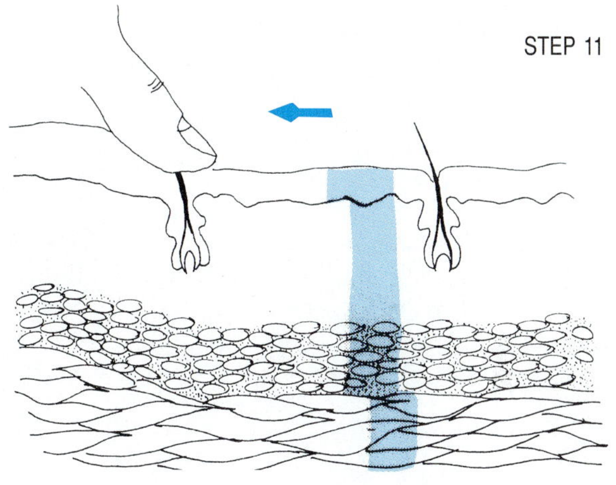

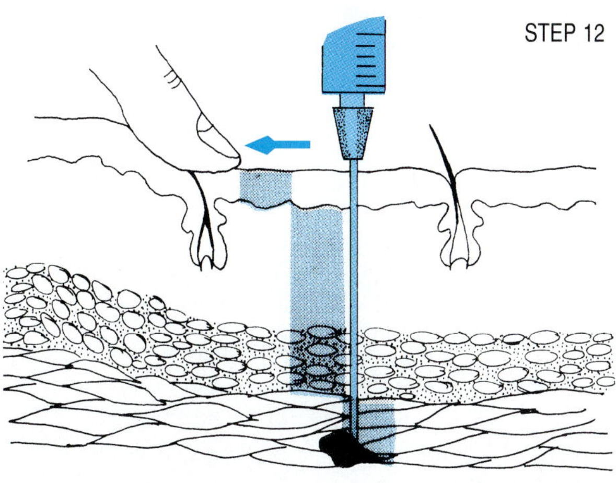

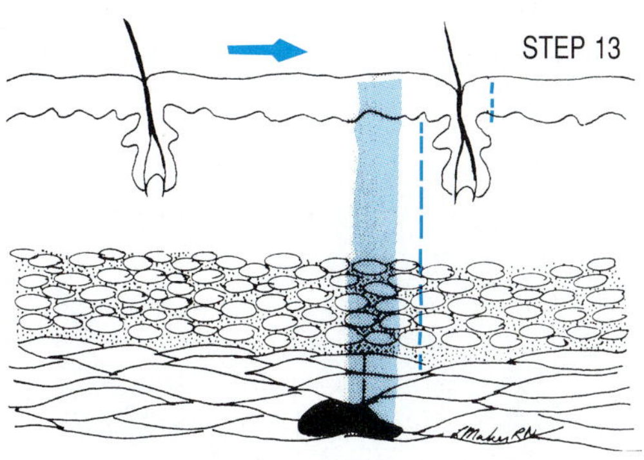

SKILL 21-15

GIVING AN INTRADERMAL INJECTION

1. Follow the five rights procedure (Box 21-4).
2. Perform the three label checks (Box 21-5).
3. Follow universal precautions (Box 12-3).
4. Wash hands.
5. Prepare medication according to standard procedure for injectables.
6. Don gloves.
7. Identify patient and explain procedure (see p. 404).
8. Select and expose inner aspect of lower arm.
9. Clean site gently with alcohol swab from center outward; let dry.
10. Two injections are made if test is for sensitivity. One injection is a control using sterile water or bacteriostatic saline; the other is substance that is to be tested.
11. Insert a 25-gauge needle with bevel up directly under skin to make a small bleb (bubble) with test solution. Insert needle at approximately a 15-degree angle (see p. 426). *Do not* inject into subcutaneous tissue. Inject control of saline into another site for comparison with test substance at designated time interval.
12. *Do not* massage site.
13. Draw a circle around skin test with a marker; label area with date, time, and name of test. Another method is to make a diagram in patient's chart to indicate location of site.
14. Remove gloves and wash hands.
15. If an indurated (hardened) erythematous area is observed, measure and record results in millimeters with metric ruler.
16. Compare control with agent; document results in chart.

A

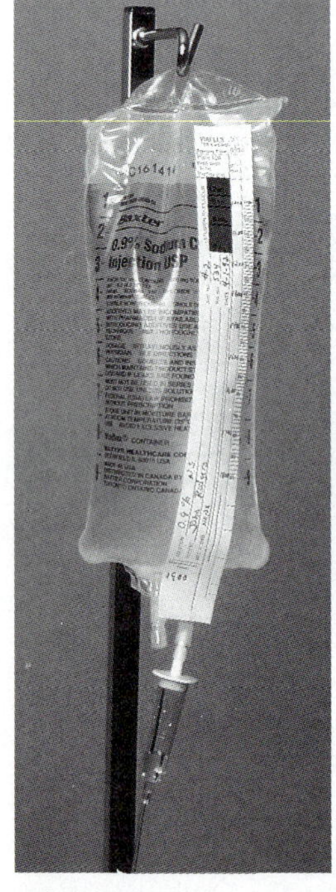

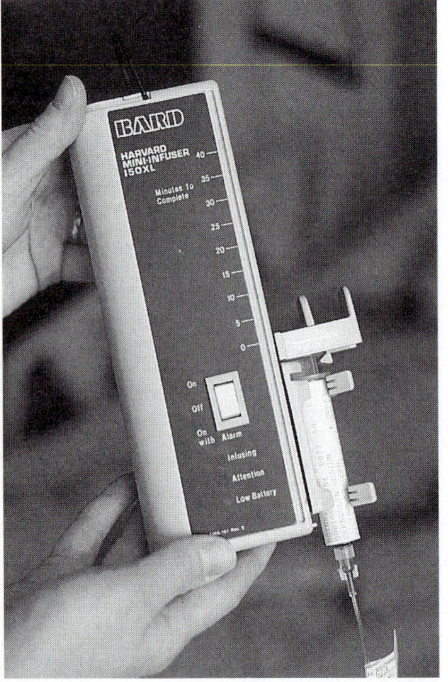

B

FIG. 21-18 Intravenous therapy. **A,** IV fluid container—gravity causes the fluid to flow. The container may be a glass bottle or plastic bag. **B,** Infusion pump and/or flow rate controller—special devices that may be attached to the IV system to mechanically control and maintain a precise rate of flow. If the pump or controller alarm sounds, the nurse will attend to the device. **C,** IPID—a small, plastic tube with a rubber seal on one end, which allows IV medication to be given intermittently. **D,** Flushing the intermittent peripheral infusion device.

C

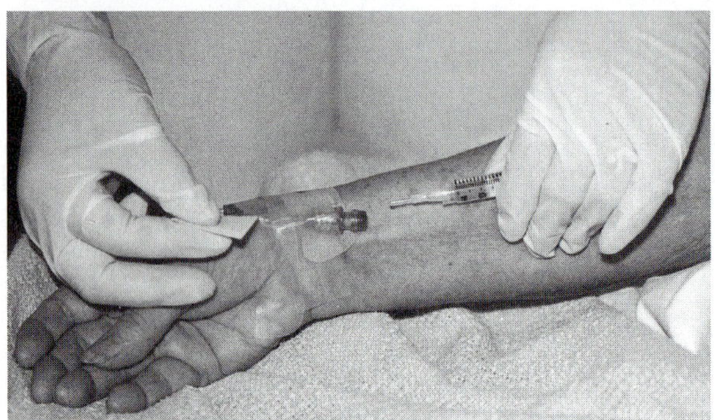

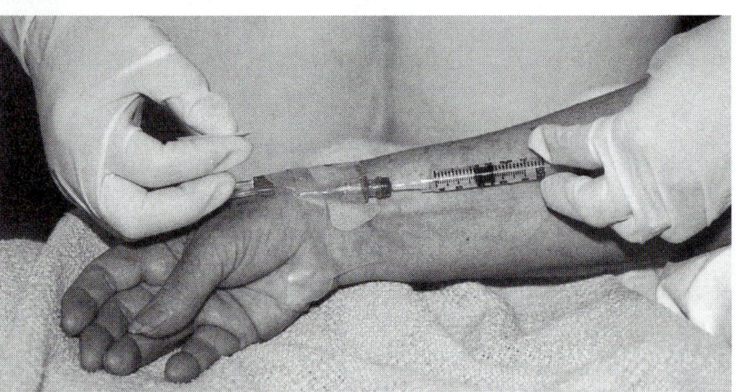

D

GIVING A SUBCUTANEOUS INJECTION

1. Follow the five rights procedure (Box 21-3).
2. Perform the three label checks (Box 21-4).
3. Follow universal precautions (Box 12-3).
4. Wash hands.
5. Prepare medication according to standard procedure for injectables.
6. Don gloves.
7. Identify patient and explain procedure (see p. 404).
8. Select and expose site (check which site was used previously and rotate site). The abdomen is the usual preferred site when administering heparin.
9. Clean site with an alcohol swab from center outward in circular motion; let dry.
10. *Method A:* Spread skin of selected site taut and hold firmly; insert needle at 45-degree angle (see p. 426) and aspirate; inject medication. Do not aspirate if heparin is being administered. *Method B:* Grasp and press together skin of selected site so that it forms roll between fingers. Insert needle at a 90-degree angle and aspirate. Do not aspirate if heparin is being given. Inject medication.
11. Withdraw needle quickly and apply an antiseptic swab or a 2 × 2 gauze sponge. Do not massage the site if heparin is administered, because this will increase local bleeding and ecchymosis will occur.
12. *Do not* recap needle; dispose directly into sharps container.
13. Remove gloves and wash hands.
14. Chart site used and amount and type of medication.

abdomen, thighs, and scapula are sites used for subcutaneous (SQ, SC, Subq) injections. The site of these injections should receive no more than 1 ml of solution and should always be carefully charted. Sites are rotated to prevent damage tissue and prevent discomfort.

Subcutaneous injections are given at a 45-degree angle if the patient is thin or at a 90-degree angle if the patient has ample subcutaneous tissue. Judgment is used in selecting sites for injection and in determining the angle of injection. Needle length is selected so that the medication will be injected into subcutaneous tissue and not muscle tissue. Usual needle length is ½ to ⅝ inch, and a 25-gauge needle is the one of choice (see Fig. 21-17 and Skill 21-16).

Intravenous Therapy

The intravenous (IV) route of administration is used more frequently as nurses assume more responsibility in IV therapy (Fig. 21-18). Advances in technology of IV equipment also enable nurses and physicians to deliver IV fluids and medications more safely.

The IV route is used to (1) provide fluid and electrolyte maintenance, restoration, and replacement; (2) administer medications and nutritional feedings, (3) administer blood and blood products, (4) administer chemotherapy to cancer patients; and (5) administer patient-controlled analgesics.

Methods of IV Administration. IV medications may be administered by several methods.

IV push. The medication is given directly into a vein or by means of a heparin or saline lock or injection port of an existing IV tubing set.

Intermittent peripheral infusion device. **Intermittent peripheral infusion devices** (IPID) (IV infusion devices with male adaptors covered by rubber diaphragms) for the administration of intermittent infusions and as an access site for emergency drugs are increasingly common (Fig. 21-18, *C*). Practitioners continue to have unanswered questions regarding the best solution to maintain the patency of intermittent infusion devices, heparin versus saline flushes.

IPIDs are devices that attach onto the needle hub. Once attached, the IPID is filled with the anticoagulant heparin or normal saline. IPID revolutionized IV therapy. They are also used in a wide variety of diagnostic tests. IPID make IV antibiotic therapy and other IV drug therapies readily accessible without causing the unnecessary pain of a restick with every dose.

Diluted heparin or normal saline is used in the IPID to keep the vein open; therefore IV medication can be administered at intervals without requiring a continuous infusion of fluid to ensure patency. A patient is able to receive IV medication without the necessity of running a fluid. This procedure is done by an RN or an LPN/LVN, depending upon the nurse practice act for each state.

The IPID, when ready for use, is flushed with 3 ml of normal saline before and after the medication. In some agencies, the IPID is then injected with diluted heparin. Flushing the IPID prevents drug incompatibility from occurring between two incompatible drugs or fluids. Disagreement exists as to the type of solution to use to keep IPIDs free of clots. Agency policies differ in flushing with normal saline or diluted heparin to maintain IPID patency.

Intermittent infusion (or piggyback). IV piggybacks (IVPB) are drug infusions that are given at intervals, such as qid (four times a day). They may be connected to heparin or saline locks or to the injection port of the IV tubing. Once the medication has infused, the piggyback is removed from the heparin or saline lock or IV tubing. Antibiotics are frequently given in this manner.

Continuous infusions. Medication is added to a bag of IV fluid and is infused over the time that the IV fluid infuses.

Electronic pumps and controllers. Pumps and controllers regulate the flow rate of infusions. Pumps deliver the fluid via pressure while controllers deliver the infusion with the aid of gravity. Controllers monitor the flow rate of fluid by a photoelectric eye (Fig. 21-19, *B*).

Patient-controlled analgesia (PCA). **Patient-controlled analgesia** (PCA) (a drug-delivery system that dispenses a preset IV dose of a narcotic analgesic into a patient's vein when the patient pushes a switch on an electric cord) (see Fig. 21-19, *A*) is administered by a programmable pump that is controlled by the patient. The nurse programs the pump according to the physician's order, which specifies the amount of narcotic the patient receives per each dose. The pump also controls the total amount of drug that may be received over a specific period. A lockout interval device automatically inactivates the system if a patient tries to increase the amount of narcotic within a preset time period.

The nurse is responsible for programming the computerized pump and for loading the morphine, Demerol, or Buprenex vial into it. The nurse is responsible for:

- Instructing the patient to press/release button when analgesia is needed
- Maintaining PCA therapy:
  - Monitoring number of dosages received by patient
  - Monitoring respirations and blood pressure of patient for signs of oversedation
  - Monitoring patient for relief of pain
  - Documenting total volume infused and remaining volume in vial every shift
  - Monitoring accuracy of infusion; checking drug infusing, dose volume, and lockout interval with physician's order

PCA medication infusion is considered by many to provide more pain relief with less medication. Also, the patient is more in control of medication administration, which may help lessen anxiety and pain. The PCA (Fig. 21-19, *A*) is an effective and efficient method for administration of analgesic medications. Dose rates and limits are programmed according to physician's orders, and the patient self-administers the medication by pressing a button.

Special PCA order sheets are used by the physician to specify the following:

1. *Type/Strength of Medication*

EXAMPLE: Morphine sulfate 1 mg/ml
or
Demerol (meperidine) 10 mg/ml

FIG. 21-19 **A,** Patient-controlled analgesia (PCA). **B,** Electronic pumps control the flow rate. (**A** Courtesy Abbott Laboratories, Abbott Park, Ill.)

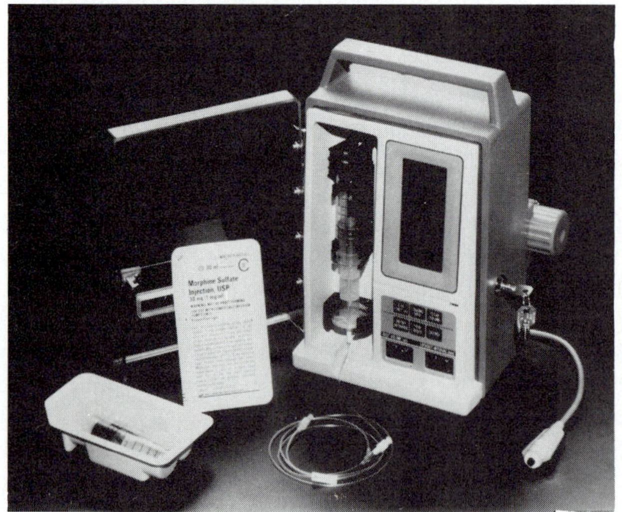

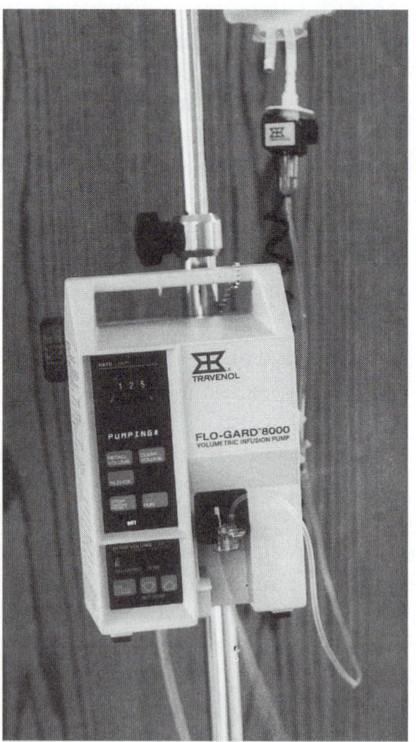

2. *Loading Dose* (an optional larger-than-usual dose to give initial pain relief)

   EXAMPLE: Range: 1.0-5.0 ml
   Usual: 1.0-2.0 ml

3. *Maintenance Dose* (dose dispensed each time patient presses control button)

   EXAMPLE: Range: 0.1-5.0 ml
   Usual: 0.5-1.0 ml

4. *Lockout Interval* (minimum time between doses)

   EXAMPLE: Range: 5-99 minutes
   Usual: 6-15 minutes

5. *Four-Hour Limit* (maximum volume delivered in 4 hours)

   EXAMPLE: Range: 5-30 ml in 5-ml increments
   Usual: 10-20 ml

Volumetric chambers. A volumetric chamber consists of IV tubing with a chamber that holds a prescribed amount of fluid; it is separate from the drip chamber. Medication such as Pitocin or lidocaine may be added to the fluid in the chamber. The delivery of the medication to the patient is carefully controlled when this method is used.

The Nurse's Responsibility in Maintaining IV Infusions. The physician orders the amount (see Fig. 20-1) and type of IV fluid and length of time that the infusion is to run. The nurse ensures that the ordered type and amount of fluid is started and that the fluid is regulated to infuse over the period ordered by the physician. An IV infusion is regulated by knowing the number of drops per minute that it will take for the entire volume of fluid to infuse over the specified time ordered by the physician.

To find the number of drops per minute (the *drip rate*), one must know which type of IV tubing will be used with the infusion. The nurse must look on the IV tubing box for the **drip factor** (an apparatus that is used to deliver measured amounts of IV solutions of specific flow rates based on the size of drops of the solution). The box will indicate whether the IV tubing is calibrated to deliver macrodrops or microdrops. Macrodrop sets will deliver 10, 15, or 20 drops per 1 ml of fluid while microdrop, or minidrop, sets will deliver 60 drops per 1 ml of fluid. The drip factor must be known to change milliliters to drops when calculating IV flow rates.

For example, a physician orders 1000 ml of D_5 ½ NS with 20 mEq KCl to be infused over an 8-hour period. How will the nurse know how many drops must drip from the drip chamber every minute for 8 hours to make the fluid run out in 8 hours? To find drops per minute, change millimeters to drops by multiplying millimeters by the drip factor (on tubing set).

EXAMPLE:

1000 ml	(total volume to be infused)
× 15	(drip factor)
5000	
1000	
15000 gtts	(drops)

Thus, 15,000 gtts will drip over 8 hours. Change hours to minutes.

EXAMPLE: 1 hr: 60 min :: 8 hr: x min

1x = 480

x = 480 min

To regulate the infusion, how many drops will need to drip over 1 minute?

EXAMPLE: 15,000 drops: 480 minutes :: X drops: 1 minute

480x = 15,000

x = 15,000 ÷ 480

x = 31 drops/min

The rate of fluid flow is regulated by adjusting the volume control clamp until 31 drops drip from the chamber in 1 minute. In 8 hours, the infusion should be completed as ordered.

EXAMPLE: The physician orders 1000 ml D_5W with 1 ampule of multiple vitamins to be infused over an 8-hour period. The drip factor on the box is 10 drips per 1 ml of fluid. Divide the amount to infuse (1000 ml) by the time period (8 hours). This will give the milliliters per hour.

$$8 \text{ hours} \overline{)\,1000 \text{ ml}} = 125 \text{ ml/hour}$$

To reduce the milliliters per hour to drops per minute, compute the following formula:

$$\frac{\text{Amount} \times \text{Drip factor}}{\text{Time}}$$

$$\frac{\text{(amount) } 125 \text{ (ml)} \times 10 \text{ (drip factor)}}{60 \text{ sec (time)}}$$

$$\frac{1250}{60} \qquad 60 \text{ sec}\overline{)\,1250} = 20/21 \text{ drops/min}$$

ANSWER: 20/21 drops/min

Monitoring IV Therapy. The nurse should check the infusion and the IV needle site at least every hour, looking at the flow of fluid, which may be altered or stopped by air in the tubing, kinked tubing, or clotted blood in the tubing. The tubing must be kept patent (open) to keep the venous site open. If the fluid flow is obstructed or significantly slowed, the needle will become occluded with coagulated blood. Another IV site will have to be selected and another venipuncture will have to be performed. The tubing must not be allowed to get air in it

GERONTOLOGICAL CONSIDERATIONS

- All phases of pharmacokinetics are affected by aging. Older persons should receive the lowest dosage of medication necessary to achieve the desired therapeutic benefits.
- Dry mouth often contributes to difficulty swallowing medications. Sipping water before attempting to swallow the medication or covering the medication with a moist food such as applesauce can facilitate swallowing.
- More precautions must be taken when administering parenteral medication to older adults because of a decreased amount of muscle and subcutaneous tissue. Sites must be examined for suitability and should be rotated. Needle length should be carefully chosen based on the selected site and a tissue assessment of the individual.
- Polypharmacy (use of excessive medications) is a problem seen in older adults. Each medication taken increases the risk of interactions or toxicity. Older persons should be taught to refrain from taking any medication unless it is approved by the primary physician.
- Accurate and current records of all prescription and over the counter medications should be kept by the older person. This list should be presented each time medical attention is sought.
- Due to decreased renal, cardiac, and/or hepatic functioning, the older adult is at greater risk of becoming adversely and possibly fatally affected by medications. Also, hospitalized older adults often have one or more chronic illnesses for which they take multiple medications.
- The nurse must be aware and observe for signs and symptoms of decreased drug excretion, cumulative effects of drugs, drug potentiations, and drug incompatibilities. Toxic, lethal, and even fatal effects must be prevented by frequent observations and careful, thoughtful assessments of the older patient.
- Some older adults do not hear, see, communicate, or move about as well as younger patients. Some may also be disoriented and may become even more disoriented at night; therefore nurses who medicate older patients must take more time to carefully assess their level of consciousness *before* and *after* medicating them.
- The nurse will carefully observe the list of medications prescribed for each patient and ascertain whether there have been any incompatibilities or incorrect dosages or whether any medications are possibly adversely affecting the patient.
- *Any* medication may cause adverse effects in the older adult, whether it is an antihistamine or a narcotic. Observe carefully for drug interactions and side effects immediately. Report and document all signs and symptoms detected. The nurse is often the first to notice a change in a patient's condition.
- The prevention of drug-related problems is the combined responsibility of the nurse, physician, pharmacist, and others who care for the patient. Communication between the health care team, the patient, *and* the patient's family must be strengthened to medicate the older adult safely and effectively.

as a result of an IV bag running dry. If bags are near completion, this should be reported to the RN or LPN/LVN, depending on the nurse state practice act.

The nurse observes the IV site every time the infusion is checked, looking for erythema, wetness, and edema. Inflammation may mean the onset of phlebitis (inflamed vein), and edema may be an extravasation (fluid infusing outside of the vein) or an infiltration of fluid into the tissue. These conditions should be reported. In addition, the following should be reported:

A patient with sudden onset of chills, fever, headache, nausea, and vomiting

An anxious, dyspneic patient with a weak and rapid pulse

These factors may indicate complications of IV therapy that require immediate medical intervention. Special considerations for older adults are highlighted in the box.

Allergic reactions may occur as a result of IV medication administration. Reactions range from a mild rash to **anaphylactic shock** (a severe, life-threatening hypersensitivity reaction). Signs and symptoms may appear suddenly or may appear as long as 30 to 60 minutes after an infusion of an IV medication. The following should be reported:

1. Respiratory distress from bronchospasms such as restlessness, dyspnea, wheezing, and cyanosis (bluish coloration of the skin)
2. Skin reactions such as pruritus (itching) or urticaria (hives)
3. Signs of circulatory collapse, such as rapidly falling blood pressure and weak and rapid (thready) pulse, vertigo
4. GI signs and symptoms such as nausea, vomiting, and diarrhea

Anaphylactic shock requires immediate intervention. The LPN/LVN should notify the RN immediately if any allergic signs or symptoms are observed.

REFERENCES AND SUGGESTED READINGS

1. Albanese J, Nutz A: *Mosby's 1995 nursing drug cards,* ed 3, St Louis, 1995, Mosby.
2. Asperhum M: *Pharmacology test,* ed 7, Philadelphia, 1992, Saunders.
3. Clark JB et al: *Pharmacologic basis of nursing practice,* ed 4, St Louis, 1993, Mosby.
4. Clayton D, Stock YN: *Basic pharmacology for nurses,* ed 10, St Louis, 1993, Mosby.
5. Clinical news, med watch and drug alert, *Nursing* 24(3):77, 1994.
6. Cohen MR et al: 12 ways to prevent medication errors, *Nursing* 24(2):34, 1994.
7. Drass J: What you need to know about insulin injections, *Nurs '92* 22(11):40, 1992.
8. *Fundamental nursing skills,* Springhouse, Penn, 1994, Springhouse.
9. Gahart BL: *Intravenous medication,* ed 8, St Louis, 1992, Mosby.
10. Goode CJ et al: Improving practice through research: the case of heparin vs. saline for peripheral intermittent infusion devices, *Med Surg Nurs* 2(1):23, 1993.
11. Hahn K: Brush up on your injection technique, *Nursing '90* 20(9):54, 1990.
12. Keen MF: Get on the right track with z-track injections, *Nursing '90* 20(8):59, 1990.
13. LaRocca C, Ottis S: *Pocket guide to intravenous therapy,* ed 2, St Louis, 1992, Mosby.
14. McConnell EA: Giving intradermal injections, *Nursing* 29(3):70, 1993.
15. McKenry LM, Salerno E: *Mosby's pharmacology in nursing,* ed 18, St Louis, 1992, Mosby.
16. *Medication administration and IV therapy manual,* ed 2, Springhouse, Penn, 1993, Springhouse.
17. Millam D: Avoiding needle-stick injuries, *Nurs '90* 20(1):61, 1990.
18. *Mosby's medical, nursing, and allied health dictionary,* ed 4, St Louis, 1994, Mosby.
19. Myers J: *Quick medication administration reference,* St Louis, 1992, Mosby.
20. Newton M, Newton D, Fundin J: Reviewing the big three injection routes, *Nurs '92* 22(2):34, 1992.
21. NPH ILITIN I: *Information for the patient (drug insert),* Indianapolis, 1992, Eli Lilly.
22. *Nursing '94 drug handbook,* Springhouse, Penn, 1994, Springhouse.
23. *Nursing procedures: student version,* 1992, Springhouse, Penn, 1992, Springhouse.
24. O'Donnell J: Drug therapy: 20 ways your role will change, *Nursing* 24(3):46, 1994.
25. Perry AG, Potter PA: *Clinical nursing skills and techniques,* ed 3, St Louis, 1994, Mosby.
26. Potter PA, Perry AG: *Basic nursing: theory and practice,* ed 3, St Louis, 1995, Mosby.
27. Potter PA, Perry AG: *Fundamentals of nursing: concepts, process and practice,* ed 3, St Louis, 1993, Mosby.
28. Reiss B, Melick M: *Pharmacological aspects of nursing care,* ed 3, Albany, NY, 1993, Delmar.
29. Senders J: Theory and analysis of typical errors in a medical setting, *Hosp Pharm* 28(6):505, 1993.
30. Sewester S: *Fact and comparison's drug information,* Philadelphia, 1992, Lippincott.
31. Skidmore LR: *Mosby's 1995 nursing drug reference,* St Louis, 1995, Mosby.
32. Stauffer S, Reilly RT: *Drug comparison handbook: generic to brand, brand to generic,* St Louis, 1992, Mosby.
33. Timby BK, Lewis LW: *Fundamental skills and concepts in patient care,* ed 5, Philadelphia, 1992, Lippincott.
34. Witmer D: Question and answer: heparin lock flush solution versus 0.9% sodium chloride injection for maintaining patency, *Am J Hosp Pharm* 50(2):241, 1993.
35. Wong DL: *Nursing care of infants and children,* ed 5, St Louis, 1995, Mosby.
36. Yanes-Eyler M: *Mosby's comprehensive review of practical nursing,* ed 10, St Louis, 1994, Mosby.

CHAPTER CHALLENGE

KEY POINTS

- The "five rights" of medication administration ensure accurate preparation and administration of medication dosages.
- Nurses administer only medications they prepare.
- The nurse never administers a medication without accurately identifying a patient.
- Medications should be charted immediately after administration.
- The nurse never leaves a prepared medication unattended.
- Failure to select injection sites by anatomical landmarks may lead to tissue, bone, or nerve damage.
- The nurse is ethically and legally responsible for ensuring that the patient receives the correct medication ordered by the physician.
- Each medication order should include the patient's name; order; date; medication name, dosage, route, and frequency of administration; and physician's signature.
- The nurse should always have a witness to the "wasting" (disposal) of part of a controlled medication, and both persons must sign the log book to indicate that the medication was wasted.
- Medications enter the body through oral, parenteral, percutaneous, and inhalation routes.
- Medications administered parenterally are absorbed more quickly than medications by other routes.
- Because of decreased renal, cardiac, or hepatic functioning, the older adult is at greater risk of becoming adversely and possibly fatally affected by medications.

STUDY QUESTIONS

1. Mr. Brown, a 71-year-old patient with hypertension, angina pectoris, anxiety, and a productive cough, is to receive the following medications at 8 AM qd. Which medication would be given *last:*
   1. Sublingual nitroglycerin
   2. Capoten tablet
   3. Robitussin cough syrup
   4. Librium
2. Ms. Wright, LPN, is asked by an RN to take an unlabeled container of solution to the operating room. Ms. Wright's best response is to say:
   1. "Of course, I'll take it right away!"
   2. "What is in the container?"
   3. "I will have the orderly take it."
   4. "I cannot transport an unlabeled container."
3. After a possible exposure to tuberculosis, a 25-year-old health worker receives a TB skin test. The skin test will be given by the following type of injection:
   1. Intramuscular
   2. Intradermal
   3. Subcutaneous
   4. Intravenous
4. Dr. Coker orders morphine sulfate gr 1/6 IM for a 28-year-old motorcyclist with multiple fractures. The nurse must choose from the following gauges of needles. Which one is most appropriate?
   1. 22
   2. 25
   3. 18
   4. 16
5. Insulin is to be given to a 55-year-old man admitted for diabetes mellitus. His insulin is to be given via subcutaneous injection. At what angle(s) may it be given:
   1. 15 degrees or 45 degrees
   2. 45 degrees or 90 degrees
   3. 15 degrees only
   4. 35 degrees only
6. The nurse must decide upon the angle used in delivering subcutaneous heparin. Her decision will be based upon:
   1. The amount of solution in the syringe
   2. The length and gauge of the needle
   3. The amount of subcutaneous tissue of the patient
   4. The needle length and the amount of subcutaneous tissue available
7. Ms. Smith complains of nausea after having a total abdominal hysterectomy. Her nurse prepares an injection of Phenergan 50 mg for IM injection. She selects a needle length of:
   1. 1-1½ inches
   2. 3/8 inch
   3. 5/8 inch
   4. ¼ inch
8. Six-month-old Jason is to be immunized for diphtheria, tetanus, and pertussis. His IM injection will be given in which muscle:
   1. Deltoid
   2. Ventrogluteal
   3. Gluteus maximus
   4. Vastus lateralis
9. Epinephrine contained in 0.3 ml is ordered for 18-year-old David who had an anaphylactic reaction to a bee sting. The nurse selected the following syringe as the best choice for delivering this volume of fluid:
   1. a 1-ml tuberculin syringe
   2. a 100 U per 1-ml syringe
   3. a 3-ml syringe
   4. a 5-ml syringe
10. Mrs. Rodrin, age 96, a nursing home patient, is to receive several medications at 2100. These medications are for emphysema, peripheral vascular disease, and arteriosclerosis. The nurse realizes that the dosages for an older person are:
    1. The same as for pediatric patients
    2. The same as average adult dosages
    3. Higher than average adult dosages
    4. Lower than average adult dosages

8

THE SURGICAL PATIENT

Nursing is the giving of yourself and getting a multitude in return. It's caring and showing kindness and understanding. It's walking into a patient's room and focusing on that patient as a person—not a room number. It's looking into that person's eyes and seeing deep inside that person—emotional as well as physical needs. It's taking care of the patient to the best of your ability, treating him with dignity and respect, and helping him "to forget his troubles" if only for a moment. The greatest reward is seeing a peacefulness and a glimmer in his eyes that lets you know you made a difference.

Kathy Beideck
Student Nurse

22

THE SURGICAL PATIENT

Elaine Kockrow
Barbara Christensen

KEY TERMS

ablative
anesthesia
asepsis
atelectasis
cachexia
catabolism
dehiscence
drainage
embolus
evisceration
extubate
exudate
granulation
incision
induration
infarct
intraoperative
palliative
paralytic ileus
patency
pathogenic
phagocytosis
primary intention
prosthesis
purulent
sanguineous
secondary intention
serosanguineous
serous
singultus
stasis
surgical asepsis
tertiary intention
thrombus

LEARNING OBJECTIVES

After reading this chapter, the student should be able to do the following:

- Define the key terms.
- Differentiate among elective, urgent, and emergency surgery.
- Explain the procedure for deep breathing, coughing, and leg exercises for postoperative patients.
- Identify factors to include in the postoperative assessment of the patient in the recovery room.
- Describe implications for parenteral fluids and assessment factors to implement for patients receiving intravenous therapy.
- Explain interventions associated with blood transfusion therapy.
- Explain the differences among primary intention, secondary intention, and tertiary intention in wound healing.
- List five principles of surgical asepsis for wound care.
- Differentiate between inflammation and infection.
- List five nursing interventions to complete when evaluating drainage from the surgical wound.
- Describe the rationale for nursing interventions designed to prevent postoperative complications.
- Discuss five areas that the nurse should review in discharge planning for the postoperative patient.

RELATED TOPICS OF INTEREST

- Cultural aspects of nursing care (Chapter 8)
- Signs, symptoms, and physical assessment (Chapter 9)
- Admission, transfer, and discharge (Chapter 11)
- Medical asepsis and infection control (Chapter 12)
- Comfort, rest, and sleep (Chapter 15)
- Basic nutrition (Chapter 18)
- Diet therapy (Chapter 19)
- Mathematics review (Chapter 20)
- Principles and practice of medication administration (Chapter 21)
- Fluids and electrolytes (Chapter 24)
- Care of the patient with a respiratory disorder (Chapter 31)

Throughout history surgery has held a mysterious aura. Ancient surgical procedures were performed by medicine men, shamans, or priests as part of healing rituals or ceremonies. Gradually, physicians became responsible for treating disease and trauma through surgical interventions. Primitive Babylonian medicine divided the practice of medicine into either surgery or internal medicine, with surgery considered the more advanced field as depicted in early writings.[8] Although modern-day surgical suites have moved surgery from the Dark Ages, patients often view the surgical process as mysterious and frightening.

PREOPERATIVE AND POSTOPERATIVE CARE: OVERVIEW

Surgery is performed for many reasons. It may be used to cure, restore function, provide relief, or diagnose. In recent years, transplant operations have also become important surgical interventions. Surgery is classified as elective, urgent, or emergency. Elective surgery is not necessary to preserve life and may be performed when the patient chooses (e.g., excising a benign cyst). Urgent surgery is required to keep additional health problems from occurring (e.g., removal of the gallbladder because of calculi). Emergency surgery is performed immediately to save the individual's life or preserve the function of a body part (e.g., perforated ulcer). Although a surgical procedure may also be labeled as either major surgery or minor surgery, all surgeries have an element of risk.

Surgery is performed for various purposes, which are diagnostic, **ablative** (an amputation or excision of any part of the body or removal of a growth or harmful substance), **palliative** (therapy designed to relieve or reduce intensity of uncomfortable symptoms without cure), reconstructive, transplant, and constructive (Table 22-1 on p. 438).

See Table 22-2 on p. 438 for frequently used surgical terminology.

Traditionally, surgical procedures were performed in a hospital setting. With the discovery of new technologies and today's emphasis on decreasing health care costs, the surgical suite may now be in a variety of settings. Although each community may use different terms for its surgery setting and process, common variations follow:

Inpatient: Patient hospitalized for surgery

One-day (same-day) surgery: Patient is admitted the day surgery is scheduled and dismissed the same day

Outpatient: Patient, not hospitalized, who is being treated; individual is either admitted to a short-stay unit or directly to the surgical suite

Short-stay surgical center ("surgicenter"): Independently owned agency; surgery performed when overnight hospitalization is not required; also called ambulatory surgical center or one-day surgery center

Short-stay unit: Department or floor where a patient's stay does not exceed 24 hours (sometimes referred to as outpatient)

Influencing Factors

Regardless of the surgical procedure scheduled, the process is a stressful experience for the patient. Observing a patient's mannerisms and listening to questions help identify the patient's feelings and concerns. Fear of the unknown can best be addressed by providing information and support; the nurse should assist patients to express their concerns so that support and reassurance can be offered.

Numerous factors affect the individual's ability to tolerate surgery.

Age. The young and the old do not tolerate major surgical treatment as well as other age-groups. Their altered metabolic needs may not respond to physiological changes quickly. Of specific concern in these age-groups is the body's response to temperature changes, cardiovascular shifts, respiratory needs, and renal function. To assist patients to return to their maximal level of health, nursing assessments and appropriate interventions should be ongoing. For considerations regarding the older adult, see the gerontological box on p. 439.

Physical Condition. Healthy patients have smoother and faster recovery periods than patients who have coexisting health problems. The nurse assesses each body system to identify actual and high-risk problems. Once problems are identified, the nurse selects measures to lessen potential postsurgical complications.

Nutritional Factors. The body uses carbohydrates, proteins, and fats to supply energy-producing glucose to its cells. Whereas carbohydrates and fats are the primary energy-producers, protein is essential to build and repair body tissue. During stressful conditions, the body's need for energy and repair increases. Nutritional needs vary with a patient's age and physical requirements; patients who maintain a sound, nutritional diet tend to recover more quickly.

A completed diet history identifies the patient's usual eating habits and nutritional patterns. Because dietary practices are influenced by a patient's ethnic, cultural, religious, and socioeconomic background, the history highlights food preferences and dislikes (see Chapter 8). With this information, foods high in energy-producing nutrients can be offered. Because surgery may decrease a patient's appetite and alter metabolic functions, the nurse observes the patient for signs of malnutrition. If malnutrition is promptly identified, tube feed-

TABLE 22-1 Classification for Surgical Procedures

Type	Description	Examples
Seriousness		
Major	Involves extensive reconstruction or alteration in body parts; poses great risks to well-being	Coronary artery bypass, colon resection, removal of larynx, resection of lung lobe, gastric resection
Minor	Involves minimal alteration in body parts; often designed to correct deformities; involves minimal risks compared with those of major procedures	Cataract extraction, facial plastic surgery, skin graft, tooth extraction
Urgency		
Elective	Is performed on basis of patient's choice; is not essential and may not be necessary for health	Bunionectomy, facial plastic surgery, hernia repair, breast reconstruction
Urgent	Is necessary for patient's health, may prevent additional problems from developing (e.g., tissue destruction or impaired organ function); not necessarily emergency	Excision of cancerous tumor, removal of gallbladder for stones, vascular repair for obstructed artery (e.g., coronary artery bypass)
Emergency	Must be done immediately to save life or preserve function of body part	Repair of perforated appendix, repair of traumatic amputation, control of internal hemorrhaging, repair of perforated ulcer, removal of embolus in artery
Purpose		
Diagnostic	Is surgical exploration that allows physician to confirm diagnosis; may involve removal of tissue for further diagnostic testing	Exploratory laparotomy (incision into peritoneal cavity to inspect abdominal organs), breast mass biopsy
Ablative	Is excision or removal of diseased body part	Amputation, removal of appendix, cholecystectomy
Palliative	Relieves or reduces intensity of disease symptoms; will not produce cure	Colostomy, debridement of necrotic tissue, resection of nerve roots
Reconstructive	Restores function or appearance to traumatized or malfunctioning tissues	Internal fixation of fractures, scar revision, breast reconstruction
Transplant	Is performed to replace malfunctioning organs or structures	Kidney, cornea, pancreas, heart, or liver transplant; total hip replacement
Constructive	Restores function lost or reduced as result of congenital anomalies	Repair of cleft palate, closure of atrial septal defect in heart

TABLE 22-2 Surgical Terminology

Term	Interpretation with Example	Term	Interpretation with Example
Anastomosis	Surgical joining of two ducts or blood vessels to allow flow from one to another; to bypass an area (e.g., Billroth I—joins together stomach and duodenum)	-ostomy	Opening is made to allow the passage of drainage (e.g., ileostomy—formation of an opening of the ileum onto the surface of the abdomen for passage of feces)
-ectomy	Surgical removal of (e.g., cholecystectomy—removal of the gallbladder)	-otomy	Opening into (e.g., thoracotomy—surgical opening into the thoracic cavity)
lysis	Destruction or dissolution of (e.g., lysis of adhesions—removal of adhesions)	-pexy	Fixation of (e.g., ceopexy—fixation or suspension of the cecum to correct its excessive mobility)
-orrhaphy	Surgical repair of (e.g., herniorrhaphy—repair of a hernia)	-plasty	Plastic surgery (e.g., mammoplasty—reshaping of the breasts to reduce, life, reconstruct)
-oscopy	Direct visualization by a scope (e.g., cystoscopy—direct visualization of the urinary tract by means of a cytoscope)		

GERONTOLOGICAL CONSIDERATIONS

- Older persons undergoing surgery have higher morbidity and mortality rates than younger persons.
- Surgery places a greater stress on older than on younger persons. The physiological status of the older individual and coexisting conditions need to be carefully evaluated before surgery. Medical management is often preferred unless a condition is life threatening.
- Older patients tend to recover more slowly from surgery. Recovery can be affected by the level of mental functioning, individual coping ability, and the availability of support systems.
- Risks of aspiration, atelectasis, pneumonia, thrombus formation, infection, and altered tissue perfusion are increased in the older adult.
- Disorientation or toxic reactions can occur in the older adult after the administration of anesthetics, sedatives, or analgesic. These reactions are often present for days after administration of the medication.
- Preoperative and postoperative teaching may require extra time. Teaching should be given at the older person's level of understanding. Directions should be repeated and reinforced frequently.

ings, intravenous therapy, or parenteral hyperalimentation can be initiated.

Psychosocial Needs. As patients and families plan for surgery, they frequently express concern about possible outcomes. Although improved health is the ultimate goal, there may be fears not easily identified or understood. Many patients fear possible anesthesia and postoperative complications—pain, disfigurement, change in body image, loss of control, disabilities, and detection of cancer—and are concerned that the surgery will not be successful. For some, there is a fear of dying. These concerns are normal; preoperative teaching lessens the fear of the unknown. See Box 22-1 for fears commonly associated with surgery and anesthesia.

There is evidence that a relationship exists between preoperative fear and postoperative behavior. The preoperative anxiety level has been shown to influence the amount of anesthesia required, the amount of postoperative pain medication needed, and the speed of recovery from surgery.

The nurse must determine each patient's perceptions, emotions, behavior, and support systems that may help or interfere with the ability to progress through the surgical period. The unhurried and understanding nurse who actively listens to the patient, the family, and significant others invites confidence and helps to promote reduction of anxiety levels (Box 22-2 on p. 440).

Box 22-1 FEARS COMMONLY ASSOCIATED WITH SURGERY AND ANESTHESIA

- **Fear of loss of control** is associated primarily with anesthesia. Patients may be concerned about their actions or verbalizations while under the effects of drugs and anesthetic. In addition, the patient becomes almost totally dependent on the health care team during the surgical experience, even for most basic needs, such as breathing and life support, while under the influence of anesthetic.
- **Fear of the unknown** is common and may result from uncertainty about the surgical outcome or may stem from a lack of knowledge regarding the surgical experience.
- **Fear of anesthesia** may include fears of unpleasant induction of or emergence from anesthesia. The patient may fear waking up during the operation and feeling pain while under the effects of anesthetic. This fear is often related to loss of control and fear of the unknown.
- **Fear of pain or inadequate postoperative analgesia** is common. Reassure the patient and significant others that the pain will be controlled.
- **Fear of death** is commonly present and constitutes a legitimate fear. Even with the great strides in surgery and anesthesia, no anesthetic or operation is perfectly safe for all patients.
- **Fear of separation** from the usual support group is often present. The patient is separated from spouse, family, or significant others as well as other support groups and is cared for by strangers during much of this highly stressful period.
- **Fear of disruption** of life patterns may be present. Surgery and recovery interfere in varying degrees with activities of daily living and social activities, as well as with work and professional activities.
- **Fear of change in body image and mutilation** is also very common. Surgery disrupts body integrity and threatens body image.
- **Fear of detection of cancer** is a frequent concern that produces a high anxiety level.

While the patient attempts to understand the approaching surgery, family members and support persons are also trying to cope. Families may have additional burdens: financial obligations, living changes, and added personal responsibilities. The patient often expresses a feeling of helplessness. In addition to nursing and medical personnel, support can be provided to patients and their families by ministerial staff, social workers, or patient advocates during this stressful time.

Socioeconomic and Cultural Needs. Rearing practices influence an individual's behaviors and beliefs. Be-

Box 22-2 HELPFUL INFORMATION FOR PREOPERATIVE PATIENTS AND FAMILIES

- Preoperative tests, reason, preparation
- Preoperative routines, sequence of events
- Special equipment needed
- Transfer to operating room (time, checking procedures)
- Recovery room
  - Place where patient will awaken
  - Frequent monitoring of vital signs
  - Return to room when vital signs stable
- Probable postoperative therapies
  Need for increased mobility as soon as possible
  Need to keep respiratory passages clear
- Anticipated treatments (e.g., IV, dressing changes, incentive spirometer)
- Pain medication routines (timing sequence, "as needed" [prn] status), other modalities of management such as patient-controlled analgesia (PCA) and epidural analgesia

cause the United States is a nation of diverse individuals, patient reactions are influenced by social, economic, religious, ethnic, and cultural values. Even geographical location affects the way an individual responds. Therefore it is important to allow patients and families to express themselves openly. By allowing each patient to share personal needs, the nurse allows the total person to be treated.

Education and Experience. As individuals age, life experiences influence problem-solving abilities and coping methods. Tailoring information to a patient's educational level permits fear to be replaced with accurate knowledge. The nurse can encourage patients to repeat or summarize what has been presented. This process validates not only what the patient heard, but also how the information was interpreted (see Chapter 4).

PREOPERATIVE PERIOD

A thorough health assessment is needed before surgery. Acute or chronic diseases hinder the body's ability to repair itself or adjust to surgical treatment. Disorders of the systems identified in Table 22-3 present high-risk conditions for surgery. Each system is further affected by the patient's age, health condition, nutritional status, and mental state.

Assessment questions to ascertain the patient's use of chemicals, alcohol, and abusive substances assist the health team to select medications tolerated by the body. Postoperative care is also adjusted to compensate, when possible, for potential complications. If a patient has been a heavy smoker, alveoli may be impaired and the patient's lung capacity reduced. Mucus and anesthesia by-products may be trapped in the lung, causing atelectasis and pneumonia. Breathing exercises and treatments for the smoker postoperatively aid in lung expansion and decrease the risk of respiratory complications.

Additional preoperative questions identify the patient's allergies, past surgeries, and infection and disease history. When questioning the patient about medication practices, the nurse asks the patient to name prescription drugs currently taken, as well as over-the-counter drugs and home remedies used. The nurse also records the patient's vital signs and height and weight before surgery to have a baseline for postoperative comparisons.

Preoperative Teaching

Patient teaching before surgery helps decrease the stress that patients feel. Because fear of the unknown is a primary stressor of preoperative patients, providing information lessens stresses associated with not knowing. Preoperative information helps to (1) lessen anxiety, (2) reduce the amount of anesthesia needed, (3) decrease postsurgical pain, and (4) reduce corticosteroid production. Although some patients ignore preoperative instruction, most patients want to help themselves deal with the situation. By decreasing postsurgical complications through preoperative teaching, wound healing occurs more rapidly.

In providing preoperative teaching, the nurse should include the patient and family and remember that basic terminology and information are easier to understand than complex explanations. The nurse should frequently stop to verify the patient's understanding of information shared, ask questions, and encourage responses. Questions that can be answered "yes" or "no" should be avoided. "Do you have any questions?" is not as clarifying as "What questions do you have?" If printed materials or videotapes are routinely used in preoperative teaching sessions, it is important to document what the patient read, heard, or saw. Older adults may have difficulty reading small print or hearing taped messages. If the patient is not a native speaker of English, an interpreter may be needed to explain information presented.

Ideally, preoperative teaching is provided 1 or 2 days before surgery, when anxiety is not as high. Although preoperative preparation varies, most institutions have an established teaching program. Preoperative teaching is began by clarifying the sequence of preoperative and postoperative events. Generally, the nurse should instruct the patient about the surgical procedure, informed consent, the method of skin preparation, and gastrointestinal cleanser to be used. The nurse reviews the time of

TABLE 22-3 Surgical Effects on Body Systems

Disease/Disorder	Surgical Effects
Cardiovascular	
Recent myocardial infarction, dysrhythmias, and congestive heart failure Hypertension Blood dyscrasias Peripheral vascular disease	Stress on the system increases workload and output. Hypotension and cardiac dysrhythmias are the most common cardiovascular complications, and early recognition and management of these complications before they become serious enough to diminish cardiac output depend on frequent assessment of the patient's vital signs. Stress of surgery causes increased demands on myocardium to maintain cardiac output. General anesthetic agents depress cardiac function.
Endocrine	
Liver disease Diabetes mellitus Thyroid disorders Adrenal insufficiency	Metabolic needs increase and the system becomes taxed. Diabetes increases susceptibility to infection and may impair wound healing from altered glucose metabolism and associated circulatory impairment. Fluctuating blood levels may cause central nervous system malfunction during anesthesia. Stress of surgery may cause decreased glucose tolerance. Liver disease alters metabolism and elimination of drugs administered during surgery and impairs wound healing because of alterations in protein metabolism.
Gastrointestinal	
Hiatal hernia Esophagitis Ulcers	Preoperative and postoperative medication may be necessary to control gastric acidity.
Esophageal varices	Risk of hemorrhage may increase due to risk of initiating hemorrhage with intubation.
Liver disease	Impaired liver function may affect metabolism and excretion of anesthetic agents.
Immune	
AIDS Allergies Immune deficiency Radiotherapy effects Chemotherapy effects	Disease slows the body's ability to fight infection. Immunological disorders increase risk of infection and delay wound healing after surgery.
Neurological	
Seizures	Patients need a check of the therapeutic levels of their medications.
Myasthenia gravis	Exclusion of the use of muscle relaxants may be warranted due to decreased ability to reverse their effects.
Cerebral vascular accident	Impaired verbal communication, defective perception of the body, paralysis, and visual disturbances place patient at high risk for injury.
Respiratory	
Bronchitis Emphysema Asthma Tumors Cystic fibrosis Chronic obstructive pulmonary disease	Lung motility is decreased and gas exchange slowed. Fever predisposes patient to fluid and electrolyte imbalances and may indicate underlying infection. Respiratory disease reduces patient's ability to compensate for acid-base alterations (see Chapter 24). Anesthetic agents reduce respiratory function, increasing risk for severe hypoventilation.
Urinary	
Nephritis Polycystic disease Renal failure Tumors	Impaired kidney function decreases excretion of anesthesia and alters acid-base balance.

the surgery and information about the recovery area. Although most patients return to their previously assigned units after surgery, a few may be transferred to an intensive care area, specialty unit, or outpatient area. If a transfer will occur, it is helpful to take the patient and family on a tour of the new unit. The nurse reinforces that vital signs, dressings, and tubes are checked every 15 to 30 minutes until the patient is awake and stable. A checklist frequently is used to provide a systematic preoperative teaching plan.

Preoperative Preparation

Preparation for surgery depends on the patient's age, physical and nutritional status, type of surgery, and the preference of the surgeon. When the surgery is performed in a short-stay or ambulatory setting, the workup normally occurs a few days in advance. If a patient is admitted to the hospital, testing may be conducted to assess for high-risk problems. If the presenting problem has been diagnosed, preparation frequently includes both in-hospital testing and evaluation of test results previously completed in the physician's office.

Laboratory Tests and Diagnostic Imaging. Testing before surgery depends on the institution's policies, physician's directives, and condition of the patient. The nurse follows standing orders to complete this overall process. Laboratory tests commonly reviewed before surgery include a urinalysis; complete blood count; and blood chemistry profile to assess endocrine, hepatic, renal, and cardiovascular functions. Serum electrolytes are evaluated if extensive surgery is planned or the patient has extenuating problems. One of the essential electrolytes examined is potassium; if potassium is not available in adequate amounts, dysrhythmias can occur during anesthesia and the patient's postoperative recovery may be slowed by general muscle weakness. A chest x-ray evaluation and electrocardiogram are used to identify disease processes or previous respiratory or cardiac damage. Additional tests are conducted to assess the organ being evaluated. Blood chemistry profile (LDH, gamma GT, alkaline phosphatase, total bilirubin) and urine bilirubin levels verify the hepatic functioning ability.

Informed Consent. The Patient's Bill of Rights (see Chapter 1) affirms that patients must give informed consent before the beginning of any procedure. In signing the consent form, the patient is competent and agrees to have the procedure that is stated on the form. Information is to be clear, the risks explained, expected benefits identified, and consequences or alternatives for the presenting problem stated. Witnesses are required, to meet the legal requirements of the state. Ideally, the surgeon discusses the surgical procedure with the patient in advance. In some institutions the surgical consent is completed in the physician's office or in the admissions department before the patient is admitted to the unit (see Fig. 2-1). The consent may not be signed by the patient if the patient has taken a narcotic or any mind-altering substance within the previous 4 hours that could alter judgment or the ability to make a reasonable, informed decision. Check the agency's policy for obtaining informed consent.

If the patient does not see or hear well, the nurse should allow additional time to explain the surgery. For individuals who are not native speakers of English, an interpreter may be used if necessary. The patient should never be coerced into signing a consent that is not understood or that contains information that differs from what was originally explained.

In an emergency the patient may not be able to give consent for surgery. Every effort is made to locate family members to assume this responsibility. Occasionally telephone permission may be obtained. In cases in which verbal consent is received, the hospital will have standard guidelines. If the patient's life is in danger and family members cannot be located, the surgeon may legally perform surgery. In cases in which family members object to surgery that the physician believes is essential, a court order may be obtained for the procedure. This practice is used very carefully, for example, when a child's life is in danger. Check agency policy.

Gastrointestinal Preparation. At midnight before surgery, the patient is usually placed on NPO status (i.e., receives nothing by mouth); this keeps the gastrointestinal (GI) tract empty when the patient is anesthetized, thereby decreasing the chance of vomiting or aspiration of emesis after surgery. An NPO sign is posted over the patient's bed, and all fluids are removed from the room. The nurse should reinforce with both the patient and family the importance of not ingesting foods or fluids. If the patient breaks the fast, the physician is notified.

While NPO, patients can have oral care. The nurse should caution the patient not to swallow fluids used during oral care. A wet cloth on the lips helps relieve dryness. If patients need to be hydrated or if special IV medications are needed, parenteral fluids or medication may be ordered. Depending on the nature of the surgery, many patients postoperatively resume foods and fluids the day of their surgeries.

Because anesthesia relaxes the bowel, a bowel cleanser may be ordered to evacuate fecal material and lessen postoperative GI problems (ileus). Frequently used evacuates are the cleansing enema or a general laxative. A GI lavage solution, GoLYTELY, an isosmotic solution, rapidly evacuates the bowel. GoLYTELY is contraindicated, however, in patients with GI obstruction, gastric retention, bowel perforation, toxic colitis, or megacolon. If a bowel preparation is used, the nurse charts the type of preparation used, the patient's tolerance to the procedure, and results. Before bowel surgery, medication (neomycin, sulfonamides, erythromycin) may be given over a period of days to detoxify and sterilize the GI tract. This lessens the chance of fecal contamination during surgery.

Skin Preparation. Preoperatively the patient may have removal of hair at the surgical site and then shower, unless contraindicated, using an antiseptic soap such as Hibiclens. There is debate about what is the best method to remove hair. A lower rate of infection occurs with either no shave or a hair clip than with any other method (electric shave, no shave but hair clipped, and razor shave). Use of a depilatory agent has also proved to have a low wound infection rate. Maintaining the skin's integrity is more important than removing hair. If shaving is used, it should be performed as close to the actual time of the surgical procedure as possible (Skill 22-1 on p. 444). Some surgical departments prepare the patient either in a surgical holding room or in the operating room itself.

Respiratory Preparation. If a general anesthetic is administered, ventilating the lungs is vital postoperatively to prevent atelectasis and pneumonia. Because the lungs do not expand fully during surgery, mucus and gases remain in the lungs until expelled. Pulmonary exercises can assist in expanding the lungs and removing these byproducts. Preoperative introduction to the use of the incentive spirometer is of great value to the patient (Skill 31-3). Before surgery the nurse should assist the patient to practice turning, coughing (Skill 22-2 on p. 445), and deep breathing (Skill 22-3 on p. 446). Since coughing increases intracranial pressure, it is usually contraindicated in cranial-related surgeries. Coughing is also contraindicated for patients having cataract surgery (Table 22-4). Some physicians believe coughing may actually cause alvedar collapse and order only incentive spirometry. Patients are frequently ambulated within a few hours after surgery to return cardiovascular and respiratory functions to normal more quickly.

Circulatory Concerns. Accompanying the need to turn, cough, and deep breathe is the need to practice leg exercises (see Skill 22-3). Because blood stasis occurs when the patient is lying flat, leg exercises should be encouraged to assist venous blood flow. With the venous blood slowing, a **thrombus** (an accumulation of platelets, fibrin, clotting factors, and cellular elements of the blood attached to the anterior wall of a vessel, sometimes occluding the lumen of the vessel) may form. If a thrombus is dislodged, it can travel as an **embolus** to the lungs, heart, or brain, where the vessel can be occluded. Without an adequate blood supply, an **infarct** (localized area of necrosis) can occur. Antiembolic stockings, Jobst pump, or Venodyne comfort stockings with intermittent external pneumonic compression system may be ordered to provide support and to prevent venous thrombus in the lower extremities (Skill 22-4 on p. 447).

Vital Signs. Vital signs mirror the body's response to anesthesia and surgery. The nurse instructs the patient before surgery that it is normal for the blood pressure, temperature, pulse, and respiration to be monitored until stable. The schedule for monitoring vital signs depends on the protocol of the hospital and the stability of the patient. Preoperative vital signs serve as the baseline for deciding when stability has returned. Guidelines for monitoring postoperative vital signs are identified on p. 451.

Genitourinary Concerns. After general anesthesia, the urinary bladder's tone is decreased. Therefore the nurse should known the patient's normal bladder habits and be able to identify when the bladder is full and distended. The nurse informs the patient preoperatively that the lower part of the abdomen will be palpated at intervals to check for bladder fullness. Once patients are awake and tolerating fluids, the nurse should encourage them to maintain an adequate intake. Occasionally a urinary catheter is inserted to monitor urinary output. This procedure is normally reserved for patients undergoing urinary surgery or who may have difficulty voiding. If a catheter is inserted, it is usually removed 1 to 2 days postoperatively to reduce the chance of bladder infection. Once it is removed, the nurse should encourage the patient to drink 8 ounces of fluids per hour while awake unless contraindicated. The nurse also monitors intake and output values until voiding returns to the patient's normal pattern.

TABLE 22-4 Surgeries for Which Coughing is Contraindicated or Modified

Surgical Site	Effect of Coughing
Intracranial	Coughing increases intracranial pressure (ICP), leading to cerebral spinal fluid leak.
Eye	Coughing increases ICP, which then increases intraocular pressure, causing pressure on suture line.
Ear	Mouth must be kept open if coughing occurs to prevent pressure backup through eustachian tube to middle ear, causing pressure on suture line.
Nose	Mouth must be kept open if coughing occurs to prevent dislodgment of clot with subsequent bleeding.
Throat	Vigorous coughing may dislodge a clot with subsequent bleeding.

SKILL 22-1

PERFORMING SURGICAL PREP

Nursing Action

1. Wash hands
2. Refer to procedure manual to verify anatomical area to be shaved according to surgery to be performed.
3. Close door, and pull curtains.
4. Explain procedure to patient
5. Position bed and patient.
6. Place towel or waterproof pad under area to be shaved.
7. Fill basin with warm water.
8. Use bath blanket to drape patient appropriately to limit exposure.
9. Adjust lighting.
10. Don gloves.
11. Lather skin well with antiseptic soap or lather and warm water, using gauze squares.
12. Hold razor at a 30- to 45-degree angle to skin (see illustration).
    a. Shave small area at a time while holding skin taut.
    b. Use short, smooth strokes.
    c. Shave hair in direction it grows.
13. Rinse razor frequently.
    a. Change blade as needed. Replace razor, if disposable razor is used.
    b. Change water as needed.
    c. Cleanse navel area with sterile cotton-tipped applicators.
14. When entire area is shaved, use washcloth and clean, warm water to cleanse area; dry skin.
15. Reassess skin for cuts or abrasions.
16. Return patient to comfortable status.
17. Clean and dispose of equipment.
18. Remove gloves.
19. Wash hands.
20. Often a patient is asked to shower with an antiseptic soap, such as Hibiclens, after the surgical shave or prep to remove any hair and for further cleansing.

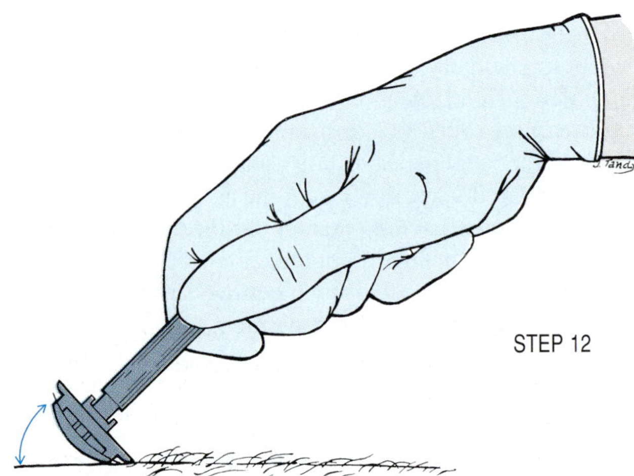

STEP 12

Sample charting

DATE	TIME	NOTES
12/8/94	8:30	Skin at surgical site shaved, including entire abdomen from nipple line to pubis. Skin intact and has no cuts or abrasions. Several small, brown nevi noted to right of umbilicus. Procedure tolerated well. Reported to K. Williams, RN.

____

(nurse's signature)

SPECIAL CONCERNS

- Small children may be easily frightened by this procedure, and it may need to be done in the operating room.
- Older adults will need detailed explanation to relieve their anxiety.
- Older adults have less subcutaneous tissue, less skin elasticity, and more delicate skin tissue. Extreme care will need to be taken when shaving the older adult.
- Older adults are usually more susceptible to infections.

TEACHING CONTROLLED COUGHING

Nursing Action

1. Wash hands.
2. Don gloves.
3. Assist patient to upright position. Place pillow between bed or chair and patient.
4. Demonstrate coughing exercise for patient (see illustration).
   a. Take several deep breaths.
   b. Inhale through nose.
   c. Exhale through mouth with pursed lips.
   d. Inhale deeply again and hold breath for count of 3.
   e. Cough two or three consecutive coughs without inhaling between coughs.
5. Abdominal or thoracic incision can be splinted before coughing with hands, pillow, towel, or rolled bath blanket (see illustration).
6. Encourage patient to practice coughing while splinting the incisional area once or twice an hour during waking hours. Assist patient as indicated.
7. Provide tissues and emesis basin for any mucus expectorated.
8. Provide washcloth and warm water for washing hands and face, provide mouth wash for oral hygiene, and return patient to comfortable position.

Sample charting

DATE	TIME	NOTES
12/8/94	2:00	Assisted to full Fowler's position. Controlled coughing completed with pillow splinting the abdominal incision. Small amount of tenacious, white mucus expectorated. No complaints of pain or discomfort noted during procedure. Oral hygiene given and returned to side-lying position. Reported to P. Barr, RN.

____
(nurse's signature)

SPECIAL CONCERNS

- Young children or older adults may not fully understand the importance of controlled coughing, and continuous reinforcement of teaching and assistance may be needed.
- Family members of a young child should be taught the procedure to assist the child. This will also help family members in meeting their needs by assisting in the care of the child.

PATIENT TEACHING

The patient should be instructed on the following:

- For the patient entering the hospital for same-day surgery, the teaching of controlled coughing may need to be taught in the physician's office, in the preoperative area, or postoperatively before the patient is discharged.
- The home health nurse may need to reinforce the importance of coughing one or two times an hour during waking hours for the first few days postoperatively.

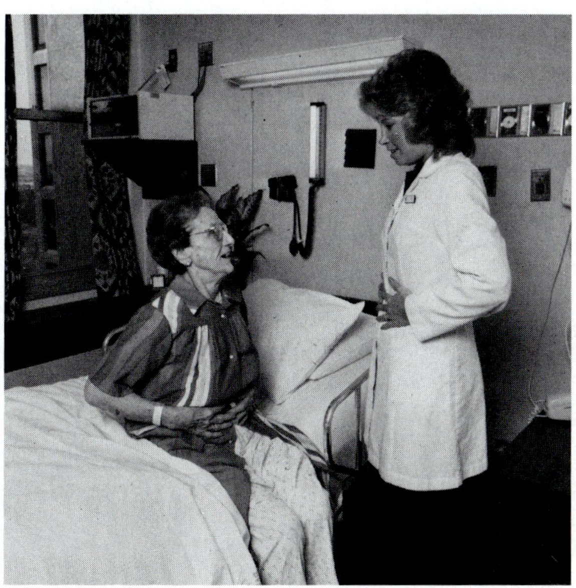
STEP 4

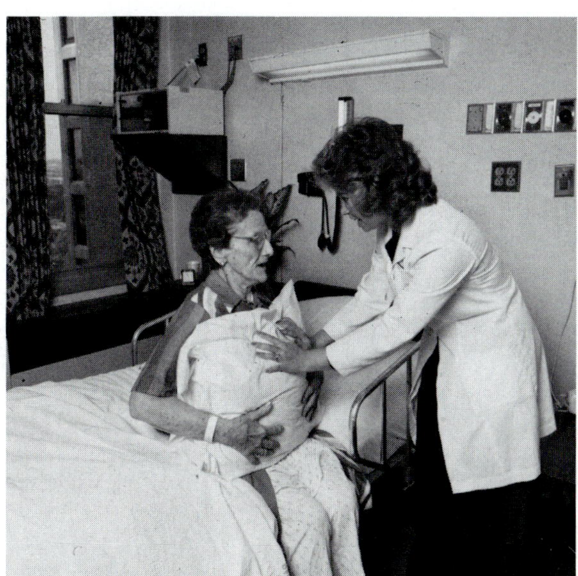
STEP 5

TEACHING POSTOPERATIVE BREATHING TECHNIQUES AND LEG EXERCISES

Nursing action

Breathing techniques

1. Wash hands.
2. Assist patient to comfortable position—sitting or standing.
3. Place pillow between patient and bed or chair.
4. Sit or stand facing patient.
5. Demonstrate taking slow, deep breaths. Avoid using shoulder and chest while inhaling. Inhale through nose.
6. Hold breath for count of 3, and slowly exhale through pursed lips.
7. Repeat exercise three to five times.
8. Have patient practice exercise.
9. Instruct patient to take 10 slow, deep breaths every 2 hours postoperatively during waking hours until up and around.
10. If patient has an abdominal or thoracic incision, instruct patient to splint incisional area, if desired, during breathing exercises.

Leg exercises

11. Lifting one leg at a time and supporting joints, gently flex and extend the leg five to ten times. Encourage medial and lateral movement of ankles 5 to 10 times (see illustrations).
12. Repeat on opposite leg. Lifting the leg and supporting the joints, gently flex and extend the leg five to ten times. Encourage medial and lateral movement of ankles 5 to 10 times.
13. Document procedure.

Sample charting

DATE	TIME	NOTES
1/8/95	1:00	Deep breathing and leg exercises taught. Return demonstration satisfactorily performed. No evidence of dyspnea noted. Instructed to practice exercises at least three more times before surgery in the AM. Reported to L. Miles, RN.

____

(nurse's signature)

SPECIAL CONCERNS

- Patients who have chronic respiratory conditions may need assistance and encouragement in carrying out these procedures.
- Special care should be taken in teaching children deep breathing exercises. Be sure to teach the family members for reinforcement.
- Older patients may need to be encouraged to practice the breathing and leg exercises; they may not fully understand the importance of the procedure.

PATIENT TEACHING

The following should be considered for the patient who requires instruction on postoperative exercise and breathing techniques:

- For the patient entering the hospital for same-day surgery, deep breathing and leg exercises may need to be taught in the physician's office, in the preoperative area, or postoperatively.
- The home health nurse may need to reinforce the importance of deep breathing and leg exercises

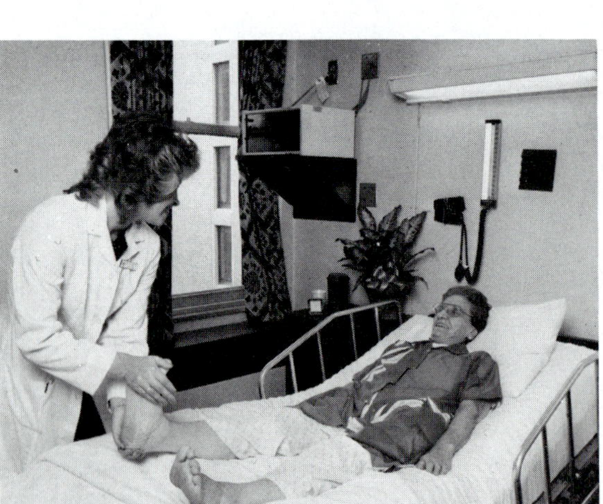

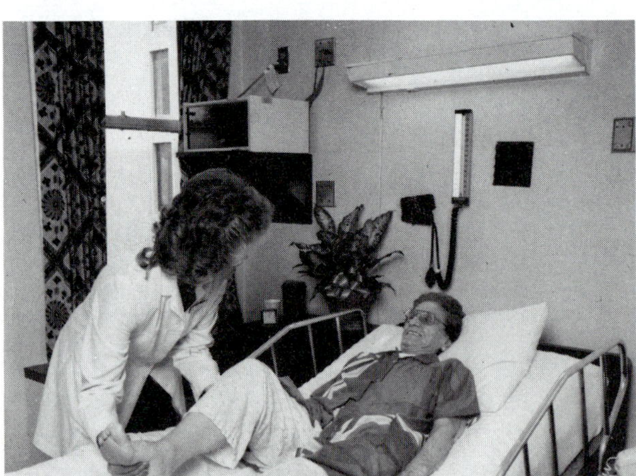

STEP 11

SKILL 22-4

APPLYING ANTIEMBOLISM STOCKINGS

Nursing action

1. Wash hands.
2. Measure thigh and calf circumference and length from groin to plantar area for full-length antiembolism stockings; measure calf circumference for knee-length antiembolism stockings; secure correct size according to measurements.
3. Assist patient to supine position.
4. turn stockings inside-out, grasp foot and heel of the stocking, and invert sock over your hand—turn leg and foot of stockings inside-out to the heel portion.
5. Remove hand and slip foot portion over patient's toes, foot, and heel, fitting patient's foot into heel and toe appropriately.
6. Pull leg portion of stocking over foot and up as far as it will go.
7. Adjust stocking to fit evenly and smoothly with no wrinkles.
8. Repeat procedure for opposite leg.
9. Assess patient periodically.
10. Assess stocking at regular intervals.
11. Document procedure.

Sample charting

DATE	TIME	NOTES
11/8/95	7:00	Knee high antiembolism stockings applied to both legs. Skin is pink and warm, and pedal pulses are present bilaterally. Reported to D. King, RN.

____
(nurse's signature)

SPECIAL CONCERNS

- Postoperative patients with abdominal or thoracic incisions will not be able to bend and pull on own stockings.
- Stockings may be difficult to fit and maintain in the obese patient and the very thin patient.
- Stockings may be difficult to apply for the elderly patients; the nurse or family members will assist the patient.

PATIENT TEACHING

The patient who will be applying antiembolism stockings should be instructed on the following:

- Patients will need to be instructed on procedure to appropriately apply antiembolism stockings.
- Nurse can teach patient appropriate care of the stockings.
- Nurse should instruct patient not to massage legs because of the risk of dislodging a blood clot.
- Patient may need to continue to apply stockings at home, if ordered by the physician, and will need to know the procedure for applying and caring for the stockings and signs of possible complications.

Surgical Wound. With today's technologies, incisions are closed in a variety of ways: suture, staples, Steri-Strips, or transparent strips. If the nurse knows the type of closure, its appearance can be explained to the patient. Some surgeries require the removal of exudate. For these patients, a drain may be in place. The nurse can explain the purpose of the drain and the need for close monitoring. Although not all incisions require dressings, the nurse will observe the wound's appearance. Wounds and drainage are described in more detail later in this unit.

Pain. Patients fear pain more than any other postsurgical complication. The nurse must impress upon the patient that pain relief is an important part of care. A variety of methods are used to reduce discomfort. If the patient is considering nontraditional analgesia (imagery, biofeedback, relaxation techniques), the nurse should review these technique and allow practice time. The majority of patients elect to obtain comfort through traditional analgesia. Postoperative pain is real, so it is important to reassure patients that addiction to analgesics very rarely occurs in the time frame needed for comfort. For the patient who is apprehensive about intermittent injections, patient-controlled analgesia (PCA) and opioids into the epidural space are safe and effective methods of postoperative pain management. When the patient is allowed oral intake, oral analgesics coupled with nontraditional methods are often effective.

Tubes. Depending on the surgery, patient teaching includes information about nasogastric tubes, wound evacuation units, and intravenous and oxygen therapy. Allowing patients to view these items and understand their purposes lessens the fear associated with each.

Preoperative Medication. Preoperative medication reduces the patient's anxiety, decreases the amount of anesthetic needed, and reduces respiratory tract secretions. The nurse should provide the patient with information on what to expect from preoperative medications. Barbiturates and tranquilizers (phenobarbital and diazepam [Valium]) are sometimes given for sedation. Narcotic analgesics (meperidine and morphine) may be administered by intermittent injection or PCA if the patient has pain before surgery; this too reduces the amount of anesthetic required. An introduction to PCA preoperatively is advantageous because the patient is better able to comprehend the concept and operation of this equipment. Anticholinergics such as atropine reduce spasms of smooth muscles and decrease gastric, bronchial, and salivary secretions. The patient frequently becomes drowsy, notices a dry mouth, and may experience vertigo after the preoperative medication is given. The nurse should ask the patient to void before receiving a preoperative medication.

If preoperative medication is given on the nursing unit, the patient must remain in bed, and the nurse raises side rails and monitors the patient every 15 to 30 minutes until the patient leaves for surgery. In many institutions the preoperative medication is given by the anesthesiologist or anesthetist in the preoperative holding area. These patients should be reassured and provided a quiet environment on the nursing unit while they are waiting to be transported to the surgical suite.

Anesthesia. **Anesthesia** means the absence of pain (*an* meaning "without" and *esthesia* meaning "awareness of feeling"). Anesthesia may be divided into three categories: general, regional, and local. General anesthesia refers to a drug-induced state in which analgesia, amnesia, muscle relaxation, and unconsciousness occur. General anesthetics may be administered by inhalation, oral, rectal, or parenteral routes, with the inhalation and intravenous routes most commonly used. Regional anesthesia refers to techniques that render only a specific region of the body insensitive to pain. Regional anesthesia provides a pain-free state with good operating conditions for certain operative procedures without producing loss of consciousness. Regional anesthesia is classified according to its induction method: nerve block, spinal anesthesia, or epidural anesthesia. Local anesthesia refers to topical application or infiltration into tissues of an anesthetic agent that disrupts sensation at the level of the nerve endings. This results in loss of sensation limited to the immediate area of application.

Preoperative Nursing Diagnoses. The nurse gathers data during assessment of the preoperative patient to identify nursing diagnoses. These diagnoses will aid the nurse in establishing a direction for care that will be provided during the preoperative, intraoperative, and/or postoperative period. The nursing diagnoses formulated during the preoperative period will allow the nurse to institute measures to ensure that care provided during all three phases of the surgical patient's care will be consistent.

The nursing diagnoses made during the preoperative period may also focus on factors that place the surgical patient at high risk for problems after surgery. For example, patients with preexisting medical disorders such as diabetes mellitus would be at high risk for impaired skin integrity. Preventive care is the key to managing the surgical patient successfully. See Box 22-3 for preoperative nursing diagnoses.

Preoperative Checklist. The nurse completes the preoperative checklist before the patient leaves the nursing unit (Fig. 22-1). If the preoperative medication is to be given on the nursing unit, the nurse completes the preoperative checklist before administering the medication.

Box 22-3 PREOPERATIVE NURSING DIAGNOSES

Airway clearance, ineffective, high risk for, related to:
- Diminished cough
- Increased pulmonary congestion

Anxiety, related to:
- Knowledge deficit of impending surgery
- Threat of loss of body part

Coping, ineffective family: compromised, related to:
- Temporary role change of patient
- Impending severity of surgery

Fear, related to:
- Impending surgery
- Anticipation of postoperative pain

Knowledge deficit, regarding implications of surgery, related to:
- Lack of experience with surgery
- Information misinterpretation

Nutrition, altered: less than body requirements, related to:
- Preoperative malnourishment

Nutrition, altered: more than body requirements, related to:
- Excess intake of food

Powerlessness, related to:
- Emergency nature of surgery

Skin integrity, impaired, high risk for, related to:
- Preoperative radiation
- Immobilization during surgery

Sleep pattern disturbance, related to:
- Fear of surgery
- Preoperative hospital routines

GPR
Great Plains Regional Medical Center

ADDRESSOGRAPH

Preoperative Assessment Form

(Please check carefully and initial)

Date January 15, 1995

1. Medical Admission Permit Signed ✓ L.H.
2. Surgical Permit Signed & Witnessed ✓ L.H.
3. Blood Transfusion Permit ✓ L.H.
4. Sterilization Permit Signed & Witnessed ✓ L.H.
5. Bone Bank Protocol Ø Recipient Ø Donor Ø
6. Authorization for Partial Abortion Ø
7. Allergies, list: penicillin
8. Identification Band ✓ L.H. Blood Bracelet ✓ L.H. Medex ✓ L.H.
9. Pre-Op Bath Done ✓ L.H. Checked By RN Fran Ranch R.N.
10. Pre-Op Bath ✓ L.H. Hospital Gown ✓ L.H. Bath Blanket ✓ L.H.
11. Remove: Dentures Ø Glasses/Contacts ✓ L.H. Jewelry/Nail Polish/Hair Pins/Make-up ✓ L.H.
12. TED stockings when ordered ✓ L.H. Side Rails Up ✓ L.H. Addressograph ✓ L.H.
13. Pre-Op Vital Signs T 98^6 P 80 R 20 BP 120/80
14. Pre-Op Medications Demerol 50 mgm and atropine 0.3 mgm Im 0900
15. Insert Foley Catheter ✓ L.H.
16. Physical Disability, such as Amputaions, Glass Eye, Etc. Ø
17. Systemic Diseases NIDDM
18. History and Physical ✓ L.H.
19. Lab Reports:
    A. Hgb on all Menstrual Age Females ✓ L.H.
    B. All Patients Age 40-60 Hgb and EKG Ø
    C. All Patients Over 60 Hgb, EKG and Chest X-ray Ø
    D. Type and Crossmatch ✓ L.H.

NURSING STAFF IDENTIFICATIION

L.H.-Lynn Huffman LPN

20. Infectious Process Present ____ Yes ____ No X
    Type of Infection ——
21. Additional Comments pre & post op. nursing interventions explained
22. Chart Signed Off Lynn Huffman LPN

FIG. 22-1 Preoperative assessment form. (Courtesy Great Plains Regional Medical Center, North Platte, Neb.)

Any **prosthesis** (an artificial replacement for a missing part of the body), contact lenses, dentures, jewelry, and other valuables are removed and either given to family members or placed in a secure area. Some hospitals allow dentures to be left in and worn to surgery and removed at a later time. The removal of dentures preoperatively is according to agency policy. If rings are worn, they should be secured with tape and the disposition of personal items charted. The patient should void before the preoperative medication is administered, or 1 hour before surgery is scheduled. Although the majority of patients become drowsy after administration of a preoperative medication, a few will either become hyperactive or demonstrate no side effects. The patient should be reminded to remain in bed and the side rails raised. The call light should be placed within reach and its location identified for the patient.

The patient is transported to the surgical area approximately 30 to 60 minutes before the scheduled procedure. Once the patient is admitted to the surgical suite, final preoperative measures are completed: the skin is prepared, an IV needle is inserted, vital signs are assessed, and chart data are reviewed. If IV therapy was not previously started, fluids are begun. An IV site is needed not only for the administration of the anesthetic, but also to hydrate body cells. The IV site is kept patent until the patient has reached a satisfactory recovery period on the surgical unit.

INTRAOPERATIVE ENVIRONMENT

Intraoperative (within the surgical suite) care centers on the care and protection of the patient. When the patient enters the operating room, the nurse identifies the patient (both verbally and by the identification band and medical records). Nursing interventions should include warm, personal contact with the patient to humanize the often cold, aseptic, and highly technical environment of the operating room. During surgery and particularly anesthesia, patients are unable to protect themselves from many sources of possible harm, and the nurse must act for the patients to prevent injury. Normal self-protective mechanisms, such as pain and withdrawal movements, are lost with the induction of anesthesia, while the protective barrier of the skin is disrupted by surgery through an incision, increasing the risk of infection. Essential elements for monitoring and protecting patient safety are a keen awareness by the nurse of the potential for harm, recognition of body areas most susceptible to injury, strict adherence to principles of positioning and asepsis, and monitoring sites for impairment or early signs of injury. Small or potentially dangerous objects such as needles and syringes should not be left near the patient. Side rails and safety straps should be used, even for the fully conscious patient; safety reminder devices may occasionally be necessary to protect the delirious, semicomatose, or disoriented patient from injury.

All persons in the operating room must be alert to contamination of sterile items and must aid in maintaining aseptic conditions. **Surgical asepsis** (protection against infection before, during, or after surgery by the use of sterile technique) is provided to prevent microbial contamination of the operative site. Maintaining a sterile environment in the surgical suite is crucial if the

TABLE 22-5 Interventions Associated with the ABCs of Immediate Recovery

Assessment Mode	Intervention
A—Airway	Maintain patency: keep head tilted up and back; may position on side with the face down and neck slightly extended Note presence or absence of gag/swallowing reflex Suction until awake and alert Provide oxygen if necessary
B—Breathing	Evaluate depth, rate, sounds, rhythm, and chest movement Assess color of mucous membranes Place hand above patient's nose to detect respirations if shallow Initiate coughing and deep breathing exercises as soon as able to respond Chart time oxygen is discontinued Monitor oxygen saturation levels (Sa_{O_2}) by pulse oximetry checks
C—Consciousness	Able to **extubate** (the process of removing endotracheal tube from airway) Patient responds to commands Patient verbalizes responses Patient reacts to stimuli
C—Circulation	Monitor T, P, R every 10 to 15 min; take axillary, tympanic, or rectal temperature if warranted Assess rate, rhythm, quality of pulse Evaluate color and warmth of skin and nail beds Check peripheral pulses as indicated Assess incision/dressing (monitor wound drainage output) Monitor IVs: solution, rate, site
S—System review	Assess neurological functions, muscle strength, and response Monitor drains, tubes; color and amount of output Check for the pressure, type, and condition of dressings Evaluate pain response; may need to give analgesic and monitor patient response Observe for allergic reactions Assess urinary output if Foley catheter is in place

wound is to remain free of contamination. The goal of surgical asepsis is to prevent or minimize postoperative wound infections. The patient is at risk for introduction of infecting organisms through catheters, drains, or the surgical wound. Standards and guidelines for surgical scrubs and skin preparation should be strictly followed. The success and ease with which the operation is accomplished greatly depend on group dynamics as professionals work to achieve common goals.

POSTOPERATIVE PERIOD

Immediate Postoperative Period

Once surgery is completed, the patient is transported to the recovery room (or postanesthesia care unit) or the intensive care area. Evaluation of the patient follows the ABCs of immediate postoperative observation: airway, breathing, consciousness, and circulation. Table 22-5 lists interventions associated with the ABCs. Most recovery room nurses use a scoring system to document patient status (Table 22-6). Vital signs are assessed every 15 minutes during the recovery period, and respiratory, and GI functions are monitored. The wound is evaluated for any **drainage** (the removal of fluids from a body cavity, wound, or other source of discharge by one or more methods). When the patient has a patent airway and stable vital signs, is conscious, and responds to stimuli, the anesthesiologist or surgeon approves the transfer of the patient back to the nursing unit. As the patient regains consciousness, relief of pain is often the first need expressed; frequently, medication is given in the recovery area. Documentation from the surgical suite and recovery room is reviewed by staff on the nursing unit to assess how well the patient tolerated the surgical process. Body temperature is carefully monitored. Hypother-

TABLE 22-6 Postanesthesia Scoring System

Postanesthesia Recovery Score	In	15	30	45	Hr	Out
Activity						
4 extremities	2	2	2	2	2	2
2 extremities	1	1	1	1	1	1
0 extremities	0	0	0	0	0	0
Respiration						
Able to deep breathe and cough freely	2	2	2	2	2	2
Dyspnea (shallow or limited breathing)	1	1	1	1	1	1
Apneic	0	0	0	0	0	0
Circulation						
BP = 20 mm Hg of preanesthesia level	2	2	2	2	2	2
Preoperative BP = 20 to 50 mm Hg of preanesthesia level	1	1	1	1	1	1
BP = 50 mm Hg of preanesthesia level	0	0	0	0	0	0
Consciousness						
Fully awake	2	2	2	2	2	2
Arousable on calling	1	1	1	1	1	1
Not responding	0	0	0	0	0	0
Color						
Normal	2	2	2	2	2	2
Pale, dusky, blotchy, jaundiced, other	1	1	1	1	1	1
Cyanotic	0	0	0	0	0	0

Dismissal criteria

Total score of 10, plus stable vital signs
A physician's order is required for discharge with lower score — Total ______

From Wetchler BV: Anesthesia for outpatient surgery, *AORN J* 34(2):282, 1981.

GPR
Great Plains Regional Medical Center
Box 1167-601 West Leota
North Platte, Nebraska 69101
308-534-9310

Postoperative Assessment Form

ADDRESSOGRAPH

Date: 1-31-95	Anesthesia Note: General	Surgeon: Dr. J. H. Christensen Other: Dr. D. Giarracco	Initials MUST Accompany Each Entry

Time received on floor: 11:30 A.M. — Amt. and type of fluid infusing upon return: D_5 1/2 NS at 125 ml/hour

TO BE COMPLETED BY PERSONNEL OBTAINING INFORMATION:					NURSING OBSERVATIONS TO BE COMPLETED BY NURSE ONLY: May include: Level of conciousenss, appearance of pt., drsg/drainage, emesis, drains, mediations, and responses, etc.		
Time	BP-P-R	Cough/ D.B.	Position R/L/B	Initial	Time		Initial
11:30	118/24 88-21					ESTIMATED BLOOD LOSS < 100 ml. — IV INTAKE 1500 ml. — OUTPUT 490 ml.	L.H.
11:45	114/78 86-22	D C B	B	L.H.		CBI 0 — HEMO-DRAINS 30 ml.	
12:00	120/76 88-23		B	L.H.	11:45	Returned from RR to 308^B per gurney	
12:15	124/80 88-22	D C B	R	L.H.		Awake and alert. Color pale. Skin cool	
12:30	122/78 86-20		R	L.H.		and dry. I.V. infusing in L antecubital	
1:00	118/74 80-18	D C B	L	L.H.		space @ 21 gtts. per minute – site	
1:30	116/72 76-17	D C B	L	L.H.		s̄ edema or erythema. Abd. dressings	
2:30	118/74 78-18	D C B	B	L.H.		dry and intact. Hemovac draining san-	
						guineous exudate. Foley catheter draining	
						clear amber urine. TED hose on. Passive	
						ROM to lower extremeties. Restless and	
						c/o severe abdominal pain.	L.H.
					12:30	Demerol 75 mgm. given IM in left	
						gluteus	L.H.
					12:45	Resting comfortably – denies pain	L.H.

NURSING STAFF IDENTIFICATION

L.H. Lynn Huffman LPN

FIG. 22-2 Postoperative assessment form. (Courtesy Great Plains Regional Medical Center, North Platte, Neb.)

mia, a core temperature of less than 98.6° F (37° C), occurs in 60% to 80% of all postoperative patients. Contributing factors include body exposure in a cold operating room, the effects of cold solutions, and as a consequence of some anesthetics. Warm blankets are usually applied to the body, especially around the feet; adding warmth around the head is helpful. A newer method is convective warming therapy, in which a disposable cover inflated with warm air from a heating unit is placed over the patient; warm air passes out through the underside, providing constantly moving warm air.

Later Postoperative Period

Immediate Assessments. When the patient returns to the nursing unit, a thorough postsurgical assessment follows. Vital signs, the intravenous and incisional sites, any tubes, and postoperative orders are reviewed. A review of each body system identifies when body functions return and provides a guideline for further assessments. Unless otherwise indicated, the nurse monitors vital signs and makes general assessments using the "times four" factor—every 15 minutes times 4; every 30 minutes times 4; every hour times 4; then every 4 hours, or until assessments are within expected ranges. The times four gauge is the maximal time that should elapse between assessments. Table 22-7 details body temperature responses to surgery. A postoperative flow sheet (Fig. 22-2) is frequently used to document the patient's progress.

Significant observations are critical for the patient after surgery. Although the patient may respond, the level of functioning is impaired. Side rails should be kept in the up position and the call light within reach. Until the patient is fully conscious, a pillow should not be placed under the head. The nurse should either position the patient on the side or raise the head of the bed to a 45-degree angle. By positioning the head higher than the chest, the chance of the patient's aspirating vomitus lessens. Because nausea and vomiting are normal in the first 12 to 24 hours, the emesis basin should remain at the bedside. If the patient vomits, the amount should be measured and carefully described in the charting. Any emesis that is red should be reported immediately. Frequently, the patient remains on NPO status for the first few hours after surgery. Fluids are introduced gradually. The usual fluid regimen ordered by the physician includes ice chips followed by clear or full liquids.

Postoperative complications can occur suddenly; therefore any change should be noted. Because the patient is often cold, additional blankets should be provided for comfort; however, sweating should not be induced. Vital signs, coupled with the patient's behavior, are first-line observations. A pulse that increases and becomes thready, coupled with a declining blood pressure, cool and clammy skin, reduced urine output, and restlessness, may signal hypovolemic shock. Hypovolemic shock in the postoperative period is frequently caused by internal hemorrhage—a life-threatening emergency (Box 22-4 on p. 454).

Incision. The incisional dressing is monitored, because bleeding or excessive drainage may also signal postoperative hemorrhage. Normally dressings are not changed but are reinforced during the first 24 hours. To accurately measure the amount of drainage, the nurse circles

TABLE 22-7 Temperature Assessment and Intervention

Cause	Assessment and Intervention
Hypothermia	
Within first 12 hr	
Response to surgery, anesthesia, and body exposure	Monitor temperature readings. Check for warmth. Provide warm blankets. Do not expose for long periods. Check orientation.
Hyperthermia	
24 to 48 hr	
Dehydration Decreased lung activity Inflammatory response to surgery	Monitor temperature readings. Monitor IV rate. Encourage fluids. Assess I&O. Have patient turn, cough, and deep breathe. Provide incentive spirometer. Assess lung sounds. Observe incision.
After day 2	
Infection: respiratory, wound, urinary, or circulatory	Monitor temperature readings. Assess lung sounds and expectoration of sputum. Evaluate incision and drainage. Monitor I&O. Encourage fluids of 6-8 oz/hr unless contraindicated. Note urine color, odor, amount, and consistency, and patient's complaints of burning on micturition. Do leg exercises q2h, and ambulate q4h.

Box 22-4 POSSIBLE CAUSES OF POSTOPERATIVE SHOCK

- Moving patient from operating table to bed
- Jarring patient (bed) during transport
- Reactions to drugs and anesthesia
- Loss of blood and other body fluids
- Cardiac dysrhythmias
- Cardiac failure
- Inadequate ventilation
- Pain

the drainage markings on the dressing and writes the time and date. A surgical incision may separate; this action of **dehiscence** (the separation of a surgical incision or rupture of a wound closure) may occur within 3 days to over 2 weeks postoperatively. Wound separation that occurs in the first 3 days is usually related to technical factors, such as the sutures. Separation from 3 to 14 days postoperatively is usually associated with postoperative complications, such as distention, vomiting, excessive coughing, dehydration, or infection. Wound separation after 2 weeks is usually associated with metabolic factors, such as **cachexia** (ill health, malnutrition, and wasting as a result of chronic disease), hypoproteinemia, increased age, or malignancy. If internal organs protrude through the incision, wound **evisceration** (protrusion of an enteral organ through a wound or surgical incision, especially in the abdominal wall) has occurred. Both wound dehiscence and evisceration require prompt attention (Fig. 22-3). If the patient feels a sudden "give," sutures may have broken.

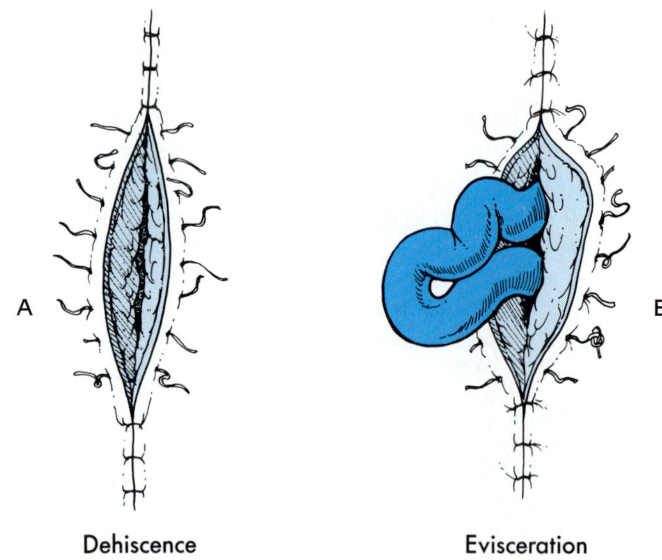

FIG. 22-3 **A,** Wound dehiscence. **B,** Evisceration.

Ventilation. Immediate postoperative hypoventilation can result from drugs (anesthetics, narcotics, tranquilizers, sedatives), incisional pain, obesity, chronic lung disease, or pressure on the diaphragm. Inadequate ventilation leads to hypoxemia. Arterial oxygenation saturation (Sao_2) can be monitored either by arterial blood gas measurements or by pulse oximetry (see Chapter 31).

Because lung ventilation is vital, the nurse assists the patient to turn, cough, and deep breathe every 1 to 2 hours until the chest is clear. Having practiced this combination preoperatively, the patient is usually able to adequately remove trapped mucus and surgical gases. To ease the pressure on the incision, the nurse helps the patient support the surgical site with a pillow, rolled bath blanket, or the heel of the hand. Analgesics, as prescribed, are given to control pain before coughing and deep breathing exercises. Early mobility and frequent position changes facilitate secretion clearance and improve the distribution of ventilation and perfusion in the lungs.

Respiratory infections are frequently caused by shallow breathing and poor coughing. The nurse should listen for wheezing or crowing sounds from patients who have undergone head or neck surgery; this response occurs when edema places pressure over the trachea, resulting in respiratory insufficiency.

If the patient feels chest pain or has a fever, productive cough, or dyspnea, **atelectasis** (an abnormal condition characterized by the collapse of lung tissue) or pneumonia may be developing. Sudden chest pain combined with dyspnea, tachycardia, cyanosis, diaphoresis, and hypotension are signs of a pulmonary embolism. The head of the bed should be raised to decrease dyspnea, and signs and symptoms must immediately be reported. Frequently oxygen therapy is instituted to assist with respirations.

Whenever air exchange is reduced, postoperative recovery slows. Medication, suctioning, and oxygen therapy may be needed to assist the patient with respiratory distress. Mechanical devices, such as incentive spirometers, are used to stimulate deep breathing. Frequently the incentive spirometer is used when the patient can deep breathe independently; the instrument visually measures the amount of air inhaled. Volume-oriented spirometers assist patients in deep breathing (Fig. 22-4). Patients are encouraged to take 10 deep breaths every hour while awake.

If respiratory complications develop, the physician may order the respiratory therapist to provide intermittent positive pressure breathing (IPPB) treatments to deliver a mixture of air and oxygen; medication can be added to enhance respirations. Chest percussion and postural drainage, a form of chest physiotherapy that combines positioning and percussion movements to

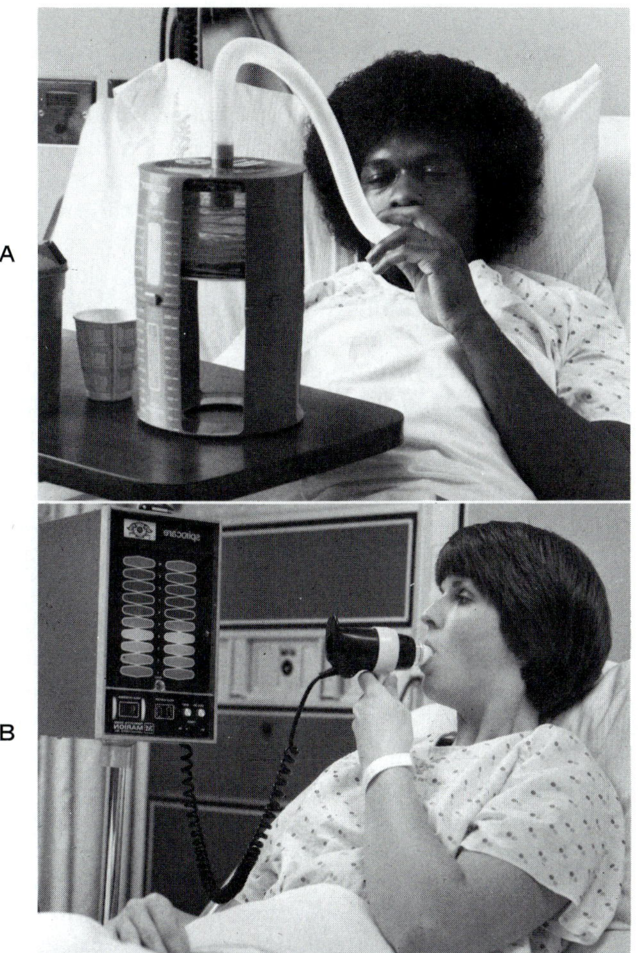

FIG. 22-4 Volume-oriented spirometer. **A,** Bellows visible to patient. **B,** Achievement light indicators.

lung areas to help dislodge and move secretions, are also utilized. Patients are not left unattended during postural drainage treatments, since they may experience respiratory distress (see Chapter 31).

Pain. Although internal organs do not have many nerve endings, a skin incision does produce painful responses. Because pain is normal postoperatively, the nurse should offer patients prescribed analgesics. The nurse should ask the patient every 3 to 4 hours if something is needed for pain because some patients will not ask for an analgesic. Within 24 to 48 hours, acute pain begins to subside. Pain medication is subsequently adjusted to meet the patient's need. In the early stages of recovery, comfort interventions help ease pain (Box 22-5). After the acute phase ends, comfort measures may be the only interventions required.

A patient's level of pain can be difficult to evaluate. There are standard pain indexes (restlessness, moaning, grimacing, diaphoresis), but some patients may not outwardly exhibit signs. Objective pain factors are detectable signs that the body is responding to "pain": vital sign changes (BP lowers in the immediate postoperative period and elevates in response to pain after about 12 hours, and pulse increases), restlessness, diaphoresis, pallor. The patient's description of discomfort represents subjective pain factors. The way the pain is affecting the patient emotionally is termed *suffering.* Pain behaviors are influenced by the patient's culture and past experiences. Behaviors include moaning, grimacing, and favoring a body area.

The effectiveness of analgesic measures differs with each person; if relief is not obtained, changing the medi-

Box 22-5 POSTOPERATIVE COMFORT MEASURES FOR PAIN

DECREASE EXTERNAL STIMULI

Darken room: close drapes.
Keep TV/radio off or low.
Monitor hall traffic/noise.
Assess staff interruptions.
Check room for noise—dripping water, buzzing lights.

REDUCE INTERRUPTIONS

Plan care to allow rest.
Post Do Not Disturb sign.
Unplug telephone.
Restrict visitors.
Pull curtains around bed.

ELIMINATE ODORS

Discuss offending odors and assess elimination.
Remove from room all dressings that are soiled with exudate.
Post No Smoking sign.
Alert housekeeping—omit room cleaning products.
Install air circulating unit.
Alert dietary department to reduce foods with odors.

NURSING INTERVENTIONS

Question normal relaxation patterns/practices.
Have patient practice deep breathing and relaxation techniques.
Plan rest periods.
Provide back rub.
Provide conversation and ask about concerns/fears.
Encourage diversional activities.
Reposition and support with pillows, bed rolls.
Check tube placement.
Offer warm fluids if indicated.
Reduce room clutter.
Provide restful environment.

cation or administration schedule may provide effective pain control. Each patient interprets pain differently and has a personal pain tolerance level; therefore, if a patient expresses pain, it is real for that person. Remember only the patient bearing the pain is an expert about that pain. McCaffery[24] states, "Pain is whatever the experiencing person says it is, existing whenever he says it does." Patients experiencing chronic pain may have more difficulty obtaining relief than individuals with acute episodes (see Chapter 15).

The success of pain management depends on the nature of the surgery, emotional state of the patient, and postoperative complications. Commonly used analgesic measures are nurse-administered narcotics, self-controlled intravenous medication administration (PCA), and pain control via the transcutaneous electric nerve stimulation (TENS) unit (Fig. 22-5). The PCA system is a pump that has a predetermined amount of analgesic contained within the unit; the system is programmed to allow only a given amount of medication to be dispensed. The patient can self-administer an analgesic by pressing a control button. The PCA system should be monitored closely every 3 to 4 hours. Attached to the skin, the TENS unit applies electric impulses to the nerve endings and blocks transmission of pain signals to the brain.

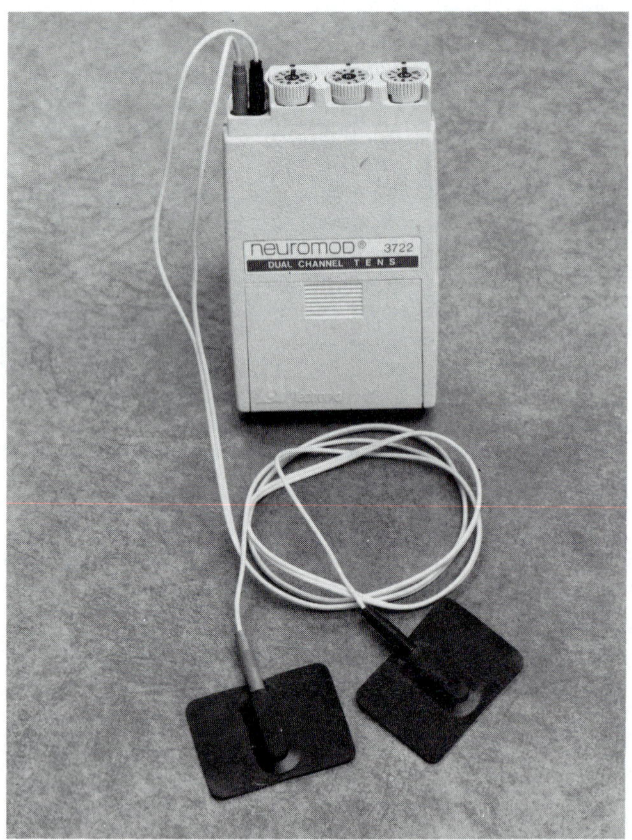

FIG. 22-5 TENS.

Urinary Function. Anesthesia retards urinary function. The bladder area is checked every 2 hours for distention. It routinely takes 6 to 8 hours for voiding to occur after surgery. If patients do not void within 8 hours, catheterization may be necessary. Catheterization should be used as a last measure. The nurse may have the patient listen to running water, place the hands in warm water, or walk to the bathroom if able, to facilitate voiding. Helping male patients stand often encourages voiding. To accurately evaluate the hydration level of the patient, intake and output are measured as long as it is deemed necessary. Usually I&O is measured while a Foley catheter is in place and the patient is receiving IV therapy. Urine measurement continues until the patient is voiding without difficulty. Fluid deficit may result from inadequate replacement of body fluids lost during surgeryor from continued fluid losses. Fluid excess may occur from large volumes of fluids replaced by IV fluids when kidney function is inadequate (evidenced by oliguria). A urine output of 30 ml per hour is considered an acceptable level postoperatively. Unless the patient has had urinary tract surgery, urine should be clear and yellow and have an ammonia odor.

Venous Stasis. Performing leg exercises every 2 hours and using antiembolic stockings aid the circulatory system, because venous **stasis** (a disorder in which the normal flow of fluid through a vessel of the body is slowed or halted) is the underlying cause of thrombus formation. Assessment of the feet and legs includes palpating for pedal pulse and noting the skin's color and temperature. If edema, aching or cramping, sensitivity, or pain occurs in the calf (Homans' sign) or leg, a thrombus should be suspected. The patient should remain in bed until the physician can do an evaluation. The nurse should teach the patient not to cross legs when in bed and encourage sitting up as another means of preventing venous stasis.

Another device that helps prevent deep vein thrombosis is the intermittent external pneumatic compression system.

Intermittent External Pneumatic Compression System. Surgical patients are at the greatest life-threatening risk of developing deep vein thrombosis and pulmonary embolism. Not only does surgery injure blood vessels, but anesthesia and inactivity cause venous stasis.

Surgery, however, is not the only risk factor. Others include pregnancy, myocardial infarction (MI), congestive heart failure, cerebral vascular accident (CVA), cancer, sepsis, and immobility.

The most effective method of decreasing the occurrence of deep vein thrombosis is with low-dose, subcutaneous heparin therapy. Heparin is an anticoagulant, but is contraindicated in trauma and general surgery patients. Antiembolism elastic stockings and ambulation have also been found useful in preventing deep vein thrombosis.

A new treatment, the external intermittent pneumatic compression system, is being used on patients who are at risk of developing deep vein thrombosis and pulmonary embolism. This device includes an air pressure pump and cuffs, one for each calf. Continuous inflation and deflation of the cuffs decreases pooling of venous blood in the legs and improves venous return to the heart. The pressure cuffs will automatically inflate to 40 mm Hg or the prescribed setting and deflate in cycles, with inflation lasting about 12 seconds and deflation lasting about 48 seconds.

This intermittent external pneumatic compression system is contraindicated for any patient with acute thrombophlebitis or deep vein thrombosis.

When ambulating the patient, the nurse should disconnect the pump tubing, but keep the cuffs in place on the calves. The device should not be disconnected for more than 30 minutes. If the patient has diagnostic examinations that require leaving the nursing unit for longer than 30 minutes, the compression pump, the cuffs, and the instructions on operation should travel with the patient.

The treatment should continue for 72 hours postoperatively, or until the patient is ambulating well. The cuffs should be removed once a day to assess for impairment of skin integrity and to provide skin care. Document the use of intermittent external pneumatic compression system and any reaction such as numbness or tingling[5] (Fig. 22-6).

Activity. Early ambulation has been a significant factor in hastening postoperative recovery and preventing postoperative complications. Numerous benefits are derived from the exercise of getting in and out of bed and walking during the early postoperative period (Box 22-6). Ambulation is usually contraindicated when there is a severe infection or thrombophlebitis.

Assessment. Before helping the patient to ambulate for the first few times after major surgery, an assessment is made of the patient's level of alertness to follow directions, cardiovascular status, and motor status:

1. Level of alertness: ask patient simple questions or to follow simple commands

Box 22-6

EFFECTS OF EARLY POSTOPERATIVE AMBULATION

INCREASED RATE AND DEPTH OF BREATHING

Prevention of atelectasis and hypostatic pneumonia
Increased mental alertness from increased oxygenation to brain

INCREASED CIRCULATION

Nutrients required for healing are more available to wound
Prevention of thrombophlebitis
Increased kidney function

INCREASED MICTURITION

Decreased pain

INCREASED METABOLISM

Prevention of urinary retention
Prevention of loss of muscle tone
Restoration of nitrogen balance

INCREASED PERISTALSIS

Promotion of expulsion of flatus
Prevention of abdominal distention and gas pain
Prevention of constipation
Prevention of paralytic ileus

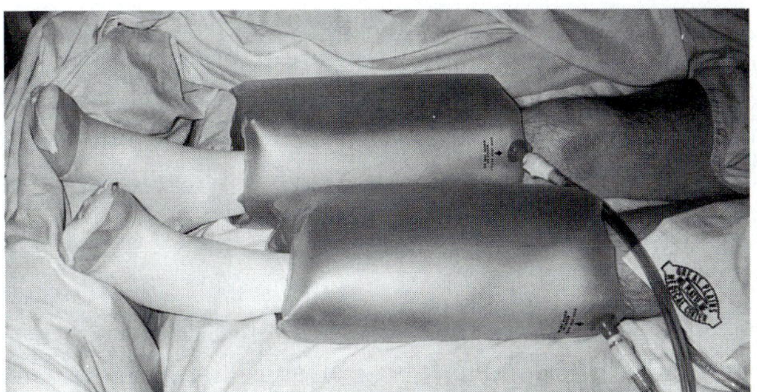

FIG. 22-6 Intermittent external pneumatic compression system.

2. Cardiovascular status
   a. Assess pulse and respiratory rate and depth while patient is supine, then after sitting
   b. Observe skin color for pallor while patient is sitting
   c. Note complaints of dizziness when patient is sitting
3. Motor status
   a. Assess muscle strength of patient's legs
   b. Assess sitting ability:
      (1) Assist patient to sitting position on side of bed
      (2) Ask patient to maintain an erect position while being gently pushed sideways

It is also important to know of any preoperative limitations to ambulation. The patient with arthritis or arteriosclerosis may take longer to move and to adjust to standing and walking. The patient who used a walker preoperatively will need assistance for a longer time before continuing to use the walker again.

Nursing interventions.

1. Encourage muscle-strengthening exercises before ambulation:
   a. Have patient bend knees, lower knees, press back of knees hard against bed.
   b. Have patient alternately contract and relax calf and thigh muscles 10 times using the following cycle: contract, relax, rest.
2. Have patient sit on side of bed (legs dangling) to become accustomed to upright position before ambulating the first time. Be sure *pulse has stabilized* (returned to baseline) before ambulation is attempted:
   a. Clamp off NG tube until patient has ambulated, then reconnect.
   b. Keep urinary tube connected to drainage bag; carry bag or pin bag to inside of robe.
   c. Attach IV bag to a movable pole.
3. Use two people to assist in ambulating a weak patient receiving IV fluids.
4. Encourage patient to walk farther at each ambulation.

The word ambulate means to move from place to place, to walk. Sitting in a chair is not ambulation. After ambulating, the patient may sit in a chair if permitted, but should be advised to stand and walk at intervals and to elevate the legs while sitting to prevent venous pooling in the extremities. Sitting in a chair for long periods is to be avoided.

Gastrointestinal Status. Abdominal distention frequently occurs after surgery. Because anesthesia and surgical manipulation slow peristalsis, it may take 3 to 4 days for bowel activity to return. Listening for bowel sounds in the lower abdomen can help gauge the return of function. Normal peristalsis is gauged by hearing 5 to 30 gurgles per minute. When listening for bowel sounds, the nurse should listen for 1 minute. If peristalsis decreases or stops, a **paralytic ileus** (a decrease in or absence of intestinal peristalsis that may occur after abdominal surgery, peritoneal trauma, and severe metabolic disease and other conditions) may have developed. If inactivity continues, an NG or nasointestinal tube to suction is usually ordered to help remove the gas formed in the stomach and small intestine. When listening for bowel sounds in patients who have an NG or nasointestinal tube, the nurse should turn off the suction machine but should *never* leave the room without turning the machine on.

Abdominal distention can be verified by measuring the patient's abdominal girth. Accurate measurement is ensured by marking on the skin the placement for the tape measure, which is at the level of the umbilicus. The nurse should assess and chart the expelling of flatus, bowel sounds, and abdominal girth. Occasionally, analgesics (meperidine) and other medications may slow peristalsis; charting the patient's GI habits aids in identifying etiological factors.

Encouraging activity (turning every 2 hours, early ambulation) assists GI activity. A rectal tube or up-and-down flush (a 250-ml tap water enema instilled into the colon; enema container lowered to withdraw air from colon; and repeat) may be ordered for ongoing distress. For the patient who has difficulty with flatus, limiting iced beverages and encouraging warm liquids may help resolve the discomfort. The patient may have fluids and food withheld until flatus is expelled. As patients return to previous eating habits, bowel function slowly resumes its preoperative state. Constipation is also a frequent problem after surgery. The same aids for abdominal distention assist in alleviating constipation. If feces are not passed within 2 to 3 days after the patient has resumed solid foods, a suppository or tap water enema may be ordered. Ambulation is encouraged to promote peristalsis.

A **singultus** (hiccup) is an involuntary contraction of the diaphragm followed by rapid closure of the glottis. Singultus results from irritation of the phrenic nerve. Since abdominal distention may be the cause, the nurse assesses the patient's abdomen for proper GI function. Although abdominal distention usually occurs from gas in the intestinal tract, the cause may be internal bleeding. The nurse should evaluate the patient for signs of shock: vital signs, skin condition, and level of consciousness.

Fluids and Electrolytes. Fluid is lost during surgery through blood loss and increased insensible fluid loss through the lungs and skin. For at least the first 24 to 48 hours after surgery, fluids are retained by the body as part of the stress response to trauma and the effect of anesthesia.

Sodium and potassium depletion can occur in the postoperative patient from the loss of blood or body fluids during surgery or the loss of GI secretion by vomiting and through NG tubes. Potassium is also lost during **catabolism** (tissue breakdown), especially after severe trauma or crush injuries. Loss of gastric secretions can result in chloride loss, producing metabolic alkalosis. Electrolytes are often added to intravenous solution in the form of potassium chloride (KCl).

Fluid tolerance and electrolyte values are closely monitored during the postoperative period. When the patient returns from the recovery room, therapy will be in progress. Until the patient is past the nausea and vomiting period and can tolerate oral fluids, parenteral therapy should be maintained. The IV line is observed for patency and ordered fluid rate, and the IV site is monitored for erythema, edema, heat, and pain. Because IV therapy may become infiltrated because of movement or inadvertent dislodgment of the needle when the patient ambulates, the site should be assessed every 1 to 2 hours or if the patient complains of discomfort. The assessment for rate of infusion is extremely important for older patients, who may experience fluid overload and pulmonary edema very quickly.

Muscles and nerves require ongoing nourishment to function adequately, and parenteral fluids contain the necessary glucose and electrolytes. Depending on the type of surgery and nutritional needs of the patient, IV therapy lasts from a few hours to a few days. As long as parenteral fluids are received, the nurse should record the patient's I&O. If there is concern about the patient's overall nutritional state, the patient should be weighed daily.

As oral fluids are introduced, patients should be encouraged to drink small amounts frequently (6 to 8 ounces per hour). The nurse reviews the diet history to note fluids normally enjoyed. Unless otherwise ordered, patients usually begin by ingesting clear liquids (7-Up, water, tea, broth, gelatin) and progress as the GI system returns to normal functioning. If the patient has difficulty drinking the amount of fluid recommended, fluids can be offered more frequently and without a straw. (A straw, while convenient, reduces the amount of fluids ingested.) Unless there are other problems (decreased renal excretion because of renal failure, age), patients should be encouraged to drink 2000 to 2400 ml in 24 hours. Because iced and carbonated beverages cause GI disturbances in some individuals, these fluids should be avoided until active peristalsis is noted. If nausea and vomiting persist, an antiemetic, such as promethazine (Phenergan), benzquinamide (Emete-Con), or prochlorperazine (Compazine), is usually ordered to be administered IM, IV, or rectally.

Postoperative Nursing Diagnoses. The nurse will determine the status of problems identified during the preoperative period. These data, combined with new relevant assessment, will be used to formulate new diagnoses. Nursing diagnoses stated before surgery may continue as a postoperative challenge. The nurse may also identify new factors that place the postoperative patient at high risk for problems occurring due to surgery, as for example, the nursing diagnosis: Pain, related to surgical incision.

The nurse will also note needs of the patient's family when making nursing diagnoses. For example, the family's inability to cope with the patient's condition necessitates the nurse's intervention. See Box 22-7 for post-

Box 22-7 POSTOPERATIVE NURSING DIAGNOSES

Airway clearance, ineffective related to:
- Diminished cough
- Retained secretions
- Prolonged sedation

Body temperature, altered, high risk for, related to:
- Lowered metabolism

Breathing pattern, ineffective, related to:
- Incisional pain
- Analgesia effects on ventilation

Communication, impaired verbal, related to:
- Endotracheal tube placement
- Airway tube placement

Coping, ineffective individual, related to:
- Constraints imposed by surgery
- Postoperative therapies

Fluid volume deficit, high risk for, related to:
- Wound drainage
- Inadequate fluid intake

Grieving, anticipatory, related to:
- Patient's critical condition

Infection, high risk for, related to:
- Surgical wound incision
- Presence of Foley catheter and wound drainage tubes

Mobility, impaired physical, related to:
- Pain
- Postoperative activity restrictions
- Casts or dressings
- Surgical incision
- NG tube placement

Oral mucous membrane, altered, related to:
- Irritation of NG or endotracheal tube
- NPO status

Self-care deficit, bathing/hygiene, dressing/grooming, feeding, toileting, related to:
- Postoperative activity restrictions
- Pain

Skin integrity, impaired, or high risk for, related to:
- Wound exudate
- Impaired mobility
- Decrease in nutritional intake

NURSING CARE PLAN: ***THE POSTOPERATIVE PATIENT***

Ms. Alonzo is a forty-year-old obese woman weighing 280 pounds admitted with choleliasis and a scheduled open cholecystectomy. Ms. Alonzo has hypertension and a history of poor wound healing.

Nursing diagnoses	Patient goals/expected outcomes	Nursing interventions
Airway clearance, ineffective, related to inability to cough deeply and retention of secretions	Patient will cough deeply with splinting of incision. Patient will expectorate mucus. Patient's temperature will be normal. Patient's lung sounds will clear after coughing.	Medicate with analgesia to control pain. Raise head of bed to full Fowler's position during exercises. Splint incision with rolled bath blanket. Have patient turn, cough, and deep breathe q1h while awake. Use incentive spirometer hourly. Take vital signs q4h and note evidence of dyspnea or restlessness. Monitor IV fluids. Offer sips of fluid qh if permissible.
Breathing pattern, ineffective, related to poor body mechanics and incisional pain	Patient will deep breathe effectively q1 to 2 h while awake. Patient will effectively use incentive spirometer. Patient will not demonstrate dyspnea or restlessness. Patient's respirations will be even and unlabored.	Encourage deep breathing q1-2h while awake. Reposition q2h; support joints and incision. Continue oxygen @ 2 L per cannula; cleanse nares q4h; post No Smoking sign. Encourage use of incentive spirometer. Record respirations q4h, noting depth, rate, quality. Assess skin and nail beds; report slow blanching color and condition q4h. Darken room; decrease stimuli, monitor pain, and offer analgesic prn.
Infection, high risk for, related to open surgical incision and draining wound	Patient's wound will not be erythematous or produce purulent exudate. Patient's temperature will remain within normal range. Patient will not complain of pain or tenderness from wound site. Patient's WBC will remain within normal range.	Use good handwashing technique. Monitor wound q4h, noting amount and color of drainage; assess skin for warmth, color, and sensation. Mark drainage on dressing q4h; reinforce prn. Report irritability, weakness, or irregular pulse. Use surgical asepsis when changing dressing. Monitor temperature q4h. Monitor WBC as ordered.

CRITICAL THINKING QUESTIONS

1. On the second postoperative day, Ms. Alonzo is taking shallow breaths and is experiencing difficulty in complying with coughing and deep breathing. Her temperature is 101.8° F, and she has adventitious breath sounds bilaterally in the bases. List several nursing interventions to assist Ms. Alonzo.
2. Ms. Alonzo is in her third postoperative day, and the nurse notes an erythematous incision with moderate amounts of purulent exudate from the Penrose drain site. The correct nursing interventions would include:
3. The signs and symptoms the nurse would note when assessing Ms. Alonzo for dehydration secondary to elevated temperature and decreased fluid intake would include:

operative nursing diagnoses. (See the nursing care plan for the postoperative patient.)

Parenteral Fluids

Healing is directly associated with well-nourished body cells. Without adequate electrolytes and nutrients, healing is hindered. For surgical patients, a patent IV site is maintained for the administration of nutrients, fluids, medications, and blood. The overall goal of fluid IV administration is to correct or prevent fluid and electrolyte imbalances. Poor tissue absorption, inadequate GI tract function, and the need for maintaining medications at optimum levels are indicators for IV therapy. IV therapy continues postoperatively until the patient tolerates fluids and oral nutrients.

Solutions. Parenteral fluids are selected for the electrolytes and nutrients provided. Three basic types of fluids exist: *isotonic, hypotonic,* and *hypertonic.* Each fluid is categorized by its total electrolyte amount and whether total osmolarity is less than, greater than, or equal to that of blood.

Parenteral solutions are chosen for their actions. *Isotonic* solutions have the same concentration of solutes (substances dissolved in a solution) as another solution. Isotonic solutions do not expand or shrink cells. Dextrose 5% in water or lactated Ringer's solution and 0.9% sodium chloride (normal saline) are examples of isotonic solutions. Their primary use is to replace fluids and provide calories. Normal saline is used to expand plasma volume and replace sodium losses, such as GI fluid loss.

Fluids that have less solute than another solution are called *hypotonic;* cells expand in a hypotonic solution. Hypotonic fluids are used to replace cellular fluids and provide water to remove body wastes. Sodium chloride (NaCl) 0.45% is an example of a hypotonic fluid.

Hypertonic fluids have a greater concentration of solute than body fluids; fluids are pulled out of cells, causing the cells to shrink. If 5% dextrose is added to normal saline or Ringer's solution (5% dextrose and 0.9% NaCl), a hypertonic solution is created. Frequently a hypertonic solution is given to provide extra calories. To help the body dilute the heavy solute concentrations found in hypertonic fluids, fluids are often administered into central veins.

Parenteral therapy is also used to administer amino acids, high concentrations of calories (hyperalimentation solutions), fat emulsions, blood products, and medications to the patient. Potassium is commonly added to the IVs of patients who have NG tubes or drainage (from ostomies or wounds) and thereby lose potassium chloride.

Regardless of the solution administered, the nurse should observe the following three guidelines: (1) monitor the solution drip rate at the ordered infusion rate, (2) infuse the amount of prescribed solution, and (3) maintain the patency of the IV needle. Monitoring the site every 1 to 2 hours is recommended, and an IV line should be assessed at least every 4 hours. During parenteral therapy, the patient's intake and output should be recorded.

Hyperalimentation, or total parenteral nutrition (TPN), provides the patient with glucose, essential amino acids, vitamins, and minerals. Roughly 1000 calories per liter of TPN therapy is supplied to patients who are unable to tolerate nutrients in the normal manner. Because of the overload TPN can exert on body systems, measurement of I&O is essential. Because hyperglycemia can occur with the high concentration of glucose, blood glucose levels should be assessed, using the Accucheck unit (glucose monitoring unit) every 4 to 6 hours. Occasionally regular insulin is ordered to help assimilate infused glucose. The jugular or subclavian vein is used as the infusion site, because TPN is highly concentrated and requires a large blood volume to help dilute it. Sterile technique (surgical asepsis) is critical whenever the site or solution is handled, to prevent the introduction of pathogens. The infusion rate of TPN solution should never be changed unless the physician orders it. To ensure a constant flow rate, TPN is administered by an infusion pump.

Intravenous Monitoring. IV sites are selected to accommodate the intended solution. Most insertion sites for postoperative patients are located in the hand or arm. A central vein, such as the subclavian vein, is used to deliver large amounts of fluids or concentrated solutions directly into the bloodstream.

Assessment of the intravenous site centers on the **patency** (a condition of being opened and unblocked) of the system. A routine should be established for checking the IV site, beginning at the solution container and ending at the site. The flow rate should be checked against the physician's order. Tubing is assessed for kinks or obstructions, and the position of the patient's hand or arm is checked. If the extremity is flexed, the vein may become occluded. Patients should be reminded to keep extremities extended. The nurse inspects and palpates the site for edema, erythema, **induration** (hardness), heat, and discomfort. A burning sensation can mean the solution is irritating the vein; the infusion rate should be slowed and monitoring should be continued. The extremity is compared with the opposite hand or arm if the site seems edematous. Edema may indicate an infiltration has occurred. It is incorrect to assume that obtaining a blood return at the IV site indicates a patent vein. Although an infiltrated IV routinely is discontinued, each institution has policies for monitoring and discontinuing IV therapy.

The flow rate is monitored according to the physician's orders. If the patient is dehydrated, in shock, or critically ill, a slow infusion rate does not provide the cardiovascular system with enough fluid. By contrast, an infusion rate that is too rapid can place too much fluid into the circulation and overload the cardiovascular, neurological, and urinary systems. Fluid overload can be fatal. Signs and symptoms associated with fluid overload include dyspnea; a rapid, weak pulse; cough; disorientation; increased or decreased blood pressure; crackles; pitting edema; weight gain; and decreased urine output. If an overload is suspected, the nurse should immediately slow the infusion rate and contact the charge nurse.

Infiltration. If edema is detected, the nurse should first loosen the tape over the insertion point. Edema that does not subside generally indicates that the catheter is out of the vein and infiltration has occurred. Discomfort or dysfunction may also indicate the solution has infiltrated. With an infiltration, the drip rate decreases in patients who have good skin turgor. When palpating the site, the nurse will find that an infiltrated area feels cool, and the skin may have a blanched appearance. If fluid seeps into the tissue and infiltration is confirmed, the solution is discontinued and another site is used to continue therapy. The site of the infiltration is monitored; usually fluid reabsorbs within 24 hours. Warm compresses should not be applied to infiltrations caused by blood and vesicants (medication that induces blistering); the agency's policy on care to be provided should be followed.

Phlebitis. Phlebitis results from mechanical irritation (the needle moves inside the vein, injuring the vessel), the low pH of some IV solutions, and highly concentrated additives. Erythema, warmth, edema, and discomfort are classic signs of phlebitis. The IV is discontinued and restarted in a different site. Reducing injurious agents, maintaining sterile technique when beginning an IV, and using in-line filters decrease vein irritation and trauma. Applying warm compresses to the inflamed area lessens discomfort.

Septicemia. If a systemic infection occurs from pathogens introduced into the circulating bloodstream, septicemia (blood poisoning) results. Signs and symptoms include a fever, chills, prostration, pain, headache, nausea, and vomiting. Antibiotic therapy is vigorously initiated if blood cultures verify a septicemic condition. Using sterile technique reduces the potential for introduction of pathogenic organisms through IV therapy.

Blood Therapy. Blood replacement therapy is most commonly used postoperatively to replace blood losses. Individuals who have personal concerns about receiving another person's blood may store their own blood with the American Red Cross before the anticipated surgery for infusion during hospitalization. The fear of receiving the HIV virus has led patients to refuse blood products (see Chapter 37 for information on HIV disease or AIDS). Testing procedures used by the American Red Cross to detect the HIV virus have dramatically reduced the incidence of its being transmitted. Plasma expanders (Plasmanate, Dextran) can be used for patients who refuse blood transfusions because of personal or religious beliefs. A drainage/reinfusion system (Fig. 22-7), Solcotrans, permits a patient's blood to be collected and reinfused after surgery. The Solcotrans system is connected to a closed wound drain intraoperatively. With a vacuum, blood is aspirated; after a maximum of 500 ml is collected, reinfusion can be done following blood transfusion procedures.

Blood transfusion reactions. If the infused blood is not compatible with the patient's blood type, a reaction results. Close monitoring is therefore crucial in assessing the patient's tolerance to the infusing blood. Vital signs are taken before beginning a blood transfusion, 15 minutes into the transfusion, and on completion. Refer to agency policy to verify protocol. Patients experiencing transfusion reactions frequently say they are "not feeling right." They may have chills, fever, low back pain, pruritus, hypotension, nausea and vomiting, decreased urine output, chest pain, and dyspnea. Frequently signs and symptoms occur within the first 15 minutes. Because signs and symptoms vary, the nurse should report any

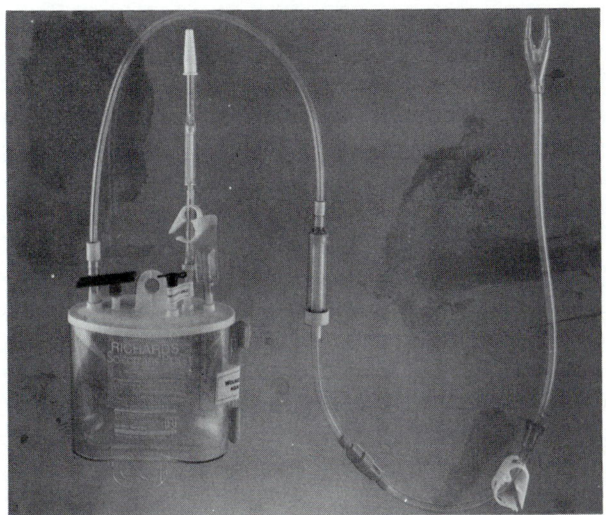

FIG. 22-7 The Solcotrans unit serves a twofold purpose: it permits drainage from surgical site and allows reinfusion of the patient's own blood—a plus in this day of widespread communicable diseases such as AIDS. (Courtesy Smith and Nephew Richards, Inc., Memphis, Tenn.)

change in the patient. If the patient is unconscious, the nurse should closely assess vital signs, urine output, and skin appearance. If a transfusion reaction is suspected, the transfusion should be stopped. The vein is kept open with 0.9% sodium chloride solution, and the physician and blood bank are notified. The nurse monitors the patient's vital signs and urine output every 15 minutes. Because transfusion reaction can be frightening, the nurse should reassure and support the patient.

If the patient is experiencing a hemolytic reaction, transfused blood is incompatible with the patient's blood type and death can occur. Although a reaction normally occurs within the first 15 minutes, it can occur anytime during the infusing process. If the reaction is severe, the patient could go into shock and die. Other types of blood transfusion reactions are febrile nonhemolytic, allergic, and anaphylactic reactions. In each type of reaction, a component within the unit of blood is incompatible with the patient's blood. The reaction can occur immediately (febrile nonhemolytic and anaphylactic) or anytime during the transfusion.

After any blood transfusion reaction, remaining blood should be returned to the blood bank for analysis. The nurse should comply with the agency's policies for monitoring blood transfusions and reactions.

Wound Care

Promoting wound healing is the focus during the postsurgical recovery phase. Various stresses affect the wound's ability to repair itself. Stress and strain (nausea, vomiting, abdominal distention, coughing, respiratory efforts) place tension against the surgical incision. During this phase, the abdominal muscles contract and cause intraabdominal pressure; if the incisional area is weak, dehiscence may occur. As the postoperative period lengthens, patient-related factors influence wound healing: age, nutritional status, physical condition, preexisting health problems, and medication habits. Other factors that may affect wound healing include preoperative skin preparation, type and severity of the surgical procedure, environment within the surgical suite, and postoperative wound care.

Surgical Wound. Wound categories result from their cause, severity of injury, amount of contamination, or the skin's integrity. For planned surgery, a wound is made by an **incision** (a cut produced surgically by a sharp instrument creating an opening into an organ or space in the body) or puncture (stab wound for a drainage system). In unplanned or emergency surgeries (traumatic injury from a knife stabbing), wound edges are brought together to aid healing. Unless a "dirty surgery" is performed (e.g., a perforated bowel, ruptured appendix), a surgical incision is cleaner than a traumatic wound.

The Centers for Disease Control and Prevention classifies wounds according to the amount of contamination involved: clean, clean-contaminated, contaminated, dirty, or infected. A *clean* wound is an uninfected surgical wound; the chance of an infection occurring postoperatively is less than 5%. A surgical incision made into the respiratory, GI, or genitourinary tract after special presurgical preparation is called a *clean-contaminated* wound. The likelihood that an infection will occur postoperatively in a clean-contaminated wound is between 3% and 11%. A *contaminated* wound results from the presence of GI products (feces with *Escherichia coli* in the colon), from an acute, nonpurulent inflammation (inflamed appendix), or when aseptic technique is broken during surgery (scalpel is reused after incising a contaminated area). A wound infection occurs 10% to 17% of the time from a contaminated wound. *Dirty* or *infected* wounds have a 27% chance of causing a wound infection. Wounds in this category (e.g., gangrenous toe) are infected before surgery.

Wound healing begins immediately after an injury and may continue for a year or longer. Although the healing process follows the same pattern, the type of wound and tissue, severity, and overall condition of the patient influence the overall process. Wound healing follows four phases: hemostasis, inflammatory, reconstruction, and maturation.[34]

Hemostasis begins as soon as the injury occurs. As blood platelets adhere to the walls of the injured vessel, a clot begins to form. Fibrin in the clot begins to hold the wound together, and bleeding subsides.

During the inflammatory phase an initial increase in blood elements (antibodies, electrolytes, plasma proteins) and water flow out of the blood vessel into the vascular space. This process causes the cardinal signs and symptoms of inflammation: redness (rubor), heat (calor), edema (tumor), pain (dolor), and tissue dysfunction. Leukocytes appear and begin to engulf bacteria, fungi, viruses, and toxic proteins. If an infection is not present, the number of leukocytes decreases. During the inflammatory phase, cells migrate, divide, and form new cells. Slowly, blood clots dissolve and the wound fills; the sides of the wound usually meet in 24 to 48 hours. As the inflammatory phase ends, new cells and capillaries fill the wound from the underlying tissue to the surface. This process seals the wound to protect it from contamination.

Collagen formation occurs during the reconstruction phase. Fibroblasts produce collagen, a gluelike protein substance that adds tensile strength to the wound and tissue. Collagen formation increases rapidly between postoperative days 5 and 25. During this phase the wound's appearance changes to an irregular, raised, purplish, immature scar. Foods rich in protein and vitamins A and C, which assist in wound repair, are encouraged during this time. If a patient is not well nourished, nutrient supplements may be ordered. Wound dehiscence most frequently occurs during the reconstructive phase.

Approximately 3 weeks after surgery, fibroblasts begin to exit the wound. The wound continues to gain strength, although healed wounds rarely return to the

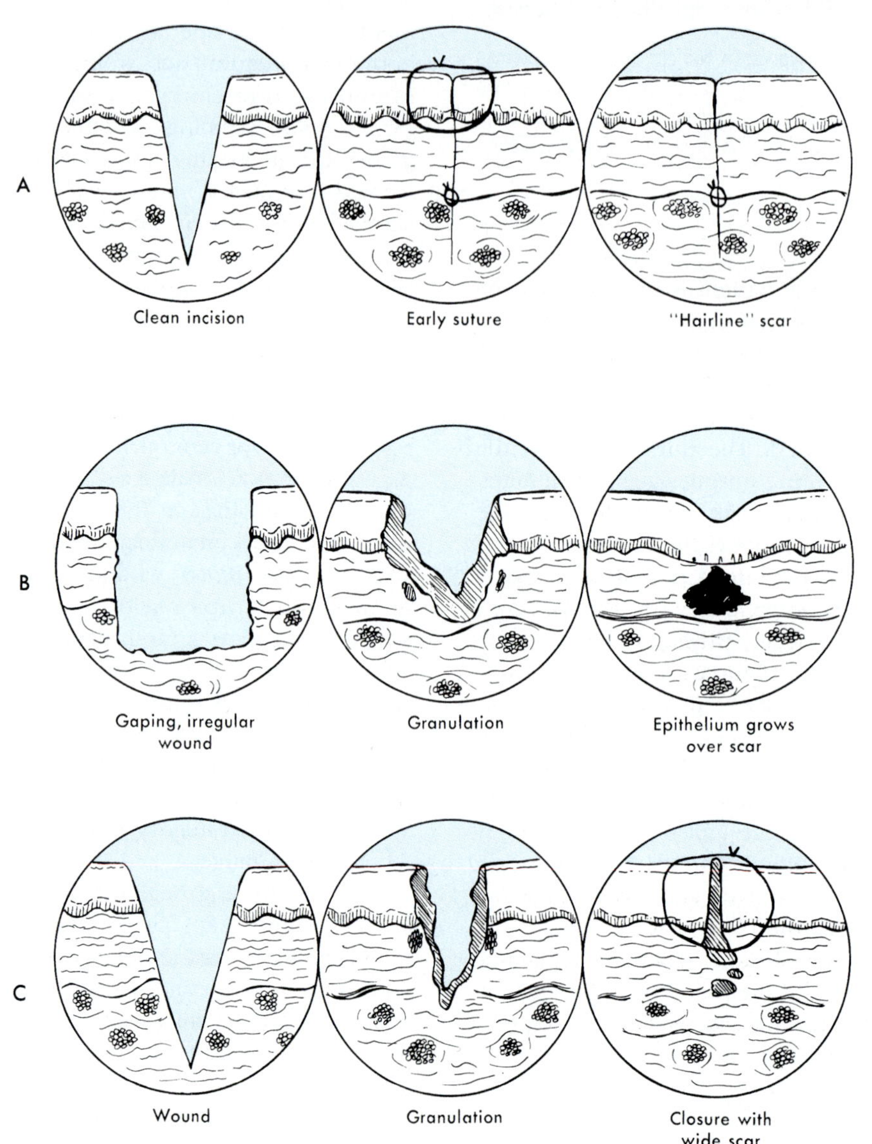

FIG. 22-8 Types of wound healing. **A,** Primary intention (primary union). **B,** Second intention (granulation). **C,** Tertiary intention (secondary suture). (From Hardy JD, editor: *Rhoads textbook of surgery: principles and practice,* ed 5, Philadelphia, 1977, Lippincott.)

strength the tissue had before surgery. Although tissue heals at varying speeds, internal wounds (stomach, colon) regain strength faster than skin wounds. Occasionally a keloid, which is an overgrowth of collagenous scar tissue, may form during this phase. The keloid's color ranges from red to pink to white. African Americans and dark-complexioned Caucasians have a higher incidence of keloid formation than other races (see Chapter 25).

Forms of Wound Healing. Three types of wound healing occur: **primary intention** (primary union), secondary intention (granulation), and tertiary (third) intention (secondary suture). Wounds that are made surgically and that have little tissue loss heal by primary intention; skin edges are close together, and minimal scarring results. Primary intention healing begins during the inflammatory phase of healing (Fig. 22-8).

Secondary intention healing occurs when skin edges are not close together (approximated) or when pus has formed. If the wound has a **purulent** (producing or containing pus) **exudate** (fluid, cells, or other substances that have been slowly exuded, or discharged, from cells or blood through small pores or breaks in cell membranes) that forms when injured or diseased tissue dies, the surgeon provides a means for its release. This is accomplished through a drainage system or by packing the wound with gauze. Slowly the necrotized tissue decomposes and escapes; the cavity begins to fill with soft, pink, fleshy projections consisting of capillaries surrounded by fibrous collagen, or **granulation** tissue. The amount of granulation tissue required depends on the size of the wound; scarring is greater in a large wound.

Healing by **tertiary intention** results if there is a delay in closing the wound and two close, granulated areas are brought together. This frequently occurs when a deep wound was not sutured or the wound breaks down. The wound is resutured when infection is no longer present.

Factors Affecting Healing. To promote healing the nurse should closely monitor fluid and nutritional needs of the patient. If the patient cannot tolerate food or fluids, TPN or NG feedings can be provided. Because patients may not be able to tolerate large meals or solid foods, dietary services can provide small, frequent feedings. Fluids, when tolerated, should be offered hourly. Unless contraindicated, the nurse should encourage an intake of 2000 to 2400 ml in 24 hours. As the patient progresses from clear to full liquids, fluids the patient enjoys should be provided. Until the patient's hydration level is stable (usually 24 to 72 hours), the patient's I&O is monitored.

The nurse assists the patient to achieve a balance between time to rest as a means to facilitate healing and activity to decrease venous stasis. When the patient is confined to bed, moving one body section at a time—head, chest, hip, legs—should be encouraged. To sit up, the patient should roll to the side and, using the elbow as a lever, push to a sitting position; this reduces the stress placed on the incision. If coughing occurs, the nurse can apply a pillow, rolled bath blanket, or the palms of the hands to the incisional area to lessen intra-abdominal pressure. Visitors may be restricted if the patient tires too easily.

Preexisting conditions, such as heart murmurs, and chronic diseases (arthritis, diabetes mellitus, hypertension) add stress to the recovering body and require ongoing monitoring. Treatment addresses the postoperative healing process and management of problems. Assessment is heightened by the need to observe signs and symptoms associated with incisional healing, as well as accompanying disorders (Table 22-8 on p. 466).

Surgical Site. The selection of the site is based on the tissue and organ involved, nature of the injury or disease process, presence of inflammation or infection, and strength of the site. If surgical procedures require a drainage system, the position of the drain also influences the placement of the incision. The surgeon's goal is to enter the cavity involved, repair the injured or diseased area, and minimize trauma as quickly as possible. Patients may be placed in positions that add stress to the tissue to facilitate the surgery. Therefore pain after surgery may be caused from strained muscles and ligaments, as well as from the surgical process.

Many options are available to the surgeon for closing the surgical incision. Common closures are sutures, staples, Steri-Strips, butterfly strips, and transparent sprays and films. A binder or bandage may be used to support the incision or secure dressings without using adhesive materials (Skill 22-5 on p. 467 and Skill 22-6 on p. 468). The nurse inspects dressings every 2 to 4 hours for the first 24 hours. The day of surgery, most wounds produce either **sanguineous** (pertaining to blood) or **serosanguineous** (thin and red composed of serum and blood) exudate. Because pressure to the surgical wound retards bleeding, wounds are usually covered by a gauze dressing. It is imperative that the nurse inspect both the dressing or incisional area and the area *under* the patient. Exudate follows the flow of gravity; therefore, depending on the contour of the body the dressing may remain dry while blood flows under the body, and hemorrhaging might go undetected.

Incision Care. Surgical wounds, because they are aseptically created, generally heal well and quickly. For psychological reasons and to prevent trauma until epithelialization occurs, the wound is usually covered initially by a dressing.

TABLE 22-8 Factors That Impair Wound Healing

Physiological Effects	Interventions
Age	
Aging alters all phases of wound healing. Vascular changes impair circulation to wound site. Reduced liver function alters synthesis of clotting factors. Inflammatory response is slowed. Formation of antibodies and lymphocytes is reduced. Collagen tissue is less pliable. Scar tissue is less elastic.	Instruct patient on safety precautions to avoid injuries. Be prepared to provide wound care for longer period. Teach home care givers wound care techniques.
Malnutrition	
All phases of wound healing are impaired. Stress from burns or severe trauma increases nutritional requirements.	Provide balanced diet rich in protein, carbohydrates, lipids, vitamins A and C, and minerals (e.g., zinc, copper).
Obesity	
Fatty tissue lacks adequate blood supply to resist bacterial infection and deliver nutrients and cellular elements.	Observe obese patient for signs of wound infection, dehiscence, and evisceration.
Impaired oxygenation	
Low arterial oxygen tension alters synthesis of collagen and formation of epithelial cells. If local circulating blood flow is poor, tissues fail to receive needed oxygen. Decreased hemoglobin (anemia) reduces arterial oxygen levels in capillaries and interferes with tissue repair.	Provide diet adequate in iron. Monitor patients' hematocrit and hemoglobin levels.
Smoking	
Smoking reduces amount of functional hemoglobin in blood, thus decreasing tissue oxygenation. Smoking may increase platelet aggregation and cause hypercoagulability. Smoking interferes with normal cellular mechanisms that promote release of oxygen to tissues.	Discourage patient from smoking by explaining its effects on wound healing.
Drugs	
Steroids reduce inflammatory response. Antiinflammatory drugs suppress protein synthesis, wound contraction, epithelialization, and inflammation. Prolonged antibiotic use may increase risk of superinfection. Chemotherapeutic drugs can depress bone marrow function, number of leukocytes, and inflammatory response.	Carefully observe patient; signs of inflammation may not be obvious.
Diabetes mellitus	
Chronic disease causes small blood vessel disease that impairs tissue perfusion. Diabetes causes hemoglobin to have greater affinity for oxygen, so it fails to release oxygen to tissues. Hyperglycemia alters ability of leukocytes to perform phagocytosis and also supports overgrowth of fungal and yeast infection.	Instruct patient to take preventive measures to avoid cuts or breaks in skin. Provide preventive foot care. Control blood sugar to reduce the physiological changes associated with diabetes.
Radiation	
Fibrosis and vascular scarring eventually develop in irradiated skin layers. Tissues become fragile and poorly oxygenated.	Closely observe patient for wound complications.
Wound stress	
Vomiting, abdominal distention, and respiratory effort may stress suture line and disrupt wound layer. Sudden, unexpected tension on incision inhibits formation of endothelial cell and collagen networks.	Control nausea with ordered antiemetics. Keep NG tubes patent and draining to avoid accumulation of secretions. Instruct patient to splint abdominal wound during coughing.

APPLYING A BANDAGE

Nursing action

1. Wash hands.
2. Position patient in comfortable position, arranging support for area to be bandaged.
3. Provide privacy.
4. Ensure that skin and/or dressing is clean and dry.
5. Separate any adjacent skin surfaces.
6. Align part to be bandaged, providing slight flexion if appropriate and not contraindicated.
7. Apply the bandage from the distal to the proximal part.
8. Apply bandage with even distribution of pressure.
9. Use proper bandage turns:
   a. Circular
      (1) Apply bandage so that each round overlaps the previous turn.
      (2) Secure in place, if appropriate.
   b. Spiral
      (1) Make two circular turns.
      (2) Continue so that each round of bandage slightly overlaps the previous round by about two thirds, progressing up the limb.
      (3) End with two circular turns, and secure with pins, tape, or clips.
   c. Spiral-reverse
      (1) Make two circular turns.
      (2) Bring bandage upward at 30-degree angle.
      (3) Place thumb of free hand on upper edge of bandage.
      (4) Fold bandage back on itself.
      (5) Continue to bandage limb, overlapping the previous turn by two thirds the width of bandage.
      (6) Perform reversal of bandage at same spot on each turn.
      (7) End with two circular turns, and secure with safety pins, tape, or clips.
   d. Recurrent
      (1) Make two circular turns with bandage.
      (2) Fold bandage back on itself, and bring it centrally over distal end to be bandaged.
      (3) Holding it with other hand, bring bandage back over the distal end to the right of center bandage.
      (4) Pass bandage from front to back and right to left, overlapping until entire area is covered.
      (5) Make two circular turns over initial turns.
   e. Figure-eight
      (1) Make two circular turns.
      (2) Carry bandage above joint and around it, then below joint and around it.
      (3) Continue above and below joint, overlapping previous turn by about two thirds the width of bandage.
      (4) End bandage above joint, making two circular turns.
10. Assess tension of bandage and circulation of extremity.
11. Position patient for comfort.
12. Document procedure.

Sample charting

DATE	TIME	NOTES
1/5/95	8:30	Elastic spiral bandage applied to right lower leg. Toes warm to touch, pink and nails blanch well. Pedal pulse strong and regular. Tolerated procedure well.

____

(nurse's signature)

SPECIAL CONCERNS

- Children will require smaller bandages.
- Older persons must be reassessed more often because circulatory complications occur more frequently.

PATIENT TEACHING

- Patient will need to be instructed on functions of bandaging.
- Patient should be taught to elevate extremity or body part if signs of impaired circulation occur (e.g., edema, decreased capillary refill).
- If bandage is applied over sterile dressing, patient must be taught procedure for changing dressing also.
- Patient and family will need to be taught the technique for applying the bandage.
- Teach family how to care for bandage.
- Patient and family will need to be taught to report changes in the affected part to the physician. Signs and symptoms of complications will need to be identified for the family.

SKILL 22-6

APPLYING A BINDER

Nursing action

1. Provide privacy for patient.
2. Assist patient to comfortable position.
3. Wash hands and don gloves.
4. Change dressing if appropriate; cleanse skin if needed.
5. Separate skin surfaces, or pad bony prominences.
6. Apply binder:
   a. Triangular binder (sling) (see Skill 51-2)
      (1) Have patient flex arm at approximately 80-degree angle, depending on purpose of binder.
      (2) Place end of triangular binder over shoulder of injured side (anterior to posterior)
      (3) Grasp other end of binder, and bring it up and over injured arm to shoulder of injured arm.
      (4) Use square knot to tie two ends together at lateral area of neck on injured side.
      (5) Support wrist well with binder; do not allow it to extend over end of binder.
      (6) Fold third triangle end neatly around elbow, and secure with safety pins.
   b. T-binder (see illustration)
      (1) Provide privacy
      (2) Don gloves.
      (3) Using appropriate binder, place the waistband smoothly under patient's waist; tails should be under patient.
      (4) Secure two ends of waistband together with safety pin.
      (5) Single tail—bring the tail up between legs to secure dressing in place. Two-rail—bring tails up one on each side of penis or large dressing.
      (6) Bring tails under and over waistband, and secure with safety pins.
   c. Elastic abdominal binder
      (1) Center binder smoothly under appropriate part of patient.
      (2) Bring ends around patient and overlap away from incision
      (3) Secure binder with Velcro or safety pins placed horizontally on abdomen.
7. Note comfort level of patients. Smooth binder to prevent wrinkles.
8. Remove gloves.
9. Document procedure.

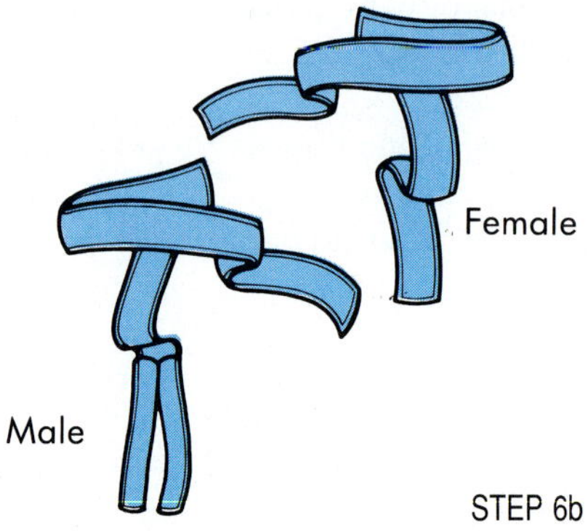

STEP 6b

Sample charting

DATE	TIME	NOTES
12/5/95	8:45	Incisional dressing dry and intact. Abdominal binder applied as ordered. Patient states, "I feel much better about getting out of bed now."

____
(nurse's signature)

SPECIAL CONCERNS

- Patients with tubes or drains who have binders applied will need to be assessed frequently to ensure patency of tubes and drainage.

PATIENT TEACHING

- Teach function of the binder to patient and family.
- Teach patient to report if binder is loose or causing pain or discomfort.
- Patient should report any breathing restrictions if binder is too tight.
- Patient will need to be taught proper application if binder will need to be applied at home.
- Patient will need to know proper care of the binder.

Incision coverings may be gauze, semiocclusive, or occlusive dressings. Gauze dressings permit air to reach the wound; semiocclusive dressings permit oxygen, but not air to pass; occlusive dressings permit neither air nor oxygen to pass. Occlusive and semiocclusive dressings are thought to promote healing by keeping wounds moist (yet sterile) so epithelial cells can slide more easily over the surface of the wound during epithelialization. Dressings over closed wounds are usually removed by the third day. Some surgeons remove dressings the first postoperative day if there are no drains present.

If an occlusive dressing is used, the tape strips are placed on all sides of the dressing. Otherwise the tape strips are placed several inches apart to allow air and/or oxygen to pass over the wound.

The nurse may use tape, ties, or bandages and cloth binders to secure a dressing over a wound site. The choice of anchoring depends on the wound size, location, presence of drainage, frequency of dressing changes, and the patient's level of activity.

When the nurse removes dressings, care is taken to avoid accidental removal or displacement of underlying drains. Because removal of dressings can be painful, it may help to give an analgesic at least 30 minutes before exposing a wound.

The nurse notes whether wound edges are closed. A surgical incision should have clean, well-approximated edges. Crusts often form along the wound edges from exudate. A puncture wound is usually a small, circular wound with the edges coming together toward the center. If a wound is open, the wound edges are separated, and the nurse inspects the condition of underlying tissue such as adipose and connective tissue. The nurse also looks for complications such as dehiscence and evisceration. The outer edges of a wound normally appear inflamed for the first 2 to 3 days, but this slowly disappears. Within 7 to 10 days a normally healing wound fills with epithelial cells, and edges close. If infection develops, the wound edges become brightly erythematous and edematous.

If a closed wound is covered by a dressing, the dressing is observed but not changed until an order is issued. Should a dressing become saturated with exudate before the order is given, the dressing over the incisional area can be reinforced by placing sterile gauze on top of the original dressing and anchoring it securely. The nurse should record and report any dressing that is reinforced. The amount of exudate observed and dressings applied are charted.

After completing an assessment of the patient's wound, the nurse identifies nursing diagnoses that will direct supportive and preventive care. Existence of a wound clearly indicates a diagnosis: Skin integrity, impaired. This diagnosis directs the nurse to initiate interventions that promote the healing process.

The patient may be at risk for poor wound healing because of preexisting conditions that impair healing (see Table 22-8). Thus, even though the patient's wound may appear normal, the nurse identifies nursing diagnoses such as Nutrition, altered or Tissue perfusion, altered that direct nursing interventions toward support of wound repair.

The nature of a wound can cause problems unrelated to wound healing. Pain and impaired mobility are problems that have implications for the patient's eventual recovery. For example, a large abdominal incision can cause enough pain to interfere with the patient's ability to turn in bed effectively. The diagnostic process box lists nursing diagnoses related to problems of wound healing (Box 22-8).

There is a trend either to leave sutured, clean wounds not dressed after surgery or to use loose dressings. These methods allow atmospheric oxygen to circulate above the wound, aiding in the healing process. In many cases if a dressing has been used for closed wounds, it is removed within 24 hours postoperatively to allow air circulation. Within 24 hours enough fibrin has usually been produced at the wound site to stop the entry of microorganisms.

Box 22-8 NURSING DIAGNOSES RELATED TO WOUND HEALING

Breathing pattern, ineffective, related to:
- Pain secondary to abdominal incision

Infection, high risk for, related to:
- Malnutrition
- Tissue loss and increased environmental exposure

Mobility, impaired physical, related to:
- Pain of surgical wound

Nutrition, altered: less than body requirements, related to:
- Inability to ingest food

Pain, acute, related to:
- Abdominal incision

Self-esteem disturbance, related to:
- Perception of scars
- Perception of surgical drains
- Reaction to surgically removed body part

Skin integrity, impaired, related to:
- Surgical incision
- Pressure
- Chemical injury
- Secretions and excretions

Skin integrity, impaired, high risk for, related to:
- Physical immobilization
- Exposure to secretions

SKILL 22-7

APPLYING A WET-TO-DRY DRESSING

Nursing action

1. Identify patient.
2. Wash hands.
3. Provide for patient privacy.
4. Explain procedure to patient.
5. Position patient.
6. Place waterproof pad appropriately.
7. Place refuse container appropriately.
8. Set up sterile field:
   a. Open barrier drape.
   b. Add sterile dressing and gauze.
   c. Add sterile basin.
   d. Pour sterile solution into basin.
   e. Ad sterile instrument set if needed.
   f. Add antiseptic swabs.
9. Loosen tapes by pulling toward incision and gently pulling skin away from tape.
10. Don clean gloves, and remove dressing and discard into refuse bag. (Refuse bag may be used for additional soiled material.)
11. Assess status of the wound.
12. Don sterile gloves.
13. Cleanse wound from incision outward, one stroke per swab, and discard.
14. Place gauze into basin.
15. Wring excess solution from dressing.
16. Place sterile (4 inch × 4 inch) gauze over open wound surfaces and press into any depressed areas.
17. Apply dry, sterile dressing (4 inch × 4 inch) over wet gauze.
18. Cover with additional dressing as needed, usually 8 inch × 10 inch abdominal dressing.
19. Secure with tape or Montgomery straps.
20. Remove gloves, and discard (see illustrations).
21. Reposition patient.
22. Discard refuse appropriately.
23. Wash hands.
24. Document status of wound, description of exudate, dressing, and solution applied, and patient response.

Sample charting

DATE	TIME	NOTES
1/5/95	11:00	Wet-to-dry dressing on left lower quadrant of abdomen removed, 2 × 3 cm of serosanguineous exudate noted on dressing. Skin around wound is pink and intact. Wet-to-dry dressing applied using ¼ strength H_2O_2 solution and normal saline. Covered with 4 × 4s and ABD pads. Patient states, "The pill before this dressing change really helped."

____
(nurse's signature)

SPECIAL CONCERNS

- Appropriately assess all wounds.
- Infected wounds cause longer hospitalization for the patient, resulting in higher cost and longer recovery time.
- It is vitally important that the nurse continually carry out appropriate technique in all patient care.

PATIENT TEACHING

- Teach the patient about healing by secondary intention.

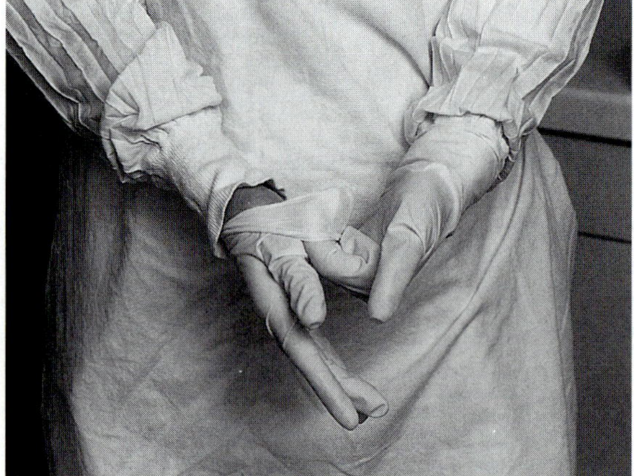

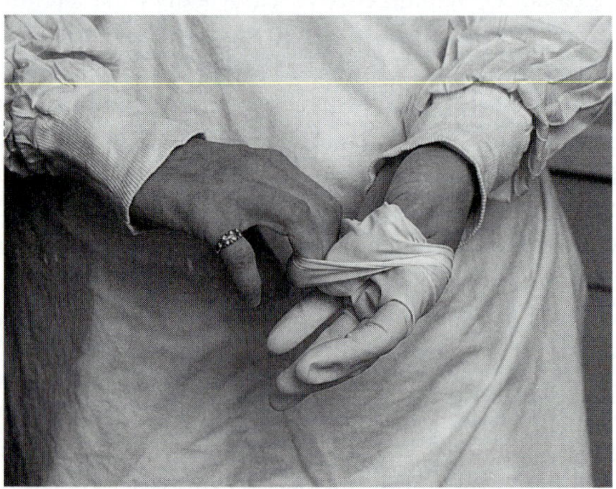

STEP 20

An open wound, while generally covered by a dressing, has packing or dressings within the cavity. Open wounds occur when an infection is present and the surgeon wants to promote drainage. As granulation takes place and the infection is treated, healing by second or tertiary intention results. Open wounds frequently leave large, uneven scars.

Sterile technique is followed whenever the wound or dressing is handled (Skill 22-7, Skill 22-8 on p. 472, and Skill 22-9 on p. 474). Sterile asepsis not only protectsthe nurse against wound drainage, but also decreases the introduction of **pathogenic** (any microorganism capable of producing disease) organisms into the wound. Using sterile **asepsis** (absence of germs) lessens the chance of the patient's acquiring a nosocomial (hospital-acquired) infection. Universal precautions should be employed when handling body secretions. Good handwashing technique and the use of sterile aseptic procedures are essential when providing surgical wound care. A gown, mask, and protective goggles are worn if soiling or splashing of wound exudate is expected.

Bandages and Binders. Bandages are available in rolls of various widths and materials, including gauze, elasticized knit, elastic webbing, flannel, and muslin. Gauze bandages are lightweight and inexpensive, mold easily around contours of the body, and permit air circulation to prevent skin maceration (the softening and breaking down of skin from prolonged exposure to moisture). Elastic bandages conform well to body parts but can also be used to exert pressure over a body part. Flannel and muslin bandages are thicker than gauze and thus stronger for supporting or applying pressure. A flannel bandage also insulates to provide warmth.

Binders are bandages that are made of large pieces of material to fit a specific body part, for example, an abdominal binder or a breast binder. Most binders are made of elastic, cotton, muslin, or flannel.

Correctly applied bandages and binders do not cause injury to underlying and nearby body parts or create discomfort for the patient (see Skills 22-5 and 22-6). For example, a chest binder must not be so tight as to restrict chest wall expansion. Before a bandage or binder is applied, the nurse's responsibilities include:

1. Inspecting the skin for abrasions, edema, discoloration, or exposed wound edges
2. Covering exposed wounds or open abrasions with a sterile dressing
3. Assessing the condition of underlying dressings and changing them if soiled
4. Assessing the skin of underlying body parts and parts that will be distal to the bandage for signs of circulatory impairment (coolness, pallor or cyanosis, diminished or absent pulses, numbness, and tingling) to provide a means for comparing changes in circulation after bandage application

Box 22-9 GUIDELINES FOR APPLYING BANDAGES AND BINDERS

1. Position body part to be bandaged in comfortable position of normal anatomical alignment. Bandages cause restriction in movement. Immobilization in normal functioning position reduces risks of deformity or injury.
2. Prevent friction between and against skin surfaces by applying gauze or cotton padding. Skin surfaces in contact with each other (e.g., between toes, under breasts) can rub against each other to cause abrasion or chafing. Bandages over body prominences may rub against skin to cause impairment of skin integrity.
3. Apply bandages securely to prevent slippage during movement. Friction between bandage and skin can cause skin impairment.
4. When bandaging extremities, apply bandage first at the distal end and progress toward the trunk (heart). Gradual application of pressure from the distal toward the proximal portion of the extremity promotes venous return and minimizes the risk of edema or circulatory impairment.
5. Apply bandages firmly with equal tension exerted over each turn or layer. Avoid excess overlapping of bandage layers. Proper application prevents unequal pressure distribution over bandaged body part. Localized pressure causes circulatory impairment.
6. Position pins, knots, or ties away from wound or sensitive skin areas. These materials can exert localized pressure and irritation.

Box 22-9 outlines the principles of bandage and binder application. After a bandage is applied, the nurse assesses, documents, and immediately reports changes in circulation, skin integrity, comfort level, and body function, such as ventilation or movement. The nurse who applies a bandage can loosen or readjust it as necessary. The nurse should have a physician's order before loosening or removing a bandage applied by a physician. The nurse explains to the patient that any bandage or binder feels relatively firm or tight. A bandage should be carefully assessed to be sure that it is properly applied and is providing therapeutic benefit, and soiled bandages should be replaced. Like a damp dressing, a bandage or binder can harbor microorganisms.

Wound Complications. Impaired wound healing, regardless of the cause, requires accurate observation and ongoing interventions. Because wound complications can be life threatening, recognizing the seriousness of signs and symptoms is vital throughout the patient's re-

SKILL 22-8

CHANGING A STERILE DRESSING

Nursing action

1. Identify patient.
2. Wash hands.
3. Provide for patient privacy.
4. Explain procedure to patient.
5. Position patient.
6. Place refuse container in convenient location away from sterile field.
7. Set up sterile field.
   a. Open sterile dressings.
   b. Use barrier drape if needed.
   c. Open sterile gloves.
   d. Dressing set if needed.
   e. Antiseptic swabs.
8. Loosen tapes by pulling toward incision and gently pulling skin away from tape.
9. Don clean gloves, and remove dressing; note color and amount of exudate and discard soiled dressing. (Refuse bag may be used for additional soiled material.)
10. Assess status of wound.
11. Don sterile gloves.
12. Cleanse wound and surrounding area with antiseptic swab, starting from incision outward, one stroke per swab (see illustrations).
13. Use sterile gauze to swab in same manner or let antiseptic air dry.
14. Cleanse drain site if applicable (see illustration).
15. Apply special-order ointment, antibiotic, debridement granules, etc., if applicable.
16. Cover wound with appropriately sized dry sterile dressing and use drain dressing, if applicable
17. Secure dressing with tape, Montgomery straps (see illustration), or binder.
18. Remove gloves appropriately.
19. Discard refuse in appropriate manner.
20. Reposition patient.
21. Wash hands.
22. Document status of wound, description of drainage, if any, dressings applied, and patient response to procedure.

Sample charting

DATE	TIME	NOTES
1/5/95	10:00	Abdominal dressing removed, 3 × 4 cm of dry, sanguineous exudate noted on dressing. Sutures remain intact with wound edges well approximated. Cleansed with hydrogen peroxide. Sterile dressing applied. Patient stated, "I have less pain in my incision today."

____
(nurse's signature)

SPECIAL CONCERNS

- Include specific interventions or techniques of dressing changes in nursing care plan to provide continuity.
- Skin surrounding wound should be protected from drainage to prevent tissue breakdown.
- Consider use of Montgomery straps when dressing requires frequent changing to prevent tape irritation of skin.
- Assess need for and provide patient teaching during dressing change.

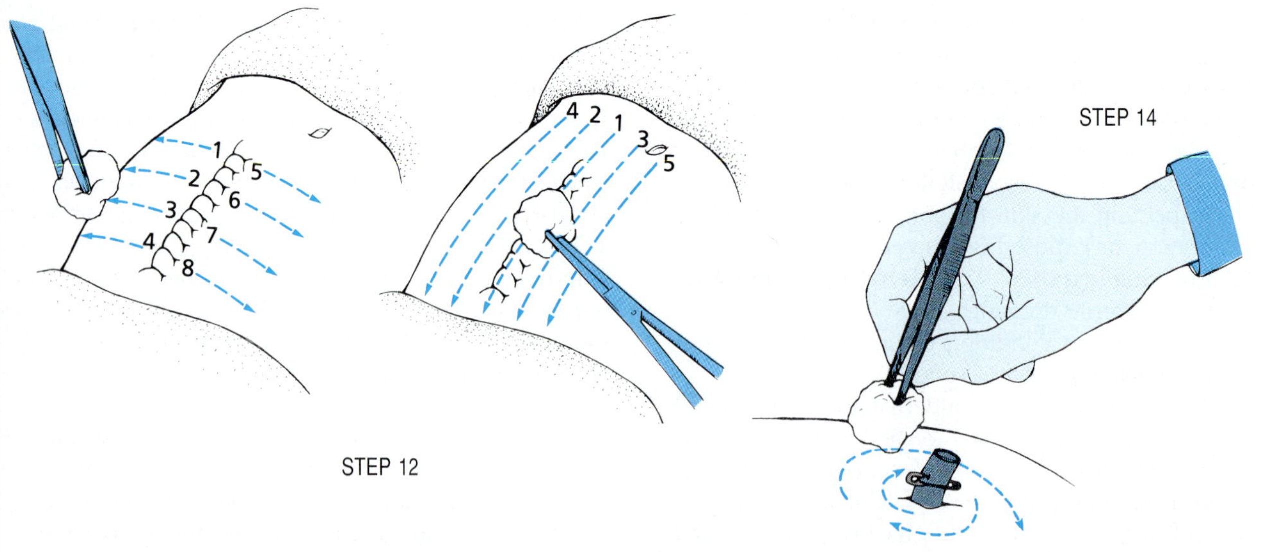

STEP 12

CHANGING A STERILE DRESSING—cont'd

SKILL 22-8

PATIENT TEACHING

When changing a dressing, the patient should be instructed on the following:

- Assist patient to accept the surgical wound by stating the progress of the wound and how healing is occurring.
- Teach the patient the importance of early ambulation after surgery.
- Teach the patient the importance of a nutritious diet in wound healing.
- Explain to patient that dressings may be required at home and how to purchase what will be needed. Inform patient of home health services if dressings need to be changed when patient is discharged per physician's order.

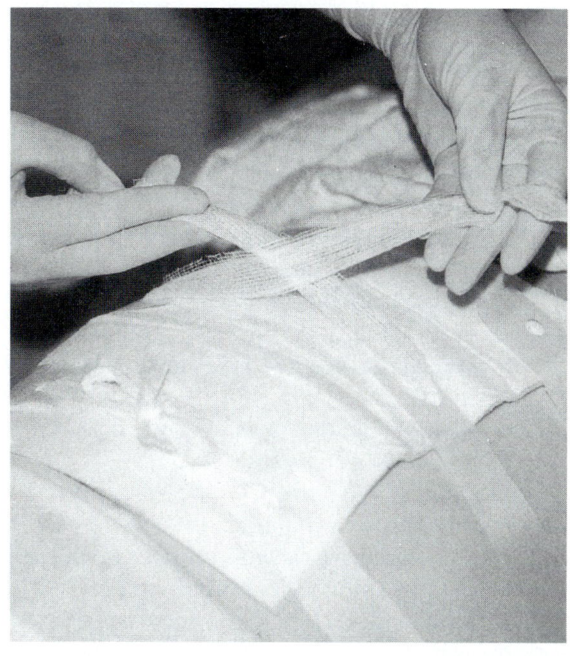

STEP 17

covery phase (Table 22-9). Additional costs of medical treatment and hospitalization for patients with wound complications increase the total cost of health care. Complications frequently result with patients who are aged, malnourished, or obese or who have infections or coexisting health conditions.

Wound bleeding may indicate a slipped suture, dislodged clot, coagulation problem, or trauma placed on blood vessels or tissue. Inspection of the wound and dressing aids in detecting increased drainage and color changes. If hemorrhage results internally, the dressing may remain dry while the abdominal cavity collects blood. The patient with increased thirst, restlessness, rapid, thready pulse, decreased blood pressure, decreased urinary output, and cool, clammy skin may be hemorrhaging. Thus monitoring vital signs, I&O, skin condition, wound site, and overall patient responses hastens the identification of hemorrhage and hypovolemic shock. Internal abdominal bleeding, if allowed to continue, causes the abdomen to become rigid and distended. If hemorrhage is not detected and stopped, hypovolemic shock can cause the circulatory system to collapse, causing death.

When wound layers separate, the patient may say that something has given way. This feeling may result after periods of sneezing, coughing, or vomiting. Evidence of serosanguineous drainage on the dressing is an important sign to assess. Dehiscence may be preceded by serosanguineous drainage. If the wound is not covered and dehiscence occurs, the patient should remain in bed and be kept NPO, told not to cough, and be reassured, and the nurse should place a sterile dressing over the area until the physician evaluates the site. When a skin su-

TABLE 22-9 Terms Associated with Wound Complications

Term	Definition
Abscess	Cavity containing pus and surrounded by inflamed tissue, formed as a result of suppuration in a localized infection
Adhesion	Band of scar tissue that binds together two anatomical surfaces normally separated; most commonly found in the abdomen
Cellulitis	Infection of the skin characterized by heat, pain, erythema, and edema
Dehiscence	Separation of a surgical incision, or rupture of a wound closure
Eviseration	Protrusion of an internal organ through a wound or surgical incision
Extravasation	Passage or escape into the tissues; usually of blood, serum, or lymph
Hematoma	Collection of extravasated blood trapped in the tissues or in an organ resulting from incomplete hemostasis after surgery

SKILL 22-9

STERILE IRRIGATION OF A WOUND

Nursing action

1. Identify patient.
2. Wash hands.
3. Provide for patient privacy.
4. Explain procedure to patient.
5. Position patient and waterproof pad appropriately.
6. Place refuse container in convenient location away from sterile field.
7. Set up sterile field:
   a. Sterile basin.
   b. Add sterile, warmed irrigation solution to basin.
   c. Open sterile dressings.
   d. Add antiseptic swabs.
   e. Open sterile gloves.
   f. Dressing set (optional).
   g. Add sterile syringe and catheter if necessary.
8. Don gown and goggles if appropriate.
9. Don clean gloves, and remove dressing; assess dressing for color and amount of exudate, and discard dressing.
10. Assess status of the wound.
11. Place collection basin appropriately.
12. Don sterile gloves.
13. Cleanse area around wound with antiseptic agent.
14. Fill irrigating syringe with solution; attach soft catheter if irrigating a deep wound with small opening.
15. Instill solution gently into wound, holding syringe approximately 1 inch (2.5 cm) above wound (see illustration). (If using catheter, gently insert into wound opening until slight resistance is met, pull back, and gently instill solution.)
    a. Solution must flow from clean area of wound to contaminated area.
    b. Pinch off catheter during withdrawal from wound.
16. Refill syringe, and continue irrigation as above until solution returns clear or prescribed amount is used.
17. Blot wound edges with sterile gauze.
18. Redress wound, if applicable, following sterile dressing change procedure.
19. Remove gloves.
20. Discard soiled material and contaminated solution appropriately.
21. Reposition patient.
22. Wash hands.
23. Document status of wound, description of exudate, type and amount of irrigating solution, equipment used, results of irrigation, dressings used, and patient response.

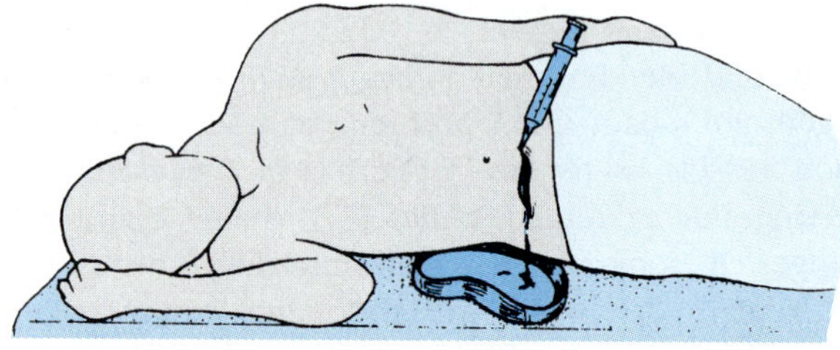

STEP 15

Sample charting

DATE	TIME	NOTES
12/6/94	12:00	Right buttock dressing removed; purulent drainage 2 cm in diameter noted. Wound remains 4 cm × 1 cm, approximately 2 cm deep. No erythema noted at wound edge. Wound irrigation with Asepto syringe using 250 ml of half-strength hydrogen peroxide solution and normal saline. Return solution clear. Temp 99.8, P 86, R 22, B/P 108/74. Patient states, "There is less pain."

(nurse's signature)

SPECIAL CONCERNS

- Patient comfort should be provided, since an irrigation can cause pain. Patient may need to be medicated before performing procedure.
- Gentleness is important in performing any type of irrigation to avoid tissue damage and pain.

PATIENT TEACHING

When performing sterile irrigation of a wound, the patient should be instructed on the following:

- Explain why wound is being allowed to heal by secondary intention.

ture breaks and dehiscence occurs, Steri-Strips or a butterfly strip may close the wound effectively. Dehiscence most frequently occurs between the fifth and twelfth postoperative day. Because most patients have been dismissed from the hospital by day twelve, patient teaching should include identification of dehiscence and the care to provide.

If an evisceration follows the dehiscence (Fig. 22-3), the patient is to remain in bed, and the wound and contents should be covered with warm, sterile saline dressings. The surgeon is notified immediately. This is a medical emergency, and the wound requires surgical repair.

Wound infection, or wound sepsis, results when the surgical wound becomes contaminated. The Centers for Disease Control and Prevention labels a wound infected when it contains purulent (pus) drainage. A surgical wound infection may develop by the fourth or fifth postoperative day, whereas a contaminated wound may show an infectious process in 2 or 3 days. A patient with an infected wound displays a fever, tenderness and pain at the wound, edema, and an elevated WBC. Purulent drainage has an odor and is brown, yellow, or green, depending on the pathogen.

A *Staphylococcus aureus* infection is the most common type of wound infection. Its incubation period is from 4 to 6 days. *Staphylococcus aureus* tends to have yellow drainage and is localized. When infection is localized, an abscess forms. In addition to experiencing the classic signs and symptoms of an infection, the patient reports a localized, throbbing pain. Treatment consists of antibiotic therapy, surgical opening (incision and drainage) of the wound, rest, heat, and elevation of the affected part. Drainage and secretion isolation usually is initiated if *S. aureus* is the causative organism.

Pathogens that live in the presence of oxygen (gram-negative bacilli) are present everywhere in the environment. The more common gram-negative bacilli are *Escherichia coli, Enterobacter, Proteus,* and *Pseudomonas aeruginosa.* Gram-negative bacilli have incubation periods of 7 to 14 days. Adequate drainage of the wound and antibiotic therapy are the primary treatments.

Streptococcal infections materialize with local tissue breakdown, gangrene, or necrotizing fasciitis. This infection produces a thin, watery pus. Signs and symptoms associated with streptococci include elevated temperature and pulse, perspiration, exhaustion, and chills. Cellulitis is an example of a streptococcal infection. Treatment consists of an antibiotic (penicillin is the medication of choice), wet compresses, rest, and elevation of the infected area.

Gas gangrene and clostridial wound infections usually occur with extensive muscle damage. Amputation of a gangrenous limb may result because of necrosis accompanied by gas bubbles in the soft tissue; this condition (gas gangrene) is caused by the exotoxins of the pathogen. Cellulitis and tetanus may also result from these pathogens. In infections, exudate cultures confirm the presence of the pathogenic organism, so that the appropriate medical therapy can follow.

Sterile Technique

Surgical asepsis or sterile technique requires a nurse to use different precautions from those of medical asepsis. Surgical asepsis requires the absence of all microorganisms, including pathogens and spores from an object. The nurse working with a sterile field or with sterile equipment must understand that the slightest break in technique results in contamination. The nurse practices surgical asepsis (for example, filling a syringe or changing a dressing on a wound) to keep microorganisms away from an area.

Although surgical asepsis is practiced in the operating room, labor and delivery area, and major diagnostic areas, the nurse may also use surgical aseptic techniques at the patient's bedside. This would include, for example, inserting IVs or urinary catheters, suctioning the tracheobronchial airway, and reapplying sterile dressings. A nurse in an operating room follows a series of steps to maintain sterile techniques, including applying a mask, protective eyewear, and a cap; performing a surgical handwashing; and applying a sterile gown and gloves. In contrast, a nurse changing a dressing at a patient's bedside may only perform a handwashing and apply sterile gloves.

Because surgical asepsis requires exact techniques, the nurse must have the patient's cooperation. Therefore, the nurse must prepare the patient before any procedure. Certain patients fear moving or touching objects during a sterile procedure, whereas others may even try to assist. The nurse explains how a procedure is to be performed and what the patient can do to avoid contaminating sterile items, including the following:

1. Avoiding sudden movements of body parts covered by sterile drapes
2. Refraining from touching sterile supplies, drapes, or the nurse's gloves and gown
3. Avoiding coughing, sneezing, or talking over a sterile area

Principles of Sterile Technique. When beginning a surgically aseptic procedure, the nurse follows certain principles to ensure maintenance of asepsis. Failure to follow each principle conscientiously endangers patients, placing them at risk for infection. The following principles are important:

1. A sterile object remains sterile only when touched by another sterile object. (This principle guides the nurse in placement of sterile objects and how to handle them.)
   a. Sterile touching sterile remains sterile; for example, sterile gloves are worn or sterile for-

ceps are used to handle objects on a sterile field.

b. Sterile touching clean becomes contaminated; for example, if the tip of a syringe or other sterile object touches the surface of a clean disposable glove, the object is contaminated.
c. Sterile touching contaminated becomes contaminated; for example, when the nurse touches a sterile object with an ungloved hand, the object is contaminated.
d. Sterile touching questionable is contaminated; for example, when a tear or break in the covering of a sterile object is found, it is discarded regardless of whether the object itself appears untouched.

2. Only sterile objects may be placed on a sterile field. All items are properly sterilized before use. The package or container holding a sterile object must be intact and dry. A package that is torn, punctured, wet, or open is unsterile.
3. A sterile object or field out of the range of vision or an object held below a person's waist is contaminated. Nurses never turn their backs on a sterile tray or leave it unattended. Contamination can occur accidentally by a dangling piece of clothing, falling hair, or an unknowing patient touching a sterile object. Any object held below waist level is considered contaminated because it cannot be viewed at all times. Sterile objects should be kept in front of the person with the hands as close together as possible.
4. A sterile object or field becomes contaminated by prolonged exposure to air. The nurse avoids activities that may create air currents, such as excessive movements or rearranging linen after a sterile object or field becomes exposed. When sterile packages are being opened, it is important to minimize the number of people walking into the area. Microorganisms also travel by droplet through the air. No one should talk, laugh, sneeze, or cough over a sterile field or when gathering and using sterile equipment. A nurse with a cold or other respiratory ailment should never perform sterile procedures unless a double mask is worn. Microorganisms traveling through the air can fall on sterile items or fields if the nurse reaches over the work area. When opening sterile packages, the nurse holds the item or piece of equipment as close as possible to the sterile field without touching the sterile surface. Minimal movement or rearranging of sterile items also reduces contamination by air transmission.
5. When a sterile surface comes in contact with a wet, contaminated surface, the sterile object or field becomes contaminated. If moisture seeps through a sterile package's protective covering, microorganisms travel to the sterile object. When stored sterile packages become wet, the nurse discards the objects immediately or sends the equipment for resterilization. When working with a sterile field or tray, the nurse may have to pour sterile solutions. Any spill can be a source of contamination unless the object or field rests on a sterile surface that cannot be penetrated by moisture. Urinary catheterization trays contain sterile supplies that rest in a sterile, plastic container. In this example, sterile solutions spilled within the container will not contaminate the catheter or other objects. In contrast, if a nurse places a piece of sterile gauze in its wrapper on a patient's bedside table and the table surface is wet, the gauze is considered contaminated.
6. Fluid flows in the direction of gravity. A sterile object becomes contaminated if gravity causes a contaminated liquid to flow over the object's surface. To avoid contamination during a surgical hand scrub, the nurse holds the hands above the elbows. This allows water to flow downward without contaminating the nurse's hands and fingers. The principle of water flow by gravity is also the reason for drying from fingers to elbows, with hands held up, after the scrub.
7. The edges of a sterile field or container are considered to be contaminated. Frequently, a nurse places sterile objects on a sterile towel or drape. Because the edge of the drape touches an unsterile surface, such as a table or bed linen, a 2.5-cm (1-inch) border around the drape is considered contaminated. The edges of sterile containers become exposed to air after they are open and are thus contaminated. After a sterile needle is removed from its protective cap or after a forcep is removed from a container, the objects must not touch the container's edge. The lip of an opened bottle of solution also becomes contaminated after it is exposed to air. When pouring a sterile liquid, the nurse first pours a small amount of solution and discards it. The solution thus washes away microorganisms on the bottle lip. Then the nurse pours a second time on the same side to fill a container with the desired amount of solution.

The nurse will assemble all the equipment necessary for a sterile procedure before the procedure has begun. In doing so the nurse avoids having to leave a sterile area unattended because some equipment is missing. A few extra supplies should be available in case objects accidentally become contaminated. If an object becomes contaminated during the procedure, the nurse should discard it immediately.

Opening Sterile Packages. Sterile items such as syringes, gauze dressings, and catheters are packaged in paper or plastic containers that are impervious to microorganisms as long as they are dry and intact. Some institutions wrap reusable supplies in a double thickness of linen or muslin. Paper packages are permeable to steam and thus allow for steam autoclaving. A disadvantage of paper wrappers is that they tear or puncture relatively easily. Sterile items are kept in clean, enclosed storage cabinets and are never in the same room as dirty equipment.

Sterile supplies have dated labels or chemical tapes that indicate the date when the sterilization expires. The tapes change color during the sterilization process. Failure of the tapes to change color means the item is not sterile. A sterile supply or piece of equipment should never be used after the expiration date. The item is either discarded or returned to the institution's supply area for resterilization.

Before opening a sterile item the nurse does a thorough handwashing. The nurse assembles the supplies at the work area, such as the bedside table or treatment room, before opening packages. A bedside table or countertop provides a large, clean working area for opening items. The work area should be above the nurse's waist level. Sterile supplies should not be opened in a confined space where a dirty object might fall on or strike them.

Sterile packaged items can be opened without contaminating the contents. Commercially packaged items are usually designed so that the nurse only has to tear away or separate the paper or plastic cover. The item is held in one hand while the wrapper is pulled away with the other. Care is then taken to keep the inner contents sterile before use. When opening items packed in linen, the nurse uses the following steps:

1. Place the item flat in the center of the work surface.
2. Remove the tape or seal indicating the sterilization date.
3. Grasp the outer surface of the tip of the outermost flap.
4. Open the outer flap away from the body, keeping the arm outstretched and away from the sterile field.
5. Grasp the outside surface of the first side flap.
6. Open the side flap, allowing it to lie flat on the table surface. Keep the arm to the side and not over the sterile surface. Do not allow flaps to spring back over the sterile contents (Fig. 22-9 on p. 478).
7. Grasp the outside surface of the second side flap and allow it to lie flat on the table surface.
8. Grasp the outer surface of the last and innermost flap.
9. Stand away from the sterile package and pull the flap back, allowing it to fall flat on the surface.
10. Use the inner surface of the cover package (except for the 1-inch border around the edges) as a sterile field to add additional sterile items. The 1-inch border can be grasped to maneuver the field on the table surface.

To open small, sterile items, the package is held in the nondominant hand while the top flap is opened and pulled away from the nurse. Using the dominant hand the nurse carefully opens the sides and top flaps away from the enclosed sterile item in the same order previously mentioned. The nurse opens items in a hand so that the item can be handed to a person wearing sterile gloves or transferred to a sterile field (Fig. 22-10 on p. 478).

Preparing a Sterile Field. When performing sterile procedures, the nurse needs a sterile work area that provides room for handling and placing of sterile items. A sterile field is an area that is free of microorganisms and is prepared to receive sterile items. The field may be prepared by using the inner surface of a sterile wrapper as the work surface or by using a sterile drape (Skill 22-10 on p. 479).

The nurse may choose to wear sterile gloves while preparing items on the field. If so, the nurse can touch the entire drape, but sterile items must be handed over by an assistant. The nurse's gloves cannot touch the outside wrappers of sterile items.

Pouring Sterile Solutions. Often the nurse must pour sterile solutions into sterile containers. A bottle containing a sterile solution is sterile on the inside and contaminated on the outside; the bottle's neck is also contaminated, but the inside of the bottle cap is considered sterile. After a cap or lid is opened, it is held in the hand or placed sterile side (inside) up on a clean surface. This means that the inside of the lid can be seen as it rests on the table surface. A bottle cap or lid should never rest sterile side down on a sterile surface because the outer edge of the cap is unsterile and would contaminate the surface. Likewise, placing a sterile cap down on an unsterile surface increases the chances of the inside of the cap becoming contaminated.

The bottle should be held with its label in the palm of the hand to prevent the possibility of the solution wetting and fading the label. Before pouring the solution into the container, the nurse pours a small amount (1 to 2 ml) into a disposable cap or plastic-lined waste receptacle. The discarded solution cleans the lip of the bottle. The edge of the bottle is kept away from the edge or inside of the receiving container.

The nurse pours the solution slowly to avoid splashing the underlying drape or field. The bottle should

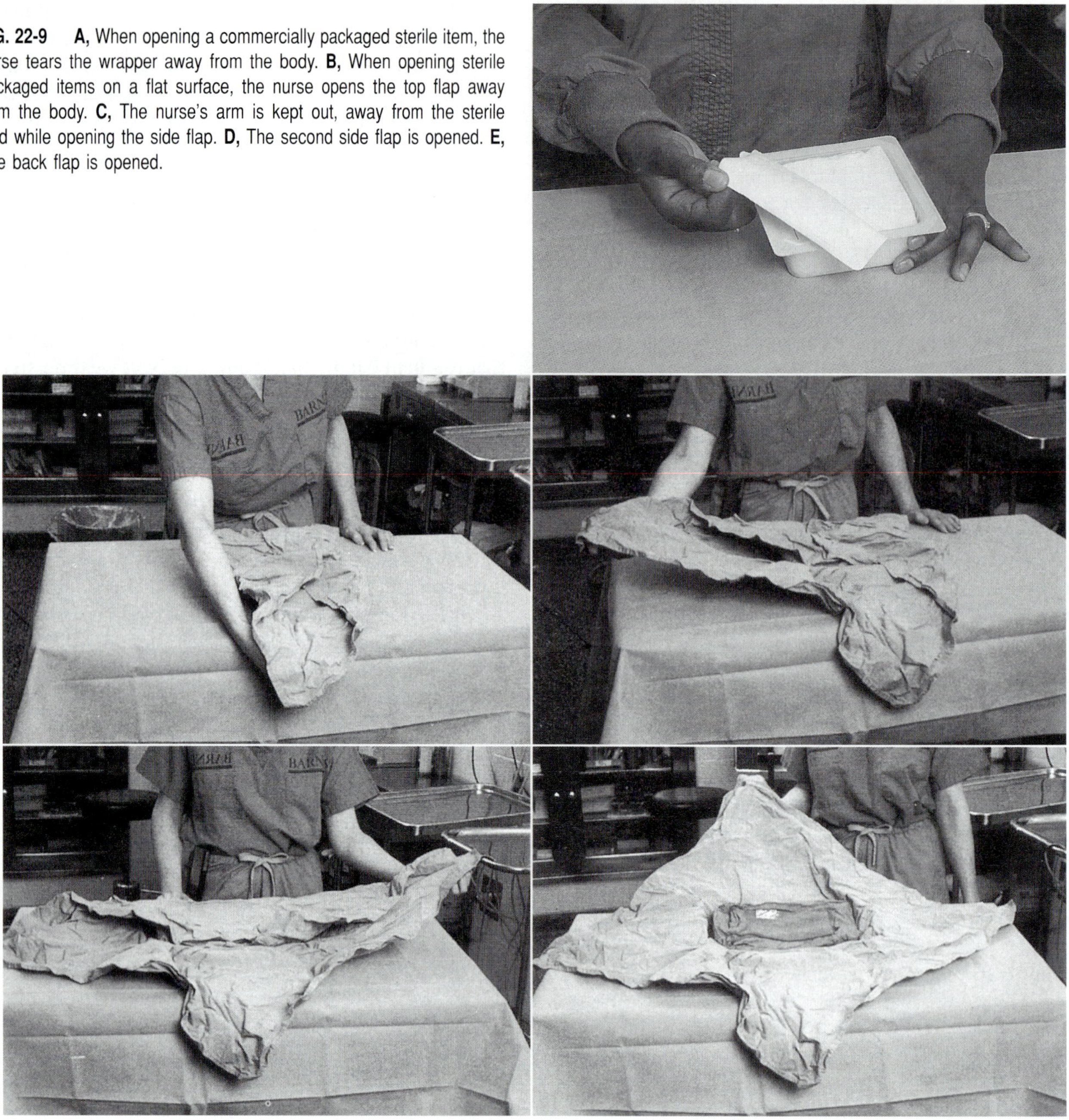

FIG. 22-9 **A,** When opening a commercially packaged sterile item, the nurse tears the wrapper away from the body. **B,** When opening sterile packaged items on a flat surface, the nurse opens the top flap away from the body. **C,** The nurse's arm is kept out, away from the sterile field while opening the side flap. **D,** The second side flap is opened. **E,** The back flap is opened.

A

B

C

D

E

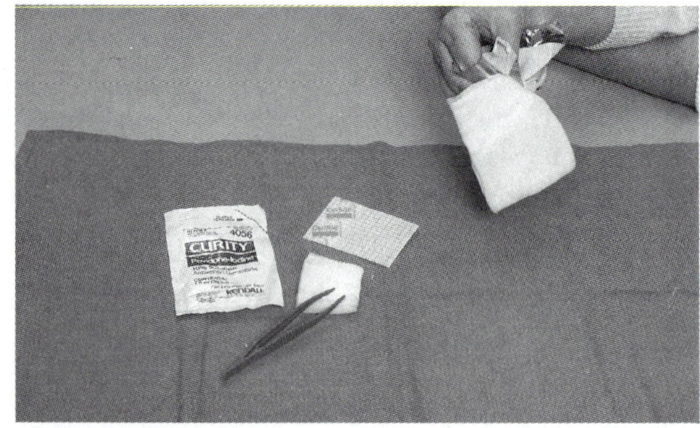

FIG. 22-10 Placing items on a sterile field.

SKILL 22-10

PREPARING A STERILE FIELD

Nursing action

1. Prepare sterile field just before planned procedure to prevent exposure of sterile field and supplies to air and contamination. Supplies are to be used immediately.
2. Select clean work surface above waist level as sterile objects held below waist are contaminated.
3. Assemble necessary equipment because preparation of equipment in advance prevents break in technique.
   a. Sterile drape
   b. Assorted sterile supplies
4. Check dates, labels, or condition of package for sterility of equipment because equipment stored beyond expiration date, or a package that is damaged, is considered unsterile.
5. Wash hands thoroughly to prevent transmission of microorganisms.
6. Place pack containing sterile drape on work surface and open as described on p. ••• to ensure sterility of packaged drape (see Fig. 22-10).
7. With fingertips of one hand, pick up folded top edge of sterile drape because the 1-inch border around drape is unsterile and may be touched.
8. Gently lift drape up from its outer cover and let it unfold by itself without touching any object. Discard outer cover with your other hand because if sterile object touches any other nonsterile object, it becomes contaminated.
9. With other hand, grasp adjacent corner of drape and hold it straight up and away from your body. Now drape can be properly placed while using two hands and the drape must be held away from unsterile surfaces.
10. Holding drape, first position the bottom half over intended work surface. This prevents the nurse from reaching over sterile field.
11. Allow top half of drape to be placed over work surface last because this creates a flat, sterile work surface.
12. Perform procedure using sterile technique to prevent wound contamination.

A 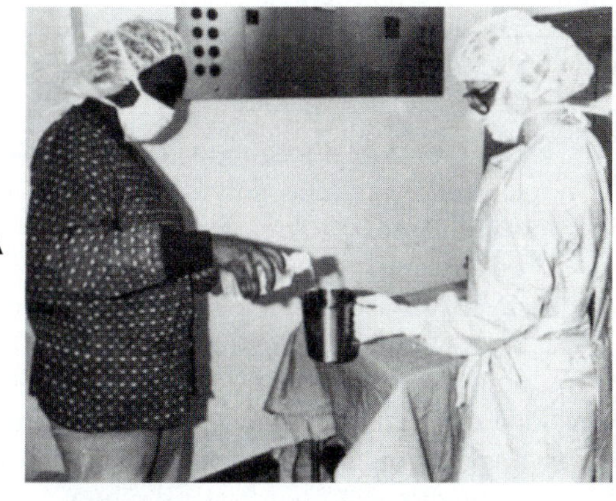

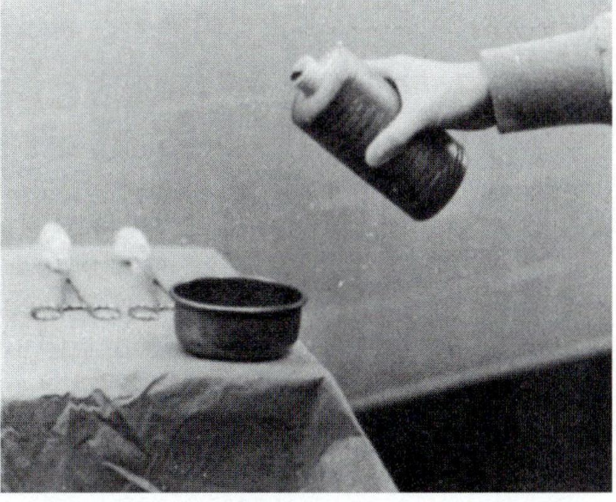 B

FIG. 22-11 **A,** Nurse stands well back from solution being poured into sterile receptacle to avoid contamination. **B,** Receptacle receiving fluid is placed near edge of sterile table to permit nurse to pour without reaching over sterile field.

SKILL 22-11

PERFORMING OPEN GLOVING

Nursing action

1. Have package of proper-sized sterile gloves at treatment area.
2. Perform thorough handwashing to remove bacteria from skin surfaces.
3. Remove outer glove package wrapper by carefully separating and peeling apart sides to prevent inner glove package from accidentally opening and touching contaminated objects.
4. Grasp inner package and lay it on clean, flat surface just above waist level. Open package, keeping gloves on wrapper's inside surface because inner surface of glove package is sterile. Sterile objects held below the waist are contaminated.
5. If gloves are not prepowdered, take packet of powder and apply lightly to hands over sink or wastebasket because powder allows gloves to slip on easily.
6. Identify right and left glove. Each glove has cuff approximately 5 cm (2 in) wide. Glove dominant hand first because gloving of dominant hand first improves dexterity. Proper identification of gloves prevents contamination by improper fit.
7. With thumb and first two fingers of nondominant hand, grasp edge of cuff of glove for dominant hand. Touch only glove's inside surface because the inner edge of cuff will lie against skin and thus is not sterile.
8. Carefully pull glove over dominant hand, leaving cuff and being sure cuff does not roll up wrist. Be sure thumb and fingers are in proper spaces. If glove's outer surface touches hand or wrist, it is contaminated.
9. With gloved dominant hand, slip fingers underneath second glove's cuff because the cuff will protect the gloved fingers. Sterile touching sterile prevents glove contamination.
10. Carefully pull second glove over nondominant hand. Do not allow fingers and thumb of gloved dominant hand to touch any part of exposed nondominant hand. Keep thumb of dominant hand abducted back because contact of gloved hand with exposed hand results in contamination.
11. After second glove is on, interlock hands together. The cuffs usually fall down after application. Be sure to touch only sterile sides so as to ensure smooth fit over fingers.

Glove disposal

12. Grasp outside of one cuff with other gloved hand; avoid touching wrist to minimize contamination of underlying skin.
13. Pull glove off, turning it inside out. Discard in receptacle so the outside of glove does not touch skin surface.
14. Take fingers of bare hand and tuck inside remaining glove cuff. Peel glove off, inside out. Discard in receptacle.

never be held so high above the container that even slow pouring will cause splashing. The bottle should be held outside the edge of the sterile field (Fig. 22-11 on p. 479).

Donning Sterile Gloves. Sterile gloves are an additional barrier to bacterial transfer. There are two gloving methods: open and closed. Nurses who work on general nursing divisions use open gloving before procedures such as dressing changes or urinary catheter insertions. The closed gloved method, which is performed when nurses wear sterile gowns, is practiced in operating rooms and special treatment areas.

The proper glove size should be selected; the glove should not stretch so tightly that it can easily tear; yet it should be tight enough that objects can be picked up easily (Skill 22-11).

Closed Gloving. Closed gloving is practiced when the nurse wears a sterile gown, such as in the operating rooms and special treatment areas. To perform the closed gloving procedure the hands are covered with gown sleeves as the nurse opens the inner sterile gloves package. With the nondominant hand inside gown cuff, pick up the glove for the dominant hand by grasping folded cuff. Extend dominant forearm with palm up and place palm of glove against palm of dominant hand. Glove fingers will point toward elbow.

Grasp back of glove cuff with nondominant hand and turn glove cuff over end of dominant hand and gown cuff (Fig. 22-12, *A*). Grasp top of glove and underlying gown sleeve with covered nondominant hand. Carefully extend fingers into glove, being sure glove's cuff covers gown's cuff. Glove nondominant hand in same manner, reversing hands (Fig. 22-12, *B*). Use gloved right hand to

A
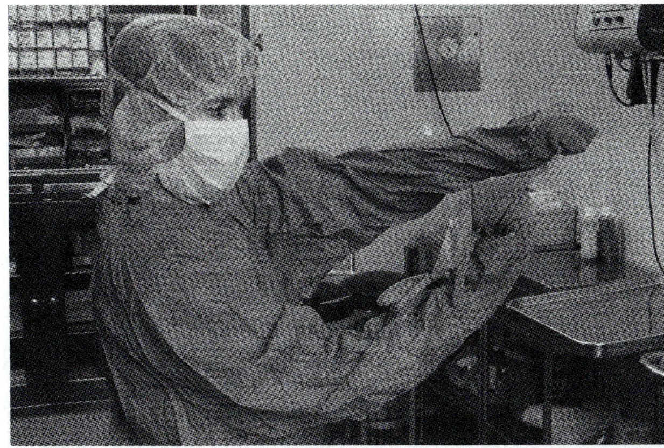

B
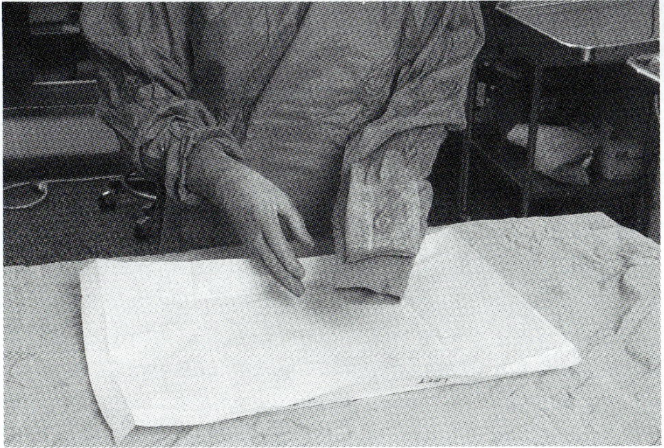

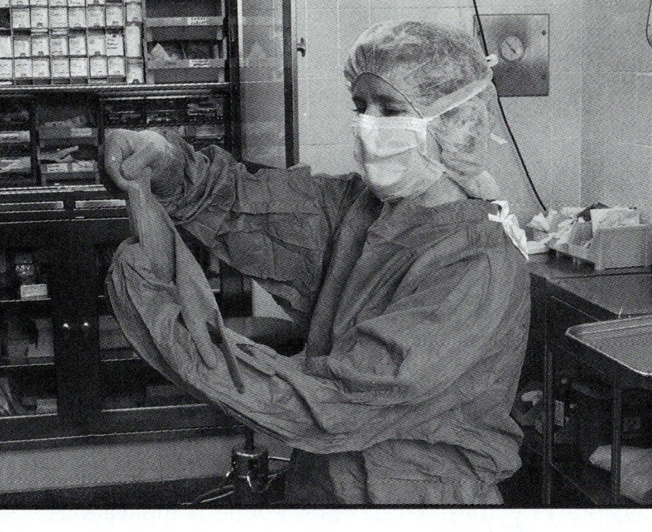
C

FIG. 22-12 **A,** Grasp back of glove cuff with nondominant hand. **B,** Glove dominant hand in same manner. **C,** Use glove right hand to pull on glove, keep hand inside sleeve.

pull on glove. Keep hand inside sleeve (Fig. 22-12, *C*).

By the use of this closed gloving procedure, the sterile barrier is maintained and contamination is avoided. The nurse is now ready to assist with sterile materials and instruments, such as are used during surgery or treatments such as wound debridement.

Drainage Systems

During surgery, tissue may be injured in a variety of ways. Not only is the diseased organ repaired or removed, but blood vessels are also cut and sutured. In addition, organs and vessels are retracted out of the surgeon's operative field during the surgical procedure. Because vessels are fragile, bruising and injury may occur. As cells are injured, inflammation begins.

Inflammation is the protective response of the patient's tissue to irritation or injury. Although this process may be chronic or acute, during surgery acute inflammation occurs. Inflammation begins as soon as the cell is traumatized by handling or by cutting. As inflammation occurs, large amounts of histamine, bradykinin, and serotonin are released, and vascular permeability takes place.

Gradually fluid from the cells clusters with leukocytes along the vessel walls, so that fibrin walls off the injury and begins to build a new cell. The amount of inflammation depends on the level of injury inflicted, size of the area involved, and physical condition of the patient. With repair, leukocytes attempt to rid the tissue of exudate from the injured cells. This process, phagocytosis, is an important function of leukocytes. **Phagocytosis** (a process by which certain cells engulf and dispose of microorganisms and cell debris) occurs when exudate from the injured cell is surrounded, engulfed, and digested by leukocytes. The leukocyte becomes the body's vacuum cleaner by removing its debris. Evidence of leukocyte action can be observed through WBC changes.

Cardinal Signs of Inflammation. Tissue involved in the inflammation process responds by becoming erythematous, hot, edematous, and painful. As the injured cell's fluid presses against surrounding tissue, there is frequently a loss of function in that area. Function generally returns when inflammation subsides. The inflammatory process normally occurs within the first 1 to 4 days after surgery. This process is the first phase in wound healing.

Drainage. Drainage is described as serous, sanguineous, or serosanguineous. **Serous** drainage is a clear, watery fluid that has been separated from its solid elements (e.g., the exudate from a blister). Serous fluid has the characteristics of serum. Serum is the clear, thin, sticky fluid portion of blood that remains after coagulation. In contrast, sanguineous drainage is fluid that contains blood. Thus serosanguineous drainage is exudate that is thin and red (usually described as pink), because it is composed of both serum and blood. If the tissue is infected, drainage may be purulent or a brown-green color. Drainage from organs has its own particular color, i.e., bile from the liver and gallbladder is green or green-brown.

The type and amount of drainage produced depend on the tissue and organs involved. Normally drainage begins as sanguineous and progresses to serosanguineous. Drainage greater than 300 ml in the first 24 hours should be treated as abnormal. By the second or third postoperative day, drainage becomes serous. When patients first ambulate, a slight drainage increase may occur. However, if drainage increases after it has decreased or the exudate becomes red or brown after it has been serosanguineous or serous, infection or wound complications should be suspected. If sanguineous drainage continues, small blood vessels may be oozing.

Not all surgical wounds drain. If drainage does occur, accurate assessments are vital. The following drainage characteristics are important to note and chart: color, amount, consistency (thick/thin), and odor. Drainage may be contained either in a drainage system or on a dressing. If a dressing is used, the amount of drainage can be monitored either by weighing the soiled dressing or by circling and dating the drainage area. Until the surgeon orders a dressing change, the soiled dressings should be reinforced.

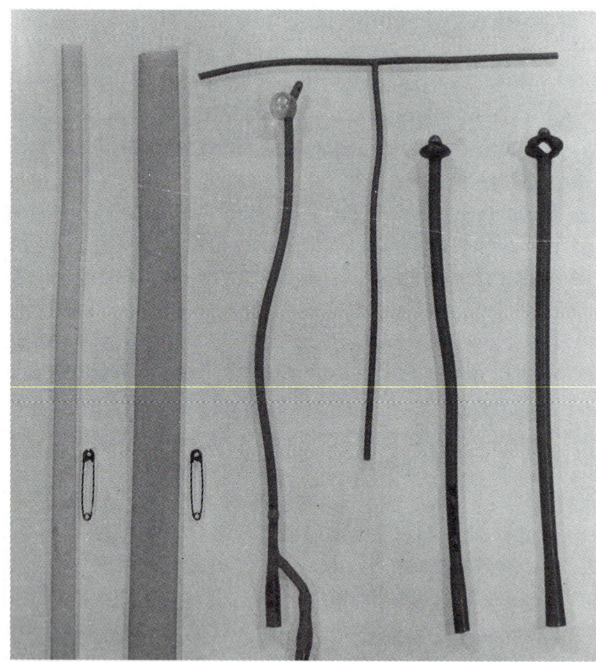

FIG. 22-13 Commonly used surgical drains. *Left to right,* penrose drains, Foley catheter, T-tube, mushroom or Pezzer, and bat-wing or Malecot.

Drainage Systems. Frequently surgical procedures are performed to remove or repair organs that lie within the body (e.g., removing the gallbladder). In these cases a mechanism is needed to assist gravity in removing exudate from the cavity. If a gastrectomy were performed using an upper abdominal midline incision, fluid would collect and remain at the surgical site. To facilitate drainage, an incision, or stab wound, is made close to the incision. The site for the stab wound is planned deliberately. It is the intent of the surgeon to drain exudate away from the incision, not toward it. If the exudate were to enter the surgical incision, contamination and infection could follow.

Gentle suction is needed in some surgeries to help gravity move the exudate. As drainage is removed, the chance of infection decreases and healing occurs more rapidly. A drainage system is chosen to fit the area to be drained, type of exudate, and amount of drainage expected (Fig. 22-13). A rubber or plastic drain may be used to remove exudate from the wound and deposit it on the skin (open drain system) or may be situated through the surgical incision or stab wound. The Penrose drain is commonly used for this purpose. When it is inserted, a sterile safety pin is placed through the drain to keep it from sliding into the wound. When the surgeon wants a gentle vacuum, a closed drainage system can be used. The portable vacuum container (e.g., Hemovac, Redi-Vacettem Snyder, Solcotrans [Fig. 22-7], Surgivac) is an expandable unit that is connected by tubes to the drainage site (Skill 22-12). As gentle suction is provided, exudate is collected in the drainage unit. The Jackson-Pratt and Davol evacuators are other types of closed drainage systems that use a bulb to provide the needed vacuum (Fig. 22-14 on p. 484).

Special drainage systems frequently are used for more difficult sites. Thoracic surgery requires negative pressure to remove drainage from the pleural space. Water-sealed systems (Emerson, Pleur-Evac) are used after chest surgery to reexpand the lung and remove exudate and air. There are various water-sealed arrangements: single-bottle, two-bottle, or three-bottle systems. Regardless of the system used, the tube from the pleural space extends under the water in one of the bottles. This allows drainage and air from the lung to be expelled under water without air moving back into the lung. In time the lung reexpands. The Pleur-Evac is a commercial drainage system that has three bottles (chambers) self-contained in one compartment. The system functions like a three-bottle system in that the unit collects drainage, maintains a seal to prevent air from entering the pleural cavity, and prevents excessive buildup of negative pressure. Water-sealed systems should never be opened to measure and discard drainage. Drainage levels are marked on the container with the date and time at the end of each shift. The previous drainage level is subtracted from the current level to obtain output mea-

SKILL 22-12

MAINTAINING HEMOVAC SUCTION AND DAVOL

Nursing action

1. Wash hands.
2. Check patient's care plan/physician order.
3. Identify patient, explain procedure, and give patient time to ask questions.
4. Bring supplies to bedside.
5. Provide for comfort and privacy.
6. Elevate bed to convenient height.
7. Drape patient, exposing only the area necessary—exposing drainage tubing insertion site. Place the Hemovac/Davol on the absorbent pad.
8. Examine drainage system (pump and tubing) for seal, patency, and stability. If not working, notify head nurse/physician.
9. Don disposable gloves.
10. Don goggles, if appropriate.
11. Remove Hemovac/Davol plug labeled "pouring spout."
12. Empty drainage into measuring device.
13. When emptying Hemovac, compress device by pushing top and bottom together with your hands.
14. Hold pump of Hemovac tightly compressed, and reinsert plug to reestablish closed drainage system. When caring for a Davol, reestablish suction by pumping bulb until balloon is completely inflated—recap drainage port. For both Hemovac and Davol keep plug out of drainage stream—hold the plug by stem—maintain sterility.
15. Observe the drainage for color, consistency, and odor.
16. Measure and record amount of drainage—rinse measuring container.
17. Position drainage system on bed, and secure system.
18. Dispose of drainage, and rinse container.
19. Remove gloves, and wash hands.
20. If specimen is ordered, send to laboratory.
21. Observe Davol/Hemovac every 2 to 4 hours to ascertain integrity of suction. Measure drainage every 8 hours or as ordered.

Sample charting

DATE	TIME	NOTES
1/31/95	7:00	Davol emptied from right lower quadrant stab wound site. 75 ml serosanguineous exudate. Balloon reinflated. Suction reestablished. Patient states, "I am not in any discomfort at present time."

____

(nurse's signature)

SPECIAL CONCERNS

- Davol/Hemovac should be observed every 2 to 4 hours to note color and amount of exudate; output should be measured and recorded every 8 hours as ordered.
- An accurate output of exudate must be recorded so the physician can determine any decrease or increase in wound exudate.
- Observe suction system to be certain Hemovac is compressed and Davol balloon is inflated to maintain proper suctioning.

PATIENT TEACHING

- Explain purpose of wound drainage system.
- Inform patient of importance of nurse measuring output.
- Instruct patient to keep Hemovac/Davol tubing clipped/pinned to gown to prevent accidental dislodgment.

SKILL 22-13

T-TUBE DRAINAGE COLLECTION

Nursing action

1. Wash hands.
2. Check patient's care plan/physician's order.
3. Identify patient, and explain procedure—give patient time to ask questions.
4. Bring supplies to bedside.
5. Provide for comfort and privacy.
6. Elevate bed to convenient height.
7. Drape patient, exposing only area necessary—place drainage bag on absorbent pad.
8. Examine drainage system for patency and for leakage.
9. Don disposable gloves.
10. Don goggles if appropriate
11. Remove plug, holding drainage spout over calibrated container.
12. Empty drainage into the measuring container—recap the drainage bag—maintain sterility.
13. Measure and record amount of drainage.
14. Rinse and replace measuring container.
15. Remove gloves, and wash hands.
16. If dressing change is required, do so at this time.
17. Position patient for comfort.

Sample charting

DATE	TIME	NOTES
1/21/95	0935	Abdominal dressings changed. Moderate amount of serosanguineous exudate T-tube in place and draining dark green liquid. 60 ml emptied from drainage bag. Incision approximated. No erythema noted. Staples in place. Assisted to bathroom. Voided 200 ml clear amber urine. Expelled moderate amount of yellow, semiformed stool. Reported to D. King, RN.

____
(nurse's signature)

SPECIAL CONCERNS

- Normal bile drainage for 24 hours is 500 ml to 1000 ml of viscous, green-brown liquid.
- Always keep the drainage bag below the level of the common bile duct to prevent contamination from backflow.
- Excessive bile leakage from wounds can indicate an occluded system; notify the physician.

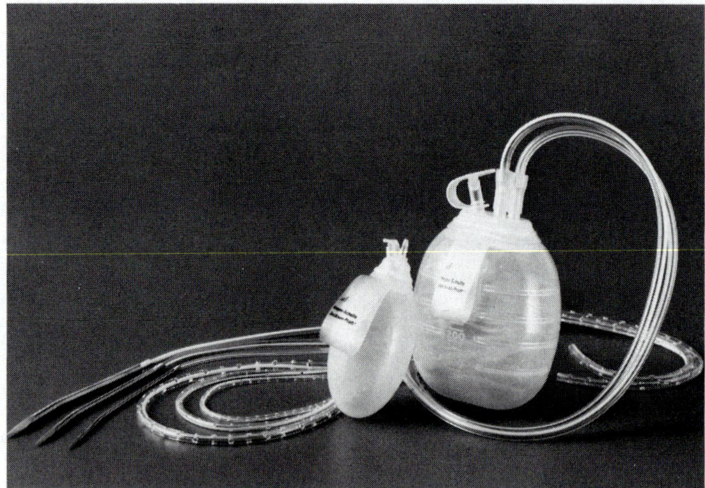

FIG. 22-14 Closed wound drainage system: Jackson-Pratt 100-ml and 400-ml reservoirs with round silicone drains and attached trocars. (Courtesy American V Mueller, American Hospital Supply Corp, Chicago, Ill.)

surement. This is documented on the patient's chart (see Chapter 31).

Various surgical drains are commonly used to facilitate drainage (Fig. 22-13). A T-tube drain is used when the common bile duct has been explored for cholelithiasis. Because edema occurs after the common bile duct is manipulated, a tube is placed in the duct to allow bile to drain (Skill 22-13). Gastric drainage can be obtained through a Levin, Salem sump, Sengstaken-Blakemore, or similar decompression tube. Similarly, the Malecot and Pezzer drains can be attached to continuous or intermittent suction to facilitate internal drainage. Intestinal decompression is accomplished by using the Cantor, Miller-Abbott, or Baker tube. While GI decompression is occurring, the patient remains NPO. Nursing interventions consist of nasal care, oral and lip care, bowel assessments, and monitoring of I&O. To ease the discomfort associated with the tube, mouth washes, ice chips, or hard candy, if allowed, is offered. When peristalsis and normal GI functions return, gastric and intestinal tubes are discontinued (see Chapter 27).

A drainage system requires close monitoring. In addition to noting the color, consistency, and amount of drainage, the tube's patency is important. A tube should not be kinked or occluded; if blood clots or exudate has slowed drainage, this should be recorded and reported. The nurse should follow hospital protocol if NG tube irrigation is indicated. If a patient has nausea, the nurse first assesses the NG tube's patency. When continuous or intermittent suctioning is attached to the drainage system, the unit should be observed for proper functioning: connections tight, machine on, visible drainage. The nurse should not disconnect, change the suction speed, or turn off a machine unless an order is received. Occasionally a drainage tube will be clamped; the nurse should report discomfort, distention, or pain experienced. It is important to properly anchor the NG tube to the patient's nose to prevent dislodgment or unnecessary discomfort. Tube guards are available that anchor the tube securely to the nose to prevent unnecessary movement of the tube. When possible, this device should be used for patient comfort rather than adhesive tape.

Containing drainage is paramount; drainage that enters a surgical incision is likely to cause an infection of the operative area. To minimize this possibility, soiled dressings should be changed. If bed clothing or linen becomes soiled, gloves should be worn during the handling of contaminated materials. Don protective goggles if there is a possibility of splash. Using sterile asepsis during dressing changes is vital to help decrease the possibility of infection. In caring for all postsurgical patients, good handwashing technique is the nurse's first line of defense; gloves, gown, and eye protectors are necessary if secretions cannot be contained. Universal precautions assist in protecting both the patient and nurse. If an infection is suspected, a wound culture is ordered to identify the bacterial agent. To control or eliminate reservoir sites for infection, the nurse eliminates sources of body fluid and exudate that might harbor microorganisms. The nurse also carefully discards articles that become contaminated with blood or infectious material. The Occupational Safety and Health Act (OSHA) of 1991 set standards for minimizing occupational exposure to bloodborne pathogens or other potentially harmful materials.

Nosocomial infections are a continual threat to the postsurgical patient. The virulence of the bacterial contamination and the resistance of the patient are the two major factors in determining whether a wound becomes infected. Because wound infections usually have an incubation period of 4 to 6 days, some patients may have been discharged when problems are noted. Patient teaching should include observations to be made so that medical treatment can be obtained if needed. Although drainage is a sign of healing, accurate assessments can signal potential wound complications.

Discharge Planning

Patients are discharged either the day of surgery or as soon postoperatively as their condition permits.

The nurse should review with the patient, the family, or significant others how to do incisional care, evaluate drainage, and change the wound dressing (Fig. 22-15).

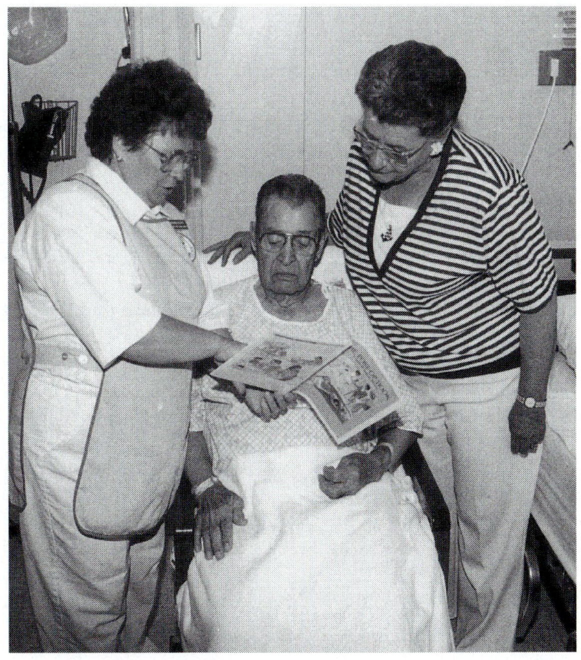

FIG. 22-15 Reviewing discharge planning instructions.

The importance of identifying signs and symptoms of a wound infection should be reinforced so prompt medical treatment is obtained. The nurse can discuss (1) how to use comfort measures and analgesics for postoperative discomfort and (2) common side effects. If GI functions have not become regular, the medical plan provided by the physician can be reviewed. The discharge plan also includes activity level, restrictive ADLs, next physician's appointment, and prescriptions. Once discharge information has been discussed, the nurse evaluates the patient's comprehension, by asking questions, requesting a return demonstration, or posing problems (for example, "If you feel a 'give' in the incisional area, what will you do?"). The patient's responses are charted on the discharge summary form.

REFERENCES AND SUGGESTED READINGS

1. Bale S, Harding KG: Using modern dressings to effect debridement, *Prof Nurs* 5:244, 1990.
2. Cahill-Wright C: Managing post-operative pain, *Nurs* '91 21(12):42, 1991.
3. Caldwell LM: Surgical outpatient concerns: what every perioperative nurse should know, *QORNJ* 53(3):761, 1991.
4. Classen DC et al: Prevention of catheter associated bacteriuria: clinical trial of methods to block three known pathways of infection, *Am J Infect Control* 19(3):136, 1991.
5. Carroll P: Using cuffs to prevent clots, *RN* 55(4), 57, 1992.
6. Cuzzell JL, Stolts NA: Wound care: trial and error yields to knowledge, *Am J Nurs* 90:53, 1990.
7. Dettebneuer PA: *Pulmonary nursing care,* St Louis, 1992, Mosby.
8. Donahue MP: *Nursing: the finest art,* St Louis, 1985, Mosby.
9. Erickson R, Yount S: Comparison of tympanic and oral temperatures in surgical patients, *Nurs Res* 40(2):90, 1991.
10. Fulk C, Hadly JC: Something for pain: new trends in epidural analgesia, *J Post Anesth Nurs* 5:247, 1990.
11. Gerberding JL: Reducing occupational risk of HIV infection, *Hosp Pract* 26(6):103, 1991.
12. Gorah L, Howry D: 25 predictions for perioperative nursing, *RN* 22(1):48, 1992.
13. Great Plains Regional Medical Center: *Admission of the patient to the recovery room policy,* North Platte, Neb, 1992, The Center.
14. Hunt TK: Basic principles of wound healing, *J Trauma* 30:5122, 1990.
15. Joint Commission on Accreditation of Healthcare Organizations: *Accreditation manual for hospitals,* Oakbrook Terrace, Ill, 1992, The Commission.
16. Kim MJ, McFarland GK, McLane AM: *Pocket guide to nursing diagnosis,* ed 5, St Louis, 1993, Mosby.
17. Kloth LC, McCulloch JM, Feedar JA, editors: *Wound healing: alternatives in management,* Philadelphia, 1990, FA Davis.
18. Leckrone L: Preparing your patient for surgery, *Nurs* 91, 21(7):46, 1991.
19. Lepczyk M et al: Effectiveness of the auscultatory method in predicting feeding tube location, *Nurs Res* 39:262, 1990.
20. Litwack K: *Post anesthesia care nursing,* ed 2, St Louis, 1995, Mosby.
21. Litwack K: What you need to know administering preoperative medications, *Nurs '91* 21(8):44, 1991.
22. Lubenow TR, IvanKovitch AD: Patient-controlled analgesia for post-operative pain, *Crit Care Nurs Clin North Am* 3(1):35, 1991.
23. Malasanos L, Barkauskas V, Stoltenberg-Allen K: *Health assessment,* ed 4, St Louis, 1990, Mosby.
24. McCaffery M, Beebe A: *Pain: clinical manual for nursing practice,* St Louis, 1989, Mosby.
25. Meeker MH, Rothrock JC: *Alexander's care of the patient in surgery,* ed 9, St Louis, 1991, Mosby.
26. Messner RL, Pinkerman ML: Preventing peripheral IV infection, *Nursing* 22(6):34, 1992.
27. Methany N: Why worry about IV fluids? *Am J Nurs* 90(6):50, 1990.
28. Miracle VA: How to perform basic airway management, *Nurs '90* 20(4):55, 1990.
29. Nightingale K: Making sense of wound closure, *Nurs Times* 86:35m, 1990.
30. Noah VA: Preop teaching is the key to PCA success, *RN* 53(5):60, 1990.
31. North A: The effects of sleep on wound healing, *Ostomy Wound Manage* 27:56, 1990.
32. Perry AG, Potter PA: *Clinical nursing skills and techniques,* ed 3, St Louis, 1994, Mosby.
33. Potter PA, Perry AG: *Basic nursing: theory and practice,* ed 3, St Louis, 1995, Mosby.
34. Potter PA, Perry AG: *Fundamentals of nursing: concepts, process, and practice,* ed 3, St Louis, 1993, Mosby.
35. Rowland MA: Myths and facts about postop discomfort, *Am J Nurs* (5):61, 1990.
36. Saltiel-Berzin R: Managing a surgical patient who has diabetes, *Nursing* 22(4):34, 1992.
37. Sommers M: Rapid fluid resuscitation, *Nurs '90* 20(1):52, 1990.
38. Timby BK, Lewis LW: *Fundamental skills and concepts in patient care,* ed 5, Philadelphia, 1992, Lippincott.
39. Timmons ME, Bower FL: The effect of structured pre-operative teaching on patient's use of patient-controlled analgesia (PCA) and their management of pain, *Orthop Nurs* 12(1):23, 1993.
40. Tucker SM et al: *Patient care standards, nursing process, diagnosis, and outcome,* ed 5, St Louis, 1992, Mosby.
41. Turner V: Standardization of wound care, *Nurs Stand* 5:25, 1991.
42. Watson DS, Karmpf G: *Monitoring the patient receiving local anesthesia,* ed 2, Denver, 1991, Association of Operating Room Nurses.
43. Way LW: *Current surgical diagnosis and treatment,* ed 9, Norwalk, Conn, 1991, Appleton & Lange.
44. Whitney R: Comparing long-term central venous catheters, *Nurs '91* 21(4):70, 1991.
45. Wild L, Coyne C: Epidural analgesia: the basics and beyond, *Am J Nurs* 92(4):26, 1992.
46. Wolcott K, McDonnell A: Malignant hyperthermia: nursing implications, *Crit Care Nurs* 10(3):8, 1990.

CHAPTER CHALLENGE

KEY POINTS

- Surgery is a highly stressful experience.
- Preoperative teaching is an individualized process and helps to reduce concerns and fears.
- Patients fear that postoperative pain will not be controlled.
- Preoperative assessments serve as postoperative guidelines.
- A consent form cannot be signed after the patient receives preoperative medication or has had a narcotic or any mind-altering substance during the previous 4 hours.
- Maintaining a patent airway is the most vital postoperative assessment.
- Postoperative complications have objective assessments.
- Ideally, preoperative teaching is provided 1 or 2 days before surgery when the patient's anxiety is not as high.
- Strict adherence to principles of aseptic technique is essential to prevent patient infection.
- General, regional, and local are the broad classifications of anesthesia.
- The most common problems encountered in the postanesthetic phase are airway obstruction, hypoventilation, hypotension, cardiac dysrhythmia, and pain.
- Early ambulation increases alertness, ventilation, muscle tone, and peristalsis; decreases pain and venous stasis; facilitates healing and voiding; and promotes increased morale.
- The Occupational Safety and Health Act (OSHA) of 1991 sets standards for minimizing occupational exposure to blood-borne pathogens or other potentially harmful materials.
- Pain management is individually managed with analgesics and comfort measures.
- Hemorrhage and shock are life-threatening conditions.
- Healing is affected by a patient's life-style, physical and mental condition, and preexisting health problems.
- Good handwashing technique and surgical sterile asepsis reduce wound infections.
- If wound dehiscence occurs, it usually happens after the third postoperative day.
- Wound drainage enhances postoperative healing but is a medium for infection.
- Discharge planning identifies home care measures to promote recovery.

STUDY QUESTIONS

1. Mr. Fletcher has cancer of the larynx and is scheduled for a laryngectomy. This is an example of which type of surgery:
   1. Minor
   2. Elective
   3. Emergency
   4. Major
2. The nurse is changing Mr. Cordos' abdominal dressings. Which of the following would indicate an acute inflammatory process in his incisional area:
   1. Skin blanching
   2. Decreased temperature
   3. Loss of sensation
   4. Localized edema
3. Mrs. Somins is being discharged, and the nurse is teaching her how to do daily dressing changes at home. The most important point to include in the teaching plan is:
   1. Discussion of surgical asepsis
   2. Good handwashing technique
   3. Instruction in sterilization
   4. Demonstration of gloving
4. To assist Mr. Brona in the prevention of postoperative pulmonary complications, preoperatively the nurse should:
   1. Ask his physician to prescribe IPPB treatment
   2. Teach him to do leg exercises
   3. Teach him to use an incentive spirometer
   4. Tell him that if he does not cough, he may need to be suctioned
5. Mr. Timmons has undergone surgery for lysis of adhesions. He is transferred from the recovery room to his own room on the surgical floor. In the immediate postoperative period when he is received on the surgical floor, the nurse should obtain blood pressure, pulse, and respiration every:
   1. 15 minutes
   2. 5 minutes
   3. 20 minutes
   4. 30 minutes

6. Mrs. Fuller had surgery for a laminectomy 2 days ago. She is receiving two units of packed red blood cells because her preoperative hemoglobin of 12.7 g has dropped to 9.1 g. She complains of a headache and nausea and vomiting during the blood transfusion. Which one of the following actions should the nurse take immediately:
   1. Check her vital signs
   2. Stop the blood transfusion
   3. Slow down the rate of blood flow
   4. Notify the physician and blood bank personnel
7. Mr. Lyons has had a small bowel resection for necrosis of a portion of the small intestine, secondary to a strangulated hernia. The fourth day postoperative he still has an NG tube in place and absence of bowel sounds. His physician is anticipating a prolonged recovery and an extended period in which Mr. Lyons will be unable to resume oral feedings. A therapy to supply extra glucose, essential amino acids, vitamins, electrolytes, and minerals for this patient is called:
   1. Isotonic solution
   2. Hyperalimentation
   3. Lactated Ringer's solution
   4. Sodium chloride (NaCl)
8. Mrs. Zohet is scheduled to have an abdominal hysterectomy in the morning. The nurse will instruct her preoperatively in the use of the incentive spirometry postoperatively to:
   1. Produce effective coughing
   2. Strengthen abdominal muscles
   3. Promote maximal lung inflation
   4. Increase circulation in the lungs
9. The nurse is changing the abdominal dressings on Ms. Lope and notes that the exudate is pink-tinged. The nurse would chart the exudate as:
   1. Purulent
   2. Serosanguineous
   3. Sanguineous
   4. Serous
10. Mrs. Kira has had a bipolar hip repair, and the nurse is to change her dressings. When cleansing the wound, the nurse should:
    1. Go over the wound twice and discard the swab
    2. Move from the outer region of the wound toward the center using one swab per stroke
    3. Start at the incisional site and move outward using one stroke per swab
    4. Use hydrogen peroxide solution followed by a normal saline rinse
11. The nurse is assessing the bowel sounds of her patient, Mr. Johnson, who has had a suprapubic prostatectomy 2 days ago. To correctly assess that he does not have bowel sounds present, the nurse would need to auscultate each quadrant for:
    1. 1 minute
    2. 3 minutes
    3. 10 minutes
    4. 15 minutes
12. Ms. Campbell is recovering from a right lobectomy. The nurse is going to assist in splinting her incision so she can cough and deep breath. The most therapeutic administration of an analgesic for Ms. Campbell would be:
    1. After the procedure so she can rest
    2. 15 minutes before the procedure
    3. 1 hour before the procedure
    4. 30 minutes before the procedure

9

THERAPEUTIC MANAGEMENT OF ADULT HEALTH DISORDERS

Anyone who has ever looked into the eyes of a person who is totally dependent on another person for his comfort and care couldn't ever walk away in indifference. "The eyes say it all!" The pain, the fear, the sorrow, the joy, the happiness, the love, and the "thank you" is all there to be seen. Nursing has helped me find an inner joy and happiness I have strived for all my life. Through my continued education, I hope to be able to give back as much as I have received. I don't need words or gestures. "The eyes say it all!"

Cathy Rowley
Student Nurse

23

INTRODUCTION TO ANATOMY AND PHYSIOLOGY

M. Christine Neff

KEY TERMS

active transport
anatomy
cell
cytoplasm
diffusion
dorsal
filtration
homeostasis
membrane
mitosis
nucleus
organ
osmosis
passive transport
phagocytosis
physiology
pinocytosis
system
tissue
ventral

LEARNING OBJECTIVES

After reading this chapter, the student should be able to do the following:

- Define the key terms.
- Use each word of a given list of anatomical terminology in a sentence.
- Define the difference between anatomy and physiology.
- Demonstrate an understanding of the body planes by labeling a diagram appropriately.
- Identify and define three major components of the cell.
- Discuss the stages of mitosis and explain the importance of cellular reproduction.
- Differentiate among tissues, organs, and systems.
- Describe the four types of body tissues.
- List the body systems, and give an example of their functions.
- Explain what will happen if cells are placed in solutions with the same or different concentrations than the cells.
- Differentiate between active and passive transport processes that act to move substances through cell membranes.

RELATED TOPICS OF INTEREST

- Fluids and electrolytes (Chapter 24)
- Anatomy and physiology of all body systems (Chapters 25 to 35)

To care for an individual with a disease process, the nurse must understand the normal functioning of the human body. To accomplish this task, the nurse must study basic human anatomy and physiology.

Anatomy is the study, classification, and description of structures and organs of the body. **Physiology** explains the processes and functions of the various structures and how they interrelate with one another. The normal, healthy human body can be compared with a finely tuned machine, with each part performing a special function to accomplish a given goal; and as with the machine, when the human body malfunctions, the repairer must understand how it functions internally.

ANATOMICAL TERMINOLOGY

To study the human body, certain terms must be mastered to specifically locate a structure. To understand the following terms, the student should consider the body in a normal anatomical position, that is, standing erect with the face and palms facing forward (Fig. 23-1).

Anterior (or **ventral**): to face forward; the front of the body. The nose is located on the anterior of the head (Table 23-1).

Posterior (or **dorsal**): toward the back. The heel is located on the posterior portion of the foot (see Table 23-1).

Cranial: toward the head. The brain is located in the cranial portion of the body.

Caudal: toward the "tail"; the distal portion of the spine. A caudal anesthetic may be given to a patient.

Superior: toward the head or above. The neck is superior to the shoulders.

Inferior: lower, below another. The foot is inferior to the ankle.

Medial: toward the midline. The sternum (breastbone) is located in the medial portion of the chest.

Lateral: toward the side. The ribs are lateral to the heart.

Proximal: nearest the origin of the structure; nearest the trunk. The elbow is proximal to the forearm.

Distal: farthest from the origin of the structure; farthest from the trunk. The fingers are distal to the hand.

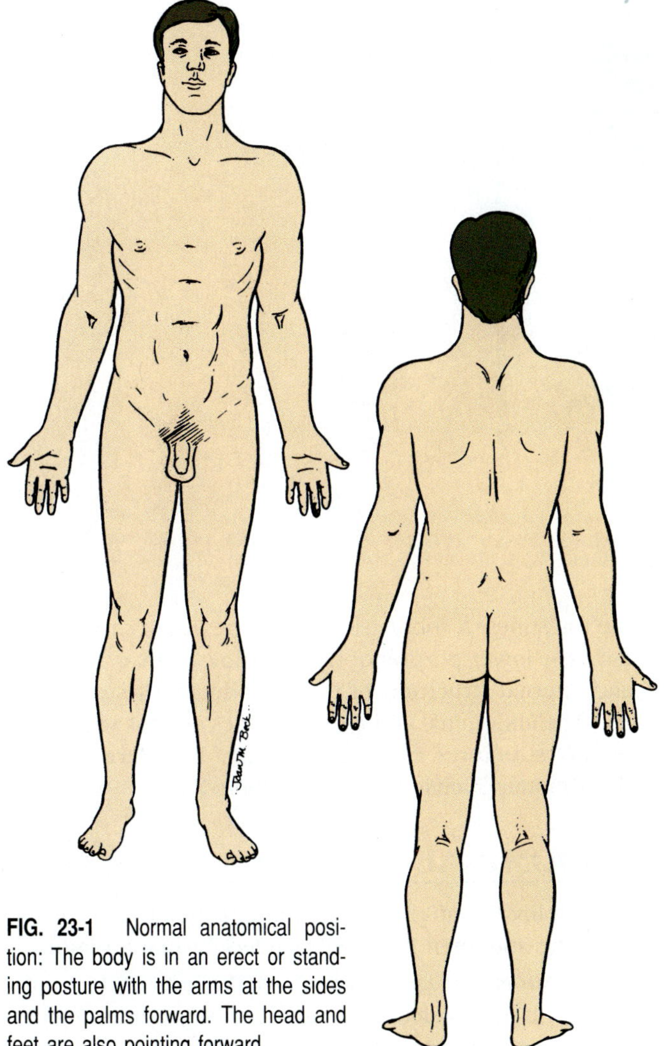

FIG. 23-1 Normal anatomical position: The body is in an erect or standing posture with the arms at the sides and the palms forward. The head and feet are also pointing forward.

BODY PLANES

To facilitate the study of the human body, it is helpful to divide it into three imaginary planes: the sagittal, the coronal, and the transverse (Fig. 23-2 on p. 492).

1. The sagittal plane runs lengthwise from the front to the back. A sagittal cut gives a right and left portion of the body. A midsagittal cut gives two equal halves.
2. The coronal (frontal) plane divides the body into a ventral (front) section and a dorsal (back) section.
3. The transverse plane cuts the body horizontally and yields a superior (upper) and inferior (lower) portion.

BODY CAVITIES

The body may be divided into two major portions: axial and appendicular. The axial portion contains the head, neck, and trunk. The appendicular portion contains the upper and lower extremities.

TABLE 23-1 Body Cavities

Body Cavity	Organ(s)
Ventral body cavity	
Thoracic cavity	
Mediastinum	Trachea, heart, blood vessels
Pleural cavities	Lungs
Abdominopelvic cavity	
Abdominal cavity	Liver, gallbladder, stomach, spleen, pancreas, small intestine, parts of large intestine
Pelvic cavity	Lower (sigmoid) colon, rectum, urinary bladder, reproductive organs
Dorsal body cavity	
Cranial cavity	Brain
Spinal cavity	Spinal cord

FIG. 23-2 Directions and planes of the body.

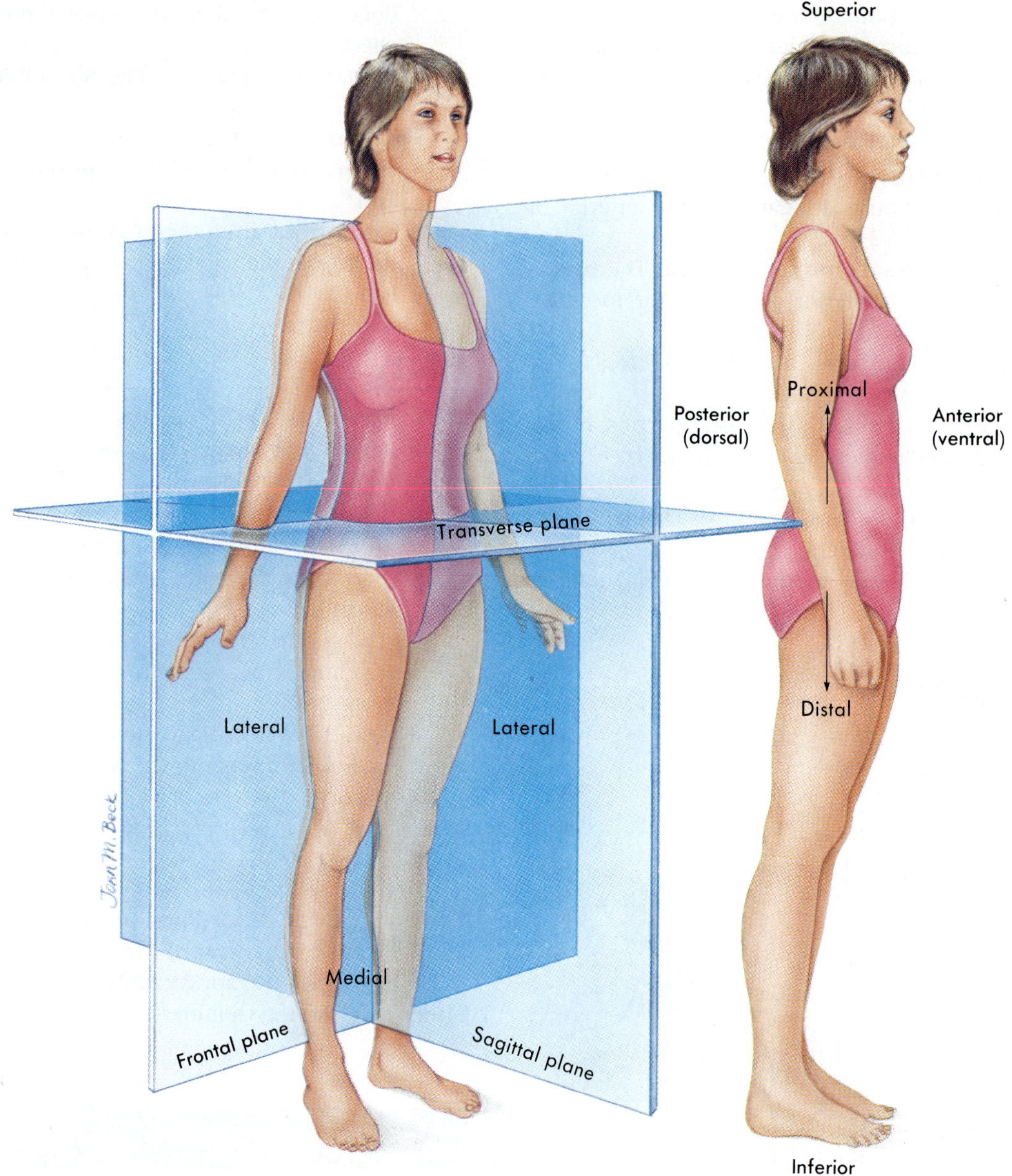

The internal body is composed of open areas, or cavities, which allow for systematic organization of the internal organs. The body cavities are divided into two large groups: the dorsal and ventral cavities. The dorsal cavity is smaller than the ventral cavity.

The dorsal cavity is composed of the cranial and spinal cavities. The cranial cavity houses the brain, whereas the spinal cavity contains the spinal cord.

The diaphragm (a muscle directly beneath the lungs) separates the ventral cavity into the thoracic (chest) and abdominal cavities (see Fig. 27-1). The thoracic cavity contains the heart and lungs. The lungs are situated in the pleural cavity (a subdivision of the thoracic cavity).

The abdominal cavity contains the stomach, kidneys, liver, gallbladder, spleen, pancreas, and a large portion of the intestines. A subdivision called the *pelvic cavity* contains the lower portion of the intestines, urinary bladder, and internal structures of the reproductive system.

The abdominal and pelvic cavities are not separated by any structures and therefore may be referred to as the abdominopelvic cavity (see Table 23-1).

ABDOMINAL REGIONS

To simplify the study and location of the abdominal organs, the abdomen has been divided into nine regions.

1. *Superior regions:* are above the level of the ninth rib and include the right hypochondriac region, the epigastric region, and the left hypochondriac region.

FIG. 23-3 Structural levels of organization in the body.

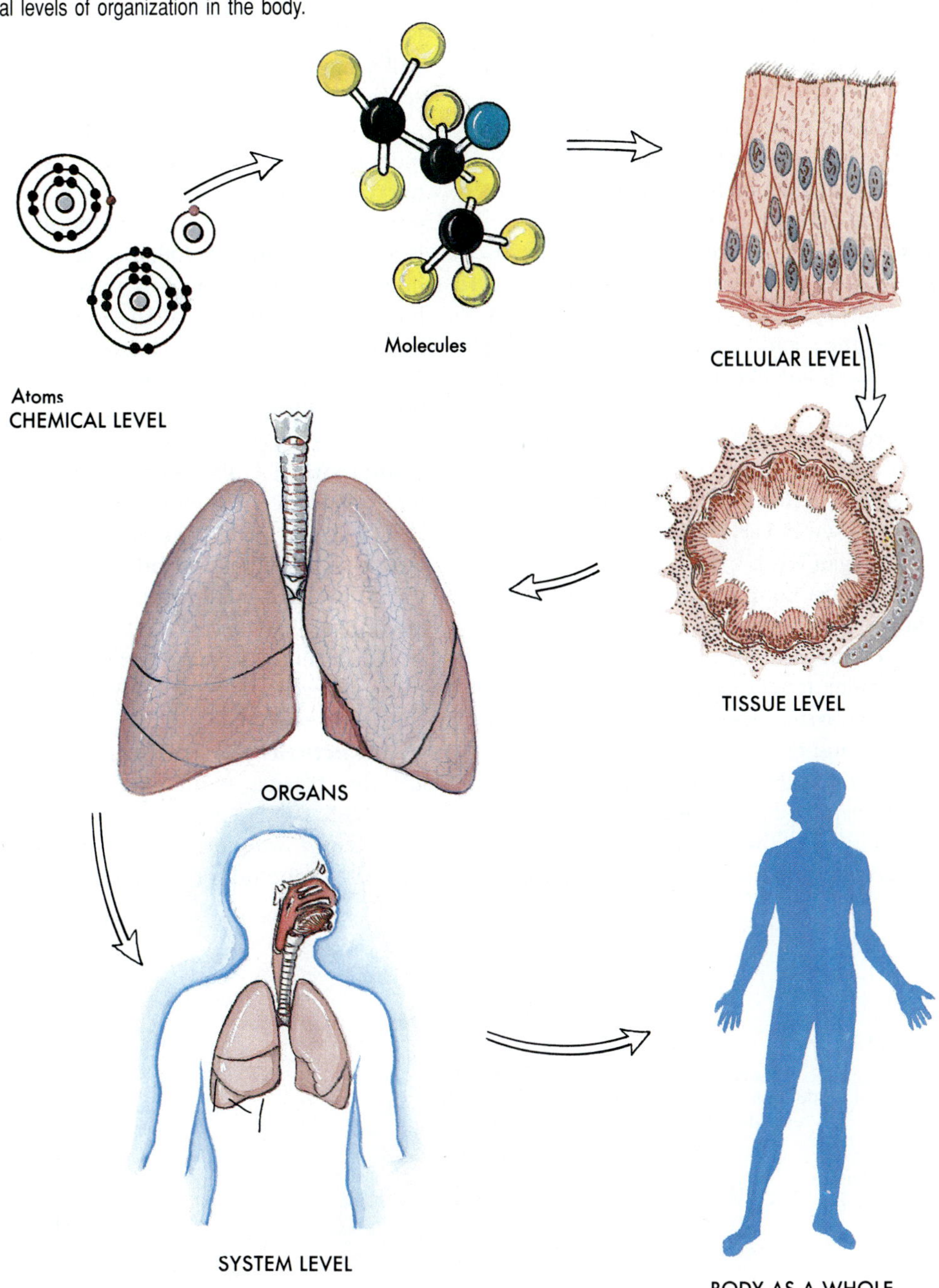

2. *Midregions:* extend inferiorly from the ninth rib to the level of the hip bones and include the right lumbar region, the umbilical region, and the left lumbar region.
3. *Inferior regions:* are below the level of the hip bones and include the right inguinal region, the hypogastric region, and the left inguinal region.

STRUCTURAL LEVELS OF ORGANIZATION

Before studying the structure and function of the human body and its many parts, it is important to think about how those parts are organized and how they might logically fit together into a functioning whole. Fig. 23-3 illustrates the differing levels of organization that influence body structure and function. Note that the levels of organization progress from the least complex (chemical level) to the most complex (body as a whole).

Organization is one of the most important characteristics of body structure. Even the word *organism,* used to denote a living thing, implies organization.

Although the body is a single structure, it is made up of billions of smaller structures. Atoms and molecules are often referred to as the chemical level of organization (see Fig. 23-3). The existence of life depends on the proper levels and proportions of many chemical substances in the cytoplasm of cells. The structural levels of organization in the body are cells, tissues, organs, and systems.

Cells are considered to be the smallest "living" units of structure and function in our body. Although long recognized as the simplest units of living matter, cells are far from simple. They are extremely complex.

Tissues are somewhat more complex than cells. By definition a **tissue** is an organization of many similar cells that act together to perform a common function. Cells are held together and surrounded by varying amounts and varieties of gluelike, nonliving intercellular substances.

Organs are more complex than tissues. An **organ** is a group of several different kinds of tissues arranged so that they can together perform a special function. For instance, the lungs shown in Fig. 23-3 are an example of organization at the organ level.

Systems are the most complex units that make up the body. A **system** is an organization of varying numbers and kinds of organs arranged so that they can together perform complex functions for the body. The organs of the respiratory system shown in Fig. 23-3 permit air to enter the body and travel to the lungs, where the eventual exchange of oxygen and carbon dioxide occurs. Organs of the respiratory system include the nose, the windpipe or trachea, and the complex series of bronchial tubes that permit passage of air into the lungs.

Cells

Nearly 300 years ago Robert Hooke discovered the first cell while examining plant fragments under the microscope. The structures reminded him of tiny, individual miniature prison cells, hence, the name **cell** (the fundamental unit of all living tissue) (Fig. 23-4). All cells are microscopic but differ widely in size and shape. Regardless of size or shape, they exhibit five unique characteristics of life—growth, metabolism, responsiveness, reproduction, and **homeostasis** (a relative constancy in the internal environment of the body, naturally maintained by adaptive responses that promote healthy survival). The human body contains trillions of these tiny powerhouses of life.

Composition Cells contain **cytoplasm,** or "living matter," a substance that exists only in cells; The protoplasm of a cell. The term *cyto-* is a combining form from the Greek and denotes a relationship to a cell. Each cell in the body is surrounded by a thin membrane, the plasma membrane. This membrane separates the cell contents from the dilute salt water solution called tissue fluid that bathes every cell in the body and a small, circular body called the *nucleus.*

Structural parts. The three main parts of a cells are the plasma membrane, the cytoplasm, and the nucleus

Plasma membrane. As the name suggests, the plasma membrane is the membrane that encloses the cy-

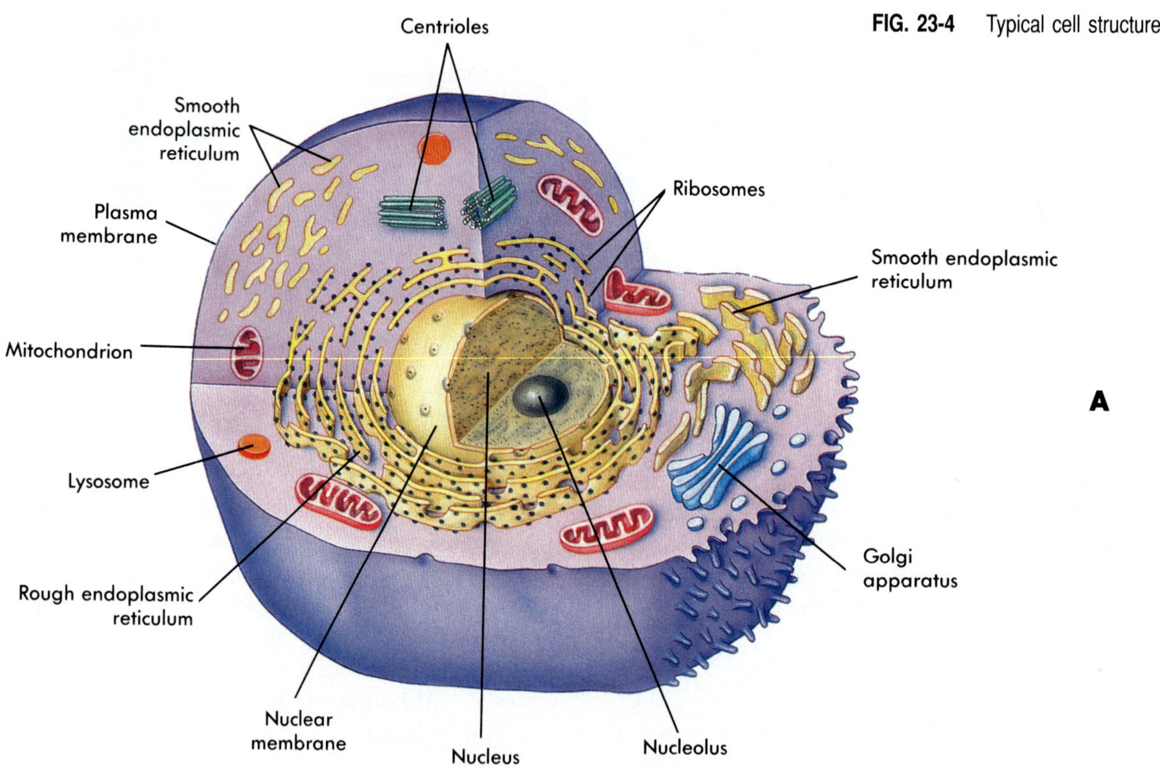

FIG. 23-4 Typical cell structure.

toplasm and forms the outer boundary of the cell. It is an incredibly delicate structure—only about 7 nm (nanometers) or 3/10,000,000 of an inch thick! Yet it has a precise, orderly structure.

Despite its seeming fragility, the plasma membrane is strong enough to keep the cell whole and intact. It also performs other life-preserving functions for the cell. It serves as a well-guarded gateway between the fluid inside the cell and the fluid around it. The plasma membrane is selectively permeable. This means the membrane permits certain substances to enter and leave at will, while not allowing other substances to cross.

Cytoplasm. Cytoplasm (protoplasm) is a sticky fluidlike substance that lies between the cytoplasmic membrane and the nucleus of the cell. Situated within the cytoplasm are numerous organelles (tiny functioning structures). These organelles were not discovered until the development of the powerful electron microscope.

Cytoplasm is composed of 70% water with traces of proteins, lipids, carbohydrates, minerals, and salts. (Table 23-2 lists major cell structures and their functions.)

Nucleus. The **nucleus** is the largest organelle within the cell. It is responsible for cell reproduction and control of the other organelles. The nucleus is surrounded by a membrane called the nuclear membrane. It contains nucleoplasm, a refined form of cytoplasm. The nucleus contains two specialized structures, the nucleolus and chromatin granules. The nucleolus is critical in the formation of protein. The chromatin granules are composed of protein and DNA (deoxyribonucleic acid). DNA contains the genetic code, or blueprint, of the body.

Endoplasmic reticulum. Throughout the cytoplasm lies a system of membranes, or canals, called the endoplasmic reticulum (ER). ER functions as a minicirculating system for the cell by carrying substances from one part of the cell to another. There are two types of ER: (1) smooth, found in cells that deal with fatty substances, and (2) rough, found in cells that manufacture proteins.

Ribosomes. Ribosomes are tiny structures floating free in the cytoplasm or attached to the rough ER. They are called protein factories because they are responsible for the production of enzymes and other proteins.

Mitochondria. The mitochondria are the powerhouses of the cells. They are bean-shaped with a foldlike interior membrane. They take food and convert it to the energy form adenosine triphosphate (ATP) for use by the cell.

Lysosomes. Lysosomes are small saclike structures containing enzymes that digest food compounds and microbes that have invaded the cell.

Golgi apparatus. The Golgi apparatus is usually located near the nucleus. It is the "packaging plant" of the cell. It packages certain carbohydrate and protein compounds into globules. Then, it moves outward toward and through the cell membrane where it breaks open and releases its contents.

Centrioles. The centrioles are paired, rod-shaped organelles. During cell division (mitosis), they aid in the formation of the spindle, a structure necessary for cell reproduction.

Protein Synthesis

Protein is a vital component of every cell in the body. To produce protein, nucleic acids exist in the cytoplasm and the nucleus of the cell.

Two important nucleic acids are (1) deoxyribonucleic acid (DNA) (Fig. 23-5 on p. 496), which is located

TABLE 23-2 Some Major Cell Structures and Their Functions

Cell Structure	Function(s)
Plasma membrane	Serves as the boundary of the cell; protein and carbohydrate molecules on outer surface of plasma membrane perform various functions (for example, they serve as markers that identify cells of each individual or as receptor molecules for certain hormones)
Endoplasmic reticulum	Ribosomes attach to rough ER to synthesize proteins; smooth ER synthesizes lipids and certain carbohydrates
Ribosomes	Synthesize proteins; they are a cell's "protein factories"
Mitochondria	Synthesize ATP; they are a cell's "powerhouses"
Lysomes	Serve as cell's "digestive system"
Golgi apparatus	Synthesizes carbohydrate, combines it with protein, and packages the product as globules of glycoprotein
Centrioles	Function in cell reproduction
Cilia	Are the short, hairlike extensions on the free surfaces of some cells capable of movement
Flagella	Are single projections of cell surfaces; much larger than cilia; the only example in humans is the "tail" of a sperm cell
Nucleus	Dictates protein synthesis, thereby playing an essential role in other cell activities, namely, active transport, metabolism, growth, and heredity
Nucleoli	Play an essential role in the formation of ribosomes

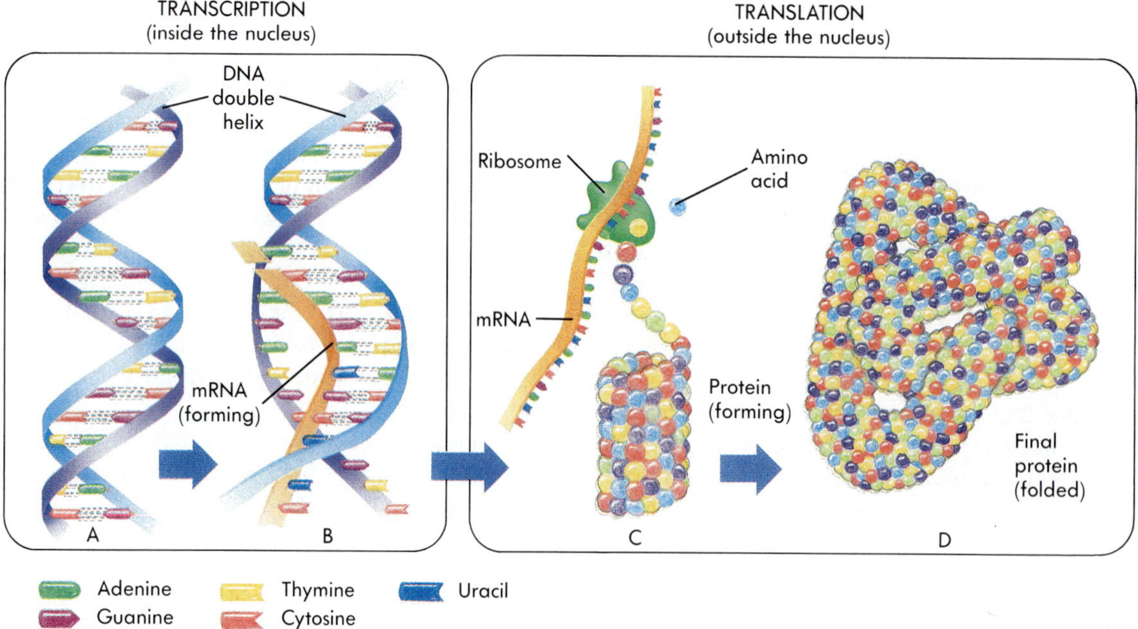

FIG. 23-5 Protein synthesis. **A,** The DNA molecule contains codons that represent a sequence of amino acids. **B,** During transcription, the DNA code is "transcribed" as an mRNA molecule forms. **C,** During translation, the mRNA code is "translated" at the ribosome, and the proper sequence of amino acids is assembled. The amino acid strand coils or folds as it is formed. **D,** The coiled amino acid strand folds again to form a protein molecule with a specific, complex shape.

in the nucleus, and (2) ribonucleic acid (RNA), which is located in the cytoplasm. The DNA encodes the message for protein synthesis and sends it to the RNA, which transports it to the ribosomes where the protein is produced. Hence, DNA is called the *chemical blueprint* and RNA is called the *chemical messenger.*

Cell Division. All cells in the body (except sex cells) reproduce by **mitosis** (type of cell division of somatic [pertaining to nonreproductive cells] in which each daughter cell contains the same number of chromosomes as the parent cell) (Fig. 23-6). The original cell divides to form two daughter cells that retain the characteristics of the original cell.

The chromosomes (spindle-shaped rods) in the nucleus of the cell carry the genes that are responsible for the organism's traits. The traits carry such hereditary factors as hair and eye color. These chromosomes are composed of DNA. Before the cell divides, the DNA must replicate itself so that each new daughter cell contains the original DNA. At the completion of cell division, the daughter cells contain both the nucleus and cytoplasm of the original cell. Each body cell in humans contains 46 chromosomes. These chromosomes exist in pairs. One member of each pair was received from the father of the offspring at the time of fertilization, and one was received from the mother. These paired chromosomes, except for the pair that determines sex, are alike in size and appearance and carry genes for the same traits.

During mitosis, the cell goes through four phases: prophase, metaphase, anaphase, and finally, telephase.

Prophase. In the nucleus the chromosomes form two strands called chromatids. In the cytoplasm the centrioles form a network of spindle fibers.

Metaphase. The nucleus membrane and nucleolus disappear and the chromosomes are aligned across the center of the cell. The centrioles are at the opposite ends of the cell and spindle fibers are attached to each chromatid.

Anaphase. The chromosomes are pulled to the opposite ends of the cell and cell division begins.

Telephase. At this final phase of cell division, the two nuclei appear and the chromosomes disperse. At the end of this phase, two new daughter cells appear.

Movement of Materials Across Cell Membranes. For a cell to survive, it must receive food and oxygen and must secrete its waste products. To accomplish this task, a number of processes allow for mass movement of substances into and out of the cells. These transport processes are classified under two general headings: *passive transport* and *active transport.*

The difference between the two categories is based on whether energy is required to effect the movement

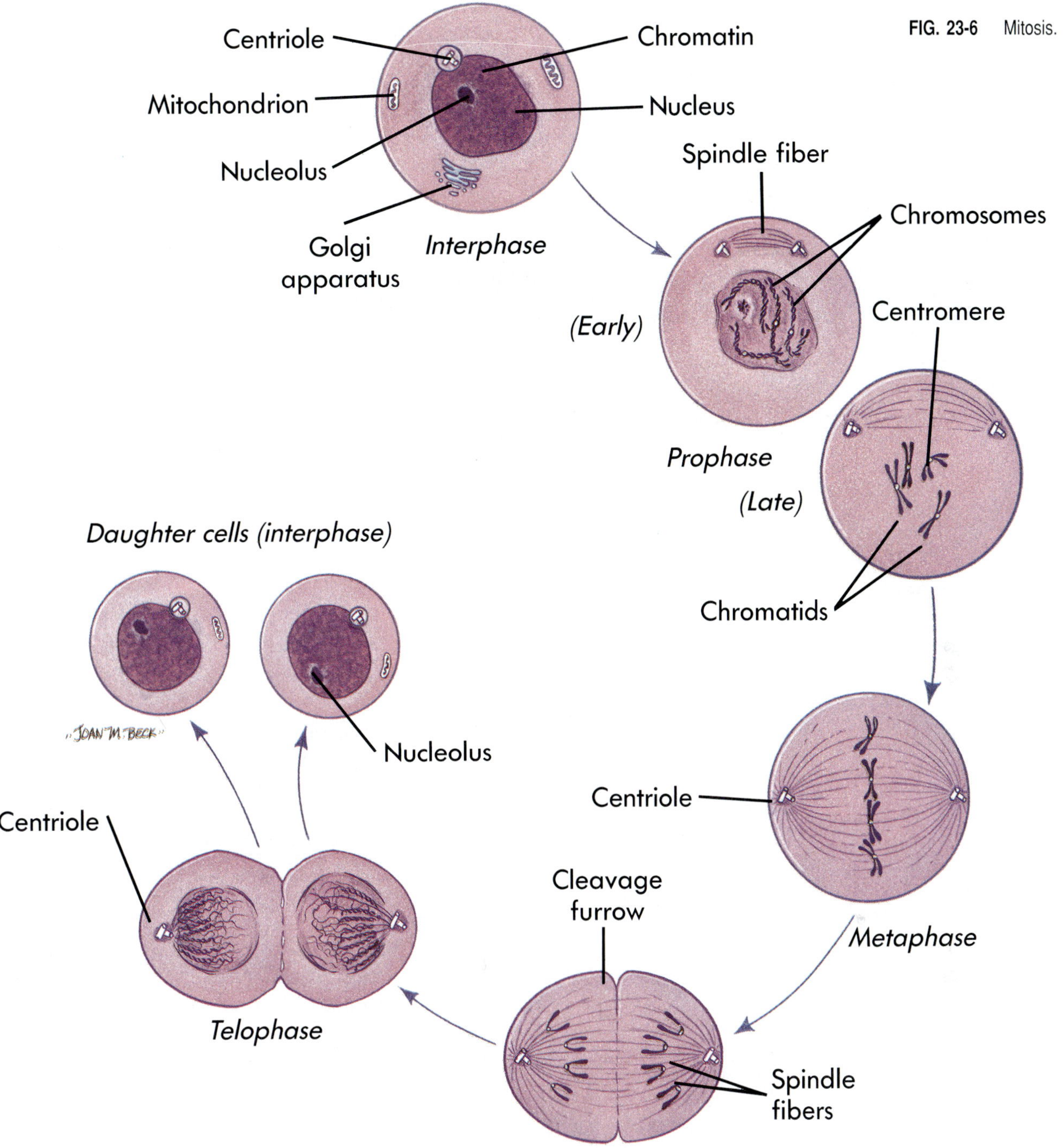

FIG. 23-6 Mitosis.

of something through the cell membrane. **Active transport** (the movement of materials across the membrane of a cell by means of chemical activity that allows the cell to admit larger molecules than would otherwise be able to enter) processes require the expenditure of energy by the cell, and passive transport processes do not. The energy required for active transport processes is obtained from an important chemical substance called adenosine triphosphate, or ATP. ATP is produced in the cell from nutrients and is capable of releasing energy that in turn enables the cell to do work. The breakdown of ATP and use of the energy that is released are required for active transport processes to occur. In **passive transport** (the movement of small molecules across the membrane of a cell by diffusion) processes, cellular energy is required to move substances from a high concentration to a lower concentration; in active transport processes cellular energy is required to move substances from a low concentration to a high concentration.

Passive transport processes. The primary passive transport processes that move through the cell membrane include the following:

1. **Diffusion:** a process in which solid particles in a fluid move from an area of higher concentra-

tion to an area of lower concentration, which results in an even distribution of the particles in the fluid (see Fig. 24-3).

2. **Osmosis:** the passage of water across a semipermeable membrane. The water moves from an area of lower concentration to an area of higher concentration (see Fig. 24-4).
3. **Filtration:** the movement of water and particles through a membrane by a force from either pressure or gravity. This membrane contains spaces through which liquid passes but that are too small to permit solid particles to pass. Movement is from areas of greater to lesser pressure. (Fig. 30-3, *B*).

TABLE 23-3 Tissues

Tissue	Location	Function
Epithelial		
Simple squamous	Alveoli of lungs	Absorption by diffusion of respiratory gases between alveolar air and blood
	Lining of blood and lymphatic vessels	Absorption by diffusion, filtration, and osmosis
Stratified squamous	Surface of lining of mouth and esophagus	Protection
	Surface of skin (epidermis)	Protection
Simple columnar	Surface layer of lining of stomach, intestines, and parts of respiratory tract	Protection; secretion; absorption
Stratified transitional	Urinary bladder	Protection
Connective*		
Areolar	Between other tissues and organs	Connection
Adipose (fat)	Under skin	Protection
	Padding at various points	Insulation; support; reserve food
Dense fibrous	Tendons; ligaments	Flexible but strong connection
Bone	Skeleton	Support; protection
Cartilage	Part of nasal septum; covering articular surfaces of bones; larynx; rings in trachea and bronchi	Firm but flexible support
	Disks between vertebrae	
	External ear	
Blood	Blood vessels	Transportation
Muscle		
Skeletal (striated voluntary)	Muscles that attach to bones	Movement of bones
	Eyeball muscles	Eye movements
	Upper third of esophagus	First part of swallowing
Cardiac (striated involuntary)	Wall of heart	Contraction of heart
Visceral (nonstriated involuntary or smooth)	In walls of tubular viscera of digestive, respiratory, and genitourinary tracts	Movement of substances along respective tracts.
	In walls of blood vessels and large lymphatic vessels	Changing of diameter of blood vessels
	In ducts of glands	Movement of substances along ducts
	Intrinsic eye muscles (iris and ciliary body)	Changing of diameter of pupils and shape of lens
	Arrector of muscles of hairs	Erection of hairs (gooseflesh) (see Fig. 23-7)
Nervous		
—	Brain; spinal cord; nerves	Irritability; conduction

*Connective tissues are the most widely distributed of all tissues.

Active transport processes. As stated, active transport is the movement of material across the membrane of a cell by means of a chemical activity that allows the cell to admit larger molecules than would otherwise be able to enter. Certain enzymes play a role in active transport, providing a chemical "pump" that helps move substances through the cell membrane. For example, insulin binds with glucose and transports the glucose into the cell. Two other active transport processes that move an object or substance through the plasma membrane and into the cytoplasm are:

1. **Phagocytosis:** (Greek for "cell-eating") permits a cell to engulf or to surround any foreign material and to digest it. This function is often performed by the white blood cells in the human body.
2. **Pinocytosis:** the process by which extracellular fluid is taken into the cell. The cell membrane develops a saclike indentation filled with extracellular fluid, then closes around it, and digests it.

Tissues

Tissues are groups of similar cells that work together to perform a specific function. The body is composed of the following four main types of tissues that compose the body's many organs:

1. Epithelial tissue
2. Connective tissue
3. Muscle tissue
4. Nervous tissue

Consult Table 23-3 for a summary of their locations and functions.

Epithelial Tissue. Epithelial cells are packed closely together and contain no blood vessels. The epithelial tissue covers the outside of the body and some of the internal structures. There are four types or forms of epithelial tissue: (1) simple squamous, (2) stratified squamous, (3) simple columnar, and (4) stratified transitional. Table 23-3 gives the locations and functions of each of these types.

Epithelial tissue serves several important functions in the body. Some of the more important are listed in the following:

1. *Protection:* Covering the body and many of its organs, it serves as a protective barrier against invasion.
2. *Absorption:* Certain specialized epithelial cells can absorb material in the body, e.g., the lining of the small intestine can absorb digested nutrients.
3. *Secretion:* Mucus is secreted in areas such as the respiratory and digestive tracts.

Connective Tissue. As the name suggests, connective tissue "connects," or joins, tissues or structures of the body. It also supports and protects body structures and exists in varying forms. It can be thin and delicate or tough and cordlike; it also exists in liquid form (blood). Mast cells, plasma cells, and white blood cells are found in connective tissue. Red blood cells are not usually found in connective tissue unless blood vessels have been injured. Unlike the closely packed epithelial tissue, the connective tissue cells are spaced among varying amounts of intercellular fluid, which is composed of protein complexes and tissue fluid.

Some of the most important forms of connective tissue are areolar connective tissue, adipose (fat) tissue, bone, cartilage, and blood. Consult Table 23-3 for the locations and functions of these tissues.

Muscle Tissue. Muscle tissue is composed of cells that contract in response to a message from the brain or spinal cord. There are three types of muscle cells: (1) skeletal (striated, voluntary), (2) cardiac (striated, involuntary), and (3) visceral (smooth, involuntary) (Fig. 23-7 on p. 500).

1. Skeletal muscle cells are striated (have a striped appearance) and attach to bones to produce voluntary movement.
2. Cardiac muscle cells are striated with fibers that branch to form many networks, or webs. These networks are found only in the walls of the heart and generally do not function at will (involuntary).
3. Visceral (smooth) muscle cells are nonstriated and have a smooth appearance. These cells appear in the viscera, or internal organs, such as the walls of the blood vessels, stomach, intestines, and uterus. Generally, they are involuntary, but some control can be exerted through the use of biofeedback techniques.

Nervous Tissue. Nervous tissue is composed of two types of cells: neurons and glial cells. The neurons are the nerve cells and are responsible for the transmission of impulses or messages. The glial cells are support cells; they support and nourish the neurons.

Neurons have three parts: (1) dendrites, which carry impulses toward the cell body; (2) cell body; and (3) axons, which carry impulses away from the cell body (see Fig. 35-2).

Membranes

Membranes are thin sheets of tissue that serve many functions in the body. They cover body surfaces, line and lubricate hollow organs, and protect and anchor organs and bones.

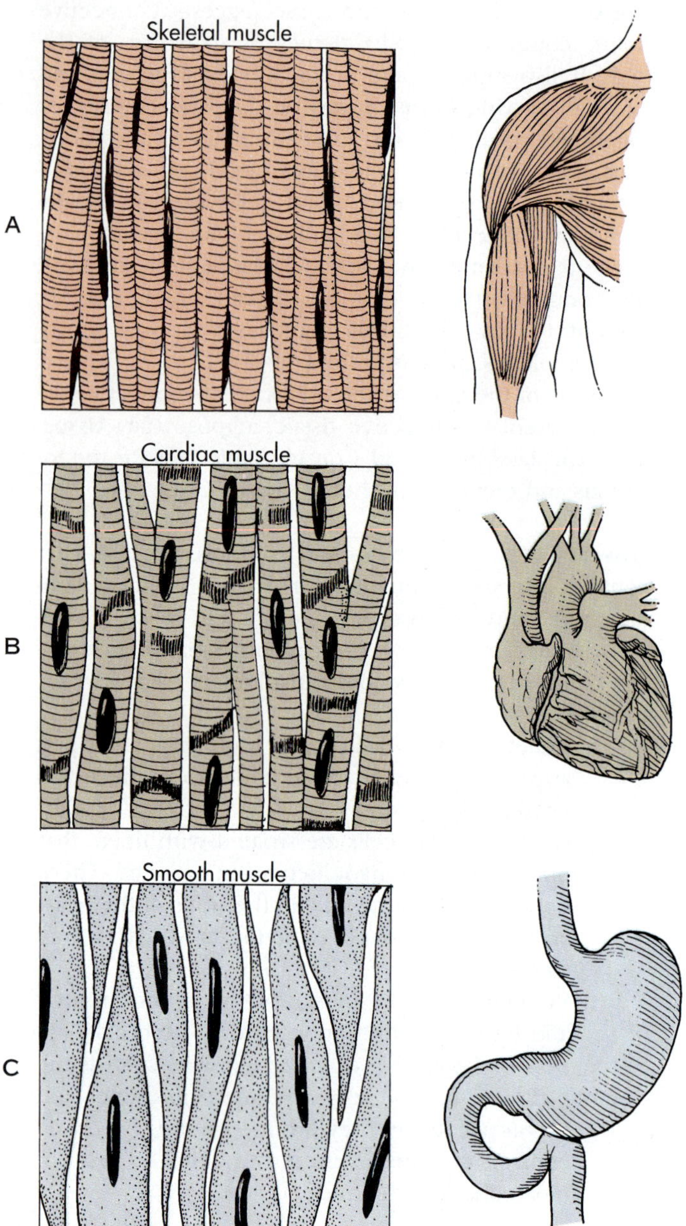

FIG. 23-7 **A,** Skeletal muscle. **B,** Cardiac muscle. **C,** Smooth muscle.

The two major types of membranes are the epithelial and the connective tissue membranes.

Epithelial Membranes. Epithelial membranes are usually composed of a thin layer of epithelial cells with an underlying layer of connective tissue for strength. Epithelial membranes may be divided into two subgroups: mucous membranes and serous membranes.

1. Mucous membranes secrete mucus (a thick, slippery material) that keeps the membranes moist and soft and protects against bacterial invasion. They line the body surfaces that open to the outside environment. Examples include the nose, mouth, urinary, respiratory, gastrointestinal, and reproductive tracts.
2. Serous membranes secrete a thin, watery fluid that prevents friction when organs rub against one another. They line the body surfaces that do not open to the outside environment. Examples include the lungs (pleura), intestines (peritoneum), and heart (pericardium).

Connective Tissue Membranes (Synovial Membrane). Connective tissue membranes are smooth, slick, and secrete synovial fluid (a thick, lubricating fluid). These membranes line the joint spaces between bones and prevent friction between the ends of the bones, thus allowing free movement of the joints.

TABLE 23-4 Ten Major Systems and Functions of the Body

System	Function
Integumentary (skin)	Covers the body and is the body's first line of defense
Musculoskeletal	Provides the body's framework and allows for movement
Circulatory	Is the major transportation system for nutrition, water, oxygen, and wastes
Digestive	Processes food and water and removes waste products
Respiratory	Delivers oxygen and removes carbon dioxide
Urinary	Removes excess water and waste products
Nervous	Contains the body's control center and is responsible for the coordination of all of the body's activities
Endocrine	Releases chemicals that regulate the body's activities
Reproductive	Enables the procreation of life
Sensory	Protects the individual by detecting changes in the environment

Organs/Systems

When several kinds of tissues are united to form a more complex function than any tissue alone, they are called organs. Examples are the heart, stomach, and kidneys. These organs are arranged together to perform a more complex function than can any organ alone in the body. When this occurs, they are then called *systems* (Table 23-4 and Fig. 23-8).

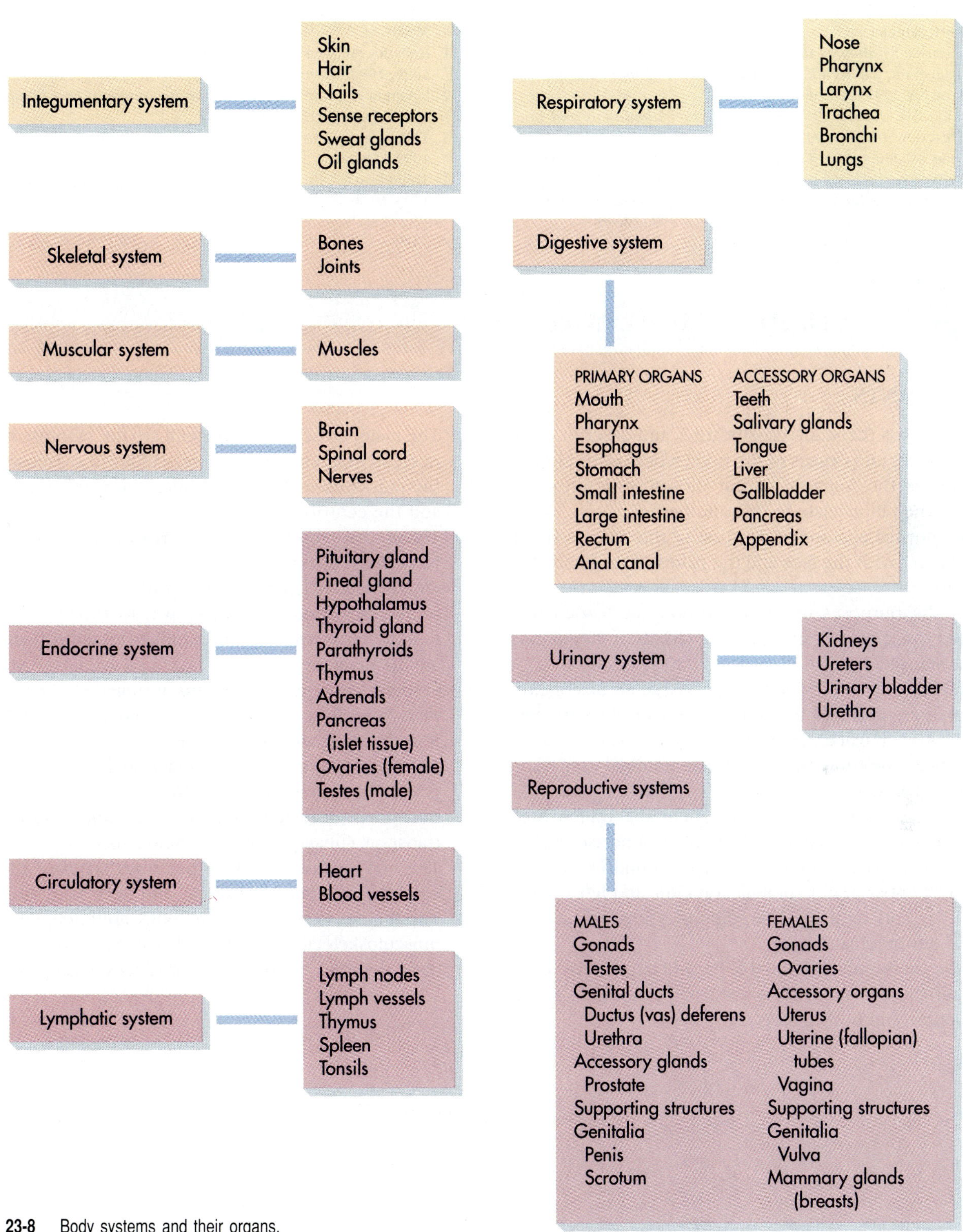

FIG. 23-8 Body systems and their organs.

REFERENCES AND SUGGESTED READINGS

1. Beare PG, Myers JL: *Principles and practice of adult health nursing*, ed 2, St Louis, 1994, Mosby.
2. Brenner BM, Rector FC, editors: *The kidney,* ed 4, Philadelphia, 1991, Saunders.
3. Gottfried SS: *Biology today*, St Louis, 1993, Mosby.
4. Hegner BR, Caldwell E: *Geriatrics: a study of maturity,* ed 5, Albany, NY, 1991, Delmar.
5. Hood GH, Dincher JR: *Total patient care: foundation and practice,* ed 8, St Louis, 1992, Mosby.
6. Long BC, Phipps WJ, Cassmeyer VL: *Medical-surgical nursing: a nursing process approach,* ed 3, 1993, Mosby.
7. McCance KL, Huether SE: *Pathophysioslogy: the biologic basis of disease in adults and children,* St Louis, 1990, Mosby.
8. Memmler RL, Cohen BJ, Wood DL: *Structure and function of the human body,* ed 5, Philadelphia, 1992, Lippincott.
9. *Mosby's medical, nursing, and allied health dictionary,* ed 4, 1994, Mosby.
10. Phipps WJ et al: *Medical-surgical nursing,* ed 4, St Louis, 1991, Mosby.
11. Seely RS, Stephen TD, Tate P: *Anatomy and physiology,* ed 2, St Louis, 1992, Mosby
12. Solomon EP: *Introduction to human anatomy and physiology,* Philadelphia, 1992, Saunders.
13. Thibodeau GA: *Structure and function of the body,* ed 9, St Louis, 1992, Mosby.
14. Thibodeau GA, Patton KT: *Anatomy and physiology,* ed 2, St Louis, 1993, Mosby.

CHAPTER CHALLENGE

KEY POINTS

- Anatomy is the study, classification, and description of structures and organs of the body, whereas physiology explains the function of the various structures and how they interrelate to one another.
- The normal anatomical position of the body is standing erect with the face and the palms of the hands forward.
- For the purposes of study, the body is divided into three imaginary planes: the sagittal, the coronal, and the transverse.
- The body can be divided into two large groups of cavities, the dorsal and the ventral. The dorsal cavity contains the cranial and spinal cavities. The ventral cavity contains the thoracic cavity, the abdominal cavity, and the pelvic cavity.
- For the purposes of study, the abdominal region is divided into nine regions: right hypochondriac region, epigastric region, and left hyponchondriac region; right lumbar region, umbilical region, and left lumbar region; and right inguinal region, hypogastric region, and left inguinal region.
- Cells are the smallest units of life and contain five characteristics: growth, metabolism, responsiveness, reproduction, and homeostasis.
- The major structures of the cell are the cytoplasm, the nucleus, the endoplasmic reticulum, the ribosomes, the mitochondria, the lysosomes, the Golgi apparatus, and the centrioles.
- Tissues are groups of similar cells that work together to perform a specific function.
- Organs are structures made up of two or more kinds of tissues organized in such a way that the tissues can together perform a more complex function than can any tissue alone.
- Systems are a group of organs arranged in such a way that they can together perform a more complex function than can any organ alone.
- To receive nutrition and oxygen and to rid itself of wastes, the cell performs these processes: passive transport (diffusion, osmosis, filtration) and active transport (phagocytosis and pinocytosis).
- The body is composed of four main types of tissues: epithelial, connective, muscle, and nervous tissues.
- The ten major systems of the body are integumentary, musculoskeletal, circulatory, digestive, respiratory, urinary, nervous, endocrine, reproductive, and sensory.

STUDY QUESTIONS

1. The anatomical terminology that refers to the distal portion of the spine:
   1. Medial
   2. Caudal
   3. Proximal
   4. Dorsal
2. The trachea, heart, blood vessels, and lungs are located in which body cavity:
   1. Dorsal
   2. Abdominopelvic
   3. Ventral
   4. Pelvic
3. A relative constancy in the internal environment of the body naturally maintained by adaptive responses that promote healthy survival:
   1. Homeostasis
   2. Mitosis
   3. Lysosomes
   4. Protein synthesis
4. A process in which solid particles in a fluid move from an area of greater concentration to an area of lesser concentration, resulting in an even distribution of the particles in the fluid, is called:
   1. Phagocytosis
   2. Pinocytosis
   3. Osmosis
   4. Diffusion
5. What is produced in the cell from nutrients and is capable of releasing energy that allows the cell to work:
   1. ATP
   2. Pinocytosis
   3. Membrane
   4. Oxytocin
6. The movement of materials across the membrane of a cell by means of chemical activity requiring the expenditure of energy by the cell is called:
   1. Passive passport
   2. Active transport
   3. Telophase
   4. Transcription
7. What type of tissue is composed of cells that contract in response to a message from the brain or spinal cord:
   1. Epithelial
   2. Connective
   3. Membrane
   4. Muscle
8. The thin sheets of tissue that secrete mucus and line the body surfaces that open to the outside environment are:
   1. Mucous membranes
   2. Serous membranes
   3. Striated, involuntary
   4. Visceral, involuntary
9. An active transport process that permits a cell to engulf or surround foreign material and digest it is called:
   1. Mitosis
   2. Pinocytosis
   3. Phagocytosis
   4. Filtration
10. A type of cell division of somatic cells in which each daughter cell contains the same number of chromosomes as the parent cell is:
    1. Flagella
    2. Mitosis
    3. ER synthesis
    4. Mitochondria

24

FLUIDS AND ELECTROLYTES

Georgeanna Temres Smith

KEY TERMS

active transport
anion
bicarbonate
buffer
calcium
cation
chloride
diffusion
electrolyte
extracellular
filtration
homeostasis
hypertonic
hypotonic
interstitial
intracellular
intravascular
ion
isotonic
magnesium
milliequivalent
osmosis
passive transport
phosphorus
potassium
sodium

LEARNING OBJECTIVES

After reading this chapter, the student should be able to do the following:

- Define the key terms.
- Describe the distribution of fluid compartments
- Describe the daily balance of intake and output.
- Explain the mechanisms by which body fluids move.
- Discuss the role of specific electrolytes in maintaining homeostasis.
- Describe the cause and effect of deficits and excesses of sodium, potassium, chloride, calcium, magnesium, phosphorus, and bicarbonate.
- Explain the role of the buffers, lungs, and kidneys in maintenance of acid-base balance.
- Describe the four major types of acid-base imbalances.

RELATED TOPICS OF INTEREST

- Basic nutrition (Chapter 18)
- Diet therapy (Chapter 19)
- Introduction to anatomy and physiology (Chapter 23)
- Care of the patient with a gastrointestinal or accessory organ disorder (Chapter 27)
- Care of the patient with a urinary disorder (Chapter 30)
- Care of the patient with a respiratory disorder (Chapter 31)
- Care of the patient with an endocrine disorder (Chapter 32)

FLUIDS (WATER)

Water has many functions. It provides an extracellular transportation route to deliver nutrients to the cells and carry waste products from the cells. Once inside the cells, it provides a medium in which chemical reactions, or metabolism, can occur. Water also acts as a lubricant for tissues. Two other important functions of water are to aid in the maintenance of acid-base balance and to assist in heat regulation by evaporation.

Water is critically important to the body. The major percentage of body weight is water. This percentage depends on several factors and varies with each individual. First, age affects the amount of water in the body. A newborn has a water content of 70% to 80% of its body weight. That percentage increases in a premature infant to as high as 90%. The infant begins to lose body fluid most rapidly in the first 6 months, and by 12 years, the proportion approaches that of an adult. The percentage of water content in the body declines from that highest percentage at birth to 50% to 60% as adults and 45% to 55% in the older person.

Another important influence on the amount of water in the body is the amount of fat in the individual. There is a correlation between water content and fat content; fat contains relatively little water. The female has proportionately more body fat than the male, which means the female has less body fluid than the male. The more obese an individual the smaller the percentage of body water. Both obese and older persons are at risk for complications of illness from dehydration or fluid shifts because of less fluid reserve in their bodies (see gerontological box). Infants are also at risk for dehydration. Over one half of an infant's fluid is **extracellular** (outside the cells) fluid (Fig. 24-1). Extracellular fluid is lost from the body more rapidly than **intracellular** (inside the cells) fluid. The very young, the very old, and the obese patients are at a higher risk for developing a fluid volume deficit. A loss of 10% of body fluid is serious in an adult, and a 20% loss is fatal. In an infant, those figures are even more significant. A loss of 5% is serious, 10% is very serious, and 15% is fatal.

GERONTOLOGICAL CONSIDERATIONS

- Older adults are at increased risk of dehydration:
  - Fat replaces lean muscle with aging, leading to a decrease in total body fluid.
  - The aging kidney is less able to concentrate urine, leading to fluid loss.
  - Decreases in mobility and diminished sense of thirst often result in decreased fluid intake.
  - Incontinent older individuals may restrict fluids to reduce the frequency of urination.
- To compensate for changes in taste, older adults may over-salt their food, resulting in electrolyte and fluid imbalance.
- Physiological changes in the skin and mucous membranes make them less reliable indicators of dehydration. Dehydration may first manifest as mild disorientation.
- Dehydration increases the risk of orthostatic hypotension.
- Decreased fluid intake increases the likelihood of constipation.
- Because the aging kidney is less efficient at excretion, administration of intravenous infusions or supplements containing sodium or potassium increase the risk of electrolyte imbalance.
- The complete blood count should be monitored carefully to detect changes in the hematocrit as it relates to hemoglobin. Decreased plasma volume elevates the hematocrit, whereas the hemoglobin level remains constant.

FLUID COMPARTMENTS

Identifying the location of fluids in the body is done by categorizing them into compartments. However, it is an abstract term, because rather than being contained in a compartment in a specific area, the fluids are in constant motion throughout the body to carry out their functions.

The body has two fluid compartments: intracellular and extracellular (Fig. 24-2 on p. 506). Even though each is specific in its location and functions, there is constant interaction between the compartments.

The fluid compartments (Tables 24-1 and 24-2 on p. 506) are as follows:

1. Intracellular
2. Extracellular
   a. Interstitial
   b. Intravascular

The intracellular fluid compartment is the larger of the two compartments. It contains the fluid inside the billions of cells within the body.

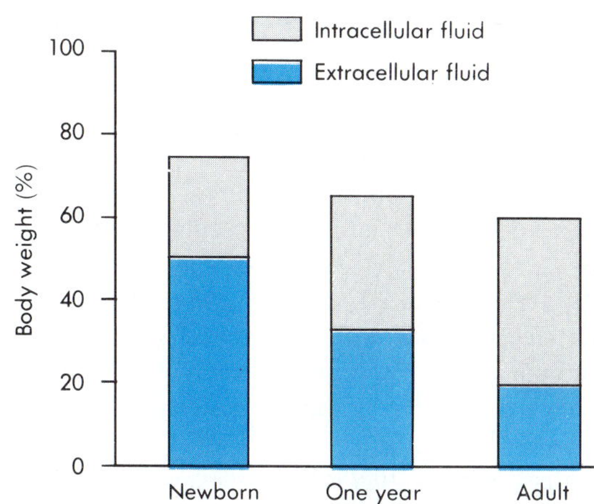

FIG. 24-1 In the newborn, more than half of total body fluid is extracellular. As the child grows, proportions gradually reach adult levels.

TABLE 24-1 Body Fluid Distribution

Compartment	Description	Fluid
Intracellular	Fluid within cells	Intracellular fluid (ICF)
Extracellular	Fluid outside cells	Extracellular fluid (ECF)
Intravascular	Fluid within blood vessels	Plasma
Interstitial	Fluid in tissues (between cells or in body spaces)	Examples: interstitial fluid, lymph, cerebrospinal fluid, intraocular fluid, GI secretions, urine, sweat, exudates

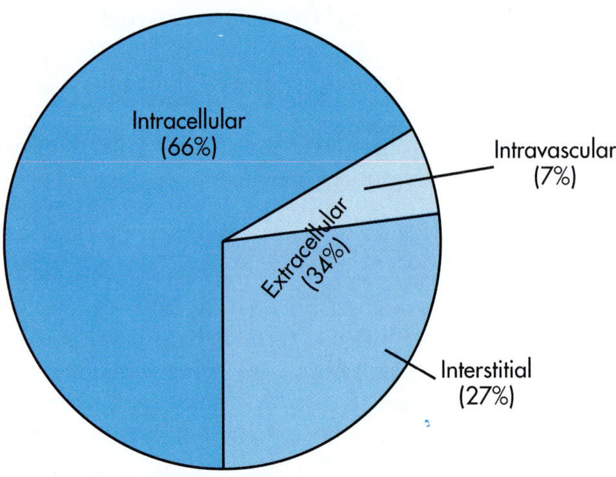

FIG. 24-2 Volumes of body fluids in each fluid compartment.

TABLE 24-2 Body Fluid Distribution

Compartment	Percent of Total Body Fluid	Fluid Volume (liters)
Extracellular fluid		
Interstitial fluid	27	11.2
Intravascular fluid (plasma)	7	2.8
Intracellular fluid	66	42.0

The extracellular compartment contains any fluid outside the cells. This compartment is further divided into the interstitial and intravascular fluid compartments.

Interstitial fluid is between the cells or in the tissues. It accounts for approximately 27% of the fluid in the patient's body. Examples of interstitial fluid include lymph, cerebrospinal fluid, and gastrointestinal (GI) secretions.

Intravascular fluid is the plasma within the vessels. The cells of the blood are considered solid particles. After the cells are removed, the liquid that remains is the plasma. It makes up the remaining 7% of our fluid volume.

The intracellular and extracellular compartments are separated by a semipermeable membrane. This membrane allows for a constant back-and-forth flow as nutrients are taken into the cell and waste products are carried out of the cell.

INTAKE AND OUTPUT

As water moves through all parts of the body, it is constantly being lost. Fluid leaves the body through the kidneys, lungs, skin, and GI tract. To maintain homeostasis, the normal daily loss must be met by the normal daily intake. **Homeostasis** is a relative constancy in the internal environment of the body, naturally maintained by adaptive responses that promote healthy survival. Daily water intake and output is about 2500 ml (Table 24-3).

Water loss is replenished in two ways—first, by ingestion of liquids and food and, second, by metabolism, both of food and in our body tissues.

Intake includes all fluids entering the body. Fluids can be liquids taken orally or consumed in food including foods that assume a liquid consistency at room temperature. Additional intake includes tube feedings and parenteral intake such as IV fluids, blood components, and total parenteral nutrition.

Liquid output includes all fluids leaving the body. Urine, diarrhea, vomitus, nasogastric suction, and chest tube drainage are examples. Drainage from surgical wounds and the drainage collected in surgical receptacles such as the Jackson Pratt, Davol, or Hemovac systems are also considered liquid output. The determination of exact amounts of fluid loss and fluid replacement is not possible as part of nursing care, so approximations are used. Because fluid intake and fluid output can be measured, the importance of accurate record keeping cannot be overstressed when determining a patient's fluid needs (Skill 24-1). A simple and accurate method of determining water balance is by weighing the patient under exact conditions, for example, same time of day, same amount of bed clothing, same type of gown, and

MEASURING INTAKE AND OUTPUT (I&O)

Nursing action/*Rationale*

1. Read physician's order *to verify procedure.*
2. Identify patient *to ensure accuracy.*
3. Explain procedure *to ensure patient's cooperation and promote patient participation.*
4. Instruct patient to inform staff of all oral intake *to ensure accurate I&O measurement.*
5. Instruct patient not to empty any output collection receptacles and to notify the nurse after elimination *to ensure accurate I&O measurement.*
6. Post signs on patient's door, bathroom door, and near patient's bed *to alert all staff and remind patient of need to measure I&O.*
7. Measure and record all fluids taken orally and all fluids administered parenterally *to ensure accurate measurement of intake.*
8. Wash hands and don gloves *to prevent transmission of microorganisms.*
9. Measure and record output in Foley drainage system, diarrhea stools, nasogastric suction, emesis, and output in surgical wound receptacles *to ensure accurate measurement and proper disposal of output.*
10. Remove gloves and wash hands *to prevent cross contamination.*
11. Compute and document I&O on patient's record *to ensure accurate documentation of total I&O.*

TABLE 24-3 Normal Fluid Intake and Loss in an Adult Eating 2500 Calories per Day (Approximate Figures)

Intake		Output	
Route	Gain (ml)	Route	Amount of Loss (ml)
Water in food	1000	Skin	500
Water from oxidation	300	Lungs	350
Water as liquid	1200	Feces	150
		Kidney	1500
TOTAL	2500	TOTAL	2500

same attached equipment, such as electrodes. Because 1 liter of fluid equals 1 kilogram (2.2 pounds), a weight change of 1 kilogram will reflect a loss or gain of 1 liter of body fluid.

MOVEMENT OF FLUID AND ELECTROLYTES

Substances entering the body begin their journey in the extracellular fluid. However, to carry out their functions, they must cross the semipermeable membrane surrounding each body cell to enter the cell. The fat and protein molecules that make up the membrane are arranged so that some substances can enter the cells and others cannot. There are several methods used to move fluids, electrolytes and other solutes, or dissolved substances from one compartment to the other.

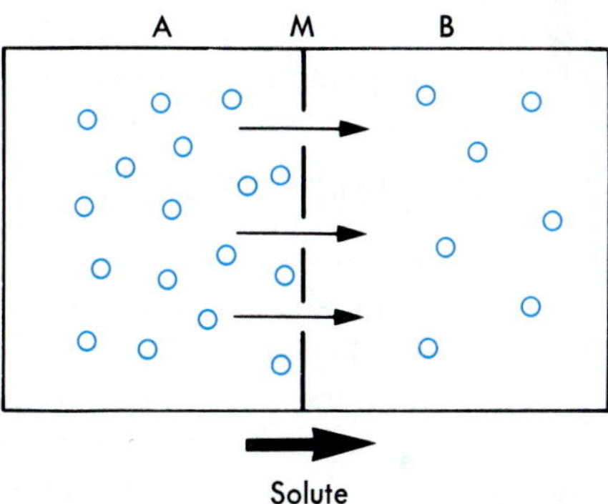

FIG. 24-3 Diffusion: solute moves through membrane *(M)* from area of greater concentration *(A)* to area of lesser concentration *(B)* until concentration on both sides is equal.

DIFFUSION

Water can move freely from one compartment to another by diffusion. **Diffusion** is the movement of particles in all directions through a solution or gas (Fig. 24-3). Diffusion occurs when ink is dropped into a glass of water. The ink will disperse in all directions until it is evenly distributed throughout the fluid. When diffusion occurs in the body, the molecules have the same action as the ink spreading through the water. With each inhalation by the patient oxygen enters the lungs and moves into the intravascular compartment and into the cells by diffusion. Oxygen can diffuse easily across the cell membrane.

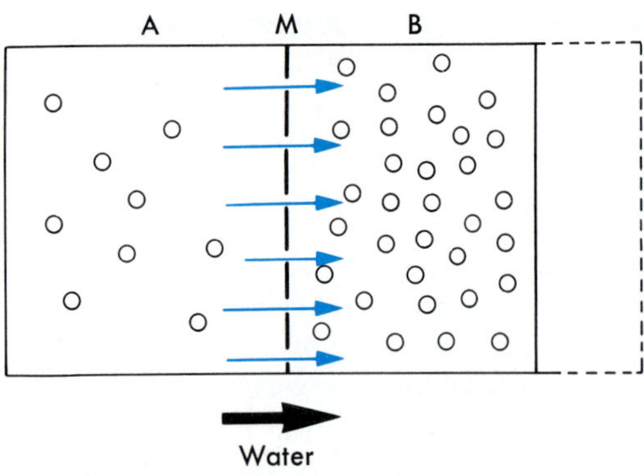

FIG. 24-4 Osmosis: water moves from area of lesser solute concentration *(A)* through a membrane *(M)* to area of greater solute concentration *(B)* until concentration of solute on both sides of the membrane is equal. Compartment *B* will have to expand *(as shown by dotted lines)* to accept the additional water.

OSMOSIS

Osmosis is the movement of water from an area of lower concentration to an area of higher concentration (Fig. 24-4). Osmosis equalizes the concentration of ions or molecules on each side of the membrane. The flow of water will continue until the number of ions or molecules on both sides of the membrane is equal. Boiling a hot dog in water is an example of osmosis. The concentration of molecules inside the hot dog is greater than in the water. The water passes through the hot dog skin, which is a semipermeable membrane, in an attempt to equalize the number of molecules on both sides of the membrane. Finally, when the hot dog can hold no more water, the skin, or semipermeable membrane, ruptures.

The red blood cells offer an example of the osmotic process in the body. If extracellular fluid is more concentrated than intracellular fluid, the fluid from the cell moves out to the extracellular fluid, causing the red blood cell to shrink. If the fluid among the compartments is in equilibrium, fluid will enter and leave the cell at the same rate and the cell size will not change. Another example is when extracellular fluid is less concentrated than the fluid in the red blood cells. Fluid moves into the cell, causing it to enlarge. The process can continue until the cell ruptures.

Solutions are classified as hypertonic, isotonic, or hypotonic according to the electrolyte concentration. The concentration of the solution will cause the cells of the body to react the same as the red blood cell. **Hypertonic** (a solution of higher osmotic pressure) solutions pull fluid from the cells, **isotonic** (a solution of same osmotic pressure) solutions expand the body's fluid volume without causing a fluid shift from one compartment to another, and **hypotonic** (a solution of lower osmotic pressure) solutions move into the cells, causing them to enlarge. Each of these actions occurs through osmosis.

FILTRATION

Filtration is the transfer of water and dissolved substances from an area of higher pressure to an area of lower pressure. An example of filtration occurs at the capillary level of the circulation. There is a force behind filtration called hydrostatic pressure, which is the force of fluid pressing outward on a vessel wall (see Fig. 30-3, *B*). The pumping action of the heart is responsible for the amount of force of the hydrostatic pressure that causes water and electrolytes to move from the capillaries to the interstitial fluid.

ACTIVE TRANSPORT

The fluid movements discussed to this point have required no energy expenditure by the body; they have been examples of **passive transport. Active transport** requires energy; it is a force that moves molecules into cells without regard for their positive or negative charge and against concentration factors that would prevent entry into the cell via diffusion. Active transport moves fluid and electrolytes from an area of lower concentration to an area of higher concentration. Adenosine triphosphate (ATP) is the energy source used to accomplish active transport. ATP energy is released in a complex metabolic process within the body's cells known as the Krebs cycle. (Krebs cycle is a sequence of enzymatic reactions involving the metabolism of carbon chains of sugars, fatty acids, and amino acids to yield carbon dioxide, water, and high-energy phosphate bonds.)

Substances actively transported through the cell membrane include sodium, potassium, calcium, iron, hydrogen, and amino acids. The movement of glucose into the cells occurs through the process of active transport. Insulin provides the transport for glucose to leave the intravascular compartment and move into the cells, where the glucose can then be used for energy.

ELECTROLYTES

As water moves through the compartments of the body, it contains substances that are sometimes called *minerals* or *salts* but are technically known as *electrolytes.* **Electrolytes** develop tiny electrical charges when they dissolve in water and break up into particles known as **ions.** Ions develop either a positive or negative electrical charge. Ions with a positive charge are called **cations.** Ions with a negative charge are called **anions.**

Examples of cations:

1. Sodium Na^+
2. Potassium K^+
3. Calcium Ca^{++}
4. Magnesium Mg^{++}

Examples of anions:

5. Chloride Cl^-
6. Bicarbonate HCO_3^-
7. Sulfate SO_4^-
8. Phosphate HPO_4^-

A balance exists between the electrolytes. For each positively charged cation, there must be a negatively charged anion.

A sample of plasma is used to measure the electrolytes. The measurement is done in milliequivalents (mEq). Rather than electrolytes being measured by their weights, they are measured by their electrical activity. A **milliequivalent** is a measure of the chemical activity or chemical combining power of an ion. The chemical activity of an electrolyte is compared with the chemical activity of hydrogen. One milliequivalent of any electrolyte has the same chemical combining power as 1 mEq of hydrogen. In each fluid compartment in the body, the cations and anions balance each other with their chemical combining power to maintain electrical neutrality, which, again, keeps the body in homeostasis.

Although the electrolytes move freely among the fluid compartments, each has a primary location. The location and function of each electrolyte become important in understanding disease processes. The body maintains homeostasis by correcting any excesses or deficiencies of the electrolytes.

Sodium

The normal blood level of **sodium** (Na^+), a cation and the most abundant electrolyte in the body, is 134 to 142 mEq/L. It is the major extracellular electrolyte, and because the plasma sample used to measure electrolyte levels comes from the extracellular fluid, the level is high. In contrast, the intracellular level of sodium is approximately 10 mEq. The major source of sodium comes from the diet. That is true of all the electrolytes. However, unlike the other electrolytes, sodium is a substance that frequently needs to be limited in the diet rather than encouraged. The kidneys are the primary excretion route for sodium. It is important to know that many electrolytes, such as sodium, not only pass into and out of the body, but also move back and forth between a number of body fluids during each 24-hour period. Fig. 24-5 shows the large volumes of sodium-containing internal secretions that are produced each day. During a 24-hour period, more than 8 liters (L) of fluid containing 1000 to 1300 mEq of sodium is poured into the digestive system. This sodium, along with most of that contained in the diet, is almost completely reabsorbed. Precise regulation and control of sodium levels are required for survival.

The functions of sodium include regulation of the water balance. Sodium controls the extracellular fluid volume mainly through osmotic pressure, because water follows the sodium in the body. It also increases cell membrane permeability. Sodium stimulates conduction of nerve impulses and helps maintain neuromuscular irritability. Sodium is important in controlling contractility of muscles, especially the heart.

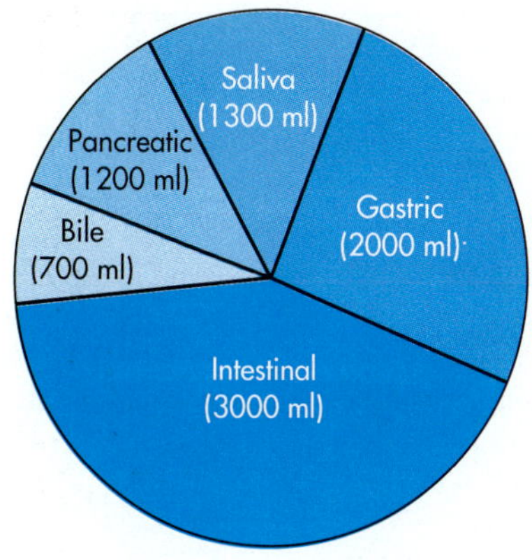

FIG. 24-5 Sodium-containing internal secretions produced every day.

Hyponatremia. A less than normal concentration of sodium in the blood is called *hyponatremia.* This can occur when there is a sodium loss or a water excess (Box 24-1 on p. 510). Hyponatremia occurs when the sodium drops below 134 mEq/L in the extracellular fluid.

When a deficiency results from sodium loss, the body attempts to compensate by decreasing water excretion. If hyponatremia occurs because of water excess, the result has a diluting effect on all of the blood components because water is being retained in the body. The signs and symptoms of hyponatremia depend on the cause and also on how rapid and severe the sodium loss. As sodium levels decrease in the extracellular fluid, water is pulled into the cells, causing them to swell, and as the fluid moves into the cells, potassium is shifted out; therefore the patient is likely to also have a potassium imbalance.

Hypernatremia. Hypernatremia is a greater than normal concentration of sodium. The sodium level exceeds 145 mEq/L. It is caused by an excess of sodium or a decrease in body water (Box 24-2 on p. 510). The body attempts to correct the imbalance by conserving water through renal reabsorption. Hypernatremia causes fluid to shift from the cells to the interstitial spaces, resulting in cellular dehydration and an interruption in cellular processes. Again, a potassium imbalance frequently occurs. In sodium retention, potassium is excreted.

Potassium

The normal blood level of potassium (K^+), the dominant intracellular cation, is 3.5 to 5.5 mEq/L. The level of potassium in the extracellular fluid is low because **potassium** is an intracellular electrolyte. Intracellular levels of potassium are 150 mEq/L. Of the body's potassium, 98% is in the cells and 2% is in the extracellular fluid.

A well-balanced diet usually provides adequate potassium. Approximately 65 mEq of potassium is re-

Box 24-1 CAUSES AND SYMPTOMS OF HYPONATREMIA

CAUSES

Loss of GI fluids
- Vomiting
- Diarrhea
- GI or biliary drainage via nasogastric tube or T-tube
- Fistulas

Loss through skin
- Diaphoresis
- Large open lesions (burns)

Shifting of body fluids
- Massive edema
- Ascites
- Burns
- Small bowel obstruction
- Lengthy hydrotherapy

SIGNS AND SYMPTOMS

Headache*
Muscle weakness
Fatigue*
Apathy
Postural hypotension*
Nausea/vomiting
Abdominal cramps

Severe or Prolonged Deficit

Shock
Mental confusion
Coma

NURSING INTERVENTIONS

Monitor I&O of patients receiving diuretic medications.
Observe for abnormal GI, renal, or skin losses.
Replace fluid loss with fluids containing sodium, not plain water.

*Most common signs and symptoms.

Box 24-2 CAUSES AND SIGNS AND SYMPTOMS OF HYPERNATREMIA

CAUSES

More water than sodium is lost from the body
An abnormally large intake of sodium
- Taking too many salt tablets
- IV saline infused too rapidly

Prepared foods: frozen, canned, smoked
- Dairy products in large amounts

SIGNS AND SYMPTOMS

Dry, tenacious mucous membranes
Low urinary output
Firm, rubbery tissue turgor

Severe or Prolonged Excess

Manic excitement
Tachycardia
Death

NURSING INTERVENTIONS

Monitor I&O
Decrease sodium intake in diet
Monitor water loss from fever, infection, increased respiratory rate

quired each day. Potassium is widely distributed in natural foods; fruits, legumes, leafy vegetables, and meat are sources of potassium (Box 24-3).

The routes of potassium excretion are the kidneys (80% to 90%) and in the feces and perspiration (10% to 20%). The kidneys control the excretion of potassium. Sodium and potassium seem to pair off against each other, and the kidneys prefer to conserve sodium, even when both electrolytes are depleted. In both normal and abnormal situations, sodium will be reabsorbed and potassium will be excreted. Because the major route of excretion of potassium is the kidneys, any condition that causes a decrease in urine output also causes a retention of potassium. A rise in potassium requires continuous monitoring. An important consideration in homeostasis is that kidney function will determine the potassium level in the body. Too little or too much potassium affects the heart muscle and can be life threatening.

The main function of potassium is regulation of water and electrolyte content within the cell. With sodium and calcium, it promotes transmission of nerve impulses and also skeletal muscle function. Potassium assists in the cellular metabolism of carbohydrates and proteins. Another function of potassium is to control the hydrogen ion concentration. When potassium moves out of the cell, sodium and hydrogen ions move in. The result is the regulation of acid-base balance.

Hypokalemia. A decrease in the body's potassium to a level below 3.5 mEq/L is known as *hypokalemia.* The major cause of potassium loss is renal excretion (Box 24-4). The kidneys do not conserve potassium and excrete it even when the body needs the potassium. The use of diuretics, such as thiazides or furosemide (Lasix), promotes hypokalemia. Conditions that cause injury to the cells, in turn, cause the release of potassium from the

Box 24-3 FOODS RICH IN POTASSIUM

FRUITS (INCLUDING JUICES)	VEGETABLES
Apricots	Asparagus
Bananas	Dried beans
Grapefruit	Broccoli
Melon	Cabbage
Cantaloupe	Carrots
Honeydew	Celery
Dried fruits, figs, dates, raisins	Mushrooms
Oranges	Dried peas
	Potatoes: white, sweet
PROTEIN FOODS	Spinach
	Squash
Beef	
Chicken	**BEVERAGES**
Liver	
Pork	Cocoa
Veal	Cola drinks
Turkey	Instant tea and coffee
Milk	
Nuts, peanut butter	

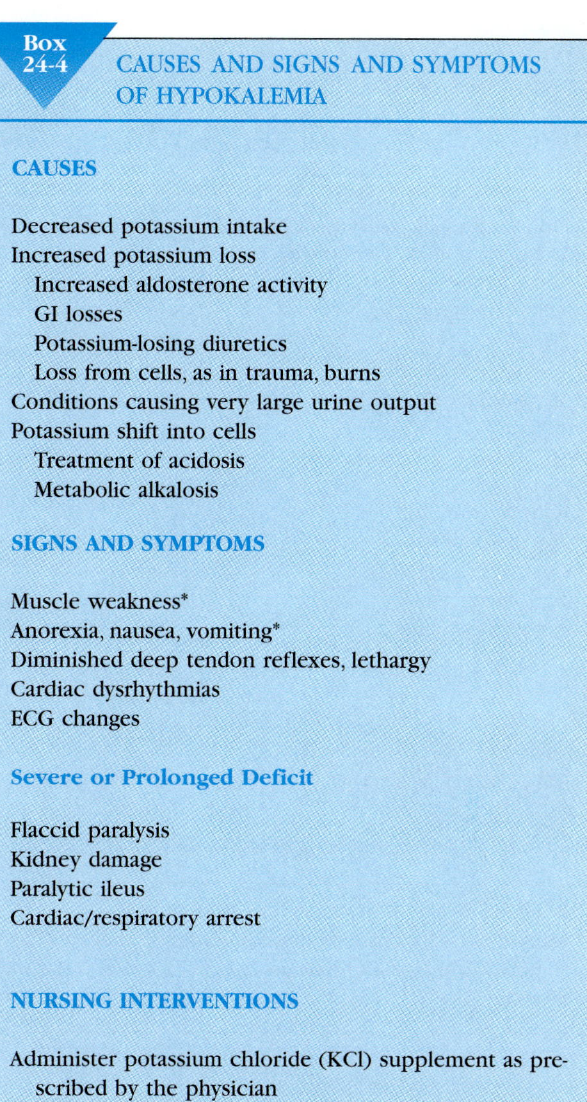

Box 24-4 CAUSES AND SIGNS AND SYMPTOMS OF HYPOKALEMIA

CAUSES

Decreased potassium intake
Increased potassium loss
- Increased aldosterone activity
- GI losses
- Potassium-losing diuretics
- Loss from cells, as in trauma, burns

Conditions causing very large urine output
Potassium shift into cells
- Treatment of acidosis
- Metabolic alkalosis

SIGNS AND SYMPTOMS

Muscle weakness*
Anorexia, nausea, vomiting*
Diminished deep tendon reflexes, lethargy
Cardiac dysrhythmias
ECG changes

Severe or Prolonged Deficit

Flaccid paralysis
Kidney damage
Paralytic ileus
Cardiac/respiratory arrest

NURSING INTERVENTIONS

Administer potassium chloride (KCl) supplement as prescribed by the physician
Encourage increased intake of foods high in potassium
Monitor I&O
Monitor telemetry

*Most common signs and symptoms.

cells to the interstitial spaces and ultimately to the kidneys. If renal function is normal, the potassium will be excreted. Because the normal amounts of potassium are so small, fluctuations have the potential to develop into serious problems. Hypokalemia can affect skeletal and cardiac function. The resulting muscle weakness causes life-threatening cardiac conduction abnormalities.

Hyperkalemia. An increase in the body's serum potassium level above 5.5 mEq/L is known as hyperkalemia. This condition is not as common as hypokalemia when renal function is normal. The major cause of potassium excess is renal disease, in which potassium cannot be excreted adequately (Box 24-5 on p. 512). When severe tissue damage occurs, potassium is released from the cells. Shock often accompanies this damage, resulting in reduced kidney output. The result is an elevated potassium level. Although hyperkalemia is less common than hypokalemia, it is often more dangerous, because of cardiac arrest, which is caused by overstimulation of the cardiac muscle.

Chloride

The normal blood level of **chloride** (Cl^-), an extracellular anion, is 96 to 105 mEq/L. It is the chief anion in interstitial and intravascular fluid. Even though chloride accounts for more than two thirds of the anions in the body, it is usually not considered alone. Chloride has the ability to diffuse quickly between the intracellular and extracellular compartments and combines easily with sodium to form sodium chloride or with potassium to form potassium chloride. It is more often linked with sodium.

The daily requirement of chloride is equal to that of sodium (3.65 to 10.85 g a day). Foods containing sodium also contain chloride. The main route of excretion is through the kidneys.

Chloride is necessary for the formation of hydrochloric acid in gastric juice. It is also a valuable electrolyte in regulating the osmotic pressure between the compartments and assisting in the regulation of acid-base balance.

Box 24-5

CAUSES AND SIGNS AND SYMPTOMS OF HYPERKALEMIA

CAUSES

Potassium intake (parenteral or oral) in excess of kidney's ability to excrete
Renal failure
Adrenal insufficiency
Potassium enters bloodstream, from injured cells with extensive trauma
Metabolic acidosis

SIGNS AND SYMPTOMS

Nausea, vomiting*
Diarrhea, colic*
Cardiac dysrhythmias*
ECG changes
Numbness, tingling

Severe or Prolonged Excess†

Flaccid paralysis
Cardiac arrest*
Anuria

NURSING INTERVENTIONS

Decrease intake of foods high in potassium
Administer Kayexalate (sodium polystyrene sulfonate) as prescribed by the physician
Monitor I&O

*Most common signs and symptoms.
†Prolonged potassium excess results in signs and symptoms similar to those of hypokalemia.

Hypochloremia. Hypochloremia usually occurs when sodium is lost, because sodium and chloride are frequently paired. The most common causes of hypochloremia are vomiting and prolonged nasogastric or fistula drainage.

Hyperchloremia. Hyperchloremia rarely occurs but may be seen when bicarbonate levels fall. The chloride anions attempt to compensate to maintain equal numbers with the cations in the body fluid. Because chloride imbalances rarely occur independently of other electrolytes, there are no specific signs and symptoms to identify a chloride imbalance.

Calcium

The normal blood level of **calcium** (Ca^{++}) is approximately 4.5 mEq/L. Of the 1200 g of calcium in the body, 99% is concentrated in the bones and teeth, where it is physiologically inactive. The remaining 1% is found in the soft tissue and the extracellular fluid. Calcium is deposited in the bones and mobilized as needed to keep the blood level constant during any period of insufficient intake. Three considerations are important in the blood calcium level:

1. The deposition and resorption of the bone
2. The absorption of calcium from the GI tract
3. The excretion of calcium in the urine and feces

Vitamin D, calcitonin, and parathyroid hormones are necessary for the absorption and utilization of calcium.

The best food sources of calcium are milk and cheese. Other sources include beans, nuts, cauliflower, lettuce, and egg yolks. The average daily intake is 200 to 2500 mg. The recommended daily allowances vary from 360 mg for infants to 1200 mg for females 15 to 18 years of age. During pregnancy, 1300 mg is required. Calcium is removed from the body via the urine and feces.

Calcium is required for the formation and maintenance of strong bones and teeth. It is also necessary for normal blood clotting. Calcium has a depressing or sedative effect on neuromuscular irritability and thus promotes normal transmission of nerve impulses, as well as helps to regulate normal muscle contraction and relaxation. It helps hold body cells together by establishing the thickness and strength of cell membranes. One of its most important functions is to act as an enzyme activator for chemical reactions in the body.

Hypocalcemia. Hypocalcemia develops when the serum level is below 4.5 mEq/L. A deficiency may be caused by a variety of problems (Box 24-6):

1. Infusion of excess amounts of citrated blood (citrates bind to the calcium)
2. Excessive loss through diarrhea
3. Inadequate dietary intake of calcium or vitamin D
4. Decreased parathyroid function
5. Pancreatic disease
6. Small bowel disease

The signs and symptoms of hypocalcemia are neuromuscular irritation and increased excitability. As neuromuscular signs and symptoms increase, tetany can occur. Tetany is a condition characterized by excessive muscle cramps, laryngeal spasms, stridor, and carpal pedal spasms.

Hypercalcemia. Hypercalcemia occurs when calcium levels exceed 5.8 mEq/L. It may occur when calcium stored in the bone enters the circulation, for example, in patients who are immobilized (Box 24-7). An increased intake of calcium or vitamin D also causes hypercalcemia. Neuromuscular activity is depressed, and renal calculi may develop because of the excretion of high levels of calcium by the kidneys.

Box 24-6

CAUSES AND SIGNS AND SYMPTOMS OF HYPOCALCEMIA

CAUSES

Excess binding of calcium ions
Large amount of citrated blood
Alkalosis
Dietary deficiency of calcium
Chronic renal failure
Pancreatic disease
Disease of small bowel
Draining intestinal fistulas
Deficiency of parathyroid hormone or vitamin D
Increased magnesium

SIGNS AND SYMPTOMS

Osteoporosis, pathologic fractures
Tingling around nose, mouth, ears, fingers, toes*
Muscle spasm of feet and hands*
Tetany
Nausea, vomiting*
Diarrhea*
Cardiac dysrhythmias, cardiac arrest
Calcium deposits in body tissues

NURSING INTERVENTIONS

Encourage intake of a diet high in calcium-rich foods
Administer calcium and vitamin D as prescribed by the physician
Monitor I&O

*Most common signs and symptoms.

Box 24-7

CAUSES AND SIGNS AND SYMPTOMS OF HYPERCALCEMIA

CAUSES

Loss from bone
- Immobilization
- Metastatic bone cancer
- Multiple myeloma

Excess intake
- Dietary
- Antacids containing calcium

Increased absorption
- Increased parathyroid hormone
- Increased vitamin D

SIGNS AND SYMPTOMS

Thirst, polyuria*
Renal stones
Decreased deep tendon reflexes
Lethargy, coma
Cardiac dysrhythmias, cardiac arrest
Decreased muscle tone*
Decreased GI motility

NURSING INTERVENTIONS

Assist in the promotion of excretion of calcium in the urine
Administer diuretics as ordered by the physician
Encourage drinking 3000-4000 ml of fluids per day
Monitor I&O

*Most common signs and symptoms.

Phosphorus

The normal blood level of **phosphorus** (HPO_4), chiefly an intracellular anion, is approximately 4 mEq/L. Phosphorus and calcium have an inverse relationship in the body: an increase in one causes a decrease in the other. As blood calcium levels increase, phosphorus levels must decrease, and vice versa. The majority (70% to 80%) of phosphorus is found in an individual's bones and teeth combined with calcium, 10% is in an individual's muscle, and the remaining 10% is in the nerve tissue of the body.

Dietary intake of phosphorus is usually 800 to 1500 mg per day. The minimum daily requirement is 800 mg. Intake should be increased during pregnancy and lactation. An adequate intake of vitamin D is necessary for the absorption of both calcium and phosphorus. Because there is a generous amount of phosphorus in many foods, a deficiency seldom occurs. Foods especially high in phosphorus include beef, pork, fish, poultry, milk products, and legumes. The kidneys are responsible for approximately 90% of the excretion of phosphorus. The remainder is excreted in the feces.

With calcium, phosphorus contributes to the support and maintenance of bones and teeth. It is important in many chemical reactions and acts as a buffer to regulate the body's acid-base balance. It promotes the effectiveness of many of the B vitamins, assists in normal nerve and muscle activity, and participates in carbohydrate metabolism.

Hypophosphatemia. Hypophosphatemia can occur from a dietary insufficiency, impaired kidney function, or maldistribution of phosphate. Muscle weakness, especially affecting the respiratory muscles, may occur.

Hyperphosphatemia. Hyperphosphatemia most commonly occurs as a result of renal insufficiency. Another cause is increased intake of phosphate or vitamin D. Signs and symptoms of tetany, numbness and tingling around the mouth, and muscle spasms develop.

Magnesium

The normal blood level of **magnesium** (Mg^{++}), the second most abundant cation in the intracellular fluid, is 1.5 to 2.4 mEq/L. Although there are only small amounts of magnesium in the blood, it is important in maintaining normal body function. The majority (60%) is found in the bone, 39% in the muscle and soft tissue, and 1% in the extracellular fluid, most of which is in the cerebrospinal fluid.

Dietary intake is usually 200 to 400 mg daily. The minimum daily requirement is 250 mg for the average adult, 150 mg for an infant, and 400 mg for a female during pregnancy and lactation. Magnesium is another electrolyte commonly distributed in foods. Whole grains, fruits, vegetables, meat, fish, legumes, and dairy products are dietary sources.

The major route of magnesium excretion is the kidneys. There is a correlation between the amount of magnesium and the amount of potassium excreted. The kidneys do not conserve potassium, but they do conserve magnesium; therefore if a magnesium deficiency develops, the body will conserve magnesium at the expense of excreting potassium.

Magnesium has not been a widely recognized electrolyte until recently. It is now linked as a cofactor in the activation of many enzymes. It also promotes regulation of serum calcium, phosphate, and potassium levels and is essential for integrity of nervous tissue, skeletal muscle, and cardiac functioning.

Hypomagnesemia. Hypomagnesemia develops when blood levels fall below 1.5 mEq/L. A decrease in magnesium often parallels decreased potassium, because if the magnesium level is low, the kidneys tend to excrete more potassium. Hypomagnesemia presents signs and symptoms of increased neuromuscular irritability similar to those observed with hypocalcemia (Box 24-8). The major causes of low magnesium are increased excretion by the kidneys, impaired absorption from the GI tract, and prolonged malnutrition.

Hypermagnesemia. Hypermagnesemia develops when blood levels exceed 2.5 mEq/L. It rarely occurs when kid-

Box 24-8 CAUSES AND SIGNS AND SYMPTOMS OF HYPOMAGNESEMIA

CAUSES

- Decreased intake
  - Prolonged malnutrition
  - Starvation
- Impaired absorption from GI tract
  - Alcoholism
  - Hypercalcemia
  - Diarrhea
  - Draining intestinal fistulas
- Conditions causing large losses of urine

SIGNS AND SYMPTOMS

- Mental changes*
  - Agitation, depression, confusion
- Paresthesias*
- Tremors
- Ataxia
- Cramps, spasticity, tetany
- Tachycardia
- Hypotension
- Dysrhythmias

NURSING INTERVENTIONS

- Increase intake of magnesium-rich foods
- Administer magnesium supplements as prescribed by the physician
- Monitor I&O

*Most common signs and symptoms.

Box 24-9 CAUSES AND SIGNS AND SYMPTOMS OF HYPERMAGNESEMIA

CAUSES

- Renal failure
- Diabetic ketoacidosis with severe water loss

SIGNS AND SYMPTOMS

- Hypotension*
- Vasodilation*
  - Heat
  - Thirst
  - Nausea/vomiting
- Loss of deep tendon reflexes
- Respiratory depression

Prolonged or Severe Excess

- Coma
- Cardiac arrest

NURSING INTERVENTIONS

- Promote urine excretion
- Administer diuretics as prescribed by the physician
- Decrease intake of foods or medications high in magnesium
- Monitor I&O

*Most common signs and symptoms.

ney function is normal. The three major causes are impaired renal function, excess magnesium administration, and diabetic ketoacidosis when there is severe water loss (Box 24-9). An excess of magnesium severely restricts nerve and muscle activity.

Bicarbonate

The normal level of **bicarbonate** (HCO_3^-), a main anion of the extracellular fluid, is 22 to 24 mEq/L. It is an alkaline electrolyte whose major function is the regulation of the acid-base balance, also called acid-alkaline balance. Bicarbonate acts as a buffer to neutralize acids in the body and maintain the 20:1 bicarbonate/carbonic acid ratio needed to keep the body in homeostasis. The kidneys selectively regulate the amount of bicarbonate retained or excreted.

ACID-BASE BALANCE

Acid-base balance means homeostasis of the hydrogen ion (H^+) concentration in the body fluids. The hydrogen ion concentration is determined by the ratio of carbonic acid (H_2CO_3) to bicarbonate (HCO_3) in the extracellular fluid. The ratio needed for homeostasis is 1 part carbonic acid to 20 parts bicarbonate. The symbol used to indicate hydrogen ion balance is pH. When pH is measured, it is the hydrogen ion concentration in the patient's body that is measured. A sample of extracellular fluid, specifically arterial blood, is used to measure an individual's pH.

Arterial blood gases will determine if a solution is acid, neutral, or alkaline. The more hydrogen ions in a solution, the more acid the solution. The fewer hydrogen ions in a solution, the more alkaline the solution. The terms *base* and *alkaline* are interchangeable: a base is an alkaline substance. An inverse relationship exists between hydrogen ion concentration and the pH level: as the hydrogen ion numbers increase, the acidity of the solution increases and the pH decreases. The opposite happens with alkalinity: the number of hydrogen ions decreases and the pH increases. A pH of less than 7.35 is acid. A pH of greater than 7.45 is alkaline. The normal pH of arterial blood is approximately 7.45, whereas the normal pH of venous blood and interstitial fluid is approximately 7.35. Between 7.35 and 7.45 is considered normal blood pH (Fig. 24-6).

There are two general types of disturbances that can cause a pH imbalance. One imbalance adds or subtracts the base substance—bicarbonate. The other imbalance adds or subtracts the acid substance—carbonic acid. The body's metabolism affects the base side of balance, so a bicarbonate imbalance causes metabolic acidosis or alkalosis. The body's respiratory system affects the acid side of the balance, so a carbonic acid imbalance causes respiratory acidosis or alkalosis. Fig. 24-7 on p. 516 shows the carbonic acid/bicarbonate ratio and pH.

The body has three systems that work to keep the pH in the narrow range of normal: the blood buffers, the respiratory system, and the kidneys. These systems are the body's three lines of defense that are constantly working to maintain a normal pH.

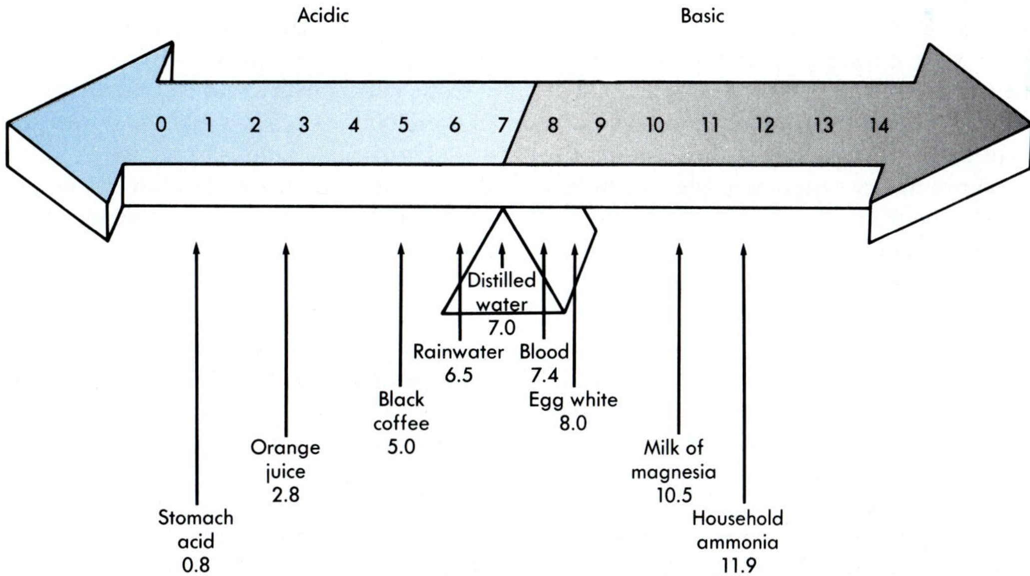

FIG. 24-6 The pH scale. A pH of 7 is considered neutral, so the scale is depicted as balancing at that point. Values to the left (below 7) are acidic (the lower the number, the more acidic). Values to the right (above 7) are basic (the higher the number, the more basic). Representative fluids and their approximate pHs are listed below the figure.

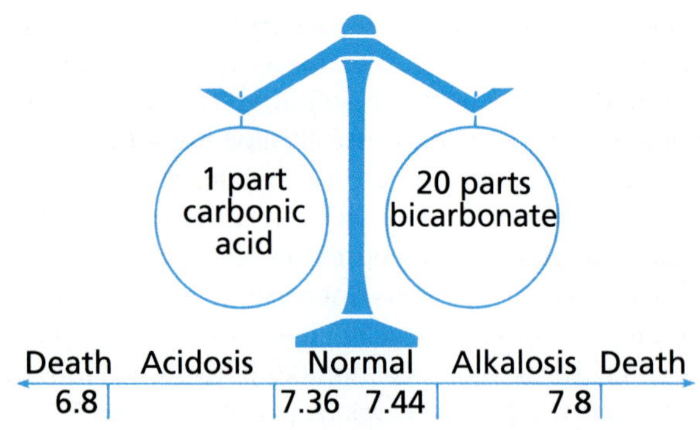

FIG. 24-7 Carbonic acid/bicarbonate ratio and pH.

The blood **buffers** can be considered chemical sponges. They circulate throughout the body in pairs, neutralizing excess acids or alkalies by contributing or accepting hydrogen ions. One buffer will dominate if the solution is too acid; the other if the solution is too alkaline. They work within a fraction of a second to prevent an excessive change in the hydrogen ion concentration. There are four major buffer systems in the body. The bicarbonate/carbonic acid system is the most important. Others are the phosphates, proteins, and hemoglobin buffer systems.

For every 1 million hydrogen ions that enter the body, the buffer systems can neutralize all but five! Once the buffer systems are exhausted, they call on the second line of defense: the lungs. By speeding up or slowing down respirations, the lungs can increase or decrease the amount of carbon dioxide in the blood. When carbon dioxide is removed from the blood, the carbonic acid level is lowered. Where it took seconds for the buffer systems to work, it takes minutes for the lungs to begin to adjust the pH. Even though the respiratory system is slower than the buffers, the lungs can eliminate large amounts of acid from the body in the form of carbon dioxide. The respiratory system regulates pH by removing carbon dioxide from the blood. Just enough carbon dioxide is retained in the blood to maintain a normal pH level. If the pH drops suddenly from the normal range of 7.35 to 7.45 to 7.0, the respiratory system can return the pH to about 7.2 to 7.3 within 1 minute. The respiratory center in the brain provides the stimulus to increase respirations; however, as the hydrogen ion concentration approaches normal, the stimulus is lost. The buffers will assist in returning the level to normal.

The third line of defense is the kidneys. The role of the lungs in coping with an imbalance is simple: we breathe either slower or faster. The kidneys have much selective control. They can excrete varying amounts of acid or base. If the acidity of blood rises above normal, the kidneys will selectively eliminate more acids so the hydrogen ion concentration increases in the blood. If the blood becomes too alkaline, the kidneys will selectively eliminate more bases, especially bicarbonate. Normal urine is acidic because the body produces excess acids in the metabolic processes that occur continuously in the body. The kidneys are the slowest of the systems, but they are efficient enough to return the pH to exactly normal. Their response takes hours to days.

The three systems work closely together to maintain a normal hydrogen ion concentration. The buffers are immediate and continuous in contributing or accepting hydrogen ions. The respiratory system can come into play within minutes, regulating the carbon dioxide level in the blood and thus controlling carbonic acid. The kidneys are the third line of defense, and although they work more slowly than the other two systems, they can eliminate either hydrogen ions or bicarbonate ions, which means they can either increase or decrease pH.

ACID-BASE IMBALANCES

Acid-base balance means homeostasis of the hydrogen ion concentration. An upset in acid-base balance results in either acidosis or alkalosis. When blood pH is below 7.35, acidosis exists; when blood pH is above 7.45, alkalosis exists. The lungs and the kidneys are the two major organs responsible for regulation of the acid and base substances in the body. When imbalances occur, they represent an imbalance in the function of the lungs, kidneys, or both.

There are four primary types of acid-base imbalances: respiratory acidosis, respiratory alkalosis, metabolic acidosis, and metabolic alkalosis.

Respiratory Acidosis

Any condition that impairs a normal ventilation causes respiratory acidosis (Box 24-10). A retention of carbon dioxide occurs with a resultant increase of carbonic acid in the blood. As pH falls and the normal 1:20 carbonic acid:bicarbonate ratio is upset, the P_{CO_2} (partial carbon dioxide) level increases. Shallow respirations result because of the retained carbon dioxide. The patient will also experience a depression of central nervous system activity. Because the lungs are responsible for the respiratory parameters of the acid-base balance, the kidneys, which are responsible for the metabolic parameters, will attempt to compensate by retaining the base substance bicarbonate.

Treatment for respiratory acidosis is aimed at improving ventilation. The primary goal is to support the patient's respirations. Intermittent positive-pressure breathing (IPPB) to assist in exhaling carbon dioxide, antibiotic for any respiratory infection, adequate hydration (2 to 3 L/day) to keep the mucous membranes moist and aid in removal of secretions, and bronchodilators to help reduce bronchial spasms may be part of the treatment regimen. Therapy is also directed at correcting the primary condition responsible for the imbalance.

Respiratory Alkalosis

Respiratory alkalosis is caused by hyperventilation (Box 24-11). Respirations that increase in rate, depth, or both can result in the loss of excessive amounts of carbon dioxide with a resultant lowering of the carbonic acid level in the blood. The pH rises because of the decrease in carbonic acid being "blown off" with each exhalation.

The common treatment for respiratory alkalosis is sedation and reassurance. If the cause is anxiety, the patient should be made aware of his abnormal breathing pattern. The patient should be instructed to breathe slowly to retain and accumulate carbon dioxide in the body. Another effective treatment is for the patient to breathe into a paper bag, which will cause rebreathing of the exhaled carbon dioxide.

Box 24-10 CAUSES AND COMMON CLINICAL SIGNS AND SYMPTOMS OF RESPIRATORY ACIDOSIS

CAUSES

- Pneumonia
- Respiratory failure
- Atelectasis
- Drug overdose
- Paralysis of respiratory muscles (Guillain-Barré syndrome, poliomyelitis, myasthenia gravis)
- Traumatic injuries to the thorax (flail chest)
- Obesity
- Airway obstruction
- Head injuries
- Cerebrovascular accident (stroke)
- Drowning
- Cystic fibrosis

COMMON CLINICAL SIGNS AND SYMPTOMS

Central Nervous System

- Lethargy
- Disorientation
- Occipital headache
- Dizziness
- Decreasing level of consciousness

Cardiopulmonary System

- Dyspnea
- Tachycardia
- Hypertension
- Cardiac dysrhythmias

Musculoskeletal System

- Tremors
- Weakness

LABORATORY DATA

- pH less than 7.35
- $Paco_2$ greater than 45 mm Hg (unless the patient has chronic obstructive pulmonary disease)
- Pao_2 normal or below 80 mm Hg, depending on severity of acidosis
- O_2 saturation normal or below 95%, depending on severity of acidosis
- HCO_3 normal in early respiratory acidosis
- K^+ above 5 mEq/L

Box 24-11 CAUSES AND COMMON CLINICAL SIGNS AND SYMPTOMS OF RESPIRATORY ALKALOSIS

CAUSES

- Anxiety
- Fear
- Anemia
- Hypermetabolic states
- Disorders of the central nervous system (head injuries, infections)
- Drugs (aspirin overdose)
- Asthma
- Pneumonia
- Inappropriate mechanical ventilator settings

COMMON CLINICAL SIGNS AND SYMPTOMS

Central Nervous System

- Anxious appearance
- Irritability
- Tingling of the extremities
- Fainting
- Dizziness

Cardiopulmonary System

- Tachypnea
- Cardiac dysrhythmias

Musculoskeletal System

- Tetany
- Muscle weakness

LABORATORY DATA

- pH 7.45 or greater
- $Paco_2$ less than 35 mm Hg
- Pao_2 normal
- O_2 saturation normal
- HCO_3 normal
- K^+ below 3.5 mEq/L

Box 24-12 CAUSES AND COMMON CLINICAL SIGNS AND SYMPTOMS OF METABOLIC ACIDOSIS

CAUSES

- Starvation
- Dehydration
- Diabetic ketoacidosis
- Renal failure
- Shock
- Diarrhea
- Drugs (methanol, ethanol, formic acid, paraldehyde, aspirin)
- Renal tubular acidosis

COMMON CLINICAL SIGNS AND SYMPTOMS

Central Nervous System

- Lethargy
- Headache
- Decreasing level of consciousness

Cardiopulmonary System

- Kussmaul respirations
- Cardiac dysrhythmias

Gastrointestinal System

- Anorexia
- Nausea
- Vomiting
- Diarrhea

Musculoskeletal System

- Weakness

LABORATORY DATA

- pH less than 7.35
- $Paco_2$ normal, or less than 35 mm Hg if lungs are compensating
- Pao_2 normal, or less than 35 mm Hg if lungs are compensating
- O_2 saturation normal
- HCO_3 below 22 mEq/L
- K^+ above 5 mEq/L

Box 24-13 CAUSES AND COMMON CLINICAL SIGNS AND SYMPTOMS OF METABOLIC ALKALOSIS

CAUSES

- Excessive vomiting
- Prolonged gastric suctioning
- Electrolyte disturbance
- Cushing's disease
- Drugs (steroids, sodium bicarbonate, diuretics)
- Hyperaldosteronism

COMMON CLINICAL SIGNS AND SYMPTOMS

Central Nervous System

- Headache
- Irritability
- Lethargy
- Decreases in level of consciousness

Cardiopulmonary System

- Atrial tachycardia
- Slow, shallow respirations with periods of apnea
- Bradycardia

Gastrointestinal System

- Nausea
- Vomiting

Musculoskeletal System

- Numbness and tingling of extremities
- Hypertonicity of muscles
- Tetany

LABORATORY DATA

- pH greater than 7.45
- $Paco_2$ normal or greater than 45 mm Hg if lungs are compensating
- Pao_2 normal
- O_2 saturation normal
- HCO_3 above 26 mEq/L
- K^+ less than 3.5 mEq/L

Metabolic Acidosis

Metabolic acidosis can result from a gain of hydrogen ions or a loss of bicarbonate, in other words, retaining too many acids (H^+ ions) or losing too many bases (HCO_3^-) (Box 24-12). Without sufficient bases, the pH of the blood falls below the normal 7.35 to 7.45. With the loss of base substances, the bicarbonate level will also drop. The effect of metabolic acidosis is hyperventilation, as the lungs attempt to compensate by blowing off carbon dioxide to lower the P_{CO_2} level. There are many causes of metabolic acidosis. Administration of sodium bicarbonate is the usual treatment for acidosis.

Metabolic Alkalosis

Metabolic alkalosis results when a significant amount of acid is lost from the body or an increase in the bicarbonate level occurs (Box 24-13). The most common cause of metabolic alkalosis is vomiting gastric content, normally high in acid. Metabolic alkalosis can occur also in patients who ingest excess amounts of alkaline agents, such as bicarbonate-containing antacids, for example, Alka-Seltzer or soda bicarbonate. Metabolic alkalosis depresses the central nervous system. Again, as with the other acid-base imbalances, treatment is aimed at the cause.

REFERENCES AND SUGGESTED READINGS

1. Cole G: *Basic nursing skills and concepts,* St Louis, 1991, Mosby.
2. Crowley LV: *Introduction to human disease,* ed 3, Boston, 1992, Jones & Bartlett.
3. Farley JM: Myths & facts . . . about electrolytes, *Nursing 89* 19(10):80, 1989.
4. Lewis SM, Collier IC: *Medical-surgical nursing: assessment and management of clinical problems,* ed 3, St Louis, 1992, Mosby.
5. Loeb S, editor: *Nursing procedures: student version,* Springhouse, Pa, 1993, Springhouse.
6. Long BC, Phipps WJ, Cassmeyer VL: *Medical surgical nursing: a nursing process approach,* ed 3, St Louis, 1993, Mosby.
7. Metheny NM: Why worry about IV fluids, *Am J Nurs* 90(6):50, 1990.
8. Potter PA, Perry AG: *Basic nursing: theory and practice,* ed 3, St Louis, 1995, Mosby.
9. Smeltzer SC, Bare BG: *Brunner and Suddarth's textbook of medical-surgical nursing,* ed 7, Philadelphia, 1992, Lippincott.
10. Terry J: The other electrolytes: magnesium, calcium, and phosphorus, *J Intravenous Nurs* 14(3):167, 1991.
11. Weldy NJ: *Body fluids and electrolytes: a programmed presentation,* ed 6, St Louis, 1992, Mosby.

CHAPTER CHALLENGE

KEY POINTS

- Water is the primary fluid in the body.
- The two fluid compartments are the intracellular and extracellular compartments. The extracellular compartment is composed of the interstitial and intravascular areas.
- Fluid movement takes place by means of three passive transport systems: diffusion, osmosis, and filtration; and one active transport system: active transport by ATP energy.
- Electrolytes are chemical compounds that carry either a positive or negative charge. Positive ions are called cations; negative ions are called anions. To maintain homeostasis, the cations and anions must balance each other in the body fluids.
- Sodium is the major extracellular cation in the body. Water follows sodium as it moves from one fluid compartment to another.
- Potassium is the major intracellular cation in the body. Imbalances in potassium, either high or low levels, may cause life-threatening cardiac conditions.
- The four acid-base imbalances are respiratory acidosis, respiratory alkalosis, metabolic acidosis, and metabolic alkalosis.
- Any process that interferes with normal ventilation and causes a decrease or an increase in the excretion of volatile acids can cause respiratory acidosis or respiratory alkalosis.
- Any process that interferes with normal production or excretion of nonvolatile hydrogen ions can cause metabolic acidosis or metabolic alkalosis.
- Respiratory acidosis or alkalosis will result when the lungs fail to regulate the carbonic acid concentration in the blood. Metabolic acidosis or alkalosis will result when the kidneys fail to regulate the bicarbonate concentration in the blood.
- If the lungs are unable to regain their ability to correct respiratory acidosis, the kidneys will respond in an attempt to correct the imbalance. If the kidneys are unable to regain their ability to correct metabolic acidosis, the lungs will respond in an attempt to correct the imbalance.

STUDY QUESTIONS

1. Mr. Kiley, age 66, has recently been experiencing excessive edema in his feet. The nurse talks with Mr. Kiley about dietary changes that might be causing the water retention associated with his edema. Which electrolyte has the greatest influence on water balance in the body?
   1. Sodium (Na^+)
   2. Potassium (K^+)
   3. Chloride (Cl^-)
   4. Calcium (Ca^{++})
2. Which regulatory system is the body's first line of defense in keeping the pH within normal limits:
   1. Buffers in the blood.
   2. Respiratory system.
   3. Renal system.
   4. Blood pressure.
3. The most accurate method for the nurse to use in determining water balance in the body is to:
   1. Weigh the patient daily at the same time each day, dressed in the same clothes, and use the same scale.
   2. Record an accurate 24-hour I&O
   3. Ask the patient to document on a form left at her bedside.
   4. Have the same nurse care for the patient each day.
4. Mrs. Wright is concerned about giving her family adequate amounts of potassium in their diets. She asks the nurse to help plan a meal containing foods with potassium. Which diet would contain foods with the most potassium?
   1. White beans and ham, green salad, and fresh fruit plate.
   2. Macaroni and cheese, corn bread, and Jell-O.
   3. Tacos, chips and salsa, and ice cream.
   4. Seafood plate, marinated vegetables, sponge cake.
5. The major route of excretion of all electrolytes from the body is via the:
   1. Skin.
   2. Lungs.
   3. Kidneys.
   4. Feces.
6. Mrs. Rogers returns from abdominal surgery with a Foley catheter. At the end of the shift, the catheter bag needs to be emptied. Before beginning the procedure, the nurse dons a pair of gloves. Mrs. Rogers asks if there is something wrong with her that requires the nurse to be so careful. The most appropriate response by the nurse is:
   1. "We can never be too careful when working in a hospital."
   2. "Your diagnosis and surgery requires us to wear gloves while doing this procedure."
   3. "It's not you, Mrs. Rogers. This is a procedure we use for all patients when we empty Foley catheter bags."
   4. "We don't always wear gloves, but I prefer to for safety reasons."
7. Fluid movement in the cells equalizes the ions or molecules on each side of the semipermeable membrane. The movement of water from an area of lower concentration to an area of higher concentration occurs through:
   1. Diffusion.
   2. Filtration.
   3. Active transport.
   4. Osmosis.
8. The largest fluid compartment in the body is the:
   1. Intracellular.
   2. Extracellular.
   3. Interstitial.
   4. Intravascular.
9. Diffusion, osmosis, and filtration are all examples of:
   1. Active transport.
   2. Passive transport.
   3. ATP energy.
   4. Krebs cycle.
10. The symbol used to indicate hydrogen ion concentration in the body is:
    1. mEq.
    2. ATP.
    3. pH.
    4. ml.

25

CARE OF THE PATIENT WITH AN INTEGUMENTARY DISORDER

Linda North

KEY TERMS

ANATOMY AND PHYSIOLOGY

ceruminous gland
corium/ dermis
epidermis
integument
melanin
sebaceous gland
sebum
sudoriferous gland

MEDICAL-SURGICAL

alopecia
autograft
contracture
Curling's ulcer
debridement
eschar
excoriation
exudate
heterograft (xenograft)
homograft (allograft)
keloid
macule
nevi
papule
pediculosis
pruritus
pustulant vesicle
rule of nines
suppuration
urticaria
verruca
vesicle
wheal

LEARNING OBJECTIVES

After reading this chapter, the student should be able to do the following:

Anatomy and Physiology

- Define the key terms.
- List and discuss the three primary functions of the integumentary system.
- Describe the differences between epidermis and dermis.
- List the three major types of glands located in the skin and discuss their functions.

Medical-Surgical

- Define the key terms.
- State the general nursing interventions for the patient with a skin disorder.
- Identify the nursing interventions needed to meet the emotional needs of a patient with a skin disorder.
- Differentiate among skin inflammations resulting from viruses, bacteria, fungi, and parasites and the appropriate therapies.
- Differentiate between type I and type II herpes.
- Discuss nursing interventions for the patient with impetigo contagiosa.
- List three nursing diagnoses for the patient with acne.
- Differentiate among types of skin tumors and medical interventions.
- State five important interventions in order of priority in the emergent phase of a major burn.
- State how to classify burns according to depth and body surface area involved.
- Identify the nursing interventions for each phase of burn care to prevent complications and promote homeostasis.
- List the primary patient and family education areas in discharge planning for the burn patient.

RELATED TOPICS OF INTEREST

- Signs, symptoms, and physical assessment (Chapter 9)
- Diet therapy (Chapter 19)

- Introduction to anatomy and physiology (Chapter 23)
- Fluids and electrolytes (Chapter 24)
- Care of the patient with a urinary disorder (Chapter 30)
- Care of the patient with an immune disorder (Chapter 36)
- Care of the patient with cancer (Chapter 38)

The skin or **integument,** a major organ, is the outer covering of the body, and together with its appendages—the hair, nails, and special glands—makes up the integumentary system. Skin is essential to life. Society has long held healthy skin in high esteem, probably because it is so easily viewed by others. People spend many hours grooming their hair, cleansing their skin, and manicuring their nails. A closer look reveals that the integument is really the body's protector—its first line of defense against infection and injury. The skin is pliable yet tough, it resists abrasions, and as it wears, it is constantly renewed from layers directly beneath it. It also insulates and cushions deeper organs. It functions in the prevention of loss of body fluids and in the regulation of body temperature. The skin also is the sensory contact with the environment: it is sensitive to heat, cold, touch, pressure, and pain.

ANATOMY AND PHYSIOLOGY

Functions of the Skin

Even though the skin covers the outside of the body, its main function is homeostasis and protection of the internal organs (Box 25-1). Daily it is subjected to temperature and humidity changes, trauma, ecchymosis, abrasions, contact with pathogens, and wear and tear. In an attempt to protect and maintain the body, the skin carries out the following functions.

Box 25-1 FUNCTIONS OF THE SKIN

Protection from environment: pathogenic organisms, foreign substances, injuries, and heat rays. The skin is the body's natural barrier against infection.
Heat regulation
Prevention of dehydration
Reservoir for food and water

Protection. Within the skin are sensory receptors that receive information about the environment. Messages about heat, cold, pain, pressure, and touch are received and relayed to the central nervous system for interpretation. Healthy skin protects the body from absorbing many chemicals and foreign substances. Additionally, as long as the skin remains intact, it provides protection from many microorganisms in the environment. Internal organs are cushioned and protected by a subcutaneous layer of adipose (fat) tissue. The skin aids in elimination and prevention of dehydration and serves as a reservoir for food and water.

Temperature Regulation. Skin assists the body in maintaining a constant temperature under varying internal and external conditions. It accomplishes this by allowing blood vessels near the surface to constrict when the environment is cold to preserve heat and allowing them to dilate when it is hot to release excess body heat. Sweat glands release moisture, which results in cooling as the moisture is evaporated. A layer of adipose tissue works as an insulator by retaining heat.

Vitamin D Synthesis. Cholesterol compounds located in the skin are converted to vitamin D when exposed to the ultraviolet rays of the sun. This vitamin is necessary for healthy bone development. Prolonged exposure to the sun's rays, which is ultraviolet radiation, should be avoided because of the increased possibility of development of skin cancer.

Basic Structure of the Skin

Skin consists of two layers: the outermost epidermis and the inner dermis or corium. Beneath these layers of skin lies the subcutaneous layer, or superficial fascia (Fig. 25-1).

Epidermis. The **epidermis** (the superficial, avascular layers of the skin, made up of an outer, dead, cornified portion and a deep, living, cellular portion) is composed of stratified squamous (from Latin *squama,* scale) epithelium. It is divided into layers, or strata. The cells of the epidermis are tightly packed and without any distinct blood supply. The innermost layer is called the *stratum germinativum;* it is the only layer of the epidermis that is able to undergo cell division and reproduce itself. It receives its blood supply and nutrition from the underlying dermis through the process called diffusion. This provides a constant new supply of cells for the upper layers and also enables the skin to repair itself from injury. As these cells are pushed to the surface, they undergo a series of changes. The internal structures of the cells are destroyed and the cells die. When they reach the outermost layer, called the *stratum corneum,* they

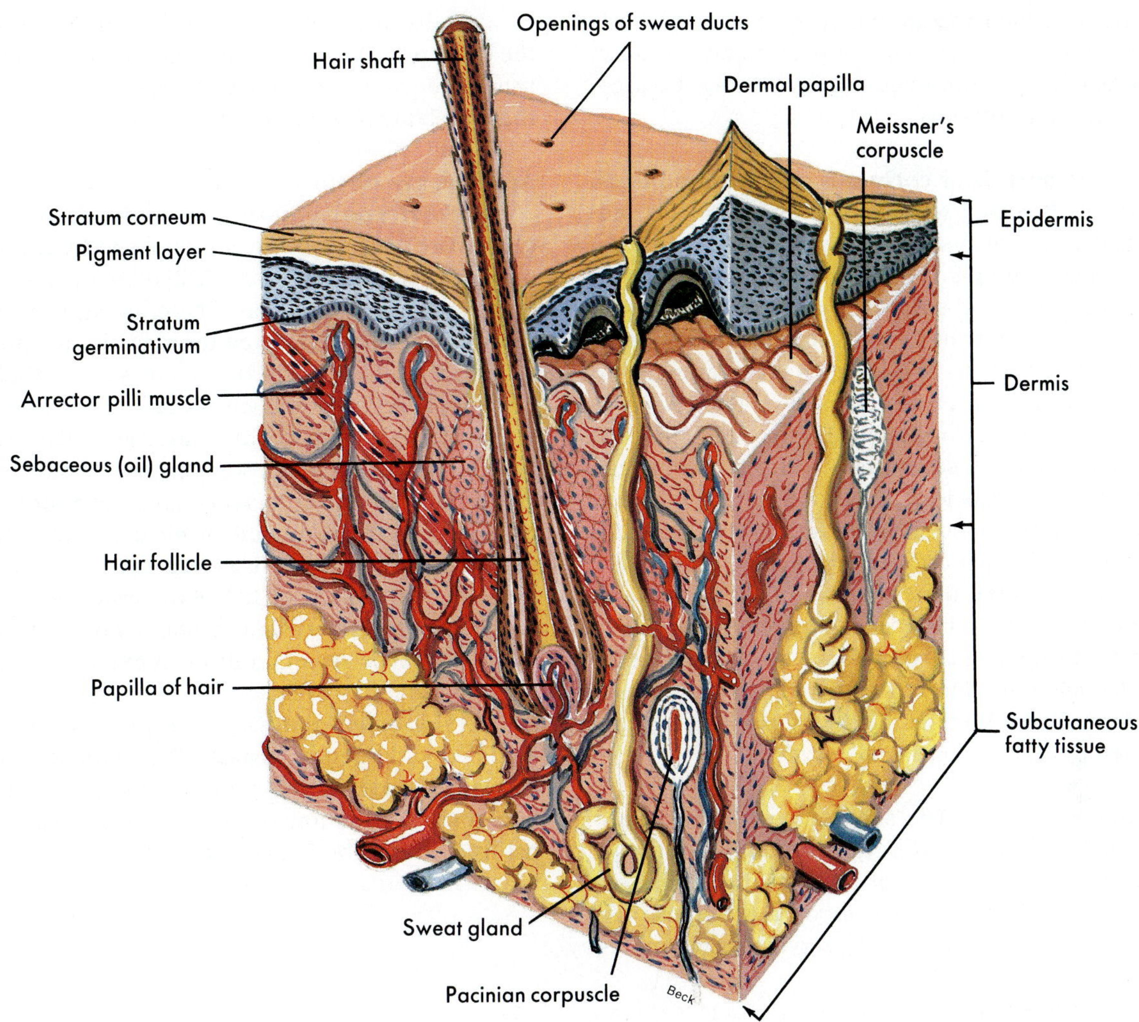

FIG. 25-1 Microscopic view of the skin in longitudinal section. The epidermis is shown raised at one corner to reveal the ridges in the dermis.

have become flat and the cell structure has become filled with a protein called *keratin* (horn), sometimes referred to as the horny layer. The keratin makes the cells dry, tough, and somewhat waterproof. There are several layers of these cells, and they are continually sloughing off, only to be replaced by new ones. From the birth of the new cell in the stratum germinativum to the death and sloughing off in the stratum corneum, the cell undergoes many changes. This whole process takes approximately 1 month. Another layer in the epidermis contains highly specialized cells called *melanocytes;* these cells give rise to the pigment called **melanin** (a black or dark brown pigment that occurs naturally in the hair and skin and in the iris and choroid of the eye), which is responsible for skin color. The greater the concentration of melanin, the darker the color of the skin. Sometimes irregular patches of concentrations of melanin occur producing "freckles." The amount of melanin a person has is inherited from the parents. Although skin color is inherited, exposure to the sun and other extraneous factors can influence skin color.

Occasionally an individual has an inherited inability to produce melanin. This results in a condition called *albinism.* An individual who has this condition is called an *albino* and has an absence of color in the skin, hair, and eyes.

Carotene, another pigment, can be found in the stratum corneum in persons of Asian descent. Carotene, along with melanin, gives rise to the yellow hue of the skin.

On the soles of the feet, palms of the hands, and tips of fingers and toes, there are series of ridges and grooves that develop in utero, during the third and fourth months of fetal development. These grooves and ridges are genetically determined and are unique to each individual. Their function is to increase gripping ability. Because they are unique, footprints and fingerprints may be used for identification purposes.

Dermis. The **dermis** or **corium** is often referred to as the true skin. It is well supplied with blood vessels and nerves and also contains glands and hair follicles. It varies in thickness throughout the body but tends to be very thick in the palms and soles. The dermis is composed of connective tissue with the cells scattered among collagen and elastic fibers. The collagen gives strength to the dermis, while the elastic connective fibers give it flexibility. The cells throughout this layer are bathed in tissue fluid called interstitial fluid. With the normal aging process the dermis loses some of its elastic connective fibers, and the subcutaneous tissue directly beneath it loses some of its adipose tissue; wrinkling of the skin results. Located in the upper portion of the dermis are small, fingerlike projections called *papillae* that project into the lower epidermal layer. They contain many capillaries that allow oxygen and nutrient exchange within the epidermal layer. Without the dermal papillae, the epidermal layer would be unable to survive.

Subcutaneous Layer. The subcutaneous layer, sometimes called the *superficial fascia,* is the layer of tissue directly beneath the dermis that connects the skin to the muscle surfaces. This layer is composed of adipose tissue and loose connective tissue. It serves several important functions:

1. It stores water and fat.
2. It insulates the body by virtue of its composition.
3. It serves as a shock absorber, protecting tissues and organs lying beneath it.
4. It serves as a pathway for nerves and vessels.

The distribution of subcutaneous tissue throughout the body provides shape and contour. A woman's body usually contains more subcutaneous tissue than a man's; thus her body is softer and more rounded.

Appendages of the Skin.

Sudoriferous glands. The **sudoriferous** (sweat) **glands** are coiled, tubelike structures located in the dermis and subcutaneous layers. The tubes open into pores on the surface of the skin. There are approximately 3 million sweat glands located throughout the integumentary system. These glands excrete sweat, resulting in cooling of the body surface. Sweat is composed of water, salts, urea, uric acid, ammonia, sugar, lactic acid, and ascorbic acid. These glands can be classified in two groups according to location and secretion. *Eccrine* glands are the most numerous and are located throughout the body. They secrete a clear, watery sweat through pores on the surface of the body. *Apocrine* glands are located in the axillary and genital region and secrete a more milky-type secretion through excretory ducts that open into the hair follicles.

Ceruminous glands. **Ceruminous glands** are modified sudoriferous glands. They secrete a waxlike substance called *cerumen* and are located in the external ear canal. It is thought that cerumen protects the canal from foreign body invasion.

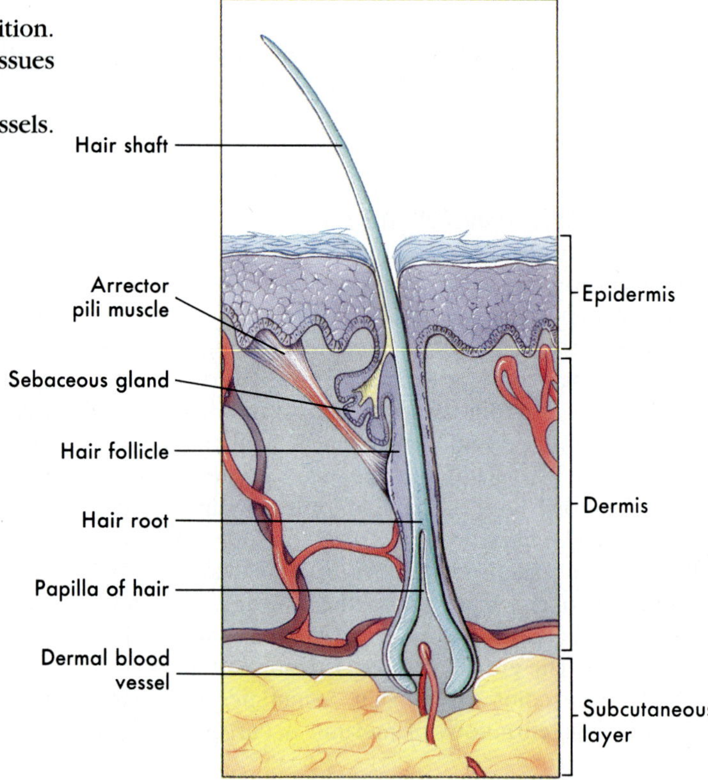

FIG. 25-2 Hair follicle. Relationship of a hair follicle and related structures to the epidermal and dermal layers of the skin.

Sebaceous glands. The **sebaceous** (oil) **glands** (one of the many sacculated [small, saclike] organs in the dermis) secrete their substance, **sebum** (the oily secretion of the sebaceous glands of the skin), through the hair follicles distributed over the body. Their function is to lubricate the skin and hair covering the body. Sebum also inhibits the growth of bacteria. During puberty, as blood levels of sex hormones increase, the amount of sebum secreted also increases.

Hair and nails.

Hair. Hair is composed of modified dead epidermal tissue, mainly keratin. It is distributed all over the body in varying amounts. The root of the hair is enclosed in a follicle deep in the dermis. The shaft of the hair protrudes from the skin. Surrounding the hair follicle is a band of muscle tissue called *arrector pili* (Fig. 25-2). A sensation of cold or fear causes these muscles to contract; the hair stands upright, and the skin surrounding it becomes dimpled. This effect is described as "hair standing on end" and "goose flesh."

Nails. Nails are also composed mainly of keratin, but it is more closely compressed. The base of the nail, the root, is composed of living cells and is mostly covered by the cuticle. Part of the root, the lunula, is exposed and looks like a white crescent. The remainder of the nail is called the *nail body.* It appears pink because of the blood vessels lying immediately beneath it (Fig. 25-3).

GENERAL ASSESSMENT

Assessment of the skin is an important nursing skill, because the skin is a patient's primary defense mechanism. The nurse needs to be aware of normal functions to accurately assess nursing problems.

The nurse should use all senses to assess the patient's skin, using the skills of inspection and palpation. The initial assessment of the patient's skin is essential; it provides baseline information that will help the nurse recognize any subsequent changes. Morning care (the bath) provides an excellent opportunity for the nurse to reassess the skin without exposure or embarrassment of the patient.

Nurses should observe the skin for color. The color of the skin depends on many physiological factors, including the following:

1. The amount of hemoglobin in the blood
2. The oxygen saturation in the blood
3. The amount of such substances as bilirubin, urea, or other chemicals in the blood
4. The quality and quantity of blood circulating in the superficial blood vessels
5. The amount of melanin in the epidermis

Assessment also includes the presence of rashes, scars, lesions, or ecchymoses, and distribution of hair. Temperature and texture should be assessed by touch using the palms of the hands to compare opposite body areas. For example, the nurse should feel both legs before stating that the left leg is cold. Using a cotton-tipped applicator to touch the soles of the foot provides a means to assess sensation. The nails should be inspected for normal development, color, shape, and thickness. Clubbing (broadening) of the fingertips indicates decreased oxygen and should be reported. The hair should

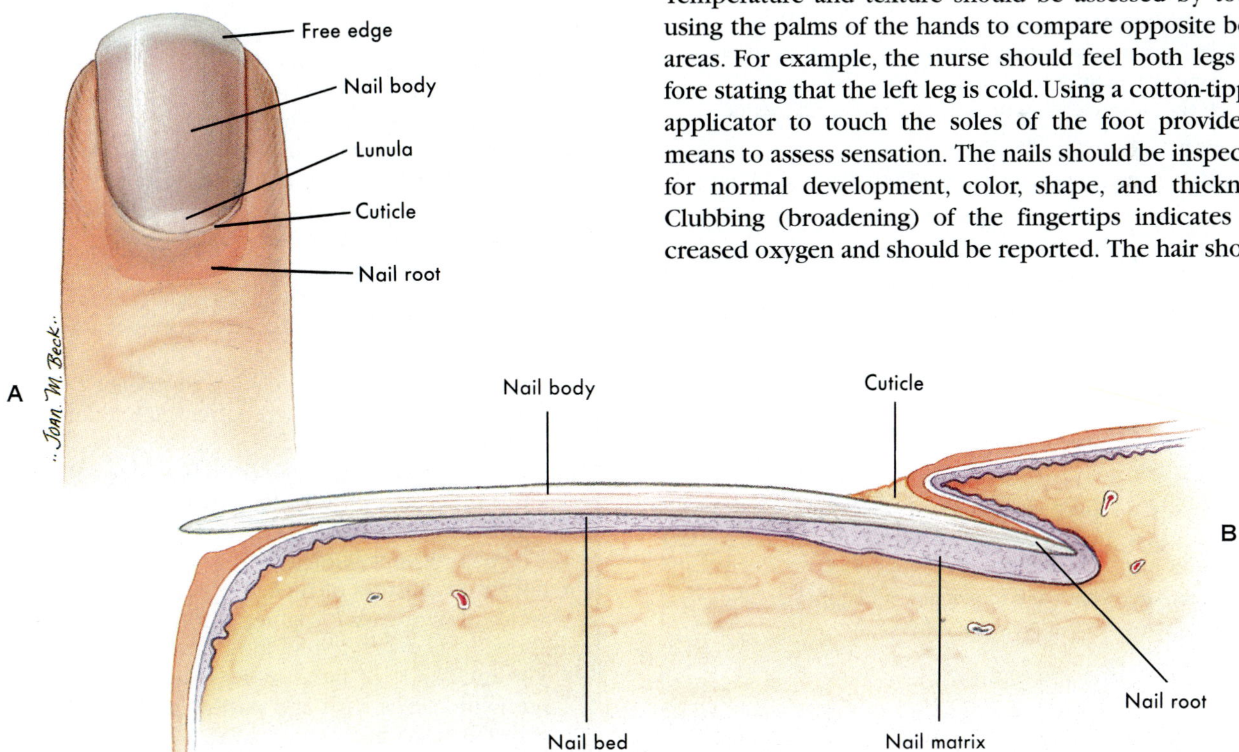

FIG. 25-3 Structure of nails. **A,** Fingernail viewed from above. **B,** Sagittal section of fingernail and associated structures.

be inspected for thickness, dryness, or dullness. Assessment also includes inspecting the mucous membranes for pallor or cyanosis. Profuse sweating or any sign of impaired skin integrity needs to be documented. The ceruminous and sebaceous glands should be inspected for overactivity or underactivity using appropriate questions, such as "How often has the wax been removed from your ears?"

If lesions are found, the exact location, length, width, diameter, and general appearance should be documented. Proper identification serves as a baseline for making evaluations of nursing interventions.

Specific types of skin lesions, their appearance, location, and duration also assist the dermatologist to diagnose a skin disorder. Primary signs and symptoms should be evaluated to identify (1) provocative and palliative factors, (2) the quality or quantity (characteristics and size) of the lesion, (3) specific region of the body, (4) severity of the signs and symptoms, and (5) the length of time the patient has had the disorder. A simple way to remember this assessment technique is to remember these letters:

P	Provocative/palliative
Q	Quality or quantity
R	Region
S	Severity
T	Time (see Box 9-4)

The aim of skin care should be prevention through patient teaching (Box 25-2). For gerontological considerations, see the gerontological box.

Well-cared-for skin is a physiological, psychological, and social asset. Well-groomed skin supports self-esteem, social acceptance, and adjustment to life in society. How a person perceives herself is important to the development of a healthy personality.

Assessment and Description of Skin Lesions

Assessment of specific skin lesions, their appearance, and location assist the dermatologist to diagnose skin disorders and the nurse to provide care. Most disorders have

Box 25-2 PREVENTION OF SKIN DISORDERS

MAINTAINING HEALTHY SKIN

1. Avoid strong or harsh soaps or detergents.
2. Keep skin well hydrated; apply lubricating lotion or cream to dry areas after bathing.
3. Avoid scraping or stripping skin surface by dry razors or removal of tape.
4. Dry damp areas (such as between toes) well to prevent maceration of skin.
5. Wear loose clothing on hot days to permit loss of heat by evaporation.

AVOIDING CAUSATIVE AGENTS

1. Avoid agents that cause skin disorders in most persons (e.g., poison ivy, excessive sunlight).
2. Avoid specific agents known to cause a skin disorder in self.
3. Use protective skin lotions when exposed to excessive sunlight.

OBSERVING SKIN CHANGES

1. Note and report changes in size, color, or general appearance of pigmented skin areas, particularly nevi.
2. Note and report changes in size and appearance of existing skin lesions.

AVOIDING SELF-TREATMENT

1. Do not use previously prescribed prescriptions on new or different skin lesions.
2. Seek medical advice when skin conditions develop.

GERONTOLOGICAL CONSIDERATIONS

- Physiological changes make the skin of the older person more fragile and susceptible to impairment.
- Aging changes include decreases in tissue fluid, subcutaneous fat, and sebaceous secretions. This results in dryness, flaking, pruritus, loss of elasticity, altered turgor, and a wrinkled appearance.
- Hyperkeratotic changes are typically seen in the nails, making them thick and difficult to care for. Podiatric care is recommended for older adults, particularly those with circulatory impairment.
- Circulatory changes and decreased mobility increase the risk of senile purpura and decubitus ulcers.
- Significant hair and scalp changes can manifest with aging:
  - Loss of pigmentation leading to graying
  - Decreased thickness and increased incidence of balding
  - Increased incidence of seborrheic dermatitis of the scalp requiring special care
  - growth of facial hair on women, which can be damaging to self-image
- Localized clusters of melanocytes surrounded by areas of decreased pigmentation result in "age spots."
- The incidence of basal and squamous cell carcinoma increases with age, particularly in individuals who have had a high level of sun exposure. Aging skin should be closely inspected for changes in the appearance of moles or warts.

only one or two types of lesions. Some of the typical clinical manifestations of skin disorders are shown (Fig. 25-4) and additional ones are listed below:

Bleb: irregular, raised area of the skin filled with a serous or seropurulent fluid; blebs can vary in size.

Bulla: larger than 1 cm in diameter; a thin-walled blister of the skin or mucous membranes containing clear, serous fluid.

Crust: dry area several layers thick; commonly called a scab.

Fissure: crack or slit in the skin.

Gumma: tumorlike lesion that resembles an abscess and is seen in late stages of syphilis.

OVERVIEW OF NURSING INTERVENTIONS FOR THE SKIN

Nursing interventions for the patient with a skin disorder involve several basic nursing procedures. The principles involved in good hygiene are the foundation for skin care. Therapeutic baths, application of hot and cold, aseptic technique, sterile technique, surgical dressing changes, and application of topical medications are used.

Therapeutic baths (Table 25-1 on p. 528) are used to stimulate circulation, remove transient bacteria, hasten **suppuration** (production of purulent matter), or improve self-esteem. Specifically for the patient requiring skin care, the bath may be performed to cleanse, disinfect, deodorize, soften, lubricate, remove parasites, or soothe **pruritus** (the symptom of itching). Special soaps,

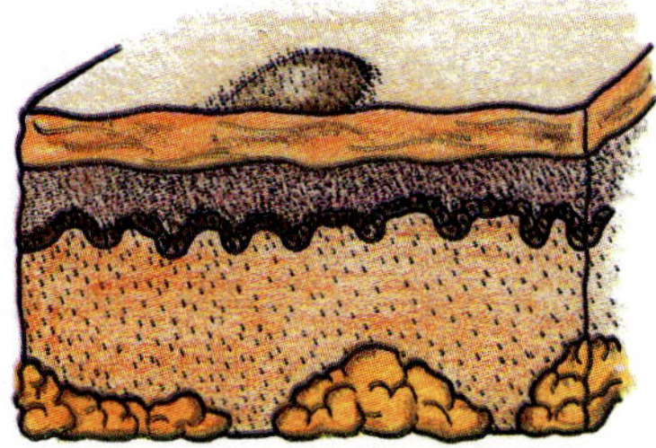

Macule flat, nonpalpable, change in skin color, smaller than 1 cm (for example, freckle, petechia).

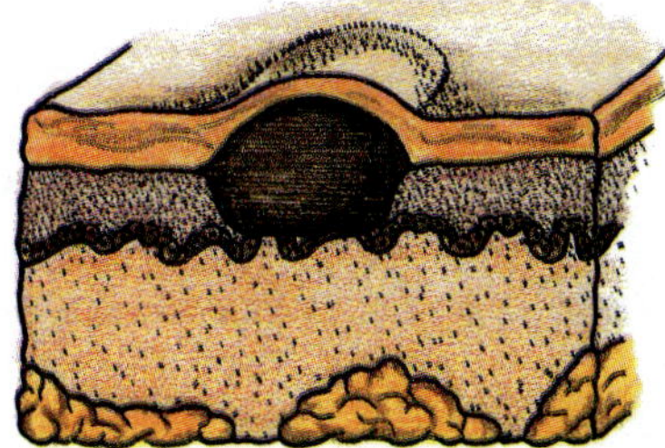

Papule: palpable, circumscribed, solid elevation in skin, smaller than 0.5 cm (for example, elevated nevus).

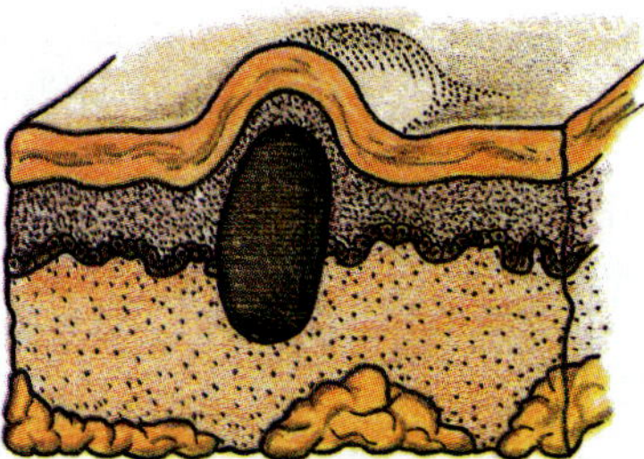

Nodule: elevated solid mass, deeper and firmer than papule, 0.5-0.2 cm (for example, wart).

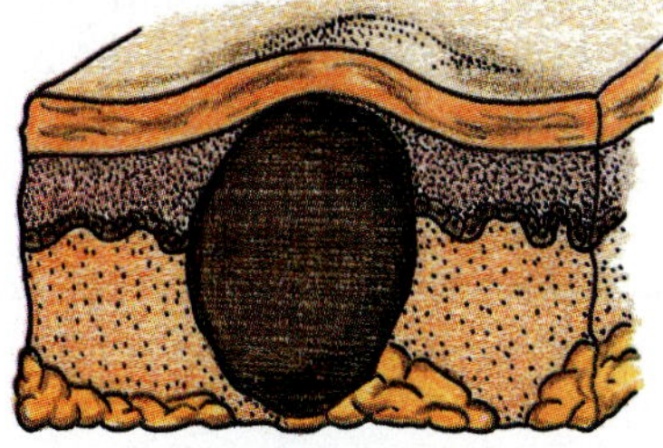

Tumor: solid mass that may extend deep through subcutaneous tissue, larger than 1-2 cm (for example, epithelioma).

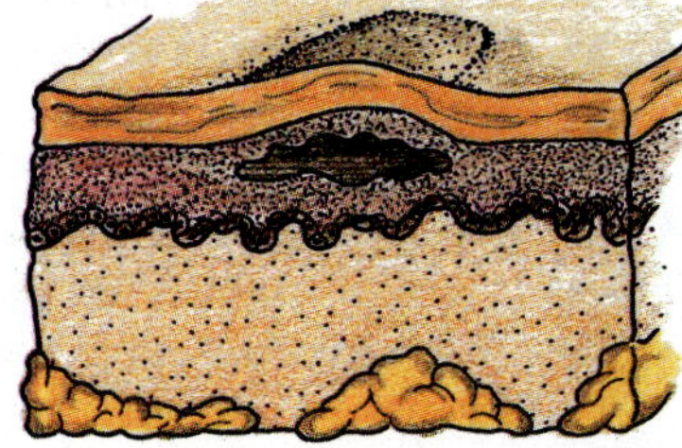

Wheal: irregularly shaped, elevated area or superficial localized edema, varies in size (for example, hive, mosquito bite).

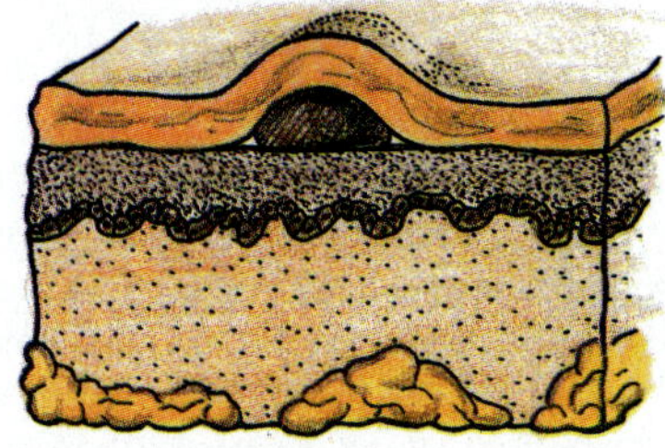

Vesicle: circumscribed elevation of skin filled with serous fluid, smaller than 0.5 cm (for example, herpes simplex, chickenpox).

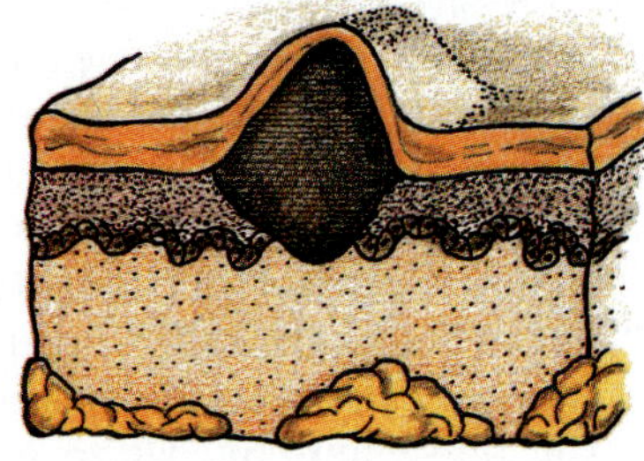

Pustule: circumscribed elevation of skin similar to vesicle but filled with pus, varies in size (for example, acne, staphylococcal infection).

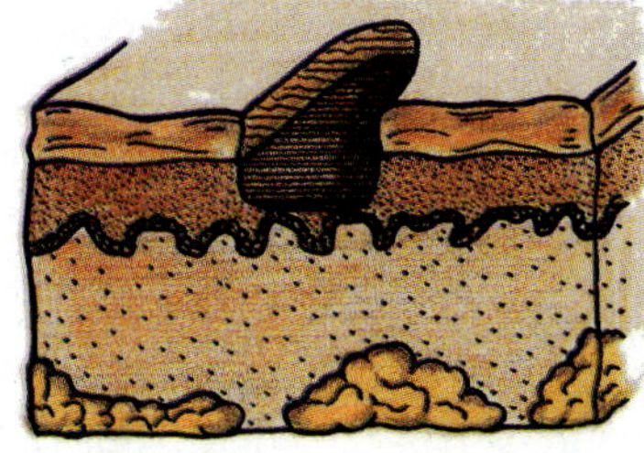

Ulcer: deep loss of skin surface that may extend to dermis and frequently bleeds and scars, varies in size (for example, venous stasis ulcer).

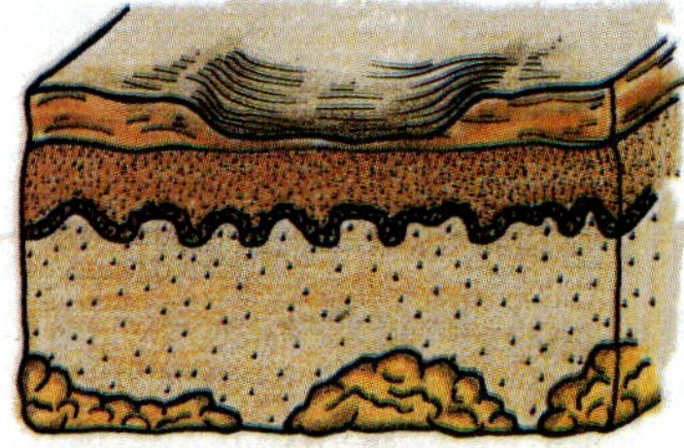

Atrophy: thinning of skin with loss of normal skin furrow with skin appearing shiny and translucent, varies in size (for example, arterial insufficiency).

FIG. 25-4 Types of skin lesions.

TABLE 25-1 Preparations Commonly Used for Baths or Soaks

Substance	Effect	Suggested Actions
Colloids: oatmeal, cornstarch, soybean powder	Antipruritic, drying	Tub surfaces become very slippery; support patient to prevent falls
Potassium permanganate	Antifungal, drying, deodorizing	Strain pulverized tablet through cheesecloth to prevent irritation; stains surfaces and linens
Burow's solution (aluminum acetate)	Antibacterial, drying	Commonly used for soaks
Sulfur bath suspension	Antibacterial	Rinse body with tepid water after bath to remove residual sulfur particles
Tar preparations	Antipruritic, moisturizing	Do not use soap with tar baths
Bath oils: Alpha-Keri, Jeri-Bath, Domol	Antipruritic, moisturizing	Tub surfaces may become slippery; support patient to prevent falls

Box 25-3 GUIDELINES FOR BATHS AND SOAKS

1. The water temperature should be comfortable to patient—usually 90° to 100° F (32 to 38° C).
2. Medication should be completely dissolved while tub is filled.
3. The soak should last 20 to 30 minutes.
4. When oils are added, patients are assisted out of the water to prevent slipping.
5. Skin is *patted* dry, not rubbed, to avoid skin irritation.
6. Creams or ointments are applied immediately after the bath to retain moisture.
7. Water should be drained from the tub before the patient gets out.
8. The door should not be locked, and the health care worker should be within hearing distance.
9. A bath mat should be used to prevent slipping.
10. Handrails may be needed in the shower or tub.
11. A seat may be needed in the tub or in the shower.
12. The patient should be shown how to use the emergency call light.
13. After a medicated bath, pour 1 cup bleach into used tub water; let stand 5 minutes; wipe sides and bottom of tub; drain tub and clean as usual.

oils, medications, and other substances are used, including oatmeal, starch, baking soda, vinegar, and bran.

The nurse responsible for bathing the patient needs to understand the rationale before the procedure is performed. Specific directions may need to be followed, such as adding the oatmeal directly under running water or to a gauze bag and placing it in the tub. The nurse's assessment of the situation is imperative if the goals of treatment are to be met.

The optimal temperature of the water ranges from 95° to 100° F (35° to 37.8° C). The tub should be thoroughly clean and full enough to cover the involved body area. Most therapeutic baths are done two to four times a day, lasting from 20 minutes to 1 hour each. When the bath is completed, the skin is patted dry, not rubbed. Safety measures should be followed to protect the patient from falling and from being chilled or burned (Box 25-3).

Heat and Cold Therapy

Local application of heat and cold to an injured body part can be therapeutic. Before using these therapies, however, the nurse must understand normal body responses to local temperature variations, assess the integrity of the body part, determine the patient's ability to sense temperature variations, and ensure proper operation of equipment. The nurse is legally responsible for safe administration of heat and cold applications.

The body can tolerate wide variations in temperature. The normal temperature of the skin's surface is 93.2° F (34° C), but temperature receptors usually adapt quickly to local temperatures between 113° and 59° F (45° and 15° C). Pain develops when local temperatures exceed these limits. Excessive heat causes a burning sensation. Cold produces a numbing sensation before pain.

The body's adaptive ability creates the major problem in protecting patients from injury resulting from temperature extremes. An individual initially feels an extreme change in temperature, but within a short time hardly notices it. This can be dangerous because this insensitivity to heat and cold extremes can result in serious tissue injury. The nurse must recognize patients most at risk for injuries from heat and cold applications (Table 25-2).

Local Effects of Heat and Cold. Heat and cold stimuli create different body responses. The choice of heat or cold therapy depends on local responses desired for wound healing.

Effects of Heat Application. Table 25-3 on p. 530 summarizes the benefits of heat application. Heat generally is quite therapeutic, improving blood flow to an injured part. If heat is applied for 1 hour or more, blood flow is increased by vasodilation (the lumen of the blood vessel widens); however, blood flow is reduced by vasoconstriction (the lumen of the blood vessel narrows) as the body attempts to control heat loss from the area. Periodic removal and reapplication of local heat restore vasodilation. Continuous exposure to heat damages epithelial cells, causing erythema, localized tenderness, and even blistering.

Effects of Cold Application. Table 25-3 also summarizes the benefits of cold application. Prolonged exposure of the skin to cold results in vasodilation. The cell's inability to receive adequate blood flow and nutrients results in tissue ischemia (decreased blood supply to a body part or organ; may be accompanied by pain and organ dysfunction). The skin initially takes on an erythematous (reddened) appearance, followed by a bluish-purple mottling with numbness and a burning type of pain. The skin's tissues can freeze from exposure to extreme cold.

Factors Influencing Heat and Cold Tolerance. The body's response to heat and cold applications depends on the following factors:

1. Duration of treatment. A person is better able to tolerate short exposure to temperature extremes.
2. Body part. Certain areas of the skin are more sensitive to temperature variations. These include the neck, inner aspect of the wrist and forearm, and perineal region. The foot and palm of the hand are less sensitive.
3. Damage to body surface. Exposed skin layers are more sensitive to temperature variations.
4. Prior skin temperature. The body responds best to minor temperature adjustments. If a body part is cool and a hot stimulus touches the skin, the response is greater than if the stimulus is warm.
5. Body surface area. A person has less tolerance to temperature changes when a large area of the body is exposed to heat or cold.
6. Age and physical condition. Tolerance to temperature variations changes with age. Patients who are very young or elderly are most sensitive to the heat and cold. If a patient's physical condition reduces the reception of sensory stimuli, tolerance to temperature extremes is high, but the risk of injury is also high.

Assessment. Before applying heat or cold therapies, the nurse assesses the patient's physical condition for signs of potential intolerance to heat and cold. The nurse first observes the area to be treated. Impairment in skin integrity, such as abrasions, open wounds, edema, bruising, bleeding, or localized areas of inflammation, increases the patient's risk of injury. Because the physician commonly orders heat and cold applications to be placed on traumatized areas, the baseline assessment provides a guide for evaluating skin changes that might occur during therapy.

Assessment also includes identification of conditions that contraindicate heat or cold therapy. An active area of bleeding should not be covered by a warm application because bleeding will continue. Warm applications are contraindicated when the patient has an acute, lo-

TABLE 25-2 Considerations Necessary to Prevent Increased Risk of Injury from Heat and Cold Applications

Consideration	Rationale
Very young patients or older patients	Thinner skin layers in children increase risk of burns. Older patients have reduced sensitivity to pain.
Open wounds, skin impairment, stomas	Subcutaneous and visceral tissues are more sensitive to temperature variations. They also contain no temperature and fewer pain receptors.
Areas of edema or scar formation	Reduced sensation to temperature stimuli occurs because of thickening of skin layers from fluid buildup or scar formation.
Peripheral vascular disease (e.g., diabetes, arteriosclerosis)	Body's extremities are less sensitive to temperature and pain stimuli because of circulatory impairment and local tissue injury. Cold application further compromises blood flow.
Disorientation or unconsciousness	Reduced perception of sensory or painful stimuli occurs.
Spinal cord injury	Alterations in nerve pathways prevent reception of sensory or painful stimuli.
Abscessed tooth or appendix	Infection is highly localized. Application of heat may cause rupture with spread of microorganisms systemically.

TABLE 25-3 Therapeutic Effects of Heat and Cold Applications

Body's Physiological Response	Rationale	Conditions Treated
Heat		
Vasodilation	Improves blood flow to injured body part; promotes delivery of nutrients and removal of wastes; lessens venous congestion in injured tissues	Inflamed or edematous body part; new surgical wound; infected wound; arthritis; degenerative joint disease; localized joint pain; muscle strains; low back pain; menstrual cramping; hemorrhoidal, perianal, and vaginal inflammations; local abscesses
Reduced blood viscosity	Improves delivery of leukocytes and antibiotics to wound site	
Reduced muscle tension	Promotes muscle relaxation and reduces pain from spasm or stiffness	
Increased tissue metabolism	Increases blood flow; provides local warmth	
Increased capillary permeability	Promotes movement of waste products and nutrients	
Cold		
Vasoconstriction	Reduces blood flow to injured part, preventing edema formation; reduces inflammation	Direct trauma (sprains, strains, fractures, muscle spasms); superficial laceration or puncture wound; minor burn; suspected malignancy in area of injury or pain; injections; arthritis and joint trauma
Local anesthesia	Reduces localized pain	
Reduced cell metabolism	Reduces oxygen needs of tissues	
Increased blood viscosity	Promotes blood coagulation at injury site	
Decreased muscle tension	Relieves pain	

calized inflammation such as appendicitis because the heat could cause a rupture. If a patient has cardiovascular problems, it is unwise to apply heat to large portions of the body because the resulting massive vasodilation may disrupt blood supply to vital organs.

Cold is contraindicated if the site of injury is already edematous. Cold further retards circulation to the area and prevents absorption of the interstitial fluid. If the patient has impairment in circulation (for example, arteriosclerosis), cold further reduces blood supply to the affected area. One other contraindication for cold therapy is shivering. Cold applications may intensify shivering and dangerously increase body temperature. The nurse also assesses the patient's response to stimuli. Reaction to light touch, pinprick, and mild temperature variations reveals the ability of the patient to recognize when heat or cold becomes excessive. If a patient has peripheral vascular disease, the nurse pays particular attention to the integrity of the extremities. For example, if the physician's order is to apply a cold compress to a lower extremity, the nurse should assess circulation to the leg by observing skin color and palpating skin temperatures, distal pulses, and edematous areas. If signs of circulatory inadequacy are present, the nurse should question the order.

Level of consciousness influences the ability to perceive heat, cold, and pain. If a patient is disoriented or unresponsive, the nurse must make frequent observations of skin integrity after therapy begins.

The nurse must also assess the condition of equipment being used. Electrical equipment should be checked for cracked cords, frayed wires, damaged insulation, and exposed heating components. Equipment containing fluids should not have leaks. The nurse also checks equipment for evenness of temperature distribution. Uneven temperature distribution suggests that the equipment is functioning improperly.

Patient Safety. Before heat or cold therapy is applied, the patient should understand its purpose, the symptoms of temperature exposure, and precautions taken to prevent injury (Box 25-4).

Applying Heat and Cold. A prerequisite to heat or cold application is a physician's order, which should include body site and the type, frequency, and duration of application. The nurse should consult the agency's procedure manual for correct temperatures.

Choice of moist or dry. Heat and cold applications can be administered in dry or moist forms. The type of

Box 25-4

SAFETY MEASURES WHEN APPLYING HEAT OR COLD THERAPY

- Do explain to the patient sensations to be felt during the procedure.
- Do instruct the patient to report changes in sensation or discomfort immediately.
- Do provide a timer, clock, or watch so that the patient can help time the application.
- Do keep the call light within the patient's reach.
- Do refer to the agency's policy and procedure manual for safe temperatures.
- Do not allow the patient to adjust temperature settings.
- Do not allow the patient to move an application or place hands on the wound site.
- Do not place the patient in a position that prevents movement away from the temperature source.
- Do not leave unattended a patient who is unable to sense temperature changes or move from the temperature source.

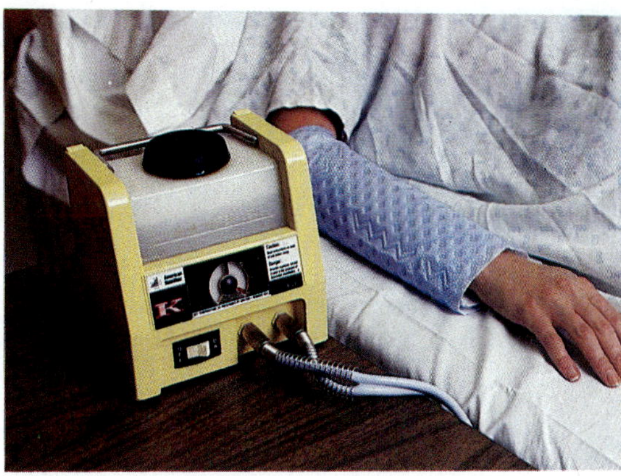

FIG. 25-5 Aquathermia pad.

wound or injury, the location of the body part, and the presence of drainage or inflammation are factors to be considered in selecting dry or moist applications.

Hot, moist compresses. For open wounds, sterile, hot, moist compresses improve circulation, relieve edema, and promote consolidation of purulent exudate. A *compress* is a piece of gauze dressing moistened in a prescribed warmed solution. A *pack* is a larger cloth or dressing applied to a larger body area.

Heat from hot compresses dissipates quickly. To maintain a constant temperature the nurse must change the compress often or apply a warm aquathermia pad or waterproof heating pad over the compress. Because moisture conducts heat, any device's temperature setting should be lower for a moist compress than for a dry application. A layer of plastic wrap or a dry towel can also be used to insulate the compress and retain heat. Moist heat promotes vasodilation and evaporation of heat from the skin's surface. For this reason a patient may feel chilly. The nurse controls drafts within the room and keeps the patient covered with a blanket or robe (Skill 25-1 on pp. 532-533).

Warm soaks. Immersion of a body part in a warmed solution promotes circulation, lessens edema, increases muscle relaxation, and can provide a means to debride wounds and apply medicated solution. A soak can also be accomplished by wrapping the body part in dressings and saturating them with the warmed solution.

The nurse positions the patient comfortably, places waterproof pads under the area to be treated, and heats the solution to about 105° to 110° F (40.5° to 43° C). After immersing the body part, the nurse covers the container and extremity with a towel to reduce heat loss. It is usually necessary to remove the cooled solution and add heat solution after about 10 minutes. The problem is to keep the solution at a constant temperature. The nurse never adds a hotter solution while the body part remains immersed. After any soak the nurse dries the body part thoroughly to prevent maceration.

Sitz baths. Sitz baths are also utilized to promote heat therapy to the pelvic region following rectal surgery, after childbirth, for painful hemorrhoids, or for vaginal inflammation (see Chapter 16).

Paraffin baths. A paraffin bath consists of a mixture of heated paraffin wax and mineral oil (1 part oil to 5 parts paraffin). Patients with painful arthritis or other joint discomforts of the hands and feet benefit most from these baths. In many institutions only physical therapists administer the applications. Patients often heat paraffin baths at home in double boilers. The bath temperature should be 128° to 130° F (53.3° to 54.4° C).

Aquathermia (water-flow) pads. A popular device in health care institutions is the aquathermia pad or water-flow pad (Fig. 25-5), used for treating muscle sprains and areas of mild inflammation or edema. The aquathermia unit consists of a waterproof plastic or rubber pad connected by two hoses to an electrical control unit that has a heating element and motor. Distilled water circulates through hollowed channels within the pad to the control unit where water is heated or cooled (depending on temperature setting). Some pads have an absorbent surface to apply moist heat. These units are safer than conventional heating pads; however, the nurse should still check for equipment malfunctions. The temperature setting is fixed by inserting a plastic key into the temperature regulator. In many institutions the central supply room sets the regulators to the recommended temperature of 105° to 110° F (40.5° to 43° C). If the distilled water in the unit runs low, the nurse simply fills

SKILL 25-1

APPLYING A HOT, MOIST COMPRESS TO AN OPEN WOUND

1. Wash hands to prevent the transmission of microorganisms.
2. Identify patient.
3. Introduce self.
4. Assess condition of exposed skin and wound on which compress is to be applied (see illustration). This assessment provides baseline for determination of changes in skin during heat application. Very thin or impaired skin is more susceptible to injury from heat.
5. Refer to physician's order for type of compress, location and duration of application, and desired temperature. This helps to ensure safe application.
6. Prepare necessary equipment and supplies; this facilitates smoothness of procedure. Materials should include the following:
   a. Prescribed solution warmed to proper temperature, approximately 110° to 115° F (43° to 46° C)
   b. Sterile gauze dressings
   c. Sterile container for solution
   d. Commercially prepared compresses (optional)
   e. Sterile gloves
   f. Petrolatum jelly, if desired
   g. Sterile cotton swabs
   h. Waterproof pad
   i. Tape or ties
   j. Dry bath towel
   k. Aquathermia or heating pad (optional)
   l. Disposable gloves
   m. Bath thermometer
   n. Bath blanket
7. Explain steps of procedure and purpose. Describe sensation to be felt (e.g., feeling of warmth and wetness). Explain precautions to prevent burning. This will minimize anxiety and promote cooperation.
8. Assist patient in assuming comfortable position in proper body alignment.
9. Place waterproof pad under area to be treated.
10. Expose body part to be covered with compress and drape patient with bath blanket. Close bedside curtains to provide privacy.
11. Assemble equipment. Pour warmed solution into sterile container. (If using portable heating source, keep solution warm. Commercially prepared compresses may remain under infrared lamp until just before use.) Open sterile packages and drop gauze into container to immerse in solution. Set aquathermia pad (if used) to correct temperature because compress must retain warmth for therapeutic benefit.
12. Put on disposable gloves. Remove any existing dressing covering wound. Dispose of gloves and dressing in proper receptacle to prevent transmission of microorganisms.
13. Apply sterile gloves. This will allow nurse to manipulate sterile dressing and touch open wound.
14. Apply sterile petrolatum jelly, if desired, with cotton swab to skin surrounding wound. Do not apply jelly on impaired skin. This will protect skin from possible burns and maceration.
15. Pick up one layer of immersed gauze and squeeze out excess water. Excess moisture macerates skin and increases risk of burns and infection.
16. Apply gauze lightly to open wound. Observe response and ask whether patient feels discomfort. In a few seconds, lift edge of gauze to assess for erythema.
17. If patient tolerates compress, pack gauze snugly against wound. Be certain all wound surfaces are covered by hot compress. This will prevent rapid cooling from underlying air currents.
18. Wrap or cover moist compress with dry bath towel. If necessary, pin or tie in place. This will insulate compress to prevent heat loss.
19. Change hot compress every 5 minutes or as ordered. This will prevent cooling and maintain therapeutic benefit of compress.
20. Apply aquathermia or waterproof heating pad over compress (optional). Keep it in place for desired duration of application (about 20 to 30 minutes). This will provide constant temperature to compress. Local application of heat for more than 60 minutes often results in vasocon-

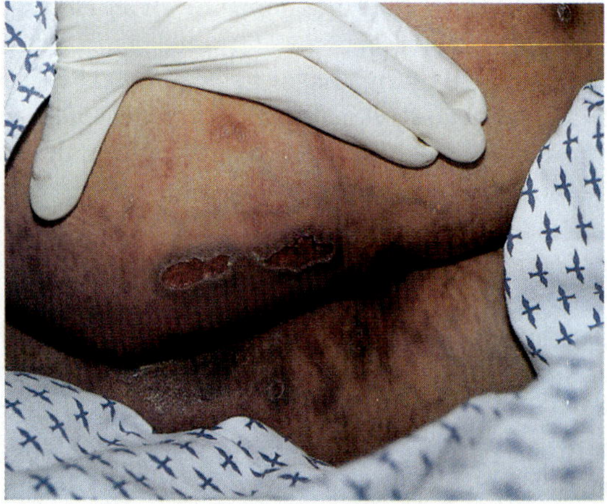

STEP 4

APPLYING A HOT, MOIST COMPRESS TO AN OPEN WOUND—cont'd

striction. Removing hot compress after 30 min and then reapplying in 15 min, if desired, maintains vasodilation and positive therapeutic effects.

21. Assess patient periodically for discomfort or burning sensation. Observe area of skin not covered by compress, because continued exposure to heat can cause burning of skin.
22. Remove pad, towel, and compress in 30 minutes. Again assess wound and condition of skin.
23. Apply dry sterile dressing as ordered, as this will prevent entrance of microorganisms into wound site.
24. Assist patient to preferred comfortable position.
25. Dispose of equipment and soiled compress. Wash hands to prevent the transmission of microorganisms.
26. Ask patient if an unusual burning sensation is noticed that was not felt before, as it may be difficult to assess burn merely by color changes if wound is inflamed or exudate is present.
27. Record type, location, and duration of application. Note temperature used in nurses' notes. This will document therapy administered.
28. Describe condition of wound and skin and patient response to document response to therapy.

the reservoir two-thirds full. Plain tap water is never added because it might leave mineral deposits in the unit.

To avoid burning the patient's skin the nurse does not place the pad directly on it. A thin towel or pillowcase fits easily over the heating pad. Tape, ties, or a gauze roll holds the pad in place. Pins are never used because they might cause a leak. The nurse assesses the patient's skin frequently for signs of burning. An application should last only 20 to 30 minutes. In some instances (for thrombophlebitis, for example) an aquathermia pad with a warm moist pack may be ordered on for 1 hour, off for 3 hours. The nurse does not allow a patient to lie on a pad. Pressure against a mattress prevents normal heat distribution. If the pad is to be applied to a region of the back, the patient should lie prone or in a lateral position.

Warm air blower. When wounds require drying (such as the donor site in split-thickness skin grafting), the nurse may use a hair dryer. The hair dryer is set on medium warm setting and then held about 8 to 10 inches in from the wound. The nurse then gently waves the device over the site for about 5 minutes or the time prescribed by the surgeon. This procedure is repeated three or four times a day until the wound is completely dry.

Heat lamps. Be certain to check agency policy in regard to the use of heat lamps. Heat lamps use infrared or regular (40 to 75 watt) light bulbs to expose superficial layers of the skin to heat. Because nothing touches the skin surface, this therapy is valuable to patients with sensitive or painful skin lesions or wounds. The lamp is used mainly to increase circulation to a wound.

After explaining the procedure, the nurse provides the patient privacy, covers any scars or stomas, cleans and dries the area to be heated, positions the lamp a safe distance from the exposed body surface, and instructs the patient not to touch the lamp's hot surface. A 60-watt bulb should be placed at least 24 in (50 centimeters [cm]) away from the area to be treated. A larger watt bulb should be about 30 in (75 cm) away. Treatments last about 20 minutes. The nurse assesses the condition of the patient's skin at least every 5 minutes for discomfort and erythema. The nurse takes precautions to protect the patient's skin.

Commercial hot packs. Commercially prepared, disposable hot packs apply warm, dry heat to an injured area. Sticking, kneading, or squeezing the pack mixes the chemicals and releases the heat. Package directions recommend the time for application.

Hot-water bottles are not recommended in acute care facilities. If they are used in the home setting, for example, extreme caution must be practiced to avoid burning the patient.

Electric heating pads. Another conventional form of heat therapy is the heating pad, which is an electric coil enclosed within a waterproof pad covered with cotton or flannel cloth. The pad is connected to an electric cord that has a temperature-regulating unit for a high, medium, or low setting. Nurses should advise patients to avoid using the high setting and to never lie on the pad. Another precaution to note is that a safety pin inserted through a pad can result in an electrical shock. Heating pads are not recommended in acute care facilities.

Cold moist and dry compresses. The procedure for applying cold, moist compresses is the same as that for warm compresses. Cold compresses should be applied for 20 minutes at a temperature of 59° F (15° C) to relieve inflammation and edema. They may be clean or sterile.

There are commercially prepared cold packs similar to the disposable hot packs for dry applications. They come in various shapes and sizes to fit different body parts. When using cold compresses, the nurse observes for adverse reactions such as burning or numbness, mottling of the skin, erythema, extreme paleness, and a bluish skin discoloration.

Cold soaks. The procedure for preparing cold soaks is the same as for warm soaks. The desired temperature for a 20-minute cold soak is 59° F (15° C). The nurse controls drafts and uses oute· coverings to protect the patient from chilling. It may be necessary to add cold water during the procedure to maintain a constant temperature.

Ice bags or collars. For a patient who has a muscle sprain, localized hemorrhage, or hematoma or who has undergone dental surgery, an ice bag is ideal to prevent edema formation, control bleeding, and anesthetize the body part. Proper use of the bag requires the following steps:

1. Fill the bag with water, secure the cap, invert to check for leaks, and pour out the water.
2. Fill the bag two-thirds full with crushed ice so that the bag can mold easily over a body part. Too heavy an ice bag will tire the body part.
3. Release any air from the bag by squeezing its sides before securing the cap because excess air interferes with conduction of cold.
4. Wipe off excess moisture.
5. Cover the bag with a flannel cover, towel, or pillowcase.
6. Apply the bag to the injury site for 30 minutes; the bag can be reapplied in an hour.

Emotional Aspects of Care

The person with a skin disorder may have a chronic or acute condition. Regardless of the severity, recovery may be a lengthy process visible to the patient—and others.

The nurse should be aware of the patient's psychosocial status; many of the skin disorders cause discolored or vesicular disfiguring, especially on the face. Patients may fear that others will be revolted by the disfiguring and reject them; this may have happened already. Patients may lose their self-esteem and sense of self-worth.

Society's reaction to a person has significant impact. Personal appearance is a primary concern to many individuals, and others may think the person is infectious and isolate him because of his appearance. The impact of a skin disease on a patient's self-concept can be detrimental because of the value society places on a person's physical characteristics.

Anxiety is a common problem in a person with a skin disorder. It is essential that the nurse provide a therapeutic environment to assist the patient to deal with anxiety in a realistic manner. One nursing intervention is to provide the patient with consistent information related to the plan of care. Second, the family and significant others should be included in the treatment plan. Family or significant others may be able to support instructions, which helps to decrease anxiety. Third, the nurse should take every opportunity to provide positive reinforcement concerning the patient's efforts and progress no matter how large or small. Referral to a psychiatric clinical nurse specialist or a support group may need to be done as soon as possible.

The nurse needs to assess patients' coping abilities by encouraging them to talk and share their feelings. Open-ended questions are used to facilitate communication. The nurse should validate or correct a patient's knowledge base. Rarely are skin diseases fatal, and very few are contagious. Nurses need to have worked through their own feelings about a patient's skin appearance before they can be a source of encouragement. The nurse's attitude and interventions should be nonjudgmental, warm, and accepting.

VIRAL DISORDERS OF THE SKIN

Herpes Simplex

Etiology/Pathophysiology. The herpetovirus *Herpesvirus hominis* is the cause of herpes simplex. Two types of the virus are known. Type 1, the more common, causes the common cold sore; type 2 is found in lesions in the genital area and is known as genital herpes. The viruses are self-limiting, and there is no cure. Type 1 is usually associated with febrile conditions.

Genital herpes can be transmitted by the mother to the baby during vaginal deliveries, causing death of the neonate. Transmission of the virus may occur by direct contact with any open lesion. The lesions are usually present for 2 to 3 weeks. The pain is most severe during the first week. Complications can be severe if the disease spreads to other body areas. The primary mode of transmission is unclean hands.

Clinical Manifestations. Type 1 herpes simplex is characterized by a **vesicle** (circumscribed elevation of skin filled with serous fluid; smaller than 0.5 cm) at the corner of the mouth, on the lips, or on the nose. It is commonly known as a *cold sore.* The involved area is usually erythematous and edematous. The vesicle then appears, ulcerates, and encrusts. When the vesicle ruptures, a burning pain is felt. General malaise and fatigue are expressed by the patient. Usual occurrence is during an acute illness or infection.

Type 2, genital herpes, produces various types of vesicles that rupture and encrust, causing ulcerations. The cervix is the most common site in women, and the penis is the most common area in men. Flulike symptoms occur 3 to 4 days after the vesicles erupt. Headache, fatigue, myalgia, elevated temperature, and anorexia are common.

Assessment. Assessment primarily involves inspection of the skin. The nurse must obtain a complete health history to support assessment data. Collection of *subjective data* will include complaints of fatigue; pruritus in the mouth for herpes simplex type 1 and in the genital area for herpes simplex type 2 (genital herpes); and complaints of a burning pain in the involved area.

Collection of *objective data* for herpes simplex type 1 will include an edematous, erythematous area at the corner of the lip. In herpes simplex type 2 the labia, vulva, or penis will appear edematous and erythematous. The vesicular lesions may rupture and develop a dried **exudate** (fluid, cells, or other substances that have been slowly exuded, or discharged, from cells or blood vessels through small pores or breaks in cell membranes).

Diagnostic Tests. Diagnosis of herpesvirus is made by laboratory assessment of cultures from the lesion. Inspection and health history also support the diagnosis.

Medical Management. Treatment is aimed at relieving symptoms. Acyclovir (Zovirax) is an antiviral agent that can alter the course of the disease. It can be administered orally, topically, or intravenously.

Nursing Interventions. Nursing interventions are primarily directed toward treatment of symptoms and prevention of the spread of the disease. Warm compresses can be used to relieve the pain and severe pruritus. The lesions should be kept dry and direct contact avoided. Analgesics such as acetaminophen (Tylenol) are effective in pain control. The specific nursing diagnoses for herpes are based on assessment data gathered.

Nursing diagnoses and interventions for the patient with herpes include, but are not limited to, the following:

NURSING DIAGNOSES	NURSING INTERVENTIONS
Pain, related to pruritus	Assess factors that precipitate pruritus. Apply local anesthetic, such as Orabase, for pain. Apply drying agent to lesions. Apply warm compresses. Have patient wear loose-fitting cotton clothing that will not constrict movement or occlude circulation.
Skin integrity, impaired, related to open lesions	Inspect lesions for drainage, color, and location. Wash hands before and after contact. Keep area dry. Administer antiviral agents as ordered. In genital herpes use of a hair dryer can promote drying of the lesions and patient comfort.
Infection, high risk for, related to break in the skin	Assess for signs of infection, such as pyrexia. The patient should be taught to practice aseptic handwashing and meticulous personal hygiene. Avoid use of occlusive ointments that prevent drying.
Knowledge deficit, related to cause and spread of the disease	Assess patient's level of understanding of the cause, treatment, and spread of the condition by using open-ended questions. Teach aseptic personal hygiene techniques. Instruct the patient that contact with the open lesions should be avoided. Stress the importance of proper follow-up care.

Patient teaching. The patient should be taught techniques to prevent the spread of the disease. He should be taught to use good hygiene in all areas of care. The complications and precipitating factors should be included in discharge planning.

Prognosis. There is no cure for the herpesvirus. Unfortunately 75% of all patients have at least one recurrence, but it is milder and of shorter duration than the primary infection.

Type I herpes simplex: healing within 10 to 14 days. May reoccur with depression of the immune system.

Type II genital herpes: lesions usually present 14 to 21 days. Approximately two thirds of infected individuals will have one to five recurrences annually.

Herpes Zoster (Shingles)

Etiology/Pathophysiology. Herpes zoster is caused by the same virus that causes chickenpox (varicella) *(Herpes varicellae)*. The lesions are located along the nerve fibers of spinal ganglia.

Herpes zoster is commonly known as *shingles.* The virus causes an inflammation of the spinal ganglia. It is believed that the virus responsible for shingles lies dormant in patients until their resistance to infections has been lowered. The virus then advances to the skin by way of the peripheral nerves. At the skin surface the virus multiplies and forms an erythematous rash of small vesicles along a spinal nerve pathway.

Clinical Manifestations. The eruption of the vesicles is proceeded by pain. The rash generally occurs in the thoracic region; the vesicles erupt in a line along the involved nerve. The vesicles rupture and form a crust, and the serous fluid in the vesicle may become purulent. The virus can also affect the lumbar, cervical, or cranial areas. The course of this painful condition is from 7 to 28 days.

The pain associated with herpes zoster is severe; most patients describe the pain as burning and knifelike. Extreme tenderness and pruritus in the area are noted. Patients with herpes zoster will request analgesic medications at frequent intervals.

Herpes zoster is usually not permanently disabling to healthy adults. The greatest risk occurs to patients who have a lowered resistance to infection, such as those on chemotherapy or large doses of prednisone, in whom the disease could be fatal.

Assessment. The assessment of the patient should include both the subjective and objective data. A good health history and thorough inspection skills are necessary to gather relevant data.

Collection of *subjective data* will include these symptoms: (1) sharp, burning pain, usually on one side only; (2) severe pruritus of the lesions; (3) general malaise; and (4) a history of chickenpox (varicella).

Collection of *objective data* includes: (1) evidence of skin excoriation related to scratching, (2) patches of vesicles on erythematous skin following a peripheral nerve pathway, and (3) demonstration of tenderness to touch.

Diagnostic Tests. The diagnostic test for herpes zoster is a culture to isolate the virus. Other diagnostic measures are physical examinations and a thorough history obtained at admission.

Medical Management. Medical interventions are directed at controlling the pain and preventing secondary complications. Analgesics are given for the pain; many times the pain requires narcotic analgesics such as codeine. Steroids may be given to decrease inflammation and edema. Lotions may be used to relieve pruritus, (Kenalog, Lidex) and corticosteroids may be used to relieve the pruritus and inflammation. Oral and intravenous acyclovir (Zovirax), administered early, reduces the pain and duration of the virus.

Nursing Interventions. Nursing interventions are directed at relieving the patient's symptoms. Pain, pruritus, and the prevention of secondary complications are the primary concerns. Tranquilizers such as lorazepam (Ativan) and hydroxyzine HCl (Atarax) are also prescribed to decrease the anxiety associated with severe pain. Analgesics are given to control pain. The nurse needs to understand and be able to apply the principles of pain management to provide nursing care. Medicated baths and warm compresses may be ordered to soothe the skin. The nurse will use aseptic technique when caring for open lesions.

Nursing diagnoses and interventions for the patient with herpes zoster include, but are not limited to, the following:

NURSING DIAGNOSES	NURSING INTERVENTIONS
Pain, acute, related to pruritus	Assess pain and pruritus for relief measures necessary. Administer medications for pain and pruritus. Stress relaxation techniques and diversional activities.
Skin integrity, impaired, related to break in skin	Assess the skin for open lesions. Assess skin for **excoriation** (an injury to the surface of the skin caused by a scratch or abrasion). Keep patient's fingernails short, and/or apply mittens. Plan a balanced diet with increased protein.
Infection, high risk for, related to tissue destruction	Assess factors that contribute to infection, such as compromised patient (one who has low resistance). Monitor for signs of infection, such as pyrexia and leukocytosis. Stress aseptic handwashing technique. Maintain aseptic technique when providing care. Limit visitors. Don gloves when caring for lesions.
Knowledge deficit, related to disease process	Assess patient's knowledge of disease and ability to learn. Identify support persons, and include them in patient's care. Provide relevant information.

Patient teaching. Patient teaching should begin with an assessment of the knowledge and readiness of the patient. Areas to cover include (1) methods for controlling the pain, (2) application of medication and wet dressings, (3) methods for inhibiting the spread of the disease, (4) techniques to prevent secondary infections, and (5) proper diet with vitamin C to promote healing.

Prognosis. The prognosis is generally good; however, older patients are more susceptible to complications such as posttherapy neuralgia, which may persist for several months after the skin lesions have cleared. Evidence indicates the herpes zoster virus remains latent in the body of a person once infected, and a person lacking varicella (chickenpox) immunity can acquire chickenpox from someone who has had the virus.

BACTERIAL DISORDERS OF THE SKIN

Impetigo Contagiosa

Etiology/Pathophysiology. Impetigo is caused by *Staphylococcus aureus,* by streptococci, or by a mixed bacterial invasion of the skin. The result is a highly contagious inflammatory disorder. Impetigo is seen at all ages but is particularly common in children.

The bacteria invade the skin. The lesions start as **macules** (small, flat blemishes that are flush with the skin surface) that develop into **pustulant vesicles** (small, circumscribed elevations of the skin, containing pus) that rupture and form a dried exudate. The crust is honey colored and easily removed. Under the dried exudate is smooth, red skin.

Clinical Manifestations. The exposed areas of the body most often affected are the face, hands, arms, and legs. The pustulant lesions are distributed randomly over the involved area. The honey-colored dried exudate ranges in size from pinpoint to the size of a nickel or larger. Impetigo is highly contagious to a person who directly contacts the exudate of a lesion. The disease may be spread by touching personal articles, linens, and clothing of the infected person.

Assessment. Collection of *subjective data* will include symptoms of (1) pruritus, (2) pain, (3) malaise, (4) spreading of the disease to different body parts, and (5) other diseases present.

Collection of *objective data* will reveal all or part of the following: (1) focal erythema, (2) pruritic areas, (3) honey-colored crust over dried lesions, (4) smooth, red skin under the crust, (5) low-grade fever, (6) leukocytosis, (7) positive culture for streptococcus or staphylococcus, and (8) purulent exudate.

Diagnostic Tests. The diagnosis is made from a culture of the exudate. The specific bacterium is identified from this culture. Inspection and symptoms make the diagnosis complete.

Medical Management. Medical treatment emphasizes the use of antiseptic soaps to remove crusted exudate and cleansing agents to thoroughly clean the involved area before application of an antibiotic cream, ointment, or lotion. Systemic antibiotics are administered either orally or by injection. Penicillin or one of its synthetic forms is commonly used. The goal is to prevent glomerulonephritis (inflammation of the glomerulus of the kidney), which may occur after streptococcal infections.

Nursing Interventions. Interventions are aimed at disrupting the course of the disease and preventing the spread of infection. Antibiotics are used to arrest the disease process. Systemic parenteral penicillin is one of the most commonly used antibiotics. The nurse should don gloves and administer special cleansing agents to wash the lesions. Antiseptics such as povidone-iodine solution (Betadine) and chlorhexidine gluconate (Hibiclens) are examples.

The lesions are usually soaked with an antiseptic solution, and the dried exudate is removed using special instruments. Topical antibiotics are applied several times a day using sterile technique.

Nursing diagnoses and interventions for the patient with impetigo include, but are not limited to, the following:

NURSING DIAGNOSES	NURSING INTERVENTIONS
Skin integrity, impaired, related to crusted, open lesions	Inspect the lesions every day for drainage, size, and extent of body area covered. Keep area clean and dry. Don gloves when giving direct patient care.
Pain, related to pruritus	Assess pain, identifying contributing factors. Administer analgesics, hot compresses, and antibiotics as directed.
Infection, high risk for, related to break in skin	Assess skin for signs of infection. Identify interventions to prevent/reduce the risk of infection. Monitor vital signs; assess for elevated temperature. Stress medical aseptic handwashing. Keep involved areas dry when providing care.
Knowledge deficit, related to the cause and spread of the disease	Assess the patient's knowledge level and readiness to learn. Demonstrate appropriate care and application of topical medications. Stress importance of individual personal items, such as linens and towels. Involve family in patient teaching.

Patient teaching. The patient and family members should be instructed in the principles of hygiene. The nurse assesses the patient's level of knowledge. When demonstrating home care techniques, reinforcement of correct information is recommended. It is imperative to stress the importance of preventing the spread of the disease by contact.

Prognosis. With proper treatment the prognosis is good.

Folliculitis, Furuncles, Carbuncles, and Felons

Etiology/Pathophysiology. Folliculitis is an infection of a hair follicle, generally from *Staphylococcus aureus* bacteria. The infection may involve one or several follicles. It often occurs after men or women shave. A stye is an example of folliculitis.

A furuncle (boil) is an inflammation that begins deep in the hair follicles and spreads to the surrounding skin. Irritation is a common predisposing factor to a furuncle.

Common locations are the posterior area of the neck, the buttocks, and the axillae.

A carbuncle is a cluster of furuncles. It is an infection of several hair follicles that spreads to surrounding tissue. Obesity, poor nutrition, untreated diabetes mellitus, and poor hygiene contribute to the formation of carbuncles.

Felons occur when the soft tissue under and around an area such as the fingernail becomes infected. The involved finger becomes erythematous, edematous, and tender to touch.

Clinical Manifestations. The involved area is usually edematous, erythematous, and painful, with pruritus commonly occurring. After several days the infected area will become localized. The exact area may get shiny, point up, and if it is a furuncle or carbuncle, the center will turn yellow. Carbuncles can have four to five cores with spontaneous rupture of the core. The pain stops immediately upon rupture of the core. A surgical incision and drain (I & D) can be performed if the core does not rupture.

Assessment. Collection of *subjective data* includes asking questions to ascertain the patient's general symptoms. Common symptoms are tenderness and pain with movement. The nurse should question the patient about a family history of diabetes mellitus or the wearing of improperly fitting clothing.

Collection of *objective data* includes noting erythema and edema in the involved area. The patient is often overweight and may use poor body hygiene techniques.

Diagnostic Tests. Diagnosis is based primarily on a thorough physical examination, health history, and inspection of the area. A culture may be done of the drainage.

Medical Management. Medical treatment is aimed at preventing the spread of the infection. Patients in the hospital are isolated, using drainage and secretion precautions. Surgical treatment may include draining the lesion and applying topical antibiotics.

Nursing Interventions. Warm soaks, two to three times a day, can be used to speed the process of suppuration. When the lesion ruptures, the hot soaks are discontinued to prevent damage of the surrounding skin and spread of the infection. Good medical asepsis should be used by the nurse while caring for these patients. In the hospital, isolation procedures for drainage and secretion should be followed. If the lesion is incised and drained, sterile technique should be used to apply topical antibiotics. The affected part needs to be immobilized to prevent pain and elevated to decrease the edema.

Nursing diagnoses and interventions for the patient with bacterial disorders include, but are not limited to, the following:

NURSING DIAGNOSIS	NURSING INTERVENTIONS
Skin integrity, impaired, related to exudate from wound	Assess wound daily for exudate and excoriation. Don gloves when providing care; use correct isolation technique. Apply skin protectant to opening.
Pain, related to edema	Assess area for any edema and tenderness. Elevate involved body part above the level of the heart. Apply hot soaks, and immobilize affected part.
Knowledge deficit, related to the disease process	Assess patient's level of knowledge and ability to learn through the use of open-ended questions. Discuss and provide written material related to the disease. Demonstrate appropriate home care.

Patient teaching. Patients should be taught not to touch the exudate. Meticulous handwashing is a must before and after contact with the lesions. Good hygiene practices should be demonstrated and return demonstrations done by the patient and family. The entire family needs individual toilet items and bath linens, and should be encouraged to use bacteriostatic soap and shampoo. Proper disposal and cleaning of contaminated articles need to be demonstrated by the nurse.

Prognosis. Patients make full recovery when the treatment plan is followed.

FUNGAL INFECTIONS OF THE SKIN

Fungal infections, which are known as *dermatophytoses,* are superficial infections of the skin. The most common types are tinea capitis, tinea corporis, tinea cruris, and tinea pedis.

Etiology/Pathophysiology. Tinea capitis is commonly known as ringworm of the scalp. *Microsporum audouinii* is the major fungal pathogen. The fungus is spread by contact with infected articles. Trauma or irritation breaks the skin and facilitates spread of the infection (Fig. 25-6).

Tinea corporis is known as ringworm of the body. It occurs on parts of the body with little or no hair.

Tinea cruris is known as jock itch. It is found in the groin area.

Tinea pedis is the most common of all fungal infections. Commonly known as athlete's foot, it is seen between the toes of persons whose feet perspire heavily.

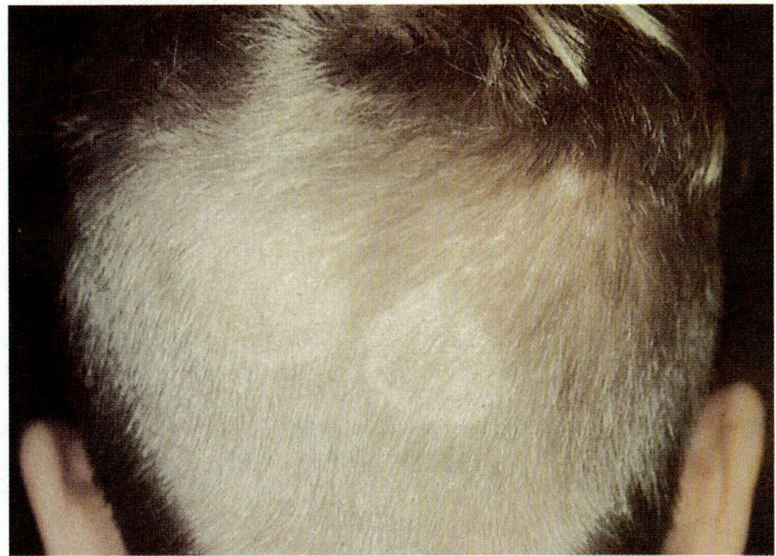

FIG. 25-6 Scalp ringworm. (From Baran R, Dawber RPR, Levene GM: *Color atlas of the hair, scalp, and nails,* London, 1991, Wolfe.)

The fungus can also be spread from contaminated public bathroom facilities and swimming pools.

Clinical Manifestations. Tinea capitis (ringworm of the scalp) is usually an erythematous, round lesion with pustules around the edges. Temporary alopecia occurs at the site, and infected hairs will turn a blue-green under a Wood's light.

Tinea corporis (ringworm of the body) produces flat lesions that are clear in the center with erythematous borders. Scaliness may also be found, and pruritus is severe.

Tinea cruris (jock itch) has brownish-red lesions that migrate out from the groin area. Pruritus and skin excoriation from scratching are found.

Tinea pedis (athlete's foot) produces more skin maceration than the others. Commonly seen are fissures and vesicles around and below the toes, with occasional discoloration of the infected area.

Assessment. The nurse's collection of the *subjective data* will include any symptoms of extreme pruritus and tenderness.

Collection of *objective data* for tinea capitis should include an inspection and location of a round lesion that is scaling and has pustules around the edges of the scalp. The involved area is erythematous and has no hair. In tinea corporis the nurse will find flat lesions with clear centers and erythematous borders on nonhairy body parts. In tinea cruris the groin area will reveal brown to red lesions that radiate outward, with skin excoriation from intense scratching. In tinea pedis the nurse will find fissures between the toes and soft skin accompanied by vesicular lesions and thick toenails.

Diagnostic Tests. The diagnosis is primarily by visual inspection. A Wood's light or Wood's lamp is an ultraviolet light used to diagnose tinea capitis. The light causes hairs infected by the fungus to become brilliantly fluorescent. No other tests are performed, but a thorough health history supports the diagnosis of all fungal infections of the skin.

Medical Management. Medical treatment involves the use of topical and/or oral antifungal drugs. Griseofulvin (Fulvicin, Grifulvin) is the most common oral drug given. Antifungal soaps and shampoos are recommended. Antifungal agents such as tolnaftate 1% (Tinactin) or Desinex can be applied directly. Treatment may last from 2 to 6 weeks. See the medications table on pp. 540-541 for a list of drugs commonly used for fungal and other integumentary infections.

Nursing Interventions. Nursing interventions for fungal infections involve two primary principles. The first is to protect the involved area from trauma and irritation by keeping it clean and dry; the second is the proper application of medications and warm compresses to alleviate the fungus.

Tinea pedis should be treated with warm soaks using Burow's solution and topical antifungal agents. Excellent foot care is stressed. The feet should be cleaned and dried thoroughly, paying special attention to the toes. Wearing sandal-type shoes or going barefoot helps decrease foot moisture. Footwear, such as stockings, needs to be of an absorbent material.

Nursing diagnosis and intervention for the patient with fungal infections include, but are not limited to, the following:

MEDICATIONS FOR THE INTEGUMENTARY SYSTEM

Medication	Trade name	Action	Side Effects	Nursing Implications
Acyclovir	Zovirax	Antiviral	Topical—burning, rash, pruritus, stinging Systemic—headache, seizures, renal toxicity, phlebitis at IV site	Topical—use glove to apply, cover lesion completely Systemic—ensure adequate hydration to prevent crystallization in kidneys administer IV dose for at least 1 hour
Alpha-Keri	Same	Emollient	Local irritation, allergic reactions	For external use only, exercise caution when using in tub to avoid slipping
Aluminum acetate solution	Burow's solution	Astringent	Local irritation, allergic reactions	For external use only, do not use with occlusive dressings
Antihistamines	Benadryl, Vistaril, Atarax, others	Blocks histamine at the H1 receptor site, inhibiting many allergic reactions	Drowsiness, dizziness, confusion, dry mouth, urinary retention	If drowsiness occurs, avoid activities that require concentration, avoid using with alcohol or other CNS depressants
Benzoyl peroxide	Many	Antiacne agent	Excessive drying of skin, allergic reactions	Discontinue use if excessive drying or peeling occurs, avoid contact with hair or fabric
Chlorhexidine gluconate	Hibiclens	Antimicrobial skin cleanser	Irritation, dermatitis, allergic reactions	For external use only, do not use on broken skin unless directed by a physician
Calamine lotion	Many	Astringent	Local irritation	For external use only
Coal tar	Many	Treatment of pruritic dermatoses, including eczema and psoriasis	Photosensitivity, dermatitis, allergic reactions	Avoid exposure to sunlight for 72 hours after use, may stain clothes and bathtub, for external use only
Corticosteroids (topical)	Lidex, Kenalog, Valisone, many others	Anti-inflammatory agent	Local irritation, maceration, superinfection, atrophy, itching, and dryness of skin (more severe local reactions and systemic effects are possible with higher doses and potency or when used with occlusive dressings)	Do not use occlusive dressings unless directed by a physician, washing or soaking area before application increases drug penetration
Crotamiton	Eurax	Scabicidal and antipruritic	Local irritation, allergic reactions	For external use only, do not aply to severely irritated skin
Curel	Same	Emollient	Local irritation, allergic reactions	For external use only
Eucerin	Same	Emollient	Local irritation, allergic reactions	For external use only
Griseofulvin	Fulvicin, Grisactin, Grifulvin, others	Antifungal agent	Hypersensitivity reactions, photosensitivity, nausea, fatigue, mental confusion	Avoid exposure to sunlight, drug absorption increased when given with meals, clinical response may appear only after full course of therapy
Isotretinoin	Accutane	Antiacne agent	Severe dryness of skin, mouth, eyes, mucous membranes, nose, and nails; skin fragility; epistaxis; joint and muscle pain; nausea; abdominal pain	Absolutely contraindicated in pregnant women of women contemplating pregnancy, female patients of childbearing age must practice contraception during therapy and 1 month before and after therapy, take drug with meals, do not take vitamin supplements containing vitamin A, avoid exposure to sunlight

MEDICATIONS FOR THE INTEGUMENTARY SYSTEM—CONT'D

Medication	Trade name	Action	Side Effects	Nursing Implications
Lindane	Kwell	Scabicide, ovicide	Local irritaion, dizziness seizures (rare)	For external use only, avoid applying to open skin lesions
Lubriderm	Same	Emollient	Local irritation, allergic reactions	For external use only, exercise caution when using in tub to avoid slipping
Methoxsalen	Oxsoralen, Oxsoralen-Ultra, 8-MOP	Skin pigmenting agent	Severe photosensitivity, nausea, nervousness, insomnia, headache, hypopigmentation	Avoid all exposure to sunlight for 8 hours after oral ingestion and for several days after topical application, wear UVA-absorbing sunglasses for 24 hours after oral ingestion, sunscreens may be used to prevent exposure to sunlight, take agent with food or milk or in divided doses, clinical response may not appear until after several months
Povidone-iodine	Betadine	Topical antimicrobial agent	Local irritation	For external use only, may stain skin and clothing
Pyrethrin	Rid, others	Pediculicide	Local irritation	For external use only, do not use for infestations of eyebrows or eyelashes
Salicylic acid	Numerous	keratolytic agent	Local irritation, erythema, scaling	For external use only; may damage clothing, plastic, wood, and other materials on contact
Tetracycline	Numerous	Antibacterial agent	Topical—stinging, burning Systemic—nausea, diarrhea, photosensitivity	Topical—slight yellowing of skin may occur Systemic—take on empty stomach; avoid concomitant administration of dairy products, laxatives, antacids, and products containing iron; avoid contact with sunlight; may cause permanent tooth discoloration when used in children
Tolnaftate	Tinactin, Aftate, others	Antifungal agent	Local irritation	For external use only

NURSING DIAGNOSIS	NURSING INTERVENTIONS
Skin integrity, impaired, related to increased moisture and pruritus	Keep involved area clean and dry. Have patients wear loose-fitting clothing and shoes. Apply medications as directed.

Patient teaching. Patient education involves teaching proper skin care and comfort measures to relieve pruritus. The nurse should review the medications to be taken and the procedures to be done at home by the patient, emphasizing that fungal skin disorders may take months to cure. General education about athlete's foot should be stressed and the many misconceptions clarified, such as wearing white socks to treat the disease.

Prognosis. Prognosis for recovery is good. Few complications result when treatment is followed.

INFLAMMATORY DISORDERS OF THE SKIN

Superficial infection of the skin is known as dermatitis. It can be caused by numerous agents, such as drugs, plants, chemicals, metals, and food. Regardless of the precipitating factor, the lesions associated with dermatitis develop along the same pattern. The nurse first observes erythema and edema, followed by the eruption of vesicles that rupture and encrust. Pruritus is always present, which promotes further skin excoriation.

Contact Dermatitis

Etiology/Pathophysiology. Contact dermatitis is caused by direct contact with agents in the environment to which a person is hypersensitive. The epidermis becomes inflamed and damaged by the repeated contact with the physical and chemical irritants. Common causes of dermatitis are detergents, soaps, industrial chemicals, and plants such as poison ivy.

Clinical Manifestations. Lesions appear first at the point of contact with the irritant. Usually the patient feels burning, pain, pruritus, and edema. The involved area is soon erythematous, with **papules** (small, raised, solid skin lesions less than 1 cm in diameter) and vesicles appearing most often on the dorsal surfaces.

Assessment. The nurse needs to thoroughly research the history of the patient's activities. The nurse may ask the patient to write a log of her activities for the 48 hours before development of symptoms.

Collection of *subjective data* usually reveals that the patient has (1) tried a new soap, (2) been traveling and using different personal items, (3) been working with plants or flowers, (4) severe pruritus, and (5) difficulty moving the involved area.

Collection of *objective data* by the nurse should find (1) erythema, (2) papules and vesicles that generally ooze and weep a clear fluid, (3) scratch marks resulting from intense pruritus, and (4) edema of the area.

Diagnostic Tests. The primary diagnostic test is accurate collection of a health history to identify the agent. Intradermal skin testing may be done to identify plants and environmental agents, and elimination diets are used to identify food allergies.

Medical Management. Medical intervention is directed at identifying the cause of the hypersensitive reaction. Symptomatic treatment for the inflammation, edema, and pruritus may include application of corticosteroids and the oral administration of antihistamines such as Benadryl.

Nursing Interventions. The primary goal is to identify the offensive agent so as to rest the involved skin and protect it from further damage. To help identify the cause, the nurse needs to describe the pattern of the reaction.

Wet dressings, using Burow's solution, help promote the healing process. To prevent infection, aseptic technique is used to apply the corticosteroids to the open lesions.

Pruritus is responsible for most of the discomfort. A cool environment with increased humidity decreases the pruritus. Cold compresses may be applied to decrease circulation to the area (vasoconstriction). Daily baths to cleanse the skin should be taken with an application of oil. Fingernails should be cut at the level of the fingertips to decrease excoriation from scratching. Clothing should be lightweight and loose to decrease trauma of the involved area.

Nursing diagnoses and interventions for the patient with inflammation of the skin include, but are not limited to, the following:

NURSING DIAGNOSES	NURSING INTERVENTIONS
Skin integrity, impaired, related to scratching	Assess for signs of scratching. Have patient keep fingernails short and wear mittens. Apply medications as directed.
Pain, related to pruritus	Assess degree of pruritus and discomfort every shift. Keep environment cool. Apply cold compresses.
Infection, high risk for, related to scratching and excoriation	Assess for signs of infection. Describe extent and location of trauma.

Patient teaching. The patient should be taught to keep an accurate history of possible predisposing offensive agents. As soon as the primary irritant has been identified, it should be avoided, as well as soaps, excessive heat, and rubbing of the area. Any time the skin is exposed to the primary irritant, the affected area should be washed thoroughly. Topical creams may be applied only as directed by a physician.

Prognosis. Removal of the offensive agent results in full recovery.

Dermatitis Venenata, Exfoliative Dermatitis, and Dermatitis Medicamentosa

Etiology/Pathophysiology. Dermatitis venenata results from contact with certain plants. Common terms used are *poison ivy* and *poison oak.* The signs and symptoms of this dermatitis include mild to severe erythema with pruritus. In this condition, on first exposure the body undergoes a sensitizing antigen formation. This results in an immunological change in certain lymphocytes. Subsequent exposure to the antigen causes the lymphocytes to release irritating chemicals, leading to inflammation, edema, and vesiculation. The lesions are mainly found on the body part exposed to the sensitizing agent.

Exfoliative dermatitis may be caused by the infestation of certain heavy metals, such as arsenic or mercury, or by antibiotics, aspirin, codeine, gold, or iodine. The skin sloughs off, and the area becomes edematous and erythematous. Severe pruritus with fever occurs, and most patients require hospitalization. Treatment is individualized. If the cause can be determined, it should be removed or treated appropriately. Care is essential to prevent secondary infection, to avoid further irritation, and to maintain fluid balance.

Dermatitis medicamentosa occurs when a person is given a medication to which he is hypersensitive. Any drug can cause a reaction, but the common agents are penicillin, codeine, and iron (Fig. 25-7).

Clinical Manifestations. Clinical manifestations range from mild to severe erythema with vesicular eruptions. In severe reactions respiratory distress may occur. Any type of lesion may be found.

Assessment. Collection of *subjective data* for dermatitis is pruritus and a burning pain in the involved area.

Collection of *objective data* reveals lesions that are white in the center and red on the periphery. Vesicles are common in dermatitis venenata. In dermatitis medicamentosa, severe dyspnea caused by respiratory distress may be noted.

Medical Management. The medical treatment for dermatitis ranges from therapeutic baths to administration of corticosteroids. The medical treatment is directed at the cause.

Nursing Interventions. In dermatitis venenata the patient should wash the affected part immediately after contact with the offending allergen. After the lesions appear, only cool, open, wet dressings should be used. However, calamine lotion is a common over-the-counter medication for pruritus.

Pruritus is the primary symptom in all dermatitis. Therapeutic baths using colloid solution, lotions, and ointments are used to help relieve the pruritus. Emotional support is necessary. The physical appearance of the patient is difficult for the patient and family members to accept.

In dermatitis medicamentosa, interventions revolve around identifying the drug and discontinuing its use. If the specific drug that is the offending allergen cannot be pinpointed, no drugs should be given. The physician must be notified. The lesions will disappear after the medication is discontinued. More specific nursing intervention is directed by individual patient symptoms. It is important to educate the patient to wear a Medic-Alert bracelet or necklace showing the name of the allergen; the patient should be instructed to notify all health care personnel of the medication allergy.

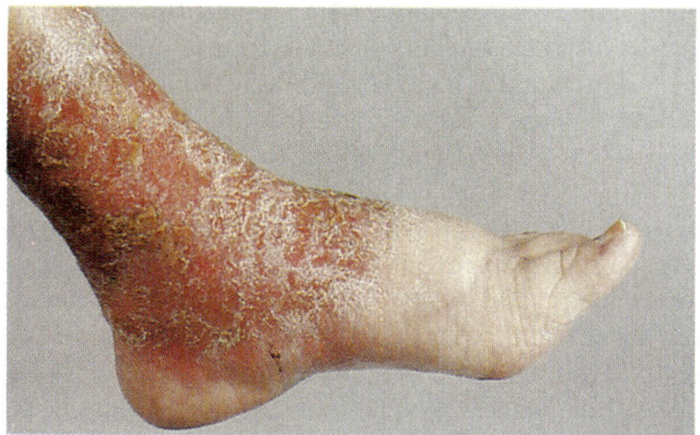

FIG. 25-7 Dermatitis medicamentosa. (From duVivier A: *Atlas of clinical dermatology,* ed 2, London, 1986, Gower.)

Nursing diagnoses and interventions for the patient with dermatitis include, but are not limited to, the following:

NURSING DIAGNOSES	NURSING INTERVENTIONS
Skin integrity, impaired, related to crusted, open lesions	Inspect the lesions every day for exudate, size, and specific body area involved. Keep area clean and dry. Don gloves when giving direct patient care.
Pain, related to pruritus	Assess pain, identifying contributing factors. Administer analgesics; cool, wet compresses; and antibiotics as directed.
Infection, high risk for, related to break in skin	Assess skin for signs of infection. Identify interventions to prevent or reduce the risk of infection. Monitor vital signs; assess for elevated temperature. Stress medical aseptic handwashing technique. Use aseptic technique, and keep involved areas dry when providing care.
Knowledge deficit, related to the cause and spread of the disease	Assess the patient's knowledge level and readiness to learn. Demonstrate appropriate care and application of topical medications. Stress importance of individual personal items, such as linens and towels. Involves patient and family in teaching.

Prognosis. Full recovery occurs when the offending agent is removed.

Urticaria

Etiology/Pathophysiology. **Urticaria** is the term applied to the presence of wheals or hives in an allergic reaction commonly caused by drugs, food, insect bites, inhalants, emotional stress, or exposure to heat or cold. The **wheals** (round elevation of the skin, white in the center with a pale red periphery) of urticaria appear suddenly.

Urticaria or hives is caused by the release of histamine in an antigen-antibody reaction.

Clinical Manifestations. The increased histamine causes the capillaries to dilate, resulting in increased permeability.

Assessment. Collection of *subjective data* includes pruritus and a burning pain.

Collection of *objective data* will identify transient wheals of varying shapes and sizes with well-defined erythematous margins and pale centers. Intense scratching may be seen, and in some cases respiration may be compromised.

Diagnostic Tests. A detailed history is the primary tool to identify the cause of hives. An allergy skin test may be performed using minute quantities of the antigen to identify the allergic substances.

Medical Management. Relief from urticaria can be achieved by administering an antihistamine and sometimes epinephrine. Identification of the cause of the urticaria is important to prevent recurrence.

Nursing Interventions. Nursing interventions are directed at helping the patient identify the cause and decreasing the discomfort from the pruritus.

Patient teaching. The patient should be taught possible causes and prevention methods. Medications should be explained thoroughly and therapeutic baths demonstrated. The signs and symptoms of an anaphylactic reaction should be covered, such as shortness of breath, wheezing, and cyanosis.

Prognosis. Patients recover fully when the offensive agent is determined and avoided.

Eczema (Atopic Dermatitis)

Etiology/Pathophysiology. Eczema is primarily a disease of infants and is associated with allergies. The common allergies are to chocolate, eggs, wheat, and orange juice.

The allergen causes histamine to be released and an antigen-antibody reaction occurs.

Clinical Manifestations. Papular and vesicular lesions appear, surrounded by erythema. The vesicles generally rupture, discharging a yellow, tenacious exudate that dries and encrusts. If the lesions become infected, the skin may depigment and become shiny with dry scales (Fig. 25-8).

Assessment. Collection of *subjective data* includes pruritus and scratching. Children are generally more fussy and irritable, and anorexia is commonly found. The skin is very sensitive to touch.

Collection of *objective data* will include vesicles and papules found on the scalp, forehead, cheeks, neck, and the surfaces of the extremities. The involved area is erythematous and very dry. Tiny cracks in the epithelium allow fluid to escape and further promote dryness. The primary signs result from the scratching from pruritus.

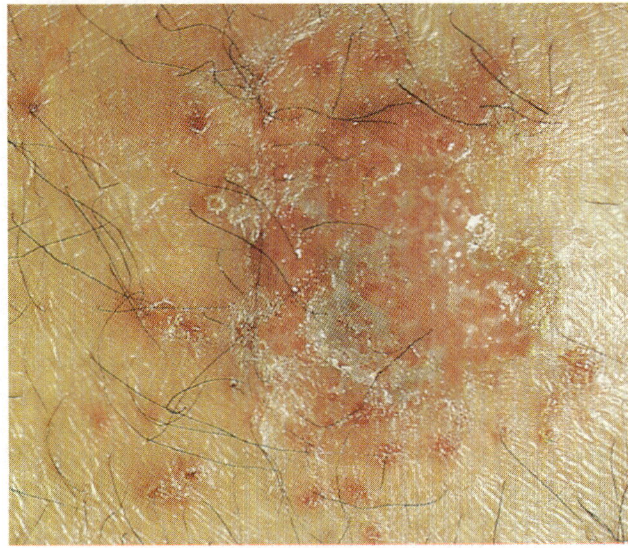

FIG. 25-8 Septic eczema. (From duVivier A: *Atlas of clinical dermatology,* ed 2, London, 1986, Gower.)

Diagnostic Tests. The diagnosis is generally made during a thorough history because heredity is a prominent factor in eczema. Diet elimination and skin testing may be used to identify the specific substance to which the patient is hypersensitive.

Medical Management. The medical treatment is concerned with reducing the amount of allergen exposure. The eruptions and pruritus can be relieved if the aggravating factor is identified and controlled. The primary goal is to break the inflammation cycle. Hydration of the skin is the key to treatment. The skin is dry because of tiny cracks that allow body fluids to escape.

The skin may be hydrated by soaking the affected area in warm water for 15 to 20 minutes and then applying an occlusive ointment to retain the water. Examples of occlusive preparations are petrolatum, corticosteroid ointments, and vegetable shortenings. The skin should be patted dry after the bath and the occlusive preparation applied immediately to the damp skin.

Nursing Interventions. Nursing interventions are directed toward treatment of symptoms for the eczematous patient. The nurse is responsible for administering the therapeutic bath and occlusive preparations as directed. Wet dressings may be used to maximize hydration of the skin. Topical steroids may be applied to relieve the discomfort of the lesions. The emotional impact experienced by eczema patients ranges from anger to depression. The nurse must provide an emotional outlet for these patients.

When the lesions begin to heal, a lotion such as Eucerin, Alpha-Keri, Lubriderm, or Curel should be applied three to four times a day to add moisture to the skin. Wet wraps and occlusive preparations only hold water already present.

Before the development of steroids, coal tar products were used to reduce the skin inflammation. Coal tar products do not decrease inflammation as quickly as steroids, but they last longer and have fewer side effects. Therefore, coal tar preparations are recommended for chronic eczema. Coal tar preparations are applied once a day at bedtime with a moisturizer. Examples of coal tar preparations are Estar-Gel and Psori-Gel.

Nursing diagnoses and interventions for the patient with eczema include but are not limited to the following:

NURSING DIAGNOSES	NURSING INTERVENTIONS
Pain, related to pruritus	Assess comfort by evaluating behavior. Apply topical medications as directed. Have patient keep fingernails short and wear cotton clothing. Administer baths, and apply occlusive preparations.
Social isolation, related to alteration in physical appearance	Assess factors that contribute to social isolation. Identify support systems for patient. Establish therapeutic relationship. Discuss situation with patient, listening carefully to expressions of concern.

Patient teaching. Patient teaching for eczematous patients should stress (1) avoidance of the agent, (2) avoidance of extreme changes in temperature, (3) how to handle dry skin, (4) no strenuous exercise in hot weather, (5) dangers of self-treatment, and (6) application of medications as directed.

The patient and family should be involved in the care; the primary concern is the chronic nature of the disease and the effect it may have on the patient's self-image and personality.

Prognosis. No definite cure exists for eczema. Eczema is a disease that requires good skin care for adequate recovery. Recurrence is common until the child reaches adolescence.

Acne Vulgaris

Etiology/Pathophysiology. Acne is an inflammatory papulopustular skin eruption that involves the sebaceous glands; it occurs primarily in adolescents. The exact cause is unknown. However, several factors that have been considered are diet, stress, heredity, and overactive hormones. Hygiene has not been found to be a significant factor in the development of acne.

Acne develops when the oil glands become occluded. At puberty androgens secreted increase the size of the oil glands, causing the sebum to combine more readily with epithelial cells and bacteria. Sebum may then occlude a hair follicle, forming a *comedo* (plural, comedones). A comedo is a blackhead. It is dark because of the effect of oxygen on sebum, not because of the presence of dirt.

Clinical Manifestations. Acne is found most often on the face, neck, upper chest, shoulder, and back. The first symptom is usually tenderness and edema in the area, followed by the comedo. The skin is oily and shiny, and the lesions last up to 10 days. Scarring results from large lesions that are traumatized when the individual tries to rupture the comedo (Fig. 25-9).

Assessment. Collection of ***subjective data*** includes asking the adolescent how acne affects life-style: Does it affect participation in activities or group communication? Most patients acknowledge that acne affects their self-image. Common locations are the face and chin. Lesions increase with emotional upsets and stress.

Collection of ***objective data*** will include noting the presence of edema in the involved area. Comedones (blackheads) are found on the face, back, and/or chest. The nurse will also observe that patients with acne do not take part in many group activities.

Diagnostic Tests. The medical diagnosis is primarily made by inspection of the lesions and a health history that supports the diagnosis. Sometimes blood samples are drawn to measure hormone levels.

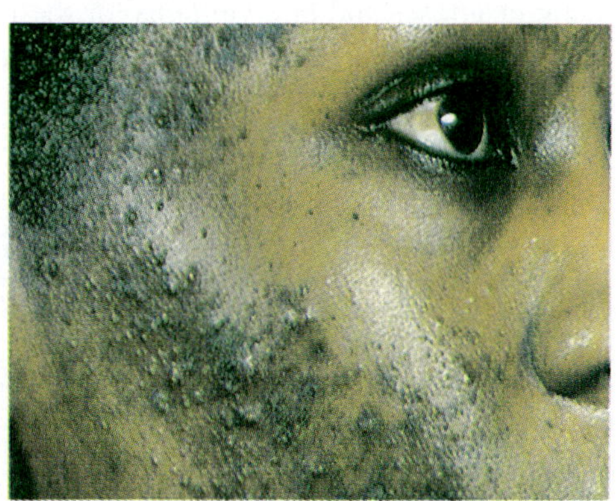

FIG. 25-9 Acne vulgaris. (From du Vivier A: *Atlas of clinical dermatology,* ed 2, London, 1986, Gower.)

Medical Management. The medical management can involve topical, systemic, or intralesional medications. Topical therapy peels away the superficial skin layer to prevent sebum occlusions. A common topical medication is benzoyl peroxide gel (like Clearasil). Effective topical therapy requires the use of special cleansing agents followed by applications of vitamin A acids, antibiotics, and sulfur-zinc lotions.

Systemic therapy may be combined with topical therapy. Systemic antibiotics such as tetracycline are used. A new drug, isotretinoin (Accutane), a form of vitamin A, is used frequently. Accutane reduces the sebum production and abnormal keratinization of gland ducts. Accutane must be prescribed with extreme caution in adolescent females, because it is destructive to fetal development during pregnancy.

Nursing Interventions. In planning nursing interventions the nurse needs to be aware that most adolescents do not comply with long-term treatment regimens. The nurse must assess and consider what acne means to them. The actual extent of the condition is not as important as the adolescent's feelings. When their faces constantly have ugly black and white lesions, it is very hard for adolescents to like themselves.

In addition to psychological concerns the nurse should focus on preventive nursing interventions. The important areas are skin care, compliance, and emotional support. Prevention stresses identification of factors that directly increase acne. Although poor hygiene may not be a cause, cleanliness decreases infection and promotes healing. The patient's hands and hair should be kept away from the face. Clothes should not restrict affected areas, and hair should be washed daily. The skin should be washed two or three times a day with a medicated soap. Cosmetics need to be water based, and products that have wax esters should be avoided. Compliance is difficult, because improvement is slow. Often 3 weeks of treatment is required before any noticeable improvement is seen by the family or friends.

Nursing diagnoses and interventions for the patient with acne vulgaris include but are not limited to the following:

NURSING DIAGNOSES	NURSING INTERVENTIONS
Skin integrity, impaired, related to occluded oil glands	Assess extent of occluded oil glands by inspecting lesions for size, color, and location. Monitor for signs of infection. Wash involved areas three to four times a day. Apply medications to decrease occlusion of oil glands.
Self-esteem disturbance, related to physical appearance	Assess primary cause of low self-esteem and extent of feelings. Assess family support. Assess patient awareness and ways to deal with the situation. Note nonverbal language to discover patient's perception of the illness. Stress the importance of not comparing oneself with others. Have patient list current success and strengths. Give positive reinforcement.
Social isolation, related to decreased self-esteem	Assess extent and feelings of isolation. Assess factors that contribute to sense of helplessness. Listen to and spend time with patient. Involve patient in support group. Focus on patient's strengths.

Patient teaching. Patient education should include the physical and emotional needs of the patient. The nurse should address diet, hygiene, stress reduction, makeup, and medications. Coping skills may need to be retaught and counseling referrals made. The extensive treatment time should be covered in minute detail, because this disease is chronic and exacerbations will occur. Keeping the adolescent communicating about feelings will decrease any long-term affects acne may have on his personality.

Prognosis. Prognosis for acne is good. However, lasting psychological effects can occur from the scarring that may result.

Psoriasis

Etiology/Pathophysiology. Psoriasis is a noninfectious skin disorder; it is a hereditary, chronic, proliferative disease involving the epidermis and can occur at any age. No specific predisposing factors are known. The skin cells divide much more rapidly than normal. The normal time for the entire skin to be replaced, through sloughing and generation of new cells, is 28 days; in psoriasis the time may decrease to 7 days. The severe scaling is a result of the rapid cell division.

Clinical Manifestations. The lesions appear as raised, erythematous, circumscribed, silvery, scaling plaques. The primary lesion is papular. The papules become plaques located on the scalp, elbows, chin, and trunk (Fig. 25-10).

Assessment. Collection of *subjective data* initially will reveal only mild pruritus. Sometimes feelings of depres-

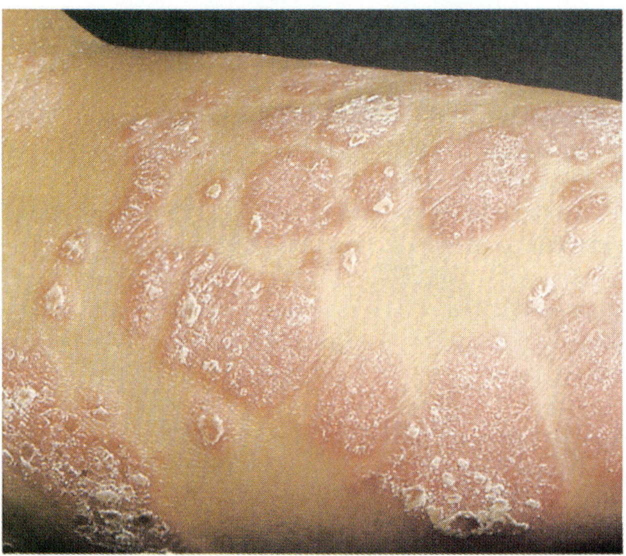

FIG. 25-10 Psoriasis. (From du Vivier A: *Atlas of clinical dermatology,* ed 2, London, 1986, Gower.)

sion, frustration, and loneliness are expressed. Observers stare and avoid contact with the patient.

Collection of *objective data* includes observing dull, erythematous, sharply outlined plaques covered with silvery scales on the elbows, knees, and scalp. Fingernails can be affected and will show pitting with yellowish discoloration.

Diagnostic Tests. No specific diagnostic tests exist for psoriasis. Primary diagnosis is made by observation of the patient and the symptoms displayed.

Medical Management. Medical management is aimed at slowing the proliferation of epithelial layers of the skin. Topical steroids and keratolytic agents are used in occlusive wet dressings to decrease inflammation. Keratolytic agents such as tar preparations and salicylic acid (Calicylic) decrease the shedding of the outer layer of the skin. Topical steroids used are hydrocortisone and Valisone.

Photochemotherapy may also be used. This treatment involves the use of a drug enhanced by exposure to light. PUVA therapy combines the use of methoxsalen (Psoralen), which is given orally, and the concurrent use of ultraviolet light A (uva); hence, the name PUVA.

Nursing Interventions. Nursing interventions include proper administration of the treatment modality. Additional rest and measures to promote psychological wellbeing, such as counseling, are necessary. The emotional needs of this patient are as important as the physical needs. Because this disease is chronic, the patient should be encouraged to focus on positive attributes.

Nursing diagnoses and interventions for the patient with psoriasis include but are not limited to the following:

NURSING DIAGNOSES	NURSING INTERVENTIONS
Skin integrity, impaired, related to proliferation of epithelial cells	Assess extent of the scaliness. Administer treatment method correctly. Use medical aseptic technique.
Self-esteem disturbance, related to appearance	Assess patient's concept of body. Help patient to focus on positive aspects. Discuss with patient ways to conceal obvious lesions.
Social isolation, related to decreased self-esteem	Assess activity pattern and social outlets. Demonstrate ways to conceal lesions with clothes. Involve patient in support group.
Infection, high risk for, related to open lesions	Assess skin for open lesions. Use surgical asepsis when caring for open lesions.

Patient teaching. The primary points should include the nature of the disease, the correct application of the treatment modality, and compliance with medical care. It should be stressed that patients should not treat themselves. The patient should be informed that the disease is not curable.

Prognosis. Psoriasis is a chronic disease. The clinical course is variable, but less than half of the patients followed for a prolonged period will have a prolonged remission; severity may range from a minimal cosmetic problem to a life-threatening emergency.

PARASITIC DISEASES OF THE SKIN

Pediculosis

Etiology/Pathophysiology. **Pediculosis** (lice infestation) is a parasitic disorder of the skin that is usually associated with poor living conditions and poor personal hygiene. This is not always the case, however; pediculosis can occur in any life-style. Lice obtain their nutrition from the blood of their victims. They leave their eggs (nits) on the skin surface attached to the shaft of the hair (Figs. 25-11 and 25-12 on p. 548).

Humans have three types of lice: the head louse, the body louse, and the pubic louse. In pediculosis capitis the head louse attaches itself to the hair shaft and lays 8 to 16 eggs per day. The eggs can be seen best at the back of the neck as gray, shiny, oval bodies.

In pediculosis corporis, the body louse is found around the neck, waist, and thighs. The louse is generally found in the seams of clothing. Severe pruritus and

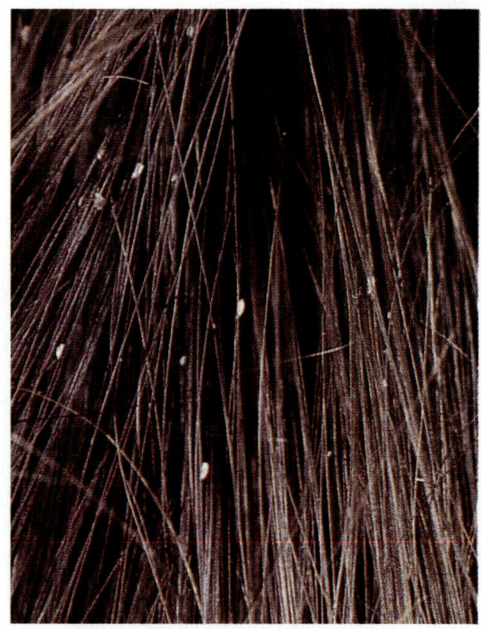

FIG. 25-11 Eggs of the pediculus attached to shafts of hair. (From du Vivier A: *Atlas of clinical dermatology,* ed 2, London, 1986, Gower.)

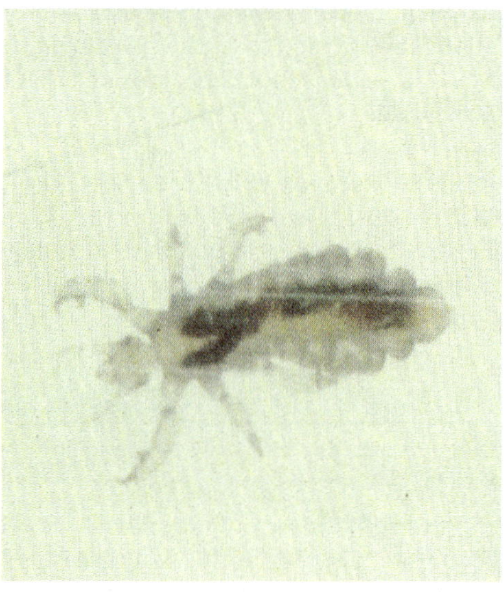

FIG. 25-12 Lice have 6 legs and are wingless. (From du Vivier A: *Atlas of clinical dermatology,* ed 2, London, 1986, Gower.)

pinpoint hemorrhages are caused from the bite of the louse.

The pubic louse, the parasite involved in pediculosis pubis, does not resemble the head or body louse. It looks like a crab with sharp pincers that attach to the pubic hair. Transmission can be by sexual contact, bed clothing, or bath towels.

Clinical Manifestations. Nits or lice can be seen on the body. Pinpoint raised red macules, pinpoint hemorrhages, and severe pruritus confirm the diagnosis. Excoriation is common because of the intense pruritus.

Assessment. Collection of *subjective data* will include complaints of pruritus in the area involved. Tenderness and difficulty wearing clothes are also noted.

Collection of *objective data* will reveal erythema, petechiae, and skin excoriation in the area.

Diagnostic Tests. The diagnostic test is a physical examination of the involved area. A health history supports the diagnosis.

Medical Management. The topical application of a pediculicide such as lindane (Kwell) or pyrethrin (RID) is used in any area the contaminated patient has contacted. The specific technique for applying these products varies but should be followed very closely to control the lice.

Nursing Interventions. The primary nursing interventions involve the application of the medication to rid the patient of the lice. Every place the patient has had contact needs to be cleaned. Health teaching stresses the transmission of the disease by contact. Assessment of the patient's emotional needs is important. Having a lice infestation carries a negative implication by society that the patient has poor hygiene practices.

Patient teaching. Nursing care focuses on identifying involved persons and appropriate health teaching. The nature and transmission of the disease are stressed. Each family member should be assessed for nits and taught measures to reduce pruritus, such as cool compresses and corticosteroid ointments. Any furniture or nonwashable materials with which the patient has come in contact should be properly cleaned to prevent reinfection.

Prognosis. The prognosis is good; proper treatment results in full recovery.

Scabies

Etiology/Pathophysiology. The cause of scabies is the female itch mite *(Sarcoptes scabiei).* The mite penetrates the skin and makes a burrow. Once under the skin, the mite lays eggs that mature and rise to the skin surface. Scabies is transmitted by prolonged contact with an infected area. Overcrowded conditions, poverty, changing sexual behaviors, and world travel have increased the incidence of scabies. Scabies now occurs in all age-groups and socioeconomic classes.

Clinical Manifestations. Scabies causes wavy, brown, threadlike lines on the body. Pruritus is severe and secondary infections are common from the excoriation caused by scratching. Locations for the threadlike lines are hands, arms, body folds, and genitalia (Fig. 25-13).

Assessment. Collection of *subjective data* includes the severe pruritus associated with scabies and the skin excoriation resulting from the scratching.

Collection of *objective data* includes finding the wavy brown lines on the body and severe erythema from the scratching.

Diagnostic Tests. Identification can be confirmed by microscopic examination of infected skin. A health history and characteristic signs and symptoms support the diagnosis.

Medical Management. Medical treatment is aimed at the elimination of the mite and prevention of complications. Drug therapy is basically the same as for pediculosis. Two additional drugs used are crotamiton (Eurax) and a 4% to 8% solution of sulfur in petrolatum.

Nursing Interventions. Nursing interventions are directed at improving skin integrity by using medical aseptic techniques to provide hygiene and to apply medications. Proper application of medication is essential to destroy the parasite. The nurse must also consider the emotional well-being of the patient. Using open-ended questions and listening skills helps the nurse to identify potential problem areas for the patient.

Patient teaching. The primary concern is to educate the family members about the transmission of scabies. Each family member needs to treat the whole body with a scabicide. Clothing, linens, and bath articles should be washed in hot water and dried in a dryer. If clothes are line dried, they should be ironed. Each member should realize the importance of compliance with the treatment. It is important that the nurse teach the family that scabies infestations can happen to anyone. The nurse must be able to use and convey a nonjudgmental attitude toward these patients.

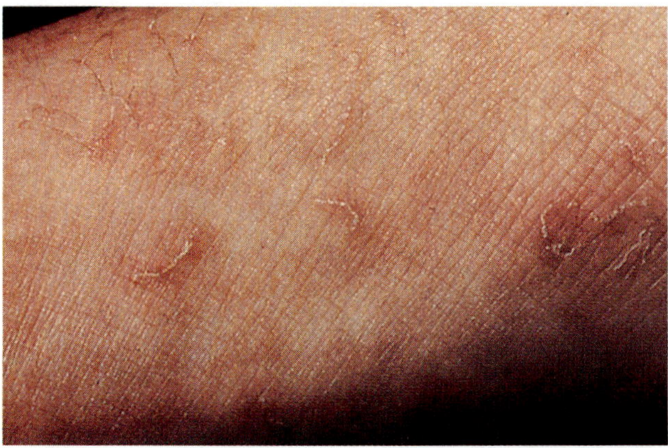

FIG. 25-13 Scabies. (From du Vivier A: *Atlas of clinical dermatology,* ed 2, London, 1986, Gower.)

Prognosis. The prognosis in good; with adequate treatment full recovery will result.

TUMORS OF THE SKIN

Overgrowth of the skin cells can develop from any layer or its appendages. The majority of skin tumors are benign. Many can be predisposing factors for skin cancer.

Clinical Manifestations. The specific signs and symptoms of skin tumors relate to the type of tumor. Keloids, which originate in scars, are hard and shiny. Angiomas resemble birthmarks, and warts (verrucae) are unattractive and located on the arms and hands. Nevi are considered to be predisposers to cancer and create anxiety in the patient when a color change is noted. Skin cancers are life threatening and occur wherever exposure to the sun may have been the greatest.

Any changes in a skin lesion should be reported to a physician. These changes could be in the size, color, border, surface, or elevation of the lesion. The development of pain, bleeding, or pruritus should also be reported.

Assessment. Collection of *subjective data* includes a good health history. The patient's risk factors should be assessed first. Life-style, occupation, family history, and geographical location are important.

Collection of *objective data* includes describing the lesion in detail. The size, location, and any pain are significant factors in determining the type of skin tumor. The appearance of the lesions can take several forms.

Diagnostic Tests. The diagnostic test for tumors of the skin is biopsy of the lesion. A health history and visual inspection support the diagnosis.

Medical Management. The primary medical intervention for skin tumors is surgical removal. Other treatment modalities are radiation therapy to decrease the size of the tumor and application of topical medications such as corticosteroids to decrease the size and inflammation.

Nursing Interventions. The potential threat of malignancy causes great concern for the patient. Careful explanations of treatments, medications, and tests help decrease anxiety. If surgery is the treatment of choice, the patient will need to be prepared for surgery.

Nursing intervention revolves around preparing the patient for the treatment needed. Most skin tumors are a threat to the patient's self-concept. Emotional care is important; the nurse should encourage the patient to verbalize feelings of fear or anxiety.

Nursing diagnoses and interventions for malignant melanoma are applicable. Although the tumors previously mentioned are not all malignant, the problems posed are the same until a definite diagnosis is made.

Patient teaching. Discharge instructions include skin care, dressing changes, and follow-up care. The nurse should involve the family in patient teaching to support the patient. The signs and symptoms of an infection should be covered for patients who have had tumors surgically removed.

Keloids

Keloids (an overgrowth of collagenous scar tissue at the site of a wound of the skin) are seen more often in African-Americans than Caucasians. Collagen tissue becomes raised, hard, and shiny. Keloids usually originate from a scar and can be located anywhere on the body. The sternum, ears, neck, and arms are common locations. Keloids are usually surgically excised but may recur. Steroids and radiation therapy are two treatment measures (Fig. 25-14).

Angiomas

An angioma develops when a group of blood vessels dilate and form a tumorlike mass. A common angioma is a birthmark, such as the port-wine birthmark. This stain is not elevated and may be found on one side of the face or any part of the body. Treatment involves electrolysis and/or x-ray therapy.

A spider angioma or telangiectasis is associated with liver disease. A group of venous capillaries dilate and branch out like a spider. Spider angiomas will usually resolve as the disease improves.

Verruca (Wart)

A **verruca** is a benign, viral, warty skin lesion with a rough, papillomatous (nipplelike) growth occurring in many forms. Verrucas may occur singly or in groups and are thought to be contagious. Common locations are the hands, arms, and fingers, but warts can occur anywhere on the body. The plantar wart develops on the sole of the foot and is extremely painful. Treatment of a wart depends on the type, location, and number. Cauterization, solid carbon dioxide, liquid nitrogen, and preparations of salicylic acid are used to remove warts from the body.

Nevi (Moles)

Nevi (singular, nevus; a pigmented, congenital skin blemish that is usually benign but may become cancerous) or moles are described as nonvascular tumors, also called *birthmarks.* There are many types of nevi, and several may become malignant, especially if traumatized. The raised, black nevus is considered one of the most threatening, and removal is recommended to prevent its becoming malignant. Any change in color, size, or texture or any bleeding or pruritus of a nevus deserves investigation.

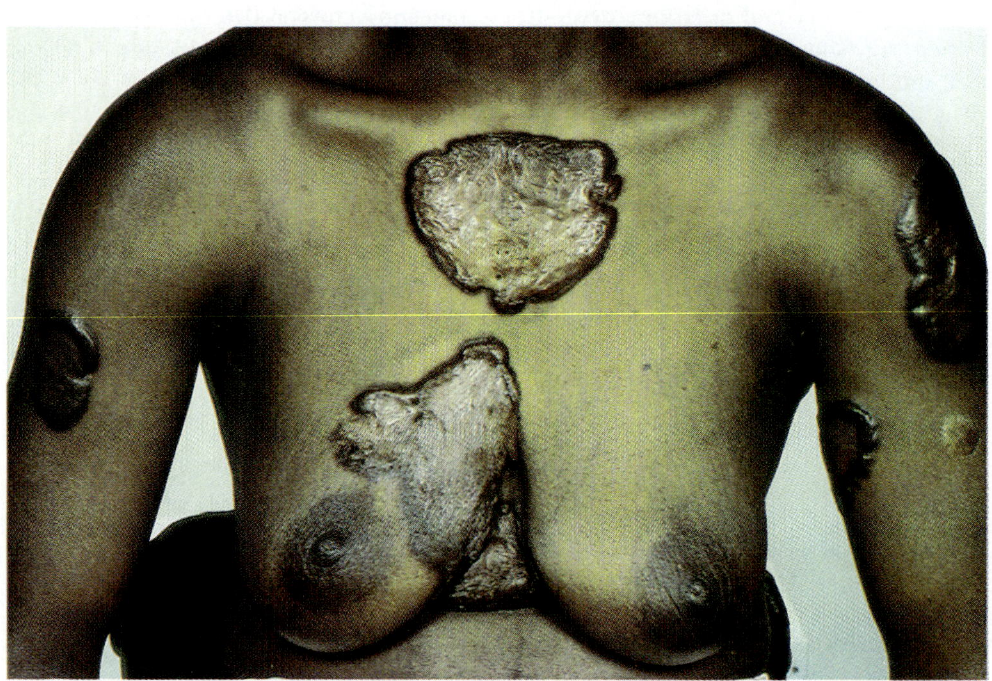

FIG. 25-14 Keloids. (From du Vivier A: *Atlas of clinical dermatology,* ed 2, London, 1986, Gower.)

Basal Cell Carcinoma

Basal cell carcinoma is one type of skin cancer. Related factors to the development of skin cancer include frequent contact with certain chemicals, overexposure to the sun, and radiation treatment. Fair-skinned people are more likely to develop skin cancer, possibly because less melanin is distributed on their skin surface.

Basal cell carcinoma is found on the face and upper trunk. It may be nodular or superficial. The nodular form is raised, firm to touch, ulcerated in the center, and has a waxy pearly border. The superficial type is raised and crusted with a raised pearly border. Local invasion destroys underlying and adjacent tissue.

Prognosis. With early detection and proper treatment, metastasis is rare, and outcome is favorable.

Squamous Cell Carcinoma

Squamous cell carcinoma occurs in body areas that have been exposed or treated with radiation. Usually the hands and head develop cancer first. The lesions are flat, nodular, and large, with some desquamation noted. Squamous cell carcinoma spreads more rapidly than other skin cancers.

Prognosis. Squamous cell carcinoma can be fatal, making early detection and treatment extremely important.

Malignant Melanoma

Etiology/Pathophysiology. A malignant melanoma is a cancerous neoplasm in which pigment cells (melano cytes) invade the epidermis, dermis, and sometimes the subcutaneous tissue. Several types of melanoma are known, and they are categorized by location and description.

Most melanomas arise from melanocytes in the epidermis, but some may appear in preexisting moles. Heredity is a factor, and any person who has a large number of moles with a variety of sizes and colors should be monitored.

The occurrence of melanoma has doubled over the past two decades, a fact associated with increased recreational exposure to the sun. The person who has a history of skin cancer is at greater risk.

Clinical Manifestations. Basically, there are four types of malignant melanomas: (1) superficial spreading melanomas, (2) malignant lentigo melanomas, (3) nodular melanomas, and (4) acral lentiginous melanomas. Superficial spreading melanomas are the most common and occur anywhere on the body. These melanomas are slightly elevated, irregularly shaped lesions, in a varying combination of hues (Fig. 25-15); common colors are tan, brown, black, blue, gray, and pink. The lentigo melanomas are usually found on the heads and necks of older persons. Characteristically these appear as tan, flat lesions that undergo changes in shape and size. The nodular melanoma grows and metastasizes faster than the other types. Nodular melanomas appear as a blueberry-type growth, varying from blue-black to pink. The patient often describes the lesion as a blood blister that fails to resolve.

Acral lentiginous melanomas occur in areas not exposed to sunlight and where no hair follicles are present. Common locations are the hands, soles, and mucous membranes of dark-skinned people.

Assessment. The collection of *subjective data* should include a thorough history related to skin cancer. Patients at greatest risk have fair complexions, blue eyes, red or blond hair, and freckles. The collection of *objective data* includes the location, color, and appearance of the lesions.

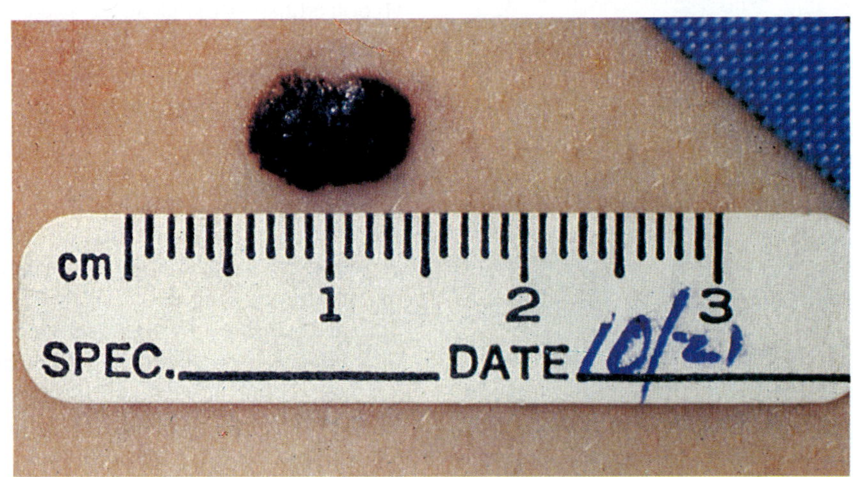

FIG. 25-15 Malignant melanoma.

Diagnostic Tests. Diagnosis primarily depends on the biopsy of the tissue. The patient is also examined thoroughly for suspicious lesions. Any lesion that is variegated in color, has an irregular border, or has an irregular surface should be monitored.

Medical Management. Medical management depends on the level of invasion and the thickness of the melanoma.

A wide excision of the primary lesion is the treatment of choice. The extent of the excision is dependent upon the size of the lesion. Skin grafts are sometimes needed.

Because melanomas tend to be radioresistant, radiation therapy is not recommended as primary treatment. It is useful for alleviating the signs and symptoms of metastatic disease of the bones, brain, and gastrointestinal tract.

Chemotherapy with agents such as cisplatin, methotrexate, and dacarbazine has some value.

Nursing Interventions. The major goals of nursing care include relief of pain, reduction of anxiety, and remission of the disease. The nurse needs to be aware that fear of the unknown is a major concern of the patient with a melanoma. Explaining procedures and diagnostic tests in terms that the patient can understand may help to decrease anxiety.

Nursing diagnoses and interventions for the patient with melanomas include but are not limited to the following:

NURSING DIAGNOSES	NURSING INTERVENTIONS
Pain, related to lesion	Assess pain using the five PQRST variables of the chief complaint. Provide nursing comfort measures, such as back rubs, to decrease pain. Administer pain medications as needed. Teach relaxation techniques.
Anxiety, related to cancer, its treatment, and prognosis	Listen to and accept expression of anger, sadness, and helplessness.
Impaired skin integrity, related to presence of lesion	Bathe patient in warm water or apply warm, moist compresses. Apply sterile dressing with antibiotic ointment when prescribed. Observe lesion or lesions for change in shape, size, and color, and for bleeding.

Patient teaching. Discharge instructions include wound care, medication, cleansing, and follow-up care. The nurse needs to assess the family's knowledge base about the seriousness and treatment of the disease.

Explain to the patient the need for regular physical examinations and regular skin self-assessment. Encourage the patient to protect skin from the sun by using sunscreens and protective clothing and limiting exposure. Medical aseptic techniques are stressed to prevent a secondary infection.

Prognosis. The key prognostic factor in malignant melanoma is the thickness of the lesion. Individuals with lesions less than 0.76 mm thick have a survival rate of almost 100%, whereas those with lesions 3 mm thick or thicker have survival rates of less than 50%. The tumor may metastasize by vascular or lymphatic spread, with rapid movement of melanoma cells to other parts of the body.

DISORDERS OF THE APPENDAGES

Alopecia

Alopecia is the loss of hair. The cause can be aging, drugs such as antineoplastics, anxiety, or disease processes. Alopecia is usually not permanent unless the loss is from aging; the hair will usually grow back but can take several months. Any time that a patient loses hair, the body image and self-esteem are threatened.

Hypertrichosis (Hirsutism)

Hypertrichosis is an excessive growth of hair in a masculine distribution. It can be hereditary or acquired as a result of hormone dysfunction and medications. The treatment is removal by dermabrasion, electrolysis, chemical depilation, shaving, plucking, or rubbing with pumice. Treatment of the specific cause will usually stop growth of more hair.

Hypotrichosis

Hypotrichosis is the absence of hair or a decrease in hair growth. Skin disease, endocrine problems, and malnutrition are associated factors. Treatment involves identifying and removing the cause.

Paronychia

Paronychia is a disorder of the nails. The nails get soft or brittle, and the shape can change as they grow into the soft tissue (ingrown nails). In paronychia an infection of the nail develops and spreads around the nail, thus giving it the nickname "runaround." Involved nails become painful as the nail loosens and separates from the tissue. Application of wet dressings or topical antibiotics may be used. Sometimes a surgical incision and drainage of the infected area are performed.

BURNS

Etiology/Pathophysiology. Each year more than 2 million people are burned. Usually 250,000 require outpatient treatment and 80,000 require hospitalization. The most significant factor is that at least half of these burns could be prevented.

Burns result from radiation, thermal energy (heat), electricity, or chemicals. Skin destruction depends on the burning agent, the temperature of the burning agent, and how long a person is in contact with the agent.

Burns first cause the capillaries in the damaged area to dilate, resulting in capillary hyperpermeability. The increased cell permeability causes the fluid to move out of the cells into the surrounding tissues, resulting in edema and vesiculation (blistering). The larger the burned area, the greater the fluid loss. The fluid loss from the intravascular area to the interstitial areas poses the greatest threat to life, because the cells become dehydrated. The blood pressure drops, and blood flow to the kidneys is decreased. Symptoms of hypovolemic shock and renal failure may develop.

The pathophysiology and care of burns may be divided into three stages. The emergent phase, stage 1, is from the onset of the injury until the patient is stabilized. In the emergent phase, hypovolemia is a major concern for up to 48 hours after a major burn. Stage 2, the intermediate/acute phase or diuretic stage, begins 48 to 72 hours after the burn injury. At this time the greatest concern is circulatory overload. The fluid shifts back from the interstitial spaces to the cells. The kidneys begin to excrete large volumes of urine; hence it is called the *diuretic stage.* Stage 3, the long-term rehabilitation phase, begins when the burn has been treated. The aim of patient care in this phase is to return the patient to normal status.

Usually the greatest fluid loss in a burn occurs in the first 12 hours. The proteins, plasma, and electrolytes shift from the vascular compartment to the interstitial compartment. Red blood cells tend to remain in the vascular system, causing increased viscosity of the blood and a falsely elevated hematocrit level. Acute dehydration is present, and renal perfusion is seriously compromised. Fluid loss causes the person to develop burn shock. Hypotension, a decreased urine output, an increased pulse, rapid, shallow respirations, and restlessness develop. The heart can no longer supply enough blood to perfuse the vital organs. The body responds by increasing the peripheral resistance. A decreased pulse pressure and an increased pulse (tachycardia) and respiratory rate (tachypnea) exemplify this. Most deaths from burns result directly from burn shock.

Fluids start to return to the vascular compartment in 48 to 72 hours. Fluid return denotes the end of the hypovolemic stage and the beginning of the diuretic stage. Reabsorption of the interstitial fluid causes an increased blood volume. As the blood volume increases, the cardiac output increases to increase renal perfusion. The result is diuresis. The patient now is at a great risk of fluid overload. The patient's vital signs, urinary output, and consciousness must be carefully monitored.

A burn victim may also have experienced smoke inhalation. Inhalation damage results from breathing the chemicals produced by the burn. The fumes produce damage to the cilia and mucosa of the respiratory tract. Alveolar surfactant is decreased, and atelectasis can occur. Breathing difficulties are not usually seen immediately but may take several hours to occur. The nurse needs to consider a patient who has sustained any burn to the upper chest, neck, and face at high risk for respiratory distress. Signs that signify respiratory difficulty are a hoarse voice or a productive cough. Other physical findings suggesting respiratory tract injury in inhalation burns include the following:

- Singed nasal hairs
- Agitation, tachypnea, flaring nostrils, or intercostal retractions
- Brassy cough, grunting, or guttural respiratory sounds
- Erythema or edema of the oropharynx or nasopharynx
- Sooty sputum

Clinical Manifestations (Table 25-4 on p. 554).Traditionally, burns have been classified as first, second, or third degree. These terms are not descriptive of the injury, because they are based only on the visual characteristics of the burn wound. The injury of a burn extends beyond what can be seen. A more accurate description is superficial thickness injuries, partial-thickness injuries, and full-thickness injuries, which graphically describes the burn and indicates the depth and severity of the tissue injury (Fig. 25-16 on p. 554).

Assessment. Factors to include in the assessment are (1) the depth of the burn, (2) the causative agent, (3) the temperature and duration of contact, and (4) the skin thickness. The patient's age and other disease processes present are equally important. The **rule of nines** is used to determine the total body surface area (BSA) involved (Fig. 25-17 on p. 555). The rule of nines divides the body into multiples of nine. The entire head is 9%; the anterior and posterior aspects of the arms are a total of 9% each; the legs are 9% anterior and 9% posterior; the chest and back are 18% each, and the perineum is 1%. The rule of nines does not take into account the different levels of growth and is not accurate for children.

The rule of nines for calculating percentage of body area burned for infants and child differs from that for adults because the surface area of the child's head is

TABLE 25-4 Causes and Factors Determining Depth of Burn Injury

Depth	Cause	Appearance	Color	Sensation
Superficial partial-thickness (first degree)	Flash flame, ultraviolet light (sunburn)	Dry, no vesicles Minimal or no edema Blanches with fingertip pressure and refills when pressure removed	Increased erythema	Painful
Deep partial-thickness (second degree)	Contact with hot liquids or solids Flash flame to clothing Direct flame Chemicals Ultraviolet light	Large, moist vesicles that will increase in size Blanches with fingertip pressure and refills when pressure removed	Mottled with dull, white, tan, pink, or cherry red areas	Very painful
Full-thickness (third degree)	Contact with hot liquids or solids Flame Chemicals Electrical contact	Dry with leathery eschar Charred vessels visible under eschar Vesicles rare but thin-walled vesicles that do not increase in size may be present No blanching with pressure	White, charred, dark tan Black Red	Little or no pain Hair easily pulls out

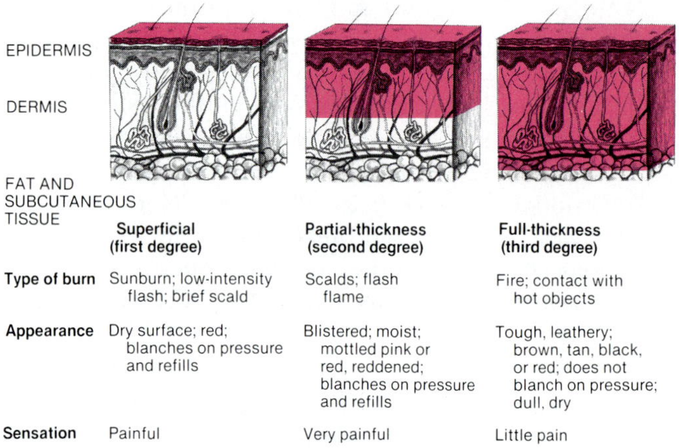

	Superficial (first degree)	Partial-thickness (second degree)	Full-thickness (third degree)
Type of burn	Sunburn; low-intensity flash; brief scald	Scalds; flash flame	Fire; contact with hot objects
Appearance	Dry surface; red; blanches on pressure and refills	Blistered; moist; mottled pink or red, reddened; blanches on pressure and refills	Tough, leathery; brown, tan, black, or red; does not blanch on pressure; dull, dry
Sensation	Painful	Very painful	Little pain

FIG. 25-16 Classification of burn depth.

greater (relative to the body) than in an adult. The child's body part and percentage of total BSA are calculated as follows:

Arm (shoulder to fingertips), 9% each
Head to neck, 18%
Anterior trunk, 18%
Posterior trunk, 18%
Leg (groin to toe), 14% each

Collection of *subjective data* will reveal the causative agent, other diseases present, the temperature and duration of contact, and patient's age.

Collection of *objective data* includes the depth of the burn, the skin thickness involved, the percentage of body surface area burned, the specific location, and any other injuries sustained. Any time a patient has a burn that involves the face, neck, or chest, the nurse needs to be observant for respiratory difficulty. It is important toidentify whether the victim has had a tetanus booster in the past 10 years to prevent complications.

The severity of the burn depends on several factors. Major burns are those that require the most skilled nursing interventions. Moderate and minor burns require fewer nursing interventions. Factors determining a major, moderate, or minor burn are the (1) percentage of the body surface area burned, (2) age of the victim, (3) specific location of the burn, (4) cause of the burn, (5) other diseases present, (6) depth of the burn, and (7) injuries sustained during the burn (Box 25-5).

Diagnostic Tests. The primary diagnostic test is a physical examination to determine the amount of burned area. Blood assessments, such as electrolytes, CBC, serum chemistries, and arterial blood gases, may be done to establish the severity of the dehydration. In inhalation burns, carboxyhemoglobin level is evaluated. Most fatalities occur among survivors with severe asphyxiation or carbon monoxide intoxication. Carbon monoxide binds to hemoglobin with greater affinity than oxygen, and therefore tissue hypoxia results.

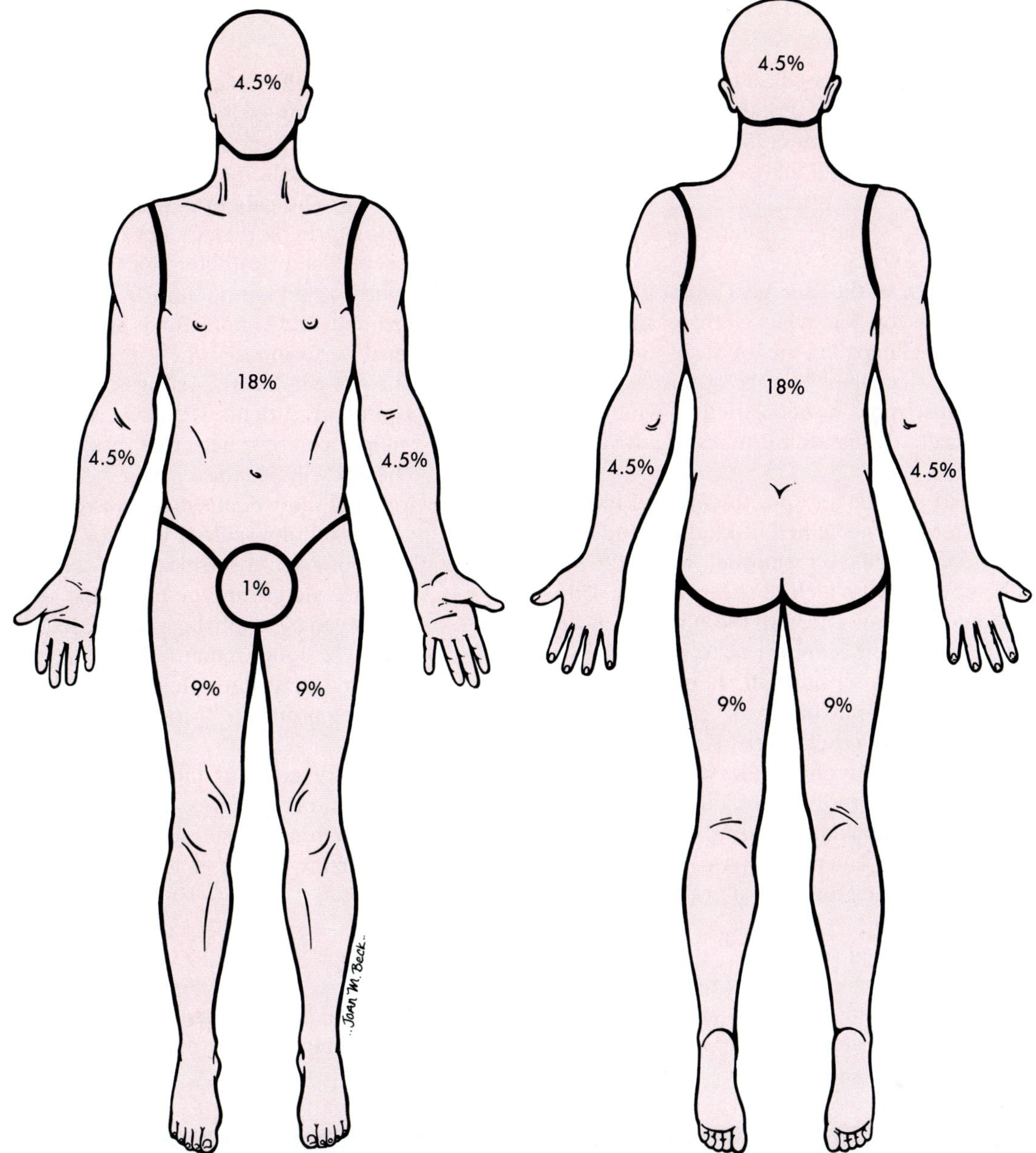

FIG. 25-17 The "rule of nines" used to estimate the amount of skin surface burned in an adult.

Box 25-5

CLASSIFICATION OF SEVERITY OF BURNS

MAJOR BURN INJURIES

Greater than 25% BSA (greater than 20% in children under 10 years and adults over 40 years of age)
Greater than 10% BSA, full-thickness
Involvement of face, eyes, ears, hands, feet, perineum
Electrical burns
Burns complicated by inhalation injury or major trauma
Burns in patients with preexisting disease (diabetes, congestive heart failure, or chronic renal failure)

MODERATE BURN INJURIES

15% to 25% BSA in adults, partial-thickness (10% to 20% BSA in children under 10 years and adults over 40 years of age)
Less than 10% BSA, full-thickness
Burns with no concurrent injury
Burns in patients with no preexisting disease

MINOR BURN INJURIES

Less than 15% BSA in adults (10% in children or the elderly)
Less than 2% BSA, full-thickness
Burns in patients with no preexisting disease

Medical Management. The medical treatment of burns is divided into three phases. Priorities exist in each phase. It is important to remember that these phases are not always clearly defined and may overlap.

Emergent Phase

The primary concern in the emergent phase is to stop the burning process by removing clothing and shoes from the victim and eliminating the source of the burn to arrest skin damage. Ice should not be applied to burns because it can cause rapid vasoconstriction, which may cause more trauma to the tissues by increasing the depth of the burn.

Step two is to provide an open airway and to control bleeding. Third, all nonadherent clothing and jewelry (rings, watches) should be removed. Fourth, the victim should be covered with a clean sheet or cloth. Fifth, the victim should be transported to the hospital. In the case of a chemical burn, it is important to rinse the skin generously with water to remove all chemicals. Electrical burns have an entry point and an exit point that need to be identified. Most electrical burns result in cardiac arrest, and the patient will require CPR (see Chapter 50).

In the hospital, the severity of the burn dictates the care given. The nurse should perform a thorough assessment every hour in the emergent phase. Patients with major burns are transferred to burn care centers or units for treatment. Patients with moderate to severe burns are treated using the following steps:

1. Establish airway—administer oxygen as ordered. Often the physician will insert an endotracheal tube to ensure a patent airway (Fig. 25-18).
2. The RN will initiate fluid therapy—intravenous fluid therapy of Ringer's lactate is begun immediately. The amount of fluid given is in accordance with the percentage of body surface area burned. The patient is weighed so the physician can determine the amount of fluids needed.
3. Insert Foley catheter for hourly output—an hourly urine output of 30 to 50 ml is recommended. Intravenous fluids are given to maintain renal perfusion.
4. The RN will insert a nasogastric tube to prevent aspiration. Patients with severe burns often develop a paralytic ileus as a result of trauma.
5. The RN will administer pain medication in small, frequent intravenous doses. Never give any medications intramuscularly in major burn victims because of poor absorption.
6. Stabilize victim, and monitor vital signs.
7. Give tetanus prophylaxis as needed.

The first 72 hours require diligent medical care to prevent death. Intravenous fluids are ordered to maintain the urine output at 30 to 50 ml per hour (Boxes 25-6 and 25-7).

The primary goals in the emergent phase are to maintain respiratory integrity and to prevent hypovolemic shock, which may result in death. (See Box 25-8 for samples of nursing diagnoses for the emergent phase of burns.)

Acute Phase

The acute phase begins when fluids begin to shift back to the intravascular compartment, usually 72 hours after

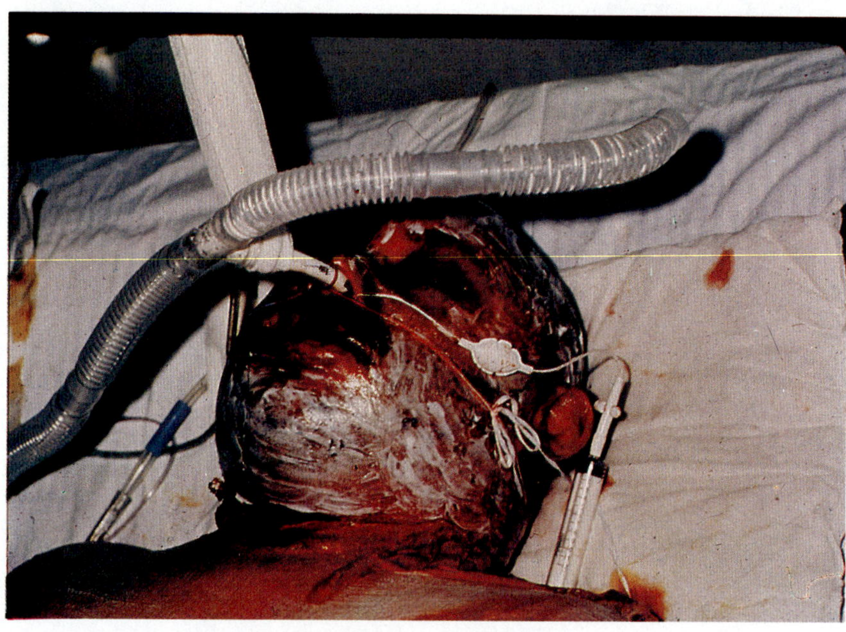

FIG. 25-18 Endotracheal intubation for patient with severe edema 5 hours after a burn injury.

the burn. During the acute phase, the patient's metabolism is increased. Urinary output increases as the fluid shifts back into the blood circulation. This will result in decreased edema in the tissues. The acute phase varies in time from 10 days to months. The two primary goals in treatment are treatment of the burn and prevention and management of complications. The most common complication and cause of death after the first 72 hours is infection. Other complications are heart failure, renal failure, **contractures** (shortening or tension of muscles that affects extension), paralytic ileus causing gastric dilation, and **Curling's ulcer** (a duodenal ulcer that develops 8 to 14 days after severe burns on the surface of the body; the first sign is usually vomiting of bright red blood).

Nursing Interventions. The data gathered should include: (1) respiratory pattern, (2) vital signs, (3) circulation, (4) intake and output, (5) patient movement, (6) bowel sounds, (7) inspection of the wound itself, and (8) mental status.

Fluid reshifting complications may also occur during the acute phase if renal damage has occurred. The patient may experience heart failure caused by the rapid increase in blood volume resulting from the return of fluid from the interstitial spaces. The primary goals in the acute phase are to maintain respiratory integrity and to prevent infection. Any erythema, odor, or exudate that is green or yellow indicates a possible infection and should be reported.

Once the patient's condition has stabilized and the diuretic or acute phase begins, a nutritional assessment should be done. Provision for adequate nutrition is the cornerstone of burn care during the acute phase. The diet needs to include increased amounts of protein, calories, and vitamins to help repair the damaged tissue. Oral intake of nutrients should be encouraged as soon as possible. The nurse monitors nutritional improvement through daily measurement of weight, serum electrolytes, and a urinalysis. Adequate nutrition decreases healing time. Skin grafts will not be successful unless nutrition is adequate. It is important that the burn patient not lose weight, because this will increase healing time.

Nursing interventions should include measures to support the patient's psychological well-being. Pain must be controlled by intravenous narcotics in small, frequent doses to ease discomfort, but not jeopardize respiratory integrity. Specific interventions include verbal support, unhurried care, truthful explanations, and effective lis-

Box 25-6

INITIAL TREATMENT OF MAJOR BURNS IN THE EMERGENCY ROOM

1. Establish airway.
2. Initiate fluid therapy by intravenous catheters.
3. Insert indwelling Foley catheter for hourly urine measurement.
4. Do circulatory assessment for circumferential occlusion resulting from eschar.
5. Insert nasogastric tube to remove stomach contents and prevent gastric distention.
6. Insert central intravenous catheter, if appropriate.
7. Manage pain by intravenous narcotics in small, frequent doses.
8. Provide tetanus prophylaxis.

Box 25-7

INDICATIONS FOR FLUID RESUSCITATION

- Burns greater than 20% BSA in adults
- Burns greater than 10% BSA in children
- Patient older than 55 or younger than 4 years of age
- Patient with preexisting disease that would reduce normal compensatory responses to minor hypovolemia (cardiac or pulmonary disease, diabetes)
- Electrical burns

Box 25-8

NURSING DIAGNOSES FOR THE EMERGENT PHASE OF BURNS

- Airway clearance ineffective, related to edema of the respiratory passages
- Fluid volume deficit (dehydration), related to shift of body fluids
- Fluid volume deficit, related to capillary hyperpermeability with fluid moving out of the cells into the interstitial area
- Anxiety, acute, related to injury
- Pain, acute, related to loss of skin
- Infection, high risk for, related to impairment of skin integrity
- Skin integrity, impaired, related to damage by the burns
- Cardiac output, decreased, related to hypovolemia
- Sensory/perceptual alterations (tactile), related to loss of skin
- Aspiration, high risk for, related to decreased peristalsis
- Swallowing, impaired, related to mucosal edema
- Communication, impaired verbal, related to breathing difficulties
- Sleep pattern disturbance, related to hospital environment

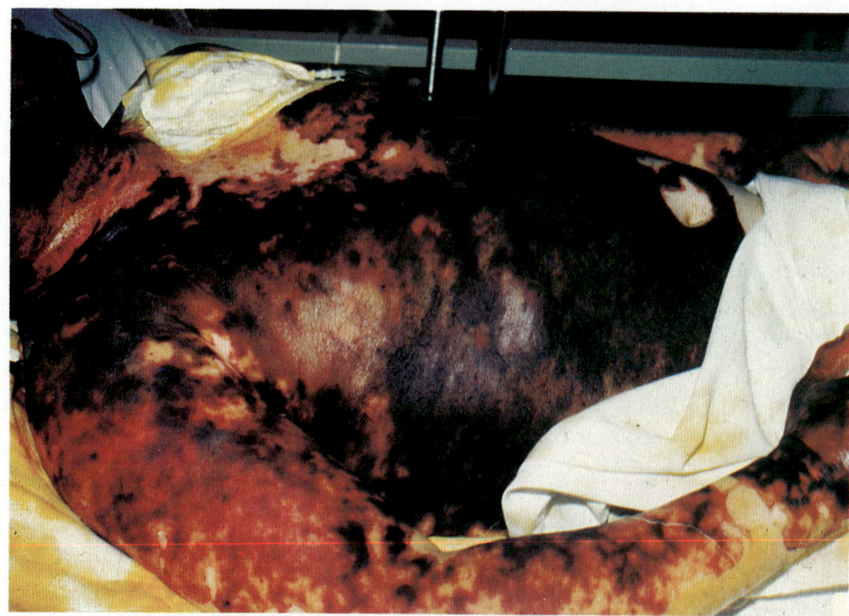

FIG. 25-19 Postburn *Pseudomas* infection.

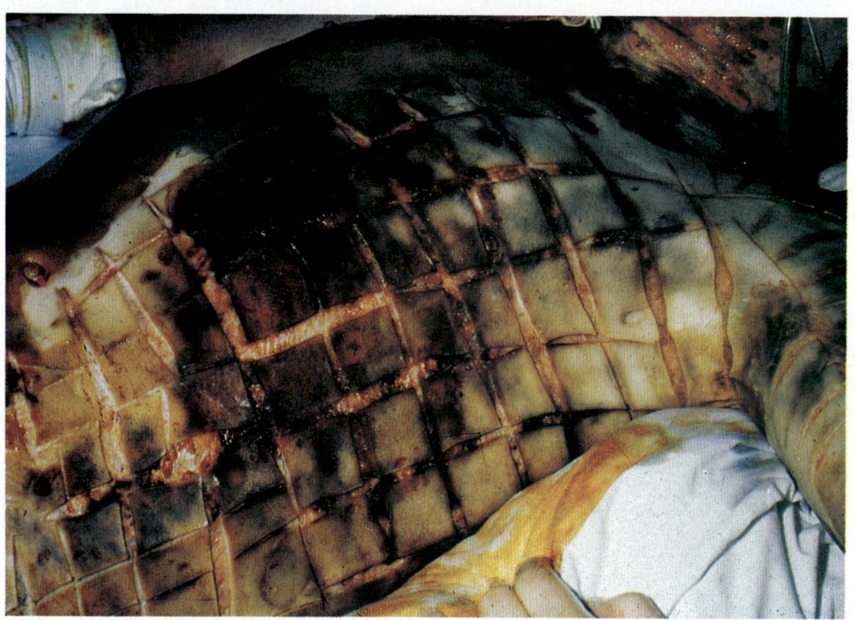

FIG. 25-20 Grid escharatomy used to alleviate circulatory and pulmonary constriction.

tening. The nurse's communication skills must be excellent.

Infection is a primary complication that should be treated at the time of the burn. Local and systemic infections are common complications at this time (Fig. 25-19). Cultures of the burn should be done at admission and periodically during care.

The burn patient does not have an intact first line of defense; the protective mechanisms are not functioning normally. The nurse should protect the patient from the environment by using protective isolation. Gowns, masks, caps, and gloves should be worn during each contact victim with major burns. Strict surgical aseptic technique is followed during dressing changes. Use of proper equipment-cleaning procedures is imperative. Hydrotherapy (whirlpool) can be a source of infection.

Wound care involves the removal of the eschar that forms. **Eschar** is a black leathery crust, a slough, that the body forms over burned tissue, which can harbor microorganisms and cause infection. It may also compromise circulatory status, and an escharotomy is often done to relieve the circulatory constriction (Fig. 25-20). Daily **debridement** (removal of damaged tissue and cellular debris from a wound or burn to prevent infection and to

TABLE 25-5 Therapeutic Positioning for the Burn Patient

Area Burned	Description of Position
Neck	No pillow Towel roll under cervical spine Neck splint
Shoulder	90 degrees' abduction, neutral rotation Elbow splint may be used to aid in maintaining position
Axilla	Abduction with 10 to 15 degrees' forward flexion and external rotation Support abducted arm by suspending from IV pole, or place on bedside table Axilla splint
Elbow	Extension Support extended arm on bedside table, foam trough Elbow splint
Hand	Hand splint
Dorsal surface	Flexion
Palmar surface	Hyperextension
Hip	Extension with neutral rotation Supine with lower extremity extended Prone lying (if medically appropriate) Trochanter roll Foam wedge along lateral aspect of thigh Knee or long leg splint
Knee	Extension Prone lying (if medically appropriate) Patient out of bed with lower extremities extended and elevated Knee splint
Ankle	Dorsiflexion Padded footboard with heels free of pressure Ankle splint

ROM to all joints should be done every 8 hours except for graft areas.

promote healing) and special cleansing help to support regeneration of the tissues. Hydrotherapy softens the eschar with water to make removal less painful. It also promotes range of motion to decrease contractures.

The specific treatment method depends on the severity of the burn. The open or exposure method is used for burns of the face, neck, ears, and perineum. The area is cleaned and exposed to air. A hard crust forms, and the regeneration of tissue occurs.

Proper positioning and range-of-motion (ROM) exercises by the physical therapist and the nurse are vital for the well-being of the burn patient (Table 25-5).

Special bed equipment is needed to prevent the burn from touching the linens. A bed cradle, a Circoelectric bed, or a Clinitron bed (Fig. 25-21) is recommended. Lights or heat lamps are used to provide additional warmth.

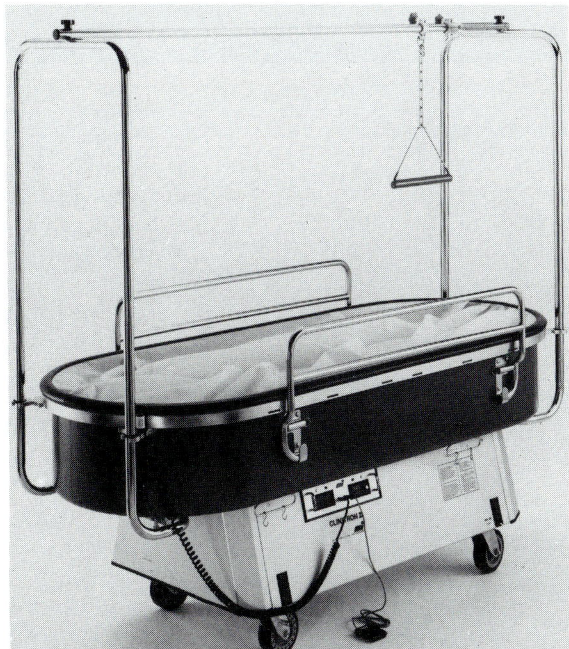

FIG. 25-21 Clinitron therapy unit.

Advantages to the open method include the following: (1) the wound can be observed more easily, (2) movement in bed is less restricted, (3) circulation of the body part is not restricted, and (4) exercises can be done more easily to prevent contractures. Disadvantages to the open method are (1) pain, chilling, (2) contamination by the health care worker, (3) unattractive appearance of the patient, which causes emotional distress, and (4) the need for strict protective isolation.

The pain can be controlled with intravenously administered narcotics in the early days of the acute phase. However, considering the long-term nature of a burn, addiction is a potential problem. Diazepam (Valium) has been found to be effective. Chilling can be controlled by keeping the room temperature 85° F (24.4° C). Humidity should be between 40% and 50%.

The closed or occlusive method involves cleaning the burn, applying the medication, and dressing the wound as ordered.

Advantages of the closed method are (1) it protects the burn area from injury and (2) it prevents contamination of the area by the health care worker. Circulation checks are important with pressure dressings.

The topical medications used to hasten healing and prevent infection vary. Topical administration is preferred, because the capillaries are coagulated by the burn. Mafenide (Sulfamylon), silver sulfadiazine (Silvadene), and silver nitrate are common drugs used in burn care. Each drug has specific advantages and disadvantages (Table 25-6 on p. 560).

Burns are not dressed in large, bulky dressings; the dressing needs to be lightweight. A single layer of gauze

TABLE 25-6 Topical Medications Used in Burn Therapy

Topical Medication	Advantages	Disadvantages
Mafenide (Sulfamylon)	Bacteriostatic against gram-negative and gram-positive organisms Penetrates thick eschar	Metabolic acidosis Pain on application Allergic rash
Silver sulfadiazine (Silvadene)	Broad antimicrobial activity against gram-negative, gram-positive, and *Candida* organisms No electrolyte imbalances Painless and somewhat soothing Not nephrotoxic	Repeated application may develop slimy, grayish appearance, simulating an infection despite negative cultures Prolonged use may cause skin rash and depress granulocyte formation
Silver nitrate	Bacteriostatic effect Lessens pain and eliminates odor Reduces evaporative water loss from burns	Electrolyte imbalances Stains everything it comes into contact with Does not penetrate eschar Pain on application
Nitrofurazone (Furacin)	Inhibits enzymes necessary for bacterial metabolism Broad spectrum of activity Effective against *Staphylococcus aureus* Not absorbed systemically Low incidence of sensitivity	Contact dermatitis in unaffected skin Urine turns a reddish color
Gentamycin sulfate (Garamycin)	Broad antimicrobial activity Painless	Ototoxicity Nephrotoxicity Development of resistant bacterial stains
Neomycin	Broad antimicrobial activity Causes miscoding in the messenger RNA of bacterial cells	Serious toxic effects Ototoxicity Nephrotoxicity
Scarlet red	Nonantiseptic (applied to gauze soaked with oil-base red dye) Drying agent Applied to donor site Promotes epithelialization	No antimicrobial effects Stains and irritates skin Infection may develop beneath scarlet red gauze, which may have systemic effects
Xeroform	Nonantiseptic Debrides and protects donor site Protects graft	Removal may be painful, because it sometimes adheres to wound Neither antiseptic nor antimicrobial
Sodium hypochlorite (Dakin's solution)	Chlorine-based solution that is bactericidal Aids in debriding wounds Aids cleaning of copious drainage	Dissolves blood clots May inhibit clotting May irritate the skin
Sutilains ointment (Travase)	Topical enzymatic agent Dissolves necrotic tissue by proteolytic action Facilitates removal of eschar and purulent drainage	Mild, transient pain on application Paresthesia, bleeding, dermatitis Dressing must be kept moist at all times

covered with medication and a single wrap of Kerlix are suggested. When applying gauze to the burn area, place gauze between skin areas that touch to prevent skin-to-skin contact.

Because having the dressing changed is very painful, pain medication should be given 30 minutes before the procedure. Most dressings are changed after hydrotherapy. An important principle to follow is to remove all old medication and eschar before new medication is applied. Failure to debride promotes infection, delays healing, and increases scarring.

Skin grafts are used as soon as possible to cover the burns. Grafting promotes healing and prevents infection. The usual timespan is during the first 3 weeks of care. There are four types of grafts. An **autograft** (surgical transplantation of any tissue from one part of the body to another location in the same individual) comes from the burn victim. A **homograft** or **allograft** (the transfer of tissue between two genetically dissimilar individuals of the same species, such as a skin transplant between two humans who are not identical twins) comes from another person such as a cadaver. A **heterograft** or **xenograft** (tissue from another species, used as a temporary graft) comes from another species such as a pig or a cow. Finally, synthetic graft substitutes are now available. The autograft is permanent, whereas the other types are temporary.

Grafts are either applied by the *pedicle method* (the tissue is left partially attached to the donor site and the other portion of the tissue is attached to the burn site) or the *free-standing method* (the tissue is completely removed from the donor site and is attached to the burn site).

Graft sites are a nursing challenge. The graft area needs as little movement as possible so as not to tear the graft. Dressings are not changed until ordered. Any movement that results in pulling the graft area can dislocate the graft. The donor site resembles a partial-thickness burn after the graft. Donor site care is as important as care of the burn site. Pain is a primary complaint after the graft and should be treated. The nurse should inspect the donor site for signs of infection, such as erythema and malodor (see patient teaching box).

The nutritional aspect of burn care is very important. Body proteins are destroyed and fluid loss occurs. The body tries to compensate by increasing metabolism to meet the body's extra demands. Enough energy is needed to maintain homeostasis, plus meet the increased need for repairing the injury.

The burn patient should eat by mouth as soon as her condition permits. Intake needs to be enough to meet the caloric and protein requirements. Protein requirements are greater than normal. Normal protein intake is 0.8 g/kg of body weight. The burned patient needs 1.5 to 3.2 g/kg of body weight (a normal 150-pound man needs 55 g of protein a day; if burned he will need 102 to 158 g of protein, depending on the extent of the burn). Daily caloric requirements range from 2000 calories to more than 6000 calories at times. Meeting these enormous requirements requires diligent nursing interventions. Foods need to be highly concentrated and offered frequently. Additional amounts of vitamins A, B, and C are needed to promote digestion, adsorption, and repair of tissue. Increased amounts of calcium, zinc, magnesium, and iron are needed. Vitamin C and zinc aid in wound healing. Added B complex vitamins aid metabolism of the extra protein and carbohydrate intake. Vitamin, mineral, and protein intake can be increased by adding concentrated oral supplements such as Ensure, Sustacal, and Carnation Instant Breakfast.

Nursing interventions to meet the extra nutritional needs present a challenge for the nurse. Most burn victims have poor appetites; therefore getting the patient to eat is difficult. Small, frequent feedings of high-calorie, high-protein, low-volume foods should be given. Some patients develop Curling's ulcer 8 to 14 days after the burn injury. The increased gastric acidity and anxiety are factors in development of the ulcer. The first sign is vomiting bright, red blood. The prophylactic treatment is often cimetidine (Tagamet), ranitidine (Zantac), or famotidine (Pepcid). See Box 25-9 for nursing diagnoses for the acute phase of burns.

PATIENT TEACHING FOR SKIN GRAFTS

1. Keep surface of healed graft moistened daily with skin lotion for 6 to 12 months. (Grafted skin does not perspire; it dries and cracks easily.)
2. Protect grafted skin from direct sunlight with a sunscreen lotion for at least 6 months.
3. Wear a strong elastic stocking for 4 to 6 months with grafts on lower extremities.
4. Report changes in the graft (hematoma, fluid, collection) to physician.

Box 25-9 NURSING DIAGNOSES FOR THE ACUTE PHASE OF BURNS

- Anxiety, acute, related to change in body image
- Fear, related to chronic illness
- Pain, chronic, related to procedures performed
- Infection, high risk for, related to open skin wounds
- Nutrition, altered; less than body requirements, related to increased metabolic demands
- Social isolation, related to perceived change in body image
- Physical mobility, impaired, related to burns
- Self-care deficit in ADLs, related to area of burn involved
- Knowledge deficit: all areas, related to expected care
- Family processes, altered, related to long-term hospitalization
- Body image disturbance related to disfigurement from burns
- Diversional activity deficit, related to confinement during care
- Coping, ineffective, individual, related to seriousness of injury and perceived role changes
- Powerlessness related to prolonged recovery, loss of income, loss of physical attractiveness

Rehabilitation Phase

Rehabilitation of the burn patient begins at admission, but the third phase of burn care begins when 20% or less of the BSA remains burned. The goal is to return the patient to a productive life. Social skills as well as physical skills are addressed. The rehabilitation process may take years.

Mobility limitations are one major concern. The patient needs a comprehensive program of positioning, skin care, exercise, ambulation, and activities of daily living. The complication of contractures is an ever-present concern in the care of a burn patient. Even though physical therapists provide most of the rehabilitative care, the nurse is responsible for determining whether the care has been provided and that continuity is maintained.

When planning the care of the person with a burn, the nurse should set short-term goals. Setting realistic expected outcomes helps to motivate patients to try to achieve more.

An ultimate goal is to restore or maintain the patient's independence. The psychological possibility of a changed body image must be addressed. The nurse should encourage the patient to verbalize fears and concerns. A social worker and/or counselor is needed. During visiting hours, the nurse can assess family interactions. Helping the family to cope with the changes in their loved one is a major part of nursing intervention.

The nursing diagnoses that apply to burn victims are numerous. The family, patient, and social role of the victim are considered. See Box 25-10 for nursing diagnoses for the rehabilitation phase of burns.

Patient teaching. Before discharge, the burn patient and family need education. Instructions should be written, complete, comprehensive, easy to understand, and realistic. Return demonstrations provide the best evaluation by the nurse that learning has taken place. The major topics to cover should be (1) wound care, (2) signs and symptoms of complications, (3) dressings, (4) skin care for the burned area, (5) exercises, (6) clothing, (7) ADLs, and (8) social skills.

Evaluation. Evaluation depends on meeting the stated goals. In evaluating the burn patient, the nurse should ask the following questions:

1. Can the patient take care of self?
2. Can the patient ambulate without difficulty?
3. Can the patient cope?
4. Can the family cope?
5. Does the patient have contractures?
6. Does the patient understand the treatment process?

Burn care is very extensive, and the exact nursing interventions for each patient are very individualized. Many times the patient must change vocations, and family relationships change. The degree of scarring, emotionally as well as physically, cannot be predicted, and the acceptance by society cannot be ascertained.

Prognosis. The factors that determine the outcome for the patient with burns are dependent upon the size of the burn, depth of the burn, age of the victim, body part involved, burning agent, and history of cardiac, pulmonary, endocrine, renal, or hepatic disease as well as other injuries sustained at time of the burn.

Box 25-10 NURSING DIAGNOSES FOR THE REHABILITATION PHASE OF BURNS

- Physical mobility, impaired, related to splinting, dressings, or pain
- Activity intolerance, related to prolonged bed rest
- Anxiety, acute to moderate, related to role change
- Body image disturbance, related to scarring
- Knowledge deficit, related to impaired home maintenance management
- Self-care deficits (ADLs), related to pain and/or fatigue
- Fear, related to impending surgery
- Disuse syndrome, high risk for, related to noncompliance
- Posttrauma response, related to the cause of the burn
- Adjustment, impaired, related to lack of ability to limited expectations of self
- Coping, ineffective individual, related to long-term rehabilitation
- Personal identity disturbance, related to inability to return to previous life-style for prolonged period
- Care giver role strain, related to prolonged recovery period
- Management of therapeutic regimen, ineffective individual, related to complexity and chronicity of rehabilitation
- Grieving, anticipatory, related to loss of wellness

REFERENCES AND SUGGESTED READINGS

1. American Cancer Society: *Cancer facts and figures, 1991,* Atlanta, 1991, The Society.
2. Anastasi JK, Rivera J: Identifying the skin manifestations of HIV, *Nursing* 22(11):58, 1992.
3. Blondell R: Parasites of the skin and hair, *Prim Care* 18(1):167, 1991.
4. Brunner L, Sudderth D: *Textbook of medical-surgical nursing,* Philadelphia, 1992, Lippincott.
5. Burgess MC: Initial management of a patient with extensive burn injury, *Crit Care Nurs Clin North Am,* 3(2):165, 1991.
6. Calistroa M: Burn care basics and beyond, *RN* 56(3):26, 1993.
7. Cuzzell JL: Clues: pain, burning and itching, *Am J Nurs* 90(7):15, 1990.
8. DeWit SC: *Keanes essentials of medical surgical nursing,* Philadelphia, 1992, Saunders.
9. DeWit S: Nursing assessment of the skin and dermatologic lesions, *Nurs Clin North Am* 25:235, 1990.
10. Ellison M, Crabtree D: Antibiotic therapy for common infections, *Prim Care* 17(3):521, 1990.
11. Gurevech I: Counseling the patient with herpes, *RN* 53(2):22, 1990.
12. Habif TP: *Clinical dermatology: a color guide to diagnosis and treatment,* ed 2, St Louis, 1990, Mosby.
13. Hegner BR, Caldwell E: *Geriatrics: a study of maturity,* ed 5, New York, 1991, Delmar.

14. Hood GH, Dincher JR: *Total patient care,* ed 8, St Louis, 1992, Mosby.
15. Jaresbery CR: Action stat! Neck and chest burns, *Nurs 90,* 20(1):33, 1990.
16. Kim MJ, McFarland G, McLane A: *Pocket guide to nursing diagnosis,* ed 4, St Louis, 1991, Mosby.
17. Levine G: Sexually transmitted parasitic diseases, *Prim Care* 18(1):101, 1991.
18. Lewis S, Collier IC: *Medical-surgical nursing: assessment and management of clinical problems,* St Louis, 1992, Mosby.
19. Long B, Phipps W, Cassmeyer L: *Medical-surgical nursing: a nursing process approach,* ed 3, St Louis, 1993, Mosby.
20. Marieb EN: *Essentials of human anatomy and physiology,* Menlo Park, Calif, 1990, Addison Wesley.
21. Memmler RL, Cohen BJ, Wood DL: *Structure and function of the human body,* ed 5, Philadelphia, 1992, Lippincott.
22. Moschella SL, Hurley HA: *Dermatology,* ed 3, Philadelphia, 1991, Saunders.
23. Phillips TJ, Dover JS: Recent advances in dermatology, *N Engl J Med* 326(3):167, 1992.
24. Phipps WJ, Long BC, Woods NF: *Medical-surgical nursing,* St Louis, ed 4, 1991, Mosby.
25. Potter PA, Perry AG: *Fundamentals of nursing: concepts, process, and practice,* ed 3, St Louis, 1993, Mosby.
26. Rosen P, Barben R, Sternbach G: *Essentials of emergency medicine,* St Louis, 1991, Mosby.
27. Sauer GC: *Manual of skin diseases,* ed 6, Philadelphia, 1991, Lippincott.
28. Scherer J: *Introductory medical-surgical nursing,* ed 5, Philadelphia, 1991, Lippincott.
29. Seidel J et al: *Mosby's guide to physical examination,* ed 2, St Louis, 1991, Mosby.
30. Solomon EP: *Introduction to human anatomy and physiology,* Philadelphia, 1992, Saunders.
31. Thibodeau GA, Anthony CP: *Structure and function of the body,* ed 9, St Louis, 1992, Mosby.
32. Thompson JM et al: *Mosby's clinical nursing,* ed 3, 1993, St Louis, Mosby.
33. Timby BK, Lewis LW: *Fundamental skills and concepts in patient care,* ed 5, Philadelphia, 1992, Lippincott.

CHAPTER CHALLENGE

KEY POINTS

- The skin, including nails, hair, and glands, makes up the integumentary system.
- The main functions of the integumentary system are protection, temperature regulation, and vitamin D synthesis.
- The two layers of true skin are the epidermis and the dermis.
- The layer of tissue directly beneath the skin is the subcutaneous layer; it is composed of adipose tissue and loose connective tissue.
- The sudoriferous (sweat) glands release perspiration through the skin.
- The sebaceous (oil) glands secrete sebum, which lubricates the skin and prevents invasion of bacteria through the skin.
- Any injury to the skin poses a threat to a person's self-concept.
- It is important to establish a therapeutic relationship to meet the psychological needs of the patient.
- Most skin disorders are not contagious and are rarely fatal. They are often chronic in nature.
- Sterile technique and isolation techniques are required with any open, draining lesion.
- Wet dressings need to be checked frequently. Constant moisture softens the skin and contributes to skin maceration.
- Application of medications must be done to clean skin.
- The nursing interventions of a skin disorder depend on the cause; however, common problems are decreased skin integrity, high risk for infection, lack of knowledge concerning the disease, and ineffective coping.
- A primary nursing intervention is patient teaching to alert the patient about the mode of transmission of the particular disease.
- The assessment of patients with skin disorders includes collection of both subjective and objective data.
- Wet dressings and baths may be done to soothe, vasoconstrict, debride, or decrease pruritus.
- Before initiating heat and cold therapy, the nurse must understand normal body responses to local temperature variations, assess the integrity of the body part, determine the patient's ability to sense temperature, and ensure proper operation of equipment.
- Malignant skin diseases need to be prevented by educating the public about causes.
- Burns can be classified by depth and body surface area involved. The pathophysiology and care of burns involve three stages, the hypovolemic/emergent phase, the diuretic/acute phase, and the long-term/rehabilitation phase.
- The three phases of burn care are overlapping, with different goals and nursing interventions in each.
- A first priority in nursing intervention for the burn patient in the emergent phase is to establish and maintain an open airway.
- The treatment method of a burn patient depends on age, body surface area involved, location, depth, and other diseases present.
- The primary causes of death in burn victims are hypovolemic shock in the first 72 hours and infection during the acute phase.

STUDY QUESTIONS

1. The layer of skin that contains blood vessels and nerves is the:
   1. epidermis
   2. dermis
   3. subcutaneous tissue
   4. melanin
2. The type of gland that secretes mainly water and salts through the pores is:
   1. sudoriferous
   2. ceruminous
   3. sebaceous
   4. arrector
3. Which gland secretes a waxlike substance and is located in the external ear canal?
   1. sebaceous
   2. ceruminous
   3. endocrine
   4. dermal
4. What is the name of the pigment that is responsible for skin color?
   1. papilla
   2. sebaceous
   3. melanin
   4. cerumen
5. What is another name for "true skin"?
   1. dermis
   2. epidermis
   3. adipose
   4. subcutaneous
6. What is the name of the band of muscle tissue that surrounds the hair shaft:
   1. pacinian
   2. arrector pili
   3. stratum
   4. papillae
7. Another name for subcutaneous tissue is:
   1. sudoriferous fascia
   2. pacinian fascia
   3. superficial fascia
   4. sebaceous fascia
8. Another name for the crescent-shaped part of the root of the fingernail is:
   1. free edge
   2. nail body
   3. cuticle
   4. lunula
9. Mr. Rodriquez, a licensed practical nurse, is collecting data regarding his patient's skin lesions. Which of the following methods would be most appropriate to use?
   1. inspection
   2. palpation
   3. auscultation
   4. percussion
10. Before applying topical medication to Timothy, a 2-year-old with impetigo, it would be most important for the nurse to:
    1. check when the dressing was last changed.
    2. remove all scabs and medication before applying new medication.
    3. be careful not to dislodge the dried exudate so as not to interrupt the granulation process.
    4. use clean technique to dress all wounds.
11. While giving Mrs. Kemlin a bath, the nurse notices a black nevus under the breast. The nurse should:
    1. use soap and water to bath the nevus.
    2. apply a bandage to prevent excoriation.
    3. document the nevus and report to the nurse in charge.
    4. document the nevus as a normal skin lesion.
12. Mr. Gordon has 30% of his body surface area burned with partial-thickness and full-thickness involvement. In order to prevent the duodenal complication of Curling's ulcer 8 to 14 days after the burn injury, the nurse could expect to administer:
    1. ranitidine (Zantac)
    2. meperidine (Demerol)
    3. acetominophen (Tylenol)
    4. atropine sulfate (Atropine)
13. In the rehabilitation phase of burn care, the nurse's primary concern is to provide interventions to:
    1. maintain skin integrity
    2. prevent impaired mobility
    3. decrease anxiety
    4. provide pain relief
14. In assessing fluid replacement in Ms. Kucera who has a moderate burn, the following would best indicate the therapeutic response to her fluid therapy?
    1. respiratory rate below 20
    2. the patient states she is not thirsty
    3. urine output of 40 cc per hour
    4. good skin turgor
15. Mr. Kordoug has partial and full-thickness burns to 25% of his body surface area. He is in danger of suffering from which type of shock?
    1. cardiogenic
    2. vasogenic
    3. neurogenic
    4. hypovolemic
16. Which of the following nursing interventions would be *most important* during the *emergent* phase of burn care?
    1. initiate fluid therapy
    2. change the dressings using aseptic technique
    3. monitor intake and output hourly
    4. establish an airway
17. The nurse has initiated measures to promote adequate *fluid balance* in the patient with a full-thickness burn. Which of the following would indicate that these measures need to be reassessed?
    1. urinary output of 200 ml in 10 hours
    2. blood pressure 120/80, pulse 84
    3. pitted edema noted in the burn area
    4. continued complaining of pain and muscle spasm

26

CARE OF THE PATIENT WITH A MUSCULOSKELETAL DISORDER

Martha E. Spray

KEY TERMS

ANATOMY AND PHYSIOLOGY

abduction
adduction
acetabulum
Achilles
acromion process
calcaneus
diaphysis
epiphysis
fibula
foramen
foramen magnum
fossa
greater trochanter
hemopoiesis
insertion
ischium
ligament
olecranon
origin
patella
pectoralis major
periosteum
sphenoid
tendon
tibia
xiphoid process

MEDICAL-SURGICAL

ankylosis
arthrocentesis
arthrodesis
arthroplasty
bipolar hip replacement (hemiarthroplasty)
blanching test
callus
Colles' fracture
compartment syndrome
crepitus
kyphosis
lordosis
ORIF
paresthesia
scoliosis
sequestrum
subluxation
tophi
Volkmann's

LEARNING OBJECTIVES

Anatomy and Physiology

After reading this chapter, the student should be able to do the following:

- Define the key terms.
- List the five basic functions of the skeletal system.
- Describe the difference between a ligament and a tendon.
- Describe three vital functions muscles perform when they contract.
- Describe the location of the major muscles of the body.
- Define the term "oxygen debt."
- List the types of body movements.

Medical-Surgical

- Define the key terms.
- Describe the following conditions: lordosis, scoliosis, and kyphosis.
- List diagnostic procedures pertinent to musculoskeletal function.
- Compare methods for assessing circulation, nerve damage, and infection in a patient who has a traumatic insult to the musculoskeletal system.
- List at least four healthy life-style measures a person can practice to reduce the risk of developing osteoporosis.
- List at least two types of skin and skeletal traction.
- List four nursing interventions appropriate for bone cancer.
- Describe the phenomenon of "phantom pain."
- Compare the medical regimens for patients suffering from "gouty arthritis," rheumatoid arthritis, or osteoarthritis.
- Discuss the nursing interventions appropriate for rheumatoid arthritis.
- Describe the nursing interventions appropriate for degenerative joint disease (osteoarthritis and ankylosing spondylitis).
- Describe the surgical intervention for arthritis of the hip and knee.
- Describe the symptoms of compartment syndrome.
- List nursing interventions appropriate for a fat embolism.
- Discuss the physiology of fracture healing (hematoma, granulation tissue, and callus formation).
- Discuss nursing interventions appropriate for a patient with a fractured hip after ORIF and bipolar hip prosthesis (hemiarthroplasty).
- Describe the nursing interventions for the patient undergoing a total hip or a total knee replacement.

RELATED TOPICS OF INTEREST

- Body mechanics (Chapter 14)
- Comfort, rest, and sleep (Chapter 15)
- Basic nutrition (Chapter 18)
- The surgical patient (Chapter 22)
- Care of the patient with a neurological disorder (Chapter 35)
- Rehabilitation nursing (Chapter 49)
- First aid (Chapter 51)

Bones and joints form the framework of the body, but the contraction and relaxation of the muscles allow movement. All movement of the body is orchestrated by the functioning of the bones, joints, and the muscles attached to the bones. This chapter will discuss the structure and function of bones and muscles and how they serve the body.

ANATOMY AND PHYSIOLOGY

Functions of the Skeletal System

The skeletal system has five basic functions: support, protection, movement, mineral storage, and hemopoiesis.

Support. The skeleton provides the body framework that supports internal tissues and organs.

Protection. The skeleton forms a firm, cagelike structure that protects many internal structures. The cranium (skull) protects the brain, the vertebrae protect the spinal cord, and the ribs and sternum (breastbone) protect the lungs and heart.

Movement. Because the skeletal muscles are attached to the bones, the bones provide leverage for movement. As a muscle contracts, it exerts pull on the bone and movement occurs.

Mineral Storage. The bones serve as a storage area for various minerals, particularly calcium and phosphorus. When the body does not receive adequate intake of these minerals, the minerals are released by the bones.

Hemopoiesis. **Hemopoiesis** (blood cell formation) takes place in the red bone marrow. The red bone marrow is spongy bone found in the ends of the long bones. A child's bones contain a proportionally larger amount of red bone marrow than an adult's. As one ages, much of the red bone marrow converts to yellow bone marrow, which is composed of fat cells.

Structure of Bones

The skeletal system is composed of 206 bones. In some areas, such as the nose, the framework is composed of both bone and cartilage. There are two basic types of bone tissue, compact and spongy. Compact bone is hard and dense; it looks smooth. Spongy bone has open areas surrounded by needlelike projections of bone tissue. These small projections contain red bone marrow.

There are four classifications of bones, based on their form and shape: long, short, flat, and irregular. Long bones are found in the extremities, short bones are found in the hands and feet, flat bones are found in the skull and sternum, and irregular bones comprise the vertebrae (backbone).

Bone Markings. In the structure and shape of bones there are various raised areas, openings, and ridges. These sites mark the areas where muscles, tendons, and ligaments are attached and where blood vessels and nerves pass. These landmarks are divided into two categories: processes (projections or prominences), which grow out from the surface of the bone, and depressions (cavities), which are indentations of the bones.

Table 26-1 identifies the bone markings. Briefly, the major structures are as follows:

1. **Acromion process:** a slightly flaring projection at the lateral end of the scapula; it forms the highest point of the shoulder
2. Mastoid process: a protuberance just behind the ear
3. **Olecranon:** the upper end of the ulna, which forms the point of the elbow
4. Iliac crest: the upper curving boundary of the ilium; it can be felt by placing the hands at the level of the waist and exerting a slight downward pressure
5. Ischial tuberosity: the large posterior part of the ischium; in erect sitting position the body rests on these tuberosities
6. Ischial spine: a small prominent area on either side of the ischium, anterior to the ischial tuberosity
7. **Acetabulum:** Latin for vinegar cup; the large, cup-shaped articular cavity at the junction of the ilium, the ischium, and the pubis, containing the ball-shaped head of the femur
8. **Greater trochanter:** a protuberance of the femur located interiorly and laterally to the head of the femur

Other important structures include the following:

1. Crests: narrow ridges of bone
2. Spines: sharp, slender projections
3. **Foramen:** round opening through a bone; of particular importance is the **foramen magnum,** located at the base of the occipital bone, which

TABLE 26-1 Identification of Bone Markings

Bone	Marking	Description
Frontal	Supraorbital margin	Arched ridge just below eyebrows
	Frontal sinuses	Cavities inside bone just above supraorbital margin; lined with mucosa; contain air
Temporal	Mastoid process	Protuberance just behind ear
	Mastoid air cells	Air-filled, mucosa-lined spaces within mastoid process
	External auditory meatus (or canal)	Opening into ear and tube extending into temporal bone
	Zygomatic process	Projection that articulates with malar (or zygomatic) bone
Occipital	Foramen magnum	Opening through which spinal cord enters cranial cavity
Sphenoid	Body	Hollow, cubelike central portion
	Sella turcica (or Turkish saddle)	Saddle-shaped depression on upper surface of sphenoid body; contains pituitary gland
	Sphenoid sinuses	Irregular, air-filled, mucosa-lined spaces within central part of sphenoid
Ethmoid	Horizontal (cribriform) plate	Olfactory nerves pass through numerous openings in this plate
	Ethmoid sinuses	Honeycombed, mucosa-lined air spaces within lateral masses of bone
Mandible	Body	Main part of body; forms chin
	Alveolar process	Teeth set into this arch
Maxilla	Alveolar process	Arch containing teeth
	Maxillary sinus	Large, air-filled, mucosa-lined cavity within body of each maxilla; largest of sinuses
Special features of skull	Sutures	Immovable joints between skull bones
	1. Sagittal	1. Joint between two parietal bones
	2. Coronal	2. Joint between parietal bones and frontal bone
	3. Lambdoidal	3. Joint between parietal bones and occipital bone
	Fontanels	"Soft spots" where ossification is incomplete at birth; allow some compression of skull during birth; also important in determining position of head before delivery; six such areas located at angles of parietal bones
	1. Anterior (or frontal)	1. At intersection of sagittal and coronal sutures (juncture of parietal bones and frontal bone); diamond shaped; largest of fontanels; usually closed by 1½ years of age
	2. Posterior (or occipital)	2. At intersection of sagittal and lambdoidal sutures (juncture of parietal bones and occipital bone); triangular in shape; usually closed by second month
Sternum	Body	Main central part of bone
	Xiphoid process	Projection of cartilage at lower border of bone
Scapula	Spine	Sharp ridge running diagonally across posterior surface of shoulder-blade
	Acromion process	Slightly flaring projection at lateral end of scapular spine; may be felt as tip of shoulder; articulates with clavicle
	Glenoid cavity	Arm socket
Humerus	Head	Smooth, hemispherical enlargement at proximal end of humerus
Ulna	Olecranon process	Elbow
Radius	Head	Disk-shaped process forming proximal end of radius; articulates with capitulum of humerus and with radial notch of ulna
Innominate (hip)	Ilium	Upper, flaring portion
	Ischium	Lower, posterior portion
	Pubic bone or pubis	Medial, anterior section
	Acetabulum	Hip socket, formed by union of ilium, ischium, and pubis
	Iliac crests	Upper, curving boundary of ilium
	Anterosuperior spine	Prominent projection at anterior end of iliac crest; can be felt externally as "point" of hip
	Ischial tuberosity	Large, rough, quadrilateral process forming posterior part of ischium; in erect sitting position body rests on these tuberosities
	Symphysis pubis	Cartilaginous, amphiarthrotic joint between pubic bones
	Obturator foramen	Large hole in anterior surface of os coxae; formed by pubis and ischium; largest foramen in body

Continued.

TABLE 26-1 Identification of Bone Markings—cont'd

Bone	Marking	Description
Innominate (hip)—cont'd	Pelvic brim (or inlet)	Boundary of opening leading into true pelvis; size and shape of this inlet has great obstetrical importance, since if any of its diameters is too small, infant skull cannot enter true pelvis for natural birth
	True (or lesser) pelvis	Space below pelvic brim; true "basin" with bone and muscle walls and muscle floor; pelvic organs located in this space
	False (or greater) pelvis	Broad, shallow space above pelvic brim inlet; name "false pelvis" is misleading, since this space is actually part of abdominal cavity, not pelvic cavity
Femur	Head	Rounded, upper end of bone; fits in acetabulum
	Greater trochanter	Protuberance located interiorly and laterally to head
	Lesser trochanter	Small protuberance located inferiorly and medially to greater trochanter
Tibia	Medial malleolus	Rounded, downward projection at distal end of tibia; forms prominence on outer surface of ankle
Fibula	Lateral malleolus	Rounded prominence at distal end of fibula forms prominence on outer surface of ankle
Tarsals	Calcaneus	Heel bone
	Talus	Uppermost of tarsals; articulates with tibia and fibula; boxed in by medial and lateral malleoli

allows the spinal cord to communicate with the brain

1. **Fossa:** a shallow depression in a bone
2. Sinus: a depression filled with air and lined with mucous membrane
3. Grooves: shallow depressions that are long and narrow, which allow the passage of nerves and blood vessels

Structure of a Long Bone. Fig. 26-1 shows a long bone; the following structures can be identified:

1. **Diaphysis:** the shaft of a long bone, composed of compact bone, yet shaped like a long, hollow tube; a strong structure but lightweight to allow movement
2. Medullary cavity: the hollow center of the bone shaft; contains the yellow bone marrow
3. **Epiphyses:** the ends of the long bones; composed of spongy bone and contain the red bone marrow
4. Articular cartilage: a thin, external covering of cartilage on each epiphysis; cushions the joint
5. **Periosteum:** a protective fibrous vascular membrane that covers the diaphysis of the bone

Articulations (Joints)

Bones cannot bend without damage. To allow movement, individual bones articulate (move) at joint sites. Bones are held together by flexible connective tissue. The joint is the point of contact between the individual bones. The structure of the individual bones depends on the function of the area. Every bone in the body (except the hyoid bone, which anchors the tongue) connects or articulates with at least one other bone.

Joints perform two important functions: they hold the bones together to form the skeleton, and they allow movement and flexibility of the skeleton.

Types of Joints. The most common way to classify joints is according to the degree of movement they permit. There are three types:

1. Synarthrosis: no movement
2. Amphiarthrosis: slight movement
3. Diarthrosis: free movement

Synarthrosis. These immovable joints are held together by fibrous connective tissue. An example is the suture lines of the skull, where the irregular edges of the bone are bound together by fibrous connective tissue.

Amphiarthrosis. These slightly immovable joints are connected by a disk of cartilage. Two examples of this type of joint are the pubic bones of the pelvis and the intervertebral joints of the spinal column.

Diarthrosis (synovial joints). These freely movable joints contain a joint capsule, joint cavity, and a layer of cartilage over the ends of the two bones (Fig. 26-2). The capsule fits over the ends of the two bones like a sleeve. It is composed of fibrous connective tissue and lined with synovial membrane, which is smooth and slippery. This membrane secretes synovial fluid, which allows free movement. Fig. 26-3 on p. 570 shows examples of diarthrotic joints: the hinge, pivot, condyloid, saddle, ball and socket, and gliding. **Ligaments** are bands of connective tissue binding joints together and connecting

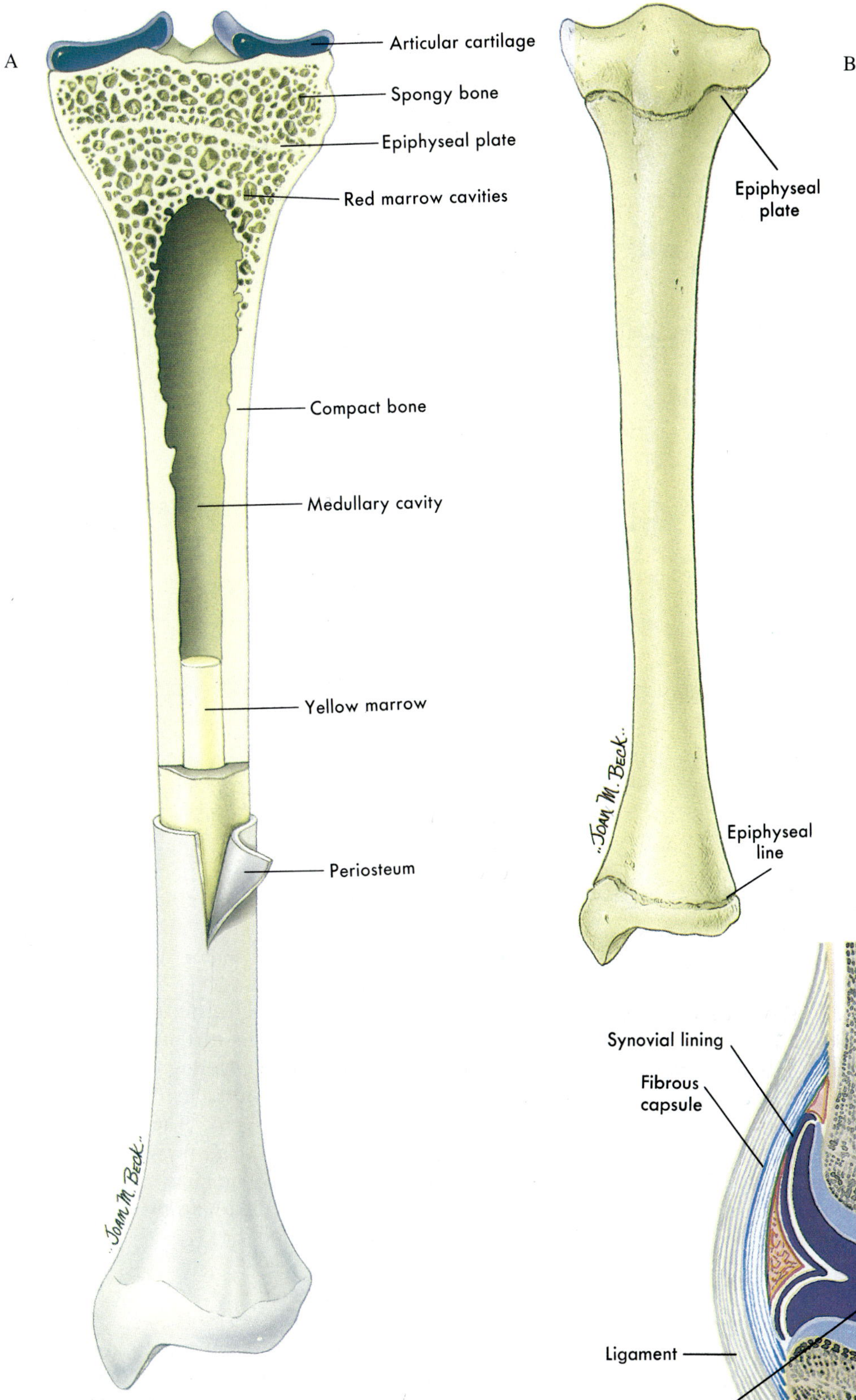

FIG. 26-1 **A,** Longitudinal section of long bone showing structural details. **B,** External view of epiphyseal lines on a juvenile long bone. The area between the epiphyses is the diaphysis.

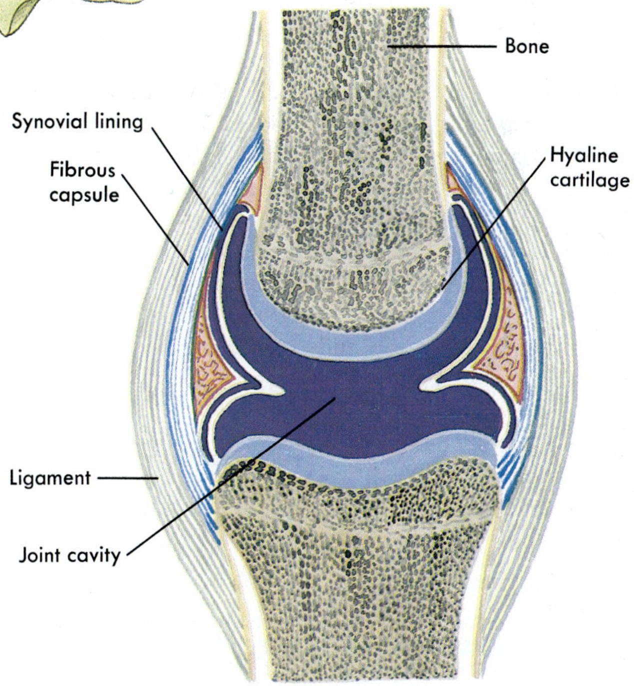

FIG. 26-2 Structure of a freely movable (diarthrotic) joint. Note these typical features: joint capsule, joint cavity lined with synovial membrane, and articular (hyaline) cartilage covering the end surfaces of the bones within the joint capsule.

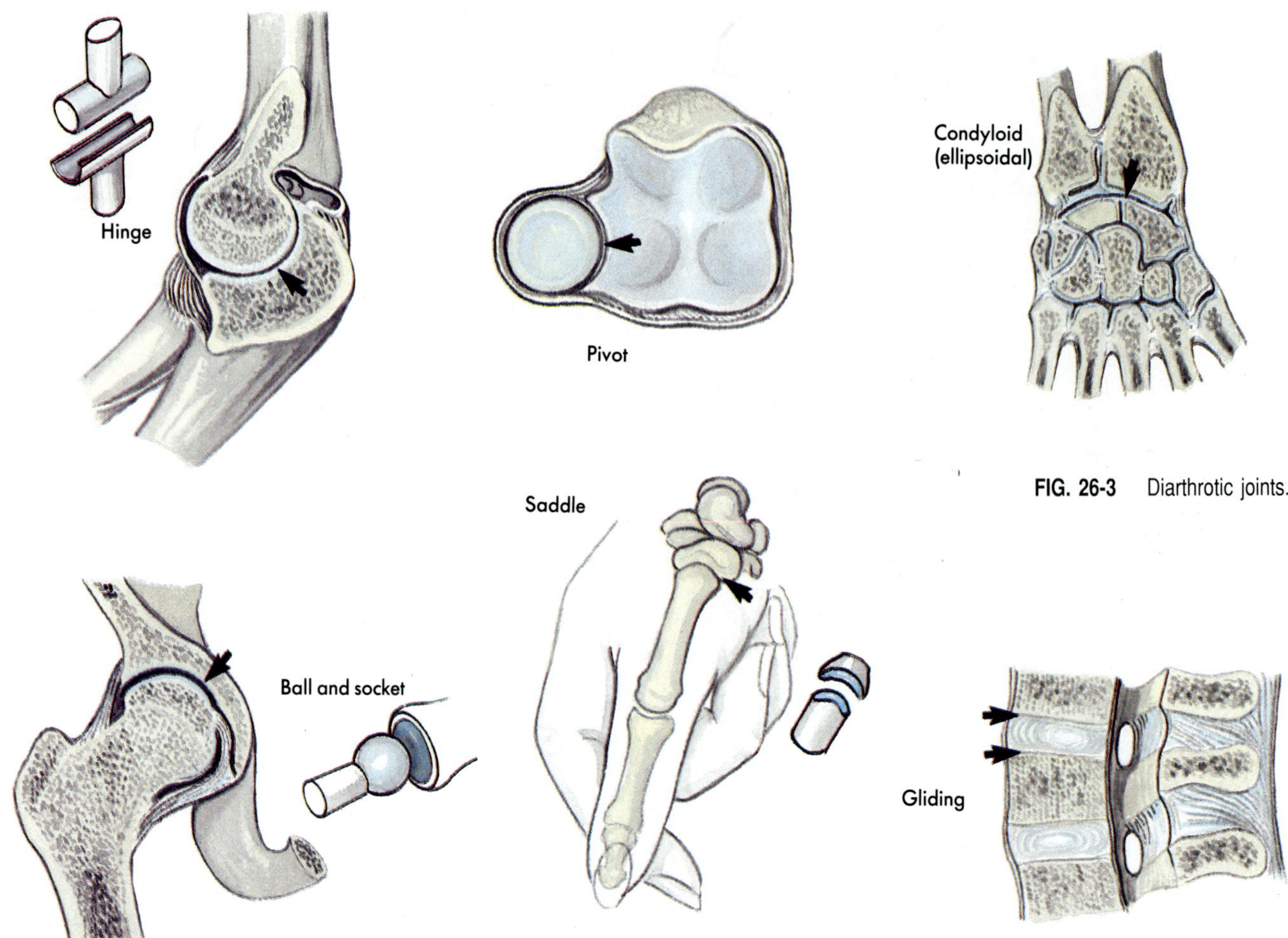

FIG. 26-3 Diarthrotic joints.

Box 26-1 MAIN PARTS OF THE SKELETON

AXIAL SKELETON	APPENDICULAR SKELETON
Skull	**Upper Extremities**
Cranium	Shoulder (pectoral) girdle
Ear bones	Arms
Face	Wrists
Spine	Hands
Vertebrae	**Lower Extremities**
Thorax	Hip (pelvic) girdle
Ribs	Legs
Sternum	Ankles
	Feet

various bones and cartilages, whereas **tendons** are white and glistening fibrous bands of tissue that attach muscle to bone. The articular cartilage covering the ends of the bones acts as a shock absorber. Bursae (small sacs of connective tissue) also cushion shock. They are located wherever pressure is exerted (e.g., between skin and bone, between tendons and bone, and sometimes between muscles). They are lined with synovial membrane and thus contain synovial fluid.

Divisions of the Skeleton

The skeleton is divided into the axial and the appendicular skeleton. The axial skeleton is composed of the skull, vertebral column, and the thorax (chest) (Box 26-1). The appendicular skeleton contains 126 bones and is composed of the upper extremities, lower extremities, shoulder girdle, and pelvic girdle (excluding the sacrum) (Box 26-1) (Fig. 26-4 and Fig. 26-5 on p. 572).

Axial Skeleton.

Skull. The skull (Fig. 26-6 on p. 573) contains 22 bones and sits on the superior portion of the vertebral

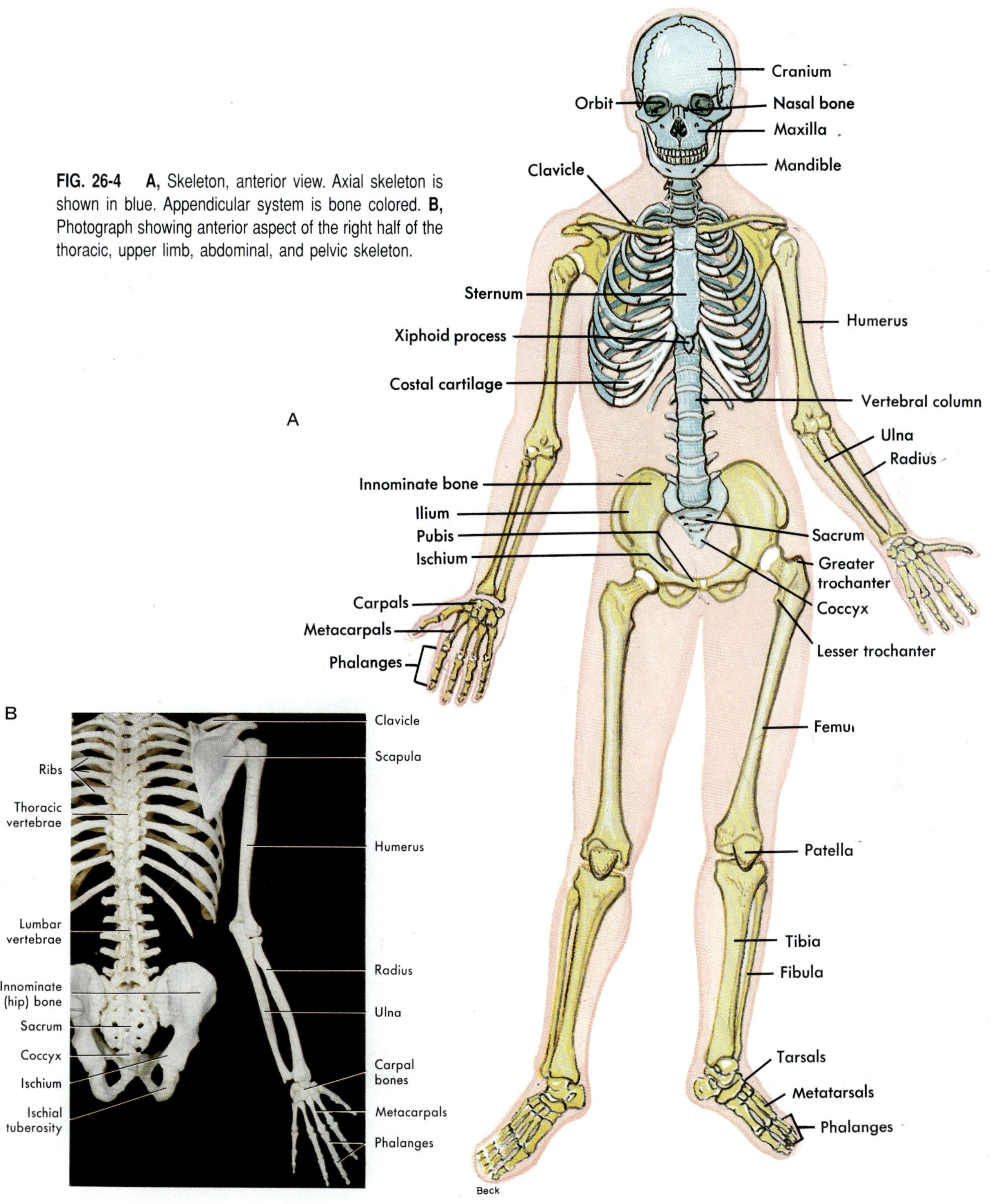

FIG. 26-4 **A,** Skeleton, anterior view. Axial skeleton is shown in blue. Appendicular system is bone colored. **B,** Photograph showing anterior aspect of the right half of the thoracic, upper limb, abdominal, and pelvic skeleton.

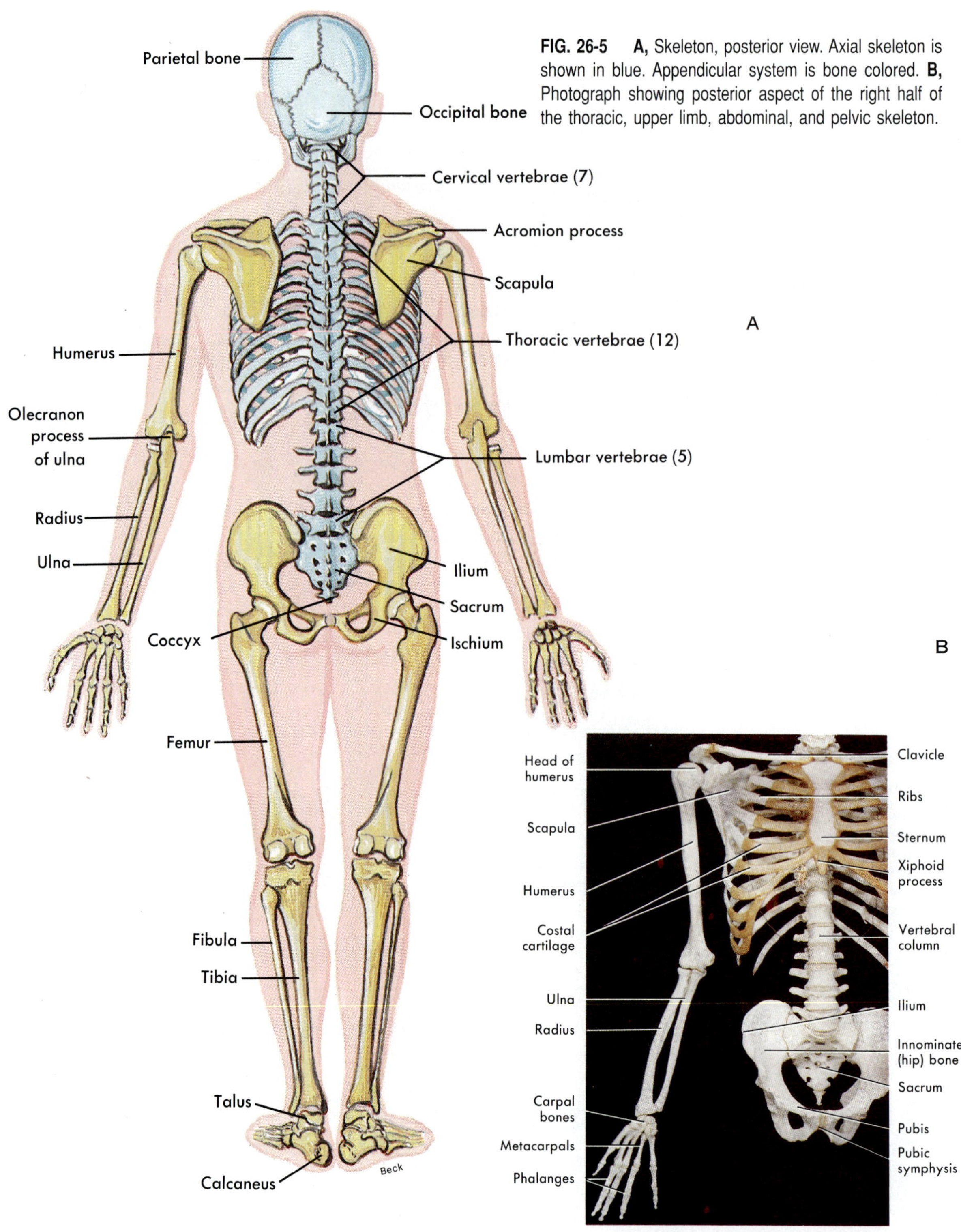

FIG. 26-5 **A,** Skeleton, posterior view. Axial skeleton is shown in blue. Appendicular system is bone colored. **B,** Photograph showing posterior aspect of the right half of the thoracic, upper limb, abdominal, and pelvic skeleton.

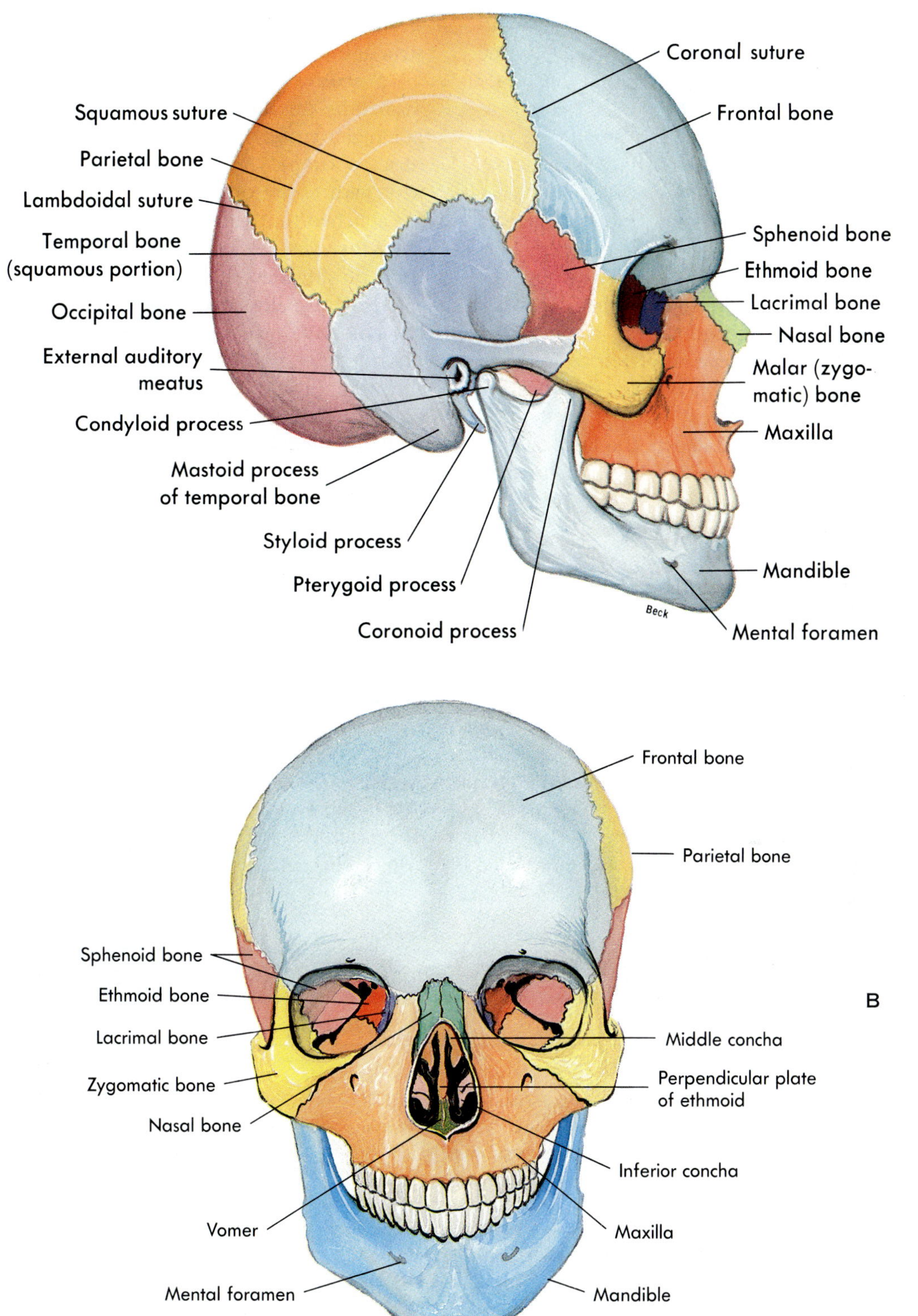

FIG. 26-6 **A,** Skull viewed from the right side. **B,** Skull viewed anteriorly.

column. Eight cranial bones enclose and protect the brain: frontal bone, parietal bones (2), temporal bones (2), occipital bone, sphenoid bone, and ethmoid bone. The remaining 14 bones are the facial bones. They are the nasal bones (2), the maxillae (2), the zygomatic bones (2), the mandible, the lacrimal bones (2), the palatine bones (2), the inferior nasal conchae (2), and the vomer (Fig. 26-6). Table 26-2 briefly describes each bone.

Vertebral column. The vertebral column (Fig. 26-7 on p. 576) supports the body and is strong and flexible. It contains a total of 26 bones: 24 single bones (vertebrae), and 2 fused bones (the sacrum and the coccyx). It is composed of five sections: cervical, thoracic, lumbar, sacral, and coccyx. The column is S-shaped and contains four curves, which develop before birth. This pattern gives flexibility and strength to the column. The first seven vertebrae are the cervical vertebrae and form the neck region. The first vertebra is called the *atlas* and allows the head to nod in a "yes" motion. The second vertebra is called the *axis* and allows the head to turn in a "no" motion. Progressing in a distal fashion, the next 12 vertebrae are called the *thoracic vertebrae.* They form the chest portion of the column, where the 12 pairs of ribs attach, and they are convex (curve outward). The next five vertebrae, the lumbar vertebrae, are the largest and heaviest of the column. They are concave (curve inward) and form the lower back. The spinal cord, which continues from the brain through the vertebral column, ends at the second lumbar vertebra. The sacrum is formed by five fused vertebrae and forms the posterior pelvis. The last section of the vertebral column is the coccyx, which is composed of four or five fused bones. It is commonly called the *tailbone.*

A single vertebra is composed of three basic parts: the body, the foramen, and the processes. The large, solid structure is the body, the opening through which the spinal column passes is the foramen, and the winglike structures are the processes.

Thorax. The thorax, or rib cage, is composed of the sternum, ribs, and the thoracic vertebrae. This cagelike structure protects the heart, lungs, and great vessels.

Sternum. The sternum (breastbone) is a flat bone formed by the fusion of three bones—manubrium (upper region), body (midportion), and **xiphoid process** (distal portion). The first seven pairs of ribs are attached to it with costal cartilage. The clavicles (collar bones) are attached to it with ligaments.

Ribs. The ribcage is composed of 12 pairs of ribs. Each rib attaches posteriorly to the vertebral column. The first 10 pairs attach anteriorly to the ribcage. The remaining two pairs seem to float free; hence the name *floating ribs.* The first 7 pairs of ribs attach directly to the sternum with costal cartilage; they are called *true ribs.* The eighth, ninth, and tenth pairs attach to the seventh rib, therefore attaching indirectly to the sternum. They are called *false ribs.*

Appendicular Skeleton. The appendicular skeleton contains 126 bones. It is composed of the bones of the limbs and the pectoral and pelvic girdles, which attach the limbs to the axial skeleton.

Pectoral girdle. The pectoral girdle is composed of the two clavicles (collarbones) and the two scapulae (shoulder-blades). It is responsible for the attachment of the upper extremities to the sternum; there is no articulation with the vertebral column. The clavicle attaches to the superior portion of the sternum, the manubrium. The distal portion of the clavicle attaches to the scapula. The scapulae are flat, triangular bones that resemble wings. The enlarged end of the spine of the scapula, the

TABLE 26-2 Bones of the Skeleton

Name	Number	Description
Cranial bones		
Frontal	1	Forehead bone; also forms front part of floor of cranium and most of upper part of eye sockets; cavity inside bone above upper margins of eye sockets (orbits) called *frontal sinus;* lined with mucous membrane
Parietal	2	Form bulging topsides of cranium
Temporal	2	Form lower sides of cranium; contain *middle* and *inner ear structures; mastoid sinuses* are mucosa-lined spaces in *mastoid process,* the protuberance behind ear; *external auditory canal* is tube leading into temporal bone
Occipital	1	Forms back of skull; spinal cord enters cranium through large opening *(foramen magnum)* in occipital bone
Sphenoid	1	Forms central part of floor of cranium; large bone at base of the skull between the occipital and ethmoid in front and the parietal and temporal bones at the side, pituitary gland located in small depression in sphenoid called *sella turcia (Turkish saddle)*
Ethmoid	1	Complicated bone that helps form floor of cranium, side walls and roof of nose and part of its middle partition (nasal septum), and part of orbit; contains honeycomb-like spaces, the *ethmoid sinuses*

TABLE 26-2 Bones of the Skeleton—cont'd		
Name	**Number**	**Description**
Face bones		
Nasal	2	Small bones that form upper part of bridge of nose
Maxillary	2	Upper jawbones; also help form roof of mouth, floor, and side walls of nose and floor of orbit; large cavity in maxillary bone is *maxillary sinus*
Zygoma	2	Cheek bones; also help form orbit
Mandible	1	Lower jawbone
Lacrimal	2	Small bone; helps form medial wall of eye socket and side wall of nasal cavity
Palatine	2	Form back part of roof of mouth and floor and side walls of nose and part of floor of orbit
Vomer	1	Forms lower, back part of nasal septum
Ear bones		
Malleus	2	Malleus, incus, and stapes are tiny bones in middle ear cavity in temporal bone; *malleus* means "hammer"—shape of bone
Incus	2	*Incus* means "anvil"—shape of bone
Stapes	2	*Stapes* means "stirrup"—shape of bone
Hyoid bone		U-shaped bone in neck at base of tongue
Vertebral column		
Cervical vertebrae	7	Upper seven vertebrae, in neck region; first cervical vertebra called atlas; second called axis
Thoracic vertebrae	12	Next twelve vertebrae; ribs attach to these
Lumbar vertebrae	5	Next five vertebrae; those in small of back
Sacrum	1	In child, five separate vertebrae; in adult, fused into one
Coccyx	1	In child, three to five separate vertebrae; in adult, fused into one
Thorax		
True ribs	14	Upper seven pairs; attach to sternum by way of *costal cartilages*
False ribs	10	Lower five pairs; lowest two pairs do not attach to sternum, therefore called *floating ribs;* next three pairs attach to sternum by way of costal cartilage of seventh ribs
Sternum	1	Breastbone; shaped like a dagger; piece of cartilage at lower end of bone called *xiphoid process*
Upper extremities		
Clavicle	2	Collarbones; only joints between shoulder girdle and axial skeleton are those between each clavicle and sternum
Scapula	2	Shoulder bones; scapula plus clavicle forms *shoulder girdle; acromion process*—tip of shoulder that forms joint with clavicle; *glenoid cavity*—arm socket
Humerus	2	Upper arm bone
Radius	2	Bone on thumb side of lower arm
Ulna	2	Bone on little finger side of lower arm; *olecranon process*—projection of ulna known as elbow or "funny bone"
Carpal bones	16	Irregular bones at upper end of hand; anatomical wrist
Metacarpals	10	Form framework of palm of hand
Phalanges	28	Finger bones; three in each finger, two in each thumb
Lower extremities		
Pelvic bones	2	Hipbones; *ilium*—upper flaring part of pelvic bone; *ischium*—lower back part; *pubic bone*—lower front part; *acetabulum*—hip socket; *symphysis pubis*—joint in midline between two pubic bones; pelvic inlet—opening into *true pelvis,* or pelvic cavity; if pelvic inlet is misshapen or too small, infant skull cannot enter true pelvis for natural birth
Femur	2	Thigh or upper leg bones; *head of femur*—ball-shaped, upper end of bone; fits into acetabulum
Patella	2	Kneecap
Tibia	2	Shinbone; *medial malleolus*—rounded projection at lower end of tibia commonly called *inner anklebone*
Fibula	2	Long slender bone of lateral side of lower leg; *lateral malleolus*—rounded projection at lower end of fibula commonly called *outer anklebone*
Tarsal bones	14	Form heel and back part of foot; anatomical ankle
Metatarsals	10	Form part of foot to which toes attach; tarsal and metatarsal bones so arranged that they form three arches in foot
Phalanges	28	Toe bones; three in each toe, two in each great toe
TOTAL	206	

acromion process, connects with the clavicle. These articulations allow a wide range of motion.

Bones of the upper extremities. The upper arm is formed by a single long bone, the humerus. It is the second longest bone in the body. It attaches to the scapula at its proximal end. This rounded head has two bony projections that are sites for muscle attachments.

The forearm is formed by two bones, the radius and the ulna. They articulate with each other and the humerus, forming the elbow. Fig. 26-8 shows the large bony process, the olecranon process; this is commonly called the *funny bone.* Distally the radius and ulna articulate with the bones of the wrist. In the anatomical position (arms at the side of the body with palms facing forward), the ulna lies medially, extending toward the little finger. The radius extends laterally, extending toward the thumb.

The wrist is formed by 8 irregular bones called the carpals. The palm of the hand is formed by 5 metacarpal bones that join the 14 finger bones, *phalanges.* Each finger contains 3 phalanges: proximal, middle, and distal. The thumb contains 2 phalanges: proximal and distal.

Pelvic girdle (pelvis). The pelvis is composed of the two large hipbones (innominate), the sacrum, and

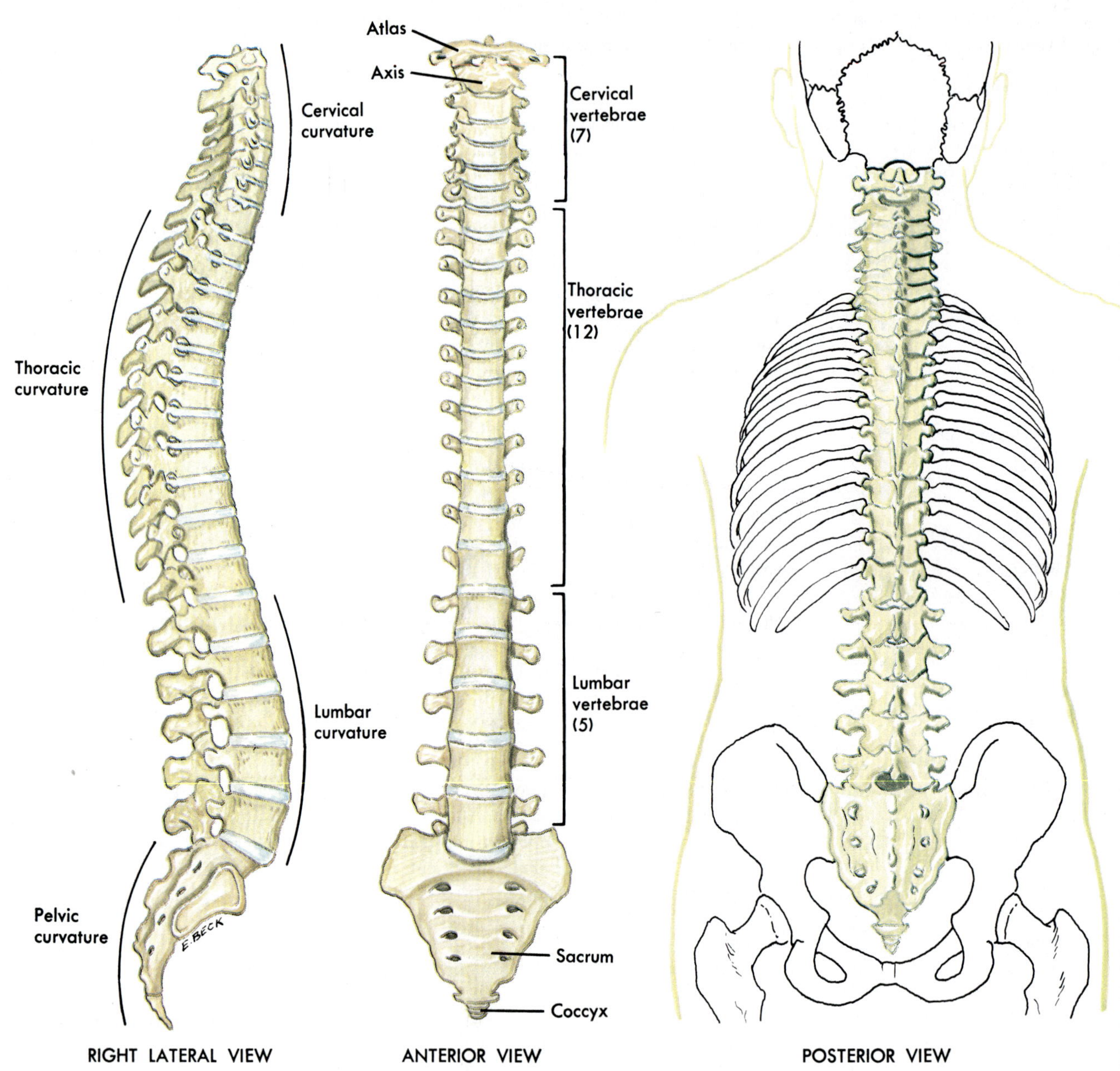

FIG. 26-7 The spinal column from three views.

the coccyx. In infancy the innominate bones are composed of three separate bones: the ilium, the ischium, and the pubis. In later years these bones fuse and become one (Fig. 26-9). The ilium is the upper, flared portion. The upper rim is called the iliac crest and is an important anatomical landmark for injection technique. It connects posteriorly with the sacrum to form the sacroiliac joint. The **ischium** (lower portion of the innominate or hip bone) is the strongest section and holds the body weight when the body is in a sitting position. The pubis forms the anterior section of the pelvis and fuses to form the symphysis pubis, a cartilaginous joint.

Bones of the lower extremities. The upper leg bone, the femur (Fig. 26-10, *A*, on p. 578), is the strongest and heaviest bone in the body. The head of the femur articulates with the hipbone in a deep socket—the acetabulum. This is an excellent example of a ball and socket joint. Distally the femur articulates with the tibia (shin). Each femur angles medially; this results in the knee joints being nearer the body's line of gravity (see Fig. 26-5). Anterior to the articulation of the upper and lower leg is the **patella** (kneecap), a small, triangular bone. The patella is surrounded by four bursae, which cushion it.

The lower leg is composed of two bones, the tibia and the fibula (Fig. 26-10, *B*). As stated, the **tibia** articulates with the femur. It is the larger of the two bones and lies medially and bears the major portion of the body weight. The **fibula** (outer and smaller bone of the lower

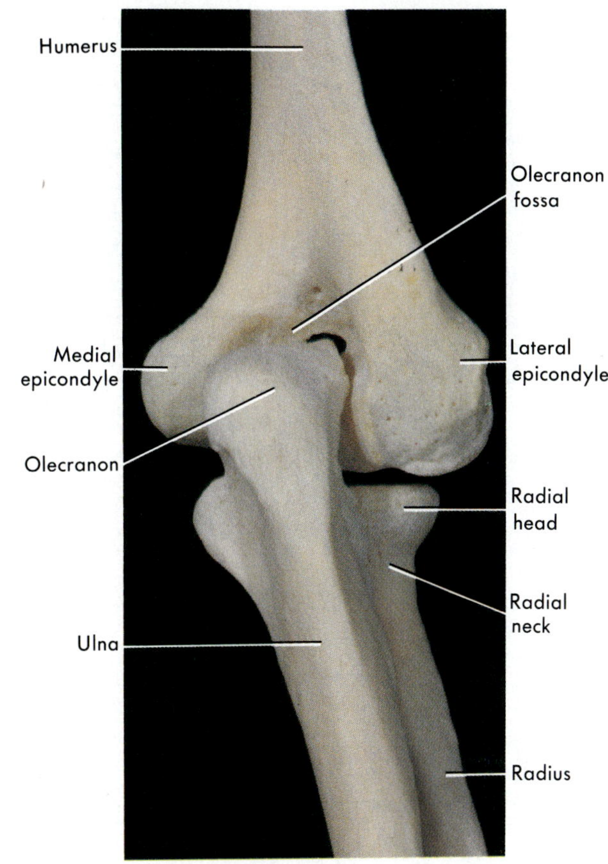

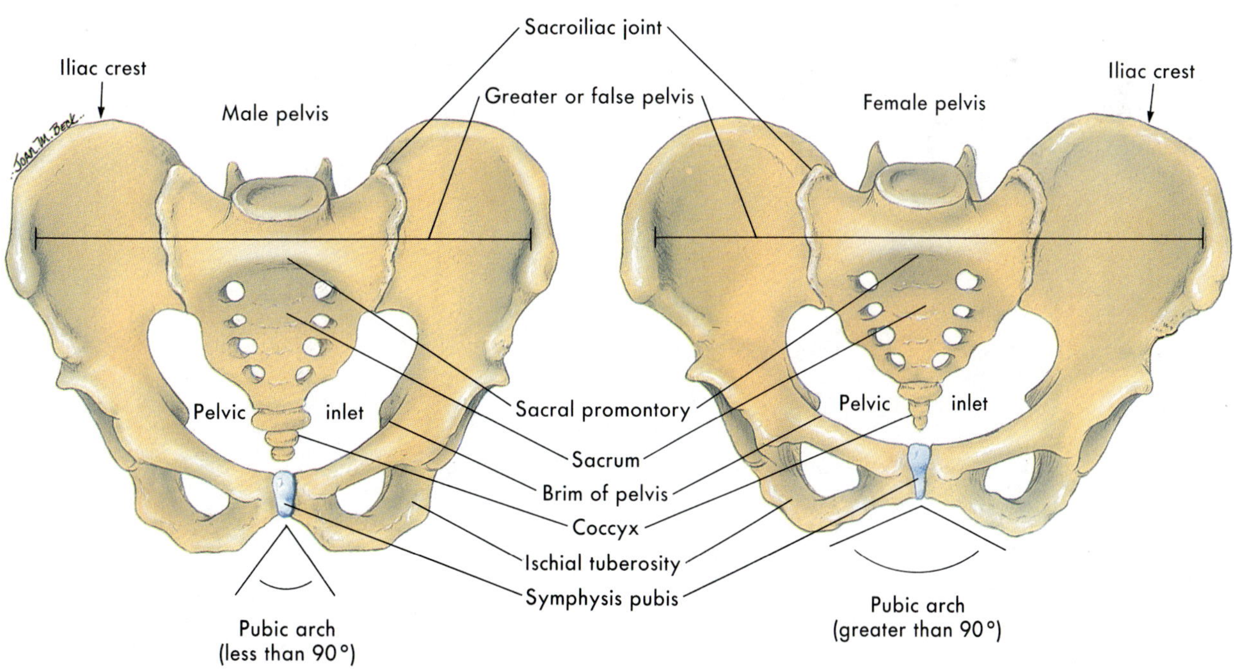

FIG. 26-9 Comparison of male and female bony pelvis.

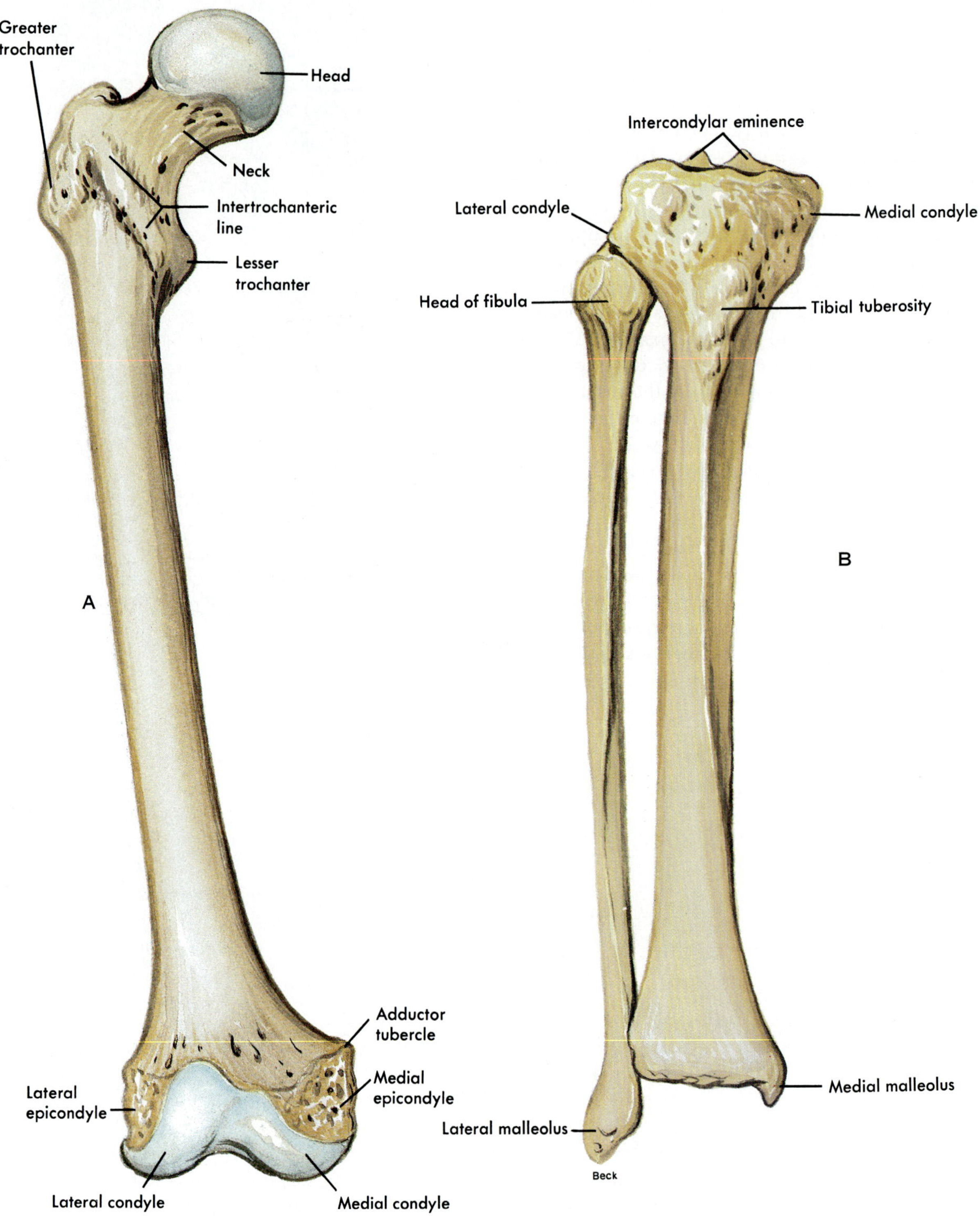

FIG. 26-10 **A,** Right femur. **B,** Right tibia and fibula.

leg), which is thin and sticklike, lies beside the tibia. It is the most slender of the long bones. The bulge on the inner aspect of the ankle is formed by the medial malleolus of the tibia; the fibula's lateral malleolus forms the lateral bulge. The length of the tibia can be easily felt along the anterior surface of the lower leg, since it is unprotected by any major muscle group.

The ankle (tarsus) is composed of seven tarsal bones. The two largest tarsals, the **calcaneus** (heelbone) and the talus (also posterior) carry most of the body weight. The talus articulates with the tibia and fibula. As a step is taken, the weight is initially carried by the talus; the weight is then transferred to the calcaneus. The foot is composed of 5 metatarsal bones (which form the instep) and 14 phalanges. There are some similarities between the feet and the hands. The great toe, like the thumb, has two bones, whereas the fingers and remaining toes have three bones. Because the foot is designed for weight bearing, it contains ligaments to bind the bones together and tendons to hold the foot in an arched position. The longitudinal arch runs from the calcaneus to the heads of the metatarsals. The transverse arch extends across the ball of the foot. These arches provide flexibility and spring motion to the gait.

Functions of the Muscular System

The bones and joints provide the framework of the body, but the muscles are necessary for movement. This motion results from contraction and relaxation of the individual muscles.

The body is composed of more than 600 muscles. They usually act in groups to execute a body movement. They comprise approximately 40% to 50% of the total body weight.

As muscles contract, they perform three vital functions: motion, maintenance of posture, and production of heat.

All body movements rely on the integrated functioning of the bones, joints, and muscles. Certain involuntary kinds of motion include activities conducted by the internal organs, such as the heart beating, the gallbladder releasing bile, and the stomach churning food. Muscle tissue is under voluntary or involuntary control. Voluntary muscle is under conscious control, whereas involuntary muscle tissue responds to internal commands without any conscious control of it.

The contraction of certain skeletal muscles gives the body proper posture. These muscles exert a pull on various bones, which allows the body to maintain a sitting or standing position.

As skeletal muscles contract, they produce body heat. It is estimated that approximately 85% of all body heat is generated by the contraction of the skeletal muscles.

Types of Muscle Tissue. Muscle tissue is categorized by location, structure, and type of nervous system control. There are three types of muscle tissue: skeletal, cardiac, and smooth muscle (see Chapter 23).

1. Skeletal muscle tissue attaches to the bones to produce movement. It is called *striated* because under the microscope it appears to have stripes running perpendicular to the length of the muscle. It is also voluntary muscle tissue because it can be consciously made to contract.
2. The heart is composed of cardiac muscle tissue, which forms the bulk of the walls of the heart. It is also striated but is under involuntary control. The heart beats 24 hours a day and does not require a conscious decision about its rate.
3. Smooth muscle tissue is composed of small, spindle-shaped cells and is nonstriated. It is responsible for the maintenance of the processes within the internal environment of the body, such as the stomach and the intestines. This muscle tissue is also involuntary.

Characteristics. Muscle tissue possesses four principal characteristics: excitability, contractility, extensibility, and elasticity.

1. Excitability is the ability of muscle tissue to respond to a stimulus. A stimulus is a change in the internal or external environment that is strong enough to initiate a nerve impulse. The point at which the nerve fiber relays the message to the muscle cell is the neuromuscular junction.
2. Contractility is the ability of the muscle to be extended (stretched). The muscle actually shortens and becomes thicker.
3. Extensibility is the ability of the muscle to be extended (stretched). Many muscle groups of the body are arranged in opposing pairs. For example, when the forearm is flexed (bent), the anterior group of muscles is contracted and the posterior group is extended.
4. Elasticity is the ability of the muscle to return to its former shape after repeated contraction or extension.

Skeletal Muscle Structure. A skeletal muscle is composed of hundreds of muscle fibers (cells). Each skeletal muscle is surrounded by a covering of connective tissue called the *epimysium.* The epimysium joins with two other inner coverings, the perimysium and the endomysium, to extend beyond the muscle to form a tough cord of connective tissue known as a *tendon.* Tendons anchor muscles to bones. As a muscle contracts, the tendon and bone corresponding to that particular muscle are pulled toward the muscle. This is how movement occurs. Tendons in the ankle and wrist are enclosed in sleeves or tubelike structures of connective tissue known as tendon sheaths. These tendon sheaths contain synovial fluid and permit the tendons to slide easily; the sheaths also keep the tendons in place. Sometimes the tendon is formed of flat, strong bands of connective tissue; it is then called an *aponeurosis.* All the tendons, ligaments, and aponeuroses of the body are composed of various sizes, shapes, and densities of connective tissue. These are collectively known as *fasciae.*

Nerve and Blood Supply. Because of the physical demands placed on the skeletal muscles, they need a constant supply of oxygen and nutrition. They are well supplied with blood vessels that carry oxygen and nutrition to the area and remove the waste products of metabolism.

Because the skeletal muscles are voluntary, they need a constant source of "information," which is supplied by nerve cells or fibers. These nerve cells continually send impulses that stimulate the muscle cells. These impulses enter at the neuromuscular junction, the point of contact between the nerve ending and the muscle fiber. As a nerve impulse passes through this junction, chemicals are released that cause the muscle to contract.

Usually one artery, two veins, and one nerve penetrate a particular muscle. Each muscle cell comes in contact with several capillaries and a portion of a nerve cell. The muscle cells, in union with the nerve cell that controls them, are called a *motor unit.*

The impulse from the nerve cell must travel across a small gap, since the nerve cell and the muscle cell do not directly touch each other. This small gap is called a *synaptic cleft* and is filled with tissue fluid. A special chemical *(neurotransmitter)* travels through the fluid to stimulate the muscle fiber. *Acetylcholine* is the specific neurotransmitter for skeletal muscle tissue. An enzyme called *cholinesterase* breaks down the acetylcholine once it has transferred the message. This allows the muscle cell to relax between impulses.

Muscle Contraction.

Muscle stimulus. Muscle cells are governed by the "all or none" law, which states that when a muscle cell is adequately stimulated or shocked, it will contract completely. Because each skeletal muscle is composed of thousands of muscle cells that react to many different nerve cells, the muscle as a whole contracts according to the "principle of graded response." The strength of the contraction of the muscle, therefore, depends on the number of individual muscle cells responding. These muscle responses allow us to tenderly brush a baby's cheek or destroy an irritating mosquito.

Muscle tone. The skeletal muscles are in a constant state of readiness for action. At any given time several muscle cells within a certain muscle are contracted; the remainder of the muscle cells are relaxed. The muscle tone provided is necessary for good posture but does not provide movement of the body. To understand the importance of muscle tone, one can observe an extremity that has become paralyzed—the muscles are flaccid, limp, or atrophied (wasted) and incapable of producing movement because the cells are no longer receiving stimuli from the nerve fibers.

Energy for contraction. An energy source is necessary for the contraction of muscle tissue. The muscle cell derives this energy from *adenosine triphosphate (ATP),* an energy-carrying molecule contained in all muscle tissue. When the muscle continues to contract and depletes the store of ATP, another energy source, glycogen, may be used. *Glycogen* (stored glucose) is found in small amounts in the skeletal muscles and in large amounts in the liver. The use of the energy sources must take place in the presence of oxygen. As the muscle contraction continues and the oxygen supply decreases, a waste product called *lactic acid* accumulates. The muscle tissue may continue to contract anaerobically (without oxygen), but the lactic acid by-product continues to accumulate. The muscle is then in a state of oxygen debt. The lactic acid that has built up causes muscle soreness. To replenish the oxygen debt, the brain stimulates the respiratory system and rapid, deep breathing occurs. This breathing pattern continues until the body has enough oxygen reserve to reverse the process.

Types of skeletal muscle contraction. The partial contraction of the muscles to maintain muscle tone has been discussed. The following is a discussion of the other major types of contraction that occur. They are isometric, isotonic, twitch, and tetanic (tetanus).

Isometric contraction. A skeletal muscle can contract without producing movement. The contraction increases the tension within the muscle but does not shorten it. The term *isometric* comes from the Greek words *isos* and *metron,* meaning equal pressure. This term refers to the fact that during relaxation and contraction the muscle length stays the same. This may be accomplished by opposing different muscles (e.g., pressing the hands together). There is no joint movement and the length of the muscle remains unchanged, but muscle strength and tone are improved. Repetition of isometric muscle contraction causes the muscles to become larger and stronger. Often, the patient who has had knee surgery is taught to use isometric exercise on the quadriceps femoris. This group of muscles covers the anterior and lateral areas of the femur and allows the individual to extend the leg.

Isotonic contraction. In an isotonic contraction the muscle shortens and can produce movement of a joint. Some examples of this type of contraction are sitting, walking, and bending the knees. Repetition of this type of contraction improves joint mobility and helps to improve muscle strength and tone.

Twitch contraction. A quick, jerky contraction in response to a single stimulus produces a muscle twitch contraction. A twitch response does not occur at the instant of the stimulation, but a fraction of a second later.

It actually occurs in three phases: the latent phase, the contraction phase, and the relaxation phase. The whole process lasts less than 1/10 of a second. The phenomenon does not occur often but can be simulated in a laboratory setting to study muscle physiology.

Tetanic contraction (tetanus). When a series of stimuli bombard the skeletal muscle tissue (20 to 30 per second), a sustained contraction will result. Normal movement is produced by incomplete, short-term tetanic contractions. The word *tetanus* comes from the Greek word *tetanos,* meaning extreme tension.

Muscle and Body Movements.

Origin and insertion. Muscles are attached, usually at a joint, to the bones by a tendon. The less movable, or fixed, end of a muscle attachment is called the **origin.** The more movable end of a muscle attachment is called the **insertion.** The fleshy part of the muscle, between the origin and insertion, is called the *belly* of the muscle. In the extremities the origin of the muscle is usually proximal and the insertion is usually distal. When muscles contract, the insertion moves toward the origin (Fig. 26-11).

Muscle action. Muscles have only one action—they pull. They are unable to push. Skeletal muscles are therefore arranged in groups and in opposing pairs at joints. The muscle that produces action is called the *prime mover.* The opposite muscle, the *antagonist,* is relaxed. For example, to touch the shoulder the biceps muscle contracts (prime mover) and pulls the radius bone upward. The triceps is relaxed (antagonist). To lower the arm, the triceps muscle contracts (prime mover) and pulls on the ulna. The biceps is relaxed and is the antagonist. Each muscle group may be either the prime mover or antagonist, depending on the desired movement. The antagonist will always relax and yield to the movement of the prime mover.

As the prime movers and antagonists perform their movements, certain muscles called *synergists* assist by steadying the movement. This helps the prime mover to function more efficiently. In some areas (e.g., the wrist), a muscle crosses two or more joints, and the contraction of the muscle will cause movement in all joints involved unless the synergists stabilize them.

Fixators stabilize the origin of a prime mover so that all the tension can be used to move the insertion bone. The fixators are specialized synergists. A prime example of a group of fixator muscles is the muscles that hold the scapula firmly against the posterior of the chest.

Types of body movements. Some muscles can move some body parts in only two directions, whereas others can move certain body parts in several directions. Some of the more common movements that the body is capable of producing are flexion, extension, abduction, adduction, rotation, supination, pronation, dorsiflexion, and plantar flexion (Box 26-2 and Tables 26-3 and 26-4 on pp. 582-583).

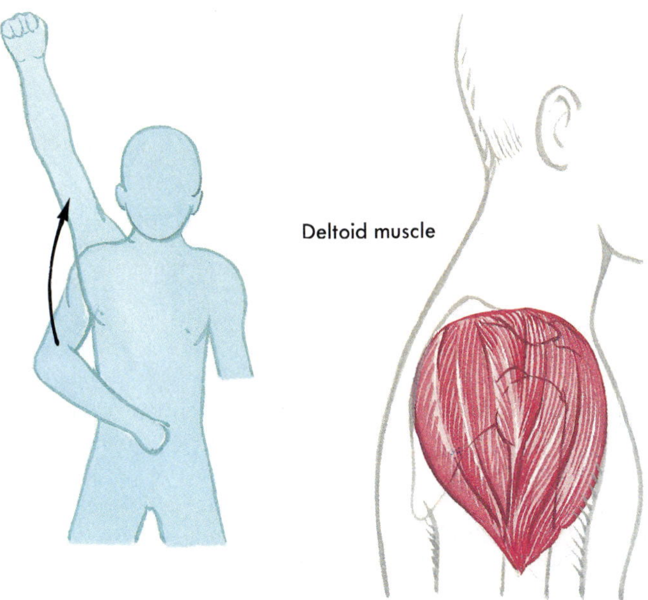

FIG. 26-11 When the deltoid muscle (shown on the figure at right) contracts, it abducts the upper arm at the shoulder joint (figure at the left).

Box 26-2 TYPES OF BODY MOVEMENT

Flexion: a movement that is allowed by certain joints of the skeleton that decreases the angle between two adjoining bones. For example, if the arm is bent at the elbow, the angle between the humerus and the ulna is decreased.

Extension (Fig. 26-12 on p. 583): a movement allowed by certain joints of the skeleton that increases the angle between two adjoining bones. For example, if the leg is extended, the angle between the femur and tibia is increased. If the extension angles more than 180 degrees, the extremity is *hyperextended.*

Abduction: a movement of an extremity away from the midline of the body.

Adduction: a movement of an extremity toward the axis of the body.

Rotation: a movement of the bone around its longitudinal axis (e.g., a pivot motion, such as shaking the head "no").

Supination: a movement of the hand and forearm that causes the palm to face upward or forward.

Pronation: a movement of the hand and forearm that causes the palm to face downward or backward.

Dorsiflexion: a movement that causes the top of the foot to elevate or tilt upward.

Plantar flexion: a movement that causes the bottom of the foot to be directed downward.

TABLE 26-3 Principal Muscles of the Body

Muscle	Function	Insertion	Origin
Muscles of the head and neck			
Frontal	Raises eyebrow	Skin of eyebrow	Occipital bone
Orbicularis oculi	Closes eye	Maxilla and frontal bone	Maxilla and frontal bone (encircles eye)
Orbicularis oris	Draws lips together	Encircles lips	Encircles lips
Zygomaticus	Elevates corners of mouth and lips	Angle of mouth and upper lip	Zygomatic bone
Masseter	Closes jaws	Mandible	Zygomatic arch
Temporal	Closes jaw	Mandible	Temporal region of the skull
Sternocleidomastoid	Rotates and extends head	Mastoid process	Sternum and clavicle
Trapezius	Extends head and neck	Scapula	Skull and upper vertebrae
Muscles that move the upper extremities			
Pectoralis major	Flexes and helps adduct upper arms	Humerus	Sternum, clavicle, and upper rib cartilages
Latissimus dorsi	Extends and helps adduct upper arm	Humerus	Vertebrae and ilium
Deltoid	Abducts upper arm	Humerus	Clavicle and scapula
Biceps brachii	Flexes lower arm	Radius	Ulna
Triceps brachii	Extends lower arm	Ulna	Scapula and humerus
Muscles of the trunk			
External oblique	Compresses abdomen	Midline of abdomen	Lower thoracic cage
Internal oblique	Compresses abdomen	Midline of abdomen	Pelvis
Transversus abdominis	Compresses abdomen	Midline of abdomen	Ribs, vertebrae, and pelvis
Rectus abdominis	Flexes trunk	Lower ribcage	Pubis
Muscles that move the lower extremities			
Iliopsoas	Flexes thigh or trunk	Ilium and vertebrae	Femur
Sartorius	Flexes thigh and rotates lower leg	Tibia	Ilium
Gluteus maximus	Extends thigh	Femur	Ilium, sacrum, and coccyx
Adductor group			
Adductor longus	Adducts thigh	Femur	Pubis
Gracilis	Adducts thigh	Tibia	Pubis
Pectineus	Adducts thigh	Femur	Pubis
Hamstring group			
Semimembranosus	Flexes lower leg	Tibia	Ischium
Semitendinosus	Flexes lower leg	Tibia	Ischium
Biceps femoris	Flexes lower leg	Fibula	Ischium and femur
Quadriceps group			
Rectus femoris	Extends lower leg	Tibia	Ilium
Vastus lateralis, intermedius, and medialis	Extend lower leg	Tibia	Femur
Tibialis anterior	Dorsiflexes foot	Metatarsals (foot)	Tibia
Gastrocnemius	Plantar flexes foot	Calcaneus (heel)	Femur
Soleus	Plantar flexes foot	Calcaneus (heel)	Tibia and fibula
Peroneus group			
Peroneus longus and brevis	Plantar flex foot	Tarsals and metatarsals (ankle and foot)	Tibia and fibula

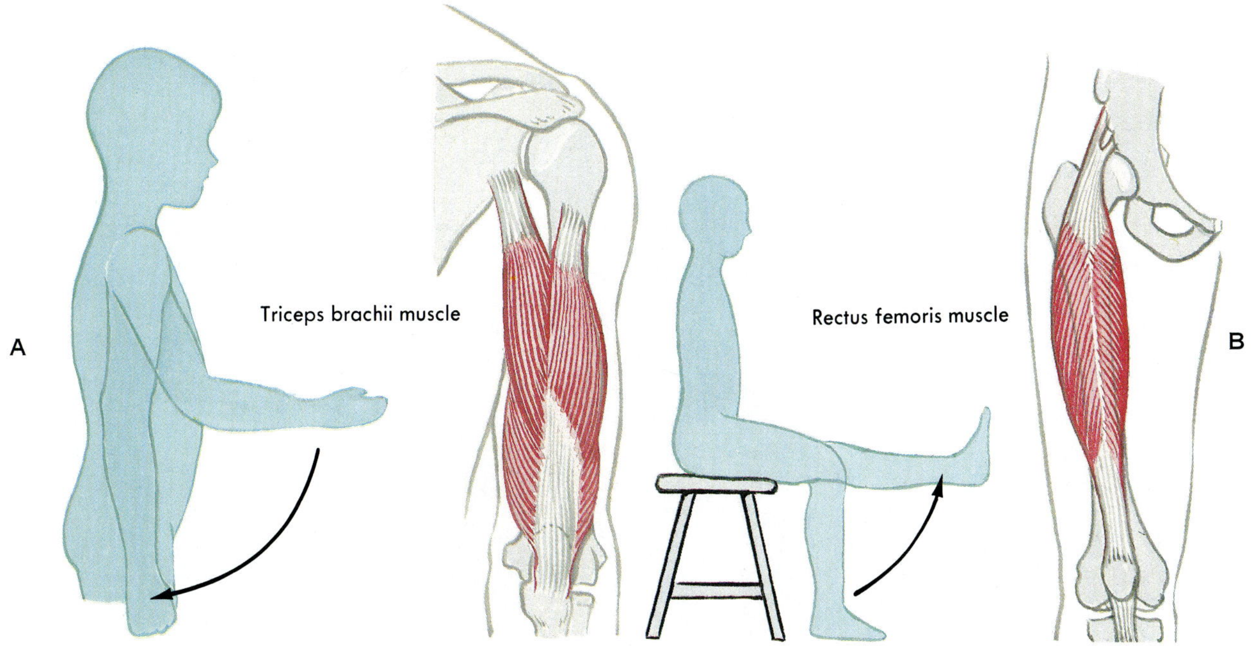

FIG. 26-12 Extension of the lower arm and lower leg. **A,** When the triceps brachii muscle (shown at the right) contracts, it extends the lower arm at the elbow joint (shown at the left). **B,** When the rectus femoris muscle (part of the quadriceps femoris muscle group) (shown at the right) contracts, it extends the lower leg at the knee joint (shown at the left).

TABLE 26-4 Muscles Grouped According to Function

Part Moved	Flexors	Extensors	Abductors	Adductors
Upper arm	Pectoralis major	Latissimus dorsi	Deltoid	Pectoralis major and latissimus dorsi contracting together
Lower arm	Biceps brachii	Triceps brachii	None	None
Thigh	Iliopsoas and sartorius	Gluteus maximus	Gluteus medius	Adductor group
Lower leg	Hamstrings	Quadriceps group	None	None
Foot	Tibialis anterior	Gastrocnemius and soleus	Peroneus longus	Tibialis anterior

Skeletal Muscle Groups. Skeletal muscles are usually classified into two broad categories: axial and appendicular. The axial muscle groups are those muscles located on the head, face, neck, and trunk. The appendicular muscle groups are all the muscles of the extremities. Figs. 26-13 and 26-14 on pp. 584-585 show the location of muscles of the trunk and extremities of the body. Fig. 26-15 on p. 586 shows the location of facial muscles. Table 26-3 groups muscles according to function and provides information about points of origin and insertion.

Muscles of the head. The muscles of the head include the facial muscles, which are responsible for facial expression, and the mastication (chewing) muscles, which prepare our food for swallowing.

Facial muscles.

Frontalis muscle: covers the frontal bone and inserts at the eyebrow. It gives movement to the forehead and permits the raising of the eyebrows.

Orbicularis oculi: encircles the eyes and permits winking, blinking, and closing of the eyes.

Orbicularis oris: encircles the lips and allows the closing of the mouth. It has been referred to as the *kissing* muscle.

Buccinator: forms the fleshy part of the cheeks. It compresses the cheek to hold food for chewing. It is referred to as the *trumpeter's muscle,* because it is the muscle that is used for whistling and blowing.

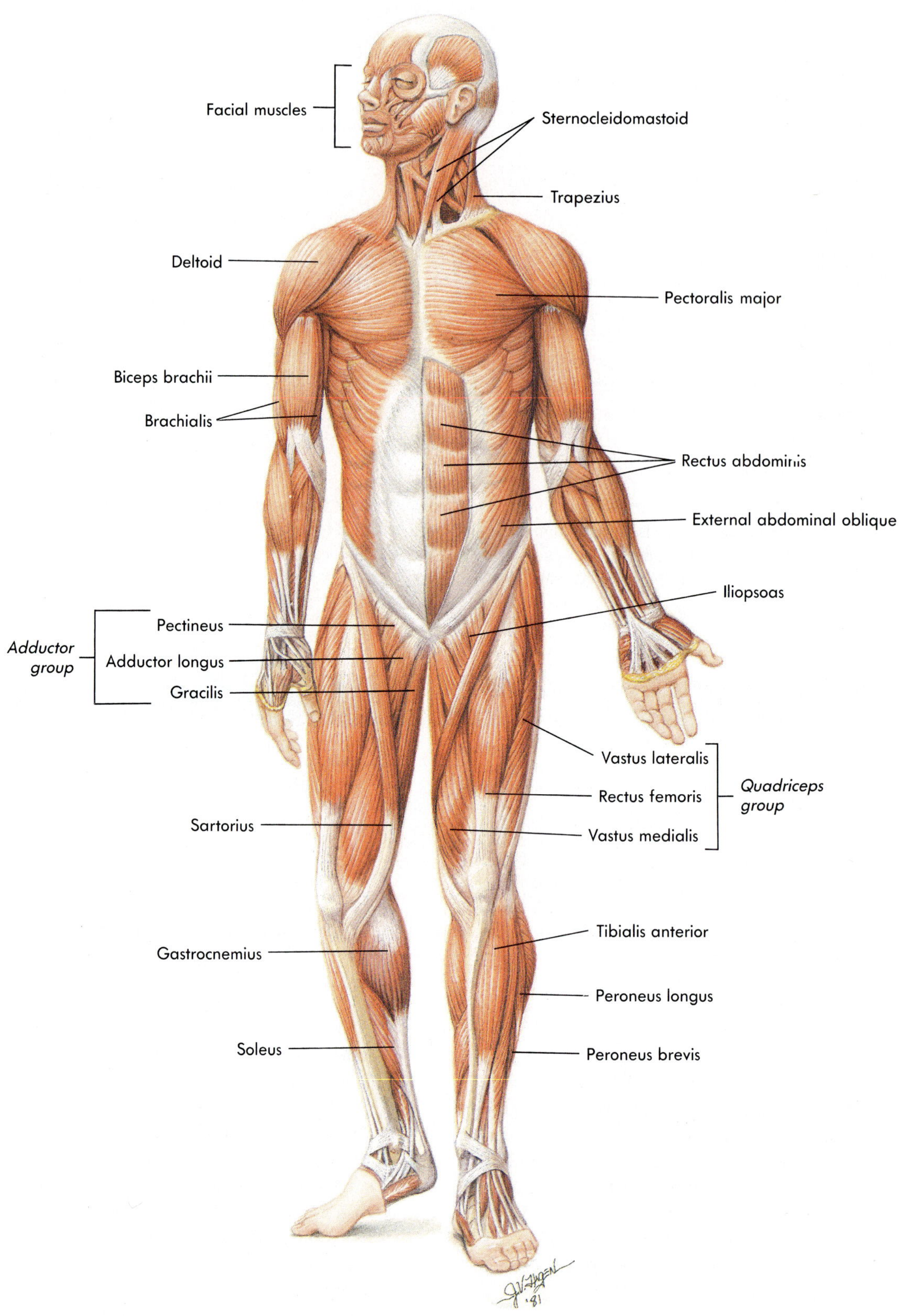

FIG. 26-13 Anterior view of the body.

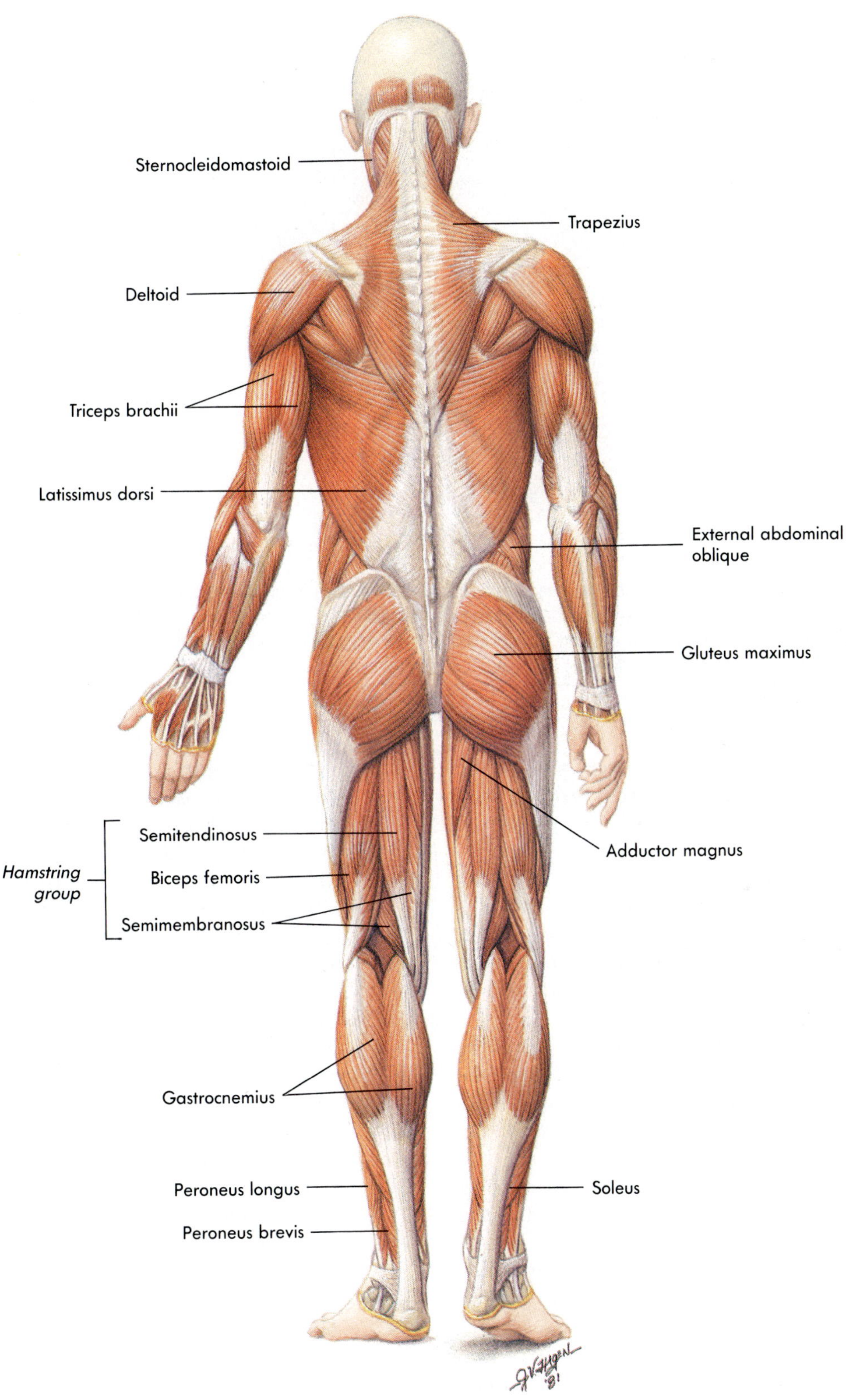

FIG. 26-14 Posterior view of the body.

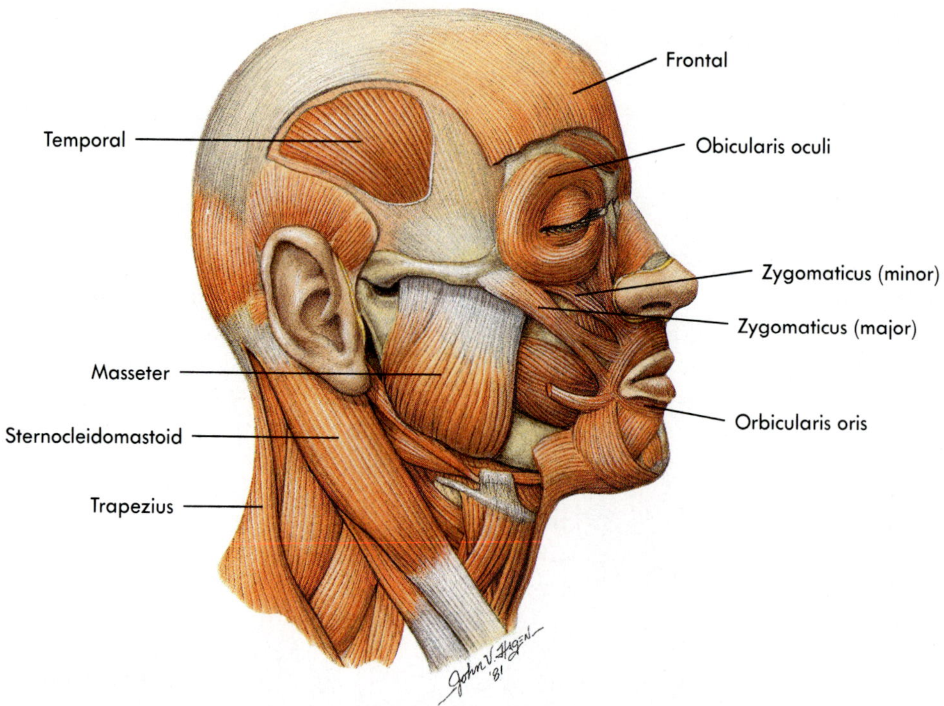

FIG. 26-15 Muscles of the head and neck. Muscles that produce most facial expressions surround the eyes, nose, and mouth. Large muscles of mastication stretch from the upper skull to the lower jaw. These powerful muscles produce chewing movements. The neck muscles connect the skull to the trunk of the body, rotating the head or bending the neck.

Zygomaticus: extends from the cheekbone to the corners of the mouth. It is referred to as the *smiling* muscle, because it draws the angle of the mouth upward.

Mastication muscles.

Masseter: extends across the angle of the jaw. It elevates the mandible during mastication.

Temporalis: extends from the temporal bone to the mandible. During mastication it elevates and retracts the mandible.

Muscles of the neck and trunk. The neck muscles are responsible for the support and movement of the neck and shoulder girdle. They are mostly strong, cordlike structures that extend inferiorly, superiorly, and obliquely.

The trunk muscles are responsible for the support and movement of the vertebral column, ribs, arms, and abdominal region.

The following is a brief discussion of the most important muscles, beginning with the anterior muscles and followed by the posterior muscles.

Anterior muscles.

Sternocleidomastoid: a pair of muscles that extend on either side of the neck from the mastoid to the sternum. As these muscles contract, the head is flexed (moved toward the chest). Contraction of one muscle rotates the head to the opposite side.

Pectoralis major: a large, fan-shaped muscle that covers the anterior chest from the sternum to the proximal end of the humerus. It acts on the shoulder joint to flex, adduct, and medially rotate it.

Diaphragm: a thin, dome-shaped muscle that separates the thoracic and abdominal cavities. The aorta, esophagus, and vena cava pass through it. It aids in respiration. During inspiration it drops down and increases the volume or space within the thoracic cavity. During expiration it moves upward and decreases the space.

Serratus anterior: a thin chest wall muscle that extends from the ribs under the arm to the scapula. The serratus anterior permits rotation of the scapula and the raising of the arm (full flexion and abduction of the arm).

Intercostal muscles: located between the individual ribs. The external intercostals raise the ribcage during inspiration, and the internal intercostals depress the ribcage during expiration. They function as secondary ventilatory muscles.

Transversus abdominis: the most interior layer of abdominal muscle. It lies horizontally across the abdomen from the iliac crests to the pubis. Constriction of this muscle compresses the abdominal contents, which assists with defecation, urination, and emesis and forces expiration.

Internal and external obliques: form the middle and outer layers of the abdominal wall. Their muscle fibers criss-cross to form a strong abdominal wall. Constriction of these muscles also compresses the abdomen with the same results as the transversus abdominis. Constriction of the one side allows the lateral movement of the vertebral column.

Rectus abdominis: a pair of superficial abdominal muscles that extend from the pubis to the sternum. They assist the transversus abdominis and the internal and external obliques with their functions.

Posterior muscles.

Trapezius: paired, fan-shaped muscles that cover the posterior neck and upper back. They are responsible for extension of the head and adduction and stabilization of the scapula. In addition, they abduct and flex the arm. The origin is the occipital bone and thoracic vertebrae; the insertion is the scapula.

Latissimus dorsi: large, flat, paired muscles that extend across the thoracic and lumbar regions of the back. They provide for extension and adduction of the humerus. They provide the power and strength for the upper arms. They are often referred to as the "swimmer's muscle." The origin sites are the spines of the thoracic vertebrae, the ilium, and the ribs; the insertion site is the humerus.

Upper extremity muscles.

Deltoid: a triangular, fleshy, muscular cap of the shoulder and upper arm. Intramuscular injections are sometimes given in this muscle (see Fig. 26-11). Contraction of this muscle abducts, flexes, extends, and rotates the arm. The origin is the clavicle and scapula; the insertion site is the humerus.

Biceps brachii: the long muscle of the upper arm on the anterior surface of the humerus. It flexes the arm and supinates the hand. In addition, it strengthens the shoulder joint. The origin is the scapula; the insertion site is the radius.

Triceps brachii: often called the *boxer's muscle* because it straightens the elbow when a blow is delivered (see Fig. 26-12, *A*). It is opposite the biceps brachii on the dorsal surface of the humerus. The origin is the scapula and humerus; the insertion is the ulna.

Lower extremity muscles.

Muscles located in the lower extremities are the longest and strongest in the body. They are responsible for locomotion and balance.

Gluteus maximus: forms the large fleshy portion of the buttocks. It is responsible for the extension and lateral rotation of the thigh. It is a common site for intramuscular injections. Its origin is the sacrum, coccyx, and ilium; the insertion is the femur.

Gluteus medius: lies interior to the gluteus maximus. It extends from the ilium (insertion) to the femur (origin). It is responsible for abduction of the hip and the rotation of the thigh medially.

Quadriceps femoris: a four-part muscle group that is located in the anterior area of the thigh. This group is responsible for the extension of the knee, particularly powerful extension, such as a kicking motion. The origin is the ilium and femur; the insertion is the tibia (see Fig. 26-12, *B*).

Hamstring group (posterior biceps and the biceps femoris): the posterior thigh muscles; their tendons can be palpated posterior to the knee bilaterally. They allow the leg to flex toward the thigh.

Adductor muscles: located on the inside, or medial, part of the thigh. They press the thighs together.

Adductor longus: the most superficial of the adductor muscles. It is a triangular muscle with its origin located at the pubis and the insertion site at the femur. It adducts and flexes the thigh.

Tibialis anterior: situated on the lateral side of the tibia. It is a thick, fleshy muscle. Its origin is the lateral side of the tibia with an insertion at the first metatarsal bone. It dorsiflexes and supinates the foot.

Iliopsoas: A short muscle that is located high on the thigh extending from the lumbar vertebrae and ilium to the head of the femur. It is a flexor muscle of the thigh.

Gastrocnemius: a large muscle located in the calf of the leg. It arises from the distal femur and its **Achilles** tendon (the common tendon of the soleus and gastrocnemius muscles; it is the thickest and strongest tendon in the body and attaches to the calcaneus. If it is severed, walking becomes very difficult because the heel cannot respond and this results in footdrop and begins near the middle of the posterior part of the leg). The gastrocnemius is often called the *toe dancer's muscle* because it is used to stand on tiptoe.

ASSESSMENT OF MUSCULOSKELETAL FUNCTION

The musculoskeletal system provides protection, support, and movement for the body. Orthopedics is the branch of medicine that deals with the prevention or correction of disorders involving locomotor structures of the body. Permanent disability and crippling will result if prompt treatment is not given to patients with musculoskeletal dysfunction. The ability to perform these functions is closely associated with the proper functioning of the nervous and circulatory systems.

Assessment of orthopedic function is necessary on all patients, but especially on those individuals who are (1) having difficulty with gait; (2) experiencing muscle weakness; (3) suffering from trauma of soft tissue and bone; (4) unable to produce movement that will enable activities for personal, economic, and social fulfillment; (5) experiencing diseases of the musculoskeletal system; or (6) chronically ill.

Assessment of posture and gait is made easily by observing the patient walking. Common posture deformities include lateral (or S) curvature of the spine known as **scoliosis;** a rounding of the thoracic spine (humpbacked appearance) known as **kyphosis;** and an increase in the curve at the lumbar space region that throws the shoulders back, making the "lordly or kingly" appearance that is known as **lordosis** (Fig. 26-16). Rigidity of the spine can result from ankylosing spondylitis, whereby the vertebrae are fused with loss of mobility, producing a rigid gait or "poker spine" appearance.

Assessment of neurological and circulatory function is important if the patient has experienced a traumatic injury; damaged blood vessels and nerves can cause permanent disabilities.

Assessing the skin for signs of coolness, pallor, or cyanosis can help the nurse determine the patient's circulatory status. A faint or absent pulse in an extremity indicates impaired circulation. Palpating the femoral, popliteal, and dorsalis pedis pulses on both extremities provides data pertinent to the lower extremities. If the pulse is not readily palpated with a light touch of the finger, a Doppler instrument can be used, which will enable the listener to hear a magnified sound of the pulsation. The absence of a pulse is serious and must be reported to the charge nurse immediately. The brachial and radial pulses are assessed to determine circulation in the upper extremities. It may be difficult to palpate a pulse when a cast or bandage makes the extremity inaccessible. It is important to reach under the cast or bandage if possible. An assessment of the pulse in the unaffected extremity is made for a comparison.

Blanching test (meaning to whiten or pale) is a test of the rate of capillary refill, which signals circulation status. This is also referred to as a *capillary nail refill test.* The nurse compresses each fingernail or toenail of the affected extremity (noting the white color as pressure is applied), releases the pressure, and notes how quickly

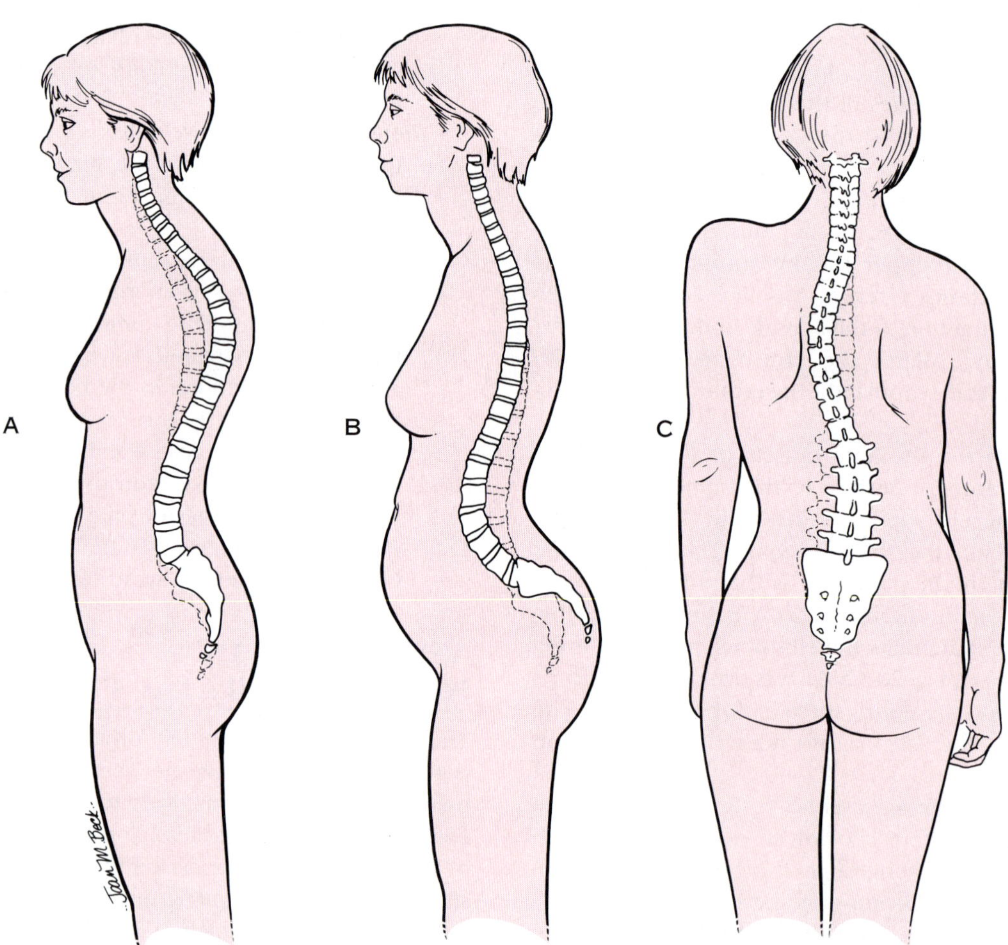

FIG. 26-16 Abnormal spinal curvatures. **A,** Kyphosis. **B,** Lordosis. **C,** Scoliosis.

the pink color returns to the nail bed. The nail bed color should return to normal within 2 seconds. If the color is slow to return, this indicates impaired circulation, and prompt attention is needed to improve circulation.

Neurovascular assessments are made on patients with musculoskeletal trauma, damage to nerves and blood vessels resulting from surgery, or tightness of bandages, splints, or casts. Impaired circulation or nerve function can cause loss of the use of an extremity; this impairment is seen more often in the extremities. Neurovascular assessment is always included as a nursing measure when caring for a patient with a cast. Immediately after a traumatic injury, postoperatively, or after casting, a neurovascular assessment is made every 15 to 30 minutes for several hours and every 3 to 4 hours thereafter, with proper documentation of the findings. Verbal complaints of numbness or tingling may result from general decreased mobility and may be relieved by flexing the fingers and toes and repositioning the extremity. However, if the numbness and tingling are not relieved by these measures and the extremity feels cool to touch, is slow in capillary refill, has diminished or absent pulses, and appears pale or cyanotic, these are significant symptoms of neurovascular impairment and the findings must be reported immediately.

Remember the 5 P's when completing assessment:

- Pulselessness
- Paresthesia (numbness or tingling sensation)
- Pallor
- Puffiness (edema)
- Pain

Effects of Bed Rest on Mineral Content in Bone. Studies done on persons confined to bed rest reveal a loss of body calcium. Men and women patients aged 18 to 80 years who were confined to bed rest for an average of 27 days because of musculoskeletal disorders of lumbar disk protrusion averaged 0.9% loss in mineral content per week from the lumbar vertebrae. This rate of loss over several weeks is a serious concern for an older individual in terms of regaining mobility; it also increases the risk of fracture. Studies done on astronauts have shown that they experienced rates of bone loss similar to bed rest rates in a weightless environment.

Diagnostic Tests

Radiographic Studies. The diagnostic study most often used for determining musculoskeletal system integrity is the radiographic, roentgenographic, or as it is more commonly known, x-ray examination or diagnostic imaging.

An x-ray examination of a joint reveals the presence of fluid, irregularity of the joint with spur formation, and changes in the size of the joint contour. It is important before x-ray examinations to ask women of child-bearing age if there is any possibility that they are pregnant, since pregnant women should not be exposed to x-ray unless in an emergency situation because of potential damage to the fetus.

Laminography or *planography* is also called *body section roentgenography.* This x-ray procedure is useful in locating small cavities, foreign bodies, and lesions that are overshadowed by opaque structures.

Scanography (a method of producing a radiograph of internal body organs by using a series of parallel beams that eliminate size distortion) is an x-ray procedure that allows accurate measurement of the bone's length.

Myelogram. Myelogram examination involves injection of a radiopaque dye into the subarachnoid space at the lumbar spine to determine the presence of herniated disk syndrome (herniated nucleus pulposus) or tumors. The test involves the same procedure as a lumbar puncture (spinal tap), as is discussed in Chapter 35. Radiographic dye will cause allergic reactions in patients with allergies to iodine and seafood or who have hay fever, asthma, or eczema. It is important that the physician be notified about such allergies so that a nonionic contrast agent can be used or medications such as steroids and/or antihistamines be given before the examination to minimize any reaction to the radiographic dye. This examination may involve the entire spine or just the cervical or lumbar area. After the myelogram, oil-based dye is removed through the spinal needle to prevent meningeal irritation. Water-soluble dye is used most often and does not need to be removed; it will be absorbed by the body and excreted in the urine.

The most common discomfort after a myelogram is headache. If water-soluble dye is used, the patient should lie quietly in a semi-Fowler's position for about 8 hours. The positioning of the patient is important to keep the dye in the lower spine. During this time, encouraging fluids will help the body absorb the dye from the spinal column. If oil-based dye is used, the patient will need to rest in a flat position for as long as 12 hours. It is important to instruct the patient to inform the nurse if there is headache, stiff neck, leg weakness, or difficulty voiding. Rare complications include seizure, infection, drowsiness, severe headache, numbness, and paralysis.

Patients needing a myelogram fear the needle will be inserted into the spinal canal and damage the cord. It is important that the nurse inform the patient that the tap is done in the lumbar region of the spine at about the fourth or fifth lumbar (L4/L5) space. The spinal cord starts at the level of the foramen magnum and ends at the second lumbar (L2) space (lower border of ribcage).

Nuclear scanning. Tests in which nuclear scanning is used are done in the nuclear medicine department, which has scanners or camera detectors that record the images on x-ray film. The dosages of radioactive isotopes are low for diagnostic tests; precautionary measures that are required for radium therapy are not necessary.

Nursing measures required when patients are scheduled for nuclear scanning procedures involve (1) obtaining written consent from the patient, (2) informing the patient that the radioactive isotopes will not affect family or visitors, and (3) following instructions as outlined by the nuclear medicine department as to special preparations for specific scans.

Magnetic resonance imaging. Magnetic resonance imaging (MRI) is used to detect pathological conditions of the cerebrum and spinal cord. It is currently used to detect herniated nucleus pulposus. The test involves the use of magnetism and radio waves to make images of cross sections of the body. MRI can give much more detailed pictures of fluid-filled soft tissue and blood vessels than any other test.

Patient preparation involves having the patient remove any metal, such as jewelry, clothing with metal fasteners, glasses, and hair clips. Patients with metal prostheses, such as heart valves, orthopedic screws, or cardiac pacemakers, cannot undergo MRI.

The machine looks like a narrow tunnel, and patients are required to lie still in this machine for 45 to 60 minutes. The patient enters the tunnel head first. This may cause anxiety and a feeling of claustrophobia. The procedure is painless; however, if the patient is extremely anxious, a sedative is given. Patients should be encouraged to use relaxation techniques, such as imagery, during the test. Because the procedure requires the patient to be motionless, relaxation techniques that require flexing and relaxing of the muscles are not appropriate.

After the test, routine vital sign measurements are taken and pretest activities can be resumed. There are no adverse effects.

Computed axial tomography (CT or CAT scan). Body sections can be examined from many different angles using a CT scanner that produces a narrow x-ray beam. Consequently, a three-dimensional picture of the structure being studied is made. The CT scanner is approximately 100 times more sensitive than the x-ray machine and should not be used unnecessarily, because of radiation exposure. Iodine contrast dye is sometimes used. CT scan is used for the head and body. It is useful in locating injuries to the ligaments or tendons and tumors of the soft tissue, and in identifying fractures in areas difficult to define by other means. Patient preparation includes (1) having the patient sign a consent form authorizing the examination if not included on the initial hospital consent form, (2) questioning the patient regarding allergies (iodine and seafood), (3) keeping the patient on NPO (nothing by mouth) status 3 to 4 hours before the test (necessary in case contrast dye is used, because the dye can cause nausea and vomiting), (4) measuring vital signs to be used as a baseline, (5) having the patient void before the test, (6) removing such articles as jewelry and hairpins, and (7) instructing the patient that he must lie still during the test and may feel warm and slightly nauseated for a few minutes when dye is injected.

Sometimes an enema to clear the colon of gas and feces is required before body scans.

After the test, the patient is observed for delayed allergic reactions (if contrast dye was used). Fluids are encouraged unless contraindicated. Pretest diet and activity can usually be resumed.

Bone scan. The bone scan test is especially valuable in detecting metastatic and inflammatory bone disease (osteomyelitis). This test involves the intravenous administration of nuclides (atomic material) approximately 2 to 3 hours before the test is scheduled. There are no food or fluid restrictions, and patients are encouraged to drink water over the next 1 to 3 hours to aid renal clearance of any radioisotope not picked up by the bone. After the patient has voided, a scanning camera reveals the degree of radionuclide uptake; areas of concentrated nucleotide uptake may represent a tumor or other abnormality. These areas of concentration can be detected days or weeks before an ordinary x-ray can reveal a metastatic lesion. The test takes approximately 30 to 60 minutes and requires the patient to lie still.

Endoscopic Examination. For an endoscopy, a lighted tube is used to visualize inside a body cavity. Although some procedures require general anesthesia, most require only local anesthesia. Emotional support and complete explanations help relieve the patient's anxiety. Preparation for an endoscopic examination is similar to surgical preparation: (1) a consent form is signed; (2) a preoperative checklist is completed with special attention to removing jewelry, dentures, and contact lenses; (3) NPO status is initiated for 6 to 12 hours before the examination; (4) premedications are given, such as atropine and a sedative; (5) the patient is encouraged to void; (6) vital signs are taken and recorded; and (7) bed rest with side rails up is maintained after the premedication is given.

Arthroscopy. Arthroscopy is an endoscopic examination that enables direct visualizing of a joint. The procedure is used to accomplish the following: (1) exploration of the joint to determine the presence of a disease process, (2) drainage of fluid from the joint cavity, and (3) removal of damaged tissue or foreign bodies from the joint.

This examination is most commonly done on the knee joint, with the synovium, articular surfaces, and meniscus (a curved, fibrous cartilage in the knee) visualized through the scope. The procedure involves insertion of a large-bore needle into the suprapatellar pouch and saline instillation into the joint. The patient may be given a general or local anesthetic agent. After the arthroscopic examination, the patient may be advised to limit activities for several days.

Aspiration. An aspiration procedure is done to obtain a specimen of body fluid. A needle is inserted into a cav-

TABLE 26-5 Laboratory Tests for Musculoskeletal Disorders

Normal Value	Possible Cause For Increase/Decrease
Calcium	
9.0-10.5 mg/dl	Increased in metastatic tumor to the bone, Addison's disease, Paget's disease of the bone, acromegaly, acute osteoporosis, hyperparathyroidism, and vitamin D intoxication Decreased in acute pancreatitis, hypoparathyroidism, vitamin D deficiency, renal failure, malabsorption, and rickets
Erythrocyte sedimentation rate (ESR)	
Males: up to 15 mm/hr Females: up to 20 mm/hr	Indicates the presence of inflammation as seen in rheumatoid arthritis and rheumatic fever One of the most objective measurements of rheumatoid arthritis severity. ESR increases as the disease worsens The ESR is a nonspecific test used to detect inflammatory, neoplastic, infectious, and necrotic processes. Increased levels are seen in multiple myeloma, acute myocardial infarctions, toxemia, and bacterial infections. Decreased levels are seen in CHF, sickle cell anemia, polycythemia vera, infectious mononucleosis, degenerative arthritis, and angina pectoris
Lupus erythematosus (LE) preparation	
No LE cells seen	Lupus erythematosus, rheumatoid arthritis, scleroderma, and drug sensitivities
Rheumatoid factor (RF)	
<60 U/ml	An immunoglobulin found in approximately 80% of adults with rheumatoid arthritis; other diseases such as systemic lupus erythematosus (SLE), may cause a positive RF
Uric acid (blood)	
Males: 2.1-8.5 mg/dl Females: 2.0-6.6 mg/dl	Increased in patients with gout, kidney failure, alcoholism, leukemias, metastatic cancer, multiple myeloma, or dehydration

ity after a local anesthetic agent is administered to the site. This procedure is performed using sterile technique. It is fairly common for the physician to take a biopsy of tissue at the same time the aspiration procedure is done. Nursing interventions are similar for all aspiration tests, with special emphasis on (1) having the consent form signed; (2) reinforcing the physician's explanation of the procedure; (3) encouraging the patient to remain immobile during the procedure; (4) having the patient void before the procedure; (5) maintaining sterile technique; (6) supporting the patient emotionally; (7) applying a sterile pressure dressing to the puncture site and maintaining the dressing until bleeding has stopped; (8) assisting with collecting, labeling, and transporting a specimen to the laboratory immediately; and (9) observing for emotional and physical distress after the procedure.

Synovial fluid aspiration. **Arthrocentesis** (the puncture of a patient's joint with a needle and the withdrawal of fluid, which is performed to obtain samples of synovial fluid for diagnostic purposes) is helpful in diagnosing trauma, systemic lupus erythematosus, gout, osteoarthritis, and rheumatoid arthritis. Normally a patient's synovial fluid is straw colored, clear, or slightly cloudy. If trauma or a disease process is present, the synovial fluid will appear cloudy, milky, sanguineous, yellow, green, or gray.

After the procedure, proper support should be given to the affected extremity. Placing the extremity on a pillow and maintaining joint rest for approximately 12 hours may be indicated. It may be necessary to apply ice to the affected joint for 24 to 48 hours unless otherwise ordered. The nurse will assess the patient for signs of infection. After the removal of the pressure dressing from the site, a Band-Aid can be used.

Electrographic Procedure. For electrographic procedures, electrodes are used to measure electrical activity in specific areas of the body.

Electromyogram (EMG). An electromyogram is a procedure that involves the insertion of needle electrodes into the skeletal muscles so that electrical activity can be heard, seen on an oscilloscope (an instrument that displays a graphic representation of electron beams on a screen), and recorded on paper at the same time. Muscles do not produce an electrical charge at rest, but with neuromuscular disorders, unusual patterns can be observed. Nerves can be observed for neuropathy and muscles for myopathy with this procedure.

Laboratory Tests

Specific laboratory tests are ordered when musculoskeletal disorders are suspended (Table 26-5).

INFLAMMATORY DISORDERS

Arthritis

Arthritis is a type of disease in which there is an inflammation of the joint. There are an estimated 50 million Americans affected by arthritis, and 4 million of these are dependent and unable to work, attend school, or participate in social functions. There are many types of arthritis, but the most common are rheumatoid arthritis, rheumatoid spondylitis, osteoarthritis (degenerative joint disease), and gout (gouty arthritis).

Rheumatoid arthritis.

Etiology/pathophysiology. Rheumatoid arthritis (RA) is the most serious form of the disease and leads to severe crippling. It is a chronic, systemic disease that affects 3% of the general population. RA can strike anyone; however, certain factors make some people more prone than others. RA usually develops between the ages of 30 and 55 years, and women seem more prone than men. There is some evidence that RA has a familial tendency.

RA can affect many organ systems (lungs, heart, blood vessels, muscles, eyes, and skin). RA is characterized by a chronic inflammation of the synovial membrane (synovitis) of the diarthrodial joints (also called synovial joints: freely movable joints in which continuous bony surfaces are covered by cartilage and connected by ligaments lined with synovial membrane).

Clinical manifestations. RA is believed to involve an immune reaction that will not shut off because of some failure in the immune system; agents that should protect the body attack joint tissues instead and cause a chronic inflammatory reaction in the synovial membrane. This in turn results in damage to the affected joint and surrounding tissue, possibly leading to gross deformity and loss of function.

RA is characterized by periods of remission and exacerbation. During remission, the symptoms actively cease. The inflammation, pain, stiffness, and edema subside, and progression of tissue damage is halted. (The patient may experience residual joint dysfunction even with remission.)

Assessment. Collection of *subjective data* includes noting the patient's complaints of malaise, muscle weakness (especially grip strength), loss of appetite, and generalized aching.

Collection of *objective data* includes observing the joints for edema, tenderness, subcutaneous nodules, limitation in range of motion (morning stiffness especially), symmetrical joint involvement, and fever.

Diagnostic tests. There is no single definite test for RA. Diagnosis is based on the patient history and findings during a physical examination. The four classic symptoms most frequently reported are morning stiffness, joint pain, muscle weakness, and fatigue. X-ray studies reveal loss of articular cartilage and change in subchondral bone. Laboratory tests are often used in confirming a diagnosis and in ruling out the presence of other diseases. They are as follows:

- *Erythrocyte sedimentation rate:* an increase indicates presence of inflammatory reaction somewhere in body
- *Rheumatoid factor (RF):* an elevation of this titer indicates abnormal serum protein concentration is present
- *Latex agglutination test:* detects presence of IgM version of rheumatoid factor, the anti-IgG antibodies
- *Red cell count:* detects anemia, often present during chronic infection
- *Synovial fluid aspiration:* normal fluid usually clear and highly viscous; however, when inflammation present, fluid is cloudy, yellow, less viscous, and contains increased protein
- *Synovial fluid biopsy:* shows changes in tissue

Medical management. The physician will order a medical regimen based on the patient's age, occupation, life-style, and joints affected. The goal of treatments is directed toward relieving pain and inflammation (see the medications table), preventing joint damage and deformities (physical therapy, traction, and splints are often used), and promoting activities of daily living by restoring or maintaining function of the affected part.

Nursing interventions. Nursing intervention is aimed at patient education to help the patient and family understand what is happening and what to expect as the disease progresses. Rest is important, since fatigue is a major problem. Sleeping 8 to 10 hours a night and taking a 2-hour nap during the day are recommended. Exercise helps prevent the joints from "freezing" and the muscles from weakening. A typical exercise program calls for two or three 10- to 15-minute daily sessions of "quiet" exercise that puts joints gently through range of motion (ROM). Heat is often used to relax and soothe muscles. Hot packs, heat lamps, and applications of hot paraffin wax are helpful. Rehabilitation is aimed at helping the patient learn ways of adapting to physical limitations and promote normal daily activities.

Nursing diagnoses and interventions for the patient with rheumatoid arthritis include but are not limited to the following:

NURSING DIAGNOSES	NURSING INTERVENTIONS
Pain, related to joint inflammation	Maintain bed rest as ordered; maintain proper body alignment Assist and teach patient to extend joints as possible and to avoid external rotation of extremities; use sand bags or trochanter rolls. Avoid use of pillows under knees. Immobilize and/or support joints.

MEDICATIONS FOR RHEUMATOID ARTHRITIS

Medication	Action	Side Effects/Toxic Effects	Nursing Implications
Salicylates			
Example: acetylsalicylic acid	Analgesic, antipyretic, antiinflammatory	Gastric irritation; dose-related salicylism; skin rash; hypersensitivity	Give with food, milk, or antacid; space q 4-6 hr to maintain antiinflammatory effect.
Nonsteroidal antiinflammatory agents (NSAIAs)			
Indomethacin (Indocin)	Analgesic, antiinflammatory	Headache; vertigo; insomnia; confusion; GI irritation	Give with food, milk, or antacid; discontinue if CNS symptoms develop and notify physician.
Ibuprofen (Motrin)	Analgesic, antiinflammatory	Same as indomethacin but believed less irritating to GI tract; fluid retention	Know that delayed absorption occurs if taken with food.
Tolmetin sodium (Tolectin)	Analgesic, antiinflammatory	Same as ibuprofen	Give with food or milk.
Naproxen (Naprosyn)	Analgesic, antiinflammatory	Same as ibuprofen; also drowsiness	Give with food, milk, or antacid; tell patient to avoid driving until dosage effect is established.
Diflunisal (Dolobid)	Analgesic, antiinflammatory	Gastric irritation; headache; vertigo; skin rash; tinnitus; fluid retention	Give with food or milk; do not use with salicylates or other antiinflammatory medications.
Piroxicam (Feldene)	Analgesic, antiinflammatory	Gastric irritation; anemia; skin rash; fluid retention; vertigo; headache	Give with food or antacid.
Potent antiinflammatory agents			
Adrenocorticosteroids (example: prednisone)	Interfere with body's normal inflammatory response	Fluid retention, sodium retention, potassium depletion; hypertension; decreased healing potential; increased susceptibility to infection; GI irritation; hirsutism; osteoporosis; fat deposits; diabetes mellitus; myopathy; adrenal insufficiency or adrenal crisis if abruptly withdrawn	Give with food, milk, or antacid; do not increase or decrease dosage without physician supervision; give in morning if given on once-a-day basis.
Phenylbutazone (Butazolidin)	Antiinflammatory; analgesic at subcortical site in brain	GI irritation; hematological toxicity; hypertension; impaired renal function	Use for short term (7-10 days); give with food or milk.
Slow-acting antiinflammatory agents			
Antimalarials			
Hydroxychloroquine (Plaquenil)	Antiinflammatory (mechanism unknown); effect not expected to be noted for 6-12 months after beginning therapy	GI disturbances; retinal edema that may result in blindness	Instruct patient to obtain eye examination before beginning therapy and every 6 months thereafter.
Gold salts—IM			
Gold sodium thiomalate (Myochrysine)	Antiinflammatory; effect not noted for 3-6 months after beginning therapy	Renal and hepatic damage; corneal deposits; dermatitis; ulcerations in mouth; hematological changes	Monitor urinalysis and CBC before each injection; report dermatitis, metallic taste in mouth, or lesions in mouth to physician.

NURSING DIAGNOSES	NURSING INTERVENTIONS
Pain, related to joint inflammation—cont'd	Administer treatments as ordered: hot packs, tub baths, ice packs, paraffin, or whirlpool. Administer acetylsalicylic acid as ordered.
Mobility, impaired physical, related to joint inflammation, edema, and pain	Assist with and teach active and/or perform passive ROM exercises after heat treatments, or apply passive ROM machine as ordered. Maintain planned rest periods. Maintain a safe environment: ■ Handrails in shower, tub, and toilet. ■ Raised toilet seat and chairs. ■ Rubber-tipped walker or cane. ■ Wheelchair in locked position when stationary.
Self-care deficits, bathing/hygiene, dressing/grooming, and feeding, related to joint inflammation, edema, and pain	Teach self-care activities. Establish and teach routine plan for ADLs. Assist with feeding prn; have patient use large-grip handles for utensils as needed. Set goals with patient; encourage short-term, easily accomplished goals. Discuss use of slip-on shoes and snaps or Velcro on clothing.

Patient teaching. As with any chronic illness, patient teaching is perhaps the most important aspect of nursing care of patients with rheumatoid arthritis. Patient teaching includes information about the following:

- Joint protection and energy conservation techniques
- Proper balance of rest and activity
- Proper use of medications, that is, names of drugs, dosages, precautions in administration, and side effects or toxic effects
- Plans for implementation of the exercise program prescribed by the physician or physical therapist
- Proper application of heat and/or cold packs
- Proper use of walking aids
- Safety measures to prevent injury
- Basics of good nutrition and importance of avoiding weight gain
- Danger of following programs that promise a "cure"

Prognosis. The course of the disease is variable but is most frequently marked by remissions and exacerbations. The prognosis is based on a variety of clinical and laboratory findings. Stage I represents early effects. Stage IV, the terminal category, includes marked joint deformity, extensive muscle atrophy, soft tissue lesions, bone and cartilage destruction, as well as fibrous or bony ankylosis.

Ankylosing Spondylitis.

Etiology/pathophysiology. Ankylosing spondylitis (AKS) is a chronic, progressive disorder of the sacroiliac and hip joints, the synovial joints of the spine, and the adjacent soft tissues. It can affect both sexes but is seen more often in young men. There is a strong hereditary tendency. Women develop a milder form of AKS, and fusion of the spine is rarely seen. It is sometimes referred to as *rheumatoid spondylitis.*

Clinical manifestations. AKS involves inflammation of the spine, and as a result, the bones of the spine grow together **(ankylosis,** fixation of a joint, often in abnormal position, usually resulting from destruction of articular cartilage and subchrondral bone).

AKS involves inflammation where the ligament or tendon attaches to the bone and does not affect the synovial membrane, as seen in rheumatoid arthritis. AKS can affect joints, such as the neck, jaw, shoulders, knees, and hips. The disease process causes the ligaments to become ossified (hardened). The cardiovascular system can be involved, and heart enlargement and pericarditis can occur. If the costovertebral joints are affected, kyphosis can occur and alter respirations. The patient may have difficulty in expanding the ribcage while breathing. Many patients with the disease also have inflammatory bowel disease. Vision loss occurs with chronic AKS, and blindness may result from the glaucoma and pupil damage.

Assessment. Collection of *subjective data* includes patient complaints of low backache, stiffness, and alternating or bilateral "sciatica pain" that lasts for a few days at a time and then subsides. Pain is more pronounced when an erect position is maintained. Inactivity causes the pain to exacerbate, and exercise gives relief. Complaints of weight loss, abdominal distention, visual problems, and fatigue are common.

Collection of *objective data* includes assessment for tenderness over the spine and sacroiliac region. Peripheral joint edema and decreased ROM may be seen. Assessment of the vital signs may indicate elevated temperature, tachycardia, and hyperpnea. Respiratory difficulties will arise if there is limited expansion of the chest, as is often seen in kyphosis.

Diagnostic tests. Patients with AKS will often have the following laboratory test results:

- Low hemoglobin and hematocrit, indicative of anemia
- Elevated ESR, common in chronic inflammatory disease
- Elevated serum alkaline phosphatase levels, seen in patients who are immobilized or have bone resorption

X-ray examination often reveals sacroiliac joint and intervertebral disk inflammation with bony erosion and joint space fusion.

Medical management. The physician usually prescribes oral analgesics and nonsteroidal antiinflammatory drugs (NSAIDs). Exercise programs (swimming and walking) are important to prevent demineralization of bone.

Surgery may be necessary to replace fused joints (hip or knee is most common). Cervical or lumbar osteotomy can be done for severe kyphosis.

Nursing interventions. Nursing intervention is aimed at maintaining alignment of the spine. Providing a firm mattress, bed board, and back brace helps provide support. Postural and breathing exercises help compensate for the possibility of impaired gas exchange caused by the changes in posture and chest cavity size. Encouraging the patient to lie on the abdomen at least 15 to 30 minutes qid helps to extend the spine. Turning and positioning q 2 hours helps to prevent decubitus ulcers.

A nursing diagnosis and interventions for the patient with ankylosing spondylitis include but are not limited to the following:

NURSING DIAGNOSIS	NURSING INTERVENTIONS
Self-esteem disturbance, related to body image change	Encourage verbalization about fears and anxiety of disease process. Deal with behavior changes: denial, powerlessness, anxiety, and dependence. Be supportive and kind but firm in setting goals. Encourage independence, and provide for tasks accomplished. Be aware of limitations, and encourage discussion of feelings and concerns.

Patient teaching. The patient should be taught the appropriate use of prescribed medications, prescribed postural exercises, and methods of applying heat to back and hips. Correct posture and prevention of complications should be promoted by the following:

- Encouraging the use of a firm mattress
- Encouraging the patient to sleep without a pillow under the head
- Encouraging respiratory exercises

Prognosis. Ankylosing spondylitis is a chronic disease occurring under the age of 30 and generally burns itself out after a course of 20 years, leaving permanent, irreversible systemic involvement.

Degenerative Joint Disease (Osteoarthritis).

Etiology/pathophysiology. Degenerative joint disease (DJD) is also known as osteoarthritis, hypertrophic arthritis, osteoarthrosis, or senescent arthritis. Almost everyone past 40 years of age has hypertrophic changes in the joints. The disease is an almost inevitable consequence of aging and is a major cause of severe chronic disability. There are two forms of osteoarthritis: primary (cause is unknown) and secondary (caused by trauma, infections, previous fractures, rheumatoid arthritis, stress on weight-bearing joints from obesity, or such occupations as coal mining or boxing).

Osteoarthritis is a nonsystemic, noninflammatory disorder that progressively causes bones and joints to degenerate.

Clinical manifestations. This disorder affects the joints of the hand, knee, hip, and cervical and lumbar vertebrae. Osteoarthritis appears to be related to aging, but researchers are unclear as to the cause. Nearly all persons older than 60 years will show osteoarthritic changes, with women being affected more often than men. The disease affects the hands in women more often, whereas in men the hips are affected.

Assessment. Collection of *subjective data* involves questioning the patient about complaints of pain and stiffness (rest usually relieves the pain in the early stages). Past illnesses, surgical procedures, or trauma may be relative, and information about excessive weight gain and occupation may be significant. Complaints of muscle spasms and reduced grip strength are common.

Collection of *objective data* includes assessment for joint edema, tenderness, instability, and deformity. *Heberden's nodes* appear on the sides of the distal joints of fingers, and *Bouchard's nodes* appear on the proximal joints of fingers—these are hard, bony, and cartilaginous enlargements. The patient's gait will reveal a limp, especially if the hips or legs are affected.

Diagnostic tests. There is no specific test to diagnose osteoarthritis. However, x-ray studies, arthroscopy, synovial fluid examination, and bone scans are used to provide information.

Medical management. The physician will order an exercise plan that is balanced with rest periods. Physical therapy using heat application helps reduce stiffness, pain, and muscle spasms. Gait enhancers, such as canes, walkers, and shoe inserts, help relieve discomfort while weight-bearing joints are used. Drug therapy involves using large dosages (10 to 15 g three to four times daily after meals) of salicylates (aspirin) or nonsteroidal anti-inflammatory drugs (such as Motrin 400 mg, four times a day). Steroids (cortisone) are sometimes used in low dosages or injected into joints to produce immediate pain relief and temporarily halt the destructive process.

Surgical intervention, such as osteotomy, may help correct malalignment. Joint replacement may be necessary to replace all or part of the joint's articulating surface. Arthroplasty of the hip and knee is the most common surgical intervention.

Nursing interventions. Nursing intervention involves encouraging the patient to maintain activities of daily living (ADLs) and adapt to limitations of the disease. Encouraging the patient to alternate sitting, walking, and standing with periods of rest can help reduce joint discomfort and deterioration. Older patients may be physically capable of turning and moving in bed but may forget to do so because of alteration in their level of orientation. Assisting the patient with a weight-reduction plan may be necessary if obesity is a problem. If splints are needed to support a painful joint, the nurse needs to assess for neurovascular impairment above and below the site of application. Gait enhancers should be checked for safety considerations, such as rubber tips on ends, proper size, and patient knowledge about use. If the patient has been taking aspirin over a period of time, GI bleeding may occur. It may be necessary for the nurse to perform a guaiac test on stool and emesis to determine the presence of occult blood.

Patient teaching. As with rheumatoid arthritis, teaching the person with osteoarthritis about the disease process and the steps to control that process is the most important aspect of nursing interventions. Patient teaching should include the same information as for rheumatoid arthritis, p. 594.

Prognosis. Degenerative joint disease (osteoarthritis) is a chronic disease that ultimately causes permanent destruction of affected cartilage and underlying bone with variable pain and disability.

Gout (Gouty Arthritis).

Etiology/pathophysiology. Gout is a metabolic disease resulting from an accumulation of uric acid in the blood. It is an acute inflammatory condition associated with ineffective metabolism of purines. Gout can be primary (linked with hereditary factors), secondary (resulting from use of certain drugs or complication of another disease), or idiopathic (unknown origin). It affects men 8 to 9 times more frequently than women and usually occurs in middle life. It does not occur before puberty in the male or before menopause in the female. It takes about 20 years for sufficient urates to accumulate in the body before causing signs and symptoms when the disease is primary. Of all persons with gout, 85% have a genetic tendency to develop the disease. **Tophi** (calculi containing sodium urate deposits that develop in periarticular fibrous tissue, typically in patients with gout) result in inflammation of the joint; it is unclear why this occurs. Typically the big toes are involved, but other joints can also be affected.

Clinical manifestations. The onset occurs at night, with excruciating pain, edema, and inflammation in the affected joint. The pain may be of short duration, returning at intervals, or it may be severe and continuous for 5 to 10 days. The patient may have repeated attacks or only one attack in a lifetime. Tophi are seen around the rim of the ear and can disfigure the ear. Surgical removal may be necessary.

Assessment. Collection of *subjective data* involves noting a complaint of pain occurring at night involving the great toe. Data collection involves a dietary history, with specific questions concerning consumption of alcohol and foods high in purine, such as organ meats (brain, kidney, liver, and heart), anchovies, yeast, herring, mackerel, and scallops.

Collection of *objective data* includes assessment of joints (especially the great toe) for signs of edema, heat, discoloration (may appear erythematous or purple), and limited movement. Vital sign data may reveal an elevated temperature and hypertension, tachycardia, and tachypnea. Careful assessment of urinary output is necessary, because tophi can form in the kidneys and alter kidney function. The patient should be assessed for the presence of tophi (typically seen on the earlobes, fingers, hands, and toes).

Diagnostic tests. Laboratory tests used to diagnose gout include serum (see Table 26-5) and urinary uric acid levels (elevation is significant); complete blood count (leukocytosis and anemia may be present); and elevated ESR. X-ray studies reveal cysts and toe bone pockets. Synovial fluid will contain urate crystals.

Medical management. Several drugs are used in the treatment of the disease. For acute attacks colchicine is administered orally or may be given intravenously. When administered orally, 0.5 mg may be given hourly for 12 doses. The drug is discontinued if GI symptoms develop or the patient has not been relieved of pain. Phenylbutazone (Butazolidin) and indomethacin (Indocin) are affective antiinflammatory drugs in treating gout. Corticosteroids can be administered orally, intravenously, or intraarticularly and will relieve signs and symptoms within 12 hours. The physician may order allopurinol (Zyloprim) to decrease the production of uric acid; probenecid (Benemid) to increase secretion of uric acid by the kidneys; and sulfinpyrazone (Anturane) to prevent the development of tophi in various parts of the body, including the kidneys.

Nursing interventions. Nursing intervention is aimed at giving medications prescribed by the physician for relief of pain and inflammation. When giving colchicine it is important to observe for side effects, such as diarrhea, nausea, and vomiting. Increasing the patient's fluid intake to at least 2000 ml daily helps eliminate the excess urinary urates. About 10% to 20% of patients with gouty arthritis have uric acid kidney stones. Careful documentation of intake and output (I&O) is necessary. Bed rest and joint immobilization are maintained during the time the patient is symptomatic. Bed cradles prevent pressure from bed linens on the affected great toe.

Nursing diagnoses and interventions for the patient with gout include but are not limited to the following:

NURSING DIAGNOSES	NURSING INTERVENTIONS
Pain, related to disease process	Maintain patient in position of comfort with foot supported and in alignment; place bed cradle over foot; no weight bearing. Apply cold packs as ordered, keeping pressure off joint. Administer analgesics and antigout and antiinflammatory agents as ordered; observe for side effects.
Knowledge deficit, related to lack of information concerning medications and home care management	Provide medication schedule, including name, dosage, purpose, and side effects. Discuss importance of diet, exercise, and rest program. Encourage follow-up visits with physician.

Patient teaching. Patient teaching is aimed at giving information about the disease and stressing the importance of keeping the serum uric acid levels within normal range by taking the prescribed medications, following the prescribed diet, and avoiding infections, lack of sleep, and stress. Colchicine, probenecid, allopurinol, and sulfinpyrazone (Anturane) are drugs that the patient may need to take for several years, even when the signs and symptoms are not present.

Prognosis. The signs and symptoms are recurrent; episodes become longer each year. The disorder is disabling and, if untreated, can progress to the development of tophi and destructive joint changes.

OTHER DISORDERS

Osteoporosis

Etiology/pathophysiology. Osteoporosis is a disorder that results in reduction in the mass of bone per unit of volume. This reduction is sufficient to interfere with the mechanical support function of the bone. The cause of osteoporosis has not been completely identified. Women between the ages of 55 and 65 years are identified as a high-risk group for postmenopausal osteoporosis, and many researchers believe that this is related to the loss of the female hormone estrogen. Studies of postmenopausal osteoporosis suggest estrogen deficiency is connected with increased bone reabsorption and sensitivity to parathyroid hormone (substance that weakens bone by increasing calcium movement from bone into extracellular fluid). Senile osteoporosis is seen in persons between ages 70 and 85 years and affects twice as many women as men. Other factors that may contribute to the condition include immobilization, use of steroids, and high intake of caffeine. Genetic (small bone structure) and environmental factors (limited exercise) can contribute to the rate of bone loss. Osteoporosis affects the vertebrae, neck of the femur, pelvis, hands, and wrists. Individuals most at risk to develop osteoporosis are small-framed, nonobese, menopausal, white females who smoke. Contributing factors are diets low in calcium throughout life, smoking, excessive coffee intake, too much protein in the diet, and a sedentary life-style.

Clinical Manifestations. The disorder develops slowly, and the first symptom is a complaint of backache. As the disease progresses, the bones become porous and brittle, which is caused by a lack of calcium.

Assessment. Collection of *subjective data* includes questioning the patient about life-style practices and complaints of pain (low thoracic and lumbar) that worsens with sitting, standing, coughing, sneezing, and straining.

Collection of *objective data* involves assessing the patient for dowager's hump (spinal deformity and height loss that develop from repeated spinal vertebral fractures) and increased lordosis, scoliosis, and kyphosis. Assessment should be done for gait impairment associated with inability to maintain erect posture.

Diagnostic Tests. The physician will order a complete blood count, serum calcium, phosphorus, and alkaline phosphatase, blood urea nitrogen, creatinine level, urinalysis, liver and thyroid function tests, and x-ray studies.

Medical Management. The physician will order a treatment regimen aimed at promoting the increase of bone density and retardation of bone loss. Calcium supplements that bring the total calcium intake to 1000 mg for men and 1500 mg for postmenopausal women are recommended. Exercise programs to improve muscle tone, such as walking, have been effective in preventing further bone loss and stimulating new bone formation. Treatment may include adequate doses of estrogen. Estrogen will not correct the condition but will help to prevent fractures.

Nursing Interventions. Nursing interventions is aimed at preventing further bone loss and fractures. A diet rich in milk and dairy products provides most of the calcium in the diet. Food and beverages that contain caffeine also contain phosphorus, which contributes to bone loss. Teaching patients relaxation techniques and encouraging them to stop smoking are recommended. Estrogen therapy is not without risk, and patients who take estrogen need information about the higher risk for thromboembolism, endometrial cancer, and possibly breast cancer. Safety measures, such as side rails, handrails, bedside commodes with seat elevators, and rubber mats in showers can prevent falls in the older patient.

Nursing diagnoses and interventions for the patient with osteoporosis include but are not limited to the following:

NURSING DIAGNOSES	NURSING INTERVENTIONS
Mobility, impaired physical, related to disease process	Provide firm mattress. Encourage ambulation with walker or cane if indicated. Assist and teach active ROM exercises q 4 hr. Monitor and maintain body alignment; fractures can occur without patient's knowledge. Handle patient carefully, and assist with and teach correct body mechanics. Administer analgesics, estrogen, calcium, and vitamin D as ordered. Provide diet high in calcium and vitamins C and D. Monitor serum calcium levels.
Knowledge deficit, related to issues of home care management	Stress importance of diet, activity, and rest; provide aerobic exercise schedule; caution patient to avoid jogging.

NURSING DIAGNOSES	NURSING INTERVENTIONS
Knowledge deficit, related to issues of home care management—cont'd	Provide medication schedule, including name, dosage, purpose, and side effects. Discuss importance of safe environment to prevent falling. Encourage reduction of caffeine, alcohol intake, and smoking.

Patient teaching. To prevent osteoporosis, women are advised to have an adequate daily intake of calcium and vitamin D, to exercise regularly, to avoid smoking, to decrease coffee intake, to decrease excess protein in the diet, and to engage in regular moderate activity such as walking, bike riding, or swimming at least 3 days a week.

After menopause the usual recommended daily allowance of 800 mg of calcium should be increased to 1500 mg. Vitamin D, which increases calcium absorption, may also need to be added to the daily regimen of postmenopausal women as per physician's orders. Follow-up visits to the physician are encouraged for direction as to medication, diet, and exercise regimen.

Prognosis. Osteoporosis is a chronic disorder in which vitamin D and calcium may help to stop the rate of bone loss. In postmenopausal women, therapy with estrogen decreases the rate of bone resorption, but bone formation does not increase. Prevention of osteoporosis should begin before bone loss, because there has been little success in therapy aimed at restoring bone.

Osteomyelitis

Etiology/Pathophysiology. Osteomyelitis (local or generalized infection of bone and bone marrow) can occur from bacteria introduced through trauma, as in the case of a compound fracture or surgery. Also, bacteria may travel by the bloodstream from another site in the body to a bone, causing the bone to become infected. Staphylococci are the most common causative agents.

Bacteria invade the bone, and degeneration of bone tissue occurs. If osteomyelitis becomes chronic, the bone tissue affected often will be weakened and predisposed to spontaneous fractures.

Clinical Manifestations. The patient with osteomyelitis is subject to contractures in the affected extremity if positioned incorrectly. It is not unusual for a new focus of infection to develop months and sometimes years after the initial infection is diagnosed.

Assessment. Collection of *subjective data* includes a complete history of injuries, surgical procedures, and diseases. An assessment includes patient's complaints of persistent, severe, and increasing bone pain and tenderness, as well as regional muscle spasm. An assessment of allergies should be done, especially to medications, since antibiotics are given long term.

Collection of *objective data* includes careful inspection of any wounds. The drainage is assessed for color, amount, and presence of odor. Vital signs are assessed for signs of infection (temperature elevation, tachycardia, and tachypnea). Assessment for edema is noted, especially in the joints with limited mobility.

Diagnostic Tests. A complete history is taken, along with physical examination. The physician will order x-ray studies and bone scan, complete blood count (leukocytosis may be present), ESR, and cultures of blood and drainage (if present).

Medical Management. Intravenous antibiotic therapy is ordered; a broad-spectrum antibiotic, such as Keflin (cephalothin) is used. Parenteral antibiotics are usually necessary for several weeks. Bed rest is usually prescribed.

For some patients surgery may be performed to remove a fragment of necrotic bone that is partially or entirely detached from the surrounding or adjacent healthy bone **(sequestrum).**

Nursing Interventions. Nursing intervention includes gentleness in moving the diseased extremity. Absolute rest of the affected part may be necessary, with careful positioning using pillows and sandbags for good alignment. During the early phase of infection, pain is extremely severe and extraordinary gentleness in moving and manipulating the infected part is essential. Often wounds are irrigated with hydrogen peroxide or other antiseptic or antibiotic solution and then covered with a sterile dressing, using strict surgical asepsis. Patients are placed on drainage and secretion precautions. Dietary planning is done with emphasis on a diet high in calories, protein, and vitamins.

Nursing diagnoses and interventions for the patient with osteomyelitis include but are not limited to the following:

NURSING DIAGNOSES	NURSING INTERVENTIONS
Injury, high risk for, related to decreased mobility and/or decrease in level of orientation	Maintain bed in low position. Keep siderails up. Maintain protective gentle restraints. Leave night-light on. Orient patient to surroundings. Assist patient in ambulation with assistive devices as needed. Maintain safe environment.
Skin integrity, impaired, related to immobility	Identify skin areas at risk: areas over bony prominences (heels, sacrum, elbows, and ischial tuberosities).

NURSING DIAGNOSES	NURSING INTERVENTIONS
Skin integrity, impaired, related to immobility—cont'd	Regularly inspect (at least q 4 hr) for signs of pressure (for example, erythema or induration). Regularly turn patient (at least q 2 hr) within limits of immobilization. Use sheepskin pads, flotation pads, Egg-Crate mattress, or Clinitron or Circ-Olectric bed. Assist patient to keep skin clean and dry, especially under casts. Massage skin with lotion q 2 to 4 hr. Encourage nutritious diet to maintain skin integrity.

Patient teaching. This includes information about the signs of infection, such as elevated temperature. Because chronic osteomyelitis may last a lifetime, it is important for the patient to be aware of the recurrence of signs and symptoms. Patients must avoid trauma to the affected bone, since pathological fractures are common.

Prognosis. Acute osteomyelitis may respond to treatment after several weeks. Chronic osteomyelitis may persist for years with exacerbations and remissions.

Herniation of Intervertebral Disk (Herniated Nucleus Pulposus)

Etiology/Pathophysiology. Herniated nucleus pulposus is a rupture of the fibrocartilage surrounding an intervertebral disk, releasing the nucleus pulposus that cushions the vertebrae above and below. This displacement puts pressure on nerve roots. Lumbar and cervical herniations are most common (see Fig. 26-17). Herniated nucleus pulposus can occur suddenly (from lifting, twisting, or trauma) or gradually (from degenerative changes [as seen with degenerative joint disease, osteoporosis, aging, and chronic diseases affected bones]). Herniations of the lumbar spine usually affect persons 20 to 45 years old; cervical herniations are seen most in persons 45 years old and older. Men are more prone to this disorder than women.

Clinical Manifestations. Low back pain that occurs with the slightest movement is the most common symptom. The pain radiates over the buttock and down the leg, following the sciatic nerve pathway *(radicular pain),* causing numbness and tingling in the affected leg.

Assessment. Collection of *subjective data* involves pain assessment and patient-stated relief measures. Pain is often exacerbated with activity. Complaints of pain in the back radiating down the leg (sciatica) are common. Complaints about activity intolerance and alteration in bowel and bladder elimination (constipation and urinary retention) are significant.

Collection of *objective data* includes observing for signs of limited spinal flexibility (limited forward bending) and gait alteration (patient may favor supporting weight on one extremity). An ineffective breathing pattern may be present and result from pain and decreased

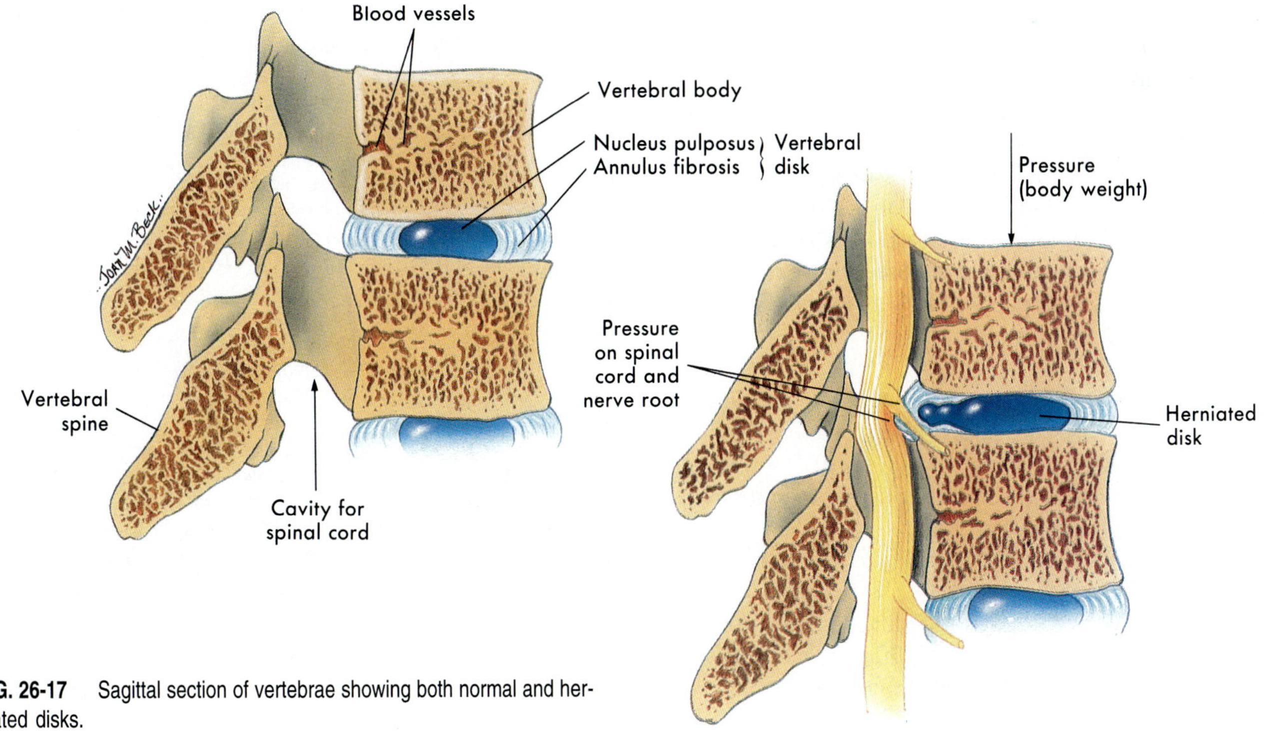

FIG. 26-17 Sagittal section of vertebrae showing both normal and herniated disks.

mobility. Assessment includes determination of bowel and bladder elimination and maintenance of traction equipment.

Diagnostic Tests. Complete history and physical examination is obtained. The physician will order x-ray studies, computed tomography, myelography, and electromyelography (to determine nerve involvement).

Medical Management. The physician will order bed rest, pain control, physical therapy (aimed at muscle strengthening and comfort), and skin traction (may be pelvic or cervical). If the patient demonstrates neurological deterioration or continued pain, a surgical procedure may be required, such as the following:

- *Laminectomy:* surgical removal of the bony arches or one or more vertebrae performed to relieve compression of the spinal cord caused by bone displacement from an injury or degeneration of a disk or to remove a displaced vertebral disk.
- *Spinal fusion (arthrodesis; the surgical immobilization of a joint; artificial ankylosis):* removal of the lamina and removal of several herniated nuclei pulposi. A portion of bone taken from the patient's iliac crest or from a bone bank is used as a bone graft in the vertebral spaces.
- *Diskectomy:* often done with a microscope. Only the extruded disk material is removed. Percutaneous lateral diskectomy is performed under local anesthesia with the surgeon cutting a window around the anulus fibrosus.
- *Chemonucleolysis:* can be done on patients who have no nerve involvement. The procedure involves administering a local anesthetic agent and then guiding a needle into the nucleus pulposus to inject chymopapain (drug that dissolves the nucleus pulposus).

Postoperative laminectomy care includes assessing the incision site for signs of infection, such as drainage, edema, odor, and temperature elevation. After a chemonucleolysis, careful assessment is noted for signs of allergic reactions to chymopapain, such as urticaria and respiratory difficulties.

Nursing Interventions. Nursing intervention is aimed at providing nursing care appropriate for the following nursing diagnoses:

- Anxiety, related to discomfort, fear of unknown, and life-style changes
- Pain (back), related to muscle spasms and painful diagnostic tests
- Constipation, colonic and urinary elimination, altered patterns, related to pain, pain medications, immobility, and neurological involvement

Nursing intervention involves giving the patient and the family information about procedures and hospital protocol to help reduce their anxiety. It is important to administer the medications prescribed on schedule and document the effectiveness of the medication. Distraction, heat or ice application (if ordered), and moving (by log rolling) and positioning the patient q 2 hr (if not contraindicated because of maintaining traction) can help promote patient comfort.

Observe dressing for bleeding or cerebrospinal fluid leakage. Apply antiembolic stockings if ordered. Careful documentation of I&O provides information about bowel and bladder function. Ensure that the patient has voided in the first 8 hours, and use nursing measures to promote voiding before resorting to catheterization. The nurse should encourage the patient to sit in a straight, firm chair for no longer than 30 minutes at one time. It is important to monitor the patient for evidence of respiratory distress and paralytic ileus and for complications seen in laminectomy patients.

Nursing diagnoses and interventions for the patient with herniated disk include but are not limited to the following:

NURSING DIAGNOSES	NURSING INTERVENTIONS
Knowledge deficit, related to home care management	Stress importance of rehabilitation plan of activity, rest, and exercise. Provide diet instructions as to type and amount, and weight maintenance (no gain) if applicable. Discuss medications: name, purpose, schedule, dosage, and side effects. Discuss signs and symptoms to report to physician: severe pain; changes in temperature, color, or sensation in extremity; and malodorous drainage from wound. Encourage follow-up visits with physician.
Powerlessness, related to decreased mobility/pain	Use active listening, and permit verbalization of anger and helplessness. Assist patient with identifying coping mechanisms that will reduce feeling of powerlessness; use those that have been successful in past. Offer positive recognition for increased activity level. Assist patient in identifying areas that can be controlled. Involve patient in decision-making process for own care.
Nutrition altered: less than body requirements; more than body requirements, related to altered mobility	Encourage diet high in protein: 150 to 300 g/day unless contraindicated. Teach patient to avoid weight gain, especially if in a molded brace. Encourage patient to eat regular meals. Give patient ample time to eat. Encourage self-feeding, but help patient or provide special assistive utensils as necessary.

NURSING DIAGNOSES	NURSING INTERVENTIONS
Nutrition altered: less than body requirements; more than body requirements, related to altered mobility—cont'd	Attend to patient's need for roughage and fluid as noted, and encourage iron and vitamins for bone repair. Position patient to facilitate comfortable intake of food and fluids.
Infection, high risk for, related to immobility and/or surgical intervention	Assess wound integrity, and observe for signs of infection or drainage. Monitor and change dressings prn; cleanse with hydrogen peroxide using surgical asepsis at least q 8 hr or per physician's protocol. Monitor temperature. Encourage coughing, turning, and deep breathing q 2 hr as indicated. Encourage ambulation as permitted.

Patient teaching. Activity out of bed may begin as early as 1 day after a simple laminectomy or 2 to 4 days after a laminectomy and fusion. The nurse should transfer the patient out of bed with as little time spent in the sitting position as possible. The patient may be permitted to walk as much as tolerated, with assistance if necessary. Braces or corsets, if prescribed, are applied before the patient gets out of bed. The nurse should encourage the patient to participate in ADLs within prescribed limits of mobility.

The patient should be instructed not to lift or carry anything heavier than 2.25 kg (5 lb) for at least 8 weeks, not to drive a car until permitted by the surgeon, and to avoid twisting motions of the trunk. Reinforce importance of follow-up visit to physician.

Prognosis. With conservative treatment, some patients will receive relief of symptoms; if neurological pathology develops, surgical intervention is needed. The prognosis is usually quite favorable.

Tumors of the Bone

Etiology/Pathophysiology. Tumors of the bone may be primary or secondary and may be benign or malignant. As with other types of tumors, the cause of bone tumors is not always known. Carcinoma of the prostate, lung, breast, thyroid, and kidney may metastasize to the bones. *Osteogenic sarcoma* is a primary malignant bone tumor that is seen most often in young people. Osteogenic sarcoma can metastasize to the lungs and to the rest of the body via the bloodstream. Osteochondroma is a type of benign tumor.

Osteogenic sarcoma is a fast-growing and aggressive tumor that affects the long bones of the body. About 50% of these tumors occur in the femur (at the distal end), affecting males between the ages of 10 and 25 more often than females.

Osteochondroma is the most common benign osteogenic tumor. This tumor is seen more often in males between the ages of 10 and 30. Osteochondromas can occur as a single tumor or as multiple tumors. They usually affect the humerus, tibia, and femur.

Clinical Manifestations. When healthy bone cells are replaced by cancer cells, the strength of the bone is altered and spontaneous fractures can occur. Anemia occurs when cancer invades the long bones and interrupts the manufacturing of red blood cells in the bone marrow. Cancerous bone tumors metastasize and invade other bones and lung tissue.

Benign bone tumors can grow large enough to put pressure on blood vessels and nerves. Benign tumors do not spread. However, they may undergo cancerous changes and become malignant.

Assessment. Collection of *subjective data* includes an awareness that malignant and benign bone tumors will cause pain in the affected bone site. Complaints of pain, especially with weight bearing, are common. The pain may result from a spontaneous fracture. The patient may also complain of tenderness at the affected side.

Collection of *objective data* includes assessment of the painful part, which may reveal edema and discoloration of the skin.

Diagnostic Tests. Diagnosis is confirmed with x-ray studies, bone scan, bone biopsy, and laboratory studies, such as complete blood cell count and platelet count (relative to bone marrow involvement); serum protein levels (elevated in multiple myeloma); and serum alkaline phosphatase level (elevation may indicate osteogenic sarcoma).

Medical Management. The physician will evaluate the tumor type, size, and location and plan the treatment accordingly.

Larger, symptomatic, benign tumors and malignant tumors require surgical intervention. The surgical procedure depends on the tumor size, location, and extent of tissue involvement. The surgery may involve (1) wide excision or resection, (2) bone curettage, or (3) leg or arm amputation.

Treatment is aimed at destroying or removing the malignant lesion. Amputation of the affected extremity followed by chemotherapy or radiation is the widely accepted protocol for treatment of malignant bone tumors.

Chemotherapy is aimed at destroying cancer cells at both primary and metastatic sites. Patients usually receive chemotherapy in cycles of 3- or 4-week intervals. Radiation therapy may be given internally and externally. It is important for the nurse to know the safety precautions and side effects of both chemotherapy and radiation therapy. (See Chapter 38 for a discussion of care of the patient with cancer.)

Nursing Interventions. Preoperatively the patient and family need complete and concise information about procedures and postoperative expectations.

Postoperative nursing interventions will include the following:

- Performing a neurovascular assessment
- Monitoring vital signs
- Administering analgesics and evaluating the effectiveness
- Providing cast care and/or dressing changes with careful documentation of drainage, odors, and signs of circulation impairment
- Cooperating with physical and occupational therapists to promote mobility and ADLs
- Educating the patient and family about home health care and early detection of tumor recurrence

Nursing diagnoses and interventions for the patient with a tumor of the bone include but are not limited to the following:

NURSING DIAGNOSES	NURSING INTERVENTIONS
Anxiety, related to fear of cancer, body image change, life-style change, and possible death	Establish therapeutic relationship: acknowledge fear and encourage patient to acknowledge and express feelings. Give accurate information about condition and therapies. Refer to resources when necessary (e.g., social worker and religious counselor).
Pain, related to soft tissue trauma, edema, and compression of nerve tissue in affected extremity	Assess type and location of pain; observe for increasing pain or dysfunction. Assist patient with changing position frequently; administer back rubs. Administer analgesics as ordered; assess effectiveness of pain relief measures. Provide diversional activities.
Mobility, impaired physical, related to surgical and medical intervention, pain, and weakness	Maintain bed rest in correct body alignment as ordered with splint and/or pillows. Assist with activity as tolerated and ordered. Ambulate with assistance if tolerated; assist to use crutches, cane, or walker if needed. Maintain planned rest periods.

Prognosis. The prognosis for bone tumors has been improved in recent years by the combination of local surgery and chemotherapy. Disease-free survival rates for patients whose osteogenic sarcoma is treated with surgery and chemotherapy appear to be greater than 50% at 5 years.

TRAUMATIC INJURIES

Traumatic injuries to the musculoskeletal system can occur in all age groups. However, aged persons may have disorders that predispose to musculoskeletal injuries. The more serious injuries involving fractures will be treated in a hospital, whereas the less serious, such as contusions, sprains, or strains, may be treated in an outpatient facility.

Contusions

Etiology/Pathophysiology/Clinical Manifestations. Contusions are the most common soft tissue injury. An injury from a blow or blunt force will cause local bleeding under the skin and possibly a hematoma (sac filled with blood). Contusions can be serious, depending on the part of the body affected. A contusion of the brain is very serious, whereas a contusion of the arm is less serious. Large areas affected by soft tissue bleeding with slow absorption of the blood have a higher potential of developing into cellulitis (an infection of the subcutaneous tissue).

Medical Management. Most contusions are treated by applying ice bags or cold compresses for 15 to 20 minutes intermittently for 12 to 36 hours for the vasoconstricting effects of cold. The involved extremity is elevated to reduce edema and suppress pain.

Prognosis. Prognosis is excellent.

Sprains

Etiology/Pathophysiology/Clinical Manifestations. This injury can result from a wrenching or hyperextension of a joint, tearing the capsule and ligaments. A sprain can involve bleeding into a joint (hemarthrosis). Common sites include the knee, ankle, and cervical spine (whiplash). Sprains are often the result of a sudden, twisting injury. Medical management is similar to that for contusions.

Prognosis. Prognosis is excellent.

Whiplash

Etiology/Pathophysiology/Clinical Manifestations. Injury at the cervical spine is known as *whiplash* and is classified under cervical disk syndrome.

Whiplash is caused by an injury that involves hyperextension, which results in compression of the anatomical structures. This type of injury usually occurs as a result of sudden acceleration or deceleration, such as rear-end car collisions that cause violent back and forth movements of the head and neck. Symptoms of a whiplash may not be obvious for a few days or even a week after the injury. Cervical fractures can accompany a whiplash injury.

Assessment. Collection of *subjective data* includes the patient's complaint of pain (the most common symptom), which usually begins in the cervical area but may radiate down the arm to the fingers and increase with cervical motion. The pain may increase sharply with coughing, sneezing, or any radical movement. Other signs and symptoms may be paresthesia (numbness or tingling), headache, blurred vision, decreased skeletal function, and weakened hand grip.

Collection of *objective data* includes edema in the cervical spine region with tightening of the muscles. Vital signs are usually within normal ranges. However, if the assessment findings indicate hypertension with widened pulse pressure and bradycardia, increased intracranial pressure (IICP) should be suspected; the findings should be reported and documented immediately. A neurological assessment is done q 15 to 30 minutes to rule out IICP. (Refer to Chapter 35 for a discussion on the care of the patient with a neurological disorder.)

Diagnostic Tests. Physical examination and x-ray studies are used to confirm the physician's diagnosis.

Medical Management. Recurrence of symptoms is common. A medical approach is most often used for treatment of whiplash. Analgesics and muscle relaxants are prescribed, along with intermittent cervical traction. Surgery may be necessary if cervical fracture with displacement occurs. (See the discussion of herniated nucleus pulposus.)

Nursing Interventions. Nursing intervention involves care of the patient with restricted activity to immobilize the cervical vertebrae to decrease irritation and provide rest for the traumatized area. This is accomplished with cervical traction. Proper assessment of traction includes the following:

- Maintaining the patient's body in proper alignment; the force or pull should be in alignment with the long axis of the bone.
- Ensuring that weights are hanging freely from the bed and are never removed without a physician's order.
- Observing the condition of the traction cords, making sure they are not weakened or frayed.
- Ensuring that all knots that are used on the rope or cord are square knots.
- Ensuring that the ropes are centered on the traction pulley.
- Ensuring that the correct weights are used, as ordered by the physician.
- Carefully observing the skin for signs of pressure and decubitus ulcer formation.

Other treatments include special exercises, heat therapy, and administration of mild analgesics as ordered by the physician to control the pain. A soft, foam rubber neck brace collar may be used for whiplash injuries to limit head movement. Careful inspection of the skin around the neck and chin is made for signs of excoriation.

Prognosis. Prognosis depends upon the extent of neurological involvement. Prognosis is excellent with minor trauma, but because the spinal canal is full of neural tissue in the cervical area, more extensive injury can produce profound disability.

Ankle Sprains

Etiology/Pathophysiology. An ankle sprain is often referred to as a twisted ankle and is caused by a wrenching or twisting of the foot and ankle (Box 26-3).

Clinical Manifestations. The ankle area will become edematous very quickly, with spasms of the muscles and pain on passive movement of the joint.

Assessment. Collection of *subjective data* includes assessment of pain and tenderness in the affected ankle that intensifies with movement of the foot or ankle.

Collection of *objective data* includes assessment of the traumatized ankle for signs of edema, limited movement and function of the joint, and ecchymosis of the soft tissue around the ankle.

Diagnostic Tests. An x-ray examination of the injured area is the only accurate way to ensure there is no bone injury.

Medical Management. Surgery may be indicated for severe sprains. The physician will suture torn ligament fibers together. If the ligaments have been torn from the bone, the surgeon will reattach them by drilling small holes in the medial malleolus (rounded bony protrusion on the medial area of the ankle).

Box 26-3 NURSING ALERT

A strain and sprain are not the same. Strains are produced by minute muscle tears and overstretching of tendons, whereas sprains are caused by a twisting of the joint.

Nursing Interventions. The injured area must be elevated and kept at rest. Application of ice for 15 to 20 minutes intermittently for 12 to 36 hours, followed after 24 hours with the application of mild heat for 15 to 30 minutes, four times daily, will promote absorption of blood and fluid from the area. Compressive dressings and splinting are used to help support the injured area. A neurovascular assessment is necessary to detect impaired tissue perfusion.

Prognosis. Prognosis is generally excellent.

Strains

Etiology/Pathophysiology/Clinical Manifestations. This injury is characterized by microscopic muscle tears as a result of overstretching muscles and tendons. An acute strain results when the muscles and tendons are overstretched in a forceful movement, such as unaccustomed vigorous exercise.

Assessment. Collection of *subjective data* involves noting the patient's complaint of sudden and severe pain away from the joint, which increases with activity. Chronic muscle strain can occur from repeated muscle overuse, and the pain may not appear for several hours after the patient has used the muscles. The patient typically complains of soreness, stiffness, and tenderness in the area.

Collection of *objective data* includes observation of stiffness, ecchymosis, and slight edema over the injury site. The most common sites are calf muscles, hamstrings, quadriceps, and the lumbosacral area. Edema can occur very rapidly in the muscle and tendon area.

Diagnostic Tests. An x-ray study is necessary to rule out bone trauma.

Medical Management. It is important to encourage exercises of the legs to prevent thrombosis development.

Surgical repair will be necessary if the muscle is completely ruptured. Analgesics and muscle relaxants are ordered by the physician. An exercise program is almost always prescribed if the strain is in the lumbosacral region. The exercises are aimed at strengthening the lower abdominal muscles.

Nursing Interventions. Nursing intervention for a strain is similar to that for a sprain. Ice application helps relieve pain, but some physicians prefer heat application rather than ice. Back strains are among the most common strains, and during exacerbation of symptoms, the patient is advised to avoid strenuous activities, use a firm chair with rigid back support, avoid wearing high heels, use a firm mattress for sleep, never sleep on the abdomen, and place a pillow under the knees to take pressure off the back.

Prognosis. Prognosis is usually very favorable.

Dislocations

Etiology/Pathophysiology. Dislocations usually involve tearing of the joint capsule; **subluxations** (partial or incomplete dislocations) involve stretching of the joint capsule. Both are temporary displacements of bones from their normal position within joints. A dislocation may be (1) congenital (e.g., congenital hip displacement), (2) caused by a disease process, or (3) caused by trauma. Stretching and tearing of ligaments and tendons, as well as fractures, can accompany a dislocation or subluxation. The displaced bone may rupture blood vessels. When subluxation occurs, the joint's articulating (movable) surfaces are partially separated.

Clinical Manifestations. Dislocation may or may not be visible. Sometimes a dislocation will change the length of an affected extremity. Pain and loss of function may be similar to that occurring with a fracture. However, dislocation partially immobilizes a joint, whereas a fracture site typically has abnormal free movement. Common dislocation sites include the shoulder, hip, and knee.

Assessment. Collection of *subjective data* includes the patient's description of the injury and pain. When the dislocation is of the shoulder, the nurse should assess for complaints of sensation loss and paresthesia.

Collection of *objective data* includes the assessment of any erythema, discoloration, edema, pain, tenderness, limitation of movement, and deformity or shortening of the extremity. The nurse should compare both sides for validation. Neurovascular assessment is important to determine if vascular or nerve injury is present in the affected area. For shoulder dislocation, the nurse should assess for an absent radial pulse, hypothermia of the hand, and wrist drop.

Diagnostic Tests. The diagnosis is based on the present complaints of discomfort, physical examination, and diagnostic x-ray examination of the injured site.

Medical Management. The physician may perform a closed reduction, which corrects the deformity through manipulation of the extremity. Surgical intervention to restore joint articulation is sometimes required.

Nursing Interventions. Nursing intervention includes measures for (1) reduction of edema and discomfort, (2) immobilization of the injured part to promote healing, and (3) patient education. Ice application is recommended for the first 24 hours after trauma. After 24 hours, heat may be used if there are no indications of bleeding. Elevation of the injured extremity on pillows and the application of elastic bandages help relieve edema. Immobilization of joints may involve application of a splint, sling, or elastic bandage. The air cast or air splint brace is an immobilization device. It is inflatable and lightweight and conforms to the extremity's size and shape. When immobilization devices are used, a neurovascular assessment is done frequently (see nursing interventions below). Analgesics should be administered as prescribed by the physician as needed. Asking the patient to rate the pain on a scale from 0 to 10 is helpful in determining pain severity. For control of extreme pain, the physician may order a narcotic, such as Demerol or morphine. For moderate to mild pain, Motrin or Tylenol may be prescribed. Positioning and repositioning the injured part can help reduce discomfort.

Nursing diagnoses and interventions for the patient for neurovascular integrity include but are not limited to the following:

NURSING DIAGNOSES	NURSING INTERVENTIONS
Tissue perfusion, altered, peripheral, related to injury/treatment Injury, high risk for, related to neurovascular impairment	Position extremities in alignment; elevate affected extremity. Compare affected extremity with unaffected extremity, using same hand for palpation. Test capillary refill (blanching test). Check each digit for sensation and motion. Document location and characteristics of pain. Palpate pedal, tibial, or radial pulses and compare to unaffected extremity. Assess for edema with pallor, cyanosis, and coldness. Elicit description of sensations from patient. Document all findings.

Patient teaching. Promoting an accident-free environment is essential. The nurse can explore areas of preventive medicine with patients. They are as follows:

- Environmental safety can include grab bars mounted in the bathroom near the toilet or tub and rubber mats or slip guards in the tub and shower. Removing throw rugs and obstacles from the floor can prevent falls. If the patient is using a gait enhancer, such as a cane, crutches, or a walker, it is important that it be used correctly. Safety precautions, such as using rubber tips on the points that make contact with the floor to prevent slippage, should be taken.
- Patients in the hospital are at risk of falling out of bed if their disease condition or medication results in disorientation. These patients need a careful assessment of their level of orientation, side rails applied to their beds, and safety reminder devices to prevent self-injury. Using a safe ladder when climbing can help prevent a fall. Wearing protective clothing while engaging in dangerous work or contact sports is also recommended.
- Appropriate health teaching should be targeted for persons at risk for musculoskeletal diseases, such as osteoporosis, which can predispose to pathological or nontraumatic fractures.

Prognosis with Treatment. Prognosis is generally excellent.

Carpal Tunnel Syndrome

Etiology/Pathophysiology. Carpal tunnel syndrome is a painful disorder of the wrist and hand, induced by compression on the median nerve between the inelastic carpal ligament and other structures in the carpal tunnel.

Carpal tunnel syndrome results from pressure on the median nerve of the wrist. The symptoms of **paresthesia** (any subjective sensation as of pricks of pins and needles) and *hypesthesia,* also called *hypoesthesia* (a decrease in sensation in response to stimulation of the sensory nerves), of the thumb, index, and middle fingers may develop spontaneously or occur as a result of disease or injury. There is a higher incidence of this condition in obese, middle-aged women and individuals employed in occupations involving repetitious motions of the fingers and hands (e.g., computer usage, basket weaving, meat carving, and typing). Carpal tunnel syndrome has become one of the three most common industrial or work-related conditions and is related to increased computer usage in all industries and departments in industries and government. Edema of the tendon sheaths caused by rheumatoid arthritis can predispose to carpal tunnel syndrome. Curiously, pregnant women may develop the syndrome during their last trimester. The reasons for this have not yet been determined, although fluid retention and edema may be contributing factors.

Clinical Manifestations. Anatomically the median nerve passes through a tunnel surrounded by the carpal bones and ligaments. When inflammation and edema of the synovial lining of the tendon sheaths occur, the tunnel space is narrowed, resulting in compression of the median nerve. The affected hand has altered ability to grasp or hold small objects. Atrophy of the thenar eminence (the padded area of the palm below the base of the thumb) is noted as the disease progresses.

Assessment. Collection of *subjective data* includes the patient's description of discomfort, such as complaints of burning pain or tingling in the hands relieved with vigorous shaking or exercising of the hands; pain may be intermittent or constant and is often more intense at night; numbness (hypesthesia) of the thumb, index, and ring fingers especially after prolonged flexion of the wrist; and inability to grasp or hold small objects.

Collection of *objective data* includes assessment of the hand, wrist, or fingers for edema, muscle atrophy, or a depressed appearance of the soft tissue at the base of the thumb on the palmar surface.

Diagnostic Tests. A conduction block at the wrist confirmed by motor nerve volicity studies is used to confirm the diagnosis.

Medical Management. If the symptoms are mild and surgery is not a desirable option, an immobilizer such as a splint can be used. Hydrocortisone acetate suspension injections can be given into the carpal tunnel for relief of mild symptoms. Surgery is indicated for severe symptoms with the occurrence of muscle atrophy. The standard surgical treatment is decompression of the median nerve by section of the transverse carpal ligament.

Nursing Interventions. If surgery is not required, the nurse will be involved with the application of an immobilizer to promote comfort. Use of a cock-up splint to relieve pressure and to lessen wrist flexion, elevation to relieve edema, ROM exercises to lessen sense of clumsiness, and restriction of twisting and turning activities of the wrist are general nursing interventions that are helpful. If surgery is required, the postoperative interventions will include the following: (1) elevating the hand and arm for 24 hours; (2) implementing and evaluating active thumb and finger motion within limits imposed by the dressing; (3) administering prescribed analgesics as needed; (4) monitoring vital signs (temperature elevation could indicate infection); and (5) checking fingers for circulation, sensation, and movement every 1 to 2 hr for 24 hr.

Patient teaching. Patients are encouraged to use the affected hand in normal activities as soon as 2 to 3 days after surgery.

Prognosis. Mild symptoms of carpal tunnel syndrome are relieved by nonsurgical treatment; severe symptoms require surgical intervention with excellent prognosis. If the patient is pregnant, relief of symptoms usually occurs after delivery.

Fractures

Etiology/Pathophysiology. A fracture is a traumatic injury to a bone in which the continuity of the tissue of the bone is broken. Descriptions of fractures by appearance can be seen in Fig. 26-18. Most fractures result from an insult to the bone, such as a forceful blow (twisting or crushing), which places more stress on the bone than it can absorb. Fractures that occur without trauma are referred to as pathological or spontaneous fractures and can be caused by a weakening of the bone because of osteoporosis, metastatic cancer and tumors of the bone, Cushing's syndrome, malnutrition, and complications of long-term steroid therapy.

Fractures may result from (1) direct force, which results in a fracture at the site of the trauma; (2) torsion, which is seen in a twisting injury where the fracture occurs at a point remote from the trauma (e.g., a forceful

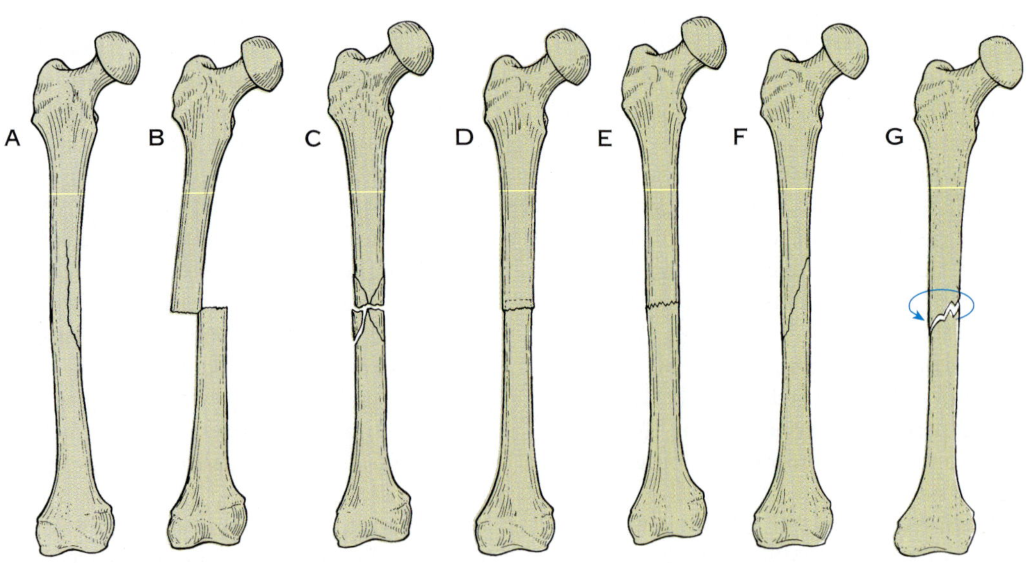

FIG. 26-18 Description of fracture by appearance. **A,** Greenstick. **B,** Complete. **C,** Comminuted. **D,** Impacted. **E,** Transverse. **F,** Oblique. **G,** Spiral.

twisting of the wrist may cause a fracture of the arm); or (3) violent contractions involving highly developed muscles (e.g., severe muscle spasms may cause a fracture in a paraplegic patient).

There are more than 150 types of fractures, which can be classified in various ways. First, they are described as either open (compound) or closed (simple) (Fig. 26-19), meaning that the fracture has occurred with protrusion of the bone through the skin or the fractured bone has not protruded through the skin. Open fractures are more serious, because they involve more soft tissue damage, require surgical treatment to repair, and are prone to infections. A bullet wound (injury is directed inward) that has fractured a bone is another example of an open fracture. A closed fracture does not involve a break in the skin. These fractures can usually be realigned by external manipulation and seldom require surgery.

A description of a fracture can be given in terms of appearance (see Fig. 26-18), such as greenstick, complete, comminuted, impacted, transverse, oblique, and spiral. They are briefly described as follows:

- *Greenstick fracture:* incomplete fracture in which the fracture line extends only partially through the bone. The bone is broken and bent but still secured at one side. This fracture is common in children, since their bones are softer and more flexible than those of adults.
- *Complete fracture:* fracture line extends entirely through the bone with the periosteum disrupted on both sides of the bone.
- *Comminuted fracture:* bone is splintered into three or more fragments at the site of the break. There is more than one fracture line. A butterfly fracture is a type of comminuted fracture.
- *Impacted fracture:* sometimes called a *telescoped* fracture, because one bone fragment is forcibly wedged into another bone fragment. In long bones this can create a shortening of the extremity.
- *Transverse fracture:* break runs directly across the bone; it is at a right angle of the bone's axis.
- *Oblique fracture:* break runs along a slant to the length of the bone; it is at about a 45-degree angle to the shaft of the bone.
- *Spiral fracture:* break coils around the bone. It is sometimes called a *torsion* fracture and will result from a twisting force.

Fractures are described as to their location on the bone, e.g., proximal, midshaft, or distal. Fractures can also be classified as to the force that caused the break. An example of this is the *marching* fracture, which can occur in the metatarsals as a result of a long march.

Physicians who have been the first to describe a type of fracture have given their names to fractures. Examples of this include the following:

- **Colles' fracture:** fracture of the distal portion of the radius within 1 inch of the joint of the wrist that commonly occurs when a person attempts to break a fall by putting the hands down.
- *Pott's fracture:* occurs at the distal end of the fibula and is characterized by chipping off of a piece of the medial malleolus with a displacement of the foot outward

Fractures are sometimes referred to as *joint* fractures if they involve or are close to a joint. *Articulation* fracture involves the surface of a joint. *Extracapsular* fracture involves a fracture near the joint but one that has not entered the joint capsule. *Intracapsular* fracture is a fracture within the joint capsule.

Fractures can also be described as to their displacement. Fig. 26-20 shows that fragments may be displaced

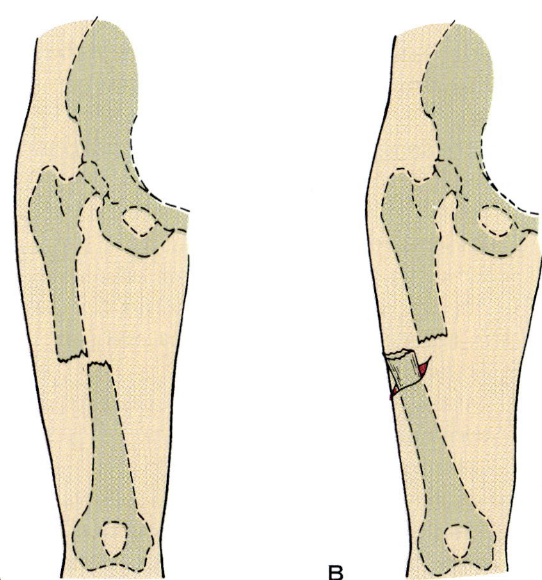

FIG. 26-19 **A,** Closed fracture. **B,** Open fracture with bone protruding through skin.

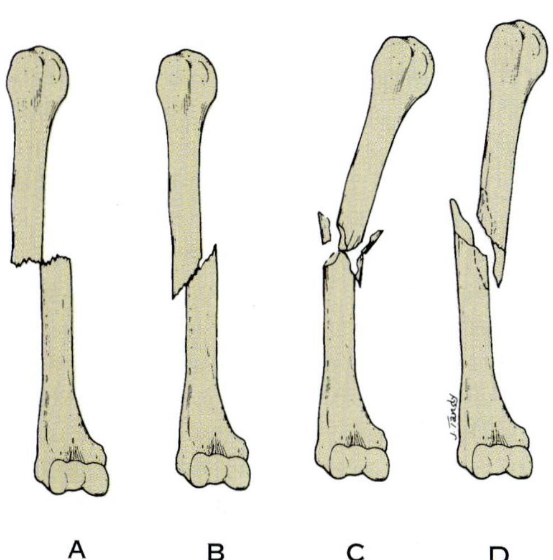

FIG. 26-20 Displacement of fragments. **A,** Sideways. **B,** Override. **C,** Angulate. **D,** Rotate.

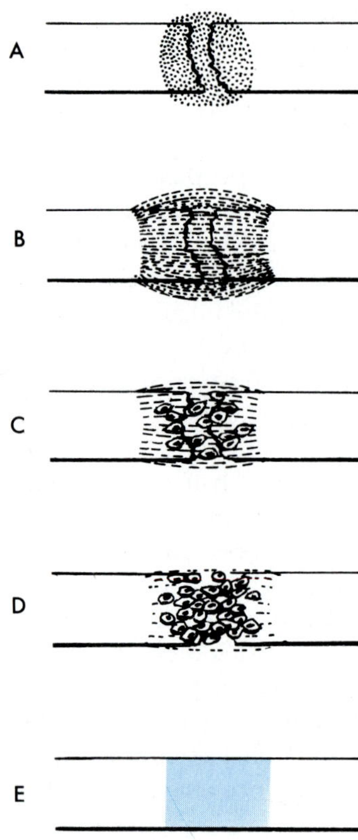

FIG. 26-21 Bone healing *(schematic representation)*.

sideways, can override the opposite fractured surface, may angulate or create a bend in the bone, and may rotate away from the fracture site. When a bone is displaced, the bone fragments can cause soft tissue damage. The patient will consequently experience severe pain, edema, and muscle spasms in the early stages of healing.

The bone is vascular; therefore when a fracture occurs, there is bleeding at the site of the fracture. A clot will form at the ends of the fractured bone (Fig. 26-21, *A*). The next phase of healing occurs when the hematoma becomes organized as fibroblasts invade the area and a fibrin meshwork is formed (Fig. 26-21, *B*). Inflammation is localized as the white cells wall off the area. Osteoblasts enter the fibrous area to help hold the union firm (Fig. 26-21, *C*). Blood vessels develop, and collagen strands start to incorporate calcium deposits. **Callus** (bony deposits formed between and around the broken ends of a fractured bone during healing) formation occurs when the osteoblasts continue to lay the network for bone buildup and osteoclasts destroy dead bone (Fig. 26-21, *D*). The collagen strengthens and continues to incorporate calcium deposits. Remodeling is the final step and occurs when the excess callus is reabsorbed and trabecular bone is laid down along the lines of stress (Fig. 26-21, *E*).

Clinical Manifestations. The signs and symptoms of fractures very according to the location and function of the involved bone, the strength of its muscle attachment, the type of fracture sustained, and the amount of related damage. Signs and symptoms are as follows:

1. Pain
2. Loss of normal function: the injured part is incapable of voluntary movements
3. Obvious deformity
4. Excessive motion at site: there is motion where motion does not usually occur
5. **Crepitus** or grating sound if limb is moved gently; no attempt should be made to determine this sign when fracture is suspected, since it may cause further damage and increase pain
6. Soft tissue edema in area of injury
7. Warmth over injured area
8. Ecchymosis of skin surrounding injured area; it may not be present for several days
9. Loss of sensation or paralysis distal to injury: indicative of nerve constricture
10. Signs of shock, related to tissue injury, blood loss, and severe pain

Assessment. Collection of *subjective data* includes the following:

- Pain at site of injury
- Loss of sensation or movement of affected part
- Determine cause of injury

Collection of *objective data* includes the following:

- Warmth, edema, and ecchymosis
- Obvious deformity
- Loss of normal function in the injured part
- Signs of systemic shock
- Signs of any circulatory, motor, or sensory impairment

Diagnostic Tests. An accurate diagnosis of the fracture is made by x-ray examination or fluoroscopy.

Medical Management. Immediate management includes the following:

1. Splinting to prevent edema of the affected part
2. Preservation of body alignment
3. Elevation of body part to limit edema
4. Application of cold packs (during first 24 hours) to reduce hemorrhage, edema, and pain
5. Administration of analgesics
6. Observation for change in color, sensation, or temperature
7. Observation for signs of shock

Secondary management is outlined as follows:

I. Simple fracture—Optimal reduction: replacing bone fragments in their correct anatomical position

A. Closed reduction: manual manipulations, moving bony fragments into position by applying distraction and pressure to distal fragments
B. Traction
C. Open reduction internal fixation **(ORIF)** is a surgical procedure allowing fracture alignment under direct visualization while using various internal fixation devices applied to the bone
D. Immobilization
   1. External fixation: cast or splint
   2. Traction
   3. Internal fixation devices such as pins, plates, screws, wires, and prostheses (Fig. 26-22)
   4. Combination of the above

II. Compound fracture
A. Surgical débridement of wound to remove dirt, foreign materials, devitalized tissue, and necrotic bone
B. Administration of tetanus toxoid
C. Culture of wound
D. Treatment with antibiotics
E. Observation for signs of osteomyelitis, tetanus, and/or gangrene
F. Closure of wound when there is no sign of infection
G. Reduction of fracture
H. Immobilization of fracture
I. Treatment of complications

Nursing Interventions. The nursing intervention of patients with fractures is essentially that given any surgical patient. The care of the patient in traction and in a cast will be discussed later in this chapter. The patient needs a well-balanced diet, but opinions differ on the value of vitamin and mineral supplements in hastening bone repair. Fluids should be encouraged. Exercise of the unaffected joints, muscle-setting exercises, skin care, and elimination are important considerations in patient care. Internal fixation has simplified nursing intervention for many patients with fractures and shortened the period of hospitalization, but many patients will require longer periods of hospitalization. If activity is restricted, the complications that result from immobility must be anticipated and prevented.

Nursing diagnoses and interventions for the patient with a fracture include but are not limited to the following:

NURSING DIAGNOSES	NURSING INTERVENTIONS
Pain, related to fracture and/or trauma	During initial stages of treatment, administer prescribed narcotic and nonnarcotic analgesic in appropriate dosages at timely intervals. Administer prescribed agents, such as diazepam (Valium), to reduce muscle spasm. Apply ice compresses as ordered to affected part. Reposition patient frequently within restrictions of the prescribed treatment. Instruct patient how to use relaxation techniques (deep breathing and imagery) to reduce tension. As pain subsides, decrease the strength and/or frequency of analgesics.

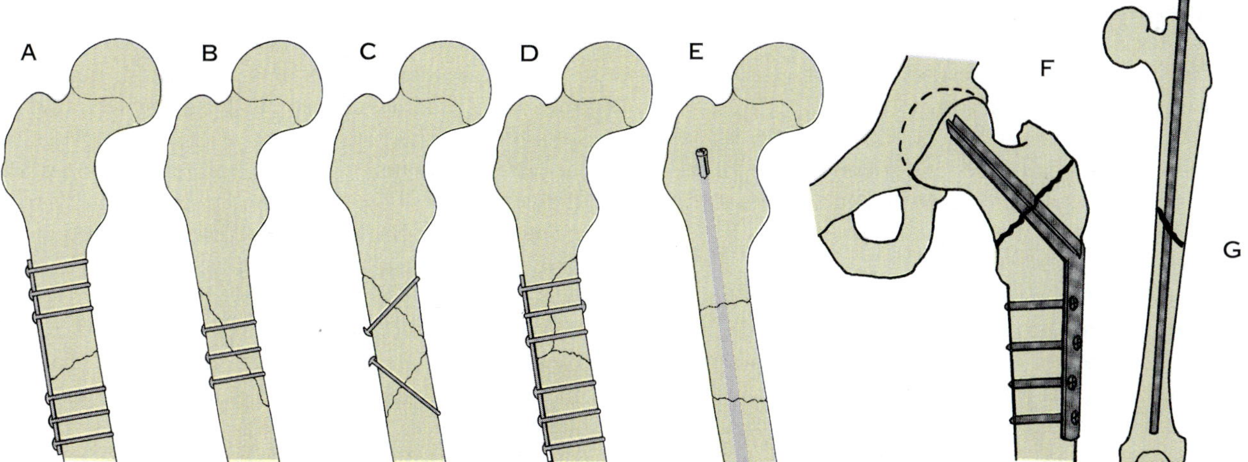

FIG. 26-22 Technique of internal fixation. **A,** Plate and six screws for transverse or short oblique fracture. **B,** Screws for long oblique or spiral fracture. **C,** Screws for long butterfly fragment. **D,** Plate and six screws for short butterfly fragment. **E,** Medullary nail for segmental fracture. **F,** Neufeld nail and screws, used in repair of intertrochanteric fracture. **G,** Küntscher nail (intramedullary rod) used in repair of midshaft femoral fracture.

NURSING DIAGNOSES	NURSING INTERVENTIONS
Mobility, impaired physical, related to injury	Allow and encourage the patient to move about to the greatest extent possible within the restrictions of the fracture reduction and the immobilizing devices. Encourage the patient to accomplish as much self-care as possible. Encourage the patient to perform muscle-toning (isometric) exercises on a regular basis, for example, quadriceps setting and gluteal setting. Encourage and assist the patient to follow through with exercise program (including ambulation) prescribed by the physician and taught by the physical therapist. Encourage and assist the patient to resume normal functioning of all ADLs (within limits of immobilization and fixation device) as soon as possible, for example, using bedside commode or toilet instead of bedpan.

Patient teaching. Patient teaching should include the following:

- How to move comfortably in bed
- How to transfer safely in and out of bed
- What weight-bearing restrictions to observe and for how long
- What activity limitations to observe and for how long
- How to properly use ambulatory assistive devices
- How to avoid edema in the affected part by proper elevation
- How to control pain or discomfort in the affected part
- What exercises to perform to maintain strength and enhance circulation
- Proper method to cleanse pins, using surgical asepsis per physician's protocol

Prognosis. The prognosis depends upon the age of the patient as well as systemic involvement. Generally the prognosis is favorable.

Fracture of the Hip.

Etiology/pathophysiology. Hip fractures are the most common type of fracture treated in the hospital. See the gerontological box for special consideration for the older adult. Women may be at a higher risk because of the potential for developing osteoporosis and because they have a longer life expectancy than men. Fractures of the hip include intracapsular fracture, when the femur is broken inside the joint, and include those of the femoral head or neck that are contained within the hip capsule (Fig. 26-23). Intracapsular fractures may disrupt the blood supply to the head of the femur, with subsequent development of avascular necrosis of the head of the femur (Fig. 26-24). Therefore, fractures of the head or proximal femoral neck may be treated with insertion of a femoral prosthesis (Fig. 26-25). The more common type of hip fracture is an extracapsular fracture, one that occurs outside the hip joint capsule. These are referred to as intertrochanteric or subtrochanteric fractures. These fractures heal well without vascular necrosis with the use of compression screws or nails because the blood supply to the fracture site comes from the surrounding vessels outside the capsule (Fig. 26-23). Side plates attached to the nails help maintain a stable reduction while healing progresses (Fig. 26-22). An intertrochanteric fracture occurs below the lesser trochanter and is frequently seen in younger patients suffering from hip trauma (see Fig. 26-23).

GERONTOLOGICAL CONSIDERATIONS

- Physiological changes of aging result in decreased joint flexibiity and muscular strength.
- Changes in bone mass, particularly in older women, increases the risk of fractures. Hip fractures and compression fractures of the spine are most common.
- Degeneratve joint disease related to "wear and tear" on joints is common. Joint replacement is increasingly common and has done much to improve mobility and the quality of life.
- Changes in the foot can occur from a lifetime of use, poorly fitted shoes, or heredity. Bunions and hammer toe are commonly seen in older adults. These may cause pain and lead to decreased mobility. Older adults should be encouraged to wear properly fitted shoes to reduce discomfort. If discomfort is severe, surgical correction may be necessary.
- The home of older adult should be checked for safety hazards such as rugs that could cause falls.
- Climbing unsteady or uneven surfaces should be avoided, since coordination and balance change with aging and falls may result.
- Older persons should be instructed in the correct use of assistive devices such as canes or walkers. They should be encouraged to use these regularly to prevent injury.

Clinical manifestations. Signs and symptoms of hip fracture are severe pain at the fracture site, inability to move the leg voluntarily, and shortening or external rotation of the leg.

Assessment. Collection of *subjective data* includes an accurate history of the events before the injury. It is important to assess the patient's level of orientation. Disorientation can occur, especially in older adults when they are in pain and anxious or are placed in an unfamiliar environment. The patient's medical and surgical history is significant, as well as any family history of bone disease. Signs and symptoms of a fracture will vary with

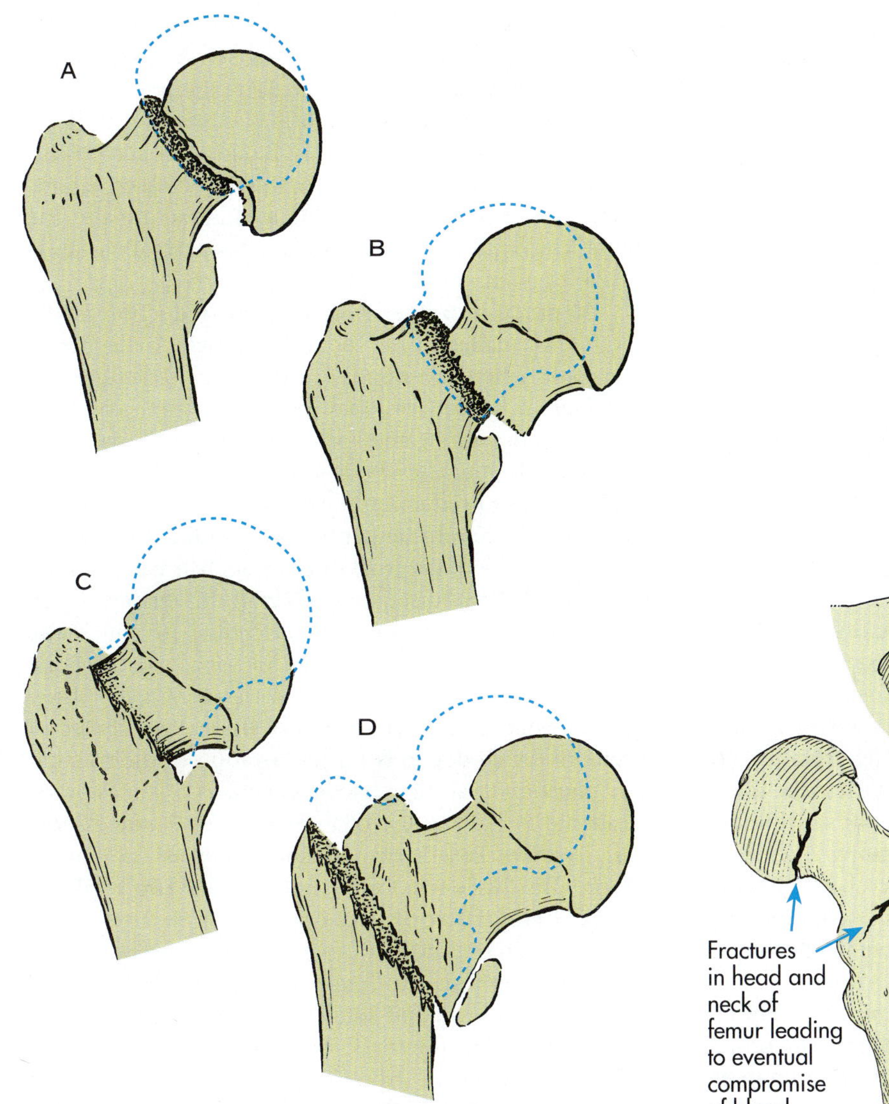

FIG. 26-23 Fractures of the hip. **A,** Subcapital fracture. **B,** Transcervical fracture. **D,** Impacted fracture of the base of the neck. **D,** Intertrochanteric fracture.

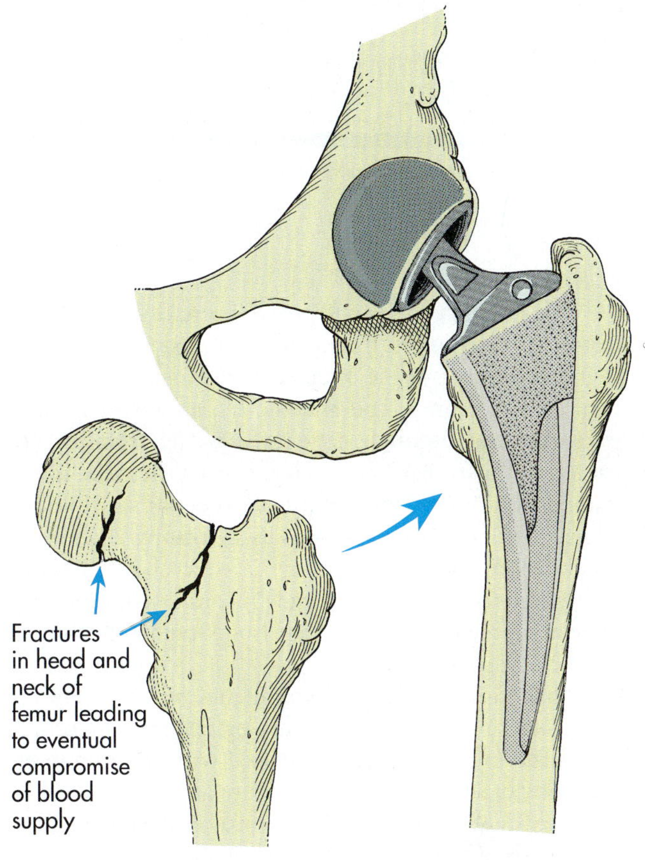

FIG. 26-25 Bipolar hip replacement (hemiarthroplasty).

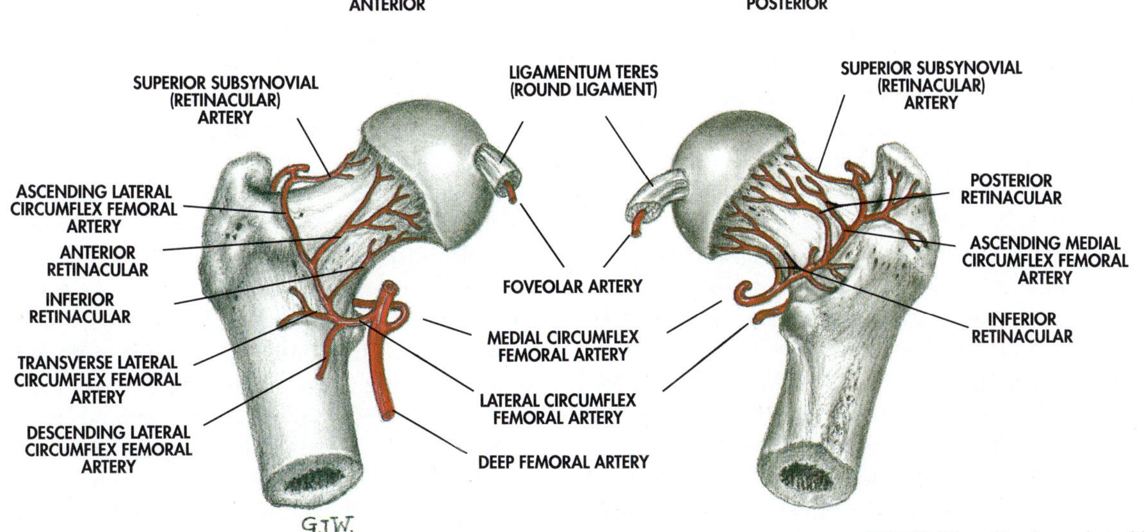

FIG. 26-24 Blood supply to hip joint.

Box 26-4 NEUROVASCULAR ASSESSMENT

Skin: coolness, pallor or cyanosis
Pulse: faintness or absence
Blanching test (capillary refill): color return within 2 seconds after pressure is released
Immobility: inability to move distal parts
Numbness or tingling: lack of relief after elevation of body part
Edema: present in varying degrees
Pain: lack of relief after elevation, administration of an analgesic, or repositioning
Sensation: decreased

Compare affected extremity with the unaffected extremity using the same hand for palpation.

the type and location of the break. There is usually some degree of discomfort. It may be more pronounced with slight movement of the affected part. Most patients will complain of pain in the affected leg after sustaining a fractured hip, although patients suffering from an impacted intracapsular fracture have very little pain, if any, immediately after the fracture. The nurse assesses edema, tenderness, muscle spasms, deformity, and loss of function. Patients may say they heard a "snap" or "pop" at the time the bone was injured. Impaired sensation may indicate nerve damage from the bone fragments "pinching" or severing the nerve.

Collection of *objective data* includes assessment for soft tissue injury with erythema or ecchymosis noted. When the injured limb is compared with the uninjured limb, obvious differences may be apparent. A change in the curvature or length of bone may indicate fracture. The nurse notes the affected leg is shorter, usually externally rotated about 90 degrees, and slightly flexed after an extracapsular hip fracture. With an intracapsular fracture the nurse notes the upper thigh is more edematous than the area below and the affected leg is shortened with external rotation. Subtrochanteric fractures cause excessive bleeding into the soft tissue, and the affected leg is shortened and rotated anteriorly. Crepitus may be felt or heard as the broken bone ends rub together. Neurovascular status of the extremity is assessed (Box 26-4). It is most important that the nurse keep the injured part at rest, because movement of a fractured bone can cause additional damage and may cause a closed fracture to become an open fracture. The data should also include an assessment of the patient's nutritional status. Both thin and obese patients are at risk for impaired skin integrity if bed rest is ordered. After the fracture is reduced, regular inspection of skin areas in contact with cast edges or traction apparatus to assess for signs of neurovascular compromise is necessary. It is also important for the nurse to note that patients suffering from any trauma are at risk for shock. Treating the shock takes precedence over treating the fracture.

Diagnostic tests. Diagnosis is confirmed by x-ray examination of the injured part. Blood tests, such as hemoglobin determination, often show decreased laboratory values because of bleeding at the fracture site; the blood glucose level may be elevated because of the stress of the trauma.

Medical management. Fracture reduction is the method of realigning the bone segments. This is necessary only when the bones are displaced. Fractures are reduced by closed or open reduction methods. Both methods are painful, and some type of anesthesia is recommended. Anesthesia also helps to relieve muscle spasms. Closed reduction involves the external manipulation of the bone fragments into position and the immobilization with external devices, such as casts, splints, or traction, as was discussed earlier in this chapter. Open reduction involves a surgical procedure in which the bone is exposed through a skin incision and the bone fragments are fixed in position with wires, nails, plates, screws, bolts, or a combination of these. The choice of fixation device depends on the location of the fracture and the potential for avascular necrosis of the femoral head and neck. The use of these devices is called *internal fixation.* Prosthetic implants, such as the Austin Moore prosthesis (Fig. 26-26) and **bipolar hip replacement (hemiarthroplasty)** (Fig. 26-25), are used to replace the femoral head and neck in fractures when the vascular supply to the femoral head may be compromised. Neufeld nail and screws are used in the repair of intertrochanteric fractures (Fig. 26-22, *F*). A Küntscher nail (intramedullary rod) is used to repair midshaft femoral fractures (Fig. 26-22, *G*). Sliding nails are used in repair of intertrochanteric fractures. Sliding nails usually permit the patient to bear weight to some degree, because they "give" slightly when subjected to weight-bearing forces without shifting their placement or penetrating the femur. Bone grafts, either autograft (patient's bone) or allograft (cadaver bone), may be used with internal fixation devices when excessive bone is lost at the fracture site. If a stable reduction cannot be achieved, the physician may do an arthroplasty (surgical reconstruction of a joint). Immobilization devices, such as casts or splints, may also be used with open reduction. An x-ray or fluoroscopic examination is needed to make an accurate diagnosis of a fracture.

Nursing interventions. Nursing intervention involves stabilizing the injured limb with a splint so that movement of the bone is limited. Open fracture will require cleansing and applying a sterile bandage to the altered skin site. Elevation of the splinted extremity will reduce edema. Tetanus immunization is given if a compound fracture is present. It is most important that the nurse remain calm and reassuring to the patient. The pa-

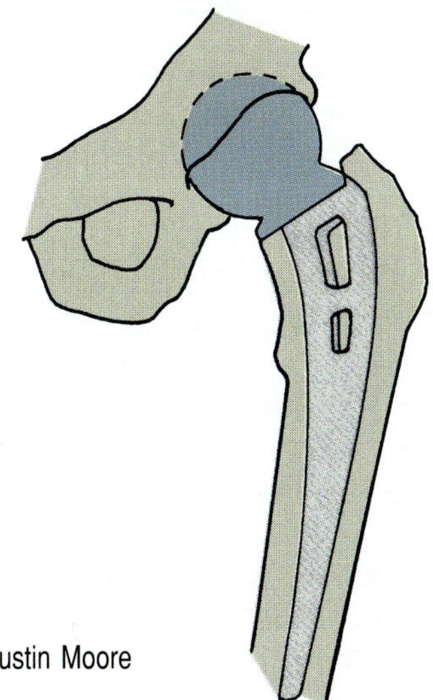

FIG. 26-26 Austin Moore prosthesis.

tient may fear severe impairment of mobility as a result of the fracture. Monitoring the vital signs at least q 4 hr will enable the nurse to detect signs of infection and shock. It is important to educate the patient to turn self (if able) frequently (q 2 hr) to prevent complications of bed rest. Encouraging the patient to help as much as possible can prevent a feeling of powerlessness. If the patient cannot manage, a turn schedule should be established (q 2 hr). Nursing intervention specific for fractured hip is concerned with prevention of shock and further complications. A major emphasis is placed on maintaining proper alignment through traction and abduction of the hip when turning a patient with a fractured hip from side to side. Some physicians do not want patients turned onto their sides for several days after surgery; others may order the patient to be turned only on the unoperated side. It is important to know what has been ordered. Educating patients about activity restrictions is most important. Patients who have had an internal fixation for a fractured hip should avoid elevating the affected extremity when sitting. The head of the bed is elevated a maximum of 45 degrees to avoid acute flexion of the hip and strain on the fixation device. Instructing the patient NOT to cross the legs is important, because crossing the legs can adduct the affected extremity and dislocate the hip.

The postoperative interventions for a patient with hip fracture repair include wound assessment with special attention to color, amount, and odor of exudate. Vital signs are assessed, as well as the suture line for approximation of skin edges and intact sutures or staples at least q 8 hr. Jackson-Pratt drainage tubes or Hemovacs are often used and must be assessed for amount and color of wound drainage at least q 4 hr. Accurate I&O findings are documented to help the physician establish the need for intravenous fluid therapy. The use of incentive spirometers is valuable in assisting the patient to perform adequate respiratory ventilation to prevent pneumonia. Turning and moving the patient on schedule will maintain skin integrity and promote circulation.

Leg manipulation during surgery and immobility afterward place the patient at risk for deep vein thrombosis and pulmonary embolism. Antiembolic stockings, Ace wraps, or pneumatic compression stockings (see Chapter 22) and foot and leg exercises increase venous flow to the heart. The stockings are removed once each shift to assess for compression points and skin integrity. Anticoagulation therapy with heparin, aspirin, or warfarin is often prescribed.

Special consideration should be taken in regard to patients who have had a prosthetic implant or bipolar hip replacement. Isometric exercises are done on the quadriceps and gluteal muscles to strengthen the muscles used for walking. Quadriceps strengthening is done 3 times a day by tensing the muscles around the knees for 5 seconds, repeating the exercise at least 9 times. Gluteal strengthening is done by tightening the muscles in the buttocks 10 times. It is important to have the patient strengthen the unaffected leg by pushing down against the footboard, holding for a count of five, releasing for a count of five, and repeating.

Nursing interventions also involve postoperative maintenance of leg abduction by using an abduction splint (a wedge-shaped foam bolster or pillow) for 7 to 10 days to prevent dislocation of the prosthesis. The abductor splint is placed between the patient's legs when in a supine position. Patients are turned with the extremities maintained in proper alignment. This can be accomplished by using the log-rolling procedure with the assistance of at least two nurses. A pillow is placed between the legs when turning the patient to maintain abduction of the legs and reduce the risk of dislocation of the prosthesis. Most physicians order the patient to be turned toward the unoperative side; the nurse should check each order by the physician. The patient is transferred from bed to chair on the unoperative side by pivoting on the unaffected leg. The injured leg is kept extended forward to avoid extreme hip flexion and possible dislocation of the prosthesis. Limit weight bearing on the hip by providing walking assists such as a walker or crutches. Provide a chair with a firm, nonreclining seat and arms; elevate the sitting surfaces as necessary with pillows or foam cushions to keep the angle of the hip within the prescribed limits when the patient is sitting.

In general, patients who have had *any* kind of internal fixation for a fractured hip should avoid elevation of the operated leg when sitting in a chair as this puts excessive strain on the fixation device.

Special considerations should be taken in regard to patients who have *internal fixation* with hip nails or pins related to hip modification in weight bearing.

- Assess ability to understand instructions and limitations.

NURSING CARE PLAN: THE PATIENT WITH A FRACTURED HIP

Mrs. Sharon Dunning, age 72, fell in her kitchen while removing cookies from the oven. She sustained a subcapital fracture of the right hip. Mrs. Dunning is scheduled in the morning for a bipolar (hemiarthroplasty) prosthesis.

Nursing diagnoses	Patient goals/expected outcomes	Nursing interventions
Tissue perfusion, altered, peripheral, related to vascular injury or interruption of arterial/venous flow secondary to edema	Patient's circulation will be maintained to fulfill body requirements.	Palpate site for warmth. Observe site for color. Apply moderate pressure to nail bed and subsequently observe speed of capillary refill. Assess pedal pulse bilaterally q 4 hr. Question patient regarding pain and paresthesia in injured part. Assist and teach patient to turn and cough q 2 hr and deep breathe q 1 hr. Apply antiembolic stockings as ordered. Monitor vital signs q 2-4 hr.
Pain, acute, related to loss of skeletal integrity and soft tissue trauma	Patient will express minimal discomfort or absence of pain.	Ask patient to rate pain/discomfort on a scale of 0-10 (0 = no pain/discomfort, 10 = worst pain). Help patient identify comfort measures that have worked in the past, such as analgesics, distraction, and relaxation. Convey acceptance of patient's report of discomfort by a willingness to provide comfort measures. Administer pain medications before activities/procedures. Offer position change, back rub, and relaxation techniques as supplements or alternatives to medication for pain relief. Provide care in an unhurried, supportive manner. Position patient toward unoperative side as ordered.
Mobility, impaired physical, related to neuromuscular/skeletal impairment, pain, and discomfort	Patient's mobility will be restored to optimal level.	Instruct and encourage the patient in active and/or passive ROM exercises to maintain or develop muscle strength and endurance. Instruct the patient in safe transfer from bed to wheelchair or commode; get patient up on noninjured side. Turn toward unoperative side. Instruct patient in correct body alignment. Encourage patient in use of trapeze. Praise efforts at mobility activities.

Skin integrity, impaired, related to immobility	Patient's skin integrity will be maintained clean, dry, and intact.	Identify early skin areas at risk, particularly areas over bony prominences (heels, sacrum, elbows, and ischial tuberosities). Regularly inspect (at least q 4 hr) for signs of pressure (for example, erythema or induration). Regularly turn (at least q 2 hr) within limits of fracture immobilization. Use sheep skin pads, flotation pads, EggCrate mattress, Clinitron, or CircOelectric bed. Assist patient to keep skin clean and dry. Massage skin with lotion q 2-4 hr. Encourage nutritious diet to maintain skin integrity.
Knowledge deficit, related to home care management	Patient and/or significant other will demonstrate understanding of home care and follow-up instructions through interactive discussion and actual return demonstration.	Stress importance of prescribed rehabilitation plan of activity, rest, and exercise. Provide diet instructions as to type and amount, and to avoid weight gain if applicable. Discuss medications: name, purpose, schedule, dosage, and side effects. Discuss signs and symptoms to report to physician: severe pain, changes in temperature, color, or sensation in extremity, malodorous drainage from wound. Stress home safety factors such as throw rugs, use of safety bars on the bathtub, elevated toilet seats. Encourage follow-up visits with physician.

CRITICAL THINKING QUESTIONS

1. The first postoperative evening, Mrs. Dunning is restless and disoriented. The nursing interventions needed to prevent dislocation of her bipolar hip prothesis would include:
2. Mrs. Dunning is in her third postoperative day, and the nurse notes an erythematous area on her coccyx. Therapeutic measures to prevent skin impairment are:
3. On Mrs. Dunning's fifth postoperative day, she complains of pain in her right calf when the nurse performs dorsiflexion. The most appropriate immediate action by the nurse would be:

- Assist to dangle at bedside on first postoperative day, then to pivot to chair with no weight on operative leg, or touch-down weight if allowed.
- Stress that operative foot should be placed on floor but weight should be borne on unoperative leg (refer to limb as either left or right leg so patient has a clear understanding) *to maintain safety in care.*
- Turn every 2 hours; prop with pillows between legs or back *to maintain position.*
- Assist with ROM exercises *to maintain muscle strength.*
- Help physical therapist walk patient with walker and limited weight to operative limb (if assistance is needed) *for comfort and safety.*
- Encourage patient and family members to walk together *for patient's safety.* Instruct family about weight-bearing techniques *for clarity and safety.*

A nursing care plan for the patient with a fractured hip is presented on pp. 614-615.

Patient teaching for hip prosthetic implant. Activity is restricted according to the fractured hip fixation device used. If a patient has a *hip prosthetic implant,* teaching includes the following:

- to avoid hip flexion beyond 60 degrees for approximately 10 days
- to avoid hip flexion beyond 90 degrees for 2 to 3 months
- to avoid adduction of the affected leg beyond midline for 2 to 3 months
- to maintain partial weight-bearing status for approximately 2 to 3 months
- to avoid positioning on the operative side in bed
- to maintain abduction of the hip by using a wedge-shaped foam bolster or pillows arranged in a wedge; this will require nursing assistance
- to see the "do not" instruction sheet for patient with hip prosthetic implant (Fig. 26-27).

Patient teaching for ORIF.

- If a stable plate and screw fixation is used to repair the fractured hip, the patient should not bear weight for 6 weeks to 3 months, to protect the fracture site.
- A telescoping nail fixation allows minimal to partial weight bearing during the first 6 weeks to 3 months.

Prognosis. Complications of hip fractures are the most common cause of death after the age of 75. Hip fractures in older adults are often complicated by the presence of other medical conditions such as diabetes mellitus; cardiac problems (e.g., congestive heart failure); and neurological disorders (e.g., cerebral vascular accidents).

A large bone such as the hip heals slowly in older patients, and this predisposes them to various complications. They are at high risk for pneumonia, deep vein

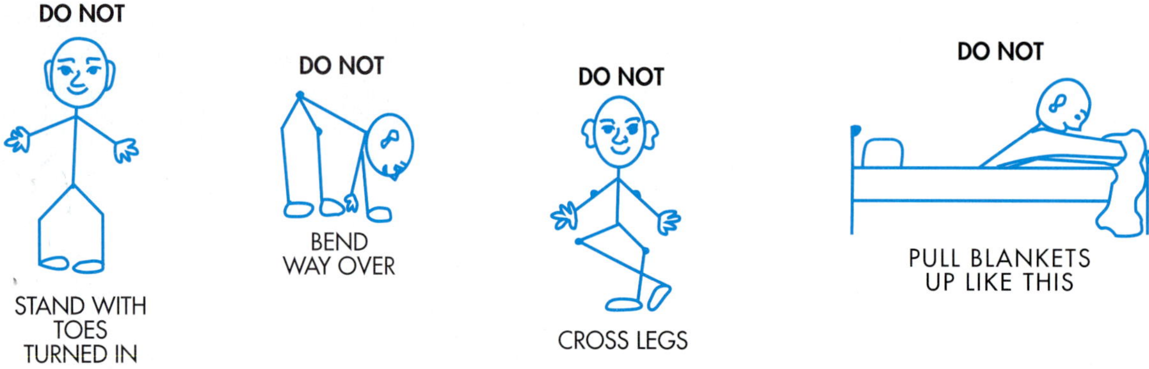
DO NOT
STAND WITH TOES TURNED IN
DO NOT
BEND WAY OVER
DO NOT
CROSS LEGS
DO NOT
PULL BLANKETS UP LIKE THIS

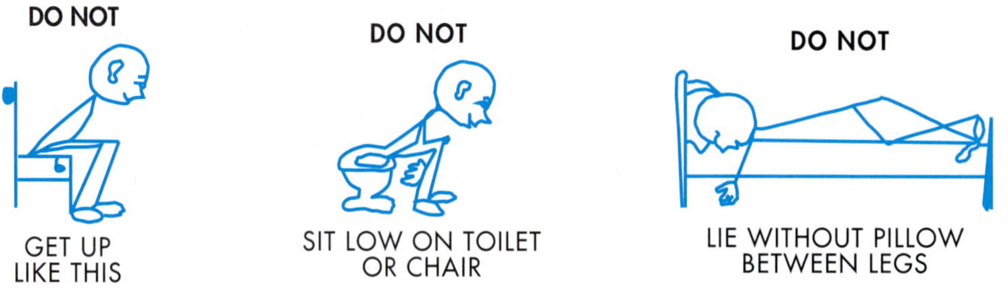
DO NOT
GET UP LIKE THIS
DO NOT
SIT LOW ON TOILET OR CHAIR
DO NOT
LIE WITHOUT PILLOW BETWEEN LEGS

FIG. 26-27 Instruction sheet for patient with bipolar hip replacement.

thrombosis, fat embolus, pulmonary embolus, decubitus ulcers, urinary retention, constipation, mental disorientation, and depression.

Fracture of the Vertebrae.

Etiology/pathophysiology. Injuries such as diving accidents or blows to the head or body can result in fractures of the vertebrae. Patients with osteoporosis and metastatic cancer are at risk for vertebral fractures. Motorcycle and car accidents (especially head-on collisions) occur more frequently with young men (ages 16 to 30 years).

Fractures of the vertebrae may involve the vertebral body, lamina, and articulating processes and may occur with or without displacement. If the fracture has displaced the vertebral structures, pressure may be placed on spinal nerves. The sharp bone fragments may also sever the spinal cord nerves, causing permanent paralysis from the point of injury downward.

Clinical manifestations. Signs and symptoms of vertebral fracture include the following:

1. Pain at site of injury
2. Partial or complete loss of mobility or sensation below level of injury
3. Evidence of fracture/fracture dislocation on routine x-ray examination, myelography, and/or CAT scans.

Assessment. Collection of *subjective data* includes assessment for pain (if fracture has altered the spinal cord, pain may not be present), numbness, tingling, and inability to move extremities from below the level of the trauma site.

Collection of *objective data* involves careful assessment of neurological function, such as pupillary reaction to light, hand grip, ability to move extremities, level of orientation, vital signs, and reaction to painful stimulation (see Chapter 35). The nurse should observe for fecal and urinary retention. The nurse should observe for signs of hemorrhage, such as hypotension, tachycardia, tachypnea, and decreased renal functioning. The continuity of traction (e.g., weights hanging free and ropes not twisted) and skin integrity (e.g., erythema, tenderness, and edema) as well as surrounding traction equipment should be assessed.

Diagnostic tests. X-ray studies are done to determine if there is compression of the vertebral bodies. A spinal cord injury may result from a fracture or dislocation of a vertebra, and if this is suspected, the physician performs a spinal tap for evaluation of the spinal fluid (presence of blood indicates trauma). Spinal fluid is normally clear in color (see Chapter 35).

Medical management. Stable injuries to the vertebrae (that are not a threat to spinal cord integrity) are treated with pain medication and muscle relaxants. Anticoagulant therapy may be ordered as a prophylaxis for thromboembolic complications. Maintaining erect posture can be enhanced by the use of a back support, corset brace, or a cast. The patient may be allowed to ambulate with assistance (gait enhancers) when discomfort subsides.

Unstable fractures that involve a degree of displacement are more serious, and treatment is aimed at fracture reduction. The fracture may be reduced by postural positioning and traction. Cranial skeletal traction is used with cervical spine fractures (see Chapter 35). A halo brace (Fig. 26-28), an external immobilization device in

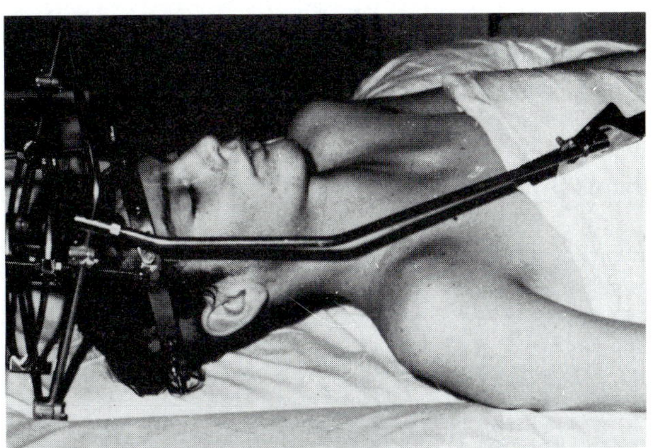
A

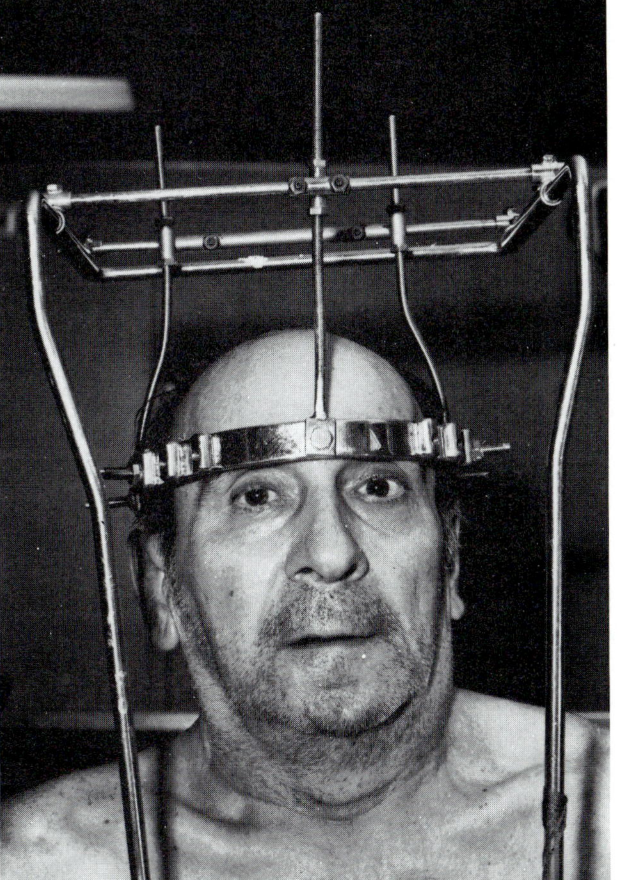
B

FIG. 26-28 **A,** Halo attached to body cast. Metal strut will be anchored firmly into body cast with additional plaster. **B,** Metal ring, or halo, that attaches to skull.

which a plaster or plastic brace that incorporates metal struts attached to pins is inserted into bone, is used to allow mobility of the patient. Pelvic traction is used for lumbar spinal fractures. An open reduction may be necessary with internal fixation using a Harrington rod. After this surgical procedure the patient is placed in a body cast. A laminectomy may be necessary.

Nursing interventions. Nursing intervention is aimed at maintaining the stability of the fracture fixation by (1) log rolling the patient for position changes; (2) following the correct procedure for turning a patient in a special bed, such as a Stryker frame or Foster bed; (3) elevating the head of the bed no more than 30 degrees; and (4) using mobilization devices for the head and back.

Nursing diagnoses and interventions for the patient with a vertebral fracture include but are not limited to the following:

NURSING DIAGNOSES	NURSING INTERVENTIONS
Powerlessness, related to decreased mobility/pain	Use active listening, and permit verbalization of anger and helplessness. Assist patient with identifying coping mechanisms that will reduce feeling of powerlessness; use those that have been successful in past. Offer positive recognition for increased activity level. Assist patient in identifying areas over which he has control. Involve patient in decision-making process for own care.
Infection, high risk for, related to immobility and/or surgical intervention	Monitor patient for signs and symptoms of infection (elevated temperature, increased pulse rate, malodorous exudate, erythema, cloudy urine, diminished breath sounds, and presence of crackles and wheezes). Monitor laboratory values, such as CBC, and blood and wound cultures. Protect patient from cross-contamination by practicing good handwashing techniques, maintaining surgical asepsis when changing dressings, and using strict surgical asepsis with catheter care. Encourage coughing, deep breathing, and leg exercises. Prevent persons with infectious processes from contact with patient.
Mobility, impaired physical, related to neuromuscular/skeletal impairment, pain, and discomfort	Maintain bed rest in correct body alignment; avoid lifting or twisting body. Place patient in immobilization device as ordered, such as cervical head halter, skeletal traction, Stryker frame, or CircOlectric bed; maintain cervical spine in extension. Assess neurovascular status q 2 hr; monitor pulse, color, temperature, sensation, and mobility of all extremities.

NURSING DIAGNOSES	NURSING INTERVENTIONS
Mobility, impaired physical, related to neuromuscular/skeletal impairment, pain, and discomfort—cont'd	Perform passive or assist with and teach active ROM exercises for all extremities q 2 hr. As fracture heals, traction is replaced with cast. Ambulate with assistance when ordered; monitor for vertigo and weakness; progress slowly.
Breathing pattern ineffective, related to location of fracture and inactivity	Assess respiratory status q 2 hr; observe for dyspnea, cyanosis, and decreased breath sounds. Auscultate chest for breath sounds q 2 hr. Provide incentive spirometer. Reposition patient q 2 hr.
Fluid volume deficit, high risk for, related to decrease of fluid intake and trauma	Monitor parenteral fluids as ordered. Monitor vital signs q 2 to 4 hr. Measure intake and output q 8 hr; observe urine output for suppression or retention. Encourage oral fluids. Auscultate bowel sounds q 4 hr; monitor for diminished sounds.

Patient teaching. Patient teaching involves teaching the patient to support the back by (1) using a firm mattress; (2) sitting in straight, firm chairs (for no longer than 20 to 30 minutes), when allowed; (3) using proper lifting techniques (using the leg muscles, not the back); and (4) doing back exercises to strengthen spinal extensor muscles.

Prognosis. Stable injuries to the vertebrae that are not a threat to spinal cord integrity have an excellent prognosis with full recovery. Unstable fractures are more serious, and prognosis is guarded when spinal cord injury is involved.

Fracture of the Pelvis.

Etiology/pathophysiology. Most pelvic fractures result from trauma involving great force, such as falls from extreme heights, automobile accidents, or crushing accidents.

When trauma is severe enough to fracture the pelvis, vital abdominal organs may also be damaged, such as the bladder, vagina, uterus, liver, spleen, intestines, or kidneys. Because the pelvis has a rich blood supply, a fracture of the pelvis can result in extensive blood loss (as much as 2 to 8 pints).

Clinical manifestations. The patient with a fractured pelvis will be unable to bear weight without discomfort. Local tenderness and edema are common at the trauma site. Hematuria (blood in the urine) may result from trauma to the bladder. Hemorrhage is by far the most life-threatening complication to a patient with a pelvic fracture.

Assessment. Collection of *subjective data* involves complaints of pelvic pain or tenderness and backache. Complaints of restlessness, anxiety, and progressive disorientation may indicate signs of shock.

Collection of *objective data* involves assessment of muscle spasms in the pelvic region; ecchymosis over the pelvis, perineum, groin, or suprapubic area; inability to raise the legs when supine; and external foot rotation on the affected side with noticeable shortening of one leg. Vital sign assessment may indicate shock (hypotension, tachycardia, tachypnea, oliguria, and diaphoresis). Careful observation for fat embolism syndrome (FES) is especially pertinent for patients with pelvic fractures. Assessing bowel sounds in all four quadrants and documenting the findings is important; large bowel and rectal lacerations are possible in patients with pelvic fractures. Assessing color and amount of urine output is necessary because of the possibility of laceration of the bladder.

Diagnostic tests. Abdominal x-ray studies are done in the supine and lateral positions. Computed tomography provides an evaluation of both the bony pelvis and intraabdominal contents. Intravenous pyelogram is performed to determine kidney damage. Interpretation of laboratory values for hemoglobin, hematocrit, urinalysis, and stool for occult blood helps determine if the patient is bleeding and if anemia is present.

Medical management. The patient often remains on bed rest for 3 weeks and then walk with crutches for about 6 weeks. If the patient has a symphysis pubis fracture and an iliac fracture on the same side, the physician will perform surgery. After surgery skeletal traction is applied for about 6 weeks to maintain the leg's position. When traction is released, the patient may ambulate without weight bearing for about 3 months. For a bilateral fracture of the pelvis, the physician may order a pelvic sling to support the fracture. To treat severe fractures that totally disrupt the pelvic ring and dislocate the sacroiliac joints, the physician may apply an external skeletal fixation device. He may also apply a spica or body cast to support the fracture.

Nursing interventions. Nursing intervention involves monitoring the patient for signs of progressive shock (hypotension, tachycardia, tachypnea, and decreased urinary output). Measuring the abdominal girth for signs of increased abdominal pressure that could result from internal hemorrhaging is done at least q 8 hr. I&O are accurately monitored for signs of hypovolemia, laceration of the bladder, and potential kidney trauma. A Foley catheter is inserted for monitoring of urine output and color. Nursing interventions appropriate for impaired mobility, impaired skin integrity, fluid volume deficit, and pain management are implemented.

A nursing diagnosis and interventions for the patient with a pelvic fracture include but are not limited to the following:

NURSING DIAGNOSIS	NURSING INTERVENTIONS
Tissue perfusion, altered, peripheral, high risk for, related to hemorrhage, hypovolemia, and/or shock.	Assess for ecchymosis over pelvis and perineum. Monitor vital signs q 15 min for evidence of shock until stable. Insert Foley catheter per physician's order to monitor color and amount of urine output. Monitor parenteral fluids per physician's order. Provide quiet, therapeutic environment. Administer oxygen per physician's order. Maintain bed rest per physician's order. Monitor bowel sounds and measure abdominal girth to ascertain possible lacerated bowel.

Patient teaching. The nurse reinforces the reasons for immobility and not bearing full weight; anxiety may prevent the patient from hearing or understanding initial explations. The nurse also explains measures for dealing with acute pain and changes in using medications as pain decreases. In addition, turning and moving techniques to prevent skin impairment are explained.

Prognosis. Hemorrhage is by far the most life-threatening complication. The long-term prognosis is dependent upon the severity of the fracture, the age of the patient, and the presence of other systemic disorders.

Complications of Fractures

Compartment Syndrome.

Compartment syndrome is a pathologic condition caused by the progressive development of arterial vessel compression and reduced blood supply to an extremity. Fractures of the forearm or tibia usually precede the onset of muscle edema within the fasciae, which form compartments for the muscles of the forearm and lower leg. When there is severe trauma, such as fractures, or compression of blood vessels as a result of a tight cast or dressing, muscle ischemia (decreased blood supply to the muscles) can occur. Irreversible muscle ischemia can occur within 6 hours as a result of compression of the arteries, nerves, and tendons entering the compartment. Paralysis and sensory loss follow, with contracture and permanent disability of the extremity seen within 24 to 48 hours.

Assessment. Collection of *subjective data* includes pain assessment. Usually the patient will complain of sharp pain, which increases with passive movement of the hand or foot. The patient experiences deep, unrelenting, progressive, and poorly localized pain unrelieved by analgesics or elevation of the extremity. Numbness or tingling in the affected extremity is common.

Collection of *objective data* involves assessment of the patient's inability to flex the fingers or toes, coolness of the extremity, and absence of pulsation in the affected extremity. Assessment of skin color for signs of pallor or cyanosis is made. Gentle palpation of the extremity will reveal slowing of the capillary refilling time (blanching). Close monitoring and proper documentation of vital signs are essential (especially temperature to detect signs of tissue necrosis) (see Box 26-4).

Medical management. The majority of these cases require a fasciotomy (incision into the fascia) to relieve pressure and allow return of normal blood flow to the area. This will be done immediately (within 30 minutes). The incision is often left open to heal by granulation (healing by second intention).

Nursing interventions. Nursing intervention includes administration of analgesics with careful documentation of relief obtained. To slow further circulatory compromise, the affected limb can be elevated, but no higher than heart level, to maintain arterial pressure. Application of cold packs and removal of any constricting material, such as an elastic bandage, are necessary. The most common complication when decompression is delayed is infection as a result of tissue necrosis. Purulent drainage from the dressing is a sign of infection and must be reported immediately. If drainage and secretion isolation are required, careful instructions should be given to the patient, who may feel isolated. Patients are encouraged to express their fears and emotional needs to the nurse. **Volkmann's contracture** is a permanent contracture (with clawhand, flexion of wrist and fingers, and atrophy of the forearm) that can occur as a result of compartment syndrome. Proper positioning and alignment can reduce the risk of this complication.

Prognosis. Compartment syndrome can result in a permanent contracture deformity of the hand or foot.

Shock. Shock can occur as a result of blood loss from a fractured bone (bone is vascular) or from severed blood vessels, seen especially in compound fractures. Pain and fear can also cause shock.

Assessment. Collection of *subjective data* includes monitoring the patient's level of consciousness. Restlessness or complaints of anxiety may suggest a decrease in cerebral perfusion, resulting in brain hypoxia. Complaints of weakness and lethargy are common.

Collection of *objective data* includes monitoring vital signs. Typical shock signs include hypotension, tachycardia, and tachypnea. As shock progresses, hypothermia will occur. There may be pallor and cool, moist skin. Oliguria (diminished urinary output) is present with shock.

Medical management. The physician's main concern will be to restore blood volume so that there can be a rapid return of oxygen to the tissues. Blood volume can be expanded with intravenous (IV) fluids (lactated Ringer's solution of 5% dextrose in saline). Whole blood, plasma, and plasma substitutes may also be given. Respiratory assistance may be given by administering oxygen. A central venous catheter may be inserted for accurate monitoring of vital signs to prevent pulmonary edema. Shock trousers may be applied. These are pneumatic trousers designed to counteract hypotension associated with internal or external bleeding and hypovolemia.

Nursing interventions. Nursing intervention includes the nurse's responsibilities in IV fluid administration. These include checking (1) the contents and IV flow rate against the physician's orders and (2) the infusion site for signs of infiltration (erythema, edema, pain, and induration [hardening of tissue]). The patient's vital signs are monitored q 15 minutes until stable. Urinary output is monitored q 1 hr. Less than 30 ml of urine per hour is indicative of decreased renal perfusion. The patient should remain flat in bed. If there are no head injuries, the lower extremities can be raised slightly to improve venous return. The Trendelenburg position should be avoided, because it tends to push the abdominal organs against the diaphragm, reducing the effectiveness of heart and lung functions. The patient must be kept warm, but external heat should be avoided. Nothing should be given by mouth, and sedatives, tranquilizers, and narcotics should be avoided. The nurse should be aware of the anxieties of the patient's family and provide them with brief explanations of the patient's condition.

Prognosis. Shock can be fatal within a few hours after injury, so immediate attention is required.

Fat Embolism. Pulmonary fat embolism syndrome involves the embolization of tissue fat with platelets and circulating free fatty acids within the pulmonary capillaries. Fat embolism is rare, but if it occurs, it can be life threatening because the fat droplets can effectively occlude capillaries of the pulmonary circulation, causing brain hypoxia and tissue death. Fat embolism should be suspected if the patient has multiple fractures or fractures of long bones and pelvis. The onset may occur within 48 hours of the injuries. Pulmonary fat embolism syndrome is the most serious complication of long bone fractures.

Assessment. Collection of *subjective data* includes assessment of mental disturbances, such as irritability, restlessness, disorientation, stupor, and coma. These symptoms can result from effects of severe hypoxemia. There may be complaints of chest pain, especially on inspiration, and complaints of localized muscle weakness, spasticity, and rigidity.

Collection of *objective data* includes assessing for tachypnea, dyspnea, hypoxemia, and auditory crackles and wheezes in the lung field. As the lung filters and traps embolic material, ventilation is disturbed. Assessment of the apical pulse is performed to detect dysrhythmias. Patients will be placed on cardiac monitoring for observation of dysrhythmias and cardiovascular collapse.

The nurse assesses the patient for petechiae (especially in the buccal membranes, conjunctival sacs, hard palate, chest, and anterior axillary folds) caused by occlusion of capillaries.

Diagnostic tests. The diagnosis is made on clinical signs and symptoms. These occur within 24 to 48 hours of injury. Blood gases are indicative of hypoxemia. Hemoglobin and hematocrit laboratory values are decreased. Fat will be present in the blood and urine. The sedimentation rate is increased, and the platelet count is decreased.

Medical management. The physician will order the administration of intravenous fluids to prevent shock and dilute free fatty acids. Steroid therapy is recommended to counteract the inflammatory response to the free fatty acids. Digoxin is often ordered to increase the patient's cardiac output. Oxygen will be administered if the Po_2 is below 70 mm Hg. Incentive spirometry is ordered to improve lung expansion and oxygenation.

Nursing interventions. Nursing intervention includes close monitoring of the patient's blood gases. Normal values include the following:

pH	7.35 to 7.45 mm Hg
Pco_2	35 to 45 mm Hg
Po_2	80 to 100 mm Hg
Sao_2	95% to 100%

Arterial hypoxia is present with fat emboli and may not be recognized clinically. If hypoxia is present, the physician will order the administration of oxygen. It is important for the nurse to check the liter flow of oxygen and educate patients and their families as to safety precautions necessary when oxygen is administered (e.g., no smoking or use of electrical equipment). Respiratory failure is the most common cause of death. Careful stabilization and immobilization of long bone fractures is an importance step in preventing fat embolism syndrome. Careful support when turning and positioning the patient can prevent the manipulation of the fracture and reduce the risk of fat embolism syndrome. An accurate record of intake, output, and daily weights is essential to monitor fluid balance.

Prognosis. Fat embolism syndrome can be life threatening.

Gas Gangrene. Gas gangrene is a severe infection of the skeletal muscle caused by gram-positive *Clostridium* bacteria, particularly *C. perfringens,* which may occur in the presence of compound fractures and lacerated wounds. These injuries can produce exotoxins that destroy tissue. The onset is usually sudden and may occur 1 to 14 days after injury. These organisms are anaerobic (grow and function without oxygen) and spore formers. They are normally found in soil and the intestinal tract of humans. As the clostridia bacteria invade devitalized tissue (especially where blood supply is diminished), they multiply and produce toxins that cause (1) hemolysis (breakdown of red blood cells and release of hemoglobin), (2) vessel thrombosis, and (3) damage to the myocardium, liver, and kidneys.

Assessment. Collection of *subjective data* includes observation of pain, which is usually sudden and severe at the site of the injury. A characteristic finding is toxic delirium.

Collection of *objective data* includes careful inspection of the skin for gas bubbles, which may be seen at the site of the wound. The various species of clostridia bacteria produce a characteristic cellulitis, in which gas is present under the skin. This causes a crepitation (crackling sensation when the skin is touched). Signs of infection may be apparent with elevated temperature, tachycardia, tachypnea, and edema around the wound. The skin around the wound becomes necrotic and ruptures, revealing necrotic muscle. There will be a foul odor from the wound discharge, which is thin and watery. Careful documentation of the patient's progress relative to antibiotic therapy is made (e.g., decline in temperature and decrease in amount of wound drainage).

Medical management. Treatment of gas gangrene involves establishing a larger wound opening to admit air and promote drainage. Antibiotics, such as penicillin G or Keflin, will be ordered intravenously and must be administered as scheduled. The patient should be observed for adverse reactions.

Prognosis. If left untreated, gas gangrene is rapidly fatal. Prompt treatment, including excision of gangrenous tissue and administration of penicillin G intravenously, saves 80% of patients. If massive gangrene develops, amputation is necessary.

Nursing interventions. Nursing intervention includes wound care using strict medical asepsis. Spore-forming bacteria are not destroyed by ordinary disinfecting methods. Therefore all contaminated equipment and linens must be autoclaved. Drainage and secretion isolation procedures are necessary to prevent the spread of the infection to other patients.

Thromboembolus.

Etiology/pathophysiology. Thromboembolus is a condition in which a blood vessel is occluded by an embolus carried in the bloodstream from the site of formation of the clot. The person suffering from pelvic and hip fractures is at high risk for this complication.

Clinical manifestations. The area supplied by an obstructed artery may tingle and become cold, numb, and cyanotic. An embolus in the lungs causes a sudden, sharp thoracic or upper abdominal pain, dyspnea, cough, fever, and hemoptysis.

Assessment. Collection of *subjective data* includes careful investigation of the patient's complaints of pain in the lower extremities (especially the calf of the leg). A complaint of tenderness over the area is common. The patient may complain of a sharp pain in the thoracic area when an embolus is in the lung.

Collection of *objective data* includes assessing for a positive Homans' sign, which is indicative of thromboembolus. Homans' sign is pain in the calf of the affected leg upon dorsiflexion of the foot. The affected area may be erythematous, warm to touch, and edematous. The nurse will assess the patient for dyspnea and presence of blood in the sputum if pulmonary embolus is present. When anticoagulant therapy is ordered, the nurse will assess for signs of bleeding, such as petechiae, epistaxis, hematuria, hematemesis, and occult or gross blood in the stool.

Diagnostic tests. A complete history is taken and a physical examination is performed. In addition to checking Homans' sign, a prothrombin time and complete blood count are obtained.

Medical management. Treatment will include administration of anticoagulants, such as heparin or warfarin. A surgical procedure known as *thrombectomy* (removal of a thrombus from a blood vessel) may be done. Oxygen therapy may be administered for thromboembolism of the lung.

Nursing interventions. Nursing intervention involves caring for the patient on activity restriction. Many times this involves bed rest with the foot of the bed elevated to aid venous return. The nurse should teach the patient to do active exercise, such as dorsiflexion (pointing backward) and plantar flexion (pointing forward) of the toes, several times each hour. This exercise is effective in stimulating circulation to the legs. Continuous hot, moist compresses are usually ordered. Antiembolic stockings are ordered while the patient is on bed rest and are maintained even after the patient is ambulatory. Assessment of lung sounds every 4 hours is indicated. It is important that the nurse adhere to the activity ordered. If the patient is receiving anticoagulants, close monitoring of prothrombin and partial thromboplastin times is necessary.

Prognosis. Obstruction of the pulmonary artery or one of its branches may be fatal. A thrombus in an extremity usually resolves with treatment and a favorable prognosis is noted (Box 26-5).

Delayed Complications. Delayed complications deal with fracture healing. A *delayed union* is a fracture that fails to heal within the usual time for fracture healing. The healing is impaired but has not completely stopped and will eventually repair itself. *Nonunion* is failure of the ends of the fractured bone to unite. A nonunion fracture fails to unite and produce a stable union after 6 to 9 months. The calcification of cartilage and bone formation do not occur. Bone grafting, prosthetic implant, internal fixation, external fixation, or a combination of these methods can be used to correct the problem of delayed or nonunion bone fractures.

Box 26-5 NURSE ALERT

Never massage a patient's lower extremities. Thromboembolus can be present without clinical signs and symptoms.

Electrical stimulation is being used by physicians as a new method of treatment in promoting healing of nonunion fractures. The use of electrical probes on bone stimulates bone production.

Prognosis. Bone production and fracture healing depend on the age and general health of the patient. Presence of other systemic diseases complicates the healing process.

NONSURGICAL INTERVENTIONS

External Fixation Devices

External fixation devices are used to hold bone fragments in normal position. Casts, skeletal and skin traction, braces, and metal pins are examples of these devices.

Skeletal Pin External Fixation. One external fixation technique immobilizes fractures by the use of pins inserted through the bone and attached to a rigid external metal frame (Fig. 26-29). This technique is becoming more popular because it provides rigid support of comminuted open fractures, infected nonunions, and infected unstable joints. However, an advantage to having the fracture open to air is the visibility of the area and accessibility for wound care. The patient can use the muscles and joints above and below the fixation and experiences less discomfort.

This procedure is performed with the patient under general anesthesia. Patients need to be reassured that the pain after the insertion of the pins is minimal. Immediately after the procedure, the extremity is placed in balanced suspension traction to help relieve the edema. Pins that are inserted through the bone are assessed at least q 8 hr with careful observation of signs of infection and loose pins. Removing dried exudate from around the pins is done 1 to 2 times daily with hydrogen peroxide or alcohol, using surgical asepsis. Patients are permitted to ambulate on crutches when soft tissue edema is relieved. They are permitted to shower when the wounds have healed but must avoid salt or chlorinated water to prevent fixator corrosion.

Casts. Casts are immobilization devices made up of layers of plaster of paris, fiberglass, or plastic roller ban-

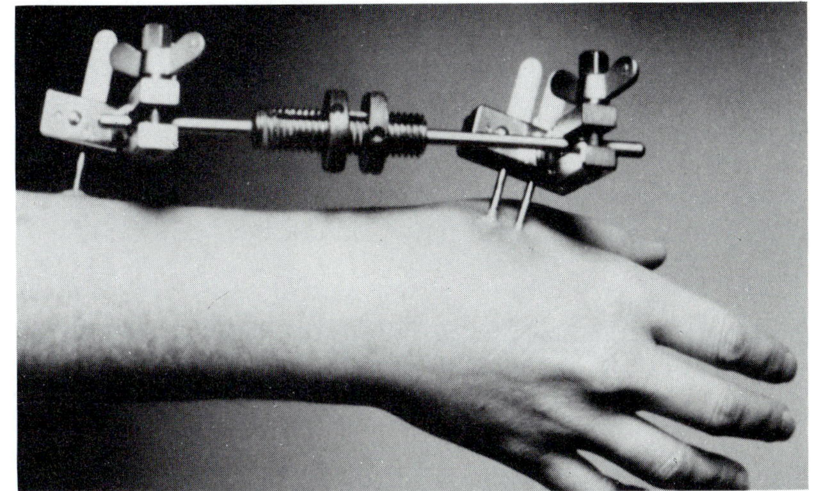

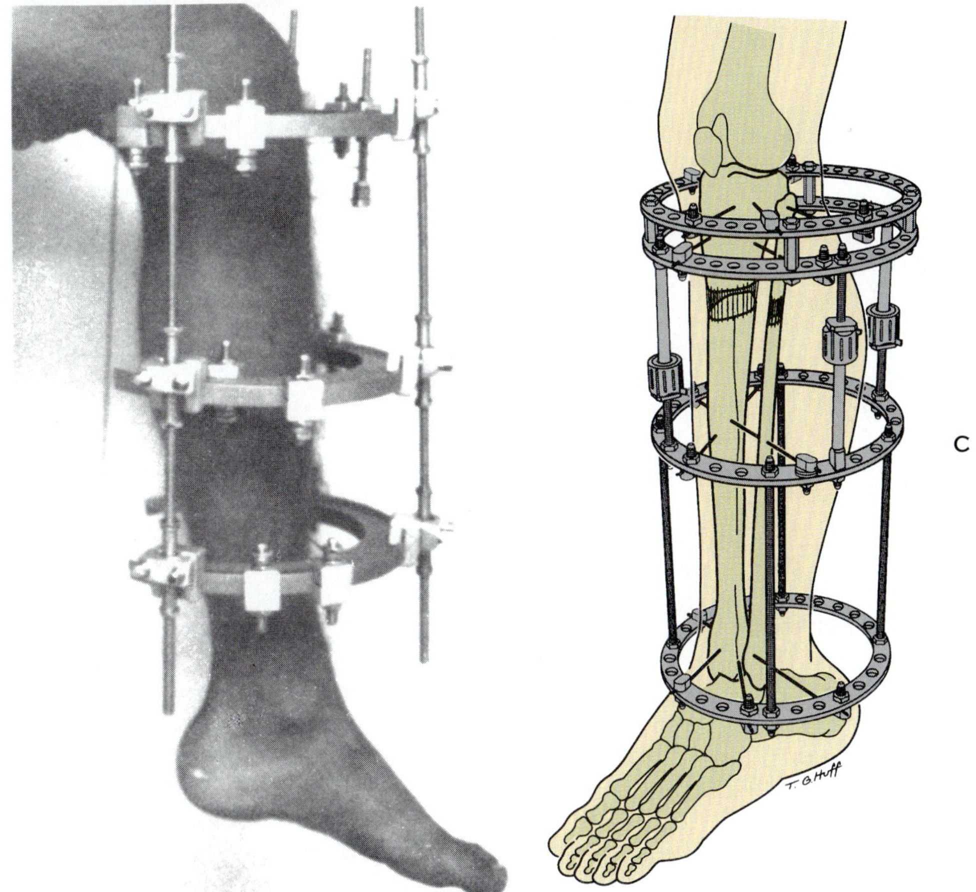

FIG. 26-29 External fixation apparatuses. **A,** Hoffman. **B,** The Monitcelli-Spinelli Circular Fixator. **C,** Ilizarov apparatus with corticotomies for lengthening lower leg.

dages. The application is similar to that for an elastic bandage. Types of casts are indicative of the part of the body immobilized. Examples include (1) short arm cast—extends from below the elbow to the proximal palmar crease; (2) long leg cast—extends from the upper thigh to the base of the toes; (3) spica cast or body cast—covers the trunk of the patient and one or both extremities (Fig. 26-30 on p. 624).

Casts are applied after the physician has properly aligned the bone through either external or internal fixation. Cast application is relatively painless except for the manipulation of the traumatized extremity. The casting procedure involves the application of a piece of Stockinette that covers the length of the extremity and area to be casted, followed by sheet wadding (pressed cotton that comes in rolled bandages), followed by the casting

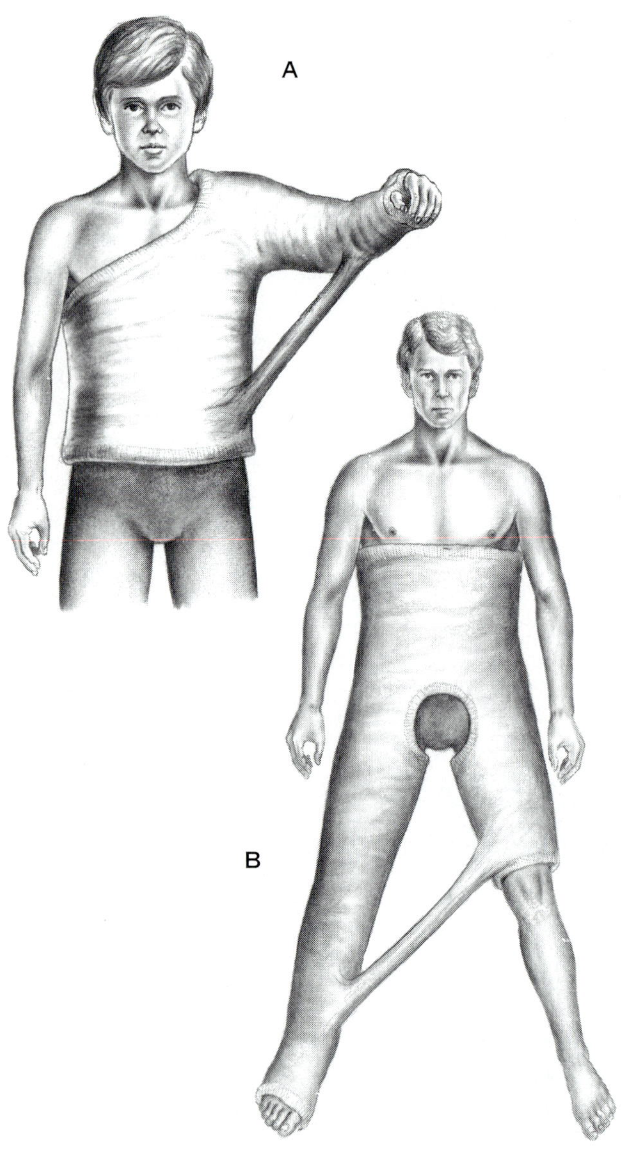

FIG. 26-30 Spica casts. **A,** Shoulder spica. **B,** One and one-half leg-hip spica.

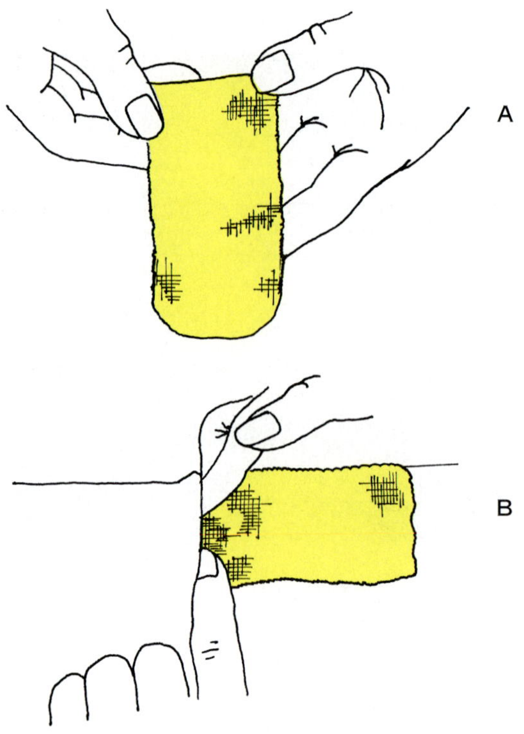

FIG. 26-31 Cast petaling. **A,** A petal is shaped from a strip of adhesive. **B,** The rounded edge of the petal is placed under the edge of the cast, and the opposite end is brought up over the edge of the cast.

material. Most physicians will bring the Stockinette up \and over the distal and proximal edge of the cast. It is important to assess these edges for rough pieces of casting that may irritate the skin. A nursing intervention to smooth out the rough edges is to "petal" the edges of the cast by placing pieces of adhesive tape (paper tape does not adhere as well as adhesive tape) cut in the shape of petals over the dried cast edges to provide a smooth surface (Fig. 26-31). Superficial burns can occur as the cast begins to set up, especially if the patient is not appropriately padded or too much fiberglass material is used.

Cast Brace. The cast brace is an alternative appliance to the traditional leg cast. It provides support and stability of the plaster cast, with additional support and mobility provided by a hinged brace. The appliance is most effective for fractures of the shaft of the femur and permits early ambulation and weight bearing. It is used approximately 2 to 6 weeks after fracture reduction.

Cast bracing is based on the concept that limited weight bearing helps promote the formation of bone. A problem encountered frequently with cast bracing is edema around the knee. Patients are instructed to elevate the leg when sitting to promote venous return. A cast shoe or walking heel incorporated into a lower extremity cast will permit weight bearing without damaging the cast (Fig. 26-32).

Assessment. Nursing assessment will be similar regardless of what kind of casting material is used. A neurovascular assessment is done q 15 to 30 minutes for several hours after casting and q 4 hr the first few days (see Box 26-4). The skin at the cast edges is observed for erythema and irritation. It is important to note any odor or drainage coming from under the cast and document the findings. Both of these signs indicate infection. The nurse should assess the patient's ability to use crutches using a three-point gait to establish normal gait and rhythm and should assess crutches for safety concerning proper fit and presence of large, rubber, suction tips on the ends.

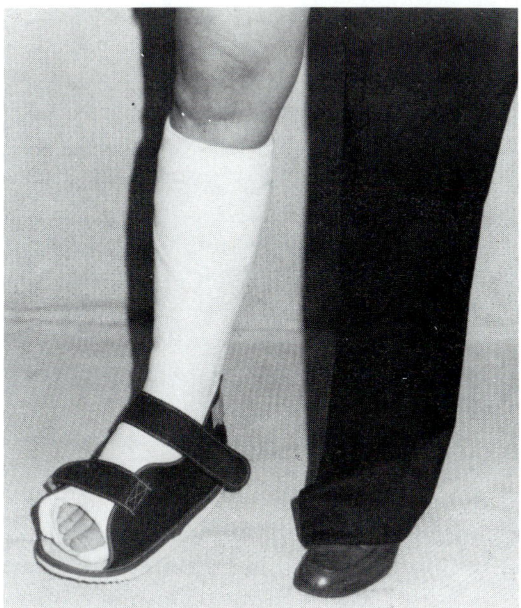

FIG. 26-32 Short leg walking cast with cast shoe.

Nursing interventions. Nursing intervention for the patient in a cast (Skill 26-1 on pp. 626-627) includes patient education concerning the prevention of infection, irritation, neurovascular pressure, and misalignment of bone ends. A wet cast must be handled gently and supported with the flat of the hand or on pillows to avoid indentations that will cause pressure on the skin and lead to skin impairment. Turning the patient frequently will aid the drying process. If a cast dryer is used, the setting should be on warm and never hot (drying a plaster of paris cast too quickly from the outside may weaken the cast). Elevating the casted extremity will reduce edema (usually elevation is recommended for 24 to 48 hours). Patients using crutches should be instructed to support their weight on the hands; weight borne on the axillae can damage the brachial plexus nerves (crutch paralysis).

Cast syndrome can occur after the application of a spica (body) cast (see Fig. 26-30, *A*) and involves acute obstruction of the duodenum. If symptoms of nausea occur, place the patient prone to relieve pressure symptoms and alert the charge nurse. Gastric decompression may be necessary, and if conventional measures fail, surgical intervention (duodenojejunostomy—making an opening into the small intestine) may be necessary.

Patient teaching. Patient teaching includes information about cleaning around the cast site with a mild soap and rinsing excessive soap so that it does not accumulate around the cast and impair the skin. A synthetic cast can be flushed with water if it becomes soiled. It must be dried afterward to prevent skin impairment and maceration (softening of the skin). Drying a synthetic cast can be accomplished by blotting it with a towel and then using a blow dryer on cool or warm setting in a sweeping motion across the cast. Proper drying may take as long as 1 hour.

Patients often complain of pruritus (itching) of the skin that is covered by a cast (especially after having the cast for a few weeks). The nurse can recommend diversional activities when the pruritus begins in addition to having the patient gently rub the area below and above the cast to retard the desire to scratch. It is important to warn patients not to stick sharp objects underneath the cast to relieve the pruritus. This may cause impairment of the skin, and serious complications can occur.

Cast Removal. Cast removal is done with an electric vibrating rather than cutting saw. Bivalving a cast may be done to relieve cast pressure. This involves splitting the cast down both sides and securing the cast pieces so that the extremity is supported (see Skill 26-1, Step 8a). Patients should be reassured that the saw poses very little risk to injuring the skin beneath the cast, even though it is noisy and has the appearance of a cutting saw. Cutting the cast can cause a very fine powder or dust to escape into the air. If this powder is inhaled over a period of time, the plaster deposits can build up in the lungs' small air sacs and cause respiratory distress. It is a safe practice for the nurse and the patient to wear a mask when casts are removed with a cast cutter.

After the removal of a cast, the buildup of secretions and dead skin on the affected extremity can be removed by gently washing and applying lotion or cream to the area. This may take several days, but the patient should be cautioned against trying to remove the devitalized material rapidly for fear of causing skin impairment. Muscle atrophy is common, especially if the extremity has been casted for several weeks. Patients should be reassured that the muscle will regain strength and size with proper exercise through either physical therapy or home exercise programs.

Traction. Traction is the process of putting an extremity, bone, or group of muscles under tension by means of weights and pulleys to (1) align and stabilize a fracture site by reducing the fractured part; (2) relieve pressure on nerves as in the case of herniated disk syndrome; (3) maintain correct positioning; (4) prevent deformities; and (5) relieve muscle spasms. The two general types of traction are skeletal and skin. Traction applied for the purpose of stabilizing a fracture will be continuous traction and must not be disconnected unless ordered by the physician. It will be easier to make the patient's bed from top to bottom when bed rest is maintained. Cervical and pelvic traction is sometimes ordered as intermittent traction to be applied as ordered by the physician.

Skeletal traction. Skeletal traction (Fig. 26-33 on p. 627) is applied directly to a bone. Wires and surgical pins are inserted through the bone distal to the fracture site while the patient is under local or general anesthesia.

SKILL 26-1

CARE OF THE PATIENT IN A CAST

1. Patient teaching
  a. Explain why the cast is being applied and how it will be applied
  b. Advise the patient that the plaster cast will feel warm as it dries
  c. Explain the extent of immobilization
  d. Explain care of the cast and expectations after discharge
  e. Instruct patient not to insert sharp objects (coat hangers or pencils) under the cast, because these may abrade the skin and lead to infection

2. Handling the new cast
(A fiberglass cast dries immediately after application; a plaster extremity cast dries in approximately 24-48 hr; a plaster spica or body cast dries in 48-72 hr [see Fig. 26-30].)
  a. Support wet cast with the flat of the hands or on pillows to avoid indentations that will cause pressure on underlying skin
  b. Place cotton blankets or other absorbent material under the cast to aid drying
  c. Expose the cast to air as much as possible to aid drying
  d. Turn the patient frequently to aid drying
  e. Use a cast dryer or hair dryer on a warm, not hot, setting to circulate air over the cast
  f. Do not apply paint, varnish, or shellac to the cast; plaster is a porous material that allows air to circulate to the skin

3. Skin care
  a. Inspect skin at edges of cast and underlying cast for erythema, skin impairment; apply petal-shaped strips of adhesive tape or moleskin around rough edges of cast (Fig. 26-31)
  b. Remove plaster crumbs from skin with a washcloth moistened with warm water
  c. Use creams and lotions sparingly as they may soften the skin and cause the cast to stick to the skin
  d. Apply waterproof material around perineal area to prevent soiling of and damage to cast and skin impairment
  e. Attend to patient's complaint of pain under the cast, particularly over bony prominences, because this may indicate pressure on the skin. If discomfort is not relieved by repositioning, report to physician. Cast pressure may need to be relieved by windowing or bivalving (cutting into halves)

4. Turning—turning to any position is generally permitted as long as the integrity of the cast is not compromised and the patient is comfortable. Do not turn by grasping the abductor bar

5. Toileting—for a long leg or hip spica cast
  a. Use a fracture pan with blanket roll or padding as support under the small of the back
  b. Elevate the head of the bed, if permitted, or place the bed in reverse Trendelenburg position

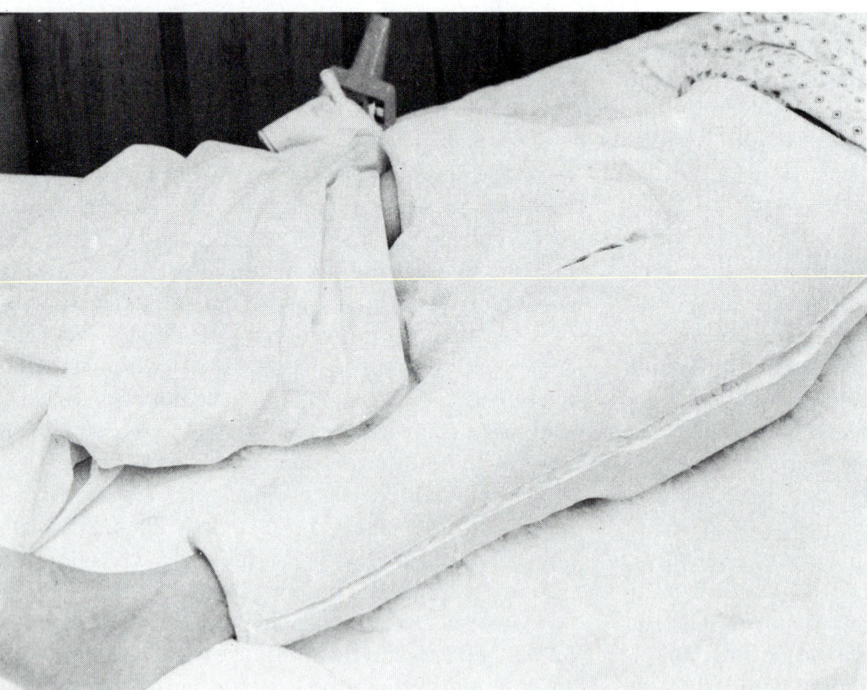

STEP 8a

CARE OF THE PATIENT IN A CAST—cont'd

6. Abdominal discomfort—cast may be "windowed" (an opening cut into it) to provide relief of abdominal distention or a port for checking bladder distention
7. Mobilization
   a. Weight bearing is at the discretion of the physician, and the amount of weight bearing will be prescribed
   b. A cast shoe or a walking heel incorporated into a lower extremity cast will permit weight bearing without damaging the cast (see Fig. 26-32)
8. Prevention of neurovascular problems (Establish baseline measurements and assess neurovascular status before cast application. Palpate distal pulses; assess color, temperature, and capillary refill of the appropriate fingers or toes; and assess neurological function, including sensation and motion in the affected and unaffected extremity.)
   a. Perform neurovascular checks every hour for at least 24 hours after cast application to detect difficulty from edema or pressure of cast on nerves or vessels. Notify physician of color changes, alterations in sensation, or motion unrelieved by position change. Cast may need to be bivalved (cut in two) to relieve pressure (see illustration)
   b. Elevate affected extremity on pillows until danger of edema is over (usually 24-48 hr)
   c. After mobilization of patient with lower extremity or upper extremity cast, avoid keeping extremity in dependent position for prolonged periods
   d. After lower extremity cast is removed, encourage patient to wear elastic stocking and elevate affected leg at rest until full mobility is regained

A

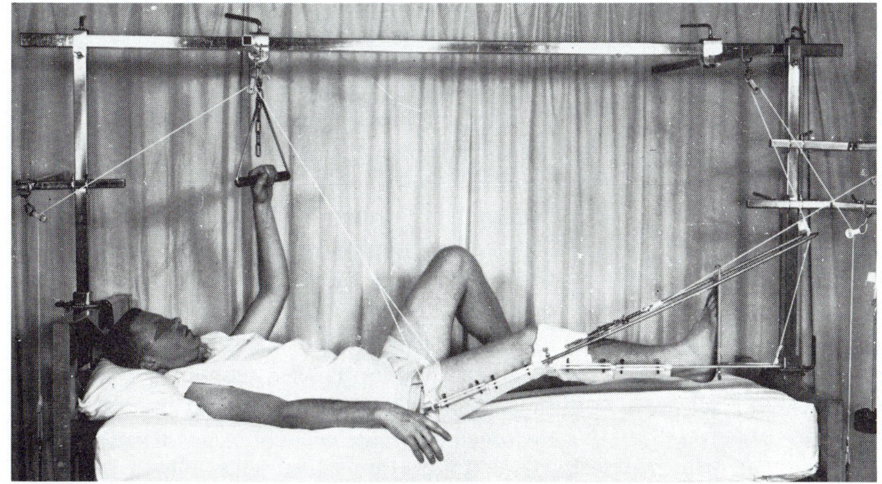

B

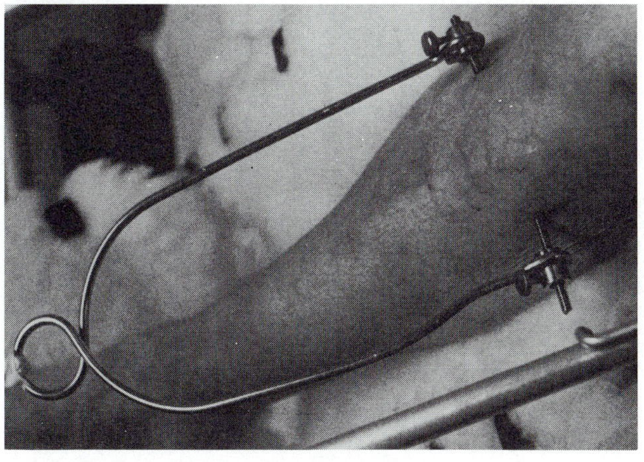

FIG. 26-33 **A,** Balanced suspension skeletal traction to the femur. **B,** Skeletal traction—pin site.

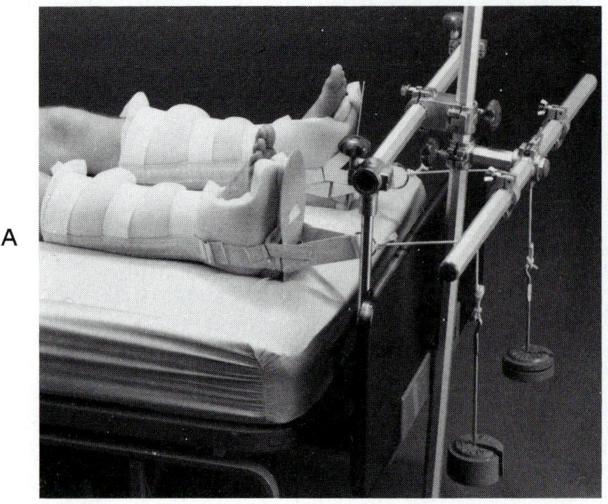

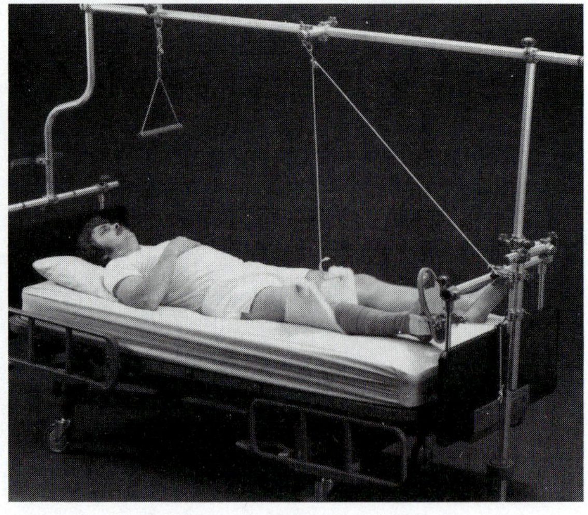

FIG. 26-34 Types of skin traction. **A,** Buck's traction. **B,** Russell traction.

The pin protrudes through the skin on both sides of the extremity, and weights are attached to a rope that is tied to a spreader bar for the purpose of traction. Skeletal traction can be used for fractures of the femur (Fig. 26-33, *A*), tibia (Fig. 26-33, *B*), humerus, and cervical spine (see Chapter 35).

Skin traction. Skin traction is accomplished by using weight that pulls on sponge rubber, moleskin, elastic bandage with adherent, or plastic materials attached to the skin below the site of the fracture, with the pull exerted on the limb. Buck's, Russell, and Bryant's are types of skin traction.

Buck's traction. Buck's traction (Fig. 26-34, *A*) is a form of traction used as a temporary measure to provide support and comfort to a fractured extremity until a more definite treatment is initiated. This traction is frequently used to maintain the reduction of a hip fracture before surgery. It can also be used to treat muscle spasms and minor fractures of the lower spine.

Russell traction. Russell traction (Fig. 26-34, *B*) is set up similar to Buck's traction. However, a knee sling is used to provide support of the affected leg. It allows more movement in bed and permits flexion of the knee joint. Russell traction is commonly used to treat hip and knee fractures.

Bryant's traction. Bryant's traction is used in pediatrics for small children with fractured femurs. Both legs are suspended at a 90-degree angle to the trunk of the body, and the weight of the lower body pulls the bone fragments of the fractured leg into alignment (see Chapter 44).

Nursing interventions. Nursing intervention of patients in traction includes the following measures:

- Maintain the patient's body in proper alignment. The force or pull on the extremities should be in alignment with the long axis of the bone.
- Ensure that weights hang freely from the bed and are *never* removed without a physician's order.
- Question patients as to their understanding of the purpose of the traction, and assess their ability to use a trapeze bar for self-movement. Elevate the foot of the bed to help prevent the patient from sliding down toward the foot of the bed.
- Observe the condition of the traction cords, making sure they are not weakened or frayed. All knots used on the rope or cord are to be square knots.
- Center the ropes on the traction pulley.
- Assess, document, and report neurovascular impairment.
- Ensure that weight used is the correct weight as ordered by the physician.
- Carefully observe the skin for signs of skin impairment. Use sheepskin heel protectors and bed pads to reduce impairment.
- If skeletal traction is used, assess the pin site for signs of infection. Cleanse the pin site q 8 hr with hydrogen peroxide or alcohol, as ordered.
- Assess the dorsalis pedis pulses bilaterally for circulatory integrity of the lower extremities.
- Inspect for loss of sensation in the dorsal area of the foot with weakness and inversion of the foot (inside surface turned outward).

Orthopedic Devices

Frames can be used for orthopedic patients to assist with turning and positioning while maintaining proper alignment. The Balkan frame is a wooden or steel attachment to the hospital bed. The frame has adjustable pulleys and a trapeze bar attached to an overhead bar.

The Bradford frame is made of rectangular steel with two pieces of canvas stretched tightly and laced to the

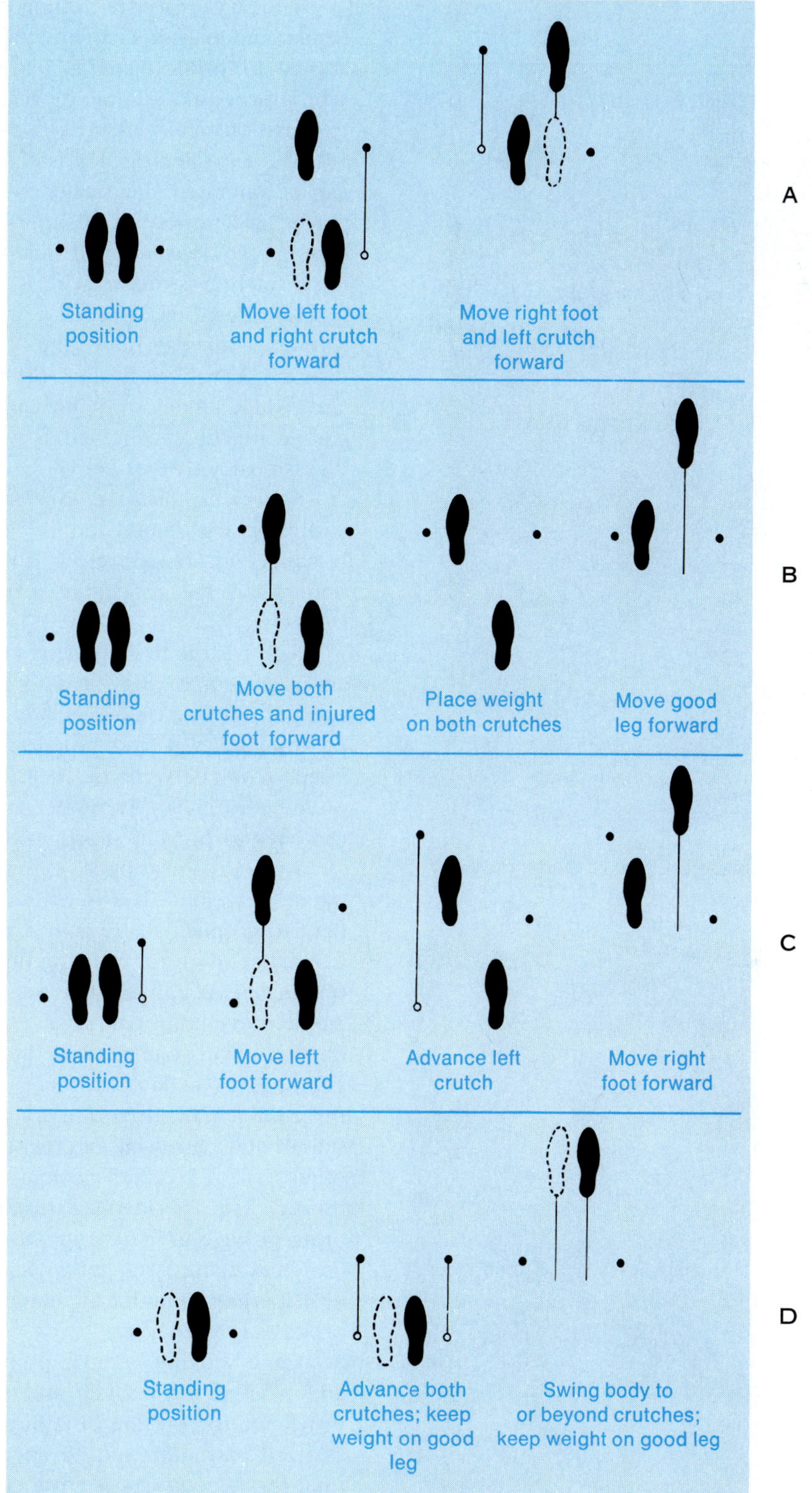

FIG. 26-35 Crutch walking. **A,** Two-point gait. **B,** Three-point gait. **C,** Four-point gait. **D,** Swing-through gait.

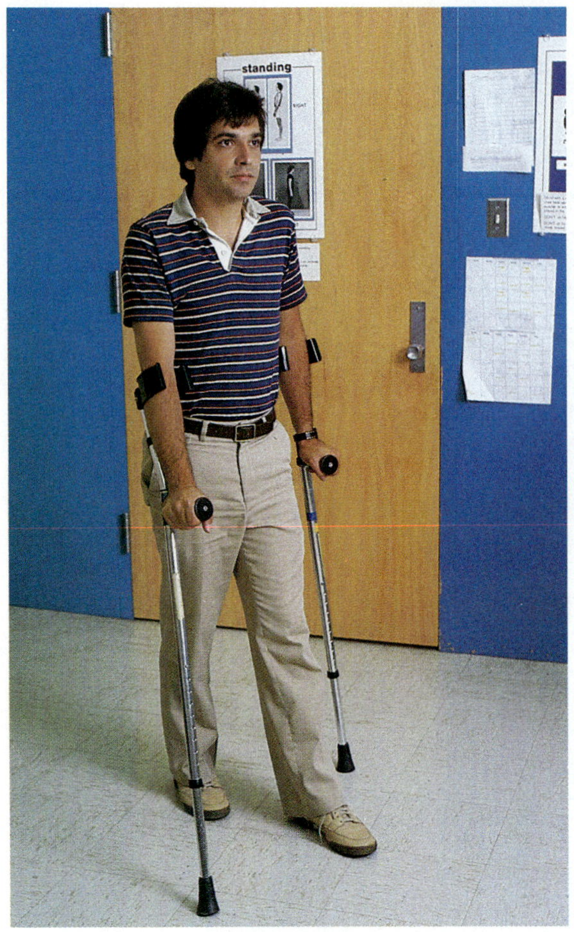

FIG. 26-36 Double adjustable Lofstrand or forearm crutches.

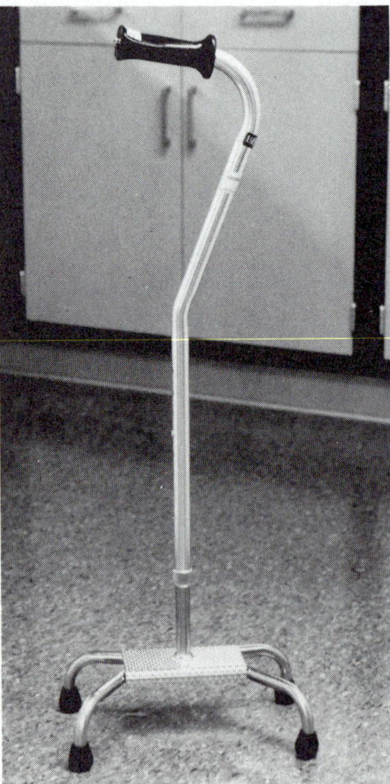

FIG. 26-37 Quad cane.

frame. A space is left in the buttocks area for toileting and hygiene.

The Stryker wedge turning frame and Foster bed are similar and assist in changing the patient's position from supine to prone. Patients may become apprehensive when turned on a frame for fear of falling, so thorough explanations and reassurances are helpful.

The CircOlectric bed is a vertical turning bed that can be operated electrically by one person and can be placed in a variety of positions. Side-to-side movement can be accomplished while maintaining proper positioning if traction is ordered.

RotoRest bed can rock a patient as much as 62 degrees, 17 times an hour. The electric-powered bed can promote decubitus healing, prevent venous thrombosis, and reduce kidney stone formation. Orthopedic traction can be attached to the bed, as well as a television set for diversional activity.

Splints, crutches, and braces are used to immobilize and assist with ambulation. There are numerous types of splints and braces, and it is important that the nurse understand the procedure for proper application for each one.

Safety is the first concern when ambulatory devices are used. Crutch safety involves (1) proper measurement (weight must be on hands, not axillae, to avoid brachial plexus paralysis), and proper measurement involves a 2-inch width between the axillary fold and the arm piece on the crutches; (2) rubber tips on the ends of the crutches to prevent slippage; and (3) adequate muscle strength in the upper extremities to support the patient's weight. The nurse should encourage the patient to do push-ups to gain strength.

Types of crutch walking depend on the number of points making contact with the floor (Fig. 26-35). For example, three-point gait involves two crutch points plus one leg making contact with the floor (patient must have strong arms to support body weight). In addition to three-point gait, there are four-point gait (slower, but stable) and two-point gait (faster; requires balance). Another type of crutch walking is swing-to or swing-through gait. This involves the patient swinging the body up to or beyond the two points of the crutch tips. Most crutch walking is taught by a physical therapist. However, it is important for the nurse to monitor the patient's progress (Fig. 26-36).

Cane walking is more popular with older patients and is used for balance and support. The patient is instructed to hold the cane in the opposite hand of the affected extremity and advance the cane at the same time the affected leg is advanced forward. An effective rubber tip on the point will help prevent any slippage (Fig. 26-37). Walkers are also used by the older adult and will assist the patient in maintaining balance. Safety concerns are the same as those for the cane (Fig. 26-38).

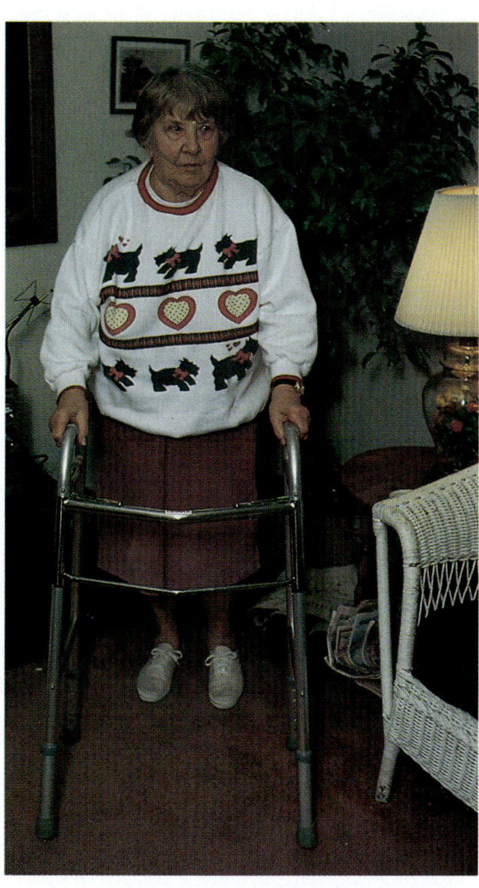

FIG. 26-38 Patient using a walker.

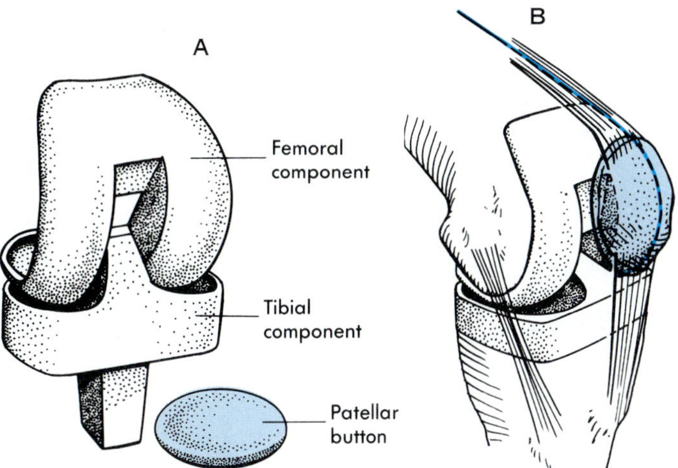

FIG. 26-39 **A,** Tibial and femoral components of total knee prosthesis. Patellar button, made of polyethylene, protects the posterior surface of the patella from friction against the femoral component when the knee is moved through flexion and extension. **B,** Total knee prosthesis in place.

SURGICAL INTERVENTION FOR MUSCULOSKELETAL DISORDERS

Surgical procedures can prevent progressive deformities, relieve pain, improve function, and correct deformities resulting from rheumatoid arthritis, osteoarthritis, and other disorders. Tendon transplants can be done to replace damaged muscles. Patients with rheumatoid arthritis may need a synovectomy (excision of synovial membrane) to maintain joint function. An osteotomy (cutting into bone to correct bone or joint deformities) can help to improve function and relieve pain. **Arthrodesis** (surgical fusion of a joint) can be performed when severe joint destruction has occurred. Total joint replacement **arthroplasty** (refers to repair or refashioning of one or both sides, parts, or specific tissue within a joint) is often required on the elbow, hip, knee, or shoulder joint to restore or increase mobility.

Knee Arthroplasty (Total Knee Replacement)

Replacement of the knee joint may be necessary to restore motion of the joint, relieve pain, or correct deformity. Fig. 26-39 shows the tibial and femoral components of a knee prosthesis. Nursing interventions for the patient undergoing total knee replacement are shown in Box 26-6 and Fig. 26-40 on p. 632.

Hip Arthroplasty (Total Hip Replacement)

A hip arthroplasty or total hip replacement is a commonly performed procedure when arthritis involves the head of the femur and acetabulum. A Vitallium cup is cemented into the arthritic acetabulum to receive the head of the femur. Total hip replacement is a recent development and was originally developed by Dr. John Charnley, a British orthopedic surgeon. There are several variations, but similar equipment is used. The Bechtol total hip system involves the use of a white plastic cup cemented in place to replace the damaged acetabulum. A stainless steel or Vitallium ball on a stem replaces the head of the femur. which is surgically removed. The stem is cemented into the femoral canal, and the new head fits precisely into the plastic acetabulum, providing friction-free movement in the joint. The cement used is a soft, surgical bone cement that hardens quickly and stabilizes the prosthesis to prevent future erosion of surrounding bone (Fig. 26-41 on p. 633).

Assessment. Collection of *subjective data* involves assessing the patient's level of orientation, since disorientation can be present in the older adult resulting from a change in the environment (home to hospital setting). Complaints of pain and numbness, tingling, or paresthesia indicate neurovascular impairment.

Collection of *objective data* includes assessment of the patient's compliance with nursing interventions to

Box 26-6

NURSING INTERVENTIONS FOR THE PATIENT UNDERGOING TOTAL KNEE REPLACEMENT

PREOPERATIVE INTERVENTIONS

Same as for any major surgery (see Chapter 22).

POSTOPERATIVE INTERVENTIONS

1. Positioning
   a. The operative leg is elevated on pillows to enhance venous return for the first 48 hours only. Pillows are placed with caution not to flex the knee.
   b. The patient may be turned from side to back to side.
2. Wound care
   a. Care of drains as for total hip replacement.
   b. Patient is assessed for systemic evidence of loss of blood (hypotension, tachycardia) if bulky compression dressing is used as it may hold large quantities of drainage before drainage is visible.
   c. Bulky dressings are removed before the patient begins active flexion.
3. Activity
   a. Passive flexion in a continuous passive motion (CPM) machine within prescribed flexion-extension limits may be started in the recovery room (see Fig. 26-40). Patient's leg should remain in machine as much as tolerated (up to 22 hours per day) to facilitate even healing of tissue. When CPM is not occurring, patient's leg is extended with no pillows under leg.
   b. Patient is encouraged to perform active dorsiplantar flexion of the ankles, quadriceps setting, and, after the drain is removed, straight leg raising exercises.
   c. Patient begins active flexion exercises three to four times a day about the fifth postoperative day.
   d. Light weight bearing with an assistive device may be started as early as the first postoperative day and increased as the patient tolerates.
   e. Sitting in a chair with the leg elevated may be started on the first postoperative day.
   f. Patient is encouraged to wear a resting knee extension splint (immobilizer) on the operated leg until able to demonstrate quadriceps control (independent straight leg raising).
4. Pain control
   a. Initial control of pain with narcotics, positioning, gradual decrease of medication to nonnarcotic analgesics as patient tolerates.
   b. Patient is encouraged to use ice to knee for 20-30 minutes before and after active flexion exercise.
5. Discharge instructions
   a. Patient must observe partial weight-bearing restriction and use ambulatory aid for approximately 2 months following discharge.
   b. Patient should continue active flexion and straight leg raising exercises at home.

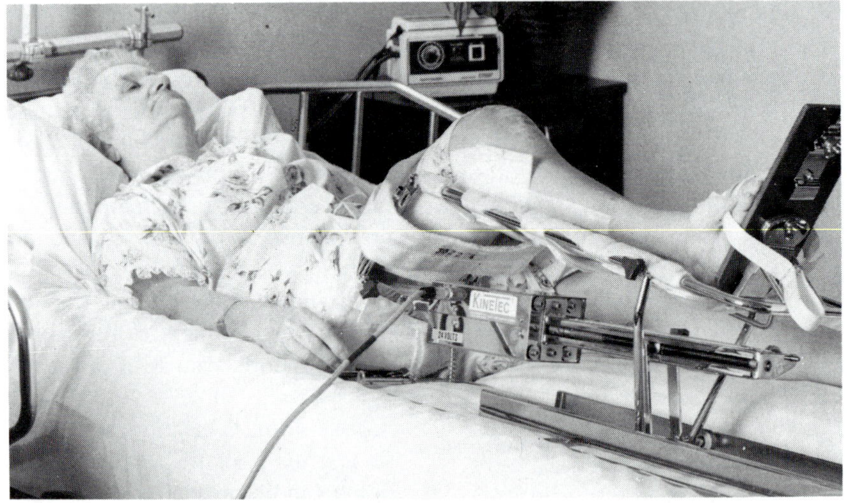

FIG. 26-40 Continuous passive ROM machine (CPM).

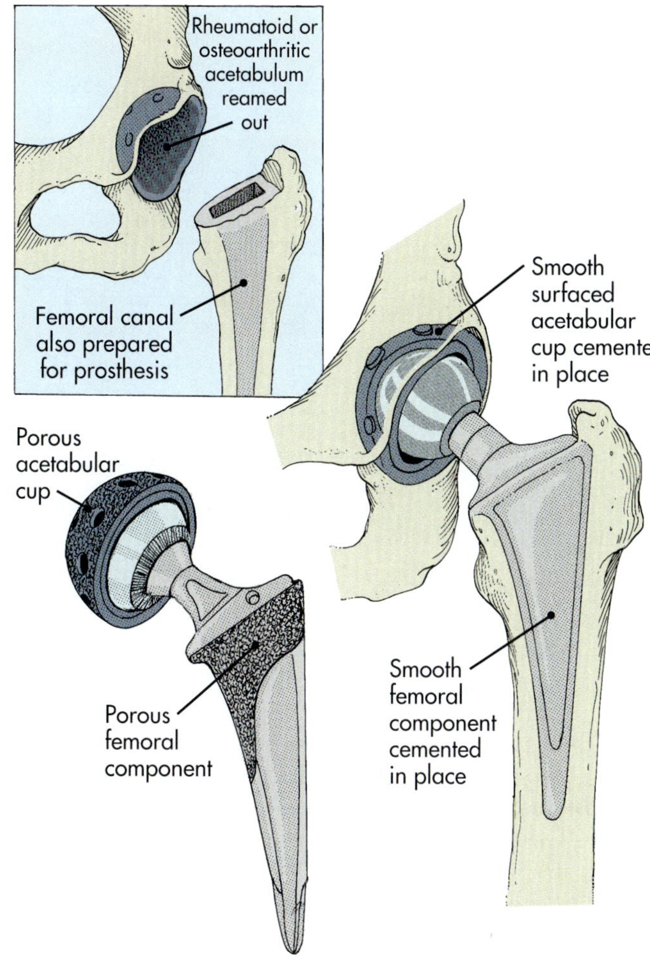

FIG. 26-41 Hip arthroplasty (total hip replacement).

promote circulation, prevent impairment of skin integrity, and prevent hypostatic pneumonia by such means as coughing, turning (to the unaffected side; additional pillows are used to keep the affected leg abducted), and deep breathing q 2 hr. Assessment of vital signs for evidence of excessive bleeding includes hypotension, tachycardia, and tachypnea. Decreased urinary output is indicative of hypovolemia. A careful assessment of the surgical wound for drainage is made at least q 4 hr. Hemovacs or other suction devices are placed in the wound during surgery to provide closed-wound suction. Assessing approximation of incision line and signs of inflammation (erythema, edema, fever, and pain) is necessary. Also included is assessing traction (if used) for correct amount of weight and proper alignment, maintaining the affected leg in an abducted position, and carefully observing for any reaction to the cement, signs of phlebitis (edema, erythema, and pain), and urinary retention (indwelling catheters may be used for the first 24 to 48 hours postoperative).

Nursing Interventions. Nursing intervention is aimed at promoting healing and facilitating mobility. The patient is taught to do isometric exercises on the quadriceps and gluteal muscles of the affected extremity by keeping the toes pointed up, flexing the ankles, and flexing and extending the knee of the unaffected extremity. Careful documentation of the patient's I&O is needed. Thigh-high antiembolism stockings are applied before or during surgery. A plan of weight bearing and physical therapy will be ordered by the physician and must be explained to the patient.

- Empty and record Hemovac drainage q 4 hr, if ordered; otherwise, empty and record as needed
- Give oxygen at 2 to 3 L per nasal cannula for 24 hours, then as needed
- Instruct patient in use of incentive spirometer q 2 to 4 hr
- Help patient do deep breathing and coughing q 2 hr
- Record I&O
- Maintain bed rest for 24 to 48 hours (varies with the security of the replacement prostheses and physician's choice)
- Change dressing after 24 to 48 hours as ordered; may reinforce dressing if necessary
- Begin clear liquids and advance to regular diet as tolerated
- Perform neurovascular checks every hour for 24 hours, then q 2 hr for 24 hours, and then q 4 hr
- Check vital signs q 4 hr
- Maintain position of operative area with splint, abduction pillow, immobilizer, and brace; turn patient to unoperative side
- Patient should be up but bearing no weight on operative limb after bed rest order expires (24 to 48 hours, depending on whether cemented or noncemented replacement was done); some physicians may permit touch-down weight bearing
- Begin physical therapy exercises on second postoperative day; exercises and schedule vary; exercises are either active or passive to all joints, excluding the operated joint, and include quadriceps setting, straight leg raising, flexion and extension, or other individually prescribed exercises for the particular joint replaced
- Patient should be up with walker or crutches four times daily; ambulation should increase as patient is able with up to 25 pounds weight to operative limb, gradually increasing to full weight bearing with crutches.
- Patient should sit in chair for 10 to 15 minutes only, two or three times daily for first week; then may sit in chair 20 or 30 minutes four times daily
- Encourage fluid intake and high-fiber foods (if tolerated) to prevent constipation; administer rectal suppository if needed to empty rectum

- Patient should wear antiembolism hose or an pneumonic stocking pump system
- Patient should use toilet riser (prevents hyperflexion of hip after total replacement)

Nursing diagnoses and interventions for the patient with a total hip replacement include but are not limited to the following:

NURSING DIAGNOSES	NURSING INTERVENTIONS
Pain, related to preoperative arthritic pain necessitating surgery and postoperative hip incisional pain secondary to bone and soft tissue trauma of surgery	Explain analgesic therapy, including medication, dose, and schedule. If patient is candidate for patient-controlled analgesic (PCA), explain concept and routine. Administer analgesics as ordered and per hospital policy/procedure. Respond quickly to pain complaints. Instruct patient to request analgesic before pain is severe. Encourage use of analgesics 30 to 45 min before therapy. Unrelieved pain hinders rehabilitation progress. Provide EggCrate mattress. Change position (within hip precautions) q 2 hr. Document all responses to analgesics.
Injury: high risk for, hip dislocation, related to improper hip joint positioning	Frequently instruct/reinforce hip positions: ■ Abduction of legs. ■ Flexion of hip <90 degrees. ■ Neutral or external rotation of affected leg. Constantly practice precautions essential to prevent dislocation of new hip joint. Dislocation can occur easily, necessitating further hospitalization and possible surgery Maintain abduction of legs and abduction splint (in and out of bed). Abduction splint between patient's legs prevents adduction of legs. Instruct patient on use of raised toilet seat (prevents hip flexion >90 degrees). Turn patient side to side in bed with pillow between legs (turn to nonoperative side unless directed differently)
Tissue perfusion altered, peripheral, high risk for, related to surgery intervention	Encourage patient to be out of bed as soon as ordered. Maintain total hip arthroplasty precautions and weight-bearing status. Encourage incentive spirometry q 1 hr while awake to increase lung expansion and prevent atelectasis, hypoxemia, pneumonia, and pulmonary embolism. Institute antiembolic devices as ordered (sequential compression device or TED hose). Antiembolic devices increase venous blood flow to heart and decrease risk of deep vein thrombosis and pulmonary embolism. Encourage leg exercises, including quadriceps sets and active ankle ROM.
Mobility, impaired physical, related to surgical procedure and discomfort	Allow patient to dangle feet at bedside several minutes before getting patient out of bed. Reinforce physical therapist's instructions for exercises and ambulation techniques and devices. Maintain weight-bearing status on affected extremity as prescribed. Consistent instructions from interdisciplinary team members promote safe, secure rehabilitation environment. Keep abduction pillow between legs while turning in bed. No sidelying on operative side. Leg is maintained in abduction when lying supine or on the nonoperative side. Use trapeze in bed to assist in mobility.

Patient teaching. Discharge instructions include the following:

- Patient must use ambulatory aid, avoid adduction, and limit hip flexion to 90 degrees for about 2 to 3 months.
- A raised toilet seat is to be obtained and used at home until flexion restrictions are removed.
- Patient may need a long-handled shoe horn and reacher to facilitate ADLs within flexion restriction.
- Patient must be made aware of the lifelong need for antibiotic prophylaxis to protect the prosthesis from bacterial infection during dental work, intrusive procedures, or surgery.

Amputation

The amputation of a portion of or an entire extremity may be necessary because of malignant tumors, injuries, impaired circulation (caused by diabetes mellitus or arteriosclerosis), congenital deformities, and infections. Most amputations are elective surgery unless the amputation is necessary because of trauma. Advances in microsurgery techniques have made it possible for surgeons to reattach severed extremities. Therefore traumatic amputations can sometimes be reversed by replantation of the part if the severed limb is kept sterile and moist in a plastic bag filled with ice water. (The part should be protected from direct contact with ice, and dry ice should not be used.)

Amputation of long bones can result in postoperative anemia. A traumatic or surgical amputation of an extremity can cause serious blood loss. Malignant bone tumors can metastasize via the bloodstream to other body systems.

Preoperative Assessment. Collection of *subjective data* includes questioning to determine the patient's understanding of the nature of the injury or disease process. Assessment of complaints of pain and symptoms of neurovascular impairment is made and documented. Assessment of the patient's level of orientation is important, since many amputations occur in the older population as a result of medical conditions that impair circulation.

Collection of *objective data* includes assessment of vital signs (temperature elevation, tachycardia, and tachypnea indicate infection). Arterial blood flow is assessed by palpation of bilateral pedal pulses and Doppler pressure measurements. Assessment is done of wound drainage for color, amount, and presence of odor. Evaluation of upper body muscle strength and nutritional status is important.

Postoperative Assessment. Collection of *subjective data* involves careful assessment of pain. *Phantom pain* (pain felt in the missing extremity as if it were still present) may occur and be frightening to the patient. Phantom pain occurs because the nerve tracks that register pain in the amputated area continue to send a message to the brain—this is normal.

Collection of *objective data* includes observing for signs of hemorrhage, such as hypotension, tachycardia, tachypnea, pallor, decreased urinary output, restlessness, and progressive loss of consciousness. Monitoring suction drainage and documenting it is important, as are assessing and protecting the remaining extremity. The nurse should observe for neurovascular impairment (done hourly in the immediate postoperative period) from tightly applied elastic wraps, dressings, or casts (see Box 26-4).

Diagnostic Tests. A complete blood count is done to determine blood dyscrasias, such as anemia and bleeding tendencies, that would influence the surgical outcome and increase postoperative complications (such as hemorrhage, delayed wound healing, and disorientation). Laboratory studies, such as blood urea nitrogen (BUN), potassium levels, and routine urinalysis, are ordered. An electrocardiogram (ECG) is ordered to detect cardiac dysrhythmias that are often present in the older patient.

Medical Management. When the amputation results from traumatic injury to an extremity, the physician's interventions will include measures to restore circulating blood volume, control pain, prevent infection in the wound, perform a plastic surgical repair at the amputation site to facilitate the use of a prosthesis, and maintain adequate urinary output.

If the amputation is an elective surgical procedure, the physician makes an assessment of the patient's physiological, psychological, and emotional status. If there is any infection present in the body (gangrene may occur in the presence of impaired circulation), treatment will include administration of antibiotics, and every attempt will be made to control the infection before any surgery is performed. The physician will discuss the possibility of the patient using a prosthesis. Much of the preoperative preparation will focus on the patient attaining a physical and emotional status conducive to wearing a prosthesis or achieving mobility through the use of a wheelchair or a gait enhancer, such as crutches or a walker.

Postoperative Nursing Interventions. Nursing intervention is aimed at prevention of deformities (contractures, especially in the joint above the amputation, or abduction deformities are common). Flexion hip contractures can be prevented postoperatively by raising the foot of the bed slightly to elevate the residual extremity (care should be taken not to flex the patient's hips by elevating the stump on a pillow), encouraging movement from side to side, and placing the patient in a prone position at least twice a day. This will stretch the flexor muscles. The nurse will be involved with teaching the patient how to strengthen remaining muscles to facilitate mobility and prevent muscle atrophy (push-ups from a prone position and sit-ups from a seated position). The application of elastic wraps to shrink and reshape the residual extremity into a cone is necessary to facilitate the proper fit and subsequent use of a prosthesis (Fig. 26-42 on p. 636). A prosthesis may be fitted as early as 2 or 3 weeks postoperatively. Because many amputations are performed in persons between 60 and 70 years of age, the patient must be observed carefully for pulmonary complications (such as pulmonary embolus) and cardiovascular collapse. Suction equipment and oxygen should be at the bedside. Patient education concerning the phenomenon of phantom-limb sensation can help relieve patient fears if patients know it is a normal physiological response. The response may be one of pain or other sensations, such as burning, tingling, throbbing, or pruritus in the amputated extremity. These sensations can last for months or decades on a consistent or intermittent basis. It is recommended that patients gently rub the residual extremity for relief. Pain medication may be necessary.

The patient should be encouraged to ventilate feelings over the loss of the extremity. The loss of an extremity results in a grieving process. The patient should be taught the importance of allowing the grieving process to occur.

For persistent, severe phantom pain, the following measures may be employed:

- Stump revision with reamputation at a higher level
- Local infiltration of the stump with procaine
- Mechanical percussion by striking the sensitive digital stump against a solid object—believed to shrink neuromas (small tumors that form in the scar tissue of the stump)
- Sympathetic nerve block

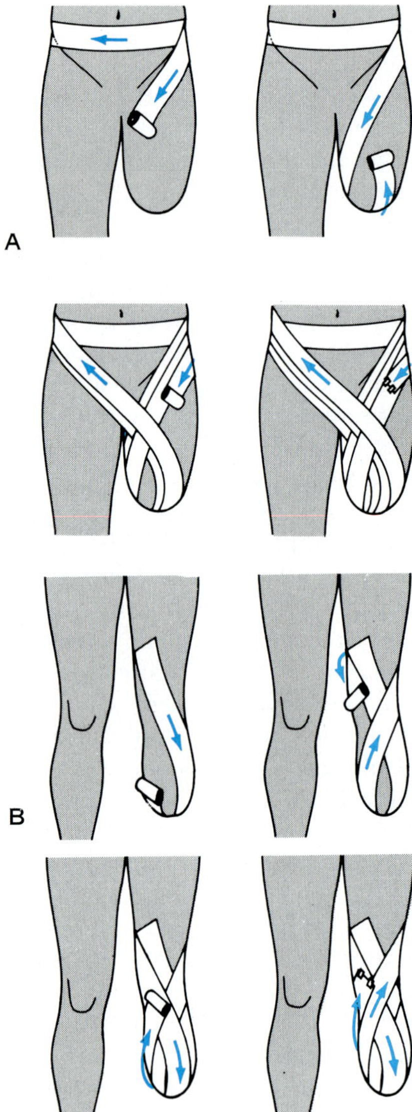

FIG. 26-42 Correct method of bandaging amputation stump. **A,** It is important to anchor bandage around patient's waist. **B,** Method for bandaging midcalf stump, where bandage need not be anchored around waist.

Nursing diagnoses and interventions for the patient undergoing an amputation include but are not limited to the following:

NURSING DIAGNOSES	NURSING INTERVENTIONS
Body image disturbances, related to loss of limb	Assess effects of amputation on body image. Allow and encourage patient to express feelings of mutilation, grief, anger, and loss to aid adaptation processes. Encourage patient to help with dressing changes and wrapping of stump as able. Teach family member wrapping techniques if necessary to increase competence and independence. Encourage family members to walk with patient to maintain strength and social contacts. Encourage grooming and wearing of personal clothing to maintain individuality and personality. Encourage activities for self-care and ambulation to maintain positive outlook and maximum strength. Encourage or arrange for social services consultation for economic and employment aid. Arrange for follow-up care referral to aid rehabilitation.
Mobility, impaired physical, related to loss of limb	Assess ability to use remaining limbs. Turn and position on side, back, and abdomen (after 24 hours) to maintain muscle and joint ROM. Teach adduction and extension exercises and help patient perform them q 4 hr to prevent abduction and flexion contractures. Assist with sitting in chair and ambulation with aid as able to maintain muscle strength. Prepare patient for physical therapy, transportation for exercises, and stump wrapping, if appropriate. Encourage family members to walk with patient during initial ambulation periods, accompanied by health professionals, to increase independence. Teach purposes of prone and extension positions to prevent contractures. Assist prosthetist with prosthesis measurements and fitting as needed to aid rehabilitation.
Pain (nerve trauma following surgery), related to surgical transection	Assess type, amount, and severity of pain. Administer narcotics as ordered q 3 hr prn for first 24 to 48 hours until surgical trauma is lessened; then administer as needed to aid pain relief. Explain causes for phantom-pain sensations and techniques to overcome them to ease concerns. Administer antibiotics as ordered to prevent infection, thereby lessening pain and scarring.

Patient teaching.

- Teach the patient and family proper positions, exercises, and ambulation techniques.
- Demonstrate stump-wrapping techniques to the patient and family.
- Explain to the patient and family that prolonged phantom-pain experiences are unusual and should receive medical attention.
- Discuss skin care with the patient and family to prevent stump irritation or impairment.
- List signs of a wound infection, and discuss these with the patient and family.

Prognosis. The prognosis for successful adaptation to an amputation is dependent upon the patient's age, the condition that resulted in amputation, other systemic disorders, emotional health, and support system.

REFERENCES AND SELECTED REFERENCES

1. Beare PG, Myers JL: *Principles and practices of adult health nursing,* ed 2, St Louis, 1994, Mosby.
2. Berne RM, Levy M: *Physiology,* ed 3, St Louis, 1992, Mosby.
3. Birchenall J, Steight M: *Care of the older adult,* ed 3, Philadelphia, 1993, Lippincott.
4. Blechman W: Osteoarthritis: are you up-to-date? *Patient Care* 26(5):99, 1992.
5. Brooks PM, Day RO: Nonsteroidal anti-inflammatory drugs: differences and similarities, *N Engl J Med* 324(24):1716, 1991.
6. Bryant B: When your patient needs back surgery, *RN* 55(7):46, 1992.
7. Dunwoody C: Pelvic fracture patient care: reflections on the past, implications for the future, *Nurs Clin North Am* 26(1):65, 1991.
8. Eden-Kilgour S, Miller B: Understanding neurovascular assessment, *Nursing* 23(8):56, 1993.
9. *Fundamental nursing skills,* Springhouse, Penn, 1993, Springhouse.
10. Gluchacki B: Recognizing compartment syndrome, *Nurs '91* 21(10):33, 1991.
11. Gordon M: *Manual of nursing diagnosis,* St Louis, 1993, Mosby.
12. Gussoni M et al: Energy cost of walking with hip a joint impairment, *Phys Ther* 10(5):295, 1990.
13. Hallal J: Back pain with postmenopausal osteoporosis and vertebral fractures, *Geriatr Nurs* 12(6):285, 1991.
14. Harkness-Hood G, Dincher J: *Total patient care: foundations and practice,* ed 8, St Louis, 1992, Mosby.
15. Hay E: That old hip: the osteoporosis process, *Nurs Clin North Am* 26(1):51, 1991.
16. Higgins RM: Replantation of digits, *Orthop Nurs* 10:11, 1991.
17. Jones-Watson P: Clinical standards in skeletal traction pin site care, *Orthop Nurs* 10:12, 1991.
18. Kane J et al: Typing system helps select total joint prosthesis, *OR Manager* 7(10):26, 1991.
19. Kelly H: Patient perceptions of pain and disability after joint arthroplasty, *Orthop Nurs* 10(6):43, 1991.
20. Kim M, McFarland GK, McLane AM: *Pocket guide to nursing diagnoses,* ed 5, St Louis, 1993, Mosby.
21. Kisner C, Colby L: *Therapeutic exercise,* ed 2, Philadelphia, 1990, FA Davis.
22. Krug B: The hip: nursing fracture patients to full recovery, *RN* April 1989, p 56.
23. Lane PL, LeBlanc R: Crutch walking, *Orthop Nurs* 9(5):31, 1991.
24. Long B, Phipps W, Cassmeyer VL: *Medical-surgical nursing: a nursing process approach,* ed 3, St Louis, 1993, Mosby.
25. Magaziner J et al: Predictors of functional recovery one year following hospital discharge for hip fracture: a prospective study, *J Gerontol* 45(3):101, 1990.
26. McFarland GK, McFarlane EA: *Nursing diagnosis and interventions: planning for patient-care,* ed 2, St Louis, 1993, Mosby.
27. McFure L: Administering analgesics: which drugs are right for your patient? *Nurs '90* 20(4):34, 1990.
28. McKenry LM, Salerno E: *Mosby's pharmacology in nursing,* St Louis, 1992, Mosby.
29. McKeon V: Estrogen replacement therapy, *Gerontol Nurs* 16(10):6, 1990.
30. Memmler RL, Cohen BJ, Wood DL: *Structure and function of the human body,* ed 5, Philadelphia, 1992, Lippincott.
31. *Mosby's medical, nursing, and allied health dictionary,* ed 4, St Louis, 1994, Mosby.
32. Mourad L: *Mosby's clinical nursing series: orthopedic disorders,* St Louis, 1991, Mosby.
33. Novicki D: Casting. II. *Podiatry Today* 19(6):83, 1992.
34. Nussman DS, Poole RC: Rescue and recovery in traumatic hip dislocation, *Am J Nurs* 9(11):34, 1991.
35. Olsen B: Self-care needs of patients in the halo brace, *Orthop Nurs* 9:27, 1990.
36. Phipps WJ, Long BC, Woods NF: *Medical-surgical nursing: concepts and clinical practices,* ed 4, St Louis, 1991, Mosby.
37. Potter PA, Perry AG: *Fundamentals of nursing: concepts, process, and practice,* ed 3, St Louis, 1993, Mosby.
38. Ross D: Acute compartment syndrome, *Orthop Nurs* 10(2):33, 1991.
39. Schellenbarger T: When you are asked about carpal tunnel syndrome, *RN* 54(7):40, 1991.
40. Seidel HM et al: *Mosby's guide to physical examination,* ed 3, St Louis, 1995, Mosby.
41. Syle D: Orthopedic complications: compartment syndrome, fat embolism syndrome and venous thromboembolism, *Nurs Clin North Am* 26(1):113, 1991.
42. Sneed N, VanBree K: Treating u ited fractures with electricity, *Gerontol Nurs* 16(8):26, 1990.
43. Solomon EP: *Introduction to human anatomy and physiology,* Philadelphia, 1992, Saunders.
44. Stanhope M, Lancaster J: *Community health nursing,* ed 3, St Louis, 1992, Mosby.
45. Swearingen P: *Medical-surgical nursing care,* ed 3, St Louis, 1994, Mosby.
46. Swearingen PL: *Pocket guide to medical-surgical nursing: nursing diagnosis and interventions,* St Louis, 1992, Mosby.
47. Thibodeau GA: *Structure and function of the body,* ed 9, St Louis, 1992, Mosby.
48. Thomas CL: *Taber's cyclopedic medical dictionary,* ed 17, Philadelphia, 1993, FA Davis.
49. Thompson JM, Bowers AC: *Clinical manual of health assessment,* ed 3, St Louis, 1992, Mosby.
50. Thompson NM et al: *Mosby's clinical nursing,* ed 3, St Louis, 1993, Mosby.
51. Tucker SM et al: *Patient care standards: nursing process, diagnosis, and outcome,* ed 5, St Louis, 1992, Mosby.
52. White AA et al: Symposium: current concepts in the management of herniated disc, *Contemp Orthop* 22:339, 1991.
53. Williamson V: Amputation of the lower extremity: an overview, *Orthop Nurs* 11(2):55, 1992.

CHAPTER CHALLENGE

KEY POINTS

- The skeletal system has five basic functions: support of the body, protection of internal organs, movement of the body, storage of minerals, and blood cell formation.
- Joints hold the bones together and allow movement and flexibility. Differences in the structure determine the amount of mobility.
- A long bone is composed of the epiphysis (end) and the diaphysis (shaft). The medullary cavity (interior of the diaphysis) contains yellow bone marrow. The epiphysis contains red bone marrow.
- The periosteum is a strong membrane that covers the bone and nourishes it.
- The skeleton is composed of two main divisions:
  - The axial skeleton—containing the skull, vertebrae, and thorax.
  - The appendicular skeleton—containing the upper and lower extremities.
- Some of the more freely movable joints are the ball and socket, hinge, pivot, and saddle.
- Bones are classified according to their shape and bone composition. They are long, short, flat, and irregular.
- The three types of muscle tissue are:
  - Smooth (involuntary) muscles, usually in the internal organs.
  - Skeletal (voluntary) muscles, attached to the bones and allow movement.
  - Cardiac (involuntary) muscles, seen only in the heart and responsible for the contraction of the chambers of the heart.
- Muscle cells are governed by the "all or none" law, which states that when a muscle cell is adequately stimulated, it will contract; otherwise there is no response.
- Muscle tissue possesses four principal characteristics:
  - Excitability—capacity to respond to a stimulus.
  - Contractility—ability to shorten and become thicker.
  - Extensibility—ability to be stretched.
  - Elasticity—ability to return to normal shape.
- The muscle tissue keeps a temporary energy store called adenosine triphosphate (ATP), which is released chemically in times of need.
- Most muscles extend over a joint and attach at the origin (an immovable bone) and at the insertion (a bone that moves readily). Tendons attach muscles to bone, whereas ligaments attach bones to bones; both are composed of fibrous connective tissue.
- An erythrocyte sedimentation rate (ESR) is the most objective laboratory test for determining the severity of rheumatoid arthritis.
- External fixation devices (such as casts, braces, metal pins, and skeletal and skin traction) are used to hold bone fragments in normal position.
- Regardless of whether the casting material is plaster of paris or a synthetic material, proper drying, cleansing, handling, and assessing are required to prevent patient complications.
- The nurse caring for a patient in traction is responsible for knowing (1) the purpose of the traction (traction applied for fractures must be continuous); (2) the equipment needed and appropriate safety measures; (3) the amount of weight ordered; and (4) the patient's knowledge regarding the traction.
- Crutches, canes, and walkers are used as gait enhancers for patients with altered mobility.
- Crutch walking involving the three-point gait is most commonly used for patients wearing leg casts.
- Osteogenic sarcoma is a common primary malignant tumor seen in young people; it can metastasize to the lungs.
- A significant postoperative nursing intervention for a patient with an amputation is proper care of the stump to facilitate the use of a prosthetic device.
- Rheumatoid arthritis affects a young population (ages 30 to 55) with crippling changes in the synovial membrane of the joints.
- Salicylates and nonsteroidal antiinflammatory agents (NSAIAs) are used to treat rheumatoid arthritis and osteoarthritis.
- Osteoarthritis is a degenerative joint disease (DJD) that affects the population over 40 years of age and causes articular cartilage degeneration.
- Arthroplasty procedures (such as hip and knee arthroplasty) are commonly performed on patients suffering from severe arthritis.
- Porous and brittle bones caused by a lack of calcium is one of the physiological changes noted in osteoporosis.
- Nursing intervention specific to the care of a patient suffering from a fractured hip involves maintaining abduction of the affected leg.
- Fractured hip fixation devices, such as hip prosthetic implant, plate and screw fixation, and telescoping nail fixation, require some degree of non-weight-bearing for 6 weeks to 3 months.
- Compartment syndrome, shock, fat embolism, gas gangrene, thromboembolus, and osteomyelitis are complications resulting from a fractured bone.
- Herniated nucleus pulposus is seen most often in the cervical and lumbar spinal region and can be treated surgically (laminectomy and spinal fusion) or medically (medication, traction, and physical therapy).

STUDY QUESTIONS

1. The end of a long bone, composed of spongy bone and containing red bone marrow, is called:
   1. Medullary cavity
   2. Diaphysis
   3. Epiphysis
   4. Olecranon process
2. The heaviest and strongest bone in the body is the:
   1. Tibia
   2. Femur
   3. Patella
   4. Radius
3. The type of muscle tissue that is voluntary:
   1. Cardiac
   2. Smooth
   3. Internal
   4. Skeletal
4. The thickest and strongest tendon in the body is the:
   1. Achilles
   2. Metacarpal
   3. Prime mover
   4. Trapezius
5. The anatomical name for the "swimmer's muscle" is:
   1. Latissimus dorsi
   2. Patella
   3. Deltoid
   4. Hamstring
6. The muscle in the upper arm that can be used as a site for intramuscular injections is the:
   1. Biceps
   2. Deltoid
   3. Patella
   4. Gluteus maximus
7. A band of connective tissue binding joints together and connecting various bones and cartilages is a:
   1. Ligament
   2. Tendon
   3. Bursa
   4. Diarthrosis
8. An example of a ball-and-socket joint is the:
   1. Knee joint
   2. Hip joint
   3. Wrist joint
   4. Ankle joint
9. Another name for the breast bone is the:
   1. Tibia
   2. Zygomaticus
   3. Mandible
   4. Sternum
10. The upper end of the ulna, which forms the point of the elbow, is the:
    1. Acromion
    2. Olecranon
    3. Acetabulum
    4. Fossa
11. JoEllen Miller, 26 years old, has been diagnosed as having rheumatoid arthritis (RA). The doctor prescribes a nonsteroidal antiinflammatory agent (NSAIA). An appropriate nursing intervention when administering NSAIAs would be to:
    1. Advise the patient to take the medicine with food
    2. Assess the patient for mental alertness
    3. Assess respiratory rate before administration
    4. Instruct the patient to take the medicine on an empty stomach
12. Mr. Sorensen is a 65-year-old male with clinical signs of gouty arthritis. He has deposits of sodium urate crystals in the tissue of the great toe. The nurse knows these deposits are referred to as:
    1. Calculi
    2. Tophi
    3. Atheroma
    4. Aschoff bodies
13. Mrs. Calland is a 65-year-old female suffering from osteoporosis. Collection of objective data involves assessing Mrs. Calland for:
    1. Radicular pain
    2. Dowager's hump
    3. Presence of a sequestrum
    4. Depressed appearance of soft tissue at base of thumb
14. Mrs. Romero is a 75-year-old retired schoolteacher who is recovering from a prosthetic implant (bipolar hip replacement) for repair of a fractured right hip. She is planning on being discharged to her home and will be seen once a week by a home health nurse. She has been receiving heparin injections subcutaneously and is to remain on the anticoagulant therapy. The most appropriate nursing diagnoses for Mrs. Romeo would include:
    1. Infection, high risk for
    2. Adjustment, impaired
    3. Nutrition, altered: less than body requirements
    4. Tissue perfusion, altered, peripheral, high risk for
15. Edith Whitmer is a 29-year-old suffering from a fractured pelvis sustained in a motor vehicle accident. She is admitted to the orthopedic unit and is being monitored closely for signs of shock and decreased urinary output. Appropriate nursing interventions include monitoring Ms. Whitmer for signs of progressive shock and:
    1. Inserting a Foley catheter per physician's order and monitoring I&O
    2. Log rolling for position change
    3. Applying Buck's traction
    4. Maintaining abduction of the hip by using a wedge-shaped foam bolster
16. Mrs. Smith, 24 years old, has been admitted to the medical unit for complaints of malaise, pain, edema,

tenderness in her joints, loss of appetite, and muscle weakness (especially grip strength). Based on the signs and symptoms the diagnosis most suspected would be:

1. Osteoarthritis
2. Rheumatoid arthritis
3. Gouty arthritis
4. Spondylitis

17. Mr. Jones is a 75-year-old retired construction worker. He has been seeing the physician for complaints of osteoarthritis. Today he is discussing concerns over his condition and asks what has caused his osteoarthritis. An appropriate response would be:

1. "You have osteoarthritis because of the difficult construction work you did for so many years."
2. "Everyone your age has arthritis; you are fortunate you are still able to walk."
3. The cause of osteoarthritis is unknown. However, almost all persons over 40 years of age have some changes in their joints."
4. "You probably did not exercise as much as you should have, and you should start vigorous exercising now to prevent further complications."

18. An appropriate nursing intervention for Mr. Smothers, a 32-year-old patient in skeletal traction, would be:

1. Provide cast care
2. Cleanse pin sites with hydrogen peroxide, and observe for signs of infection
3. Place patient on drainage and secretion precautions
4. Encourage the patient to sit in a straight, firm chair for no longer than 20 minutes at each time

19. Mike Thomas is an 8-year-old soccer player who has a greenstick fracture of his left tibia. Mike's mother asks the nurse what a greenstick fracture is. The most appropriate nursing response would be:

1. "It is a fracture that extends through the bone with disruption of the periosteum and usually affects males."
2. "It is when the bone splinters into three or more pieces."
3. "It is a fracture that telescopes."
4. "It is an incomplete break where the fracture line extends only partially through the bone."

20. Mr. Learn is a 45-year-old who suffered a knee injury while playing football with his son. He is scheduled for an arthroscopic examination and asks the nurse to explain the procedure. The most appropriate nursing response would be:

1. "Your physician will insert a small scope into your knee joint to visualize the joint for damaged tissue."
2. "The test involves the use of magnetism and radio waves to make images of cross sections of the body."
3. "The x-ray technician will inject your knee joint with an atomic material and take an x-ray of your affected knee."
4. "The physician will insert needle electrodes into the knee muscle so that electrical activity of the knee can be documented."

27

CARE OF THE PATIENT WITH A GASTROINTESTINAL OR ACCESSORY ORGAN DISORDER

Mary Lynne Todd Acheson

KEY TERMS

ANATOMY AND PHYSIOLOGY

adenosine triphosphate (ATP)
alimentary canal
amino acid
anabolism
bolus
catabolism
chemical digestion
chyme
deciduous
dentin
enamel
enzyme
gingiva
impaction
jaundice
mastication
mechanical digestion
mesentery
Oddi's sphincter
pepsin
peristalsis
ruga
villus

MEDICAL-SURGICAL

achalasia
achlorhydria
anastomosis
ascites
asterixis
cachexia
carcinoembryonic antigen (CEA)
dehiscence
dysphagia
esophageal varices
evisceration
exacerbation
flatulence
hematemesis
hepatic encephalopathy
intussusception
leukoplakia
lumen
melena
occlusion
occult blood
paracentesis
parenchyma
pathognomonic
pruritus
regurgitation
remission
steatorrhea
stoma
tenesmus
volvulus

LEARNING OBJECTIVES

After reading this chapter, the student should be able to do the following:

Anatomy and Physiology

- Define the key terms.
- List in sequence each of the component parts or segments of the alimentary canal and identify the accessory organs of digestion.
- Discuss the function of each digestive and accessory organ.
- Describe the process of digestion of fats, carbohydrates, and protein and give the end products of each process.
- Describe the peritoneum and list its two prominent extensions.

Medical-Surgical

- Define the key terms.
- Discuss nursing interventions for six diagnostic examinations for patients with disorders of the gastrointestinal tract.
- List the medication therapy for the patient with a peptic ulcer.
- List five signs and symptoms of gastrointestinal bleeding.
- Differentiate among irritable bowel syndrome, ulcerative colitis, and Crohn's disease.
- Identify nursing interventions for preoperative and postoperative care of the patient with gastric resection.
- Identify five nursing interventions for the patient with a stoma for fecal diversion.
- State the purpose of nasogastric suctioning.
- Differentiate between the nursing interventions for a patient with a laparoscopic cholecystectomy and those for a patient with an open abdominal cholecystectomy.
- State the five types of viral hepatitis.
- List the subjective and objective data for the patient with viral hepatitis.
- State the signs and symptoms caused by the liver's inability to metabolize bilirubin.
- Discuss specific teaching content for the patient with cirrhosis of the liver.
- Describe the medical management of and nursing interventions for the patient with acute pancreatitis.

RELATED TOPICS OF INTEREST

- Signs, symptoms, and physical assessment (Chapter 9)
- Specimen collection and diagnostic examination (Chapter 17)
- Basic nutrition (Chapter 18)
- Diet therapy (Chapter 19)
- The surgical patient (Chapter 22)
- Care of the patient with an endocrine disorder (Chapter 32)
- Care of the patient with cancer (Chapter 38)

ANATOMY AND PHYSIOLOGY

Digestive System

Although it is understood that food is necessary for existence, not everyone understands (1) what happens to food once it is chewed and swallowed, (2) how food is prepared for its trip to each individual cell, and (3) the many changes that food undergoes, both chemically and physically. This chapter will discuss these changes and their impact on the body.

The digestive tract, or **alimentary canal** (a musculomembranous tube, extending from the mouth to the

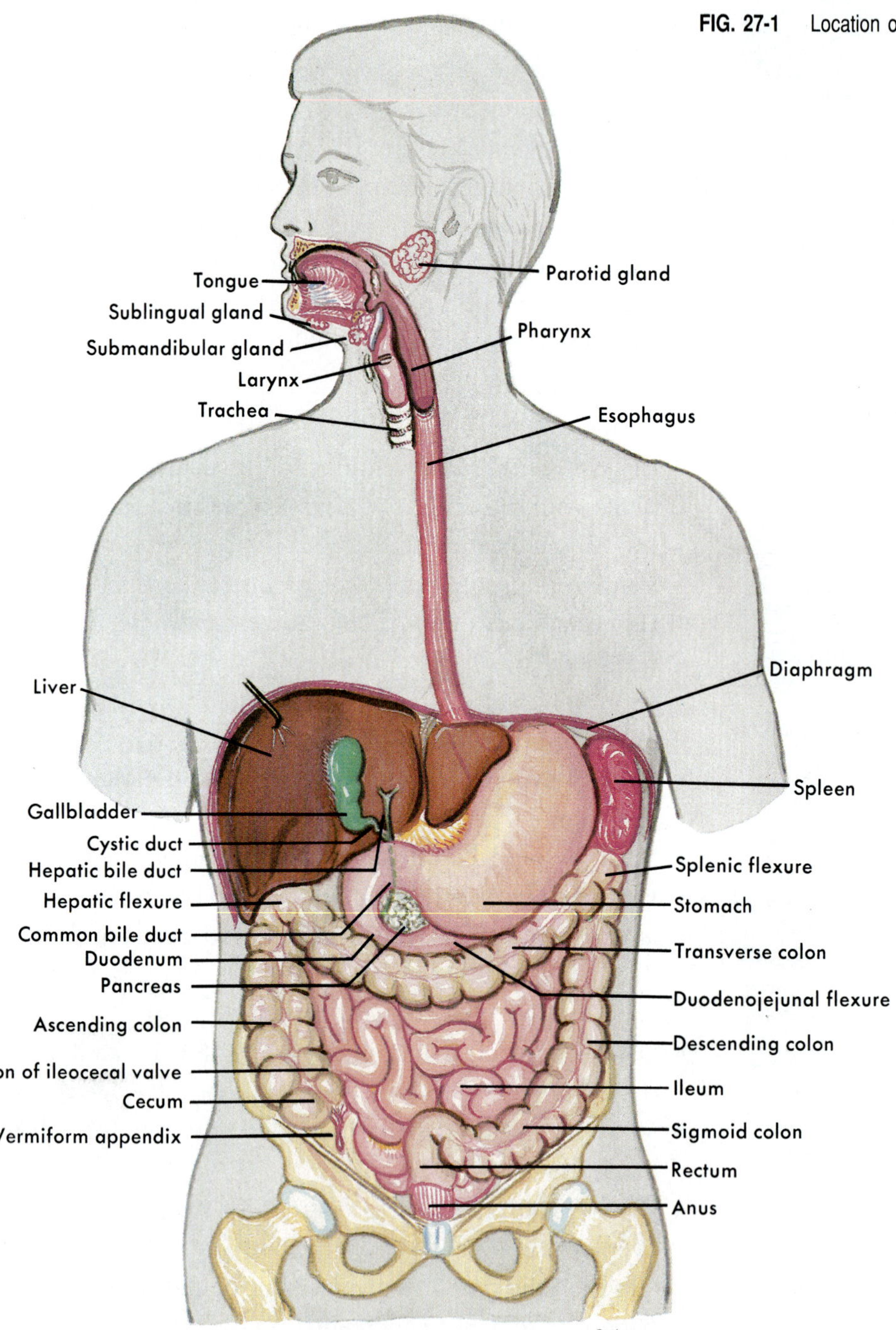

FIG. 27-1 Location of digestive organs.

anus), is approximately 30 feet long. During **peristalsis** (the coordinated, rhythmic, serial contraction of smooth muscle that forces food through the digestive tract, bile through the bile duct, and urine through the ureter), the tract shortens to approximately 15 feet. The tract begins at the mouth and continues through the body trunk to exit at the anus. It consists of the mouth, pharynx, esophagus, stomach, small intestine, large intestine, and anus (Fig. 27-1).

The alimentary canal is composed of four layers of specialized tissue. They are as follows:

1. Mucosa (mucous membrane): innermost layer, which secretes mucus
2. Submucosa: layer of connective tissue rich in blood vessels and nerves, which plays a regulatory role
3. Smooth muscle layer: circular and longitudinal layer, which aids in peristalsis
4. Fibrous connective tissue with a thin outer serous membrane

Accessory organs aid in the digestive process but are not considered part of the digestive tract. They release chemicals into the system through a series of ducts. The teeth, tongue, salivary glands, liver, gallbladder, and pancreas are considered accessory organs. These will be discussed in detail in the chapter.

Box 27-1 ORGANS OF THE DIGESTIVE SYSTEM

MAIN ORGANS

Mouth
Pharynx (throat)
Esophagus (foodpipe)
Stomach
  Fundus
  Body
  Lesser curvature
  Greater curvature
  Pylorus
Small intestine
  Duodenum
  Jejunum
  Ileum
Large intestine
  Cecum
Large intestine—cont'd
  Colon
    Ascending colon
    Transverse colon
    Descending colon
    Sigmoid colon
Rectum
Anal canal

ACCESSORY ORGANS

Teeth and tongue
Salivary glands
  Parotid
  Submandibular
  Sublingual
Liver
Gallbladder
Pancreas
Vermiform appendix

Organs of the Digestive System (Box 27-1)

Mouth. The mouth (buccal cavity) marks the entrance to the digestive system. The roof of the mouth is composed of the hard and soft palates. The hard palate is formed by bony structures; the soft palate is composed of muscle and covered by mucous membrane. The soft palate is posterior to the hard palate and contains muscle, blood vessels, nerves, and mucous glands. The uvula, a small, cone-shaped tag of tissue, extends from the middle of the posterior edge of the soft palate. It protects the entrance to the nasal cavity during swallowing. The lateral walls of the mouth are formed by the cheeks.

The floor of the mouth contains a muscular appendage, the tongue. The anterior portion of the tongue is attached to the floor of the mouth by the *frenulum,* a fold of mucous membrane. The tongue is involved in chewing, swallowing, and the formation of speech. Tiny elevations, *papillae,* contain the taste buds. They differentiate among the bitter, sweet, sour, and salty sensations.

Digestion begins in the mouth. Here the teeth mechanically shred and grind the food and the **enzymes** (complex proteins, produced by living cells, that are capable of inducing chemical changes in other substances without being changed themselves) begin the chemical breakdown of carbohydrates. In addition, the oral cavity, the tongue, and the teeth play a role in speech production.

Teeth. Everyone has two sets of teeth during his lifetime. The first set (**deciduous** [any one of the set of 20 teeth that appear normally during infancy, consisting of four incisors, two canines, and four molars in each jaw], baby teeth) begins to erupt at 6 months of age; the deciduous teeth continue to appear until 2 years of age. These remain until the age of 6 years. By this time the jawbone has grown sufficiently to accommodate the larger, permanent teeth that replace the deciduous teeth.

The permanent teeth are structured to last a lifetime. Generally, by 12 years of age all the deciduous teeth have been replaced by permanent teeth. By adulthood, permanent teeth will number 32. Each tooth is designed to carry out a specific task. Immediately to the center of the mouth lie the incisors, which are structured for biting and cutting. Posterior to the incisors are the canines, pointed teeth used for tearing and shredding food. The molars are to the rear of the jaw (Fig. 27-2 on p. 644). These teeth have four cusps (points) and are used for **mastication** (to crush and grind food). The last set of molars to erupt, one superior and one inferior bilaterally, is referred to as *wisdom teeth.* They usually do not erupt until age 18. Often the jaw will not accommodate the extra molars and they remain embedded in the jawbone. This results in a condition called **impaction** (condition of being tightly wedged into a part, or eruption of a tooth blocked by other teeth), and the wisdom teeth must be surgically removed.

Tooth construction. Each tooth develops in a socket (alveolus) deep in the jaw, which is really an extension of the mandible and maxilla. The **gingivae** (gums) cover the area and extend partially into the

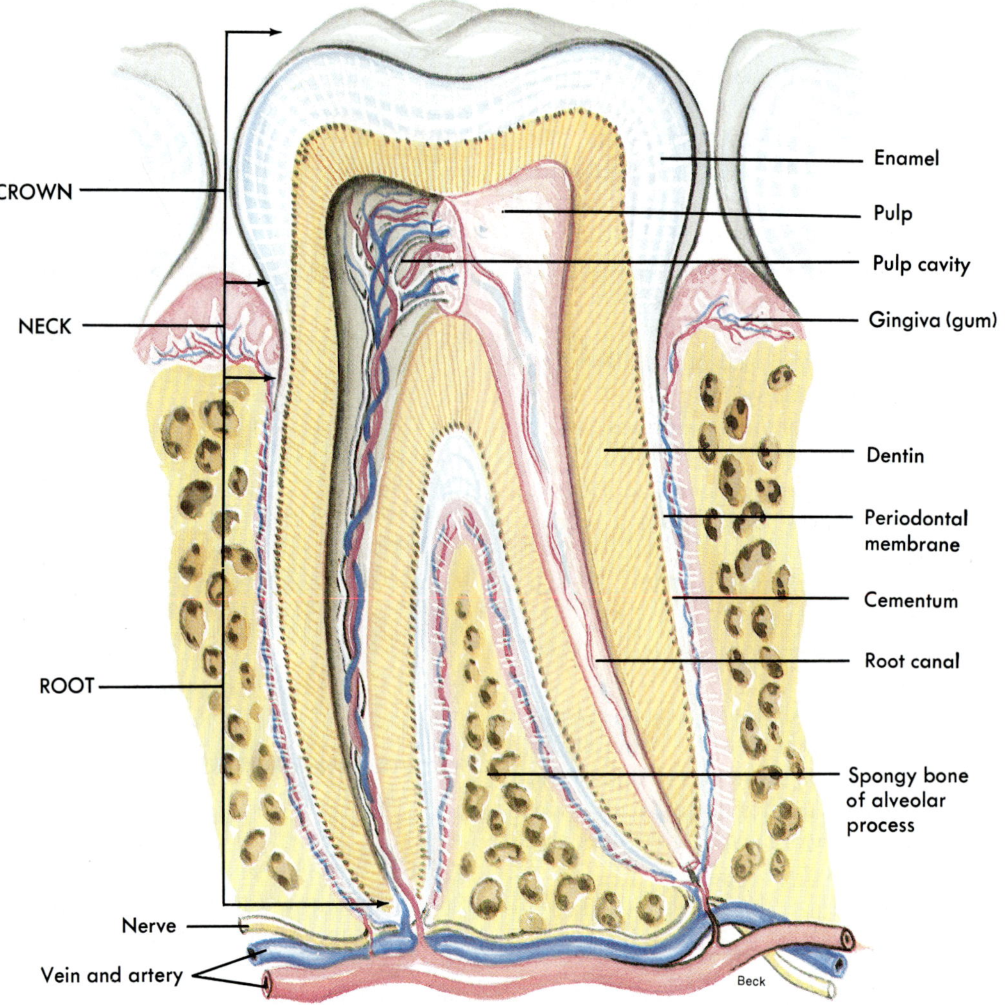

FIG. 27-2 A molar tooth sectioned to show its bony socket and details of its three main parts: crown, neck, and root. Enamel (over the crown) and cementum (over the neck and root) surround the dentin layer. The pulp contains nerves and blood vessels.

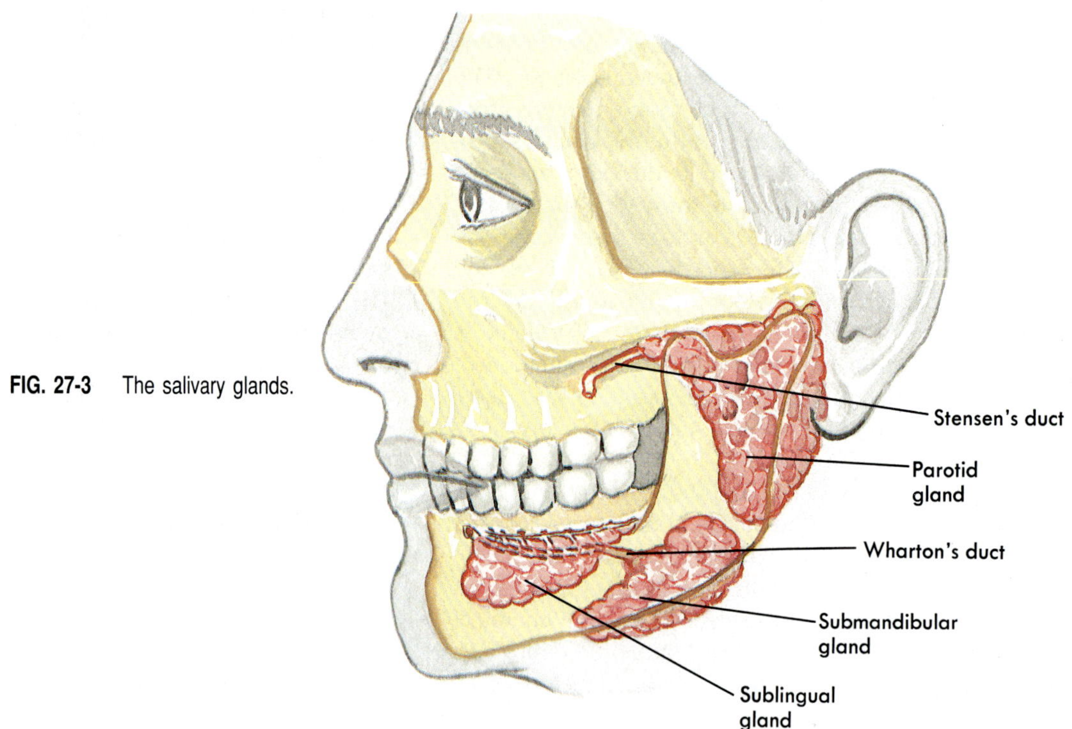

FIG. 27-3 The salivary glands.

socket. The portion of the tooth above the gum line is the crown; the portion below the gum line is the root. The neck of the tooth is the junction between the crown and the root.

The centermost part of the tooth is the pulp cavity; it contains the blood vessels and nerves. Surrounding the pulp is the **dentin** (a calcified tissue that gives shape and structure to the tooth). The outer covering of the tooth is the **enamel,** the hardest material in the body. It protects the inner structures of the tooth from wearing away and from exposure to the many acids in foods.

Salivary glands. There are three pairs of salivary glands (Fig. 27-3). They secrete a fluid called *saliva,* which is approximately 99% water with enzymes and mucus. The largest pair, the parotid glands, lies just anterior to the ear near the jawline. These are the glands that become edematous and hurt with epidemic parotitis (mumps). Their ducts (Stensen's ducts) open into the oral cavity just superior to the upper second molars. The second set, the submandibular glands, is found inferior to the tongue in the posterior part of the mouth. Their ducts (Wharton's ducts) are found posterior to the lower central incisors bilateral to the frenulum. The third set of glands, the sublingual glands, lies immediately anterior to the submandibular glands. Their ducts open onto the floor of the mouth directly inferior to the tongue.

Normally these glands secrete enough fluid (saliva) to keep the mucous membrane of the mouth moist. Once food enters the mouth, the secretion increases to lubricate and dissolve the food and to begin the chemical process of digestion. The salivary glands secrete about 1000 to 1500 ml of saliva daily. The major enzyme is salivary amylase (ptyalin), which is responsible for the initiation of carbohydrate metabolism. Another enzyme, lysozyme, destroys bacteria, which protects the mucous membrane from infections and protects the teeth from decay. After food has been ingested, the salivary glands continue to secrete saliva, which cleanses the mouth.

Esophagus. The esophagus is a muscular, collapsible tube, which is approximately 10 inches long. It articulates the laryngopharynx with the opening to the stomach. It passes through the diaphragm via an opening called the *esophageal hiatus* (a weakness in this area results in a condition called *hiatal hernia*). The esophagus is a passageway for the **bolus** (food broken down and mixed with saliva and ready to be swallowed) to pass to the stomach. No digestion takes place here. Peristalsis moves the bolus through the tube in 5 to 6 seconds.

Stomach. The stomach is located in the left upper quadrant of the abdomen, directly inferior to the diaphragm (Fig. 27-4). When the stomach is empty, the inner lining

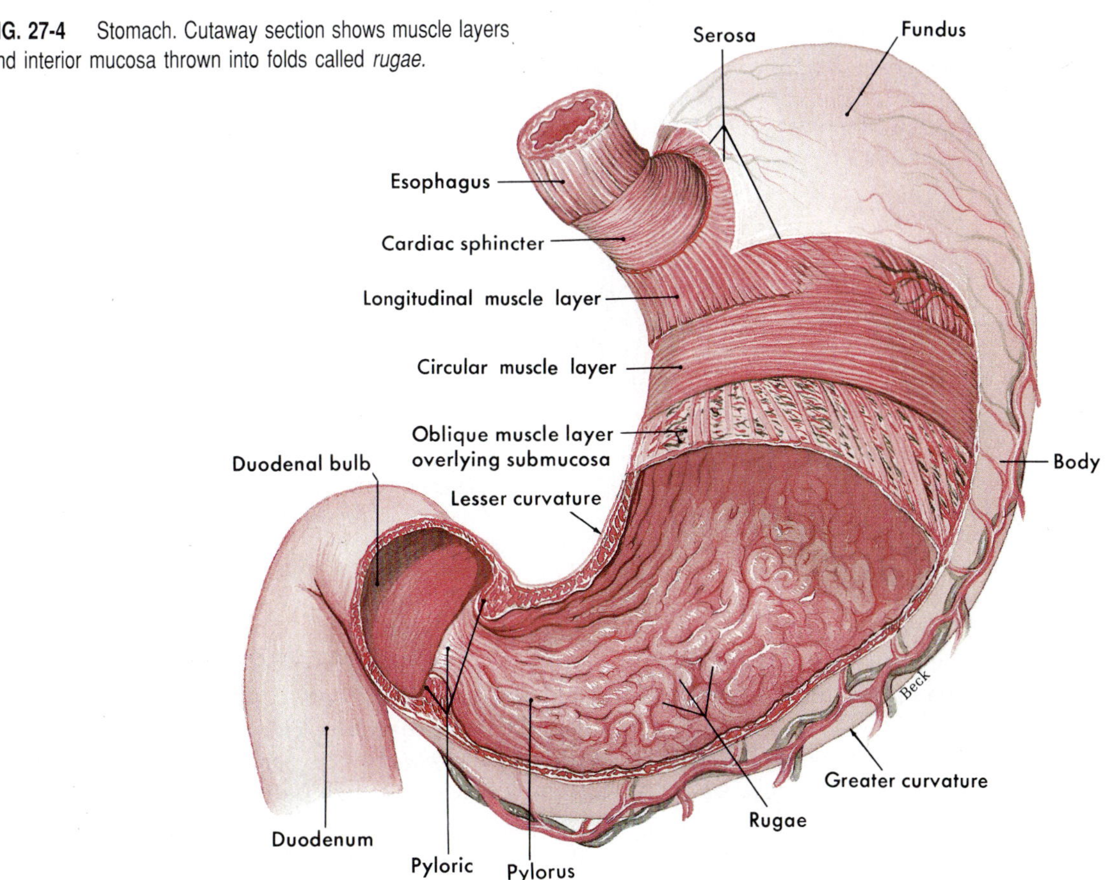

FIG. 27-4 Stomach. Cutaway section shows muscle layers and interior mucosa thrown into folds called *rugae.*

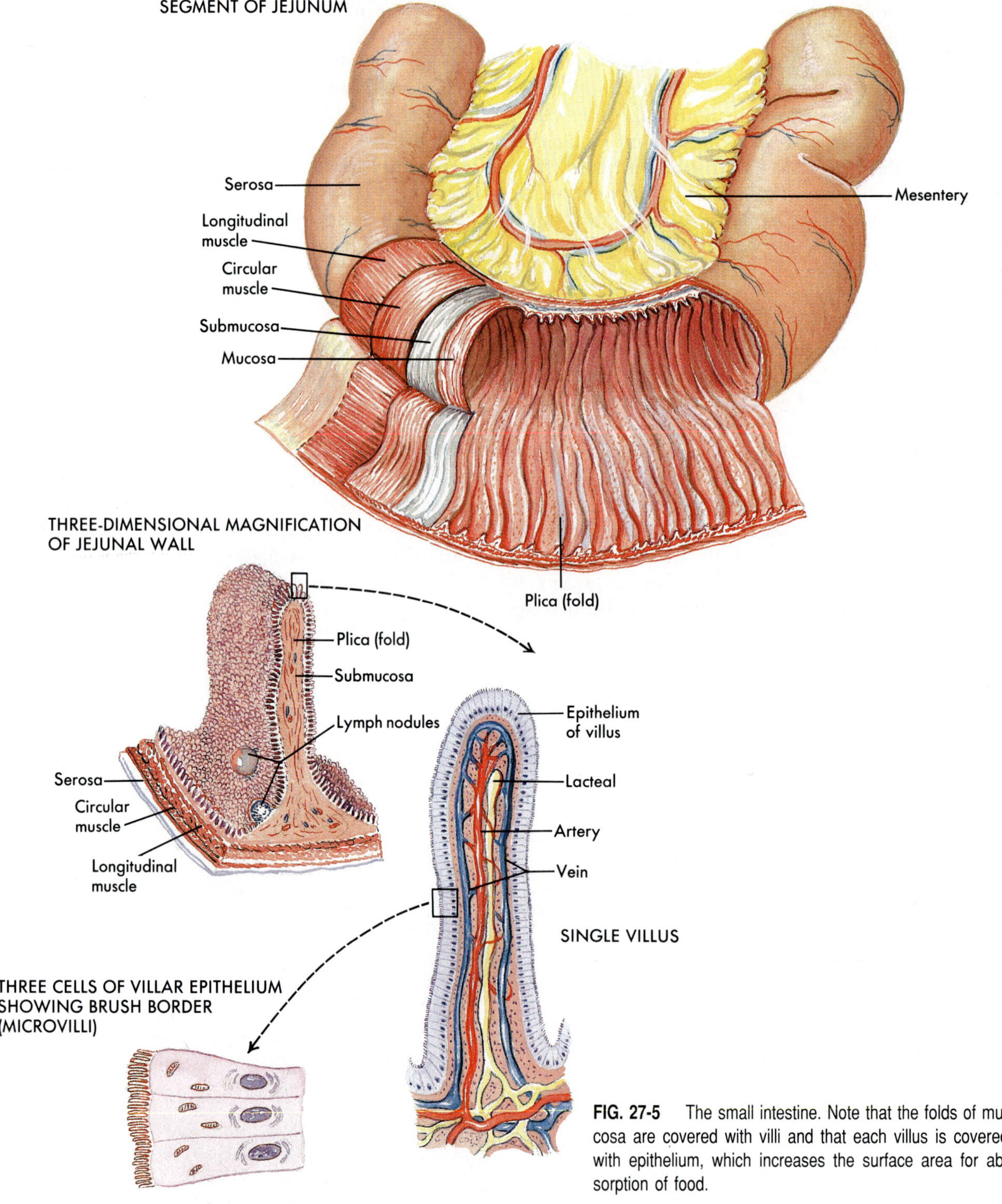

FIG. 27-5 The small intestine. Note that the folds of mucosa are covered with villi and that each villus is covered with epithelium, which increases the surface area for absorption of food.

collapses into **rugae** (folds or creases, especially of the folds of mucous membrane seen on the internal surface of the stomach).

When the stomach is filled, it stretches to the size of a football and holds approximately 1 liter. It receives its blood supply from the celiac artery. The stomach is divided into three major sections: (1) fundus—superior section, (2) body—middle section, and (3) pyloric portion—inferior section. The outer angle of the stomach is called the *greater curvature,* and the inner angle is called the *lesser curvature.* The entrance to the stomach is the *cardiac sphincter* (so named because of the proximity to the heart); the exit is the *pyloric sphincter*.

As the food leaves the esophagus, it enters the stomach through the relaxed cardiac sphincter. The sphincter then contracts, preventing esophageal reflux (splash ing, or return flow), which can be irritating. This condition is sometimes referred to as *heartburn.*

Once the bolus has entered the stomach, the muscular layers of the stomach churn and contract to mix and compress the contents with the gastric juices and water. The gastric juices are a group of secretions that are released by the gastric glands. Digestion of protein begins in the stomach. Hydrochloric acid softens the connective tissue in meat, kills bacteria, and activates **pepsin** (the chief enzyme of gastric juices that converts proteins into proteoses and peptones). Mucin is released to protect the stomach lining. Intrinsic factor (a substance secreted by the gastric mucosa) is produced to allow for the intestinal absorption of vitamin B_{12}. After the stomach has completed its work, the food has been broken down into a viscous semiliquid substance called **chyme.** The chyme is sent through the pyloric sphincter into the duodenum, for the next phase of digestion.

Small Intestine. The small intestine (Fig 27-5), is a 20-foot-long tube; it is 1 inch in diameter. It begins at the pyloric valve and ends at the ileocecal valve. It is divided into three major sections: duodenum, jejunum, and ileum. The inner mucous membrane lining contains the intestinal glands, which secrete the intestinal juices (enzymes). Most of digestion is accomplished here—as much as 90%. The intestinal juices finish the metabolism of carbohydrates and proteins. Bile and pancreatic juices enter the duodenum. The bile from the liver breaks fat molecules into smaller droplets, which enables the digestive juices to complete their process. Pancreatic juices contain water, protein, inorganic salts, and enzymes. Pancreatic juices are essential in breaking down proteins into their amino acid components, in reducing dietary fats to glycerol and fatty acids, and in converting starch to simple sugars.

The inner surface of the small intestine falls into numerous folds called *plicae.* These folds contain millions of tiny, fingerlike projections, clustered over the entire mucous surface of the small intestine, called **villi.** They are responsible for the absorption of the products of digestion into the bloodstream. They increase the absorption area of the small intestine 600 times. Inside each villus is a rich capillary bed, along with modified lymph capillaries called *lacteals.* The lacteals are responsible for the absorption of metabolized fats.

Large Intestine. Once the small intestine has finished with its specific tasks, the ileocecal valve, which separates the cecum from the ileum, opens and releases the contents into the large intestine. This tube is larger in diameter (2 inches) but shorter (5 feet) than the small intestine. It is composed of the cecum; appendix; ascending, transverse, descending, and sigmoid colons; rectum; and anus (Fig. 27-6 on p. 648). The process of digestion is completed here in the terminal portion of the digestive tract. Basically the large intestine has four major functions: (1) completion of absorption; (2) manufacture of certain vitamins; (3) formation of feces; and (4) expulsion of feces.

Just inferior to the ileocecal valve is the cecum, a blind pouch approximately 2 to 3 inches long. Dangling from the cecum is a small, wormlike, tubular structure, the vermiform appendix. It is composed of lymphoid tissue. To date there is no known function for the appendix. It is common for the appendix to become inflamed, resulting in a condition known as *appendicitis,* which requires prompt surgical attention to prevent infection of the surrounding tissues. The open end of the cecum connects the small and large intestine. The colon is divided into four portions: (1) ascending, (2) transverse, (3) descending, and (4) sigmoid. The ascending colon continues upward on the right side of the abdomen to the inferior area of the liver. This right colonic area is called the *hepatic flexure.* It then crosses to the left side of the abdomen, forming the transverse colon. The transverse colon continues inferior to the spleen. This left colonic area is called the *splenic flexure.* The descending colon passes downward on the left side of the abdomen to the level of the iliac crest. The sigmoid colon begins here and continues toward the midline to the level of the third sacral vertebra.

Bacteria in the large intestine change the chyme into fecal material by releasing the remaining nutrients. The bacteria are also responsible for the synthesis of vitamin K, needed for normal blood clotting, and the production of some of the B-complex vitamins. Once formed, these vitamins are absorbed from the large intestine and enter the blood.

No villi are present in the mucosa of the large intestine; as a result, much less surface area is available for absorption, and the efficiency and speed of movement of substances through the wall of the large intestine are slower than in the small intestine. Only mucus is secreted by the large intestine, since most of the digestive process has already taken place in the small intestine. As the fecal material continues its journey, the remaining water is absorbed into the bloodstream by osmosis. Sodium and other salts are absorbed by active transport. Normal passage of material through the large intestine takes about 3 to 5 days.

Rectum. Finally, the waste products have been prepared for expulsion from the body, metabolism and absorption have been completed, and feces has been formed. The last 8 inches of the large intestine forms the rectum, which appends to the exit—the anal canal, which terminates with the anus. Under usual conditions the anus remains closed. It contains an internal sphincter composed of smooth muscle (involuntary) and an external sphincter composed of skeletal muscle (voluntary). With the urge to defecate, these sphincters relax and feces is expelled. The rectum carries the feces from the colon to the anal canal and functions as an excretory canal.

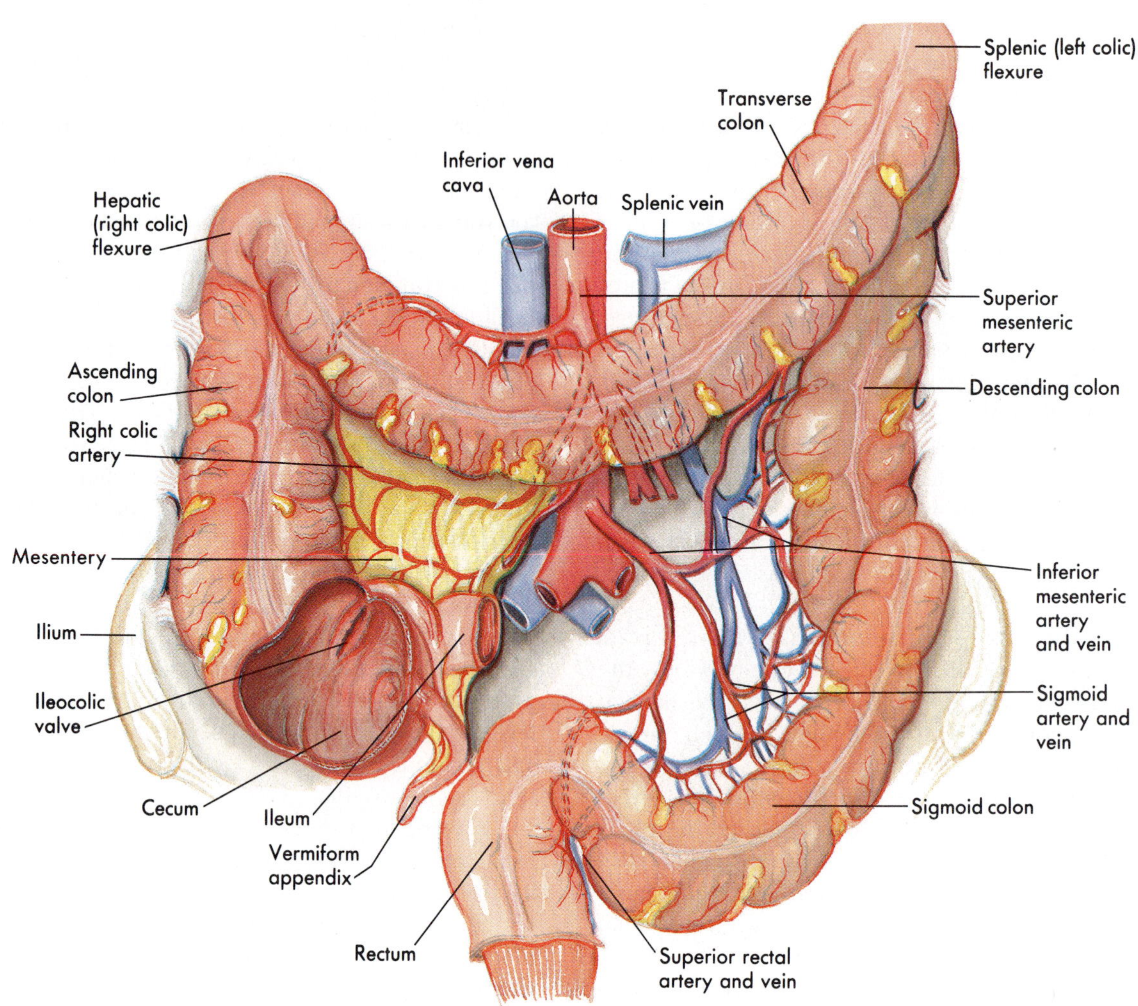

FIG. 27-6 Divisions of large intestine.

Normally, the two sphincter muscles stay contracted to keep the anus closed except during defecation. Often after a person has a CVA (stroke), the voluntary anal sphincter at first becomes paralyzed. This means that the individual has no control over bowel movements. Normally, as the rectum becomes distended with stool, the urge to defecate becomes apparent. The brain sends a message to the anal sphincters, they relax, and stool is expelled.

Accessory Organs of Digestion

Liver. The liver is the largest glandular organ in the body and one of its most complex. It is completely covered by a tough fibrous sheath, Glisson's capsule. In the adult it weighs 3 pounds. It is located just inferior to the diaphragm, covering most of the right upper quadrant and extending into part of the left epigastrium. It is divided into the right and left lobes. Approximately 1500 ml of blood is delivered to the liver every minute by the portal vein and the hepatic artery. At any given moment the liver holds about 1 pint of blood or approximately 13% of the total blood supply of the body. Oxygenated blood is carried by the hepatic artery, and the portal vein delivers deoxygenated blood that is rich in nutrients that have been absorbed from the small intestine.

The cells of the liver produce a product called *bile*, a yellow-brown or green-brown liquid. It consists mostly of water, salts, cholesterol, and bile pigments. Bile is necessary for the metabolism of fats. The liver releases 500 to 1000 ml of bile daily. The bile travels to the gallbladder through the right and left hepatic ducts. If it is not needed, the bile backs up into the cystic duct to be stored in the gallbladder for later use.

Bilirubin is the main bile pigment. It is released as red blood cells are broken down by the liver. When it reaches the intestines, the bilirubin is broken down and its products give feces its color.

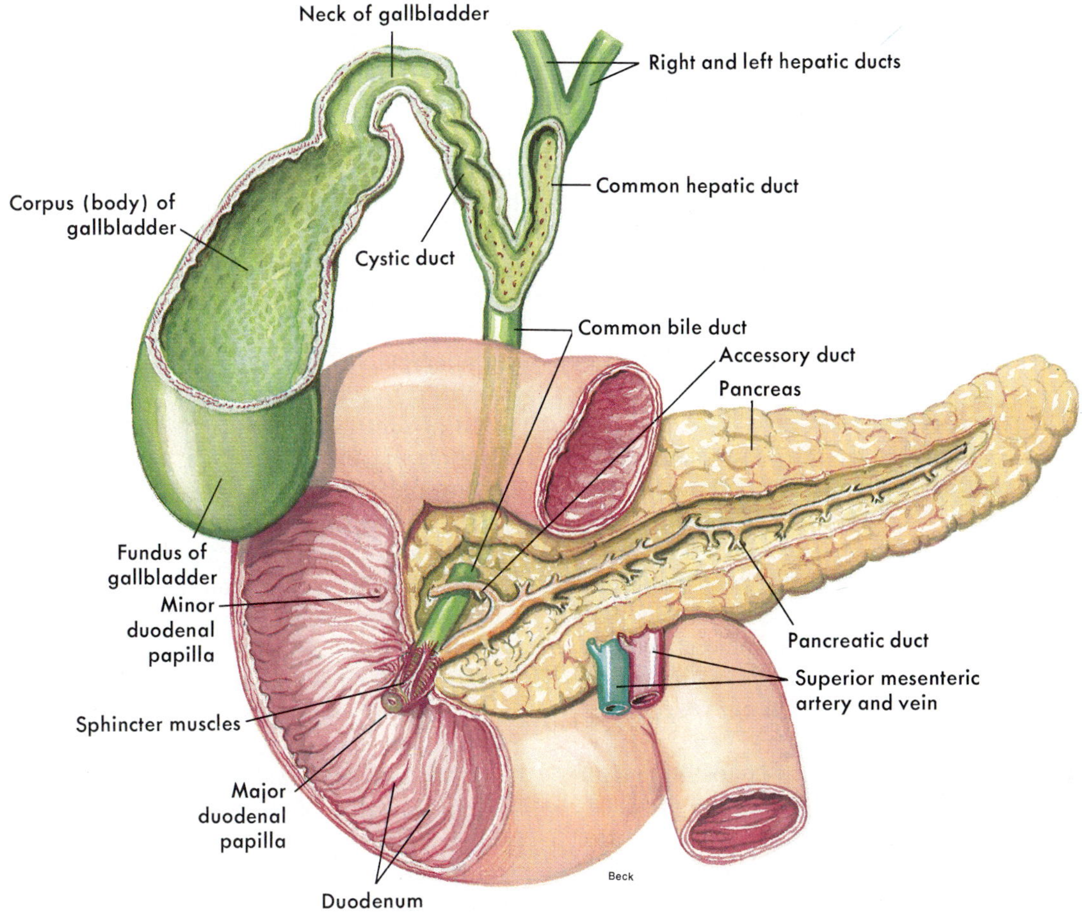

FIG. 27-7 The gallbladder and bile ducts. Obstruction of the hepatic or common bile duct by stone or spasm occludes the exit of the bile from being ejected into the duodenum.

In addition to the production of bile, some of the many other functions of the human liver are the following:

1. It manufactures heparin, prothrombin, and fibrinogen—all necessary for blood coagulation management.
2. It manufactures cholesterol.
3. It manufactures albumin, which helps maintain normal blood volume.
4. It filters out old red blood cells and certain bacteria.
5. It detoxifies alcohol, nicotine, and other poisons and certain drugs.
6. It converts poisonous ammonia to urea.
7. It is one of the main sources of body heat.
8. It stores copper, vitamin B_{12}, and fat-soluble vitamins A, D, E, and K.
9. It stores sugar in the form of glycogen for later use by the body.
10. It participates with the kidneys to activate vitamin D.
11. It breaks down nitrogenous wastes (from protein metabolism) to urea, which the kidneys can then excrete from the body.

Gallbladder. The gallbladder (Fig 27-7) is an ovoid, muscular sac, about 3 to 4 inches long. It is located on the right inferior surface of the liver. Because the small intestine needs bile only a few times a day, the gallbladder stores and concentrates it. When chyme, containing fat, enters the first portion of the small intestine (duodenum), the gallbladder contracts and releases bile through the cystic duct into the common bile duct. A circular muscle called **Oddi's sphincter** is located at the opening of the common bile duct into the duodenum at the papilla of Vater. When open, this sphincter empties bile into the duodenum under the influence of cholecystokinin, an enzyme.

If a stone occludes the common bile duct, bile refluxes into the hepatic ducts and then into the liver. This puts pressure on the liver to release bilirubin into the bloodstream. This results in **jaundice** (yellow discoloration of the skin, sclerae, and mucous membranes), which is caused by greater than normal amounts of bilirubin in the blood.

It is important to remember that bile is produced by the liver and stored and concentrated by the gallbladder. It is then released into the duodenum for the metabolism of fats. It travels from the liver through the right and left hepatic ducts through the cystic duct to the gallbladder. Once the gallbladder contracts, bile travels down the cystic duct to the common bile duct and then into the duodenum. The system of passageways is referred to as the *biliary ductal system* or *biliary apparatus.*

Pancreas. The pancreas is an elongated gland that lies posterior to the stomach (see Fig. 27-7 and Chapter 32). It is an active organ that is involved in both endocrine and exocrine duties. In this chapter the discussion of the pancreas is limited to the exocrine activities. It involves the production of digestive enzymes that are transported through an excretory duct of Wirsung to the duodenum. This pancreatic duct connects to the common bile duct from the liver and gallbladder and empties through a small orifice in the duodenum called the *papilla of Vater.*

Each day the pancreas produces 1000 to 1500 ml of pancreatic juice to aid in digestion. This pancreatic juice contains the digestive enzymes protease (trypsin), lipase (steapsin), amylase (amylopsin), which are important because of their ability to digest the three major components of chyme—proteins, fats, and carbohydrates. In addition, it contains an alkaline substance, sodium bicarbonate, which has the ability to neutralize the hydrochloric acid in the gastric juices that enter the small intestine from the stomach (Table 27-1).

Occasionally the pancreas becomes diseased, resulting in pancreatic digestive juices actually digesting the pancreas. This serious condition is called *acute pancreatitis.*

Peritoneum. The peritoneum is a serous membrane that covers most of the abdominal organs. It is the largest membrane in the body; the heart and lungs are also covered with serous membrane. The peritoneum is composed of squamous epithelium with a supportive layer of connective tissue. The walls of the abdominal cavity are covered with the parietal (of or pertaining to the outer wall of a cavity or organ) peritoneum, and the abdominal organs are covered with visceral (the internal organs enclosed within a body cavity, primarily the abdominal organs) peritoneum. The space between these two layers is called the *peritoneal cavity.* It has a thin coating of serous fluid. This allows the two layers of the membranes to slide against each other during breathing and digestive movements (Fig. 27-8). Some organs that lie on the posterior wall of the abdomen have only an anterior covering of peritoneum; the kidneys and pancreas are examples. They are referred to as *retroperitoneal* organs. If an organ within the abdominal cavity becomes infected, the infection can spread easily to the membrane, resulting in a condition called *peritonitis.*

TABLE 27-1 Chemical Digestion

Digestive Juices and Enzymes	Enzyme Digests	Resulting Product*
Saliva		
Amylase (ptyalin)	Starch (polysaccharide)	Maltose (a disaccharide, or double sugar)
Gastric juice		
Protease (pepsin) plus hydrochloric acid	Proteins, including casein	Proteoses and peptones (partially digested proteins)
Lipase (of little importance)	Emulsified fats (butter, cream, and so on)	**Fatty acids and glycerol***
Pancreatic juice		
Protease (trypsin)	Proteins (either intact or partially digested)	Proteoses, peptides, and **amino acids***
Lipase (steapsin)	Bile—emulsified fats	**Fatty acids and glycerol***
Amylase (amylopsin)	Starch	Maltose
Intestinal juice (succus entericus)		
Peptidases	Peptides	**Amino acids***
Sucrase	Sucrose (cane sugar)	**Glucose and fructose*†** (Simple sugars of monosaccharides)
Lactase	Lactose (milk sugar)	**Glucose and galactose*** (simple sugars)
Maltase	Maltose (malt sugar)	**Glucose*** (grape sugar)

*Substances in boldface type are end products of digestion, that is, completely digested foods ready for absorption.
†Glucose is also called *dextrose;* fructose is called *levulose.*

Usually it can be resolved with antibiotic therapy, but the individual is very ill with severe abdominal pain and elevated temperature.

Extensions. The peritoneum lies in large folds throughout the abdominal cavity, surrounding the various organs. These large folds contain blood vessels, lymph vessels, and the nerves that supply the abdominal organs. The peritoneum anchors the organs to each other and also to the abdominal walls. The first extension of the peritoneum, which is called the **mesentery,** is shaped like a giant, pleated fan. Its smaller edge attaches to the lumbar region of the posterior abdominal wall, and its long, loose, outer edge encloses most of the small intestine, anchoring it to the posterior abdominal wall. The mesocolon attaches the large intestine to the posterior abdominal wall. The mesocolon carries the blood supply to the intestines (see Fig. 27-8).

Two other extensions are called the *lesser* and *greater omenta.* They too arise from the peritoneal folds. The lesser omentum arises from the lesser curvature of the stomach and suspends the stomach and duodenum from the liver. The greater omentum arises from the greater curvature of the stomach and is attached to the duodenum, stomach, and large intestine. It contains large quantities of adipose tissue. It descends over the intestines, and because spotty deposits of fat give it a lacy appearance, it has been nicknamed the *fatty lace apron.* The greater omentum also contains many lymph nodes, which, in the presence of infection, will attempt to resolve the infection and prevent its spread to the peritoneum (see Fig. 27-8).

Regulation of Food Intake

The hypothalamus, a portion of the diencephalon of the brain, contains two centers that have an impact on eating habits. The first area is called the *feeding center.* When it is stimulated, an individual will eat even if not hungry. The second center is the *satiety center,* and when stimulated it signals the individual to stop eating. These centers work in conjunction with other areas of the brain to balance eating patterns. Many other factors also impact eating styles. For example, distention of the stomach activates the satiety center, decreasing the appetite. Cool temperatures increase appetite. Warm temperatures decrease it. In addition to the many controls within our bodies, life-styles, eating habits, emotions, and genetic factors all influence intake of food and blend together to influence each individual's body build.

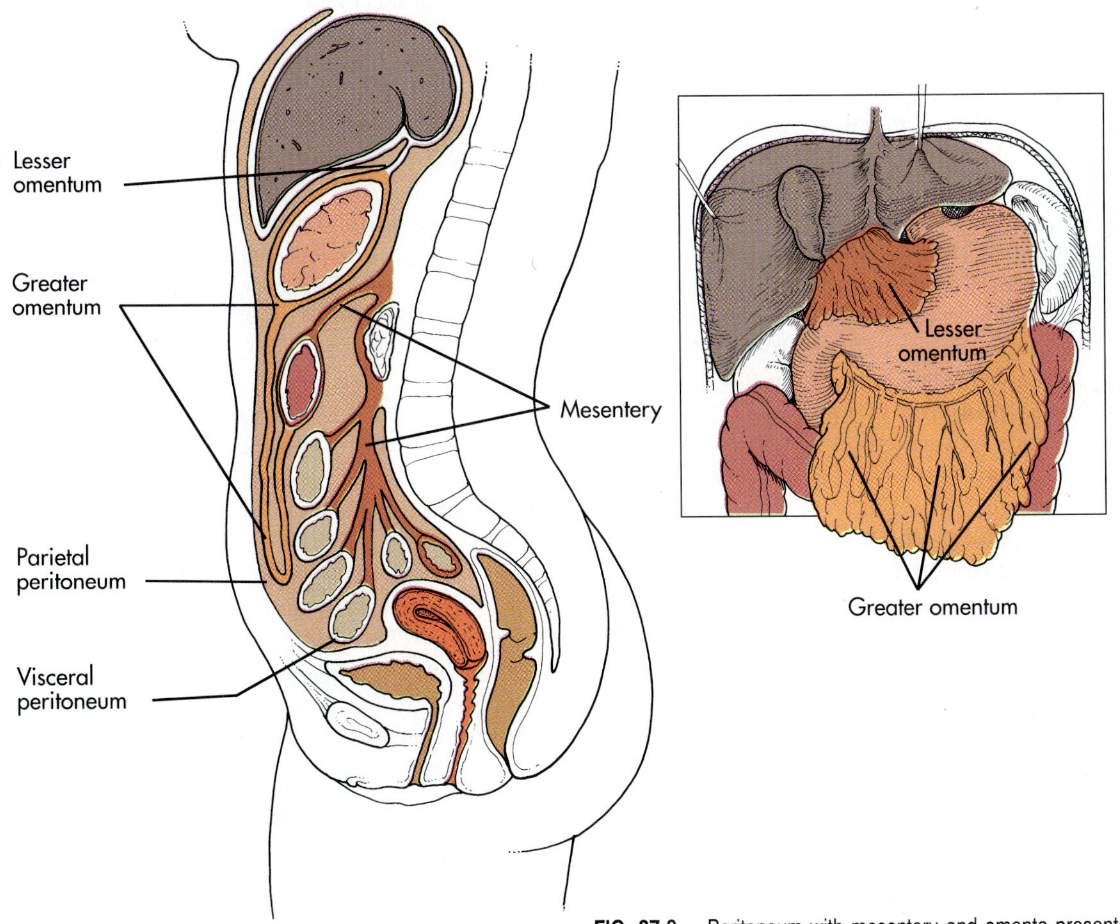

FIG. 27-8 Peritoneum with mesentery and omenta presentation.

Digestion. Once food is ingested into the digestive system, two major types of processes take place to prepare the food for use by the cells. The first is **mechanical digestion** (the food is broken into smaller particles and propelled through the gastrointestinal system to become mixed with the various enzymes). In mechanical digestion the chemical structure of the food is not altered—only the physical size of the product is changed to prepare it for chemical digestion.

The second process is **chemical digestion** (see Table 27-1) (the series of reactions that breaks the proteins, fats, and carbohydrates into molecules that the cells can readily use). The speed of the process is enhanced by the presence of the various enzymes throughout the digestive tract. It starts with the enzyme in saliva and ends with the intestinal enzymes.

Metabolism. Metabolism is the total of all chemical processes that take place in living organisms, resulting in growth, generation of energy, elimination of wastes, and activation of other bodily functions as they relate to the distribution of nutrients in the blood after digestion.

Metabolism can be divided into two phases. The first is **catabolism,** in which chemical compounds are broken into simpler forms with the release of energy. This energy provides the cells strength to perform their various activities. Catabolism is the destructive phase of metabolism; it releases usable forms of energy. The second phase, **anabolism,** is the building aspect, in which the energy released from catabolism allows the cells to build more complex, usable forms of nutrients. For example, fats are converted to phospholipids, which in turn form the plasma membrane. Anabolism is the building and repairing phase of metabolism.

The amount of energy used by the body at rest is called the *basal metabolic rate (BMR).* It is the amount of energy necessary for vital body functions, such as respiration and circulation, to continue. When foods are metabolized, they give off different amounts of energy. This energy value is measured in units called *kilocalories (kcal).* The more active the body is, the more kilocalories it needs to maintain homeostasis. Any excess is stored for later use.

Fats yield 9 kilocalories per gram (kcal/g), proteins yield 4 kcal/g, and carbohydrates also yield 4 kcal/g (see Chapter 18). If the number of grams of a specific food is determined, this number is easily converted to caloric value. For example, a banana contains 25 g of carbohydrates. Because carbohydrates contain 4 kcal/g, multiplying 4×25 shows that a banana contains 100 calories. Many books and pamphlets are available that list the caloric value of foods.

Carbohydrate Digestion and Metabolism. Most carbohydrates that are ingested are in the form of complex sugars (polysaccharides). They must be converted to simple sugars (monosaccharides) to be absorbed and used by the cells. This process begins in the mouth with the enzyme *salivary amylase* (ptyalin). Because food passes quickly through the mouth, salivary amylase only initiates the process of conversion. It continues to work on carbohydrates in the stomach for 15 to 20 minutes until hydrochloric acid, released by the stomach, stops the process. As chyme passes to the small intestine, the process begins again with the release of pancreatic amylase from the pancreas and the three major enzymes from the small intestine—maltase, sucrase, and lactase. Once the carbohydrates have been changed to glucose, they can enter the cell wall. Once inside the cell, a series of processes takes place that releases energy for cell use. Approximately one half of the energy is stored as **adenosine triphosphate (ATP)** (an enzyme involved in obtaining energy for cellular metabolism), which can be released instantaneously by the cell as needed. A certain amount of glucose is stored in the liver in the form of glycogen. When the body needs this reserve, the liver breaks the glycogen down to glucose and releases it into the bloodstream for immediate use.

Fat Digestion and Metabolism. Most fat (lipid) digestion and metabolism occur in the small intestine. Bile, which is produced by the liver and stored in the gallbladder, is released through the cystic duct into the duodenum. It mechanically breaks the large fat globules into small droplets. Pancreatic lipase, an enzyme found in pancreatic juice, chemically converts the droplets into a usable form of fatty acids and glycerol. The fatty acids and glycerol are then absorbed into the lymph system through the lacteals in the villi of the small intestine and are then transported to the liver. The liver uses some lipids for energy and releases the rest for use by cells.

Lipids are necessary for the proper absorption of the fat-soluble vitamins (A, D, E, K), for cushioning of the internal organs, as a reserve energy source, and as part of many cell structures.

Protein Digestion and Metabolism. Protein breakdown begins in the stomach with the release of the enzyme *pepsin.* It converts the protein to a usable form called **amino acids** (the building blocks of which proteins are constructed and the end products of protein digestion).

Protein conversion is completed in the small intestine where the enzymes *trypsin* and *chymotrypsin* are found in the pancreatic juice. As the amino acids are freed, they are absorbed by the villi of the small intestine and sent to the liver for dispersal throughout the body. Amino acids (protein) are the chief structural components of the body. Twenty amino acids are necessary for human metabolism or growth, but because some are supplied by food and the others can be produced by the body, the ones provided by food are called *essential.* Muscle tissue, some chromosomes, enzymes, and some hormones are composed of amino acids.

ASSESSMENT OF THE GASTROINTESTINAL SYSTEM AND ACCESSORY ORGANS

Laboratory and Diagnostic Examinations

See Table 17-1 for summary list.

Upper Gastrointestinal Study (Upper GI Series, UGI).

Rationale. The upper GI study consists of a series of x-ray films of the lower esophagus, stomach, and duodenum, using barium sulfate as the contrast medium. A UGI series will detect any abnormal conditions of the upper GI tract, any tumors, or other ulcerative lesions.

Nursing interventions. The patient should maintain NPO status after midnight. The nurse should explain to the patient the importance of rectally expelling all the barium after the examination. Stools will be light in color until all the barium is expelled. Eventual absorption of fecal water may cause a hardened barium impaction. Increasing fluid intake is usually effective. Milk of magnesia (60 ml) is commonly given after the examination unless contraindicated.

Tube Gastric Analysis.

Rationale. The contents of the stomach are aspirated to determine the amount of acid produced by the parietal cells in the stomach. The analysis is done to determine the completeness of a vagotomy, confirm hypersecretion or **achlorhydria** (an abnormal condition characterized by the absence of hydrochloric acid in the gastric juice), estimate acid secretory capacity, or assay for intrinsic factor.

Nursing interventions. The patient should receive no anticholinergic medications for 24 hours before the test and should maintain NPO status after midnight so the gastric acid secretion will not be altered. The nurse should inform the patient that smoking is prohibited before the test because nicotine stimulates the flow of gastric secretions.

The nurse or radiology personnel will insert a nasogastric tube into the stomach to aspirate gastric content. Specimens should be labeled properly and sent to the laboratory immediately. The nasogastric tube is removed as soon as specimens are collected. The patient may then eat if indicated.

Esophagogastroduodenoscopy (EGD, UGI Endoscopy, Gastroscopy).

Rationale. Endoscopy enables direct visualization of the upper GI tract by means of a long, fiberoptic, flexible scope. The esophagus, stomach, and duodenum are examined for tumors, varices, mucosal inflammations, hiatal hernias, polyps, ulcers, strictures, and obstructions. Also, the endoscopist can remove polyps, coagulate sources of active GI bleeding, and perform sclerotherapy of esophageal varices through endoscopy. Areas of narrowing can be dilated by the endoscope itself or by passing a dilator through the scope. Camera equipment may be attached to the viewing lens, and the existing pathological condition can be photographed.

Not only can the esophagus, stomach, and duodenum be evaluated by endoscopy, but by the use of a longer fiberoptic scope, the upper small intestine can be evaluated. This is referred to as *enteroscopy.*

Nursing interventions. The nurse should explain the procedure to the patient. The patient should maintain NPO status after midnight. The nurse should obtain the patient's signature on a consent form and should also complete a preoperative checklist (see Chapter 22) for the endoscopic examination. Because the patient's pharynx has been anesthetized (by spraying) with lidocaine HCl (Xylocaine), the nurse should not allow the patient to eat or drink until the gag reflex returns (usually about 2 to 4 hours). The nurse should assess for any signs and symptoms of perforation, including abdominal pain and tenderness, guarding, oral bleeding, melena, and hypovolemic shock.

Barium Swallow.

Rationale. This barium contrast study is a more thorough study of the esophagus than that provided by most UGI examinations. As in most barium contrast studies, defects in luminal filling and narrowing of the barium column indicate tumor, scarred stricture, or esophageal varices. With a barium swallow, anatomical abnormalities, such as hiatal hernia, are easily recognized. Left atrial dilation, aortic aneurysm, and paraesophageal tumors (such as bronchial or mediastinal tumors) may cause extrinsic compression of the barium column within the esophagus.

A product called Gastrografin is now used in place of barium for patients where bleeding from the GI system may occur and surgery is being considered. Gastrografin facilitates imaging through x-ray, but if the product escapes from the GI tract, unlike barium, it is absorbed by the surrounding tissue. Complications can occur if barium leaks from the GI tract.

Nursing interventions. The patient should maintain NPO status after midnight. Food and fluid in the stomach will prevent the barium from accurately outlining the GI tract, and the radiographic results may be misleading. The nurse should explain to the patient the importance of rectally expelling all barium. Stools will be light in color until this occurs. Eventual absorption of fecal water may cause a hardened barium impaction. Increasing fluid intake is usually effective. Milk of magnesia (60 ml) is usually given after the examination unless contraindicated.

Esophageal Function Studies (Bernstein Test).

Rationale. The Bernstein test, an acid-perfusion test, is an attempt to reproduce the symptoms of gastroesophageal reflux. It aids in differentiating esophageal pain caused by esophageal reflux from that caused by angina pectoris. If the patient suffers pain with the instillation of hydrochloric acid into the esophagus, the test is positive and indicates reflux esophagitis.

Nursing interventions. The nurse should avoid sedating the patient, because the patient's participation is essential for swallowing the tubes, swallowing during acid clearance, and describing any discomfort during the instillation of hydrochloric acid. The patient is NPO for 8 hours before the examination, and any medications that may interfere with the production of acid, such as antacids and analgesics, are withheld.

Examination of Stool for Occult Blood.

Rationale. Tumors of the large intestine grow into the **lumen** (the cavity or channel within a tube or tubular organ) and are subjected to repeated trauma by the fecal stream. Eventually the tumor ulcerates and bleeding occurs. Usually the bleeding is so slight that gross blood is not seen in the stool. If this **occult blood** (blood that is obscure or hidden from view) is detected in the stool, a benign or malignant GI tumor should be suspected.

Occult blood in the stool may occur also in ulceration and inflammation of the upper or lower GI system. Other causes include swallowing blood of oral or nasopharyngeal origin.

Stool may be obtained by digital retrieval by the nurse or physician. However, the patient is usually asked to collect stool in an appropriate container.

Nursing interventions. The nurse should instruct the patient to keep the stool specimen free of urine or toilet paper, because either can contaminate the specimen and alter the test results. The nurse or patient should don gloves and use tongue blades to transfer the stool to the proper receptacle.

Sigmoidoscopy (Lower GI Endoscopy).

Rationale. Endoscopy of the lower GI tract allows visualization and, if indicated, access to obtain biopsy specimens of tumors, polyps, or ulcerations of the anus, rectum, and sigmoid colon. Because the lower GI tract is difficult to visualize radiographically, the direct visualization afforded through sigmoidoscopy is beneficial. Microscopic review of tissue specimens obtained using this procedure can provide the diagnoses of many lower bowel disorders.

Nursing interventions. The nurse should explain the procedure to the patient. The patient should sign a consent form for the procedure. The nurse administers enemas as ordered on the evening before and/or the morning of the examination to ensure optimum visualization of the lower GI tract. After the examination the nurse observes the patient for evidence of bowel perforation (abdominal pain, tenderness, distention, and bleeding).

Barium Enema Study (Lower GI Series).

Rationale. The barium enema (BE) study consists of a series of x-ray films of the colon used to demonstrate the presence and location of polyps, tumors, and diverticula. Positional abnormalities (such as malrotation) can also be detected. Therapeutically, the BE study may be used to reduce nonstrangulated ileocolic **intussusception** (infolding of one segment of the intestine into the lumen of another segment) in children.

Nursing interventions. The nurse may administer cathartics such as magnesium citrate or other cathartics designated by institution policy the evening before the BE. A cleansing enema (Skill 27-1) may also be administered the evening before or the morning of the BE if directed by physician's order or hospital policy. Milk of magnesia (60 ml) may be ordered after the BE to stimulate evacuation of the barium.

After the BE study, the patient should be assessed for complete evacuation of the barium. Retained barium may cause a hardened impaction. Stool will be light in color until all the barium has been expelled.

Colonoscopy.

Rationale. With the development of the fiberoptic colonoscope, a high percentage of patients can have the entire colon from anus to cecum examined. Therefore with colonoscopy the detection of lesions in the proximal colon, which would otherwise be undetected by sigmoidoscopy, is possible. Benign and malignant neoplasms, mucosal inflammation or ulceration, and sites of active hemorrhage can also be visualized. Biopsy specimens can be obtained and small tumors removed through the scope with the use of cable-activated instruments. Actively bleeding vessels can be coagulated.

Patients who have had cancer of the colon are at high risk for developing a subsequent colon cancer; patients who have a family history of colon cancer are at high risk. For these patients colonoscopy allows early detection of any primary or secondary tumors.

Nursing interventions. The patient signs a consent form. The nurse explains the procedure to the patient. The patient is instructed regarding dietary restrictions: usually a clear liquid diet is permitted 1 to 3 days before the procedure to decrease the residue in the bowel, and then NPO status is maintained for 8 hours before the procedure. The nurse administers a cathartic, enemas, and premedication as ordered to decrease the residue in the bowel. GoLYTELY (Box 27-2), an oral or nasogastric (NG) colonic lavager, is an osmotic electrolyte solution that is now commonly used as a cathartic. It is a polyethylene glycol solution. If taken orally, instruct the patient to drink the solution rapidly: 8 oz (240 ml) every 15 minutes until he has consumed enough solution to make the colonic contents a light yellow liquid. If it is given per lavage, it must be given rapidly. Taking the solution slowly will not clean the colon efficiently.

SKILL 27-1

ADMINISTERING AN ENEMA

1. Introduce self.
2. Identify patient.
3. Wash hands.
4. Explain procedure.
5. Prepare solution. There are several types of enema solution. Cleansing enemas include tap water, normal saline, low-volume hypertonic solution, and soapsuds solution. (Considering the reports of soap damage to colonic mucosa, it seems prudent to use alternatives such as saline, plain tap water or a prepackaged enema.[36])
6. Arrange equipment at bedside.
7. Pull curtain and close door to provide privacy.
8. Assist patient to the left Sims' position. When giving an enema to a patient who is unable to contract the external sphincter, position the patient on the bedpan. Giving the enema with the patient sitting on the toilet is unsafe because the inserted rectal tubing can abrade the rectal wall.
9. Place waterproof pad under patient.
10. Place bath blanket over patient, and fanfold linen to foot of bed; adjust patient's gown to keep it from being soiled while it still provides privacy.
11. Don gloves.
12. Clamp tubing 7 inches (28 cm) from end; fill container with correctly warmed solution (usually 1000 ml* at 105° F) and any additives (read disposable package instructions). Release clamp, allowing solution to flow through tubing to remove any air from the tubing; reclamp.
    *Suggested maximum volumes:
    Infant: 150 to 250 ml
    Toddler: 250 to 350 ml
    School-aged child: 300 to 500 ml
    Adolescent: 500 to 750 ml
    Adult: 750 to 1000 ml
13. Lubricate 4 inches (10 cm) at end of the tubing; spread patient's buttocks to expose anus; while rotating tube, gently insert it 3 to 4 inches (7 to 10 cm).
14. Elevate container 12 to 18 inches (30 to 45 cm) above level of anus to allow solution to flow at adequate rate.
15. Release clamp; allow solution to flow slowly while holding clamp; solution should flow for 5 to 10 min (the higher the solution container, the more rapid the rate of flow).
16. Lower container or clamp tubing if patient complains of cramping; encourage slow, deep breathing.
17. Clamp and remove tube when enough solution has been administered. Encourage patient to retain solution at least 5 min; retention of solution promotes peristalsis and enhances defecation.
18. When patient can no longer retain solution, assist to bedpan, bedside commode, or bathroom; remind patient not to flush toilet.
19. Provide for patient hygiene; assist patient to bed or chair.
20. Dispose of equipment and supplies. Remove gloves; wash hands.
21. Record procedure and observations.
22. Report abnormalities.

FOR COMMERCIALLY PREPARED ENEMA

- Remove cover from tip of enema (tip is prelubricated); insert entire tip into anus.
- Squeeze container until it is empty. Most containers hold about 250 ml.

Box 27-2 GOLYTELY BOWEL PREP

1. Give patient one Reglan 10-mg tablet, as prescribed, orally 30 min before proceeding with Step 2.
2. Administer the GoLYTELY solution* (prepared by pharmacy) per physician's orders:
    a. 240 ml orally q 15 min or
    b. 30 ml/min via NG tube. Use a Travasorb enteral feeding container and a size 10 feeding tube.

Administer until stools are clear yellow.

*Administer a minimum of 1 gallon of solution over a 2-hour period.

After colonoscopy, the nurse checks for evidence of bowel perforation (abdominal pain, guarding, distention, tenderness, excessive rectal bleeding, or blood clots) and examines stools for gross blood. Assess for hypovolemic shock.

Stool Culture (Stool for Culture and Sensitivity [C & S]; Stool for Ova and Parasites [O & P]).

Rationale. The feces (stool) can be examined for the presence of bacteria, ova, and parasites (a plant or animal that lives upon or within another living organism at whose expense it obtains some advantage). Many bacteria (such as *Escherichia coli*) are indigenous in the bowel. Bacterial cultures are usually done to detect enteropathogens (such as *Staphylococcus aureus, Salmonella, Shigella or Clostridium difficile*).

When a patient is suspected of having a parasitic infection, the stool is examined for ova and parasites (O & P). Usually at least three stool specimens are collected on subsequent days.

Nursing interventions. If an enema must be administered to collect specimens, only normal saline or tap water should be used. Soapsuds or any other substance could affect the viability of the organisms collected.

Stool samples for O & P are obtained before barium examinations. The patient is instructed not to mix urine with feces. The nurse dons gloves to collect the specimen. The specimen should be taken to the laboratory within 30 minutes of collection in specified container.

Obstruction Series (Flat Plate of the Abdomen).

Rationale. The obstruction series is a group of x-ray studies performed on the abdomen of patients who have suspected bowel obstruction, paralytic ileus, perforated viscus (any large interior organ in any of the great body cavities), or abdominal abscess. This series usually consists of at least two x-ray studies. The first is an erect abdominal x-ray study that should include visualization of the diaphragm. X-ray images are examined for evidence of free air under the diaphragm, which is **pathognomonic** (sign or symptom specific to a disease condition) of a perforated viscus. This x-ray study is used also to detect air-fluid levels within the intestine.

Nursing interventions. For adequate visualization, the nurse should ensure that this study is scheduled before any barium studies.

Diagnostic Studies Used in the Assessment of the Hepatobiliary and Pancreatic Systems.

Serum bilirubin test. Normal values are as follows:

Direct bilirubin: 0.1-0.3 mg/dl
Indirect bilirubin: 0.2-0.8 mg/dl
Total bilirubin: 0.1-1.0 mg/dl
Total bilirubin in newborns: 1-12 mg/dl

Rationale. Total serum bilirubin determination measures both direct, or conjugated (water-soluble), and indirect, or unconjugated (water-insoluble), bilirubin. Total serum bilirubin level is the sum of the direct and indirect bilirubin levels. Testing for bilirubin in the blood provides valuable information for diagnosis and evaluation of liver disease, biliary obstruction, erythroblastosis fetalis, and hemolytic anemia.

Nursing interventions. The nurse should keep the patient on NPO status until after the blood specimen is drawn.

Liver enzyme tests. The normal values* are as follows:

AST (aspartate aminotransferase; formerly serum glutamic-oxaloacetic transaminase [SGOT]): Adult 5-40 IU/L (AST level is elevated in myocardial infarctions, hepatitis, acute pancreatitis, hepatic necrosis, acute renal disease, and acute hemolytic anemia)

ALT (alanine aminotransferase; formerly serum glutamate pyruvate transaminase [SGPT]): Adult/child 5-35 IU/L (ALT level is elevated in hepatitis, cirrhosis, hepatic necrosis, and hepatic tumors and by hepatotoxic drugs)

LDH (lactic dehydrogenase): 45-90 U/L (Increased values in myocardial infarction, pulmonary infarction, hepatic disease, hemolytic anemia, and skeletal muscle disease.

Alkaline phosphatase: Adult 30-85 ImU/ml (alkaline phosphatase level is elevated in obstructive disorders of the biliary tract, cirrhosis, primary and metastatic tumors, metastatic tumor in bones, and healing fractures)

Gamma GT (gamma glutamyltransferase): male and female over age 45—8 to 38 U/L; female under age 45—5 to 27 U/L. (Levels are elevated in liver cell dysfunction such as hepatitis and cirrhosis, with the use of hepatotoxic drugs, and in myocardial infarction [MI] [4-10 days after], congestive heart failure, and alcohol ingestion.)

Rationale. The liver is a storehouse of many enzymes. Injury or diseases affecting the liver will cause release of these intracellular enzymes into the bloodstream, and their levels will be elevated. Some of these enzymes are produced also in other organs, and injury or disease affecting these other organs will also cause an elevated serum level. Therefore although elevation of these serum enzymes is found in pathological liver conditions, the test is not specific for liver diseases alone.

Nursing interventions. The nurse should assess the venipuncture site for bleeding.

Serum protein test. The normal value are as follows:

---

*U/L = units per liter; IU/L = international units per liter; ImU/ml = international milliunits per milliliters.

Total protein: 6-8 g/dl
Albumin: 3.2-4.5 g/dl
Globulin: 2.3-3.4 g/dl
Albumin globulin (A/G ratio): 1.2-2.2 g/dl

Rationale. One way to assess the functional status of the liver is to measure the products that are synthesized there. One of these products is protein, especially albumin. When disease affects the liver cell, the hepatocyte loses its ability to synthesize albumin and the serum albumin level is markedly decreased.

Low serum albumin levels may result also from (1) excessive loss of albumin into urine (as in nephrotic syndrome) or into third-space volumes (as in ascites) or (2) protein-caloric malnutrition.

Nursing interventions. The nurse should assess the venipuncture site for bleeding.

Oral Cholecystography (Gallbladder Series, GB Series, Cholecystogram).

Rationale. The oral cholecystogram provides x-ray visualization of the gallbladder after the oral ingestion of a radiopaque, iodinated dye. Adequate visualization of the gallbladder requires concentration of the dye within the gallbladder. Oral cholecystogram is less accurate than the gallbladder ultrasound. The following factors are necessary for adequate dye concentration:

1. Ingestion by the patient of the correct number of dye tablets the evening before the examination
2. Adequate absorption of the dye from the GI tract; vomiting or diarrhea will preclude absorption of the dye
3. Abstinence from food (especially a fatty meal) on the morning of the test
4. Uptake from the portal system and excretion of the dye by the liver
5. Patency of the cystic duct
6. Concentration of the dye within the gallbladder

Nursing interventions. Before the administration of the dye, the nurse should make certain the patient is not allergic to iodine, to prevent adverse or allergic reaction to dye. This rarely occurs because the dye is not administered intravenously. If no allergy to iodine is present, the nurse administers six iopanoic acid (Telepaque) tablets orally, one every 5 minutes, beginning after the evening meal. The patient is on NPO status from midnight. The patient may be given a high-fat meal or beverage to stimulate emptying of the gallbladder after the test has begun. No other food or fluids will be allowed until the examination is complete.

Intravenous Cholangiography (Intravenous Cholangiogram, IVC).

Rationale. In this study intravenously administered radiographic dye is concentrated by the liver and secreted into the bile duct. IVC allows visualization of the hepatic and common bile ducts and also the gallbladder if the cystic duct is patent. IVC is used to demonstrate stones, stricture, or tumor of the hepatic duct, common bile duct, and gallbladder.

Operative Cholangiography. In operative cholangiography, the common bile duct is directly injected with radiopaque dye. Stones appear as radiolucent shadows, and tumors cause partial or total obstruction of the flow of dye into the duodenum. By visualization of the biliary duct structures, the surgeon is provided with a "road map" of a commonly difficult anatomical area. This reduces the possibility of inadvertently injuring the common duct.

If common duct stones are suspected, not only must a cholecystectomy be performed, but also a common duct exploration (CDE). When intraoperative cholangiography is used routinely, CDE is performed only on those with positive cholangiography.

T-tube Cholangiography (Postoperative Cholangiography).

Rationale. T-tube cholangiography is performed to diagnose retained ductal stones postoperatively in the patient who has had a cholecystectomy and a common bile duct exploration and to demonstrate good flow of contrast of bile into the duodenum. The test is performed through the use of a T-shaped rubber tube that the surgeon places in the bile duct during the operation. Through the end of the T-tube that exits through the abdominal wall, dye can be injected and x-ray films taken.

Nursing implications. The nurse should protect the patient from sepsis by connecting the T-tube (if left in place) to a sterile closed-drainage system. If the T-tube is removed, the T-tube tract site should be kept covered with a sterile dressing to prevent bacteria from entering the ductal system.

Nursing interventions. Before the administration of the dye, the nurse should ensure that the patient is not allergic to iodine. Preparation of the patient also includes NPO after midnight and until the examination is completed. The nurse administers a cleansing enema on the morning of the examination, if ordered.

Ultrasound Examination of the Liver, Gallbladder, and Biliary System (Echogram of the Liver, Gallbladder, and Biliary System).

Rationale. Ultrasound is a radiological technique in which deep structures of the body are visualized by recording the reflections (echoes) of ultrasonic waves directed into the tissues. This diagnostic test is not effective in examining all tissue because ultrasound waves do not pass through structures that contain air, such as the lungs. Although fasting is preferred, it is not necessary for ultrasonography. Because this study requires no contrast material and has no associated radiation, it is especially useful for patients who are allergic to contrast and for pregnant patients. Ultrasound is used with increasing frequency to corroborate data already obtained by "questionable positive" cholangiograms, liver scans, and oral cholecystograms.

Nursing interventions. The patient is NPO from midnight. If the patient has had recent barium contrast studies, the nurse should request an order for cathartics. Ultrasound cannot penetrate barium, and the study will not be adequate.

Gallbladder Scanning (Hepatobiliary Imaging, HIDA Scanning).

Rationale. Through the use of technetium (Tc) (technetium 99), the biliary tract can be evaluated in a safe, accurate, and noninvasive manner. The primary use of this study is in the diagnosis of acute cholecystitis. This procedure is superior to oral cholecystography, ultrasonography, and CT scanning of the abdomen for the detection of acute cholecystitis.

Nursing interventions. The nurse should assure the patient that exposure to radioactivity is minimal because only tracer doses of the radioisotopes are used. The patient is NPO from midnight until the examination is complete.

Liver Biopsy.

Rationale. Liver biopsy is a safe, simple, and valuable method of diagnosing pathological liver conditions. For this study a specially designed needle is inserted through the skin and abdominal wall and into the liver. A piece of liver tissue is removed for microscopic examination. The tissue sample is placed into a correctly labeled specimen bottle containing formalin and sent to the pathology department. Percutaneous liver biopsy is used in the diagnosis of various liver disorders, such as cirrhosis, hepatitis, drug-related reactions, granuloma, and tumor.

Nursing interventions. The nurse should explain the procedure to the patient and obtain the patient's signature on a consent form. Food and fluids are withheld 4 to 8 hours before the test. The nurse ensures that platelet and prothrombin tests have been ordered and any abnormal values are reported to the physician. After the procedure the nurse observes the patient for symptoms of bleeding. Vital signs are monitored every 15 minutes for 1 hour, then every 30 minutes for 4 hours, and then every 4 hours for 24 hours.

Some pain is common. When leakage involves a large quantity of blood or bile, the peritoneal reaction is great and the resulting pain is severe. The nurse assesses for pneumothorax (collapsed lung) caused by improper placement of the biopsy needle into the adjacent chest cavity. The nurse should report these signs and symptoms immediately to the physician. The patient should remain on bed rest for 24 hours.

Liver Scanning (Radioisotope Liver Scanning).

Rationale. This radionuclide procedure is used to outline and detect structural changes of the liver. A radionuclide is given intravenously. Later, a gamma-ray detecting device (Geiger counter) is passed over the patient's abdomen. This records the distribution of the radioactive particles in the liver. The spleen can also be visualized by the detector when technetium 99 sulfur is used.

Nursing interventions. The patient should be NPO from midnight. The nurse should assure patients that they will not be exposed to a large amount of radioactivity, because only tracer doses of isotopes are used.

Blood Ammonia.

Normal value: 47-65 μmol/L.

Rationale. Ammonia, a by-product of protein metabolism, is normally converted by the liver into urea and then secreted by the kidneys (see blood urea nitrogen [BUN]). With severe liver dysfunction or when the blood flow to the liver is altered, the blood ammonia level rises and the BUN level decreases. The blood ammonia level is primarily used as an aid in diagnosing hepatic encephalopathy or coma. Elevated blood ammonia levels suggest liver dysfunction as the cause of these signs and symptoms.

Nursing interventions. The nurse should list on the laboratory requisition any antibiotics the patient is currently taking. Certain broad-spectrum antibiotics such as neomycin can cause a decreased ammonia level, thus giving inaccurate test results.

Hepatitis Virus Studies (Hepatitis-Associated Antigen [HAA]). A normal laboratory test result will be negative for the presence of the antigen.

Rationale. Hepatitis is an inflammation of the liver caused by a virus. Five viruses are now recognized that can cause this disease: hepatitis A virus, hepatitis B virus, hepatitis C virus, hepatitis D virus, and hepatitis E virus. Hepatitis A and B have been recognized for years, but hepatitis C, D, and E were identified only recently. The individual hepatitis viruses can be detected by different antigen and antibody levels, and different incubation periods must be considered.

Nursing interventions. The nurse should use universal precautions and should handle the serum specimen as if it were capable of transmitting viral hepatitis. Health care personnel will don gloves when handling any blood or body fluids and will wash hands carefully after handling all equipment.

Serum Amylase Test.

Normal value: 25-125 U/L.

Rationale. The serum amylase test is an easily and rapidly performed test for pancreatitis. Damage to pancreas cells (as in pancreatitis) or obstruction to the pancreatic ductal flow (as in pancreatic carcinoma) will cause an outpouring of this enzyme into the intrapancreatic lymph system and also into the free peritoneum. Blood vessels draining the free peritoneum and absorbing the lymph pick up this excess amylase. An abnormal rise in the serum level of amylase is the result, and it will occur within 12 hours of the onset of pancreatic disease. Because amylase is rapidly cleared by the kidney, serum levels may return to normal within 48 to 72 hours.

Nursing interventions. The nurse should note on the laboratory requisition if the patient is receiving IV dextrose or any medications, because these can cause a false negative result.

Urine Amylase Test. The normal value for this study is 3 to 35 IU/hr.

Rationale. Because the kidney rapidly clears amylase, disorders affecting the pancreas will cause elevated amylase levels in the urine. Levels of amylase in the urine remain elevated for 7 to 10 days after the onset of disease. This fact is important if the diagnosis of pancreatitis is to be made in patients who have had symptoms for 3 days or longer.

Nursing interventions. The nurse should record the exact times of the beginning and end of the collection period. A 2-hour spot urine or 6-hour, 12-hour, or 24-hour collection can be performed, depending on the physician's order. The collection begins after the patient empties the bladder and discards that specimen. All subsequent urine is collected, including the voiding at the end of the collection period. The specimen should be kept on ice or refrigerated until it is sent to the laboratory.

Ultrasound Examination of the Pancreas.

Rationale. Through the use of reflected sound waves, ultrasonography of the pancreas provides diagnostic information of this rather inaccessible abdominal organ. Ultrasound examination of the pancreas is mainly used to establish the diagnosis of carcinoma, pseudocyst, pancreatitis, and pancreatic abscess. Because ultrasound abnormalities persist from several days to weeks, the diagnosis of pancreatitis can be supported by this study even after the serum amylase and lipase levels have returned to normal. Furthermore, follow-up ultrasound study can be used to monitor the resolution of pancreatic inflammation and the response of a tumor to therapy.

Nursing interventions. Fluids and foods are withheld for 8 hours before the examination, but fasting is not mandatory to obtain accurate results. If the patient's abdomen is distended with gas or if the patient has had a recent barium examination, this study should be postponed, because gas or barium will interfere with sound wave transmission.

Computed Tomography of the Abdomen (CT Scan of the Abdomen).

Rationale. CT scan of the abdomen is a noninvasive, accurate x-ray procedure used to diagnose pathological pancreatic conditions, such as inflammation, tumor, cyst formation, ascites, aneurysm, and cirrhosis of the liver. The recognizable cross-sectional image produced by a CT scan is especially important for studying the pancreas, because this organ is retroperitoneal and well hidden by the overlying peritoneal organs.

Nursing interventions. Fluids and food are withheld from midnight until the examination is complete; however, this test can be performed on an emergency basis on patients who have recently eaten. If possible, the nurse should show the patient a picture of the machine and encourage the patient to verbalize fears, since some patients suffer claustrophobia when enclosed in the machine.

Endoscopic Retrograde Cholangiopancreatography of the Pancreatic Duct (ERCP of the Pancreatic Duct).

Rationale. Not only can the biliary system be visualized by ERCP, the pancreatic duct can be seen also. During the test a fiberoptic duodenoscope is inserted through the oral pharynx, through the esophagus and stomach, and into the duodenum. Dye is injected for radiographic visualization of the common bile duct and pancreatic duct. ERCP of the pancreas is a sensitive and reliable procedure for detecting clinically significant degrees of pancreatic dysfunction. It can also be used to evaluate obstructive jaundice, remove common bile duct stones, and place biliary and pancreatic duct stents to bypass obstruction. Localized pancreatic duct narrowing indicates tumor. Chronic pancreatitis is demonstrated by multiple areas of ductal narrowing, which can be visualized by ERCP.

Nursing interventions. Food and fluids are withheld for 8 hours before the examination, and the patient's signature on a consent form is obtained. The nurse should tell patients that the test takes approximately 1 to 2 hours, during which time they must lie completely motionless on a hard x-ray table. Remaining still for this period of time may be uncomfortable for the patient. After the procedure, keep the patient NPO until gag reflex returns; assess for abdominal pain, tenderness, and guarding. Assess for signs and symptoms of pancreatitis, which is the most common ERCP complication. These signs and symptoms include increasingly intense abdominal pain, nausea, vomiting, and diminished or absent bowel sounds. Assess for hypovolemic shock.

DISORDERS OF THE MOUTH

Common disorders of the mouth and esophagus that interfere with adequate nutrition include poor dental hygiene, infections, inflammation, and cancer.

Dental Plaque and Caries

Etiology/Pathophysiology. Dental decay is an erosive process that results from the action of bacteria on carbohydrates in the mouth, which in turn produces acids that dissolve tooth enamel. Most Americans (95%) experience tooth decay sometime in their life span. Dental decay can be caused by one of several factors, among which are the following:

- The presence of dental plaque, a thin film on the teeth made of mucin and colloidal material found in saliva and often secondarily invaded by bacteria
- The strength of acids and the ability of the saliva to neutralize them
- The length of time the acids are in contact with the teeth
- Susceptibility of the teeth to decay

Medical Management. Interventions include treatment of dental caries by removal of affected areas of the tooth and replacement with some form of dental material. Treatment of periodontal disease centers on removal of plaque from the teeth. If the disease has advanced, surgical interventions of the gingivae and alveolar bone may be necessary.

Nursing Interventions and Patient Teaching. Proper technique for brushing and flossing the teeth at least twice a day is the nurse's primary focus of teaching for these patients. Plaque forms continuously and must be removed periodically through regular visits to the dentist. The patient must understand the importance of prevention through continuous care. Because carbohydrates create an environment in which caries develops and plaque accumulates more easily, proper nutrition is included in patient teaching. When the patient is ill, the normal cleansing action of the mouth is impaired. Illnesses, drugs, and irradiation all interfere with the normal action of saliva. If the patient is unable to manage oral hygiene, the nurse must assume this responsibility.

Nursing diagnoses and interventions for the patient with dental plaque and caries include but are not limited to the following:

NURSING DIAGNOSES	NURSING INTERVENTIONS
Knowledge deficit, related to inability to prevent dental caries and periodontal disease	Assess and observe the oral cavity for moisture, color, and cleanliness. Stress importance of meticulous oral hygiene. Explain need to see dentist at least yearly for examination.
Noncompliance, related to hygiene and dietary restrictions	Brush teeth bid and prn with toothpaste or powder, baking soda, or mouthwash. Rinse with water or mouthwash. Cleanse mouth with equal parts of hydrogen peroxide and water prn for halitosis. Teach oral hygiene to patient.

Prognosis. The prevention and elimination of dental plaque and caries are directly related to oral hygiene, dental care, nutrition, and heredity. All but heredity are controllable characteristics. The prognosis is more favorable for persons who brush, floss, regularly visit the dentist for removal of affected areas, eat low-carbohydrate foods, and drink fluoridated water.

Candidiasis

Etiology/Pathophysiology. This condition is any infection caused by a species of *Candidia,* usually *Candida albicans. Candida* is a fungal organism normally present in the mucous membranes of the mouth, intestinal tract, and vagina and is also found on the skin of healthy people. This infection is also referred to as *thrush* and *moniliasis.*

This disease appears more commonly in the newborn infant who becomes infected while passing through the birth canal. In the older individual, candidiasis may be found in patients with leukemia, diabetes mellitus, or alcoholism, and in the person who has been on antibiotics (chlortetracycline or tetracycline) or steroids for long periods or who is in a general weakened state.

Clinical Manifestations. Candidiasis appears as small white patches on the mucous membranes of the mouth and tongue. There may be one or more lesions on the mucosa, depending on the duration of the infection. If the patch or plaque is removed, painful bleeding can occur.

Medical Management. Treatment may include 1 to 4 ml of nystatin (Mycostatin) dropped in the infected infant's mouth several times a day. For the adult, half-strength hydrogen peroxide/saline mouth rinses may provide some relief. For treatment of adult *Candida* vaginal infection, nystatin vaginal tablets (100,000 units dissolved) inserted into the vagina twice a day is effective. Ketoconazole taken systemically appears to be equally effective.

Nursing Interventions. The nurse must use meticulous handwashing to prevent spread of infection. The infection may be spread in the nursery by carelessness of nursing personnel. Handwashing, care of feeding equipment, and cleanliness of the mother's nipples are important to prevent spread. The nurse should cleanse the mouth of any foreign material, rinsing the mouth and lubricating the lips. The mouth should be inspected using a flashlight and tongue blade.

Prognosis. If the host has a strong defense system and medical treatment is initiated early in the course of the disease, the prognosis is good.

Carcinoma of the Oral Cavity

Etiology/Pathophysiology. The lips, the oral cavity, the tongue, and the pharynx are prone to develop malignant lesions. The largest number of these tumors are squamous cell epitheliomas that grow rapidly and metastasize to adjacent structures more quickly than do most malignant tumors of the skin. In the United States oral cancer accounts for 4% of the cancers in males and 2% in females.

Tumors of the salivary glands occur primarily in the parotid gland and are usually benign. Tumors of the submaxillary gland have a high incidence of malignancy. These malignant tumors grow rapidly and may be accompanied by pain and impaired facial function.

Kaposi's sarcoma is a malignant skin tumor that occurs primarily on the legs of men between 50 and 70 years of age. Recently it has been seen with increased frequency as a nonsquamous tumor of the oral cavity in patients with AIDS. The lesions are purple and nonulcerated. Irradiation is the treatment of choice.

Cancer or neoplasm is characterized by the uncontrolled growth of anaplastic cells that tend to invade surrounding tissue and to metastasize to distant body sites.

The tumor seen with cancer of the lip is usually called an *epithelioma.* It occurs most frequently as a chronic ulcer of the lower lip in men. The cure rate for cancer of the lips is high because the lesion is easily apparent to the patient and to others. Metastasis to regional lymph nodes has occurred in only 10% of persons when diagnosed. In some instances a lesion may spread rapidly and involve the mandible and the floor of the mouth by direct extension. Occasionally the tumor may be a basal cell lesion that starts in the skin and spreads to the lip.

Cancer of the anterior tongue and floor of the mouth may seem to occur together because their spread to adjacent tissues is so rapid. Metastasis to the neck has already occurred in more than 60% of patients when the diagnosis is made because of the tongue's abundant vascular and lymphatic drainage. Recent investigation has revealed a higher incidence of cancers of the mouth and throat among persons who are heavy drinkers and smokers. Also, data show that the mortality for young males between the ages of 10 and 20 has doubled over the past 30 years as a result of the use of smokeless tobacco (snuff). This combination of high alcohol consumption and smoking or chewing tobacco causes an apparent breakdown in the body's defense mechanism. Predisposing factors include exposure to the sun and wind, but more important is the progression of leukoplakia to an epidermoid lip cancer.

Clinical Manifestations. **Leukoplakia** (a white firmly attached patch on the mouth or tongue mucosa) may appear on the lips and buccal mucosa. These nonsloughing lesions cannot be rubbed off by simple mechanical force. They can be benign or malignant. A small percentage develop into squamous cell carcinomas, and biopsy is recommended if the lesions persist for longer than 2 weeks. They occur most frequently between the ages of 50 and 70 years and appear more commonly in men.

Assessment. Collection of *subjective data* includes understanding that malignant lesions of the mouth are usually asymptomatic. The patient may feel only a roughened area with the tongue. As the disease progresses, the first complaints may be (1) difficulty in chewing, swallowing, or speaking; (2) edema, numbness, or loss of feeling in any part of the mouth; and (3) earache, faceache, and toothache, which may become constant. Cancer of the lip is associated with discomfort and irritation caused by the presence of a nonhealing lesion that may be raised or ulcerated. Malignancy at the base of the tongue produces less obvious symptoms: slight dysphagia, sore throat, and salivation.

Collection of *objective data* includes observing for premalignant lesions, including leukoplakia (white patches). Unusual bleeding in the mouth, some blood-tinged sputum, lumps or edema in the neck, and hoarseness may be observed.

Diagnostic Tests. Indirect laryngoscopy is an important diagnostic test for examination of the soft tissue. This procedure is especially important for men 40 years of age or older who have dysphagia and a history of smoking and alcohol ingestion. Radiographic evaluation of the mandibular structures is also an essential part of the head and neck examination to rule out the presence of cancer. Excisional biopsy is the most accurate method for a definitive diagnosis. Oral exfoliative cytology is a means of screening intraoral lesions. A scraping of the lesion provides cells for cytological examination. The chance for a false negative finding is about 26%.

Medical Management. Treatment depends on the location and staging of the malignant tumor. Stage I oral cancers are treated by surgery or radiation. Stages II and III cancers require both surgery and radiation. Treatment for stage IV cancer is usually palliative. The survival rate for patients with oral cancers averages less than 50%.

Small, accessible tumors can be excised surgically and include a glossectomy, removal of the tongue; hemiglossectomy, removal of part of the tongue; mandibulectomy, removal of the mandible; and total or supraglottic laryngectomy, removal of the entire larynx or the portion above the true vocal cords.

Large tumors usually require more extensive and traumatic surgery. In a functional neck dissection of neck cancer with no growth in the lymph nodes, the lymph nodes are removed but the jugular vein, sternocleidomastoid muscle, and spinal accessory nerve are preserved. In radical neck dissection, all these structures are removed and reconstructive surgery is necessary after tissue resection. These patients may have drains in the incision sites that are connected to suction to aid healing and reduce hematomas. A tracheostomy may also be performed, depending on the degree of tumor invasion.

Because of the location of the surgery, complications can occur. These include airway obstruction, hemorrhage, tracheal aspiration, facial edema, fistula formation, and necrosis of the skin flaps. Neurological complications can occur because of nerves being severed and manipulated during surgery.

Radiation may be in the form of external radiation by use of roentgenograms or other radioactive substances or in the form of internal radiation by means of needles or seeds. The purpose of radiation therapy is to shrink the tumor. It can be given preoperatively or postoperatively, depending on the physician's preference and the patient's disease process. In more advanced cases, chemotherapy may be combined with radiation postoperatively to make the patient more comfortable. Other treatment options include laser excision.

Nursing Interventions. It is important that the nurse have a holistic approach to the patient. This includes being aware of the patient's level of knowledge regarding the disease, the emotional response and coping abilities, and the spiritual needs. The nursing interventions must be individualized to the patient, beginning with the preoperative stage, through the postoperative stage, and are complete after the patient's rehabilitation in the home environment. Family members, hospice members, close friends, social workers, and pastoral care staff may be necessary for information and support during this potentially fatal disease.

Nursing diagnoses and interventions for the patient with oral cancer include but are not limited to the following:

NURSING DIAGNOSES	NURSING INTERVENTIONS
Nutrition, altered: less than body requirements, related to oral pain or postoperative tissue loss (mucous membranes)	Monitor the patient for changes in the character and quantity of mucus after radiation therapy. Provide meticulous oral hygiene. Observe for temporary or permanent loss of taste and the need for alternative routes for nutrition by monitoring daily weights.
Body image and personal identity disturbance, related to disfiguring appearance of an oral lesion or reconstructive surgery	Provide alternative methods for communication if dysarthria (difficult, poorly articulated speech, resulting from interference in the control over muscles of speech) results from radiation treatment. Provide information to the patient and family to help with difficult decisions related to surgery, radiation, or chemotherapy. Be a support person to the patient and family.

Patient teaching. Prevention centers on avoidance of predisposing factors: excess exposure to sun and wind on the lips, elimination of smoking or chewing tobacco, and maintenance of good oral and dental care. There is a high correlation between the incidence of cancer of the mouth and cirrhosis of the liver associated with alcohol intake. Early detection of oral cancer can help increase the patient's chance of survival. Any person with a mouth lesion that does not heal within 2 to 3 weeks is urged to seek immediate medical care. Preoperative and postoperative care must be taught to the surgical patient, with full explanations regarding speech loss and alternate methods of nutritional intake. Explanation of tracheostomy care and other tubes the patient may be discharged with will relieve anxiety and encourage the patient's control over the situation.

Prognosis. Staging and biological characterization of the neoplasm provide prognostic information. The prognosis of carcinoma in the oral cavity is directly related to the size of the primary tumor, the involvement of regional nodes, and the presence or absence of metastasis. The patient's immunological response and general condition also influence the prognosis and the choice of therapy.

Carcinomas of the lip can be detected early by the person, the physician, or the dentist during examination and the prognosis for cure is high. If the carcinoma is difficult to detect, as on the anterior tongue and floor of the mouth, it will be in the more advanced stage when detected and the prognosis will be bleak. The 5-year survival rate for cancer of the oral cavity and pharynx is 53% for whites and 34% for blacks.

DISORDERS OF THE ESOPHAGUS

Carcinoma of the Esophagus

Etiology/Pathophysiology. This disorder is a malignant epithelial neoplasm that has invaded the esophagus and has been diagnosed as the presence of a squamous cell carcinoma or an adenocarcinoma.

Of esophageal cancers, 90% are squamous cell carcinomas, which are associated with both alcohol intake and tobacco use and possibly long-standing **achalasia** (an abnormal condition characterized by the inability of a muscle to relax, particularly the cardiac sphincter of the stomach). Of cancers of the esophagus, 6% are adenocarcinomas and are associated with reflux esophagitis. Environmental carcinogens, nutritional deficiencies, chronic irritation, and mucosal damage have all been considered as causes of esophageal cancer. Unfortunately, because of the location, esophageal cancer is usually at a late stage when discovered and treatment is aimed toward comfort and control rather than cure. Carcinoma of the bronchus, stomach, or breast may metastasize to the esophagus. The prevalent age group for esophageal cancer is 55 to 70 years. It occurs more commonly in men.

Clinical Manifestations. The most common clinical symptom is progressive **dysphagia** (difficulty in swallowing) over a 6-month period, with the sensation of food sticking in the throat.

Assessment. Collection of *subjective data* includes noting that initially the patient may have difficulty in swallowing when bulky foods are eaten; later it occurs with soft foods and finally with liquids and even saliva. Another symptom is *odynophagia* (painful swallowing). Pain is an unusual symptom and indicates local extension of the malignancy.

Collection of *objective data* includes the nurse observing the patient for **regurgitation** (a backward flowing or the casting up of undigested food), vomiting, hoarseness, chronic cough, and iron-deficiency anemia. Weight loss may be directly related to the tumor or a side effect of treatment or the inability to swallow.

Diagnostic Tests. A barium swallow examination with fluoroscopy and endoscopy is used to detect esophageal cancer. A biopsy and cytological examination provide a high degree of accuracy in the final diagnosis.

Medical Management. Tumor staging must be addressed to determine tumor size and patient management. In advanced cases, surgery is offered for palliative purposes to relieve dysphagia and restore continuity of the alimentary tract. An aggressive approach provides excellent palliation (therapy designed to relieve or reduce intensity of uncomfortable symptoms but not to produce a cure), increased longevity, and a chance for a cure. Standard resection seems to give as good a result as a radical procedure.

Radiation therapy may be curative and/or palliative. Special problems associated with radiation therapy include the development of an esophagotracheal fistula (an abnormal passage between two internal organs). Aspiration from the fistula and edema from the radiation must be anticipated. Chemotherapy using a single drug or a combination of drugs is considered a palliative treatment of advanced cancer of the esophagus. Because of the extreme toxicity of these drugs, side effects of respiratory and liver dysfunction, nausea and vomiting, leukopenia, and sepsis can be anticipated. The following four types of surgical procedures can be performed:

1. Esophagogastrectomy—Resection of a lower esophageal section with a proximal portion of the stomach, followed by **anastomosis** (a surgical joining of two ducts or blood vessels to allow flow from one to the other) of the remaining portions of esophagus and stomach
2. Esophagogastrostomy—Resection of a portion of the esophagus with anastomosis to the stomach
3. Esophagoenterostomy—Resection of the esophagus and anastomosis to a portion of the colon
4. Gastrostomy—Insertion of a catheter into the stomach and suture to the abdominal wall; performed when it is assumed that the patient will not be able to take food orally because of inoperable cancer of the esophagus interfering with swallowing

Nursing Interventions. Nursing diagnoses and interventions for the patient with esophageal carcinoma include but are not limited to the following:

NURSING DIAGNOSES	NURSING INTERVENTIONS
Breathing pattern, ineffective, related to incisional pain and proximity to the diaphragm	Monitor respirations carefully because of proximity of incision to diaphragm and patient's difficulty in carrying out breathing exercises.
Nutrition, altered: less than body requirements, related to dysphagia, decreased stomach capacity, gastrostomy tube	Monitor I&O and daily weights to determine adequate nutritional intake. Assess patient to determine which foods patient can and cannot swallow to select and prepare edible foods.
Infection, high risk for, related to poor nutritional status, weakness, and impaired healing process	Assess for signs of infection: low-grade temperature, abnormal breath sounds, and increased pulse and respiratory rates.
Skin integrity, impaired, high risk for, related to gastrostomy tube or fistula output	Inspect skin frequently for leakage from gastrostomy tube or from fistula formation.

Patient teaching. The nurse should discuss with the patient and family all aspects of care, including surgery, radiation, and chemotherapy if necessary. Psychological adjustment of the patient who cannot ingest food orally, whether temporary or permanent, is difficult. Step-by-step explanations of all diagnostic tests, medications, procedures, and the treatment plan will help to decrease the patient's anxiety. The nurse should support the patient with this serious diagnosis by allowing time for questions.

Prognosis. In carcinoma of the esophagus, the disease is usually well advanced by the time symptoms exist. The delay between the onset of early symptoms and the time when the patient seeks medical advice is often 12 to 18 months. High mortality rates among these patients are affected by the following issues: (1) The patient is generally older, (2) the tumor has usually invaded surrounding structures, (3) the malignancy tends to spread to nearby lymph nodes, and (4) the location of the esophagus in relation to the heart and lungs makes these organs accessible to the extension of the tumor.

The esophagus, with its extensive lymphatic network, facilitates the rapid spread of malignant cells to varying local and distant sites. Carcinoma of the esophagus has a current survival rate of 20%. The only prognostic variable is the stage of disease (an indication of the importance of early diagnosis).

Achalasia

Etiology/Pathophysiology. Achalasia, also called *cardiospasm,* is an abnormal condition characterized by the inability of a muscle to relax, particularly the cardiac sphincter of the stomach.

Although the cause is unknown, nerve degeneration, esophageal dilation, and hypertrophy are thought to contribute to the disruption of the normal neuromuscular activity of the esophagus. This results in decreased motility of the lower portion of the esophagus, absence of peristalsis, and dilation of the lower portion. Thus little or no food can enter the stomach, and in extreme cases, the dilated portion of the esophagus can hold as much as a liter or more of fluid. This disease may occur in persons of any age, but it is more prevalent in those between 20 and 50 years.

Clinical Manifestations. The primary symptom of achalasia is dysphagia. The patient has a sensation of food sticking in the lower portion of the esophagus. As the condition progresses, the patient complains of regurgitation of food, which relieves prolonged distention of the esophagus. There may be some occurrence of substernal chest pain.

Assessment. The nurse should observe for loss of weight, poor skin turgor, and weakness.

Diagnostic Tests. Radiological studies show esophageal dilation above the narrowing at the cardioesophageal junction. The diagnosis is confirmed by manometry, which shows the absence of primary peristalsis. Esophagoscopy is also used to confirm the diagnosis.

Medical Management. The conservative treatment of achalasia includes drug therapy and forceful dilation of the narrowed area of the esophagus. Anticholinergics, nitrates, and calcium channel blockers reduce lower esophageal sphincter pressure.

Dilation is done by first emptying the esophagus. Then a dilator with a deflated balloon is passed down to the sphincter. The balloon is inflated and remains so for 1 minute; it may need to be reinflated one or two times.

A cardiomyotomy is the preferred surgical approach. In this procedure the muscular layer is incised longitudinally, down to but not through the mucosa. Two thirds of the incision is in the esophagus, and the remaining one third is in the stomach; this permits the mucosa to expand so that food can pass easily into the stomach.

Nursing Interventions. Nursing interventions for esophageal surgery are presented in Box 27-3.

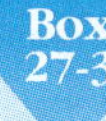

Box 27-3 NURSING INTERVENTIONS FOR THE PERSON EXPERIENCING ESOPHAGEAL SURGERY

PREOPERATIVE NURSING INTERVENTIONS

1. Encourage improved nutritional status.
   a. High-protein, high-calorie diet if oral diet is possible.
   b. Total parenteral nutrition may be necessary for severe dysphagia or obstruction.
2. Give meticulous oral hygiene; breath may be malodorous.
3. Give preoperative preparation appropriate for thoracic surgery.
4. Give prescribed antibiotics before esophageal resection or bypass, as ordered.

POSTOPERATIVE NURSING INTERVENTIONS

1. Promote good pulmonary ventilation.
2. Maintain chest drainage system as prescribed.
3. Maintain gastric drainage system.
   a. Small amounts of blood may drain from nasogastric tube for 6 to 12 hours after surgery.
   b. Do not disturb nasogastric tube (to prevent traction on suture line).
4. Maintain nutrition.
   a. Start clear fluids at frequent intervals when oral intake is permitted.
   b. Introduce soft foods gradually to several small meals of bland foods.
   c. Have patient maintain semi-Fowler's position for 2 hours after eating and while sleeping if heartburn (pyrosis) occurs.

Nursing diagnoses and interventions for the patient with achalasia include but are not limited to the following:

NURSING DIAGNOSES	NURSING INTERVENTIONS
Nutrition altered: less than body requirements, related to difficulty in swallowing both liquids and solids	Encourage fluids with meals to increase lower esophageal sphincter pressure and push food into stomach. Monitor liquid diet for 24 hours after dilation procedure.
Anxiety, related to continuous dilation process with threat of complications	Monitor for signs of esophageal perforation (chest pain, shock, dyspnea, fever) after dilation. Provide calm, nonstressful environment. Reinforce physician's explanation of disease process. Encourage verbalization of fears; assist patient with identifying stressors and positive coping behaviors.

Patient teaching. Home care and follow-up care should be discussed in preparation for dismissal. A family member or support person should be included if possible, and patient should be an active participant in the planning. The following teaching should be included:

1. Explain need for high-calorie, high-protein diet, and provide printed material describing same.
2. Explain need to elevate head while sleeping and to avoid bending and stooping.
3. Discuss medications if prescribed: name, dosage, time of administration, purpose, and side effects.
4. Discuss methods of avoiding constipation by using high-fiber foods if tolerated and natural laxatives.
5. Explain importance of follow-up care with physician.
6. Discuss symptoms of recurrence or progression of disease and need to report these to physician.

Prognosis. Esophageal motility is not restored by dilation procedure, but the open sphincter relieves the dysphagia in about 80% of cases, and the esophageal lumen is reduced in size. Surgical separation, in addition to bag dilation, permits normal peristalsis to return in approximately 10% of patients with achalasia.

DISORDERS OF THE STOMACH

Gastritis (Acute)

Etiology/Pathophysiology. Gastritis is an inflammation of the lining of the stomach. Acute gastritis refers to a temporary inflammation associated with alcoholism, smoking, and stressful physical problems, such as burns, major surgery, food allergens, presence of viral, bacterial, or chemical toxins, chemotherapy, or radiation therapy. Changes in the mucosal lining interfere with acid and pepsin secretion. Acute gastritis is often a single occurrence that resolves when the offending agent is removed.

Clinical Manifestations. If the condition is acute, fever, epigastric pain, nausea, vomiting, headache, coating of the tongue, and loss of appetite may occur. If the condition results from ingestion of contaminated food, the intestines are usually affected and diarrhea may occur.

Assessment. Collection of *subjective data* involves observing for anorexia, nausea, discomfort after eating, and pain, although some patients with gastritis have no symptoms.

Collection of *objective data* includes observing for vomiting, hematemesis, and melena caused by gastric bleeding.

Diagnostic Tests. Testing the stools for occult blood, noting WBC differential increases related to certain bacteria, evaluating serum electrolytes, and observing for elevated hematocrit related to dehydration all aid in the diagnosis.

Medical Management. If medical treatment is required, antiemetics, such as prochlorperazine (Compazine) or trimethobenzamide (Tigan), may be prescribed. Antacids and cimetidine (Tagamet) or ranitidine (Zantac) may be given in combination. Antibiotics are given if the cause is a bacterial agent. Intravenous fluids are used to correct fluid and electrolyte imbalances. Patients who experience GI bleeding from hemorrhagic gastritis require fluid and blood replacement and nasogastric lavage.

Nursing Interventions. The nurse records the patient's I&O. Foods and fluids are withheld orally as prescribed until the signs and symptoms subside. The nurse should monitor the patient's tolerance to oral feedings. The nurse will monitor the intravenous feedings as prescribed.

Nursing diagnoses and interventions for the patient with gastritis include but are not limited to the following:

NURSING DIAGNOSIS	NURSING INTERVENTIONS
Fluid volume deficit, related to vomiting, diarrhea, and blood loss	Keep patient NPO or on restricted food and fluids as ordered, and advance as tolerated. Monitor laboratory data for fluid and electrolyte imbalances (potassium, sodium, and chloride). Record I&O.

Patient teaching. Patient education should include an explanation of (1) the effects of stress on the mucosal lining of the stomach, (2) how salicylates and nonsteroidal antiinflammatory medications and particular foods may be irritating; and (3) how life-styles that include alcohol and tobacco may be harmful. The nurse should be able to assist the patient in locating self-help groups in the community to deal with these stressful behaviors.

Prognosis. Because of the many classifications and causes of gastritis, prognosis is variable. Generally, prognosis is good in individuals who are willing to change their life-styles and follow a medical regimen.

Peptic Ulcers

Peptic ulcers are ulcerations of the mucous membrane or deeper structures of the GI tract. They most commonly occur in the stomach and duodenum. The term *peptic ulcer* refers to ulcers that are the result of acid and pepsin imbalances.

Peptic ulcer disease remains a major health problem and affects more men than women. The older adult reflect an increase in this disease, perhaps as a result of the use of nonsteroidal antiinflammatory drugs. Symptoms are common between the ages of 25 to 50, with the peak occurrence at age 40. Peptic ulcers require the presence of gastric acid and result from two major causes: an excess of gastric acid (duodenal ulcers) or a decrease in the natural ability of the GI mucosa to protect itself from acid and pepsin (gastric ulcers).

A common belief is that persons exhibiting certain traits such as tenseness or a striving for perfection or success are more likely to develop peptic ulcers. Conclusive evidence to support this belief is lacking.

Types of Peptic Ulcers.

Gastric ulcers.

Etiology/pathophysiology. The most common site of a gastric ulcer is in the distal half of the stomach. The cause of gastric ulcers is not clear. There is a relationship between diet, genetic predisposition, ingestion of excessive amounts of salicylates, and use of tobacco and increased incidence of gastric ulcers. Once the gastric mucosal barrier is damaged, acid secretion is stimulated. Without intervention, the cells die, erosion occurs, and ulcers develop. Gastric mucosal damage can occur in some individuals within 1 hour after the ingestion of acetylsalicylic acid. Reflux of duodenal contents (bile acids) also causes severe gastric mucosal damage. Gastric ulcers may occur on the surface of a gastric tumor because of interference with the blood supply.

Duodenal ulcers.

Etiology/pathophysiology. The term *duodenal ulcer* is given to a group of disorders that may or may not be caused by hypersecretion. Excessive production or excessive release of gastrin and/or increased sensitivity to gastrin is found in 40% of people with these ulcers. In the other 60%, the amount of acid produced is normal but perhaps the buffering ability is lacking in the duodenum. Risk factors include *Helicobacter pylori* infection, NSAIDs, cigarette smoking, and coffee. Recently, the organism *Helicobacter pylori* has been implicated in the possible development of duodenal ulcers. Ulceration occurs when the acid secretion exceeds the buffering factors.

Clinical manifestations. Both gastric and duodenal ulcers may have similar symptoms but differ in timing, degree, or factors that worsen or alleviate the symptoms. Pain is the characteristic symptom and is described as dull, burning, boring, or gnawing; it is located in the midline of the epigastric region.

Assessment. Collection of *subjective data* requires an awareness that in gastric ulcer patients, the pain is closely associated with food intake and usually does not awaken the patient at night like the pain experienced by those with duodenal ulcers. Nausea, eructation, and distention are common complaints, termed *dyspepsia.* All these subjective symptoms intensify if the complications of perforation and obstruction are manifested.

Collection of *objective data* includes observing for hemorrhage, a common complication with gastric ulcers; more gastric ulcers bleed than do duodenal ulcers. Duodenal ulcers are more apt to have chronic bleeding and are more prone to perforate than gastric ulcers.

When GI bleeding occurs, one sign is vomiting blood **(hematemesis)** that has a coffee grounds appearance as a result of action of the gastric acid on the hemoglobin molecule. There may be presence of **melena** (tarlike, fetid-smelling stool containing undigested blood) when the blood becomes black and tarry as it passes through the digestive tract. In extreme cases, bright red blood may be passed rectally. Both salicylates and alcohol aggravate bleeding in patients with a history of peptic ulcers.

Bleeding from a gastric ulcer is more difficult to control than bleeding from a duodenal ulcer. Hemorrhage, with accompanying symptoms of shock, occurs when the ulcer erodes into a blood vessel. Surgical intervention is indicated if the patient remains unstable after receiving blood over several hours.

Perforation occurs when the ulcer crater penetrates the entire thickness of the wall of the stomach or duodenum. The release of gastric acid, pancreatic enzymes, or bile causes signs and symptoms of pain, emesis, fever, hypotension, and hematemesis.

Diagnostic tests. Fiberoptic endoscopy can detect both gastric and duodenal ulcers. This is called *esophagogastroduodenoscopy.* The lesion can be viewed, biopsy performed, and cell washings taken for cytological examination. The patient is sedated but remains conscious throughout the endoscopy procedure. Local anesthetics are used to anesthetize the throat, decrease the gag reflex, and minimize pain during the procedure. No liquids or food are allowed for 1 to 2 hours or until the patient can swallow. Radiological studies (UGI) are not as specific for small lesions but are still commonly used. Hematest of feces for detecting occult blood in the intestinal tract may also be used for diagnosis.

Medical management. The physician may order a nasogastric tube to be inserted to remove gastric content and blood (see p. 672 for a discussion of nursing interventions for nasogastric tubes). Surgery is indicated usually for complications: perforation, penetration, obstruction, or intractability (no longer responding to medical management).

Scar tissue builds up with repeat episodes of ulceration and healing, causing obstruction, particularly at the pylorus. The patient may present with gastric dilation, vomiting, and distention. When fluid and electrolyte balance is achieved, surgical intervention is possible.

The primary treatment for peptic ulcers is to reduce signs and symptoms by decreasing or neutralizing the

MEDICATIONS FOR GASTROINTESTINAL DISORDERS

Medication	Trade Name	Action	Side Effects	Nursing Implications
Antacids (aluminum, calcium, and magnesium salts and sodium bicarbonate are all used)	Maalox, Mylanta, Titralac, Alternagel, others	Neutralizes gastric acid, aluminum and calcium antacids also bind phosphates in renal failure patients	Aluminum—constipation, hypophosphatemia; calcium—constipation, rebound hyperacidity, hypercalcemia; magnesium—diarrhea, hypermagnesemia; sodium bicarbonate—sodium and water retention, alkalosis, rebound hyperacidity	Monitor serum electrolytes with long-term use, do not give antacid simultaneously with other medications because absorption of the other medication may be affected, best to separate administration by 2 hours
Antispasmodics (includes atropine, scopolamine, hyoscyamine, dicyclomine, clidinium, others)	Donnatal Bentyl, others	Anticholinergic agents that decrease GI motility by relaxing GI smooth muscle	Dry mouth and skin, constipation, paralytic ileus, urinary retention, tachycardia, drowsiness, dizziness, confusion, altered vision	Avoid using other CNS depressants or alcohol concomitantly, avoid driving or other potentially hazardous tasks until accustomed to sedating effects
Bismuth subsalicylate	Pepto-Bismol	Antidiarrheal agent, also used in peptic ulcer disease due to *Helicobacter pylori*	Fecal impaction, tinnitus	May turn stools dark gray-black, avoid use with aspirin, consult physician if diarrhea is accompanied by high fever or lasts more than 2 days
Cimetidine	Tagamet	H_2 receptor antagonist, inhibits gastric acid secretion	Confusion, headache, gynecomastia, bone marrow suppression (rare)	Increases serum levels and clinical effects of oral anticoagulants, theophylline, phenytoin, some benzodiazepines, and propranolol (these medications may require dosage reduction)
Dimenhydrinate	Dramamine, others	Antiemetic agent, blocks central vomiting center	Drowsiness, dry mouth, constipation	Avoid use with other CNS depressants and alcohol, avoid driving or other hazardous activities until accustomed to sedating effects
Diphenoxylateatropine	Lomotil	Antidiarrheal agent (diphenoxylate—narcotic, atropine—anticholinergic)	Drowsiness, sedation constipation, dry mouth, urinary retention	Avoid use with other CNS depressants and alcohol, avoid driving or other hazardous activities until accustomed to sedating effects, do not use in infectious diarrhea
Famotidine	Pepcid	H_2 receptor antagonist, inhibits gastric acid secretion	Headache, dizziness, constipation thrombocytopenia, (rare)	Unlike cimetidine, does not affect serum levels of hepatically metabolized drugs (warfarin, phenytoin, theophylline)

Continued.

MEDICATIONS FOR GASTROINTESTINAL DISORDERS—cont'd

Medication	Trade Name	Action	Side Effects	Nursing Implications
Kaolin-pectin	Kaopectate	Antidiarrheal agent	Constipation	Shake well before using
Ketoconazole	Nizoral	Antifungal agent	Gynecomastia, impotence, hepatotoxicity, abdominal pain	Requires acid environment for absorption; do not use with antacids, H_2 receptor blockers, or omeprazole; do not use with terfenadine, astemizole, or loratadine—has caused dysrhythmias and death; monitor liver function tests often; monitor serum levels and clinical effects of warfarin, cyclosporine, and theophylline
Lactulose	Chronulac, Cephulac, others	Acidifies colonic contents, thus decreasing absorption of ammonia from gut, also has cathartic laxative properties, primary use in hepatic encephalopathy	Nausea, vomiting, diarrhea	Titrate dose to 3-4 loose stools per day, monitor for dehydration and improvement in mental status
Loperamide	Imodium	Antidiarrheal agent	Drowsiness, dry mouth constipation	Monitor for dehydration, do not use in infectious diarrhea
Mesalamine	Rowasa, Asachol	GI antiinflammatory agent	Abdominal cramps and gas, rash, headache, dizziness,	Swallow tablets whole, give enema at bedtime, retain 6-8 hours
Misoprostol	Cytotec	Prostaglandin analog that acts as gastric mucosal protectant, protects against NSAID-induced ulcers	Diarrhea, nausea, vomiting flatulence, uterine cramping	Absolutely contraindicated in pregnant women, women of childbearing age must use reliable contraception
Nizatidine	Axid	H2 receptor antagonist, inhibits gastric acid secretion	Drowsiness, headache, dizziness, sweating, thrombocytopenia (rare)	Does not affect serum levels of hepatically metabolized drugs (warfarin, phenytoin, theophylline)
Nystatin	Mycostatin, Nilstat, others	Antifungal agent, available as oral suspension and topical product	Oral—nausea, vomiting, diarrhea topical—local irritation	Long-term therapy may be needed to clear infection, use for entire course
Olsalazine	Dipentum	GI antiinflammatory agent	Diarrhea, abdominal pain and cramps, nausea, allergic reactions, arthralgia, rash, anaphylaxis	Take with food, notify physician if severe diarrhea occurs
Omeprazole	Prilosec	Proton pump inhibitor, totally eradicates gastric acid production	Headache, dizziness, abdominal pain, nausea, vomiting, rare bone marrow suppression	Inhibits hepatic metabolism of warfarin, phenytoin, benzodiazepines, and other drugs metabolized by liver, do not crush or chew capsule contents

MEDICATIONS FOR GASTROINTESTINAL DISORDERS—cont'd

Medication	Trade Name	Action	Side Effects	Nursing Implications
Prochlorperazine	Compazine	Antiemetic agent, blocks central vomiting center	Drowsiness, extrapyramidal symptoms, orthostatic hypotension, constipation, dry mouth, urinary retention	Avoid use with other CNS depressants and alcohol, avoid driving and other activities until accustomed to effects; may cause hypotension when given IV, do not use in patients with Parkinson's disease
Propantheline	Pro-Banthine	Antisecretory and antispasmodic agent, slows GI motility through anticholinergic activity	Drowsiness, confusion, dry mouth, constipation, urinary retention, tachycardia, blurred vision	Avoid use with other CNS depressants or alcohol, avoid driving or other activities until accustomed to effects; may cause hypotension when given IV, do not use in patients with Parkinson's disease
Ranitidine	Zantac	H_2 receptor antagonist, inhibits gastric acid secretion	Headache, abdominal discomfort, granulocytopenia and thrombocytopenia (both rare)	Minimal effect on serum levels of hepatically metabolized drugs (phenytoin, warfarin, theophylline)
Sucralfate	Carafate	Gastric mucosal protectant agent, adheres to site of ulcer	Constipation, hypophosphatemia	Do not give with other drugs, coating action may interfere with the absorption of other drugs, separate by 2 hours
Sulfasalazine	Azulfidine	GI antiinflammatory agent	Nausea, vomiting, abdominal pain, photosensitivity, rash, Stevens-Johnson Syndrome (rare), renal failure, bone marrow suppression (rare), allergic reactions, anaphylaxis	Ensure adequate hydration to prevent crystallization in kidneys, avoid exposure to sunlight, women on oral contraceptives need to use alternative methods because of decreased effectiveness of oral contraceptives, may increase effect, monitor CBC, renal function, take with meals
Vasopressin	Pitressin	Synthetic pituitary hormone with antidiuretic effects on kidney (used to treat diabetes insipidus), also a potent vasoconstictor (used to treat bleeding esophageal varices)	Hypertension; ischemia to heart, mesenteric organs, and kidneys; angina, myocardial infarction, water retention, hyponatremia	Use with caution in older patients or patients with known coronary artery disease, use caution in patients with known congestive heart failure, discontinue if chest pain develops, monitor urine output, serum sodium

normal gastric acidity with drug therapy. The types of drugs most commonly used include the following (see medications table on pp. 667-669):

- Antacids: neutralize or reduce the acidity of the stomach contents; these are Maalox, Gaviscon, Rolaids, Tums, Mylanta, and Riopan.
- Histamine H_2 receptor blockers: decrease acid secretions by blocking the histamine H_2 receptors; these include cimetidine (Tagamet), ranitidine (Zantac), famotidine (Pepcid), and nizatidine (Axid). Do not give histamine receptor antagonists within 2 hours of antacids.
- Proton pump inhibitor: antisecretory agent to inhibit secretion of gastrin by the parietal cells of the stomach; this includes omeprazole (Prilosec, Liosec).
- Mucosal healing agents: heal ulcers without antisecretory properties, possibly by adhering to the proteins in the ulcer base; this includes sucralfate (Carafate) and misoprostol (Cytotec).

Research shows that treating the *Helicobacter pylori* organism with bismuth compounds and antibiotics results in lower relapse rates of ulcers at 1 year. Such therapy may have great implications for duodenal ulcers. Further research will be forthcoming in this area.

Diet therapy to promote healing includes diets high in fat and carbohydrates and low in protein and milk products. However, most patients do not understand or choose not to follow this regimen. Therefore it is recommended that smaller meals taken more frequently throughout the day decrease the degree of gastric motor activity. Bland diets do not promote patient compliance. Because caffeinated and decaffeinated coffee, tobacco, alcohol, and aspirin aggravate the mucosal lining of the stomach and duodenum, an effort should be made to change the life-style of the patient with ulcers.

Surgery is usually indicated for complications. Surgical intervention has decreased drastically with more effective diagnosis and medical treatment. Types of surgical procedures include the following:

- Antrectomy: removal of the entire antrum, the gastric-producing portion of the lower stomach, to eliminate the main stimuli to acid production.
- Gastroduodenostomy (Billroth I) (Fig. 27-9, *A*): fundus of the stomach is directly anastomosed to the duodenum; used to remove ulcers or cancer located in the antrum of the stomach.
- Gastrojejunostomy (Billroth II) (Fig. 27-9, *B*): duodenum is closed, and the fundus of the stomach is anastomosed into the jejunum; used to remove ulcers or cancer located in the body of the fundus.
- Total gastrectomy: removal of the entire stomach; rarely used for patients with gastric cancer.
- Vagotomy: removal of the vagal innervation to the fundus, decreasing acid produced by the parietal cells of the stomach (Fig. 27-10).

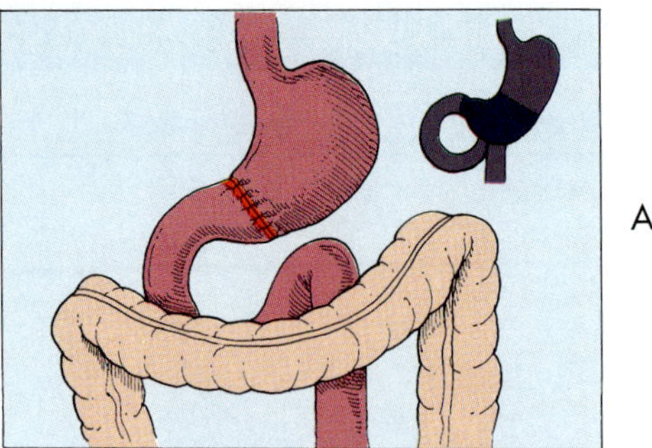

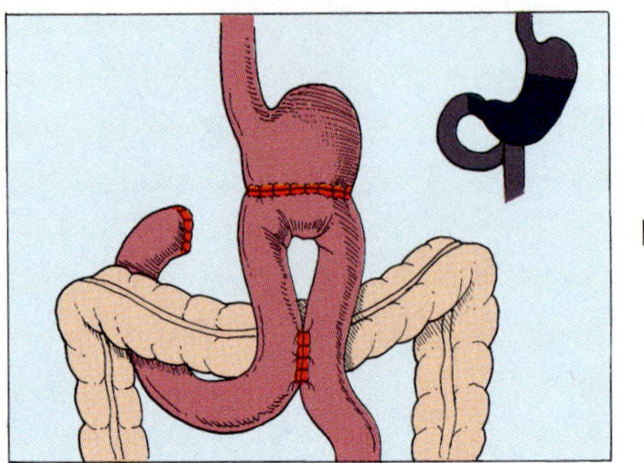

FIG. 27-9 Types of gastric resections with anastomoses. **A,** Billroth I. **B,** Fillroth II.

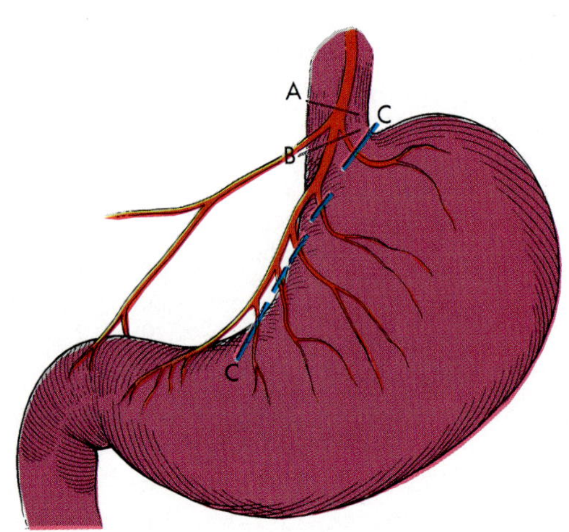

FIG. 27-10 Types of vagotomies. *A,* Truncal. *B,* Selective. *C,* Proximal or parietal cell.

- Pyloroplasty: surgical enlargement of the pylorus to provide drainage of the gastric contents.

The decision as to which procedure to use is difficult; the choice depends on physician preference and results of diagnostic testing. Regardless of the procedure selected, postoperative complications can occur.

Bleeding may occur up to 7 days after gastric surgery. Abdominal rigidity, abdominal pain, restlessness, an elevated temperature, increase in pulse, decrease in blood pressure, and leukocytosis are all possible indica-

TABLE 27-2 Purposes of NG Intubation

Purpose	Description	Type of Tube
Decompression	Removal of secretions and gaseous substances from GI tract; prevention or relief of abdominal distention	Salem sump, Levin, Miller-Abbott (see Fig. 27-11, *B*)
Feeding (gavage) (see Chapter 19)	Instillation of liquid nutritional supplements or feedings into stomach for patients unable to swallow fluid	Duo, Dubhoff, Levin
Compression	Internal application of pressure by means of inflated balloon to prevent internal GI hemorrhage	Sengstaken-Blakemore
Lavage	Irrigation of stomach in cases of active bleeding, poisoning, or gastric dilation	Levin, Ewald, Salem sump (see Fig. 27-11, *A*)

tions of postoperative bleeding. The amount and type of drainage from the incision must be noted. Surgical intervention may be necessary to correct the bleeding.

The *dumping syndrome* is a rapid gastric emptying causing distention of the duodenum or jejunum produced by a bolus of hypertonic food. Increased intestinal motility and peristalsis and changes in blood glucose levels occur. Diaphoresis, nausea, vomiting, epigastric pain, explosive diarrhea, borborygmi (noises made from gas passing through the liquid of the small intestine), and dyspepsia may be reported by patients. The dumping syndrome can occur after gastric resection procedures. Treatment includes eating six small meals daily that are high in protein and fat and low in carbohydrates, eating slowly, and avoiding fluids during meals. Treatment also includes (1) anticholinergic agents to decrease stomach motility and (2) reclining for approximately 1 hour after meals.

There are several other complications after gastric surgery that present serious health threats. Diarrhea is common and usually responds to conservative treatment of controlled diet and antidiarrheal agents. Lomotil, Imodium, paregoric, or codeine is often used. Reflux esophagitis and nutritional deficits, including weight loss, malabsorption, anemia, and vitamin deficiency, can also be life threatening.

Pernicious anemia is a serious potential complication in any patient who has had a total gastrectomy or extensive resections. This is caused by a deficiency of the intrinsic factor, produced exclusively by the stomach, that aids intestinal absorption of vitamin B_{12}. It is recommended that all patients with a partial gastrectomy have a blood serum vitamin B_{12} level measured every 1 to 2 years so that replacement therapy can be instituted before anemia appears. The most common cause of anemia after gastric surgery is iron deficiency. Iron-deficiency anemia is caused by impaired absorption in the duodenum and proximal jejunum as a result of rapid gastric emptying. Replacement therapy consists of oral iron in the ferrous form.

Nursing interventions. Nasogastric tube insertion, irrigation, and GI suctioning are often performed while a patient is feeling ill and uncomfortable. In addition to being skilled and knowledgeable in performing these procedures, the nurse is responsible for allaying the patient's fears and anxieties. Eliciting patient cooperation not only makes the procedures easier but also helps reduce patient discomfort.

An understanding of the following points will enable the nurse to help patients through the experience of GI intubation:

- For most patients, GI intubation is a new and frightening experience.
- Inability to chew, taste, and swallow food and liquids may contribute to patient anxieties during GI intubation.
- A patient with a nasogastric (NG) or intestinal tube is usually on NPO status.
- The presence of an NG or intestinal tube is a constant irritant to the nasopharynx and nares, requiring frequent care to the mouth and nose.
- A patient with a GI tube may be afraid that moving will dislodge the tube. The nurse must implement frequent position changes to enhance tube functioning and prevent complications of immobility.

An NG tube is inserted through the nose, pharynx, and esophagus into the stomach (Skill 27-2 on pp. 672-674). Various tubes are available, depending on the purpose (Table 27-2 and Fig. 27-11 on p. 677).

During insertion the tube may enter the trachea rather than the stomach. Before instilling liquids through the tube or attaching the tube to suction, the nurse should determine that the tube is in the stomach (see Skill 27-2, Steps 27 and 28). Skills 27-3 to 27-5 on pp. 674-675 present various aspects of NG tube care.

Text continued on p. 677.

SKILL 27-2

INSERTING NASOGASTRIC TUBE

1. Inspect condition of patient's oral cavity. This determines need for special nursing measures for oral hygiene after tube placement.
2. Palpate patient's abdomen. This determination will later serve as comparison after tube is inserted.
3. Check medical record for physician's order, type of NG tube to be placed, and whether tube is to be attached to suction or drainage bag. Procedure requires physician's order. Adequate decompression depends on suction.
4. Prepare equipment and supplies:
   a. 14 or 16 Fr NG tube (smaller lumen for child)
   b. Water-soluble lubricating jelly
   c. Stethoscope
   d. Tongue blade
   e. Flashlight
   f. Asepto bulb or cone-tip syringe
   g. Nose guard
   h. Safety pin and rubber band
   i. Clamp
   j. Suction container
   k. Suction machine
   l. Bath towel
   m. Glass of water with straw
   n. Facial tissues
   o. Normal saline
   p. Tincture of benzoin (optional)
   q. Nonsterile gloves
5. Identify patient and explain procedure. This prevents error and gains patient's cooperation to facilitate passage of tube.
6. Wash hands and don gloves to prevent transmission of microorganisms.
7. Position patient in high Fowler's position with pillows behind head and shoulders. Raise bed to its highest horizontal level. This promotes patient's ability to swallow during procedure. Good body mechanics prevents injury to nurse or patient.
8. Assemble all equipment at bedside and place on your side of bed. Pull curtain around bed or close room door to provide privacy. Procedure should be organized to limit patient discomfort.
9. Stand at right side of bed if right-handed and left side if left-handed. This allows easiest manipulation of tubing.
10. Place bath towel over patient's chest; give tissues to patient. This prevents soiling of gown. Tube insertion through nasal passages may cause tearing.
11. Instruct patient to relax and breathe normally while occluding one naris. Repeat this action for other naris. Select nostril with greater air flow, as the tube passes more easily through naris that is more patent.
12. Measure distance to insert tube: Measure distance from tip of nose to earlobe to xiphoid process of sternum (see illustration). Tube

STEP 12

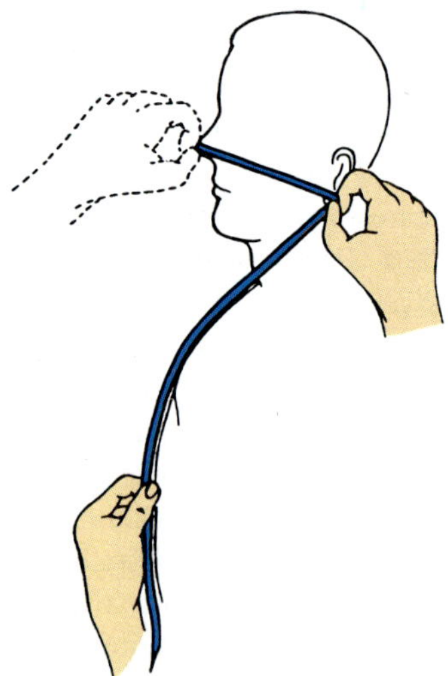

STEP 16

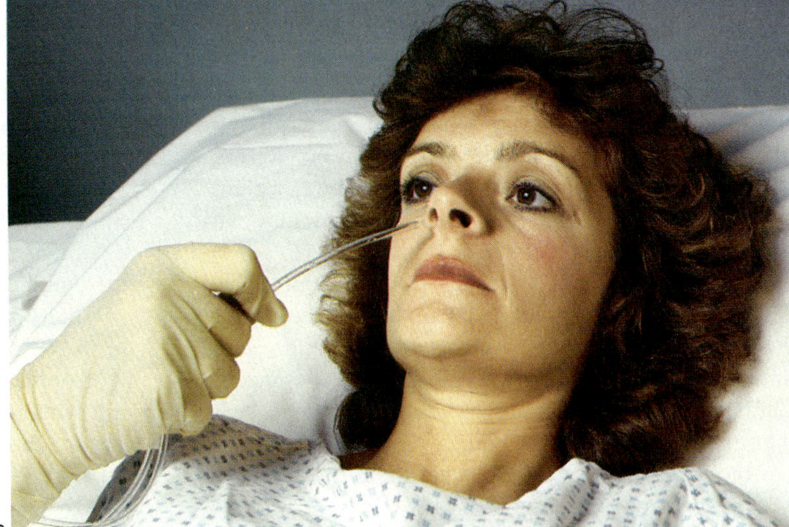

INSERTING NASOGASTRIC TUBE—cont'd

should extend from nares to stomach; distance varies with each patient. This measurement provides distance from nose to stomach in 98% of patients.

13. Mark length of tube to be inserted with piece of tape or note distance from next tube marking.
14. Curve 4 to 6 inches (10 to 15 cm) of end of tube tightly around index finger; release. Curving tube tip aids insertion.
15. Lubricate 3 to 4 inches (7.5 to 10 cm) of end of tube with water-soluble lubricating jelly. This minimizes friction against nasal mucosa.
16. Initially instruct patient to extend neck back against pillow; insert tube slowly through naris with curved end pointing downward (see illustration). This facilitates initial passage of tube through naris and maintains clear airway for open naris.
17. Continue to pass tube along floor of nasal passage, aiming down toward ear. When resistance is felt, apply gentle downward pressure to advance tube (do not force past resistance). This will minimize discomfort of tube rubbing against upper nasal turbinates. Resistance is caused by posterior nasopharynx. Downward pressure helps tube to curl around corner of nasopharynx.
18. If resistance continues, withdraw tube, allow patient to rest, relubricate tube, and insert into other naris, because forcing against resistance can cause trauma to mucosa. Help relieve anxiety.
19. Continue insertion of tube until just past nasopharynx by gently rotating tube toward opposite naris:
    a. Stop tube advancement, allow patient to relax, and provide tissues. This relieves anxiety; tearing is natural response to mucosal irritation.
    b. Explain that next step requires swallowing because tube is about to enter esophagus.
20. With tube just above oropharynx, instruct patient to flex head forward and dry swallow or suck in air through straw. Advance tube 1 to 2 inches (2.5 to 5 cm) with each swallow. If patient has trouble swallowing and is allowed fluids, offer glass of water. Advance tube with each swallow of water because the flexed position closes off upper airway to trachea and opens esophagus. Swallowing closes epiglottis over trachea and helps to move tube into esophagus. Swallowing water reduces gagging or choking.
21. If patient begins to cough, gag, or choke, stop tube advancement. Instruct patient to breathe easily and take sips of water. Tubing may accidentally enter larynx and initiate cough reflex. Gagging is eased by swallowing water.
22. If patient continues to cough, pull tube back slightly.
23. If patient continues to gag, check back of pharynx using flashlight and tongue blade.
24. After patient relaxes, continue to advance tube desired distance. Tip of tube should be in the stomach to decompress properly.
25. Ask patient to talk. Patient would be unable to talk if tube is passed through vocal cords.
26. Check posterior pharynx for presence of coiled tube as the tube is pliable and can coil up in back of pharynx instead of advancing into esophagus.
27. Attach cone-tipped syringe to end of tube. Aspirate gently back on syringe to obtain gastric contents. (Insufflation of air into tube followed by auscultation of sounds is no longer considered most effective in determining tube placement. Sounds transmitted by insufflation of air may be transmitted from pleural space to upper abdomen giving false impression of placement [Metheny et al, 1988].) Check agency's policy for preferred method.
28. Measure pH of aspirate with color-coded pH paper with range of whole numbers from 1 to 11. Gastric aspirates have decidedly acidic pH values, preferably 4 or less.
29. If tube is not in the stomach, advance another 1 to 2 inches (2.5 to 5 cm) and repeat Step 27 to check for tube placement.
30. After tube is properly inserted, clamp end or connect it to suction. Intermittent suction is most effective for decompression. Tube is often clamped for short periods of time, such as during ambulation.
31. Secure tube to nose with a nasal guard. Avoid putting pressure on nares (see illustration).
32. Fasten end of tube to gown by looping rubber band around tube in slip knot. Pin rubber band to gown. This reduces pressure on nares if tube moves. Pinning provides slack for movement.
33. Unless physician orders otherwise, head of bed should be elevated 30 degrees as this helps pre-

Continued.

SKILL 27-2

INSERTING NASOGASTRIC TUBE—cont'd

vent esophageal reflux and minimizes irritation of tube against posterior pharynx.

34. Remove gloves and dispose of appropriately
35. Wash hands to reduce transmission of microorganisms.
36. Record in nurses' notes time and type of tube inserted, tolerance to procedure, confirmation of placement, character and amount of gastric contents and whether tube is clamped or connected to suction.

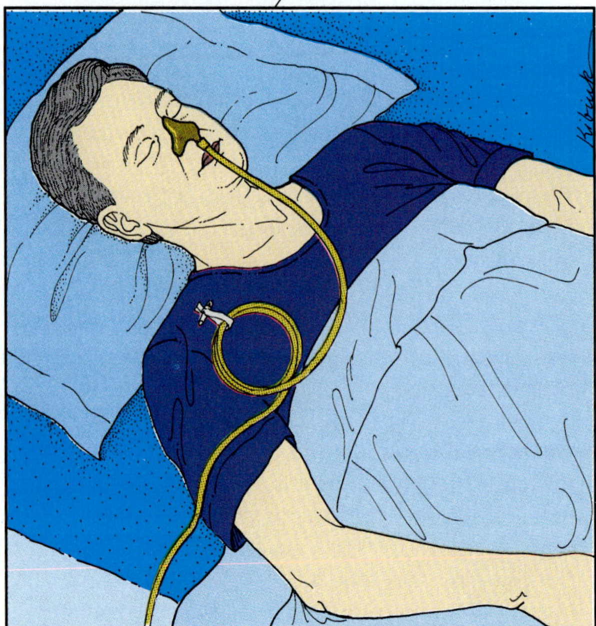

STEP 31

SKILL 27-3

GASTRIC AND INTESTINAL SUCTIONING CARE

1. Introduce self.
2. Identify patient.
3. Wash hands.
4. Explain procedure.
5. Check suction apparatus:
   a. For suction machine (Gomco)
      1. Machine is plugged in securely.
      2. Light is blinking on and off.
      3. Tubing connections are tight.
      4. Setting is correct.
   b. For wall suction
      1. Pressure gauge connections are tight.
      2. Pressure indicated on gauge is as ordered or according to agency policy.
      3. Suction is set at *intermittent* or *continuous* as ordered.
6. Ensure that tubing is not kinked and that patient is not lying on tubing.
7. Pin NG tube to patient's gown with enough slack to allow movement.
8. Verify that drainage is moving through tubing to drainage collection bottle.
9. For Salem sump tube, see that vent is pointing upward; vent pointing downward could promote drainage through vent via gravity.

   Listen at opening of blue air vent; hissing sound indicates air vent is patent. If no hissing sounds are heard, instruct patient to cough or reposition to the right or left Sims' or supine position. It may be necessary to momentarily disconnect the NG tube from the suction tubing; be certain to reconnect immediately.
10. Don gloves, and measure amount of drainage in bottle, noting color; empty if becoming full and at end of each shift.
11. Remove gloves (dispose of appropriately), and wash hands.
12. Record procedure and observations.
13. Report abnormalities.

SKILL 27-4

NASOGASTRIC TUBE IRRIGATION

1. Introduce self.
2. Identify patient.
3. Wash hands.
4. Explain procedure.
5. Arrange equipment at bedside.
6. Pull curtain and close door to provide privacy.
7. Don gloves.
8. Verify that tube is in place.
   a. Attach syringe to tube, and aspirate gastric contents.
9. Pour normal saline into container; draw up 30 ml (or amount ordered) into bulb or piston syringe.
10. Connect syringe to NG tube; keeping syringe in upright position, gently instill 30-ml saline (or ordered amount); do not use force.
11. If resistance is met, change patient's position and repeat attempt; if resistance continues, check with RN or physician.
12. Withdraw fluid into syringe, and measure; continue irrigating with ordered amount of saline until purpose of irrigation has been accomplished.
13. Reconnect NG tube to suction.
14. Note amount of saline instilled and withdrawn.
15. Dispose of equipment.
16. Remove gloves; wash hands.
17. Record procedure and observations (include type and amount of solution used and character and volume of aspirate).
18. Report abnormalities.

SKILL 27-5

NASOGASTRIC TUBE REMOVAL

1. Introduce self.
2. Identify patient.
3. Wash hands.
4. Explain procedure.
5. Arrange equipment at bedside.
6. Pull curtain and close door to provide privacy.
7. If tube is attached to suction, turn off suction machine and disconnect tubing; remove nose guard; and unfasten pin from gown.
8. Place towel or waterproof pad across patient's chest, and give patient tissues.
9. Don gloves.
10. Have patient take deep breath and hold breath; pinch tube with fingers or clamp (to prevent aspiration from any leakage); quickly and smoothly remove tube while patient is holding breath. (If patient begins to gag, continue to remove tubing as the tubing is causing the patient to gag.)
11. Place tubing in plastic bag or towel.
12. Provide oral and nasal care; make patient comfortable.
13. Dispose of tube and equipment; measure drainage; note color; write down for documentation later.
14. Remove gloves; wash hands.
15. Record procedure and observations. Include removal of NG tube, patient's tolerance of procedure, presence of bowel sounds, and any abdominal distention.
16. Report abnormalities. (Inspect condition of nares, nose, and oral cavity.)
17. Palpate abdomen periodically, noting any distention; auscultate abdomen for bowel sounds.

NURSING CARE PLAN: ***THE PATIENT WITH GASTROINTESTINAL BLEEDING***

Mr. Dennison, a 33-year-old stockbroker, is admitted with pain in the epigastric region and copious hematemesis. He appears anxious; his skin is cool and clammy, and he is breathing rapidly. This patient has a history of recurrent episodes of vomiting blood that has a coffee-ground appearance. He denies the presence of passing blood rectally but admits his stools have changed in consistency.

Nursing diagnoses	Patient goals/expected outcomes	Nursing interventions
Gas exchange, impaired, related to weakened condition, hemorrhage	Patient will demonstrate normal respiratory rate. Patient will breathe deeply and cough with assistance. Patient will not demonstrate rales or rhonchi.	Assess emergency ABCs of Airway, Breathing, and Circulation. Encourage the patient to breathe deeply and cough q 4 hr or more often if needed. Explain importance of gas exchange in preventing infection in the lungs. Monitor patient's breathing by assessing breath sounds in all lobes of the lung. Document, and notify physician of any abnormalities. Administer O_2 as ordered.
Fluid volume deficit, high risk for, related to hemorrhage, vomiting, and diarrhea	Patient will have normal fluid balance as evidenced by balanced I&O within 48 hr, including stable weight. Blood pressure, pulse, and respiratory rate will be within normal limits. Patient will have normal tissue turgor.	Accurately record I&O q 1 hr until stable: emesis, urine, and stool. Document fluid losses for possible imbalance; urine output less than 30 ml/hr may indicate hypovolemia. Monitor for signs and symptoms of dehydration and fluid electrolyte imbalance (dry mucous membranes, poor skin turgor, thirst, decreased urinary output, and changes in behavior) q 15 min until stable, then q 2 hr. Document characteristics of output. Test all emesis and fecal output for presence of blood as ordered. Prepare to assist with inserting an NG tube. Irrigate NG tube with cool saline as ordered to promote clotting; irrigation removes old blood from the stomach.
Anxiety, related to hospitalization and illness	Patient will demonstrate decrease in anxiety as evidenced by ability to sleep and/or rest at frequent intervals, verbalization of feelings, and blood pressure and pulse within normal limits.	Assess physiological components of anxiety: restlessness, increased pulse and respirations, diaphoresis, and elevated blood pressure at least q 8 hr. Provide concise explanations for all procedures; prepare patient for surgery if indicated. Develop rapport with patient and family members with each contact.

Tissue perfusion, altered, related to blood and fluid loss	Patient will demonstrate adequate renal perfusion as evidenced by urine output greater than 30 ml/hr. Patient will have normal blood pressure, pulse, and respirations. Patient will be oriented ×3.	Assess for signs and symptoms of hypoxia continually: cyanosis, dyspnea, and disorientation. Assess for urine output less than 30 ml/hr; insert Foley catheter as ordered. Monitor hemoglobin and hematocrit values on each laboratory report; normal ranges are Hgb: 12-18 g/dl and Hct: 37%-52% Assess vital signs q 15 min or q 1-2 hr if stable.

CRITICAL THINKING QUESTIONS

1. Mr. Dennison has a nasogastric tube that is draining sanguineous fluid. He complains of severe fatigue and epigastric pain. He is pale and drawn, with a hemoglobin level of 5.1 g/dl. Mr. Dennison puts his light on and requests the nurse to assist him to the bathroom for a bowel movement. The appropriate interventions to ensure the safety of Mr. Dennison would be:
2. During assessment of Mr. Dennison, the signs and symptoms that would indicate a fluid volume deficit would be:
3. Mr. Dennison verbalizes to the nurse that he fears he may die. He appears anxious and tremulous. To assist in decreasing his fears, the most therapeutic approach would be:

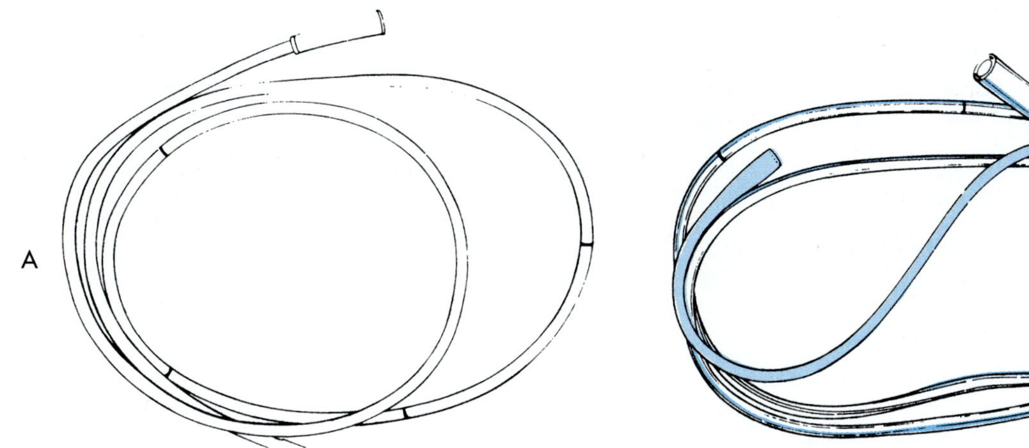

FIG. 27-11 Nasogastric tubes. **A,** Levin tubes. **B,** Salem sump tube.

Nursing interventions depend on the stage of the ulcer disease. The emphasis on patient care should always be on prevention and early detection of pain in the epigastric region, hematemesis, melena, or tenderness and rigidity of the abdomen. See the therapeutic dialogue and the nursing care plan for the patient with GI bleeding.

THERAPEUTIC DIALOGUE

Nurse: You look like you are resting better, Mrs. Snodgrass. How have you been feeling? *(Reaffirming a relationship that was begun yesterday.)*

Patient: Hello, Mrs. Fuller. My stomach pain is much better. The medicine helped.

Nurse: If you are comfortable, perhaps you and your husband have some questions about why you are here. *(Trying to determine if the patient is receptive to patient teaching. A knowledge deficit was suspected on admission.)*

Patient: I was scared when I started to vomit blood. It has happened before but not this much. Where does the blood come from?

Nurse: You have a diagnosis of GI bleed with questionable duodenal ulcer. That means you have bleeding in the gastrointestinal system, either in the stomach or in some part of the intestine. *(The nurse begins with the admitting diagnosis and explains one thing at a time, making sure the patient verbalizes understanding before continuing.)* Do you understand what I have said so far?

Patient: Well, I understand where the bleeding is coming from, but why am I bleeding there?

Nurse: We are not sure yet, Mrs. Snodgrass, but you are scheduled for a procedure that will allow the doctor to actually look at the surface of the stomach and a portion of the intestine. It is called an endoscopy, and it will be done tomorrow morning. Did someone explain this to you? *(The nurse answers the question openly and honestly and uses the answer to lead into further patient education.)*

Nursing diagnoses and interventions for the specific stages of ulcer care include but are not limited to the following:

NURSING DIAGNOSES	NURSING INTERVENTIONS
Peptic ulcer disease Knowledge deficit, related to medications, diet, and signs and symptoms of bleeding or perforation	Provide verbal and written instruction on exact dosage and time intervals for medications and if medication is taken with or without food. Have dietician provide instructions on therapeutic diet. Explain that repeat episodes are not uncommon; listen carefully for aggravating factors.
Pain, related to gastric acid on ulceration of gastric or duodenal mucosa	Give prescribed histamine H_2 receptor antagonists—cimetidine (Tagamet), ranitidine (Zantac), famotidine (Pepcid), or nizatidine (Axid)—with meals and at bedtime. Give prescribed antacid 1 and 3 hours after meals. Teach relaxation measures as appropriate. Instruct patient on side effects of antacid drugs (constipation or diarrhea) and importance of contacting physician if this occurs.
Nutrition, altered: less than body requirements, related to pain, dyspepsia	Explain to patient reason for six meals and avoidance of foods that irritate mucosa lining.
Noncompliance related to treatment and behavior modification	Teach patient to report pain of sudden and severe onset and passage of blood by emesis or rectally. Teach effects of aspirin, smoking, and alcohol on ulcer formation.
Anxiety, related to disease process	Help patient identify risk behaviors: anxiety, restlessness, and insomnia; and available resources for behavior modification.
Gastric surgery Fluid volume deficit, high risk for, related to hemorrhage	Monitor for hypotension and tachycardia, sudden and severe abdominal pain, shallow respirations, vomiting, rigid and tender abdomen, and diminished bowel sounds. Monitor vital signs; record accurate I&O; note weight gain or loss Monitor temperature and oral mucous membranes for dryness; provide oral hygiene (toothbrushing or mouthwash); apply lubricant to lips and nares prn. Monitor parenteral fluids as ordered by physician.
Noncompliance, related to risk behaviors (use of tobacco/alcohol) and dietary patterns	Assess patient's level of knowledge regarding food and other irritants to mucosal lining. Teach preventive measures, such as quitting smoking. Explain need for small and frequent meals. Caution patient to avoid high-fiber foods, sugar, salt, caffeine, and alcohol, as well as milk. Remind to take fluids between meals, not with meals. Explain to eat slowly and chew food well. Discuss importance of adequate rest and exercise.
Nutrition, altered: less than body requirements, related to preoperative and postoperative food and fluid restrictions	Maintain NPO status. Connect NG tube to intermittent suction apparatus. Note color and amount of gastric output q 4 hr. Do not reposition tube. Maintain patency of tube by irrigation with measured amounts of saline *only* if ordered; NOTE: After gastrectomy, output will be minimal. Monitor parenteral fluids with electrolyte additives as ordered. Measure intake and output. When bowel sounds return, administer clear liquids as ordered. Progress to small, frequent meals of soft food as ordered. Avoid milk, since it may cause dumping syndrome.

Patient teaching. It is necessary for the nurse to form a trusting relationship with the patient because of the severity of the condition and the long-term treatment of the patient with an ulcer. The family should be included with the patient for understanding and support, and the patient should be involved in goal setting if compliance is to be obtained.

The patient should be aware that if severe and sudden pain occurs, medical attention should be sought immediately. Assistance should be given to the patient in describing signs and symptoms of weakness, anorexia, nausea, diarrhea, constipation, anxiety, or restlessness. When medications are prescribed, the patient must fully understand (1) why the drugs are taken in large doses (30 ml), seven times daily (1 and 3 hours after a meal and at bedtime) or at the specific times ordered and (2) the side effects that are known (diarrhea and constipation). Preventive teaching includes identifying risk behaviors in the patient's life-style, such as the use of tobacco and alcohol and engaging in stress-related activities. Dietary needs should emphasize six smaller meals daily and avoidance of any foods that cause noticeable stomach discomfort.

If surgery is required, procedures should be explained thoroughly, including the reasons for them. The nurse should explain immediate postoperative care, including deep breathing, coughing, position changes, the need for frequently monitoring vital signs, intravenous tubing, NG tubing, catheters, and other drainage tubes, and the use of patient-controlled analgesia or other medications for pain relief. The ability of the patient to eat normally after healing will depend on the type of surgery and when peristalsis returns. The nurse should help the patient to realize that repeat episodes of symptoms are not unusual and to seek medical care if they recur.

Prognosis. Recurrence of an ulcer is possible and may happen within 2 years in about one third of all patients. The likelihood of recurrence is lessened by eliminating foods that aggravate the condition. If symptoms recur, the prognosis is better in patients who resume antacid medications hourly and seek further medical treatment.

Cancer of the Stomach

Etiology/Pathophysiology. The incidence of gastric cancer has declined significantly in western Europe and the United States. In the 1940s, gastric cancer was the most common malignant disease in the United States. The most common neoplasm or malignant growth in the stomach is adenocarcinoma. The primary location is in the pyloric area. Because of the location, the tumor may metastasize to lymph nodes, liver, spleen, pancreas, or esophagus. Gastric cancer is more common in people 50 to 70 years of age.

The cause is not known, but numerous factors are associated with the disease. These include history of polyps, pernicious anemia, hypochlorhydria (deficiency of hydrochloride in stomach's gastric juice), gastrectomy, chronic atrophic gastritis, and gastric ulcer. Because the stomach has prolonged contact with food, an association exists between cancer in this part of the body and diets high in salt, preservatives, and carbohydrates and low in fresh fruits and vegetables.

Clinical Manifestations. The patient may be asymptomatic in early stages of the disease.

Assessment. Collection of *subjective data* may include complaints of vague epigastric discomfort or indigestion and postprandial (meal) fullness; 10% of patients have complaints of an ulcerlike pain that does not respond to therapy. Anorexia and weakness are also common.

Collection of *objective data* may include weight loss, bleeding in the stools, hematemesis, and vomiting after drinking fluids or eating meals.

Diagnostic Tests. The tumor is diagnosed by x-ray studies (GI series), endoscopic/gastroscopic examinations with biopsy, stool occult blood tests, and gastric analysis. Carcinoembryonic antigen (CEA) is usually elevated in advanced gastric cancer.

Medical Management. The most therapeutic management of stomach cancer is surgical removal. Unfortunately, the purpose of the surgery may be an exploratory celiotomy to determine involvement or to make the patient more comfortable. A partial or total gastric resection is the choice for an extensive lesion. Surgery for advanced gastric cancer carries high morbidity (the condition of being diseased) and mortality rates.

Wound healing may be disrupted by **dehiscence** (a partial or complete separation of the wound edges) or by **evisceration** (when the patient's viscera protrude through the disrupted wound) (see Fig. 22-7). Dehiscence and evisceration may be caused by problems in suturing the wound or by poor tissue integrity. Some of the factors that may predispose a wound to dehiscence are excessive coughing, straining, malnutrition, obesity, and infection. Nursing interventions for the patient who has experienced dehiscence include instructing the patient to remain quiet and to avoid coughing or straining. The patient should be positioned to remove further stress on the wound. If evisceration occurs, the patient is kept on bed rest and the protruding viscera is loosely covered with a warm sterile saline dressing. The surgeon should be notified immediately, since treatment consists of reapproximating the wound edges (see Chapter 22).

Chemotherapy has greater response and longer survival rates than radiation. Radiation combined with chemotherapy have been more effective. These treatment modalities are often used with surgery.

Nursing Interventions. The nurse should provide further clarification of the disease and the surgical intervention to the patient and family. The preoperative preparation includes improving the patient's nutritional status by monitoring hyperalimentation and providing supplemental diet feedings. Postoperative teaching is necessary to relieve anxiety and promote understanding of drainage tubes, feeding tubes, dressing changes, weakness, medications, and other routine care.

Nursing diagnoses and interventions for the patient with cancer of the stomach include but are not limited to the following:

NURSING DIAGNOSES	NURSING INTERVENTIONS
Breathing pattern, ineffective, related to pain, exploration of chest and abdominal cavities, and abdominal distention	Place patient in semi-Fowler's position to aid ventilation. Encourage and assist with gentle turning and repositioning. Encourage patient to turn, breathe deeply, and cough at least q 2 hr until patient is ambulating well; splint incision before patient coughs; encourage ambulation.
Injury, high risk for, related to aspiration, infection, hemorrhage, anastomotic leak into abdominal cavity, and anemia/vitamin deficiency	Monitor closely for elevated temperature, bleeding from incision, pallor, dyspnea, cyanosis, tachycardia, increased respirations, and chest pain. Monitor laboratory results and activity tolerance because of possible anemia. Change dressings, using sterile technique.

Patient teaching. Because care encompasses so many areas, instruction should be (1) planned according to the patient's needs and level of understanding, (2) given when the patient is free of pain and rested, and (3) communicated both verbally and in print. Surgery, chemotherapy, radiation therapy, continued nutritional needs, pain relief, and support groups for psychosocial needs should be explained.

Weight loss will indicate the need for additional caloric intake and can be measured by daily weights compared with the patient's normal weight before illness. Prevention of skin excoriation around the feeding tube is important. Hypermotility or diarrhea that follows radiation therapy can be treated with medication. Alternative methods of care for the debilitated patient and family may include referral for hospice care.

Prognosis. The prognosis for patients with gastric cancer is poor. About 60% have clinical findings at the time of diagnosis, resulting in a low cure rate.

PATIENTS WITH INTESTINAL DISORDERS

Intestinal Infections

Etiology/Pathophysiology. Intestinal infections are the invasion of the alimentary canal (both the small and large intestine) by pathogenic microorganisms that reproduce and multiply. The infectious agent can enter the body by several routes. The most common entry is through the mouth by contaminated food or water. Some intestinal infections occur as a result of person-to-person contact. Fecal-oral transmission occurs through poor handwashing after elimination. In active homosexual males, "gay bowel syndrome" is introduced by single-cell protozoal infections.

Bacterial flora grow naturally in the intestinal track and help the immune system combat infection. Their presence can be altered through long-term antibiotic therapy. The impaired immune response in some individuals delays the body's attempt to destroy invading pathogens.

Infectious diarrhea causes secretion of fluid into the intestinal lumen. Clostridial and *Salmonella* bacteria are associated with intestinal infections. These bacteria produce toxic substances, and the mucosal cells respond by secreting water and electrolytes, causing an imbalance. The amount of fluid secreted exceeds the ability of the large intestine to reabsorb the fluid into the vascular system.

Sigmoidoscopic or colonoscopic examination and stool specimens are used in the diagnosis of a specific type of inflammation or colitis called *antibiotic-associated pseudomembranous colitis (AAPMC).* This type of colitis is a complication of treatment with a wide variety of antibiotics, including lincomycin, clindamycin, ampicillin, erythromycin, tetracycline, cephalosporins, and aminoglycosides. A *Clostridium difficile* test is ordered on the stool specimen to aid in the diagnosis of AAPMC in both inpatients and outpatients. The identification of characteristic lesions of AAPMC is done on tissues obtained through endoscopy examination.

Treatment with antibiotics results in the inhibition of normal bacterial growth in the intestine. This inhibition of normal flora can lead to the overgrowth of other bacteria such as *C. difficile.* Under the right conditions, *C. difficile* produces two toxins, A and B. The literature states that both toxin A and toxin B are produced by *C. difficile* at the same time and that these two toxins cause the tissue damage seen in AAPMC disease. The incidence of *C. difficile* toxin found in the stool has ranged from 1% to 2% in a normal population to 10% in hospital inpatients and up to 85% to 90% in patients with proven AAPMC. The *C. difficile* test used alone is not conclusive but does aid in the diagnosis of AAPMC.

Since the level of *C. difficile* antigens associated with the disease state may vary, a negative *C. difficile* test result alone may not rule out the possibility of *C. difficile*–associated colitis. The nurse must monitor signs and symptoms of the disease such as the duration of antibiotic treatment and duration and severity of diarrhea. These observations, with the presence of colitis or pseudomembranes, are all factors the physician must consider when diagnosing AAPMC disease.

Clinical Manifestations. Diarrhea is the most common manifestation of an intestinal infection. The fecal output has increased water content, and if the intestinal mucosa is directly invaded, the feces may contain blood and mucus.

Assessment. Collection of *subjective data* includes noting complaints of diarrhea, rectal urgency, **tenesmus** (ineffective and painful straining with defecation), nausea, and abdominal cramping.

Collection of *objective data* may include a fever greater than 102° F (38.8° C) and vomiting. History taking will provide useful information regarding number and consistency of bowel movements, recent use of antibiotics, recent travel, food intake, and exposure to noninfectious causes of diarrhea. Noninfectious diarrhea may be caused by heavy metal poisoning, shellfish allergy, and ingestion of toxic mushrooms and fish toxins. Diarrhea from noninfectious causes is usually characterized by a short incubation period (minutes to hours after exposure).

Diagnostic Tests. The key laboratory test for patients with intestinal infections is a stool culture. Another laboratory test that may be included is a blood chemistry study to monitor changes in the patient's fluid and electrolyte status.

Medical Management. Usually the treatment of intestinal infections is conservative, letting the body limit the infection. Antibiotics may be given in cases of prolonged or severe diarrhea with a stool positive for leukocytes. If fluid and electrolyte replacement is necessary to offset the losses from diarrhea, the oral route is usually sufficient. The intravenous route is indicated if the patient cannot take sufficient fluids orally.

The use of antidiarrheals and antispasmodic agents may actually increase the severity of the infection by prolonging the contact time of the microbe with the intestinal wall. Kaolin and pectin (Kaopectate) may be used to increase stool consistency. Bismuth subsalicylate (Pepto-Bismol) can effectively decrease intestinal secretions and decrease the diarrhea volume. These medications require large doses to be effective (30 to 60 ml every 30 minutes to 1 hour), and their use remains controversial.

Nursing Interventions. The nurse must do a thorough assessment to determine the seriousness of the intestinal infection. Determining the onset of the disease and the number of people exposed is important, because the majority of GI infections are communicable and represent a community health problem. The nurse must also assess for fluid imbalance. This assessment should include measurement of postural changes in blood pressure, skin turgor, mucous membrane hydration, and urine output.

Nursing diagnoses and interventions for the patient with intestinal infections include but are not limited to the following:

NURSING DIAGNOSES	NURSING INTERVENTIONS
Fluid volume deficit, related to excessive losses from diarrhea and vomiting	If oral intake can be tolerated, apple juice, clear carbonated beverages, clear broth, plain gelatin, and water should be offered. If intravenous feedings are required, these fluids should have electrolytes added.
Pain: abdominal, related to intestinal inflammation and diarrhea	Discontinue oral feedings if intestinal stimulation occurs. Bed rest may decrease abdominal peristalsis.
Nutrition, altered: less than body requirements, related to decreased intake and decreased absorption	Monitor for decreasing episodes of diarrhea. Monitor blood pressure, mucous membranes, and urinary output. Monitor weight loss if symptoms are severe.
Skin integrity, impaired, anal, related to excoriation from diarrhea	Promote hygiene and prevent additional excoriation by offering soothing ointments, sitz baths, and perineal washes after bowel movements.

Patient teaching. The nurse should instruct the patient to report the number, color, and consistency of bowel movements, abdominal cramping, and pain. The patient and family should understand the importance of handwashing after bowel movements to interrupt the fecal-oral route of transmission. Those family members responsible for food preparation should be made aware of the importance of proper methods of food preparation and storage to reduce the growth of infecting organisms.

Prognosis.

Intestinal infections. The body may be able to successfully defend against the infection without intervention. In severe cases, medications and fluid replacement assist the body and the cure rate is good.

Antibiotic-associated pseudomembranous colitis. The prognosis of AAPMC is better when the disease is diagnosed early and the antibiotics are changed. This allows the normal growth of bacteria in the intestine to resume.

Irritable Bowel Syndrome

Etiology/Pathophysiology. Irritable bowel syndrome (IBS; also called *mucous colitis* and *spastic colon*) is a disorder with episodes of alterations in bowel function. IBS is extremely common, occurring in about 20% of community populations. A small number of these people (5%) have severe symptoms that are difficult to manage. The cause of IBS may be a low pain threshold to intestinal distention caused by abnormal intestinal sensory neural circuitry.

The patient with IBS may have associated psychological problems. In patients without psychological problems, the symptoms are attributed to spastic and uncoordinated muscle contractions of the colon, usually related to ingestion of excessively coarse or highly seasoned foods. However, there is also (1) a correlation of panic attacks in patients with IBS and (2) an association of chronic low abdominal (pelvic) pain and a history of childhood sexual abuse.

Clinical Manifestations. Alterations of bowel function include abdominal pain relieved after a bowel movement, more frequent bowel movements with pain onset, a sense of incomplete evacuation, flatulence, and constipation, diarrhea, or both. Functional diarrhea is increased by stress; usually weight loss does not occur. The physical examination is generally normal, and nocturnal symptoms are rarely present. The symptoms of IBS are deceptive in nature and are frustrating to manage.

Assessment. Collection of *subjective data* for the patient with IBS includes complaints of abdominal distress, pain at onset of bowel movements, abdominal pain relieved by defecation, and feelings of incomplete emptying after defecation. Collection of *objective data* includes mucus in stools, visible abdominal distention, and frequent or unformed stools.

Diagnostic Tests. A complete blood count and erythrocyte sedimentation rate may uncover iron deficiency anemia from GI blood loss or other indirect evidence of inflammatory bowel disease. A stool occult blood test and blood chemistry abnormalities may suggest organic GI disease. Both gross and microscopic examination of rectal or colonic mucosa may yield a conclusive diagnosis.

Medical Management.

Diet and bulking agents. Increasing dietary fiber increases stool bulk and frequency of passage and also bloating. Adequate fiber is more reliably provided with bulking agents than with diet unless the patient is a strict vegetarian. The bulking agents seem to be most effective in the treatment of constipation-predominant IBS, although they may alleviate mild diarrhea. If a patient consistently has exacerbation of symptoms after certain foods, those foods should be avoided.

Medication. Anticholinergic drugs relieve abdominal cramps. Milk of magnesia may be prescribed if constipation does not respond to augmented fiber or if the patient cannot tolerate it. Mineral oil, in sufficient doses, is cheaper, "gasless," and generally effective. Opioids can be quite effective in diarrhea-predominant IBS. Antianxiety drugs may help patients suffering from panic attacks associated with IBS. Antidepressants may be used sparingly for diarrhea-predominant IBS in patients with severe pain who have not responded to other measures. Simple, short-term psychotherapy has shown long-term beneficial effects in some patients with IBS.

Nursing Interventions. Most patients with IBS learn to cope with their symptoms sufficiently well to live with reasonable comfort. It is the nurse's role to assist in identifying the 5% of patients with IBS who need management. Nurses skilled in history taking, listening skills, nutrition planning, and understanding the relationship of psychological effects on the body can assist the patient in setting goals to manage the disease. The nurse should emphasize the importance of keeping a daily log showing diet; number and type of stools; presence, length, severity, and duration of pain; side effects of medication; and life stressors that aggravate the disorder. This information will assist in the diagnosis and treatment of IBS.

Nursing diagnoses and interventions for the patient with an irritable bowel include but are not limited to the following.

NURSING DIAGNOSES	NURSING INTERVENTIONS
Pain, related to diet consumed and bowel evacuation	Logging the type of food for fiber content, consistency of stool, degree of pain.
Knowledge deficit, related to the effect of fiber content on a spastic bowel	Patient teaching regarding the relationship of fiber to both constipation and diarrhea. Patient teaching regarding the use of bulking agents.

Patient teaching. IBS carries many personal feelings that the patient must recognize and be comfortable with before a plan of care can be established. Therefore it is important to establish a strong relationship with the patient before patient teaching begins. Patient teaching includes diet management and ways to control anxiety in daily living. The goal of patient teaching is to empower the patient to help control the disorder. Community resources for counseling should be provided to the patient if the nurse has observed a relationship of psychological problems to increased or decreased elimination accompanied by pain and discomfort.

Prognosis. Approximately 95% of these patients are successfully managed. Compliance with a diet low in residue and a nonstressful daily regimen contribute significantly to a good prognosis.

Chronic Inflammatory Bowel Disease

Ulcerative colitis and Crohn's disease are chronic, episodic, inflammatory diseases. These disorders afflict young adults with education, careers, and the raising of families ahead of them. Ulcerative colitis and Crohn's disease appear more often in women, in the Jewish population, and in the nonwhite population; there seems to be a familial tendency.

The causes of ulcerative colitis and Crohn's disease are unknown, although theories exist. These include both genetic and environmental factors, including viral infection, allergies to certain foods, immunological factors, and psychosomatic disorders. Inflammatory bowel diseases are characterized by **exacerbations** (increase in the severity of the disease or any of its symptoms) and **remissions** (a decrease in the severity of the disease or any of its symptoms).

The two diseases require similar nursing interventions but different surgical interventions. Other similarities and differences exist (Table 27-3). Patients have been known to have features of both diseases, making a definite diagnosis difficult.

Ulcerative Colitis.

Etiology/pathophysiology. The incidence of ulcerative colitis is twice that of Crohn's disease. The common enteric bacterium *E. coli* may play a role. Psychosomatic factors may cause, aggravate, or be a result of inflammatory bowel disease. The social isolation and frustration that accompany this chronic illness cause difficulties in effectively coping with daily life.

Ulcerative colitis is confined to the mucosa and submucosa of the colon. The disease can affect segments of the entire colon, depending on the staging (phases or periods in the course of the disease). This disease usually starts on the left side of the colon and progresses to the right side. Tiny abscesses form, which grow and produce purulent drainage, sloughing of the mucosa, and subsequent ulceration. Capillaries become friable and bleed, causing the characteristic diarrhea containing pus and blood. Pseudopolyps are common in chronic ulcerative disease and may become cancerous. With healing and the natural formation of scar tissue, the colon may lose elasticity and absorptive capability.

Clinical manifestations. Pathological findings differ in particular individuals, but diarrhea is a predominant sign. It is not uncommon for a patient with ulcerative colitis to have as many as 15 to 20 liquid stools a day, containing blood, mucus, and pus. With severe diarrhea there may be losses of sodium, potassium, bicarbonate, and calcium ions. Abdominal cramps may occur before the bowel movement. The feeling of the urge to defecate lessens as scarring within the bowel progresses. This results in involuntary leakage of stool.

Complications of ulcerative colitis include toxic megacolon (toxic dilation of the large bowel). This life-threatening complication occurs in less than 5% of patients. The bowel becomes distended and so thin that perforation could happen at any time. Clinical manifestations of toxic megacolon include a temperature of 104° F (40° C) or more and abdominal distention. In those who have had chronic ulcerative colitis for 10 to 15 years, carcinoma of the colon occurs in 40% to 50% of cases with total colonic involvement. Surgical interventions for treatment of this complication are usually necessary.

Assessment. Collection of *subjective data* for the patient with ulcerative colitis includes complaints of rec-

TABLE 27-3 Comparison of Ulcerative Colitis and Crohn's Disease

Factor	Ulcerative Colitis	Crohn's Disease
Cause of disorder	Unknown; possible cause is enteric bacterium *E. coli*	Unknown; possible cause is an altered immune state
Area of involvement	Usually confined to mucosa or submucosa of the colon	Primarily the small intestine but can affect the colon
Area of inflammation	Mostly mucosal	Transmural (pertaining to the entire thickness of the wall of an organ)
Extent of involvement	Diffuse areas, contiguous (sharing a boundary or edge)	Segmental areas, noncontiguous
Character of stools	Blood present No fat 15-20 liquid stools daily	No blood present Steatorrhea (fat in stool) 3-4 semisoft stools daily
Major complication	Toxic megacolon	Malabsorption
Major complaint	Rectal bleeding Abdominal cramping	Right lower abdominal pain with mass present
Reason for surgery	Poor response to medical therapy Complications	Complications
Response to surgery	Curative	Noncurative, high recurrence rate
Cancer potential	Increased risk	Risk increases with age

tal bleeding and abdominal cramping. Lethargy, a sense of frustration, and loss of control result from painful abdominal cramping and the unpredictable bowel movements.

Collection of *objective data* for the patient with ulcerative colitis includes weight loss, abdominal distention, fever, tachycardia, leukocytosis, and observation of frequency and characteristics of stools.

Diagnostic tests. Barium studies of the intestine, sigmoidoscopy and colonoscopy with possible biopsy, and checking the stool for melena aid the physician in diagnosis. Additional studies include radiologic examination of the abdomen, determination of serum electrolytes and albumin levels and liver function, and other hematological studies.

Medical management. The medical interventions chosen depend on the phase of the disease and the individual response to therapy. Common treatment modalities include medication, diet intervention, and stress reduction.

Drug therapy. The four major categories of drugs used are (1) those that affect the inflammatory response, (2) antibacterial drugs, (3) drugs that affect the immune system, and (4) antidiarrheal preparations.

- Sulfasalazine (Azulfidine) containing acetylsalicylic acid is the drug of choice for mild chronic ulcerative colitis. It affects the inflammatory response and provides some antibacterial activity.
- Nonsulfa drugs include olsalazine (Dipentum), given orally, and mesalamine (Rowasa), given by retention enema.
- Corticosteroids are antiinflammatory drugs effective in relieving symptoms of moderate and severe colitis; they can be given systemically or topically.
- Antidiarrheal agents are recommended over anticholinergic agents because anticholinergic drugs can mask obstruction or contribute to toxic colonic dilation. Loperamide (Imodium) may be used to treat cramping and diarrhea of chronic ulcerative colitis. Azathioprine (Imuran) is also beneficial.

Diet therapy. Diet therapy that excludes milk products and highly spiced foods has been effective in approximately 20% of the patients. A high-protein, high-caloric diet is recommended for persons who are nutritionally deficient. Hyperalimentation may be used for nutrition, fluid, and electrolyte replacement in severe cases.

Stress control. Ulcerative colitis is aggravated by stress. Identifying the factors that cause stress is the first step in controlling the disease. Working with the patient to find healthful coping mechanisms is part of the holistic approach in nursing interventions.

Surgical intervention. If an acute episode does not respond to treatment, if complications occur, or if the risk of cancer becomes greater because of the presence of chronic ulcerative colitis, surgical intervention is indicated (Box 27-4). Most surgeons prefer a conservative approach, removing only the diseased portion of the colon. The operations of choice may be a single-stage total proctocolectomy with construction of internal reservoir and valve (Kock's pouch, or Kock's continent ileostomy) (Fig. 27-12), total proctocolectomy with ileoanal anastomosis with or without construction of an internal reser-

Box 27-4 SURGICAL INTERVENTIONS

Colon resection: Removal of a portion of the large intestine and anastomosis of the remaining segment
Ileostomy: Surgical formation of an opening of the ileum onto the surface of the abdomen, through which fecal matter is emptied
Ileoanal anastomosis: Removal of the colon and rectum but the anus is left intact along with the anal sphincter; anastomosis is formed between the lower end of the small intestine and the anus
Proctocolectomy: Removal of anus, rectum, and colon; ileostomy is established for the removal of digestive tract wastes
Kock's pouch (Kock's continent ileostomy): Surgical removal of the rectum and colon (proctocolectomy) with formation of a reservoir by suturing loops of adjacent ileum together to form a pouchlike structure, nipple valve, and stoma

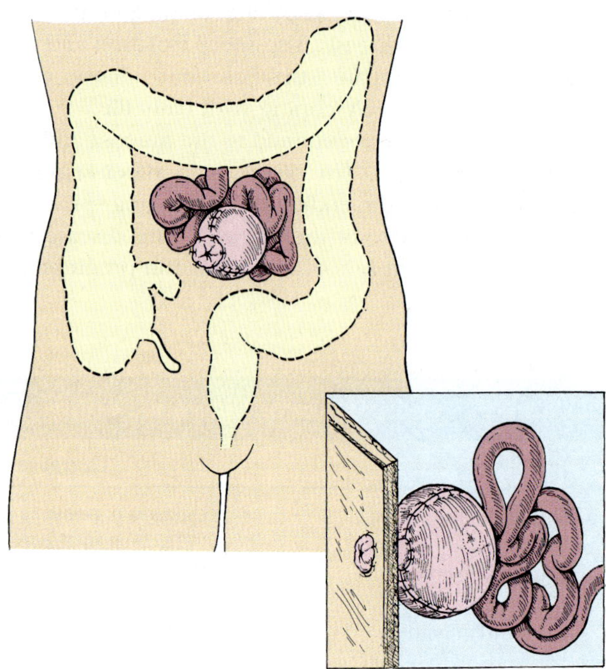

FIG. 27-12 Kock's pouch (Kock's continent ileostomy).

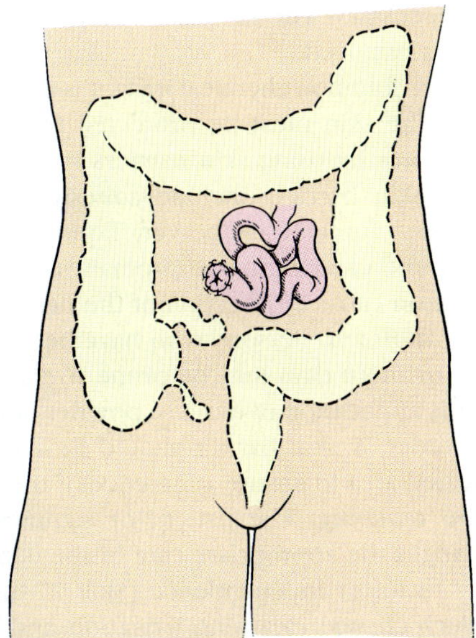

FIG. 27-13 Ileostomy with absence of resected bowel.

voir, and temporary ileostomy. In the case of a poor-risk patient, a subtotal colectomy may be performed with ileostomy (Fig. 27-13). After the patient's recovery (approximately 2 to 4 months), removal of the rectum or construction of an internal reservoir can be done.

Today some patients view a permanent ileostomy as more forbidding than the disease itself. These surgical procedures are not without risk, and the patient may want to live with the disease and long-term risk of cancer rather than undergo the procedure.

Nursing interventions. Areas of nursing intervention include a thorough assessment of the patient's bowel elimination, knowledge level, support systems, coping abilities, nutritional status, pain, and ability to understand the disease process and treatment required. Patients need a complete understanding of the plan of care so that they can make informed choices. Prevention of future episodes is a goal for the ulcerative colitis patient.

Preoperative care for these patients includes (1) selection of stoma site, (2) performing additional diagnostic tests if cancer is suspected, (3) allocation of time to accept that previous treatments were unsuccessful in curing the disease, and (4) preparation of the bowel for surgery. The bowel is prepared 2 or 3 days preoperatively. A bland to clear liquid diet is ordered, and a bowel prep of laxatives, GoLYTELY (an oral or NG colonic lavage/electrolyte solution), and enemas as ordered (see Skill 27-1). Antibiotics, such an erythromycin and neomycin, are given to decrease the number of bacteria in the bowel.

Postoperative nursing interventions depend on the type of procedure performed and the individual's response. Areas of concern are bowel and urinary elimination, fluid and electrolyte balance, tissue perfusion, comfort/pain, nutrition, gas exchange, infection, and in the case of ostomy construction, assessment of the ileostomy and peristomal skin integrity.

Nursing diagnoses and interventions for the patient with chronic inflammatory bowel disease include but are not limited to the following:

NURSING DIAGNOSES	NURSING INTERVENTIONS
Knowledge deficit, related to lack of information about disease and treatment	Actively listen for 15 minutes daily. Explain disease process to patient and/or family. Instruct patient on dosage of medications and side effects.
Anxiety, related to unknown disease outcome	Examine stressors in patient's life and realistic ways to reduce them. Use regularly scheduled pain medication rather than prn administration to manage pain.
Nutrition, altered: less than body requirements, related to bowel hypermotility and decreased absorption	Provide small frequent meals, which will help patients with poor appetite or intolerance to larger amounts. Eliminate foods that aggravate condition.
Diarrhea, related to bowel irritability	Keep bedpan or commode nearby; use room deodorizer to control odor. Offer support to patient during diagnostic and treatment phase.
Powerlessness, related to loss of control of body function	Assist weakened patient with activities of daily living (bathing, oral hygiene, shaving, and other grooming needs). Offer choices to patient, when possible, to facilitate patient control.

Nursing diagnoses for the surgical patient may be focused on potential ineffective individual coping, disturbance in self-esteem, and body image disturbance. Nursing interventions include reinforcement of the physician's explanation of the surgical procedure and expected outcomes. Providing reading material and demonstrating the care of an ostomy pouch when the patient demonstrates readiness will reduce anxiety. A visitor from the United Ostomy Association can provide hope, as a recovered and productive role model. The nurse should not expect *immediate* patient acceptance of the stoma; acceptance will be gradual. The nurse should be supportive and should encourage the patient to verbalize fears. See Box 27-5 on p. 686 for postoperative nursing interventions.

Peristomal area integrity. The nurse should assess the peristomal skin for impairment of integrity. Four primary factors contributing to loss of peristomal skin integrity are allergies, mechanical trauma, chemical reactions, and infection.

Allergies to pouches, adhesives, skin barriers, powders and paste, or belts are evident at areas of contact. The skin may appear erythematous, eroded, weeping, and bleeding. Avoidance of the irritant by changing the type of pouch, tape, or adhesive may resolve the problem.

Mechanical trauma caused by pressure, friction, or stripping of adhesives and skin barriers can be avoided by less frequent changes of the pouch, using adhesive tape sparingly, and wearing a belt only when the patient feels it is necessary. The skin must be protected when the pouch is removed.

The most common chemical irritant is the stool from the stoma. The skin must be protected from these digestive enzymes by using skin barriers before applying the pouch. Skin barriers include adhesives (Stomahesive), powders (Stomahesive power), liquid skin barriers (Skin Prep), and caulking paste (Stomahesive paste).

A common cause of infection of the peristomal skin is *Candida albicans.* Persons who have been on antibiotics for 5 or more days may be prone to this problem. Treatment is application of nystatin powder or cream, by physician order. A skin barrier should be applied over the medicated area to ensure adherence of the adhesive.

Patient teaching. The patient or significant other must be taught the appropriate care of the ileostomy or colostomy to foster independence (Skill 27-6). This includes pouch change, cleansing, irrigation, and skin care. A list of foods that are known to commonly cause problems of constipation, diarrhea, blockage, odors, and flatus is helpful. A list of resource people, phone numbers, where to obtain supplies, and what to ask for should be sent home with the patient.

Prognosis. The prognosis in patients with chronic ulcerative colitis is directly related to the number of years they have had the disease. This is due to the increased incidence of carcinoma when the colon is extensively involved over a length of time. The disease carries a higher mortality rate in patients who have the disease 15 to 20 years.

Box 27-5 POSTOPERATIVE NURSING INTERVENTIONS

1. Monitor NG suction for patency until bowel function is resumed. Accurately record color and amount of output. Irrigate NG tube prn. Apply water-soluble lubricant to nares. Assess bowel sounds, being certain to turn off NG suction when auscultating bowel sounds.
2. Initiate ostomy care and teaching when bowel activity begins. Nurse should be sensitive to patient's pain level and readiness for teaching of ostomy care.
3. Observe **stoma** (an artificial opening of an internal organ on the surface of the body) for color and size (should be erythematous and slightly edematous).
4. Select pouch that has skin-protective barrier, accordion flange to ease pressure applied to new incisional site, adhesive backing, and pouch opening no more that 1/16 inch larger than stoma. Stomas change in size over time and should be measured before new supplies are ordered.
5. Empty pouch when it is approximately one-third full to prevent breaking seal, resulting in pouch leakage.
6. Explain that initial dark green liquid will change to yellow-brown as patient is allowed to eat.
7. Teach patient to care for the stoma; this includes having patient look at stoma and gradually assist with emptying, cleaning, and changing pouch; teach patient that normal grieving occurs after loss of rectal function. Be supportive of patient's concerns.
8. Promote independence and self-care to decrease state of denial.
9. Instruct on follow-up home care, including changing pouch every 5 to 7 days. Using antacids, skin protective paste, and liquid skin barrier may be appropriate if skin excoriation is observed.
10. Patient may shower or bathe with or without pouch on.
11. Patient should avoid lifting objects over 10 lb.
12. A special diet is not necessary, but fluids should include 8 to 10 glasses of water a day, food should be chewed well, and certain gas-forming foods should be limited or avoided.
13. Sexual relationships can be resumed when physician feels it is not harmful to the surgical area. Counseling may be appropriate if patient has fear of resuming this activity.

Crohn's Disease.

Etiology/pathophysiology. Crohn's disease, although not as prevalent as ulcerative colitis, is increasing in incidence. Crohn's disease is also known as *regional enteritis, transmural colitis,* or *granulomatous colitis.* The cause of the disease is not known, but there seems to be a strong association between Crohn's disease and altered immune mechanisms. It most often affects persons 15 to 30 years of age.

Clinical manifestations. As the name *regional enteritis* implies, only one segment of the bowel may be involved, or segments of healthy tissue may alternate with multiple segments of diseased tissue. The inflammation, fibrosis, scarring, and transmural (pertaining to the entire thickness of the wall of an organ) characteristics of Crohn's disease primarily occur in the small intestine, mainly in the ileum. In some patients, the disease may involve the colon without any changes in the small intestine.

Malabsorption is the major problem when the small intestine is involved. Megaloblastic anemia results from decreased absorption of vitamin B_{12} in the small intestine. Fluid and electrolyte disturbances with acid-base imbalances can occur, particularly with a depletion of sodium or potassium associated with diarrhea or with ex-

PERFORMING COLOSTOMY/ILEOSTOMY CARE

1. Introduce self.
2. Identify patient.
3. Wash hands.
4. Explain procedure.
5. Arrange supplies/equipment at bedside or in bathroom (see illustration).
6. Pull curtain and close door to provide privacy.
7. Position patient so that stoma is easily accessible and patient is comfortable.
8. Don gloves.

NOTE:

As many of the following steps as possible should be performed by the patient with the nurse teaching and assisting as needed. Independence will come. Be alert to signs of patient readiness.

9. Unfasten and remove belt; carefully remove wafer seal from skin (adhesive solvent may be needed).
10. Place reusable pouch in bedpan or disposable pouch in plastic bag.
11. Cleanse skin with warm water; pat dry to avoid rubbing and skin impairment.
12. Measure stoma using measuring device.
13. Place toilet tissue over stoma; use gauze for ileostomy to prevent expelled stool from causing skin impairment; note color and viability of stoma. If using Skin Prep, apply to skin and allow to dry.
14. Apply protective skin barrier about 1/16 inch from stoma (Stomahesive, Hollihesive, Karaya paste or powder).
15. Apply protective wafer with flange, cutting an opening in the center of wafer 1/16 inch larger than stoma.
16. Gently attach pouch to flange by compressing the two together.
17. If Karaya seal pouch is used, moisten seal with a few drops of warm water until seal is sticky.
18. Remove tissue or gauze from stoma and backing from protectant; center opening over stoma, and press against skin for 1 to 2 minutes, smoothing outward with fingers.
19. Fold bottom edges of pouch over one time to fit clamp. Secure clamp.
20. If belt is used, attach at this time.
21. Assist patient to comfortable position in bed or chair; remove equipment from bedside.
22. Empty, wash, and dry reusable pouch.
23. Dispose of soiled supplies in plastic bag; remove gloves; wash hands.
24. Record procedure and observations (type of pouch, skin barrier, amount and appearance of feces, and condition of stoma and surrounding skin).
25. Report abnormalities.

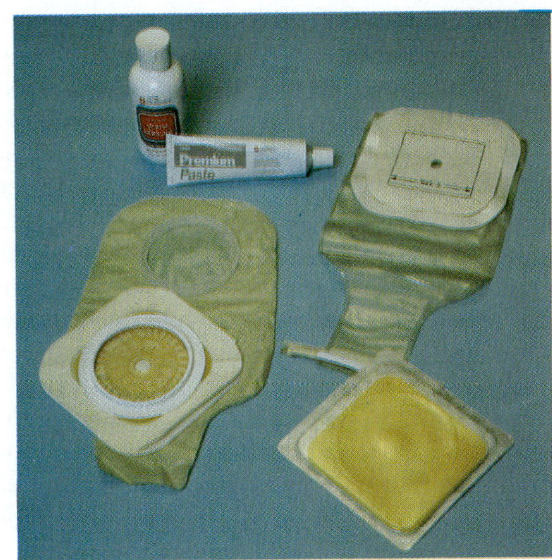

STEP 5

cessive small intestine drainage through fistulas that may be associated with the pathological process.

Assessment. Collection of *subjective data* for the patient with Crohn's disease includes noting the patient's list of vague complaints, including weakness, loss of appetite, sleeplessness due to diarrhea, and pain and stress. Right-lower-quadrant abdominal pain is characteristic of the disease and may be accompanied in the same area by a tender mass of thickened intestines.

Collection of *objective data* for the patient with Crohn's disease includes complaints of diarrhea—three or four semisolid stools daily, containing mucus and pus but no blood. **Steatorrhea** (excess fat in the feces) may also be present if the ulceration extends high in the small intestine. Intestinal fistulas or poor absorption of bile salts by the ileum may cause stools to become watery. Fever and unexplained anemia may also occur. Anal diseases, such as fissures or fistulas in the anus, are common manifestations.

Diagnostic tests. The diagnostic tests for Crohn's disease are essentially the same as for ulcerative colitis, that is, x-ray studies, endoscopy, stool examination, and blood tests. Sigmoidoscopy helps differentiate ulcerative colitis from Crohn's disease. Endoscopy helps in the diagnosis of diseases of the small intestine but colonoscopy is rarely used for ulcerative colitis because of the possible complications of hemorrhage and perforation. Blood tests for anemia may also be ordered.

Medical management. Treatment of the patient must be individualized depending on the age of the patient, the location and severity of the disease, and the type of complications that may be present. Medication, diet intervention, stress reduction, and surgery are used to manage Crohn's disease.

Diet. Bowel symptoms and diarrhea are minimized by excluding from the diet (1) lactose-containing foods in patients suspected of having lactose intolerance; (2) *Brassica* vegetables (cauliflower, broccoli, asparagus, cabbage, and Brussels sprouts); (3) caffeine, beer, monosodium glutamate, and sugarless (sorbitol-containing) gum and mints; and (4) highly seasoned foods, concentrated fruit juices, carbonated beverages, and fatty foods.

Diets high in protein (100 g/day) are recommended for patients with hypoproteinemia caused by mucosal loss, malabsorption, maldigestion, or malnutrition. Elemental diets have been shown to induce remission in 90% of patients with Crohn's disease. Free elemental diets may help patients with diarrhea because they require minimal digestion and reduce stool volume. Such elemental dietary preparations include Criticare, Travasorb-HN, and Precision High Nitrogen. Hyperalimentation has been shown to be more effective in patients with Crohn's disease than in those with ulcerative colitis.

Medications. Corticosteroids continue to be the preferred medical treatment of active Crohn's disease when there is small intestinal involvement. Sulfasalazine (Azulfidine) is effective in active Crohn's disease, especially when there is colonic involvement. Antibiotics have been used for treating microabscess formation as a complication of Crohn's disease, rather than in treating the actual disease process. Antidiarrheal agents (Lomotil and Imodium) and antispasmodics (Donnatal and Bentyl) have proven effective but are used with caution because of side effects. Particular problems with inadequate vitamin B_{12} absorption result when the terminal ileum is resected; lifelong replacement of vitamin B_{12} is then necessary.

Complications of inflammation with fibrous scarring, obstruction, fistula formation in the small intestine, abscesses, and perforation are indications for surgical excision and anastomosis. If surgery is performed, resection is preferred because bypass has a greater failure rate.

Two types of surgery used in Crohn's disease are (1) segmental resection of diseased bowel with anastomosis of ileum with the remaining ascending or transverse colon and (2) bypass of the diseased bowel by anastomosis of ileum to the colonic area free of disease, leaving the diseased bowel intact. Complications of malabsorption occur with both types of surgery. Surgery is performed only in selected instances for Crohn's disease because of a high rate of recurrence.

Nursing interventions. Nutrition, fluid balance, elimination, medications, psychological aspects, and sexuality must be considered in caring for the patient with Crohn's disease. Total parenteral nutrition may be ordered in cases of severe disease and marked weight loss. Tube feedings that allow rapid absorption in the upper GI tract are begun, and then oral intake of a low-residue, high-protein, high-caloric diet is gradually introduced. Vitamin supplements are frequently necessary, and vitamin B_{12} is given when there is a marked loss of ileum. When anemia is present, iron dextran (Imferon) is given by Z-track injection, since oral intake of iron is ineffective because of the intestinal ulceration.

Oral diets of 2500 ml/day to replace loss of fluids and electrolytes caused from diarrhea are not uncommon. Weight is monitored for losses or gains. The condition of the skin and all fluid I&O are monitored daily. A urinary output of at least 1500 ml/day is desired.

When the person is hospitalized, a bedside commode or a bedpan must be accessible at all times because of the urgency and frequency of stools. Emptying the bedpan immediately and deodorizing the room maintain an aesthetic environment. The anal region may become excoriated from frequency of stools. The anal area should be examined regularly and kept clean using medicated wipes (Tucks) and sitz baths. These nursing interventions will promote comfort and hygiene for the patient.

Instructions and information for the patient related to medications include the following:

- Take sulfasalazine in equally divided doses.
- Take medication with a full glass (240 ml) of water.
- If gastric upset occurs, take medication after meals or with food.
- Report side effects to physician (headache, photosensitivity, rash or peeling of skin, aching of joints, unusual bleeding or ecchymosis, jaundice, continuous nausea, vomiting).
- Male infertility may be a side effect but is completely reversed on discontinuation of the medication.

Emotional support. Most patients with Crohn's disease require emotional support from nurses, physicians, aides, stomal therapists, and others. The support groups sponsored by the Crohn's and Colitis Foundation of America (formerly the National Foundation of Ileitis and Colitis) have played a major part in helping these patients. Tranquilizers, antidepressants, and psychology or psychiatry services may be required in the management of the disease. Current evidence suggests that Crohn's disease is not caused by psychological stress but that psychiatric disturbances are the result of the nature of the symptoms and chronicity of the disease.

Nursing diagnoses and interventions for patients with Crohn's disease include but are not limited to the following:

NURSING DIAGNOSES	NURSING INTERVENTIONS
Anxiety, related to inability to cure disease	Explore with the patient factors that aggravate the disease. Explain the relationship of diet to the disease.
Powerlessness, related to exacerbations and remissions	Assist the patient in listing factors that can be controlled: diet, stressors, medication compliance, self-monitoring of symptoms.
Nutrition, altered: less than body requirements, related to bowel hypermotility and decreased absorption	Emphasize the importance of weighing daily, following special diets, and assessing energy levels.
Sexuality patterns, altered, related to impotency	Explain the undesired side effect of medications on the male. Discuss alternative methods of sexual gratification until drug is discontinued and potency returns.

Patient teaching. The patient must understand the effects of diarrhea and rapid emptying of the small intestine on the nutritional needs of the body. This will lead to acceptance of special diets and the ability to retain some personal control of the disease.

The patient must also understand the relationship of emotional feelings to Crohn's disease. Identifying resources for emotional support in the family and community and among health professionals will promote coping skills and mental hygiene.

Prognosis. Crohn's disease has a high rate of recurrence, especially in patients under 25 years of age. The rate of recurrence after surgery is 50% for the first 5 years and 75% in 10 years. Prognosis depends on the extent of involvement, duration of illness, and success of medical interventions. No known therapy will maintain a patient with Crohn's disease in remission.

Acute Abdominal Inflammations

Appendicitis.

Etiology/pathophysiology. Appendicitis is the inflammation of the vermiform appendix, usually acute, which if undiagnosed leads rapidly to perforation and peritonitis.

Appendicitis is most apt to occur in teenagers and young adults and is more common in males.

The vermiform appendix is a small tube in the right lower quadrant of the abdomen. The lumen of the proximal end is shared with that of the cecum, whereas the distal end is closed. The appendix fills and empties regularly in the same way as the cecum. However, the lumen is tiny and is easily obstructed. If it becomes obstructed and inflammation occurs, pathogenic bacteria *(E. coli)* begin to multiply in the appendix and infection develops with the formation of pus. If distention and infection are severe enough, the appendix may rupture, releasing its contents into the abdomen. The infection may be contained within an appendiceal abscess or may spread to the abdominal cavity, causing generalized peritonitis.

Clinical manifestations. Light palpation of the abdomen will elicit rebound tenderness. The abdomen musculature overlying the right lower quadrant may feel tense as a result of voluntary rigidity. The patient will often be lying on the back or side with knees flexed in an attempt to decrease muscular strain on the abdominal wall.

Assessment. Collection of *subjective data* includes the most common complaint of constant pain in the right lower quadrant of the abdomen around McBurney's point (exactly halfway between the umbilicus and the crest of the right ilium). The pain may be accompanied by nausea and anorexia.

Collection of *objective data* includes vomiting, a low-grade fever (99 to 102° F [37.2 to 38.8° C]), an elevated white blood count, rebound tenderness, a rigid abdomen, and decreased or absent bowel sounds.

Diagnostic tests. A white blood count (WBC) with differential will be ordered. Approximately 90% of persons will have a WBC above 10,000/mm^3, and approximately 75% will have a neutrophil count above 75%. A flat film of the abdomen is helpful for diagnosis. When diagnosis is difficult, Hypaque contrast studies, ultrasound, and laparoscopy may be used.

Medical management. Emergency surgical intervention is the treatment of choice for acute appendicitis. It may be performed as an incidental procedure when a patient is having another abdominal surgical procedure. Because mortality correlates with perforation and perforation correlates with duration of symptoms, early diagnosis and appendectomy are essential for the lowest acceptable morbidity and mortality. Antibiotic therapy is given both prophylactically and when perforation is likely. Complications that can occur include infection, intraabdominal abscess, and mechanical small bowel obstruction.

Nursing interventions. The nursing interventions of the patient include following general preoperative procedure. The nurse should explain diagnostic tests and possible surgical procedures to relieve anxiety. Other interventions include bed rest, NPO status, comfort measures for pain relief so that symptoms will not be masked by medication, and fluid and electrolyte replacement. The temperature, blood pressure, pulse, and respirations are monitored and documented every hour because of the threat of perforation with peritonitis.

SKILL 27-7

INSERTING A RECTAL TUBE

1. Introduce self.
2. Identify patient.
3. Wash hands.
4. Explain procedure.
5. Arrange equipment at bedside.
6. Pull curtain and close door to provide privacy.
7. Have patient assume side-lying position, and arrange gown and top linens to prevent soiling yet covering patient.
8. Place waterproof pad under buttocks.
9. Don gloves, and lubricate tube well with petrolatum or water-soluble lubricant.
10. Expose anus, and insert tube 4 to 6 inches (10 to 15 cm) in the same manner as for an enema (see Procedure 27-5).
11. Insert drainage end into receptacle, or use commercially prepared set.
12. Instruct patient to lie quietly to prevent dislodgement of tube; leave tube in place no more than 30 minutes. If flatulence persists, the nurse should notify the physician.
13. Remove tube and assist patient to bedpan, bedside commode, or toilet as necessary; stimulation of peristalsis may result in bowel movement.
14. Provide for patient hygiene; assist patient to bed or chair.
15. Dispose of equipment and supplies; remove gloves, and wash hands.
16. If flatulence, abdominal discomfort, or distention continues, reinsert tube prn or as ordered by physician. (Continued use of rectal tubes can cause irritation and eventual excoriation (skin impairment) of the anus and rectal mucosa.)
17. Record procedure and observations.
18. Report abnormalities.

No narcotics are given during diagnosis to prevent masking of symptoms; sedatives may be given if necessary. In some cases an ice bag to relieve pain is given; *no* heat is applied, since this may increase circulation to the appendix and lead to rupture. A cleansing enema is usually not ordered because of the danger of rupture. Postoperatively, a rectal tube may be inserted for relief of flatus (Skill 27-7). General postoperative care is performed (see Chapter 22).

Nursing diagnoses and interventions for the patient with appendicitis include but are not limited to the following:

NURSING DIAGNOSES	NURSING INTERVENTIONS
Knowledge deficit, related to disease process and surgery	Explain definition of diagnosis, diagnostic tests as they are ordered, and possible surgical intervention.
Fluid volume deficit, related to vomiting	Monitor patient for signs of dehydration and fluid and electrolyte imbalance (poor skin turgor, flushed dry skin, coated tongue, oliguria, confusion, and abnormal sodium, potassium, and chloride levels).
Pain, related to inflammation	Provide support to patient and family through listening and explanation of tests and procedures; explain need to withhold medications. Monitor increase in amount of pain experienced, rebound tenderness, and abdominal rigidity. Take vital signs frequently (q 15 min).

NURSING DIAGNOSES	NURSING INTERVENTIONS
Infection, high risk for, related to rupture of appendix	Monitor incision site for pain, tenderness, and edema. Maintain sterile asepsis for dressing changes. Monitor temperature for elevation q 4 hr.

Patient teaching. Patient teaching may include the reason for intravenous fluids with gradual advancement of diet from clear liquids to general as peristalsis returns. If antibiotics or oral medications are continued postoperatively, the patient should understand the name, purpose, and side effects of each medication. If complications occur necessitating an NG tube or drainage tubes, the nurse should ensure the patient understands the reason for these interventions.

Prognosis. The rate of cure through surgical intervention is high in patients with appendicitis. The patient's prognosis is altered if peritonitis complicates this diagnosis.

Diverticular Disease of the Colon.

Etiology/pathophysiology. Diverticular disease has two clinical forms, *diverticulosis* and *diverticulitis.* Diverticulosis is the presence of pouchlike herniations through the muscular layer of the colon, particularly the sigmoid colon (Fig. 27-14). Diverticulitis is the inflammation of one or more diverticula.

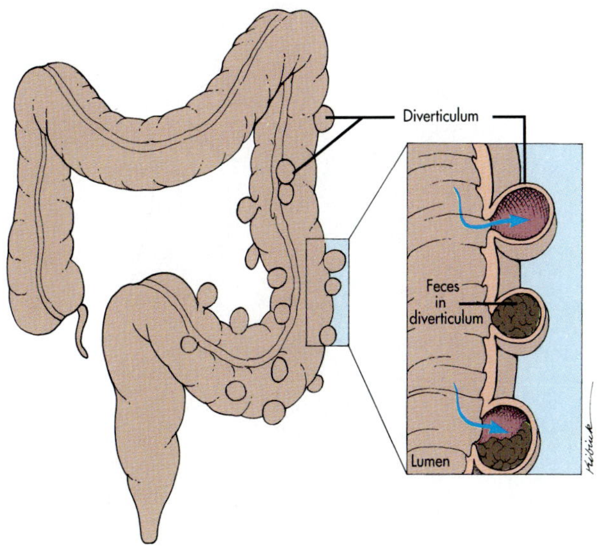

FIG. 27-14 Diverticulosis.

Diverticulosis affects increasing numbers of people over 50 years of age and may be the result of the modern, highly refined, low-residue diet. The penetration of fecal matter through the thin-walled diverticula causes inflammation and abscess formation in the tissues surrounding the colon. With repeated inflammation, the lumen of the colon narrows and may become obstructed. When one or more diverticula become inflamed, diverticulitis results, which is a complication of diverticulosis. This inflammation can lead to perforation, abscess, peritonitis, obstruction, and hemorrhage.

Clinical manifestations. When diverticula perforate and diverticulitis develops, the patient will complain of mild to severe pain in the lower left quadrant of the abdomen and will have fever and an elevated white blood cell count and sedimentation rate. If the condition goes untreated, septicemia and septic shock can develop. This patient will be hypotensive and have a rapid pulse. Intestinal obstruction can occur, and the patient will experience abdominal distention, nausea, and vomiting.

Assessment. Collection of *subjective data* includes an awareness that the patient with diverticulosis may not display any problematic symptoms. Subjective complaints of constipation and diarrhea accompanied by pain in the left lower quadrant are common to some. Other common symptoms include increased flatus and chronic constipation alternating with diarrhea, anorexia, and nausea.

Collection of *objective data* may include abdominal distention, low-grade fever, vomiting, and blood in the stool.

Diagnostic tests. Hypaque contrast studies are preferred over barium enema for diagnostic studies because there is less chance of bowel rupture. Both will visualize the outpouchings along with the distortions and narrowing of the lumen. Colonoscopy may be beneficial in diagnosing certain cases and is especially helpful in ruling out carcinoma.

Medical management. The treatment of diverticulosis depends on the cause. If muscle atrophy is responsible for the disease, a low-residue diet, stool softeners, and bed rest are traditional interventions. When increased intracolonic pressure and muscle thickening are causes, a high-fiber diet of bran, fruits, and vegetables is recommended. Sulfa drugs have been used to treat uncomplicated signs of inflammation. Microperforation resulting in localized abscess is treated with a combination of antimicrobials effective against gram-negative, gram-positive, and anaerobic organisms. Analgesics are given intramuscularly for pain. Patients with acute attacks of diverticulitis that do not respond to antibiotics and bed rest may require hospitalization with NG drainage, parenteral fluids, and intravenous antibiotics.

Surgical treatment is advised if long-term problems do not respond to medical management and is mandatory if complications, such as hemorrhage, obstruction, abscesses, or perforation, occur. In elective surgery a thorough bowel preparation is most important. Laxatives, enemas, or intestinal lavage by GoLYTELY (see Box 27-2), as discussed, are given to cleanse the bowel, depending on the surgeon's preference. Antibiotics are given orally and parenterally.

In cases of perforation, abscess, peritonitis, or fistula, resection of the bowel with a temporary colostomy is needed. Either the one-stage procedure (resection of the affected bowel with anastomosis and no diverting colostomy) or the two-stage procedure (resection of the diseased bowel with diverting colostomy) is performed.

The bowel diversion can be accomplished by the Hartmann's procedure (Fig. 27-15 on p. 692) where the descending colon is resected, the proximal end is brought to the abdominal wall surface, and the distal bowel is sealed off for later anastomosis. The second procedure is the double-barrel colostomy, where the bowel is brought up through the abdominal surface, or loop colostomy (Figs. 27-16 and 27-17 on p. 692). The bowel can be opened at the time of surgery or postoperatively. Removal of the affected bowel segment and reanastomosis of the bowel are done during the initial procedure.

Closure of the temporary colostomy is the desired goal in the case of diverticular disease. Usually this is done from 6 weeks to 3 months after the initial surgical procedure. Again, the bowel must be prepared for closure by a liquid diet, laxatives, antibiotics, intestinal lavage as mentioned, and a cleansing colostomy irrigation of the proximal and, in the case of the loop or double-barrel colostomy, distal end of the stoma.

Nursing interventions. Nurses should remember that when the distal loop is irrigated, irrigating solution and bowel contents will usually return from both the dis

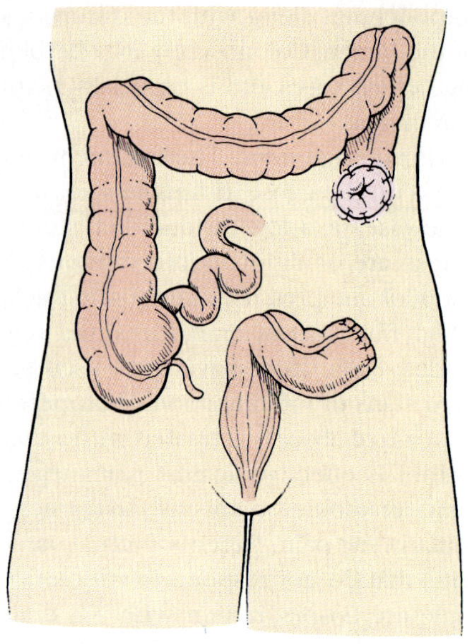

FIG. 27-15 Hartmann's pouch.

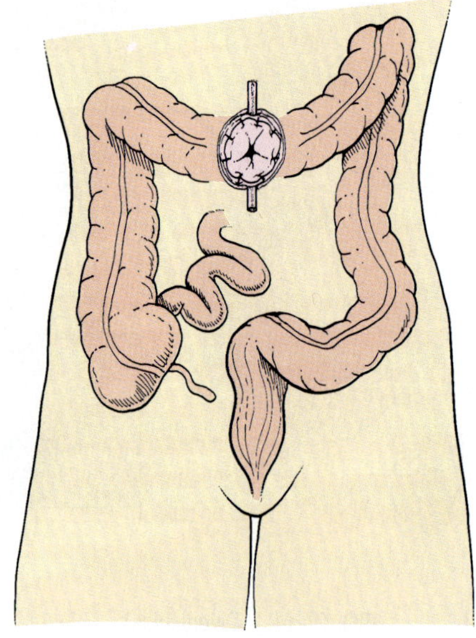

FIG. 27-17 Transverse loop colostomy with rod/butterfly.

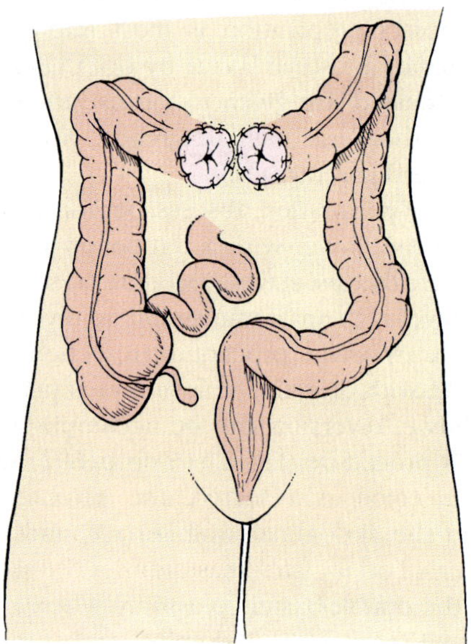

FIG. 27-16 Double-barrel transverse colostomy.

tal opening and rectum, so placement of the patient on the toilet or bedpan is important during the procedure.

The return of bowel activity after closure may take several days. The patient will again have intravenous fluids and an NG tube for the first few days postoperatively.

Nursing interventions include patient teaching of the disease process and surgery, if planned. The nutritional status must be assessed and discussion and reinforcement given as needed. The nurse should determine the nature of the pain the patient is having so that interventions of comfort measures or medication can be administered to provide relief. The patient and family should be included in the goals of the teaching plan.

Nursing diagnoses and interventions for the patient with diverticular disease include but are not limited to the following:

NURSING DIAGNOSES	NURSING INTERVENTIONS
Knowledge deficit, related to disease process and treatment	Instruct patient and significant others in disease process and signs and symptoms of acute diverticulitis attack.
Nutrition, altered: less than body requirements, related to decreased oral intake	Instruct in dietary roughage (for prevention) or bland, low-residue diet (for inflammatory phase).
Pain, related to inflammation of bowel	Administer proper diet to prevent aggravation; administer analgesics as ordered for pain. Provide uninterrupted periods of rest.
Anxiety, related to concerns about surgery	Explain diagnostic tests, reason for surgery if necessary, and possibility of temporary colostomy and what this means. Spend additional time listening to patient.
Infection, high risk for, related to abscesses, perforation, purulent drainage, and fecal material	Observe wound and drain sites frequently for signs of infection. Perform meticulous wound care if wound is left open for drainage. Monitor for elevated temperature q 4 hr.

Patient teaching. When a colostomy is performed, the patient or significant other should be able to verbalize and demonstrate understanding of the ostomy care to the nurse. The teaching of colostomy care should not be rushed and must be done when the patient is free of pain and receptive to learning. A family member may be taught to help until the patient is able to assume self-care, keeping in mind that the ultimate goal is patient independence. A home care referral may be needed so that the teaching process can continue after discharge.

Prognosis. With diverticulosis, the prognosis is good. Most patients have few symptoms except for occasional bleeding from the rectum. Diverticulitis has a good prognosis, with 25% of patients needing bowel resection of the affected part in acute cases to reduce mortality and morbidity.

Peritonitis.

Etiology/pathophysiology. Peritonitis is an inflammation of the abdominal peritoneum. This condition occurs after fecal matter seeps from the rupture site, causing bacterial contamination of the peritoneal cavity. Some examples may be diverticular abscess and rupture, acute appendicitis with rupture, and strangulated hernia. Chemical irritation can also cause peritonitis. Blood, bile, necrotic tissue, pancreatic enzymes, and foreign bodies are examples of these chemical irritants.

Clinical manifestations. Generalized peritonitis is an extremely serious condition characterized by severe abdominal pain. The patient usually lies on the back with the knees flexed to relax the abdominal muscles; any movement is painful. The abdomen is usually tympanic and extremely tender to the touch.

Assessment. Collection of *subjective data* includes observing for severe abdominal pain; any movement is painful. Nausea and vomiting occur, and as peristalsis ceases, constipation occurs with no passage of flatus. Chills, weakness, and abdominal tenderness (local and diffuse, often rebound) are also manifested.

Collection of *objective data* includes noting a weak and rapid pulse, fever, and lowered blood pressure. Leukocytosis and marked dehydration occur, and the patient can collapse and die.

Diagnostic tests. A fat plate of the abdomen is ordered to ascertain if free air is present under the diaphragm as a result of visceral perforation. A CBC with differential is ordered to determine the degree of leukocytosis present. A blood chemistry profile to determine renal perfusion and electrolyte balance is done.

Medical management. Aggressive therapy includes correction of the contamination or removal of the chemical irritant by surgery, and parenteral antibiotics. Nasogastric intubation is ordered to prevent GI distention. Intravenous fluids and electrolytes will prevent or correct imbalances. Early treatment to prevent severe shock from the loss of fluid into the peritoneal space is essential.

Nursing interventions. Nursing interventions for the patient with peritonitis include the following:

1. Place patient on bed rest in semi-Fowler's position to help localize purulent exudate in lower abdomen or pelvis.
2. Give oral hygiene to prevent drying of mucous membranes and cracking of lips from dehydration.
3. Monitor fluid and electrolyte replacement.
4. Encourage deep breathing exercises; patient tends to have shallow respirations as a result of abdominal pain or distention.
5. Use measures to reduce anxiety.
6. Use meticulous surgical asepsis for wound care.

Patient teaching. The nurse should instruct the patient of the importance of ambulation, coughing, deep breathing, and leg exercises. If the patient has a draining wound at discharge, she should be taught surgical asepsis for dressing changes. A nutritious diet is encouraged. The patient should be instructed not to lift more than 10 pounds until instructed by the physician to do so. The importance of the patient's keeping physician follow-up appointments is stressed.

Prognosis. The mortality rate of generalized peritonitis is 40% with the use of antibiotics and intensive support systems. Age, type of contamination, and tissue perfusion negatively affect the prognosis.

Hernias

Abdominal Hernia.

Etiology/pathophysiology. Most hernias result from congenital or acquired weakness of the abdominal wall or postoperative defect, coupled with increased intraabdominal pressure from coughing, straining, or an enlarging lesion within the abdomen.

The different types of hernias include abdominal, femoral or inguinal, hiatal, and umbilical. A femoral or inguinal hernia is caused by a weakness in the lower abdominal wall opening through which the spermatic cord emerges in men and the round ligament emerges in women. A hiatal hernia (esophageal hernia or diaphragmatic hernia) results from a weakness of the diaphragm (see discussion on hiatal hernia). An umbilical hernia is when the rectus abdominis muscle is weak, and the bowel protrudes against the umbilicus.

A hernia may be reducible (can be returned to its original position by manipulation) or irreducible (cannot be returned to its body cavity). An incarcerated hernia is when the intestinal flow is obstructed. The hernia is strangulated when the blood supply is occluded. Immediate surgical intervention is performed when a hernia strangulates, to prevent anaerobic infection in this affected area.

Factors such as age, wound infection, malnutrition, obesity, increased intraabdominal pressure, or abdominal distention affect formation of hernias after surgical incisions. Fewer hernias occur with transverse incisions than with longitudinal incisions. Also, upper abdominal incisions are associated with fewer hernias than lower abdominal incisions.

Assessment. Collection of *subjective data* includes palpation of the hernia area, revealing the contents of the sac as soft and nodular (omentum) or smooth and fluctuant (bowel). At no time should the nurse attempt to reduce the sac in the ring, since this can lead to complications, such as rupture of the strangulated contents.

Both subjective and objective signs and symptoms depend on where the hernia occurs. With an inguinal hernia, the patient may complain of pain, urgency, and the presence of a mass in the groin region.

Collection of *objective data* includes visibility of a protruding mass or bulge around the umbilicus, in the inguinal area, or near an incision; this is the most common objective sign. If complications such as incarceration or strangulation follow, there may be bowel obstruction, vomiting, and abdominal distention.

Diagnostic tests. The diagnosis is aided by palpation of the weakened wall. X-ray films of the suspected area are diagnostic tests that may be ordered.

Medical management. Hernias that cause no discomfort can be left unrepaired unless strangulation or obstruction follows. The patient should be taught to seek medical advice promptly if abdominal pain, distention, changing bowel habits, temperature elevation, nausea, and/or vomiting occurs. If the hernia can be reduced manually, a truss or firm pad placed over the patient's hernia site and held in place with a belt prevents the hernia from protruding and holds the abdominal contents in place.

Elective surgery for hernia repair may be done because of the inconvenience to the patient or constant risk of strangulation. A procedure to close the hernia defect by approximating adjacent muscles or using a synthetic mesh is done on either an inpatient or outpatient basis.

Nursing interventions. The nursing interventions of the patient with an abdominal hernia require observation of the hernia's location and size; the patient may be limited in activity and the type of clothing worn. Tissue perfusion to the area should be observed.

Open abdominal surgery may be necessary for the patient with a strangulated hernia. The patient should be prepared for a long hospitalization, which may include NG suctioning, intravenous antibiotics, fluid and electrolyte replacement, and parenteral pain medication until peristalsis returns.

Postoperatively the patient should be monitored for urinary retention, wound infection at the incision site, and with inguinal hernia repair, scrotal edema. If scrotal edema is present, it may be decreased by elevating the scrotum on a rolled pad, applying an ice pack, and providing a supportive garment (jockstrap or Jockey shorts). The patient should deep breathe every 2 hours, but many physicians discourage coughing. The nurse should verify the postoperative orders. The patient should be taught support of the incision by splinting the area with pillow or pad. This support along with analgesics will help to relieve pain.

Nursing diagnoses and interventions for the patient with a hernia include but are not limited to the following:

NURSING DIAGNOSES	NURSING INTERVENTIONS
Knowledge deficit, related to disease process	Instruct patient to observe and report hernias that become nonreducible, begin to become edematous, or produce increased pain. Abdominal distention and change in bowel habits should be reported also.
Pain, related to tissue edema	Explain reason to avoid prolonged standing, lifting, or straining. Instruct patient to support weakened area by use of truss or manually as needed (as when coughing).
Tissue perfusion, altered, related to strangulation/incarceration of hernia	Monitor patient for increased pain, distention, changing bowel habits, temperature elevation, nausea, and vomiting. Report changes in appearance and signs and symptoms to physician.

Patient teaching. Follow-up care includes teaching the patient to limit activities and avoid lifting heavy objects or straining with bowel movements for 5 to 6 weeks. Also the patient should immediately report to the physician any erythema or edema of the surgical area or increased pain or drainage.

Hiatal Hernia. Hiatal hernia is a protrusion of the stomach and other abdominal viscera through an opening in the membrane or tissue of the diaphragm (Fig. 27-18). A hiatal hernia is the most common problem of the diaphragm that affects the alimentary tract. A hiatal hernia

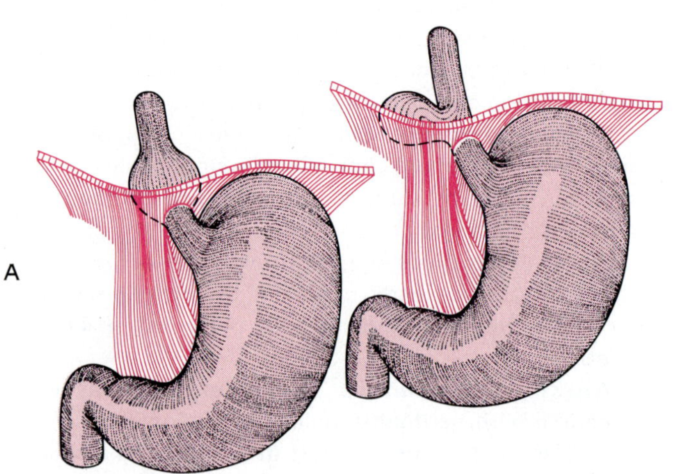

FIG. 27-18 Hiatal hernia. **A,** Sliding hernia. **B,** Rolling hernia.

is an anatomical condition and not a disease. This condition occurs in about 40% of the population, and most people display few, if any, symptoms. The major difficulty in symptomatic patients is gastroesophageal reflux, and these patients complain of pyrosis (heartburn) after overeating. Complications of strangulation, infarction, or ulceration of the herniated stomach are serious and require surgical intervention. Factors contributing to the development of these hernias include obesity, trauma, and a general weakening of the supporting structures as a result of aging (see gerontological box).

Medical management. The physician may select one of the following procedures:

- A posterior gastropexy, where the stomach is returned to the abdomen and sutured in place.
- Transabdominal or transthoracic fundoplication, where the fundus is wrapped around the lower part of the esophagus and sutured in place (Fig. 27-19).

GERONTOLOGICAL CONSIDERATIONS

- Loss of teeth and resultant use of dentures can interfere with chewing and lead to digestive complaints.
- Dysphagia is commonly seen in the older adult population and may be caused by changes is the esophageal musculature or by neurological conditions.
- Hiatal hernias and esophageal diverticuli are significantly increased with aging because of changes in musculature of diaphragm and esophagus.
- There is decreased secretion of hydrochloric acid (hypochlorhydria and achlorhydria) from the parietal cells of the stomach. This results in an increased incidence of pernicious anemia and gastritis in the aged population.
- Peptic ulcers are common, but often the symptoms are vague and go unrecognized until there is a bleeding episode. Medications such as aspirin, NSAIDs, and steroids that are taken for the chronic degenerative joint conditions common with aging should be used with caution because they can contribute to ulcer formation.
- Frequency of diverticulosis and diverticulitis increases dramatically with aging and can contribute to malabsorption of nutrients.
- Constipation is a problem for many older persons. Inactivity, changes in diet and fluid intake, and medications can contribute to this problem. Bowel elimination should be monitored and a bowel regimen established to prevent bowel impaction.
- Incidence of cholelithiasis increases with aging. Older individuals with histories of this should be observed closely for changes in the color of urine and stool or other signs and symptoms.

Nursing interventions. Nursing care of the patient after surgery is similar to that after gastric surgery or thoracic surgery, depending on the procedure performed (see Chapter 22).

Prognosis. The prognosis for hernias is good because surgical intervention is usually successful. This, of course, can be altered if the patient is a poor surgical risk or if other complications exist.

Intestinal Obstruction

Etiology/Pathophysiology. An intestinal obstruction results in failure of the contents of the intestine to pass through the lumen of the bowel (Fig. 27-20 on p. 696). Some conditions do not cause occlusion, but decrease peristalsis. This is referred to as *paralytic ileus.*

Most obstructions occur in the ileum, which is the narrowest segment of the small intestine. Adhesions (see Fig. 27-20, *A*) or incarcerated hernias cause 90% of all obstructions. Other causes include impacted feces, tumor of the bowel, intussusception (see Chapter 44) (prolapse of one segment of bowel into the lumen of another segment), **volvulus** (see Fig. 27-20, *B*) (a twisting of bowel onto itself), or the strictures of inflammatory bowel disease. Residues from foods high in fiber, such as raw coconut or fruit pulp, can also obstruct the small bowel.

When the small intestine becomes obstructed, the normal process of secretion and reabsorption of 7 to 8 L of electrolyte-rich fluid is interrupted. Large amounts of fluid, bacteria, and swallowed air build up in the bowel proximal to the obstruction. Water and salts shift from the circulatory system to the intestinal lumen, causing distention and further interference with absorption. Increased capillary permeability results, allowing bacterial movement across the bowel.

Clinical Manifestations. The signs and symptoms of intestinal obstruction vary with the site and degree of ob-

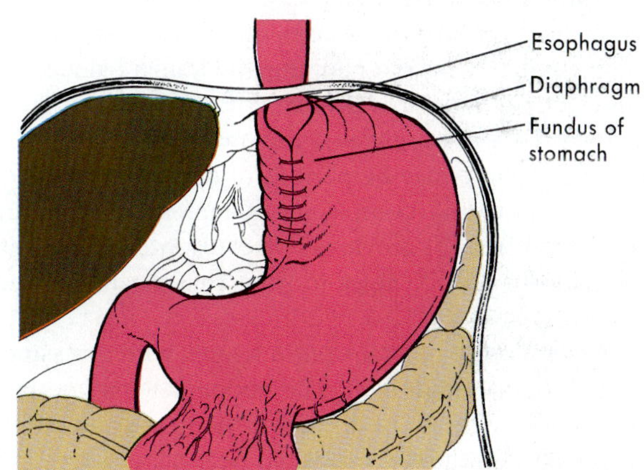

FIG. 27-19 Nissen fundoplication for hiatal hernia showing fundus of stomach wrapped around distal esophagus and sutured to itself.

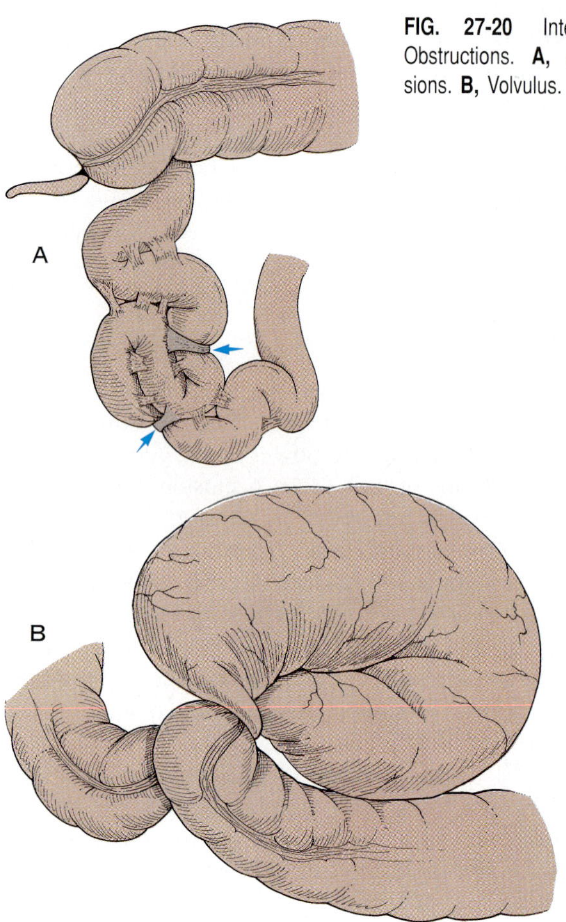

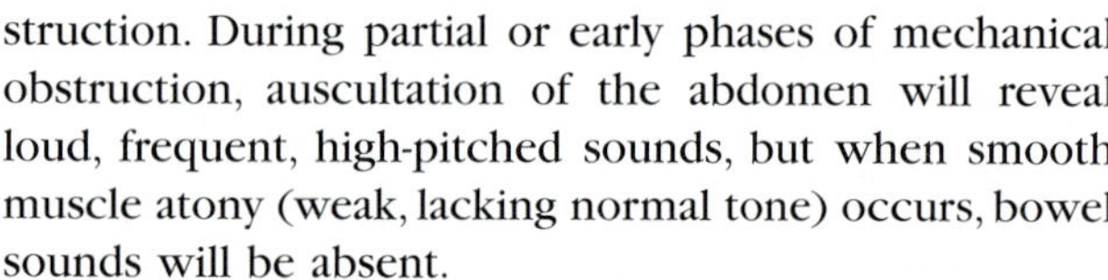

FIG. 27-20 Intestinal Obstructions. **A,** Adhesions. **B,** Volvulus.

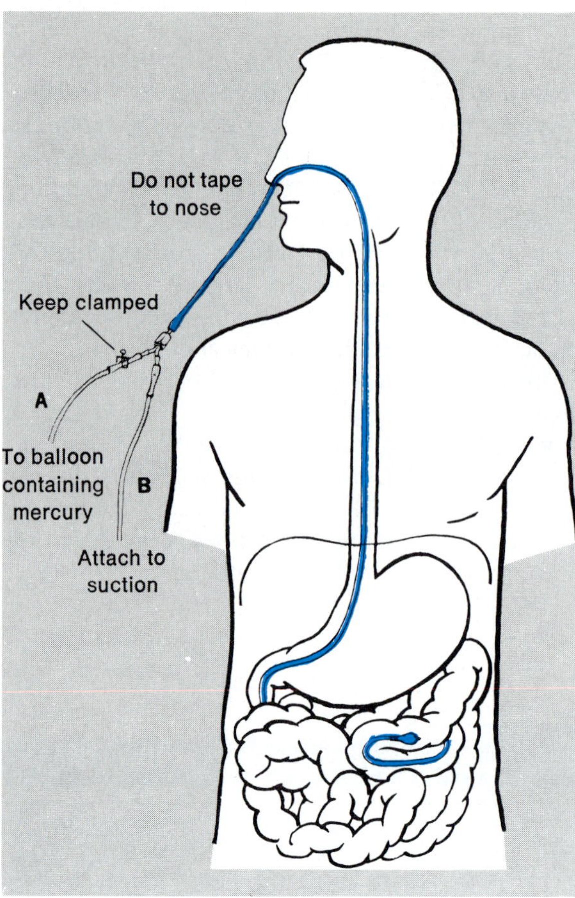

FIG. 27-21 Intestinal decompression tube in place. Note that tube is not taped to nose. *A,* Arm of Y-tube leading to balloon containing mercury or air must be kept clamped. *B,* Arm of Y-tube is attached to rubber tubing leading to suction.

struction. During partial or early phases of mechanical obstruction, auscultation of the abdomen will reveal loud, frequent, high-pitched sounds, but when smooth muscle atony (weak, lacking normal tone) occurs, bowel sounds will be absent.

Assessment. Collection of *subjective data* should include information about the pattern of the patient's pain, including onset, frequency, and characteristics. Complaints of early intestinal obstruction of the small intestine include spasms of cramping abdominal pain as peristaltic activity increases proximal to the obstruction. As the obstruction progresses, the intestine becomes fatigued and there may be periods of decreased or absent bowel sounds and complaints of increased abdominal pain. Any history of previous bowel disorders or abdominal surgeries and changes in bowel elimination should be noted.

Collection of *objective data* begins with assessment of the patient's abdomen. The abdominal surface is inspected for evidence of distention, hernias, scars indicating previous surgeries, or visible peristaltic waves. The increased peristaltic activity produces an increase in auscultated bowel sounds. Other objective data include vomiting, signs of dehydration caused by the fluid shift, abdominal tenderness and muscle guarding, and decreased blood pressure.

Obstruction of the colon causes less severe pain than obstruction of the small intestine, marked abdominal distention, and constipation. The patient may continue to have bowel movements. The colon distal to the obstruction continues to empty.

Diagnostic Tests. X-ray examination reveals the level of obstruction and its cause. The fluid and electrolyte balance can be monitored through laboratory test results. Elevated blood urea nitrogen (BUN) and decreased serum sodium, potassium, and magnesium are common. The patient's hemoglobin and hematocrit may be increased because of hemoconcentration associated with the fluid volume deficit.

Medical Management. Treatment includes the evacuation of intestinal contents by means of an intestinal tube. An NG or nasojejunal tube will be inserted to decompress the intestine. The use of a long nasointestinal tube with a mercury weight at the distal portion of the tube helps relieve an obstruction (Fig. 27-21). Surgical repair is necessary to relieve mechanical obstructions caused by adhesions and hernias. Fluid and electrolyte balances are restored by carefully monitored intravenous infusion. Nonnarcotic analgesics are usually prescribed to avoid the decrease in intestinal motility that often accompanies the administration of narcotic analgesics.

Nursing Interventions. Unless surgery is indicated, the nursing intervention consists of careful monitoring of fluids and electrolytes, observation of the function of tubes used to decompress and relieve distention, and the administration of analgesics.

For the patient with intestinal obstruction undergoing surgery, the preoperative preparation will include explanations of the procedure at a level the patient can understand. Emotional support for the patient will be important because the patient is experiencing not only the stressors of pain and vomiting, but also the added stressor of emergency surgery.

The postoperative nursing interventions are similar to those for any patient who has had abdominal surgery (see Chapter 22). The nurse should place the patient in Fowler's position for greater diaphragm expansion and should encourage the patient to breathe through the nose and not swallow air, which would increase distention and discomfort. She should encourage deep breathing and coughing. Nasointestinal suctioning will be continued until bowel activity returns. The nurse should assess for bowel sounds and abdominal girth to help to determine the return of peristalsis. Some patients may require temporary bowel diversion via a double-barrel or loop colostomy to manage the obstruction.

Nursing diagnoses and interventions for the patient with an intestinal obstruction include but are not limited to the following:

NURSING DIAGNOSES	NURSING INTERVENTIONS
Pain, acute, related to increased peristalsis	Reposition patient frequently to help intestinal tube advance. Irrigate suction tubing with sterile saline to keep tube patent. Explain purpose of all procedures. Provide comfort measures. Administer analgesics as ordered.
Fluid volume deficit, related to increased losses from vomiting and shift of fluids	Monitor for signs of dehydration, decreased blood pressure, change in laboratory values, and decreased urine output. Record and report frequency, amount, and nature of emesis. Record urine output.
Gas exchange, impaired, related to abdominal distention	Observe for changes in size, tenderness, and bowel sounds in abdomen. Note any change in respiratory pattern and increased anxiety. Monitor arterial blood gas returns, reporting changes as they occur.

Patient teaching. Follow-up teaching focuses on prevention and includes dietary management, prevention of constipation, and recognition of early symptoms of recurrence and the need to seek prompt medical care. For the patient with a temporary ostomy, follow-up care will be necessary as plans are made for closure of the stoma.

Prognosis. The prognosis depends on early detection of the obstruction and the type and cause of the obstruction, as well as the success of medical interventions. The prognosis is poorer in patients who develop complications such as hypovolemic shock.

Cancer of the Colon

Etiology/Pathophysiology. Malignant neoplasms that invade the epithelium and surrounding tissue of the colon and rectum are the second most prevalent internal cancers in the United States.

In the colon, 45% of growths are seen in the sigmoid and rectal areas, 25% in the cecum and ascending colon, and the remaining 30% in the transverse splenic flexure, hepatic flexure, and descending colon. Cancer occurs with the same frequency in men and women, with the highest incidence in the ages of 60 years and older.

The cause of colorectal cancer remains unknown, but certain conditions appear to be more prone to malignant changes. These conditions are termed *predisposing* or *risk factors.* Particular diseases over time, including ulcerative colitis and diverticulosis, increase the risk of colorectal cancer. Neoplastic polyps or adenomas may undergo malignant change and become frank carcinomas. Recent research has isolated a gene that causes colon cancer in certain families. History taking and regular check-ups are important preventive measures. Other factors implicated in colorectal cancer include lack of bulk in the diet, high fat intake, and high bacterial counts in the colon. It is theorized that carcinogens are formed from degraded bile salts, and the stool that remains in the large bowel for a longer period as a result of too little fiber to stimulate its passage may overexpose the bowel to these carcinogens. There is also a theory that the increased transit time for low-fiber foods to pass through the intestine is related to malignancy. These factors have encouraged diet changes; decreased animal fat and increased high dietary fiber found in fruits, vegetables, and bran may have a protective effect and act as a primary preventive measure.

Clinical Manifestations. Signs and symptoms of cancer of the colon vary with the location of the growth.

Assessment. Collection of *subjective data* includes complaints of a change in bowel habits alternating between constipation and diarrhea, excessive flatus, and cramps. Constipation is more likely produced by de-

SKILL 27-8

DIGITAL EXAMINATION WITH REMOVAL OF FECAL IMPACTION

1. Introduce self.
2. Identify patient and explain procedure.
3. Wash hands.
4. Arrange equipment at bedside.
5. Pull curtain and close door to provide privacy.
6. Place patient in left Sims' position, and place waterproof pad under patient's buttocks.
7. Place the bedpan on the bed close to the patient's buttocks.
8. Arrange patient's gown and top linen to prevent soiling yet exposing only what is necessary.
9. Don gloves; lubricate forefinger well with petrolatum or water-soluble lubricant to reduce irritation. (Use the index finger of your dominant hand.)
10. Insert finger gently; slowly but gently move finger into and around the fecal mass; as pieces of the mass are broken off, remove them to bedpan. This procedure can be very uncomfortable for the patient. Excess rectal manipulation may cause irritation to the mucosa, bleeding, and stimulation of the vagus nerve, which results in a reflex slowing of the heart rate.
11. Continue procedure until impaction is removed.
12. Stop procedure for a few minutes if patient complains of severe discomfort, to give patient opportunity to rest. (Reassess the patient's heart rate and observe for signs of fatigue.)
13. After removal is complete, wash and dry perineal area. (Assist the patient to toilet or position on the bedpan if urge to defecate develops.)
14. Remove waterproof pad and equipment; reposition patient.
15. Dispose of supplies; clean and return equipment.
16. Remove gloves; wash hands.
17. Record procedure and observations.
18. Report abnormalities. This procedure may be followed by enemas or cathartics—check the physician's order.

scending colon cancer, while ascending colon cancer may occur with no change in bowel habits (Skill 27-8). The other complaint may be rectal bleeding, with the color varying from dark to bright red, depending on the location of the neoplasm. Later stages of colon cancer may include subjective symptoms of abdominal pain, nausea, and **cachexia** (weakness and emaciation associated with general ill health and malnutrition).

Collection of *objective data* includes observing for vomiting, weight loss, abdominal distention or ascites, unexplained anemia, and test results that are compatible with the diagnosis.

Diagnostic Tests. Early diagnosis of the tumor, including identifying the type of cells involved, is the most important factor in treating the disease. Digital examination can identify 15% of colorectal cancers. Proctosigmoidoscopy with biopsy can enable detection of 66% of these tumors.

A baseline colonoscopy at age 30 should be performed on those who have a family history of colon cancer. The colonoscopy should be repeated every 4 years if one family member is affected or every 3 years if two first-degree relatives are affected.

The fecal occult blood examination followed by proctosigmoidoscopy remains the most reliable tool for screening. Other laboratory and diagnostic studies include an upper GI series, radiological abdominal series, barium enema, hemoglobin, hematocrit, electrolytes, and the blood test for **carcinoembryonic antigen (CEA).** Active malignancy growth within the body can be assayed by a blood test when cancer and metastasis are suspected. The CEA is a glycoprotein antigen in adenocarcinomas of the GI tract. Antibodies to this antigen are measured. Because the CEA level can be elevated in benign and malignant diseases, it is *not* considered a specific test for colorectal cancer. Its use is limited to determining the prognosis and monitoring the patient's response to antineoplastic therapy.

Medical Management. Medical treatment includes radiation, chemotherapy, and surgery. Radiation therapy is often used before surgery to decrease the chance of cancer cell implantation at the time of resection. Radiation can both reduce the size of the tumor and decrease the rate of lymphatic involvement. There are few side effects from radiation before surgery, but there are complications.

Postoperatively those patients at high risk for recurrence or persons whose disease has progressed may receive radiation administered over 4 to 6 weeks (see Chapter 38 for a discussion of radiation).

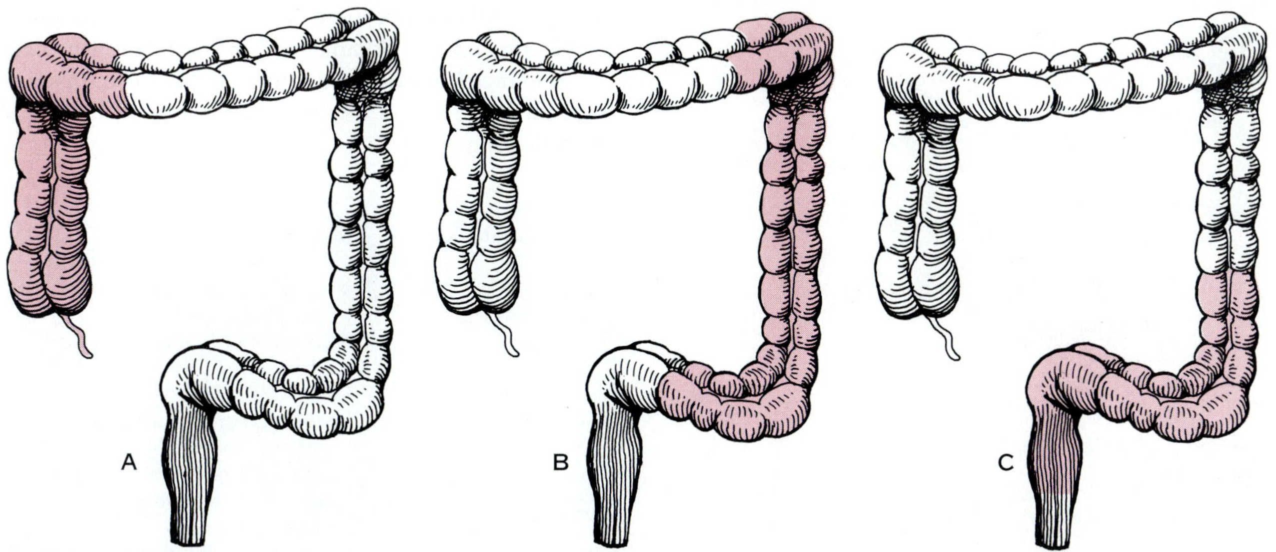

FIG. 27-22 Bowel resection. **A,** Right hemicolectomy. **B,** Left hemicolectomy. **C,** Anterior rectosigmoid resection.

Chemotherapy is given (1) to patients with systemic disease that is incurable by surgery or radiation alone, (2) to patients in whom undetectable metastasis is suspected, or (3) for palliative therapy to reduce tumor size or relieve symptoms of the disease, such as obstruction or pain. Physician opinion and individual patient response regarding use of chemotherapy for colorectal cancer vary (see Chapter 38 for a discussion of chemotherapy).

Surgical interventions for treatment depend on the location of the tumor, presence of obstruction or perforation of the bowel, possible metastasis, the patient's health status, and the surgeon's preferences. When obstruction has not occurred, a portion of the bowel on either side of the tumor is removed and an end-to-end anastomosis is done between the divided ends. When obstruction of the bowel occurs, the commonly used procedures are as follows:

- One-stage resection with anastomosis.
- Two-stage resection with (1) resection by bringing the ends of the bowel to the surface and creating a temporary colostomy and mucus fistula or Hartmann's pouch (see Fig. 27-15), (2) a double-barrel colostomy (see Fig. 27-16), or (3) a temporary loop colostomy (see Fig. 27-17), for closure later.

Surgical procedures for colorectal cancer include the following:

- Right hemicolectomy: resection of ascending colon and hepatic flexure (Fig. 27-22, *A*); ileum anastomosed to transverse colon.
- Left hemicolectomy: resection of splenic flexure, descending colon, and sigmoid colon (Fig. 27-22, *B*); transverse colon anastomosed to rectum.
- Anterior rectosigmoid resection: resection of part of descending colon, the sigmoid colon, and upper rectum (Fig. 27-22, *C*); descending colon anastomosed to remaining rectum.

In carcinoma of the rectum every effort is made by the surgeon to preserve the sphincter. An end-to-end anastomosis is often used. If the surgeon is unable to do an anastomosis, an abdominoperineal resection may be done. This refers to removal of the colon and rectum by way of the abdomen and the perineum. The proximal end of the descending colon is brought through the abdominal wall to form a permanent colostomy (Fig. 27-23 on p. 700).

Nutritional status is important because of the threat of infection and postoperative healing process that may follow a compromised state as a result of constipation, diarrhea, nausea, vomiting, and possible obstruction.

Nursing Interventions. The assessment of bowel and urinary elimination, fluid and electrolyte balance, tissue perfusion, nutrition, pain, gas exchange, infection, and peristomal skin integrity was discussed previously.

Preoperative care. The patient will have some type of bowel preparation, which usually includes 2 or 3 days of liquid diets, a combination of laxatives, GoLYTELY, or enemas and oral antibiotics to sterilize the bowel. The antibiotic of choice may be neomycin, kanamycin, or erythromycin; each suppresses anaerobic and aerobic organisms in the colon.

Other aspects of preoperative care include instruction in turning, coughing, and deep breathing; wound splinting; and leg exercises. The patient should know that he will have intravenous lines, a Foley catheter, a NG tube, and abdominal dressings after surgery.

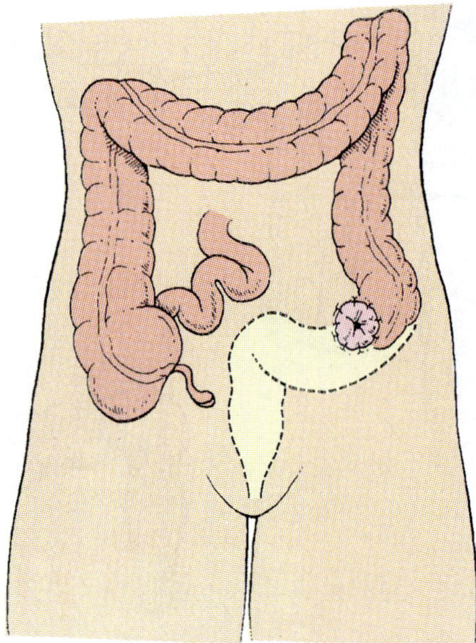

FIG. 27-23 Descending/sigmoid colostomy.

If a stoma is to be created, the enterostomal therapist should be notified so that the stoma site can be marked before surgery. The stoma should be placed at the best site for the patient.

Postoperative care. The patient should be assessed for stable vital signs and return of bowel sounds. The dressings should be checked for drainage or bleeding and changed as needed per the physician's order. The NG tube and Foley catheter should be monitored for flow and amount and color of output. Accurate I&O records must be kept to maintain the fluid and electrolyte balance. Other postoperative care includes coughing, deep breathing, early ambulation, adequate nutrition, pain control, and meticulous wound and stoma care.

Paralytic ileus, a common complication of abdominal surgery, produces the classic signs of increased abdominal girth, distention, nausea, and vomiting. Interventions include decompression of the bowel with an NG tube, NPO status, and increased patient activity.

Long-term complications of abdominal resection with permanent colostomy are urinary retention or incontinence, pelvic abscess, failure of perineal wound healing or wound infection, and sexual dysfunction.

In addition to monitoring the stoma (an artificial opening of an internal organ on the surface of the body) for color, size, location, and the condition of the peristomal skin, the nurse must watch for possible complications. Common stoma complications in the immediate postoperative period are necrosis and abscess. Necrosis results from a compromised blood flow to the stoma, causing the stoma to appear pale and dusky to black. Abscess caused by stoma placement too close to the wound, retention sutures, and drains must be assessed promptly. All complications must be reported promptly to the surgeon and documented in the medical record.

Nursing diagnoses and interventions for the patient with cancer of the colon include but are not limited to the following:

NURSING DIAGNOSES	NURSING INTERVENTIONS
Nutrition, altered: less than body requirements, related to vomiting and/or anorexia, surgical intervention, and depression	Maintain NPO status as ordered. Monitor parenteral fluids. Monitor patency and function of NG tube. Measure I&O. Monitor vital signs and serum electrolytes, Hct, and Hgb. Provide high-protein, high-carbohydrate, high-calorie, low-residue diet as allowed and tolerated.
Powerlessness, related to loss of control of bowel elimination	Involve the patient in decision making where possible. Foster independence in daily activities as soon as possible. Explain whether surgical procedure is temporary.
Coping, ineffective individual/family, related to illness/surgery and prognosis	Plan time for patient's verbalization. Listen carefully. Demonstrate a sincere interest in patient and family. Involve significant other in health teaching and decision making. Explain all procedures and treatments. Reinforce physician's explanations of disease process and prognosis. Assess present coping patterns, and identify strengths and weaknesses.
Knowledge deficit, related to home care needs and chemotherapy and/or radiotherapy	Provide information about diet, activity, and rest. Discuss medications: name, dosage, purpose, time of administration, and side effects. Explain side effects of chemotherapy and ways of managing them using other members of health team. Encourage follow-up visits with physician. Refer to community resource agencies as necessary.
Body image disturbance, related to loss of normal body function (colostomy)	Allow time for grieving. Assist patient and significant other in accepting ostomy. Allow time for and encourage verbalization. Answer all questions, and explain treatment and procedure. Provide care in positive manner; always avoid facial expressions connoting distaste. Observe for signs of denial, grief, or anger. Provide privacy and safe environment. Encourage self-care and independence when patient demonstrates readiness.

Patient teaching. The patient with a permanent end colostomy can be taught two forms of colostomy management: (1) emptying and cleansing the pouch as

PERFORMING A COLOSTOMY IRRIGATION

SKILL 27-9

1. Introduce self.
2. Identify patient.
3. Wash hands and explain procedure.
4. Pull curtain and close bathroom door to provide privacy.

NOTE: As many of the following steps as possible should be performed by the patient with the nurse teaching and assisting as needed. Independence will come. Be alert to signs of patient readiness.

5. Arrange equipment at bedside or in bathroom.
6. Position patient:
   In bathroom—have patient sit on toilet or on chair in front of toilet.
   In bed—have patient lie comfortably with head elevated slightly.
7. Don gloves.
8. Remove pouch, cleanse skin, and place irrigation sleeve over stoma; attach belt if using; place end of sleeve in toilet.
9. Close clamp on irrigating tubing; fill irrigating container with 1000 ml tepid water (or as otherwise ordered). Container may be hung on a hook at patient's shoulder level. Allow a small amount of water to flow through tubing.
10. Attach cone to tubing; lubricate cone; insert cone into stoma through top of sleeve (see illustration).
11. While holding cone in place, allow solution to flow slowly into colon (500 - 1000 ml slowly over 15 min.). If patient complains of cramping, stop flow without removing cone until cramps subside. (Solution container should be hung 18 inches above the stoma.)
12. After all solution is instilled, remove cone and close top of sleeve.
13. Instruct patient to sit about 15 to 20 min while returns flow into toilet.
14. Drain sleeve; rinse and remove it.
15. Observe patient and results of irrigation; flush toilet.
16. Perform colostomy care (see Skill 27-5).
17. Clean and dry irrigation equipment; dispose of nonreusable supplies; remove gloves, and wash hands.
18. Assist patient to comfortable position.
19. Record procedure and observations (including characteristics of feces and tolerance of procedure).
20. Report abnormalities.

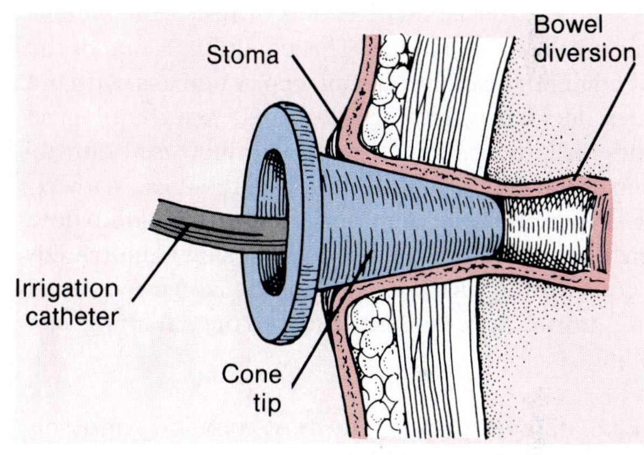

needed and (2) managing colostomy irrigation (Skill 27-9). Factors to consider in planning patient teaching are past bowel habits, location of colostomy, age of the patient, general health of the patient, and the patient's personal preference.

Nerves that control the bladder may be damaged when a large amount of tissue is removed in the abdominoperineal resection. When the Foley catheter is removed after surgery, the patient may be unable to void or empty the bladder completely. If the problem does not resolve, the patient may need a Foley catheter and a urology consultation.

When a large amount of tissue is removed, as in the abdominoperineal resection, and a cavity is left as sanctuary for bacteria, there is increased risk of infection. The drain site is monitored for increased pain, erythema, and purulent drainage, and body temperature is monitored for elevation. The perineal wound may be closed in one of three ways. The closed wound with a drain to suction has a high risk for abscess formation. The semiclosed wound is partially closed with either a Davol or Penrose drain that is left in place longer, with the drain shortened over time by the physician or nurse. The open wound, where packing is used and later removed, may need irrigating, and sitz baths may be required to facilitate healing. Changes in exudate color and odor and temperature elevation should be reported to the physician and documented.

Sexual dysfunction by both men and women is related to removal of the rectum. Contributing factors may be partial to complete disruption of the nerve's supply to the genital organs, psychological factors, or decreased activity associated with age. When a comfortable relationship exists between the nurse and the patient, the topic of sex can be introduced more effectively. Exploring the patient's and the partner's fears and providing information on penile prosthesis surgery and simple suggestions to both partners will help decrease anxiety concerning intercourse. Counseling may be necessary if the patient's and spouse's perceptions of body image have been altered. Support groups are available to the cancer patient in most communities. Above all, the nurse's silent communication of touch and eye contact can give the patient a message that he is accepted and valued.

Prognosis. The 5-year survival rate for patients with localized disease is 87% for those with colon tumors and 79% for those with rectal tumors. These rates are reduced by half with regional or distant involvement. Only distant metastases prevent the possibility of a cure.

Hemorrhoids

Etiology/Pathophysiology. Hemorrhoids are varicosities (dilated veins) that may occur outside the anal sphincter as external hemorrhoids or inside the sphincter as internal hemorrhoids. This condition is one of the most common health problems seen in humans, with the greatest incidence from ages 20 to 50 years. Etiological factors include straining at stool with increased intraabdominal and hemorrhoidal venous pressures. With repeated increased pressure and obstructed blood flow, permanent dilation occurs. Factors causing hemorrhoids are constipation, diarrhea, pregnancy, congestive heart failure, portal hypertension, and prolonged sitting and standing.

Clinical Manifestations. The most common symptoms associated with enlarged, abnormal hemorrhoids are prolapse and bleeding. The bright red bleeding and prolapse usually occur at time of defecation.

Assessment. Collection of *subjective data* includes noting the patient's complaints of constipation, **pruritus,** severe pain when dilated veins become thrombosed, and bleeding from the rectum that is not mixed with feces.

Collection of *objective data* includes observing external hemorrhoids and palpating internal hemorrhoids on examination. Because bleeding and constipation are signs of cancer of the rectum, all patients with these symptoms should have a thorough examination to rule out cancer.

Medical Management. Conservative interventions include the use of bulk stool softeners, such as Metamucil, bran, and natural food fibers, to relieve straining. Topical creams with hydrocortisone relieve pruritus and inflammation, and analgesic ointments, such as dibucaine (Nupercainal), relieve pain. Sitz baths are usually given to relieve pain and edema and promote healing.

The rubber-band ligation is a popular and easy method of treatment. Tight bands are applied with a special instrument in the physician's office, causing constriction and necrosis. The destroyed tissue sloughs off in about 1 week, and discomfort is minimal. Sclerotherapy (a needle is inserted at the apex of the hemorrhoid column and a sclerosing agent is injected), cryotherapy (tissue destruction by freezing), infrared photocoagulation (destruction of tissue by creation of a small burn), laser excision, and operative hemorrhoidectomy are additional interventions.

Hemorrhoidectomy, the surgical removal of hemorrhoids, can be performed if other interventions fail to relieve the distressing signs and symptoms. After removal of the hemorrhoid, wounds can be left open or closed, although closed wounds are reported to heal faster. Although this surgery is not considered a major procedure, pain may be acute, requiring narcotics and analgesic ointments. Complications of hemorrhoidectomy include hemorrhage, local infection, pain, urinary retention, and abscess.

Nursing Interventions. Rectal conditions can be embarrassing to the patient, and the nurse's direct but concerned attitude can decrease this embarrassment. The nurse can assess the knowledge level by asking patients about their condition, what they have been told about treatment, and what treatments have been done before surgery and why.

The nurse should assess the patient with a prolapsed hemorrhoid for edema, thrombosis, and ischemia. Ischemic tissue will be dark red to necrotic (black). A low-bulk diet can produce chronic constipation, and this should be explained to the patient.

For the surgical patient, vital signs should be taken frequently for the first 24 hours to rule out internal bleeding. Early ambulation and a soft diet facilitate bowel elimination. The patient may have a great deal of anxiety concerning the first defecation, and this should be discussed.

Nursing diagnoses and interventions for the patient with hemorrhoids include but are not limited to the following:

NURSING DIAGNOSES	NURSING INTERVENTIONS
Pain, related to edema, prolapse, and surgical intervention	Instruct patient to wash anal area after defecation and pat dry. Sitz baths or local heat applied to site may be soothing. Use of local anesthetics (Nupercainal ointment or Tucks pads) may give relief. Reinforce need for high-residue diet.

NURSING DIAGNOSES	NURSING INTERVENTIONS
Pain, related to edema, prolapse, and surgical intervention—cont'd	Instruct patient on manual reduction of external hemorrhoids. Apply ice packs to hemorrhoids if thrombosed to prevent edema and pain. Use a cushion for sitting postoperatively.
Tissue perfusion, altered, gastrointestinal, related to postoperative hemorrhage	Inspect site frequently first 24 hours. Check vital signs on regular postoperative routine. Avoid rectal tubes and rectal temperatures. Assess Hgb and Hct levels.
Anxiety, related to previous experiences, fear of first bowel movement postoperatively, and lack of knowledge regarding diet	Establish a supportive relationship with patient. Explain need for high-residue diet. Administer laxatives and oil retention enema as ordered. Give analgesic before first bowel movement and a sitz bath after for pain relief.

Patient teaching. The patient is advised to include in the diet bulk-forming foods, such as fresh fruit, vegetables, and bran cereals, as well as 8 to 10 glasses of fluid a day unless contraindicated. If the patient is anemic, discussion of foods high in iron, such as red meats, liver, and dark green leafy vegetables, can be included. Moderate exercise and establishing a routine time for a daily bowel movement should be emphasized. The patient should also be instructed to report any signs of infection or delayed healing.

Prognosis. There are several preferred methods of treatment for hemorrhoids. Both conservative modes of treatment and surgical intervention for hemorrhoids have good prognostic rates.

Anal Fissure and Fistula

Anal fissure is a linear ulceration or laceration of the skin of the anus. Usually it is the result of trauma caused by hard stool that overstretches the anal lining. The fissure is aggravated by defecation, which initiates spasm of the anal sphincter, pain, and at times, slight bleeding. If the lesion does not heal spontaneously, the tract is excised surgically.

An anal fistula is an abnormal opening on the cutaneous surface near the anus. Usually this is from a local crypt abscess and also is common in Crohn's disease. A perianal fistula may or may not communicate with the rectum. It results from rupture or drainage of an anal abscess. This chronic condition is treated by a fistulectomy (removal) or fistulotomy (opening of the fistula tract).

The postoperative care required for repair of an anal fissure or fistula is similar to that for the patient who has had a hemorrhoidectomy.

Prognosis. The prognosis for anal fissures and fistulas is good. This favorable prognosis is found in patients treated with conservative measures as well as in those who have surgical intervention.

DISORDERS OF THE LIVER, BILIARY TRACT, AND EXOCRINE PANCREAS

The liver, gallbladder, and exocrine pancreas are all organs that assist with digestion.

Disorders of the Liver

Cirrhosis.

Etiology/pathophysiology. Cirrhosis is a chronic, degenerative disease of the liver in which the lobes are covered with fibrous tissue, the **parenchyma** (tissue of an organ as distinguished from supporting or connective tissue) degenerates, and the lobules are infiltrated with fat. The fibrous (scar) tissue restricts the flow of blood to the organ, which contributes to its destruction. Hepatomegaly (enlargement of the liver) and, later, liver contraction cause loss of the organ's function.

There are several forms of cirrhosis, caused by different factors. Laennec's cirrhosis, more commonly found in the Western world, affects more men than women and is found in patients with a history of chronic ingestion of alcohol. Postnecrotic cirrhosis, found worldwide, is caused by viral hepatitis, exposure to hepatotoxins (i.e., industrial chemicals), or infection. Primary biliary cirrhosis is found more often in women and results from destruction of the bile ducts. Secondary biliary cirrhosis is caused by chronic biliary tree obstruction caused by gallstones, a tumor, or biliary atresia in children. There are other types of cirrhosis, the cause of which is not always known.

With repeated insults, the liver can progress through the following stages: destruction, inflammation, fibrotic regeneration, and hepatic insufficiency. Although liver cells have a great potential for regeneration, repeated scarring decreases their ability to be replaced. As the blood supply continues to be diminished and the scar tissue increases, the organ atrophies.

Functions of the liver are altered in several ways. The liver's ability to synthesize albumin is reduced as a result of liver cell damage. The obstruction of the portal vein as it enters the liver results in portal hypertension, or increased pressure in the veins that drain the gastrointestinal tract. This increased pressure causes **ascites** (an accumulation of fluid and albumin in the peritoneal cavity). The damaged liver cannot metabolize protein in the usual manner; therefore protein intake may result in an elevation of blood ammonia levels. Reduced synthesis of protein and the leaking of existing protein result in hypoalbuminemia (reduced protein or albumin level in the blood), which reduces the blood's ability to regain fluids through osmosis. Protein must be present in adequate amounts to create colloidal osmotic pressure and "attract" the fluid to pass back into the blood vessels after it escapes in the capillaries. As fluid leaves the blood and the circulating volume decreases, the receptors in the brain signal the adrenal cortex to increase secretion of aldosterone to stimulate the kidneys to retain sodium and water. The normal liver inactivates the hormone *aldosterone,* but the damaged liver allows its effect to continue (hyperaldosteronism). Retention of fluid and sodium results in increased pressure in blood vessels and lymphatic channels, resulting in portal hypertension. Ascites is thus a result of portal hypertension, hypoalbuminemia, and hyperaldosteronism.

Hepatic insufficiency gradually causes veins in the upper part of the body to distend, including the esophageal vein. Esophageal varicosities develop, which may rupture, causing severe hemorrhage.

Clinical manifestations. Clinical manifestations of cirrhosis of the liver differ, depending on whether the patient is in the early or the later stages of disease. In the early stages, the liver is firm and therefore easier to palpate, and abdominal pain may be present because of rapid enlargement that produces tension on the fibrous covering of the organ. Later stages of the disease present manifestations of dyspepsia, changes in bowel habits, gradual weight loss, ascites, enlarged spleen, and *spider telangiectases* (dilated superficial arterioles). These later manifestations are the result of scarring of liver tissue that produces chronic failure of liver function and also fibrotic changes that cause obstruction of the portal circulation.

When enough cells of the liver become involved to interfere with its function and obstruct its circulation, the GI organs and the spleen become congested and cannot function properly. Anemia occurs because of the body's decreased ability to produce RBCs and platelets. The cirrhotic liver cannot absorb vitamin K or produce the clotting factors VII, IX, and X. This causes the patient with cirrhosis to have bleeding tendencies.

Assessment. Collection of *subjective data* in the *early stages* may include the patient describing symptoms as "flulike," including loss of appetite, nausea and vomiting, general weakness, fatigue, indigestion, abnormal bowel function (either constipation or diarrhea), flatulence, and abdominal discomfort. The anatomical area most commonly affected is in the epigastric region or the right upper quadrant of the abdomen.

Collection of *subjective data* in the *later stages* includes noting those subjective symptoms listed under early stages but they are more intense. The patient may complain of dyspnea and severe fatigue that interfere with the ability to carry out routine activities.

Collection of *objective data* in the *early stages* may include observing low hemoglobin, fever, jaundice, and loss of weight.

Collection of *objective data* in the *later stages* may include noting epistaxis, purpura, hematuria, spider hemangioma, and bleeding gums. Late symptoms are ascites, hematological disorders, splenic enlargement, and hemorrhage from esophageal varices or other distended GI veins. The patient may also appear mentally disoriented, unable to understand, and display different behaviors or speech patterns. Any prolonged interference with gas exchange leads to hypoxia, coma, and ultimately death.

Diagnostic tests. There are many diagnostic tests to aid in the diagnosis of cirrhosis. Abnormal electrolyte values, elevated serum bilirubin, AST (SGOT), ALT (SGPT), LDH, and gamma GT, decreased serum albumin, elevated ammonia, abnormal CBC, low blood glucose (hypoglycemia) from impaired gluconeogenesis, prolonged prothrombin time, and abnormal urinalysis may give evidence of poor liver functioning. Visualization through endoscopic retrograde cholangiopancreatography (to detect common bile duct obstruction), esophagoscopy with barium esophagography to visualize varices, scans and biopsy of the liver, and ultrasonography are used to diagnose cirrhosis. **Paracentesis** (a procedure in which fluid is withdrawn from the abdominal cavity) will relieve ascites and also provide fluid for laboratory examination.

Medical management. When possible causes have been identified, the initial treatment is to eliminate these causes, decrease the buildup of fluids in the body, prevent further damage to the liver, and provide individual supportive care to the patient. Eliminating alcohol, hepatotoxins (i.e., acetaminophen [Tylenol]), or environmental exposure to harmful chemicals is essential to prevent further damage to the liver. Diet therapy is aimed at correcting malnutrition, promoting the regeneration of functional liver tissue, and compensating for the liver's inability to store vitamins, while avoiding fluid retention and hepatic encephalopathy. A well-balanced, high-calorie (2500 to 3000 calories/day), moderate high-protein (75 g of high-quality protein/day), low-fat, low-sodium (200 to 1000 mg/day) diet with additional vitamins and folic acid will usually meet the needs of the patient with cirrhosis and improve deficiencies that exist (with impending liver failure, restrict protein and fluids).

Antiemetics may be prescribed to control nausea or vomiting. The patient must be monitored closely for toxicity that develops quickly when the poorly functioning liver cannot clear these drugs from the system. Diphenhydramine (Benadryl) or dimenhydrinate (Dramamine) may be given, whereas prochlorperazine maleate (Compazine), hydroxyzine pamoate (Vistaril), or hydroyzine hydrochloride (Atarax) should be avoided.

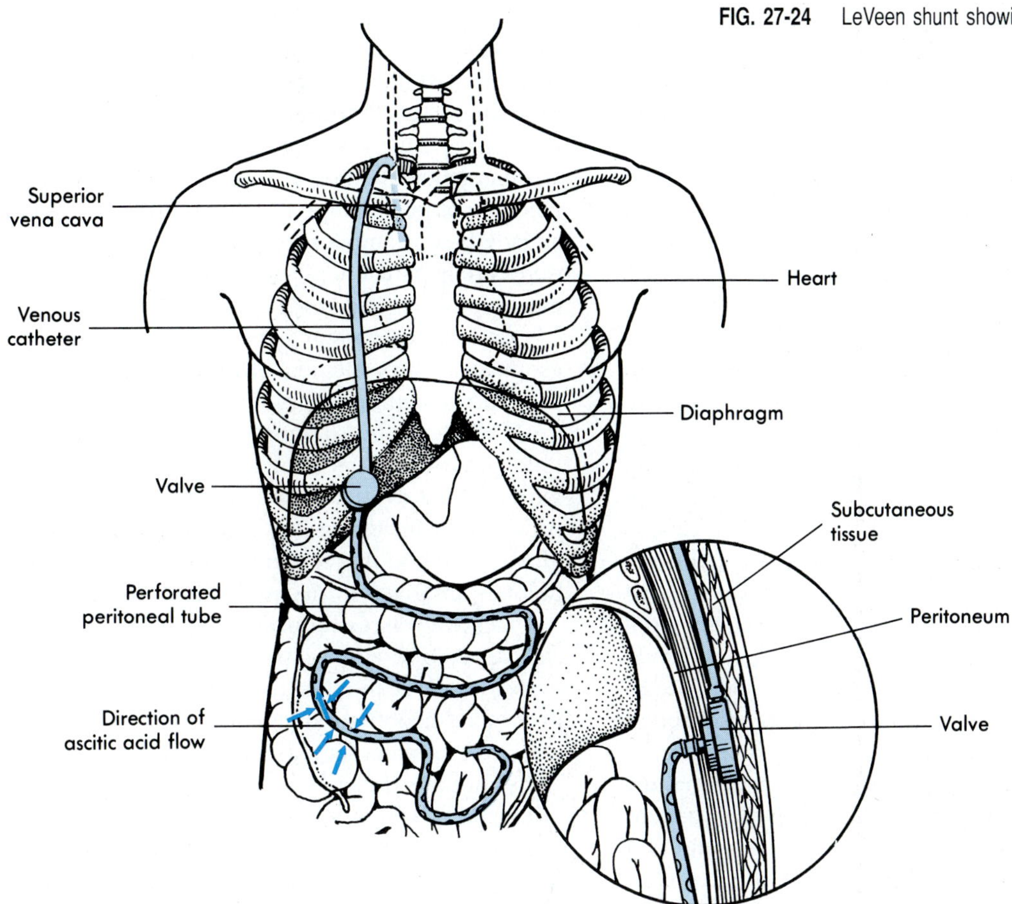

FIG. 27-24 LeVeen shunt showing placement of catheter.

Complications and treatment. Ascites is the presence of excessive fluid in the peritoneal cavity. The severity of fluid retention will determine the treatment. Initially the patient will be placed on bed rest with accurate monitoring of I&O. The patient's diet will be restricted for amount of fluid (500 to 1000 ml) and sodium (200 to 100 mg). Diuretic therapy may be added if the diet does not control the ascites and edema. Spironolactone (Aldactone) 300 to 1000 mg/day may be used to obtain the desired diuresis. Other diuretics may be added, including furosemide (Lasix) or hydrochlorothiazide (HydroDIURIL). Vitamin supplements may include vitamin K, vitamin C, and folic acid. Salt-poor albumin may be administered in an attempt to restore plasma volume if the intravascular volume is decreased significantly. Complications of diuretic therapy include plasma volume deficit, decreased renal function, and electrolyte imbalance.

Another method of treatment for ascites and edema is the LeVeen continuous peritoneal jugular shunt, introduced in 1962 (Fig. 27-24). This procedure allows the continuous shunting of ascitic fluid from the abdominal cavity through a one-way, pressure-sensitive valve into a silicone tube that empties into the superior vena cava. The patient with this shunt must be monitored carefully for complications, which include congestive heart failure, leakage of the ascitic fluid, infection at the insertion sites, peritonitis, septicemia, and shunt thrombosis.

Paracentesis is a temporary method of removing fluid by withdrawing fluid from the abdominal cavity by either gravity or vacuum. An incision is made in the skin, and a hollow trocar, cannula, or catheter is passed through the incision and into the cavity. The fluid is removed over a period of 30 to 90 minutes to prevent sudden changes in blood pressure, which could lead to syncope. The patient is monitored closely for signs of hypovolemia and electrolyte imbalances. A dressing is applied over the insertion site, and the nurse observes for bleeding and drainage.

Portal hypertension is an increased venous pressure in the portal circulation caused by compression or by occlusion in the portal or hepatic vascular system. In most instances, portal hypertension that develops from cirrhosis is irreversible.

Esophageal varices (a complex of longitudinal, tortuous veins at the lower end of the esophagus) enlarge and become edematous as the result of portal hypertension. They are especially susceptible to ulceration and hemorrhage. Varices can rupture as a result of anything that increases the abdominal venous pressure, such as coughing, sneezing, vomiting, or the Valsalva maneuver. Rupture may occur slowly over several days or suddenly and without pain. An endoscopy may be performed to identify the varices or to rule out bleeding from other sources.

Therapeutic management of a ruptured esophageal varix is a medical emergency. The patient's airway must be maintained, the bleeding varix controlled, and IV lines established for fluids and blood replacement as needed. The hormone *vasopressin,* administered intravenously or directly into the superior vena cava, is used to decrease or stop the hemorrhaging. If the vasopressin drip does not stop or control bleeding, a Sengstaken-Blakemore tube with openings at the tip may be inserted. This triple-lumen tube has a lumen for inflating the esophageal balloon, one for inflating the gastric balloon, and one for gastric lavage (Fig. 27-25). The tube is passed through the nose, and when it is in place, the balloon in the stomach or the one in the esophagus or both are inflated to press against the bleeding vessels and control the hemorrhage. The gastric aspiration is attached to low, intermittent suction. When either balloon is inflated, a Levin tube is passed into the esophagus through the mouth and attached to low suction to drain the saliva that cannot drain into the stomach. The balloon must be deflated periodically to prevent necrosis. The patient is allowed nothing by mouth, and the head of the bed should be elevated 30 to 45 degrees to help prevent aspiration of stomach contents and help the patient breathe.

Gastric lavage will be performed to remove any swallowed blood from the stomach. Iced, isotonic saline solutions for the lavage are used by some to facilitate vasoconstriction. Endoscopic sclerotherapy may also be used to control the bleeding.

Patients suffering from portal hypertension and esophageal varices may benefit from surgical shunting procedures that divert blood from the portal system to the venous system. The portacaval shunt diverts blood from the portal vein to the inferior vena cava. The splenorenal shunt requires the removal of the spleen, and the splenic vein is anastomosed to the left renal vein. The mesocaval shunt involves anastomosis of the superior mesenteric vein to the inferior vena cava. These procedures have a high mortality. They may be performed in an emergency situation to control acute esophageal varix bleeding or in a therapeutic situation when a patient has already bled. Complications of surgical shunting procedures are hepatic encephalopathy, gastrointestinal bleeding, ascites, and liver failure.

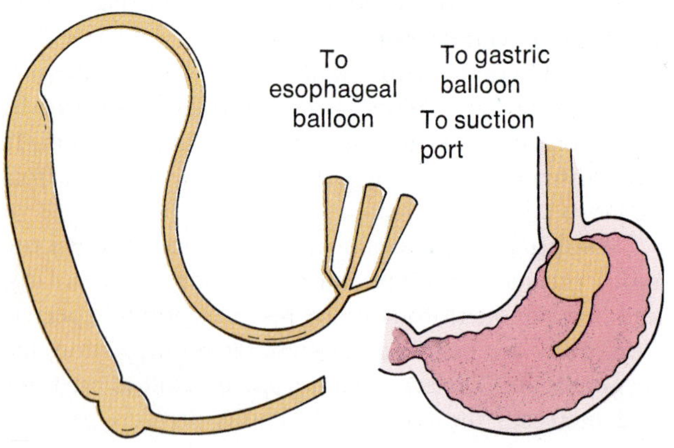

FIG. 27-25 Sengstaken-Blackmore tube.

Care of the patient who has hemorrhaged from an esophageal varix includes maintenance of oxygen content levels within the blood, blood transfusions with fresh whole blood to supply the body with more clotting factors, and electrolyte replacements as needed without fluid overload. The buildup of ammonia can be prevented with the use of cathartics and enemas to remove any blood that has entered the intestinal tract. Antibiotics are given to destroy colonic bacteria.

Hepatic encephalopathy is a type of brain damage caused by liver disease and consequent ammonia intoxication. It is thought to be the result of a damaged liver being unable to metabolize substances that can be toxic to the brain, such as ammonia. The patient's signs and symptoms progress from inappropriate behavior, disorientation, flapping tremors, and twitching of the extremities to stupor and coma. Treatment of the patient with hepatic encephalopathy is to give supportive care that will prevent further damage to the liver. Protein in the diet and drugs that are normally detoxified by the liver are avoided until the liver regains adequate function. Medications may be given to cleanse the bowel and help decrease the serum ammonia. Lactulose (Chronulac) decreases the bowel's pH, thus decreasing the production of ammonia by bacteria within the bowel. Lactulose may be administered orally or as a retention enema. It also functions as a cathartic. Neomycin inhibits protein synthesis in bacteria, thereby decreasing the production of ammonia. **Asterixis** (a hand flapping tremor) is when the patient stretches out an arm and hyperextends the wrist with the fingers separated, relaxed, and extended. A rapid, irregular flexion and extension (flapping) of the wrist will occur in the patient who is acutely ill.

Nursing interventions. The nurse should check vital signs every 4 hours and more often if evidence of hemorrhage is present. The patient should be observed for GI hemorrhage as evidenced by hematemesis, melena, anxiety, and restlessness.

Most patients will require a well-balanced, moderate high-protein, high-carbohydrate diet with adequate vitamins. With impending liver failure, protein and fluids will be restricted. Sodium restriction is frequently necessary, and this can make providing a palatable diet more difficult. Frequent oral hygiene and a pleasant environment should be provided to help the patient to increase food intake.

A major nursing focus for many patients is helping them to deal with alcoholism. This requires trust that the health team is interested in the patient's well-being. Patients must admit that they have drinking problems. Confrontation may sometimes be used to help patients accept the problems. Patients are often referred for counseling for their alcoholism.

Because of pruritus, malnutrition, and edema, the patient with cirrhosis is prone to skin lesions and decubitus formation. Preventive nursing interventions to avoid impairment of skin integrity, such as Eggcrate mattresses, frequent turning, back rubs, and massage of bony prominences, should be initiated. The nurse should apply soothing lotion to relieve pruritus.

The nurse should observe the patient's mental status and report changes, such as disorientation, headache, or lethargy. It is important for the nurse to assist in activities of daily living as needed to promote good hygiene while conserving energy. The nurse observes for edema by measuring ankles daily and observes for ascites by measuring abdominal girth. An accurate I&O is recorded, as well as daily weight.

Nursing diagnoses and interventions for the patient with cirrhosis include but are not limited to the following:

NURSING DIAGNOSES	NURSING INTERVENTIONS
Tissue perfusion, altered, gastrointestinal related to impaired blood coagulation or hemorrhage from portal hypertension	Monitor patient for signs of bleeding: gums, injection sites, decrease in BP, increase in pulse, hematemesis, and melena. Monitor Hgb and Hct. Monitor parenteral fluids and/or blood transfusions. Administer vitamin K and neomycin as ordered. Instruct patient to avoid straining with stools and to avoid vigorous toothbrushing. Monitor gastric output—color and consistency.
Thought processes altered, related to potential increase of serum ammonia and hepatic coma	Observe frequently for changes in mental status: lethargy, drowsiness, and confusion. Monitor neurological status for decreased motor ability. Provide safe environment: side rails up, bed in low position, and safety reminder devices if necessary. Avoid use of sedatives, tranquilizers, and narcotics.
Nutrition, altered: less than body requirements, related to inadequate diet, vomiting, or anorexia	Provide small, frequent feedings of prescribed diet; the amount of protein, carbohydrates, and fat will depend on the patient's ability to metabolize these nutrients; salt may be restricted. Assist and encourage patient to eat, and consider preferences in food choices. Dietician to follow patient and assist in making healthy choices.

Patient teaching. The patient with cirrhosis must understand the need for adequate rest and avoiding infections. Activity must be planned around complete bed rest until strength is regained. Turning the patient at least every 2 hours and providing range-of-motion exercises will help avoid infection and prevent thrombophlebitis. The nurse should instruct the patient to use a soft-bristled toothbrush, use an electric razor, blow nose cautiously, and avoid straining at stools to prevent bleeding as a result of a lack of vitamin K and certain clotting factors. Soap, perfumed lotion, and rubbing alcohol should be avoided because they will cause further drying of the skin. If pruritus and dryness of skin are present, diphenhydramine (Benadryl) may be administered. The nurse should explain the relationship of the therapeutic diet to the diagnosis and ability of the liver to function.

Community resources for home health care and detoxification programs may help the patient and family deal with problems that arise after discharge. Help the patient and family identify community resources available for alcohol rehabilitation. Because of the seriousness of the disease, the patient and family need understanding and support throughout the treatment.

Prognosis. The prognosis for cirrhosis of the liver is related to the cause of the disease, the susceptibility of the individual, and the extent of the involvement. Fibrosis of the cirrhotic liver cannot be cured, but its progression may be halted or slowed by proper management by the physician and the patient.

Hepatitis.

Etiology/pathophysiology. Hepatitis is an inflammation of the liver resulting from several causes, including viral agents, bacterial agents, or exposure to toxic substances.

The five types of viral hepatitis are caused by distinct but similar viruses that produce almost identical signs and symptoms but vary in their incubation period, mode of transmission, and prognosis. Hepatitis A, formerly called *infectious hepatitis,* is the most common form today and is a short-incubation virus (10 to 40 days). Hepatitis B, formerly called *serum hepatitis,* is a long-incubation virus (28 to 160 days). A third virus, known as *hepatitis C,* has an incubation period of 2 weeks to 6 months, commonly 6 to 9 weeks. Hepatitis D (also called *delta virus*) causes hepatitis as a coinfection with hepatitis B and may progress to cirrhosis and chronic hepatitis. The incubation period is 2 to 10 weeks. Hepatitis E (also called *enteric non-A-non-B hepatitis*) is transmitted through fecal contamination of water, primarily in developing countries. It is rare in the United States. The incubation period is 15 to 64 days. Health officials are required by law to report all cases of viral hepatitis to the Centers for Disease Control and Prevention (CDC) in Atlanta.

The modes of transmission of the five types of viral hepatitis are:

- Hepatitis A spreads by direct contact, through the oral-fecal route, usually by food or water contaminated with feces. Up to 50% of all people in the United States have been infected by the time they reach adulthood, most of them suffering minimal symptoms or no symptoms at all.
- Hepatitis B is transmitted by contaminated serum by blood transfusion, the use of contaminated needles and instruments, needle sticks, IV drug use, and dialysis, and by direct contact with body fluids from the infected persons, such as breast milk and sexual contact.
- Hepatitis C is transmitted through needle sticks, blood transfusions, and IV drug use and by unidentified means. In the past, hepatitis C could not be detected in banked blood, so it was more easily transmitted through transfusion. A new blood screening test is expected to greatly reduce the number of cases of transfusion-related hepatitis C.
- Hepatitis D is transmitted the same way as hepatitis B; it appears as a coinfection of hepatitis B.
- Hepatitis E is transmitted by the fecal/oral route; it spreads through the fecal contamination of water.

The basic pathological findings in the five forms of viral hepatitis are identical. A diffuse inflammatory reaction occurs, and liver cells begin to degenerate and die. As the liver cells degenerate, the normal functions of the liver slow down. The outcome of the disease may be affected by the virulence of the virus, the preexisting condition of the liver, and the health care given when the disease is diagnosed.

Clinical manifestations. The clinical manifestations for viral hepatitis vary greatly: some patients are asymptomatic, whereas others develop hepatic failure or hepatic encephalopathy.

Assessment. Collection of *subjective data* includes patients' reports of general malaise, aching muscles, photophobia, lassitude, headaches, and chills. Abdominal pain, dyspepsia, nausea, diarrhea, and constipation are reported also. The patient may complain of pruritus from the presence of bile on the skin. The patient will complain of tenderness in the liver and will remain fatigued for several weeks.

Collection of *objective data* includes observing hepatomegaly (enlarged liver), enlarged lymph nodes, weight loss, and rhinitis. Jaundice appears because of the damaged liver's inability to metabolize bilirubin; the resultant signs noted are yellowish skin, discoloration of the sclera and mucous membranes, dark amber urine, and clay-colored stools. It is not uncommon for relapses to occur in the convalescent stage.

Diagnostic tests. Changes in the liver caused by viral hepatitis cause elevated direct bilirubin, gamma GT, AST (SGOT), ALT (SGPT), LDH, and alkaline phosphatase, a prolonged prothrombin time, and in severe hepatitis, a decreased serum albumin. Leukopenia is common in these patients, and hypoglycemia is present in approximately 50% of the patients with hepatitis. Serum is examined for the presence of HAA (hepatitis-associated antigen) A, B, C, or D. No test is available for E.

Medical management. There is no specific treatment for patients with viral hepatitis other than supportive therapy for existing signs and symptoms and preventing the transmission of the disease. The patient's care can be in the hospital when bilirubin concentrations in the blood are >10 mg/dl and for those with a prolonged prothrombin time, but usually the patient is cared for at home. Bed rest for several weeks is commonly prescribed.

Alcohol in the diet is not allowed for at least 1 year, and the patient may need supportive care from the community to facilitate compliance. Most patients will tolerate small, frequent meals of a low-fat, high-carbohydrate diet. Hydroxyzine (Atarax) or trimethobenzamide (Tigan) may be given 30 minutes before meals for patients with nausea. If the patient is dehydrated, intravenous fluids will be given with additions of vitamin C for healing, vitamin B complex to assist the damaged liver's inability to absorb fat-soluble vitamins, and vitamin K to combat prolonged coagulation time. Avoid all unnecessary medications, particularly sedatives.

Gamma globulin or immune serum globulin should be given as soon as possible to persons who have been in direct contact with a person with hepatitis A during the infectious period (2 weeks before and 1 week after onset of symptoms). The dosage of 0.02 ml/kg of body weight, given intramuscularly, is effective in preventing hepatitis A in 80% to 90% of the cases.

Individuals who have been exposed to hepatitis B virus via a needle puncture or sexual contact should be protected with hepatitis B immune globulin (HBIG). A dose of 0.06 ml/kg of body weight is administered intramuscularly as quickly after exposure as possible. This dose is repeated 1 month later.

Persons identified as being at high risk for developing hepatitis B should be vaccinated if they are not already immune. These persons include the following:

- All health care personnel (personnel at highest risk are emergency room, operating room, intensive care unit, and dialysis personnel, phlebotomists, and laboratory technicians)
- Persons with high-risk life-styles (drug addicts, homosexuals, and prostitutes)
- Infants born to mothers who are hepatitis B surface antigen (HBsAg) positive

The protection program consists of three vaccinations: an initial vaccination, a vaccination 1 month later, and a third vaccination 6 months after the first injection. The hepatitis B vaccine has been shown to provide protection for 3 to 5 years in approximately 90% of the persons treated.

Because B, C, and D hepatitis are spread mainly through blood transfusions, blood products should be used only when necessary. The blood used should be screened for elevated ALT (SGPT) and anti-hepatitis B core (anti-HBc), anti-hepatitis C, and anti-hepatitis D.

Nursing interventions. The care of the patient with viral hepatitis includes ensuring rest, maintaining adequate nutrition, providing adequate fluids, and caring for the skin. The care of the patient with hepatitis continues over time, and support and patient education are necessary throughout the entire illness.

Preventing the transmission of the disease is of primary importance in caring for the patient with viral hepatitis. The patient, family, and health care providers must be knowledgeable about routes of transmission of the virus and take steps to avoid such transmission. Proper personal hygiene and good sanitation will help prevent the spread of hepatitis A. Patients should be given a thorough explanation of the reasons for the precautions and should be instructed in the proper handling of their own secretions and body wastes and in thorough methods of handwashing. Gown and gloves should be worn when handling excreta, giving enemas, taking rectal temperatures, handling food wastes, handling needles, disposing of urine, or carrying out any other procedure or hygiene measure that involves direct contact with the patient's body fluids.

When the patient has hepatitis B, utmost care must be taken in handling syringes, needles, and other instruments that are contaminated with the patient's serum. Disposable equipment and dishes should be used and isolation precautions taken. Special handling of blood, body fluids such as saliva, semen, and vaginal secretions is essential to prevent the transmission of hepatitis B. Use enteric precautions for 7 days after onset of hepatitis A. Use universal precautions for all patients.

Nursing diagnoses and interventions for the patient with hepatitis include but are not limited to the following:

NURSING DIAGNOSES	NURSING INTERVENTIONS
Injury, high risk for, related to poor nutrition and prolonged clotting times	Pad side rails if necessary. Assist weakened patient with activities. Encourage use of electric razors and soft toothbrush.
Nutrition, altered: less than body requirements, related to inadequate intake associated with current anorexia, nausea, vomiting, and altered metabolism of nutrients by the liver	Provide diet high in carbohydrates and low in fats, and encourage total fluid intake of 2500 to 3000 ml daily. Monitor I&O. Monitor daily weight. Note color and consistency of stool and color and amount of urine. Administer antiemetics as ordered. Offer support and understanding. Promote adequate rest.
Pain, related to pruritus as a result of elevated bilirubin levels	Avoid soap and rubbing alcohol on patient's skin. Pat skin dry; use soft clothes, bed linens, and towels. Provide moisturizing lotions. Administer antihistamines for severe pruritus as ordered.

Patient teaching. When the patient with viral hepatitis can be cared for at home, the family will need to be taught necessary precautions. Sexual activity should be avoided during the acute stage of hepatitis B, C, and D. Patients with hepatitis must wash hands thoroughly following toileting, must disinfect articles soiled with feces (boil 1 minute), and must not prepare foods for others during symptomatic disease.

If possible, separate bathroom facilities should be used by the patient. Personal care items and drinking glasses should not be shared. The patient's clothes should be laundered separately in hot water. Contaminated items should be disposed of properly.

The patient and family should be aware of signs and symptoms associated with hepatitis, including light-colored stools, dark-colored urine, jaundice, fever, GI disturbances, unusual bleeding that might be indicative of a prolonged prothrombin time, and tenderness or pain in the abdomen. The danger of alcohol use and its effect on the liver should be clearly understood.

Prognosis. The prognosis of hepatitis differs with the causative agent. Recovery from hepatitis A is high, with a mortality rate of 0.5%.

Mortality from hepatitis B has been reported to be as high as 10%. Hepatitis B is one of the most serious forms of hepatitis, often progressing to cirrhosis, chronic hepatitis, liver cancer, and death. Hepatitis C often progresses to chronic hepatitis, cirrhosis, and death. Hepatitis D may progress to cirrhosis and chronic hepatitis. It has a high mortality rate. Hepatitis E has a 10% mortality rate in pregnant women; otherwise it is not believed to be fatal.

Recovery from acute toxic hepatitis is rapid if the hepatotoxin is identified early and removed or if exposure to the agent has been limited. However, the prognosis is poor if there is a prolonged period between exposure and the onset of signs and symptoms because there are no effective antidotes.

Liver Abscesses.

If an infection develops anywhere along the GI tract, there is danger that the infecting organisms may reach the liver through the biliary system, portal venous system, or hepatic arterial or lymphatic systems. Most bacteria are promptly destroyed, but occasionally some gain a foothold. If the disease progresses, it can become life threatening. In the past the mortality rate was 100% because of the vague clinical symptoms, inadequate diagnostic tools, and inadequate surgical drainage of the abscess. Today, medical management is more successful.

Etiology/pathophysiology. If the body is not successful in destroying bacteria, the bacterial toxins attack neighboring liver cells, and the neurotic tissue produced serves as a protective wall for the organism. Meanwhile, leukocytes migrate into the infected area. The result is an abscess cavity full of a liquid containing living and dead leukocytes, liquefied liver cells, and bacteria. Pyogenic (pus-producing) abscesses of this type may be single or multiple.

Clinical manifestations. Patients with liver abscess present vague signs and symptoms. Fever accompanied by chills, abdominal pain, and tenderness in the right upper quadrant of the abdomen are common complaints.

Assessment. Collection of *subjective data* includes chills, complaints of dull abdominal pain, abdominal tenderness, and discomfort.

Collection of *objective data* includes fever, hepatomegaly (abnormal enlargement of the liver), jaundice, and anemia.

Diagnostic tests. The diagnosis is established by demonstrating a space-occupying lesion in the liver radiographically (x-ray, ultrasound, CT, and liver scan). Amebic (microscopic, single-celled parasite) liver abscess can also be confirmed by amebic serology (laboratory examination of antigen-antibody reaction of amebae in serum).

Medical management. Usually liver abscess can be managed by medical therapy. Treatment includes intravenous antibiotic therapy that is specific to the organism identified.

Percutaneous (performed through the skin) drainage of liver abscess is reserved for patients who are not responding to medical therapy or are at high risk for rupture. Open surgical drainage has been the standard in patients whose liver abscesses have ruptured into the peritoneal space, but some of these patients are now being managed with percutaneous drainage. All patients will require a full course of antibiotic therapy.

Nursing interventions. Continuous monitoring and supportive care are indicated because of the seriousness of the patient's condition. Monitoring objective and subjective symptoms is important. If signs and symptoms increase in depth and severity, the physician should be notified.

The patient's individualized response to drug therapy is determined by a decrease in fever, tenderness and rigidity of the abdomen, chills, and discomfort. If percutaneous or open surgical drainage is instituted, the nurse must observe the drainage for amount, color, and consistency.

Nursing diagnoses and interventions for the patient with a liver abscess include but are not limited to the following:

NURSING DIAGNOSES	NURSING INTERVENTIONS
Body temperature, altered, high risk for, related to infectious state	Check temperature as ordered by physician or as indicated by the patient's worsening condition and report findings to physician. Encourage fluids to prevent dehydration. Monitor IV fluids. Explain how fever and drainage can deplete fluids in the body. Record I&O. Monitor oral mucous membranes and skin turgor during assessment.
Knowledge deficit, related to relationship of infection to nutritional needs	Explain the body's need for added calories and protein to fight infection. Weigh patient daily for weight gain or loss to determine adequate nutritional intake.

Patient teaching. In addition to the relationship of infection and nutrition, the nurse may need to teach preoperative and postoperative procedures (see Chapter 22) if the patient requires percutaneous or open surgical drainage. A thorough explanation and assessment for the patient's understanding are necessary to determine adequacy of teaching skills. Anxiety in the seriously ill patient decreases as the knowledge base increases and the patient feels more in control of the situation.

Prognosis. The prognosis for patients with liver abscesses was very poor in the past with a mortality rate of 100%. The prognosis today is much improved because of advanced diagnostic tests, including the CT and liver scans, and aggressive medical and nursing interventions.

Cholecystitis and Cholelithiasis

Etiology/Pathophysiology. Disorders of the biliary system are common in the United States and are responsible for the hospitalization of more than a half million people a year. The two most common conditions are cholecystitis and cholelithiasis (Box 27-6). These two diseases are seen more commonly in women than men, in Native Americans and Caucasians than in Orientals and African-Americans, and in obese people, pregnant women, people with diabetes, multiparous women, and women who use birth control pills.

Cholecystitis can be caused by an obstruction, a gallstone, or a tumor. More than 90% of the cases of cholecystitis are caused by gallstones. The exact cause of stone formation in the gallbladder and the common bile duct is not known. However, an alteration in lipid metabolism and the role of female sex hormones are related to the disease.

Box 27-6 DEFINITIONS

chole pertaining to bile
cholang pertaining to bile ducts
cholangiography x-ray examination of bile ducts
cholangitis inflammation of bile duct
cholecyst pertaining to gallbladder
cholecystectomy removal of gallbladder
cholecystitis inflammation of gallbladder
cholecystography x-ray examination of gallbladder
cholecystostomy incision and drainage of gallbladder
choledocho pertaining to common bile duct
choledocholithiasis stones in common bile duct
choledochostomy exploration of common bile duct
cholelith gallstone
cholelithiasis presence of gallstones

When an obstruction, gallstone, or tumor prevents bile from leaving the gallbladder, the trapped bile acts as an irritant, causing cellular infiltration of the gallbladder wall after 3 to 4 days. A typical inflammatory response occurs, and the gallbladder becomes enlarged and edematous. The vascular occlusion along with bile stasis causes the mucosal lining of the gallbladder to become necrotic. Initially the bile in the gallbladder is sterile. The bacterial growth is caused by the ischemia and occurs usually within a few days. There is danger of rupture of the gallbladder and spread of infection to the hepatic duct and liver. When the disease is severe enough to interfere with the blood supply, the gallbladder wall may become gangrenous.

Clinical Manifestations. The condition may be acute, with a sudden onset of nausea and vomiting and severe, colicky pain in the right upper quadrant of the abdomen, or chronic, evidenced by several milder attacks of pain and a history of fat intolerance. Many patients with gallstones are asymptomatic, and the gallstones are discovered only during an examination for another problem.

Assessment. Collection of *subjective data* includes complaints of indigestion after eating foods high in fat. The pain of acute cholecystitis is abrupt in onset, reaches a peak intensity quickly, and remains at that level for 2 to 4 hours. It localizes in the right-upper-quadrant epigastric region. The pain radiates around the midtorso to the right scapular area. Anorexia, nausea, vomiting, and **flatulence,** (excess formation of gases in the stomach or intestine) are also noted. The patient may experience increased heart and respiratory rates and become diaphoretic, leading the individual to think she is having a heart attack. These symptoms are decreased or absent in the patient with chronic cholecystitis.

Collection of *objective data* may include a low-grade fever and an elevated leukocyte count, as well as mild jaundice, stool that contains fat (steatorrhea), and clay-colored stool caused by a lack of bile in the intestinal tract. The urine may be dark amber and contain urobilinogen as the kidneys try to remove the excess bilirubin from the bloodstream.

Diagnostic Tests. There are a number of diagnostic studies that are performed to confirm a diagnosis of cholecystitis and cholelithiasis. Fecal studies, serum bilirubin tests, ultrasound of the gallbladder and biliary system, and oral cholecystogram may be done. Operative cholangiography is when the common bile duct is directly injected with radiopaque dye and is most commonly done at the time of gallbladder surgery.

Medical Management. If the attack of cholelithiasis is mild, the patient is treated conservatively. Bed rest is prescribed an NG tube is inserted and connected to low suction, and the patient is placed on no fluids by mouth (NPO). This allows the GI tract and thus the gallbladder to rest. Intravenous fluids are given to rehydrate the patient and replace drainage from the NG tube.

Antispasmodic and analgesic drugs may be given to decrease the patient's pain. Meperidine (Demerol) is commonly used, because there is decreased incidence of spasms of the sphincter of Oddi with this drug. Antibiotics may be given (1) prophylactically to prevent infection, (2) to treat an already present infection, and (3) after perforation, should it occur. A diet that is low in fat and cholesterol may be prescribed. Avoidance of foods that are spicy is also suggested.

Lithotripsy. Extracorporeal shock wave lithotripsy (ESWL) is used to treat a patient who has mild or moderate symptoms caused by a few stones. The patient is treated by a machine that discharges a series of shock waves through water or a cushion that breaks the stone into fragments. The natural flow of bile carries the stone fragments out of the gallbladder into the intestine for eventual excretion. Nursing intervention after the procedure is similar to that for patients undergoing liver biopsy.

Surgical intervention. A cholecystectomy (removal of the gallbladder) is usually the treatment of choice. The gallbladder is removed, and the cystic duct, vein, and artery are ligated. A laparoscopic cholecystectomy and open abdominal cholecystectomy are the two surgical procedures. A Jackson-Pratt drain, Davol, or a Penrose drain may be inserted if an open cholecystectomy is performed. If the stones are in the common bile duct and edema is present, a biliary drainage tube, or T-tube, will be inserted to keep the duct open and al-

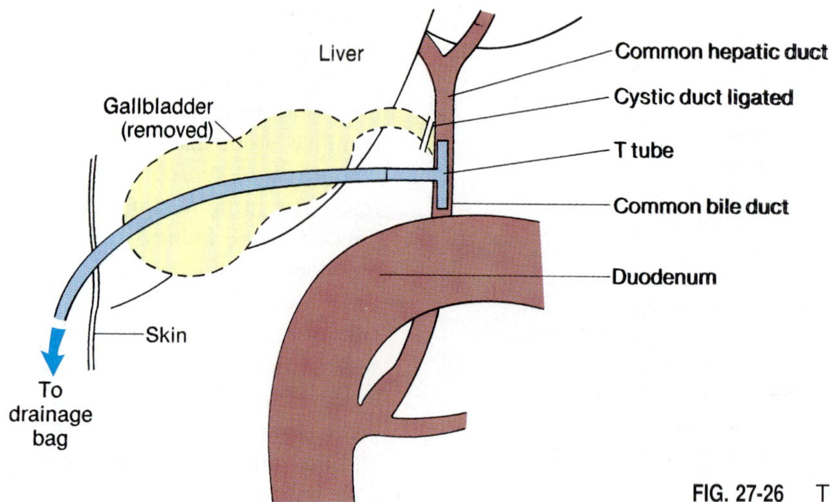

FIG. 27-26 T-Tube in common bile duct.

low drainage of the bile until the edema resolves. The short end of the tube is placed in the common bile duct, and the longer end of the tube is brought to the surface through a stab wound. The long end is attached to a closed drainage system (bile bag) that is placed below the level of the common bile duct (Fig. 27-26).

The T-tube also provides a route for postoperative cholangiography if desired (T-tube cholangiogram). The cholangiogram assesses the patency of the common bile duct. The T-tube will be removed 24 hours after the cholangiogram if the edema is resolved and the common bile duct appear normal. The 24-hour period allows the dye to drain out of the common bile duct. If the edema does not resolve in this time, the patient may be discharged with the T-tube in place.

Laparoscopic cholecystectomy. The newest operative procedure, which is now the most common treatment for cholecystitis and cholelithiasis, is done by way of endoscopy. It is called a *laparoscopic cholecystectomy,* and a laser or cautery is used to remove the gallbladder. This procedure involves removing the gallbladder through one of four small punctures in the abdomen, and is a relatively minor procedure compared with the standard surgical treatment. The first laparoscopic cholecystectomy was performed in the United States in 1988. Laparoscopic cholecystectomy offers several advantages over the common open abdominal cholecystectomy, including the following:

1. It is less invasive, and thus there is less chance of wound infection or respiratory impairment, a shorter healing time, and a shorter recuperative time.
2. There is no unsightly scar.
3. There is less pain and thus more rapid return to normal activities.

When a medical history, physical examination, and blood studies are complete, an ultrasound is done to locate gallstones and detect any dilation of the hepatic bile ducts. If *choledocholithiasis* (stones in common bile duct) is confirmed, a sphincterectomy and stone extraction are performed before laparoscopic surgery.

It is important to obtain informed consent for endoscopic and open cholecystectomy in case converting from one procedure to the other is necessary. The conversion may be necessary if extensive adhesions, gallstones within the common bile duct, unusual vascular or ductal anatomy, unsuspected pathology of the abdomen, or excessive bleeding complicates the endoscopic procedure.

During surgery, the abdominal cavity is inflated with 3 to 4 L of carbon dioxide to improve visibility. The surgeon removes the deflated gallbladder through a laparoscope. If the organ contains excessive amounts of bile or gallstones, which can prevent it from collapsing, its contents will be aspirated first.

Postoperative care for laparoscopic cholecystectomy. A small number of patients report minor discomfort at the laparoscopic insertion site or mild shoulder pain resulting from diaphragmatic irritation secondary to abdominal stretching or residual carbon dioxide. Oral analgesics or antiinflammatory agents relieve these symptoms.

Oral liquids and a light meal are given the first night after surgery. There will be four bandages at the puncture site on the abdomen. Vital signs are routinely assessed. The patient is ambulatory the first postoperative night.

One of six patients is discharged the day of surgery. Most patients are discharged the next day. Patients are usually able to resume moderate activity within 48 to 72 hours.

Patient teaching. Before discharge, patients should be able to eat without difficulty and walk and should have no abdominal distention, evidence of bleeding, or bile leakage. They are instructed to report immediately any severe pain, tenderness in the right upper quadrant, increase in abdominal girth, leakage of bile-colored drainage from the puncture sites, increase in pulse, or symptoms of low blood pressure. Patients are instructed that they usually can return to work in 3 days and can resume full activity after 1 week.

Although there are contraindications for endoscopic cholecystectomies, most patients are able to choose this less painful, less expensive procedure.

Nursing Interventions. Nursing interventions begin with careful assessment of the characteristics of pain (if it is present) and any signs of jaundice of the skin, sclera, and mucous membrane. The patient's urine and stool should be observed for alterations in the presence of bilirubin.

When the patient is treated conservatively, the nursing interventions center on keeping the patient comfortable by carefully administering the medications prescribed and monitoring the patient's response to the medication. The patient on NPO status because of the presence of an NG tube must be monitored closely for amount, color, and consistency of output. The NG tube should be connected to low suction, and the nasal area should be inspected for irritation and necrosis from the tube. Antiemetics may be administered if nausea persists.

IV infusions are observed for patency, correct rates, and entry sites that are free from erythema and edema. I&O are measured and described carefully.

Preoperative care includes teaching the patient to turn, cough, and deep breathe and to use an incentive spirometer to facilitate air movement in and out of the lungs to prevent pneumonia. By understanding how to splint the abdomen with the hands or a bath blanket before attempting a cough, practicing repositioning in the hospital bed, and assuming a sitting position from a standing or lying position, the patient will be able to follow postoperative instructions more easily. If an open cholecystectomy is anticipated, explaining the NG tube, intravenous tubing, and urinary catheter and their functions will help relieve patient anxiety. The patient should be familiar with any medications that may be used to relieve pain and nausea, and should understand that vitamin K and antibiotics are given preoperatively to prevent hemorrhage and infection.

Postoperative care for open cholecystectomy includes monitoring vital signs and observing dressings frequently and carefully for exudate or hemorrhage. The dressings will usually require reinforcement at the drain site. The patient is placed in semi-Fowler's position to facilitate drainage. A Jackson-Pratt or Penrose drain or Davol, which promotes drainage and prevents pressure and fluid accumulation under the diaphragm, must be monitored for patency. Initially there should be less than 50 ml of serosanguineous exudate during an 8-hour period. The surgeon should be notified if the drainage is excessive, contains bile, or is bright red.

The patient will need encouragement to perform deep breathing and coughing because of the location of the incision. Pain medication should be given frequently in the early postoperative period to facilitate movement and deep breathing. The patient is usually dangled the night of surgery and ambulated the first postoperative day. The patient's neurological status is monitored by checking the ability to be aroused easily, orientation to the environment and family, and ability to move extremities equally on command.

Fluid balance is maintained with intravenous therapy; potassium is usually added to compensate for loss from surgery. The nurse should check the NG tube for proper drainage and may irrigate with physiological saline solution. Usually 30 ml of solution is sufficient to determine the tube's patency. The patient is given nothing by mouth while the NG tube is in place, although sips of water or ice chips may be allowed to keep the mouth moist. The nurse should check the physician's order before giving ice or fluids to the patient, and the patient should be allowed to rinse the mouth frequently. Glycerin or petroleum jelly should be applied to the lips, and the naris through which the tube is passed should be cleansed and lubricated. A tube guard is placed on the nose and to the NG tube to maintain tube placement.

The nurse will be responsible for the care of the T-tube if one is placed. The drainage bag for the T-tube is placed below the level of the common bile duct to prevent the reflux of bile. The bag must be positioned so the tube is not kinked or bile cannot drain from the liver. The position of the bag and tube and the color and amount of exudate must be checked frequently during the first 24 hours and recorded. A gauze roll should be placed under the tube, anchoring it to the patient's abdomen and preventing tension and pull on the tube caused by the weight of the bag. The tube will drain as much as 500 ml during the first 24 hours. The amount should decrease as the edema resolves and bile begins flowing through the common bile duct. The nurse must be careful not to dislodge the T-tube when the patient's dressings are changed as prescribed by the physician.

After oral intake is resumed, the physician may order the tube clamped for 1 to 2 hours before meals and unclamped 1 to 2 hours after the patient eats, to aid in the digestion of the fat. The patient may show signs of distress while the tube is clamped, which include abdominal pain, nausea, vomiting, light brown urine, and clay-colored stools. If distress occurs, the tube should be unclamped immediately. The time that the T-tube remains clamped will be increased as the patient tolerates the procedure. The tube may be left in place for as long as 10 days. The physician will remove the tube when the common bile duct is patent for drainage of bile.

Bowel sounds should be checked every 8 hours to determine the return of peristalsis. A clear liquid diet is usually ordered 24 to 48 hours postoperatively and increased as tolerated. When solid food is started, it will usually be low in fat. Flatulence or nausea after eating certain foods may persist after surgery, and the patient should be instructed to experiment with different foods.

The patient who undergoes a cholecystectomy must be observed for complications. These include jaundice, from an occluded common duct, and hemorrhage, indicated by a decrease in blood pressure, a rise in pulse, and increased exudate at the dressing site. An elevated temperature could indicate peritonitis or wound infection. Pancreatitis may occur after cholecystectomy.

Patients at high risk of not surviving a cholecystectomy may need a cholecystostomy (forming an opening into the gallbladder through the abdominal wall). This can be done using a local anesthetic. The opening will provide a means of removing purulent exudate and possibly the stone. It also allows drainage of the bile.

Nursing diagnoses and interventions for the patient with open cholecystectomy or cholecystostomy include but are not limited to the following:

NURSING DIAGNOSES	NURSING INTERVENTIONS
Breathing pattern, ineffective, related to pain of high abdominal incision and failure to splint area with coughing and movement	Assist patient to cough and to take 10 deep breaths hourly. Instruct patient on splinting techniques. Turn q 2 hr. Administer analgesics as ordered to facilitate deep breathing and movement. Ambulate as early as possible.
Impaired skin integrity, high risk for, related to wound drainage and accidental obstruction of bile drainage	If T-tube is present: Maintain patency and prevent tension on tube. Promote drainage by placing patient in low to semi-Fowler's position. Observe, describe, and record amount and character of exudate at least q 8 hr. Empty bag when half full. Clamp tube as ordered by physician 3 to 4 days postoperatively. Reinforce primary dressing, and observe exudate; change and apply sterile, dry dressing as ordered; use Montgomery straps to secure if drainage is profuse. Cleanse skin thoroughly at insertion site before applying sterile dressing. Apply skin barriers for added protection prn; Betadine ointment may be used as antimicrobial agent.
Fluid volume deficit, high risk for, related to intolerance for diet, nausea and vomiting, presence of NG tube, and amount of bile drainage	Maintain intravenous fluid therapy as ordered. Maintain patency of NG tube, if present. Record I&O. Monitor drainage on dressings if present.
Fluid volume deficit, high risk for, related to intolerance for diet, nausea and vomiting, presence of NG tube, and amount of bile drainage—cont'd	Reinforce dietary instruction for fat-restricted diet. Observe color of skin, sclera, and mucous membrane for jaundice, and signs of bile flow obstruction. Administer bile or bile salts if ordered.

Patient teaching. Dietary teaching is necessary for the patient who is treated conservatively for cholecystitis, as well as the patient who undergoes surgery. The patient who is treated conservatively must remain on continuous dietary restrictions of fatty foods. Foods to avoid include fried foods, cream, whole milk, butter, margarine, peanut butter, nuts, chocolate, pastries, and gravies. For the postsurgical patient, instruction is given to try small amounts of foods that previously caused discomfort and gradually eliminate those that continue to do so. The patient can usually resume a normal diet without difficulty.

The patient should understand that stones may recur elsewhere in the biliary system. The patient should be able to identify the signs of complications that should be reported. These include jaundice cause d by occlusion or stricture of a duct, hemorrhage and/or leakage of bile, elevated temperature, pain, and dietary intolerance associated with another attack. The patient should also be able to demonstrate care of the T-tube, if present on discharge, identify activity restrictions, and identify a date for return visit to the physician.

Prognosis. With prompt treatment of cholecystitis and cholelithiasis, the prognosis is excellent. Laparoscopic surgery has further decreased the number of complications. The prognosis is not as favorable in patients who develop pancreatitis.

Pancreatitis

Etiology/Pathophysiology. Pancreatitis is an inflammatory condition of the pancreas that may be acute or chronic. Although the exact cause of pancreatitis remains unknown, many predisposing factors have been identified. Acute or chronic pancreatitis is generally the result of damage to the biliary tract, as by alcohol, trauma, infectious disease, or certain drugs. Alcoholism and biliary tract disease are the two factors most commonly associated with pancreatitis.

In the pathophysiological process of pancreatitis, the enzymes cannot flow out of the pancreas because of **occlusion** (an obstruction or closing off) of the duct by edema, stones, or scar tissue. The pancreatic enzymes build up and increase pressure within the duct. The duct ruptures, releasing enzymes that begin digesting the pancreas (autodigestion). In chronic pancreatitis, atrophy of the acinar tissue allows replacement of fibrotic tissue, and necrosis of the pancreas occurs.

The development of pseudocysts or abscesses in pancreatic tissue is a serious complication. After autodigestion occurs, the pancreas and occasionally surrounding organs form walls around cystic fluid, including pancreatic enzymes, and necrotic debris. These pseudocysts can develop into an abscess.

Clinical Manifestations. Manifestations include severe abdominal pain radiating to the back. The pain is sometimes relieved by assuming a forward position, taking the stomach weight off the pancreas. Jaundice may be noted if the common bile duct is obstructed.

Assessment. Collection of *subjective data* may include noting that patients exhibit extreme symptoms or none at all. When symptoms are evident, it is difficult to distinguish the symptoms of pancreatitis from other abdominal disorders. The most specific complaint is abdominal pain that radiates to the back. The pain can be excruciating. This pain is caused by the enlargement of the pancreatic capsule, an obstruction, or the chemical irritation from the enzymes. The pain is usually decreased by flexing the trunk, leaning forward from a sitting position, or by assuming the fetal position and is increased by eating or lying down. Other complaints include anorexia, nausea, malaise, and restlessness.

Collection of *objective data* may include noting the presence of low-grade fever, vomiting in 70% to 90% of patients, jaundice if the common bile duct is obstructed, weight loss, steatorrhea, and tachycardia.

Diagnostic Tests. Both acute and chronic pancreatitis are diagnosed by radiological studies (abdominal CT scan and ultrasound), endoscopy, and laboratory analysis of the amount of pancreatic enzymes in the blood. Laboratory tests will reveal an increased serum amylase during the first few days and then increased urine amylase thereafter. Leukocytosis, an elevated hematocrit, hypocalcemia, hypoalbuminemia, and hyperglycemia may also be present. Pancreatic insulin production may be diminished if the islets of Langerhans become infected, and some patients develop diabetes mellitus.

Medical Management. Teatment is medical unless the precipitating cause is biliary tract disease; then surgery may be indicated. Food and fluids are withheld to avoid stimulating pancreatic activity, and IV fluids are administered. The patient is on NPO status, and an NG tube is inserted to decrease pancreatic stimulation, treat or prevent nausea and vomiting, and decrease abdominal distention. A common complaint is constant, severe pain, and meperidine (Demerol) 75 to 125 mg every 3 to 4 hours is administered. Morphine may cause spasms of the sphincter of Oddi and should be avoided.

Parenteral anticholinergic medication, such as atropine or propantheline (Pro-Banthine), will help decrease pancreatic activity. Antacids or antihistamine H_2 receptor antagonists, such as cimetidine (Tagamet), may be given to prevent stress ulcers caused by decreased gastric pH. Antibiotics are prescribed by some physicians to counteract secondary infections.

If the patient has severe acute pancreatitis, hyperalimentation may be required to maintain an adequate state of nutrition. As the patient improves, further attacks may be prevented by maintaining a bland, low-fat, high-protein, high-carbohydrate diet. The diet must be free of alcohol and gastric stimulants, such as coffee. Oral hypoglycemic agents or insulin may be needed if there is destruction of the islets of Langerhans.

Nursing Interventions. The presence and location of pain are important to determine, as well as what aggravates or relieves the pain. Keeping the patient as comfortable as possible involves proper administration of pain medications. The patient is usually on bed rest with bathroom privileges to decrease the flow of pancreatic enzymes. Nutritional needs are met by intravenous feedings as long as necessary. The patient who is addicted to alcohol may go through withdrawal while in the hospital. The nurse must be prepared to protect the patient from injury and provide supportive care to the patient and family. All replacement fluids and medications must be monitored carefully for proper administration.

Nursing diagnoses and interventions for the patient with pancreatitis include but are not limited to the following:

NURSING DIAGNOSES	NURSING INTERVENTIONS
Pain, related to stimulation of nerve endings caused by enlargement of pancreatic capsule, obstruction, or chemical irritation from enzymes	Administer medications as prescribed, and monitor relief. Restrict diet as necessary to prevent aggravation of pain (free from fats, alcohol, caffeine). Use alternative comfort measures: repositioning, positive imagery, and providing time for listening. Monitor NG tube for functioning to prevent abdominal distention.
Nutrition, altered: less than body requirements, related to inadequate intake associated with current anorexia, nausea, vomiting, and loss of enzymes necessary for the digestive process	Administer intravenous fluids or hyperalimentation as ordered. Weight patient daily at same time and using same scale. Record I&O, including NG tube output. Administer antacids and antiemetics as prescribed. Instruct patient in a diet that is bland, low in fat, and high in protein and carbohydrate.

Patient teaching. The patient will remain on a bland, low-fat, high-calorie, high-carbohydrate diet after discharge. Alcohol and beverages or foods containing caffeine will not be allowed if full recovery is desired. The patient should also understand the disease process and the severity of the disease and related complications.

Prognosis. The prognosis of pancreatitis depends on the course and complications of the disease. In most patients, acute pancreatitis is mild, requiring less than 1 week of hospitalization. However, 5% to 25% of patients have a more complicated course. Interestingly, complications can occur with mild, acute, chronic, or severe pancreatitis. Mortality rates for acute necrotizing pancreatitis range from 10% to 50%.

Cancer of the Pancreas

Although once considered relatively rare, pancreatic cancer is now the fourth leading cause of cancer death in men and the sixth leading cause in women. A major factor in the high death rate from pancreatic cancer is the difficulty in diagnosing it at an early curable stage. This disease usually occurs after middle age, with peak incidence about the age of 60.

Etiology/Pathophysiology. The cause of cancer of the pancreas is unknown, but it is diagnosed more often in cigarette smokers, persons exposed to chemical carcinogens, and persons with diabetes mellitus and pancreatitis. Diets high in meat, fat, and coffee consumption are also linked to pancreatic cancer.

The cancer may originate in the pancreas or be the result of metastasis from cancer of the lung, stomach, duodenum, or common bile duct. Most often the head of the pancreas is involved and causes jaundice by compressing and obstructing the common bile duct. As the cancer spreads, the posterior wall of the stomach, the duodenal wall, the colon, and the common bile duct may be invaded. Biliary obstruction and gallbladder dilation are subsequent complications. It is not uncommon for the tumor to grow rapidly and invade the vascular and lymphatic systems. Many patients live only 3 to 6 months after diagnosis is confirmed.

Clinical Manifestations. The insidious onset of the disease with initially vague symptoms generally accounts for delays in diagnosis. Pain occurs in about 85% of the patients. About half of the patients develop diabetes mellitus if islet cells are involved.

Assessment. A psychosocial history during patient assessment may reveal at-risk populations. These populations include engineers, coal and gas-plant employees, chemists, and workers exposed to betanaphthyl and benzidine. Collection of *subjective data* includes anorexia, fatigue, nausea, flatulence, a change in stools, and steady, dull, and aching pain in the epigastrium or referred to the back. The pain is usually worse at night.

Collection of *objective data* includes weight loss, often gradual and progressive, which is one of the earliest signs. Jaundice usually is progressive and may occur late. Pruritus accompanies the jaundice. Many patients have recent onset of diabetes mellitus.

Diagnostic Tests. Diagnosis at the early stages of cancer of the pancreas is attempted by radioimmunoassay for circulating CEA and tumor-associated antigen. Other diagnostic studies include duodenal endoscopy to obtain specimens for cytologic examination, endoscopic retrograde cholangiopancreatography (ERCP), pancreatic scans, and arteriography. A definite diagnosis before surgery is difficult.

Medical Management. Often, malignant tumors of the pancreas are inoperable by the time diagnosis is made. Treatment of pancreatic cancer is primarily surgical and has been associated with a high mortality rate. Cancer of the head of the pancreas is usually treated by pancreatoduodenectomy; the Whipple procedure involves resection of the antrum of the stomach, duodenum, and varying amounts of the pancreas. Anastomoses are constructed between the stomach, common bile duct and pancreatic ducts, and the jejunum.

Another procedure is total pancreatectomy with resection of parts of the GI tract. Subtotal pancreatic resection has complications of postoperative pancreatic fistulas and is not recommended. Combination therapy using radiation and chemotherapy may be used to relieve symptoms but is not considered curative.

Nursing Interventions. Pancreatic surgery is radical surgery that requires critical care nursing. The major aspects of postoperative care are focused on maintaining fluid and electrolyte balance, preventing hemorrhage, preventing respiratory complications, and monitoring endocrine and exocrine functions of the pancreas.

Nursing diagnoses and interventions for patients with cancer of the pancreas include but are not limited to the following:

NURSING DIAGNOSES	NURSING INTERVENTIONS
Fluid volume deficit, high risk for, related to possible hemorrhage and drainage	Maintain patency of GI tubes to relieve distention and compression at the surgical site. Measure I&O and weight daily. Replace pancreatic enzymes to enhance fat digestion and control amount of fat in diet. Administer insulin if necessary.

NURSING DIAGNOSES	NURSING INTERVENTIONS
Skin integrity, impaired, high risk for, related to drainage from wound	Monitor for excoriation and infection; use skin barriers and disposable postoperative pouches and appliances to prevent enzymatic contact with the skin and to aid in the accurate collection and measurement of pancreatic drainage.

Patient teaching. The patient is facing a life-threatening illness, and family members and close friends are important for the patient's well-being. If the patient has an inadequate support system, it is important to use the resources that are available. The hospital chaplain or personal minister, social worker, dietician, physician, and nurse can become a support system for the patient. These members of the health care team can provide active listening and a caring attitude for this patient.

Prognosis. The prognosis for patients with cancer of the pancreas is very poor. Median survival after diagnosis is only 4 to 8 months. The 5-year survival rate remains less than 1%. Resection of the tumor improves median survival to 17 to 20 months, but the 5-year survival rate remains less than 10%.

REFERENCES AND SUGGESTED READINGS

1. Aach R et al: The ABCs of viral hepatitis, *Patient Care* 26(13):34, 1992.
2. Anagnostakos NP, Tortora GJ: *Principles of anatomy and physiology,* ed 5, New York, 1987, Harper & Row.
3. Beare PG, Myers JL: *Principles and practice of adult health nursing,* St Louis, 1990, Mosby.
4. Belcher A: *Cancer nursing: Mosby's clinical nursing series,* St Louis, 1992, Mosby.
5. Boyer MJ: *Study guide to Brunner/Sudarth's textbook of medical-surgical nursing,* ed 7, Philadelphia, 1992, Lippincott.
6. Brunner LS, Suddarth DS: *Textbook of medical-surgical nursing,* ed 7, Philadelphia, 1992, Lippincott.
7. Bryant G: When the bowel is blocked, *RN,* 55(1):58, 1992.
8. Butler L: Hepatitis: a nurse's story, *RN,* 55(4):66, 1992.
9. Centers for Disease Control: Hepatitis B virus: a comprehensive strategy for eliminating transmission in the United States through universal childhood vaccination, *MMWR* 40(RR-13):1, 1992.
10. Driscoll D: Perinatal transmission of hepatitis B, *RN* 55(4):65, 1992.
11. Fong E, Ferris EB, Skelly EG: *Body structures and functions,* ed 7, New York, 1989, Delmar.
12. Gardner S, Sessner R: Upper GI bleeds, *RN* 55(12):42, 1992.
13. Gauwitz D: Endoscopic cholecystectomy: the patient, *Nurs 90* 20(12):58, 1990.
14. Hampton B, Bryant R: 1992 Ostomies and content diversions, *Nurs Manage,* St Louis, 1992, Mosby.
15. Heeg J, Coleman D: Hepatitis kills, *RN* 55(4):60, 1992.
16. Lancaster S, Stockbridge J: PV shunts relieve ascites, *RN* 55(8):58, 1992.
17. Hegner BR, Caldwell E: *Geriatrics: a study of maturity,* ed 5, New York, 1991, Delmar.
18. Hennessy K: National support and gastrointestinal disease, *Nurs Clin North Am* 24(2):372, 1989.
19. Hood GH, Dincher JR: *Total patient care,* ed 8, St Louis, 1992, Mosby.
20. Kiyosawa K et al: Hepatitis C in hospital employees with needlestick injuries, *Ann Intern Med* 115(5):367, 1991.
21. Kohn CL, Keithley JH: Enteral nutrition: potential complications and patient monitoring, *Nurs Clin North Am* 24(2):••, 1989.
22. Krasner D: Six steps to successful stoma care, *RN* 56(7):32, 1993.
23. Long B, Phipps W, Cassmeyer V: *Medical-surgical nursing: a nursing-process approach,* ed 3, St Louis, 1993, Mosby.
24. Marieb EN: *Human anatomy and physiology,* Reading, Mass, 1989, Benjamin/Cummings.
25. Martin F: When the liver breaks down, *RN* 55(8):52, 1992.
26. Marx J: Viral hepatitis: unscrambling the alphabet, *Nursing* 23(1):34, 1993.
27. Memmler RL, Choen BJ, Wood DL: *Structure and function of the human body,* ed 5, Philadelphia, 1992, Lippincott.
28. Metheny NM, Spies M, Eisenberg P: Measures to test placement of nasogastric and nasointestinal feeding tubes: a review, *Nurs Res* 37:324, 1988.
29. Monroe D, Jaffe E: Patient teaching for x-ray and other diagnostics, *RN* 53(4):52, 1990.
30. Pagana K, Pagana T: *Mosby's diagnostic and laboratory test reference,* St Louis, 1992, Mosby.
31. Phipps W et al: *Medical-surgical nursing: concepts and clinical practice,* ed 4, St Louis, 1991, Mosby.
32. Potter PA, Perry AG: *Fundamentals of nursing: concepts, process, and practice,* ed 3, St Louis, 1993, Mosby.
33. Rake R: *1993 Conn's current therapy,* Philadelphia, 1993, Saunders.
34. Renkes J: GI endoscopy: managing the full scope of care, *Nursing* 23(6):50, 1993.
35. Roberts M: Assessing and treating volvulus, *Nursing* 22(2):56, 1992.
36. Schmelzer M et al: Say nope to soap, *Am J Nurs* 93(3):21, 1993.
37. Seidel HM et al: *Mosby's guide to physical examination,* ed 2, St Louis, 1991, Mosby.
38. Steven C et al: Epidemiology of hepatitis C virus: a preliminary study in volunteer blood donors, *JAMA* 263(1):49, 1990.
39. Surratt S et al: Troubleshooting a sump tube, *Am J Nurs* 93(1):42, 1993.
40. *Taber's cyclopedic medical-dictionary,* ed 17, Philadelphia, 1993, Davis.
41. Thompson C: Managing acute pancreatitis, *RN* 55(3):52, 1992.
42. Thompson J et al: *Mosby's clinical nursing,* ed 3, St Louis, 1993, Mosby.
43. Tucker SM et al: *Patient care standards: nursing process, diagnosis, and outcome,* ed 5, St Louis, 1992, Mosby.
44. Webber-Jones J: Declog a feeding tube, *Nursing* 22(4):62, 1992.
45. Wetlis D et al: Gallstone: alternatives to surgery, *RN* 15(4):44, 1990.
46. Wyngaarden JB, Smith LH, Bennett JC: *Cecil's textbook of medicine,* ed 19, Philadelphia, 1992, Saunders.

CHAPTER CHALLENGE

KEY POINTS

- The digestive tract begins with the mouth, extends through the thoracic and abdominal cavities, and ends with the anus.
- The major processes of digestion and absorption take place in the small intestine.
- The large intestine is responsible for the preparation and evacuation of the waste products—feces.
- Mechanical digestion is the physical breakup of large particles of food.
- Chemical digestion refers to the series of reactions that breaks the protein, fats, and carbohydrates into simpler chemical forms.
- Diet therapy has an important role in the treatment of GI disorders.
- Treatment of esophageal disorders often involves providing the patient with a means of eating, in addition to treating the disorder.
- Common causes of gastric disorders are alcohol, tobacco, aspirin, and antiinflammatory agents.
- Duodenal ulcers are the most common type of peptic ulcer disease.
- New surgical procedures are available as alternatives to the traditional ileostomy and colostomy.
- A nursing goal for the patient with an ileostomy or colostomy is fostering patient independence in daily care when the patient demonstrates readiness.
- Keeping the surgical area free of contamination is of primary importance after rectal surgery.
- The approximate location of GI bleeding may be determined by the characteristics of the emesis or fecal material.
- The nurse explains the purpose of any diagnostic procedure, how the procedure is performed, and the preparation necessary for the procedure and assists in the patient's understanding of the results.
- Individuals with inflammatory bowel disease have a greater risk of developing cancer of the bowel.
- Early detection of cancer in the GI system facilitates early treatment and a better prognosis.
- An NG tube is inserted to keep the stomach empty until peristalsis is resumed after a general anesthetic or any condition that interferes with peristalsis.
- Effective postoperative care begins with patient teaching during the preoperative period.
- Cholecystectomy (removal of the gallbladder by means of laparoscopic or open abdominal procedure) is one of the most commonly performed surgical procedures.
- Clinical manifestations of acute pancreatitis include severe abdominal pain radiating to the back; the pain is sometimes relieved when the patient assumes a forward position, taking the weight of the stomach off the pancreas.
- The most common cause of cirrhosis of the liver is alcohol ingestion.
- Pancreatic disorders may cause diabetes mellitus because of interference with insulin production.
- The nurse must be aware of the effect of medications on the GI system and how this may affect the patient.
- Planned nursing interventions must be individualized according to each patient's and family's unique needs.
- Prevention of the spread of viral hepatitis is a primary concern of health care professionals.
- If an infection develops anywhere along the GI tract, there is danger that the infecting organism may reach the liver through the biliary system, portal venous system, or hepatic arterial or lymphatic system.
- An important aspect of nursing interventions in patients with hepatitis and cirrhosis of the liver is the relief of pruritus.

STUDY QUESTIONS

1. Because the small intestine needs bile only a few times a day, bile is stored and concentrated in the:
   1. pancreas
   2. gallbladder
   3. liver
   4. small intestine
2. Although food is digested throughout the alimentary canal, up to 90% of digestion is accomplished in the:
   1. gallbladder
   2. mouth
   3. small intestine
   4. large intestine
3. Calcified tissue that gives shape and structure to the tooth is called:
   1. enamel
   2. dentin
   3. pulp
   4. gingivae
4. The exit from the stomach is called the:
   1. cardiac sphincter
   2. pyloric sphincter
   3. lesser curvature
   4. greater curvature

5. The intrinsic factor is a gastric secretion necessary for the intestinal absorption of vitamin:
   1. B_1
   2. B_{12}
   3. C
   4. K
6. Which organ manufactures heparin, prothrombin, and fibrinogen?
   1. gallbladder
   2. liver
   3. pancreas
   4. salivary gland
7. The digestive enzyme present in saliva is called:
   1. ptyalin
   2. sucrase
   3. lipase
   4. trypsin
8. What is the largest membrane of the body that covers most of the abdominal organs?
   1. ampulla of Vater
   2. peritoneum
   3. mesentery
   4. omentum
9. Another name for the buccal cavity is the:
   1. stomach
   2. liver
   3. mouth
   4. vermiform appendix
10. In preparing the patient for endoscopic examination of the upper GI tract, the patient's pharynx is anesthetized with Xylocaine. Nursing interventions include:
    1. allowing fluids up to 4 hours before exam
    2. withholding anticholinergic medications
    3. prohibiting smoking before the test
    4. keeping patient NPO until gag reflex returns
11. Liver biopsy is a safe, simple, and valuable method of diagnosing pathological liver conditions. However, the nurse must anticipate possible complications, including which one of the following nursing diagnoses:
    1. pain, related to leakage of blood and bile into peritoneal cavity
    2. noncompliance, of medications, related to testing procedure
    3. social isolation, related to tissue sample being removed for biopsy
    4. sleep pattern disturbance, related to lack of information on hospital protocol
12. Mr. Sones, 35 years of age, has been admitted with a diagnosis of peptic ulcers. The nurse recognizes the following drugs as those most commonly used in these patients to decrease acid secretions:
    1. Maalox and Kayexalate
    2. Tagamet and Zantac
    3. Erythromycin and Flagyl
    4. Dyazide and Carafate
13. Mrs. Powell is scheduled in the morning for a hemicolectomy for removal of a cancerous tumor of the ascending colon. The physician has ordered intestinal antibiotics preoperatively to:
    1. decrease the bulk of colon contents
    2. reduce the bacteria content of the colon
    3. soften the stool
    4. prevent pneumonia
14. Nurses, as well as other health care providers, are at risk for hepatitis B. For prophylaxis to be most effective in these workers:
    1. prophylaxis must be instituted before exposure
    2. prophylaxis can be instituted either before or after exposure
    3. prophylaxis must be instituted after exposure
    4. prophylaxis instituted before or after exposure is effective forever
15. Mrs. Lydia Bailey is a 78-year-old female who was admitted during the evening shift with a tentative diagnosis of cancer of the esophagus. The nurse in her initial assessment finds the patient's major complaint is:
    1. dysphagia
    2. malnutrition
    3. pain
    4. regurgitation of food
16. Mr. Bockus, a 78-year-old patient, is admitted with common bile duct obstruction related to cancer of the pancreas. The nurse would expect the following clinical manifestations:
    1. brown-colored feces
    2. pinkish skin color
    3. straw-colored urine
    4. jaundice
17. Knowledge deficit is a commonly used nursing diagnosis when patients need information regarding their conditions and diagnostic tests. Before a gastroscopy, the nurse should inform the patient that:
    1. fasting for 6 to 8 hours is necessary before the examination
    2. a general anesthetic will be used
    3. after gastroscopy, she may eat or drink immediately
    4. it is necessary to be an inpatient in the hospital

18. In evaluating the care of Ms. Kucera, a young executive admitted with bleeding peptic ulcer, the nurse focuses on nursing interventions. A nursing intervention associated with this type of patient is:
    1. checking the blood pressure and pulse rates each shift
    2. frequently monitoring hemoglobin and hematocrit levels
    3. observing vomitus for color, consistency, and volume
    4. checking the patient's low-residue diet

19. Mr. Lavern, the staff nurse on the surgical floor, is aware of pulmonary complications that frequently follow upper abdominal incisions. These are most frequently related to:
    1. aspiration
    2. pneumothorax if the chest cavity has been entered
    3. shallow respirations to minimize pain
    4. not forcing fluids

28

CARE OF THE PATIENT WITH A CARDIOVASCULAR DISORDER

Barbara Christensen
Elaine Kockrow

KEY TERMS

ANATOMY AND PHYSIOLOGY

aorta
artery
arteriole
atria
capillary
diastole
mediastinum
myocardium
septum
systole
vein
vena cava
ventricles
venule

MEDICAL-SURGICAL

aneurysm
angina pectoris
arteriosclerosis
atherosclerosis
bradycardia
cardioversion
congestive heart failure (CHF)
coronary artery disease (CAD)
defibrillation
dysrhythmia
embolus
endarterectomy
hypoxemia
intermittent claudication
ischemia
myocardial infarction
occlusion
orthopnea
peripheral
pleural effusion
polycythemia
pulmonary edema
tachycardia

LEARNING OBJECTIVES

After reading this chapter, the student should be able to do the following:

Anatomy and Physiology

- Define the key terms.
- Discuss the location, size, and position of the heart.
- Identify the chambers of the heart.
- List the functions of the chambers of the heart.
- Identify the valves of the heart and their locations.
- Explain what produces the two main heart sounds.
- Trace a drop of blood through the heart and lungs.
- Describe the differences among veins, arteries, and capillaries.
- Trace the path of blood through the coronary, systemic, pulmonary, and hepatic portal circulations.

Medical-Surgical

- Define the key terms.
- Compare nonmodifiable risk factors in coronary artery disease (CAD) with factors that are modifiable in life-style and health management.
- List diagnostic tests used to evaluate cardiovascular function.
- Describe five cardiac dysrhythmias.
- Compare etiology/pathophysiology, signs and symptoms, medical management, and nursing interventions for patients with angina pectoris, myocardial infarction, or congestive heart failure.
- Specify patient teaching for patients with cardiac dysrhythmias, angina pectoris, MI, CHF, and valvular heart disease.
- List the signs and symptoms of pulmonary edema.
- Discuss nursing interventions for the patient with pulmonary edema.
- Identify risk factors associated with peripheral vascular disorders.
- Describe the effects of aging on the peripheral vascular system.
- Compare and contrast signs and symptoms associated with arterial and venous disorders.
- Discuss nursing interventions for arterial and venous disorders.
- Compare essential (primary) hypertension and secondary hypertension.
- Discuss the importance of patient education for hypertension.
- Discuss appropriate patient education for thrombophlebitis.

RELATED TOPICS OF INTEREST

- Communication (Chapter 4)
- The nursing process (Chapter 5)
- Signs, symptoms, and physical assessment (Chapter 9)
- Basic nutrition (Chapter 18)
- Diet therapy (Chapter 19)
- Care of the patient with a gastrointestinal or accessory organ disorder (Chapter 27)
- Care of the patient with a respiratory disorder (Chapter 31)
- Cardiopulmonary resuscitation (Chapter 50)

ANATOMY AND PHYSIOLOGY

The cardiovascular (circulatory) system is the transportation system of the body. It delivers oxygen and nutrition to the cells to support their individual activities and transports the cells' waste products to the appropriate organ for disposal.

In ancient times the blood was referred to as the "river of life" or "fluid of life." Some even believed it had magical properties. All knew it was necessary to maintain life. This chapter discusses the structure and function of the blood vessels and the heart.

Heart

The heart is a remarkable organ, not much bigger than the fist (Fig. 28-1). It is responsible for pumping 1000 gallons of blood every day through the closed circuit of blood vessels. It beats 100,000 times a day and transports the blood 60,000 miles through a network of blood vessels. The heart is a hollow organ composed mainly of muscle tissue with a series of one-way valves.

The heart is located in the chest cavity between the lungs in a region called the **mediastinum** (the mass of

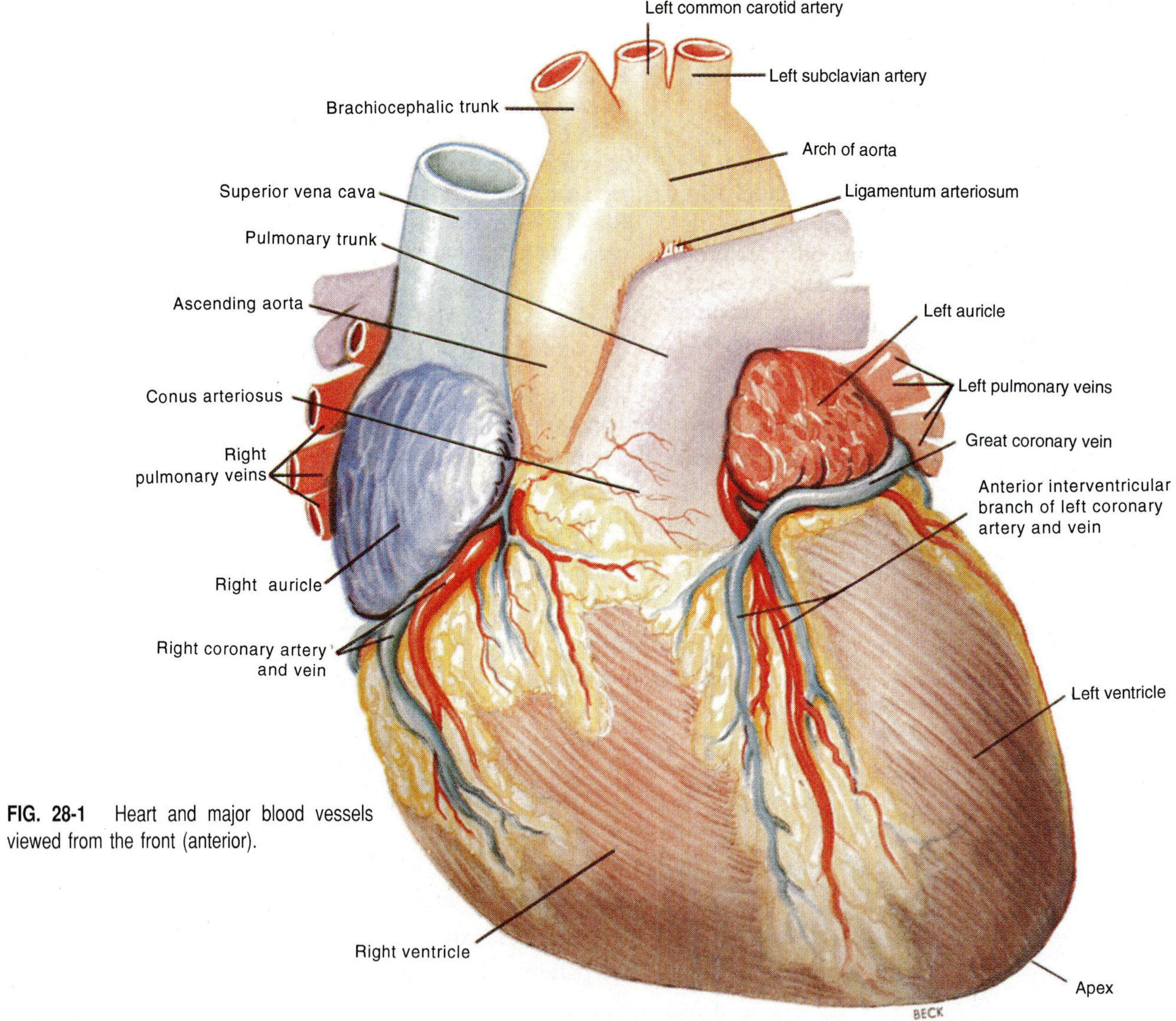

FIG. 28-1 Heart and major blood vessels viewed from the front (anterior).

organs and tissues separating the lungs; it contains the heart and its large vessels, the trachea, and the esophagus). Two thirds of the heart lies left of the midline (Fig. 28-2). The lungs lie to either side of it. The wider base of the heart lies superiorly and beneath the second rib. The apex, or narrow part, of the heart lies inferiorly, slightly to the left between the fifth and sixth ribs near the diaphragm.

Heart Wall. The heart is composed of three layers: epicardium, myocardium, and endocardium. The total structure is covered by a two-layered serous membrane called the *pericardium.* The inner layer is the *visceral pericardium,* which adheres to the heart, whereas the outer layer, the parietal pericardium, anchors the heart within the chest wall. Between the two thin membranes is a serous fluid that allows friction-free movement of the heart as it contracts and relaxes.

The **myocardium** (a thick, contractile, middle layer of uniquely constructed and arranged muscle cells that forms the bulk of the heart wall; the middle layer) is the thickest and strongest layer of the heart. It is composed of cardiac muscle tissue. The contraction of this tissue is responsible for the pumping of the blood.

The *endocardium* (innermost layer) is composed of a thin layer of connective tissue. This structure lines the interior of the heart, the valves, and the large vessels of the heart.

Heart Chambers. The heart is divided into a right and left half by a muscular partition called the **septum** (Fig. 28-3 on p. 724). There are four chambers: two **atria** (a chamber or cavity such as the upper chambers of the heart) and two **ventricles** (a small cavity; either of the two lower chambers of the heart that, when filled with blood, contract to propel the blood into the arteries). The upper chambers are the right and left atria, and the lower chambers are the left and right ventricles. The septum dividing the atria is called the *interatrial septum,* and the septum dividing the ventricles is called the *interventricular septum.* In the normal healthy heart there is no opening between the right and left sides of the heart. Each chamber of the heart and its function will be discussed in the text that follows.

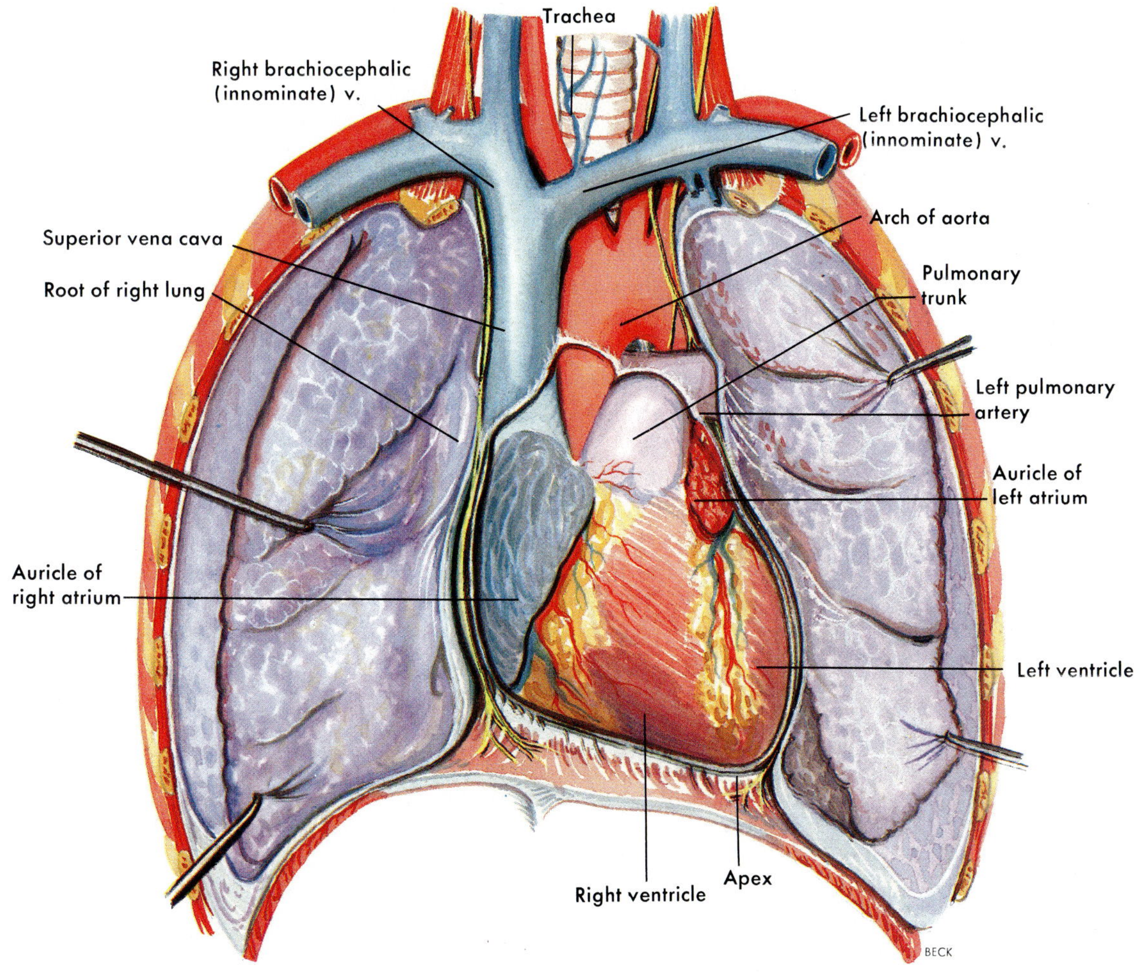

FIG. 28-2 Anatomical relationship of the heart to other structures in the thoracic cavity.

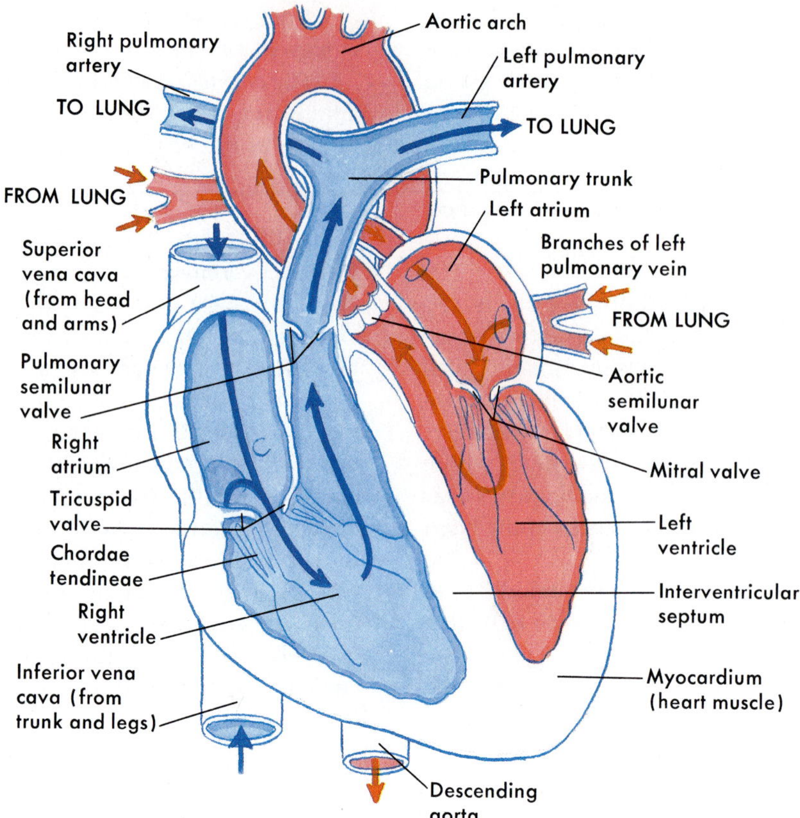

FIG. 28-3 Cutaway view of the front section of the heart showing the four chambers, the valves, the openings, and the major vessels. *Arrows* indicate the direction of blood flow; the blue areas represent unoxygenated blood, and the red areas represent oxygenated blood.

Right atrium. The upper right chamber, the right atrium, receives deoxygenated blood from the entire body. The superior vena cava returns blood from the head, neck, arms, and trunk. The inferior vena cava returns blood from the lower body. The coronary sinus returns it from the heart muscle.

Right ventricle. The right ventricle is the lower right chamber, and it receives blood from the right atrium. It should be remembered that this blood is deoxygenated. The right ventricle pumps it to the lungs via the pulmonary artery to release carbon dioxide and receive oxygen.

Left atrium. The left atrium is the upper left chamber of the heart. It receives the oxygenated blood from the lungs via the four pulmonary veins.

Left ventricle. The left ventricle is the lower left chamber of the heart. It receives the oxygenated blood from the left atrium. It is the thickest, most muscular section of the heart and pumps the oxygenated blood out through the aorta to all parts of the body. The heart actually functions as two separate pumps: the right side receives deoxygenated blood and pumps it to the lungs, and the left side receives the oxygenated blood from the lungs and pumps it throughout the body.

Heart Valves. Located within the heart are four *valves* that keep the blood moving forward and prevent backflow. The heart has two *atrioventricular (AV) valves.* They are located between the atria and ventricles. The right AV valve is located between the right atrium and right ventricle. It is called the *tricuspid* valve because it contains three flaps, or cusps. The left AV valve is composed of two cusps (bicuspid) and is commonly called the *mitral valve.* It is located between the left atrium and the left ventricle. Both the bicuspid and tricuspid valves open to allow blood to flow from the atria to the ventricles and then close rapidly to prevent backflow. Small, cordlike structures, chordae tendineae, connect the AV valves to the walls of the heart and work with papillary muscles located in the walls of the ventricles to make a tight seal to prevent backflow when the ventricles contract.

The two remaining valves, the *semilunar valves,* are located at the points where the blood exits the ventricles. The pulmonary semilunar valve is located between the right ventricle and the pulmonary artery. Blood is pushed out of the right ventricle and travels to the lung via the pulmonary artery. The aortic semilunar valve is located between the left ventricle and the aorta.

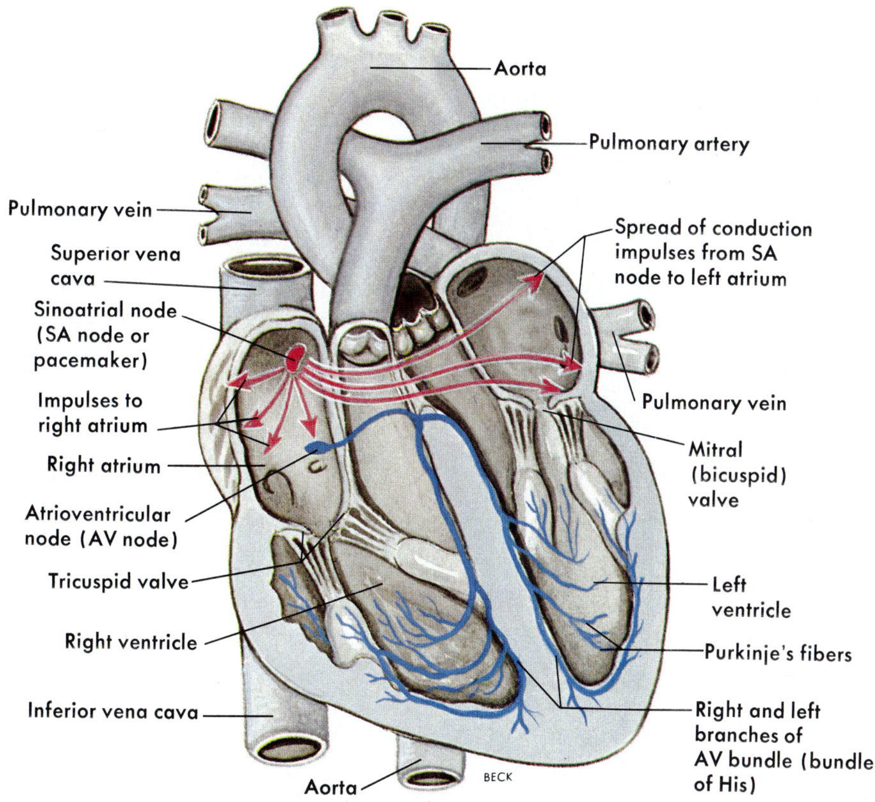

FIG. 28-4 The conduction system of the heart. The SA node in the wall of the right atrium sets the basic pace of the heart's rhythm, so it is called the *pacemaker.*

When the left ventricle contracts, the blood is forced into the aorta and the semilunar valve closes. Both of the semilunar valves are composed of three cusps that resemble a half moon, hence the name *semilunar.*

Electrical Conduction System. Heart muscle tissue contains an inherent ability to contract in a rhythmic pattern. This ability is called *automaticity.* If heart muscle cells are removed and placed under a microscope, they continue to beat. In addition, they have the ability to respond to a stimulus the same as nerve cells. This unique property is called *irritability.* Automaticity and irritability are two characteristics that affect the functions of the conduction system. Hormones, ion concentration, and changes in body temperature also affect the following functions:

- Conduction of messages around the heart
- Initiation of heartbeat
- Coordination of beating patterns between the atria and the ventricles

The heartbeat is initiated in the sinoatrial (SA) node, which is located in the upper part of the right atrium just below the opening of the superior vena cava (Fig. 28-4). Because it regulates the beat of the heart, it is known as the *pacemaker,* and it causes contraction of the atria. Impulses are passed to the AV node, which is located in the base of the right atrium. The impulses are slowed by the AV node to allow the atria to complete contraction and to allow the ventricles to fill. The impulse then passes to a group of conduction fibers called the *bundle of His (AV bundle)* and break into right and left branches to travel to smaller branches called the *Purkinje fibers,* which surround the ventricles. The message travels rapidly through the ventricles and causes contraction. This causes emptying of the ventricles.

Brief description of the impulse pattern: SA node → AV node → bundle of His → right and left bundle branches → Purkinje fibers

Cardiac Cycle. The cardiac cycle refers to a complete heartbeat. The two atria contract while the two ventricles relax. When the ventricles contract, the two atria relax. The phase of contraction is called **systole** (Fig. 28-5 on p. 726), and the phase of relaxation is called **diastole** (the period of time between contraction of the atria or the ventricles during which blood enters the relaxed chambers from the systemic circulation and the lungs—Fig. 28-6 on p. 726). Complete diastole and systole of both atria and ventricles are a cardiac cycle; this takes an average of 0.8 second.

The heart sounds *(lubb* and *dubb)* are produced by closure of the valves. The first sound, lubb (long and low

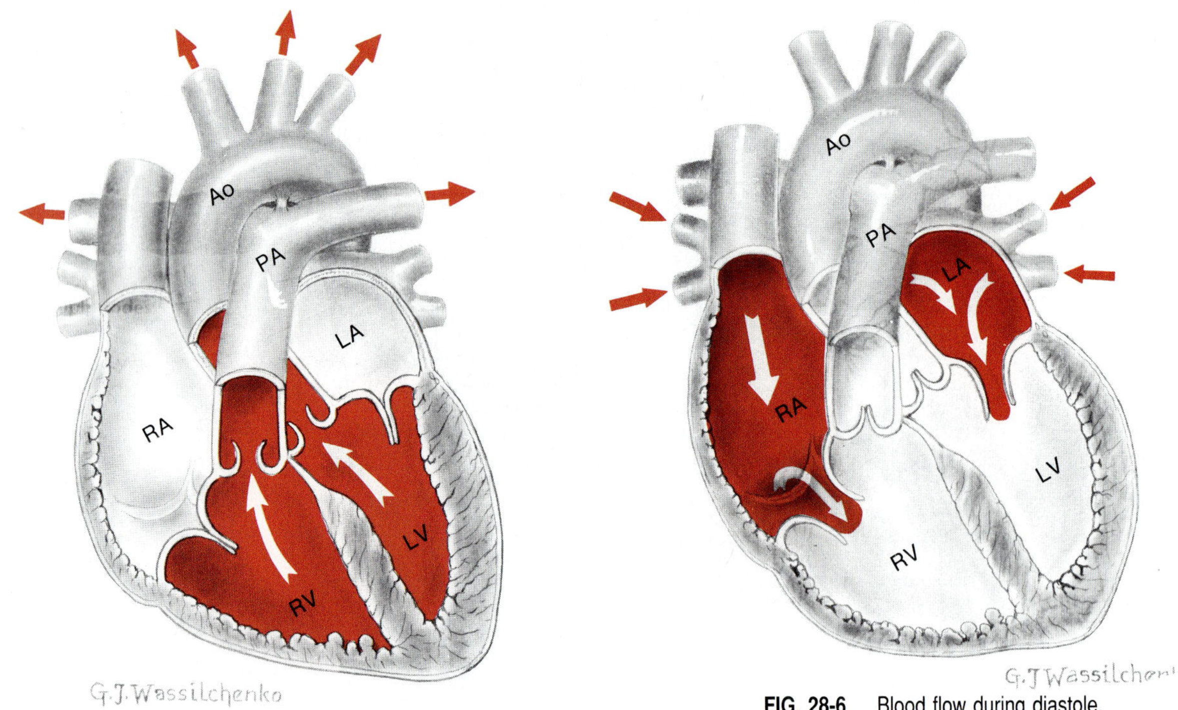

FIG. 28-5 Blood flow during systole.

FIG. 28-6 Blood flow during diastole.

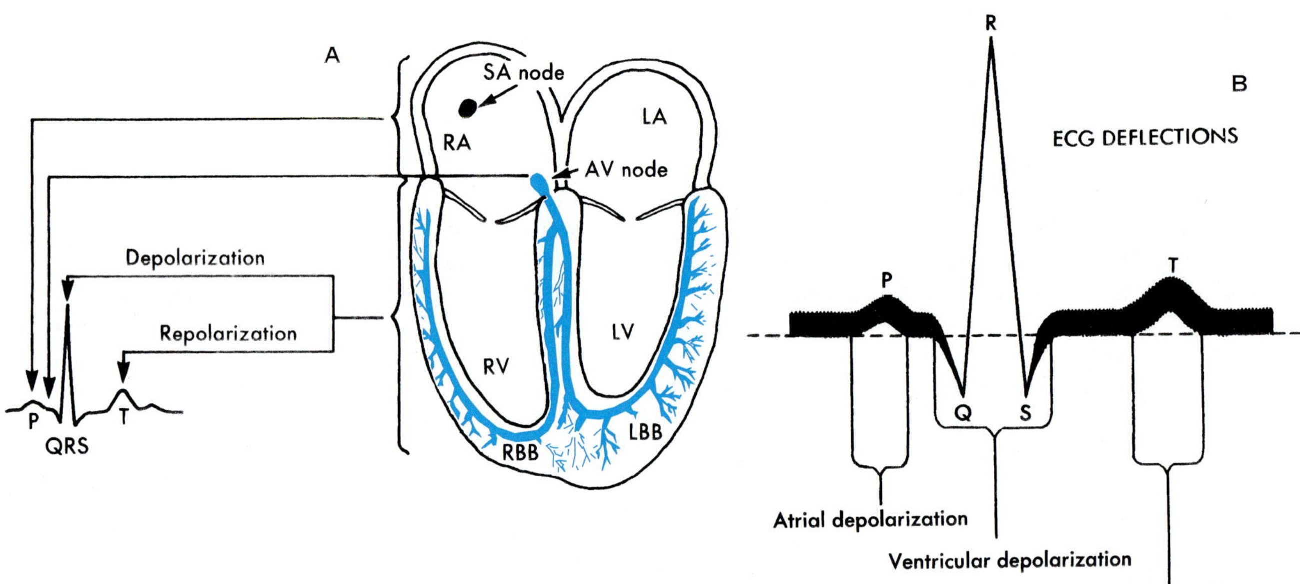

FIG. 28-7 Normal ECG deflections. **A,** P wave, QRS complex, and T wave. **B,** Relationship of ECG to cardiac muscle activity. *RBB,* Right bundle block; *LBB,* left bundle block.

pitched), is heard when the AV valves close. The second sound, dubb (short, sharp sound), is heard when the semilunar valves close. Occasionally a murmur (swishing sound) can be heard. This can be a normal functional phenomenon produced by rapid filling of the ventricles or an abnormal condition produced by ineffective closure of the valves.

Electrocardiogram. As the heart goes through its cycle, tiny electrical currents are produced that can be measured and are of clinical value in diagnosing the condition of the heart. A normal tracing is shown in Fig. 28-7.

Each electrocardiogram (ECG) has three distinct waves, or deflections: the *P wave,* the *QRS complex,* and the *T wave.* When the heart contracts, the electrical ac-

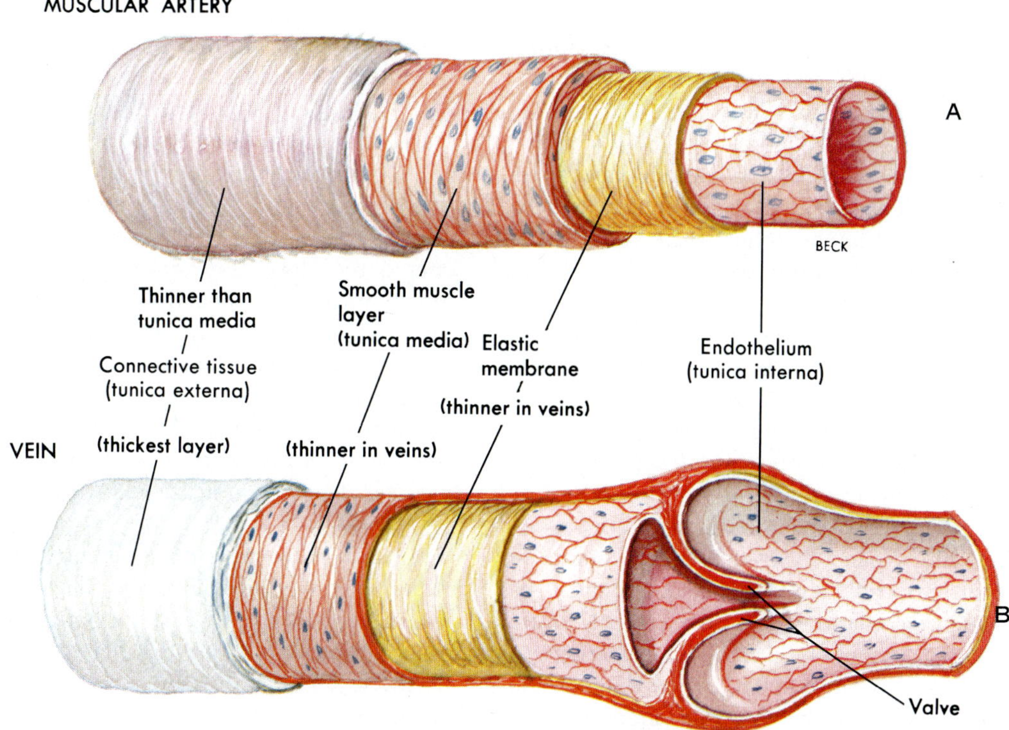

FIG. 28-8 Artery and vein. Schematic drawing of an artery **(A)** and a vein **(B)** shows comparative thicknesses of the three layers: the outer layer or tunica externa, the muscle layer or tunica media, and the tunica interna lined with endothelium. Note that the muscle and outer layers are much thinner in veins than in arteries and that veins have valves.

tivity is called *depolarization. Repolarization* is the relaxation phase. The P wave represents the depolarization of the atria. The QRS complex represents the depolarization of the ventricles. The T wave represents the repolarization of the ventricles. Atrial repolarization is not represented but does occur; it is covered by the large QRS interval and cannot be seen on the ECG tracing.

Interpreting ECG tracings requires special knowledge. Interpretation is usually done by a physician, although many nurses have a basic understanding of ECGs. To interpret them, the reader considers the shapes of the waves and the time intervals between them. Many nurses, especially those working in critical care units, can identify changes in the tracing patterns.

Blood Vessels

There are three main types of blood vessels organized to carry blood to and from the heart. **Capillaries** (tiny blood vessels joining arterioles and venules) connect the **arteries** (large vessels carrying blood in a direction away from the heart) to the **veins** (vessels that convey blood from the capillaries to the heart). The veins return the blood to the heart. The heart delivers the blood to the arteries, which branch into tiny arteries called **arterioles** (blood vessels of the smallest branch of the arterial circulation), which deliver the blood to the tissues. Within the tissues, microscopic vessels, capillaries, form an extensive (50,000 miles) network that allows exchanges of products and byproducts between the tissues and blood. The capillaries then join with tiny veins, **venules,** that link with the larger veins and return to the heart.

A summary of the pattern:
Artery → arteriole → capillary → venule → vein

Structure of Vessels. The walls of the vessels consist of three layers, or tunics: tunica externa or adventitia (outermost); tunica media (middle); and tunica interna or intima (innermost). The tunica externa is composed of connective tissue rich in elastic and collagen fibers. This layer is very thin in arteries but is the thickest layer of veins. The tunica media is composed of smooth (involuntary) muscle. The muscle layer is much thicker in arteries than in veins because the thicker muscle layer in the artery wall must be able to resist great pressures generated by ventricular systole. In arteries, the tunica media plays a critical role in maintaining blood pressure and controlling blood distribution (Fig. 28-8, *A*). This smooth muscle is controlled by the autonomic nervous system. The tunica interna is composed of flat epithelial cells, which allows the blood to flow freely. Veins have a unique structural feature: they are equipped with one-way valves that prevent the backflow of blood (Fig. 28-8, *B*).

Capillaries are microscopic and contain only the tunica interna. This allows for exchange of nutrients, oxygen, and carbon dioxide and other waste products as they pass among the cells in the tissues.

Functions of Vessels. Arteries, veins, and capillaries have different functions. Arteries and arterioles distribute blood from the heart to capillaries in all parts of the body. In addition, by constricting or dilating, arterioles help maintain arterial blood pressure at a normal level. Venules and veins collect blood from capillaries and return it to the heart. They also serve as blood reservoirs because they can expand to hold a larger volume of blood or constrict to hold a much smaller amount. Capillaries function as exchange vessels. For example, nutrients and oxygen move out of the blood in capillaries into interstitial fluid and on into cells. Carbon dioxide and other substances move in the opposite direction (that is, into the capillary blood vessels from the cells). Fluid is also exchanged between capillary vessels and interstitial fluid.

Circulation

Coronary Blood Supply. To sustain life, the heart must pump blood throughout the body on a regular, ongoing basis. As a result, the heart muscle or myocardium requires a constant supply of blood containing nutrients and oxygen to function effectively. The delivery of oxygen- and nutrient-rich arterial blood to cardiac muscle tissue and the return of oxygen-poor blood from this active tissue to the venous system is called the coronary circulation (Fig. 28-9).

Blood flows into the heart muscle by way of two small vessels that are surely the most famous of all the blood vessels—the right and left coronary arteries. The word *coronary* means resembling or being a crown. The coronary arteries form a crown around the myocardium (see Figs. 28-1 and 28-9).

The openings into these small vessels lie behind the flaps of the aortic semilunar valves (see Fig. 28-9).

The coronary arteries bring oxygen and nutrition to the myocardium. Once the circulation is completed and the carbon dioxide and waste products have been collected, the blood flows into a large coronary vein and, finally, into the coronary sinus, which empties into the right atrium. These two main arteries have many tiny branches that serve the heart. If an artery becomes occluded, these branches provide collateral circulation (alternate routes) to nourish the heart muscle. If the occlusion is severe, surgery and other procedures may be needed. These treatments will be discussed later.

Systemic Circulation. Systemic circulation occurs when blood is pumped from the left ventricle of the heart through all parts of the body and returns to the right atrium. When the oxygenated blood leaves the left ventricle, it enters the largest artery (2.5 cm or 1 inch in diameter) of the body, the **aorta** (the main trunk of the systemic arterial circulation composed of four parts: the ascending aorta, the arch, the thoracic portion of the descending aorta, and the abdominal portion of the descending aorta) (Fig. 28-10). As the blood flows through the artery branches, the branches become smaller in diameter (arterioles). The blood continues to flow into the capillaries. The capillaries surround the cells, and the exchange of oxygen, nutrients, and carbon dioxide and other waste products occurs. The blood proceeds to the tiny venules, then to the larger veins, and finally returns to the right atrium via the largest vein, the **vena cava** (one of two large veins returning blood from the peripheral circulation to the right atrium of the heart) (Fig. 28-11).

The blood is now deoxygenated and needs to be replenished with oxygen. It is important to note that the upper portion of the vena cava (superior vena cava) re-

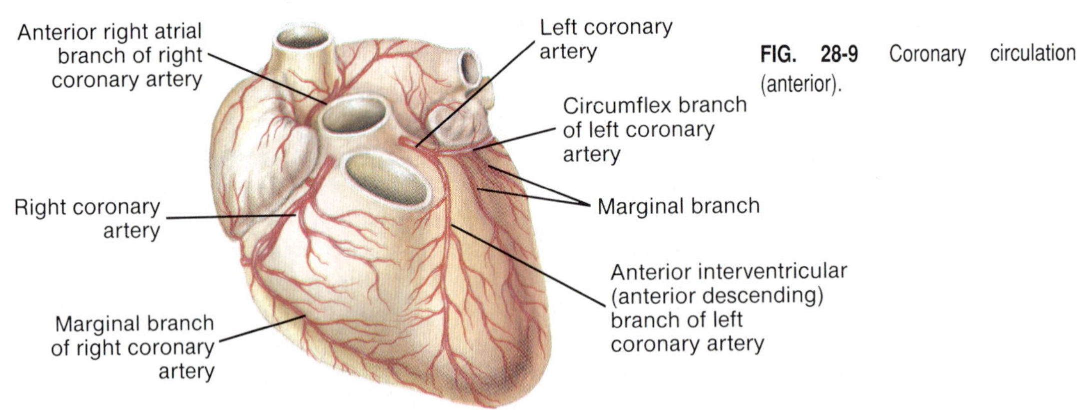

FIG. 28-9 Coronary circulation (anterior).

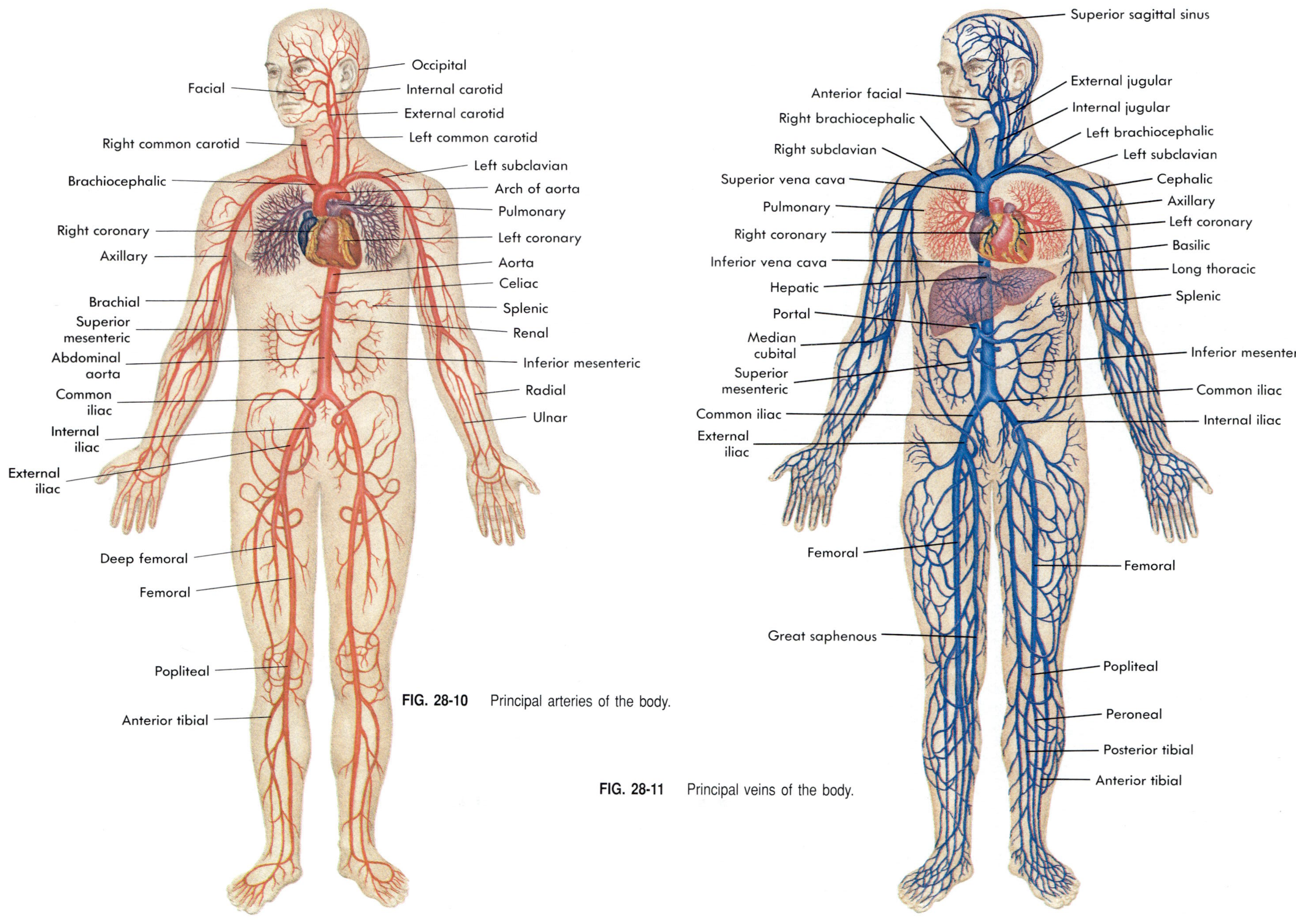

FIG. 28-10 Principal arteries of the body.

FIG. 28-11 Principal veins of the body.

turns deoxygenated blood from the head, neck, chest, and upper extremities. The inferior vena cava returns deoxygenated blood from parts of the body below the diaphragm. To study the names and locations of the major arteries and veins of the body, see Figs. 28-10 and 28-11 on p. 729.

Pulmonary Circulation. The deoxygenated blood will now pass through pulmonary circulation to pick up the needed oxygen. Blood is pumped from the right atrium to the right ventricle, where it leaves the heart to travel via the pulmonary artery to the lungs. Once the blood reaches the lungs, it travels through arterioles to the capillaries. The microscopic capillaries surround the alveoli (air sacs), where oxygen diffuses into the bloodstream. The capillaries then connect with the venules and finally with the four pulmonary veins, which return the oxygenated blood to the left atrium of the heart. It is then pumped to the left ventricle and to the aorta, and systemic circulation is then repeated.

The blood circulation pattern: Superior vena cava/inferior vena cava → right atrium → tricuspid valve → right ventricle → pulmonary semilunar valve → pulmonary artery → capillaries in the lungs → pulmonary veins → left atrium → bicuspid valve → left ventricle → aortic semilunar valve → aorta

See Fig. 28-12 for the blood circulation pattern through the body.

Hepatic Portal Circulation. Blood flowing through the liver takes a special route called hepatic portal circulation. Veins from the spleen, stomach, pancreas, gallbladder, and intestines do not pour their blood directly into the inferior vena cava as do the veins from other abdominal organs. Instead, they send their blood to the liver by means of the hepatic portal vein (Fig. 28-13). The blood then must pass through the liver before it reenters the regular venous return to the heart. Blood leaves the liver by way of the hepatic veins, which drain into the inferior vena cava. As noted, blood normally flows from ar

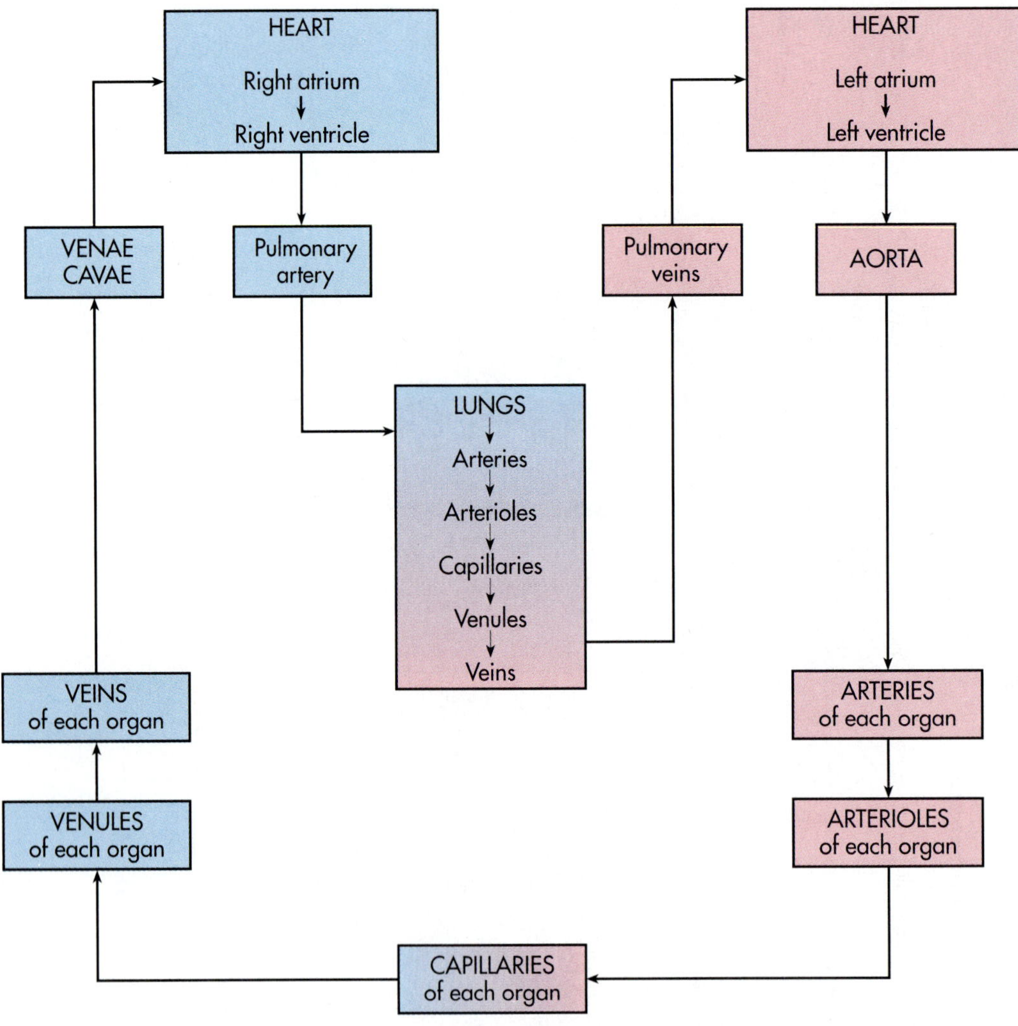

FIG. 28-12 Route of circulating blood.

teries to arterioles to capillaries to venules to veins and back to the heart. Blood flow in the hepatic portal circulation, however, does not follow this typical route. Venous blood, which would ordinarily return directly to the heart, is sent instead through a second capillary bed in the liver. The hepatic portal vein (Fig. 28-13) is located between two capillary beds—one set in the digestive organs and the other in the liver. From the liver capillary beds, the path of blood returns to its normal route.

The detour of venous blood through a second capillary bed in the liver before its return to the heart serves some valuable purposes. For example, when a meal is being absorbed, the blood in the portal vein contains a higher-than-normal concentration of glucose. Liver cells remove the excess glucose and store it as glycogen; therefore blood leaving the liver usually has a normal blood glucose concentration. Liver cells also remove and detoxify various poisonous substances that may be present in the blood. The hepatic portal system is an excellent example of how "structure follows function" in helping the body maintain homeostasis.

From the liver the blood then empties into the hepatic veins, which empty into the inferior vena cava, which returns blood to the right atrium of the heart.

DISORDERS OF THE CARDIOVASCULAR SYSTEM

Cardiovascular disorders continue to be a major health care problem in the United States. Public awareness, modifications in life-styles, and improvements in medical treatment have contributed to a decline in overall deaths since the 1970s. The nurse's role in caring for patients with cardiovascular disorders includes an awareness of the prevalence of cardiac disease, knowledge of risk factors and the disease process, implementation of nursing interventions, and patient teaching.

Normal Aging Patterns

By the time an individual reaches the age of 65, any number of physiological changes have reduced the efficiency

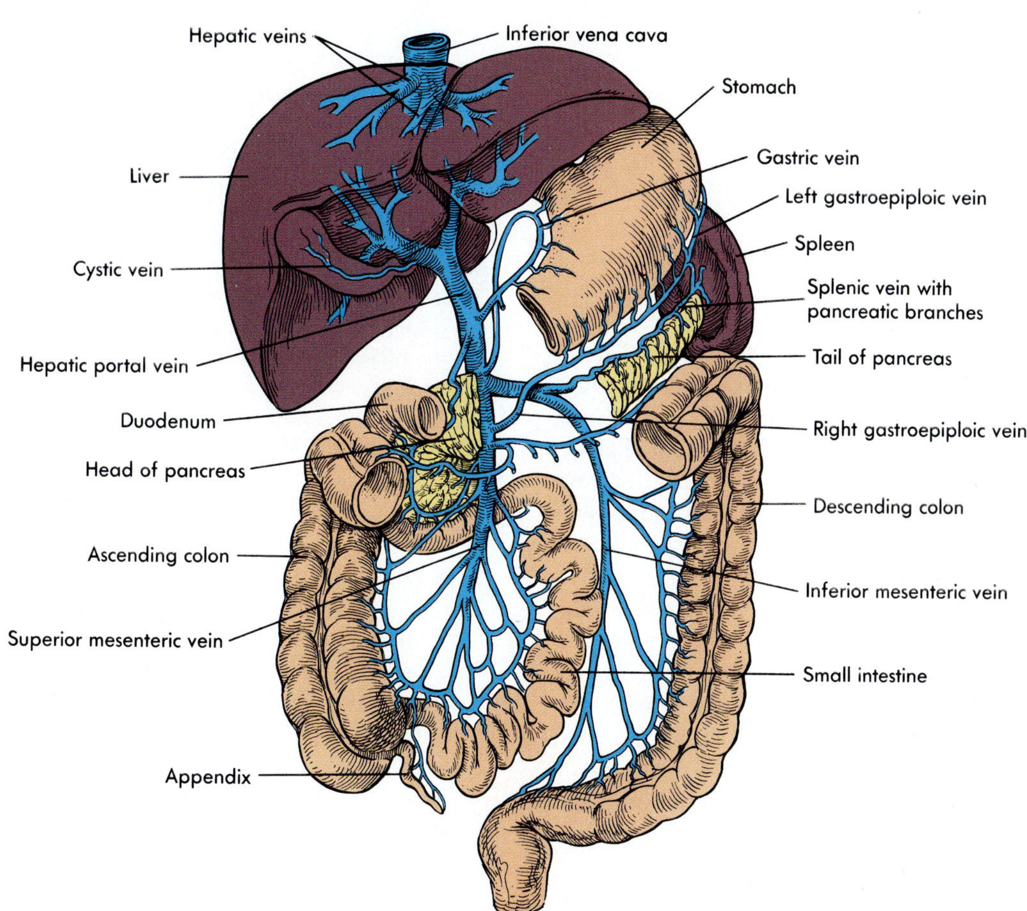

FIG. 28-13 Hepatic portal circulation. In this very unusual circulation, a vein is located between two capillary beds. The hepatic portal vein collects blood from capillaries in visceral structures located in the abdomen and empties it into the liver. Hepatic veins return blood to the inferior vena cava.

of the heart as a pump. Decreased cardiac muscle mass may occur due to atrophy of muscle cells. Myocardial stiffness and a decrease in cardiac compliance occur due to increasing amounts of connective tissue. The aorta and major coronary arteries develop atherosclerosis and become less elastic. There is a decrease in the heart's ability to contract forcefully and quickly. Increased amounts of connective tissue in the electrical pathways of the heart may slow conduction and heart rate response, especially in conjunction with exercise. The heart valves become more susceptible to fibrosis and calcification, causing them to become more rigid. Yet the heart still is very capable of functioning adequately unless there is underlying cardiac disease. Considerations for older adults are listed in the gerontological box.

GERONTOLOGICAL CONSIDERATIONS

- Changes in the cardiac musculature lead to reduced efficiency and strength, resulting in decreased cardiac output.
- Disorientation, syncope, and decreased tissue perfusion to organs and other body tissues can occur as a result of decreased cardiac output.
- Aging causes sclerotic changes in blood vessels and leads to decreased elasticity and narrowing of the lumen. Arterial pathology resulting from the aging process causes hypertension because of the increased cardiac effort needed to pump blood through the circulatory system.
- Progressive coronary artery changes can lead to the development of collateral coronary circulation. This can modify the severity of signs and symptoms seen in myocardial infarction. Angina symptoms may be less pronounced, and dyspnea may replace angina as a key symptom of acute infarction.
- Congestive heart failure can result from rapid intravenous infusion.
- Edema secondary to congestive heart failure may cause tissue impairment in the immobile older adult. Immobility leads to venous stasis and increases the risk of venous thrombosis and embolus formation.
- Older adults with cardiac disease often receive several medications, which are often prescribed at lower doses than for younger adults. Even with lower doses of medications, the older adult should be observed closely for signs of toxicity, since the rate of drug metabolism and excretion decreases with age.
- Independent older adults with cardiac conditions should receive adequate teaching regarding medication, diet, and warning signs of complications. They should be encouraged to maintain regular contact with the physician and to seek care at the first sign of problems.

Assessment of the Cardiovascular System

The nurse begins assessment of the patient with a cardiovascular disorder by performing a physical assessment and by obtaining a complete health history.

The physical assessment includes level of consciousness, vital signs, lung sounds (crackles, wheezes), bowel sounds, apical and pedal pulses, capillary refill, skin color (pallor, cyanosis), turgor, temperature and moisture, and presence of edema.

The history includes a description of symptoms, when they occurred, their course and duration, location, precipitating factors, and relief measures. Specific signs and symptoms the nurse should be aware of include the following:

- *Pain*—The character, quality, radiation, and associated symptoms must be noted. Have patient rate pain on a scale of 1 to 10. Chest pain is the primary complaint when patients give symptoms of heart disease. The patient may use the following terms to describe the pain: dull, sharp, pressure, squeezing, crushing, viselike, grinding, or radiating. Precipitating onset is noted. Pain originating from cardiac muscle **ischemia** (decreased blood supply to a body organ or part) is anxiety-producing. It may lead to other signs and symptoms such as nausea, vertigo, or diaphoresis. Chest pain is significant in indicating cardiac ischemia or damage.
- *Palpitations*— Characterized by rapid, irregular, or pounding heartbeat, palpitations may be associated with cardiac **dysrhythmias** (any disturbance or abnormality in a normal rhythmic pattern) or cardiac ischemia. Patients may begin to notice the heartbeat and describe it as "pounding" or "racing." This can be frightening for the patient.
- *Cyanosis*—A bluish discoloration of the skin and mucous membranes caused by an excess of deoxygenated hemoglobin in the blood, cyanosis results from decreased cardiac output and poor peripheral perfusion.
- *Dyspnea*—Characterized by difficulty breathing or shortness of breath. Dyspnea with activity should also be noted. This symptom is referred to as exertional dyspnea and is commonly associated with decreased cardiac function.
- *Orthopnea*—Orthopnea is an abnormal condition in which a person must sit or stand in order to breathe deeply or comfortably.
- *Cough*—Characterized by a fluid accumulation in the lungs. It may be dry or productive. The patient may describe it as irritating or spasmodic. Dyspnea may be associated with it. The production of sputum should be observed for frothiness or hemoptysis (this characteristic will be discussed in pulmonary edema).

- *Fatigue*—Characterized by feeling exhausted accompanied by activity intolerance is associated with decreased cardiac output. The patient may be unable to perform activities of daily living (ADLs). Depression may accompany this or be a result of it.
- *Syncope*—Syncope or fainting is a brief lapse of consciousness caused by transient cerebral hypoxia. It is usually preceded by a sensation of lightheadedness. It can result from a sudden decrease in cardiac output to the brain as a result of dysrhythmia (bradycardia or tachycardia) or decreased pumping action of the heart.
- *Diaphoresis*—The secretion of sweat, especially profuse secretion; is associated with clamminess. It is a result of decreased cardiac output and poor peripheral perfusion.
- *Edema* or weight gain of more than 3 lb in 24 hours may be indicative of heart failure.

Risk Factors for Cardiovascular Disorders

Risk factors have been identified through research methods that indicate predispositions to developing cardiovascular disease. An accumulation of more than one risk factor is indicative of increasing risk for developing cardiovascular disease. Risk factors are classified as those that are nonmodifiable and those that are modifiable (Box 28-1).

Box 28-1 RISK FACTORS ASSOCIATED WITH CARDIOVASCULAR DISORDERS

NONMODIFIABLE	MODIFIABLE
Family history	Smoking
Age	Hyperlipidemia
Sex	Hypertension
Race	Diabetes
	Obesity
	Sedentary life-style
	Stress
	Use of oral contraceptives
	Psychosocial factors: type A personality

Nonmodifiable Factors. An important aspect of caring for the patient with a cardiovascular disorder is understanding the risk factors for cardiovascular disease and incorporating them into patient teaching. The nonmodifiable risk factors associated with cardiovascular disorders include the following.

Family history. Familial tendency to develop cardiovascular disease has been documented in the literature. A family member such as a parent or sibling who has a cardiovascular problem before 50 years of age places the patient at greater risk for developing cardiovascular disease.

Age. Normal physiological changes that occur with aging as well as past life-style habits increase the patient's risk for developing cardiovascular disease with advancing age. Approximately 50% of all myocardial infarctions (MIs; heart attacks) occur in persons over the age of 65.

Sex. Men are at a greater risk of developing cardiovascular disease than women. Women are affected following menopause because of the decrease in estrogen. The incidence of cardiovascular disease in women is increasing. Factors believed to be responsible are increased social and economic pressures on women and changes in life-style, including an increased incidence of smoking and use of oral contraceptives. There is a growing awareness of women's increased risk factors by the medical association.

Race. Black males have a higher incidence of hypertension than do whites.

Modifiable Factors.

Smoking. Individuals who smoke have a two to three times greater risk of developing cardiovascular disease. This is proportional to the number of cigarettes smoked. Individuals who quit smoking decrease their risk. The nicotine content of cigarettes and the production of carbon monoxide place a greater demand on the heart and interfere with oxygen supply.

Hyperlipidemia. Hyperlipidemia is elevated concentrations of any or all lipids in the plasma. The ratio of high-density lipoproteins (HDL) to low-density lipoproteins (LDL) is the best predictor for the development of cardiovascular disease. Density levels vary according to the protein-fat ratio:

VLDL (very-low-density lipoproteins) = more fat than protein (primarily triglycerides)
LDL (low-density lipoproteins) = equal fat and protein (approximately 50%) with moderate amounts of phospholipids cholesterol
HDL (high-density lipoproteins) = more protein than fat (may serve a protective function, removing cholesterol from tissues)

A diet high in saturated fat, cholesterol, and calories contributes to hyperlipidemia. Therefore, dietary control is an important factor in modifying this risk factor. An overall serum cholesterol level of 200 mg/dl or less is desired. Levels above 200 mg/dl increase the risk of developing cardiovascular disease.

Hypertension. Hypertension is blood pressure higher than 140/90 mm Hg, particularly elevated systolic pressures, that increase an individual's risk of developing cardiovascular disease. Adhering to medical therapy for control of elevated blood pressure helps to modify the individual's risk.

Diabetes mellitus. Cardiac disease has been found to be more prevalent in the individual with diabetes mellitus. This is thought to be related to elevated blood glucose levels, but the relationship is not clear. Adherence to medical therapy for regulating blood glucose levels helps to modify the individual's risk.

Obesity. Excess body weight increases the workload of the heart. It also contributes to the severity of other risk factors. A weight-reduction program and maintaining an ideal body weight help to modify the individual's risk.

Sedentary life-style. Lack of regular exercise has been correlated with increased risk of developing cardiovascular disease. Regular aerobic exercise can improve the heart's efficiency as well as contribute to lowering blood glucose levels, improving the ratio of HDLs to LDLs, reducing weight, lowering the blood pressure, reducing stress, and improving overall feelings of well-being.

Stress. The stress response of the body releases catecholamines that increase the heart rate. The vasoconstriction that thus occurs may be a contributing factor to developing cardiovascular disease. Stress reduction measures may be important in modifying an individual's risk.

Oral contraceptives. The use of oral contraceptives has been linked to the development of cardiovascular disease. The relationship has not been clearly identified. Oral contraceptive use in conjunction with other risk factors is not recommended.

Psychosocial factors. The coronary-prone, or Type A, personality has been demonstrated to be more characteristic of persons who will develop CAD. The characteristics of this personality trait include aggressiveness, competitiveness, and an urgent sense of time. When the Type A personality is combined with other risk factors such as age, high lipid levels, and smoking, the risk of heart disease increases.

Diagnostic Tests

Diagnostic tests to evaluate cardiovascular function are as follows.

Diagnostic Evaluation. The nursing responsibilities are to physically prepare the patient for diagnostic procedures and to explain the examination to the patient. Cardiovascular function is evaluated through diagnostic examinations.

Diagnostic imaging. X-ray examination of the chest provides a film record of heart size, shape, and position and outline of shadows. Lung congestion is also shown, indicating heart failure, perhaps in the earliest stages.

Fluoroscopy, the action-picture x-ray, allows observation of movement. It is invaluable in pacemaker or intracardial catheter placement.

An angiogram is a series of x-rays taken after injection of radiopaque dye into an artery or vein. The circulatory process aids in diagnosis of vessel occlusion, pooling in various heart chambers, and congenital anomalies.

Arteriography, or visualization of coronary arteries, is used to determine the extent of coronary occlusion by use of a radiopaque catheter threaded into areas suspected of occlusion.

An aortogram visualizes the abdominal aorta and the major leg arteries by use of dye injected through the femoral artery. X-ray visualization is employed. Aneurysms and many other abnormalities can be diagnosed. Contrast media to visualize the aortic arch and branches may also be employed.

Cardiac catheterization and angiography. Cardiac catheterization is an invasive procedure used to visualize the heart's chambers, valves, great vessels, and coronary arteries.

The passage of a catheter into the heart chambers through a peripheral vessel is used to measure (1) pressure within the heart and (2) blood-volume relationship to cardiac competence. Valvular defects, occlusion, and congenital anomalies are determined. Blood samples are obtained. Contrast dye may be injected to allow better heart and vessel visualization (angiography). Because iodine is in the contrast medium, sensitivity to iodine is determined before injection to avoid allergic reaction, which could be a dangerous complication of this procedure. Cardiac catheterization is performed under sterile surgical conditions, and its invasive characteristic requires a prior signed consent and standard preoperative teaching. This procedure aids in diagnosis, in prevention of progression of cardiac conditions, and in accuracy in evaluation and treatment of the critically ill patient.

Electrocardiography. The electrocardiogram (ECG/EKG) is a graphic study of the electrical activities of the myocardium to determine transmission of cardiac impulses through the muscles/conduction tissue. Rhythmic disturbance, myocardial damage, and hyperkalemia (elevated serum potassium) can be determined by the physician through ECG.

A standard ECG has 12 electrodes, or leads: six are placed on the chest in different positions and six on the limbs. A conductive gel is used to enhance the contact and transmission. The patient is in a supine position. However, ambulatory ECGs and exercise/stress test ECGs require position variation. The machine, an electrocardiograph or galvanometer, records the energy wave of each heartbeat through a vibrating needle on graph paper, which feeds through the machine at a standard rate. Each ECG waveform represents a single electrical impulse as it travels through the heart (see Fig. 28-7).

The ECG tracing is "read" or interpreted by a cardiac specialist (cardiologist) as well as by internal medicine specialists, family practitioners, pediatricians, and emergency room physicians. The reading can also be displayed on the fluorescent screen (oscilloscope) of a cardiac monitor. A graphic tracing may be printed out by the monitor.

Ambulatory ECGs, can be used to monitor heart rhythm over prolonged periods—12, 24, or 48 hours—and compared with various activities or symptoms as recorded in a diary kept by the patient. A Holter monitor (small portable recorder) is attached to the patient by one to four leads, with a 2-pound tape recorder carried on a belt or shoulder strap. The monitor operates continuously to record the patterns and rhythms of the patient's heartbeat. In conjunction with the diary of activities and symptoms kept by the patient, the physician can note various events, times, and medication peaks that affect or precipitate dysrhythmias. An ambulatory ECG is particularly useful for patients whose clinical symptoms indicate heart disorder but may have normal ECG tracings on standard testing.

Cardiac monitors. It is common practice to continually assess the cardiac electrical activity of patients who are known or suspected to have dysrhythmias or who are prone to develop dysrhythmias. This assessment is performed with a cardiac monitor, which displays information from conductive electrodes that recognize the electrical activity of the heart and relay it to a video display screen. The electrodes are placed on the chest.

Most monitors provide a visual display of cardiac electrical activity and the correct heart rate. Preset alarms warn of heart rates that exceed or drop below limits considered acceptable for each patient.

Acutely ill persons in intensive care settings are increasingly monitored by battery-powered ECG transmitters that do not require direct connection of the patient to the oscilloscope. This monitoring is called telemetry, which is the electronic transmission of data to a distant location. The electrodes placed on the patient's chest are attached to a transmitter carried by the patient in a pocket or pouch. The transmitter sends a radio signal to a receiver, usually located at the nurse's station.

Patients need telemetry monitoring for various reasons, including a history of cardiac disease, angina pectoris, suspected dysrhythmias, a change in medications, surgery, an electrolyte abnormality, or unexplained syncope. Many of these patients are monitored in a centralized area such as an intermediate care or step-down unit (with monitors at the nurse's station). But remote telemetry means the patient is on a medical/surgical unit and is being monitored at a separate location, called the home unit, which is usually on a critical care unit.

Remote telemetry patients are usually stable. But even a stable patient's condition can change rapidly, and telemetry allows continuous heart monitoring to detect abnormalities.

Attachment to a cardiac monitor does not significantly alter a patient's need for nursing interventions. Placement of the monitoring electrodes on the anterior thorax (chest) rather than the extremities leaves the patient relatively free to carry on usual activities. Special attention should be paid to the electrode site to ensure a constant tight seal between the electrode and the skin and to note the development of any skin impairment. The nurse should also check the telemetry pack for integrity of the lead wires and test the monitoring device's battery with a battery tester. The nurse must also inform the monitoring area whenever the patient is moved off the unit for a diagnostic test because the patient may go outside the monitor's range. Another important safety measure is never to remove telemetry and allow the patient to shower unless the physician has written the order to allow a shower. The patient could be subject to severe dysrhythmia, which would not be detected if the telemetry were removed during showering.

Exercise/stress ECG is another form of monitoring the heart's capability. It is accomplished in a laboratory setting during the performance of a prescribed exertion by the patient. Tasks include use of treadmills, stair climbing, aerobic exercise, and other forms of exertion. Monitored carefully, the patient is coaxed to a limit of exertion to evaluate ischemia, dysrhythmia, and the extent of cardiac capability under extreme circumstances, thus setting the limit of exercise tolerance in cardiac disease.

Echocardiography uses high-frequency ultrasound directed at the heart. The echo, or reflected sound, is graphically recorded. Size, shape, and position of cardiac structures are outlined. The focus of this diagnostic effort is to detect pericardial effusion (the escape of fluid from blood vessels because of seepage, usually into a body cavity), ventricular function, cardiac tumors, valvular function, and congenital heart disorder.

Phonocardiography is the mechanical or electronic registration of heart sounds. It involves the use of electrically recorded, amplified sounds. Special microphones attached to the patient's chest pick up cardiac sounds produced by pressure changes in the heart and great vessels. The sounds are graphically recorded on special phonograph paper so that a permanent record is available. Phonocardiography can be helpful in determining the exact timing and characteristics of murmurs and extra heart sounds.

Vectocardiography is a study of the direction and magnitude of the electrical forces of the heart's action by a continuous series of loops (vectors) that represent the cardiac cycle. It records heart action in a three-dimensional loop—a variation of the standard 12-lead ECG.

Positron emission tomography (PET) is a computerized radiographic technique that uses radioactive substances to examine the metabolic activity of various body structures. In PET studies the patient either inhales or is injected with a biochemical radioactive substance. Specific color-coded images reveal organs' metabolic functions. Used for the last decade to study dementia, stroke, epilepsy, and tumors, PET is proving its merit in the diagnosis and treatment of cardiac disease. PET's ability to distinguish between viable and nonviable myocardial tissue allows physicians to identify the most appropriate candidates for bypass surgery or angioplasty. PET is also able to accurately detect coronary artery disease (CAD)—noninvasively—in an asymptomatic patient, prompting early intervention that can salvage potentially ischemic myocardium when ischemia is present.

Thallium scanning. Thallium 201 is an intracellular ion that is actively transported into normal cells. If the cell is ischemic or infarcted, the thallium will not be picked up and a "cold spot" image is produced. Since the thallium concentrates in tissue with normal blood flow, tissue with inadequate perfusion appears as dark areas on scanning. The radioisotope is injected intravenously while the patient exercises on a treadmill. In patients who cannot tolerate physical exercise, dipyridamole (Persantine) is given before the thallium to physiologically simulate exercise-induced stress.

Laboratory Examination. History and physical examination as well as blood studies aid the physician in diagnosing and monitoring the cardiovascular disease process. The nurse's responsibility is to prepare the patient by explaining the tests and the preparation required for each test.

Blood cultures to detect growth of bacteria in the blood are crucial to the diagnosis of bacterial endocarditis.

A *complete blood count (CBC)* is a determination of the red and white blood cells per cubic millimeter as well as of white blood cell differential, platelets, hemoglobin, and hematocrit. Low hemoglobin indicates decreased ability to carry oxygen to the cells as well as the condition of anemia; elevated white blood cell (leukocyte) count indicates infection or inflammation; and elevated red blood cell (erythrocyte) count indicates that the body is compensating for chronic **hypoxemia** (an abnormal deficiency of oxygen in the arterial blood) by stimulating red blood cell production by the bone marrow, leading to secondary **polycythemia** (abnormal increase in the number of red blood cells in the blood). Chronic hypoxemia is often noted in congestive heart failure.

Coagulation studies are useful in monitoring the patient receiving anticoagulant drug therapy, which is prescribed for patients with myocardial infarction with congestive heart failure. Coagulation studies are also important in patients who have chronic atrial fibrillation or a patient with atrial fibrillation who is to undergo **cardioversion** (the restoration of the heart's normal sinus rhythm by delivery of a synchronized electric shock through two metal paddles placed on the patient's chest). These studies include prothrombin time (PT) and partial thromboplastin time (PTT).

Erythrocyte sedimentation rate (ESR) is used to monitor or rule out inflammatory conditions of the heart. The sedimentation rate is elevated with myocardial infarction and bacterial endocarditis and decreases when healing begins. The level of the ESR also indicates the extent of inflammation and infection in rheumatic fever.

Serum electrolyte tests focus on the body's balance of sodium, potassium, and calcium, necessary for myocardial muscle function. Sodium (Na^+) is necessary for maintaining fluid balance. Potassium (K^+) is required for relaxation of cardiac muscle, and calcium (Ca^{++}) is necessary for contraction of cardiac muscle. The physician compares serum electrolyte levels with ECG changes.

Serum lipids are associated with vascular disease, particularly CAD. Cholesterol and triglycerides bound to plasma proteins are found in the blood as lipoproteins. Density levels vary according to the protein-fat ratio: Serum lipids are associated with risk of cardiovascular disease. An elevated HDL is desired, but LDL or VLDL increases the risk for cardiovascular disease (see p. 733).

Arterial blood gases monitor oxygenation (Po_2, CO_2) and acid-base balance (pH). This test is useful in patients with unstable cardiac conditions to determine the blood oxygenation process and for evaluation of patients in cardiac failure.

Cardiac Dysrhythmias

A dysrhythmia or arrhythmia refers to any cardiac rhythm that deviates from normal sinus rhythm. Normal sinus rhythm originates in the sinoatrial (SA) node and is characterized by:

- Rate: 60 to 100 beats/minute
- P waves: precede each QRS complex—atrial depolarization
- P-R interval: interval between atrial and ventricular repolarization
- QRS complex: ventricular depolarization
- T wave: ventricular repolarization
- Rhythm: regular

A dysrhythmia is the result of an alteration in the formation of impulses through the SA node to the rest of the myocardium, an alteration in the conduction system, or both. Signs and symptoms of dysrhythmia vary as does treatment, depending on the type and severity of the dysrhythmia. A short overview of each dysrhythmia follows.

Types of Dysrhythmias.

Sinus tachycardia. Sinus **tachycardia** is a rapid regular rhythm, originating in the SA. It is characterized by a heartbeat of 100 or more per minute.

Causes of sinus tachycardia may include exercise, anxiety, fever, medications, hypothermia, heart failure, excessive caffeine, tobacco, and shock. Tachycardia acts to increase the amount of oxygen delivered to the cells of the body by increasing the amount of blood circulated through the vessels.

Clinical manifestations include occasional palpitations. Many patients are asymptomatic. Other signs and symptoms may include hypotension and angina, if cardiovascular disease is also present.

Medical treatment is directed at the primary cause. This is a normal rhythm and is not usually caused by a cardiac problem.

Sinus bradycardia. Sinus **bradycardia** is a slow rhythm originating in the SA node. It is characterized by a pulse rate of less than 60 beats per minute. Some sources use a rate of 50 or below as an indication of bradycardia. Causes of sinus bradycardia may include sleep, vomiting, intracranial tumors, myocardial infarction (MI), drugs, vagal stimulation, endocrine disturbances, and hypothermia. Often found in association with MI, it is a beneficial rhythm because it reduces myocardial oxygen demand. This may be a normal rate and rhythm for an athlete.

Clinical manifestations include fatigue, lightheadness, and syncope. Some patients are asymptomatic.

Medical management is directed toward the primary cause of the problem and maintaining cardiac output. Atropine may be prescribed to increase the heart rate. A temporary or permanent implantable pacemaker is sometimes necessary (Figs. 28-14 and 28-15).

Premature atrial tachycardia. Premature atrial tachycardia is the sudden onset of a rapid heartbeat. It originates in the atria. It is characterized by a pulse rate of 150 to 250 beats per minute.

Causes of premature atrial tachycardia include drugs, alcohol, mitral valve prolapse, emotional stress, smoking, and hormone imbalance. The cause is typically not associated with heart disease.-

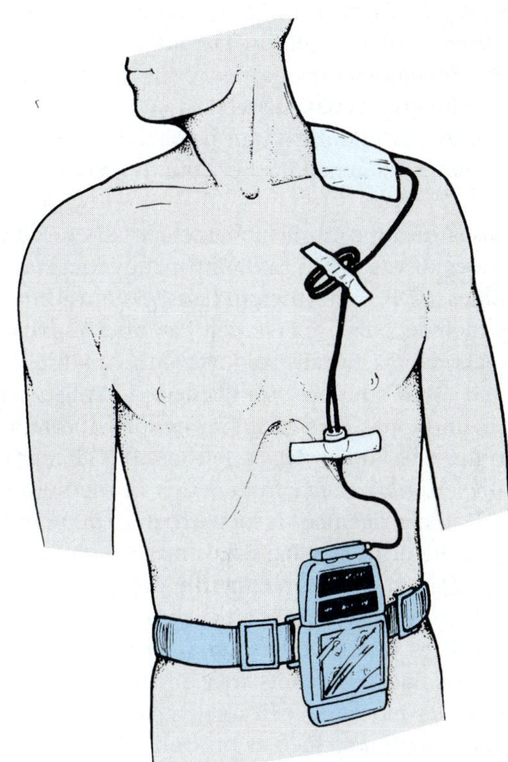

FIG. 28-14 Temporary external pacemaker.

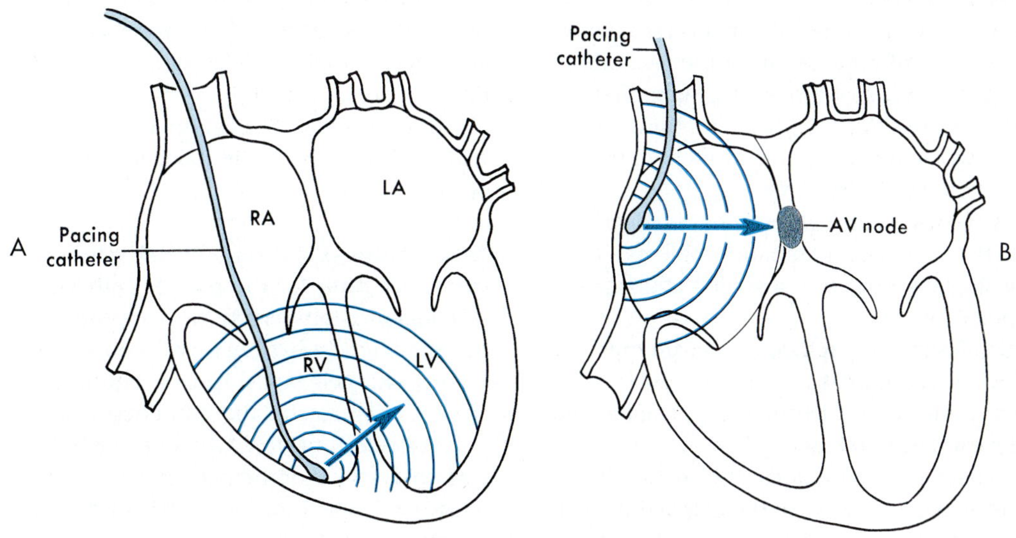

FIG. 28-15 **A,** Ventricular pacing. Impulses are initiated in ventricle. **B,** Atrial pacing. Impulses are initiated in atrium and travel to ventricles by normal conduction system.

Clinical manifestations include palpitations, lightheadness, dyspnea, and anginal pain.

Medical management first looks at how well the patient tolerates the dysrhythmia and at the overall clinical picture. Then the focus is aimed at decreasing the heart rate and eliminating the underlying cause. Specific treatments may include carotid sinus pressure, digitalis, calcium channel blockers, propranolol, quinidine, and cardioversion.

Atrial fibrillation. Atrial fibrillation is a very rapid production of atrial impulses. The atria beat chaotically and are not contracting properly due to disorganized atrial impulses. It is characterized by an atrial rate of 350 to 600 beats per minute. If untreated, the ventricular response rate will generally be 100 to 180 beats per minute.

Causes of atrial fibrillation include atherosclerosis, mitral valve disease, CHF, cardiomyopathy, congenital abnormalities, COPD, and thyrotoxicosis. Clinical manifestations include pulse deficit, palpitations, dyspnea, and pulmonary edema. Because of ventricular rhythm irregularity and atrial contractions, decreased cardiac output is noted. In the presence of mitral stenosis, thrombi may form in the atria and cause embolisms, thus affecting the lungs or periphery (away from center of the body).

Medical management is focused on treating the irritability of the atria, slowing the ventricular response to atrial stimulation, and correcting the primary cause. The goal of therapy is to prevent atrial thrombi from becoming embolisms in the body, such as in the lungs or periphery. Specific treatments may include digitalis, calcium channel blockers such as verapamil (Calan, Isoptin), antidysrhythmics such as procainamide (Procan SR, Pronestyl), quinidine, anticoagulants such as heparin or coumadin, and cardioversion. Cardiac output may be impaired, resulting in heart failure, angina, and shock.

Atrioventricular block. Atrioventricular block occurs when there is a defect in the AV junction that slows or impairs conduction of impulses from the SA node to the ventricles. Three types of blocks are seen: first degree, second degree, and third degree. The third-degree block indicates a worsening of the impairment in the AV junction and a complete heart block.

Causes of AV block include atherosclerotic heart disease, MI, and CHF as the most common problems. Other causes may be digitalis toxicity, congenital abnormality, drugs, and hypokalemia.

Clinical manifestations include no symptoms for first-degree block; vertigo, weakness, and irregular pulse for second-degree block; and hypotension, angina, and heart failure for third-degree block.

Medical management evaluates the patient's response and determines the cause of the dysrhythmia. Atropine and isoproterenol may be prescribed. A pacemaker may be necessary (see Fig. 28-15).

Premature ventricular contractions. Premature ventricular contractions (PVCs) are early ventricular beats that occur in conjunction with the underlying rhythm. The characteristics of the underlying rhythm remain the same except for the PVC itself and the regularity of the rhythm.

PVCs may originate from more than one location in the ventricles and be caused by irritability of the ventricular musculature, exercise, stress, electrolyte imbalance, digitalis toxicity, hypoxia, and MI.

Clinical manifestations depend on the frequency of PVCs and their effect on the ability of the heart to pump blood effectively. Some patients are asymptomatic; others may experience palpitations, weakness, and lightheadness. Other symptoms are associated with decreased cardiac output.

Medical management focuses on treating the cause and prescribing antidysrhythmics such as lidocaine, procainamide, or bretylium (Bretylate, Bretylol).

PVC may be a single event or may occur several times in a minute or in pairs or strings. PVCs that last long enough to cause ventricular tachycardia may lead to a patient's death.

Ventricular fibrillation. Ventricular fibrillation occurs when the ventricular musculature of the heart is quivering. This can be fatal very quickly. This medical emergency is characterized by rapid and disorganized ventricle pulsation.

The cause is usually myocardial ischemia or infarction. Other causes are untreated ventricular tachycardia, electrolyte imbalances, digitalis or quinidine toxicity, and hypothermia.

Clinical manifestations are the result of no cardiac output and include loss of consciousness, lack of a pulse, loss of blood pressure and respirations, possible seizures, and sudden death if untreated.

Medical management is focused on providing emergency treatment, including CPR, **defibrillation** (the termination of ventricular fibrillation by delivering a direct electrical countershock to the patient's precordium), and medications such as lidocaine (Xylocaine), bretylium, or procainamide.

If ventricular fibrillation is not terminated rapidly with defibrillation, brain damage will occur due to lack of blood flow.

Assessment of Cardiac Dysrhythmias. Collection of *subjective data* for the patient with a cardiac dysrhythmia includes observing for symptoms associated with the specific dysrhythmia. Symptoms may include palpitations, skipped beats, nausea, lightheadedness, vertigo, anxiety, dyspnea, fatigue, and chest discomfort.

Collection of *objective data* includes immediate visual observation of the patient when ECG monitoring indicates a dysrhythmia. Signs may include syncope, irregular pulse, tachycardia, and tachypnea. The patient's response to the dysrhythmia is important to implementing interventions. Vital signs and observation for signs of decreased cardiac output should be noted.

Diagnostic Tests for Cardiac Dysrhythmias. ECG monitoring, telemetry, and Holter monitoring are commonly utilized to confirm the diagnosis of cardiac dysrhythmias.

Nursing Interventions for Cardiac Dysrhythmias. Nursing interventions focus on symptomatic relief, promotion of comfort, relief of anxiety, emergency action as needed, and patient teaching.

Assess level of patient's anxiety and degree of understanding, noting both verbal and nonverbal expressions regarding diagnosis, procedures, and treatments.

Provide explanation for the diagnostic and/or monitoring devices in use. Nursing interventions include monitoring heart rate and rhythm. Administer antidysrhythmic agents as ordered and monitor response. Maintain quiet environment; administer sedation or pain medication as ordered. Administer oxygen as ordered.

Nursing diagnoses and interventions for the patient with cardiac dysrhythmias include but are not limited to the following:

NURSING DIAGNOSES	NURSING INTERVENTIONS
Pain, related to ischemia	Administer medication(s) as ordered. Teach relaxation techniques. Institute position change and support. Administer prescribed oxygen.
Cardiac output, decreased, related to cardiac insufficiency	Monitor heart rate and rhythm. Reduce cardiac workload by encouraging bed rest. Elevate head of bed 30 to 45 degrees for comfort. Restrict activities as ordered; plan care to avoid fatigue. Administer antidysrhythmic agents as ordered. Monitor for signs of drug toxicity.
Coping, ineffective individual, related to fear of and uncertainty about disease process	Assist patient with identifying strengths and coping skills. Supply emotional support. Teach relaxation techniques. Assess level of coping ability and family support level. Explain purpose of care as related to specific dysrhythmia.

Patient teaching. Explain any prescribed dietary restrictions, such as the need to avoid products that have caffeine (e.g., coffee, certain teas, soft drinks, chocolate). Explain importance of avoiding or stopping smoking or use of nicotine products. Instruct the patient regarding medication therapy and its purposes, desired effects, and dosage and the side effects to report to the physician. Explain the reason for and method of taking pulse rate and rhythm. Explain the need to exercise to tolerance, to avoid strenuous and/or isometric activity, and to check with the physician regarding limitations and allowances. Instruct the patient regarding energy conservation for ADLs: regular rest periods between activities and for 1 hour after meals; when possible, sit rather than stand when performing a task; stop activity or task if symptoms such as fatigue, dyspnea, or palpitations begin.

Cardiac Arrest

The sudden cessation of cardiac output and circulatory process is termed cardiac arrest. Conditions leading to cardiac arrest are severe ventricular tachycardia, ventricular fibrillation, and ventricular asystole. Because of the manifestation of anaerobic tissue cell metabolism and respiratory and metabolic acidosis caused by the absence of O_2-CO_2 exchange, immediate initiation of cardiopulmonary resuscitation (CPR) is indicated to prevent major organ damage. Signs and symptoms of cardiac arrest include abrupt loss of consciousness with no response to stimuli, gasping respirations followed by apnea, absence of pulse (radial, carotid, femoral, and apical), absence of blood pressure, pupil dilation, and development of pallor and cyanosis.

Initiation of CPR is done by the first person to discover the condition. The aim is to reestablish circulation and ventilation. Prevention of severe damage to the brain, heart, liver, and kidneys as a result of anoxia is of primary concern. The *ABCs* of CPR should be remembered: *A—open A*irway; *B*—restore *B*reathing; and *C*—restore *C*irculation (see Chapter 50).

After successful CPR, the patient is on continuous ECG monitoring. Chest x-ray examination and hemodynamic testing are done, as are arterial blood gas and cardiac enzyme studies. Urinary output is monitored closely. Vital signs are taken every 15 minutes until stable. The ultimate medical intervention is to correct the underlying cause of the arrest.

Artificial Cardiac Pacemaker. Pacemakers are battery-operated generators that initiate and control the heart rate by delivering an electrical impulse via an electrode to the myocardium. The batteries can last 16 years or longer. Implantation of myocardial electrodes is initiated when a patient has a symptomatic AV block. The use of pacemakers has expanded to include treatment of symptomatic *brachydysrhythmia* (slow and irregular heartbeat) and *tachydysrhythmia* (irregularity of heartbeat combined with rapid rate).

A pacemaker maintains the normal cardiac rhythm by electrically stimulating the heart muscle.

A permanent pacemaker is placed when a patient has irreversible complete heart block, causing severe decrease in cardiac output. A temporary pacemaker is used for cardiac support following some MIs or open heart surgery.

Catheter-like electrodes are placed within the area to be paced: atrium, ventricle, or both (see Fig. 28-15).

Nursing Interventions. After placement of a pacemaker, the nurse closely monitors heart rate and rhythm by apical pulse and by ECG patterns. Vital signs and level of consciousness are checked frequently until stable. The insertion site is observed for erythema, edema, and tenderness, which could indicate the presence of infection. The patient may be on bed rest with the arm on the pacemaker side immobilized for the first 8 to 12 hours, and then allowed to resume normal activity.

Patient teaching. The patient should be informed of the necessity to continue medical management, and the nurse should advise that medical-alert identification as well as pacemaker information should be carried. The nurse should emphasize the importance of reporting signs and symptoms of pacemaker failure: weakness, vertigo, chest pain, and pulse changes.

The patient should be taught potentially hazardous situations to avoid. Each pacemaker manufacturer can provide a list of devices that should be avoided by patients with pacemakers (e.g., older model microwave ovens). The patient should be told to avoid holding electrical equipment (such as blowdryers or battery-operated toothbrushes) next to the pacemaker. This may cause interference, placing the pacemaker in a fixed mode and interfering with its functioning. The patient should be taught to move away from any device that may cause untoward symptoms such as vertigo.

The heart rate of the pulse generator for the pacemaker is set according to the clinical condition of the patient and the desired therapeutic goal. With rare exceptions, the rate is set between 70 and 80 beats per minute. If the heart rate falls below the preset level, notify the physician.

The nurse teaches the patient how and when to take a radial pulse. The pulse should be taken at the same time each day as well as when symptoms of vertigo or weakness occur. The following are important to remember when teaching the patient with a pacemaker:

- List symptoms to expect and to report to physician.
- Promote understanding of medication administration.
- Explain treatment outcomes.
- Explain importance of maintaining prescribed diet and fluid amounts.
- Explain importance of not smoking.

Prognosis. The patient can expect to lead a reasonably normal life with full resumption of most activities as prescribed by the physician.

DISEASES AND DISORDERS OF THE HEART

Coronary Atherosclerotic Heart Disease

The coronary arteries arise from the base of the aorta just below the semilunar valves (see Fig. 28-9). These arteries curve and angle in an attempt to adequately supply the heart muscle with oxygen and nutrients. The shapes, contours, and arrangements of the vessels allow for easy entrapment of substances that interfere with blood flow.

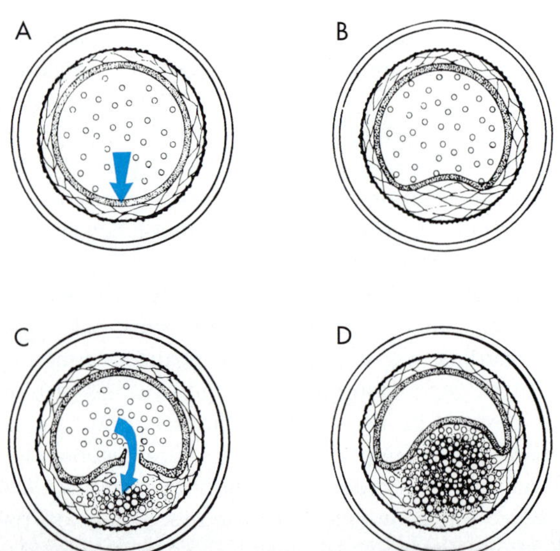

FIG. 28-16 Progressive development of coronary atherosclerosis. **A,** Injury to intimal wall. **B,** Lipoprotein invasion of smooth muscle cells. **C,** Development of fatty streak and fibrous plaque. **D,** Development of complicated lesion.

Coronary artery disease (CAD) is the term used to describe a variety of conditions that obstruct blood flow in the coronary arteries. **Atherosclerosis** (a common arterial disorder characterized by yellowish plaques of cholesterol, lipids, and cellular debris in the inner layers of the walls of large and medium-size arteries) is the primary cause of coronary atherosclerotic heart disease (CAHD). The lumen (a cavity or channel within any organ of the body) of the vessel narrows as the disease progresses. Blood flow to the heart is obstructed when this process occurs in the coronary arteries.

Atherosclerosis, the basic underlying disease affecting coronary lumen size, is characterized by changes in the intimal (the innermost layer of a structure, such as the lining membrane of an artery) lining of the arteries. The severity of the disease is measured by the degree of obstruction within each artery and by the number of vessels involved. Obstructions exceeding 75% of the lumen of one or more of the three coronary arteries increase the risk of death.

The basic physiological changes of the atherosclerotic process result in problems with myocardial oxygen supply and demand. When the myocardial oxygen demand exceeds the supply delivered by the coronary arteries, ischemia results (Fig. 28-16). The artery walls also become less elastic and less responsive to blood flow.

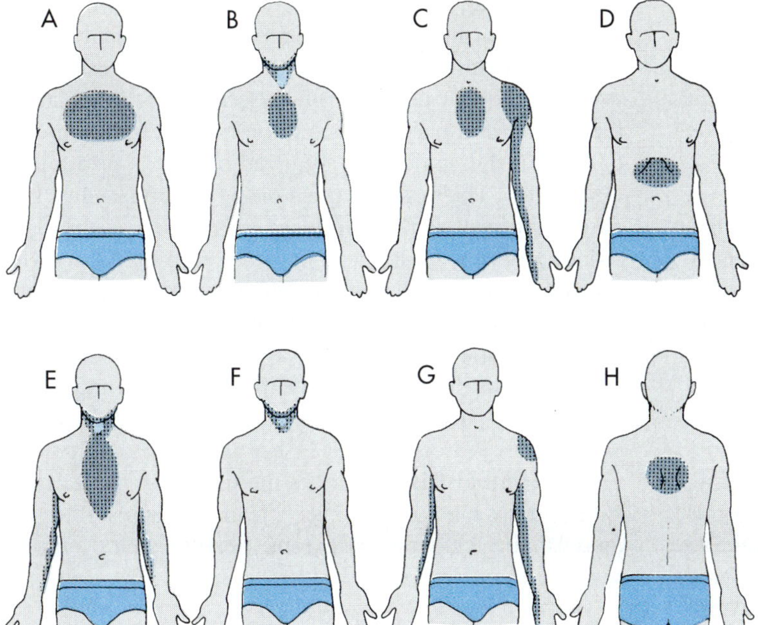

FIG. 28-17 Sites to which ischemic myocardial pain may be referred. **A,** Upper chest. **B,** Beneath sternum radiating to neck and jaw. **C,** Beneath sternum radiating down left arm. **D,** Epigastric. **E,** Epigastric radiating to neck, jaw, and arms. **F,** Neck and jaw. **G,** Left shoulder and inner aspect of both arms. **H,** Intrascapular.

Angina Pectoris

Etiology/Pathophysiology. Angina means a spasmodic, cramplike choking feeling. Pectoris refers to the breast or chest area. **Angina pectoris** is used to denote the paroxysmal (marked, usually episodic, increase in symptoms) thoracic pain and choking feeling caused by anoxia (lack of oxygen) of the myocardium.

Angina pectoris occurs when the cardiac muscle is deprived of oxygen. Atherosclerosis of the coronary arteries is the most common cause. The narrowed lumina of the coronary arteries are unable to deliver oxygen-rich blood to the myocardium. When the myocardial oxygen demand exceeds the supply, *ischemia* (decreased blood supply to a body organ or part, often marked by pain and organ dysfunction) of the heart muscle occurs, resulting in chest pain or angina. Typically angina occurs with an increased cardiac workload brought on by exposure to intense cold, exercise, unusually heavy meals, emotional stress, or any other strenuous activity.

Clinical Manifestations. Pain is the outstanding characteristic of angina pectoris (Fig. 28-17). The patient usually describes the pain as a heaviness or tightness of the chest. At times it is thought to be indigestion. The pain is often substernal (below the sternum) or retrosternal (behind the sternum). Pain may radiate to other sites, or it may occur in only one site. The pain often radiates down the left inner arm to the little finger and also upward to the shoulder and jaw. It may also be described as a pressure or a squeezing sensation, but it is *not* usually described as a sharp pain. Sometimes a patient will experience posterior thoracic or jaw pain only. Other, less common signs and symptoms may accompany the episode of chest pain, such as dyspnea, anxiety, apprehension, diaphoresis, and nausea. The signs and symptoms of angina are often very similar to those of MI. Anginal pain is believed to be a temporary lack of oxygen and blood supply to the heart. It is often relieved by rest or medication such as nitroglycerine, which dilates the coronary arteries and increases the flow of oxygenated blood to the myocardium.

Assessment. Collection of *subjective data* includes noting the patient's statements regarding the location, intensity, radiation, and duration of pain. The patient may express a feeling of impending death. Precipitating factors that resulted in the development of symptoms should be assessed. Determine what relief measures were used currently as well as in the past. Identify whether there have been any changes in the frequency or severity of symptoms that might indicate a progressive worsening of the ischemia.

Collection of *objective data* includes noting the patient's behavior, such as rubbing the left arm or pressing a fist against the sternum. Monitor vital signs and note changes or abnormalities. Increases in pulse rate, blood pressure, and respiratory rate may be noted. Identify the presence of diaphoresis or anxiety.

Diagnostic Tests. The diagnosis of angina pectoris is frequently made on the basis of the patient's history.

The electrocardiogram may reveal findings of ischemia and rhythm changes. Holter monitoring is utilized to correlate activity with precipitating factors. The exercise stress test is used to determine ischemic changes in a controlled environment. Thallium 201 scanning and PET are used to diagnose ischemic heart disease. Electrocardiogram changes are monitored while the patient exercises on a treadmill. Coronary angiography may be done to determine the extent of CAD.

Medical Management. The focus of medical management is to control symptoms by reducing cardiac ischemia. Cardiovascular risk factors are identified and corrected if possible. Precipitating factors, such as exposure to intense cold, strenuous exercise, smoking, heavy meals, and emotional stress, are identified and avoided. Medication therapy to dilate coronary arteries and decrease the workload of the heart consists of vasodilators (nitrates, especially nitroglycerin), β-adrenergic blocking agents, and calcium channel blockers. If angina is present, give nitroglycerin sublingually. Repeat dosage in 5 minutes if pain does not subside. Repeat two or three times at 5-minute intervals. Call physician if pain has not subsided after third nitroglycerin tablet.

Surgical management of the patient with CAHD may consist of performing a coronary artery bypass graft (CABG), which is a method of bypassing occluded vessels by suturing one end of the graft to the aorta and the other end below the area of the occlusion in the coronary artery (Fig. 28-18). Any number of grafts can be done, depending on the areas of occlusion in the coronary arteries. Blood flows to the myocardium through the grafts and bypasses the occluded coronary arteries. The grafts are usually taken from sections of the saphenous veins in the legs, or the internal mammary (breast) artery is utilized.

Another surgical procedure for management of the patient with CAHD is percutaneous transluminal coronary angioplasty (PTCA). PTCA is an invasive procedure performed in the cardiac catherization laboratory. The technique widens the narrowing in a coronary artery without surgery. Percutaneous denotes that the procedure is performed through the skin; transluminal means that it is within the lumen of the artery. Fluoroscopy is used to guide a catheter from the femoral or brachial artery to the coronary arteries to be treated. Inflation of a balloon in the catheter is achieved once it is positioned (Fig. 28-19). The outward push of the balloon against the narrowing wall of the coronary artery reduces the constriction until it no longer interferes with blood flow to the heart muscle. Vessel patency is reestablished by angioplasty (vessel repair). This procedure may take 1 to 2 hours, with the patient usually awake but mildly sedated. Postprocedure nursing interventions are to continually monitor the patient, as with any surgical recovery. Attention to the area of catheter insertion focuses on hemorrhage potential. The patient is monitored in the cardiac care unit, usually for 1 to 2 days prior to dismissal to the medical/surgical unit. The total hospitalization stay is several days.

Nursing Interventions. Nursing interventions are based on the individual needs of the patient. They focus on achievement of five major patient outcomes.

- Promoting comfort—Reduce or remove any known factors that are contributing to increased pain. Assess for causes of decreased pain tolerance, such as anxiety, fatigue, or lack of knowledge. Fatigue from increased oxygen demands with a decreased oxygen supply increases pain perception. Promote measures to reduce fatigue, such as providing rest periods. Provide a calm environment to decrease stress and anxiety. Administer sublingual vasodilators, such as nitroglycerin, as ordered.
- Promoting tissue perfusion—Instruct patient to avoid becoming overly fatigued and to stop activity immediately in the presence of chest pain, dys-

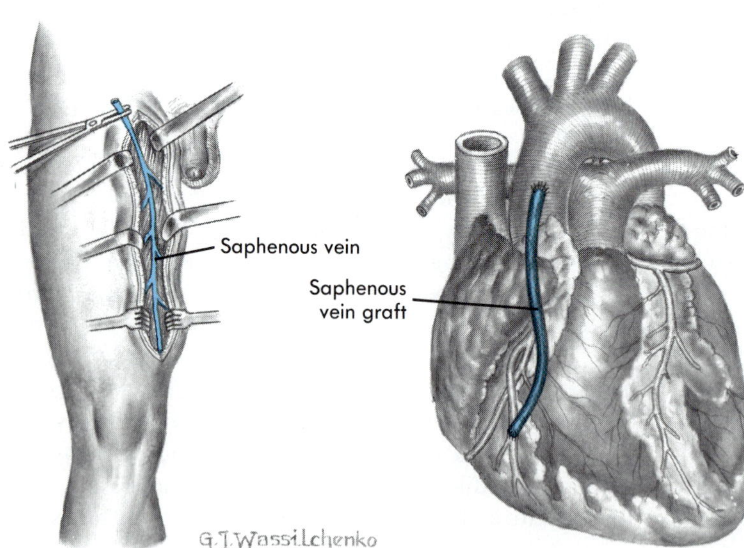

FIG. 28-18 Saphenous vein graft.

pnea, syncope, or vertigo, which indicate low tissue perfusion.

- Promoting activity and rest—Augment (boost or embellish) the patient's activity tolerance by encouraging slower activity or shorter periods of activity with more rest periods. Most people with angina pectoris are able to tolerate mild exercise such as walking or playing golf, but exertion such as running or climbing stairs rapidly causes pain. Anginal pain occurs more easily in cold weather. The key is to avoid overexertion.
- Promoting relief of anxiety and feeling of well-being—Assist the patient to reduce the level of anxiety. The patient should minimize emotional outbursts, worry, and tension. Persons with angina may need continuing help in accepting situations as they find them. Supportive family members, a spiritual advisor, business associates, and friends can sometimes be of assistance. Relaxation techniques and music therapy may be beneficial to the person with angina pectoris. Support peer groups and behavioral change programs are available. An optimistic outlook helps to relieve the work of the heart. Many persons who learn to live within their limitations live out their expected life span despite the disease.
- Teaching patient and family—Delay teaching until the patient is ready. The patient needs to be relatively free of pain and excessive anxiety in order to learn. Promote a positive attitude and active participation of patient and family to encourage compliance. The teaching plan should include information concerning medications, approaches to minimize the events that trigger angina pectoris, effects of exercise on reduction of myocardial oxygen needs, and the need for regular medical follow-up (see the patient teaching box on p. 744).

Nursing diagnoses and interventions for the patient with angina pectoris include but are not limited to the following:

NURSING DIAGNOSES	NURSING INTERVENTIONS
Pain, related to myocardial ischemia	Administer O_2 as ordered. Administer prescribed nitroglycerin. Repeat every 5 minutes, three times. If pain is unrelieved, notify physician. Monitor blood pressure and pulse before and after administration of nitroglycerin. Promote rest. Maintain diet as ordered; if chest pain occurs during eating or immediately after, advise small feedings rather than two or three large meals. Balance rest with activity. Instruct patient to stop activity at the first sign of chest pain or other symptoms of cardiac ischemia.

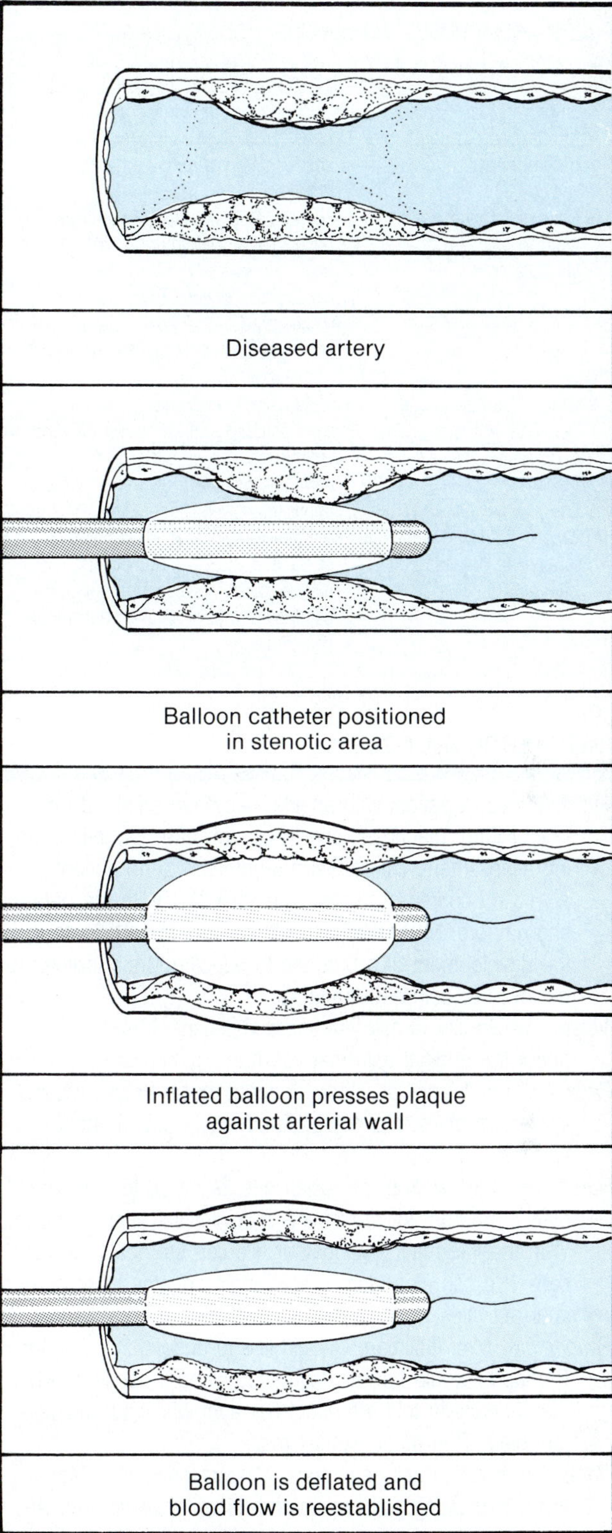

FIG. 28-19 Coronary angioplasty procedure.

NURSING DIAGNOSES	NURSING INTERVENTIONS
Tissue perfusion, altered cardiovascular, related to narrowing of coronary arteries	Administer prescribed oxygen. Instruct patient that nitroglycerin may need to be taken before exercise or sexual activity to prevent cardiac ischemia.
Activity intolerance, related to pain, sedentary life-style	Encourage less strenuous or shorter periods of activity interspersed with rest. Avoid exercise in cold weather. Take prescribed nitroglycerin before activities that will increase the workload of the heart.
Anxiety, related to change in health status, fear of death, threat to self-esteem	Provide calm environment. Instruct patient to utilize stress-reducing techniques. Provide information to decrease anxiety about unanswered questions.
Knowledge deficit, related to disease process and treatment	The nurse will assist in the formulation of a teaching plan that includes information about medications, reducing risk factors, pacing activity, and medical follow-up.

THERAPEUTIC DIALOGUE

Mrs. Martinez, a patient with angina, has been admitted for further care, diagnosis, and treatment. After the initial nursing assessment, Nurse Gallman interviews the patient about the course of her anginal episodes. With the data she gathers, Nurse Gallman will be able to participate in the development of a program to educate Mrs. Martinez to minimize or control the attacks.

Nurse: I would like to ask you some questions, Mrs. Martinez, about the anginal pain that you are experiencing.

Patient: I already told Dr. Mack all about those attacks when I visited his office. His nurse Miss Nichols has all those records.

Nurse: Yes, I know. Your physician has asked us to help you plan a program for preventing or minimizing these attacks. With the information we gather, we can set goals for your care. We can also identify how angina relates to some of your activities.

Patient: OK, Mrs. Gallman, I would like to understand it better. Perhaps I would be less frightened when it happens. My friend Jeanette told me about her aunt who had angina—she died. That really worries me.

Nurse: We hope to decrease some of your fears, Mrs. Martinez, by helping you understand. First, when do your attacks usually occur?

Patient: Oh, mostly after a real busy day, you know—shopping, or after gardening or house cleaning. But a few times, I had problems after my sister-in-law Lisa visited. She and Tom—he's my husband—always seem to get into upsetting discussions. They never got along well. She upsets us both—she criticizes everything!

Nurse: Have you noticed if a big meal is related to the pain?

Patient: No, not really. . . . Well, only when my sister-in-law is there. We hardly ever eat big meals anymore, except when she comes. She expects to be fed well. Tom and I have cut down a lot. Big meals upset our systems—and then her—that harping on old problems and how she thinks we should run our lives! She upsets me so!

Nurse: Mrs. Martinez, I think we must talk more on how to handle stressful problems like Lisa. But first, could you describe the pain for me: Does it come on suddenly? How long does it last? What does it feel like?

PATIENT TEACHING FOR ANGINA PECTORIS

Use of nitrate medications

Use nitroglycerin prophylactically to avoid pain known to occur with certain activities.

Burning sensation on tongue indicates nitroglycerin is activated.

Throbbing sensation in head and flushing may occur.

Sit and stand slowly after taking nitroglycerin.

Place nitroglycerin tablets under the tongue at the onset of anginal pain; second tablet can be taken after 5 minutes and third tablet after another 5 minutes if pain is unrelieved.

Call physician if pain does not subside after third nitroglycerin tablet; go to nearest emergency department; do not drive yourself.

Always carry nitroglycerin.

Store nitroglycerin in dark bottle and keep in dry place.

Replenish nitroglycerin supply every 6 months or before expiration date.

Remove all old nitrate ointment before application of new cream.

Ways to minimize precipitating events

Avoid overexertion.

Try to reduce stress and anxiety, which cause blood vessels to constrict.

Avoid overeating, as it places an increased workload on the heart.

Avoid cold weather (constricts coronary vessels to conserve body heat, hence anginal pain can develop more easily).

Dress warmly in cold weather.

Avoid hot, humid conditions (increases workload of heart).

Walk downhill and with wind, since walking uphill and against wind increases workload of heart.

Effects of exercise program in reduction of myocardial oxygen needs

Engage in regular exercise program.

Exercise conditions heart muscle and can decrease oxygen demand during exertion.

Space exercise period with rest periods.

Take nitroglycerin before exertion.

Need for regular medical follow-up

Patient: Oh, no—not all of a sudden. It is just dull at times, like a stomach upset. But then, it travels up in my chest and gets really heavy—like a pressure. Sometimes, it makes my face and teeth hurt; and my arm, too—this one *(left)*—all the way down to my little fingers. If it's a really bad attack, I sometimes feel like I am going to vomit.

Nurse: On a scale of 1 to 10, how would you rate most of your angina attacks?

Patient: Probably 5 to 6 would be the average, but sometimes it's a 10.

Nurse: Does your heart beat faster?

Patient: Oh, yes, and I just have to sit down and be quiet or I can't catch my breath. That's when I take the nitroglycerin. I carry it with me all the time now—in this special little container.

Nurse: I see. And how long does it take for the pain to stop after you take the medicine?

Patient: I used to think it took forever, but Tom—he times it for me—says it lasts about 15 to 20 minutes. I relax a little, and it passes.

Nurse: What about the weather, Mrs. Martinez? Have you noticed that it affects your attacks in any way?

Patient: I don't know if it is all those clothes or the weather, but I get more pains if I get out in the cold.

Nurse: Do you or your husband smoke?

Patient: Not anymore. I gave up cigarettes when this angina started on me. I noticed the difference, too. Now, I can't even stay in a room if people are smoking. I also cut down on coffee when I retired. Dr. Mack said that the caffeine isn't good for the angina. All the good things, they have to go when you get old!

Nurse: Maybe with some understanding of how certain activities and influences affect your condition, you can find new "good things" for you to enjoy just as much. Soon we will talk again. There are some effective coping methods to decrease your stress when Lisa visits that we can explore.

Patient teaching. Promote a positive attitude and provide an environment conducive to teaching the patient and the family. Establish the readiness of the patient to learn. See box on patient teaching.

Prognosis. The prognosis for the patient with angina pectoris may be grave. Attacks may be intermittent. With proper rest and care, recovery is possible.

Myocardial Infarction

Etiology/Pathophysiology. **Myocardial infarction** is an occlusion of a major coronary artery or one of its branches with subsequent necrosis of myocardium caused by atherosclerosis or an **embolus** (a foreign object, a quantity of air or gas, a bit of tissue, or a piece of a thrombus that circulates in the bloodstream until it becomes lodged in a vessel). An obstruction by atherosclerotic process or an embolus may interrupt the blood supply. Coronary **occlusion** (a blockage in a canal, vessel, or passage of the body) is the general term for occlusion of a coronary artery. The occlusion may also be caused by the formation of a thrombus. This is generally referred to as a coronary thrombosis. The occlusion leads to tissue ischemia. Ischemia to the myocardium lasting more than 35 to 45 minutes produces cellular damage and necrosis (Fig. 28-20). The ability of the cardiac muscle to contract and pump blood is impaired. The final extent of damage to the surrounding tissues is dependent on the ability to develop collateral circulation. Collateral circulation is the development of new vessels within the heart to compensate for the loss of circulation from the occluded artery. The location of the occlusion and the extent of the tissue damage affect the patient's response to the injury. The soft, necrotic area is gradually replaced by fibrous tissue as the healing process occurs.

Clinical Manifestations. An asymptomatic MI may occur. This is referred to as a silent MI. Many of the symptoms of MI are associated with irreversible ischemia, but they are similar to the signs and symptoms of angina pectoris. The symptoms for an MI are more severe and last longer than an angina attack. Pain is the foremost symptom of MI (see Box 28-2 on p. 746).

The pain location and radiation to other sites are depicted in Fig. 28-17. It is often described as crushing or-

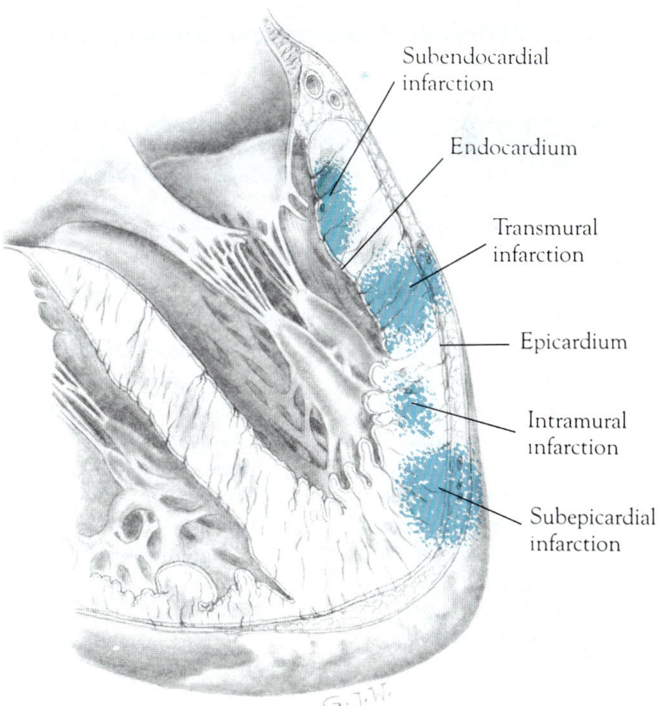

FIG. 28-20 Location of infarctions in ventricle wall.

viselike, an oppressive sensation as though a heavy object is sitting on the chest. The pain is retrosternal (behind the sternum) and in the heart region. It often radiates down the left arm and to the neck, jaws, teeth, and epigastric area. It may occur suddenly, or it may build up over a few minutes. It may occur in conjunction with intense emotion, during exertion, or at rest. The pain is prolonged and more intense than angina pain. It lasts longer than 30 minutes and can last several hours. It is *not* relieved by changes in body position, nitroglycerin, or rest. Other signs and symptoms may occur in conjunction with the pain. These include nausea, shortness of breath, dizziness, weakness, diaphoresis, pallor, ashen color, and a sense of impending doom. See Table 28-1 for comparison of signs and symptoms and the medical management of angina pectoris and MI.

Assessment. Collection of *subjective data* includes the onset, location, quality, duration, and radiation of pain. Shortness of breath, dizziness, weakness, and anxiety or fear may be expressed. Identify precipitating factors. Inquire about measures the patient may have tried to relieve the pain.

Collection of *objective data* includes observation of the patient's behavior to determine apprehensiveness

Box 28-2 SIGNS AND SYMPTOMS OF MYOCARDIAL INFARCTION

SUBJECTIVE DATA (SYMPTOMS)	OBJECTIVE DATA (SIGNS)
Heavy pressure or squeezing in center of chest behind sternum	Pallor
Pain is retrosternal and in heart region, often radiating down the left arm and to the neck, jaw, and teeth	Erratic behavior
Anxiety	Hypotension, shock
Dyspnea	Cardiac rhythm changes
Weakness, faintness	Vomiting
Nausea	Fever
	Diaphoresis

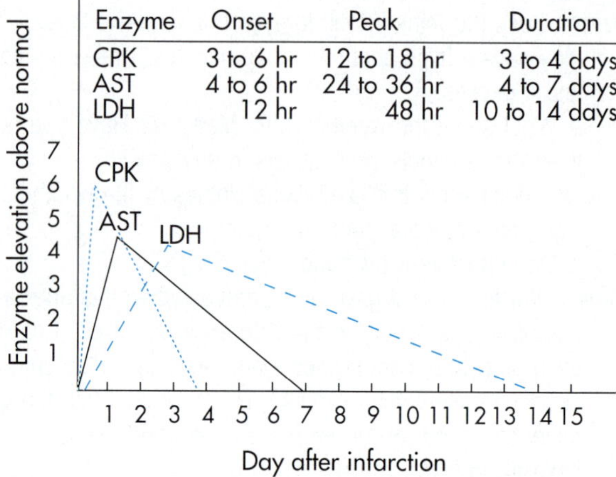

FIG. 28-21 Patterns of serum enzyme levels after myocardial infarction.

TABLE 28-1 Coronary Artery Disorders

Signs and Symptoms	Medical Management	Signs and Symptoms	Medical Management
Angina pectoris		**Myocardial infarction**	
Chest pain (substernal, retrosternal), may radiate to neck, jaw, left arm, and shoulder; great anxiety, fear of approaching death; face pale, ashen; pulse variable, usually tense and quick; blood pressure elevated during an attack; usually brought on by exertion, emotional upsets; relieved by rest, nitroglycerin	Avoidance of precipitating factors Reduction of modifiable risk factors Medications: nitrates, beta-adrenergic blocker agents, calcium channel blockers Oxygen therapy ECG monitoring	Severe, crushing chest pain; prolonged heavy pressure or squeezing pain in center of chest, may spread to shoulder, neck, arm, 4th and 5th finger on left hand, teeth, and jaw; may radiate as with angina; not relieved with rest, nitroglycerin; may be associated with dyspnea, diaphoresis, apprehension, nausea, and vomiting; signs and symptoms of cardiogenic shock may develop	Relief of pain (O_2, morphine and/or other analgesics ECG monitoring Thrombolytic therapy to dissolve clot Reduction of O_2 demand (rest) Prevention of complications (through use of stool softeners, anticoagulants) Treatment of complications (dysrhythmias, CHF)

and anxiety. Typical vital signs reveal hypotension, pulse abnormalities such as tachycardia, a barely perceptible pulse, and early temperature elevation. Note the presence of diaphoresis; vomiting; ashen color; cool, clammy skin; "labored respirations;" and cardiac dysrhythmias. If possible ascertain the presence of risk factors. A respiratory assessment should also be made.

Diagnostic Tests. Diagnostic tests are used to confirm the diagnosis of MI. Blood tests are initially obtained. An elevated white blood cell count (WBC) of 12,000 to 15,000/mm^3 is associated with severe infarcts. The increase begins a few hours after the onset of pain and lasts for 3 to 7 days. The ESR rises during the first week and may remain elevated for several weeks.

ECG findings that indicate MI include ST segment elevation and the development of Q waves. In time the ST segment returns to normal and the T wave inverts. These ECG changes are important in confirming the diagnosis of MI. A chest x-ray is done to note size and configuration of the heart. More complex tests are occasionally done, including cardiac fluoroscopy, myocardial imaging (thallium scan), PET, and MUGA scanning (multiple-gated cardiac blood pool imaging). These tests may be done in conjunction with other tests to diagnose MI and determine the severity of CAD.

Specific serum enzymes are released into the vascular system when infarcted cardiac muscle cells die (Fig. 28-21).

Cardiac enzyme studies. Cell membrane damage or necrosis causes the release of certain enzymes into the blood. Amounts found in the blood content are commonly elevated with an incidence of MI, defibrillation, trauma, and drug therapy (steroids, morphine, and antibiotics). Specific enzymes and elevation values follow.

Creatine phosphokinase (CPK or CK) is a muscle enzyme found in the brain, skeletal muscle, and myocardium. Isoenzymes of CK relate to the specific tissue and differentiate the sources.

MEDICATIONS FOR MYOCARDIAL INFARCTION

Classification	Agent	Action
Vasopressors	Dopamine (Intropin)	Raise systemic arterial pressure and cardiac output.
Anticoagulants	Heparin Warfarin (Coumadin)	Reduce incidence of clotting.
Analgesics	Morphine	Control pain.
Tranquilizers	Diazepam (Valium)	Decrease anxiety and restlessness.
Thrombolytic agents	Streptokinase (Streptase)	Use of thrombolytic (pertaining to dissolution of blood clots) agents when acute MI symptoms are less than 6 hr, preferably 30 min to 1 hr, duration; these agents restore blood flow and therefore limit infarct size in certain patients.
Tissue plasminogen activator (TPA)	Alteplase, recombinant Activase	
Nitrates	Nitroglycerin Isosorbide	Dilate blood vessels, increase coronary artery blood supply, and decrease oxygen demands.
β-Adrenergic blockers	Propranolol (Inderal) Nadolol (Corgard) Metoprolol (Lopressor)	Block β-adrenergic stimulation and decrease myocardial oxygen demands.
Calcium channel blockers	Nifedipine (Procardia) Diltiazem (Cardizem) Verapamil (Calan, Isoptin)	Dilate blood vessels, increase coronary artery blood supply, and decrease myocardial oxygen demands.
Salicylates	Aspirin	Decrease platelet adhesion and thus decrease thrombosis formation.
Antidysrhythmics	Lidocaine (Xylocaine) IV	Treat ventricular dysrhythmias.
Stool softeners	Surfak Colace	Reduce straining at stool, prevent constipation produced by decreased mobility and use of constipating narcotics.
Diuretics	Furosemide (Lasix)	Control edema.
Electrolyte replacement	Slow-K	May be necessary when diuretics are used.

- CK isoenzyme I (BB) originates from brain tissue.
- CK isoenzyme II (MB) originates from myocardial tissue.
- CK isoenzyme III (MM) originates in skeletal muscle.

CK MB
Normal range: 75 U/L; MI range: 10-25 times normal
Onset: 3-6 hours; peak: 12-18 hours; duration: 3-4 days (see Fig. 28-21.)

Lactic dehydrogenase (LDH) is composed of five isoenzyme components. Subunit LDH is found in cardiac muscle. An elevation of LDH and CK isoenzyme II (MB) in the serum is indicative of an MI.

Medical Management. The focus of medical management is to prevent further tissue injury and limit the size of the infarction. Intervention is designed to facilitate cardiac tissue perfusion and reduce the workload of the heart. Promoting tissue oxygenation, relieving pain, preventing complications, improving tissue perfusion, and preventing further tissue damage are all important medical considerations.

Medications such as morphine and Valium are used to alleviate pain and anxiety. See the medications table on p. 747 for medications commonly prescribed for the patient with myocardial infarction. Oxygen is prescribed to facilitate cardiac tissue perfusion. Attention is given to respiratory difficulties, fluid overload, and cardiac dysrhythmias.

Medical therapy is also directed toward limiting the size and extent of injury by attempting to reperfuse (the reinstitution of blood flow to an area that was ischemic) the occluded coronary artery. Fibrinolytic agents such as streptokinase, (streptase), anistreplase, and tissue plasminogen activator (TPA) such as alteplase are currently used to attempt reperfusion. Thrombolytics salvage heart muscle by minimizing infarct size and maximizing heart function. They lyse (decompose or dissolve) the clot in the occluded coronary artery, reopening the vessel and allowing perfusion (the passage of fluid through a specific organ) of the heart muscle. To be effective reperfusion must be attained within 3 to 5 hours following the onset of symptoms. It is most effective in the first 30 minutes to 1 hour. Before a thrombolytic is administered, a thorough history must be obtained. There are certain conditions that would exclude the use of thrombolytics: active internal bleeding, suspected aortic dissecting aneurysm, recent head trauma, history of hemorrhagic cerebrovascular accident within the past year, or a surgery within the past 10 days.

TABLE 28-2 Cardiogenic Shock

Cardiogenic shock is an acute and serious complication of MI and congestive heart failure. It is characterized by low cardiac output and peripheral vascular system collapse. Left ventricular function is severely decreased, resulting in an inadequate blood supply to the vital organs. Immediate detection and treatment are necessary to prevent irreversible shock and death. Cardiogenic shock proves fatal in 80% of cases.

Clinical Manifestations	Signs and Symptoms	Medical Management	Nursing Interventions
Decreased cardiac output Myocardial ischemia Cerebral hypoxia Impaired tissue perfusion Renal circulation decreased Anaerobic metabolism with lactic acidosis Peripheral vascular system collapse Shock	Dysrhythmias, chest pain Anxiety, agitation, restlessness, disorientation Urinary output diminished or absent Lactic acid accumulation in blood Tachycardia, thready pulse, tachypnea Decreased blood pressure Narrowed pulse pressure Cyanosis, cold moist, pale clammy skin Decreased peripheral pulses Capillary refill time decreased Hypoactive bowel sounds	Recognition and control of life-threatening signs and symptoms Oxygenation promotes tissue perfusion Parenteral fluid acts as a volume expander Drug therapy Vasopressors: Raise arterial blood pressure Inotropics and cardiac glycosides: Increase cardiac contraction and strengthen and correct dysrhythmias Adrenergic drugs: Dopamine (Intropin) at therapeutic levels increases cardiac output and blood pressure Sodium bicarbonate: Combats lactic acidosis	Monitor vital signs every 15-20 min during acute stage and every 2 hr when stabilized. Administer O_2 as ordered. Use semi-Fowler's position. Monitor acid-base balance. Monitor urine output hourly to determine adequate kidney perfusion. Allow nothing by mouth. Initiate bed rest to minimize energy expenditure. Administer medications as ordered. Provide comfort measures.

Complications commonly associated with MI include ventricular fibrillation, cardiogenic shock (Table 28-2), congestive heart failure, and dysrhythmias. Other complications may occur, such as ventricular aneurysm, pericarditis, and embolism.

Nursing Interventions. Administer oxygen for 24 to 48 hours and longer if pain, hypotension, dyspnea, or dysrhythmias persist.

Administer medications as prescribed:

- Morphine sulfate for relief of pain and apprehension and to produce vasodilation. Provisions for comfort and rest are essential to reduce stress and increase myocardial oxygen perfusion.
- Anticoagulants (heparin or warfarin) may be prescribed to decrease incidence of thrombophlebitis and pulmonary embolism.
- Administer stool softener as prescribed to prevent rectal straining. Valsalva's maneuver causes changes in blood pressure and heart rate, which may trigger ischemia, dysrhythmias, or cardiac arrest.

Instruct the patient to avoid excessive fatigue and to stop activity immediately in the presence of chest pain, dyspnea, or faintness. Plan nursing interventions to promote rest and minimize unnecessary disturbances.

Monitor vital signs; document rate and rhythm of pulse.

The patient is usually placed on bed rest with commode privileges for 24 to 48 hours. Assist with ADLs. During this period sedation with Valium or an equivalent may be prescribed to relieve anxiety and restlessness and to promote sleep. After the first 24 to 48 hours, patients are usually encouraged to increase their activity gradually, depending on the size of the infarction. During this period the patient is continually monitored for signs of dysrhythmias, cardiac pain, and changes in vital signs.

Diet is usually withheld until stabilization. Liquid diet is progressed as tolerated to regular diet with modifications. A low-fat, low-sodium, easily digested diet is desirable. Caffeine is withheld to prevent stimulation of the heart rate.

Prevention of complications is a primary objective. Antiembolic stockings are used. Ongoing assessment of cardiac status, dyspneic condition, and pulse change (rate, rhythm, and volume) is made and reported.

During hospitalization, many patients experience denial, depression, and anxiety. Anxiety varies in intensity, depending on the severity of the threat as perceived by the patient and on the patient's success in coping.

Nursing diagnoses and interventions for the patient with an MI include but are not limited to, the following:

NURSING DIAGNOSES	NURSING INTERVENTIONS
Pain, acute chest, related to myocardial ischemia	Assess original pain; assess location, duration, radiation, and onset of new symptoms.
Pain, acute chest, related to myocardial ischemia—cont'd	Administer prescribed analgesics (usually morphine sulfate, which relieves pain, reduces anxiety, causes vasodilation of vascular smooth muscle, and reduces myocardial workload). Maintain bed rest and reduced patient activity. Administer O_2 as prescribed. Record patient's response to pain-relief measures. Employ alternative methods of pain relief. Provide calm, restful environment for the patient.
Tissue perfusion, altered cardiovascular, related to decreased cardiac output	Administer prescribed oxygen. Maintain bed rest to decrease cardiac workload. Monitor ECG for dysrhythmic complications. Monitor for complications that decrease cardiac output, such as shock or congestive heart failure. Monitor vital signs, including apical pulse.
Activity intolerance, related to ventricular dysfunction, pain	Maintain initial bed rest. Progress activity gradually, per physician's order. Have patient participate in cardiac rehabilitation program, per physician's order. Balance rest periods with activity. Utilize antiembolic stockings, per physician's order.
Anxiety, related to change in health status, fear of death	Assess for signs and verbal expressions of anxiety and coping mechanisms used. Promote restful sleep patterns. Reassure through patient education, enlisting family support, and allowing positive and negative expression of feelings. Remain with patient during periods of highest anxiety; offer reassurance; use calm, but concerned voice. Administer antianxiety agents as needed, per physician's order. Initiate relaxation techniques, e.g., deep breathing, visual imagery, soft rhythmic music. Encourage participation in cardiac rehabilitation program.
Constipation, high risk for, related to opiate analgesics, immobility	Administer stool softener per physician's order. Instruct the patient not to strain or hold the breath while having a bowel movement. This is to avoid the Valsalva maneuver, which causes changes in heart rate, blood pressure, and cardiac rhythm. Encourage fluid intake within acceptable range.
Cardiac output, decreased, related to conduction defects (dysrhythmias) and decreased myocardial pumping action	Assess and monitor vital signs every 4 hr. Maintain bed rest with head of bed elevated 30 degrees for first 24 to 48 hr to reduce myocardial oxygen demand.

NURSING DIAGNOSES	NURSING INTERVENTIONS
Cardiac output, decreased, related to conduction defects (dysrhythmias) and decreased myocardial pumping action—cont'd	Monitor intravenous feedings; infuse according to physician's order. Administer prescribed medications such as antidysrhythmias, nitrates, and beta blockers. Auscultate breath sounds and heart rate every 4 hr; increase activity level as prescribed by physician's orders.
Knowledge deficit, related to disease process and therapeutic plan for recovery	Develop a teaching plan to provide information regarding disease process, activity limits, medications, dietary restrictions, risk factor modification, and when to notify the physician (see patient teaching box).

Patient teaching. Patients and their family members need teaching to reassure them of recovery. Over 85% of all patients with an uncomplicated MI return to work. Education should cover resuming sexual activities. Once patients with an uncomplicated MI are able to climb two flights of stairs without difficulty, they are usually able to resume sexual activities. Approximately 80% of all postcoronary patients will be able to resume sexual activity without serious risks. The other 20% need not abstain totally, but their sexual activity should be limited according to their cardiac capacity.

Participation in a cardiac rehabilitation program should be discussed before discharge from the hospital. A monitored exercise program and continuing education are provided with outpatient cardiac rehabilitation. The physician may prescribe cardiac rehabilitation during the inpatient and outpatient phase of recovery following an MI (patient teaching box).

Prognosis. It is imperative that medical care be instituted without delay. Many myocardial infarction patients not treated prior to reaching the hospital die. Delaying specific therapy may cause loss of life. The prognosis also depends on the area and extent of the damage and the presence of complications.

PATIENT TEACHING FOR A MYOCARDIAL INFARCTION

- Teach the effects of MI, the healing process, and treatment regimen
- Teach the effect of medications in the treatment of MI
- Teach the association between risk factors and coronary artery disease
- Teach to identify nonmodifiable risk factors
- Teach to identify modifiable risk factors (especially cigarette smoking)
- Teach the effect of dietary restrictions on CAHD: 2 g sodium, 1500 calories, low cholesterol, no caffeine, fluid restrictions
- Teach the patient to avoid foods high in sodium, saturated fats, and triglycerides. Review alternative ways of seasoning foods to avoid cooking with salt. Explain need to limit intake of eggs, cream, butter, and foods high in animal fat
- Teach the effect of activity on the heart and need to participate in a progressive activity plan
- Refer the patient to social support groups as indicated
- Teach resumption of sexual activity (if appropriate)
  - Abstention from sexual intercourse as directed, usually for 4 to 6 weeks (sexual closeness, for example, cuddling, may be started earlier as desired)
  - Reporting to physician the following symptoms occurring during or following intercourse:
    - Dyspnea or increased heart rate continuing for more than 15 minutes after intercourse
    - Extreme fatigue
    - Chest pain during intercourse
    - Palpitations for more than 15 minutes after intercourse
    - Insomnia after intercourse

Congestive Heart Failure

Etiology/Pathophysiology. When the heart is no longer able to pump enough blood to meet the demands of the body, it is referred to as heart failure or cardiac insufficiency. **Congestive heart failure (CHF)** is an abnormal condition characterized by circulatory congestion as a result of the heart's inability to act as an effective pump. Circulatory congestion and compensatory mechanisms occur. Congestive heart failure may develop after an MI, in response to prolonged hypertension, or in relation to valvular heart disease or inflammatory heart disease. Other factors associated with CHF include infection, stress, hyperthyroidism, anemia, and fluid replacement therapy. CHF is the most common diagnosis for the hospitalized patient over age 65.

Because the left ventricle is most often affected by coronary atherosclerosis and hypertension, heart failure usually begins there. If untreated the condition progresses to right-sided failure. Right ventricular failure can occur separately from left ventricular failure, but its appearance is more often a consequence of left-sided failure. The signs and symptoms of heart failure are the result of decreased cardiac output from impaired cardiac pumping power and congestion that involves the pulmonary system, the venous system, or both.

Left ventricular failure. When the left ventricle is unable to pump enough blood to meet the demands of the body, major consequences occur. The first is the signs and symptoms of decreased cardiac output. The second is pulmonary congestion. Increased pressure in the left side of the heart backs up into the pulmonary system and the lungs become congested with fluid. Fluid leaks through the capillaries and permeates air spaces in the lungs. If during each heartbeat the right ventricle pumps out just one more drop of blood than the left, then within only 3 hours the pulmonary blood volume will have expanded by 500 ml. Pulmonary edema and **pleural effusion** (an abnormal accumulation of fluid in the thoracic cavity between the visceral and parietal pleurae) occur. Signs and symptoms of this condition include dyspnea, orthopnea, pulmonary crackles, hemoptysis, and cough.

Right ventricular failure. Right ventricular failure occurs when the right ventricle is unable to pump effectively against increased pressure in the pulmonary circulation. Most often the increased pressure is the result of blood backing up from a failing left ventricle, but right ventricular failure can also be a result of chronic pulmonary disease and pulmonary hypertension. Inability of the right ventricle to pump blood forward into the lungs results in congestion. The right ventricle of the heart is unable to adequately empty its blood volume and thus cannot accommodate all the venous blood that is normally returned to the right side of the heart. Venous blood is reflected backward into the systemic circulation. Increased venous volume and pressure force fluid out of the vasculature into interstitial tissue (peripheral edema). Edema is a sign of increased interstitial fluid and appears in dependent areas of the body such as the sacrum when supine and the feet and ankles while in an upright position. The edema may progress to pitting edema. As right ventricular failure continues, edema may progress up the legs into the thighs, external genitalia, and lower trunk. To check for edema, press down on the tissue for several seconds and lift the finger. If the depression does not fill almost immediately, pitting edema is present (Fig. 28-22 and Table 28-3).

One liter of fluid equals 1 kilogram (2.2 pounds); a weight gain of 2.2 pounds will signify a gain of 1 liter of body fluid. The liver may become congested, and fluid can accumulate in the abdomen (ascites). Distended neck veins may be observed when the patient is in a sitting position.

Clinical Manifestations. Manifestations of congestive heart failure are those associated with decreased cardiac output, left ventricular failure, and right ventricular failure (Box 28-3 on p. 752).

Assessment. Collection of *subjective data* includes complaints of dyspnea, **orthopnea** (an abnormal condition in which a person must sit or stand in order to breath deeply or comfortably), cough, and the precipitating factors and methods for relief. Also listen to patient's statements that relate to fatigue, anxiety, weight gain from fluid retention, and edema. Document any pain, anginal or abdominal, and the patient's stated ability to perform ADLs.

Collection of *objective data* includes noting presence of dyspnea, orthopnea, edema (site, degree of pitting), abdominal distention secondary to ascites, weight gain, adventitious breath sounds, abnormal heart sounds (gallop and murmurs), activity intolerance, and jugular vein distention. Blood flow to the kidneys is diminished, resulting in oliguria. Oxygen deficit in tissues results in cyanosis and general debilitation.

Diagnostic Tests. Diagnosis is based on presenting signs and symptoms of congestive heart failure and is confirmed by various diagnostic tests. A chest x-ray reveals pulmonary vascular congestion, pleural effusion,

TABLE 28-3 Pitting Edema Scale

Scale	Degree	Response
1+ Trace	Slight	Rapid
2+ Mild	0-0.6 cm (0-¼ in)	10-15 sec
3+ Moderate	0.6-1.3 cm (¼-½ in)	1-2 min
4+ Severe	1.3-2.5 cm (½-1 in)	2-5 min

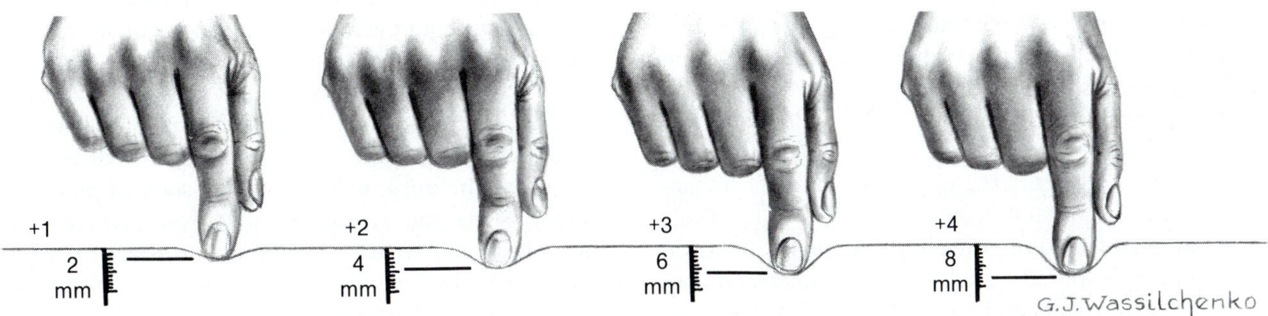

FIG. 28-22 Scale for pitting edema depth.

Box 28-3 SIGNS AND SYMPTOMS OF CONGESTIVE HEART FAILURE

DECREASED CARDIAC OUTPUT

Fatigue
Angina pain
Anxiety
Oliguria
Decreased gastrointestinal motility
Pale, cool skin
Weight gain

LEFT VENTRICULAR FAILURE

Dyspnea
Cough
Frothy, blood-tinged sputum
Orthopnea
Pulmonary crackles (moist popping and cracking sounds heard most often at the end of inspiration)
Evidence of pulmonary vascular congestion with pleural effusion, as seen on chest x-ray

RIGHT VENTRICULAR FAILURE

Edema in feet, ankles, sacrum; may progress up the legs into thighs, external genitalia, and lower trunk
Anorexia, nausea, and abdominal distention
Liver congestion
Ascites
Distended jugular veins

and cardiomegaly (cardiac enlargement). ECG reveals cardiac dysrhythmias. Echocardiography is done to determine valvular heart disease, presence of pericardial fluid, and CHF. Gated pool imaging is used to evaluate left ventricular function, and pulmonary artery catheterization is done to assess right and left ventricular function.

Laboratory tests include sodium and potassium levels. Blood chemistry will reveal elevated blood urea nitrogen (BUN) and creatinine due to decreased glomerular filtration; liver function values (ALT, AST, alkaline phosphatase) will be mildly elevated. Arterial blood gases may reveal hypoxemia.

Medical Management. The objectives of medical management include the following:

- Increasing cardiac efficiency with digitalis and vasodilators for expanded output; angiotension converting enzyme inhibitors (ACE inhibitors) such as captopril (Capoten), enalapril (Vasotec), ramipril (Altace), benazepril (Lotensin), and lisinopril (Prinivil) decrease peripheral vascular resistance and have proven to extend the lives of patients with CHF as well as lengthen time between admissions (see the medications table)
- Lowering oxygen requirements of the body systems through bed rest, with head of bed elevated to 45 degrees to reduce myocardial oxygen demand and decrease circulating volume returning to heart
- Providing oxygen to the tissues through oxygen therapy if patient is hypoxic
- Treating edema and pulmonary congestion with diuretics and a sodium-restricted diet
- Weighing patient daily to monitor fluid retention

Once the workload of the heart is decreased and diuresis of engorged tissues and organs is achieved, the activity ability of the patient will increase. These objectives are achieved by medication therapy and bed rest. Medication therapy with digoxin, ACE inhibitors, thiazide, and loop diuretics is a common initial treatment (see the medications table).

Nursing Interventions. Nursing interventions focus on promoting oxygenation to the tissues, balancing rest and activity, promoting nutritional balance and a low-salt diet, decreasing stress and anxiety, maintaining skin integrity, and patient teaching (see nursing care plan on pp. 754-755).

In acute congestive heart failure, administration of oxygen and medication should be of first concern. Decreasing oxygen requirements through complete bed rest will slow the heart rate and increase cardiac and respiratory reserves. Anxiety produced from the effects of signs and symptoms and the fear of a life-threatening situation can be allayed by reassurance and explanation. Accurate interventions, observation, and reporting reduce the threat of such complications as embolus, thrombophlebitis, MI, and pulmonary edema.

In chronic heart failure or after the acute crisis, complete bed rest and freedom from stress should be maintained. This decreases cardiac workload. Fowler's position relieves pulmonary congestion by lowering venous return to the cardiopulmonary system, and dyspnea becomes less prevalent. Relieving respiratory distress lessens oxygen requirements and aids in adequately supplying oxygen to tissues and organs.

Nursing interventions include measures to prevent disease progression and complications. Vital signs are monitored for changes. Signs of respiratory distress will be noted. The nurse will observe for signs of pulmonary edema. Signs and symptoms of left-sided versus right-sided heart failure are carefully monitored. Urinary output is typically low, and edema is soft and pitting; legs are elevated to decrease edema.

The nurse should also note increase in abdominal girth and total body weight as indicators of fluid reten-

Medications for Congestive Heart Failure

Agent	Action	Nursing Interventions
Cardiac glycosides		
Digitalis preparations, such as digoxin (Lanoxin)	Strengthen cardiac force and efficiency. Slow heart rate. Increase circulation, effecting diuresis.	Monitor apical pulse to ensure rate above 60; monitor for toxicity (nausea, vomiting, anorexia, dysrhythmia, bradycardia, tachycardia, headache, fatigue, and blurred or colored vision).
Diuretics		
Thiazides, such as chlorothiazide (Diuril), hydrochlorothiazide (Esidrix and Hydrodiuril)	Increase renal secretion of sodium. Are safe for long-term use. Block sodium and water reabsorption in kidney tubules.	Monitor electrolyte depletion; weigh daily to ascertain fluid loss.
Sulfonamides (loop diuretic), such as furosemide (Lasix)	Act rapidly for less responsive edema.	Administer in AM, to prevent nocturia. Monitor for electrolyte depletion. Consider sulfa allergy (furosemide).
Aldosterone antagonist (potassium-sparing), such as spironolactone (Aldactone)	Relieve edema and ascites that do not respond to usual diuretics. Block sodium-retaining and potassium-excreting properties of aldosterone.	Monitor for gastrointestinal irritation and hyperkalemia.
Potassium supplements		
Potassium (K-Lyte)	Restore electrolyte loss.	Monitor blood potassium levels.
Sedatives and analgesics		
Temazepam morphine (Restoril)	Promote rest and comfort. Relieve chest and abdominal pain. Lessen dyspnea.	Monitor rest and sleep benefits.
Nitrates		
Nitroglycerin (Cardabid)	Dilate arteries. Reduce blood pressure.	Monitor blood pressure.
Ace inhibitors		
Captopril (Capoten) Enalapril (Vasotec) Vamipril (Altace) Benazepril (Lotensin) Lisinopril (Prinivil)	Act as antihypertensives and reduce peripheral arterial resistance	Observe patient closely for a precipitous drop in blood pressure within 3 hr after initial dose; monitor blood pressure closely. Monitor blood potassium levels.

tion common in heart failure. The nurse will auscultate lung fields to determine the presence of crackles and wheezes, coughing, and complaints of dyspnea. Restful sleep may be possible only in the sitting position or with the aid of extra pillows. Activity intolerance accompanied by extreme fatigue and anxiety is usually noted.

See Box 28-4 on p. 756 for guidelines for nursing interventions for the patient with CHF.

Patient teaching. Patient teaching includes information about medications, diet restrictions, oxygen therapy if indicated, balancing rest and activity, signs and symptoms of cardiac congestion, and when to notify the physician. See the patient teaching box on p. 756 for teaching the patient with CHF.

Prognosis. Congestive heart failure is a chronic condition. With treatment advances, many people now survive for years with damaged hearts.

Pulmonary Edema

Etiology/Pathophysiology. **Pulmonary edema** (the accumulation of extravascular fluid in lung tissues and alveoli, caused mostly by CHF) is an acute and extensive, life-threatening complication of congestive heart failure. Fluid from the left side of the heart backs up into the pulmonary vasculature and results in extravascular fluid accumulation in the interstitial space and alveoli. This causes the patient to "drown" in the secretions.

NURSING CARE PLAN: *CARE OF THE PATIENT WITH CONGESTIVE HEART FAILURE*

Mr. Dravland is a 61-year-old clinic administrator. He was admitted to the hospital with the diagnosis of congestive heart failure. He has a history of hypertension and coronary artery disease. Six months ago he had a myocardial infarction. He has felt tired for the past 3 weeks and has been experiencing increased dyspnea. He has noticed some swelling in his ankles and is concerned about gaining 5 pounds in the last week as well as increasing intolerance to exertion. The nursing admission history revealed:

- Mr. Dravland has not been taking his antihypertensive medication regularly. He didn't like the side effects and stopped taking the medication, but he was too embarrassed to call his doctor
- Vital signs revealed an elevated blood pressure
- Shortness of breath during activities and when lying down
- Pitting edema of both ankles
- Crackles bilaterally in the lungs

Nursing diagnoses	Patient goals/expected outcomes	Nursing interventions
Cardiac output, decreased, related to cardiac insufficiency	Patient will have decreased dyspnea with activities and when lying in bed.	Maintain initial bed rest with stress-free environment. Maintain semi-Fowler's to high Fowler's position. Explain and encourage gradual increases in activity to prevent a sudden increase in cardiac workload. Monitor respirations, lung sounds, heart sounds, and vital signs q 4 hr. Administer digitalis, diuretics, ACE inhibitors, vasodilators, beta blockers, and antihypertensive medication as prescribed.
Fluid volume excess, related to cardiovascular, pulmonary, and systemic congestion	Patient will have decreased edema, weight, and dyspnea.	Monitor I&O and weigh daily. Assess abdominal girth, dependent edema, and presence of neck vein distention. Assess respiratory status for crackles, dyspnea, orthopnea, and cough. Maintain a low-sodium (2-g) diet and fluid intake restrictions per physician's order. Administer diuretic and postassium replacements as prescribed.
Gas exchange impaired, related to pulmonary edema	Patient will have decreased adventitious lung sounds and decreased dyspnea with activity and at rest.	Administer prescribed oxygen. Maintain semi-Fowler's or high Fowler's position while patient is in bed. Assess respiratory status for crackles, dyspnea, orthopnea, and cough.
Noncompliance with therapeutic regimen, related to side effects of medication and lack of understanding	Patient will adhere to prescribed treatment and feel comfortable talking to health professionals about problems.	Explore previous noncompliance to determine reasons from patient's perspective.

Activity intolerance, related to dyspnea, peripheral edema, and fatigue	Patient will complain of less dyspnea at rest and with activity and will adjust to and compensate for physical disabilities; patient will learn to conserve energy.	Plan activities to conserve energy. Encourage rest as soon as patient starts to tire. Teach patient how to participate in physical activities without exhausting himself. Administer oxygen as needed. Encourage participation with ADLs as tolerated and gradually progress activity levels as symptoms permit.
Knowledge deficit, related to lack of understanding of importance of complying with prescribed treatment		Develop trusting relationship. Explain possibility of alternatives if one method of treatment is not working. Encourage questions and discussion about treatment plan.
Skin integrity, impaired, high risk for, related to edema and poor tissue perfusion	Patient's skin will remain intact during hospitalization.	Maintain adequate nutrition. Utilize prophylactic measures to prevent skin impairment, particularly over edematous areas. Assess skin frequently. Alternate positions every 2 hours or more often to promote tissue circulation and prevent skin impairment.
Anxiety, related to change in health status, life-style changes, fear of death, or threat to self-concept	Patient will be able to verbalize anxieties. Patient will demonstrate reduction of anxiety by enjoying periods of rest and sleep.	Identify coping techniques. Provide information to decrease fears. Identify support systems. Provide calm, relaxing environment. Administer antianxiety medications per physician's orders as needed. Help patient cope with life-style changes. He may feel anxious due to changes in body image, family and social roles, and finances. Focus on progress patient is making in managing his condition. Encourage patient to participate in health care decisions, and allow him to ventilate anger and frustration.

CRITICAL THINKING QUESTIONS

1. Mr. Dravland is experiencing severe dyspnea, with the presence of crackles bilaterally in all lung fields. His pulse is 108, and respirations are 33. His nurse enters the room to perform his morning ADLs; the nursing interventions that would be most beneficial would include:
2. On assessing Mr. Dravland's skin, the nurse notes 4+ pitting edema in his lower extremities. She also notes a weight gain of 6 pounds in the past 24 hours. For therapeutic diuresing to occur, the medical management would include:
3. Mr. Dravland puts his light on to request assistance to ambulate. The nurse notes subclavicular retractions and cyanosis of his nailbeds. The most appropriate nursing action by the nurse would be:

Box 28-4 GUIDELINES FOR NURSING INTERVENTIONS FOR THE PATIENT WITH CONGESTIVE HEART FAILURE

Provide oxygenation
- Administer oxygen by nasal cannula at 2-6 L/min as prescribed for dyspnea
- Patient should be well supported in semi-Fowler's or high Fowler's position

Encourage bed rest
- Reinforce importance of conservation of energy and planning for activities that avoid fatigue

Encourage activity within prescribed restrictions; monitor for intolerance to activity (dyspnea, fatigue, increased pulse rate that does not stabilize)

Assist with ADLs as necessary; encourage independence within patient's limitations

Provide diversional activity that will assist in conservation of energy

Monitor for signs of fluid and potassium imbalance; record daily weights, I&O

Provide skin care, particularly over edematous areas; use prophylactic measures to prevent skin impairment

Assist in maintaining an adequate nutritional intake while observing prescribed dietary modifications (sodium restrictions)

Monitor for constipation; give prescribed stool softeners

Give prescribed medications
- Digitalis (take apical pulse before administration)
- Diuretics (assess for hypokalemia)
- Vasodilators, ACE inhibitors, beta blockers
- Medications to reduce anxiety and promote sleep

Provide patient/family opportunities to discuss their concerns

Teach patient about the disorder and self-care

PATIENT TEACHING FOR CONGESTIVE HEART FAILURE

Monitor for signs and symptoms of recurring congestive heart failure and report these signs and symptoms to the physician or clinic:

Weight gain of 1-1.5 kg (2-3 lb) over a short period of time (about 2 days)

Shortness of breath

Orthopnea

Swelling of ankles, feet, or abdomen

Persistent cough

Frequent nighttime urination

Avoid fatigue and plan activity to allow for rest periods.

Plan and eat meals within prescribed sodium restrictions.

Avoid salty foods

Avoid drugs with high sodium content (e.g., some laxatives and antacids, Alka-Seltzer)—read the labels.

Eat several small meals rather than three large meals per day.

Take prescribed medications.

If several medications are prescribed, develop a method to facilitate accurate administration.

Digitalis: check own pulse rate daily; report a rate of less than 60/min to physician.

Diuretics

Weight self daily at same time of day.

Report weight gain to physician.

Eat foods high in potassium and low in sodium (such as oranges, bananas).

Vasodilators

Report signs of hypotension (light-headedness, rapid pulse, syncope) to physician.

Avoid alcohol when taking vasodilators.

Report to physician for follow-up as directed.

Clinical Manifestations. The patient exhibits signs of severe respiratory distress when pulmonary edema occurs. Frothy sputum is produced from air mixing with the fluid in the alveoli; the sputum is blood-tinged from blood cells that have exuded into the alveoli.

Assessment

See Box 28-5 for signs and symptoms of pulmonary edema.

Diagnostic Tests. Diagnosis is made through signs and symptoms and is supported by chest x-ray and arterial blood gas studies. Pao_2 and $Paco_2$ may reveal respiratory alkalosis or acidosis.

Medical Management. Medical management involves simultaneous interventions to promote oxygenation, improve cardiac output, and reduce pulmonary congestion. Without emergency treatment, respiratory failure may occur (Table 28-4).

Nursing Interventions. Interventions include administering oxygen. Place patient in an upright position with legs in a dependent position to decrease venous return to the heart, relieving pulmonary congestion and dyspnea. Monitor arterial blood gases and administer drugs as ordered. Auscultate lung sounds often. Provide emotional support; remain with patient. Explain all procedures. Monitor vital signs, fluid I&O, and serum electrolytes. Assist in applying rotating tourniquets as ordered.

TABLE 28-4 Medical Management for Acute Pulmonary Edema

Intervention	Rationale
Patient in high Fowler's position or over side of bed with arms supported on bedside table	Promotes expansion of lungs; legs in dependent position causes venous pooling and reduction in venous return (preload)
Morphine sulfate, 10-15 mg intravenously	Decreases patient anxiety; slows respirations; reduces venous return
Oxygen at 40%-70% by face mask; intubation as needed	Promotes oxygenation; increased tidal volume also promotes removal of secretions from alveoli
Rapid digitalization if patient not previously taking digitalis	Increases the force of myocardial contraction and increases cardiac output; reduces heart rate; converts rapid rate dysrhythmias such as atrial fibrillation
Aminophylline, 250-500 mg (diluted), given intravenously over approximately 30 min	Relieves bronchospasm and wheezing; acts as diuretic
Diuretics: Furosemide (Lasix)	Reduces pulmonary edema by decreasing the fluid in the lungs and increasing excretion through the kidneys
Rotation of tourniquets (infrequently used), manually or by machine; pressure applied to three limbs at a time; cuff inflation slightly above patient's diastolic blood pressure; cuff inflated for 45 min followed by 15 min free of compression	Reduces cardiopulmonary overload by temporarily pooling blood in the extremities

Nursing diagnoses and interventions for the patient with pulmonary edema include but are not limited to the following:

NURSING DIAGNOSES	NURSING INTERVENTIONS
Fluid volume excess, related to fluid accumulation in pulmonary vessels	Administer diuretics as ordered. Carefully monitor I&O. Weigh patient at same time each day. Assist with rotating tourniquets as ordered.
Gas exchange, impaired, related to fluid in lungs	Assess for signs of hypoxia, such as restlessness, disorientation, and irritability. Monitor arterial blood gases per physician's order. Administer oxygen as per physician's order. Position patient in high Fowler's position with legs in dependent position or sitting and leaning forward on overbed table to facilitate breathing.
Anxiety, related to fear of suffocation and death	Promote optimal air exchange to decrease anxiety. Assess level of anxiety and coping mechanisms. Deliver nursing interventions in a supportive, kind, and proficient manner. Assess support systems available to patient, and mobilize resources.

Prognosis. Pulmonary edema is a grave, life-threatenting condition that is usually responsive to aggressive interventions.

Box 28-5 SIGNS AND SYMPTOMS OF PULMONARY EDEMA

Restlessness	Tachycardia
Vague uneasiness	Pallor or cyanosis
Agitation	Cough productive of large quantities of blood-tinged, frothy sputum
Disorientation	Audible wheezing, crackles
Diaphoresis	Cold extremities
Severe dyspnea	
Tachypnea	

Valvular Heart Disease

Etiology/Pathophysiology. Normal heart valves function to maintain the direction of blood flow through the right atrium, right ventricle, lungs, left atrium, left ventricle, and to the rest of the body. Heart valves operate by passively opening and closing in response to pressure changes in the heart. The tricuspid valve is located between the right atrium and right ventricle. The pulmonic valve allows blood to flow through the pulmonary artery into the lungs. The mitral valve is located between the left atrium and the left ventricle. The aortic valve allows blood to flow from the left ventricle into the aorta. Valvular disease occurs when the valves are compromised and do not open and close properly. Two problems occur when valves are compromised: *stenosis* is a thickening of the valve tissue, which causes the valve to become narrow, and *insufficiency* occurs when the valve is unable to close completely.

A prominent factor in the development of valvular disease is a history of rheumatic fever. Clinical symptoms of valvular heart disease tend to occur 10 to 40 years after an episode of rheumatic fever. Because the blood volume and workload of the heart are greater on the left than on the right, the valves affected more frequently are the mitral and aortic. Valvular heart disorders include mitral stenosis, mitral insufficiency, aortic insufficiency, aortic stenosis, tricuspid insufficiency, and tricuspid stenosis.

Clinical Manifestations. Signs and symptoms seen in valvular disorders are related to decreased cardiac output.

Assessment. Collection of *subjective data* includes noting patient's statement of a history of rheumatic fever and of an inability to perform activities and ADLs without fatigue or weakness. Assessment includes the patient's statement of chest pain, its quality, duration, and onset, as well as precipitating factors and measures that provided relief. The patient may complain of having had heart palpitations. The patient may verbalize feelings of lightheadedness, dizziness, or fainting. The history may include a patient statement of weight gain. Dyspnea, exertional dyspnea, and nocturnal (nighttime) dyspnea as well as orthopnea are often reported, depending on the degree of heart failure.

Collection of *objective data* includes observing for a heart murmur and noting the character and the presence of any adventitious breath sounds (crackles, wheezes) as well as the presence of any edema, pitting or nonpitting.

Diagnostic Tests. The diagnostic tests used to confirm a diagnosis of valvular heart disease are chest x-ray, ECG, echocardiogram, and cardiac catheterization.

Medical Management. Medical management includes activity limitations, sodium-restricted diet, diuretics, digoxin, and antidysrhythmics.

Surgical intervention is usually indicated for a patient whose life-style is severely affected by valvular heart disease. There are two basic surgical procedures: repair of the valve pathology or replacement of the valve.

When medical therapy no longer alleviates clinical symptoms or when there is diagnostic evidence of progressive myocardial failure, surgery is often performed. The surgery may include the following:

- Open mitral commissurotomy—A surgical splitting of the fused mitral valve leaflet for treating stenosis of the mitral valve.
- Valve replacement—Replacement of the stenosed or incompetent valve with a bioprosthetic or mechanical valve; commonly used valves include tilting discs, porcine (pig) heterografts (tissue taken from one species and grafted onto another), homografts (a graft of tissue obtained from a member of the same species as the individual receiving it), and ball-in-cage valves.

Nursing Interventions. Nursing interventions are focused on assisting with ability to perform ADLs, relieving specific symptoms associated with decreased cardiac output, and promoting comfort.

The nursing interventions include administering the prescribed medications (diuretics, digoxin, and antidysrhythmics). Also included in nursing interventions are recording I&O, daily weight, respiratory rate and rhythm, as well as auscultation of breath sounds, heart sounds, and blood pressure. Assessment also includes a check for capillary perfusion, pedal pulses, and presence of edema. A sodium-restricted diet for fluid control is maintained.

Maintain therapeutic oxygen therapy as prescribed. Design with the patient a plan for rest periods and identify those ADLS that are fatiguing and with which the patient will need some assistance.

Nursing diagnoses and interventions for the patient with valvular heart disease include but are not limited to the following:

NURSING DIAGNOSES	NURSING INTERVENTIONS
Activity intolerance, related to weakness, fatigue, and dyspnea	Balance activities with rest periods. Identify fatiguing activities, and obtain assistance as needed. Utilize oxygen as prescribed by physician.
Fluid volume excess, related to decreased cardiac output	Administer prescribed oxygen, digoxin, diuretics, antidysrhythmics. Monitor I&O. Weigh patient daily. Perform respiratory assessment. Perform cardiovascular assessment. Inspect for presence of edema. Obtain vital signs routinely. Maintain sodium-restricted diet.

Patient teaching. Patient teaching focuses on medications, dietary management, activity limitations, diagnostic tests, surgical interventions, and postoperative care as appropriate for each individual patient. Discuss with the patient the disease process and associated symptoms to report to the physician. Explain to the patient antibiotic prophylaxis to prevent infectious endocarditis. Explain the importance of notifying the dentist, urologist, and gynecologist of valvular heart disease. Discuss with the patient the need to maintain good oral hygiene, daily care, and regular visits to the dentist.

Prognosis. The prognosis of valvular heart disease is variable, depending on the specific pathology. The prognosis after surgery is fair to good with amelioration (improvement) of signs and symptoms but often without resolution of all abnormalities.

INFLAMMATORY HEART DISORDERS

All cardiac tissues are susceptible to inflammation, and heart failure can be a serious and rapid result of the inflammatory process.

Rheumatic Heart Disease

Etiology/Pathophysiology. Rheumatic heart disease, a result of rheumatic fever, is an inflammatory disease that predominantly results from a delayed childhood reaction to inadequately treated childhood pharyngeal or upper respiratory tract infection (group A β-hemolytic streptococci).

Ineffective treatment of infection results in delayed reaction and inflammation of the cardiac tissues as well as the central nervous system, joints, skin, and subcutaneous tissues. Of the individuals affected with rheumatic fever, 90% are between the ages of 5 and 15. The onset of rheumatic fever is usually sudden, often occurring in from 1 to 5 symptom-free weeks after recovery from pharyngitis (sore throat) or from scarlet fever. However, rheumatic fever may progress with symptoms and go undiagnosed and untreated. Years later the patient may develop clinical manifestations of valvular heart disease.

Rheumatic heart disease can affect the pericardium, myocardium, or endocardium. The affected tissue develops small areas of necrosis, which heal leaving scar tissue. The heart valves are typically the most affected and become fibrous and incompetent. Valvular heart disease may be the result.

Clinical Manifestations. Fever, increased pulse, epistaxis, anemia, joint involvement, and nodules on joints and subcutaneous tissue may be noted. Carditis can develop. When valvular involvement occurs, signs and symptoms are specific to each condition.

Assessment. Collection of *subjective data* may reveal joint pain (polyarthritis), as well as abdominal pain. There is also lethargy and fatigue.

Collection of *objective data* includes skin manifestations of small erythematous circles and wavy lines on the trunk and abdomen that appear and disappear rapidly (erythema marginatum). The nurse may observe involuntary, purposeless movement of the muscles if Sydenham's chorea (St. Vitus' dance), a disorder of the central nervous system, is present. Heart murmur may be auscultated if carditis with valve involvement is present. Rheumatic heart disease is characterized by heart murmurs resulting from stenosis or insufficiency of the valves.

Diagnostic Tests. Diagnosis is made through signs and symptoms and supported by laboratory study results. An echocardiogram is done to determine the extent of damage to the valves and myocardium. An echocardiogram shows cardiac dysrhythmia. Cardiac murmurs or friction rub can be heard. There is no specific diagnostic test for rheumatic fever. Sedimentation rate and leukocyte count will be elevated. The development of serum antibodies against the streptococci (measured by antistreptolysin-O [ASO] titer) may be present. C-reactive protein, elevated in a specimen of blood, is abnormally high.

Medical Management. Intervention is more effective when approach is by preventive measures. Rapid treatment for pharyngeal infection, usually with prolonged antibiotic therapy, is desired. Penicillin is the antibiotic most commonly preferred. Bed rest is necessary in the acute phases, as is restriction of normal activity. Symptomatic treatment and care are given. Aspirin for joint pain and inflammation is accompanied by application of gentle heat. A well-balanced diet, following the Food Pyramid guidelines, is supplemented by vitamins B and C and high-volume fluid intake. In some patients, surgical commissurotomy or valve replacement is necessary.

Nursing Interventions. Signs and symptoms largely determine the type of nursing interventions. Bed rest during the initial attack is recommended, especially if carditis is present. If polyarthritis is present, the nurse helps minimize joint pain by proper positioning the patient. After the acute stage, the child or young adult is treated at home. A schedule of daily events is reviewed with the patient and the parents.

Nursing interventions are carried out quickly and skillfully to minimize discomfort and prevent tiring the child. Throughout the course of the disease the patient and family benefit from emotional support and appropriate diversions (see Chapter 44).

Patient teaching. The focus of teaching is to facilitate an understanding of the disease process, signs and symptoms, gradually increasing activity levels, and medications, including prophylactic use of antibiotics to prevent recurrence. The importance of a nutritional diet needs emphasis as well as when to notify the physician if signs and symptoms develop. Patients with a history of rheumatic fever or evidence of rheumatic heart disease should receive daily prophylactic penicillin by mouth or monthly intramuscular injections of penicillin to prevent streptococcal infection, at least during childhood and adolescence. Patients with evidence of deformed heart valves should be given prophylactic antibiotics before surgery and all dental procedures.

Prognosis. Prognosis depends upon involvement of the heart; carditis can result in a serious heart disease. Valvular heart disease may result.

Pericarditis

Etiology/Pathophysiology. Pericarditis is the inflammation of the membranous sac surrounding the heart. It may be manifested as an acute or a chronic condition. Trauma or bacterial, viral, or fungal infection is associated with acute pericarditis. It may occur as a complication of systemic lupus erythematosus, scleroderma, azotemia, or MI. Fibrosis of the pericardial sac develops in the chronic form.

Fibrous constriction and thickening of the pericardium occur gradually, causing compression severe enough to prevent normal filling during diastole. Surgical removal of the pericardium may be necessary to restore normal cardiac output.

Clinical Manifestations. Pericarditis differs clinically from other inflammatory conditions of the heart in that the presentation of debilitating pain—much like that of MI—is common. Orthopneic positioning may promote relief. Dyspnea, fever, chills, diaphoresis, and leukocytosis are observed. Pericardial friction rub, grating, scratching, and leathery sounds are detected, as is dysrhythmia.

Decreased heart function to the level of cardiac failure can occur when the heart is compressed by excess fluid in the pericardial sac. Normally, only a few drops of fluid are found in the pericardial sac, yet 150 to 200 ml may develop with incidence of pericarditis. When pericardial effusion restricts heart movement (cardiac tamponade), a pericardial tap (pericardiocentesis) may be performed to remove excess fluid and restore normal heart function.

Assessment. Collection of *subjective data* includes the patient's description of muscle aches, fatigue, and dyspnea. Excruciating chest pain is said to originate precordially and radiate to the neck and shoulders with severe and sudden onset.

Collection of *objective data* includes noting expressed substernal chest pain that radiates to the shoulder and neck, obvious by orthopneic positioning and facial grimace on inspiration. Elevated temperature accompanies chills and may be followed by diaphoresis. A nonproductive cough is often present. Verbalizing anxiety, anticipation of danger, or uneasiness is common. Vital sign changes include a rapid and forcible pulse and rapid, shallow breathing. Pericardial friction rub heart sounds become muffled, and dysrhythmia may be noted by the physician's assessment.

Diagnostic Tests. ECG changes (dysrhythmia) will be noted. Echocardiography will show the presence of pericardial effusion. Laboratory studies will show leukocytosis (10,000 to 20,000/mm^3 will be present), and the sedimentation rate will be elevated. Chest x-ray examination will show cardiac enlargement and pericardial effusion.

Medical Management. Analgesia for comfort and relief of pain reassures the anxious patient. Oxygen and parenteral fluids are usually given. The physician prescribes salicylates for increased temperature, antibiotics for infection, and antiinflammatory agents (indomethacin) and corticosteroids for a persistent inflammatory process. These medicines require nursing knowledge of untoward effects and nursing implications in the control of this condition. Surgical intervention—pericardial fenestration (pericardial window) or pericardiocentesis (pericardial tap)—may be performed to provide continuous drainage of pericardial fluid. Complications may include atelectasis and introduction of infectious agents.

Nursing Interventions. Vital signs are carefully evaluated, and lung and heart sounds are auscultated.

The nurse will provide supportive measures and observe for complications in the patient with pericarditis. Bed rest is maintained to promote healing and decrease the cardiac workload. The head of the bed is elevated 45 degrees to decrease dyspnea. Hypothermia treatment may be necessary to reduce elevated temperature. The nurse may remain with the patient if anxiety is present. Explain all procedures thoroughly.

Nursing diagnoses and interventions for the patient with inflammatory heart conditions include but are not limited to the following:

NURSING DIAGNOSES	NURSING INTERVENTIONS
Cardiac output, decreased, related to inflammatory process	Maintain bed rest with head of bed elevated 45 degrees. Assess vital signs q 2-4 hr as indicated by patient's condition. Administer medications as ordered. Monitor I&O. Provide planned rest periods.
Nutrition, altered, less than body requirements, related to loss of appetite	Assess for anorexia and weight loss; weigh daily; compare values. Encourage intake of foods high in protein and caloric value; provide supplemental feedings.

NURSING DIAGNOSES	NURSING INTERVENTIONS
Pain, related to inflammatory process	Assess and record pain, type and quality. Administer analgesics according to need, as ordered. *(Pain is what the patient says it is.)* Use comfort measures to provide physical and emotional support.
Fluid volume excess, related to ineffective myocardial pumping action	Restrict sodium in diet as prescribed; monitor I&O. Weigh daily; compare values. Administer diuretic therapy as ordered; monitor electrolyte values. Observe respiration and pulse quality. Assess for dyspnea and peripheral edema.
Knowledge deficit, related to disease process	Discuss disease process and symptoms to be reported. Discuss need for ongoing medical care. Explain necessity for rest, avoidance of fatigue, diversion, and program of structured exercise. Stress importance of avoiding potential for exposure to infections and seeking treatment if symptoms arise. Discuss medications, side effects, purpose, and administration techniques. Stress need for overall good health maintenance, proper medical supervision, and dietary restrictions.

Prognosis. The prognosis is fair in early stages but extremely grave if purulent and fibrinous stages develop.

Endocarditis

Etiology/Pathophysiology. Endocarditis is an infection or inflammation of the inner membranous lining of the heart, particularly the heart valves. Classified on the basis of cause, it may result from invasion of an organism (bacterial endocarditis) or may be the result of injury to the lining. Endocarditis may develop after cardiac surgery, which in itself is traumatic.

Persons at risk include patients with rheumatic heart disease, congestive heart disease, or degenerative heart disease. In some cases endocarditis is preceded by intrusive procedures such as dental procedures, minor surgery, gynecological examinations, or insertion of indwelling urinary catheters. Other persons at high risk include those who "mainline" street drugs, because of the possibility of bacteremia from contaminated needles and syringes.

Bacteria, most commonly *Streptococcus viridans* or *Staphylococcus aureus, Staphylococcus epidermidis,* and enterococci, are deposited on the heart lining or valves. As the organism embeds into the tissue, a vegetative growth perforates the chambers or valve leaflets. Fibrin and calciferous growths of the vegetation may ulcerate and scar the valves or may break away, causing emboli, infection, or abscess in organs where they may lodge. The kidneys and spleen are often affected.

Clinical Manifestations. Occurring in acute or subacute form, signs and symptoms progress either rapidly, in dangerous sequence during the acute phase, or gradually, with damage occurring over a long period.

Assessment. Collection of *subjective data* includes noting patient complaints of influenza-like symptoms with recurrent fever, undue fatigue, chest pain, headaches, and joint pain.

Collection of *objective data* may reveal the significant signs of petechiae in the conjunctiva, mouth, and legs and anemia. Weight loss may occur. Pulse is rapid. Murmurs can be detected.

Diagnostic Tests. ECG changes and chest x-ray examination denote evidence of CHF and heart enlargement. Echocardiography determines the extent of valvular damage. Laboratory findings indicate leukocytosis and increased sedimentation rate. Blood cultures determine the the causative organism, and sensitivity tests indicate the effective antibiotic needed for medical management.

Medical Management. Management relies on bed rest to decrease the heart's workload. After the blood cultures, massive doses of antibiotics are administered—usually parenterally—to combat the organism. Antibiotic therapy is often as long as a month, or in the case of some organisms, as long as 2 months.

Prophylactic antibiotic treatment is recommended for individuals who are considered at "high risk" for developing bacterial endocarditis. Previous valve surgery, preexisting valvular heart disease, or congenital abnormalities may require patients to take "bacterial endocarditis precautions." This involves antibiotic therapy as prescribed by the physician before any invasive procedure such as dental work or minor surgery.

Surgical repair of diseased valves or prosthetic valvular replacement may be necessary if the patient's condition is severe.

Nursing Interventions. The nursing interventions are based primarily on the signs and symptoms. Observation for petechiae, location of pain, vomiting, and fever is a nursing responsibility. If these signs and symptoms are observed, they should be reported at once.

During the acute phase, it is essential to maintain the patient on bed rest and provide a calm, quiet environment. Vital signs should be taken every 4 hours, including apical pulse. When activity or ambulation begins, assess pulse before and after to determine the effects on the heart muscle.

Ensuring adequate nutrition is important. Frequently patients have a decreased appetite in conjunction with the disease process. The nurse should provide attractive meals with supplemental between meal nourishment. Promoting rest and comfort and preventing further inflammation and infection are the focus of nursing interventions while the patient is hospitalized.

Patient teaching. Patient teaching focuses on identifying causes, bacterial endocarditis precautions, dietary requirements and gradually increasing activity levels as well as teaching regarding the need for prophylactic antibiotics before any invasive procedure if the patient has preexisting valvular heart disease.

Prognosis. Before the advent of antibiotics, patients with bacterial endocarditis could be expected to live approximately 1 year; prompt treatment with intensive antibiotic therapy will now cure about 90% of patients with this condition.

Myocarditis

Inflammation of the myocardium may originate from rheumatic heart disease; viral, bacterial, or fungal infection; or endocarditis or pericarditis. The cause may be unknown.

Signs and symptoms will vary according to the site of manifestation. However, cardiac enlargement, murmur, gallop, and tachycardia are typically seen in myocarditis. Cardiomyopathy may develop as a complication. Involvement and enlargement of the myocardium may result in dysrhythmias.

Therapy is symptomatic and primarily follows the same approach as that of endocarditis: bed rest, oxygen, antibiotics, antiinflammatory agents, careful assessments, and correction of dysrhythmias.

Recovery may occur; however, cardiomyopathy may develop. As a result, the disease may have a long, benign course, or it may result in sudden death during exercise.

DISORDERS OF THE PERIPHERAL VASCULAR SYSTEM

Peripheral vascular disease refers to any abnormal condition that affects the blood vessels outside the heart and the lymphatic vessels. The word **peripheral** means pertaining to the outside, surface, or surrounding area.

The peripheral vascular system consists of arteries, capillaries, and veins. This system supplies oxygen-rich blood to the upper and lower extremities of the body, and returns blood and carbon dioxide from those areas to the heart and lungs. Disorders of the peripheral vascular system occur when circulation to the upper and lower body extremities is compromised.

Normal Aging Patterns

Degenerative changes occur in the vascular system as part of the normal aging process. These changes affect the walls of the blood vessels and predispose persons to problems in the transport of blood and nutrients to the tissues. The inner walls of the blood vessels (tunica interna) become thick and less compliant. A decrease in the elasticity of the middle walls of the blood vessels (tunica media) causes less flexibility. These changes markedly decrease the elasticity and flexibility of the vessels and therefore increase peripheral vascular resistance, causing a rise in blood pressure. This may ultimately lead to an elevation in overall blood pressure. These changes may increase a person's susceptibility to peripheral vascular disease (see gerontological box on p. 732).

Risk Factors for Peripheral Vascular Disorders

Risk factors for peripheral vascular disorders are similar to those for cardiovascular disorders (see Box 28-1).

An important aspect of caring for the patient with a peripheral vascular disorder is understanding the risk factors and incorporating them into patient teaching.

Age. As a person ages, arteriosclerotic changes occur in the peripheral vascular system, which leads to increased peripheral vascular resistance and decreased blood flow to the tissues.

Gender. Men are more susceptible to arteriosclerotic changes. This decreases after menopause when the effects of estrogen are no longer present.

Smoking. Smoking is one of the major contributing factors in the development of peripheral vascular problems. The nicotine in cigarettes causes vasoconstriction and spasms of the arteries, contributes to an elevation in blood pressure, and reduces circulation to the extremities. The carbon monoxide inhaled in cigarette smoke reduces oxygen transport to the tissues.

Hypertension. Increased blood pressure causes wear and damage to the inner arterial walls of the blood vessels, resulting in a buildup of fibrous tissue. This in turn leads to further narrowing of the vessel and increased resistance to blood flow.

Hyperlipidemia. An elevation in serum cholesterol and triglycerides contributes to the buildup of plaque inside the blood vessels.

Obesity. Excessive body weight and body fat contribute to the severity of other risk factors. Extra weight in relation to bone structure and height places an increased workload on the heart and blood vessels and may contribute to congestion in the venous system.

Lack of Exercise. Decreased activity may compromise the peripheral vascular system due to a lack of muscle tone. The contraction and relaxation of muscles facilitate the return of blood in the veins to the heart and lungs. Benefits that result from regular physical activity, such as weight and stress reduction and improved vascular tone, are not realized in the sedentary individual.

Emotional Stress. Stress contributes to increased blood pressure, increased production of cholesterol, and increased vasoconstriction of the blood vessels.

Diabetes Mellitus. Uncontrolled elevated serum glucose levels may contribute to the atherosclerotic process, although the exact mechanism by which diabetes mellitus contributes to the development of peripheral vascular disorders is unknown. Elevated serum glucose levels may result in circulatory disorders.

Family History. A family history of atherosclerosis increases an individual's risk.

Assessment

Arterial Assessment. The first symptom of decreased arterial circulation is pain. The pain that initially occurs is from arterial insufficiency and ischemia. Arterial insufficiency occurs when not enough blood is available or able to flow through the arteries to body tissues. Ischemia occurs when the tissue does not receive enough oxygen-rich blood to function normally. Ischemic pain in the lower extremities is usually characterized by a dull ache in the calf muscles. It is often accompanied by leg fatigue and cramping. The pain is brought on by exercise and relieved by rest. It is referred to as **intermittent claudication** (a weakness of the legs accompanied by cramplike pains in the calves caused by poor circulation of the blood to the leg muscles). Pain may also be felt in the thighs and buttocks. As arterial disease progresses and becomes chronic, pain occurs even at rest. Burning, tingling and numbness of the legs may occur at night while the patient is lying down.

Other assessments the nurse makes include palpating and comparing pulses in the extremities. Pulses may be weak, thready, or absent in the affected extremity due to decreased blood flow. The nurse checks the affected extremity and compares it with the unaffected extremity for color, temperature, skin characteristics, and capillary refill time (Box 28-6).

Venous Assessment. Decreased venous circulation leads to edema. When the venous system is not sufficiently returning blood from the tissues to the heart and lungs (venous insufficiency), excess fluid is left in the tissues of the affected extremity (edema). The nurse will assess for edema in the affected extremity and compare it with the unaffected extremity. Venous insufficiency may lead to changes in the pigmentation of the skin. The nurse assesses the skin for darker pigmentation, dryness, and scaling in the affected extremity. Chronic edema and stasis of blood from venous insufficiency may lead to ulceration of the tissues. These ulcers are referred to as stasis ulcers. Peripheral pulses are usually present with venous insufficiency. Pain, aching, and cramping associated with venous disorders are usually relieved by activity and/or elevating the extremity. Refer to Table 28-5 on p. 764 for a comparison of signs and symptoms associated with arterial and venous disorders.

Box 28-6 CAPILLARY REFILL TIME

1. Apply pressure to a toenail or fingernail for several seconds until it blanches (the area loses its color).
2. Relieve the pressure.
3. Note the amount of time it takes for the color to return.
   - The color should return almost instantly, in less than 2 seconds.
   - When there is an arterial disorder, the time it takes for the color to return will be greater than 2 seconds.

Diagnostic Tests.

Diagnostic tests for peripheral vascular disorder include noninvasive procedures and invasive procedures.

Noninvasive procedures include the following:

- Treadmill test—This is an exercise test used to determine blood flow in the extremities after exercising. It is used to identify pain associated with exercise such as claudication.
- Plethysmography—Changes in blood volume are assessed in the veins of the calf or other body extremities by using a plethysmograph.
- Digital subtraction angiography (DSA)—Initially an intravenous contrast solution visible to radiography is administered. This allows blood vessels in the extremities to be visualized by radiography by using an image intensifier video system and a television monitor.
- Doppler ultrasound—A Doppler ultrasound flowmeter is used to measure blood flow in arteries or veins. This is helpful in assessing intermittent claudication, obstruction of deep veins, and other disorders of peripheral veins and arteries.

Invasive procedures include the following:

- Phlebography or venography, a radiographic visualization of veins. A contrast medium is administered through a catheter placed in a foot vein. Films are taken to detect filling defects. Venography is used to assess the condition of the deep leg veins and to diagnose deep vein thrombosis.

TABLE 28-5 Comparisons of Signs and Symptoms Associated with Arterial and Venous Disorders

Signs and Symptoms	Arterial Disorder	Venous Disorder
Pain	Aching to sharp cramping brought on by exercise; relieved by rest	Aching to cramping pain; relieved by activity and/or elevating extremity
Pulses	Diminished or absent	Usually present
Edema	Usually absent	Usually present; increases at the end of the day and when extremity is in a dependent position
Skin changes	Cool or cold Dry, shiny Hairless Pallor develops with elevation; becomes erythematous with dangling	Warm, thick, and toughened Darkened pigmentation Stasis ulcers

- 125 I-fibrinogen uptake test—This test is used for looking at acute calf vein thrombosis. When thrombus formation occurs, large amounts of fibrinogen are present at the site of clot formation. When fibrinogen is tagged with^{125} I and given intravenously, it can be detected in the bloodstream by a gamma ray detector. This test is costly and time consuming, but accurate.
- Angiography is done by injection of a contrast medium intravascularly and then visualizing the arteries using radiography.

Arterial Disorders

Arteriosclerosis and Atherosclerosis. **Arteriosclerosis** (a common arterial disorder characterized by thickening, loss of elasticity, and calcification of arterial walls, resulting in a decreased blood supply) is the underlying problem associated with peripheral vascular disorders. Arteriosclerosis and atherosclerosis are frequently used interchangeably.

Atherosclerosis is characterized by yellowish plaques of cholesterol, lipids, and cellular debris in the inner layers of the walls of large and medium-size arteries. The result of atherosclerosis is narrowing of the artery. Nutrients and oxygen to the tissue can be reduced, resulting in ischemia to the tissue cells. Since this is a form of arteriosclerosis, the arterial wall also loses its elasticity and becomes less responsive to change in blood volume and pressure. Plaque, once formed in the arteries, is thought to be irreversible. Lesions in the arteries formed from plaque may completely occlude an artery. Atherosclerosis can progress to obstruction, thrombosis, aneurysm development, and rupture.

When the need for oxygen in the tissues exceeds the supply, ischemia occurs and may result in cell death and/or tissue necrosis. The degree of reduction in blood flow and oxygen determines the amount of ischemia and necrosis that may occur in the tissues. Specific peripheral vascular disorders that stem from arteriosclerosis and atherosclerosis will be discussed individually in this chapter.

Hypertension. Hypertension will be considered with peripheral vascular disorders. Hypertension is a risk factor in atherosclerosis, which leads to peripheral vascular disease.

Etiology/pathophysiology. Hypertension or high blood pressure occurs when there is a sustained elevated systolic blood pressure of greater than 140 mm Hg and/or a sustained elevated diastolic blood pressure of greater than 90 mm Hg. See Table 28-6 for classifications of high blood pressure. A diagnosis is not based on a one-time elevated blood pressure reading, but after averaging two or more elevated blood pressure readings taken on separate occasions. Although there is no way of predicting in whom high blood pressure will develop, hypertension can be detected easily.

Approximately 60 million Americans have hypertension and an additional 25 million have borderline hypertension. It has been estimated that up to 50% of the adult population in the United States have undiagnosed hypertension. It is difficult to determine exact numbers because most individuals are symptom-free.

Blood pressure is the pressure exerted by the blood on the wall of any blood vessel. Systolic blood pressure is the greatest force caused by the contraction of the left ventricle of the heart. Diastolic blood pressure occurs during the relaxation phase between heartbeats. Blood flow is determined by the amount of blood the heart pumps with each contraction and how fast the heart beats. Peripheral vascular resistance is affected by the diameter of the blood vessel and the viscosity of the blood. Blood flow and peripheral vascular resistance play an important role in regulating blood pressure. Increased pe-

TABLE 28-6 Classifications of High Blood Pressure*

Category	Range (mm Hg)
Normal BP	<140/80
Borderline	140 to 159/85 to 89
Isolated systolic hypertension	≥160
Mild hypertension	90 to 104 (diastolic BP)
Moderate hypertension	105 to 114 (diastolic BP)
Severe hypertension	115 or greater (diastolic BP)

*Represents the average of two or more measurements taken on two separate occasions.
From 1984 Report of Joint National Committee on Detection, Evaluation, and Treatment of High Blood Pressure, *Arch Intern Med* 144:105, 1984.

ripheral vascular resistance resulting from vasoconstriction or narrowing of peripheral blood vessels is a common factor in hypertension.

Vasoconstriction and vasodilation are controlled by the sympathetic nervous system and the renin-angiotensin system of the kidney. Stimulation of the sympathetic nervous system and the release of epinephrine and/or norepinephrine cause blood vessel constriction and increased peripheral vascular resistance. The activation of the renin-angiotensin system occurs with decreased blood flow to the kidney. Renin leads to the formation of angiotensin, which is a potent vasoconstrictor. Angiotensin stimulates the secretion of aldosterone, leading to the retention of sodium and water. The result is an increased blood pressure via these physical mechanisms.

There are two main types of hypertension: essential (primary) hypertension and secondary hypertension. The occurrence of hypertension increases with age and other risk factors.

Essential (primary) hypertension. Essential (primary) hypertension makes up 90% to 95% of all diagnosed cases. Although there is no generally accepted cause of essential hypertension, several theories have been suggested to explain the mechanisms involved, including arteriolar changes, sympathetic nervous system activation, hormonal influence (renin-angiotensin-aldosterone system stimulation), and genetic factors. For a long time many experts believed that an increase in systolic blood pressure was a normal part of aging. In fact, some adhered to the theory that "100 mm Hg plus the patient's age" was a tolerable systolic blood pressure in the older adult. Treatment for hypertension was based primarily on the diastolic reading and isolated systolic hypertension (ISH) often was not treated.

The Systolic Hypertension in the Elderly Program (SHEP) study results, published in 1991, reported that ISH is now believed to raise the risk of cardiovascular disease and strokes in both middle-aged and older people. It is actually a better overall predictor of cardiovascular morbidity and mortality than diastolic pressure in these two age groups. (Diastolic pressure remains the better predictor of coronary artery disease in people under age 45.) ISH is defined as an elevated systolic blood pressure of 140 mm Hg or more with a diastolic blood pressure below 90 mm Hg. The value of treating ISH in older patients has only recently been established, but now those findings are being widely circulated.[44]

Prognosis. With prolonged untreated essential hypertension, the elastic tissue in the arterioles is replaced by fibrous tissue. This process leads to decreased tissue perfusion, especially in the target organs—the heart, kidney, and brain—resulting in deterioration of major organs. Coronary artery disease and cerebrovascular accident, the great causes of death and disability, are much more frequent in those who have elevated blood pressure than those who are normotensive. With treatment, the prognosis is usually good. Risk factors that contribute to the development of essential hypertension are listed in Box 28-7.

Secondary hypertension. Secondary hypertension is attributed to an identifiable medical diagnosis.

Box 28-7 RISK FACTORS THAT CONTRIBUTE TO DEVELOPMENT OF ESSENTIAL HYPERTENSION

NONMODIFIABLE RISK FACTORS

- Age—Risk increases as age advances past 30 years
- Gender—Men are more at risk than women
- Race—Twice as high in African-Americans as in Caucasians
- Family History—Risk increases with a family history of hypertension

MODIFIABLE RISK FACTORS

- Smoking—Nicotine constricts blood vessels
- Obesity—Associated with increased blood volume
- High-Sodium Diet—Increases water retention, which increases blood volume
- Elevated Serum Cholesterol—Leads to atherosclerosis and narrowing of blood vessels
- Oral Contraceptives/Estrogen Therapy—May contribute to elevated blood pressure
- Alcohol—Increases plasma catecholamines (biologically active amines, epinephrine, and norepinephrine), which leads to blood vessel constriction
- Emotional Stress—Stimulates the sympathetic nervous system, which leads to blood vessel constriction
- Sedentary Life-style—Regular exercise over time contributes to lowering blood pressure

TABLE 28-7 Causes of Secondary Hypertension

Condition/Disorder	Mechanisms
Renal vascular disease	Kidney disease (glomerulonephritis, renal failure, physiological changes related to type of disease) affects renin and sodium and results in hypertension.
Diseases of the Adrenal Cortex	Atherosclerotic changes in renal arteries cause increase in peripheral vascular resistance.
Primary aldosteronism	Increase in aldosterone causes sodium and water retention and increases blood volume.
Cushing's syndrome	Increase in blood volume.
Pheochromocytoma	Excess secretion of catecholamines increases peripheral vascular resistance.
Coarctation of the aorta	Causes marked elevated blood pressure in upper extremities with decreased perfusion in lower extremities.
Head trauma or cranial tumor	Increased intracranial pressure reduces cerebral blood flow and stimulates medulla oblongata to raise blood pressure.
Pregnancy-induced hypertension	Cause unknown; generalized vasospasm may be a contributing factor.

Conditions associated with secondary hypertension are given in Table 28-7.

Prognosis. In most instances, secondary hypertension will subside when the primary disease process is treated or corrected.

Malignant hypertension. Malignant hypertension is a severe, rapidly progressive elevation in blood pressure (diastolic pressure greater than 120 mm Hg) that causes damage to the small arterioles in major organs (heart, kidneys, brain, eyes). A primary distinguishing finding is inflammation of arterioles (arteriolitis) in the eyes. This type of hypertension is most common in black males under age 40.

Prognosis. Unless medical treatment is successful, the course is rapidly fatal. The most common causes of death are MI, congestive heart failure, stroke, or renal failure.

Clinical manifestations. Hypertension is essentially a disease without symptoms until vascular changes occur in the heart, brain, or kidneys. Signs and symptoms usually occur as a result of advanced hypertension. These signs and symptoms may include awakening with a headache, blurred vision, and spontaneous epistaxis (nosebleed). With prolonged hypertension, chemical manifestations affect the brain, heart, and kidneys. Ultimately, decreased blood flow to these major organs as a result of prolonged hypertension may lead to angina pectoris, MI, congestive heart failure, renal failure, stroke, and cerebral hemorrhage.

Assessment. Collection of *subjective data* regarding symptoms, history of hypertension, and knowledge level data may include:

1. Assess for morning headache in the occipital area, blurred vision
2. Assess for presence of risk factors (see Box 28-7)
3. Assess for knowledge level of hypertension; definition, meaning of systolic and diastolic readings, complications of hypertension, possible concerns regarding treatment

Collection of *objective data* would include the following:

1. Measuring the blood pressure in both arms in supine and sitting positions. Previous blood pressure results would be used to compare reading. Two or more blood pressure measurements are taken on two separate occasions.
2. Measuring height and weight and record
3. Assessing and recording heart sounds
4. Palpating and recording peripheral pulses

Diagnostic tests. Diagnostic tests associated with hypertension are those that evaluate the functions of the brain, heart, and kidneys. The results indicate the effects of hypertension on these organs and provide baseline information for future reference. These tests include:

- Serum levels of sodium, potassium, calcium, hemoglobin, hematocrit
- Creatinine, BUN (blood urea nitrogen), urinalysis, intravenous pyelography (effect on kidneys)
- Chest x-ray, ECG, and possible echocardiography (effect on heart)

Medical management. Medical management is directed at controlling the hypertension and preventing complications. The goal is to keep the blood pressure at less than 140/90 mm Hg. Treatment is based on the severity of the hypertension, associated risk factors, and damage to major organs. Antihypertensive medications are utilized along with nonpharmacological measures to lower blood pressure.

Nonpharmacological measures include:

- Diet: weight control, reduction of saturated fats, and low sodium
- No smoking
- Decreased alcohol intake
- Regular aerobic exercise
- Relaxation techniques/stress management

Nursing interventions/patient teaching. The main focus of nursing interventions is to maintain blood pressure management through patient teaching about hypertension, risk factors, and drug therapy. Patient compliance is improved with education about side effects of medications, dietary instruction, exercise, and stress-reduction techniques (Box 28-8).

A nursing diagnosis and interventions for the patient with hypertension include but are not limited to the following:

NURSING DIAGNOSIS	NURSING INTERVENTIONS
Knowledge deficit, related to disease process and therapeutic management	Assess level of understanding. Implement teaching plan for hypertension: ■ Disease process, risk factors ■ Prescribed medications and side effects; proper dosage and administration; necessity of taking medication even when blood pressure readings are normal ■ Dietary restrictions ■ Exercise program ■ Relaxation techniques ■ Sexual dysfunction as a potential side effect of adrenergic inhibitors ■ Compliance with therapy and follow-up appointments Encourage the patient to report promptly any problems to health care professionals for counseling.

Box 28-8 MEASURES TO INCREASE COMPLIANCE WITH ANTIHYPERTENSIVE THERAPY

1. Be sure that patient understands that absence of symptoms does not indicate control of blood pressure; remind patient that symptoms do not occur until advanced stages of the disease.
2. Advise patient against abrupt withdrawal of medication; rebound hypertension can occur.
3. Encourage patient to discuss unpleasant side effects of medication with a health care professional.
4. If remembering to take medications is a problem, discuss alternate ways to remember, such as taking them with certain meals or placing medication in separate containers labeled with times of day.
5. Suggest patient participate in an exercise program with a friend or pay for the program (more likely to participate "to get money's worth").
6. Include family and significant others in the teaching process to provide support and promote adherence to regimen.
7. Explain reason for regular health care follow-up (high blood pressure is a chronic disorder).
8. Contact patients who consistently cancel follow-up appointments.

Arteriosclerosis Obliterans.

Etiology/pathophysiology. Arteriosclerosis obliterans is a disorder in which there is a narrowing or an occlusion of the intima and media of the blood vessel walls. Plaque formation, as a result of the arteriosclerotic process, forms on the internal wall of the blood vessel, causing partial or complete occlusion of the blood vessel. The result is little or no blood flow to the affected extremity. The artery is unable to supply blood and oxygen to the tissues whether the patient is exercising or at rest. Signs and symptoms associated with tissue ischemia then occur.

Clinical manifestations. Pain is the first symptom that occurs from tissue ischemia. The pain generally occurs in the affected extremity in conjunction with sustained activity (see Table 28-5). This is due to the demand of the tissue exceeding the available blood supply. The process of activity → ischemia → pain in an affected extremity is referred to as claudication. The pain of claudication subsides with rest; therefore it is frequently referred to as intermittent claudication (a weakness of the legs accompanied by cramplike pains in the calves caused by poor circulation of the blood to the muscles). A burning pain at rest or at night is manifested when the disease process is severe. Symptoms of coldness, numbness, and tingling may be associated with the pain.

Assessment. Collection of *subjective data* focuses on pain associated with intermittent claudication. Does the pain occur with activity, and is it relieved by rest? Is pain occurring at rest?

Collection of *objective data* includes assessment of pulses in the affected extremity, which may be weak or absent, and comparison with pulses in the unaffected extremity. Other assessment factors may include pallor, hairless, shiny skin that is dry and cool to touch. Chronic arterial occlusion may show assessment findings of rubor (discoloration or erythema [redness] caused by inflammation) or cyanosis, arterial ulcers, cellulitis, or gangrenous changes in the affected extremity.

Diagnostic tests. A variety of tests are useful to diagnose arteriosclerosis obliterans. Treadmill testing, digital subtraction angiography, Doppler ultrasound, magnetic resonance imaging (MRI), and angiography may be likely choices.

Medical management. Medical management is focused on preventing complete arterial occlusion. The most frequently used medications to treat obstructive arterial disorders include anticoagulants, fibrinolytics, and vasodilators. The use of vasodilators is controversial; most studies indicate that these drugs are not effective. Anticoagulants are used to prolong clotting time, thus preventing extension of a clot and inhibiting further clot formation. Heparin and coumadin are the most commonly administered anticoagulants. Fibrinolytics or thrombolytics are useful in dissolving existing thrombi. Streptokinase (Streptase) is frequently a drug of choice.

Surgical intervention for advanced disease includes embolectomy (removal of embolism) or endarterectomy (surgical removal of the lining of an artery, usually performed on any diseased or occluded major artery, e.g., carotid, femoral, or popliteal), arterial bypass, percutaneous transluminal angioplasty (PTA), or amputation.

Nursing interventions/patient teaching. Nursing interventions will be based on assessment findings and nursing diagnoses. Interventions include but are not limited to the following:

- promoting comfort, tissue perfusion, and activity
- maintaining skin integrity
- preventing infection and injury
- teaching the patient and family proper care and management of risk factors

NURSING DIAGNOSES	NURSING INTERVENTIONS
Activity intolerance, related to ischemic pain and/or immobility	Prevent hazards of immobility by turning, positioning, and deep breathing, isometric, and range-of-motion exercises. Encourage program of balanced exercise and rest to promote circulation. Instruct the patient to use pain or intermittent claudication as a guide to limiting activity during exercise.
Tissue perfusion, altered peripheral, related to decreased arterial blood flow	Place patient's legs in a dependent position relative to the heart to improve peripheral bloodflow. Avoid raising feet above heart. Promote vasodilation by providing warmth to extremities and keeping room warm. Teach the patient to avoid vasoconstriction from nicotine, caffeine, stress, or chilling. Teach the patient to avoid constrictive clothing such as garters, tight stockings, or belts. Administer prescribed medications. Teach the patient to avoid crossing the legs.
Skin integrity, impaired, high risk for, related to decreased oxygenation to tissues	Teach the patient and family proper skin and foot care: ■ Inspect feet daily; wash and dry gently with mild soap and warm water; use clippers not scissors for nail care; wear wool or cotton socks; use lamb's wool between toes; and use lanolin on dry areas. ■ Avoid the use of heat on feet. ■ Wear comfortable shoes that are not restrictive to circulation and that do not cause feet to perspire. Do not go barefoot. ■ Seek medical help for corns, calluses, and ingrown toenails. ■ Notify the physician at the first signs of injury or skin impairment. ■ Utilize a foot cradle or a padded foot board to promote healing and protect skin.

Prognosis. In advanced disease, the ischemia may lead to necrosis, ulceration, and gangrene (particularly of the toes and distal foot) because of the decreased circulation.

Arterial Embolism.

Etiology/pathophysiology. Arterial emboli are blood clots in the arterial bloodstream. They may originate in the heart from an atrial dysrhythmia, MI, valvular heart disease, or congestive heart failure. Other foreign substances such as a detached arteriosclerotic plaque or tissue may result in arterial emboli. The danger of an embolus is when it lodges in and occludes a blood vessel. Blood flow to the area distal to the lodged embolus is impaired and ischemia occurs. Signs and symptoms depend on the size of the embolus and the amount of circulation that is compromised.

Clinical manifestations. Sudden loss of blood flow to tissues causes severe pain. Distal pulses are absent and the affected extremity may become pale, cool, and numb. Necrotic changes may occur. Shock may result if the embolus occludes a large artery.

Assessment. Collection of *subjective data* includes determining the onset of pain and numbness and the location, quality, and occurrence of these symptoms.

Collection of *objective data* includes assessing pulses in the affected extremity. Comparison of both extremities to determine skin temperature and color is of great importance.

Diagnostic tests. Doppler ultrasonography and angiography are indicated to obtain a diagnosis.

Medical management. Medications used to treat obstructed arteries include anticoagulants and fibrinolytics or thrombolytics. Anticoagulants are utilized to prevent further clot formation and inhibit extension of a clot. Thrombolytics or fibrinolytics are used to dissolve an existing clot. See the medication table on p. 747 for more information on anticoagulants and fibrinolytics.

Endarterectomy (the surgical removal of the intimal lining of an artery) may be selected as the treatment of choice (Fig. 28-23). This involves stripping arteriosclerotic plaques from the intima or inner media of arteries affected by atherosclerosis. Balloon catheters and other instruments are used to accomplish this. Removal of plaques and thrombi increases blood flow and lessens the danger of complications from further emboli.

Embolectomy is another treatment utilized when larger arteries are obstructed. It is the surgical removal of a blood clot. Surgery must be done within 6 to 10 hours of the event to prevent necrosis and loss of the extremity. Endarterectomy and embolectomy may be done together to deal with the existing emboli and prevent recurrence.

Nursing interventions. Nursing interventions are similar to those for arteriosclerosis obliterans in terms of preventing further arterial problems. During the acute phase the patient must be monitored for changes in skin

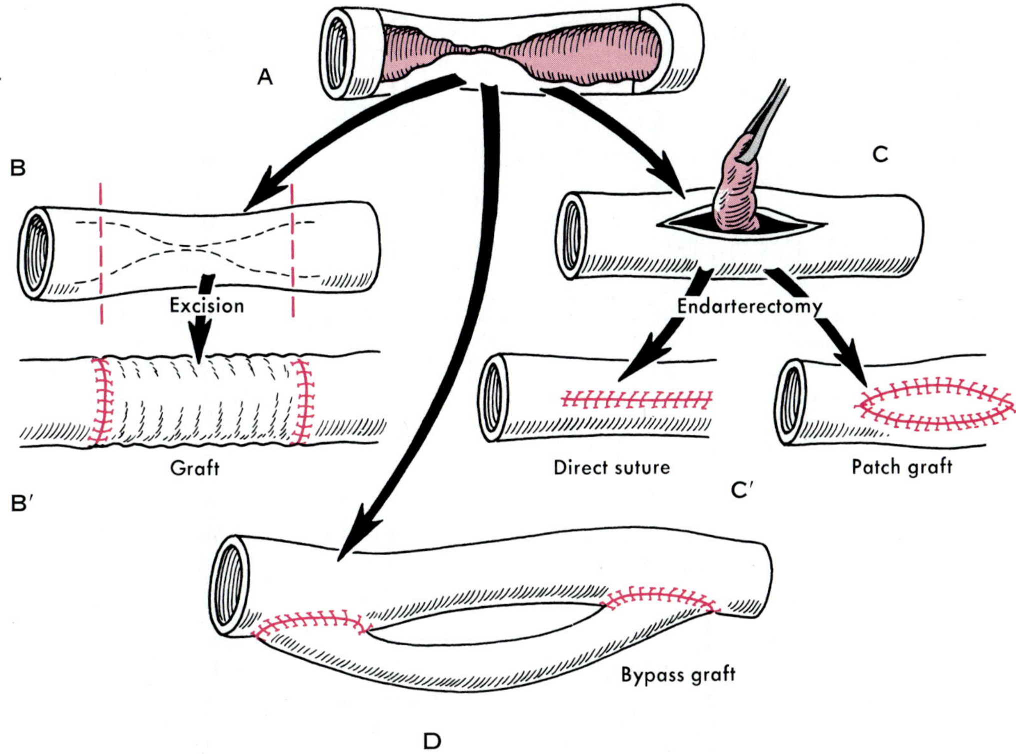

FIG. 28-23 **A,** Obstructed artery. Methods of restoring arterial blood flow include excision **(B),** graft **(B′);** endarterectomy **(C),** direct suture and patch graft reconstruction **(C′);** and bypass graft **(D).** (Redrawn from Fairbain JF et al: *Peripheral vascular disease,* Philadelphia, 1972, Saunders.)

color and temperature of the extremity distal to the embolus. Increasing pallor, cyanosis, and coolness of the skin indicate worsening or occlusion of arterial circulation to the extremity. Keep the extremity warm, but do not apply direct heat.

Nursing diagnoses and nursing interventions for the patient having an embolectomy and/or endarterectomy include but are not limited to the following postoperative nursing interventions:

NURSING DIAGNOSES	NURSING INTERVENTIONS
Tissue perfusion, altered peripheral, related to decreased arterial blood flow	Monitor skin color and temperature distal to the graft site every hour. Assess sensation and movement in the distal extremity. Assess peripheral pulses in the involved extremity: ■ Sudden absence of pulse may indicate thrombosis. ■ Mark location of peripheral pulse with a pen to facilitate frequent assessment. ■ Use a Doppler if pulses of involved extremity are nonpalpable and compare with pulses of noninvolved extremity. Monitor extremity for edema. Check incision for erythema, edema, and exudate.
Tissue perfusion, altered peripheral, related to decreased arterial blood flow—cont'd	Monitor and immediately report signs of complications, such as increasing pain, fever, changes in drainage, absent or weakening pulse, change in skin color, limitation of movement, or paresthesia. Promote circulation: ■ Reposition patient every 2 hr. ■ Tell patient not to cross legs. ■ Use a footboard and overbed cradle to keep linens off extremity. ■ Encourage progressive activity when permitted. Avoid sharp flexion in area of graft. Monitor for signs of bleeding secondary to anticoagulation therapy.
Knowledge deficit, related to anticoagulant therapy	Teach patient general action and side effects of prescribed drug; to avoid taking medications with aspirin, which also has anticoagulant effect. Instruct patient to take anticoagulant at same time every day; and to not stop taking it until advised by physician. Have patient check for signs of bleeding (gum bleeding, epistaxis [nosebleed], ecchymosis [bruising], cuts that do not stop bleeding with direct pressure, blood in urine or stool); report promptly to health care professional.

NURSING DIAGNOSES	NURSING INTERVENTIONS
Knowledge deficit, related to anticoagulant therapy—cont'd	Encourage patient to wear a Medic Alert bracelet or carry an identification card containing the drug name, drug dosage, and physician's name in case of emergency. Have patient report for prescribed blood tests (PTT, PT) used to adjust drug dosage. Tell patient not to add dark green and yellow vegetables to diet (contain vitamin K, which counteracts the anticoagulant drug effect). Instruct patient to restrict alcohol intake (increases anticoagulant effect).

Patient teaching. Patient teaching is the same as for arteriosclerosis obliterans, with an emphasis on anticoagulant therapy.

Prognosis. Prognosis depends upon the size of the embolus, the presence of collateral circulation, and the proximity to a major organ.

Arterial Aneurysm.

Etiology/pathophysiology. An **aneurysm** is an enlarged, dilated portion of an artery. Aneurysms may be the result of arteriosclerosis, trauma, or a congenital defect. Aneurysms of the lower extremities commonly affect the popliteal artery. Other areas predominantly affected are the thoracic and abdominal aorta as well as coronary and cerebral arteries. An aneurysm starts with a weakened arterial wall that becomes dilated from blood flow and pressure in the area. The pathological effect of this condition is differentiated according to shape and site of presentation (Fig. 28-24).

Clinical manifestations. Thrombi form at the site of an aneurysm and break off, causing emboli that may occlude distal portions of the artery. The patient may be asymptomatic. A large pulsating mass may be the only identifiable factor.

Assessment. Collection of *subjective data* by the nurse reveals a patient whose condition has no subjective symptoms unless the aneurysm is large and impinges upon other structures, which can result in pain and inequality of pulses.

Collection of *objective data* includes palpation of a large pulsating mass at the site of the aneurysm.

Diagnostic tests. Fluoroscopy, chest x-ray studies, CT scan, ultrasound, and arteriography are utilized to diagnose the presence of an aneurysm.

Medical management. Aneurysms are monitored for complications such as rupture, formation of thrombi, and ischemia. Control of hypertension is the first priority of care. Surgical intervention may be utilized. The blood vessel may be ligated or grafts may be used to replace the section of the artery that contains the aneurysm or to bypass the aneurysm.

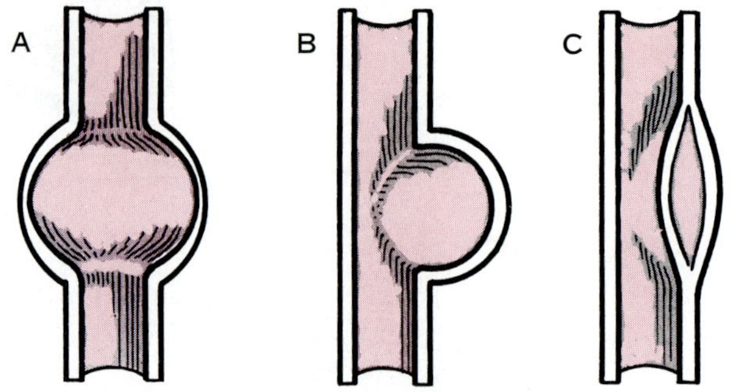

FIG. 28-24 Types of aneurysms. **A,** Fusiform. **B,** Saccular. **C,** Dissecting.

A fusiform aneurysm (all the walls of the blood vessel dilate more or less equally, creating a tubular swelling) can be removed and repair made with a graft of synthetic fiber, such as Dacron or Teflon, or with another vessel taken from another region of the patient's body. Saccular aneurysms (a yielding of a weak area on one side of the vessel and not involving the entire circumference, usually due to trauma; is attached to the artery by a narrow neck) can be removed, and the vessel suture or a patch graft can be used to replace the deformity (Fig. 28-25).

In repair of a popliteal aneurysm, popliteal blood flow is more enhanced when a homograft/allograft (the transfer of tissue between two genetically dissimilar individuals of the same species, as a tissue transplant between two humans who are not identical twins) is used.

Nursing interventions. Initial nursing interventions include monitoring the status of an existing aneurysm.

Postoperative nursing diagnoses and interventions for the patient with arterial aneurysm include but are not limited to the following:

NURSING DIAGNOSES	NURSING INTERVENTIONS
Tissue perfusion, altered peripheral, related to decreased arterial blood flow	Assess circulation (especially extremities) by pedal pulse checks and capillary refill assessments. Be alert for complications.
Pain, related to pressure on surrounding tissue	Assess level of pain and related symptoms. Administer analgesia as ordered. Assess source of pain, and report to physician.
Anxiety, related to feelings of impending death	Examine coping ability. Provide active listening and genuine interest. Maintain therapeutic environment. Administer antianxiety medications as ordered.

Patient teaching. Since aneurysm formation is most commonly associated with atherosclerosis, patient teach-

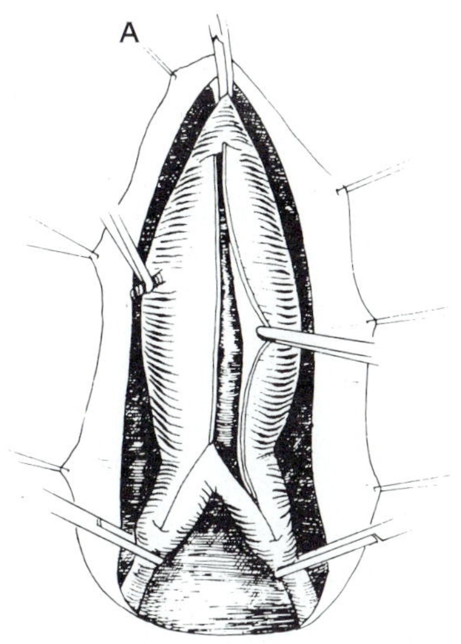

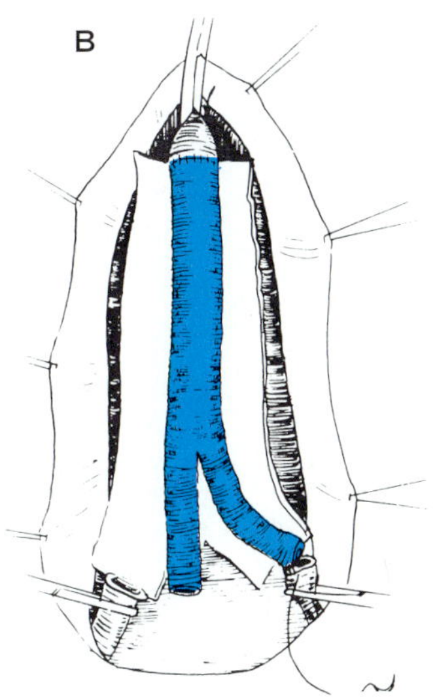

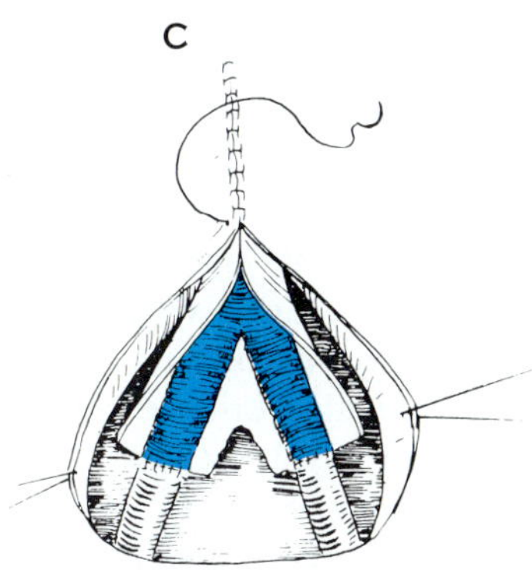

FIG. 28-25 Abdominal aneurysm. **A,** Aneurysm of aorta and iliac arteries. **B,** Bifurcation graft used to replace the excised aneurysm. **C,** Closure of the posterior peritoneum over the graft and suture line. (Redrawn from Crawford ES et al: *Surg Clin North Am* 46:963, 1966.)

ing is focused on risk factor management, including control of hypertension as well as promotion of tissue perfusion, maintenance of skin integrity, and prevention of infection and injury.

Prognosis. An aneurysm may rupture and cause hemorrhage, resulting in death without emergency surgical intervention. With surgical intervention, the prognosis is often good.

Thromboangiitis Obliterans (Buerger's Disease).

Etiology/pathophysiology. Thromboangiitis obliterans (Buerger's disease) is an occlusive vascular condition in which the small and medium-size arteries become inflamed and thrombotic. The cause is not fully understood, but men between the ages of 20 and 40 who smoke are usually those affected with the disorder. Men are affected 75 times more often than women. The disorder develops in the small arteries and veins of the feet and hands. The wrists and lower legs may also be involved. Occlusion of the arteries leads to ischemia, pain, and in later stages, infection and ulceration.

Clinical manifestations. The main characteristic is inflammation of vessel walls. The most common symptom is pain with exercise affecting the arch of the foot, also called instep claudication. When the hands are involved, the pain is usually bilaterally symmetric (equal). Pain may occur at rest and be frequent and persistent, particularly when it occurs in the patient who also has atherosclerosis. The skin in the affected extremity may be cold and pale, and ulcers and gangrene may be present. A sensitivity to cold is an outstanding clinical manifestation. An early sign of Buerger's disease may be superficial thrombophlebitis.

Assessment. Collection of *subjective data* includes information about pain, claudication, and sensitivity to cold in affected extremities and risk factor assessment.

Collection of *objective data* includes presence of pulses, skin color, and temperature in the affected extremities.

Diagnostic tests. Diagnostic tests may include arteriography, digital subtraction angiography, Doppler ultrasound, and exercise testing.

Medical management. The goal of medical management is directed at preventing disease progression. Modifying risk factors and smoking cessation are a major focus. Smoking causes vasoconstriction and decreases blood supply to the extremities. Exercise to develop collateral circulation is encouraged. Surgical intervention, such as amputation of gangrenous fingers and toes, may be indicated. A sympathectomy (a surgical interruption of part of the sympathetic nerve pathways) to alleviate pain and vasospasm may also be performed.

Nursing interventions. Nursing interventions are focused on managing risk factors, promoting tissue perfusion, providing comfort measures, and patient teaching. Care of the extremities to prevent necrosis and gangrene includes hydration and cleanliness. Well-fitting shoes and socks alleviate pressure.

Patient teaching. The hazards of cigarette smoking and its relationship to thromboangiitis obliterans are the primary focus of patient teaching. The goal is to have the patient quit smoking. None of the palliative treatments are effective if the patient does not stop smoking. Nowhere are the cause and effect of smoking so dramatically presented as with Buerger's disease.

Prognosis. Buerger's disease is a chronic condition. Amputation may be necessary if the condition progresses to gangrene with chronic infection and extensive tissue destruction.

Raynaud's Phenomenon/Raynaud's Disease.

Etiology/pathophysiology. Raynaud's phenomenon or disease is caused by intermittent arterial spasms.

There are intermittent attacks of ischemia of the body, especially the fingers, toes, ears, and nose, caused by exposure to cold or by emotional stimuli.

The attacks usually occur secondary to such other conditions as scleroderma (a relatively rare autoimmune disease affecting blood vessels and connective tissue), rheumatoid arthritis, systemic lupus erythematosus, drug intoxication, and occupational trauma. The condition is called Raynaud's disease when there is a history of signs and symptoms for at least 2 years with no progression and no evidence of an underlying cause. It commonly affects women between the ages of 20 to 40 and is more prevalent during the winter months. The exact cause is unknown. It is thought that emotional stress, alterations in the nervous system and immunological system, and hypersensitivity to cold may play a role in the development of signs and symptoms. Few arterial changes occur initially, but as the disease progresses, the intimal wall thickens and there is hypertrophy of the medial wall.

Clinical manifestations. The patient typically complains of chronically cold hands and feet. During arterial spasms, pallor, coldness, numbness, cutaneous cyanosis, and pain occur. Chronic Raynaud's disease may result in ulcerations on the fingers and toes.

Assessment. Collection of *subjective data* includes determining underlying disease processes, risk factor evaluation, and complaints of cold hands and/or feet. Assessing the patient's perception of pain, numbness, tingling, and burning associated with arterial spasm would be included.

Collection of *objective data* would include assessment of pallor, coldness, blanching, cyanosis, and finally reactive hyperemia (increased blood in part of the body, caused by increased blood flow) with erythema following an arterial spasm. The fingers and toes would be inspected for the presence of ulceration because of circulatory inadequacy and residual waste products.

Diagnostic tests. A cold stimulation test is used to diagnose Raynaud's disease. Skin temperature changes are recorded by a thermistor attached to each finger. The patient's hand is submerged in an ice water bath for 20 seconds, and ongoing temperatures are recorded. A comparison is made for baseline data.

Medical management. Medical therapy is aimed at prevention. Drug therapy may be prescribed to reduce pain and promote circulation. Medications may consist of vasodilators, calcium antagonists, and vascular smooth muscle relaxants to promote circulation and reduce pain. Biofeedback techniques have been utilized to increase skin temperature and thereby prevent spasms. Surgical interventions may include sympathectomy for symptomatic relief. If the disease is advanced, with ulcerations and gangrene, the involved area may have to be amputated.

Nursing interventions. Nursing interventions are similar to those for other arterial disorders: promoting tissue perfusion, maintaining comfort, and preventing injury and infection. Risk factor management includes stress-reduction techniques.

Patient teaching. Nursing diagnoses and interventions stress patient teaching for the patient with Raynaud's disease, including but not limited to the following:

NURSING DIAGNOSIS	NURSING INTERVENTIONS
Knowledge deficit, related to effects of cigarette smoking, stress reduction, and avoiding exposure to cold	Develop teaching plan to include the following: ■ Effects of smoking on vasoconstriction and arterial blood flow. ■ Techniques for smoking cessation—stop smoking programs, biofeedback, hypnosis. ■ Techniques for stress reduction: massage, imagery, music, exercise, lifestyle changes. ■ Ways of avoiding exposure to cold: layer clothing, wear mittens and warm socks during winter months, use caution when cleaning the refrigerator and freezer, wear gloves when handling frozen foods, avoid occupations that require constant exposure to cold.

Prognosis. Prognosis for Raynaud's phenomenon, which occurs secondary to other conditions, depends on recognition and treatment of the underlying disease. Raynaud's disease may be controlled by protecting the body and extremities from the cold and using of mild sedatives and vasodilators. Attacks persist but can be controlled. No serious disability develops, but this condition is sometimes associated with the development of rheumatoid arthritis or scleroderma.

Venous Disorders

Venous disorders occur when there is an interruption of blood flow returning from the tissues to the heart. Changes in smooth muscle and connective tissue make the veins less distensible. The valves in the veins may malfunction, causing backflow of blood. The major venous disorders are thrombophlebitis and varicose veins (Table 28-8).

Thrombophlebitis.

Etiology/pathophysiology. Thrombophlebitis is inflammation of a vein in conjunction with the formation of a thrombus. It occurs more frequently in women and affects people of all races. The incidence increases with aging. Other factors associated with the development of thrombophlebitis include venous stasis, hypercoagulability (excessive clotting) of the blood, and trauma to the blood vessel wall. Immobilized patients, who have had surgical procedures involving pelvic

TABLE 28-8 Venous Disorders

Signs and Symptoms	Medical Management/Nursing Interventions
Thrombophlebitis	
Entire extremity may be pale, cold, and edematous. Area along vein may be erythematous and feel warm to touch. Homans' sign: pain in calf on dorsiflexion. Superficial veins feel indurated (hard) and thready or cord-like and are sensitive to pressure. Difference in circumference of extremities.	Maintain bed rest during acute phase. Apply warm, moist heat to reduce discomfort and pain. Elevate extremity, but pillows are not used and knees are never bent unless the foot of the bed is elevated. Assess circulation of the affected extremity, skin condition, and pulses in all extremities. Measure calf circumference daily and record. Use antiembolism stocking on unaffected extremity. Administer heparin and coumadin as per physician's orders. Administer vasodilator to combat arterial spasms and improve circulation as per physician's orders. Administer fibrinolytics (streptokinase) to resolve the thrombus as per physician's orders. Begin exercise program after acute phase as per physician's orders.
Varicose veins	
Veins appear as darkened, tortuous, raised blood vessels; more pronounced on prolonged standing. Feeling of heaviness in legs. Fatigue. Pain and muscle cramps. Edema. Ulcers on skin.	Conservative treatment: ■ Elevate legs 10-15 minutes at least every 2 to 3 hr. ■ Wear elastic stockings. ■ Unna's paste boot recommended for older or debilitated person with cutaneous ulcers (see Fig. 28-26). ■ Avoid standing for long periods of time. ■ Avoid anything that impedes venous flow, such as garters, tight girdles, crossing the legs, and prolonged sitting. ■ Weight reduction if obese. ■ Injection of sclerosing solutions for small varicosities. Surgery: ■ Venous ligation and stripping.

blood vessel manipulation, such as total hip replacement or pelvic surgery, or patients with MI are prone to thrombophlebitis. Thrombophlebitis develops in deep veins as well as superficial veins. Thrombophlebitis usually occurs in an extremity, most frequently a leg. A dislodged deep vein thrombus can be carried to the lungs in the bloodstream and cause a pulmonary embolus.

Clinical manifestations. Pain and edema occur when the vein is obstructed. The size of the calf or thigh may increase in circumference. Active dorsiflexion of the foot may result in calf pain. This is referred to as Homans' sign and may be indicative of thrombophlebitis. Thrombophlebitis of the superficial veins may show signs of inflammation such as erythema, warmth, and tenderness along the course of the vein.

Assessment. Collection of *subjective data* includes characteristics of pain in the affected extremity, noting onset and duration, and any history of venous disorders.

Collection of *objective data* includes inspecting the extremity and determining color and temperature (pale and cold if vein is occluded; erythematous and warm if superficial vein is inflamed). Both legs are measured for circumference and comparison and to detect edema.

Diagnostic tests. Diagnostic tests include venography, Doppler ultrasonography, and impedance plethysmography.

Medical management. Superficial thrombophlebitis is usually treated with bed rest, moist heat, and elevation of the legs. Some physicians believe that complete immobilization is necessary to prevent emboli formation; other believe that clots are sufficiently adhered to vein walls and that mobility improves general circulation and prevents further venous stasis. Drug therapy may include nonsteroidal antiinflammatory drugs (NSAIDs). Deep vein thrombophlebitis requires hospital treatment. The patient is placed on bed rest during the acute phase to prevent embolus. Anticoagulants such as heparin intravenously and oral warfarin (Coumadin) are routinely given. Fibrinolytics and vasodilators may be prescribed. The affected extremity is elevated periodically above heart level to prevent venous stasis and to reduce edema. Specific orders depend on the physician's preference.

When the patient begins to ambulate, elastic stockings (antiembolism stockings) are used to compress the superficial veins, increase blood flow through the deep veins, and prevent venous stasis.

Surgery is indicated only when conservative measures have been unsuccessful. A thrombectomy or the transvenous placement of a grid or umbrella in the vena cava may be done to prevent the flow of emboli into the lungs.

Nursing interventions. The major emphasis for the patient with thrombophlebitis is preventing complications, promoting comfort, and patient teaching about the disease and prevention of recurrence.

Nursing diagnoses and interventions for the patient with thrombophlebitis include but are not limited to the following:

NURSING DIAGNOSES	NURSING INTERVENTIONS
Pain, related to inflammatory process	Maintain initial bed rest. Provide warm, moist heat; be aware that edematous sites burn easily. Administer prescribed analgesics.
Tissue perfusion, altered peripheral, related to decreased venous blood flow	Confine patient to bed in acute phase. Elevate affected extremity according to physician's orders. Check circulation frequently (monitor pedal pulses, capillary refill). Administer prescribed NSAIDs, anticoagulants, and/or fibrinolytics. Measure calf or thigh circumference daily. Assess site for signs of inflammation and edema. Have patient wear elastic stockings when ambulatory. Implement graded exercise program as ordered.
Knowledge deficit, related to disease process and risk factors	Develop a teaching plan to prevent venous stasis, including the following: ■ Avoid prolonged sitting or standing; begin weight reduction if obese. ■ Avoid crossing the legs at the knee, tight stockings, or garters. ■ Elevate legs when sitting. ■ Do flexion-extension exercises of feet and legs when sitting or lying down to promote circulation and venous return. ■ Do not massage extremities because of danger of embolization of clots (thrombus breaking off and becoming an embolus). ■ Take prescribed medication.

Patient teaching. See previous nursing diagnosis and interventions.

Prognosis. A major risk during the acute phase of deep vein thrombophlebitis is dislodgment of the thrombus, which can migrate to the lungs, causing a pulmonary embolus.

Varicose Veins.

Etiology/pathophysiology. A varicose vein is a tortuous, dilated vein with incompetent valves.

The highest incidence of varicose veins occurs in women aged 40 to 60. Approximately 15% of the adult population is affected. Causes of varicose veins include congenitally defective valves, an absent valve, or a valve that becomes incompetent. External pressure on the legs from pregnancy or obesity can place a strain on the vessels, and they become elongated and dilated. Poor posture, prolonged standing, and constrictive clothing may also contribute to this problem. The great and small saphenous veins of the legs are most often affected. The vessel wall weakens and dilates, stretching the valves and resulting in an inability of the vessel to support a column of blood. Pooling of blood in the veins or varicosities are the result. Chronic blood pooling in the veins is referred to as venous stasis. Hemorrhage can occur if there is trauma to a varicose vein.

Clinical manifestations. Varicose veins may be primary or secondary. Primary varicosities have a gradual onset and affect superficial veins. Secondary varicosities affect the deep veins and result from chronic venous insufficiency or venous thrombosis. Often there are no symptoms except the appearance of darkened veins on the patient's legs. Symptoms include fatigue, dull aches, cramping of muscles, and a feeling of heaviness or pressure arising from decreased blood flow to the tissues. Signs and symptoms such as edema, pain, changes in skin color, and ulceration may occur from venous stasis.

Assessment. Collection of *subjective data* includes gathering information about predisposing factors: a family history of varicose veins, pregnancy, or other conditions that could cause pressure on the veins. Also to be included are symptoms the patient is experiencing such as aches, fatigue, cramping, heaviness, and pain.

Collection of *objective data* includes inspecting the legs for varicosities, edema, color, and temperature of the skin and observing for ulceration.

Diagnostic tests. Trendelenburg's test is done to diagnose the ability of the venous valves to support a column of blood by measuring venous filling time. The patient lies down with the affected leg raised to allow for venous emptying. A tourniquet is applied above the knee, and the patient stands. The direction and filling time of the veins are recorded both before and after the tourniquet is removed. When the veins fill rapidly from a backward blood flow, the veins are determined to be incompetent.

Medical management. Mild signs and symptoms may be controlled with elastic stockings, rest periods, and leg elevation. Sclerotherapy consists of injection of a sclerosing solution at the sites of the varicosities. It is done as an outpatient procedure and produces permanent obliteration (complete occlusion of a part) of collapsed veins and good cosmetic results. Elastic bandages are applied for continuous pressure for 1 to 2 weeks. Surgical intervention is indicated for pain, progression of varicosities, edema, stasis ulcers, and cosmetic reasons. Surgery consists of vein ligation and stripping. The great saphenous vein is ligated (tied) close to the femoral junction.The great and small saphenous veins are stripped out through small incisions made in the inguinal area, above and below the knee and the ankle. The incisions are covered with sterile dressings, and an elastic bandage is applied and is to be worn for at least 1 week.

Nursing interventions. Nursing interventions focus on care of the patient following a surgical procedure, including maintaining comfort, maintaining peripheral circulation and venous return, and patient teaching regarding varicosity prevention and maintenance.

Nursing diagnoses and interventions for the patient with varicose veins include but are not limited to the following:

NURSING DIAGNOSES	NURSING INTERVENTIONS
Activity intolerance, related to pain	Keep patient flat in bed for first 4 hr postoperatively. Medicate patient 30 min before ambulation. Elevate leg to promote venous return when lying or sitting.
Tissue perfusion, altered peripheral, related to impaired venous blood return	Monitor for signs and symptoms of bleeding postoperatively. If bleeding occurs, apply pressure to the wound, elevate the leg, and notify the physician. Keep elastic bandage snug and wrinkle free; do not remove bandage for daily dressing change. Encourage deep-breathing exercises and early ambulation to facilitate venous return. Encourage dorsiflexion exercises while in bed or sitting to facilitate venous return.
Knowledge deficit, related to disease process, measures to avoid venous stasis and promote venous return	Develop teaching plan to include: ■ Avoid anything that can increase pressure above the knees, e.g., crossing the legs, sitting in chairs that are too high, wearing garters and knee-high stockings. ■ Begin regular exercise to promote venous return by contraction of leg muscles. ■ Avoid prolonged sitting or standing. ■ Elevate legs when sitting. ■ Maintain ideal weight. ■ Wear elastic stockings for support for activities that require prolonged standing or when pregnant.

Patient teaching. See above Nursing Diagnoses and Interventions.

Prognosis. Varicosities are chronic conditions; the affected person must know how to prevent venous stasis and encourage venous return.

Venous Stasis Ulcers.

Etiology/pathophysiology. Venous stasis ulcers or leg ulcers occur from chronic deep vein insufficiency and stasis of blood in the venous system of the legs. Other causes include severe varicose veins, burns, trauma, sickle cell anemia, diabetes mellitus, neurogenic disorders, and hereditary factors. A leg ulcer is an open, necrotic lesion that results when an inadequate supply of oxygen-rich blood and nutrients reaches the tissue. The result is cell death, tissue sloughing, and skin impairment. Decreased circulation to the area contributes to the development of infection and prolonged healing.

Clinical manifestations. Varying degrees of pain may be reported, ranging from mild discomfort to a dull, aching pain relieved by elevation of the extremity. The skin is visibly ulcerated and has a dark pigmentation. Edema may be present. Ulcerations often occur around the medial aspect of the ankle. Pedal pulses are present.

Assessment. Collection of *subjective data* includes onset and duration of pain and successful relief measures. Predisposing factors such as thrombophlebitis, venous insufficiency, and/or diabetes mellitus are noted.

Collection of *objective data* would include inspection of ulcerated areas, size, location, and condition of skin, color, and temperature. Palpate pedal pulses, and observe for presence of edema.

Diagnostic tests. Diagnostic tests utilized to confirm venous insufficiency and stasis are venography and Doppler ultrasonography.

Medical management. Management is focused on promoting wound healing and preventing infection. Debridement of necrotic tissue, antibiotic therapy, and protection of the ulcerated area are usual treatments. Debridement may be mechanical, such as applying wet-to-dry dressing to the wound. The dressing is applied damp; when dry, it is removed, pulling off the debris that has adhered to the dressing. Debridement can be chemical, which is the use of enzyme ointments such as fibrinolysin deoxyribonuclease (Elase) placed over the ulcer to break down necrotic tissue. Surgical debridement using a scalpel is done when other measures are not successful. Protection of ulcerated areas may be accomplished with the use of an Unna paste boot (Fig. 28-26 on p.776). This boot protects the ulcer and provides constant and even support to the area. A moist, impregnated gauze is wrapped around the patient's foot and leg. It hardens into a "boot" that may be left on for 1 to 2 weeks, although it may be changed more often if there is copious drainage.

Nursing interventions. Nursing interventions focus on promoting wound healing, promoting comfort, maintaining peripheral tissue perfusion, preventing infection, and patient teaching.

Nursing diagnoses and interventions for the patient with venous stasis ulcers include but are not limited to the following:

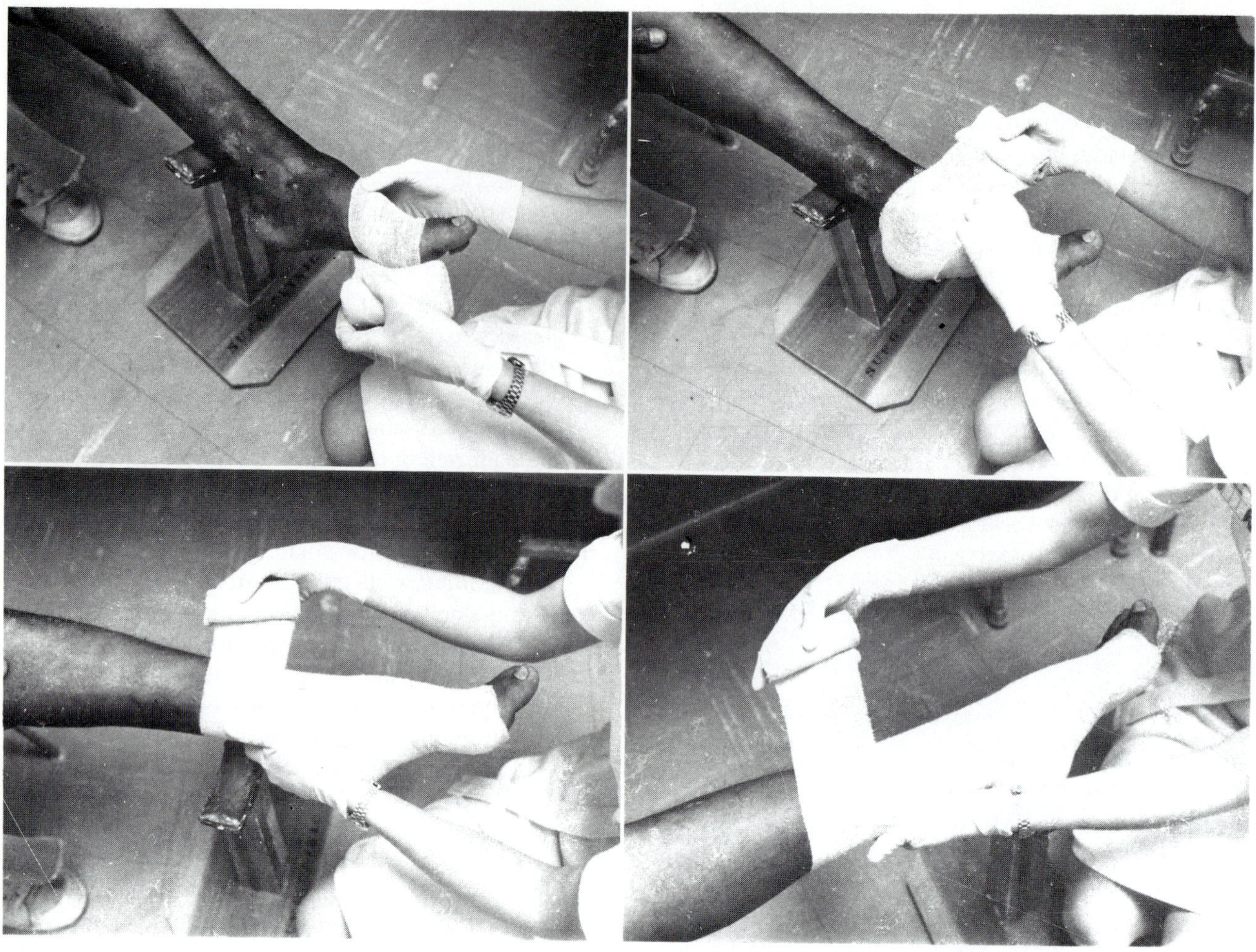

FIG. 28-26 Nurse applying Unna paste boot using specially impregnated gauze. Note ulcers on inferior aspect of patient's foot.

NURSING DIAGNOSES	NURSING INTERVENTIONS
Skin Integrity, impaired, related to open ulceration	Perform dressing changes per physician's order, using wet-to-dry technique, topical drug treatments, Unna boot therapy. Assess wound for signs and symptoms of infection. Provide antibiotic therapy as prescribed. Encourage nutritional intake to promote wound healing.
Tissue perfusion, altered (peripheral), related to insufficient venous circulation	Elevate extremities when sitting or lying to promote venous return and decrease incidence of edema and venous stasis. Use overbed cradle to protect extremities from pressure of bed linens. Use cotton between toes to prevent pressure on a toe ulcer. Assess level of discomfort.
Pain, related to leg ulcers	Administer prescribed analgesic and anti-inflammatory medication as needed.
Knowledge deficit, related to proper care of leg ulcers, dressing changes, and prevention of venous stasis	Develop a teaching plan to include the following: ■ Signs and symptoms of infection and when to notify the physician. ■ The procedure for aseptic dressing changes and use of supplies and equipment. Assess the patient's ability to perform procedure correctly. ■ Avoid venous stasis by refraining from prolonged sitting, standing, leg crossing, or girdle use.

Patient teaching. Patient teaching focuses on preventing infection, maintaining peripheral tissue circulation, avoiding venous stasis, and proper wound care and dressing changes. See previous nursing diagnoses and interventions.

Prognosis. Venous stasis ulcers are a chronic condition caused by chronic venous insufficiency and delayed healing. Most venous ulcers heal with therapy.

REFERENCES AND SUGGESTED READINGS

1. American Heart Association: *Heart facts,* Dallas, 1991, The Association.
2. Baker JD: Assessment of peripheral arterial occlusive disease, *Nurs Clin North Am* 3(3):493, 1991.
3. Berne RM, Levy MN: *Cardiovascular physiology,* ed 6, St Louis, 1992, Mosby.
4. Blank C, Irwin G: Peripheral vascular disorders; assessment and interventions, *Nurs Clin North Am* 25(4):777, 1990.
5. Braunwall E et al: *Harrison's principles of internal medicine,* ed 12, New York, 1991, McGraw-Hill.
6. Canobbio MM: *Cardiovascular disorders: Mosby's clinical nursing series,* St Louis, 1990, Mosby.
7. Carpenito LJ: *Nursing diagnoses: application to clinical practice,* ed 4, Philadelphia, 1991, Lippincott.
8. Cronn A: Beating the clot: saving the heart with thrombolytic drugs, *Nursing* 23(8):34, 1993.
9. Curtin Capasso V, Cote K: The management of patients undergoing arterial reconstructive surgery, *Med Surg Nurs* 2(1):11, 1993.
10. D'Agincourt L: PETS metabolic potency wins its clinical respect, *Diag Imaging* 11(1):68, 1992.
11. Daley R, editor: Dilated cardiomyopathy: a clinical update, *Crit Care Nurs Currents* 10(1):1, 1992.
12. Dault LH et al: Helping your patient through a cardiac catheterization, *Nursing* 22(2):52, 1992.
13. Deglin J, Vallerand A, Russin M: *Davis's drug guide for nurses,* ed 2, Philadelphia, 1991, FA Davis.
14. Downs F: How to make a difference, *Nurs Res* 40:323, 1991.
15. Drew BJ: Using cardiac leads: the right way, *Nursing* 22(2):50, 1992.
16. Dykes PC: Minding the five Ps of neurovascular assessment, *Am J Nurs* 93(6):38, 1993.
17. Editors of Nursing 91 and Gleason B: Teaching your patient about his antianginal drugs, *Nursing* 21(1):65, 1991.
18. Fellows E, Jocz AM: Getting the upper hand on lower extremity arterial disease, *Nursing* 21(8):34, 1991.
19. Finesilver C, Metzle DJ: Right ventricular infarction: the critically different MI, *Am J Nurs* 91(4):32, 1991.
20. Gleason B: After myocardial infarction: how to teach a patient in denial, *Nursing* 21(5):48, 1991.
21. Gleason B: Loosening the grip of anginal pain, *Nursing* 21(1):33, 1991.
22. Hitchins M: Telemetry: who's watching the monitor, *Crit Care Nurs* 8:100, 1992.
23. Johannsen JM: Update: guidelines for treating hypertension, *Am J Nurs* 93(3):42, 1993.
24. Joint National Committee on Detection, Evaluation and Treatment of High Blood Pressure: *1992 report,* National Heart, Lung and Blood Institute, US Department of Health and Human Services Publication, 1992.
25. Kinney MR et al: *Comprehensive cardiac care,* ed 7, St Louis, 1991, Mosby.
26. Letterer RA et al: Learning to live with congestive heart failure, *Nursing* 22(5):34, 1992.
27. Long BC, Phipps WJ, Cassmeyer VL: *Medical-surgical nursing: a nursing process approach,* ed 3, St Louis, 1993, Mosby.
28. Luquire R, Houston S: Cardiomyopathy: how to buy time, *RN* 56(5):29, 1993.
29. McMillan J, Lettle-Longeway C: Right ventricular infarction, *Focus Crit Care* 18(2):158, 1991.
30. Miller et al: Regimen compliance two years after myocardial infarction, *Nurs Res* 39(6):333, 1990.
31. Mitzger B, Therrien B: Effect of position on cardiovascular response during the Valsalva maneuver, *Nurs Res* 39(4):198, 1990.
32. *Mosby's medicine, nursing, and allied health dictionary,* ed 4, St Louis, 1994, Mosby.
33. Norton M, Letizia M, Jennrich JA: Right ventricular infarction: review of pathophysiology, medical treatment and nursing care, *Med-Surg Nurs* 2(3):203, 1993.
34. Pagana KD, Pagana TJ: *Mosby's diagnostic and laboratory test reference,* St Louis, 1992, Mosby.
35. Phipps WJ et al: *Medical-surgical nursing: concepts and clinical practice,* ed 4, St Louis, 1991, Mosby.
36. Scalzo T: Managing a patient on remote telemetry, *Nursing* 22(3):57, 1992.
37. Schultz SJ et al: Preparing your patient for a cardiac PET scan, *Nursing* 21(9):63, 1991.
38. Solomon J: Managing a failing heart, *RN* 54(8):46, 1991.
39. Sommers MS: The shattering consequences of CPR, *Nursing* 22(7):34, 1992.
40. Smith CE: Assessment under pressure: when your patient says "My chest hurts," *Nursing* 21(11):67, 1991.
41. Thomas CL: *Taber's cyclopedic medical dictionary,* ed 17, Philadelphia, 1993, FA Davis.
42. Thompson JM et al: *Mosby's clinical nursing,* ed 3, St Louis, 1993, Mosby.
43. Trottier D, Kochar M: Around-the-clock blood pressure monitoring: how to get good results, *Nursing* 22(1):67, 1992.
44. Trottier DJ, Kochar MS: Managing isolated systolic hypertension, *Am J Nurs* 93(10):50, 1993.
45. Tucker SM et al: *Patient care standards, nursing process, diagnosis and outcome,* ed 5, St Louis, 1992, Mosby.
46. Weikart C: New eye into the heart, *RN* 56(10):37, 1993.
47. Witherell CL: Questions nurses ask about pacemakers, *Am J Nurs* 90(12):20, 1990.
48. Wright S: Pathophysiology of congestive heart failure: *J Cardiovasc Nurs* 4(3):1, 1990.

CHAPTER CHALLENGE

KEY POINTS

- The cardiovascular system is composed of the heart, blood vessels, and lymphatic structures.
- The functions of the cardiovascular system are to deliver oxygen and nutrients to the cells and to remove carbon dioxide and waste products from the cells.
- The heart is a large pump (the size of a human fist) that propels blood through the circulatory system.
- The heart is composed of four chambers—two atria and two ventricles.
- There are two coronary arteries; they supply the heart with nutrition and oxygen.
- The electrical pattern of impulse starts with the sinoatrial node (SA node), which is the pacemaker of the heart; it initiates the heartbeat. This impulse travels to the atrioventricular node (AV node). From here the impulse travels to a bundle of fibers called the bundle of His and finally to the Purkinje fibers.
- There are three kinds of blood vessels organized for carrying blood to and from the heart: the arteries, veins, and capillaries.
- Systemic circulation carries oxygen and nutrients to the body tissues.
- Pulmonary circulation sends deoxygenated blood from the right side of the heart to the lungs, picks up the oxygen, and returns the blood to the left side of the heart.
- Hepatic circulation diverts the blood from systemic circulation to the liver to store excess amounts of sugar and to detoxify any poisonous substances.
- Risk factors for developing coronary artery disease (CAD) are classified as nonmodifiable and modifiable.
- Nonmodifiable risk factors for CAD include advancing age, being of the male gender or black race, and a positive family history of CAD.
- Major nonmodifiable risk factors for CAD include cigarette smoking, hyperlipidemia, diabetes mellitus, and hypertension. A diet high in cholesterol and saturated fats contributes to risk factors.
- An important aspect of caring for the patient with a cardiovascular disorder is understanding the risk factors and incorporating them into patient teaching.
- Major diagnostic tests to evaluate cardiovascular function may include chest x-ray, arteriography, cardiac catheterization, electrocardiography (ECG), telemetry, stress test, positron emission tomography (PET), and thallium scanning.
- Common laboratory examinations to evaluate cardiovascular function are blood cultures, complete blood count (CBC), prothrombin time (PT), partial thromboplastin time (PTT), erythrocyte sedimentation rate (ESR), serum electrolytes, lipids (VLDL, LDL, HDL), and arterial blood gases (ABGs).
- Coronary artery disease (CAD) is the term used to describe a variety of conditions that obstruct blood flow in the coronary arteries.
- When the myocardial oxygen demand exceeds the myocardial oxygen supply, ischemia of the heart muscle occurs, resulting in chest pain or angina.
- Patient teaching to minimize the pain of angina pectoris will include nitroglycerin before exertion, small feedings rather than two or three larger meals, exercise periods with rest periods, stopping activity at first sign of chest pain, avoiding exposure to extreme weather conditions, ceasing to smoke, and seeking a calm environment.
- The subjective data of a patient with myocardial infarction (MI) may include heavy pressure or squeezing pressure in the chest, retrosternal pain radiating to left arm and jaw, anxiety, and nausea.
- Major objective data for the patient with MI include pallor, hypertension, cardiac rhythm changes, vomiting, fever, and diaphoresis.
- Possible nursing diagnoses for the patient with MI may include pain (acute), tissue perfusion (altered), activity intolerance, decreased cardiac output, anxiety, and constipation.
- Congestive heart failure (CHF) refers to the congested state of the heart, lungs, and systemic circulation as a result of the heart's inability to act as an effective pump.
- It is important for the nurse to realize that 1 liter of fluid equals 1 kilogram (2.2 pounds); a weight gain of 2.2 pounds will signify a gain of 1 liter of body fluid.
- Signs and symptoms of CHF with left ventricular failure include dyspnea; cough; frothy, blood-tinged sputum; pulmonary crackles; and evidence of pulmonary vascular congestion with pleural effusion.
- Signs and symptoms of CHF with right ventricular failure include edema in feet, ankles, and sacrum, which may progress into the thigh and external genitals; liver congestion; ascites; and distended jugular veins.
- Medical management of CHF includes increasing cardiac efficiency with digitalis, vasodilators, and ACE inhibitors; lowering oxygen requirements through bed rest; providing oxygen to the tissues through oxygen therapy if the patient is hypoxic; treating edema and pulmonary congestion with a diuretic and a sodium-restricted diet; and weighing daily to monitor fluid retention.

- Nursing interventions for the patient with valvular heart disease include administering the prescribed medications (diuretics, digoxin, and antidysrhythmics); monitoring I&O and daily weight; auscultating breath sounds and heart sounds; blood pressure; and assessing capillary perfusion, pedal pulses, and presence of edema.
- Patient teaching for the patient with valvular heart disease includes dietary management, activity limitations, and the importance of antibiotic prophylaxis before invasive procedure.
- Peripheral vascular disease refers to any abnormal condition that affects the blood vessels outside the heart and the lymphatic vessels.
- Arteriosclerosis is the underlying problem associated with peripheral vascular disorders.
- Hypertension occurs when there is a sustained elevated systolic blood pressure >140 mm Hg and/or sustained elevated diastolic blood pressure of >90 mm Hg on two or more such readings.
- The main focus of nursing interventions for the patient with hypertension is to maintain blood pressure management through patient teaching, risk factor recognition, and drug therapy as well as dietary management, exercise, and stress-reduction techniques.
- An aneurysm is an enlarged, dilated portion of an artery and may be the result of arteriosclerosis, trauma, or a congenital defect.
- The hazards of cigarette smoking and its relationship to thromboangiitis obliterans (Buerger's disease) are the primary focus of patient teaching.
- The two major venous disorders are thrombophlebitis and varicose veins.
- Thrombophlebitis results in calf pain upon dorsiflexion of the foot, which is referred to as Homans' sign.
- Patient teaching to avoid thrombophlebitis includes: avoid prolonged sitting or standing, reduce weight if obese, dorsiflexion-extension exercises of feet and legs, do not cross legs at the knees, and elevate legs when sitting.

STUDY QUESTIONS

1. The blood that is pumped out of the left ventricle contains:
   1. A full supply of oxygen
   2. Impurities that must be removed by the liver
   3. A high percentage of carbon dioxide
   4. All the wastes to be delivered to the organs of excretion
2. The heart contracts in the following patterns:
   1. Right atrium, left atrium, then the ventricles
   2. Both atria, then both ventricles
   3. Right atrium, right ventricles, then the left atrium, left ventricles
   4. Ventricles, then atria
3. The interior lining of the heart, the valves, and the large vessels of the heart is called the:
   1. Endocardium
   2. Myocardium
   3. Pericardium
   4. Epicardium
4. Valve flaps prevent the backflow of blood from the pulmonary artery into the:
   1. Lung
   2. Right atrium
   3. Right ventricle
   4. Left atrium
5. Skeletal muscles help the veins with the upward movement of blood when the muscles:
   1. Dilate
   2. Contract
   3. Inhibit nerve stimulation
   4. Stimulate nerve endings
6. Veins need valves for the purpose of:
   1. Pumping blood through the veins
   2. Filtering out any thrombi in the pulmonary circulation
   3. Keeping venous blood flowing in the direction of the right atrium
   4. Keeping oxygenated blood flowing in the direction of the right atrium
7. The type of circulation that occurs when blood is pumped from the left ventricle of the heart through all parts of the body is called:
   1. Coronary circulation
   2. Systemic circulation
   3. Pulmonary circulation
   4. Portal circulation
8. The normal period in the heart cycle during which the muscle fibers lengthen, the heart dilates, and the cavities fill with blood, roughly the period of relaxation, is called:
   1. Systole
   2. Pulse pressure
   3. Diastose
   4. Diastole
9. Within the various tissues, tiny microscopic vessels form an extensive network (50,000 miles) that allows for exchange of oxygen, carbon dioxide, and nutrients. These vessels are called:
   1. Arteries
   2. Veins
   3. Lymphatics
   4. Capillaries
10. The right atrium receives blood from the:
    1. Superior and inferior venae cavae
    2. Pulmonary veins, pulmonary arteries

3. Superior and inferior venae cavae and coronary sinus
4. Membranous septum, coronary sinus

11. When Mr. Jorgen is receiving heparin therapy, the nurse should:
    1. Observe him for cyanosis
    2. Remember that a sedimentation rate is ordered for monitoring blood coagulation
    3. Give the injection intramuscularly
    4. Observe emesis, urine, and stools for blood
12. Mr. Steadmen, age 72, is admitted to the medical floor with a diagnosis of CHF. In CHF, an increase in abdominal girth, increase in total body weight, and pitting edema are indications of:
    1. Fluid retention
    2. Electrolyte imbalance
    3. Disorganized ventricle pulsation
    4. AV node dysfunction
13. Timmy Coble, 10 years old, is diagnosed with rheumatic fever. Of all the manifestations that may be seen in rheumatic fever, the one that may lead to permanent complications is:
    1. Sydenham's chorea
    2. Erythema marginatum
    3. Subcutaneous nodules
    4. Carditis
14. Mrs. Lambertz, age 67, has a diagnosis of hypertension. She is being dismissed from the hospital. Her teaching should include:
    1. Instruction in consuming a bland diet
    2. Encouragement to take medicines until blood pressure is controlled
    3. Encouragement to begin a vigorous exercise program
    4. Education on continuing to take antihypertensive medications as prescribed
15. Mr. Michaels is an 86-year-old patient who is receiving D 5½ NS per IV at 83 ml per hour on the pump. It is vitally important that the IVs of elderly patients be monitored carefully because:
    1. These patients do not get dehydrated very easily
    2. They may get a fluid overload of the circulatory system
    3. Of the increased risk of infection in the veins
    4. Of the danger of thrombophlebitis developing in the peripheral system
16. Mr. Mesnis is a 34-year-old patient with a history of IV drug use. He is diagnosed with acute bacterial endocarditis. Nursing interventions for this patient would include:
    1. Early ambulation and activity progression
    2. Bed rest for several weeks
    3. Low-calorie diet
    4. Dilution of blood by increased fluid intake
17. Mr. Kucera is a 62-year-old patient with a history of angina pectoris. To decrease the pain from angina pectoris, Mr. Kucera should:
    1. Take a cardiac glycoside at first symptom of cardiac pain
    2. Be careful to avoid taking more than 3 or 4 nitroglycerin pills daily
    3. Take nitroglycerin sublingually QID
    4. Take nitroglycerin sublingually at the first sign of chest discomfort
18. Mrs. Jones has an arterial occlusive disorder. Patient teaching for arterial occlusive disorders would include:
    1. Encouraging the patient to ambulate frequently
    2. The importance of avoiding exposure to cold and chilling
    3. Teaching self-massage of the legs with lotion
    4. Maintaining a reduced-calorie diet
19. Mr. Regon has just returned to the floor from the ICU, where he was treated for a myocardial infarction. He makes the following statement, "I might as well have died because now I won't be able to do anything." Which of the following statements would be the nurse's most appropriate response:
    1. "Don't worry about it; everything will be all right."
    2. "You shouldn't be thinking about that; you are doing so well."
    3. "You think you will not be able to do anything."
    4. "Take life one day at a time."
20. Mrs. Rogers, age 75, is diagnosed with congestive heart failure. The nursing diagnosis of activity intolerance, related to dyspnea and fatigue, would be appropriate. Choose the appropriate nursing intervention in keeping with this diagnosis:
    1. Plan frequent rest periods
    2. Allow patient to shower
    3. Encourage patient to perform all ADLs
    4. Set a goal to increase patient exercise daily to improve cardiac output

29

CARE OF THE PATIENT WITH A BLOOD OR LYMPHATIC DISORDER

Barbara Lauritsen Christensen
Elaine Kockrow

KEY TERMS

ANATOMY AND PHYSIOLOGY

basophil
cisterna chyli
differential white blood cell count
eosinophil
erythrocyte
hematocrit
hemoglobin
hemostasis
lacteal
leukocyte
lymphocyte
monocyte
neutrophil
phagocytosis
thrombocyte

MEDICAL-SURGICAL

anemia
aplasia
disseminated intravascular coagulation
erythrocytosis
extravasation
hemarthrosis
hemophilia A
heterozygous
homozygous
idiopathic
leukemia
lymphangitis
lymphedema
myeloproliferative
pancytopenic
pernicious
Reed-Sternberg cell
thrombocytopenia

LEARNING OBJECTIVES

After reading this chapter, the student should be able to do the following:

Anatomy and Physiology

Define the key terms.

- Describe the components of blood.
- Differentiate among the functions of erythrocytes, leukocytes, thrombocytes, and the lymphatic system.
- Discuss the several factors necessary for the formation of erythrocytes.
- Describe what the leukocyte differential means.
- Describe the blood clotting process.
- List the names of the basic blood groups.
- Describe the difference between lymph and blood.
- Describe the generalized functions of the lymphatic system and list the primary lymphatic structures.

Medical-Surgical

- Define the key terms.
- List common diagnostic tests for evaluation of blood and lymph disorders, and discuss the significance of the results.
- Apply the nursing process to the care of the patient with disorders of the hematological and lymphatic systems.
- Compare and contrast the different types of anemia in terms of pathophysiology, assessment, and nursing interventions.
- Compare and contrast the disorders of coagulation (thrombocytopenia, hemophilia, DIC) in terms of pathophysiology, assessment, and nursing interventions.
- Discuss medical management of patients with hemophilia and DIC.
- List six signs and symptoms associated with hypovolemic shock.
- Discuss important aspects that should be presented in patient teaching and home care planning for the patient with pernicious anemia.
- Discuss the prognoses for patients with acute and chronic leukemia.
- Discuss the primary goal of nursing interventions for the patient with lymphedema.
- Differentiate between Hodgkin's Disease and non-Hodgkin's lymphomas and related medical management and nursing interventions.

RELATED TOPICS OF INTEREST

- Basic nutrition (Chapter 18)
- Diet therapy (Chapter 19)
- Care of the patient with a gastrointestinal or accessory organ disorder (Chapter 27)
- Care of the patient with a cardiovascular disorder (Chapter 28)
- Care of the patient with a respiratory disorder (Chapter 31)
- Care of the patient with an immune disorder (Chapter 36)
- Cardiopulmonary resuscitation (Chapter 50)

ANATOMY AND PHYSIOLOGY

This chapter presents transportation and protection, two of the body's most important functions. Without transportation and protection for the cells, the homeostasis of the body would be threatened. The systems that provide these vital services for the body are the circulatory and lymphatic systems. This chapter discusses the primary transportation fluid—blood—and presents an overview of the lymphatic system. Blood not only performs vital transportation services, but it also provides much of the protection necessary to withstand foreign invaders. The lymphatic system helps maintain fluid balance, and lymphoid tissues help protect the internal environment.

All of us live in a hostile and dangerous environment. Each day we are faced with potentially harmful toxins, disease-causing bacteria, viruses, and even cells from our own bodies that have been transformed into cancerous invaders. Fortunately, we are protected from this staggering variety of differing biological enemies by a remarkable set of defense mechanisms.

Characteristics of Blood

In ancient times blood was referred to as the "river of life," or "fluid of life." Some even believed it had magical properties. All knew it was necessary to maintain life.

Blood is a viscous (thick), red fluid that contains red blood cells, white blood cells, and platelets, which are suspended in a light yellow fluid called *plasma.* Plasma constitutes 55% of the blood's volume; the remaining 45% is composed of the blood cells and platelets.

Blood is slightly alkaline, with a pH range of 7.35 to 7.45. It has a sodium chloride (NaCl) concentration of 0.9%. The average adult blood volume is 5 to 6 quarts (liters), or 10 to 12 pints.

The blood performs three critical functions. First, it transports oxygen and nutrition to the cells and waste products away from the cells. Second, it regulates the acid-base balance (pH) with buffers, aids with body temperature because of its water content, and controls the water content of its cells as a result of dissolved sodium ions. Third, it protects the body against infection with special cells and prevents blood loss with special clotting mechanisms.

The individual components of the blood are discussed in the following sections.

Red Blood Cells. **Erythrocytes** (red blood cells [RBCs]) give blood its rich color. The mature RBC contains cytoplasm and the red pigment, **hemoglobin** (Hg) (a complex protein-iron compound in the blood that carries oxygen to the cells from the lungs and carbon dioxide away from the cells to the lungs). The normal hemoglobin level is, male: 14 to 18 g/dl; female: 12 to 16 g/dl. The average life span of an RBC is 120 days. An erythrocyte is the major cellular element of the circulating blood; its principal function is to transport oxygen and carbon dioxide. The hemoglobin molecule is composed of globin surrounded by four iron compounds called *heme.* When the RBC passes through the lungs, the hemoglobin combines chemically with the oxygen to form *oxyhemoglobin,* which travels to the body cells where the oxygen is released. The hemoglobin, in turn, picks up carbon dioxide and chemically forms *carboxyhemoglobin,* which returns to the lungs where it releases the carbon dioxide and picks up more oxygen to repeat the cycle (Fig. 29-1).

Erythrocytes are continuously produced in the red bone marrow, principally in the vertebrae, ribs, sternum, and proximal ends of the humerus and femur. RBC formation in the adult begins from large nucleated stem cells that develop into a stage in which a fine reticular network known as reticulocytes develops. This reticular structure is lost before the cells enter circulation as mature erythrocytes. A mature RBC does not contain a nucleus. Reticulocytes normally constitute about ½% to 2% of circulating blood.

The proper formation of erythrocytes depends upon several factors, among them healthy conditions of the bone marrow; dietary substances such as iron and copper, plus essential amino acids; certain vitamins, especially vitamin B_{12}; and folic acid. A feedback mechanism controls the rate at which red blood cells are matured and released into the bloodstream. This feedback mechanism is energized when the amount of oxygen delivered to the tissues by RBCs is decreased. The decreased oxygen triggers the release of an enzyme, the renal erythropoietic factor, in the kidneys. Erythropoietin is carried to the bone marrow where it initiates the development of mature RBCs. The increased number of red blood cells allows more oxygen to be delivered to the tissues, and as a result, the signal to increase RBC production is shut off.

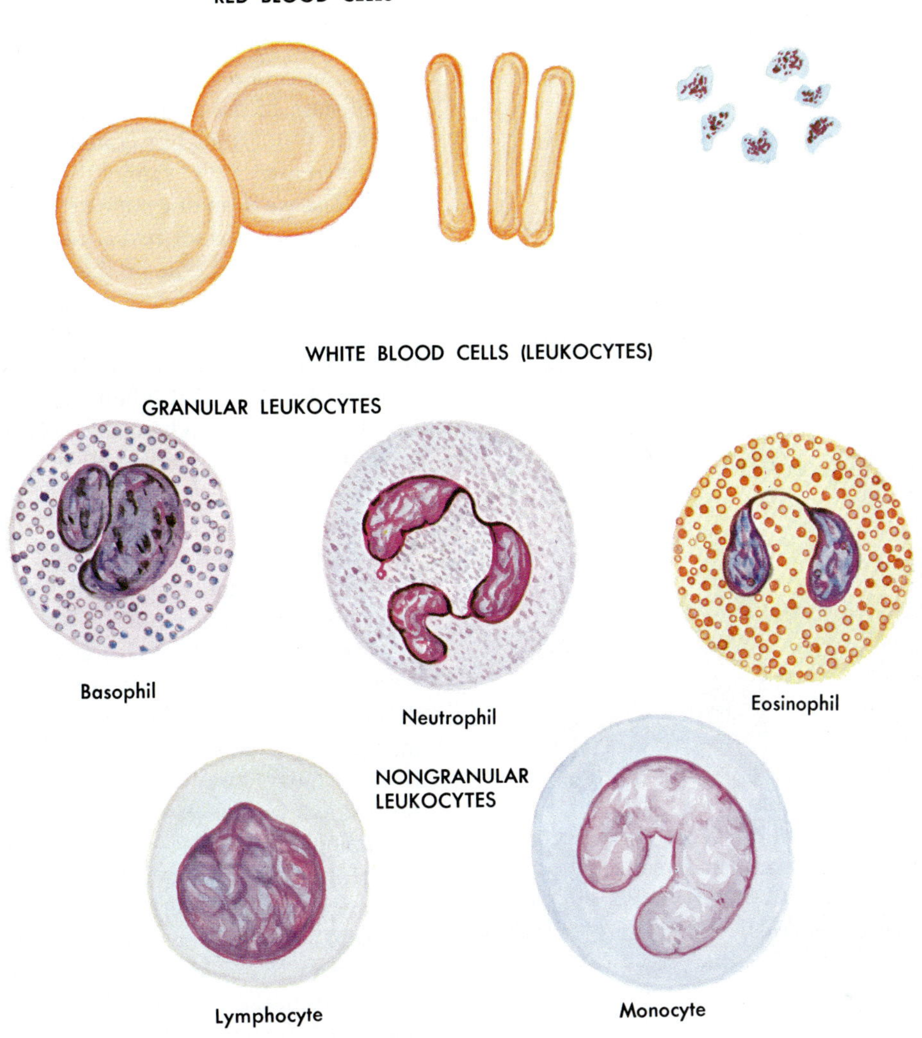

FIG. 29-1 Human blood cells. There are approximately 30 trillion blood cells in the adult. Each cubic millimeter of blood contains from 4½ to 5 million RBCs, 5000 to 10,000 WBCs, and 150,000 to 400,000 platelets.

New erythrocytes are produced at a rate of slightly more than 1% a day. The body needs to produce approximately 2,400,000 RBCs per second to maintain this concentration of blood. An RBC lives about 120 days.

A common laboratory test called the **hematocrit** (a measure of the packed cell volume of red cells, expressed as a percentage of the total blood volume) can tell a physician a great deal about the volume of RBCs in a blood sample. If whole blood is placed in a special hematocrit tube and then "spun down" in a centrifuge, the heavier formed elements will quickly settle to the bottom of the tube. During the hematocrit procedure, RBCs are forced to the bottom of the tube first. The WBCs and platelets then settle out in a layer called the buffy coat. In Fig. 29-2 on p. 784 the buffy coat can be seen between the packed RBCs on the bottom of the hematocrit tube and the liquid layer of plasma above. Normally between about 42% to 52% of the blood volume in males and between 37% to 47% in females consists of RBCs. For a patient with anemia, the percentage of RBCs drops, and for a patient with polycythemia (increased RBC), it increases dramatically (see Fig. 29-2).

If hemoglobin falls below the normal level, as it does in anemia, an unhealthy chain reaction begins: less hemoglobin, less oxygen transported to cells, slower breakdown and use of nutrients by cells, less energy produced by cells, decreased cellular functions. If one understands the relationship between hemoglobin and energy, one can understand that an anemic person's chief complaint will probably be feeling "so tired all the time."

Erythrocytes number 4.5 to 5 million per cubic millimeter (mm^3) of blood. As they age and are no longer useful, they are removed from the bloodstream and destroyed by the liver and the spleen. Hemoglobin is bro-

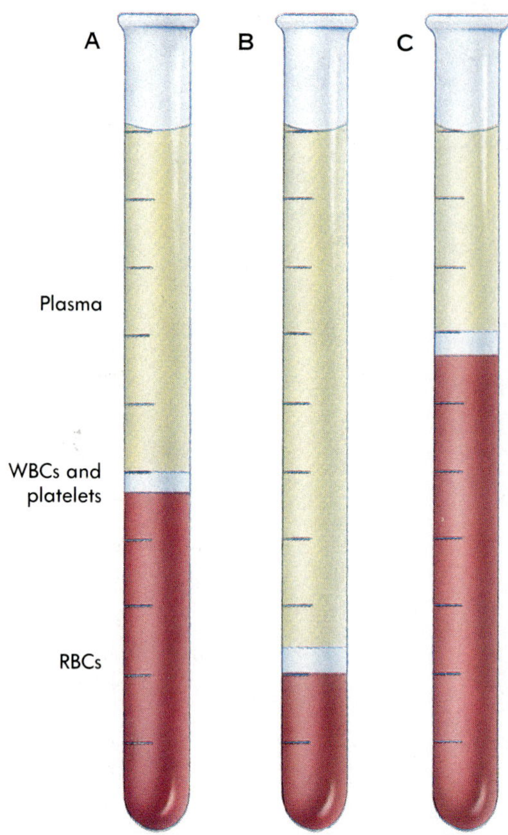

FIG. 29-2 Hematocrit tubes showing normal blood, anemic blood, and polycythemic blood. Note the buffy coat located between the packed RBCs and the plasma. **A,** A normal percentage of RBCs. **B,** Anemia (a low percentage of RBCs). **C,** Polycythemia (a high percentage of RBCs).

ken down, and proteins and iron are stored and utilized in the formation of new erythrocytes. The iron-containing portion (hematin) produces bilirubin. Bilirubin is a waste product and is eventually excreted in the bile by the liver.

White Blood Cells. Unlike the erythrocytes, the **leukocytes** (white blood cells [WBCs]) have nuclei, are colorless, and live from a few days to several years. They are primarily involved in body defenses, such as destruction of bacteria and viruses. They number 5000 to 10,000/mm^3 of blood. Some WBCs can actually leave the bloodstream and move through tissue spaces to fight foreign invaders, such as bacteria.

There are two broad categories of white cells: granulocytes (granule-containing) and agranulocytes (granule-free). The three types of granulocytes are neutrophils, eosinophils, and basophils. The agranulocytes include the lymphocytes and monocytes. A **differential white blood cell count** is an examination in which the different kinds of WBCs are counted and reported as percentages of the total examined. They also may be reported as absolute (actual number).

Because leukocytes respond predictably to symptoms of infection and recovery, they are a reliable gauge of the state of the body's defenses. That's why the differential WBC is such a common blood test. Although the differential WBC cannot, by itself, be used to diagnose a disease or to discriminate between a bacterial and viral infection, it does reveal activity that points to occult (hidden) infection or that signals the intensity of chemotherapy.

The granulocytes develop from the red bone marrow and contain granules in their cytoplasm. The granules are demonstrated when the cells are stained with Wright's stain (a chemical solution). **Neutrophils** (granular circulating leukocytes essential for **phagocytosis**)—(the process by which bacteria, cellular debris, and solid particles are destroyed and removed) ingest bacteria and dispose of dead tissue. They also release lysozyme, an enzyme that destroys certain bacteria. The normal value of neutrophils is 60% to 70%.

Mature neutrophils have a short life span—about 7 hours—after which they die, along with the bacteria and debris they have engulfed. Bone marrow thus needs to manufacture neutrophils constantly; normally, it stores about a 6-day supply. Because neutrophils respond in proportion to the severity of the infection, an overwhelming infection may deplete marrow reserves. When this happens, the marrow releases immature polys, called bands, that are in the final stages of development. When the band count exceeds 8% of the total number of polys, the marrow has used up its reserve. The presence of excess bands in the peripheral blood is called a shift to the left (that is, a shift toward immature cells) and indicates severe infection.

Eosinophils are WBCs that play a role in allergic reactions and are effective against certain parasitic worms. Normal values of eosinophils are 1% to 4%. **Basophils** are WBCs that are essential to the nonspecific immune response to inflammation because of their role in releasing histamine (vasodilator) during tissue damage or invasion. Normal values of basophils are 0.5% to 1%. **Monocytes** are WBCs that function similarly to neutrophils; they circulate in the bloodstream and move into tissue, where they engulf foreign antigens and cell debris. They are useful in removing dead bacteria and cells in the recovery stage of acute bacterial infections. Normal values of monocytes are 2% to 6%. The **lymphocytes** are WBCs that are responsible for antibody formation, a special protein that combats foreign invaders, or antigens. They set up the antigen-antibody process, which protects the body. There are two groups of lymphocytes, B cells and T cells. The function of the B cells is to search out, identify, and bind with specific antigens. T cells, when exposed to an antigen, divide rapidly and produce large numbers of new T cells that are sensitized

TABLE 29-1 What the Differential Tells You

	Normal Values			
	Relative (Percent of Total WBC)	Absolute (Actual Number) $\times 10^9$/L (in/mm3)	Elevated	Depressed
Neutrophils (granulocytes)	60%-70%	3.0-7.0 (3000-7000)	Infection Physiological stressors Myelocytic leukemia Catecholamines Glucocorticoids Diabetic ketoacidosis Renal failure Tissue breakdown	Cancer chemotherapy Viral infection (some, not all) Aplastic anemia Infection in the immunocompromised adult Malnutrition
Eosinophils (granulocytes)	1%-4%	0.05-0.4 (50-400)	Parasitic infection Allergic reaction Eczema Leukemia, myelogenous Autoimmune disease Addison's disease	Possible elevated adrenal steroid production
Basophils (granulocytes)	0.5%-1%	0.025-0.1 (25-100)	Granulocytic and basophilic leukemia	Hyperthyroidism Stress Prolonged steroid therapy
Lymphocytes (agranulocytes)	20%-40%	1.0-4.0 (1000-4000)	Viral illness Infectious mononucleosis Lymphocytic malignancy Chronic inflammation Autoimmune disease Thyrotoxicosis	HIV infection Hodgkin's disease Aplastic anemia Steroid use Renal failure Systemic lupus erythematosus
Monocytes (agranulocytes)	2%-6%	0.1-0.6 (100-600)	Viral infections Bacterial and parasitic infections Lymphoma Multiple myeloma	Not associated with specific disorders

From Gawbikowski J: White cells at war, *Am J Nurs* 92(3):44, 1992.

to that antigen. They work together with the B cells to destroy the foreign antigen. Normal values of lymphocytes are 20% to 40% (Table 29-1).

Thrombocytes (Platelets). **Thrombocytes** (platelets) are the smallest cells in the blood. They are circular cell fragments, which do not contain nuclei. They have a life span of 5 to 9 days and number 150,000 to 400,000/mm^3 of blood. They are produced in the red bone marrow and function in the process of hemostasis (the prevention of blood loss). They assist in clotting formation, which seals off a break in the continuity of the walls of the blood vessels.

Hemostasis. **Hemostasis** is a body process that arrests the flow of blood and prevents hemorrhage. Three actions take place: (1) vessel spasm, (2) platelet plug formation, and (3) clot formation (Fig. 29-3 on p. 786). When a vessel has a tear or rupture, the smooth muscle in the walls of the vessel causes it to contract. Platelets rush to the area and attempt to seal the area, which is effective in small vessel tears. The third process, clot formation, is more detailed and occurs in larger injuries.

Once the platelets reach the injured area and attempt to plug it, a series of reactions involving clotting factors (proteins in the blood) takes place (Fig. 29-4 on p. 786). Thromboplastin is released by the injured tissues and initiates a series of chemical reactions that lead to clot formation. The thromboplastin chemically reacts, along with calcium ions (present in the blood), to convert prothrombin (manufactured in the liver and present in the blood) to thrombin. The thrombin links with fibrinogen (present in the blood) to form fibrin. Fibrin molecules are long, thin strands that collect red blood cells and platelets at the injury site. This action forms a clot. Vitamin K stimulates the liver cells to increase the

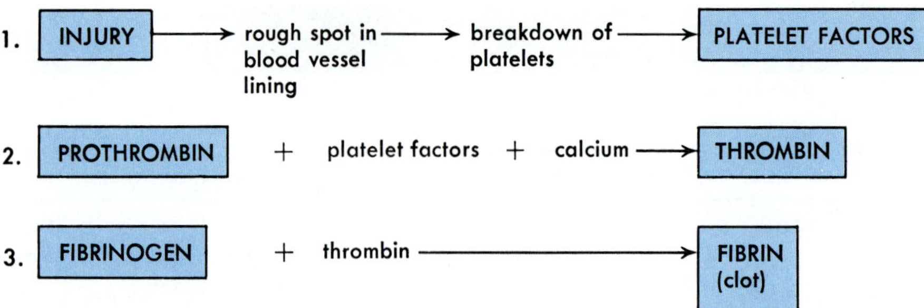

FIG. 29-3 Diagram showing the main steps in blood clotting—a process far more complex than is indicated here.

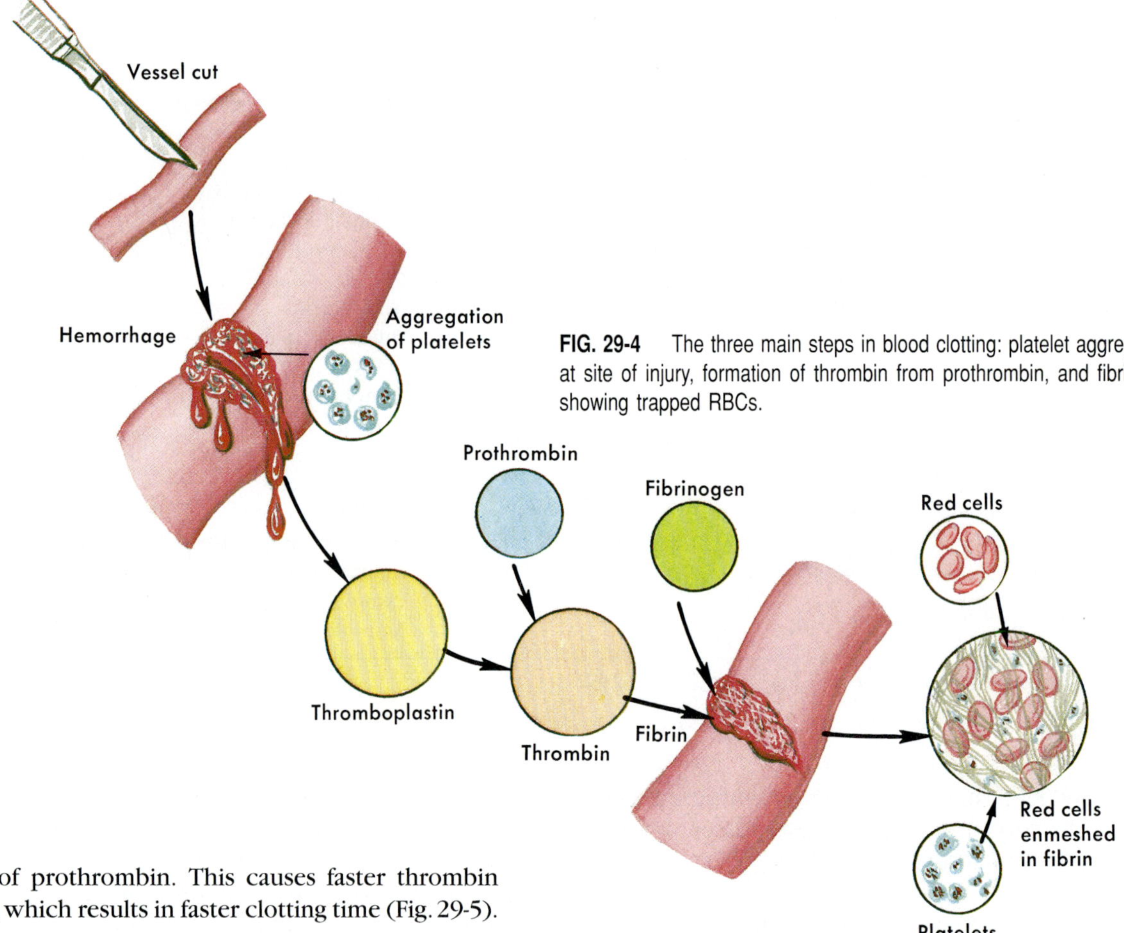

FIG. 29-4 The three main steps in blood clotting: platelet aggregation at site of injury, formation of thrombin from prothrombin, and fibrin clot showing trapped RBCs.

synthesis of prothrombin. This causes faster thrombin formation, which results in faster clotting time (Fig. 29-5).

Summary of this process:

Injury . . . hemorrhage . . . grouping of platelets . . . thromboplastin released . . . (reacts along with calcium ions) . . . converts prothrombin . . . to thrombin . . . links with fibrinogen . . . forms fibrin . . . traps RBCs and platelets . . . FORMS CLOT

Blood Types (Groups). A person's blood group or type is determined genetically and inherited from the parents. Blood types are determined according to the presence or absence of specific proteins (antigens) on the outer surface of the RBCs. In certain types of blood the antigens on the RBCs are accompanied by other proteins found in the blood plasma (antibodies).

The word *antibody* can be defined in terms of what causes its formation or in terms of how it functions. Defined the first way, an antibody is a substance made by the body in response to stimulation by an antigen. Defined according to its functions, an antibody is a substance that reacts with the antigen that stimulated its formation. Many antibodies react with their antigens to clump or agglutinate them. In other words, they cause their antigens to stick together in little clusters.

Every person's blood is one of the following blood types in the ABO system of typing:

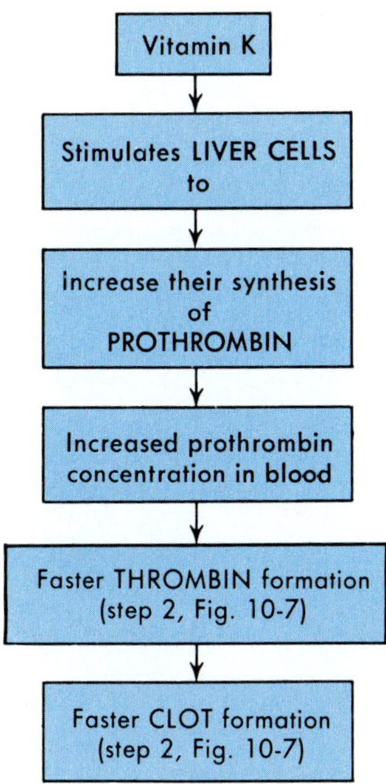

FIG. 29-5 How vitamin K acts to accelerate blood clotting.

Type A
Type B
Type AB
Type O

Suppose one has type A blood (as do about 41% of Americans). The letter A stands for a certain type of antigen (a protein) in the plasma membrane of one's RBCs since birth. Because one is born with type A antigen, the body does not form antibodies to react with it. In other words, one's blood plasma contains no anti-A antibodies. It does, however, contain anti-B antibodies. For some unknown reason, these antibodies are present naturally in type A blood plasma. The body did not form them in response to the presence of the B antigen. In summary, then, in type A blood the RBCs contain type A antigen and the plasma contains anti-B antibodies.

Similarly, in type B blood, the RBCs contain type B antigen, and the plasma contains anti-A antibodies. In type AB blood, as its name indicates, the RBCs contain both type A and type B antigens, and the plasma contains neither anti-A nor anti-B antibodies. The opposite is true of type O blood; its RBCs contain neither type A nor type B antigens, and its plasma contains both anti-A and anti-B antibodies.

Harmful effects or even death can result from a blood transfusion if the donor's RBCs become agglutinated by antibodies in the recipient's plasma. If a donor's RBCs do not contain any A or B antigen, they of course cannot be clumped by anti-A or anti-B antibodies. For this reason the type of blood that contains neither A nor B antigens—namely, type O blood—can be used in an emergency as donor blood without the danger of anti-A or anti-B antibodies clumping its RBCs. Type O blood has therefore been called *universal donor* blood. Similarly, blood type AB has been called *universal recipient* blood because it contains neither anti-A nor anti-B antibodies in its plasma. Therefore it does not clump any donor's RBCs containing A or B antigens. In a normal clinical setting, however, all blood intended for transfusion is typed and cross-matched carefully to the blood of the recipient for a variety of factors. Fig. 29-6 on p. 788 shows the results of combinations of donor and recipient blood.

There are two types of reactions that can occur: agglutination and hemolyzation. In agglutination the donor cells clump together because of the antibodies; this occludes the arteries and can result in death. In the second process, hemolyzation, the antibodies cause the RBCs of the recipient to rupture and release their cell contents; this can also lead to death.

Rh Factor. In 1940 a genetic factor was discovered when research was being conducted on the blood of the rhesus monkey, hence the name Rh factor. People who have the Rh factor, which is located on the surface of the RBCs, are said to be Rh positive; people who do not have the factor are said to be Rh negative. Of the population, 85% have the factor; 15% do not.

Normally human plasma does not contain Rh antibodies. They develop in response to an individual receiving the wrong type of blood. This occurs if an Rh-negative person receives a transfusion of Rh-positive blood. In approximately 2 weeks, Rh antibodies are produced and remain in the blood. If the person then receives more Rh-positive blood, a severe reaction occurs because the Rh-positive antibodies react with the donor blood. It hemolyzes the red blood cells, causing them to rupture and lose their contents.

Rh incompatibility is seen more commonly in pregnancy. For example, the father has Rh-positive blood, the mother has Rh-negative blood, and the baby has inherited Rh-positive blood from the father. Before or during childbirth, a small amount of blood from the baby can intermingle with the blood of the mother (transplacental bleeding). If she should become pregnant again and carry another Rh-positive baby, the antibodies that she has produced could cross to the baby and cause hemolysis of the baby's RBCs. This condition in the baby is known as erythroblastosis fetalis.

Fortunately there is a means to prevent this sequence of events. The mother's blood is tested for antibodies, and she can receive an intramuscular dose of RhoGAM—a desensitization drug. This enables her to carry the next infant without Rh incompatibility.

Lymphatic System

The lymphatic system is a subdivision of the cardiovascular system. It consists of the lymphatic vessels, the lymph fluid, and the lymph tissue. This system has three

Recipient's blood		*Reactions with donor's blood*			
RBC antigens	Plasma antibodies	Donor type O	Donor type A	Donor type B	Donor type AB
None (Type O)	Anti-A Anti-B				
A (Type A)	Anti-B				
B (Type B)	Anti-A				
AB (Type AB)	(none)				

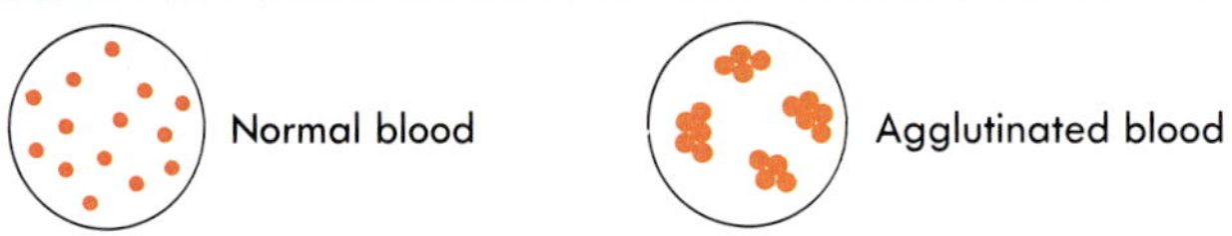

FIG. 29-6 Results of different combinations of donor and recipient blood. The left columns show the recipient's blood characteristics and the top row shows the donor's blood type.

basic functions: (1) maintenance of fluid balance, (2) production of lymphocytes, and (3) absorption and transportation of lipids from the intestine to the bloodstream.

Lymph and Lymph Vessels. Maintaining the constancy of the fluid around each body cell is possible only if numerous homeostatic mechanisms function effectively together in a controlled and integrated response to changing conditions. The circulatory system provides a key role in bringing many needed substances to cells and then removing the waste products that accumulate as a result of metabolism (see Chapter 28). This exchange of substances between blood and tissue fluid occurs in capillary beds. Many additional substances that cannot enter or return through the capillary walls, including excess fluid and protein molecules, are returned to the blood as lymph. Lymph is a specialized fluid formed in the tissue spaces and transported by way of specialized lymphatic vessels to eventually reenter the circulatory system. In addition to lymph and the lymphatic vessels, the lymphatic system includes lymph nodes and specialized lymphatic organs such as the thymus and spleen (Fig. 29-7).

Lymph forms in this way: blood plasma filters out of the capillaries into the microscopic spaces between tissue cells because of the pressure generated by the pumping action of the heart. There, the liquid is called interstitial fluid or tissue fluid. Much of the interstitial fluid goes back into the blood by the same route it came out (that is, through the capillary membrane). The remainder of the interstitial fluid enters the lymphatic system before it returns to the blood. The fluid, now called lymph, enters a network of tiny blind-ended tubes distributed in the tissue spaces. These tiny vessels, called lymphatic capillaries, permit excess tissue fluid and some other substances such as dissolved protein molecules to leave the tissue spaces.

Lymphatic and blood capillaries are similar in many ways. Both types of vessels are microscopic and both are formed from sheets consisting of a cell layer of simple squamous epithelium called *endothelium.* The flattened endothelial cells that form blood capillaries, however, fit tightly together so that large molecules cannot enter or exit from the vessel. The "fit" between endothelial cells forming the lymphatic capillaries is not as tight. As a result, they are more porous and allow larger molecules,

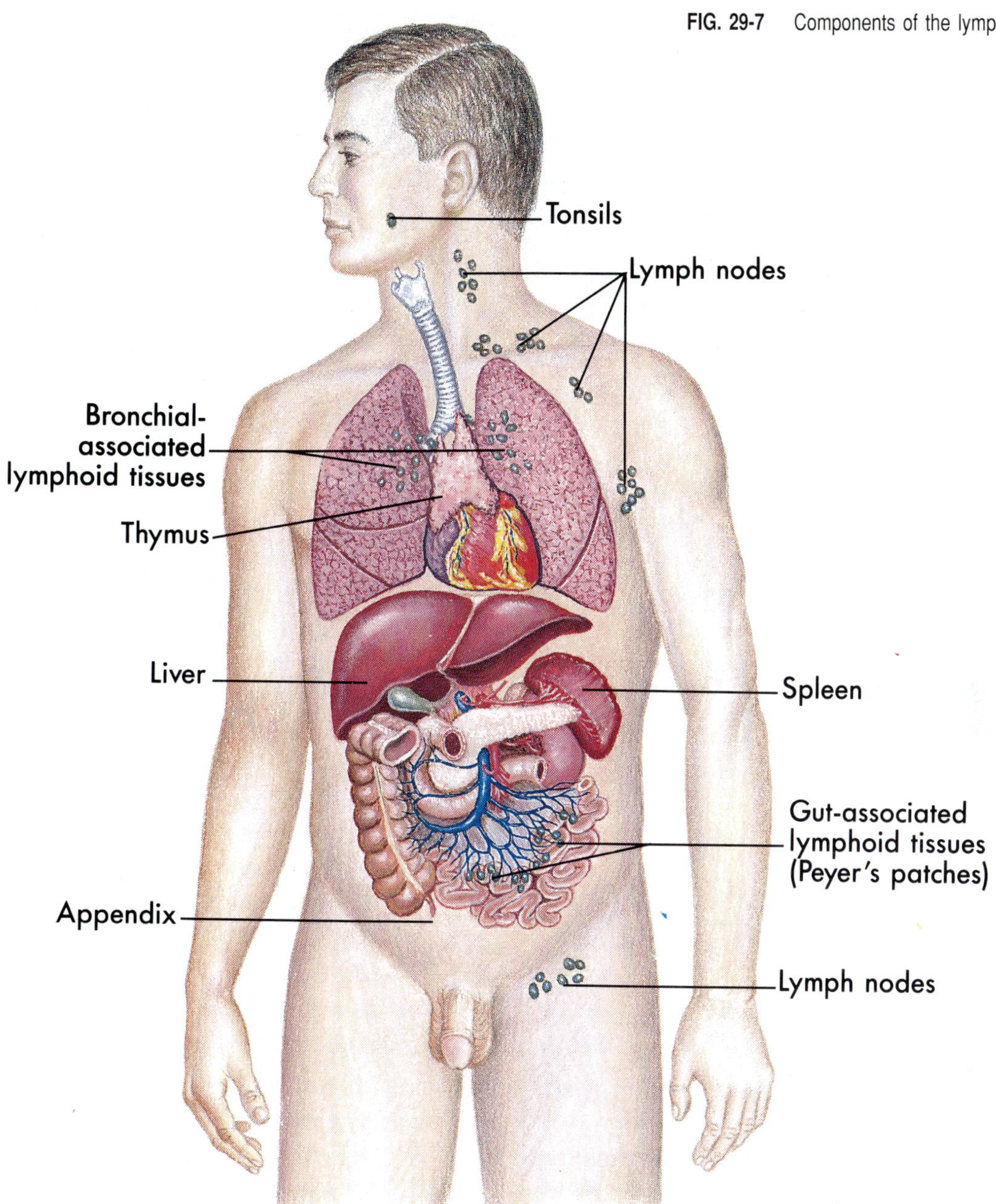

FIG. 29-7 Components of the lymphatic system.

including proteins and other substances, as well as the fluid itself, to enter the vessel and eventually return to the general circulation. The movement of lymph in the lymphatic vessels is one way. Unlike blood, lymph does not flow over and over again through vessels that form a circular route.

Lymph flowing through the lymphatic capillaries next moves into successively larger and larger vessels called lymphatic venules and veins and eventually empties into two terminal vessels called the right lymphatic duct and the thoracic duct, which empty their lymph into the blood, which travels to the right subclavian vein to the superior vena cava and finally to the right atrium of the heart. The lymph can travel in only one direction: from the organs toward the heart—never away from the heart. Lymph from about three fourths of the body eventually drains into the thoracic duct, which is the largest lymphatic vessel in the body. Lymph from the right upper extremity and from the right side of the head, neck, and upper torso flows into the right lymphatic duct (Fig. 29-8 on p. 790). The lymphatic vessels have a "beaded" appearance, caused by the presence of valves that assist in maintaining a one-way flow of lymph. The thoracic duct in the abdomen has an enlarged pouchlike structure, the **cisterna chyli,** that serves as a storage area for lymph moving toward its point of entry into the venous system (Fig. 29-9 on p. 790).

Lymphatic capillaries in the villi of the small intestine are called **lacteals.** They transport fats obtained from food to the bloodstream (see Fig. 27-5).

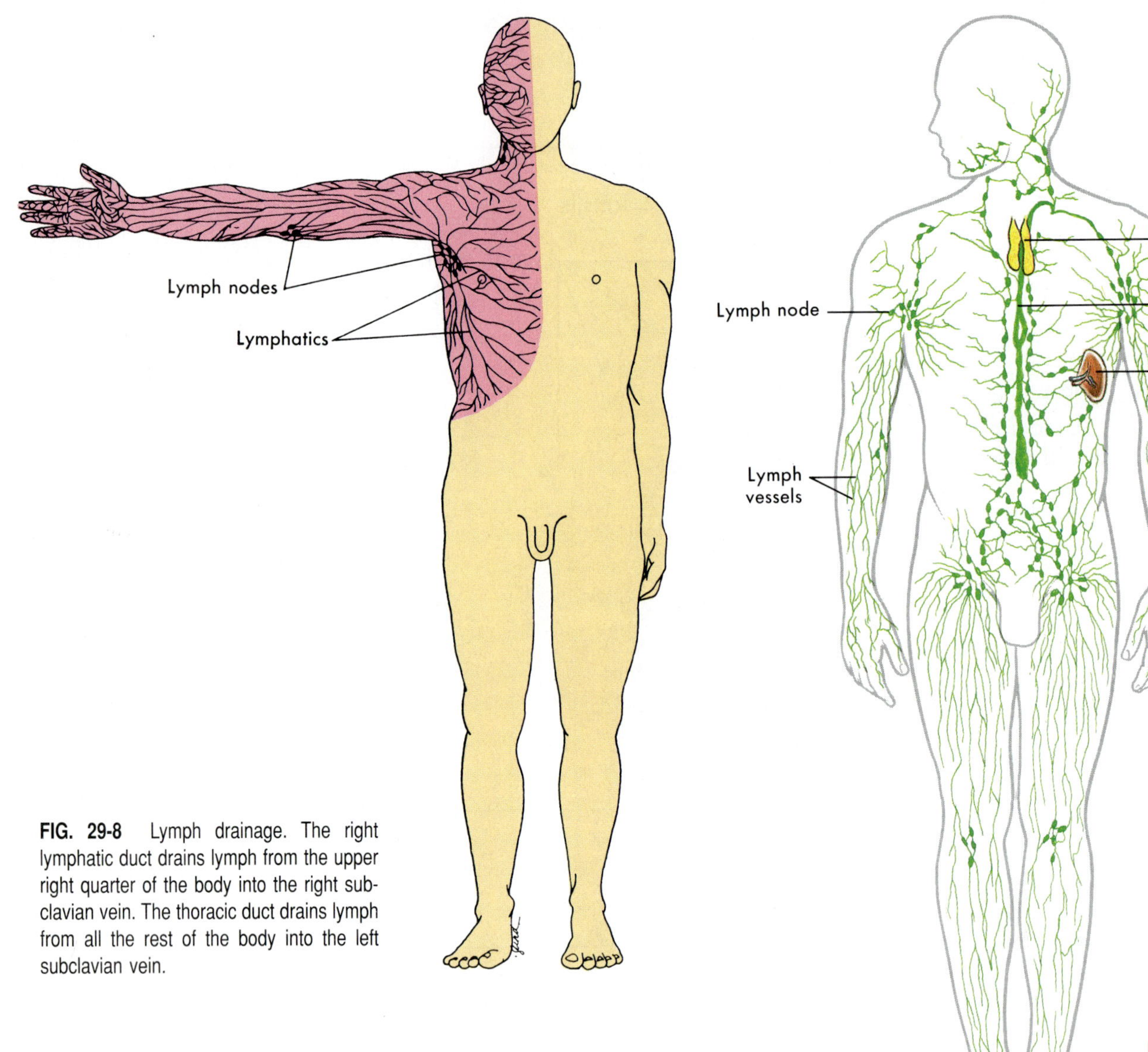

FIG. 29-8 Lymph drainage. The right lymphatic duct drains lymph from the upper right quarter of the body into the right subclavian vein. The thoracic duct drains lymph from all the rest of the body into the left subclavian vein.

FIG. 29-9 Lymphatic system.

Lymphatic Tissue.

Lymph nodes. Lymph nodes (glands) have two functions: (1) to filter impurities from the lymph (much like an oil filter in a car) and (2) to produce lymphocytes (WBCs). The body contains 500 to 600 lymph nodes. They are small, bean-shaped structures, usually appearing in groups. They range in size from 1 to 25 mm (0.04 to 1 inch) in length. These groups are most numerous in the axillary, groin, abdomen, thorax, and cervical regions (see Figs. 29-7 and 29-9).

As lymph moves from its origin in the tissue spaces toward the thoracic or right lymphatic ducts and then into the venous blood, it is filtered by moving through lymph nodes, which are located in clusters along the pathway of lymphatic vessels. Some of these nodes may be as small as a pinhead, and others may be as large as a lima bean. Except for a comparatively few single nodes, most lymph nodes occur in groups or clusters in certain areas. Figs. 29-7 and 29-9 show the locations of the clusters of clinical importance. The structure of the lymph nodes makes it possible for them to perform two functions: defense and WBC production (lymphocytes).

Defense function: biological filtration. Lymph nodes perform biological filtration, a process in which cells alter the contents of the filtered fluid. Biological filtration of bacteria and other abnormal cells prevents local infections from spreading. When passing through the node, lymph is filtered so that injurious particles such as bacteria, soot, and cancer cells are removed and prevented from entering the blood and circulating all over the body. Clusters of lymph nodes allow a very effective biological filtration of lymph flowing from specific body areas (Fig. 29-10).

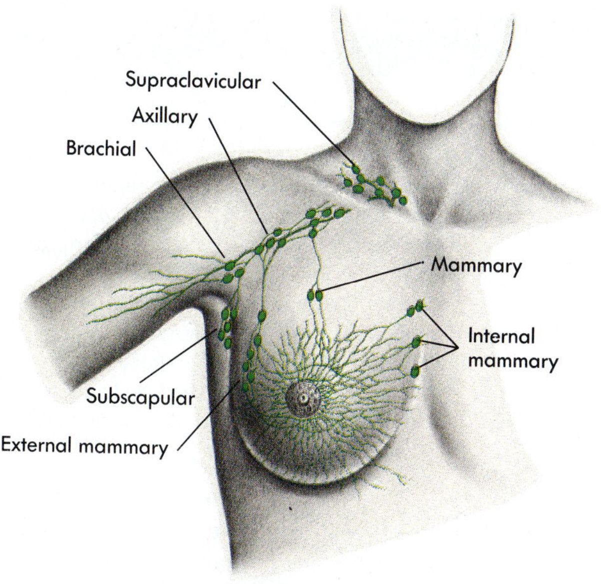

FIG. 29-10 Lymphatic drainage of the breast. Note the extensive network of nodes that receive lymph from the breast.

Tonsils. The tonsils are masses of lymphatic tissue embedded in the mucous membrane of the oral cavity and the pharynx. The pharyngeal tonsil (adenoid) is located in the posterior wall of the nasopharynx. The lingual tonsils are located on either side of the soft palate at the base of the tongue. The palatine tonsils are located on either side of the soft palate in the pharynx. These tonsils are removed when a tonsillectomy is performed.

The tonsils protect the body against invasion of foreign substances by producing lymphocytes and antibodies. They also trap bacteria and may become enlarged. The tonsils are larger in children. They begin to atrophy (shrink) at about age 7.

Spleen. The spleen is a soft, highly vascular, roughly ovoid organ, located in the upper left quadrant of the abdominal cavity, just below the diaphragm (see Fig. 29-7). It is protected by the lower three ribs. The spleen is 12.5 to 16 cm (5 to 6 inches) long and 5 to 7.5 cm (2 to 3 inches) wide. It is considered part of the lymphatic system because it contains lymphatic nodules.

The spleen stores 1 pint of blood, which can be released in emergencies, such as hemorrhage, in less than 60 seconds. This large accumulation of blood gives it a unique deep purple color.

The main functions of the spleen are (1) to serve as a reservoir for blood; (2) to form lymphocytes, monocytes, and plasma cells; (3) to destroy worn-out red blood cells; and (4) to remove bacteria by phagocytosis (engulfing and digesting), (5) to produce red blood cells before birth (the spleen is believed to produce red cells after birth only in cases of extreme hemolytic anemia).

Thymus. The thymus is located in the upper thorax posterior to the sternum and between the lungs in the mediastinum (see Fig. 29-7). The thymus gland functions in utero (before birth) and a few months after birth to develop the immune system. The thymus is responsible for the development of the T lymphocytes of the cell-mediated immune response before they migrate to the lymph nodes and the spleen (see Chapter 36). At puberty the thymus gland atrophies (shrinks) and eventually becomes replaced with fat and connective tissue.

DISEASES AND DISORDERS OF THE HEMATOLOGICAL AND LYMPHATIC SYSTEMS

The hematological and lymphatic systems include the blood and the organs of blood production—the bone marrow and lymphatic tissue. The blood is the only organ in the body that exists in a fluid state. As such, it is the liaison between body organs and systems, carrying oxygen, nutrients, antibodies, hormones, and other substances related to body functions. Blood also transports cellular wastes and protects the body from infection.

Disorders of blood production, bone marrow, or lymphatic tissues will affect virtually all body systems. Disturbances in this delicate balance can produce life-threatening signs and symptoms or occurrences, severe pain, and incapacitation.

Assessment

The nursing data collection is from diverse sources: patient and family observation, physical examination, and diagnostic evaluation results (Table 29-2 on p. 792).

Collection of *subjective data* is vague and nonspecific at the disease process onset: malaise, fatigue, and weakness. History of illness, easy bruising, bleeding tendencies with petechiae, and ecchymosis may be related. Integumentary changes, including pruritus, nonhealing cuts and bruises, draining lesions, jaundice, and palpable subcutaneous nodules may be reported. Edema and tenderness in lymph node regions may be accompanied by pain, sometimes severe. Gastrointestinal (GI) complaints are noted, as well as cardiovascular and respiratory changes. Neurological complaints may include headache, numbness, tingling, paresthesia, and behavioral alteration. Gerontological considerations are listed in the box on p. 793.

Collection of *objective data* uses a system-by-system approach to confirm patient complaints. Manipulation of joints can reveal stiffness and hematoma and may produce pain. Oral cavity examination can reveal lesions, ulcers, signs of bleeding, or gingivitis. Cardiovascular and respiratory assessments include breath and heart sound variations and pain or dyspneic positioning. Anxiety is noted, as well as observation of diminished comprehensive ability. Listening and an unhurried interview may reveal many symptoms not previously mentioned.

TABLE 29-2 Diagnostic Blood Studies

Blood Test	Normal Values	Description	Clinical Significance
CBC with differential			
RBC	Males: 4.7-6.1 million/mm^3 Females: 4.2-5.4 million/mm^3	Actual cell count	Increased in dehydration, polycythemia, at high altitudes, and with hypoxia; decreased in anemia, leukemia, and posthemorrhage
Hgb	Males: 14-18.0 g/dl Females: 12-16 g/dl		Increased in polycythemia, dehydration, chronic obstructive lung disease; decreased in anemias and after hemorrhage
Hct	Males: 42%-52% Females: 37%-47%		Increased with severe burns, shock, severe dehydration, and polycythemia; decreased with severe blood loss, leukemia, and anemias
WBC with differential			
WBC	5000-10,000/mm^3	Actual cell count	Increased neutrophils with a number of bacterial infections, inflammatory but noninfectious diseases (collagen disorder, rheumatic fever, and pancreatitis); increased with infectious diseases (usually of bacterial origin) and with trauma, or leukemia; decreased by chemotherapy, radiation, aplastic anemia, and agranulocytosis
Neutrophils	60%-70%	Percentages of WBCs	Increased with burns, crushing injuries, diabetic acidosis, and infections; decreased in bone marrow failure (e.g., following antineoplastic chemotherapy or radiation therapy or in agranulocytosis), dietary deficiencies, and autoimmune diseases
Eosinophils	1%-4%	Percentages of WBCs	Increased eosinophils found with allergic and parasitic disorders
Basophils	0.5%-1%	Percentages of WBCs	Increased basophils are uncommon and are found with some forms of acute leukemia
Lymphocytes	20%-40%	Percentages of WBCs	Increased in infectious mononucleosis, measles, certain viruses, infectious hepatitis, and lymphocytic leukemia; decreased in AIDS, lupus erythematosus, and Hodgkin's disease
Monocytes	2%-6%	Percentages of WBCs	Increased in the recovery phase of bacterial infections, chronic inflammatory conditions, and monocytic leukemia
Erythrocyte sedimentation rate (ESR)	Male: 0-15 mm/hr Female: 0-20 mm/hr	Rate at which RBCs settle out of a tube of unclotted blood in 1 hr	Increased in tissue destruction; indicates infection when results are compared with elevation in WBC count. ESR is a fairly reliable indicator of the course of disease and can therefore be used to monitor disease therapy, especially for inflammatory autoimmune diseases
Reticulocyte count	0.5% to 2%	Number of reticulocytes in whole blood	Increased in bone marrow hyperactivity and hemorrhage; decreased in hemolytic disease
Platelet count	150,000-400,000/mm^3	Actual cell count	Increased in granulocytic leukemia; decreased in thrombocytopenia or aplastic anemia
Prothrombin time	11-12.5 sec	Rapidity of blood clotting	Detects plasma clotting defects, screens for coagulation, and monitors warfarin (Coumadin) therapy; possible critical values >20 sec

TABLE 29-2 Diagnostic Blood Studies—cont'd

Blood Test	Normal Values	Description	Clinical Significance
Partial thromboplastin time	60-70 sec	Fibrin clot formation	Detects coagulation defects of the intrinsic system and deficiency of plasma clotting. The appropriate dose of heparin can be monitored by the PTT; possible critical values >100 sec
Bleeding time	1-9 min (Ivy method)	Amount of time for a small stab wound to stop bleeding	Prolonged in hemorrhagic disease or with coagulation factor defect
Clotting time	3-9 min	Amount of time for blood in a tube to clot	Prolonged with deficiency in coagulation factors or vitamin K; used to monitor anticoagulant therapy

GERONTOLOGICAL CONSIDERATIONS

- The subjective symptoms of hematological disorders (e.g. fatigue, weakness, dizziness, and dyspnea) may be mistaken for normal changes of aging or attributed to other disease processes commonly seen in the older adult.
- The most common blood disorders are forms of anemia.
- Decreased production of intrinsic factor in the aging gastric mucosa results in an increased incidence of pernicious anemia.
- Many older adults suffer from conditions, such as colonic diverticuli, hiatal hernia, or ulcerations, that can cause occult bleeding. Older adults with these conditions should be observed for iron deficiency anemia.
- Age-related problems such as altered dentition, limited financial resources, difficulty in food preparation, and poor appetite resulting from emotional upset or depression can cause an increased incidence of iron deficiency anemia.
- Severe or persistent anemia can place additional stress on the aging or diseased heart.
- Administration of blood products should be done with caution, since the older adult is at increased risk of developing congestive heart failure. Careful assessment of cardiopulmonary function and intake and output are essential.
- Oral administration of iron preparations increases the risk of GI irritation and constipation in the older adult.
- Ingestion of large amounts of aspirin and other antiinflammatory medications commonly taken by the older adult increases the risk of gastrointestinal bleeding and can lead to alteration in clotting.
- Chronic lymphocytic leukema is the most common form seen with aging. This form of leukemia usually progresses slowly in the older adult and is rarely treated.

Diagnostic and Laboratory Tests

Complete Blood Count. The complete blood count (CBC) is an important part of routine screening and hospital admission. It involves several tests, each of which assesses the three major cells formed in the bone marrow. The CBC detects many disorders of the hematological system and provides data for the diagnosis and evaluation of disorders in other body systems. A CBC includes red and white cell counts, hematocrit and hemoglobin levels, erythrocyte indices, differential white cell count, and examination of the peripheral blood cells (see Table 29-2). No special patient preparation is required, other than explaining to the patient that a blood sample will be taken from the hand or arm and that the sample will be evaluated for infection or anemia in the body.

Red Cell Indices. Red cell indices are measurements of the size and hemoglobin content of erythrocytes. This measurement provides information about the average volume or size of a single RBC (mean corpuscular volume [MCV]). Mean corpuscular hemoglobin, (MCH), is a measure of the average amount (weight) of hemoglobin within an RBC. Mean corpuscular hemoglobin concentration (MCHC) is a measure of the average concentration or the percentage of hemoglobin within a RBC.

Peripheral Smear. The peripheral smear often accompanies the differential WBC count and permits examination of the size, shape, and structure of individual RBCs and platelets. This information is useful in differentiating various forms of anemias and blood dyscrasias.

Schilling Test. The Schilling test is a laboratory blood test for diagnosing pernicious anemia. The test measures the absorption of radioactive vitamin B_{12}, before and after parenteral injection of the intrinsic factor, by examination of the urinary excretion of vitamin B_{12}. Normal findings are excretion of 8% to 40% of radioactive vitamin B_{12} within 24 hours.

Gastric Analysis. Gastric analysis is useful in determining pernicious anemia. In pernicious anemia, the gastric secretions are minimal and the pH remains elevated, even after injection of histamine.

Lymphangiography. This is a radiological examination used to detect lymph node metastatic involvement. Contrast medium is injected into a lymphatic vessel of the foot or hand, followed by radiological visualization of the lymphatic system.

Bone Marrow Aspiration or Biopsy. When the diagnosis is not clearly established by peripheral blood smears or when further information is needed, this procedure is specific for establishing the diagnosis and for treatment response. The most common site for bone marrow aspiration or biopsy is the iliac crest. Examination is made of cells: types, numbers, and maturation. The procedure is possible because normal bone marrow is soft and semifluid and can therefore be removed by aspiration through a needle. Bone marrow aspiration is most commonly performed in persons with marked anemia, neutropenia (decreased number of WBCs), acute leukemia, and thrombocytopenia (decreased number of platelets).

Disorders Associated with Erythrocytes

Anemia. **Anemia** is a disorder characterized by RBC and hemoglobin and hematocrit levels below normal range; anemias also exhibit increased RBC destruction (hemolytic anemia). Anemia causes delivery of insufficient amounts of O_2 to tissues and cells. Erythrocytes are classified according to size, shape, and color. Hemoglobin content is expressed as normochromic or hypochromic anemia, whereas RBC size is usually expressed as macrocytic, microcytic, or normocytic.

Etiology/pathophysiology. Anemia can be caused by many factors. Anemias may be divided into those that are the result of blood loss, impaired production of RBCs, increased destruction of RBCs, or nutritional deficiencies. Hemorrhage or blood loss accounts for temporary anemia, whereas nutritional deficit can be the cause of long-term iron-deficiency anemia. Marrow failure is linked to a disease process, toxic exposure, tumor, or unknown causes. A decrease in RBC production or destruction results in a lower number of circulating red blood cells. Bone marrow hematopoietic function manifests the inability to produce the needed quantity.

Loss of the O_2-carrying element in the blood results in supply-demand imbalance in vital organs. Peripheral circulation compensates by shunting blood to vital organs, thus causing hypoxic status in other body parts. Rapid hematopoietic effort causes blood cell irregularities (immature RBCs) and inability to produce RBCs, with resultant decrease of RBC count.

Clinical manifestations. Although each type of anemia has its specific signs and symptoms, some are also typical of all anemias. These signs and symptoms arise from decreased O_2-carrying capacity. The following are typical:

- Anorexia
- Cardiac dilation
- Disorientation
- Dyspepsia
- Dyspnea
- Exertional dyspnea
- Fatigue
- Headache
- Insomnia
- Pallor (mucous membranes and skin)
- Palpitation
- Systolic murmur
- Tachycardia
- Vertigo

Assessment. Collection of *subjective data* commonly includes expressions of weakness, dyspnea, fatigue, and vertigo. Anorexia and dyspepsia may accompany headache and insomnia, but the patient does not link these complaints to the condition unless questioning leads to this conclusion.

Collection of *objective data* includes observing signs of bleeding or shock (hypovolemic anemia). Laboratory values show low RBC count and hematocrit and hemoglobin levels. Pallor of skin and mucous membranes is present, and cardiac symptoms are noted and related to anemia. If anemia is a long-term presentation, the patient may have ulcerations of the extremities.

Diagnostic tests. Blood studies will show RBC count and hemoglobin and hematocrit levels to be below normal. Serum iron, total iron-binding capacity, and serum ferritin levels are below normal. Reticulocyte count is increased because of immaturity of RBCs. Bone marrow study will show a deviation from normal findings. Peripheral blood smears enable identifications of abnormalities of shape and color of cells. A Schilling test reveals malabsorption of vitamin B_{12}.

Medical management. Intervention depends on the cause. Correction of the disease process may correct or lessen the anemic condition. Transfusion is appropriate for blood loss, as is replacement of iron and vitamin B_{12} if these are deficient. Treatment is often specific to the particular anemia.

Nursing interventions. Nursing diagnoses and interventions for the patient with anemia include but are not limited to the following:

NURSING DIAGNOSES	NURSING INTERVENTIONS
Tissue perfusion, altered, related to cardiovascular function	Observe vital signs and peripheral pulses for circulatory change. Monitor fluid and electrolyte status. Monitor cardiac and pulmonary status. Check skin and mucous membranes for hematoma, hemorrhage, and ecchymosis. Assess skin integrity.

NURSING DIAGNOSES	NURSING INTERVENTIONS
Gas exchange, impaired, related to RBC, hemoglobin, and hematocrit deficit	Evaluate ability to manage ADLs, related to O_2 decrease. Assess activity response, dyspnea, and heart rate. Observe for cyanosis, hypoxia, and hypercapnia. Maintain bed rest as necessary and provide ROM exercise. Administer oxygen as ordered. Explain activity-oxygen deficit relationship.
Activity intolerance, related to O_2 deficit, secondary to decreased hemoglobin and hematocrit	Plan care to provide optimum rest. Assist in identifying factors causing intolerance. Assess ability to perform ADLs, ambulation, and exercise. Assess potential for injury caused by mobility impairment. Teach performing at own rate of ability, to reduce energy expenditure.

Patient teaching. Considerations for education will be tailored to the individual conditions and needs.

Types of Anemia

Hypovolemic Anemia (Blood Loss Anemia).

Etiology/pathophysiology. RBC and other component deficiencies caused by an abnormally low circulating blood volume from hemorrhage is classified as secondary anemia. Blood loss of 1000 ml or more in an adult can be severe. It is usually related to internal or external hemorrhage caused by a surgical procedure, GI bleeding, menorrhagia, trauma, or severe burns.

The loss of blood decreases the amount of circulating fluid and hemoglobin, and decreases the amount of oxygen carried to the tissues of the body. The tissues must have oxygen to survive. The average adult has an approximate total blood volume of 6000 ml (6 liters; 12 pints) and can tolerate a loss of up to 500 ml. If the loss approaches 1000 ml, acute complications, such as hypovolemic shock, may occur. The rapidity of blood loss is related to the severity and number of signs and symptoms. RBC count and hematocrit drop to half the normal range, resulting in hypovolemic shock.

Clinical manifestations. Signs and symptoms include those associated with hypovolemia and hypoxemia; weakness, stupor, irritability, and pale, cool, moist skin may be observed. Vital signs demonstrate hypotension, tachycardia, and hypothermia. Decreased hemoglobin and hematocrit levels may not be evident until several hours after blood loss has occurred. The severity of the patient's signs and symptoms correlates with the severity of the blood loss.

Assessment. Collection of *subjective data* commonly includes complaints of thirst, weakness, irritability, and restlessness.

Collection of *objective data* includes decreased blood pressure; rapid, weak, thready pulse; and rapid respirations. Cold, clammy skin with pallor is noted. Oliguria is often evident. Mental disorientation as well as physical collapse with prostration can occur.

Diagnostic tests. RBC, hemoglobin, and hematocrit levels are severely decreased, often to half the normal values.

Medical management. In the case of massive hemorrhage, measures are taken to control the bleeding, treat for shock, and replace the volume of circulating fluid with blood transfusion, plasma, dextran (volume expander), or other IV therapy. Oxygen therapy is ordered to restore decreased available oxygen caused by decreased hemoglobin in the blood.

Nursing interventions. The nurse will monitor blood and fluid restoration and identify blood loss sites to control the bleeding. Patients should be kept flat and warm. Vital signs should be taken at frequent intervals. Care should be taken to prevent injury to a restless or disoriented patient. Intake and output (I&O) are measured, with careful monitoring of urine output for oliguria caused by decreased renal perfusion.

Patient teaching. If the cause of the hemorrhage is a chronic problem, the patient should be taught to monitor bleeding amounts, occasion, and associated factors and to report to the physician immediately for treatment.

Prognosis. Without treatment, death will result. With aggressive treatment, the prognosis is favorable.

Pernicious anemia.

Etiology/pathophysiology. **Pernicious** refers to the causing of great injury, destruction, deadly, or fatal. Without treatment, pernicious anemia would be fatal. This type of anemia is the result of a metabolic defect: the absence of an intrinsic factor secreted by the gastric mucosa. It is a progressive, megaloblastic, macrocytic anemia affecting mainly older adults. The intrinsic factor is essential for absorption of vitamin B_{12} (cyanocobalamin).

Because the intrinsic factor is not available to combine with vitamin B_{12}, transport of this necessary vitamin to the ileum is prevented. Deficiency of the vitamin affects growth and maturity of all body cells. There is deficiency in the maturation of RBCs in the marrow. The erythrocyte membrane becomes fragile and ruptures easily. This vitamin is related to nerve myelination and, if it is absent, progressive demyelination and degeneration of nerves and white matter occur.

Clinical manifestations. Extreme weakness is noted with dyspnea, fever, and hypoxia. As the condition progresses, weight loss is apparent, as is slight icterus (jaundice) with pallor. The skin may appear a pale lemon-yellow color because of the excessive destruction of the RBCs, which causes the bile pigments to increase in the blood serum. Edema of the legs occurs, as do intermittent constipation and diarrhea.

Assessment. Collection of *subjective data* will include noting the patient's complaints of palpitations, nausea, flatulence, and indigestion. There is soreness and burning of the tongue. Weakness and difficulty swallowing (dysphagia) may occur. Neurological symptoms may develop, including tingling of the hands and feet and loss of sense of body position.

Collection of *objective data* includes observation of a smooth and erythematous tongue, with infection about the teeth and gums. Cerebral signs include mental disorientation, personality changes, and behavior problems. Severe neurological impairments can result, which may include partial or total paralysis that results from destruction of the nerve fibers of the spinal cord.

Diagnostic tests. The Schilling test shows malabsorption of vitamin B_{12}. Bone marrow aspiration reveals abnormal RBC development.

Medical management. Cyanocobalamin (vitamin B_{12}) injections, folic acid supplement, and iron replacement are ordered. If the anemia is severe, the patient may be transfused with packed red blood cells. Injections of vitamin B_{12} must be continued during the patient's lifetime. Treatment is individualized, but one injection every 2 months may keep the patient free of signs and symptoms.

Nursing interventions. The nursing interventions will depend to some extent on the stage of the disease. Symptomatic approach in nursing intervention is appropriate. When the patient is confined to the hospital, vital signs should be checked every 4 hours. Special mouth care should be performed several times daily. The diet should be high in protein, vitamins, and minerals.

Patients are especially sensitive to cold, and additional lightweight, warm blankets may be needed. Interventions should conserve energy and prevent injury.

Nursing diagnoses and interventions for the patient with pernicious anemia include but are not limited to the following:

NURSING DIAGNOSES	NURSING INTERVENTIONS
Injury, high risk for, related to sensory and motor losses, alteration in mental status	Use bed rest, with side rails up as needed, to prevent patient fatigue and falls caused by weakness. Assist with ambulation to avoid falls. Use bed cradle or footboard to prevent pressure on lower extremities. Apply heat with extreme caution to avoid burning the skin. Support patient with patience and reassurance to reduce irritability and depression.
Nutrition, altered: less than body requirements, related to sore mouth and tongue, diarrhea, and/or constipation	Administer vitamin B_{12} and other medications prescribed to promote production of erythrocytes. Encourage diet high in vitamins, iron, and protein to promote production of healthy erythrocytes.
Nutrition, altered: less than body requirements, related to sore mouth and tongue, diarrhea, and /or constipation—cont'd	Provide meticulous and frequent oral hygiene to promote improved appetite and prevent infection. Offer small, frequent feedings to prevent digestive overload. Observe for diarrhea or constipation and treat as prescribed to avoid fluid and electrolyte imbalance and discomfort.
Gas exchange, impaired, related to inadequate numbers of and impaired functioning of erythrocytes	Provide bed rest, with side rails up, to decrease cardiopulmonary workload. Monitor pulse, blood pressure, and rate and quality of respirations to assess adequacy. Observe mood, appropriateness of behavior, and orientation to determine mental status. Ask patient to report dyspnea and palpitations. Monitor laboratory reports to determine oxygenation of blood.

Patient teaching. Patient knowledge in regard to the disease process and the importance of following lifetime therapy of vitamin B_{12} is essential if the disease is to be controlled. Discuss the importance of a diet high in vitamin B_{12}. Activity adjustment when signs and symptoms are present may lessen the patient's stress. The need for assistance with ADLs and for frequent rest periods should be impressed on the patient and significant persons involved in the care.

Prognosis. This condition, if untreated, can be considered terminal. With treatment the patient may be asymptomatic.

Aplastic Anemia.

Etiology/pathophysiology. Aplastic anemia (**aplasia** [in hematology, a failure of the normal process of cell generation and development]) is a condition that develops without known cause, but it is thought to be congenital. It is an immunological injury resulting in a decrease of bone marrow function. Secondary aplastic anemia is directly related to exposure to viral invasion, medications, chemicals, radiation, or chemotherapy, where the hematopoietic tissue is replaced by fatty marrow, causing a defect in RBC production.

Depression of erythrocyte production results in lowered hemoglobin and RBCs. Leukopenia and thrombocytopenia may develop. Persons with aplastic anemia are usually **pancytopenic;** that is, all three major blood elements (red cells, white cells, and platelets) from the bone marrow are reduced or absent.

Clinical manifestations. Repeated infections with high fevers may occur, along with fatigue, weakness, and general malaise. Dyspnea and palpitations occur. Mortality is high from complications of infection and hemorrhage. Bleeding tendencies are reported: petechiae, ecchymoses, bleeding gums, and epistaxis occur, as well as GI and genitourinary system bleeding.

Assessment. Collection of *subjective data* includes a history of exposure to chemicals such as insecticides and drugs in addition to a family history of aplastic anemia. The patient is questioned about the ability to carry out activities of daily living (ADLs) without fatigue.

Collection of *objective data* includes monitoring the patient for pallor, signs of infection, and bleeding tendencies. Also, dyspnea and tachycardia may be noted.

Diagnostic tests. Bone marrow study (aspiration biopsy) shows hypoplastic or aplastic fatty deposits, a decrease in cellular elements, and depressed hematopoietic activity. Peripheral blood smears show that blood cells may be normocytic and normochromic.

Medical management. The cause of aplastic anemia must be identified promptly and removed or discontinued. Bone marrow suppression is expected with certain antineoplastic medications or radiation therapy, and frequent monitoring of laboratory values should be done to maintain control.

Blood transfusions are avoided if possible, to prevent iron overloading and the development of antibodies to tissue antigens. Platelet transfusions that are HLA (human lymphocyte antigen) matched are used to treat serious bleeding in the thrombocytopenic patient. The cautious use of blood transfusion is necessary to minimize the risk of rejection for the bone marrow transplant candidate.

A splenectomy may be required in patients with hypersplenism when that is the cause of destruction of normal platelets. Steroids and androgens are sometimes used to stimulate the bone marrow. Antithymocyte globulin has recently become an important therapy for patients who are not candidates for bone marrow transplantations. Bone marrow transplantation is the treatment of choice in patients under the age of 50 who have a compatible donor. Granulocytic-macrophage colony-stimulating factor (GM-CSF) is used as biological response modifier treatment for aplastic anemia.

Bone marrow transplant. This procedure is indicated in certain conditions and diseases such as immunodeficient states, cancer, leukemia, and recurrent aplastic anemia. A matched donor and recipient are essential to avoid rejection or complications. Specimens from twins, siblings, or self (autologous) while in remission are preferred.

After emotional and physical preparation, blood studies are done to set baselines and to assess the patient's status. A pathogen-free environment is established, with the patient placed on protective isolation with monitoring for fever or infection. Medication therapy used in the preparation may include immunosuppressants, antibiotics, and antianxiety agents.

Bone marrow transplants are used increasingly in hematological malignancies after large doses of chemotherapy or radiation therapy. The amount of chemotherapy or radiation that can ordinarily be administered is limited because of its toxicity to the bone marrow. By transplanting bone marrow after these therapeutic modes, much larger therapeutic doses can be administered.

Bone marrow is obtained by multiple marrow aspirations under general or spinal anesthesia, usually yielding 500 to 800 ml of marrow. The marrow is cyropreserved (frozen) until used. Shortly after chemotherapy (with or without radiation therapy) is completed, the patient receives the donated marrow through an intravenous (IV) catheter. This infusion of marrow is called the *rescue process.* The marrow travels through the bloodstream to the bone marrow, where it begins to manufacture new leukocytes, erythrocytes, and thrombocytes. The infused marrow repopulates the marrow of the patient after several weeks. There is great risk of toxicity to the patient, including infections, marrow rejection, and graft-versus-host disease. Medications supporting graft acceptance include cyclosporine (immunosuppressant) and chemotherapy (to prevent graft-versus-host complication).

Nursing interventions. Proper observation and care after bone marrow study are essential. Patients with aplastic anemia are highly susceptible to infection, and thus nursing interventions should be toward prevention. Strict aseptic techniques must be adhered to for dressing changes and IV site care. Meticulous care to prevent impaired skin and mucous membrane integrity includes avoiding intramuscular injections and avoiding administration of rectal medications or rectal temperatures. Protective devices, such as an Egg Crate mattress, are indicated. In the presence of thrombocytopenia, the nurse should observe carefully for any signs of bleeding and prevent even the slightest trauma. The patient's urine and stool should also be monitored for occult or gross blood.

Splenectomy. The surgical excision of the spleen may be performed to treat blood dyscrasias with incidence of splenomegaly; to treat trauma to the spleen; or to remove a diseased spleen. Preoperative assessment includes cardiovascular observation, respiratory function determination, and GI evaluation. Postoperatively, these observations are compared with the patient's baseline evaluations, and the patient is observed for any infection or inflammation. Potential complications include infection, hemorrhage, shock, and paralytic ileus. Parenteral therapy and nasogastric (NG) suction are maintained and observed. Management of the patient's postoperative pain is addressed. Movement and positioning to prevent infection or pneumonia are also maintained.

Nursing diagnoses and interventions for the patient with aplastic anemia include but are not limited to the following:

NURSING DIAGNOSES	NURSING INTERVENTIONS
Activity intolerance, related to inadequate tissue oxygenation	For hypoxia: Place the patient in a sitting position; observe respiration rate, pulse, and dyspnea; observe skin color and temperature; assist with care; plan rest periods; administer oxygen as needed; monitor laboratory values to improve gas exchange. Assist with ADLs as necessary. Encourage patient to engage in activities on a progressive basis as fatigue decreases in response to therapy. Help patient explore feelings associated with fatigue.
Infection, high risk for, related to increased susceptibility	Maintain reverse isolation to avoid exposure to pathogens. Observe for increase in temperature, pulse, and respirations as signs of infection. Observe the patient for "sniffles," sore throat, anorexia, and pain on urination. Administer antibiotics as ordered to combat specific pathogens. Encourage mobility, turning, coughing, deep breathing, and increased fluids to reduce susceptibility to infection.
Fluid volume deficit, high risk for, related to inadequate platelet count and impaired clotting.	Handle the patient gently to avoid trauma. Give injections only if necessary and apply pressure afterward to prevent **extravasation** (the escape of fluids into surrounding tissue). Observe for changes in vital signs and for bleeding (e.g., urine, stool, gums, or nose) to identify internal blood loss. Avoid constipation to prevent tissue irritation and possible bleeding. Apply ice bag or manual pressure to promote vascular constriction and clotting. Monitor blood studies such as RBC, Hgb, and Hct levels to determine status of intravascular volume. Observe for petechiae and ecchymosis as signs of intradermal bleeding.

Patient teaching. All persons with aplastic anemia need to know how to protect themselves from excessive bleeding. Assist the patient to maintain a balance between rest and activity. Discuss with the patient how to avoid infection, especially of the respiratory or urinary tract.

Prognosis. Prognosis is guarded; the object of care is to produce remission and prolong survival.

Iron Deficiency Anemia.

Etiology/pathophysiology. Iron deficiency anemia is a condition in which the RBCs contain decreased levels of hemoglobin.

The most common cause of iron deficiency anemia is excessive iron loss. In adults, the most common source is chronic intestinal or uterine bleeding; however, iron deficiency anemia can also be caused by bleeding from gastric or duodenal ulcers, esophageal varices, hiatal hernias, colonic diverticula, and tumors. Menstrual blood losses and blood losses related to pregnancy are common causes of iron deficiency anemia in young adult women. Rarely, excessive losses occur through microhemorrhages into lung tissue or from intestinal parasites. Even without excessive blood loss, iron deficiency anemia can also result when the body's demand for iron exceeds its absorption, which commonly occurs in infants, young adolescents, and pregnant women. Less commonly, iron deficiency anemia results from malabsorption of iron caused by diseases such as celiac disease and sprue. Subtotal gastrectomy may lead to iron deficiency caused by *achlorhydria* (loss of hydrochloric acid), occult bleeding, and decreased iron in postgastrectomy diets. Deficiency caused by poor dietary intake is rare in middle-aged adults.

Clinical manifestations. The symptoms of iron deficiency anemia are fatigue, weakness, and shortness of breath. Signs and symptoms typical of heart failure may also occur.

Assessment. Collection of *subjective data* includes noting that peculiar to iron deficiency anemia are GI symptoms, such as glossitis (manifested by inflammation and soreness of the tongue) and *pagophagia* (the desire to eat ice, clays, or starches).

Collection of *objective data* includes noting the signs, including pallor and tachycardia. Fingernails may be fragile and assume the shape of the head of a spoon with a central depression and raised borders. Mucous membranes of the mouth may be inflamed (stomatitis), and lips may be erythemic with cracking at the angles.

Diagnostic tests. The peripheral blood counts show that RBC and hemoglobin levels and the hematocrit are decreased; serum iron levels are low.

Medical management. Iron salts such as ferrous sulfate are administered. The hematocrit should rise 5% to 15% in 3 weeks and the hemoglobin 2 to 5 g/dl. For the body to incorporate 100 mg of iron per day, 900 mg should be administered daily. Iron is administered orally or by injection. Ascorbic acid has been shown to enhance iron absorption. Food sources of iron include meat, fish, poultry, eggs, green leafy vegetables, whole grains, and dried beans. See Box 29-1 for food sources of these nutrients.

When the patient cannot tolerate oral preparations of iron, parenteral iron therapy is used. The Z-tract method of giving Imferon intramuscularly is preferable, to prevent skin staining (see Chapter 21).

Nursing interventions. Because the treatment course is directed toward diagnosis and alleviating the cause, the patient interview is important. Medication therapy for iron replacement is initiated as ordered. Assist to plan for rest periods when fatigue is present.

Box 29-1 FOOD SOURCES OF IRON, FOLIC ACID, AND VITAMIN B_{12}

IRON

Organ meats: liver, kidney, heart, and tongue
Muscle meats, especially dark meat from poultry
Eggs
Shellfish
Whole-grain breads and cereals
Iron-enriched or fortified breads and cereal
Dark green vegetables: spinach, Swiss chard, kale, greens (dandelion, beet, and turnip)
Dried fruits: apricots, dates, figs, prunes, and raisins
Legumes and nuts

FOLIC ACID

Green leafy vegetables
Asparagus, broccoli
Organ meats: liver and kidney
Whole-grain breads and cereals
Enriched and fortified breads and cereals

VITAMIN B_{12}

Organ meats: liver and kidney
Muscle meats
Milk and cheese
Eggs

Patient teaching. Education about nutritional needs relative to the condition may prevent this anemia. Foods high in iron include organ meats, white beans, leafy vegetables, raisins, molasses, dried fruit, and egg yolk.

Explanation of the side effects of iron therapy is essential to alleviate distress and to extend the therapy for the necessary time (see patient teaching box). Reporting signs and symptoms to the physician requires knowledge of those that are significant. Diarrhea or nausea is significant, but black, tarry stools are not (expected with iron therapy).

Prognosis. Prognosis is usually good with correction of the underlying cause and compliance with the medical treatment.

Sickle Cell Anemia.

Etiology/pathophysiology. Sickle cell anemia is the most common genetic disorder in the United States. Sickle cell anemia occurs predominantly in the African-American population. A sickle cell is an abnormal, crescent-shaped RBC containing hemoglobin S—a defective hemoglobin molecule. This anemia is a severe, chronic, incurable condition that occurs in persons **homozygous** (having two identical genes) for hemoglobin S (Hgb-S). Sickle cell crisis is an episode of acute "sickling" of erythrocytes, which causes occlusion and ischemia in distal blood vessels. Sickling indicates a clumping or aggregation of these misshapen RBCs, which lodge in small vessels. Sickle cell trait is the **heterozygous** (having two different genes) form of sickle cell anemia whereby the individual has both Hgb-S and hemoglobin A in the RBCs. Signs and symptoms do not occur with this trait. However, the genetic implication is notable. Approximately one of every 10 African-Americans has sickle cell trait and about one out of every 500 has sickle cell anemia. Tissue hypoxia and ischemia occur, causing pain and edema as a result of inflammation. Fragile RBC destruction thus inhibits the oxygen-carrying function.

Clinical manifestations. Usually the patient is asymptomatic for the first year of life. However, periods of crisis then occur, accelerating the signs and symptoms. There are definite physical and probable emotional factors (stress) that precipitate a painful episode. Physical factors include events that cause dehydration or change the oxygen tension in the body, such as infection, overexertion, weather changes (cold), ingestion of alcohol, and smoking. Loss of appetite and irritability with weakness follow minor infections. Abdominal enlargement with pooling of blood in the liver, spleen, and other organs may accompany jaundice. Joint and back pain are noted, as is edema of extremities. Complications include multisystem failure, infarctions, hemorrhage, and retinal damage leading to blindness.

PATIENT TEACHING FOR IRON ADMINISTRATION

- Iron preparations supplement iron stores. Dosages are determined by the elemental iron content of the preparation. Iron supplements may be contraindicated in peptic ulcer disease. Side effects include GI upset (nausea, vomiting), constipation or diarrhea, and green to black stools. Elixir may stain teeth.
- Take iron with or after meals to avoid gastric upset. Do not administer with antacids.
- If a dose is missed, continue with schedule. Do not double a dose.
- Iron may interfere with absorption of oral tetracycline antibiotics. Do not take within 2 hours of each other.
- Dilute liquid iron preparations in juice or water, and administer with a straw to avoid staining of teeth.
- Drink juice (preferably orange juice) to promote absorption.
- Check for constipation or diarrhea. Record color (iron turns stools green to black) and amount of stool.
- Iron is toxic, and caution must be taken to store iron preparations out of a child's reach.

Assessment. Collection of *subjective data* begins with assessing the patient's knowledge and feelings about the disease and factors that appear to participate crisis or exacerbate signs and symptoms. Fatigue may be reported when anemia is severe. Data pertaining to pain characteristics are appropriate when pain is present.

Collection of *objective data* includes observing for abdominal enlargement, and jaundice, as well as edema of extremities and signs of hemorrhage.

Diagnostic tests. Hemoglobin electrophoresis in the patient with sickle cell anemia is specific for detecting sickle cell crisis or anemia. In the patient with sickle cell anemia, more than 80% of hemoglobin as shown by electrophoresis is hemoglobin S and not hemoglobin A. A stained blood smear detects anemia only. Hematocrit and hemoglobin levels are below normal values. WBCs are increased with infection.

Medical management. Persons with mild sickle hemoglobin syndromes do not require treatment. In persons with high concentrations of sickle hemoglobin and frequent painful crises, treatment is required. Therapy includes rest, hydration, oxygen, analgesics for pain, and treatment for infections. Transfusion therapy may be given; blood products generally used are packed RBCs.

Nursing interventions. Supportive treatment follows sign and symptom presentation: hydration and analgesia during crises and dilution of blood with increased fluid intake to reverse sickling. Monitoring the transfusion therapy for evidence of transfusion reaction is vital. Attention to fever and infection is important. Genetic counseling is indicated.

Nursing diagnoses and interventions for the patient with sickle cell anemia include but are not limited to the following:

NURSING DIAGNOSES	NURSING INTERVENTIONS
Pain, related to thrombotic crisis	Place patient in proper anatomical alignment, and protect joints. Position patient by slow, gentle handling. Apply warmth with soaks or compresses to relieve discomfort. Give analgesics as ordered.
Skin integrity, impaired, related to altered circulation to tissues, resulting in hypoxia and inadequate nutrition	Remove constrictive clothing to enhance circulation. Maintain room and body warmth to avoid discomfort or chilling. Initiate ROM exercises; support joints at rest and with movement to stimulate circulation. Inspect extremities for adequate circulation. Palpate for arterial pulses to assess patency of arterial circulation. Monitor blood studies for gas exchange and hematology as indicators of adequate tissue perfusion. Place patient on bed rest to decrease resistance to peripheral circulation.
Skin integrity, impaired, related to altered circulation to tissues, resulting in hypoxia and inadequate nutrition—cont'd	Elevate affected part(s) to enhance venous return. Implement cleaning procedure (use hydrogen peroxide or saline solution) to remove drainage and necrotic tissue. Apply sterile dressing or expose affected area to air to promote healing. Apply heat with lamp or cradle as ordered to enhance circulation and healing. Observe response to evaluate effectiveness of therapy. Cut patient's nails and discourage scratching to avoid injury.
Injury, high risk for, related to joint edema and bone fragility	Change the patient's position frequently with joint support to avoid trauma. Initiate ROM exercises and physical activity to maintain muscle tone. Encourage the patient to eat foods high in calcium, protein, and vitamins to enhance bone integrity. Observe for pain, edema, or abnormal alignment as signs of trauma.
Knowledge deficit, related to disease process, complications, activity, and nutrition	Teach prevention of exacerbation by: Avoiding infection, dehydration, and O_2 deficiency. Avoiding exertion beyond limitations. Maintaining optimum health status. Eating a high-calorie, high-protein, well-balanced diet and maintaining maximum fluid intake. Instruct to report to physician: Joint or abdominal pain. Fever or infection, hemorrhage, and hematuria Explain medication goals and importance of ongoing care. Identify disease process.

Patient teaching.

- Alert the patient to the need for family testing to determine the presence of Hbg-S; genetic counseling is available for carriers.
- Explain how to avoid sickle cell crises: avoid high altitudes, flying in unpressurized planes, dehydration, cold temperatures, iced liquids, and vigorous exercise; use stress-reduction methods.
- Explain to the patient that young pregnant women have a high risk for developing pulmonary and/or renal complications.
- Practice ROM exercises with patient and encourage regular physical activity to prevent bone demineralization. Explain the need for balance between rest (physical and mental) and activity, such as ROM and isometric exercises.
- Discuss principles of good nutrition, such as the importance of protein, calcium, vitamins, and adequate fluids.

- Alert the patient to the signs and symptoms of increased intracranial pressure, to the need to blow the nose gently, to avoid coughing, and to avoid straining on elimination.
- Demonstrate to the patient how to monitor oral intake, urinary output, and urine protein.
- Advise the patient to avoid trauma and extremes in temperature; patients should not smoke and should protect extremities from injury because of impaired circulation.

Prognosis. Prognosis is guarded. In addition to hemolytic anemia, painful crises occur and there are multiple infarctions of most organ systems.

Polycythemia Vera (Erythrocytosis).

Etiology/pathophysiology. This is a **myeloproliferative** (excessive bone marrow production) disorder with hyperplasia of bone marrow, which manifests with an increase in circulating erythrocytes, granulocytes, and platelets. It is a stem cell abnormality of unknown cause. Polycythemia vera is characterized by **erythrocytosis** (an abnormal increase in the number of circulating red cells). Secondary to pulmonary and heart disease, polycythemia vera is also thought to be associated with prolonged high altitude exposure. Bone marrow output of RBCs increases in response to hypoxic tissue conditions, causing viscosity of the blood, which impedes flow.

Multiorgan system disease is affected by hyperplastic bone marrow elements. Because of the increased erythrocyte mass, hypervolemic and hyperviscous (sticky) occurrence is 2 to 3 times normal. The sluggish circulatory process predisposes to infarctions of vital organs.

Clinical manifestations. This disorder is of gradual onset and has a progressive course of some length. It mainly affects men in middle age. Venous distention and platelet dysfunction cause esophageal varices, epistaxis, GI bleeding, and petechiae.

Assessment. Collection of *subjective data* includes noting patient complaints of sensitivity to hot and cold and pruritus. Headaches, vertigo, tinnitus, and blurred vision are often present.

Collection of *objective data* includes noting eczema and dermatological changes. The skin may develop an erythemic appearance. Elevated blood pressure accompanies left ventricular hypertrophy and angina.

Diagnostic tests. Arterial blood gases show O_2 concentration lower than normal. Plasma and red cell volume are increased. Hemoglobin, hematocrit, reticulocytes, and erythrocytes are increased. The basal metabolic rate (BMR) is increased without thyroid function alteration.

Medical management. Repeated phlebotomy decreases blood viscosity: removal of 500 to 2000 ml of blood until hematocrit maintains at 45%; the repeat of this procedure if hematocrit rises above 50%. If radiation or chemotherapy follows, patient stability is maintained.

Nursing interventions. Nursing diagnoses and interventions for the patient with polycythemia vera include but are not limited to the following:

NURSING DIAGNOSES	NURSING INTERVENTIONS
Tissue perfusion, altered, cardiopulmonary, cerebral, GI, and/or peripheral, related to hyperviscosity of fluid and potential bleeding	Have patient maintain position of comfort. When patient is on bed rest, do not raise knee gatch. Provide active or passive ROM exercises q 2 to 4 hr. Check peripheral pulses and color and temperature of extremities q 4 to 6 hr. Report early signs or symptoms of thrombosis or bleeding to physician If patient has bleeding tendency, avoid invasive procedures when possible. Avoid trauma; provide soft-bristled toothbrush. Encourage avoidance of sodium-rich foods to reduce fluid retention.
Activity intolerance, related to ischemia	Encourage adequate exercise and mobility to prevent stasis. Explain disease course and signs and symptoms expected.

Patient teaching. The nurse should alleviate knowledge deficit of this condition if it exists. The nurse should emphasize the importance of medical and nutritional regimen compliance. Diet teaching includes emphasis on avoiding foods that contain iron, while increasing calories and protein (because of BMR increase).

Signs and symptoms that need medical supervision include those of thrombosis (pain, edema, or erythema), and this must be stressed to the patient. Because this is a chronic illness, emotional support is imperative.

Prognosis. Polycythemia vera is a chronic, life-shortening disorder. Permanent cure cannot be achieved today, but remission of many years can be produced.

Disorders Associated with Leukocytes

Agranulocytosis.

Etiology/pathophysiology. This potentially fatal condition of the blood is characterized by a severe reduction in the number of granulocytes (basophils, eosinophils, and neutrophils). The white blood count is extremely low (leukopenia) as is the differential neutrophil count—less than 200/mm^3 (neutropenia).

Adverse medication reaction or toxicity is the primary cause of agranulocytosis. However, neoplastic disease, chemotherapy, and radiation therapy are often cited as causative. Viral and bacterial infections are possible causes of the condition. Heredity is also considered.

A suppression of the bone marrow by the causative agent reduces the number and production of white blood cells. Leukocytes, formed in the bone marrow, provide body protection against microorganisms. This protection is ineffective when bone marrow suppression has occurred.

Clinical manifestations. Fever, chills, headache, and fatigue are symptoms associated with infection and inflammatory process. Ulcerations of mucous membranes—the mouth, nose, pharynx, vagina, and rectum—are also found. Bronchial pneumonia and urinary tract infections are complications that occur in the later stages.

Assessment. Collection of *subjective data* includes noting the common complaints of fever, extreme fatigue, and prostration. All medications taken, whether prescription or over-the-counter, are considered as possible causes of the condition.

Collection of *objective data* includes observing fever over 100.6° F (38.1° C). Erythema and pain from ulcerations may occur. Ulcerations are cultured for microorganisms. Lung and bronchial auscultation reveals crackles and rhonchi because of trapped exudates.

Causative chemical agent

- Antihistamines
- Analgesics (Butazolidin)
- Antithyroid drugs (propylthiouracil)
- Antiepileptics (phenytoin)
- Antibiotics (chloramphenicol, penicillin derivatives, cephalosporins)
- Sulfonamides and derivatives
- Phenothiazides (Thorazine, Prolixin, Sparine, Compazine)
- Diuretics

Diagnostic tests. Leukocytes with neutrophils differential will be below normal. A bone marrow study will show depression of activity.

Medical management. The main objective of treatment is to alleviate the factors responsible for bone marrow depression and to prevent or treat infection. Blood cultures may be done when fever is elevated, and cultures may be ordered if ulceration occurs. Transfusions are often ordered. Protective isolation may also be instituted.

Nursing interventions. A patient with a compromised WBC system is highly susceptible to life-threatening infections. Nursing interventions are directed toward protecting the patient from potential sources of infection, and conscientious monitoring to detect the earliest signs of infection is necessary so that prompt therapy may be started. Meticulous washing of the hands by medical and nursing personnel and strict asepsis are mandatory.

Nursing diagnoses and interventions for the patient with agranulocytosis include but are not limited to the following:

NURSING DIAGNOSES	NURSING INTERVENTIONS
Infection, high risk for, related to depressed WBC (leukocytes) production	Maintain scrupulously clean patient environment. Be certain no person with any type of infection is allowed in contact with the patient. Observe for signs and symptoms of infection, such as elevated temperature and chills. Wash hands meticulously and use strict asepsis for procedures. Enforce protective isolation to protect patient from pathogens. Provide high-protein, high-vitamin, high-calorie diet to maintain nutritional status. Encourage patient to take fluids to promote hydration. Monitor heart rate, respirations, blood pressure, and temperature to assess for signs of infection. Observe for any patient restlessness and irritability as possible signs of infection. Observe the patient for extreme fatigue, sore throat or mouth, and fever as signs of infection. Observe WBC count. Use cooling measures (cooling blanket and tepid baths) to reduce fever if present. Administer antibiotics as ordered to combat specific pathogens. Use stool softeners as ordered to prevent intestinal stasis as site for infection. Provide perineal care to maintain hygiene and prevent infection.
Pain, related to ulceration or inflammatory process	Relieve pain through analgesia, ice collar, or warm saline gargles. Maintain patient on bed rest for malaise and prostration. Support body parts in proper alignment.
Knowledge deficit, related to disease rarity	Teach causative agents. Inform of methods to reduce infection potential. Address diet for healing and comfort: high-vitamin (especially C), high-calorie, and soft or liquid diet as tolerated.

Patient teaching.

- Discuss with the patient the use of frequent, thorough oral hygiene to treat or prevent mouth and pharyngeal infection.
- Explain the need for a soft, bland diet high in protein, vitamins, and calories.
- Encourage a balance between rest and activity to prevent fatigue and generalized weakness.
- Explain the need to avoid crowds, people with infectious diseases, and cold or hot environments;

also teach signs and symptoms of infection and appropriate interventions.

Prognosis. Agranulocytosis is a potentially fatal condition because of the possibility of a life-threatening bacterial infection.

Leukemia.

Etiology/pathophysiology. **Leukemia** is a malignant disorder of the hematopoietic system, in which an excess of leukocytes accumulates in the bone marrow and lymph nodes. The cause, while unknown, is attributed to genetic origin, a virus, or exposure to radiation or chemotherapeutic agents that are toxic to bone marrow.

Bone marrow is replaced by rapidly developing white cells with abnormal numbers and forms of immature cells found in the circulation and infiltrated into the lymph nodes, spleen, and liver. Organ enlargement occurs. Hematopoietic function is disturbed by incompetent bone marrow. Increased susceptibility to infection results.

Classification. Leukemia is classified according to the type of proliferating cells, the clinical course, and the duration of the disease. Classification includes those affecting precursors (a substance that precedes another substance) of the granulocytes, lymphocytes, and monocytes. Examples include lymphocytic, myelogenous, or monocytic leukemia, and they are classified as to acute or chronic form.

Clinical manifestations. Signs and symptoms correlate with other disorders or conditions, including anemia (pallor, fatigue, malaise, decreased activity tolerance), thrombocytopenia (petechiae, epistaxis, easy bruising, occult blood in stool or urine), and leukopenia (fever, upper respiratory and urinary infections). Enlarged lymph nodes may be the first sign of the disease in some persons.

Diagnostic tests. The white blood count is low, elevated, or excessively elevated. Bone marrow biopsy shows immature leukocytes. Chest x-ray examination may show mediastinal node and lung involvement and bone changes. Lymph node biopsy reveals excessive blasts (immature cells).

Assessment. Collection of *subjective data* includes noting patient complaints regarding symptoms that may seem unrelated at first. Pain in bones or joints as well as abnormalities of skin (petechiae, ecchymoses) and mucous membranes (bleeding) are often noticed. Fatigue, malaise, and irritability are usually present.

Collection of *objective data* includes noting those signs listed in clinical manifestations. Infections are common. Occult blood is shown in laboratory specimens of urine and stool.

Medical management. The goal of treatment is to achieve remission or to control the symptoms. Treatment is aimed at eradicating the leukemia with chemotherapy or bone marrow transplant. Drug toxicity observation is imperative (Box 29-2).

Box 29-2 CHEMOTHERAPEUTIC AGENTS COMMONLY USED IN LEUKEMIA THERAPY

Amsacrine	Doxorubicin
Asparaginase	6-Mercaptopurine
Busulfan	Methotrexate
Chlorambucil	Prednisone
Cyclophosphamide	6-Thioguanine
Cytarabine	Vincristine
Daunorubicin	

Tremendous progress in the treatment of leukemia has been made during the past decade. This has come about with the use of a complex combination of medications and radiation therapy. Bone marrow transplantation may be selected as the treatment of choice in patients with suitable donors if the initial remission of the acute leukemia has been induced. Before the transplant the patient's bone marrow cells and leukemic cells must be killed by massive chemotherapy and total body irradiation. The patient may succumb to infection, hemorrhage, or graft-versus-host disease (see p. 797).

In chronic leukemia, which occurs almost entirely in adults and develops slowly, the desired objectives of treatment depend on the kind of cells that are involved. Medications commonly used include chlorambucil (Leukeran), hydroxyurea, corticosteroids, and cyclophosphamide (Cytoxan). Irradiation of lymph nodes is often used, and blood transfusion may be given if anemia is severe. Although medications are not curative in chronic leukemia, they help to prolong life. See the medications table and Chapter 44.

Nursing interventions. Prevention of infection by protective isolation and teaching the avoidance of infectious agents is of utmost importance. Leukopenia can be fatal. The usual inflammatory process to control infection is decreased. Therefore frequent observation for signs and symptoms of infection is necessary. Thrombocytopenia-induced hemorrhage may be life threatening. Therefore prevention of this condition through safe, gentle care is a primary consideration. Pain may be controlled through analgesia as ordered and by comfort measures. Coping mechanisms may be strained because of pain, change of body image, or fear of death, and therefore support of patient and family is promoted through a positive nurse-patient-family relationship and referral to community support groups.

MEDICATIONS FOR BLOOD AND LYMPHATIC DISORDERS

Medication	Trade Name	Action	Side Effects	Nursing Implications
Cyanocobalamin (vitamin B_{12})	Cobex, Vitamin B_{12}	Needed for adequate nerve functioning, protein and carbohydrate metabolism, normal growth, RBC development, cell reproduction	Flushing, diarrhea, itching, rash, hypokalemia	Assess GI functions and potassium levels at beginning of treatment; stress need for patients with pernicious anemia to return for monthly injections; give intramuscularly only.
Folic Acid (vitamin B_9)	Folvite	Needed for erythropoiesis; increases RBC, WBC, and platelet formation in megaloblastic anemias	Pruritus, rash, general malaise, bronchospasm, slight flushing	Know that drug may be administered by deep intramuscular, subcutaneous, or intravenous routes; do not mix with other medications in same syringe for intramuscular injections.
Ferrous sulfate	Feosol, Fer-In-Sol	Replaces iron stores needed for RBC development	Nausea, constipation, epigastric pain, black and red tarry stools, vomiting, diarrhea, discolored urine, staining of teeth	Know that between-meal dosing preferable but can be given with some foods, although absorption may be decreased; give tablets with orange juice to promote iron absorption; to avoid staining teeth, give elixir iron preparations through straw; know that oral iron may turn stools black.
Iron dextran	Imferon	Is released into the plasma and carried by transferrin to the bone narow, where it is incorporated into hemoglobin	Stained skin at site of injection, fever, chills, headache, sweating, discolored urine, diarrhea	Administer 0.5-ml test dose by preferred route before therapy; wait at least 1 hour before giving remaining portion.
Desmopressin acetate	DDAVP, Concentraid	Promotes reabsorption of water by kidneys and increase in plasma factor VIII levels, which increases platelet aggregation, resulting in vasopressor effect	Nasal irritation, congestion, drowsiness, headache, flushing, nausea, abdominal cramps, heartburn, vulval pain, hypertension	Avoid overhydration; assess pulse and blood pressure when giving drug subcutaneously; monitor factor VIII antigen levels and APTT.
Filgrastim (G-CSF)	Neupogen	Stimulates proliferation and differentiation of neutrophils	Fever, alopecia, skeletal pain, nausea, vomiting, diarrhea, mucositis, anorexia	Monitor CBC and platelet count before treatment and twice weekly; refrigerate, do not freeze, avoid shaking; store at room temperature for at least 6 hours; discard any vial that has been at room temperature for more than 6 hours.

Patient teaching. Procedures, meaning of treatments, and care plans should be discussed by the nurse and the patient. The nature of the disease and previous information the patient has received should be discussed. Community resources for support and information are invaluable for education of the patient and family. Expectations of physical abilities, remission, and future plans should be examined. Continuation of medical regimen is encouraged, as is avoidance of situations where infection can be transmitted. Medication and diet information is important.

Prognosis. Perhaps more dramatically than in any other malignant disorder, chemotherapy has improved the prognosis of children with acute lymphocytic leukemia (ALL). Untreated patients have a median survival time of 4 to 6 months. With current therapy of vincristine and prednisone, and an anthracycline drug (daunorubicin or doxorubicin), the median survival rate is about 5 years, and approximately 50% of children with ALL can now be cured. In acute myelogenous leukemia (AML), remission can be achieved in up to 75% of cases; however, relapse will eventually occur in most cases. Only about 20% to 25% of adults with AML experience a 5-year remission.

Overall survival for chronic lymphocytic leukemia is variable. In early stages, median survival rate ranges from 10 to 12½ years; in advanced stages, survival is approximately 18 months.

See the nursing care plan on pp. 806-807 for the patient with leukemia.

Coagulation Disorders

Overview.

Etiology/pathophysiology. Release of blood from the vascular system results from trauma or vessel damage, vessel inadequacy, disturbance of function of platelets or clotting factors, or liver disease (impairment of clotting mechanisms).

The clotting mechanism is a hemostatic chain reaction. Vasoconstriction inhibits capillary leakage; hematoma compression provides pressure. Body reaction occurs: arterial blood pressure lowers. Any manifestation that alters this process predisposes to hemorrhage. The affected mechanism may be vascular, platelet dysfunction, or plasma coagulation factor alteration. The disorder may be congenital or acquired, possibly secondary to other disease or to medication toxicity.

Clinical manifestations. Skin and mucous membrane manifestations include petechiae and ecchymoses. Epistaxis and gingival bleeding are common. Circulatory hypovolemia is noted through hypotension, pallor, cool, clammy skin, and tachycardia. GI tract bleeding is common, with abdominal flank pain caused by internal bleeding. The central nervous system involvement ranges from altered response and malaise to loss of consciousness or affected speech.

Assessment. Collection of *subjective data* includes noting a history of bleeding after surgical or dental procedures. The exposure to toxic or hazardous agents or to radiation may be revealed. Complaint of headache, extremity pain, easy bruising, oronasal bleeding, and numbness is noted. Medications taken may lead to suspicion of toxicity (aspirin).

Collection of *objective data* involves observation of pain upon pressure of abdomen, revealing liver and spleen tenderness, and perhaps enlargement. Examination of emesis and stool may show signs of bleeding. Joint examination exhibits motion pain.

Diagnostic tests. The platelet count will be low. The RBC count will be low with decreased hemoglobin. Coagulation time is altered. Bone marrow studies show abnormal cells.

Medical management. The underlying cause is assessed and corrected, and replacement transfusions may be ordered. Heparin therapy or medication toxicity is considered as a possible cause. Infections and complications are treated or prevented.

Nursing interventions. Many times, medical intervention depends on accurate reporting of signs and symptoms and nursing observations. In disorders of coagulation the nurse should monitor vital signs to note any signs of hypovolemic shock. Gentle movement of the patient is necessary to prevent trauma to the tissues. The nurse will monitor IV infusions and transfusions as ordered.

Platelet Disorders.

Thrombocytopenia.

Etiology/pathophysiology. A deficiency of the number of circulating platelets or change in the function of platelets alters the process of coagulation. **Thrombocytopenia** is an abnormal hematological condition in which the number of platelets is reduced. Decreased production occurs in aplastic anemia, leukemia, and tumors. Decreased platelet survival occurs in the presence of antibody destruction, infection, or viral invasion. Increased platelet destruction is caused by disseminated intravascular coagulation. Splenomegaly results from entrapment of blood in the spleen.

The most common cause of increased destruction of platelets is thrombocytopenic purpura, which may be drug-induced or **idiopathic** (cause unknown, referred to as idiopathic thrombocytopenic purpura [ITP]). If the cause is medication-induced (Box 29-3 on p. 808), the patient's platelet counts usually return to normal 1 to 2 weeks after the medication is withdrawn. ITP occurs most commonly in the second and third decades of life, and it is caused by the production of an autoantibody (immunoglobulin G [IgG]) directed against a platelet antigen.

NURSING CARE PLAN: THE PATIENT WITH LEUKEMIA

Mrs. Mogis is a 26-year-old patient diagnosed with acute lymphatic leukemia. She is married and the mother of a 3-year-old daughter. Mrs. Mogis has been receiving chemotherapy and is immunocompromised, with a differential WBC revealing a neutrophil count of 22%. Her hemoglobin is 8.8 g/dl, and her platelets are 55,000 mm^3. Her mouth appears edematous, and she complains of oral tenderness.

Nursing diagnoses	Expected goals/outcomes	Nursing interventions
Infection, high risk for, related to leukopenia	Patient will remain free of infection. Patient or care giver will identify measures to prevent or control infection. Patient or care giver will verbalize and report signs and symptoms of infection.	Inspect all body sites for infection at least daily; NOTE and report fever, sore throat, purulent exudate, chills, cough, burning with urination, erythema, edema, tenderness, and pain. Monitor vital signs. Obtain cultures as ordered. Monitor WBC counts and culture reports. Administer antibiotics on time as ordered. Promote and maintain hygiene integrity of skin and mucous membranes. Use aseptic technique in treatments. Teach the patient and family: Necessity of avoiding crowds/patients with infections while WBC count <1000 mm^3. Personal hygiene measures. Signs and symptoms of infection.
Injury, high risk for, related to thrombocytopenia	Patient will be free from bleeding. Patient will exhibit control of bleeding episodes. Patient or caregiver will demonstrate measures to prevent or control bleeding.	Monitor platelet counts. Assess patient for bleeding. Institute bleeding precautions. Teach patient measures to prevent or control bleeding.
Oral mucous membrane, altered: stomatitis, related to chemotherapy, leukemia infiltrates	Patient will be free from stomatitis. Patient or care giver will demonstrate oral hygiene regimen. Patient or care giver will verbalize symptoms to report to physician.	Assess oral cavity: note color, moisture, and presence and descriptions of lesions. Assess for signs of infection. Implement oral hygiene regimen: use salt rinses, dilute peroxide rinses, use soft toothbrush or sponge-tipped applicator. Encourage bland, nonirritating diet. Use artificial saliva and lip lubricants as ordered for comfort.

Activity intolerance related to anemia	Patient will demonstrate self-care measures within ability to perform.	Monitor Hgb and Hct. Assess for signs and symptoms of anemia. Assess ability to perform self-care. Promote frequent rest periods and provide assistance to decrease energy expenditure. Monitor transfusion of RBCs as ordered. Teach signs of anemia and measures to conserve energy.
Coping, individual and family, ineffective, related to diagnosis and disease process	Patient and family will demonstrate measures to effectively cope.	Assess coping capabilities of patient and significant others. Discuss disease process and expectations. Alleviate knowledge deficit. Encourage questions and self-expression: listen actively, demonstrate compassion, reassure with touch and personal contact. Assess fear of threat of death: allow time for personal expression, and provide one-on-one discussion opportunity.
Knowledge deficit, related to diagnosis and treatment	Patient demonstrates knowledge related to diagnosis of leukemia and prescribed treatments.	Provide written materials to reinforce teaching. Repeat information as frequently as needed. Note patient's response to teaching. Teach signs and symptoms of disease process and side effects of treatments. Inform patient of resources available for health care, both in hospital and at home. Teach signs and symptoms that should be reported to a nurse or physician (e.g., elevated temperature, bleeding, nausea/vomiting, pain, drainage). Teach importance of proper nutrition and hydration.

CRITICAL THINKING QUESTIONS

- What would you do if you noted a visitor who had an obvious upper respiratory infection approaching Mrs. Mogis's room?
- What nursing intervention would be most appropriate in providing therapeutic oral hygiene for Mrs. Mogis?
- State your choice of a bath and ADLs that would be most beneficial for Mrs. Mogis.

Box 29-3 MEDICATIONS WITH THROMBOCYTOPENIC EFFECTS

Aspirin
Digitalis derivatives
Furosemide
Nonsteroidal antiinflammatory agents (azathioprine, D-penicillamine, phenylbutazone, ibuprofen, indomethacin)
Oral hypoglycemics
Penicillins
Quinidine
Rifampicin
Sulfonamides
Thiazides

Bleeding occurs from many capillaries. Thrombocytopenia is the most common cause of bleeding disorders. It is related to bone marrow defect associated with neoplastic disease or immune response to drugs.

Clinical manifestations. The major signs of thrombocytopenia observable by physical examination are petechiae and ecchymoses on the skin. Petechiae occur only in platelet disorders. The severity of signs and symptoms correlates with the platelet count. As the level drops below 150,000/mm^3, the risk for bleeding from mucous membranes and in cutaneous sites and internal organs increases. Significant risk for serious bleeding occurs once the count is below 20,000/mm^3.

Assessment. Collection of *subjective data* includes questioning the patient about recent viral infections (they may produce a transient thrombocytopenia), medications in current use, and extent of alcohol ingestion.

Collection of *objective data* includes observing the patient for petechiae and ecchymoses throughout the skin. Epistaxis and gingival bleeding may be noted.

Diagnostic tests. The tests include complete laboratory studies to ascertain the characteristics of all blood cells, which include platelet count, peripheral blood smear, and bleeding time. In addition, a bone marrow examination is performed to determine the presence of immature platelets. Examination also reveals presence or absence of primary bone marrow abnormalities, such as neoplastic invasion or aplastic anemia.

Medical management. The primary treatments are corticosteroid therapy and splenectomy. Other treatments may include gamma globulin or immunosuppressive drugs. Transfusions with platelet concentrates may be used in persons with thrombocytopenic bleeding.

Nursing interventions. The nurse will support the medical treatment regimen, using specific interventions for specific disease causes. If medication toxicity is the cause, the medication is discontinued. Infections are prevented by meticulous asepsis and gentle handling of the patient. Plasma and platelet infusion and whole blood transfusions are monitored closely for reaction and effects on patients' conditions.

Nursing diagnoses and interventions for the patient with thrombocytopenia include but are not limited to the following:

NURSING DIAGNOSES	NURSING INTERVENTIONS
Tissue perfusion, altered: cerebral, cardiopulmonary, renal, GI, peripheral, related to bleeding	Monitor vital signs and neurological status. Assess for bleeding and fluid imbalance. Check patient's urine, stool, and emesis for blood. Monitor invasive diagnostic procedure sites for bleeding. Maintain comfort measures and bed rest. Avoid trauma and infection. Observe patient receiving parenteral fluids and blood components carefully for untoward signs. Monitor potential sites of hemorrhage.
Pain, related to hemorrhage	Assess discomfort and pain level. Assess patient's ability to cope and response to pain. Administer analgesia as ordered, and note patient response. Provide education.

Patient teaching. An understanding of the disease process and causative agents is necessary in forming a knowledge base for self-care and prevention of trauma or infection. Instructions on signs and symptoms, as well as preventive measures, must be given: avoiding trauma and constipation and checking for presence of blood. The nurse should stress the importance of notifying the physician of signs and symptoms of bleeding.

Prognosis. Prognosis is variable, depending upon the underlying case. In ITP, treatment may need to be administered for a period of 3 to 4 weeks before a complete response is seen.

Clotting Factor Defects.

Hemophilia.

Etiology/pathophysiology. This hereditary coagulation disorder is characterized by a disturbance of the clotting factors. **Hemophilia A,** the more common type, which represents 85% of the total incidence, lacks antihemophilic factor VIII, which is needed to convert prothrombin to thrombin through thromboplastin component. Hemophilia B (Christmas disease) exhibits a deficiency of factor IX with absence of plasma thromboplastin component (a plasma protein), resulting in nonformation of thromboplastin.

Hemophilia is an X-linked hereditary trait that affects mainly males; females are carriers. A decrease in the formation of prothrombin activators occurs as a result of the decrease in clotting factors.

The patient used to be at high risk for AIDS because of the need for cryoprecipitate concentrates and contamination with HIV virus. A number of persons with hemophilia A have developed AIDS from transfusions of factor VIII concentrate. This problem should be eliminated with the testing of all blood donors for evidence of HIV virus and, more recently, with the knowledge that heat treatment of factor VIII concentrates destroys the AIDS virus.

Clinical manifestations. Internal or external hemorrhage occurs with large ecchymoses into tissue—especially muscles, which may show deformity, and joints, which become ankylosed. **Hemarthrosis,** or bleeding into a joint space, is a hallmark of severe disease and usually occurs in the knees, ankles, and elbow. Pain, edema, erythema, and fever accompany hemarthrosis. Small cuts can prove fatal; blood loss from simple dental procedures may be significant. Pain from the hemorrhage damage is significant.

Assessment. Collection of *subjective data* includes noting reports by patient and family of incidents of ecchymoses and hemorrhage from even the slightest trauma. Pain is associated with joint motion.

Collection of *objective data* includes noting the presence of blood in subcutaneous tissues, urine, or stool and noting edematous or immobile joints.

Diagnostic tests. Factors VIII and IX are absent or deficient. Coagulation profiles reveal a normal platelet count, bleeding time, and prothrombin time (PT). The partial thromboplastin time (PTT) is prolonged. Laboratory personnel must be notified of the patient's disorder to alleviate further incidents of trauma as a result of diagnostic procedures (e.g., venipuncture).

Medical management. Minimizing bleeding and relieving pain are the main focuses of care. Transfusions and administration of factor VIII or IX concentrate may be prophylactic or used to stop the hemorrhage. Two different clotting factor concentrates made from human plasma can be used. One, cryoprecipitate, is a clotting factor concentrate rich in factor VIII. Its use is waning due to risk, although small, of viral disease transmission. Additionally, home administration of cryoprecipitate is difficult because of the need to store it at low temperatures. The second human-derived product, factor VIII concentrate, is most typically used. A wide variety of products of this type are available, and are all freeze-dried concentrates of factor VIII prepared from pooled plasma from thousands of donors. These products are specially treated to inactivate any viral contamination (such as HIV or hepatitis viruses). Factor IX concentrates are also available and prepared in a similar fashion.

Because human plasma products still carry a very slight risk of infection transmission and require human donors, scientists have used genetic engineering to manufacture factor VIII. This product, recombinant factor VIII, is advantageous because of viral safety, unlimited supply, and lower cost. Recombinant factor VIII should soon become commercially available for widespread use.

Nursing interventions. The nurse will control hemorrhages in emergency situations by pressure and cold application to the site. Support and reassurance are imperative. Education of the patient and entire family is significant because many persons may be involved in the patient care. The nurse will monitor transfusions of factor VIII concentrate. The supportive care measures include pain management and genetic counseling.

Nursing diagnoses and interventions for the patient with hemophilia include but are not limited to the following:

NURSING DIAGNOSES	NURSING INTERVENTIONS
Tissue perfusion, altered, related to blood loss from coagulation deficit	Assess for extent of hemorrhage. Prevent further hemorrhage or extension. Monitor vital signs and laboratory reports. Apply cold compresses to bleeding areas. Assess for anxiety, shock, disorientation, and decreased urinary output. Teach safety precautions to prevent trauma.
Pain, related to hemorrhage into tissues	Administer analgesia as ordered. Move patient gently and slowly, supporting joints. Prevent deformity through support, splints, and physical therapy. Administer warm soaks (avoid hot to alleviate extension of hematoma) as ordered.
Coping, individual and family, ineffective, related to long-term illness	Discuss disease process, altered lifestyle, and acceptance. Suggest genetic counseling. Encourage independence. Encourage compliance with medical regimen. Assess parental knowledge or guilt feelings. Be an active listener.
Fluid volume deficit, related to bleeding	Monitor vital signs and level of consciousness for evidence of acute hemorrhage. Monitor blood component therapy as ordered to control bleeding. Monitor I&O. Apply ice pack to affected joint or traumatized area to control bleeding. Administer analgesics to relieve joint pain. Assess amount, consistency, and frequency of bleeding: Nose Joints Skin Stool and urine Pad counts Monitor laboratory tests to monitor degree of blood loss. Avoid trauma, such as falls, bumps, or injections.

Patient teaching. Avoiding injury and controlling bleeding are significant points. Physical activity within limits and avoiding trauma should be discussed by the nurse. Wearing of medical alert identification is encouraged. Supervision of young patients, as well as informing playmates, teachers, and others, is important. Emergency care teaching includes immobilization of affected part, ice application, and notifying the physician. Diet to prevent obesity, which puts excess pressure on joints, is discussed. Regular dental care and preventive dental and medical measures are important aspects for the nurse to cover. Overprotection can sometimes be a factor to discuss. No aspirin or any other medication should be taken except with the physician's knowledge.

Prognosis. Before the appearance of the HIV virus, the average life span of the person with hemophilia was near normal. Although estimates of prevalence of HIV in the hemophiliac population vary widely, the majority of severe hemophiliacs who received clotting factor concentrates before 1984 are seropositive for HIV. Now, with the development of methods to heat-inactivate the virus, the risk of contracting HIV from clotting factor concentrates is almost nil. With the methods to control HIV transmission, the average life span is near normal.

von Willebrand's disease.

Etiology/pathophysiology. This inherited bleeding disorder is characterized by abnormally slow coagulation of blood and spontaneous episodes of GI bleeding, epistaxis, and gingival bleeding caused by a mild deficiency of factor VIII. It is common in postpartum periods, as menorrhagia, and after surgery or trauma. Although similar to hemophilia, it is not limited only in males.

Treatment includes administration of cryoprecipitate containing factor VIII, fibrinogen, or fresh plasma. Desmopressin (DDAVP) is becoming the treatment of choice in mild hemophilia. This drug is a synthetic of the human antidiuretic hormone, vasopressin. It acts by causing an increase in factor VIII release from storage sites in the body. Desmopressin is often administered prophylactically to patients with mild hemophilia who require surgery or dental extractions. Observation and nursing intervention for hemophilia A and B can easily be adapted to von Willebrand's disease.

Prognosis. Prognosis is usually good.

Disseminated intravascular coagulation (DIC).

Etiology/pathophysiology. **Disseminated intravascular coagulation** (DIC) is a grave coagulopathy resulting from the over stimulation of clotting and anticlotting processes in response to disease or injury, including septicemia, obstetrical complication, malignancies, tissue trauma, transfusion reaction, burns, shock, and snake bites (Box 29-4).

Plasma clotting factors are depleted during widespread clotting within small vessels. This in turn leads to a bleeding disorder and thrombosis. The primary disorder initiates generalized intravascular clotting, which in turn overstimulates fibrinolytic mechanisms; as a result the initial hypercoagulability is followed by a deficiency in clotting factors with subsequent hypocoagulability and hemorrhaging.

Box 29-4 PRECIPITATING CAUSES OF DIC

OBSTETRICAL

- Abruptio placentae
- Retained dead fetus
- Amniotic fluid embolism
- Retained placenta
- Toxemia
- Hydatidiform mole (intrauterine mass of grapelike chorionic villi)
- Acute fatty liver of pregnancy

NEOPLASTIC

- Carcinomas
- Acute leukemias
- Adenocarcinomas
- Sarcomas
- Polycythemia vera
- Pheochromocytoma (a vascular tumor of the adrenal medulla)

HEMATOLOGICAL

- Blood transfusion reaction
- Sickle cell crisis
- Thalassemia major (genetic hemolytic anemia; occurs in people of Mediterranean origin)

TRAUMA

- Burns
- Multiple injury
- Transplant rejection
- Surgery, particularly if extracorporeal (heart-lung machine used) circulation was used
- Heat stroke
- Fat emboli
- Snake bite
- Aspirin poisoning

OTHER

- Acute infectious process/sepsis
- Hepatitis
- Glomerulonephritis
- Purpura
- Cirrhosis
- Shock
- Necrotizing enterocolitis
- Systemic lupus erythematosus
- Anaphylaxis

From Young LM: DIC: the insidious killer; *Crit Care Nurs* 10(9):27, 1990.

Clinical manifestations. Bleeding is noted in mucous membranes, venipuncture or surgical sites, GI and urinary tracts, and generally from all orifices, and ranges from occult to profuse. Dyspnea, hemoptysis, and diaphoresis with cold, mottled digits are observed.

Assessment. Collection of *subjective data* includes noting patient complaints of bone and joint pain. Visual changes occur.

Collection of *objective data* includes observing for occult or obvious bleeding. Purpura on the chest and abdomen, reflecting fibrin deposits in capillaries, is a common first sign of DIC. Skin and mucosa color and petechiae are noted. Abdominal tenderness may be shown. GI bleeding, hematuria, pulmonary edema, pulmonary embolism, hypotension, tachycardia, absence of peripheral pulses, restlessness, convulsions, or coma may be present.

Diagnostic studies. The coagulation profile shows prolonged clotting. The platelet count shows marked thrombocytopenia. Other tests show hypofibrinogenemia and factors V and VIII deficit.

Medical management. In keeping with the medical therapeutic approach, the underlying cause is addressed and corrected and transfusion replacement and cryoprecipitate are ordered. Heparin therapy will block the subsequent formation of microemboli by inhibiting thrombin activity. It has no effect, however, on existing clots. The goal underlying the administration of heparin is to stop the rapid overproduction of microemboli and thus allow for reperfusion of vital organs and replenishment of clotting factor supplies.

Nursing interventions. Protection from bleeding and trauma and pressure to sites of hemorrhage are essential nursing measures. Support and reassurance may aid in relieving high stress levels. Patients are monitored in a quiet, nonstressful environment. The side rails are padded, and foam or cotton swabs are used for mouth care. Monitoring of vital signs and administration of transfusions and cryoprecipitate are necessary.

Nursing diagnoses and interventions for the patient with DIC include but are not limited to the following:

NURSING DIAGNOSES	NURSING INTERVENTIONS
Injury, high risk for bleeding and/or fluid deficit, related to depleted coagulation factors, adverse effects of heparin (excess heparin, insufficient heparin)	Monitor Hct and Hgb. Examine skin surface for signs of bleeding; note petechiae, purpura, hematomas, oozing of blood from IV sites, drains, and wounds, and bleeding from mucous membranes Observe for signs of bleeding from GI/ and genitourinary tracts. Note any hemoptysis or blood obtained during suctioning. Observe for changes in mental status; institute neurological checklist (mental status changes may occur with the decreased fluid volume or with decreasing Hgb).
Injury, high risk for bleeding and/or fluid deficit, related to depleted coagulation factors, adverse effects of heparin (excess heparin, insufficient heparin)—cont'd	Monitor vital signs. Observe for signs of orthostatic hypotension (drop of >15 mm Hg when changing from supine to sitting position indicates reduced circulating fluids). Avoid IM injections; any needle stick is a potential bleeding site. Apply pressure to oozing site. Prevent trauma to catheter/tubes by proper taping, minimum pulling.
Tissue perfusion, altered peripheral, high risk for, related to DIC with peripheral thromboembolus formation in capillaries and arterioles resulting in possible interruption of arterial flow and hypovolemia	Assess color, warmth, movement, and sensation of extremities (acute occlusion results in a numb, cold limb, with pain aggravated by movement of the limb). Assess peripheral pulses and mark with skin marker if diminished; use Doppler as needed to assess for pulses. Assess blood pressure. Elevate extremities to promote venous return and prevent edema formation, which could further add to a decrease in peripheral perfusion. Monitor fluids and medications as needed to prevent hypotension, which will lead to a further decrease in perfusion to extremities.

Patient teaching.

- Discuss with the patient and family signs and symptoms of the syndrome, which should be reported immediately to the nurse or physician.
- Assist patient in learning to administer heparin therapy subcutaneously if prescribed.
- Assist the patient and family to avoid mechanical trauma such as from a hard toothbrush, blade razor, rough nose blowing, or contact sports.

Prognosis. Mortality in DIC varies because of varying degrees of severity. Death is usually a result of either uncontrolled hemorrhage or irreversible end organ damage or both.

Lymphatic Disorders

Lymphagitis.

Etiology/pathophysiology. **Lymphangitis** is an inflammation of one or more lymphatic vessels or channels that usually results from an acute streptococcal or staphylococcal infection in an extremity.

Clinical manifestations. Lymphangitis is characterized by fine, red streaks from the affected area to the groin or axilla. The infection is usually not localized, and edema is diffuse. Chills, fever, and local pain accompany headache and myalgia. Septicemia may occur; lymph nodes enlarge.

Medical management. Administration of penicillin or other antimicrobial drugs controls the infection. Hot, moist heat—soaks or packs—brings comfort.

Nursing interventions. Aseptic technique promotes healing. Rest and extremity elevation may relieve the pressure.

Prognosis. With treatment, the prognosis is usually good.

Lymphedema.

Etiology/pathophysiology. **Lymphedema** is a primary or secondary disorder characterized by the accumulation of lymph in soft tissue and edema. The accumulation of lymph in soft tissue is caused by obstruction, an increase in the amount of lymph, or removal of the lymph channels and nodes. The condition may be hereditary.

If the lymphatic drainage function is disturbed, an inflammatory process may result.

Clinical manifestations. Massive edema and tightness cause pressure and pain in the affected extremities. It progresses toward the trunk and is aggravated by (1) standing; (2) pressure, as with pregnancy or premenstruation; (3) obesity; and (4) warm, humid environments.

Assessment. Collection of *subjective data* includes the nurse noting the patient's complaints of pain and pressure. Medical history of varicosities, pregnancy, or modified radical mastectomy is important.

Collection of *objective data* includes observation of the extremities for edema and palpation of pedal pulses.

Diagnostic test. Lymphangiography is used to differentiate from venous disorders.

Medical management. Diuretics and antimicrobials are administered as ordered. Mechanical management includes use of compression pumps and elastic sleeves or stockings on the affected limb. Diet restrictions include limiting sodium and avoiding spicy foods, which would precipitate thirst.

Nursing interventions. The primary goal of care is to increase lymphatic drainage and avoid trauma. Elevation of the extremities while asleep and periodically during the day will facilitate draining the tissues. Massage toward the trunk followed by active exercise (e.g., walking) decreases the edema. Avoidance of constrictive clothing, shoes, or stockings (except elastic stockings) is advisable. Meticulous skin care must be maintained, and every effort must be made to prevent infections.

An important nursing intervention is the provision of emotional support for the patient. Body image disturbance related to the appearance of the lymphedematous extremity should be addressed. Emphasizing that lymphedema need not prevent the individual from engaging in routine activity may increase self-esteem.

A nursing diagnosis and interventions for the patient with lymphedema include but are not limited to the following:

NURSING DIAGNOSIS	NURSING INTERVENTIONS
Skin integrity impaired, related to impaired lymphatic drainage	Protect engorged tissues. Consider physical therapy or ROM exercises (aids lymphatic flow). Examine skin for impaired skin integrity. Gently handle affected parts. Apply skin-protecting moisturizers or emollients. Teach application of supportive stockings or elastic sleeves.

Patient teaching. The patient should be made aware of the progression of the condition and of the cause. If the disorder is long-term and ongoing, coping with its effects must be approached. Rationale behind nursing interventions must be explained to enhance the ongoing medical regimen. If unsightly results are permanent, the patient must consider acceptance rather than social isolation.

Prognosis. There is no cure for the disorder, but signs and symptoms can be controlled with compliance to treatment.

Malignant Lymphoma.

Etiology/pathophysiology. This condition is a neoplastic disorder of lymphoid tissue. Malignant lymphoma is starting to be characterized as a neoplasm of the immune system. The cause is unknown, but a viral source is suspect. This group includes non-Hodgkin's lymphoma (NHL). In most cases of NHL, the cause is unknown, but patients who have received immunosuppressive agents have a more than 100 times greater chance of developing NHL. This is probably due to the immunosuppressive agents, activating tumor viruses. A herpes-like virus is suspected, but a definite relationship has not been established. It is more common in males over 60 years of age, Caucasians, and those of Jewish ancestry.

Tumors usually start in lymph nodes and spread to lymphoid tissue in the spleen, liver, GI tract, and bone marrow. Involvement of lymphoid tissue also results in malabsorption and bone lesions.

Clinical manifestations. Painless, enlarged lymph nodes are found in the cervical area, and fever, weight loss, anemia, pruritus, and susceptibility to infection develop. Pressure symptoms in the involved areas are noted. Pleural effusion, bone fractures, and paralysis are complications.

Assessment. Collection of *subjective data* includes frequent patient complaints of fatigue, malaise, and anorexia. Fever and diaphoresis are noted also.

Collection of *objective data* includes examination of the abdomen for splenomegaly. Enlarged lymph nodes are also evident.

Diagnostic tests. A bone scan reveals fractures, lesions, and tumor infiltration. Blood studies show hypercalcemia. A Coombs' test is positive for antiglobulin. Biopsies of lymph nodes, liver, and bone marrow are done for specific evidence of a pathological condition.

Medical management. Once the diagnosis is made, the extent of the disease (staging) will be determined. Accurate staging is crucial to determine the treatment regimen. The therapeutic regimen for NHLs includes chemotherapy and radiation. Some chemotherapy agents used are cyclophosphamide (Cytoxan), vincristine (Oncovin), prednisone, doxorubicin (Adriamycin), bleomycin, and methotrexate. In general, radiotherapy is the initial treatment when the disease has a localized presentation. Chemotherapy is the mainstay of treatment of NHLs that are not localized. Bone marrow transplantation may be indicated. Tumor necrosis factor (TNF) is currently being used. Tumor necrosis factor has direct cell toxicity and stimulates the immune system. Interferon is currently being investigated as a treatment option. Older patients have difficulty tolerating the aggressive chemotherapy treatments. This population is increasing and new approaches are being examined.

Nursing interventions. Supportive care of the patient during radiation and chemotherapy is primary in nursing management. Observation for complications follows. Further intervention is similar to that for Hodgkin's disease.

Patient teaching. Explanations of the extensive workup in diagnosis and its importance of staging the disease for determining the treatment plan are an important focus of patient teaching in the diagnostic period.

Prognosis. The prognosis is influenced by the staging classification.

Hodgkin's Disease.

Etiology/pathophysiology. Hodgkin's disease is a malignant disorder characterized by painless, progressive enlargement of lymphoid tissue. It affects males twice as frequently as females, and the age incidence curve is bimodal (two separate populations). There is a peak early in life, in the second and third decades, and a peak later in life, in the sixth and seventh decades. The two peaks in incidence have been suggested as separate diseases. The first incident peak suggests a viral etiology. Beginning as an inflammatory or infectious process, it develops into a neoplasm. The exact cause is unknown. Hodgkin's disease is thought to be an immune disorder (T cell disease). Infectious etiology has been investigated, especially regarding oncovirus.

Lymphoid tissue enlargement is first noticed in the cervical nodes and spleen and is characterized by abnormal or atypical cells. **Reed-Sternberg cells** (atypical histiocytes) are large, abnormal, multinucleated cells in the lymphatic system found in Hodgkin's disease. These cells increase in number, replacing normal cells.

Clinical manifestations. Anorexia, weight loss, and extreme pruritus are outstanding complaints associated with this condition. Low-grade fever and night sweats occur. Anemia and leukocytosis follow with development of complications of respiratory infections.

Assessment. Collection of *subjective data* includes noting the common complaints of malaise and appetite loss. Pruritus is severe. Bone pain occurs later.

Collection of *objective data* includes palpating enlarged lymph nodes—cervical and supraclavicular. Splenomegaly, hepatomegaly, and abdominal tenderness are found. Excoriation of skin and evidence of scratching from pruritus are noted. Edema of the face and neck may be noticed. Weight and nutritional status are recorded.

Diagnostic tests. Treatment depends on diagnosis of the stage or extent of involvement. Blood studies show anemia (normocytic, normochromic), WBC increase, and an abnormal erythrocyte sedimentation rate. Chest x-ray examination may reveal a mediastinal mass. Lymphangiograms can detect retroperitoneal node involvement. Lymph node biopsy that includes laparoscopy for retroperitoneal nodes is done. CT scan and ultrasound examination can indicate an enlarged spleen or liver. The presence of Reed-Sternberg cells remains a hallmark for the presence of Hodgkin's disease.

Medical management. Treatment depends on the staging process (Box 29-5 on p. 814).

In general, radiation therapy is used against the localized forms (Stages I and II), and chemotherapy is used against the generalized forms (Stages III and IV).

Combination chemotherapy and radiation has been used. The most commonly used combination is the MOPP regimen, which consists of mechlorethamine (nitrogen mustard), vincristine, procarbazine, and prednisone. Bone marrow transplantation and biological response modifiers are treatment options.

Nursing interventions. The nurse will plan care according to the staging process level. Awareness of side effects of radiotherapy or chemotherapy is important in preparing the patient to deal effectively with the conditions. Comfort measures with focus on skin integrity are carried out. Soothing baths with antipruritic medication (as ordered) can be effective. Fever and perspiration may be controlled with medication and attention to increased fluid intake plus necessary linen changes to prevent further skin problems. Extensive tests must be explained to the patient because there is a tendency toward impatience and anxiety.

Nursing diagnoses and interventions for the patient with Hodgkin's disease include but are not limited to the following:

NURSING DIAGNOSES	NURSING INTERVENTIONS
Skin integrity impaired, related to pruritus and jaundice	Assess condition of skin and level of discomfort. Administer skin care by baths and keep patient clean and dry. Apply calamine lotion, cornstarch, sodium bicarbonate, and medicated powders to relieve pruritus. Maintain adequate humidity and cool room to decrease pruritus. Monitor vital signs for fever; assess for perspiration and change linen, keeping it wrinkle free.
Pain, related to pruritus	Assess level and intensity of pain and ability of patient to cope. Administer medication for specific condition involved in discomfort. Use active and passive exercise, positioning for comfort. Teach relaxation techniques and diversional activity. Allow verbalization; be an active listener.
Infection, related to immune system ineffectiveness	Protect the environment and teach the importance of possible reverse isolation. Use meticulous handwashing. Prevent contamination by infectious visitors. Maintain hygiene and cleanliness of area. Monitor vital signs, I&O, respiratory status, and skin integrity.
Anxiety and fear, related to unknown outcome	Instruct patient on symptoms, disease progression, and treatment regimen. Encourage open communication and venting feelings. Encourage questions and problem solving.

Patient teaching. Understanding the disease is important to enable personal interaction in regard to self-care and retaining independence. The impact on the patient's life, as well as the effect on significant others, is a prime consideration of patient attitude and adjustment. Realistic approaches to the illness and therapies are imperative. Guidance toward counseling for stress management can be helpful. Special nutritional consideration for excess weight loss or undernourished condition is made.

Prognosis. The prognosis is steadily improving. It is dependent upon the stage of the disease. The prognosis for untreated patients is about 5 years; those diagnosed and treated in stage I or II have a 95% cure rate, whereas those in stage III or IV have a poor prognosis.

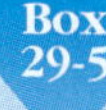

Box 29-5 ANN ARBOR CLINICAL STAGING: CLASSIFICATION OF HODGKIN'S DISEASE

STAGE I

- Abnormal single lymph nodes
- Regional or single extralymphatic organ or site

STAGE II

- Two or more abnormal lymph nodes on the same side of the diaphragm
- Localized involvement of extralymphatic organs or sites

STAGE III

- Abnormal lymph node regions on both sides of diaphragm
- May be accompanied by spleen involvement
- May be accompanied by localized involvement of extralymphatic organs or sites

STAGE IV

- Diffuse and disseminated involvement of one or more extralymphatic tissues and/or organs—with or without lymph node involvement

THERAPEUTIC DIALOGUE

Mr. Loris is a 25-year-old male with a recent diagnosis of Hodgkin's disease. When the nurse enters Mr. Loris's room, she notes he appears tense and drawn.

Nurse: You seem tense and preoccupied.

Mr. Loris: Why did this have to happen to me? I just got married and things were going so well. Dr. Mack said I would have to have radiation, then chemotherapy. I've heard that can make me sterile.

Nurse: The diagnosis of Hodgkin's disease certainly is worrisome for you and your wife.

Mr. Loris: Why do I feel so sad? I just want to cry?

Nurse: That is a very natural response; you are grieving because of loss of a totally healthy body as well as concern over the possibility of being sterile.

Mr. Loris: I don't know what to say to my wife.

Nurse: Are you frightened about how she might respond if you would become sterile?

Mr. Loris: Yes, I am scared; maybe I won't seem as masculine as I now am. I read somewhere about a male being able to store his sperm in a sperm bank before taking radiation and chemotherapy.

Nurse: Dr. Mack will be stopping in to see you tonight. Would you like to discuss this option with him at that time?

Mr. Loris: I think I will ask Sarah to come up this afternoon and see what she thinks about all of this.

Nurse: It is OK for you to let your loved ones know you are afraid.

Mr. Loris: I need to let Sarah know my feelings.

Nurse: Your desire to have an open communication with Sarah is helpful to both of you. I'll stop by and visit with you later.

REFERENCES AND SUGGESTED READINGS

1. Beare PG, Myers JL: *Adult health nursing,* ed 2, St Louis, 1994, Mosby.
2. Berkey KM, Hanson HI, Hanson S: *Pocket guide to family assessment and interventions,* St Louis, 1991, Mosby.
3. Bullough B, Bullough V: *Nursing in the community,* St Louis, 1990, Mosby.
4. Christensen PJ, Kenny JW: *The nursing process: application of theories, frameworks, models,* ed 3, St Louis, 1990, Mosby.
5. Cookfair J: *Nursing process and practice in the community,* St Louis, 1991, Mosby.
6. Dutcher JP: *Modern transfusion therapy,* Boca Raton, Fla, 1990, CRC Press.
7. Erickson JM: Blood support for the myelosuppressed patient, *Semin Oncol Nurs* 6:61, 1990.
8. Flyge HA: Meeting the challenge of neutropenia, *Nursing* 23(7):60, 1993.
9. Ford REN: *Psychosocial and ethical issues in bone marrow transplantation.* In Kasprisin CA, Snyder L, editors: *Bone marrow transplantation: a nursing perspective,* Arlington, Va, 1990, American Association of Blood Banks.
10. France-Dawson M: Sickle cell conditions and health knowledge, *Nurs Stand* 4:30, 1990.
11. Fuller AK: Platelet transfusion therapy for thrombocytopenia, *Semin Oncol Nurs* 6:123, 1990.
12. Gawbikowski J: White cells at war, *Am J Nurs* 92(3):44, 1992.
13. Grau PA: Are you at risk for hepatitis B? *Nurs '91* 21(3):44, 1991.
14. Gronewald S et al, eds: *Cancer nursing principles and practice,* ed 3, Boston, 1993, Jones & Bartlett.
15. Gulanick M et al: *Nursing care plans: nursing diagnosis and intervention,* ed 3, St Louis, 1994, Mosby.
16. Harovas J, Anthony H: Your guide to trouble free transfusions, *RN* 56(11):26, 1993.
17. Hepatitis B finger-stick infections from the *N Engl J Med* 326(11):721, 1992.
18. Heymann SJ et al: How safe is safe enough? New infections and the U.S. blood supply, *Ann Intern Med* 117:612, 1992.
19. Hood GH, Dincher JR: *Total patient care,* ed 8, St Louis, 1992, Mosby.
20. Kim MJ, McFarland GK, McLane AM: *Pocket guide to nursing diagnoses,* ed 5, St Louis, 1993, Mosby.
21. Kodish E et al: Bone marrow transplantation for sickle cell disease, *N Engl J Med* 325(19):1349, 1991.
22. Kresivic DM, Kralik K: Understanding therapeutic plasma exchange, *Nurs '90* 20(4):68, 1990.
23. Lacher M, Redman JR: *Hodgkin's disease: the consequence of survival,* Philadelphia, 1990, Lea & Febiger.
24. Lewis SM, Collier IC: *Medical-surgical nursing: assessment and management of clinical problems,* ed 3, St Louis, 1992, Mosby.
25. Long BC, Phipps WJ, Cassmeyer VL: *Medical-surgical nursing: a nursing process approach,* ed 3, St Louis, 1993, Mosby.
26. *Mosby's medical, nursing, and allied health dictionary,* ed 4, St Louis, 1994, Mosby.
27. Memmler RL, Cohen BJ, Wood DL: *Structure and function of the human body,* ed 5, Philadelphia, 1992, Lippincott.
28. Pagana KD, Pagana TJ: *Mosby's diagnostic and laboratory test reference,* St Louis, 1992, Mosby.
29. Pavel JN: Red blood cell transfusions for anemia, *Semin Oncol Nurs* 6:17, 1990.
30. Phipps WJ, Long BC, Woods NF: *Medical-surgical nursing: concepts and clinical practice,* ed 5, St Louis, 1995, Mosby.
31. Poulton R: Home care program for hemophiliacs, *Md Nurs* 9:5, 1990.
32. Querin JJ, Stahl LD: 12 simple, sensible steps for successful blood transfusions, *Nurs '90* 20(10):68, 1990.
33. Rayflied S, Theriot BL: Maximizing safe blood transfusions, *Adv Clin Care* 5:17, 1990.
34. Seidel HM et al: *Mosby's guide to physical examination,* ed 3, St Louis, 1995, Mosby.
35. Thibodeau GA: *Structure and function of the body,* ed 9, St Louis, 1992, Mosby.
36. Thompson JM et al: *Mosby's clinical nursing,* ed 3, St Louis, 1993, Mosby.
37. Urba WJ, Longo DL: Hodgkin's disease, *N Engl J Med* 326(10):678, 1992.
38. Whitman M, McDaniel RW: Preventing lymphedema: an unwelcome sequel to breast cancer, *Nursing* 23(12):36, 1993.
39. Young LM: DIC: the insidious killer, *Crit Care Nurse* 10(9):27, 1990.

CHAPTER CHALLENGE

KEY POINTS

- Blood is a thick, red fluid composed of plasma, red blood cells, white blood cells, and platelets, which are suspended in a light yellow fluid called plasma.
- The blood performs several critical functions: it transports oxygen and nutrition to the cells and waste products away from the cells; it regulates acid-base balance (pH) with buffers; and it protects the body against infection and prevents blood loss with special clotting mechanisms.
- Excess bands in the peripheral blood are called shifts to the left (that is, a shift toward immature cells) and indicate severe infection.
- Every person's blood is one of the following blood types in the ABO system of typing: type A, type B, type AB, type O.
- The lymphatic system is a vast, complex network of capillaries, thin vessels, valves, ducts, nodes, and organs that helps to protect and maintain the internal fluid environment of the entire body by producing, filtering, and conveying lymph and by producing various blood cells.
- The tonsils are composed of lymphoid tissue and are responsible for the filtering of bacteria.

- The thymus gland is composed of lymphoid tissue in utero (before birth) and the early years of life. It aids in the development of the immune system.
- The spleen is also composed of lymphoid tissue and has many functions, such as filtering out old RBCs, storing a pint of blood, producing antibodies, and phagocytosis of bacteria.
- Anemia may be caused by blood loss, impaired RBC production, increased RBC destruction, or nutritional deficiency.
- Weakness and fatigue are major symptoms of anemia. They result from decreased oxygenation from decreased levels of hemoglobin and increased energy needs required by increased RBC production.
- Sickle cell anemia is a hemolytic anemia with a genetic basis; a sickle cell crisis occurs when the RBCs become deoxygenated and sickle-shaped, thus causing stasis and obstruction of the microvasculature, leading to organ infarction and necrosis.
- Ingestion of iron compounds or IM Z-track imferon is part of the therapy for iron-deficiency anemia.
- Thrombocytopenia is a decrease in the number of circulating platelets and leads to bleeding; persons with thrombocytopenia need to learn how to prevent injury and hemorrhage.
- Hemophilia is a hereditary coagulation disorder, hemophilia A is a lack of coagulation factor VIII, and hemophilia B is a lack of factor IX. Maintenance therapy consists of blood factor replacement therapy and prevention of injury.
- Disseminated intravascular coagulation (DIC) is a coagulation disorder characterized initially by clotting and secondarily by hemorrhage. It results from an alteration in the balance between clotting factors and fibrinolytic factors; the person is usually critically ill.
- Persons with alterations of WBCs are at high risk of infection, because leukocytes are a major factor in the body's defense against invading microorganisms.
- The leukemias are malignant disorders characterized by uncontrolled proliferation of WBCs and their precursors; the cause is unknown, but several theories have been proposed.
- Leukemias may be lymphocytic or myelogenous, and acute or chronic. Acute leukemias have a rapid onset and a short course, if untreated; chronic leukemias have a more insidious onset and longer course. The major therapies for leukemias are chemotherapy and bone marrow transplantation.
- Lymphomas are malignant disorders of the lymphatic system. Persons with Hodgkin's disease have defective cellular immunity and are therefore at high risk for infection. Non-Hodgkin's lymphoma is a group of lymphoid malignancies. Chemotherapy and radiation are the primary medical treatment for lymphomas.

STUDY QUESTIONS

1. Another name for a red blood cell is:
   1. Leukocyte
   2. Monocyte
   3. Erythrocyte
   4. Platelet
2. The test for a measure of the packed cell volume of red cells expressed as a percentage of the total blood volume is:
   1. Hematocrit
   2. Erythrocyte sedimentation rate
   3. Reticulocyte
   4. Differential
3. The gland that plays a role in the development of the body's immune system is the:
   1. Tonsils
   2. Thymus
   3. Spleen
   4. Liver
4. A granular circulating leukocyte essential for phagocytosis by which bacteria, cellular debris, and solid particles are destroyed and removed is called a(n):
   1. Basophil
   2. Lymphocyte
   3. Neutrophil
   4. Eosinophil
5. The enlarged pouchlike structure in the thoracic duct that serves as a storage area for lymph moving toward its point of entry into the venous system is the:
   1. Cisterna chyli
   2. Lacteal
   3. Inferior vena cava
   4. Right lymphatic duct
6. The complex protein-iron compound in the blood that carries oxygen to the cells from the lungs and carbon dioxide away from the cells to the lungs is:
   1. Leukocyte
   2. Thrombocyte
   3. Hemoglobin
   4. Erythrocyte
7. The type of blood that is called the universal donor blood is:
   1. Type A
   2. Type B
   3. Type AB
   4. Type O
8. Lymph is a material that is obtained from:
   1. A special protein that combats foreign invaders
   2. Tissue fluid
   3. The breakdown of red and white blood cells
   4. Fluid absorbed from the large intestine

9. An intestinal lymphatic that takes up chyle and passes it to the lymph circulation and to the thoracic duct and to the blood vascular system is:
   1. Lactiferous ducts
   2. Laminae
   3. Lambda
   4. Lacteal
10. The spleen is located in which quadrant of the abdominal cavity:
   1. Upper right
   2. Upper left
   3. Lower left
   4. Lower right
11. Mrs. Walters is immunosuppressed by chemotherapy. She has a WBC of $1500/mm^3$, with neutrophils of 20%. Which of the following statements indicates she understands home care instructions relating to her immune system:
   1. Take antibiotics prophylactically
   2. Take large doses of vitamins
   3. Avoid individuals with infections
   4. Use only sterile bed linens
12. Mr. Rappaport's platelets have dropped to $18{,}000/mm^3$. The most appropriate nursing intervention is to:
   1. Provide oral hygiene 4 times per day
   2. Institute bleeding precautions
   3. Order a high-protein diet
   4. Request an order for nasal oxygen
13. Mrs. Brase tells the nurse that her husband, admitted with advanced leukemia, is talking about dying and expressing fears of death. She asks for suggestions for helping with her husband. Which of the following responses by the nurse is best:
   1. "Mr. Rappaport will probably die of another disease before he dies of leukemia."
   2. "Mr. Rappaport is expressing a readiness to be admitted to a hospice."
   3. "Talk of death is natural at this time but will diminish as he feels better."
   4. "It's normal to want to talk about death; what we can do is be supportive by listening."
14. Which of the following statements is the most accurate instruction for a patient who is to undergo a bone marrow aspiration:
   1. "There will be no pain, just perhaps a slight discomfort."
   2. "You will be under general anesthesia during the procedure."
   3. "There will be a brief, sharp pain during the aspiration."
   4. "There will be no pain during the procedure but some afterward."
15. Mrs. Jacobson is a 27-year-old housewife and mother of two children. She is being seen by the nurse at the health maintenance organization for signs of fatigue. She has a history of iron-deficiency anemia. Which of the following data from the nursing history indicates that the anemia is not currently managed effectively:
   1. Pallor
   2. Poor skin turgor
   3. Heart rate 68, weak pulse
   4. Respirations 18 and regular
16. An important nursing care goal to establish for Mrs. Jackson, who has iron-deficiency anemia, is:
   1. Use birth control to avoid pregnancy
   2. Increase fluids to stimulate erythropoiesis
   3. Decrease fluids to prevent sickling of RBCs
   4. Alternate periods of rest and activity to balance oxygen supply and demand
17. The nurse instructs Mrs. Jackson about foods rich in iron. Which of the following foods should be included in the diet:
   1. Fresh fruit and milk
   2. Cheeses and processed lunch meats
   3. Dark green vegetables and organ meats
   4. Fruit juices and cornmeal breads
18. Which of the following statements by the patient with pernicious anemia would indicate that she has understood the teaching:
   1. "I'll be glad when I can stop the injections and take only oral medicine."
   2. "I'll have to take B_{12} shots for the rest of my life."
   3. "After a while I'll no longer need to take shots, just the pills."
   4. "I was glad to hear that pills are available to treat me."
19. Mr. Grenes is admitted with polycythemia vera. He has a hemoglobin of 20 g/dl. A probable treatment which will be ordered is:
   1. Whole blood transfusion
   2. Platelet transfusion
   3. Phlebotomy with removal of 800 ml of blood
   4. Vitamin B_{12} injection

30

CARE OF THE PATIENT WITH A URINARY DISORDER

Alita K. Sellers
Carolyn Edwards

KEY TERMS

ANATOMY AND PHYSIOLOGY
albuminuria
antidiuretic hormone (ADH)
Bowman's capsule
calyx
creatinine
cortex
glomerulus
glycosuria
hematuria
hilus
ketoaciduria
medulla
nephron
trigone
ureter

MEDICAL-SURGICAL
anasarca
anuria
asthenia
azotemia
bacteriuria
costovertebral angle
cytological evaluation
dialysis
diuresis
dysuria
hydronephrosis
ileal conduit
micturition
nephrotoxin
nocturia
oliguria
prostatodynia
pyuria
residual urine
retention
urolithiasis

LEARNING OBJECTIVES

Anatomy and Physiology

After reading this chapter, the student should be able to do the following:

- Define the key terms.
- Describe the structures of the urinary system and their functions.
- Discuss the nephron and its function.
- List the three processes involved in urine formation.
- Discuss the normal versus abnormal components of urine.
- Name three hormones and their influence on nephron function.

Medical-Surgical

- Define the key terms.
- Describe the alterations in renal function associated with disorders of the urinary tract.
- Select nursing diagnoses for care alterations in urinary function.
- Prioritize the special needs of the patient with urinary dysfunction.
- Appraise the changes in body image created when the patient experiences an alteration in urinary function.
- Identify the effects of aging on urinary system function.
- Adapt teaching methods for the patient with urinary diversion.
- Discuss the impact of renal disease on family function.
- Incorporate pharmacotherapeutic and nutritional considerations into the nursing care plan of the patient with a urinary disorder.

RELATED TOPICS OF INTEREST

- Medical asepsis and infection control (Chapter 12)
- Comfort, rest, and sleep (Chapter 15)
- Specimen collection and diagnostic examination (Chapter 17)
- Diet therapy (Chapter 19)
- The surgical patient (Chapter 22)
- Fluids and electrolytes (Chapter 24)
- Care of the patient with a cardiovascular disorder (Chapter 28)
- Care of the patient with a respiratory disorder (Chapter 31)
- Care of the patient with an endocrine disorder (Chapter 32)
- Care of the patient with a neurological disorder (Chapter 35)

ANATOMY AND PHYSIOLOGY

Daily, the cells throughout the body metabolize ingested nutrients. This process provides energy for the body, and produces waste products. As protein breaks down, nitrogenous wastes—urea, ammonia, and **creatinine** (an important nitrogenous compound produced by metabolic processes in the body)—are produced. Excretion of these waste products is the primary function of the kidneys. The kidneys also assist in regulating the body's water, electrolytes, and acid-base balance. To perform these tasks the kidneys filter the blood. The urinary system is probably the most important system in maintaining homeostasis.

The urinary system is composed of (1) two kidneys, which produce urine after filtering the wastes from the blood; (2) two ureters, which transport the urine from the kidneys to the bladder; (3) one bladder, which collects and stores the urine; and (4) one urethra, which transports the urine from the bladder to the outside of the body for elimination (Fig. 30-1).

This chapter will explore the filtering process, the composition of urine, and the pathway of urine removal from the body.

Kidneys

The kidneys lie behind the peritoneum (retroperito neal), just below the diaphragm on each side of the vertebral column. They are dark red, bean-shaped organs that are 4 to 5 inches (10 to 12 cm) long, 2 to 3 inches (5 to 7.5 cm) wide, and about 1 inch (2 cm) thick. Because of the size and shape of the liver, the right kidney lies slightly lower in the posterior abdominal cavity than the left kidney. The kidneys are surrounded by a layer of adipose tissue that anchors them in place. Near the center of the medial border is a notch or indentation called the **hilus** where the ureter, blood vessels, and nerves enter or exit the kidney.

Gross Anatomical Structure. The outer covering of the kidney is composed of a strong layer of connective tissue called the *renal capsule.* Directly beneath the renal capsule is the renal **cortex** (the outer part of the kidneys; the word "cortex" comes from the Latin word for "bark" or "rind," so the cortex of an organ is its outer layer), which is soft and granular (Fig. 30-2 on p. 820). It contains 1.25 million renal tubules. These tubules are part of the microscopic filtration system. Immediately be-

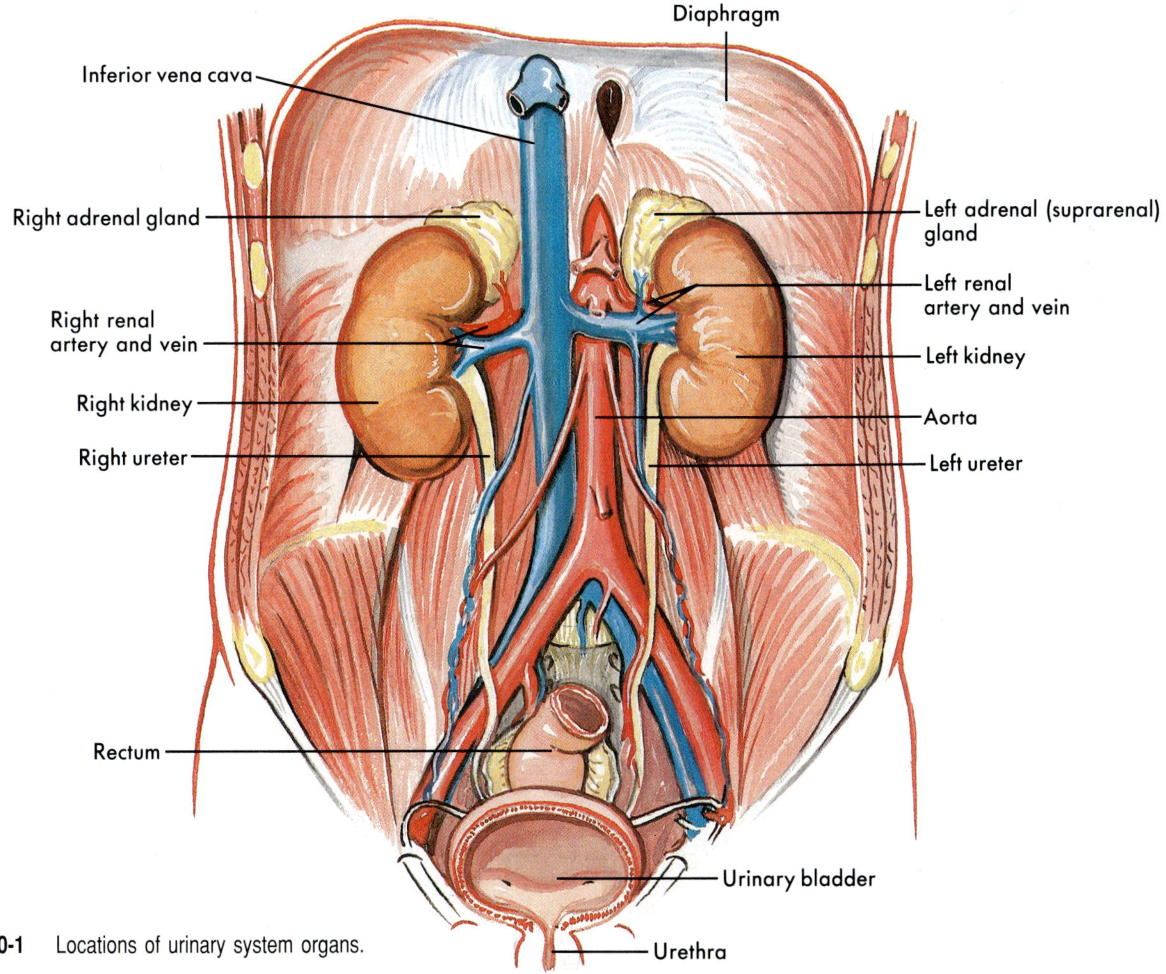

FIG. 30-1 Locations of urinary system organs.

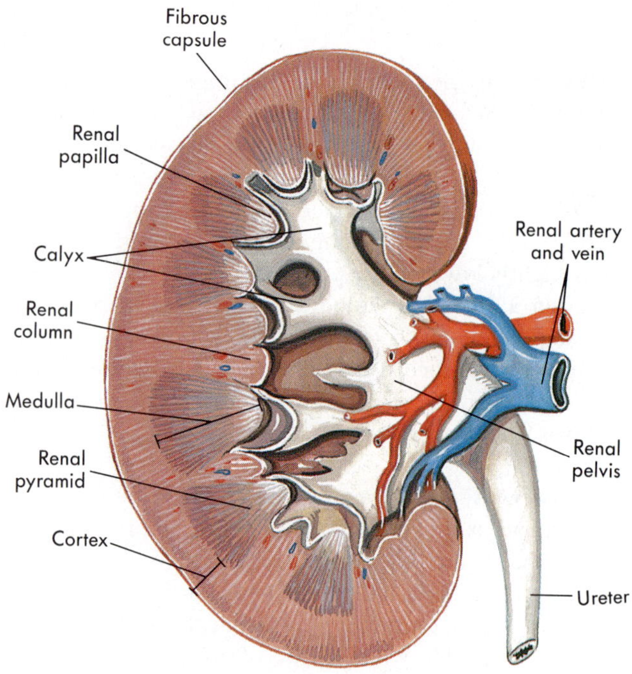

FIG. 30-2 Coronal section through right kidney.

neath the cortex is the medulla, which is a darker color. The **medulla** (the most internal part of a structure or organ, as the renal medulla) contains the triangular pyramids. Continuing inward, the narrow points of the pyramids (papillae) empty urine into the calyces. The **calyces** are cuplike extensions of the renal pelvis that guide urine into the renal pelvis. The innermost region is called the *renal pelvis,* and each pyramid empties into a calyx in this region. The renal pelvis is really an expansion of the upper end of the ureter; the ureter in turn drains the finished product, urine, into the bladder.

Microscopic Structure.

Nephron. Each kidney contains more than 1 million nephrons. The **nephron** is a structural and functional unit of the kidney, resembling a microscopic funnel with a long stem and two convoluted sections (Fig. 30-3). It is responsible for filtering the blood and processing the urine. The nephron has three major functions: (1) controlling body fluid levels by selectively removing or retaining water; (2) assisting with the regulation of the pH of the blood, and (3) removing toxic wastes from the blood. Approximately 60 times a day the body's entire volume of blood is filtered through the kidneys. Basically, the nephron consists of two main structures: the renal corpuscle and the renal tubule.

The renal corpuscle contains a tightly bound network of capillaries in a cluster and enveloped in a thin wall (**glomerulus;** plural, glomeruli) that are held inside a cuplike structure of a renal tube **(Bowman's capsule).** The renal arteries (right and left) branch off the abdominal aorta and enter the kidney at the hilus. The renal arteries continue branching until blood is delivered to the glomerulus by the afferent arteriole. The blood leaves the glomerulus through the efferent arteriole. Blood finally reaches the renal veins and flows into the inferior vena cava. Fig. 30-3 shows that the afferent arteriole is much larger than the efferent arteriole. This blood flow pattern increases the pressure within the glomerular capillaries. Blood pressure (hydrostatic pressure) determines the glomerular filtration rate (GFR). Those substances that move along this pressure gradient, leaving the glomerulus and entering Bowman's capsule, are now referred to as filtrate. This process is indiscriminate as to the quantity of substances that are filtered. This results in the first step of urine production—glomerular filtration. This filtrate contains blood plasma without the blood proteins and blood cells. The process continues as Bowman's capsule extends into the renal tubules. The efferent arterioles also connect to the peritubular capillaries that surround the renal tubules (Fig. 30-3).

The second step of the urine formation process is reabsorption. As the filtrate leaves the Bowman's capsule, it enters a long, coiled, twisting tubule that descends in the center, much like a hairpin. The first segment of the tubule system is the proximal convoluted tubule; the second segment is the loop of Henle (a hairpinlike curve); and the third segment is the distal convoluted tubule. The system is completed by the emptying of filtrate into the collecting tubules.

Reabsorption begins as soon as the filtrate reaches the tubule system. The filtrate contains important products needed by the body; water, glucose, and ions must be reabsorbed for body use. In fact, 99% of the filtrate is returned to the blood (Fig. 30-4).

Tubular secretion, the third step of urine formation, is responsible for removing substances from the blood and adding it to the filtrate (urine). Some of the substances secreted are potassium and hydrogen ions, creatinine, urea, and ammonia. Certain drugs, such as penicillin, are also removed by tubular secretion. Secretion also helps to maintain blood pH. This secretion process occurs primarily in the distal convoluted tubules.

In summary, the three phases of urine formation (Table 30-1 on p. 822) and the location of the processes are as follows:

1. *Filtration* of water and blood products occurs in the glomerulus of Bowman's capsule.
2. *Reabsorption* of water, glucose, and needed ions back into the blood occurs primarily in the proximal convoluted tubules, loop of Henle, and distal convoluted tubules. Peritubular capillaries bring blood to the area. This process reclaims important substances needed by the body.
3. *Secretion* of certain ions, nitrogen waste products, and drugs occurs primarily in the distal convoluted tubule. This process is the reverse of reabsorption; the substances move from the blood to the filtrate.

FIG. 30-3 Cross section from the four segments of the renal tubule are shown.

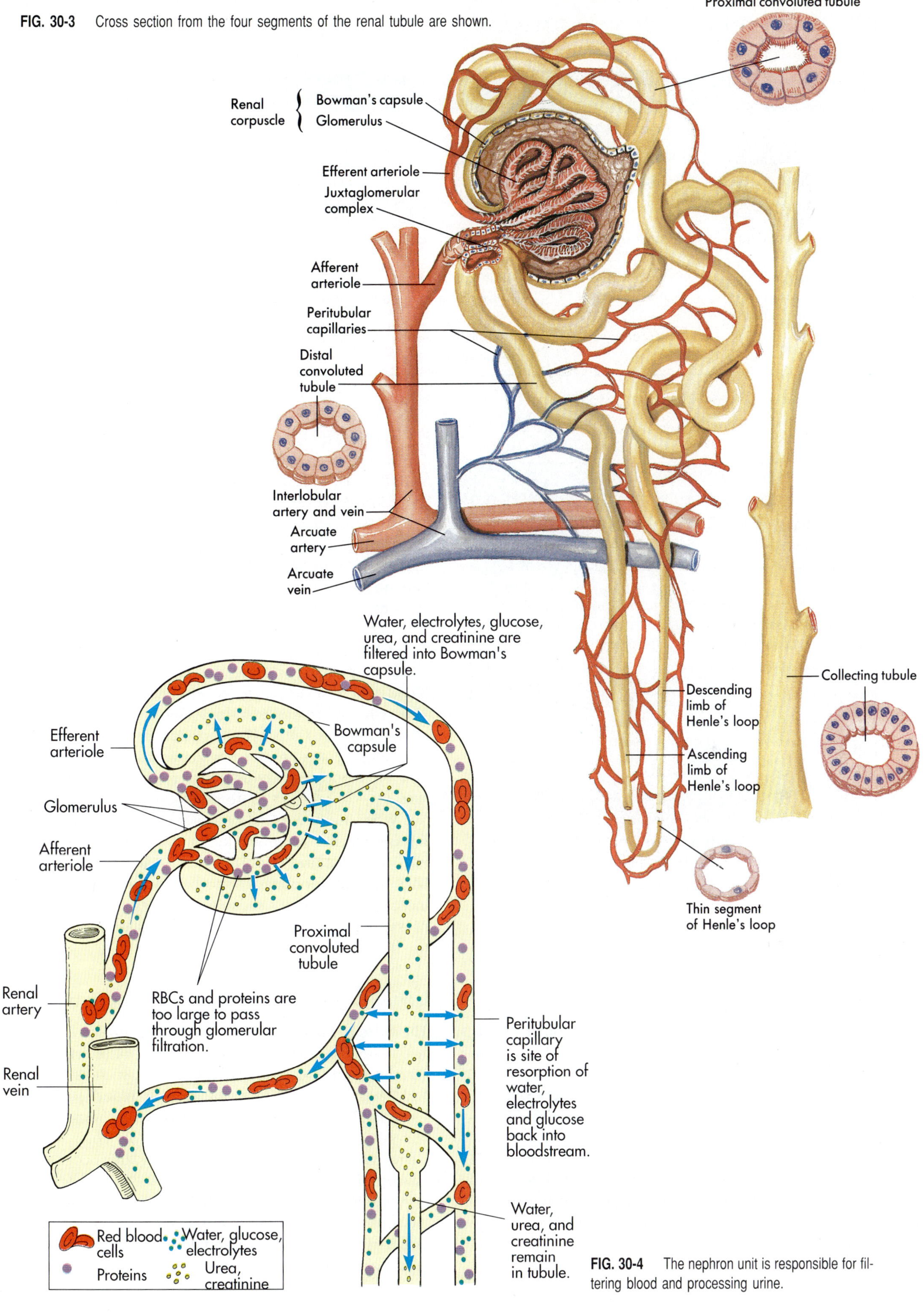

FIG. 30-4 The nephron unit is responsible for filtering blood and processing urine.

TABLE 30-1 Functions of Parts of the Nephron in Urine Formation

Part of Nephron	Process in Urine Formation	Substances Moved and Direction of Movement
Glomerulus	Filtration	Water and solutes (e.g., sodium and other ions, nitrogen waste products, urea, uric acid, creatinine, glucose, and other nutrients) filter through the glomeruli into Bowman's capsule
Proximal convoluted tubule	Reabsorption	Water and solutes
Loop of Henle	Reabsorption	Sodium and chloride ions
Distal convoluted and collecting tubules	Reabsorption	Water, sodium, and chloride ions
	Secretion	Ammonia, potassium ions, urea, uric acid, creatinine, hydrogen ions, and some drugs

Box 30-1 MAJOR FUNCTIONS OF THE KIDNEYS

Urine formation: Glomerular filtration, tubular reabsorption, and secretion

Fluid and electrolyte control: Maintain correct balance of fluid and electrolytes within a normal range by excretion, secretion, and reabsorption

Acid-base balance: Maintain pH at normal range by directly excreting H^+ ions and forming bicarbonate for buffering

Excretion of waste products: Direct removal of metabolic waste products contained in the glomerular filtrate

Blood pressure regulation: Regulate blood pressure by controlling the circulating volume and renin secretion

RBC production: Erythropoietin secreted by kidneys stimulates bone marrow to produce RBCs

Regulation of calcium-phosphate metabolism: Vitamin D activation regulated by kidneys

Hormonal influence on nephron function. When the body has suffered increased fluid loss through hemorrhage, diaphoresis, vomiting, diarrhea, or other means, the blood pressure drops, which decreases the amount of filtrate produced by the kidneys. The posterior pituitary gland releases **antidiuretic hormone (ADH)** (a hormone that decreases the production of urine by increasing the reabsorption of water by the renal tubules), which prevents excess water loss in the urine. ADH causes the cells of the distal convoluted tubules to increase their rate of water reabsorption. This returns water to the bloodstream, which increases the blood pressure to a more normal level and causes the urine to become very concentrated.

When there is decreased blood volume, decreased sodium ions, or increased potassium ions in the blood, the adrenal cortex releases the hormone *aldosterone.* This causes increased sodium retention, which results in increased potassium excretion. Since water follows sodium, the tubules increase water reabsorption and blood volume improves. Urine volume is influenced not by the amount of filtrate but rather by the degree of reabsorption of water.

If blood pressure is low, the cells of the juxtaglomerular apparatus release the enzyme renin into the blood where it activates the glycoprotein angiotensin. The *renin-angiotensin* system affects the reabsorption of water and sodium. When arterial pressure falls, intrarenal angiotensin promotes water and sodium reabsorption and blood vessel constriction to normalize the pressure.

When the kidneys do not get enough oxygen, they release another hormonelike substance that acts as an enzyme to produce erythropoietin. Erythropoietin stimulates the red bone marrow to produce red blood cells, increasing the blood's capacity to carry oxygen and thus preventing anemia. See Box 30-1 for major functions of the kidneys.

Urine Composition and Characteristics

The word *urine* comes from one of its components, uric acid. Daily the body forms 1000 to 2000 ml of urine; this amount is influenced by several factors, such as mental and physical health, oral intake, and blood pressure. Urine is 95% water; the remainder is nitrogenous wastes and salts. It is usually a transparent yellow color with a characteristic odor. Normal urine is yellow because of urochrome, a pigment resulting from the body's destruction of hemoglobin. Urine is slightly acidic, with a pH of 4.6 to 8.0. Healthy urine is sterile, but at room temperature it rapidly decomposes and develops the odor of ammonia as a result of the breakdown of urea.

Urine Abnormalities

A urinalysis, which studies the physical, chemical, and microscopic properties of urine, can give important diagnostic information. If the body's homeostasis has been compromised, certain substances may spill into the urine. Some of the more common substances include:

1. *Albumin:* The presence of albumin in the urine **(albuminuria)** indicates possible kidney disease, increased blood pressure, or possibly irritation of the kidney cells from heavy metals.
2. *Glucose:* The presence of sugar in the urine **(glycosuria)** most often indicates a high blood glucose level. This condition is seen with diabetes mellitus, because the pancreas is not producing enough insulin to metabolize the glucose. The blood glucose level increases above the renal threshold (the point at which the kidney tubules can no longer reabsorb), and the glucose spills into the urine.
3. *Erythrocytes:* The presence of erythrocytes in the urine **(hematuria)** usually indicates infections, tumors, or kidney disease. Occasionally an individual may have a kidney stone and the irritation produces hematuria.
4. *Ketone bodies:* The presence of ketone bodies in the urine, **ketoaciduria** (also called ketonuria), occurs when excessive quantities of fatty acids are oxidized in the liver. This condition may be seen with diabetes mellitus, low carbohydrate intake, starvation, or any other metabolic condition in which fats are rapidly catabolized.
5. *Leukocytes:* The presence of leukocytes (white blood cells) occurs when there is an infection in the urinary tract. A sterile urine specimen for culture and sensitivity identifies the specific organism. The individual may then be treated with antibiotics.

Ureters

Once the urine has been formed in the nephrons, it passes to the paired ureters. **Ureters** are actually extensions of the kidney pelvis and extend 10 to 12 inches (25 to 30 cm) to the lower part of the urinary bladder. The walls of the ureters are composed of three layers of tissue: (1) the mucosa (inner layer) protects the lining of the ureter from the acidic urine; (2) the muscle (middle layer) creates peristaltic waves every 1 to 5 minutes—this propels the urine into the bladder (the more urine produced, the closer the peristaltic waves); and (3) the fibrous coat (outer layer), which is a protective layer with fibrous extensions that anchor the ureters.

As the ureters leave the kidneys, they are retroperitoneal and pass under the urinary bladder before entering it. This anatomical position prevents backflow of urine, because pressure in the urinary bladder compresses the ureters.

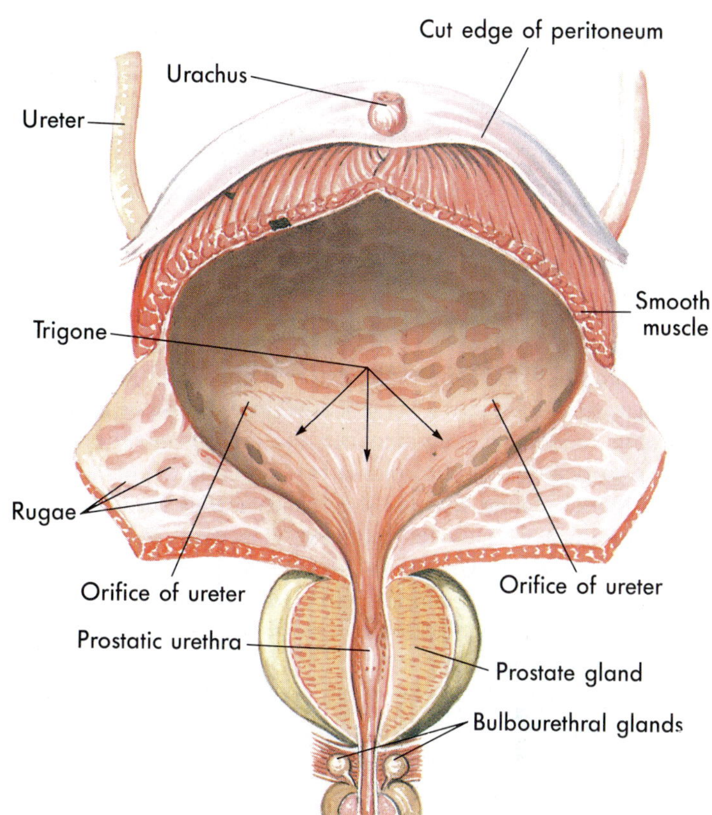

FIG. 30-5 The male urinary bladder, cut to show the interior. Note how the prostate gland surrounds the urethra as it exits the bladder.

Urinary Bladder

The urinary bladder (Fig. 30-5) is a temporary storage pouch for urine. It is composed of collapsible muscle and is located anterior to the small intestine and posterior to the symphysis pubis. The lower portion, continuous with the urethra, is called the neck; its upper tip, connected to the umbilicus by the umbilical ligament, is called the apex. The region between the two openings of the two ureters and the urethra is the **trigone.** The musculature of the bladder consists of interlacing smooth muscle fibers that run longitudinally, obliquely, and transversely. Collectively these muscle fibers are referred to as the detrusor muscle. As the bladder fills with urine, it rises into the abdominal cavity and can actually be palpated. Under normal conditions the bladder can distend to hold 750 to 1000 ml of urine. When the bladder contains approximately 250 ml of urine, the individual has a conscious desire to urinate. This is because the stretch receptors become activated and a message is sent to the spinal cord. A moderately full bladder holds about 470 ml (1 pint) of urine.

Two sphincters, the internal and external, control the release of the urine. The internal sphincter is composed of involuntary muscle, and as the bladder becomes full, the stretch receptors cause contractions, pushing the urine past the internal sphincter. The urine then presses on the external sphincter, which is composed of skeletal or voluntary muscle. Although an individual feels the urge to void, it can be controlled. As the bladder continues to fill, the message will be sent at intervals, until it becomes necessary to respond to the message and urinate.

Urethra

The urethra is the terminal portion of the urinary system. It is a small tube that carries urine by peristalsis from the bladder out of its external opening, the urinary meatus. In females it is embedded in the anterior wall of the vagina and exits between the clitoris and the vaginal opening. It is approximately ¼ inch in diameter and 1½ inches long. Because the urinary orifice (urinary meatus) is very close to the anus, it is fairly easy for *Escherichia coli* (*E. coli*) in the stool to enter the urinary meatus and cause a urinary infection. Females should be taught to cleanse anterior to posterior to decrease possible contamination.

In males the urethra is approximately 8 inches long. It leaves the urinary bladder, passes through the prostate gland, and extends the length of the penis. The urinary orifice is in the center of the distal surface or the glans penis. In the male the urethra serves two functions: a passageway for urine and a passageway for semen.

GERONTOLOGICAL CONSIDERATIONS

- Urinary frequency, urgency, nocturia, and incontinence are common with aging. These occur because of weakened musculature in the bladder and urethra, diminished neurological sensation combined with decreased bladder capacity, and the effects of medications such as diuretics.
- Urinary incontinence is a leading reason for institutional placement of older adults.
- Urinary incontinence can lead to a loss of self-esteem and result in decreased participation in social activities.
- Older women are particularly at risk for stress incontinence because of hormonal changes and weakened pelvic musculature.
- Older men are particularly at risk for urinary retention because of prostatic hypertrophy.
- Urinary tract infections in older adults are often associated with invasive procedures such as catheterization, diabetes, and neurological disorders.
- Inadequate fluid intake, immobility, and conditions that lead to urinary stasis increase the risk of infection in the older adult.
- Frequent toileting and meticulous skin care can reduce the risk of skin impairment secondary to urinary incontinence.

The mucous membrane that lines the urethra is continuous with the bladder, ureters, and kidney pelves. This anatomical feature is important, because infection can spread easily throughout the system.

Normal Aging Patterns

With aging the kidneys lose part of their normal functioning capacity; in fact, by the age of 70 the filtering mechanism is only 50% as efficient as at age 40. This occurs because of decreased blood supply and loss of nephrons.

In the aging female the bladder loses tone and the perineal muscles may relax; this can result in stress incontinence. In the aging male the prostate gland may become enlarged (this occurs in 75% of men by the age of 70) and leads to constriction of the urethra. Incomplete emptying of the bladder in both sexes increases the possibility of urinary infection. Assessing the amount, color, and odor of the urine may detect early symptoms. For specific considerations, see the gerontological box.

CARE OF THE PATIENT WITH A URINARY DISORDER: GENERAL CONSIDERATIONS

Assessment of Urinary Function

Assessment of the urinary tract is included in baseline data for all patients. Assessment of the urinary tract is emphasized in special circumstances: (1) persons who may be at high risk for renal disease, such as individuals exposed to **nephrotoxins** (substances with specific destructive properties for the kidneys, such as aminoglycoside antibiotics [gentamicin, kanamycin], heavy metal [lead, mercury, cisplatin], solvents and chemicals [arsenic, ethylene glycol, carbon tetrachloride], NSAIDs, radiopaque contrast media) and those experiencing systemic changes from altered health states, such as pregnancy, diabetes mellitus, or hypertension; (2) conditions that may directly compromise renal function, including trauma, fluid depletion, or retention; and especially (3) patients with active or suspected renal disease.

The subject of urinary problems is a delicate one to approach, perhaps because the urinary system is closely associated with the reproductive system and cultural taboos surrounding sexuality. Often the patient's self-image and sexual performance are affected by altered urinary function. It is important for the nurse to be sensitive to the patient's feelings, guiding the interview to ensure accurate assessment while maintaining the patient's dignity. The nurse uses inspection, auscultation, percussion, and palpation to assess the urinary system.

Collection of Subjective and Objective Data. The nursing assessment should include the patient's description of urine, urination patterns, sensation associated with urination, such as burning or pain, and difficulty starting or maintaining the urine stream. Advancing renal disease causes systemic changes, particularly in the respiratory and circulatory systems. The nurse assesses for signs and symptoms of fluid overload or depletion. The skin provides easily assessed clues about the patient's state of hydration. Dryness and pruritus occur from electrolyte imbalance and the buildup of waste products. Mucous membranes become dry if the patient fails to maintain adequate hydration. Uremic frost, the white sediment deposited on the skin from azotemia, may be present; however, this is seen less frequently because more effective management measures are now available.

Geriatric patients should be assessed for the effects of aging on renal functioning. Faulty renal circulation from generalized arteriosclerosis and a decrease in the number of functioning nephrons diminish the efficiency of the kidneys. Decreased bladder capacity, weakened musculature and sphincter tone, diminished innervation, and enlarged prostate in men interfere with sensation and bladder control. The role of the nurse in completing a physical assessment may vary widely in different care settings.

The nurse records the subjective and objective data findings for the nursing assessment. When possible, the patient's or family's own words should be recorded in quotation marks to describe the patient complaints; then objective assessment findings are documented, both normal and abnormal. The nurse selects NANDA-approved nursing diagnoses that describe the patient's problems. Suggested nursing diagnoses are included within the discussion of the urinary tract disorders and should be augmented with general medical/surgical principles where appropriate.

Diagnostic Tests

Diagnostic tests for urinary tract conditions include laboratory tests, diagnostic imaging, and endoscopic procedures. Nursing responsibilities vary according to the studies performed. Nurses need to be aware of specific patient variables that may influence test results: state of hydration, nutritional status, or trauma.

Urinalysis. The most common urinary diagnostic study is the urinalysis. Table 30-2 provides a description of normal and abnormal constituents in the urine and possible factors that will influence test results. A urinalysis may be done in relation to conditions of other body systems because of the role of the kidneys in maintaining homeostasis. Urinalysis is completed on a clean-catch or catheterized specimen. A clean-catch urine specimen is obtained after cleansing the area surrounding the urinary meatus with an antiseptic solution. The patient voids a small amount into a nonsterile container, discards it, and continues to void into the sterile specimen container. The inside of the sterile specimen container and the lid must not be touched, because contamination alters test results. If it is necessary to obtain a catheterized specimen, aseptic technique must be maintained. If an indwelling catheter is in place, aseptic technique is used to obtain a urine sample through the port on the drainage tubing. A urine specimen for culture may be obtained using these same procedures to confirm suspected infections, to identify causative organisms, and to determine appropriate antimicrobial therapy (see Chapter 17). Cultures are also obtained for periodic screening of urine when the threat of a urinary tract infection (UTI) persists. A sample of urine that has been properly collected and stored is considered to be normal if it contains 10,000 or fewer organisms per milliliter. Organisms

TABLE 30-2 Urinalysis

Constituent	Normal Range	Variation Factors
Color	Pale yellow to amber	Diabetes insipidus, biliary obstruction, medications, foods
Turbidity	Clear to slightly cloudy	Phosphates, WBCs, bacteria
Odor	Mildly aromatic	Medication, bacteria, food
pH	4.6 to 8	Stale specimen, food intake, infection, homeostatic imbalance
Specific gravity	1.005 to 1.030	State of hydration, diabetes insipidus
Glucose	Negative	Diabetes mellitus, medications, food intake
Protein	Negative	Renal damage that allows protein to escape through the glomeruli, muscle exertion, fever, severe dehydration
Bilirubin	Negative	Liver disease with obstruction or damage
Hemoglobin	Negative	Trauma, renal disease
Ketones	Negative	Diabetes mellitus, diet, febrile disease
Red blood cells	2 to 3/HPF	Blood dyscrasias, renal disease, bladder disease (cystitis, cancer), anticoagulant drugs, trauma
White blood cells	4 to 5/HPF	Renal disease, lower urinary tract disease
Casts	Rare	Renal disease; found in large numbers in nephritis
Bacteria	Negative	Urinary tract infection

of this magnitude are the result of normal urethral flora and do not signify UTI. A UTI is diagnosed when bacterial counts in a properly collected and stored sample reach 100,000 or more organisms per milliliter and when the organisms are of one or very largely one bacterial type.

There are various reagent strips available to test urine for abnormal substances. The strips are a quick reference that can be used in a clinic setting or at home. Easy-to-follow instructions accompany the specific reagent strips.

Since the kidneys excrete substances in varying amounts and rates during a 24-hour period, the nurse may be responsible for collecting a 24-hour urine sample. The first voiding is discarded and the time noted at the beginning of the 24-hour urine collection. For the next 24 hours all urine is collected and placed in a special laboratory container. Common substances measured to monitor kidney filtration include total urine protein, creatinine, and electrolytes. Depending on the test ordered, the specimen container may contain special chemicals (preservatives) and/or the urine may need to be kept cold. The nurse should follow the institutional procedure manual.

Blood Urea Nitrogen. Blood urea nitrogen (BUN) is a laboratory test used to determine the kidney's ability to rid the blood of the nonprotein nitrogen (NPN) waste, urea, which results from protein breakdown (catabolism). The acceptable serum range for BUN is 10 to 20 mg/dl. For a more accurate test result, the patient should receive nothing by mouth (NPO) for 8 hours before blood sampling. If the BUN is elevated, preventive nursing measures should be instituted to protect the patient from possible disorientation or convulsions (see Chapter 35).

Creatinine Clearance. Creatinine, a nonprotein nitrogen (NPN) substance, is present in blood and urine. Creatinine is generated during muscle contraction and then excreted by glomerular filtration. Levels are directly related to muscle mass and are usually measured for a 24-hour period. During the testing period, excessive physical activity should be avoided. A fasting blood sample is drawn at the onset of testing and another at the conclusion. All urine in the 24-hour period is collected, since any deviation will alter test results. An elevation in serum levels with a decline in urine levels indicates renal disease. Normal ranges are: serum—0.5 to 1.1 mg/dl, urine—97 to 137 ml/min (male), 88 to 128 ml/min (female).

Phenolsulfonphthalein. Excretory ability of the renal tubules is assessed by the phenolsulfonphthalein (PSP) test. The PSP test provides much the same data as the creatinine clearance test and is now being performed less often. The red dye, PSP, is injected intravenously, and at intervals urine samples are obtained. Normally 60% to 75% of the dye is excreted in the urine after 2 hours.

Concentration and Dilution. A noninvasive examination to assess the kidney's ability to concentrate and dilute urine is done by withholding fluids and then giving the patient large amounts of fluids. Urine samples are taken during the test to check the specific gravity. Specific gravity will decrease with increased hydration in normal kidney function. With kidney damage the specific gravity does not change regardless of fluid intake.

Assessment of *osmolality*, which measures the weight of the solute compared with its own weight, may be preferred over specific gravity. Regardless of the measurement used, the same testing procedure is followed. Plasma osmolality may be done in conjunction with the urine sampling when pituitary disorders are suspected.

Urine Uric Acid Analysis. A urine uric acid analysis is a 24-hour urine collection to measure the body's production and consequent excretion of uric acid. The test determines the effectiveness of medication or the need for medication changes for patients who repeatedly form uric acid **urolithiasis** (formation of urinary calculi). There are no pretest preparations other than explaining the procedure for a 24-hour urine collection. Although dietary intake is not usually restricted during the test, it may influence the test results. The normal uric acid serum range is 2.0 to 8.5 mg/dl. The normal uric acid urine range is 250 to 750 mg/24 hours. The uric acid level may be altered in the presence of conditions such as multiple myeloma, chronic glomerulonephritis, gout, and polycythemia vera.

Kidney-Ureter-Bladder (KUB) Radiography. A KUB radiograph assesses the general status of the abdomen and evaluates the size, structure, and position of the urinary tract structures. No special preparation is necessary. The nurse should explain that the procedure involves changing position on the x-ray table, which may be uncomfortably firm. Abnormal findings related to the urinary system may indicate tumors, calculi, glomerulonephritis, cysts, and other conditions.

Excretory Urography or Intravenous Urography (IVU). IVU evaluates structures of the urinary tract, filling of the renal pelvis with urine, and transport of urine via the ureters to the bladder. Many institutions use the term *intravenous pyelogram* (IVP) when referring to IVU. It is vital that the nurse determine whether the patient has an allergy to iodine (or iodine-containing foods such as iodized salt, saltwater fish, seaweed products, vegetables grown in iodine-rich soils), since it is the base of the radiopaque dye that will be injected into a vein for this and other radiological examinations. If the patient has previously had an allergic reaction, the physician may order a corticosteroid or an antihistamine to be administered before testing or, as an alternative, may order ultrasonography.

Because kidneys and ureters are positioned in the retroperitoneal space, gas and stool in the intestines interfere with radiographic visualization. Preparation usually includes a light supper, a non-gas-forming laxative, and NPO 8 hours before testing. In planning the testing regimen, the nurse should schedule urography before barium-based studies. When the dye is injected, the patient will experience a warm, flushing sensation and a metallic taste. During the procedure vital signs will be monitored frequently. X-ray films will be taken at various intervals to monitor movement of the dye. Abnormal findings may indicate structural deviations, hydronephrosis, calculi within the urinary tract, polycystic kidney disease, tumors, and other conditions.

Retrograde Pyelography. Retrograde pyelography involves examination of the lower urinary tract with a cystoscope under aseptic conditions. The urologist injects radiopaque dye directly into the ureters to visualize the upper urinary tract. Urine samples can be obtained directly from the renal pelvis. Additional retrograde studies include the following:

- *Retrograde cystography:* Radiopaque dye is injected through an indwelling catheter into the urinary bladder for visualization of the urinary bladder to evaluate its structure or to determine the cause of recurrent infections.
- *Retrograde urethrography:* A catheter is inserted and dye injected as with the cystography to assess the status of the urethral structure.

Voiding Cystourethrography. Voiding cystourethrography is used in conjunction with other diagnostic studies to detect abnormalities of the urinary bladder and urethra. Preparation includes an enema before testing. An indwelling catheter is inserted into the urinary bladder, and dye is injected to outline the lower urinary tract. X-ray films are taken, and the catheter is then removed. The patient will be asked to void while x-ray films are being taken. Some patients may experience embarrassment or anxiety related to the procedure and should be given the opportunity to express their feelings. Structural abnormalities, diverticula, and reflux into the ureter may be detected.

Endoscopic Procedures. Endoscopic procedures are visual examinations of hollow organs using an instrument with a scope and light source. Because of the invasive nature of the procedure, an informed consent is necessary, and because the procedure is most often performed in the surgical suite, preoperative preparation is indicated (see Chapter 22). The urologist performs the procedure.

Cystoscopy is a visual examination to inspect, treat, or diagnose disorders of the urinary bladder and proximal structures. Patient preparation includes a description of the procedure. Usually the procedure is carried out using a local anesthetic after the patient has been sedated. Patient safety is paramount when the patient is sedated.

The patient will be placed in lithotomy position for the procedure, which may produce embarrassment and anxiety. The thought of a scope being passed while the patient is awake may intensify these feelings. The nurse should provide an opportunity for the patient to verbalize feelings.

The scope is passed under aseptic conditions after a local anesthetic, such as procaine, is instilled into the urethra. The patient will experience a feeling of pressure as the scope is passed. Continuous fluid irrigation of the bladder is necessary to facilitate visualization. Care after the procedure includes hydration to dilute the urine. The first voiding after the procedure should be monitored, assessing time, amount, color, and any **dysuria** (painful urination). The nurse can expect the first voiding to occasionally be blood tinged due to the trauma of the procedure.

The urologist can perform a brush biopsy via a ureteral catheter during a cystoscopy. A nylon brush is inserted through the catheter to obtain specimens from the renal pelvis or calyces. Nephroscopy (renal endoscopy) is done using the percutaneous (effected through the skin) route and provides direct visualization of the upper urinary structures. The urologist can obtain biopsy or urine specimens or remove calculi.

Renal Angiography. Renal angiography aids in evaluation of blood supply to the kidneys, evaluates masses, and detects possible complications after kidney transplantation. The patient should have oral intake withheld the night before the procedure. Because the procedure requires the passing of a small radiopaque catheter into an artery, usually the femoral or axillary artery, to provide a port for the injection of radiopaque dye, when the procedure is completed, the patient will need to lie flat in bed for several hours to minimize the risk of bleeding. The puncture site should be assessed for bleeding or hematoma formation, and the pressure dressing at the site should be maintained. Circulatory status of the involved extremity will be assessed every 15 minutes for 1 hour, then every 2 hours for 24 hours.

Renal Venogram. A renal venogram will provide information about the kidney's venous drainage. Access for the radiopaque catheter is the femoral vein. The patient will be monitored afterward for bleeding at the puncture site.

Computed Tomography. Computed tomography (CT scan) differentiates masses of the kidney. Images are obtained by a computer-controlled scanner. A radiopaque dye may be injected to enhance the image. The nurse informs the patient that the table on which she is placed and the machine "taking pictures" will move at intervals and that it is very important to lie still. The CT body-scanning unit will take multiple cross-section pictures at several different sites, creating a three-dimensional "map" of the kidney structure. Visualization of the adrenals, bladder, and prostate may also be done.

Magnetic Resonance Imaging (MRI). MRI uses nuclear magnetic resonance as its source of energy to obtain a visual assessment of body tissues. There is no special preparation of the patient for MRI other than removal of all metal objects that might be attracted by the magnet. Patients with metal prostheses, such as heart valves, orthopedic screws, or cardiac pacemakers, cannot undergo MRI.

It should be emphasized that the examination area will be confining and that a repetitive "pounding" sound will be heard (somewhat like the sound of a muffled jackhammer). MRI can be used for various diagnoses of pathological conditions of the renal system.

Renal Scan. A radionuclide tracer substance that will be taken up by renal tubular cells or excreted by the glomerular filtrate is injected intravenously. A series of computer-generated images will then be made. The scan will provide data related to functional parenchyma (the essential parts of an organ that are concerned with its function). No special preparation is needed. The nurse must check facility policy concerning the disposal of the patient's urine for the first 24 hours. The pregnant nurse should refrain from caring for this patient during this time.

Ultrasonography. Ultrasonography is a diagnostic tool that uses the reflection of sound waves to produce images of deep body structures. The nurse should inform the patient that to carry out the procedure, a conducting jelly will be applied to the skin over the area to be studied to improve the transmission of sound waves. The sound waves are of a very high frequency that is inaudible to the human ear and will be converted into electrical impulses that will be photographed for study.

Ultrasonography of the kidney will visualize size, shape, and position of the kidney and delineate any irregularities in structure. Deviations from normal findings may indicate tumor, congenital anomalies, cysts, or obstructions. No special preparations are necessary.

Renal Biopsy. The kidney can be biopsied by an open procedure similar to other surgical procedures on the kidney or by the less invasive method of needle biopsy, also called a *percutaneous biopsy.* The patient should understand that pain may be experienced during the procedure and that directions, such as holding the breath, must be followed. Bed rest is instituted for 24 hours after the procedure. Mobility is restricted to bathroom privileges for the next 24 hours, and gradual resumption of activities is allowed after 48 to 72 hours.

Urodynamic studies are indicated when neurological disease is or is suspected of being an underlying cause of incontinence. The studies evaluate detrusor reflex. The patient may experience embarrassment and slight discomfort. During cystometrogram a catheter is inserted into the bladder, then connected to a cystometer, which measures bladder capacity and pressure. The patient will be asked about sensations of heat, cold, and urge to void and will be instructed at times to void and change position.

Cholinergic and anticholinergic medications may be administered during urodynamic studies to determine their effects on bladder function. (A cholinergic drug, such as Urecholine, stimulates the atonic bladder; an anticholinergic, such as atropine, brings an overactive bladder to a more normal level or function.)

Associated testing includes rectal electromyography, which involves placement of an electrode and urethral pressure profile, which necessitates the use of a special catheter connected to a transducer to evaluate urethral pressures.

Medication Considerations in Patient Care

The kidneys filter a wide range of water-soluble products from the blood, including medications. The kidney's effectiveness in removing certain medications from the blood may be affected by various conditions, such as renal disease, changes in the pH of urine, and age. Patients with renal disease will be administered reduced doses of medications to minimize further damage or drug toxicity. Alteration in urinary pH affects the absorption rate of certain medications. Older patients may have decreased physiological functioning, diminishing the kidneys' capacity for excretion of drugs. Diminished kidney function interferes with the filtration of water-soluble medications. The medications included in this discussion are not inclusive but are intended to be representative of those medications used in the management of renal and urinary disorders.

Medications That Enhance Urinary Output (Diuretics). Diuretics are administered to enhance urinary output. This action is achieved by increasing the kidney's filtration of sodium, chloride, and water at different sites in the kidney. Diuretics are used in the management of a variety of disorders, such as congestive heart failure and hypertension. Diuretics are classified by chemical form, as well as the site and type of action on the kidney. Box 30-2 lists generic or selected trade name diuretics (also see Table 30-3 on pp. 830-831).

The most widely used diuretics are the thiazide diuretics. Acting on the distal tubule, thiazide diuretics interfere with the reabsorption of chloride, sodium, and

Box 30-2 GENERIC (SELECTED TRADE) NAME DIURETICS

- Loop diuretics
  Furosemide (Lasix), bumetanide (Bumex)
- Osmotic diuretics
  Mannitol (Osmitrol)
- Potassium-sparing diuretics
  Spironolactone (Aldactone)
- Thiazides
  Chlorothiazide (Diuril)
  Hydrochlorprothiazide (HydroDIURIL)
- Thiazide-related products
  Chlorthalidone (Hygroton)

water. Thiazides have a rapid onset and extended action, with few side effects. This group of medications is used primarily to treat hypertension and edema associated with a variety of disorders, including renal problems such as end-stage renal disease. Adverse actions of these medications result largely from the changes in electrolytes that occur with **diuresis** (secretion and passage of large amounts of urine). Care must be taken to compensate for the loss of electrolytes, particularly potassium. Potassium chloride and dietary supplements are frequently prescribed with these medications. Commonly used thiazide diuretics include chlorothiazide (Diuril) and hydrochlorprothiazide (HydroDIURIL).

Carbonic anhydrase inhibitors are weak diuretics and are not widely used. Acetazolamide (Diamox) is the most commonly used of the group. Carbonic anhydrase inhibitors interfere with the bonding of water and carbon dioxide by carbonic anhydrase, an enzyme present in red blood cells.

A third type of diuretic, the loop diuretics, acts by inhibiting the absorption of sodium and chloride in the loop of Henle. This group contains the strongest diuretic agents; they are used in a variety of disorders, including nephrotic syndrome, congestive heart failure, and pulmonary edema. The side effects of loop diuretics are the signs and symptoms associated with rapid fluid loss: vertigo, hypotension, and possible circulatory collapse, as well as decrease in serum potassium (hypokalemia). Frequently prescribed loop diuretics are furosemide (Lasix) and bumetanide (Bumex).

A fourth type of diuretic is the osmotic diuretic. An osmotic diuretic is easily filtered by the kidney but poorly reabsorbed in the renal tubules. As large amounts of filtrates accumulate, the osmotic pressure rises in the tubule; reabsorption of water decreases and urine flow increases with excretion of electrolytes. Mannitol is the most commonly administered medication in this group. Osmotic diuretics are used to manage edema, promote systemic diuresis in cerebral edema, decrease intraocular pressure, and improve renal function in acute renal failure. In acute renal failure osmotics are used to attempt to prevent irreversible failure, but they are contraindicated in advanced stages of renal failure.

Lastly, the potassium sparing diuretics are weak and consequently are used in combination with other diuretics. Although the actions of these medications are varied, they all conserve potassium that is usually lost with sodium in diuresis. Spironolactone (Aldactone) is perhaps the most commonly prescribed of this group.

Patients receiving diuretics often have disease conditions such as congestive heart failure and pulmonary edema. Therefore nursing interventions include monitoring for signs and symptoms of fluid overload: changes in pulse rate, respirations, cardiac sounds, and lung fields. Daily morning weights should be recorded for the patient receiving diuretics. Accurate intake and output (I&O) records should be kept, and blood pressure, pulse, and respirations should be documented 4 times a day until the medication is regulated and the vital signs stabilize. BUN, serum electrolytes, and urine are assessed as ordered. Diet instruction to the patient and family should include a warning to avoid overuse of salt in cooking or as a table additive. A number of salt substitutes are currently on the market; however, the long-term effects of those potassium preparations are not known and could further complicate the renal patient's condition. The use of most diuretics, with the exception of the potassium-sparing diuretics, requires adding daily potassium sources (e.g., baked potatoes, raw bananas, apricots, or navel oranges). In some cases it is necessary for the physician to order potassium supplements to be taken in combination with the diuretic.

Medications That Act on the Bladder. Few medications are used specifically for treatment of conditions of the urinary tract. Oxybutynin chloride (Ditropan), a strong antispasmodic, is used for the treatment of bladder spasms, reducing the frequency of the bladder contractions. It is also used for the patient with a neurogenic bladder to inhibit the sensation to void.

Bethanechol chloride (Urecholine), a parasympathetic nerve stimulant, is used to treat nonobstructive urinary retention by contracting the detrusor muscle of the bladder. Side effects are of parasympathetic nerve stimulation: increased gastric motility with nausea, vomiting, and diarrhea; skin flushing; perspiration; headache; decreased cardiac output; and hypotension.

Phenazopyridine hydrochloride (Pyridium) is a urinary analgesic and a smooth muscle stimulant. It anesthetizes the mucous lining of the ureters and bladder as the medication is excreted from the body. It is used for the relief of discomfort associated with a urinary tract infection, such as burning, frequency, and urgency, or diagnostic procedures or treatments that irritate the urinary mucosa, for example, endoscopy. Use of this medi-

TABLE 30-3 Characteristics of Major Diuretic Classes

Action	Site	Route	Peak	Effect on Electrolytes
Thiazide diuretics				
Impair sodium and chloride reabsorption, leading to excretion of electrolytes and water	Distal convoluted tubule and ascending loop of Henle	Oral (injectable solution not advised except in an emergency)	Oral: onset 1-2 hr, peak 4-6 hr	Hypokalemia (extreme potassium depletion in blood), hyponatremia (decreased sodium concentration in blood), hypercalcemia (excessive amount of calcium in blood)
Loop or high-ceiling diuretics				
Inhibit tubular reabsorption of sodium and chloride	Primarily the ascending loop of Henle and possible sites in proximal and distal tubules	Oral; injectable solution	Oral: onset 30-60 min, peak 1-6 hr Injectable: onset 5-10 min, peak 15-30 min	Hypokalemia, hypochloremia (decrease in chloride in the blood), hyponatremia, hypocalcemia (abnormally low blood calcium), hypomagnesemia (decreased magnesium in the blood)
Potassium-sparing diuretics				
Inhibit sodium reabsorption and potassium secretion	Distal tubule	Oral	Onset 1-4 hr, peak 4-6 hr; maximum diuretic effect 2-3 days and persisting	Hyperkalemia (excessive amount of potassium in the blood)
Osmotic diuretics				
Increase plasma osmotic pressure, causing redistribution of fluid toward the circulatory vessels	Proximal tubule, descending loop of Henle, and collecting tubule	Oral or IV	Onset 30-60 min; diuresis 1-3 hr	Hypernatremia (excess of sodium in the blood)
Carbonic anhydrase inhibitor diuretics				
Interfere with enzyme carbonic anhydrase	Proximal tubule	Oral; injectable	Onset 1-2 hr, peak 2-4 hr, effect sustained 8-12 hr	Hypokalemia, hyponatremia, hyperchloremia

cation is contraindicated after bladder surgery. The patient should be informed that the urine will be reddish-orange. If the scleras of the patient's eyes become yellow, the medication should be discontinued and the physician notified.

Medications That Are Used for Urinary Tract Infections. Certain antimicrobial agents are administered primarily for the treatment of infections within the urinary tract. These agents lower the pH in the urine, creating a poor environment to support growth of bacteria. The appropriate medication is selected according to Gram-stain sensitivity of the organism causing the infection. Cinoxacin (Cinobac) is used for recurrent UTIs caused by *E. coli*, *Proteus mirabilis*, and other gram-negative microbes. Side effects include gastrointestinal (GI) irritation with loss of appetite, nausea, vomiting, abdominal cramping, and diarrhea. Allergic signs and symptoms are skin rash, urticaria, and perineal burning.

Methenamine mandelate (Mandelamine) is nonspecific and suppresses gram-negative and gram-positive organisms in urine of low pH. Methenamine mandelate is used for patients with chronic, recurrent urinary tract infections as a preventive measure after the use of antibiotics that clear the infection. Although side effects are rare, they include nausea, vomiting, skin rash, and urticaria (hives). Nalidixic acid (NegGram) is an antibiotic; its use is contraindicated in renal impairment.

Examples	Effects on Acid-Base Balance	Use	Considerations
Chlorothirazide (Diuril), hydrochlorprothiazide (HydroDIURIL) Thiazide-related: Chlorthalidone (Hygroton)	Hypochloremic (deficiency of the chloride content of the blood) alkalosis	Manage systemic edema, control mild to moderate hypertension	Contraindicated in anuria; may take 1 month to achieve full antihypertensive effect
Furosemide (Lasix), bumetanide (Bumex)	Hypochloremic alkalosis	Severe edema associated with CHF, relief of acute pulmonary edema; effective in patients with impaired renal function	Most potent action of all diuretics, thereby lead to significant electrolyte depletion; effective in patients with impaired renal function.
Spironolactone (Aldactone)	Minimal	Manage systemic edema, control mild to moderate hypertension	Monitor BUN; contraindicated in hyperkalemia, impaired renal function, use with other potassium-sparing medications
Mannitol (Osmitrol)	Minimal	Prevent/treat oliguric phase of acute renal failure	Assess cardiovascular system prior to mannitol administration because of high risk of inducing CHF; avoid extravasation (to escape from a vessel into tissues) which may lead to tissue irritation/necrosis
Acetazolamide (Diamox)	Hyponatremic acidosis; metabolic acidosis possible if given with salicylates	Limited usefulness: treat drug-induced CHF edema	Mild diuretic, also used to lower intraocular pressure

Nalidixic acid is used to treat gram-negative microbes, such as *E. coli* and *P. mirabilis*. The common side effects are drowsiness, vertigo, weakness, nausea, and vomiting. Nitrofurantoin (Furadantin, Macrodantin) is effective against both gram-positive and gram-negative microbes (e.g., *Streptococcus faecalis, E. coli*, and *Proteus*) in the urinary tract only. Common side effects are loss of appetite, nausea, and vomiting. Norfloxacin (Noroxin) is a broad-spectrum antibiotic effective against gram-positive and gram-negative organisms: *E. coli, P. mirabilis, Pseudomonas, Staphylococcus aureus, Staphylococcus epidermidis,* and others. Because of expense, however, its use is typically reserved for the treatment of organisms that are resistant to other agents. The most common side effects are vertigo, headache, and nausea. Patient teaching includes a warning that the urine will turn dark yellow to brown in color.

Nursing Interventions. Precautions should be taken in the nursing interventions of patients receiving antibiotics for UTIs. The nurse should (1) report use of any other medications, since a number of medications are contraindicated because of negative drug interactions; (2) administer medications with food or milk to lessen GI upset; (3) hydrate the patient to produce daily urinary output of 2000 ml, unless contraindicated; (4) instruct the patient to take all the medication, even though the symptoms may subside quickly; (5) soothe skin impairment with cornstarch or a bath of bicarbonate of soda or very diluted vinegar; (6) observe the patient receiving NegGram for visual disturbances and offer appropriate assistance for ambulation or transfer; (7) monitor the patient receiving nitrofurantoin for signs of allergic response (e.g., erythema, chills, fever, and dyspnea)—if these signs or symptoms develop, medication should be discontinued and the physician notified (trial doses of this medication may be used to detect possible allergic reaction before administering full dosage); (8) report continuing signs of infection; (9) maintain acidic pH in urine to enhance medication action; and (10) be aware that use of these medications is contraindicated in patients with impaired renal function.

Nutritional Considerations

The nutritional needs of the patient with a urinary tract disorder vary with each disease process. Unique nutritional problems of the patient with a urinary tract disorder will be discussed with each disorder. The presence of other systemic disease, such as diabetes mellitus, complicates the therapeutic diet of the patient with a urinary tract disorder. Some general guidelines include the following: (1) provide foods from each of the Food Pyramid groups; (2) provide adequate hydration, with modifications according to physician order (unless the patient is on fluid restriction, daily fluid intake is 2000 ml to aid in flushing the urinary tract; some physicians prefer that the fluid be water only); (3) restrict certain foods for patients who are prone to calculi formation; (4) avoid excess sodium intake; and (5) increase calories to maintain weight, if necessary. The patient receiving renal dialysis is on a special diet with many restrictions specific to individual needs (see also Chapters 18 and 19).

Maintaining Adequate Urinary Drainage

Urine clears the body of waste materials and aids in the balance of electrolytes. Conditions that interfere with urinary drainage may therefore create a health crisis. It is important to reestablish urine flow as soon as possible to prevent the buildup of toxins in the bloodstream. Patients at risk for difficulty with urine elimination include patients who have undergone surgical procedures of the bladder, prostate, or vagina; patients with primary urological problems, such as urethral stricture; and those who are critically ill with multisystem problems.

Urinary catheters are used to maintain urine flow, to divert urine flow to facilitate healing postoperatively, to introduce medications by irrigation, and to dilate or prevent narrowing of some portions of the urinary tract. Catheters may be used for intermittent or continuous urinary drainage. Urinary catheters may be introduced into the bladder, ureter, or kidney. The type and size of urinary catheter used are determined by the location and cause of the urinary tract problem. Catheters are measured by the French (F) system. Urethral catheters range in size from 14 to 24 F for adult patients. Ureteral catheters are usually 4 to 6 F. The physician always inserts ureteral catheters. The nurse is usually responsible for the insertion of indwelling urethral catheters.

Types of Catheters. Different types of catheters are used for different purposes. The *coudé catheter* with a tapered tip is selected for ease of insertion when enlargement of the prostate gland is suspected. The curved stylet is used to assist the physician in the insertion of a urethral catheter in a male patient. The *Foley catheter* is designed with a balloon near its tip so the balloon may be inflated after insertion, holding the catheter in the urinary bladder for continuous drainage. *Malecot* and *Pezzer* or *mushroom catheters* are used to drain urine from the renal pelvis of the kidney. The *Robinson catheter* has multiple openings in its tip to facilitate intermittent drainage. *Ureteral catheters* are long and slender to pass into the ureters. The *whistle-tip catheter* has a slanted, larger orifice at its tip to be used if there is blood in the urine. The *cystostomy, vesicostomy,* or *suprapubic catheter* is introduced through the abdominal wall above the symphysis pubis. This catheter is used to divert urine flow from the urethra as needed to treat injury to the bony pelvis, urinary tract, or surrounding organs; strictures; or obstruction. The catheter is inserted via surgical incision or puncture of the abdominal and bladder walls with a trocar cannula. The catheter is connected to a sterile closed drainage system and secured to avoid accidental removal; the wound is covered with a sterile dressing. When the lower urinary tract has healed, the patient's ability to void is tested by clamping the catheter so the patient can try to void naturally. When the measured residual urine is consistently less than 50 ml, the catheter is usually removed and a sterile dressing is placed over the wound.

An *external (Texas* or *condom) catheter* is not a catheter but a drainage system connected to the external male genitalia. This noninvasive appliance is used for the incontinent male to minimize skin irritation from urine. The appliance is removed daily for cleansing and inspection of the skin. Use of the external catheter allows for a more normal life-style for the patient.

Nursing Interventions. Nursing interventions for the patient with a urinary drainage system include employing a number of principles to prevent and detect infection and trauma (Skills 30-1 to 30-4 on pp. 833-839):

1. Follow aseptic technique to avoid introduction of microorganisms from the environment. Never rest the collecting bag on the floor.
2. Record I&O. For precision monitoring, such as hourly urine output, add a urometer to the drainage system. If urine output falls to less than 50 ml per hour, first check the drainage system for proper placement and function.

CATHETERIZATION: MALE OR FEMALE

1. Wash hands.
2. Introduce self.
3. Identify patient by checking identification band.
4. Explain procedure and prepare equipment.
5. Close door and draw curtains to provide privacy.
6. Don nonsterile gloves.
7. Place waterproof absorbent pad under patient's buttocks.
8. Position patient.
   a. Male: supine position with thighs slightly abducted allows relaxation of muscles and easy access to urinary meatus.
   b. Female: dorsal recumbent position with knees flexed and feet about 2 feet apart allows relaxation of muscles and easy access to urinary meatus.
9. Drape patient with bath blanket, covering upper body and shaping over both knees and legs, leaving genital area exposed.
10. Provide good light.
11. Arrange supplies and equipment on bedside table.
12. Wash perineal area with warm soapy water and wash cloth.
13. Rinse and dry area.
14. Remove disposable gloves and place in paper bag.
15. Wash hands.
16. Open packaging using sterile technique.
17. Don sterile gloves.
18. If indwelling catheter is used, test balloon by injecting normal saline or sterile water into balloon lumen until balloon is inflated, then aspirate saline or sterile water.
19. Add antiseptic to cotton balls; open lubricant container. Lubricate catheter about 3.5 to 5 cm (1½ to 2 in) for female; about 15 to 18 cm (6 to 7 in) for male.
20. Nurse wraps edges of sterile towel around gloved hands to protect them from contamination while placing towel under edge of patient's buttocks.
21. Cleanse perineal area using forceps to hold cotton balls soaked in antiseptic solution.
   a. Male (see illustration)
      (1) Grasp penis at shaft below glans with one hand; continue to hold throughout insertion of catheter.
      (2) With other hand, use forceps to hold cotton balls soaked in antiseptic solution.
      (3) Cleanse meatus in circular motion to decrease introduction of organisms into bladder.
      (4) Repeat cleansing two more times using sterile cotton balls each time.
   b. Female (see illustration)
      (1) Spread labia minora with thumb and index finger of nondominant hand to expose meatus; continue to hold throughout insertion of catheter.
      (2) With other hand, use forceps to hold cotton balls soaked in antiseptic solution.
      (3) Cleanse area from clitoris toward anus, using a different sterile cotton ball each time—first to the right of the meatus, then to the left of meatus, then down the center over meatus.
      (4) Contamination occurs when the labia come together. If this should happen, repeat cleansing sequence.
22. Pick up catheter with free sterile-gloved hand, near the tip; hold remaining part of catheter coiled in hand; place distal end in basin.
23. Insert catheter gently, about 15 to 18 cm (6 to 7 in) for male or 3.5 to 5 cm (1½ to 2 in) for female. If inserting an indwelling catheter: when urine flow is established, insert catheter 3.5 cm (1½ inches) further, inflate balloon with 10 ml

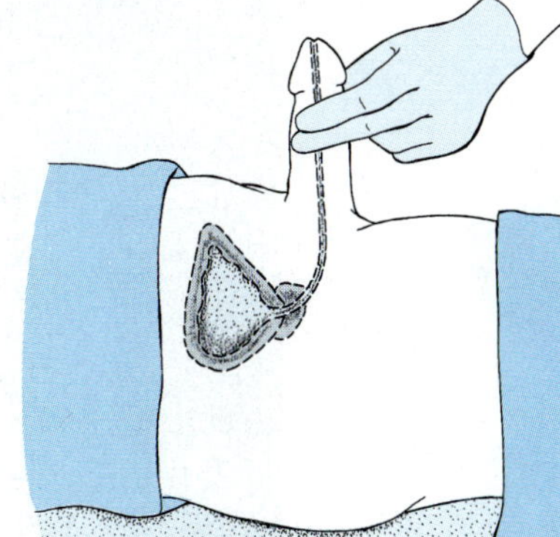
STEP 21a

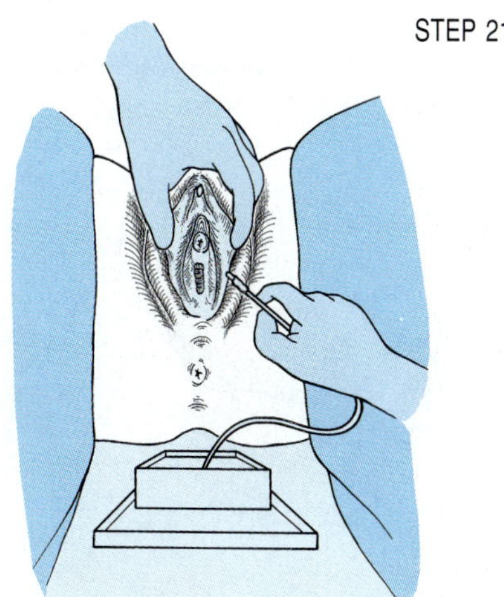
STEP 21b

Continued.

CATHETERIZATION: MALE OR FEMALE—cont'd

sterile water, watch patient's face for grimacing (a sign that balloon is inflating in urethra; if this occurs, deflate balloon and reposition catheter as above), gently pull back on catheter until resistance is felt as balloon rests at orifice of urethra.

24. Collect urine specimen, if needed, by placing open lumen end of catheter into specimen container.

25. Type of catheter
   a. Indwelling catheter
      (1) Inflate balloon with required amount of normal saline or sterile water (see illustration).
      (2) Pull gently to feel resistance.
      (3) Attach end of catheter to collecting tube of drainage system, holding drainage bag below the level of bladder (most catheters are presealed to the collecting tube of the drainage system).
      (4) Attach collection bag to side of bed (see illustration).
      (5) Secure catheter to patient to minimize tension and trauma to urethral opening.
         (a) Male
            Tape catheter to top of thigh or apply leg strap; allow slack for body movement.
         (b) Female
            Tape catheter to inner thigh or apply leg strap; allow slack for body movement.
      (6) Clip drainage tubing to bed linen; allow slack for body movement.
   b. Straight catheter
      (1) Hold coiled catheter in hand with opening over basin.
      (2) Empty bladder (approximately 700 to 1000 ml) unless institution policy differs.
      (3) Withdraw catheter slowly.

26. Dry perineal area.

27. Dispose of equipment and linen according to universal precautions.

28. Remove gloves and wash hands.

29. Reposition patient, remove drape, and cover patient.

30. Label urine specimen with patient's name, date, physician's name, and other pertinent information.

31. Check flow of urine and drainage tubing setup.

32. Open door or drapes.

33. Check patient for comfort level, catheter tubing placement, and whether patient has any questions.

34. Send urine specimen, if obtained, to laboratory.

35. Document procedure.

36. Report any unusual findings immediately.

Sample charting

Date	Time	Notes
11/14/95	8:45	Foley catheter, #16 with 5-cc balloon inserted without resistance; connected to continuous drainage system and secured to bed frame; 300-ml clear, amber urine returned; catheter taped to right thigh. Urine flow continuous. Patient teaching initiated; tolerated procedure well. Urine specimen sent to laboratory. Reported findings to Sammy Hansen, RN, BSN.

____
(nurse's signature)

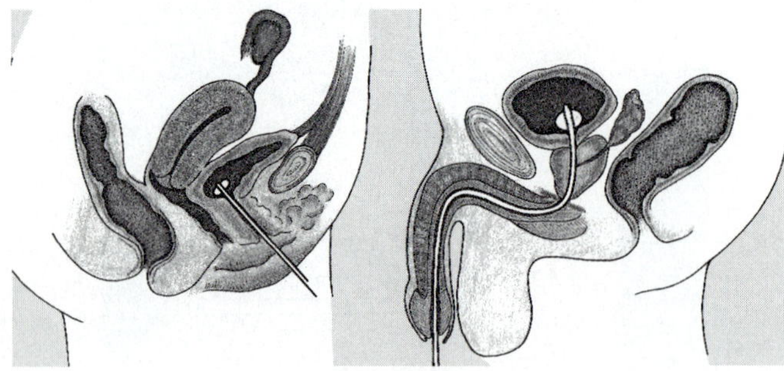

STEP 25a(1)

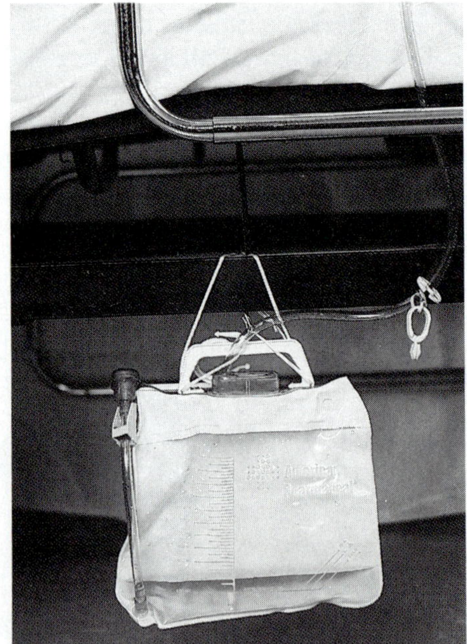

STEP 25a(4)

CATHETERIZATION: MALE OR FEMALE—cont'd

SPECIAL CONCERNS

The following should be considered when caring for a patient with a catheter:

- Maintain universal precautions.
- Position patient for continuing flow of urine.
- Position constant drainage system to ensure flow of urine.
- Monitor color and character of urine.
- Never disconnect the catheter except to irrigate; irrigate only with physician's order.
- Maintain closed drainage system to prevent contamination.
- Never elevate drainage bag above level of the patient's bladder or cavity being drained; teach the patient to carry the drainage bag at arm's length while ambulating.
- Attach drainage bag to bed frame; do not attach to side rails.
- Never allow drainage tubing or bag to touch floor.
- Check tubing for kinks or occlusions.
- Check drainage system for leaks or holes in plastic.
- Empty drainage bag at least q 8 hr.
- Keep accurate record of output.
- Be sensitive to patient's feelings regarding catheter and constant drainage system.
- Determine level of understanding of need for catheter and limitation of movement with catheter.
- Maintain adequate fluid intake, contingent on the patient's overall condition; this is essential to ensure free-flowing urine.
- If patient is uncircumcised male, reposition foreskin over the glans penis to prevent trauma.
- Assess the urine in the drainage tubing, *not* the accumulation in the collecting bag. If the drainage tubing becomes cloudy or stained, change the tubing to aid accurate observation of the urine.
- Note that procedure outlined is for standardized catheters, 16 or 18 F. If a smaller catheter is needed for a pediatric patient or if a larger catheter is necessary for the patient with dilated urinary meatus, consult the hospital procedure manual for modification of techniques. Be particularly careful to adequately lubricate the catheter and to calculate the appropriate depth of insertion.

PATIENT TEACHING

The catheterized patient should be instructed on the following:

- Caution patient not to lie on drainage tubing.
- Explain the side effects of a nonfunctioning catheter.
- Explain the importance of holding the catheter bag at arm's length while ambulating.
- Teach the need to report untoward signs and symptoms, such as a burning sensation, pressure in the bladder, elevated temperature, and chills.
- Answer patient's questions about procedure.

3. Adequately hydrate the patient to flush the urinary tract.
4. Do not open the drainage system after it is in place except to irrigate the catheter, and then only with a specific order from the physician. It is important to maintain a closed system to prevent urinary infections.
5. Perform catheter care twice daily and as needed, using universal precautions. Each institution has a specific protocol for catheter care. Cleanse perineum with mild soap and warm water, rinse well, and pat dry. At times an antiseptic solution or ointment may be ordered to use at the catheter insertion site. Betadine ointment may be the agent of choice to place at the meatus and around the catheter to prevent infection.
6. Check the drainage system daily for leaks.
7. Avoid placement of the urinary drainage bag above the level of the catheter insertion, which would cause urine to reenter the drainage system and contaminate the urinary tract.
8. Prevent tension on the system or backflow of urine while transferring the patient.
9. Ambulate the patient if possible to facilitate urine flow. If the patient's activity must be restricted, turn and reposition every 2 hours.
10. Avoid kinks or compression of the drainage tube that may cause pooling of the urine within the urinary tract. Gently coil excess tubing, secure with a clamp or pin to avoid dislodging the catheter, and release the tubing before transferring or repositioning the patient.

SKILL 30-2

CATHETER CARE

1. Wash hands
2. Introduce self.
3. Identify patient by checking identification band.
4. Explain procedure to the patient and prepare equipment.
5. Close door and draw curtains to provide privacy.
6. Don nonsterile gloves.
7. Place waterproof disposable pad under patient's buttocks and to the side from which catheter care will be given.
8. Position patient.
   a. Male: supine position
   b. Female: dorsal recumbent position
9. Drape patient with bath blanket exposing perineal area. Remove nonsterile gloves.
10. Open sterile supplies, using sterile technique, and arrange on bedside table.
11. Don sterile gloves.
12. Place sterile drape over patient's perineum.
13. Hold cotton balls over container and pour antiseptic solution over them. Place in sterile basin or container.
14. With one hand expose urethral meatus:
    a. Male: retract foreskin, then hold penis erect.
    b. Female: gently retract labia minora away from urinary meatus, and hold in position.
15. Observe meatus, catheter, and surrounding tissue to assess normal or abnormal condition. Determine presence or absence of inflammation, edema, malodorous exudate, color of tissue, burning sensation.
16. Wash the area at the meatus and around catheter with cotton balls:
    a. Male:
       (1) With one cotton ball cleanse around meatus and catheter in a circular motion.
       (2) Repeat two more times, using different cotton balls each time.
    b. Female:
       (1) With one cotton ball swab to one side of labia minora from anterior to posterior of anal area.
       (2) Repeat with second cotton ball on opposite side.
       (3) Repeat with third cotton ball down middle over meatus and around catheter; do not bring cotton ball up once descent has begun.
17. Discard soiled cotton balls in other basin in container.
18. With forceps, pick up cotton ball soaked in antiseptic solution or mild soap and water, cleanse around catheter from urethral opening to approximately 10 cm (4 inches) to clean catheter of exudate.
19. Dispose of equipment and linen, according to universal precautions; remove gloves.
20. Retape or strap catheter to thigh to prevent trauma and pain from tension and pulling.
21. Reposition patient.
22. Check flow of urine through tubing.
23. Wash hands.
24. Document procedure.
25. Report any unusual findings immediately.

Sample charting

Date	Time	Notes
11/4/95	10:00	Catheter care given. Large amount of dried, yellow exudate around catheter at meatus. No erythema or edema noted. Catheter draining clear amber urine. T 99.4 (po), P 88, R 22. Reported findings to D. McClellan, RN.

____
(nurse's signature)

PATIENT TEACHING

The catheterized patient should be instructed on the following:

- Explain the need for the patient to drink fluids.
- Explain the need for meticulous catheter care.
- Answer patient's questions about procedure.

SPECIAL CONCERNS

The following should be considered when caring for the patient with a catheter:

- Maintain universal precautions.
- Provide intake for patient.
- Maintain I&O record.
- Check patient's temperature every 4 hours for 24 hours if odor or exudate is present.
- Adequate fluid intake, dependent on the patient's overall condition, is essential to ensure free-flowing urine.
- If patient is uncircumcised male, reposition foreskin over the glans penis to prevent trauma.
- Assess the urine in the drainage tubing, *not* the accumulation in the collecting bag. If the drainage tubing becomes cloudy or stained, change the tubing to aid accurate observation of the urine.
- See Skill 30-1.

SKILL 30-3

CATHETER IRRIGATION: OPEN, INTERMITTENT, CONTINUOUS

1. Wash hands.
2. Introduce self.
3. Identify patient by checking identification band.
4. Explain procedure to patient and prepare equipment.
5. Close door and draw curtains to provide privacy.
6. Don nonsterile gloves.
7. Place waterproof absorbent pad under patient's buttocks and to the side from which bladder irrigation will be done.
8. Position patient
   a. Male: supine position
   b. Female: dorsal recumbent position
9. Drape patient with bath blanket, exposing perineal area and remove nonsterile gloves.
10. Open method
    a. Pour sterile irrigating solution (sterile normal saline is used as an irrigating solution unless otherwise specified) into sterile graduated container, and recap solution bottle.
    b. Don sterile gloves.
    c. Place sterile basin between patient's legs, close to perineal area.
    d. Disconnect catheter from drainage system, and plug drainage tubing with sterile plug.
    e. Draw 30 ml of sterile solution in syringe.
    f. Cleanse catheter end with antiseptic swab.
    g. Place tip of syringe into end of catheter and gently inject solution.
    h. Withdraw syringe and allow solution to drain into basin by gravity.
    i. If solution does not return, turn patient on side facing nurse to facilitate drainage.
    j. Repeat injection of solution until amount ordered is injected and returned.
    k. Remove plug from drainage tubing, and connect tubing to catheter.
    l. Measure solution to determine amount returned and amount of urine expelled.
11. Intermittent method (repeat steps 1 through 8 as described)
    a. Pour sterile irrigating solution (sterile normal saline is used as in irrigating solution unless otherwise specified) into graduated container.
    b. Draw up sterile solution into syringe.
    c. Clamp catheter below injection port.
    d. Cleanse swab port with antiseptic.
    e. Insert needle of syringe into port.
    f. Inject solution into catheter slowly to avoid bladder spasm and to dislodge clots, sediment, or other material.
    g. Remove syringe and clamp.
12. Continuous method
    a. Set up irrigating solution by attaching tubing to bag.
    b. Clamp off tubing so no solution flows through.
    c. Hang bag on IV pole.
    d. Open clamp, and allow solution to flow through tubing.
    e. Cleanse irrigating lumen on end of triple-lumen catheter.
    f. Connect irrigating solution tubing to catheter lumen.
    g. Restore flow as ordered, calculate drip.
    h. Deduct solution from urine in drainage bag when emptying.
13. Collect soiled material and waterproof absorbent pad; discard into plastic bag.
14. Remove bath blanket; place in laundry hamper.
15. Remove gloves, and discard into plastic bag.
16. Reposition patient.
17. Check flow of urine through drainage tubing.
18. Wash hands.
19. Record urine output on I&O record.
20. Answer patient's questions about procedure.
21. Document procedure.
22. Report any unusual findings immediately.

Sample charting

Date	Time	Notes
11/6/95	8:30	Continuous catheter irrigation maintained with 1000 ml normal saline at 20 gtts per min. Urine return light pink; with several small, dark-red clots. Teaching reinforced with reminder to drink water and keep catheter tubing over leg. Tolerating procedure well. Reported findings to Karen Williams, RN, MA.

____
(nurse's signature)

PATIENT TEACHING

The catheterized patient should be instructed on the following:

- Explain the need for the patient to drink fluids.
- Identify the side effects that may occur, and explain the need to report them immediately.
- Answer patient's questions about procedure.

Continued.

SKILL 30-3

CATHETER IRRIGATION: OPEN, INTERMITTENT, CONTINUOUS—cont'd

SPECIAL CONCERNS

The following should be considered when caring for the patient with a catheter:

- Maintain universal precautions.
- Provide intake for patient.
- Maintain I&O record.
- Inject solution slowly into bladder, and allow to drain by gravity so as not to cause trauma or collapse bladder.
- If catheter will not irrigate with gentle pressure, report to charge nurse.
- Sterile normal saline is used as the irrigating solution unless otherwise specified.
- Assess the urine in the drainage tubing, *not* the accumulation in the collecting bag. If the drainage tubing becomes cloudy or stained, change the tubing to aid accurate observation of the urine.

11. Gently inspect the entry site of the catheter for blood or exudate that may indicate trauma or infection. Observe the color and composition of the urine to note any blood or sediment. During drainage of the collection bag note the presence of malodor.
12. Collect specimens from the catheter by cleansing the drainage port with alcohol, then withdrawing the urine by using a sterile needle and a sterile 10-ml syringe using universal precautions. Send the urine specimen immediately to the laboratory (see Chapter 17).

After the urinary catheter is removed, the patient may experience difficulty voiding until bladder tone and sensation return. If the patient complains of urinary retention, the nurse should institute the following measures:

1. If necessary, urination may be stimulated by running water, placing the patient's hands in water, or pouring water over the perineum. If the last method is attempted, the amount of water used should be subtracted in calculating the correct amount voided.
2. If the patient's condition permits, it is preferable for a female to sit on a bathroom stool or commode, and preferable for a male to stand to void.

The patient may experience some dribbling of urine after voiding as a result of dilation of the sphincter from the catheter. The time, amount, and color of the urine output should be recorded.

Nursing diagnoses and interventions for the patient with a urinary catheter include but are not limited to the following:

NURSING DIAGNOSES	NURSING INTERVENTIONS
Trauma, high risk for, related to insertion and maintenance of the catheter	Lubricate catheter. Secure catheter to leg. Move drainage bag when transferring patient.
Trauma, high risk for, related to insertion and maintenance of the catheter—cont'd	Provide adequate fluids. Administer urinary analgesic as ordered. Allow enough slack in tubing for patient to move about freely while in bed.
Infection, high risk for, related to invasive use of catheter	Use aseptic technique. Complete meticulous catheter care. Keep drainage system closed and patent. Avoid placement of drainage bag above level of catheter insertion (meatus) Avoid reflux of urine. Encourage adequate fluid intake. Administer antimicrobials as ordered.

Patient teaching. The patient should be instructed about proper transfer from bed, chair, or stretcher and taught the principles of catheter care. Fluid intake should be encouraged to flush the urinary system.

Self-Catheterization. Self-catheterization may be the intervention of choice for the patient who experiences spinal cord injury or other neurological disorders that interfere with urinary elimination. Intermittent self-catheterization promotes independent function for the patient. At home there is less risk of cross-contamination than in the hospital, so the catheterization procedure can be safely modified as a clean technique, although the nurse will instruct the patient using strict surgical asepsis in the hospital because of the risk of infection there. The need for the patient to be alert for signs of infection and to have periodic evaluations by the physician should be emphasized. Institutional guidelines for catheter insertion technique should be followed.

Bladder Training. Bladder training involves developing the use of the muscles of the perineum to improve voluntary control over voiding; bladder training may be modified for different problems. In preparation for the removal of a urethral catheter, the physician may order

DISCONTINUING A FOLEY CATHETER

1. Wash hands.
2. Introduce self.
3. Identify patient by checking identification band.
4. Explain the procedure to the patient and prepare equipment.
5. Close door and draw curtains.
6. Place waterproof absorbent pad under patient's buttocks and to the side in which catheter will be removed.
7. Arrange supplies on bedside table.
8. Don sterile gloves.
9. Wash meatus and around catheter with sterile cotton balls soaked in antiseptic solution as per Skill 30-2.
10. Collect urine specimen, if ordered. Clamp off drainage between catheter and drainage tubing for about 15 minutes before collecting specimen. Leave drainage tubing intact and clamp tubing with rubber band. This allows adequate amount of urine (about 5 to 10 ml) for specimen collection. Cleanse port with antiseptic solution. Insert 22-gauge needle attached to 10-ml syringe into port of catheter. Urine will return in syringe when nurse pulls back on plunger. Place urine into correctly labeled sterile specimen container.
11. Untape catheter from patient's thigh.
12. Deflate balloon by:
    a. Cleansing valve outlet with antiseptic solution on a swab.
    b. Inserting the barrel of a syringe into the tube extension used for inflating the catheter.
    c. Aspirating the total amount of fluid used to inflate the balloon.
13. Carefully withdraw catheter out of meatus.
14. Inspect the catheter to be certain it is intact; report promptly to charge nurse if it is not.
15. Observe color of urine and condition of meatus. Check for abnormalities, infection, or other unusual effects.
16. Wash meatus with cotton balls soaked in antiseptic solution.
17. Remove urine from urinary drainage bag, and record amount of urine on intake and output sheet.
18. Dispose of equipment and linens, according to universal precautions.
19. Remove gloves and wash hands.
20. Label urine specimen with patient's name, date, and other pertinent information, and send to the laboratory.
21. Explain to the patient the effects of catheter removal and need to drink fluids. Explain the need for the nurse to measure the voided urine. Check to see if the patient has questions.
22. Document procedure.
23. Report any unusual findings immediately.

Sample charting

Date	Time	Notes
11/26/95	14:30	#16 Foley catheter removed intact after 10 ml of solution aspirated from balloon valve. Patient c/o slight burning sensation. 350-ml clear amber urine in drainage bag. Patient teaching included encouragement for patient to drink fluids and need to measure urine output. Reported findings to Pam Barr, RN, BSN.

____

(nurse's signature)

SPECIAL CONCERNS

The following should be considered when discontinuing the catheter:

- Maintain universal precautions.
- Provide fluid intake for patient.
- Provide easy access to bedpan, urinal, bedside commode, or bathroom with urine collection device.
- Provide nurse call signal within reach.
- Maintain I&O record.
- Check patient's temperature q 4 hr for 24 hours.
- When patient voids, check time, amount, color, and consistency.

PATIENT TEACHING

The patient should be instructed on the following when the Foley catheter has been removed:

- Explain to patient that it will take time for the urinary bladder to reestablish voluntary control of urine.
- Describe how to collect and measure urine output and the need for same.
- Explain the need for the patient to drink fluids.
- Tell the patient that it is common to feel some burning or discomfort in the meatal area when first voiding.
- Identify the side effects that may occur, and explain the need to report them immediately.

a clamp/unclamp routine to improve bladder tone. For the patient with stress incontinence, the muscles of the perineum are exercised to assist in stopping urine flow. The nurse instructs the patient to perform *Kegel* or *pubococcygeal exercises* by tightening the muscles of the perineal floor. The patient can perhaps develop awareness of the appropriate muscle group by trying to stop the flow of urine during voiding. Having identified the correct muscles and the feeling of their contraction, the patient can be directed to tighten the muscles of the perineum, holding that tension for 10 seconds, then relaxing for 10 seconds. The exercises should be done initially in groups of 10, building to groups of 20, four times a day. Because muscle control develops gradually, it may take 4 to 6 weeks to develop control of leakage.

For habit training, a voiding schedule is established. The nurse monitors the patient's voiding for a few days to identify patterns or schedules voiding times to correlate with the patient's activities. Typical voiding times are on arising, before each meal, and at bedtime. The patient is assisted to void as scheduled. After a few days, the scheduled voiding pattern is evaluated by identifying its effectiveness in keeping the patient continent. The schedule is modified until continence is established. Fluid intake and medications may influence voiding patterns (that is, the patient may need to void 30 minutes after the ingestion of coffee or furosemide in response to the diuretic effect). Reduction of fluid intake during the hours preceding bedtime may aid in keeping the patient dry during sleep.

Prognosis. The outcome of patient treatment and nursing care planning/intervention for the patient with urinary disorders is dependent on multiple variables: age, preexisting health conditions, general health status, complications, compliance, and available family and community support.

Alterations in Voiding Patterns

Urinary Retention.

Etiology/pathophysiology. Urinary **retention** is the inability to void even with an urge to void. It may be acute or chronic. With urinary retention the patient may not be able to empty the bladder, creating urinary stasis and increasing the possibility of infection.

Urinary retention may occur from a variety of causes: secondarily in response to stress; interference with the sphincter muscles during surgery to the perineum; occlusion of the urethra by calculi, infection, or tumor; medication side effects; or perineal trauma secondary to vaginal delivery. With chronic urinary retention the bladder capacity may be exceeded and the urine may overflow the bladder, causing incontinence.

Clinical manifestations. The signs and symptoms of urinary retention are sometimes vague and easily overlooked. The bladder becomes increasingly distended and may be palpated above the symphysis pubis. Urinary retention may cause the patient considerable discomfort and anxiety.

Assessment. Collection of *subjective* data includes noting patient complains of frequency with or without symptoms of burning, urgency, and nocturia, and occasionally acute discomfort. Initial symptoms may not seem to be directly associated with urinary retention.

Collection of *objective data* includes assessing urinary bladder distention: palpable ovoid (egg-shaped) bladder, arising suprapubically, voiding frequently, voiding small amounts, and episodes of incontinence. Patients with diminished sensorium, as from spinal cord injury or organic brain disorder, may show signs of restlessness and irritability without direct complaints about difficulty voiding.

Medical management. Mechanical methods, such as the use of urinary catheters or the surgical release of obstructions, may be necessary for the treatment of urinary retention. Urinary analgesics and antispasmodics are administered as prescribed to enhance patient relaxation.

Nursing interventions. The primary goal of nursing intervention is the reinstitution of normal voiding patterns. Regardless of the pathological findings and medical intervention, the nurse can greatly aid in the reinstitution of adequate voiding by supporting the patient's efforts with a private, relaxed environment. Bladder training approaches may assist the patient to empty the bladder. Warm showers or sitz baths may promote relaxation of the abdominal, gluteal, and sphincter muscles. Warm beverages may help the patient relax. If possible, the patient should be permitted whatever position is preferred for voiding: for the female sitting on a commode or bathroom stool is best; for the male standing may be more natural.

When continence is established, the patient may be catheterized intermittently to determine whether the bladder is emptying. The patient should void, and the amount should be measured. Immediately after the voiding the patient should be catheterized and the amount measured. The amount retained in the bladder is **residual urine** and should be less than 50 ml. If the underlying pathological condition remains unchanged, this patient may still be at risk for again developing retention. It is therefore important to teach the patient and/or primary caretaker to be observant for signs and symptoms of urinary retention and to notify the physician immediately if they return.

A nursing diagnosis and interventions for the patient with urinary retention include but are not limited to the following:

NURSING DIAGNOSIS	NURSING INTERVENTIONS
Urinary elimination, altered patterns of, related to sensory/motor impairment, neuromuscular impairment, or mechanical trauma	Establish urinary drainage. Develop voiding schedule. Teach Kegel exercises. Assist with skin care. Suggest use of protective clothing. Engage patient in social activities. Teach importance of adequate fluid intake.

Urinary Incontinence.

Etiology/pathophysiology. Urinary incontinence is the involuntary loss of urine from the bladder. The patient may be totally incontinent, have dribbling, or experience leakage while lifting or sneezing (stress incontinence).

Incontinence may arise as a complication of many disorders, such as infection within the urinary tract, loss of sphincter control, or sudden change in the pressure within the abdomen. Incontinence may be permanent, as with spinal cord trauma, or temporary, as with pregnancy. Women with weakened structures of the pelvic floor are prone to stress incontinence. Although incontinence may occur in patients of any age, loss of control of urination is a particular problem for the older adult.

Clinical manifestations. The cardinal sign of urinary incontinence is the involuntary loss of urine, which may or may not be the primary reason the patient seeks treatment.

Assessment. Collection of subjective data includes seeking information concerning the patient's inability to control the urine. A woman may complain of urine leaking when she coughs, sneezes, or lifts heavy objects.

Collection of objective data includes the nurse being alert for clues that the patient is experiencing difficulty controlling the flow of urine. The assessment guidelines should be followed to clarify the patient's complaints.

Medical management. The management of incontinence depends on the underlying cause. If the problem arises from a disorder within the neck of the bladder, surgical repair may be necessary. The patient may require temporary or permanent urinary diversion or management with an indwelling catheter.

Nursing interventions. Bladder training exercises should be taught to improve the tone of the perineal muscles. Use of protective undergarments may help keep the patient and the patient's clothing dry. For the female patient, Kegel exercises are helpful. Ten repetitions five times a day is helpful. Many patients who are incontinent have low self-esteem. The nurse can be supportive by listening, encouraging the patient to express feelings, and providing kind reassurances. Never scold!

Fluids are an important part of the care plan for any incontinent patient. Without fluids, urine may become more concentrated, irritating the bladder mucosa and increasing the urge to urinate.

Neurogenic Bladder.

Etiology/pathophysiology. Neurogenic bladder means the loss of voluntary voiding control, resulting in urinary retention or incontinence. Neurogenic bladder is caused by a lesion of the nervous system that interferes with normal nerve conduction to the urinary bladder. The lesion may be caused by a congenital anomaly, such as spina bifida, a neurological disease, such as multiple sclerosis, or trauma, as in spinal cord injury. The two types of neurogenic bladder are *spastic* and *flaccid*.

Spastic (reflex or automatic) bladder is caused by a lesion above the voiding reflex arc (upper motor neuron) that results in a loss of sensation to void and a loss of motor control. The bladder wall then atrophies, decreasing bladder capacity. Release of the urine occurs on reflex, with little or no conscious control.

A flaccid (atomic, nonreflex) bladder, caused by a lesion of a lower motor neuron, continues to fill and distend, with pooling of urine and incomplete emptying. Because of the accompanying loss of sensation, the patient may not even experience discomfort that would indicate retention.

Clinical manifestations. Identification of the disease process is the first step in assessing the potential problem of neurogenic bladder. Prevention of complications is a major concern; infection occurs from urinary stasis and repeated catheterization. Retention of urine may lead to backup of urine (reflux) into the upper urinary tract and to the distention of the structures of the urinary tract. Renal failure is the leading cause of death in patients with neurogenic bladder.

Assessment. Collection of *subjective data* includes noting patient complains consistent with the pathophysiology of the neurogenic bladder.

Collection of *objective data* involves investigating the urinary status of the patient at risk for neurogenic bladder; this includes patients with a congenital anomaly, a neurological disease, or a spinal cord injury. The patient with a spastic bladder will experience urinary incontinence, whereas the patient with a flaccid bladder will describe infrequent voiding. Signs of a UTI may not be evident due to the patient's decreased nerve sensation.

Diagnostic tests. Diagnostic testing is completed to assess the type and extent of damage to the urinary tract; chemistry studies monitor change in BUN and creatinine levels. X-ray studies outline structural changes that occur.

Medical management. Patients identified at high risk for neurogenic bladder should be closely monitored.

Assessment of urinary function should be started early in the course of treatment and antibiotics should be given to treat signs of infection. The patient is aided by the use of parasympathomimetic medication [for example, bethanechol chloride (Urecholine)] to increase the contractility of the bladder. It may be necessary for the patient to use intermittent self-catheterization or a urinary collection system if continence is not achieved.

Nursing interventions. The goal for management of the patient with neurogenic bladder is to establish urinary elimination and prevent complications. Because of the disturbance of neurological function, it may not be possible to reinstate normal voiding function. The patient with a spastic bladder may be placed on a bladder training program, with self-stimulation used every 2 hours to empty the bladder: the patient tries to initiate voiding using bladder compressions achieved by applying pressure to the abdomen suprapubically or by digital stimulation of the anal sphincter. Residual urine is then measured by catheterization. As the patient becomes more proficient in emptying the bladder, the times between the catheterizations are increased until voiding is achieved independently.

It is important to educate the patient to be alert for signs of the bladder becoming distended.

Management of the patient with a flaccid bladder is similar. The patient may be placed on a 2-hour voiding schedule for bladder training. Issues of self-esteem are crucial for this patient to remain in social settings. The nurse should provide a supportive, sensitive environment for the patient to discuss ways to adapt to an altered self-image.

Urinary Tract Infections. A UTI is the presence of microorganisms in any urinary system structure. **Bacteriuria** (presence of bacteria in the urine) is the most common of all nosocomial infections; most are associated with the use of urinary catheters. UTIs are common in older patients, related to bladder obstruction, insufficient bladder emptying, decreased bactericidal secretions of the prostate, and increased perineal soiling in females. Immobility and sensory and multiple organ impairment may increase the probability of infection in the older adult. UTIs are common in children, second only to respiratory infections. Females are more susceptible to UTIs than males because the urethra is short and proximal to the vagina and rectum.

Etiology/pathophysiology. UTIs are caused by pathogens that enter the urinary tract, with or without the presence of symptoms. Normally the flushing of the urinary tract with urine is sufficient to keep pathogens washed away. However, some conditions interfere with this process; urinary obstruction, ureterovesical or urethrovesical reflux, sexual intercourse, and catheterization may introduce bacteria into the urinary system. Many chronic health states predispose the patient to a UTI: diabetes mellitus, multiple sclerosis, spinal cord injuries, hypertension, and diseases of the kidney.

Changes in urinary tract homeostasis allow the concentration of bacteria and increase the risk of infection. The patient with a compromised immune system does not seem to be predisposed to UTI infections but once the infection is established will have difficulty recovering. Risk of infection also increases with age, sexual activity, and impaired innervation. Infections of the lower urinary tract increase the risk of infection of the upper urinary tract.

Gram-negative microorganisms, such as *E. coli*, *Klebsiella*, *Proteus*, or *Pseudomonas*, that commonly infect the urinary tract are usually from the gastrointestinal tract and ascend through the urinary meatus. Normally the body's defenses keep infections in check and clear them from the system before signs and symptoms appear. If there is incomplete emptying of the bladder or reflux of urine, the retained urine supports growth of bacteria.

Clinical manifestations. The common signs and symptoms associated with UTI are urgency, frequency, burning on urination, and microscopic to gross (visible without aid of microscope) hematuria. UTIs are identified by the location of the infection: urethritis (urethra), cystitis (urinary bladder), and pyelonephritis (kidney). Infections of the bladder are said to be *lower* UTIs, whereas infections of the kidneys are *upper* UTIs.

Assessment. Collection of *subjective data* includes noting patient complaints of pain or burning on urination, urgency, frequency, and **nocturia** (excessive urination at night). The patient may also have related **asthenia** (a general feeling of tiredness and listlessness). Abdominal discomfort, perineal pain, or back pain may be present, depending on the extent of the disease process and site of infection.

Collection of *objective data* involves palpation of the lower abdomen, which may produce discomfort over the urinary bladder. Urine may be cloudy or blood tinged.

Diagnostic tests. Urine culture and bacteriology tests confirm the diagnosis. For patients with repeated UTIs or systemic disease, more detailed urological studies, such as an IVU and a voiding cystogram, are completed to assess the extent of involvement and damage to the structures of the urinary tract. Microscopic inspection of the urine often reveals bacteria, hematuria (blood in the urine), and **pyuria** (pus in the urine). Prostatitis is confirmed by patient history and culture of prostatic fluid or tissue.

Medical management. The goal of medical management is to eliminate bacteria from the urinary tract, thereby relieving symptoms, preventing damage to renal structures, and preventing spread of infection to other body systems. Antiinfective medications are prescribed in either oral or parenteral single or multiple doses, depending on the severity of the infection, microbial sensitivity, cost, and the medications the patient can tolerate. Urinary antiseptics, such as methenamine mandelate (Deltamine) or methenamine hippurate (Hip-Rex), may be used prophylactically in recurrent infections. Some of these medications are instilled directly into the bladder (Skill 30-5 on p. 844). If the infection is complicated by obstruction, that obstruction should be removed. If the patient experiences neurogenic bladder or other retention, the use of intermittent catheterization permits urinary drainage.

Nursing interventions. Nursing intervention should be supportive, with patient education for adequate hydration and hygiene. Because there is a strong tendency for these infections to recur by either reinfection or persistent infection, patient education must include early detection. Comfort measures include a regimen of antiinfective agents, urinary analgesics, such as phenazopyridine HCl (Pyridium), adequate fluid intake, and perineal care. If treatment is effective, the patient should receive relief quickly. Infection may spread from the urinary system to other parts of the body. *Urosepsis* is septic poisoning due to retention and absorption of urinary products in the tissues.

Urethritis.

Etiology/pathophysiology. Urethritis, inflammation of the urethra, is classified by the presence or absence of gonorrhea. Nongonorrheal urethritis is called *nonspecific urethritis* (NSU). NSU may be caused by monilial or trichomonal infections in women. Bacteria are present normally in the urethra but do not cause problems unless the integrity of the mucous membrane or tissues is interrupted, as when a catheter is in place or trauma has occurred.

Clinical manifestations. The clinical manifestations include inflammation of the urethra with pus formation in the mucus-forming glands within the lining of the urethra. Gonorrheal urethritis is evidenced by acute infection of the mucous membrane of the urethra that causes a purulent exudate from the meatus; the patient feels discomfort and burning on urination.

Assessment. Collection of *subjective data* should be done with an awareness that the patient may be asymptomatic or may complain of dysuria, urethral pruritus, and urethral discharge. Women may complain of vaginal discharge or vulvar irritation.

Collection of *objective data* includes inspecting the urethra for purulent exudate or inflammation.

Diagnostic tests. These are usually limited to a Gram stain of the exudate to identify the pathogen.

Medical management. The first step in medical management is prevention of injury to the urethra during catheterization or sexual intercourse. Comfort measures include a regimen of antibiotics, adequate fluid intake to flush the system, and special care of the perineum using clean technique.

Nursing interventions. These should focus on patient education: avoid sexual activity until the infection clears; take all medications, especially antibiotics, to ensure the infection is resolved; use condoms for some protection from reinfection; and instruct sexual partners to be evaluated for urethritis to prevent continuing infections.

Cystitis.

Etiology/pathophysiology. Cystitis is an inflammation of the wall of the urinary bladder, usually caused by urethrovesical reflux, introduction of a catheter or similar instrument, or perhaps contamination from feces.

Cystitis is most common in women, due to ease of entrance of pathogens through the short urethra, even during voiding.

The most common microorganism causing acute cystitis is *E. coli.* Conflicting data exist about the role of bubble baths, clothing, and hygiene in increasing the risk of cystitis in women. Cystitis in men usually occurs secondary to another infection, such as prostatitis or epididymitis.

Clinical manifestations. The common signs and symptoms associated with cystitis are dysuria, urinary frequency, and pyuria.

Assessment. Collection of *subjective data* includes assessment of the lower abdomen, which may produce discomfort over the urinary bladder. Patient complaints include burning on urination, dysuria (painful or difficult urination), frequency, urgency, and nocturia.

Collection of *objective data* includes a clean-catch or catheterized urinalysis with culture and sensitivity to aid in confirming the diagnosis and in determining the appropriate treatment.

Diagnostic tests. Microscopic inspection of the urine often reveals bacteria, hematuria, and pus. A voiding cystogram may be used to identify reflux of urine into the bladder. Diagnosis is confirmed by a clean-catch, midstream urinalysis that reveals a bacterial count greater than 100,000 organisms/ml. The most commonly found organism is *Staphylococcus* or *Candida*.

Medical management. For cystitis without the complications of obstruction or other underlying pathological conditions, medical management consists of single-dose or short-term therapy with an antiinfective agent (see the section, Medication Considerations in Patient Care). If the treatment is effective, the patient should receive relief quickly. A repeat urinalysis 1 to 3 days after initiation of the medication confirms the effectiveness of the intervention.

Nursing interventions. This should focus on teaching because there is a strong tendency for these infections to recur by either reinfection or persistent infection. The patient should be encouraged to drink 2000 ml of fluid per day. Accurate I&O should be recorded.

SKILL 30-5

BLADDER INSTILLATION

1. Wash hands.
2. Introduce self.
3. Identify patient by checking identification band.
4. Explain procedure to the patient and prepare equipment.
5. Close door and draw curtains to provide privacy.
6. Don nonsterile gloves.
7. Place waterproof absorbent pad under patient's buttocks and to the side from which bladder instillation will be done.
8. Position patient
   a. Male: supine position
   b. Female: dorsal recumbent position
9. Drape patient with bath blanket, exposing perineal area.
10. Remove nonsterile gloves.
11. Open sterile supplies using sterile technique, and arrange on bedside table.
12. Pour sterile prescribed medication or solution into sterile graduated container.
13. Don sterile gloves.
14. Place sterile basin between patient's legs, close to perineal area.
15. Disconnect catheter from drainage system, and plug drainage tubing with sterile plug to prevent infection.
16. Draw up prescribed amount of medication or solution into syringe.
17. Cleanse end of catheter with antiseptic swab.
18. Place tip of syringe into end of catheter, and inject solution slowly.
19. Clamp off end of catheter with sterile plug for period of time ordered to allow medication or solution to be absorbed by bladder.
20. Unclamp end of catheter, and allow remaining medication or solution to drain out by gravity.
21. Remove plug from drainage tubing, and connect tubing to catheter.
22. Reposition patient.
23. Measure solution to determine amount returned and amount of urine expelled.
24. Dispose of equipment and linen according to universal precautions; remove gloves.
25. Check flow of urine through drainage tubing.
26. Record urine output on intake and output record.
27. Answer patient's questions about procedure.
28. Wash hands.
29. Document procedure.
30. Report any unusual findings immediately.

Sample charting

Date	Time	Notes
12/14/94	6:30	Penicillin 500 mg in 25 ml sterile water at room temperature instilled into urinary bladder via Foley catheter for 10 minutes. 20 ml returned. Solution returned clear. Tolerated procedure well. Encouraged fluids. Performed by P. Johnson, LPN.

____
(nurse's signature)

SPECIAL CONCERNS

The following should be considered when preparing to perform a bladder instillation:

- Provide intake for patient.
- Maintain careful I&O record.
- Triple-lumen catheter does not require disconnecting catheter from drainage tubing.
- Inject solution slowly into bladder, and allow to drain by gravity so as not to cause trauma or collapse bladder.

PATIENT TEACHING

The patient receiving a bladder instillation should be instructed on the following:

- Explain the need for the patient to drink fluids.
- Identify the side effects that may occur, and explain the need to report them immediately.

Patient teaching. Teaching must include early detection. Long-term prophylaxis with low doses of medication may be necessary. Currently available is a simple urine test, Chem Strip LN, which allows the patient to test the urine at the first sign of infection and to call the physician for a prescription.

Prognosis. Successful treatment is contingent upon the patient's ability to maintain adequate flushing of the urinary tract and completion of the antiinfective cycle.

Prostatitis.

Etiology/pathophysiology. Prostatitis, defined as inflammation and/or infection of the prostate gland, is actually a group of diseases. Bacterial prostatitis is caused by infectious organisms such as *Pseudomonas* and *Streptococcus faecalis* traveling up the urethra. Nonbacterial prostatitis may result from a variety of reasons related to occlusion of the urethra (e.g., enlargement of the prostate gland).

Prostatodynia (pain in the prostate gland) presents with neither inflammation nor infection but demonstrates the other symptoms typical of prostatitis.

Clinical manifestations. The patient experiences a burning sensation, discomfort in the perineum, dysuria, frequency, and urgency. Edema of the prostate gland may serve as an obstruction, causing urinary retention as a complication to the prostatitis. Pooling of urine may also foster stone formation. Other complications are epididymitis, pyelonephritis, and bacteremia. Although the patient may be asymptomatic, the symptoms of acute bacterial prostatitis are often the same as a UTI with pain in the low back, perineum, or rectum. Because of a potential for relapse, the condition may become chronic.

Diagnostic tests. Diagnosis is confirmed by patient history and culture of prostatic fluid or tissue.

Assessment. Collection of *subjective data* includes noting complaints of chills and low back and perineal pain. Chronic bacterial prostatitis causes dysuria, urgency, frequency, nocturia, and pain in the lower abdomen or back, perineum, or genitalia.

Collection of *objective data* involves assessing for elevated temperature and palpation of the prostate gland by the physician by rectal examination, which may reveal the prostate to be firm, edematous, and tender.

Medical management. If the condition is infectious, management focuses on control of the infection and prevention of the complications of abscess formation or bacteremia. Broad-spectrum antiinfective therapy is administered for 4 to 12 weeks, because prostatitis is often difficult to cure. Intravenous antibiotic administration may be necessary to achieve sufficiently high medication levels in the blood and tissues.

Nursing interventions. Regardless of the pathological basis, comfort measures used are analgesics, sitz baths, and stool softeners to reduce pain, edema, spasm, and straining pressure in the pelvis.

Patient teaching. Teaching includes the medication regimen and avoiding alcohol, caffeine, and spicy foods. Sexual arousal and intercourse should be avoided in acute prostatitis; however, intercourse may be beneficial in the treatment of chronic prostatitis. Follow-up with the physician is crucial because of the likelihood that the disorder will become chronic.

Prognosis. Prostatitis is difficult to cure and requires long periods of antibiotic treatment. The patient may not see the need of continuing antibiotic therapy after the initial symptoms have subsided. It is imperative that he understand the importance of taking all the antibiotic prescribed.

Pyelonephritis.

Etiology/pathophysiology. Pyelonephritis is an inflammation of the structures of the kidney—the renal pelvis, renal tubules, and interstitial tissue. Pyelonephritis is almost always caused by *E. coli*.

Pyelonephritis is usually seen in association with pregnancy; chronic health problems, such as diabetes mellitus or polycystic or hypertensive kidney disease; insult to the urinary tract from catheterization; or infection, obstruction, or trauma. Careful management of these disorders is important to prevent pyelonephritis.

The kidney becomes edematous and inflamed, and the blood vessels are congested. The urine may be cloudy and contain pus (pyuria), mucus, and blood. Small abscesses may form in the kidney.

Clinical manifestations. Acute pyelonephritis may be unilateral or bilateral, causing chills, fever, prostration, and flank pain. Repeated episodes of pyelonephritis lead to a chronic disease pattern with atrophy of the kidney as the nephrons are destroyed. Studies have also shown that chronic pyelonephritis may develop in association with other renal diseases unrelated to infection processes. **Azotemia** (the retention in the blood of excessive amounts of nitrogenous compounds) develops if enough nephrons are nonfunctional.

Assessment. Collection of *subjective data* includes noting that in acute pyelonephritis the patient will become acutely ill, with malaise and pain in the **costovertebral angle** (CVA) [one of two angles that outline a space over the kidneys]). CVA tenderness to percussion is a common finding in pyelonephritis. In the chronic phase, the patient may show unremarkable symptoms, such as nausea and general malaise.

Collection of *objective data* includes assessing the patient for signs of infection: elevated temperature, chills, and pus in the urine. Systemic signs occur as a result of the chronic disease: elevated blood pressure and gastrointestinal irritation such as vomiting and diarrhea.

Diagnostic tests. Diagnosis is confirmed by bacteria and pus in the urine and leukocytosis. A clean-catch or catheterized urinalysis with culture and sensitivity identifies the pathogen and determines appropriate antimicrobial therapy. An IVU will identify the presence of obstruction or degenerative changes caused by the infectious process. Assessment of BUN and creatinine levels of the blood and urine may be used to monitor kidney function.

Nursing interventions. A nursing diagnosis and interventions for the patient with pyelonephritis include but are not limited to the following:

NURSING DIAGNOSIS	NURSING INTERVENTIONS
Urinary elimination, altered patterns of, related to infection, and fluid volume excess, secondary to (2°) fluid retention and electrolyte imbalance	Monitor body temperature. Observe urine for cloudy appearance, high specific gravity, and hematuria. Assess flank pain and tenderness over affected kidney. Weigh daily. Institute strict I&O monitoring. Observe for changes in fluid and electrolytes as evidenced by alteration in mental status, cardiac dysrhythmias, increase in blood pressure, thirst, and fluid retention. Enhance patient comfort with a warm shower, back rubs, and a warm, soothing environment. Use antimicrobial agents singly or in combination to control bacterial growth, as prescribed. Administer urinary analgesics as ordered.

Patient teaching. The patient should be taught to identify the signs and symptoms of infection—elevated temperature, flank pain, chills, fever, nausea and vomiting, urgency, fatigue, and general malaise. The patient should also be taught indications, dose, length of course, and side effects of the medications. The nurse should emphasize the importance of follow-up care with the physician on a routine basis and when signs of infection arise.

Prognosis. Prognosis is dependent upon early detection and successful treatment. Baseline assessment for every patient must include urinary assessment because pyelonephritis may occur as a primary or secondary disorder.

Obstructive Disorders of the Urinary Tract

Urinary Obstruction.

Etiology/pathophysiology. Obstruction at any point within the urinary tract can adversely affect function and alter structure. Causes of obstruction include strictures, kinks, cysts, tumors, calculi, and prostatic hypertrophy. Obstruction may lead to: alterations in blood chemistry; infection that thrives as a result of urine stasis; ischemia due to compression; or atrophy of renal tissue.

Clinical manifestations. The patient may be unaware of any problems initially if the obstruction is partial, allowing urine to drain and kidney function to remain within normal limits. With prostatic hypertrophy the obstructive process may be so gradual that the patient ignores the vague symptom of dull flank pain and seeks medical attention only when urination becomes acutely difficult. Acute pain occurs as the musculature is stretched by increasing pressure from urine accumulation and as muscular contractions increase in an attempt to move urine past the obstruction. This classic symptom is found with renal calculi and is renal colic.

Assessment. Collection of *subjective data* includes noting the initial complaint of the continued need to void, although the patient may be able to void small amounts. Pain may range from dull flank pain to acute, incapacitating pain. Nausea often accompanies acute pain.

Collection of *objective data* includes noting on physical assessment if the bladder is palpable suprapubicly because of urine retention. The affected kidney may also be palpable. Retention with overflow occurs when the patient is unable to completely empty the urinary bladder and it quickly refills, causing the urge to void again. The nurse should assess time and amount of voidings.

Diagnostic tests. As a quick evaluation the physician may order a KUB radiograph. Renal ultrasonography or IVU will provide definitive information about structural changes. Other diagnostic tests may include visual examinations with the aid of endoscopy, and blood chemistry profile.

Medical management. Initial intervention will be to establish urine drainage and relieve discomfort. Conservative measures include insertion of an indwelling catheter, pain medication (usually narcotic), and an anticholinergic agent to decrease smooth muscle motility. It may be necessary to establish urine drainage surgically by inserting a catheter directly into the bladder through the abdominal wall (suprapubic cystostomy), into a ureter (ureterostomy), or into the kidney (nephrostomy).

Nursing interventions. These procedures require observation for hemorrhage, maintaining aseptic care of the surgical site, and providing a safe environment to prevent injury and infection.

Prognosis. The prognosis is variable, depending on the cause of the obstruction. If surgical correction is successful, the prognosis is excellent.

Hydronephrosis.

Etiology/pathophysiology. **Hydronephrosis** (the dilation of the renal pelvis and calyces) may occur either unilaterally or bilaterally. Hydronephrosis is caused by obstructions in the urinary tract. An obstruction may be located in the lower urinary tract, in the ureters, or in the kidneys. The location of the obstruction will determine whether one or both kidneys are affected.

An obstruction generates pressure from accumulated urine that cannot flow past the obstruction. This pressure may cause functional and anatomical damage to the renal system. The renal pelvis and ureters dilate and hypertrophy. This pressure, if prolonged, causes fibrosis and loss of function in affected nephrons. If the condition is left untreated, the kidney may be destroyed.

Clinical manifestations. Hydronephrosis can occur without any symptoms as long as kidney function is adequate and urine can drain. The amount of pain is proportional to the rate of stretching. Slowly developing hydronephrosis may cause only a dull flank pain, whereas a sudden occlusion of the ureter, such as may occur from a calculus, causes a severe stabbing (colicky) pain in the flank of the abdomen. Nausea and vomiting, which often accompany hydronephrosis, are caused by a reflex reaction to the pain and will usually subside when the pain is controlled.

Assessment. Collection of *subjective data* involves questioning the patient about the presence of pain, including location, intensity, and character, and about the presence of nausea. The patient's voiding pattern should be discussed: frequency, difficulty starting a stream of urine, dribbling at the end of **micturition** (voiding), nocturia, and burning on urination. Any history of obstructive disorders should be noted.

Collection of *objective data* includes assessing patients suspected of having hydronephrosis for vomiting, hematuria, urinary output, dyspnea, edema, a palpable mass in the abdomen, bladder distention on palpation, and tenderness over the kidneys or bladder.

Diagnostic tests. A urinalysis and serum renal function studies are obtained. X-ray examinations may include cystoscopy, retrograde pyelogram, IVU, KUB radiograph, CT scan, and/or ultrasound evaluation. Sometimes a renal biopsy is performed.

Medical management. Management is usually conservative if the condition is not severe. Surgical intervention is used to relieve the obstruction and preserve renal function. If the kidney is severely damaged, a nephrectomy may be necessary. If infection is present, antiinfective medications are administered: penicillin in combination with a sulfonamide (Gantrisin) or a sulfamethoxazole (Septra, Bactrim). Narcotics, such as morphine and meperidine, in combination with antispasmodic drugs, such as propantheline (Pro-Banthine) and belladonna preparations, are usually necessary to relieve severe, colicky pain.

Nursing interventions. Nursing interventions for the patient with hydronephrosis will include administering medications as ordered, monitoring intake (intravenous and oral) and output, observing for signs and symptoms of infection, and monitoring vital signs. The nurse will need to encourage the patient to take fluids and will also assess the patient for pain. Any drainage tubes will need to be kept open and anchored to avoid inadvertent displacement. If a catheter is present, regular catheter care will be necessary. If surgery has been performed, the dressing must be observed, because drainage of urine may continue for some time. The area should be kept clean and dry to avoid excoriation of the skin. All procedures should be explained to the patient and family.

Patient teaching. Patient teaching should include an explanation of the abnormality, along with the signs and symptoms of infection or obstruction. Measures to prevent infection should be explained, such as adequate fluid intake, perineal hygiene daily with mild soap and water (drying thoroughly), and regular emptying of the bladder.

Prognosis. Prognosis is directly proportional to the degree of urinary system destruction and the need for surgical intervention.

Urolithiasis. Urolithiasis (urinary stones) can form in any area of the urinary tract. Urolithiasis is a general term that encompasses all urinary calculi, but they are also named specifically to indicate where they are located or formed: nephrolithiasis (stones in the kidney), ureterolithiasis (stones in the ureter), and cystolithiasis (stones in the bladder). Other descriptive terms are *calculi* (stones) and *lithiasis*, which means the formation of stones.

Etiology/pathophysiology. Urolithiasis develops from minerals that have precipitated out of solution and adhere, forming stones that vary in size and shape. The event that initiates stone formation remains elusive, but some individuals are known to be predisposed: persons who are immobile, hyperparathyroid, or have recurrent UTIs.

Clinical manifestations. Size and degree of mobility of the stone influence symptomatology. The patient with renal colic will seek care immediately, whereas a person with a less mobile stone may not seek assistance until signs of infection or hydronephrosis occur.

Assessment. Collection of *subjective data* may include the patient with mobile calculi complaining of intractable pain (pain that is unrelieved by ordinary medical and surgical measures and is usually accompanied by nausea and vomiting). The patient describes the pain as starting in the flank and radiating into the groin, the genitalia, and the inner thigh. The patient with a less mobile stone will have signs and symptoms associated with urinary infection or hydronephrosis.

Collection of *objective data* includes the nurse assessing for the presence of hematuria (gross or microscopic on urinalysis), and vomiting.

Diagnostic tests. Diagnostic tests include KUB, IVU, ultrasound, cystoscopy, and urinalysis. Other tests may be ordered to determine stone content, presence of infection, and alterations in blood chemistry that may influence stone formation. Twenty-four-hour urine examination may be done to detect abnormal excretion of calcium oxalate, phosphorus, and uric acid.

Medical management. Antiinfective agents may be administered in the presence of infection or prophylactically. If stones are not passed, invasive techniques may be indicated. Stones in the lower tract can be removed by cystoscopy with stone manipulation or by surgical incision (Fig. 30-6). Terminology describes the location: ureterolithotomy, pyelolithotomy, and nephrolithotomy. Chemolytic agents, either alkylating or acidifying agents, may be instilled to dissolve stones. Extracorporeal shockwave lithotripsy is an alternative to surgery. The patient is submerged in a special tank of water and ultrasonic shock waves are used to pulverize the stone. Urine must still be strained, even if a catheter is in place. Renal colic may still occur as the patient passes the stone fragments. Long-term management may include dietary adjustments to influence the urine pH or to decrease availability of certain substances to discourage stone formation. Moderate reduction of calcium phosphorus and purine containing foods may be beneficial when stones are caused by metabolic abnormalities. Some foods to be avoided include cheese, greens, whole grains, carbonated beverages, nuts, chocolate, shellfish, and organ meat (see also Chapters 18 and 19). Adequate daily fluid intake of 2000 ml will help cleanse the urinary tract (unless clinically contraindicated). Some physicians encourage diets that alter the urine pH, to produce a less favorable environment for stone formation. Drug therapy will be specific to stone composition: in calcium stone formation, sodium cellulose phosphate binds with ingested calcium and prevents its absorption; aluminum hydroxide gel will bind with excess phosphorus, allowing intestinal excretion rather than urinary excretion; allopurinol (Zyloprim) reduces serum urate levels, thereby facilitating reabsorption of urate crystals.

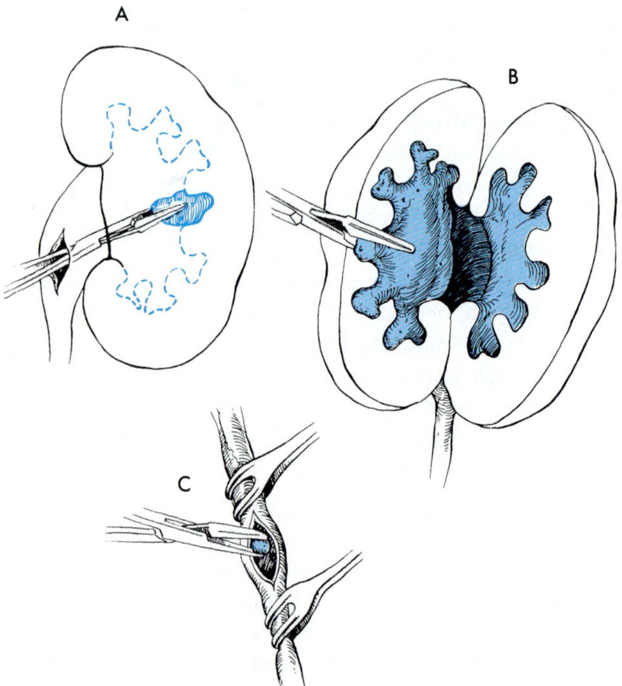

FIG. 30-6 Location and methods of removing renal calculi from upper urinary tract. **A,** Pyelolithotomy, removal of stone through renal pelvis. **B,** Nephrolithotomy, removal of staghorn calculus from renal parenchyma (kidney split). **C,** Ureterolithotomy, removal of stone from ureter.

Nursing interventions. Stones are more likely to be passed if the patient remains active and increases fluid intake. If pain is so severe as to require narcotic medication, the nurse must exercise discretion in allowing the patient out of bed. If nausea inhibits oral intake, the physician may order supplemental intravenous fluids. All urine will be strained. Because stones may be any size, even the smallest "speck" must be saved for assessment. The nurse should encourage fluids and administer analgesics as ordered. Pain should be monitored for passage of stone. Urine should be assessed for possible hematuria. BUN and creatinine should be monitored for indication of continuing urinary obstruction.

Nursing diagnoses and interventions for the patient with urolithiasis include but are not limited to the following:

NURSING DIAGNOSES	NURSING INTERVENTIONS
Pain, acute, related to mobility of calculi	Develop pain management plan. Provide comfort measures. Provide diversional activities. Determine nature, intensity, location, duration, and alleviating factors of pain. Note for nonverbal signs of pain (restlessness, wrinkled brow, clenched fists, elevated BP, and tachycardia). Monitor urine for flow, color, and amount. Provide nonpharmacological comfort measures: ■ Assist patient with assuming a comfortable position. ■ Teach relaxation techniques. ■ Provide diversional activity. ■ Provide a restful environment. ■ Encourage fluids to dilute urine and flush stones. ■ Assist patient with ambulation, if tolerated, to promote movement of stones. Administer antispasmodics and analgesics as ordered. Monitor and document pain relief and side effects of medications.
Infection, high risk for, related to obstruction	Monitor and report signs and symptoms of infection (elevated temperature, chills, flushed). Provide nutrition/fluids. Discuss life-style factors that predispose to infection. Check temperature q 4 hr and report if above 101° F (38.5° C). Note character of urine: report if cloudy and malodorous. Use handwashing technique: teach and encourage patient to do the same. Instruct patient to avoid persons with infections.

Patient teaching. The nurse should instruct the patient about measures to prevent stone formation, obstruction, and infection. Prescribed diet, including fluid intake, should be discussed, as well as home medications (their purpose, dose, refills, and side effects). The patient should avoid inactivity by walking frequently. The need for follow-up with the physician should be emphasized, including keeping scheduled appointments and reporting difficulty of urination.

Although opinions vary greatly as to benefits of dietary restrictions, the nurse may be responsible for clarifying diet instructions. Fluid intake should be encouraged to at least 3000 ml of fluid in 24 hours unless contraindicated. Persons who are calcium stone formers may need to curtail their intake of dietary calcium (dairy products, antacids, and so on) to within minimum RDA guidelines. Persons who form oxalate stones should limit oxalate-containing foods (beans, deep-green leafy vegetables, cocoa, and so on).

Prognosis. Prognosis is related to the location of the stone and the extent of invasive procedures necessary to remove the stone. A certain population is categorized as "stone formers" and consequently are at high risk for recurrence.

Renal Tumors.

Etiology/pathophysiology. More common in men than in women, renal tumors are primarily adenocarcinomas that develop unilaterally and are often quite large when first detected. Renal cell carcinoma as a primary malignant tumor appears to arise from cells of the proximal convoluted tubules. Risk factors include smoking, familial incidence, and preexisting renal disorders, such as adult polycystic kidney disease and renal cystic disease secondary to renal failure. Transitional cell tumors of the renal pelvis cause hematuria and can be confirmed by cytological study.

Clinical manifestations. The most common signs and symptoms are intermittent, painless hematuria, misleading the patient to defer seeking medical attention. Other signs and symptoms appear after the malignant process has advanced: weight loss, dull flank pain, a palpable mass in the flank area, and gross hematuria. Metastatic-related signs and symptoms include respiratory distress and bone pain.

Assessment. Collection of *subjective data* includes a patient history of blood in the urine, which "comes and goes." When the bleeding occurs, there is usually no associated pain. In advanced stages of the illness, the patient will experience weight loss, fatigue, and dull flank pain.

Collection of *objective data* involves a physical assessment that reveals a mass in the patient's flank area in the advanced stages of the illness. Hematuria may be obvious, as well as signs related to the systemic metastasis.

Diagnostic tests. Urinalysis will reveal hematuria in most patients. IVU will detect a renal mass, and ultrasonography will define composition of the mass in most instances. If indicated, other tests will be used to evaluate the status of other body systems; these include scans, MRI, and renal arteriography.

Medical management. Patients with localized disease usually respond well to radical nephrectomy. Radiation therapy and chemotherapy have proved to be of only minimal benefit.

Nursing interventions. Care of the patient with surgery of the urinary tract will be addressed on pp. 864-868.

Nursing diagnoses and interventions for the patient with renal tumors include but are not limited to, the following:

NURSING DIAGNOSES	NURSING INTERVENTIONS
Coping, ineffective individual, related to powerlessness	Encourage patients to express feelings of frustration, anger, fear, and uncertainty. Actively listen. Observe for behavioral and emotional signs of grieving (denial, anger, crying, withdrawal, dependency). Support realistic hope: answer questions honestly. Provide assistance from other professionals to help patient with emotional changes (social worker, clergy, psychologist, psychiatrist). Assist patient with identifying strengths and coping skills. Inquire as to how patient usually decreases tension and anxiety.
Knowledge deficit, related to limited information	Adapt teaching to patient's level of knowledge. Involve significant others in teaching process. Instruct patient on name of medications, dosage, schedule, purpose, and side effects. Teach patient to drink fluids generously unless contraindicated. Instruct patient to maintain mobility as tolerated. Instruct patients to avoid persons with infections.

Patient teaching. The patient should be instructed about community resources, support groups, and home health care. The nurse should emphasize the importance of follow-up care, including following discharge instructions and keeping return appointment.

Prognosis. A positive prognosis would rely on early detection.

Renal Cysts.

Etiology/pathophysiology. A single renal cyst may occur without clinical significance, but multiple cysts interfere with kidney function. The most clinically significant problems arise with *polycystic kidney disease*, which may be acquired or inherited. A patient with long-standing renal insufficiency or a dialysis patient may develop polycystic disease. Kidney function is compromised by the pressure of the cysts on kidney structures, secondary infections, and tissue scarring caused by rupturing of the cysts. The patient may progress to end-stage renal disease (ESRD).

Clinical manifestations. Symptoms are influenced by the degree of kidney structure involvement. The most common site is the collecting ducts, which fill with urine and/or blood. As the disease progresses, fewer nephrons are available to maintain normal kidney function.

Assessment. Collection of *subjective data* includes noting the most common symptoms of abdominal and flank pain, followed by headache, gastrointestinal complaints, voiding disturbances, and a history of recurrent UTIs.

Collection of *objective data* involves an initial assessment that includes observation for systemic changes. The nurse should closely monitor blood pressure, which is usually elevated, and hematuria. Document the degree of patient complaints and response to intervention.

Diagnostic tests. Diagnosis is established by family history, physical examination, excretory urography, and imaging of cysts on x-ray examination or sonography. Blood chemistry results, such as urea and creatinine levels, are used to monitor the level of kidney function.

Medical management. There is no specific treatment for polycystic kidney disease. Medical treatment is aimed at relief of pain and symptoms of the disease. Heat and analgesics may relieve some of the discomfort caused by the enlarging kidneys. If the patient bleeds, heat should be discontinued and the patient should be placed on bed rest. Hypertension is treated vigorously with antihypertensive agents, diuretics, and fluid and dietary modifications. Because infections are common, antibiotics are often prescribed. As the disease progresses, dialysis or renal transplantation may be required.

Nursing interventions. Individual complaints and the severity of the disease process will influence nursing interventions. Patients and family members need to be given information about the availability of genetic counseling. The nurse should emphasize the need to report any changes in health status to the physician.

Prognosis. Prognosis with a single cyst is favorable but guarded with polycystic disease because of the chronic nature of the disease.

Tumors of the Urinary Bladder.

Etiology/pathophysiology. Tumors of the urinary bladder range from benign papillomas to invasive carcinomas. The bladder is the most common site of cancer in the urinary tract, occurring more often in men than in women. Papillomas have the potential to become cancerous and are removed when detected.

Clinical manifestations. The patient may delay seeking medical attention, because the primary sign of bladder cancer is painless, intermittent hematuria.

Assessment. Collection of *subjective data* may include symptoms such as changes in voiding patterns, signs of urine obstruction, or renal failure, depending on the extent of the disease process.

Collection of *objective data* includes assessing the patient's understanding of current health status, which will aid the nurse in planning teaching interventions. Accurate documentation of the time and amount of voiding, including the urine character, is indicated.

Diagnostic tests. Diagnostic tests include cystoscopy to obtain tissue samples for **cytological evaluation** (study of cells). Kidney function tests will assist in evaluation of overall renal status.

Medical management. The patient with local disease may be treated by removing the tissue by burning with an electric spark (fulguration), laser, instillation of chemotherapy agents, or radiation therapy. These individuals need to be closely monitored with cytology studies and cystoscopy, since recurrence is as high as 60%. A partial or total cystectomy may be performed to remove invasive lesions. With complete removal of the urinary bladder, urinary diversion is necessary. (See pp. 864-868 for a discussion of ileal conduit or sigmoid conduit.)

Nursing interventions. The importance of follow-up care for the patient with papilloma must be emphasized. Care of the patient with bladder cancer will be influenced by the extent of the disease process, medical treatment, coincidental illness, and the patient's response to treatment. Observation of voiding patterns and urine character are necessary to monitor response to these therapies.

Patient teaching. Patient teaching is indicated so that the patient can return to optimum performance of activities of daily living. Suggested interventions are addressed under surgical interventions, pp. 866 and 868.

Prognosis. There is a direct relationship between the prognosis and the extent of the disease process when diagnosed. The other most important aspect in recovery is the patient's adaptability to any changes in urinary elimination as a result of treatment.

Conditions Affecting the Prostate Gland

Benign Prostatic Hypertrophy.

Etiology/pathophysiology. The prostate gland encircles the male urethra at the base of the urinary bladder (see Fig. 30-5). Its function is secretion of an alkaline fluid that helps neutralize seminal fluid and increases sperm motility. Benign prostatic hypertrophy (BPH), enlargement of the prostate gland, is common in men older than 50 years. The cause is unclear but may be influenced by hormonal changes. The prostate enlarges, exerting pressure in the urethra and vesical neck of the urinary bladder, which prevents complete emptying.

Clinical manifestations. The patient will have symptoms associated with urinary obstruction, inward pressure on the urethra by the enlargement of the prostate. Other clinical manifestations include complications of urinary obstruction, such as urinary tract infection, hematuria, oliguria, and signs of renal insufficiency.

Assessment. Collection of *subjective data* includes the patient describing the urine stream as difficult to start, slow, and painful, with complaints of frequency and nocturia (awakened by urgency to void two or more times). Collectively these symptoms may be referred to as *prostatism* (any condition of the prostate gland that causes retention of urine in the bladder).

Collection of *objective data* involves the nurse's eliciting information to aid in determining the severity of the obstruction, in particular voiding patterns.

Diagnostic tests. On rectal examination, the physician may palpate the enlarged prostate gland, which has an elastic consistency. The hypertrophied prostate is symmetrically enlarged with a uniform, boggy presentation. Severity of the process can be determined through detecting alterations in blood chemistry, measuring residual urine, or by cystoscopy and/or IVU. Cytological evaluation will determine whether the process is benign or malignant.

Nursing interventions. Initial management is aimed at relieving the obstruction, usually by insertion of a Foley catheter. Care must be taken to avoid rapid decompression of the bladder to prevent rupture of mucosal blood vessels. Usually no more than 1000 ml of urine should be removed from a distended bladder initially. Physician's orders should be followed for the individual patient.

Prostatectomy (removal of the prostate gland) is indicated to relieve and/or prevent further obstruction of the urethra. The physician will choose the surgical approach for the prostatectomy after thorough appraisal of the patient. Preoperatively the physician may order an enema to reduce the possibility of the patient's straining to defecate after surgery, which could cause bleeding. Other preoperative preparations are standard, as noted in Chapter 22. There are four surgical techniques by which a prostatectomy may be done; they are presented in Box 30-3. They are (1) transurethral prostatectomy, (2) suprapubic prostatectomy, (3) perineal prostatectomy, and (4) retropubic prostatectomy (Fig. 30-7 on p. 852).

With BPH, a transurethral resection of the prostate (TURP) is less invasive and less stressful for the patient, especially the older patient or the patient with coincidental illness. Removal of the tissue is done through the urethra. With this procedure the outer capsule of the prostate gland is left in place, maintaining the continuity between the bladder and the lower urethra (Fig. 30-9, *A*). Care of this patient is centered on observation of urine character and maintaining patency of the Foley catheter.

Box 30-3 FOUR PROSTATECTOMY TECHNIQUES

1. *Transurethral prostatectomy* is done by approaching the gland through the penis and bladder using a resectoscope, a surgical instrument with an electric cutting wire for resection and cautery, to resect the lobes away from the capsule (Fig. 30-7, *A*).
2. *Suprapubic prostatectomy* is accomplished by an incision through the abdomen; the bladder is opened, and the gland is removed from above with the finger (Fig. 30-7, *B*).
3. *Perineal prostatectomy* requires an incision through the perineum between the scrotum and the rectum (Fig. 30-7, *C*).
4. *Retropubic prostatectomy* is the method in which a low abdominal incision is made, but the bladder is not opened. The gland is removed by making an incision into the capsule encasing the gland (Fig. 30-7, *D*).

The patient who has a TURP may have continuous closed bladder irrigation or intermittent irrigation to prevent occlusion of the catheter with blood clots, which would cause bladder spasms. The patient and family need to know that hematuria is expected after prostatic surgery. Vital signs and urine color will be monitored every 2 hours for the first 24 hours to detect early signs of complications. With continuous bladder irrigation (CBI) the urine will be light red to pink, and with intermittent irrigation the urine will be a clear, cherry red color. Continuous irrigation is achieved by using a three-way catheter (one lumen for irrigation fluid, one for urine drainage, and one to the retention balloon) or by using two catheters (Foley and suprapubic—one for irrigation fluid and one for urine drainage). The irrigation solution is usually normal saline. To determine urine output, the nurse will subtract the amount of irrigation fluid used from the Foley catheter output to obtain actual urine. This is reported as "actual urine output." Catheter drainage tubes should be checked frequently for kinks that would occlude urine flow and cause bladder spasms. The patient should be advised not to try to void around the catheter, since this will contribute to bladder spasms. Hemorrhage is always a possibility. Belladonna and opium (B&O) suppositories are helpful to relieve bladder spasms but are not used in the retropubic approach because rectal stimulation is contraindicated.

Routine postoperative care is instituted. Prolonged sitting is to be avoided, because the resulting increased intraabdominal pressure may cause the operative site to bleed. The catheter will be removed when the urine becomes clear. The patient is informed that he may experience frequency, voiding small amounts with some dribbling initially. He should be instructed to void with the

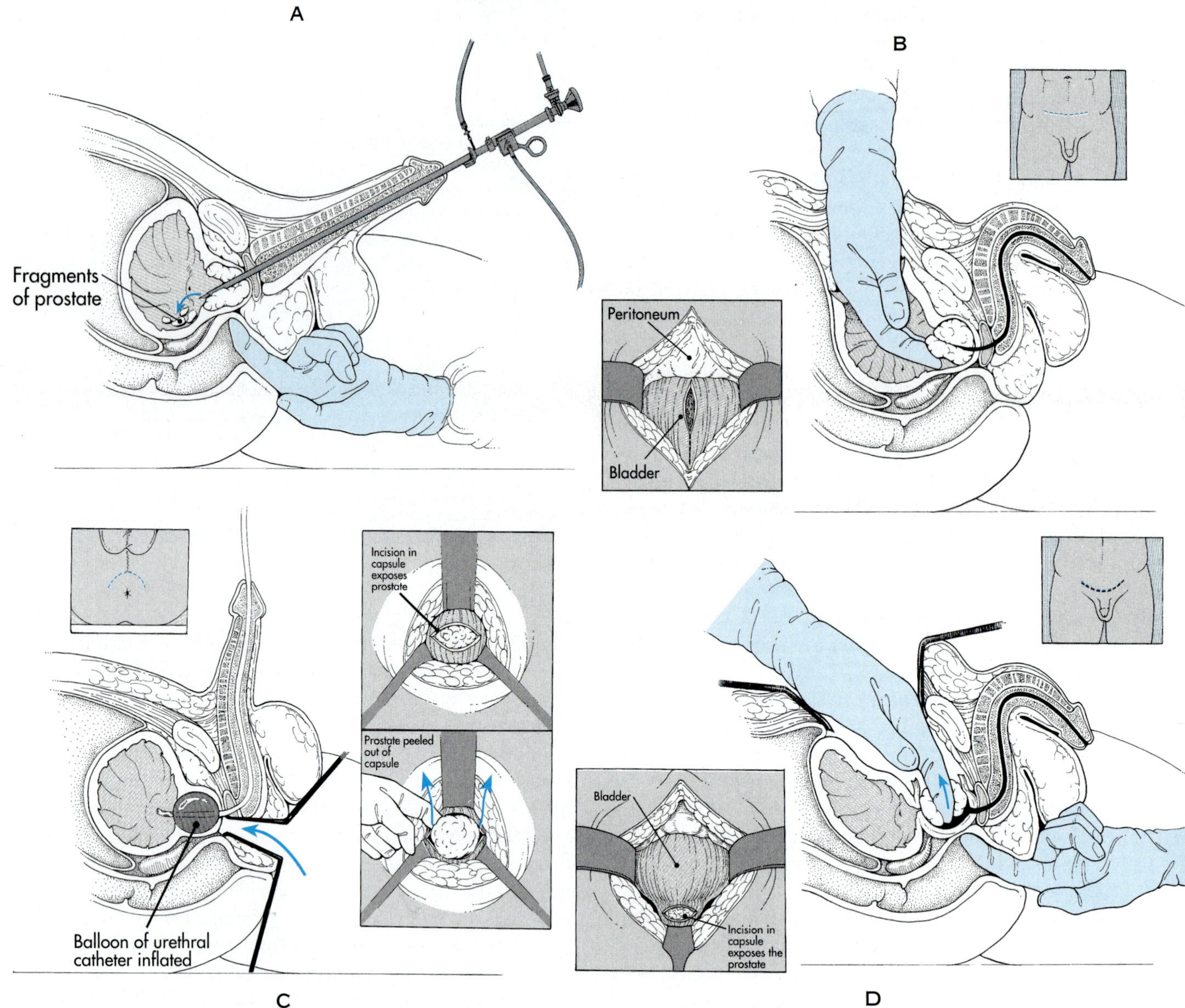

FIG. 30-7 Four types of prostatectomies. **A,** Transuretheral resection of prostate gland by means of resectoscope. Note enlarged prostate gland surrounding urethra and tiny pieces of prostatic tissue that have been cut away. **B,** Suprapubic. **C,** Radical perineal. **D,** Retropubic prostatectomy.

first urge to prevent increased bladder pressure against the operative site.

Some physicians may request that samples of the most recent voidings be saved for assessment. When the patient voids, the nurse records the time, amount, and color of each voiding.

A suprapubic or abdominal approach will require dressing observations and changes. When a suprapubic catheter is present, it will be cared for in the same manner as the Foley catheter.

Prognosis. Prognosis is favorable without residual effects; the length of time for cessation of dribbling is very individualized.

Cancer of the Prostate.

Etiology/pathophysiology. Prostatic cancer is common in men older than 50 years. This insidious cancer usually starts as a nodule on the posterior portion of the prostate; thus symptoms are not present initially. When the tumor causes urinary symptoms, the cancer is in advanced stages. At this point metastasis is common; frequent sites are the pelvic lymph nodes and bone. Regular rectal examinations and PSA measurement to detect abnormalities of the prostate gland leads to early treatment and an increased survival rate.

Clinical manifestations. The patient will have signs and symptoms related to urinary obstruction. Other signs and symptoms will be determined by the presence and/or degree of metastasis.

Assessment. Collection of *subjective data* involves understanding that the patient with prostatic cancer may have no symptoms until the disease is advanced. The patient may seek medical intervention for BPH, which often accompanies prostate cancer, or when he experiences back pain or sciatica that occurs from metastatic changes in the bony pelvis. The patient may complain of dysuria, frequency, and nocturia.

Collection of *objective data* includes noting metastatic changes seen in the lymph glands of the pelvis and in the bones of the lower spine, pelvis, and hips with associated signs. Hematuria may or may not be present, depending on the stage of the malignancy.

Diagnostic tests. On rectal examination by the physician, the involved area of the prostate gland will feel firm and fixed with hardened nodules typically in the posterior lobe of the gland. Definitive diagnosis is made by cytological examination. Prostate cells can be obtained by needle aspiration. Serum acid phosphatase will be elevated when the disease process extends beyond the prostatic capsule.

Measurement of prostate-specific antigen (PSA) and prostatic acid phosphatase (PAP) should be done to help determine the stage of the disease. Both of these tests rise in response to tissue manipulation and remain elevated: the PSA for 12+ days, the PAP for 1 to 2 days.[48] It is important, therefore, to secure the blood sample before physical examination.

PSA is increasing considerably the odds of early diagnosis. PSA, normally secreted and disposed of by the prostate, increases in the bloodstream in cancer of the prostate as well as in the harmless condition of benign prostatic hypertrophy (BPH). Elevated PSA levels mean further diagnostic evaluation is needed. In cases when PSA levels are high but a digital exam is normal, the imaging technique of transrectal ultrasound is proving increasingly helpful in detecting cancer tumor of the prostate gland too small to be palpated rectally.[59] The normal PSA level is less than 4 ng/ml.Other tests, such as a bone scan and serum alkaline phosphatase will be performed to assess the degree of metastasis.

Medical management. Treatment is based on the stage of the cancer—whether it has spread beyond the wall of the prostate, and to what extent—and the age of the patient. In the older male with an estimated remaining life span of 5 or 10 years, controlling the disease with radiation or hormone therapy may be enough. In many cases, particularly in men over 70 years of age, prostate cancer grows slowly, and hormone therapy can hold the disease at bay for several years.

Localized prostate cancer can be cured by radiation therapy or surgery. Radiation therapy (35 treatments, one a day for 5 weeks) also is used when the cancer has spread to just outside the gland, in an attempt to destroy cancer cells and shrink the prostate.

The operation to remove the prostate is called a radical prostatectomy. Radical prostatectomy by the perineal approach is used in patients with early-stage clinical disease and is considered one of the most effective ways of eradicating the tumor. This procedure involves removing the entire prostate, including the true prostatic capsule, seminal vesicles, and a portion of the bladder neck. The remaining portion of the bladder neck is reanastomosed to the urethra. The retropubic approach often is used first, because it provides access to the pelvic lymph nodes (pelvic lymphadenectomy) and affords more urinary control and less stricture formation.

A nerve-sparing prostatectomy procedure is being used for the retropubic and perineal approach in an attempt to prevent impotence and reduce the likelihood of urinary incontinence. This procedure is not guaranteed, because the extent of surgical resection needed to confine the disease is not known before the surgery. The three goals of a radical prostatectomy are removing all the tumor, preserving urine control, and preserving sexual function. Extent of sexual function may not be known for 6 to 12 months postoperatively.[61] This patient will need emotional support related to the cancer and the possibility of impotence as a result of the surgery. Preoperative teaching should include an opportunity for the patient and his partner to discuss optional treatments and mortality rate.

When the capsule of the prostate gland is removed, as with the perineal approach, there is no longer a connection between the bladder and the lower urethra. The area where these two structures are reconnected is usually supported by placement of a Foley catheter. Extreme care must be taken not to cause tension on the catheter, which would disturb the surgical area. The catheter will remain indwelling for several postoperative days.

In cases of advanced cancer, hormonal manipulation with estrogen therapy may be used in an attempt to alter the tumor growth by blocking androgen production. Palliative therapy for patients with metastatic disease also may include orchiectomy (removal of the testes). Bilateral orchiectomy may be used to eliminate 95% of testosterone production, a step that is useful in managing metastatic disease. The patient may receive relief from such symptoms as pain or obstruction, but may, however, experience feminization, increased incidence of cardiac disease, thrombophlebitis, pulmonary embolus, and cerebrovascular accident. Additional therapies are instituted to treat these side effects.

Radiation therapy may be used in advanced stages of the illness as primary or palliative treatment. Management of disseminated disease with cytotoxic drugs has been marginally successful.

Because cure for cancer of the prostate is possible only when the tumor is discovered early, it is important to teach all male patients over the age of 40 to have annual or biannual rectal examinations and yearly PSA serum levels.

Nursing interventions. Postoperative nursing management is similar to that for perineal surgery, with special attention to maintenance of bowel and bladder function while keeping the surgical wound clean and avoiding pressure on the perineum and wound. Adequate fluid intake, modification of dietary selections, and perineal exercises may be used to promote regulation of bowel and bladder function. Extreme care must be taken to prevent trauma to the perineum to avoid possible perforation of the perineum, causing a fistula. Rectal temperature-taking, enemas, and use of rectal tubes are therefore forbidden. Extreme care must be taken not to create tension on the Foley catheter, which would disturb the surgical area. The nurse observes the color of the urine for signs of bleeding. The patient will also have a tissue drain inserted during surgery to promote drainage from the wound in the perineum. Initially, there may be some small amount of urine from the drain, but this should cease in 1 or 2 days. Surgical asepsis should be followed during dressing changes. Irrigation of the perineum may be ordered to cleanse the wound and soothe the patient. Comfort measures and analgesics should be administered as ordered for pain control in the lower back, pelvis, upper thighs, and operative site.

Patient teaching. Another possible complication of the surgery is urinary incontinence. The nurse should teach the patient how to keep himself clean. He may need an opportunity to discuss feelings of depression about his altered body function. Modification of life-style and maintenance of confidence are important for his return to preillness function.

- Emphasize the need for adequate fluid intake, exercise, and rest.
- Instruct the patient in pain-relieving measures (e.g., exercise, warmth, and medication).
- Tell the patient to notify the physician or the nurse if any signs and symptoms of renal insufficiency appear.
- Discuss alternate expressions of sexuality, the value of sexual counseling, and the possibility of recovering some or all of sexual function after treatment is completed.

Prognosis. There is a direct correlation between prognosis and the extent of the disease process when diagnosed. Grading of the tumors (well, moderately, or poorly differentiated) correlates with the prognosis; the more poorly differentiated the tumor, the poorer the prognosis. Pathologists use a system called *Gleason score* to rank cell differentiation. A low score—2, through 4—is good. A high score—7 through 10—is not.[60] The treatment goal for localized disease process is cure, and palliation is used for extended disease process.

Urethral Strictures

Etiology/Pathophysiology. A urethral stricture is a narrowing of the lumen of the urethra that interferes with urine flow. Narrowing may be congenital or acquired. Acquired strictures may be caused by chronic infection, trauma, or tumor or as a complication of radiation treatment of the pelvis.

Clinical Manifestations. Signs and symptoms include dysuria, weak stream, splaying (spreading out) of the urine stream, nocturia, and increasing pain with bladder distention. In the presence of infection, fever and malaise may be apparent.

Assessment. Collection of *subjective data* includes noting a patient complaint of difficulty initiating the urine stream and the stream seeming to spray more than usual or even seeming to "fork."

Collection of *objective data* includes assessing for signs that may indicate an infectious process and gathering information to describe the infectious process to describe the extent of the stricture and possible presence of an obstruction.

Diagnostic Tests. Diagnosis can be confirmed by a voiding cystourethrogram, which demonstrates stricture. Additional diagnostic studies help evaluate damage caused by the obstruction.

Medical Management. Correction of the stricture may be achieved by dilation with metal sounds or surgical release (internal urethrotomy).

Nursing Interventions. Care includes adequate hydration to decrease discomfort when voiding and monitoring of urine output. Mild analgesics should be sufficient to relieve discomfort. Sitz baths may relieve discomfort and encourage voiding. Reconstruction (urethroplasty) of the urethra may require temporary urinary diversion (see care guidelines, p. 832). After the procedure, a splinting catheter will support the suture line. Care must be taken not to cause tension on the catheter.

Prognosis. Prognosis after surgical correction or dilation is favorable.

Urinary Tract Trauma

Etiology/Pathophysiology. Any patient with a history of traumatic injury should be assessed for involvement of the urinary tract. Such injuries may include contusions or rupture of the urinary structures. A patient who has undergone abdominal surgery should also be observed for incidental injury sustained during the operation. Traumatic invasion of the urinary tract may be evident in open wounds to the lower abdomen, such as with gunshot or stab wounds. Contusion or laceration of the urethra may lead to urethral stricture and possible impotence in males secondary to soft tissue, blood vessel, and nerve damage.

Clinical Manifestations. Urine output should be monitored hourly for amount and color, and any evidence of hematuria should be reported. The patient is assessed for abdominal pain and tenderness, which may indicate internal hemorrhage, peritonitis, or seepage of urine into the tissues.

Assessment. Collection of *subjective data* involves understanding that the trauma patient may be unable to relate any symptoms that would aid in the assessment of urinary tract involvement. If the patient is able to respond, any reference to the signs of hematuria is extremely important.

Collection of *objective data* includes a comprehensive assessment of the trauma patient reviewing all body systems. Assessment related to the urinary tract includes hourly measurement of I&O, observation of urine character or difficulty voiding, evaluation of complaints of abdominal, flank, or referred shoulder pain, and evaluation of abdominal distention and girth.

Diagnostic Tests. Diagnosis of traumatic involvement of the urinary tract may be aided by KUB radiograph, IVU, urinalysis, excretory urogram, and cystoscopy.

Medical Management. Surgical intervention will be necessary for correction of tears or rupture of the integrity of the urinary tract, to reinstate urine flow. If damage to the structures is severe, removal of the kidney or bladder may be necessary with the creation of urinary diversion as discussed later in this chapter.

Management of possible hemorrhage and prevention of infection are necessary preoperatively and postoperatively.

Nursing Interventions. Nursing responsibility centers on identifying individuals at risk and detecting variations in assessment findings that indicate trauma to the urinary tract. The nurse should document and report all findings.

Prognosis. Prognosis depends on the extent and location of the trauma.

NONINFECTIOUS DISORDERS OF THE URINARY SYSTEM

Nephrotic Syndrome

Etiology/Pathophysiology. Nephrotic syndrome (nephrosis) is a group of signs characterized by marked proteinuria, hypoalbuminemia, and edema. Several events may precipitate the signs of nephrotic syndrome; the primary form of nephrosis occurs in the absence of glomerulonephritis or systemic disease, with the inciting event being an upper respiratory infection or allergic reaction.

Physiological changes in the glomeruli interfere with selective permeability. Blood protein is allowed to pass into the urine (proteinuria), causing a loss of serum protein (hypoalbuminemia). This decreases serum osmotic pressure, thus allowing fluid to seep into interstitial spaces, and edema occurs.

Clinical Manifestations. The patient has severe generalized edema **(anasarca),** anorexia, fatigue, and altered renal function.

Assessment. Collection of *subjective data* includes noting patient complaints of loss of interest in eating, a constant feeling of being tired, foamy urine from the presence of protein, and decreased urine output (oliguria).

Collection of *objective data* includes the nurse assessing the degree of fluid retention by monitoring daily weight, intake and output, respiratory effort, and level of consciousness. The patient may relate problems with "swelling" of his face, hands, and feet. Skin integrity is assessed to determine special needs.

Diagnostic Tests. Blood chemistry findings include hyperalbuminuria, hypoalbuminemia, and hyperlipidemia. Renal biopsy provides identification of the type and extent of tissue change. Other diagnostic testing will be performed to identify the specific underlying cause.

Medical Management. Medical management depends on the extent of tissue involvement and may include the use of (1) corticosteroids (Prednisone) to control systemic symptoms, (2) potassium-sparing antihypertensives, such as spironolactone (Aldactone), or (3) antineoplastic agents (used for immunosuppressive effect). Potent loop diuretics (furosemide [Lasix], bumetanide [Bumex]) as well as thiazide diuretics (hydrochlorothiazide [HydroDIURIL], chlorthalidone [Hygrotin]) are used to relieve edema. Hypoproteinemia may be treated with normal serum albumin and protein-rich nutrition replacement therapy.

Nursing Interventions. Nursing intervention includes monitoring of fluid balance (weight, measuring abdominal girth, I&O), bed rest in the presence of extreme edema (recumbent position may initiate diuresis), and assessing for electrolyte imbalance. Skin care is very important as is a gradual increase in activity as the edema is resolved.

Diet includes protein replacement using foods that provide high biological value (meat, fish, poultry, cheese, eggs) and restriction of sodium to decrease edema. Blood pressure is often elevated and should be monitored closely for changes.

Patient teaching. As the patient begins to convalesce, the teaching plan includes the following:

- Medication regimen: type, dosage, side effects, and need to finish prescription (as appropriate)

- Nutrition teaching
- Self-assessment of fluid status: weight, presence of edema
- Signs and symptoms requiring immediate attention (increase in edema, fatigue, headache, infection)
- Need for follow-up care

Prognosis. In approximately 25% of children and 50% to 75% of adults who develop nephrosis the disease progresses to renal failure within 5 years. In other individuals (particularly children) there may be remissions or nephrotic syndrome may exist in a chronic form. Other than treating the underlying illness, little can be done to prevent a recurrence of nephrosis.

Nephritis

Formerly called *Bright's disease*, nephritis encompasses a number of kidney disorders characterized by inflammation of the kidney, involving the glomeruli, tubules, or interstitial tissue and abnormal function. Included in this group of disorders are acute and chronic glomerulonephritis.

Acute Glomerulonephritis.

Etiology/pathophysiology. The health history commonly reveals that the onset of acute glomerulonephritis was preceded by an infection, such as a store throat or skin infection (most commonly *β-hemolytic streptococcus*) 2 to 3 weeks earlier, or other preexisting multisystem diseases, such as systemic lupus erythematosus. The infectious disease process triggers an immune response on the affected kidney structure, resulting in inflammation of glomeruli that allows excretion of red blood cells and protein in the urine. The condition is common in children and young adults.

Clinical manifestations. It is not unusual for family members to first note that the individual has "swelling" of the face, especially around the eyes, and a pale coloring. Some patients may be acutely ill with a multitude of symptoms, while others may be diagnosed on routine examination with only vague symptoms.

Assessment. Collection of *subjective data* includes noting the patient relating symptoms indicative of anorexia, nocturia, malaise, and exertional dyspnea.

Collection of *objective data* includes assessment of skin integrity and general condition of skin; the presence, degree, and nature of edema with associated difficulty in breathing on exertion, when recumbent, or as evidenced by changes in lung and heart sounds (unusual heart sounds, crackles over lung fields, distention of neck veins); hematuria with changes in urine color from "cola" to frank sanguineous; or changes in voiding, decrease in amount of urine output, or dysuria.

Diagnostic tests. Diagnostic tests will reveal elevation of BUN, serum creatinine, potassium, erythrocyte sedimentation rate (ESR), and antistreptolysin-O titer (ASO titer). Urinalysis will show red blood cells, casts, and/or protein.

Medical management. Medical management includes treatment of primary symptoms while preventing complications to cerebral and cardiac function. Serum electrolyte levels (sodium and potassium) may indicate a need to adjust dietary intake of sodium and potassium. Level of consciousness should be monitored when the BUN is elevated. Bed rest and fluid intake adjustments are guided by urinary output until diuresis is adequate.

A prophylactic antimicrobial agent, such as penicillin, may be administered for several months after the acute phase of the illness to protect against recurrence of infection. Diuretics may be prescribed to control fluid retention and antihypertensives to reduce blood pressure.

Nursing interventions. Nursing intervention will be guided by individual patient needs, focusing on relief of symptoms and prevention of complications. Dietary intake will include protein restrictions, with carbohydrates providing a source of energy.

Nursing interventions include monitoring I&O and vital signs. Level of activity will be determined by the degree of edema, hypertension, proteinuria, and hematuria because excessive activity may increase these signs.

Patient teaching. Because of the long-term nature of glomerulonephritis, patient teaching is important. Proteinuria and hematuria may exist microscopically even when other symptoms subside. Although fatigue may be present, these patients usually feel well; therefore, they often must be convinced of the need to continue prescribed treatment and to return for follow-up care. Teaching includes the following:

- Nature of the illness and effect of diet and fluids on fluid balance and sodium retention.
- Diet teaching regarding prescribed sodium and fluid restrictions (provide written information regarding sodium content of foods, as necessary).
- Medication regimen (dose, frequency, side effects, need to continue as per physician instructions).
- Need to pace activities with rest if fatigue is present.
- Avoidance of trauma and infection (may exacerbate the illness).
- Signs and symptoms indicating need for medical attention (hematuria, headache, edema, hypertension).
- Importance of follow-up health care.

Prognosis. The prognosis of acute poststreptococcal glomerulonephritis is generally good; however, some patients develop chronic glomerulonephritis and ESRD, requiring dialysis or renal transplantation.

Chronic Glomerulonephritis.

Etiology/pathophysiology. With chronic glomerulonephritis there is usually no indication of an inciting event. Occasionally the patient with acute glomerulonephritis will progress to a chronic phase. Because other chronic illnesses, (e.g., diabetes mellitus or systemic lupus erythematosus) may mask the symptoms of renal degeneration, many patients will not seek medical attention until renal function is compromised. Chronic glomerulonephritis is characterized by slow, progressive destruction of glomeruli with related loss of function. The kidney will atrophy (actually decrease in size).

Clinical manifestations. Signs and symptoms may include malaise, morning headaches, dyspnea with exertion, visual and digestive disturbances, edema, weight loss, and fatigue. Physical findings include hypertension, anemia, proteinuria, anasarca, and cardiac and cerebral manifestations.

Assessment. Collection of *subjective data* includes the patient complaints of fatigue and a decreased ability to perform ADLs as a result of dyspnea and decreasing ability to concentrate. Investigate complaints of morning headaches: location, pattern, and character; note presence of any visual disturbance.

Collection of *objective data* includes the nurse's clarifying outward manifestations of the headache and respiratory effort that may interfere with daily task performance. Assess mental functioning, irritability, slurred speech, ataxia or tremors. Careful assessment of the degree of edema will be documented, noting specific location and response to pressure by pressing the fingers into the edematous area and observing for pitting (see Chapter 28). Note skin color, ecchymoses (irregularly formed hemorrhagic areas of the skin) or rash, dry skin, and scratching. Observe urine color and amount. Monitor vital signs, including a chest assessment for cardiac and pulmonary signs of fluid retention: unusual heart sound, crackles over lung fields, distention of neck veins.

Diagnostic tests. Early disease shows albumin and RBCs in the urine, although renal function test results are within normal limits. With advanced destruction of nephrons the specific gravity becomes fixed and blood levels of nonprotein nitrogen wastes (creatinine and urea) increase. Creatinine clearance may be as low as 5 to 10 ml/minute compared with the normal range of 97 to 137 ml/min in men and 88 to 128 ml/min in women.

Medical management. Medical management includes control of secondary side effects as discussed with acute glomerulonephritis, with the use of renal dialysis and possible kidney transplantation to provide elimination of wastes from the body.

Nursing interventions. Nursing interventions for the patient with chronic glomerulonephritis represent a special challenge. This patient has already suffered major damage to the kidney filtration system. It is crucial that the patient's condition not be further compromised by infection or other complications. Changes in vital signs and diagnostic tests are monitored to aid in choosing proper nursing interventions. Interventions parallel those noted with nephrotic syndrome and acute glomerulonephritis. Chronic glomerulonephritis may progress to ESRD, necessitating related nursing interventions. Interventions are listed in Box 30-4.

A nursing diagnosis and interventions for the patient with chronic glomerulonephritis include but are not limited to the following:

NURSING DIAGNOSIS	NURSING INTERVENTIONS
Fluid volume excess, related to decreased urine output secondary to renal dysfunction	Assess understanding of therapeutic interventions. Monitor and report signs and symptoms of fluid excess (hypertension, CHF, weight gain, edema). Measure and document I&O q hr.

Box 30-4 NURSING INTERVENTION GUIDELINES FOR THE PATIENT WITH NEPHRITIS

ACTIVITY

Bed rest until edema and blood pressure are reduced
Encourage quiet diversional activities
Ambulate gradually with assistance
Space activity to lessen fatigue

FLUID BALANCE MAINTENANCE

Implement dietary restrictions
Monitor I&O
Document reactions to medication

DIET THERAPY

Protein restrictions to decrease nitrogenous wastes
Sodium restrictions to prevent further fluid retention
Increase calories for energy source

DRUG THERAPY

Prophylactic antibiotics
Antihypertensives
Diuretics
Drug interactions, side effects to expect and report

HEALTH MAINTENANCE

Recovery may be extended
Urine will be monitored for albumin and RBCs by physician
Teach early signs of fluid retention
Signs and symptoms may resolve and then become worse
Normal activities may be resumed after urine is clear for a month, though the patient is not considered cured until the urine is free of albumin and RBCs for 6 months

NURSING DIAGNOSIS	NURSING INTERVENTIONS
Fluid volume excess, related to decreased urine output secondary to renal dysfunction—cont'd	Note amount and character of urine: report decreased urine output to physician. Weigh patient daily at the same time with the same clothing and same scale. Restrict sodium as ordered. Replace fluids according to fluid loss as ordered. Provide ice chips to control thirst. Administer diuretics as ordered. Monitor electrolytes and report abnormal laboratory values, and signs and symptoms of electrolyte imbalances.

Patient teaching. The focus for patient teaching must be preventive health maintenance, emphasizing a health-promoting life-style, with prevention and early treatment of infections.

Prognosis. Some persons with minimal impairment in renal function continue to feel well and show little progression of disease. With other individuals the progression of renal deterioration may be slow but steady and end in renal failure. In still other individuals the progression of disease is rapid.

Renal Failure

An acute or chronic state, renal failure is characterized by the inability of the kidneys to excrete wastes, concentrate urine, and conserve or eliminate electrolytes. Predisposing concurrent illnesses include burns, trauma, congestive heart failure, volume depletion, and renal disease. Nursing interventions to prevent the development of renal failure include adequate hydration, prevention of infections, monitoring for signs and symptoms of shock, and teaching drug side effects to report immediately.

Acute Renal Failure.

Etiology/pathophysiology. Kidney function may be altered by interference with the kidney's ability to be selective in filtering blood or by an actual decrease in blood flow to the kidneys. A number of medical conditions can lead to acute renal failure (ARF), such as hemorrhage, trauma, infection, and decreased cardiac output. The course of ARF is divided into phases. In the **oliguric** (a diminished capacity to form and pass urine, less than 500 ml every 24 hours, so that the end products of metabolism cannot be excreted efficiently) *phase,* BUN and serum creatinine levels rise while urine output decreases.

Some patients may experience the nonoliguric form, usually caused by nephrotoxic antibiotics, with which urinary output may exceed 2 liters per day. The oliguric phase may last from several days to 4 to 6 weeks.

In the *diuretic phase*, blood chemistry levels begin to return to normal and urine output increases. Return to normal or near-normal function occurs in the *recovery phase*.

Clinical manifestations. The patient may experience anorexia, nausea, vomiting, edema, and associated signs and symptoms of diminished renal function.

Assessment. Collection of *subjective data* includes the patient report of experiencing lethargy, loss of appetite, nausea, and headache.

Collection of *objective data* involves physical findings that will depend on the progression of the disease process. The nurse assesses for dry mucous membranes, poor skin turgor, urine output of less than 400 ml/24 hr, vomiting, diarrhea, and anasarca. If the disease is in the severe stage, assessment findings may include central nervous system manifestations of drowsiness, muscle twitching, and convulsions.

Diagnostic tests. Physical assessment, history, and elevated blood chemistry tests such as BUN and creatinine (azotemia) will confirm diagnosis. After the patient is stabilized, further studies may be done to assess for residual damage.

Medical management. Measures include administration of fluids and osmotic preparations to prevent decreased renal perfusion, manage fluid volume, and treat electrolyte imbalances. Renal dialysis may be necessary to manage systemic fluid shifts, especially cardiac and respiratory, and may be effective in removing some nephrotoxins.

Diet should be protein sparing, high in carbohydrate, and low in potassium and sodium. Drug therapy may include diuretics to initiate diuresis: furosemide (Lasix), hydrochlorothiazide (Hydrodiuril), or mannitol. Potassium-lowering agents are used to remove potassium through the gastrointestinal tract: sodium polystyrene sulfonate (Kayexalate) is administered orally or as a retention enema. Sodium bicarbonate is used to cause potassium to move into the cell from blood plasma. Blood pressure is controlled by antihypertensives (clonidine [Catapres], hydralazine [Apresoline]). Antibiotics that are not dependent on kidney excretion are used to eradicate or prevent infection. Whatever combination of drug therapy is utilized, dosage and administration times will require adjustment according to the level of kidney function.

Nursing interventions. Accurate documentation of urine output is necessary to identify the level of renal function. Azotemia may be revealed by blood chemistry studies. The patient with azotemia must be observed for changes in level of consciousness. Fluid status, vital signs, and response to therapies must be closely monitored. Frequent skin care with tepid water to remove urea crystals will be comforting. Dialysis presents special nursing challenges (see p. 860-864).

Patient teaching. Teaching includes the following:

- Cause of renal failure and problems with recurrent failures.

- Identification of preventable environmental or health factors contributing to the illness (such as hypertension, nephrotoxic drugs).
- Teach dietary restrictions and medication regimen.
- Signs and symptoms of infection and of returning renal failure to be reported to physician.
- Instruct patient concerning activity.
- Need for ongoing follow-up care.

Prognosis. Recovery from an episode of ARF depends on the underlying illness, condition of patient, and careful supportive management given during the period of kidney shutdown. The leading cause of death is infection, such as of the urinary tract, lungs, and peritoneum. Infection develops in approximately 80% of patients with ARF. The incidence of GI bleeding, the second most frequent cause of death, is about 25%. Mortality from fluid overload and acidosis has been reduced as a result of dialysis and other forms of therapy. There is potential for recovery of renal function in patients who survive the acute episode of tubular insufficiency. Although kidney tissue may regenerate more completely after toxic injury than ischemia, both forms usually show return to normal or near-normal renal function.

For those in whom ARF has been caused by glomerular disease or severe infection of kidney tissue, the prognosis may not be as favorable. Return of renal function is determined by the extent of scarring and destruction of functional renal tissue that has occurred during the acute episode of kidney failure.

Chronic Renal Failure (End-Stage Renal Disease).

Etiology/pathophysiology. Chronic renal failure or end-stage renal disease (ESRD) exists when the kidneys are unable to regain normal function. As many as 80% of nephrons may be severely impaired before loss of renal function is detected. The most common causes of ESRD are pyelonephritis, chronic glomerulonephritis, glomerulosclerosis, chronic urinary obstruction, severe hypertension, diabetes mellitus, gout, and polycystic kidney disease. Whatever the cause, dialysis or kidney transplantation will be needed to maintain life.

ESRD represents a significant health problem worldwide, resulting in the death of thousands, and financial crisis for the patients and their families. The government does actively help defray costs through the Medicare program. ESRD develops slowly over an extended period as a result of kidney disease or other disease processes that compromise renal blood perfusion.

Clinical manifestations. The onset of signs and symptoms may be so gradual and the signs and symptoms so vague that the patient is unable to identify when the problems started. When questioned, the patient may be able to relate occurrences that seemed insignificant at the time. The clinical picture is usually unique to the individual. Common symptoms are headache, lethargy, asthenia (decreased strength or energy), anorexia, pruritus, elimination changes, **anuria** (urinary output less than 100 to 250 ml/day), muscle cramps or twitching, impotence, characteristic dusky, yellow-tan, or gray skin color from retained urochrome pigments, and signs and symptoms characteristic of central nervous system involvement, such as disorientation and mental lapses.

Other associated conditions are responsible for many of the symptoms. Azotemia develops as excessive amounts of nitrogenous compounds build in the blood. Anemia occurs when the production of renal erythropoietin is decreased as a result of loss of kidney function. Acidosis, hypertension, and glucose intolerance may be present as a result of the insult to homeostasis.

Assessment. Collection of *subjective data* will include noting patient complaints of joint pain and edema, severe headaches, nausea, anorexia, intermittent chest pain, weakness, and in particular, fatigue, intractable singultus (hiccups), decreased libido, menstrual irregularities, impaired concentration.

The clinical consequences of renal failure are far reaching, affecting nearly every body system.

Collection of *objective data* involves a nursing assessment that may yield unremarkable results, except for signs and symptoms that support the patient complaints. Uremic encephalopathy affects the central nervous system. Usually the first sign is a reduction in alertness and awareness. Respirations will become Kussmaul (abnormally deep, very rapid sighing respirations) in character and coma develops. The accumulation of urates results in halitosis with a urine odor and "uremic frost" on the skin in the form of a white powder.

Diagnostic tests. Diagnosis of ESRD is confirmed by elevated BUN of at least 50 mg/dl and serum creatinine levels greater than 5 mg/dl, electrolyte imbalance (including a decreased number of bicarbonate and magnesium and an increased number of potassium, sodium, and phosphatase ions), and other indicators related to the underlying cause. Renal function studies assess the degree of damage and/or level of renal function.

Medical management. Medical management is instituted to delay the onset of ESRD as long as possible. Renal dialysis is initiated when necessary, and the patient may be prepared for renal transplantation. Medications are used, as with acute renal failure, to control systemic changes resulting from a shift in fluid and electrolyte balance, acidosis, possible hyperkalemia, possible seizure activity, hypertension, and infection. Drug therapy may include anticonvulsants to control seizure activity (phenytoin [Dilantin], diazepam [Valium]); antianemics, vitamin supplements to counteract nutritional deficiencies, antiemetics (prochlorperazine [Compazine]), antipruritics (cyproheptadine [Periactin]), biological response modifiers to stimulate red cell production (epoetin alpha [Epogen]) to treat anemia caused by a reduced production of erythropoietin, and other medications as needed to meet individual needs.

Nursing interventions. Nursing interventions focus on restoring homeostasis. Measures to control fluid and electrolyte balance vary greatly, according to unique needs of the individual patient. Nutritional therapy is aimed at reserving protein stores and preventing production of additional protein waste products that the kidney would have to clear. High biological proteins are used to provide the essential amino acids.

Box 30-5

NURSING INTERVENTION GUIDELINES FOR THE PATIENT WITH RENAL FAILURE

FLUID AND ELECTROLYTE BALANCE

Assess I&O (hourly may be indicated)
Weigh daily (same time, same clothing, same scale)
Assess overt (open to view) signs of hydration status (edema, turgor)
Assess covert (hidden) signs of hydration status (breath sounds, laboratory studies, and so on)

NUTRITION

Provide prescribed diet
Guide patient food selection
Plan fluid intake per shift within prescribed limits and according to patient preference
Reinforce diet instructions as indicated

COMFORT AND SAFETY

Provide quiet environment (sound and lighting)
Space nursing interventions to conserve patient energy
Medicate as needed for comfort
Skin care to alleviate discomfort resulting from pruritus
Mouth care as needed
Maintain asepsis during procedures
Prevent exposure to pathogens

COPING BEHAVIORS

Listen (patient and significant other)
Refer to pastoral care or religious support group if indicated
Provide private times with significant others
Offer interview with social services

DOCUMENTATION AND REPORTING

Document all relevant findings
Maintain open communications with supervisory staff
Adjust nursing care plan as indicated to meet changing patient needs
Dietary restrictions: food exchange, measuring fluids, food diary
Health promotion/illness prevention measures

The diet is high in calories from carbohydrates and fats from polyunsaturated sources (to maintain weight and spare protein), at least 2500 to 3000 calories daily. Other dietary restrictions are related to the patient's degree of acidosis. Potassium is retained; therefore foods high in potassium are restricted. Sodium is controlled at a level sufficient to replace sodium loss without causing fluid retention.

Nursing interventions for ARF are also instituted for ESRD. Emphasis is placed on emotional support for the patient who faces role changes and invasive treatments such as dialysis and/or kidney transplantation. Box 30-5 offers guidelines for supporting the patient with renal failure. Fluid balance is of prime importance. The patient may have fluid equal to the amount excreted in the urine plus about 300 to 600 ml to compensate for ***insensible*** (imperceptible) ***fluid loss*** (fluid lost through the lungs, perspiration, and feces). Salt substitutes are not advised, because most contain potassium. If seizure activity occurs, safety measures need to be instituted to provide for patient protection (see Chapter 35). See the nursing care plan for the patient with ESRD.

Patient teaching. Patient teaching should emphasize food exchanges and fluid intake within restrictions.

Care of the patient requiring dialysis. **Dialysis** (a medical procedure for the removal of certain elements from the blood by virtue of the difference in their rates of diffusion through an external semipermeable membrane or, in the case of peritoneal dialysis, through the peritoneum) mimics kidney function, helping to restore balance when normal kidney function is interrupted temporarily or permanently. Dialysis involves either diffusion of wastes, drugs, or excess electrolytes or osmosis of water across a semipermeable membrane into a dialysate fluid that is prescribed specific to individual patient needs. Dialysis is achieved by the process of hemodialysis or peritoneal dialysis.

Hemodialysis. Hemodialysis requires an access to the patient's circulatory system to route blood through the artificial kidney (dialyzer) for removal of wastes, fluids, and electrolytes and then return the blood to the patient's body. Temporary methods include subclavian or femoral catheters or an external shunt placed in the nondominant forearm. In ESRD, access can be achieved by constructing a direct or a graft arteriovenous fistula (Fig. 30-8 on p. 863). Hemodialysis is usually scheduled three times a week for 3 to 6 hours. Patients can be maintained on dialysis therapy and their lives prolonged pending the possibility of a kidney transplantation.

MEDICAL MANAGEMENT. Medical management includes continuation of previously instituted therapies. Blood levels of drugs excreted by the kidney must be closely monitored to maintain therapeutic levels and to prevent toxic accumulations. Medication may include antihypertensives, cardiac glycosides, antibiotics, and antidysrhythmics. The patient is instructed not to take over-the-counter medications without consulting the physician.

NURSING CARE PLAN THE PATIENT WITH END-STAGE RENAL DISEASE

Barry Johnson, a 37-year-old high school basketball coach, visited his family doctor with complaints of weight loss, decreasing strength, increasing inability to concentrate, and morning headaches. Examination revealed severe hypertension, yellow-gray skin color, and pale mucous membranes. After diagnostic studies reveal chronic glomerulonephritis with ESRD, Mr. Johnson is admitted to the hospital to stabilize his condition.

Nursing diagnoses	Patient goals/expected outcomes	Nursing interventions
Fluid volume excess, related to compromised renal regulatory mechanism resulting in sodium and water retention	Patient will achieve near-normal level of fluid volume as evidenced by decreasing edema and maintenance of skin integrity.	Monitor signs of fluid imbalance: daily weight, skin turgor, edema, I&O, blood blood pressure, respiratory rate and quality. Identify sources of fluids and electrolytes: foods, fluids, medications—oral and IV. Teach patient to plan nutritional intake within prescribed limits for diet and fluids. Provide fluids within prescribed limits.
Nutrition, altered: less than body requirements, related to dietary restrictions, anorexia, GI distress	Patient weight will stabilize within normal limits for this patient.	Assess baseline nutritional needs. Provide clean, quiet, odor-free environment during meals. Complete mouth care before meals. Assist in food selection within dietary restrictions. Provide six small feedings throughout the day. Teach meal and fluid planning within dietary restrictions. Use a food diary to monitor nutritional intake and deficiencies. Ask family to bring favorite foods from home, within dietary restrictions. Foster independence by having patient feed self. Administer antiemetics 30 min before meal times to control nausea. Monitor intake with calorie count prn. Enhance food flavor with herbs instead of salt or salt substitutes.
Coping, ineffective individual, related to personal vulnerability associated with diagnosis	Patient will verbalize acceptance of situation.	Establish rapport with patient and family. Foster demonstration of feelings. Suggest utilization of hospital and community resources. Maintain open communications between health care providers and patient/significant others. Give positive feedback as patient uses new coping skills.

Continued.

Powerlessness, related to chronic illness	Patient will participate in decision making to help determine his own plan of care.	Support patient's expression of feelings about self and illness. Validate patient's feelings of powerlessness when they surface. Explain rationale for all procedures/treatments according to patient's understanding and desire to be informed. Request patient input to plan when and how care should be done. Negotiate with patient when changes are necessary in the schedule (e.g., testing, treatment therapies). Modify the environment to facilitate participation in self-care. Develop consistent approach among all health care providers.
Knowledge deficit, related to limited exposure to renal disease information	The patient will verbalize an increase knowledge of disease process.	Evaluate readiness to learn treatment regimen. Provide unhurried time with patient. Listen to patient's concerns to formulate a teaching plan. Provide information at patient's level of understanding. Pace teaching to patient's capacity to process information. Communicate teaching plan with all health care providers to support consistency.
Noncompliance to therapeutic regimen, related to complexity of life-style changes.	The patient will modify ADLs to adhere to therapeutic regimen.	Discuss with patient and significant others rationale for therapeutic regimen (diet, medications, exercise) Discuss with patient what constitutes compliant behavior. Collaborate with patient in evaluation of current life-style practices. Explore alternative behaviors to meet new life-style requirements. Teach consequences of compliant versus noncompliant behavior. Use community resources to support patient and family adaptation.
Self-esteem, situational low, related to inability to concentrate	Patient will use behaviors that generate self-confidence	Support patient's verbalization of feelings about self. Assist patient in identifying personal strengths. Explore with patient ways to compensate for inability to concentrate: write journal notes, make lists, use tape recorder, ask significant others to reinforce memory. Reinforce health-promoting practices.

CRITICAL THINKING QUESTIONS

1. Mr. Johnson complains of loss of appetite as well as a limited choice of foods to eat. Helpful suggestions to improve his nutritional status would include:
2. Mr. Johnson establishes a therapeutic nurse-patient relationship with Nurse Jones. He confides that he is having marital problems partly due to his inability to have a satisfactory sexual relationship with his wife. An appropriate response by the nurse would be:
3. The nurse notes Mr. Johnson's disinterest in his therapeutic regimen of diet, medications, and fluid restrictions. He states, "What's the use? I will never be well again." Therapeutic interventions would include:

Box 30-6 NURSING INTERVENTION GUIDELINES FOR THE PATIENT UNDERGOING HEMODIALYSIS

PATIENT TEACHING

Reinforce explanation of dialysis procedure
Inform of community resources
Explain dietary restrictions
Self-care, general

MONITORING DURING DIALYSIS

Maintain asepsis and universal precautions
Weigh before and after treatment
Vital signs every 30-60 min (B/P in arm without fistula)
Maintain orientation (thought processes may be altered)
Hemorrhage resulting from heparin use during dialysis
Equipment (interruption of procedure)

ACTIVITY

Diversions (reading, television, sleep)
Comfort (reclining, sitting, lying)
Dietary intake (may be hungry or nauseated)

CARE AFTER DIALYSIS OR BETWEEN TREATMENTS

Schedule fluid intake within restrictions
Monitor signs of fluid and electrolyte imbalance
Assess the access site for signs of infection, adequate circulation
Post signs regarding location of access site; do not take blood pressure or perform a venipuncture on arm with access site
Assess, document, and report changes in general status
Skin care (bathe with tepid water to remove urea deposit)

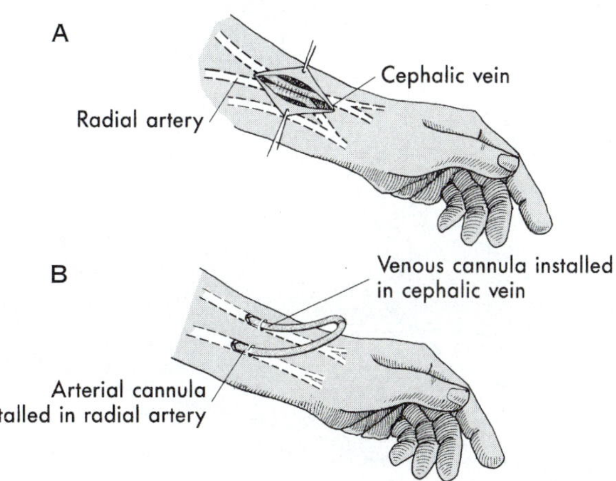

FIG. 30-8 Frequently used means for gaining vascular access for hemodialysis include: **A,** arteriovenous fistula and, **B,** external arteriovenous shunt.

NURSING INTERVENTIONS. Nursing interventions are dictated by individual patient conditions. The patient receiving renal dialysis may have other acute or chronic problems. Most patients are dialyzed on an outpatient basis. General nursing care guidelines are noted in Box 30-6 and the ESRD Nursing Care Plan on pp. 861-863.

Peritoneal dialysis. Peritoneal dialysis can be performed with a minimum of equipment and by the patient who is ambulatory. Unlike hemodialysis, peritoneal dialysis is performed 4 times a day, 7 days a week. One exchange cycle usually requires 30 to 40 minutes. The principle of osmosis and diffusion through a semipermeable membrane is the same as in hemodialysis, but the peritoneum is used as the semipermeable membrane instead of the artificial kidney. Peritoneal dialysis is contraindicated for those individuals with systemic inflammatory disease, previous abdominal surgery, and chronic back pain, among others.

The physician places a catheter into the peritoneal space under aseptic conditions (Fig. 30-9). The dialyzing fluid is then instilled for a predetermined period and then drained. The ESRD patient may be maintained on peritoneal dialysis, continuous ambulatory peritoneal dialysis (CAPD), or continuous cycle peritoneal dialysis (CCPD). The patient is taught how to do the dialysis, which allows for more freedom. Although hemodialysis can also be done at home, it is much more expensive and confining than CAPD.

NURSING INTERVENTIONS. Common complications associated with peritoneal dialysis guide nursing interventions. Hypotension may occur with excessive sodium and fluid removal. Peritonitis may arise from sepsis. Pain and/or hemorrhage may accompany instillation of the dialysate. Box 30-7 lists nursing intervention guidelines for peritoneal dialysis.

Nursing diagnoses and interventions for the patient undergoing dialysis include but are not limited to the following:

NURSING DIAGNOSES	NURSING INTERVENTIONS
Fluid volume deficit, related to dialysis or inadequate fluid intake; fluid volume excess, related to retention or noncompliance with fluid restriction	Weigh every morning. Assess skin turgor. Monitor vital signs and laboratory studies. Measure I&O. Restrict fluid intake.
Infection, high risk for, related to invasive techniques	Identify sources of potential infection. List signs of infection.
Role performance altered, related to chronic illness, treatment, side effects	Encourage verbalization of self-concept. Assist in identifying personal strengths. Assist patient and significant others with clarifying expected roles and those that must be relinquished or altered. Support grief work if lost role has occurred.
Sexuality patterns altered related to altered body function	Encourage verbalization of sexual concerns. Inform physician of patient concerns.

PROGNOSIS. The patient with effective medical management can be maintained indefinitely on dialysis.

Surgical Procedures for Urinary Dysfunction

If damage to the urinary system cannot be corrected by medical management, surgical intervention may be necessary for temporary or permanent resection of the affected organ, such as when kidney function is lost. Dialysis is a viable management alternative, but a kidney transplant is preferable. It may become necessary for the patient to have a live or cadaver kidney replace the damaged kidney. Common surgical interventions and nursing intervention priorities are listed in Table 30-4. Preoperative and intraoperative management measures are the same as for major abdominal surgery and general anesthesia (see Chapter 22). Suggested nursing diagnoses include those for abdominal surgery.

Nephrectomy. Nephrectomy is the surgical removal of the kidney. Postoperative management for surgical removal of the kidney is based on the prevention and detection of hemorrhage by monitoring vital signs, especially pulse and blood pressure; observation for restlessness, GI complications of nausea, vomiting, and abdominal distention; and establishment of adequate urinary drainage. I&O are recorded. If the thoracic cavity is opened during surgery, the patient will have chest tubes (see Chapter 31). Pain may compromise respiratory efficiency. Analgesics are administered as ordered to facilitate lung expansion and the patient's activity level. The patient is repositioned every 2 hours and ambulated as ordered. Dressings are changed according to the physician's order, and the amount and color of exudate are recorded.

Patient teaching. This includes instructing the patient to avoid heavy lifting, maintain hydration of 2000 ml each day unless contraindicated, monitor output, avoid use of alcohol, and avoid respiratory infections and hazardous activities that may cause assault to the remaining kidney.

Prognosis. Complete recovery from nephrectomy is expected in the absence of any complication.

Nephrostomy. Nephrostomy is an incision to drain the pelvis of the kidney. Catheters are used to drain the wound. Care must be given to prevent obstruction of the catheters with blood clots postoperatively. The amount of drainage from the catheters is measured and recorded,

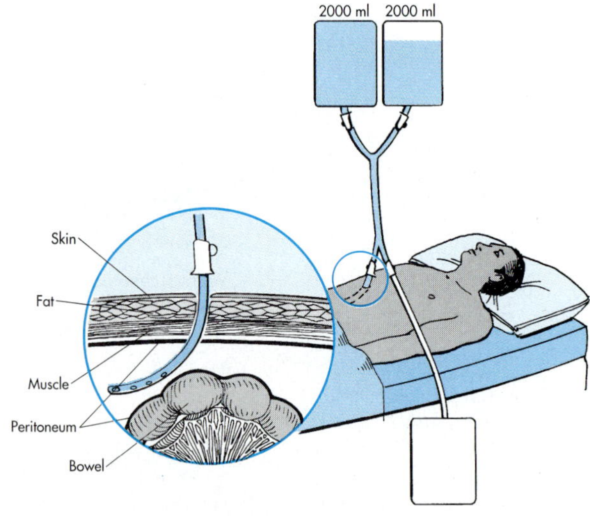

FIG. 30-9 Patient receiving peritoneal dialysis. Dialysis fluid is being inserted into peritoneal cavity.

and dressings are changed frequently, keeping the skin clean using surgical asepsis. The patient is turned and positioned to the affected side when ordered to facilitate drainage and assist in respiratory ventilation. Never clamp a nephrostomy catheter (tube); acute pyelonephritis may result. Irrigation of a nephrostomy catheter is usually done by the physician with no more than 10 ml of sterile normal saline.

Kidney transplantation. There are special considerations for nursing interventions for a kidney transplantation recipient. Preoperative nursing intervention is complicated by the patient's fear and anxiety about transplantation and about possible rejection of the implanted organ. The patient is dialyzed until surgery can be satisfactorily completed. In surgery the nonfunctioning kidney remains in place and the donor kidney is positioned in the iliac fossa anterior to the crest of the ileum. The ureter is anastomosed into either the patient's ureter or bladder (Fig. 30-10).

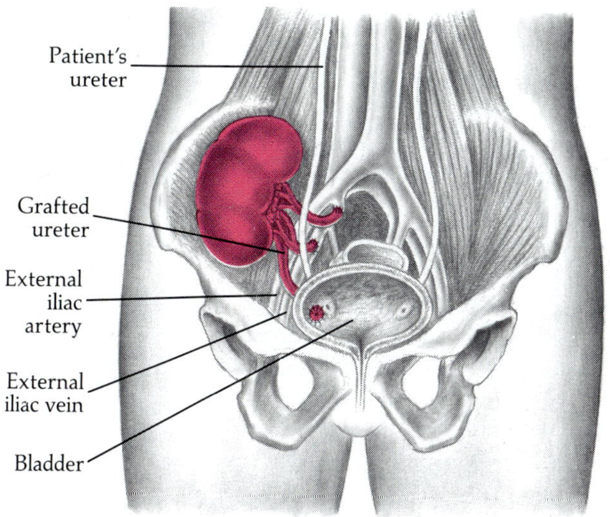

FIG. 30-10 Renal transplantation.

Postoperatively the patient is assessed for signs of rejection and infection: apprehension, generalized edema, fever, increased blood pressure, oliguria, edema, and/or tenderness over the graft site. An immunosuppressive therapeutic agent, such as cyclosporine (Sandimmune), is used alone or in conjunction with steroids. Cyclosporine is considered the most effective drug to date in suppressing the immune system's efforts to reject tissue while leaving the recipient sufficient immune activity to combat infection. Immunosuppressive therapy increases the risk for infection and possible steroid-induced bleeding.

Box 30-7 NURSING INTERVENTION GUIDELINES FOR THE PATIENT UNDERGOING PERITONEAL DIALYSIS

PATIENT TEACHING

Explanation of procedure
Signs of complications
Diet and/or fluid restrictions
Medication (schedule in relation to dialysis time)
Dialysate should be body temperature to lessen discomfort

MONITORING DURING DIALYSIS

Weigh before and after procedure
Hemorrhage (smoky, pink, or red-tinged dialysate)
Type of dialysate (tailored to patient needs)
Amount and timing of dialysate instillation
Vital signs

CARE BETWEEN DIALYSES

Signs of peritonitis (pain, fever, cloudy fluid)
Strict aseptic care of catheter site
Weigh daily

TABLE 30-4 Surgical Interventions and Nursing Intervention Priorities

Surgical Intervention	Nursing Intervention Priorities
Nephrostomy—surgical procedure in which an incision is made on the flank of patient so that a catheter can be inserted into the kidney pelvis for drainage	Meticulous skin care, assessment for hemorrhage, accurate I&O
Nephrectomy—surgical removal of the kidney	Assessment for hemorrhage, promotion of respiratory effort, accurate I&O
Cystectomy—surgical removal of the bladder	Promotion of urinary drainage via ileoconduit, I&O
Ureterosigmoidostomy—surgical procedure in which a ureter is implanted in the sigmoid colon of the intestinal tract	Meticulous skin care, monitoring of electrolyte imbalance, assessment of signs and symptoms of infection
Cutaneous ureterostomy—surgical implantation of the terminal ends of the ureter under the skin	Meticulous skin care, assessment of urinary obstruction, accurate I&O

Patient teaching. Home follow-up becomes a life pattern for the transplantation patient. Patient education is extensive: diet, fluids, daily weights, strict I&O measurement, prevention of infection, and avoidance of activities that may compromise the integrity of the urinary tract. Community support groups, sponsored by the National Association of Patients on Hemodialysis and Transplantation, Inc., assist the patient and family to adapt to living with dialysis and transplantation. The National Kidney Foundation has a written protocol for the procurement of organs for donation.

Prognosis. Successful transplantation parallels the individual patient's general health status and compliance to the treatment plan. Transplantation offers the only possibility of return to a normal life-style for ESRD patient.

Urinary Diversion. Several types of procedures are used to divert the flow of urine when required for treatment of bladder cancer, invasive cancer of the cervix, neurogenic bladder, and congenital anomalies. Often a cystectomy is done to surgically remove the bladder.

The cystectomy patient presents a unique challenge because of the need to create an artificial port for urine elimination. The most common urinary diversion procedure is the ileal conduit (Bricker's procedure or ileal loop). In an **ileal conduit** procedure the ureters are implanted into a loop of the ileum that is isolated and brought to the surface of the abdominal wall (Fig. 30-11). Occasionally a segment of the sigmoid colon is isolated and used instead of the ileum (sigmoid conduit). The integrity of bowel function is maintained with the

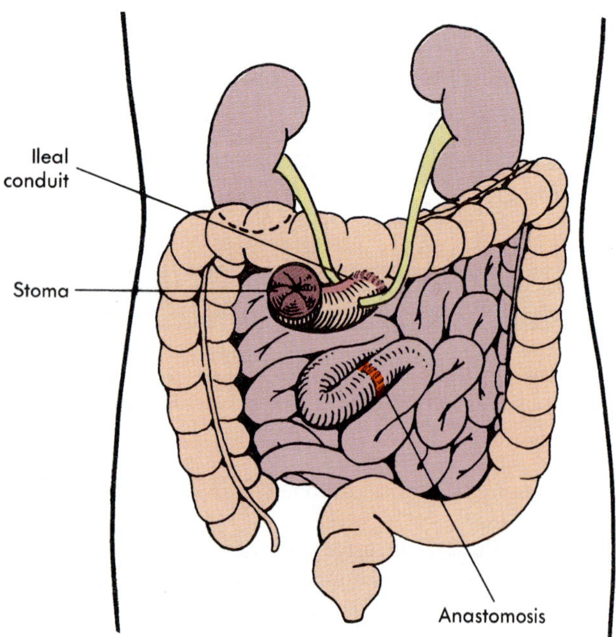

FIG. 30-11 Ileal conduit or ileal loop.

anastomosis of the remaining intestine. A drainage bag (urostomy bag or appliance) is fitted over the stoma to contain the constant drainage of urine. Continual urine drainage prevents increased pressure within the conduit that would cause backflow to the kidneys, compromise the circulatory integrity of the conduit, or rupture the surgical anastomosis. Decreased urine output and low abdominal pain may signal the onset of such problems. Complications of this procedure are wound infection, dehiscence, urinary leakage, ureteral obstruction, small bowel obstruction, stomal gangrene, contraction of the stoma, pyelonephritis, renal calculi, and/or a compromised respiratory status secondary to incisional pain.

Postoperatively, urine flow is measured hourly. Output below 30 ml per hour should be reported to the physician immediately. A healthy stoma will appear moist and pink and may even bleed slightly. The skin around the stoma should be inspected daily for signs of bleeding, excoriation, and infection. Any odor of urine about the patient may indicate an infection or leak of urine from the drainage bag. Large quantities of water should be ingested to flush the ileal conduit. There will be mucus present in the urine from the intestinal secretions.

Care of the patient with an ileal conduit is a nursing challenge because of the continual drainage of urine through the stoma.

To change the urostomy bag, the urostomy bag is drained and removed. The skin is cleansed with water, and the new appliance is applied as outlined in the institution's standards of care. (See Skill 30-6 for a discussion on stomal care.) When the peristomal skin is healed, the bag is emptied at 2- to 3-hour intervals and a straight drainage tube connected to a drainage bag is used at night. A permanent urostomy bag can be left in place 4 to 7 days if it remains sealed. The nurse should recommend that the patient have two bags so one can be worn while the other is washed. Some patients prefer to use disposable bags. Odor is controlled by using deodorant drops or tablets in the urostomy bag; avoiding odor-producing foods, such as beans, onions, cabbage, asparagus, high-fiber wheat, simple sugars, and milk in the lactose-intolerant patient; and cleansing the urostomy bag with a vinegar and water rinse and thoroughly drying.

Patient teaching. Patient teaching centers on the task of life-style adaptation: care of the stoma, nutrition, fluid intake, maintaining self-esteem in light of altered body image, modifying sexual activities, and early detection of complications. Patient teaching begins with appliance selection, sizing the stoma, and changing the appliance. The home health nurse can assist the patient in modifying care to the home environment and by providing support during this stressful adjustment period.

The continent ileal urinary reservoir, or Kock pouch, is created by implantation of the ureters into a segment of the small intestine that has been surgically removed from the rest of the bowel and anastomosed to the ab-

SKILL 30-6

PERFORMING UROSTOMY CARE

1. Introduce self.
2. Identify patient.
3. Wash hands.
4. Explain procedure.
5. Arrange supplies at bedside or in bathroom.
6. Pull curtain and close door to provide privacy.
7. Position patient so that stoma is easily accessible and patient is comfortable.
8. Don gloves.

NOTE:

As many of the following steps as possible should be performed by the patient with the nurse teaching and assisting as necessary. Independence will come. Allow time for grieving for a lost body part. Be alert to signs of patient readiness.

9. Empty urine into graduated pitcher; write down amount for later documentation.
10. Carefully remove wafer seal from skin (adhesive solvent may need to be used) and place pouch in plastic bag.
11. Cleanse skin with warm water, and pat dry to avoid rubbing and causing skin impairment.
12. Measure stoma using measuring device; note color and viability of stoma.
13. Place gauze over stoma to prevent urine from contacting skin.
14. If using Skin Prep, apply to skin and allow to dry; apply protective stoma paste about 1⁄16 inch from the stoma.
15. Apply protective wafer with flange, cutting an opening in the center of wafer 1⁄16 inch larger than stoma.
16. Gently attach pouch to flange by compressing the two together.
17. If belt is used, attach at this time. Be certain belt is on the level with stoma. Applying belt above or below stoma can break appliance's seal or can cause belt to rub or injure stoma.
18. Attach pouch to gravity drainage tubing if ordered.
19. Assist patient to comfortable position.
20. Clean and store equipment.
21. Dispose of soiled supplies in plastic bag; remove gloves; wash hands as per universal precautions.
22. Record procedure and observations.
23. Report abnormalities to charge nurse or physician.

SPECIAL CONCERNS

- Avoid touching the stoma with adhesive solvents to prevent irritating the stoma.
- Wick the urine with an absorbent, lint-free material to prevent a constant flow of urine while changing the appliance.
- Remove hair from the stomal area with scissors or an electric razor to prevent hair follicles from becoming irritated when the pouch is removed.
- Suggest that the procedure be performed in the morning before fluids are consumed and when urine flows more slowly.
- Tell the patient that when applied properly, the appliance should remain in place 3 to 5 days.

PATIENT TEACHING

- Teach the patient to empty appliance through the drain valve when it is one-third to one-half full to prevent the weight of the urine from loosening the seal around the stoma.
- Teach the patient to connect the appliance to a urine-collection container at night to prevent urine from stagnating in the appliance.
- Teach the patient sanitary and dietary measures that can protect the peristomal skin and control odor.
- Offer positive reinforcement and written instructions.

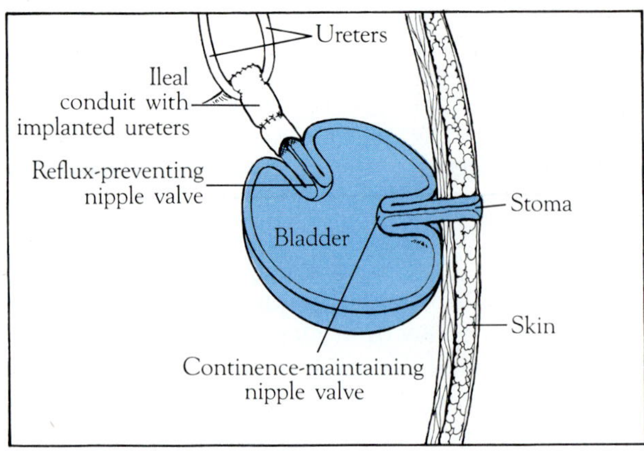

FIG. 30-12 Kock pouch.

dominal wall. Control of urine flow is achieved by the use of a nipplelike valve that prevents leakage of urine. To drain the urine from the reservoir, the patient inserts a catheter through the valve at regular intervals, thus minimizing the reabsorption of waste materials from the urine and reflux into the ureters (Fig. 30-12).

Prognosis. Although the patient may fully recover without recurrence, the day-to-day challenges of managing a urinary diversion will be permanent.

THERAPEUTIC DIALOGUE

Tom Jones, student nurse, enters Barry Johnson's room to complete the initial morning assessment and finds him crying while struggling to get out of bed.

Mr. Jones: Mr. Johnson, what is wrong? *(General lead, allows patient to describe)*

Mr. Johnson: Oh, nothing!

Mr. Jones: (Therapeutic silence, remains attentive, gives time)

Mr. Johnson: Nothing is going right. I might as well be dead!

Mr. Jones: What is wrong? (General lead, he didn't answer, encourages description)

Mr. Johnson: I was trying to get up to take a shower, but I'm so weak I can't get myself out of bed.

Mr. Jones: That must be frustrating. *(Voicing the implied)*

Mr. Johnson: That's an understatement! Look at me! I'm 37 years old; I should be in my prime but instead I'm losing weight; can't do my job because I can't concentrate. How am I suppose to feel?

Mr. Jones: It must be frightening to experience all these changes. It would be understandable for you to be scared. *(Validating feelings)*

Mr. Johnson: I am scared! What if I never get better? I read this article about someone younger than I am who had the same thing and he died when he had to go on dialysis.

Mr. Jones: What do you think will happen to you? *(General lead, encourages description without prescribing response)*

Mr. Johnson: Well, I don't know. The doctor keeps avoiding my questions and I see myself being less able to do anything. Maybe I am afraid—afraid of dying.

Mr. Jones: (Therapeutic silence, allows time for reflection)

Mr. Johnson: Well, I never thought I'd say that—being afraid to die. It doesn't seem so frightening to say. I guess I didn't trust myself to be honest with myself or anyone else.

Mr. Jones: Being honest with yourself is an important step to understanding. *(pause)* It seems, too, that you may not have accurate information about your illness. Let's plan to talk with your doctor about what you can reasonably expect—things you will be able to do, limitations, and things that you can do to enhance your physical and emotional health. *(Summarizing and goal-setting for individualized patient teaching and discharge planning)*

Mr. Johnson: That sounds great, Mr. Jones. I really do want to do whatever I can to improve my chances of a better life. Would you help me get up to shower?

REFERENCES AND SUGGESTED READINGS

1. Abrams AC: *Clinical drug therapy,* ed 3, Philadelphia, 1991, Lippincott.
2. American Cancer Society: *Cancer facts and figures 1991,* Atlanta, 1991, The Society.
3. American Cancer Society: *Cancer manual,* ed 8, Boston, 1990, The Society.
4. Bender P: Deceptive distress in the elderly, *Am J Nurs* 92(10):28, 1992.
5. Brenner MB, Rector FC, editors: *The kidney,* ed 4, Philadelphia, 1991, Saunders.
6. Brundage DJ: *Renal disorders,* St Louis, 1992, Mosby.
7. Brunner LS, Suddarth DS, Bare BG: *Textbook of medical-surgical nursing,* ed 7, Philadelphia, 1991, Lippincott.
8. CA Cancer J Clin 42:4, 1992.
9. Chambers JK: Renal insufficiency implications for care of the medical-surgical patient, *Med-Surg Nurs* 2(1), 1993.
10. Clark JB, Queener SF, Karb VB: *Pharmacologic basis of nursing practice,* ed 4, 1993, St Louis, Mosby.
11. *Clinical practice guideline: urinary incontinence in adults,* March 1992, US Department of Health & Human Services.
12. Dunn SA: How to care for a dialysis patient, *Am J Nurs* 93(6):26, 1993.
13. Faller NA: Clean intermittent catheterization, *Ostomy Wound Manage* 38(7):29, 1992.
14. Fischbach FT: *A manual of laboratory and diagnostic tests,* ed 4, Philadelphia, 1992, Lippincott.
15. Fox F: Recurring urinary tract infections: incident and risk factors, *Am J Public Health* 80(3):331, 1990.
16. Gillenwater JY: *The 1991 year book of urology,* St Louis, 1991, Mosby.
17. Graham-Macaluso MM: Complications of peritoneal dialysis: nursing care plans to document teaching, *ANNA J* 18(5):459, 1991.
18. Haskell CM: *Cancer treatment,* ed 3, Philadelphia, 1990, Saunders.
19. Hood GH, Dincher JR: *Total patient care: foundations and practice,* ed 8, St Louis, 1992, Mosby.
20. Ignatavicius DD, Bayne MV: *Medical-surgical nursing,* Philadelphia, 1991, Saunders.
21. Jacobson JR, Striker GE, Klahr S: *The principles and practice of nephology,* St Louis, 1991, Mosby.
22. Kalatrieder DL et al: Can remainders curb incontinence? *Geriatr Nurs* 11(1):17, 1990.

23. Karb VB, Queener SF, Freeman JB: *Handbook of drugs for nursing practice,* St Louis, 1992, Mosby.
24. Kim MJ, McFarland GK, McLane AM: *Pocket guide to nursing diagnoses,* ed 5, St Louis, 1993, Mosby.
25. Kuhn MM: *Pharmacotherapeutics: a nursing process approach,* ed 2, Philadelphia, 1991, FA Davis.
26. Lederer JR et al: *Care planning pocket guide,* ed 3, Redwood City, Calif, 1990, Addison-Wesley.
27. Levinsky NG, Retlig RA: The Medicare End-Stage Renal Disease Program, *N Engl J Med* 324(16):1143, 1991.
28. Lewis SM, Collier IC: *Medical-surgical nursing: assessment and management of clinical problems,* ed 3, St Louis, 1993, Mosby.
29. Long BC, Phipps WJ, Cassmeyer VL: *Medical-surgical nursing: a nursing process approach,* ed 3, St Louis, 1993, Mosby.
30. Malseed ZK: *Pharmacology drug therapy and nursing considerations,* ed 3, Phildelphia, 1990, Lippincott.
31. Martin JP: Transrectal ultrasound: a new screening test for prostatic cancer, *Am J Nurs* 91(2):69, 1991.
32. McCance KL, Huether SE: *Pathophysiology: the biologic basis of disease in adults and children,* St Louis, 1990, Mosby.
33. McCormick KA et al: Urinary incontinence in adults, *Am J Nurs* 92:10, 1992.
34. McHenry LM, Salerno E: *Mosby's pharmacology in nursing,* ed 18, St Louis, 1992, Mosby.
35. Moore MC: *Pocket guide to nutrition and diet theory,* St Louis, 1993, Mosby.
36. Moore S et al: Bladder cancer: new methods, new management, *Am J Nurs* 93(5):32, 1993.
37. Morton PG: *Health assessment in nursing,* ed 2, Springhouse, Penn, 1993, Springhouse.
38. *Mosby's medical, nursing, and allied health dictionary,* ed 4, 1994, St Louis, Mosby.
39. Neuman DK et al: Restoring urinary continence, *Am J Nurs* 91(1):28, 1991.
40. Nill JV: What's wrong with this peristomal skin? *Am J Nurs* 91(12):44, 1991.
41. Pagana KD, Pagana TJ: *Diagnostic testing and nursing implications: a case study approach,* ed 4, 1994, St Louis, Mosby.
42. Pagana KD, Pagana TJ: *Mosby's diagnostic and laboratory test reference,* 1992, St Louis, Mosby.
43. Palmer MH et al: Risk factors for urinary incontinence one year after nursing home admission, *Res Nurs Health* 14:405, 1991.
44. Phipps WJ et al: *Medical-surgical nursing: concepts and clinical practice,* ed 4, St Louis, 1991, Mosby.
45. Potter PA, Perry AG: *Fundamentals of nursing: concepts, process, and practice,* ed 3, St Louis, 1993, Mosby.
46. Power I, Williams D: Urinary incontinence: helping a patient regain control, *Nursing* 22(12):46, 1992.
47. Schroder SA, Tierney LM, editors: *Current medical diagnosis and treatment,* Norwalk, Conn, 1991, Appleton & Lange.
48. Shipley WU et al: Cancer of the prostate. In *Cancer manual,* ed 8, Boston, 1990, American Cancer Society.
49. Spender RT et al: *Clinical pharmacology and nursing management,* ed 4, Philadelphia, 1993, Lippincott.
50. The Staff: *Fundamental nursing skills,* Springhouse, Penn, 1992, Springhouse.
51. Thomas CL: *Taber's cyclopedic medical dictionary,* ed 17, Philadelphia, 1993, FA Davis.
52. Thompson JM et al: *Mosby's clinical nursing,* ed 3, 1993, St Louis, Mosby.
53. Toto KH: Acute renal failure: a question of location, *Am J Nurs* 92(11):44, 1992.
54. Tucker SM et al: *Patient care standards, nursing process, diagnosis and outcome,* ed 5, St Louis, 1992, Mosby.
55. Webber-Jones J: Performing clean, intermittent self-catheterization, *Nursing* 8:56, 1991.
56. Weber J: *Nurses' handbook of health assessment,* ed 2, Philadelphia, 1993, Lippincott.
57. Wever J: *Nurse's handbook of health assessment,* ed 2, Philadelphia, 1993, Lippincott.
58. Williams SR: *Essentials of nutrition and diet therapy,* ed 6, St Louis, 1994, Mosby.
59. Willis D: Taming the overgrown prostate, *Am J Nurs* 92(2):34, 1992.
60. Wong DL: *Nursing care of infants and children,* ed 5, St Louis, 1995, Mosby.
61. Worthington JF: Outlining prostate cancer, *Hopkins Medical News* 15(2):20, 1992.

CHAPTER CHALLENGE

KEY POINTS

- The kidneys lie retroperitoneally, just below the diaphragm.
- The functioning unit of the kidney is the nephron.
- The kidneys rid the body of wastes and excess electrolytes, maintain water and electrolyte balance, and maintain acid-base balance.
- Kidney function is achieved by the processes of filtration, secretion, and reabsorption.
- Assessment of the urinary tract is included in baseline data for all patients.
- The subject of urinary problems is an embarrassing topic for many patients. The nurse must be sensitive to the patient's feelings and be supportive.
- Aging may have a negative influence on urinary function, but many problems can be corrected.
- Hydration status is monitored by daily weights, I&O, laboratory studies, inspection of the skin and mucous membranes, and level of consciousness.
- A large percentage of nosocomial infections involve the urinary tract.
- Proper care of urinary catheters will decrease the chance of urinary tract infections.
- Surgical intervention may be indicated for urinary dysfunction that cannot be corrected by medical management.
- Dialysis, which mimics kidney function, may be used temporarily or as a long-term therapy.
- Dietary fluid and medication modifications may be necessary for the patient with urinary dysfunction.

STUDY QUESTIONS

1. After the physician explains the urinary diversion procedure to Mr. Clinton, he continues to ask the nurse questions. The best response by the nurse would be:
   1. "Tell me what you know about the surgery."
   2. "The doctor will answer any questions you have tomorrow."
   3. "Mr. Clinton, please don't worry about your surgery. We will take good care of you."
   4. "Why don't you talk to your wife and try to forget about the surgery for a while."
2. The patient receiving potassium-depleting diuretic therapy is encouraged to include the following group of foods in the diet:
   1. Liver, eggs, dark green vegetables
   2. Corn flakes, wheat breads, corn grits
   3. Tomatoes, citrus fruits, broccoli
   4. Cottage cheese and other cheese products
3. Which of the following nursing diagnoses should receive first priority in planning care of the patient with ESRD:
   1. Health maintenance, altered
   2. Fluid volume excess
   3. Denial, ineffective
   4. Role performance, altered
4. Mr. Cordova, age 72, is taking a diuretic called Bumex. Which of these findings would suggest that the Bumex is having the desired effect:
   1. Decreased bacteremia
   2. Decreased confusion
   3. Increased diuresis
   4. Increased albuminuria
5. Ms. Jorgens is scheduled for an intravenous urography examination. Before the procedure, it is essential to obtain information from Ms. Jorgens regarding any allergy to:
   1. Sweet potatoes
   2. Dairy products
   3. Saltwater fish
   4. Wheat products
6. Mr. Lemley, a 42-year-old construction worker, is admitted with a diagnosis of recurrent urolithiasis. He has been medicated with meperidine (Demerol) 100 mg and promethazine HCl (Phenergan) 25 mg. Mr. Lemley is very restless and wants to walk. The nurse's first priority at this time is to:
   1. Encourage fluid intake
   2. Monitor urinary output
   3. Obtain a medical history
   4. Maintain a safe environment
7. Which of these observations of the older patient's urinary function would the nurse expect to find as a result of the aging process:
   1. Intermittent changes in urine concentration
   2. Changes in voiding patterns
   3. Decreased urine output
   4. Changes in color, volume, odor
8. The nurse explains to Mr. Rote that he will not be permitted oral intake for at least 8 hours before the intravenous urography examination in order to:
   1. Enhance the effects of the dye
   2. Increase urine dilution
   3. Reduce bladder distention
   4. Prevent visualization disturbances
9. Mr. Langford is admitted with ESRD. He has a greatly elevated blood urea nitrogen of 85 mg/dl. With excessive elevation of the blood urea nitrogen level, Mr. Langford should be assessed for:
   1. Dysuria
   2. Dystrophy
   3. Dehydration
   4. Disorientation
10. Which of the following findings on a routine urinalysis report would indicate an abnormal result:
    1. Turbidity clear
    2. pH 6.0
    3. 3+ protein
    4. Bilirubin negative
11. During a follow-up visit after being diagnosed with chronic glomerulonephritis, Mrs. Webb asks why she has anemia when her problem is with her kidneys. The nurse understands that one factor is:
    1. The acid-base imbalance suppresses red bone marrow
    2. The healthy kidney produces erythropoietic factor
    3. The healthy kidney eliminates red blood cells
    4. Increasing BUN levels destroy red blood cells
12. During the interview Mr. Redman begins to cry when relating the reason for his hospital admission. The best response for the nurse would be to:
    1. Continue the interview as though nothing has happened
    2. Wait quietly until he can continue
    3. Tell him not to worry about crying
    4. Leave so he can be alone

31

CARE OF THE PATIENT WITH A RESPIRATORY DISORDER

Barbara Christensen
Elaine Kockrow

KEY TERMS

ANATOMY AND PHYSIOLOGY
alveolus
bronchiole
chemoreceptor
cilia
hemoglobin
hilum (hilus)
larynx
pharynx
pleural effusion
surface tension
surfactant
trachea
tracheostomy

MEDICAL-SURGICAL
acute coryza
adventitious
atelectasis
bronchoscopy
cor pulmonale
crackle
cyanosis
dyspnea
embolism
empyema
epistaxis
exacerbation
extrinsic
hemoptysis
hypercapnia
hypoventilation
hypoxia
intrinsic
orthopnea
pleural friction rub
pneumothorax
sibilant wheeze
sonorous wheeze
stertorous
tachypnea
thoracentesis
virulent

LEARNING OBJECTIVES

After reading this chapter, the student should be able to do the following:

Anatomy and Physiology

- Define the key terms.
- List and define the parts of the upper and lower respiratory tract.
- Describe the purpose of the respiratory system.
- Differentiate between external and internal respiration.
- List the ways in which oxygen and carbon dioxide are transported in the blood.
- Discuss the mechanisms that regulate respirations.

Medical-Surgical

- Define the key terms.
- List five nursing interventions to assist patients with retained pulmonary secretions.
- Identify those signs and symptoms that indicate a patient is experiencing hypoxia.
- Identify four strategies the nurse can teach patients to decrease the risk of infection.
- Differentiate between tuberculosis infection and tuberculosis disease.
- List three medications commonly prescribed for the patient with tuberculosis.
- Differentiate between medical management of the patient with emphysema and the patient with asthma.
- Discuss why low-flow oxygen is required for patients with emphysema.
- Compare/contrast nursing observations and interventions for the patient with chronic obstructive pulmonary disease (COPD) and the patient with pneumonia.
- List three nursing observations/interventions pertaining to the care of the patient with closed chest drainage.
- Discuss nursing interventions for the patient with a laryngectomy.
- State three possible nursing diagnoses for the patient with altered respiratory function.
- Identify nursing interventions relevant to psychosocial concerns of the patient with altered respiratory function.
- Discuss three risk factors associated with pulmonary emboli.

RELATED TOPICS OF INTEREST

- Signs, symptoms, and physical assessment (Chapter 9)
- Vital signs (Chapter 10)
- Specimen collection and diagnostic examination (Chapter 17)
- The surgical patient (Chapter 22)
- Care of the patient with a cardiovascular disorder (Chapter 28)
- Care of the patient with a blood or lymphatic disorder (Chapter 29)
- Care of the patient with an endocrine disorder (Chapter 32)
- Care of the patient with a neurological disorder (Chapter 35)
- Cardiopulmonary resuscitation (Chapter 50)

ANATOMY AND PHYSIOLOGY

If an individual has experienced choking or has had to struggle for breath, the sensation of panic is a reminder that one cannot live without oxygen. For the millions of cells throughout the body to carry out their specialized activities, it is mandatory that they have a continuous supply of oxygen. External respiration, or breathing, allows the exchange of oxygen and carbon dioxide between the lungs and the environment. As air is inhaled, it is warmed, moistened, and filtered to prepare it for use by the body. The respiratory system works with the cardiovascular system to deliver the oxygen to the cells, where it is used to provide the cells with energy to carry out metabolism. Internal respiration refers to the exchange of oxygen and carbon dioxide at the cellular level. Oxygen enters the cells while carbon dioxide leaves the cells. These gases diffuse across the cell membranes into the bloodstream. The cardiovascular system plays the role of transporter. Failure of the respiratory or cardiovascular system has the same result: rapid death of the cells from oxygen starvation. Fig. 31-1 shows the structural plan of the respiratory organs.

Upper Respiratory Tract

Nose. Air enters the respiratory tract through the nose. The air is filtered, moistened, and warmed as it enters the two nasal openings (nares) and travels to the nasal cavity. The nasal septum separates the nares. This entire area is lined with mucous membrane, which is vascular. This provides the warmth and moisture necessary. Normally a liter of moisture is secreted by this membrane every day.

Lateral to the nasal cavities are the three scroll-like bones called *turbinates* or *conchae* (Fig. 31-2), which cause the air to move over a larger surface area. This increase in surface area allows the air more time for warming and moisturizing. Lining the nasal cavities are tiny hairs, which trap dust and other foreign particles and prevent them from entering the lower respiratory tract.

Communicating with the nasal structures are the paranasal sinuses (Fig. 31-3 on p. 874). They are called the *frontal, maxillary, sphenoid,* and *ethmoid cavities.* They are hollow areas, which makes the skull lighter. It is believed they give resonance to the voice. They are lined with mucous membrane continuous with the nasal cavity. Because of this, nasal infections can cause sinusitis, which is uncomfortable and difficult to treat.

The receptors for the sense of smell are located in the mucosa of the nasal cavities. They are the nerve endings of the olfactory nerve, the first cranial nerve. The nasolacrimal ducts, or tear ducts, communicate with the upper nasal chamber. Hence when an individual cries, there are copious nasal secretions.

Pharynx. The **pharynx** (a tubular structure about 5 inches [13 cm] long that extends from the base of the skull to the esophagus and is situated just in front of the cervical vertebrae), or throat, is the passageway for both air and food. At the distal end of the pharynx, food passes to the esophagus. The pharynx is divided into three subdivisions: (1) nasopharynx (most superior portion); (2) oropharynx (posterior to mouth); and (3) laryngopharynx (directly superior to larynx).

The eustachian tubes enter either side of the nasopharynx, connecting it to the middle ear. Because the inner linings of the pharynx and the eustachian tubes are continuous, an infection of the pharynx can spread easily to the middle ear. This is very common in children.

In the mucous membrane of the pharynx are masses of lymphatic tissue called the tonsils. The adenoids (pharyngeal tonsils) are in the nasopharynx, whereas the palatine tonsils are in the oropharynx. Inflammation of these structures is referred to as *tonsillitis,* also very common in children. Physicians now recognize the importance of tonsils because of their lymphatic properties and thus their role in body defense mechanisms. Fewer tonsillectomy procedures are being performed.

Larynx. The **larynx** (Fig. 31-4, *A* on p. 875), or organ of voice, is supported by nine areas of cartilage and connects the pharynx with the trachea. The largest area of cartilage is composed of two fused plates and is called the *thyroid cartilage* or *Adam's apple.* It is the same size in females and males until puberty. At puberty, it produces a large projection in the neck of the male due to its enlargement. The epiglottis, a large, leaf-shaped area of cartilage, protects the larynx when swallowing. It covers the larynx tightly to prevent food from entering the trachea and directs the food to the esophagus (Fig. 31-4, *B*.)

The larynx contains the vocal cords, which are muscular folds of tissue that extend from the lateral walls. During expiration air rushes over the vocal cords, which

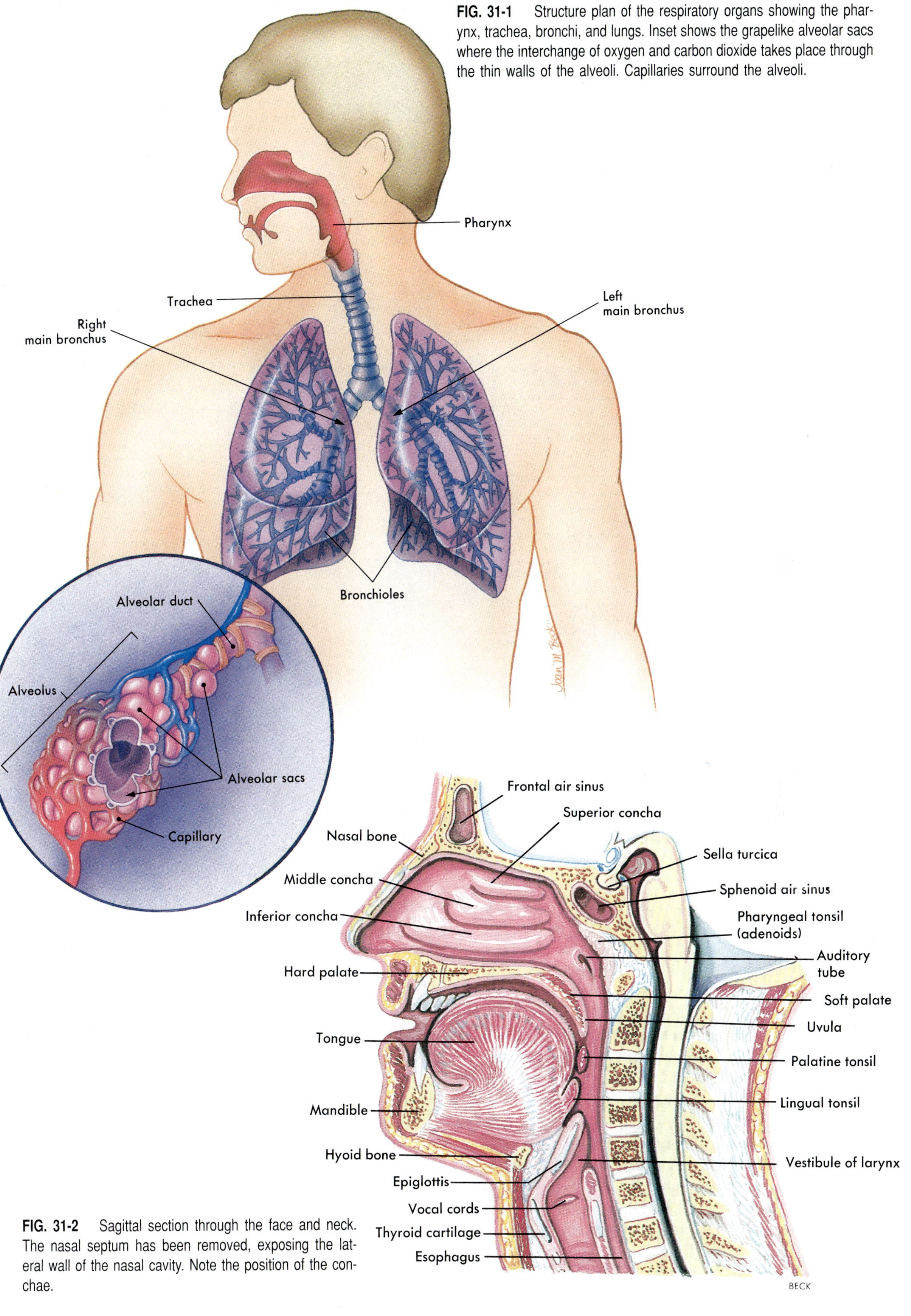

FIG. 31-1 Structure plan of the respiratory organs showing the pharynx, trachea, bronchi, and lungs. Inset shows the grapelike alveolar sacs where the interchange of oxygen and carbon dioxide takes place through the thin walls of the alveoli. Capillaries surround the alveoli.

FIG. 31-2 Sagittal section through the face and neck. The nasal septum has been removed, exposing the lateral wall of the nasal cavity. Note the position of the conchae.

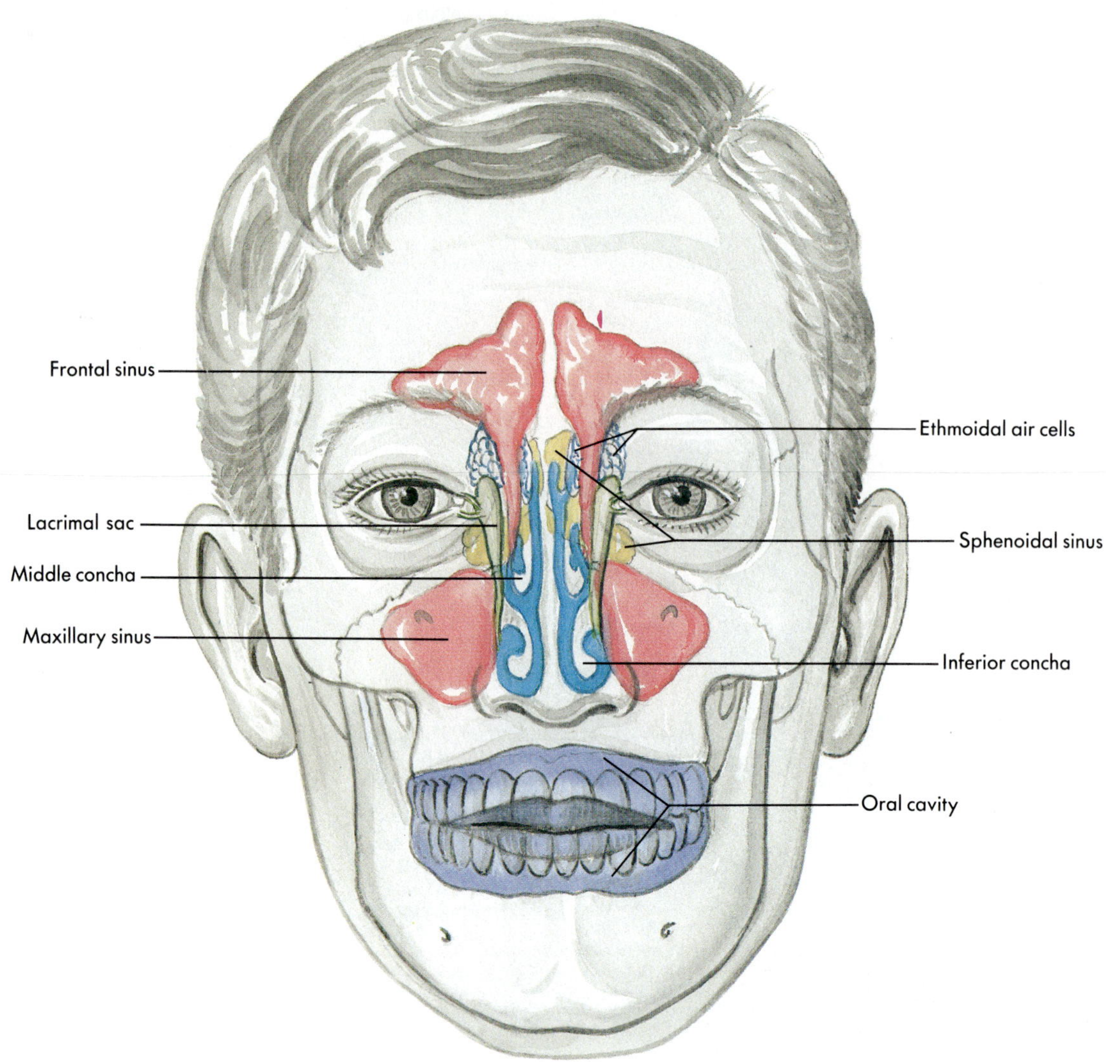

FIG. 31-3 Projections of paranasal sinuses and oral nasal cavities on the skull and face. Note the direct connection between the sinuses and the nasal cavity.

causes them to vibrate. This enables speech to occur. The opening between the vocal cords is the glottis. The size of the vocal cords varies, which accounts for differences in pitch. Because the male usually has larger vocal cords, his voice is deeper than the female's.

Trachea. The **trachea,** or windpipe, is a tubelike structure that extends approximately 5 inches (11 cm) to the midchest, where it divides into the right and left bronchi. It lies anterior to the esophagus and connects the larynx with the bronchi. The ventral (anterior) surface of the tube is covered in the neck by the isthmus (narrow connection) of the thyroid gland. It contains C-shaped cartilaginous rings that keep it from collapsing. The open part of the C-shape lies posterior to the column, anterior to the esophagus, which allows for expansion of the esophagus during swallowing while still maintaining patency of the trachea. This is necessary for uninterrupted breathing. The entire structure is lined with mucous membrane with tiny **cilia** (small, hairlike processes on the outer surfaces of small cells, aiding metabolism by producing motion or current in a fluid) that sweep dust or debris upward toward the nasal cavity. Any large particles initiate the cough reflex, which is a protective mechanism that aids in the evacuation of foreign material. Sometimes, because of an airway obstruction, it becomes necessary to perform a **tracheostomy** (a surgical opening into the trachea through which an indwelling tube may be inserted). Once this procedure is completed, the individual breathes through the tracheal opening rather than the nose. The opening is below the larynx, so the air cannot pass over the vocal cords. The vocal cords cannot vibrate, and speech becomes physiologically impossible.

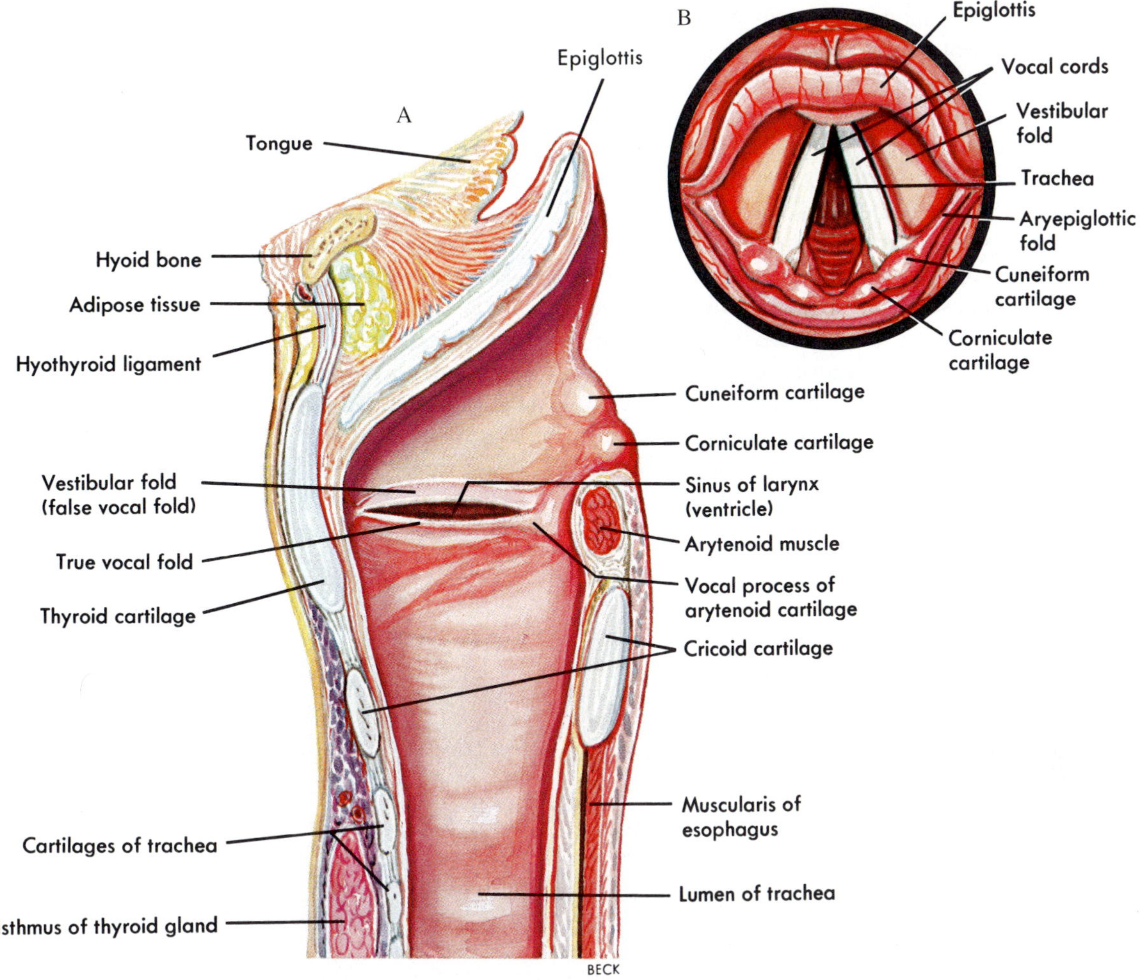

FIG. 31-4 **A,** Sagittal section through the larynx. **B,** Larynx and vocal cords as viewed from above through a laryngeal mirror.

Lower Respiratory Tract

Bronchial Tree. As the trachea enters the lungs, it divides into the right and left bronchi. The right bronchus enters into the right lung. It is larger in diameter and more vertical in descent. The left bronchus enters the left lung. It is smaller in diameter and slightly horizontal in position. Because of this design, foreign objects that are aspirated generally enter the right bronchus.

The large bronchi continue to divide into smaller structures called **bronchioles** (a small airway of the respiratory system extending from the bronchi into the lobes of the lung). These structures continue to divide into smaller, tubelike structures called terminal bronchioles or alveolar ducts. All these structures are lined with ciliated mucous membrane, as is the trachea.

The end structures of the bronchial tree are called alveoli. These saclike structures resemble a bunch of grapes. A single grapelike structure is called an **alveolus** (a combing form meaning "trough, channel, cavity") (see Figs. 31-1 and 31-5). It is in this terminal structure of the bronchial tree that gas exchange takes place. Each alveolus is surrounded by a blood capillary, where diffusion of carbon dioxide and oxygen occurs.

Main bronchi and bronchioles. As stated, the lungs contain a right primary bronchus and a left primary bronchus. The bronchi consist of three layers of tissue. The outer layer is composed of fibrous tissue reinforced with cartilage. The middle layer is composed of smooth muscle. The innermost layer is mucous membrane coated with cilia. The bronchi connect the trachea to the smaller tubules, the bronchioles.

As the bronchi divide into the smaller structures, bronchioles, they lose the outer cartilage and fibrous tissue. Their walls are thinner and contain elastic tissue. It has been estimated that there are more than a million bronchioles in each lung. This branching and continual division of tubules make these structures resemble a tree with its branches—hence the name bronchial tree.

Alveoli. The terminal structure of the bronchial tree is the alveolus, a small, grapelike structure. Alveoli are contained in small sacs called the alveolar sacs. The walls of the individual alveoli are composed of a single layer of cells with elastic fibers intertwined. This enables them to contract and relax with breathing. Alveoli are very effective in gas exchange, mainly because they are extremely thin-walled; each alveolus lies in contact with a blood capillary. In addition, each alveolus is coated with a thin covering of **surfactant** (certain lipoproteins that reduce the surface tension of pulmonary fluids, allowing the exchange of gases in the alveoli of the lungs and contributing to the elasticity of pulmonary tissues). Surfactant reduces the **surface tension** (the tendency of the surface of a liquid to minimize the area of its surface by contracting; this property affects the exchange of gases in the pulmonary alveoli) of the alveolus and prevents it from collapsing after each breath (Fig. 31-5). There are millions of alveoli in the lungs; they give shape and form to the lungs. They are filled with air, and lung tissue would float if put in water.

This tiny, grapelike structure is the most important feature of the respiratory system. It is here the oxygen diffuses into the cardiovascular system.

In the cardiovascular system the vessels get smaller and smaller until they reach the smallest structure, called a capillary, which is microscopic. In the lungs these capillaries surround the alveoli. Because the walls of the capillaries are thin and the walls of the alveoli are also thin, diffusion allows the oxygen to pass from the alveoli into the capillaries (see Fig. 31-5). Once the oxygen enters the capillaries, it attaches itself to the red blood cells, more specifically, the hemoglobin portion of the red blood cells. The oxygen then continues in the bloodstream to the heart to be transported to the cells throughout the body.

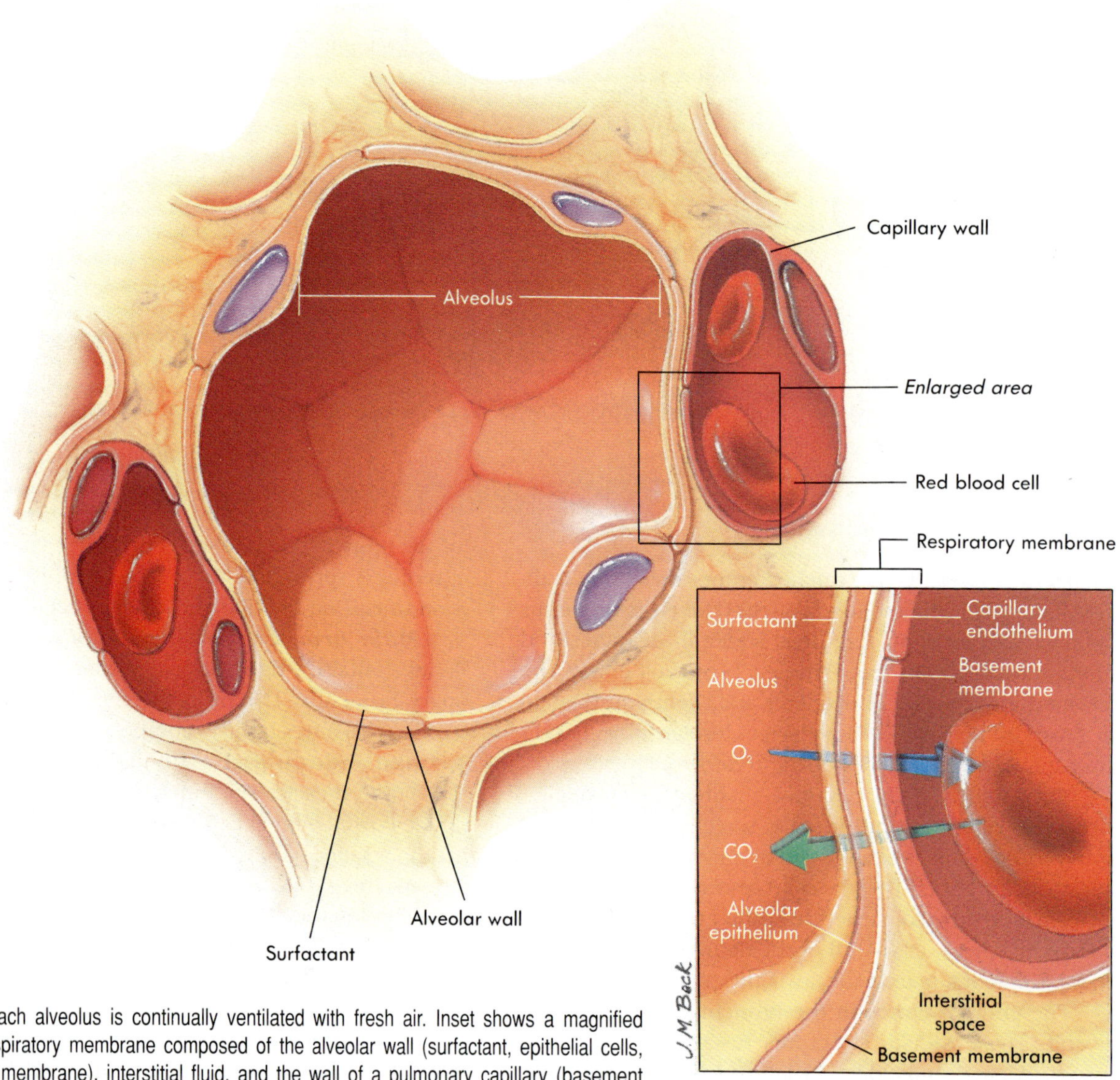

FIG. 31-5 Each alveolus is continually ventilated with fresh air. Inset shows a magnified view of the respiratory membrane composed of the alveolar wall (surfactant, epithelial cells, and basement membrane), interstitial fluid, and the wall of a pulmonary capillary (basement membrane and endothelial cells). The gases, CO_2 (carbon dioxide) and O_2 (oxygen), diffuse across the respiratory membrane.

Mechanics of Breathing

Thoracic Cavity. The lungs occupy almost all the thoracic cavity except the centermost area, the mediastinum, which contains the heart and great vessels. This cavity, the interpleural space, is enclosed by the sternum, ribs, and thoracic vertebrae.

Lungs. The lungs are large, paired, spongy, cone-shaped organs (Fig. 31-6). They weigh approximately 2½ pounds. The right lung contains three lobes; the left lung contains only two lobes. Located approximately 1 inch (2 cm) above the first rib is the narrow part—the apex, or superior, subclavicular part—of each lung. The broad, inferior part—the base of the lungs—lies on the diaphragm. The **hilum** (a depression or pit at that part of an organ where vessels and nerves enter) is the medial portion and contains the pulmonary artery, pulmonary vein, main bronchus, and lymph nodes.

The lungs receive their blood supply through the pulmonary veins and pulmonary arteries, which come directly from the heart. The pulmonary artery comes from the right ventricle of the heart and brings deoxygenated blood to the lungs. It then flows through the thousands of tiny lung capillaries that are near the air-filled alveoli. External respirations or the exchange of gases between the blood and alveolar air occurs by diffusion.

Diffusion is a passive process that results in movement down a concentration gradient; that is, substances move from an area of high concentration to an area of low concentration of the diffusing substance. Blood flowing through lung capillaries is low in oxygen. Oxygen is continually removed from the blood and used by the cells of the body. By the time it enters the lung capillaries, it is "low" in oxygen content. Because alveolar air is rich in oxygen, diffusion will cause movement of oxygen from the area of high oxygen concentration (capillary blood).

Diffusion of carbon dioxide also occurs between blood in lung capillaries and alveolar air. Blood flowing

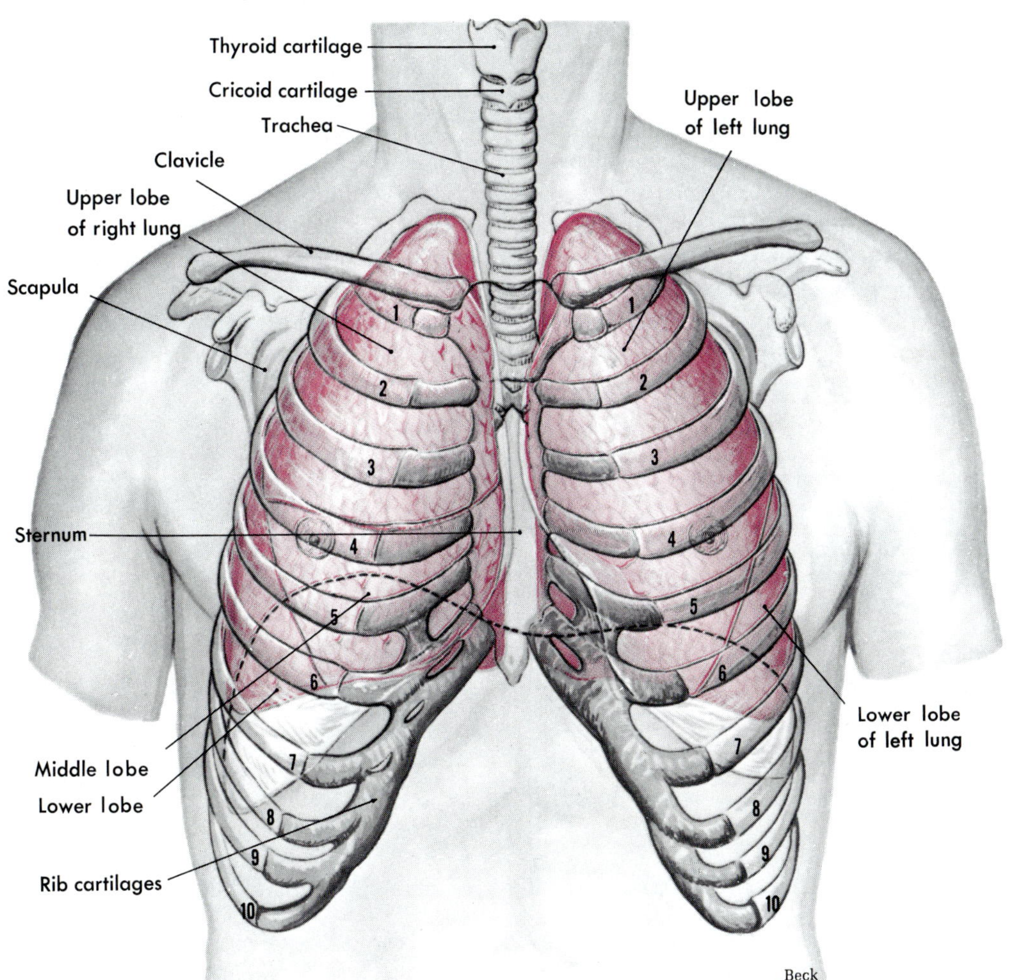

FIG. 31-6 Projection of the lungs and trachea in relation to rib cage and clavicles. Dotted line shows location of dome-shaped diaphragm at the end of expiration and before inspiration. Note that apex of each lung projects above the clavicle. Ribs 11 and 12 are not visible in this view.

through the lung capillaries is high in carbon dioxide. As body cells remove oxygen from circulating blood, they add the waste product carbon dioxide to it. As a result, the blood in pulmonary capillaries eventually becomes low in oxygen and high in carbon dioxide. Diffusion of carbon dioxide results in its movement from an area of high concentration in the pulmonary capillaries to an area of low concentration in alveolar air. Then from the alveoli, carbon dioxide leaves the body in the expired air (see Figs. 31-1 and 31-5).

The capillaries surround the alveoli. The blood becomes rich with oxygen, goes to the pulmonary veins, returns to the left atrium, and continues to the left ventricle. It is then transported throughout the body.

The surface of each lung is covered with a thin, moist, serous membrane composed of tough endothelial cells. It is called the *visceral pleura.* The walls of the thoracic cavity are also covered with the same type of membrane, called the *parietal pleura.* The pleural cavity around the lungs is an airtight vacuum that contains negative pressure. The pressure within the lungs is atmospheric and is higher than in the pleural cavity. The negative pressure assists in keeping the lungs inflated. The visceral and parietal pleurae produce a serous secretion, which allows the lungs to slide over the walls of the thorax during breathing. Usually the body produces the exact amount needed. If too much serous secretion is produced, it results in an accumulation of fluid in the pleural space, **pleural effusion.** This causes the pleural space to become distended and puts pressure on the lungs, making it difficult for the patient to breathe. The physician may decide to remove this fluid. In this case, a thoracentesis will be performed. A needlelike instrument is inserted into the pleural space, and the fluid is removed (see Chapter 17).

Another condition that could result is *pleurisy.* In this condition the pleura becomes inflamed and produces too little fluid. With each breath the patient experiences sharp chest pain.

Pressure Changes. For breathing to occur, changes of pressure within the thoracic cavity must take place. Immediately preceding inspiration the air pressure inside the lungs is equal to the atmospheric pressure. For inspiration to occur, the lungs must have less pressure than the atmosphere. To achieve this, the volume of the lungs must be increased. The lungs need to expand for inspiration. This expansion causes an increase in lung volume and decreases the pressure in the lungs. To accomplish this (1) the external intercostal muscles contract and lift the ribs upward and outward; (2) the diaphragm contracts, which flattens and lowers its dome; and (3) the sternum is pushed forward, increasing the anteroposterior diameter. All these activities occur simultaneously. They result in increased lung volume and decreased atmospheric pressure. As a result, the outside air rushes into the lungs (inspiration).

For expiration to take place, all structures relax; it is a passive process. The sternum drops back, the ribs move down, and the diaphragm moves up. These movements decrease the diameter of the thoracic cavity and return it to its resting state (Fig. 31-7).

Respiratory Movements/Ranges. The rhythmic movements of the chest walls, ribs, and associated muscles

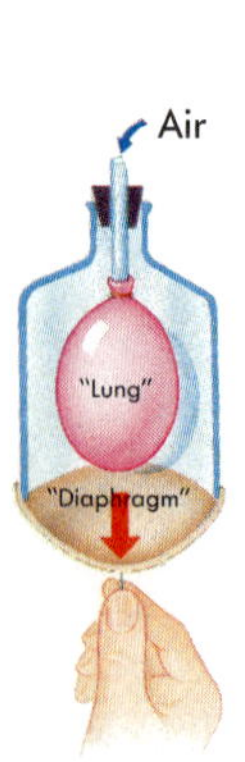

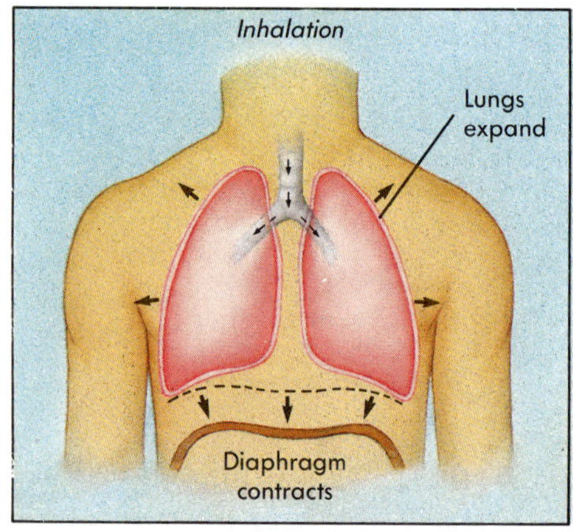

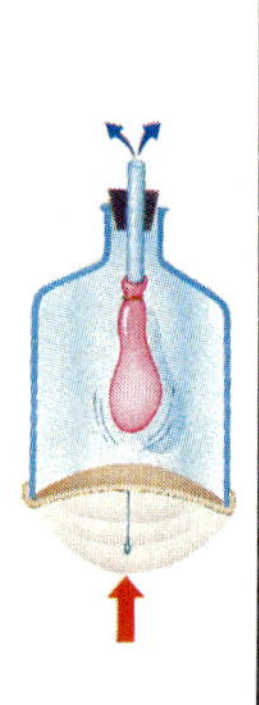

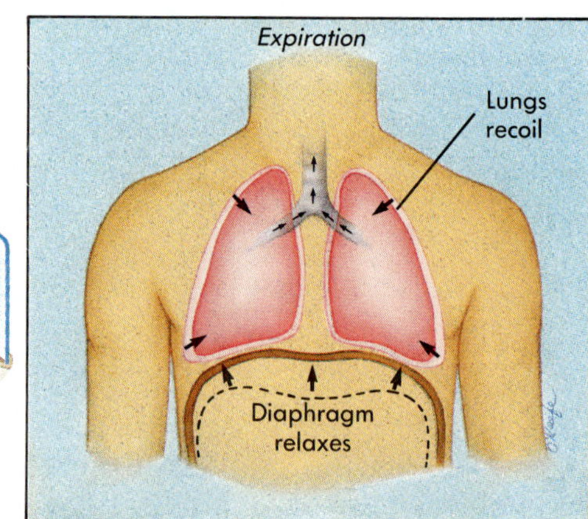

FIG. 31-7 During inspiration, or inhalation, the diaphragm contracts, increasing the volume of the thoracic cavity. This increase in volume results in a decrease in pressure, which causes air to rush into the lungs. During expiration, the diaphragm returns to an upward position, reducing the volume in the thoracic cavity. Air pressure increases then, forcing air out of the lungs. *Insets* show the classic model, in which a jar represents the rib cage, a rubber sheet represents the diaphragm, and a balloon represents the lungs.

when air is inhaled and exhaled make up the respiratory movements. The combination of one inspiration and one expiration makes one respiration, or respiratory movement. At rest the normal inspiration lasts about 2 seconds and expiration about 3 seconds.

Room air when inhaled contains about 21% oxygen; exhaled air contains 16% oxygen and 3.5% carbon dioxide. This represents the actual amount of oxygen used from a single breath.

When air enters the respiratory system, it must travel through the bronchial tree. As the tubes become smaller, the air moves more slowly until it reaches the alveoli, where it moves only by diffusion. Because the walls of the alveoli are thin and moist, the exchange of oxygen and carbon dioxide occurs readily.

The normal range of respirations for an adult at rest is about 14 to 20 breaths per minute. This rate can be affected by many variables: age, sex, activity, disease, and body temperature. For example, the respiratory rate for a newborn is 40 to 60 breaths per minute; early school age, 22 to 24 breaths; teenagers, 20 to 22 breaths; adults, 14 to 20 breaths. The normal range for females is usually slightly higher than for males.

Members of the health care team should assess all factors influencing the patient's respirations and should count the respirations without patient awareness to prevent alterations in the breathing pattern (see Chapter 10).

Regulation of Respiration

Nervous Control. The medulla oblongata and pons of the brain are responsible for the basic rhythm and depth of respirations. This rhythm can be modified according to the demands of the body. Other parts of the nervous system help to coordinate the transfer from inspiration to expiration. These areas are the pneumotaxic area, in the upper pons, and the apneustic area, in the lower pons (see Chapter 35).

Because the respiratory center can relay messages to the cerebal cortex, there is also some voluntary control, which allows alteration of breathing patterns. Breath can be held for a short period, but as the carbon dioxide level in the blood increases, the inspiratory area of the brain is stimulated, messages are sent to the inspiratory muscles, and breathing resumes on an involuntary basis. This mechanism makes it impossible to kill oneself by holding the breath.

Stretch receptors located in the walls of the bronchioles and alveoli respond to overinflation, as well as extreme deflation. Impulses alerting the status of inflation travel along the vagus nerve, and appropriate action is taken to prevent injury to the lung tissues. The phrenic nerve arises in the cervical plexus, enters the thorax, and passes to the diaphragm. The phrenic nerve contains sensory and motor fibers. It is generally known as the motor nerve to the diaphragm and helps innervate the diaphragm.

Chemoreceptors (sensory nerve cells activated by chemical stimuli) located in the carotid and aortic bodies are specialized receptors that are sensitive to increases in blood carbon dioxide level and decreases in blood oxygen level. They also can sense and respond to increasing blood acid levels. The carotid body receptors are found at the point where the common carotid arteries divide, and the aortic bodies are small clusters of chemosensitive cells that lie adjacent to the aortic arch near the heart. When stimulated by increasing levels of blood carbon dioxide, decreasing oxygen levels, or increasing blood acidity, these receptors send nerve impulses to the respiratory regulatory centers, which in turn modify respiratory rates.

Chemical Stimuli. Carbon dioxide is considered the chemical stimulant for regulation of respiration, but it is actually the hydrogen ions that maintain the control. In the bloodstream carbon dioxide combines with water to form carbonic acid, which immediately converts to hydrogen ions and bicarbonate ions. It should be remembered that the more hydrogen ions a solution contains, the more acidic it becomes. Therefore the more carbon dioxide in the blood, the more acidic the blood becomes. After exhalation the blood becomes more alkaline. The normal pH of blood is 7.35 to 7.45—a narrow range. Deviation from this range causes the patient to develop either alkalosis or acidosis.

Most of the oxygen transported to the cells is bound to the **hemoglobin** (a complex protein-iron compound in the blood that carries oxygen to the cells from the lungs and carbon dioxide away from the cells to the lungs) portion of the red blood cells. Normally this is a weak bond and is easily broken at the cellular level. Once the cells use the oxygen, carbon dioxide is given off and must return to the lungs. For carbon dioxide to reach the lungs, it must travel on the bicarbonate ion. After reaching the lungs, carbon dioxide is exhaled with expiration.

Respiratory Measurements. A device called a spirometer is used to provide diagnostic information about the respiratory capacity of the lungs. The patient breathes into the device, and a tracing is made of the breathing ability (see p. 882).

Tidal volume refers to the amount of air inhaled and exhaled at rest. This is about 500 ml, or 1 pint. Vital capacity refers to a maximum inhalation followed by a maximum exhalation. This is 4500 to 5000 ml in an adult with healthy lung tissue. Total lung capacity refers to the total volume of air contained in the lungs after maximum inspiration. On the average this is about 6000 ml. Residual volume is the amount of air that remains in the lungs after maximum exhalation.

Modified respiratory movements. Such emotions as laughing, crying, sobbing, yawning, and sighing can be expressed. Respirations can also remove foreign matter from the respiratory tract by sneezing and coughing. Most of these responses are involuntary, but some of these movements can be initiated voluntarily. The most common movements are listed as follows:

- Cough: A deep breath is taken and the glottis closes. This results in a strong expiration, which forces the glottis open. In turn, air passes through the upper respiratory passageways with significant force.
- Sneeze: Air is forced through the nasal cavities instead of the oral cavity. The uvula closes the oral cavity, which aids in redirecting the forced air. A sneeze can clear the upper respiratory passageways.
- Sigh: A deep inspiration is followed with a short, forceful expiration.
- Yawn: A deep breath is taken with the mouth wide open, causing all the alveoli to ventilate, which does not happen with normal breathing.
- Sob: A series of convulsive inspirations are taken, immediately followed by a single, prolonged expiration. The glottis closes earlier than normal, and only a little air can reach the lungs.
- Cry: Normal inhalation is followed by exhalation with many short, convulsive movements. Facial grimaces are also present.
- Laugh: Same movements occur as with crying, distinguished only by the individual's facial expression.
- Singultus (hiccups): A sharp inspiratory sound is caused by stimulation or irritation of the phrenic nerve (which serves the diaphragm) when the diaphragm contracts and the glottis closes.

ASSESSMENT OF RESPIRATORY FUNCTION

The function of the respiratory system is gas exchange (oxygen and carbon dioxide) at the alveolar/capillary level. This function depends on the lungs' capability for contraction and expansion, which in turn is influenced by musculoskeletal and neurological functions.

The respiratory system is always included in a physical assessment of the patient's general health. Certain types of patients require more extensive assessments: those with acute or chronic respiratory or cardiac conditions, those with a history of respiratory impairment related to trauma or allergic reactions, or those who have recently undergone surgery or anesthesia. Because physical and emotional responses are often correlated, the nurse should also inquire about any accompanying anxiety or stress. This information should be obtained in an unhurried, matter-of-fact manner.

The respiratory assessment will include collection of *subjective data.* During the interview the patient should be encouraged to describe any symptoms, such as shortness of breath, dyspnea on exertion, or cough. **Dyspnea,** or difficulty breathing, is a subjective experience that only the patient can accurately describe. Data should include onset, duration, precipitating factors, and relief measures, such as position and use of over-the-counter or prescribed medications. If the patient has reported a cough, the nurse will ask for a description of the cough: productive or nonproductive; harsh, dry, or hacking; and color and amount of mucus expectorated. This information should be recorded as direct quotes from the patient when possible.

The nurse will then gather *objective data.* Assessment begins with observation. The patient's expression, chest movement, and respirations all provide valuable visual clues. There may be times when the patient cannot verbalize distress, but the wide-eyed, anxious look on the patient's face reflects the fear of suffocating. Flaring nostrils indicate that the patient is struggling to breathe, which is usually a late sign of respiratory distress. Initial observation by the nurse will yield information on the patient's skin color and turgor. The nurse will note any obvious respiratory distress, wheezes, or **orthopnea** (an abnormal condition in which a person must sit or stand in order to breathe deeply or comfortably).

To continue this assessment, the nurse will auscultate all lung fields, anteriorly and posteriorly, noting the presence of **adventitious** sounds (abnormal sounds superimposed on breath sounds, including sibilant wheezes [formerly called simply *wheezes*], sonorous wheezes [formerly called simply *rhonchi*], crackles [formerly called *rales*], and pleural friction rubs) (Fig. 9-6). **Sibilant wheezes** are musical or whistlelike sounds, caused by the rapid movement of air through narrowed bronchioles. **Sonorous wheezes** are low-pitched, loud, coarse, snoring sounds. They are often heard on expiration. **Crackles** are popping sounds that are created when air is forced through respiratory passages narrowed by fluid, mucus, or pus. They are associated with inflammation or infection of the small bronchi, bronchioles, and alveoli. They can be heard on inspiration, expiration, or both. **Pleural friction rubs** are low-pitched, grating or creaking lung sounds that occur when inflamed pleural surfaces rub together during respiration[41] (Table 31-1). The nurse can also assess chest movement. Note if the chest expands equally on both sides; chest expansion on one side only may indicate serious pulmonary complications. The nurse should note retraction of the chest wall between the ribs and under the clavicle during inspiration. This can signal late-stage respiratory distress. Another important aspect in collecting objective data is to be alert for signs and symptoms of hypoxia (Box 31-1).

Diagnostic Tests

A variety of tests are used to evaluate respiratory status and identify respiratory conditions. Other tests include diagnostic imaging, laboratory work, and more invasive measures. Nurses should be familiar with these tests so they can adequately prepare the patient.

Chest Roentgenogram. Usually referred to as chest x-ray, chest roentgenograms are an essential diagnostic tool for evaluating disorders of the chest. A chest x-ray provides visualization of the lungs, ribs, clavicles, humeri, scapulae, vertebrae, heart, and major thoracic vessels. This test gives information on alterations in size and location of the pulmonary structures and blood flow, as well as identifies the presence of lesions, infiltrates, foreign bodies, or fluid. A chest x-ray also identifies whether a disorder involves the lung parenchyma (the tissue of an organ as distinguished from supporting or connective tissue) or the interstitial spaces. Chest x-rays can also confirm pneumothorax, pneumonia, pleural effusion, and

Box 31-1 SIGNS AND SYMPTOMS OF HYPOXIA

- Apprehension, anxiety, restlessness
- Decreased ability to concentrate
- Decreased level of consciousness
- Increased fatigue
- Vertigo
- Behavioral changes
- Increased pulse rate; as hypoxia advances, bradycardia results
- Increased rate and depth of respiration; as hypoxia progresses, shallow, slow respirations develop
- Elevated blood pressure; if O_2 deficiency is not correct, blood pressure will decrease
- Cardiac dysrhythmias
- Pallor
- Cyanosis
- Clubbing
- Dyspnea

TABLE 31-1 Adventitious Breath Sounds

Type	Characteristics	Comments
Crackles (rales)	Brief, not continuous; more common in inspiration; wet or dry crackling sound; not cleared by coughing	Caused by fluid, mucus, or pus in the small airways and alveoli
Fine crackles	As described above; high-pitched, sibilant crackling at end of inspiration	Found in diseases affecting bronchioles and alveoli
Medium crackles	As described above; medium pitch, more sonorous, moisture sound during midinspiration	Associated with diseases of small bronchi
Coarse crackles	As described above; loud, bubbly sound in early inspiration	Associated with diseases of small bronchi
Sonorous wheezes (rhonchi)	Deep, running sound that may be continuous; usually louder in early expiration	Caused by air moving through narrowed tracheobronchial passages (e.g., secretions, tumor, spasm); cough may alter sound if caused by mucus in trachea or large bronchi
Sibilant wheezes (wheezes)	High-pitched, musical, whistlelike sound during inspiration or expiration; sound may consist of several notes or one, and may vary from one minute to the next	Caused by narrowed bronchioles; bilateral wheeze often result of bronchospasm; unilateral, sharply localized wheeze may result from foreign matter or tumor compression
Pleural friction rub	Dry, creaking, grating, low-pitched sound with a machinelike quality during both inspiration and expiration; loudest over anterior chest	Sound originates outside respiratory tree, usually caused by inflammation; over the lung fields it suggests pleurisy; over the pericardium it suggests pericarditis with a pericardial friction rub. To distinguish the two, ask the patient to hold the breath briefly. If the rubbing sound persists, it is a pericardial friction rub because the inflamed pericardial layers continue rubbing together with each heartbeat; a pleural rub would stop when breathing stops

pulmonary edema. The chest x-ray examination can be performed at different angles for greater clarification. The nurse should have the patient wear a hospital gown tied in back. Pins must not be used. Any article of clothing containing metal, such as a bra with metal hooks, or jewelry must be removed, since the metal will produce a shadow on the film.

Computed Tomography. Computed tomography (CT) scans of the lungs take pictures of small layers of pulmonary tissue, usually to identify a pulmonary lesion. These views can be diagonal or cross-sectional, with a scanner rotating at various angles. Although this test is painless and noninvasive and results in little radiation exposure, patient teaching is necessary before the procedure to offer explanations and allay anxiety.

Pulmonary Function Testing (PFT). Pulmonary function tests are performed to assess the presence and severity of disease in the large and small airways. PFT is composed of various procedures to obtain information on lung volume, ventilation, pulmonary spirometry, and gas exchange. Lung volume tests refer to the volume of air that can be completely and slowly exhaled after a maximum inhalation (vital capacity [VC]). Inspiratory capacity (IC) is the largest amount of air that can be inhaled in one breath from the resting expiratory level. Total lung capacity (TLC) is calculated to determine the volume of air in the lung after a maximal inhalation. Ventilation tests evaluate the volume of air inhaled or exhaled in each respiratory cycle. Pulmonary spirometry tests evaluate the amount of air that can be forcefully exhaled after maximum inhalation. These tests require the use of a spirometer.

One of the most important tools for diagnosing respiratory diseases is gas exchange, which identifies the capacity for carbon dioxide to be diffused. This component of PFT determines the degree of function in the pulmonary capillary beds in contact with functioning alveoli.

Mediastinoscopy. A mediastinoscopy is a surgical endoscopic procedure in which an incision is created in the suprasternal notch, allowing the endoscope to be passed into the upper mediastinum. This is performed to gather a sample of lymph nodes for biopsy for tumor diagnosis. Because these lymph nodes receive lymphatic drainage from the lungs, they are of diagnostic value for carcinoma. This procedure is performed in the operating room, and the patient usually receives a general anesthetic agent.

Laryngoscopy. Laryngoscopy can be performed for either direct or indirect visualization of the larynx. Indirect laryngoscopy is probably the most common procedure for assessment of respiratory difficulties; this entails the use of a laryngeal mirror in the awake patient's mouth for visualization. This procedure can be used for biopsy or polyp excision.

Direct laryngoscopy requires local or general anesthesia and exposes the vocal chords with a laryngoscope passed down over the tongue.

Bronchoscopy. A **bronchoscopy** is performed by passing a bronchoscope into the trachea and bronchi. By use of either a rigid bronchoscope or a flexible fiberoptic bronchoscope, the instrument of choice in most cases, the larynx, trachea, and bronchi can be visualized (Fig. 31-8). Diagnostic bronchoscopic examination includes observation of the tracheobronchial tree for (1) abnormalities, (2) tissue biopsy, and (3) secretions collected for cytological (cell) or bacteriological examination. A local anesthetic agent may be used, but an intravenous general anesthetic agent is usually given. The patient is treated as a surgical patient. Nursing interventions for patients after bronchoscopy are as follows:

1. Patient is on NPO status until gag reflex returns, usually about 2 hours after the procedure.
2. Patient is in semi-Fowler's position and turns on either side to facilitate removal of secretions, unless the physician specifies another position.
3. Patient is monitored for signs of laryngeal edema or laryngospasms, such as stridor or increasing dyspnea.

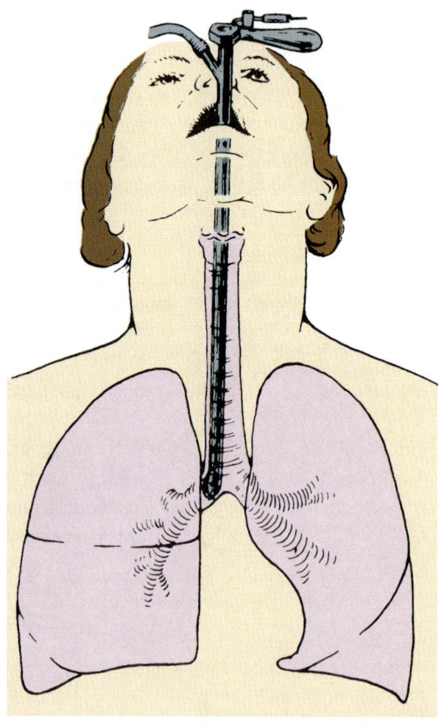

FIG. 31-8 Bronchoscope inserted through the trachea into bronchus.

4. If lung tissue biopsy is taken, sputum is monitored for signs of hemorrhage. NOTE: Blood-streaked sputum can be expected for a few days after biopsy.

Sputum Specimen. Sputum samples frequently are obtained for microscopic evaluation, such as Gram stain and culture and sensitivity (Box 31-2). For the range of sputum characteristics, see Box 31-3.

Cytology Studies. Cytology tests can be performed on any body secretion, such as sputum or pleural fluid, to detect the presence of abnormal or malignant cells.

Thoracentesis. **Thoracentesis** is the surgical perforation of the chest wall and pleural space with a needle for the aspiration of fluid for diagnostic or therapeutic purposes or for the removal of a specimen for biopsy. Indications for a thoracentesis include the following:

1. Removal of fluid for diagnostic purposes
   a. The pleural fluid can be examined for specific gravity, white blood cell count, red blood cell count, protein, and glucose.
   b. The fluid can be cultured for pathogens and checked for the presence of abnormal or malignant cells.
   c. The gross appearance of the fluid, the quantity obtained, and the location of the site of the thoracentesis should be recorded.
2. Biopsy of the pleura
3. Removal of fluid when it is a threat to patient safety or comfort
4. Instillation of medication into the pleural space

Nursing interventions for the patient undergoing thoracentesis include the following:

1. Explain the procedure; obtain a written consent; every means should be used to relieve the patient's anxiety.
2. The procedure is usually carried out in the patient's room. The patient sits on the edge of the bed with the head and arms resting on a pillow placed on an overbed table. Patients who cannot sit up should be turned to the unaffected side with the head of the bed elevated 30 degrees (see Chapter 17).
3. Vital signs, general appearance, and respiratory status should be monitored throughout the procedure. Usually no more than 1300 ml of pleural fluid should be removed within a 30-minute period because of the risk of intravascular fluid shift with resultant pulmonary edema.
4. After thoracentesis, the patient is positioned on the unaffected side.

The specimen should be labeled and sent immediately to the laboratory as per physician's orders.

Box 31-2 GUIDELINES FOR SPUTUM SPECIMEN COLLECTION

1. Explain to the patient that the sputum must be brought up from the lungs. Patients who have difficulty producing sputum or who have very tenacious sputum may be dehydrated. Encourage fluid intake.
2. Collect specimens before meals to avoid possible emesis from coughing.
3. Instruct patient to inhale and exhale deeply three times, then inhale swiftly, cough forcefully, and expectorate into the sterile sputum container. Usually early morning samples are collected on 3 consecutive days.
4. If your patient can't raise sputum spontaneously, a hypertonic saline aerosol mist may help to produce a good specimen. Instruct the patient to take several normal breaths of the mist, inhale deeply, cough, and expectorate.
5. Instruct patient to rinse mouth with water before expectorating into sterile specimen bottle to decrease sputum contamination.
6. Notify staff as soon as a specimen is collected so it can be properly labeled and sent to the laboratory without delay.
7. Sputum samples can also be obtained indirectly, such as with nasotracheal suctioning with a catheter or transtracheal aspiration. Care must be taken to ensure that the suction catheters remain sterile. A physician's order must be obtained for endotracheal suctioning.

Box 31-3 RANGE OF SPUTUM CHARACTERISTICS

COLOR

Clear
White
Yellow
Green
Brown
Red
Pink-tinged
Streaked with blood

CONSISTENCY

Frothy
Watery
Tenacious

ODOR

None
Malodorous

BLOOD

All the time
Occasionally
Early morning

Box 31-4 GUIDELINES FOR INTERPRETING ABGS

1. Examine each value by itself.

NORMAL ABGs

pH	7.35-7.45
$Paco_2$	35-45 mm Hg
Pao_2	80-100 mm Hg
HCO_3	21-28 mEq/L
O_2 saturation	≥95%

2. Determine whether the pH reflects acidity or alkalinity.

pH of 7.35 and lower = acidity.
pH of 7.45 and higher = alkalinity.

3. Which other value corresponds with that condition?

NOTE: $Paco_2$ reflects respiratory factors; HCO_3 reflects metabolic factors.

CO_2 is a potential acid, so CO_2 of greater than 45 = more acidity.
HCO_3 is a basic (alkaline) substance, so HCO_3 higher than 45 = more alkalinity.

EXAMPLE: A patient with acute exacerbation of COPD has the following ABGs:

pH	7.42
$Paco_2$	49 mm Hg
Pao_2	50 mm Hg
HCO_3	31 mEq/L
O_2 saturation	84%

Because the pH is within a normal range, this is a compensated respiratory problem. The kidneys have increased the amount of bicarbonate they put into the blood to bring the pH to a normal level.

Arterial Blood Gases (ABGs). Blood gas analysis is an essential test in diagnosing and monitoring patients with respiratory disorders. This test yields definitive information on the patient's respiratory status and metabolic balance. The procedure is performed at the bedside. A heparinized syringe and needle are used to withdraw 3 to 5 ml of arterial blood, usually from the radial artery. Other possible sites include femoral or brachial arteries. After the sample is obtained, the nurse must place direct pressure on the puncture site for a minimum of 5 minutes to prevent hematoma formation and blood loss. If the patient is on anticoagulants, maintain pressure for 20 minutes or longer until bleeding stops. Place the capped syringe in a basin of crushed ice and water to preserve the gas and pH levels of the specimen. Send the properly labeled specimen to the laboratory immediately.

The blood gas values (Box 31-4) assess the patient's metabolic (acid-base) status by measuring the pH. Carbon dioxide tension is measured by $Paco_2$ and will assess the patient's ventilation. The metabolic evaluation is assessed by measuring the bicarbonate (HCO_3). Oxygen saturation (Pao_2 and O_2) is also measured.

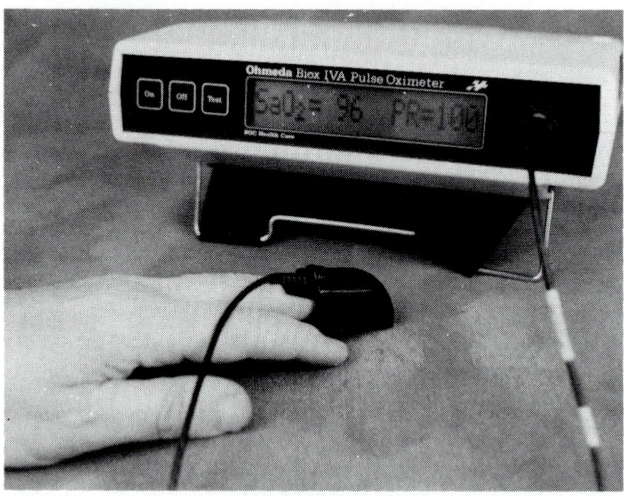

FIG. 31-9 Portable pulse oximeter displays oxygen saturation and pulse rate. (Courtesy Ohmeda, Boulder, Colo.)

Pulse Oximetry. Pulse oximetry is a noninvasive method of providing continuous monitoring of Sao_2 (saturation of oxygen) for assessment of gas exchange. The system consists of a probe that looks like a large clothespin and is applied to a finger, toe, earlobe, or the bridge of the nose. The probe has a light-emitting sensor that shoots narrow beams of red and infrared light through the tissue and a light-receiving sensor that measures the amount of light being absorbed by oxygenated and deoxygenated hemoglobin in pulsating arterial blood. The probe is connected to a computer with a monitor that displays hemoglobin oxygen saturation and pulse rates (Fig. 31-9). A pulse oximeter will beep if the patient's Sao_2 registers outside of the limits set in response to the physician's order.

For decades, physicians have relied on ABG analysis to evaluate gas exchange and oxygen transport. As valuable as this test is, ABG results reflect a patient's oxygenation status only one moment in time. Today, pulse oximetry permits continuous, noninvasive monitoring of Sao_2. Oximetry technology allows the nurse to assess minute-to-minute changes in arterial saturations, intervene before hypoxemia produces obvious and serious signs and symptoms, and evaluate the patient's response to treatment.

An Sao_2 of 90% to 100% is needed to adequately replenish O_2 in plasma. The ability of hemoglobin to feed oxygen to the plasma weakens significantly when the Sao_2 drops below 85%. An Sao_2 under 70% is considered life-threatening.

Arterial oxygen saturation can be quickly and noninvasively determined through pulse oximetry. Severe circulatory problems may diminish the accuracy of the reading. If oximetry results seem questionable, the physician will usually order ABG tests.

DISORDERS OF THE UPPER AIRWAY

Epistaxis

Etiology/Pathophysiology. The underlying cause of **epistaxis** (a bleeding from the nose) is congestion of the nasal membranes, leading to capillary rupture. This condition is frequently caused by injury and occurs more frequently in men.

Epistaxis can be either a primary disorder or secondary to other conditions. It can be related to menstrual flow in women, as well as hypertension. Other causes include local irritation of nasal mucosa, such as dryness, chronic infection, or trauma (i.e., injury, vigorous nose blowing, or nose picking). A prime consideration of epistaxis is the many capillaries in the nasal passages.

Clinical Manifestations. The primary observation is the presence of bright red blood draining from one or both nostrils. With a severe nasal hemorrhage adults can lose as much as 1 liter of blood per hour, but this loss is not prolonged. Exsanguination (loss of blood to the point at which life can no longer be sustained) from the usual epistaxis is rare.

Assessment. Collection of *subjective data* includes interviewing the patient and asking the patient to relate the duration and severity of bleeding and identification of precipitating factors, if possible.

Collection of *objective data* involves the nurse assessing the presence of bleeding from one or both nostrils. She will also need to determine whether the bleeding is occurring in the anterior or posterior portion of the nasal passageway. The nurse will assess the patient's blood pressure; temperature, pulse, and respirations (TPR); and any evidence of hypovolemic shock. Severe bleeding results in a drop in blood pressure, which may cause the bleeding to stop.

Diagnostic Tests. A hemoglobin and hematocrit determination will aid in establishing an estimate of the blood loss. PT and PTT will assist in identifying contributing factors, such as a bleeding tendency and clotting abnormalities. A rhinoscopy may be performed to locate the bleeding site as well as possible causes and treatment. This procedure involves inserting a lighted nasal speculum into the nasal cavity.

Medical Management. There are many possible treatments for epistaxis, including nasal packing with cotton saturated with 1:1000 epinephrine to promote local vasoconstriction. Cautery can be either electrical (in which the bleeding vessel is burned [cauterized]) or chemical (a silver nitrate stick is applied to the site of the bleeding). Posterior packing of the nasal cavity may be needed, or use of a balloon tamponade. This is done by inserting a Foley-like catheter into the nose and inflating the balloon after it is placed posteriorly. Traction is then placed on the catheter so the vessel in the area is compressed. Also, some physicians will prescribe antibiotics (penicillin) after the bleeding is controlled to minimize risk of infection.

Nursing Interventions. Nursing interventions include applying pressure on the bridge of the nose by compressing the soft tissue of the nose against the septum with a finger to decrease blood flow to the area. Firm pressure should be maintained for at least 5 to 10 minutes, and it may be necessary for as long as 30 minutes.

Nursing diagnoses and interventions for the patient with epistaxis include but are not limited to the following:

NURSING DIAGNOSES	NURSING INTERVENTIONS
Tissue perfusion, altered, cerebral and/or cardiopulmonary, related to blood loss	Assess vital signs and level of consciousness q 15 min and report any changes. Document estimated blood loss.
Aspiration, high risk for, related to bleeding	Elevate head of bed; place patient in Fowler's position with the head forward; patient should be encouraged to let the blood drain from the nose. Pinch nostrils; have the patient breathe through the mouth; apply ice compresses over the nose (however, the primary benefit of the application of ice is that it requires the patient to remain still); assist patient to clear secretions. Maintain airway patency. Instruct patient to expectorate any blood or clots rather than swallow them, which could cause nausea and vomiting.
Fear, related to perceived blood loss and difficulty swallowing	Instruct patient to mouth breathe to promote optimal air exchange, because anxiety will be increased when patient feels unable to breathe. Decrease sense of fear by staying with patient and offering reassurance in a calm manner. Promote patient's dignity by providing privacy.

Patient teaching. The patient (and the family, if possible) should be instructed not to pick, scratch, or otherwise irritate the nares. To prevent recurrent hemorrhage, the patient is warned not to blow the nose vigorously and to avoid dryness of the nose. The patient and/or family should be instructed regarding the risks of foreign objects inserted in the nose (this is especially important in pediatric patients). The use of a vaporizer to keep nasal mucous membranes moist should be encouraged as well as the use of saline or nasal lubricants.

Prognosis. With treatment, prognosis is good.

Deviated Septum and Nasal Polyps

Etiology/Pathophysiology. Common conditions that cause nasal obstruction include nasal polyps or deviated septum caused by congenital abnormality or, more likely, injury.

The septum deviates from the midline and can cause a partial obstruction of the nasal passageway. Nasal polyps are tissue growths on the nasal tissues that are frequently caused by prolonged sinus inflammation; allergies are often the underlying cause.

Clinical Manifestations. The major manifestations of nasal septal deviations and polyps are **stertorous** (pertaining to a respiratory effort that is strenuous and struggling, provoking a snoring sound) respirations, dyspnea, and sometimes postnasal drip.

Assessment. Collection of *subjective data* includes establishing the presence of previous injuries or infections, allergies, and sinus congestion. The patient will offer complaints of dyspnea.

Collection of *objective data* involves the nurse attempting to identify the condition and its location. The rate and character of the patient's respirations must be noted.

Diagnostic Tests. Sinus x-ray studies will depict the presence of shadowy sinuses when nasal polyps are present, and a shift of the nasal septum will be evident with a septal defect. A deviated septum may also be present on visual examination.

Medical Management. These conditions frequently require surgical correction, such as a submucous resection in which obstructive portions of cartilage or bone are removed from the nasal septum. Nasoseptoplasty may be done to reconstruct the nasal septum, and is replacing submucous resection as the operation of choice for deviated nasal septum, or nasal polypectomy may be done to remove the polyps. Actions include nasal packing to control bleeding, for 24 hours, and then maintaining nasal mucosa hydration with nasal irrigation of saline or application of a light layer of petroleum to the external nares to prevent drying. Medications include (1) corticosteroids (prednisone), which will cause polyps to decrease or disappear, and (2) antihistamines for allergy signs and symptoms, to decrease congestion in both septal deviations and polyps. Antibiotic agents (penicillin) may be used in both conditions to prevent infection. Analgesics (acetaminophen [Tylenol]) may be given to relieve the headache that occurs with septal deviation.

Nursing Interventions. Nursing interventions are generally aimed at maintaining airway patency and preventing infection. Postoperative intervention for nasal surgery will include monitoring closely for infection or hemorrhage and maintaining patient comfort.

Nursing diagnoses and interventions for the patient with deviated septum and nasal polyps include but are not limited to the following:

NURSING DIAGNOSES	NURSING INTERVENTIONS
Airway clearance, ineffective, related to nasal exudate	Document patient's ability to clear secretions, and note respiratory status. Elevate head of bed, and apply ice compresses to the nose to decrease edema, discoloration, discomfort, and bleeding. Change nasal drip pad as needed, documenting color, consistency, and amount of exudate.
Injury, high risk for, related to trauma to bleeding site associated with vigorous nose blowing	Assess and report exudate (as stated above). Instruct patient against blowing nose in immediate postoperative period, because this could increase bleeding, edema, and ecchymosis.

Patient teaching. The patient should be instructed to contact the physician if bleeding or infection develops. The patient should be instructed to use nasal sprays and drops judiciously because of the possible rebound effect on nasal mucous membranes. The patient should be reminded to avoid nose blowing, vigorous coughing, or Valsalva maneuver (technique in which the patient holds the breath and bears down as if straining during a bowel movement) for 2 days postoperatively. The nurse should assure the patient that facial ecchymosis and edema may persist for several days after surgery.

Prognosis. With surgical correction, the prognosis is excellent.

Upper Airway Obstruction

Etiology/Pathophysiology. Upper airway obstruction is precipitated by a recent respiratory event, such as traumatic injury to the airway or surrounding tissues. Common airway obstructions include dentures, aspiration of vomitus or secretions, and the most common airway obstruction in an unconscious person, the tongue.

Altered physiology includes any condition that could produce airway obstruction, such as laryngeal spasm caused by tetany resulting from hypocalcemia. Another cause may be laryngeal edema caused by injury.

Clinical Manifestations. The main signs are stertorous respirations, altered respiratory rate and character, and apneic periods.

Assessment. Collection of *subjective data* is limited because a patient is unable to talk when the airway is obstructed. The nurse therefore must make a prompt and accurate assessment of objective data.

Collection of *objective data* includes the nurse promptly assessing for signs of **hypoxia** (an inadequate, reduced tension of cellular oxygen; see Box 31-1), **cyanosis** (slightly bluish, grayish, slatelike, or dark purple discoloration of the skin resulting from the presence of abnormal amounts of reduced hemoglobin in the blood), stertorous respirations, and wheezing or stridor (harsh, high-pitched sounds during respiration, caused by obstruction). As hypoxia progresses, the respiratory centers in the brain (medulla oblongata and pons) are depressed, resulting in bradycardia and shallow, slow respirations.

Diagnostic Tests. Because this is a medical emergency, no diagnostic tests are needed. This condition is diagnosed by a prompt and accurate assessment.

Medical Management. The patient may require an emergency tracheostomy to remove the obstruction. Depending on the cause of the obstruction, an artificial airway may need to be inserted to maintain patency. Examples of artificial airways include pharyngeal, endotracheal, and tracheal.

Nursing Interventions. The most immediate nursing intervention will be that of opening the airway and restoring patency. This may be accomplished by properly repositioning the patient's head and neck, or it may require further maneuvers. The head-tilt/chin-lift practice is recommended by the American Heart Association because this technique minimizes further damage in the presence of a suspected cervical neck fracture. With a foreign body airway obstruction, the Heimlich maneuver is used (see Chapter 50).

Nursing diagnoses and interventions for the patient with an airway obstruction include but are not limited to the following:

NURSING DIAGNOSES	NURSING INTERVENTIONS
Airway clearance, ineffective, related to obstruction in airway	Reestablish and maintain secure airway. Administer oxygen as ordered. Suction as needed, and assess patient's ability to mobilize secretions. Monitor vital signs and breath sounds closely.
Aspiration, high risk for, related to partial airway obstruction	Monitor respiratory rate, rhythm, and effort. Assess patient's ability to swallow secretions by elevating the head of the bed. Assess and document breath sounds. Facilitate optimal airway and *functional* swallowing by elevating head of bed. Note amount, color, and characteristics of secretions. Suction as needed.

Patient teaching. The best goal of education is prevention. The patient and family should be taught how to assess for airway patency. Appropriate use of the Heimlich maneuver should be provided. Rationale for all treatments and procedures should be explained.

Prognosis. With immediate medical and nursing intervention, the prognosis is good; without emergency intervention, the condition is life threatening.

Cancer of the Larynx

Etiology/Pathophysiology. Squamous cell carcinoma of the larynx is increasing in frequency. Occurring most often in people over age 60, 90% of laryngeal cancers occur in men. It appears to be correlated to heavy smoking and alcohol use, chronic laryngitis, vocal abuse, and family history. Because of the increase in the number of women who are heavy smokers, their incidence of carcinoma of the larynx is increasing.

Laryngeal cancer limited to the true vocal cords is slow growing because of decreased lympatic supply; however, elsewhere in the larynx there is an abundance of lymph tissue, and cancer in these tissues spreads rapidly and metastasizes early to the deep lymph nodes of the neck.

Clinical Manifestations. Progressive or persistent hoarseness is an early sign. Any person who is hoarse longer than 2 weeks should seek medical treatment. Signs of metastasis to other areas include pain in the larynx radiating to the ear, difficulty swallowing (dysphagia), a feeling of a lump in the throat, and enlarged cervical lymph nodes.

Assessment. Collection of *subjective data* includes assessing the onset and duration of symptoms. A complaint of referred pain to the ear (otalgia), as well as difficulty breathing (dyspnea) or swallowing, should be noted.

Collection of *objective data* includes examining sputum for the presence of blood **hemoptysis** (expectorating blood from the respiratory tract).

Diagnostic Tests. Visual examination of the larynx with direct laryngoscopy is done to determine the presence of laryngeal cancer. A health history will be helpful in making the diagnosis, and a biopsy and microscopic study of the lesion will be definitive.

Medical Management. Treatment will be determined by the extent of tumor growth. Radiation therapy or surgery is often performed. If the tumor is limited to the true cord without limitation of cord movement, then radiation therapy is the best course of treatment. Surgical intervention is considered when extension of the tumor fixes one of the cords or extends upward or downward

TRACHEOSTOMY CARE AND SUCTIONING

1. Check physician's orders.
2. Assess patient's tracheostomy for sanguineous exudate, edema, and respiratory obstruction.
3. Obtain supplies and equipment, and take to bedside.
4. Explain procedure.
5. Wash hands.
6. Pull curtain around bed and close door to room.
7. Position patient in semi-Fowler's position.
8. Provide paper and pencil for patient; because patient cannot speak, this offers means of communication.
9. Position self at head of bed facing patient. Always face patient while cleaning a tracheostomy. Observe for respiratory difficulty and coughing, which might expel cannula.
10. Place towel or prepackaged drape under tracheostomy and across chest.
11. Prepare equipment and supplies on over bed table.
    a. Open suction catheter, leaving it in its wrapper to maintain sterility and attach to suction machine.
    b. Pour cleansing solution in one basin and rinsing solution in another basin. The first basin should have hydrogen peroxide to cleanse mucus and secretions from inner cannula. The second basin should contain normal saline to rinse cannula. If basins are prepackaged and under sterile gloves, use one-glove technique to remove basins and pour solution with ungloved hand.
    c. Turn on suction machine.
    d. Apply other sterile glove. Keep dominant hand sterile.
12. Unlock and remove inner cannula, and place in hydrogen peroxide cleansing solution. Placing fingers on tabs of outer cannula prevents movement that may irritate surrounding tissue and cause pain and coughing. NEVER remove outer cannula. If it is expelled by patient, use hemostat to hold tracheostomy open and call for assistance. A sterile packaged hemostat as well as an extra sterile tracheostomy set should always be available at the bedside.
13. Suction inner aspect of outer cannula.
    a. Withdraw sterile rinsing solution through catheter by placing thumb over suction control to moisten catheter.
    b. Ask patient to take several deep breaths or if patient is receiving oxygen, remove oxygen immediately before suctioning.
    c. Remove thumb from suction control or pinch catheter with gloved thumb and index finger; insert catheter 5 to 6 inches. (Depth of catheter should be length of outer cannula and extend approximately 1 to 2 inches beyond distal end.)
    d. Apply intermittent suction by placing thumb on and off suction control, and gently rotate catheter as it is withdrawn.
    e. Suction for at least 10 to 15 seconds. Do not suction longer than 15 seconds. (Holding your own breath until uncomfortable may provide same effect of not breathing that patient experiences.)
    f. Studies have shown adverse effects of saline lavage on oxygenation. Researchers speculate that saline acts as a barrier to gas exchange and thus reduces oxygenation. The theoretical advantage for instilling saline—to loosen secretions—also has not been supported. Little or no evidence that saline is distributed beyond the main stem bronchi has been found.[49]
    g. Allow patient to rest between each episode of suctioning. If patient was previously receiving oxygen, it may be reapplied at the prescribed rate. Suctioning can be exhausting and frightening for patient. Resting helps to regain depleted oxygen and renew strength.
    h. Rinse catheter with sterile solution, and repeat suction if needed.
    i. Turn off suction, and dispose of catheter.
14. Apply second sterile glove, if one-gloved technique is used, or apply new pair of sterile gloves.
15. Clean inner cannula:
    a. Use pipe cleaners and brush to clean inside and outside of inner cannula.
    b. Place inner cannula in sterile normal saline solution.
    c. Inspect inner and outer areas of inner cannula.
    d. Insert inner cannula and lock in place.
16. Clean skin around tracheostomy and tabs of outer cannula with hydrogen peroxide. Use wipes that are free of lint around the tracheostomy opening. Inhaled lint irritates the respira-

TRACHEOSTOMY CARE AND SUCTIONING—cont'd

tory passages and may cause undue coughing. Special tracheostomy dressings are available.

17. Thoroughly rinse cleansing solution from skin; place dry, sterile dressing around tracheostomy face plate.
18. Change cotton tapes (always do this last to prevent risk of cannula being expelled); attaching clean tape is done only when needed:
    a. Untie one side of cotton tape from outer cannula, and replace with clean one. Obtaining assistance of another person who will stabilize the tracheostomy tube while one set of ties is removed and replaced is advisable. This will provide more room for threading the clean ties.
    b. Bring clean tape under back of neck. (Securely hold tracheostomy tube in place to prevent movement of cannula that could stimulate coughing and expel cannula.)
    c. Untie other side from outer cannula and replace with clean tape.
    d. Tie ends of two clean cotton tapes together and position knot at side of neck. (Avoid placing knot at back of neck, which can cause pressure and discomfort to cervical vertebrae.)
19. Provide mouth care.
20. Remove gloves.
21. Adjust top linens, and position patient in comfortable position.
22. Place call light, paper, and pencil within easy reach.
23. Dispose of soiled supplies in appropriate area.
24. Wash hands.
25. Reassess patient's tracheostomy for signs of bleeding, edema, and respiratory obstruction.
26. Record in nurse's notes: tracheostomy care performed, patient's response, respiratory assessment, suction performed, any adverse reactions, and condition of tracheal stoma. If oxygen is administered, note flow and method used.

Skill 31-2 describes how to care for a tracheostomy or T-piece. The T-piece is the large plastic tubing fastened over the tracheostomy.

CARE OF PATIENT WITH CUFFED TRACHEOSTOMY TUBE

1. Follow steps 1 to 11.
2. Suction patient.
3. Connect syringe to pilot balloon valve (see illustration).
4. Position stethoscope in sternal notch or above tracheostomy tube, and listen for minimal amount of air leak at end of inspiration (see illustration).
5. Remove all air from cuff if no air leak is auscultated; this releases excessive air pressure.
6. While listening with stethoscope, slowly inflate cuff with 0.5 to 1 ml of air at a time. When no air leak is heard, stop injecting air and slowly withdraw up to 0.5 ml of air until air leak is auscultated with stethoscope.
7. If excessive air leak is heard, slowly add air as in step 6.
8. Remove stethoscope and cleanse diaphragm with alcohol swab.
9. Do not leave syringe attached to pilot balloon valve; remove syringe and either discard in proper container or store per agency's policy.
10. Reposition patient.
11. Wash hands.
12. Document as in Step 26.

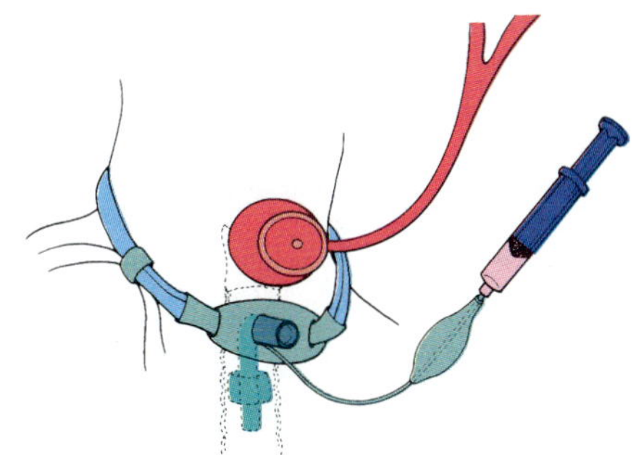

STEP 3

SKILL 31-2

CARING FOR A TRACHEOSTOMY COLLAR AND T-PIECE/TUBE

1. Wash hands.
2. Position the patient for comfort, usually in a semi-Fowler's position.
3. Inspect the rate of flow and the solution level for humidification often during the course of the patient's oxygen therapy.
4. Provide nose and mouth care to keep the mucosa lubricated, moist, clean, and fresh during the course of the patient's therapy.
5. Secure the collar or T-piece at the neck over the tracheostomy (see illustration).
6. Adjust the oxygen flow rate according to the physician's order.
7. Adjust the temperature of the humidified oxygen.
8. Use large-lumen tubing from the oxygen source to the patient.
9. Condensation occurs within the tracheostomy collar or T-piece, so observe frequently (see illustration).
10. The collar or T-piece and tubing should be removed frequently to be drained and cleaned to prevent the patient from aspirating the moisture. (Excessive water accumulates more frequently at higher humidities.)
11. As moisture collects, suction the tracheostomy and provide tracheostomy care as often as necessary.
12. Mist should always be visible.

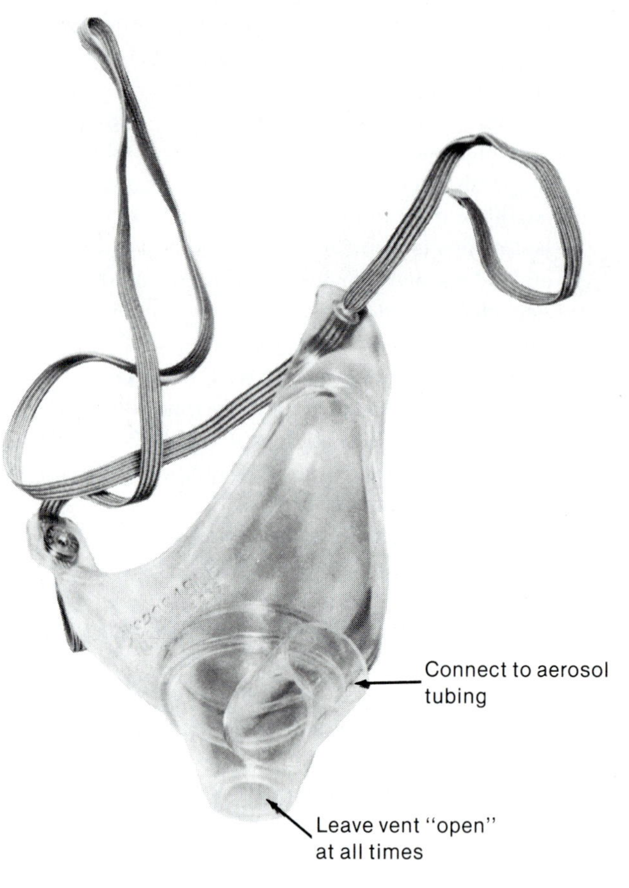

STEP 9

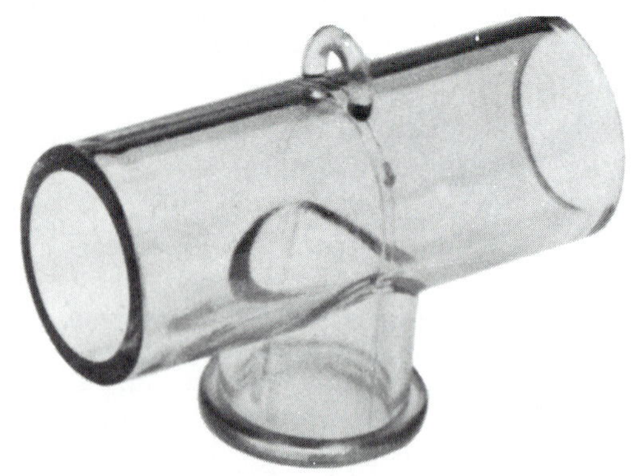

STEP 5

from the larynx, and it may include either a total or partial laryngectomy or a radical neck dissection. A partial laryngectomy is done to remove the diseased vocal cord and possibly a portion of thyroid cartilage, requiring the placement of a temporary tracheostomy (Skill 31-1 on pp. 888-889), which will be closed when the edema has decreased. A total laryngectomy is performed when the cancer of the larynx is advanced and requires the placement of a permanent tracheostomy. Because the patient can no longer breathe through the nose, the sense of smell is absent. The voice is also absent, because the larynx is removed. There is no connection between the patient's mouth and trachea.

A radical neck dissection to remove cervical lymph nodes is often done in conjunction with a total laryngectomy in those patients in whom risk of metastasis to the neck from carcinoma of the larynx is high. This surgery entails removal of the submandibular salivary gland, sternocleidomastoid muscle, spinal accessory nerve, and the internal jugular vein, which results in one-sided shoulder droop.

Nursing Interventions. Airway maintenance through proper suctioning techniques is important (Skill 31-3 on pp. 892-893). Skin integrity surrounding the tracheal opening should be assessed; the nurse should be alert for signs of infection.

The nurse should monitor I&O balance and assist with tube feedings as ordered. The nurse should explain to the patient that the tube feedings are temporary and that when healing occurs in a few weeks, normal eating may begin again. The nurse should weigh the patient daily and assess hydration status for the need for additional fluids; note skin turgor and observe for diarrhea.

Because of neck and facial disfigurement and loss of voice, a thorough psychosocial assessment and resultant interventions will be beneficial. The nurse should encourage communication through writing and facial and hand gestures. Often no one else can give a patient reassurance that speech can be regained as well as a fellow patient who has undergone the same surgical intervention. Many cities have a Lost Chord Club or a New Voice Club, and the members are willing to visit hospitalized patients.

Care of the tracheostomy. The term *tracheostomy* means "an artificial opening made by a surgical incision into the trachea." After the surgical procedure is performed, the physician inserts a tracheostomy tube into the opening and secures it in place by cotton tapes around the patient's neck. This procedure is performed to provide the patient with a patent airway. Sterile gauze is placed around the opening under the flange of the outer tube for skin protection. Use wipes that are free of lint around the tracheostomy opening. Inhaled lint irritates respiratory passages and may cause undue coughing. The primary nursing responsibilities are to maintain a patent airway, keep the inner cannula clean, prevent impairment of surrounding tissue, and provide a means of communication for the patient. An endotracheal (Fig. 31-10) or tracheostomy tube provides a direct route for introduction of pathogens into the lower airway, increasing the risk of infection. It is essential that the following preventive nursing interventions be consistently implemented:

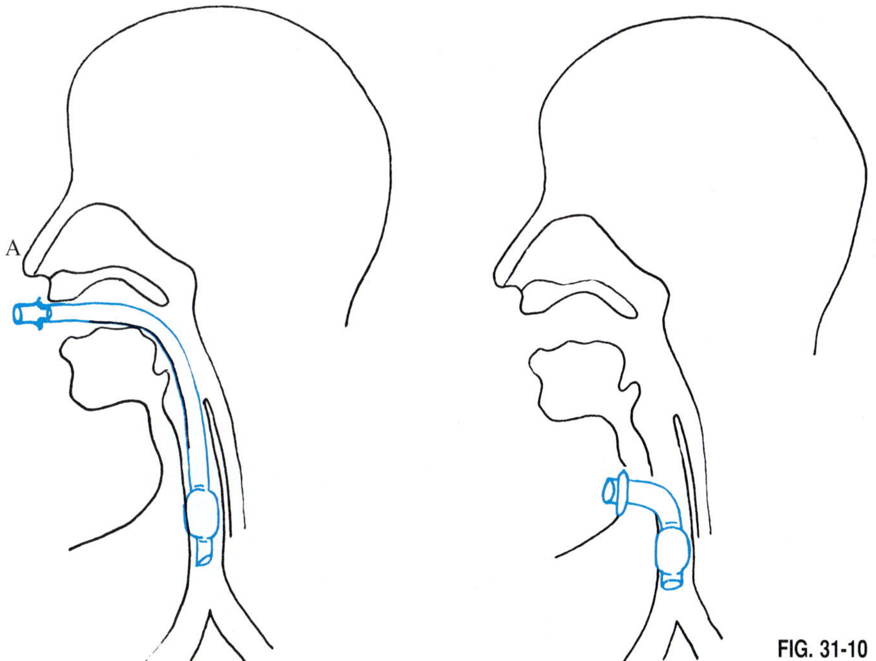

FIG. 31-10 **A,** Position of endotracheal tube. **B,** Position of tracheostomy tube.

CLEARING THE AIRWAY

1. Check physician's order.
2. Assess need for suctioning: gurgling respirations, restlessness, vomitus in mouth, and drooling are indications.
3. Explain procedure to patient. Explain that coughing, sneezing, or gagging is expected.
4. Assemble equipment.
5. Wash hands.
6. Provide privacy.
7. Position patient.
   a. If patient is alert and conscious, place in semi-Fowler's position with head to one side (placing head to one side promotes drainage of secretions and facilitates insertion of the suction catheter).
   b. If patient is unconscious, place in side-lying position facing nurse.
8. Place towel lengthwise under patient's chin and over pillow.
9. Pour sterile normal saline solution into sterile container.
10. Don sterile gloves on dominant hand.
11. Turn on suction machine, and select appropriate suction pressure. Never suction with any more vacuum pressure than needed to remove the secretions, and use the smallest catheter that will remove the secretions well.

Common vacuum settings for wall suction units

Infants	50-95 mm Hg
Children	95-110 mm Hg
Adults	110-150 mm Hg

Common catheter sizes

Infant	6-8 French
Children	8-10 French
Adults	12-16 French

12. Aspirate solution through catheter by placing thumb over open end of connector or over vent to (1) check patency of suction catheter and suction pressure and (2) moisten catheter for ease of insertion.
13. Remove thumb from Y-connector opening or pinch catheter with thumb and index finger; if using suction catheter with vent, remove thumb from vent opening. This prevents injury to mucous membrane while catheter is being inserted.
14. Insert catheter.

OROPHARYNGEAL SUCTIONING

a. Gently insert Yankauer or tonsillar tip suction catheter (see illustrations) into one side of mouth.
b. Glide Yankauer toward oropharynx without suction.
c. Move Yankauer around mouth until secretions are cleared.
d. Encourage patient to cough—this moves secretions from lower airway into mouth and upper airway.
e. Rinse Yankauer with water in cup or basin until connecting tubing is cleared of secretions.
f. Repeat procedure as is necessary.

NASOPHARYNGEAL SUCTIONING

g. Holding catheter with thumb and index finger, place nasal catheter near patient's earlobe to tip of nose. Do not touch side of face, nose, or earlobe. This marks catheter for correct length of insertion at that point. From earlobe to tip of nose approximates depth of insertion.

Length of insertion

Adults	16 cm
Older children	8-12 cm
Infants and young children	4-8 cm

h. Lubricate catheter with water-soluble jelly. Water-soluble lubricant dissolves and thus buildup that may hinder airway is prevented.
i. Hold catheter to observe its natural curvature and gently insert catheter into one side of nasal passage.

NASOTRACHEAL SUCTIONING

j. Holding catheter with thumb and index finger, place nasotracheal catheter near earlobe to tip of nose and extend to trachea to measure for correct length of insertion (see illustrations). Do not touch side of face, nose, or earlobe; maintain sterility.

STEP 14a

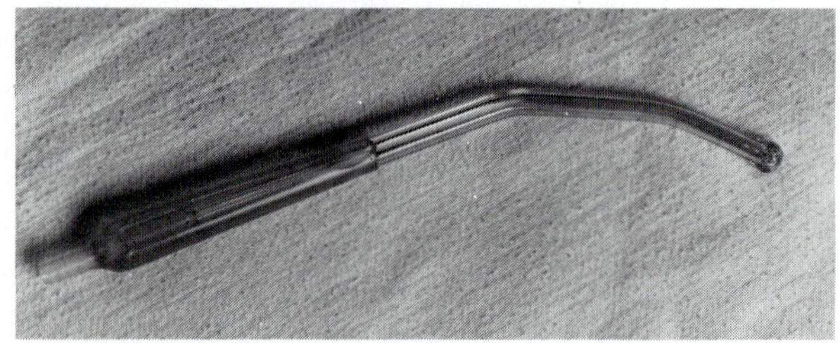

CLEARING THE AIRWAY—cont'd

Length of insertion

Adults	20-24 cm
Older children	14-20 cm
Young children and infants	8-14 cm

k. Lubricate catheter with a water-soluble jelly. This facilitates gliding catheter past nasal turbinates.

l. Ask patient if either side of nose is obstructed and use unobstructed side. Hold catheter to observe its natural curvature, and gently insert catheter into one side of nasal passage.

m. Stimulate coughing reflex, or ask patient to cough to guide catheter into trachea. If no cough reflex is present or if patient cannot assist, insert catheter when patient inhales; this avoids displacement of catheter into esophagus.

15. Apply suction by placing thumb over suction opening; rotate catheter gently as catheter is withdrawn.
16. Observe patient closely, and limit suction to 10 to 15 seconds.
17. Repeat suctioning if needed.
18. Allow 1 to 2 minutes' rest between suctioning if procedure must be repeated. If oxygen is administered by nasal cannula, mask, or other means, reapply oxygen during rest period. This provides rest and comfort and allows patient to regain oxygen supply. Time allowed for patient to rest between suctioning can vary from 1 to 2 minutes to 20 to 30 seconds, depending on patient's ability to tolerate procedure.
19. When suctioning is complete, suction between cheeks and gum line and under tongue; suction mouth last to prevent contaminating catheter.
20. If patient is alert and can cooperate, request patient to deep breathe and cough.
21. Place catheter in solution, and supply suction, which flushes secretions from catheter and tubing to maintain patency if procedure needs to be repeated.
22. Discard catheter: wrap catheter around gloved hand; pull glove off hand and over catheter. This reduces the spread of microorganisms and prevents direct contact with equipment and secretions.
23. Wash hands.
24. Place sterile, unopened catheter at patient's bedside to provide quick access to suction equipment if patient needs suctioning immediately.
25. Provide mouth care.
26. Observe patient's breathing patterns. Observe for decrease in anxiety, fatigue, vital signs, and level of consciousness and color.
27. Document in nurses' notes: date, time, and method of suctioning, and color, odor, amount, and consistency of secretions. Include respiratory assessment after suctioning, and patient's response.

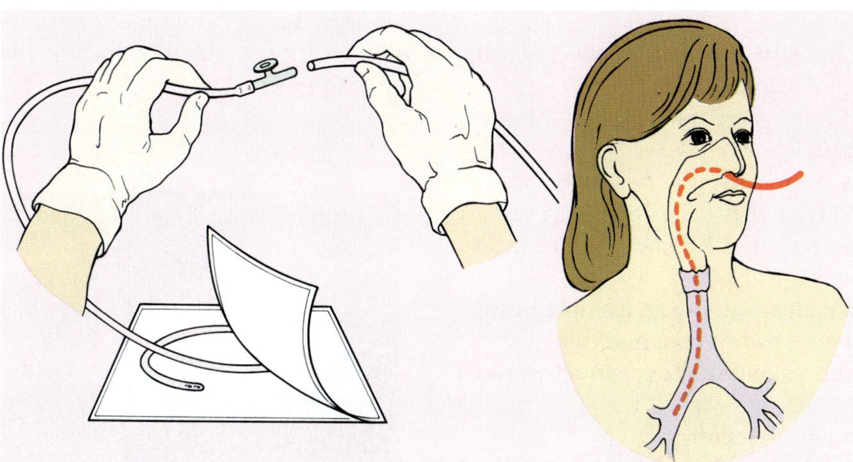

STEP 14a, cont'd

1. **Minimize infection risk**
   a. Assess the patient regularly for excess secretions, and suction as often as necessary.
   b. Provide constant airway humidification.
   c. Change all respiratory therapy equipment every 8 hours.
   d. Remove water that condenses in equipment tubing.
   e. Provide frequent mouth care (apply moisturizing agents to dry cracked lips).
   f. Maintain nutritional levels.
      (1) Patients' with endotracheal tubes are allowed nothing by mouth. Nourishment should be provided parenterally or by gastrointestinal feedings.
      (2) Patients with a tracheostomy tube are usually able to swallow and have a normal oral intake. Some experts prefer that the cuff be inflated while the patient is eating to prevent aspiration. Others believe that the inflated cuff bulges into the esophagus and makes swallowing more difficult. Nursing assessment or physician orders will determine which technique is used.
      (3) Ensure adequate ventilation and oxygenation
         (a) Assess lung sounds regularly.
         (b) Turn and reposition the patient every 2 hours for maximum ventilation and lung expansion.
         (c) Assess the effects of respiratory therapy frequently.
      (4) Provide safety and comfort
         (a) Assess tube placement at regular intervals—tracheostomy tubes are secured around neck with tapes or specially designed ties.
         (b) Change the tapes or ties whenever soiled to decrease skin irritation.
         (c) Always keep a spare tracheostomy tube at the bedside.
2. **Minimize sensory deprivation**
   a. Organize questions so that the patient can use a simple yes or no response by nodding the head or using hand signals
   b. See whether the patient can use an erasable board (Magic Slate) or note pad to communicate.
   c. Always talk to the patient and explain all procedures.
   d. Reorient the patient frequently.
   e. Encourage family and friends to talk to patient.
   f. Keep a call light (or tap bell) within patient's reach.

The tubes used to maintain this artificial airway are commonly referred to as *tracheostomy tubes.* The tracheostomy tube is usually made of metal or plastic. Previously, the more common tracheostomy tube had three parts: outer cannula, inner cannula, and obturator. The obturator was placed within the outer cannula, with the round, blunt end protruding through the distal end of the cannula. This provided a smooth, rounded edge and made insertion less traumatic to the tissues and trachea. Once the outer cannula was in place, the obturator was removed and the inner cannula was inserted within the outer cannula and locked in place.

With today's knowledge and new materials, a single cannula tracheostomy is more commonly used. This type of tracheostomy is referred to as the *cuffed tracheostomy tube* (Fig. 31-11). It is made of plastic and has an inflatable cuff around the middle of the distal portion of the tube. The physician may order a cuffed tracheostomy tube to be used initially until the healing process of the tracheal stoma is complete. The cuffed tube (Fig. 31-12) is commonly used for temporary use, to hold the tube in place during special treatments, such as ventilation or IPPB, and to prevent aspiration during such activities as eating or taking medications.

Although nursing care of patients with endotracheal (Fig. 31-12) and tracheostomy tubes is similar, patients with tracheostomies have additional nursing care needs. Analgesics and sedatives are given judiciously so as not to depress the respiratory center. The patient is suctioned as often as necessary, possibly every 5 minutes during the first few postoperative hours (when respirations are noisy and pulse and respiratory rates are increased, the patient needs to be suctioned). Patients who are conscious can usually indicate when they need to be suctioned. A patient who is able to expectorate secretions will require suctioning less frequently. The amount of mucus subsides gradually and suctioning will be less frequent. However, the patient remains apprehensive and needs constant attendance.

Nursing diagnoses and interventions for the patient with a tracheostomy tube include but are not limited to the following:

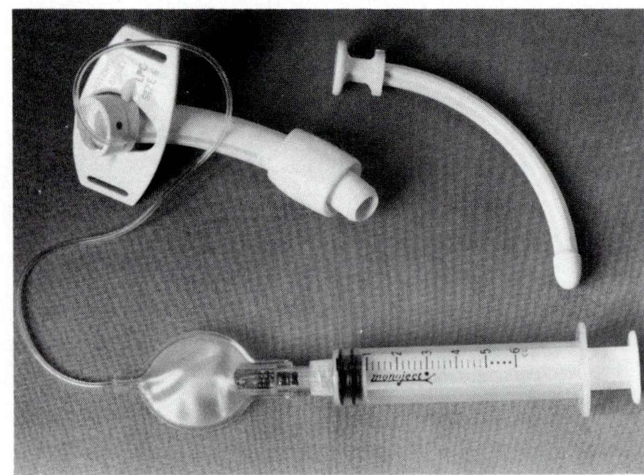

FIG. 31-11 Tracheostomy tube and inner cannula.

NURSING DIAGNOSES	NURSING INTERVENTIONS
Airway clearance, ineffective, related to secretions or other obstruction	Suction secretions as needed. Provide tracheostomy care according to protocol; ensure the availability of emergency equipment (oxygen and tracheostomy tray). Offer small, frequent feedings, and give liquid or pureed food as tolerated to prevent choking. Teach patient stoma protection. Assess respiratory rate and characteristics q 1 to 2 hr. Maintain head of bed elevated at 30 degrees or higher. Turn, cough, and encourage deep breathing q 2 to 4 hr. Auscultate lung sounds. Provide constant humidity. Suction laryngectomy tube prn, using aseptic technique; instruct patient to inhale as catheter is advanced. Clean inner cannula of laryngectomy tube q 2 to 4 hr and prn, using a solution of normal saline and hydrogen peroxide. Suction trachea prn.
Anxiety, related to inability to speak, isolation, mutilating surgery, diagnosis of cancer, and drooling	Keep call light within easy reach at all times. Locate patient close to nurses' station. Answer call light/bell as quickly as possible. Check patient frequently. Keep oral suction catheter beside patient to suction oral cavity. Encourage significant other to support patient.
Anxiety, related to inability to speak, isolation, mutilating surgery, diagnosis of cancer, and drooling—cont'd	Encourage patient to care for own tracheostomy when feasible. Provide information about alternative methods of communication.
Communication, impaired verbal, related to removal of larynx	Provide patient with implements for communication, including pencil, paper, Magic Slate, picture books, or electronic voice device. Keep call light/bell by patient's hand at all times. Ask patient questions that require only a yes or no response, if possible, to avoid fatigue and frustration. Refer patient to local support groups (e.g., Lost Chord Club) and the local chapter of the American Cancer Society. Assist with speech rehabilitation. Review instructions about esophageal and electroesophageal speech. Reinforce need for regular follow-up with speech pathologist and surgeon after discharge.
Self-esteem disturbance, related to disfiguring surgery	Assist patient to identify past strengths and coping mechanisms. Assess patient's body image concept, and note nonverbal responses to changes that have taken place. Allow time for the grieving process. Provide patient with tissues to absorb oral secretions. Provide oral care, including mouthwash or half-strength hydrogen peroxide q 2 hr.

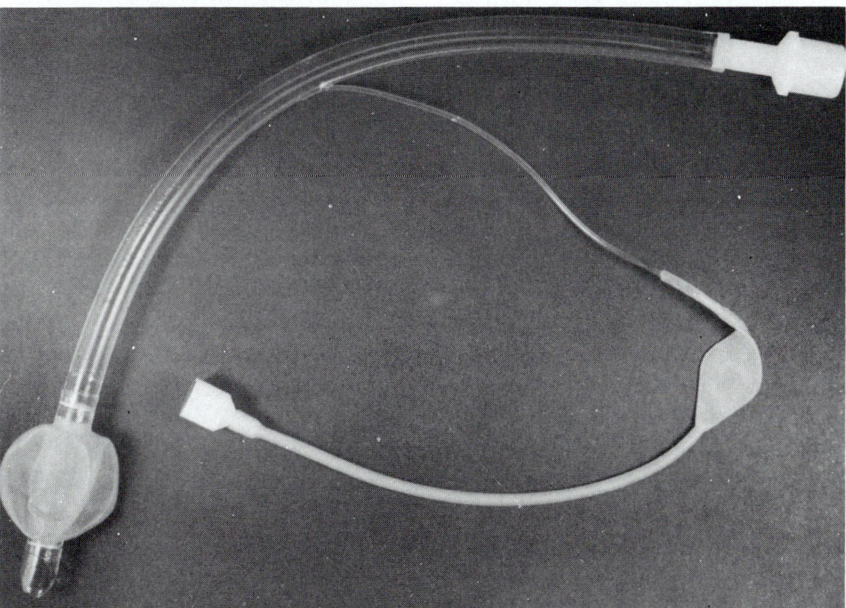

FIG. 31-12 Forregar high-volume, low-pressure cuffed endotracheal tube. Cuff shown here is not inflated. Low-pressure cuff is preferred because it is less likely to cause tracheal damage.

Patient teaching. Techniques of airway maintenance, such as oxygen usage, deep breathing, and coughing, should be explained. The importance of dietary management in relationship to airway maintenance should be discussed. Optimal communication should be encouraged through speech rehabilitation and community support groups.

Prognosis. If tumor is limited to the true cord, the cure rate is 80% to 90%. The prognosis in primary supraglottic and subglottic cancer is poor.

RESPIRATORY INFECTIONS

Acute Rhinitis (Common Cold, Acute Coryza)

Etiology/Pathophysiology. Acute rhinitis or **acute coryza,** known as the *common cold,* is an inflammatory condition of the mucous membranes of the nose and accessory sinuses. It is characterized most typically by edema of the nasal mucous membrane. The common cold is usually caused by one or more viruses; however, it may become complicated by a bacterial infection. Signs and symptoms usually are evident within 24 to 48 hours after exposure. Sinus congestion causes increased sinus drainage, leading to postnasal drip. The postnasal drip causes throat irritation, headache, and earache. Most persons with colds contaminate their hands when coughing or sneezing, thus contaminating everything they touch. Others become infected when touching the telephone, computer, or anything else that has been touched by the person with a cold. Also, many colds are believed to be spread through shaking hands with a person who has a cold.

Clinical Manifestations. An increased amount of thin, serous nasal exudate and a productive cough are two of the most common signs. Sore throat and fever are often present. If the infection remains uncomplicated, it generally subsides in a week.

Assessment. Collection of *subjective data* includes the patient's complaints of sore throat, dyspnea, and congestion of varying duration.

Collection of *objective data* includes noting the color and consistency of the nasal exudate. A visual exam of the throat may reveal erythema, edema, and local irritation. The nurse will also document the presence and duration of fever.

Diagnostic Tests. Throat and sputum cultures will indicate the presence and nature of microorganisms.

Medical Management. Medical management is aimed at accurate diagnosis and prevention of complications. No specific treatment is available for the common cold. Among the medications used are (1) aspirin or acetaminophen for analgesia and reduction of temperature (aspirin is not used in infants, children, and adolescents because of the danger of developing Reye's syndrome); (2) a cough suppressant for a dry, nonproductive cough; or (3) an expectorant for a productive cough. If the presence of a secondary bacterial infection is confirmed, an antibiotic agent (e.g., erythromycin) is prescribed.

Nursing Interventions. Nursing interventions are aimed at promoting comfort. Such measures include encouraging fluids and applying warm, moist packs to sinuses.

Nursing diagnoses and interventions for the patient with acute rhinitis include but are not limited to the following:

NURSING DIAGNOSES	NURSING INTERVENTIONS
Airway clearance, ineffective, related to nasal exudate	Encourage fluids to liquify secretions and aid in their expectoration. Use vaporizer to moisten mucous membranes and prevent further irritation.
Infection, high risk for, related to retained pulmonary secretions	Check temperature q 2 to 4 hr. Promote rest and comfort. Encourage coughing and deep breathing q 2 hr.
Health-seeking behaviors: illness prevention, related to preventing exacerbation or spread of infection	Remind patient and family of health maintenance behaviors to decrease risk of illness, such as adequate fluid and nutritional management and sufficient rest. Teach importance of hygiene measures to decrease spread of infection.

Patient teaching. The patient should be taught correct hand washing technique and proper disposal of tissues used for nasal secretions. The nurse should instruct the patient to limit exposure to others during the first 48 hours and to check the temperature every 4 hours.

Prognosis. Signs and symptoms are resolved in 2 to 10 days. Even though the common cold does not cause death, its economic importance is vast because it is the greatest cause of absenteeism in industry and schools.

Acute Follicular Tonsillitis

Etiology/Pathophysiology. Acute follicular tonsillitis can be an acute inflammation of the tonsils. It is the result of an air- or food-borne bacterial infection, often *Streptococcus.* It can also be viral, but this occurs less often. If it is caused by group A β-hemolytic streptococci, sequelae such as rheumatic fever, carditis, and nephritis must be considered. It appears to be most common in school-age children. Signs and symptoms of tonsillitis include sore throat, fever, chills, and anorexia. The tonsils become enlarged and often contain purulent exudate.

Clinical Manifestations. Acute follicular tonsillitis manifests itself clinically with enlarged, tender, cervical lymph nodes. Fever may be present with chills, general muscle aching, and malaise. Laboratory data reveal an elevated white blood cell count.

Assessment. Collection of *subjective data* includes monitoring the severity of throat pain and the possibility of referred pain to the ears. Headache or joint pain should be noted.

Collection of *objective data* includes a visual examination that shows increased throat secretions and enlarged, erythematous tonsils.

Diagnostic Tests. Throat cultures will identify the causative microorganism, most commonly β-hemolytic streptococci. A complete blood count will be done to determine if the white blood count is elevated. It is not uncommon for the white blood count to be 10,000 to 20,000 per cubic millimeter.

Medical Management. If antibiotics to which the offending organism is sensitive are administered early, infection subsides. Until recently tonsillectomy/adenoidectomy was the surgical intervention of choice. When this procedure is performed, the tonsils and adenoids are surgically excised. This procedure occurs only in persons who have recurrent attacks of tonsillitis. The procedure is usually performed from 4 to 6 weeks after an acute attack has subsided. Either general or local anesthesia is used. When a tonsillectomy/adenoidectomy is performed, hemostasis is of utmost importance, because the patient can lose a large amount of blood through hemorrhage without demonstrating any outward signs of bleeding. The physician may be able to control minor postoperative bleeding by applying a sponge soaked in a solution of epinephrine to the site. The patient who is bleeding excessively often is returned to the operating room for surgical treatment to stop the hemorrhage.

Medications used in tonsillitis include analgesics and antipyretics, such as acetaminophen, and antibiotic agents, such as penicillin. Warm saline gargles are also beneficial.

Nursing Interventions. One of the primary nursing goals for acute tonsillitis is to provide meticulous oral care, which will promote comfort and assist in combating infection. An important postoperative nursing intervention is to observe and report if the patient exhibits frequent swallowing, because this is often a subtle but reliable indication of excessive bleeding.

Postoperative care for tonsillectomy includes maintaining intravenous fluids until the nausea subsides, at which time the patient may begin drinking ice cold liquids. Red liquids are discouraged so they do not mask presence of bleeding. The diet will be advanced to custard and ice cream and then to a normal diet as soon as possible. An ice collar should be applied to the neck for comfort and to reduce bleeding by vasoconstriction. Vital signs must be monitored to assess for hemorrhage, postoperative fever, or other complications. Comfort measures are important, and emotional support is essential. This surgery is less common today because the role of lymphoid tissue in the body's immune mechanism has been determined.

Nursing diagnoses and interventions for the patient with acute follicular tonsillitis include but are not limited to the following:

NURSING DIAGNOSES	NURSING INTERVENTIONS
Pain, related to inflammation/irritation of throat	Assess degree of pain and need for pain medication. Document effectiveness of medication, and offer pain medication as ordered. Maintain bed rest, and promote rest. Offer warm saline gargles, ice chips, and ice collar as needed.
Fluid volume deficit, high risk for, related to inability to maintain usual oral intake because of painful swallowing	Assess hydration status by noting mucous membranes, skin turgor, and urine output. Encourage increased oral intake: cold liquids, sherbet, and ice cream will be best tolerated; carbonated drinks may be taken if patient tolerates; avoid offering fruit juices, because they may burn throat.

Patient teaching. The patient or family should be instructed that the patient should complete the entire course of the prescribed antibiotic. If patient has had surgery (tonsillectomy and adenoidectomy [T&A]), dietary instruction should be offered regarding appropriate foods and liquids. The nurse should teach the patient to avoid attempting to clear the throat immediately after surgery (may initiate bleeding) and to avoid coughing, sneezing, or vigorous nose blowing for 1 to 2 weeks. Some surgeons no longer prescribe aspirin for pain after tonsillectomy, as it increases the tendency to bleed; acetaminophen or other aspirin substitute is usually ordered. The nurse should remind the patient to avoid overexertion and should ascertain that the patient and family know how to reach the physician in case of increased pain, fever, or bleeding.

Prognosis. Tonsillitis is usually self-limited, but serious complications, such as sinusitis, otitis media, mastoiditis, rheumatic fever, nephritis, or peritonsillar abscess, may occur.

Laryngitis

Etiology/Pathophysiology. Laryngitis often occurs secondary to other respiratory infections. Laryngeal inflammation is a common disorder that can be either chronic or acute. Acute laryngitis may cause severe respiratory distress in children under 5 years of age because the relatively small larynx of the young child is subject to spasm when irritated or infected and readily becomes partially or totally obstructed.

Acute laryngitis often accompanies viral or bacterial infections. Other causes include excessive use of the voice or inhalation of irritating fumes. Chronic laryngitis is usually associated with inflammation of laryngeal mucosa or edematous vocal cords.

Clinical Manifestations. Clinical manifestation include hoarseness of varying degrees or even complete voice loss. The throat will feel scratchy and irritated, and the patient may have a persistent cough.

Assessment. Collection of *subjective data* includes the patient reporting progressive hoarseness and a cough that may be productive or may be dry and nonproductive. The nurse should attempt to identify any precipitating factors such as excessive voice use or increased exposure to inhaled irritants.

Collection of *objective data* includes the nurse evaluating the patient's voice quality as well as the characteristics (color, consistency, and amount) of sputum produced.

Diagnostic Tests. Laryngoscopy will reveal abnormalities (edema, drainage) of vocal cords and erythematous laryngeal mucosa.

Medical Management. If due to a virus, there is no specific therapy; if bacterial, medications include antibiotics (such as erythromycin). Analgesics/antipyretics for comfort, antitussives to relieve cough (such as Phenergan with codeine), and throat lozenges to promote comfort and decrease irritation are useful.

Nursing Interventions. General interventions include use of warm or cool mist inhalation via vaporizer. The patient should be encouraged to rest the voice by limiting verbal communication.

Nursing diagnoses and interventions for the patient with laryngitis include but are not limited to the following:

NURSING DIAGNOSES	NURSING INTERVENTIONS
Pain, related to throat irritation	Assess level of pain, and offer medications to promote comfort. Use steam inhalation as ordered.
Verbal communication, impaired, related to edematous vocal cords	Instruct patient on the importance of resting the voice. Provide other means for communication (written word, gestures). Anticipate patient's needs whenever possible.

Patient teaching. If the patient receives antibiotic agents, the nurse should instruct him to finish the entire prescribed course. The patient should be reminded of the need to limit use of the voice. Patients who smoke should be encouraged to quit and also to limit exposure to irritating fumes.

Prognosis. Prognosis is good in adults. In the infant and young child respiratory obstruction can result in respiratory distress.

Pharyngitis

Etiology/Pathophysiology. Pharyngitis may be either chronic or acute. It is the most common throat inflammation and frequently accompanies the common cold. Pharyngitis is usually viral in origin but can be caused by hemolytic streptococci, staphylococci, or other bacteria. There is increased evidence of gonococcal pharyngitis caused by the gram-negative diplococcus *Neisseria gonorrhoeae.* A severe form of acute pharyngitis often is referred to as *strep throat,* because the streptococcus organism is commonly the cause. This disorder is contagious for 2 or 3 days after the onset of signs and symptoms.

Clinical Manifestations. Pharyngitis manifests itself clinically by a dry cough, tender tonsils, and enlarged cervical lymph glands. The throat appears erythematous, and soreness may range from slight scratchiness to severe pain with difficulty swallowing.

Assessment. Collection of *subjective data* includes any reported pharyngeal discomfort, presence of fever, or any difficulty swallowing.

Collection of *objective data* includes palpating for enlarged, edematous glands and associated tenderness and noting elevated temperature.

Diagnostic Studies. Throat cultures will be done to document presence or absence of a bacterial infection.

Medical Management. Commonly ordered medications include antibiotics, such as penicillin or erythromycin, to (1) treat severe infections or (2) prevent superimposed infections, particularly in persons who have a history of rheumatic fever or bacterial endocarditis. Analgesics/antipyretics, such as acetaminophen, are used to promote comfort.

Nursing Interventions. The nurse should offer throat rinses/gargles and encourage oral intake. The importance of adequate rest and use of a vaporizer to increase humidity should be emphasized.

Nursing diagnoses and interventions for the patient with pharyngitis include but are not limited to the following:

NURSING DIAGNOSES	NURSING INTERVENTIONS
Oral mucous membrane, altered, related to edema	Provide warm saline gargles to promote comfort. Assess level of pain, and offer medications as ordered. Encourage oral intake of fluids. Offer frequent oral care.
Fluid volume deficit, high risk for, related to decreased oral intake as a result of painful swallowing.	Observe and record patient's hydration status. Monitor I&O, and patient's temperature. Maintain IV therapy if indicated.

Patient teaching. The nurse should perform and document medication teaching: the importance of completing the entire prescribed course of antibiotics and any side effects of medications. The patient should be instructed to avoid exposure to inhaled irritants and to use preventive measures, such as using a vaporizer and maintaining adequate fluid intake.

Prognosis. Signs and symptoms will usually resolve in 4 to 6 days unless secondary complications develop.

Sinusitis

Etiology/Pathophysiology. Sinusitis can be chronic or acute, involving any sinus area, such as maxillary or frontal. This infection can be either viral or bacterial in origin and often is a complication of pneumonia or nasal polyps.

The underlying pathophysiology begins with an upper respiratory infection that leads to a sinus infection.

Clinical Manifestations. The patient with sinusitis often complains of a constant, severe headache with pain and tenderness in the particular sinus region. Frequently there is a purulent exudate.

Assessment. Collection of *subjective data* includes the patient reporting a decreased appetite or nausea. The patient may also complain of generalized malaise, headache, and pain in the sinus region.

Collection of *objective data* involves the nurse assessing vital signs, particularly temperature, and also assessing the character and amount of drainage.

Diagnostic Tests. Sinus x-ray studies are frequently done to depict cloudy or fluid-filled sinus cavities. A simple way to diagnose sinusitis is with transillumination. This procedure involves shining a light in the mouth with the lips closed around it; infected sinuses will look dark, and normal sinuses will transilluminate.

Medical Management. Nasal windows or other surgical incisions can be created to allow better drainage and removal of diseased mucosal tissue. One of the most common surgical procedures to relieve chronic maxillary sinusitis is the Caldwell-Luc operation, which is a radical antrum operation involving the creation of an incision under the lip to remove diseased mucosal and bone tissue.

Medications used to treat sinusitis include antibiotic agents (penicillin), analgesics to relieve headache (acetaminophen [Tylenol], possibly with codeine), antihistamines (azatadine [Optimine]) to reduce congestion and secretions, and vasoconstrictors in the form of nasal sprays (Afrin) to reduce local vascular congestion.

Nursing Interventions. Steam inhalation and warm, moist packs will facilitate drainage and promote comfort.

Nursing diagnoses and interventions for the patient with sinusitis include but are not limited to the following:

NURSING DIAGNOSES	NURSING INTERVENTIONS
Breathing pattern, ineffective, related to nasal congestion	Assess respiratory status frequently, noting any changes; mouth breathing may be necessary because of nasal airway/sinus discomfort.
Pain, related to sinus congestion	Document comfort level. Assess need for pain medication, and document patient response. Elevate head of bed to promote drainage of secretions. Apply warm, moist packs four times/day to promote secretion drainage and provide relief.

Patient teaching. The aim of patient education is to prevent reoccurrence or complications of sinus infection. The patient should be instructed to be alert to signs and symptoms of sinusitis so early treatment can be obtained.

Prognosis. Prognosis for uncomplicated sinusitis is good; complications include cavernous sinus thrombosis and spread of infection to bone, brain, or meninges, which can result in meningitis, osteomyelitis, or septicemia.

DISORDERS OF THE LOWER AIRWAY

Acute Bronchitis

Etiology/Pathophysiology. Usually acute bronchitis is secondary to an upper respiratory infection, but it can be related to exposure to inhaled irritants. Inflammation of the trachea and bronchial tree causes congestion of the mucous membranes, which results in retention of tenacious secretions. These secretions can become a culture medium for bacterial growth.

Clinical Manifestations. Acute bronchitis manifests itself by a productive cough, diffuse rhonchi/wheezes, dyspnea, chest pain, and low-grade temperature. Generalized malaise and headache are also common symptoms.

Assessment. Collection of *subjective data* includes the patient's complaints of feeling poorly and experiencing headache and aching tightness in the chest.

Collection of *objective data* involves a nursing assessment that includes monitoring vital signs frequently, checking breath sounds, and noting the presence of wheezes or basilar crackles.

Diagnostic Tests. The usual diagnostic aids include a chest x-ray examination to ensure clear lung fields and sputum specimen to determine the presence of associated bacterial infections.

Medical Management. A quick recovery is promoted by preventing further infectious complications. The physician may order sputum cultures periodically to ascertain that there is no secondary infection.

Medications that are frequently prescribed are cough suppressants (codeine), antitussives (dextromethorphan [Pertussin]), antipyretics (Tylenol), and bronchodilators (terbutaline [Brethine]). Antibiotics, such as ampicillin, may be ordered to combat an infectious process or to prevent its occurrence.

Nursing Interventions. The goal of nursing interventions is to facilitate recovery and prevent secondary infections. Such actions include placing the patient on bed rest to conserve energy, using a vaporizer to add humidity to inhaled air, and increasing fluid intake.

Nursing diagnoses and interventions for the patient with acute bronchitis include but are not limited to the following:

NURSING DIAGNOSES	NURSING INTERVENTIONS
Infection, high risk for, related to retained pulmonary secretions	Assess for signs/symptoms of infection: fever, dyspnea, color and characteristics of sputum production. Administer antipyretics and antibiotics as ordered.
Airway clearance, ineffective, related to tenacious pulmonary secretions	Assess patient's ability to move secretions; also note an increase in retained pulmonary secretions. Facilitate airway clearance by elevating head of bed and liquefying secretions by use of humidifier and adequate fluid intake (3000 to 4000 ml/day). Suction as needed. When offering fluids, avoid dairy products, which tend to produce more tenacious secretions.
Fatigue, related to prolonged coughing periods	Encourage rest periods between activities. Assess support systems and available resources; refer as necessary.

Patient teaching. The patient should be instructed on measures that will prevent exacerbation or recurrence of infection. Such measures include stressing the importance of increasing oral fluid intake, incorporating rest periods between activities, and teaching the patient the signs that may indicate worsening infection (purulent sputum and increased dyspnea). Medication teaching would involve emphasizing the importance of adhering to prescribed medication regimen and using analgesics and antipyretics to reduce fever and malaise. The nurse should teach the patient to limit exposure to others, who may spread infection, and to avoid smoking or other irritating fumes.

Prognosis. Prognosis for acute bronchitis is good.

Legionnaires' Disease

Etiology/Pathophysiology. The causative microorganism of this disease is *Legionella pneumophila,* first identified in 1976 when it caused a pneumonia outbreak at a convention of the American Legion in Philadelphia, Pennsylvania. *Legionella pneumophila* is a gram-negative bacillus not previously recognized as an agent of human disease. This organism thrives in water reservoirs, such as in air conditioners and humidifiers, and is transmitted through airborne routes. The *Legionella* microbe can progress in two different forms—influenza or Legionnaires' disease, which characteristically results in life-threatening pneumonia. This pneumonia causes lung consolidation and alveolar necrosis. The disease progresses rapidly (less than 1 week) and can result in respiratory failure, renal failure, bacteremic shock, and ultimately, death.

Clinical Manifestations. Clinical manifestations include markedly elevated temperature, headache, nonproductive cough, diarrhea, and general malaise.

Assessment. Collection of *subjective data* includes noting the patient's complaints of dyspnea, headache, and chest pain on inspiration.

Collection of *objective data* includes many significant signs associated with this infectious process. A markedly elevated temperature (102° to 105° F [38.8° to 40.5° C]) bears close watching and immediate interventions. Another sign the patient will exhibit is a nonproductive cough with difficult and rapid breathing. Auscultation of lungs will reveal crackles or wheezes. Because of the high fever and extreme respiratory effort, tachycardia and signs of shock may be present. Hematuria may develop, indicative of resulting renal impairment.

Diagnostic Tests. Diagnostic tests to confirm *Legionella pneumophila* infection are cultures of blood, sputum, and pulmonary tissue or fluid. Chest x-ray studies will show patchy infiltrates and small pleural effusions.

Medical Management. The physician may need to place the patient on assisted ventilation, which requires intubating the patient through an oral or nasal airway or directly via the trachea. Close observation for disease progression is required.

The patient may also require temporary renal dialysis because of acute kidney failure.

To control and compensate for impaired/ineffective respiratory function, the patient will require oxygen therapy, possibly even mechanical ventilation. The patient will need adequate IV fluid therapy to maintain hydration and electrolyte status.

Antibiotic agents (erythromycin) will be given early in the course of the disease and for a prolonged period to treat the infection. Rifampin is also of benefit. Antipyretics will be administered to reduce the patient's temperature. The patient may also require vasopressors (dopamine or dobutamine) and analgesics to treat shock signs and promote comfort.

Nursing Interventions. The patient will be maintained on bed rest, and I&O will be monitored.

Nursing diagnoses and interventions for the patient with Legionnaires' disease include but are not limited to the following:

NURSING DIAGNOSES	NURSING INTERVENTIONS
Tissue perfusion, altered, cardiopulmonary or renal, related to lack of oxygen	Monitor and report signs and symptoms of impending shock (decreased blood pressure and increased pulse). Administer vasopressor drugs as ordered. Maintain hydration status and urinary output. Assess changes in level of consciousness. Assist with acute hemodialysis if indicated.
Breathing pattern, ineffective, related to respiratory failure	Assess signs and symptoms of respiratory failure. Note respiratory rate, rhythm, and effort. Be alert to cyanosis and dyspnea. Assist with oxygen therapy or mechanical ventilation as ordered. Facilitate optimal ventilation—patient in semi-Fowler's position if condition tolerates; suction as needed. Have patient cough and deep breathe q 2 hr if able. Identify associated factors, such as ineffective airway clearance, pain, and altered level of consciousness.
Fluid volume deficit, high risk for, related to hypovolemic shock	Administer prescribed IV solution. Monitor I&O. Be alert to signs of impending renal failure—decreased urinary output and hematuria.

Patient teaching. Because of the many alarming actions necessary to treat this disease and its complications, patient and family education is important. The nurse should instruct the patient and family on the purpose of respiratory support—oxygen therapy or ventilator assistance—and how to use these procedures for the greatest benefit. Explanations should be provided of all procedures before their implementation. The purpose of hemodialysis and why it is required should be explained. The nurse should stress the importance of controlling the patient's temperature and fluid and electrolyte status. Emotional support should be offered to the patient and family as needed.

Prognosis. Legionnaires' disease is a severe, often fatal disease. The mortality has been 15% to 20% in a few localized epidemics.

Tuberculosis

Etiology/Pathophysiology. In 1882, Koch identified the tubercle bacillus *(Mycobacterium tuberculosis)* as the causative agent for tuberculosis (TB).

TB is a chronic pulmonary and extrapulmonary (outside of the lung) infectious disease acquired by inhalation of a dried droplet nucleus containing a tubercle bacillus into the alveolar structure of the lung. It is characterized by stages of early infection (frequently asymptomatic), latency, and a potential for recurrent postprimary disease. It most commonly affects the respiratory system, but other parts of the body such as gastrointestinal and genitourinary tracts, bones, joints, nervous system, lymph nodes, and skin may become infected.

Tuberculosis infection is different from tuberculosis disease. It is important to differentiate *infection* with TB from *active disease.* Although infection always precedes the development of active disease, only about 10% of infections progress to active disease. Tuberculosis infection is characterized by the presence of mycobacteria in the tissue of a host who is free of clinical signs and symptoms and who demonstrates the presence of antibodies against the mycobacteria. Tuberculosis disease is manifest as pathological and functional signs and symptoms indicating destructive activity of mycobacteria in host tissue. Transmission is primarily by inhalation of minute dried-droplet nuclei (each containing a single tubercle bacillus), coughed or sneezed into the air by a person whose sputum contains **virulent** (the power of microorganism to produce disease) tubercle bacilli.

A common misconception about TB is that it is easily transmitted. In fact, most people exposed to TB do not become infected. The body's first line of defense, the upper airway, prevents most inhaled TB organisms from ever reaching the lungs. If the inhaled particles are small enough, the organisms can survive in the upper respiratory tract, reach the alveoli, and establish infection.

Less commonly, transmission may occur by ingestion or by invasion of the skin or mucous membranes.

TB had been epidemic in the Western world and was responsible for one third of the deaths of young adults in Europe. Following Koch's discovery, improvement in living conditions, sanitation, and the development of effective drug therapy and treatment brought about a steady decline in mortality attributable to TB. Shortly after the centennial of Koch's work, eradication of the disease in the United States was considered a realistic goal by the year 2010.

A decade later, there is less reason for optimism. Approximately 10 to 15 million Americans are infected with the TB bacillus, and TB case rates in the United States rose by 18% from 1985 to 1991. Most alarming, a growing percentage of new cases of TB are resistant to the drugs that are traditionally used to fight the disease.[19]

TB has been particularly prevalent among persons infected with the human immunodeficiency virus (HIV). The status of the host's immune system is the major determinant for the development of active TB. The disease occurs most often in individuals with incompetent immune systems, such as HIV-infected persons, the older adult, people receiving immunosuppressive therapy, and the malnourished.

Hospitals are a high-risk setting for TB transmission, and health care workers are at high occupational risk for TB infection. Until recently, the vulnerability of hospital workers to TB infection had not been emphasized. This complacency is changing with the wide publicity accompanying the increase of TB (see Box 31-5 for high-risk groups).

In the lung, pulmonary macrophages ingest TB bacteria. Macrophages engulf the organisms, but do not kill them. Instead, they surround them and wall them off in tiny, hard capsules called tubercles. Macrophages activate lymphocytes and within 2 to 10 weeks, activated lymphocytes usually control the initial infection in the lung and nonpulmonary sites. Nonmultiplying tubercle bacilli can survive, often more than 50 years, in human tissue.

Most people who become infected with the TB organism do not progress to the active disease stage. They remain asymptomatic and noninfectious. They will have a positive tuberculin skin test, and chest x-rays will be negative. These people still retain a lifelong risk of developing reactivation TB if the immune system is compromised.

Clinical Manifestations. The clinical manifestations are insidious. Generally there is fever, weight loss, weakness, and a productive cough. Later in the disease daily recurring fever with chills, night sweats, and hemoptysis are seen.

Assessment. Collection of *subjective data* includes the patient reporting loss of muscle strength and weight loss.

Box 31-5 HIGH-RISK GROUPS TO SCREEN FOR TB

- HIV-infected persons
- Close contacts (especially children and adolescents) of persons with active infectious TB
- Persons with conditions that increase the risk of active TB after infection, such as silicosis, diabetes, chronic renal failure, history of gastrectomy, weight 10% below ideal body weight, prolonged corticosteroid or other immunosuppressive therapy, some hematological disorders (leukemia and lymphomas, for example), and other malignancies
- Persons born in countries with a high prevalence of TB
- Substance abusers, such as alcoholics, IV drug users, and cocaine or crack users
- Residents of long-term care facilities, nursing homes, prisons, mental institutions, homeless shelters, and other congregate housing settings
- Medically underserved low-income populations, including racial and ethnic minorities, homeless people, and migrant workers
- Health care workers and others who provide service to any high-risk group

Collection of *objective data* includes evaluating and recording the amount, color, and characteristics of sputum produced.

Diagnostic Tests. Diagnostic evaluation for pulmonary TB includes a Mantoux tuberculin skin test. The tuberculin skin test is used to identify persons infected with the TB organism. A positive reaction can detect infection 2 to 10 weeks after exposure to the tubercle bacillus. To read the test 48 to 72 hours later, measure and record the subsequent induration (an area of hardened tissue); do not measure the erythema (redness). A negative reaction is <5 mm. If the patient is infected with tuberculosis (whether active or dormant), lymphocytes will recognize the purified protein derivative antigen in the skin test and cause a local indurated reaction. Generally, the larger the reaction, the greater the likelihood that the person is infected with the TB organism. However, a negative reaction doesn't rule out infection. An infected person whose immune system has been weakened by disease, drugs, or old age may have a limited or negative reaction. If the test is negative and the physician strongly suspects tuberculosis, a "second-strength" tuberculin test can be used. If this test is then negative, the patient does not have tuberculosis. Other diagnostic tests that are used to confirm the diagnosis of pulmonary tuberculosis are Chest x-ray and evaluation of sputum specimens for mycobacterial organisms. Sputum specimens can be rapidly smeared, stained, and screened for the presence of acid-fast organisms. Mycobacteria are one of the few organisms that are characteristically acid-fast. Three positive acid-fast smears constitute a presumptive diagnosis of TB and indicate the need for treatment. The diagnosis of tuberculosis is confirmed if TB bacilli grow in culture, a process that may take 6 to 8 weeks. All patients with tuberculosis must be reported to the appropriate public health authority for case follow-up and investigation of contacts.

Medical Management. Drug therapy is the mainstay of tuberculosis treatment. Infectiousness declines rapidlyonce drug therapy is initiated, even before sputum smears become negative. Cough frequently also declines with drug therapy. If a patient has a definite clinical response to therapy (for example, signs and symptoms such as cough and fever are improved), respiratory isolation is sometimes discontinued after 2 weeks of treatment. If there is any question of infectiousness, hospitalized patients remain in respiratory isolation for the duration of their hospital stay.

Compared with most other infectious diseases, treatment for TB is lengthy, typically 6 to 9 months, and sometimes longer for extrapulmonary disease. If treatment isn't continued for a long period of time, some of the TB organisms will survive and the patient will be at risk for a relapse.

Treatment therapy now involves multiple drugs to which the organisms are susceptible. If only one drug is given, the patient may become resistant to it. When two or more drugs are used, each helps prevent the emergence of organisms resistant to the other. The drugs that are used to treat tuberculosis are categorized as first-line drugs and second-line drugs. First-line drugs are isoniazid (INH); rifampin (rifampicin); rifampin and isoniazid (Rifamate), a fixed combination of 300 mg rifampin and 150 mg isoniazid per capsule; pyrazinamide; ethambutol; and streptomycin. Second-line drugs are ethionamide, para-aminosalicylate sodium (PAS), cycloserine, capreomycin, kanamycin, and amikacin. See medication table on pp. 904-905.

The monitoring of patients with TB is critically important; the failure to complete prescribed medication treatment accounts for most treatment failures. To ensure compliance and to help prevent the development of drug-resistant strains of the tubercle bacillus, there may be circumstances when it may be necessary for the health care worker to watch the patient take the medications.

Nursing Interventions. If TB is suspected, permission to place the patient in acid-fast bacilli (AFB) isolation precautions should be requested immediately. These precautions would include the use of isolation rooms with a negative air pressure so that air flows into, rather than out of, the room. Doors and windows must be kept closed to maintain airflow control. Room air should be exhausted directly to the outside and not recirculated to other rooms. Also included in AFB isolation precautions is the use of particulate respiration masks (because AFB particles pass through standard masks). Although TB is not easily transmitted, it is more easily transmitted in closed spaces and in areas with poor ventilation and no environmental controls.

Perhaps the simplest, most effective, technique for stopping TB at the source is kindly insisting that patients cover their noses and mouths when coughing or sneezing.

In order to assist the patient's compliance to the prescribed medication regimen, the nurse must develop a supportive relationship with the patient.

Nursing interventions are focused on preventing complications and illness transmission.

Nursing diagnoses and interventions for the patient with tuberculosis include but are not limited to the following:

NURSING DIAGNOSES	NURSING INTERVENTIONS
Breathing pattern, ineffective, related to pulmonary infectious process	Monitor breathing for evidence of dyspnea or signs and symptoms of pneumothorax. Evaluate degree of respiratory effort, and assist as needed. Assess expectorated sputum for hemoptysis. Assist immobile patient to turn, cough, and deep breathe q 2-4 hr to prevent pooling of secretions.
Infection, high risk for (patient contacts), related to viable *Mycobacterium tuberculosis* in respiratory secretions	Obtain specimen for culture (incorrect collection and handling may destroy or contaminate specimen, thus interfering with diagnostic results). Employ AFB isolation until antimicrobial therapy is successfully initiated for sputum-positive patients, to prevent transmission of organisms. Employ drainage and secretion precautions until wounds from patient with extrapulmonary tuberculosis stop draining to prevent transmission of organism. Instruct the patient to cough and sneeze into tissue and properly dispose of to prevent organism transmission.
Nutrition: altered, less than body requirements, related to infection	Offer high-protein, high-carbohydrate diet to provide adequate calorie intake to meet increased nutritional needs during infection. Encourage adequate intake by offering small, frequent feedings in a pleasant atmosphere.

Patient teaching. The nurse should teach the patient techniques of proper disposal and handwashing re-

MEDICATIONS FOR RESPIRATORY DISORDERS

Medication	Trade Name	Action	Side Effects	Nursing Implications
Acetylcysteine	Mucomyst	Mucolytic agent, also used as antidote in acetaminophen overdose	Nausea, vomiting, rhinorrhea, mucorrhea, bronchospasm	Store product in refrigerator, bad taste may be masked by mixing with soft drink when using as antidote
Aminoglycosides (gentamicin, tobramycin, streptomycin, kanamycin, others)	Many	Broad spectrum antibiotic, interferes with protein synthesis in bacteria	Renal impairment or failure, ototoxicity	Monitor BUN and serum creatinine frequently, to enhance toxicities use with other nephrotoxic agents, ensure adequate hydration, adjust doses based on serum concentrations
Aminophylline	Many	See theophylline	See theophylline	See theophylline
Azatadine	Optimine, also available in numerous combination allergy and cold preparations	Antihistamine, blocks allergic response through histamine receptor blockade	Drowsiness, confusion, dry mouth, constipation, urinary retention, blurred vision, increased viscosity of respiratory secretions	Avoid use with alcohol or other CNS depressants, avoid driving and other hazardous activities
$Beta_2$ receptor agonists (isoetharine, isoproterenol, terbutaline, albuterol, metaproterenol, others)	Bronkosol (isoetharine), Isuprel (isoproterenol), Brethine (terbutaline) Proventil, Ventolin (albuterol), Alupent (metaproterenol)	Beta-2 receptor agonists, cause bronchodilation	Anxiety, headache, insomnia, dizziness, restlessness, tachycardia, palpitations, angina or chest pain, cardiac dysrhythmias	Use with caution in cardiac disease, proper use of metered dose inhaler is crucial to achieve therapeutic response, instruct patients carefully and thoroughly
Corticosteroids (prednisone, methylprednisolone, hydrocortisone, others)	Deltasone, others (prednisone), Medrol, others (methylprednisolone), Cortef, others (hydrocortisone)	Antiinflammatory agent	Short-term—sodium and water retention, hypokalemia, hyperglycemia, euphoria Long-term—osteoporosis, increased susceptibility to infection, poor wound healing, bruising, thinning of skin, Cushingoid weight distribution, cataracts, glaucoma, peptic ulcer disease, myopathy, muscle weakness, suppression of endogenous glucocorticoid production	Do not discontinue medication abruptly, dosage must be slowly tapered down, patient should carry identification on person signaling steroid use, take with food or milk to minimize upset
Epinephrine	Adrenalin, many others	$Beta_1$ and $beta_2$ receptor agonist, causes bronchodilation and cardiac stimulation, $alpha_1$ agonist activity may cause vasoconstriction	Tachycardia, palpitations, angina, chest pain, myocardial infarction, cardiac dysrhythmias, hypertension, restlessness, agitation, anxiety	Use with extreme caution in cardiac disease, do not use OTC cough or cold preparations, do not use discolored preparations
Ethambutol	Myambutol	Antitubercular agent	Optic neuritis, blurred vision or decreased visual acuity, hyperuricemia, exacerbation of gout, drowsiness, confusion, GI effects, hepatotoxicity, thrombocytopenia	Patient should have baseline visual examination at start of therapy, emphasize that long-term therapy is required for cure

Medication	Trade Name	Action	Side Effects	Nursing Implications
Isoniazid (INH)	Nydrazid, others	Antitubercular agent	Peripheral neuropathy, hepatotoxicity, SLE-like syndrome, hyperglycemia, bone marrow suppression	Monitor liver function, emphasize that long-term therapy is required, instruct patient to report numbness or tingling of extremities
Oxymetazoline	Afrin, others	Vasoconstrictor, used for nasal congestion	Local nasal irritation, dryness, rebound congestion	Do not use for more than 4 consecutive days to minimize rebound congestion
Para-aminosalicylate sodium (PAS)	Many	Antitubercular agent	Nausea, vomiting, diarrhea, abdominal pain, hypersensitivity reactions, hepatotoxicity, leukopenia, thrombocytopenia	Take with food, discard if discolored, use with caution in peptic ulcer disease or congestive heart failure, emphasize that long-term therapy is required
Potassium iodide	Many, also available in numerous combination preparations	Expectorant, mucokinetic agent	Hypersensitivity, rash, metallic taste, burning in mouth or throat, GI irritation, headache, parotitis, hyperkalemia	Do not use in pregnant women, mix with fruit juice to mask taste
Pyrazinamide	Many	Antitubercular agent	Hyperuricemia, exacerbation of gout, hepatotoxicity	Monitor liver function tests and serum uric acid levels, instruct patient not to use alcohol, emphasize that long-term therapy is required
Rifampin	Rifadin, Rimactane	Antitubercular agent	Flu-like syndrome, hematopoietic reactions, hepatotoxicity, rash, red-orange coloration of bodily fluids, shortness of breath, heartburn, sore mouth and tongue, dizziness, confusion	Give on empty stomach; emphasize that long-term therapy is required; may accelerate metabolism of other drugs, including theophylline, oral contraceptives, and warfarin; instruct patient that body fluids may be discolored; may cause permanent staining of soft contact lenses
Theophylline (aminophylline is a salt of theophylline)	Many	Bronchodilator	Anxiety, restlessness, insomnia, headache, seizures, tachycardia, cardiac dysrhythmias, nausea, epigastric pain, hematemesis, gastroesophageal reflux, tachypnea	Do not crush sustained release preparations, contents of pellet-containing capsules may be sprinkled over food, avoid caffeine, use with caution in peptic ulcer disease or cardiac dysrhythmias, metabolism affected by other medications (erythromycin, ciprofloxacin, cimetidine, rifampin), monitor serum concentrations

lated to coughing and sneezing. These measures will decrease the spread of infection. The nurse should explain the vital importance of adhering to the medication regimen as ordered and the need for prolonged treatment. The patient should be instructed on medication, dosage, frequency, and possible side effects. The nurse should emphasize the need to report hemoptysis, dyspnea, vertigo, or chest pain. The patient should be reminded to maintain adequate fluid and nutritional requirements.

Prognosis. Although infection always precedes the development of the disease, only about 10% of infections progress to active disease. Active TB requires a long course of drug ingestion—6 to 9 months minimum, and often longer—to result in an arrest of the disease. As many as 50% of patients fail to complete therapy as prescribed. Numerous drug-resistant tuberculosis cases have been reported in HIV-infected persons with TB. These infections were characterized by rapid disease progression, with 4 to 16 weeks from diagnosis to death and mortality rates of 72% to 89%.

Nonmultiplying tubercle bacilli can survive more than 50 years in human tissue and can become reactivated when the patient has a compromised immune system.

Pneumonia

Etiology/Pathophysiology. Pneumonia is an inflammatory process of the respiratory bronchioles and the alveolar spaces that is caused by an infection. It can also be caused by oversedation, inadequate ventilation, or aspiration.

Pneumonia can occur in any season, but is most common during winter and early spring. Persons of all ages are susceptible, but pneumonia is more common among infants and the elderly. Pneumonia is often caused by aspiration of infected materials into the distal bronchioles and alveoli. Certain individuals are especially susceptible, including persons whose normal respiratory defense mechanisms are damaged or altered (those with chronic obstructive pulmonary disease, influenza, or tracheostomy and those who have recently had anesthesia); persons who have a disease affecting antibody response; and persons with alcoholism, in whom there is increased danger of aspiration; and persons with delayed white blood cell response to infection. Increasingly, nosocomial pneumonia (acquired in the hospital) is a cause of morbidity and mortality.

Pneumonia is a communicable disease; the mode of transmission is dependent on the infecting organism. Pneumonia is classified according to the offending organism rather than the anatomical location (lobar or bronchial) as was the practice in the past.

Pneumonia can be caused by bacteria, viruses, mycoplasma, fungi, and parasites. Currently, about half of pneumonia cases are caused by bacteria and half by virus. Up to 96% of bacterial pneumonia is caused by four organisms, *Streptococcus pneumoniae* (pneumococcal), hemolytic streptococcus type A, *Staphylococcus aureus,* and *Haemophilus influenzae* (type b). Nonbacterial or atypical pneumonia is caused by *Mycoplasma pneumoniae, Legionella pneumophila* (Legionnaire's disease), and *Pnemocystis carinii* pneumonia.

Aspiration pneumonia syndrome occurs most commonly as a result of aspiration of vomitus when the patient is in an altered state of consciousness owing to a seizure, drugs, alcohol, anesthesia, acute infection, or shock. Aspiration pneumonia may be acquired through foreign body aspiration or may follow aspiration of toxic materials such as toxic fluids like gasoline or kerosene.

The causative agents of bacterial aspiration pneumonia include *Staphylococcus aureus, Escherichia coli, Klebsiella pneumoniae, Pseudomonas aeruginosa,* and *Proteus.*

The pathophysiology of pneumonia depends on the causative agent. Bacterial pneumonia is marked by an alveolar suppurative (process of pus formation) exudate with consolidation of infection. Mycoplasmal and viral pneumonia produce interstitial inflammation with no consolidation or exudate. Fungal and mycobacterial pneumonias are marked by patchy distribution that may undergo necrosis with the development of cavities. Aspiration pneumonia presents with various physiological responses depending upon the pH of the aspirated substance.

An overview of the pathophysiology is as follows: (1) pulmonary cilia cannot remove accumulating secretions from the respiratory tract; (2) these retained secretions then become infected; (3) inflammation of some part of the respiratory tract develops, leading to a localized edema; (4) this causes decreased oxygen/carbon dioxide exchange. This process can begin in the bronchi or in the lobe of one lung, and it can become more extensive.

Clinical Manifestations. There are many significant signs and symptoms seen in pneumonia. A productive cough is very common; color and consistency of sputum will vary depending on the type of pneumonia present. Severe chills, elevated temperature, and increased heart and respiratory rates may accompany the painful, productive cough. For special considerations for older adults, see gerontological box.

Clinical manifestations are dependent on the type of pneumonia:

- **Streptococcal, pneumococcal**—Sudden onset; chest pain; chills; fever; headache; cough; rust-colored sputum; crackles and possibly friction rub; hypoxemia as blood is shunted away from area of consolidation; cyanosis; area of consolidation visible on chest x-ray; sputum culture needed to determine causative agent

GERONTOGICAL CONSIDERATIONS

- Signs and symptoms of pneumonia are often atypical in older adults. Fever, cough, and purulent sputum may be absent. Generalized signs and symptoms such as lethargy, disorientation, dyspnea, tachypnea, chills, chest pain, and vomiting, as well as an unexpected exacerbation of coexisting conditions, should be viewed with suspicion, since they may indicate pneumonia in the older adult.
- Adequate hydration is very important for the older person with pneumonia. It helps liquify secretions and promotes expectoration.
- Many older adults have difficulty expectorating. This slows resolution of congestions and increases the difficulty of obtaining sputum specimens. Because deep breathing and coughing are difficult, the older person may require suctioning to remove respiratory secretions. This should be done with discretion, since too-frequent suctioning can stimulate increased production of secretions.
- Older adults, particularly those living in an institution, should have routine skin tests for tuberculosis. Many older adults were exposed to tuberculosis during their childhood and have positive results on skin tests. These individuals should receive routine chest x-ray studies. Older adults who have histories of inactive tuberculosis should be watched for recurrence of active tuberculosis. Signs and symptoms are often vague and include loss of appetite and weight loss.
- Older immigrants and immunosuppressed older adults should be watched closely for drug-resistant strains of tuberculosis.
- Provided that there is no serious disease of the respiratory tract, the older person is generally able to maintain adequate ventilation and oxygenation.
- However, changes of aging do have an impact on respiratory function:
  - Drier mucous membranes and decreased number of cilia affect the older individual's ability to humidify inhaled air and trap debris. These, in turn, increase the risk for inflammation and irritation of the upper respiratory tract.
  - Kyphosis and calcification of costal cartilage are common changes. These restrict expansion of the thoracic cavity and lead to a barrel-chested appearance.
  - Intercostal muscles and the diaphragm lose elasticity, resulting in a decreased ability to breathe deeply and cough.
  - The elasticity of airways and alveoli decreases, alveoli thicken, and pulmonary blood flow decreases, resulting in increased risk for impaired gas exchange.
- Years of exposure to air pollution, smoke, and mechanical irritants increase the risk for respiratory disease in older adults, particularly those who have emphysema and chronic bronchitis.
- Inactivity and immobility increase the risk of stasis pooling of respiratory secretions. This increases the risk of pneumonia.
- Neurological damage as a result of cerebrovascular accidents, Parkinson's disease, and other conditions are increasingly common in the older adult. Any neurological disorder that decreases the gag or swallow reflexes increases the risk of aspiration of fluids and food, with resultant trauma to the respiratory tract.
- Cor pulmonale with right-sided congestive heart failure, as well as left-sided congestive heart failure with pulmonary congestion, are common complications of chronic obstructive pulmonary disease in the older adult.

- **Staphylococcal**—Many of same signs as streptococcal; sputum copious and salmon colored
- **Klebsiella**—Many of the same signs and symptoms as streptococcal; onset more gradual; more bronchopneumonia (inflammation of the terminal bronchioles and alveoli) visible on chest x-ray; if treatment delayed beyond second day after onset, patient will become critically ill; mortality high
- **Haemophilus**—Commonly follows upper respiratory infection; low-grade fever; croupy cough; malaise; arthralgias; yellow or green sputum
- **Mycoplasmal**—Gradual onset; headache; fever; malaise; chills; cough severe and nonproductive; decreased breath sounds and crackles; chest x-ray clear; white blood cell count normal
- **Viral**—Signs and symptoms generally mild; cold symptoms; headache; anorexia; fever; myalgia (tenderness or pain in muscles); irritating cough that produces mucopurulent or bloody sputum; bronchopneumonic type of infiltration on chest x-ray; white blood cell count usually normal; rise in antibody titers

Assessment. Collection of *subjective data* includes obtaining the patient's description of the history, onset, and duration of cough. The patient may complain of fever and night sweats.

Collection of *objective data* involves nursing assessment measures, including checking the level of consciousness and vital signs, especially temperature and respirations, every 2 hours or as ordered. The color, consistency, and amount of sputum produced should be noted. The nurse should inspect the thorax to determine the patient's use of accessory muscles in respiratory effort and note any cyanosis or dyspnea. The nurse will observe and document if the patient needs to use abdominal muscles or intercostal muscles to adequately breathe. On auscultation, the nurse will hear crackles on inspiration and possibly a pleural effusion.

Diagnostic Tests. Blood and sputum cultures will help in identification of organisms. Sputum for culture and sensitivity should be collected before initiation of antibiotic therapy, to identify the causative agent. Chest x-ray studies will reveal changes in density, primarily in the lower lobes. White blood cell count will be normal or even low in viral or mycoplasmal pneumonia, whereas it will be elevated in bacterial pneumonia. Pulmonary function tests may be done to determine whether lung volume is decreased and ABG values will be determined to identify altered gas exchange. Pulse oximetry will be ordered to monitor oxygen saturation of arterial blood levels. Oximetry is invaluable for rapid and continuous assessment of oxygen needs.

Medical Management. If an accumulation of pus in the pleural space (empyema) occurs, the physician will insert a chest tube for drainage. The physician will also prescribe oxygen therapy and physiotherapy—chest percussion and postural drainage. Patients should be encouraged to cough and deep breathe to maximize ventilatory capabilities.

Commonly prescribed medications include antibiotics—penicillin, erthromycin, cephalosporin, and tetramycin—depending upon causative organism and sensitivity. Analgesics and antipyretics (Tylenol or aspirin), expectorants, and bronchodilators are often prescribed. Humidification with humidifier or nebulizer if secretions are tenacious and copious is useful. Oxygenation is prescribed if the patient has oxygen saturation of less than 90%. Venturi mask or nasal prongs are commonly used.

A vaccine is now available for the most common and important bacterial pneumonia, streptococcal pneumonia.

Nursing Interventions. Nursing strategies are aimed at assisting the patient to conserve energy. The nurse should allow rest periods and should facilitate optimal air exchange by placing the patient in high Fowler's position. Place the patient on the side with the "good lung down." The "good lung down" position benefits those with unilateral pulmonary pathology, including unilateral pneumonia. In pneumonia and many other pulmonary problems, Pa_{O_2} rises when the healthy lung is dependent or "good lung down." When the unimpaired lung is down, this better ventilated lung also is vastly better perfused. Studies have revealed that hypoxia worsened when patients were placed on their back or side with the affected (sick) lung down.[50]

Nursing interventions also include assessing the patient to identify inability to move secretions. If inability is identified, assist with appropriate measures (such as coughing, positioning, suctioning, and liquefying secretions). Promptly administer bronchodilators, mucolytics, and expectorants per protocol as prescribed to dilate bronchioles and remove secretions. Carefully and frequently auscultate chest for quality of breath sounds and adventitious sounds. Note cough and sputum characteristics and document. Provide hydration to liquefy secretions and replace fluids.

Nursing diagnoses and interventions for the patient with pneumonia include but are not limited to the following:

NURSING DIAGNOSES	NURSING INTERVENTIONS
Breathing pattern, ineffective, related to inflammatory process and pleuritic pain	Assess ventilation, including evaluation of breathing rate, rhythm, and depth; chest expansion; presence of respiratory distress such as dyspnea, shortness of breath, nasal flaring, pursed-lip breathing, or prolonged expiratory phase; and use of accessory muscles. Auscultate lungs for crackles, wheezes, and pleural friction rub. Identify contributing factors such as airway clearance or obstruction problem or weakness. Encourage increased fluid intake to 1½ to 2 L/day, unless contraindicated, to liquefy secretions for easier expectoration. Maintain patient in position that facilitates ventilation (head of bed in semi-Fowler's position or patient sitting and leaning forward on overbed table). Instruct patient in proper pulmonary hygiene routines that will promote easy and effective breathing, facilitate removal of secretions from tracheobronchial tree, and minimize pulmonary congestion, which would lead to superinfections (an infection occurring during antimicrobial treatment for another infection). Assess patient for fatigue in relation to attempts to breathe. Protect patient from known sources of secondary infection.
Gas exchange, impaired, related to alveolar-capillary membrane changes secondary to inflammation	Assess patient to identify signs, such as restlessness, disorientation, and irritability, that may indicate body's response to altered blood gas states (hypoxia). If necessary and with physician consultation, administer oxygen by nasal cannula or Venturi mask to maintain oxygen saturations above 90%. Monitor serum electrolytes that may change owing to alterations in oxygenation and metabolism. Carefully monitor body temperature, which may fluctuate owing to alterations in metabolism or infection.

NURSING DIAGNOSES	NURSING INTERVENTIONS
Fatigue, related to debilitated state	Assess patterns of fatigue. Assess factors related to fatigue and strategies for dealing with them. Assess support systems and available resources. Administer treatments or medications to relieve discomfort. Enhance patient's ability to rest between specified activities.
Health maintenance, altered, related to pneumonia	Provide strict isolation for patient with pneumonia caused by *Staphylococcus.* Adhere to strict handwashing to prevent spread of disease.
Nutrition, altered: less than body requirements, related to debilitated state	Help patient choose foods that are easy to chew and swallow. Assist with eating if patient is too weak or too hypoxic. Offer in-between-meal nourishment. Provide oxygen while eating as ordered. Provide high-protein diet; administer vitamins as ordered.

Patient teaching. The nurse should teach the patient and family the following:

- Deep breathing and coughing techniques
- The importance of handwashing to prevent the spread of the disease
- Facts about and the importance of prescribed medications such as antibiotics, including the action, dosage, frequency of administration, and side effects
- Information regarding the specific type of pneumonia the patient has, treatment, anticipated response, possible complications, and probable disease duration
- That a change in health status must be reported to the patient's health care providers (indicators of change may include a change in sputum characteristics of color, decreased activity tolerance, fever despite the antibiotics, increasing chest pain, or a feeling that things are not getting better)
- The importance of consuming large quantities of fluid
- Adaptive exercise and rest techniques
- That streptococcal pneumonia (pneumococcal) vaccine is available

Prognosis. The disease usually resolves within 2 to 3 weeks with proper treatment. However, pneumonia is the most common cause of death from infectious disease in North America. It is also considered to be the major cause of disease and death in critically ill patients. Despite the use of antibiotics, pneumonia still accounts for 27.7 of every 100,000 deaths.

Bacterial aspiration pneumonia has a poor prognosis even with antibiotic therapy. It may cause extensive lung damage, resulting in lung abscess or empyema. Mortality is 70% with *Pseudomonas aeruginosa,* 45% with *Escherichia coli,* 35% to 50% with *Klebsiella pneumoniae,* and 15% to 50% with *Staphylococcus aureus.*

Pleurisy

Etiology/Pathophysiology. Pleurisy is an inflammation of the visceral and parietal pleura. Pleurisy can be caused by either a bacterial or viral infection. The underlying physiological change is an inflammation of any portion of the pleura. It may occur spontaneously but more frequently results as a complication of pneumonia, pulmonary infarctions, viral infections of the intercostal muscles, pleural trauma, or early stages of tuberculosis or lung tumor.

Clinical Manifestations. One of the first symptoms of pleurisy may be a sharp inspiratory pain, often radiating to the shoulder or abdomen of the affected side. The pain felt in pleurisy is caused by stretching of the inflamed pleura. If pleural effusion develops, pain subsides and fever and dry cough occur. Other signs and symptoms include dyspnea, cough, and elevated temperature.

Assessment. Collection of *subjective data* is awareness of a patient's complaint of chest pain on inspiration. The patient may also report an elevated temperature.

Collection of *objective data* includes the nurse's assessment of the nature of inspiratory pain, noting its radiation points. The nurse should monitor vital signs, especially temperature, every 2 or 4 hours. Respiratory rate and rhythm should be monitored and documented, noting dyspnea. On auscultation of the lungs the nurse will hear a pleural friction rub.

Diagnostic Tests. The presence of a pleural friction rub may be considered to be diagnostic. Chest x-ray examination is of limited value in diagnosing pleurisy unless there is the presence of a pleural effusion if fluid accumulates.

Medical Management. The physician may inject an anesthetic block around the vertebra to block the intercostal nerves, thus relieving pain. Prescribed medications may include antibiotics (penicillin) to combat the infection and analgesics (Demerol or morphine) to decrease pain when the patient takes deep breaths and coughs. Antipyretics (Tylenol) are used for fever. Oxygen may be administered.

Nursing Interventions. The patient should be positioned comfortably on the affected side to splint the chest, and heat may be applied to the area.

Nursing diagnoses and interventions for the patient with pleurisy include, but are not limited to, the following:

NURSING DIAGNOSES	NURSING INTERVENTIONS
Pain, related to stretching of the pulmonary pleura as a result of fluid accumulation	Assess patient's pain level and need for pain medication; administer as needed, documenting effectiveness. Assist with splinting affected side when patient coughs and deep breathes.
Gas exchange, impaired, related to pain on inspiration and expiration	Assess patient's level of consciousness, noting an increase in restlessness or disorientation, which may indicate ineffective breathing. Auscultate lungs for wheezes, crackles, and pleural friction rub. Reposition patient q 2 hr to prevent pooling of secretions and to promote optimal lung expansion. Elevate head of bed to facilitate optimal ventilation.

Patient teaching. The patient should be instructed to be alert to signs and symptoms of exacerbation—purulent sputum production, further increase in temperature, and increased pain. The nurse should teach the patient to effectively cough every 2 hours and to splint the affected side.

Prognosis. Prognosis is usually excellent. Complications of atelectasis or secondary infection such as pneumonia may develop.

Pleural Effusion/Empyema

Etiology/Pathophysiology. Once the pleural lining is inflamed (as in pleurisy), fluid can accumulate in the pleural space. This accumulation of fluid is known as pleural effusion. Pleural effusion is rarely a disease by itself but occurs as a secondary problem when the physiological pressure in the lungs and pleurae is disturbed. If the fluid becomes infected, it is called **empyema.**

The pathophysiology of pleural effusion lies in the alteration of pressure gradients or surface characteristics of capillaries. Empyema may be acute or can become chronic. In acute empyema there is inflammation of the affected area with a thin layer of fluid. If this goes untreated, the fluid thickens and the pleura becomes scarred and fibrosed, losing its elasticity.

Clinical Manifestations. Pleural effusion is generally associated with other disease processes, such as pancreatitis, cirrhosis of the liver, congestive heart failure, kidney disease, or carcinoma involving altered capillary permeability. Empyema is usually seen as a result of bacterial infection, as in pneumonia, tuberculosis, or blunt chest trauma. The patient may have a persistent fever in spite of receiving antibiotics.

Assessment. Collection of *subjective data* includes the patient verbalizing complaints of dyspnea and air hunger. The patient may also disclose feelings of fear and anxiety related to decreased levels of oxygen.

Collection of *objective data* in both pleural effusion and empyema includes the nurse's assessment of signs and symptoms of respiratory distress, such as nasal flaring, tachypnea, dyspnea, and decreased breath sounds. Breath sounds and vital signs, especially temperature, should be assessed frequently.

Diagnostic Tests. Effusions or pleural fluid will be evident on chest x-ray examination. Often a thoracentesis (needle inserted into pleural space to aspirate excess fluid) will be done not only to obtain a specimen for culture to identify the causative agent, but to relieve the dyspnea and discomfort.

Medical Management. Usually this condition requires a thoracentesis to remove fluid from the pleural space. A possible danger resulting from this procedure is removing fluid too rapidly; less than 1300 to 1500 ml at one time is recommended.

A chest tube may be inserted for continuous drainage and medication instillation. This tube will be sutured into place and covered with a sterile dressing.

The patient may have a thoracic drainage system in use. To prevent the lung from collapsing, a closed system is used, which maintains the lung cavity's normal negative pressure. With this procedure one or, more commonly, two thoracotomy tubes are inserted into the pleural space and are attached to a closed-system, water-seal drainage. One catheter is inserted through a stab wound in the anterior chest wall; this is referred to as the *anterior tube.* It is used to remove air from the pleural space. The second tube is inserted through a stab wound in the posterior chest and is referred to as the *posterior tube.* It is primarily for the drainage of serosanguineous fluid or purulent exudate. The posterior (lower) tube may be larger in diameter than the anterior (upper) tube to prevent it from becoming occluded with exudate or clots (Fig. 31-13).

When chest tube drainage is initiated, a 2-L clear glass bottle may be used, although other commercial devices (Fig. 31-14) are available. Approximately 300 ml of sterile water, or enough to fill the bottle 1 to 2 cm from the bottom, is added so the end of the glass rod is under water to maintain water-seal drainage and prevent air from entering the pleural cavity (Fig. 31-15).

Nursing Interventions. General nursing measures include placing the patient on bed rest. The patient may be receiving oxygen therapy; if so, frequent oral care will help prevent drying of mucous membranes. Also, the nurse should encourage effective coughing and deep breathing techniques and respiratory treatments. If the patient has had a thoracentesis, a large sterile dressing will be applied, and the nurse will assess the dressing for drainage, noting color and amount.

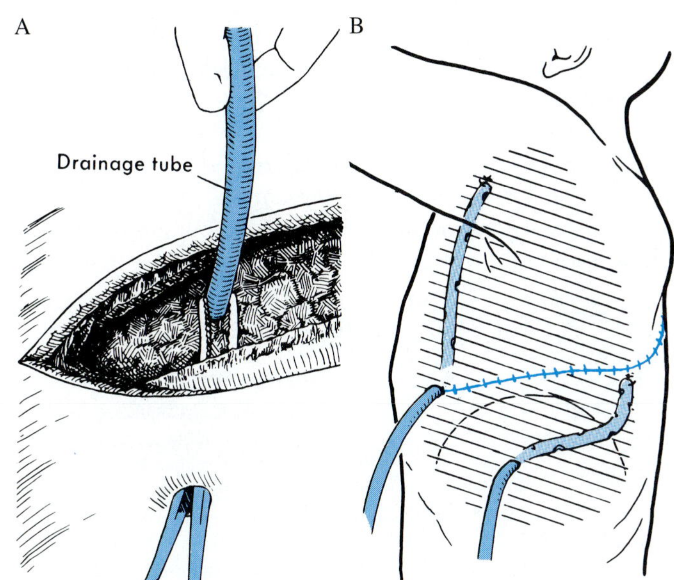

FIG. 31-13 **A,** Drainage tube inserted into pleural space. **B,** Note that upper and lower tubes are placed well into pleural space.

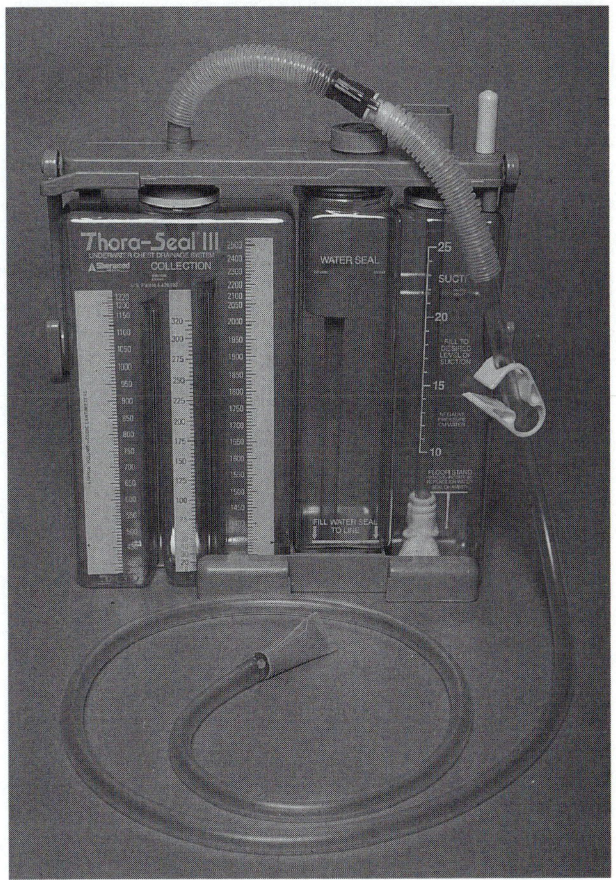

FIG. 31-14 Pleur-evac, a disposable, commercial chest drainage system. (Courtesy Deknatel.)

The nurse must assure that patency of the chest tube system is maintained so that it can drain fluid adequately. Areas of concern for maintaining chest tubes and closed chest drainage bottles are the following:

1. Proper system function: ensuring that the water in the water-seal chamber fluctuates when suction is applied; there should not be any bubbling in the water seal, because this indicates an air leak.
2. Potential atelectasis resulting from hypoventilation: assessing for increased dyspnea; checking chest x-ray studies frequently to compare degree of lung consolidation.
3. Increased air in the pleural space: noting any air leaks in the system; ensuring tubing is secure and remains patent.
4. Complication of infection; noting an increase in white blood cells, elevated temperature, and presence of purulent drainage.

While the chest tube is in place, the nurse will usually position the patient on the unaffected side to keep the tube from becoming kinked; however, the patient may assume any position of comfort in bed. There is no contraindication to ambulation with a chest tube in place, as long as the water-seal bottle remains below the level of the chest. The nurse must facilitate coughing and deep breathing procedures at least every 2 hours and auscultate breath sounds frequently. The nurse will document the amount and characteristics of pleural fluid drainage by marking and documenting the drainage level on the container at the end of each shift. Write date and hour on container so that amount of drainage can easily

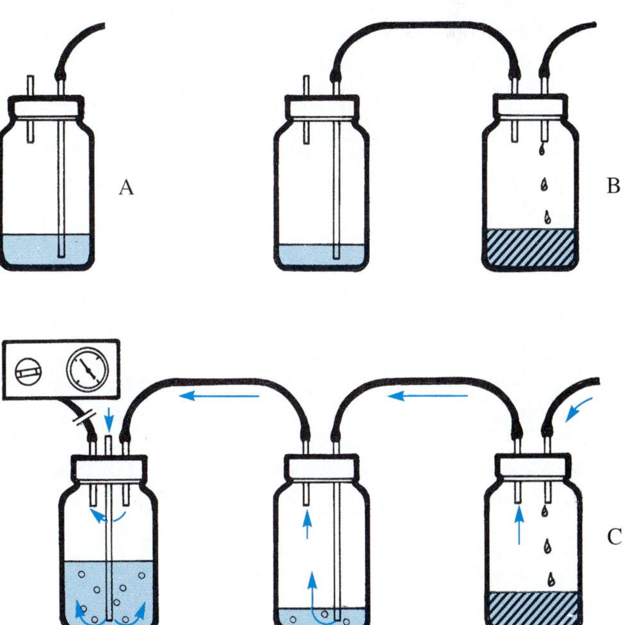

FIG. 31-15 Water-sealed, closed chest drainage system. **A,** One-bottle system. **B,** Two-bottle system. **C,** Three-bottle system with suction.

Box 31-6

MAINTAINING CHEST TUBES AND CLOSED CHEST DRAINAGE BOTTLES

1. Mark water level in bottles with strip of adhesive tape or felt-tip pen so that amount of drainage can easily be determined. Write date and hour on container.
2. Watch for and correct dependent loops, which allow fluid to collect in tubing and impede removal of air and fluid from pleural space.
3. Be sure that tip of chest tube is 1 inch (1 to 2 cm) under water so that if the bottle accidentally tips over, the tube will remain under water.
4. Check the glass rod in the bottle for fluctuation frequently. If the column of water is not fluctuating:
   a. Be sure patient is not lying on tubes.
   b. Check connections to be sure chest tube system is intact.
   c. Ask patient to cough or change position to see if fluctuation is restored.
   d. Fluctuation will stop when lung is reexpanded. Call the surgeon if the tubes are not patent (column of fluid not fluctuating).
5. Keep two hemostats at the bedside so that the chest tube can be clamped if a bottle is accidentally broken. When a bottle is broken, the chest catheter should be clamped (if there is a written order) and then reconnected to a sterile setup as soon as possible. Sterile water should be used in the bottles. As soon as the system is reconnected with the tip of the tube under water, the clamp should be removed. Except in case of an emergency such as a broken bottle, most thoracic surgeons prefer that tubes not be clamped, and a specific order is written if clamping is desired.
6. Never clamp chest tubes unless a bottle breaks (a rare occurrence) or without a written order. When chest tubes are clamped, air (positive pressure) may be trapped in the pleural space and further collapse the lung. If a patient is being transported from one place to another, such as to the radiology department, tubes should not be clamped
7. Never lift chest tube bottles above the level of the patient's chest, as this allows fluid to be pulled into the pleural space.
8. The water-seal bottles should be placed on the floor so that they will not be broken by a lowered siderail. When a Hi-Lo bed is being used, care is taken not to lower the bed onto the bottles.
9. If additional suction is being used, check frequently to be sure it is functioning at the prescribed level of negative pressure.

be determined (Box 31-6). The nurse can usually prevent a chest tube from being accidentally removed by careful attention to securing connections and positioning drainage tubes.

The patient will receive antibiotic agents and the nurse should administer them as ordered.

Nursing diagnoses and interventions for the patient with pleural effusion/empyema include but are not limited to the following:

NURSING DIAGNOSES	NURSING INTERVENTIONS
Gas exchange, impaired, related to ineffective breathing pattern	Assess for changes in level of consciousness, such as disorientation, restlessness, or irritability, because these may indicate increasing hypoxia as a result of ineffective breathing. Monitor arterial blood gases and pulse oximetry. Encourage coughing and deep breathing to rid secretions and facilitate lung expansion. Reposition patient q 2 hr to prevent pooling of secretions. Assess for atelectasis.
Self-care deficit, related to mobility restriction	Assess patient's ability to care for self, and assist when needed. Encourage increasing activity level when fever is reduced.

Patient teaching. The nurse should explain all procedures before their implementation. The patient should be prepared emotionally for chest tube insertion. The patient and family should be taught about his condition and the healing process. The nurse should instruct the patient on effective coughing and deep breathing techniques.

Prognosis. The prognosis, is variable, depending on the patient's overall health status.

Atelectasis

Etiology/Pathophysiology. **Atelectasis** (an abnormal condition characterized by the collapse of lung tissue, preventing the respiratory exchange of carbon dioxide and oxygen) occurs from occlusion of air (blockage) to a portion of the lung. Atelectasis is a common postoperative complication resulting from shallow breathing. All or part of the lung collapses, usually as a result of **hypoventilation** (an abnormal condition of the respiratory system that occurs when the volume of air that enters the alveoli and takes part in gas exchange is not adequate for the metabolic needs of the body), which then leads to bronchial obstruction caused by mucus accumulation. Accumulation of secretions, a foreign body, or a tenacious plug of mucus may completely occlude a bronchus, closing off all air to a portion of the patient's lung. Atelectasis can also be the result of compression of lung tissue caused by emphysema, pneumothorax, or tumor.

The altered physiology depends on the site and degree of occlusion. If the main stem bronchus is obstructed, there will be severe ventilatory compromise. When a small bronchiole becomes obstructed, as with secretion accumulation, there are fewer signs and symptoms because the respiratory system will try to compensate. However, in either case, atelectasis can lead to stasis pneumonia (because the retained secretions are rich in nutrients for the growth of bacteria) as well as lung damage.

Clinical Manifestations. The patient will display dyspnea, **tachypnea** (an abnormally rapid rate of breathing), pleural friction rub, restlessness, hypertension, and elevated temperature.

Assessment. Collection of *subjective data* includes the patient complaining of severe shortness of breath (dyspnea) requiring much effort, which results in fatigue. The patient may also verbalize a feeling of air hunger and resulting anxiety.

Collection of *objective data* includes the nurse noting decreased breath sounds and crackles on auscultation. The nurse should assess vital signs frequently because hypertension will be present at first, followed by hypotension. Respiration rate and amount of effort required for breathing should be noted. The patient may exhibit altered levels of consciousness caused by hypoxia.

Diagnostic Tests. Serial chest x-ray studies (frequently repeated x-ray examinations of same area done for comparison) will demonstrate atelectatic changes. Arterial blood gases will reveal a $Pa{O_2}$ of less than 80 mm Hg initially; this generally improves within the first 24 hours. Pulse oximetry will reveal oxygen saturation levels below 90%. $Pa{CO_2}$ will be normal or low, because of hypoventilation. A bronchoscopy may reveal a bronchial obstruction.

Medical Management. Atelectasis frequently requires chest tube insertion as an attempt to reexpand the lung. Ventilation maintenance through intubation is frequently required.

Nursing Interventions. Postoperatively, patients should be reminded to cough, deep breathe, and change positions every 2 hours. Administer analgesia to relieve pain and facilitate ventilatory effort. Assist patient to move and clear secretions; provide emotional support. Early ambulation is encouraged. Incentive spirometry (Skill 31-4 on p. 914) and respiratory treatments with intermittent positive pressure breathing (IPPB) may be ordered, as well as oxygen therapy. Chest physiotherapy with postural drainage will be administered (Skill 31-5 on p. 915). The patient may require suctioning; saline lavage often helps loosen secretions for easier removal. Prescribed medications may include bronchodilators (Proventil) to dilate the bronchioles and facilitate secretion removal, antibiotics to prevent infection, and mucolytic agents (acetylcysteine) to reduce the viscosity of the secretions.

Nursing diagnoses and interventions for the patient with atelectasis include but are not limited to the following:

NURSING DIAGNOSES	NURSING INTERVENTIONS
Airway clearance, ineffective, related to inability to clear secretions	Assess patient's ability to move secretions, and assist if needed. Such measures are: reposition patient q 2 hr; encourage coughing and deep breathing, and suction as needed; liquify secretions using IPPB with nebulizer as ordered. Position patient as much as possible on unaffected side to promote maximum ventilation to affected side. Encourage adequate hydration to liquify secretions. Auscultate breath sounds frequently, documenting and reporting any changes. Assess color, consistency, and amount of secretions removed via either coughing or suction.
Coping, ineffective individual, related to invasive medical regimen	Assess the patient's ability to comply with the prescribed regimen and to cooperate with care givers. Identify patient's emotional support systems.

Chest percussion and vibration. *Chest percussion* involves striking the chest wall over the area being drained. The hand is positioned so that the fingers and thumb touch and the hand is cupped. Percussion on the surface of the chest wall sends waves of varying amplitude and frequency through the chest. The force of these waves can change the consistency of the sputum or dislodge it from the airway walls. Chest percussion is performed by alternating hand motion against the chest walls. Percussion is performed over a single layer of clothing and not over buttons, snaps, or zippers. The single layer of clothing prevents slapping the patient's skin. Thicker material lessens the vibrations from percussion.

Percussion is contraindicated in patients who have bleeding disorders, osteoporosis, or fractured ribs. Caution should be taken to percuss the patient's lung fluids and not the scapular regions, or trauma may occur to the patient's skin and underlying musculoskeletal structures.

Vibration is a fine, shaking pressure applied to the chest wall only during exhalation. This technique is

SKILL 31-4

THE USE OF SPIROMETRY

Spirometry, referred to as *incentive spirometry,* is a procedure in which a device (spirometer) is used at the bedside at regular intervals to encourage the patient to deep breathe. Inspired measurement can be seen and used to encourage the patient to attain the established goal.

There are three primary purposes for the use of the incentive spirometer:

- To prevent or treat atelectasis
- To improve lung expansion
- To improve oxygenation

Incentive spirometry encourages patients to breath in their normal inspiratory capacities. Because of postoperative pain, a postoperative inspiratory capacity of one half to three fourths of the preoperative volume is acceptable.

There are two general types of incentive spirometers:

Flow-oriented inspiratory spirometer This type of incentive spirometer is inexpensive and measures inspiration but not volume. It contains one or more clear plastic cylinder chambers that contain freely movable, colored, light-weight plastic balls. The patient is instructed to place the mouthpiece in the mouth and inhale slowly and deeply, which raises the balls in the cylinders. The patient is encouraged to keep the colored balls floating as long as possible. The cylinders are marked to measure the degree of elevation so that the degree of elevation and the length of time the patient can maintain elevation can be recorded (see Fig. 22-4).

Volume-oriented spirometer This form of incentive spirometer maintains a known volume of inspiration. The patient is encouraged to breathe with normal inspired capacity.

1. Check the physician's orders.
2. Assess patient's respiratory status and lung sounds. Indications for spirometry are (a) asymmetrical chest wall movement, (b) increased respiratory rate, (c) increased production of sputum, and (d) diminished lung expansion postoperatively.
3. Explain procedure, and instruct patient in the correct use of the spirometer. Frequently this is accomplished by the respiratory therapist. However, it may be the nurse's responsibility to follow up and promote proper technique.
4. Obtain supplies and equipment.
5. Wash hands.
6. Place prescribed incentive spirometer at the bedside.
7. Place patient in semi-Fowler's or high Fowler's position.
8. Place tissues, emesis basin, and bedside trash bag within easy reach.
9. Instruct patient to completely cover mouthpiece with lips.
10. Instruct patient to (a) inhale slowly until maximum inspiration is reached, (b) hold breath 2 or 3 seconds, and (c) slowly exhale.
11. Instruct patient to relax and breathe normally for a short time. This prevents patient from hyperventilating and provides a resting period to prevent fatigue.
12. Instruct and encourage the patient to gradually increase depth of inspiration.
13. Offer mouthwash after spirometry is completed.
14. Store spirometer in an appropriate place, such as the bedside table, until next scheduled time.
15. Position patient as desired or as ordered.
16. Place call light within easy reach.
17. Wash hands.
18. Assess respiratory status, and evaluate patient's response to spirometry.
19. Document in nurses' notes: patient's respiratory status before and after incentive spirometry, type of spirometry, and any adverse effects from the procedure.

thought to increase the velocity and turbulence of exhaled air, facilitating secretion removal. Vibration increases the exhalation of trapped air and may shake mucus loose and induce a cough. Vibration is not recommended in infants and young children.

Postural drainage. Postural drainage is the positioning technique that draws secretions from specific segments of the lung and bronchi into the trachea. Coughing or suctioning normally removes secretions from the trachea. The procedure for postural drainage can include most lung segments (see Skill 31-4). Because patients may not require postural drainage of all lung segments, the procedure is based on clinical assessment findings. For example, patients with left lower lobe atelectasis may require postural drainage of only the affected region, whereas a child with cystic fibrosis may require postural drainage of all lung segments. (See Skill 31-5 for performing postural drainage.)

Patient teaching. The nurse should instruct the patient on proper techniques for effective coughing and

PERFORMING PULMONARY PHYSIOTHERAPY (POSTURAL DRAINAGE)

1. Check physician's orders. (For best results postural drainage should be performed before meals and at bedtime.)
2. Assess respiratory status and lung sounds. This determines location of secretions before postural drainage and provides a baseline to note effectiveness of procedure.
3. Explain the procedure.
4. Obtain supplies and equipment.
5. Wash hands; don gloves.
6. Provide privacy.
7. Position patient according to the lung area to be drained (see illustration): provides gravitational drainage of secretions. Placing pillows for support will help provide comfort for the patient.
8. Place paper tissues and emesis basin within easy reach to collect secretions expectorated by patient.
9. Encourage deep breathing and coughing at intervals: facilitates bringing secretions toward the oropharynx where they can be expectorated or suctioned.
10. Cover patient with a light-weight blanket to prevent chilling.
11. Offer assistance with oral hygiene to provide comfort and reduce nausea if present.
12. Measure secretions if ordered; note color, amount, and consistency.
13. Position patient as desired or ordered after procedure.
14. Dispose of secretions and soiled tissues in appropriate area.
15. Remove gloves; wash hands.
16. Assess respiratory status, and evaluate patient's response.
17. Document in nurses' notes: patient's respiratory status before and after postural drainage; any secretions expectorated, including amount, color, and other characteristics; any adverse effect; and the patient's response to the treatment.

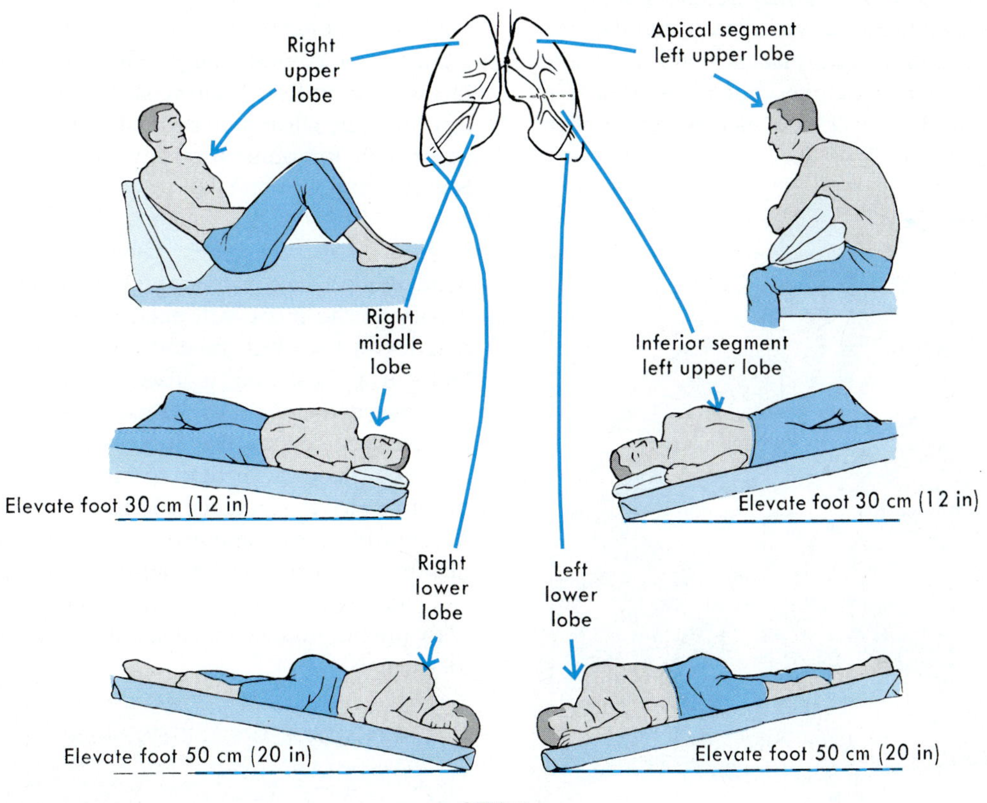

STEP 7

deep breathing, as well as other measures to facilitate optimal air exchange, such as increasing movement and changing position. Medication teaching should address the rationale for prescribed medications, as well as side effects.

Prognosis. Prognosis is dependent upon age and preexisting illness of the patient.

Pneumothorax

Etiology/Pathophysiology. **Pneumothorax** is a collection of air or gas in the pleural space, causing the lung to collapse. It can be secondary to a ruptured bleb on the lung surface (as in emphysema) or a severe coughing episode. It can be caused by a penetrating chest injury where the pleural lining is punctured, or a spontaneous pneumothorax can occur suddenly without an apparent cause (Fig. 31-16).

When the pleural space is penetrated, air enters, thus decreasing the normal negative pressure. Consequently the lung cannot remain fully inflated.

Clinical Manifestations. The patient may present with a recent chest injury. There will be decreased breath sounds on the affected side and a sudden, sharp chest pain with dyspnea. The patient may be diaphoretic and exhibit an increased heart rate, tachypnea, and dyspnea. There will be a cessation of normal chest movements on the affected side. With a pneumothorax resulting from penetrating injury, there will be a sucking sound heard on inspiration.

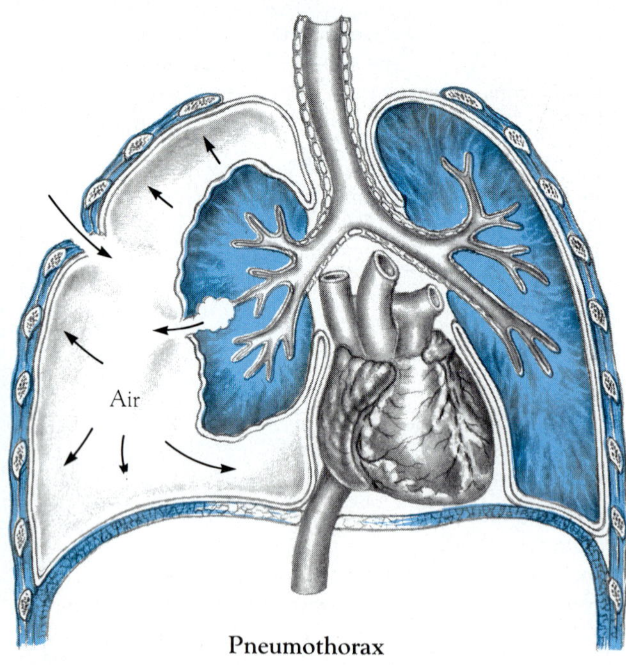

FIG. 31-16 Pneumothorax: complete collapse of the right lung.

As positive pressure increases in the pleural space, the lung collapses. Because lung tissue no longer expands, the mediastinum may shift to the unaffected side (mediastinal shift), placing increased pressure on large vessels and resulting in decreased venous return.

Assessment. Collection of *subjective data* may include reporting a recent penetrating chest injury or severe coughing episode. The patient may also complain of shortness of breath of sudden onset and may indicate feelings of anxiety associated with air hunger.

Collection of *objective data* involves a nursing assessment that includes frequent vital signs, noting any change in respiratory and cardiac rate and rhythm. On auscultation the nurse will note bilateral unequal breath sounds, diminished on the affected side. Color, characteristics, and amount of sputum should be noted.

Diagnostic Tests. Important findings to aid in diagnosis will come from the patient's history. For example, the patient may report a recent chest injury or a precipitating respiratory condition, such as chronic obstructive pulmonary disease (COPD). Chest x-ray examination will reveal decreased lung expansion. Arterial blood gases will show a decrease in pH and Pa_{O_2}, with an increased Pa_{CO_2}.

Medical Management. Surgery may be done to insert a chest tube (thoracotomy). The chest tube is inserted in the fifth and sixth intercostal spaces at the midaxillary line. The chest tube is attached to a water seal drainage system. Intermittent positive pressure may be administered.

Nursing Interventions. General measures include maintaining airway patency and providing adequate oxygenation. The nurse will need to assess and document patency of the chest tube system, keeping it free from kinks. If a chest tube is inserted, the nurse must note the color and amount of drainage and assess integrity of the drainage system. The nurse will monitor blood pressure and place the patient in high Fowler's position to promote airway clearance and lung expansion. Pain may be controlled by administering appropriate analgesics, but the use of respiratory depressants is avoided.

Nursing diagnoses and interventions for the patient with pneumothorax include but are not limited to the following:

NURSING DIAGNOSES	NURSING INTERVENTIONS
Breathing pattern, ineffective, related to nonfunctioning lung	Assess respiratory rate and rhythm, and note any signs of respiratory distress, such as dyspnea, use of accessory muscles, nasal flaring, and anxiety. Provide chest tube care, maintaining secure placement.

NURSING DIAGNOSES	NURSING INTERVENTIONS
Breathing pattern, ineffective, related to nonfunctioning lung—cont'd	Facilitate ventilation by elevating head of bed, and administer oxygen as ordered. Suction as needed to remove secretions. Encourage adaptive breathing techniques to decrease respiratory effort. Encourage rest periods interspersed with activities.
Fear, related to feeling of air hunger	Assess patient's feelings of fear related to health concerns and feeling of air hunger. Identify positive coping methods, and support their use. Determine support systems available to patient.
Gas exchange, impaired, related to inability to breathe deeply	Assess for signs of hypoxia, i.e., restlessness, disorientation, and irritability. Monitor arterial blood gases and pulse oximetry. Monitor fluid and electrolyte status and I&O, being alert to changes caused by altered oxygenation.

Patient teaching. The nurse should explain the rationale for treatments—oxygen therapy and chest tube drainage—before their implementation. Effective breathing techniques and the need for ongoing medical care should be reinforced. The nurse should instruct the patient to limit exposure to people who may have infections, such as upper respiratory infection or influenza. The patient is advised not to smoke but to drink fluids copiously, to avoid fatigue and strenuous activity, and to report any signs and symptoms of recurrence, such as chest pain, difficulty breathing, or fever, to the physician.

Prognosis. The lung will usually reexpand within several days. The chest tube is removed by the physician when a chest x-ray shows that the lungs are completely expanded.

Lung Cancer

Etiology/Pathophysiology. The incidence of lung cancer has been steadily increasing during the past 50 years in both men and women. In 1986 cancer of the lung surpassed breast cancer to become the number one cancer killer of women. Thus lung cancer is now the leading cause of death from cancer in both men and women. Lung cancer causes 21% of cancer deaths in women and 34% of cancer deaths in men. Tumors may result from metastasis anywhere in the body or may appear as primary tumors. Metastasis from the colon and kidney is common. Metastasis to the lung may be discovered before the primary lesion is known, and sometimes the location of the primary lesion is not determined during the person's life. It has been linked primarily with cigarette smoking. A history of smoking, especially for 20 years or more, is considered to be a prime risk factor. Approximately 80% of lung tumors are linked to cigarette smoking. "Passive smoking" (breathing in sidestream smoke) brings as many, if not more, carcinogens into the body as inhaled smoke.[3] Occupational exposures, such as asbestos or chrome, are also risk factors. It is suspected that air pollutants may increase risk.

The mortality of persons with lung cancer depends primarily on the specific type of cancer and the size of the tumor when detected. Squamous cell carcinoma is the most common, followed by adenocarcinoma; undifferentiated small cell (oat cell) carcinoma is the least common. Most people who develop the disease are over 50 years of age.

Clinical Manifestations. If the lesion is located peripherally, there are few symptoms and it may not be discovered until visualized on a routine chest x-ray examination. If the peripheral lesion perforates the pleural space, a pleural effusion will result and severe pain will occur. Central lesions originate from a larger branch of the bronchial tree. These lesions cause obstruction and erosion of the bronchus. Signs and symptoms are hemoptysis, dyspnea, fever, and chills. Auscultation may reveal wheezing on the affected side as well. Phrenic nerve involvement causes paralysis of the diaphragm.

As the disease progresses, metastasis may occur, along with weight loss. Primary lung tumors usually metastasize to the liver or to nearby structures, such as the esophagus, heart pericardium, skeletal bone, and brain.

Assessment. Collection of *subjective data* includes the patient's complaints of a chronic cough and of hoarseness. The patient may also report weight loss and extreme fatigue. The nurse should interview the patient regarding a family history, especially a history of cigarette smoking and of exposure to occupational irritants.

Collection of *objective data* includes assessing the cough, noting color (especially blood streaked) and consistency of sputum, as well as frequency, duration, and precipitating factors. Also the nurse should assess the characteristics of the cough (moist, dry, hacking) and effect of body position and should identify with the patient what, if anything, helps to relieve the cough. The lungs should be auscultated to determine if unilateral wheezing is present. Invasion of the superior vena cava causes edema of the neck and face and is called *superior vena cava syndrome.*

Diagnostic Tests. Chest x-ray studies and CT scan of the chest are used to identify the location and size of the tumor. Bronchoscopy with biopsy or brushings and sputum for cytology will indicate the presence of malignant cells. A mediastinoscopy may be done to determine whether spread of the tumor to the lymph nodes has occurred. Scalene lymph node biopsy is also done to determine metastasis. This biopsy is performed in the supraclavicular area.

Medical Management. The treatment of lung cancer depends on the type and stage of lung cancer. Unfortunately, most patients are not diagnosed early enough for curative surgical intervention. It is estimated that one third of the patients are inoperable when first seen, and one third are found to be inoperable on exploratory thoracotomy. Of the third who are operable, the surgical mortality is 10% for pneumonectomy and 2% to 3% for lobectomy. A pneumonectomy is the most common surgical treatment. This consists of removing the entire lung. Because there is no lung left to require reexpansion, drainage tubes usually are not necessary. The fluid remaining in that area will consolidate eventually, which will help prevent a mediastinal shift. A lobectomy is performed when one lobe is involved rather than the entire lung. If only a portion of a lobe of a lung is involved, a segmental resection is done. Both a lobectomy and segmental resection require chest tube insertion to facilitate lung reexpansion. (For water-seal drainage, see Figs. 31-14 and 31-15.) Radiation therapy and chemotherapy are often done in conjunction with surgery to enhance recovery. In small oat cell cancer of the lung, chemotherapy alone or combined with radiation has largely replaced surgery as a treatment of choice. A large percentage of these patients experience remission; in some cases the remission has been long lasting. At present about one third of the patients who have surgery experience tumor spread.

Nursing Interventions. Nursing intervention is often directed at postsurgical interventions, including facilitating recovery and preventing complications by promoting effective airway clearance through frequent repositioning, coughing, and deep breathing. The nurse will assess vital signs frequently, auscultating breath sounds. After routine postoperative vital signs check, the patient will be checked every 2 hours to ascertain stability; as progress is made, the patient will be checked every 4 hours.

Prescribed medications are primarily antineoplastic agents to prevent or reduce tumor growth. Medications will be given also for symptomatic relief: narcotic analgesics for pain control, antipyretics for fever, and antiemetics for nausea.

Nursing diagnoses and interventions for the patient with lung cancer include but are not limited to the following:

NURSING DIAGNOSES	NURSING INTERVENTIONS
Airway clearance, ineffective, related to lung surgery	Facilitate optimal breathing by placing patient in a sitting position. Assist with position changes frequently. Promote coughing and deep breathing, providing necessary splinting. Encourage early ambulation to mobilize secretions.
Nutrition, altered: less than body requirements, related to fatigue and dyspnea	Encourage patient to eat by serving meal in calm, unhurried manner, offering assistance as needed. Provide pleasant environment for meals. Determine dietary preferences, and encourage family to bring special favorites. Offer small, frequent meals and nutritious snacks. Administer antiemetics before meals to prevent nausea. Monitor I&O and patient's weight to determine nutritional status and needs.
Mobility, impaired physical, related to dyspnea	Assess patient's ability to ambulate, and assist as needed. Encourage range-of-motion exercise to maintain muscle strength. Exercise (including movement of the shoulder on the affected side) is important. Encourage conservation of energy, and assess for signs of fatigue.
Activity intolerance, related to generalized weakness	Observe response to activity. Identify factors contributing to intolerance (e.g., stress, side effects of medications). Assess patient's sleep patterns. Plan rest periods between activities. Perform activities for patient until patient can perform them. Provide progressive increase in activity as tolerated. Provide oxygen as ordered. Problem solve with patient to determine methods of conserving energy while performing tasks.
Fear, related to cancer, treatment, and prognosis	Monitor changes in communication patterns with others. Monitor expressions such as worthlessness, anxiety, powerlessness, abandonment, or exhaustion. Listen and accept expressions of anger without personalizing reaction. Encourage patient to identify problem, redefine situation, obtain needed information, generate alternatives, and focus on solutions.

Patient teaching. The nurse should teach the patient effective coughing techniques. The patient and family should be instructed regarding nutritional needs and importance of maintaining physical mobility. If the patient smokes, encourage quitting and encourage family members to stop also. Encourage eating a diet high in protein and calories. The nurse should also instruct the patient and family regarding signs and symptoms that could indicate recurrence of metastasis, such as fatigue, weight loss, increased coughing or hemoptysis, central nervous system changes, and arm or shoulder pain. Identify resources in the community, such as the American Cancer Society and the American Lung Association, that can assist the patient and family with information, support groups, and equipment needed.

Prognosis. Only 13% of lung cancer patients live 5 years or longer after diagnosis. The survival rate is 40% for cases detected in a localized stage; only 20% of lung cancers are discovered that early. Survival rates have improved only slightly over the past 10 years.

Pulmonary Edema

Etiology/Pathophysiology. Pulmonary edema is an accumulation of serous fluid in interstitial lung tissue and alveoli resulting from:

- Severe left ventricular failure resulting from a weakened myocardium due to a myocardial infarction
- Inhalation of irritating gases
- Rapid administration of intravenous fluids (whole blood, plasma, or fluids)
- Barbiturate or opiate overdose

Cardiogenic pulmonary edema usually accompanies underlying cardiac disease in which the failure of the left ventricle causes pooling of fluid to back up into the left atrium and into pulmonary veins and capillaries. The most common cause of pulmonary edema is increased capillary hydrostatic pressure from left ventricular failure.

As the pulmonary capillary pressure exceeds the intravascular pressure, serous fluid is rapidly forced into the alveoli. Fluid rapidly reaches the bronchioles and bronchi, and patients literally begin to drown in their own secretions. As oxygen decreases, the person shows signs of severe respiratory distress.

Pulmonary edema is acute and extensive and may lead to death unless treated rapidly.

Clinical Manifestations. The primary signs and symptoms of pulmonary edema are dyspnea and related breathing disturbances. Labored respirations, tachypnea, tachycardia, cyanosis, and, especially, pink (or blood-tinged), frothy sputum are the most obvious signs. The patient may also exhibit restlessness or agitation because of the altered tissue perfusion and resulting hypoxia and respiratory failure.

Assessment. Collection of *subjective data* includes noting the patient's complaints of severe dyspnea and a feeling of impending death.

Collection of *objective data* involves the nurse assessing for signs of respiratory distress. Such signs include nasal flaring and sternal retractions with inspiration, as well as rapid, stertorous respirations, hypertension, tachycardia, restlessness, and disorientation. On auscultation the nurse will most likely hear wheezing and crackles. On physical examination the nurse will often note a sudden weight gain caused by fluid retention, decreased urinary output as a result of retained fluid in the pulmonary vasculature, and a productive cough of frothy, pink sputum.

Diagnostic Tests. Chest x-ray examination will reveal fluid infiltrates, indicating alveolar edema, increased pleural space fluid (pleural effusion), and enlarged heart (cardiomegaly). Arterial blood gases are altered, with varying Pa_{O_2} and Pa_{CO_2} levels. There may be respiratory alkalosis or acidosis. Sputum cultures are done periodically to rule out a bronchopulmonary infection.

Medical Management. The physician will order oxygen therapy and may intubate the patient for adequate ventilation support. Rotation of tourniquets, infrequently used, can be done manually or by machine. Pressure is applied to three limbs at a time; cuff inflation is slightly above patient's diastolic blood pressure; the cuff is inflated for 45 minutes followed by 15 minutes free of compression. Medications will include diuretics to reduce alveolar and systemic edema by increasing urinary output (furosemide [Lasix]) and a narcotic analgesic, usually morphine sulfate, to decrease respiratory rate, lower the patient's anxiety level, and reduce venous return. Bronchodilators (aminophylline or theophylline) will be given to increase ventilation, and medications such as cardiotonic glycosides (digoxin [Lanoxin]), will be used to treat underlying causative conditions.

Nursing Interventions. An important nursing measure is accurate assessment and documentation to identify changes in the patient's condition. This includes assessment of respiratory status and frequent monitoring of I&O, vital signs, arterial blood gases, pulse oximetry, and electrolyte values. The nurse maintains oxygenation therapy as ordered—commonly delivered by Venturi mask at 40% to 70% concentration. Mechanical ventilation may be required; in this case the intubated patient needs oral care and tracheostomy care according to protocol. Optimal air exchange must be facilitated by maintaining the patient in high Fowler's position. A patent IV line must be maintained, usually at a very slow rate to keep the vein open for medication administration (i.e., 30 ml/hr) per infusion pump. This prevents adding even more fluid to the overloaded patient. The patient requires extremely close monitoring of cardiac status and accurate measuring and recording of I&O.

Nursing diagnoses and interventions for the patient with pulmonary edema include but are not limited to the following:

NURSING DIAGNOSES	NURSING INTERVENTIONS
Gas exchange, impaired, related to excess fluid in pulmonary vessels interfering with oxygen diffusion	Be alert to any signs indicating altered ventilation, such as restlessness, irritability, disorientation, or apprehension. Monitor arterial blood gases, and notify physician of any change. Monitor vital signs frequently, including cardiac rhythm.

NURSING DIAGNOSES	NURSING INTERVENTIONS
Gas exchange, impaired, related to excess fluid in pulmonary vessels interfering with oxygen diffusion—cont'd	Administer oxygen therapy as ordered, and document patient response. Administer diuretics, bronchodilators, morphine sulfate, cardiotonic glycosides, and other medications as ordered.
Fluid volume excess, related to altered tissue permeability	Assess indicators of patient's fluid volume status, such as breath sounds and skin turgor. Monitor I&O accurately. Monitor electrolyte values closely, and notify physician of alterations. Administer diuretics as ordered, and note patient response. Weigh patient daily on same scale at same time of day with same amount of bed linen and patient clothing. Provide low-sodium diet to prevent excess fluid retention.
Fatigue, related to increased respiratory effort	Allow adequate rest periods interspersed with nursing interventions. Relate level of fatigue to patient activity, and modify accordingly. Encourage energy conservation; limit visitors as needed. Identify and promote patient's support systems.

Patient teaching. The patient should be taught effective breathing techniques. Medication teaching regarding actions, side effects, and dosage of prescribed medications should be given to the patient and family. The patient and family should be instructed on a low-sodium diet and referred to the dietician for follow-up. The nurse should emphasize to the patient and family the signs and symptoms to observe that would indicate alteration in health, such as productive cough (noting the color and characteristics of sputum), activity intolerance, or the presence of dyspnea.

Prognosis. The prognosis for acute pulmonary edema is guarded and may lead to death unless treated rapidly.

Pulmonary Embolus

Etiology/Pathophysiology. The most common pulmonary perfusion abnormality, pulmonary **embolism** (PE), is caused by the passage of a foreign substance (blood clot, fat, air, or amniotic fluid) into the pulmonary artery or its branches, with resulting obstruction of the blood supply to lung tissue and subsequent collapse. Pulmonary embolism usually occurs in patients identified to be at risk, such as the following:

- Those with prior thrombophlebitis
- Those who have recently had surgery, been pregnant, or given birth
- Women who are taking contraceptives on a long-term basis
- Those with a history of congestive heart failure, obesity, or immobilization from fracture; immobilization appears to be a key consideration

Venous stasis, venous wall injury, and increased coagulability of blood cause the formation of a venous thrombus. The thrombus (usually in the deep veins of the lower extremities) dislodges and travels to the pulmonary artery where it becomes lodged. At the site of the embolus, lung tissue is ventilated but perfusion is inadequate because of the occlusion. As a result of this, arterial hypoxia develops.

Clinical Manifestations. A pulmonary embolus manifests itself by a sudden, sharp abdominal or thoracic pain associated with dyspnea and hemoptysis. The respiratory rate will be rapid. In small areas of infarction, presenting signs and symptoms are a small amount of hemoptysis, pleuritic chest pain, elevated temperature, and increased white blood cell count. In large areas of infarction, symptoms include hypoxia, hypotension, and tachypnea. Lung sounds will be diminished, and crackles may be present.

Assessment. Collection of *subjective data* includes noting the patient's report of presence and degree of dyspnea and chest pain. Nursing assessment will also include identifying the presence of associated risk factors.

Collection of *objective data* involves the nurse assessing for pleuritic pain and noting the nature of the patient's cough. Further assessment includes breath sounds, vital signs, and being alert for tachycardia and tachypnea. On auscultation the nurse will note any dullness in lung sounds and the presence of a pleural friction rub. In assessing the psychological response of the patient, the nurse will document the presence and degree of anxiety, which is often correlated to air hunger.

Diagnostic Tests. Arterial blood gases will be significantly altered, depicting hypoxia and respiratory alkalosis. Initially, the chest x-ray is normal. After 24 hours, the x-ray may reveal small infiltrates secondary to atelectasis. Chest x-ray examination also will show an enlarged main pulmonary artery. CT scans of the lung may be helpful unless the patient has a history of congestive heart failure or chronic obstructive pulmonary disease, in which case an evaluation of the ventilation/perfusion ratio will be more definitive.

Medical Management. When there are multiple pulmonary emboli present, an umbrella filter may be placed in the inferior vena cava to retain the emboli, preventing their migration to other parts of the body.

The physician will prescribe anticoagulant therapy to prevent clot formation. Initially heparin will be administered intravenously, by way of either continuous infusion on a pump or intermittent boluses. The effectiveness of heparin is determined by monitoring partial thromboplastin time (PTT) values, which should be maintained at 1½ to 2 times the control (or normal) values. In the event of overheparinization resulting in profound bleeding, the treatment is intravenous administration of protamine sulfate. Heparin therapy is gradually tapered (it may take several days) while oral anticoagulation (warfarin [Coumadin]) is initiated. Effectiveness of warfarin therapy is determined by monitoring prothrombin time (PT) values, with the goal being 1¼ to 1⅕ times the control (or normal) values. Vitamin K reverses the effects of warfarin. Fresh frozen plasma may be required in cases of severe bleeding.

Some physicians prefer to use fibrinolytic agents, such as urokinase or streptokinase.

Nursing Interventions. General nursing interventions include applying TED hose and elevating the lower extremities. The nurse should check peripheral pulses and frequently measure bilateral calf circumference to check for occlusion caused by a clot. The head of the bed may be slightly elevated, and oxygen will be administered by mask or nasal cannula to facilitate optimal gas exchange. The patient will promote lung expansion by coughing and deep breathing.

Related nursing interventions will include assessing for signs of bleeding—epistaxis, hemoptysis, bleeding from gums or rectum, and ecchymosis. Other general nursing interventions will include placing the patient on bed rest for the first few days and gradually increasing activity.

Nursing diagnoses and interventions for the patient with pulmonary embolus include but are not limited to the following:

NURSING DIAGNOSES	NURSING INTERVENTIONS
Gas exchange, impaired, related to alteration in pulmonary vasculature	Assess sensorium and vital signs q 2 hr or as needed, noting any changes indicative of altered oxygenation/ventilation. Elevate head of bed 30 degrees to improve ventilation. Administer oxygen as ordered. Monitor arterial blood gases frequently, reporting any increase or decrease of $Paco_2$ and Pao_2 of more than 10 mm Hg. Be alert to any dysrhythmias.
Physical mobility, impaired, related to fatigue associated with dyspnea	Encourage the patient to reduce the effort of breathing by using effective breathing techniques. Place TED hose on patient for continuous wear; remove at least q 8 hr. Deliver passive range of motion, and assist with position changes q 2 hr.
Protection, altered, related to risk of prolonged bleeding or hemorrhage secondary to anticoagulation therapy	Monitor vital signs for indicators of profuse bleeding or hemorrhage resulting from anticoagulant therapy: hypotension, tachycardia, and tachypnea. At least once a shift check stool, urine, sputum, and vomitus for occult blood using agency-approved method for testing per protocol. At least once a shift inspect wounds, oral mucous membranes, any entry site of an invasive procedure, and nares for evidence of bleeding. To prevent hematoma formation, avoid giving IM injection unless it is unavoidable. Teach patient the necessity of using sponge-tipped applicators and mouthwash for oral care to minimize the risk of gum bleeding. Instruct patient to shave with an electric rather than a bladed razor.

Patient teaching. Medication teaching is a major nursing concern. Often oral anticoagulation becomes a lifelong regimen that bears close monitoring, so the nurse must assess the patient's present knowledge base and expand on it. Preventive measures are also important, especially in the postoperative period. The nurse should teach the patient techniques to reduce venous pooling (which could precipitate thrombophlebitis), such as position changes and wearing nonrestrictive clothing. The patient must be told to avoid crossing the legs while in a sitting or lying position and also to avoid standing in one place for a prolonged period, because these activities increase venous pooling. The nurse should teach the rationale and application procedure for antiembolism hose. Explain that patient should put them on in the morning before getting out of bed. The patient and family should be instructed on signs and symptoms of pulmonary embolism to report to the physician, such as chest pain and dyspnea. Blood-tinged sputum or blood in the urine, which could result from anticoagulant therapy, should also be reported.

Prognosis. Early diagnosis and appropriate treatment reduce mortality to under 10%. Although most pulmonary emboli resolve completely and leave no residual deficits, some patients may be left with chronic pulmonary hypertension.

Adult Respiratory Distress Syndrome (ARDS)

Etiology/Pathophysiology. ARDS is not a disease but a complication that occurs as a result of other disease processes. There are many causes of ARDS, which results from either a direct or indirect pulmonary injury. Possible causes include viral or bacterial pneumonia, chest trauma, aspiration, or any type of shock. Drug overdoses, renal failure, and pancreatitis are also known to be causative factors, as well as COPD, neuromuscular defects with Guillain-Barré syndrome, and myasthenia gravis.

Regardless of the cause of ARDS, there is a certain sequela of events in the body's response that remains the same. The surface of the alveolar capillary membrane becomes altered, causing increased permeability, which then allows fluid to leak into the interstitial spaces and alveoli. This creates pulmonary edema and hypoxia. The alveoli lose their elasticity and collapse, which causes the blood to be shunted through the impaired alveoli, hence interfering with oxygen transport. The damaged capillaries allow plasma and red blood cells to leak out, resulting in hemorrhage.

Clinical Manifestations. ARDS manifests itself in 12 to 24 hours postinjury, resulting in lung tissue damage or hypovolemic shock, and 5 to 10 days after sepsis development, the patient will experience respiratory distress with altered breath sounds. There may be altered sensorium as a result of an elevated $Paco_2$ and decreased Pao_2. Additional signs will be cardiovascular in nature: tachycardia, hypotension, and decreased urinary output.

Assessment. Collection of *subjective data* involves a nursing assessment that will include background information and a history of the present illness (obtained from family members, because the patient is usually too ill to give details).

Collection of *objective data* involves the nurse being an astute observer of any change in the patient's condition, no matter how small or gradual. The nurse must make an accurate and thorough initial assessment so such changes will be quickly recognized. Initial assessment includes identifying and documenting respiratory rate, rhythm, and effort. Signs of dyspnea should be noted, such as nasal flaring, sternal and subclavicular retractions, or cyanosis. The nurse should auscultate the lungs and document the presence of crackles or wheezing and should maintain close observation of vital signs. Frequent assessment of the level of consciousness, with particular attention to increased restlessness or lethargy, is necessary.

Diagnostic Tests. Pulmonary function tests will be done to determine the ease or difficulty of oxygen in crossing the alveolar capillary membrane. Arterial blood gases will show definitive changes: the Pao_2 will be decreased (less than 70 mm Hg), the $Paco_2$ will be increased (greater than 35 mm Hg), and the bicarbonate ion will be decreased (less than 22 mEq/L). Initially, HCO_3 increases in an attempt to buffer the elevated $Paco_2$ level, thereby maintaining pH in the normal range. The pH will be elevated initially but will steadily decrease as the patient's condition deteriorates. A chest x-ray examination will depict thickened bronchial margins and possibly diffuse infiltrates.

Medical Management. The medical plan focuses on supportive treatment by maintaining adequate oxygenation and treating the cause—drug overdose, infections, or inhaled toxins. Medications commonly used to treat associated conditions include corticosteroids to treat pulmonary edema, aiding in restoring lung tissues to their normal structure and function. Morphine sulfate is commonly given to sedate restless patients and decrease respiratory rate. When the patient is intubated and ventilator dependent, a neurological blocking agent, such as Pavulon, may be administered to suppress the patient's own respiratory effort, relying on the controlled ventilator assistance.

Other medications may include cardiotonic glycosides (digoxin) to enhance cardiac function and antibiotic agents to prevent the complication of infection.

Nursing Interventions. The goal of nursing interventions is to provide adequate oxygenation and ventilation and to treat the multisystem responses caused by ARDS. Nursing intervention includes knowledge of mechanical ventilator settings and effects. Nursing intervention correlated to this is pertinent to intubated patients, such as suctioning, providing oral care, and assessing for signs of inadequate ventilation. Arterial blood gases as well as pulse oximetry should be monitored closely and any changes reported.

Also, an accurate, ongoing assessment of cardiac function is important. The nurse should be alert for and document any rate or rhythm changes. The RN will notify the physician of any changes.

The nurse should assess vital signs and identify the presence of an elevated temperature so that cultures can be obtained to treat infections.

Nursing diagnoses and interventions for the patient with ARDS include but are not limited to the following:

NURSING DIAGNOSES	NURSING INTERVENTIONS
Gas exchange, impaired, related to tachypnea	Monitor arterial blood gases, and report any increase or decrease of $Paco_2$ and Pao_2 of more than 10 to 15 mm Hg. Address any factors that would contribute to restlessness and anxiety, because they increase the body's oxygen demand and will exacerbate the patient's already serious condition. Administer oxygen per order, assessing and recording patient response. Monitor electrocardiogram changes. Report any changes in vital signs and any change in patient's level of response, no matter how small or gradual.

NURSING DIAGNOSES	NURSING INTERVENTIONS
Breathing pattern, ineffective, related to respiratory distress	Assess respiratory rate, rhythm, and effort, being alert to signs of dyspnea, such as cyanosis and dyspnea. Facilitate optimal ventilation by proper positioning. Maintain airway patency by encouraging frequent coughing and deep breathing if able, or suctioning as needed.

Patient teaching. The nurse should teach the patient effective breathing techniques, emphasizing the importance of frequent position changes and coughing and deep breathing. If the patient is intubated, the nurse should explain all procedures before their implementation and should explain the importance of working *with* the ventilator and not trying to breathe independently. The patient should be reassured that the ventilator will breathe for him and that those breaths will be more effective than his own. The nurse should explain to the patient and family the importance of using rest and activity appropriately. Explanations of the purpose and side effects of all medications should be offered.

Prognosis. ARDS affects an estimated 150,000 persons each year, and one half of these will die despite supportive therapy.

OXYGEN THERAPY

The goal of oxygen therapy is to prevent or to relieve hypoxia. Any patient with impaired tissue oxygenation can benefit from controlled oxygen administration. Oxygen is not a substitute for other treatment, however, and should be used only when indicated. Oxygen should be treated as a drug. It is expensive and has dangerous side effects. As with any drug, the dosage or concentration of oxygen should be continuously monitored. The nurse should routinely check the physician's orders to verify that the patient is receiving the prescribed oxygen concentration. The five rights of medication administration also pertain to oxygen administration (see Chapter 21).

The element oxygen is a colorless, odorless, and tasteless gas that will not burn or explode. However, if combined with other factors, such as an electrical spark or fire, oxygen will support combustion and ignite. Nurses should follow all the following safety precautions:

1. Place "No Smoking" and "Oxygen in Use" signs in conspicuous locations.
2. Instruct patient, family, and visitors that smoking is not permitted, because oxygen supports combustion.
3. Avoid the use of electrical appliances, such as razors, blankets and heating pads.
4. Secure portable oxygen delivery systems, such as cylinders, to prevent falling or accidentally being tipped over.
5. Avoid placing oxygen cylinders near sources of heat, such as lamps or radiators.
6. Avoid clothing that is non-fire resistant.
7. Ensure that all electrical equipment is functioning appropriately and is well grounded. Avoid frayed, tangled, or cluttered cords, and do not overload circuits with too many appliances.
8. Know the institution's fire procedure and location of fire extinguishers.
9. Administer oxygen as ordered by a physician; the physician determines the method of administration and the flow rate of oxygen.

Oxygen therapy is frequently initiated by a respiratory therapist, who is a health care professional licensed to deliver treatment that will improve a patient's ventilation and oxygenation needs. Among the treatments often performed by a respiratory therapist is intermittent positive-pressure breathing (IPPB) therapy. This is delivered by a mechanical device that hyperinflates lungs by applying positive pressure to the airways.

The signs and symptoms manifested by patients who might require oxygen will vary according to the degree of oxygen deficiency (see Box 31-1). See Skill 31-6 on pp. 924-927 for O_2 administration.

Transtracheal Oxygen Delivery

A newer method of oxygen delivery is the transtracheal catheter, which is inserted directly into the trachea between the second and third tracheal cartilages. Transtracheal oxygen delivery was pioneered by Heimlich.

Unlike a tracheostomy tube, a transtracheal catheter (Fig. 31-17) does not interfere with drinking, eating, or

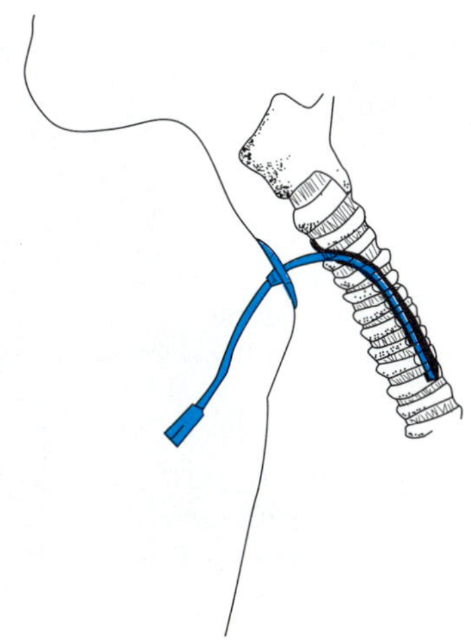

FIG. 31-17 A transtracheal catheter may be inserted into the trachea between the second and third tracheal cartilages.

SKILL 31-6

OXYGEN ADMINISTRATION

1. Check physician's order.
2. Assess patient for signs of hypoxia and respiratory distress.
3. Assess patient's airway, and suction any secretions obstructing airway (see Skill 31-2).
4. Obtain supplies and equipment.
5. Explain procedure and necessity of precautions to take during oxygen therapy.
6. Place "No Smoking/Oxygen in Use" signs in conspicuous places.
7. Wash hands.
8. Provide privacy.
9. Position patient in Fowler's or semi-Fowler's position unless otherwise ordered, to allow for appropriate lung expansion.
10. Fill humidifier container to designated level, if used; use sterile, distilled water or as prescribed; this provides moisture to prevent drying of the nasoorpharyngeal mucosa.
11. Attach flow meter to humidifier, and insert in proper oxygen source; most institutions have a central source of oxygen with a specially designed outlet. Flow meter must be properly secured to oxygen source.
12. Administer oxygen therapy:

    Nasal cannula: A simple two-prong plastic device that is used to deliver low concentration of oxygen. A nasal cannula allows patient to eat and talk normally and is appropriate for all age groups. Caution should be observed in proper placement of prongs to prevent oxygen from coming in direct contact with nasal mucosa. Oxygen has drying effect on mucosa and interferes with moistening and warming air inhaled through nasal passage, making breathing uncomfortable for patient. It is nurse's responsibility to maintain method, flow rate, comfort, and safety of a patient receiving oxygen therapy.

    a. Attach nasal cannula to oxygen tubing (if it is not preattached), and then attach to flow meter.
    b. Place prongs in cup of water. Adjust flow meter to 6 to 10 L to flush tubing and prongs with oxygen. This determines patency and removes any microscopic particles that may be in the tubing. If water bubbles, tubing and prongs are patent. Wipe off water.
    c. Adjust flow rate to the prescribed amount.
    d. Place a nasal prong into each naris of the patient (see illustration). Place prongs of nasal cannula into patient's nares to direct flow of oxygen into patient's upper respiratory tract. Adjust liter flow per physician's order; usually 2 L/min is prescribed.
    e. Adjust straps of the cannula over the ears and tighten under the chin. The fit should be snug and comfortable to prevent displacement of prongs.
    f. Place padding between strap and ears. Lamb's wool, gauze, or cotton balls may be used to prevent irritation.
    g. Provide slack of tubing, and secure to patient's garment to reduce risk of prongs' causing pressure on the nares and displacement as patient moves or is repositioned.
    h. Maintain regular assessment.
        - Check cannula q 8 hr for possible obstruction.
        - Observe external nasal area, nares, and superior surface of both ears for skin impairment q 6 to 8 hr.
        - Check nares and prongs, and cleanse with cotton-tipped applicator as needed.
        - Check physician's orders for prescribed flow rate q 8 hr.
        - Maintain solution in humidifier container, if used, at appropriate level at all times.

    Nasal catheter: Administration of oxygen through a nasal catheter is less preferred than the use of the nasal cannula because it can traumatize the nasal mucosa on insertion, causing discomfort to patient.

    i. Attach nasal catheter to oxygen tubing, and then attach tubing to flow meter.
    j. Place catheter in cup of water, and turn on flow meter to 6 to 10 L to flush tubing. Wipe off water.

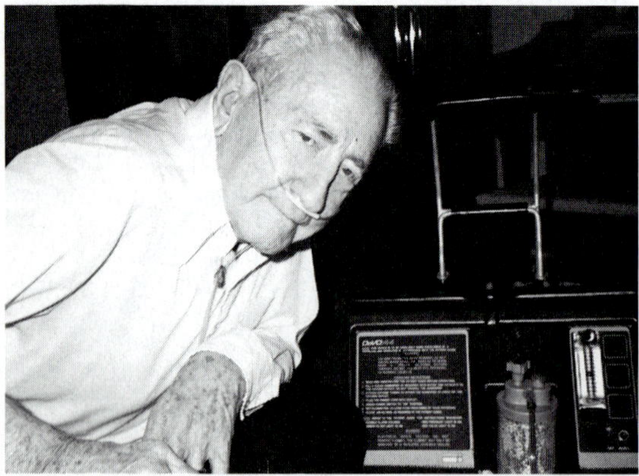

STEP 12d

OXYGEN ADMINISTRATION—cont'd

k. Adjust flow rate to prescribed amount; usually 2 L/min is ordered.

l. Determine depth of insertion by using nasal catheter to measure from patient's earlobe to tip of nose. Marking place on catheter will assure nurse of proper length of insertion.

m. Cover tip of catheter with water-soluble lubricant to reduce friction and trauma to nasal mucosa as catheter is inserted. Vaseline is never used because of danger of lipid pneumonia.

n. Hold catheter to observe its natural curvature, and gently insert catheter into one side of nasal passage.

o. Inspect mouth to visualize tip of catheter.

p. Withdraw catheter approximately 1 cm (½ in), or until it is no longer visible.

q. Tape catheter in place—may be taped to bridge of nose or side of cheek.

r. Provide slack of tubing, and secure to patient's garment.

s. Maintain regular assessments.
- Alternate placement of catheter by using opposite nasal passage q 8 hr.
- Observe external nasal area and nares for skin impairment q 6-8 hr.
- Check nares, and cleanse with cotton-tipped applicator.
- Check physician's orders for prescribed flow rate q 8 hr.
- Maintain solution in humidifier container at proper level at all times.
- Change catheters at least once daily or q 8 hr at the most.

Face mask: Depending on patient's respiratory condition, physician may prescribe oxygen to be administered by oxygen mask (see illustration). The mask is designed to fit snugly over patient's nose and mouth. There are different types of masks that may be used to meet patient's needs, such as Ventimask (see illustration), nonrebreathing mask, and aerosol mask.

t. Adjust flow rate of oxygen per physician's order. Usually 6 to 10 L/min, which is measured in percentages, is prescribed. Respiratory therapist is usually responsible for maintaining proper flow. Observe for fine mist or bubbling in humidifier.

u. Allow patient to hold mask, and place your hand over patient's hand if possible. Placing mask over patient's face may cause feeling of suffocation and apprehension. This action allows patient to become accustomed to mask and to have some control of placing it on face.

v. Place mask over bridge of nose; then cover mouth.

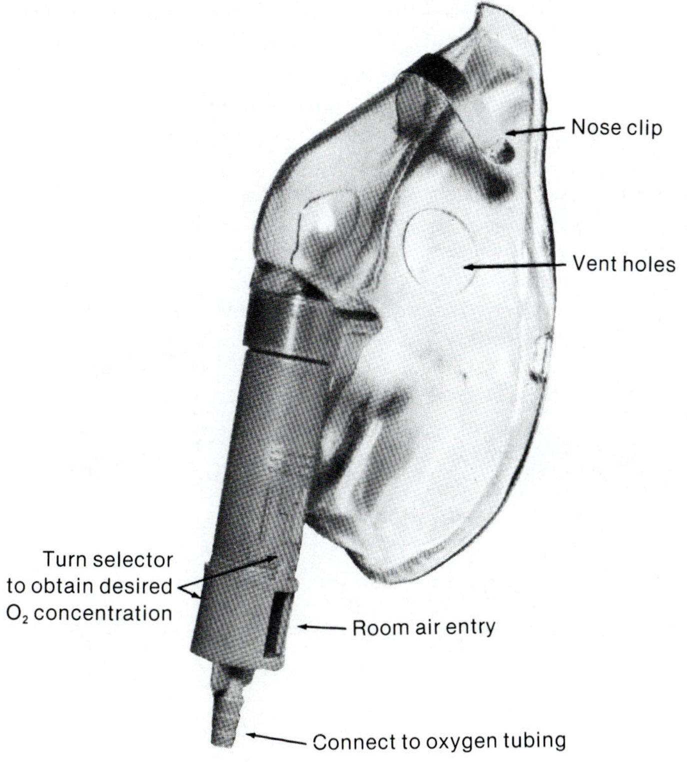

STEP 12t

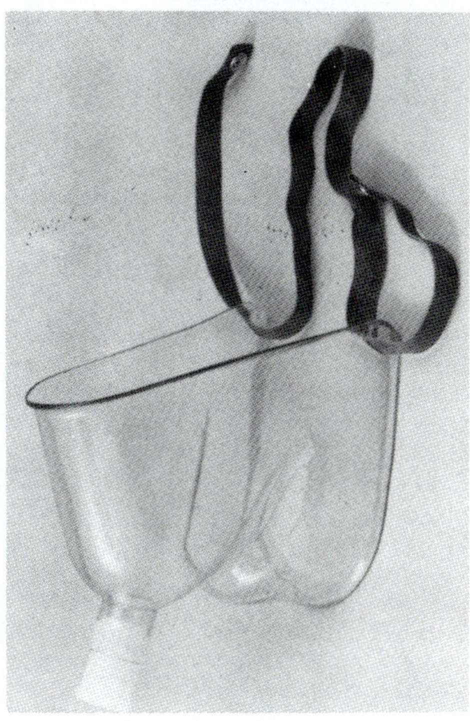

STEP 12z

OXYGEN ADMINISTRATION—cont'd

w. Adjust straps around patient's head and over ears. Place cotton ball or gauze over ears under elastic straps.

x. Observe reservoir bag if one is attached to mask. This ensures mask is fitting appropriately by expanding and collapsing with patient's breathing. Complete collapse indicates oxygen flow should be increased.

y. Maintain regular assessments:
- Remove mask and clean skin and dry q 1-2 hr.
- Check physician's orders for prescribed flow rate q 8 hr.
- Maintain solution in humidifier container, if used, at appropriate level at all times.

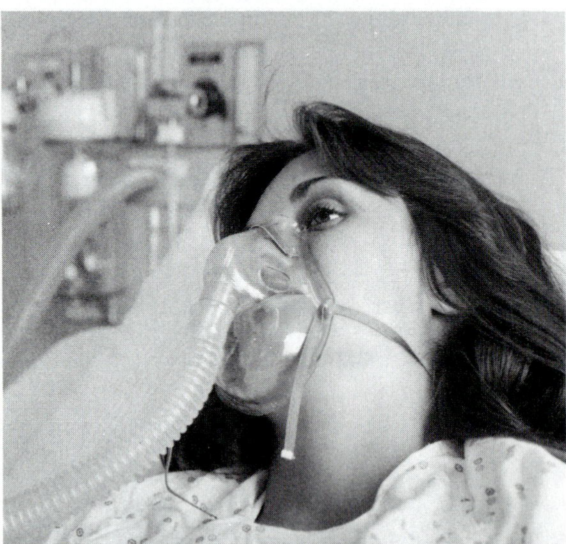

STEP 12z, cont'd

z. If face tent is used (see illustration), a mist should always be present.

Oxygen tent: An oxygen tent provides fine mist, constant temperature, and high concentration and flow rate of oxygen. Mist is produced by humidification of oxygen confined within clear plastic canopy. Canopy encloses upper torso of patient. Psychological effect of covering patient's head may increase anxiety and therefore increase feeling of suffocation. Reassurance must be provided to relieve anxiety before placing patient in oxygen tent. Children requiring oxygen therapy are in respiratory distress, which increases oxygen requirements. Severely anxious children may be less frightened if they see someone close by and if they are reassured that they will not be left alone. Because the canopy is clear, it allows the patient to have visual contact with nursing staff and visitors. Some visual distortion of persons and objects can be expected when patient looks through canopy, and this should be explained (see illustration). Because moisture accumulation frequently occurs from humidification of oxygen, the nurse's primary responsibility is to keep the patient warm and dry to prevent chilling. Clothing and bed linens may need to be changed more frequently. The tent also provides constant temperature, which is usually 70° F. Temperature may be adjusted for comfort of patient but should not exceed 10° over recommended temperature. The oxygen tent is designed more specifically for the pediatric patient; however, it may also be used for the adult.

STEP 12aa

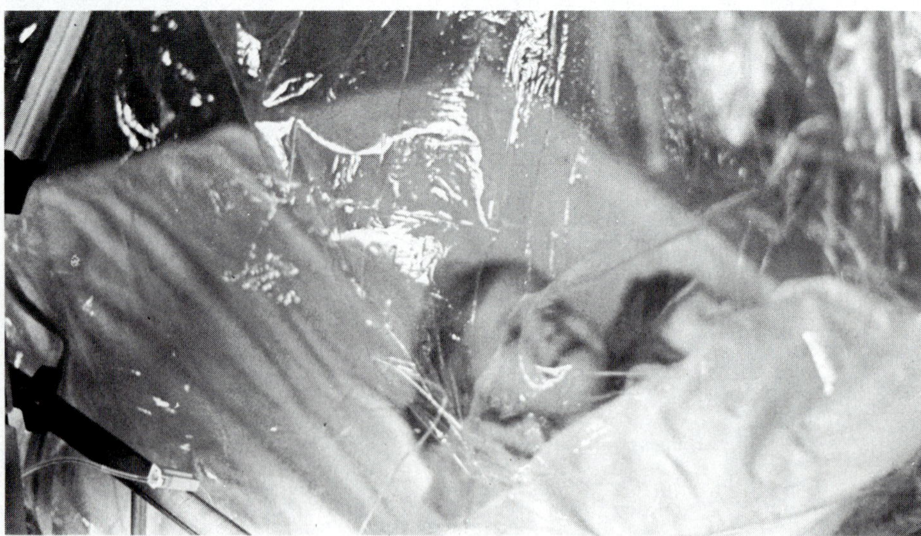

OXYGEN ADMINISTRATION—cont'd

aa. Place oxygen machine at head of bed for ease of draping canopy over head of bed and patient and to place humidifier where mist will be inhaled by patient.

ab. Fan fold top sheet to patient's waist; may be used to secure front edge of canopy or to cover patient later if needed.

ac. Set temperature to 70° F, recommended setting unless ordered otherwise; temperature is regulated by a thermostat.

ad. Turn machine on, and adjust flow rate to 10 to 12 L/min. Leave machine on until it registers appropriate temperature and oxygen concentration.

ae. Placement of canopy:
- Lift canopy over patient, and tuck back of canopy under head of mattress.
- Tuck sides of canopy under sides of mattress at head of bed.
- Place folded bath blanket lengthwise across patient's thighs.
- Place lower, front edge of canopy to conform to shape of patient's thighs; place this edge of canopy within folded bath blanket.
- Tuck folded bath blanket and canopy under sides of mattress to secure it and prevent leakage of oxygen.

af. Use zipper openings to provide care and administer medications: prevents large amounts of oxygen escaping and maintains control of temperature and humidity.

ag. Maintain regular assessments.
- Check temperature, flow rate, and humidity at least q 4 hr.
- Assess patient's response.
- Check patient's clothing frequently, and change bed linens as needed.
- Mist within the tent should always be visible.

13. Wash hands.
14. Document in nurses' notes: date, time, flow rate, method of oxygen delivery, temperature being maintained (if tent is used), respiratory assessment, patient's response, any changes in physician's orders, and any adverse reactions or side effects.

SKILL 31-6

talking. The nasal cannula delivers oxygen only during inhalation, but the transtracheal oxygen delivery system delivers oxygen throughout the respiratory cycle. No oxygen is lost to the atmosphere; therefore oxygen delivery is less expensive. Additional humidification is unnecessary because the nasopharynx, the area in most need of supplemental humidity, is bypassed. This allows the flow rate to be decreased for some patients. Those patients who require 2 L/min with a cannula will only need 1 L/min with a transtracheal catheter. The low flow rates enable patients to use portable oxygen delivery systems longer between refills. It is recommended for those patients with congestive heart failure (CHF) and COPD.

This method is especially adapted for home use. It allows the individual to be active. It may even be concealed under a shirt and tie. The transtracheal tract opening should be inspected regularly for erythema, edema, or excessive exudate. (Small amounts of clear exudate are expected.) The area is cleaned twice daily with a cotton-tipped applicator. To remove dried exudate, hydrogen peroxide may be used to wash the neck. The transtracheal tract (like a tracheostomy) never truly heals as long as it is kept open for oxygen delivery. If replacement is delayed more than 30 minutes, the opening may seal.

A small oxygen tube (an 8 or 9 French catheter) is inserted through the transtracheal tract opening. Oxygen is administered through the small oxygen tube. The tube is removed for cleaning. Oxygen is then administered through the nose. Clean technique is used. The transtracheal oxygen catheter may need cleaning several times a day. An extra transtracheal oxygen catheter is kept at the bedside. Avoid reusing a transtracheal catheter after 3 months. Catheters tend to become brittle with extended use.

CHRONIC OBSTRUCTIVE PULMONARY DISEASE

Chronic obstructive pulmonary disease (COPD) is a progressive and irreversible condition that is characterized by diminished inspiratory and expiratory capacity of the lungs. It is a chronic respiratory condition that obstructs the flow of air to or from the patient's bronchioles. COPD includes emphysema, chronic bronchitis, asthma, and bronchiectasis. All diseases included in COPD are characterized by *chronic air flow limitation,* a new term that accurately describes the underlying pathology.

Emphysema

Etiology/Pathophysiology. Emphysema symptoms usually develop when the patient is in the 40s, with disability increasing by age 50 to 60. This condition is characterized by changes in the alveolar walls and capillaries: thus emphysema is primarily an alveolar disease.

A component of pulmonary connective tissue, lung elastin, is destroyed by an enzyme, which then causes decreased pulmonary surface area available for gas exchange. The bronchi, bronchioles, and alveoli become inflamed as a result of chronic irritation. Because of bronchiole lumen narrowing, air becomes trapped in the alveoli during expiration, causing alveolar distention (see Fig. 31-18). The alveoli then rupture and scar, losing their elasticity. Oxygen in the arterial blood decreases, and CO_2 increases. This process is worsened by cigarette smoking and other inhaled irritants. Cigarette smoking is by far the most common cause of emphysema and chronic bronchitis. There is a lag of 30 to 35 years, on average, between taking up smoking and onset of signs and symptoms. The patient is disabled because all available energy must be used for breathing. Emphysema or other obstructive lung diseases can lead to **cor pulmonale,** an abnormal cardiac condition characterized by hypertrophy of the right ventricle of the heart as a result of hypertension of the pulmonary circulation. Cor pulmonale results in the presence of edema in the lower extremities as well as in the sacral and perineal area, distended neck veins, and enlargement of the liver with ascites. These signs result from the development of right-sided congestive heart failure (cor pulmonale), one of the complications of emphysema.

Clinical Manifestations. The primary symptom of emphysema is dyspnea on exertion. Initially there is little sputum production, but later it becomes copious. The patient will eventually appear barrel chested (an increased anteroposterior diameter caused by overinflation) and begin using accessory muscles for breathing (Fig. 31-19). Spontaneous pursed-lip breathing and chronic weight loss with emaciation ensue.

Assessment. Collection of *subjective data* includes a nursing assessment that details a history of onset of symptoms. The nurse should note duration and intensity of dyspnea, cough, and sputum production (documenting color and amount). Also the patient's reported history of smoking and exposure to inhalants, and family history of respiratory disorders should be determined.

Collection of *objective data* includes assessment of presenting signs, such as tachycardia, tachypnea, peripheral cyanosis, and clubbing of fingers. The most outstanding feature of clubbing is a lateral and longitudinal curvature of the nails accompanied by soft tissue enlargement, presenting a bulbous (bulb-shaped), shiny appearance.

Diagnostic Tests. Pulmonary function tests will be done to measure total lung capacity, which will be de-

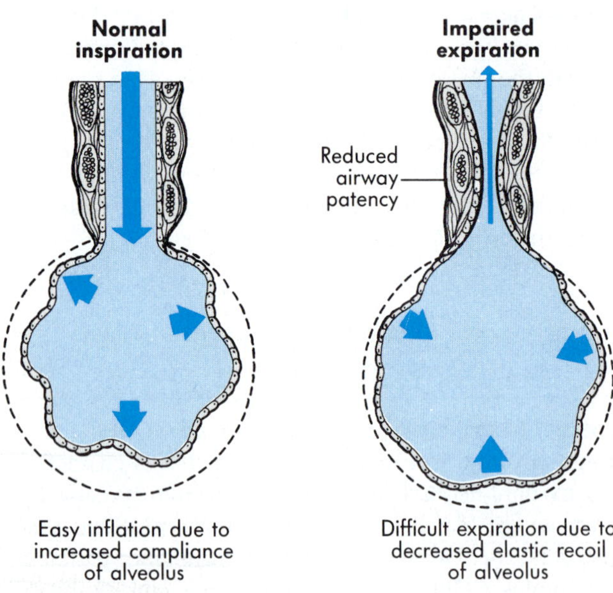

FIG. 31-18 Mechanisms of air trapping in emphysema. Damaged or destroyed alveolar walls no longer support and hold open the airways, and alveoli lose their property of passive elastic recoil. Both of these factors contribute to collapse during expiration.

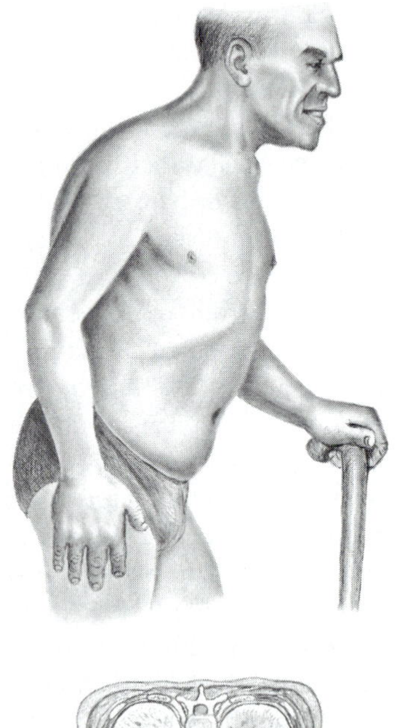

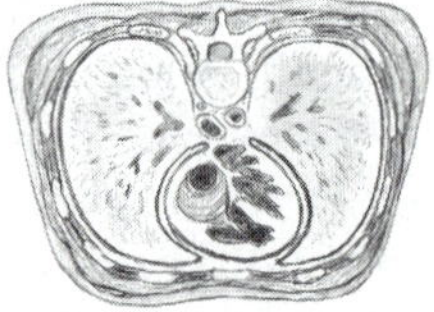

FIG. 31-19 Barrel chest. Note increase in AP diameter.

creased with COPD. Residual volume is increased, as are compliance and airway resistance. Ventilatory response is decreased. Pulse oximetry is useful in assessing oxygen saturation in arterial blood.

Arterial blood gases will reveal a decreased Pao_2, and $Paco_2$ will often be increased. A chest x-ray examination will show hyperinflation of the lungs, widened intercostal spaces, and flattened diaphragm with increased anteroposterior diameter (associated with barrel chest). Hematology studies should be done to determine if a positive $alpha_1$-antitrypsin assay exists (an enzyme deficiency causing airway abnormalities resulting in emphysema). Complete blood count will reveal elevated erythrocytes and hemoglobin and hematocrit levels (polycythemia, as a compensatory response to chronic hypoxia).

Medical Management. The medical plan will include long-term management with home oxygen therapy and chest physiotherapy as needed. In an acute exacerbation the patient may require mechanical ventilation.

Prescribed medications will include bronchodilators (theophylline or aminophylline, isoproterenol [Isuprel], terbutaline [Brethine], metaproterenol [Alupent], albuterol (Proventil), and isoetharine [Bronkosol]) to enlarge the bronchioles for greater oxygenation and ease of secretion clearance, and corticosteroids to decrease pulmonary inflammation and obstruction. Corticosteroids are usually prescribed only during an acute exacerbation because of the many side effects seen in long-term steroid therapy. Antibiotics are frequently ordered to reduce the risk of infection related to retained pulmonary secretions. Diuretics will assist with fluid removal. During an acute exacerbation, severe dyspnea can produce considerable anxiety, restlessness, or irritability in the patient. In these cases, a central nervous system (CNS) depressant, specifically, a narcotic, sedative, or tranquilizer, may be prescribed. The patient with COPD must be carefully monitored because of the high risk for respiratory failure from CNS depressants. The patient should be carefully evaluated for hypoxemia before a CNS depressant is prescribed.

Nursing Interventions. Nursing intervention will be directed at attempting to decrease the patient's anxiety and promote optimal air exchange. Such measures include elevating the head of the bed and administering *low-flow* (1 to 2 L by nasal cannula) oxygen as ordered (see Skill 31-5). (This is extremely important for COPD patients, because a higher flow of oxygen delivery can be dangerous, since it diminishes the brain's respiratory [regulatory] center and can cause respiratory failure.) The nurse should assist with chest physiotherapy, which includes percussion, vibration, and postural drainage. All three techniques will help loosen secretions to be expectorated; it sometimes takes several hours after chest physiotherapy before the patient can expectorate loosened secretions (see Skill 31-4). Increasing oral intake of fluids will liquify secretions, thus aiding in their removal. Additionally, the use of a humidifier will enhance this process. Frequent oral care will promote comfort. The nurse should allow sufficient rest periods and should assist the patient in ADLs to prevent decrease in oxygen saturation levels.

The nurse can assist the patient in maintaining nutritional intake by advising rest for 30 minutes before eating. This will conserve energy and decrease dyspnea.

The patient with emphysema has a markedly increased need for protein and calories to maintain an adequate nutritional status. A high-protein, high-calorie diet should be divided into five or six small meals a day. Oral fluid intake should be maintained at 2 to 3 L/day unless contraindicated (because of congestive heart failure, for example). Instruct the patient to drink fluids between meals, rather than with meals, to reduce gastric distension and pressure on the diaphragm. Perform frequent oral hygiene to freshen the patient's mouth after coughing exercises and before meals.

Nursing diagnoses and interventions for the patient with emphysema include but are not limited to the following:

NURSING DIAGNOSES	NURSING INTERVENTIONS
Airway clearance, ineffective, related to narrowed bronchioles	Assess patient's ability to mobilize secretions, intervening as needed. Encourage coughing and deep breathing, frequent position changes, and increased oral intake (up to 2000 ml/day). Elevate head of bed; suction as needed. Assist with respiratory treatments. Auscultate lungs, reporting any changes in lung sounds.
Anxiety, related to feeling of dyspnea	Promote optimal air exchange to decrease anxiety. Assess patient's anxiety level, noting ability to cooperate with treatment regimen. Explain all procedures before their implementation. Encourage effective breathing techniques. Assess support systems available to patient, and mobilize resources.
Activity intolerance, related to imbalance between oxygen supply and demand, secondary to inefficient work of breathing	Organize care so that periods of activity are interspersed with periods of at least 90 min of undisturbed rest. Assist patient with active ROM exercises to build stamina and prevent complications of decreased mobility. Monitor patient's respiratory response to activity. Activity intolerance is indicated by excessively increased respiratory rate (e.g., increased more than 10 breaths/minute above patient's baseline) and depth, dyspnea, and use of accessory muscles of respiration.

NURSING CARE PLAN: ***THE PATIENT WITH EMPHYSEMA***

Mr. Oden is a 91-year-old patient admitted with an exacerbation of COPD. His respirations are 32 and labored. He has nasal flaring and his nail beds are cyanotic. He has a barrel chest and digital clubbing. He states he has a productive cough and "can't get my air." It is noted he expectorates tenacious yellow mucus. He appears anxious during the assessment.

Nursing diagnoses	Patient goals/expected outcomes	Nursing interventions
Airway clearance, ineffective, related to tenacious secretions	Patient will maintain patent airway as evidenced by decreased rhonchi, wheezes, tachypnea, dyspnea, and ABG values within limits (for this patient).	Assess lung sounds q 2-4 hr. Encourage turning, coughing, and deep breathing q 2-4 hr. Suction prn. Explain all medications used in inhalation therapy, and assist with treatment. Monitor effectiveness.
Breathing pattern, ineffective, related to decreased lung expansion secondary to chronic air flow limitations	Following treatment intervention, patient's breathing pattern improves as evidenced by reduction in or absence of dyspnea.	Assess for indicators of respiratory distress (i.e., agitation, restlessness, decreased level of consciousness, and use of accessory muscles of respiration). Auscultate breath sounds; report a decrease in breath sounds or an increase in adventitious breath sounds. Instruct patient in the use of pursed-lip breathing, which provides internal stability to the airways and may prevent airway collapse during expiration. Administer bronchodilator therapy as prescribed. Monitor patient's response to prescribed O_2 therapy. Be aware that high concentrations of O_2 can depress the respiratory drive in individuals with chronic CO_2 retention.
Infection, high risk for, related to retained tenacious secretions	Patient will be free from infection as evidenced by normal temperature and WBC, and sputum will be clear in color and decreased in amount.	Record TPR q 4 hr and more often if needed. Administer antipyretic prn. Change position q 4 hr. Encourage fluids, and record I&O every shift.
Anxiety, related to dyspnea	Patient will experience decreased anxiety as evidenced by verbalization of needs and concerns and statements of preference for more therapeutic coping methods.	Assess level of anxiety, and attempt to reduce by using calm, therapeutic interactions. Teach anxiety reduction techniques: pursed-lip breathing and controlled respirations. Assess family interactions; monitor as needed.

CRITICAL THINKING QUESTIONS

1. Mr. Oden turns on his light and states that he is "unable to get his air." The nurse notes subclavicular retractions and a respiratory rate of 36. His oxygen is flowing at 1 L per nasal cannula. Nursing interventions that will decrease his dyspnea include:
2. While the nurse is performing an assessment on Mr. Oden, he states, "I'm so tired of fighting to breathe that I wish I could just go to sleep and never wake up." An appropriate response would be:
3. During vital signs assessment, the nurse notes that Mr. Oden's temperature is 102° F, the pulse rate is 110 and the respiratory rate is 44. The nurse knows that Mr. Oden's COPD places him at a high risk for:

NURSING DIAGNOSES	NURSING INTERVENTIONS
Infection, high risk for, related to retained pulmonary secretions	Assess for indications of infection—sputnum color, amount, and odor—as well as vital signs. Emphasize importance of reducing risk for secondary infection by decreasing exposure to others.

Patient teaching. The nurse should instruct the patient and family (1) on the importance of not smoking and of reducing exposure to other inhaled irritants and (2) effective breathing techniques (i.e., pursed-lip breathing) and relaxation exercises for anxiety control. Teach the patient about the dangers of increased oxygen intake to a patient dependent on hypoxic drive for ventilation. Also, the nurse should teach the patient and family (1) how to prevent infection and (2) symptoms that should be reported to the physician. See the therapeutic dialogue and the nursing care plan for the patient with emphysema.

Prognosis. Emphysema is usually irreversible. COPD is the fourth leading cause of death in the United States.

THERAPEUTIC DIALOGUE: PATIENT WITH EMPHYSEMA

Charles Oden, a 91-year-old man, lives at home with Annetta, his wife of 38 years. He was admitted to the hospital with acute **exacerbation** (an increase in the seriousness of a disease or disorder as marked by greater intensity in the signs or symptoms of the patient) of emphysema. Mr. Oden has a 24-year history of emphysema, with progression of signs and symptoms. Signs and symptoms that he manifests are exertional dyspnea, expectoration of copious amounts of tenacious mucus, fatigue, and fear of suffocation.

Mr. Oden: Will it always be like this? I am so short of air.

Nurse: Are you frightened?

Mr. Oden: I am not afraid of dying, but I worry about having to fight for my air.

Nurse: (Gently touches Mr. Oden's arm) Try taking slow, deep breaths, and concentrate on remaining calm.

Mr. Oden: Sometimes I can't even get to the bathroom and do my business—much less help Annetta with the dishes or even fill the bird feeder.

Nurse: Do you feel you are becoming a burden?

Mr. Oden: I have to be good to Annetta. I want to have something left to give her.

Nurse: I notice you are breathing more easily. I will be back to check on you, and perhaps we can continue this conversation.

Chronic Bronchitis

Etiology/Pathophysiology. Chronic bronchitis is characterized by a recurrent or chronic productive cough for a minimum of 3 months a year for at least 2 years. It is caused by physical or chemical irritants or an infection of bacterial or viral origin. Cigarette smoking is by far the most common cause of chronic bronchitis. The underlying process is an impairment of cilia, so they can no longer move secretions. Mucous gland hypertrophy causes hypersecretion, altering cilia function. There is an increased susceptibility to infection. Chronic infection causes airway scarring, which causes obstruction. This increased airway resistance leads to bronchospasm. There is an altered oxygen-carbon dioxide exchange hypoxia (an inadequate, reduced tension of cellular oxygen) and **hypercapnia** (greater than normal amounts of carbon dioxide in the blood).

Clinical Manifestations. Primary signs include a productive cough, most pronounced in the mornings (this is often overlooked by cigarette smokers). There is also increased dyspnea and use of accessory muscles.

In the later stages of the disease, cyanosis develops, often accompanied by right ventricular failure. The patient with chronic bronchitis often has a characteristic reddish-blue skin color, resulting from polycythemia, cyanosis, and dependent edema, which is associated with right ventricular failure.

Assessment. Collection of *subjective data* includes obtaining a detailed history of smoking or exposure to irritants, as well as family history of respiratory disorders. Also, the patient's current medication and treatment regimen should be determined.

Collection of *objective data* includes assessing the patient's productive cough, noting characteristics and amount of sputum. The nurse should assess the severity of dyspnea and presence of wheezing and should note the patient's level of restlessness. Also, when vital signs are checked, special attention should be paid to tachycardia, tachypnea, and elevated temperature.

Diagnostic Tests. A CBC will show increased erythrocytes, hemoglobin, hematocrit, and white blood cell count. ABG values will reveal respiratory acidosis, hypoxia, and hypercapnia. Pulse oximetry is valuable to assess oxygen saturation levels in arterial blood. There will be an alteration in pulmonary function studies that reveals airflow limitation on expiration, increased airway resistance and residual volume, and often electrolyte abnormalities. Oximetry levels should be monitored on all patients with hypoxia.

Medical Management. The medical plan is aimed at minimizing the disease progression and facilitating optimal air exchange by reducing spasms and secretions.

Prescribed medications will include bronchodilators (theophylline or aminophylline, isoproterenol (Isuprel), terbutaline (Brethine), metaproterenol (Alupent), isoetharine (Bronkosol), albuterol (Probentil), and mucolytics to enhance airway patency. Antibiotic agents (erythromycin) are commonly ordered.

Nursing Interventions. The nurse should provide adequate hydration to liquify secretions and aid in their removal. The patient must be suctioned as needed and maintained on low-flow oxygen. The nurse should offer frequent oral hygiene and provide rest periods. The nutritional needs are similar to the patient with emphysema.

Nursing diagnoses and interventions for the patient with chronic bronchitis include but are not limited to the following:

NURSING DIAGNOSES	NURSING INTERVENTIONS
Breathing pattern, ineffective, related to retained pulmonary secretions	Assess degree of dyspnea, noting nasal flaring, sternal retractions, and pursed-lip breathing. Instruct on effective breathing techniques. Suction as needed.
Fatigue, related to increased respiratory effort	Assess degree of fatigue, and with patient, use problem-solving techniques to explore techniques for decreasing fatigue. Provide treatments in calm, unhurried manner. Identify support systems, and refer if needed. Encourage adequate periods of rest.

Patient teaching. The nurse should teach the patient effective breathing techniques and instruct the patient and family on avoidance of infection exposure. Instruct the patient to notify the physician at the first sign of a respiratory infection. Usually the best indication of such an infection is a change in the color, consistency, or amount of sputum. Medication teaching should be provided, including action, rationale, and side effects. The nurse should stress the importance of increasing fluid intake. The patient and family should be encouraged not to smoke and to avoid using powders and aerosols.

Prognosis. Chronic bronchitis is usually irreversible. COPD is the fourth leading cause of death in the United States, after heart disease, cancer, and traumatic injuries.

Asthma

Etiology/Pathophysiology. Asthma is a broad clinical syndrome and an airway pathology. It involves episodic increased tracheal/bronchial responsiveness to various stimuli, resulting in widespread narrowing of the airways, which usually improves either spontaneously or with treatment. It is classified as extrinsic or intrinsic. **Extrinsic** is caused by external factors, such as environmental allergens (pollens, dust, feathers, animal dander, foods, etc.); **intrinsic** is from internal causes, not fully understood but often triggered by respiratory infection. Recurrence of attacks is greatly influenced by secondary factors, by mental or physical fatigue, and by emotional factors.

Asthma can result from an altered immune response or increased airway resistance and altered air exchange. An acute asthma attack is caused by an antigen-antibody reaction in which histamine is released. There are three mechanisms involved: (1) recurrent, reversible obstruction of airflow in the bronchioles and smaller bronchi secondary to bronchospasm; (2) increased capillary permeability resulting in edema of mucous membranes with increased narrowing of airways; and (3) increased mucus secretion.

Clinical Manifestations. Mild asthma is manifested by dyspnea on exertion and wheezing and is usually controlled by medications. An acute asthma attack usually occurs at night and will include tachypnea, expiratory wheezing, use of accessory muscles, and nasal flaring. There will also be increased anxiety and diaphoresis. The patient will exhibit a productive cough of copious, thick mucus. Asthma can be triggered by external factors, such as dust, mold, or lint, or precipitated intrinsically by a respiratory infection or exercise.

Status asthmaticus is a severe, unrelenting attack that fails to respond to usual treatment. Symptoms of an acute attack are present, and the trapped air leads to exhaustion and respiratory failure.

Assessment. Collection of *subjective data* includes noting that the patient may report asthma-related factors: medications, self-care regimen, precipitating factors, and anxiety.

Collection of *objective data* includes the nurse assessing the presence of cyanosis, the amount of respiratory effort, and vital signs. The patient may assume a "hunched forward" position in an attempt to get more air. The nurse should auscultate the lungs for wheezing.

Diagnostic Tests. To diagnose asthma the physician will order ABG and pulmonary function tests. The chest x-ray examination will reveal lung hyperinflation related to air trapping, and a flat diaphragm related to increased intrathoracic volume. A sputum culture should be obtained from the patient to rule out any secondary infection. A CBC will reveal an increased eosinophil count in the differential, which is indicative of an allergic response. If the patient has been taking theophylline, a blood sample should be drawn to determine whether the prescribed dose of theophylline is maintained at a therapeutic level; the acceptable therapeutic range is 10-20 μg/ml. This will also reduce the risk of complications as a result of toxicity.

Medical Management. Medications will include bronchodilators (epinephrine), methylxanthines (theophylline), IV aminophylline in a loading dose, subcutaneous terbutaline (Brethine), or the latter two may be given simultaneously and then in a maintenance dose for 48 to 72 hours; aminophylline blood levels should be monitored. Steroids (prednisone or Deltasone) are prescribed to decrease pulmonary inflammation and enhance airway patency. Aerosol therapy includes 1 to 2 inhalations of 0.5 ml isoetharine (Bronkosol) in 2.5 ml of saline. Antibiotic agents (ampicillin) are commonly administered prophylactically. Once the acute event is over, the medical plan includes identification of precipitating factors and promoting optimal health. Elimination of allergen or countermeasures, such as desensitization or hyposensitization, are desirable.

Nursing Interventions. Nursing intervention includes ensuring adequate fluid intake and optimal ventilation. Measures to facilitate these goals include incorporating rest periods into activities and interventions, elevating the head of the bed, teaching effective breathing techniques, such as pursed-lip breathing, and providing oxygen therapy as ordered. The nurse should monitor vital signs and electrolytes. Kind and empathetic emotional support is vital.

Nursing diagnoses and interventions for the patient with asthma include but are not limited to the following:

NURSING DIAGNOSES	NURSING INTERVENTIONS
Breathing pattern, ineffective, related to narrowed airway	Assess ventilation, and be alert for signs of increasing dyspnea, such as using accessory muscles, nasal flaring, dyspnea, pursed-lip breathing, or prolonged expiration. Maintain position to facilitate ventilation, such as elevated head of bed or leaning on overbed table. Administer prescribed medications. Assist with administration of respiratory treatments. Provide care in calm, unhurried manner. Attempt to minimize exposure to dust and other irritants by maintaining clean environment and use of humidifier. Maintain adequate hydration.
Health maintenance, altered, related to possible allergens in the home	Implement mutual problem-solving to explore with patient and family what stimulants may be in home environment, such as allergens. Facilitate allergy testing if needed. Teach the patient and family importance of avoiding exposure to known irritants.

Patient teaching. The nurse should educate the patient and family to identify signs and symptoms and precipitating factors, to avoid recurrent attacks. The patient should be instructed on relaxation techniques to use to manage anxiety. The importance of health maintenance measures, such as adequate fluid intake and effective breathing techniques, should be stressed.

Prognosis. Asthma is the leading cause of chronic illness in childhood. If status asthmaticus is not reversed, death will ensue.

Bronchiectasis

Etiology/Pathophysiology. Bronchiectasis is a gradual, irreversible process that involves chronic dilation of bronchi and that eventually destroys bronchial elastic and muscular elements. This pulmonary muscle tone is gradually lost after one or, as is generally the case, repeated pulmonary infections in children and adults.

This condition is usually secondary to failure of normal lung tissue defenses (as caused by cystic fibrosis, foreign body, or tumor). It occurs as a complication of recurrence of an inflammation/infection process that gradually alters the pulmonary structures.

Clinical Manifestations. Signs and symptoms occur after a respiratory infection. The signs and symptoms usually seen are dyspnea, cyanosis, and clubbing of fingers. There are paroxysms of coughing upon arising in the morning and when lying down. This severe coughing produces copious amounts of foul-smelling sputum. Fatigue, weakness, and a loss of appetite are also noted.

Assessment. Collection of *subjective data* includes noting the patient's report of difficulty breathing, weight loss, and fever.

Collection of *objective data* includes the nurse hearing fine crackles and wheezes in the lower lobes on auscultation. The patient will exhibit a prolonged expiratory phase and increased dyspnea. Hemoptysis is seen in 50% of the patients.

Diagnostic Tests. Chest x-ray examination will be essentially normal, but inflammation and mediastinal shift may be the result of overinflation of specific lobes. Sputum cultures can rule out the presence of a bacterial infection. CBC may show the presence of polycythemia, caused by pulmonary insufficiency (hypoxia). Pulmonary function tests will show a decreased forced expiratory volume.

Medical Management. Oxygen will be ordered at low flow volume. The patient may require surgery if there is no response to more conservative measures, such as medications, chest physiotherapy, and adequate hydration. If surgery is needed, the affected area will be removed (lobectomy).

Medications include mucolytic agents (acetylcysteine [Mucomyst]), as well as antibiotics and bronchodilators (theophylline or aminophylline).

Nursing Interventions. General nursing interventions include using a cool mist vaporizer to provide humidity and increasing oral intake of fluids to aid in secretion removal. The nurse should assess vital signs and lung sounds every 2 to 4 hours. The patient should be suctioned as needed and assisted to turn, cough, and deep breathe every 2 hours. The nurse should assist with chest physiotherapy.

Nursing diagnoses and interventions for the patient with bronchiectasis include but are not limited to the following:

NURSING DIAGNOSES	NURSING INTERVENTIONS
Airway clearance, ineffective, related to retained pulmonary secretions	Assess patient's ability to mobilize secretions, assisting as needed. Encourage postural drainage and coughing; suction if needed. Encourage frequent position changes to facilitate secretion mobility and removal. Maintain adequate hydration. Administer mucolytic agents as ordered, and note patient response.
Physical mobility, impaired, related to decreased exercise tolerance	Assess patient's activity tolerance, and promote adaptive techniques, such as incorporating rest periods into activities. Promote a gradual increase of activity, noting patient tolerance. Problem solve with patient and family to identify methods of energy conservation and ways to implement them into life-style.

Patient teaching. The nurse should teach the patient and family environmental awareness (avoidance of smoke, fumes, and irritating inhalants). Smoking should be discouraged and appropriate rest/exercise practices should be taught. The nurse should perform medication teaching, including dosage, rationale, and side effects. The patient and family should be instructed on signs and symptoms of a secondary infection. The nurse should ensure that the patient knows how to reach the physician after discharge.

Prognosis. Bronchiectasis is a chronic disease. Surgical removal of a portion of the patient's lung is the only cure.

Cystic Fibrosis

Etiology/Pathophysiology. Cystic fibrosis is a genetic disorder of the exocrine glands that causes production of excessively thick mucus. It is thought to be related to an enzyme deficiency and is a multisystem disease affecting the respiratory system, pancreas, and sweat glands. The most common cause of death is progressive respiratory infections.

Bronchial obstruction occurs because of tenacious mucus, resulting in atelectasis and hyperinflation. This progresses to hypoxia, hypercapnia, and acidosis. The occurrence of mucostasis leads to pulmonary infection in the patient.

Clinical Manifestations. The patient will present with respiratory distress: congestion, tachypnea, and dyspnea. Crackles and wheezes will be heard on auscultation. The patient with cystic fibrosis will have a barrel chest and clubbing of fingers and toes. The patient will also demonstrate a productive cough, cyanosis, and possibly a headache or altered sensorium or level of consciousness.

Assessment. Collection of *subjective data* involves the nurse obtaining the patient's history and noting the present medication regimen, need for life-style alterations, and previous treatments or surgery. The nurse should determine the effectiveness of the patient's support systems and determine if intervention is needed.

Collection of *objective data* involves the nurse assessing the patient's respiratory status and effort, vital signs, appetite, and evidence of malnutrition.

Diagnostic Tests. The diagnosis of cystic fibrosis is made by a sweat chloride level greater than 60 mEq/L (normal amount is 1 to 60 mEq/L) and is commonly diagnosed during childhood. Other diagnostic tests include chest x-ray studies (which may reveal disseminated infiltrates), pulmonary function tests, and sputum examination. Some physicians will also order ABG tests. Decrease or absence of pancreatic enzymes can also confirm cystic fibrosis.

Medical Management. The goal of the medical plan is to decrease the occlusion of the bronchi by mucus. The patient may require surgery, such as a resection of blebs, or a tracheostomy to permit airway clearance and mechanical ventilation.

Prescribed medications include mucolytic agents, to combat the tenacious secretions, and expectorants (potassium iodide), to assist with their clearance. Bronchodilators, such as theophylline, are commonly ordered to facilitate airway patency. Antibiotic agents are frequently ordered (1) to treat infection or (2) prophylactically. A multivitamin supplement should be given.

Nursing Interventions. Because cystic fibrosis is a multisystem disease, the nursing interventions are broad and address many systems. Interventions pertinent to respiratory symptoms will be addressed here. The nurse will determine that the patient's immunizations are current or, if needed, update as ordered. The nurse will assist with aerosol treatments and administer oxygen as ordered. A thorough dietary review must be completed, and the nurse can assist in planning a diet with increased calories and protein and decreased fat content. The nurse will also assist with the development of a network for psychosocial support.

Nursing diagnoses and interventions for the patient with cystic fibrosis include but are not limited to the following:

NURSING DIAGNOSES	NURSING INTERVENTIONS
Airway clearance, ineffective, related to tenacious pulmonary secretions	Determine patient's ability to mobilize secretions and assist as needed with chest physiotherapy. Administer medications as ordered, noting effectiveness. Provide adequate hydration to liquify secretions. Auscultate breath sounds frequently and report any changes. Assess productive cough, noting color, amount, and characteristics.
Nutrition, altered: less than body requirements, related to altered digestion of fat, protein, and carbohydrates	Accurately weigh patient daily. Monitor I&O, skin turgor and tone. Offer small, frequent, high-caloric, high-protein, low-fat feedings. Administer prescribed pancreatic enzyme at mealtime. Be alert to signs of malnutrition.
Family coping: potential for growth, related to chronic illness of family member	Assess and support patient/family's knowledge of disease and treatments. Explain all procedures. Identify coping skills, and support their use. Assist with contacting support systems as needed.

Patient teaching. The nurse should teach the patient effective breathing techniques and adaptive exercise/rest practices. The importance of up-to-date immunizations and the necessity of adhering to the prescribed medical/dietary regimen should be stressed.

Prognosis. Median survival is approximately 20 years of age, and males survive much longer than females. The reason for this is unknown.

REFERENCES AND SUGGESTED READINGS

1. American Cancer Society: *Cancer facts and figures 1991,* Atlanta, 1992, The Society.
2. Assessing the lungs: adapted from *Clinical Skill Builders, Rapid Assessment,* 1991, Springhouse Corporation, *Nurs '91* 21(11):32C, 1991.
3. Belcher AE: Cancer nursing: Mosby's clinical nursing series, St Louis, 1992, Mosby.
4. Bolgiano CS et al: Administering oxygen therapy: what you need to know, *Nurs '90* 20(6):47, 1990.
5. Boutolte J: TB: the second time around and how you can help to control it, *Nursing* 23(5):42, 1993.
6. Carroll P: Nursing the thoracotomy patient, *RN* 55(6):34, 1992.
7. Carroll PL: What's new in chest-tube management, *RN* 54(5):34, 1991.
8. Caruthers DD: Infectious pneumonia in the elderly, *Am J Nurs* 90(2):46, 1990.
9. Centers for Disease Control: Guidelines for preventing the transmission of tuberculosis in health care settings, with special emphasis on HIV-related issues, *MMWR* 39:1, 1990.

10. Centers for Disease Control and Prevention: Many hospitals unprepared as MDR−+B reported nationwide, *Hospital Infection Control* 20(2):17, 1993.
11. Centers for Disease Control and Prevention: National action plan to combat multidrug-resistant tuberculosis, *MMWR* 41(RR-11):6, 1992.
12. Crowe M, Ultrino C: Psychosocial implication of lung cancer, *J Pract Nurs* 40:36, 1990.
13. Dettenmeir PA: *Pulmonary nursing care,* St Louis, 1992, Mosby.
14. Dolin JT: *Critical care nursing: clinical management through the nursing process,* Philadelphia, 1991, FA Davis.
15. Dooley S et al: Multidrug-resistant tuberculosis, *Am J Int Med* 117(3):257, 1992.
16. Dowling PT: Return of tuberculosis: screening and preventive therapy, *Am Fam Physician* 43(2):457, 1991.
17. Ehrhardt BS, Graham M: Pulse oximetry: an easy way to check oxygen saturation, *Nurs '90* 20(3):50, 1990.
18. Eid N et al: Chest physiotherapy in review, *Respir Care* 36(4):270, 1991.
19. Elpern EH, Girzadas AM: Tuberculosis update: new challenges of an old disease, *Med-Surg Nurs* 2(3): 1993.
20. Finesilver C: Perfecting the art of respiratory assessment, *RN* 55(2):22, 1992.
21. Graham NM et al: Prevalence of tuberculosis positivity and skin anergy in HIV seropositive and seronegative intravenous drug users, *JAMA* (3)267:369, 1992.
22. Haln K: Tips for giving oxygen therapy, *Nurs '90* 20(2):70, 1990.
23. Iserman MD, Chon DL, Sbarbaro JA: Directly observed treatment of tuberculosis, *N Engl J Med* 328:576, 1993.
24. Lavin J, Haidorfer C: Anergy testing: a vital weapon, *RN* 9:31, 1993.
25. Lewis Mantik S, Collier Cox I: *Medical-surgical nursing: assessment and management of clinical problems,* ed 3, St Louis, 1992, Mosby.
26. Long BC et al: *Medical-surgical nursing: a nursing process approach,* ed 3, St Louis, 1993, Mosby.
27. McConnell EA: Minimizing respiratory problems, *Nursing* 21(1):34, 1991.
28. McMahon Casey K: Fighting MDR-TB, *RN* 56(9):27, 1993.
29. *Mosby's dictionary of medicine, nursing, and allied health,* ed 4, St Louis, 1994, Mosby.
30. Orse AJ: Asthma: the danger is real, *RN* 54(4):58, 1991.
31. Pagana KD, Pagana TJ: *Mosby's diagnostic and laboratory test reference,* St Louis, 1992, Mosby.
32. Phipps WJ et al: *Medical-surgical nursing: concepts and clinical practice,* ed 4, St Louis, 1991, Mosby.
33. Potter P, Perry AG: *Fundamentals of nursing: concepts, process and practice,* ed 3, St Louis, 1993, Mosby.
34. Reinke LF et al: Transtracheal oxygen therapy and alternative delivery approach, *Pers Respir Nurs* 3(3):3, 1992.
35. Ruppel G: *Manual of pulmonary function testing,* ed 6, St Louis, 1994, Mosby.
36. Scalan CL: *Egan's fundamentals of respiratory therapy,* ed 6, St Louis, 1995, Mosby.
37. Schmitz TM: The semi-prone position in ARDS: five case studies, *Crit Care Nurs* 11(5): 1991.
38. Seidel HM et al: *Mosby's guide to physical examination,* ed 3, St Louis, 1995, Mosby.
39. Sornesso G: Are you ready to use pulse oximetry? *Nurs '91* 21(8):60, 1991.
40. Springhouse Staff: *Nursing procedures,* Springhouse, Penn, 1992, Springhouse.
41. Stiesmeyer JK: Pulmonary assessment: a four step approach, *Am J Nurs* 93(8):22, 1993.
42. Swearingen PL: *Manual of medical-surgical nursing,* ed 3, St Louis, 1994, Mosby.
43. Thompson JM et al: *Mosby's clinical nursing,* ed 3, St Louis, 1993, Mosby.
44. Timby BK, Lewis LA: *Fundamental skills and concepts in patient care,* ed 5, 1992, Philadelphia, Lippincott.
45. Weilitz P: *Pocket guide to respiratory care,* St Louis, 1991, Mosby.
46. Whitney E: Chronic bronchitis and emphysema, *Nursing* 22(3):34, 1992.
47. Wilson EB, Malley N: Discharge planning for the patient with a new tracheostomy, *Crit Care Nurs* 10(7):73, 1990.
48. Wilson SF, Thompson JM: *Respiratory disorders,* St Louis, 1990, Mosby.
49. Winslow EH: Working smart: save the saline, *Am J Nurs* 93(10):16, 1993.
50. Yeau EMJ: How position affects oxygenation: good lung down? *Am J Nurs* 92(3):27, 1992.

CHAPTER CHALLENGE

KEY POINTS

- When air is inhaled, it is warmed, moistened, and filtered to prepare it for use by the body.
- The most important structure of the respiratory system is the alveolus; it is here that actual air exchange occurs.
- For breathing to occur, pressure changes must occur within the thoracic cavity.
- The combination of one inspiration plus one expiration equals one respiration, or one respiratory movement.
- The primary function of the respiratory system is to exchange oxygen and carbon dioxide at the alveolar-capillary level.
- The ability of the lungs to expand and contract depends on musculoskeletal and neurological functions, as well as physiological conditions affecting the respiratory system.
- When obtaining a nursing history, the nurse will assess onset and duration of present signs and symptoms, previous respiratory conditions, current medications, family history, and exposure to irritants.
- Activity tolerance is frequently altered as a result of decreased oxygenation/ventilation.
- Anxiety can exacerbate pulmonary disorders, increasing the body's need for oxygen.
- Breathing exercises can improve ventilation.

- Effective breathing techniques include elevating the head and chest to maintain airway patency; deep breathing and coughing exercises to facilitate lung expansion; and pursed-lip breathing to decrease the effort of breathing.
- Adequate fluid intake and humidity help moisten secretions, thus aiding in their clearance.
- A thorough psychosocial assessment and resultant interventions are necessary for the patient with a laryngectomy, because of loss of voice and neck and facial disfigurement.
- Chest drainage serves a twofold purpose: it (1) drains air, blood, or fluid from the pleural space and (2) restores negative pressure. It requires a water seal to prevent air from reentering the pleural space.
- Techniques used in chest physiotherapy include percussion, vibration, and postural drainage.
- Nursing interventions after thoracic surgery that assist in preventing complications by promoting effective airway clearance are (1) frequent repositioning, (2) coughing, and (3) deep breathing.
- Studies have revealed that hypoxia worsens when patients are placed on their backs or sides with the affected (sick) lung down.
- *Low-flow* oxygen therapy is required for patients with COPD, because higher oxygen concentrations depress the body's own respiratory regulatory centers.
- Hospitals are a high-risk setting for TB transmission, and health care workers are at high occupational risk for TB infection.
- Patients with respiratory disorders must reduce exposure to infection, because infection will further increase the body's oxygen demands.
- Chronic obstructive pulmonary disease includes emphysema, chronic bronchitis, asthma, and bronchiectasis.
- Transmission of tuberculosis is primarily by inhalation of minute droplet nuclei (each containing a single tubercle bacillus) coughed or sneezed by a person whose sputum contains tubercle bacilli.
- Pulse oximetry is a noninvasive method providing continuing monitoring of Sa_{O_2} (saturation of oxygen).
- The definitive diagnostic test to confirm cystic fibrosis is a sweat chloride test.

STUDY QUESTIONS

1. Rapid and deeper respirations are stimulated by the respiratory center of the brain when:
   1. Oxygen saturation levels are >90%
   2. Carbon dioxide levels increase
   3. The alveoli contract
   4. The diaphragm contracts and lowers its dome
2. Once oxygen enters the capillaries, it attaches itself to:
   1. Leukocytes
   2. Thrombocytes
   3. Reticulocytes
   4. Hemoglobin
3. The tendency of molecules of a substance (gaseous, liquid, or solid) to move from a region of high concentration to one of lower concentration is the passive process in which the exchange of gases between the blood capillary and alveolar area occurs. This process is called:
   1. Osmosis
   2. Filtration
   3. Diffusion
   4. Transport
4. Paralysis of the diaphragm would cause respiratory difficulty because it would make it impossible:
   1. For the intercostal muscles to contract
   2. To increase the up and down size of the chest cavity
   3. For the alveolar muscles to relax
   4. For subclavicular retraction to occur
5. Each alveolus is coated with a thin lipoprotein covering that prevents it from collapsing after each breath; this covering is:
   1. LDH
   2. Isoenzyme
   3. Surfactant
   4. Sebum
6. The walls of the thoracic cavity are lined with a serous membrane composed of tough endothelial cells called:
   1. Visceral pleura
   2. Apnestic serosa
   3. Pneumotaxic serosa
   4. Parietal pleura
7. Hollow areas, which make the skull lighter, give resonance to the voice, and communicate with the nasal structures, are the:
   1. Parietal, temporal, sphenoid, and ethmoid sinuses
   2. Occipital, frontal, ethmoid, and paranasal sinuses
   3. Frontal, maxillary, sphenoid, and ethmoid sinuses
   4. Olfactory, maxillary, ethmoid, and sphenoid sinuses
8. An obstruction in which of the following anatomical areas would prevent any oxygen from reaching lung tissue:
   1. The left bronchus
   2. The trachea
   3. The right bronchioles
   4. The alveolar sac

9. The exchange of oxygen and carbon dioxide in external respiration takes place in the:
   1. Lungs
   2. Bronchioles
   3. Capillaries and the body cells
   4. Alveoli and pulmonary capillaries
10. Foods and fluids are kept out of the trachea by a thin, leaf-shaped structure that covers the entrance of the larynx when the individual swallows. This is called the:
   1. Uvula
   2. Epifascial
   3. Epilate
   4. Epiglottis
11. Mr. Kilo, age 73, is diagnosed with chronic bronchitis. He is very dyspneic and must sit up to breathe. An abnormal condition in which there is discomfort in breathing in any but an erect sitting position is:
   1. Orthopnea
   2. Dyspnea
   3. Orthropsia
   4. Cheyne-Stokes
12. Ms. Cordilla, age 45, is being evaluated to rule out pulmonary tuberculosis. Which finding is most closely associated with TB?
   1. Leg cramps
   2. Night sweats
   3. Skin discoloration
   4. Green-colored sputum
13. The health care workers caring for Ms. Cordilla, who is diagnosed with active tuberculosis, are instructed in methods of protecting themselves from contracting tuberculosis. The Centers for Disease Control and Prevention currently recommends that health care workers who care for TB-infected patients:
   1. Ask the patient to wear a mask while in isolation
   2. Wear a surgical mask
   3. Wear a small-micron, fitted filtration mask
   4. Receive the BCG vaccine
14. Sally Jones is an 8-year-old who has just undergone a tonsillectomy. The most significant observation is:
   1. Temperature of 99.4° F
   2. Hoarseness of the voice
   3. Complaints of throat pain
   4. Frequent swallowing
15. The physician ordered a blood culture and sputum specimen to be obtained for Mr. Cordova, a patient who has pneumonia. These diagnostic tests should be collected:
   1. After initiation of antibiotic therapy
   2. The morning following admission
   3. Before initiation of antibiotic therapy
   4. At the first elevated temperature
16. Ms. Vira, age 62, has just returned to her room following a bronchoscopy. No food or fluids should be given after the examination until:
   1. Total absence of blood-streaked sputum
   2. The head nurse gives the order
   3. Her gag reflex returns
   4. She is up and about and steady on her feet
17. Mr. Martinez was in a motor vehicle accident and has a lacerated pleura secondary to fractured ribs. To promote reexpansion of his lung, what type of thoracic drainage system was used:
   1. Open system to promote negative pressure
   2. Closed system to maintain the lungs' normal negative pressure
   3. Closed system to maintain the lungs' positive pressure
   4. Closed system to allow air to enter the pleural cavity for reexpansion
18. Mr. Romar, 45 years old, is a second-day postoperative patient recovering from thoracic surgery. A very therapeutic nursing intervention would include:
   1. Splinting the anterior and posterior chest
   2. Splinting the anterior chest
   3. Placing the patient in a supine position
   4. Allowing the patient to sleep uninterrupted for 8 hours
19. Mr. Alney, age 71, is admitted with an exacerbation of COPD. He has dependent edema and ascites as well as dyspnea. A complication that may occur in COPD, in which some of the capillaries surrounding the alveoli are destroyed resulting in pulmonary hypertension, blood returning to the right side of the heart, and signs/symptoms of right-sided CHF is:
   1. Pulmonary edema
   2. Cor pulmonale
   3. Tetralogy of Fallot
   4. Acyanotic heart disease
20. Mr. Fletcher, age 52, had a laryngectomy due to cancer of the larynx. Dismissal instructions are given to Mr. Fletcher and his family. Which response, by written communication from Mr. Fletcher or verbal response by the family, will be a signal to the nurse that the instructions need to be reclarified:
   1. Report swelling, pain, or excessive drainage
   2. The suctioning at home must be a clean procedure not sterile
   3. Cleanse skin around stoma bid, use hydrogen peroxide and rinse with water, pat dry
   4. It is acceptable to take over-the-counter medications now that condition is stable

32

CARE OF THE PATIENT WITH AN ENDOCRINE DISORDER

Sylvia Long Baldwin

KEY TERMS

ANATOMY AND PHYSIOLOGY

adrenal gland
adrenalin
adrenocorticotropic hormone (ACTH)
androgen
antagonist
antidiuretic hormone (ADH)
calcitonin
endocrine gland
estrogen
exocrine gland
follicle-stimulating hormone (FSH)
glucagon
graafian follicle
hormone
hypercalcemia
insulin
luteinizing hormone (LH)
negative feedback
nodule
oxytocin
parathyroid gland
parathyroid hormone
pituitary gland
progesterone
prolactin
somatotropin
testosterone
tetany
thymus gland
thyroid gland
thyroid-stimulating hormone (TSH)

MEDICAL-SURGICAL

Chvostek's sign
dysphagia
endocrinologist
glycosuria
hirsutism
hyperglycemia
hypocalcemia
hypoglycemia
hypokalemia
idiopathic hyperplasia
ketoacidosis
ketone body
lipodystrophy
neuropathy
polydipsia
polyphagia
polyuria
Trousseau's sign
turgor
type I diabetes mellitus
type II diabetes mellitus

LEARNING OBJECTIVES

After reading this chapter, the student should be able to do the following:

Anatomy and Physiology

- Define the key terms.
- List and describe the endocrine glands and their hormones.
- Explain the action of the hormones on their target organs.
- Define the negative feedback system.
- Describe how the hypothalamus controls the anterior and posterior pituitary glands.

Medical-Surgical

- Define the key terms.
- List four clinical manifestations of diabetes insipidus.
- List three tests used in the diagnosis of hyperthyroidism.
- Give the clinical manifestations for patients with acromegaly, giantism, pheochromocytoma, hyperparathyroidism, and hypoparathyroidism.
- Explain how to test for Chvostek's sign and Trousseau's sign.
- List two significant complications that may occur after thyroidectomy.
- Differentiate between the clinical manifestations of Cushing's syndrome and those of Addison's disease.
- Explain the interrelationship of diet, exercise, and medication in the control of diabetes mellitus.
- Describe the proper way to draw up and administer insulin.
- Differentiate among the signs and symptoms of diabetic ketoacidosis (DKA), hyperglycemic hyperosmolar nonketotic coma (HHNC), and hypoglycemic reaction.
- List four nursing interventions that foster self-care in the activities of daily living of the patient with diabetes mellitus.

RELATED TOPICS OF INTEREST

- Cultural aspects of nursing care (Chapter 8)
- Specimen collection and diagnostic examination (Chapter 17)
- Diet therapy (Chapter 19)
- Principles and practice of medication administration (Chapter 21)
- The surgical patient (Chapter 22)
- Care of the patient with a reproductive disorder (Chapter 33)

- Care of the patient with a neurological disorder (Chapter 35)
- Normal pregnancy (Chapter 39)

There are two broad categories of glands: exocrine and endocrine. **Exocrine glands** secrete through a series of ducts; examples of exocrine glands are the sebaceous and sudoriferous glands of the skin. Their secretions usually serve protective or functional purposes. **Endocrine glands** are ductless; that is, they release their secretions directly into the bloodstream. These secretions have a regulatory function.

The endocrine system is composed of a series of ductless glands whose work is closely related to the nervous system. Both systems control homeostasis through communications within the systems. The nervous system exerts its control very rapidly through miles of nerve fibers. The endocrine system communicates more slowly through the use of **hormones,** which are chemical messengers that travel through the bloodstream to their target organ. When the hormone reaches its target, a metabolic change occurs.

The total weight of all the endocrine glands is less than half a pound, yet they exert a very powerful influence. The slightest change in hormonal levels can upset the metabolic balance of the entire body. Hormones can increase or decrease a normal body process by exerting an effect on its target organ. Too much or too little of a given hormone can interfere with the action of the other hormones, and for this reason they are somewhat interrelated. The endocrine glands (Fig. 32-1) have a generalized effect on the patient's metabolism, growth and development, reproduction, and many other body activities.

The amount of hormonal release is controlled by a **negative feedback** (in physiology, a decrease in function in response to stimuli) system. Information is constantly being exchanged between the target organ and the pituitary gland via the bloodstream regarding the impact of the hormone on the target organ. For example, after food is ingested, the blood sugar (glucose) level increases. In response, the pancreas releases insulin into the blood to metabolize the glucose. As the blood glucose level drops, further release of insulin is inhibited. Because these responses are opposite to the stimulus, this mechanism is called negative feedback.

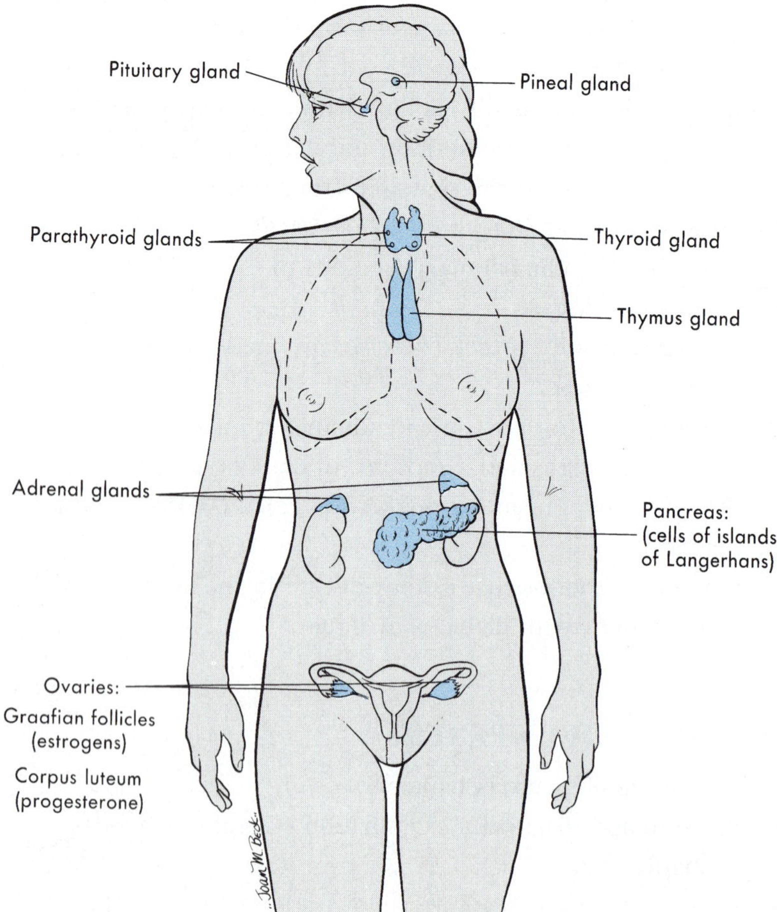

FIG. 32-1 Location of the endocrine glands in the female. Thymus gland is shown at maximal size at puberty.

Hormones are composed of protein or steroids. Protein hormones attach themselves to the cell walls of the target organ and cause a change within the cell as a result of their outside influence. Steroid hormones pass through the cell wall and combine with receptors within the cytoplasm, causing the nucleus to respond with change. Therefore protein hormones indirectly cause change within the target organ cells, whereas steroid hormones impart a direct change within the cell by actually entering the cell itself.

PROSTAGLANDINS

Prostaglandins, discovered in the early 1930s, are a group of hormone substances with one distinct difference: they are produced throughout the body by various tissues and localize their effect on that particular tissue. Most other hormones are produced by a specific organ and travel through the bloodstream to their target tissue. Prostaglandins also exert their effect on hormones that have traveled to the target tissue; they can increase or decrease the effect of these hormones.

ENDOCRINE GLANDS AND HORMONES

Pituitary Gland

The **pituitary gland** (hypophysis), the size of a small pea, is one of the most powerful glands in the body. It has been called the "master gland," because through the negative feedback system it exerts its control over the other endocrine glands. It is important to remember, however, that it works closely with the hypothalamus of the brain.

The pituitary is located in the cranial cavity in a small saddlelike depression in the sphenoid bone (the sella turcica). It is divided into two segments, each with specialized hormones. The first segment is called the *anterior pituitary* (adenohypophysis); the second is called the *posterior pituitary* (neurohypophysis). The gland is connected to the hypothalamus by a stalklike projection called the *infundibulum.* The hypothalamus actually produces the hormones of the posterior pituitary and releases them for storage in the posterior pituitary gland; they are in turn released from the posterior pituitary as a result of nerve impulses received from the hypothalamus.

Anterior Pituitary Gland

Six major hormones are secreted by the anterior pituitary gland. It constitutes about 75% of the total weight of the pituitary gland. Five of the hormones are called *tropic* hormones because they are responsible for the stimulation of other endocrine glands. Prolactin, the remaining hormone, causes the mammary glands to produce milk. These hormones and their functions are shown in Fig. 32-2 and Fig. 32-3 on p. 942 and are discussed below.

1. **Somatotropin**—*human growth hormone (HGH).* HGH speeds up the cells' anabolism of amino acids, which results in the formation of tissue proteins. This process stimulates the systemic growth of the body. A deficiency of this hormone results in a small but proportioned individual. This hormone can be administered in controlled situations to enable the individual to reach a more normal physical stature.
2. **Prolactin**—*lactogenic hormone.* Prolactin functions in the pregnant woman to develop the mammary glands for milk production. After de-

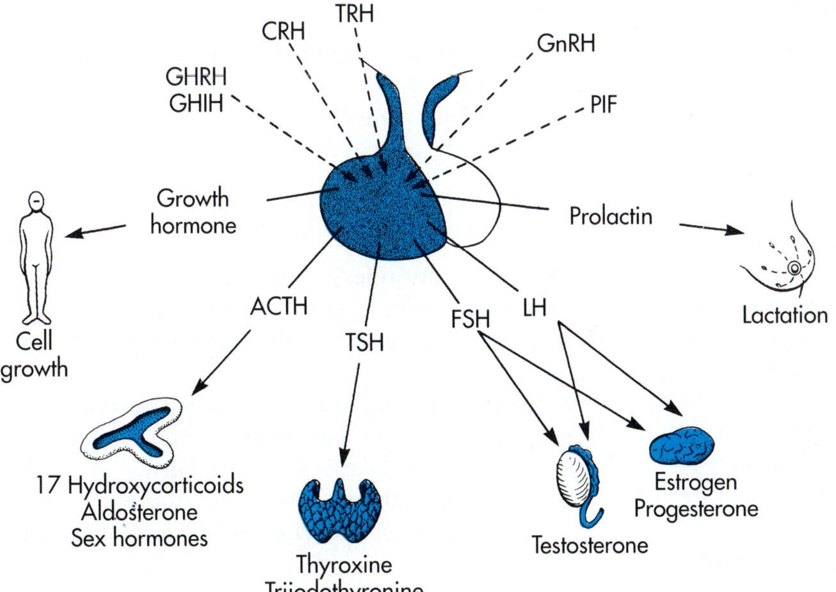

FIG. 32-2 Relationships among hormones of the hypothalamus, anterior pituitary glands, and target tissues are depicted. Only five released or inhibitory hormones have been chemically identified: growth hormone–releasing hormone (*GHRH*); growth hormone–inhibitory hormone (somatostatin)(*GHIH*); thyrotropin-releasing hormone (*TRH*); corticotropin-releasing hormone (*CRH*); and gonadotropin-releasing hormone (*GnRH*). Dopamine is thought to be a prolactin-inhibiting factor (*PIF*). Each anterior pituitary hormone is shown with its respective target tissues: body cells (*GH*); adrenal cortex (*ACTH*); thyroid (*TSH*); testes and ovaries (*FSH* and *LH*); and breasts (*prolactin*).

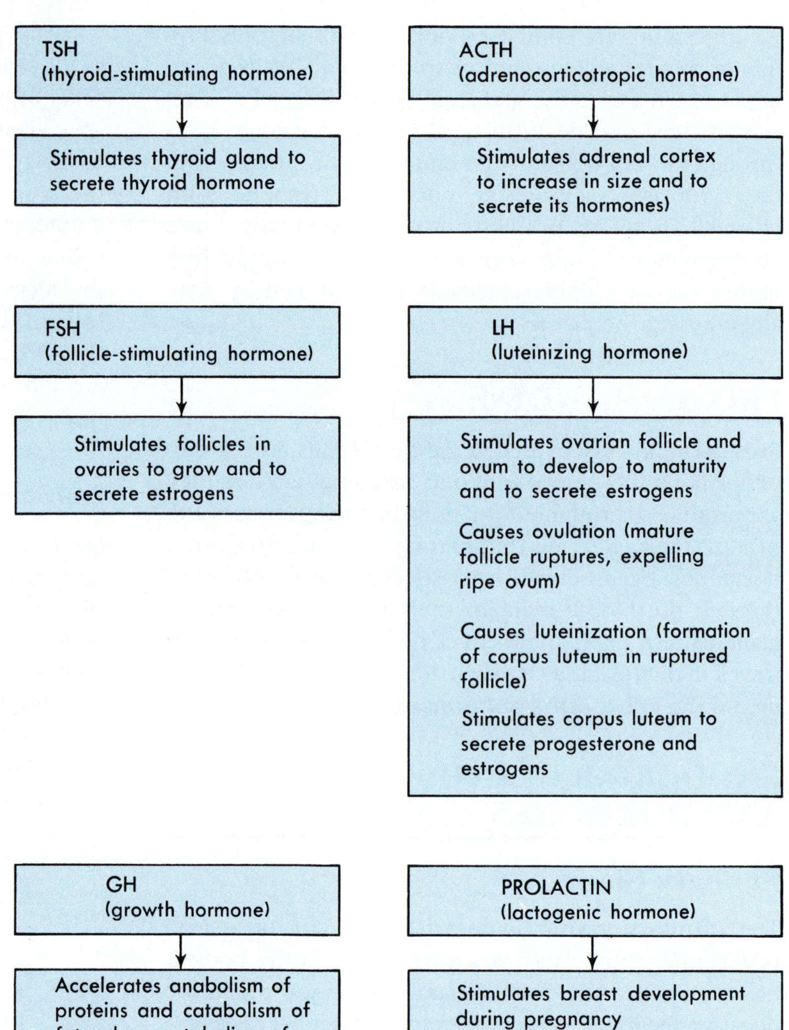

FIG. 32-3 Names and functions of anterior pituitary hormones.

livery, the suckling of the infant stimulates the continuation of the production of milk. The actual release of milk is controlled by oxytocin, a hormone in the posterior lobe.

3. **Adrenocorticotropic hormone (ACTH).** ACTH stimulates the endocrine activity of the cortex portion of the adrenal glands. It operates on the negative feedback system.
4. **Thyroid-stimulating hormone (TSH).** TSH acts on the thyroid gland to increase thyroid hormone secretion; it also operates on the negative feedback system.
5. **Follicle-stimulating hormone (FSH).** FSH stimulates the growth of the graafian follicle that leads to ovulation in the female. In the male, FSH leads to the development of the sperm cells.
6. **Luteinizing hormone (LH).** LH initiates ovulation and release of the egg, followed by the formation of the corpus luteum (yellow body), which in turn produces the hormones estrogen and progesterone. In the male LH is called *interstitial cell-stimulating hormone (ICSH);* it causes the interstitial cells of the testes to produce sperm.

Posterior Pituitary Gland

Two hormones are released by the posterior pituitary; however, these were originally produced in the hypothalamus. They are stored in the posterior pituitary until needed by the body.

1. **Oxytocin.** Oxytocin promotes the release of breast milk and stimulates uterine contractions during labor. It can be used clinically to induce labor; it may also be used to increase uterine tone and prevent hemorrhage immediately after delivery.
2. **Antidiuretic hormone (ADH).** ADH causes the kidneys to conserve body water by decreasing

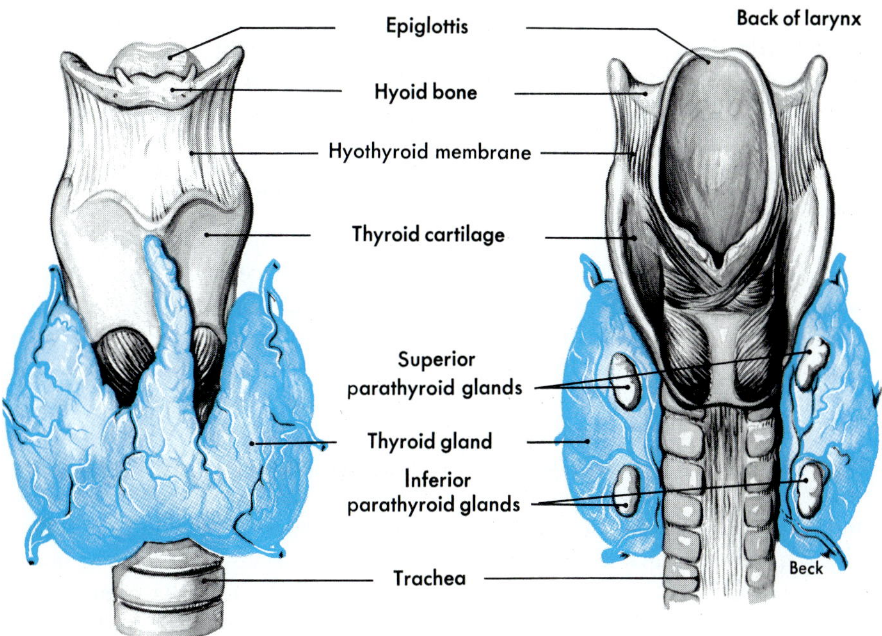

FIG. 32-4 Thyroid and parathyroid glands. Note their relations to each other and to the larynx and trachea.

the amount of urine produced. It also causes constriction of the arterioles in the body, which results in increased blood pressure. (This hormone is sometimes referred to as *vasopressin* because of its effect on blood pressure.) Alcohol consumption inhibits the secretion of ADH, which results in increased urinary output. This is possibly the reason for thirst when one has drunk too much alcohol.

Thyroid Gland

The **thyroid gland** is butterfly shaped, with one lobe lying on either side of the trachea (Fig. 32-4). It lies just below the larynx. The lobes are connected in the center by a mass of tissue called the *isthmus.* The gland is very vascular and receives approximately 80 to 120 ml of blood per minute.

The thyroid gland secretes thyroxine (T_4) and triiodothyronine (T_3). Thyroxine molecules contain four atoms of iodine, whereas triiodothyronine molecules contain three. T_4 is the most abundant of these hormones, and T_3 converts to T_4 when it reaches the liver and the lungs; therefore these hormones will be discussed together. Adequate oral intake of iodine is necessary for the formation of thyroid hormones. When thyroid hormones combine with plasma proteins, they are referred to as *protein-bound iodine (PBI).*

These hormones have three main regulatory functions: (1) growth and development, (2) metabolism, and (3) activity of the nervous system. Their function is controlled by the release of TSH from the pituitary gland.

Calcitonin is a hormone also released by the thyroid gland. This hormone works as an **antagonist** (any agent that exerts an opposite action to that of another) of the parathyroid hormone. It decreases blood calcium levels by causing calcium to be stored in the bones. It prevents **hypercalcemia,** a condition in which there is too much calcium in the blood. Administration of calcitonin has been used in conjunction with calcium intake to treat postmenopausal osteoporosis.

Laboratory tests are performed to monitor the function of the thyroid gland. Blood tests called T_3 and T_4 thyroid function tests are performed by mechanically tracing radioactive T_4 in the body and observing the speed at which it enters the thyroid gland. Another frequently used test, the protein-bound iodine test, estimates the amount of circulating iodine in the blood.

Parathyroid Glands

The **parathyroid glands** are located on the posterior surface of the thyroid gland (Fig. 32-4). Usually there are four of them, but sometimes there are as many as 10. These glands secrete parathyroid hormone (parathormone).

As an antagonist to calcitonin from the thyroid, **parathyroid hormone** tends to increase the concentration of calcium in the blood. It also regulates the amount of phosphorus in the blood. Under its influence, two changes occur in the kidneys: it increases the removal of calcium and magnesium from the urine that is being produced and accelerates the elimination of phosphorus in the urine.

The delicate balance of blood calcium is extremely important for normal body function. When blood calcium levels are low, the nerve cells become excited and stimulate the muscles with too many impulses, resulting in spasms **(tetany).** When the blood calcium levels are abnormally high, heart function becomes impaired and can result in cardiac arrest.

Adrenal Glands

The **adrenal glands** (suprarenal glands) are small, yellow masses that lie directly atop the kidneys. The adrenal glands have two separate parts, much the same as the pituitary gland. Each part functions independently of the other. Both glands contain an outer section, the *adrenal cortex,* and a small inner section, called the *adrenal medulla.* Each gland is covered by a thin, fibrous capsule; directly beneath the capsule is a thick layer of fatty connective tissue.

Adrenal Cortex

The adrenal cortex (outer layer) is divided into three separate layers or zones. Each zone is composed of a certain type of cells and secretes a particular hormone. All three of the hormones secreted by the adrenal cortex are steroids. They are (1) mineralocorticoids, (2) glucocorticoids, and (3) sex hormones (androgens). Fifteen percent of the cortical volume lies directly beneath the connective tissue and is called the *zona glomerulosa.* It secretes a group of hormones called *mineralocorticoids.* As their name suggests, they are primarily involved in water and electrolyte balance and indirectly in the management of blood pressure. Aldosterone, the principal mineralocorticoid, regulates sodium and potassium levels by exerting its effects on the kidney tubules. It decreases the level of potassium and increases the level of sodium in the bloodstream. The retention of sodium causes retention of water, which leads to an increase in blood volume and blood pressure.

The second group of hormones (glucocorticoids) are secreted by the middle layer, the *zona fasciculata.* The most important hormone of this group is cortisol, responsible for about 95% of glucocorticoid activity. It is involved in glucose metabolism and provides extra reserves of energy in times of stress. The secretion of glucocorticoids is regulated by the hormone ACTH, which is released by the pituitary. In times of stress large amounts of cortisol are released, initiating the process of *gluconeogenesis* in which amino acids are converted to glucose. This takes place in the liver, and the newly formed glucose is released in the bloodstream. The glucocorticoids exhibit antiinflammatory properties and many times are administered for such conditions as rheumatoid arthritis.

The inner zone, called the *zona reticularis,* releases the sex hormones. Small amounts of **androgens** (male sex hormones) and **estrogens** (female sex hormones) are secreted by this layer. In the adult the release of these hormones from the adrenals is a relatively small amount, and their impact on the system is insignificant.

Adrenal Medulla

The cells composing the adrenal medulla arise from the same type of cells as those of the sympathetic nervous system. Two hormones are released by the medulla during times of stress. Epinephrine **(adrenalin)** and norepinephrine can cause the heart rate and blood pressure to increase, the blood vessels to constrict, and the liver to release glucose reserves for immediate energy. This is a systemic preparation of the body for "the flight or fight" response that is needed in times of crisis. This whole process happens very quickly, because the messages are sent via the sympathetic nerve fibers. Once the message is received, the medulla pours epinephrine and norepinephrine into the bloodstream.

Pancreas

The pancreas is an elongated gland that lies posterior to the stomach. It is a very active organ in that it is composed of both endocrine and exocrine tissue. The exocrine activity involves production of digestive enzymes, which are transported through ducts to the small intestine. The islets of Langerhans, responsible for the endocrine activity of the pancreas, are tiny clusters of cells capable of producing hormones. These clusters number over a million and are microscopic. They secrete two major hormones: insulin and glucagon. The majority of the islet cells are *beta cells,* and they secrete **insulin** (a naturally occurring hormone secreted in response to increased levels of glucose in the blood). The remaining islet cells are called *alpha cells,* and they secrete the hormone glucagon. Both hormones have an impact on the amount of glucose circulating in the blood but are antagonists (have the opposite effect).

Many hormones, such as glucagon, epinephrine, and the glucocorticoids, cause an increase in the blood glucose levels. Insulin is the only hormone that causes a decrease in blood glucose levels. When the proper amount of insulin is released, blood glucose levels remain between 65 and 120 mg/dl. If the pancreas is unable to produce an adequate amount of insulin, the blood glucose level rises dramatically and may even spill into the urine. The circulating glucose cannot be metabolized, and the body begins to rely on fats and proteins for energy. At this point the body becomes dysfunctional, with serious complications.

On the other hand, when glucose levels are too low, the alpha cells of the islets release the hormone **glucagon.** Its target organ is the liver. The liver has stored glycogen as a reserve form of glucose. Glucagon stimulates the liver to break down the stored glycogen to glucose, which is released into the bloodstream. It also promotes an increase in the fatty acid levels in the blood by releasing fat stores from adipose tissue. This provides nutrients for glucose production.

These two hormones, glucagon and insulin, though antagonists, work together to keep glucose levels within normal ranges. When glucose ranges fall below normal, glucagon acts to raise it; when glucose ranges are too high, insulin is released to lower it.

Female Sex Glands

Deep in the lower abdominal region, lying to the upper right and left of the uterus, lie the almond-shaped ovaries, the two major sex glands of the female. The ovaries begin their production of hormones at puberty. At this time, the gonadotropin hormones stimulate the ovaries to release estrogen and progesterone in a rhythmic pattern—the menstrual cycle. The **graafian follicle** (mature ovarian vesicle that ruptures during ovulation to release the ovum) secretes the hormone estrogen. Estrogen is responsible for the development of the secondary sex characteristics: the appearance of axillary and pubic hair and the maturation of the reproductive organs. It also prepares the uterus monthly for the possibility of pregnancy. When the egg that has matured in the graafian follicle has been released at the midpoint of the menstrual cycle, a structure called the *corpus luteum* (yellow body) forms and releases progesterone. **Progesterone** is a female hormone that maintains the preparation of the reproductive organs that was initiated by estrogen. Progesterone prepares the uterus to accept a fetus and maintain the pregnancy. If pregnancy occurs, progesterone levels remain high. If no pregnancy occurs, progesterone and estrogen levels fall, initiating the menstrual flow.

The placenta is a temporary endocrine gland that forms and functions during pregnancy. During this time the ovaries become inactive, and the placenta releases the estrogen and progesterone needed to maintain the pregnancy.

A more in-depth discussion of these hormones can be found in Chapters 33 and 39.

Male Sex Glands

Suspended outside the body in a saclike structure, the scrotum, lie the two oval sex glands called the *testes.* The interstitial cells of the testes produce the hormone **testosterone.** It is responsible for the development of the secondary sex characteristics, including the appearance of axillary and pubic hair and the maturation of the reproductive organs. In addition, testosterone is responsible for the deepening of the voice, the appearance of a beard, and the development of muscle and bone mass. Unlike the female, whose eggs are present at birth, the male must continually produce sperm to remain fertile. Testosterone is necessary for sperm formation. If the levels of this hormone fall below normal ranges, sterility results.

Thymus Gland

The **thymus gland** lies in the upper thorax, posterior to the sternum (see Fig. 32-1). It produces the hormone thymosin, which plays an active role in the immune system. T lymphocytes (a type of white blood cell) are stimulated to carry out immune reactions to certain types of antigens. The thymus gland programs this information into the T lymphocytes in utero and during the first few months of life.

Pineal Gland

The pineal gland is a small, cone-shaped gland located in the roof of the third ventricle of the brain (see Fig. 32-1). It secretes the hormone melatonin, which seems to inhibit reproductive activities by inhibiting the gonadotropic hormones. This is particularly important in preventing sexual maturation until the child's body has reached adult size. After adulthood has been reached, the pineal gland possibly has an impact on the rhythm of the menstrual cycle. It may also stimulate the adrenal cortex to secrete aldosterone.

DISORDERS OF THE PITUITARY GLAND (HYPOPHYSIS)

Acromegaly

Etiology/Pathophysiology. An overproduction of somatotropin (growth hormone, GH) in the adult causes acromegaly, a condition that affects an estimated 250 persons in the United States each year. The cause either may be **idiopathic hyperplasia** (increase in number of cells without a known cause) of the anterior lobe of the pituitary gland or may be attributed to tumor growth. Unfortunately, growth changes that occur in acromegaly are irreversible, even with adequate medical or surgical intervention.

Clinical Manifestations. The subsequent overabundance of growth hormone produces many changes throughout the patient's body, including enlargement of the cranium and lower jaw, with separation and malocclusion of the teeth, bulging forehead, a bulbous nose, thick lips, enlarged tongue, and generalized coarsening of the facial features. The hands and feet become enlarged (Fig. 32-5 on p. 946), as do the heart, liver, and spleen; muscle weakness usually develops. Joints may hypertrophy and become painful and stiff. Male patients may become impotent, and female patients may develop a deepened voice, increased facial hair growth, and amenorrhea. If a tumor is present, pressure on the optic

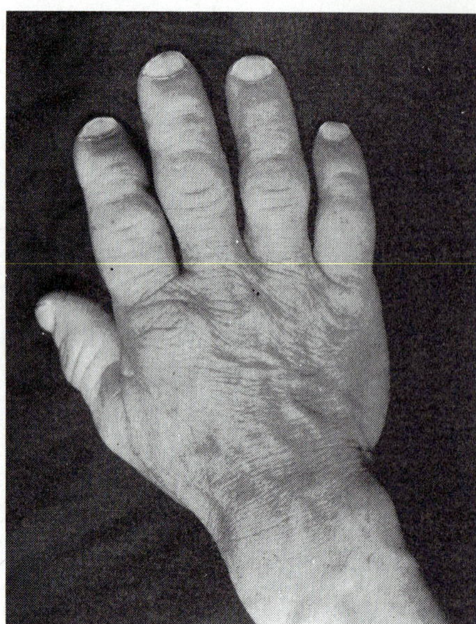

FIG. 32-5 Hand showing characteristic of an acromegalic condition.

nerve may cause partial or complete blindness. Severe headaches commonly occur.

Assessment. Collection of *subjective data* includes determining the presence of headache and/or visual disturbances and any precipitating factors. Muscle weakness and its effect on the patient's ability to perform activities should be evaluated. Patients should be encouraged to verbalize emotional responses to sexual problems (such as impotence in males and masculinization in females).

Collection of *objective data* includes ongoing assessment of bone enlargement and joint involvement, evidenced by gait changes and increasing inability to perform other activities. The interval between doses of pain medication should be evaluated. Changes in vital signs that may herald the onset of early congestive heart failure include dyspnea, tachycardia, weak pulse, and hypotension.

Diagnostic Tests. Diagnosis of acromegaly is based on the patient's history and the clinical manifestations, as well as computed tomography (CT) scan and cranial x-ray evaluation. Laboratory tests confirm the presence of elevated serum GH levels. The patient's oral intake is restricted ror 8 hours before this test.

Medical Management. In the past, estrogens were administered to these patients. Newer medical treatments include bromocriptine mesylate (Parlodel) and somatostatin analogs, especially in patients who are not candidates for surgery or radiation therapy. These drugs are used in an attempt to suppress growth hormone secretion. Surgical treatment may include either cryosurgery (the use of subfreezing temperatures to destroy tissue) or transsphenoidal removal of tumor tissue. New irradiation procedures using proton beam therapy have been used to destroy GH-secreting tumors. Proton beam treatment uses very low doses of radiation, and therefore is much less destructive to adjacent tissues, such as the hypothalamus and temporal lobes, than conventional radiation therapy.

Nursing Interventions. Nursing interventions are mainly supportive. If there is muscle weakness, joint pain, or stiffness, patients should be assessed for ability to perform activities of daily living. The presence of headache may impair the patient's ability to socialize and may also impede education. Worsening headache may indicate tumor progression. The diet should be soft and easy to chew, since jaw muscles and the temporomandibular joint may be involved. The patient should be encouraged to chew thoroughly, and the nurse should allow adequate time during meals, assisting when necessary. Fluids should be encouraged often. Nonnarcotic analgesics may be given for pain relief. Visual impairment may increase the risk of injury for these patients, so care should be taken to prevent stumbling into furniture or dropping objects.

As the body undergoes change, the patient may develop problems with self-esteem and may feel physically unattractive. There may be difficulties in communicating with significant others, and this may lead to disturbances in individual or family coping methods. Other complications of acromegaly are related to the enlargement of the liver, spleen, and heart. Cardiac dysrhythmias may develop, and the patient may experience heart failure. Abdominal girth may increase as a result of weight gain and inactivity, and respiratory difficulty may occur.

Nursing diagnoses and interventions for the patient with acromegaly include but are not limited to the following:

NURSING DIAGNOSES	NURSING INTERVENTIONS
Self-esteem, chronic low, related to irreversible body changes	Convey respect and nonjudgmental acceptance of the patient as a person. Help the patient set achievable short-term goals.
Activity intolerance, related to physical weakness	Assess patient's current activity level and priorities for activity performance. Discuss with patient alternate ways of performing activities.
Trauma, high risk for, related to muscle weakness	Assist patient to identify hazards in the environment. Help patient develop a plan to increase ambulation, asking for assistance as needed.

Patient teaching. The patient should remain under the supervision of a physician so that any complications can be diagnosed promptly and treated adequately. The patient should be taught exercises that can be performed at home, such as active range of motion of joints of the extremities and of the neck, to help prevent muscle atrophy and loss of movement.

Prognosis. Even with adequate medical or surgical treatment, the physical changes are irreversible, and the patient is prone to develop complications.

Gigantism

Etiology/Pathophysiology. Gigantism usually results from an oversecretion of GH as a result of hyperplasia of the anterior pituitary, and this hyperplastic tissue may develop into a tumor. Another possible cause is a defect in the hypothalamus, which directs the anterior pituitary to release excess amounts of GH.

Clinical Manifestations. When overproduction of GH occurs in a child before closure of the epiphyses, there is an overgrowth of the long bones, which results in the attainment of great height, accompanied by increased muscle and visceral development. There is an increase in weight, but body proportions are usually normal. Despite their size, these patients are usually quite weak. Other kinds of gigantism may be caused by certain genetic disorders or by disturbances in sex hormone production. Once identified, these children should be referred for further medical evaluation and follow-up.

Assessment. Collection of *subjective data* includes assessment of the patient's understanding of the disease process, as well as the ability to verbalize emotional responses.

Collection of *objective data* requires frequent measurement of height. The patient's use of adaptive coping measures should be assessed, as well as family interactions.

Diagnostic Tests. The GH-suppression test (also called the *glucose-loading test)* may be done to evaluate GH levels. In the patient with gigantism, baseline levels of GH will be high.

Medical Management. Medical management of children with gigantism may include surgical removal of tumor tissue or irradiation of the anterior pituitary gland, with a subsequent replacement of pituitary hormones as indicated. The physician will then observe the child for development of related complications, such as hypertension, heart failure, osteoporosis, thickened bones, and delayed sexual development.

Nursing Interventions. Nursing interventions primarily include early identification of children who are experiencing increased growth rates compared with other children in their age group. There are potential problems with self-image, especially if the child is a preteen who is a great deal taller than peers. Girls usually suffer more emotional trauma in this situation than boys do. The nurse must be understanding and compassionate and accentuate the positive aspects of being tall.

Nursing diagnoses and interventions for the patient with gigantism include but are not limited to the following:

NURSING DIAGNOSES	NURSING INTERVENTIONS
Self-esteem, chronic low, related to irreversible body changes	Be genuinely interested in and concerned about the patient. Help patient to identify problems in relating to others.
Coping, ineffective individual, related to personal vulnerability	Assess patient's coping behaviors, stresses, and adaptive skills. Provide positive feedback.
Coping, ineffective family: compromised, related to prolonged disease	Provide adequate and correct information to patient and significant others. Help patient and family to identify strengths and weaknesses in interpersonal relationships.

Patient teaching. Early diagnosis of these patients is essential, because proper medical management can retard the height a child will reach. The importance of regular visits to the pediatrician or pediatric **endocrinologist** (a physician who specializes in endocrinology) ,should be stressed to the parents.

Prognosis. The expected life span of these patients is longer now, with new medical and surgical advances. However, their life expectancy is shorter than that of the average individual.

Dwarfism

Etiology/Pathophysiology. A condition in which there is a deficiency in growth hormone is called *hypopituitary dwarfism.* Most cases are idiopathic, but a small number can be attributed to an autosomal-recessive trait. In some cases there is also a lack of ACTH, TSH, and the gonadotropins.

Clinical Manifestations. The most common clinical manifestation of dwarfism is that the child is a great deal shorter than peers. These patients usually appear well proportioned and well nourished but appear younger than their chronological age. There may be problems with dentition as the permanent teeth erupt, because the jaws are underdeveloped. Sexual development is usually normal but delayed. Many dwarfs are able to reproduce normal offspring, unless there is an accompanying deficiency in gonadotropins. Because only a small number of children who experience short stature or delayed growth suffer from dwarfism, it is crucial that the diagnostic workup be thorough.

Assessment. Collection of *subjective data* includes assessment of the patient's understanding of the disease process, as well as emotional responses to it. A family history of dwarfism may reveal previously successful coping strategies. The patient should be encouraged to verbalize feelings. Normal intelligence is displayed by most of these children. The child's growth pattern should be compared with that of siblings and other relatives at comparable age periods. The child's history usually reveals a normal birth weight. It is important to determine when the child's growth retardation was first noted.

Collection of *objective data* includes regular measurement of height and weight to determine responses to GH and other hormones that may be administered. Current height and weight should be compared with standard growth charts.

Diagnostic Tests. Diagnostic tests include x-ray evaluation of the wrist for bone age and a skull series to rule out a pituitary tumor. Definitive diagnosis is based on finding decreased plasma levels of GH. The patient's oral intake should be restricted after midnight for this test.

Medical Management. Medical treatment involves replacement of GH by injection, as well as the addition of other specific hormones as needed to correct deficiencies. If a tumor is the cause of dwarfism, surgery is usually indicated.

Nursing Interventions. Particular care should be exercised to identify children with growth problems. The physician will correlate the onset of growth retardation with symptoms of headache, visual disturbances, or behavior changes that might indicate tumor, so the nurse should be alert for these. The nurse should be careful not to make the parents feel guilty about any delay in seeking medical attention for their child.

Nursing diagnoses and interventions for the patient with dwarfism include but are not limited to the following:

NURSING DIAGNOSES	NURSING INTERVENTIONS
Body image disturbance, related to negative self-perception	Encourage patient to verbalize feelings about body. Respect patient's need for privacy while performing personal hygiene.
Knowledge deficit: therapeutic regimen, related to age level and learning ability	Explain diagnostic and therapeutic measures, considering patient's level of understanding. Praise patient's efforts to cooperate with plan of treatment.

Patient teaching. The child should be encouraged to wear age-appropriate clothing and engage in activities with peers, because major problems with self-esteem can occur in dwarfism. The child's abilities and strengths should be emphasized, not physical size.

Prognosis. Most of these patients lead fairly normal lives, and many become parents of normal children. Complications experienced are often of the musculoskeletal and cardiovascular systems.

Diabetes Insipidus

Etiology/Pathophysiology. Diabetes insipidus (*diabetes:* "sievelike, siphonlike"; *insipidus:* "tasteless") is a transient or permanent metabolic disorder of the posterior pituitary in which antidiuretic hormone (ADH) is deficient. The condition may be either primary or secondary to others, such as head injury, intracranial tumor, intracranial aneurysm, or infarct. Infections, such as encephalitis or meningitis, have been known to cause diabetes insipidus.

Clinical Manifestations. Diabetes insipidus is characterized by marked polyuria and intense polydipsia. The urine is very dilute, looking much like water, with a low specific gravity (1.001 to 1.005), the normal being 1.005 to 1.030. Urinary output may exceed 10 L in a 24-hour period, whereas the average is 1.5 L. The patient craves cold or iced water and may drink 4 to 40 L of fluid daily, yet may become severely dehydrated and have increased levels of sodium in the blood. Even when unconscious after surgery or head trauma, these patients continue to produce copious quantities of urine.

Assessment. Collection of *subjective data* includes evaluation of the patient's understanding of the relationship of symptoms (such as thirst and polyuria) to the underlying cause. The patient should be able to verbalize the importance of *not* restricting oral fluids. The severity of thirst should be assessed. The patient may be very embarrassed about the constant need to drink and then empty the bladder and may voluntarily restrict social contacts and work activities. The patient is weak, tired, and lethargic.

Collection of *objective data* to be assessed includes skin **turgor** (the normal resiliency of the skin) and color and specific gravity of the urine, and intake and output (I&O) should be carefully monitored. The skin is dry, turgor is poor, and there is loss of body weight. Constipation may occur. The patient should be weighed daily in the early morning, before breakfast. The nurse should determine the presence of nocturia.

Diagnostic Tests. Diagnosis is based on clinical manifestations, as well as urinary specific gravity and urinary ADH measurement. The fluid deprivation (water deprivation) test may be ordered to determine how well the pituitary is producing ADH and to help rule out other causes. A CT scan and x-ray evaluation of the sella turcica (the "Turkish saddle"-shaped depression in the sphenoid bone that houses the pituitary gland) may be done.

Medical Management. Medical treatment involves administration of ADH preparations, intramuscularly, subcutaneously, or by nasal spray. Coffee, tea, and other beverages containing caffeine are usually eliminated from the diet because of their possible diuretic effect.

Nursing Interventions. Because of the potential for fluid volume deficit, the urinary output of pediatric and unconscious patients should be carefully monitored. Skin turgor should be assessed frequently, as should the condition of oral mucous membranes. The patient should be weighed daily. Oral fluids should not be limited in an effort to reduce urinary output.

Nursing diagnoses and interventions for the patient with diabetes insipidus include but are not limited to the following:

NURSING DIAGNOSES	NURSING INTERVENTIONS
Fluid volume deficit, high risk for, related to excessive urine production	Assess for signs and symptoms of dehydration (dry mouth, poor skin turgor, soft eyeballs, lowered BP, rapid pulse). Measure urinary output. Obtain daily weight.
Skin integrity, impaired, high risk for, related to altered state of hydration	Inspect skin for erythema, cyanosis, vesicles, and lesions. Prevent pressure on skin and skeletal prominences by turning and ambulating patient, use of sheepskin, Egg-crate mattress, or other measures. Increase fluid intake up to 2600 ml/day if possible. Encourage patient to eat food adequate in calories, protein, and vitamin C to promote healthy skin.

Patient teaching. The patient should be instructed to wear medical alert jewelry, such as a necklace or bracelet, stating the diagnosis of diabetes insipidus. It is important that the patient remain under medical supervision for monitoring of the metabolic state, because the condition may worsen with time.

Prognosis. The prognosis depends on the etiology. Those patients who survive will usually be dependent on medication for the rest of their lives.

Syndrome of Inappropriate Antidiuretic Hormone (SIADH)

SIADH occurs when the pituitary gland releases too much ADH. In response to ADH, the kidneys reabsorb more water, decreasing urine output and expanding the body's fluid volume. The patient experiences hyponatremia, hemodilution, and fluid overload without peripheral edema.

Etiology/Pathophysiology. ADH regulates the body's water balance. Synthesized in the hypothalamus, ADH is stored in the posterior pituitary gland. When released into the circulation, it acts on the kidney's distal tubules and collecting ducts, increasing their permeability to water. This decreases urine volume because more water is being reabsorbed and returned to the circulation, which increases blood volume.

When the body's system of checks and balances malfunctions—whether from a tumor, medication, unrelated disease process, or some other cause—ADH may be released continuously, causing SIADH.

ADH is released in response to stress. Be alert to patients who have the following risk factors and who are also in pain or undergoing stressful procedures:

- Medications
  - General anesthetics
  - Narcotics
  - Barbiturates
  - Thiazide diuretics
  - Oral hypoglycemics
  - Oxytocin
- Malignancies
  - Oat-cell cancer of the lung
  - Duodenal cancer
  - Pancreatic cancer
- Nonmalignant pulmonary diseases
  - Tuberculosis
  - Lung abscess
  - Pneumonia
- Nervous system disorders
  - Head trauma
  - Cerebral vascular thrombosis
  - Cerebral atrophy
  - Acute encephalitis
  - Meningitis
  - Guillain-Barré syndrome
- Miscellaneous
  - Hypothyroidism
  - Lupus erythematosus

Clinical Manifestations. Clinically, SIADH is characterized by hyponatremia and water retention that progresses to water intoxication. The severity of the patient's condition depends on how hyponatremic he becomes and how rapidly fluid accumulates. Most signs and symptoms appear when serum sodium levels fall below 125 mEq/L.

Assessment. Collection of *subjective data* includes vague complaints. Hyponatremia triggers the earliest symptoms, which being rather nonspecific could indicate other disorders. These symptoms include weakness, muscle cramps, anorexia, nausea, and headache.

Collection of *objective data* includes assessment for hyponatremia. Hyponatremia may trigger diarrhea. The patient may also be disoriented and irritable, and may demonstrate a weight gain. Fluid intake will exceed urine output. The patient will not develop peripheral edema, because excess fluid is accumulating in the vascular system and not in the interstitial spaces.

As water intoxication progresses and serum becomes more hypotonic, brain cells expand (become edematous). So later signs of SIADH are neurological. The patient will become progressively lethargic, with marked personality changes. The patient will have seizures, and the deep tendon reflexes will diminish or disappear altogether.

Diagnostic Tests. Laboratory tests will show hyponatremia (sodium < 135 mEq/L). The blood urea nitrogen and creatinine will be low to normal. Urine specific gravity will be greater than 1.032, and urine sodium will be elevated.

Medical Management. The physician will order fluid restriction. Initially fluids may be restricted to 800 to 1000 ml of fluid per day. However, with severe hyponatremia fluids may be restricted to 500 ml per day.

Daily fluid intake should equal fluid output. If fluid restriction is adequate, a gradual increase in serum sodium along with a decrease in body weight will be shown.

A hypertonic saline infusion will be ordered to correct sodium imbalance and to pull water out of edematous brain cells.

Medications such as demeclocycline (Declomycin), a tetracycline derivative, 300 mg orally qid may be ordered. The physician may also prescribe lithium carbonate. Both of these drugs interfere with the antidiuretic action of ADH and cause polyuria. Diuretics such as furosemide (Lasix), 40 to 80 mg orally daily in divided dosages or 20 to 40 mg IV daily, may be prescribed.

Treatment must also be directed at eliminating the underlying problem. Surgical resection, radiation, or chemotherapy may be indicated for malignant neoplasms. If the causative factor is a medication, it is discontinued.

The loss of potassium and other electrolytes from diuresis should be monitored closely as well as I&O to prevent hypovolemia.

Nursing Interventions. Nursing interventions for SIADH focus on a continual assessment of the patient's condition to determine if his condition is improving, not deteriorating. Every 3 to 4 hours a neurological examination is performed, and the patient's hydration status is assessed. Auscultate lung sounds every 2 to 4 hours to check for crackles that would indicate overhydration. Report and document any changes immediately.

Serum electrolytes, urine sodium, and urine specific gravity are observed carefully because overcorrection can cause hypernatremia.

A daily weight is necessary at the same time and on the same scales. I&O are closely monitored; output is the guide to regulating intake.

The nursing goal is to control the patient's intake and to minimize discomfort. Explain why fluids are being restricted; allow the patient to divide allotted fluids and to choose the fluids, if possible. Fluids should be high in sodium (milk, orange or tomato juice, and beef or chicken broth). Salty foods should be avoided (potato chips or bacon, for example) because they will make the patient more thirsty.

Frequent mouth care is essential to maintain the integrity of oral mucous membranes. Steps must be taken to prevent skin impairment. Keep the patient and family members informed with simple explanations, such as that pain and anxiety can aggravate SIADH. If nausea is present (due to water intoxication), obtain an order for an antiemetic to be administered 30 minutes before meals.

Nursing diagnoses and interventions for the patient with SIADH include but are not limited to the following:

NURSING DIAGNOSES	NURSING INTERVENTIONS
Fluid volume excess, related to decreased urine output	Obtain daily weight, same scales, same time. Assess and record I&O. Monitor laboratory results. Administer medications as ordered. Maintain dietary and fluid restrictions (fluids should be high in sodium; avoid salty foods). Monitor IV infusions (e.g., 5% sodium chloride over several hours)
Oral mucous membrane, altered, high risk for, related to fluid restrictions of 1000 ml per 24 hours	Provide frequent oral care; avoid alcohol-based mouth washes and lemon glycerin swabs. Provide water-soluble lubricant for lips. Allow patient to choose fluids and to divide the allotted amount (e.g., one half in morning, one third in evening, and the remainder during the night). Offer simple explanation for fluid restrictions. If ordered, administer antiemetics 30 min before meals.
Thought processes, altered, related to fluid excess	Assess orientation to time, place, and person. Maintain a stable and safe environment. Reduce confusing environmental stimuli. Explain rationale for disturbance in thought processes to family members. If appropriate, request that a family member stay with the patient.

Patient teaching. Patient teaching should be an ongoing part of nursing care. Be certain the patient understands the treatment plan, the rationale behind it, and the expected outcome. The teaching should include information about signs and symptoms of SIADH, and that the physician should be alerted if any changes are noted. SIADH can recur following discharge.

Prognosis. SIADH is potentially dangerous but treatable. If signs and symptoms are recognized early and intervention is appropriate, the prognosis is good; without treatment, coma and death occur.

DISORDERS OF THE THYROID AND PARATHYROID GLANDS

Hyperthyroidism

Etiology/Pathophysiology. Hyperthyroidism, also called *Graves' disease,* exophthalmic goiter, and thyrotoxicosis, is a condition in which there is increased activity of the thyroid gland, with overproduction of the thyroid hormones thyroxine (T_4) and triiodothyronine (T_3). As a result, all the patient's metabolic processes are exaggerated. Although the exact cause of hyperthyroidism is unknown, it may result from extreme physical or emotional stress. It may occur during pregnancy, in adolescence, and in the presence of infection. There may be a genetic basis or autoimmune factors. The condition affects an estimated 0.4% of women but is seen much less often in men.

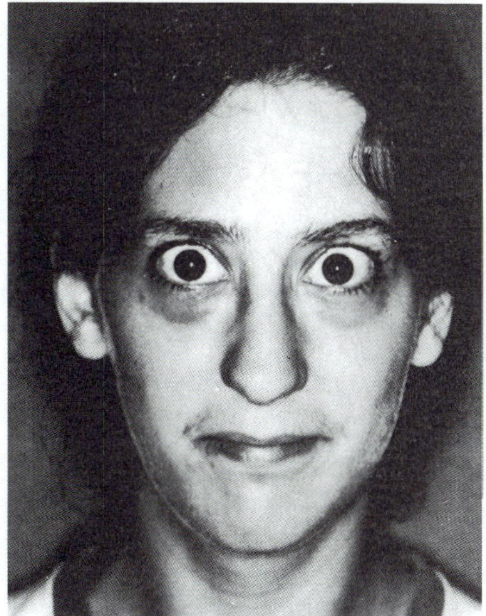

FIG. 32-6 Exophthalmia of Graves' disease.

Clinical Manifestations. Clinical manifestations are numerous and varied and are mild to severe. There is usually visible edema of the anterior portion of the neck as a result of enlargement of the thyroid. In severe cases, exophthalmos (bulging of the eyeballs) may occur, usually attributable to periorbital edema (Fig. 32-6).

Assessment. Collection of *subjective data* includes assessment of the ability to concentrate and the presence of memory loss. The patient may complain of dysphagia or may be hoarse. There is usually weight loss, even in the presence of a voracious appetite. The patient appears very nervous, jittery, and excitable and may experience insomnia. These patients are emotionally labile and may overreact to stressful situations.

Collection of *objective data* includes assessment of changes in the vital signs. The pulse is usually rapid, blood pressure is elevated, and a bruit may be auscultated over the thyroid. The skin is warm and flushed, and the hair is fine and soft. Female patients may cease to menstruate. Elevated body temperature may be accompanied by intolerance to heat, with profuse diaphoresis. The presence of tremors of the hands should be noted. Behavior changes may include hyperactivity and clumsiness. Daily weighing usually shows weight loss.

Diagnostic Tests. Diagnostic tests usually include those in Box 32-1 on p. 952.

Medical Management. Medical management for hyperthyroidism may include administration of drugs that block the production of thyroid hormones, such as propylthiouracil or methimazole (Table 32-1 on p. 952). This may be followed after the acute stage by a therapeutic dose of radioactive iodine (^{131}INaI or ^{125}INaI), based on the patient's age, clinical manifestations, and estimated weight of the thyroid. This is done in an effort to destroy some of the hypertrophied thyroid tissue. The patient will usually begin to notice a decrease in symptoms within 6 to 8 weeks after the dose of the drug. An unfortunate sequela of this treatment in most patients is the development of hypothyroidism. For this reason, the patient must have adequate follow-up medical supervision. ^{131}I is not a radiation hazard to the nonpregnant patient but is absolutely contraindicated during pregnancy. Pregnant nurses should not care for this patient for several days.

Surgical treatment for hyperthyroidism is subtotal thyroidectomy, a procedure in which approximately five sixths of the thyroid is removed. Surgery is usually delayed, if possible, until the patient is in a normal-thyroid (euthyroid) state, because of the risk of excess bleeding during thyroidectomy, as well as postoperative thyroid crisis. Patients who have only mild hyperthyroidism will rarely be admitted to the acute care hospital. They will be followed by the physician in an office or clinic setting. However, the hospital nurse may come in contact with the patient because of admission for a different condition and will also care for these patients before and after thyroidectomy.

Nursing Interventions. The hyperthyroid patient has a need for more nutrients because of increased metabolism, so diet therapy usually consists of food high in calories, vitamins (especially the B vitamins), minerals, and

Box 32-1

DIAGNOSTIC TESTS FOR HYPERTHYROIDISM

T_3 (serum triiodothyronine). Measures the T_3 level in the blood serum. Normal is 110-230 ng/dl. As with the thyroxin (T_4 test), the serum T_3 is an accurate measurement of thyroid function. T_3 is less stable than T_4. An elevated T_3 determination is clinically important in the patient who has a normal T_4 level but has all the signs and symptoms of hyperthyroidism. In this patient the test may identify T_3 thyrotoxicosis.

T_4 (serum thyroxine). Measures the T_4 level in the blood serum. Normal is 4 to 11 μg/dl. Some medications such as oral contraceptives, steroids, estrogens, and sulfonamides may be withheld for several hours before the T_3 and T_4 tests, but food and fluids are not withheld. Elevated levels of these tests usually indicate hyperthyroidism.

RAIU (radioactive iodine uptake test). Radioactive iodine, ^{131}I, is given by mouth to the fasting patient. After 2, 6, and 24 hours, a scintillator is held over the thyroid to measure how much of the isotope has been removed from the bloodstream. A hyperactive thyroid may remove up to 90% of the drug. This test may be affected by prior ingestion of iodine-containing substances or foods. It is necessary to obtain a signed consent form for this test. Also, any allergy to iodine should be noted on the request form, along with medications currently being taken. No radiation precautions are necessary.

Thyroid scan. ^{131}I is given to the patient either orally or intravenously. If an IV dose is given, the scan may be done in 30 to 60 minutes. A scintillation camera positioned over the patient's thyroid sends images that are received on an oscilloscope and may be printed out on special paper. A consent form must be signed for this test. No radiation precautions are necessary. Thyroid-stimulating hormone (TSH) is suppressed in hyperthyroidism. Normal is 2 to 10 μU/ml.

TABLE 32-1 Medications Commonly Used to Treat Hyperthyroidism and Hypothyroidism

Medication	Common Side Effects
Hyperthyroidism	
Iodine or iodine products (potassium or sodium iodide with strong iodine solution, SSKI, Lugol's solution)	Nausea, vomiting, diarrhea, abdominal pain
Radioactive iodine (^{131}INaI or ^{125}INaI)	Sore throat, edema or pain in neck, temporary loss of taste, nausea, vomiting, painful salivary glands
Methimazole (Tapazole), propylthiouracil (Propyl-Thoracil, PTU)	Rash or pruritus, vertigo, nausea, vomiting, loss of taste, paresthesias, abdominal pain
Hypothyroidism	
Levothyroxine sodium (Levothroid, Synthroid, Eltroxin) Liothyronine sodium (Cytomel, Tertroxin) Liotrex (Euthroid, Thyrolar) Thyroglobulin (Proloid) Thyroid (Armour Thyroid, Thyro-Teric, Westthroid)	Nervousness, irritability, tremors, insomnia, tachycardia, hypertension, palpitations, cardiac dysrhythmias, vomiting, diarrhea, nausea, appetite changes, weight loss, menstrual irregularities, leg cramps, fever

carbohydrates. Between-meal snacks are offered. Food should be soft and easily swallowed if there is **dysphagia** (difficulty in swallowing). Coffee, tea, and colas should be avoided because of their stimulant effect. Preoperative nursing interventions for the patient who is scheduled for a thyroidectomy should stress keeping the environment as stable as possible to prevent emotional strain. Visitors may have to be limited to ensure adequate time for the patient to rest. The room should be quiet and cool, not above 23° C (74° F). The nurse should encourage food and fluids to help replace electrolytes lost from perspiration. Attention should be paid to skin integrity for patients who are perspiring profusely. Keep the skin clean and dry, and change the patient's gown and bed linen as needed. Preoperative teaching is extremely important for this patient, and should include instructions on how to properly support the head while turning in bed or rising to a sitting or standing position. The nurse (or patient) should place both hands behind the head and maintain anatomical position while the rest of the body is being moved. The patient is also taught to deep breathe, but the physician will determine whether coughing is to be done postoperatively, since coughing puts a strain on the suture line. The nurse should inform the patient that a period of "voice rest" may be enforced for 48 hours postoperatively and that pencil and paper will be provided for writing notes instead of talking. Voice checks may be done every 2 to 4 hours, as ordered by the physician. The nurse asks the patient to say "ah" and checks for excessive hoarseness or voice changing. Slight hoarseness is to be expected and should not be cause for alarm. Approximately 12.4% of patients suffer some damage to the laryngeal nerve during surgery, but this is not always permanent.

Postoperative management of this patient includes keeping the bed in semi-Fowler's position, with pillows supporting the head and shoulders. The patient should be cautioned to avoid hyperextending the head to prevent excess tension on the incision, which is usually made in a naturally appearing horizontal crease in the anterior neck. There should be a suction apparatus and tracheotomy tray available for emergency use. A cool mist humidifier at the bedside may help soothe the throat and prevent coughing. Vital signs should be checked frequently, with special attention paid to the rate and depth of respirations and observation for any dyspnea (shortness of breath or difficulty in breathing) related to edema in the operative site. Before any liquid is given orally, the nurse must be sure the swallowing and cough reflexes have returned. The nurse must be alert for signs of internal or external bleeding; early internal bleeding may be evidenced by restlessness, apprehension, an increased pulse rate, a decreased blood pressure, and a feeling of fullness in the neck. Later, cyanosis may develop, signaling an obstructed airway, and the surgeon must be notified immediately. The dressing on the neck should be inspected frequently for obvious external bleeding. The nurse should also check for bleeding at the sides and back of the neck and on top of the patient's shoulders, because oozing blood may pool there as a result of gravity. Most surgeons will allow a dressing to be reinforced as needed and loosened slightly if the patient complains that it is too tight.

Postoperatively, the diet initially will consist of clear, cool liquids, progressing to soft food as tolerated. This is followed by a regular diet as soon as possible in an effort to help the patient regain lost weight and correct any nutritional deficiencies.

In addition to hemorrhage, there are two significant postoperative complications after thyroidectomy for which the nurse must be ever watchful. The first is tetany. One possible cause of tetany is the inadvertent removal of one or more of the parathyroid glands during surgery. Another is edema in the operative area, which causes an occlusion of parathyroid release into the bloodstream, resulting in a low serum calcium level, the symptoms of which include numbness and tingling in the fingertips and toes and around the mouth. There may be carpopedal spasms (muscle spasms in the wrists and feet) and increased pulse, respirations, and blood pressure, accompanied by anxiety and agitation. Laryngeal spasm and stridor may occur. **Chvostek's sign** will be positive (an abnormal spasm of the facial muscles elicited by light taps on the facial nerve in patients who are hypocalcemic), and **Trousseau's sign** may also be positive (a test for latent tetany in which carpal spasm is induced by inflating a sphygmomanometer cuff on the upper arm to a pressure exceeding systolic blood pressure for 3 minutes; a positive test may be seen in hypocalcemia and hypomagnesemia). The condition may, if untreated, progress to convulsions or lethal cardiac dysrhythmias. Emergency treatment of tetany is the intravenous administration of calcium gluconate, which should always be available postoperatively.

The other serious complication after thyroidectomy is thyroid crisis, or thyroid storm. Fortunately, it occurs rarely, and can usually be attributed to manipulation of the thyroid during surgery, which causes the release of large amounts of thyroid hormones into the bloodstream. If thyroid crisis occurs, it usually does so within the first 12 hours postoperatively. In thyroid crisis, all the signs and symptoms of hyperthyroidism are exaggerated. Additionally, the patient may develop nausea, vomiting, severe tachycardia, severe hypertension, and occasionally hyperthermia up to 41° C (106° F). Extreme restlessness, cardiac dysrhythmias, and delirium may also occur. The patient may develop congestive heart failure and may die. Emergency treatment of thyroid crisis includes intravenous administration of fluids, sodium iodide, and corticosteroids; antipyretics; and oxygen as needed. Prompt, adequate treatment usually results in dramatic improvement within 12 to 24 hours.

Nursing diagnoses and interventions for the patient having a thyroidectomy include but are not limited to the following:

NURSING DIAGNOSES	NURSING INTERVENTIONS
PREOPERATIVE	
Hyperthermia, high risk for, related to increased metabolism	Assess body temperature at regular intervals. Regulate environment (room temperature, linens, clothing) to help keep patient comfortable.
Nutrition altered: less than body requirements, related to increased metabolism	Encourage patient to eat prescribed diet, avoiding caffeine. Assess daily weight and food intake.
Thought processes altered, related to physiological changes and sleep deprivation	Explain procedures slowly; give a limited number of instructions and repeat if needed. Decrease stimuli to minimize distractions and help patient concentrate.
Skin integrity impaired, related to nutritional status	Carefully assess skin daily. Keep linens dry and wrinkle free.
POSTOPERATIVE	
Swallowing impaired, related to postoperative edema	Ensure swallowing and cough reflexes present before oral intake. Encourage patient to drink slowly and chew food thoroughly.

NURSING DIAGNOSES	NURSING INTERVENTIONS
Breathing pattern, ineffective, high risk for, related to postoperative edema and pain	Monitor rate and depth of respirations. Assess breath sounds and skin color. Encourage slow, deep breaths at least once an hour. Position to maximize respiratory effort.
Pain, related to surgical incision	Administer analgesics as ordered, and monitor relief. Use comfort measures (e.g., relaxation techniques, gentle backrub, distraction techniques).
Infection, high risk for, related to invasive surgical procedure	Use sterile technique when changing dressing on neck and during other invasive procedures. Assess body temperature every 4 hr, and report elevation to physician.

NURSING DIAGNOSES NURSING INTERVENTIONS

Patient teaching. Patient education after thyroidectomy includes stressing the importance of follow-up medical supervision. Thyroid function tests are done periodically to determine resolution of the hyperthyroid condition, as well as the possible development of hypothyroidism, a sequela that occurs in approximately 43% of surgical cases. Before leaving the hospital, the patient should be taught proper care of the incision site and symptoms that might indicate development of an infection, in which case the surgeon must be notified immediately. Discuss with the patient the need for a high-calorie, high-protein, high-carbohydrate diet until weight is stable.

Prognosis. With adequate, appropriate medical or surgical treatment, these patients usually have a normal life expectancy. However, exophthalmos, if present, may remain to a lesser degree in some unfortunate persons.

Hypothyroidism

Etiology/Pathophysiology. Hypothyroidism is the clinical state that occurs when the thyroid fails to secrete sufficient hormones, resulting in a slowing of all the body's metabolic processes. It may be caused by a condition of the thyroid itself or by a failure of the pituitary gland to furnish sufficient TSH for proper stimulation of thyroid secretion. It is sometimes an unfortunate sequela of the medical or surgical treatment of hyperthyroidism. It occurs most often in women aged 30 to 60 and is believed to be more common in the older adult than previously thought. Severe hypothyroidism in adults is called myxedema (Fig. 32-7). Congenital hypothyroidism is called cretinism (Fig. 32-8) and is estimated to occur in 1 of every 4000 to 5000 newborns.

Clinical Manifestations. Clinical manifestations range from mild to severe and depend on the degree of thyroid hormone deficiency present. There is a slowing of all the body's metabolic processes, resulting in decreased production of body heat, intolerance to cold, and weight gain. Atherosclerotic changes may result in coronary artery disease.

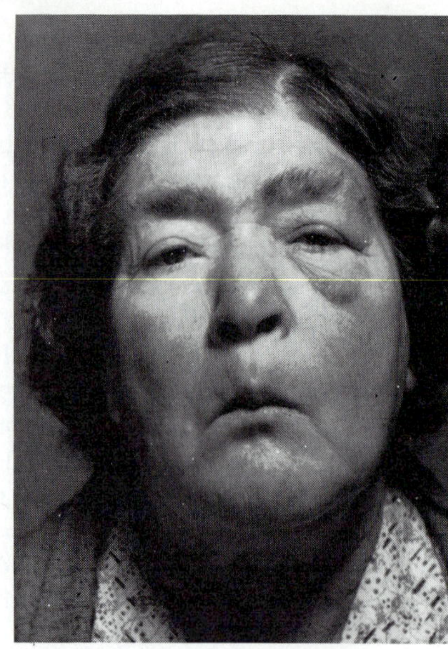

FIG. 32-7 Person with myxedema.

Assessment. Collection of *subjective data* includes the patient's mental and emotional status, because he may display depression or paranoia, impaired memory, and general slowing of thought processes. There may be hearing and speech deficits. The patient is lethargic, forgetful, and irritable. Because of the body's slowed metabolism, anorexia and constipation may develop. Both sexes may experience decreased libido and reproductive difficulty. Female patients suffer from menstrual irregularities and may have difficulty conceiving or completing a pregnancy. Many experience spontaneous abortion, and this contributes to emotional distress and anxiety. The nurse should assess the patient's adaptive coping methods.

Collection of *objective data* includes assessment of the skin and hair. The hair thins and may fall out; the skin becomes thickened and dry. Facial features may enlarge to give the patient an edematous appearance. A masklike facial expression is common. The voice is characteristically low and hoarse. Decreased metabolism usually causes bradycardia, decreased blood pressure and respirations, and exercise intolerance. The patient's ability to perform activities may decrease because of weakness, clumsiness, and ataxia. The respiratory rate must be closely assessed after administration of any central nervous system depressant. The abdomen should be evaluated for distention, because *myxedema ileus* may occur.

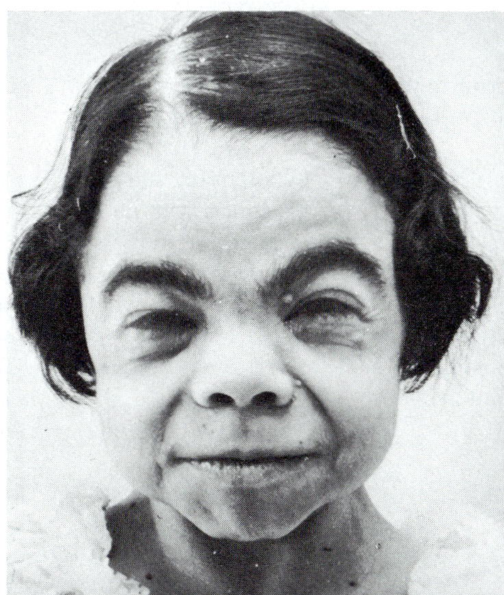

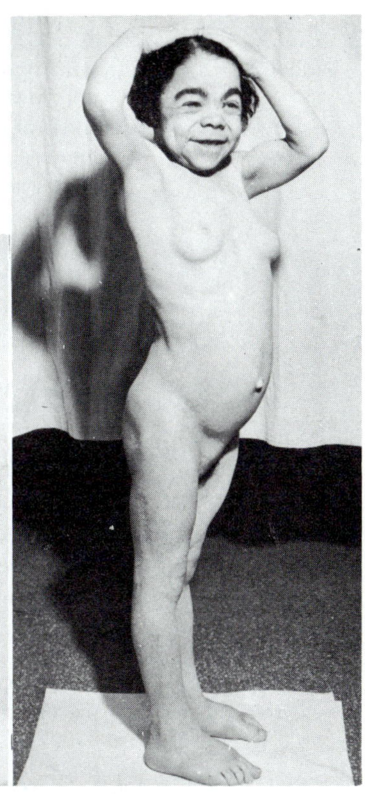

FIG. 32-8 Adult cretin (33 years old, untreated). Note characteristic cretinoid features, dwarfism (height 44 inches), absent axillary and scant pubic hair, poorly developed breasts, protruding abdomen, and small umbilical hernia.

Diagnostic Tests. The diagnosis of hypothyroidism is based on the physical examination and history and on appropriate laboratory tests, such as TSH, T_3, and T_4. Low levels of T_3 and T_4 are the underlying stimuli for TSH. Therefore a compensatory elevation of TSH occurs in patients with primary hypothyroid states and low levels of T_3 and T_4 are present. Subclinical cases may go undiagnosed for years, so the nurse should be aware of subtle clues while interviewing and caring for the patient. Recent research has suggested that mild hypothyroidism exists in approximately 5% of the population, more often in women. In children, when T_4 replacement begins before epiphyseal fusion, the chance for normal growth is greatly improved.

Medical Management. The treatment for hypothyroidism is replacement therapy, with desiccated animal thyroid (Armour Thyroid), thyroglobulin (Proloid), or synthetic products such as levothyroxine sodium (Levothoroid) or liothyronine sodium (Cytomel) by mouth (Table 32-1). These drugs are usually given in the morning to enhance utilization of nutrients ingested during the daily meals. The patient will initially be given a low dose, with increases as necessary till the desired effect is achieved. A maintenance dose will then be established. The nurse should watch the patient for adverse effects of drug therapy, which mimic the signs and symptoms of hyperthyroidism. There is usually a dramatic change in the patient within a short time after replacement therapy begins (see medications table on p. 956).

Nursing Interventions. Nursing interventions for the hospitalized severely hypothyroid patient center mainly on symptomatic relief. The room must be kept at least 20° to 23° C (68° to 74° F), and the patient should not be chilled during the bath or other procedures. Extra time should be allowed for physical care, so that the patient does not feel rushed. Accurate records of bowel elimination must be kept, since constipation may be severe. Stool softeners, bulk laxatives, or enemas may be ordered. A high-protein, high-fiber, low-calorie diet is given. Concentrated carbohydrates such as sweets should be avoided, to help prevent excess weight gain. The patient should be encouraged to take increased oral fluids. The nurse should watch for chest pain or dyspnea, accompanied by changes in the rate or rhythm of the heart, because this may indicate development of cardiac involvement. Since most hypothyroid patients are more susceptible to the effects of sedatives, hypnotics, and anesthetics, the nurse must be alert for possible adverse effects if these agents are given for this condition.

Nursing diagnoses and interventions for the patient with hypothyroidism include but are not limited to the following:

MEDICATIONS FOR ENDOCRINE DISORDERS

Medication	Trade Name	Action	Side Effects	Nursing Implications
Bromocriptine	Parlodel	Inhibits prolactin secretion, lowers serum levels of growth hormone, dopamine receptor agonist	Nausea, headache, dizziness, abdominal cramping, orthostatic hypotension	Give with meals to prevent GI effects, change positions carefully to prevent orthostatic hypotension; contraindicated with hypersensitivity to ergot derivatives
Calcium salts (gluconate, lactate, chloride gluceptate)	Many	Calcium electrolyte replacement	Hypercalcemia, phlebitis, necrosis, and burning at IV site; bradycardia, hypotension, and dysrhythmias with rapid IV administration	Monitor cardiac status and blood pressure and for extravasation when giving IV
Fludrocortisone	Florinef	Adrenal cortical steroid with mineralocorticoid activity, promotes sodium and water retention	Hypertension, edema, sweating, rash, hypokalemia	Monitor for hypokalemia and fluid retention/depletion, do not discontinue abruptly, patient should carry identification signaling use
Levothyroxine (T4)	Synthroid, Levothyroid, others	Thyroid hormone replacement	Most are due to therapeutic overdose and include anxiety, insomnia, headache, hypertension, tremors, angina, dysrhythmias, tachycardia, menstrual irregularities	Give in AM to minimize insomnia, use caution in older adult or patients with coronary artery disease, monitor for signs of overdose, do not switch brands unless instructed
Mitotane	Lysodren	Adrenal cytotoxic agent, reduces production of adrenal steroids	Anorexia, nausea, vomiting, diarrhea, lethargy, somnolence, vertigo, rash	Tell patient to use contraception and caution when driving or performing tasks requiring alertness, monitor for dehydration
Potassium iodide (SSKI)	Many	Blocks release of thyroid hormone in thyroid storm and hyperthyroidism, also used as an expectorant	Hypersensitivity reactions, rash, metallic taste, burning in mouth or throat, GI irritation, headache, parotitis, hyperkalemia	Should not be used in pregnant women, mix with fruit juice to mask taste
Somatostatin analogs (octreotide)	Sandostatin	Intestinal hormone analog that suppresses activity of GI hormones (gastrin, insulin, VIP, glucagon, secretin, and growth hormone); used for carcinoid tumors, Vipomas, and high-output fistulas	Nausea, diarrhea, abdominal pain, headache, injection site discomfort, hyperglycemia, hypoglycemia	SQ is the preferred route of administration, but may also be given IV
Vasopressin (antidiuretic hormone)	Pitressin	Synthetic pituitary hormone with antidiuretic effects on the kidney (used to treat diabetes insipidus), also a potent vasoconstrictor (used to treat bleeding esophageal varices)	Nasal irritation and congestion with nasal preparations; hypertension; ischemia to heart, mesenteric organs, and kidneys; angina; myocardial infarction; water retention; hyponatremia	Use with caution in older patients or patients with coronary artery disease, use caution with CHF, discontinue if chest pain develops, monitor urine output and serum sodium

NURSING DIAGNOSES	NURSING INTERVENTIONS
Cardiac output, decreased, related to decreased metabolism	Assess pulse, BP, skin color, and temperature. Schedule nursing activities around patient's activity cycle, with rest periods as needed to conserve energy.
Constipation, colonic, related to decreased peristaltic action	Assess frequency and character of stools. Encourage oral fluid intake and high-fiber food intake.
Thought processes, altered, related to decreased metabolic state	Assess level of orientation to person, place, and time. Explain procedures slowly and simply, reinforcing them as necessary.

Patient teaching. Regular checkups are essential, because drug dosage may have to be adjusted from time to time. The patient should understand the desired effects of the medication and also the major adverse effects that might occur. The patient should be instructed to eat well-balanced meals of high-fiber foods, such as fruits, vegetables, and whole-grain cereals and breads; there should be adequate intake of iodine, in foods such as saltwater fish, milk, and eggs; fluids should be increased to help prevent constipation. The patient and family should be told that mental and physical slowness may still be present but should improve with thyroid replacement therapy.

Prognosis. Most hypothyroid patients do well with proper medical supervision, although they will probably have to take medication for the rest of their lives.

Simple (Colloid) Goiter

Etiology/Pathophysiology. A simple, or colloid, goiter develops when the thyroid gland enlarges in response to low iodine levels in the bloodstream or when it is unable to utilize iodine properly. When the blood level of T_3 is too low to signal the pituitary to decrease TSH secretion, the thyroid gland then responds by increasing the formation of thyroglobulin (colloid), which accumulates in the thyroid follicles and causes enlargement of the gland (Fig. 32-9). Most cases of simple goiter can be attributed to insufficient dietary intake of iodine, leading to this overgrowth of thyroid tissue.

Clinical Manifestations. There are usually no manifestations of overt thyroid dysfunction, and the diagnosis is made essentially using the patient's physical manifestations.

Assessment. Collection of *subjective data* focuses on assessing the patient's emotional response to the unsightly enlargement of the thyroid, and the patient

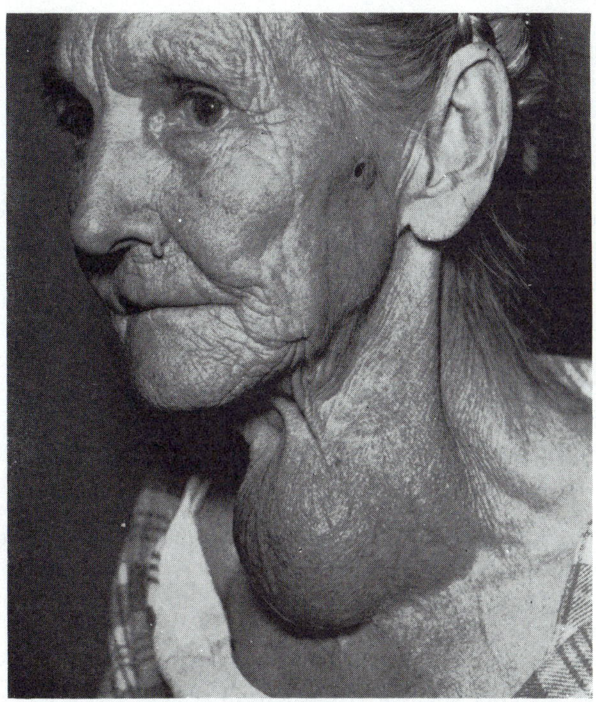

FIG. 32-9 Simple goiter.

should be encouraged to verbalize emotional responses. The patient may only complain of symptoms of dysphagia, hoarseness, or dyspnea related to the pressure of the enlarged gland against the esophagus and trachea. Dysphagia may contribute to difficulty ingesting adequate food and fluids. The patient should be assessed for increasing dyspnea. The patient's understanding of the need for medication, diet therapy, and medical follow-up should be determined.

Collection of *objective data* includes assessment of increased goiter size, voice changes, and adequacy of food and fluid intake. The thyroid may be only slightly enlarged, or it may be so enlarged that surgery must be done to improve respiration or swallowing.

Medical Management. Surgery may sometimes be performed for cosmetic effect, because this type of goiter can be very unsightly and damaging to the patient's self-image and self-esteem. If thyroidectomy is done, most of the gland is removed. Medical treatment consists of oral administration of potassium iodide, as well as foods high in iodine.

Nursing Interventions. Nursing interventions after thyroidectomy (previously discussed) are aimed at prevention of complications such as bleeding, tetany, and thyroid crisis. Nursing diagnoses and interventions for the patient with simple (colloid) goiter include but are not limited to the following:

NURSING DIAGNOSES	NURSING INTERVENTIONS
Noncompliance, high risk for, related to therapeutic regimen	Provide opportunities for patient to ventilate feelings about treatment plan. Correct misconceptions, and reinforce previous medical instructions. Stress importance of taking prescribed medications, having regular checkups, and avoiding any identified goitrogenic foods.
Body image disturbance, high risk for, related to altered physical appearance	Develop open and trusting relationship so patient will express feelings. Discuss ways to disguise thyroid enlargement (e.g., scarves, high collars, make-up).

Patient teaching. The nurse should stress the importance of adequate dietary intake of iodine by the patient. Medical supervision is recommended at regular intervals.

Prognosis. Most patients can expect to live a normal life after adequate treatment of goiter.

Cancer of the Thyroid

Etiology/Pathophysiology. Cancer of the thyroid is a relatively rare malignancy, affecting approximately 25 of each 1 million people in the United States each year. However, more cases are expected, because between 1949 and 1960 many infants and children through adolescence were irradiated to shrink enlarged thymus tissue, tonsils, or adenoids and to treat severe cases of acne vulgaris. Cancer of the thyroid occurs more frequently in females and in Caucasians. The incidence rises as age increases. Most malignancies of the thyroid are papillary, well-differentiated adenocarcinoma, a type of cancer that grows slowly, is usually contained, and does not spread beyond the adjacent lymph nodes. Cure rates after thyroidectomy in these cases are excellent. Other cancers, follicular and anaplastic, though much more rare, have extremely low cure rates.

Clinical Manifestations. The principal clinical manifestation of thyroid cancer is the presence of a firm, fixed, small, rounded mass or **nodule** that is felt during palpation of the gland. This nodule is painless. Only in rare instances have the symptoms of hyperthyroidism been seen.

Assessment. The collection of *subjective data* includes an assessment of the patient's use of adaptive coping methods to deal with the diagnosis, as well as an observation of the support system composed of the patient's significant others. The patient's understanding of the importance of medical follow-up should be assessed also.

Collection of *objective data* to be assessed includes progression of enlargement of the tumor area preoperatively, response to ^{131}I therapy, and skin involvement in the neck and torso after radiation therapy.

Diagnostic Tests. Diagnosis of papillary thyroid cancer is suspected when a thyroid scan shows a "cold" nodule, indicating decreased uptake of ^{131}I. Benign adenomas and follicular cancers are usually visualized as "hot" nodules because of their increased uptake of the isotope. Thyroid function tests usually yield normal results. To confirm the diagnosis a thyroid needle biopsy may be done, but this should be attempted only by a skilled practitioner, since seeding of adjacent tissues may occur during the procedure. Metastasis can then result, with the prognosis becoming much more grave.

Medical Management. Treatment of thyroid cancer is a total thyroidectomy, with subsequent lifelong thyroid hormone replacement therapy. If metastasis is present at the time of the initial surgery, a radical neck dissection may be performed. In addition, radiation therapy, chemotherapy, and administration of ^{131}I may be done.

Nursing Interventions. Nursing interventions for the patient after thyroidectomy (discussed previously) are instituted. Nursing diagnoses and interventions for the patient with cancer of the thyroid include but are not limited to the following:

NURSING DIAGNOSES	NURSING INTERVENTIONS
Anxiety, related to situational crisis	Encourage patient to discuss feelings about upcoming surgery. Monitor level of anxiety. Maintain a calm environment; try to decrease stressors.
Coping, ineffective individual, related to personal vulnerability in crisis	Help patient identify previously successful coping methods. Teach new coping methods as needed.

Patient Teaching. The patient should be aware of the importance of proper medical follow-up to monitor thyroid hormone replacement therapy and to help ensure prompt diagnosis of any future metastatic lesions. Before discharge from the hospital, the patient should be taught proper care of the surgical incision.

Prognosis. The prognosis after treatment for thyroid cancer depends on the type of tumor involved. For papillary carcinoma, the prognosis is excellent; for follicular and anaplastic carcinomas, the prognosis is much less favorable.

Hyperparathyroidism

Etiology/Pathophysiology. Hyperparathyroidism involves overactivity of the parathyroid glands, with increased production of parathormone. The cause of this condition may be a primary hypertrophy of one or more of the tiny parathyroid glands, usually in the form of an adenoma. It may also result from chronic renal failure, pyelonephritis, or glomerulonephritis. Parathyroid carcinoma is a rare condition, with rapid progress and a very grave prognosis. Hyperparathyroidism usually occurs in adults between 30 and 70 years of age, and twice as often in women.

Clinical Manifestations. The primary clinical manifestation is hypercalcemia. This occurs as calcium leaves the bones and accumulates in the bloodstream. As a result, the bones become demineralized and may cause skeletal pain, pain on weight bearing, and pathological fractures (fractures that result from slight or no trauma to diseased bone). The high level of calcium in the blood may lead to the formation of kidney stones.

Assessment. Collection of *subjective data* includes assessment of the severity of skeletal pain, the degree of muscle weakness, and the effectiveness of analgesics. It is important to determine nursing measures that contribute to the patient's comfort and mobility. As neuromuscular function decreases, there is generalized fatigue, drowsiness, apathy, nausea, and anorexia; the degree of anorexia and nausea should be assessed. There may be constipation, personality changes, disorientation, and even paranoia. Symptoms that may indicate calculus formation are renal colic and dull back pain.

Collection of *objective data* includes careful observation for any skeletal deformity or abnormal movement of bone that might indicate a pathological fracture. The urine should be observed for quantity and the presence of hematuria and stones. There may be vomiting and weight loss. Hypertension and cardiac dysrhythmias may present significant problems. Changes in the serum calcium level may cause bradycardia and other cardiac irregularities. The level of consciousness may decrease, resulting in stupor or coma.

Diagnostic Tests. X-ray examination may reveal skeletal decalcification. Blood parathyroid hormone (PTH) levels are increased, as are alkaline phosphate levels. The patient should receive nothing by mouth for 8 to 12 hours before these tests. The serum calcium level is elevated, while the serum phosphorus level is decreased. A differential diagnosis should be made to rule out multiple myeloma, Cushing's syndrome, vitamin D excess, and other causes of hypercalcemia.

Medical Management. The treatment for hyperparathyroidism is surgical removal of an existing tumor, or removal of one or more parathyroid glands.

Nursing Interventions. Preoperative nursing interventions include helping restore fluid and electrolyte balance by encouraging increased oral fluid intake and by carefully monitoring the IV fluid therapy. The patient's intake and output should be monitored, because diuretics may be used. Furosemide (Lasix) is the diuretic of choice. Thiazide diuretics are not used, because they decrease renal excretion of calcium and thus increase the hypercalcemic state. Urine may be strained, since development of kidney calculi is not uncommon. Daily serum calcium levels may be ordered. The diet should be low in calcium, eliminating milk and other dairy products. Cranberry juice may be helpful in promoting acidic urine, thereby lessening the possibility of calculus formation. Some antacids are high in calcium and should not be used. The patient's pain should be accurately assessed and prescribed analgesics administered as needed. Postoperatively, the patient will be cared for in the same manner as after a thyroidectomy, with careful monitoring of intake and output. These patients commonly retain fluid in the tissues after surgery and will often have decreased urinary output. It is important to avoid overhydration at this point. The patient should be assessed frequently for signs of **hypocalcemia** (a deficiency of calcium in the blood serum), such as tetany, cardiac dysrhythmias, and carpopedal spasms. In the event that tetany does occur, calcium gluconate is usually administered intravenously.

Nursing diagnoses and interventions for the patient with hyperparathyroidism include but are not limited to the following:

NURSING DIAGNOSES	NURSING INTERVENTIONS
Activity intolerance, related to neuromuscular dysfunction	Assist patient to identify factors that increase or decrease activity tolerance and to eliminate or reduce painful, fatiguing activities. Encourage the patient to follow prescribed, individualized activity or exercise program.
Pain: skeletal, joint; renal colic, related to physiological variables	Assess factors that cause or worsen pain, and help patient adjust body mechanics or activity. Encourage adequate fluid intake, while assessing cardiac and renal output.
Trauma, high risk for, related to environmental agents	Assess for and eliminate potentially harmful factors in patient's environment. Instruct patient to use appropriate safety measures (e.g., walker, shower aids, siderails).

Patient teaching. The patient should be taught the principles of good body mechanics so that pathological fractures may be prevented during ambulation. The patient is reassured that bone pain should gradually decrease as electrolyte balance is restored and the condition is alleviated. The patient should be encouraged to participate in mild exercise as prescribed by the physician to regain muscle strength and a feeling of normal well-being. The nurse should teach the patient how to check the urine for the presence of stones or blood and how to monitor the pulse for any changes. The home environment should be evaluated and a plan developed for changes that may be necessary to prevent accidents.

Prognosis. With proper medical or surgical treatment, the patient can lead a fairly normal life. In patients with parathyroid carcinoma, the prognosis is very grave.

Hypoparathyroidism

Etiology/Pathophysiology. Hypoparathyroidism occurs when there is decreased parathyroid hormone, resulting in decreased levels of serum calcium. Idiopathic hypoparathyroidism is a rare condition, thought to be either autoimmune or familial in origin. Most commonly the cause is the inadvertent removal or destruction of one or more of the tiny parathyroid glands during thyroidectomy.

Clinical Manifestations. Decreased parathyroid hormone levels in the bloodstream cause an increased serum phosphorus level and a decreased serum calcium level, resulting in neuromuscular hyperexcitability, involuntary and uncontrollable muscle spasms, and hypocalcemic tetany. Severe hypocalcemia may result in laryngeal spasm, stridor, cyanosis, and an increased possibility of asphyxia. In some patients, there is calcification of the basal ganglia in the brain, causing a Parkinson-like syndrome with bizarre posturing and spastic movements.

Assessment. Collection of *subjective data* includes assessment of neuromuscular activity for symptoms such as dysphagia and numbness or tingling in areas of the skin. The patient may feel anxious, irritable, or depressed. The patient may experience headaches and nausea. Abdominal or flank pain may occur if a renal calculus attempts to pass down the ureter into the bladder. The effectiveness of narcotics used to relieve renal colic must be assessed.

Collection of *objective data* to be assessed includes the appearance of positive Chvostek's sign or Trousseau's sign. If laryngeal spasm and stridor should occur, cyanosis may appear. Cardiac output may decrease as a result of hypocalcemia, and the patient may develop dysrhythmias. Tetanic spasms of the extremities may be observed.

Diagnostic Tests. Diagnostic laboratory studies confirm the presence of decreased serum calcium with increased urinary calcium, and increased serum phosphorus with decreased urinary phosphorus. Other possible causes of hypocalcemia, such as vitamin D deficiency, kidney failure, and acute pancreatitis, should be ruled out.

Medical Management. The immediate treatment of hypoparathyroid tetany is intravenous administration of calcium gluconate or calcium chloride (10%). This drug is very irritating to the vessel wall and should always be given very slowly, with a rate not to exceed 1 ml/min. The patient may complain of a hot feeling of the skin or tongue. If given too rapidly, intravenous calcium can precipitate cardiac arrest. Care should be taken that none of the drug escapes the vein and extravasates into the tissues, as sloughing may occur. After the initial IV dose, calcium may be continued in a slow IV infusion until tetany is controlled; then it is given orally. Vitamin D is usually also given orally to help increase the absorption and blood level of calcium.

Nursing Interventions. Any patient receiving calcium, especially intravenously, must be monitored for signs of hypercalcemia. The most common clinical manifestations of this are vomiting, disorientation, anorexia, abdominal pain, and weakness. The nurse should assess the patient for respiratory distress, renal involvement, and adverse reactions to calcium therapy, such as bradycardia, syncope, and hypotension. Calcium should be used cautiously in digitalized patients, because it may cause digitalis toxicity. Cimetidine (Tagamet) interferes with normal parathyroid functioning and should also be used carefully in these patients. The diet should contain foods high in calcium, such as dairy products, dark green vegetables, soybeans, and canned fish with the bones included. High-calcium snacks should be offered.

Nursing diagnoses and interventions for the patient with hypoparathyroidism include but are not limited to the following:

NURSING DIAGNOSES	NURSING INTERVENTIONS
Injury, high risk for, related to postoperative hypocalcemia	Assess for signs and symptoms of hypocalcemia (e.g., muscle spasms, laryngeal stridor, convulsion). Institute prescribed calcium therapy if need arises.
Nutrition, altered: less than body requirements, related to calcium intake	Give calcium replacement agents as scheduled. Monitor Chvostek's and Trousseau's signs. Arrange for dietitian to discuss dietary sources of calcium. Assess patient's intake of high-calcium foods.

Patient teaching. The patient should be taught the early symptoms of hypocalcemia and instructed to notify the nurse or physician if they occur. It is important that periodic blood levels of calcium and phosphorus be drawn while the patient is hospitalized. The patient should be taught to monitor the pulse for changes, as well as proper maintenance of fluid balance and the use of calcium supplements at home.

Prognosis. For most patients, fairly normal life-style and life expectancy are possible.

DISORDERS OF THE ADRENAL GLANDS

Adrenal Hyperfunction (Cushing's Syndrome)

Etiology/Pathophysiology. Cushing's syndrome (hypercortisolism) is a rare condition in which the plasma levels of adrenocortical hormones are increased. It occurs in only about 10 people in a million and is three times more common in women than in men. This syndrome may be caused by hyperplasia of adrenal tissue resulting from overstimulation by the pituitary hormone ACTH, by a tumor of the adrenal cortex, by ACTH-secreting neoplasms outside the pituitary (such as oat-cell carcinoma of the lung), and occasionally by overuse of corticosteroid drugs. The body's protective feedback mechanism fails, with resultant excess secretion of the adrenal hormones: glucocorticoids, mineralocorticoids, and sex hormones.

Clinical Manifestations. This overabundance of hormones produces the signs and symptoms commonly associated with Cushing's syndrome, including moonface and buffalo hump. The arms and legs become thin as a result of muscle wasting. **Hypokalemia** (a condition in which an inadequate amount of potassium, the major intracellular cation, is found in the circulating bloodstream) is usually present. There is usually protein in the urine, as well as increased urinary calcium excretion, which may lead to the development of renal calculi. Osteoporosis results from abnormal calcium absorption, and kyphosis may develop. The patient is very susceptible to all kinds of infections, but the symptoms of these may be masked and not detected until the infection has progressed to a point that may be life threatening.

Assessment. Collection of *subjective data* includes assessment of the patient's ability to concentrate. Patients may feel irritable, and mental changes may develop. Some patients experience emotional instability, with severe mood swings, and occasionally a psychosis. Depression is very common, and the possibility of suicide is an ever-present concern for the nurse, who must be alert to subtle changes in the patient's affect, and must keep the environment free from objects with which the patient may inflict self-harm. Patients of both sexes may experience loss of libido and alterations in self-esteem; there may be concerns about sexual dysfunction. The patient should be encouraged to verbalize concerns about altered body image. Severe backache is often present and may signal a compression fracture of a vertebral body. The severity of back pain should be assessed, as well as nursing measures that contribute to the patient's comfort. Appetite usually increases, so the patient's understanding of special dietary restrictions should be assessed, as well as the understanding of the importance of medical follow-up.

Collection of *objective data* includes observation of the skin for the presence of ecchymoses and petechiae. The skin becomes thin and fragile and wound healing is delayed. There may be weight gain and abdominal enlargement, with development of striae, and this increased girth may contribute to difficulty with mobility. Weight should be monitored, because peripheral edema and associated hypertension are common. Impaired carbohydrate metabolism results in hyperglycemia. Women may experience **hirsutism** (excessive body hair in a masculine distribution), menstrual irregularities, and deepening of the voice. Elevated body temperature may signal the presence of an undetected infection.

Diagnostic Tests. Diagnosis is usually based on the clinical appearance of the patient and on the results of laboratory tests. Plasma cortisol levels are usually elevated. Plasma ACTH levels may be increased or decreased, depending on the location of a tumor. Skull x-ray evaluation may detect an erosion of the sella turcica in the presence of a pituitary tumor. Adrenal angiography will aid in diagnosing an adrenal tumor. Twenty-four-hour urine tests for 17-ketosteroids and 17-hydroxysteroids show increased levels present. Abdominal CT scan and ultrasound may help localize an abdominal tumor.

Medical Management. Treatment is directed toward the causative factor. If an adrenal tumor is present, adrenalectomy is usually indicated for its removal. Pituitary tumors may be irradiated or removed surgically by transsphenoidal microsurgery. If the patient is unable to undergo surgery because of inoperable cancer elsewhere in the body or another preexisting serious condition, mitotane (Lysodren) therapy may be used. This cytotoxic agent is toxic to the adrenal glands and is given for at least 3 months, during which time the patient must be monitored for symptoms of hepatotoxicity, such as jaundice, gastrointestinal upsets, and pruritus. The diet should be lowered in sodium to help decrease edema. Reduced calories and carbohydrates will help control hyperglycemia, and foods high in potassium will help correct hypokalemia.

Nursing Interventions. Important nursing interventions include gentle handling to prevent skin impairment or excessive ecchymosis, as well as frequent assessment for areas of erythema, edema, or early signs of infection. The patient should be encouraged to turn frequently and ambulate as tolerated to eliminate undue pressure on bony prominences. Elbow and heel protectors and an Eggcrate mattress pad may help prevent decubiti in the bedridden patient. The patient should be encouraged to participate as fully as possible in normal ADLs, interspersing personal hygiene tasks with rest periods to prevent overtiring.

Nursing diagnoses and interventions for the patient with Cushing's syndrome include but are not limited to the following:

NURSING DIAGNOSES	NURSING INTERVENTIONS
Knowledge deficit, related to therapeutic regimen	Assess patient's understanding of prescribed medication and diet. Encourage patient to wear Medic Alert jewelry and carry wallet identification cards.
Activity intolerance, related to weakness and immobility	Assess patient's current activity tolerance, and identify priorities for energy expenditures. Plan activity and rest periods with patient.
Fluid volume excess, related to compromised regulatory mechanisms	Monitor daily weight, intake, and output. Encourage compliance with salt restriction.
Self-esteem disturbance, related to abnormal physical changes	Allow patient to verbalize negative feelings about body changes. Help patient set realistic goals based on physical tolerance.

Patient teaching. The patient's mental attitude is extremely important. The nurse should encourage verbalization of concerns and should also be watchful for the development of depression and the presence of suicidal thoughts. Patients should be helped to understand their prescribed medication, such as mitotane (Lysodren), as well as possible side effects. It is important for the patient to wear a Medic Alert bracelet or necklace and to carry a wallet card stating the diagnosis of Cushing's syndrome. There may be a major life-style change to which the patient must adjust, and the aid of a social worker may be enlisted. Before adrenalectomy, the patient should be taught the importance of avoiding stress and avoiding infections. Postoperative teaching includes proper wound care and the symptoms of Addison's disease, which is sometimes an unavoidable sequela after this type of surgery.

Prognosis. Depending upon whether the etiology of the disease was benign or malignant, and whether the treatment was successful or unsuccessful, the patient with Cushing's syndrome can expect to have major life-style changes, possibly with many complications and a shortened life expectancy.

Adrenal Hypofunction (Addison's Disease)

Etiology/Pathophysiology. Adrenocortical insufficiency occurs when the adrenal glands do not secrete adequate amount of glucocorticoids and mineralocorticoids. It may initially be seen as Addison's disease, a rather rare primary condition; it may result from adrenalectomy, pituitary hypofunction, or long-standing steroid therapy. Addison's disease can result from idiopathic adrenal atrophy, cancer of the adrenal cortex, or tuberculosis. Deficiencies in aldosterone and cortisol produce disturbances of the metabolism of carbohydrates, fats, and proteins, as well as sodium, potassium, and water. This results in electrolyte and fluid imbalance, dehydration, water loss, and hypovolemia.

Clinical Manifestations. Clinical manifestations are directly related to imbalances in adrenal hormones, nutrients, and electrolytes.

Assessment. Collection of *subjective data* to be assessed includes the presence of nausea, anorexia, and craving for salt. Postural hypotension may be associated with vertigo, weakness, and syncope, resulting in reluctance to attempt normal activities. The patient may complain of severe headache, disorientation, abdominal pain, or lower back pain, which could represent early symptoms of adrenal crisis. This patient tolerates stress poorly, feels anxious and apprehensive, and may thus suffer under emotional trauma more easily than a normal person would. It is important to assess emotional status and allow the patient to ventilate feelings about altered self-image. The nurse should also assess the patient's overall understanding of the disease process and the importance of medical treatment and follow-up.

Collection of *objective data* includes observation of changes in the color of the mucous membranes and the skin, with the appearance of darkly pigmented areas commonly observed. There is usually weight loss, which may be accompanied by vomiting and diarrhea. Hypoglycemia may contribute to the patient's fatigue; the nurse should assess the patient's ability to perform ADLs. An abnormally low or abnormally high body temperature, hyponatremia, and hyperkalemia are signs of impending adrenal crisis.

See Table 32-2 for a nursing assessment comparison of Cushing's syndrome and Addison's disease.

Diagnostic Tests. Laboratory studies show decreased serum sodium, increased serum potassium, and decreased serum glucose. A 24-hour urine specimen shows decreased levels of 17-ketosteroids and 17-hydroxysteroids. Fasting plasma cortisol levels and aldosterone levels are low. A glucose tolerance test may yield abnormal results.

TABLE 32-2 Nursing Assessment of Patients with Cushing's Syndrome or Addison's Disease

Area of Assessment	Clinical Manifestations in Cushing's Syndrome	Clinical Manifestations in Addison's Disease
Cardiovascular	Mild to moderate hypertension	Postural hypotension, vertigo, syncope
Neurological	Impaired memory and concentration, insomnia, irritability	Lethargy, headache
Musculoskeletal	Muscle weakness, muscle wasting in extremities, back and rib pain, kyphosis	Muscle weakness, fatigue, muscle aches, muscle wasting
Integumentary	Skin thin; frequent petechiae and ecchymoses, hyperpigmentation, poor wound healing	Hyperpigmentation, decreased body hair
Self-care and hygiene	Tires easily	Tires easily; very susceptible to infections of all kinds
Nutrition/fluid balance	Increased appetite, moderate weight gain, edema, buffalo hump, moonface, obesity of trunk, hyperglycemia; need for decreased salt intake, reduced calories and carbohydrate intake, increased potassium intake	Nausea and vomiting, fluid and electrolyte imbalance, dehydration, weight loss, hypoglycemia; need for increased salt and decreased potassium intake

Medical Management. Medical treatment involves the prompt restoration of fluid and electrolyte balance, as well as replacement of the deficient adrenal hormones. Fludrocortisone (Florinef) is usually the drug of choice. The diet should be high in sodium and low in potassium.

Nursing Interventions. The nurse should carefully assess the circulatory status of the patient, keep accurate intake and output records, and record daily weight. Skin turgor should be checked and fluids offered frequently. Vital signs are monitored at regular intervals, with particular attention paid to the temperature and blood pressure. The patient is also monitored for response to prescribed steroid drugs and any adverse effects promptly reported to the physician. The environment must be kept as free from stressors as possible. Visitors and hospital personnel should be screened for the presence of infectious disease and excluded from the patient's room. This patient should be continually assessed for signs of developing adrenal (addisonian) crisis, in which there may be a sudden, severe drop in blood pressure, nausea and vomiting, an extremely high temperature, and cyanosis, progressing to vasomotor collapse and possibly to death. Emergency treatment is intravenous administration of corticosteroids in a solution of saline and glucose.

Nursing diagnoses and interventions for the patient with Addison's disease include but are not limited to the following:

NURSING DIAGNOSES	NURSING INTERVENTIONS
Infection, high risk for, related to altered metabolic processes	Assess environment for stressors. Screen visitors and personnel for contagious disease. Monitor temperature routinely. Stress importance of medications.
Tissue perfusion, altered peripheral, related to electrolyte imbalance	Monitor vital signs and intake and output. Have patient make position changes slowly; monitor for vertigo, visual changes.
Sleep pattern disturbance, related to anxiety and fatigue	Decrease amount of external stimuli. Use comfort measures (e.g., backrub, dark room, relaxation techniques). Do not disturb patient when sleeping.
Fluid volume deficit, high risk for, related to electrolyte imbalance	Assess skin turgor for dehydration. Encourage compliance with increased dietary salt.

Patient teaching. Before discharge from the hospital, the patient must be taught the importance of adhering to the prescribed drug therapy, having regular medical checkups, and immediately reporting all illnesses, even a cold, to the physician. The patient should understand the importance of avoiding stress, one of the major precipitating factors in adrenal crisis, and should be encouraged to eliminate excess stressors. Other factors include overexertion, diarrhea, infection, decreased intake of salt, exposure to cold, and surgery. The nurse should teach the patient to wear a Medic Alert bracelet or necklace and to carry a wallet card.

Prognosis. With long-term steroid therapy, adequate medical care, and follow-up, this patient has a fair prognosis.

Pheochromocytoma

Etiology/Pathophysiology. A pheochromocytoma is a chromaffin cell tumor, usually found in the adrenal medulla, that causes excessive secretion of epinephrine and norepinephrine. These tumors occur most often in adults between the ages of 20 and 60 and are almost always benign; only about 10% are malignant.

Clinical Manifestations. The principal manifestation of pheochromocytoma is hypertension, which may be intermittent but is usually persistent. Hypertensive crisis episodes may occur, during which the blood pressure may fluctuate widely, sometimes as high as 300/175. Signs and symptoms may be triggered by an identifiable factor, such as overexertion or emotional trauma, or they may occur for no apparent reason. Extreme hypertension may result in cerebrovascular accident, kidney damage, and retinopathy. Cardiac damage may occur, resulting in congestive heart failure.

Assessment. Collection of *subjective data* to be assessed during hypertensive crisis includes the presence of severe headache and palpitations. The patient may feel nervous, dizzy, and dyspneic and may experience paresthesias. There may be nausea and intolerance to heat. Anxiety is common, and the patient may have trouble sleeping. The nurse should question the patient about the occurrence of symptoms in relation to identifiable factors such as excess stress or overexertion and should assess the coping methods identified.

Collection of *objective data* includes frequent measurement of blood pressure and respiratory rate for increases and of pulse for tachycardia. There may be tremors, diaphoresis, dilated pupils, glycosuria, and hyperglycemia. The nurse should assess responses to prescribed medications.

Diagnostic Tests. A 24-hour urine test (the vanillylmandelic acid [VMA] test) will be used to diagnose pheochromocytoma. VMA is the main urinary metabolite of epinephrine and norepinephrine. A test that may be used to confirm the results of the VMA test is the total urine catecholamine test, which also requires a 24-hour specimen. Elevations of these metabolites will confirm the diagnosis. CT scan of the adrenal glands, along with IVP (intravenous pyelogram), may help in locating the tumor. Oral intake is restricted for 8 hours before IVP, and laxatives are usually administered the evening before the test.

Medical Management. Treatment is usually surgical removal of the tumor, if possible, and sometimes removal of the adrenal gland as well. Preoperatively, the patient may be given alpha-adrenergic blocking agents such as phentolamine mesylate (Regitine) or phenoxybenzamine HCl (Dibenzyline) in an effort to control hypertension. Metyrosine (Demser) may be given to help inhibit catecholamine production, and the drug must be continued on a long-term basis if the tumor is inoperable.

Nursing Interventions. Postoperative care is carried out in the same manner as for any major abdominal surgery, with the following special concerns. If the patient has undergone adrenalectomy, large amounts of hydrocortisone will be given. The patient must be watched carefully for fluctuations in blood pressure caused by adrenal manipulation during surgery, with subsequent release of epinephrine and norepinephrine. These fluctuations may be severe and life threatening if cardiovascular collapse occurs. The patient should avoid excess stress and must be allowed adequate time to rest; sedatives may be given to ensure this. A careful I&O record should be kept and intravenous solutions administered exactly as ordered. Vasopressors and corticosteroids may be given. The diet should be free from stimulants, such as coffee, tea, and soft drinks containing caffeine.

Nursing diagnoses and interventions for the patient with pheochromocytoma include but are not limited to the following:

NURSING DIAGNOSES	NURSING INTERVENTIONS
Tissue perfusion, altered: cardiopulmonary, renal, related to hypertension	Monitor BP and pulse and record I&O. Eliminate smoking and caffeine-containing beverages.
Activity intolerance, related to hypertension	Assist with gradual position changes from lying to sitting or standing. Limit activity as needed, to prevent increased hypertension.
Anxiety, related to situational crisis	Help patient identify stressors. Assess previous satisfactory coping methods with patient. Encourage patient to verbalize feelings of powerlessness and loss of control.

Patient teaching. Follow-up 24-hour urine tests (VMA, catecholamines) may be done to determine return to normal levels. When this goal is achieved, the patient is pronounced cured and may resume normal activities. If the tumor is inoperable, it is important that the patient remain under lifelong medical supervision, and the importance of compliance with prescribed treatment is stressed. Medic Alert jewelry should be worn and a wallet card carried. The patient should be taught self-monitoring of blood pressure and instructed when to call the physician if elevation occurs.

Prognosis. The prognosis after successful removal of the causative tumor is good; for an inoperable tumor, the prognosis depends on adequate medical management of hypertension.

DISORDERS OF THE PANCREAS

Diabetes Mellitus

Etiology. Diabetes mellitus, or DM (*diabetes:* "to pass through"; *mellitus:* "sweet or related to honey"), is a systemic metabolic disorder that involves improper metabolism of carbohydrates, fats, and proteins. This condition may be caused by a decrease or absolute lack of insulin production by the beta cells of the islets of Langerhans in the pancreas or by the decreased activity of the insulin that is secreted. There are several types of DM, but in each type, hyperglycemia is present as the principal clinical manifestation. Although the exact cause of DM is unknown, a number of factors have been demonstrated as contributing to its development: genetic predisposition, viruses (such as coxsackievirus B, rubella, and mumps), the aging process, diet and life-style, and ethnicity. Obesity is felt to be a major factor. Recent research has suggested that the T lymphocytes may play a role in the development of autoimmune destruction of the pancreatic insulin-producing cells.

Types of Diabetes Mellitus. There are two main types of diabetes mellitus: **type I** (insulin-dependent **diabetes mellitus** or IDDM) and **type II** (non-insulin-dependent **diabetes mellitus** or NIDDM). Type I was formerly called juvenile diabetes, or juvenile-onset diabetes. Type II was formerly called adult-onset diabetes, or maturity-onset diabetes. Other types of DM patients include those diagnosed with such conditions as pancreatitis, genetic syndromes, malnutrition, chemical- or drug-induced disease, and pregnancy. There are some distinct differences between type I and type II diabetes (Table 32-3). In type I (IDDM), destruction of beta cells in the pancreatic islets results in deficient insulin *production,* but the patient retains normal sensitivity to insulin action. In type II (NIDDM), the main problem seems to be an abnormal resistance to insulin *action.* Regardless of the type of DM, all these patients have impaired glucose tolerance. Only 5% to 10% of all people with diabetes have type I, but since they do not produce adequate amounts of endogenous (produced by the body) insulin, they must take regular injections of exogenous (from outside the body) insulin or they will die.

About 90% of people with diabetes in the United States have type II, with a high incidence among Blacks, Hispanics, and American Indians, especially members of the Pima tribe.

There are about 6 million diagnosed cases of type II diabetes in the United States, with an estimated equal number of undiagnosed cases. Cases of type II diabetes are usually diagnosed after age 30, and 80% of these patients are overweight, with a familial history of diabetes. They are usually able to secrete sufficient amounts of insulin, but their body tissues are unable to properly utilize it. These patients can usually achieve good control of their disease by diet and oral hypoglycemics, using insulin only when first diagnosed and during times of illness, surgery, or other periods when the body's insulin level is out of control.

Pathophysiology. In normal metabolism, the end-products of digestion (glucose, fatty acids and glycerol, and amino acids) are absorbed into the venous circulation and carried to the liver, where they may then be either used immediately or stored for later use. The liver can change glycerol and fatty acids into glucose, and glucose into triglycerides, as needed. Fatty acids may also be changed into **ketone bodies** (normal metabolic products, such as β-hydroxybutyric acid and aminoacetic acid, from which acetone may arise spontaneously), which serve as fuel for the muscles of the body and as an energy source for the brain. Glucose storage takes place in the form of glycogen in the liver. Free glucose in the bloodstream can always be used by the brain and

TABLE 32-3 Comparison of Diabetes Mellitus Type I (IDDM) and Diabetes Mellitus Type II (NIDDM)

Factor	Type I	Type II
Age at onset	Usually 30 years or younger	Usually more than 30 years
Body weight	Normal or underweight	80% are overweight
Symptoms at onset	Sudden; polydipsia, polyuria, weight loss, weakness, fatigue; glycosuria, hyperglycemia; acidosis, progressing to DKA	Gradual; may be asymptomatic at onset; later, may develop signs and symptoms of type I; others include slow wound healing, blurred vision, pruritus, boils or other skin infections; vaginal infections in women
Treatment	Diet, exercise, and insulin	Diet and exercise *or* diet, exercise, and oral hypoglycemic agents *or* diet, exercise, oral hypoglycemic agents, and insulin during times of illness
Incidence of complications	Frequent	Frequent
Psychosocial and sexual concerns	Irritability; altered body image; mood swings, depression; menstrual irregularities; hirsutism; decreased libido	Altered body image; amenorrhea; decreased libido; poor tolerance to stress

kidney, since it is not necessary for insulin to be present to enable glucose molecules to enter the brain cells or the glomeruli. But insulin *must* be present for muscle cells and other body cells to be able to utilize glucose. Glycogen can be changed back into glucose as needed by the body for energy. In the patient with diabetes, lack of proper amounts of insulin, or its inadequate utilization, impairs the use of glucose by the body. Thus the excess glucose accumulates in the bloodstream, and **hyperglycemia** (greater than normal amounts of glucose in the blood) exists. To rid the body of this abnormal amount of glucose, the kidneys will excrete it in the urine. This is called **glycosuria** (abnormal presence of a sugar, especially glucose, in the urine), a condition that necessitates an extra amount of water for proper dilution of the urine. The patient then develops **polyuria** (excretion of an abnormally large quantity of urine), and also experiences **polydipsia** (excessive thirst). Often the patient is unable to drink enough fluid to compensate for polyuria and may become dehydrated. Even though there is excess glucose available in the bloodstream, it cannot be utilized by the body tissues without the help of insulin. So the cells are not properly nourished, and **polyphagia** (eating to the point of gluttony) develops. In spite of increased food intake, metabolism remains faulty, and the patient loses weight. Since carbohydrates cannot be utilized properly, proteins and fats are broken down and ketone bodies used excessively for heat and energy. Because ketone bodies are acid substances, the patient may develop acidosis. Diabetic **ketoacidosis** (acidosis accompanied by an accumulation of ketones in the body), formerly called diabetic coma, may develop, and the patient could die.

Clinical Manifestations. The clinical manifestations of type I diabetes mellitus include the three classic "polys": polyuria, polydipsia, and polyphagia. As ketone bodies accumulate in the bloodstream, imbalances of sodium, potassium, and bicarbonate result. Type II diabetics, most of whom are older than age 30, experience very different signs and symptoms. In the early stages of the disease, the patient may be asymptomatic but later may complain of symptoms associated with type I, plus a number of others. These patients may not seek medical care until a severe complication such as kidney involvement, retinopathy, or gangrene occurs.

Assessment. Collection of *subjective data* to be assessed includes hunger, thirst, and nausea. In addition to frequent urination of large amounts, the patient may complain of nocturia, weakness, and fatigue. There may be blurred vision, seeing halos around lights, and headache. Symptoms such as cold extremities, cramping pain in the calves and feet during exercise or walking, decreased sensation to pain and temperature in the feet, and numbness and tingling of the lower extremities may occur. There may be pruritus. Male patients may become impotent. The patient may verbalize negative feelings about his or her body and the ability to cope with the illness. The nurse should assess coping methods, as well as the patient's knowledge about the disease process. Misunderstandings and lack of interest may result in inadequate skills to manage the necessary diabetic lifestyle, such as diet planning, injections, and exercise programs. The patient's understanding of the importance of compliance with prescribed medical treatment should be assessed, as well as the patient's willingness to obtain adequate follow-up.

Collection of *objective data* includes assessment of the skin, since slow wound healing, boils, carbuncles, and ulcerations are common. Women with DM may experience frequent vaginal infections, and vaginal discharge is often bothersome. In type I patients, weight loss and muscle wasting may be seen, but many type II patients remain obese. The skin on the lower extremities may appear shiny and thin, with less hair present. The legs and feet may feel cold to the touch, and there may be ulcerated areas. Gangrene of the toes is a dreaded sign. The nurse should assess the patient's ability to perform blood and/or urine testing and proper injection of insulin.

Diagnostic Tests. Diagnosis of DM is made on the basis of clinical manifestations, plus the patient's history and laboratory findings. The patient with random blood glucose over 200 mg/dl should be further evaluated. The glucose tolerance test is especially reliable as a diagnostic tool (Box 32-2). Blood tests commonly done include those in Box 32-2.

Since 1982 the American Diabetes Association (ADA) has recommended self-monitoring blood glucose (SMBG) instead of urine testing in any patient with IDDM. This is accomplished in a number of ways. Blood from a fingerstick may be placed on a reagent strip and compared with a color chart, or it may be placed into a reflectance meter. Another type of meter uses a glucose sensor instead of a meter, and test strips are not used; instead, a drop of blood is placed directly into the machine. SMBG is the monitoring tool of choice because it provides an accurate picture of current blood glucose levels. Its use in NIDDM patients is usually limited to stabilization of glucose control after initial diagnosis and during periods of instability of control, such as infections. SMBG is more expensive than urine testing but is felt to result in fewer hospitalizations for the patient, so it is probably more cost effective on a long-term basis. If overall achievement of control is accomplished and complications are reduced proportionally, the cost then becomes negligible.

Urine tests are definitely not as reliable as blood tests but may still be done in some agencies. However, this diagnostic tool is now almost obsolete. Usually urine tests are done with dipsticks that measure the percentages of glucose and/or acetone in a urine sample. The patient may be instructed to test the urine at home. There are several methods of accomplishing this, but regardless of which is employed, a double-voided specimen should be tested each time. Urine that has accumulated in the bladder for several hours will be much less accurate in determining the true amounts of glucose and ketones than a fresh specimen will. In the older person with diabetes, the point at which glucose will be spilled into the urine is higher than that of a younger person. In other words, the "renal threshold" is higher, and blood glucose may actually be very high, yet the urine will test negative for glucose. To obtain a specimen for testing, the patient should empty the bladder completely, than 30 to 60 minutes later, void again, and perform the test on this specimen. If the patient has an indwelling catheter, the tubing should be drained into the collection bag, then clamped for 30 minutes, after which a specimen is drawn from the port with a sterile syringe and needle to prevent contamination of the closed system. Some of the products used to test the urine for glucose only are Clinitest tablets (Ames), Chemstrip bG (Bio-Dynamics), Tes-tape (Lilly), and Diastix (Ames). Acetone testing products include Ketostix (Ames) and Acetest tablets. Ketodiastix (Ames) may be used to test for both glucose and acetone. The manufacturer's directions on all packages of these products and others must be followed exactly, because inaccurate results may occur otherwise. The results from glucose testing are usually recorded in percentages, ranging from 0% to 5%. The amount of acetone is represented by a color change, in shades of pink to purple, recorded as negative to large amounts. Testing for acetone should be done routinely when glucose in the urine is 1% or more and also during illness or during periods of high stress, because the presence of acetone in the urine indicates the possibility of impending ketoacidosis.

Box 32-2

DIAGNOSTIC TESTS FOR DIABETES MELLITUS

Fasting blood sugar (FBS). After an 8-hour fast, blood is drawn. The normal is 60 to 110 mg/dl of venous blood.

Oral glucose tolerance test (OGTT). After an 8- to 12-hour fast, a venous blood specimen is drawn and a urine sample is collected and discarded. Then the patient is given a measured amount of carbohydrate solution orally. Blood and urine samples are obtained at 30 minutes, 1 hour, and 2 hours after ingestion of the solution. The test may continue for up to a total of 4 hours, as ordered by the physician. In nondiabetic patients, blood sugar returns to normal in about 2 hours. In diabetic patients this does not occur; values will remain higher than normal for a longer time. Blood samples are drawn by the laboratory technician and urine samples are collected by the nurse, if this test is done on a hospital inpatient. The patient may usually have water orally during the testing time to facilitate the collection of urine samples. The nurse must properly label each timed specimen.

Serum insulin. Absent in IDDM; normal to high in NIDDM.

Postprandial (after a meal) blood sugar (PPBS). A fasting patient is given a measured amount of carbohydrate solution orally. An alternate method is to have the patient eat a measured amount of foods containing carbohydrates, fats, and proteins. A blood sample will be drawn 2 hours after completion of the meal. Elevated plasma glucose over 160 mg/dl may indicate the presence of DM.

Patient self-monitoring of blood glucose (SMBG). A blood sample is obtained by the fingerstick method, by either the patient or the nurse, and tested using a dipstick or machine.

Glycosylated hemoglobin (Hb A_{1c}). This blood test measures the amount of glucose that has become incorporated into the hemoglobin within an erythrocyte; these levels are reported as a percentage of the total hemoglobin. Since glycosylation occurs constantly during the 120-day life span of the erythrocyte, this test reveals the effectiveness of diabetes therapy for the preceding 8 to 12 weeks. Glycosylated hemoglobin levels remain more stable than plasma glucose levels, and are evaluated by one venipuncture every 6 to 8 weeks. Normal Hb A_{1c} is approximately 5% of the total.

Medical Management. Medical treatment for DM, no matter what type, consists mainly of *diet, exercise, and medication,* the major goal being to achieve control of the disease and prevent complications. It is hoped that the patient will assume a large part of the responsibility for self-care, with emphasis on optimal wellness instead of illness. Since 1921, when Charles Best and Frederick Banting first isolated insulin, medical science has made many dramatic strides in the care of the patient with diabetes, but physicians depend on the help obtained from other members of the health care team, especially nurses. Every newly diagnosed patient must undergo an intensive and extensive education program to learn proper diet, medication routines, home testing of blood and urine, and the role of exercise. The importance of the nurse as a teacher cannot be overemphasized.

Diet. Diet therapy for the patient with diabetes is aimed at helping to achieve a normal blood glucose level and attaining or maintaining ideal body weight, while ensuring proper growth and/or body maintenance. The services of a dietitian should be enlisted for each newly diagnosed diabetic. The menu must be individualized, taking into consideration the patient's age, weight, activity level, life-style, ethnic background, and food preferences.

TABLE 32-4 Commercially Available Forms of Insulin

Type of Insulin	Manufacturer	Strength (units/ml)	Source	Impurities (PPM)	Onset (hr)	Peak (hr)	Duration* (hr)	Glycosuria†	Hypoglycemia†
Fast-acting insulin injection									
Humulin R (human)	Lilly	100	Semisynthetic	—	0.5-4	2.5-5	5-16	Early AM(1)	Before lunch(3)
Novolin R (human)	Novo Nordisk	100	Semisynthetic	—	0.5-4	2.5-5	5-16	Early AM	Before lunch
Regular (purified pork) insulin	Novo Nordisk	100	Pork	<10	0.5	2.5-5	8	Early AM	Before lunch
Regular insulin	Novo Nordisk	100	Pork	<25	0.5-1	3-6	6-8	Early AM	Before lunch
Regular Iletin I	Lilly	100	Beef and pork	<25	0.5-1	3-6	6-8	Early AM	Before lunch
Regular Iletin II (Beef)	Lilly	100	Beef	<10	0.5-1	3-6	6-8	Early AM	Before lunch
Regular Iletin II (Pork)	Lilly	100, 500	Pork	<10	0.5-1	3-6	6-8	Early AM	Before lunch
Velosulin	Novo Nordisk	100	Pork	<10	0.5	1-3	8	EarlyAM	Before lunch
Velosulin (human)	Novo Nordisk	100	Semisynthetic	—	0.5	1-3	8	Early AM	Before lunch
Prompt insulin zinc suspension									
Semilente Iletin I	Lilly	100	Beef and pork	<25	0.5-1	4-6	12-16	Early AM	Before lunch
Semilente insulin	Novo Nordisk	100	Beef	<25	0.5-1	4-6	12-16	Early AM	Before lunch
Intermediate-acting isophane insulin suspension (NPH)									
Humulin N (human)	Lilly	100	Semisynthetic	—	1-4	4-12	16-28	Before lunch(2)	3 PM to supper(3)
Insulatard (NPH)	Novo Nordisk	100	Pork	<10	1.5	4-12	24	Before lunch	3 PM to supper
Insulatard (NPH) human	Novo Nordisk	100	Semisynthetic	—	1.5	4-12	24	Before lunch	3 PM to supper
Novolin N (human)	Novo Nordisk	100	Semisynthetic	—	1-4	4-12	16-28	Before lunch	3 PM to supper
NPH Insulin	Novo Nordisk	100	Beef	<10	1-1.5	8-12	24	Before lunch	3 PM to supper
NPH (purified pork) insulin	Novo Nordisk	100	Pork	<10	1.5	4-12	24	Before lunch	3 PM to supper
Isophane insulin suspension and insulin injection									
Humulin 70/30	Lilly	100	Semisynthetic	—	0.5	4-12	24	Before lunch	3 PM to supper
Mixtard	Novo Nordisk	100	Pork	<10	0.5	4-8	24	Before lunch	3 PM to supper
Novolin 70/30 (human)	Novo Nordisk	100	Semisynthetic	—	0.5	4-12	24	Before lunch	3 PM to supper
Insulin zinc suspension									
Humulin L	Lilly	100	Semisynthetic	—	1-4	7-15	16-28	Before lunch	3 PM to supper
Lente Iletin I	Lilly	100	Beef and pork	<25	1-1.5	8-12	24	Before lunch	3 PM to supper
Lente Iletin II	Lilly	100	Beef or pork	<10	1-1.5	8-12	24	Before lunch	3 PM to supper
Lente insulin	Novo Nordisk	40, 100	Beef	<10	1-1.5	8-12	24	Before lunch	3 PM to supper
Lente (purified pork) insulin	Novo Nordisk	100	Pork	<10	2.5	7-15	22	Before lunch	3 PM to supper
Novolin L (human)	Novo Nordisk	100	Semisynthetic	—	1-4	7-15	16-28	Before lunch	3 PM to supper
Extended insulin zinc suspension									
Humulin U Ultralente	Lilly	100	Semisynthetic	—	4-8	12-18	24-28	Supper to bedtime	2 AM to breakfast
Ultralente Iletin I	Lilly	100	Beef and pork	<25	4-8	16-18	36†	Supper to bedtime	2 AM to breakfast
Ultralente insulin	Novo Nordisk	100	Beef	<25	4-8	16-18	36†	Supper to bedtime	2 AM to breakfast

*The times listed are averages based on a newly diagnosed diabetic patient. Factors modifying these times include patient variation, site and route of administration, and dosage.
†Most frequently occurs when insulin is administered (1) at bedtime the previous night; (2) before breakfast the previous day; (3) before breakfast the same day.

The ability to choose and pay for groceries, prepare food, and properly store leftovers must be assessed. After discharge from the hospital, detailed dietary instructions will be of no use to the patient who does not have money, cooking skills, and appliances necessary to comply with them. If the patient is living with the family, the person who will be planning and preparing the meals must be educated along with the patient, and this person should be taught how to fit the patient's dietary needs into the family menus. The physician and dietitian will decide the proper amounts of each nutrient in the dietary prescription. Diets are based on ADA recommendations, and patients may obtain additional information and menus from that organization at no cost.

Quantitative diabetic diets consist of measured amounts of food in the Food Pyramid, with 50% to 60% of total kilocalories from carbohydrates, 12% to 20% of total kilocalories from proteins, and no more than 30% of total kilocalories from fats. Complex carbohydrates and polyunsaturated fats are best for these patients to use. Concentrated carbohydrates such as candy or other sweets should not be used by the diabetic for whom an ADA diet is prescribed. Results of recent studies have shown that different carbohydrate foods affect the blood glucose level in different ways; this varying effect is termed the *glycemic index*. So, for the person with diabetes, emphasis may be placed not only on the amount of carbohydrate eaten but on the glycemic index of those foods.

The *qualitative* diet is unmeasured and more unstructured, stressing moderation when selecting food from the Food Pyramid and reducing the use of simple carbohydrates, saturated fats, and alcohol. This diet may be used for the patient whose blood glucose levels are not extremely high, for the pediatric patient, or for the patient who is noncompliant with the ADA diet.

Insulin-dependent patients are usually given midafternoon and bedtime snacks in addition to their regular three meals a day. It is important that food intake be evenly distributed throughout the day, taking insulin dosage and exercise into consideration. The patient who plans to engage in strenuous exercise may be able to eat more food, because exercise increases the absorption rate of insulin, thereby enabling muscles to utilize glucose more effectively. (For further information on diabetic diets, see Chapter 19.)

Diabetics should do a fingerstick blood glucose level test before each meal and at bedtime until their disease is under control. Thereafter, they usually test once or twice a day, as directed by the physician, unless they become ill or their diabetes becomes uncontrolled. Urine testing may be done at home, instead of blood testing, but should be on a regular basis, such as before meals, using a double-voided specimen each time.

The patient may need follow-up visits with a dietitian as well as with the physician. Obese patients with NIDDM are encouraged to lose weight, because many are then able to control their diabetes with only diet and exercise, eliminating the need for medication. The patient with IDDM should try to attain and maintain ideal weight, because better control of the condition usually results. Good control of DM is desirable in helping to prevent complications.

Exercise. The patient with diabetes should exercise regularly. The physician will help determine the best type of exercise for each patient. Exercise is beneficial, not only because it aids in promoting proper utilization of glucose, but also because it is important to the overall functioning of the cardiovascular system and will increase the patient's feeling of well-being.

Medications. Insulin and oral hypoglycemics are the drugs of choice for patients with diabetes (Table 32-4). Insulin administration is necessary for all patients with type I and in patients with type II who cannot be controlled on diet or oral hypoglycemics alone. Insulin may be obtained from the pancreatic tissue of pigs or cows and has recently been produced synthetically employing recombinant DNA techniques using *Escherichia coli* bacteria (Fig. 32-10). Insulin is a hormone and is absorbed into the patient's bloodstream. There are many types and brands of insulin. A number of different chemicals can be added to insulins to potentiate their action, and these types cannot be administered intravenously. Only regular insulin can be given intravenously. Insulin is given subcutaneously, and in rare instances, such as in DKA, is given intramuscularly to some patients. When giving insulin, the nurse must be careful to inject into the *subcutaneous pocket* (space between the fat and muscle layers) only, avoiding depositing the medication directly into the fat or muscle (Fig. 32-11 on p. 970). Insulin is packaged in vials containing 40, 100, or 500 U/ml. Syringes are calibrated by units, and may be 30 U (0.3 ml), 50 U (0.5 ml), or 100 U (1 ml) size (see Fig. 32-10).

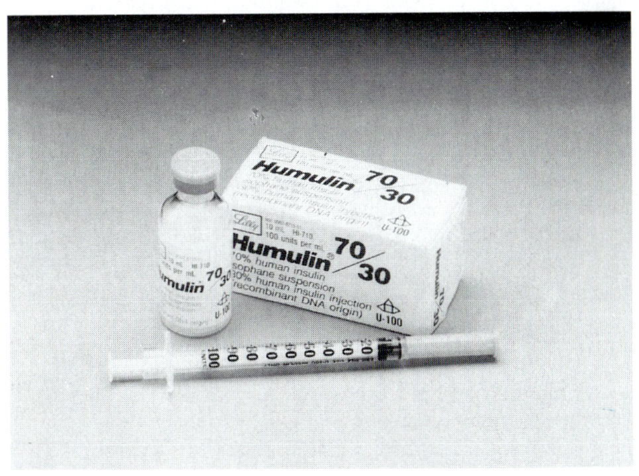

FIG. 32-10 U-100 insulin and disposable U-100 insulin syringe.

Needles are very fine, usually 25- to 32-gauge, to be as atraumatic to the tissue as possible. Regardless of the units in a vial or on a syringe, the nurse *must* be sure that these match before drawing up a dose of insulin. Needles and syringes used now in the hospital are of the disposable type. However, some older patients may still be using glass syringes and metal needles in the home, sterilizing them by boiling. An open bottle of insulin currently being used does not have to be kept in the refrigerator. In fact, it is now believed that insulin should be administered at room temperature, not straight from the refrigerator, to help prevent insulin **lipodystrophy** (abnormality in the metabolism or deposition of fats). Extra bottles are stored in the refrigerator.

Box 32-3 offers guidelines for preparation of a dose of insulin, one or two types at a time.

Patients who self-inject insulin at home may want to have a family member oversee the procedure. Nurses administering insulin injections should always have the dose drawn up in the syringe checked by another licensed person to prevent medication errors. The patient with diabetes should ideally be taught self-injection technique before discharge from the hospital. However, some patients are unable to perform this because of physical problems or intellectual incapacity, visual disturbances, or age. In these cases, family members or others have to administer the injections. Before discharge, either the pa-

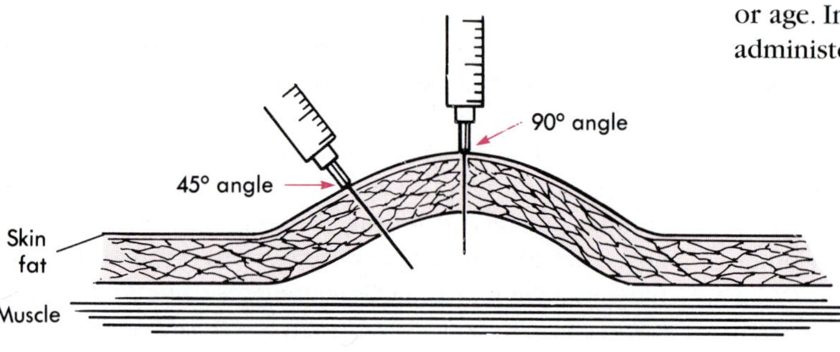

FIG. 32-11 Insulin is injected into the pocket between subcutaneous fat and muscle occurring when the skin is pinched up. The angle of injection may be 45 or 90 degrees.

Box 32-3 PREPARATION OF INSULIN

1. Thoroughly wash hands with warm water and soap.
2. Assemble all equipment needed, such as needle and syringe unit, prep sponge, and insulin.
3. Turn the insulin vial onto its side and gently rotate between the hands several times to be sure it is mixed. The precipitate should be evenly blended. This does not need to be done with regular insulin because it has no precipitate. Never shake insulin vigorously, because this creates air bubbles.
4. Clean the rubber stopper on the vial with a prep sponge.
5. Remove the needle cover and draw in the same amount of air as units of insulin to be injected.
6. Insert the needle into the rubber stopper of the vial and then inject air; invert the bottle with the syringe unit attached, making sure the tip of the needle is below the level of the insulin so air will not be drawn into the syringe.
7. Pull back slowly on the plunger, a few units past the desired dose of insulin.
8. Inspect for air bubbles in the syringe; if any are seen, gently tap the barrel until they rise to the top, then push back into the vial with plunger, to the level of the desired dose of insulin.
9. Holding onto the barrel and plunger, remove the syringe unit and put the needle cover back on. Check insulin dose with a second licensed nurse. Proceed with injection procedure.

TWO INSULINS

1. Follow steps 1 through 5 at left.
2. Insert the desired amount of air into the vial of the longer-acting insulin first.
3. Inject the desired amount of air into the shorter-acting insulin vial; leave the syringe unit in this vial, invert, and proceed through steps 6 through 9 but do not inject yet. *Set the vial of shorter-acting insulin out of reach to prevent accidental reuse.*
4. Insert the needle into the vial of longer-acting insulin, being careful to hold onto the plunger so none of the insulin in the syringe enters that vial.
5. Slowly pull the plunger to the level of the combined total of both types of insulin desired (e.g., regular 10 U, NPH 30 U, totalling 40 U). Do not pull extra units into the syringe! Take special care not to get any air bubbles into the syringe, because they will displace some of the insulin and make the dose incorrect. If this happens, you will have to discard the whole syringeful and start all over again. Check insulin dose with a second licensed nurse.
6. If the dose is correct, proceed with the injection procedure.

tient or the significant other, or both, must display the ability to correctly draw up and inject insulin. In a newly diagnosed patient, regular insulin may be injected before each meal. After reasonable control of hyperglycemia is achieved, the dosage schedule may be changed to once a day, in the morning before breakfast, with the type of insulin being intermediate- or long-acting. See Table 32-4 for types of insulin. Sometimes diabetic patients take two doses of insulin, in divided doses given before breakfast and before the evening meal. The nurse should be alert for signs of **hypoglycemia** (a less than normal amount of glucose in the blood, usually caused by administration of too much insulin, excessive secretion of insulin by the islet cells of the pancreas, or dietary deficiency) at the peak of action of whatever type of insulin the patient is taking and the patient should be instructed to notify a member of the nursing staff if any of the following signs of hypoglycemic (insulin) reaction occurs: faintness, sudden weakness, excessive perspiration, irritability, hunger, palpitations, trembling, or drowsiness.

After appropriate blood or urine testing, the patient will choose an injection site. The subcutaneous pocket is the desired layer into which insulin should be injected. Insulin should *not* be injected into the muscle, because it enters the bloodstream too quickly and could cause hypoglycemia. Site selection is crucial, as is site rotation. Patients may find it easier to keep track of their injection sites by recording each injection on a numbered chart (Fig. 32-12).

Because of differing anatomical absorption rates of insulin, it is currently recommended that injections should be given in all the available areas in a site, such as the thigh, before moving to another site. In this way the diabetic may take eight or more injections, spaced 1 to 1½ inches apart, thus allowing the tissues in other sites to recover more fully before being used again. This technique helps prevent lipodystrophy and lipoatrophy, conditions that can lead to unsightly lumps under the skin and inhibition of insulin absorption. If the patient engages in heavy exercise, an injection site may be chosen where movement will not be as great, because exercise may increase insulin absorption. The technique for insulin injection is described in Box 32-4 on p. 972.

There are several new delivery systems now available to the person who finds injections emotionally and/or physically uncomfortable. These include automatic injectors, the jet stream (needleless) injector, the Insuflon indwelling insulin delivery service, and the button infuser.

Another method of insulin administration is continuous subcutaneous insulin infusion (CSII) using the external infusion pump. This small, battery-operated, computerized device is worn on the user's body, usually in a pocket or on a belt. It is attached to a thin tubing with a needle on the end, which is inserted into the subcutaneous tissue. A continuous, or basal, rate of regular insulin (e.g., Humulin BR) delivery can be programmed, with bolus doses administered as needed. For carefully selected and properly educated patients, the pump offers improved flexibility in life-style, improved control of blood glucose and Hb A_{1c} levels, as well as freedom from multiple daily injections. Properly disassembled, insulin pumps such as the H-Tron V100 (Disetronic) can even be worn during bathing or while swimming. The insertion site is usually the abdomen, but the buttocks, thighs, arms, and sections of the back may be used, with the insertion site covered by a clear occlusive dressing, which is usually changed every other day.

Oral hypoglycemics are compounds that stimulate the beta cells in the pancreatic islets to produce insulin.

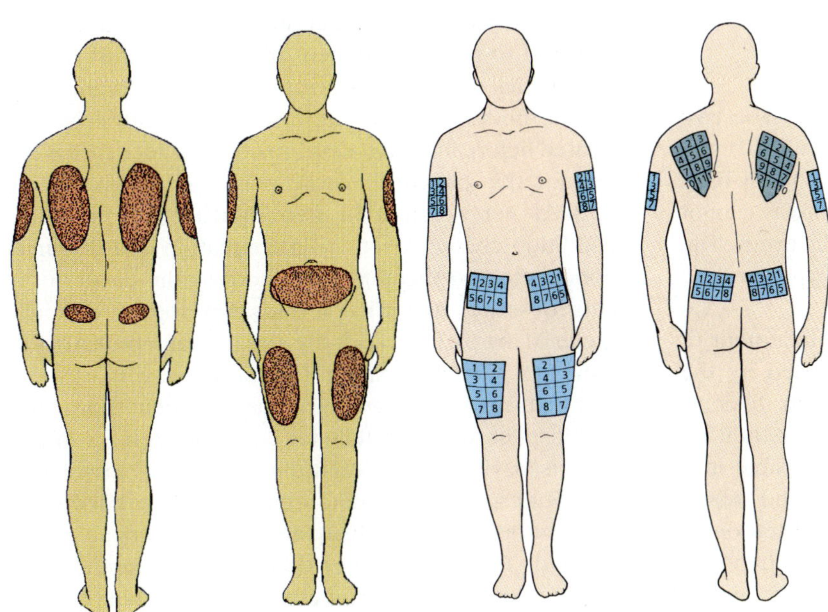

FIG. 32-12 Rotation of sites for insulin injections.

Box 32-4 TECHNIQUE FOR INSULIN INJECTION

1. Follow steps 1 through 9 or 1 through 6 from Box 32-3, as before, to prepare the insulin dose.
2. Don disposable gloves.
3. Clean the injection site with a prep swab, using a circular motion. Allow the alcohol to dry. Place the swab between the last two fingers of the hand not used to inject the insulin.
4. Pick up the syringe and remove the needle cover and lay it aside. Hold the syringe like a dart.
5. Using the other hand, gently pinch up at least a 2-inch fold of tissue (not just the skin!).
6. Quickly insert the needle into the top (apex) of the fold, entering the *subcutaneous pocket.* The "soft spot" technique is to insert the needle about 1 inch to the side of the apex of the fold, into softer tissue, entering the pocket. The needle should be inserted at a 90-degree angle unless the patient is very thin and has little subcutaneeous tissue. In that case, the angle may be reduced by up to 45 degrees.
7. Release the skin fold and use that hand to steady the barrel of the syringe. Pull back on the plunger to check for blood. If any is seen, remove the syringe unit and start over with a second dose of insulin.
8. If no blood is seen, inject the insulin over a period of 3 to 5 seconds.
9. Place the alcohol swab against the needle hub, at the injection site, and pull the syringe unit straight out in one swift motion. Gently press on the injection site for a few seconds, but *do not massage the site.*
10. Carefully place the entire unit, uncapped, into the sharps container provided.
11. Record the injection site and insulin dose on a chart or other documentation sheet and store insulin and other supplies properly.

These drugs are *not* an oral form of insulin. The two groups of hypoglycemics are the biguanides (DBI) and the sulfonylureas (Table 32-5). Biguanides are rarely used now because of their toxicity. The sulfonylureas cannot be taken by persons who are allergic to sulfa drugs. The main side effect of oral hypoglycemics is hypoglycemic reaction.

Another drug that may be used in the treatment of DM is glucagon, a hormone normally secreted by the alpha cells of the pancreas. It stimulates the liver to change stored glycogen into glucose, which is then released into the bloodstream. Glucagon is available in a purified, crystallized form for reconstruction and subcutaneous, intramuscular, or intravenous administration in the event of loss of consciousness as a result of hypoglycemic reaction. The usual dose is 0.5 to 1.0 mg for adults, with smaller doses for children. Some form of oral protein and carbohydrate, such as milk and crackers, should be given after the patient regains consciousness. A commercially prepared kit containing glucagon is carried by many people with diabetes, along with concentrated carbohydrate such as candy or glucose gel.

The surgical treatment of DM, type I (IDDM), is still an experimental area. Two procedures are now available to selected patients. One is pancreas transplant, a procedure first performed at the University of Minnesota in 1966. The other is implantation of an insulin-infusion pump under the skin. Much research into these two surgical procedures is currently being conducted, as is pancreatic islet transplant between identical twins. Today, many people have benefited from pancreatic transplant.

Nursing Interventions. Persons with diabetes may be hospitalized as a direct result of their disease process, or they may have a different primary diagnosis. The main focus of nursing interventions must always be on the primary diagnosis, but the nurse must remember that the patient is also diabetic and is susceptible to a number of complications in addition to all those experienced by nondiabetic patients.

Daily routine for the patient with diabetes includes accurate monitoring of blood glucose levels, either by fingerstick specimens or by laboratory testing. Urine testing, when done, should be on a second-voided specimen each time. Careful attention to diet is important, and the nurse should note the amount of food eaten at each meal and record it accurately. If the patient with type I DM is not hungry, is nauseated, or cannot eat for any other reason, the next dose of insulin may be withheld and administered later, as determined by the physician. If the patient does not like the types of food on the meal tray, the dietitian should be consulted and a visit arranged.

Good skin care is essential for the person with diabetes, because poor circulation, so common in diabetes, can lead to the development of skin problems. Any abnormalities such as cuts, scratches, or lesions anywhere on the body should be reported to the physician and treated before infection develops. Special foot care is crucial for this patient, because poor circulation and decreased nerve sensation **neuropathy** (any abnormal condition characterized by inflammation and degeneration of the peripheral nerves) increase the danger of ulcers or other abnormal lesions developing into gangrene. Many patients seek the services of a podiatrist for their foot care. The patient should thoroughly wash the feet with soap and water every day, dry them thoroughly, and inspect them carefully for cracks, blisters, or foreign objects, paying special attention to the area between the toes. Foot soaks or powders are not recommended. Clean socks should be worn daily, and tight garters should be avoided. The toenails should be clipped straight across so the edges do not become ingrown. The nurse should

TABLE 32-5 Sulfonylureas

Generic and Brand Name	Usual Daily Dose	Onset of Action (hr)	Peak of Action (hr)	Duration of Action (hr)
Acetohexamide (Demylor)	250-1500 mg	1	4-5	12-18
Chlorpropamide (Diabinese, Glucamide)	100-500 mg	1	3-6	24-60
Glipizide (Glucotrol)	5-40 mg	1	2-6	12-24
Glyburide (DiaBeta, Micronase)	1.25-20 mg	1	2-4	16-24
Glyburide (Glynase)	0.75-12 mg	1	2-4	16-24
Tolazamide (Tolinase)	100-1000 mg	4-6	4-8	12-24
Tolbutamide (Orinase, Oramide)	500-3000 mg	½-1	3-5	6-12

never trim the toenails of a patient with diabetes without a physician's written order. No hot water bottles or heating pads should be put on the feet, because burns may occur and not be felt. Sturdy, properly fitting shoes should be worn, and the patient should not go barefoot at any time. The physician should be notified immediately of any injury to the toes or feet.

The patient who is receiving insulin should be watched very carefully for development of hypoglycemia, especially when the particular kind of insulin being injected is at its peak of action. Hypoglycemia is seen much less frequently in patients receiving oral hypoglycemics, but it can occur.

The emotional aspects of diabetes are numerous, and many patients experience a period of denial after the initial diagnosis. Some patients become very depressed. Since this disease affects all age groups, nursing interventions must be tailored to fit the needs of each patient. The gerontological box highlights considerations for the older adult. Patients with diabetes must have help in working through their feelings, so the nurse must be a good listener and be supportive at all times. The patient who does not satisfactorily resolve any major problems in accepting the diagnosis of DM may be noncompliant with the treatment plan.

The nurse who supervises the patient in a home setting must encourage the patient to take the prescribed medication faithfully, eat the right kinds of food, test blood and/or urine correctly, and exercise regularly. If a family member is going to be responsible for the patient's care, the nurse must make sure that the caregiver is functioning adequately in this role. Some patients live alone and do very well caring for themselves, with occasional visits from a home health or public health nurse. Others who have visual disturbances, circulatory problems, or other conditions may need daily visits and more actual nursing intervention, such as help with hygiene, arrangements for meals, and administration of insulin injections. See the nursing care plan for the patient with diabetes mellitus on pp. 974-975.

GERONTOLOGICAL CONDSIDERATIONS

- Diabetes mellitus is the most common endocrine disorder seen in older adults.
- Glucose tolerance decreases with aging, and blood glucose levels tend to increase.
- The classic signs and symptoms of diabetes may not be obvious in the older adults.
- Dietary management may be complicated by a variety of social, economic, and financial factors.
- Hormone supplements must be administered with caution, since side effects are more likely to occur.
- Older adult diabetics are at increased risk for infection and should be counseled to receive proper immunizations and seek regular medical attention for even minor symptoms.

Acute complications. One of the acute complications of DM is coma, which may be attributed to three different causes. The first type of coma can occur during diabetic ketoacidosis (DKA), which results from inadequate amounts of insulin present or from inadequate insulin utilization. The second type, hyperglycemic hyperosmolar nonketotic coma (HHNC), involves no acidosis or ketonemia, but results from excess glucose presence, diuresis, and dehydration without adequate fluid replacement. The third type may occur during hypoglycemic reaction, which results from an excess amount of insulin available, with an inadequate amount of glucose present. These three complications are compared and contrasted in Table 32-6 on p. 976. Emergency care of the patient experiencing DKA or hypoglycemia is found in Box 32-5 on p. 975 and Box 32-6 on p. 976.

Another acute complication faced by the patient with diabetes is the development of infections of any kind. The presence of hyperglycemia and ketonemia hinders the phagocytic action of leukocytes. An infection can therefore become more severe and last longer, with poor wound healing taking place. The possibility of DKA increases in the presence of infection, and control of the

NURSING CARE PLAN: ***THE PATIENT WITH DIABETES MELLITUS***

Mrs. Toren is an obese, 52-year-old married woman with NIDDM diagnosed 3 years ago. She was referred to a short-term ambulatory diabetes education program by her physician for instruction on insulin administration since blood glucose control had not been achieved with dietary measures.

The nursing history identified the following:

She sees referral as necessary but perceives it and inability to control weight and blood glucose as a personal failure.

She maintains inconsistent sleep/activity schedule. (Works 8 PM to 8 AM Saturday and Sunday with 2 to 4 hours sleep during day; rises at 8 AM and retires at 11 PM on other days.)

She has accurate knowledge about dietary modifications and has participated successfully in several weight-reduction programs with 20- to 40-pound weight loss each time.

She does not exercise consistently.

She has monitored blood glucose once or twice on self (self-monitoring of blood glucose [SMBG]).

She states that work is important to her; satisfactions are derived from work and group socialization, and it "keeps me busy."

She fears that her husband will die suddenly at home. Two years ago she had performed CPR when he had a cardiac arrest at home. Realizes that she maintains work schedule "to keep me from worrying about my husband."

Objective data included blood glucose, 220 mg/dl; weight, 200 lb; BP 134/84.

Collaborative nursing actions include teaching Mrs. Toren those measures that will help her achieve control of blood glucose (insulin, diet, and exercise) and to detect, prevent, and treat hypoglycemic reactions. The nurse reported Mrs. Toren's work schedule to the physician and asked for insulin dosage alterations on weekends. The physician was unaware of her work schedule and stated that blood glucose control could not be optimum with this schedule.

Nursing diagnoses	Patient goals/expected outcomes	Nursing interventions
Knowledge deficit: self-injections, self-blood glucose monitoring, related to lack of exposure	Patient will independently administer insulin to self. Patient will perform SMBG accurately. Patient will use measurements obtained by SMBG to achieve blood glucose below 140 mg/dl. Patient will be able to detect and treat hypoglycemia.	Support patient as necessary to self-inject insulin. Observe patient's skill in SMBG; correct as necessary. Review with patient the effect of activity, dietary intake, and insulin on blood glucose. Instruct patient on frequency and timing of SMBG. Review with patient signs and symptoms and treatment measures. Refer to dietitian for modification of diet necessary with insulin and for verification of diet knowledge.

Health maintenance, altered, related to ineffective coping skill	Patient will state at least one change that will improve blood glucose control.	Teach patient effects of stress, lack of exercise, and activity pattern on blood glucose. Explore with patient willingness and ability to change behaviors: sleep/activity, coping, and exercise. Engage patient in mutual problem solving; refrain from prescribing. Explore sources for long-term support in learning more effective coping skills; suggest support groups: 1. For spouses of patients with myocardial infarction 2. For weight loss and *maintenance* of weight loss 3. Available at work in health service program Suggest to patient that she seek a trial period on day shift on week ends.

CRITICAL THINKING QUESTIONS

1. Mrs. Torean has received Humulin 25 units subcutaneously at 7:30 AM. She has eaten her ADA diet at breakfast and lunch. At 3:00 PM, she complains of being hungry, nervous, and tremulous. The immediate nursing intervention would include:
2. Mrs. Torean states, "I need to lose about 40 pounds, and I'm considering joining a weight-reduction club." Helpful suggestions by the nurse for Mrs. Torean would include:
3. In discharge planning, the nurse notes that Mrs. Torean has poorly fitting shoes. Important discharge teaching for foot care for Mrs. Torean would include:

Box 32-5

EMERGENCY CARE FOR DIABETIC KETOCIDOSIS (DKA)

Usual Treatment During Acute Stage

An IV is started, using an 18-gauge needle, and fluid replacement is begun, usually with normal saline. Regular insulin (the only kind that can be given IV) may be added to the IV fluid, but is usually hung separately, as a piggy-back infusion, using 100 units regular insulin in 500 ml normal saline. The infusion is administered with a pump controller. The infusion rate is adjusted to obtain/maintain desired blood glucose levels.

- IV replacement of potassium to help move insulin into cells
- Oxygen administration; insertion of nasogastric tube: connected to intermittent suction
- Cardiac monitoring; central venous pressure (CVP) and Swan-Ganz monitoring if available
- Foley catheter usually inserted with intake and output monitored hourly
- Vital signs and neurological status assessed frequently
- Hourly determination of blood glucose level (Accu-check method or venous sample)

Nursing Interventions During and After DKA

- Keep airway patent.
- Maintain patent intravenous infusion at prescribed rate.
- Keep accurate intake and output record.
- Do accurate blood testing for glucose and urine testing for acetone.
- Monitor vital signs frequently, and assess cardiac status on monitor.
- Assess level of consciousness frequently, and perform neurological checks as ordered.
- Assess the causation of DKA.

TABLE 32-6 Comparison of Diabetic Ketoacidosis, Hypoglycemic Reaction, and Hyperglycemic Hyperosmolar Nonketotic Coma

Assessment	Ketoacidosis (DKA)	Hypoglycemic Reaction	Hyperglycemic Hyperosmolar Nonketotic Coma (HHNC)
Type of diabetes	Type I (IDDM)	Type I (IDDM) or type II (NIDDM)	Type II (NIDDM)
Cause	Inadequate insulin present	Too much insulin or oral hypoglycemic agent present	Inadequate insulin or oral hypoglycemic agent present
Patient history	Omitted or insufficient dose of insulin, stress, GI upsets, dietary noncompliance	Reduced food intake, delayed meal, too much exercise	Reduced fluid/food intake with increased urine output resulting in *severe* dehydration
Onset of symptoms	Hours to days	Minutes to hours	Days
Previous diagnosis as having diabetes	Almost always	Yes; on medication	Usually type II, on hypoglycemic agent
Age of patient	Usually younger patient	Usually younger patient	Usually elderly patient
Apperance of skin	Hot, dry	Cool, moist	Hot, dry; body temperature elevated
Breath	Fruity (from acetone)	Normal	Normal
Mucous membranes	Dry	Moist	Very dry
Respirations	Deep; may have Kussmaul respirations (air hunger) as a result of metabolic acidosis	Rapid, shallow	Normal
Neurosensory	Drowsiness to coma	Impaired consciousness, personality changes, may lose consciousness	Lethargy, decreased consciousness, may lose consciousness
Blood pressure	Low	Normal	Decreased
Glycosuria and ketonuria	Present	Absent	Glycosuria present; no ketonuria
Polyuria and polydipsia	Present	Absent	Present
Hunger	Absent; may have nausea/vomiting	Present; may be nauseated	Absent
Blood glucose level	Usually 300-800 mg/dl	Usually below 50 mg/dl	600-2000 mg/dl; serum osmolality very increased
Emergency treatment	Insulin, usually regular	Glucose (oral or intravenous) or glucagon (sub-q, IM, or IV)	Large amounts of intravenous fluids; regular insulin

Box 32-6

EMERGENCY CARE FOR HYPOGLYCEMIC REACTION

Immediate Treatment: If Conscious

Give patient 10 to 20 g of oral glucose in some form, such as 4 oz orange juice or regular soft drink (*not* diet drink), half of any kind of candy bar; commercially prepared concentrated dextrose tablets or glucose paste; 1 tube Cake Mate Icing gel (small); 2 tsp sugar or honey; 6 jelly beans or gumdrops; 5 or 6 Lifesavers or other roll candy; 4 animal crackers; 1 granola bar.

Immediate Treatment: If Unconscious

Squeeze one tube of glucagon gel between teeth and gums, in buccal space, or give glucagon 0.5 to 1.0 mg subcutaneously or intramuscularly; get patient to hospital. Hospitalized patients may receive IV bolus of 20 ml of 50% glucose or 50 ml of 20% glucose; glucagon may be given intravenously. May need IV 10% or 20% glucose at 100 ml/hr to follow.

Nursing Interventions During and After Hypoglycemic Episode

- Stay with the patient; check vital signs and do fingerstick blood glucose levels.
- Monitor for worsening of condition, or relief of symptoms.
- If patient becomes unconscious, administer glucagon buccal, subcutaneously, intramuscularly, or intravenously.
- Be sure patient ingests food such as milk, crackers with peanut butter (6), or 1 slice cheese and 6 crackers after symptoms terminate.
- Observe closely for 1 to 2 hours after cessation of symptoms.
- Notify physician about the hypoglycemic reaction.
- Assess reason the reaction may have occurred.

disease is harder to achieve. Patients with diabetes are often hospitalized for treatment of infections that might be handled on an outpatient basis for the nondiabetic patient.

Long-term complications. Long-term complications of diabetes include blindness, cardiovascular problems, and renal failure. Diabetes causes more cases of blindness in the United States than any other disease process. Diabetic retinopathy involves progressive changes in the microcirculation of the retina, resulting in hemorrhages, scar tissue formation, and various degrees of retinal detachment. New surgical techniques such as laser beam coagulation of retinal vessels may improve vision for selected patients with early diagnosis. Vascular changes in patients with diabetes, especially capillary changes, contribute to the development of renal sclerosis, often progressing to end-stage renal disease (ESRD). Many of these patients have to undergo either peritoneal dialysis or hemodialysis as a result. Diabetes contributes to accelerated atherosclerotic changes in the blood vessels, resulting in myocardial infarction, stroke, and the development of gangrene in the lower extremities. Many people with diabetes have to undergo amputation as a result of this. Additionally, nervous system manifestations (diabetic neuropathy) are commonly seen, which cause pain and decreased sensation in the extremities and contribute to the development of diabetic gangrene. Many men with diabetes experience problems with impotence or premature ejaculation. Patients of either gender may have orthostatic hypotension and bladder or bowel dysfunction.

THERAPEUTIC DIALOGUE

Mr. Garcia is a 67-year-old Hispanic male who was diagnosed 18 months ago with NIDDM. He has done well on a regimen of diet, exercise, and oral hypoglycemic medication *(DiaBeta 2.5 mg daily).* Three days ago he dropped a brick on his right foot while remodeling his fireplace and was treated in the emergency room. He is being seen today for a follow-up visit with his internist. The office nurse, Mrs. Buchanan, will first talk with him and assess his condition.

Nurse: Good morning, Mr. Garcia. How are you doing this morning?

Mr. Garcia: Much better, thank you. My foot still gives me a little trouble when I walk very far, but the swelling is down. I've been watching for red streaks, like they told me to in the emergency room, but so far there is only this scraped place and a bruise on the top of my foot *(shows nurse the area).*

Nurse: That's good. What kind of treatment are you using for your injured foot?

Mr. Garcia: I'm washing my foot twice a day with soap and water, and putting Neosporin ointment on the scrape, and then putting on a Bandaid.

Nurse: That sounds as if it should be adequate. Now let me get a close look at both feet. *(Thoroughly examines the injured area, as well as the rest of the right foot; then examines the left foot.)* The skin on your feet looks a little dry, Mr. Garcia, and your toenails are getting quite thick and long. Do you have any problems cutting them?

Mr. Garcia: I sure do! It's pretty hard for me to see exactly where I need to clip them sometimes, and I'm afraid I'll cut my toe, so I usually just let them go until my wife can help me. She's scared of cutting me, so she usually doesn't get them short enough.

Nurse: I understand. Proper foot care is very important for any patient with diabetes to prevent complications such as infection or tissue injury that could become very serious. Dr. Miller usually refers his patients to a podiatrist when they are having problems such as yours. A podiatrist specializes in care of the feet, and can properly trim your toenails as needed, as well as care for any corns or calluses that may develop.

Mr. Garcia: That sounds like a really good idea. I sure don't want to wind up like my cousin and some other people I've seen, having to have a toe or my whole foot amputated! Can you give me the name of a good podiatrist?

Nurse: Yes, I can. (*Hands pamphlet to Mr. Garcia.*) This pamphlet stresses the importance of foot care, and on the back page has the names of four podiatrists Dr. Miller recommends. You can choose the one you prefer. Now, I'm going to get Dr. Miller so that he can examine you.

Mr. Garcia: Thanks, Mrs. Buchanan. It's really good not to have to worry about cutting those toenails anymore!

Nursing diagnoses and interventions for the patient with diabetes mellitus include but are not limited to the following:

NURSING DIAGNOSES	NURSING INTERVENTIONS
Knowledge deficit: management of diabetes mellitus, related to lack of exposure	Assess level of understanding of disease process. Institute diabetic teaching plan. Have patient participate in planning daily routine, anticipating discharge and home care.
Powerlessness, related to chronic illness	Provide opportunities for patient to express feelings about self and illness. Encourage patient's participation in all aspects of self-care. Provide positive reinforcement. Maintain calm, confident attitude.
Tissue perfusion altered: peripheral, renal, related to reduced arterial blood flow	Assess peripheral pulses, skin color, temperature, capillary refill. Teach patient to avoid pressure against popliteal area and to avoid constricting hose and socks.
Fluid volume deficit, high risk for, related to excessive loss through physiological routes	Assess skin turgor for dehydration. Encourage intake of noncaloric liquids. Monitor I&O.

NURSING DIAGNOSES	NURSING INTERVENTIONS
Nutrition altered: potential for more than body requirements, related to excessive intake	Arrange consultation with dietitian and reinforce the dietary prescription.
	Allow patient to verbalize concerns about diet.
Skin integrity impaired, high risk for, related to internal factors	Assess feet daily for skin changes and pressure areas.
	Instruct patient regarding proper foot care.
	Encourage good hydration and nutritional status.
Coping, ineffective individual, related to personal vulnerability	Assist patient to assess personal strengths and weaknesses, current stressors, and stress-management skills.
	Encourage maximal self-care. Assist patient in determining realistic goals.
	Refer patient to appropriate agencies and services (local support groups, American Diabetes Association).
Therapeutic regimen (individual), ineffective management of, related to health beliefs	Instruct in proper self-injection of insulin; have patient perform return demonstration.
	Reinforce instructions regarding availability of glucose and glycogen sources.
	Remove potentially hazardous objects from environment.
Noncompliance (diabetic management), high risk for, related to patient's value system	Establish therapeutic relationship so patient can express negative feelings.
	Correct misconceptions about treatment regimen.
	Assist patient in setting long-term goals for lifetime optimal disease management.
	Involve significant others whenever possible, and encourage communication between them and the patient.

Patient teaching. There are many important areas of education for the person with diabetes, including the importance of proper administration of insulin or oral hypoglycemics, as well as their side effects (see Therapeutic Dialogue); the signs and symptoms of hyperglycemia and hypoglycemia; methods of testing blood glucose levels and of urine testing for glucose and acetone; planning and preparing the prescribed diet; and personal hygiene, emphasizing skin and foot care. The nurse should stress the interrelationship among diet, medication, and exercise. The patient should be instructed to visit the dentist regularly and have an annual examination by an ophthalmologist. Because infections and illnesses of any kind could result in loss of diabetic control, the patient should be instructed to notify the physician at the first sign of any illness. Special plans for travel include providing extra insulin vials and syringes, carrying food and some form of concentrated carbohydrate, and arranging for SMBG or urine testing. Provisions for adequate rest time must be made, because exhaustion may lead to changes in the overall condition.

Before discharge from the hospital, the patient should verbalize an understanding of how complications may be prevented and display an interest in maintaining optimal wellness. The nurse should stress the importance of regular medical checkups. The social aspects of DM cannot be ignored. Patients need to learn about life-style adjustment and should wear Medic Alert jewelry and carry medical information wallet cards at all times. Decisions such as whether to attempt pregnancy should be thoroughly explored by women with diabetes. Above all, the patient must accept the responsibility for self-care and recognize that making the right choices can affect life expectancy as well as the quality of life. A current trend is for hospitals to employ a diabetes nurse specialist to develop and implement patient and staff education.

Prognosis. Although the life expectancy for the person with diabetes is usually decreased, current research and recent advances have led to the hope of a much better prognosis. Early diagnosis and prompt, accurate treatment are essential in promoting longevity. Quality of life has been enhanced by better ways to control hyperglycemia and by earlier recognition of developing complications.

REFERENCES AND SUGGESTED READINGS

1. Anagnostakos NP, Tortora GJ: *Principles of anatomy and physiology,* ed 5, New York, 1987, Harper & Row.
2. Borders L et al: Reuse my syringe? *Diabetes Forecast* 43(11):28, 1990.
3. Brancati FL et al: The excess incidence of diabetic end-stage renal disease among Blacks, *JAMA* 268(21):3079, 1992.
4. Chipps E: Transsphenoidal surgery for pituitary tumors, *Crit Care Nurse* 12(1):30, 1992.
5. Christensen MH et al: How to care for the diabetic foot, *Am J Nurs* 91(3):50, 1991.
6. Cole G: *Basic nursing skills and concepts,* St Louis, 1991, Mosby.
7. Davis ED, Chesnaky P: Site rotation, *Diabetes Forecast* 45(3):54, 1992.
8. Dellasega C: Self-care for the elderly diabetic, *J Gerontol Nurs* 16(1):16, 1990.
9. Doeren E, Friedman N: Urine testing: still in style, *Diabetes Forecast* 45(9):62, 1992.
10. Drass J: What you need to know about insulin injections, *Nursing* 22(11):40, 1992.
11. Feldman V: Reacting to the reaction, *Diabetes Forecast* 45(12):40, 1992.
12. Fong E, Ferris EB, Skelly EG: *Body structures and functions,* ed 7, New York, 1989, Delmar.
13. Garvey WT, Brechtel G: Oral agents and the road this far, *Diabetes Forecast* 44(11):42, 1991.
14. Graves L III: Diabetic ketoacidosis and hyperglycemic hyperosmolar nonketotic coma, *Crit Care Nurs Q* 13(3):50, 1990.
15. Greene LB, Johns S: Can you solve this assessment puzzle? *RN* 53(11):64, 1990.
16. Hahn K: Brush up on your injection technique, *Nurs 90* 20(9):54, 1990.
17. Halloran TH: Nursing responsibilities in endocrine emergencies, *Crit Care Nurs Q* 13(3):74, 1990.
18. Handerhan B: Recognizing adrenal crisis, *Nursing* 22(4):33, 1992.

19. Hanis CL et al: Mortality of Mexican Americans with NIDDM, *Diabetes Care* 16(1):82, 1993.
20. Hegner BR, Caldwell E: *Geriatrics: a study of maturity,* ed 5, New York, 1991, Delmar.
21. Hood GH, Dincher JR: *Total patient care,* ed 8, St Louis, 1992, Mosby.
22. Howard BV et al: Risk factors for coronary heart disease in diabetic and nondiabetic native Americans: the strong heart study, *Diabetes* 41(2):4, 1992.
23. Isley WL: Thyroid disorders, *Crit Care Nurs Q* 13(3):39, 1990.
24. Jewler D: Screening for diabetes, *Diabetes Forecast* 44(7):56, 1991.
25. Kestel F: Using blood glucose meters: what you and your patient need to know, *Nursing* 23(3):34, 1993.
26. Kestel F: Using blood glucose meters: what you and your patient need to know. *Nursing* 23(4):50, 1993.
27. Lindaman C: SIADH: is your patient at risk? *Nursing* 22(6):60, 1992.
28. Liu QZ: Insulin treatment, endogenous insulin concentration, and ECG abnormalities in diabetic Pima Indians, *Diabetes* 41(9):1141, 1992.
29. Long BC, Phipps WJ, Cassmeyer V: *Medical-surgical nursing: a nursing process approach,* ed 3, St Louis, 1993, Mosby.
30. Marieb EN: *Human anatomy and physiology,* Reading, Mass, 1989, Benjamin Cummings.
31. Memmler RL, Cohen BJ, Wood DL: *Structure and function of the human body,* ed 5, Philadelphia, 1992, Lippincott.
32. Mercer ME: About diabetes insipidus, *Nursing* 20(5):20, 1990.
33. Mettler FA Jr et al: Thyroid nodules in the population living around Chernobyl, *JAMA* 268(5):616, 1992.
34. Nyhlin KT: Diabetic patients facing long-term complications: coping with uncertainty, *J Adv Nurs* 15(9):1021, 1990.
35. Pagana KD, Pagana TJ: *Mosby's diagnostic and laboratory test reference,* St Louis, 1992, Mosby.
36. Peragallo-Dittko V: Straight shooting: a critical look of injection technique, *Diabetes Self-Management* 9(3):3, 1992.
37. Peterson A, Drass J: Managing acute complications of diabetes, *Nursing* 21(2):34, 1991.
38. Radak J: Who gets diabetes? *Diabetes Forecast* 43(12):38, 1990.
39. Reasner CA: Adrenal disorders, *Crit Care Nurs Q* 13(3):67, 1990.
40. Roberts A: The thyroid gland and its disorder in later life, *Nurs Times* 86(28):63, 1990.
41. Sage R: A fine design for foot care, *Diabetes Forecast* 44(11):72, 1991.
42. Saltiel-Berzin R: Managing a surgical patient who has diabetes, *Nursing* 22(4):34, 1992.
43. Solomon EP: *Introduction to human anatomy and physiology,* Philadelphia, 1992, WB Saunders.
44. Sparks SM, Taylor CM: *Nursing diagnosis reference manual,* ed 2, Springhouse, Pa, 1993, Springhouse.
45. Steil CF, Deakins DA: Oral hypoglycemics: what you and your patient need to know, *Nursing* 22(11):34, 1992.
46. Steil CF, Deakins DA: Today's insulins: what you and your patient need to know, *Nursing* 20(8):34, 1990.
47. Stewart J: Treating hypoglycemia: knowing when to say when, *Diabetes Forecast* 44(8):54, 1991.
48. Thibodeau GA: *Structure & function of the body,* ed 9, St Louis, 1992, Mosby.
49. Tomky D: Insulin pumps, *Diabetes Forecast* 44(10):28, 1991.
50. Valentine V: Choices available for insulin delivery, *Diabetes in the News* 11(6):42, 1992.
51. Wakelee-Lynch J: Transplanting islet cells, *Diabetes Forecast* 45(1):28, 1992.
52. Weakland BS, Conboy D: Nancy's secret, *Nursing* 21(5):57, 1991.
53. Williams SR: *Basic nutrition and diet therapy,* ed 9, St Louis, 1992, Mosby.
54. Winer N: Pheochromocytoma, *Crit Care Nurs Q* 13(3):14, 1990.
55. Winter WE, Atkinson MA: Getting to the root of type I diabetes, *Diabetes Forecast* 45(5):34, 1992.
56. Yen PK: Following the new diabetic diet, *Geriatr Nurs* 11(6):303, 1990.
57. Yucha C, Suddaby P: David could have died of thirst, yet he never felt thirsty, *Nursing* 21(7):42, 1991.

CHAPTER CHALLENGE

KEY TERMS

- Endocrine glands are ductless glands that release chemicals (hormones) into the bloodstream to regulate body activities.
- The pituitary gland located in the brain is the master gland of the endocrine system.
- Hormones have a generalized effect on metabolism, growth and development, and reproduction.
- The endocrine glands regulate themselves by a series of negative feedback messages.
- The hormones secreted by the endocrine glands affect tissues of the entire body, and an imbalance in their levels may contribute to pathological changes in many different systems.
- Acromegaly and gigantism, disorders of the pituitary gland, result in growth changes that may lead to negative effect on the patient's self-image and self-esteem.
- Diabetes insipidus is a disorder of the posterior pituitary and must not be confused with diabetes mellitus, a disorder of the pancreas.
- Clinically, SIADH is characterized by hyponatremia and water retention that progresses to water intoxication.
- When caring for the hyperthyroid patient, the nurse must provide for adequate rest periods and be sure that fluid and food intake meets the patient's nutritional needs.
- The emotions of the hyperthyroid patient are very labile, so the nurse must try to eliminate sources of stress from the environment, to help prevent emotional trauma.
- ^{131}I should not be administered to a pregnant patient because of the risk of danger to the fetus; pregnant nurses should not care for these patients.
- Three postoperative complications may be life threatening to the thyroidectomy patient: hemorrhage, tetany, and thyroid crisis.
- The hypothyroid patient may experience sluggish mental and physical functioning, so the nurse must be patient and allow adequate time for nursing routines.

- The prognosis for papillary adenocarcinoma of the thyroid is excellent, because few of these tumors metastasize.
- When administering intravenous calcium chloride to any patient, the nurse must be careful that none of the drug extravasates, because tissue sloughing may result.
- The extreme hypertension often seen in patients with pheochromocytoma may result in CVA.
- Depression is very common in the patient who suffers from Cushing's syndrome; the nurse must be alert for suicidal thoughts and suicide attempts by this patient.
- The three main facets of medical treatment for the patient with diabetes mellitus are diet, exercise, and medication.
- IDDM is usually first diagnosed in persons under the age of 30; NIDDM is more commonly found after age 30, and the incidence increases with the aging process.
- The older person with diabetes may have a very high blood glucose level before excreting any into the urine because of an increased renal threshold for glucose.
- The diabetic diet must be individualized, taking many factors into consideration, such as age, life-style, food preferences, and the ability to cook and store food.
- The person with IDDM must have access to a source of quick glucose at all times, in the event of a hypoglycemic reaction.
- The nurse must become familiar with the clinical manifestations of DKA/HH, and hypoglycemic reaction to properly assess diabetic patients, as well as educate them in self-care.
- Patients on insulin therapy and oral hypoglycemics must be observed carefully during the time of peak action of the medication, and treatment must be initiated promptly if hypoglycemia develops.
- DKA can result in seizures, brain damage, or death for the diabetic patient.

STUDY QUESTIONS

1. The hormones responsible for "flight or fight" are:
   1. estrogen and testosterone
   2. FSH and LH
   3. Epinephrine and norepinephrine
   4. calcitonin and parathormone
2. The hormones responsible for blood calcium levels are:
   1. calcitonin and parathormone
   2. estrogen and progesterone
   3. melatonin and FSH
   4. thyroxine and parathormone
3. The master gland of the body is the:
   1. thyroid gland
   2. adrenal gland
   3. pineal gland
   4. pituitary gland
4. Which hormone stimulates uterine contractions?
   1. thyroxine
   2. follicle-stimulating hormone
   3. oxytocin
   4. luteinizing hormone
5. What hormone is responsible for male secondary sex characteristics?
   1. estrogen
   2. progesterone
   3. testosterone
   4. adrenalin
6. Mary Peterson is a 29-year-old secretary who received ^{131}I yesterday in an attempt to slow the progression of her hyperthyroid condition. For which of the following personnel would participating in her direct bedside care be dangerous?
   1. The 19-year-old first-semester nursing student
   2. A 34-year-old staff nurse who is new to the unit
   3. The 22-year-old aide who is 6 weeks pregnant
   4. A 49-year-old RN just returning from sick leave
7. Ms. Cronkin is a 35-year-old patient who is the first night postoperative from having had a thyroidectomy. She experiences signs and symptoms of postoperative tetany. The nurse should implement the physician's order and immediately administer:
   1. sodium iodide po
   2. potassium chloride IV
   3. magnesium sulfate IM
   4. calcium gluconate IV
8. Mrs. Chan is a 47-year-old mother of three who had successful cranial surgery to remove a pituitary tumor 3 days ago, leaving her with partial left hemiparesis and diabetes insipidus. Which of the following nursing diagnoses is of the greatest priority postoperatively?
   1. Fluid volume deficit, high risk for, related to excessive loss via the urinary system
   2. Hopelessness, related to development of chronic illness (hemiparesis and diabetes insipidus)
   3. Oral mucous membrane alteration, high risk for, related to dehydration
   4. Coping, ineffective family: compromised, high risk for, related to chronic illness
9. Fred Jenkins is a 34-year-old construction worker recently diagnosed as having acromegaly. Because of the pathophysiology of his condition, Mr. Jenkins' laboratory data will probably show elevated levels of:
   1. FSH
   2. LH
   3. TSH
   4. GH

10. Assessing Ms. Cronkin, a postoperative thyroidectomy patient, the nurse should check for damage to the laryngeal nerve. Which of the following is most likely to suggest that damage may have occurred?
    1. The patient complains of a slight sore throat.
    2. The patient's voice tone has changed slightly.
    3. The patient is unable to swallow fluids.
    4. The patient is becoming increasingly hoarse.
11. To help Mr. Rodriques, a newly diagnosed patient with IDDM, meet the goal of maintaining blood glucose control, which of the following is of greatest priority in the plan of care?
    1. Teach the patient the effect of diet, exercise, and insulin on the blood glucose level.
    2. Refer the patient to the hospital dietitian for intense education about his dietary needs.
    3. Instruct the patient on SMBG, observe return demonstrations, and correct his technique as needed.
    4. Review with the patient the desired effects of his medication, as well as possible side effects.
12. James Thompson is a 22-year-old male who has been an insulin-dependent diabetic for the last year. Which of the following statements demonstrates his need for more teaching?
    1. "If I want to lose weight, all I have to do is increase my dose of insulin."
    2. "I can have an occasional beer if it's calculated into my diet."
    3. "I will maintain better control of my blood sugar if I eat regular meals."
    4. "It is important that I eat properly, exercise regularly, and take my insulin injections."
13. To meet the goal of prevention of injury to Mr. Cordos, an IDDM patient, which of the following nursing interventions is most important to include in the care plan?
    1. Assess peripheral pulses and capillary refill in the lower extremities.
    2. Instruct the patient in the proper technique for self-injection of insulin.
    3. Stress the importance of keeping the skin on the feet soft and supple.
    4. Remove potentially hazardous objects from the patient's environment.
14. An hour ago, you administered morphine sulfate 15 mg IM to Ms. Mason, who had a thyroidectomy this morning. Now you observe she is slightly difficult to arouse, with respirations 12/min. You are correct to think that:
    1. Ms. Mason has been oversedated, and you should call her physician immediately.
    2. Ms. Mason may be developing airway problems caused by edema in her neck.
    3. Ms. Mason has probably been relieved of postoperative pain and is able to rest.
    4. Ms. Mason may be having an unusual reaction to the morphine, indicating an allergy.
15. Mark Anderson, age 45, has been admitted to your hospital unit with the primary medical diagnosis of Addison's disease (adrenal hypofunction). Assessment reveals the presence of postural hypotension, fatigue, nausea, vomiting, and poor skin turgor. Which of these nursing diagnoses is of greatest priority at this time?
    1. Infection, high risk for
    2. Body temperature, altered, high risk for
    3. Injury, high risk for
    4. Fluid volume deficit, high risk for

33

CARE OF THE PATIENT WITH A REPRODUCTIVE DISORDER

Elaine Kockrow
Barbara Christensen

KEY TERMS

ANATOMY AND PHYSIOLOGY

areola
Bartholin's gland
cervix
Cowper's gland
epididymis
external genitalia
fallopian tube
fundus
hymen
labia majora
menarche
prepuce
seminal vesicle
Skene's gland
spermatogenesis
vagina
zygote

MEDICAL-SURGICAL

amenorrhea
candidiasis
carcinoma in situ
chancre
Chlamydia trachomatis
circumcision
climacteric
colporrhaphy
colposcopy
cryptorchidism
culdoscopy
curettage
dysmenorrhea
endometriosis
epididymitis
fistula
hypermenorrhea
laparoscopy
mammography
menorrhagia
metrorrhagia
panhysterosalpingo-oophorectomy
Papanicolaou (Pap) smear test
phimosis
procedentia
quadrantectomy
trichomoniasis
tylectomy

LEARNING OBJECTIVES

After reading this chapter, the student should be able to do the following:

Anatomy and Physiology

- Define the key terms.
- List and describe the functions of the organs of the male and female reproductive tracts.
- Discuss menstruation and the hormones necessary for a complete cycle.

Medical-Surgical

- Define the key terms.
- Discuss the impact of illness on the patient's sexuality.
- List nursing interventions for patients with menstrual disturbances.
- Discuss nursing interventions for the patient undergoing diagnostic studies related to the reproductive system.
- Discuss the importance of the Papanicolaou smear test in early detection of cancer.
- Discuss four important points to be addressed in discharge planning for the patient with pelvic inflammatory disease (PID).
- List four nursing diagnoses pertinent to the patient with endometriosis.
- Identify the clinical manifestations seen with a vaginal fistula.
- Discuss the four major areas of postoperative concerns in the nursing interventions for a patient undergoing hysterectomy.
- Identify four nursing diagnoses pertinent to ovarian cancer.
- Describe six important points to emphasize in the teaching of breast self-examination.
- Compare five surgical approaches for cancer of the breast.
- Discuss nursing interventions for the patient after a mastectomy.
- List several discharge planning instructions for the mastectomy patient.
- Describe nursing interventions for the patient with prostatitis.
- Distinguish between hydrocele and varicocele.
- Discuss the importance of monthly testicular self-examination beginning at 15 years of age.
- Discuss patient education related to prevention of sexually transmitted diseases.

RELATED TOPICS OF INTEREST

- Care of the patient with a urinary disorder (Chapter 30)
- Care of the HIV-positive or AIDS patient (Chapter 37)
- Care of the patient with cancer (Chapter 38)
- Normal pregnancy (Chapter 39)
- Normal labor and delivery (Chapter 40)
- Care of the mother and newborn (Chapter 41)
- Care of the mother and newborn at risk (Chapter 42)

Conception and birth are made possible through the dynamics of the normally functioning male and female reproductive systems. Reproduction of like individuals is necessary for the continuation of the species. The male and female sex glands (gonads) produce the gametes (sperm and ova) that unite to form a fertilized egg (zygote), the beginning of a new life.

ANATOMY AND PHYSIOLOGY

Male Reproductive System

The organs of the male reproductive system include the testes, the penis, a ductal system, and the accessory glands (Fig. 33-1 on p. 984). These structures have various functions: producing and storing sperm, depositing sperm for fertilization, and developing the male secondary sex characteristics.

Testes (Testicles). The two oval testes (gonads) are enclosed in a saclike structure, the scrotum, which lies suspended from the exterior abdominal wall. This keeps the temperature in the testes below the normal body core temperature, which is necessary for viable sperm production and storage.

Each testis is divided into lobules by a fibrous tissue called the *tunica albuginea.* Each lobule contains one to three coiled seminiferous tubules that produce the sperm cells. After puberty millions of sperm cells are produced daily. Small clusters of interstitial cells surround the seminiferous tubules throughout the testes. These cells (cells of Leydig) are responsible for the production of the male sex hormone *testosterone.* Testosterone is responsible for the development of male secondary sex characteristics.

Ductal System.

Epididymis. Sperm produced in the seminiferous tubules immediately travel to a network of ducts called the *rete testis.* These passageways contain cilia that sweep the sperm out of the testes into the **epididymis,** a tightly coiled tube structure that lies superior to the testes and extends posteriorly. The immature sperm are stored here to mature and gain strength to enable them to fertilize the ovum. This maturing process can last from a few hours to 10 days. If the sperm are not used after 4 weeks, they are reabsorbed into the body. With sexual stimulation the walls of the epididymis contract, forcing the sperm along the seminiferous tubules of the testes to the vas deferens.

Ductus deferens (vas deferens). The ductus deferens is approximately 18 inches (46 cm) long and rises along the posterior wall of the testes. As it moves upward it passes through the inguinal canal into the pelvic cavity and loops over the urinary bladder. The ductus deferens, nerves, and blood vessels are enclosed in a connective tissue sheath called the *spermatic cord.*

If a man elects to be sterilized for birth control management, it is a simple procedure to make small slits on either side of the scrotum and sever the ductus deferens. This procedure is called a *vasectomy.* It renders the man sterile because sperm can no longer be expelled.

Ejaculatory duct and urethra. Behind the urinary bladder, the ejaculatory duct connects with the ductus deferens. The ejaculatory duct is only 1 inch (2.5 cm) long. It unites with the urethra to pass through the prostate gland. The urethra extends the length of the penis, ending at the bulb of the penis with the urinary meatus. The urethra carries both sperm and urine, but because of the urethral sphincter it does not do so at the same time.

Accessory Glands. The ductal system transports and stores sperm. The accessory glands, which produce the liquid portion, seminal fluid (semen), include the seminal vesicles, prostate gland, and the Cowper's glands. The thick, alkaline fluid makes up 60% of the volume of the semen. Alkalinity protects the sperm from the acid condition of the vagina and increases the motility of the sperm. With each ejactulation (2 to 5 ml), approximately 200 to 500 million sperm are released. Although it takes only one sperm to unite with one egg to cause fertilization, it takes many sperm to break down the outer coating of the egg (zona pellucida) to allow entry of the single sperm.

Seminal vesicles. The **seminal vesicles** are paired structures that lie at the base of the bladder and produce 60% of the volume of semen. In addition to its alkalinity, the seminal fluid is high in fructose, a sugar that provides nourishment and energy for the sperm. The fluid is released into the ejactulatory duct to meet with the sperm.

Prostate gland. The single, doughnut-shaped prostate gland surrounds the neck of the bladder and urethra; it secretes 20% of the volume of the thick, alkaline semen. It is a firm structure about the size of a chestnut,

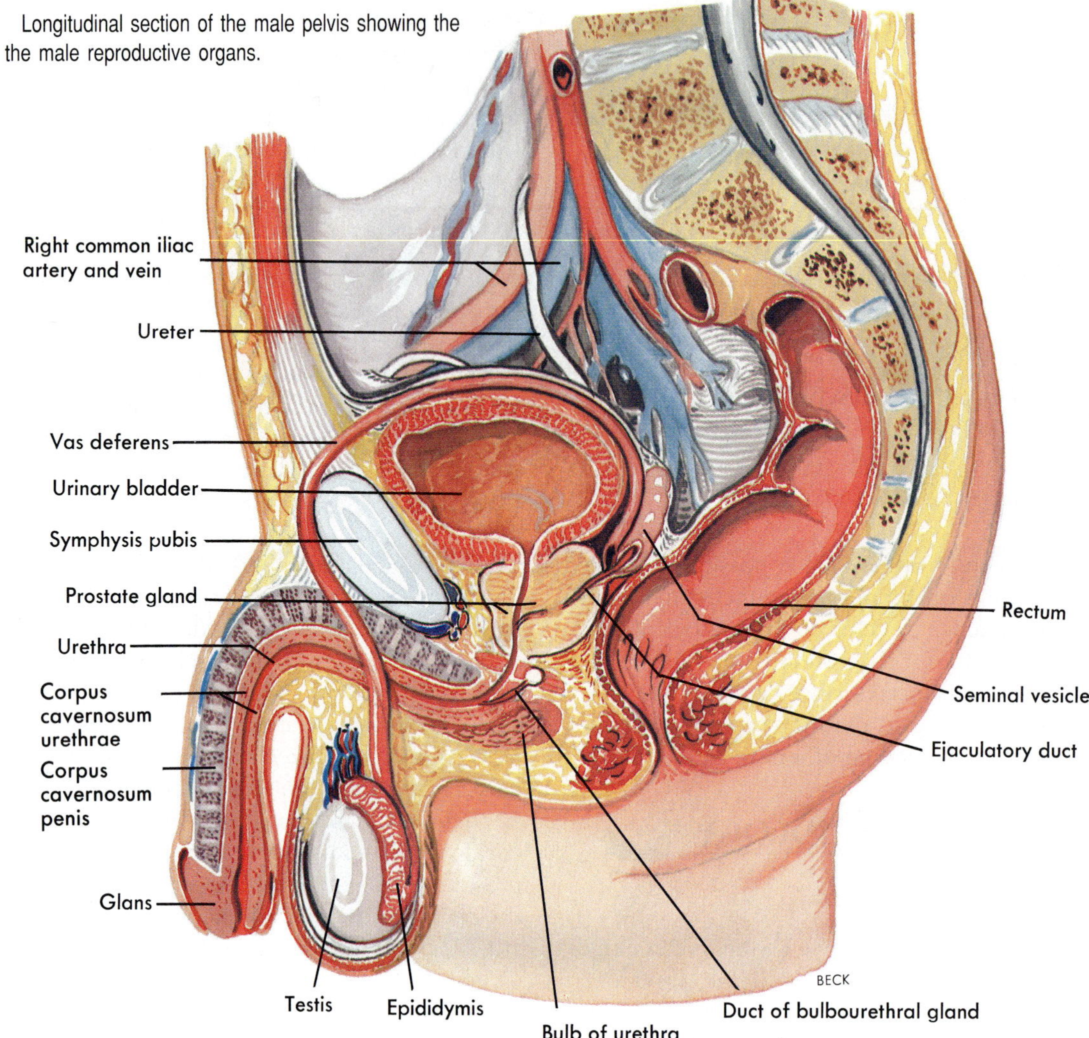

FIG. 33-1 Longitudinal section of the male pelvis showing the location of the male reproductive organs.

composed of muscular and glandular tissue. The ejaculatory duct passes obliquely through the posterior part of the gland. With the aging process the prostate gland often hypertrophies, leading to difficulty in urination, because the gland surrounds the urethra.

Cowper's glands. **Cowper's glands** (bulbourethral glands), the two pea-sized glands beneath the bulb of the male urethra, secrete a clear mucus that drains into the urethra. They correspond to the Bartholin glands in the female. This fluid contributes to the total volume of the semen and also provides lubrication during sexual intercourse.

Urethra and Penis. The male urethra serves the twofold purpose of conveying urine from the bladder and carrying the reproductive cells and secretions to the outside. The cylindrical penis is the organ of copulation. The shaft of the penis ends with an enlarged tip called the *glans penis.* The skin covering the penis lies in folds around the glans; this tissue is called the **prepuce** or foreskin. This excess tissue is sometimes removed in a surgical procedure called *circumcision* to prevent phimosis (a tightness of the prepuce of the penis that prevents the retraction of the foreskin over the glans).

Three masses of erectile tissue containing many sinuses fill the shaft of the penis. With sexual stimulation the sinuses fill with blood, causing the penis to become erect. After the penis ejaculates the semen, it returns to its flaccid state.

Sperm. At puberty, **spermatogenesis** (the process of development of spermatozoa) begins and continues throughout life. The mature sperm consists of three distinct parts: (1) the head, which contains the enzyme hyaluronidase, (2) the midpiece, which carries on metabolism to provide energy for locomotion, and (3) the tail or flagellum, which propels the sperm. Mature sperm, once deposited in the female reproductive system, live approximately 48 hours. If they come in contact with a mature egg, the enzyme on the head of the sperm bombards the egg in an attempt to break down the coating

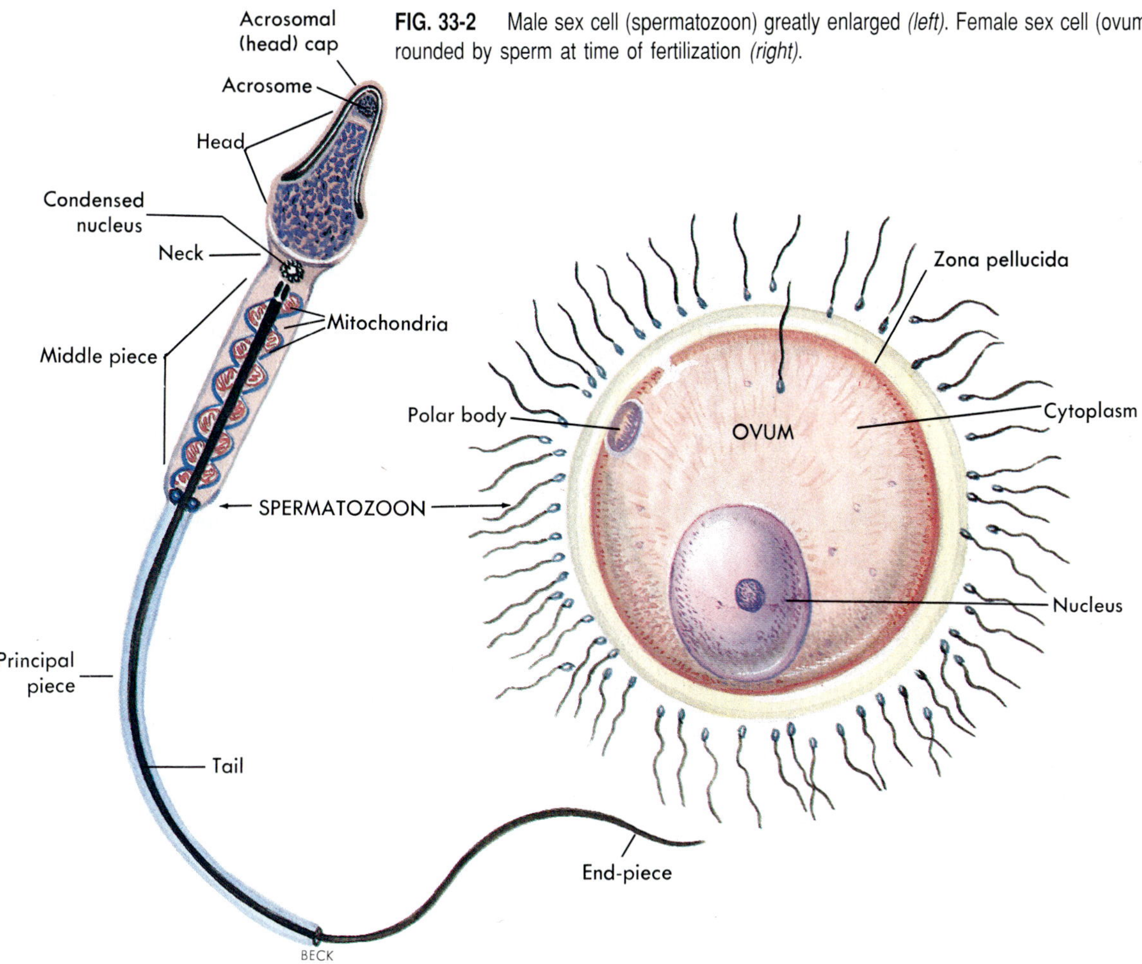

FIG. 33-2 Male sex cell (spermatozoon) greatly enlarged *(left)*. Female sex cell (ovum) surrounded by sperm at time of fertilization *(right)*.

of the egg (zona pellucida) (Fig. 33-2). It takes thousands of sperm to break the coating, but only one sperm enters and causes fertilization, and the remaining sperm disintegrate.

Female Reproductive System

The organs of the female reproductive system include the ovaries, uterus, fallopian tubes, and vagina (Figs. 33-3 and 33-4 on p. 986). These organs, along with a few accessory structures, produce the ovum, house the fertilized egg, maintain the embryo, and nurture the newborn infant. The ability to conceive and nurture this new human being requires the intricate balance of many hormones and the menstrual cycle.

Ovaries. The paired ovaries (gonads) are the size and shape of almonds. They are covered with epithelium and are located bilateral to the uterus, immediately inferior to the fallopian fimbriae. They are supported by the ovarian and broad ligaments. At puberty they release the female sex hormones estrogen and progesterone and release a mature egg during the menstrual cycle. Each ovary contains 30,000 to 40,000 microscopic ovarian follicles.

At puberty, the female's body prepares for ovulation (Fig. 33-5 on p. 987) and the possibility of pregnancy each 21 to 45 days. The normal or usual cycle is 28 days. This series of preparations is called the menstrual cycle and will be discussed in detail later in the chapter.

The ovaries prepare an egg (ovum) in a pocket- or envelope-shaped structure called a *graafian follicle.* The cells of the follicle walls secrete estrogen. When an ovum has ripened, the follicle ruptures and releases the ovum from the surface of the ovary into the abdominal cavity. The fingerlike projections of the fallopian tubes, fimbriae, sweep the ovum into the fallopian tubes. Once this mature ovum has been expelled, the follicle is transformed into a solid glandular mass called the *corpus luteum,* which means "yellow body." This structure secretes both estrogen and progesterone. Normally the corpus luteum shrinks and is replaced by scar tissue called *corpus albicans.*

Fallopian Tubes (Oviducts). The **fallopian tubes** are a pair of ducts opening at one end into the upper por-

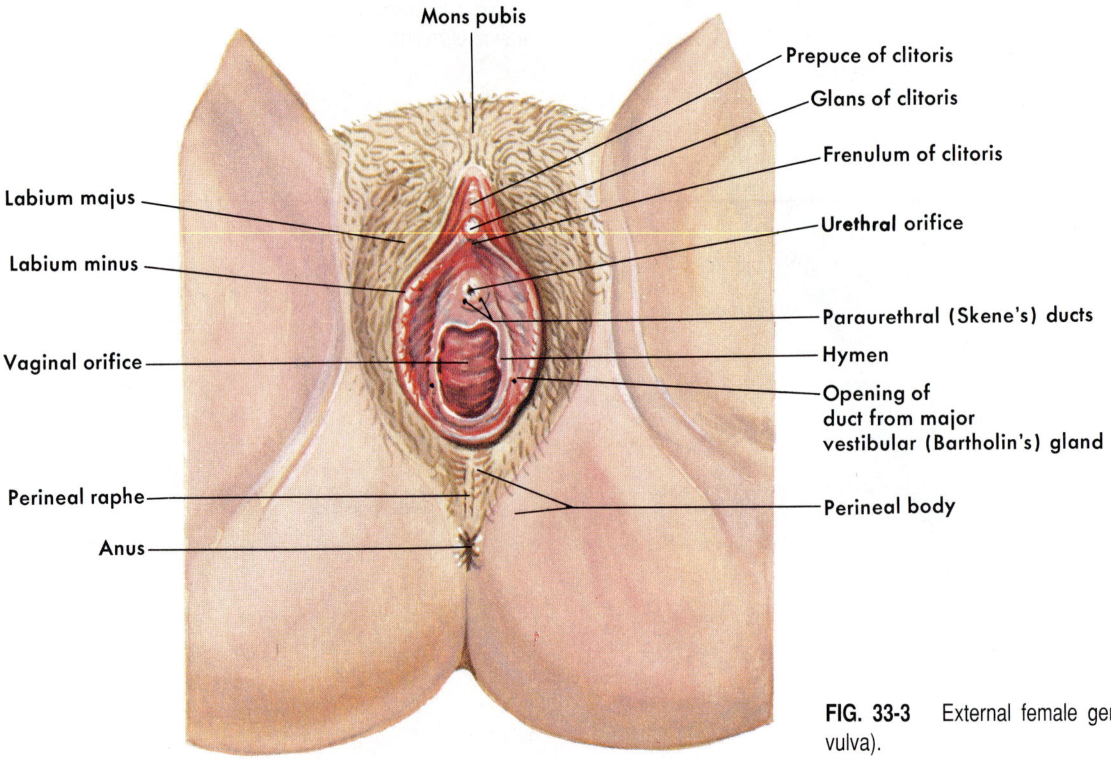

Mons pubis
Prepuce of clitoris
Glans of clitoris
Frenulum of clitoris
Labium majus
Urethral orifice
Labium minus
Paraurethral (Skene's) ducts
Vaginal orifice
Hymen
Opening of duct from major vestibular (Bartholin's) gland
Perineal raphe
Perineal body
Anus

FIG. 33-3 External female genitals (the vulva).

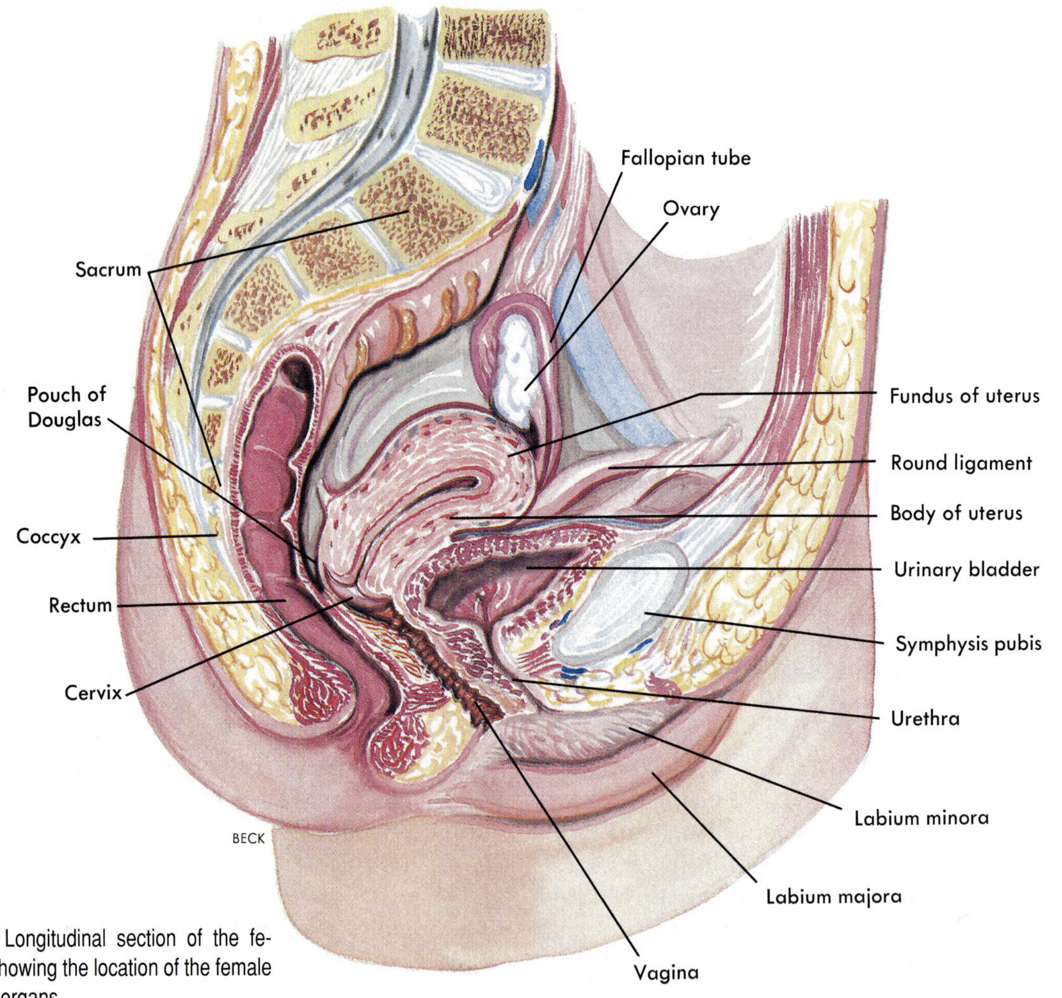

FIG. 33-4 Longitudinal section of the female pelvis showing the location of the female reproductive organs.

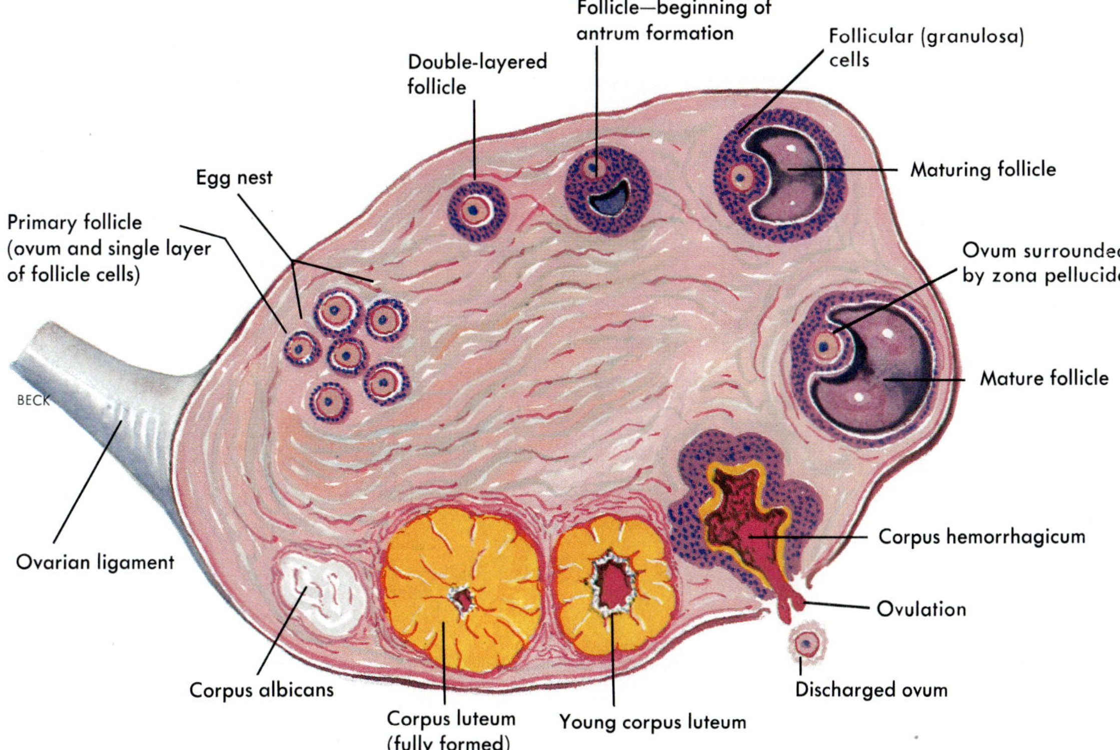

FIG. 33-5 Mammalian ovary showing successive stages of ovarian (graafian) follicle and ovum development. Begin with the first stage (egg nest) and follow around clockwise to the final stage (corpus albicans).

tion (fundus) of the uterus and the other end into the peritoneal cavity, over the ovary. They are approximately 4 inches (12 cm) long with fimbriae at the distal ends. The entire inner surfaces of the tubes are lined with cilia. They are composed of three layers of tissue: (1) mucosa, the inner layer, (2) muscle, the middle layer, and (3) serosa, the outer layer. When the graafian follicle of the ovary ruptures and releases the mature ovum, the fimbriae sweep the mature ovum into the fallopian tube. Fertilization takes place in the outer third of this tube, and the fertilized ovum **(zygote)** is moved along the tube by the combination of muscular peristaltic movements and the sweeping action of the cilia. If the mature ovum is not fertilized, it disintegrates. In about one of every 250 pregnancies, the zygote imbeds in the fallopian tube rather than sweeping along to the uterus. The condition is called *ectopic pregnancy* and results in the rupturing of the fallopian tube, a medical emergency.

Uterus. The uterus is shaped like an inverted pear and measures 3 inches (7.5 cm) by 2 inches (5 cm) by 1 inch (2.5 cm) in the nonpregnant state. It is situated between the urinary bladder and the rectum and is supported by the broad and round ligaments. It consists of three layers of tissue: (1) endometrium, the inner layer, composed of mucous membrane, (2) myometrium, the middle layer, composed of muscle tissue, and (3) perimetrium, the outer layer, composed of serous membrane.

The uterus is divided into three major portions (Fig. 33-6 on p. 988). The upper, rounded portion of the uterus, the **fundus,** is the insertion site of the fallopian tubes. The larger midsection is called the *corpus* or body. The smaller, narrower lower portion of the uterus is called the **cervix.** Part of the cervix actually descends into the vaginal vault. During pregnancy the uterus is capable of enlarging up to 500 times its size.

The uterus is a remarkable organ. Each month it prepares for implantation of a fertilized ovum. If pregnancy does not occur, the lining sloughs off with menstruation. If pregnancy does occur, it allows for development of the fetus for 9 months. At the end of this period it goes through a series of contractions (labor) and expels the infant. To prevent hemorrhage after childbirth, it contracts sharply. Because the muscle fibers run in all directions and the blood vessels are intertwined between them, this clamping action prevents bleeding.

Vagina. The **vagina** is a thin-walled, muscular, tubelike structure of the female genitalia, which is approximately 3 inches (7.5 cm) long. It is located between the urinary

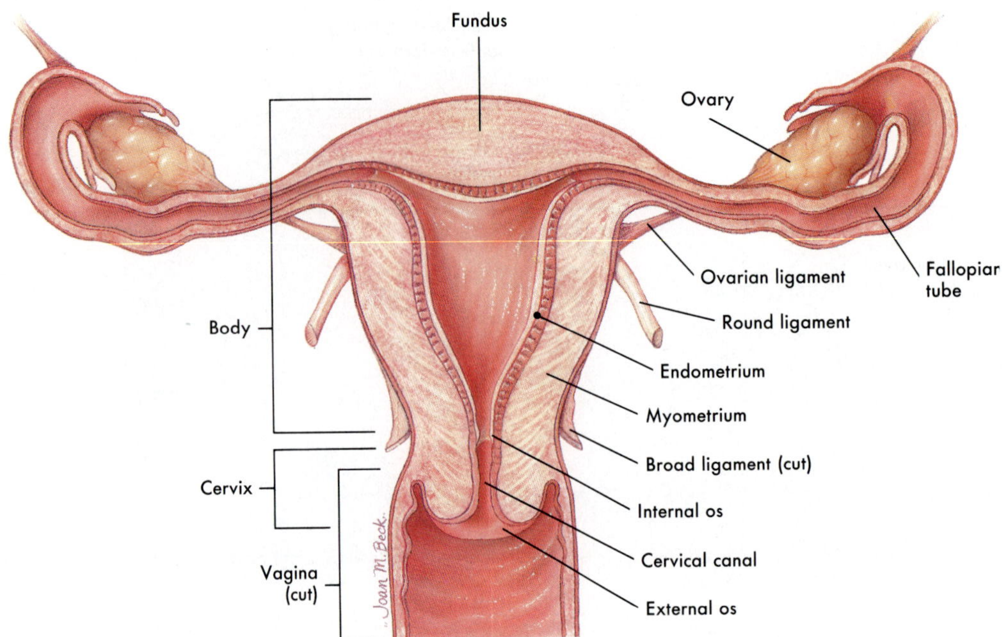

FIG. 33-6 Sectioned view of the uterus showing relationship to the ovaries and vagina.

bladder and the rectum. The superior portion articulates to the cervix of the uterus; the inferior portion opens to the outside. The vagina is lined with mucous membrane, which is responsible for most of the lubrication during sexual activity. The walls of the vagina normally lie in folds called *rugae.* This enables the vagina to stretch to receive the penis during intercourse and to allow the passage of the infant during the birth process.

The external opening of the vagina is covered by a fold of mucous membrane, skin, and fibrous tissue called the **hymen.** For centuries the hymen was a symbol of virginity, but it is now realized that rigorous exercise or insertion of a tampon for menstrual flow may tear the hymen. If the hymen has remained intact, it is ruptured with coitus (intercourse).

External Genitalia. The reproductive structures located outside the body are the **external genitalia** or vulva. Included are the mons pubis, labia majora, labia minora, clitoris, and vestibule (see Fig. 33-3).

Located superior to the symphysis pubis is a mound of fatty tissue, covered with coarse hair. This structure is the mons pubis. Extending from the mons pubis to the perineal floor are two large folds of tissue called the **labia majora** (large lips). These structures protect the inner structures and are also covered with pubic hair. In addition, the labia majora contain sensory nerve endings and an assortment of sebaceous (oil) and sudoriferous (sweat) glands. Directly beneath the labia majora lie the labia minora (small lips); these are smaller folds of tissue, devoid of any pubic hair, that merge anteriorly to form the prepuce of the clitoris.

The clitoris is comparable to the male penis. It too is composed of erectile tissue that becomes engorged with blood during sexual stimulation. It is the center of sexual excitement for the female.

The space enclosing the structures located beneath the labia minora is called the vestibule. It contains the clitoris, urinary meatus, hymen (if present), and the vaginal opening.

Accessory Glands. Bilateral to the urinary meatus lie the paraurethral or **Skene's glands,** the largest glands that open into the urethra. They contain ducts that open just within the urethral orifice. These glands are responsible for the secretion of mucus and are similar in function to the prostate gland in the male. Bilateral to the vaginal opening are two small, mucus-secreting glands called the greater **Bartholin's** (vestibular) **glands.** These glands secrete a mucuslike secretion that lubricates the area for sexual intercourse. Their secretion is similar to the fluid released by the bulbourethral glands in the male.

Perineum. The area enclosed by the posterior end of the labia (fourchette) and the anterior portion of the anus is called the *obstetrical perineum;* the area enclosing the region containing the reproductive structures is referred to as the *general perineum.* The perineum is diamond shaped and starts at the symphysis pubis and extends to the anus. Sometimes with childbirth, the phy-

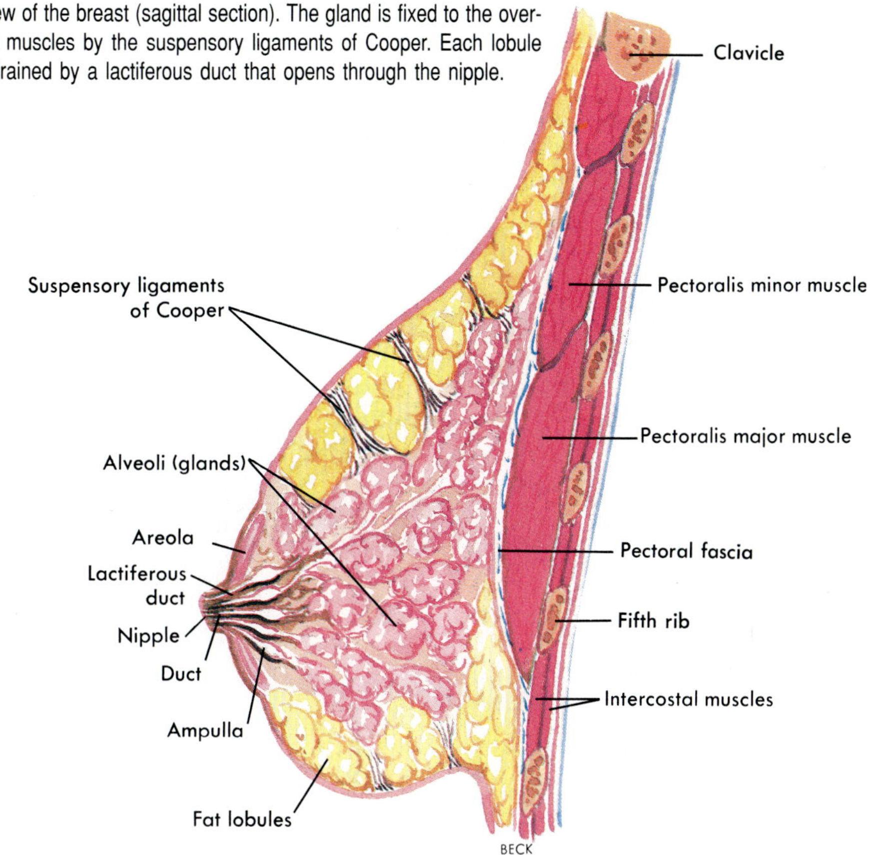

FIG. 33-7 Lateral view of the breast (sagittal section). The gland is fixed to the overlying skin and pectoral muscles by the suspensory ligaments of Cooper. Each lobule of secretory tissue is drained by a lactiferous duct that opens through the nipple.

sician clips the perineum extending from the fourchette in a procedure called an *episiotomy* to prevent tearing of tissue with childbirth.

Mammary Glands (Breasts). The breasts are attached to the pectoral (chest) muscles by connective tissue and to the skin and deep fascia by ligaments of Cooper (suspensory ligaments) (Fig. 33-7). Breast tissue is identifiable in both sexes. During puberty several things occur to the female breasts that change the size, shape, and ability to function.

Each breast contains 15 to 20 lobes that are separated by adipose tissue. The amount of adipose tissue is responsible for the size of the breast. It is important to realize that size of the breast has no impact on the ability of the breast to function—to produce and eject milk. Within each lobe there are many lobules that contain milk-producing cells (alveoli or acini); these lobules lead directly to the lactiferous ducts that empty directly into the nipple.

The nipple is composed of smooth muscle that allows it to become erect. The dark pink or brown tissue surrounding the nipple is called the **areola.** Small papillae on the areola are called the *tubercles of Montgomery.* These structures are sebaceous glands that secrete oil to keep the nipple supple, to prevent it from drying and cracking.

Milk production does not start until the woman has given birth. At this time, under the influence of prolactin, the milk is formed. The hormone *oxytocin* allows the milk to be released. The amount of milk produced is directly related to the stimulus of the suckling infant. The more the infant nurses, the more milk is produced.

Menstrual Cycle. At puberty, the female reproductive system, under the influence of hormones, prepares itself for the possibility of pregnancy. The major changes occur within the uterus. The inner lining, the endometrium, is prepared to receive and nurture a fertilized ovum. It will nurture this egg, allowing it to grow through embryonic and fetal stages and finally to the birth of the infant.

Menarche, the first menstrual cycle, usually begins around the age of 12 years. Each month, for 30 to 40 years, an ovum matures and is released about 14 days before the next menstrual flow. This, on average, occurs every 28 days. If fertilization occurs, menstrual cycling subsides and the body adapts to the developing fetus (see Chapter 39).

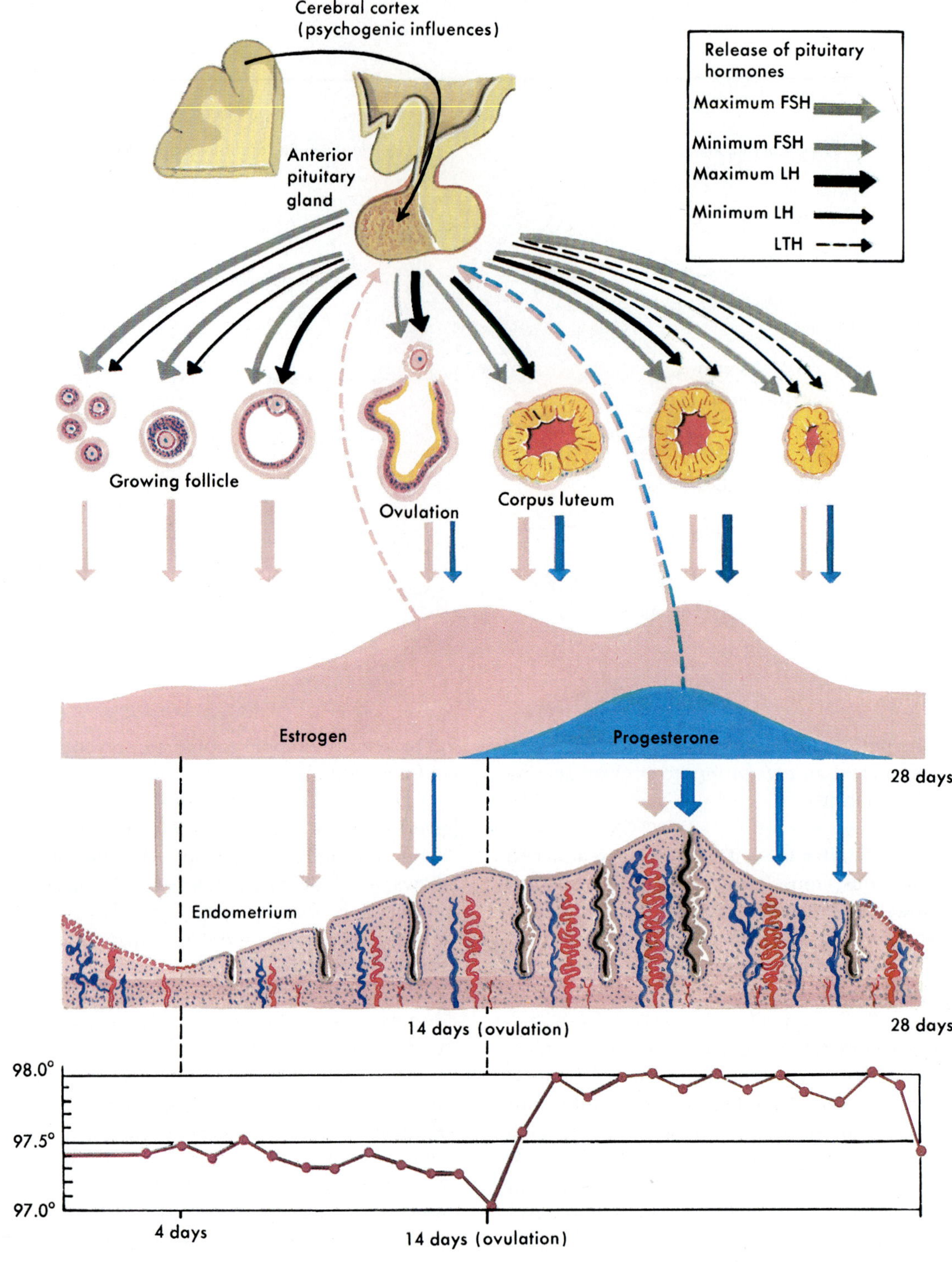

FIG. 33-8 Diagram illustrating the interrelationships among the cerebral, hypothalamic, pituitary, ovarian, and uterine functions throughout a usual 28-day menstrual cycle. The variations in basal body temperature are also illustrated.

Generally speaking, the menstrual cycle can be divided into three phases: menstrual, preovulatory, and postovulatory. For our discussion, we will use the 28-day cycle to explore what happens (Fig. 33-8). On days 1 through 5 of the cycle the endometrium sloughs and is accompanied by 1 to 2 ounces of blood loss. The anterior pituitary begins to release follicle-stimulating hormone (FSH); as the level of FSH increases, the egg matures within the graafian follicle. From days 6 through 13 (preovulatory phase) estrogen is released from the maturing graafian follicle. This estrogen causes the vascularization and thickening of the uterine lining. On day 14 the anterior pituitary releases luteinizing hormone (LH), which causes the rupture of the graafian follicle and the release of the mature ovum. During days 15 through 28 (postovulatory phase) the developing corpus luteum releases estrogen and progesterone, which maintains the vascularization of the uterus if pregnancy does occur. If this is the case, the corpus luteum continues to release estrogen and progesterone to maintain the uterine lining until the placenta is formed, which then takes over the job of hormonal release. If pregnancy does not occur, the corpus luteum lasts for 8 days and then disintegrates. At this point the hormone level decreases over several days and menstruation starts again.

Effects of Normal Aging Patterns on the Reproductive System

Menopause occurs in the normal female between the ages of 35 to 60 years. The average age is 51. Whether it occurs earlier or later, menopause should not be considered abnormal. Cigarette smoking and living at high altitudes are associated with early menopause. During this time the menstrual flow ceases and hormonal levels decrease. This is the period when a woman may experience "hot flashes" (a sudden warm feeling) that are caused by the decrease in estrogen production. Changes also occur in the reproductive organs. The vagina loses elasticity. The breasts and vulva lose some adipose tissue, which results in decreased tissue turgor. The bones may also become brittle and prone to osteoporosis.

In the male there is no menopausal period. Sperm production decreases but does not cease. In later years, testosterone production decreases, but not dramatically.

Basically, as long as the older individual is healthy, there is nothing in the aging process that prohibits normal sexual function. Factors that affect the reproductive system in the older adult are highlighted in the gerontological box.

GERONTOLOGICAL CONSIDERATIONS

Women

- Many older women are reluctant to seek medical care for problems of the reproductive system. This may be related to cultural factors, embarrassment or lack of knowledge. Routine gynecological examination should continue as part of the physical examination even after menopause.
- Certain forms of cancer of the reproductive tract are more common with aging. Any vaginal bleeding should be reported to the physician promptly, as should pelvic pain, pruritus, or skin lesions in the genital region.
- Decreased level of estrogen with aging and systemic disease such as diabetes predispose older women to vaginitis.
- Breast cancer risk increases over age 40. Breast examination should continue throughout the lifespan. The American Cancer Society recommends an annual mammogram for women over age 50.

Men

- Decreased production of testosterone results in changes in the male reproductive system, but the ability to procreate can continue until the eighth decade. Sexual interest often continues late into life.
- Chronic health problems such as diabetes or hypertension and many medications can result in impotence in older men.
- Prostate enlargement is increasingly common with each decade after age 40. Although this enlargement is most often benign, cancer of the prostate is a serious condition most often seen in older men. Ultrasonography of the prostate is particularly useful in diagnosing prostatic cancer when combined with rectal examination and prostatic/specific antigen (PSA).

HUMAN SEXUALITY

Sexuality and sex are two different things. Sexuality is often described as the sense of being female or male. It has biological, psychological, social, and ethical segments. *Sexuality* influences life experiences, and sexuality is influenced by life experiences. The term *sex* has a more limited meaning. It usually describes the biological aspects of sexuality such as genital sexual activity. Sex may be used for pleasure or reproduction. As a result of life's changes or by personal choice, sexual activity may be absent from a person's life for brief or prolonged periods.

The process by which people come to know themselves as females or males is not clearly understood. Being born with female or male genitalia and subsequently learning female or male social roles seem to be factors; yet this does not explain differences of sexuality and sexual behavior. These variations are more understandable if the nurse remembers that sexuality is intertwined with all aspects of self.

Biological identify or the differences between men and women are established at conception and are further influenced at puberty from the effects of hormones. Gender identity is the sense of being feminine or masculine. As soon as the infant is born and sometimes before, the outside world labels the child as *girl* or *boy*. Adults adjust their behavior to relate to a female or male baby. These varied patterns of interaction influence the infant's developing sense of gender identity.

Children will explore and seek to understand their own bodies. Combining this information with the way in which they are treated, they begin to create an image of themselves as a boy or as a girl. By age 3 children are aware that they will remain a boy or a girl, and no outward change in their appearance will alter this. This understanding is part of the development of self-concept.

Gender role is the manner in which a person acts as female or male. Many believe that society influences female and male behavior and is thus the primary source of femaleness or maleness. Because gender role behavior is encouraged, differences among individual's sexual behaviors develop. Most likely, as with the other human behaviors, sexual behavior is a combination of many interacting biological and environmental factors.

Cultural factors can be key ingredients in defining sex roles. Some cultures tightly dictate roles as feminine or masculine (for example, the male is the bread winner, and the female is the care giver). Other groups may be more flexible in role definition and encourage men or women to explore a variety of roles without labeling the behavior as *feminine* or *masculine*.

Sexual orientation is the clear and persistent erotic preference of a person for one sex or the other. There are heterosexual, homosexual, and lesbian as well as bisexual individuals. The origins of sexual orientation are still not understood. Biological theorists describe them in genetic terms, which means they are determined at conception. Psychological theorists attribute orientation to early learning experiences, and believe that cognitive processes decide sexual orientation. Still other theorists state that genetics and environment are the major influences in the development of the sexual partner preference.

For some people the inward sense of sexual identity does not match the biological body. These people are known as transsexuals. Researchers do not clearly understand how this mismatch occurs. Transsexuals do not see their sexual identity as a choice but as clear and persistent orientation dating back to early childhood. Most homosexual men and women define themselves as satisfied with their gender and social roles. They simply have a persistent desire for their same sex.

A transvestite is most often a heterosexual male who periodically dresses like a woman. This is usually done in private and kept secret even from those who are closest to them.

Because sexuality is linked to every aspect of living, any sexual choice involves personal, family, cultural, religious, and social standards of conduct. Ideas about ethical sexual conduct and emotions related to sexuality form the basis for sexual decision making. The range of attitudes about sexuality extends from a traditional view of sex only within marriage to the point of view that allows individuals to determine what is right. Sexual choices that overstep a person's ethical standard may result in internal conflicts.

Sexual decisions may be based solely on religion; others view any sexual act between consenting adults in private as moral. People will always differ in beliefs about sexual ethics. The debate over sexuality-related issues such as abortion, contraception, sources of sex education, sexual variations, and premarital or extramarital intercourse will continue.

Because wellness includes sexual health, sexuality should be a part of the health care program. Yet sexual assessment and interventions are not always included in health care. The area of sexuality can be emotional for nurses and patients. See Box 33-1 for factors that can interfere with promotion of patient's sexual health.

Nurses can deal with personal attitudes by accepting their existence, exploring their sources, and finding ways to work with them. Professional behavior does not have to compromise the personal sexual ethics of nurses or patients. Professional behavior must guarantee that patients receive the best health care possible without diminishing their self-worth. Promotion of self-education and honest examination of sexual beliefs and values can help in reducing sexual bias.

Giving patients information about sexuality does not mean agreement. Patients need accurate, honest information about the effects of illness on sexuality and the ways that it contributes to wellness. Nurses need to provide this information.

Although there is no single approach to taking a sexual history, application of certain principles contrib-

Box 33-1 FACTORS THAT CAN INTERFERE WITH PROMOTING SEXUAL HEALTH

- Lack of information
- Conflicting values system—attitudes and beliefs
- Anxiety (Are specific attitudes, feelings, and actions "normal"?)
- Guilt
- Lack of comfort with sexuality
- Invasion of privacy
- Lack of regard for hospitalized patients' need for time alone with significant other
- The manner in which the patient is touched
- Fear of being judged
- Lack of understanding of the effects of illness and treatment on sexual functioning

utes to both the patient's and the nurse's comfort. (See Box 33-2 for requirements for taking a sexual history.)

Some principles to follow that contribute to a comfortable atmosphere for nurse and patient are:

- Obtain sexual history early in nurse-patient relationship, which indicates permission for patients to discuss sexual concerns.
- Avoid overreacting or underreacting to patient's comments, which aids in truthful data collection.
- Use language that the patient understands; both patient and nurse may need to define their terms to ensure accurate data gathering.
- Move from the less sensitive to more sensitive areas. This will promote patient-nurse comfort.
- Terminate the sexual history by inquiring if the patient has additional questions or concerns.

A brief assessment can be included in the nursing history by means of three questions (Box 33-3). The questions may be adapted to deal with illness, hospitalization, life events, or any other relevant matter that may influence or interfere with sexual health.

The questions may also be adjusted to draw out the patient's expectations of changes resulting from procedures, medications, or surgery. It is often unnecessary for the nurse to ask the last two questions because many patients voice their concerns about masculinity, femininity, and sexual functioning without further encouragement.

Nurses may intervene with sexual problems among patient populations through four strategies: educating patient groups likely to have sexual concerns, providing anticipatory guidance throughout the life cycle, promoting a milieu conducive to sexual health, and validating normalcy about sexual concerns.

Several self-help groups and other organizations publish easy-to-read pamphlets on sexuality (Box 33-4). These pamphlets can often be purchased for a nominal fee and given to patients. Most pamphlets can be obtained directly from state or local chapters. Chapters of other self-help groups can be contacted about availability of sexuality resources for patients. Some groups publish newsletters that address sexuality.

Nurses can also write their own pamphlets for patients. Although this requires some effort, it may provide additional incentive for staff to address sexuality. Once developed, these pamphlets can be made available to others.

Box 33-2 REQUIREMENTS FOR TAKING A SEXUAL HISTORY

- Provision of privacy—a closed room
- An atmosphere of trust—ensure confidentiality
- Comfort on the part of nurses with their own sexuality

Box 33-3 BRIEF SEXUAL HISTORY

1. Has your (illness, pregnancy, or hospitalization) interfered with your being a (husband, wife, significant other, father, mother)?
2. Has your (abortion, heart attack) changed the way you see yourself as (woman, man)?
3. Has your (colostomy, mastectomy, hysterectomy) changed your ability to function sexually (or your sex life)?

Illness and Sexuality

Illness may cause changes in one's self-concept and an inability to function sexually. Medications, stress, fatigue, and depression also affect sexual functioning. Alcohol abuse can lead to a reduced sex drive and inadequate sexual functioning.

Disinterest or lack of desire for sexual activity generally occurs with patients at the time they are preoccupied with symptoms of illness. Most often these sexual symptoms disappear as patients recover from the acute phase of illness and sexual activity is resumed. However, some illnesses, such as diabetes mellitus, end-stage renal disease, spinal cord injuries, and heart disease, may cause patients some concerns or actual inabilities with sexual function.

Changes in the nervous system, circulatory system, or genital organs may lead to sexual health problems. The patient with spinal cord injuries can experience an interruption of the peripheral nerves and spinal cord reflexes that involve sexual responses. Spinal cord-injured men and women have reported organsm in spite of complete denervation of all pelvic structures. They reported that the orgasm was satisfying and led to a comfortable resolution stage of sexual excitement for many of them.

Box 33-4 SELF-HELP ORGANIZATIONS THAT PUBLISH SEXUALITY PAMPHLETS

National Multiple Sclerosis Society: *Sexuality and MS*
American Arthritis Foundation: *Living and loving*
American Cancer Society: *Sexuality for the man with cancer, Sexuality for the woman with cancer*
American Diabetes Association: several pamphlets and articles for men and women with diabetes mellitus

Sexual dysfunction of the diabetic patient can occur when the disease is not well controlled. The dysfunction generally disappears when the lack of control is diagnosed and treated. Impotence is found in approximately half of the men who have diabetes and is generally related to poor control of the diabetes. Sexual counseling is important to (1) provide accurate information about the sexual aspects of the disorder, (2) dispel the patient's faulty assumptions and expectations, and (3) give advice designed to optimize the level of sexual self-esteem and dispel the guilt that is frequently found with both partners.

A mastectomy results in both physical and emotional trauma. The resultant disfigurement is only one of multiple problems that are being faced. Patients must grapple with these problems as well: (1) how to cope with cancer, (2) how the operation will affect the relationship with the spouse or significant other, (3) how they can relate to the strangeness of their own body, and (4) how their sexual life will be affected. Problems that arise with pelvic irradiation for cancer of the cervix are much harder to treat than those of mastectomy, because the entire physiology of the vagina is altered by the radiation and there is a true loss of function. With the mastectomy the function that is lost is the ability to nurse an infant. The goal for the patient and partner is to face the issue straightforwardly, so that both partners can acknowledge the diagnosis and true feelings can be acknowledged and discussed. If feelings are repressed—not verbalized or shared—both the patient and the significant other may suffer.

For the patient undergoing a mastectomy, her sexual self-concept and intimate physical interactions can and will be affected. Two variables that influence a woman's sexual function are (1) sufficient self-love and acceptance and (2) positive attitudes and feelings about sexuality. The male partner should be persuaded to face his own feelings so that he is able to offer support to his partner. Therapeutic counseling before surgery can aid the patient's and partner's acceptance and recovery after surgery.

HEALTH HISTORY

Health history data should be relevant to the developmental age of the patient. Information about reproductive health and sexuality can form a large portion of the data collection. This history is as important as the physical and mental information as a basis for determining appropriate nursing diagnoses and interventions. Data collected about sexual health, sexual relations, birth control methods, sexually transmitted disease, and the use of chemical substances provide an opportunity to clarify any misconceptions, myths, and hearsay that may be revealed during history taking.

Data Collection: Female

Data collection for adolescent and adult women focuses on the reproductive tract and the menstrual, gynecological, and obstetrical history.

The menstrual history includes the time of menarche (onset of menstrual flow) to the climacteric (cessation of menstrual cycle), as to: (1) age of onset, (2) date of last menstrual flow, (3) usual amount and volume of flow (number of pads used per day), (5) presence of **dysmenorrhea** (painful menstruation), **menorrhagia** (excessive flow), **amenorrhea** (absence of flow), or **metrorrhagia** (excessive spotting between cycles), and (5) other difficulties during menses.

The gynecological assessment includes data on (1) vaginal discharge (odor, color, frequency, and duration), (2) vaginal pruritus (itching), (3) vaginal irritation with coital activity, (4) date and results of the last Papanicolaou (Pap) test, (5) types of birth control methods or kinds of contraceptives used, and (6) family history of cancer of the reproductive system.

If the female has conceived, information should be collected as to gravidity (number of pregnancies) and parity (number of births), abortions, miscarriages, and stillbirths. Assessment of the breast includes (1) tenderness of the breast areas, (2) pain, (3) masses in any specific areas, (4) presence of nipple discharge, (5) knowledge and frequency of breast self-examination, and (6) date of last mammogram, if applicable.

Data Collection: Male

The data collected from the male adolescent and the adult male include (1) urological history of voiding difficulties and/or any discharge from the penis, (2) characteristics of the urine (odor, color, amount, and frequency), (3) information on prostate and/or testicular problems, (4) frequency of PSA testing if applicable, (5) masses or lesions on genitalia, (6) frequency of testicular self-examination, (7) frequency of professional testicular examination, (8) nature of measures to prevent infections, and (9) birth control measures. In addition, the nurse should note concerns about sexual health and the climacteric voiced by the patient.

DIAGNOSTIC TESTS FOR PROBLEMS OF THE REPRODUCTIVE SYSTEM

Diagnostic Tests for the Female

The pelvic examination is performed by a physician and is advantageous for visualization and palpation of the vulva, perineum, vagina, cervix, ovaries, and uterine surfaces. During the pelvic examination specimens are frequently obtained for diagnostic purposes. The pelvic examination progresses from the visualization and/or palpation of the external genital organs for edema and irritations to inspection for abnormalities of the internal organs. To visualize internal organs the physician inserts a vaginal speculum. The physician may do a rectovaginal examination to evaluate abnormalities or problems of the rectal area and the posterior internal organs (Box 33-5).

Colposcopy (*colpo,* a combining form meaning or pertaining to "the vagina," *scopy,* combining form meaning "observation") provides direct visualization of cervix and vagina. The patient is prepared for a pelvic examination. The vaginal speculum is inserted, followed by the insertion of the colposcope for inspection of the area. The color of the tissue, presence of growths and lesions, and condition of the vascularity are observed and specimens obtained as necessary.

Culdoscopy is another diagnostic procedure that provides visualization of the uterus and adnexa (uterine appendages, ovaries, fallopian tubes) and small intestine. The patient is given a local, spinal, or general anesthetic. After the anesthetic is administered, the patient is assisted to a knee-chest position. The culdoscope is passed through the vaginal wall in back of the cervix. The area is examined for tumors, cysts, and endometriosis. During the procedure conization (removal of eroded or infected tissue) may be done. This procedure is generally done on an outpatient basis.

Laparoscopy (the examination of the abdominal cavity with a laparoscope through a small incision made beneath the umbilicus) provides direct visualization of the uterus and adnexa. Preparation of the patient includes insertion of a Foley catheter to maintain bladder decompression for an open view. The procedure is usually done with a general anesthetic. The cervix is grasped by forceps and a lighted laparoscope is inserted through the incision. Carbon dioxide may be introduced to distend the abdomen for easier visualization. If a biopsy is to be done or organs are to be manipulated, a second incision may be made in the lower abdomen to allow for instrument insertion. The ovaries and fallopian tubes may be observed for masses, ectopic pregnancy, adhesions, and pelvic inflammatory disease. Tubal ligations may be done using this procedure.

Box 33-5 ENDOSCOPIC PROCEDURES FOR VISUALIZATION OF PELVIC ORGANS

Colposcopy Visualization of vagina and cervix under low-power magnification

Culdoscopy Insertion of a culdoscope through posterior vaginal vault into cul-de-sac of Douglas for visualization of fallopian tubes and ovaries

Hysteroscopy Insertion of a hysteroscope through the cervix for visualization of inside of the uterus

Laparoscopy Insertion of a laparoscope (under local anesthesia) through small incision in abdominal wall (inferior margin of umbilicus), which is insufflated with carbon dioxide; permits visualization of all pelvic organs

Papanicolaou (Pap) smear test (a simple smear method of examining stained exfoliative peeling and sloughing off of tissue or cells) is most widely known for its use in the early detection of cervical cancer. Scrapings of secretions and cells are taken from the cervix and spread on a glass slide. The slide is sprayed with a fixative and sent to the laboratory for analysis. It is important that slides be properly labeled. The label should give the date, time of the last menstrual period, and whether the woman is taking estrogens or birth control pills. Annual tests should be performed for women who (1) are over 40 years of age, (2) are in high-risk categories for cervical cancer, (3) have had previous positive reports, and (4) are sexually active women under 20 years of age. If a Pap test is positive or suggests a malignancy, a cervical biopsy is done to confirm the diagnosis.

Biopsies are procedures in which samples of tissues are taken for evaluation to confirm or locate a lesion. Tissue is aspirated by special needles or removed by forceps or through an incision.

A *cervical biopsy* is done to evaluate suspicious cervical lesions and to diagnose cervical cancer. The biopsy is generally done without anesthesia. For direct visualization the colposcope is inserted through the vaginal speculum, the cervical site is selected and cleansed, and tissue is removed. The area is packed with gauze or a tampon to check the blood flow.

A *breast biopsy* is performed to differentiate benign or malignant tumors. Breast biopsy is indicated for patients with palpable masses, suspicious areas appearing from mammography, and persistent encrusted, purulent, inflamed, or sanguineous discharge from the nipples. The procedure is performed by needle biopsy, under local anesthetic, or by open biopsy with general or local anesthetic. In a needle biopsy, fluid is aspirated from the breast and is expelled into a specimen bottle. Pressure is placed on the site to stop bleeding. When bleeding has ceased, an adhesive bandage is applied. In an open biopsy, an incision is made in a portion of the breast to expose the mass; tissue portions are incised, or the whole mass may be incised. Specimens of selected tissue may be frozen and stained for rapid diagnosis. The wound is sutured and a bandage is applied. The incision site should be observed for bleeding, tenderness, and erythema.

An *endometrial biopsy* is performed to collect tissue for diagnosis of endometrial cancer and analysis for infertility studies. The procedure is generally performed at the time of menstruation when the cervix is dilated and cells are more easily obtained. The cervix is locally anesthetized, a curette is inserted, and tissue is obtained from selected sites of the endometrium.

Conization of the cervix is indicated when eroded or infected tissue is to be removed or there is a need for confirmation of cervical cancer. A cone-shaped section is removed when the mass is confined to the epithelial tissue. After surgery the area is packed with gauze to control bleeding. The patient is observed for bleeding and is generally discharged from the hospital the same day.

Dilation and **curettage** (scraping of material from the wall of a cavity or other surface, performed to remove tumors or other abnormal tissue for microscopic study) is a procedure performed to obtain tissue for biopsy, to correct cervical stricture, and/or to treat dysmenorrhea. The patient is prepared for general anesthesia. While the patient is anesthetized, the cervix is dilated and the inside of the uterus scraped with a curette. A packing may be inserted for hemostasis and a perineal pad is applied for absorption of drainage.

Cultures and smears are collected to examine and identify infectious processes, presence of abnormal cells, and hormonal changes of the reproductive tissue. Specimens collected for smears are prepared by spreading the collected smear on a glass slide and covered with a second slide or sprayed with a fixative. Specimens should be handled with aseptic technique and caution should be observed to avoid transfer and spread of organisms. Cultures are taken from exudates of the breast, vagina, rectum, and/or urethra. Sexually transmitted diseases and mastitis are diagnosed by isolation of the causative organisms.

Shiller's iodine test is used for the early detection of cancer cells and to guide the physician in doing a biopsy. An iodine preparation, applied to the cervix, produces a brown stain for normal vaginal cells. Glycogen, which is present in normal cells, will stain brown when the iodine solution is applied. Abnormal or immature cells do not absorb the stain. This method of detection is valuable but is not entirely reliable, because normal cells sometimes lack glycogen, and malignant tissue at times will contain glycogen. After the procedure the patient should wear a perineal pad to avoid staining of the clothing.

Radiographic examinations are performed to detect abnormal tissue, locate abnormal structures, and observe patency of ducts.

Hysterograms and *hysterosalpingograms* are studies for visualizing the uterine cavity to confirm (1) tubal abnormalities (adhesions and occlusions), (2) presence of foreign bodies, (3) congenital malformations, and (4) traumatic injuries. The patient is placed in the lithotomy position. A speculum is inserted in the vagina, a cannula is inserted through the speculum into the cervical cavity, and a contrast medium is injected through the cannula. As the contrast medium progresses through the cavity, the uterus and fallopian tubes are viewed by the fluoroscope and films are taken.

Mammography is radiography of the soft tissue of the breast to allow identification of various benign and neoplastic processes, especially those not palpable on physical examination. It is believed that the average breast tumor is present for 9 years before it is palpable. Mammography is helpful as a screening procedure for those with a family history of breast cancer. It is recommended by the American Cancer Society that baseline mammograms be performed on women between the ages of 35 and 39; every 1 to 2 years for women 40 to 49 years of age; and yearly for women 50 years of age and beyond.

At the time the procedure is scheduled, the nurse advises the patient to refrain from using body powders, deodorants, and ointments on the breast areas, because this could cause false-positive results. Before the procedure the patient is provided with a patient gown and asked to remove jewelry and upper garments. The patient is asked to sit or stand in an upright position and rest one breast on the x-ray table. A compressor is placed on the breast, and the patient is asked to hold her breath as an anterior view is taken. The machine is rotated and again the breast is compressed and a lateral view is taken. The procedure is repeated on the other breast. The patient may be asked to wait until the x-ray films are read. Xeromammography involves recording of the radiographic images on a selenium-coated plate and transferring the images to a special paper. This process enables enhancement of edges and sharpening of images.

Magnetic resonance imaging (MRI) provides excellent visualization of tissue without the use of a contrast medium or ionizing radiation. It is not as readily available or economical as other diagnostic methods.

In *pelvic ultrasonography,* high-frequency sound waves are passed into the area to be examined and images are formed on a screen—similar to an x-ray film. Ultrasound is useful in detecting foreign bodies (such as IUDs), distinguishing between cystic and solid tumor bodies, evaluating fetal growth and viability, detecting fetal abnormalities, and detecting ectopic pregnancy. Generally it is noninvasive, safe, and painless. Fluids are encouraged. The nurse should explain that a full bladder is essential to the accuracy of the test.

Tubal insufflation (Rubin test) involves transuterine insufflation of the fallopian tubes with carbon dioxide (Fig. 33-9). The procedure enables evaluation of the patency of the fallopian tubes and may be part of a fertility study. Tubal insufflation takes approximately 30 minutes and is usually performed on an outpatient basis. If the tubes are open, the gas enters the abdominal cavity. A high-pitched bubbling can be heard through the abdominal wall with the stethoscope as the gas escapes

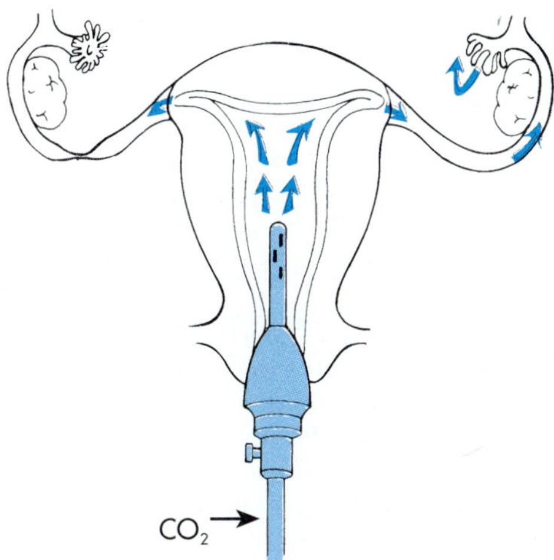

FIG. 33-9 Rubin test. Carbon dioxide escapes into abdominal cavity through patent left uterine tube.

from the tubes. The patient may complain of shoulder pain from diaphragmatic irritation; an x-ray film will show free gas under the diaphragm. If the tubes are occluded, gas cannot pass from the tubes, and pain will not be reported.

All pregnancy tests, regardless of method, are based on detection of human chorionic gonadotropin (HCG), which is secreted in the urine after the fertilization of the ovum. Regardless of method, it is important to know that the tests do not indicate whether the pregnancy is normal. False positives may occur.

Diagnostic Tests for the Male

Testicular biopsy is a means to detect abnormal cells and the presence of sperm. The testing can be done by aspiration or through an incision. The anesthetic used depends on the choice of technique. Postbiopsy care consists of comfort measures with a scrotal support, ice pack, and analgesic medications. Warm sitz baths for edema may be helpful. The nurse should instruct the patient to call the physician if bleeding occurs.

Semen analysis can be performed to substantiate the effectiveness of a vasectomy, to detect semen on the body or clothing of a suspected rape victim, and to rule out paternity. The procedure is generally one of the first tests to be performed on the male patient to evaluate fertility. Collection of semen for evaluation of fertility may be by manual stimulation, coitus interruptus, or the use of a condom.

Prostatic smears are obtained to detect and identify microorganisms and tumor cells in the prostate. The physician massages the prostate by way of the rectum, and the patient voids into a sterile container prepared with additive preservative. The specimen is collected and a smear is prepared in the laboratory. It is possible to detect some cases of cancer and even tuberculosis of the prostate gland by this method.

In *cystoscopy* the prostate and bladder of the male can be examined by passing a lighted cystoscope through the urethra to the bladder. The examination is usually performed without anesthesia, but a local anes-

Box 33-6 NURSING INTERVENTIONS FOR THE PATIENT UNDERGOING DIAGNOSTIC STUDIES

1. Explain the examination carefully.
2. Provide privacy.
3. Obtain a signed consent when necessary.
4. Prepare the skin for surgery according to agency protocol.
5. Assess the patient for allergies.
6. As appropriate, request that the patient partially or completely disrobe and remove all jewelry. Provide gown and/or drape.
7. Give preexamination instructions; NPO status if indicated.
8. Encourage verbalization and discussion of fears.
9. Administer preexamination medication as ordered by physician.
10. Occasionally it will be necessary to advise patients to go without medications for 24 hours. A medication history should be obtained.
11. If the specimen is to be collected at home, stress the importance of handling all specimens precisely as directed.
12. It may be necessary to monitor vital signs.
13. Be attentive during examination; offer support as necessary.
14. Relay any immediate concerns to the physician as appropriate.
15. Guide patients to follow any postexamination instructions.
16. Inform the patient that some discomfort can be expected. Minor discomfort can be relieved by mild analgesics such as aspirin or Tylenol, but if pain becomes more intense, the physician should be notified. Most discomfort is temporary.
17. When pertinent, tell patients to rest and to avoid any heavy lifting following the examination for 24 hours as directed by the physician.
18. When relevant, advise the patient to avoid douching or intercourse until the site is healed. Consult the physician.
19. Caution patients to report any bleeding from an incisional area.
20. Advise the patient to avoid the use of tampons as directed by the physician.
21. Inform the patient how test results may be obtained.

thetic may be instilled into the bladder. This can be done for both men and women to detect bladder infections and tumors.

Other diagnostic studies for men include the rectal digital examination and the prostatic-specific antigen (PSA), a highly sensitive blood test. PSA, which is normally secreted and disposed of by the prostate, shows up in the blood stream in cancer as well as in a harmless condition called *benign prostatic hyperplasia (BPH)* or *prostate enlargement.* Elevated PSA levels in the blood stream means something needs to be checked. Still other studies are the alkaline phosphatase (ALP) test and the acid phosphatase (ACP) test. The ACP test is being used less frequently since the PSA test was developed (see Chapter 30). These specific tests are useful in diagnosing benign prostatic hypertrophy, prostatic cancer, bone metastasis in prostatic cancer, as well as other disease conditions. See Box 33-6 on p. 997 for nursing interventions for patients undergoing diagnostic tests.

THE REPRODUCTIVE CYCLE

Menarche

Menarche, the beginning of menses, designates the first menstrual cycle. Menarche is a sign of puberty in the young female and that the body is capable of supporting pregnancy.

The menarche occurs from 9 to 17 years of age, the average age being 12.5 years. The cycle length varies from 24 to 32 days, the average cycle lasting 29 days. The duration of the flow is from 1 to 8 days, the average being 3 to 5 days. The amount of flow is from 10 to 75 ml, the average being 35 ml per cycle.

The nurse should help patients promote reproductive and sexual health. Nurses may have the opportunity to instruct or counsel women about personal hygiene. Personal cleanliness is a health habit that should be promoted for all patients and implemented in each care plan. This is especially meaningful during menstruation. See Box 33-7 for health teaching for menstruation.

Box 33-7 HEALTH TEACHING FOR MENSTRUATION

1. Knowledge of the physiological process
2. Factors that may alter the menstrual cycle: stress, fatigue, exercise, acute or chronic illness, changes in climate, or working hours and pregnancy
3. Personal hygiene
   a. Wear pads during early period of heavy flow
   b. Change tampons frequently to decrease risk of toxic shock syndrome
   c. Consult physician if tampons cause discomfort
   d. Take a daily shower for comfort (warm baths may relieve slight pelvic discomfort)
   e. Keep perineal area clean and dry; cleanse from anterior to posterior
   f. Cotton underwear preferred
      Nylon panty hose and tight-fitting slacks cause retention of moisture and should not be used for extended periods of time
   g. Feminine hygiene products, such as vaginal sprays and suppositories, may contribute to a feeling of cleanliness.
   h. A daily douche is not recommended, because it changes the protective bacterial flora of the vagina and predisposes the woman to infection
4. Exercise
   a. Exercise is not contraindicated and may help prevent discomfort
   b. Modify exercise if fatigue occurs
5. Diet
   a. Restrict salt intake if fluid retention is present
   b. Consult a physician if fluid retention persists after menstruation
6. Discomfort
   a. For mild discomfort take aspirin or acetaminophen (Tylenol), apply warmth, and rest
   b. For prolonged, severe discomfort, consult a physician

Disturbances of Menstruation

Because of the relationship between the menstrual cycle and the body's mechanisms of hormonal secretion, a decrease or increase in the activity of the hormonal glands can disturb menstruation. The most common disturbances include the following:

Amenorrhea: absence of menstrual flow
Dysmenorrhea: painful menstruation
Abnormal uterine bleeding
Hypermenorrhea/menorrhagia: excessive bleeding (amount and duration)
Metrorrhagia: bleeding between menstrual periods

Another disturbance of the menstrual cycle is premenstrual syndrome. This will be discussed later.

Suggested nursing diagnoses are anxiety, ineffective coping, fear, pain, knowledge deficit, and low self-esteem. Nursing interventions are based on specific behaviors, symptoms, and treatments.

Amenorrhea. Amenorrhea (absence of menstrual flow) is normal before puberty, after menopause, during pregnancy, and sometimes during lactation. Menstrual flow may also be absent or suppressed as a result of hormonal abnormalities or surgical interventions such as a hysterectomy (surgical removal of the uterus).

Etiology/pathophysiology. Amenorrhea is classified as *primary* when menarche has not occurred by the age of 17 to 18 years. The cause may be a congenital defect. *Secondary* amenorrhea means that there has been an initial menarche but flow has ceased for at least

3 months or there has been an absence of vaginal fluid for 12 months, coupled with a history of irregular bleeding. Causes for secondary amenorrhea may be normal pregnancy; frequent, vigorous exercise, as in women athletes; or an emotional disorder such as depression, anorexia (lack of appetite), or bulimia (an insatiable craving for food, often resulting in episodes of continuous eating followed by purging).

Assessment. Early diagnosis and prompt management are necessary if more serious reproductive and genital problems are to be prevented. The nurse should urge the sexually active woman to see a physician as soon as a menstrual period is missed. Maintaining health during pregnancy is vital for both the mother and the fetus. Women who suspect their amenorrhea is caused by menopause can be examined by a physician to confirm this.

Obtaining a family history is important. Emotional factors (behaviors) that may influence the menstrual cycle should be assessed. A menstrual history should include (1) the number of periods missed and (2) whether amenorrhea was present previously. Recent use of medications and drugs needs to be determined.

Diagnostic tests. Beyond the preliminary workup and when pregnancy is not a possibility, the diagnostic study for primary and secondary amenorrhea is the same. This study includes the following:

Pelvic examination
Blood, urine, and hormonal analysis
Determination of existing tumors
Papanicolaou (Pap) smear

Medical management. Treatment is based on the underlying cause and must be determined on an individual basis. It may mean hormonal therapy, or, as in a majority of cases, surgical intervention may be necessary.

Nursing interventions. Nursing diagnoses and interventions for women with amenorrhea but are not limited to the following:

NURSING DIAGNOSIS	NURSING INTERVENTIONS
Coping, ineffective individual, related to lack of menstrual flow	Acknowledge patient's feelings. Provide emotional support. Refer to counseling as necessary Explain diagnostic procedures. Provide information, privacy, or consultation as indicated for sexual concerns.

Patient teaching. The nurse should encourage compliance with treatment and emphasize the importance of follow-up visits with the physician for treatment, therapy, and further evaluation of treatment efficacy.

Dysmenorrhea. Uterine pain with menstruation, commonly called "menstrual cramps," is dysmenorrhea. Primary dysmenorrhea that is not associated with pelvic disorders usually develops when ovulatory function is established (under 20 years of age), and there is no underlying organic disease. Often it will disappear or decline after pregnancy or by the late twenties. Secondary dysmenorrhea is painful menstruation caused by organic disease such as pelvic inflammatory disease (PID) or endometriosis and most often occurs in women over 20 years of age.

Studies in industry and schools have shown dysmenorrhea to be the greatest single cause of absenteeism among women. It is one of the most common health problems for which women seek treatment.

Etiology/pathophysiology. The causes of dysmenorrhea can be related to endocrine imbalance, increase in prostaglandin secretions, or chronic illnesses, fatigue, and anemia.

A recent theory proposes that hypercontractility of the uterus resulting from higher-than-normal levels of prostaglandins may be the cause of dysmenorrhea. Whatever the cause, the symptoms and pain are real. Conditions that cause general debilitation, such as inadequate diet and exercise, anemia, and fatigue, are often related to dysmenorrhea.

Assessment. Many women have systemic symptoms of breast tenderness, abdominal distention, nausea and vomiting, headache, vertigo, palpitations, and excessive perspiration.

The nurse should assess the woman for colicky and cyclic pain and, infrequently, dull pain in the lower pelvis that radiates toward the perineum and back. This pain may be experienced 24 to 48 hours before menses or at the onset of menses.

Family history is important, because dysmenorrhea has been reported to be significantly increased among mothers and sisters of women with dysmenorrhea.

Secondary dysmenorrhea is suspected if the symptoms begin after 20 years of age. It has been described as a steady or cramping pain and may be specific to the site of pelvic disorder.

Diagnostic tests. Diagnostic studies to rule out organic causes for dysmenorrhea include pelvic examination, laparoscopy, dilation and curettage, and hysterosalpingography.

Medical management. Treatment of secondary dysmenorrhea is aimed at the cause. Surgical and medication intervention may be appropriate, depending on the severity and type of pathological condition.

If no organic cause is found, the nurse should instruct the woman to exercise and eat nutritious foods, especially those high in fiber, and to avoid constipation (see Chapter 19).

Local applications of heat and mild analgesics are prescribed. Medications for dysmenorrhea include aspirin, which causes vasodilation of blood vessels, and prostaglandin inhibitors such as ibuprofen (Motrin) and naproxen sodium (Anaprox). Oral contraceptives may be used to suppress ovulation by inhibiting prostaglandin levels (see medication table on pp.1000-1001).

MEDICATIONS FOR REPRODUCTIVE DISORDERS

Medication	Trade Name	Action	Side Effects	Nursing Implications
Oral contraceptives (estrogen-progesterone combinations)	Ortho Novum, Norlestrin, Ovral, Triphasil	Inhibit ovulation by suppressing gonadotropins FSH and LH and alters genital tract to inhibit sperm penetration and inhibit implantation	Nausea, cramps, diarrhea, appetite change, acne, rash, increased BP, thrombophlebitis, edema, dysmenorrhea, bleeding irregularities, depression, fatigue, breast changes, cholestatic jaundice, optic neuritis	Monitor glucose, thyroid function, and liver function tests; check Homan's sign for clot detection; monitor blood pressure; discontinue if patient if pregnant.
Conjugated equine estrogen	Premarin	Needed for proper functioning of female reproductive system, affects release of gonadotropins, inhibits ovulation, and is involved in adequate calcium use in bone structure	Nausea, peripheral edema, enlargement of breasts, breast tenderness, anorexia, vomiting, diarrhea, headache, thrombophlebitis, dizziness, depression	Check urine glucose in diabetic patient; notify physician of weight gain of 5 pounds or greater per week (patient may need diuretic); monitor blood pressure; check liver function test; check Homan's sign for possible clots; give IV product slowly to prevent flushing.
Butoconazole	Femstat Cream	Same as clotrimazole	Same as terconazole	Same as clotrimazole.
Clotrimazole	Mycelex-7, Gyne-Lotrimin, Femcare	Interferes with fungal DNA replication, binds sterols in fungal cell membrane	Rash, urticaria, stinging, burning, peeling, blistering skin fissures, abdominal cramps, bloating, urinary frequency	Watch for allergic reactions; note therapeutic response-decrease in size and number of lesions); use gloves for application; know that it can be used through menstrual cycle; avoid use of other vaginal creams or suppositories during therapy.
Miconazole nitrate	Monistat-3, Monistat-7	Same as clotrimazole	Vulvovaginal burning, itching, pelvic cramps, rash, urticaria, stinging, burning, contact dermatitis	Same as clotrimazole.
Tioconazole ointment	Vagistat-1	Same as Miconazole but 2 to 8 times more potent	Vulvovaginal burning, itching, soreness, swelling	Same as clotrimazole.
Metronidazole	Flagyl, Protostat	Direct-acting amebicide/trichomonacide binds, degrades DNA in organism	Rash, headache, dizziness, fatigue, convulsions, blurred vision, nausea, vomiting, diarrhea, pseudomembranous colitis, albuminuria, neurotoxicity, metallic taste, disulfiram type of reaction with alcohol	Watch for allergic reactions and superinfection; check stool for parasites; give oral form with food; watch for vision problems; tell patient not to drink alcohol during therapy.

MEDICATIONS FOR REPRODUCTIVE DISORDERS—cont'd

Medication	Trade Name	Action	Side Effects	Nursing Implications
Nystatin	Mycostatin	Same as clotrimazole	Rash, urticaria, stinging, burning	Same as clotrimazole.
Terconazole	Terazol-7, Terazol-3	Same as clotrimazole	Vulvovaginal burning, itching, pelvic cramps, rash, urticaria, stinging, burning	Same as clotrimazole.
Nystatin	Nilstat, Mycostatin, O-V statin	Interferes with fungal DNA replication, causes fungal cell membrane permeability	Rash, stinging, burning, urticaria, nausea, vomiting, anorexia, diarrhea	Watch for allergic reaction; use gloves for topical application; For vaginal preparation, tell patient that she may need light-day pads.
Topical amphotericin B	Fungizone—cream, lotion, ointment	Binds to ergosterol, altering cell membrane permeability in susceptible fungi	Urticaria, stinging, burning, dry skin, pruritis, contact dermatitis, staining of nail lesions	Cover lesion completely after cleansing and drying well; use gloves to prevent further infection; watch for allergic reactions; tell patient that it may cause skin and clothing discoloration.
Medroxyprogesterone acetate	Provera Amen, Cycrin, Depo-Provera	Inhibits secretion of pituitary gonadotropins, which acts to prevent follicular maturation and ovulation; stimulates growth in mammary tissue	Bleeding irregularities, breast tenderness, masculinization of fetus, edema, cholestatic jaundice, thrombophlebitis, anorexia, acne, mental depression, weight gain or loss	Notify physician of weight gain of 5 pounds or greater per week; monitor blood pressure at beginning of treatment and periodically thereafter check liver function test; discontinue if patient is pregnant.
Transdermal estrogen system	Estraderm	Same as conjugated equine estrogen	Same as conjugated equine estrogen	Same as conjugated equine estrogen.
Testosterone propionate	Testosterone Propionate	Increases weight by building body tissue; increases potassium, phosphorus, chloride, and nitrogen levels; increases bone development	Acne, flushing, gynecomastia, edema, hypercalcemia, nausea, cholestatic hepatitis, aggressive behavior, headache, anxiety, mental depression, androgenic and anabolic activity	Check weight daily; monitor blood pressure; monitor growth rate in children; check electrolyte (potassium, sodium, chloride, calcium) and cholesterol levels; monitor liver function test.
Danazol	Danocrine	Synthetic androgen, causes atrophy of endometrial tissue; decreases FSH and LH, which leads amenorrhea and anovulation	Fluid retention, virilization, androgenic effects, weight gain, amenorrhea, dizziness, headache, rashes, hepatic impairment	Check weight; monitor I & O; check for edema; give with food or milk to decrease GI upset.
Acyclovir ointment	Zovirax	Antiviral agent that interferes with DNA synthesis needed for viral replication	Mild pain with transient burning;stinging, pruritus, rash, vulvitis	Apply ointment every 3 hr or 6 times daily around the clock; cover all lesions; use gloves when applying for self-protection.

Nursing interventions. Nursing diagnoses and interventions for women with dysmenorrhea include but are not limited to the following:

NURSING DIAGNOSES	NURSING INTERVENTIONS
Knowledge deficit, related to lack of education concerning disease process and treatment	Present information on orientation to the hospital setting, disease process, procedures to be performed, medications, and treatments.
	Prepare for informational question and answer sessions according to patient needs.
	Teach procedures patient must know how to perform.
	Obtain feedback.
	Be certain learning has taken place. (Reinforce teaching as needed.)
	Develop a trusting relationship.
	Involve patient in care.
Pain, related to biological agent	Assess nature of pain.
	Observe nonverbal cues.
	Encourage pain reduction techniques as appropriate.
	Explore best method for controlling pain (medication, positioning, comfort measures such as backrub or use of heat or cold, etc.).
	Monitor vital signs.
	Provide quiet environment, calm activities.
	Promote wellness; discuss with significant other(s) ways in which they can assist the patient.

Patient teaching. The nurse should instruct women to maintain good posture, to exercise, and to practice good nutrition and should encourage a positive attitude. Women who are unable to engage in normal activities because of dysmenorrhea should be urged to seek health care.

Abnormal Uterine Bleeding. Abnormal uterine bleeding may take many forms. Two of these will be discussed: hypermenorrhea and metrorrhagia.

Hypermenorrhea is excessive bleeding at the time of the regular menstrual flow. In younger women it may be attributable to endocrine disturbances but in older women it is usually indicative of inflammatory disturbances or uterine tumors. Emotional or psychological problems may also affect uterine bleeding. The severity of hypermenorrhea is usually estimated in terms of numbers of pads or tampons used in excess of those used for the regular menstrual flow.

Metrorrhagia is the appearance of uterine bleeding between the regular menstrual periods or after menopause. It merits early diagnosis and treatment, because it may be indicative of cancer or benign tumors of the uterus.

Diagnosis is made by a routine speculum and pelvic examination. Also used to diagnose gynecological causes of hypermenorrhea and metrorrhagia are the endometrial biopsy and dilation and curettage (D&C).

The nurse should (1) assess for bleeding, pain, vaginal secretions, and psychosocial concerns; (2) encourage the woman to express her feelings; (3) explain the importance of recording dates, type of flow, and number of sanitary pads or tampons used; (4) teach the patient pain-relieving techniques; and (5) explain the importance of sharing concerns with her partner.

Women of all ages need to be educated about the importance of follow-up care when abnormal uterine bleeding is initially detected.

Premenstrual Syndrome (PMS). PMS occurs in 30% to 50% of females between the ages of 25 to 45 years. It differs from dysmenorrhea because it has no relation to ovulation.

Etiology/pathophysiology. It is believed that PMS is related to the neuroendocrine events occurring within the anterior pituitary gland. It is known that there is a loss of intravascular fluid into the body tissues, which causes water retention, bloating, and weight gain.

The syndrome occurs 7 to 10 days before the menstrual period and usually subsides within the first 3 days after the onset of the menstrual flow.

Intake of sodium and use of alcohol, tobacco, and caffeine should be evaluated as possible causes.

Clinical manifestations. Symptoms are multiple and vary among individuals and may be behavioral or physical. Behavioral symptoms include irritability, lethargy (inactivity), fatigue, sleep disturbances, and depression. Headache, vertigo, backache, acne, paresthesia (burning, tingling) of hands and feet, and allergies, if present, may become worse. There are many symptoms that may appear alone or in combination with other symptoms. Some women accept the symptoms as being normal and only after the symptoms become severe do they seek medical help.

Assessment. Collection of *subjective data* needs to be specific as to the symptoms and combination of symptoms that occur with each woman. Each patient is asked to maintain a log for three consecutive menstrual cycles of symptoms and activities that relate to the menstrual period. The collected information can be analyzed and symptoms treated accordingly.

Collection of *objective data* pertinent to the syndrome, especially the inability to perform activities of daily living in the multiple roles as wife, mother, and career person, should be assessed by the nurse.

Diagnostic tests. Diagnostic tests include evaluation of estrogen and progesterone levels to rule out hormonal imbalances and determination of glucose levels; low levels may lead to irritability. Dietary analysis may reveal the need for adjustments or alterations.

Medical management. PMS has no single treatment and no specific medication. Some physicians prescribe analgesics, diuretics, and progesterone. The patient's diet should be reviewed. A diet high in complex carbohydrates, moderate in protein, and low in refined sugar and sodium should be eaten, especially during the premenstrual interval. The consumption of caffeine (in tea, coffee, or caffeine-containing beverages), chocolate, and alcohol and smoking should be reduced or eliminated. Regular exercise 3 or 4 times a week for 30 minutes is encouraged, especially during the premenstrual interval. Because fatigue may exaggerate PMS symptoms, adequate rest, sleep, and relaxation are helpful (see Chapter 18).

Nursing interventions. Nursing diagnoses and interventions for the woman with premenstrual syndrome include but are not limited to the following:

NURSING DIAGNOSIS	NURSING INTERVENTIONS
Anxiety, related to PMS	Encourage verbalization of feelings. Acknowledge existence of the syndrome and its symptoms. Encourage the patient to keep a menstrual symptom calendar to document the cycle and nature of the symptoms. Encourage the patient to plan activities during the symptom-free part of her cycle. Administer supplements of vitamin B_6, calcium, and magnesium as prescribed. Encourage daily exercise and relaxation. Encourage self-help groups and the reading of self-help literature (group support tends to reduce stress). Provide emotional support with a nonjudgmental and caring manner. Assist in identifying possible sources of anxiety. Assist in identifying coping mechanisms.

Patient teaching. The patient should assume responsibility for following a dietary plan of eating small meals and eliminating or restricting sugar, alcohol, caffeine, and nicotine, which may minimize the symptoms of PMS.

Climacteric. The **climacteric** is the phase of the aging process of women and men who are making a transition from a reproductive phase to a nonpreproductive stage of life. The phase occurs in middle adulthood and marks the onset of a decrease in hormone secretion, cessation of ovulation and menses, and physical changes.

Menopause. The female climacteric is called *menopause.* Female menopause is the normal cessation of the menstrual cycle, which appears on an infrequent cycle for a period of time that usually does not exceed 2 years. As long as the menstrual cycle occurs, no matter how infrequently, ovulation continues and the potential for conception exists.

Etiology/pathophysiology. Menopause is the normal decline of ovarian function resulting from the aging process. Menopause begins in most women between 35 and 60 years of age, the average age being 51, and is characterized by infrequent ovulation, decreased menstrual function, and eventually cessation of the menstrual flow.

Menopause may be artificially induced by such procedures as irradiation of the ovaries and surgical removal of both ovaries. Each of these has one common consequence, namely, cessation of menstruation. However, surgical removal or irradiation of the ovaries results in menopause with all its physiological changes whereas ovaries left intact after hysterectomy will continue to function provided the age of climacteria has not yet been reached.

Decline in ovarian function produces a variety of symptoms, such as a decrease in the frequency, amount, and duration of the menstrual flow, spotting, amenorrhea, and polymenorrhea (increased number of menstrual periods). Symptoms can last from a few months to several years before menstruation ceases permanently. Menopause is not considered to be completed until 1 year after the last menstrual period.

Clinical manifestations. Physical changes that occur in the body systems do not generally develop until after permanent cessation of menstruation. Changes of the reproductive system include shrinkage of vulval structures, atrophic vulvitis, shortening of the vagina, and dryness of the vaginal wall. There is a pelvic relaxation of supporting structures as a result of the decrease in estrogen. Cystitis and urinary frequency and urgency may appear as changes of the urinary system. There is a loss of skin turgor and elasticity, increase in subcutaneous fat, decrease in breast tissue, and thinning of hair of the axilla, head, and pubis. About 25% of postmenopausal women develop osteoporosis.

Assessment. Collection of *subjective data* should include family history. The nurse should determine whether family members and/or significant others are aware of the transition and if they are supportive. Emotional illness, if present, should be noted. "Hot flashes" caused by glandular imbalances may become prominent. Other symptoms may include fatigue, vertigo, headache, nausea, dyspareunia, palpitations, and chest and neck pain. With some there is an emotional feeling of being unwanted and some may fear growing old. Both could cause depression.

Collection of *objective data* includes an awareness that some patients may display frequent crying spells and/or outbursts of anger. The use of contraceptives should be explored. Frequency, amount, and duration of the menstrual flow need to be assessed. Diaphoresis, weight gain, and vomiting, as well as tachycardia, may occur. The nurse can note many of these disturbances.

Diagnostic tests. Tests include analysis of hormonal levels. Other diagnostic testing may be indicated by symptoms. Some examinations are performed to rule out possible conditions such as cancer.

Medical management. Typically, estrogen therapy is administered cyclically, usually in the form of conjugated equine estrogens (Premarin) taken orally from days 1 to 25; from days 15 to 25 medroxyprogesterone acetate (Provera) is taken. Thereafter, this cycle is repeated. A transdermal estrogen system (Estraderm) in the form of skin patches is also currently being evaluated as a long-term modality for osteoporosis. Estrogen therapy is contraindicated in thromboembolic disease, in undiagnosed vaginal bleeding, and with estrogen-dependent tumors of the uterus or breast. It is used cautiously in cases of underlying cardiovascular or severe hepatic or renal disease. It may increase the risk of endometrial carcinoma. Characterized by decreased bone mineral content and bone calcium, osteoporotic problems include back pain, decreased height and mobility, and fractures of the spine, arm, upper femur and ribs (see Chapter 26).

Some physicians recommend calcium supplements, which are available in many forms, but the generic calcium carbonate products are the most cost effective.

Nursing interventions. Education regarding menopause should occur before its onset. Many women appreciate opportunities made by nurses to discuss menopause. An exercise program should be set up that includes both movement and weight bearing. Walking is an excellent weight-bearing exercise. Other exercises include bicycling, stationary cycling, and aerobic dancing.

Nursing diagnoses and interventions for the patient with menopause include but are not limited to the following:

NURSING DIAGNOSES	NURSING INTERVENTIONS
Self-esteem disturbance, related to concerns about femininity, sexuality, and aging	Encourage patient and/or significant others to verbalize concerns. Confirm accurate information. Correct information related to self-concept issues. Avoid value judgments. Refer patient to couple, family, and/or sex therapy as appropriate. Provide understanding and support as appropriate.
Knowledge deficit regarding patient's physiological and psychological changes, related to climacteric and menopause	Explain the process of climacteric and menopause, depending on the patient's ability to comprehend. Explain importance of keeping fit, eating a well-balanced diet, getting adequate rest and sleep, avoiding stress and fatigue, and continuing contraception until indicated by physician. If estrogen replacement therapy is ordered, inform patient about side effects. Instruct patient to report any vaginal bleeding occurring 6 months or more after last menstrual period. Inform patient of the availability of water-soluble lubricants if needed before coitus.

Patient teaching. The nurse should emphasize that the climacteric is normal and self-limiting, and menopause is not the end of the patient's sex life. A nutritious diet and weight control will improve physical condition, and an exercise program promotes vitality. Interest and participation in activities will help decrease anxiety and tension. Skin creams and lotions can be used to prevent drying, pruritus, and cracking skin. The nurse should encourage the woman to perform breast self-examination monthly and monitor calcium intake. Contraceptives should be used for 1 year after the last menstrual period. The patient can obtain a prescription for treatment of pruritus or burning of the vulva. Women can practice Kegel exercises daily (Box 33-8) to strengthen pelvic muscles. A water-soluble lubricant such as K-Y jelly can be used to prevent dyspareunia (painful intercourse). The side effects of any medications or hormonal therapy should be explained. The nurse should emphasize that an annual physical examination is important for maintaining good health.

Male climacteric. The climacteric is less pronounced in men and may not even be apparent in many men.

Etiology/pathophysiology. The appearance of the climacteric phase is gradual and occurs between the ages of 55 and 70. There is a gradual decrease of testosterone levels and seminal fluid production. The impact is largely psychological, possibly because of the recognition of some reduction of sexual activity and interests.

Clinical manifestations. Manifestations are mostly physiological changes. Erections require more time and are not as full or firm. The prostate gland enlarges, and secretions diminish; seminal fluid decreases. The physical changes occur as the man grows older, and the most noticeable signs are thinning and loss of hair from the head, chest, axillae, and pubis. There may be some flushing and chilling. Muscle tone is decreased.

Assessment. Collection of *subjective data* generally reveals that the man is at the peak of his career or possibly considering retirement. He interprets the decreased

Box 33-8 KEGEL EXERCISES

Kegel exercises are performed to help strengthen and tighten muscles that support the pelvic organs. These muscles (pelvic floor) are used to stop the flow of urine. To perform Kegel exercises while standing or sitting, tighten the pelvic floor muscles as hard as you can. Hold for 5 seconds, then release. Repeat at least 10 times. This exercise can be done many times throughout the day. Practice while urinating: try to stop the flow of urine by tightening the pelvic muscles.

sexual needs as a loss of productivity and sexual power. Therefore the assessment should invite verbalization of emotions with coping mechanisms.

Collection of *objective data* includes assessment of behaviors that may be causing the man to be stressed and concerned. Changes that he has noted regarding his life-style and feelings of loss of self-worth should be expressed.

Diagnostic tests. Diagnostic tests include a complete physical examination to rule out abnormalities of structure and function.

Nursing interventions. Nursing diagnoses and interventions for men experiencing male climacteric include but are not limited to the following:

NURSING DIAGNOSIS	NURSING INTERVENTIONS
Coping, ineffective individual, related to situational crisis (climacteric)	Show understanding and concern. Assist the patient in identifying how the problem affects his life and future, his family, and significant others. Encourage the patient to verbalize whether factors could be influencing the way he sees the problem. Assist the patient in identifying strengths and coping skills and the nature and strength of situational support. Collect data about current and potential sources of support. Assist the patient in planning alternative solutions. Give positive reinforcement.

PATIENT TEACHING. The patient should be informed that the climacteric is normal. The nurse should encourage patients to verbalize their fears and to seek counseling if stress increases.

Impotence. Impotence is the inability of an adult man to achieve penile erection. Several forms are recognized: functional impotence (psychological basis), anatomical impotence (results from a physical defect of genital structures), and atonic impotence (involves disturbed neuromuscular function). Some neurological abnormalities that affect erectile function are tabes dorsalis, caused by advanced syphilis; congenital spinal cord anomalies, such as spina bifida; spinal cord tumors; amyotrophic lateral sclerosis (Lou Gehrig's disease); multiple sclerosis; or cord compression caused by a herniated disc. The nurse can best understand impotence by developing a broad understanding of the factors that contribute to the condition.

Medical management. Medical treatment is based on careful assessment of the causative factors. It is known that such medications as antihypertensive, antidepressive, and antianxiety agents, as well as some cardiac agents, may cause impotence. Illicit or abused substances such as alcohol, cocaine, and nicotine are also known to cause impotence. Such disease conditions as diabetes mellitus or end-stage renal, heart, and chronic obstructive pulmonary disease may also be causative factors in impotence.

There are mechanical devices available for the patient with impotence. Surgical implantation of a penile prosthesis may be performed as a "day-stay" procedure or may require hospitalization for 5 or more days, depending on the patient and the type of device used (Fig. 33-10).

Nursing interventions. The nurse is responsible for teaching the patient to administer hormonal medication (testosterone) and to watch for side effects. The nurse should advise the patient to take oral hormonal replacement drugs with meals to prevent nausea.

The nurse should advise the patient about signs and symptoms of infection of the implant, including tenderness of the penis, fever, dysuria, and signs of urinary tract infection. The nurse should educate the patient to seek medical attention promptly if infection occurs.

Infertility.

Etiology/pathophysiology. Infertility is defined as the inability to conceive after 1 year of sexual inter-

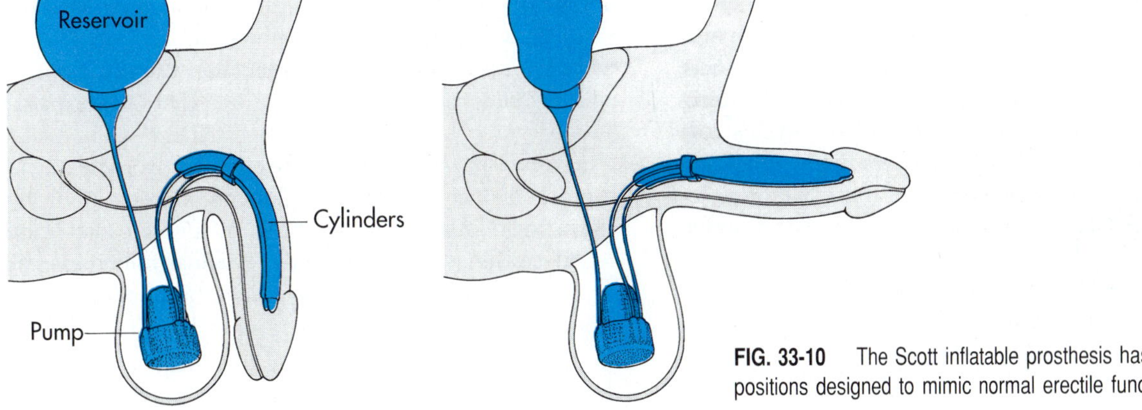

FIG. 33-10 The Scott inflatable prosthesis has erect and flaccid positions designed to mimic normal erectile function.

course without birth control measures. Primary infertility refers to couples who have never conceived. Secondary infertility refers to couples who have conceived but now are not able to do so.

The age of the woman has a significant bearing on her ability to conceive. The most fertile time of a woman's life is between the twentieth and twenty-ninth year. The most fertile time of a man's life is in his late teens and early twenties. A man's fertility does not decrease much as he grows older, but a woman's fertility drops dramatically as she ages.

Infertility may be caused by impaired sperm or ovum production or an occlusion within the reproductive system that prevents the sperm and ova from meeting. Infections of the reproductive tract, such as pelvic inflammatory disease, and sexually transmitted diseases, such as syphilis, are frequently associated with infertility. Because the man may be the infertile partner in 40% of cases of infertility, the quality and quantity of the sperm must be analyzed. The primary causes of infertility of the female are tubal insufficiency and ovarian and uterine conditions such as endometriosis or congenital defects.

Assessment. Collection of *subjective* and *objective data* includes physical examination and health histories for both partners, to make the infertility assessment and prepare a plan of treatment.

Diagnostic tests. Specific testing is necessary to rule out systemic diseases such as diabetes mellitus, neoplasms, hepatic and renal diseases, and viral conditions. Genetic defects and disorders of the testes are explored. Diagnostic testing can produce a great deal of anxiety and stress. This testing may continue for fairly long periods with or without favorable results. Male testing is somewhat simpler and most of the time is not as expensive. If there is reason to suspect infertility or sterility of the man, it is appropriate to test him first. Male infertility testing includes semen analysis, which measures the quantity and quality of semen, volume of sperm cells, sperm motility, and sperm density; and endocrine imbalance testing, which explores possible disruption of the pituitary gonadotropins and testosterone production.

Female testing focuses on the ovulation process and reliability of the reproductive organs. Female infertility testing includes (1) basal body temperature to assess ovulation; (2) endometrial biopsy, which confirms ovulation and endometrial cyclic changes; (3) endocrine studies to detect the nature of the functioning of the adrenal and thyroid glands with anovulation cycles; (4) Rubin's insufflation test, which determines tubal patency; and (5) hysterosalpingography and hysterography to assess the position and alignment of the reproductive organs.

Male and female interaction studies include the (1) Huhner test, which examines the cervical mucus for motile sperm cells after intercourse at midmenstrual cycle; (2) immunological or immunoglobin (antibody) testing for detection of spermicidal antibodies in the sera of the woman; and (3) testing both the man and woman for normalcy of their sex chromosomes.

Medical management. Medical treatment for any infertile couple depends on the cause of the infertility.

Medications causing dysfunctions can be discontinued and/or adjusted. Artificial creams, oils, and lubricants and douching can be discontinued. The man whose sperm production is low may need testosterone, vitamins, and nutritional counseling. He may need to avoid wearing jockey shorts and avoid hot tubs and saunas that may keep his testicles too warm. The woman who has endocrine deficiencies may be treated to gain the necessary balances. Surgery may be necessary to reconstruct anatomical defects.

Nursing interventions. Patients who are infertile experience guilt, disappointment, and alterations in self-esteem. Many also experience the inability to conceive as a loss and demonstrate typical grief reactions. The nurse must be sensitive to these feelings and help patients identify their reactions and coping strategies. During counseling the nurse also provides information about alternatives or options for parenting.

Prognosis. Approximately 50% of couples who undergo assessment and treatment for infertility are likely to conceive.

INFECTIONS OF THE FEMALE REPRODUCTIVE TRACT

Infections of the female reproductive tract are most commonly found in the vagina, the cervix, the fallopian tubes, and the adjacent areas. The vagina is lubricated and protected by flora containing Döderlein's bacilli, acid pH, and secretions from the vaginal and cervical cells.

Causative organisms of vaginal infections are multiple. The most common organisms that cause infection are *Escherichia coli, Candida albicans,* and *Trichomonas vaginalis.* Infections are more likely to occur when the flora and the acidity of the vagina are disturbed by administration of medication (birth control pills and antibiotics), stress, malnutrition, douching, aging, and disease. Yeast organisms grow best in an acid pH (−4.7), whereas *Trichomonas* and organisms causing nonspecific vaginitis flourish on a pH (5+) that is more alkaline.

Organisms are often introduced from external sources by way of unclean douche nozzles, poor hygiene, inadequate handwashing, neglected nail care, soiled clothing, and intercourse. Vaginal infections can be sexually transmitted, and unless both partners are treated, the infection returns.

Simple Vaginitis

Etiology/Pathophysiology. Vaginitis is a common vaginal infection. It is usually caused by *E. coli,* an organism found in feces and the rectum. It may be caused by staphylococcal and streptococcal organisms, *T. vaginalis* (a flagellated protozoan), *C. albicans* (a yeastlike fungus), and *Gardnerella* bacillus.

Vaginitis is an inflammation of the vagina. If the patient changes perineal pads and/or tampons infrequently, an irritation of the vaginal tract and inner groin occurs. This creates a medium suitable for organism growth. Examination of the vaginal walls will show a profuse foamy (bubbly) exudate if the cause of the vaginitis is *T. vaginalis.* If *C. albicans* is the causative agent, a thick, cheese-like discharge results. Bacterial vaginitis produces a milk-like discharge with a foul odor.

Clinical Manifestations. The exudate in vaginitis is yellow, white, or grayish white, curdlike, and generally accompanied by pruritus, burning, and edema of the surrounding tissue. Voiding and defecation generally intensify the symptoms.

Assessment. Collection of *subjective data* includes assessment of menstrual history, age at menarche, length of cycles, duration and nature of flow, any dysfunctions, birth control methods, medications taken, family history of diabetes mellitus, previous vaginal infections, and sexually transmitted diseases. Sexual practices and information about signs of infection in the sex partner should be elicited. Dysuria may occur as a consequence of local irritation of the urinary meatus.

Collection of *objective data* includes observation for excoriations of the skin caused by scratching, in which case secondary infection may result. The specific type of exudate is observed.

Diagnostic Tests. Diagnostic tests include direct visual examination of the vagina, culture of the organism, and bimanual examination to assess for inflammation of the vagina and its surrounding tissues.

Medical Management. Vaginal infection can be treated by a variety of methods. The major goals are to cure the infection, prevent reinfection, prevent complications, and prevent infection of the sexual partner or partners. Douching is frequently prescribed for treatment, as well as local applications of vaginal suppositories, ointments, and creams (Skill 33-1 on p. 1008).

Nursing Interventions. The nurse should advise the patient of the importance of handwashing before and after vaginal application of medications. Applications of heat in the form of douches, perineal irrigations, or sitz baths may be administered.

Nursing diagnoses and interventions for the patient with vaginitis include but are not limited to the following:

NURSING DIAGNOSES	NURSING INTERVENTIONS
Pain, related to vaginal discharge	Flush vaginal flora with acid douche (15 ml white vinegar with 1000 ml water) as ordered. Antibiotic creams may be applied after douche as ordered. Sitz bath for edema.
Infection, high risk for, related to invasion of pathogenic organisms	Cleanse perineum with witch hazel cleansing pads after defecating and voiding as ordered.
Knowledge deficit, related to good personal body hygiene	Provide appropriate teaching.
Infection, high risk for, related to sexually transmitted disease	Administer medication and treatments as ordered. Teach preventive methods, such as use of condoms
Sexual dysfunction, related to discomfort and pain	Recommend that partner be checked for infection and treated as necessary to avoid reinfection.

Patient teaching. Most patients with vaginal infection are directed to abstain from sexual intercourse during the period of treatment. The male partner's use of a condom until symptoms of infection disappear may be advised. The patient is also instructed that her sexual partner should be treated.

Prognosis. With proper treatment, the prognosis is good.

Senile Vaginitis or Atrophic Vaginitis

This condition occurs in women after menopause and upon aging. Low estrogen levels cause the vulva and vagina to atrophy and become susceptible to the invasion of bacteria. The exudate causes pruritus, edema, and skin irritations. Estrogen, vaginal suppositories, and ointments may be applied.

Cervicitis

Cervicitis, infection of the cervix, is one of the most common diseases of the reproductive system. The infection occurs from vaginal infection or sexually transmitted disease, such as *Chlamydia trachomatis* infection, gonorrhea, herpes II, or trichomoniasis. The infection often follows childbirth or abortion when lacerations occur. Therapy is specific to the causative organisms. Symptoms are backaches, whitish exudate, and menstrual irregularities. If cervicitis remains untreated, the tissues are continually irritated and the infection may spread to other pelvic organs. Personal hygiene and frequent warm tub

SKILL 33-1

PERFORMING A VAGINAL IRRIGATION (DOUCHE)

1. Review physician's order.
2. Identify patient.
3. Explain procedure to patient.
4. Suggest elimination.
5. Obtain and prepare supplies:
   Douche kit (bag, tubing, and nozzle)
   1000 to 1500 ml of irrigating solution at 100.5° to 110° F (40.5° to 43.3° C)
   Bedpan
   Disposable gloves; goggles is splashing is likely
6. Assist patient onto bedpan; head of bed may be raised slightly for patient's comfort. Inspect perineal area. If necessary, don gloves, and perform perineal care.
7. Don clean gloves; don goggles, if splashing is likely.
8. Allow sufficient solution to run through tubing to expel air and to moisten nozzle; allow some solution to flow onto patient's perineal area to test degree of warmth of solution.
9. Separate labia while directing some solution to flow over outer area.
10. Insert nozzle downward and backward. *Gently* rotate nozzle within vagina during irrigation.
11. Position container of irrigation solution at height that will not allow the solution to instill too quickly (18 to 24 inches [45 to 60 cm] above patient's hips).
12. Instruct patient to tighten her perineal muscles as if to suppress urination, and then relax: repeat four or five times throughout irrigation.
13. When all solution has been instilled, remove nozzle, allowing the patient to expel remaining solution.
14. Dispose of equipment per agency's policy.
15. Dispose of gloves, and wash hands.
16. Perform any necessary comfort measures.
17. Document observations and patient's reaction.

baths can minimize odor and discomfort. Local applications of vaginal suppositories, ointments, and creams are usually prescribed.

Pelvic Inflammatory Disease

Pelvic inflammatory disease (PID) is any acute, subacute, recurrent, or chronic infection of the cervix (cervicitis), uterus (endometritis), fallopian tubes (salpingitis), and ovaries (oophoritis) that has extended to the connective tissues lying between the broad ligaments.

Etiology/Pathophysiology. The most common causative organisms are *Neisseria gonorrhoeae, Streptococcus, Staphylococcus, Chlamydia,* and tubercle bacilli. PID can follow the insertion of a biopsy curette or an irrigation catheter, abortion, pelvic surgery, sexual intercourse, or infection during pregnancy. The condition may occur with or without gonorrheal infection and may be mild or severe.

When conditions or procedures alter or destroy the cervical mucus, bacteria ascend into the uterine cavity. Pelvic examination and movement of the reproductive organs are painful. PID is very serious, because it may cause adhesions and sterility. Sexually active women with more than one partner are at higher risk for PID.

Clinical Manifestations. The patient is usually hospitalized to isolate the organism and plan the treatment. The patient and those assisting with the care should be informed of all precautions that are necessary and be instructed to use universal precautions. The use of goggles is recommended if any splashing is likely. Signs and symptoms are temperature elevation, chills, severe abdominal pain, malaise, nausea and vomiting, and malodorous purulent vaginal exudate.

Assessment. Collection of *subjective data* relates to the severity of the disorder, pain, time of onset, and frequency—primary infection or continuous reinfection. Sexual history, pelvic examinations, and pelvic procedures are important, because they may reveal the origin of the pathogen.

Collection of *objective data* invites assessment of the knowledge of the patient, level of discomfort, and coping mechanisms used. The patient should be assessed for fever and the amount and characteristics of vaginal discharge.

Diagnostic Tests. Diagnostic tests include Gram stains of secretions from the endocervix, urethra, and rectum. Culture and sensitivity testing identifies organisms and is helpful in selection of antibiotics for treatment. Laparoscopy or ultrasound visualization of the pelvic inflammation may be necessary to confirm the extent of infection. The leukocyte count and erythrocyte sedimentation rate are also assessed to confirm an infectious process.

Medical Management. The goal of treatment is to control and eradicate the infection by preventing the infection from spreading to other body systems. Treatment includes systemic antibiotics administered intravenously and/or intramuscularly.

Nursing Interventions. Nursing interventions include (1) following the medical plan of treatment; (2) monitoring vital signs and progress of treatment; (3) providing fluids to avoid dehydration; (4) performing palliative measures for comfort in bathing, changing of perineal pads, personal hygiene, and warm douches; (5) providing patient support with a positive, nonjudgmental attitude, and (6) positioning the patient in Fowler's position to facilitate drainage.

Nursing diagnoses and interventions for the patient with PID include but are not limited to the following:

NURSING DIAGNOSES	NURSING INTERVENTIONS
Pain, related to infection process	Manage pain with analgesics as ordered; assess effectiveness of pain relief measures. Provide comfort measures.
Fluid volume deficit, high risk for, related to inadequate intake, fatigue, pain, and fluid losses caused by elevated temperature	Maintain parenteral fluids as ordered. Provide adequate oral intake of fluids as prescribed. Monitor I&O.
Coping, ineffective individual, high risk for, related to condition	Provide emotional support. Encourage verbalization of feelings. Provide therapeutic environment for the patient.
Health maintenance, altered, high risk for, related to insufficient knowledge of condition and complication	Patient teaching includes understanding of the significance of pelvic inflammatory disease and the importance of complying with medication therapy.

Patient teaching. Discharge planning should include patient teaching and instructions for (1) contracting the physician if a low-grade fever persists or purulent vaginal discharge occurs; (2) understanding the significance of the pelvic inflammatory condition; (3) understanding compliance with medication therapy; (4) handwashing technique and practices of body hygiene with bathing, avoidance of tampons, frequent changing of perineal pads, and clean clothing; (5) understanding the importance for the sexual partner to be examined and treated to avoid recurrence of the PID; and (6) recognizing that intercourse is sometimes very painful after an occurrence of PID and that sexual activity should be avoided until advised by a physician.

Prognosis. Women with PID are usually of childbearing age. If severe or chronic PID is present, infertility may result from adhesions in the fallopian tubes. With adequate treatment, the prognosis is good.

Toxic Shock Syndrome

Etiology/Pathophysiology. Toxic shock syndrome (TSS) was first identified in the 1970s. It is an acute bacterial infection caused by *Staphylococcus aureus* and usually occurs in women who are menstruating and using tampons (particularly superabsorbent tampons). Women at greatest risk are those who insert tampons with their fingers instead of with inserters, women with chronic vaginal infections, and women with genital herpes. TSS can also occur in nonmenstruating women.

Clinical Manifestations. Often the woman will have flulike symptoms for the first 24 hours. Between days 2 and 4 of the menstrual period the patient may have an elevated temperature (up to 102° F [39° C]), vomiting, diarrhea, myalgia, hypotension, and signs suggesting the onset of septic shock. Sore throat, headache, and a red macular palmar or diffuse rash followed by desquamation of the skin, hands, and feet may develop, urinary output is decreased, and the blood urea nitrogen (BUN) level is elevated. Disorientation may occur from dehydration and release of toxins. Pulmonary edema and inflammation of mucous membranes may occur.

Assessment. Collection of *subjective data* includes determining whether the patient has recently used tampons, and how long she used a single tampon before changing it. Information should be obtained about myalgia, sore throat, headache, and fatigue.

Collection of *objective data* includes assessing for edema. The palms and soles should be assessed for the presence of an erythematous rash. Desquamation and sloughing occur within 1 to 2 weeks after the rash. The patient's level of consciousness should be noted. The presence of hypotension is a sign of TSS. Nonpurulent inflammation of the conjunctiva and hyperemia of the oropharynx and vagina are also signs of TSS.

Diagnostic Tests. Blood tests will demonstrate leukocytosis, thrombocytopenia, and elevated levels of bilirubin, urea nitrogen, creatinine, SGOT (AST), SGPT (ALT), and CPK. Blood and urine cultures should be taken along with throat cultures when appropriate, and vaginal and genital specimens should be evaluated.

Medical Management. Treatment of TSS varies because of the range in types of and severity of symptoms. Antibiotic therapy is given according to the results of the culture and sensitivity tests performed. Parenteral therapy is given to maintain proper fluid balance. Laboratory data are evaluated for electrolyte imbalance caused by vomiting and diarrhea, elevated BUN suggesting renal involvement, and elevated enzymes suggesting liver dysfunction.

Nursing Interventions. When the patient is hospitalized, bed rest is prescribed and antibiotics are administered. Close monitoring of vital signs and fluid status is important. If there is respiratory distress, oxygen therapy is instituted.

Nursing diagnoses and interventions for the patient with TSS include but are not limited to the following:

NURSING DIAGNOSES	NURSING INTERVENTIONS
Anxiety, related to TSS	Encourage patient to verbalize fears. Provide quiet, therapeutic environment. Provide support and understanding.
Fluid volume deficit, high risk for, related to vomiting and diarrhea	Monitor amount, frequency, and characteristics of vomitus and diarrhea. Assess tissue turgor for evidence of dehydration. Assess patient for dry mucous membranes, and monitor parenteral fluids with electrolytes as ordered. Monitor I&O.
Pain, related to myalgia	Provide comfort measures. Administer analgesics as ordered.

Patient teaching. Since the use of tampons during menstruation has been linked to TSS, it is recommended that superabsorbent tampons not be used. If tampons are used, they should be alternated with the use of pads. Tampons should be changed frequently (every 4 hours) and should be inserted carefully to avoid abrasions. Patients who have had TSS should not use tampons. The patient should be taught to wash hands thoroughly before inserting a tampon. Women who are menstruating and develop a sudden high fever accompanied by vomiting and diarrhea should be counseled by the nurse to seek immediate medical attention. If the woman is wearing a tampon, she should remove it immediately.

Prognosis. TSS is a rare and sometimes fatal disease. Prognosis depends on the severity of the disease and how quickly therapeutic measures to combat shock and renal failure, if present, are instituted.

DISORDERS OF THE FEMALE REPRODUCTIVE SYSTEM

Endometriosis

Endometriosis is a condition in which endometrial tissue appears outside the uterus.

Etiology/Pathophysiology. Endometrial tissue can be found on the ovaries, fallopian tubes, and uterus, within the abdominal cavity, and in the vagina (Fig. 33-11). The spread of the tissue is believed to be through the lymphatic circulation, by menstrual backflow to the fallopian tubes and pelvic cavity, or through congenital displacement of the endometrial cells.

The tissue responds to the normal stimulation of the ovaries, bleeds each month, and forms an endometrial crust, which causes an endometrial cyst. This cyst may rupture and cause further reproduction of tissue.

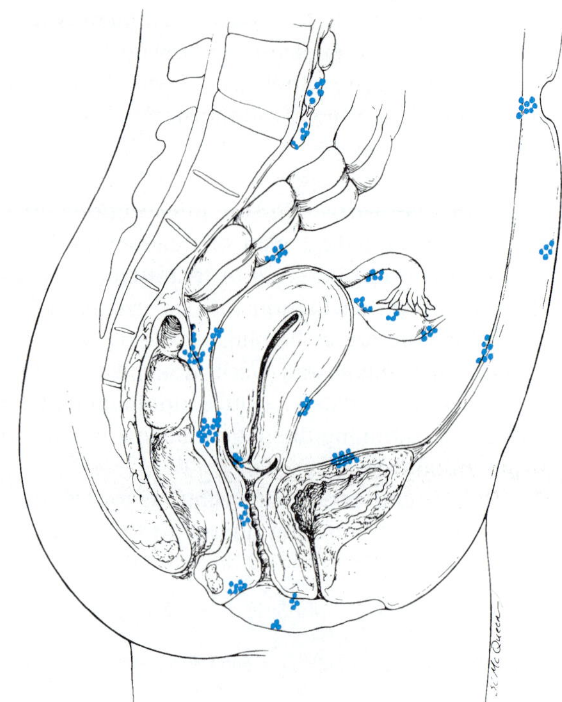

FIG. 33-11 Common sites of endometriosis.

Clinical Manifestations. Symptoms are lower abdominal and pelvic pain with or without pain in the rectum. It may be unilateral or bilateral and may radiate to the lower back, legs, and groin. Symptoms are more acute during menstruation and subside after menstruation. There is some evidence that women have a greater chance (about 7 times greater) of developing endometriosis if a sister or mother has it. The highest incidence of endometriosis is among white women 25 to 35 years of age who are in the higher socioeconomic classes and who postpone childbearing until the later reproductive years. Women who have not conceived or lactated are at greater risk. Pregnancy is encouraged, because it is believed that an interruption of the menstrual cycle will slow the progress of the disorder. Pregnancy is also advised for women who want children, because a complication of endometriosis is infertility.

Assessment. Collection of *subjective data* includes obtaining a history of the patient's symptoms, including pelvic pain with menstruation, aching, cramping, a bearing-down sensation in the pelvis, or lower back dyspareunia (sexual intercourse is accompanied by pain). The type of pain may indicate the presence of ripe cysts that are about to rupture or may indicate the formation of infected tissue. The patient may reveal a history of menstrual irregularities such as amenorrhea.

Collection of *objective data* involves noting signs, which appear 5 to 7 days before menses and last 2 to 3 days. Signs may include abnormal uterine bleeding.

Diagnostic Tests. Laparoscopy with a biopsy of the lesions may confirm the diagnosis. Regular pelvic examinations are recommended to monitor progression.

Medical Management. Medical treatment consists of high-dose antiovulatory medications to inhibit ovulation and induce a state physiologically similar to pregnancy and thus suppress menstruation. Synthetic androgens such as danazol may be prescribed to arrest proliferation of the endometrium and prevent ovulation, producing atrophy of the displaced endometrium. Occasionally women have spontaneous disappearance of endometriosis. Some women who become pregnant are asymptomatic after pregnancy. When involvement is severe, surgery may be necessary. A laparoscopy may be performed to remove endometrial implants and adhesions. Lasers may be used to vaporize the small implants of endometrial tissue. A total hysterectomy, oophorectomy, and salpingectomy may also be done.

Nursing Interventions. The nurse should reinforce the physician's explanation of the expected results of treatment, instruct the patient regarding the dosage, frequency, and side effects of prescribed medications, and emphasize the importance of regular checkups and of reporting abnormal vaginal bleeding. The nurse should also encourage the patient to verbalize her concerns. The nurse should assist the patient with comfort measures and help her with adaptive responses to self-concept.

Nursing diagnoses and interventions for the patient with endometriosis include but are not limited to the following:

NURSING DIAGNOSES	NURSING INTERVENTIONS
Pain, related to displaced endometrial tissue	Institute comfort measures to cope with pain, such as medications and warm compresses to abdomen. Maintain bed rest when pain is most severe.
Anxiety, related to unpredictable nature of the illness	Provide emotional support during symptoms by encouraging verbalization of concerns, making correct responses, and giving referrals to appropriate resources. Assist to develop effective coping mechanisms.
Sexual dysfunction, related to painful intercourse or infertility	Emphasize importance of communicating fears and concerns that lead to anxiety.
Health maintenance, altered, related to insufficient knowledge of condition and medication therapy	Instruct patient to take medications as prescribed and rationale for same.

Patient teaching. The nurse who is caring for a patient who has endometriosis should reinforce the physician's explanation of the expected results of treatment, teach pain-relieving techniques to the patient, instruct the patient regarding the dosage and frequency and possible side effects of any prescribed medications, and emphasize the importance of regular checkups and the importance of reporting any abnormal vaginal bleeding.

Prognosis. Approximately half of women with endometriosis are infertile. If a young woman has endometriosis, she is usually advised to have a family early because the fertility rate is low. Menopause stops the progress of endometriosis.

Vaginal Fistula

A **fistula** is defined as an abnormal opening between two organs.

Etiology/Pathophysiology. Vaginal fistulas are caused by an ulcerating process resulting from cancer, radiation, weakening of tissue by pregnancies, and surgical interventions.

Vaginal fistulas are named for the organs involved (Fig. 33-12):

Urethrovaginal fistula: opening between the urethra and vagina

Vesicovaginal fistula: opening between the bladder and vagina

Rectovaginal fistula: opening between the rectum and vagina

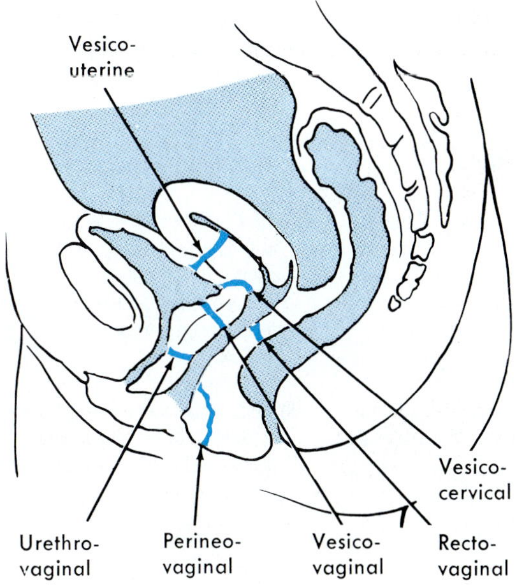

FIG. 33-12 Types of fistulas that may develop in vagina and uterus.

Clinical Manifestations. Fistulas are recognized by their exudate, which has a distinct odor of urine or feces. Generally a bladder infection is present. The vesicovaginal fistula causes a constant trickling of urine into the vagina; a rectovaginal fistula allows feces and flatus to enter the vagina.

Assessment. Collection of *subjective data* includes the patient's understanding of the exudate that occurs as well as of any causative factors. The patient will report the presence of urine or feces from the vagina.

Collection of *objective data* that should be assessed includes any behaviors that indicate stress, anxiety, and pain. The patient may express feelings of disturbance in self-esteem because of the condition. The nurse should observe for urine or feces on the perineal pad.

Diagnostic Tests. Diagnostic testing includes methylene blue instillation in bladder, and an intravenous pyelogram and/or cystoscopy to assist in the location of the fistula. Pelvic examination is performed.

Medical Management. Healing is promoted by an increase in vitamin C and protein in the diet. The patient is given oral or parenteral antibiotics. If the organ tissue is healthy, a surgical approach is recommended. The surgical approach may be similar to anterior or posterior colporrhaphy, which will be discussed later in the chapter. Fistulas that are difficult to repair or very large may require urinary or fecal diversion.

Nursing Interventions. Soiling from leakage of urine or stool into the vagina is disturbing for the patient. Sitz baths, deodorizing douches, perineal pads, and protective undergarments will be necessary. If the fistula is repaired surgically, a Foley catheter will be inserted postoperatively to prevent strain on the suture line caused by a full bladder.

Nursing diagnoses and interventions include but are not limited to the following:

NURSING DIAGNOSES	NURSING INTERVENTIONS
Impaired skin integrity, related to exudate	Teach how to care for the skin with douches, creams, and sitz baths.
Sexual dysfunction, related to pain during sexual activity	Offer support and understanding of distress toward sexual activities and self-esteem.
Coping, ineffective individual, related to abnormal vaginal exudate	Actively listen. Teach patient douche cleansing and meticulous care of perineal area. Encourage adaptive coping behaviors.
Fear, related to concern about outcome of surgical therapy or medical treatment	Encourage verbalization of fears. Answer questions honestly.

Prognosis. Vaginal fistulas may close spontaneously but frequently need to be repaired surgically. If so, 4 to 6 months are required for the inflammation to subside before surgery can be attempted.

Relaxed Pelvic Muscles

The most common problems resulting from relaxed pelvic muscles are displaced uterus with prolapse and/or procidentia, cystocele, urethrocele, rectocele, enterocele, and malpositions of the uterus.

Displaced Uterus. Normally the uterus lies with the cervix at a right angle to the long axis of the vagina, and the body of the uterus is inclined slightly forward. A displaced uterus is usually congenital, but may be caused by childbirth. Backward displacement may be retroversion or retroflexion. Retroversion position places the cervix at the normal axis, but the body of the uterus is directed toward the sacrum. In retroflexion the angle of the body of the uterus is on the cervix. The patient has backache, muscle strain, leukorrheal discharge, and heaviness in the pelvic area and tires easily. Treatment consists of a pessary and possible uterine suspension.

Uterine Prolapse and Procidentia.

Etiology/pathophysiology. **Procidentia** (uterine prolapse) is a herniation of the uterus into the vagina and at times beyond the vulva (Fig. 33-13). When the uterus loses its support, the organ descends and prolapses into the vaginal canal. In uterine procidentia there is a protrusion of the uterus, vaginal wall, rectum, and bladder.

Obstetrical trauma, overstretching of the uterine muscle support system, coughing, straining, and lifting heavy objects contribute to uterine prolapse and procidentia.

Clinical manifestations. The woman with uterine prolapse or procidentia may complain of urinary incontinence, retention, constipation, backache, and vaginal exudate from the increased pressure exerted by the prolapsed uterus. The symptoms may increase with coughing or prolonged standing.

Medical management. A vaginal pessary may be of some help, but the surgical correction is generally a vaginal hysterectomy with anterior and posterior repair. It is also called an anteroposterior colporrhaphy.

Cystocele and Rectocele.

Etiology/pathophysiology and clinical manifestations. When the tissue, muscles, and ligaments that support the uterus and perineum have been stretched and weakened by childbearing, multiple births, and/or cervical tears, the organs gradually move into other positions. The relaxation of the tissues, muscles, and ligaments of the bladder causes a displacement of the blad-

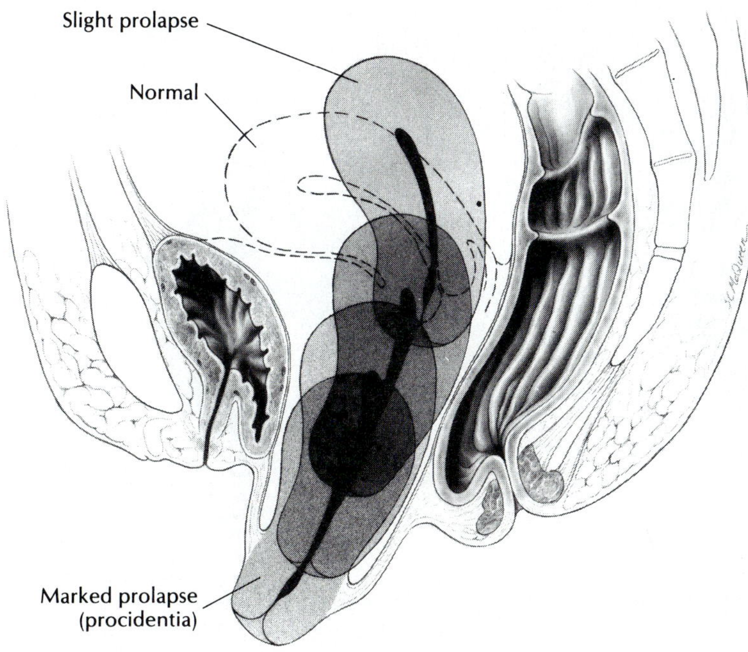

FIG. 33-13 Prolapse of the uterus. (Redrawn from Symmonds RE: *Relaxations of pelvic supports.* In Benson RC, editor: *Current obstetric and gynecologic diagnosis and treatment,* ed 5, Los Altos, Calif, 1984, Lange.)

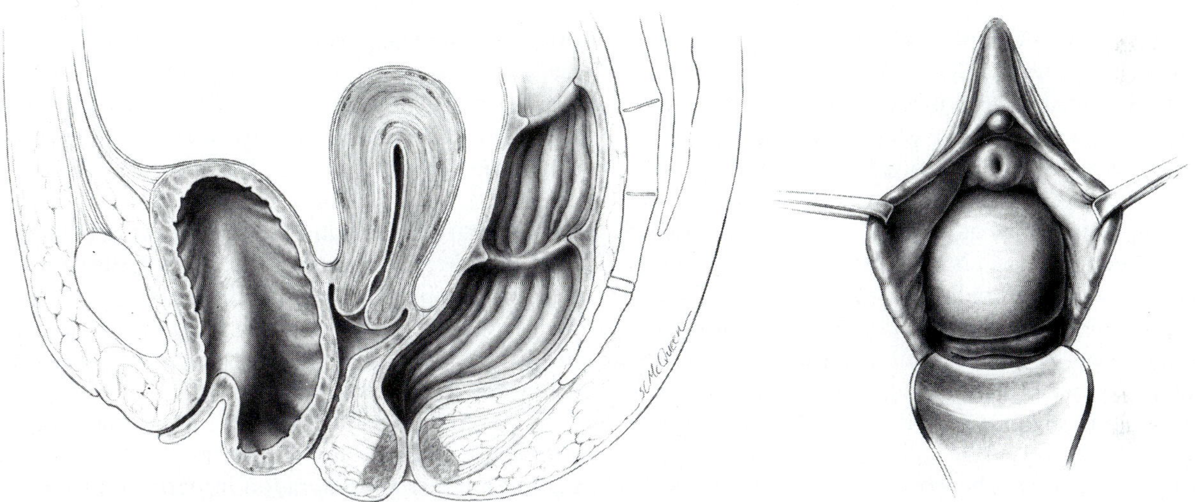

FIG. 33-14 Side and direct view of cystocele. (Redrawn from Symmonds RE: *Anatomy of the female reproductive system.* In Benson RC, editor: *Current obstetric and gynecologic diagnosis and treatment,* ed 5, Los Altos, Calif, 1984, Lange.)

der into the vagina. This is referred to as a *cystocele* (Fig. 33-14). Clinical symptoms are urinary urgency, frequency, and/or incontinence; fatigue; and pelvic pressure. A large cystocele prevents complete emptying of the bladder, which leads to bacterial growth and infection.

The relaxation of the supporting tissues to the rectum causes the rectum to move toward the posterior vaginal wall and form a rectocele (Fig. 33-15 on p. 1014). The rectocele causes constipation, rectal pressure, heaviness, and hemorrhoids.

Medical management. Correction of cystocele and rectocele is surgical repair involving shortening of the muscles that support the bladder and repair of the rectocele. This is known as anterior posterior or anteroposterior **colporrhaphy.** It is sometimes referred to as an A&P repair.

Nursing interventions. Preoperative and postoperative nursing interventions include the following. Preoperative care for colporrhaphy is especially important in ensuring as clean an operative area as possible. Patients may be given a cathartic followed by enemas to

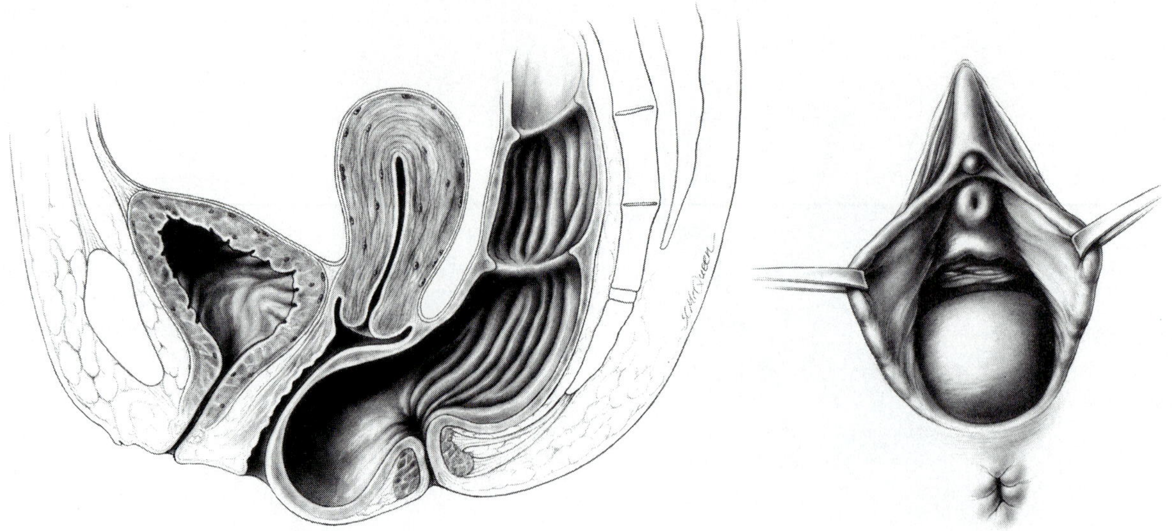

FIG. 33-15 Side and direct views of rectocele. (Redrawn from Symmonds RE: *Relaxations of pelvic supports.* In Benson RC, editor: *Current obstetric and gynecologic diagnosis and treatment,* ed 5, Los Altos, Calif, 1985, Lange.)

be sure the bowel is completely empty. A liquid diet for 48 hours before surgery will help keep the bowel empty. A cleansing vaginal douche is given the evening before and the morning of surgery. Postoperative care includes checking vital signs and observing for hemorrhage. A retention catheter is usually inserted into the bladder to keep it empty and prevent pressure on sutures. It is important to keep the fecal residue as soft as possible; some physicians order only liquids for several days, or they may order mineral oil to be given every night. An oil retention enema may be ordered, but cleansing enemas are not given. The patient's perineal area is cleansed carefully using surgical asepsis. Early ambulation is also encouraged.

Patient teaching. The patient should be advised against standing for long periods or lifting heavy objects. Coitus must be avoided until healing occurs, usually about 6 weeks.

Prognosis. With surgical correction, the prognosis is good.

Benign Tumors of the Uterus

Etiology/Pathophysiology. Fibroid tumors are benign tumors arising from the muscle tissue of the uterus. It has been estimated that 20% to 25% of women over 30 years of age develop uterine fibroid tumors (myomas). Their growth is stimulated by ovarian hormones.

The size and number of myomas vary. Most are found in the body of the uterus, but some occur in the cervix or may involve the broad ligaments.

Clinical Manifestations. The symptoms are primarily pressure from an enlarging pelvic mass, pain (including dysmenorrhea), abnormal uterine bleeding, and abnormally long or heavy bleeding (menorrhagia) with menstrual periods. If the fibroid tumor becomes large enough to cause pressure on other structures, there may be backache, constipation, and urinary symptoms.

Assessment. Collection of *subjective data* includes asking the patient about the presence of pain with menstruation or abnormally heavy flow. The patient is asked to describe her symptoms, which may include pelvic fullness or heaviness, constipation, urinary frequency or urgency, and menorrhagia.

Collection of *objective data* includes assessing the patient for excessive heavy discharge of blood by observing the number and saturation of perineal pads.

Diagnostic Tests. Diagnostic studies may include a pregnancy test, D&C, laparoscopy, and ultrasonography.

Medical Management. The treatment of fibroid tumors depends on the symptoms and the age of the patient, whether more children are desired, and how near to menopause the woman is. Myomectomy is the procedure of choice during childbearing years. If there is severe bleeding or obstruction, a hysterectomy may be necessary.

Nursing Interventions and Patient Teaching. For preoperative and postoperative nursing interventions for the patient who has a hysterectomy, see pp. 1015-1016 and Chapter 22. The nurse caring for a patient with fibroid tumors should reinforce the physician's explanation of the treatment plan—either a total hysterectomy or pelvic examination at regular intervals to monitor the status of the fibroid tumor. The nurse instructs the patient about the dosage and frequency of prescribed medications and possible side effects. The patient with menorrhagia should be taught to include adequate iron in her diet to prevent iron deficiency anemia from the extra blood loss. The importance of regular checkups to monitor the status of the fibroid tumor should be emphasized, and the nurse can encourage the patient to express her feelings and assist her with coping mechanisms.

Nursing diagnoses and interventions for the patient with fibroid tumors include but are not limited to the following:

NURSING DIAGNOSES	NURSING INTERVENTIONS
Pain, related to fibroid tumors	Assess pain location, onset, and duration. Administer analgesics as ordered. Provide comfort measures as needed.
Self-esteem disturbance, related to the presence of fibroid tumors	Encourage verbalization of concerns. Be an active listener.

Prognosis. Fibroid tumors of the uterus tend to disappear spontaneously with menopause. They rarely become malignant. Infertility may result from a myoma that obstructs or distorts the uterus or fallopian tubes. Myoma in the body of the uterus may cause spontaneous abortions, and those near the cervical opening may make the delivery of a fetus difficult and may contribute to postpartum hemorrhage.

Ovarian Cysts

Etiology/Pathophysiology. Ovarian cysts are benign tumors that arise from dermoid cells of the ovary or from a cystic corpus luteum or graafian follicle.

Clinical Manifestations. Ovarian cysts enlarge and are palpable on examination. They may cause no symptoms, or they may result in a disturbance of menstruation, a feeling of heaviness, and slight vaginal bleeding.

Medical Management. The cysts are usually removed by an ovarian cystectomy.

Nursing Interventions. Nursing interventions are similar to those for the patient having an abdominal hysterectomy.

Prognosis. The prognosis is good; ovarian cysts do not become malignant.

Hysterectomy

A hysterectomy involves the removal of the uterus, including the cervix. This procedure may be done for many conditions, such as dysfunctional uterine bleeding, endometriosis, malignant and nonmalignant tumors of the uterus and cervix, and disorders of pelvic relaxation and uterine prolapse.

Various terms are used to describe the removal of the uterus. A total hysterectomy is the removal of the entire uterus. The vagina remains intact, and intercourse is possible even though childbearing is not. Estrogens are still released. Menopause will occur naturally because the ovaries are still present. A total abdominal hysterectomy with bilateral salpingooophorectomy (TAH-BSO) is the removal of the uterus, fallopian tubes, and ovaries. It is sometimes called **panhysterosalpingooophorectomy.** A radical hysterectomy also includes the removal of the pelvic lymph nodes. If the ovaries are removed with these surgeries, there is a surgically induced menopause.

Vaginal Hysterectomy. A vaginal hysterectomy may be done for a prolapsed uterus. It is not used nearly as often as the abdominal approach. The vaginal approach is selected for the patient who cannot tolerate abdominal surgery or prolonged anesthesia. There is no abdominal incision. The patient is placed in a lithotomy position, and the uterus is removed through the vagina. Advantages of the vaginal entrance are that there is no wound dehiscence, there is less pain, complications are less likely, hospitalization is shorter, and there is no abdominal scar. The most important disadvantage is that there is a limited view of the operative field for visualizing intrapelvic and intraabdominal organs. Other disadvantages are risk of bleeding and postoperative infection.

Abdominal Hysterectomy. An abdominal hysterectomy is preferred when there is a need to explore the pelvic cavity and if the fallopian tubes and ovaries are to be removed. There are three procedures for an abdominal hysterectomy, named according to the extent of the surgery performed. *Subtotal hysterectomy* refers to the removal of the corpus (the larger upper portion or body) of the uterus and leaves the cervical stump in place. *Total hysterectomy* is the removal of the entire uterus, including the cervix, but leaving the fallopian tubes and ovaries in place. *Total hysterectomy with bilateral salpingo-oophorectomy* or *hysterosalpingo-oophorectomy* involves the removal of the entire uterus plus the fallopian tubes and the ovaries.

Nursing Interventions.

Preoperative interventions. When the physician has explained the surgery to the patient, the nurse can reinforce the explanation and answer questions the patient might have. The nurse should encourage verbalization of fears. Additional preoperative instructions are given to help the woman prepare for recovery postoperatively. The nurse should instruct the patient how to turn, cough, and deep breathe.

Before a vaginal or abdominal hysterectomy, the colon is emptied to prevent postoperative distention. The patient may be on a low-residue diet for several days preoperatively. Enemas may be given the evening before surgery.

The bladder may be decompressed to prevent trauma during surgery. The indwelling catheter will generally remain in place for 1 or 2 days after surgery.

An antiseptic vaginal douche may be ordered to decrease microbial invasion of the surgical site.

If the surgeon anticipates excessive manipulation of the intestines, a nasogastric tube may be inserted to prevent abdominal distention. The patient should be instructed about the purpose of the tube and that it will be kept in place for a few days after surgery.

Surgical preparation of the skin includes the surgical prepping of the abdomen, pelvis, and perineum. The patient will sign a consent form, and oral intake will be restricted after midnight.

Postoperative interventions. Postoperative nursing interventions focus on monitoring vital signs and preventing urinary retention, intestinal distention, and venous thrombosis. If a retention catheter was inserted, it should be kept patent and connected to closed drainage. Meticulous catheter care is performed to prevent bladder infection. If no retention catheter is in place, the patient is checked frequently for bladder distention; an accurate urine output is recorded. The incidence of urinary retention is greater after a hysterectomy than after any other type of surgery, because some trauma to the bladder unavoidably occurs. If the patient does not have a catheter and is unable to void, catheterization every 8 hours may be necessary. Occasionally the patient will have residual urine. The physician often orders catheterization of the patient to check for residual urine; 50 ml or less is within the normal range.

A nasogastric tube may be inserted. A small up-and-down flush enema (Harris) may be ordered to help relieve distention. Early ambulation is very helpful to return the bowel to normal function. When bowel sounds have returned and flatus is being expelled, the patient is allowed liquids by mouth and a gradual increase in return to solid foods.

Patients undergoing pelvic surgery are more susceptible to venous stasis and thrombophlebitis because of trauma to blood vessels. The patient is usually permitted to be out of bed on the first postoperative day, but the nurse should encourage the patient to dangle her legs and to sit on the side of the bed before standing and walking to prevent the effects of postural hypotension. Antiembolic stockings may be used to prevent thrombus or embolus formation, and legs should be exercised frequently when the patient is in bed. Many physicians prescribe the use of intermittent pneumonic compression cuffs for the calves to prevent venous stasis (see Chapter 22). The patient should avoid bending her knees. These activities could cause pooling of blood in the pelvic cavity, resulting in stasis in the lower extremities. The patient at risk for thromboembolic disease may receive low-dose heparin to prevent thrombus formation.

Analgesics such as meperidine (Demerol) may be ordered for relief of pain. Slight vaginal drainage may occur for 1 or 2 days, but any unusual bleeding should be reported to the physician.

The nurse will observe the abdominal dressing on the patient with an abdominal hysterectomy for evidence of hemorrhage. Surgical asepsis is carried out for the dressing change. The patient usually receives intravenous feedings for several days postoperatively. The rate of flow and the condition of the IV site are carefully monitored.

Nursing diagnoses and interventions for the patient who has had a hysterectomy include but are not limited to the following:

NURSING DIAGNOSES	NURSING INTERVENTIONS
Knowledge deficit, related to preoperative and postoperative period	Obtain feedback of patient's knowledge of surgery and preoperative and postoperative procedures. Clarify any misconceptions related to outcome of the surgical procedure, such as fear of sexual dysfunction, mood swings, and loss of femininity. Provide education related to surgical menopause. Provide emotional support to patient and her partner.
Urinary elimination, altered patterns, related to postsurgical sensorimotor impairment	Connect indwelling catheter to closed gravity drainage. Give meticulous catheter care as indicated. Record color and amount of urinary output. Promote micturition at regular intervals when catheter is removed. Catheterize for residual urine as ordered.
Self-esteem disturbance, high risk for, related to body image change and value of reproductive organs	Encourage verbalization with significant others. Relate importance of communicating anything that causes anxiety. Reinforce correct information and provide factual information to correct any misconceptions.
Pain, related to abdominal incision	Assess postoperative pain. Administer analgesics as ordered. Assist patient in splinting abdominal incision while coughing and ambulating.
Tissue perfusion, altered, peripheral, related to pelvic surgery, thrombophlebitis	Ensure that bed is not elevated in the knee gatch position. Assess proper placement of antiembolic stockings every 4 hr as ordered. Assist in passive and active leg exercises every shift. Encourage ambulation. Assess legs for erythema, increased tenderness, severe cramping, positive Homans' sign every shift.

Patient teaching. Before the patient's discharge, the physician will explain to the woman and her partner that there should be no sexual intercourse for 4 to 6 weeks after surgery. If there has been an abdominal incision, there may be further restrictions on heavy lifting (nothing over 10 pounds), walking up and down stairs, and prolonged riding in the car. Riding in the car may cause pelvic pooling and development of a thrombus in the legs.

The patient should know that vaginal drainage is normal for about 2 to 4 weeks after an abdominal hysterectomy.

The patient should avoid wearing any tight clothing such as a girdle or knee-high hose, which might constrict circulation to the surgical site and cause venous stasis.

There are several signs and symptoms of infections that should be reported by the patient to the physician if they occur: (1) erythema, edema, exudate, or increased tenderness along the surgical incision; (2) increased malodorous vaginal exudate; (3) a temperature of 101° F (38.3° C) or more; and (4) any problems with urinating, such as difficulty starting to void, voiding too often, voiding small amounts, or a burning sensation while urinating (indicative of a bladder infection).

CANCER OF THE FEMALE REPRODUCTIVE TRACT

Cancer is the second most common cause of death in women, and malignant tumors of the reproductive tract represent a significant portion of the total number of deaths from cancer.

Ovarian cancer is the fifth most frequently occurring cancer in women. Uterine cancer, principally arising in the cervix, is the sixth most common cancer of women, ranking behind cancer of the (1) breast, (2) colon and rectum, (3) endometrium, (4) lung, and (5) ovary. Cervical cancer often affects women in their reproductive years, and with the diagnostic Pap smear the cancer can be detected in its early stages. Unfortunately, only 10% to 15% of women in the United States obtain a Pap smear each year.

Endometrial cancer is primarily a disease of women over 50 years of age, but the incidence among younger women is increasing. Most cases of ovarian cancer occur in women over 50, but malignant neoplasms of the ovaries may occur at all ages.

Cancer of the Cervix

Cancer of the cervix is usually a squamous cell carcinoma. Unless treated in its early stages, the tumor invades the vagina, pelvic wall, bladder, rectum, and regional lymph nodes.

Etiology/Pathophysiology. Women who become sexually active in their teens are at a higher risk for cancer of the cervix, as are those who have had multiple sexual partners, those who have multiple births, and those of lower socioeconomic status. There is an increased incidence of cervical carcinoma in young women whose mothers took diethylstilbestrol (DES) during pregnancy as treatment to prevent spontaneous abortion.

Viral and chronic infections and erosions of the cervix are most likely significant in the development of cancer. **Carcinoma in situ** is a preinvasive, asymptomatic carcinoma that can only be diagnosed by microscopic examination of cervical cells. Once it is diagnosed, it can be treated early without radical surgery. Carcinoma in situ of the cervix is essentially 100% curable.

Clinical Manifestations. Most cervical cancer is silent in the early stages and offers few symptoms. The two chief symptoms are leukorrhea and irregular vaginal bleeding or spotting between menses. Bleeding often occurs after coitus or after menopause. Bleeding at first appears as very slight, but as the disease progresses, the bleeding increases in amount. The vaginal exudate becomes watery and then increases as a dark, bloody exudate that has an offensive odor caused by necrosis and infection of the tumor mass. As the cancer progresses, the bleeding may become constant and increasing in amount. With advanced stages there is severe pain in the back and upper thighs and legs.

Assessment. Collection of *subjective data* includes the nurse urging women to have regular health appraisals and pelvic examinations, so that cancer of the cervix can be detected in its earliest stages. The patient will present no symptoms in the early stages of cancer of the cervix. If the tumor becomes more invasive, the patient will experience back and leg pain, weight loss, and malaise.

Collection of *objective data* includes assessing the patient for abnormal vaginal discharge by observing the sanitary pads. The vaginal exudate may be watery to dark red and malodorous. The number and saturation of the perineal pads should be noted. If the tumor becomes more invasive, the patient will be assessed for anemia, fever, and the presence of lymphedema.

Diagnostic Tests. The following tests are performed to determine the presence of cervical cancer: (1) Pap smear, (2) Schiller's test, (3) physical examination, (4) cervical biopsy, and (5) additional diagnostic studies, such as CT scan, chest x-ray evaluation, intravenous pyelogram, cystoscopy, sigmoidoscopy, or liver function studies to determine the extent of invasion.

Medical Management. Carcinoma in situ is treated by removal of the affected area. This removal can be accomplished by a variety of techniques, including electrocautery, cryosurgery (use of subfreezing temperature to destroy tissue), laser, conization, and hysterectomy. Conization is the removal of a cone-shaped section of the cer-

vix. This surgery is particularly useful to preserve childbearing function.

Early carcinoma of the cervix can be treated with a hysterectomy or intracavitary radiation (see Chapter 38).

A radical hysterectomy with pelvic lymph node dissection may be required for more extensive lesions. The treatment plan is tailored to each patient based on the extent of the disease.

Nursing Interventions. Nursing interventions should include verbal reassurance. In advanced cancer of the cervix, the nurse should position the patient comfortably, change her position slowly, maintain the patient's body alignment, provide pain relief measures, change the patient's dressings and sanitary pads frequently, and assess color, odor, and amount of drainage. The skin is assessed for impairment. (See p. 1016) regarding nursing interventions for the patient having a hysterectomy.)

Nursing diagnoses and interventions for the patient with cancer of the cervix include but are not limited to the following:

NURSING DIAGNOSES	NURSING INTERVENTIONS
Fear, related to diagnosis of cancer	Assist patient with recognizing and clarifying fears and with developing coping strategies for those fears. Be an active listener.
Skin integrity, impaired, related to drainage	Assist and teach patient to perform perineal care every 3 to 4 hr. Keep skin dry. Change sanitary pads every 3 to 4 hr or more frequently if needed.
Self-esteem disturbance, related to body image change and value of reproductive organs	Encourage patient's comments and questions about condition. Encourage verbalization with significant others. Provide factual information to correct any misconceptions.
Pain, chronic, related to complication of metastasis	Assist patient in assuming a position of comfort. Administer analgesics as ordered. Keep patient pain free.

Patient teaching. The nurse can both educate and encourage patients to assume responsibility for their health by having a yearly Pap smear. The nurse should encourage patients to seek prompt medical assistance for any abnormal vaginal exudate.

Prognosis. The prognosis is good if the cancer is treated in the early stages. It usually takes 2 to 10 years for squamous cell carcinoma to become invasive beyond the basement membrane and metastasize. Therefore early diagnosis and treatment are vital for survival.

Cancer of the Endometrium

Etiology/Pathophysiology. Cancer of the endometrium (uterine cancer) usually affects postmenopausal women. Endometrial cancer is usually an adenocarcinoma. The tumor is more likely to be localized, but may spread to the cervix, bladder, rectum, and surrounding lymph nodes. It is the most common malignancy of the female genital tract. Those in high-risk groups are women with a history of irregular menstruation, difficulties during menopause, obesity, hypertension, diabetes mellitus, those who have not had children, and those with a family history of cancer of the uterus. Women who have used high-level estrogen birth control pills and estrogen replacement therapy to treat menopausal symptoms have a greater likelihood of developing endometrial cancer.

The tumor in situ is slow growing. Invasion and metastasis occur later, with spread to the cervix and myometrium and ultimately to the vagina, pelvis, and lungs.

Clinical Manifestations. About 50% of patients with postmenopausal bleeding have cancer of the uterus. In premenstrual or postmenopausal women, any abnormal bleeding or spotting should be reported.

Assessment. Collection of *subjective data* includes the nurse assisting the patient in identifying and reporting changes in reproductive or sexual health. The patient may report abdominal pressure and pelvic fullness. The patient will have a history of postmenopausal bleeding and leukorrhea. Pelvic and back pain and postcoital bleeding are late signs and symptoms.

Collection of *objective data* includes the nurse observing the patient for color and amount of vaginal exudate on perineal pads. The nurse will assess the patient for complaints of pain and enlarged lymph nodes.

Diagnostic Tests. Pelvic and rectal examination and D&C are used to diagnose cancer of the endometrium.

Medical Management. Treatment of cancer of the endometrium depends on the stage of the tumor and the woman's health. Surgery, radiation, or chemotherapy may be used to remove the tumor and/or treat metastasis. For early cancer of the endometrium, a total abdominal hysterectomy and bilateral salpingo-oophorectomy are done. Intracavitary radiation followed by a hysterectomy and bilateral salpingo-oophorectomy may be done for the early stage of endometrial cancer (stage I). Patients with stage II disease may receive pelvic irradiation to cause shrinkage and help prevent spread. Afterward the patient will undergo a hysterectomy. Patients with stage III and IV disease are uncommon, and treatment is tailored for each patient based on extent of disease.

Nursing Interventions. See p. 1016 concerning care of the patient undergoing a hysterectomy; also see Chapter 38 for care of the patient with intracavitary radiation.

Patient teaching. Health teaching and follow-up after discharge should emphasize the need for regular physical examination by the physician and the importance of compliance with the prescribed treatment plan.

Prognosis. Cancer of the endometrium is primarily a slow-growing adenocarcinoma. Metastasis occurs late, and the sign of irregular vaginal bleeding often appears early enough to allow for cure of the disease. Stage I tumors have the highest 5-year survival rate (about 77%).

Cancer of the Ovary

Etiology/Pathophysiology. Ovarian cancer, the fifth most common cause of cancer death in women, is the leading cause of gynecological death in the United States. Women between the ages of 50 and 59 have the greatest number of cases of ovarian cancer, but it can occur at any age. In the early stages the tumors are asymptomatic and when detected usually have spread to other pelvic organs. Females at high risk are those who are infertile, anovulatory, nulliparous, and habitual aborters. Other high risk factors include high fat diet and exposure to industrial chemicals such as asbestos and talc. Ovarian cancer commonly spreads by peritoneal seeding of the cancer cells. Common sites of metastasis are the peritoneum, omentum, and bowel surfaces.

Clinical Manifestations. In the early stages the symptoms may cause vague abdominal discomfort, flatulence, and mild gastric disturbances. As the tumor progresses, abdominal girth enlarges from the presence of ascites, and there is flatulence with distention. Other symptoms that can be present are urinary frequency, nausea, vomiting, constipation, and weight loss.

Assessment. Collection of *subjective data* includes awareness that cancer of the ovary is difficult to detect. The patient will report symptoms of abdominal discomfort, gastric disturbances (such as nausea and constipation), and urinary frequency.

Collection of *objective data* includes the nurse observing any increase in the abdominal girth. The patient may void at frequent intervals because of pressure on the bladder. The patient may be dyspneic related to ascites and pressure on the diaphragm.

Diagnostic Tests. Women should have annual pelvic examinations after menopause so that changes indicating ovarian cancer can be found at an early and potentially curable stage. Ovarian cancer is diagnosed by palpation of a pelvic mass and aspiration of ascitic fluid and detection of cancer cells in the fluid. A laparotomy is performed to determine the stage. A blood test to determine cancer antigen 125 (CA-125) is used to identify women with ovarian cancer. In ovarian cancer, the CA-125 level is elevated (see Chapter 38).

Medical Management. Treatment often involves surgery alone or with radiation or chemotherapy (see Chapter 38). Surgery may be a total abdominal hysterectomy with bilateral salpingooophorectomy and omentectomy (excision of portions of the peritoneal folds).

Nursing Interventions. Nursing interventions for any patient with ovarian cancer include management similar to that for patients undergoing abdominal hysterectomy and receiving chemotherapy and external radiation. (See Chapter 38.)

Because ovarian cancer is generally at an advanced stage at the time of diagnosis, despite the woman's feeling well, support and encouragement to comply with the treatment regimen are important nursing interventions. As the disease progresses, the nurse will become involved in activities to increase the patient's comfort.

Nursing diagnoses and interventions for the patient with cancer of the ovaries include but are not limited to the following:

NURSING DIAGNOSES	NURSING INTERVENTIONS
Pain, chronic, related to metastatic process	Establish trusting relationship with patient. Monitor and document pain characteristics. Administer prescribed analgesics every 3 to 4 hr to control pain. Provide environment conducive to comfort and rest.
Breathing pattern, ineffective, related to ascites and pressure on diaphragm	Maintain patient in semi-Fowler's position. Observe for respiratory distress. Administer oxygen as prescribed. Assist the patient to turn, cough, and deep breathe every 2 to 4 hr. Monitor vital signs.
Fluid volume excess, related to ascites	Monitor IV fluids. Maintain accurate I&O. Weigh patient daily. Observe for signs of edema. Measure abdominal girth daily.
Coping, ineffective family: compromised, related to poor prognosis	Assess present coping abilities. Encourage and allow time for verbalization of feelings. Support patient's coping strengths, and discuss alternative coping measures. Involve patient and significant others in nursing interventions and procedures.
Urinary elimination, altered patterns of, related to pressure of tumor on bladder	Measure I&O to monitor for fluid balance. Inspect urine for bleeding to detect evidence of infection or bladder wall irritation. Inspect abdomen for distention to determine effectiveness of bladder emptying. Ambulate patient as tolerated to promote urinary elimination. Catheterize only as necessary to avoid infection.

Prognosis. More than 60% of women with ovarian cancer are diagnosed with advanced disease. The 5-year survival rate for stage I tumors is 55% to 90%; for stage II tumors, the survival rate is 0 to 40%, and it is extremely poor for stages III to IV.

PROBLEMS OF THE FEMALE BREAST

Fibrocystic Breast Condition

Etiology/Pathophysiology. Fibrocystic breast condition involves benign tumors of the breasts, usually occurs in women 30 to 50 years of age, and is rare in postmenopausal women. This suggests that the occurrence is related to ovarian activity.

The cysts are characterized by numerous cellular changes, with an abnormal amount of epithelial hyperplasia and cystic formation within the mammary ducts. The cysts rarely become malignant, but the risk of breast cancer does increase for women who have fibrocystic breast condition; therefore the cysts are observed with great caution.

Clinical Manifestations. Cystic lesions are often bilateral and multiple. The cysts are soft, well differentiated, tender to touch, and freely movable. The lumpiness and tenderness are more apparent before menses.

Diagnostic Tests. The disorder is diagnosed by mammography or ultrasound and confirmed by biopsy. As a therapeutic measure, the cyst is aspirated by needle and syringe to empty the secretions, and the fluid is sent to the laboratory for cytological examination. Aspiration produces a turbid; nonhemorrhagic; yellow, greenish, or brownish fluid.

Medical Management. When cysts recur in the same area and repeated aspirations are ineffective, surgical excision of the cyst may be done.

Conservative treatment is the usual approach to fibrocystic breast condition. The usefulness of eliminating methylxanthines from the diet (coffee, tea, cola) is still controversial, but it is the least expensive therapy. Many women have reported a lessening of symptoms after altering their diet, even though findings by palpation and mammogram were not significantly changed. Danocrine (danazol) may be prescribed to inhibit FSH and LH production, thereby decreasing ovarian production of estrogen. Danocrine may cause weight gain, hot flashes, menstrual irregularities, hirsutism, and deepening of the voice. Vitamin E may also be prescribed, but its efficacy has not been proved.

Patient Teaching. The nurse should instruct the patient to perform breast self-examination 1 week after menses and be able to recognize the presence of cysts and note any changes.

Acute Mastitis

Acute mastitis is an acute bacterial infection usually caused by *Staphylococcus aureus* or streptococci. It is most often observed during lactation and late pregnancy. The infection may result from inadequate cleanliness of the breasts, a nipple fissure, or infection in the infant. The breasts are tender, inflamed, and engorged, causing the milk flow to be obstructed.

Treatment involves application of warm packs, support to the area by a well-fitting brassiere (which also supplies comfort), and systemic treatment with antibiotics.

Chronic Mastitis

Chronic mastitis tends to develop in women between 30 and 50 years of age and is more common in those who have had children, have had difficulty with inverted and cracked nipples, and have had problems with nursing their infants. A traumatic blow to the breasts allows the fat to necrose in the area and form abscesses. There is an increased fibrosis of the tissue, which causes cysts to form. The cysts are tender, painful, and palpable on examination. The disorder is generally unilateral and benign and most frequently occurs in obese women. Treatment is the same as for acute mastitis.

Breast Cancer

Breast cancer is the most common malignancy affecting women in the United States. Approximately one of every nine women will develop breast cancer during her lifetime. The incidence of breast cancer in men is rare—less than 1%. The American Cancer Society predicted 150,000 women would be diagnosed with breast cancer in 1991 and that 44,300 would die. Women consider this disease their most serious health problem. Older women (those over 65 years of age) have twice the incidence of breast cancer as women age 45 to 64. In women over 55, 50% more patients have metastatic disease at presentation than do younger women. Vital to the process of detection are monthly breast self-examination, breast imaging with mammography and other diagnostic studies to detect small tumors before they can be palpated, and periodic breast examinations by a physician.

Etiology/Pathophysiology. The cause of breast cancer is unknown. The high incidence occurring in women implies hormonal cause. Predisposing factors for women at high risk are shown in Box 33-9.

Other possible risks that influence cancer formation are exposure to heavy radiation, immunodeficiency (reduced protection against disease), estrogen therapy, high dietary fat intake, and fibrocystic breast condition.

Breast cancer is usually an adenocarcinoma, arises from the epithelium and develops in the lactiferous ducts, and infiltrates the parenchyma (the tissue of an organ other than the supporting or connective tissue). The cancer occurs most often in the upper outer quadrants of the breasts of women who have not given birth or breast-fed a child. A slow-growing breast cancer may take up to 8 or 9 years to become palpable or to have reached the size of a small pea. Metastasis is by the lymphatic system and blood stream (Fig. 33-16). The most common sites for metastasis are bone, lungs, pleura, breast site, central nervous system, and liver, in that order. When referring to estimated growth rate of breast cancer, the term "doubling time" indicates the time it takes malignant cells to double in number. Assuming that the doubling is constant and that the neoplasm originates in one cell, a carcinoma with a doubling time of 100 days may not reach clinically detectable size, 1 cm, for 8 years. Rapid-growing cancers have a much shorter preclinical course and a greater tendency to metastasize to regional nodes or more distant sites by the time a breast mass is discovered.

Clinical Manifestations. Breast tumors are usually small, solitary, irregularly shaped, firm, nontender, and nonmobile. There may be a change in skin color, tenderness present, puckering and/or dimpling (peau d'orange—appearance of an orange skin) of tissue, nipple discharge, and/or retraction of the nipple and axillary tenderness.

Box 33-9

PREDISPOSING FACTORS FOR FEMALES AT HIGH RISK FOR BREAST CANCER

1. Gender: being a female introduces a high risk
2. Age: higher incidence occurs with women over age 40 and in the postmenopausal phase of life
3. Race: Caucasian in the middle or upper socioeconomic class
4. Genetics: women whose mother and sisters have developed cancer
5. Menarche: occurred before the age of 12
6. Parity (total number of pregnancies): decreased for women if birth is before 18 years; increased for women who are not sexually active and infertile women, women who become pregnant after the age of 35
7. Menopause: late menopause after the age of 55
8. Other cancer: had other cancer such as endometrial, ovarian, and colon; if cancer has appeared in one breast, it is more likely to occur in the other breast

More than 90% of breast cancers are detected by the patient. Breast self-examinations should be performed at monthly intervals, preferably 1 week after menses. Breast examination for the postmenopausal woman should be done on the same day each month (Fig. 33-17 on p. 1022). If there are questionable findings, the patient should immediately contact her physician. The points in Box 33-10 on p. 1022 should be used in teaching breast self-examination.

Diagnostic Tests. Diagnosis of tumors is generally made by physical examination combined with mammography or ultrasound, and if necessary, confirmed by biopsy. If the screening mammogram indicates a problem or if the woman has a breast mass, a xeromammogram may be done. The xeromammogram provides a uniform image of the breast, giving a wide exposure.

A biopsy is an incisional procedure done in the operating room. The patient may be scheduled for removal of the breast if the biopsied tissue confirms malignancy. This type of scheduling reduces performing surgery twice and may be the choice of many women. Frequently patients prefer to have a discussion with physician and family regarding the biopsy report and to discuss alternative modes of treatment before a mastectomy is performed. Radiographic studies may be obtained before or after the biopsy to detect possible metastasis to the brain, chest, liver, and bones. Further confirmation may be needed to determine the status of lymph nodes of the axillary and the supraclavicular areas (see Fig. 33-16).

Medical Management. The intervention for treatment of breast cancer depends on the stage of the tumor, the age and health status of the patient, the hormonal sta-

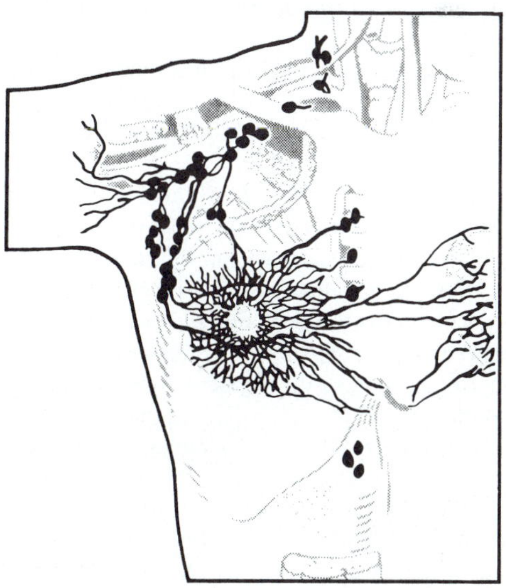

FIG. 33-16 Lymphatic spread of breast cancer. (From American Cancer Society: *A cancer source book for nurses,* New York, 1981, The Society.)

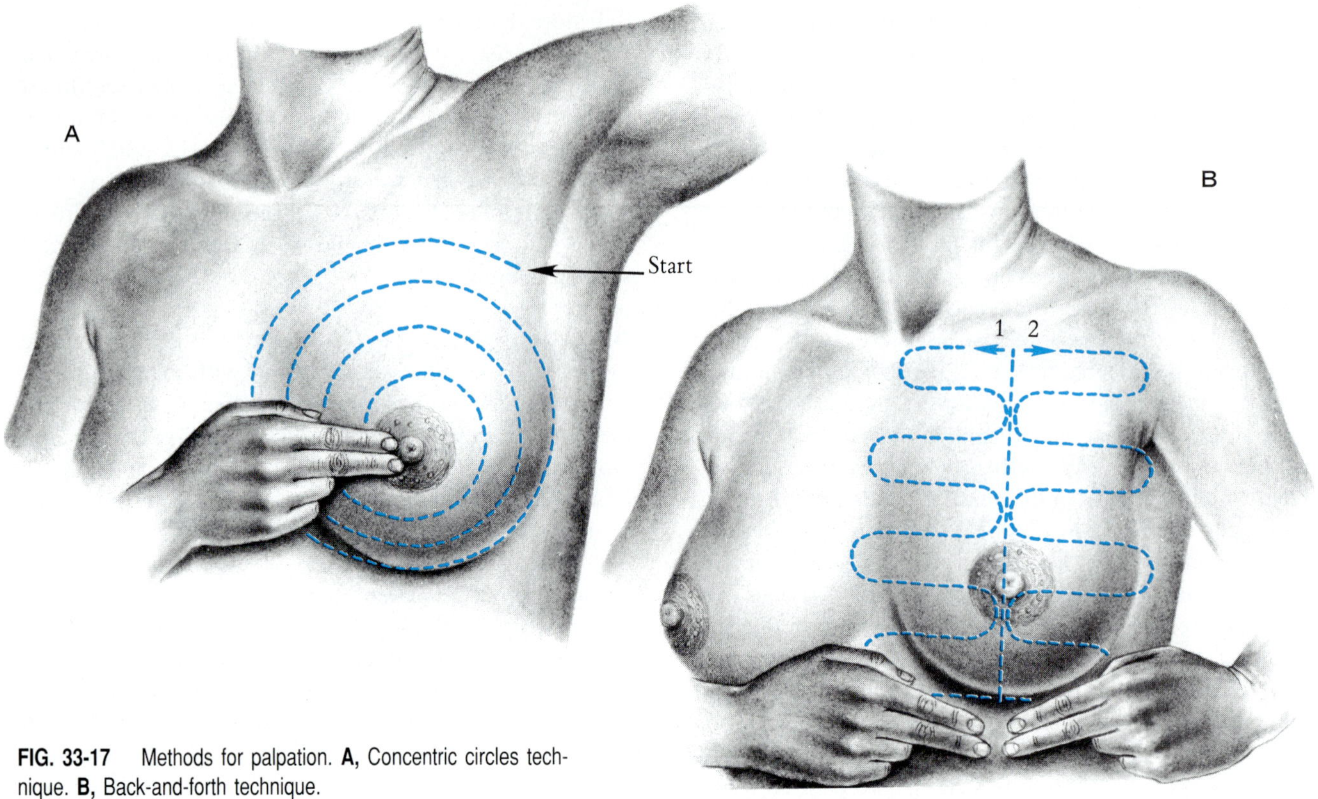

FIG. 33-17 Methods for palpation. **A,** Concentric circles technique. **B,** Back-and-forth technique.

Box 33-10 BREAST SELF-EXAMINATION

1. The majority of breast lumps are not cancer.
2. Cancerous breast lesions are treatable.
3. Breasts should be examined each month for premenopausal women 7 to 8 days after conclusion of the menstrual period when they are least congested, and on the same day of each month for postmenopausal women.
4. Visual inspection and palpation should be done.
5. Visual inspection should be done when the woman is stripped to the waist and looking in a mirror, using the following arm positions: arms at rest at sides, hands on hips and pressed into hips, contracting chest muscles; hands over the head (torso in upright position); hands over head (torso leaning forward).
6. Palpation may be done in the shower when the soap and water assist the hands to glide over the skin. However, the examination of large breasts and axillae is better done in a supine position rather than a standing position.
7. The entire breast should be examined in a systematic way, moving clockwise, with a circular motion. Always include the axillae in the examination.
8. Specific examination of the nipple, through compression for discharge, and the areola, through palpation, should not be forgotten:
9. Any breast change should be reported to the physician.

tus, and the presence of estrogen receptors in the tumor. Radiation, chemotherapy, and surgery alone or in combination are the most common modes of treatment of cancer of the breasts (see Chapter 38).

Staging. After breast surgery and axillary dissection, the staging process is completed. The universal staging and classification system for breast cancer agreed on in 1987 is the tumor, node, metastasis (TNM) system (Box 33-11). Staging depends on size of the tumor, size and presence or absence of nodal malignancy, and presence or absence of distant metastasis. Tumors are classified from stage 0 to stage IV.

Surgical interventions. Surgery plays a vital role in the management of breast cancer. Tissue biopsy, inspection and biopsy of lymph nodes in the axillary areas, radiological examinations, and laboratory reports are aids in making the decision that surgery should be performed. Several surgical approaches may be selected for the removal of the breast carcinoma (Fig. 33-18). Types of approaches include the following:

1. A lumpectomy (**tylectomy,** tumorectomy) is the removal of a circumscribed area with the tumor. This surgery is usually done when the tumor is small and is on the peripheral area of the breast. The breast contour and muscle support are preserved if possible. The patient and physician may decide to use local irradiation of the breast to destroy potentially microscopic cancer cells.
2. A partial mastectomy **(quadrantectomy)** is another form of segmental mastectomy in which

Box 33-11 TNM STAGING

Stage 0: tumor in situ that has no nodal or metastatic involvement and is noninvasive
Stage I: tumor is 1 to 2 cm or smaller, with no nodal or metastatic involvement
Stage II: tumors 2 to 5 cm, with or without nodal involvement and no metastasis
Stage III: tumors 5 to 10 cm, usually with lymph node involvement and no metastasis
Stage IV: denotes any size tumor, with or without nodal involvement and with distant metastasis

the quadrant of the breast in which the tumor is located is removed. In most instances, axillary nodes are dissected through a separate incision. Augmental surgery may be required at a later time, because this surgery can be disfiguring.

3. A subcutaneous mastectomy is the removal of malignant breast tissue, leaving the breast skin surface and nipple in place. At this time a prosthesis can be implanted if surgical conditions are considered appropriate.
4. A simple mastectomy is the removal of the entire breast. The skin flap is retained to cover the incised area. Both pectoralis major and pectoralis minor muscles are left intact.
5. A modified radical mastectomy is performed when the tumor is 4 cm or larger, if it is invasive, or if the patient and physician decide this procedure is in the patient's best interest. In this operation all breast tissue, overlying skin, nipple, and pectoralis minor muscle are removed, as are samples of axillary lymph nodes, and fascia under the breast. The pectoralis major muscle remains intact.
6. A radical mastectomy involves removal of the breast, major and minor pectoral muscles, all lymph nodes, fat, and fascia. A skin graft may be used to cover the incised area. This type of surgery is seldom done in the United States, because refined techniques of pathological evaluations, radiation therapy, and chemotherapy have made it unnecessary in most cases.

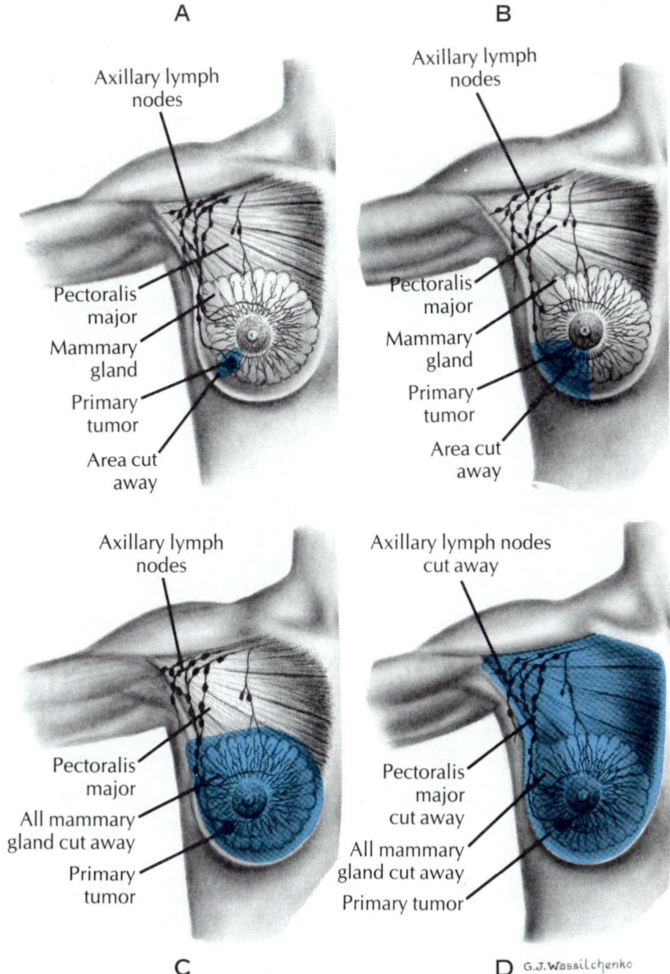

FIG. 33-18 Four ways to deal surgically with cancer of the breast. **A,** Lumpectomy (tylectomy). **B,** Quadrantectomy (segmental resection). **C,** Total (simple) mastectomy. **D,** Radical mastectomy.

Nursing Interventions. The physician will discuss with the patient and family the rationale for mastectomy and the manner of coping with the cosmetic effects of and psychological response to the operation. Patients often have questions about possible alternatives to standard or modified mastectomy.

The patient may be confused with so many options of therapy and surgical interventions. During this time the nurse plays an active role as listener and reinforcer of information provided by the physician and providing responses that can encourage and assist the patient to verbalize her concerns and recognize her feeling about the surgery. The emotional preparation of the patient may be more important than the physical preparation. Often there is anticipatory grieving for the loss of a body part.

Preoperative preparation enlists the participation of patient, support group, and nursing staff so that progressive care can continue, beginning at admission through surgery, recovery, and the postoperative period. The essential admission assessment provides data that are helpful in planning care by the nurse and patient. Nursing diagnoses can be developed and a plan of care individualized for the patient according to her needs. (See the nursing care plan on pp. 1024-1026.)

It is important for the nurse to assess and identify the members of the patient's support system to know

NURSING CARE PLAN: THE PATIENT UNDERGOING MASTECTOMY

Ms. Christian, age 52, was diagnosed with ductal cell carcinoma of the left breast. She has undergone a left modified radical mastectomy.

Nursing diagnoses	Patient goals/expected outcomes	Nursing interventions
Fear, related to the cancer diagnosis and surgical intervention	Patient will be able to state fears.	Encourage patient to talk about specific fears and feelings about each fear.
	Patient will be able to state a positive improvement in coping.	Provide a calm supportive environment. Provide information on coping mechanisms. Encourage consultation with resource persons (e.g., psychologist, clergy, nurse specialist, and Reach to Recovery). Use support of family/significant others. Encourage use of comfort measures, such as music.
	Patient can describe type of surgical procedures. Patient can recite postoperative interventions that will occur.	Encourage patient's comments and questions about surgery and postoperative care.
Infection, high risk for, related to surgical incision and presence of drain	Skin will remain free of signs and symptoms of infection.	Assess skin integrity. Instruct on signs and symptoms of infection.
	Vital signs and WBC values will be maintained within normal limits.	Assess and report abnormal vital signs and elevated WBC; skin changes and comfort level. Observe and record amount of exudate. Check drainage tubing for patency.
Pain, acute, related to incision	Patient will verbalize site and nature of pain; will relate comfort increase. Patient will demonstrate willingness to participate in self-care activities. Patient will interact positively with staff and significant others. Patient will demonstrate relaxed facial expression and body movements.	Assess attitude toward pain; record verbal and nonverbal cues. Give analgesics as prescribed on a regular basis for first 24 hours, then as necessary. Explore methods for controlling pain, e.g., medications, visual imagery, controlled breathing, and diversionary activities; monitor effectiveness. Position patient on back or unaffected side in semi-Fowler's position. Encourage frequent changes in position while in bed and early ambulation.
Mobility, impaired physical, related to surgery, pain, and discomfort	Patient's mobility will be restored to optimum level. Patient will willingly participate in exercise program. Patient will verbalize comfort levels. Patient will regain ROM of affected arm.	Assist in activity progression from sitting to ambulating. Encourage participation in exercise program for affected arm. Turn and reposition every 2 hours or as needed; position for body alignment. Encourage bilateral use of arms in activities, such as personal hygiene.

Body image disturbance, related to surgical procedure	Patient will verbalize acceptance of altered body image as evidenced by absence of weeping, irritability, verbalization of discomfort with present body, and attempting difficult physical or mental tasks despite limitations. Patient demonstrates interest in her personal appearance. Patient will verbalize plans to resume former activities.	Encourage patient's comments and questions about surgery, progress, and prognosis. Encourage patient to discuss change in her body with husband or significant other. Reinforce correct information, and provide factual information to correct any misconceptions. Relate importance of communicating anything that causes anxiety. Encourage patient to verbalize and explore feelings regarding impact missing body part might have on patient's functioning as a sexual partner and in activities of daily living. Encourage a patient to continue activities associated with femininity, such as fixing hair, using make-up, wearing own apparel. Encourage patient to look at and touch the changed body part when she demonstrates readiness. Encourage use of rehabilitation services (e.g., Reach to Recovery, Wellness Community).
Knowledge deficit, related to home care management	Patient and family will demonstrate understanding of home care and follow-up instructions through discussion and return demonstration.	Assess current level of learning and determine needs.
	Patient will exhibit increased interest in exercise program as shown by verbal and nonverbal cues and will demonstrate correct method of postoperative arm exercises.	Explain importance of exercise to tolerance; instruct patient to stop at point of pain.
	Patient will verbalize the necessity of healing to occur before a permanent prosthesis is worn.	Discuss types of prosthesis available; instruct to not wear permanent prosthesis until incision is healed.
	Patient will verbalize/demonstrate how to change dressing on her incision. Patient will identify and recite signs/symptoms of infection.	Teach care of incision. Discuss signs and symptoms to report to physician: erythema, pain, edema, drainage, elevated temperature. Emphasize need to gradually resume activities of daily living. Explain that incision and/or chest wall may feel numb.
	Patient will verbalize/demonstrate procedure for breast self-examination. Patient will verbalize specific precautions to prevent infection and lymphedema in affected arm.	Instruct patient to examine remaining breast once a month. Caution patient to avoid injections, vaccinations, taking of BP, taking of blood samples, or insertion of IV line in affected area. Emphasize importance of follow-up outpatient care.

CRITICAL THINKING QUESTIONS

1. Ms. Christian confides in her nurse that she feels ugly and unattractive and refuses to look at her incision. A helpful approach by the nurse could include:
2. In assessing Ms. Christian, the nurse notes her holding her left arm guardedly in an adducted position. She does not use it for ADLs. Effective patient teaching would include:
3. Discharge teaching for Ms. Christian to prevent trauma and infection of her left arm would include:

their strengths and concerns about the pending treatment and interventions. Support does not always need to come from the immediate family and close circle of friends. Outside support and resources can come from coworkers, religious groups, oncology clinicians, psychologists, and Reach to Recovery support groups. It is important to openly discuss the patient's fears, and this is often done by the nurse who has established a therapeutic relationship with the patient and family.

Reach to Recovery volunteers have been a source of information, encouragement, and support for the female with breast cancer. The organization is based on the premise that rehabilitation for a woman with breast cancer should include communication with, and support from, another who has shared a similar situation and who has learned to cope and resume her normal activities.

Nursing interventions for patients who undergo surgery of the breast include monitoring vital signs and observing for symptoms of shock or hemorrhage, since many large blood vessels are involved in the procedure. Drains such as a Davol or Hemovac may be placed in the axilla to facilitate drainage and prevent formation of a hematoma. Postoperative dressings are usually constrictive and bulky and may tend to embarrass respiratory effort as well as cause pain and discomfort. When the vital signs are stable, the patient is placed in a 45-degree Fowler's position to promote drainage. The position should be changed frequently, and deep breathing and coughing are encouraged.

Some patients may experience incisional pain for several days after surgery and when doing arm exercises. There may be complaints of numbness and referred pain in the arm of the operative area. The pain radiates to the shoulder and the back because of severance of peripheral nerves. Most of the nerves regenerate, but there are cases of residual numbness. Analgesics may be given as the patient feels she needs it. Care must be exercised to prevent oversedation. It is important for the patient to deep breathe and cough to prevent postoperative atelectasis.

Physicians differ in opinion about the best positioning of the affected arm. Some physicians place the affected arm in the dressing and place it in a sling for a couple of days postoperatively. Some physicians believe slings should be avoided. If the arm is not restricted by dressings, it may be elevated on a pillow with the hand and wrist higher than the elbow and the elbow higher than the shoulder joint. This will facilitate the flow of fluids by the lymph and venous routes and prevent lymphedema.

Usually the patient is allowed to ambulate on the first postoperative day. Assistance to move out of bed will be needed to have the patient learn to maintain balance because of breast removal and bulky dressings. If a modified radical mastectomy has been the surgical intervention, the defense mechanisms are lessened by the removal of lymph nodes.

Patients should be taught not to have any procedures involving the arm on the affected side—blood pressure readings, injections, IV infusion of fluids, or blood drawing, which may cause edema or infection, and to guard against infections from burns, needle pricks (sewing), and gardening injuries. Removing lymph nodes and channels increases the risk of developing lymphedema, even years after surgery. Referral to physical therapy may be indicated to control lymphedema if it develops. The patient should be instructed to avoid sleeping on the involved arm. Clothing on the affected arm should be nonconstricting. Braclets and watches should be worn on the unaffected arm (Box 33-12).

The longer the edema persists, the more difficult it is to manage. Diuretics and low-sodium diets are often prescribed. If the edema persists, elastic stockinette is measured for precise fit to avoid venous flow constriction. The sleeve is applied from the wrist to the shoulder and worn when the patient is out of bed. When the patient is sleeping, the arm is positioned to aid venous flow. If the lymphedema is severe, the physician may order Jobst extremity therapy. There is an automatic inflation and deflation of a pneumomassage sleeve that can be placed on the arm. The compression pump is strictly contraindicated when there is evidence of acute phlebitis, perivascular lymphangitis, or cellulitis.

Isometric exercises are helpful for increasing the circulation and development of the collateral lymph system. Opening and clenching fingers and squeezing a rub-

Box 33-12 HAND AND ARM CARE AFTER BREAST SURGERY

1. Prevention of infection
   a. Wear gloves when cleaning with harsh detergent.
   b. Wear gloves when gardening.
   c. Avoid injections, vaccinations, and venipuncture in involved arm.
   d. Use cuticle remover in preference to cutting cuticles.
   e. Sew with a thimble.
   f. Avoid chapped hands; use lanolin cream daily.
   g. Take care when using equipment that might cut, scrape, or abrade.
   h. Shave underarms with an electric razor.
   i. Avoid insect bites; use insect repellent.
2. Prevention of constricting circulation
   a. Do not take blood pressure in involved arm.
   b. Wear loose clothing; avoid tight bra straps or tight sleeves.
   c. Wear watch or jewelry on uninvolved arm.
   d. Carry purse on uninvolved arm or shoulder.
3. Prevention of burns
   a. Wear padded mitts to reach in oven; use potholders.
   b. Prevent sunburn; use sunscreens with SPF of 15; cover arms during prolonged exposure.
4. Prevention of drag or pull
   a. Carry heavy packages on uninvolved arm.
   b. Avoid motions that increase centrifugal force.
5. Immediately report any signs of erythema, edema, warmth, or pain.

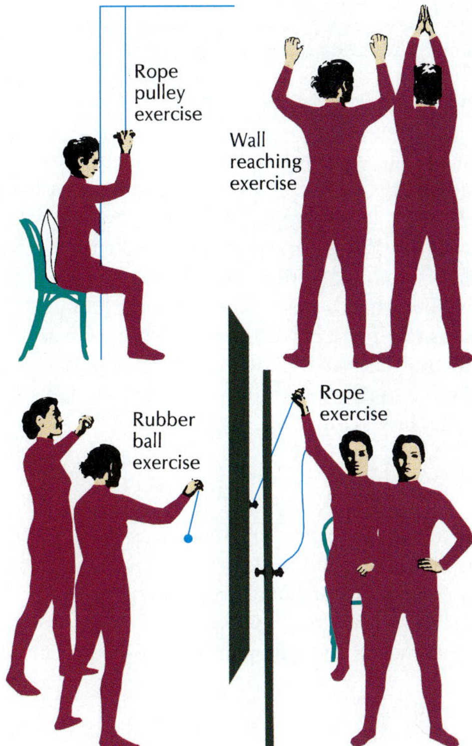

FIG. 33-19 Exercises after mastectomy.

ber ball can be started in the first few postoperative days. This activity provides extension and flexion of the wrist and elbow. The activity is equivalent to sewing, knitting, typing, and playing piano when at home.

Preventing muscle contractures. Specific exercises may be ordered to restore the muscle strength and full range of motion of the affected area. Gentle exercises started early in the postoperative course help to decrease muscle tension and to regain muscle function more quickly. The nurse or the therapist should instruct the patient and encourage the continuation of the exercises on discharge. Many of the exercises may be incorporated into activities of daily living as normal daily tasks are assumed (Fig. 33-19; see also Box 33-13 on p. 1028).

Exercising can be painful but can be accepted as a challenge by the patient with the support group encouraging her. The challenge can be met and the results of muscular strengthening achieved.

Body image acceptance. After losing a breast, many patients experience grief over the loss of a body part. This acute grief is like a crisis and may last 4 to 6 weeks or longer. Grief makes the fact of loss real. The process of grieving is essential for personal adaptation to the loss. The nurse can assist the patient to find helpful coping mechanisms. When deep breathing exercises are started immediately after surgery and the patient has been able to splint the area, and while exercising her arm, the woman will recognize the absence of the breast through touch. Dressing changes and incision cleansing with patient involvement make the absence real. Being involved and responsible for the dressing and incision allows a more personal approach to the patient. At this time support by the nurse is very important. The nurse can provide a mirror or seat the patient in front of the mirror so that the patient can see the operative site being cleansed and dressed. The nurse must be very sensitive to the patient and be alert for signs of readiness by the patient to become involved in care and accepting of the loss of the body part. The incisional area may be erythematous and edematous, but the discoloration will gradually lessen and the site will become more comfortable. The patient should be encouraged to apply and massage cocoa butter or a cream to make the incisional line softer. The patient should be counseled that it takes time to accept the loss and heal emotionally as well as physically.

Prosthesis. A breast prosthesis should not be worn unless authorized by the physician. There are many breast forms available. Forms are made of gels and

Box 33-13 POSTMASTECTOMY ARM EXERCISES

EXERCISE: CLIMBING THE WALL

1. Stand facing wall with toes 6 to 12 inches from wall.
2. Bend elbows and place palms of hands against wall at shoulder level.
3. Move both hands parallel to each other up the wall as far as possible until incisional pull or pain occurs.
4. Move both hands down to starting position.
5. Goal is complete extension with elbow straight.
6. Activities that use the same action: reaching top shelves, hanging out clothes, washing windows, hanging curtains, setting hair.

EXERCISE: ELBOW PULL-IN

1. Extend arms sideways to shoulder level.
2. Clasp hands behind neck.
3. Pull elbows forward until they touch.
4. Return to position 2.
5. Unclasp hands and extend arms sideways at shoulder level.
6. Lower arms to side.

EXERCISE: BACK SCRATCH

1. Place hand of unoperated side on hip for balance.
2. Bend elbow of affected arm, placing back of hand on small of back.
3. Work hand up the back slowly until fingers reach opposite shoulder blade.
4. Lower arm and straighten both arms.

EXERCISE: ROPE PULL

1. Attach a rope over a shower rod, hook, or over top of an open door.
2. Sit on a chair (with door between legs if using a door) and grasp each end of rope.
3. Alternately pull on each end, raising affected arm to a point of incisional pull or pain.
4. The goal is to raise the affected arm almost directly overhead.

molded silicone. Most forms are covered with soft fabric and are light in weight and feel like breast tissue. In selecting a breast form there is a shape for each type of breast, because each body is different and each surgery is different. Forms have been developed that can be fitted for a right or left breast, slanted for the breast that was slanted or a full breast with an outer curve that simulates the extension of the breast under the axilla and upward on the chest. It is advisable to have a skilled fitter from a reliable company to fit the prosthesis.

A well-fitted brassiere is essential before choosing the shape form. If the woman is very active and desires a pocket or restraining cup, the brassiere needs to be equipped for it. Brassieres can be purchased with these adaptions. Some available forms can be worn against the skin with no underpadding or bra cups. Most forms can be washed with water and mild detergent to keep the form clean and supple. Many prostheses are waterproof and can be worn swimming; when wet they do not "weigh down" the wearer with heaviness.

When the patient is being fitted with a prosthesis, the best assurance that the fit is right is when:

1. The brassiere fits snugly around the rib cage
2. The prosthesis fills the bottom of the bra cup
3. The prosthesis projects the same as the remaining breast, with form bulk and nipples in position
4. The breasts are separated when the bra is centered
5. The top of the bra cup is filled and appears like the other breast

Breast Reconstruction. The patient whose disease is limited to the breast may benefit from reconstructive surgery. The benefits of breast reconstruction include avoidance of an external prosthesis that has potential for slipping, greater choice of clothing (including lower necklines), and loss of self-consciousness about appearance. For many women breast reconstruction is beneficial in improving self-esteem. Breast reconstruction can produce psychological benefits and provide many women with a renewed sense of wholeness and a return to a normal state. The most important indicators for reconstruction are the patient's motivation and desire for the procedure. The prime determinant for the procedure is the clinical status of the patient. Goals for reconstruction are to select the simplest type that meets the patient's needs and expectations to match the opposite breast in size, shape, and contour.

Breast reconstruction can be performed immediately after surgery or at a later time. An increasing number of women are electing immediate reconstruction; this may prolong the initial hospitalization but eliminates the need for a second hospitalization and contributes to self-esteem. Others wait until they have completed adjuvant chemotherapy or radiation to be sure that the area is disease free.

Breast implant. If the remaining skin is sufficient to cover an implant, surgery may consist of placing a permanent silicone implant under the pectoralis muscle. Possible complications of silicone implants include infection, deflation, a false mammography result, and silicone leaks.

It has also been suggested that the silicone filling or the implant covering can lead to autoimmune or connective tissue disease. Although most surgeries have not resulted in complications, differing opinions regarding the safety of breast implants led the Food and Drug Administration (FDA) in early 1992 to issue some recommendations. Breast implants were permitted after breast

TABLE 33-1 Prognosis and Nodal Involvement in Breast Cancer

Lymph Nodes Involved	Metastatic Recurrence
1 to 3 nodes	50%-60% metastasis
4 to 10 nodes	75%-85% metastasis
> 10 nodes	Even worse prognosis

cancer surgery because of the offsetting positive contribution to recovery, but a moratorium was imposed on breast implants solely for cosmetic purposes until data establishing safety could be provided.

Latissimus dorsi flap graft. A latissimus dorsi graft is a free flap graft in which an "island" of latissimus muscle, fat, and skin is transferred to the breast area, where it provides adequate cover for an implant.

Transabdominal island flap. The transabdominal island flap (TAIF) method creates a breast that better approximates breast tissue than the silicone implant. TAIF surgery involves transferring a section of abdominal skin and fat and part of the rectus abdominis muscle to the breast area by tunneling under the skin. The tissue is then shaped as a new breast. TAIF involves more extensive surgery than the implant procedure and usually requires a week-long hospital stay.

Nipple reconstruction is usually performed as a separate procedure after the breast reconstruction has been completed. Nipple construction is generally from available tissue at the site or harvested tissue from the opposite breast. New techniques allow the nipple to be created from tissue and subcutaneous tissue of the breast mount. Areola reconstruction is provided by obtaining pigmented skin from the upper thigh or by using skin from the lateral chest area.

Prognosis. The 5-year survival rate for localized breast cancer is 85% for white women and 79% for black women. After the disease spreads beyond the breast, the survival rate drops dramatically. Breast cancer is the leading cause of cancer deaths among women 15 to 54 years of age.[3] The most important prognostic factor is the stage of the disease (see Box 33-11). See Table 33-1 for node involvement and metastasis.

INFLAMMATORY DISORDERS OF THE MALE REPRODUCTIVE SYSTEM

Prostatitis

Etiology/Pathophysiology. Prostatitis is an acute or chronic infection of the prostate gland. It is commonly a result of bacterial invasion from the urethra. The causative organisms include *Escherichia coli, Klebsiella, Proteus, Pseudomonas, Streptococcus,* and *Staphylococcus.*

Bacterial invasion originates in the bloodstream and/or from a descending infection from the kidneys.

Clinical Manifestations. Symptoms include sudden onset of chills and fever. There is urgency and frequency of urination, dysuria (pain on urination), cloudy urine, perineal fullness, low back pain, arthralgia (pain in the joints), and myalgia (pain in the muscles). When the gland is palpated, there is tenderness, edema, and firmness. In chronic prostatitis, many patients may appear to be asymptomatic, but generally the same symptoms exist as in the acute phase with a lesser degree of intensity.

Diagnostic Tests. Diagnostic testing includes culture and sensitivity tests of the urethra, prostatic fluid, and urine for organism identification and appropriate antibiotic therapy. Prostatic fluid is collected by prostate massage and expression of fluid. The pH of the fluid is generally elevated. A rectal examination done by the physician reveals gland tenderness and edema.

Medical Management. Medical management includes antibiotic therapy and periodic digital massage of the prostate by the physician to increase the flow of infected prostatic secretions. Heat may be applied by means of sitz baths.

Nursing Interventions. Nursing interventions primarily focus on symptoms and include (1) a full explanation of antibiotic therapy and the need for compliance with treatment, which may be lengthy in chronic prostatitis; (2) supportive care such as bed rest to relieve strain and pain of the perineum and suprapubic area, sitz baths to promote muscle relaxation, and stool softeners to prevent straining on defecation; (3) monitoring I&O, and (4) encouraging follow-up for evaluation of the inflammation.

Nursing diagnoses and interventions for the patient with prostatitis include but are not limited to the following:

NURSING DIAGNOSES	NURSING INTERVENTIONS
Pain, acute, related to disease process	Assess type and location of pain; provide analgesics as ordered. Bed rest to promote comfort. Provide nonpharmacological comfort measures; 1. Assist patient with assuming comfortable position. 2. Provide diversional activity. 3. Provide a restful environment.
Self-esteem disturbance, high risk for, related to fear of impotence and embarrassment	Encourage patient to express feelings. Actively listen. Encourage adaptive coping behaviors.
Knowledge deficit, related to illness and outcome	Instruct patient in necessity to comply with taking prescribed medication and to follow orders for activity level.

Prognosis. Recurrent episodes of acute prostatitis may cause fibrotic tissue to form; the fibrosis causes a hardening of the prostate gland that may initially be confused with carcinoma.

Epididymitis

Etiology/Pathophysiology. **Epididymitis** is an infection of the cordlike excretory duct of the testicle. It is one of the common infections of the male reproductive tract. The causative organisms are *Staphylococcus aureus, E. coli, Streptococcus* species, and *Neisseria gonorrhoeae.* The inflammation is associated with urethral strictures, cystitis, and prostatitis.

Symptoms can occur after trauma to the genital area, after instrumentation of the urethra and cystocopy, and after physical exertion or prolonged sexual activity.

Clinical Manifestations. Severe pain appears suddenly in the scrotum and radiates along the spermatic tube. Edema appears and the patient develops a "duck walk" or "waddling gait" because of the sensitivity and pain that walking stimulates. The scrotal area becomes tender. Pyuria (pus in urine) is present. Chills and fever are noted.

Diagnostic Tests. Diagnostic testing includes examining the first daily flow of urine and sending a midstream specimen to the laboratory to check for pyuria. The epididymis is massaged by the physician and a fluid expression specimen is sent to the laboratory. Physical examination of the scrotum is performed. The WBC is monitored for leukocytosis.

Medical Management. Medical management includes a regimen of bed rest and support of the scrotum. Cold may be applied for relief of edema and discomfort, and the appropriate antibiotic is administered. If abscess formation occurs, incision and drainage (I&D) of the scrotum may be required.

Nursing Interventions. Nursing interventions for patients with epididymitis include (1) bed rest during the acute phase of illness, (2) support of the testicular area, with scrotal support by elevation of the scrotum on a folded towel during bed rest and athletic support when ambulatory, (3) ice compresses to the area in the initial phase to hasten recovery, and (4) explaining the need for compliance with antibiotic therapy until all signs of inflammation have disappeared.

Prognosis. The infection can be bilateral and may recur. Bilateral epididymitis can cause sterility. Untreated epididymitis leads to necrosis (death of tissue) of testicular tissue; in addition, abscesses can form, and septicemia can develop, which can be fatal.

DISORDERS OF MALE GENITAL ORGANS

Phimosis

Etiology/Pathophysiology. **Phimosis** is a condition in which the prepuce is too small to allow retraction of the foreskin over the glans. Phimosis is often congenital but may be acquired as a result of local inflammation or disease. The condition is rarely severe enough to obstruct the flow of urine but may contribute to local infection because it does not permit adequate cleansing treatment.

Medical Management. A surgical procedure **(circumcision)** may be performed in which a part of the foreskin is removed, leaving the glans penis uncovered.

Nursing Interventions. After a circumcision a sterile petrolatum gauze dressing is applied and changed after each voiding. The nurse should always observe the patient for unusual bleeding and obstruction of urine flow.

Hydrocele

Etiology/Pathophysiology. A hydrocele is an accumulation of fluid between the membranes covering the testicle and the membrane enclosing the testicle. The scrotum slowly enlarges as the fluid accumulates. Pain occurs if the hydrocele develops suddenly. Most hydroceles occur in males over the age of 21. The actual cause is not known, but it may develop as a result of trauma of the area, orchitis (inflammation of the testes), or epididymitis.

Medical Management. Treatment includes aspiration of fluid from the sac or surgical removal of the sac to avoid constriction of the circulation of the testicles. After aspiration the pain is relieved and the scrotum can be examined more easily.

Nursing Interventions. Nursing interventions consist of maintaining bed rest, scrotal support with elevation, ice to edematous areas, and frequent changes of dressings to avoid skin impairment.

Prognosis. With treatment, prognosis is good.

Varicocele

Varicocele occurs when the veins within the scrotum become dilated. Obstruction and malfunctioning of the veins cause engorgement and elongation, which do not allow adequate drainage of the blood. The symptoms are a pulling sensation that causes a dull aching and pain accompanied by edema of the scrotal area. The treatment is surgical removal of the obstruction. Nursing interventions include bed rest with scrotal support, ice to the incisional site, and medication for discomfort as ordered.

Prognosis. Varicocele is often seen in men with low fertility. Ligation of the spermatic vein has been shown to improve semen quality.

CANCER OF THE MALE REPRODUCTIVE TRACT

The more common tumors of the male reproductive tract involve the testis, prostate gland, and penis. Most tumors of the male reproductive system are malignant.

Men should be taught to do testicular self-examination. The examination takes 3 minutes and should be done monthly. The best time to do a testicular self-examination is after the man has had a warm shower and the scrotal skin is relaxed. Each testicle should be rolled gently between the thumb and fingers of both hands, examining for lumps or nodules. If any lumps or nodules are found, a physician should be consulted promptly.

Cancer of the Testis

Etiology/Pathophysiology. Cancer of the testis is the second most common malignancy in men 25 to 35 years of age and is the most common cause of death in this age group. The causes are unknown. The incidence of this cancer is higher in men with **cryptorchidism** (failure of testes to descend into the scrotum). Other associated factors are testicular atrophy and scrotal trauma. The most common type of testicular cancer is seminoma, which usually spreads slowly through the lymphatics. Embryonal tumors include the spermatic cord and metastasize early to the lungs.

Clinical Manifestations. The signs and symptoms of early disease include an enlarged scrotum, and a firm, painless, smooth mass in the testicular area is noted. At times the patient may speak of a feeling of heaviness. Diagnosis is generally revealed when the patient complains of the presence of the mass or at the time of a routine physical examination.

Medical Management. Radical inguinal orchiectomy is usually the treatment of choice. This is the removal of the testis, epididymis, a portion of the gonadal lymphatics, and their blood supply. The remaining testis provides enough testosterone to maintain the man's sexual characteristics. He may have a lower sperm count of decreased sperm mobility. Surgery is generally followed by radiation and/or chemotherapy. Often a retroperitoneal lymph node dissection is performed to remove affected nodes and to assist in determining the tumor stage. Staging a testicular tumor helps determine treatment.

Box 33-14 TESTICULAR SELF-EXAMINATION (TSE)

Perform TSE after a bath or shower when scrotum is warm and most relaxed.

Grasp testis with both hands and palpate gently between thumb and fingers. The testis should feel smooth and egg-shaped and be firm to touch.

The epididymis, found behind the testis, should feel like a soft tube (Fig. 33-20).

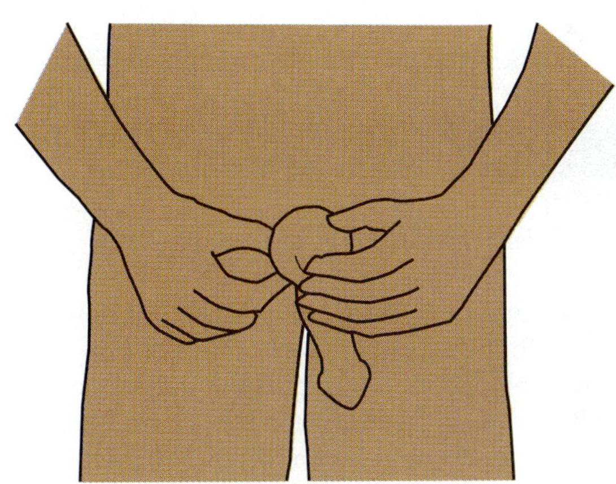

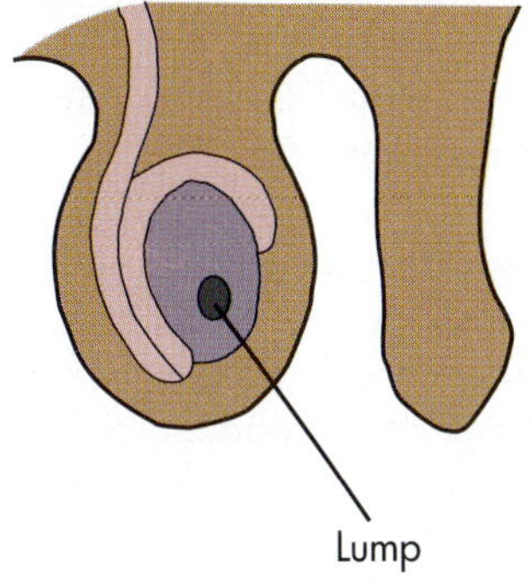

FIG. 33-20 Testicular self-examination.

Nursing Interventions and Patient Teaching. The priority for care of patients who have or are at risk for a tumor of the testis is early detection by testicular self-examination. Young men should be taught to perform self-examination monthly beginning at 15 years of age. The scrotum is checked for color, contour, and skin breaks. The left side is usually longer because the left testicle is suspended from a longer spermatic cord. Each testicle is gently palpated by grasping the scrotum in the center with the thumb and index finger (Box 33-14 and Fig. 33-20). Normal testicles are firm but somewhat resilient, smooth, and mobile. If a testicle is indurated (hardened), carcinoma is suspected.

Prognosis. With the advent of tumor markers (which indicate the presence of disease and enable the physician to monitor its response to treatment), refined surgery, and effective chemotherapy, the cure rate is as high as 90%.

Cancer of the Penis

Etiology/Pathophysiology. Cancer of the penis is rare. It generally appears in men over 50 years of age. Men who have not been circumcised, have not maintained good personal hygiene, or have had sexually transmitted diseases are at risk.

Clinical Manifestations. The tumor is painless, and a wartlike growth or ulceration on the gland under the prepuce is present. It is common for mestastasis to occur to the inguinal nodes and adjacent organs.

Diagnostic Tests. Biopsy confirms the diagnosis.

Medical Management. Surgical intervention requires removal of as little tissue as possible, but it may be necessary to do a partial or total amputation of the penis as well as remove the adjacent tissue and inguinal lymph nodes. When mestastasis involves the bladder and rectum, more radical surgery may be needed, and outlets for urinary or fecal elimination are provided by creating an ileoconduit and a colostomy. The surgeon may place a suprapubic catheter into the bladder as a means of draining the urine from the bladder.

Nursing Interventions. Nursing interventions include providing emotional support. If amputation of the penis is required, the patient faces the psychological trauma associated with loss of sexuality and loss of ability to urinate through the penis. Nursing interventions include monitoring urine output by suprapubic catheter or if an ileoconduit was performed, monitoring urine in the urostomy bag. Elevation of the scrotum controls edema. The nurse will provide comfort measures to control pain.

See Chapters 30 and 38 for a discussion of cancer of the prostate.

SEXUALLY TRANSMITTED DISEASES

Today, despite sweeping advances in the diagnosis and treatment of communicable diseases, the incidence of infections transmitted through intimate or sexual activities continues to increase worldwide.

Sexually transmitted diseases (STDs), *previously called venereal diseases,* are infections that are usually transmitted during intimate sexual contact. They may have other routes of transmission (e.g., an infected mother to her newborn), occur with or without symptoms, and have long periods of asymptomatic infectivity.

Any sexually active person may be at risk for a sexually transmitted disease. Persons who have frequent sexual contact with multiple partners are at very high risk. Common characteristics of these individuals are young, single, urban, poor, male, and homosexual. Because some STDs persist and are infectious for long periods (herpes genitalis and AIDS), even persons in mutually monogamous sexual relationships are at some risk. The proliferation of acquired immunodeficiency syndrome (AIDS) since the late 1970s has produced an urgent reason to educate sexually active individuals to the risk of unprotected sexual contact.

As of 1993, the Centers for Disease Control (CDC) reported 300,000 cumulative cases of AIDS in the United States and estimated that another 1 million people were infected with human immunodeficiency virus (HIV), the causative organism of AIDS. These are sobering statistics indeed. The number of people contracting the traditionally defined STDs (e.g., syphilis, gonorrhea) is even greater. Gonorrhea is estimated to infect 250 million people worldwide and nearly 3 million in the United States each year. Annual syphilis incidence is about 50 million cases worldwide and 50,223 in the United States. No reliable statistics exist for the "new generation" STDs, such as trichomoniasis, herpes simplex virus (HSV), venereal warts, scabies, and others; these are probably even more prevalent. In addition, bowel pathogens such as *Salmonella,* amoebae, hepatitis B, and the herpesviruses may be sexually transmitted.

Despite the physical and emotional discomfort, the possibility of long-term disability (infertility, chronic infectivity), and advances in diagnosis and treatment that sharply decrease the period of infectivity, STDs continue to be among the world's most common communicable diseases. Four main factors are responsible: (1) unprotected sex, (2) antibiotic resistance, (3) treatment delay, and (4) sexual behavior patterns and permissiveness. The following is a discussion of some of the more commonly diagnosed sexually transmitted diseases.

Herpes Genitalis

Etiology/Pathophysiology. Herpes genitalis or herpes simplex virus (HSV) is an infectious viral disease, characterized by recurrent episodes of acute, painful, erythematous, vesicular eruptions (blisters) on or in the genitalia or rectum.

The two closely related forms are designated types I and II. Most persons are infected in infancy with type I during feeding or kissing by adults. There are infrequent recurrences around the lips. A prior infection with HSV I confers relative immunity to HSV II. This immunity may enable persons infected with HSV I to be completely resistant or have a less dramatic HSV II infection.

HSV II is usually acquired sexually after puberty in the genital or anal regions.

Clinical Manifestations. Signs appear as fluid-filled vesicles after the incubation period and in women usually occur on the cervix, which is considered the primary site, but may also be seen on the labia, rectum, vulva, vagina, and skin and on the glans penis, foreskin, and penile shaft of men. Other lesions may appear on the mouth and anus. Vesicles may rupture and develop into shallow, painful ulcers; they are erythematous with marked edema and tenderness. Lymph nodes may become involved. Initial lesions last from 3 to 10 days, and recurrent lesions have a duration of 7 to 10 days. The infection may be accompanied by fever, malaise, dysuria, and in women, leukorrhea. Sites are painful in the presence of fever, stress, or emotional upset or when exposed to intense heat. Complications are rare.

Medical Management. Diagnosis is based on the physical examination and the patient history. The diagnosis is confirmed by appearance of the virus on tissue cultures. Ointments such as acyclovir inhibit the virus. Antibacterial agents combat secondary infections.

Nursing Interventions and Patient Teaching. The nurse should advise the patient that genital lesions should be kept clean and dry. Hands should be washed thoroughly after touching a lesion. Loose, absorbent underclothing is usually more comfortable than close-fitting clothing. Sitz baths decrease lesional discomfort and enhance urinary and bowel elimination. The patient should be taught that sexual intercourse during the active lesion phase increases the risk of transmission and may also be painful. Future sexual partners and health care providers should be advised of recurring or latent infections. The nurse should teach the role of stress, poor nutrition, and insufficient rest related to recurrences of signs and symptoms. Women patients need a yearly Pap test and should inform their physician in the event of future pregnancies so that the course of the disease can be monitored closely; there is a possibility of spontaneous abortion. The nurse should provide the patient with nonjudgmental support and with the contact number of the local herpes support group if one exists.

Prognosis. Herpes genitalis is a recurrent disease with no cure.

Syphilis

Etiology/Pathophysiology. The coiled spirochete *Treponema pallidum* causes syphilis. Congenital syphilis occurs in about 1 in 10,000 pregnancies, generally in minority populations. The age group with the highest incidence is 20 to 40 years. The incidence of syphilis has increased dramatically. In 1990, the 50,223 reported cases of primary and secondary syphilis were the single largest yearly total since 1948. This epidemic is occurring primarily among young, heterosexual, minority populations and may be related to cocaine use and exchange of sex for drugs, especially crack cocaine.

Syphilis is the third most frequently reported communicable disease in the United States, exceeded only by varicella (chickenpox) and gonorrhea. Transmission occurs primarily through sexual contact during the primary, secondary, and latent stages of the disease. Prenatal infection from the mother to the fetus is possible. The organism thrives in the warm parts of the body and can be destroyed by soap and water. The spirochete penetrates intact skin as well as openings in the mucous membrane of the genital organs, rectum, and mouth.

Clinical Manifestations. Each stage of syphilis has its peculiar signs and symptoms: primary, secondary, latent, and tertiary syphilis. The signs and symptoms of syphilis range from the clean-based **chancre** (painless erosion or papule that ulcerates superficially with a scooped-out appearance) of primary syphilis to the skin rashes of secondary syphilis. Moist, raised, gray to pink lesions of the genital or perirectal skin, enlarged lymph nodes, fever, fatigue, or infections of the eyes, bones, liver, or meninges may occur. In the late stages of syphilis, dementia, pain or loss of sensation in the legs and destruction of the aorta occur. Destructive inflammatory masses can appear in any organ. In tertiary or late-stage syphilis the heart and blood vessels (cardiovascular syphilis) and the central nervous system (neurosyphilis) are frequently involved. Tabes dorsalis, paresis, and various psychoses may result.

Diagnostic Tests. Diagnostic tests that are available include the Venereal Disease Research Laboratory (VDRL) slide test and rapid plasma reagin (RPR) test. All patients should be checked for gonorrhea as well.

Medical Management. Penicillin is the drug of choice of syphilis, but the treatment regimen varies according to the stage of the disease. A dose that ensures an adequate blood level for more than 7 days is needed. When the patient is allergic to penicillin, erythromycin or tetracycline is used. Report disease to infection control authorities as prescribed by local health agencies.

Nursing Interventions. Nursing interventions, other than the routine implications for patients with STDs, include monitoring for drug reaction to penicillin, stressing good handwashing technique with the patient, encouraging follow-up visits with the physician, and informing the patient that he or she should absolutely not engage in sexual intercourse until cured.

Prognosis. Syphilis can be successfully treated at any stage of the disease, but treatment may be prolonged in latent and late syphilis. Although syphilis can be cured in late stages, damage to the body is more difficult to manage. Untreated syphilis will go from primary to secondary latent and eventually to tertiary stage.

Gonorrhea

Etiology/Pathophysiology. Gonorrhea is caused by *Neisseria gonorrhoeae,* a gram-negative diplococcoid bacterium, and almost exclusively follows sexual contact. It is the most commonly reported communicable disease in the United States. It is estimated that at least 2 million unreported cases occur each year. The disease is most common in the 20 to 24 age group, closely followed by the 15 to 19 age group. Those who are at risk are sexually active individuals and women who use birth control pills or who are otherwise susceptible to infections. Gonorrhea is primarily an infection of the genital or rectal mucosa but is not limited to the genital organs; it can infect the mouth and the throat through oral sex with an infected partner. It may also infect the eyes. Three times as many males are infected as females. The incubation period of gonorrhea is 3 to 5 days.

Clinical Manifestations. Some infected males may be asymptomatic after the incubation period but in a short time develop signs and symptoms of urethritis, dysuria, infection with a purulent discharge, and edema of the affected area. Most females remain asymptomatic but may show a greenish-yellow discharge from the cervix. Other female signs and symptoms, which may vary depending on the infected site, are urinary frequency, purulent discharge from the urethra, pruritus, burning and pain of the vulva, vaginal engorgement and erythema, abdominal pain and distention, muscular rigidity, and tenderness. As the infection spreads, nausea, vomiting, fever, and tachycardia may develop. Other signs and symptoms that appear may include pharyngitis, tonsillitis, rectal burning, pruritus, and purulent rectal discharge.

Diagnostic Tests. Diagnosis is determined by cultures from the site of infection. Cultures isolate the organism and establish an identification. An important concern in treatment for gonorrhea is coexisting chlamydial infection (see pp. 1035-1036). This infection has been documented in up to 45% of gonorrhea cases when adequate chlamydial cultures are performed. It is important to test for syphilis as well.

Medical Management. Therapy for gonorrhea presents a greater problem than that for syphilis because the gonococcus tends to develop resistance to antibiotics. It is also believed that inadequate therapy is common in the United States. Several drug regimens are in use. Emphasis is on single-dose treatment because it avoids the need for follow-up and patient cooperation.

The treatment regimen recommended by the CDC is as follows:

1. Ceftriaxone (Rocephin) 250 mg IM in a single dose
2. Alternative therapy, including spectinomycin (Trobicin) 2 g IM once, ampicillin 3.5 g PO in a single dose or amoxicillin 3 g PO in a single dose

Spectinomycin is recommended by the CDC for the treatment of persons with resistant strains of *N. gonorrhoeae.*

Nurses need to be alert to changes in CDC recommendations. Report disease to infection control authorities as prescribed by local health agency.

Nursing Interventions and Patient Teaching. The nurse should advise patients that loose, absorbent underclothes, changed frequently after perineal/penile cleansing, will enhance comfort. Sitz baths decrease lower abdominal discomfort and dysuria. The patient should avoid infecting sexual partners and be taught that sterility may occur as a result of gonorrhea.

The nurse should obtain laboratory specimens as ordered. Alternative methods of birth control can be discussed as appropriate. The nurse encourages notification of present and past sexual partners of the diagnosis and the need for them to promptly seek medical care.

Prognosis. With treatment, gonorrhea is curable, but reoccurrence is common. The inflammation may clear up without serious results, or it may become chronic and produce urethral stricture. It may produce complications such as prostatitis, epididymitis, orchitis, arthritis, and endocarditis. It can result in sterility in the female. No case of acute gonorrhea in the female should be considered cured until three consecutive negative smears of the cervix and Bartholin's and Skene's glands are obtained.

Trichomoniasis

Etiology/Pathophysiology. Trichomoniasis is a sexually transmitted disease caused by the protozoan *Trichomonas vaginalis,* which affects about 15% of sexually active females and 10% of sexually active males. The incubation period is 4 to 28 days. Trichomoniasis is usually transmitted by sexual intercourse, and at times by dirty douche nozzles and douche containers and moist washcloths. Occasionally the newborn develops an infection from an infected mother. *T. vaginalis* thrives when the vaginal mucosa is more alkaline than normal. Frequent douching and use of oral contraceptives and antibiotics raise the normal pH of the vagina.

Clinical Manifestations. Most males and females are asymptomatic. The male signs and symptoms are mild to severe transient urethritis, dysuria, frequency of urination, pruritus, and purulent exudate. Approximately 70% of infected females are asymptomatic; signs and symptoms when present include profuse, frothy, gray, green, or yellow, malodorous discharge; pruritus; edema; tenderness of vagina; dysuria; frequency of urination; spotting; menorrhagia; and/or dysmenorrhea. Signs and symptoms may persist for a week to several months. Signs and symptoms may be more pronounced after menstruation and/or during pregnancy.

Diagnostic Tests and Medical Management. Diagnosis is based on the microscopic examination of the vaginal discharge that identifies *T. vaginalis.* Treatment for both males and females is oral metronidazole (Flagyl) in small doses for 7 days or one large single dose. The patient should avoid alcoholic beverages, because alcohol can cause a reaction with signs and symptoms of disorientation, headache, cramps, vomiting, and possible convulsions. Metronidazole can cause the urine to turn dark brown.

Nursing Interventions. The nurse should counsel the patient to avoid alcohol during treatment, inform patients that their urine may turn dark orange or brown, and counsel patients to avoid douches, sprays, and powders. The patient should be taught how to disinfect douche nozzles, applicators, diaphragms, and the toilet area. The nurse encourages the patient to wear loose-fitting clothing and cotton underwear, encourages follow-up visits with the physician, and discusses the need to contact sex partners to encourage their treatment.

Prognosis. With treatment trichomoniasis is curable. Reinfection is common if sexual partners are not treated simultaneously. Chronic infection may develop in untreated cases.

Candidiasis

Etiology/Pathophysiology. **Candidiasis** (candidosis, moniliasis) is a mild fungal infection that appears in men and women. Candidal infections are usually caused by *Candida albicans* and *Candida tropicalis.* The fungi are a part of the normal flora of the gastrointestinal tract, mouth, vagina, and skin. The infection often occurs when the glucose level rises from diabetes mellitus or when resistance is lowered from diseases such as carcinoma. Radiation, immunosuppressant drugs, hyperalimentation, antibiotic therapy, and oral contraceptives may predispose individuals to candidiasis. The male and female display signs of scaly skin, erythematous rash, and at time exudates that appear under the breasts, between the fingers, and in the axillae, groin, and umbilicus.

Clinical Manifestations. If the mother is infected, a newborn can contract oral *thrush* during delivery. The infant may display a diaper rash. Nails become edematous and have a darkened, erythematous nail base from which there is purulent exudate. Thrush may appear on the mucous membranes of the mouth and cause edema and engorgement. The infant may have an edematous tongue that can cause respiratory distress. The female patient may have a cheesy, tenacious white discharge accompanied by pruritus, and an inflamed vulva and vagina. The male presents signs of an infected penis with purulent exudate. Systemic infections are represented by chills, fevers, and general malaise.

Diagnostic Tests and Medical Management. Diagnosis is based on evidence of the *Candida* species on a Gram stain of collected specimens from scraping of the vagina and penis, from pus, and from exudate from the mouth. Treatment consists of treating and improving any underlying condition, such as controlling diabetes mellitus, discontinuing antibiotics and oral contraceptives, and catheter therapy. Nystatin (Mycostatin) is effective for superficial candidiasis; topical amphotericin B is effective for skin and nail infections.

Nursing Interventions. The nurse should emphasize the use of prescribed ointments, sprays, and creams as indicated for each part of the body affected. Teaching includes the method for inserting vaginal suppositories (to be inserted high into the vagina when in a dorsal recumbent position) and remaining on the back for 30 minutes to allow suppository absorption. Sexual partner(s) should be encouraged to have examination and treatment. Good handwashing techniques should be taught to avoid reinfection or the transfer of the fungi. The nurse encourages pregnant women to accept treatment to prevent infection of the newborn at the time of delivery.

Prognosis. The condition of candidiasis is curable with the use of the prescribed treatment.

Chlamydia

Etiology/Pathophysiology. ***Chlamydia trachomatis,*** a gram-negative, intracellular bacterium, causes several commonly sexually transmitted diseases. Cervicitis and urethritis are most common, but like the gonococcus, *Chlamydia* organisms also cause epididymitis in men and salpingitis in women. Chlamydial infections may be the most commonly occurring sexually transmitted disease in the United States. Chlamydial infections are responsible for about 20% to 30% of diagnosed pelvic inflammatory disease cases. It is estimated that about 11,000 women each year become involuntarily sterilized and 36,000 suffer ectopic pregnancies as a result of this organism. Chlamydia is highest in young, promiscuous, indigent, unmarried women who live in the inner city and in those who have a prior history of an STD. Because it is not a reportable disease, the actual number of cases is unknown. It is estimated that each year 3 to 4 million Americans suffer from epidemic chlamydial infections.

Although both men and women may have asymptomatic infection, women are more likely to be asymptomatic carriers despite deep pelvic infections, such as infection of the fallopian tubes and pelvic inflammatory disease (PID).

Clinical Manifestations. In men signs and symptoms may include a scanty white or clear exudate, burning or pruritus around the urethral meatus, urinary frequency, and mild dysuria. Signs and symptoms of cervicitis in women may include one or more of the following: vaginal pruritus or burning, dull pelvic pain, low-grade fever, vaginal discharge, and irregular bleeding.

Diagnostic Tests. A recently developed test, the fluorescein-labeled monoclonal antibody test, provides a ready basis for diagnosis. Treatment can be initiated promptly based on a confirmed diagnosis.

Medical Management. The drug of choice for treatment of chlamydial infection is tetracycline. Pregnant patients or patients who are allergic to tetracycline can be treated with erythromycin. Penicillin, the drug of choice to treat gonorrhea, may temporarily suppress the multiplication of chlamydia, but usually does not provide a cure.

Nursing Interventions. Patients' physical symptoms are commonly complicated by their emotional responses to STDs. Complaints of depression, anger, fear, and guilt are common and need to be addressed if education and treatment are to be effective. Outcome is also influenced by educational and income level, primary language, health insurance coverage, and support network. The focus of patient education is on prevention (Box 33-15).

Prognosis. With treatment chlamydial infection is curable. Reinfection occurs if sexual partners are not treated simultaneously. It is estimated that each year 11,000 women with untreated chlamydial infections become involuntarily sterilized. Chlamydial infections can be transmitted to infants during delivery, causing conjunctivitis and pneumonia.

Box 33-15 PREVENTION OF SEXUALLY TRANSMITTED DISEASES

- Individuals should reduce the number of partners they have sex with—preferably to one person.
- Avoid contact with individuals known to be infected or who are at high risk of infection.
- Avoid contact with the genital area if signs and symptoms develop.
- Hands and the genital-rectal area should be washed before and immediately after having intercourse.
- Special attention must be given to washing the foreskin.
- A mouthwash or gargle with hydrogen peroxide (1 part to 3 parts of water) or Listerine antiseptic may slightly reduce the risk of oropharyngeal STD infection.
- Use barrier (condom) contraceptives with new partners.
- Use a water-based lubricant.
- Void after intercourse.
- Avoid excess douching.
- If an STD infection is suspected, seek medical help immediately.
- Individuals with multiple sex partners should seek an STD examination twice a year or more if needed.

Acquired Immunodeficiency Syndrome

Acquired immunodeficiency syndrome (AIDS) is the ultimately fatal, advanced stage of a chronic retroviral infection that gradually destroys the cell-mediated immune system. For a more detailed discussion on this STD, see Chapter 37.

FAMILY PLANNING

Methods of Contraception

Advances in drug therapy and family planning technology have made available a range of options for individuals wishing to prevent or plan conception. Birth control planning involves moral, religious, cultural, and personal values, and the nurse should be sensitive to these factors when discussing birth control with patients.

There are several types of birth control procedures or devices that can be employed. The selection of the particular method should be based on the health of the individual, effectiveness of the method, cost, ease of use, and age and parity (total number of pregnancies) of the patient. Willingness of the patient to comply with use and preference of the couple are two additional factors taken into consideration when selecting a method of contraception. The nurse can help by reinforcing information given by the physician and encouraging patients to seek more information, directing them to the source.

Contraceptive methods and products can be categorized as surgical, hormonal, barrier, and behavioral. Surgical and hormonal methods will be addressed here.

Surgical Methods. Sterilization is a permanent, effective method of birth control that can be performed for men or women. Many states have laws regulating this method of birth control; in some states the husband and wife must both sign a release for the operative procedure. Persons who have not had children are often advised against sterilization.

Vasectomy is the operation performed on a man to terminate the passage of sperm through the vas deferens (Fig. 33-21). There are several ways to perform this procedure, and it can generally be done in the physician's office, in same-day surgery centers, or in ambulatory surgical units.

Although the procedure is intended to be permanent, the patient may wish to reverse the procedure because of remarriage or death of a child. This procedure is known as *vasovasotomy.* Research is being considered to develop a device that permits a reversible vasectomy.

Sperm counts will be required for 6 weeks or until semen is tested free of sperm. The nurse should advise the patient that until the semen tests free of sperm, the ability to impregnate exists.

Tubal ligation (Fig. 33-22) is the surgical sterilization approach for women. There are various approaches used to accomplish this procedure, some of which are ligation, clips, bands or rings, and coagulation. This intervention can be performed through the abdomen or through the vagina. Regardless of method, only a short hospitalization is required. After surgery, ova will not pass through the fallopian tubes. The menstrual cycle, however, will remain normal because the ovaries continue to produce estrogen. Reconstruction of the tubes is possible, with a 50% success rate. A tubal ligation may be performed at the same time other abdominal surgeries are done. The abdominal approach to the tubal ligation is often called *Band-Aid surgery* because a very small incision requiring only a Band-Aid is necessary.

The nurse should advise the patient that she will be allowed up after recovery from anesthesia. She may even be discharged the same day. Postoperative discomfort is minor. There may be abdominal cramping and perhaps a transitory headache. The patient should avoid strenuous exercises and lifting. If there is a vaginal discharge or if spotting appears, the patient should wear a perineal pad.

Hysterectomy (removal of the uterus) and oophorectomy (removal of the ovaries) are other surgical procedures that will cause the woman to be sterile. These were discussed on p. 1015.

Hormonal Contraceptives. Oral contraceptives (birth control pills) are hormonal contraceptives taken orally. Birth control pills are a popular and easy form of contraception that is close to 100% effective. The pill, which is taken by the woman, inhibits release of follicle stimulating hormone (FSH), and subsequently the menstrual cycles are anovulatory (the ovaries do not release ova).

Birth control pills have the advantage of being easy to take, not requiring use of a contraceptive device before intercourse, and being highly effective. They are prescribed by the physician, and the woman should have a yearly physical examination while taking birth control pills. The woman must remember to take the pill daily. If she forgets to take one, she is usually advised to take two the next day. If she misses more than two pills she should stop taking the pills for that cycle, wait 7 days, and then restart the regimen. It is advisable to use another form of contraception for that cycle. The pills should be stored carefully. The pills are affected by high humidity and should be kept in a dry place; extreme heat should be avoided because heat can decrease the potency of the pills.

Some women experience various side effects when using the pills, particularly during the first few months. The signs and symptoms are usually similar to those during the first trimester of pregnancy: nausea, vomiting, weight gain, and breast swelling. The nurse advises pa-

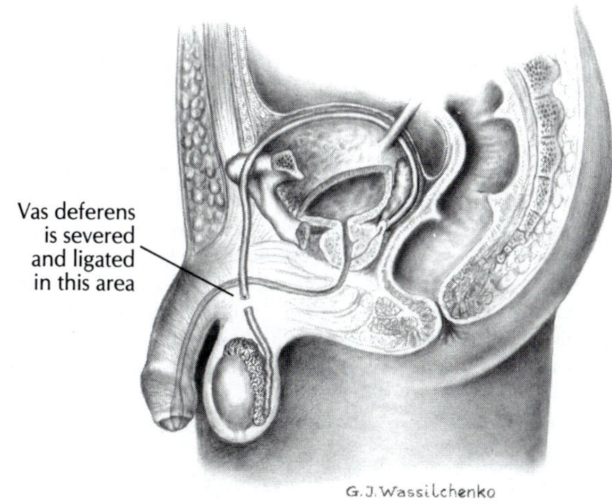

FIG. 33-21 Vasectomy. Sperm duct severed (and ligated).

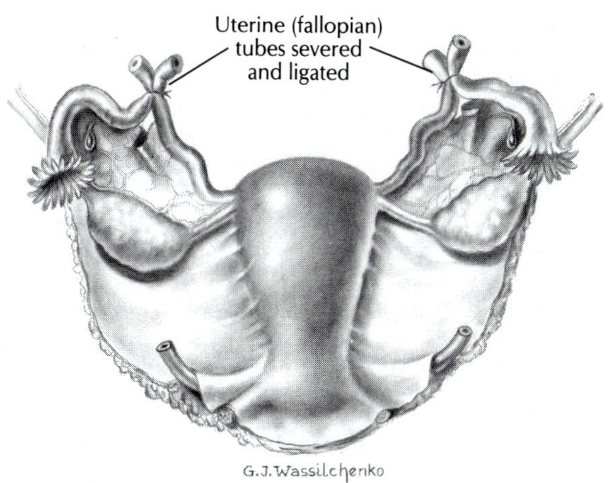

FIG. 33-22 Tubal ligation. Oviduct ligated and severed.

tients to take the pills after a meal to lessen the nausea. It will be helpful to take the pills at the same time each day. Women taking birth control pills are more susceptible to vaginal infections.

Oral contraceptives have been demonstrated to have a relationship to certain cardiovascular disorders; consequently women with hypertension, thromboembolic diseases, or a history of circulatory disease, varicosities, or diabetes mellitus should be discouraged from using birth control pills. Smoking increases the risk of cardiovascular and cerebrovascular complications in women taking birth control pills.

Other side effects are often related to birth control use. As research findings are published, more information is available to use in considering birth control pills as a method for contraception. The nurse is in a position to assist the patient to interpret the information for her individual needs.

Some research has been conducted in the use of male contraceptives. Under investigation in the United States and elsewhere are antispermatogenic agents that create temporary infertility by interfering either with spermatogenesis or with the sperm's ability to fertilize ova. These agents can be given by injection or taken orally.

REFERENCES AND SUGGESTED READINGS

1. Anagnostakos NP, Tortora GJ: *Principles of anatomy and physiology,* ed 5, New York, 1987, Harper & Row.
2. Beare PG, Myers JD: *Principles and practice of adult health nursing,* St Louis, 1992, Mosby.
3. Belcher AE: *Cancer nursing,* St Louis, 1992, Mosby.
4. Centers for Disease Control, staff and outside experts: Pelvic inflammatory disease: guidelines for prevention and management, MMWR 40(RR-5):1, 1991.
5. Davies K: Genital herpes: an overview, *J Obstet Gynecol Neonatal Nurs* 19(5):401, 1990.
6. Debuona BA et al: Sexual behavior of college women in 1975, 1986 and 1989, *N Engl J Med* 322(12):321, 1990.
7. Deitch KV, Smith JE: Symptoms of chronic vaginal infection and microoscopic condyloma in women, *J Obstet Gynecol Neonatal Nurs* 19(2):133, 1990.
8. Dulaney PE et al: A comprehensive education and support program for women experiencing hysterectomies, *J Obstet Gynecol Neonatal Nurs* 19(4):319, 1990.
9. Dupont WD, Page DL: Menopausal estrogen replacement therapy and breast cancer, *Arch Intern Med* 151(1):67, 1991.
10. Fong E, Ferris EB, Skelly EG: *Body structures and functions,* ed 7, New York, 1989, Delmar.
11. Gurevich I: Counseling the patient with herpes, *RN* 53(2):22, 1990.
12. Hegner BR, Caldwell E: *Geriatrics: a study of maturity,* ed 5, New York, 1991, Delmar.
13. Hood GH, Dincher JR: *Total patient care,* ed 8, St Louis, 1992, Mosby.
14. Jossens MOR, Sweet RL: Pelvic inflammatory disease: risk factors and microbial etiologies, *J Obstet Gynecol Neonatal Nurs* 22(2): 169, 1993.
15. Keller ML, Jadack RA, Mims LF: Perceived stressors and coping response in persons with recurrent genital herpes, *Res Nurs Health* 14:421, 1991.
16. Keresztes PA, Dan AJ: Estrogen and cardiovascular disease, *Cardiovas Nurs* 28(1):1, 1992.
17. Lauver D et al: Spontaneous causal searching and adjustment to abnormal Papanicolaou test results, *Nurs Res* 39(5):305, 1990.
18. Lethbridge DJ: Choosing and using contraception: towards a theory of women's contraception self-care, *Nurs Res* 40(5):276, 1991.
19. Lindow KB: Premenstrual syndrome: family impact and nursing implications, *J Obstet Gynecol Neonatal Nurs* 20(2):135, 1991.
20. Long BC, Phipps WJ, Cassmeyer VL: *Medical-surgical nursing: a nursing process approach,* ed 3, St Louis, 1993, Mosby.
21. Love SM: Fibrocystic diseases, *Patient Care* 24(7):65, 1990.
22. Malasanos L et al: *Health assessment,* ed 4, St Louis, 1990, Mosby.
23. Marchbanks PA, Lee C, Peterson B: Cigarette smoking as a risk factor for pelvic inflammatory disease, *Am J Obsetet Gynecol* 162(3):639, 1990.
24. Marieb EN: *Human anatomy & physiology,* Reading, Mass, 1989, Benjamin/Cummings.
25. Martin FL: When the solution is a prosthesis, *RN* 53(3):32, 1990.
26. Memmler RL, Cohen BJ, Wood DL: *Structure and function of the human body,* ed 5, Philadelphia, 1992, Lippincott.
27. Moorhouse MF, Doenges ME: *Nursing diagnosis, care planning, and documentation,* Philadelphia, 1990, FA Davis.
28. Murata, JM: Abnormal genital bleeding and secondary amenorrhea: common gynecologic problems, *J Obstet Gynecol Neonatal Nurs* 19(1):26, 1990.
29. Ornitz AW, Brown MA: Family coping and premestrual symptomatology, *J Obstet Gynecol Neonatal Nurs* 22(1):49, 1993.
30. Peterson HB et al: Pelvic inflammatory disease: key treatment issues and options, *JAMA* 266(18):2505, 1991.
31. Phipps WJ, Long BC, Woods NF: *Medical-surgical nursing: concepts and clinical practice,* ed 4, St Louis, 1991, Mosby.
32. Potter PA, Perry AG: *Fundamentals of nursing: concepts, process, and practice,* ed 3, St Louis, 1993, Mosby.
33. Reznichek CG, Reznichek R: The problem most women won't talk about: impotence, *RN* 54(2):28, 1990.
34. Ricket B: Estrogen replacement: making informed choices, *RN* 55(9):26-32, 1992.
35. Seidel HM et al: *Mosby's guide to physical examination,* ed 2, St Louis, 1991, Mosby.
36. Sexually transmitted diseases in the 1990's (editorial), *N Engl J Med* 325(19):1368, 1991.
37. Solomon EP: *Introduction to human anatomy and physiology,* Philadelphia, 1992, Saunders.
38. Stampfer MJ et al: Postmenopausal estrogen therapy and cardiovascular disease, *N Engl J Med* 325:756, 1991.
39. Thibodeau GA: *Structure and function of the body,* ed 9, St Louis, 1992, Mosby.
40. Thompson J et al: *Mosby's clinical nursing,* ed 3, St Louis, 1993, Mosby.
41. Those other STDs (editorial), *Am J Public Health* 81(10):1250, 1991.
42. Timby BK, Lewis LW: *Fundamental skills and concepts in patient care,* ed 5, Philadelphia, 1992, Lippincott.
43. Tinkle MB: Genital human papillomavirus infection: a growing health risk, *J Obstet Gynecol Neonatal Nurs* 19(6):501, 1990.
44. Touchstone D, Daves D: Consider chlamydia, *RN* 55(9):32, 1992.
45. Tucker S et al: *Patient care standards,* ed 5, St Louis, 1992, Mosby.
46. Velduis JD: Management of amenorrhea, *Hosp Pract* 23(11A):40, 1988.
47. Wilbur JE et al: The relationship of energy expenditure to physical and psychologic symptoms in women at midlife, *Nurs Outlook* 40(6):269, 1992.
48. Woods NF: Human sexuality in health and illness, ed 3, St Louis, 1984, Mosby.
49. Worthington JF: Outliving prostate cancer, *Hopkins Medical News* 15(2):20, 1992.

CHAPTER CHALLENGE

KEY POINTS

- All patients are sexual, and their total health is affected by their emotions, behaviors, beliefs, attitudes, and knowledge of sexuality.
- Sperm are produced in the seminiferous tubules and stored in the epididymis.
- Testosterone, the male sex hormone, is responsible for male secondary sex characteristics.
- Seminal fluid is produced in the seminal vesicles, prostate gland, and Cowper's glands.
- In the female, each month an egg matures in the graafian follicle, which is located in the ovary.
- The acini cells in the mammary glands produce milk after the birth of a child.
- The menstrual cycle prepares the uterus and causes ovulation to occur each month.
- Because of the relationship between the menstrual cycle and the body's mechanisms of hormonal secretion, a decrease or increase in the activity of the hormonal glands can disturb menstruation.
- Early diagnosis and prompt management are necessary if reproductive and genital problems of a more serious nature are to be prevented.
- Health teaching for patients with menstrual disturbances includes a knowlege of the physiological process, factors that alter menstruation, personal hygiene, exercise, diet, and pain management.
- Discharge planning is vital to prevent reinfection after pelvic inflammatory disease.
- Pregnancy is encouraged in the patient with endometriosis, because it will slow the progress of the disorder; infertility is a complication as the condiditon continues.
- Postoperative nursing interventions for the patient having a hysterectomy include monitoring vital signs and prevention of urinary retention, intestinal distention, and venous thrombosis.
- It is important to educate women in the necessity of having a yearly Papanicolaou smear examination of the cervix as a method of early detection of cervical cancer.
- It is a nursing responsibility to teach breast and testicular self-examination.
- Several surgical approaches may be selected for the removal of breast carcinoma: lumpectomy, partial mastectomy, simple mastectomy, modified radical mastectomy, and radical mastectomy.
- Discussion of hand and arm care, prevention of muscle contractions, body image acceptance, and fitting for a prosthesis are all areas to be addressed in discharge planning for a patient after a mastectomy.
- Nursing interventions for a patient with prostatitis include the need for compliance with treatment, supportive care such as bed rest and sitz baths, and monitoring intake and output.
- A hydrocele is an accumulation of fluid between the membranes covering the testicle and the membrane enclosing the testicle, whereas a varicocele occurs when the veins within the scrotum become dilated.
- Young men should be taught to perform testicular self-examination beginning at 15 years of age.
- Any sexually active person may be at risk for a sexually transmitted disease.
- The focus of patient education related to sexually transmitted diseases is on prevention.

STUDY QUESTIONS

1. Mrs. McIntosh, a 61-year-old patient, visits her physician because of an increase in her abdominal girth and dyspnea over the past month as a result of pressure on her diaphragm. She is diagnosed as having cancer of the ovaries. These two clinical manifestations result from:
   1. development of ascites
   2. metastasis to the bowel
   3. dilation of the alveoli
   4. bladder distention
2. Elizabeth Manuel is a 30-year-old premenopausal female who is asking the nurse the most appropriate time of the month to do her self-examination of the breasts. The most appropriate reply by the nurse would be:
   1. during her menstruation
   2. 7 to 8 days after conclusion of the menstrual period
   3. the same day of each month
   4. the 26th day of the menstrual cycle
3. Ms. Fernando is a 52-year-old patient who has ductal cell carcinoma of the left breast. She is in the first postoperative day after having had a modified radical mastectomy. A Davol drain is in place in the left axillary region. The main purpose of this drain is to:
   1. control numbness of her left incisional site
   2. improve her ability to perform range-of-motion exercises on her affected side
   3. facilitate drainage and prevent formation of a hematoma

4. prevent postoperative phlebitis in her affected arm

4. David Cosogoma is a 35-year-old patient who has received a vasectomy. Teaching for this patient should include the following information:
   1. the procedure is reversible if he later changes his mind
   2. he should abstain from sexual intercourse until the incision is completely healed
   3. he should apply warm compresses to the scrotum 4 times a day
   4. he should return to the physician at regular intervals for sperm counts

5. Mrs. Brodbeck is a 44-year-old patient who is admitted for an abdominal hysterectomy. She is instructed that she will have a Foley catheter in place postoperatively. She asks the nurse how many days she will have the catheter in place. The best response by the nurse would be that:
   1. the indwelling catheter will probably remain in place for 1 week
   2. the indwelling catheter will be removed after you are fully awake from the anesthesia
   3. the indewlling catheter will generally remain in place 1 to 2 days after surgery
   4. the indwelling catheter will remain in place for a few days postdischarge

6 Mrs. Pinkerton is a 60-year-old patient who has had a vaginal hysterectomy for a prolapsed uterus. The nurse is very aware that patients undergoing pelvic surgery are more susceptible to certain postoperative complications, and thus adjusts postoperative interventions to prevent:
   1. wound dehiscence
   2. wound infection
   3. atelectasis and hypostatic pneumonia
   4. venous stasis and thrombophlebitis

7. Mrs. Ludeman, 49 years of age, is an obese diabetic who has had a total abdominal hysterectomy. On the third postoperative day, Mrs. Ludeman complains of increased pain in the operative site. She states, "It feels like something suddenly popped." With the symptoms presented, it would be likely that when the nurse removes the abdominal dressing she may note that:
   1. the wound has purulent exudate
   2. dehiscence has occurred
   3. the wound is indurated and tender to touch
   4. the wound is well approximated

8. Miss Barr is a 20-year-old patient who goes to the physician's office with vaginal pruritus, burning, dull pelvic pain, and purulent vaginal discharge. A diagnostic test reveals she has chlamydia. The nurse goes over the medication schedule carefully with Miss Barr. Another very important nursing intervention to achieve satisfactory patient outcome would be to:
   1. encourage her to have her sexual partner(s) seek medical care as soon as possible to avoid reinfection of the patient
   2. recommend she abstain from sexual contact while lesions are present
   3. provide social and emotional support because the edematous, draining lymph nodes may be disturbing to Miss Barr's self-image
   4. educate Miss Barr that the causative organism is a spirochete that gains entrance into the body during intercourse

9. Mrs. McKellips is a 40-year-old patient with a right modified radical mastectomy with wide resection of the axillary lymph nodes. Which of the following is contraindicated in the postoperative care for Mrs. McKellips:
   1. encouraging turning, coughing, and deep breathing
   2. taking the blood pressure in her right arm
   3. drawing a circle around the drainage on the pressure dressing
   4. administering meperidine IM every 4 hours as needed

10. John Piper is a 23-year-old who is diagnosed with gonorrhea. Because of statements made in his patient interview, the nurse has established a nursing diagnosis of noncompliance. Which is the most effective way to overcome noncompliance for this patient:
   1. telephone follow-up
   2. case finding
   3. single-dose treatment of Rocephin IM
   4. extensive patient education program

11. The nurse is teaching a group of teenagers about contraception and sexually transmitted diseases. The nurse asks the students if they know which is the most prevalent of the sexually transmitted diseases. In a discussion they are surprised to learn it is:
   1. syphilis
   2. chlamydial infections
   3. gonorrhea
   4. herpes genitalis

12. Ms. Tysdal is a 73-year-old patient who comes to the physician's office with the complaint of constant seepage of feces from her vagina, causing her embarrassment due to soilage and odor. She is presenting signs of:
   1. rectovaginal fistula
   2. vesicovaginal fistula
   3. urethrovaginal fistula
   4. rectocele

34

CARE OF THE PATIENT WITH AN EYE OR EAR DISORDER

Patricia Helmer Oles
Karen H. Richardson

KEY TERMS

ANATOMY AND PHYSIOLOGY

accommodation
aqueous humor
canal of Schlemm
cerumen
choroid
cochlea
conjunctiva
cornea
crystalline lens
eustachian tube
incus
iris
malleus
pinna
proprioceptors
pupil
refraction
retina
sclera
semicircular canals
stapes
tympanic membrane
vitreous humor

MEDICAL-SURGICAL

astigmatism
audiometry
cataract
conjunctivitis
cryosurgery
diabetic retinopathy
enucleation
exophthalmos
glaucoma
hyperopia
keratoplasty
labyrinthitis
mastoiditis
mydriatic
myopia
myringotomy
radial keratotomy
retinal detachment
Snellen test
stapedectomy
strabismus
tinnitus
tympanoplasty
vertigo

LEARNING OBJECTIVES

Anatomy and Physiology

After reading this chapter, the student should be able to do the following:

- Define the key terms.
- List the major sense organs, and discuss their anatomical position.
- List the parts of the eye, and define the function of each part.
- Compare and contrast the function of the rods and cones.
- List the three divisions of the ear, and discuss the function of each.

Medical-Surgical

- Define the key terms.
- Discuss the effects of noise pollution on the internal structures of the ear.
- Describe two changes in the sensory system that occur as a result of the normal aging process.
- Identify factors influencing assessment of the eye and ear.
- Describe the techniques used in assessment of the eye and ear.
- Identify the purposes and procedures of diagnostic tests of the eye and ear.
- Describe major eye inflammations and appropriate nursing interventions.
- Compare the nature of cataracts, glaucoma, and retinal detachment and appropriate nursing interventions for each.
- Identify the nursing interventions associated with medical-surgical treatments of the eye and ear.
- Differentiate between conductive and sensorineural hearing loss.
- List communication tips for hearing- and sight-impaired persons.
- Give patient instructions regarding care of the eye and ear in accordance with written protocol.
- Describe appropriate nursing interventions for the patient having ear surgery.

RELATED TOPICS OF INTEREST

- Diet therapy (Chapter 19)
- Principles and practice of medication administration (Chapter 21)
- The surgical patient (Chapter 22)
- Care of the older adult (Chapter 45)

The sensory system constantly gathers information through millions of receptors scattered throughout the body and delivers it to the brain for interpretation. This process allows humans to survive safely by allowing appropriate responses to external stimuli. The five major senses are taste, touch, smell, sight, and hearing. The sense of balance (equilibrium) is linked with hearing, because the sensors are located within the ear.

ANATOMY OF THE EYE

The eye is a marvelous spherical structure, only 1 inch (2.5 cm) in diameter. The eye contains 70% of the sensory structures of the body. The optic tracts contain more than 1 million nerve fibers that carry messages from the eye to the brain, where they are interpreted. Only a small portion of the eye is visible externally; the remainder is enclosed in the skeletal bones of the face and cushioned by layers of fat. The skeletal bones surrounding the eyeball include the frontal, zygomatic, sphenoid, ethmoid, and lacrimal bones.

Accessory Structures of the Eye

The accessory structures of the eye—the eyebrows, eyelids, eyelashes, and lacrimal apparatus—function mainly as protective devices. In addition, six extrinsic eye muscles control gross eye movement and allow the eyes to focus on any object in the visual field. These six muscles are the superior, inferior, medial, and external rectus muscles and the superior and inferior oblique muscles. Superior to the eyes are the eyebrows, which are composed of coarse hair; they protect the eyes from perspiration and foreign objects and shade the eyes from direct rays of the sun.

The upper and lower eyelids protect the anterior portion of the eye. As a reflex in response to danger, they close automatically. They close with sleep to keep the eye moist. Blinking spreads lubricating secretions over the eye when an individual is awake. Lashes protrude from both the upper and lower lids to shade the eye and prevent debris from entering it.

The structures of the lacrimal apparatus (Fig. 34-1) manufacture and drain tears to keep the eyeball moist and sweep away debris that might enter the eye.

Tears are composed of a watery secretion that contains salts, mucus, and a bactericidal enzyme called *lysozyme.* The lacrimal glands are located superior and lateral to each eye. Blinking causes tears to flow medially to the lacrimal ducts, which empty into the lacrimal sacs. The lacrimal sacs in turn empty into the nasolacrimal ducts and drain into the nasal cavity.

The six extrinsic eye muscles are controlled by the third or oculomotor, fourth or trochlear, and sixth or abducent cranial nerves. They are attached to the sclera or white part of the eye. The eyes are able to move laterally, medially, superiorly, and inferiorly. Occasionally, children develop a condition commonly called *lazy eye,* which involves a weak or elongated eye muscle and is characterized by visual disturbances. It is corrected with eye exercises or surgical shortening of the muscle.

The **conjunctiva** (Fig. 34-2) is a thin mucous membrane that lines the inner aspect of the eyelids and the anterior surface of the eyeball to the edges of the cornea. Sometimes the blood vessels of the conjunctiva become dilated because of irritation or congestion, and the individual is said to have "bloodshot" eyes.

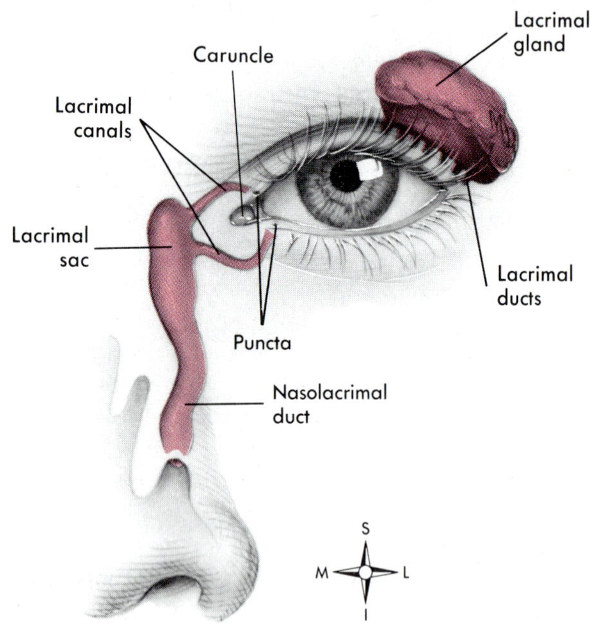

FIG. 34-1 Lacrimal apparatus.

Structure of the Eyeball

The eyeball (Fig. 34-2) is composed of three layers or tunics. The outermost layer is the fibrous tunic, composed of thick, white, opaque connective tissue called the **sclera** or white of the eye. The sclera covers the posterior five sixths of the eyeball. The sclera gives shape to the eyeball and because of its toughness protects the inner eye structures. Posteriorly, it is pierced by the optic nerve and, with the transparent cornea, makes up the outermost of three tunics covering the eyebulb. The central anterior portion of the sclera, the **cornea,** is transparent and covers the colored portion of the eye, the iris. The cornea is the eye's window to the world, allowing light rays to enter the inner portion of the eye. The cornea is dense, uniform in thickness, and nonvascular, and it projects like a dome beyond the sclera. The degree of corneal curvature varies in different individuals and in the same person at different ages. The curvature is more pronounced in youth than in advanced age. Located at the border or junction of the sclera and cornea

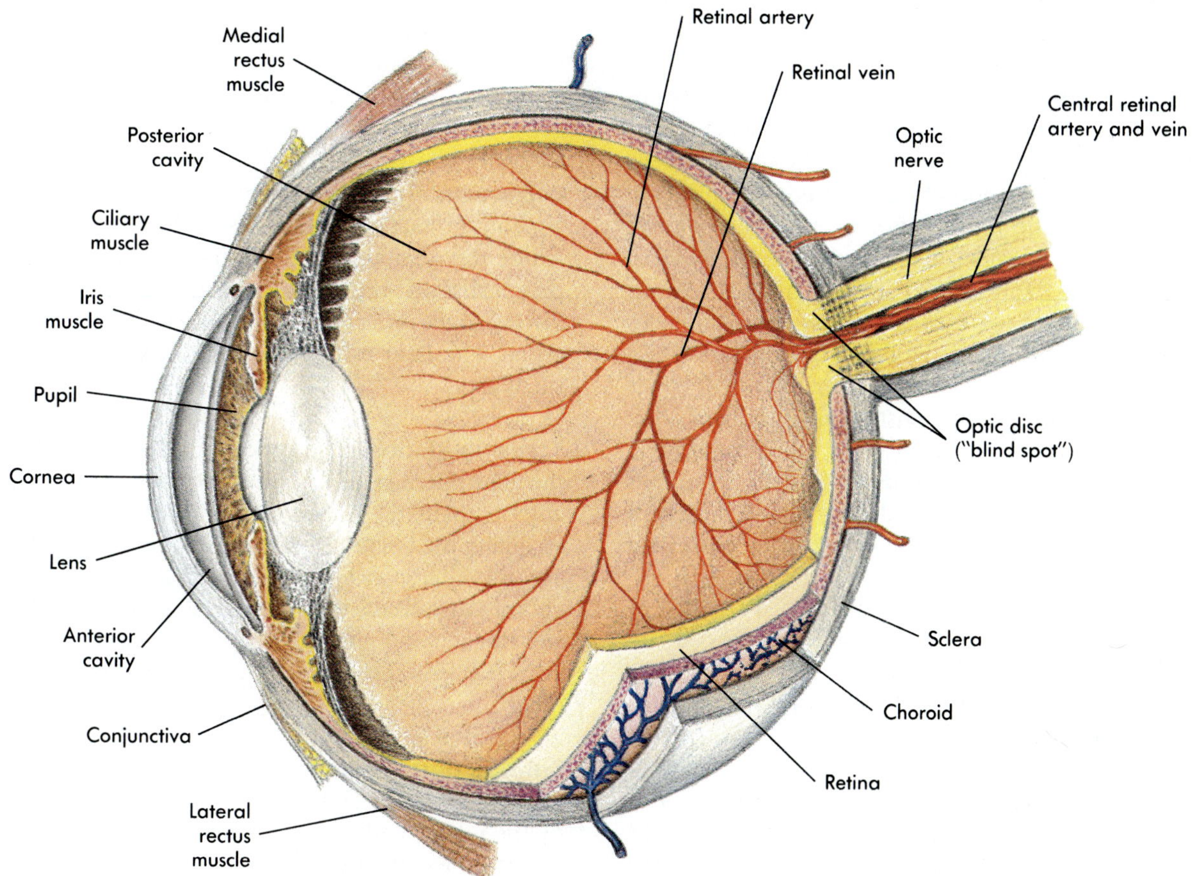

FIG. 34-2 Horizontal section through the left eyeball. The eye is viewed from above.

is a special structure called the **canal of Schlemm.** It is a tiny venous sinus at the angle of the anterior chamber of the eye, which drains the aqueous humor and funnels it into the bloodstream. This aids in controlling intraocular pressure (the pressure within the eyeball).

The middle layer is the vascular tunic. It contains the choroid, the ciliary body, and the iris. The posterior portion of the middle layer is called the **choroid,** which is a thin, dark brown membrane that lines most of the internal area of the sclera. It is highly vascular and supplies nutrients to the retina. The choroid contains a large amount of pigment, which absorbs light rays and prevents them from reflecting outside the eye. The anterior portion of the vascular tunic forms the ciliary body, which is an intrinsic muscular ring that holds the lens in place and changes the shape of the lens for near or far vision. The ciliary body also attaches to the **iris,** a pigmented intrinsic muscular ring that resembles a doughnut. A circular opening in the iris of the eye, located slightly to the nasal side of the center of the iris, is the **pupil.** The color of the iris varies from shades of blue to brown; this is determined by the amount of pigment the iris contains and is an inherited characteristic. The iris lies between the cornea and the lens and regulates the amount of light entering the eye, much like a camera lens. The periphery of the iris is continuous with the ciliary body and is connected to the cornea by the pectinate ligament. The iris divides the space between the lens and the cornea into an anterior and posterior chamber. Two sets of smooth muscles control the iris, which in turn affects the pupil. In bright light the circular muscle fibers of the iris contract and the pupil contracts; in dim light the radial muscle fibers of the iris contract and the pupil dilates.

The innermost tunic of the eye is the **retina,** a 10-layered, delicate, nervous tissue membrane of the eye, continuous with the optic nerve, that receives images of external objects and transmits impulses through the optic nerve to the brain and lies only in the posterior portion of the eyeball. Located within the retina are specialized sensory cells called *rods* and *cones* (photoreceptors). They are responsible for the conversion of light to nerve impulses, which are transported through the optic nerve to the brain, where, in the visual area of the cerebral cortex located in the occipital lobe, they register as visual sensations. Dim light can stimulate the rods, but fairly bright light is necessary to stimulate the cones. Rods are the receptors for night vision and cones for daytime vision. Rods are also responsible for peripheral vision. There are three kinds of cones; each is sensitive to a different color: red, green, or blue. Scattered throughout the central portion of the retina, these three types of cones allow distinction of different colors. Cones are concentrated in the *fovea centralis,* the area of most acute vision. This is a small, depressed area in the posterior portion of the retina. Color pigments that are sensitive to light allow the rods and cones to function. Vitamin A is responsible for the production of these pigments. The absence of any of these three types of cones causes color blindness. The most common type of color blindness is red-green blindness. Color blindness is an inherited condition occurring primarily in males. The rods and cones are scattered throughout the retina, except where the optic nerve exits the eye. This area is called the *optic disc* or *blind spot.*

Chambers of the Eye

The eye is divided into two chambers by the **crystalline lens,** a transparent, colorless structure in the eye, biconvex in shape, enclosed in a capsule, and held in place just behind the pupil by the suspensory ligament. The function of the crystalline lens is to focus light rays so that they form a perfect image on the retina. Anterior to the crystalline lens is the anterior chamber. It is filled with a clear, watery fluid **(aqueous humor)** similar to blood plasma. It is continually secreted by the ciliary bodies of the choroid. To maintain normal intraocular pressure this fluid is reabsorbed into the venous system at the iridocorneal angle by means of the sinus venosus (called the canal of Schlemm). Aqueous humor is constantly being formed, drained, and replaced in the anterior cavity. Aqueous humor helps maintain the shape of the eyeball, keeps the retina attached to the choroid, and refracts light.

The posterior chamber is filled with **vitreous humor,** a transparent, jellylike substance filling the cavity behind the crystalline lens of the eye. Vitreous humor gives shape to the eyeball, keeps the retina attached to the choroid, and also refracts light. It differs from the aqueous humor not only in composition but also in production. It is formed during embryonic development and is not continually replaced.

PHYSIOLOGY OF VISION

Light must travel through the cornea, aqueous humor, pupil, crystalline lens, vitreous humor, and finally to the rods and cones of the retina. The image is transported via the optic nerve to the visual center of the cerebral cortex of the brain.

Image Formation of the Retina

Four basic processes are necessary to form an image: (1) refraction of light rays, (2) accommodation of the lens, (3) constriction of the pupil, and (4) convergence of the eyes.

Refraction. **Refraction** is the bending of light rays. The aqueous humor, crystalline lens, and vitreous humor constitute the refracting media of the eye. Light is bent as it passes through these colorless structures of the eye, allowing light from the environment to focus on the retina. The light from a large area can be focused on a small area.

Accommodation. The process of **accommodation** is the adjustment of the eye for various distances; thus it is able to focus the image of an object on the retina by changing the curvature of the lens. For near vision to occur, the ciliary muscle must contract, which pulls the choroid toward the lens, thus causing the lens to shorten and thicken and giving it a convex appearance. This allows the lens to bend light rays toward the fovea centralis.

Constriction. The amount of light entering the eye is regulated by the pupil; the size of the pupil is controlled by the dilator and constrictor muscles of the iris. To assist with accommodation, constriction of the diameter of the pupil must occur to prevent light from entering the periphery of the lens. If light entered the periphery, it would not focus on the retina and the image would be blurred.

Convergence. Convergence is the movement of both eyes medially to allow light rays from an object to hit the same points on both retinas. The extrinsic eye muscles control this movement. As the object becomes closer, the eyes turn toward the nose; this allows binocular vision (seeing the same object with both of the eyes).

ANATOMY AND PHYSIOLOGY OF THE EAR

The external ear (pinna or auricle) reveals only a portion of the complex organ of hearing. Within the ear lie many structures that allow hearing and interpretation of sound and assist in maintaining equilibrium (balance). Anatomically, when examining the ear from the external structures to the internal structures, one finds three distinct divisions: the external ear, middle ear, and inner ear (Fig. 34-3). The external and middle ears deal exclusively with sound waves, while the inner ear deals with sound waves and equilibrium.

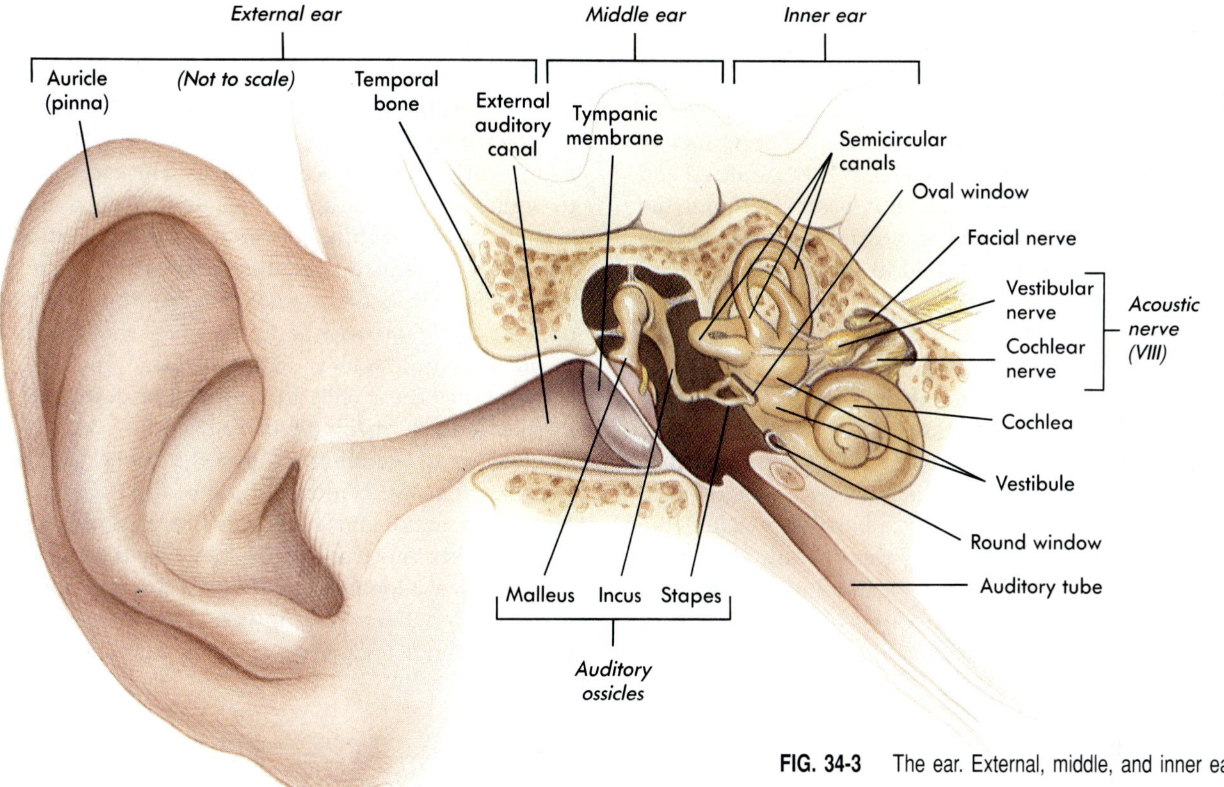

FIG. 34-3 The ear. External, middle, and inner ears.

External Ear

The external ear is composed of the auricle or **pinna** (outer flap of tissue and cartilage), the external auditory canal, and the **tympanic membrane** (eardrum), a thin, semitransparent membrane. The tympanic membrane separates the external and the middle ear and transmits sound vibrations to the internal ear by means of the auditory ossicles. The external ear is designed to collect sound waves and channel them to the middle ear. The upper part of the pinna is composed of elastic cartilage, while the lower part, the lobe, is mainly soft fleshy tissue. The whole structure is attached to the head by ligaments and muscles. The center opens into the external auditory canal.

The external auditory canal, or meatus, is a tube 1 inch (2.5 cm) long that terminates at the tympanic membrane. The walls of the canal are composed of bone lined with cartilage; this cartilage is continuous with the cartilage of the pinna. The epithelium (skin) covering the canal is thin and very sensitive. It contains cilia (tiny hairs) and specialized sebaceous (oil) glands called *ceruminous glands.* They secrete **cerumen** (ear wax), which protects the lining from infection. The cilia, in combination with the cerumen, also prevent foreign objects from entering the ear. Because the canal is composed of epithelium, it is subject to the same irritations and infections as the skin covering the body. Foreign objects must not be inserted into the canal, because the skin is delicate and the tympanic membrane could be ruptured.

Middle Ear

The middle ear, or tympanic cavity, is a small, air-filled chamber located within the temporal bone. The **eustachian** (auditory) **tube** is lined with mucous membrane that joins the nasopharynx and the middle ear cavity. This tube equalizes the air pressure on either side of the tympanic membrane. When one swallows or yawns, the tube allows air to enter the middle ear, which equalizes the middle-ear and external-ear pressure. Because the pharynx, eustachian tube, and middle ear are all covered with a continuous mucous membrane, infection can travel very easily from the throat to the middle ear. This is often seen in young children. The posterior wall of the middle ear opens into the mastoid process, an area filled with air spaces, which also aids in equalization of air pressure. Infection of the middle ear, if untreated, can spread to the mastoid process.

Extending along the middle ear chamber are three small bones (ossicles) that carry sound waves from the external ear to the inner ear. These three small bones are named according to their shape: The **malleus** (hammer), **incus** (anvil), and **stapes** (stirrup). The internal surface of the tympanic membrane is connected to the first of these three bones, the malleus. The malleus transfers sound waves to the incus, which in turn transfers them to the stapes. The stapes pushes against the oval window, a small membrane that marks the beginning of the inner ear. When sound waves cause the tympanic membrane to vibrate, that movement is transmitted and amplified by the ear ossicles as it passes through the middle ear. Movement of the stapes against the oval window causes movements of fluid in the inner ear.

Internal Ear

The most important portion of the ear, the inner ear or labyrinth, is a series of canals. Structurally, it contains the bony labyrinth, which is lined with the membranous labyrinth. The bony labyrinth is filled with a fluid called *perilymph* and contains three subdivisions called the **semicircular canals** (any of three bony, fluid-filled loops in the osseous labyrinth of the internal ear; associated with the sense of balance), vestibule, and cochlea. The membranous labyrinth is a series of sacs and tubes that contain a thicker fluid called *endolymph.* The endolymph and perilymph have different chemical compositions, but they are both fluids and both conduct sound waves through the inner ear system.

The **cochlea** resembles a snail's shell and contains the *organ of Corti,* the organ of hearing. It contains many hearing receptors or hair cells. These cells respond to sound waves by stimulating the cochlear nerve (a branch of the eighth cranial nerve—the vestibulocochlear nerve), which transmits the message to the brain. These hair cells may become damaged from noise pollution (i.e., high-intensity sounds such as those produced by jet engines, factory equipment, and rock and roll bands). Once these cells are damaged or destroyed, hearing becomes permanently damaged.

Deeper in the inner ear, past the cochlea, is the *vestibule* or the oval central portion of the bony labyrinth. The vestibule contains receptors that respond to gravity. They provide information on which way is up and which way is down, allowing an individual to remain in an upright position. Extending upward from the vestibule are three semicircular canals responsible for maintaining bal-

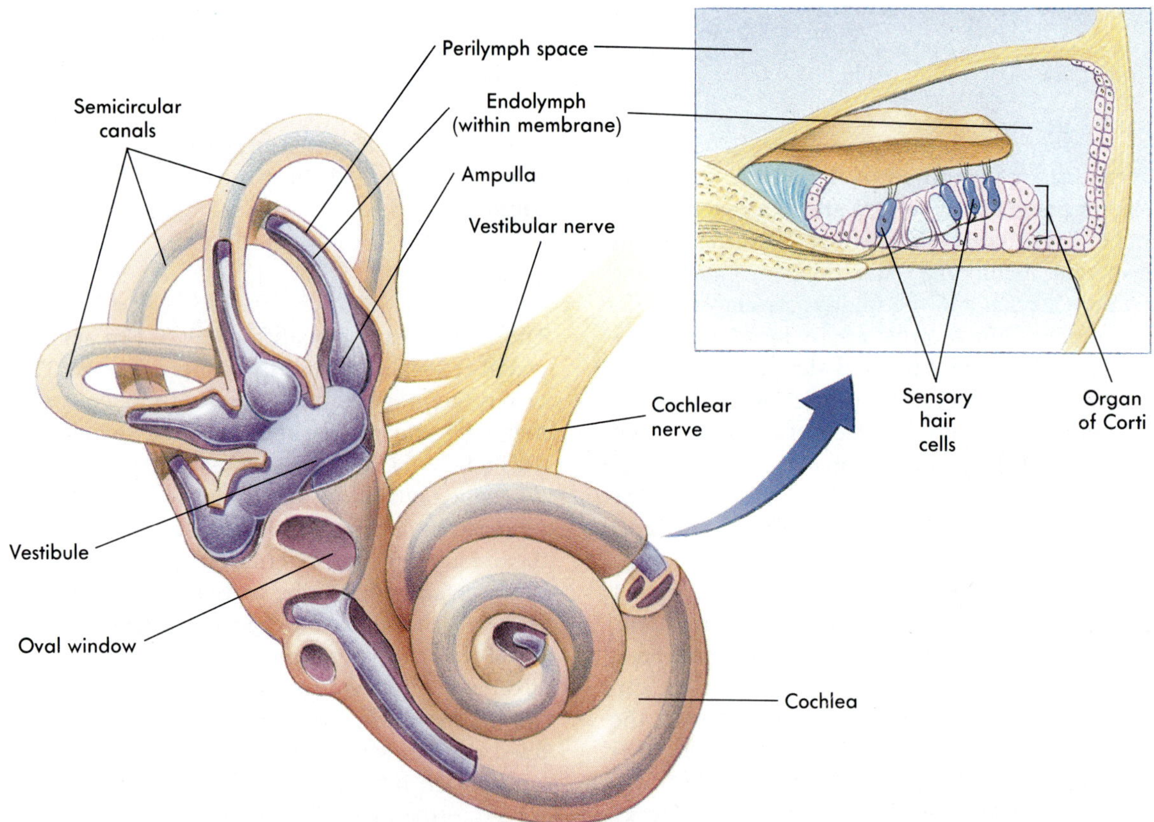

FIG. 34-4 The inner ear. The bony labyrinth (orange) is the hard outer wall of the entire inner ear, and includes semicircular canals, vestibule, and cochlea. Within the bony labyrinth is the membranous labyrinth (purple), which is surrounded by perilymph and filled with endolymph. Each ampulla in the vestibule contains a crista ampullaris that detects changes in head position and sends sensory impulses through the vestibular nerve to the brain. *Inset* shows a section of the membranous cochlea. Hair cells in the organ of Corti detect sound and send the information through the cochlear nerve. The vestibular and cochlear nerves join to form the eighth cranial nerve.

ance and equilibrium. They contain sensory hair cells and endolymph. The motion of the endolymph stimulates the hair cells, which stimulates the receptors; then the message is sent to the brain for interpretation (Fig. 34-4).

OTHER SPECIAL SENSES

Taste and Smell

On the tongue of the average adult there are approximately 10,000 taste buds; some are also located on the inner aspect of the cheeks. Taste buds are the receptors for four basic sensations. They respond only to substances in solution; otherwise, they are not activated. The four taste sensations and the locations of the taste buds that detect them are as follows:

- *Sweet:* located in the tip of the tongue, they respond to sugar and other sweet substances.
- *Sour:* located on the sides of the tongue, they respond to acid content of foods.
- *Salty:* located on the tip of the tongue, they respond to metal ions contained in foods.
- *Bitter:* located on the posterior portion of the tongue, they respond to alkaline or basic ions contained in foods.

The taste receptors send their messages to the taste center of the cerebral cortex of the brain. It is important to note that the sense of taste works very closely with the sense of smell for the identification of various foods. The senses of touch and sight are also involved.

The receptors for the sense of smell (*olfactory receptors*) are located in the roof or upper part of the nasal cavity. The olfactory receptors, embedded in the epithelium, each send cilia into the nasal chamber. On inhalation, an odor comes in contact with the olfactory receptors, and the message is then sent to the brain. Memory for certain odors is long-standing; certain odors stimulate certain memories (e.g., pine scent, Christmas; talcum powder, infants). All persons have special memories that come to mind when certain odors are smelled. The body is not able to regenerate olfactory cells; once they are damaged, the sense of smell is impaired.

Touch

The receptors for touch (*tactile receptors*) are located throughout the integumentary system. They respond to touch, pressure, and vibration. The most abundant receptors are the *Meissner's corpuscles* and *pacinian corpuscles*. Meissner's corpuscles, found in the fingertips, interpret fine touch and vibration. The pacinian corpuscles are located throughout the body but particularly in the joints, mammary glands, and external genitalia of both sexes. They are sensitive to pressure and vibration. Other receptors, free nerve endings, are located throughout the body and interpret painful stimuli and temperature.

Position/Movement

Proprioception (sense of position) maintains the proper position of the body. **Proprioceptors** (any sensory nerve ending, such as those located in muscles, tendons, and joints, that responds to stimuli originating from within the body regarding movement and spatial position) work in conjunction with the semicircular canals and vestibule of the inner ear to maintain proper coordination. They orchestrate the body for running, walking, dancing, and many other activities. Once they receive information from the environment, they send it to the cerebellum for interpretation. Proprioceptors allow one to sense the position of the different parts of the body and be aware of the movement of each.

NORMAL AGING PATTERN OF THE SENSORY SYSTEM

As an individual ages, the crystalline lens of the eye hardens and becomes too large for the eye muscles, thus causing a loss of accommodation, which often requires the need for bifocals or trifocals. The crystalline lens loses some of its transparency and becomes more opaque, and glare begins to become a problem. Concurrently the pupil becomes smaller and decreases the amount of light that reaches the retina, and one needs brighter lighting to read.

The aging ear loses the ability to hear high frequencies and to distinguish consonant sounds, probably as a result of deterioration of the nerve fibers and breakdown of the cells in the organ of Corti.

The remaining senses undergo slight changes that decrease their reaction or threshold time, which results in slower response or diminished sensation. The gerontological box on p. 1048 highlights specific considerations for the older adult.

CARE OF THE PATIENT WITH AN EYE DISORDER

Nursing Considerations

An initial consideration in caring for the patient with an eye disorder would include review of the following items:

Eye pain, pruritus, excessive tearing, floaters, light flashes, discharge, visual changes, or blind spots
History of allergies
Current medication for the eye disorder
Side effects of medications, if any
Use of glasses or contact lenses
Adequacy of current eyewear prescription
Personal habits related to care of eyewear

Once the information has been gathered and communicated, the nurse assists with the eye examination. The results of the initial examination are compared with normal findings (Table 34-1 on p. 1048).

GERONTOLOGICAL CONSIDERATIONS

- Multiple changes in vision that normally occur with aging include:
  - Changes in accommodation, resulting in increased difficulty focusing on close objects (presbyopia), which leads to difficulty reading or doing other close work
  - Decreased color perception and discrimination, particularly with shades of blue, green, and violet
  - Poor adaptation to changes in light, resulting in "night blindness" and increased sensitivity to glare
  - Alterations in depth perception, leading to increased risk of falls
  - Decreased secretion of tears, resulting in complaints of dryness or pruritus, which leads to a high risk for irritation of the cornea
  - Increased incidence of moving particles or "floaters" that interfere with visually based tasks
- Older adults experience an increased incidence of eye disorders, including cataracts, retinal detachment, macular degeneration, and glaucoma.
- A third of all individuals over the age of 70 have significant hearing loss.
- Hearing loss in older adults is most often sensorineural and involves loss of the high frequencies. Hearing loss results in the distortion of speech, which can lead to failure to respond to directions or inappropriate behaviors often misinterpreted as disorientation.
- Hearing loss can lead to social isolation when the older adult is unable to understand and participate in normal conversation.
- A decreased number of receptors in the nasal cavities and papillae of the tongue results in changes in smell and taste. Most affected are the sweet and salty tastes.
- Medications often affect the taste of food and can contribute to altered nutrition.

TABLE 34-1 Normal Findings of the Adult Eye

Area Examined	Findings
Eyelids	Blink reflex to light or touch intact. Lid margins just above corneala borders.
Eyeball	Eyeball does not protrude beyond supraorbital bridge of frontal bone. Eyeball is usually moist; moisture may be diminished in the older adult.
Conjunctivae	*Palpebral* (eyelid): Pink, uniform blood vessels without discharge.
	Bulbar: Clear, tiny red vessels; in the older adult, the bulbar conjunctiva may lose luster.
Sclera	Generally white. May have yellow-tan dots in a dark-skinned individual.
Cornea	Transparent, smooth, convex. In the older adult, a gray ring around cornea (*arcus senilis*) may be present as a result of lipid deposits.
Iris	Round, intact, bilateral coloration. In the older adult, color may be paler and shape less regular.
Pupil	Equal, round, reactive to light and accommodation. Response to light is equal bilaterally. In the older adult constriction response may be slower.
Internal eye (including retina, vessels, and optic disc)	Retina is intact.
	Vessel structure is intact and bilaterally similar in pattern. Optic disc has well-defined border.
Visual acuity	
Distant vision	20/20 (able to read line 20 of eye chart at a distance of 20 feet).
Near vision	Able to read newspaper print at 14 inches.
Peripheral vision	Side vision is 90 degrees from central visual axis. Upward 50 degrees; downward 70 degrees.
Eye movement	Coordinated eye movement bilaterally.
Color perception	Able to properly identify eye colors of major groups: red, blue, and green.

Diagnostic Testing

Once the initial eye examination is completed, the patient may require additional diagnostic testing. The major diagnostic eye tests, including the **Snellen test,** are explained in Table 34-2.

Additional eye tests may be required to assist in the diagnosis. The Amsler grid is used to detect a defect of the macular area of the retina. The tangent screen evaluates central and peripheral fields of vision. The Goldmann perimetry test detects and evaluates the progression of glaucoma (an abnormal condition of elevated pressure within the eye because of obstruction of the

TABLE 34-2 Major Diagnostic Eye Tests

Purpose	Equipment	Procedure	Patient Teaching
Snellen test*			
Assessment of visual acuity; used as screening test	Snellen chart; eye patch/cover	1. Patient stands or sits 20 ft from chart. 2. Covers one eye. 3. Asked to read above or below the 20/20 line. 4. Repeats step 3 using the other eye. 5. Findings are documented.	1. Explain test. 2. If findings are abnormal (i.e., other than 20 ft required to read the chart line), encourage patient to seek further eye testing.
Color vision			
Prerequisite for driver's license	Color chart or machine	1. Color dots are reflected on a background of mixed colors. 2. Patient identifies color patterns on the test field. 3. Finding are documented.	1. Explain procedure. 2. Encourage patient to seek further testing when results indicate inaccurate recognition of color patterns.
Refraction			
Measurement of visual acuity to determine refractory errors such as: *myopia* (nearsightedness), *hyperopia* (farsightedness), *presbyopia* (inability to focus on close objects), and *astigmatism* (blurred vision)	Retinoscope or sample lenses	1. Ophthalmologist/optometrist asks patient to indicate clear/blurred vision with each lens change in the retinoscope.	1. Explain procedure. 2. Examiner discusses results with patient and encourages appropriate corrective measures.
Ophthalmoscopy			
Evaluation of underlying structures of the eye; routine screening	Ophthalmoscope; **mydriatic** (causing pupillary dilatation) drops to dilate the pupil	1. Mydriatic drops applied. Mydriatic drops are contraindicated in patients with narrow-angle glaucoma. 2. As pupil dilation occurs, the room is darkened. 3. Patient is instructed to remain still and focus on a stationary object. 4. Examiner uses ophthalmoscope to view internal eye structure. 5. Findings are documented.	1. Explain procedure. 2. Instruct patient that effects of the drops will last no longer than 1 hr. 3. Sunglasses are required when outside or in brightly lit room until pupils return to normal size. 4. Examiner discusses results with patient and encourages corrective measures.
Tonometry (see Fig. 34-9)			
Measurement of intraocular pressure to detect tumors and glaucoma	Tonometer Topical anesthetic may be used	1. Examiner places tonometer on cornea. 2. Pressure readings are obtained. 3. Findings are documented.	1. Explain procedure. 2. Encourage patient to relax to avoid false high readings. 3. Eyes are not to be rubbed for approximately 30 min to avoid corneal irritation. 4. Contact lenses may be reinserted 2 hr after completion of test.

*Eye chart test for visual acuity: letters, numbers, or symbols are arranged on the chart in decreasing size from top to bottom.

outflow of aqueous humor), which affects peripheral vision. Exophthalmometry measures the degree of forward placement of the eye, known as **exophthalmos** (an abnormal condition characterized by a marked protrusion of the eyeballs). Slit-lamp examination is done to examine the conjunctiva, lens, vitreous humor, iris, and cornea. The Schirmer test evaluates the function of the major lacrimal glands. Fluorescein angiography is used to examine the microvascular structures of the eye and assess patency of the lacrimal system.

DISORDERS OF THE EYE

Blindness and Near Blindness

Etiology/Pathophysiology. Blindness is a loss of visual acuity that ranges from partial to total loss of sight. It may be congenital or acquired.

The World Health Organization (WHO) has determined that in the United States there are approximately 1 million people who are legally blind. Legal blindness refers to individuals with a maximal visual acuity of 20/200 with corrective eyewear and/or visual field sight capacity reduced to 20 degrees. (The normal visual field range is 180 degrees.)

Categories have been established to help determine the exact extent of the vision loss and what assistance measures are appropriate for the individual. These categories range from low vision loss (20/70 to 20/200) to three categories of blindness (20/400, 20/1200, and no light perception).

Congenital blindness results from various birth defects. Acquired blindness in adults occurs as a result of such disorders as diabetic retinopathy, glaucoma, cataracts, and retinal degeneration; acute trauma is also a common cause.

Clinical Manifestations. The degree of vision loss will depend on the extent of trauma or disease. Symptoms may include diplopia, pain, presence of floaters and flashes of light, and pruritus or burning of eyes. Additional physical manifestations of the visually impaired patient include loss of peripheral vision, halos (colored circles around the cornea), a sense of orbital pressure, bulging of the eye(s), and any difference in the appearance of an eye structure, such as the pupil.

The wide variety of emotional symptoms associated with blindness may range from fear, anxiety, disorientation, depression, helplessness, and hopelessness to acceptance.

Assessment. Collection of *subjective data* may include noting the patient complaint of blurred vision as an early symptom of an eye disorder. It is important to determine the onset, severity, and duration of the symptoms, as well as any factors that relieve symptoms.

Collection of *objective data* may include observing squinting and rubbing of the eyes. It is important to note the patient's compensation measures, such as use of a magnifying glass. The use and effectiveness of assistive eyewear are also determined.

Emotionally the patient may experience poor interpersonal communication skills and coping mechanisms. Because self-care skills may be impaired, a blind individual may prefer isolation, causing additional physical and emotional difficulties.

Diagnostic Tests. An ophthalmoscopic examination is performed first. Other tests may include color and light vision tests and peripheral vision tests.

Medical Management. Corrective eyewear (contact lenses and glasses) is the first method of medical management for a partially sighted individual. If the visual defect results from an inflammatory disorder, medication is prescribed, appropriate to the causative agent.

Additional assistive devices for a visually impaired patient include canes, Seeing Eye dogs, magnifying systems, and telescopic lenses. The patient should be evaluated by an eye specialist to determine which devices are best suited. Some of the more technologically complex devices are expensive and may not be covered by insurance.

Canes are the most frequently used device for the partially or totally blind person. They are lightweight and portable and allow the patient simple maneuvering. The drawback to their use is that overhead objects are not usually detected. The newer laser canes provide more information about objects in front and at head and foot levels, but these are not readily available and are expensive. Seeing Eye dogs allow the blind person mobility that would otherwise be difficult. Trained dogs steer the patient away from obstacles, both aerial and stationary.

Surgical correction of the visual defect may provide eyesight. New laser surgeries provide excellent results in selected cases.

Nursing Interventions. The nurse might falsely assume that patients should be in the acceptance phase if the blindness has been present for years. This is not necessarily the case. Complications of long-term blindness may result in physical and emotional problems. Physically, the patient may be malnourished from diminished self-care cooking skills. The patient may also have secondary infections related to poor hygiene practices. Assistance with activities of daily living (ADLs) is a primary focus of patient care. Adequate time should be provided to allow the patient to assist in self-care. Emotional aspects of nursing care include appropriate communication (Box 34-1).

The impact of vision loss affects not only the patient, but also family, friends, and the community. Coping

Box 34-1 GUIDELINES FOR COMMUNICATING WITH BLIND PERSONS

- Talk in a normal tone of voice.
- Do not try to avoid common phrases in speech, such as "See what I mean?"
- Introduce yourself with each contact (unless well known to the person).
- Explain any activity occurring in the room.
- Announce when you are leaving the room so the blind person is not put in the position of talking to someone who is no longer there.

mechanisms differ among individuals. It is a nursing responsibility to educate, assist, counsel, and prevent complications. A comprehensive approach to patient care is essential with blind individuals. Use of government and community resources is absolutely necessary; individuals should be encouraged to contact the Department of Health and Human Services for resources and assistance. When a total approach is taken, the patient's successful adjustment to home, work, and society is possible. Blind individuals are capable of leading a full and active life and need to be treated as such.

Nursing diagnoses and interventions for the patient with blindness or near blindness include but are not limited to the following:

NURSING DIAGNOSES	NURSING INTERVENTIONS
Fear related to blindness	Determine the patient's level of fear. Orient the patient to use persons and the environment. Use therapeutic touch. Avoid loud sounds that may startle the patient.
Injury, high risk for, related to new environment	Use protective devices, such as side rails and canes. Alter surroundings to afford safety—clear passageways, nonslip rugs, and so on.
Self-care deficit, feeding, related to new routine	Describe the meal tray contents; arrange foods by texture and temperature; describe the location of the foods by the clock method (e.g., orange juice at 11:00 position, spoon at 9:00).

Patient teaching. The patient will require instruction on ambulatory safety. Aspects to include in the instructions are walking slowly, using verbal clues from the walking companion, and encouraging the patient to touch objects or borders.

The walking companion should precede the patient by about 1 foot and have the patient's hand on the companion's elbow to provide security. For both short-term and long-term blindness, if total vision is affected, a description of the surroundings is appropriate.

Prognosis. Blindness and near-blindness disorders have been reduced due to emphasis on early diagnosis and treatment. Laser surgery treatment has provided patients with advanced technology to reduce and limit complications.

Early childhood vision screening in the schools has contributed to the early diagnosis and treatment of refractory errors. Permanent visual loss may occur if strabismus and astigmatism are not treated at the preschool level. Physician monitoring of intermittent follow-up care is crucial until 10 years of age. New technology in eyewear significantly reduces refractory error problems in the adult. Radial keratotomy for myopia improves vision markedly and is under continued study for long-term complications.

Refractory Errors

Astigmatism and Strabismus.

Etiology/pathophysiology. Common refractory errors (**astigmatism**, **strabismus**, **myopia**, and **hyperopia**) are described in Table 34-3 on p. 1052.

Clinical manifestations. Refer to Table 34-3.

Assessment. Refer to Table 34-3.

Diagnostic tests. Common tests used in the diagnosis of refractory errors include ophthalmoscopy, retinoscopy, visual acuity tests, and refraction tests.

Medical management. Many refractory errors are treated with the use of corrective eyewear. Although corrective eyewear is the more common treatment, the preferred treatment is surgical correction.

Nursing interventions. The hospitalized patient wearing corrective eyewear requires daily assistance in cleansing and maintenance. If eyeglasses are worn, the lenses are washed daily with a mild or diluted glass cleaner and rinsed before drying with a soft cloth. Screw fittings should be checked to make sure they are secure. Contact lenses are cared for based on the manufacturer's directions. Safety should be maintained when corrective eyewear is not worn.

A nursing diagnosis and interventions for the patient with astigmatism, strabismus, myopia, and hyperopia include, but are not limited to the following:

NURSING DIAGNOSIS	NURSING INTERVENTIONS
Fear and/or anxiety, related to sensory/perceptual changes (visual)	Explain all procedures and diagnostic tests. Orient patient to the environment, offer reassurance and understanding, and identify anyone entering the room to prevent startling the patient.

TABLE 34-3 Common Refractory Errors

Description	Etiology/pathophysiology	Clinical manifestations	Assessment
Astigmatism			
Defect in the curvature of the eyeball surface	May be hereditary or a muscular deficit Occurs when the light rays cannot be focused clearly on a point on the retina because the spherical curve of the cornea is not equal in all meridians	Blurring of vision	*Collection of subjective data:* Complaints of eye discomfort, difficulty in focusing, blurred vision
Strabismus			
Inability of the eyes to focus in the same direction; commonly called *cross-eyed* *Esotropia*: eye turns in the direction of the nose *Exotropia*: eye turns outward	May result from neurological or muscular dysfunction or may be inherited Only one eye can fix on an object, since the optic axes do not focus simultaneously	Eyeball position is not symmetrical	*Collection of subjective data:* States difficulty following objects *Collection of objective data:* One eye, rather than both eyes, focuses or follows an object
Myopia			
Condition of nearsightedness	Elongation of the eyeball or an error in refraction so that parallel rays are focused in front of the retina	Inability to see objects at a distance	*Collection of subjective data:* Difficulty seeing faraway objects *Collection of objective data:* Snellen test
Hyperopia			
Condition of farsightedness	May result from error of refraction in which rays of light entering the eye are brought into focus behind the retina	Inability to see objects at close range	*Collection of subjective data:* Difficulty seeing near objects *Collection of objective data:* Snellen test

Patient teaching. The patient should be encouraged to see an optometrist or ophthalmologist yearly to keep the eyewear prescription current. The patient should be instructed on the use and care of eyewear; complications may result if the patient does not follow use and care instructions (see the patient teaching box).

Myopia.

Etiology/pathophysiology. Refer to Table 34-3.

Clinical manifestations. Refer to Table 34-3.

Assessment. Refer to Table 34-3.

Diagnostic tests. Commonly, diagnosis of myopia follows a visit to the physician due to the patient's inability to see distant objects clearly. Following routine examinations (see Table 34-3), the patient will be assessed for corrective lenses or corrective refractory surgery.

Medical management. The majority of patients are prescribed corrective eyeglasses or contact lenses. Patients who are unable or unwilling to wear corrective eyewear for occupational or cosmetic reasons may elect surgical correction.

Surgical management. Refractory surgery is effective in treating the cause of visual problems, instead of correcting symptoms. Patients are selected based on the degree of myopia, the shape of the cornea, and absence of medical conditions such as severe diabetes, glaucoma, or pregnancy. The usual age for correction is between 20 to 60 years. A surgical procedure called **radial keratotomy** (RK), developed in 1978, makes microscopic incisions on the surface of the cornea outside the optical area. These eight spokelike incisions flatten the cornea to a more normal curvature, thus reducing or eliminating myopia.

Nursing interventions. The postoperative patient will leave the hospital or clinic shortly after surgery. An eyepatch will be placed on the operative site until the next morning. Patients can be up and around at home. Due to visual limitations patients will need assistance. If

PATIENT TEACHING FOR CONTACT LENS CARE

DO

- Wash and rinse hands thoroughly before handling a lens.
- Keep fingernails clean.
- Remove lenses from their storage case one at a time, and place on the eye.
- Start with the same lens (left or right) each time of insertion.
- Use lens placement technique learned from eye specialist.
- Use proper lens care products.
- Wear lenses daily, and follow the prescribed wearing schedule.
- Remove a lens if it becomes uncomfortable.
- Keep regular appointments with the eye specialist.
- Remove lenses during sunbathing, showering, or swimming.

DO NOT

- Use soaps that contain cream or perfume for cleansing lenses.
- Let fingernails touch lenses.
- Mix up lenses.
- Exceed prescribed wearing time.
- Use saliva to wet lenses.
- Use homemade saline solution or tap water to wet or clean lenses.
- Borrow or mix lens care solution.

pain is experienced, the physician will prescribe oral analgesics. The patient will be seen the next day for physician follow-up. Postoperative physician checkups are scheduled at 1 week and then monthly for 1 year.

A nursing diagnosis and interventions for the patient with myopia include but are not limited to the following:

NURSING DIAGNOSIS	NURSING INTERVENTIONS
Injury, high risk for, related to visual changes	Reinforce physician's postoperative instructions. Orient the patient to the environment. Remove obstacles in the patient's environment.

Patient teaching. Instruct the patient preoperatively to stop wearing hard contact lenses 1 to 2 days before the surgical evaluation. Encourage rest the first day postoperatively. Inform the patient that if pain persists after the first postoperative day, the physician should be notified. Instruct the patient that infection is a rare complication of the procedure. Teach the patient that vision is assessed regularly to evaluate functional vision without corrective eyewear. Patients are advised that postoperative visual acuity is not always 20/20 without glasses. The goals of operative interventions are improving ADLs and allowing the possibility of driving a vehicle without glasses during the day. As a result of a slightly dilated pupil, the patient may experience a glare or halos from lights, which may require that glasses be worn for night driving.

Hyperopia.

Etiology/pathophysiology. Common refractory errors are included in Table 34-3.

Clinical manifestations. Refer to Table 34-3.

Assessment. Refer to Table 34-3.

Diagnostic tests. Common tests utilized in the diagnosis of hyperopia include ophthalmoscopy, retinoscopy, visual acuity tests, and refraction tests.

Medical management. The main treatment for farsightedness is corrective eyewear, either contact lenses or glasses. There are a variety of lenses available on the market, including hard, soft, and gas-permeable lenses.

Nursing interventions. The nurse should emphasize the importance of proper care of contact lenses. Eyeglasses should properly fit the bridge of the nose to eliminate slippage and uneven level of each lens.

A nursing diagnosis and interventions for the patient with hyperopia include, but are not limited to the following:

NURSING DIAGNOSIS	NURSING INTERVENTIONS
Knowledge deficit related to lack of experience with corrective eyewear	Answer all questions the patient might have on eyewear maintenance. Obtain literature on lens care. Encourage physician follow-up as directed.

Patient teaching. Patient teaching should include the following instructions:

- Washing the hands is essential whether applying or removing contact lenses.
- Clean the lens as directed by the manufacturer.
- Keep the lens storage kit clean.
- Avoid potential corneal abrasions.
- Report any signs of photophobia, dryness, excessive burning or tearing.

Inflammatory and Infectious Disorders of the Lid

Hordeolum, Chalazion, and Blepharitis. The most commonly seen infections and inflammatory disorders of the lid are listed in Table 34-4 on p. 1054.

TABLE 34-4 Common Infections/Inflammatory Disorders of the Lid

Description	Etiology/Pathophysiology	Clinical Manifestations	Assessment
Hordeolum (Stye)			
Acute infection of eyelid margin or sebaceous glands of the eyelashes	Frequently caused by the *Staphylococcus* organism One or more pustules may form	Abscess localized to base of eyelashes, with edema of lid	*Collection of subjective data:* Localized tenderness and pain resulting from edema; pain diminished after pustule ruptures *Collection of objective data:* Raised, erythematous area on eyelid; pustule exudate
Chalazion			
Inflammatory cyst on the meibomian gland at the eyelid margin; may require weeks to develop into a cyst	May be caused by infection; associated with diabetes mellitus, gout, and anemia	Discomfort, mass on eyelid, edema, visual disturbance	*Collection of subjective data:* Pressure felt as eyelid closes over cornea; patient may describe vision changes *Collection of objective data:* Cyst formation; eyelid edema
Blepharitis			
Inflammation of eyelid margins	Ulcerative: caused by bacterial infection, usually staphylococcal organisms Nonulcerative: caused by psoriasis, seborrhea, or allergic response	Pruritus, erythema of eyelid, eyelid pain, photophobia Excessive tearing may occur in nonulcerative type	*Collection of subjective data:* Eye pruritus; lids adhere together during sleep *Collection of objective data:* Eyes erythematous; patient rubs eyes; sensitivity to light; tear spillage

SKILL 34-1

APPLICATION OF WARM MOIST EYE COMPRESSES

Nursing action

1. Identify patient.
2. Refer to physician's order.
3. Assess condition of both eyes.
4. Prepare necessary equipment and supplies.
5. Explain procedure to patient.
6. Assist patient to comfortable position.
7. Provide privacy.
8. Place towel/waterproof pad under patient's head.
9. Don gloves.
10. Use sterile technique when infection or ulceration is present; clean technique may be used for allergic reactions.
11. Use separate equipment for bilateral eye infections.
12. Change gloves and wash hands before treating each eye.
13. Temperature of compresses should not exceed 120° F (49° C).
14. Change compresses frequently over 10 to 20 minutes.
15. Do not exert pressure on eyeball.
16. Sterile petrolatum may be used on skin *around* eyes, if desired, to protect skin.
17. If sterility is not necessary, moist heat may be applied by means of a clean washcloth.
18. Remove and dispose of equipment.
19. Remove gloves, and wash hands.
20. Record type, temperature, and duration of application.
21. Describe condition of eyes before and after treatment and patient's response to treatment.

Clinical manifestations. Refer to Table 34-4.

Assessment. Refer to Table 34-4.

Diagnostic tests. The eyelid margin is examined. Culture and sensitivity tests of any drainage may be ordered. Visual disturbances are also noted.

Medical management. Antiinfective agents are prescribed. Localized incision and drainage of a cyst or stye may be performed under local anesthesia. Warm normal saline compresses are ordered for 10 to 20 minutes two to four times a day.

Nursing interventions. A primary objective of nursing care for the patient with an infectious or inflammatory process of the lids is prevention of the spread of infection. Care should be taken when applying compresses (Skill 34-1). Handwashing is essential before contact with the eye.

Patient teaching. Instructions should be provided on the use of prescribed drops or ointments (see Skill 21-6). The patient is taught the use of warm compresses and informed about specific hygiene practices, such as keeping hands clean and away from the eyes and replacing mascara after 3 to 6 months, since the oils decompose and may harbor bacteria. The patient is cautioned to avoid irritating fumes or smoke, which may cause the patient to rub the eyes, leading to further infection. The use of eye makeup is discouraged until all inflammation subsides.

Prognosis. The inflammatory and infectious phases of these conditions respond favorably, in the majority of patients, to topical antimicrobials. Incision and drainage of cystlike formations result in minimal complications and risk to the patient.

Conjunctivitis.

Etiology/pathophysiology. **Conjunctivitis** is an inflammation of the conjunctiva resulting from bacterial or viral infection, allergy, or environmental factors. It is commonly called *pink eye.*

Acute bacterial conjunctivitis is usually transmitted by direct contact with a contaminated object. Pneumococcal, staphylococcal, streptococcal, gonococcal, and chlamydial organisms are the major causative agents. The hands are the most common transmitter of bacteria from the contaminated object to the eye. The eye, because of its warmth, moisture, and extensive vascularization, provides the bacteria with an excellent medium for multiplication. Conjunctivitis represents about two thirds of the 1 million cases per year of eye inflammation and infection. The disease is usually self-limiting, leaving no permanent impairment.

Viruses of the respiratory or intestinal tract may result in a secondary infection of the eye. The two more common viral agents are *Chlamydia trachomatis* and type 1 herpes simplex. Trachoma, a highly contagious form of conjunctivitis, is caused by a strain of the *C. trachomatis* virus. Transmission is by direct contact with an ocular discharge. It is rare in the United States but is a major cause of blindness in the Far East and Mediterranean countries.

Clinical manifestations. The inflammatory process that results from the contamination produces erythema of the conjunctiva, edema of the lid, and a crusting discharge on the lids and cornea. This infection, if untreated, leaves the eyelid scarred with granulations that invade the cornea, resulting in loss of vision.

Assessment. Collection of *subjective data* includes an awareness that during allergy seasons and because of exposure to environmental irritants, the patient may report pruritus, burning, and excessive tearing.

Collection of *objective data* includes observing eyes that are erythematous, with edema of the lid. A dried exudate may be noted.

Diagnostic tests. The conjunctiva is scraped for bacteria and stained for microscopic examination.

Medical management. Medical treatment is similar to that for blepharitis.

Nursing interventions. The lid and lashes are cleansed of exudate with normal saline. Warm compresses are applied two to four times a day. When allergies are present, cold saline compresses may be ordered for control of edema and pruritus. Eye irrigations with normal saline or lactated Ringer's solution may be prescribed to remove secretions. Topical antibiotics and adrenocortical steroid medications are administered. Eyepads are contraindicated, because they enhance bacterial growth.

Nursing diagnoses and interventions for the patient with conjunctivitis include but are not limited to the following:

NURSING DIAGNOSES	NURSING INTERVENTIONS
Pain related to pruritus, secondary to inflammatory process	Apply warm or cold compresses. Administer prescribed eye medications; ensure proper installation of eyedrops and ointments; administer eye irrigation as prescribed. Administer analgesics as ordered.
Sensory/perceptual alterations (visual), high risk for, related to edema and exudate	Assess patient's limitations in visual sensory perception. Implement safety measures as appropriate.

Patient teaching. The patient and family should be instructed to avoid contact with the eyes or soiled materials when an infection is present. Individual washcloths and towels are to be used. The patient is instructed to wash hands if contact is made with the eyes and before any treatments and is also taught to perform and describe treatments such as irrigations, compresses, and medication administration. The patient should avoid noxious fumes or smoke and should not wear contact lenses during the suppuration period.

Prognosis. Conjunctivitis responds successfully to topical antimicrobials. Patient teaching reduces the risk of continued exposure and reinfection. Although highly contagious, the disease is self-limiting, leaving no chance of permanent visual impairment unless a chronic condition develops.

Inflammatory and Infectious Disorders of the Cornea and Sclera

Keratitis.

Etiology/pathophysiology. Keratitis, an inflammation of the cornea, may result from injury, irritants, allergies, viral infection, or diseases such as congenital syphilis, smallpox, and some nervous disorders. It may be superficial and involve the epithelial layer only or invade the subepithelial layer and the endothelial membrane. The layers of the eye are innervated, and thus when inflammation is present, pain will be acute. Ulcers may form in the eye membrane layers, resulting in scattered scarring of the corneal surface.

Pneumococcus, Staphylococcus, Streptococcus, and *Pseudomonas* are the most common types of bacterial causes of keratitis. The viral agent most often responsible for corneal inflammation is the herpes simplex virus. Keratitis can be triggered by stress, illness, and exposure to ultraviolet light. The condition may be associated with the use of ophthalmological steroid medications. Overuse or abuse of topical steroids may injure epithelial cells.

Another form of keratitis is acanthamoebic keratitis. The *Acanthamoeba* organism is found in the soil, airborne dust, fresh water, and the noses and throats of healthy humans. This organism is often found to be resistant to antimicrobial agents. Contact lens wearers are more susceptible, because traditional cleaning agents for lenses include rinsing with clean or distilled water. People who swim frequently are at greater risk, because the amoeba is not killed by usual methods of disinfection, such as chlorine.

Clinical manifestations. Severe eye pain is the most common symptom that differentiates this disease from other eye inflammatory diseases. If uncontrolled, keratitis may result in blepharospasms and vision loss. Other symptoms include photophobia, tearing, edema, and visual disturbances.

Assessment. Collection of *subjective data* includes noting the severity and duration of the pain, the extent of light sensitivity, and any vision loss.

Collection of *objective data* includes assessing the patient for facial grimacing, lacrimation, and photophobia.

Diagnostic tests. Depending on the causative agent, a variety of diagnostic tests may be ordered, including culture and sensitivity tests, fluorescein staining, and Gram staining. Ophthalmoscopic examination is also performed.

Medical management. Medical management includes topical antibiotic therapy. Systemic antibiotics may be prescribed for severe cases. Cycloplegic-mydriatic drugs may be ordered, which paralyze the ocular muscles of accommodation and dilate the pupil. Analgesics are used to control pain associated with acute inflammation. Pressure dressings may be ordered to relax the eye muscle and decrease discomfort. These dressings are often applied to both eyes, since the eyes move together. Warm or cold compresses two to four times daily are prescribed for symptomatic relief. Epithelial debridement of loose tissue may be performed. Surgical management involves a corneal transplant, known as *keratoplasty.*

Nursing interventions. The focus of nursing interventions for keratitis includes control of pain, safety, and prevention of complications.

Nursing diagnoses and interventions for the patient with keratitis include but are not limited to the following:

NURSING DIAGNOSES	NURSING INTERVENTIONS
Infection, high risk for, related to inflammatory process	Assess eye exudate to determine whether isolation is required. Administer eye and systemic medications to control and prevent the spread of infection.
Pain, related to inflammatory process	Administer topical anesthetics if ordered to reduce spasms. Apply pressure dressing to the eye(s) to rest the muscle activity. Apply warm or cold eye compresses (as ordered) bid to qid to control pain.
Injury, high risk for, related to visual disturbances	Instill topical anesthetic medications for pain reduction. Ensure safety measures, such as moving needed objects close to the patient, orienting the patient to the environment, and using side rails if the patient is hospitalized. Assist patient in ambulation as indicated.

Patient teaching. The nurse should provide information on self-care of a corneal abrasion. The patient must also learn to wash the hands before instilling medication and to prevent infection by not rubbing the eyes. The patient is instructed to note any change in discharge or increase in pain and to notify the physician immediately.

Prognosis. Topical antimicrobial therapy, when begun promptly after diagnosis by culture, results in rapid healing and minimal visual impairment. Chronic keratitis may develop if treatment is delayed. Corneal tissue may become necrotic, leading to deeper ulceration and vision loss due to opaque scarring of the cornea. Keratoplasty has limited success because healing is slow due to the avascularity of the cornea.

Noninfectious Disorders of the Lacrimal Gland

Diagnostic tests. The definitive test for dry eye is the *Schirmer test*. Normal results should indicate 10 to 15 mm of wet paper.

Medical management. Medical management for dry eye includes artificial tear replacement. Many nonprescription products are available for this purpose.

Estrogen therapy may be prescribed for postmenopausal women. Medications that may cause dry eye as a side effect are limited, if possible. If an infection accompanies the dry eye syndrome, antibiotic therapy will be prescribed.

As many environmental irritants as possible are eliminated. If contact lenses cause local irritation and dry eye, a change in the prescription or type of lens is advised.

Results of the fluorescein staining test for excessive tear disorder are considered normal if the dye disappears from the lacrimal cul-de-sac within 1 minute.

When excessive tearing results from environmental irritants, the patient is encouraged to eliminate the noxious element. Filtering machines are available to control pollen and dust levels in the environment.

Surgical repair of an injured punctal sac by correctly aligning the eyelid margin or by probing an obstructed punctum (opening to the tear duct) to allow for tear reabsorption is the advised method of treatment.

Nursing interventions. A nursing diagnosis and interventions for the patients with dry eye and excessive tearing include but are not limited to the following:

NURSING DIAGNOSIS	NURSING INTERVENTIONS
Injury, high risk for, related to inflammatory process	Note lubrication of eye surfaces. Document level of discomfort. Instill medications as ordered.

Patient teaching. The patient should be instructed on instilling eye medications, and appropriate hygiene practices should be reinforced. Instructions are given on avoiding irritants.

Prognosis. Eye drops alleviate the majority of symptoms due to dry eye. Long-term use of artificial tears results in no adverse reactions. Control of medical conditions minimizes discomfort and complications. Surgical repair of the punctal sac is a safe procedure and has a good prognosis.

Noninfectious Disorders of the Lid

Ectropion and Entropion.

Etiology/pathophysiology. Two noninfectious conditions cause an abnormal turning of the eyelid margins: ectropion and entropion.

Ectropion is the outward turning of the eyelid margin. There are two types—atonic and cicatricial. In the older patient, it is common for the orbicularis oculi muscle to be relaxed. This condition is atonic ectropion.

Cicatricial ectropion involves either eyelid margin. The most common causes are eyelid laceration and burns of the conjunctival tissue.

Entropion is an inward turning of the eyelid. The lower eyelid margin is the most frequently involved. The conjunctival membrane lining the eyelid and part of the eyeball are exposed. Entropion is caused by atrophy of the eyelid tissue, spasms of the orbicularis oculi muscle, or scarring of the tarsal plate (dense connective tissue that stiffens the eyelid) resulting from congenital origin or trauma. Varying degrees of atonia exist in the older adult orbicularis; this is considered common.

Clinical manifestations. Ectropion and entropion are characterized by abnormal direction of the eyelid, with tear spillage and corneal dryness.

Assessment. Collection of *subjective data* includes noting the degree of vision loss and determination of tear loss and/or dryness of the cornea.

Collection of *objective data* includes observing the extent to which the patient can perform ADLs and the presence of any eyelid margin inflammation.

Diagnostic tests. The physician determines these conditions through a visual and ophthalmological examination.

Medical management. Medical intervention consists of topical medications to reduce conjunctival and corneal inflammation or drying. Surgery is the preferred treatment. Resection of the tarsal plate, removal of the scarred tissue, or tightening of the orbicularis oculi muscle is the choice for permanent repair.

Nursing interventions. Interventions for ectropion and entropion involve monitoring the medical treatment and reporting its progress. If the eyelid is surgically repaired, the patient should be monitored for safety considerations.

A nursing diagnosis and interventions for the patient with ectropion or entropion include but are not limited to the following:

NURSING DIAGNOSIS	NURSING INTERVENTIONS
Sensory/perceptual alterations (visual), related to edema and exudate	Caution the patient regarding loss of depth perception and peripheral vision. Assist the patient with self-care activities. Observe the intactness of the eye patches. Provide safety through the use of side rails. Note any eyelid margin inflammation. Change dressings as ordered. Instill medications as prescribed.

Prognosis. Early diagnosis and treatment of eyelid disorders reduce the risk of conjunctival and cornea inflammation and scarring. Monitoring of treatment reduces the need for surgical intervention and minimizes visual disturbances.

Noninfectious Disorders of the Lens

Cataracts.

Etiology/pathophysiology. A **cataract** is an opacity, or clouding, of the lens. The lens is normally clear and transparent. As one ages, there is a gradual opacification of the lens. When a cataract develops, the lens becomes foggy and decreases vision. If a large enough portion of the lens becomes opaque, light cannot reach the retina. Cataracts are not contagious or result from cancer, as some individuals believe. This is false information and the patient needs to be educated about the pathophysiology of the condition.

Cataracts may be congenital or acquired from systemic disease, trauma, toxins, intraocular inflammation, and aging. Senile cataracts, associated with the older adult, are the most common type.

Clinical manifestations. Symptoms of a cataract include blurring of vision, diplopia, photosensitivity, and difficulty in driving at night; no pain is associated with cataract formation. There is an opacity in the center portion of the lens (Fig. 34-5).

Assessment. Collection of *subjective data* includes noting blurring of vision as often the first symptom to be expressed by the patient. The nurse should note any subjective complaints, such as "hazy" or "fuzzy" vision.

Collection of *objective data* involves observing the patient for difficulty in reading, noting whether the patient brings newsprint close to the eyes. Sensitivity to light should also be noted.

Diagnostic tests. Ophthalmoscopic examination is the primary evaluative method.

Medical management. Medical intervention involves monitoring the patient for changes in vision associated with an increasing size of the cataract. Surgery is the only definitive method of treatment and can be performed at any age. It may be done using local or general anesthesia. There are two methods of surgery: intracapsular and extracapsular extraction.

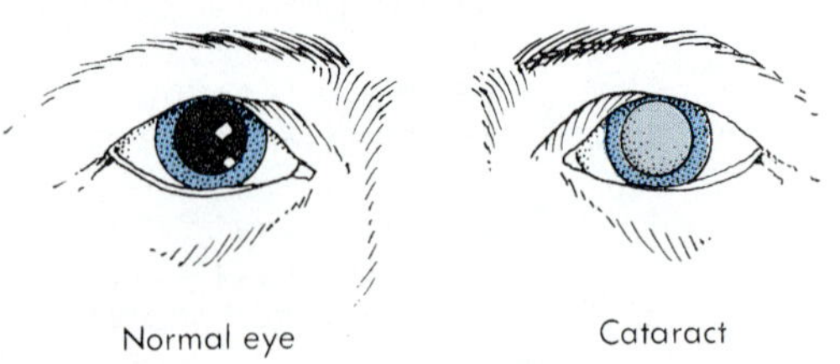

FIG. 34-5 Cataract, visible in the left eye as white opacity of the lens, is seen through the pupil.

Intracapsular surgery involves removing the lens and its entire capsule. The extracapsular method, the most common form of treatment, removes the lens and anterior capsule without removing the posterior capsule. Healing is rapid with this method.

During surgery, the physician may implant a synthetic (not from a human donor) intraocular lens (Fig. 34-6) in the anterior or posterior chamber. When intraocular lenses are not implanted, the physician will prescribe external lenses or glasses. Special contact lenses provide the patient many options for comfort.

Nursing interventions. Preoperative and postoperative nursing care is a primary nursing responsibility (see the nursing care plan).

Cataract symptoms usually develop slowly and can easily be detected. Annual examinations, especially for persons 40 and older, should be encouraged. If a cataract is treated early, blindness is usually prevented. Surgery provides about a 90% success rate of acceptable levels of vision.

Patient teaching. The nurse should reinforce postoperative instructions and observe the patient's correct use of eye medications and eye patches before discharge. The nurse should assess the patient's knowledge of contact lens use and care. Safety measures appropriate to vi-

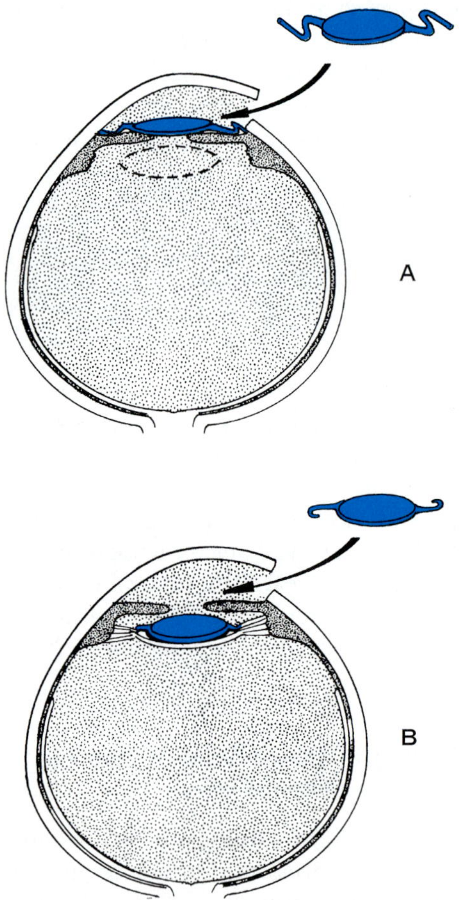

FIG. 34-6 Intraocular lens. **A,** Anterior lens implant in front of the iris. **B,** Posterior lens implant behind iris.

NURSING CARE PLAN: ***THE PATIENT WITH AN EYE DISORDER***

Mrs. Jorgensen is an 82-year-old widow who lives alone. She has developed bilateral cataracts and is admitted to same-day surgery for right cataract extraction with lens implantation.

Nursing diagnoses	Patient goals/expected outcomes	Nursing interventions
Injury, high risk for, related to altered visual acuity	Patient will not have any evidence of injury.	*Preoperative* Instill eye drops as prescribed. Administer preoperative medications or sedatives as ordered. Explain postoperative procedures to expect, such as patches and eye drops. *Postoperative* Instill mydriatic/cycloplegic and corticosteroid eye drops as prescribed. Instruct patient to avoid sudden head movement, heavy lifting, bending over, coughing, sneezing, vomiting, or straining with elimination, which cause increased intraocular pressure. Maintain prescribed eye patch/shield in position during specified hours. Remove environmental barriers to ensure safety. Keep side rails up at all times. Plan all care with patient: explain routines of what will happen and when. Visit frequently, and announce yourself on entering room. Assist with and teach deep breathing exercises. Check with physician for any special positioning and/or precautions. (If turned, position patient on the unaffected side.) Elevate head of bed 30 degrees as ordered. Assist with and teach active and passive ROM exercises q 4 hr. Increase activities and ambulation as ordered; assist as needed. Teach self-care activities, and assist as needed.

Continued.

Sensory/perceptual alteration (visual), related to trauma/disease of the eye	Patient will attain maximum functioning within limits of visual impairment.	Determine nature of visual symptoms, such as degree of vision loss or pain. Note eye and/or lid inflammation, edema, or appearance changes. Determine the patient's visual limitations. Provide self-care assistance and unit orientation. Reinforce discharge instructions for the patient and family regarding home care follow-up. Maintain safety precautions regarding physical environment. Encourage the patient to wear prescribed glasses during activity. Reinforce that limitations in vision will be present during the healing phase, especially with peripheral and depth perception.
Knowledge deficit, related to unfamiliarity with the eye disorder	Patient and/or family will obtain adequate knowledge related to care of the eye.	Reinforce preoperative/postoperative instructions on eye care. Reinforce correct technique regarding medication administration. Demonstrate and request return demonstration on eye patch dressing changes. Observe the patient's knowledge of contact lens use and care. Reinforce safety precautions that should be observed as a result of vision loss. Encourage the patient to report any sudden symptoms of severe pain, sudden vision loss, or signs of infection. Encourage the patient to carry identification regarding date of recent eye surgery.
Anxiety/fear, related to visual impairment	Patient will experience less anxiety/fear.	Observe level of patient/family anxiety. Note patient's coping mechanism related to vision loss. Encourage ventilation of feelings and concerns. Support patient/family's positive actions toward adapting to visual limitations.

CRITICAL THINKING QUESTIONS

1. Mrs. Jorgensen puts her call light on and tells the nurse that she has severe pain and pressure in her right eye. The initial response by the nurse would include:
2. To minimize the risk of injury to Mrs. Jorgensen's operative eye, discharge planning would include:
3. In visiting with Mrs. Jorgensen, the nurse finds that she enjoys embroidery and knitting. Mrs. Jorgensen states that she is looking forward to resuming her handiwork. Appropriate patient teaching would be:

PATIENT TEACHING AFTER EYE SURGERY

- Sleep on unaffected side for the prescribed time (3 to 4 weeks) to prevent pressure on operated eye.
- Wash hands before instilling eyedrops or changing eyepad.
- If an eyepad is required:
  - Use two oval eyepads, to provide snug but gentle pressure to prevent blinking against resistance.
  - Apply tape (paper or silk) diagonally from above nose to lower cheek.
- Apply metal eye shield at night to protect eye.
- Use glasses indoors and sunglasses with side sections outdoors to protect eyes from foreign substances and ultraviolet light until healing occurs.
- Avoid rubbing or pressing on the eye (creates pressure and may dislodge sutures).
- Avoid showers and shampooing hair (soap may irritate eye) for specified period as instructed; the time period differs from 1 day to up to 2 weeks.
- Avoid bending at the waist or lifting heavy objects for at least 1 month to prevent increased intraocular pressure (IOP) or adhesions of the iris.
  - To pick up objects from floor, kneel while keeping head erect.
  - To put on stocking or to tie shoes, sit and raise foot to reach hand while keeping the head erect.
  - Long pick-up "forceps" can facilitate picking up small objects from the floor without having to bend over.
- Avoid straining with bowel movements or with other activities, and avoid violent coughing (increases IOP).
- Limit reading (back and forth movement may loosen stitches); television is usually permitted.
- Report signs of edema, discharge, or pain to physician (may indicate infection or hemorrhage).

sion alterations should be discussed, and the patient should be encouraged to notify the physician of any complications such as pain, erythema, drainage, or sudden visual changes. If sudden pain occurs, the nurse should call the physician. See therapeutic dialogue and the patient teaching box for postoperative eye surgery teaching.

Prognosis. Gradual loss of lens transparency can result in risk of injury to the patient because of vision loss. Patients must be carefully monitored for degeneration of the lens. The condition may be accompanied by secondary glaucoma, which further reduces visual acuity. Surgical intervention is advised to improve vision. Complications may recur years after cataract surgery and should be reported to the ophthalmologist.

THERAPEUTIC DIALOGUE

Mrs. Bemus, age 71, has been experiencing decreasing vision for the past 5 years. She seeks medical attention and is told that surgery will be required to correct her condition. While talking to the patient, the nurse senses her reluctance to comply with postoperative treatment.

Patient: I'm too old to go through all the routines that the doctor wants me to. It involves too much.

Nurse: I know that surgery is a concern for you. You must have many emotions that you are feeling right now. It's understandable that you have concerns about your recovery.

Patient: There's so much to think about and remember.

Nurse: The doctor and our staff are here to help make your recovery as easy as possible for you. Tell me what bothers you the most.

Patient: What if I go home and fall? I could reinjure my eye or break something, like my hip.

Nurse: There are several things that you and your family can do to prevent any injury to yourself. The doctor and staff will explain these things very carefully to you.

Patient: I'm afraid I'm too old to learn.

Nurse: (Touching the patient) The staff will provide as much time and support as you need to help you learn. I have a feeling that you will surprise yourself at how well you do!

Patient: My doctor thinks I'll have no problems. *(After a few seconds)* Maybe the doctor and you are right.

Nurse: I suggest you talk to the doctor about your feelings. Together, we'll help you in any way we can.

Patient: I guess anything's possible! Thanks for your understanding. Being old isn't easy. Yet, as my husband used to say: "You're never too old to learn!"

Disorders of the Retina

Diabetic Retinopathy.

Etiology/pathophysiology. **Diabetic retinopathy** is a disorder of retinal blood vessels characterized by capillary microaneurysms, hemorrhage, exudates, and the formation of new vessels and connective tissue.

Diabetic retinopathy usually appears 10 years after onset of diabetes mellitus. The incidence increases in relationship to the length of time the patient has had the disease. The disorder occurs more frequently in patients with long-standing, poorly controlled diabetes mellitus.

The initial stage of diabetic retinopathy may last for several years. The blood vessels in the retina begin to widen and become tortuous. Microaneurysms then develop at the periphery and small hemorrhages develop. These may disappear but leave in their place scars that can decrease vision. Increased capillary permeability causes protein exudate.

As the disease progresses, new blood vessels form on the retina and into the vitreous. These new vessels rupture, causing decreased vision. Absorption of some of the blood can occur, which will improve vision until another hemorrhage occurs. Significant vision loss will eventually occur as these hemorrhages continue. Vitreous contraction and full detachment can occur as the vessels and surrounding tissue become fibrous.

Clinical manifestations. Symptoms include microaneurysms, which can only be identified by ophthalmoscopy in the initial stage. In the advanced stages, the patient will have progressive vision loss and the presence of "floaters," which are minute products of the hemorrhage.

Assessment. Collection of *subjective data* must include assessing the length and control of diabetes mellitus. The patient will have varying degrees of vision loss, from decreased vision to blindness. The patient's knowledge of therapy should be assessed.

Collection of *objective data* involves noting that in the early stages there are no symptoms; as the disease progresses, vision is diminished.

Diagnostic tests. Indirect ophthalmoscopy shows dilated and tortuous vessels and narrowing or obliteration of the arteries. Opacities, hemorrhages, and microaneurysms can be seen.

Slit-lamp examination provides magnification of the lesions.

Medical management. Surgical intervention includes photocoagulation and/or vitrectomy. Photocoagulation destroys new blood vessels, seals leaking vessels, and helps to prevent retinal edema by use of a laser beam. (See the discussion of photocoagulation on pp. 1071-1072.) A vitrectomy may be performed when photocoagulation is not possible.

Nursing interventions. Nursing diagnoses and interventions for the patient with diabetic retinopathy include but are not limited to the following:

NURSING DIAGNOSES	NURSING INTERVENTIONS
Fear, related to unfamiliarity with procedure	Determine patient's knowledge of purpose and procedure of photocoagulation.
Anxiety, related to lack of knowledge	Assure the patient that the procedure is painless and takes approximately 15 to 20 minutes. Explain that a family member or friend must be available to drive the patient home.

Patient teaching. The patient should follow the same instructions at home as for the patient undergoing eye surgery (see patient teaching box).

Prognosis. The best treatment of diabetic retinopathy is early detection. Frequent eye examinations reduce the complication of vision loss, and modern laser technology is a highly effective method of reducing further damage to the retina and improving vision.

Macular Degeneration.

Etiology/pathophysiology. Macular degeneration is a condition of the aging retina characterized by slow, progressive loss of central and near vision. There are two types of macular degeneration. The first, called the *wet type*, has new vessel growth in the macular region that occurs suddenly. The macula becomes displaced, and scarring occurs.

The second, known as the dry type, is the more common. Degenerative changes are the cause: lipid deposits occur, followed by slow atrophy of the macular region, including the retina.

Clinical manifestations. The main symptom of macular degeneration is gradual and variable bilateral loss of central vision. One eye may have a greater loss than the other eye. Color perception may also be affected.

Assessment. Collection of *subjective data* includes noting that the patient may have difficulty distinguishing colors correctly. The nurse should assess for visual disturbances and coping mechanisms for the loss.

Collection of *objective data* includes the nurse noting the degree to which the patient can centrally view objects.

Diagnostic tests. Indirect ophthalmoscopy is used to detect opacity, hemorrhage, and new blood vessel formation. In addition, retinal detachment or other abnormalities can be seen.

Medical management. Photocoagulation may be used, but only if the areas of new vessels have not grown into the macula. This procedure may be useful in the wet type if treatment is begun within the first few days after onset of symptoms. There is no treatment for the dry type.

Nursing interventions. The patient needs patience and understanding in order to cope with the continuing loss of sight. The nurse needs to assist the patient through the process of acceptance of loss of sight. Maintaining safety is important because only peripheral vision exists.

A nursing diagnosis and interventions for the patient with macular degeneration include but are not limited to the following:

NURSING DIAGNOSIS	NURSING INTERVENTIONS
Sensory/perceptual alterations (visual), related to disease process	Note the extent of visual loss and the level of difficulty with ADLs; assist the patient to develop ways of performing these activities. Determine the patient's support systems and elicit help, if available.

Patient teaching. The nurse instructs the patient about the disease process, stressing that peripheral vision will be maintained. The patient is provided ways to maintain as much independence as possible, and family and friends can learn the areas in which to assist.

Prognosis. Early diagnosis of macular degeneration is critical to prevent blindness. Ophthalmic laser surgery is of limited benefit because of the gradual and progressive course of the disorder. Photocoagulation is preventive, not curative.

Retinal Detachment.

Etiology/pathophysiology. **Retinal detachment** is a separation of the retina from the choroid in the posterior area of the eye (Fig. 34-7). This usually results from a hole in the retina that allows vitreous humor to leak between the choroid and the retina.

The immediate cause may be severe trauma to the eye, such as a contusion or penetrating wound. In most cases, however, retinal detachment is the result of internal changes related to aging and sometimes inflammation of the eye. Retinal detachment may also occur in debilitated patients when there is sudden severe physical exertion.

As the detachment progresses, there is an interruption in the transmission of visual images from the retina to the optic nerve. The result is a progressive loss of vision to complete blindness.

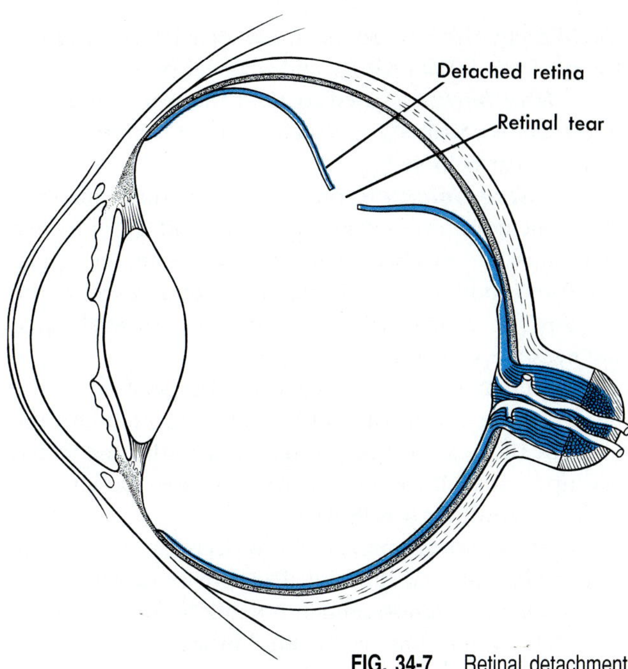

FIG. 34-7 Retinal detachment.

Clinical manifestations. Symptoms include a sudden or gradual development of flashes of light, followed by floating spots and loss of a specific field of vision.

Assessment. Collection of *subjective data* includes noting patient complaints of flashing lights unilaterally and floaters. There is a progressive vision restriction in one area. If the tear is acute and extensive, the patient will describe a sensation of a "curtain being drawn" across the eye. Because the retina does not contain sensory nerves that relay sensations of pain, the condition is painless.

Collection of *objective data* includes observing the patient for the ability to perform ADLs. The level of anxiety associated with coping is also assessed.

Diagnostic tests. Indirect ophthalmoscopy is used to detect pallor of the retina as well as the detachment. Three-mirror gonioscopy provides a magnified view of any retinal lesions. Slit-lamp examination magnifies the lesions.

Medical management. The treatment of choice is early corrective intervention. One of four procedures may be performed.

Photocoagulation is used to burn localized tears or breaks that may have occurred in the posterior portion of the eyeball. This causes an eventual sealing of the tear or break.

Cryosurgery is used to "freeze" the borders of a retinal hole with a frozen-tipped probe. The probe is applied to the scleral surface directly over the retinal hole area. The hole seals when the resultant inflammatory process produces scarring.

Diathermy is used to burn a retina break using an ultrasonic probe. The probe is applied to the scleral surface directly over the retinal break. Sealing occurs from the resultant inflammatory and scarring process.

Scleral buckle is used to hold the retina and choroid together. Scarring can then occur and permanently seal the tear or hole.

Nursing interventions. Postprocedure management includes cycloplegic-mydriatic and antiinfective eye drops. Eye patches are applied over only the operative eye or both eyes, providing the required rest of the eye for 1 to 2 days. Safety measures are essential, since the eyes are patched.

Depending on the procedures, the position of the head postoperatively may vary. If air is injected into the vitreous, the head will be positioned with the unaffected eye upward with the patient lying on the abdomen or sitting forward for 4 to 5 days.

Dark glasses are prescribed to decrease the discomfort of *photophobia* (abnormal sensitivity to light).

A nursing diagnosis and interventions for the patient with retinal detachment include but are not limited to the following:

NURSING DIAGNOSIS	NURSING INTERVENTIONS
Anxiety, related to visual alterations	Allow the patient the opportunity to discuss feelings and fears about the possible loss of vision. Answer questions honestly and correct any misunderstandings. Explain the reasons for restrictions of activities and for procedures.

Patient teaching. Temporary restrictions of reaching, work, and activity should be discussed with the patient (see patient teaching box).

Prognosis. Retinal detachment requires treatment: the degree of restoration of sight depends on the extent and duration of separation. Maximum vision is achieved within 3 months after surgery. Unless replaced, a detached retina slowly dies after several years of detachment. Blindness from retinal detachment is irreversible.

PATIENT TEACHING FOR RETINAL DETACHMENT

- Return to sedentary activity in 2 weeks; no heavy lifting or active physical activity for 6 weeks, or as instructed by physician.
- Check with physician concerning shampooing of hair.
- Limit reading for 3 weeks (or as instructed by physician).
- Use correct technique for administration of eye medications.
- Report to ophthalmologist any signs of further detachment (flashes of light, increase in "floaters," blurred vision).
- Report for medical follow-up visits as instructed.

Disorders of Intraocular Pressure

Glaucoma.

Etiology/pathophysiology. **Glaucoma** is an abnormal condition of elevated pressure within an eye because of obstruction of the outflow of aqueous humor. It is associated with a progressive loss of peripheral vision.

Glaucoma is found in persons who are middle-aged and older. Approximately 12% to 15% of all blindness in the United States results from glaucoma. It is seldom seen in persons under 35 years of age but may occur in infancy.

Glaucoma occurs when there is an obstruction of the aqueous humor drainage that increases the intraocular pressure (Fig. 34-8). Damage to the optic nerve results.

Open-angle glaucoma, also known as chronic simple glaucoma, is a common form of the disease. The course of the disease is slowly progressive and results from degenerative changes. It is often bilateral.

Closed-angle glaucoma, also known as acute glaucoma, occurs if there is an abrupt angle change of the iris, causing rapid vision loss and dramatic symptoms.

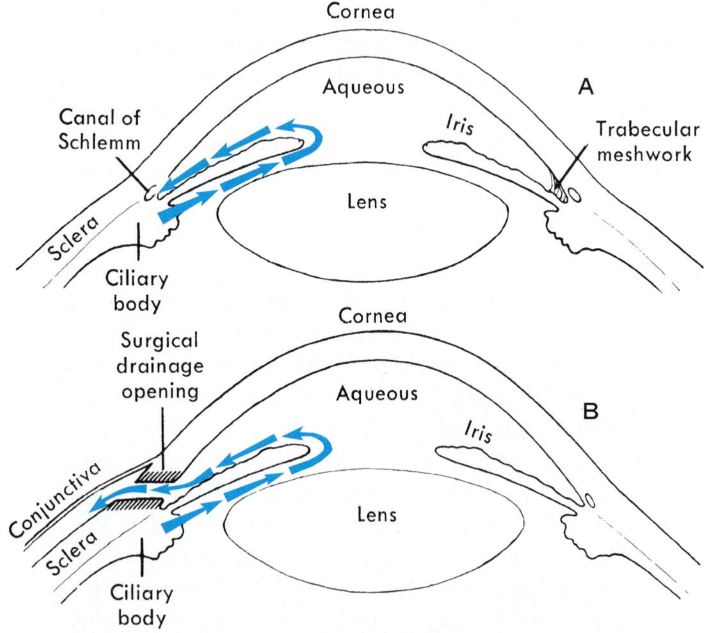

FIG. 34-8 **A,** Originating from ciliary processes, aqueous humor flows through the pupil into the anterior chamber and normally leaves the eye by way of the canal of Schlemm. **B,** In glaucoma, normal aqueous outflow is occluded. Purpose of glaucoma surgery is to create a new channel through which aqueous humor leave the eye.

Clinical manifestations. In open-angle glaucoma, the patient has no signs or symptoms during the early stages of the disease. As the symptoms become apparent, they include tunnel vision, eye pain, difficulty adjusting to darkness, halos around lights, and inability to detect colors. Intraocular pressures will be elevated.

Closed-angle (acute) glaucoma produces severe pain, decreased vision, and nausea and vomiting. The sclera is erythematous, and the pupil is enlarged and fixed. The patient sees colored halos around lights. There is an acute increase in the intraocular pressure.

Assessment. Collection of *subjective data* includes noting the time of day when the eye pain occurs. Frequency, intensity, and duration of the pain are also assessed. Complaints of peripheral vision loss, maladaptation to darkness, and halos seen around lights are noted. Severity of headaches and presence of nausea and vomiting are determined.

Collection of *objective data* includes noting a need for frequent eyeglass prescription changes. Elevated intraocular pressures are also present.

Diagnostic tests. Tonometry is used to test for intraocular pressure (Fig. 34-9). A patient with glaucoma would test above the normal range of 10 to 22 mm Hg. Visual field studies will show a decline in the patient's peripheral vision.

Medical management. Open-angle glaucoma is medically treated by the use of beta-blockers, miotics, and carbonic anhydrase inhibitors (see medication table on pp. 1066-1067). A beta-blocker, such as Betoptic, will reduce intraocular pressure. Miotics, such as pilocarpine, constrict the pupil and draw the iris away from the cornea, allowing aqueous humor to drain out of the canal of Schlemm. Carbonic anhydrase inhibitors, such as Diamox, decrease the production of aqueous humor. The result is a lowering of intraocular pressure. Surgery is done when medications do not control the pressure and consists of a trabeculectomy or laser trabeculoplasty. *Trabeculectomy* is the removal of corneoscleral tissue, usually the canal of Schlemm and trabecular meshwork. This produces an increase in the outflow of aqueous humor. Laser trabeculoplasty produces openings in the trabecular meshwork.

Closed-angle glaucoma is medically treated with osmotic diuretics, such as mannitol, carbonic anhydrase inhibitors, and miotics. Surgical treatment includes a peripheral iridectomy or an iridotomy. A peripheral iridectomy is the removal of part of the iris. The procedure is performed with the patient under general anesthesia; this often restores drainage of the aqueous humor. Postoperatively the patient is observed for signs and symptoms of local hemorrhage or excessive pain. An iridotomy is an incision into the iris of the eye to create an opening for aqueous flow. A local or general anesthetic may be used. Postoperatively the dressing is observed for signs of drainage.

Nursing interventions. Nursing interventions involve protecting the patient's safety, monitoring compliance to therapy, and reinforcement of discharge instructions (see the nursing care plan).

Patient teaching. The areas of education are covered in the patient teaching box.

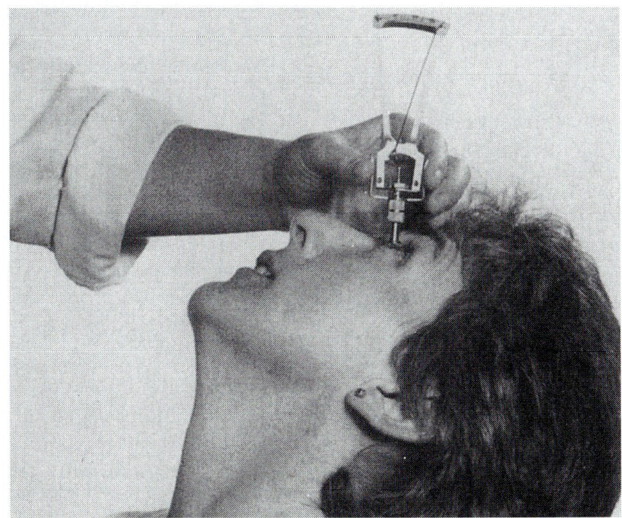

FIG. 34-9 Measurement of intraocular pressure with the Schiotz tonometer.

PATIENT TEACHING FOR GLAUCOMA

- Medical supervision will be required for the rest of life.
- Eye drops *must* be continued as long as prescribed even in the absence of symptoms; usually treatment is life long.
  - Blurred vision decreases with prolonged use.
  - Avoid driving for 1 to 2 hours after administration of miotics.
- To prevent complications:
  - Press lacrimal duct for 1 minute after eye drop insertion to prevent rapid systemic absorption.
  - Have reserve bottle of eye drops at home.
  - Carry eye drops when away from home.
  - Carry card identifying glaucoma and the eye drops solution prescribed.
- Bright lights and darkness are not harmful.
- There is no apparent relationship between vascular hypertension and ocular hypertension.
- Report any reappearance of symptoms immediately to ophthalmologist.
- If admitted to hospital for a different medical condition, alert the staff of continued need for prescribed eye drops.
- Avoid the use of mydriatic or cycloplegic drugs (e.g., atropine) that dilate the pupils.

MEDICATIONS FOR EYE DISORDERS

Medication	Trade Name	Action	Side Effects	Nursing Implications
Sulfacetamide sodium	Sulamyd	Broad-spectrum bacteriostatic antifective agent used in treatment of ocular infections such as conjunctivitis, corneal ulcers, trachoma, and chlamydial infections	Pruritus, edema, erythema, other eye irritations	Know that it is contraindicated in sulfonamide hypersensitivity and that purulent exudate may inactivate drug; do not use silver preparations concurrently; use proper ophthalmic technique; comply with full course of treatment, store properly; discard solution if it discolors; warn patient to avoid sharing washcloths and towels with family members.
Betaxolol hydrochloride	Betoptic	Beta adrenergic blocking agent that reduces formation and possibly increases outflow of aqueous humor; is used in treatment of open-angle glaucoma to lower intraocular pressure; is used only in special circumstances with patients who have heart conditions	Insomnia, irritation of eyelids, stinging on instillation, occasional tearing, photophobia, systemic effects, possible disorientation, bradycardia, weakness, dyspnea	Know pregnancy cautions; do not touch dropper on eye; use proper administrative technique; give proper dosage; keep container tightly closed; determine intraocular pressure 4 weeks after treatment; use cautiously in patients with history of heart failure or with diabetes mellitus.
Timolol maleate	Timoptic	Beta adrenergic blocking agent that reduces aqueous formation and possibly increases aqueous outflow, is used in treatment of open-angle glaucoma and hypertension, is used only in special circumstances for patients who have heart conditions	Ocular sensitivity, severe irritation of eye or eyelid, systemic effect of cardiac failure, chest pain, disorientation, diarrhea, dizziness, exacerbation of asthma	Know that it may mask hypoglycemia; measure intraocular pressure after 4 weeks of treatment; avoid abrupt cessation; use cautiously in bronchial asthma and heart conditions, know pregnancy and breastfeeding cautions; use proper administration technique; use correct amount; keep container tightly closed.
Dexamethasone	Decadron	Steroid used in treatment of ocular inflammation; risk-benefit determination in cataracts and glaucoma	Local irritation, retardation of corneal healing, blurred vision, eye pain, secondary eye infection	Know that it may mask infection; use for only short term in children; tell patient not to wear contact lens during treatment; shake bottle before using; use proper administration technique; check with physician before using for future eye conditions; check with physician if condition does not improve in 5 to 7 days.

MEDICATIONS FOR EYE DISORDERS—cont'd

Medication	Trade Name	Action	Side Effects	Nursing Implications
Acetazolamide	Diamox	Blocks action of carbonic anhydrase, thereby promoting excretion of sodium, potassium, bicarbonate, and water; is adjunct in open-angle glaucoma; lowers intraocular pressure or hepatic or adrenocortical impairment	Diarrhea, weakness, discomfort, urinary frequency, loss of appetite, nausea, vomiting, numbness in hands, contraindication in severe renal hepatic or adrenocortical impairment	Know pregnancy and lactation cautions; give with food; give accurate dosage; in diabetes, know that it may increase blood and urine glucose levels; caution drowsiness; monitor I&O and weight daily.
Pilocarpine hydrochloride	Pilocar Isopto Carpine	Cholinergic drug that causes contraction of sphincter muscles of iris, resulting in mitosis, is used to reduce intraocular pressure in treatment of open-angle glaucoma; is used as adjunct with carbonic anhydrase inhibitors	Muscle tremors, nausea and vomiting, dyspnea, wheezing, bronchial spasms, local irritation	Encourage patient to have periodic intraocular pressure determinations; use proper administration technique; use exact dosage; monitor for blurred vision or changes in vision; use cautiously in bronchial asthma and hypertension; apply light finger pressure on lacrimal sac 1 min after instillation of drops.
Cyclopentolate hydrochloride	Cyclogyl	Anticholinergic agent that produces mydriasis and cycloplegia; is a risk-benefit consideration with angle-closure glaucoma; is a diagnostic agent	Ataxia, behavioral disturbances, tachycardia, disorientation, fever	Prevent contamination of dropper; give proper dosage; warn patient of increased sensitivity to light and suggest sunglasses; know that it is contraindicated in narrow-angle glaucoma; use cautiously in older adult.
Osmitrol	Mannitol	Osmotic diuretic that causes decrease in intraocular pressure	Fluid and electrolyte imbalance, chest pain, tachycardia, chills and fever, difficult urination	Administer by intravenous infusion; know pregnancy caution; know that duration of action is 1 to 3 hr; monitor vital signs at least hourly and I&O, weight, and potassium levels daily.
Polyvinyl alcohol	Liquifilm Forte	Tearlike lubricant for relief of dry eyes and eye irritations	Headache, burning, blurred vision, eye pain	Teach patient to instill; warn patient not to touch dropper to eye; to avoid contamination of solution, warn patient not to touch tip of container to eye.
Gentamicin sulfate	Garamycin	Disrupts protein synthesis; aminoglycoside Bactericidal antibiotic used in treatment of blepharitis conjunctivitis	Pruritus, erythema, edema, ocular discomfort, blurred vision (may occur for few minutes after application)	Comply with full course of therapy; if no improvement occurs after a few days, check with physician.

Prognosis. Today's method of medical and surgical management provides the patient with an excellent prognosis for a full recovery. Complications are few if care is early in the course of the condition. When glaucoma is ignored or noncompliance to therapy is noted, blindness may occur. Regular eye examinations are required to detect and monitor for increased intraocular pressure. Generally, once damage has occurred, the condition is irreversible. Surgery and medication help to lessen the complications from glaucoma.

Injuries to the Eye

Corneal Injuries.

Etiology/pathophysiology. Corneal injuries result from injuries to corneal layers of the eye. The cornea is the convex, transparent outermost layer of the eye. It is composed of five layers of tissue and is uniform in nature. The cornea is nonvascular; therefore no bleeding occurs from injury unless subcorneal structures are involved. The cornea is kept moist by tear production and is protected from daily insult by the eyelid.

Foreign bodies are the most common cause of corneal injury. Dust particles, propellants, and eyelashes may lodge in the conjunctiva or cornea. The eyes blink in response to the irritant, and further irritation occurs from the upper lid closing frequently, thus moving the foreign body into deeper layers or a wider area of the cornea.

Burns often occur in the home and workplace. When burns affect the eye, it is considered a medical emergency. Depending on the chemical causing the burn, the damage may be superficial or deep. Chemical irritants such as acids and alkylines and metal flashes from acetylene blowtorches cause significant pain, depending on the depth of chemical erosion.

Abrasions and lacerations are usually superficial scratches that occur from injuries to the eye, such as fingernails or clothing. They may be painful, depending on the depth of the abrasion.

Penetrating wounds are the most serious corneal injuries. Eye structures may be injured permanently, resulting in total blindness. Infection may result from the introduction of microorganisms on the penetrating object.

Clinical manifestations. Foreign bodies produce pain on eyeball movement or when the eyelid moves over the eyeball during blinking. Excessive tearing, erythema of the conjunctiva, and pruritus may occur.

Acute pain and burning are the primary symptoms with any topical burn to the eye.

Abrasions and lacerations produce mild to severe pain, depending on the depth of corneal involvement. The pain may be transitory and slight, or spasmodic and deep.

Penetrating wounds result in varying degrees of pain. If underlying structures are involved, pain may be absent because the nerves have been severed.

Assessment.

Foreign bodies. Collection of *subjective data* includes noting the time and type of injury. The patient is assessed for the degree and severity of eye pain and vision loss. The patient should be asked about any first-aid treatment provided.

Collection of *objective data* includes observation of the foreign body and extent of damage. When the intracapsular area has been penetrated, fluid will be leaking from the eye.

Burns. Collection of *subjective data* includes determining the degree of pain. It is important to assess the substance causing the burn and any first-aid treatment that has been provided. Vision loss is determined by the physician.

Collection of *objective data* includes noting the extent of the burn in and around the eye, including eyelashes and eyebrows, and assessing the condition of the eyeball.

Abrasions and lacerations. Collection of *subjective data* includes assessing the patient for the degree of pain following the incident and how the injury occurred. Treatments used at the time of injury are noted.

Collection of *objective data* includes assessing the degree of damage of the eyeball and surrounding structures, and any vision loss is noted.

Penetrating wounds. Collection of *subjective data* includes noting the time and causative factors related to the injury. Presence and severity of pain are assessed. Determine any first-aid treatment rendered.

Collection of *objective data* includes determining the type and size of the penetrating object. Fluid leakage from the eye is noted. The damage to surrounding structures is assessed.

Diagnostic tests. Tests include visual and ophthalmoscopic examination, fluorescein staining, peripheral vision tests, and slit-lamp examination.

Medical management. Foreign bodies are medically treated with a flush of normal saline when the object is near the sclera and conjunctiva; it can then be removed by a clean swab or tissue. Cotton is not to be used, because it may scratch the cornea. If the object is not easily flushed away, the individual must see an ophthalmologist to have the object removed. Antibiotic topical eye ointments are ordered.

Burns are medically treated with a prolonged, 15- to 20-minute or longer tap water flush immediately after burn exposure. This will help prevent scar formation. The eyelids are separated during the flush procedure. The patient is then treated in a local emergency department or physician's office for follow-up care. Home remedy first-aid treatment should not be done. Topical anti-infective agents are ordered for the eye. Abrasions and lacerations of the eye are medically cleaned with a normal saline solution. Antibiotic therapy, usually topical, is prescribed.

See Box 34-2 for eye safety measures and Table 34-5 for first-aid for eye injuries.

Immediately after a penetrating wound injury, both the eyes should be covered while transporting the patient to the hospital because both eyes work in synchrony. Covering the eyes prevents the eye from involuntarily moving with the other eye. A shield reduces further injury but must not touch the foreign object. A Styrofoam cup provides adequate coverage and is readily available. The foreign object should not be removed except by a trained physician.

Nursing interventions.

Foreign bodies. The nurse will assist with the required irrigation of the eye (Skill 34-2 on p. 1070).

Burns. The nurse will assist with the flushing process and providing eye medications as ordered.

Abrasions and lacerations. The nurse will assist with cleaning the eye as ordered and providing general first-aid (see Table 34-6).

Penetrating wounds. The nurse should note whether the pupil on the affected side becomes irregular. This results when the iris of the affected eye moves to occlude the wound area. Infection potential is high; therefore topical and systemic antibiotics are ordered. If the wound is small, self-healing occurs. If the wound is large or deep, enucleation of the eye may be performed.

Effective and immediate therapy is crucial for any injury to the eye. If treatment is interrupted, ineffective, or not sustained, permanent eye damage will occur. The most frequent complications include infection, vision disturbances, and blindness.

A nursing diagnosis and interventions for the patient with an eye injury include but are not limited to the following:

NURSING DIAGNOSIS	NURSING INTERVENTIONS
Pain, related to inflammatory process	Note the level of pain, using a grade of 1 to 10. Administer ordered local and/or systemic analgesics; administer antiinfective topical agents, and apply warm or cool compresses as ordered.

Patient teaching. The nurse should ensure that the patient can apply ointments and dressings, if ordered. The patient is instructed in the use of other therapy devices, such as warm or cool compresses. Proper handwashing techniques are taught. Dark sunglasses are to be worn by the patient if cycloplegic or mydriatric eye drops are used. Instruct the patient to avoid future epi-

Box 34-2 EYE SAFETY MEASURES

- Avoid frequent rinsing of eyes with unprescribed solutions.
- Discard any ophthalmic solution that is cloudy, is discolored, has been open for ≥3 months, or contains particles.
- Avoid self-treament of an eye inflammation with a medication prescribed for a previous eye disorder.
- To avoid eye strain:
  - Use a good light for reading or doing work that requires careful visual focus.
  - When reading or focusing eyes for long periods, look at distant objects for a few minutes at repeated intervals to rest eyes.
  - Avoid rubbing eyes.
  - Wash hands before touching eyes.
  - Wear safety glasses when engaging in activities that could injure the eyes.
  - Wear dark glasses for prolonged exposure to very bright light (such as sunlight or snow or water).
  - Flush eyes with copious amount of water when any irritating substances are accidentally introduced.
  - Do not attempt to remove foreign bodies from the cornea; cover eye and seek medical attention.
  - If a speck of dust blows in eye, pull upper lid over lower lid and let the tears wash the speck to the inner canthus or lower lid, where it may be safely removed.

TABLE 34-5 First-Aid for Eye Injuries

Injury	Interventions
Burns: chemical, flame	Flush eye immediately for 15 to 20 minutes or longer with cool water or any available nontoxic liquid; seek medical assistance.
Loose substance on conjunctiva: dirt, insects	Lift upper lid over lower lid to dislodge substance, produce tearing; irrigate eye with water if necessary; do not rub eye; obtain medical assistance if above interventions fail.
Contact injury: contusion, ecchymosis, laceration	Apply cold compresses if no laceration present; cover eye if laceration present; seek medical assistance.
Penetrating objects	Do not remove object; place protective shield over eye (e.g., paper cup); cover uninjured eye to prevent excess movement of injured eye; seek medical assistance.

SKILL 34-2

EYE IRRIGATION

Nursing action

1. Review physician's order.
2. Identify patient.
3. Wash hands.
4. Assess condition of both eyes.
5. Prepare supplies and equipment.
6. Explain procedure.
7. Provide privacy.
8. Place patient lying toward side to be irrigated to prevent fluid from flowing into other eye.
9. Place towel under patient's head.
10. A plastic squeeze bottle is used unless very large amounts of fluid are needed.
11. Don gloves.
12. Gently direct the irrigating fluid along the conjunctiva from the *inner* to the *outer* canthus (see illustration).
13. Avoid directing a forceful stream onto the eyeball.
14. Avoid touching any eye structures with irrigation equipment.
15. A piece of gauze may be wrapped around the gloved index finger to raise upper lid for better cleaning if heavy discharge is present.
16. Place an emesis basin at side of face to collectirrigating fluid.
17. Gently dry the eyelids.
18. Remove and discard gloves.
19. Wash hands.
20. Document procedure: duration, type and amount of solution, and characteristics of drainage. Record assessment before and after procedure. Note patient's response.

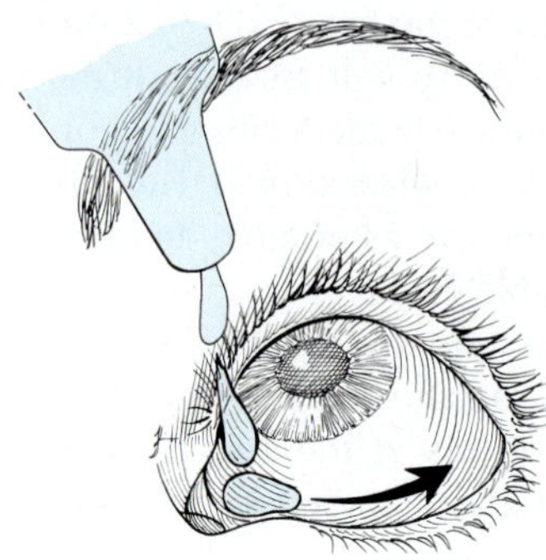

STEP 12

sodes of chemical or environmental hazards. The patient should understand discharge instructions, including the need for follow-up physician visits and symptoms to report. The nurse should determine the patient's knowledge about the progress of therapy.

Prognosis. Immediate and appropriate treatment reduces the severity and complications of eye injuries. The chosen treatment must be monitored to prevent permanent eye damage and vision problems. Superficial corneal abrasions usually heal without incident. Deeper abrasions or burns may result in permanent visual loss due to scarring.

SURGERIES OF THE EYE

Enucleation

Eye **enucleation** is the surgical removal of the eyeball. It is often necessary after severe eye trauma but may be done for other reasons, such as malignant tumors. Surgical methods vary from removal of the entire eyeball or the eyeball contents to removal of the eyeball and all underlying structures.

Nursing Interventions. Preoperative care includes determining the patient's feelings about the surgical intervention. It may be a welcome relief from pain and pressure of a malignancy. For other patients it is a disfiguring surgery that leads to a drastic change in life-style. Other nursing responsibilities include therapeutic dialogue between the physician and patient regarding the exact nature of the surgery. If a prosthesis (commonly called "glass eye") is used, the nurse should ensure that the patient understands its care.

Postoperatively a pressure dressing is applied over the socket of the eye to control hemorrhage. The nurse observes the dressing at least every hour for the first 24 hours. The patient is questioned about any pain on the affected side of the head or any headache, which might indicate hemorrhage or infection. These findings should be reported to the physician immediately. Routine postoperative procedures of coughing and turning on the affected side are discouraged to prevent sutures from dislodging.

Prognosis. Patients who undergo enucleation surgery are excellent candidates for prosthetic replacements. A prosthetic eye may be worn once healing occurs, usually in 4 to 6 weeks.

Keratoplasty (Corneal Transplant)

Keratoplasty is the excision of the corneal tissue, followed by surgical implantation of a cornea from another human donor. It is done to replace damaged cornea resulting from trauma, ulceration, or congenital deformities of the cornea. The surgery can be successful if the area of implantation is small. The possibility of donor rejection is high when large amounts of tissue replacement are required. Rejection normally begins about 3 weeks after surgery. Medications to suppress rejection (e.g., cyclosporine) may be ordered. If the cornea is perforated from ulcer formation or from surgical implantation, vision will be destroyed.

Corneal grafts are taken usually within 5 hours after death from a donor who is ideally between 25 and 35 years old. An appropriate donor is an individual who died of injury or acute disease. The corneas of persons with chronic or communicable diseases, such as hepatitis, AIDS, or cancer, are not appropriate for transplantation. The donor eye should have normal light perception and projection. The donor tissue is best used within 48 hours after removal. The nurse is often the individual most accessible to the family when questions of organ donation occur. Responsibilities would include notification of appropriate supervisory personnel.

Keratoplasty is performed with the patient under local or general anesthesia. The transplanted tissue is sutured into place to maintain graft alignment and a watertight wound.

Nursing Interventions. Preoperatively the nurse encourages the patient to express fears related to surgery and gives instructions in the use of protective eyeglasses if eye medication is used, causing dilation. The nurse maintains safety in the environment by use of safety devices and orienting the patient to each new environment. The surgical areas are cleansed and prepared as ordered, usually with an antiseptic solution. Preoperative teaching includes deep breathing and turning to reduce any complications associated with surgery. Coughing is discouraged, because sutures may break. Dietary restrictions, if ordered, should be maintained; a light breakfast may be allowed if the surgery is done with the patient under a local anesthesia. Prescribed medications are administered.

Postoperatively the nurse ensures that correct postoperative positioning is maintained; the patient is usually positioned on the back or nonoperated side until the physician allows turning to the operated side. Activity restrictions as ordered are reinforced to prevent injury to the eye. Safety measures are employed until the patient is able to ambulate safely. Anyone coming into the room should announce his or her presence. The patient should avoid bending, lifting, and straining for approximately 1 month to prevent intraocular pressure or suture tension.

Progressive activity should be prescribed by the physician. Regular postoperative visits with the eye surgeon should be encouraged. The nurse should report any severe or progressive pain to the surgeon immediately, as well as any complaints of erythema, loss of vision, or photophobia that would occur with corneal rejection. Systemic and ophthalmic medications are administered. Strict surgical asepsis must be maintained during dressing changes. Staff, the patient, and the family must wash hands thoroughly before any contact with the eye area. The patient should be instructed to avoid the use of such irritants as powder, perfume, and propellants, which might cause sneezing and displacement of sutures. The patient should not rub the eye area, or contamination of the site or suture displacement may result. The patient's diversional activities should be assessed; television is usually permitted, but reading is limited because of the side-to-side movement of the eyes. The lateral motion of the eye may cause loosening of sutures. If an eye patch or a metal eyecup shield is ordered, the nurse can demonstrate care. The eye patch is applied snugly to inhibit the blink reflex and allow the eye to rest. The metal eyecup shield is used during the night to protect the eye from trauma. Discharge instructions should be obtained from the physician regarding use of eyewear.

Prognosis. The cornea is avascular, therefore healing is slow. Incidence of infection is increased as a result. The transplanted donor tissue may be rejected. Incidence of rejection is reduced if the donor is a family member with similar tissue type.

Photocoagulation

Using a laser, a small, intense beam of light is directed into a small spot on the retina. Conversion into heat energy occurs and coagulation of tissue protein occurs, which is called *photocoagulation.*

Photocoagulation is a nonsurgical procedure usually performed on an outpatient basis. Without surgical intervention, the structures of the eye remain undisturbed and only the sealing of leakage and offending tissue destruction occurs.

Photocoagulation is useful in diabetic retinopathy to cauterize hemorrhaging vessels. It cannot increase visual acuity but can prevent further loss. Usually no hospitalization or postoperative medical management is required.

Nursing Interventions. Postoperative assessment for patients who have undergone photocoagulation therapy includes assessment of vision. There may be a constriction of peripheral fields, and central vision may temporarily be decreased. A decrease in night vision and a headache resulting from the laser's bright light may also occur.

Prognosis. Photocoagulation is used to prevent eye damage and is not curative. Minimal destruction of tissue occurs with photocoagulation. The procedure is nonsurgical; therefore, infection risk is minimal.

Vitrectomy

A vitrectomy is the removal of excess vitreous fluid caused by hemorrhage and replacing it with normal saline. Any scar tissue may also be removed.

Postoperative management includes the prescription of topical eye medication for 4 to 6 weeks. Acetaminophen or acetaminophen with codeine is prescribed for pain management.

A pressure patch to the operative eye is placed immediately after surgery. Ice packs to reduce inflammation are ordered.

Nursing Interventions. The patient is required to maintain a position on the abdomen or sitting forward resting the nonoperated side of the head on a table to allow air that is in the eye to float against the retina. These positions are maintained for 4 to 5 days. This is not required if oil has been injected into the eye during the vitrectomy instead of normal saline.

Dark glasses are prescribed postoperatively to decrease the discomfort of photophobia.

Postoperative assessment includes assessment of the eye patch, ice packs, and abnormal vital signs, especially fever. The dressing should be assessed for bleeding.

Patient teaching. The aspects of patient education are detailed in the patient teaching box on p. 1061.

Prognosis. The procedure has limited benefits and continues to be investigated as to its benefits versus complications.

CARE OF THE PATIENT WITH AN EAR DISORDER

Nursing Considerations

Once the history and general assessment have been done, the nurse should focus on aspects related to the ear. Additional information would include the following:

- Occurrence of ear drainage, tinnitus, vertigo, wax buildup, pressures, pain, and pruritus
- Behavioral clues indicating hearing loss (Box 34-3)
- History of medications used for ear disorders, specifically those known to be ototoxic
- Current medications for the ear disorder
- Side effects of medication, if any
- Associated speech pattern abnormalities
- Use of assistive hearing devices
- Home remedies that cause ear trauma

Box 34-3 BEHAVIORAL CLUES INDICATING HEARING LOSS

Any adult who
- Is irritable, hostile, hypersensitive in interpersonal relations
- Has difficulty in hearing upper frequency consonants
- Complains about people mumbling
- Turns up volume on television and radio
- Asks for frequent repetition and answers questions inappropriately
- Loses sense of humor, becomes grim
- Leans forward to hear better; face serious and strained
- Shuns large- and small-group audience situations
- May appear aloof and uninterested
- Complains of ringing in the ears
- Has an unusually soft or loud voice
- Repeatedly asks, "What did you say?"

The nurse communicates the gathered data to the appropriate personnel and documents the findings in the patient record. The next step in the assessment process is to prepare the patient for the initial otoscopic diagnostic evaluation.

Diagnostic Testing

Otoscopy. With an otoscope the examiner can visualize the external auditory canal and the eardrum, or tympanic membrane. Normally, the tympanic membrane is disk shaped and pearl gray or pale pink in color. This is the initial examination of the ear, performed before other testing. One responsibility of the nurse is to explain to the patient the purpose and procedure of otoscopy. The patient should be reassured that otoscopy is a painless test requiring only about 1 to 2 minutes, with slight pulling of the ear upward and backward during the procedure.

Tuning Fork Tests. The two most common tests using tuning forks are the Weber and Rinne tests. These tests are used to determine hearing loss as well as data related to the type of loss.

The Weber test is a method of assessing auditory acuity, especially useful in determining whether defective hearing in an ear is a conductive loss caused by a middle ear problem or a sensorineural loss, resulting from a disorder in the inner ear or auditory nerve system. The test is performed by placing the stem of a vibrating tuning fork in the center of the patient's forehead, or on the maxillary incisors. The loudness of the sound is equal in both ears if hearing is normal. If the person has a sensorineural loss in one ear, the unaffected ear perceives the sound as louder. When conductive hearing loss is present, the sound is louder in the affected ear, but it does not hear ordinary background noise conducted through the air and receives only vibrations by bone conduction (Fig. 34-10).

The Rinne test is a method of distinguishing conductive from sensorineural hearing loss. The test is performed with tuning forks placed ½ inch (1.25 cm) from the external auditory meatus and again with the vibrating stem placed over the mastoid bone. While one ear is tested, the other is masked (Fig. 34-11). In sensorineural loss the sound is heard longer by air conduction, while in conduction hearing loss the sound is heard longer by bone conduction.

Nursing responsibility in both the Weber and Rinne tests includes explanation of the purpose and procedure of the tests. The nurse should stress that the patient will need to concentrate and indicate through the use of hand signals in which ear or ears the sound is heard in the Weber test and when no longer heard in the Rinne test. In addition, the nurse should assure the patient that the test is painless and requires only a few minutes.

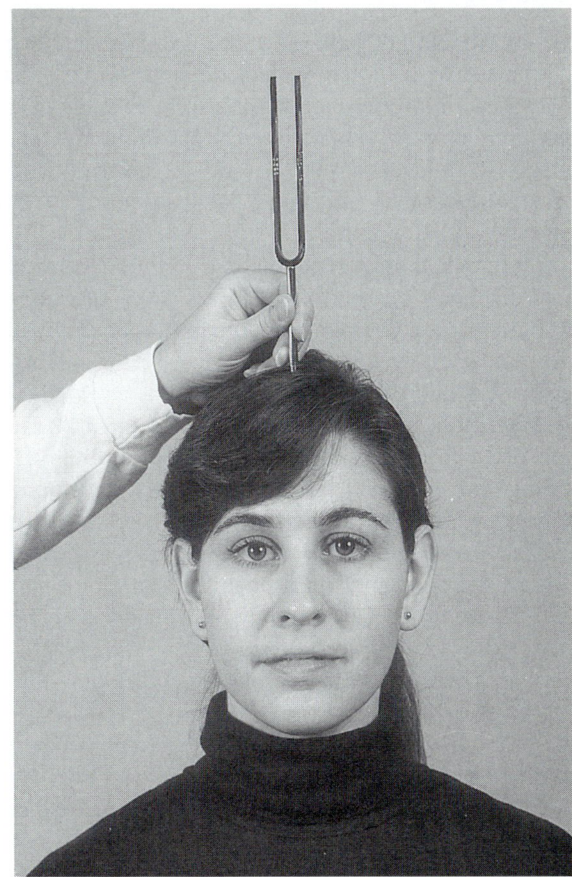

FIG. 34-10 Weber tuning fork test.

Audiometric Testing. **Audiometry** is a test of hearing acuity. Various audiometric tests determine the lowest intensity of sound at which an individual can perceive an auditory stimulus (hearing threshold), hear different frequencies, and distinguish different speech tones.

Nursing responsibilities include providing the patient with the purpose and procedure of each test. Any required responses by the patient should be reviewed.

Vestibular Tests. Vestibular testing measures balance and equilibrium. The Romberg and past-point tests are used for patients complaining of dizziness or disequilibrium.

The *Romberg test* measures the patient's ability to perform specific tasks with eyes open and then with eyes closed. The normal response is maintaining balance throughout the entire test. An abnormal response is indicative of loss of the sense of position (in which the patient loses the balance when standing erect, feet together, and eyes closed).

Past-point testing measures the patient's ability or inability to place a finger accurately on a selected point on some other part of the body. The inability to correctly perform the test indicates a lack of coordination in voluntary movements.

The nurse's responsibility is to explain the purpose and procedure of each test. Safety measures are taken to prevent patient injury during the Romberg test if the patient cannot maintain balance.

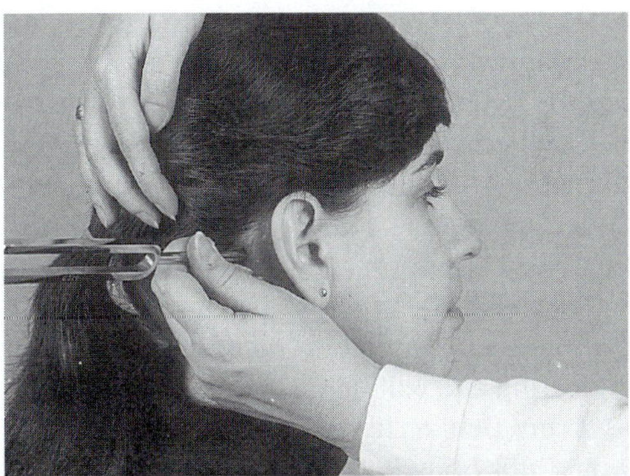

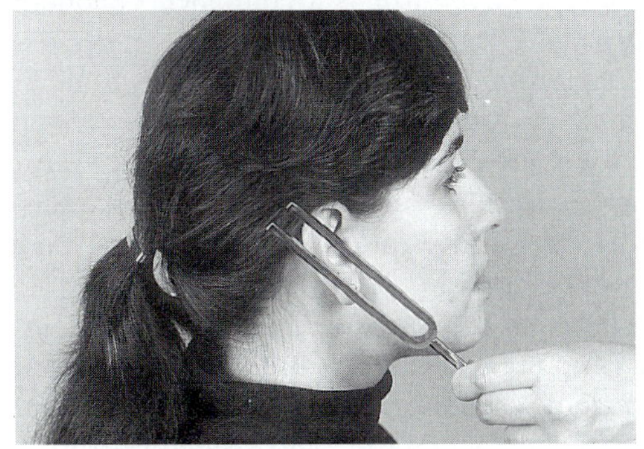

FIG. 34-11 Rinne tuning fork test.

Disorders of the Ear

Loss of Hearing (Deafness). Deafness is characterized by a partial or complete loss of hearing. Any ear disorder can cause interference with hearing to some degree. Interference with sound wave transmission can be caused by fluid accumulation and inflammations, fixation of the ossicles, and inner ear disorders that interfere with sound vibrations.

More than 6 million people in the United States have some degree of bilateral hearing loss. More than 50% of these people are over 65 years of age. Recognition, diagnosis, and early treatment may help to prevent further impairment and damage.

The implications of hearing loss are great. Hearing is needed to develop speech and conceptual ability; thus hearing loss may well affect personality development and intelligence test responses when the hearing impairment is severe and congenital. This may have implications for the person's education and socialization. As the loss of hearing increases, the person may socially withdraw because of the inability to understand and be understood; this could lead to isolation and depression.

Types of hearing loss. There are six types of hearing loss: conductive, sensorineural, mixed, congenital, simulated, and central.

In *conductive hearing loss*, sound is inadequately conducted through the external or middle ear to the sensorineural apparatus of the inner ear. A common cause is buildup of cerumen. Sensitivity to sound is diminished, but clarity or interpretation of the sound is not changed. When increased volume compensates for the loss, then hearing is normal; therefore a hearing aid can be helpful.

In *sensorineural hearing loss* sound is conducted through the external and middle ear in a normal way, but a defect in the inner ear results in its distortion, making discrimination difficult. This type of hearing loss is usually caused by trauma, infectious processes, presbycusis (hearing loss caused by aging), or exposure to ototoxic drugs. Destruction of cochlear hair by intense noise may also cause sensorineural loss. Amplifying sound, such as with a hearing aid, will help some people with this type of loss. Many people have an intolerance to loud noise and would not be helped by a hearing aid.

Mixed hearing loss is a combined conductive and sensorineural hearing loss.

Congenital hearing loss is present from birth or early infancy. Anoxia or trauma during delivery may be causes. Rh incompatibility may also be a cause. The mother's exposure during pregnancy to syphilis or rubella and the use of ototoxic drugs during pregnancy may also be causes.

Simulated hearing loss is a loss of hearing in which there is no organic cause. It is also known as functional psychogenic or nonorganic hearing loss. *Central hearing loss* occurs when the brain's auditory pathways are damaged, as in cerebrovascular accident.

Clinical manifestations. Clinical manifestations may vary, depending on the degree of deafness. Symptoms may range from such subtle clues as requests for repeating information to more obvious signs of nonresponse.

Assessment. Collection of *subjective data* includes noting the onset and progression of the condition, deficit in one or both ears, family history, history of head trauma, exposure to noise, current medications, visual or speech disorders, and any other ear symptoms.

Collection of *objective data* must include an assessment of behavioral clues that indicate a hearing difficulty. (See Box 34-3 for behavioral clues indicating difficulty hearing.)

Diagnostic tests. Conductive hearing loss produces lateralization of sound to the deaf ear in the Weber test. Results of the Rinne test show that sounds transmitted through bone conduction are heard longer than or equal to sounds transmitted through air conduction.

Sensorineural hearing loss produces lateralization of sound to the better ear in the Weber test. Results of the Rinne test show that air-conducted sounds are heard longer than bone-conducted sounds, but not twice as long.

Audiometric testing determines the type of hearing loss and the degree of impairment.

Medical management. Medical management depends on the type of impairment. Surgical procedures may be required. Hearing aids or cochlear implants may be used when appropriate. Cochlear implantation is performed in individuals with profound bilateral sensorineural hearing loss who receive no measurable assistance

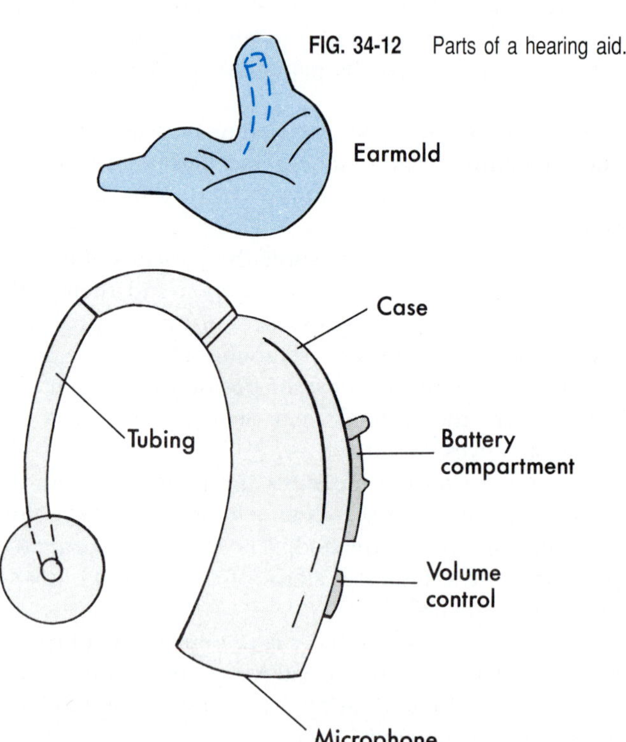

FIG. 34-12 Parts of a hearing aid.

from lip reading with a properly fitting hearing aid. The electrical activity of hearing is initiated by hair cells in the organ of Corti and sent to the brain along nerve fibers that make up the auditory nerve. In most deaf individuals, these hair cells are damaged. The goal of cochlear implantation is to bridge the gap created by the hair cell loss and directly stimulate the remaining neurons. Studies have shown that even when there is a complete loss of hair cells, a percentage of cochlear neurons remains. A small computer changes the spoken words into electrical impulses that are transmitted to an implanted cochlear coil.

Nursing interventions. Patients with partial hearing loss may benefit from a hearing aid (Fig. 34-12). The patient is assisted in caring for the hearing aid as detailed in Box 34-4.

A nursing diagnosis and an intervention for the patient with hearing loss include but are not limited to the following:

NURSING DIAGNOSIS	NURSING INTERVENTION
Sensory/perceptual alterations (auditory), related to disease process	Facilitate communication with the patient by following the interventions provided in Box 34-5.

Patient teaching. The nurse assists the patient in learning to care for a hearing aid, if prescribed. The patient can be instructed to request that others speak slowly or more clearly and repeat if necessary.

Prognosis. Surgical repair of the injured structures increases the likelihood of restoring partial or complete hearing, especially when implants are used. Complications of surgery are rare. Technical advances have also improved the quality of hearing. Microtechnology has reduced the size of hearing aids until they are almost undetectable.

Box 34-4 CARE OF THE HEARING AID

- Wash earmold or plug daily in mild soap and water, using a pipe cleaner to cleanse the cannula.
- Dry earmold or plug thoroughly before reconnecting it to the receiver.
- Keep an extra battery and cord available at all times.
- When hearing aid is not in use, turn aid off and open battery compartment.
- If hearing aid whistles, reinsert earmold.
- If hearing aid fails to work:
  - Check the on-off switch
  - Inspect earmold for cleanliness
  - Examine battery for tightness of fit
  - Examine cord plug for tightness of insertion
  - Examine cord for breaks
  - Replace battery and/or cord

Inflammatory and Infectious Disorders of the Ear

External Otitis.

Etiology/pathophysiology. External otitis or otitis externa is an inflammation or infection of the external canal or the auricle of the external ear and is sometimes called *swimmer's ear.* External otitis may be acute or chronic.

Box 34-5 FACILITATING COMMUNICATION FOR PERSONS WITH IMPAIRED HEARING

- Get the person's attention by raising an arm or hand.
- Start with the light on your face; this will help the person speech read.
- Face the person when speaking.
- Speak clearly, but do not overaccentuate words.
- Speak in a normal tone; do not shout or raise the pitch of voice. Shouting overemploys normal speaking movements and may cause distortion and be too loud for the person with sensorineural damage. If the person has conductive loss only, sometimes making the voice louder without shouting is helpful.
- If the person does not seem to understand what is said, express it differently. Some words are difficult to "see" in speech reading, such as *white* or *red.*
- Move closer to the person and toward the better ear if the person does not hear you.
- Write out proper names or any statement that you are not sure was understood.
- Do not chew gum or cover the mouth when talking to a person with limited hearing.
- Observe for inattention that may indicate tiredness or lack of understanding.
- Use phrases to convey meaning rather than one-word answers. State the major topic of the discussion first and then give details.
- Do not show annoyance by careless facial expression. Persons who are hard of hearing depend more on visual clues for acceptance.
- Encourage the use of a hearing aid if the person has one; allow the person to adjust it before speaking.
- If in a group, repeat important statements and avoid asides to others in the group.
- Avoid the use of the intercommunication system as this may distort sound and cause poor communication.
- Do not avoid conversation with a person who has hearing loss.

Adapted from Conover M, Cober J: *Nurs Clin North Am* 5:497, 1970.

External otitis can be caused by allergy, bacteria, fungi, viruses, and trauma. Allergic reaction can stem from nickel or chromium in earrings. In addition, chemicals in hair sprays, cosmetics, hearing aids, and medications, especially sulfonamides and neomycin, are common sources of allergy. Common bacterial agents are *Staphylococcus aureus, Pseudomonas aeruginosa,* and *Streptococcus pyogenes.* Frequently the viruses herpes simplex and herpes zoster are implicated. The external ear may also be affected by eczema, psoriasis, and seborrheic dermatitis. Fungi such as *Aspergillus* and *Candida* may also be causes. External otitis is more prevalent during hot, humid weather.

Trauma from cleaning or scratching the ear canal with a foreign object, such as a cotton swab, bobby pin, or finger, may result in irritation and possible introduction of infectious organisms. Certain activities allow moisture to become trapped in the ear, creating medium for infection; these include use of earphones, hearing aids, earplugs, earmuffs, and stethoscopes. Excessive swimming may wash out the protective cerumen, remove skin lipids, and lead to secondary infection.

Malignant external otitis is a rare, lethal form caused by *Pseudomonas* and occurring mostly in patients with diabetes. It is a bone-destroying infection that quickly involves all surrounding ear structures.

Clinical manifestations. The acute inflammatory or infectious process produces pain with movement of the auricle or chewing, and often the entire side of the head aches. Erythema, scaling, pruritus, edema, watery discharge, and crusting of the external ear may occur.

With chronic external otitis there is usually pruritus, but no pain with movement of the auricle. A discharge is also present.

Assessment. Collection of *subjective data* includes determining the onset, duration, and severity of pain, which is crucial to the assessment of inflammatory disease of the ear. The patient should be questioned about any home remedies used to treat infections. Knowledge of preventive measures is also assessed.

Collection of *objective data* includes noting a discharge, which may be watery or yellow and tenacious with a fetid odor. The discharge will be black if from a fungal infection. There may be a partial loss of hearing or the feeling that the ear is occluded if the ear canal is edematous or is obstructed by adenoids. Palpation of the external ear may produce pain.

Diagnostic tests. A culture of the exudate is obtained to identify bacterial, viral, or fungal organisms.

Medical management. Oral analgesics such as codeine may be used if the pain is severe. Corticosteroids (1% hydrocortisone) may be used to reduce edema and to allow antibiotics to penetrate. A wick is inserted into the ear canal to prevent loss of medication from the canal and maintain continuous absorption of the medicine. The physician orders frequency of the wick change. Antimicrobial agents such as antibiotic or antifungal ear drops may be used. The most commonly used contain 0.5% neomycin or 10,000 U/ml of polymyxin B. Systemic antibiotics are used only if the infection is severe. The specific antibiotic used will be based on the results of the culture.

Nursing interventions. The ear canal is carefully cleansed (Skill 34-3). Heat may be applied to the external ear for pain relief. An adequate method of communication is implemented. Ear drops are instilled (see Skill 21-7).

Acute external otitis may become a chronic problem. If the infection remains untreated and enters the brain, death can occur.

A nursing diagnosis and interventions for the patient with external otitis include but are not limited to the following:

NURSING DIAGNOSIS	NURSING INTERVENTIONS
Pain, related to inflammatory process	Apply warm compresses as ordered. Administer prescribed analgesics, and instill ordered ear medications.

Patient teaching. The nurse ensures that the patient has the knowledge to prevent further infection and can care for the infected ear.

Prognosis. External otitis responds favorably to topical antibiotic and corticosteroid ear drops. Systemic antibiotics are rarely required unless cellulitis is present. The rare malignant external otitis media has a mortality of 50% to 75% unless the condition is treated.

Otitis Media.

Etiology/pathophysiology. Otitis media, an inflammation or infection of the middle ear, is the most common disorder of the middle ear. Acute otitis media is most often caused by *Haemophilus influenzae* or *Streptococcus pneumoniae.* Chronic otitis media is usually caused by gram-negative bacteria, such as *Proteus, Klebsiella,* and *Pseudomonas.* In addition, allergy, mycoplasma, and several viruses may be factors.

Otitis media occurs more frequently in children, especially at 6 to 36 months of age, in the winter and early spring. Children's shorter and straighter eustachian tubes provide easier access of the organisms for the nasopharynx to travel to the middle ear.

The patient usually has had a recent upper respiratory infection. The infection ascends via the eustachian tube and involves the lining of the entire middle ear. Usually only one ear is affected.

Viral infections frequently cause a serous otitis media. Retraction of the tympanic membrane occurs with a buildup of sterile serous exudate. If there is a secondary bacterial infection, purulent exudate collects behind the tympanic membrane, causing it to bulge. This is called *purulent otitis media.*

EAR IRRIGATION

Nursing Action

1. Review physician's order.
2. Identify patient.
3. Wash hands and don gloves.
4. Assess condition or external ear structures and canal for erythema, edema, and exudate.
5. Arrange supplies and equipment. Provide privacy.
6. Explain steps of procedure, and advise patient of sensations that might be experienced: vertigo, fullness, and warmth.
7. Assist patient to either a side-lying or a sitting position with head tilted toward affected ear. Position emesis basin under ear. (Patient may help hold basin).
8. Place towel under patient's shoulder just under ear and emesis basin.
9. Inspect auditory canal for any accumulation of cerumen or debris. Remove with cotton applicator and solution.
10. Check irrigating solution for proper temperature (body temperature 98.6° F [37° C]). Test temperature of solution by sprinkling a few drops on inner wrist. Fill bulb syringe with appropriate volume.
11. Straighten auditory canal for introduction of solution. In infants, pull auricle (or pinna) down and back. In adults, pull auricle up and back.
12. With tip of syringe just above canal, irrigate gently by creating steady flow of solution against roof of canal (see illustration). *Do not occlude canal with tip of syringe.*
13. Continue irrigation until all debris has been removed or all solution has been used.
14. Assess patient for vertigo or nausea. Onset of symptoms may require temporary cessation of procedure.
15. Dry off auricle, and apply cotton ball loosely to auditory meatus.
16. Position patient on side of affected ear for 10 minutes.
17. Remove equipment and gloves. Wash hands.
18. Return to patient to assess character and amount of drainage, and determine patient's level of comfort.
19. Record in nurse's notes patient's response to irrigation and note type, temperature, and volume of solution used and character of exudate. Record assessment of the ear canal before and after irrigation.
20. Return to patient after 10 minutes to remove cotton ball and reassess drainage. Patient may resume normal level of activity.

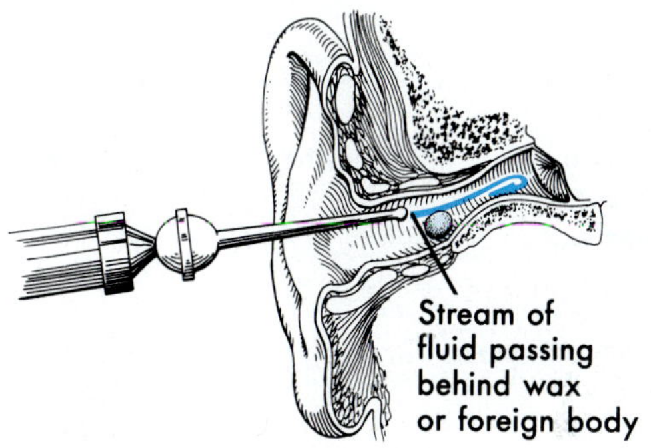

STEP 12

Clinical manifestations. The patient will experience a sense of fullness in the ear and also have severe, deep throbbing pain behind the tympanic membrane. This severe pain may disappear if the tympanic membrane ruptures. Hearing loss, **tinnitus** (a subjective noise sensation heard in one or both ears), and fever may also be present.

Assessment. For information on collection of *subjective data,* refer to the discussion of external otitis, p. 1076.

Collection of *objective data* is the same as for external otitis, with the exception of noting pain on palpation of the external ear.

Diagnostic tests. A culture of the purulent drainage is obtained to identify the causative organisms.

Medical management. Antibiotic therapy is based on results of the culture. Analgesics such as codeine are prescribed for severe pain. Sedatives are prescribed for children to provide rest and pain relief. Local heat is used and nasal decongestants are ordered. See the medication table on pp. 1078-1079 for drugs used in the treatment of otitis media and other ear disorders.

Needle aspiration of secretions collected behind the tympanic membrane may be necessary. Myringotomy—a surgical incision of the tympanic membrane to relieve pressure and release purulent exudate from the middle ear—may be required.

Nursing interventions. Inner ear pressure may cause discomfort, requiring pain medication to be prescribed. Sedatives may be ordered for young children.

Hearing loss may also occur. Effective communication is essential. Parents of young patients should be alerted to the fact and their help enlisted in monitoring the level of loss.

MEDICATIONS FOR EAR DISORDERS

Medication	Trade Name	Action	Side Effects	Nursing Implications
Carbamide peroxide	Debrox	Cerumen removal	Contact dermatitis	Do not use if eardrum is perforated or if there is ear discharge. Is not recommended for children. Avoid eyes. Reevaluate if edema, erythema, or pain persists. Use proper administration technique by allowing drops to enter ear canal and not touching dropper.
Colistin/neomycin/hydrocortisone/thonzonium	Coly-Mycin S Otic	Antibiotic/steroid/detergent indicated for susceptible disease of external auditory canal, mastoidectomy, and otitis media fenestration	Ototoxicity in prolonged use Contact dermatitis Hypersensitivity, including puritus, skin rash, erythema, and edema	Do not heat bottle above body temperature With herpes simplex, do not use if patient is infected. Do not use if eardrum is perforated. Use for 10 days only. Keep dropper from touching skin. Check with physician if signs and symptoms worsen or do not improve after 1 week. Shake well before using. Use cotton plug to keep moist; change plug daily.
Triethanolamine polypeptide oleate condensate	Cerumenex	Cerumen removal	Contact dermatitis	Fill ear canal. Insert cotton plug after 15 to 30 min. Irrigate ear canal with warm water.
Amoxicillin trihydrate	Amoxil	System penicillin antibiotic used in acute otitis media	Anaphylaxis Skin rash Diarrhea	Use caution during pregnancy and lactation. Take for full treatment period. Consult with physician if no improvement occurs in a few days. Take on full or empty stomach. Check with physician about treating diarrhea. Do not give if patient has penicillin or cephalosporin allergy.
Cefaclor	Ceclor	Second generation cephlosporin used to treat amoxicillin-resistant otitis media	Anaphylaxis Skin rash Joint pain Fever Diarrhea Abdominal cramping	Use proper administration technique if suspension is given. Store suspension in refrigerator. Give on full or empty stomach. Give full course of therapy. Tell patient not to use alcohol. Do not give if patient has penicillin or cephalosporin allergies.

MEDICATIONS FOR EAR DISORDERS—cont'd

Medication	Trade Name	Action	Side Effects	Nursing Implications
Meclizine hydrochloride	Antivert	Anticholinergic antihistamine that acts as antiemetic, antivertigo agent Treatment and prophylixis Possible effectiveness for diseases affecting vestibular system	Drowsiness Blurred vision Dry mouth	Use caution during pregnancy and breastfeeding. Give with food, water, or milk. Tell patient to avoid alcohol and CNS depressants. Is not recommended for children under 12.
Dimenhydrinate	Dramamine	Anticholinergic antihistamine used in treatment of vertigo	Blurred vision Drowsiness Shortness of breath Painful urination Disorientation	Know that antihistamines may inhibit lactation. Give no CNS depressants. Give with food or milk. Use caution during pregnancy in early months.
Antipyrine/ benzocaine	Auralgan	Analgesic Local anesthetic Otitis media adjunct to cerumen removal	Contact dermatitis	Use caution during pregnancy and lactation. Date bottle and discard after 6 mo from first use. Do not use if eardrums are perforated. Warm bottle. Position patient on side and fill ear canal. Use cotton plug. Wash dropper before replacing in bottle.
Acetic acid	Vo Sol Hydrochloride Otic	Antibacterial Antifungal Astringent Superficial infections of external auditory canal	Contact dermatitis Transient stinging	Clean ear first. Use cotton plug for first 24 hr. Contact physician if condition worsens or no improvement occurs after 5 to 7 days. Do not wash dropper; doing so may dilute medication.
Sulfamethoxazole trimethoprim	Bactrim	Systemic antibacterial Acute otitis media No sulfonamide allergy	Fever Itching Skin rash Photosensitivity Dizziness	Is not recommended when breastfeeding or during pregnancy Emphasize importance of proper dental care. Know that blood glucose levels may be affected in patients using oral antidiabetic agents. Maintain adequate fluid intake. Advise patient to avoid sun exposure. Complete treatment. With pediatric suspension, shake well.
Polymixin B/neomycin/ hydrocortisone	Cortisporin	Antibiotic and steroid used same as Coly-Mycin S	Ototoxicity in prolonged use Contact dermititis pruritus Erythema Edema	Use caution during pregnancy and lactation. Do not use if eardrum is perforated. Keep dropper from touching skin. Shake well before using. Use cotton plug to keep moist; change plug daily.

Chronic otitis media caused by repeated attacks of acute otitis media may result in a permanent perforation of the tympanic membrane. The result is a slight to moderate conductive hearing loss.

A growth called *cholesteatoma* occurs when a tympanic membrane perforation allows squamous epithelium of the external auditory canal to enter and grow in the middle ear. Enlargement is slow, but the mass can expand into the mastoid antrum and destroy adjacent structures.

Mastoiditis, which is an infection of one of the mastoid bones, may develop. It is usually an extension of a middle ear infection that was untreated or inadequately treated. Signs of mastoiditis should be reported immediately, including earache, fever, headache, malaise, and large amounts of purulent exudate.

A nursing diagnosis and interventions for the patient with otitis media include but are not limited to the following:

NURSING DIAGNOSIS	NURSING INTERVENTIONS
Skin integrity, impaired, related to edema and exudate	Note and report any outer ear purulent exudate. Keep ear clean and dry; sterile cotton may be used to absorb drainage, if ordered. Monitor temperature, and report changes.

PATIENT TEACHING FOR EAR INFECTION

Prevention of Further Infection

- Protect ear canal during showers (cotton with petrolatum in external canal; use a shower cap over ears).
- Avoid swimming during infection or following a perforated eardrum; avoid swimming in contaminated water when infection is healed.
- Continue antibiotic therapy for prescribed number of days, even when symptoms disappear.
- Get adequate and early treatment of upper respiratory tract infections and allergic conditions.

Care of Infected Ear

- Use correct ear drop insertion or ear irrigations, as prescribed.
- Wash hands before and after changing cotton plugs to prevent secondary infection.
- Keep external ear clean and dry to protect skin from drainage.

Signs Requiring Medical Attention

- Fever
- Return of ear pain or discharge

Patient teaching. The nurse should ensure that the patient and parents are aware of the necessity to complete the entire course of antibiotic therapy. Children are to be fed upright to prevent nasopharyngeal flora from entering the eustachian tube. The patient is instructed to blow the nose gently and not forcefully. If a myringotomy has been performed, the patient and parents are instructed to change the cotton in the outer ear at least twice a day (see the patient teaching box).

Prognosis for otitis media. Middle ear infections usually resolve completely with systemic antibiotic therapy. Chronic or untreated otitis media may lead to sound transmission hearing loss, which is successfully treated with tympanoplasty.

Prognosis for mastoiditis. The infection is difficult to treat and may require antibiotic therapy, intravenously, for several days. Since children are most often affected, immediate treatment of the infection is crucial. Residual hearing loss may follow the infection. If early decalcification is present, intense antibiotic therapy and myringotomy can usually cure mastoiditis; if it has progressed to further destruction, simple mastoidectomy is necessary (see patient teaching box).

Labyrinthitis.

Etiology/pathophysiology. **Labyrinthitis** is an inflammation of the labyrinthine canals of the inner ear. Labyrinthitis is the most common cause of **vertigo** (the sensation that the outer world is revolving about oneself or that one is moving in space). A common cause is a viral upper respiratory infection that spreads into the inner ear; other causes include certain drugs and foods. The vestibular portion of the inner ear may be destroyed by streptomycin. Tobacco and alcohol may also be causative factors. A rarer form of labyrinthitis is caused by bacteria. It is usually associated with middle ear and mastoid infections.

Clinical manifestations. Severe and sudden vertigo are the most common symptoms of labyrinthitis. Also present are nausea and vomiting, nystgamus, photophobia, headache, and ataxic gait.

Assessment. Collection of *subjective data* should include noting the frequency and duration of the vertigo, as well as any safety measures taken by the patient during an attack. Other symptoms, such as hearing ability, ringing in the ears, and nausea, are assessed. Because fear is associated with the attacks, the patient's feelings should be explored.

Collection of *objective data* includes noting vomiting as well as any jerking movement of the eyeballs, unilaterally or bilaterally. The color and moisture of skin are assessed to determine the extent of autonomic response.

Diagnostic tests. Electronystagmography may show a diminished or absent nystagmus with stimulation. Audiometric testing shows a low-tone sensorineural hearing loss.

Medical management. There is no specific treatment for labyrinthitis. Usually antibiotics and dimenhydrinate (Dramamine) or meclizine HCl (Antivert) for vertigo are prescribed. If nausea and vomiting persist, parenteral fluids are administered.

Nursing interventions. It is important to note the frequency and degree of vertigo. Antibiotics and medications for vertigo are administered. Fluid intake is assessed to ensure dehydration does not occur.

A nursing diagnosis and interventions for the patient with labyrinthitis include but are not limited to the following:

NURSING DIAGNOSIS	NURSING INTERVENTIONS
Injury, high risk for, related to altered sensory perception (vertigo)	Keep side rails up. Note presence of vertigo before patient ambulates. Supervise ambulation. Caution the patient not to attempt ambulation alone and to call for assistance.

Patient teaching. The nurse instructs the patient concerning vertigo using the information in the patient teaching box.

Prognosis. Labyrinthitis usually resolves itself with little or no hearing impairment.

Obstructions of the Ear.

Etiology/pathophysiology. Ear canal obstruction is usually caused by impaction or excessive secretion of cerumen or by foreign bodies, including insects. Children often place beans, beads, pebbles, and small toys in their ears. Usually those objects are found on routine examination.

Obstruction by cerumen can be caused when excessive amounts are produced by overactive glands, or from impaction of cerumen in narrow or tortuous ear canals.

Clinical manifestations. The obstruction may cause the ear to feel occluded. There may be presence of tinnitus or "buzzing," pain in the ear, and slight hearing loss.

Assessment. Collection of *subjective data* includes interviewing the patient about any possible foreign bodies being introduced into the ear and any home remedies used to remove the object. If the patient is a child, determination is made of risk factors causing ear obstructions, such as beads or nuts.

Collection of *objective data* involves the nurse noting any presence of a foreign body in the external ear canal. Children are observed for tugging of the pinna.

Diagnostic tests. Otoscopic examination provides visualization of the cause of the obstruction.

PATIENT TEACHING FOR VERTIGO

- Nature of the disorder
  - Physiological basis for the vertigo
  - Avoidance of any known precipitating factors
  - Rationale for a low-salt diet
- Actions to take during an attack
  - Lie down immediately, and call for help if necessary at the first signs of an attack
  - If driving when an attack occurs, pull over immediately to the curb
  - Lie immobile, and hold head in one position until vertigo lessens
- Ask for assistance when ambulating if dizzy
- Take prescribed medications as instructed even if no recent attacks have occurred; check with physician before discontinuing any medication
- Symptoms requiring medical attention: changes in symptoms or nature of attacks

Medical management. Medical management includes removal of cerumen by irrigation or cerumen spoon. Foreign objects are removed with forceps, if possible. Insects are smothered with drops of an oily substance and removed with forceps. Medications, such as carbamide peroxide 6.5%, may be used to soften cerumen. Surgical removal of the foreign object may be necessary.

Nursing interventions. The nurse assists with the irrigation of the ear (see Skill 34-4). Medications are instilled into the ear as ordered.

A nursing diagnosis and interventions for the patient with obstructions of the ear include but are not limited to the following:

NURSING DIAGNOSIS	NURSING INTERVENTIONS
Sensory/perceptual alterations (auditory), related to presence of foreign body causing obstruction	Note the presence and amount of hearing impairment and/or tinnitus. Assure the patient or parents that once the obstruction is removed, any hearing loss or tinnitus should disappear.

Patient teaching. The nurse informs the patient and parents about the danger of placing objects in the ears. The nurse also reinforces the method for preventing cerumen obstruction through the instilling of 1 to 2 drops of an oily substance at night. This is followed by hydrogen peroxide in the morning and cleaning with a soft cotton wick.

Prognosis. Ear canal obstructions due to cerumen and foreign bodies resolve completely with treatment. Vertigo may be experienced temporarily until the ear canal dries. Disorientation in the older adult may occur from the cerumen impaction and temporary loss of hearing.

Noninfectious Disorders of the Ear

Otosclerosis.

Etiology/pathophysiology. Ostosclerosis is a condition characterized by chronic progressive deafness caused by the formation of spongy bone, especially around the oval window, with resulting ankylosis (immobility of a joint) of the stapes, causing tinnitus and then deafness.

The cause is unknown, although about half of the patients with the disease have a family history of the disease. Women are affected twice as often as men. Frequently pregnancy triggers a rapid onset of this condition. Previous ear infections are not believed to be related to otosclerosis.

Gradual replacement of normal bone, in the otic capsula, by highly vascular otosclerotic bone occurs. This replacement bone is described as spongy. Calcification of the area follows, and conductive hearing loss is then produced.

Clinical manifestations. The patient with otosclerosis will experience a slowly progressive conductive hearing loss and will describe a low- to medium-pitched tinnitus. The deafness is usually first noted between the ages of 11 and 20.

Assessment. Collection of *subjective data* includes noting the degree and progression of hearing loss or tinnitus as well as mild dizziness to vertigo. Family history for the disease is assessed.

Collection of *objective data* includes assessment of behavioral clues related to hearing loss as in Box 34-3.

Diagnostic tests. Otoscopy will reveal a normal eardrum. A pink blush called *Schwartz's sign* may be seen through the ear; this is indicative of a high degree of vascularity in active otosclerotic bone. The result of the Rinne test shows sounds transmitted by bone conduction lasting longer than by air conduction in the affected ear. The Weber test results are the reverse from normal hearing. Audiometric testing shows a lateralization of sound more to the affected ear. The Weber test in otosclerosis would result in a lateralization of sound to the affected ear. Audiometric testing may show minimal to total hearing loss. Tympanometry may reveal evidence of stiffness in the sound conduction system. Hearing loss ranges from mild in the early stages to total loss in the later stages.

Medical management. Otosclerosis is usually treated with a stapedectomy to restore hearing (see stapedectomy, p. 1083). When a stapedectomy is not indicated, an air conduction hearing aid may be prescribed.

Nursing interventions. Nursing diagnoses and interventions of otosclerosis are specific to poststapedectomy care. (See pp. 1083 and 1085).

Patient teaching. Refer to the discussion on ear surgery, p.1086.

Prognosis. Patients report varying degrees of success with hearing following stapedectomy surgery. For some patients stapedectomy is successful in permanently restoring hearing. A hearing aid may further enhance sound conduction to more normal levels.

Ménière's Disease.

Etiology/pathophysiology. Ménière's disease is a chronic disease of the inner ear characterized by recurrent episodes of vertigo, progressive unilateral nerve deafness, and tinnitus.

Ménière's disease is most common in women between the ages of 50 and 60 years. The cause is unknown, although occasionally the condition follows middle ear infection or trauma to the head.

There is an increase in endolymph fluid, either from increased production or decreased absorption. This causes increased pressure in the inner ear labyrinth. Attacks of severe vertigo, tinnitus, and progressive deafness result from this increased pressure. Usually one ear only is involved.

Clinical manifestations. The patient experiences recurrent episodes of vertigo with associated nausea and tinnitus, and hearing loss may be present. During an attack, vomiting, diaphoresis, and nystagmus may occur. These attacks last from a few minutes to several hours. Sudden movements often aggravate the symptoms.

Assessment. Collection of *subjective data* includes noting the frequency and severity of the vertigo attack. History and knowledge of the disorder and circumstances that precipitate an attack are noted. Assessment is made of actions taken by the patient during an attack and the degree of relief those actions provide.

Collection of *objective data* includes determining unilateral or bilateral hearing loss. The nurse observes the patient for associated signs during an attack.

Diagnostic tests. Audiologic tuning fork tests show a sensorineural deficit. Vestibular testing shows lack of balance.

Medical management. There is no specific therapy for Ménière's disease. Fluid restriction, diuretics, and a low-salt diet are prescribed in an attempt to decrease fluid pressure.

Dimenhydrinate (Dramamine), meclizine HCl (Antivert), and diphenhydramine (Benadryl) are prescribed for use between attacks. In acute attacks the medications may be given intravenously. Atropine is also given for its anticholinergic effect during these acute attacks.

For preservation of hearing, surgical procedures may be performed. Approximately 5% to 10% of the patients with Ménière's disease require surgery. These surgeries and subsequent nursing interventions are discussed in Table 34-6.

Nursing interventions. The nurse should maintain the prescribed low-salt diet and administer diuretics as

TABLE 34-6 Surgery for Ménière's Disease

Type	Description	Residual	Postoperative Nursing Interventions
Surgical destruction of labyrinth	Extraction of membranous labyrinth by suction; access to inner ear through external canal (stapes and incus removed)	Destroys remaining hearing	Bed rest and NPO until vertigo subsides in 1 to 3 days Avoid sudden movement of head for 1 to 2 weeks Take action to prevent falls from unsteadiness for 1 to 3 weeks
Endolymphatic subarachnoid shunt	Insertion of drain tube from endolymphatic sac into subarachnoid space; access through mastoid	Preserves hearing in 60% to 70% of patients	Monitor for vertigo (rare)
Cryosurgery	Application of intense cold to lateral semicircular canals to decrease sensitivity or to create an otic-periotic shunt; access through mastoid	Preserves hearing in 80% of patients	Monitor for dizziness for 2 days Take action to prevent falls from unsteadiness for 2 to 3 weeks
Vestibular nerve section	Dissection of cranial nerve VIII (vestibular portion); access through mastoid or through cranial drilling over roof of internal auditory canal	Preserves hearing in 90% of patients	Same as for surgical destruction of labyrinth

ordered. The patient may have some auditory deficit, which will require alternate methods of communication. If the patient's tinnitus becomes distressing, an increase in background noise, such as music, may provide relief.

A nursing diagnosis and interventions for the patient with Ménière's disease include but are not limited to the following:

NURSING DIAGNOSIS	NURSING INTERVENTIONS
Injury, high risk for, related to sensory-perceptual alterations (vertigo)	Keep side rails up. Assist with ambulation, and instruct the patient to call for assistance before attempting to ambulate. Have the patient sit or lie down when vertigo occurs. Have the patient move slowly and avoid turning the head suddenly. Administer medications, as prescribed. Position patient on unaffected side. Stand in front of patient, and prevent head turning. Avoid bright or glaring lights around patient. Place all needed supplies so that patient does not have to turn head.

Patient teaching. The nurse provides information about a low-salt diet and taking diuretics. The patient should be warned to avoid reading when vertigo or tinnitus is present. The patient is instructed to avoid smoking to prevent vasoconstriction. The patient should learn to identify precipitating factors and the proper actions to take when an attack occurs: (1) sit or lie down immediately, (2) stop the care and pull over to the side of the road, and (3) keep medication available at all times. See nursing care plan on p. 1084 for patient with Ménière's disease.

Prognosis. There are usually several yearly attacks until the disease either resolves itself or progresses to complete deafness in the affected ear.

SURGERIES OF THE EAR

Stapedectomy

Stapedectomy is the removal of the stapes of the middle ear and insertion of a graft and prosthesis. The stapes that has become fixed is replaced so that vibrations can again transmit sound waves through the oval window to the fluid of the inner ear. This is performed to restore hearing in the treatment of otosclerosis.

Using a local anesthetic, the surgeon removes the stapes, and the opening into the inner ear is covered with a graft of body tissue. One end of a small plastic tube or piece of stainless steel wire is attached to the graft, while

NURSING CARE PLAN ***THE PATIENT WITH MÉNIÈRE'S DISEASE***

Ms. Lucas is a 66-year-old patient admitted with Ménière's disease. She complains of dizziness, nausea, ringing in the ears, and an unsteady gait. She is accompanied by her husband of 35 years.

Nursing diagnoses	Patient goals/expected outcomes	Nursing interventions
Anxiety, related to effects of disorder	Patient will experience decreased signs of anxiety.	Encourage patient to explore concerns about decreased hearing and effects of vertigo attacks and to take action in relation to the concerns. Explore patient's knowledge of the disorder and correct misunderstandings. Encourage realistic hope about expected hearing ability as described by physician. Refer patient to necessary support services, such as social worker or audiologist.
Sensory/perceptual alterations: vestibular, auditory, related to disease process	Patient will describe actions to avoid vertigo. Patient will interact with others accurately.	Help patient identify avoidable actions that precipitate vertigo attacks. Encourage patient to move slowly and not turn head suddenly when vertigo is present. If tinnitus is distressing, increase background noises such as music. If hearing is decreased: a. Use measures to facilitate communication with hearing impaired. b. Refer patient to audiologist, if appropriate.
Injury, high risk for, and trauma, related to vertigo	Patient will not sustain injury.	Keep side rails up when patient with vertigo is in bed. Assist with ambulation as needed. Encourage patient to sit or lie down and to remain immobile if signs of dizziness occur. Teach patient to stop car at side of road immediately at first signs of dizziness while driving.
Bathing/hygiene, dressing/grooming, feeding, toileting, self-care deficit, potential, related to sensory/perceptual disturbances	ADL needs will be met. Patient will function as independently as condition permits.	Provide desired foods and fluids if nausea is present. Assist with hygiene as needed while encouraging independence; place hygiene supplies so that patient does not have to turn head. Provide sufficient time for ADLs so patient can move slowly.

Ineffective coping, individual, related to anxiety	Patient will identify coping pattern and resultant effects. Patient will describe alternative coping behaviors.	Make decisions regarding safety of patient and others when patient is unable to do so. Assist patient to identify usual coping behaviors and the consequences of the behaviors. Assist patient to identify personal strengths. Teach patient alternative coping behaviors (see Chapter 46).
Knowledge deficit, related to unfamiliarity with treatment	Patient will describe nature of disorder, therapy, and safety measures.	Teach patient about the disorder, therapy, and need for medical follow-up. Teach patient ways to protect self from injury and to prevent vertigo attacks when possible.

CRITICAL THINKING QUESTIONS

1. Ms. Lucas states that she would prefer going to the bathroom without the assistance of a nurse. The appropriate response by the nurse would be:
2. Ms. Lucas tells the nurse that she is very depressed because of her very unpleasant symptoms and wonders if she will ever feel well again. A therapeutic reply would be:
3. The nurse notes an unpleasant odor from Ms. Lucas; her hair is unkempt, and she has poor oral hygiene. The nurse is preparing to give her a warm, therapeutic bed bath. Ms. Lucas states, "I feel too dizzy to take a bath." To promote personal hygiene and patient compliance, the nurse would:

the other end is attached to the two remaining bones of the middle ear, the malleus and the incus.

Nursing Interventions. Postoperative management consists of an external ear packing to ensure healing; the packing is left in place 5 or 6 days. The patient should remain in bed for approximately 24 hours, depending on physician preference. Gradual activity, when allowed, is provided. The patient is kept flat with the operative side facing upward to maintain the position of the prosthesis and graft; therefore the nurse makes certain that the patient is not turned. Headache and dizziness are expected early in the postoperative period. The patient's hearing does not improve until the edema subsides and the packing is removed by the physician.

Possible complications of the stapedectomy include infection of the external, middle, or inner ear. Displacement or rejection of the prosthesis or graft may occur, or perilymph fluid may leak around the prosthesis into the middle ear, causing ringing in the ears and vertigo.

Nursing diagnoses and interventions are provided on p.1086.

Prognosis. As edema decreases, sound conduction will improve to more normal levels.

Tympanoplasty

Tympanoplasty is any of several operative procedures on the eardrum or ossicles of the middle ear designed to restore or improve hearing in patients with conductive hearing loss. These operations may be used to repair a perforated eardrum, for otosclerosis, or for dislocation or necrosis of a small bone of the middle ear.

Nursing Interventions. Postoperative management consists of bed rest until the next morning. The head of the bed is elevated 40 degrees, and the operative side faces upward. Medications include narcotic analgesics; tetracycline HCl (Achromycin) as an antiinfective agent; and meclizine HCl (Antivert) for vertigo.

Postoperatively the presence of bleeding, the amount, color, and consistency of drainage, and temperature must be noted and reported. Complaints of vertigo when the patient is getting out of bed should be noted; with sudden movements, nausea and vertigo may occur. Keep the head of the patient's bed elevated 40 degrees. Possible complications include infection and displacement of the graft.

Nursing diagnoses and interventions are provided in the discussion of myringotomy, which follows.

PATIENT TEACHING FOR EAR SURGERY

- Change cotton in ear daily as prescribed
- Open mouth when sneezing or coughing and blow nose gently one side at a time for 1 week (to prevent increased ear pressure and infection)
- Keep ear dry for 6 weeks (to prevent infection)
  - Do not wash hair for 1 week
  - Protect ear when outdoors using two pieces of cotton (use petrolatum jelly on outer ball)
  - Protect ear with shower cap when bathing
- Wear ear protectors as necessary for exposure to loud noises
- Follow activity guidelines
  - No physical activity for 1 week
  - No exercises or active sports for 3 weeks
  - Return to work in 1 week (3 weeks for strenuous work)
- Avoid exposure to persons with upper respiratory tract infections
- Avoid airplane flights for at least 1 week (to prevent effects of pressure changes)

Prognosis. Improved hearing will be noted if there is no involvement of the ossicles.

Myringotomy

Myringotomy is a surgical incision of the eardrum. It is performed to relieve pressure and release purulent exudate from the middle ear. The procedure is done under either local or general anesthetic.

A myringotomy may be performed in one of two ways. Using a myringotomy knife, the surgeon makes a curved incision in the drumhead. In the second procedure, a heated wire loop is touched for about 1 second to the drumhead, producing a 2-mm hole.

Nursing Interventions. Pus and fluid may drain immediately, requiring suctioning. Cotton placed in the ear absorbs drainage, which may continue several days.

The incision usually heals quickly with little scarring. Disruption of hearing does not usually occur.

Postoperative management includes cotton in the ear for absorption of drainage. Cotton should be changed frequently to avoid recontamination of the surgical area. Medications commonly used are tetracycline (Achromycin) and polymyxin B (Neosporin) ear drops as antiinfective agents. Tylenol with codeine may be used for pain.

Postoperatively the nurse monitors for signs of drainage and bleeding and reports any occurrence. Incisional pain or hearing impairment should be noted.

Nursing diagnoses and interventions for the patient after a myringotomy include but are not limited to the following:

NURSING DIAGNOSES	NURSING INTERVENTIONS
Mobility, impaired physical, related to surgical procedure	Note patient's ability to comply with bed rest order. Keep the patient's operative side up; do not allow the patient to be turned.
Activity intolerance, high risk for, related to pain and vertigo	Keep side rails up. When movement is allowed, begin gradually. Administer prescribed medications for pain and vertigo as needed.
Injury, high risk for, related to sensory-perceptual alterations (auditory)	Note and report any drainage or bleeding. Assist with ambulation when it is allowed.

Patient teaching. Provide the information in the patient teaching box and ensure understanding.

Prognosis. Once pressure is relieved, hearing is restored to more normal levels unless scarring is present.

REFERENCES AND SUGGESTED READINGS

1. Allen M: Adjusting to visual impairment, *J Ophthalmic Nurs Technol* 9(2):47, 1990.
2. Beare PG, Myers JL: *Principles and practice of adult health nursing,* ed 2, St Louis, 1994, Mosby.
3. Berne RM, Levy M: *Physiology,* ed 3, St Louis, 1992, Mosby.
4. Bocking H et al: Artificial eyes, *Nurs Times* 86(8):40, 1990.
5. Boyd-Monk H: Assessing acquired ocular diseases, *Nurs Clin North Am* 25(4):811, 1990.
6. Boyd-Monk H: Eye trauma in the workplace, *AAOHN J* 38(10):487, 1990.
7. Bradley S: The signs of silence: communicating with deaf and hearing-impaired patients, *J Emerg Med Serv* 16(8):26, 1991.
8. Brinkman K: Why can't your patient hear you? *RN* 54:45, 1991.
9. Burrell LD: *Adult nursing in hospital and community settings,* Norwalk, Conn, 1992, Appleton & Lange.
10. Cleveland PJ, Morris J: Ménière's disease: the inner ear out of balance, *RN* 53(8):28, 1990.
11. Cohen EJ, Krachmer JH: Red eyes and contact lenses, *Patient Care* 26(9):143, 1992.
12. Craven RF, Hirnle CJ: *Fundamentals of nursing: human health and function,* Philadelphia, 1992, Lippincott.
13. Danyluk AW, Paton D: Diagnoses and management of glaucoma, *Clin Symp* 43(4):21, 1991.
14. Estey A, Jeremy P, Jones M: Developing printed materials for patients with visual deficiencies, *J Ophthalmic Nurs Technol* 9(6):247, 1990.
15. Farrell TA: Minimizing the systemic effects of glaucoma medications, *Geriatrics* 46(5):61, 1991.
16. *Fundamental nursing skills,* Springhouse, Penn, 1994, Springhouse.
17. Gordon M: *Manual of nursing diagnosis: 1993-1994,* St Louis, 1993, Mosby.
18. Grimes MR et al: Worldwide blindness, *Nurs Clin North Am* 27(3):807, 1992.
19. Igratavichius DD, Bayne MV: *Medical-surgical nursing: a nursing process approach,* Philadelphia, 1991, Saunders.
20. *Illustrated manual of nursing practice,* ed 2, Springhouse, Penn, 1994, Springhouse.

21. Ing MR: Infection following strabismus surgery, *J Ophthalmic Nurs Technol* 10(5):211, 1991.
22. Javitt JC et al: Undertreatment of glaucoma among black Americans, *N Engl J Med* 325(20):1418, 1991.
23. Jinks MJ: Counseling older adults with hearing impairment, *J Pract Nurs* 41(3):43, 1991.
24. Kim MJ et al: *Pocket guide to nursing diagnoses,* ed 5, St Louis, 1993, Mosby.
25. Lehne RA: *Pharmacology for nursing care,* Philadelphia, 1990, Saunders.
26. Lewis SM, Collier IC, Cox I: *Medical-surgical nursing: assessment and management of clinical problems,* ed 3, St Louis, 1992, Mosby.
27. Long BC, Phipps WJ, Cassmeyer VL: *Medical-surgical nursing: a nursing process approach,* ed 3, St Louis, 1993, Mosby.
28. Martinelli AM: Glaucoma: classification, treatment options, patient care, *AORN J* 54(4):743, 1991.
29. McCance KL, Huether SE: *Pathophysiology: the biologic basis for disease in adults and children,* ed 2, St Louis, 1994, Mosby.
30. McConnell E: How to irrigate the eye, *Nurs '91* 21(3):28, 1991.
31. McFarland GK, McFarlane EA: *Nursing diagnosis and intervention: planning for patient care,* ed 2, St Louis, 1993, Mosby.
32. McKenry LM, Salerno E: *Mosby's pharmacology in nursing,* St Louis, 1992, Mosby.
33. Memmler RL, Cohen BJ, Wood DL: *Structure and function of the human body,* ed 5, Philadelphia, 1992, Lippincott.
34. Milder B, Rubin ML: *The fine art of prescribing glasses: without making a spectacle of yourself,* ed 2, Gainsville, Fla, 1991, Triad.
35. *Mosby's medical, nursing, and allied health dictionary,* ed 4, St Louis, 1994, Mosby.
36. Mulrow CD: Screening for hearing impairment in the elderly, *Hosp Pract* 26(2A):79, 1991.
37. Newell F: *Ophthalmology: principles and practice,* ed 7, St Louis, 1992, Mosby.
38. Pagana KD, Pagana TJ: *Mosby's diagnostic and laboratory tests reference,* ed 2, St Louis, 1992, Mosby.
39. Palumbo MV: Hearing access 2000: increasing awareness of the hearing impaired, *J Gerontol Nurs* 16(9):26, 1990.
40. Phipps WJ et al: *Medical-surgical nursing: concepts and clinical practices,* ed 4, St Louis, 1991, Mosby.
41. Potter P: *Pocket guide to physical assessment,* ed 3, St Louis, 1994, Mosby.
42. Potter PA, Perry AG: *Basic nursing: theory and practice,* ed 3, St Louis, 1995, Mosby.
43. Potter PA, Perry AG: *Fundamentals of nursing: concepts, process, and practice,* ed 3, St Louis, 1993, Mosby.
44. Powell MA: Conjunctivitis versus iritis: question and answer, *J Am Acad Nurse Pract* 2(3):125, 1990.
45. Reiss BS, Evans ME: *Pharmacological aspects of nursing care,* ed 3, Albany, NY, 1990, Delmar.
46. Roeser RJ, Adams RM, Watkins S: Cerumen management in hearing conservation: The Dallas (Texas) Independent School District Program, *J Sch Health* 61(1):47, 1991.
47. Sands J: *Clinical manual of medical-surgical nursing,* ed 2, St Louis, 1991, Mosby.
48. Seidel HM et al: *Mosby's guide to physical examination,* ed 2, St Louis, 1995, Mosby.
49. Skidmore-Roth L: *Mosby's 1995 drug reference,* St Louis, 1995, Mosby.
50. Smith D: *Clinical nursing skills,* Norwalk, Conn, 1992, Appleton & Lange.
51. Solomon EP: *Introduction to human anatomy and physiology,* Philadelphia, 1992, Saunders.
52. Swearingen P: *Medical-surgical nursing care,* ed 3, St Louis, 1994, Mosby.
53. Swearingen PL: *Pocket guide to medical-surgical nursing: nursing diagnoses and interventions,* St Louis, 1992, Mosby.
54. Thibodeau GA: *Structure and function of the body,* ed 9, St Louis, 1992, Mosby.
55. Thomas CL: *Taber's cyclopedic medial dictionary,* ed 17, Philadelphia, 1993, FA Davis.
56. Thompson JM, Bowers AC: *Clinical manual of health assessment,* ed 3, St Louis, 1992, Mosby.
57. Thompson JM et al: *Mosby's clinical nursing,* ed 3, St Louis, 1993, Mosby.
58. Tolson D, Swan I: Gentle persuasion: hearing impairment, *Nurs Times* 87(23):29, 1991.
59. Tucker SM et al: *Patient care standards: nursing process, diagnosis, and outcome,* ed 5, St Louis, 1992, Mosby.

CHAPTER CHALLENGE

KEY POINTS

- The five major senses are taste, touch, smell, sight, and hearing/balance.
- Seventy percent of the sensory structures of the body are located in the eye.
- The accessory structures of the eye are the eyebrows, eyelids, eyelashes, and the lacrimal apparatus.
- The three tunics of the eyeball are the fibrous tunic (sclera), the vascular tunic (choroid), and the retina.
- The two chambers of the eye are the anterior chamber (which contains aqueous humor) and the posterior chamber (which contains vitreous humor).
- Image formation at the retina requires four basic processes: refraction, accommodation, constriction, and convergence.
- The photoreceptors of the retina are the rods and cones. The rods control vision in dim light and the cones control vision in bright light. The cones are also responsible for color vision.
- Light entering the eye must travel through the cornea, aqueous humor, pupil, crystalline lens, vitreous humor, and finally, the retina.
- The ear is divided into external, middle, and inner ears.
- The external ear flap is called the *pinna* (auricle); it extends into the external ear canal.
- The middle ear contains the ossicles and the entrance of the eustachian tube and ends with the tympanic membrane.
- The internal ear contains the vestibule, cochlea, and semicircular canals.
- The organ of Corti is the organ of hearing; it is located within the cochlea.
- The semicircular canals are responsible for the sense of balance and equilibrium.
- The tastebuds differentiate four basic tastes: sweet, sour, salty, and bitter. Food must be in solution for interpretation, because a chemical reaction occurs.

- Normal aging causes decreased hearing and sight as a result of normal changes of the structures.
- Individuals with chronic disease or who are over 40 should be examined yearly to detect eye abnormalities or so that changes in therapy may be prescribed.
- Refractory errors include the conditions hyperopia (farsightedness), presbyopia (farsightedness related to the aging process), and astigmatism (objects waver).
- Ranges of 20/20 to 20/40 vision are considered normal, whereas 20/200 is defined as legal blindness.
- Cataracts are an opacity of the lens and may be removed by intracapsular or extracapsular extraction.
- Glaucoma is a slow, progressive disorder involving increased intraocular pressure. It is related to occlusion of aqueous humor drainage.
- Loss of hearing may result from infection, trauma, or use of ototoxic drugs, or may be a congenital condition.
- Conductive hearing loss is a decrease in amplification, whereas sensorineural hearing loss is interference within the inner ear.
- Prevention of serious complications of ear disorders, such as infections, mastoiditis, and brain abscess, requires early detection and treatment.
- Injury, high risk for, is the primary nursing diagnosis for the patient experiencing vertigo, which occurs in labyrinthitis and Ménière's disease.
- An essential communication tip for speaking to the hearing impaired is to face the patient and to speak clearly without shouting.

STUDY QUESTIONS

1. Another name for the incus, malleus, and stapes is:
   1. tympanic membrane
   2. ossicles
   3. pinna
   4. major structures
2. The organ of hearing is the:
   1. semicircular canals
   2. Organ of Cortii
   3. tympanic membrane
   4. oval window
3. The structure that maintains balance is the:
   1. organ of Corti
   2. oval window
   3. semicircular canals
   4. tympanic membrane
4. Another name for the tympanic membrane is:
   1. pinna
   2. eardrum
   3. oval window
   4. cerumen
5. The innermost covering of the eyeball is the:
   1. retina
   2. sclera
   3. cornea
   4. macula
6. The structures responsible for color vision are the:
   1. rods
   2. cones
   3. iris
   4. lens
7. The structure that is the eye's window is the:
   1. iris
   2. cornea
   3. sclera
   4. lens
8. The name of the waxy substance that protects the lining of the ear canal from infection is:
   1. cerumen
   2. stapes
   3. endolymph
   4. ossicles
9. The taste buds on the tongue that respond to sugar and other sweet substances are located on the:
   1. posterior portion of the tongues
   2. tip of the tongue
   3. sides of the tongue
   4. inferior portion of the tongue
10. The tiny venous sinus located at the junction of the sclera and cornea that aids in controlling intraocular pressure is the:
    1. retina
    2. choroid
    3. canal of Schlemm
    4. lacrimal gland
11. Mrs. Rollands is to have a laser treatment to cauterize hemorrhaging vessels caused by diabetic retinopathy. The name of the procedure is:
    1. enucleation
    2. scleral buckle
    3. photocoagulation
    4. trabeculoplasty
12. The parents of Tim, age 11 years, want to know more about Tim's conductive hearing loss. The nurse would explain that:
    1. sound is delivered through the external and middle ear, but a defect in the inner ear results in distortion of sound
    2. sound is inadequately delivered through the external or middle ear to the inner ear
    3. there is no organic cause, but a functional problem exists
    4. the brain's auditory pathways are damaged
13. Ms. Jones has impaired hearing. To facilitate communication, the nurse would:
    1. face Ms. Jones when speaking
    2. overaccentuate words to make the communication more effective
    3. shout to allow Ms. Jones to hear
    4. use one-word answers when speaking
14. Mr. Martinez tells the nurse he has dizziness. He states that the doctor used another term. The correct term is:
    1. tinnitus
    2. labyrinthitis
    3. sensory neural
    4. vertigo
15. Mrs. Rodriquez is diagnosed with an inner ear problem. The major symptom would be:
    1. echoing
    2. intense pain
    3. vertigo
    4. loss of hearing
16. Evaluation of the eye as it adjusts to seeing objects at various distances is called:
    1. PERRLA
    2. refraction
    3. focusing
    4. accommodation
17. Mrs. Onidas has tunnel vision, eye pain, difficulty in adjusting to darkness, halos seen around lights, and failure to detect colors. These indicate:
    1. chronic glaucoma
    2. cataracts
    3. entropion
    4. detached retina

35

CARE OF THE PATIENT WITH A NEUROLOGICAL DISORDER

Elizabeth Schenk

KEY TERMS

ANATOMY AND PHYSIOLOGY
action potential
axon
central nervous system
dendrite
motor (efferent) neurons
neuromuscular junction
neuron
neurotransmitter
peripheral nervous system
sensory (afferent) neurons
synapse

MEDICAL-SURGICAL
agnosia
aneurysm
aphasia
apraxia
aura
Bobath approach
bradykinesia
cerebrovascular accident (CVA)
diplopia
dysarthria
dysphagia
flaccid
Glasgow coma scale
global cognitive dysfunction
hemianopia
hemiplegia
hyperreflexia
nystagmus
postictal period
proprioception
unilateral neglect

LEARNING OBJECTIVES

After reading this chapter, the student should be able to do the following:

Anatomy and Physiology

- Define the key terms.
- Name the two structural divisions of the nervous system.
- List the parts of the neuron, and describe the function of each part.
- Discuss the main function of each neurotransmitter.
- Describe the "all or none" law and its impact on the nervous system.
- Discuss the difference between a motor neuron and a sensory neuron.
- List the main parts and coverings of the brain.
- Discuss the parts of the peripheral nervous system and how the system works with the central nervous system.
- Name the 12 cranial nerves, and list the areas they serve.

Medical-Surgical

- Define the key terms.
- List physiological changes that occur in the nervous system with aging.
- Discuss the Glasgow coma scale.
- Explain three parts of the neurological assessment.
- Explain the importance of prevention in problems of the nervous system, and give at least one example of prevention.
- List five signs and symptoms of increased intracranial pressure and why they occur, as well as nursing interventions that decrease intracranial pressure.
- Give examples of two degenerative neurological diseases and two diseases related to infection of the nervous system, and explain the pathophysiology involved.
- State two complications of brain surgery and the signs and symptoms seen with each complication.
- Explain the mechanism of injury to the brain that occurs with cerebrovascular accident and traumatic brain injury.
- Discuss nursing interventions to assist in the rehabilitation of the patient with a cerebrovascular accident.
- Discuss patient teaching and home care planning for the patient with multiple sclerosis or Parkinson's disease.
- Discuss the pathophysiology of Guillain-Barré syndrome, trigeminal neuralgia, and Bell's palsy.

RELATED TOPICS OF INTEREST

- Comfort, rest, and sleep (Chapter 15)
- Care of the patient with an eye or ear disorder (Chapter 34)
- Care of the HIV-positive or AIDS patient (Chapter 37)
- Care of the patient with cancer (Chapter 38)
- Care of the older adult (Chapter 45)
- Mental health concepts (Chapter 46)
- Rehabilitation nursing (Chapter 49)

The nervous system is responsible for communication and control within the body. It interprets or processes the information received and sends information to the appropriate area of the brain or spinal cord, from which a response is generated. The nervous system is the body's link with the environment. It works in conjunction with the endocrine system to maintain the body's homeostasis. The nervous system reacts in split-seconds, whereas the hormones secreted by the endocrine glands work more slowly in initiating a response.

ANATOMY AND PHYSIOLOGY

Structural Divisions

There are two main structural divisions of the nervous system (Fig. 35-1). The first division, the central nervous system (CNS), is composed of the brain and the spinal cord. It occupies a central or medial position in the body and is responsible for interpreting incoming sensory information and issuing instructions based on past experi-

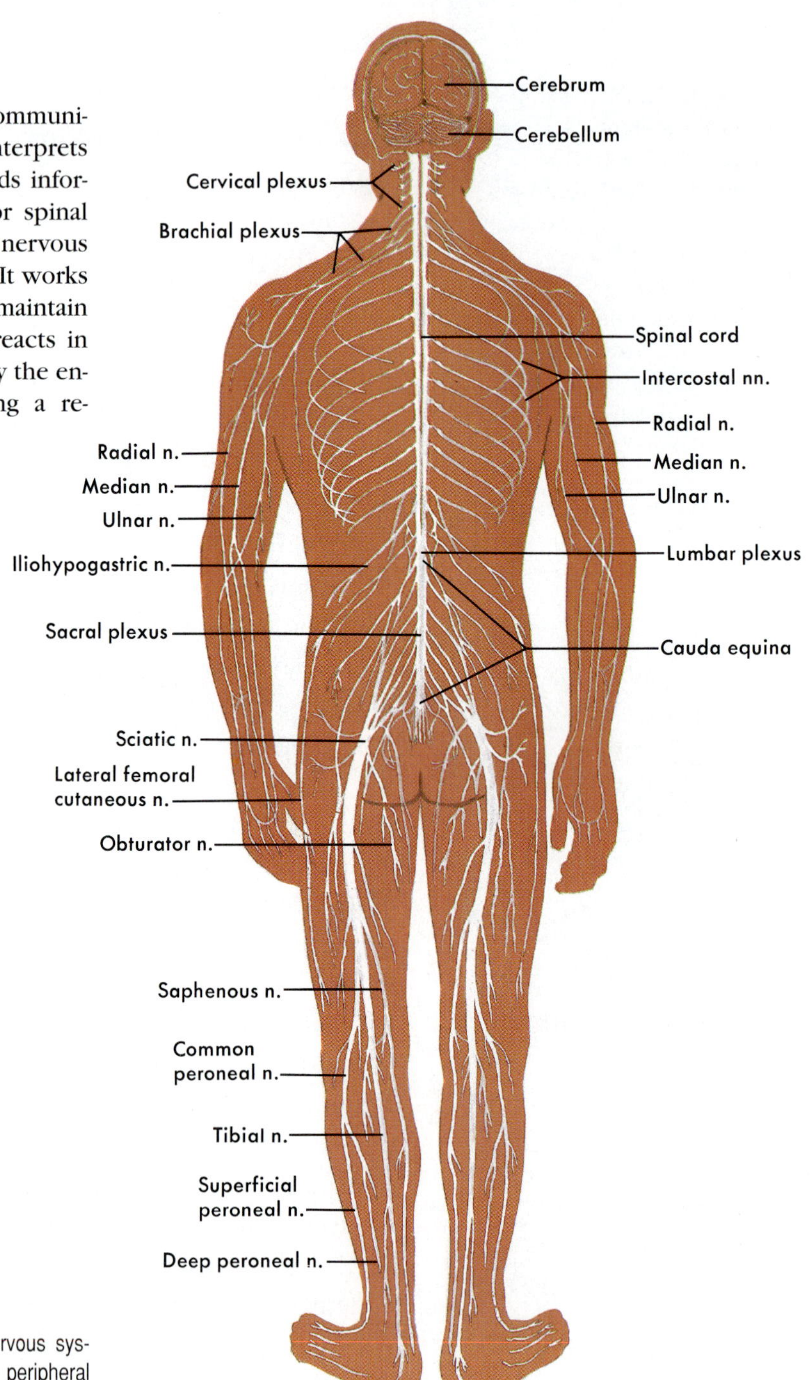

FIG. 35-1 The central and peripheral divisions of the nervous systems. The CNS consists of the brain and spinal cord. The peripheral nervous system is composed of the cranial and spinal nerves.

ences. The second component is the peripheral nervous system, which lies outside the CNS. It is composed of the motor and sensory nerves and ganglia outside the brain and spinal cord, consisting of 12 pairs of cranial nerves, 31 pairs of spinal nerves, and their various branches in body organs. The cranial nerves carry impulses to and from the brain, whereas the spinal nerves carry impulses to and from the spinal cord.

Sensory (afferent) neurons conduct sensory impulses from the periphery of the body to the brain or spinal cord via the dorsal spinal roots. **Motor (efferent) neurons** transmit nerve impulses from the brain or from the spinal cord to muscular or glandular tissue.

The peripheral nervous system contains two main divisions: the somatic nervous system and the autonomic nervous system. The somatic nervous system sends messages from the CNS to the skeletal muscles (voluntary muscles). The autonomic system transmits messages from the CNS to smooth muscle, cardiac muscle, and certain glands. The autonomic system is sometimes called the *involuntary nervous system,* because its action takes place without conscious control.

Cells of the Nervous System. There are two broad categories of cells within the nervous system. The first category, the neurons, are the transmitter cells. They carry the messages to and from the brain and spinal cord. The second category, the neuroglia or glial cells, are the support cells to the neurons. They support and protect the neurons while producing cerebrospinal fluid, which bathes the structures of the CNS.

Neuron Structure. A **neuron** (nerve cell) is the basic nerve cell of the nervous system and is a separate unit composed of three main structures: the cell body, the axon, and the dendrites (Fig. 35-2). The cell body contains a nucleus surrounded by cytoplasm. The **axon** is a cylindric extension of a nerve cell that conducts impulses away from the neuron cell body. The **dendrites** are branching structures that extend from the cell body and receive impulses. Between each neuron is a gap (space) called the **synapse,** defined as the region surrounding the point of contact between two neurons or between a neuron and an effector organ, across which nerve impulses are transmitted through the action of a neurotransmitter.

All neurons are governed by the "all or none law," which means there is never a partial transmission of a message—the impulse is either strong enough to elicit a response or too weak to generate the message.

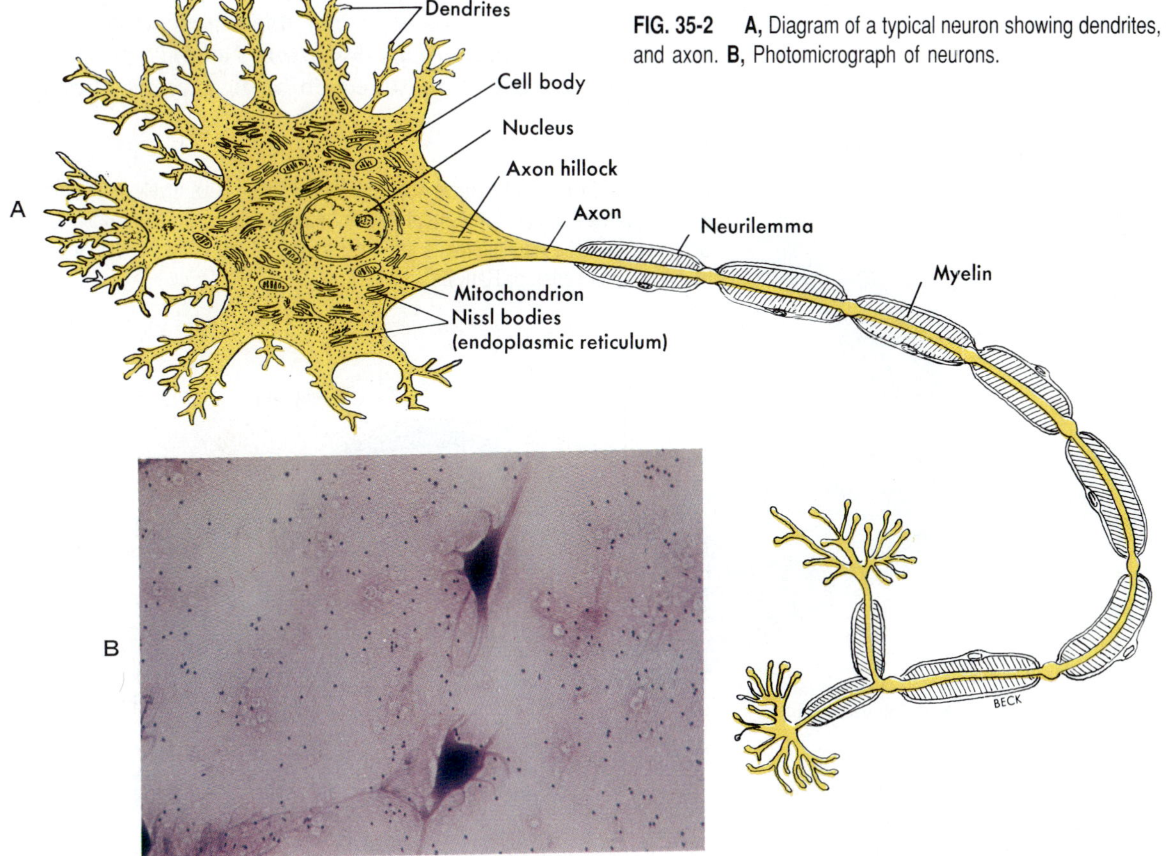

FIG. 35-2 **A,** Diagram of a typical neuron showing dendrites, cell body, and axon. **B,** Photomicrograph of neurons.

Neuromuscular Junction. The area of contact between the ends of a large myelinated nerve fiber and a fiber of skeletal muscle is called the **neuromuscular junction.** This area of contact is necessary for functioning of the body. The neurotransmitters act to make sure that the neurological impulse passes from the nerve to the muscle.

Neurotransmitters. Numerous chemicals called **neurotransmitters** modify or result in the transmission of impulses between synapses. The most well-known neurotransmitters are acetylcholine, norepinephrine, dopamine, and serotonin.

Acetylcholine plays a role in nerve impulse transmission; it spills into the synapse area and speeds the transmission of the impulse. The enzyme *cholinesterase* is then released to deactivate the acetylcholine once the message or impulse has been sent. This happens rapidly and continuously as each impulse is relayed.

Norepinephrine has an impact on maintaining arousal (awakening from a deep sleep), dreaming, and regulation of mood (e.g., happiness, sadness).

Dopamine primarily effects motor function; it is involved in gross subconscious movements of the skeletal muscles. It also plays a role in emotional responses. In Parkinson's disease there is a decrease in dopamine levels, and the individual suffers from tremors, or involuntary, trembling muscle movements. (This will be discussed in detail later in the chapter.)

Serotonin, another neurotransmitter, induces sleep, affects sensory perception, controls temperature, and has a role in control of mood.

In the past few years another group of chemical messengers has been discovered; they are known as *neuropeptides.* Some neuropeptides function as neurotransmitters, but generally they increase or decrease the response of the other neurotransmitters. In 1975 enkephalins were discovered; they are the body's natural pain relievers. Enkephalins are thought to inhibit the pain impulses and bind with the same receptors as chemicals such as morphine and other narcotics.

Chemical endorphins have been isolated in the pituitary and have several functions. They suppress pain and are linked with memory and learning, sexual activity, and many more functions.

Neuron coverings. Many neuron fibers (axons and dendrites) are covered with a white, waxy, fatty material called *myelin* (Fig. 35-3). Myelin increases the rate of transmission of impulses and protects and insulates the fibers. Axons leaving the CNS are wrapped in layers of myelin with indentations called nodes of Ranvier. These nodes further increase the rate of transmission, because the impulse can jump from node to node.

In the peripheral nervous system, the myelin is produced by Schwann cells. The outer membrane of the Schwann cells gives rise to another layer called the neurilemma. The neurilemma is a very important layer, because it helps to regenerate injured axons. Thus regeneration of nerve cells occurs only in the peripheral nervous system. Cells damaged in the CNS result in permanent damage (paralysis), because they do not have neurilemma and are not able to regenerate.

Neuron classification. Neurons are classified according to the direction of the message they transmit.

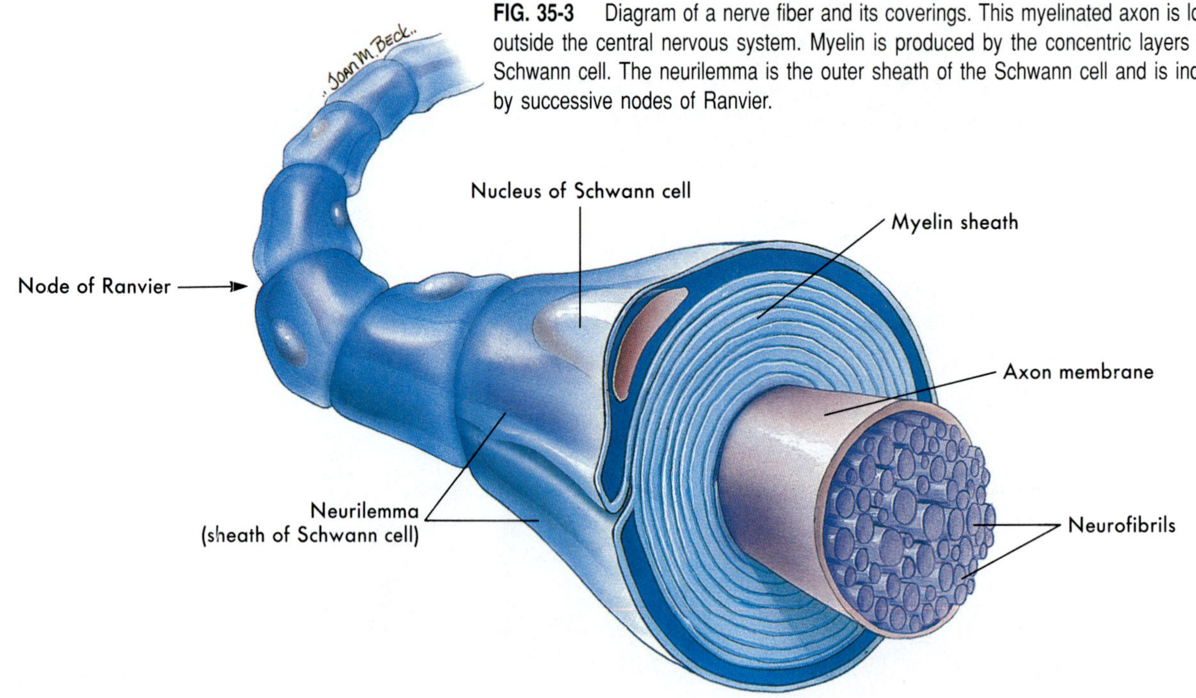

FIG. 35-3 Diagram of a nerve fiber and its coverings. This myelinated axon is located outside the central nervous system. Myelin is produced by the concentric layers of the Schwann cell. The neurilemma is the outer sheath of the Schwann cell and is indented by successive nodes of Ranvier.

Sensory (afferent) neurons transmit messages to the brain and spinal cord. Motor (efferent) neurons transmit messages away from the brain and spinal cord. The sensory neurons carry information for interpretation; the motor neurons carry information for response to the interpreted information.

Nerve fibers. Groups or bundles of nerve fibers wrapped in connective tissue and lying outside the CNS are called *nerves.* Groups of nerve cell bodies that lie outside the CNS are called *ganglia.*

Inside the CNS the terminology changes. The bundles of nerve fibers are called *tracts* and the cell bodies are called *nuclei.*

Nerve Impulses. A nerve cell impulse is the ability of the cell to change the electrical charge on the cell membrane and transmit the electrical current along the cell membrane. Because of positive and negative ions concentrated on either side of the membrane, the inside of the membrane at rest is negative as compared with the outside. A nerve impulse is a local reversal in the charge on the cell membrane that then spreads along the membrane like an electrical current. The neuron has the ability to respond to a stimulus and convert it into a nerve impulse; this is called *irritability.* The nerve cell also has the ability to transmit the impulse to other neurons; this is called *conductivity.*

Nerve cell impulses are stimulated by pressure, temperature, and chemical changes and are governed by the "all or none" law.

Transmission of nerve impulses. In the resting phase the cell membrane of the nerve cell is negatively charged. During this period, the predominant extracellular ion is sodium and the predominant intracellular ion is potassium. An impulse brings about a sudden shift in the sodium and potassium across the cell membrane and reverses the electrical charge. This sudden change is called an **action potential** or action current (an electric impulse consisting of a self-propagating series of polarizations and depolarizations transmitted across the cell membranes of a nerve fiber during the transmission of a nerve impulse and across the cell membranes of a muscle cell during contraction or other activity of the cell). Once the impulse has been transmitted, the cell membrane returns very rapidly to its former state.

Central Nervous System

The **central nervous system,** one of the two main divisions of the nervous system composed of the brain and spinal cord, functions somewhat like a computer but is much more complex. The cranium protects the brain and the vertebral column protects the spinal cord.

Brain. Specialized cells in the brain's mass of convoluted, soft, gray or white tissue coordinate and regulate the functions of the CNS. The brain is one of the largest organs, weighing approximately 3 lb (6.6 kg). It is divided into four principal parts: the cerebrum, the diencephalon, the cerebellum, and the brain stem (Fig. 35-4 and Fig. 35-5 on p. 1094).

Cerebrum. The cerebrum is the largest part of the brain. It is divided into the right and left hemispheres. The outer portion of the cerebrum is composed of gray

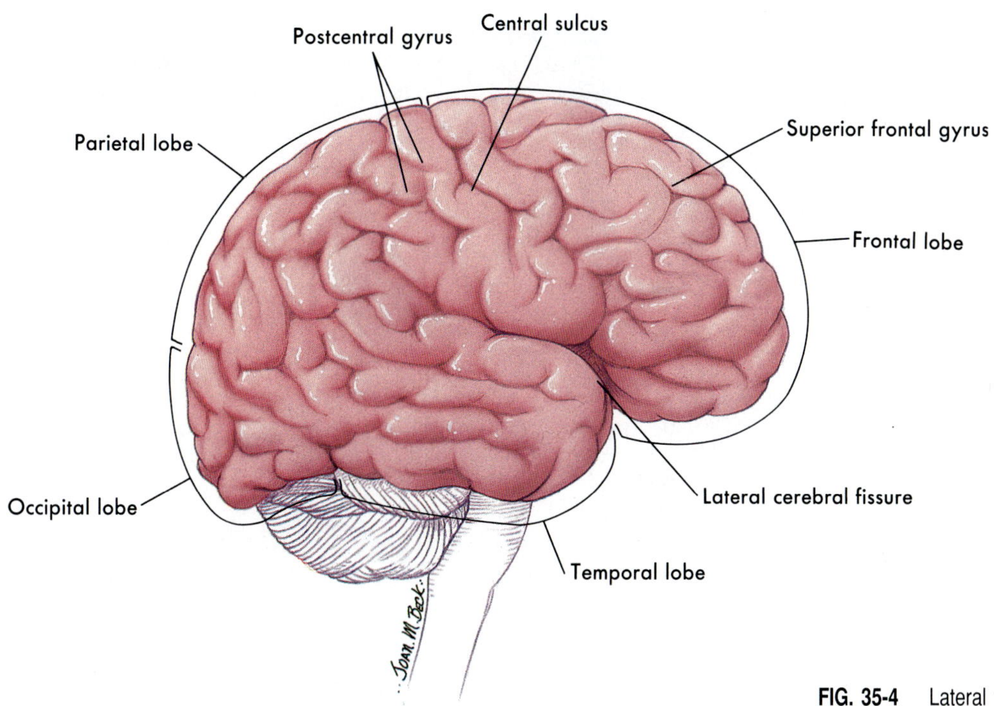

FIG. 35-4 Lateral view of the brain.

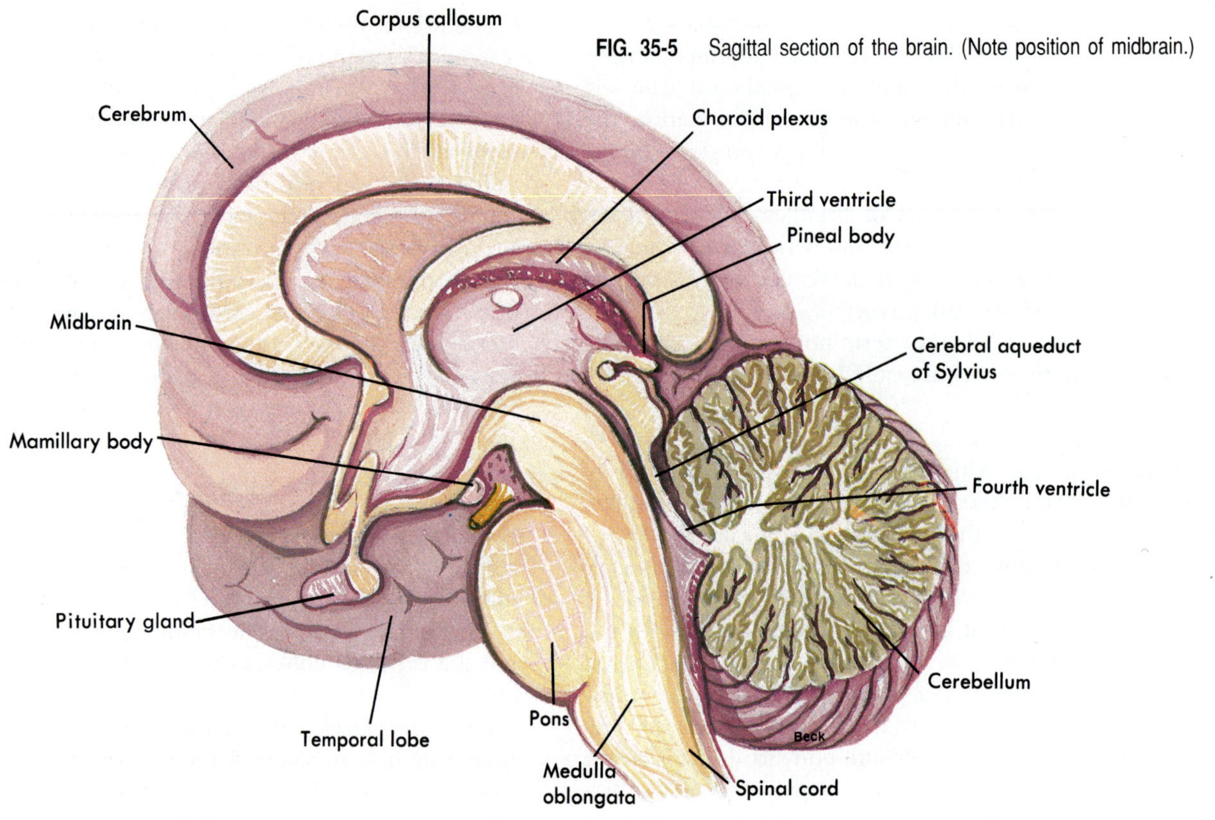

FIG. 35-5 Sagittal section of the brain. (Note position of midbrain.)

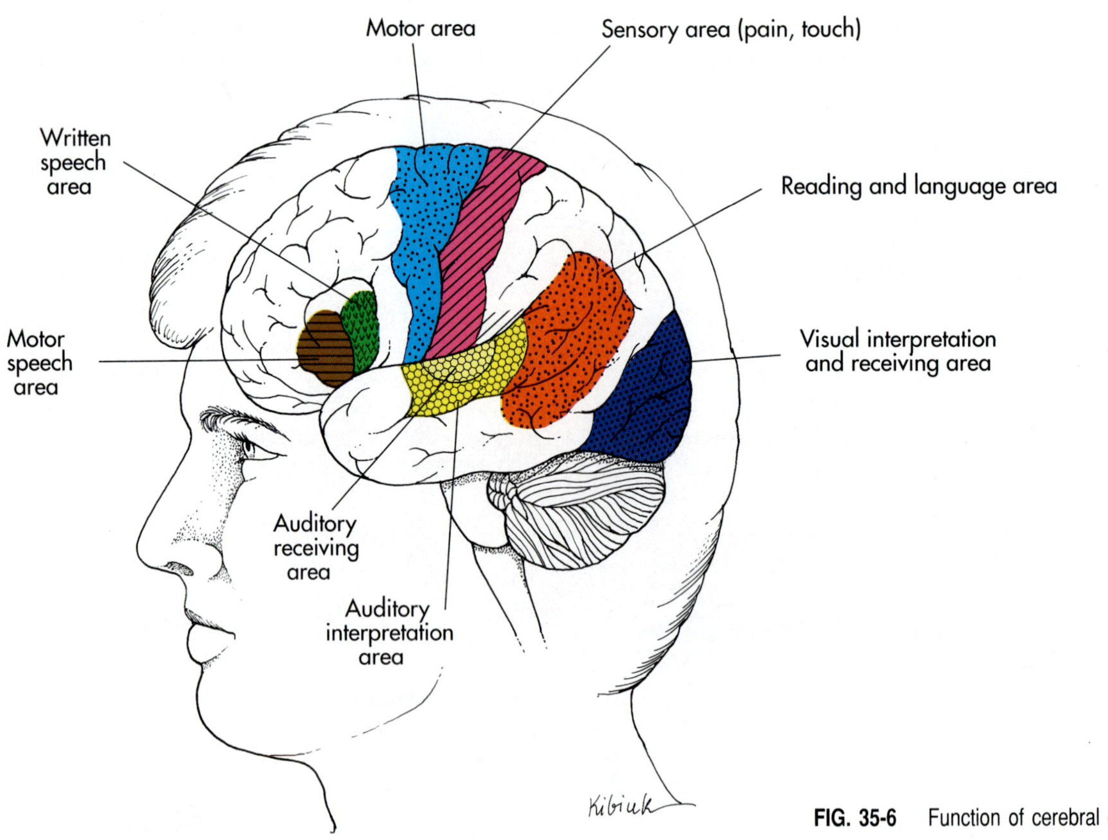

FIG. 35-6 Function of cerebral cortex.

Box 35-1 CEREBRUM FUNCTIONS

FRONTAL LOBE

Written speech (ability to write)

Motor speech (ability to speak)

Motor ability—directs movements of body; the left side of the brain controls the right side of the body, and the right side of the brain controls the left side of the body

Intellectualization—the ability to form concepts, to think

Judgment formation

PARIETAL LOBE

Contains the sensory area; the impulses from the skin, such as touch, pain, and temperature, are interpreted

Ability to recognize body parts

Ability to determine left from right

Determination of shapes, sizes, and distances takes place here

TEMPORAL LOBE

Memory storage

Integration of auditory stimuli; this lobe receives and interprets impulses from the ear

OCCIPITAL LOBE

Contains the visual area for interpreting impulses from the retina of the eye

Understanding of the written word

matter and is called the *cerebral cortex.* It is arranged in folds that are called *gyri* (convolutions); the grooves are called *sulci* (fissures) (see Fig. 35-4). A deep fissure divides the right and left hemispheres; it is called the *longitudinal fissure.* A bridge or connecting structure, the corpus callosum, links the two hemispheres. Other fissures divide the hemispheres into four lobes that are named for the bones lying over them: the frontal lobe, the parietal lobe, the temporal lobe, and the occipital lobe (see Chapter 26 for the location of cranial bones). The interior of the cerebrum is composed of white matter consisting of bundles of nerve fibers (tracts). Throughout the white matter are small islands of gray matter called *basal ganglia.* The basal ganglia play an important role in body movement and posture. The functions of the four lobes of the cerebrum are described in Box 35-1 (Fig. 35-6).

Diencephalon. The diencephalon is often called the *interbrain:* it lies directly beneath the cerebrum. It contains the thalamus and the hypothalamus. The thalamus, an oval structure with two lobes, is approximately 1 inch (3 cm) in diameter; it composes four fifths of the diencephalon. The thalamus serves as a relay station for some sensory impulses while interpreting other sensory messages, such as pain, light touch, and pressure.

The hypothalamus, which lies below the thalamus, plays a vital role in the control of body temperature, fluid balance, appetite, and certain emotions, such as fear, pleasure, and pain. Both the sympathetic and parasympathetic divisions of the autonomic system are under control of the hypothalamus, as is the pituitary gland. Thus the hypothalamus influences the heartbeat, the contraction and relaxation of the walls of the blood vessels, hormone secretion, and other vital body functions (Box 35-2 on p. 1096).

Cerebellum. The cerebellum lies posterior and inferior to the cerebrum. It is the second largest portion of the brain. The cerebellum contains two hemispheres with a convoluted surface much like the cerebrum. Structurally it resembles a small head of cauliflower.

The cerebellum is mainly responsible for coordination of skeletal muscles and maintenance of balance, equilibrium, and muscle tone. Sensory messages from the semicircular canals in the inner ear send their messages to the cerebellum (see Fig. 35-5).

Brain stem. The brain stem is located at the base of the brain and contains the midbrain, pons, and medulla oblongata. These structures serve to connect the spinal cord and the cerebrum (see Box 35-2). The brain stem carries all nerve fibers between the spinal cord and the cerebrum.

Midbrain. The midbrain forms the superior portion of the brain stem. It is responsible for motor movement, the relay of impulses, and auditory and visual reflexes. It is the origin of cranial nerves III and IV.

Pons. The pons connects the midbrain to the medulla oblongata. The word *pons* means "bridge." It is the origin of cranial nerves V through VIII. The pons is composed of myelinated nerve fibers and is responsible for sending impulses to the structures that are inferior and superior to it. It also contains a respiratory center that complements respiratory centers located in the medulla.

Medulla oblongata. The medulla oblongata is the distal portion of the brain stem. It is the origin of cranial nerves IX through XII. The medulla contains the cardiac center that regulates the heartbeat and force of the contraction. It also contains the respiratory center that controls the rhythm of breathing. A vasomotor center regulates the diameter of the blood vessels, which aids in control of the blood pressure. The medulla also controls the coordination of swallowing, coughing, sneezing, vomiting, and hiccuping (singultus).

Box 35-2

INTERBRAIN AND BRAIN STEM FUNCTIONS

DIENCEPHALON (THALAMUS AND HYPOTHALAMUS) (INTERBRAIN)

Receives sensory impulses (pain, temperature, and touch)

Acts as relay station

Controls pain threshold

Acts in synthesis of vasopressor and oxytocin

Helps maintain wakeful state

Controls temperature

Generates emotional response

BRAIN STEM

Midbrain

Motor movement

Relay of impulses

Postural reflex patterns

Auditory reflexes

Righting reflex

Some control of vision

Origin of cranial nerves III and IV

Pons

Pneumotaxic center (rhythmicity of respirations)

Connection between the medulla, midbrain, and cerebellum

Origin of cranial nerves V, VI, VII, and VIII

Medulla Oblongata

Cardiac, vasomotor, and respiratory center

Center for cough, swallowing, and singultus

Role in reticular activating system

Origin of cranial nerves IX, X, XI, and XII

Coverings of the brain and spinal cord. The brain and spinal cord are surrounded by three protective coverings (membranes) called the meninges (Fig. 35-7). The outermost covering, the dura mater, is a tough, fibrous membrane that adheres to the skull. The middle layer, the arachnoid membrane, resembles a spiderweb with cerebrospinal fluid (CSF) filling its spaces. The innermost layer, the pia mater, is a thin, vascular layer with many blood vessels that provides oxygen and nourishment to the nervous tissue. These three layers protect the brain and spinal cord and also bathe it in cerebrospinal fluid.

Ventricles. The ventricles (four in all) are spaces or cavities located in the brain (Fig. 35-8). Each hemisphere of the cerebrum has a lateral ventricle. These connect to the third ventricle in the diencephalon. The fourth ventricle is dorsal to the pons. CSF is formed continuously from fluid filtering out of the blood in a network of capillaries called the *choroid plexus* (Fig. 35-9). The choroid plexus lines the roofs of the ventricles. The CSF flows from the lateral ventricles down through the interventricular foramen (Monro) into the third ventricle; it continues down the aqueduct of Sylvius into the fourth ventricle. Openings in the roof of the fourth ventricle allow the fluids to flow into the subarachnoid spaces around the brain and the spinal cord. The flow of fluid is from the blood in the choroid plexuses, through the ventricles, the central canal, the subarachnoid spaces, up into arachnoid granulations projecting up into venous sinuses, and returning to the venous circulation.

The CSF is clear and resembles plasma. It contains proteins, glucose, urea, and salts; it also contains certain substances that form a protective barrier that prevents some (but not all) harmful substances from entering the brain and spinal cord. This fluid cushions the brain and spinal cord, protecting them from trauma.

In a 24-hour period, the choroid plexus secretes about 500 to 570 ml of CSF. Only about 125 to 150 ml is circulating at any given time. It delivers nutritive substances and removes waste and toxic substances from the cells of the CNS.

Spinal Cord. The spinal cord is a 17- to 18-inch (45- to 48-cm) cord that extends from the brain stem to the sec-

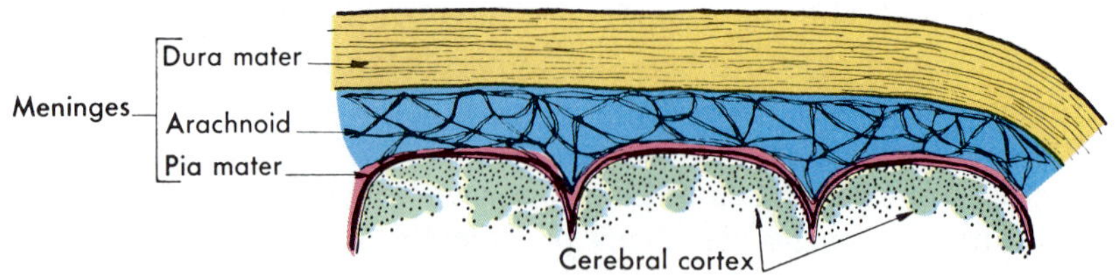

FIG. 35-7 Schematic drawing showing the structure of the meninges around the brain.

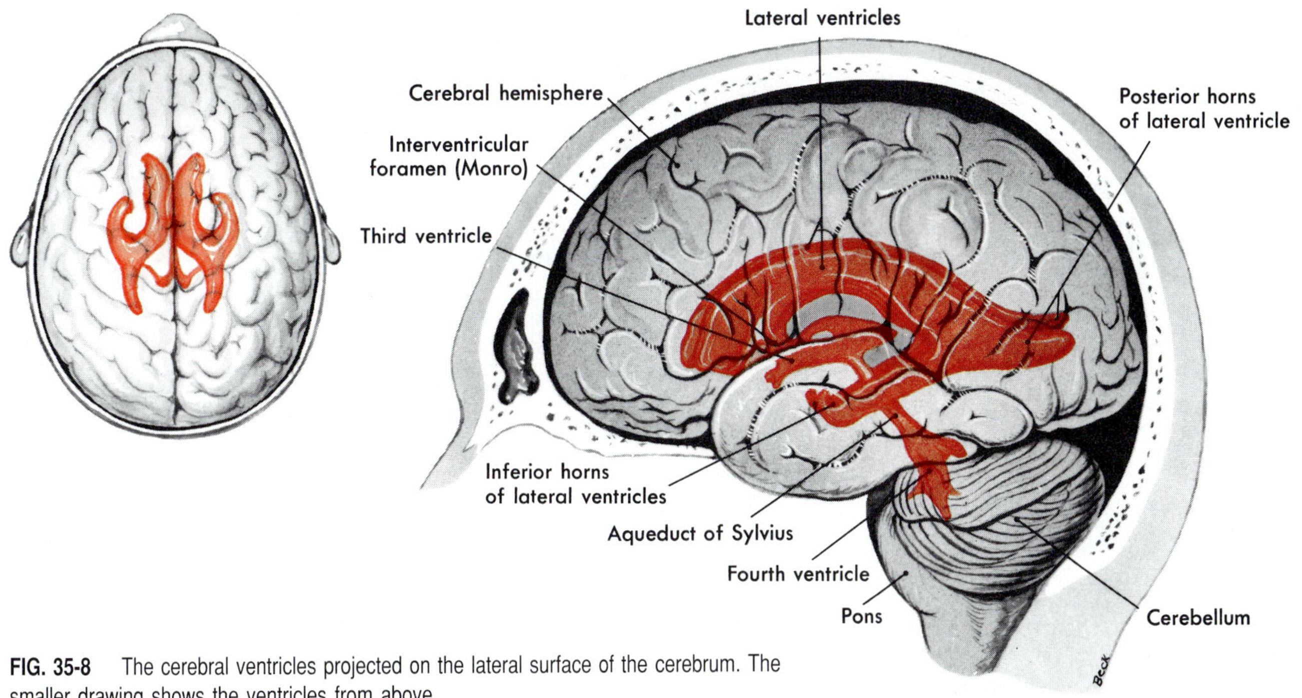

FIG. 35-8 The cerebral ventricles projected on the lateral surface of the cerebrum. The smaller drawing shows the ventricles from above.

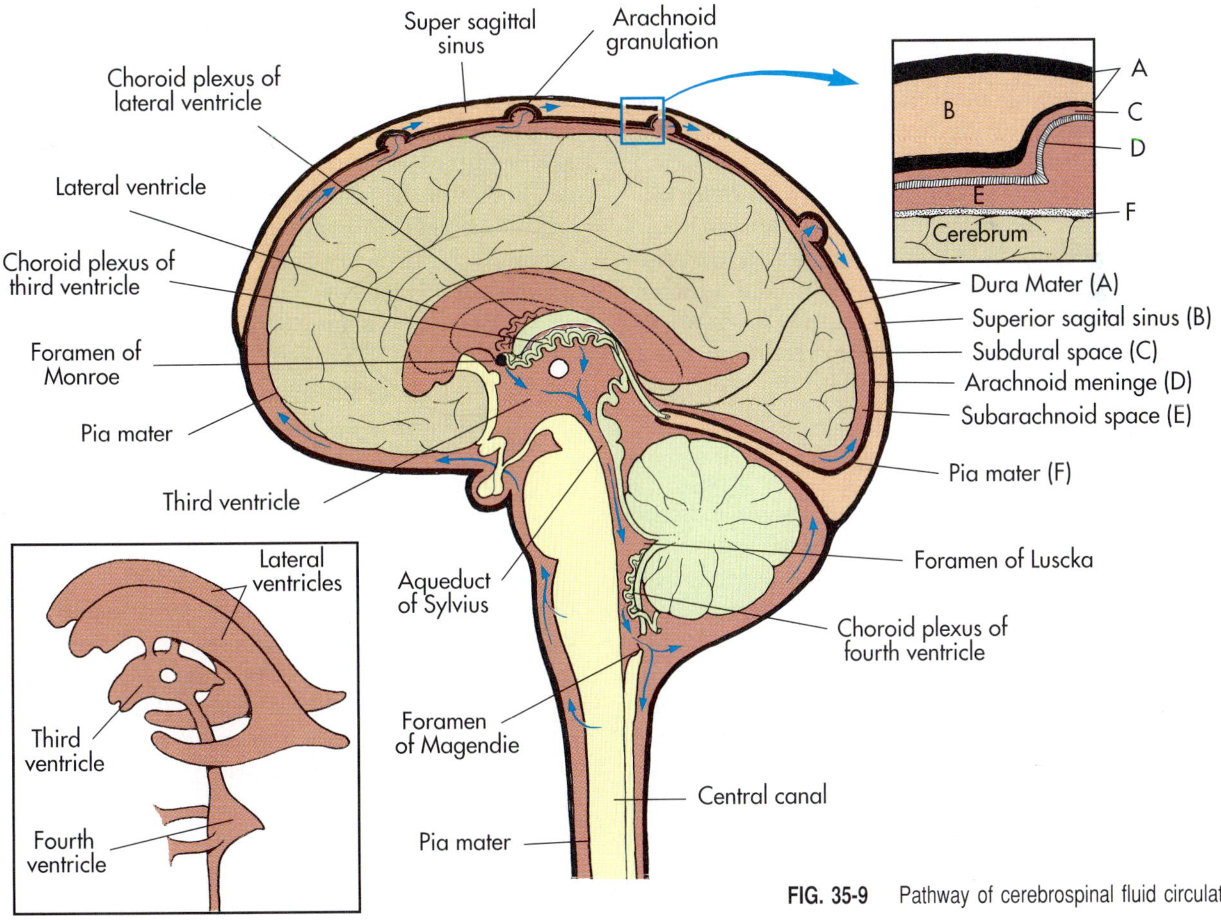

FIG. 35-9 Pathway of cerebrospinal fluid circulation.

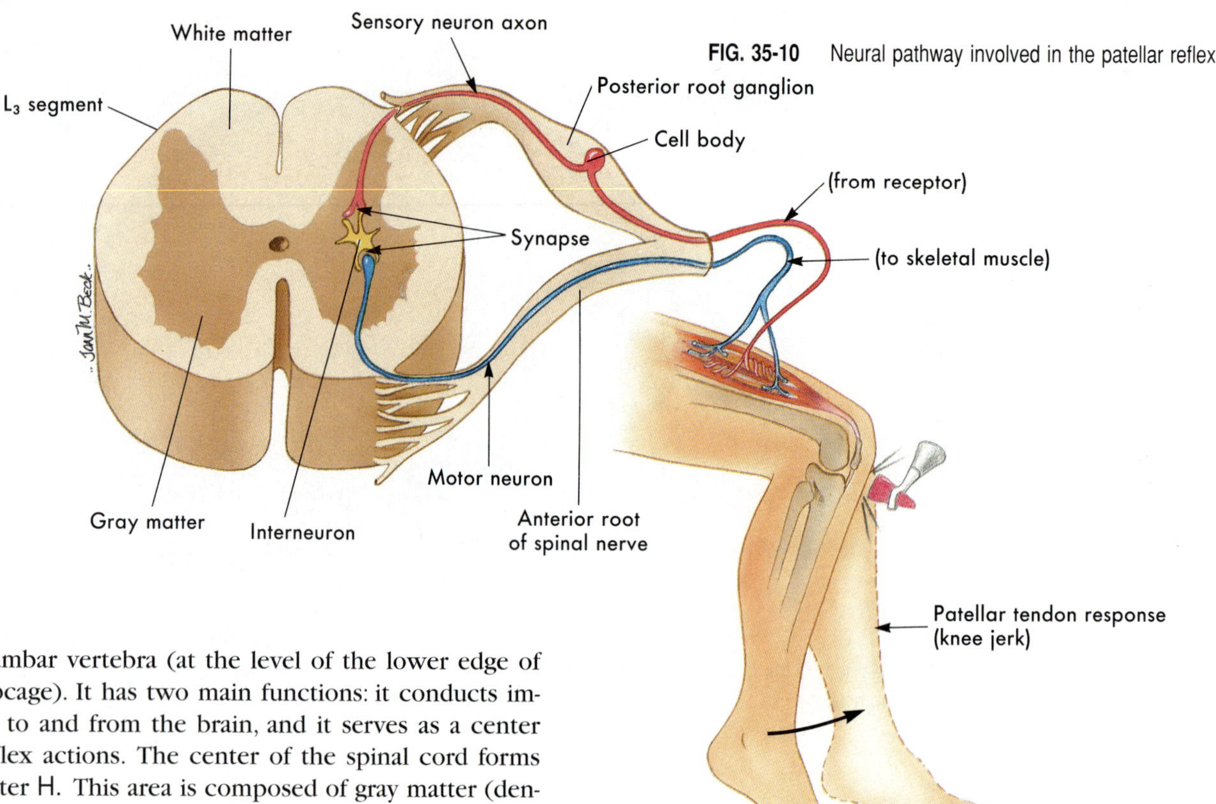

FIG. 35-10 Neural pathway involved in the patellar reflex.

ond lumbar vertebra (at the level of the lower edge of the ribcage). It has two main functions: it conducts impulses to and from the brain, and it serves as a center for reflex actions. The center of the spinal cord forms the letter H. This area is composed of gray matter (dendrites and cell bodies of neurons), while the outer portion is composed of white matter (myelinated nerve fibers).

The white matter contains the spinal tracts (groups of axons that carry the messages). The ascending tracts carry the messages to the brain, and the descending tracts carry the messages away from the brain.

The spinal cord is responsible for certain reflex activities (e.g., knee jerk) (Fig. 35-10). A sensory neuron sends the information to the cord, a central neuron (located in the cord) interprets the impulse, and a motor neuron sends the message back to the muscle or organ involved. Thus a message is sent, interpreted, and acted upon without traveling to the brain.

Peripheral Nervous System

The **peripheral nervous system** is the motor and sensory nerves and ganglia outside the brain and spinal cord, and is composed of 31 pairs of spinal nerves, 12 pairs of cranial nerves, and the autonomic nervous system.

Spinal Nerves. The 31 pairs of spinal nerves are all mixed nerves. This means they transmit sensory information to the spinal cord through afferent neurons and motor information from the CNS to the various areas of the body through efferent neurons. The spinal nerves are named according to the corresponding vertebra (e.g., C1, C2). Each spinal nerve has two attachments to the spinal cord. The dorsal root attaches posteriorly and consists of afferent fibers (sensory), while the ventral root attaches anteriorly and consists of efferent fibers (motor). Each dorsal root has an enlarged area composed of gray matter (dorsal root ganglion), which consists of the cell bodies of the sensory neurons.

As the spinal nerves leave the spinal cord, they develop several branches (plexuses). The most important plexuses are as follows:

1. Cervical plexus, which serves the shoulders, neck, and diaphragm
2. Brachial plexus, which serves the arms, wrists, and hands
3. Lumbar plexus, which serves the lower abdomen, buttocks, and anterior thighs and legs
4. Sacral plexus, which serves the lower trunk and posterior surface of the thighs and legs

Cranial Nerves. There are 12 pairs of cranial nerves, which attach to the posterior surface of the brain, mainly the brain stem (Fig. 35-11). The cranial nerves are always written in Roman numerals (e.g., I, II, III). All 12 pairs conduct impulses between the head, neck, and brain, excluding the vagus nerve (X), which also serves organs in the thoracic and abdominal cavities. Table 35-1 lists the names of the cranial nerves, where the impulses are conducted, and their functions.

Autonomic Nervous System. This portion of the nervous system controls the activities of the smooth muscle,

FIG. 35-11 Undersurface of the brain showing attachments of the cranial nerves.

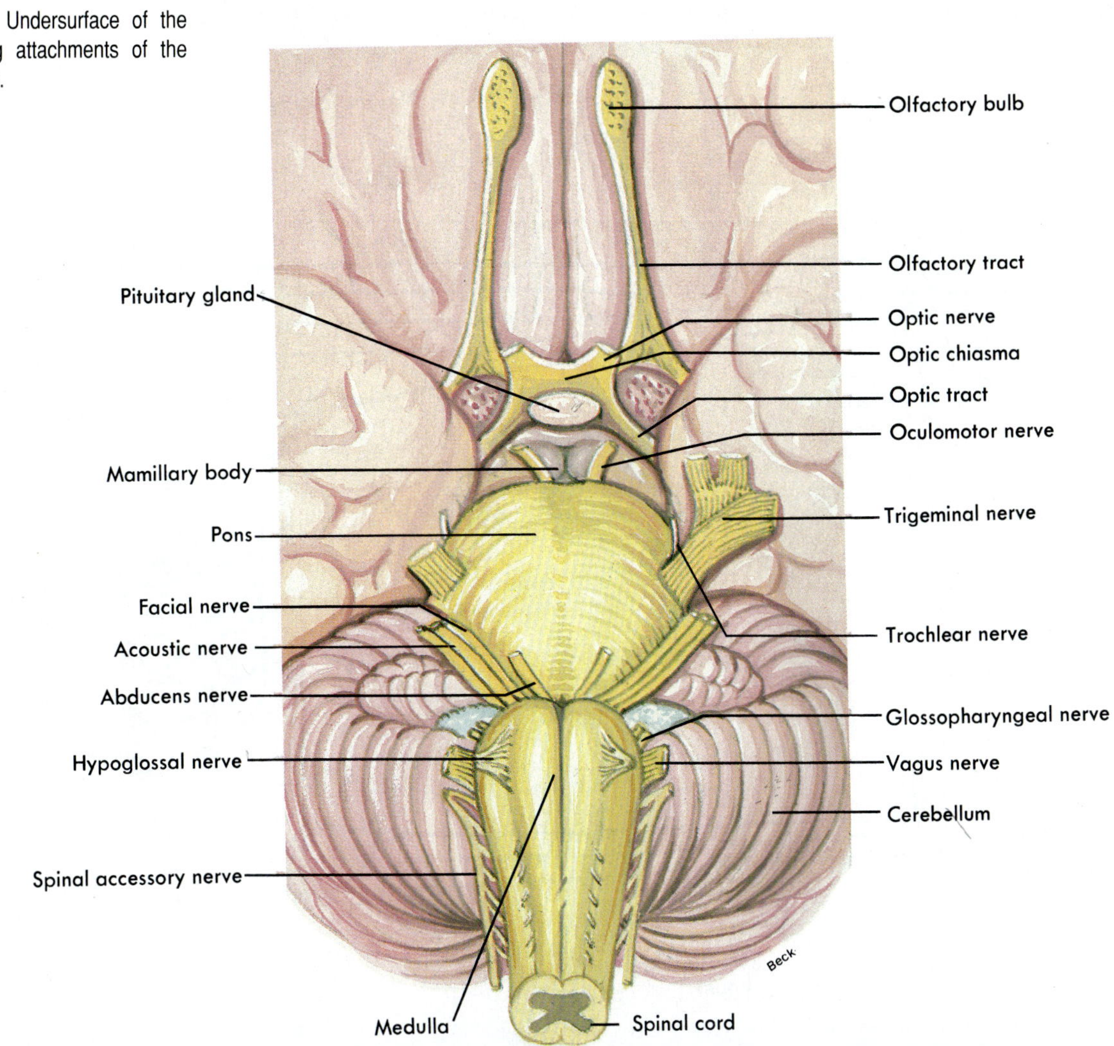

TABLE 35-1 Cranial Nerves

	Nerve*	Conducts Impulses	Functions
I	Olfactory	From nose to brain	Sense of smell
II	Optic	From eye to brain	Vision
III	Oculomotor	From brain to eye muscles	Eye movements
IV	Trochlear	From brain to external eye muscles	Eye movements
V	Trigeminal (or trifacial)	From skin and mucous membrane of head and from teeth to brain; also from brain to chewing muscles	Sensations of face, scalp, and teeth, chewing movements
VI	Abducens	From brain to external eye muscles	Turning eyes outward
VII	Facial	From taste buds of tongue to brain; from brain to face muscles	Sense of taste; contraction of muscles of facial expression
VIII	Acoustic	From ear to brain	Hearing; sense of balance
IX	Glossopharyngeal	From throat and taste buds of tongue to brain; also from brain to throat muscles and salivary glands	Sensations of throat, taste, swallowing movements, secretion of saliva
X	Vagus	From throat, larynx, and organs in thoracic and abdominal cavities to brain; also from brain to muscles of throat and to organs in thoracic and abdominal cavities	Sensations of throat, larynx, and of thoracic and abdominal organs; swallowing, voice production, slowing of heartbeat, acceleration of peristalsis
XI	Spinal accessory	From brain to certain shoulder and neck muscles	Shoulder movements; turning movements of head
XII	Hypoglossal	From brain to muscles of tongue	Tongue movements

*The first letter of the words of the following sentence are the first letters of the names of cranial nerves: "On Old Olympus' Towering Tops A Finn And German Viewed Some Hops." Many generations of students have used this or a similar sentence to help them remember the names of cranial nerves.

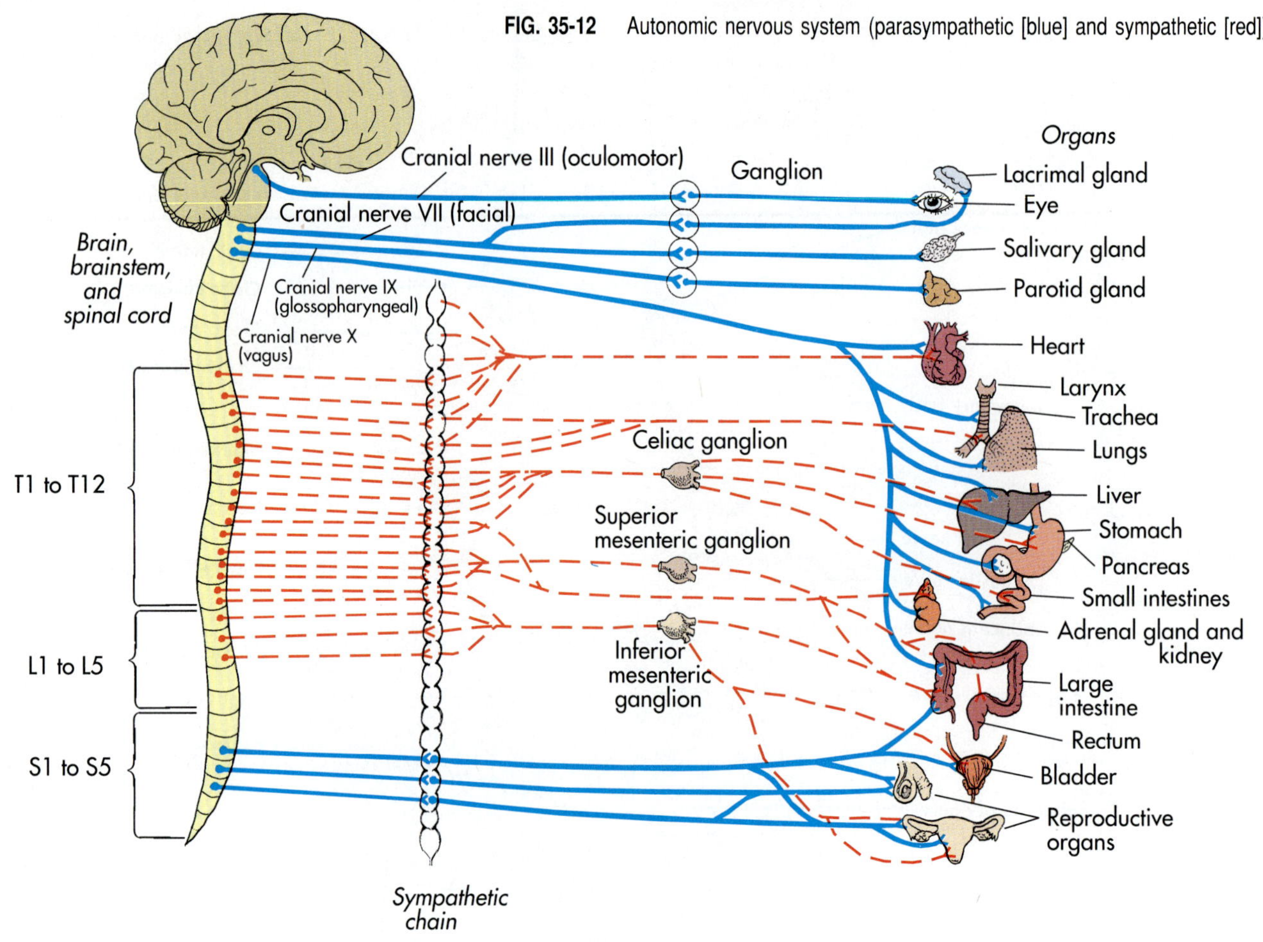

FIG. 35-12 Autonomic nervous system (parasympathetic [blue] and sympathetic [red]).

TABLE 35-2 Autonomic Functions

Visceral Effectors	Parasympathetic Control	Sympathetic Control
Heart muscle	Decreases rate and strength of heartbeat	Increases rate and strength of heartbeat.
Respiratory tract	Constriction of bronchial tubes	Dilation of bronchial tubes to allow more oxygen to enter
Smooth muscle		
Of most blood vessels	None	Constricts blood vessels and increases blood pressure
Of blood vessels in skeletal muscles	None	Dilates blood vessels
Of digestive tract	Increases peristalsis	Decreases peristalsis; inhibits defecation
Of anal sphincter	Inhibits—opens sphincter for defecation	Stimulates—closes sphincter
Of urinary bladder	Stimulates—contracts bladder	Inhibits—relaxes bladder
Of urinary sphincters	Inhibits—opens sphincter for urination	Stimulates—closes sphincter
Of eye		
Iris	Stimulates circular fibers—constriction of pupil	Stimulates radial fibers—dilation of pupil
Ciliary	Stimulates—accommodation for near vision (bulging of lens)	Inhibits—accommodation for far vision (flattening of lens)
Of hairs (pilomotor muscles)	No parasympathetic fibers	Stimulates—"goose pimples"
Glands		
Adrenal medulla	None	Increases epinephrine secretion
Sweat glands	None	Increases sweat secretion
Digestive glands	Increases secretion of digestive juices	Decreases secretion of digestive juices
Salivary glands	Increases flow and fluidity of saliva	Decreases flow and fluidity of saliva

cardiac muscle, and all of the glands. The autonomic nervous system is not a separate nervous system but a subdivision of the peripheral nervous system.

It is misleading to think of this system as the "automatic" system, although most of its activity is performed on an unconscious level. Its primary function is to maintain internal homeostasis; for example, it strives to maintain a normal heartbeat, a constant body temperature, and a normal respiratory pattern.

To maintain this homeostasis, the autonomic system has two divisions: the *sympathetic nervous system* and the *parasympathetic nervous system.* These two divisions are antagonistic—one slows an action, while the other accelerates the action. For example, the sympathetic system increases the heartbeat, whereas the parasympathetic system decreases the heartbeat (see Fig. 35-12).

Table 35-2 lists the antagonistic functions of the sympathetic and parasympathetic nervous systems. It is important to note that both these systems function simultaneously, but they have the ability to dominate each other as the need arises. In times of stress, the sympathetic system takes over to prepare the body for "flight or fight." The heartbeat increases, the blood pressure increases, and the adrenal glands increase their secretions. To calm the body after the crisis, the parasympathetic system becomes dominant, slowing the heartbeat and decreasing the blood pressure and adrenal hormone output.

CARE OF THE PATIENT WITH A NEUROLOGICAL DISORDER

The clinical picture for the patient with neurological problems is often complex. Understanding these conditions requires knowledge of the anatomy and physiology of the nervous system. The nervous system coordinates and controls all activities of the body by acting as an electrical conductance system. It performs four basic functions, including the receiving of information (stimuli) over sensory (afferent) pathways, the communicating of information between distal parts of the body, the processing of information received at conscious and reflex levels to determine responses, and the transmitting of information over motor (efferent) pathways to body organs. This is done via the neuron, which is the basic unit of the nervous system.

Changes in the Nervous System with Aging

The effects of aging on the nervous system are variable. The changes that occur include a loss of brain weight and a substantial loss of neurons (1% a year after age 50), with the cortex losing cells faster than the brain stem. The remaining cells undergo structural changes. There is also a general decline in interconnections of dendrites, a reduction in cerebral blood flow, and a decrease in brain metabolism and oxygen utilization. The neurons may contain senile plaques, neurofibrillary tangles, and the age pigment lipofuscin. There is often an altered sleep/wakefulness ratio, a decrease in the ability to regulate body temperature, and a decrease in the velocity of nerve impulses. The blood supply to the spinal cord is decreased, resulting in decreased reflexes.

Normal changes in the nervous system associated with aging are *not* the same as senility, organic brain disease, or Alzheimer's disease. Many older persons reach old age with no functional deterioration of the nervous system. However, these normal changes may make care of the older patient a challenge. An example is the rehabilitation of older patients (see gerontological box).

Prevention of Neurological Problems

Many conditions of the nervous system have no known cause. Other neurological problems can be prevented or their effects reduced by modifying life-style factors. Neurovascular diseases occur in part as a result of defined risk factors. These are the same factors that also increase

GERONTOLOGICAL CONSIDERATIONS

- As neurons are lost with aging, there is a deterioration in neurological function, resulting in slowed reflex and reaction time.
- Tremors that increase with fatigue are commonly observed in adults.
- The sense of touch and the ability for fine motor coordination diminish with aging.
- Most older persons possess the ability to learn, but the speed of learning is slowed. Short-term memory is more affected by aging than long term memory.
- The incidence of physiological dementia or organic brain syndrome, including Alzheimer's disease, Pick's disease, and multiinfarct dementia, increases with aging.
- The incidence of cerebrovascular accident increases with age. The prognosis is affected by the location and extent of the cerebral damage. Rehabilitation potential after a stroke is often reduced by advanced age and coexisting medical problems.
- Nerve irritation resulting from arthritis, joint injuries, or spinal cord compression can cause chronic pain or weakness.
- Dementia is not a normal consequence of aging but may be a result of many reversible conditions, including anemia, fluid and electrolyte imbalance, malnutrition, hypothyroidism, metabolic disturbances, drug toxicity, and hypotension.

the risk of cardiac disease and include high blood pressure, high blood cholesterol levels, cigarette smoking, obesity, stress, and lack of exercise.

The avoidance of cigarette smoking has been found to decrease the incidence of lung cancer. This is significant for the nervous system, because cancer of the lung often metastasizes to the brain.

Prevention of neurological problems resulting from trauma is a major challenge. These injuries include the fairly common diagnoses of spinal cord injury and head injury, which occur frequently in young persons. Patient teaching regarding avoiding such injuries should include the following:

- Avoidance of drug and alcohol use
- Safe use of motor vehicles—use of automobile seat belts, helmets with motorcycles and snowmobiles
- Safe swimming practices—avoidance of diving in shallow water
- Safe handling and storage of firearms
- Use of hardhats in dangerous construction areas
- Use of protective padding as needed for sports[60]

Neurological diseases, such as meningitis or a brain abscess, that occur as a result of infection can sometimes be prevented by prompt treatment of ear and sinus infections. The practice of safe and responsible sex is important, because some neurologically related diseases, such as syphilis and AIDS, are spread by sexual contact. Safe practices include abstinence, monogamy, and the use of condoms. Treatment for drug abuse, especially intravenous use, is important, as in the prevention of AIDS.

Neurological Assessment

History. A comprehensive history is essential to the diagnosis of neurological disease. This includes specifics about symptoms experienced, as well as the patient's understanding and perception of what is happening. Obtaining information from family members and/or significant others may also be extremely helpful. The same format should be followed routinely to make sure information is complete.

For patients with suspected neurological conditions, the presence of many symptoms or subjective data may be significant. These include the following:

- Headaches, especially ones that first occur after middle age, or ones that change in character; headaches that are worse in the morning or awaken a person from sleep are especially significant
- Clumsiness or loss of function in an extremity
- Change in visual acuity
- Any new or worsened seizure activity
- Numbness or tingling in one or more extremities
- Pain in an extremity or other part of the body
- Personality changes or mood swings
- Extreme fatigue or tiredness

Mental Status. Assessment of the neurological patient's mental status is important. An examination of mental status generally includes orientation (person, place, and time), mood and behavior, general knowledge (such as the names of the presidents of the United States), and short-term and long-term memory. The patient's attention span and ability to concentrate may also be assessed.

It is important to document mental status in specific terms. For instance, it is better to document "oriented to name, date, and hospital" than to document "oriented."

Level of Consciousness. A decreasing level of consciousness is the earliest sign of increased intracranial pressure. Restlessness, disorientation, and lethargy may be seen first. Observations are recorded in terms of behavior and signs—not labels such as "disoriented." One way of classifying level of consciousness is in Table 35-3.

Glasgow coma scale. A quick, practical, and standardized system for assessing the degree of conscious impairment in the critically ill and for predicting the duration and ultimate outcome of coma, particularly with head injuries, is the **Glasgow coma scale** (Fig. 35-13). It was developed in 1974 and consists of assessment of three parts of the neurological assessment: eye opening, best motor response, and best verbal response.

The stronger the stimulus needed to obtain a response, the lower the patient's score. The number value assigned to each part of the scale is added to yield an objective score. The score for a patient who is not neurologically impaired is 14 to 16, depending on the system used. The lowest possible score is 3. Generally, any score of 7 or less is commonly accepted as a definition of coma. The scale has a high degree of consistency even when used by staff of varied experience.

Language and Speech. It is important to assess the language and speech capability of the neurological patient. Speech is a function of the dominant hemisphere, which

TABLE 35-3 Levels of Consciousness

Level	Description
Alert	Responds appropriately to auditory, tactile, and visual stimuli
Disorientation	Disoriented, unable to follow simple commands, thinking slowed, inattentive
Stupor	Responds to verbal commands with moaning or groaning, if at all
Semicomatose	Is an impaired state in consciousness, characterized by obtundation and stupor, from which a patient can be aroused only by energetic stimulation
Comatose	Unable to respond to any external stimuli; loss of brain functions

is on the left side of the brain for all right-handed people and most left-handed people. **Aphasia** is an abnormal neurological condition in which the language function is defective or absent because of an injury to certain areas of the cerebral cortex. These areas are Broca's area in the frontal lobe and Wernicke's area in the posterior part of the temporal lobe.

It includes all areas of language, including speech, reading, writing, and understanding. Aphasia has been subdivided as follows:

1. Sensory aphasia or receptive aphasia—inability to comprehend the spoken word or written word
2. Motor aphasia—inability to use symbols of speech (also called expressive aphasia)
3. Global aphasia—inability to understand the spoken word, as well as to speak

Anomia is a form of aphasia characterized by the inability to name objects. **Dysarthria** is defined as difficult, poorly articulated speech that usually results from interference in the control over the muscles of speech. The general cause is damage to a central or peripheral nerve.

Cranial Nerves. Assessment of cranial nerve function is another important part of the neurological assessment. The 12 pairs of nerves emerge from the cranial cavity through openings in the skull. (See Table 35-1 for specifics of cranial nerve classification and assessment.)

Motor Function. Evaluation of motor status of the neurological patient will detect abnormalities in the normal functioning of nerves and muscles. Motor function disturbances are the most commonly encountered neurological symptom. In general, the parts of the motor status examination include gait and stance, muscle tone, coordination, involuntary movements, and the muscle stretch reflexes.

Damage to the nervous system often causes a serious problem in mobility. A loss of function is called *paralysis;* a lesser degree of movement deficit is called *paresis.*

Injury or disease of motor neurons causes alterations of muscle strength, tone, and reflex activity. The specific signs and symptoms vary according to whether the lesion involves an upper motor neuron or a lower motor neuron. Muscles may be **flaccid** (weak, soft, and flabby and lacking normal muscle tone), with absent deep tendon reflexes, or they may be spastic, with increased reflexes. With some muscle problems, the affected muscle shows small, localized, spontaneous and involuntary contractions called fasciculations. With other problems, clonus (a forced series of alternating contractions and partial relaxation of a muscle) may occur.

Sensory and Perceptual Status. The sensory examination is the most difficult part of the neurological evaluation. Specific alterations in sensation that should be assessed include pain, touch, temperature, and **proprioception,** the sensation pertaining to stimuli originating from within the body regarding spatial position and muscular activity or to the sensory receptors that they activate. This sensation gives one the ability to know the position of the body without looking at it and the ability to "know" objects by the sense of touch.

Unilateral neglect, a condition in which an individual is perceptually unaware of and inattentive to one side of the body, may also occur. Another perceptual

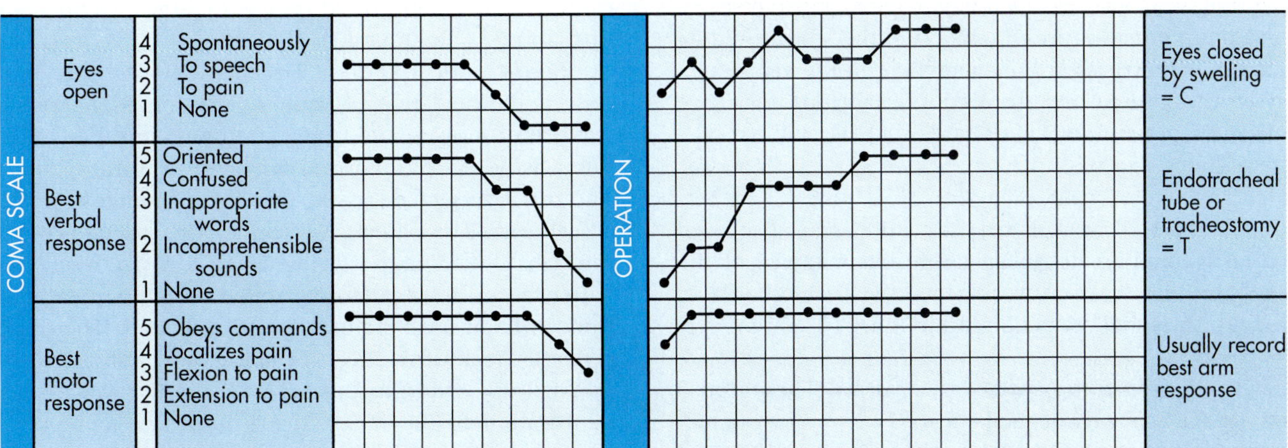

FIG. 35-13 Glasgow Coma Scale, demonstrating measurement of level of consciousness. Record *C* if eyes are closed by edema; record *T* if endotracheal tube or tracheostomy tube is in place. Notice change in patient's condition just before and after surgery.

problem is **hemianopia,** which is characterized by defective vision or blindness in half of the visual field.

In clinical settings it is usually not feasible or necessary to complete the total neurological examination during shift-to-shift assessments of the patient. In many settings, however, such as intensive care units, the neurological checks may be done as frequently as every hour. Factors that are the most important include orientation, level of consciousness, muscle strength, ability to speak, involuntary movements, and any abnormal posturing.

Laboratory Tests

Blood and Urine Tests. Assessment of the neurologically impaired patient includes a variety of blood and urine tests. A culture of the urine may rule out infection involving the urinary tract. Other urine testing may indicate the presence of diabetes insipidus. Urine drug screens may be done to rule out drug use as a cause of lethargy or to identify specific drugs ingested.

Arterial blood gas values may be an important diagnostic tool in monitoring the oxygen content of the blood. The gases may be altered with neurological diseases such as Guillain-Barré syndrome, in which breathing patterns may be altered. Blood tests that are routinely done may help narrow the diagnosis of neurological disorder.

Cerebrospinal Fluid. Examination of the CSF can yield information about many neurological conditions.

Normally there are up to 10 lymphocytes per milliliter of spinal fluid. An increase in the number of cells may indicate an infection, such as tuberculosis or a viral infection. Bacterial infections such as tuberculous meningitis often lower the CSF glucose level, as well as the chloride levels. A culture or smear examination is done to determine the causative organism in meningitis. Spinal fluid protein is elevated when degenerative diseases or a brain tumor is present. Blood in the spinal fluid indicates hemorrhage from somewhere in the ventricular system. A protein electrophoresis evaluation may give evidence of neurological diseases such as multiple sclerosis (Table 35-4).

TABLE 35-4 Normal Characteristics of Cerebrospinal Fluid (CSF)

Determination	Value
Specific gravity	1.007
pH	7.35 to 7.45
Chloride	120 to 130 mEq/L
Glucose	50 to 75 mg/dl
Pressure	80 to 200 mm water
Total volume	80 to 200 ml (15 ml in ventricles)
Total protein	15 to 45 mg/dl (lumbar)
	10 to 25 mg/dl (cisternal)
	5 to 15 mg/dl (ventricular)
Gamma globulin	6% to 13% of total protein
Cell count	
RBC	None
WBC	0-10 cells (all lymphocytes and monocytes)

Other Tests. Plain skull x-ray films of the head and vertebral column are useful in ruling out fractures of the skull and cervical vertebrae. Since the development of the CT scan, skull x-ray films are not used as extensively as before.

Computed tomography (CT) scan. The purpose of the CT scan, also called the *CAT scan,* is to detect pathological conditions of the cerebrum and spinal cord using a technique of scanning without radioisotopes. There is no special physical preparation of the patient for the test. A CT scan takes 20 to 30 minutes if done without contrast medium and about 60 minutes if the scan is also done with contrast. The procedure is painless, except for the slight discomfort that occurs when an intravenous line is started for the injection of the contrast dye. There is also some discomfort in lying still, and possible feelings of claustrophobia as a result of the head being positioned in the head holder. If contrast medium is used, it is important for the nurse to document and report to the physician any history of allergy to iodine and seafood, because iodine is present in the contrast medium.

During the procedure, the patient lies supine with the head positioned within a rubber head holder to prevent air gaps between the machine and the scalp. The head is scanned in two planes simultaneously and at various angles. Each image that appears is a specific layer of brain tissue. The computer displays a printout that indicates areas of increased densities (e.g., tumors or thrombi) (see Chapter 17).

Brain scan. Like the CT scan, the brain scan's purpose is the detection of pathological conditions of the cerebrum. It uses radioactive isotopes and a scanner. There is no special physical preparation of the patient. The procedure takes approximately 45 minutes for the actual scan. The patient is injected with a radioisotope (mercury or sodium pertechnetate [Tc 99m]). While the patient lies still, a scanner is passed over the brain area. Concentrated areas of uptake are reflected. There are generally no adverse effects from the procedure and only minimal discomfort associated with the intravenous administration of the radioactive isotopes. If mercury is used as the isotope indicator, a mercurial diuretic (meralluride [Mercuhydrin]) is administered several hours before the procedure to allow a greater concentration of the mercury to be circulated to brain tissue, since meralluride minimizes the uptake of mercury by the kidneys.

MRI scan. The magnetic resonance imaging (MRI) scan uses magnetic forces to image body structures. It has relevance in the nervous system as a way to detect pathological conditions of the cerebrum and spinal cord. Because the scan involves a magnetic force, the patient should be cautioned to remove watches, credit cards, and any metal from the clothing before entering the scanning room. The patient should also be questioned about the presence of any metal in the body that would preclude the use of the scan, such as orthopedic appliances, aneurysm clips, and pacemakers.

During the procedure the patient lies supine with the head positioned in a head holder. The test takes 45 to 60 minutes. The procedure is painless, except for discomfort in lying still and possible feelings of claustrophobia. The patient should be warned that the machine makes different and somewhat loud noises during the scanning procedure.

PET scan. Another evaluative measure that is similar to the CT scan and MRI scan is the positron emission tomography (PET) scan. In this procedure the patient receives an injection of deoxyglucose with radioactive fluorine. The area in question is scanned, and a color composite picture is obtained. Shades of color give an indication of the level of glucose metabolism; this then can be translated into indications of a pathological state. As with the CT scan, discomfort is minimal. The patient should be aware of the need to lie still for the duration of the scan, usually about 45 minutes.

Lumbar puncture. A lumbar puncture is often performed as part of the diagnostic workup of the patient who may have a neurological problem. It is contraindicated in patients who might have increased intracranial pressure, because the withdrawal of fluid may cause the medulla oblongata to herniate downward into the foramen magnum.

A lumbar puncture is done to obtain CSF for examination or relief of pressure or to allow the introduction of dye or medication. It is a common procedure, usually done in the patient's room. The procedure takes 10 to 15 minutes. Slight pain and pressure may be felt as the dura is entered. A sharp, shooting pain down one leg may occur, caused by the needle coming close to a nerve.

The patient is usually positioned on the side with the knee and head flexed at an acute angle. This allows for maximal lumbar flexion and separation of the interspinous spaces. After anesthetizing the area with a local anesthetic, the physician inserts the needle below the level of the spinal cord, at the L4-L5 or L5-S1 interspace. The inner needle is removed to allow for drainage and measurement of spinal fluid. The level-of-fluid column in the manometer is used to measure the pressure. Fluid may be collected for various tests or to relieve pressure. The first specimen of spinal fluid may contain blood from slight bleeding at the site of the puncture. This specimen should not be sent for cell count.

After the procedure, the patient lies flat in bed for several hours. The site of the puncture should be assessed for any leakage, as evidenced by moisture on the bandage or around the puncture site. Headache is fairly common and is thought to be caused by the loss of spinal fluid through the dura mater. If a headache develops, bed rest, analgesics, and ice to the head may help.

Electroencephalogram. The electroencephalogram (EEG) is used to provide evidence of focal or generalized disturbances of brain function by measuring the electrical activity of the brain. There is no special preparation for this test, but the patient is encouraged to be quiet and rest before the procedure, unless it is to be a sleep-deprived EEG. With this, the patient is kept awake the night before the test, and the EEG is usually done first thing in the morning. The EEG usually takes about 1 hour to complete. The hair and scalp of the patient should be clean. The electrodes are placed on the scalp with collodion in a set pattern to cover all scalp areas. There is no pain associated with an EEG.

The basic resting rhythm of the EEG is affected by opening the eyes or altering attention. Recordings are sometimes made while the patient is asleep or sleep deprived, when the seizure threshold may be lowered. Comparisons are made of different patterns of the recordings (Fig. 35-14 on p. 1106). After the test the patient should be allowed to rest. The patient should be assisted if necessary in washing the hair and removing the collodion from the scalp.

Myelogram. The myelogram is commonly used to identify lesions in the intradural or extradural compartments of the spinal canal by observing the flow of radiopaque dye through the subarachnoid space. The two types of dyes most commonly used are metrizamide and iophendylate (Pantopaque) dye. Before the procedure the patient's baselines of lower extremity strength and sensation are assessed and documented. The patient is informed that the procedure takes about 2 hours. The patient should also be told that there may be slight discomfort as the dura is entered and that she may be asked to assume a variety of positions during the procedure.

If the patient is scheduled for a metrizamide myelogram, certain drugs should not be allowed for 24 to 48 hours before the scan because they lower the seizure threshold, one of the side effects of the dye. These drugs include the phenothiazines, tricyclic antidepressants, CNS stimulants, and amphetamines.

The patient is usually positioned on the side with both knees and the head flexed at an acute angle to allow maximal flexion of the lumbar area for ease in performing the lumbar puncture. After the puncture is performed, the inner needle is removed to allow drainage of CSF, measurement of pressure, and collection of specimens. The dye is instilled and the needle is removed. The patient is then turned to various positions so the spinal cord can be visualized while fluoroscopic and ra-

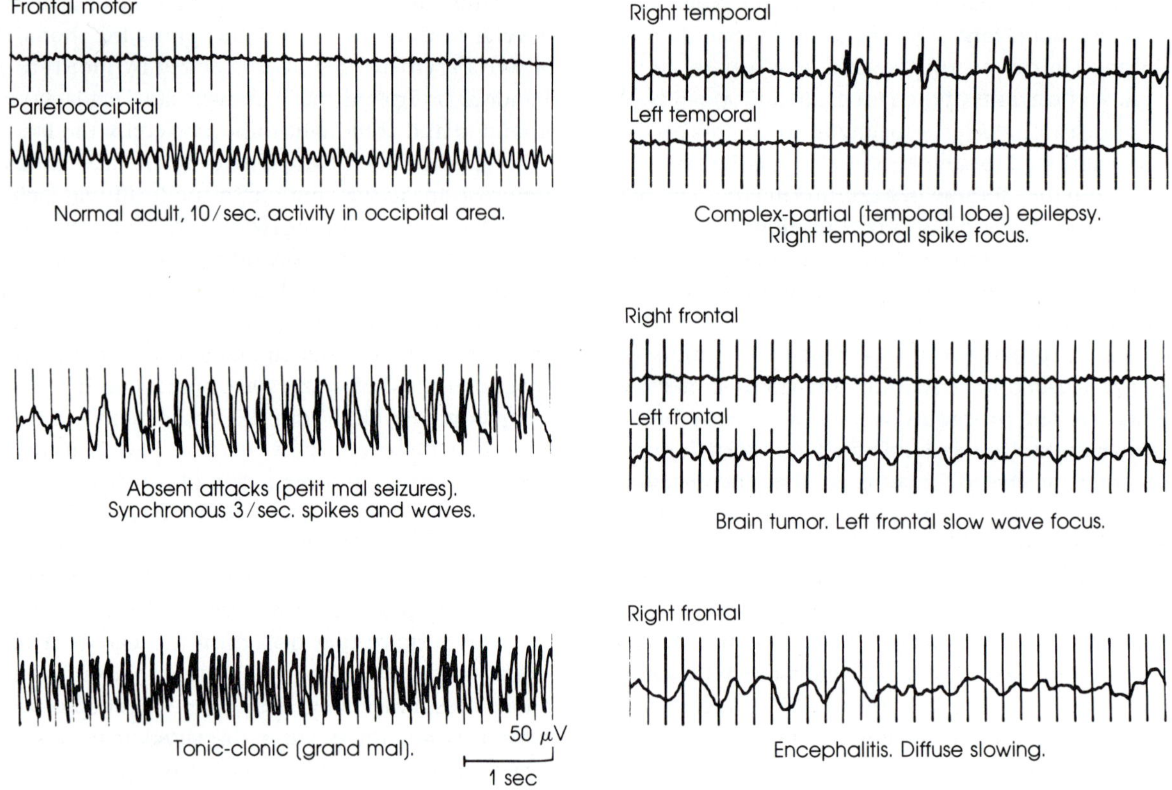

FIG. 35-14 Tracings of electroencephalogram. The normal tracing is demonstrated, as are several pathological states.

diopaque films are taken. After the procedure is completed, Pantopaque dye must be removed via another lumbar puncture to prevent serious irritation of the meninges. Metrizamide dye does not have to be removed. The patient usually undergoes a CT scan 4 to 6 hours after a metrizamide myelogram.

Care after the procedure varies, depending on the dye used. With a Pantopaque myelogram, the patient lies flat in bed overnight. No pillow is used, and the head of the bed is not elevated. The site of the puncture should be observed for any leakage of CSF, and the strength and sensation of the lower extremities should be assessed. Headache is fairly common after the procedure.

If the patient has had a myelogram using metrizamide dye, the head and thorax must remain elevated to at least 30 to 50 degrees for at least 8 hours and then elevated to at least 30 degrees for another 24 hours. Fluid intake is encouraged to assist in absorption of the dye. Common side effects with this dye include nausea, vomiting, and seizures, as well as nonspecific behavior changes. The peak risk for these side effects is 4 to 6 hours after completion of the procedure. The site of the puncture and strength and sensation of the lower extremities are assessed. The patient must avoid the use of the same drugs that were restricted before the procedure for 24 to 48 hours, because they lower the seizure threshold. Despite the side effects, the advantages of the metrizamide myelogram are many. The dye is less viscous and allows better visualization of smaller areas than that obtained with a myelogram using Pantopaque dye.

Angiogram. The angiogram (cerebral arteriography) is a fairly common procedure used to visualize the cerebral arterial system by injecting radiopaque material. It allows the detection of arterial aneurysms, vessel anomalies, ruptured vessels, and displacement of vessels by tumors or masses.

Before the procedure the patient is usually given clear liquids, although in some institutions all oral intake is restricted. The patient must be assessed for any allergy to iodine because the dye contains iodine. If the femoral approach is to be used, it is helpful to assess and mark the locations of the bilateral pedal pulses. If the carotid artery is used, the neck circumference is measured as part of the baseline data. Immediately before the procedure, baseline vital signs and pulses are measured, and a neurological check is performed and recorded.

The test takes approximately 2 to 3 hours. The patient may experience discomfort in lying still for that period of time. When the dye is injected, most patients complain of feeling extremely hot and seeing flashes of light.

The patient is positioned supine on the x-ray table. A local anesthetic agent is used to anesthetize the area of the puncture site. The catheter is introduced percutaneously and introduced into the relevant vessels. At times, the catheter may be inserted directly into the carotid or vertebral arteries. After all the injections are done, the catheter is withdrawn and pressure is applied to the puncture site for at least 15 minutes.

After the procedure, bed rest is ordered for a specified time, usually 4 to 6 hours. Vital signs are checked frequently (at times as often as every 15 minutes), and a neurological check is performed with every vital sign check. The site of the puncture is assessed frequently for the presence of a hematoma. With a femoral stick, the pulses distal to the site are checked for evidence of arterial occlusion. With a carotid stick, the patient is assessed for any difficulty breathing or swallowing or an increase in the girth of the neck.

The patient undergoing this procedure is at risk for cerebral vascular accident, as well as an increase in intracranial pressure. Any change in level of consciousness or other parts of the neurological assessment should be promptly reported.

Digital subtraction angiography. In digital subtraction angiography (DSA), abnormalities of the cerebrovascular system are identified using a process that removes overlying structures from the image, so that clinically significant details can be displayed in an enhanced way. Often the same vessels used for an angiogram are used with the DSA. Care of the patient before and after the procedure is the same as that for the patient undergoing angiography.

Electromyogram. An electromyogram (EMG) is used to measure the contraction of a muscle in response to electrical stimulation. It provides evidence of lower motor neuron disease, primary muscle disease, and defects in the transmission of electrical impulses at the neuromuscular junction, such as in myasthenia gravis. There is no special preparation for the test. The test takes approximately 45 minutes for one muscle study. The patient needs to know that there will be discomfort when the electrode is inserted into the muscle and when the electrical current is used. The muscle may ache for a short time after the procedure.

During the test, an electrode is inserted into selected skeletal muscles. An electric current is passed through the electrode, and the machine graphs the variations of muscle potentials (voltage). After the procedure it is important to assess the patient for signs of bleeding at the site of the electrode insertion. The patient may need an analgesic for discomfort and a rest period.

Echoencephalogram. An echoencephalogram uses ultrasound to depict the intracranial structures of the brain. It is especially helpful in detecting ventricular dilation and a major shift of midline structures in the brain as a result of an expanding lesion. The preparation of the patient, the actual procedure, and aftercare are similar to those of the brain scan.

Other tests. Several other tests are used to detect neurological problems of the ventricles and cisternal system. These include the ventriculogram and the pneumoencephalogram. Both tests use air as a contrast; it is inserted into the ventricular system. The ventriculogram is usually performed in the operating room under general or intravenous anesthesia. The pneumoencephalogram is done rarely since the advent of less-invasive procedures such as the CT scan. After either procedure the patient is often quite uncomfortable, with a headache and nausea. Side effects are common until the air is absorbed, usually in 24 to 48 hours.

Common Neurological Problems

Headaches.

Etiology/pathophysiology. Headache is a common neurological complaint; its significance is variable and it can result from many different causes. The source of recurring headache should be determined through careful physical examination with appropriate neurological assessment. Some tumors may produce no symptoms except for headache for a long period.

The exact mechanism of head pain is not known. Although the skull and brain tissues are not able to feel sensory pain, pain arises from the scalp and its blood vessels and muscles and from the dura mater and its venous sinuses. Pain also arises from the blood vessels at the base of the brain and from cervical cranial nerves. Blood vessels may dilate and become congested with blood. Headaches can be classified as vascular, tension, and traction-inflammatory. Vascular headaches include migraine, cluster, and hypertensive headaches. Tension headaches may arise from psychological problems of tension or stress or from medical problems such as cervical arthritis. Traction-inflammatory headaches include those caused by infection, intracranial or extracranial causes, by occlusive vascular structures, and by temporal arteritis.

Clinical manifestations. Headache pain may be made worse by stress or tension. Knowledge of the patient's perception of the effect of stress on the pain is important in planning effective interventions.

Migraine headaches are unusual in that there are prodromal (early signs and symptoms of a developing condition or disease) signs and symptoms that occur before the acute attack. These may include any of the following: visual field defects, experiencing unusual smells or sounds, disorientation, paresthesias, and in rare cases, paralysis of a part of the body. During a migraine headache, signs and symptoms may include nausea, vomiting, sensitivity to light, chilliness, fatigue, irritability, diaphoresis, edema, and other signs of autonomic dysfunction.

Assessment. Collection of *subjective data* includes the patient's understanding of the headache, possible causes, and any precipitating factors. It is important to determine what measures relieve the symptoms, as well as the location, frequency, pattern, and character of the pain. This includes the site of return of the headache, time of day, and intervals between the headaches. The initial onset of the headache, presence of any symptoms that occur before the headache or associated symptoms, the presence of allergies, and any family history of similar headache patterns are also important to assess.

Collection of *objective data* includes any behaviors indicating stress, anxiety, or pain. Changes in the ability to carry out activities of daily living (ADLs), an abnormally raised body temperature, and the presence of sinus drainage may be important. Abnormalities noted during the physical examination portion of the neurological assessment should also be documented. (See therapeutic dialogue.)

THERAPEUTIC DIALOGUE

Nurse: Can you describe your problem to me?
Patient: It's a pain in my head.
Nurse: When did this pain start?
Patient: About a month ago.
Nurse: Did anything else happen at that same time?
Patient: My daughter left home for college.
Nurse: How did you feel about that?
Patient: I was really upset. She was my baby. I can't believe that she's gone.
Nurse: Was there anything else that you noticed at the same time? Like an increased temperature or nasal drainage?
Patient: No, I don't think so.
Nurse: What made the headache worse?
Patient: Thinking about my loneliness.
Nurse: What made the headache better?
Patient: Sleeping or taking a Valium.
Nurse: Have you had trouble sleeping or noticed that your appetite was worse?
Patient: I wake up early in the morning. I don't feel much like eating.
Nurse: Have you lost weight?
Patient: About 10 pounds in the last month.
Nurse: Can you tell me what the pain feels like?
Patient: It's a pain that goes through my whole head. It throbs and gets worse in the evening.
Nurse: What do you think is the cause of the headache?
Patient: I guess maybe I'm upset that my daughter left.

Diagnostic tests. It is important to evaluate headaches that are not transient. Usual testing includes a neurological examination, a CT scan (MRI or PET scan may also be done), a brain scan, skull x-ray films, and a lumbar puncture. A lumbar puncture is not done, however, if there is evidence of increased intracranial pressure or if a brain tumor is suspected, because quick reduction of pressure produced by removal of the spinal fluid may cause brain herniation. In these situations, a CT scan is done first.

Medical management

Dietary counseling. Some foods may cause or worsen headaches. These include foods containing tyramine, nitrates, or glutamates. One example of this is monosodium glutamate (MSG), often used in the preparation of Chinese foods. Other substances that may provoke headaches include vinegar, chocolate, yogurt, alcohol, fermented or marinated foods, ripened cheese, cured sandwich meat, caffeine, and pork.

Psychotherapy. Patients with headaches may respond to psychotherapy. This is not to say that the headache pain is not physiological in nature, but counseling can help the patient to develop awareness of stress factors and to deal with the pain. The patient may need help in expressing feelings about intractable headache pain.

Medications. Medications are often used to treat headache. These will be described in terms of their use for migraine, cluster, and tension headaches.

MIGRAINE HEADACHES. Acetylsalicylic acid (aspirin) may be helpful after a migraine headache has developed. Ergotamine tartrate preparations taken early in the attack may prevent progression of the headache. These drugs are usually successful in treating migraines. Ergotamine tartrate preparations act by constricting cerebral blood vessel walls and reducing cerebral blood flow. They can be given orally, sublingually, rectally, or by injection. These preparations are also available in combinations with other drugs, such as caffeine, phenobarbital, and belladonna. Side effects of ergot preparations include nausea, vomiting, numbness and tingling, muscle pain, and changes in heart rate. They cannot be taken by pregnant women because they stimulate contractions of the uterine smooth muscle.

Other drugs that may be used include nonnarcotic analgesics, such as phenacetin, acetaminophen, or propoxyphene (Darvon). Codeine may be prescribed. Propranolol hydrochloride (Inderal) has been used in the prophylactic treatment of migraine and other vascular headaches.

CLUSTER HEADACHES. Because the pain associated with vascular cluster headaches is often extremely severe, narcotic analgesics, sometimes given intramuscularly, are used. Patients with cluster headaches usually feel fine between attacks, so no analgesic is needed during these times.

TENSION HEADACHES. Nonnarcotic analgesics are often used to treat tension headaches. These include acetaminophen, propoxyphene, phenacetin, and aspirin. Narcotics are avoided because these drugs are often subject to abuse; it is much better to counsel patients to develop other ways to relieve headaches.

Nursing interventions. Since stress and emotional upsets may precipitate some headaches and worsen others, relaxation and rest should be facilitated. This includes relaxation techniques, planned sleeping hours, and regular rest periods. The patient may need the nurse to assist with this. Alcohol should not be used to relieve tension, because it may become addicting and has been found to be a significant cause of cluster headaches. Regular physical exercise may also help to prevent headaches, especially ones caused by tension.

If a patient is suffering from a severe headache, the nurse should plan nursing interventions so that only essential activities take place. Interventions should be grouped so that the patient has adequate time to rest.

Comfort measures. Other treatments that may be helpful for a patient with a headache include cold packs applied to the forehead or base of the skull. Pressure applied to the temporal arteries may be helpful. Persons with migraine headaches, especially, are usually most comfortable lying in a dark room with minimal auditory stimulation.

Identifying triggering factors. Triggering factors associated with severe and recurring headaches may include fatigue, alcohol, stress, seasonal climate changes, hunger, allergies, and menstruation. The nurse may need to help the patient identify these factors. They can be assessed through ongoing observation of the patient's personality, habits, and ADLs, as well as career plans, work habits, family relationships, coping mechanisms, and relaxation activities. A diary or journal kept by the patient may be helpful in determining these factors.

Nursing diagnoses and interventions for the patient with headache include but are not limited to the following:

NURSING DIAGNOSES	NURSING INTERVENTIONS
Anxiety, related to pain	Provide quiet environment. Encourage verbalization of concerns. Provide diversional activities.
Pain, acute or chronic, related to disease process	Administer analgesics as ordered. Provide comfort measures. Maintain nonstressful environment. Encourage pain reduction techniques as appropriate: rocking movements, external warmth, breathing patterns.

Patient teaching. Teaching is an important part of the nursing intervention of the patient with headaches. Topics include (1) avoidance of factors that trigger headaches, (2) relaxation techniques including biofeedback, (3) importance of maintaining regular sleep patterns, (4) medications to be used (including dose, actions, and side effects), and (5) the importance of follow-up care.

Prognosis. With proper treatment the person with headaches can expect to live a normal life. Changes in life-style may need to occur, especially during acute episodes of headache pain. The person may have to adjust to periodic headaches and will need to rest until the headache resolves.

Neurological Pain.

Etiology/pathophysiology and clinical manifestations. Neurological pain, other than headache, is common. The transmission of pain is not fully understood, but patients may experience disabling pain either caused by a disorder within the nervous system or caused peripherally at a distant part of the body.

The transmission of pain impulses is not fully understood. Neurological pain may arise from lesions involving the peripheral cutaneous nerves, the sensory nerve roots, the thalamus, and the central pain tract (lateral spinothalamic) at some level. Each produces characteristic pain. Pain receptors are not adaptable, and pain impulses continue at the same rate as long as the stimulus is present. They are specific for pain only. Pain receptors can be activated by cellular damage, certain chemicals such as histamine, heat, ischemia, muscle spasm, and sensations of cold and pruritus that go beyond a specific level of intensity.

Pain that is described as unbearable and does not respond to treatment is classified as *intractable.* It is chronic and often debilitating, and may prevent the patient from functioning in ADLs.

Assessment. The perception of pain is highly subjective. Collection of *subjective data* includes the patient's understanding of the pain, any precipitating factors, and measures that relieve stress, including medication. The site, frequency, and nature of the pain are important, as well as the usual coping patterns of the patient when under stress. The presence of associated symptoms and measures that make the pain worse are important subjective data.

The quality of pain and its distribution are important factors to assess. Pain may vary from mild to excruciating.

Collection of *objective data* may be limited when assessing neurological pain. Objective factors that should be assessed are any behavioral signs indicating pain or stress, a change in the ability to carry out ADLs, any muscle weakness or wasting, vasomotor responses (such as flushing), abnormalities of spinal reflexes, and abnormalities noted during the sensory examination.

Diagnostic tests. Diagnostic tests for the patient in pain may include electrical stimulation used to define the pain to a greater degree. Psychological testing may be part of the workup. If back or neck pain is present, a myelogram is usually performed.

Medical management

Nonsurgical methods of pain control. Neurological pain sometimes responds to other methods of pain control. These include transcutaneous electrical nerve stimulation (TENS) and spinal cord stimulation. Both techniques use electrodes applied near the site of pain or on or around the spine (see Chapter 22). The stimulator is used to modify the sensory input by blocking or changing the painful sensation with a stimulus that is perceived to be less painful or nonpainful. Acupuncture has also been used to treat patients with neurological pain.

NERVE BLOCK. A nerve block is used to control intractable pain. It involves the injection of a local anesthetic, alcohol, or phenol close enough to a nerve to block the conduction of impulses. Sources of pain often treated with a nerve block include trigeminal neuralgia, cancer, or peripheral vascular disease. The duration of effect is from several months to several years.

MEDICATIONS. Medications are often used to treat patients with neurological pain. These often include nonnarcotic analgesics such as acetaminophen, propoxyphene (Darvon), phenacetin, and acetylsalicylic acid. Narcotics may be prescribed, as well as muscle relaxants, but these drugs may lead to abuse. The emphasis should be on helping the patient learn other measures to control the pain.

Surgery. In cases of intractable pain that does not respond to more conservative measures, surgery may be necessary to reduce or abolish pain. Neurosurgical procedures that may be done include neurectomy, rhizotomy, cordotomy, and percutaneous cordotomy.

These procedures all have potential complications that need to be considered before the decision is made to perform surgery. For example, a patient who undergoes a cordotomy may be expected to have difficulties with postural hypotension, ability to feel hot or cold, and possibly motor and bowel function. Temporary edema of the cord from the procedure may lead to temporary paralysis or leg weakness.

Nursing interventions

Comfort measures. A patient with neurological pain may be very uncomfortable and should be assisted to assume a position of comfort. For example, the patient with back pain should avoid movements that cause direct or indirect movement of the spinal cord. The patient may find lying in a supine position uncomfortable. The nurse should help the patient find a comfortable position and may need to actively assist the patient in turning or moving. Straining when having a stool can intensify pain, and a stool softener may be needed. The nurse should offer prune juice and a high-fiber diet and encourage up to 2000 ml a day or more of fluids.

Promotion of rest and relaxation. As with headache, stress and emotional upsets may precipitate or exacerbate neurological pain. Rest and relaxation should be facilitated, with planned sleeping hours and rest periods as needed.

Some patients with pain, especially intractable pain, may respond well to psychotherapy. This does not mean that the pain does not have a physiological basis, but counseling can help the patient develop awareness of what makes the pain worse and how to cope with the discomfort.

Nursing diagnoses and interventions for neurological pain are the same as those listed previously for headache, with the addition of the following:

NURSING DIAGNOSES	NURSING INTERVENTIONS
Disuse syndrome, high risk for, related to lack of use of a body part as a result of pain	Explain need for regular exercise program to maintain joint mobility: ROM exercises to all body joints q 2 to 4 hr. Be positive and reassuring in approach.
Self-care deficit, feeding, bathing/hygiene, dressing/grooming, related to pain	Provide basic ADL needs as necessary, but encourage patient to begin to participate at ability level. Provide sufficient time for ADLs. Facilitate use of self-help devices as needed. Provide for total hygiene as indicated.

Patient teaching. Teaching is an important part of the nursing interventions of the patient with neurological pain. Teaching should include at least the factors that are taught to the patient with headache. Also important is the awareness of physical methods such as positioning the body to increase comfort and the structuring of the home and work setting to keep stressors at a minimum.

Prognosis. As with headache pain, neurological pain can in most cases be treated adequately. Life-style changes may be helpful in allowing the person to live a full life.

Increased Intracranial Pressure.

Etiology/pathophysiology and clinical manifestations. Increased intracranial pressure is a complex grouping of events that occurs because of multiple neurological conditions. It often occurs suddenly, can progress rapidly, and often requires surgical intervention. It is a potential complication in many neurological conditions and can rapidly lead to death if not arrested and reversed.

Specific causes of increased intracranial pressure include space-occupying lesions that increase tissue volume, cerebrospinal problems, and cerebral edema. An increase in any one of the contents of the cranium is usually accompanied by a reciprocal change in the volume of one of the others. This is because the cranial vault is rigid and nonexpandable. The buildup of pressure may occur slowly over weeks or rapidly, depending on the cause. Usually one side of the brain will be more involved, but both sides of the brain will eventually be involved.

As the pressure increases within the cranial cavity, it is first compensated for by venous compression and cerebrospinal displacement. As the pressure continues to rise, the cerebral blood flow decreases and inadequate perfusion of the brain occurs. This inadequate perfusion starts a vicious cycle that causes the P_{CO_2} to increase and the P_{O_2} and the pH to fall. These changes cause vasodilation and cerebral edema. This edema leads to further increased intracranial pressure, which causes increased compression of neural tissue and an even greater increase in intracranial pressure.

When the pressure buildup is greater than the brain's ability to compensate, pressure is exerted on surrounding structures where the pressure is lower. This movement of pressure is called *supratentorial shift* and can result in herniation.

As a result of herniation of the brain, the brain stem is compressed at various levels, which in turn compresses the vasomotor center, the posterior cerebral artery, the oculomotor nerve, the corticospinal nerve pathway, and the fibers of the ascending reticular activating system. The life-sustaining mechanisms of consciousness, blood pressure, pulse, respiration, and temperature regulation are all impaired.

Assessment. The detection of increased intracranial pressure must occur early while it is still reversible. The ability to make accurate observations, interpret observations intelligently, and record observations carefully is most important for the nurse working with patients with increased intracranial pressure.

Collection of *subjective data* for a diagnosis of increased intracranial pressure includes the patient's understanding of the condition, presence of any visual changes (**diplopia** or double vision), and a change in the ability to think. The diplopia usually results from paralysis or weakness of one of the muscles that controls the eye movement. It often occurs fairly early in the process of increased intracranial pressure. The presence of nausea or pain, especially headache, is also important. The headache is thought to result from venous congestion and the tension in the intracranial blood vessels as the cerebral pressure rises. Headache that occurs with increased intracranial pressure usually increases in intensity with coughing, straining at stool, or stooping. It is usually present in the early morning and may awaken the patient from sleep.

Collection of *objective data* includes a change in the level of consciousness. A decreasing level of consciousness is an early sign of increased intracranial pressure. This may include disorientation, restlessness, or lethargy. Observations are recorded in terms of behaviors and signs and symptoms, not in terms of labels. It is important to chart what is seen, not what is inferred.

Pupillary signs may also change with increased intracranial pressure. Pupillary responses are controlled by cranial nerve III (oculomotor nerve). As the brain herniates, the nerve is compressed with the top part of the nerve being affected first. The *ipsilateral pupil* (when the lesion is in one hemisphere) remains dilated and is incapable of constricting. The pupil appears larger than that of the affected side and does not react to light. As the intracranial pressure increases and both halves of the brain become affected, bilateral pupil dilation and fixation occur. Dilating pupils that respond slowly to light are a sign of impending herniation. A pupil that is fixed and dilated is sometimes called a "blown pupil" and is an ominous sign that *must* be reported to the physician immediately (Fig. 35-15).

Changes in the blood pressure and pulse are seen with increasing intracranial pressure. Herniation causes ischemia of the vasomotor center, which excites the vasoconstrictor fibers, causing the systolic blood pressure to rise. If the intracranial pressure continues to increase, diastolic blood pressure may fall, resulting in a widening pulse pressure.

Pressure in the vasomotor center also increases the transmission of parasympathetic impulses through the vagus nerve to the heart, causing a slowing of the pulse. A widened pulse pressure, increased systolic blood pressure, and bradycardia are together called *Cushing's response.* It is considered an important diagnostic sign of late-stage increased intracranial pressure.

Brain herniation produces respiratory problems that are variable and related to the level of the brain stem compression or failure. The breathing pattern may be deep and stertorous (snorelike) or periodic (Cheyne-Stokes) respirations. *Ataxic* breathing may also occur; this is an irregular and unpredictable breathing pattern with random, shallow, and deep breaths and occasional pauses. It is seen in patients with medulla oblongata damage. As intracranial pressure increases to fatal levels, respiratory paralysis occurs.

Failure of the thermoregulatory center because of compression occurs later with increased intracranial pressure. It results in high, uncontrolled temperatures. This hyperthermia increases the metabolism of brain tissue.

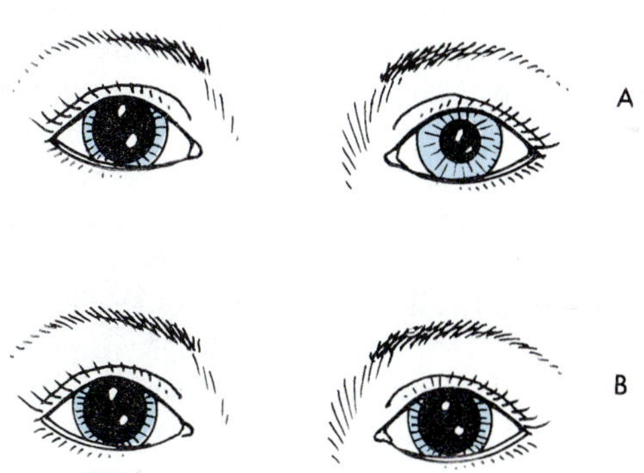

FIG. 35-15 **A,** Unequal pupils, also called *anisocoria.* **B,** Dilated and fixed pupils indicative of severe neurological deficit.

Compression of the upper motor neuron pathway (corticospinal tract) interrupts transmission of impulses to the lower motor neuron, and progressive muscle weakness occurs. The presence of Babinski sign, hyperreflexia, and rigidity are additional signs of decreased motor function. Seizures may occur. Herniation of the upper part of the brain stem may produce characteristic posturing when the patient is stimulated. The worsening of motor problems is significant, because it means that the intracranial pressure is continuing to increase.

Vomiting and singultus are two objective signs that may be seen with increased intracranial pressure. The vomiting is often projectile in nature. Singultus is caused by compression of the vagus nerve (cranial nerve X) that occurs as brain stem herniation occurs.

One last objective sign is papilledema, which is detected with the use of an ophthalmoscope (usually a physician's function). As intracranial pressure increases, the pressure is transmitted to the eyes through the CSF and to the optic disc. As the optic disc becomes edematous, the retina is also compressed. The damaged retina cannot detect light rays. Visual acuity is lessened as the blind spot enlarges. *Papilledema* is also called a *choked disc.*

Diagnostic tests. The diagnosis of increased intracranial pressure is usually made with a CT or MR scan, which can show actual structural hernation and shifting of the brain. Most of the time, however, acute increased intracranial pressure is a medical emergency and there is little time for diagnostic tests. The diagnosis must be made on the basis of frequent and careful observation and neurological testing. *The presence of even subtle changes can be very significant.*

In some postoperative or critically ill patients, internal measuring devices are used to diagnose increased intracranial pressure. One of the most common requires the placement of a hollow screw through the skull into the subarachnoid space. The device is connected to a transducer and oscilloscope for continuous monitoring. Waveforms are produced that indicate the intracranial pressure.

Medical management. The prevention of increased intracranial pressure may not be possible, but prevention of further increases in pressure with resulting damage to the brain is crucial. The medical treatment of the patient with increased intracranial pressure depends on the cause of the pressure. For example, surgery may be done to remove a tumor. If surgery is not possible, efforts are made to reduce the pressure through the use of drug therapy or other measures.

Mechanical decompression. Rapidly rising intracranial pressure can be relieved by mechanical decompression. This may include a craniotomy, in which a bone flap is removed and then replaced, or a craniectomy, in which the bone flap is removed and not replaced. The craniectomy is often done when pressure is high. Other means of decompression may include drainage of the ventricles or any subdural hematoma.

Endotracheal intubation may be necessary. With the use of controlled ventilation, the P_{CO_2} can be lowered to below normal, which causes a slightly alkalotic pH. The decrease in the P_{CO_2} and the increase in pH will decrease vasodilation and decrease intracranial pressure.

Medications. Three types of medications are usually administered to patients with increased intracranial pressure: osmotic diuretics, corticosteroids, and anticonvulsants. Osmotic diuretics are also called hyperosmolar drugs. They draw water from the edematous brain tissue. An example of this type of medication is mannitol. It begins to reduce increased intracranial pressure within 15 minutes, and its effects last for 5 to 6 hours. Glycerol is another osmotic diuretic that is sometimes used.

The corticosteroid that is usually given is dexamethasone. With this drug, monitoring of blood glucose levels is important because steroids can affect carbohydrate metabolism and glucose utilization.

Anticonvulsants are given to prevent seizures. Phenytoin (Dilantin) is the most commonly given drug. It can be given intravenously but is usually not given intramuscularly because of poor absorption. Narcotics and other drugs that cause respiratory depression are avoided.

Internal monitoring devices. Internal monitoring devices are being used more frequently to diagnose and monitor increased intracranial pressure. Three basic monitoring systems are used: the ventricular catheter, subarachnoid bolt or screw, and epidural sensor. These monitoring devices produce pressure waves that can be evaluated to indicate the status of increased intracranial pressure.

Nursing interventions

Therapeutic measures. Therapeutic measures to reduce venous volume may be implemented. These include the following:

1. Elevate head of the bed to 30 to 45 degrees to promote venous return.
2. Place neck in neutral position (not flexed or extended).
3. Position patient to avoid flexion of the hips, waist, and neck as well as rotation of the head, especially to the right.
4. Instruct patient to avoid isometric or resistive exercises.
5. Restrict fluid intake.
6. Implement measures to help patient avoid Valsalva maneuver (any forced expiratory effort against a closed airway, such as straining to have a stool).
7. Have a Foley catheter in place if the patient is not alert because of the large amount of urine that is produced.
8. Perform suctioning only as necessary and only oropharyngeally.

9. Administer oxygen via mask or cannula to improve cerebral perfusion.
10. Use hypothermia blanket to control body temperature (increased body temperature increases brain damage).

Nursing diagnoses and interventions for the patient with increased intracranial pressure may include but are not limited to the following:

NURSING DIAGNOSES	NURSING INTERVENTIONS
Breathing pattern, ineffective, related to neuromuscular impairment	Maintain patent airway; avoid flexion of neck. Administer oxygen and humidification as ordered. Provide oral nasopharyngeal airway as indicated for managing secretions; suction oropharynx prn.
Sensory/perceptual alteration: visual, tactile, related to altered cerebrovascular perfusion	Maintain method of communication. Maintain safe environment. Anticipate needs of patient.
Injury, high risk for, related to physiological effects of sustained elevations in intracranial pressure	Elevate head of bed 30 degrees. Maintain body position: avoid semiprone or prone position. Avoid compression of neck veins. Check blood pressure, pulse, and respiration q 30 min. Perform neurological check q 30 min using Glasgow Coma Scale; report any findings below 8 to physician.

Patient teaching. The patient with increased intracranial pressure is often unresponsive. However, information about procedures that are being done should be shared with the patient and the family. This may help both be as cooperative as possible.

Prognosis. The prognosis for the patient with increased intracranial pressure depends on the cause and rapidity with which it is treated. The nurse assumes a very important role in monitoring the patient for signs and symptoms of increased pressure. After herniation of the brain has begun as a result of pressure, there is little chance for complete reversal without significant brain damage.

Alterations in Muscle Tone and Motor Function.

Etiology/pathophysiology. Motor function disturbances are the most commonly encountered neurological signs and symptoms. Damage to the nervous system often causes serious problems in mobility.

Clinical manifestations. Injury or disease of motor neurons results in alterations of muscle strength, tone, and reflex activity. Muscle tone may be described as *flaccid* (weak, soft, and flabby and lacking normal muscle tone) or *hyperreflexic* (increased reflex actions). The specific clinical manifestations differ according to the location of the neurological lesion.

Assessment. Collection of *subjective data* for patients with motor problems includes the patient's understanding of the problem and possible causes. The initial onset of the symptoms, measures that improve symptoms, and the presence of clumsiness or incoordination or abnormal sensation are important to assess. If the lesion occurs suddenly, as in spinal cord injury from trauma, subjective symptoms may be minimal. If the motor deficit develops slowly, subjective symptoms may be so subtle that they are at first ignored.

Collection of *objective data* includes coordination, muscle strength, muscle tone, and the presence of any muscle atrophy. Reflexes are often checked, as well as the presence of clonus or fasciculations and the ability to move muscles. Any abnormal gait is significant, as well as a change in the ability to carry out ADLs.

Diagnostic tests. One of the most common procedures for detecting pathological conditions of muscle is the electromyogram. It detects the various types of electrical activity and abnormal patterns that may appear in resting muscle in the presence of pathology.

Medical management. Patients with motor problems may have problems with spasticity. Muscle relaxants may be used to decrease tone and involuntary movements. Some commonly prescribed medications include baclofen (Lioresal), dantrolene sodium (Dantrium), and diazepam (Valium). Baclofen has been used intrathecally to reduce spasticity. Common side effects of these drugs include drowsiness and vertigo. These side effects are increased by the use of alcohol or other depressants.

Some patients may have severe swallowing difficulty **(dysphagia).** This commonly results from obstructive or motor disorders of the esophagus and is commonly associated with neurological problems. The patient with dysphagia often requires prefeeding and feeding exercises.

In patients at severe risk for aspiration, a video fluoroscopy with barium may be done to rule out aspiration. The procedure requires the patient to swallow a small amount of liquid or semisolid barium while a fluoroscopic examination is being done.

For patients with paralysis, the eye on the affected side of the body may need to be protected if the lid remains open and there is no blink reflex. The patient is at high risk for corneal scratches or irritation. Irrigation with a physiological solution of sodium chloride may be used, followed by eye drops. An eye pad may be used to keep the eye closed, although an eye shield is preferable.

Nursing interventions

Safety needs. Patients with paralysis have significant safety needs. This includes protection from falling, including the use of side rails when the patient is in bed and a chair restraint when the patient is in a chair, especially if balance cannot be maintained. If the patient also has a sensory problem, which often accompanies paralysis, the danger to a part of the body may not be realized. An example is the patient with a CVA who is not aware that a hemiplegic arm is hanging over the side of the wheelchair arm.

The eye on the affected side of the body should be cleaned and assessed for signs of infection on a regular basis, usually at least three times a day. The patient must also learn to inspect affected body parts for injury.

Skin over bony prominences needs to be inspected regularly for signs of pressure. Paralyzed persons are at risk for skin impairment and should be taught to turn themselves in bed and to reposition themselves in the bed or chair independently, if possible. If the patient is unable to turn independently, the nurse carries out this function. Usually the patient is turned from one side to another or from one side to the back to the other side. Repositioning also includes weight shifts, done by the patient or by staff. These weight shifts may include controlled leaning from one side to another or push-ups done by the patient. If the patient is not able to do the activity, she is taught to take the responsibility to remind the staff when it is time to do the weight shift.

Paralyzed or weakened areas should be inspected at least daily for any signs of skin impairment. A mirror is often used to assist in the assessment of skin by the patient. With this, the patient is able to visualize all skin areas and is not as dependent on staff or family.

Activity needs. The extremities of a person who has an acute motor problem may be flaccid at first. Spasticity of muscles develops gradually. The joints then become flexed and fixed in useless, deformed positions unless preventive measures are taken.

The nurse should carefully place the extremities in a normal anatomical position to prevent deformity. Counterpositioning may be helpful. In **hemiplegia** (paralysis of one side of the body) the affected upper extremity is pulled inward at the shoulder joint and the wrist drops; in the lower extremity the knee flexes and the foot drops. In counterpositioning the nurse positions the patient so that the shoulder and upper arm are in abduction, the elbow is flexed, the wrist is dorsiflexed, the knee is in neutral position, and the foot is dorsiflexed. If the person is supine, a pillow can be placed between the upper arm and body to hold the arm in abduction. Physical therapists and occupational therapists can provide splints and braces that can aid in positioning.

In positioning, footboards may be used to prevent footdrop, although some feel that these contribute to increased spasticity and should not be used routinely for patients who have muscle spasms. High-topped tennis shoes or other devices, such as splints or braces, can help prevent footdrop, if therapy is initiated early. In some hospitals, casts are applied to patients' lower extremities to prevent footdrop or to reverse contractures. The presence of the cast impedes spasticity. A sling or hook harness may be useful to support the affected arm to prevent shoulder subluxation.

The prone position is excellent for patients who are able to tolerate it. Not only is the chance of skin impairment decreased with this position, but it also causes extension of the hip and knee joints, and the ankles by means of gravity. A pillow placed under the chest may help patients comfortably assume this position.

Positioning of the paralyzed person is extremely important. Complications such as footdrop and flexion contractures of the knee seriously limit mobility. As a result, the level of self-care and independence is diminished. Most joint deformities in a paralyzed person are preventable with early and continuing nursing interventions.

In addition to positioning, interventions for the person with paralysis include range-of-motion (ROM) exercises to all joints. These may be passive (carried out by the nurse) or active (carried out by the patient). Passive ROM is indicated at least three times daily for all joints that the patient cannot voluntarily move.

Nutritional needs. Patience and persistence are often necessary in giving food and fluids to the patient with hemiplegia. Important nursing measures include avoiding foods that cause choking, checking the affected side of the mouth for accumulation of food and resultant poor hygiene, not mixing liquids and solid foods, and encouraging the patient to take small bites. If the patient has dentures, they should be worn. The patient should sit at a 90-degree angle with the head up and chin slightly tucked. The head should not be extended and the patient should be encouraged to tip the head toward the unaffected side while swallowing. Assistive devices for feeding include utensils with universal cuffs, covered plastic cups, scoop dishes, plate guards, and Asepto syringes. (See Chapter 45.) These enable the patient to be less dependent on the staff. These devices are usually available through therapists in most hospitals.

Activities of daily living. During the acute rehabilitative phases of a motor problem, patients with paralysis are taught how to carry out daily activities to the extent that they are able. A variety of devices are available to assist with dressing and grooming. The occupational therapist becomes involved in many of these activities, including homemaking. It is important to stress the concept of the rehabilitative team in managing these patients. The patient is taught to compensate for weakness or paralysis. It is important for the nurse to give the patient the time to do activities on her own if she is able. It is often easier and faster to do things for the patient, but this defeats the purpose of rehabilitation.

Psychological adjustments. The person with paralysis may need assistance in adjusting to body changes. The loss of the ability to function independently is traumatic, and the patient may have fears of rejection, as well as loss of self-esteem and concerns about the future. A grief reaction similar to that described in the stages of dying and death may occur. At times, the patient may relate to the paralyzed part of the body as though it were not a part of her and may have nicknames for the body part. Nursing interventions are essential in helping the patient cope with the loss of function and change in body image. This includes praising the patient for achievements, encouraging expression of fears and grief, and helping him see that there is life after disability. It might be helpful to have the patient visited by someone with the same disability who has been successfully rehabilitated.

Nursing diagnoses and interventions for the patient with alterations in muscle tone and motor function include but are not limited to the following:

NURSING DIAGNOSES	NURSING INTERVENTIONS
Mobility, impaired physical, related to neuromuscular impairment	Perform active or passive ROM exercises q 4 hr to all extremities, neck, hands, fingers, wrists, elbows, knees. Provide physical therapy as ordered: massage and stretching exercises. Maintain planned rest periods. Encourage ambulation to tolerance. Arrange for necessary assistive devices for home care needs.
Grieving, anticipatory, related to perceived or actual loss of body function	Provide emotional support; actively listen to patient's concerns about body image changes. Encourage communication with family and/or significant other. Deal with feelings of frustration, helplessness, and powerlessness associated with loss of motor function.
Disuse syndrome, high risk for, related to impaired functioning of body part	Perform hand, finger, foot exercises; assist in active and passive ROM exercises q 2 to 4 hr. Assist patient with using supportive devices as indicated: overhead trapeze, braces, walker, cane. Encourage use of involved side when possible. Instruct patient to use unaffected extremity to support weaker side (e.g., lift involved left leg with right leg or lift involved left arm with right arm).
Skin integrity, impaired or high risk for, related to pressure on bony prominences	Administer skin care q4h; keep skin meticulously clean, dry, lotioned, and massaged. Use Eggcrate mattress. Assess skin for erythema or excoriation q 2 hr. Turn q 2 hr. Encourage nutritional diet and adequate fluid intake.

Patient teaching. Teaching is an extremely important part of caring for the person with motor problems. Appropriate teaching activities include the following: safety needs, skin care, activity needs (ROM and positioning), medications (dosage, action, times, and side effects), the importance of good nutrition, activities of daily living, bowel and bladder care, and the importance of follow-up care. Written instructions are helpful to reinforce teaching and for the patient to refer to when he returns home. Family members should be taught, to prepare them for when they will need to assume some of the care for the patient.

Alterations in Sensory and Perceptual Function.

Etiology/pathophysiology. The presence of a lesion anywhere within the sensory system pathway, from the receptor to the sensory cortex, alters the transmission or perception of sensory information. The parietal cortex is of major importance in interpretation of sensation. Loss of, decrease in, or increase in sensation of pain, temperature, touch, and proprioception results in difficulty in daily functioning. Any alteration lessens the patient's ability to be completely protected from inadvertent injury.

One specific loss is proprioception, or the ability to know the position of the body and its parts without directly looking at the part. **Agnosia** is a total or partial loss of the ability to recognize familiar objects or persons through sensory stimuli as a result of organic brain damage.

Assessment. Collection of *subjective data* includes the patient's understanding of the sensory disturbance, measures that relieve symptoms (including medications), and the presence of symptoms that occur with the sensory problem. An example is the person who experiences weakness of a hand and at the same time feels numbness and tingling. The onset of the sensory problem and the specific site in the body are important information to collect.

Collection of *objective data* includes noting the patient's ability to perform purposeful movements or to recognize familiar objects.

Medical management. Refer to medical management for alterations in the patient's muscle tone and motor function.

Nursing interventions. The most important nursing intervention for the patient with sensory dysfunction is teaching the patient protective measures in relation to the sensory deficit or alteration. This includes helping the patient to learn to inspect parts of the body that have no feeling or protect sensitive body parts from the discomfort of linen rubbing over them. If a patient has a deficit in one sense, he should be taught to compensate with another (e.g., the patient who learns to lip read because of a hearing deficit; the patient with hemianopia who is taught to scan the printed page).

Nursing diagnoses and interventions for the patient with a sensory or perceptual problem are the same as those for the patient with a motor problem, with the addition of but not limited to the following:

TABLE 35-5 Characteristics of Seizures

Incidence	Characteristics	Clinical Signs	Aura	Postictal Period
Grand mal				
Are most common	Generalized, characterized by loss of consciousness for several minutes	Aura Cry Loss of consciousness Fall Tonic-clonic movements Incontinence	Yes Flashing lights Smells Spots before eyes (scotomata) Vertigo	Yes Need for sleep 1 to 2 hr Headache common
Petit mal				
Usually occur during childhood and adolescence Frequency decreases as child gets older	Sudden impairment in or loss of consciousness with little or no tonic-clonic movement Occurs without warning Has tendency to appear a few hours after arising or when person is quiet	Sudden vacant facial expression with eyes focused straight ahead All motor activity ceases except perhaps for slight symmetrical twitching about eyelids Possible loss of muscle tone Consciousness returns	No	No
Psychomotor				
Occur at any age	Sudden change in awareness associated with complex distortion of feeling and thinking and partially coordinated motor activity Longer than petit mal	Behaves as if partially conscious Often appears intoxicated May do antisocial things such as exposing self or carrying out violent acts Autonomic complaints, such as shivering, may occur Urinary incontinence	Yes Complex hallucinations or illusions	Yes Confusion Amnesia Need for sleep
Jacksonian-focal				
Occur almost entirely in patients with structural brain disease	Depends on site of focus May or may not be progressive	Commonly begin in hand, foot, or face May end in grand mal seizure	Yes Numbness Tingling Crawling feeling	Yes
Myoclonic				
May antedate grand mal by months or years	May be very mild or may have rapid, forceful movements	Sudden involuntary contraction of muscle group, usually in extremities or trunk No loss of consciousness	No	
Akinetic				
Not common	Peculiar generalized tonelessness	Person falls in flaccid state Unconscious for minute or two	Rarely	No

NURSING DIAGNOSIS	NURSING INTERVENTIONS
Injury, high risk for, related to sensory/perceptual alteration	Maintain safe environment. Teach patient to protect body parts that have decreased sensation. Teach patient to inspect body parts for possible injury. Protect patient from sustaining injury from hot liquid or heating pads.

Patient teaching. The teaching for a patient with a sensory deficit is essentially the same as that for the patient with a motor deficit (see p. 1115).

Specific Neurological Disorders

Functioning of the neurological system can be interrupted for a variety of reasons. These include conduction abnormalities, degenerative diseases, vascular problems, infection, tumors, trauma, and cranial and peripheral nerve disorders. Selected disorders in each area will be discussed.

Conduction Abnormalities.

Epilepsy or seizures

Etiology/pathophysiology. The incidence of epilepsy has been recorded throughout history. Seizures occur in all races and affect men and women equally. There is no apparent geographical distribution. In many the onset of seizures is before the age of 20, but it can begin at any age. The incidence is about 1 in every 200 to 300 persons.

Clinical manifestations. Seizures can be classified according to the varied features of the attack. This includes grand mal (major or generalized), petit mal, psychomotor, Jacksonian or focal, and miscellaneous (myoclonic and akinetic) seizures. See Table 35-5 for a description of seizures.

Epilepsy can be defined as a transitory disturbance in consciousness or in motor, sensory, or autonomic function with or without a loss of consciousness. It is associated with sudden, excessive, and disorderly discharges in the neurons of the brain that result in the sudden, violent, involuntary contraction of a group of muscles. The patterns or forms of seizures vary and depend on the area of the brain from which the seizure arises. Seizures occur for a variety of reasons, including hypoglycemia, infection, and electrolyte imbalance.

The excessive neuronal discharges may result in a tonic convulsion, with alternate contraction and relaxation of opposing muscle groups. This gives the characteristic tonic-clonic jerking movements of the body. Seizures are followed by a rest period of variable length, called the **postictal period.** During this period the patient usually feels groggy and acts disoriented. Complaints of headache and muscle aches are common. Usually the patient sleeps after a seizure and may experience amnesia for the event.

When recurrent, generalized seizure activity occurs at such frequency that full consciousness is not regained between seizures, it is called status epilepticus. This is a medical emergency and requires medical and nursing interventions to prevent death from brain damage resulting from prolonged hypoxia and exhaustion. The nursing interventions always involve ensuring that there is a patent airway and that the patient is protected from injury. Medications used to stop the seizure activity may be of such volume that the patient is rendered unconscious. The nurse must then assume total care of the patient's needs. A Foley catheter will usually be inserted and the patient will have an intravenous line. The patient may be intubated and receiving ventilatory support. The skin should be protected from injury. Care should be used with safety reminder devices if the patient is awake and active so that they do not cause injury if she begins to have a seizure.

Assessment. Collection of *subjective data* includes the patient's awareness of the disorder and any precipitating factors. The presence of an aura preceding a seizure is important to consider. An aura occurs in about 50% of all patients with grand mal seizures. **Aura** is defined as a sensation, as of light or warmth, that may precede an attack of migraine or an epileptic seizure. The exact character of the aura varies from person to person and is specific to the individual. Awareness of an aura allows the person to be aware of the impending seizure and seek safety and privacy.

Collection of *objective data* includes the number of seizures occurring within a specific time, the character of the seizure, and any behaviors noted and injuries suffered. The character of the seizure should be described as completely as possible, including duration, the nature of the patient's movements, whether the patient was incontinent, any cries or sounds that were made, and the level of alertness.

Diagnostic tests. The most common test used to evaluate seizures is the EEG. It allows a specific diagnosis of the nature of the seizure. This test was described earlier in the chapter (see Fig. 35-14).

Medical management

MEDICATIONS. Treatment of patients with a seizure disorder almost always includes the use of one or more of the anticonvulsant drugs (Table 35-6 on p. 1118). The choice of medication depends on the type of seizure. Failure to take the prescribed medication or to take an adequate dose is often the cause of failure in treatment. Blood levels may be checked to provide an accurate check on the therapeutic level of the medications taken. If medication is not effective, surgical removal of the brain tissue where the seizure occurs may be done.[30]

ACTIVITIES OF DAILY LIVING. Until seizures are controlled, activities such as driving a car, operating machinery, or

TABLE 35-6 Anticonvulsants Used to Prevent and Control Seizures

Drug	Use Related to Seizure Type	Toxic Effects
Phenytoin sodium (Dilantin)	Grand mal, focal, psychomotor	Ataxia, vomiting, nystagmus, drowsiness, rash, fever, gum hypertrophy, lymphadenopathy
Phenobarbital (Luminal)	Grand mal, focal, psychomotor	Drowsiness, rash
Primidone (Mysoline)	Grand mal, focal, psychomotor	Drowsiness, ataxia
Ethosuximide (Zarontin)	Petit mal, psychomotor, myoclonic, akinetic	Drowsiness, nausea, agranulocytosis
Trimethadione (Tridione)	Petit mal	Rash, photophobia, agranulocytosis, nephrosis
Diazepam (Valium)	Grand mal and status epilepticus, mixed	Drowsiness, ataxia
Carbamazepine (Tegretol)	Grand mal, psychomotor	Rash, drowsiness, ataxia
Valproic acid (Depakene)	Petit mal, absence of seizures	Nausea, vomiting, indigestion, sedation, emotional disturbance, weakness, altered blood coagulation
Clonazepam (Clonopin)	Petit mal, akinetic, myoclonic, grand mal seizures	Drowsiness, ataxia, hypotension, respiratory depression
Mephenytoin (Mesantoin)	Grand mal, focal, psychomotor	Ataxia, nystagmus, pancytopenia, rash

swimming should be avoided. Maintaining adequate rest and good nutrition is also important. Alcohol use should be avoided. If the patient is receiving long-term phenytoin (Dilantin) therapy, good hygiene practices for the mouth and teeth are important because of the side effect of edematous and enlarged gums (gingival hyperplasia). The patient should wear a medical alert bracelet or tag.

Nursing interventions

CARE DURING A SEIZURE. The primary goals of the nurse and the family caring for a patient having a seizure are protection from aspiration and injury and observation and recording of the seizure activity. The patient should never be left alone. If the patient is sitting or standing, she should be lowered to the floor in an area away from furniture and equipment. Support and protect the head; turn to side if possible to maintain airway. If there is time, clothing may be loosened around the neck. No effort should be made to restrain the patient during the seizure. The nurse should not try to pry open the jaw to place a padded tongue blade. Padded side rails may be used, especially if seizures often occur during sleep.

Nursing diagnoses and interventions for the patient with seizures may include but are not limited to the following:

NURSING DIAGNOSES	NURSING INTERVENTIONS
Airway clearance, ineffective, related to mucus accumulation in oropharyngeal area during seizure	Place patient in side-lying position to prevent aspiration and ensure airway patency. Suction secretions prn.
Anxiety, related to threat to self-concept, powerlessness	Instruct in and encourage use of relaxation exercises, deep breathing techniques.

NURSING DIAGNOSES	NURSING INTERVENTIONS
Anxiety, related to threat to self-concept, powerlessness—cont'd	Encourage verbalization of fears. Provide restful environment. Provide emotional support.
Injury, high risk for, related to rapid onset of altered state of consciousness and seizure activity	Pad side rails. If patient is out of bed during seizure activity, assist to the floor and remove objects that may harm her. Maintain patent airway. Inform patient of seizure and reorient if necessary.

PATIENT TEACHING. Teaching for the patient with a seizure disorder usually includes the use of medications, including dose, action, and side effects, as well as the importance of avoiding alcohol. Safety measures to avoid injury, good oral hygiene, the importance of adequate rest and diet, and the importance of taking medications even if the patient is seizure free should be emphasized. Any restrictions on activities, the importance of follow-up care, and how to access community resources are taught. The patient should be encouraged to avoid excessive stress and to wear a medical alert tag or bracelet.

Prognosis. The majority of patients with seizures are able to control them with medications and can lead a normal life. With most seizure disorders, the number and intensity of seizures stay constant. However, in patients who experience a first seizure as a result of a brain tumor or another brain pathology, the prognosis is more uncertain.

Degenerative Diseases. The term *degenerative diseases* is used to refer to neurological disorders in which there is a premature aging of nerve cells, which is caused by suspected metabolic disturbance or for which the cause is unknown. Three diseases will be discussed: multiple sclerosis, Parkinson's disease, and Alzheimer's disease.

Multiple sclerosis

Etiology/pathophysiology. Multiple sclerosis (MS) is a common degenerative neurological disease that affects many people. The cause is unknown, although genetics have been implicated, because there is a higher rate of the disease among relatives. A recent discovery by researchers is that people with the first signs and symptoms of MS have a proliferation of a certain type of immune cell called *gamma/delta T cells* in their spinal fluid in the initial phases of MS. These cells are not found in patients who have had the disease for a long time. T cells are the "field commanders" of the immune system, which usually defend the body from outside attackers. In MS, however, something goes wrong and induces the T cells to attack the body. Persons living in temperate climates have an increased risk of the disease. Viral and immunological causes for the disease have also been suggested.

The onset of signs and symptoms is usually between the ages of 20 and 40. The course of the disease is estimated to be 12 to 25 years. The highest number of persons with MS live in the Great Lakes area, the Pacific Northwest, and the North Atlantic states.

Multiple foci of *demyelination* are distributed randomly in the white matter of the brain stem, spinal cord, optic nerves, and cerebrum. During the demyelination process, the myelin sheath and the sheath cells are destroyed, causing an interruption or distortion of the impulse so that it is slowed or blocked. There is evidence of partial healing in areas of degeneration, which explains the transitory nature of early signs and symptoms.

Clinical manifestations. Because of the wide distribution of areas of degeneration, the variety of signs and symptoms in MS is greater than in other neurological diseases. These include visual problems, urinary incontinence, fatigue, weakness or incoordination of an extremity, sexual problems such as impotence in men, and swallowing difficulties. The majority of persons have early remissions that may last for a year or more. Exacerbations may be aggravated or precipitated by fatigue, chilling, or emotional disturbances.

Assessment. Collection of *subjective data* includes the patient's understanding of the disease. The presence of eye problems such as diplopia, scotomata (spots before the eyes), and blindness is important. The patient may also talk about weakness or numbness of a part of the body, fatigue, emotional instability, bowel and bladder problems, vertigo, or loss of joint sensation. In men, the presence of impotence is significant. Pain is not a common symptom.

Collection of *objective data* includes documented abnormalities in neurological testing that may include **nystagmus** (involuntary, rhythmic movements of the eye; the oscillations may be horizontal, vertical, rotary, or mixed), muscle weakness and spasms, changes in coordination, or a spastic, ataxic gait. There may be evidence of behavior changes such as euphoria, emotional lability, or mild depression. Urinary incontinence, difficulty in swallowing, and intention tremors of the upper extremities may be present.

Diagnostic tests. Examination of the CSF in patients with multiple sclerosis usually shows elevated gamma globulin and a proliferation of gamma/delta T cells in the initial phase as well as an increased number of WBC. A CT scan may show enlargement of the ventricles. The MRI scan has been found very helpful in the diagnosis of MS.

Medical management

MEDICATIONS. There is no specific treatment for MS, although many different remedies have been tried. Favorable results often occur with the use of adrenocorticotropic hormone (ACTH) and the corticosteroids such as prednisone (Deltasone) or dexamethasone (Decadron). These may be given orally, intramuscularly, or intravenously. The effects of ACTH and the steroids on the demyelinating process are unknown. If steroids are used in high doses at the start of an exacerbation, the episode seems to resolve more rapidly. If spasticity is a problem, drugs such as diazepam (Valium), dantrolene sodium (Dantrium), and baclofen (Lioresal) may be helpful in preventing or decreasing the spasms. Betaseron (Interferon beta-1b) subcutaneously every other day is indicated for use in ambulatory patients with relapsing-remitting multiple sclerosis to reduce the frequency of clinical exacerbations. Many research studies are being conducted in the search for more effective medications to use in the treatment of MS.

ELIMINATION. Urinary frequency and urgency may respond to propantheline bromide (Pro-Banthine). Cholinergic drugs such as bethanechol chloride (Urecholine) can sometimes help the patient with a neurogenic bladder by exerting a direct antispasmodic effect on smooth muscles. Because urinary tract infections are a major problem in MS, some patients are given prophylactic doses of medications such as trimethoprim and sulfamethoxazole (Bactrim, Septra) or nitrofurantoin (Macrodantin). Cystometric studies can be helpful in defining the specific bladder problem.

The patient should be encouraged to drink adequate fluids (at least 2000 ml a day). If the patient suffers from constipation, a stool softener such as docusate sodium (Colace) may be used, as well as prune juice.

Nursing interventions

NUTRITION. A well-balanced diet with high-fiber foods and adequate fluids is important. Obesity will make it more difficult for the patient to meet daily needs and maintain mobility. The patient who is obese should be referred to the dietitian and be placed on a calorie-restricted diet that will help the patient lose weight slowly, while receiving adequate nutrition.

SKIN CARE. It is important to teach the patient with MS and/or the caregiver frequent turning to avoid skin impairment. Devices to relieve pressure, such as Egg-Crate or air mattresses, may be helpful. Because of sensory involvement, the patient may not feel discomfort that signals the need to change position.

ACTIVITY. Patients with MS are encouraged to exercise regularly, but not to the point of fatigue. Daily rest periods may be helpful. During an acute exacerbation, patients are often kept as quiet as possible; this includes bed rest.

One side of the body is often more affected than the other. The patient must learn to stabilize the gait by leaning toward the less-involved side. If the foot slaps forward when he is walking, the patient should be taught to put the foot down in a pronounced fashion and roll the weight forward on the side of the foot.

CONTROL OF ENVIRONMENT. Hot baths should be avoided, because they often increase weakness. Traveling in hot weather should be planned to prevent travel during the warmest part of the day. If at all possible the patient should be in air-conditioned surroundings during the summer.

Persons with MS do best in a peaceful and relaxed environment. They may have slowness of speech and slowness in the ability to respond, as well as sudden explosive emotional outbursts of crying or laughing. The patient and family will need support in terms of this behavior.

Nursing diagnoses and interventions for the patient with MS may include but are not limited to the following:

NURSING DIAGNOSES	NURSING INTERVENTIONS
Powerlessness, high risk for, related to physical limitations imposed by progressive physical deterioration, loss of body control, and/or threat to physical integrity	Provide emotional support, thorough explanations, and reassurance. Be alert to emotional changes and mood swings. Encourage patient's participation and expression of needs and feelings. Maintain planned rest periods. Encourage self-care as indicated. Provide physical care as indicated.
Nutrition, altered: less than body requirements	Maintain high-calorie, high-vitamin, high-protein diet. Assist patient in selection of beneficial foods. Serve meals attractively and maintain pleasant surroundings. Promote small, frequent meals. Report alterations in eating and drinking patterns to physician.
Self-care deficit: bathing/hygiene, dressing/grooming, feeding, toileting, related to limitations in physical mobility imposed by disease process	Administer oral hygiene before meals. Assist with or provide physical hygiene as indicated by physical ability. Maintain appropriate bathing temperatures. Administer oral hygiene q 4 hr and prn. Catheterize intermittently as indicated; teach self-catheterization when possible. Plan bladder dysfunction program as appropriate for spasticity or flaccidity. Institute bowel control program (establish regular bowel routine, avoid constipation). Assist in dressing/grooming as indicated. Provide nutritious, attractive meals.
Body-image disturbance, related to neurophysiological deficits resulting from disease process	Be supportive of patient's emotional needs relating to changes in body image. Acknowledge concerns about body image. Encourage participation in MS support groups. Emphasize need for diversional activities, such as reading, watching television, hobbies, and games.
Knowledge deficit, related to disease process	Explain nature of disease, emphasizing that this is not a hereditary condition. Explain that warm weather and hot baths may increase weakness. Emphasize importance of avoiding fatigue and becoming overworked or emotionally stressed, since these may be precipitating factors in exacerbation. Explain importance of exercising regularly and the need to maintain rest periods. Discuss need for patient support when ambulating with walker, cane, or braces as indicated. Explain importance of maintaining skin integrity. Explain importance of avoiding persons with infections. Encourage independence and self-care to point of tolerance.

PATIENT TEACHING. Teaching is important for both the patient with MS and significant others. In late stages of the disease the care functions usually have to be assumed by someone other than the patient. Important points include those for the patient with motor and sensory problems (see p. 1115). In addition, it is important to teach about the importance of spacing activities and avoiding temperature extremes, and the potential for emotional lability. The nurse should make sure that the patient and/or family has the address of the nearest MS society or support group.

Prognosis. The prognosis is variable. Some patients have MS for many years with few deficits, whereas other patients quickly become debilitated. The ability of the patient to conserve energy and avoid stress may help prevent exacerbations. Exacerbations are treated and usually resolve.

Parkinson's disease

Etiology/pathophysiology. Parkinson's disease (parkinsonism) is one of the more common diseases of the nervous system. It may also be referred to as *idiopathic Parkinson's* or *spasmus agitans.* It was first described by James Parkinson in 1817. The mean age of onset is 60 years, and the prevalence increases with age. The incidence is about 130 per 100,000 population. It affects both sexes equally, as well as all races.

Etiological factors in Parkinson's disease include viral, toxic, vascular, and genetic causes. Some believe that arteriosclerosis may be a causative factor. Drug-induced parkinsonian syndromes occur with drugs that interfere with the synthesis or storage of dopamine or interfere with the striatal dopamine receptors. These drugs include reserpine (Serpasil), phenothiazines, butyrophenones (haloperidol), and cocaine.

Clinical manifestations. In Parkinson's disease, there is no true paralysis and no loss of sensation. Some of its characteristics indicate upper motor neuron involvement. It is characterized by muscular tremors and rigidity. Defects in judgment and emotional instability may occur, but intelligence is not impaired. A decrease in blinking is seen. All signs and symptoms increase with fatigue.

Assessment. Parkinson's disease starts with subtle symptoms and progresses slowly. Collection of *subjective data* includes symptoms of fatigue, presence of incoordination, judgment defects, emotional instability, and heat intolerance. The patient's understanding of the disease should be assessed.

Collection of *objective data* includes the presence of tremor, which is the outstanding sign of the disease. This has been described as a pill-rolling motion of the fingers or a resting tremor. **Bradykinesia** (an abnormal condition characterized by slowness of voluntary movements and speech) is present with rigidity and loss of postural reflexes. Muscle rigidity leads to a masklike appearance of the face and slowed, monotonous speech; drooling; moist, oily skin; and a shuffling, propulsive gait that the patient may not be able to stop until meeting an obstruction. Swallowing may be abnormal, and the patient may be constipated. There may be a scaly, erythematous rash, particularly near the ears and eyebrows and in the scalp and nasolabial folds.

Diagnostic tests. There is no specific diagnostic test for Parkinson's disease. The clinical examination and history and the patient's response to medication confirm the diagnosis. If there is a history of chronic dementia, the CT scan may show cerebral atrophy. The EEG may show minimal slowing, and the upper GI evaluation may show decreased motility.

Medical management

MEDICATIONS. Treatment for Parkinson's disease is based on easing of the signs and symptoms of the disease. There are several different drugs that may be used that have had a dramatic effect on the course of the disease:

- Trihexyphenidyl hydrochloride (Artane)
- Benztropine mesylate (Cogentin)
- Procyclidine hydrochloride (Kemadrin)
- Biperiden lactate (Akineton Lactate; injection)
- Levodopa (Dopar)
- Amantadine hydrochloride (Symmetrol)
- Carbidopa-levodopa (Sinemet)
- Selegiline hydrochloride (Eldepryl)

After prolonged treatment with some of the drugs, side effects may increase, and the effectiveness of the medication may decrease. It may be helpful to admit the patient to the hospital, during which all drugs are withdrawn for a time. The medications are then restarted, and often smaller doses produce favorable results. Complications such as aspiration can occur during this time, because withdrawal of the drugs causes immobility and rigidity. See the medications table on pp. 1122-1123.

SURGERY. Surgery that involves destroying portions of the brain that control the rigidity or tremor has been found helpful with some patients. Newer experimental surgery includes transplanting part of the adrenal gland into the brain. Medications are discontinued several days preoperatively so that signs and symptoms will be at their maximum at the time of surgery.

Another new treatment approach for Parkinson's disease involves human fetal dopamine cell transplants. Some studies have shown that this procedure is more effective than adrenal medullary transplants. The subject of using fetal tissue, however, is filled with controversy.

Nursing interventions

ACTIVITY NEEDS. Special attention should be paid to posture. Lying on a firm bed without a pillow may help prevent the spine from bending forward. Holding the hands folded behind the back when walking may help to keep the spine erect and prevent the arms from falling stiffly at the sides. The patient cannot be hurried, because it will make the bradykinesia worse.

FEEDING. When the disease is advanced, aspiration is a real concern. Care should be taken during feeding. Unless the disease is well controlled by medication, drooling can be a problem and increases with general excitement. When patients are dressed, garments with generous pockets for an ample supply of tissues will help them to be less conspicuous.

MEDICATIONS FOR NERVOUS SYSTEM DISORDERS

Medication	Trade Name	Action	Side Effects	Nursing Implications
Amantadine hydrochloride	Symmetrel	Treats some Parkinson's disease and drug-induced extrapyramidal reactions, although its action in treatment of Parkinson's disease is unknown	Nausea, vomiting, vision changes, dysrhythmias, disorientation, orthostatic hypotension, depression, fatigue	Tell patient to drink no alcohol; administer no CNS depressants; know pregnancy cautions; tell patient not to cease taking medication without conferring with physician and not to deviate from prescribed dosage; for best absorption, instruct patient to take after meals if orthostatic hypotension occurs; instruct patient not to stand or change positions too quickly.
Baclofen	Lioresal	Reduces transmission of impulses from spinal cord to skeletal muscles, is antispasicity agent for treatment of spinal spascity resulting from multiple sclerosis or spinal cord injury	Drowsiness, dizziness, disorientation, light headedness, hypotension, urinary frequency, possible increase in blood glucose level	Be aware of pregnancy; give oral form with meals or milk to prevent gastrointestinal distress; watch for increased incidence of seizures in patients with epilepsy; tell patient to avoid activities that require alertness until CNS effects of drugs are known.
Trihexphendidyl hydrochloride	Artane	Blocks central cholinergic receptors, helping to balance cholinergic activity of basal ganglia; is antidyskinetic and anti-Parkinson; controls some mild cases adjunct to more potent drugs, controls extrapyramidal reactions caused by drugs	Skin rash, eye pain, nervousness, headaches, tachycardia, urinary hesitancy, urine retention, dry mouth, disorientation	Do not give antacids or antidiarrheal agents within 1 hour of giving medication; give with food; caution patient to rise slowly; use cautiously in patients with narrow-angle glaucoma and hypertension; warn patient to avoid activities that require alertness until CNS effects of drugs are known; tell patient to relieve dry mouth with cool drinks, ice chips, and hard candy.
Pyridostigmine bromide	Mestinon	Inhibits destruction of acetylcholine released from parasympathetic and somatic efferent nerves; causes acetylcholine to accumulate, promoting increased stimulation of receptor; is used in myasthenia gravis and by the oral route for senility associated with Alzheimer's disease	Headache, seizures, bradycardia, hypotension, bronchospasm, increased bronchial secretions	Know that it is difficult to judge optimum dosage; monitor and document patient's response after each dose when using for myasthenia gravis; stress importance of taking drug exactly as ordered, on time, and in evenly spaced doses.

MEDICATIONS FOR NERVOUS SYSTEM DISORDERS—cont'd

Medication	Trade Name	Action	Side Effects	Nursing Implications
Benztropine mesylate	Cogentin	Blocks central cholinergic receptors, helping to balance cholinergic activity in basal ganglia; is indicated in treatment of mild cases of Parkinson disease and control of extrapyramidal reactions	Dizziness, drowsiness, depression, orthostatic hypotension, palpitation, tachycardia	Know importance of following prescribed dosage; discontinue drug slowly; tell patient to drink no alcohol, tell patient of breast feeding warnings; give with food; tell patient to rise slowly and notify physician of severe allergic reactions; do not give with antacids.
Tacrine hydrochloride	Cognex	Is reversible cholineterase inhibitor, is used for treatment of mild-to-moderate dementia of Alzheimer's type	Bradycardia, nausea and vomiting, loose stools, ataxia, CNS disturbance, anorexia, agitation, increased serum transaminase levels, jaundice	Know risk of ulcers; monitor liver enzyme weekly for first 18 weeks; increase dosage at 6-week intervals; do not use NSAIDs concomitantly; know that it potentiates theophylline.
Levodopa	Dopar Larodopa	Is antiparkinson agent (mechanism of action is unknown); increases balance between cholinergic and dopaminergic activity to allow more normal body movements and alleviate signs and symptoms	Aggressive behavior, involuntary grimacing, head and body movements, depression, suicidal tendencies, orthostatic hypotension, nausea, vomiting darkened urine, excessive and inappropriate sexual behavior	Know that it is contraindicated in narrow-angle glaucoma; monitor patients receiving antihypertensive and hypoglycemic agents; advise patient to change positions slowly and dangle legs; protect drug from heat, light, moisture.
Carbidopa/ levodopa	Sinemet	Increases levels of dopamine and levodopamine; is antiParkinson agent; improves modulation of voluntary nerve impulses transmitted to the motor cortex (lower dosage is needed than with single-dose therapy; efficiency may increase 75% when caridopa and levodopa are used in combination).	Mental depression, mental changes, nausea and vomiting, orthostatic hypotension, dizziness, uncontrollable body movements	Give with food; give only as directed, know that effectivness may take months; warn patient of breastfeeding and pregnancy cautions; caution patient about drowsiness and getting up too fast; know that lying may affect control of blood glucose and darken urine.
Selegiline hydrochloride	Eldepryl	Is MAO inhibitor treatment adjunct to levodopa and levodopa/carbidopa; may slow Parkinsons disease and need for increased medication; may prolong life span of persons with Parkinson's disease	Severe orthostatic hypotension, increased tremors, chorea, restlessness, grimacing, nausea and vomiting, slow urination, increased sweating, alopecia	Advise patient not to take more than 10 mg daily there is no evidence that a greater amount improves effectiveness and it may increase adverse reactions); warn patient not to drink alcohol and little coffee; give with food; tell patient to rise slowly and notify physician of side effects; tell patient not to take over-the-counter cold remedies; monitor blood pressure and respirations

ELIMINATION. The patient with Parkinson's disease may feel urgency and hesitancy in voiding. Measures appropriate for the patient with multiple sclerosis also apply to these patients.

Chronic constipation may be a real concern. The patient should be on a diet high in fiber and roughage for bulk. The nurse should encourage oral fluid intake, and stool softeners, suppositories, and prune juice are often helpful. Mild cathartics such as milk of magnesia are used if required.

Nursing diagnoses and interventions for the patient with Parkinson's disease are the same as those for the patient with MS, with the addition of, but not limited to, the following:

NURSING DIAGNOSES	NURSING INTERVENTIONS
Constipation, related to decreased intestinal motility	Encourage fluids to 3000 ml daily unless contraindicated. Encourage diet high in fiber and roughage. Stool softeners and suppositories are helpful. Discourage enemas because they further decrease motility. Offer prune juice.
Aspiration, high risk for, related to disease process	Ensure that when patient is eating, he sits at 90-degree angle with head up and chin slightly tucked, avoiding extending the head. Do not mix liquids and solid foods. Encourage patient to take small bites.

PATIENT TEACHING. Education for the patient with Parkinson's disease should include the importance of taking medications on the prescribed time schedule. The importance of good skin care must be stressed, as well as the importance of keeping active so that the patient remains as mobile as possible. Proper positioning should be demonstrated to the patient and family if they will be taking care of the patient. Proper feeding techniques to reduce the risk of aspiration should be taught to the family and patient. (See interventions for High Risk for Aspiration)

Prognosis. The prognosis for the patient with Parkinson's disease is usually quite good. If the patient takes medication as prescribed, signs and symptoms can be controlled for a long period.

Alzheimer's disease

Etiology/pathophysiology. Alzheimer's disease is a degenerative disorder that affects the cells of the brain and causes impaired intellectual functioning. It is a common cause of dementia in the older person and affects men and women in equal numbers. One person in 20 will develop Alzheimer's disease by age 65; 1 in 10 will have it by age 75; and 1 in 3 will have it by age 90. Alzheimer's may strike persons in their forties and fifties. The cause is unknown. The changes in the brain of patients with Alzheimer's disease include plaques in the cortex and fibrillary degeneration within pyramidal ganglion cells. These changes were first discovered in 1907 by the German neurologist Alois Alzheimer.

Clinical manifestations. The progression of Alzheimer's disease is commonly divided into four stages. In the early stage a person with Alzheimer's has relatively mild memory lapses and may have difficulty in using the correct word. The attention span is decreased, and there may be disinterest in surroundings. In the second stage the person has more obvious memory lapses, especially with short-term memory, and usually may be disoriented to time. Loss of personal belongings is common, as is confabulating (making up stories) to explain the loss of memory. By the time a person reaches the third stage, there is total disorientation to person, place, and time, and motor problems such as **apraxia** (an impairment in the ability to perform purposeful acts) interfere with the ability to carry out daily functions. Wandering is common. In the terminal stage, severe mental and physical deterioration is present. Total incontinence is common.

There may be some variations in these stages. However, all persons with Alzheimer's disease experience a steady deterioration in their physical and mental status, usually lasting 7 to 15 years until death occurs.

Assessment. Memory loss is the first symptom usually noticed in Alzheimer's disease, combined with the inability to carry out normal activities. Other evidence may be the presence of agitation and/or restlessness. It is important to rule out other conditions such as pernicious anemia, drug reactions, depression, or hormonal imbalances.

Diagnostic tests. There is no diagnostic test specific for Alzheimer's disease. A CT scan may be used to rule out other pathological conditions. A family history of Alzheimer's disease is significant. At times the diagnosis can only be confirmed at the time of autopsy.

Medical management. The case of the patient with Alzheimer's disease can be frustrating for the physician, because the treatment options are so limited. Often medications make the condition worse. Drugs such as lorazepam (Activan) or haloperidol (Haldol) in small doses may be necessary to lessen agitation and unpredictable behavior. Tacrine hydrochloride (Cognex) is being used in the treatment of mild to moderate dementia of the Alzheimer's type with some benefit.

Nursing interventions. Nursing interventions are directed toward maintaining adequate nutrition. This can be a challenge, because often the patient will not sit still long enough to eat. Finger foods may be helpful, as well as letting the patient eat while walking. Frequent feedings with high nutritive value are important. Encouraging fluids up to at least 2000 ml a day is also helpful, (see nursing care plan, pp. 1125-1126).

Safety demands a special mention. Because of memory problems, patients with this disease often do dangerous things, such as walking outside while not

NURSING CARE PLAN: THE PATIENT WITH ALZHEIMER'S DISEASE

Mrs. Akers is a 65-year-old widow who has been a seamstress. She has a progressive history of memory loss, paranoia, disorientation, and agitation. She was diagnosed as having Alzheimer's disease 2 years ago. Her family kept her at home until 6 months ago, when she was admitted to a long-term care institution.

The nursing history and data obtained indicated the following:

1. She is incontinent of urine about 50% of the time.
2. She usually sleeps for about 3 to 4 hours a night.
3. She is incontinent of stool.
4. She tends to wander if not observed.
5. She is disoriented as to time and place and her environment; she often thinks the nurses are her children.
6. Her health is good except for the Alzheimer's disease.
7. Her verbal expression is good.
8. Her weight is in the 70th percentile for her height.

Nursing diagnoses	Patient goals/expected outcomes	Nursing interventions
Anxiety, related to cognitive impairments	Patient will express minimal anxiety.	Assess cause of anxiety. Use calm, undemanding, unhurried approach. Encourage exercise. Keep nursing interventions consistent and simple. Minimize patient's choices in care. Teach relaxation techniques.
Communication, impaired verbal, related to motor or cognitive deficits	Patients will be able to express needs.	Maintain calm atmosphere; avoid rushing. Listen carefully to patient. Speak slowly and distinctly. Try to anticipate patient's needs. Encourage speech therapy.
Incontinence, functional, related to condition and cognitive impairment	Patient will be continent.	Take patient to bathroom regularly. Encourage adequate fluid intake (at least 2000 ml/day.) Determine patient's preference for fluid. Place sign on door indicating "Toilet" or "Bathroom." If patient has urgency, ensure proximity to bathroom. Simplify closures on clothing. Avoid fluids before bedtime. Use disposable protective perineal garments (Attends).
Self-care deficit: feeding, dressing/grooming, bathing/hygiene, related to cognitive deficit	Patient will have minimal deficit in self-care.	Use nonverbal cues or demonstration as adjunct to verbal cues. Provide few choices (e.g., in choosing clothes). Do not hurry patient; assist as needed.

Continued.

Nutrition, altered: less than body requirements, related to agitation	Patient will maintain weight.	Provide properly balanced diet. Administer diet as ordered; present one course at a time (e.g., salad first, then entree). Assist patient in cutting food. Provide finger food when possible. Offer frequent snacks. Attempt to redirect to eating. Weigh at least monthly. Consult with dietitian.
Injury, high risk for, re lated to cognitive prob lems	Patient will remain free of injury.	Provide constant supervision. Remove safety hazards. Have patient wear well-fitting tie shoes. Use safety reminder devices only when necessary. Introduce all care givers by name each time; repeat on regular basis. Give single, simple instructions. Use exercise to tire patient. Use medication only as needed.
Sleep pattern disturbance, related to agitation	Patient will sleep 6 hr per night.	Avoid use of caffeine. Control disturbances and noise. Maintain quiet environment: close doors; pull drapes and dividers; decrease stimuli. Provide night lights, soft music. Coordinate nursing functions to allow for rest periods and fewer interruptions at night. Maintain balance of activity and rest. Increase activity to tolerance. Limit sleep during daytime. Provide comfort measures. Use medication only as necessary. Wear colored uniforms if white causes patient agitation.
Coping, ineffective family: compromised, related to long-term deteriorating effects of disease process	Family and/or significant others will demonstrate ability to cope with disease process.	Provide emotional support. Refer family to support groups. Refer to social services for financial concerns and potential placement. Refer to home care services for in-home assistance for home maintenance management problems. Ensure that family is informed about disease process and physician's instructions for supportive care.

CRITICAL THINKING QUESTIONS

1. Mrs. Akers continuously wanders about the long-term care facility. She is unable to sit at the table for an entire meal. She has lost approximately 20 lb in the past 3 months. Helpful measures to improve her nutritional status would include:
2. To assist Mrs. Akers to obtain a better sleep pattern, helpful interventions include:
3. Mrs. Akers has difficulty in maintaining good personal hygiene. Methods for assisting Mrs. Akers to maintain personal hygiene would include:

dressed, turning on stoves, wandering away, and setting fires. Measures that the family can take include removing burner controls from the stove at night, double-locking all doors and windows, and keeping the person under constant supervision. One very frustrating part of the disease is that many patients sleep for only short periods and are awake most of the night.

PATIENT TEACHING. Most of the time education is directed at the family, because by the time the condition is diagnosed there is usually serious mental impairment. The family should be helped to set a realistic schedule that also allows them time for rest and relaxation. If necessary, the family may need to consider placing the patient in a long-term care facility. The family should be put in touch with the local support group for Alzheimer's disease.

Prognosis. There currently is no effective treatment to stop the progression of Alzheimer's disease. The disease progresses at a variable rate. Ultimately, most patients die from respiratory or other infections. Special Alzheimer's units and family and nursing approaches may help the patient stay as productive and safe as possible.

Vascular Problems. Interference with function because of vascular conditions is a common cause of neurological impairment. Two conditions will be discussed in this section: cerebrovascular accident and intracerebral hemorrhage.

Cerebrovascular accident (CVA)

Etiology/pathophysiology. **Cerebrovascular accident** is an abnormal condition of the blood vessels of the brain, characterized by occlusion, an embolus, or cerebrovascular hemorrhage, resulting in ischemia of the brain tissue normally perfused by the damaged vessels. CVA (or stroke) is the most common disease of the nervous system and is ranked as the third leading cause of death in the United States, with about 200,000 deaths annually. Strokes affect persons in all age groups, but the greatest number of persons are between 75 and 85 years of age. Strokes leave many persons with residual effects.

CVAs are caused by a number of pathological processes; these include thrombosis, embolism, and hemorrhage. Many underlying factors are also contributing causes: atherosclerosis, heart disease, hypertension, kidney disease, peripheral vascular disease, and diabetes mellitus. Other risk factors include obesity, high serum cholesterol, cigarette smoking, stress, and a sedentary lifestyle. Oral contraceptives also increase the risk of stroke.

Clinical manifestations. Permanent damage can result from a CVA because of anoxia of the brain. The type of permanent deficits will depend on the area of the brain that is affected. The area of the brain affected depends on which cerebral vessels are involved. The vessel most commonly affected is the middle cerebral artery. Frequently, the patient is unconscious and may experience convulsions. Both unconsciousness and convulsions result from generalized ischemia and the brain's response to abrupt hypoxia.

CEREBRAL THROMBOSIS. Thrombosis is the most common cause of CVA, and the most common cause of cerebral thrombosis is atherosclerosis. Additional disease processes that cause thrombosis are hypotension and other types of vascular injury such as arteritis. CVA resulting from thrombosis is seen most often in the 60- to 90-year-old age group. Thrombi usually occur in larger vessels and are associated with damage to the vessel wall. The internal carotid arteries are a common source of thrombi.

Symptoms of this type of CVA tend to occur during sleep or soon after arising. This is thought to result partly from the fact that recumbency causes a lowering of blood pressure, which can lead to brain ischemia. Postural hypotension may also be a factor. Neurological signs and symptoms frequently worsen for the first few hours after a CVA.

CEREBRAL EMBOLISM. Embolism is the second most common cause of CVA. Persons who have CVAs resulting from embolism are usually younger. The emboli most commonly originate from a thrombus in the heart, often caused by rheumatic heart disease with mitral stenosis and atrial fibrillation or myocardial infarction.

Emboli usually affect small vessels and are commonly found at points of bifurcation in blood vessels. They most frequently occur in the midcerebral artery.

CEREBRAL HEMORRHAGE. Intracerebral or intracranial hemorrhages include bleeding into the brain itself or bleeding into the subarachnoid space. The bleed causes damage by destroying and replacing brain tissue. Intracranial hemorrhages are the third most common cause of CVAs. The peak incidence of aneurysms occurs in persons who are 35 to 60 years of age. Women are more frequently affected than men.

An aneurysm is often the cause of hemorrhage. An **aneurysm** is a localized dilation of the wall of a blood vessel usually caused by atherosclerosis and hypertension or, less frequently, by trauma, infection, or a congenital weakness in the vessel wall. It ruptures as a result of a small hole that occurs in a part of the aneurysm. The hemorrhage spreads rapidly, producing localized damage and irritation to the cerebral vessels. The bleeding usually stops when a plug of fibrin platelets is formed. The hemorrhage begins to absorb within 3 weeks. Recurrent rupture is a risk 7 to 10 days after the initial hemorrhage.

TRANSIENT ISCHEMIC ATTACK. Transient ischemic attack (TIA) refers to an episode of cerebrovascular insufficiency with temporary episodes of neurological dysfunction that vary in severity. The most common deficit is contralateral weakness of the lower face, hands, arms, and legs; transient dysphasia; and some sensory impairment. Between attacks the neurological status is normal.

The major importance of TIAs is that they warn the patient of the existence of an underlying pathological condition. At least one third of patients who experience TIAs will have a CVA in 2 to 5 years.

Assessment. Collection of *subjective data* that are important with a patient experiencing a CVA includes the description of the onset of symptoms, the presence of headache, any sensory deficit, such as numbness or tingling, the inability to think clearly, and the presence of visual problems. In the case of a hemorrhage the headache may be described as sudden and explosive. The patient's ability to understand the condition should be assessed.

Collection of *objective data* includes the presence of hemiparesis or hemiplegia, any change in the level of consciousness, signs of increased intracranial pressure, respiratory status, and the presence of aphasia. The exact clinical picture varies, depending on the area of the brain affected. When the middle cerebral artery is affected, as is most common, the signs and symptoms seen include contralateral paralysis or paresis, contralateral sensory loss, dysphasia or aphasia if the dominant hemisphere is involved, spatial-perceptual problems, changes in judgment and behavior if the nondominant hemisphere is involved, and contralateral (homonymous) hemianopia.

Diagnostic tests. A lumbar puncture is often performed; blood in the spinal fluid will indicate a hemorrhage. A CT scan may show an area of decreased density, and a brain scan will show an area of diminished perfusion. Following TIAs, a cerebral angiogram or digital subtraction angiogram (DSA) may be done.

Medical management. If the patient has had a stroke as a result of an aneurysm, surgery may be necessary to prevent a rebleed. The surgery consists of a craniotomy and tying off or clipping of the aneurysm. If the base of the aneurysm is too large for these procedures to be done, it may be coated with a liquid, adherent, plastic substance that hardens to form a firm support for the weakened vessel wall.

After a TIA, a carotid endarterectomy may be performed. This includes cleaning out the occluded carotid artery. It may be useful in preventing a stroke.

In an attempt to prevent further thrombosis or emboli, the physician may prescribe warfarin (Coumadin) and heparin if it is certain that the cause is cerebral thrombosis. The use of anticoagulants is controversial. Some patients may be treated with various types of vasodilating agents, although the effectiveness of this type of therapy is not well established. Drugs to reduce intracranial pressure, such as dexamethasone (Decadron), may be given. Suppositories such as bisacodyl (Dulcolax) are generally prescribed to be given daily or every other day. However, some physicians order stool softeners, laxatives, or enemas.

Fluids may be restricted for the first few days after a CVA in an effort to prevent edema of the brain. The patient will be fed intravenous fluids, or a nasogastric tube may be inserted and tube feedings begun.

The length of time the patient remains in bed depends entirely on the type of CVA suffered and the judgment of the physician in regard to early mobilization. Some physicians prescribe fairly long periods of rest after CVAs, whereas others believe in early mobilization, a day or two after the accident has occurred.

Nursing interventions. Goals in the initial phase are directed toward survival needs of the patient and prevention of further complications. Neurological assessment is done at regular intervals but at least once each shift to detect changes in status and any complications such as worsening stroke. Some patients may be unconscious as a result of increased intracranial pressure and will need total care (see pp. 1112-1113).

Because nutrition is a concern and the patient may have great difficulty in swallowing at first, tube feedings may be necessary, as well as intravenous fluids unless the patient is more alert. See the section on motor and sensory problems for a discussion of techniques to assist in feeding the patient with dysphagia.

If the patient is responsive after the onset of the stroke, the nurse needs to help the patient assume as much self-care as possible. This includes assisting with teaching the patient one-handed dressing techniques and one-handed feeding techniques. It is important to reinforce teaching by other members of the patient's health team.

The patient with a CVA may be incontinent at first. It is important to remove the urinary catheter (if there is one) as soon as possible to prevent urinary tract infection. The patient should be put on a bladder training program to assist in regaining continence. This usually includes taking the patient to the bathroom every few hours and encouraging fluids (at least 2000 ml per day). The patient's normal bowel pattern before the stroke needs to be assessed and included in the nursing care plan if possible. If the patient has difficulty with communication, the use of a picture of a bathroom or toilet can be useful.

Return of motor impulses and movement in involved extremities occurs in stages, lasting from hours to months. Recovery may also halt at a specific stage and progress no further. Return of function is significant for functional use of extremities but also increases the possibility of contractures. Appropriate nursing interventions to prevent contractures include passive exercise, active exercise, strength-building of the unaffected side, and early ambulation to promote the return of muscle function. (See pp. 1113-1114.)

One approach to positioning of the patient with a stroke is the **Bobath approach** (a treatment approach designed to normalize muscle tone by providing as many sensations of normal muscle tone, posture, and movement as possible). The goal of the treatment is to redirect short-term memory toward an appreciation of normal movement of the paralyzed side by incorporating techniques of weight-bearing, counterrotation, and protraction of the shoulder girdle and pelvis. The reader is referred to a rehabilitation nursing text for further description of this technique. Nurses in rehabilitation settings are often taught this approach.

Patients may experience a loss of proprioception with a stroke. This may include apraxia and agnosia (a total or partial loss of the ability to recognize familiar objects or persons). The nurse can assist the patient with activities by repeating directions and demonstrating care. If the patient has hemianopia, which is common, the patient should be approached from the nonparalyzed side for care. The patient should be taught to scan past midline to the side where there is the deficit. These patients may also fail to recognize that they have a paralyzed side. This is called *unilateral neglect.* This patient must be taught to inspect this side of the body for injury and to protect it from harm. These patients often show poor judgment and may move impulsively or unsafely. They need to be observed for this and safety precautions should be taken if needed until the patient can learn to compensate for this lack of judgment. Crying or emotional lability is common.

It is important to foster the patient's sense of self-esteem. The nurse must always treat the patient as an adult, not as a child. The patient's successful efforts and gains in self-care should be praised and reinforced.

COMMUNICATION PROBLEMS. Many CVA patients have speech problems, including dysarthria and aphasia. The patient may be frustrated and should be approached in an unhurried manner. Often, the patient does much better with communication when not feeling pressured to speak. The nurse may find that giving the patient a communication board is helpful. The nurse should wait for the patient to communicate, rather than using prompting or finishing the sentence before the patient has a chance to find the appropriate word. Inability to articulate does not mean that the patient has decreased cognitive abilities.

The nursing diagnoses and interventions for the patient who has had a CVA include but are not limited to the following:

NURSING DIAGNOSES	NURSING INTERVENTIONS
Airway clearance, ineffective, related to inability to maintain secretions	Position body and head to avoid obstruction of airway and provide optimal secretion removal. Suction secretions prn. Provide oral or nasopharyngeal airway to maintain airway patency. Auscultate chest for breath sounds q 2 h to 4 hr. Administer oxygen/humidification as ordered. Monitor arterial blood gases and hemoglobin.

NURSING DIAGNOSES	NURSING INTERVENTIONS
Body image disturbance, related to neurophysical deficits	Determine patient's perception of change in body image and subsequent threat to self. Encourage verbalization (if able) of anger, fear, frustration, or anxiety about altered functioning of body part. Encourage patient to look at and touch changed body part. Assist family in adapting to change by providing resources, encouraging verbalization, and including family members in care. Assess own attitudes and values related to physical appearance. Teach patient and family the stages of grief and importance of grief work.
Communication, impaired verbal, related to ischemic injury	Speak slowly and distinctly. Phrase questions that can be answered by yes or no (or by signals). Try to anticipate patient needs. Provide call signal within reach of unaffected hand. Begin speech therapy as soon as possible.
Tissue perfusion, altered cerebral, related to ischemic injury	Maintain bed rest, with head of bed elevated 15 to 60 degrees. Check q 15 to 30 min to assess alterations in circulatory status; immediately report any sudden changes in blood pressure or pupillary or neurological status. Check rectal temperature q 2 to 4 hr; hypothermia or cooling measures may be needed. Maintain parenteral fluid as ordered.
Home maintenance management, impaired, related to individual family member, lack of finances, or family organization	Refer patient and family to services of social worker. Involve patient (if possible) and family members in problem-solving solutions to individual needs. Arrange for necessary assistive devices through home health. Encourage expression of feelings and discuss concerns.
Incontinence, total, related to cognitive problems	Monitor urinary output and signs of retention or incontinence. Assure patient that urinary problems will probably improve. Provide catheter care if retention catheter is needed initially. Offer bedpan or urinal after meals and at regular intervals. Provide fluids to maximum amount prescribed; provide greater amounts before 4 PM. Use disposable adult diaper or external urinary system as indicated.
Injury, high risk for, related to changes in sensory-perceptual function	Maintain seizure precautions. Maintain safe environment. Use side rails with padding as indicated. Maintain quiet environment. Use soft safety reminder devices as indicated. Maintain bed in low position.

NURSING DIAGNOSES	NURSING INTERVENTIONS
Knowledge deficit related to disease process	Teach patient and family prescribed therapy to be carried out at home, plans for increased patient independence, professional and community resources necessary to achieve long-term goals, and plans for follow-up care.
Mobility, impaired physical, related to neuromuscular impairment	Encourage active ROM and exercises of unaffected extremities. Encourage patient to move in bed as able. Teach patient how to sit up on side of bed and to transfer to chair when permitted. Support activities initiated by physical therapy staff. Encourage ambulation when possible and provide support. Provide shoe support for transfer and ambulation.
Nutrition, altered: less than body requirements, related to impaired ability to swallow	Provide IV fluids and tube feedings as prescribed during initial period. Assess ability to swallow before initiating feedings. Position patient with head elevated and turned to unaffected side when feeding patient. Provide foods initially that are easier to swallow (soft or pureed foods except for mashed potatoes). Use training cup or feeding syringe for fluids as necessary. Inspect mouth for food trapped in cheek pockets. Be patient when feeding patient and provide directions for swallowing, as needed. Encourage patient to feed self as soon as possible; provide self-help devices as necessary.
Self-care deficit, bathing/hygiene, related to impaired physical mobility and alteration in cognitive process	Administer skin care q 4 hr. Use oil-based lotions. Inspect area over bony prominences q 4 hr for any skin impairment. Maintain body alignment. Provide physical hygiene as indicated. Encourage patient to assist as able. Praise efforts at personal hygiene.

PATIENT TEACHING. The teaching for a patient with a CVA includes teaching the patient about techniques to compensate for the deficits suffered as a result of the stroke. In this the nurse functions as part of the rehabilitation team. This rehabilitation must start at the time of admission to the acute care facility. The patient will probably be attending occupational and physical therapy and may need speech therapy.

If the patient is receiving medication (e.g., for hypertension), it is important to teach the patient and/or family about side effects and the schedule for taking the medication. Plans for follow-up should be discussed. The patient and/or family may be referred to a stroke club for support.

The patient's family needs to be taught techniques to enhance safety and communication. If the patient has a problem with dysphagia, the family needs to be taught appropriate techniques. Because of the chronicity of caring for the stroke patient there is a high risk for care giver stress. Referral to an appropriate stroke support group is needed. Instructions should be written out for the patient or family to refer to after discharge. Most rehabilitation centers will also include therapeutic leaves as a way to test the family's skills and knowledge. Each pass or leave has specific goals, and feedback is obtained from the family about additional teaching that may be needed. The family and patient should also be educated about the perceptual problems associated with stroke, along with techniques that compensate for these deficits (e.g., writing down instructions for the patient who has trouble carrying out an activity alone).

PROGNOSIS. The prognosis for patients with a stroke depends on the size of the lesion in the brain as well as the patient's premorbid status. With therapy, significant functional gains can be made, even when paralysis or weakness continues. Many patients are able to return home and even remain independent after a CVA.

Cranial and Peripheral Nerve Disorders.

Trigeminal neuralgia

Etiology/pathophysiology. Trigeminal neuralgia is one specific kind of peripheral nerve problem. It is caused by degeneration of or pressure on the nerve, and its etiology is unknown. It is also called *tic douloureux.* It usually affects persons in middle or late adulthood and is slightly more common in women.

Clinical manifestations. Trigeminal neuralgia is characterized by excruciating, burning pain that radiates along one or more of the three divisions of the fifth cranial nerve (Fig. 35-16). The second and third divisions are most commonly affected. The pain typically extends only to the midline of the face and head because this is the extent of the tissue supplied by the offending nerve. There are areas along the course of the nerve known as *trigger points,* and the slightest stimulation of these areas may initiate pain. Persons with trigeminal neuralgia try desperately to avoid triggering them.

Medical management. Carbamazepine (Tegretol) is the drug of choice for the treatment of trigeminal neuralgia pain. Nicotinic acid, thiamine chloride, analgesics, and even cobra venom have been tried with little success. Absolute alcohol may be injected into the peripheral branches of the trigeminal nerve. This provides relief for weeks to months.

Permanent relief of pain is obtained only by surgery that consists of inserting a fine needle through the cheek and injecting an alcohol solution or surgically resecting

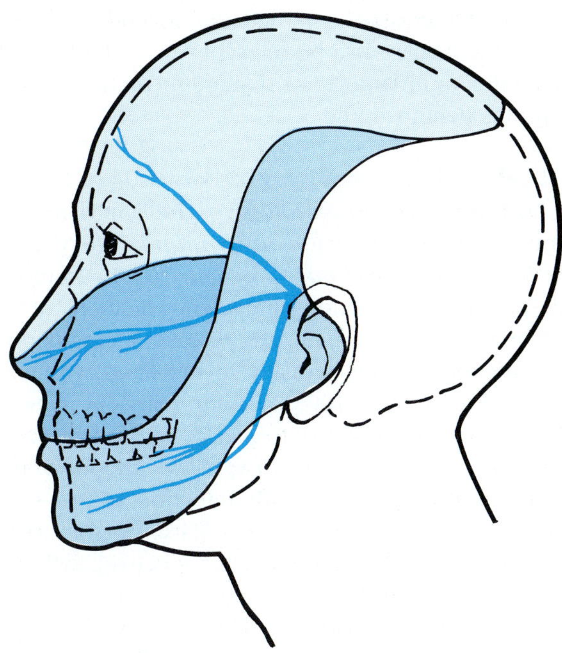

FIG 35-16 Pathway of trigeminal nerve and facial areas innervated by each of the three main divisions of this nerve.

the sensory root of the trigeminal nerve. This is not always successful. Within 24 hours after a fifth nerve resection, many patients develop herpes simplex of the lips (cold sores). Usually these lesions heal in approximately a week.

Nursing interventions. It is common for patients with trigeminal neuralgia not to have eaten properly for some time because eating causes pain. They may be undernourished and dehydrated. They may not have washed, shaved or combed the hair for some time. Oral hygiene often has been neglected. Measures to increase comfort for patients before surgery or for patients being treated nonsurgically are in Box 35-3.

Prognosis. The acute pain seldom lasts more than a few seconds or a minute or two, but will be excruciating. The onset of pain can occur at any time during the day or night and may recur several times daily for weeks at a time. Some patients will have more or less continuous discomfort and sensitivity of the face. Permanent relief of pain is obtained only by surgery.

Bell's palsy (peripheral facial paralysis)

Etiology/pathophysiology. Bell's palsy is thought to be caused by an inflammatory process involving the facial nerve (VII) anywhere from the nucleus in the brain to the periphery. Other theories of cause include local ischemia and edema or emotional trauma with resultant vasoconstriction. Any of the three branches of the facial nerve may be affected. The disorder can be unilateral or bilateral.

Box 35-3 COMFORT MEASURES FOR PATIENTS WITH TIC DOULOUREUX

1. Keep room free of drafts.
2. Avoid walking briskly to bedside of patient.
3. Place bed out of traffic area to prevent jarring of bed.
4. Avoid touching the patient's face.
5. Do not urge patients to wash or shave the affected area or to comb the hair.
6. Avoid hot or cold liquids, which trigger pain.
7. Puree food and ensure that it is lukewarm. If necessary, suggest that food be taken through straw.

Clinical manifestations. With Bell's palsy there is usually an abrupt onset of numbness or a feeling of stiffness or drawing sensation of the face. Unilateral weakness of the facial muscles usually occurs, resulting in inability to wrinkle the forehead, close the eyelid, pucker the lips, or retract the mouth on that side. The face appears asymmetric, with drooping of the mouth and cheek. Other symptoms that may occur include the following:

1. Loss of taste
2. Reduction of saliva on affected side
3. Pain behind the ear
4. Ringing in ear or other hearing loss

Medical management and nursing interventions. There is no specific therapy for Bell's palsy. Electrical stimulation or warm moist heat along the course of the nerve may help. Steroids given early in the course may speed recovery. Protection of the eye when the eyelid does not close is important. Massage of the affected areas is sometimes recommended. Exercises may be prescribed for 5 minutes 3 times a day. These include wrinkling the brow and forehead, closing the eyes, and puffing out the cheeks.

Prognosis. Some 80% of patients recover fully in weeks or months, although recovery may take as long as a year, with recovery of taste being the first sign of improvement. Recovery of taste within the first week signals a good chance for full recovery of motor function. This favorable prognostic sign also holds true if paralysis remains incomplete within the first 5 to 7 days.

Infection and Inflammation.

Etiology/pathophysiology. Interference with function because of infection or inflammation is a common occurrence. Some specific conditions include meningitis, encephalitis, brain abscess, Guillain-Barré syndrome, herpes zoster, neurosyphilis, and AIDS. Only Guillain-Barré syndrome, meningitis, and AIDS will be discussed in this chapter.

The nervous system may be affected by a variety of organisms and may suffer from toxins of bacteria and viruses. These toxins reach the nervous system from a variety of sources, including adjacent bones, blood, or lymph. Meningitis can occur as a result of an invasive procedure such as surgery.

Assessment. Subjective and objective assessments are important in any patient who has infection of the nervous system. Collection of *subjective data* includes a history of infection, such as an upper respiratory infection, and the presence of discomfort that may include headache or stiff neck. The initial onset of symptoms, any difficulty in thinking, and the presence of weakness may be important. The patient's understanding of the condition should be assessed.

Collection of *objective data* includes behavioral signs indicating discomfort or disorientation, as well as an inability to carry out ADLs. The physical assessment part of the neurological assessment may reveal abnormalities; the presence of a fever, vomiting, abnormal CT results, seizures, altered respiratory patterns, tachycardia, and meningeal irritation is significant. The patient's level of consciousness and orientation should be assessed.

Diagnostic tests. Many of the infections of the nervous system can be diagnosed by examining the CSF. A CT scan or an EEG may also be done.

Nursing interventions. Nursing diagnoses and interventions for the patient with an infection/inflammation are the same as for those for the patient who has had a CVA, with the addition of but not limited to the following:

NURSING DIAGNOSES	NURSING INTERVENTIONS
Hyperthermia, related to inflammatory response to CNS infection	Assess temperature q 2 h and prn. Provide cooling measures prn; avoid cooling to point of shivering. Administer antipyretics as ordered. Administer antibiotics as ordered. Monitor parenteral fluids as ordered. Control exposure to extremes in temperature. Assess TPR q 2 hr as indicated.
Thought processes, altered, related to neurophysiological response to infection	Protect patient from self-injury. Provide soft safety reminder devices to prevent injury. Introduce self to patient and establish rapport to prevent agitation. Relate date, time of day, and recent activities. Speak in kind tone, using short, simple sentences. Maintain a therapeutic environment.

Patient teaching. Education for the patient with an infection includes teaching about the disease process, the treatments involved, and the expected outcomes. If the patient is seriously ill, the initial teaching focuses on the family. Other aspects of teaching for motor and sensory problems may also be relevant for the patient with an infection or inflammation, depending on the signs and symptoms demonstrated.

Guillain-Barré Syndrome (Polyneuritis).

Etiology/pathophysiology. Guillain-Barré syndrome is also called *acute inflammatory polyradiculopathy* or *postinfectious polyneuritis.* It results in widespread inflammation and demyelination of the peripheral nervous system. The disease affects persons of all ages and is seen equally in men and women. It affects 1.5 people in 100,000 each year. The cause is unknown but is thought to be a viral agent or an autoimmune reaction. More than half of the individuals affected have had a nonspecific infection 10 to 14 days before the onset of the disease. Many persons developed the signs and symptoms after receiving swine flu vaccine in the early 1980s.

Clinical manifestations There is variation in the pattern of the onset of weakness as well as in the rate of progression of signs and symptoms. The progression may stop at any point. The patient may have difficulty swallowing, breathing, and speaking if cranial nerves VII, IX, and X are involved. Symmetrical muscle weakness and lower motor neuron paralysis are present. The paralysis usually starts in the lower extremities and moves upward to include the thorax, upper extremities, and face. Respiratory failure may occur if the intercostal muscles are affected. A fluctuating blood pressure may occur as a result of effects on the autonomic nervous system.

Diagnostic tests. Guillain-Barré syndrome is diagnosed by elimination of other reasons for the signs and symptoms as well as by the characteristic muscle weakness. A CT scan may be ordered to rule out tumors or a stroke. Changes in the respiratory status may aid in the diagnosis. A lumbar puncture may be done. A history of a recent infection is considered important.

Medical management. Adrenocortical steroids are used to treat the signs and symptoms of Guillain-Barré syndrome. It has also been found that plasma exchanges lead to decreased severity and length of symptoms. Patients who develop respiratory failure require mechanical ventilation and may require a tracheostomy. Arterial blood gas monitoring is used to assess the respiratory status. If the patient has severe paralysis and is expected to have a long recovery period, a gastrostomy tube may be placed to provide adequate nourishment.

Nursing interventions. Close monitoring of respiratory function is important and necessary. If the patient requires mechanical ventilation, the nurse must be aware that cognition (the mental faculty or process by which knowledge is acquired) is not impaired and that the patient will require reassurance. The patient may also require nutritional maintenance intravenously or through a nasogastric tube. Attention to the prevention of complications, such as contractures, decubitus ulcers, and loss of ROM is important to allow complete recovery. Vital signs and the motor strength of the patient should be assessed frequently. The patient must be monitored for signs of hypoxia.

Prognosis. Of the persons suffering from Guillain-Barré syndrome, 85% will regain complete function. The recovery period may vary from weeks to years. Those not recovering completely have some degree of permanent neurological deficit. Generally, recovery from the disease occurs in the reverse order of how the paralysis or weakness occurred.

Meningitis.

Etiology/pathophysiology and clinical manifestations. Meningitis is an acute infection of the meninges. It is usually caused by one of several organisms, including pneumococci, meningococci, staphylococci, streptococci, *Haemophilus influenzae,* and viral aseptic agents. The effect of the bacteria in the subarachnoid space is an inflammatory reaction in the pia mater and arachnoid and in the CSF. Pus accumulates, and the bacteria may injure nervous tissue.

Meningitis can be classified as bacterial or aseptic. The incidence of bacterial meningitis is higher in fall and winter, when upper respiratory tract infections are common. Pathological changes that can occur include hyperemia of the meningeal vessels, edema of brain tissue, increased intracranial pressure, a generalized inflammatory reaction with exudation of white blood cells into the subarachnoid spaces, and associated hydrocephalus (in infants) caused by exudate occluding the ventricles.

Two abnormal signs that occur with meningitis are *Kernig's sign* (inability to extend the legs completely without extreme pain) and *Brudzinski's sign* (flexion of the hip and knee when the neck is flexed). The onset of meningitis is usually sudden and is characterized by severe headache, stiffness of the neck, irritability, malaise, and restlessness. Nausea, vomiting, and delirium develop, as well as increased temperature, pulse rate, and respirations.

Diagnostic tests. Meningitis is diagnosed by examining the CSF. A culture and sensitivity test is done to ascertain the pathogenic organism. A CT scan of the head and an EEG are also ordered.

Medical management. Treatment of meningitis consists of massive doses of antibiotics. Multiple antibiotics are often used. The medication is usually given intravenously or intrathecally (directly into the spinal canal). Hyperosmolar agents or steroids may be needed to decrease intracranial pressure. Anticonvulsants may be given to prevent seizures.

Nursing interventions. Respiratory isolation is required until the pathogen can no longer be cultured from the nasopharynx. This is usually accomplished after 24 hours of effective antibiotic therapy. Other nursing interventions include the general care given a critically ill patient who may be irritable, disoriented, and unable to take fluids. Dehydration is common, and the patient almost always has an intravenous line. The room is kept darkened and noise is kept to a minimum, since any increase in sensory stimulation may cause a seizure. If the patient is disoriented, safety precautions need to be taken, including safety reminder devices if needed.

Prognosis. With most cases of meningitis, the prognosis for complete recovery is good. The prognosis depends on the quickness with which antibiotics were administered. With severe cases of meningitis, there may be residual neurological damage or death.

Acquired Immunodeficiency Syndrome.

Etiology/pathophysiology. Acquired immunodeficiency syndrome (AIDS) is a disease that has serious implications for the nervous system, with more than 40% of AIDS patients having neurological signs and symptoms. Patients develop neurological signs and symptoms either as a result of infection with HIV itself or as a result of associated infections. See Chapter 37 for a discussion of AIDS.

Clinical manifestations. Patients with AIDS may have ADC (AIDS dementia complex), which is known as subacute encephalitis. This may be manifested as difficulty in concentrating or a recent memory loss, which may progress to a **global cognitive dysfunction** (generalized impairment of intellect, awareness, and judgment). Patients may also experience opportunistic infections such as meningitis, herpes simplex, cytomegalovirus, toxoplasmosis, and cryptococcal meningitis. Primary malignant lymphomas of the CNS may also develop.

Diagnostic tests. The diagnostic tests used to determine whether a neurological problem is related to AIDS include serological studies, a lumbar puncture, and CT scan. At times, a cerebral biopsy may be necessary to make the differential diagnosis.

Medical management. Treatment of the patient with neurological problems related to AIDS depends on the nature of the infection. Various methods of treatment have included administration of antiviral, antifungal, and antibacterial agents. Radiation has been used on the affected part of the brain. Experimental therapies including iron dextran (Imferon) have been attempted. Mortality remains high despite aggressive therapy.

Nursing interventions. The patient is likely to be disoriented, and may need to be reoriented frequently. Safety measures such as padded side rails may be necessary to prevent injury to the patient, who may have seizures.

The patient may experience pain and have difficulty sleeping. It is important to administer medications to the patient as needed and to structure activities to avoid waking him. The patient may also have visual problems associated with the disease, and the nurse must be careful to orient the patient to nursing interventions.

Most patients with AIDS experience depression and powerlessness about the nature of the disease. They may isolate themselves from others. Patients should be encouraged to talk about their fears and concerns, be assisted to find emotional support, and be referred to a support group. The nurse needs to maintain a nonjudgmental attitude.

The patient may be incontinent of bowel and bladder. It is important to encourage an active bowel and bladder program. If the patient is experiencing diarrhea, it is important to keep the rectal area as clean and dry as possible and administer antidiarrheals if ordered. The patient may also have difficulty with nausea. Foods that the patient likes should be offered in small, frequent meals. Tube feedings or hyperalimentation may be needed if the patient agrees.

Prognosis. The prognosis for the patient with AIDS is terminal, often within a short time. Currently, there is little that can be done to substantially lengthen life. After a patient experiences neurological complications, AIDS is usually fairly well advanced.

Tumors.

Intracranial tumors

Etiology/pathophysiology and clinical manifestations. Intracranial tumors include both benign and metastatic lesions. All areas and structures of the brain can be affected. Primary intracranial tumors, or *neoplasms,* arise from the cells of brain tissue and the primary and pineal glands. These tumors include gliomas, meningiomas, pituitary tumors, and neuromas. Metastatic tumors also occur frequently in the brain. Brain tumors are named for the tissues from which they arise (see Chapter 38).

Assessment. Collection of *subjective data* includes the patient's understanding of the diagnosis, as well as changes in personality or judgment and the presence of abnormal sensations or visual problems. Complaints of unusual odors may be present with tumors of the temporal lobe. Headache, hearing loss, or the inability to carry out daily activities is also important to assess.

Collection of *objective data* includes motor strengths, gait, the level of alertness and consciousness, and orientation. The pupils are assessed for response and equality. The presence of seizures in an adult is significant. Speech abnormalities, cranial nerve abnormalities, and signs and symptoms of increased intracranial pressure are also significant.

Diagnostic tests. No one procedure is entirely diagnostic of brain tumors, but a CT scan is often the basis for the diagnosis. Other tests that may be performed include the brain scan, MRI, PET scans, and the EEG. Arteriography may also be done.

Medical management. The general method of treatment for intracranial tumors includes surgical removal when feasible, radiation, and chemotherapy. The choice of therapy is determined by the tumor type and site. A combination of methods is often used.

SURGERY. A surgical opening through the skull is called a *craniotomy.* Following removal of the bone, an incision is made into the meninges, and the tumor is removed. The removed bone is carefully preserved and may be replaced at the end of surgery if there is no indication of infection or increased intracranial pressure. The removal of part of the skull without replacement is called *craniectomy.*

Nursing interventions. Preoperative preparation of both the patient and the family is important. Specific fears may be related to a permanent change in appearance, dependency, and possible death. A baseline neurological assessment is important. Treatments and procedures, including the shaving of hair, are explained. Usually hair is shaved in the operating room. It is then given to the patient who may choose to have it made into a wig. The family needs to be prepared for the appearance of the patient after surgery.

Postoperative care is determined by the patient's condition. Most patients spend one or two nights in an intensive care unit, under close nursing observation, with frequent neurological checks. The patient should be assessed carefully for indications of increased intracranial pressure. The patient may have residual motor or sensory problems as a result of the tumor or surgery. (The interventions needed are listed on p. 1115.)

Nursing diagnoses and interventions for the patient with a brain tumor are the same as those for the patient who has had a CVA, with the addition of but are not limited to the following:

NURSING DIAGNOSES	NURSING INTERVENTIONS
Anxiety, related to unknown outcome of disease process	Observe for signs of increasing anxiety. Assist in identifying coping skills. Maintain a calm, unhurried manner. Teach relaxation exercises and techniques. Administer tranquilizers and sedatives as ordered. Allow for verbal expression of anger. Use touch, reassurance, and positive body language.
Pain, related to pressure on brain	Assess type and location of pain. Administer analgesics as ordered and assess effectiveness of pain relief measures; narcotics such as morphine, which depress respirations, are not used. Turn and change position q 2 to 4 hr. Provide back rubs and skin care. Maintain planned rest periods. Assist patient with alternate comfort measures.

NURSING DIAGNOSES	NURSING INTERVENTIONS
Sensory/perceptual alterations: visual, auditory, kinesthetic, tactile, related to compression/displacement of brain tissue	Maintain method of communication. Provide for social interaction. Maintain safe environment. Provide orientation and appropriate level of stimuli.
Thought processes, altered, related to altered circulation and/or destruction of brain tissue	Protect patient from self-injury. Provide soft safety reminder devices as indicated. Assist patient in self-care activities. Speak in kind tone using short, simple sentences. Give one direction at a time. Relate date, time of day, and recent activities. Maintain a therapeutic environment. Keep equipment and personal possessions in same place. Encourage socialization.

Prognosis. The outlook for the patient with a brain tumor depends on whether the tumor was benign or malignant and on the size and location of the mass. Tumors that infiltrate the brain usually result in a decreased life span. With radiation and chemotherapy, patients with malignant tumors may be assisted in living longer.

Trauma. Interference with neurological function can occur as a result of trauma. Parts of the nervous system commonly subjected to trauma include the craniocerebrum, the spinal cord, and peripheral nerves. Only the first two will be discussed in this chapter.

Craniocerebral trauma

Etiology/pathophysiology. Craniocerebral trauma, or head injury, causes death or serious disability in people of all ages. Head injury is the second most common cause of neurological injuries and the major cause of death between ages 1 and 35. Causes of head injury include motor vehicle and motorcycle accidents, falls, industrial accidents, assaults, and sports trauma.

Craniocerebral trauma may result in injury to the scalp, skull, and brain tissues. Injuries vary from minor scalp wounds to concussions and open fractures of the skull with severe damage to the brain. The amount of obvious damage is not indicative of the seriousness of the trouble. Effects of severe head injury include cerebral edema, sensory and motor deficits, and increased intracranial pressure.

Injuries to the brain can result from direct or indirect trauma to the head. Indirect trauma is caused by tension strains and shearing forces transmitted to the head by stretching of the neck. Direct trauma occurs when the head is directly injured. This results in an *acceleration-deceleration* injury, with rotation of the skull and its contents. Bruising or contusion of the occipital and frontal lobes and the brain stem and cerebellum may occur.

Clinical manifestations. Head injuries may be open or closed. Open head injuries result from skull fractures or penetrating wounds. The amount of injury with this type of wound is determined by the velocity, mass, shape, and direction of the impact. A skull fracture (linear, comminuted, depressed, or compound) may also occur. Fractures of the base of the skull are more serious because of their location near the medulla.

Closed head injuries include concussions (a violent jarring of the brain against the skull), contusions, and lacerations. Lacerations of the scalp bleed profusely because of the large vascularity in the region. Hemorrhage resulting from craniocerebral trauma may occur in the following sites: scalp, epidural, subdural, intracerebral, and intraventricular. Epidural and subdural hematomas require careful and continuous observation by the nurse. Epidural hematomas form as blood collects rapidly between the dura and skull. If lethargy or unconsciousness develops after the patient regains consciousness, an epidural hematoma may be suspected and needs immediate treatment.

A subdural hematoma forms as venous blood collects below the dura. Because the bleeding is under venous pressure, the hematoma formation is relatively slow. The clot will cause pressure on the brain surface and will displace brain tissue. If a patient who has been conscious for several days after head injury loses consciousness or develops neurological signs and symptoms, a subdural hematoma should be suspected. Subdural hematomas may be classified as acute, subacute, or chronic.

Assessment. Collection of *subjective data* includes the patient's understanding of the injury and the resulting pathological processes. Determining how the injury happened and whether the patient has headache, nausea, or vomiting is important. Abnormal sensations and a history of a loss of consciousness and of bleeding from any orifice should be noted.

Collection of *objective data* includes the status of the respiratory system, level of alertness and consciousness, and size and reactivity of the pupils; these should be checked frequently. The nurse also assesses the patient's orientation, motor status, vital signs, the presence of bleeding or vomiting, and abnormal speech patterns.

Medical management. Immediate care of the patient with a head injury is directed toward lifesaving measures and the maintenance of normal body function until recovery is ensured. It is extremely important to maintain a patent airway and ensure adequate oxygenation. Suctioning may be necessary (but never through the nose because of the possibility of a skull fracture), as well as the administration of oxygen. Arterial blood gas levels are checked.

Medications are used to reduce cerebral edema and increased intracranial pressure, which are common problems in patients with head injuries. Medications include mannitol and dexamethasone. Codeine or other analgesics that do not depress the respiratory system are used for pain control. Anticonvulsants may be given to prevent seizures. Measures to control elevated temperatures are taken because hyperthermia increases brain metabolism, resulting in brain damage.

Nursing interventions

PREVENTION OF INFECTION. The patient's ears and nose are checked carefully for signs of blood and serous drainage, which indicate that the meninges are torn and spinal fluid is escaping. No attempt should be made to clean out the orifice. If there is evidence of drainage from the nose, the patient should not cough, sneeze, or blow the nose. If there is a question about whether drainage is CSF, a Tes-Tape will show a positive reaction for sugar. Meningitis is a possible complication when communication with the meninges and the nose or ears occurs.

EMOTIONAL SUPPORT. It is not uncommon that the patient with a head injury shows a loss of memory and loss of initiative. Behavioral problems associated with a lack of judgment and restlessness may also occur. Restlessness in the head-injured patient may be caused by the need for a change of position, pain, or the need to empty the bladder. These patients need firm but gentle care, with specific guidelines for what behavior is allowed. It is not helpful to argue with the patient. It may be helpful to redirect his attention. Memory aids such as a log book or written schedule can be very useful in assisting him with orientation.

The length of convalescence will depend on the amount of brain damage and how rapid the recovery is. Many patients with head injury will recover physically but will have behavioral and psychological problems that make it difficult for them to function independently. (See Chapter 49.)

Nursing diagnoses and interventions for the patient with a head injury are the same as for the patient with has had a CVA, with the addition of but are not limited to the following:

NURSING DIAGNOSIS	NURSING INTERVENTIONS
Social interaction, impaired, related to cognitive and affective deficits from neurophysiological trauma	Encourage and support verbalization about feelings, medical conditions, and current treatment; listen nonjudgmentally. Build trust through consistency and keep promises. Involve patient in plan of care. Give full attention to patient during verbal interactions and recognize qualities to promote self-esteem.

PATIENT TEACHING. A patient with a head injury may be seen in the emergency room but not be admitted to the hospital. Such a patient needs to be taught about observations for complications. Teaching for patients with a head injury and who have residual deficits severe enough to require rehabilitation is similar to that needed for patients with motor or sensory problems.

Prognosis. The outcome for a patient with a head injury is often unpredictable. The extent of damage or recovery is not positively correlated with the amount of damage seen in surgery or on CT scan. Even minor head injuries can result in residual effects. The person with a head injury is more prone to injuries and problems related to the brain damage (see Chapter 49).

Spinal cord trauma

Etiology/pathophysiology. Spinal cord injury from accidents is a common and increasing cause of serious disability and death. Approximately 10% of traumatic injuries to the nervous system involve the spinal cord. Most persons involved with spinal cord injuries are males between the ages of 18 and 25. Automobile, motorcycle, diving, surfing, and other athletic accidents and gunshot wounds are major causes of spinal cord injury.

The soft tissue of the spinal cord is protected by the vertebral column. Injuries that occur to this column include a simple fracture, compressed or wedged fracture, comminuted or burst fractures, or dislocation of the vertebrae (Fig. 35-17). As a result the cord is often damaged. Severe traumatic lesions of the spinal cord may result in total transection of the spinal cord or a tearing of the cord from side to side at a particular level, with a complete loss of spinal cord function. This total transection is also called a *complete cord injury.* With this type of injury, all voluntary movement below the level of the trauma is lost. A partial transection or *incomplete injury* involves a partial transection or injury of the cord. Quadriplegics are patients who sustain injuries to one of the cervical segments of the spinal cord. Paraplegics are those whose lesions are confined to the thoracic, lumbar, or sacral segments of the spinal cord. The signs and symptoms of an incomplete injury are variable (Table 35-7).

Clinical manifestations

SPINAL SHOCK. Initially, in most spinal cord injuries, there is a period of flaccid paralysis and a complete loss of reflexes below the trauma. Sensory and autonomic functions are also lost. This is called *areflexia* or spinal shock and is temporary. During this time the patient may need temporary respiratory support.[33]

AUTONOMIC DYSREFLEXIA. One complication of spinal cord injury that is extremely important to understand is autonomic dysreflexia or **hyperreflexia** (a neurological condition characterized by increased reflex actions). It occurs in patients with cord injuries above the sixth tho-

Box 35-4 EMERGENCY CARE FOR AUTONOMIC DYSREFLEXIA OR HYPERREFLEXIA

- Place patient in sitting position to decrease blood pressure.
- Check patency of catheter for kinking. If catheter is occluded, insert new catheter immediately.
- Check return for impaction.
- If it is necessary to remove impaction, an anesthetic ointment should be used.
- Administer ganglionic blocking agent such as hexamethonium or a vasodilator such as nitroprusside (Nipride) as ordered if conservative measures are not effective.
- Continue monitoring blood pressure.
- Send urine for culture if no other cause is found; urinary infection can lead to symptoms of autonomic dysreflexia.

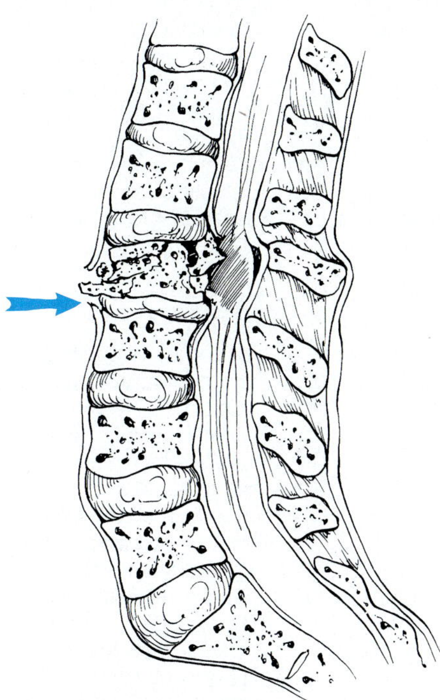

35-17 Damage to spinal cord and distortion of adjacent structures that may occur in traumatic injuries to spine.

racic vertebra and most commonly in patients with cervical injuries. *Autonomic dysreflexia* occurs as a result of abnormal cardiovascular response to stimulation of the sympathetic division of the autonomic nervous system as a result of stimulation of the bladder, large intestine, or other visceral organs. The clinical signs include bradycardia, hypertension, diaphoresis, "goose flesh," severe headache, and nasal stuffiness. Patients tend to develop individual signs and symptoms of this condition and are soon able to recognize them.

The most common cause of this condition include a distended bladder or a fecal impaction. It is a medical emergency that requires immediate treatment to prevent a CVA, blindness, or death (Box 35-4).

TABLE 35-7 Muscle Function After Spinal Cord Injury

Spinal Cord Injury	Muscle Function Remaining	Muscle Function Lost
Above C4	None	All, including respiration
C5	Neck Scapular elevation	Arms Chest All below chest
C6-C7	Neck Some chest movement Some arm movement	Some arm, fingers Some chest All below chest
Thoracic	Neck Arms (full) Some chest	Trunk All below chest
Lumbosacral	Neck Arms Chest Trunk	Legs

SEXUAL FUNCTION. In most cases men experience impotence, decreased sensation, and difficulties with ejaculation. Impairment of fertility is common. The experience of orgasm is described as different than before the injury. Women with spinal cord injury are able to continue to perform sexually, although perception of sexual pleasure is usually altered.

Assessment. Collection of ***subjective data*** includes information about the nature of the injury, presence of any dyspnea, and unusual sensations. The presence of pain, any loss of consciousness, and the absence of sensation on sensory examination are important to assess.

Collection of ***objective data*** includes the level of alertness and consciousness, orientation, pupil size and reactivity, motor strength, skin integrity, and bowel and bladder status, including distention. It is important to assess for other injuries, such as fractured bones or head injury.

Diagnostic tests. X-ray films are often taken first to detect any cervical vertebra fracture or displacement. A spinal tap or myelogram may also be done to detect occlusion. A CT scan and MRI scan may be helpful to rule out spinal cord injury.

Medical management. Immediate care after spinal cord injury is directed toward realignment of the bony column in the presence of fractures or dislocations. The measures involved may include simple immobilization, skeletal traction, or surgery for spinal decompression. Skeletal traction may include Crutchfield tongs (Fig. 35-18), halo traction, (see Chapter 26), or a Stryker or Foster frame. Bracing may be used for thoracic or lumbar injuries. Often a surgical decompression is not performed until after a period of skeletal traction if the injury involves the cervical region.

Nursing interventions

MOBILITY. Throughout all stages of hospitalization of the patient with a spinal cord injury, nursing and medical interventions are directed toward restoration of structural or body integrity. All efforts are taken to ensure that the skin is intact, that contractures do not develop, and that ROM is maintained. Early mobilization is important. When patients, especially quadriplegics, begin to sit up, it may be necessary to wrap the legs with thromboembolism stockings to encourage venous return. Slowly increasing the angle of sitting up is essential to prevent hypotension. A recliner wheelchair is usually necessary.

URINARY FUNCTION. Usually a Foley catheter is inserted initially; later bladder training is started (see Chapter 30). Intermittent catheterization is often used. Fluid intake that exceeds 2000 ml per day is encouraged.

BOWEL FUNCTION. Patients are usually started on a bowel program early in their hospital stay. At first bisacodyl (Dulcolax) suppositories are given as regular intervals—usually every other night. This is followed by digital stimulation to further stimulate peristalsis. The goal is to eliminate the need for suppositories. Other aids to bowel programs are the use of adequate fluids (usually at least 2000 ml per day), stool softeners, and prune juice.

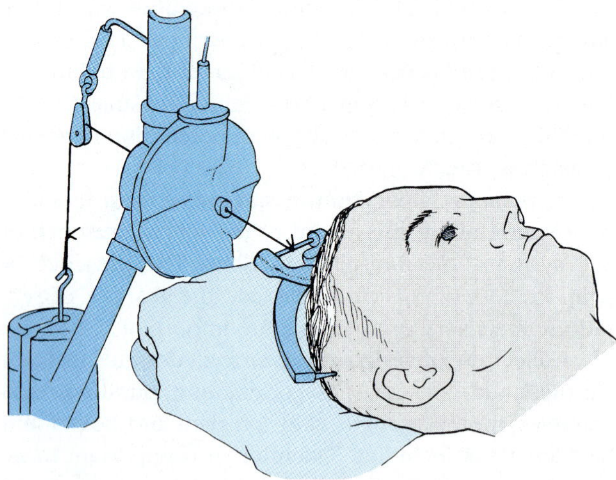

FIG 35-18 Patient with Crutchfield tongs inserted into skull to hyperextend head and neck.

Nursing diagnoses and interventions for the patient with a spinal cord injury are the same as those for the patient with a motor or sensory problem, with the addition of but not limited to the following:

NURSING DIAGNOSES	NURSING INTERVENTIONS
Breathing pattern, ineffective, related to neurogenic or traumatic injury	Maintain patent airway. Auscultate breath sounds. Be cognizant of assisted ventilation and oxygenation being ordered, as well as measurement of vital capacity to ensure adequate ventilation. Be aware that tracheostomy may be indicated. Maintain nasal and oropharyngeal airway and suction as needed.
Dysreflexia, related to neurophysiological trauma to spinal cord above sixth thoracic vertebra	See Box 35-4 for emergency interventions.
Knowledge deficit, related to diagnosis and potential home management	Ensure that patient and significant other are informed about disease and prognosis. Prepare for chronicity and duration of rehabilitative process. Discuss medications: name, dosage, route, side effects, and purpose. Refer to appropriate rehabilitative and counseling resources.
Powerlessness, related to actual or perceived body image changes	Encourage communication between patient and family or significant others. Encourage independence when possible; be aware of limitations. Involve patient in decision-making process when formulating care plan. Help patient set small, realistic goals. Give positive reinforcement for independent functioning. Assist patient in identifying areas that can be self-controlled. Support all verbalization of feelings, especially anger.
Urinary elimination, altered patterns of, related to sensory-motor impairment	Check carefully for voiding and for distention of the bladder. Teach patient intermittent self-catheterization if indicated. Teach patient Credé's maneuver as indicated (see Chapter 30). Use Foley catheter if indicated; administer meticulous aseptic technique in changing catheters. Teach patients signs of infection. Encourage patient to have a genitourinary checkup at least yearly. Maintain fluid intake of 3 to 4 L daily unless contraindicated. Use adult diapers if necessary.

PATIENT TEACHING. Teaching of the patient with a spinal cord injury includes education about autonomic dysreflexia and about sexual functioning after spinal cord injury. Other teaching points are found in the sections of this chapter dealing with the patient with motor or sensory problems.

Prognosis. In cases of a complete spinal cord injury, there is almost no chance of return of any function. However, the paraplegic or quadriplegic patient can live a satisfying life with adaptations and assistance. Care will be necessary to prevent infections, such as urinary tract or respiratory infections. With patients with incomplete cord lesions, the amount of return of function is variable and often unpredictable.

REFERENCES AND SUGGESTED READINGS

1. Anagnostakos NP, Tortora GJ: *Principles of anatomy and physiology,* ed 5, New York, 1987, Harper & Row.
2. Anderson S: Guillain-Barré syndrome: giving the patient control, *J Neurosci Nurs* 24(3):158, 1992.
3. Andrus C: Intracranial pressure: diagnosis and nursing management, *J Neurosci Nurs* 23:85, 1991.
4. Aumick J: Head trauma: guidelines for care, *RN* 54(4):27, 1991.
5. Backman D: The diagnosis and management of common neurologic sequelae of closed head injury, *J Head Trauma Rehabil* 7(2):50, 1992.
6. Baggerly J: Sensory perceptual problems following stroke: the "invisible" deficits, *Nurs Clin North Am* 26(4):997, 1991.
7. Barker E: Action stat SCI, *Nurs '90* 20(11):33, 1990.
8. Barker E: Neurological assessment, *RN* 55(4):28, 1992.
9. Barker E et al: Cranial nerve assessment, *RN* 55(5):62, 1992.
10. Besidin R et al: Managing advanced Alzheimer's disease, *Patient Care* 25(18):75, 1991.
11. Borgman M et al: Nursing care of the stroke patient using Bobath principles: an approach to altered movement, *Nurs Clin North Am* 26(4):28, 1991.
12. Boss B: Managing communication disorders in stroke, *Nurs Clin North Am* 26(4):985, 1991.
13. Bozzacco V: Long-term psychosocial effects of spinal cord injury, *Rehabil Nurs* 18(2):82, 1993.
14. Bruckbauer E: Recognizing poststroke depression, *Rehabil Nurs* 16(4):212, 1991.
15. Buelow J: A correlational study of disabilities, stressors, and coping methods in victims of multiple sclerosis, *J Neurosci Nurs* 23:247, 1991.
16. Chase J: Spinal stenosis: when arthritis is more than arthritis, *Nurs Clin North Am* 26(1):53, 1991.
17. Chipps E: Transsphenoidal surgery for pituitary tumors, *Crit Care Nurse* 12(1):30, 1993.
18. Curry K et al: The relationship between extended periods of immobility and decubitus ulcer formation in the acutely spinal cord injured individual, *J Neurosci Nurs* 24(4):185, 1992.
19. DiIorio C, Price M: Swallowing: an assessment and practice guide, *Am J Nurs* 90:38, 1990.
20. Dittmar S: *Rehabilitation nursing: process and application,* St Louis, 1989, Mosby.
21. Dodson E et al: Are you up-to-date on seizures? *Patient Care* 25(11):162, 1991.
22. Dykes PC: Minding the five Ps of neurovascular assessment, *Am J Nurs* 93(6):38, 1993.
23. Edwards D et al: Hyperthermia treatment for malignant astrocytomas: nursing implications, *J Neurosci Nurs* 23:34, 1991.
24. Emich-Herring B, Wood P: A team approach to neurological based swallowing disorders, *Rehabil Nurs* 15:242, 1990.
25. Farkkila M et al: Plasma exchange therapy reduces the nursing care needed in Guillain Barré Syndrome, *J Adv Nurs* 17(6):672, 1992.
26. Finocchiaro D, Hersfeld, S: Understanding Alzheimer's disease, *Am J Nurs* 90(9):56, 1990.
27. Fong E, Ferris EB, Skelly EG: *Body structures and functions,* ed 7, New York, 1989, Delmar.
28. Hall G: This hospital patient has Alzheimer's, *Am J Nurs* 91(10):45, 1991.
29. Hall M et al: Multidisciplinary approaches to management of acute head injury, *J Neurosci Nurs* 24(4):199, 1992.
30. Hansberry J et al: Managing chronic pain with a permanent epidural catheter, *Nurs '90* 20(10):53, 1990.
31. Hartshorn JC et al: Impact of epilepsy on quality of life, *J Neurosci Nurs* 24(1):24, 1992.
32. Hegner BR, Caldwell E: *Geriatrics: a study of maturity,* ed 5, New York, 1991, Delmar.
33. Hickey J: Myasthenic crisis: your assessment counts, *RN* 54(5):54, 1991.
34. Hodges K, Root L: Surgical management of intractable seizure disorder, *J Neurosci Nurs* 23:93, 1991.
35. Hood GH, Dincher JR: *Total patient care,* ed 8, St Louis, 1992, Mosby.
36. Hubsky E et al: Fatigue in multiple sclerosis: guidelines for nursing care, *Rehabil Nurs* 17(4):176, 1992.
37. Jopp M et al: Using self-care theory to guide nursing management of the older adult after hospitalization, *Rehabil Nurs* 18(2):91, 1993.
38. Kirby N: The individual with high quadriplegia, *Nurs Clin North Am* 24(1):179, 1989.
39. Larsen P: Psychosocial adjustment in MS, *Rehabil Nurs* 15:242, 1990.
40. Leahy N: Complications in the acute stages of stroke: nursing's pivotal role, *Nurs Clin North Am* 26(4):971, 1991.
41. Long B, Phipps W, Cassmeyer V: *Medical-surgical nursing: a nursing process approach,* ed 3, St Louis, 1993, Mosby.
42. Loughery L: Carol gave up fighting . . . until her nurse stepped in, *Nursing* 21(8):50, 1991.
43. Lower J: Rapid neuro assessment, *Am J Nurs* 92(6):38, 1992.
44. Luchka S: Working with ICP monitors, *RN* 54(3):34, 1991.
45. Marieb EN: *Human anatomy & physiology,* Reading, Mass, 1989, Benjamin/Cummings.
46. Marr J: The experience of living with Parkinson's disease, *J Neurosci Nurs* 23(5):325, 1991.
47. Mauss-Clum N et al: Locked in syndrome: a team approach, *J Neurosci Nurs* 23(5):273, 1991.
48. Memmler RL, Cohen BJ, Wood, DL: *Structure and function of the human body,* ed 5, Philadelphia, 1992, Lippincott.
49. Mocsny N: Toxoplasmic encephalitis in the AIDS patient, *Rehabil Nurs* 18(1):20, 1993.
50. Morgan S: A passage through paralysis, *Am J Nurs* 92(4):54, 1992.
51. *Mosby's medical, surgical, and allied health dictionary,* ed 4, St Louis, 1994, Mosby.
52. North B et al: Living in the halo, *Am J Nurs* 92(4):54, 1992.
53. Olson E et al: The hazards of immobility, *Am J Nurs* 90(3):43, 1990.
54. Pagana KD, Pagana TJ: *Mosby's diagnostic and laboratory test reference,* St Louis, 1992, Mosby.
55. Penrose N: Guillain-Barré syndrome: a case study, *Rehabil Nurs* 18(2):88, 1993.
56. Phipps M: Assessment of neurologic deficits in stroke: acute-care and rehabilitation implications, *Nurs Clin North Am* 26(4):957, 1991.
57. Piazza D et al: Hope, social support, and self-esteem of patients with spinal cord injuries, *J Neurosci Nurs* 24(4):224, 1991.
58. Purath J: Assessing headache pain, *RN* 54(10):26, 1991.
59. Rankin J: The nursing diagnosis: swallowing, impaired and bedside assessment of swallowing in neurologically involved case, *J Neurosci Nurs* 24(2):117, 1992.

60. Rice M: Minor head injury: is anybody listening? *J Neurosci Nurs* 24(3):173, 1992.
61. Savoy S, Gianino J: Intrathecal baclofen infusion: an innovative approach for controlling spinal spasticity, *Rehabil Nurs* 18(2):105, 1993.
62. Schererr A: How HIV attacks the CNS, *Am J Nurs* 90(5):66, 1990.
63. Shaid E et al: Focusing on dementia, *J Gerontol Nurs* 18(7):39, 1992.
64. Sherman D: Managing an acute HI, *Nurs '90* 20(4):46, 1990.
65. Snyder M, ed: *A guide to neurological and neurosurgical nursing,* ed 2, New York, 1991, Delmar.
66. Solomon EP: *Introduction to human anatomy and physiology,* Philadelphia, 1992, Saunders.
67. Steele C et al: Myths & facts . . . about Alzheimer's disease, *Nursing* 22(4):25, 1992.
68. Stevenson J: Family stress related to home care of Alzheimer disease patients and implications for support, *J Neurosci Nurs* 22:179, 1990.
69. Stewart-Amidei C: An ounce of prevention . . . head and spinal cord injury prevention programs, *J Neurosci Nurs* 22(5):273, 1990.
70. Sullivan J: Neurologic assessment, *Nurs Clin North Am* 25:795, 1990.
71. Thibodeau GA: *Structure and function of the body,* ed 9, St Louis, 1992, Mosby.
72. Vos H: Making headway with intracranial hypertension, *Am J Nurs* 93(2):28, 1993.
73. Weiss J: Multiple sclerosis: will it come between us? Sexual concerns of clients and their partners, *J Neurosci Nurs* 24(4):190, 1992.

CHAPTER CHALLENGE

KEY POINTS

- The nervous system is the body's link with the environment. It allows the interpretation of information and appropriate action to occur.
- The two main structural divisions of the nervous system are the central nervous system and the peripheral nervous system.
- The central nervous system is composed of the brain and the spinal cord.
- The peripheral nervous system is composed of the nerve cells lying outside of the central nervous system. It is composed of the somatic nervous system and the autonomic nervous system.
- A nerve cell is composed of three parts: the dendrite, the cell body, and the axon. The space between each nerve cell is called the synapse.
- All neurons are governed by the "all or none" law, which means there is never a partial transmission of a message. The impulse must be strong enough to elicit a response, or the impulse is not transmitted.
- Myelin is a white, waxy, fatty material that covers neuron fibers. It increases the rate of transmission of impulses and protects and insulates the fibers.
- Another material that covers neuron fibers is found only in the peripheral nervous system. It is called neurilemma, and it helps to regenerate injured axons.
- The brain and spinal cord are protected by the bony coverings (skull and vertebral column), the cerebrospinal fluid, and the three meninges (pia mater, arachnoid, and dura mater).
- The cerebrum is the largest part of the brain and contains five major areas: motor, sensory, visual, speech, and auditory. The cerebrum governs the ability to reason and make judgments.
- The diencephalon lies beneath the cerebrum and contains the thalamus and hypothalamus. The thalamus serves as a relay station, while the hypothalamus has several roles, such as temperature control, water balance, and appetite.
- The cerebellum is the second largest portion of the brain and is responsible for coordination of skeletal muscles and maintenance of balance and equilibrium.
- The peripheral nervous system is composed of the cranial nerves, the spinal nerves, and the autonomic nervous system.
- The autonomic nervous system contains two subdivisions: the sympathetic nervous system and the parasympathetic nervous system. The sympathetic nervous system "speeds" things up and the parasympathetic nervous system "slows" things down.
- Normal changes of aging are not the same as senility, Alzheimer's disease, or organic brain damage.
- The source of any headache should be determined through neurological testing, because it may be a symptom of a serious pathological condition.
- A lumbar puncture should not be done if there is evidence of increased intracranial pressure because of the danger of brain herniation.
- Any increase in the volume of one of the contents of the cranium (brain, blood vessels, and cerebrospinal fluid) results in increased intracranial pressure, because the cranial vault is rigid and does not expand.
- Classic signs of increased intracranial pressure include restlessness, disorientation, headache, contralateral hemiparesis, an ipsilaterally dilated pupil, and visual changes that include blurring and diplopia.
- Nursing intervention measures can significantly influence intracranial pressure.

- Epilepsy is a transitory disturbance in consciousness or in motor, sensory, or autonomic functions with or without loss of consciousness, caused by sudden, excessive, and disorderly electrical discharges of the brain.
- Early signs and symptoms of multiple sclerosis are usually transitory.
- Cerebrovascular accident is the most common disease of the nervous system and can be caused by thrombus, embolus, or hemorrhage.
- Helpful nursing interventions for the patient with Alzheimer's disease include using nonverbal clues or demonstrations as adjuncts to verbal cues, providing very few choices, and not hurrying the patient.
- Trigeminal neuralgia (tic douloureux) is characterized by excruciating, burning pain that radiates along one or more of the three divisions of the fifth cranial nerve.
- With Bell's palsy, there is usually an abrupt onset of numbness or a feeling of stiffness or a drawing sensation of the face.
- Of the persons suffering from Guillain-Barré syndrome, 85% will retain complete function.
- Approximately 40% of patients with AIDS have neurological symptoms that result from infection from HIV itself or from associated complications of AIDS.
- Many patients with head injury may recover physically, but they will have behavioral and psychological problems that make it difficult for them to function independently.
- The signs and symptoms of intracranial tumors result from both local and general effects of the tumor.
- Autonomic dysreflexia in the patient with spinal cord injury is a medical emergency that demands quick nursing interventions.
- The first sign of increased intracranial pressure may be a lessening of the state of consciousness.
- It is important to document patients' behaviors in terms of what is seen, not what is inferred.

STUDY QUESTIONS

1. The central nervous system works with what system to maintain homeostasis in the body:
   1. endocrine
   2. integumentary
   3. musculoskeletal
   4. reproductive
2. Special chemicals that assist in the transmission of a message are called:
   1. dendrites
   2. axons
   3. neurotransmitters
   4. cell bodies
3. The neuron has special structures that receive impulses and transmit them to the cell body. They are called:
   1. axons
   2. dendrites
   3. cell bodies
   4. neurotransmitters
4. The nodes of Ranvier:
   1. increase the speed of message transmission
   2. decrease the speed of message transmission
   3. increase regeneration of the nerve cell
   4. decrease regeneration of the nerve cell
5. Another name for the "interbrain," which contains the hypothalamus and thalamus, is the:
   1. cerebrum
   2. cerebellum
   3. diencephalon
   4. brain stem
6. Which part of the brain is mainly involved in coordination of skeletal muscles, maintenance of balance, and control of muscle tone?
   1. cerebrum
   2. cerebellum
   3. diencephalon
   4. brain stem
7. Which part of the brain contains the respiratory center?
   1. medulla oblongata
   2. thalamus
   3. hypothalamus
   4. cerebrum
8. The covering of nerve tissue that allows regeneration is the:
   1. myelin
   2. nodes of Ranvier
   3. neurilemma
   4. pia mater
9. What structure is responsible for the transmission of messages to the brain and the spinal cord?
   1. afferent neurons
   2. efferent neurons
   3. nerve fibers
   4. nerve impulses
10. The largest part of the brain is:
    1. the medulla oblongata
    2. the cerebellum
    3. the cerebrum
    4. the pons

11. Sue Brown, a nursing student, is caring for a patient with a head injury. What nursing intervention is *contraindicated* in the presence of an acute head injury:
    1. Suctioning through the nose
    2. Elevating head of bed 30 degrees
    3. Turning from side to side
    4. ROM exercises
12. Mrs. Smith, an 85-year-old, is admitted to a nursing home. The nurse knows that she can expect to see some normal aging changes in Mrs. Smith. An abnormal aging change of the neurological system is:
    1. Altered sleep/wakefulness ratio
    2. Senile changes in mental ability
    3. Reduction in cerebral blood flow
    4. Decrease in weight of the brain
13. Timothy Jones, a 17-year-old adolescent, is admitted with a head injury sustained while driving a three wheeler on his ranch. He is demonstrating a decreased level of consciousness. The physician orders a Glasgow Coma Scale every 3 hours. The Glasgow Coma Scale is a simple instrument to use in a systematic assessment of level of sconsciousness. It is based on the patient's response in three major areas. They are:
    1. verbal, sensation, motor
    2. eye, motor, verbal
    3. verbal, pain, reflexes
    4. eye, pain, verbal
14. Jack Thomas is a 26-year-old patient who suffered a spinal cord injury that has left him a quadriplegic. Mr. Thomas at times has problems with autonomic dysreflexia. Which of the following signs or symptoms is not indicative of autonomic dysreflexia:
    1. Hypotension
    2. Diaphoresis
    3. Bradycardia
    4. Severe headache
15. Mr. Lambert has a history of grand mal seizures. Patients with these seizures often experience a warning feeling before a seizure. This is called:
    1. Convulsion
    2. Tonicity
    3. Postictal
    4. Aura
16. Robert Jones has advanced Parkinson's disease. Which of the following is often a complication seen in patients with Parkinson's disease?
    1. Total paralysis
    2. Increasing spasticity
    3. Sjögren's syndrome
    4. Aspiration pneumonia
17. Mr. Josea was admitted for observation after being thrown out of his vehicle and sustaining a head injury. He has been alert and oriented, but after several days he becomes less responsive. What should be suspected?
    1. Ruptured aneurysm
    2. Skull fracture
    3. Herniation of the medulla oblongata
    4. Epidural hematoma
18. Mr. Eyten is a 46-year-old patient with a 13-year history of progressively deteriorating multiple sclerosis. Which of the following nursing interventions would NOT be appropriate for Mr. Eyten:
    1. Taking the patient to the bathroom frequently
    2. Giving a hot bath to ensure cleanliness
    3. Encouraging fluids to prevent urinary infection
    4. Using a suppository to help evacuate the bowel
19. Ms. Willard is a 32-year-old patient with a spinal cord injury at C6. She often has signs and symptoms resulting from autonomic dysreflexia. Which of the following is NOT a cause of her autonomic dysreflexia?
    1. Kinked catheter
    2. Bowel impaction
    3. Urinary infection
    4. Postural hypotension

36

CARE OF THE PATIENT WITH AN IMMUNE DISORDER

Iva L. Mueller
Barbara Christensen
Elaine Kockrow

KEY TERMS

adaptive immunity
allergen
antigen
attenuated
autoimmune
autologous
cellular immunity
humoral immunity
hypersensitivity
immunity
immunization
immunocompetent
immunodeficiency
immunogen
immunology
immunosuppressive
immunotherapy
innate immunity
lymphokine
proliferation

LEARNING OBJECTIVES

After reading this chapter, the student should be able to do the following:

- Define the key terms.
- Describe the two major types of immunity: innate and adaptive.
- Review the mechanisms of immune response.
- Differentiate between humoral and cellular immunity.
- Explain the terms *immunocompetent, immunodeficient,* and *autoimmunity.*
- Discuss the hypersensitivity diseases.
- Outline the immediate aggressive treatment in anaphylaxis.
- Discuss the causation of autoimmune disorders.
- Discuss the nursing interventions and patient teaching for myasthenia gravis.
- Describe the nursing care plan for a patient with systemic lupus erythematosus.
- Explain an immunodeficiency disease.

RELATED TOPICS OF INTEREST

- The surgical patient (Chapter 22)
- Introduction to anatomy and physiology (Chapter 23)
- Care of the patient with an integumentary disorder (Chapter 25)
- Care of the patient with a respiratory disorder (Chapter 31)
- Care of the HIV-positive or AIDS patient (Chapter 37)
- Care of the patient with cancer (Chapter 38)

NATURE OF IMMUNITY

The word *immune* is derived from the Latin word *immunis,* meaning "free from burden." Immunology is an evolving science that essentially deals with the body's ability to distinguish self from nonself. This distinction is accomplished through a complex network of highly specialized cells and tissues that collectively are called the *immune system.*

The immune system has three main functions: (1) to protect the body's internal environment against invading organisms, (2) to maintain homeostasis by removing damaged cells from the circulation, and (3) to serve as a surveillance network for recognizing and guarding against the development, growth, and dissemination of abnormal cells. When the immune system responds appropriately to a foreign stimulus, the body's integrity is maintained; this is called *immunocompetence.* If the immune response is too weak or too vigorous, homeostasis is disrupted, causing a malfunction in the system, or immunoincompetence. Disruption of the homeostatic balance of the immune system can cause a number of diseases to manifest. Inappropriate responses of the immune system have been classified into four categories: (1) hyperactive responses against environmental antigens (e.g., allergy); (2) inability to protect the body, as in immunodeficiency disorders (e.g., acquired immunodeficiency syndrome [AIDS]); (3) failure to recognize the body as self, as in autoimmune disorders (e.g., systemic lupus erythematosus); and (4) attacks on beneficial foreign tissue (e.g., organ transplant rejection or transfusion reaction).

Resistance to disease is referred to as **immunity** (the quality of being insusceptible to or unaffected by a particular disease or condition). There are two major subclassifications of immunity: innate (natural) and adaptive (acquired) immunity (Fig. 36-1). Innate immunity is nonspecific, whereas adaptive immunity is specific. The study of the immune system is **immunology.**

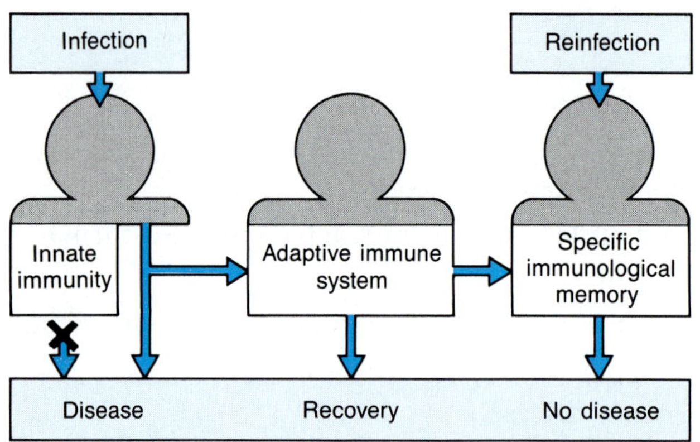

FIG. 36-1 When an infectious agent enters the body, it first encounters elements of the innate immune system. These may be sufficient to prevent disease, but if not, a disease will result, and the adaptive immune system is activated. The adaptive immune system produces recovery from the disease and establishes a specific immunological memory, so after reinfection with the same agent, no disease results. The individual has acquired immunity to the infectious agent.

Innate or Natural Immunity

The body's first line of defense, **innate immunity,** provides physical and chemical barriers to invading pathogens and protects locally against the external environment. The innate system is composed of the skin and mucous membranes, cilia, stomach acid, tears, saliva, sebaceous glands, and secretions and flora of the intestine and vagina. These organs, tissues, and secretions provide biochemical and physical barriers to disease. The first line of defense provides nonspecific immunity to the individual (Table 36-1).

Adaptive or Acquired Immunity

If the components of innate or natural immunity fail to prevent invasion or to destroy a foreign pathogen, the adaptive immune response is summoned to assist in the

TABLE 36-1 Innate and Adaptive Immunity

Characteristics	Innate	Adaptive
Physical barriers	Physical defense: skin and mucous membranes	None
Response mechanisms	Nonspecific: mononuclear phagocytic system; inflammatory response	Specific immune response: humoral immunity, cellular immunity
Soluble factors	Chemical defense: lysozyme, complement, acute phase proteins, interferon	Antibodies, lymphokines
Cells	Phagocytes, natural killer (NK) cells	T lymphocytes, B lymphocytes
Specificity	None	Present
Memory	None	Present

battle. This is the body's second line of defense against disease. **Adaptive immunity** (provides a specific reaction to each invading antigen and has the unique ability to remember the antigen that caused the attack) protects the internal environment. The systemic immune system is composed of highly specialized cells and tissues, including the thymus, spleen, bone marrow, blood, and lymph (Fig. 36-2). Adaptive or acquired immunity includes both humoral and cell-mediated immunity. The characteristics of an adaptive immune system are specificity (specific) and memory. This specific immunity results from the production of antibodies in the cells. Antibodies develop naturally after infection or artificially after vaccinations. Another function of the immune system is to maintain homeostasis by removing damaged elements from the system. The third function is to provide the body with a surveillance network to guard against development, growth, and dissemination of tumor cells.

The cells of the immune system are the macrophages and the lymphocytes. When organisms pass the epithelial barriers, phagocytes become activated. Phagocytes also have the ability to migrate through the bloodstream to the tissues for the body's second line of defense against disease. Phagocytes engulf and destroy microorganisms that pass the skin and mucous membrane barriers. These cells also assist in the immune response by carrying antigens to the lymphocytes.

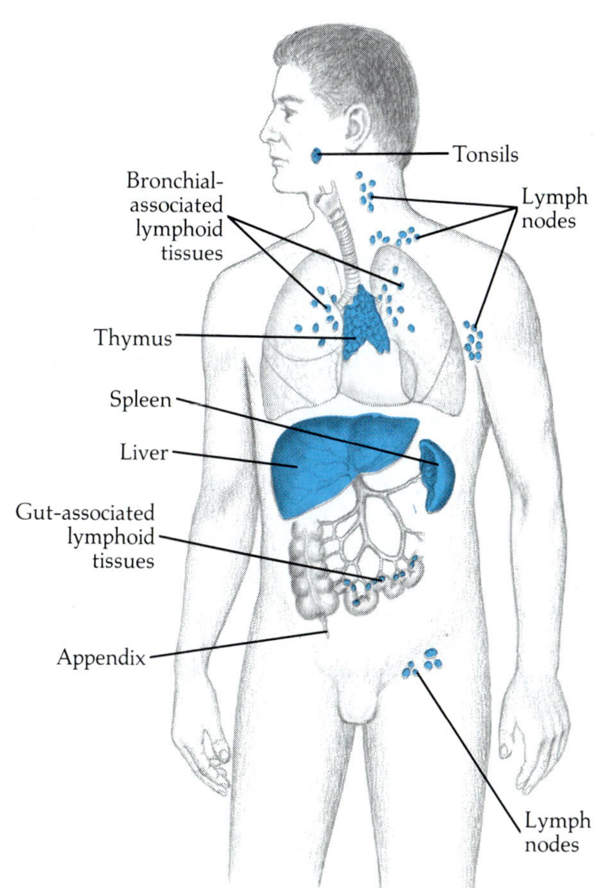

FIG. 36-2 Organization of the immune system.

Lymphocytes include the T and B cells (Fig. 36-3 on p. 1146) and the large, granular lymphocytes also known as *NK* or *natural killer cells*. Approximately 70% to 80% of the lymphocytes are T cell lymphocytes. When activated, T cells release a substance called **lymphokine** (one of the chemical factors produced and released by T cells that attracts macrophages to the site of infection or inflammation and prepares them for attack).

In addition to these functions, in the antigen-antibody reaction, T cells cooperate with the B cells to produce antibodies but do not produce antibodies themselves. T cells are responsible for cell-mediated immunity and provide the body with protection against viruses, fungi, and parasites. T cells also provide protection in allograft (transfer of tissue between two genetically dissimilar individuals of the same species) and against malignant cells.

B cells comprise approximately 20% to 30% of the lymphocyte population. B cells cause the production of antibodies and proliferate (increase in number) in response to a particular **antigen** (a substance recognized by the body as foreign that can trigger an immune response). An antigen is usually a protein that causes the formation of an antibody and reacts specifically with that antibody. B cells migrate to the peripheral circulation and tissues and eventually are filtered from the lymph and stored in the lymphoid tissue of the body.

The initial formation of B cells does not require antigen stimulation or any other environmental stimuli. However, B cell **proliferation** (reproduction or multiplication of similar forms) depends on antigen stimulation. B cells are responsible for humoral immunity. B cells produce antibodies and provide protection against bacteria, viruses, and soluble antigens. See Table 36-1 for innate and adaptive immunity presentation.

Humoral Immunity

Humoral immunity (one of the two forms of immunity that respond to antigens, such as bacteria and foreign tissue) is mediated by the B cells. B cells produce antibodies in response to antigenic challenge. On first exposure to a given antigen, a primary humoral response is initiated. This response is generally slow compared with that to subsequent antigen exposures. Memory B cells cause antibody proliferation at a much more rapid rate once the body has experienced a primary antigen exposure. It does not matter if primary exposure is caused by antigen or **immunization** (a process by which resistance to an infectious disease is induced or increased) agent; the memory response is more rapid and more sustained after initial exposure.

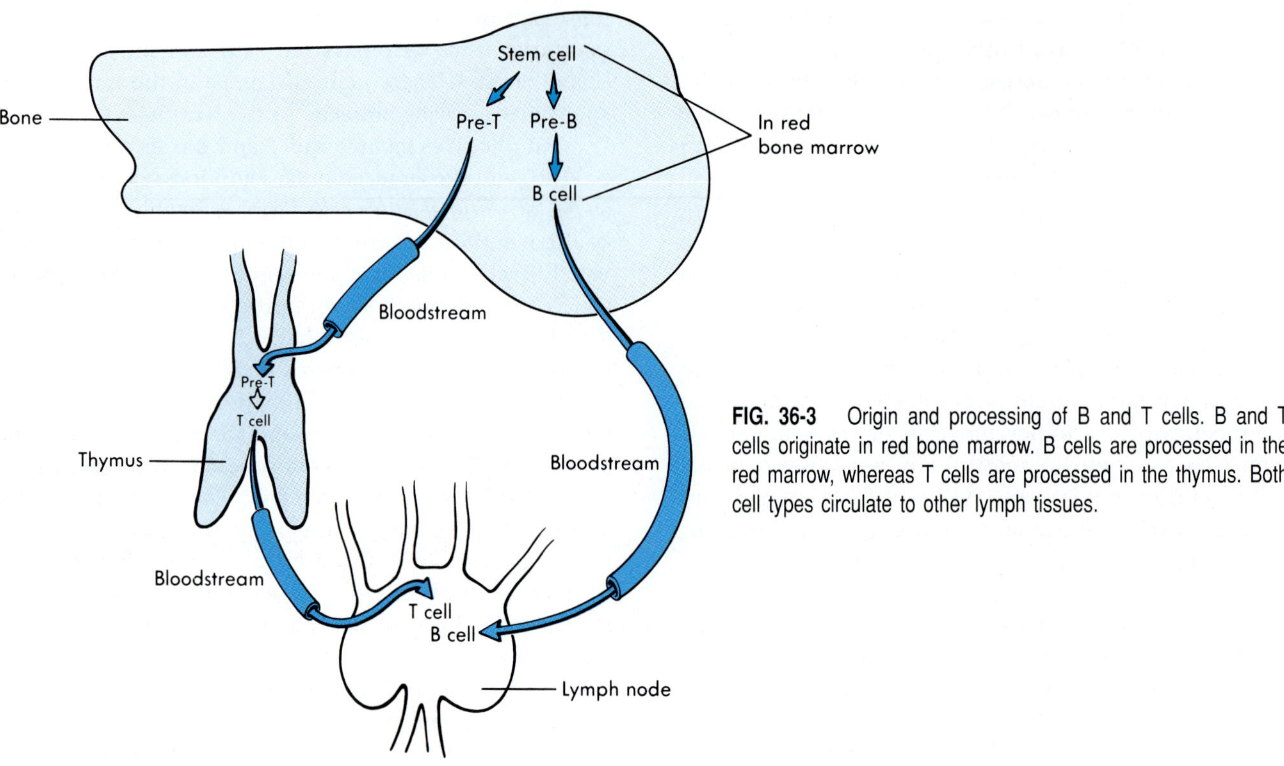

FIG. 36-3 Origin and processing of B and T cells. B and T cells originate in red bone marrow. B cells are processed in the red marrow, whereas T cells are processed in the thymus. Both cell types circulate to other lymph tissues.

Box 36-1

THE FOUR R'S OF THE IMMUNE RESPONSE

Recognize self from nonself. Normally the body recognizes its own cells as nonantigenic; therefore an immune response generally is triggered only in response to agents that the body identifies as foreign. In autoimmune disorders the ability to differentiate self from nonself is disrupted, and the immune system attacks the body's own cells as if they were foreign antigens.

Respond to nonself invaders. The immune system responds in part by producing antibodies that target specific antigens for destruction. New antibodies are produced in response to new antigens. Deficits in the ability to respond can result in immunodeficiency disorders.

Remember the invader. The ability to remember antigens that have invaded the body in the past is the immune system's memory. This characteristic allows a quicker response if subsequent invasion by the same antigen occurs.

Regulate its action. Self-regulation allows the immune system to monitor itself by "turning on" when an antigen invades and "turning off" when the invasion has been eradicated. Regulation prevents the destruction of healthy or host tissue. The inability to regulate could result in a chronic inflammation and damage to the host tissue.

Antigen is presented to the T cell helper population by the macrophage. Most are then taken to the B cells, and assisted by helper T cells, the B cells initiate production of antibodies. Suppressor T cells maintain the humoral response at a level appropriate for the stimulus.

Antibodies produced by one's own body are said to provide active immunity. Antibodies formed by another in response to a specific antigen and administered to an individual will provide only temporary or passive immunity.

Even though humoral immunity is mediated by the B cell population, helper T cells and suppressor T cells have a function and are vital to the **immunocompetent** (the ability of an immune system to mobilize and deploy its antibodies and other responses to stimulation by an antigen) person. Both the number and functions of the helper and suppressor T cells help determine the strength and persistence of an immune response. The normal ratio of helper T cells to suppressor T cells is 2:1 in the body. When this ratio is disrupted, autoimmune and immunodeficient diseases occur.

Exposure to antigen and response with antibody may activate either (1) the humoral complement system, which results in breakdown of the bacteria and release of lysosomes to destroy bacteria, or (2) the antigen/antibody reaction, which results in degranulation mast cells and release of histamine, which produces the symptoms

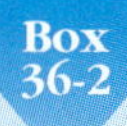
Box 36-2

REVIEW OF THE MECHANISMS OF IMMUNE RESPONSE

- The skin and mucous membranes are natural barriers to infectious agents. When these barriers are crossed, the immune response is begun in the immunocompetent host.
- The first time an antigen enters the body, the antigen is processed by macrophages and presented to lymphocytes. Responses of B cells to the antigen in humoral immunity require interaction with T helper cells, which assist B cells in responding to the antigen by proliferating, synthesizing, and secreting the appropriate antibody. Antigens are then neutralized by antibodies or can form immune complexes or be phagocytosed by macrophages or neutrophils.
- Humoral immunity is not effective against intracellular organisms. Once the organisms have penetrated the host's cells, the antibody cannot function. Cellular immunity is the primary defense against intracellular organisms. In cellular immunity the antigen is processed by macrophages and recognized by T cells. T cells produce lymphokines, which further attract macrophages and neutrophils to the site for phagocytosis, or cytotoxic killer T cells can respond directly.
- Any B cell or T cell lineage could lead to immunodeficiency, as well as to defects in the complement or phagocytic systems.

of allergy. Antigen is referred to as **allergen** (a substance that can produce a hypersensitive reaction in the body but is not necessarily inherently harmful) when symptoms of allergy occur. Antigen is referred to as **immunogen** (any agent or substance capable of provoking an immune response or producing immunity) when immunity results.

COMPLEMENT SYSTEM

The word *complement* became part of the terminology of immunology at the turn of the century, when researchers recognized that blood plasma contained a substance necessary to complete the destruction of bacteria. The complement system is a system of approximately 25 serum enzymatic proteins that interact with one another and with other components of the innate (natural) and adaptive (acquired) immune systems. Normally, complement enzymes are inactive in plasma and body fluids. When an antigen and antibody interact, the complement system is activated. Complement functions in a "step by step" series much like the clotting mechanism, but with a different purpose. The complement system can destroy the cell membrane of many bacterial species, and this action attracts phagocytes to the area.

CELLULAR IMMUNITY AND CELL-MEDIATED IMMUNITY

Cellular immunity, also called *cell-mediated immunity* (the mechanism of acquired immunity characterized by the dominant role of small T cells), results when T cells are activated by an antigen. Whole cells become sensitized in a process similar to that which stimulates the B cells to form antibodies. Once these T cells have been sensitized, they are released into the blood and body tissues where they remain indefinitely. On contact with the antigen to which they are sensitized, they will attach to the organism and destroy it. Cellular immunity is involved in resistance to infectious diseases caused by viruses and some bacteria, delayed hypersensitivity reactions, some aspects of resistance to cancer, certain autoimmune diseases, graft rejection in organ transplants, and certain allergies (Box 36-1).

Hypersensitivity reactions are cell-mediated responses of the body. For review, see Box 36-2 on the mechanisms of immune response.

GENETIC CONTROL OF IMMUNITY

More is being discovered about the genetic role in immunity. There is a genetic link to both well-developed immune systems and poorly developed or compromised immune systems.

The immune system develops at different rates and at different times in fetal and early life. For humans, the bone marrow provides the continuous service of stem cells and all the other cells involved in the immune response.

TOLERANCE

Immunological tolerance is the development of nonreactivity toward particular antigens and as such is the reverse of immunity. Tolerance is enhanced by immunosuppressive drugs. The fundamental basis of the immune system is tolerance to "self" tissues and lack of tolerance to foreign tissue or antigen, marked by an appropriate immune response. Failure of the appropriate response may be marked by a failure to respond against foreign protein or a hypersensitivity reaction.

IMMUNE RESPONSE

There are two ways of assisting the body to develop immunity: immunization and immunotherapy. The theory behind immunization is to have controlled exposure to a disease-producing pathogen, developing antibody production while preventing disease. The first immunization is credited to Edward Jenner (1796), who observed that individuals who had had cowpox became immune to the disease. The idea of administering "attenuated (weakened) microbes" developed, and the scientific approach was applied by Louis Pasteur. Vaccines and toxoids are altered, **attenuated** (the process of weakening the degree of virulence of a disease organism), in such a way as to reduce their degree of power without losing their ability to produce antibodies. In immunization, the immune system mounts a greater response to a second encounter with an antigen. The vaccine, or toxoid, stimulates humoral immunity, which provides protection from disease for months to years.

Immunotherapy (a special treatment of allergic responses that administers increasingly large doses of the offending allergens to gradually develop immunity) consists of injecting a person with a very diluted antigen (allergen) to which the patient has a type I hypersensitivity. The strength of the dilution is increased over a long period, and weekly injections are given over a 1- to 3-year period. The theory behind immunotherapy is to assist the individual to build a tolerance to the allergen without developing fever or increased signs and symptoms. *Desensitization* is another term used for immunotherapy. It is indicated for patients with clinically significant disease for whom avoidance of the allergen or treatment with medication is inadequate. It is considered safe in properly selected patients but does present problems, which include a lengthy, expensive process and a potential for severe anaphylaxis.

Immunotherapy may be coseasonal, preseasonal, or perennial. Perennial therapy is most widely accepted, since it allows for a higher cumulative dose, which produces a better effect. Perennial therapy usually begins with 0.05 ml of a 1:10,000 dilution and increases to 0.5 ml in a 6-week period. The amount given again decreases to 0.05 ml while the dilution lessens to 1:1000 to begin the next series. The amount increases each week until a 0.5 ml dose is given. The next cycle begins with a 0.05 ml dose of 1:100 dilution. Over another 6-week period, the amount administered will increase to 0.5 ml. Perennial therapy is administered subcutaneously. The patient must always be observed for at least 20 minutes after administration, since hypersensitivity reaction or anaphylaxis may occur. The treatment protocol for anaphylaxis with immunotherapy is generally accepted to be 0.3 ml of 1:1000 epinephrine hydrochloride (Adrenalin Chloride) subcutaneously every 15 minutes for three doses.

Most patients begin immunotherapy at the physician's office, and subsequent weekly injections are given until the maintenance level is reached. Home administration by the patient or a family member is acceptable once maintenance level is reached. Interrupted regimens because of illness may place the patient at risk for reaction. The physician should be consulted before administering a dose of diluted allergen if illness or interruption of time schedule has occurred while the patient is on maintenance immunotherapy.

Alterations in the Immune Response

Failure of the immune system occurs in several ways and expresses itself in mild to severe form. There are many points at which the system can malfunction while attempting to provide the body with protective defense.

It is thought that failures occur because of genetic factors, developmental defects, infection, malignancy, injury, drugs, or altered metabolic states. For considerations concerning the older adult, see the gerontological box.

Severity of altered immune response disorders ranges from mild to chronic to life threatening and is categorized as follows:

I Hypersensitivity disorder: involves allergic response and tissue rejection

II Immunodeficiency disease: involves altered and failed immune response

III Autoimmune disease: involves extensive tissue damage resulting from an immune system that seemingly reverses its function to one of self-destruction

GERONTOLOGICAL CONSIDERATIONS

- Older adults are at increased risk for inflammation and infections resulting from changes in natural defense mechanisms.

  Pathogens are able to enter through breaks in the fragile, dry skin, increasing the risk of skin infections.

  Decreased movement of respiratory secretions increases the risk of respiratory infections.

  Decreased production of saliva and gastric secretions increases the risk of gastrointestinal infections.

  Decreased tear production increases the risk of eye inflammation and infections.

  Structural changes in the urinary system that lead to urinary retention or stasis increase the risk of urinary tract infection.
- Signs and symptoms of infection tend to be more subtle than in younger individuals. Because older persons have decreased body temperature, fever may be more difficult to detect. Changes in behavior such as lethargy, fatigue, disorientation, irritability, and loss of appetite may be early signs of infection.
- Functioning of the immune system appears to decrease somewhat with advanced age. Specific data on this is not conclusive, but research is continuing.
- The older adult's immune system continues to produce antibodies and therefore immunization for diseases such as pneumonia and influenza is recommended.
- Older individuals who have chronic illnesses are generally at increased risk for infection.

See Box 36-1 for the four R's of the immune response.

HYPERSENSITIVITY DISORDERS

Hypersensitivity (an abnormal condition characterized by an excessive reaction to a particular stimulus) disorders arise when harmless substances, such as pollens, danders, foods, and chemicals, are recognized as foreign. The body mounts an immune response in much the same way it does to any foreign protein. The result, however, differs. The host becomes sensitive after first exposure, and on subsequent exposure the allergic individual exhibits a hypersensitivity reaction. Chronic exposure leads to chronic allergy response, which ranges from mild to incapacitating signs and symptoms.

Hypersensitivity disorders are believed to be a genetic defect that allows increased production of IgE (immunoglobulin E—a humoral antibody). Exposure to antigen may occur by inhalation, ingestion, injection, or touch (contact). Signs and symptoms occur as a result of histamine release and may be local (gastrointestinal, skin, respiratory, conjunctival) or systemic (anaphylaxis). The exact mechanism and pathway of these inflammatory responses are not clearly understood.

It is known that a combination of interrelated factors occurs with increased severity of symptoms. These factors include those found in Box 36-3.

Diagnostic Tests

Hypersensitivity illnesses are diagnosed largely through patient history and physical examination. Laboratory studies are supportive tools for diagnosis and therapy.

Box 36-3 FACTORS INFLUENCING HYPERSENSITIVITY

Host response to allergen. The more sensitive the individual, the greater the allergic response.

Exposure amount. Generally, the greater the amount of allergen the individual is exposed to, the greater the chance of severe reaction.

Nature of the allergen. Most allergy reactions are precipitated by complex, high-molecular-weight protein substances.

Route of allergen entry. Most allergens enter the body via gastrointestinal and respiratory routes. Injections of venoms and medications hold a more severe threat of allergic response.

Repeated exposure. Generally, the more the individual is exposed, the greater the response.

A thorough history is the most important diagnostic tool. A detailed history is taken, listing (1) onset, nature, and progression of signs and symptoms; (2) aggravating and alleviating factors; and (3) frequency and duration of signs and symptoms. Environmental, household, and occupational factors are assessed. Common offenders include pollens, spores, dusts, food, drugs, and insect venoms. Many but not all offenders are seasonal in nature. Signs and symptoms generally vary from mild upper respiratory manifestations, such as sneezing and excessive nasal secretions, to watery, itching eyes. Skin signs and symptoms are often eczema-like or urticarial. Diarrhea may be a gastrointestinal complaint in some individuals. More severe signs and symptoms include those of the lower respiratory tract, such as coughing, wheezing, chest discomfort, breathing difficulties, and shock. Shock would soon be followed by cardiovascular collapse and respiratory arrest. The complete history will assist in accurate diagnosis.

The physical examination should include a thorough assessment of the skin, middle ear, conjunctiva, nasooropharynx, and chest.

Laboratory studies are usually not necessary unless allergic signs and symptoms are severe and protracted. A complete blood count (CBC), skin testing, total serum IgE levels, and a specific IgE level for a particular allergen may be ordered. The latter test is called *RAST* (radioallergosorbent test).

Overview of Medical Management

Treatment of hypersensitivity disorders includes (1) symptom management with medications, (2) environmental control, and (3) immunotherapy. The most effective treatment is environmental control, which includes avoidance of the offending allergen.

Pollens are seasonal and can be avoided at season peaks with air conditioning and limiting time spent outdoors. Mold spores can be reduced by maintaining dry conditions and using air filters. House dust can be controlled by damp dusting, use of air filters, and decreased use of carpet and overstuffed furniture. Most other offending allergens can simply be avoided (food, drugs, chemicals, and stinging insects).

Medications are used to treat and alleviate signs and symptoms. Antihistamines compete with histamine by attaching to the cell surface receptors and blocking histamine release. Antihistamines therefore must be initiated soon after exposure or taken on a regular basis. Drowsiness, mucous membrane dryness, and occasionally central nervous system excitation are side effects of the earlier antihistamines. Examples of these include pseudoephedrine (Actifed), diphenhydramine (Benadryl) chlorpheniramine (Chlor-Trimeton), and brompheniramine (Dimetapp). A more recent member, terfenadine (Seldane), does not cause the drowsiness and is therefore more desirable for those who experience drowsiness with antihistamine use.

Overview of Nursing Interventions

Assessment. Assessment should involve predominantly the integumentary, gastrointestinal, respiratory, and cardiovascular systems. The nurse should be aware of the seasonal nature of the complaints.

Collection of *subjective data* includes pruritus, nausea, and uneasiness.

Collection of *objective data* includes sneezing, excessive nasal secretions, lacrimation, inflamed nasal membranes, skin rash or areas of raised inflammation, diarrhea, cough, wheeze, impaired breathing, and hypotension (Table 36-2).

Nursing Diagnoses. Nursing diagnoses for patients with atopic illness include (1) high risk for injury, related to exposure to allergen; (2) activity intolerance, related to malaise; and (3) high risk for infection, related to inflammation of protective mucous membranes.

Patient teaching. Patient teaching should revolve around the specific diagnosis. The patient should be informed regarding seasonal avoidance of the offending allergens and should understand the therapeutic medication plan. The nurse will focus on health promotion and health teaching for self-care management.

Urticaria

Etiology/Pathophysiology. Urticaria (hives) occurs as a local allergic response, generally to foods. Offending foods may include oranges, strawberries, nuts, tomatoes, and shellfish. Food coloring may precipitate symptoms in some individuals.

Clinical Manifestations. The pruritic lesions are IgE-mediated tissue responses and are pale raised wheals. The wheals are transient and may disappear and then recur elsewhere on the body. They may involve any part of the body, including skin, mouth, and larynx, and may cause respiratory and GI tract signs and symptoms.

Nursing Interventions. Allergic urticaria is self-limiting, and treatment other than allergen avoidance may not be necessary. Local application of Caladryl or calamine lotion may be used. Antihistamines and epinephrine may be used to hasten relief of more extensive reactions.

Prognosis. With treatment, the prognosis is excellent.

Angioedema

Etiology/Pathophysiology. Angioedema is a form of urticaria. It occurs in the subcutaneous tissue, whereas urticaria is a skin and mucous membrane lesion. Angioedema is caused by the same offenders that cause urticarial lesions.

Angioedema is characterized by local edema of an entire area, such as an eyelid, a thumb, or a lip. Seldom does more than a single edematous area appear at one time.

Medical Management. Treatment to relieve angioedema may include the use of antihistamine drugs—epinephrine or corticosteroids.

Nursing Interventions. A cold pack or cold compress may be used.

Prognosis. With treatment, the prognosis is excellent.

Allergic Rhinitis and Allergic Conjunctivitis (Hay Fever)

Etiology/Pathophysiology. These atopic allergic conditions are a result of antigen/antibody reactions occurring in the nasal membranes, nasopharynx, and conjunctiva from inhaled or contact allergens. Many infants, children, and adults have these seasonal or perennial conditions, resulting in absences from school and work.

TABLE 36-2 Summary of Hypersensitivity Reactions and Hypersensitivities (Allergies)

Disorder	Signs and Symptoms
Anaphylactic shock	Initial pruritus and sneezing, apprehension; edema of face, hands, and other body parts; dyspnea, wheezing, shock
Urticaria	Skin lesions: pale elevated centers on an erythematous background (wheal); pruritus
Atopic	
Allergic rhinitis (hay fever)	Sneezing, pruritus, lacrimation (watery eyes); thin secretions draining from nose
Allergic asthma	Wheezing, coughing, dyspnea (see Chapter 31)
Atropic dermatitis	Pruritus, vesicles, oozing and crusting lesions, scaling

Rhinitis and conjunctivitis occur as the result of antigen/antibody reaction. Ciliary action slows, mucosal gland secretion increases, leukocyte (eosinophil) infiltration occurs, and because of increased capillary permeability and vasodilation, local tissue edema results.

Common allergens causing allergic rhinitis and conjunctivitis (hay fever) are tree, grass, and weed pollens, mold spores, fungi, house dusts, mites, and animal danders. Other allergens include some foods, drugs, and insect stings.

Clinical Manifestations. Acute ocular manifestations include edema, photophobia, excessive tearing, blurring of vision, and pruritus.

Individuals with rhinitis complain of excessive secretions or inability to breathe through the nose because of congestion and/or edema.

Serious otitis media symptoms can occur if the eustachian tubes are occluded. These symptoms occur more in childhood, with the individual complaining of ear fullness, ear popping, or decreased hearing.

Assessment. The initial complaints of seasonal rhinitis and conjunctivitis include severe sneezing, congestion, pruritus, and lacrimation (watery eyes). Cough, epistaxis, and headache may also occur. More chronic signs and symptoms include headache, severe nasal congestion, postnasal drip, and cough. If these are not treated, chronic sufferers eventually develop secondary infections, such as otitis media, bronchitis, sinusitis, and pneumonia.

Medical Management. Treatment goals are to relieve signs and symptoms and prevent infections and other complaints, such as malaise, extreme fatigue, and severe headaches. Avoiding the allergen is effective. Perennial use of antihistamines is recommended. Changing from one antihistamine to another seasonally may help to impede tolerance to any one medication.

Decongestants may be added and used intermittently for 3 to 5 days if congestion occurs. Common over-the-counter decongestants, such as phenylephrine, pseudoephedrine, chlorpheniramine, and phenylpropanolamine, are contained in familiar products, such as Actifed, Triaminic, and Robitussin.

Long-term, consistent use of topical or nasal corticosteroids is highly recommended. Included are beclomethasone (Vancenase, Beconase), dexamethasone (Decadron, Turbinaire), and flunisolide (Nasalide). Corticosteroids require a prescription. For information about drugs used to treat immune disorders, see the medications table on p. 1152.

Pressure headaches may require narcotic analgesics until signs and symptoms are relieved. Hot packs over facial sinuses offer relief if headache is related to sinus congestion.

Box 36-4 CONTROL OF ENVIRONMENTAL ALLERGENS

1. Use air conditioner and air filters; change furnace filter monthly.
2. Use synthetic overstuffed furniture, pillows, and mattresses—no kapok or feathers.
3. Avoid wool clothing. Use garment bags to decrease dust.
4. Damp dust floors.
5. Avoid dried plants.
6. Avoid drying laundry outdoors during seasonal peaks of allergens.
7. Avoid outdoor exposure during seasonal peaks of offending pollens, especially on windy days.
8. Have no fur-bearing pets.
9. Avoid gardening, lawn mowing, and damp, musty places.

Box 36-5 SELF-CARE MANAGEMENT AND COMFORT MEASURES TO RELIEVE SYMPTOMS

Congestion. Keep head of bed elevated 45 degrees to facilitate drainage. Humidify air. Use decongestant as directed.

Eye discomfort. Apply warm compress. Use synthetic "tears." Avoid sprays, makeup, or other irritating contactants.

Headaches. Administer analgesics. Apply hot pack over facial sinuses.

Fatigue. Plan rest periods. Be aware of potential interference to activity that may occur related to drug therapy.

Nursing Interventions. These illnesses are self-limiting, so the nurse focuses on health promotion and maintenance teaching to provide for self-care management.

Patient teaching. The nurse's responsibilities in patient education are as follows:

1. Teach patient ways to avoid allergen (Box 36-4).
2. Teach patient self-care management through symptom control (Box 36-5).
3. Teach medication action and usage; assess for medication effectiveness.

Atopic Dermatitis

Etiology/Pathophysiology. Atopic dermatitis (eczema) is an inflammatory skin response to certain aller-

MEDICATIONS FOR IMMUNE DISORDERS

Medication	Trade Name	Action	Side Effects	Nursing Implications
Diphenhydramine	Benadryl	Is antihistamine	Drowsiness, confusion, nasal stuffiness, dry mouth, photosensitivity, urine retention	Use cautiously with CNS depressants, including alcohol; give with food; know that it is safe hypnotic for older adults; tell patient to avoid driving or hazardous activity due to drowsiness.
Terfenadine	Seldane	Is antihistamine	Dysrhythmias, headache, dry mouth and throat	Do not use with ketoconazole (Nizoral), erythromycins, clarithromycin (Biaxin), azithromycin (Zithromax) because it may cause dysrhythmias and death; know that it is less sedating than most; instruct patient not to exceed prescribed dose; monitor for dysrhythmias.
Dexamethasone	Decadron, Turbinaire	Is corticosteroid (inhaled)	Nasal irritation, rebound congestion, hypertension, headache, seizure, fluid retention	Do not use for extended period; use cautiously with diabetes and peptic ulcers; know that it is not effective for acute episodes; tell mothers not to breastfeed while using.
Flunisolide	Nasalide, Rhinalar	Is corticosteroid (inhaled)	Headache, transient nasal burning, epistaxis, nausea, vomiting	Know that it is not effective for acute episodes; use regularly; teach care and cleaning of inhaler; if symptoms do not improve in 3 weeks, consult physician.
Epinephrine	Adrenalin, Sus-phrine, Epi-pen	Is bronchodilator	Nervousness, tremor, headache, hypertension, tachycardia, ventricular fibrillation, CVA	Do not use with MAO-inhibitor; use cautiously in patients with hyperthyroid, hypertension, diabetes, and heart disease.
Edrophonium chloride	Tensilon, Enlon, Reversol	Is cholinergic	Respiratory paralysis, bronchospasms, headaches, seizures, weakness, hypotension, abdominal cramps, salivation, urination, lacrimation, diarrhea.	Have atropine available for antidote; know that it has rapid onset and short duration; monitor vital signs; know that it is used to diagnose myesthenia gravis.
Pyridostigmine	Mestinon, Regonal	Is cholinergic	Respiratory paralysis, bronchospasms, headaches, seizures, weakness, hypotension, abdominal cramps, salivation, urination, lacrimation, diarrhea.	Have atropine available for antidote; monitor vital signs closely; know that it is used to treat myesthenia gravis; stress importance of compliance.

genic offenders. It is characterized by dry, erythematous, raised pruritic lesions, often occurring facially and at the antecubital and popliteal spaces.

Clinical Manifestations. Atopic dermatitis occurs in individuals with a strong family history of allergy. Allergens may be contactant or ingested.

Assessment. Generally, in contact dermatitis the allergic manifestation occurs locally where the contact occurred, such as nettle rash on fingertips or on the leg that brushed the plant. Eczema occurs on the face and at the antecubital spaces. Both are manifestations of antigen/antibody reaction and are IgE mediated.

Medical Management, Nursing Interventions, and Patient Teaching. Treatment modalities include hot moist packs, emollients, and topical steroid creams. The nursing diagnosis is skin integrity, impaired. Intervention includes skin care and application of topical medication.

Patient education should include avoidance of the allergen, application of a thin layer of steroid cream after skin cleansing or hot moist packs, and prevention of skin impairment through use of lotions and emollients and decreased use of soaps and dry heat.

Anaphylaxis

Etiology/Pathophysiology. The most severe allergic reaction that is IgE-mediated is anaphylaxis, or systemic reaction to allergens. The antigens causing anaphylaxis include (1) venoms; (2) drugs, such as penicillin and aspirin; (3) contrast media dyes; (4) insect stings; and (5) some foods.

Clinical Manifestations. In anaphylaxis, the reaction occurs very rapidly after exposure, from seconds to a few minutes. Fatal reactions are associated with a fall in blood pressure, laryngeal edema, and bronchospasm, leading to cardiovascular collapse, myocardial infarction, and respiratory failure.

In anaphylaxis, massive release of mediators initiates events in target organs throughout the body. Skin and GI signs and symptoms may occur, although respiratory and cardiovascular signs and symptoms predominate. Anaphylactic reactions are classified as mild, moderate, and severe.

Assessment. Early recognition of signs and symptoms and early treatment may prevent severe reactions and even death. Generally, the more rapid the onset, the more severe the outcome. Overall, the individual may have a feeling of uneasiness that increases to a sense of foreboding and leads to a fear of impending death. The skin may or may not be involved. Urticaria and pruritus may be present in mild and moderate anaphylaxis, whereas cyanosis and pallor may be seen in severe reactions. Upper respiratory signs and symptoms range from congestion and sneezing to edema of the tongue and larynx with stridor and occlusion of the upper airways. Lower respiratory signs and symptoms will follow, including bronchospasm, wheezing, and severe dyspnea. GI signs and symptoms will increase from nausea, vomiting, and diarrhea to dysphagia and involuntary stools. The patient may have cardiovascular signs and symptoms, such as tachycardia and hypotension. Signs and symptoms may increase, and the patient may display coronary insufficiency, vascular collapse, dysrhythmias, shock, cardiac arrest, respiratory failure, and death.

Medical Management. Immediate aggressive treatment is the goal in anaphylaxis. At the first sign, 0.5 ml of epinephrine (Adrenalin Chloride) 1:1000 is given subcutaneously. It may be repeated at 15-minute intervals as prescribed by the physician. Benadryl 50 to 100 mg may be given IM or IV as indicated for allergic signs and symptoms. If moderate to severe signs and symptoms occur, IV therapy may be initiated to prevent vascular collapse and the patient may be intubated to prevent airway obstructions. Oxygen may be administered by mask. Aminophylline may be given to relieve bronchospasm.

Nursing Interventions. These measures include the following:

1. Assess vital signs continuously.
2. Assess intake and output.
3. Assess respiratory status, including dyspnea, wheezing, and decreased breath sounds.
4. Assess circulatory status, including dysrhythmias, tachycardia, and hypotension.
5. Assess mental status, including anxiety, malaise, confusion, and coma.
6. Assess skin status, including erythema, urticaria, cyanosis, and pallor.

Box 36-6 COMMON ALLERGENS CAUSING ANAPHYLAXIS

DRUGS	VENOMS	FOODS
Vaccines	Honeybees	Peanuts
Allergen extracts	Wasps	Brazil nuts
Enzymes	Hornets	Cashew nuts
Penicillins		Berries
Sulfonamides		Shellfish
Dextrans		Egg albumin
Hormones		
Contrast media		
Anesthetic agents		

7. Assess GI status, including nausea, vomiting, diarrhea, and incontinence.

The diagnosis is most often made by a history of signs and symptoms. Looking at and listening to the anxious patient should be leading clues in suspecting anaphylaxis.

An alert diagnostician will question the patient about recent exposure to known antigens that cause anaphylaxis (Box 36-6 on p. 1153). Most laboratory studies would not be beneficial.

Nursing diagnoses for the patient with anaphylaxis include but are not limited to the following:

NURSING DIAGNOSES	NURSING INTERVENTIONS
Injury, high risk for, related to exposure to allergen	Maintain airway. Administer medications as ordered.
Breathing patterns, ineffective, related to edema, bronchospasm, and increased secretions	Administer oxygen if ordered. Administer prescribed medications. Monitor vital signs. Suction if necessary.
Cardiac output, decreased, related to increased capillary permeability and vascular dilation	Monitor IV fluid infusions as ordered. Monitor vital signs. Monitor I&O. Obtain complete allergy history. Document signs and symptoms, interventions, and response.

Patient teaching. The nurse's responsibilities in patient education are as follows:

1. Reassure patient during procedures.
2. Teach patient avoidance of allergen.
3. Teach the use of Medic-Alert identification.
4. Teach patient preparation and administration of epinephrine subcutaneously.

Prognosis. If left untreated, the signs and symptoms can lead to death in a relatively short time

Transfusion Reactions

Transfusion reactions are a hypersensitivity disorder and are best illustrated by reactions that occur with mismatched blood.

Careful selection of blood donors is important in prevention of transfusion reaction, followed by careful type and cross-matching of blood from donor to recipient. Storage of blood and administration protocol are important in blood reaction prevention. Blood and blood components should be refrigerated at specific temperatures until ½ hour before administration. Blood must be administered within 4 hours after refrigeration; blood components within 6 hours after refrigeration. Donor and recipient numbers are specific and must be thoroughly checked and the patient identified with an armband. All blood and blood products are administered through microaggregate filters. The nurse should monitor for adverse effects.

Transfusion reactions are labeled mild, moderate, and severe. The most severe reactions occur within the first 15 minutes, moderate reactions within 30 to 90 minutes, and mild reactions may be delayed to late in the transfusion or hours to several days after transfusion.

Mild transfusion reaction signs and symptoms include dermatitis, diarrhea, fever, chills, urticaria, cough, and orthopnea. Treatment includes (1) stopping the transfusion and (2) administering saline, steroids, and diuretics as ordered. Transfusion may continue at a slower rate. In moderate reactions, in which fever, chills, urticaria, and wheezing occur after the first 30 minutes of administration, the transfusion is stopped and saline is continued. Antihistamines and epinephrine may be given. The physician decides if the transfusion is to continue. With severe reaction, the transfusion is stopped and saline is given to provide venous access. It is recommended that the blood or blood product be returned to the laboratory for immediate testing if any type of reaction occurs (see Chapter 22).

The best method for prevention of transfusion reaction is **autologous** (pertaining to a tissue occurring naturally and derived from the same individual) transfusion, or use of one's own blood, for replacement therapy. Weeks to months in advance of expected need, the patient donates blood to be frozen and stored for personal use.

DELAYED HYPERSENSITIVITY DISEASE

Delayed hypersensitivity reactions occurring 24 to 72 hours after exposure are mediated by T cells accompanied by release of lymphokines. Delayed reaction contact dermatitis, such as after contact with poison ivy, is one example. Tissue transplant rejection is another example. Only transplant rejection will be discussed.

Transplant Rejection

Transfer of healthy tissue or organs from a donor to recipient has been done for many years. The immune process that protects the body from foreign protein is the same process at work in tissue transplant rejection. Knowledge of the function of the immune system enabled medical experts to find a way to control the rejection process. It is now possible to prepare the body before tissue transplant for grafting to be successful.

Autograft, or transplantation of tissue from one site to another on an individual, is successful. It is used after trauma and in reconstructive surgery.

Isograft is transfer of tissue between genetically identical individuals, such as identical twins.

Allograft is a term applied to the transplantation of tissue between members of the same species. Because few humans are born with an identical twin, allograft is the most common form of tissue transplant.

Antigenic determinants on the cells lead to graft rejection via the immune process. Therefore before transplantation, recipient tissue is as closely matched as possible to donor tissue antigenic determinants. Tissue matching leads to a better chance of success.

Tissue rejection does not occur immediately after transplantation. It takes several days for vascularization to occur. Seven to ten days after blood supply is adequately established, sensitized lymphocytes appear in sufficient numbers for sloughing to occur at the site.

Graft rejection is slowed through use of chemical agents that interfere with the immune response process. Included are corticosteroids, cyclosporine A, and azathioprine. This chemical therapy is referred to as **immunosuppressive** (the administration of agents that significantly interfere with the ability of the immune system to respond to antigenic stimulation by inhibiting cellular and humoral immunity) therapy.

Infection is a threat to the immunosuppressed patient. Meticulous aseptic technique is required when caring for these individuals. Prophylactic antibiotic therapy may be advisable, and good skin care is necessary. Visits to the bedside are limited in frequency for both staff and family. Persons with infection are not allowed at the bedside.

IMMUNODEFICIENCY DISEASES

The first evidence of **immunodeficiency** (an abnormal condition of the immune system in which cellular or humoral immunity is inadequate and resistance to infection is decreased) disease is an increased susceptibility to infection. The problem can manifest as recurrent infection or chronic infection. Unusually severe infection with complications or incomplete clearing of an infection may also indicate an underlying immunodeficiency.

Defects in genes leading to immunodeficiency provide a hereditary link to the diseases.

Agammaglobulinemia

Etiology/Pathophysiology. Agammaglobulinemia is a primary immunodeficiency disease of B cell deficiency occurring in boys. This severe deficiency illness is characterized by severe, recurrent, pyogenic infections.

Most primary immunodeficiency diseases are believed to be caused by single genetic defects. Secondary immunodeficiency disease is acquired. An example is AIDS (see Chapter 37 for further discussion).

Multiple Myeloma

Etiology/Pathophysiology. Multiple myeloma, a neoplastic immunodeficiency disease, occurs most frequently after age 40 and affects twice as many men as women. Onset is gradual and insidious and often goes unrecognized for years while the individual experiences frequent, recurrent bacterial infections. This increased susceptibility to infection follows disturbances of antibody formation by abnormal plasma cells. Suppression of normal antibody levels is seen in this plasma cell tumor disease. Incidence of multiple myeloma has increased and now approaches that of Hodgkin's disease.

Clinical Manifestations. The disease process will show a proliferation of malignant plasma cells and development of single or multiple bone marrow tumors. This is followed by bone destruction with dissemination into lymph nodes, liver, spleen, and kidneys.

The skeletal system symptoms typically involve the ribs, spine, and pelvis. Individuals complain of bone pain that increases with movement. Some develop pathological fractures accompanied by severe pain.

In the individual with multiple myeloma, disruption of production of erythrocytes, platelets, and leukocytes occurs because of crowding of the marrow by the abnormal proliferation of plasma cells. This leads to increased infection, anemia, and increased potential for bleeding. Calcium and phosphorus drain from bones, leading to hypercalcemia and renal problems.

Assessment. Collection of *subjective data* includes assessment of the patient's complaints of pain, including location, intensity, and duration. The patient's understanding of the disease, verbalization of discouragement, hopelessness, and desires for emotional and spiritual support should be addressed.

Collection of *objective data* includes assessing the patient's facial expression for signs of increased pain with movement, the ability to perform activities of daily living (ADLs), increased body temperature, increased potential for bleeding, changes in urine characteristics, and effectiveness of medication administration.

Diagnostic Tests. Diagnosis of multiple myeloma is made with x-ray studies, bone marrow biopsy, and laboratory examination of blood and urine.

X-ray examinations reveal widespread demineralization and osteoporosis. Bone marrow studies reveal large numbers of immature plasma cells, which normally account for only 5% of marrow population. Bence Jones protein appears in the urine.

Medical Management. Treatment is symptomatic, since multiple myeloma is not curable. Radiation and chemotherapy are initiated to both reduce tumor size and impede tumor growth. Radiation is used in small doses. The antineoplastic drugs of choice are the alkylating agents, such as melphalan (Alkeran) and cyclophosphamide (Cytoxan). Bone marrow depression occurs as a side effect, and therefore the CBC is monitored during treatment.

Hypercalcemia and pain also should be addressed. Hospitalization to administer corticosteroids and fluids may be required.

Nursing Interventions. Care of the patient with multiple myeloma should focus on pain relief, prevention of infection and bone injury, and maintenance of hydration. Attention to the psychosocial, emotional, and spiritual needs is also indicated.

Nursing diagnoses and interventions for the patient with multiple myeloma include but are not limited to the following:

NURSING DIAGNOSES	NURSING INTERVENTIONS
Injury, high risk for, related to osteoporosis	Protect from bone injury; use log roll, turning sheet.
Pain, related to disease process	Administer analgesics as ordered. Assess contributing factors.
Fluid volume deficit: actual, related to impaired renal function	Increase fluid intake to 3000-4000 ml/day. Maintain I&O record.
Infection, high risk for, related to stasis of body fluids and immunosuppression	Administer antibiotics as ordered. Maintain aseptic technique. Monitor vital signs.
Spiritual distress, related to intense suffering	Listen to patient complaints of anger, concern, alienation from God; refer to religious counselor or significant others who could provide support.

Patient teaching. The nurse's responsibilities in patient education are as follows:

1. Teach patient to avoid traumatic bone injury.
2. Teach patient pain control modality.
3. Teach patient importance of hydration.
4. Teach patient prevention of infection.
5. Assist patient to identify spiritual resources.

Prognosis. This disease is usually progressive and generally fatal.

AUTOIMMUNE DISORDERS

Autoimmune (pertaining to the development of an immune response [autoantibodies or cellular immune response] to one's own tissues) disorders are failures of the tolerance to "self." Autoimmune disorders may be described as an immune attack on the self and result from the failure to distinguish "self" protein from "foreign" protein.

As a person ages, the probability of failure in any system occurs. It is not clearly understood what happens when autoimmune responses occur.

Whatever the cause, autoimmune disorders exist. There are many illnesses now believed to be in this classification. Included are pernicious anemia, Guillain-Barré syndrome, scleroderma, Sjögren's syndrome, rheumatic fever, rheumatoid arthritis, ulcerative colitis, and male infertility. These conditions are discussed elsewhere in the text. The following are autoimmune diseases.

Myasthenia Gravis

Etiology/Pathophysiology. Myasthenia gravis is an unpredictable autoimmune disorder occurring primarily in women in the 18- to 25-year-old age group and men in the 50- to 60-year-old age group. It is not considered hereditary, and the incidence is somewhere between 2 and 10 in every 100,000 population.

The defect is thought to be an alteration in neuromuscular transmission that causes muscular weakness. The postsynaptic acetylcholine receptors on the muscle cell's plasma membrane for an unknown reason are no longer recognized as "self" and therefore elicit an antigenic effect. Myasthenia so limits muscle contraction that a severe patient weakness occurs with increased activity.

Clinical Manifestations. Myasthenia gravis occurs in both ocular (pertaining to the eye) and generalized forms. In ocular myasthenia gravis, the signs and symptoms include ptosis (eyelid droops) and diplopia (double vision). The generalized variety may vary from mild to severe signs and symptoms. The patient may complain initially of ptosis and diplopia. Skeletal weakness, dysarthria (difficult or inarticulate speech), and dysphagia (difficult swallowing) may follow. In more severe cases or as the disease progresses, the patient will complain of severe ocular, pharyngeal, and respiratory muscle weakness. Bowel and bladder sphincter weakness occurs with severe loss of muscle control.

There may be a tendency for the head to fall forward, and there may be weak, nasal-sounding speech. Upper extremity involvement is to be anticipated, and occasionally the lower extremities are weak. Muscle atrophy does not occur, reflexes are normal, and cerebral function remains intact. Dyspnea and severe respiratory weakness are very problematic. Periods of exacerbation and remission are expected.

Assessment. Collection of *subjective data* includes the complaints of weakness; double vision; eye, throat, and respiratory muscle weakness; dyspnea; swallowing difficulties; and urinary and bowel incontinence. The patient may or may not complain of upper and/or lower extremity weakness.

Collection of *objective data* includes ptosis, nasal-sounding speech, and loss of muscle control.

Complications with myasthenia gravis include respiratory distress, pneumonia, choking, and swallowing difficulties.

Diagnostic Tests. A detailed history and physical examination may suggest an autoimmune disorder.

The IV anticholinesterase test is a reliable diagnostic tool. Edrophonium chloride (Tensilon) or neostigmine bromide (Prostigmin Bromide) is administered intravenously, and the patient response is carefully evaluated. Muscle function improves dramatically in a short time with patients who have the illness.

Actual diagnosis can be made partly on the basis of electromyography (EMG).

Medical Management. Anticholinesterase drugs, such as neostigmine (Prostigmin) and pyridostigmine (Mestinon), may be administered. These medications allow acetylcholine to accumulate at synapses and promote nerve impulse transmission.

Corticosteroids may be used as adjunct therapy.

Immunosuppressants, such as azathioprine (Imuran) and cyclophosphamide (Cytoxan), are also used.

Physical therapy, such as range-of-motion exercises, may be beneficial in muscle function. Braces, splints, walkers, and canes may assist the patient in achieving some independence.

Nursing Interventions. Nursing interventions for the patient with myasthenia gravis include nursing diagnosis, interventions, and teaching related to muscle weakness and disturbance in self-esteem.

Nursing intervention is aimed at assessing respiratory status and minimizing complications.

Nursing diagnoses and interventions for the patient with myasthenia gravis include but are not limited to the following:

NURSING DIAGNOSES	NURSING INTERVENTIONS
Mobility, impaired physical, related to muscle weakness	Plan activities and rest to reduce fatigue. Assess functional ability.
Breathing pattern, ineffective, related to muscle weakness	Elevate head of bed. Suction airway as indicated. Supervise use of durable medical equipment.
Urinary elimination, altered patterns, related to decreased muscle control	Establish urinary program. Provide incontinence aids. Palpate bladder. Catheterize intermittently.
Injury, high risk for, related to trauma	Assess muscle strength and gross and fine motor coordination.
Communication, impaired verbal, related to muscle weakness	Provide slate board and picture board. Validate nonverbal communication.
Self-care deficit, bathing/hygiene, related to spasticity or muscle weakness	Determine individual strengths and skills. Assist with necessary adaptations.
Self-esteem disturbance: situational low self-esteem, related to powerlessness	Assess patient interaction with significant others; encourage expression of feelings.
Swallowing impaired, related to muscular weakness, choking	Provide for food and fluids more easily swallowed; remain with patient during meals.

Patient teaching. The nurse's responsibilities in patient education are as follows:

1. Teach safety measures; teach use of assistive mobility devices, braces, and walkers.
2. Teach good posture and use of accessory muscles; assist patient with learning breathing exercises.
3. Instruct in use of laxatives or stool softeners; schedule social activities within time frame of bowel program.
4. Teach use of Credé method to express urine from the bladder and Valsalva maneuver to increase intraabdominal pressure; teach self-catheterization program; stress need for adequate fluid intake.
5. Identify need for safety devices; discuss need for and sources of supervision and available day care programs.
6. Teach alternate communication skills; refer to speech therapy.
7. Refer to occupational therapy and respite care.
8. Teach learning strategies for dealing with feelings and acceptance of strengths and weaknesses.
9. Consult with physician and/or dietary department regarding optimum diet plan.

Prognosis. Myasthenia gravis is a chronic disease. Rest and medications can improve but not eliminate the signs and symptoms. Some cases are mild, but others are rapidly fatal; death results from respiratory failure. The course is variable. Prolonged remission may occur.

Systemic Lupus Erythematosus

Lupus is the Latin word for wolf. This term has been used since 1230 AD to describe the cutaneous skin changes that resemble the zygomatic erythremia of a red wolf.

Etiology/Pathophysiology. Systemic lupus erythematosus (SLE) is systemic multisystem, autoimmune response inflammatory disorder characterized by autoantibodies, directed against autologous (origin within self) tissues and serum protein factors. SLE is distinguished by an inflammatory lesion that affects several organ systems, specifically the skin, joints, kidneys, and serous membranes.

SLE is chronic and incurable and is multicausal. Although the origin of the syndrome remains a mystery, increasing evidence suggests that immunological, hormonal, genetic, and possibly viral factors may contribute to the onset of this disease, which is most prevalent in women of childbearing age. Nine times more women than men are affected by this disorder, and three times as many African-Americans as Caucasians are affected. About 10% of cases occur later in life. Survival rates have increased to longer than 15 years after diagnosis with this disorder.

TABLE 36-3 Pathogenic Occurrences and Clinical Manifestations in Body Systems of Persons with SLE

Musculoskeletal	Inflammation of vessels, tendons, and muscle tissue occurs because of deposits of fibrin. Polyarthralgia and polyarteritis occur in approximately 90% to 95% of patients.
Gastrointestinal	Ulceration occurs on mucosal membranes because of degeneration of collagen tissue, with GI manifestations of hemorrhage, abdominal pain, pancreatitis, cholecystitis, and bowel infarction.
Renal	Glomerular sclerosis and glomerulonephritis occur.
Hematological	Cells are destroyed, and interference with coagulation occurs because of circulating antibodies. Anemia, leukopenia, lymphopenia, thrombocytopenia, and elevated erythrocyte sedimentation rate result.
Cardiovascular	Pericarditis is the most common cardiac manifestation. It often is the first clinical problem the patient manifests. Pericardial rub, commonly associated with pericarditis, can lead to dysrhythmias; vasculitis in the small vessels may occur.
Pulmonary	Pleurisy and pleural effusions resulting from inflammation of the pleura are relatively common.
Cutaneous	Classic characteristics include the erythematous butterfly rash over the bridge of the nose and on the cheeks and linear erythema along the eyelids (Fig. 36-4). Other features may include bullae, patchy areas of purpura, urticaria, and subcutaneous nodules.
Neurological	Mental and neurological signs and symptoms occur in 35% to 40% of patients with SLE. Signs and symptoms relate to the central nervous system, not to the peripheral nerves. Mental and behavioral changes may occur, as well as seizures, headaches, and cerebrovascular accidents.

Box 36-7 DIAGNOSTIC TESTS FOR SYSTEMIC LUPUS ERYTHEMATOSUS

- Antinuclear antibody (ANA)
- DNA antibody
- Complement
- CBC
- Erythrocyte sedimentation rate (ESR)
- Sedimentation rate
- Coagulation profile
- Rheumatoid factor (RF)
- Rapid plasma reagin (RPR)
- Skin and renal biopsy
- C-reactive protein (CRP)
- Coombs test
- LE cell prep (lupus erythematosus cell preparation)
- Urinalysis
- Chest x-ray study

SLE is a serious illness despite advances in treatment. The cause remains unclear, and more than one factor is likely. Genetic predisposition seems apparent in most instances, coupled with an inciting agent or factor.

T suppressor cells are decreased in the person with SLE. In addition, T suppressor cells that are present function in a limited manner. Antibodies develop against other antigens.

Clinical Manifestations. Clinical manifestations are nephritis, pericarditis, synovitis, organic brain syndromes, peripheral neuropathies, anemia, leukopenia, thrombocytopenia, coagulopathies, immunosuppression, and dermatitis.

Refer to Table 36-3 for pathogenic occurrences and clinical manifestations in body systems.

Diagnostic Tests. Diagnostic tests for SLE are given in Box 36-7.

Many of these test results are positive in the presence of inflammatory disease. No single test is considered conclusive for diagnostic purposes. However, positive results of one or more diagnostic tests along with at least three other criteria may lead to the diagnosis of SLE. This would include the following criteria:

1. Erythema butterfly rash over the nose and cheeks and along the eyelids; alopecia (hair loss) with frontal alopecia seen more frequently in women; other skin features are bullae, patchy areas of purpura, thickening of epidermis
2. Photosensitivity
3. Oral ulcers
4. Polyarthralgias and polyarthritis
5. Pleuritic pain, pleural effusion, pericarditis, and vasculitis
6. Renal disorders as evidenced by the presence of protein and/or cellular casts in the urine
7. Neurological signs, such as seizures of unknown cause
8. Hematological disorders, such as hemolytic anemia, leukopenia, lymphopenia, or thrombocytopenia, in absence of other diagnostic reasons

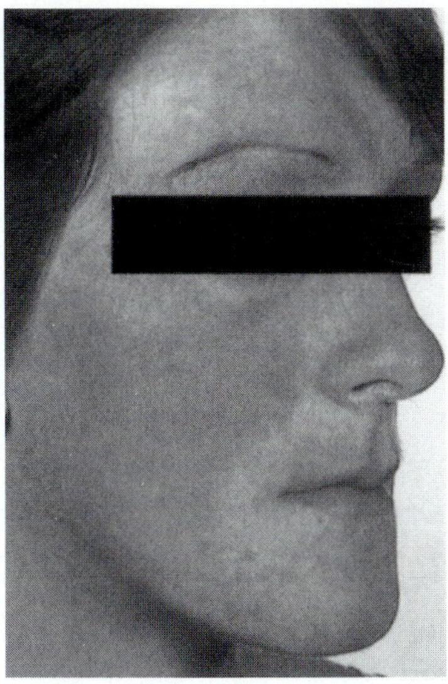

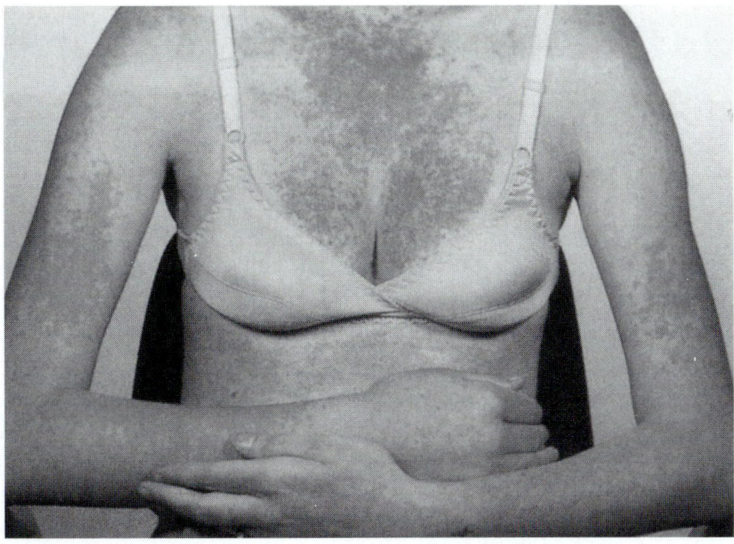

FIG. 36-4 Erythematous butterfly rash of person with SLE.

9. Immunological disorder identified with positive LE prep or antinuclear antibody (ANA) or double-stranded DNA (ds-DNA)
10. Positive ANA in absence of patient use of drugs known to cause drug-induced lupus erythematosus

Medical Management. SLE is best treated symptomatically. Attempts to induce remission of the disease, to alleviate exacerbations early, and to prevent untoward complications are goals of therapy, as are therapeutic management of the signs and symptoms of the syndrome and suppression of inflammation.

Drug therapy includes use of nonsteroidal antiinflammatory agents, such as acetylsalicylic acid (ASA) and indomethacin (Indocin), antimalarial drugs (hydroxychloroquine [Plaquenil] or chloroquine) and corticosteroids, such as prednisone, in low doses given several times a day. Methylprednisolone may be used intravenously in cases of exacerbation.

Peak amounts of steroids are given to achieve remission. Doses are then decreased slowly until a maintenance dose is reached.

Topical corticosteroid creams are used for the rash of SLE.

Antineoplastic drugs such as azathioprine (Imuran), cyclophosphamide (Cytoxan), or chlorambucil (Leukeran) may be used therapeutically to achieve remission or to control the signs and the symptoms of the patient's illness.

Antimalarial drugs (hydroxychloroquine [Plaquenil]) are used to control discoid and other skin lesions and rheumatic manifestations. Because retinal toxicity may occur at high doses, patients should receive pretreatment and annual ophthalmic examinations.

Antiinfective agents are used both to treat and to prevent infections in the patient with SLE.

Peritoneal dialysis or hemodialysis may be indicated in patients who have moderate to severe renal involvement.

Analgesics and diuretics may be used to treat symptoms often found in individuals with SLE.

Supportive therapy, such as balanced diet, a balance of rest and activity, and reduction of exposure to the sun, may also be indicated.

Nursing Interventions. Because SLE is a multisymptom disease, a thorough assessment is indicated. The plan of care should be individually tailored to include (1) skin care, including teaching avoidance of direct sunlight and use of protective clothing and sunscreen; (2) balancing rest and activity; (3) assisting the patient to recognize changes in condition; (4) early recognition of signs and symptoms of infection; (5) stress reduction and management; and (6) balanced nutrition and reduction of sodium intake. Because the disease is one of exacerbation and remissions, each exacerbation will intensify the patient's stress and subsequently decrease the patient's ability to cope. The nurse should provide psychosocial, emotional, and spiritual support for the patient.

Patients with impaired immune system function must endure the consequences of chronic and/or incurable disease. A caring and gentle approach to patient care, as well as understanding, will help lessen the burden and stress of these illnesses. See the nursing care plan on pp. 1160-1161 for the patient with SLE.

Patient Teaching. The nurse's responsibilities in patient education are as follows:

NURSING CARE PLAN: ***THE PATIENT WITH SLE***

Miss Thompson, age 34, is suffering from an acute exacerbation of systemic lupus erythematosus. She is admitted to the medical unit with severe joint pain, butterfly rash, generalized edema, and Sjögren's syndrome.

Nursing diagnoses	Patient goals/expected outcomes	Nursing interventions
Skin integrity, impaired, related to skin rash (butterfly across face), hair loss, skin atrophy, discoid lesions involving other parts of the body	Patient will verbalize understanding of skin care regimen and positioning schedule. Patient will demonstrate behaviors to promote skin healing. Patient will experience improved wound/lesion healing.	Assess and monitor skin and mucous membranes and describe lesions' size, characteristics, and changes noted. Monitor for signs of infection. Assess nutritional status and areas at risk for pressure. Measure I&O. Encourage oral hygiene. Develop positioning schedule. Use appropriate devices, such as air mattress, Egg Crate mattress, sheepskin, or foam padding, where indicated. Provide optimum nutrition. Encourage patient to keep sun exposure at minimal by wearing long-sleeved blouses or shirts and wide-brim hats and by using sunscreens with a sun protection factor (SPF) of 15. Teach skin care maintenance.
Fear, related to separation from support system (hospitalization, treatments, and threat of death)	Patient will acknowledge fear. Patient will use effective coping measures. Patient will demonstrate problem solving and use resources effectively.	Assess signs of denial, depression. Listen to patient concerns. Allow patient to express feelings freely. Make certain patient receives accurate information about SLE. Teach exercises in visualization and relaxation. Provide emotional support, and work with patient to identify resources for support and coping mechanisms that have proved helpful in the past. Encourage participation in local chapter of Lupus Foundation of America.
Self-care deficit, bathing/hygiene, related to weakness and restricted activity	Patient will verbalize importance of personal hygiene.	Assist in ADLs.

Body image disturbance, related to baldness, skin pattern pathologies	Patient will verbalize understanding of altered body image. Patient will have a positive, accepting, and realistic body image. Patient will perform self-care activities within level of own ability. Patient will identify personal community resources that can provide assistance.	Assess patient's perception of body image; investigate what aspects are not pleasing and how changes are perceived as deviating from social norms. Teach patient ways to improve body image (e.g., improved personal hygiene, wearing make-up, change in clothes, protecting self from sun). Encourage family members and significant others to maintain open communication with patient. Record emotional changes. Set limits on maladaptive behavior.

CRITICAL THINKING QUESTIONS

1. Miss Thompson has painful, edematous joints that greatly decrease her mobility. She has 4+ pitting edema to the lower extremities secondary to the loss of protein through her glomerulus. The most appropriate nursing interventions to decrease Miss Thompson's pain level and to increase her mobility would be:
2. On entering the room, the nurse notes Miss Thompson crying. She verbalized that her lifestyle is severely altered because she is unable to be in the sun to work in her beloved garden. What nursing interventions would be most beneficial?
3. Miss Thompson confides she fears that this severe increase in her symptoms will lead to an early death. The initial response to this statement which would be of greatest assistance would be:

1. Provide the patient and family with information about SLE, and encourage them to contact the local chapter of the Lupus Foundation of America.
2. Teach the patient and family side effects of all medications and ways to manage these side effects.
3. Teach the patient and family the importance of avoiding contact with persons who may have contagious infections. Avoid crowds when on high-dose steroids.
4. Teach the importance of skin care:
   a. Instruct patient to avoid dryness and the use of irritating soaps and shampoos.
   b. Encourage use of hypoallergenic make-up. Encourage the wearing of a wig, scarf, or turban if the patient is sensitive about significant hair loss.
   c. Teach photosensitive patients to avoid sun exposure.
5. Teach methods of maintaining activity level.
6. Teach the importance of regular follow-up health care, including physical and blood examinations.
7. Teach the importance of balanced diet.
8. Instruct patient with renal involvement about end stage renal failure and available treatment options as per physician's orders.
9. Teach patient to carry a medical alert identification at all times.
10. Direct patient and family to appropriate and available resources.
11. Instruct patient to avoid birth control pills or intrauterine devices (IUDs) (Preferred method of contraception is diaphragm and foam, as per physician's orders.)

Prognosis. There is no known cure for SLE. Management of the disease depends on the nature and severity of the manifestations and the organs affected. Earlier treatment modalities have contributed toward a better prognosis.

REFERENCES AND SUGGESTED READINGS

1. Ammann A: *Antibody (B-cell) immunodeficiency disorders*. In Stites DP, Terr AL, editors: *Basic and clinical immunology,* ed 7, San Mateo, Calif, 1991, Appleton & Lange.
2. Blansfield J: Emergency autotransfusion in hypovolemia, *Crit Care Nurs Clin North Am* 2:195, 1990.
3. Bradley-Springer L: Human immunodeficiency virus infection in the health care worker, *J Assoc Nurses AIDS Care* 4(1):37, 1993.
4. Carson H: Subacute cutaneous bypass, *Bay Area Lupus Foundation Newsletter* 13(2): 1990.
5. Cassidy JT, Petty RE: *The textbook of pediatric rheumatology,* ed 2, New York, 1990, Churchill Livingston.
6. Clark C: Nursing care for multiple sclerosis, *Orthop Nurs* 10(1):21, 1991.
7. Colletti M et al: *Immunologic system*. In Thompson J et al: *Mosby's clinical nursing,* ed 3, St Louis, 1993, Mosby.
8. Dietary guidelines for the patient with systemic lupus erythematosus, *Bay Area Lupus Foundation Newsletter* 13(2):79, 1990.
9. Draggo SS: Banking your own blood, *Am J Nurs* 92(3):61, 1992.
10. Freedman S et al: Bone marrow transplant: overview and nursing implications, *Crit Care Nurs Q* 13(4):83, 1991.
11. Golub ES, Green DR: *Immunology: a synthesis,* ed 2, Sunderland, Mass, 1991, Sinauer.
12. Harvey CJ, Verklan T: Systemic lupus erythematosus: obstetric and neonatal implications, *NAACOGS Clin Issues Perinatal Women's Health Nurs* 1(2):177, 1990.
13. Hood GH, Dincher JR: *Total patient care,* ed 8, St Louis, 1993, Mosby.
14. Hotter AN: Wound healing and immunocompromise, *Nurs Clin North Am* 25(1):193, 1990.
15. Jackson SA: The immune system: basic concepts for understanding transplantation, *Crit Care Nurs Q* 13(4):83, 1991.
16. Kim MJ et al: *Pocket guide to nursing diagnosis,* ed 5, St Louis, 1993, Mosby.
17. Lancaster L, editor: *American Nephrology Nurses Association care curriculum for nephrology nursing,* ed 2, Pitman, NJ, 1990, The Association.
18. Leach M: Anemia: nursing care and intervention, *Prof Nurse* 454, 1991.
19. Legun LA: Systemic lupus during pregnancy, *Patient Care Teaching* 20(9):86, 1990.
20. Lewis S, Collier I: *Medical-surgical nursing,* St Louis, 1992, Mosby.
21. Long BC, Phipps WJ, Cassmeyer VL: *Medical-surgical nursing: a nursing process approach,* ed 3, St Louis, 1993, Mosby.
22. Malasanos L et al: *Health assessment,* ed 4, St Louis, 1990, Mosby.
23. Mirabelli L: Caring for patients with rheumatoid arthritis, *Nursing 90* 22(9):67, 1990.
24. *Mosby's medical, nursing, and allied health dictionary,* ed 4, 1994, St Louis, Mosby.
25. Mudge-Grout CL: *Immunologic disorders,* Mosby's clinical nursing series, St Louis, 1993, Mosby.
26. National Blood Resource Education Program's Nursing Education Working Group: Autologous transfusion, *Am J Nurs* 91(6):47, 1991.
27. Norman PS: Immunotherapy of IgE-mediated disease, *Hosp Pract* 25(4):81, 1990
28. Pagana-Deska K, Pagana TJ: *Mosby's diagnostic and laboratory reference,* St Louis, 1992, Mosby.
29. Phipps WJ et al: *Medical-surgical nursing: concepts and clinical practice,* ed 4, St Louis, 1991, Mosby.
30. Rate NS: *Alterations in immunity and inflammation.* In McCance L, Huether S, editors: *Pathophysiology: the biologic basis for disease in adults and children,* St Louis, 1990, Mosby.
31. Seidel HB, Dains J, Benedict GW: *Mosby's guide to physical examination,* St Louis, 1991, Mosby.
32. Stites DP, Terr AT, editors: *Basic and clinical immunology,* ed 7, San Mateo, Calif, 1991, Appleton & Lange.
33. Thomas CL: *Taber's cyclopedic medical dictionary,* ed 17, 1993, Philadelphia, FA Davis.
34. Thompson JM et al: *Mosby's clinical nursing,* ed 3, St Louis, 1993, Mosby.
35. Warkentin TE, Kelton JG: Current concepts in the treatment of immune thrombocytopenia, *Drugs* 40(4):531, 1990.

CHAPTER CHALLENGE

KEY POINTS

- The two major forms of immunity are innate and acquired or adaptive.
- T lymphocytes, B lymphocytes, and macrophages are the three major cells active in acquired immunity.
- B lymphocytes produce antibodies.
- T lymphocytes do not produce antibodies, but assist the B cell.
- T lymphocytes release lymphokines.
- Macrophages trap, process, and present antigen to T lymphocytes.
- Autoimmune disorders are failures of the tolerance to "self."
- Supportive therapy, such as balanced diet, balance of rest and activity, and reduction of exposure to the sun, is indicated in chronic debilitating syndromes, such as SLE.
- Muscular weakness that impairs respiratory function and bowel and bladder function and results in a high risk for injury is a key factor in myasthenia gravis.
- Infection is a primary threat to the immunosuppressed patient. Aseptic technique is required when caring for these patients. Good skin care is necessary.
- Careful selection of blood donors and careful typing and cross-matching of blood are important in prevention of transfusion reaction.
- Early recognition of signs followed by early treatment may decrease the severity of allergic reaction.
- Avoidance of the offending allergen is an important teaching concept related to atopic allergy.

STUDY QUESTIONS

1. Mrs. Curtis is a 54-year-old insurance agent. She has had SLE for 13 years. She is admitted to the hospital for management of an exacerbation. The medical plan includes bed rest and corticosteroids. The nurse instructs Mrs. Curtis about the use of corticosteroids. Which of the following statements indicates Mrs. Curtis understands how to use this drug? Mrs. Curtis states she will:
   1. Use the medication when she has pain
   2. Take the medication on an empty stomach
   3. Take the medication exactly as prescribed
   4. Discontinue the medication when the rash on the face disappears
2. Mr. Torgis is recovering from having a kidney transplant. The nursing intervention of this immunosuppressed patient should include:
   1. Prophylactic antibiotic therapy
   2. Meticulous aseptic technique
   3. Restriction of all visitors
   4. Administration of antineoplastic medication therapy
3. Innate or natural immunity is:
   1. The body's first line of defense against disease and protects locally against the external environment
   2. The body's second line of defense against disease and protects the internal environment
   3. Mediated by B cells to produce antibodies in response to antigenic challenge
   4. An immunity that is specific
4. Ms. Kinis is a 26-year-old patient with a history of numerous allergies. The nurse's most important teaching concept is:
   1. Immunotherapy regimen
   2. Avoidance of the allergen
   3. Antihistamine administration
   4. Adrenalin administration
5. Humoral immunity is mediated by:
   1. T cells
   2. B cells
   3. Macrophages
   4. Myeloblasts
6. Cellular immunity develops when which cells are activated by an antigen:
   1. T cells
   2. B cells
   3. Neutrophils
   4. Monoplasts
7. Desensitization is another term for:
   1. Autoimmune disorders
   2. Adaptive immunity
   3. Immunotherapy
   4. Immunodeficiency disease
8. After a bee sting, Mrs. Wortham's face becomes edematous and she begins to wheeze. Based on this assessment, the nurse would be prepared to administer:
   1. Aminophylline
   2. Benadryl
   3. Epinephrine
   4. Valium
9. The nurse gave an intramuscular penicillin injection to her patient. Which of the following would be a sign of a systemic anaphylactic response:
   1. Increased blood pressure
   2. Rhinitis
   3. Urticaria
   4. Wheezing
10. The family of Mr. Jorgensen, a 68-year-old patient with multiple myeloma who has been receiving chemotherapy for 2 weeks, complains that he does not seem to be improving. Which of the following responses by the nurse would be most appropriate:
    1. The drugs are not always helpful.
    2. It may take several weeks before any improvement is noted.
    3. Radiation therapy may also be needed before you'll see any changes.
    4. Don't give up hope; spontaneous remissions are known to occur.
11. Mrs. Rodweiges is a 38-year-old patient who is receiving two units of packed cells at 15 macrodrops per minute. Fifteen minutes after the start of the transfusion the nurse notes the following vital signs: pulse 110, respirations 28, BP 98/58, and temperature 101° F. The patient is shivering. The nurse's next action would be to:
    1. Slow the infusion rate
    2. Stop the infusion
    3. Administer aspirin as ordered for elevated temperature
    4. Report the findings to the nurse manager

37

CARE OF THE HIV-POSITIVE OR AIDS PATIENT

Virginia F. Wilkinson

KEY TERMS

acquired immunodeficiency syndrome (AIDS)
Centers for Disease Control and Prevention (CDC)
ELISA
HIV disease
HIV infection
human immunodeficiency virus (HIV)
Kaposi's sarcoma (KS)
lymphocyte
opportunistic
phagocyte
***Pneumocystis carinii* pneumonia (PCP)**
receptor
retrovirus
seroconversion
seronegative
surveillance
virulent
Western blot

LEARNING OBJECTIVES

After reading this chapter, the student should be able to do the following:

- Define the key terms.
- Describe the agent that causes AIDS.
- Relate the January 1993 CDC definition of AIDS.
- Explain the difference among HIV infection, HIV disease, and AIDS.
- Describe the progression of HIV infection.
- Discuss how HIV is transmitted and how it is not transmitted.
- Describe patients who are at risk for HIV infection.
- Discuss the use of effective prevention messages in counseling patients.
- Discuss the issues related to HIV antibody testing.
- Define the nurse's role in the prevention of HIV infection.
- Discuss the nurse's role in assisting the HIV-infected patient with coping, reducing anxiety, minimizing social isolation, and assisting with grieving.
- Describe the multidisciplinary approach in caring for a patient with HIV disease.
- List signs and symptoms that might be indicative of HIV disease.
- List opportunistic infections associated with AIDS.
- Implement a plan of care for the patient with AIDS.

RELATED TOPICS OF INTEREST

- Signs, symptoms, and physical assessment (Chapter 9)
- Medical asepsis and infection control (Chapter 12)
- Care of the patient with a reproductive disorder (Chapter 33)
- Care of the patient with an immune disorder (Chapter 36)
- Loss, grief, dying, and death (Chapter 52)

HISTORY OF AIDS

As the epidemic of acquired immunodeficiency syndrome (AIDS) in the United States enters its second decade, nurses are faced with the unique challenges associated with this dreaded communicable disease. AIDS was first reported in 1981 as a unique condition characterized by a breakdown in the body's immune system. Affected individuals were vulnerable to infections that a healthy immune system ordinarily could destroy. ***Pneumocystis carinii* pneumonia (PCP)** (an unusual pulmonary disease caused by a parasite that is primarily associated with persons who have suppressed immune systems) and **Kaposi's sarcoma (KS)** (a rare cancer of the skin or mucous membranes characterized by blue, red, or purple raised lesions) were occurring at alarming rates in clusters of young homosexual men in New York and California. The **Centers for Disease Control and Prevention (CDC)** (an agency of the U.S. government that provides facilities and services for the investigation, identification, prevention, and control of disease) soon learned that this condition was also affecting injecting drug users and persons with hemophilia and later learned that it also affected heterosexual men and women.[16]

In 1985 researchers isolated a virus believed to be the agent responsible for AIDS. Different investigators gave different names to the virus: AIDS-related virus (ARV), lymphadenopathy-associated virus (LAV), and human T lymphotropic virus type III (HTLV III). All appear to be the same or close members of the same family, and in 1986 the virus was named **human immunodeficiency virus (HIV)** (a retrovirus that causes AIDS).

Since the first cases of AIDS were reported in 1981, the CDC has revised the case definition 3 times to more accurately reflect the disease. The most recent revision was implemented January 1, 1993, and adds conditions more applicable to women and injecting drug users (see Table 37-1). Since HIV selectively infects and destroys cells that display CD4 molecules on their surface (primarily T_4 lymphocytes), the new definition includes all HIV-infected persons who have CD4 counts of 200 or fewer (as opposed to the normal 600 to 1200 cells/mm^3). Three clinical conditions, pulmonary tuberculosis, recurrent pneumonia, and invasive cervical cancer, were also added. The definition is for reporting and surveillance so that the disease can be monitored with a consistent approach for public health purposes.[11]

Acquired immunodeficiency syndrome (AIDS) (an acquired condition that impairs the body's ability to fight disease) is the end stage of a continuum of **HIV infection** (the state in which HIV enters the body and under favorable conditions multiplies, producing injurious effects to the body) (Fig. 37-1 on p. 1166 and Fig. 37-5). HIV infection may exist for years without symptoms before it progresses to **HIV disease** (symptomatic HIV infection not severe enough for a diagnosis of AIDS; examples of signs and symptoms of HIV disease are persistent, unexplained fever; night sweats; diarrhea; weight loss; and fatigue). *HIV disease* is a diagnostic term used for the spectrum of clinical illness and progressive deterioration of the immune system resulting from HIV infection and replaces the previously used terms *AIDS-related complex (ARC)* and *AIDS*. *AIDS* has been defined for surveillance and reporting purposes but is not used alone to diagnose serious disease caused by HIV infection.

IMPACT OF AIDS NATIONWIDE AND WORLDWIDE

Reporting of HIV and AIDS

Cases of AIDS are reported to each state health department and to the CDC. The case is reported in the state of residence at the time of the diagnosis. HIV infection is not a reportable condition in all states, and information reported varies according to state laws and regula-

TABLE 37-1 1993 Revised Classification System for HIV Infection and Expanded AIDS Surveillance Case Definition for Adults and Adolescents ≥ 13 Years of Age*

	Clinical Categories		
CD4 + T-Cell Categories	(A) Asymptomatic, Acute (Primary) HIV, or PGL	(B) Symptomatic, Not (A) or (C) Conditions	(C) AIDS-Indicator Conditions†
(1) ≥ 500/μL	A1	B1	C1
(2) 200-499/μL	A2	B2	C2
(3) <200/μL AIDS-indicator T-cell count	A3	B3	C3

PGL, Persistent generalized lymphadenopathy.
*HIV-infected persons classified in A3, B3, or any C cell meet the 1993 AIDS surveillance case definition.
†Includes opportunistic diseases, pulmonary tuberculosis, recurrent pneumonia, and invasive cervical cancer.
From Centers for Disease Control and Prevention.

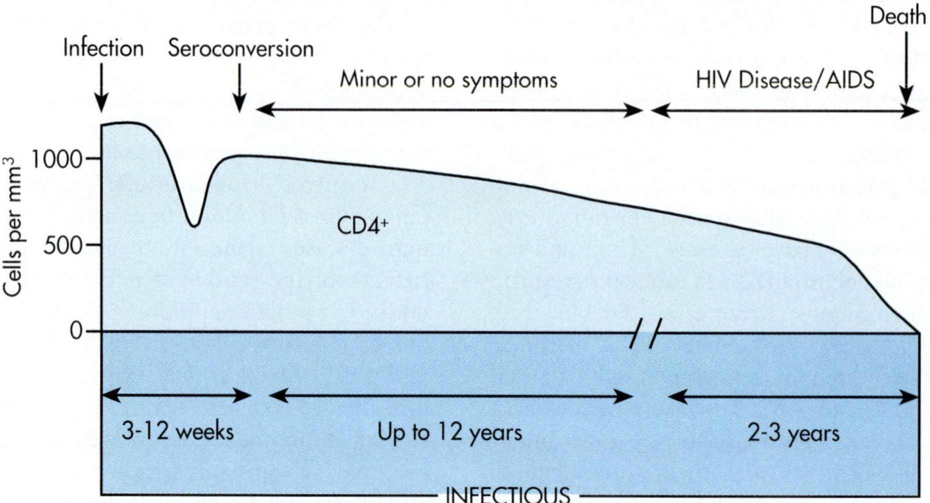

FIG. 37-1 The progression from initial HIV infection to AIDS. Seroconversion from HIV antibody negative to HIV antibody usually occurs within 3 to 12 weeks after infection with HIV. Signs and symptoms may not occur for many years, the average being 8 to 10 years. HIV infection results in symptomatic HIV disease as the virus progressively compromises the immune system by depleting the CD4 cells; when the cells are 200 or less and/or opportunistic diseases occur, HIV disease progresses to AIDS, the end stage of HIV infection. The person infected with HIV is infectious at any stage. (Adapted from *Science,* May 1993, Robin Weiss.)

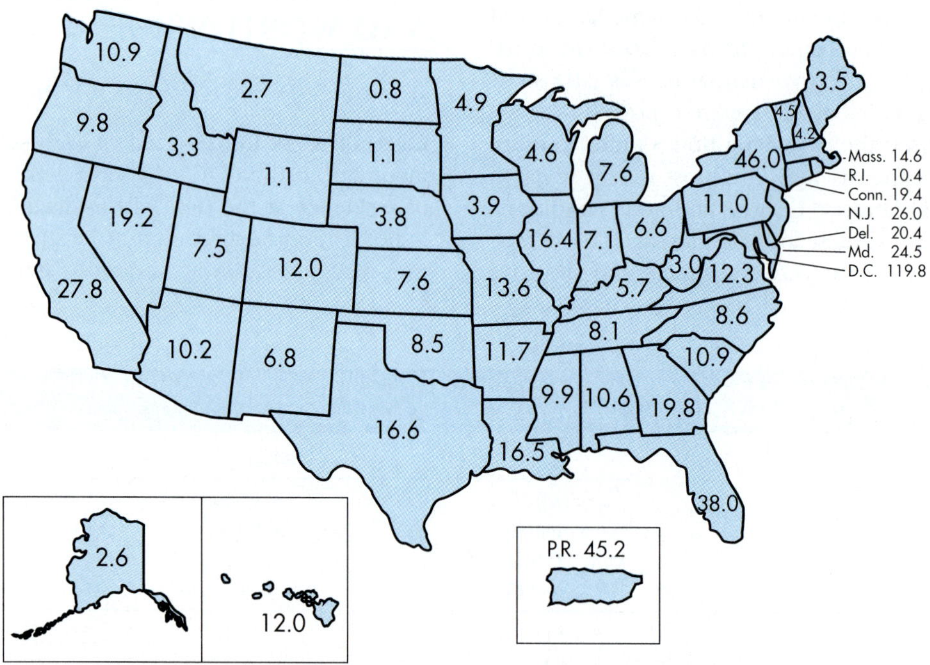

FIG. 37-2 AIDS annual rates per 100,000 population for cases reported in 1992, United States. (From *CDC HIV/AIDS Surveillance Report,* February 1993.)

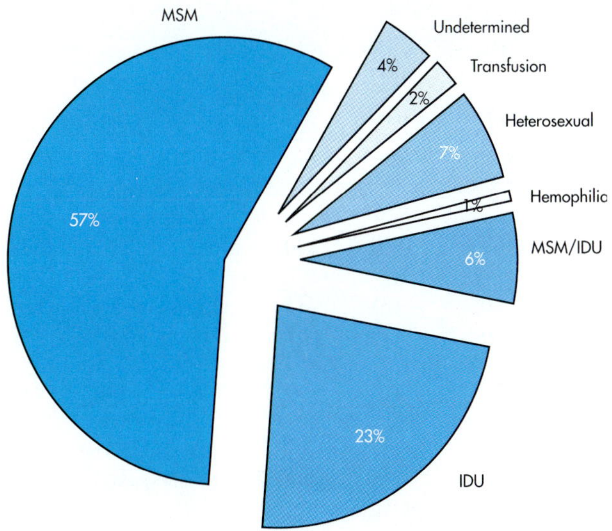

FIG. 37-3 Percentage of adult cases of AIDS in the United States by risk exposure from January 1981 to December 1992. *MSM,* Men who have sex with men; *IDU,* injecting drug users. (From CDC NE Department of Health, HIV/AIDS Prog.)

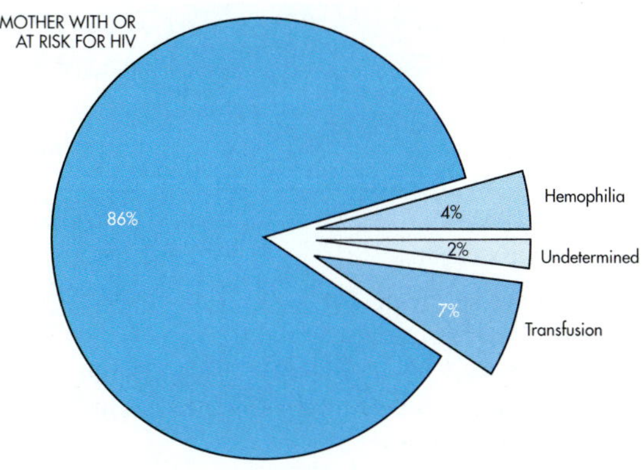

FIG. 37-4 Percentage of AIDS cases in children in the United States by risk exposure from January 1981 to December 1992. (From CDC NE Department of Health, HIV/AIDS Prog.)

tions, so the AIDS case **surveillance** (the exercise of continuous scrutiny of and watchfulness over the distribution and spread of infections and related factors that is of sufficient accuracy and completeness to be pertinent to effective control) system continues to be the most consistent source for monitoring the impact of HIV infection.

U.S. cases, which have been reported from all 50 states, the District of Columbia, and four U.S. territories, exceeded 300,000 by mid-1993. The CDC estimates that there are over 1 million people infected with HIV in the United States who are not yet reported as having AIDS (Fig. 37-2). The CDC and most state health departments publish quarterly HIV and AIDS surveillance reports that include cases by age (see gerontological box), sex, risk category, ethnic group, state, and time period.

Trends

The distribution of AIDS cases varies greatly among geographical areas, racial and ethnic groups, and other subpopulations. Men make up 80% of the cases, reflective of the large number of cases in homosexual and bisexual men, but that percentage is a decrease from 1989 when men were 90% of the total. Women and children constitute the fastest-growing segment of the population with AIDS. The number of cases attributed to heterosexual contact increased from the 120 reported in 1985 to 4114 in June 1992. Reported cases attributed to heterosexual contact with a partner at risk for HIV infection are increasing faster than any other category of AIDS cases—up 5% between 1989 and 1992. The increase in this category is most pronounced in women (Figs. 37-3 and 37-4).[9]

AIDS takes a disproportionate toll on the African-American and Hispanic populations. African-Americans comprise 12% of the U.S. population, but constitute 30% of the reported AIDS cases. Hispanics represent 17% of the AIDS cases and only 7% of the U.S. population. Over half of the female AIDS cases are in black women, and over 53% of pediatric AIDS cases are among black children. Hispanic children represent over 24% of the pediatric AIDS cases (Table 37-2 on p. 1168).[33]

The World Health Organization (WHO) estimates that as of mid-1993 over 13 million individuals worldwide have been infected with HIV, with 3 million being women. There are over 2 million cases of AIDS reported worldwide (Box 37-1 on p. 1168).[31]

GERONTOLOGICAL CONSIDERATIONS

- Because of the modes of transmission, HIV is not a common disease in older adults. An occasional case resulting from contaminated blood transfusion before screening for HIV or the use of contaminated needles may be seen.
- Most individuals who are HIV positive develop AIDS within a short period and die of complications at a young age. There is, however, a group of asymptomatic individuals of middle and late middle age who are infected with HIV, which could result in an HIV-positive geriatric population in the near future.

TABLE 37-2 Adult and Adolescent AIDS Cases*

	White, Not Hispanic		Black, Not Hispanic		Hispanic		Asian/Pacific Islander		American Indian/ Alaska Native		Total	
	No.	(%)	No.	(%)	No.	(%)	No.	(%)	No.	(%)	No.	(%)
Male exposure category												
Men who have sex with men	99,016	(79)	25,547	(43)	16,342	(46)	1161	(80)	240	(64)	142,626	(64)
Injecting drug use	8895	(7)	21,100	(36)	13,613	(38)	50	(3)	42	(11)	43,786	(20)
Men who have sex with men and inject drugs	9044	(7)	4407	(7)	2334	(7)	36	(2)	61	(16)	15,899	(7)
Hemophilia/coagulation disorder	1619	(1)	159	(0)	166	(0)	24	(2)	9	(2)	1983	(1)
Heterosexual contact	1121	(1)	4392	(7)	881	(2)	14	(1)	4	(1)	6419	(3)
Recipient of blood transfusion, blood components, or tissue	2170	(2)	490	(1)	307	(1)	60	(4)	2	(1)	3036	(1)
Other/undetermined†	2962	(2)	3040	(5)	1784	(5)	103	(7)	16	(4)	7965	(4)
Male subtotal	124,827	(100)	59,135	(100)	35,427	(100)	1448	(100)	374	(100)	221,714	(100)
Female exposure category												
Injecting drug use	2901	(42)	7860	(54)	2784	(48)	19	(13)	35	(57)	13,626	(50)
Hemophilia/coagulation disorder	32	(0)	8	(0)	3	(0)	—		—		43	(0)
Heterosexual contact	2275	(33)	5191	(36)	2280	(40)	54	(38)	15	(25)	9835	(36)
Receipt of blood transfusion, blood components, or tissue	1201	(17)	419	(3)	271	(5)	45	(31)	5	(8)	1944	(7)
Other/undetermined	518	(7)	1073	(7)	407	(7)	25	(17)	6	(10)	2037	(7)
Female subtotal	6927	(100)	14,551	(100)	5745	(100)	145	(100)	61	(100)	27,485	(100)
Total	131,754		73,686		41,172		1591		435		249,199	

*By Sex, Exposure category, and Race or Ethnicity, Reported through December 1992, United States.
†*Other* refers to seven health care workers who developed AIDS after occupational exposure to HIV-infected blood, as documented by evidence of seroconversion, and to two patients who developed AIDS after exposure to HIV within the health care setting, as documented by laboratory studies.

Box 37-1 REPORTED CASES OF AIDS

United States AIDS cases	253,448
United States AIDS deaths	171,890
World AIDS cases	Over 2 million

Data from the World Health Organization and the Centers for Disease Control and Prevention, cumulative reported cases through December 1992.

EPIDEMIOLOGY OF HIV

HIV the Agent

HIV is a member of the retrovirus family. Like all viruses, it must live in a host cell; it cannot live or replicate (reproduce or duplicate) outside a host cell. As a **retrovirus,** it is composed of genetic material called RNA (ribonucleic acid), instead of the more common DNA (deoxyribonucleic acid) found in most living cells. Retroviruses carry their genetic code in RNA rather than DNA material and replicate in a reverse manner. A human cell divides by copying DNA into RNA. Retroviruses must copy their RNA into DNA to divide and replicate (Fig. 37-5). HIV is a fragile virus outside the human body. It is destroyed by heat and light and ordinary cleaning solutions such as household bleach.

When HIV enters the body, its primary target is the immune system. The immune system is a complex set of responses that recognizes and defends the body against foreign invaders. Phagocytes and lymphocytes are key players in the immune response. **Phagocytes** are white blood cells that are able to surround, engulf, and digest microorganisms and cellular debris. **Lymphocytes** are white blood cells that occur in two forms, B cells and T cells. The function of B cells is to search out,

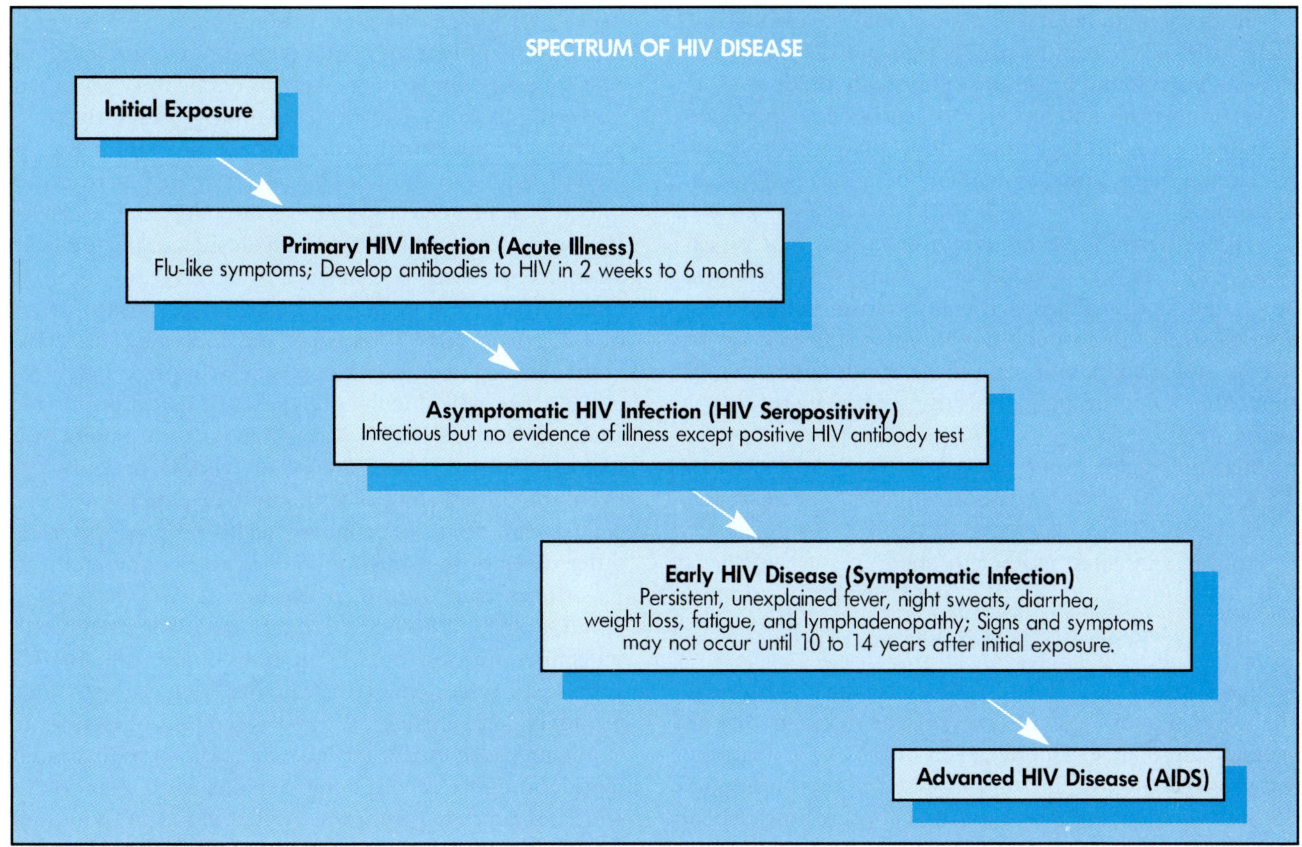

FIG. 37-5 Spectrum of HIV disease.

identify, and bind with specific antigens. T cells have several functions but primarily mediate (cause a change to occur in) cellular immune responses. Each lymphocyte has **receptors** (molecules that recognize or respond to specific invaders) on its surface that match one of the millions of foreign invaders in the body. When the invader attaches to its matching receptor, the inactivation or destruction begins. In addition to receptors, T lymphocytes have CD4 and CD8 molecules on their surface. Helper T cells (a subset of T cells essential for activating antibody production by B cells and initiating many other immune responses) carry the CD4 molecule and suppressor, or killer, T cells (a subset of T cells that kill body cells infected by viruses or transformed by cancer) carry the CD8 molecule. When HIV enters the body, it circulates in the blood until it touches a cell with the CD4 receptor on its surface. T cells have numerous CD4 receptors and are, therefore, most readily infected by HIV. Cells in the nervous system and the skin have CD4 receptors and can be infected with HIV, but because they express CD4 to a lesser degree, they may be less readily infected. As HIV infection progresses, there is a loss of helper T cells while the suppressor or killer T cells persist. Consequently, in an HIV-infected person the CD4:CD8 ratio (normally 1.5:1 to 2:1) falls to as low as 0:1. As T cell numbers decrease, the immune system loses its ability to detect and destroy infectious diseases and cancer cells, which results in HIV disease and AIDS. The exact way HIV damages the immune system is still unknown.[43]

Modes of Transmission

After more than a decade of study and research about HIV, a great deal is known about how HIV is transmitted and how it is not transmitted. Considerable fear and misinformation have been generated about HIV, possibly more than any other disease in this century. It is imperative that patients, families, and health care providers be knowledgeable about transmission and behaviors that put them at risk.

The transmission of HIV is dependent on the presence of the virus, behaviors that put individuals at risk of being exposed to the virus, the infectiousness of the virus, and the susceptibility of the uninfected individual who is exposed. Considering these factors, HIV can be transmitted at any stage of an individual's infection or at any point of the HIV disease continuum[37] (see Fig. 37-1).

Blood, semen, vaginal secretions, and breast milk are the body fluids that most readily transmit HIV. Although HIV has been found in various other body fluids such as saliva, urine, tears, and feces, there has been no evidence of transmission through these body fluids. Body fluids containing blood could potentially be a means of transmission.

HIV is transmitted by certain behaviors, *not* by casual contact such as hugging, dry kissing, shaking hands, or sharing food or utensils. It is not transmitted by mosquitoes, in the air through coughing or sneezing, or by sharing office space and equipment. Studies consistently show, after a decade, that HIV is transmitted by three major means:

1. Anal and vaginal intercourse
2. Injecting drugs with HIV-contaminated needles/paraphernalia
3. From HIV-infected mother to child

Routes of Transmission

Sexual Exposure. Transmission can occur through exchange of semen, vaginal secretions, or blood in anal or vaginal intercourse. Openings or microscopic tears in the tissue allow a point of entrance for the virus into the bloodstream. Studies show that the greatest risk is through unprotected receptive anal intercourse, because the rectum is not well lubricated and is a tighter orifice, making tissue trauma more likely. Ulcerating genital diseases such as herpes and syphilis are believed to increase the risk of sexual transmission of HIV. The transmission of HIV from an infected male to an uninfected female is estimated to be 18 times more likely than that from an infected female to an uninfected male. Oral-genital transmission occurs rarely.

Parenteral Exposure.

Injecting drug use. The most common mode of parenteral (not in or through the digestive system) exposure is through the sharing of needles and paraphernalia among injecting drug users (IDU). Injecting drug use refers to all drug use that involves the use of needles, including street drugs and steroids. The intravenous drug user usually draws back a small amount of blood into the syringe to be sure that the needle is in the vein, and then injects the drug. The needle and the syringe, both containing small amounts of infected blood, are then passed on to the next person, resulting in cross-infection. The health of drug users is often already compromised because of poor nutrition and poor hygiene; the long-term effects of drug use make them more susceptible to HIV infection.

Occupational. Occupational exposure to infected blood and body fluids occurs most frequently through a percutaneous (performed through the skin, e.g., needlestick) route. Even though exposures occur through both mucous membrane and cutaneous contact, studies show that transmission is more likely to occur through percutaneous exposure. The CDC continues to investigate reports of occupational exposure, not only from the infected patient to the health care provider but from the infected health care provider to the patient. The risk of HIV transmission following a needlestick exposure from an infected source is estimated to be very low, approximately 1 in 250 (0.3%). In comparison, the risk of hepatitis B virus (HBV) transmission following an HBV-contaminated needlestick exposure is approximately 3% to 30%. The only documented cases of HIV transmission from an infected health care provider to a patient was that of a dentist in Florida who infected six patients.[17,18] Even after the testing of thousands of patients who received care from an infected health care provider, no other cases of transmission have been documented.

Blood and blood products. HIV-contaminated blood, tissue, and blood products were sources of HIV transmission prior to 1985. In 1985 blood tests for HIV antibodies, treatment (i.e., heat treatment) of the blood products to inactivate HIV, and screening of donors to eliminate those at risk for HIV infection were instituted. Blood products received by persons with hemophilia were concentrated from the pooled blood of thousands of donors, any one of whom could have been infected with HIV. About 3% of the cumulative cases of AIDS are attributed to HIV transmission from contaminated blood, tissue, and blood products received prior to 1985. As a result of advanced technology in blood testing and treatment and increased donor screening, the blood supply is now considered safe. However, an infected donor who is not eliminated through the screening process would not be detected by the testing for HIV antibodies if the donor is newly infected and **seroconversion** (the development of detectable levels of antibodies in which there is a change in serological tests from negative to positive as antibodies develop in reaction to an infection) has not occurred. Rarely would this happen as seroconversion usually occurs in 95% of persons within 3 months and 99% of persons within 6 months, but the possibility makes screening for donors at risk for HIV infection very important.

Perinatal Exposure. An infected mother can transmit HIV to her baby in utero or perinatally during delivery. It is estimated that 30% of infected mothers transmit HIV to their infants. Breastfeeding is also but less commonly associated with transmission of HIV. An infected mother should be counseled about the risk of transmitting HIV through breastfeeding. Even though the risk may be small, the recommendation would be not to breastfeed unless other circumstances prevail, such as inaccessibility to formula.

PREVENTION

HIV disease/AIDS is preventable. However, prevention takes the cooperation and efforts of public health care providers, medical providers, nurses in all areas, communities, families, churches, and schools, to name only a few. Education is our only vaccine. Many patients admitted to acute-care facilities have unrecognized HIV infection or are at risk for HIV infection. Nurses have a responsibility to assess each patient's risks for HIV infection and counsel those at risk about HIV testing, behaviors that put them at risk, and how to eliminate or reduce those risks. The nurse needs to feel comfortable with HIV transmission and prevention issues, sexual terms, terminology related to drug use, and risk reduction techniques. The local or state health department has resources for training and providing prevention messages. HIV counseling and testing are important factors in the prevention of HIV. Box 37-2 lists important functions of HIV counseling and testing.

Prevention counseling should be sensitive to issues of sexual identity, developmentally appropriate (i.e., information and services should be provided at a level of comprehension that is consistent with the age and the learning skills of the person being served), and culturally and linguistically specific (i.e., information should be presented in dialect and terminology consistent with the patient's language and style of communication).

Risk Assessment

Risk assessment should be patient-centered so that the patient understands and takes "ownership" of the risk for HIV infection. The assessment needs to include a thorough sexual and drug use history done in a forthright, nonjudgmental, empathetic manner. Patients need to be assessed for disease manifestations, such as sexually transmitted diseases, which would be indicative of risky behaviors. Risk assessment should be a continual process in patient care.[2]

HIV infection in women has frequently been overlooked for several reasons. First, in the United States, the disease occurred mostly in men, and treatment models were developed from the progression of the disease in men. Second, providers did not assess risk in women, and women did not seek counseling and testing because of denial or ignorance so intervention has not been implemented effectively. The CDC case definition, implemented January 1, 1993, includes at least one female specific disease, cervical carcinoma. Women need to be assessed for different manifestations, such as the common initial presenting condition for HIV-positive women, vaginal candidiasis.[25]

Box 37-2 MAJOR FUNCTIONS OF HIV COUNSELING

The CDC identifies the following major functions of HIV counseling and testing:

- Providing a convenient opportunity for persons to learn their current HIV serostatus.
- Allowing persons to receive prevention counseling to help initiate behavior changes to avoid HIV infection or, if already infected, to prevent transmission of HIV to others.
- Helping persons obtain referrals to receive additional prevention, medical care, and other needed services, such as drug treatment, family planning, and support.
- Providing prevention services and referrals for sex and needle-sharing partners of HIV-infected persons.

Data from Centers for Disease Control: Recommendation for HIV testing services for inpatients and outpatients in acute-care hospital settings and technical guidance on HIV counseling, *MMWR* 42(RR-2), January 1993.

Risk Reduction

Risk reduction counseling should be an interactive process resulting in a negotiated plan based on the patient's circumstances, skills, and needs. Risk reduction is an ongoing process, and the nurse needs to be aware of and to use every opportunity to reinforce and support positive preventive choices. Box 37-3 on p. 1172 lists prevention options to use during risk reduction counseling.

Occupational Exposure

The relative risk of HIV transmission in the health care setting is very low. As of December 1992, the CDC had reported that 33 health care workers had seroconverted to HIV positive following occupational exposures, primarily needlestick injuries. Infection control is an essential component of good health care for all patients, regardless of their diagnosis. Universal precautions should be used with all blood and body fluids to prevent the transmission of bloodborne pathogens such as HIV and HBV. HBV is a more **virulent** (the power of a microorganism to produce a disease) virus, is found in greater concentrations in blood and body fluids, and lives outside the body for longer periods. HBV is transmitted by the same routes as HIV.[14,36] (Also see Chapter 12).

BARRIERS TO PREVENTION

There are numerous barriers to prevention, not the least of which is denial that there is a risk, that is, the attitude that "it won't happen to me." Because the virus infected the gay population first in the United States, many other

Box 37-3 PREVENTION OPTIONS

SEXUAL

No Risk

- Abstinence from sexual contact in which there is exchange of semen, vaginal secretions, or blood.
- Partners who are in a mutually monogamous (the state of having one mate) relationship in which neither partner is at risk of infection through injection drug use and in which neither partner was previously exposed to HIV through drug use or sexual contact.

Reduced Risk

- Limiting the number of partners, even though there would potentially be a risk if there were sexual contact with one infected partner.
- Protective measures through consistent and correct use of latex condoms with a spermicide in every act of sexual intercourse in which there would be exchange of semen, vaginal secretions, or blood.[37] The correct use of condoms is as follows:
  -Put on the condom as soon as erection occurs and before any sexual contact (anal, vaginal, or oral).
  -Leave space at the tip of the condom.
  -Use only water-based lubricants.
  -Hold the condom firmly to keep it from slipping off and withdraw from the partner immediately after ejaculation.

INJECTION DRUG USE

No Risk

- Stop the use of injectable drugs. Drug treatment opportunities should be provided.
- If drugs are going to be injected, use sterile needles and equipment.

INJECTION DRUG USE—cont'd

Reduced Risk

- If needles and equipment are going to be shared, instructions on cleaning should be given.
- Fill the syringe with sodium hypochlorite 5.25% (e.g., Clorox) bleach two times, empty two times. Fill the syringe with clean water two times and empty two times. Inactivation of HIV requires a 30-second exposure to 100% bleach.[42]

PERINATAL

No Risk

- Avoidance of pregnancy or abortion are the only certain ways to prevent transmission of HIV to a fetus or infant.
- A woman of child-bearing age of unknown HIV status should be counseled about behaviors that would put her at risk for HIV infection and about behaviors that would put her partner or spouse at risk for HIV infection. If risk factors are determined in either case, both individuals should be counseled about testing for HIV.

Reduced Risk

- Adherence to birth control measures, including use of condoms, to avoid pregnancy.

subpopulations have ignored their risks.[16] Fear and misinformation are also significant barriers. Some individuals are so fearful that they will no longer give blood, and they will not eat at a restaurant if they think a gay food handler is employed. Fear and misinformation reinforce the need for consistent, accurate information about the virus, the risks of transmission, and HIV disease itself.

Cultural and community attitudes, values, and norms can affect the success of prevention efforts. A community may be opposed to HIV/AIDS education in the local school district because of the fear that values will be compromised. Those values may include views on sexuality, abstinence, use of condoms, drug use, and giving instruction on cleaning needles and syringes. Community organizations, churches, educators, and leaders can determine what the expectations or norms of that community will be. Cooperative efforts are essential for successful prevention of HIV transmission. The issues related to the HIV epidemic—sex, death, and homosexuality—are not easy issues for most cultures or communities.

Prevention of HIV transmission requires a commitment to change behaviors that put one at risk. Education to alter behavior change is a long-term process. Health care providers need to take every opportunity to educate their patients on how to avoid or reduce the risk for HIV infection. Collective efforts will have the greatest impact.

Fear of alienation and discrimination are additional barriers to prevention. In some cases, individuals are reluctant to even pick up a pamphlet about HIV because they fear someone will believe they are gay or a drug user. There is evidence that people will not go to a physician or to a counseling and testing site for HIV testing because they fear being seen. Fear of discrimination includes fear of losing family, friends, prestige, jobs, housing, and insurance.

INTERVENTION

Persons at risk for HIV infection should be encouraged to know their HIV status. Existing evidence strongly supports the efficacy (effectiveness) of some preventive measures taken to postpone the onset of disease as well as the influence of educational messages in reducing the transmission of HIV.

The individual needs to understand the following implications of an HIV test:

- The individual's blood is tested with an enzyme-linked immunosorbent assay **(ELISA)** (an antibody test that detects the presence of HIV antibodies). If the ELISA is positive for HIV, then the same blood is tested a second time with an ELISA. If the second ELISA is positive, the blood is tested with the **Western blot** (a laboratory blood test to detect the presence of antibodies to a specific antigen), which is a more specific, confirmatory test. The person should be told a test is positive for HIV only after this sequence.[10]
- The series of tests confirms the presence of antibodies to HIV and does not mean the person has AIDS. The test is not a diagnostic test for AIDS. AIDS is diagnosed using the 1993 CDC definition presented previously.
- A **seronegative** (the blood test does not detect HIV antibodies) test is not an assurance that the patient is free of infection because seroconversion may not have occurred.
- A seronegative test does not mean that the patient is free from risk of infection. If the patient continues risky behavior such as unprotected sexual intercourse with an HIV-infected partner or using HIV-contaminated needles or paraphernalia, transmission may occur.

Linkages for Intervention

Patients who are HIV seropositive need to be linked to various points of intervention, depending on the patients' needs. Patients often deny the infection and neglect their mental and physical health as well as continue behaviors that put themselves and others at risk. Interventions need to be sustained as the emotional impact of such news can override any initial information provided. Providers need to reinforce safer behaviors and the need for medical and emotional support. Any person notified of HIV-positive results has a further need for psychological and emotional support. Types of assistance include family planning, drug treatment, behavior modification counseling, treatment for sexually transmitted disease, treatment for tuberculosis, immunizations, prophylactic treatment to prevent opportunistic infections, financial assistance, mental health evaluation, spiritual support, social services, dental care, and nutritional assistance. The seropositive patient should be told not to donate blood, tissues, organs, or semen. Identification of sexual and needle-sharing partners should be elicited, and they should be notified of their potential exposure, either by the patient or by the local or state health department.

CLINICAL MANIFESTATIONS

Stages of HIV Infection

HIV infection encompasses a full spectrum of disease progression, AIDS being only one part. A mononucleosis-like syndrome, known as *seroconversion illness*, occurs in about 20% of HIV-infected individuals. Acute signs and symptoms include fatigue, fever, sweats, headache, muscle and joint pain, diarrhea, and rash and can occur within 5 days to 3 months of infection, although most often they occur within 2 to 4 weeks.

After seroconversion, persons may be asymptomatic for months or years, during which time they look and feel well. Other persons may experience vague or subtle signs and symptoms, and still others may develop a variety of signs and symptoms that become chronic in nature but not necessarily debilitating. The average time from seroconversion to the diagnosis of AIDS is 10 years; however, for some individuals it is much longer and for some it is only a few months. The reasons for these variations are still somewhat unknown, even though general health and well-being play an important part.

Symptomatic HIV infection includes a variety of signs and symptoms as a result of immune deficiency (Box 37-4). As HIV infection progresses, the immune sys-

Box 37-4 SIGNS AND SYMPTOMS OF HIV INFECTION

Abdominal pain
Chills and fever
Cough (dry or productive)
Diarrhea
Disorientation
Dyspnea
Fatigue
Headache
Lymphadenopathy (any disorder of the lymph nodes or lymph vessels)
Malaise
Muscle/joint pain
Night sweats
Oral lesions
Shortness of breath
Skin rash
Sore throat
Weight loss

TABLE 37-3 Symptomatic Stages of HIV Infection

HIV Disease	Signs and Symptoms	Common Treatments	Nursing Interventions
Opportunistic diseases			
Candida albicans infection (fungal infection)	Loss of appetite Creamy-white plaques in the mouth and throat Sore throat Difficulty swallowing Skin lesions Rectal or vaginal pain Rectal lesions	Nystatin Ketoconazole Clotrimazole Fluconazole	Promote oral hygiene and avoidance of tissue trauma. Promote food and fluid intake. Monitor for bleeding lesions of oral and rectal mucous membranes.
Cryptococcus meningitidis (fungal infection)	Fever Severe headache Sleepiness Stiff neck Change in mental status Nausea Blurred vision	Amphotericin B Fluconazole	Monitor vital signs. Relieve symptoms, e.g., headache. Assure safety. Assistance in ADLs. Assess for depression.
Cryptosporidium (protozoan infection)	Severe, watery diarrhea Nausea or vomiting Abdominal cramping Fever Weakness	Antidiarrhea medication Intravenous fluid therapy	Promote good nutrition: proper hydration and diets low in residue. Provide skin care, cleansing with mild soap, application of moisture creams, air mattress. Assess for electrolyte imbalances and dehydration.
Cytomegalovirus (CMV) retinitus, gastritis (herpesvirus)	Loss of vision Fever Fatigue Fatigue/severe malaise Weight loss Copious diarrhea Abdominal pain	Ganciclovir Foscarnet	Assess for changes in vision. Use dim lighting. Institute patient teaching related to vision change. Encourage grief counseling. Assess for safe ADLs. Identify local services for visually impaired.
Herpes simplex (virus)	Weeping skin lesions (oral, genital, or perirectal) Rectal bleeding Rectal discharge Pain associated with lesions	Acyclovir (Zovirax)	Assess for intact skin or lesions. Promote comfort. Prevent infection: use separate washcloth, wear gloves, avoid tub baths.
Mycobacterium avium complex (bacteria)	Fever Severe weight loss Abdominal pain Diarrhea Abnormal food absorption	Rifampin Ethambutol Ciprofloxacin Amikacin	Promote good food and fluid intake. Provide skin care. Relieve symptoms.

Mycobacterium tuberculosis (bacteria)	Weight loss Fever Weakness Shortness of breath Nausea/vomiting	INH (isoniazid) Rifampin Pyrazinamide Ethambutol	Minimize effects of fever, weakness. Promote adequate food and fluid intake. Promote comfort. Monitor vital signs. Assist with oxygen therapy. Assess for signs and symptoms of respiratory failure. Note respiratory rate, rhythm. Be alert for cyanosis and dyspnea. Facilitate optimal ventilation; have patient in semi-Fowler's position.
Pneumocystis carinii pneumonia (PCP) (protozoa)	Fever Chills Night sweats Cough Shortness of breath Weight loss Weakness	Bactrim Septra Pentamidine Dapsone Trimethoprim	Monitor vital signs, activity, and fatigue levels. Relieve symptoms. Monitor for side effects of medications. Maintain adequate ventilation and comfort. Promote ADLs while preventing fatigue. Maintain hydration status, fluid intake. Minimize anxiety, exertion, and environmental pollutants.
Malignant neoplasm			
Kaposi's sarcoma (KS) (neoplasm)	Brown or purple cutaneous lesions on the skin or mouth Internal lesions, pulmonary Edema, secondary to lymphatic occlusion by KS lesions Shortness of breath (dyspnea) Cough Diarrhea	Limited with the exception of pulmonary KS Radiation therapy for management of lesions	Skin care of lesions. Prevention of effects of edema. Maintain skin integrity. Gentle massage with creams and oils to promote comfort.
Nervous system disorders			
HIV dementia complex and central nervous system disorders	Cognitive changes Gait disturbance Progressive weakness Speech problems Lethargy Forgetfulness Incontinence Visual problems Disorientation Depression	Rule out treatable causes	Maintain stable environment. Provide understandable information. Monitor changes in mental status and functions. Promote ADLs. Assess patient's capabilities for ADLs. Assess for self-destructive behavior. Assess family and community resources. Demonstrate caring, concern, and respect.

Adapted from HIV/AIDS Curriculum, Mountain-Plains Regional AIDS Education and Training Center.

tem loses its ability to fight infectious agents and cancer cells. Even in the asymptomatic period, a gradual decrease in the CD4 cells occurs. CD4 and CD8 counts are important laboratory indicators of disease progression. As indicated earlier, a normal CD4 count is 600 to 1200 cells/mm^3, and a normal CD4:CD8 ratio ranges from 1.5:1 to 2:1. In an HIV-infected person the CD4:CD8 ratio often falls to as low as 0:1. The helper T lymphocytes carrying the CD4 molecule decrease while the suppressor T lymphocytes carrying the CD8 molecule persist, resulting in a deterioration of the immune system. A CD4 count of less than 500 is indicative of a suppressed immune system, and a count of less than 200 cells/mm^3 generally indicates a more severely suppressed immune system and the onset of **opportunistic** (caused by normally nonpathogenic organisms in a host whose resistance has been decreased by such disorders as AIDS) diseases such as *Pneumocystis carinii* pneumonia (PCP) and Kaposi's sarcoma (Table 37-3 on pp. 1174-1175).[7]

AIDS, the end stage of HIV infection, is characterized by a severely compromised immune system that is unable to fight opportunistic diseases, including infections and cancers that would not be debilitating to a noncompromised host (Table 37-3). The nervous system is often affected. Persons with a diagnosis of AIDS have been known to survive 5 or more years, but premature death seems to be inevitable.

Treatment

Prophylactic treatments are usually prescribed when the CD4 count is less than 500 cells/mm^3. Zidovudine (AZT, Retrovir) has been shown to prolong life, decrease the risk and severity of opportunistic infections, and improve neurological symptoms. Drugs such as acyclovir, interferon, didanosine (dideoxyinosine) and dideoxycytidine used in combination with AZT are being evaluated. Like zidovudine, didanosine inhibits HIV replication. In studies, didanosine increased CD4 cell counts, a sign of improvement. But it is unknown at this time whether didanosine also halts the progression of HIV infection (as zidovudine does), reducing the incidence of opportunistic infections and prolonging survival. So zidovudine is still considered the drug of choice for HIV infection. However, the latest research is less favorable than earlier reports regarding zidovudine. Didanosine is a useful alternative in patients who cannot tolerate zidovudine. The nurse needs to be aware of the side effects of as well as the nursing considerations in administration of these drugs. See the medication table for other drugs used to treat HIV infection.

Many opportunistic infections respond to treatment, but most cannot be cured. Maintenance treatment is often prescribed to prevent recurrence or for primary prevention of opportunistic diseases. Examples are aerosol pentamidine to prevent the occurrence of *Pneumocystis carinii* pneumonia (PCP) for patients with CD4 counts of less than 200 cells/mm^3 and INH (isoniazid) for patients with a positive Mantoux test (tuberculin skin test) who have no history of treatment for tuberculosis.[26]

The clinical trials being conducted by the National Institutes of Health as well as universities, pharmaceutical companies, and other agencies may be important considerations for persons with HIV disease. Patients with HIV disease may be able to participate in these clinical trials or may benefit from the results of the research studies. Nontraditional therapies are commonly used by persons with HIV disease for many reasons, some of which include: the limitations and side effects of approved treatments, the patient's determination to find a "cure" or at least some comfort, mistrust of the health care system, and the easy access to nontraditional therapies. Patients should be asked about what other therapies they may be using, and the therapies should be evaluated objectively.

NURSING INTERVENTIONS

The nurse needs to establish a comfort level in interacting with gay men and drug users before caring for persons with HIV disease. Patients with HIV disease need to be treated in a nonjudgmental, empathetic, and caring manner regardless of their sexual preference or drug-using history. The nurse must see the patient as a unique individual with a need to be cared for with compassion, consideration, and dignity. Knowledge of HIV transmission and competence in Universal Precautions will minimize fear of caring for the HIV-infected patient.[5]

Health care needs can be unpredictable and assessment difficult because of the clinical diversity of HIV infection. HIV disease may require alternating periods of long-term and acute care. The patient may fear isolation in the community or with family and friends because of the stigma of the disease.[16]

The nursing interventions for the patient with HIV disease will vary from simple nursing care to complex procedures related to the multiple physical and psychosocial problems of the disease. The psychosocial implications for the patient with HIV disease are generally complex. Patients with HIV disease have considerably more psychosocial problems than patients with other terminal illnesses. They face uncertainty, isolation, fear, and depression. The condition has no cure, it is contagious, it is fatal, and it has media attention. The stigma of the disease because of its association with drug use, homosexuality, and sexual transmission is a major concern. The patient often fears abandonment and isolation from family and friends or already has experienced it. The patient is usually young and may have limited financial resources. The patient may be gay and may be strug-

MEDICATIONS FOR AIDS

Medication	Trade Name	Action	Side Effects	Nursing Implications
Dapsone (DDS)	Avlosulfon, Dapsone	Leprostatic	Convulsions, megaloblastic anemia, exfoliative dermatitis, photosensitivity, headache, anxiety, disorientation, abdominal pain, anorexia, blurred vision, photophobia	Monitor renal and liver functions; administer with meals; compliance is very important because therapy may be long term.
Ganciclovir	Cytovene	Antiviral	Granulocytopenia, thrombocytopenia, irreversible neutropenia, anemia, eosinophilia, hemorrhage, coma, hematuria, retinal detachment, retinitis	Use contraception during treatment; have regular eye examinations during therapy, assess ISO; ensure that patient is adequately hydrated before and during therapy because drug is excreted through kidney.
Foscarnet sodium	Foscavir	Antiviral	Seizures, coma, paralysis, cardiac arrest, pseudomembranous colitis, eye changes, esophageal ulcerations, hepatitis, granulocytopenia, leukopenia, pulmonary embolism, thrombosis, anemia, leukocytosis, renal failure, pneumothorax, respiratory depression (Because Foscavir is nephrotoxic; it can worsen renal impairment.)	Monitor liver and renal function; monitor respirations, electrolyte levels, and heart; notify physician of all side effects; increase intravenous fluids to reduce renal toxicity.
Co-Trimoxazole (SMZ-TMP)	Bactrim, Septra	Antiinfective	Hepatitis, enterocolitis, leukopenia, neutropenia, hemolytic anemia, thrombocytopenia, Stevens-Johnson syndrome, renal failure, allergic myocarditis	Check sulfa allergy before initiating therapy; push fluids while on therapy; obtain specimen for culture and sensitivity tests before first dose; tell patient to take medication exactly as prescribed.
Fluconazole	Diflucan	Antifungal	Nausea, vomiting, diarrhea, cramping, increased alanine aminotransferase (ALT) and aspartate aminotransferase (AST)	Monitor renal and liver function; know that long-term therapy may be required; know that the incidence of adverse reactions appears to be greater in HIV-infected patients.
Amphotercin-B	Fungizone	Antifungal	Convulsions, permanent renal damage, acute liver failure, ototoxicity, hemorrhagic gastroenteritis, arthralgia, thrombocytopenia, agranulocytosis, leukopenia, eosinophilia, nausea and vomiting, anorexia, headache, rash, chills	Avoid use with other nephrotoxic drugs if possible; monitor renal and liver functions; watch for hypokalemia; report tinnitus or other hearing changes.

Continued.

MEDICATIONS FOR AIDS—cont'd

Medication	Trade Name	Action	Side Effects	Nursing Implications
Epoetin-Alpha	Epogen, Procrit	Hematopoietic agent	Seizures, headache, nausea, vomiting, diarrhea, rash, iron deficiency, elevated platlet count, hypertension	Monitor blood count and blood pressure.
Zidovudine	AZT, Retrovir	Antiviral	Granulocytopenia, anemia, fever, headache, malaise, insomnia, dizziness, confusion, nausea, vomiting, diarrhea, anorexia, mouth ulcers, taste changes, hearing loss	Get blood counts every 2 weeks: does not cure AIDS but only reduces symptoms; report sore throat, lymph node swelling, malaise, or fever to physician; remind patients that they must comply with 4-hour dosage schedule.
Acyclovir	Zovirax	Antiviral	Convulsions, tremors, confusion, dizziness, headache, bone marrow depression, nausea, vomiting, diarrhea, increased ALT and AST, vaginitis, acute renal failure, rash, itching	Avoid during pregnancy: does not cure infection but lessens symptoms; take around clock; report hematuria, weakness, and fatigue to physician; monitor blood counts and liver function.
Dideoxyinosine (DDI), Didanosine	Videx	Antiviral	Pancreatitis, diarrhea and vomiting, liver abnormalities, dry mouth, increased ALT and AST, peripheral neuropathy, seizures, central nervous system depression, leukopenia, granulocytopenia, anemia, alopecia	Monitor blood count and liver function; report tingling of extremities and abdominal pain; administer on empty stomach; tell patient to chew tablets thoroughly before swallowing and drink at least 1 oz of water with each dose; teach patients receiving a sodium-restricted diet that each two-tablet dose contains 529 mg of sodium.
Dideoxycytidine (DDC)	Zalcitabine	Antiviral	Pancreatitis, diarrhea and vomiting, liver abnormalities, dry mouth, increased ALT and AST, peripheral neuropathy, seizures, central nervous system depression, leukopenia, granulocytopenia, anemia, alopecia	Monitor blood count and liver function; report tingling of extremities and abdominal pain; make certain patient understands that drug does not cure HIV infection and that opportunistic infections may still occur despite continued use.
Pentamidine Isethionate	Nebupent, Pentam 300	Antiprotazoal	Thrombocytopenia, anemia, leukopenia, acute renal failure, pancreatitis, electrocardiographic abnormalities, increased ALT and AST, metallic taste, hypotension, dizziness, confusion, hallucinations	Have patient lie down for treatment and monitoring of blood pressure; Administered via intravenous, intramuscular, or inhalation routes; know that pain and induration occur universally with intramuscular injection; Administer deep intramuscular injection.

gling with his own sexuality and acceptance from his family and community. The patient may be a young, single woman with children who has no financial resources or family support. She may be more concerned about her children than her own physical or emotional needs. Nurses need to establish support for their own feelings of sympathy and helplessness in the difficult situation so often accompanying the patient with HIV disease or AIDS. Words are one way to convey caring; listening is another important tool; however, the nurse may find it difficult to know what to say. The nurse can develop a good therapeutic relationship with the patient by allowing the patient to assist and participate in the planning of care and decisions regarding care.[18] (See the Therapeutic Dialogue.)

THERAPEUTIC DIALOGUE

Nurse: I need to take a look at the abscess on your anus.

Patient: Do you have to? I take care of it myself, and I do a portable sitz bath after every stool. I keep it real clean.

Nurse: I'm sure it bothers you to have people look . . . *(Recognizes patient's sensitivity)*

Patient: Well, everybody wants to look. I've shown it so many times, I guess one more wouldn't hurt. I get so tired of it though. *(Does not look at nurse while speaking)*

Nurse: Have you had the abscess a long time? *(Gives patient space by verbalizing rather than going directly to the exam)*

Patient: Yeah, it's been draining for almost 2 months now, but it isn't as painful and it doesn't drain so much anymore.

Nurse: Well, if it's ok with you, I could look at it today, and then later on I would be able to tell you how much improvement is made. If not, I could wait and assess it on my next visit, whichever you'd rather. *(This allows the patient to help make the decision. Nurse looks directly at the patient to show she is not uncomfortable.)* Actually, I wouldn't have to assess it every visit. *(Allows patient some control over his plan of care)*

Patient: Well go ahead. Be sure you wear gloves because it's draining some. Be careful, it hurts if you press on it. Some nurses are rough. *(Patient shows concern for the caregiver while expressing own needs)*

Nurse: There are signs of improvement. No deep redness . . . there is still some deeper pink color around the open area. Obviously you are doing a good job with the sitz baths. *(Nurse shows concern and regard for the patient)*

A multidisciplinary care approach seems to be the most appropriate method to care for patients with HIV disease because of their complex needs. The patient should be the primary member of the multidisciplinary team, along with the primary care physician, social worker or case manager, and the nurse. Other team members may include a dentist, dietitian, mental health worker, substance use counselor, as well as members of the patient's family or significant others.

The disease affects primarily young people at the most productive time in their lives. It is a time when they are expected to take control of their own lives, and they want to have an active role in the decision making and planning for their own care. They may experience bouts of serious, debilitating illness and then recover enough to function effectively for an unpredictable period. Persons with HIV disease often prefer to stay at home as long as possible, and some prefer to die at home. Long-term care in an inpatient setting is not very compatible with the social needs of the young patient. Prolonged care is expensive, and many patients with HIV disease do not have health insurance. Alternative care is an important consideration in the care plan of the patient with HIV disease. Volunteers through churches and AIDS service organizations are known to provide support and care services for the patient and families. Friends, family, and significant others are important resources to be considered when planning care for the patient with HIV disease.[36]

Infection control is essential for the patient with a challenged immune system. The patient's room needs to be damp mopped and dusted daily to minimize the exposure to airborne organisms. Incontinent diarrhea is a common occurrence requiring additional cleaning. Food needs to be adequately cleaned and cooked to destroy any potentially infectious organisms. The patient needs to be instructed and supported in good personal hygiene and skin care. Showers are recommended whenever possible. The patient with chronic diarrhea requires frequent cleansing with a gentle soap and application of lotion to prevent skin impairment. The patient who is more debilitated may need an air mattress, frequent turning, and application of emollients to prevent skin impairment.[29] Guidelines for the care of the patient with HIV infection/AIDS are given in Box 37-5 on p. 1180. The most important infection control factor in protecting the immunocompromised patient from infections is consistent good handwashing techniques by care givers, visitors, and the patient. Visitors and care providers need to monitor their own health to avoid exposing the patient to unnecessary pathogens, particularly airborne illness (see Chapter 12). Nursing interventions for patients with the various HIV diseases and treatments are described in Table 37-3 and the care plan on pp. 1181-1182.[30]

Assisting With Coping

Individuals who are exposed to HIV infection, but who are without symptoms or complications of infections or cancers, live with a great deal of uncertainty and anxiety interspersed with denial and hopefulness. The role of the nurse in this stage of the disease process is to provide continued education about AIDS, as well as to assist in realistic goal setting. Patients are encouraged to participate in their own care and to maintain positive relationships.

As the HIV infection progresses through the clinical complications of infections and cancers, patients experience multiple losses, including loss of energy, self-care deficit requiring assistance with activities of daily living (ADLs), and loss of independence, employment, finances, and hope. The reality of death emerges. Nursing interventions focuses on a philosophy of facing life a day at a time and living each day to the fullest extent possible by resolving multiple conflicts. This may be a time for strengthening personal and spiritual relationships.

Empathic listening and the ability to help patients find meaning in life become critical nursing interventions. Assisting families and significant others in providing support to the terminally ill patient despite their own anger and grief is a unique nursing challenge. Such care, although emotionally draining for the nurse, can provide positive feelings of professional accomplishment.

The diagnosis of HIV infection, with its social stigma, poor prognosis, and lethal nature, is indeed a cata-

Box 37-5

CARING FOR THE PATIENT WITH HIV INFECTION/AIDS

PREVENT INFECTION

1. Wash hands frequently and use emollient for patient and caregiver.
2. Use a gentle liquid soap (such as Castile); avoid bar soaps, which may irritate skin.
3. Provide for daily showering or basin bath; avoid tub bath if rashes are present.
4. Use a separate wash cloth for lesions.
5. Use soft toothbrushes; nonabrasive toothpaste; and mouth rinses with sodium bicarbonate, saline, or lemon and hydrogen peroxide before meals and at bedtime.
6. Use measures to prevent skin impairment, such as turning sheets, sheepskin, eggcrate or air mattresses.
7. Elevate and support areas of edema.
8. Observe biopsy sites and IV insertion sites daily for signs of infection.
9. Change dressings at least every other day; avoid plastic occlusive dressings.
10. Avoid sources of microbes, such as uncooked plants or ingestion of fresh fruits and vegetables.
11. Carry out measures to prevent spread of infection: use gloves for contact with bodily secretions, double plastic bags to dispose of bodily secretions, use bleach and water (1 : 10) for cleaning contaminated areas.

MODIFY ALTERATIONS IN BODY TEMPERATURE

1. Administer prescribed antibiotics, IV fluids, or antipyretics.
2. Encourage fluid intake >2500 ml.
3. Maintain daily I & O records.
4. Weigh daily.
5. Provide tepid sponge baths and linen changes as necessary.
6. Instruct patient in deep-breathing and coughing exercises to prevent atelectasis and additional fever.

PROMOTE GOOD NUTRITION

1. Provide instruction for high-calorie, high-protein, high-potassium, low-residue diet.
2. Encourage high-calorie, high-potassium snacks.
3. Suggest foods that are easy to swallow (gelatin, yogurt, puddings) when dysphagia is present.
4. Avoid foods that are spicy or acidic, rare meats, and raw fruits and vegetables.
5. Provide oral care before patient eats.
6. Encourage patient to get out of bed and sit up for meals if possible.
7. Avoid odors by aerating room.
8. Make appropriate dietary consultations.

PROMOTE SELF-CARE

1. Assess realistic functional ability.
2. Plan, supervise, and assist with ADLs as necessary.
3. Encourage patient to be as active and independent as possible.
4. Assist patient with range-of-motion exercise to prevent contractures.
5. Provide equipment such as assistive eating devices, walkers, and commodes to promote patient independence.
6. Pace activities and schedule rest periods to prevent fatigue.

PROVIDE COUNSELING

1. Assess and support patient coping mechanisms.
2. Explore with patient and significant others normalcy of grief.
3. Assist patient and significant others in acknowledging and planning for anticipated losses.
4. Provide information as desired and necessary, depending on patient's ability to understand.
5. Suggest appropriate religious support.
6. Facilitate participation in support groups or individual counseling as pertinent.

NURSING CARE PLAN THE PATIENT WITH AIDS

Mrs. Jules, a 32-year-old woman with AIDS, was admitted to the medical unit with *Pneumocystis carinii* pneumonia. Her temperature is 103°, her pulse is 110, and respirations are 38. She has diarrhea and anorexia and is in a cachexic state. She has coarse crackles bilaterally in all lung fields.

Nursing diagnoses	Patient outcomes/expected outcomes	Nursing interventions
Airway clearance, ineffective, related to infection, secretions	Airway will be patent. Patient will verbalize preventive measures. Patient will experience improved vital signs and breathing.	Elevate head of bed; change position every 2 hr; encourage deep breathing, coughing, exercises. Give medications as ordered. Assess for increased signs of respiratory distress. Teach patient contributing causes and prevention.
Nutrition, altered: less than body requirements, related to inadequate food intake and abdominal cramping with food ingestion	Patient will experience increase in body weight and appetite. Patient will report a decrease in abdominal cramping with use of antispasmodics.	Assess ability to chew. Note food intolerances; provide diet modifications and dietary supplements. Encourage foods that appeal to the patient. Provide frequent oral care. Weigh weekly. Assess needs for parenteral nutrition.
Activity intolerance, related to weakness	Patient will report measurable increase in activity tolerance.	Identify activities that are too strenuous; plan care with rest periods. Provide for progressive activity as patient tolerates. Inform patient when evidence of progress occurs.
Diarrhea, related to inflammation, irritation, or malabsorption	Patient will verbalize understanding of causative factors. Patient will experience improved bowel function. Patient will tolerate increased variety of foods. Patient will maintain adequate hydration.	Assess onset and pattern of diarrhea: record frequency, amount, characteristics. Assess for fecal impaction. Promote relaxation and decreased stress. Limit caffeine, high-fiber foods, milk, and fruits. Increase fluid intake. Record I & O if indicated. Apply skin barrier if needed to protect from skin impairment. Place disposable protective perineal garment if patient is incontinent.

Social isolation, related to altered state of wellness, alterations in physical appearance, and inability to engage in satisfying personal relationships	Patient will express increased sense of self-worth. Patient will demonstrate a trust in the health care provider. Patient will participate in community support group.	Assess patient's feelings about self. Identify support systems available to the patient, including family, friends, and community support groups. Establish a therapeutic relationship; spend time with patient; listen carefully; encourage verbalization of feelings. Involve patient with others having similar circumstances.
Skin integrity, impaired, related to disruption of skin surface, trauma	Patient will demonstrate behaviors to promote healing. Patient will experience improvement of wounds and lesions.	Inspect skin on a daily basis; describe lesions and changes observed; monitor for signs and symptoms of infections; keep area clean with mild soap and water. Perform and instruct in aseptic/clean technique for dressing changes and proper disposal of soiled dressings. Provide soaks if ordered; expose wound to air if indicated. Teach skin care.

CRITICAL THINKING QUESTIONS

1. Mrs. Jules is restless and complains of a feeling of suffocation. She attempts to drink a glass of water and begins to cough violently, becoming cyanotic. The immediate nursing intervention would be:
2. In performing ADLs for Mrs. Jules, the most beneficial type of bath would be:
3. As Mrs. Jules' condition improves, she tells the nurse of her depression because of the loss of her support system of family and friends. Present a therapeutic dialogue between the nurse and patient.

strophic event for patients and care givers. Patients experience a variety of intense emotions that threaten self-esteem and predispose to depression and feelings of powerlessness. Anxiety is a response that pervades the entire HIV illness continuum. Anxiety and denial often accompany the initial diagnosis and intensify with physical decline and loss of independence, job, and finances. Anxiety may become incapacitating as death becomes a reality. Nursing interventions to promote effective coping focus on exploring and strengthening healthful coping strategies and maintaining sources of psychological support.

Reducing Anxiety. Individuals experiencing the anxiety of HIV infection are often in a state of crisis. Continued clarification and education about the HIV infection, complications, and treatment are critical. Every effort should be made to include the patient in planning medical and nursing interventions. An assessment of past coping styles and support systems should be made early and continually reevaluated. Healthful patterns of coping, such as talking or relaxation and meditation, are encouraged. Relationships with family, friends, and lovers should be maintained and may be strengthened through the HIV crisis. Conversely, past conflicts, especially among family members, may persist and intensify during the HIV crisis.

Occasionally anxiety, denial, depression, and even grief may persist for extended periods, interfering with daily functioning, productive communication and relationships, and even the ability to make decisions. The nurse must be able to assess normal periods of anxiety, depression, and grief, as well as refer patients and significant others for psychological evaluation and counseling for ineffective coping patterns. Although reactions of anxiety and depression are normal, professional intervention is necessary whenever they preclude communication and daily functioning for an extended time (usually longer than 3 months). Patients with HIV infection and depression should be assessed for suicidal ideation because this phenomenon occasionally occurs in terminally ill patients who are experiencing anxiety and fear of further pain and physical decline. Early recognition of depression is critical because some cases of depression and anxiety may respond to medications and psychotherapy.

Individuals with diffuse anxiety often feel they have little control over their daily existence. A schedule of activities that patients develop with guidance from health care professionals may decrease anxiety and feelings of powerlessness. Opportunities for spiritual support and comfort should be explored. Significant others may also experience anxiety. Community support groups for patients and significant others may offer additional sources of support and contribute to healthful coping. Planned, uninterrupted time with only the nurse, patient, and significant other may create a supportive environment that decreases anxiety and promotes healthful coping.

Support Interactions to Minimize Social Isolation. The psychosocial aspects of AIDS are devastating. Because at present no cure exists for the HIV infection, the diagnosis of HIV infection, like a diagnosis of cancer, brings potential denial, fear, depression, and anger. The social stigma of AIDS, based on associations with homosexuality, intravenous drug abuse, and sexual transmission, cannot be minimized. One of the earliest issues that HIV-infected individuals face is sharing the information with significant others. Tremendous fear of family anger, rejection, or abandonment is a real concern.

Often families and friends who are struggling with their own anxieties and fears abandon the patient. When this happens, the nurse should try to assist the patient to find other sources of social support. In some cities there are support groups for patients and separate groups for significant others. HIV-infected individuals who have been exposed by contaminated blood or unknowingly through heterosexual relationships may feel unique and experience intense anger and hostility. These patients are usually supported by their families and friends. They can be isolated by other persons who do not understand that HIV and AIDS are not spread by casual contact.

Assist With Grieving

As with patients with other terminal illnesses, patients diagnosed with the HIV infection may experience strong emotions of fear, anger, denial, or quiet depression. Some patients benefit from individual empathic listening and exploring feelings, fears, and treatment options. Other patients may benefit from support groups with patients experiencing similar feelings. Significant others, including family and lovers, experience their own feelings of fear, anger, and embarrassment. Individual counseling and support groups may be helpful for loved ones who will need to be a source of support for the patient. Practical issues such as employment disability, housing discrimination, insurance coverage, and preparation for death also need to be addressed. Referral to social workers and appropriate community agencies can alleviate many concerns that plague acutely and terminally ill patients. Continued participation in religious services and the support of fellow worshippers and clergy should not be overlooked as a source of healthy coping. Many members of the clergy are experienced in grief counseling and can be helpful to patients and significant others.

Confidentiality

Respect for the patient's right to confidentiality is particularly important for the patient with HIV disease. The diagnosis of HIV disease needs to be carefully protected and shared only with the care givers who need to know for purposes of providing care and treatment. Otherwise, the patient should be in control of who is told of the diagnosis. The nurse should have the utmost respect for the patient's right to confidentiality, meaning the patient or the diagnosis is not discussed at mealtime, during breaks, or with coworkers, friends, or family.

HIV disease/AIDS has taught health care providers to be more aware of the human condition so that they can deal with their own prejudices, judgments, and concerns. Health care providers are challenged by the patient with HIV disease or AIDS, whose needs and suffering require more than nursing skill, education, and technology. A spirit of compassion stemming from a genuine willingness to serve the needs of another is essential in caring for the patient with AIDS.

REFERENCES AND SUGGESTED READINGS

1. Anastasi JK: Caring for patients with diarrhea. Half of HIV positive patients will develop diarrhea. Learn how to cope, *Nursing* 23(8):68, 1993.
2. Bellet PS, Maloney MG: The importance of empathy as an intervening skill in medicine, *JAMA* 266(13):1831, 1991.
3. Bender B: Outpatient management of patients infected with human immunodeficiency virus, *J Fam Pract* 34(4):464, 1992.
4. Bradley-Springer L: Human immunodeficiency virus infection, *J Assoc Nurses AIDS Care* 4(1):37, 1993.
5. Breault A, Polifroni E: Caring for people with AIDS: nurses' attitudes and feelings, *J Adv Nurs* 17:21, 1992.
6. Catania JA, Coater TJ: Prevalence of AIDS related risk factors and condom use in the United States, *Science* 258(5085):1101, 1992.
7. Centers for Disease Control: Guidelines for the performance of CD4+ T-cell determinations in persons with human immunodeficiency virus infection, *MMWR* 41(RR-8):1, 1992.
8. Centers for Disease Control: *HIV/AIDS prevention training,* Bull No 25, February 1993.
9. Centers for Disease Control: *HIV/AIDS surveillance:* U.S. AIDS cases reported through December 1992, 1993.
10. Centers for Disease Control: Interpretive criteria used to report Western blot results for HIV-1-antibody testing: United States, *MMWR* 40(40):692, 1991.

11. Centers for Disease Control: 1993 revised classification for HIV infection and expanded surveillance case definition for AIDS among adolescents and adults, *MMWR* 41 (RR-17), December 1992.
12. Centers for Disease Control: Purified protein derivative (PPD)—tuberculin anergy and HIV infection: guidelines for anergy testing and management of anergic persons at risk of tuberculosis, *MMWR* 40(RR-5):27, April 1991.
13. Centers for Disease Control: Recommendation for HIV testing services for inpatients and outpatients in acute-care hospital settings and technical guidance on HIV counseling, *MMWR* 42 (RR-2), January 1993.
14. Centers for Disease Control: Recommendations for preventing transmission of human immunodeficiency virus and hepatitis B virus to patients during exposure from invasive procedures, *MMWR* 40 (RR-8), July 1991.
15. Centers for Disease Control: The second 100,000 cases of acquired immunodeficiency syndrome—United States, June 1981-December 1991, *MMWR* 41:28, January 1992.
16. Centers for Disease Control: Update: acquired immunodeficiency syndrome—United States, 1981-1990, *MMWR* 40:358, July 1991.
17. Centers for Disease Control: Update: investigations of persons treated by HIV-infected health workers—United States, *MMWR* 42:329, May 1993.
18. Centers for Disease Control: Update: transmission of HIV infection during invasive dental procedures—Florida, *MMWR* 40:377-381, July 1991.
19. De Horritz J, Sadoresky R: Initial clinical assessment and management of HIV, *RN* 56(5):34, 1993.
20. Ferrell JA, Boyle JS: Bereavement experiences: caring for a partner with AIDS, *J Community Health Nurs* 9(3):127, 1992.
21. Flaskerud JH: HIV disease and levels of prevention, *J Community Health Nurs* 9(3):137, 1992.
22. Fredericks CM: Helping Ben live and die his way, *Nursing* 22(9):59, 1992.
23. Gauthier AM: Would you divulge confidential information about a patient's HIV status? *Nursing* 22(10):59, 1992.
24. Gollub EL, Stein ZA: Commentary: the new female condom: item 1 on a women's AIDS prevention agenda, *Am J Public Health* 83(4):498, 1993.
25. Greenspan A, Gastro K: Heterosexual transmission of HIV infection, *Siecus Report* 19(1), October/November 1990.
26. Jewett J, Hecht F: Preventive health care for adults with HIV infection, *JAMA* 269(9):1144, 1993.
27. Kelley PK et al: The new face of AIDS, *Am J Nurs* 93(3):26, March 1993.
28. Kling C, Reily WD: Transcending AIDS, *Hospice,* p 24, Summer 1992.
29. Long B, Phipps W, Cassmeyer V: *Medical-surgical nursing: a nursing process approach,* ed 3, St Louis, 1993, Mosby.
30. Maier D et al: *HIV/AIDS curriculum: Mountain-Plains Regional AIDS Education and Training Center,* ed 4, September 1992.
31. Merson M: Slowing the spread of HIV: agenda for the 1990s, *Science* 260:1266, 1993.
32. Mudge-Grout CL: *Immunologic diseases,* St Louis, 1992, Mosby.
33. National Commission on AIDS: *The challenge of HIV/AIDS in communities of color,* Washington, DC, December 1992.
34. Otten Jr MW et al: Changes in sexually transmitted disease rates after HIV testing and posttest counseling, Miami, 1988 to 1989, *Am J Public Health* 83(4):529, 1993.
35. Piette JD et al: The effects of immune status and race on health service use among people with HIV disease, *Am J Public Health* 83(4):510, 1993.
36. Ragsdale D, Kotarba J, Merrow J: Quality of life of hospitalized person with AIDS, *Image J Nurs Sch* 24(4):, 1992.
37. Roper WL, Peterson HB, Curran JW: Commentary: condoms and HIV/STD prevention: clarifying the message, *Am J Public Health* 83(4):501, 1993.
38. Rosenberg Z, Fauci A: Activation of latent HIV infection, *J NIH Res* 2:41, July 1992.
39. Sandi MA, Volberding PA: *Medical management of AIDS,* Philadelphia, 1990, Saunders.
40. Smeltzer SW: Women and HIV infection, *Image J Nurs Sch* 23(4):249, 1991.
41. Tannenbaum I: Women and HIV, *RN* 56(5):34, 1993.
42. US Department of Health and Human Services: Role of bleach in human immunodeficiency virus prevention programs for injecting drug users, *HIV/AIDS Prevention Bulletin,* April 19, 1993.
43. Weiss R: How does HIV cause AIDS? *Science* 260:1273, 1993.
44. Wofsy C: Clinical manifestations of HIV in women, *AIDS File* 5(3):3, 1991.

CHAPTER CHALLENGE

KEY POINTS

- HIV, a retrovirus, is the agent that causes HIV disease and AIDS.
- Education is our only "vaccine" for preventing HIV disease and AIDS.
- Women and children constitute the fastest growing segment of the population with AIDS.
- AIDS is the end stage of HIV infection.
- When HIV enters the body, its primary target is the immune system.
- HIV is transmitted by three major routes:
  1. Anal and vaginal intercourse
  2. Injecting drugs with contaminated needles/works
  3. From infected mother to child
- Blood, semen, vaginal secretions, and breast milk are the body fluids that most readily transmit HIV.
- Nurses have a responsibility to assess each patient's risks for HIV infection and counsel those at risk about testing, behaviors that put them at risk, and how to eliminate or reduce those risks.
- A positive HIV antibody test does not mean the patient has AIDS.
- A multidisciplinary care approach in which the patient is a primary member of the team is the most appropriate method to care for patients with HIV disease because of their complex needs.
- As HIV infection progresses, the immune system loses its ability to fight infectious agents and cancer cells.
- Patients at risk for HIV infection should be encouraged to know their HIV status.
- Whether or not signs and symptoms are present, a person infected with HIV virus can transmit the virus.
- Barriers to HIV prevention include denial, fear, misinformation, and cultural and community norms.
- CD4 counts are important markers of disease progression and the status of the immune system.
- The stigma of HIV disease, because of its association with drug use, homosexuality, and sexual transmission, is a major concern.
- The 1993 expanded case definition of AIDS includes all HIV-infected persons who have CD4 T-lymphocyte counts of less than 200 cells/mm^3; includes all persons who have one or more of these three clinical conditions—pulmonary tuberculosis, recurrent pneumonia, or invasive cervical cancer; and retains the 23 clinical conditions listed in the 1987 AIDS case definition.

STUDY QUESTIONS

1. Jane Smith, age 28, has been informed by her physician that she has AIDS, and she asks the nurse, "What causes AIDS?" The nurse's response should be that:
   1. It is caused by the common herpes, the same virus that causes cold sores
   2. The agent that causes AIDS is the human immunodeficiency virus
   3. Cytomegalovirus is the cause of AIDS, a virus to which most people have been exposed
   4. AIDS is caused by *Cryptococcus,* an infectious agent that is usually not a problem except when the body's immune system is unable to fight infections
2. Mrs. Jones' husband asks the nurse to move his wife to another room because, "I heard the woman in the bed next to my wife has HIV and I'm afraid my wife will catch it. They use the same phone and the same bathroom." The nurse's response should be that HIV is not transmitted by casual contact, such as sharing phones or the toilet seat; it is spread only through contact with the following body fluids:
   1. Blood, vaginal secretions, semen, and breast milk
   2. Tears, saliva, sweat, and blood
   3. Urine, feces, vomit, and blood
   4. Sweat, semen, vaginal secretions, and saliva

3. Mr. Conley, a patient in the emergency room, was told by the physician that he will be tested for HIV. How would the lab determine whether Mr. Conley's blood was seropositive for HIV?
   1. By two positive ELISA tests and a positive Western blot test
   2. By a positive Western blot test
   3. By two positive ELISA tests
   4. By a positive ELISA test
4. Mr. Conley has been told by his physician that his HIV test results are positive. The nurse has a responsibility to discuss the major routes of HIV transmission with him. Which of the following routes of transmission would she discuss:
   1. Food, water, air
   2. Mosquitoes, hot tubs, dirty toilets
   3. Intercourse, sharing needles, mother-to-child
   4. Receiving blood, intercourse, kissing
5. A colleague says to you, "Jane is not at risk for HIV, she has been married for 10 years and has two children. We don't need to assess her risks." The most appropriate response would be:
   1. You are correct, the greatest risk is with gay men.
   2. The fastest-growing segments of the population with AIDS are women and children. We need to assess her risks.
   3. We don't need to be concerned about married women like Jane; she's in a monogamous relationship.
   4. We'll just review her chart and see if she has any past history that would be indicative of risks.
6. In reviewing the chart of Mr. Brown, who has HIV disease, what would be an important marker to determine the progression of his HIV disease?
   1. Weight loss
   2. CD4 counts
   3. Presence of Kaposi's sarcoma
   4. Fever/chills
7. Ms. Romeo has been informed by her physician that she is infected with HIV. She asks the nurse, "How long do I have to live?" The nurse's most appropriate response would be:
   1. A patient with HIV infection can be expected to develop signs and symptoms of HIV disease within 6 months.
   2. Some people with HIV infection live up to 12 years without symptoms.
   3. AIDS usually occurs within 2 years after infection.
   4. Most people with HIV infection live up to 10 years after infection.
8. Jim was admitted with *Pneumocystis carinii* pneumonia and learned for the first time that he is HIV positive. He questions the nurse, "How does HIV cause this pneumonia?" The nurse's response should be:
   1. HIV attacks the respiratory system, making the lungs more susceptible to other organisms.
   2. HIV attacks the immune system, a system that protects the body from foreign invaders, making it unable to fight organisms such as the one causing your pneumonia.
   3. HIV attacks the circulatory system, decreasing the blood and oxygen supply to the lungs, making them more susceptible to organisms such as the one causing your pneumonia.
   4. HIV attacks the digestive system, decreasing the absorption of essential nutrients, making the body unable to maintain its oxygen and energy sources.
9. Jason, a patient treated for chlamydia, says, "I don't have sex with anyone who looks like they have AIDS." The nurse, in the process of informing him about the transmission of HIV, should confirm that HIV can be transmitted:
   1. At the time of seroconversion
   2. After the development of HIV disease
   3. From the time someone is infected until death
   4. After the diagnosis of AIDS
10. Jason, after being treated for chlamydia, is assessed for risks of HIV. The nurse discovers that Jason has had other sexually transmitted diseases and has had multiple male partners in the last 6 months. The nurse's most appropriate response would be to:
    1. Counsel Jason about abstinence and monogamous relationships
    2. Counsel Jason about the importance of knowing his HIV status and what the HIV test results mean
    3. Omit counseling because Jason was counseled about risk reduction when he had his last STD
    4. Reinforce risk reduction, including the use of condoms with every act of sexual intercourse, and counsel Jason about knowing his HIV status

38

CARE OF THE PATIENT WITH CANCER

Joyce E. Myers
Janice Bridges Flynn

KEY TERMS

alopecia
autologous
benign
biopsy
cachexia
carcinogen
carcinoma
differentiated
immunosurveillance
leukopenia
malignant
mammogram
metastasis
neoplasm
oncology
palliative
Papanicolaou test
sarcoma
stomatitis
thrombocytopenia

LEARNING OBJECTIVES

After reading this chapter, the student should be able to do the following:

- Define the key terms.
- List seven risk factors for the development of cancer.
- State seven warning signs of cancer.
- Indicate the incidence of cancer as one of the leading causes of death in the United States.
- Define terminology used to describe cellular changes, characteristics of malignant cells, and types of malignancies.
- Describe the major categories of chemotherapeutic agents.
- Describe the process of metastasis.
- Explain common reasons for delay in seeking medical care when a diagnosis of cancer is suspected.
- List common diagnostic tests used to identify the presence of cancer.
- Explain why biopsy is essential in confirming a diagnosis of cancer.
- Define the systems of tumor classification: *grading* and *staging*.
- Discuss six general guidelines for the use of pain relief measures for the patient with advanced cancer.
- Describe the nursing interventions for the individual undergoing surgery, radiation therapy, chemotherapy, immunotherapy, or bone marrow transplantation.

RELATED TOPICS OF INTEREST

- Diet therapy (Chapter 19)
- The surgical patient (Chapter 22)
- Care of the patient with a reproductive disorder (Chapter 33)
- Care of the patient with an immune disorder (Chapter 36)
- Loss, grief, dying, and death (Chapter 52)
- Hospice care (Chapter 53)

Oncology is the sum of knowledge regarding tumors; it is the branch of medicine that deals with the study of tumors. Oncology nursing is the care of people with cancer. Until the recognition of AIDS, probably no other medical diagnosis produced as much fear as cancer. The American Cancer Society indicates that in a lifetime, cancer will affect three of four families in the United States. Approximately one out of three Americans will someday develop cancer. Of every five deaths in the United States from all causes, one is from cancer. Cancer is the second leading cause of death.

Cancer is not one disease, but a group of diseases characterized by uncontrolled growth and spread of abnormal cells. Early detection and prompt treatment can cure some cancers and slow the progression of others. If not detected and/or controlled, cancer can result in death. Overall, cancer affects people of all ages, but occurs more frequently in the aged and the very young. More children, ages 3 to 14, die of cancer than of any other disease.

Lung cancer is the leading cause of cancer-related death in both men and women. Other cancers, such as breast and prostate, occur more often than lung cancer but have a better cure and survival rate due to early detection and treatment (Fig. 38-1).

PREVENTION AND DETECTION OF CANCER

Carcinogenesis and the Primary Prevention of Cancer

Carcinogenesis is the term used for the various factors that are possible origins of cancer. Primary prevention of cancer consists of changes in life-style habits to eliminate or reduce exposure to **carcinogens,** which are substances known to increase the risk for the development of cancer.

Risk factors include the following:

1. *Smoking:* According to the American Cancer Society, smoking is the most preventable cause of death from lung cancer. It is estimated that about 87% of people who develop lung cancer are smokers. Other cancers associated with smoking

CANCER INCIDENCE BY SITE AND SEX*

Male	Female
PROSTATE 132,000	BREAST 180,000
LUNG 102,000	COLON & RECTUM 77,000
COLON & RECTUM 79,000	LUNG 66,000
BLADDER 38,500	UTERUS 45,500
LYMPHOMA 27,200	LYMPHOMA 21,200
ORAL 20,600	OVARY 21,000
MELANOMA OF THE SKIN 17,000	MELANOMA OF THE SKIN 15,000
KIDNEY 16,200	PANCREAS 14,400
LEUKEMIA 16,000	BLADDER 13,100
STOMACH 15,000	LEUKEMIA 12,200
PANCREAS 13,900	KIDNEY 10,300
LARYNX 10,000	ORAL 9,700
ALL SITES 565,000	ALL SITES 565,000

*Excluding nonmelanoma skin cancer and carcinoma in situ.

CANCER DEATHS BY SITE AND SEX

Male	Female
LUNG 93,000	LUNG 53,000
PROSTATE 34,000	BREAST 46,000
COLON & RECTUM 28,900	COLON & RECTUM 29,400
PANCREAS 12,000	PANCREAS 13,000
LYMPHOMA 10,900	OVARY 13,000
LEUKEMIA 9,900	UTERUS 10,000
STOMACH 8,000	LYMPHOMA 10,000
ESOPHAGUS 7,500	LEUKEMIA 8,300
LIVER 6,600	LIVER 5,700
BRAIN 6,500	BRAIN 5,300
KIDNEY 6,400	STOMACH 5,300
BLADDER 6,300	MULTIPLE MYELOMA 4,500
ALL SITES 275,000	ALL SITES 245,000

FIG. 38-1 Comparison of cancer incidence and deaths by site and sex (1992 estimates). (Redrawn from American Cancer Society: *Cancer facts and figures,* Atlanta, 1993, The Society.)

are: bladder, kidney, mouth, pharynx, larynx, esophagus, pancreas, uterine, and cervix.

2. *Dietary habits:* When it comes to preventing cancer, is diet really important? Experts believe diet is very important. According to the National Institutes of Health, over one third of cancer deaths in 1992 may be related to diet. Diet plays a role in the development of cancer of the colon, rectum, and breast. A diet high in fiber and low in fat is recommended for prevention (Box 38-1). To teach Americans how to improve their diets, the National Cancer Institute (NCI) has launched a program called "5 a Day for Better Health." It aims to show how easy it is to add at least five servings of fruits and vegetables to the daily diet as a way of reducing the risks of cancer. Obesity is a risk factor for breast, prostate, gallbladder, ovarian, and uterine cancers.[7]
3. *Exposure to radiation:* Excessive exposure to the ultraviolet rays of the sun is a factor in the development of basal and squamous cell skin cancers and melanoma. Sunlamps and tanning booths also emit ultraviolet rays and have the same risks as sunlight. In addition, the effects of radiation commonly used for medical diagnosis and treatment are known to be carcinogenic. (Exposure should be limited and monitored.)
4. *Exposure to environmental and chemical carcinogens:* Some of these include fumes from rubber and chlorine, dust from cotton and coal, dust from nickel, chromate, asbestos, and vinyl chloride. There is a greater incidence of bladder cancer among people who live in urban areas and among those who work with dyes, rubber, or leather.
5. *Smokeless tobacco:* Use increases the risk of cancer of the mouth, larynx, throat, and esophagus.
6. *Frequent heavy consumption of alcohol:* This may result in oral cancer and cancer of the larynx, throat, esophagus, and liver.

Detection of Cancer

Detection of cancer includes the following measures:

1. Planned periodic examinations and the recognition of cancer's warning signals (Box 38-2), which enable the individual to obtain medical attention early. Early detection provides the time needed to diagnose and initiate treatment before cancer has reached an advanced stage.
2. Colorectal tests (men and women)
   a. Digital-rectal examination every year after age 40
   b. Hematest stool for blood every year after age 50
   c. Proctosigmoidoscopy every 3 to 5 years after age 50
3. Prostate cancer detection
   a. Prostate-specific antigen (PSA) test yearly for men over 50
   b. Yearly digital examination for men over 40
4. Pelvic examination for women must include a Papanicolaou test: annually after 18 years of age.
5. Breast cancer detection
   a. Monthly self-examination (men and women)
   b. Part of physical examination (men and women)
   c. **Mammogram** (x-ray study of the breast; use of radiography of the breast to diagnose breast cancer) baseline needed age 35 to 39; then ev-

Box 38-1 FOODS TO REDUCE CANCER RISK

- Vegetables from the cabbage family, such as:
  broccoli
  cauliflower
  brussels sprouts
  all types of cabbage and kale
- Vegetables high in β-carotene, such as:
  carrots squash
  peaches broccoli
  apricots
- Rich sources of vitamin C, such as:
  grapefruit red and green peppers
  oranges broccoli
  canteloupe tomatoes
  strawberries
- The National Cancer Institute has recommended including at least five servings of fruits and vegetables in the daily diet.
- Lean meat, fish, skinned poultry
- Low-fat dairy products, including white cheese rather than yellow
- Avoid salt-cured, smoked, or nitrite-cured foods

Box 38-2 CANCER'S SEVEN WARNING SIGNALS

If you have a warning signal, see your doctor.

1. Change in bowel or bladder habits
2. A sore that does not heal
3. Unusual bleeding or discharge
4. Thickening or lump in breast or elsewhere
5. Indigestion or difficulty in swallowing
6. Obvious change in wart or mole
7. Nagging cough or hoarseness

ery 1 or 2 years, based on findings; every year after age 50 (women only). Mammography can detect a mass before it can be felt.

It is reported that 4 of 10 patients (40%) who are diagnosed with cancer today will be alive 5 years after diagnosis. If other problems are not also present, such as heart disease, accidents, and old age, the expected survival rate may increase to 51%.[7]

Beginning at the high school years, all women should be taught to examine their breasts each month, 2 or 3 days after the menstrual period ends. After menopause, a woman should choose a day to help remind her, such as the first day of each month. A woman needs to become familiar with the appearance and feel of her breasts. This will help her identify any change from one month to the next. Any abnormality, such as a discharge from nipples, puckering, dimpling, or scaling of the skin and the palpation of lump or thickness, is significant.

The following is a guide in examining the breasts:

1. Inspect the breasts before a mirror; raise arms behind head and also place hands on hips with shoulders and elbows pulled forward; gently squeeze the nipples to determine if any discharge is present.
2. While bathing, when the breasts and hands are wet, slide the fingers over the skin to check each breast with the opposite hand; use the flat surface of two or three fingers; this is a good practice for men, as well as women.
3. In the lying-down position, place a towel or small pillow under the shoulder of the breast being examined to flatten the breast and make it easier to feel; use the flat surface of two or three fingers of the hand opposite the side being examined; gently palpate each breast, moving in at least three circles of different distances from the nipple at different points, such as 1 o'clock, 2 o'clock, 3 o'clock, and continuing to the 12 o'clock position.

The upper, outer tail of the breast that extends to the axilla and the entire axillary area must also be checked (see Chapter 33).

Nurses should teach breast self-examination to all patients, emphasizing that any problem identified should be brought to the attention of a physician. Any delay is a waste of valuable time if cancer is present.

Men should be taught to check the scrotum for enlargement, thickening, or the presence of a lump felt in the testicles. This should be done monthly, after a warm bath or shower. It should be emphasized that a physician must be contacted to determine the significance in any changes from the normal, smooth consistency of the testes (see Chapter 33). Men over 50 should be advised to have a PSA (prostate-specific antigen) and rectal exam once a year. Symptoms of blood in the urine, a weak flow of urine, or problems urinating should be reported to the physician.

A common reason for delay in diagnosing cancer is because early malignant changes do not produce pain. Cancer may be insidious in onset and may often be far advanced before the individual experiences any symptoms.

PATHOPHYSIOLOGY OF CANCER

Normal cells divide and make new cells that are like the parent cells. When malignant cells change, they become unlike parent cells. They are not differentiated or recognizable as being the same in size or shape as normal cells. Cancer cells can divide and multiply but not in a normal manner. Instead of limiting their growth to meet specific needs of the body, they continue to reproduce in a disorderly and unrestricted manner. The cellular features of cancer cells are a local increase in the number of cells, loss of normal cellular arrangement, variation in cell shape and size, increased nuclear size, increased mitotic activity, and abnormal mitosis and chromosomes.

Neoplasm is the term for uncontrolled or abnormal growth of cells. Neoplasms may be **benign** (not recurrent or progressive) or **malignant** (growing worse, resisting treatment; said of cancerous growths [Table 38-1]). The growths are also called *tumors,* which means swelling or enlargement. They may be localized or invasive. Benign tumors may become serious because of localized increase in growth with damage to surrounding tissues, such as a benign brain tumor. Malignant neoplasms may progress and destroy surrounding tissues. They may also metastasize from the primary site of origin to distant sites.

Metastasis (the process by which tumor cells are spread to distant parts of the body) is the term used to describe the movement of cancer cells from the primary site to a secondary site. Once cancer cells have moved

TABLE 38-1 General Characteristics of Neoplasms

Benign Tumors	Malignant Tumors
Slow, steady growth	Rate of growth varies—usually rapid
Remains localized	Metastasizes
Usually contained within a capsule	Rarely contained within a capsule
Smooth, well-defined, movable when palpated	Irregular; more immobile when palpated
Resembles parent tissue	Little resemblance to parent tissue
Crowds normal tissue	Invades normal tissue
Rarely recurs after removal	May recur after removal
Rarely fatal	Fatal without treatment

to another area of the body, secondary tumors may grow in that area. Metastasis can occur by the following mechanisms:

1. Direct spread of tumor cells by diffusion to other body cavities.
2. In the circulation by way of the blood and lymphatic channels.
3. Transplantation or the direct transport of tumor cells from one site to another. Transplantation may occur accidentally during surgery or other procedures when cancer cells are "carried" on instruments or gloves.

In addition to the identified carcinogenic factors that may cause malignant cellular changes, certain viruses have been suspected. There is also evidence to suggest that there are genetic factors that result in the predisposition to the development of cancer.

The body's immune system is responsible for recognizing and destroying malignant cells. The immune system may be weakened by cancer-producing substances, tumor cells, and the aging process.

Some T cells are responsible for **immunosurveillance** (the immune system's recognition and destruction of newly developed abnormal cells). When a cell becomes malignant, it carries a tumor-specific antigen on its membranes that is recognized as nonself and destroyed. If T cell function is suppressed by age, drugs (e.g., corticosteroids), poor nutrition, alcohol, serious infections, or certain disease processes (e.g., neoplastic invasion of bone and lymph tissue), the risk of cancer increases. To suppress T cell rejection of a transplanted organ, steroids and other drugs are administered. The resultant loss of immunosurveillance increases the risk of certain cancers.

Description, Grading, and Staging of Tumors

Tumors are described according to the parent tissue of the specific location in the body. **Carcinoma** is the term used for malignant tumors composed of epithelial cells, with a tendency to metastasize. **Sarcoma** refers to the malignant tumor of connective tissues such as muscle or bone usually presenting as a painless swelling. Sarcoma may affect the bones, bladder, kidneys, liver, lungs, parotids, and spleen.

Tumors are classified grade 1 to grade 4 by the degree of malignancy. Grade 1 is the most differentiated tumor (most like the parent tissue) and the least malignant. Grade 4 is the least **differentiated** (unlike parent tissue) tumor and highly malignant.

The tumor, node, metastasis (TNM) system of staging cancer is used to indicate tumor size, spread to lymph nodes, and extent of metastasis (Box 38-3). This system is used to direct treatment, predict prognosis, and contribute to cancer research by ensuring reliable comparison of different patients.

A tumor may be named for its location, its cellular makeup, or the person by whom it was identified.

Exfoliative (shedding of something) cytology (**Papanicolaou** [Pap] smear **test**) is a means of studying cells that the body has shed during the normal sequence of growth and replacement of body tissues. If cancer is present, cancer cells are also shed. It is used most commonly to detect cancers of the cervix, but it may be used for tissue specimens from any organ.

The results of the Pap test may be reported as:

Class 1 Absence of atypical or abnormal cells

Class 2 Atypical cytology but no evidence of malignancy (may indicate infection or inflammation)

Class 3 Cytology suggestive of but not conclusive for malignancy

Class 4 Cytology strongly suggestive of malignancy

Class 5 Cytology conclusive for malignancy

Except for a *Class 5 report,* abnormal Pap test reports require additional examination of tissue to confirm a diagnosis.

Box 38-3 TNM CANCER STAGING CLASSIFICATION SYSTEM

T* subclasses

TX—tumor cannot be adequately assessed
TO—no evidence of primary tumor
TIS—carcinoma in situ
T1, T2, T3, T4—progressive increase in tumor size and involvement

N† subclasses

NX—regional lymph nodes cannot be assessed
NO—no regional lymph node metastasis
N1, N2, N3—increasing involvementof regional lymph nodes

M‡ subclasses

MX—not assessed
MO—no (known) distant metastasis
M1—distant metastasis present, specify site(s)

Histopathology

G1—well-differentiated grade
G2—moderately well-differentiated grade
G3—poorly differentiated grade
G4—undifferientated

From American Joint Committee for Cancer: *AJCC Manual for Staging of Cancer,* ed 4, Philadelphia, 1992, JB Lippincott.
*T—Primary tumor.
†N—Regional lymph nodes.
‡M—Distant metastasis.

DIAGNOSIS OF CANCER

Persons who show signs of cancer should undergo diagnostic testing to confirm or rule out the diagnosis. The only definite way to determine the presence of malignant cells is to obtain tissue **biopsy** (the removal of a small piece of living tissue from an organ or other part of the body for microscopic examination to confirm or establish a diagnosis, establish prognosis, or follow the course of a disease).

In general, the purpose of a biopsy is to obtain a sample of tissue for pathological examination. The three types of biopsy are incisional, excisional, and needle/aspiration (see Fig. 38-2). *Incisional* biopsy is the removal of a portion of tissue for examination (e.g., the bite biopsy performed during endoscopy). *Excisional* biopsy is the removal of the complete lesion, with little or no margin of surrounding normal tissue removed (e.g., polypectomy). Another example of excisional biopsy is the dissection of peripheral lymph nodes (e.g., those of the axilla for staging of breast cancer or those of the peritoneal region for staging of various abdominal cancers). *Needle/aspiration* biopsy is the aspiration of fluid or tissue by means of a needle (e.g., breast biopsy is performed with an aspiration needle). *Transcutaneous aspiration* biopsy has eliminated most of the exploratory laparotomies for diagnosing metastatic cancer of the liver or for primary inoperable pancreatic cancer. Organs accessible to thin-needle biopsy under guidance of palpation include breasts, skin, thyroid, prostate, palpable lymph nodes, and salivary glands.

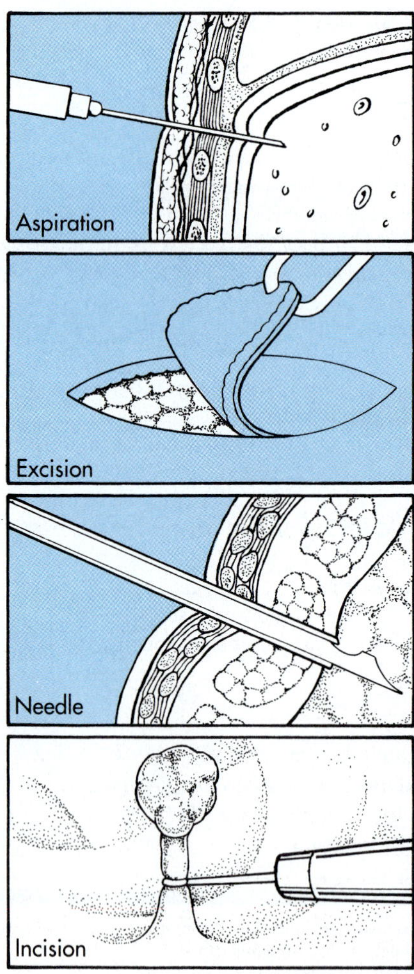

FIG. 38-2 Types of biopsy.

Cells or tissue can also be obtained using an endoscope to directly visualize an internal structure through a body cavity or through a small incision. Endoscopes are rigid or flexible tubes containing a magnifying lens and a light. Endoscopes vary in diameter and length according to the structure being examined; that is, the bronchoscope is used to visualize the tracheobronchial tree; upper gastrointestinal (GI) endoscopy allows direct visualization of the upper GI tract (esophagus, stomach, duodenum); the colonoscopy is used to visualize the entire colon; the sigmoidoscope is used to examine the sigmoid colon, rectum, and anus.

Other diagnostic studies determine the depth of the specific lesion and identify other structures that may have been invaded. These include x-ray and scanning procedures. Commonly ordered x-ray studies are the chest x-ray, mammography, bone scan, GI series, barium enema, and intravenous pyelogram.

Bone scanning involves several steps. First, a radioactive material is injected into a vein in the arm. The patient is encouraged to drink water over the next 1 to 3 hours to aid renal clearance of any radioisotope not picked up by the bone. Areas of concentrated uptake may represent a tumor or abnormality. These areas of concentration can be detected days or weeks before an ordinary x-ray can reveal a lesion. Bone scanning is indicated to detect metastatic tumor; all malignancies capable of metastasis may reach the bone, especially those malignancies of the breasts, kidneys, lungs, prostate, thyroid, and urinary bladder.

Tomography is the special technique of making multiple x-ray films at different depths of a specific area, organ, or structure. The details of each thin section can be clearly visualized.

Computed tomography (CT scan) uses x-rays and a computed scanning system to produce and record images of specific structures at different angles. The entire body can be scanned to detect the presence of any abnormal lesion. CT scan is especially helpful to detect small lesions that may not be seen by radiographs or tomography.

Radioisotope studies require the injection or ingestion of a radioactive substance. A scanning device is used to identify the distribution of the substance in different areas of the body. Concentration of the radioisotope in a specific organ, such as the thyroid or brain, identifies tumor in that location (may be primary or metastatic).

Ultrasound testing is a noninvasive procedure using high-frequency sound waves to examine internal structures of the body. As a transducer is moved over the area being studied, an ultrasound beam is directed through the tissues, which reflects back to the transducer where the sound waves are converted into electrical impulses, which produce an image on a display screen. Ultrasound can show the size, consistency, and shape of the structure being studied and is most helpful in distinguishing between cystic and solid tumors. Ultrasound is not used to examine bones or air-filled organs. The procedure is painless. Persons having ultrasonography will feel the transducer moving over their skin and may need to hold the breath for brief periods and to remain still while the procedure is being done.

Magnetic resonance imaging (MRI) is a painless diagnostic procedure that does not involve any exposure to radiation. As the person reclines on a narrow surface that moves into a cylindrical tunnel containing magnetic coils, radio frequency energy waves produce signals that are processed by a computer and displayed as images on a video monitor. The images can be recorded on film or magnetic tape for permanent storage. This test is currently used in the diagnosis of intracranial and spinal lesions and of cardiovascular and soft tissue abnormalities. The procedure also provides information about changes within cells of soft tissues, arteries, veins, the brain, and spinal column.

The person having MRI must not have any magnetic materials on the body during the test. (No jewelry may be worn.) MRI cannot be done if the person has any metallic implants in the body, such as a pacemaker, an orthopedic nail, or an aneurysm screw.

The person having the test can talk to those performing the test by means of a microphone placed inside the scanner tunnel. The person will hear the sound waves thumping on the magnetic field, and must lie still while the test is being done, which may take longer than an hour to obtain the images needed.

Commonly used laboratory tests include:

1. *Measurement of acid phosphatase and alkaline phosphatase levels in the blood.*

   Acid phosphatase is elevated if cancer is in the prostate gland. Alkaline phosphatase is elevated if there is metastasis to the bone or liver.
2. *Serum calcitonin level*

   Calcitonin is a hormone secreted by the thyroid gland in response to a rising serum calcium level. The level is increased in the blood of people who have cancer of the thyroid. It may be elevated with breast cancer and oat cell cancer of the lung. Calcitonin stimulation testing may be used in addition to the baseline level testing to confirm a diagnosis. It is essential that the person having this test does not eat or drink during the night before the test.
3. *Carcinoembryonic antigen (CEA) serum level*

   Normally, production of CEA stops before birth, but may begin again if a neoplasm develops. This test cannot be used as a general indicator of cancer because there are other reasons why the level may be elevated. The level is elevated in people who smoke. It is found in increased amounts in the blood of people with colorectal cancer. The test may assist in the evaluation of cancer treatment where a rising CEA may indicate tumor recurrence or metastatic disease. This test is used less frequently recently because research has found it less accurate than was previously thought.
4. *Prostate-specific antigen (PSA) and CA-125*

   There are many different blood studies (markers) currently being evaluated to determine their usefulness in cancer screening and diagnosis. Two examples are the PSA for prostate cancer and CA-125 for ovarian cancer. PSA is a biological marker, specific for cellular activity in the prostate gland.

   PSA, the gold standard tumor marker for prostate cancer, is increasingly important in the diagnostic assessment and follow-up of patients with the disease. PSA also plays an important role in staging prostate cancer and in monitoring for recurrence. The American Cancer Society began recommending its use for screening asymptomatic men in November 1992.

   Although PSA levels usually are elevated when cancer is present, PSA alone does not diagnose prostate cancer. Other common conditions such as benign enlargement of the prostate can also elevate PSA. The finding of elevated PSA requires further evaluation to assess the cause of the high levels. This may involve an ultrasound of the prostate gland.

   The PSA assay requires a physician's interpretation. There is no specific level of PSA that signals the presence or absence of prostate cancer. The test is produced by different manufacturers, and the different products yield different results. Men with benign prostate enlargement will have different normal levels than men with normal-sized prostate glands.

   To determine what role PSA might play in screening asymptomatic men, the American Cancer Society in 1987 undertook its National Prostate Cancer Detection Project, a long-term study of 2425 men at 10 clinical centers across the United States. This study looked at the impact of PSA and two other screening methods, digital rectal examination (DRE) and transrectal ultrasound (TRUS), alone and in combination in early detection of prostate cancer.

   The American Cancer Society currently recommends that asymptomatic men over the age of 40 be screened for prostate cancer via DRE and men over age 50 should undergo annual PSA and

DRE. If the result of either is suspicious, further evaluation is necessary.

A PSA is done by collecting a sample of the patient's blood before prostate palpation. The normal range for a man over the age of 40 is 0 to 4 ng/ml. Although the PSA is used in screening to detect prostate cancer, it is used most widely to determine the effectiveness of cancer treatment and to assess the recurrence of prostate cancer. A rising PSA following surgery for cancer of the prostate suggests the cancer has recurred.

The CA-125 is a cancer antigen detected in the blood and peritoneal ascites. The normal range is 35 U/ml. CA-125 may be elevated in gynecological cancers (including ovarian cancer) and cancer of the pancreas.

A monoclonal antibody has been developed that reacts with this antigen, giving physicians a method to measure the amount of CA-125 present in blood samples. The amount of CA-125 in the blood is a useful test to monitor whether a cancer is growing or regressing.

CA-125 has been touted as a way to detect primary ovarian cancer. Although a detection test for ovarian cancer is desirable, unfortunately, CA-125 does not fit this category. CA-125 is useful mainly to signal a recurrence of ovarian cancer. Other conditions, such as endometriosis, hepatitis, pelvic inflammatory diseases, or pregnancy, may cause increased levels of CA-125 in blood.

5. *Stool examination for blood*

   The cause of blood in the stool must be identified to rule out the possibility of cancer. The guaiac test is commonly used to detect occult (hidden) blood in the stools. Names of other commonly used tests for occult blood in the stool are Hematest, Occultest, and Hemoccult test. Early detection self-tests are available for home use. If blood is found, the person should seek immediate medical attention. For accurate test results for the presence of blood, it is essential that the person not have any of the following foods or medications for 4 days before the test:

Red meat	Aspirin
Turnips	Vitamin C
Melons	

   The test must be performed on three consecutive bowel movements.

People must be urged to follow through with diagnostic tests recommended as a result of initial tests.

CANCER THERAPIES

Surgery

By the time it is decided that surgery is needed to remove a cancerous lesion, cancer cells may already have spread to other areas. The goal of surgery is to remove all malignant cells. This includes the removal of the tumor, surrounding tissue, and regional lymph nodes that may be present. Surgery in conjunction with chemotherapy and/or radiation therapy may increase the destruction of cancer cells. The effects of cancer drugs and radiation treatments administered before, during, and after surgery are being investigated. A surgical cure may result from a well-isolated lesion removed in the very early stages, such as in cancer of the skin, testicle, breast, or cervix. Surgery may be performed for many reasons—preventive, diagnostic, curative, and **palliative** (therapy designed to relieve or reduce intensity of uncomfortable symptoms but that does not produce cure).

Surgery may be performed to remove polyps in the colon before they undergo any malignant changes. Occasionally, prophylactic mastectomy is done to prevent breast cancer in those identified to be at very high risk because of family history or other factors.

A radical surgical approach to operable tumors is no longer routinely used, because a greater variety of surgical procedures, more sophisticated staging techniques, and more advanced treatment options are available. The more conservative surgical management of breast cancer is an excellent example of this trend.

If the cancerous lesion has already metastasized, surgery may provide palliation by relieving some of the associated problems, such as obstruction, ulceration, hemorrhage, or pain.

The pituitary, adrenals, ovaries, or testes may be surgically removed to help control the growth and spread of malignancies caused by hormonal stimulation.

Reconstructive surgery may be needed to improve body functions and appearance after some types of surgery, such as modified radical mastectomy. Breast reconstruction is an option for women whose disease and treatment enable the surgeon to implant a prosthesis or to transplant tissue from other areas of the body to create a more natural breast. When this is anticipated, preoperative counseling by the surgeon and the nurse will help the patient consider the long-range outcome instead of the immediate, initial surgical procedure.

Nursing Considerations. If the nurse is not present when the physician explains recommendations for care, she must ask the physician what has been told to the patient and the family. This is essential to reinforce the information given by the physician. Patients and families are usually frightened and may not remember all that the physician has explained to them. For considerations for the older adult, see the gerontological box.

The patient should have confidence and trust in those responsible for her care. Positive feelings and attitudes promote relaxation and help reduce anxiety and fear. The nurse should encourage the patient to ask the physician any questions concerning potential risks as a result of a given treatment (see therapeutic dialogue). A

GERONTOLOGICAL CONSIDERATIONS

- There are more cases of cancer among older adults than people of any other age group.
- The incidence of cancer increases with aging, possibly as a result of decreased effectiveness of the immune system and changes in deoxyribonucleic acid (DNA).
- The types of cancers seen in older adults are prostate, lung, breast, and colon-rectum cancer. Cancers of the skin, urinary bladder, vagina, and vulva are seen primarily in older adults. Chronic lymphocytic leukemia and multiple myeloma are seen more frequently in older adults than in younger people.
- Many of the early signs and symptoms of cancer may be misdiagnosed as normal changes of aging. The importance of routine medical screening and self-examination should be stressed to the aging adult.
- Because of fear or past experience, older persons may adopt a fatalistic frame of mind after hearing the diagnosis of cancer. Use of the terms *tumor* or *growth* may be more acceptable.
- The type of treatment for cancer should be based on the older person's wishes and overall state of health. Older individuals, their family members, and significant others should be presented with all options so that informed decisions regarding treatment can be made.

patient needs to feel comfortable with the decision to follow through with the physician's recommendations.

The following are guidelines to assure that patients get the information they need:

- Be present when the patient and his physician are discussing treatment decisions.
- If it seems necessary, clarify explanations of treatments, including benefits and side effects, and help the patient formulate questions and voice concerns.
- Afterwards, talk to the patient and his family about the information the doctor presented, and assess their understanding of the treatment, as well as their goals and needs.
- Report any apparent misunderstandings, unrealistic expectations, or other problems to the doctor.
- Talk to the patient to verify that his problem was resolved.
- Accept and support the patient's choice, regardless of your opinion.

The use of laser beams is increasing as an alternative for some surgical procedures. The laser beam vaporizes tissue with little bleeding and low risk of infection. Currently the major uses of laser surgery are in ophthalmology, gynecology, urology, neurosurgery, and otolaryngology. The chief discomfort while undergoing laser surgery is that the person must lie very still while the laser is in use.

Preparing the patient for a surgical procedure must include an explanation of what to expect postoperatively. Preoperative teaching is discussed in Chapter 22.

Whatever the surgical procedure, the patient's nutritional status, both before and after surgery, has been found to be a significant factor in the amount of surgery that can be tolerated, the rate of recovery from the surgery, and the adequacy of wound healing.

When surgery may result in a changed body image, such as mastectomy, laryngectomy, or formation of an ostomy, the patient may benefit from talking with another person who has had the same type of surgery. The American Cancer Society sponsors support groups. They also specially prepare volunteers to visit individuals who need these types of surgical procedures. *Reach to Recovery,* the *Lost Chord Club,* and the *Ostomy Club* are some of the special groups that are available in some local communities.

THERAPEUTIC DIALOGUE

Nurse: Good afternoon, Mrs. Smith. My name is Jan Jones, and I will be your nurse this evening. How are you feeling? *(introduction and general lead)*

Patient: I'm feeling all right now. It's tomorrow I'm dreading.

Nurse: You are dreading tomorrow? *(restatement)*

Patient: Yes. My doctor told me he has to remove my entire breast and even cut under my arm to remove any lymph nodes that may be malignant. I dread the thought that I will look so different.

Nurse: You are anxious about the fact that you may look different. *(reflection)*

Patient: I will be embarrassed to undress in front of my husband. He may think I am no longer attractive.

Nurse: Have you had a chance to discuss your feelings with your husband? *(clarifying)*

Patient: No, he is out of town and will be back tonight. I guess I could talk to him tonight. Maybe he will accept it better than I think.

Nurse: We'll talk more after you have had a chance to talk to him about your feelings. Is there anything else on your mind that you would like to talk about now? *(showing acceptance and general lead)*

Radiation Therapy

Radiation therapy can be used to cure or control cancer that has spread to local lymph nodes or to treat tumors that cannot be removed.

Radiation may be used preoperatively to reduce the size of a tumor. Postoperative radiation may be indicated to destroy malignant cells not removed by surgery. Radiation may be used to slow the growth of malignant tumors.

Radiation may be delivered externally or internally. External therapy may be directed toward superficial lesions or may be targeted to deeper structures within the

Box 38-4

INSTRUCTIONS FOR NURSING INTERVENTIONS FOR PATIENTS TREATED WITH (UNSEALED INTERNAL RADIATION) I-131 FOR THYROID CANCER

1. Nurses should spend as little time as possible for ordinary nursing care. The patient must be as self-sufficient as possible. The patient is radioactive and exposes the nurse to radiation while she is caring for the patient. The radioactive I-131 leaves the patient through urine and perspiration. Therefore, the patient contaminates everything he touches and can spread contamination to the nurse in this way.

PRECAUTIONS THAT WILL REDUCE EXPOSURE TO THE NURSE:

A. Limit the time spent in the room. Work quickly and only enter as necessary.
B. When in the room, maintain as much distance from the patient as possible. A few feet distance makes a lot of difference in the exposure to the nurse.
C. Wear shoe covers and disposable, fluid proof gloves, and avoid contact with all surfaces in the room.
D. When leaving the room:
   1. Wash hands with gloves on.
   2. Remove one shoe cover at the door, step that foot out, and drop that shoe cover into the trash.
   3. Remove the other shoe cover and step that foot out and drop that shoe cover into the trash.
   4. Remove gloves and drop them into the trash.
   5. Do not remove shoe covers or gloves from the room. All trash must stay in the room.
E. Always wear the dosimeter while in the room, and log the exposure you receive at each visit. (The dosimeter, log, and instructions are outside the door.)

2. NO VISITORS are allowed.
3. The patient is confined to the room.
4. Nothing is to leave the room unless checked for contamination and released by the Radiation Safety Officer (RSO) or his designate. All trash and laundry are to remain in the special containers.
5. Pregnant nursing or Nuclear Medicine personnel will not enter the area.
6. Shoe covers and fluid-proof disposable gloves (nonsterile type) are to be worn when entering the room. (Gowns will be available.)
7. The dosimeter is to be worn in the room, and exposure is to be logged when leaving the room.
8. All clothes and bed linens used by the patient should be placed in the laundry bag provided and should be left in the patient's room to be checked by the Radiation Safety Officer or his designee.
9. No housekeeping is allowed until the room is officially released.
10. Food is delivered only by nursing. It is delivered to the door and picked up by the patient. Mail, flowers, etc., are delivered in the same way.
11. Only disposable items may be used in the care of these patients, whenever possible. These items should be placed in the designated waste container. Contact the Radiation Safety Officer or his designee for proper disposal of the contents of the designated waste container.
12. Except in emergencies, urine collection or blood draws are not allowed after the patient has been dosed with I-131. The urine and blood are radioactive.
13. The patient is to flush the toilet three times after each use, and males should sit down to void.
14. If the nurse helps to collect the excreta, disposable gloves should be worn. Afterwards, hands should be washed with the gloves on and again after the gloves are removed. The gloves should be placed in the designated waste container for disposal by the Radiation Safety Officer or his designee.
15. Utmost precautions must be taken to see that no urine or vomitus is spilled on the floor or the bed. If any part of the patient's room is suspected to be contaminated, notify the Radiation Safety Officer or his designee in the Nuclear Medicine Department.
16. If a nurse, attendant, or anyone else knows or suspects that his or her skin or clothing, including shoes, is contaminated, notify the Radiation Safety Officer or his designee immediately. This person should remain in an area adjacent to the patient's room and should not walk about the hospital. If the hands become contaminated, wash them immediately with soap and water.
17. If a therapy patient should need emergency surgery or should die, notify the Radiation Safety Officer or the Nuclear Medicine Department *immediately*.
18. Vomiting within 24 hours after oral administration, urinary incontinence, or excessive sweating within the first 48 hours may result in contamination of linen and floor. In any such situation, or if radioactive urine and/or feces is spilled during collection, call the Radiation Safety Officer or his designee. Meanwhile, handle all contaminated material with disposable gloves and avoid spreading contamination.
19. All vomitus will be kept in the patient's room for disposal by the Radiation Safety Officer or his designee *only* if the patient has vomited over the bed or the surrounding area. Otherwise, it will be flushed down the toilet with at least three volumes of water or more after it. Feces need not be routinely saved, unless ordered on the chart. The same toilet should be used by the patient at all times and it should be well flushed (at least three times).
20. The patient may not be discharged without prior approval of the radiation safety officer or his designate. The room may not be remade or used or entered by unauthorized people until released by the radiation safety officer. Nothing may leave the room unless checked for contamination and released by the radiation safety officer.

Courtesy Great Plains Regional Medical Center Nuclear Medicine Dept, North Platte, Neb.

body. Normal cells are better able to recover from the damage caused by radiation than are cancer cells. Because malignant cells lack the capacity for repair, more cancer cells than normal cells are damaged by radiation. However, normal cells do have a maximum dose of radiation that they can tolerate before irreversible damage occurs. Treatment plans are designed to minimize the radiation dose to normal structures. Meticulous planning and recording of dose are essential.

External Radiation Therapy. When external radiation is planned, the specific area on the body is marked to indicate the port for external radiation to be directed. These markings must not be washed off. If the area becomes wet while bathing, pat the area with an absorbent towel to dry the skin. Help the patient to understand the need to protect this area. Also instruct the patient to avoid the use of any ointments, lotions, or powder on this area. The physician may approve specific lotions or creams for drying skin. The patient should be told to protect the radiated area from direct sunlight and to avoid applications of heat or cold, since these would increase erythema, drying, and pruritus of the skin, which is common over an irradiated area.

A diet high in protein and calories and a fluid intake of 2 or 3 quarts of fluid per day must be encouraged. The person undergoing radiation therapy should be assured that lethargy and fatigue are not uncommon during treatment and that frequent rest periods are helpful.

Some 60% of all people with cancer are treated with radiation therapy at some point. For many of these, radiation therapy is the only therapy needed to destroy the cancer.

Internal Radiation Therapy. General principles to be followed when caring for the patient treated with internal radiation are the following:

1. Assemble materials, and plan ahead to provide several nursing interventions at the same time when entering the patient's room.
2. Stand at the greatest distance away from the site where an internal radiation device is in the patient's body.
3. Limit the time needed for close contact near the site being irradiated. If direct, prolonged care is needed, nurses should wear a lead apron.

Unsealed internal radiation is administered intravenously or orally so that it is distributed throughout the patient's body. Special precautions must be taken to prevent exposure to radiation from direct contact with the patient or from contact with any of his body tissue or fluid (Box 38-4).

Radioactive implant (brachytherapy) is the insertion of *sealed radioactive materials* temporarily or permanently into hollow cavities, within body tissues, or on the body's surface. The radioactive source delivers a specific radiation dose continuously over hours or days. A highly concentrated radiation dose is delivered in or near a tumor. This technique is generally combined with a course of external radiation therapy to increase the dosage to a specific site. Certain organs, such as the uterus and vagina, are natural receptacles for the placement of an applicator that can be loaded with radioactive material. Radioactive needles, wires, seeds, beads, or catheters may be inserted directly into tumor tissue.

Children younger than 18 years and pregnant women should not be allowed to visit implant patients. Approved visitors should be advised regarding the recommended limit of time and safe distance to stay with the patient. Visitors shall be instructed to limit visits to 10 minutes when with the patient, always standing as far away from the pelvic area as possible.

When cancer of the cervix is treated with the use of an applicator containing a radioactive material, the applicator is placed in the vagina. The following special nursing measures are indicated:

1. Place "Radiation in Use" sign on the patient's door.
2. Prevent dislodgment. Keep patient on strict bed rest. Instruct the patient not to turn from side to side or onto the abdomen. Do not raise the head of the bed more than 30 to 45 degrees.
3. Do not give a complete bed bath while the applicator is in place, and do not bathe the patient below the waist. Do not change bed linen unless necessary.
4. Encourage the patient to do active range-of-motion (ROM) exercises with both arms and mild foot and leg exercises to minimize the hazards of immobility. Patient will wear antiembolism stockings (TED hose).
5. Monitor vital signs every 4 hours, observing for elevations in temperature, pulse, and respirations. A temperature above 100° F (37.7° C) should be reported to the physician.
6. Observe for and report the development of any rash or skin eruption, excessive vaginal bleeding, or vaginal discharge.
7. Keep accurate intake and output (I&O) record. Encourage a fluid intake of at least 3 L daily. An indwelling catheter is in place to reduce the size of the bladder and decrease effects of radiation on the bladder. Check to be sure it is draining well.
8. Serve diet as ordered—usually a low-residue diet to minimize peristalsis and bowel movement, which might lead to dislodgment of applicator.
9. Check position of applicator every 4 hours.
10. Keep long-handled forceps and a special lead container in the patient's room for use by the radiologist, should the implant become dislodged. *Never touch a dislodged applicator or any other materials that have fallen out of the*

patient. These may contain the radiative sources. Any bed linens, dressings, or pads that have been changed for the patient must be checked with a radiation survey meter before they are removed them from the patient's room.

11. After the applicator is removed, the indwelling catheter is usually removed and a douche and enema are generally prescribed.
12. Precautions are no longer needed after removal. Encourage ambulation and gradual resumption of activities.
13. Sexual intercourse is usually delayed for 7 to 10 days.
14. Instruct the patient to notify the physician of nausea, vomiting, diarrhea, frequent or painful urination, or a temperature above 100° F (37.7° C).

The nurse should follow the principles of time limits and safe distance when caring for the patient with a radiation implant. Directions supplied by the hospital related to the radioactive substance being used should be followed. Generally, it is recommended that the nurse spend no more than 10 minutes at a time in the room of a patient with an implant. The nurse should stand at least 6 feet away from the patient when not giving direct care and stand as far away from the pelvic area as possible when the cervical implant is in use.

Chemotherapy

Chemotherapy drugs are used to reduce or slow the growth of metastatic cancer. Most chemotherapeutic agents work by interfering with the cells' ability to multiply or reproduce. Drugs that interfere with a cell's *replication* (process of duplicating, reproducing) process damage the cell and cause cellular death. Both malignant and normal cells are affected by chemotherapy. Cells that multiply rapidly are affected the most, such as cells of the *hematopoietic system, hair follicles,* and the *GI system*. Most of the side effects from chemotherapeutic agents result from the destruction of normal cells in the above systems. Common side effects are given below by system.

Hematopoietic System.

Leukopenia. **Leukopenia** (reduction in the number of circulating white blood cells due to depression of the bone marrow), a common problem for patients receiving chemotherapy, can lead to life-threatening infections. Lack of neutrophils, the type of white blood cell (WBC) most often suppressed in the differential WBC, is called *neutropenia.* Without enough neutrophils, the body's first line of defense collapses, opening the way for pneumonia, septicemia, or another potentially overwhelming infection.

The nurse needs to protect the patient against pathogens, monitor the patient for signs of infection, and respond aggressively if infection occurs. Monitor the patient's vital signs every 4 hours and notify the physician if temperature starts to rise. A temperature of 100° F (38° C) or more is considered a sign of impending infection.

The nurse should take the following systematic approach to assessing the patient for infection[15]:

1. *Assessing the mouth*

   Stomatitis, an inflammation of the oral mucosa, is one of the most common complications of chemotherapy and can easily lead to severe swallowing problems and systemic infections. Use a penlight and tongue blade to look for lesions, ulcers, or white plaque.

   Teach the patient the importance of performing regular, but gentle, mouth care. Have the patient use a soft toothbrush and rinse the mouth with normal saline or sodium bicarbonate solution every 2 to 4 hours. A sponge-tipped applicator (Toothette) may help prevent bleeding gums, a common adverse effect of chemotherapy and radiation.

   To reduce the risk of an oral *Candida* infection, the physician may order prophylactic antifungal medications such as oral nystatin (Mycostatin) suspension, clotrimazole (Lotrimin) lozenges, or fluconazole (Diflucan). A soft or liquid diet may also be ordered
2. *Assessing the skin*

   A rash or eruption may indicate that the patient has an infection or is predisposed to one.

   Bacteria may flourish in skin folds, such as in the groin and axillae, so clean these areas twice a day with soap and water. Water-soluble moisturizers may be used to keep the patient's skin from drying. To prevent cuts, advise the patient to shave with an electric razor.

   Vascular access sites are common gateways to infection. Central and peripheral intravenous (IV) catheters should all be monitored carefully. Check for edema, drainage, erythema, or pain around catheter entry sites.

   Organisms can also grow along catheter tracts and infect the blood, resulting in septicemia. Signs and symptoms of a catheter tract infection include tenderness around the catheter site and referred pain in the shoulder.

   Administer oral drugs whenever possible. Try to avoid subcutaneous (SC) or intramuscular (IM) injections because they can cause abscesses in patients with neutropenia. Excessive bleeding is also a risk for these patients because of the potential for associated decreases in platelets and other formed elements in the blood.

   Puncturing the skin is sometimes unavoidable, as when the patient needs a bone marrow biopsy, for example. After a biopsy, carefully assess the site, swab it with an antibacterial solution (such as povidone-iodine [Betadine]), and apply an occlusive dressing until the skin heals.

3. *Assessing for pulmonary function*

   Be aware many neutropenic patients with lung infections do not have common signs and symptoms, such as sputum production or infiltrates demonstrable on chest x-rays. Therefore, be alert for other indications of an impending infection, including changes in lung sounds, respiratory rate and rhythm, and breathing effort. The patient may also complain of pain during inspiration or expiration.

   To help prevent a lung infection, encourage the patient to be as active as able and to perform deep-breathing and coughing exercises. Using an incentive spirometer can help by maximizing ventilatory capacity.

4. *Assessing urinary and bowel function*

   Changes in urinary function can also warn of infection in a neutropenic patient. Assess for decreased urinary output, changes in the urine's odor or color, hematuria, or glycosuria—all possible signs of infection. The patient may also complain of urinary frequency, urgency, or pain.

   To reduce the risk of urinary infection, avoid bladder catheterization. If catheterization is absolutely indicated, follow strict aseptic technique when inserting the catheter and perform catheter care according to the agency's guidelines.

   Also routinely assess the patient's bowel function. Assess stool samples for color, consistency, and the presence of blood, and ask the patient to report any changes in bowel habits.

   Does the patient need to strain when defecating? If so, the physician may prescribe a stool softener such as docusate (Colace). Straining can cause ulcerations or fissures in the rectum, creating ports of entry for bacteria. Avoid enemas, rectal medications, and rectal thermometers, which can break the mucosal lining. Be aware that neutropenia predisposes to rectal abscesses. If the patient complains of perirectal pain, the physician should be notified immediately.[15]

A recent breakthrough in treating patients with neutropenia is commercially made colony-stimulating factors (CSFs), the only therapy that can actually prevent or manage neutropenia. The two types of CSFs are granulocyte colony-stimulating factors (G-CSF) (filgrastim [Neupogen]) and granulocyte-macrophage colony-stimulating factors (GM-CSF) (sangramostim [Leukine or Prokine]). These CSFs are given subcutaneously or intravenously.

Although CSFs are extremely expensive, they are used prophylactically for patients at high risk for neutropenia, such as patients with a history of developing severe or prolonged neutropenia after chemotherapy.

Anemia. Anemia is a reduction in the number of circulating red blood cells due to depression of the bone marrow.

Fatigue is a major problem for persons with anemia because of the decreased oxygenation to tissues from the decreased hemoglobin. For the hospitalized patient, plan care so that there is a balance between activities and rest to prevent increased oxygen expenditure and hypoxemia. Persons at home need to plan ADLs to allow rest periods.

Thrombocytopenia. **Thrombocytopenia** is a reduction in the number of circulating platelets, due to the depression of the bone marrow.

The following are patient teaching measures to prevent injury/hemorrhage due to decreased platelets:

- Use soft toothbrush or swab for mouth care.
- Keep mouth clean and free of debris.
- Avoid intrusions into rectum (for example, rectal medications, enemas).
- Use electric shaver.
- Apply direct pressure for 5 to 10 minutes if any bleeding occurs.
- Avoid contact sports, elective surgery, and tooth extraction.
- Avoid picking or blowing nose forcefully.
- Avoid trauma, falls, bumps, cuts; avoid contact sports.
- Avoid use of aspirin or aspirin preparations.
- Use adequate lubrication and gentleness during sexual intercourse.

Integumentary System.

Alopecia. **Alopecia** is loss of hair due to the destruction of hair follicles.

Alopecia may occur by two mechanisms. If the hair roots are atrophied, alopecia occurs readily. The hair falls out either falls out spontaneously or during hair combing, often in large clumps. If the hair shaft is constricted because of atrophy or necrosis, the hair will break off very near the scalp. The root remains in the scalp and a patchy, thinning pattern of hair loss occurs. Hair loss may also occur on other parts of the body. Loss of leg, arm, pubic, axillary, and facial hair is seen less often, although loss of eyebrows and eyelashes may occur.

The pattern and extent of hair loss cannot be accurately predicted for a given patient. When the treatment is given with a drug known to cause alopecia, the patient needs to be told that severe hair loss can begin within a few days or weeks of treatment and that partial or complete baldness can quickly ensue. Drug-induced alopecia is never permanent. The patient may experience a change in hair color or texture when regrowth occurs. Occasionally, hair growth may return while chemotherapy treatment continues. Given this perspective, coupled with the goal of disease control or cure, most patients tolerate the hair loss with minimal distress. However, many patients have difficulty adjusting to the

MEDICATIONS FOR CANCER

Medication	Trade Name	Action	Side Effects	Nursing Implications
Ondansetron	Zofran	Antiemetic	Headache, diarrhea, constipation, abdominal pain, transient increase in aspartate aminotransferase (AST) and/or alanine aminotransferase (ALT)	Dilute intravenous dose with D_5W or NaCl and give total dose (approximately 32 mg) 30 min before chemotherapy. Give 8 mg orally before chemotherapy and three times a day for 2 days.
Granisetron	Kytril	Antiemetic	Headache, constipation, somnolence, diarrhea, mild changes in blood pressure	Administer dose over 5-min period, beginning 30 min before chemotherapy. Know that granisetron (Kytril) is given once a day in a 5-min infusion, whereas ondansetron (Zofran) is given in three 15-min infusions.
Prochlorperazine	Compazine	Antiemetic	Extrapyramidal symptoms, orthostatic hypotension, ocular changes (blurred vision), dry mouth, constipation, urine retention, photosensitivity	Use cautiously with other CNS depressants (alcohol) and medications that decrease blood pressure, as well as patients with liver disease. Decrease dose in older adults. Do not exceed recommended dose. Protect from light.
Diphenoxylate/ Atropine	Lomotil	Antidiarrheal	Sedation, dizziness, dry mouth, urinary retention, rash	Watch for physical dependence. Know that it should work within 48 hr. Give naloxone as antidote for respiratory depression.
Morphine	Roxanol, MS Contin	Narcotic analgesic	Decreased respiratory rate, euphoria, seizures, physical dependence, hypotension, bradycardia, miosis, drowsiness, dizziness, urinary retention, constipation, rash	Use cautiously with other CNS depressants (alcohol). Monitor respirations, heart rate, and mental status closely. Have naloxone available as antidote. Do not give sustained release tablets for acute pain.
Hydromorphone	Dialudid	Narcotic analgesic	Decreased respiratory rate, euphoria, seizures, physical dependence, hypotension, bradycardia, miosis, drowsiness, dizziness, urinary retention, constipation, rash	Use cautiously with other CNS depressants (alcohol). Monitor respirations, heart rate, and mental status closely. Have naloxone available as antidote. Do not give sustained release tablets for acute pain. Have Dialudid-HP (10 mg/ml) available for chronic pain.
Naproxen	Naprosyn, Anaprox	Nonsteroidal antiinflammatory agent (NSAID)	Agranulocytosis, headache, dizziness, drowsiness, peripheral edema, visual disturbances, gastrointestinal upset (occult blood loss and peptic ulcers), prolonged bleeding time, tinnitus	Know that concurrent use of alcohol, acetylsalicylic acid, and/or steroids will increase chance of gastrointestinal bleeding. Know that it may interact with warfarin sodium (Coumadin). Avoid use in patient allergic to acetylsalicylic acid. Give with food. Advise patient that it may take 4 weeks to show benefit.

change in body image due to hair loss. The hair is very much a part of the self-image.

To meet the patient's needs, an education program, written materials, and educational sessions with a hairstylist are valuable services for the patient. Provide sincere concern and emotional support for the patient.

Gastrointestinal System.

Stomatitis. **Stomatitis** is a mouth inflammation due to destruction of normal cells of the oral cavity.

Stomatitis may range from an erythema of the oral mucosa to mild or severe ulceration. Methotrexate, 5-fluorouracil (5-FU), doxorubicin, dactinomycin, and bleomycin are the chemotherapeutic drugs that most frequently cause stomatitis. Patients may also develop a superimposed *Candida* infection of the mouth and esophagus, and oral nystatin is usually prescribed. Good mouth care is important.

Nausea, vomiting, diarrhea. These are disorders of the GI tract due to the breakdown of normal GI cells.

Nausea and vomiting are among the most uncomfortable and distressing side effects of chemotherapy. The onset and duration vary greatly among patients and with the drug given. For the ambulatory patient, nausea may interfere with the ability to continue daily work. Persistent vomiting may result in fluid and electrolyte imbalance, general weakness, and weight loss. Decline of nutritional status renders the patient more susceptible to infection and perhaps less able to tolerate therapy. Such physiological symptoms can accompany or precipitate psychological responses that might include depression and withdrawal. Every effort must be made to minimize chemotherapy-induced nausea and vomiting.

Antiemetics vary in success. Tetrahydrocannabinol (THC) taken in pill form produces an antiemetic effect in some patients who have not benefited from the commonly prescribed prochlorperazine (Compazine). Metoclopramide (Reglan), ondansetron (Zofran), and granisetron (Kytril) are often helpful for persons receiving chemotherapy, and lorazepam (Ativan) is often effective in producing a relaxed state during which an individual is less sensitive to nausea-inducing stimuli. See the medications table for information about specific drugs.

It is imperative that patients receive antiemetic drugs to control the side effects of nausea and vomiting while undergoing chemotherapy. The patient may receive antiemetics orally, intramuscularly, rectally, intravenously as well as via pumps like those used in patient-controlled analgesia. With the advent of new antiemetic medications such as ondansetron (Zofran) and ganisetron (Kytril), chemotherapy-induced nausea and vomiting are much less severe.

Changes in bowel habits commonly occur, but usually do not require intervention. If diarrhea becomes marked or persists, an antidiarrheal medication such as diphenoxylate with atropine (Lomotil) may be prescribed.

Combinations of chemotherapy agents, as well as chemotherapy combined with other treatments, have increased the number of cures, remissions, and palliative outcomes.

Many of the problems experienced by people undergoing chemotherapy are the same as those that may result from radiation therapy (depending on the target site and amount of radiation). The nurse must help the patient realize that some of the problems are the result of therapy and not a sign that the cancer is increasing.

Nursing diagnoses and interventions for the patient undergoing chemotherapy include but are not limited to the following:

NURSING DIAGNOSES	NURSING INTERVENTIONS
Tissue integrity, impaired: oral mucous membrane, related to stomatitis (inflammation of the mouth); xerostomia (decreased salivation)	Assist with frequent, careful oral hygiene and hydration; use very soft toothbrush. Provide meticulous mouth care. Give soothing oral lozenges; use ice chips and frequent sips of ice water; avoid hot beverages; use lip balm for dryness.
Nutrition, altered: less than body requirements, related to anorexia (from changes in taste and smell); nausea/vomiting; dysphagia (difficulty in swallowing); aspiration; diarrhea; malabsorption; cachexia (general ill health and malnutrition, marked by weakness and emaciation, usually associated with a serious disease such as cancer)	Provide adequate, easily digestible, soft, bland diet; avoid spicy foods. Keep room free of odors and clutter. Give small, frequent, highly nutritional meals to meet the extra demands created by energy used by malignant cells; allow extra time to eat.
Fatigue, related to anemia	Arrange rest periods before meals and at frequent periods throughout day. Provide slow, individualized schedule for activities; wheelchair/walker may conserve energy.
Fluid volume deficit, related to nausea and vomiting	Administer antiemetic as needed before treatments known to cause nausea and vomiting. Provide clean environment with fresh air and no odors. Administer IV therapy as ordered. Monitor I&O, daily weight, and electrolytes. Assess tissue turgor.
Infection, high risk for, related to weakened immune system; leukopenia	Protect against infections—especially from other people. Avoid crowds. Observe and promptly report to physician any signs of inflammation at injection sites or insertion sites of any peripheral or central IV lines. Use sterile technique whenever possible. Initiate reverse isolation as indicated.

NURSING DIAGNOSES	NURSING INTERVENTIONS
Infection, high risk for, related to weakened immune system; leukopenia—cont'd	Monitor temperature, leukocyte count. Discourage fresh-cut flowers. Avoid indwelling catheters, performing rectal procedures, or examinations. Administer antibiotics as prescribed.
Trauma, high risk for, related to fatigue, increasing weakness, and thrombocytopenia	Protect from injuries that may result in bleeding; inspect for evidence of bleeding or bruising; use smallest needles for injections.
Self-esteem disturbance: situational low self-esteem, related to changes in appearance if cachexia is experienced as a result of advanced cancer	Encourage active participation in planning and care for self; assist with hair care to maintain attractive appearance. Maintain supportive, nonjudgmental attitude.
Diversional activity deficit, related to decreased energy as a result of anemia	Provide time for viewing or listening to favorite TV or radio programs. Encourage hobby or games with others. Encourage visitors and conversation regarding current events. Encourage participation in activities, such as church, the theater, or shopping at stores (conserve energy). Encourage eating out in a favorite restaurant for special occasions. Encourge patient to arrange short drives to favorite location, such as beach, parks, lakes.
Pain, related to late-stage problems resulting from progressive cancer	Assist to develop and maintain trusting relationship with care givers. Provide medications as ordered before pain intensifies. Provide comfort measures, such as good alignment and frequent position changes. Encourage relaxation by use of soft music and quiet environment.
Knowledge deficit, related to prognosis and expected outcome of disease	Be realistic and honest in discussions regarding the future as per physician's guidance. Assist to identify and fulfill planning for personal business and family matters with awareness of shortened life-expectancy if a poor prognosis has been established.
Anxiety/fear, related to the diagnosis of cancer	*Listen* with genuine interest and concern.
Tissue integrity, impaired, related to damage to integumentary tissue: alopecia	Be alert to the fact that alopecia is very traumatic to the patient's self-image. Give reassurance that problem is usually not permanent. Assist to choose an attractive wig to have when needed.
Activity intolerance, related to fatigue, decreased mobility, and effects of disease	Change position frequently (at least every 2 hr). Provide ROM exercises every 8 hr. Pace activities; provide adequate rest.
Skin integrity, impaired, related to decreased mobility and altered nutritional status.	Massage over bony prominences each time position is changed. Use alternating air pressure mattress. Keep sheet smooth (no wrinkles). Inspect carefully for potential development of decubitus.
Coping, ineffective individual and family, related to feelings about diagnosis of cancer, change in body image, feelings of powerlessness/inability to control outcome of disease	Encourage communication/sharing of feelings among family members. Assess patient's coping behavior, and determine its effectiveness. Reassure patient that mood changes are temporary. Encourage use of resources, such as support groups.

Chemotherapy has proven effective in treatment of many cancer patients. Many cancer patients can be cured with chemotherapy, while others will experience cancer-free intervals and/or control of cancer pain. Nurses must learn about each drug being administered to anticipate the expected side effects and plan the nursing interventions needed.

There are safety guidelines to be followed by the care giver for the preparation and administration of chemotherapeutic agents, since they may be absorbed into the skin or inhaled. The major types of chemotherapeutic agents used to treat cancer are given in Table 38-2. See Chapter 29 for additional chemotherapeutic agents.

Immunotherapy

When conventional treatment for cancer is not sufficient, immunotherapy (also called *biological response modifiers*) may be recommended. This therapy is given to stimulate the body's natural immune system. The immune system has the ability to control cancer cells. Experiments have demonstrated the body does have a defense mechanism against cancer. Some of the agents that stimulate the body's natural immune system include Bacille Calmette-Guérin (BCG), interferons, interleukin-2 (IL-2), and specific malignant cell antibodies produced in the laboratory from actual tumor cells from a patient's body. When these agents are used, nurses must accurately observe and record patient responses and promptly report potential adverse reactions. Much is yet to be learned about immunotherapy. This treatment is still in the experimental stage. New techniques for treating cancer are being developed, and the future may hold new hope for otherwise terminally ill people.

Bone Marrow Transplantation

Bone marrow transplantation (BMT) following treatment with high-dose chemotherapy or radiation is being used in patients with a variety of malignancies. This is a "rescue" technique that allows administration of necessary but normally toxic doses of drugs and/or radiation.

Most transplantation bone marrow is obtained by multiple needle aspirations from the posterior iliac crest while the patient is under general or spinal anesthesia. The anterior iliac crest and sternum may also be used.

TABLE 38-2 Agents Used in Cancer Chemotherapy

Classification	Mode of Action	Example	Common Side Effects
Alkylating agents	Interfere with DNA replication; cell cycle nonspecific	Cyclophosphamide (Cytoxan) Cisplatin (Platinol) Chlorambucil (Leukeran)	Bone marrow depression, nausea and vomiting, alopecia
Antimetabolites	Damage cell in "S" phase; cell-cycle specific	5-Fluorouracil (5-FU) Mercaptopurine/6-MP (Purinethol) Methotrexate (mexate)	Bone marrow depression, nausea, diarrhea
Antibiotics	Inhibit DNA and RNA synthesis; cell-cycle nonspecific	Bleomycin (Benoxane) Doxorubicin (Adriamycin)	Bone marrow depression, organ toxicity
Plant alkaloids	Inhibit cell division; cell-cycle specific	Vinblastine (Velban) Vincristine (Oncovin)	Bone marrow depression, peripheral nerve toxicity
Hormones, steroids	Alter hormonal environment that promotes cancer growth	Estrogens (DES) Androgens (Testosterone propionate) Adrenocorticosteroids (prednisone)	Feminizing effects in men, masculinizing effects in women, potentially toxic to most body systems
Hormone inhibitors	Bind at receptor sites	Aminoglutethimide (Cytadren) Tamoxifen (Nolvadex)	Hot flashes, nausea, vomiting, adrenal insufficiency

The amount of marrow extracted ranges from 600 to 2500 ml for the average adult. After processing, the marrow is given to the patient intravenously through a transfusion bag, or it can be frozen (cryopreservation). Marrow may be kept for 3 or more years. When the bone marrow is infused, it is via a central line without a filter over a period of 1 to 4 hours.

Bone marrow may be removed from an individual for personal use (**autologous;** indicating something that has its origin within an individual, especially a factor present in tissues or fluids) at a later time, or an individual may be given bone marrow removed from another person. Both kinds of bone marrow transplantations are being used in the treatment of cancer; however, autologous transplants are more widely used. The patient is still at high risk for developing infection during the process of autologous transplant, since the immune defenses have been weakened by the removal of the bone marrow and by the chemotherapy or radiation. These patients are cared for in special bone marrow units so they can be monitored closely.

Effects to prevent infections include protective isolation or laminar airflow rooms; prophylactic systemic antibiotics and antiviral agents (primarily acyclovir); and routine cultures of blood, urine, throat, and stool. Despite these and other interventions, the patient can become septic in hours, with multisystem failure.

Survival after bone marrow transplantation depends on the patient's age, remission, status, and clinical status at the time of transplantation.

Nurses should communicate genuine concern for cancer patients. This includes reinforcing information explained to patients by their physicians regarding the expectations of their specific treatments. Patients may become discouraged by toxic side effects and other problems they experience while undergoing conventional cancer therapies. Nurses should allow extra time to listen to patients with cancer express their feelings and to encourage them to follow the guidelines of conventional medical practice that offer the most hope.

The number of cancers that are being cured is rising daily. In 1992, 452,000 or 4 of 10 cancer patients were reported to be free of the disease for 5 years or more after having chemotherapy/radiation treatments alone or combined with other therapies.[2]

ADVANCED CANCER

Pain Management

Patients with cancer may have pain at any point during the course of the disease and its treatment. In fact, of the 4 million people throughout the world who die from cancer each year, 70% experience pain as a primary symptom. Unfortunately, many people believe that pain is an early symptom of cancer and do not seek diagnosis until pain occurs. Pain is almost without exception a late symptom of cancer and indicates tumor obstruction, pressure on nerves, invasion of bone, phantom sensation, peripheral neuropathy, and neuralgia.

It is estimated that 85% of patients with cancer pain can be managed effectively with appropriate therapy. The American Cancer Society, the American Pain Society, the World Health Organization, and the Oncology Nursing Society, as well as many other organizations, consider pain control to be a major issue in the management of a person with cancer.

One of many challenges facing the nurse who cares for the patient with pain is the assessment of the pain. The nurse must accept the definition of pain as whatever the person experiencing the pain says it is, existing whenever the patient says it does.[23]

This approach is frustrating to many nurses and physicians, who may doubt the presence and nature of the patient's pain when there are no physiological parameters by which to measure it. The nurse must gather data and properly assess the patient. It is of extreme importance not to be judgmental concerning the patient's complaints of pain.

Narcotics (opioids) used in the management of cancer pain include morphine (the prototype), hydromorphone, and methadone. Sustained-release morphine in an oral form, such as MS Contin or Roxanol SR, has been found to be of particular value in the management of the terminally ill person with pain. Administering narcotics via transdermal method, IV drips, intrathecally, and epidurally enhances the analgesic effect of the opioids. Avoiding the peaks and valleys of pain relief with bolus injections provides a more constant analgesic effect for patients with cancer pain. The need for around-the-clock dosage is clear. Fixed dosage schedules with adequate doses for pain relief provide more constant blood levels and predictable pain relief. Some patients have breakthrough pain that requires additional doses, but the fixed dosage schedule should be maintained. Side effects of the narcotics that require monitoring and intervention by the nurse include constipation, vomiting, and respiratory and central nervous system depression.

Patient self-control methods include distraction, massage, relaxation, biofeedback, hypnosis, and imagery. Many patients respond positively to the opportunity for self-care in the management of pain and indicate that such self-control measures enhance the effectiveness of other prescribed pain interventions.

The nurse's unique contributions to pain management are acting as key link between the patient and the health care team, the amount of time spent with the patient, the ability to assess the patient's response to the pain and its management, and the role of patient and family educator. In addition, the nurse should be able to articulate a concise pain assessment, and anticipate and address patient, family, and health care provider misconceptions about pain management. For example, many patients and their families have opioid phobia, the irrational and undocumented fear that even appropriate use of narcotics causes addiction. This fear of addiction among both health care providers and the public seems to be a major reason for the undertreatment of pain. Fear of addiction should not enter into pain relief for the terminally ill. The nurse must understand and be able to articulate the necessity of opioids in terminally ill patients. The nurse must use pain management strategies appropriately to enable patients and their families to accept the therapeutic value of drugs such as narcotics. Patients should not be subjected to the severe suffering of controllable pain.

General guidelines for the use of pain relief measures are:

1. Use a variety of pain relief measures.
2. Use pain relief measures before the patient's pain becomes severe.
3. Include pain relief measures that the patient believes will be helpful.
4. Determine the patient's ability or willingness to participate actively in the use of pain relief measures.
5. Rely on patient behavior that indicates pain severity rather than relying on known physical stimuli.
6. Encourage the patient to try a pain relief measure at least two times before abandoning it as ineffective.
7. Have an open mind as to what may relieve the patient's pain, including nonpharmacological measures.
8. Keep trying to relieve the pain; do not become discouraged and do not stop working with the patient.

Chemical means of pain management include the use of narcotics and nonnarcotics. Nonnarcotic analgesics of value in the treatment of certain levels of cancer pain are acetaminophen, aspirin, and nonsteroidal anti-inflammatory drugs such as ibuprofen, indomethacin, and naproxen.

Adequate rest, sleep, diversion, and other meaningful activities will also help in the management of the patient's pain.

Fear and anxiety increase as a result of pain. Many cancer patients believe increased pain is a sign their condition is worsening and death is imminent. Pain increases their fear, and the cycle of pain continues.

The combination of (1) appropriate pain relief methods, (2) the opportunity to make personal and spiritual peace if there are unresolved conflicts in relationships with others, and (3) someone to listen and offer comfort is probably the most effective pain reliever known. The patient with advanced cancer often experiences **cachexia**, which is a profound state of ill health, malnutrition, and wasting. Positioning, giving meticulous skin care, offering nutritious fluids and foods, and taking other comfort measures to promote relaxation and rest will also help to reduce pain and severe fatigue.

Caring for the Patient

The patient and the family may become irritable and angry with care givers when suffering and progressive problems are experienced. Nurses should understand that these feelings are not directed toward them personally but have emerged from the circumstances associated with the patient's disease. A display of anger toward the staff may be caused by deep-seated frustration or anxiety. Understanding and continued warm, responsive caring are the best approaches. The patient may not hear the explanations that have been given when feelings are at a high level. By listening and administering kind and gentle nursing care, the nurse may communicate more effectively than with words. Touch may also be appropriate to add the dimension of another human being's awareness of the emotional distress being experienced.

Nurses are in the enviable position being able to make cancer's effect less traumatic through sensitivity and creativity. Nurses need to understand how much each patient needs a sense of control—some need it more than others. The health care system encourages dependency by stripping away most traces of a patient's identity. An adult is told when to get out of bed, have a drink, wash up, even urinate. The nurse should be aware of the dynamics of what is happening to the patient, and provide as many avenues of control by the patient as possible. It is important that nurses learn the art of talking to patients, not at patients. Stay watchful, for the family and the patient's sake.[33]

Terminal Prognosis

Coping with the multiple problems experienced when one has advanced cancer can lead to a sense of helplessness and hopelessness in spite of all efforts. The patient and the family may look forward to death as a relief from unrelenting suffering.

Spiritual activities may provide mental and emotional strength in spite of physical deterioration. The patient may ask the nurse to read the Bible or to pray together, or the patient may request that a minister, priest, or rabbi visit. Spiritual strength may help the patient and the family to cope with continuing problems encountered in the cancer experience.

The hospital social worker assists the patient/family in planning to meet the immediate needs for home care. Arrangements for any special supplies and equipment are made before discharge. The nurse plays a major role in teaching the patient and at least one family member or significant other how to continue any special care needed at home, such as dressing changes, irrigations, the management of a feeding tube, or the care of a central venous line for administration of parenteral nutrition or medications.

Throughout the hospital stay, nurses must take advantage of time available to promote self-care to the extent possible. Assessment of readiness to learn and ability to assume active participation in caring for self is a major responsibility of nurses. Advanced clinical nursing specialists may need to be consulted to provide individualized guidelines for teaching patients. Plans for patient education must be written on the nursing care plan. Evidence of the patient's comprehension of and ability to handle self-care must be documented, and assistance needed from others must be planned and provided for accordingly. Continuity of care is the goal in discharge planning. Hospice services can be arranged in most communities for those who have advanced cancer. There are free-standing hospices, hospices within a hospital or skilled nursing facility, or at-home arrangements. The primary focus of hospice is enhancing the quality of life for the individual, not prolonging life. Efforts are directed toward relief from pain and other problems. Skilled professional care and voluntary support services are provided to assist the patient and family to live life to the fullest each day. See Chapter 53 for a discussion about hospice care.

REFERENCES AND SUGGESTED READINGS

1. American Cancer Society: *Cancer facts and figures,* Atlanta, 1991, The Society.
2. American Cancer Society: *Cancer facts and figures, 1992,* Atlanta, 1992, The Society.
3. Baird S et al: *Cancer nursing: a comprehensive textbook,* Philadelphia, 1991, Saunders.
4. Belcher AE: *Cancer nursing: Mosby's clinical nursing series,* St Louis, 1992, Mosby.
5. Berwich M et al: The role of the nurse in skin cancer prevention, screening, and detection, *Semin Oncol Nurs* 7(1):64, 1991.
6. Bower CL: Three cancer complications that can't wait, *Nursing* 23(10):34, 1993.
7. Brown H: The twenty-first century and the control of cancer, *Oncol Nurs Forum* 17(4):497, 1990.
8. Brunner L et al: *Textbook of medical-surgical nursing,* ed 7, Philadelphia, 1992, Lippincott.
9. Burrell L: *Adult nursing in hospital and community settings,* Norwalk, Conn, 1992, Appleton & Lange.
10. Cancer update 92, *Nursing* 22(3):62, 1992.
11. Cancer update 93, *Nursing* 23(4):59, 1993.
12. *Chemotherapy and you,* US Department of Health and Human Services, National Cancer Institute, 1990.
13. Derby S: Ageism in cancer care of the elderly, *Oncol Nurs Forum* 18(5), 1991.
14. Fischbach F: *Laboratory and diagnostic tests,* Philadelphia, 1992, Lippincott.
15. Flyge HA: Meeting the challenge of neutropenia, *Nursing* 23(7):60, 1993.
16. Holdbrook-West E: Did Henry deserve more from us? *RN* 96(10):42, 1993.
17. Holmes F et al: Biology of cancer and aging, *Cancer Supplement* 68(11):2525, 1991.
18. Kim MJ, McFarland GK, McLane AM: *Pocket guide to nursing diagnosis,* ed 5, St Louis, 1993, Mosby.
19. Laszlo J, Cotanch P: Managing chemotherapy induced nausea and vomiting, *Cancer Supplement* 70(4), 1992.
20. Litley LL, Scott HB: Taxol for ovarian cancer: what you need to know, *Am J Nurs* 93(12):46, 1993.

21. Long BC, Phipps WJ, Cassmeyer VL: *Medical-surgical nursing: a nursing process approach,* ed 3, St Louis, 1993, Mosby.
22. Mach C: Assessment of the autologous bone marrow transplant patient according to Orem's self-care model, *Cancer Nurs* 15(6):429, 1992.
23. McCaffery M, Beebe A: *Pain: clinical manual for nursing practice,* St Louis, 1989, Mosby.
24. McKenry L, Salerno E: *Pharmacology in nursing,* St Louis, 1992, Mosby.
25. Meyer C: Oncology nurses: doing the unexpected, *Am J Nurs* 93(5):79, 1993.
26. *Mosby's medical, nursing, and allied health dictionary,* ed 4, St Louis, 1994, Mosby.
27. New drugs: a dose a day can keep enemies at bay, *Am J Nurs* 94(7):55, 1994.
28. Oberst M et al: Self-care burden, stress appraisal and mood among persons receiving radiotherapy, *Cancer Nurs* 14(2), 1991.
29. Otto S: *Oncology nursing,* St Louis, 1991, Mosby.
30. Pagana KD, Pagana TJ: *Mosby's diagnostic and laboratory test reference,* 1992, Mosby.
31. Phipps WJ et al: *Medical-surgical nursing: concepts and clinical practice,* ed 4, St Louis, 1991, Mosby.
32. Preisler H, Raza A: The role of emerging technology in the diagnosis and staging of neoplastic disease, *Cancer* 69(6):1520, 1992.
33. Strong B: Advice from a cancer patient, *Nursing* 22(5):46, 1992.
34. Studua K et al: Basic cancer concepts, *Cancer Nurs* 15(6):437, 1992.
35. Swongen A et al: *Nursing pharmacology,* ed 2, Philadelphia, 1991, Lippincott.
36. Thomas CL: *Taber's cyclopedic medical dictionary,* ed 17, Philadelphia, 1993, FA Davis.
37. Thompson JM et al: *Mosby's manual of clinical nursing,* ed 3, St Louis, 1993, Mosby.
38. Tucker SM et al: *Patient care standards: nursing process, diagnosis, and outcome,* ed 5, St Louis, 1992, Mosby.
39. Volunteers of the American Cancer Society: *Testicular health,* Georgia Division, Inc, 16-003 GA Div Health Service, 1990.
40. Ward S et al: Patients' reactions to completion of adjuvant breast cancer therapy, *Nurs Res* 41(6):362, 1992.

CHAPTER CHALLENGE

KEY POINTS

- It is currently estimated that one of every five people in the United States will get cancer, and of the people who do, more than 50% may die from the disease within 5 years.
- There is strong evidence that what people eat or drink or their life-style habits predispose to the development of cancer.
- It is important to have periodic physical examinatins and to seek medical attention promptly if one of the warning signs of cancer develops.
- A common reason for a delay in diagnosing cancer is because early malignant changes are not accompanied by pain.
- Seeking medical attention when any warning signs occur is also frequently delayed because people fear the possible diagnosis of cancer and hope the signs and symptoms will just go away.
- The diagnosis of cancer has a profound effect on family members, as well as on the patient. Shock, disbelief, denial, anger, and fear are experienced. The feelings are accompanied by a high degree of anxiety and a sense of helplessness.
- Most of the side effects from chemotherapeutic agents result from destruction of normal cells from the hematopoietic system, hair follicles, and the gastrointestinal system.
- The American Cancer Society sponsors organized support groups for individuals with the same types of cancer. Some of these are *Reach to Recovery,* the *Lost Chord Club,* and the *Ostomy Club.* Prepared volunteer visitors are available in most communities to visit a newly diagnosed patient on the approval of the responsible physician.
- Spiritual strength assists the patient and the family to cope with the problems experienced as a result of cancer. Based on the patient's preference, religious counsel may be helpful.
- The American Cancer Society, the American Pain Society, the World Health Organization, and the Oncology Nursing Society consider pain control to be a major issue in the management of a person with cancer.
- The concepts of rehabilitation should be applied in planning care for the patient with cancer that will promote the highest level of functioning possible.

STUDY QUESTIONS

1. Ms. Niembers, a 61-year-old patient, is receiving chemotherapy. Ms. Niembers becomes anemic with petechiae and ecchymoses scattered over her upper trunk, especially her arms. Which of the following side effects is Ms. Niember experiencing:
   1. Bone marrow suppression
   2. Cardiac suppression
   3. Liver toxicity
   4. Pulmonary toxicity
2. Before the insertion of a cervical implant, the nurse tells Mrs. Peters what to expect while it is in place. Which statement is accurate:
   1. "Nurses will always be available, but they will spend only short periods of time at your bedside."
   2. "Personal cleanliness is essential, so you will be given a complete bedbath each day."
   3. "Pain or discomfort is a common side effect of this type of radiation."
   4. "Your bed linens will be completely changed each day to minimize radioactive contamination."
3. Tom Jones, a 24-year-old patient, has been receiving chemotherapy for acute lymphoblastic leukemia. Which of the following statements would indicate Tom understands discharge teaching concerning leukopenia:
   1. "I am cured and have no limitations."
   2. "My family can catch leukopenia, so I need to be careful not to get too close to any of them."
   3. "I should avoid close contact with persons who might give me an infection."
   4. "I need to be careful not to cut myself when shaving, because I may not be able to stop the bleeding."
4. Ms. Ramus, a 42-year-old patient, has palpated a small lump on her left breast during her monthly breast self-examination. She has scheduled an appointment with her physician. Which of the following tests will be used to make a definite diagnosis of a benign or malignant tumor of her breast:
   1. Biopsy
   2. Mammography
   3. Tomography
   4. Ultrasound
5. Mr. Romero, age 58, is instructed by the nurse in the correct preparation for laboratory testing of his stools for occult blood. Which of the following will he be instructed to avoid for 4 days prior to testing:
   1. Aspirin and vitamin C
   2. B complex vitamins
   3. Fat-soluble vitamins
   4. Antibiotics
6. The nurse educator is discussing the importance of the reduction of carcinogens in primary prevention of cancer. Which risk factor is considered significant in the cause of several types of cancer:
   1. Diet low in fat
   2. Occasional moderate use of alcohol
   3. High pollen count in the environment
   4. Smoking
7. A therapeutic approach by the nurse to assist Mr. Burrows, a terminally ill cancer patient, in the management of his pain is that:
   1. Antiinflammatory agents are effective analgesics for severe pain
   2. Narcotics should be withheld because they are addictive
   3. Pain is what the patient says it is
   4. One can increase one's tolerance for pain
8. Mrs. Lusus, 42 years old, is receiving chemotherapy known to cause alopecia. Which of the following plans is most appropriate:
   1. Suggesting that she buy a wig before she loses her hair
   2. Encouraging her to have a permanent to give her hair body to prevent hair loss
   3. Instructing her to brush her hair vigorously to strengthen the roots
   4. Teaching her to rub her scalp with hydrogen peroxide to prevent scalp irritation from hair loss
9. Which of the following statements by Ms. Jorgensen, a chemotherapy patient with a low WBC count, a low platelet count, and an Hgb of 5.6 would indicate the need for further teaching:
   1. "I check my mouth and teeth after each meal."
   2. "I've been very constipated and need an enema."
   3. "My husband and I have been using a vaginal lubrication before intercourse."
   4. "My lips are dry and cracking; I need some lubricant."
10. Mr. Limus, a 62-year-old patient receiving radiation therapy, has red, dry skin in the area of treatment. The nurse instructs Mr. Limus about care of the skin in the marked area. Which of the following indicates Mr. Limus has understood the instructions? He states he will:
    1. Use an astringent after washing the site
    2. Use rubbing alcohol to prevent breakdown
    3. Keep the area as dry as possible
    4. Apply lotion to keep the skin soft

10

MATERNAL AND NEONATAL NURSING

I think this excerpt from a letter to my Dad states my feelings on why I want to be a nurse! "The other day at clinicals, Dad, I was scheduled to be in Physical Therapy, but I was transferred to OB (Maternity Ward) instead. As fate would have it, there was a girl who had a baby, and the baby was born dead. Sometimes, Dad, I question why I was put on this earth, what is my purpose? Well, I was quite certain of that on this particular day. This may sound awkward, but it felt so good just to be able to help these people through such a grave misfortune. I try to remember how so many people help us in our lives and just to be able to reciprocate somehow is such a great reward. I thought I might just become a pretty good nurse after all, Dad. I look forward to when I'll have such complete confidence of that.

Nancy J. Von Opitz
Student Nurse

39

NORMAL PREGNANCY

Gloria E. Wold

KEY TERMS

amniocentesis
antepartal
ballottement
blastocyst
chorionic villi
ectoderm
ectopic pregnancy
endoderm
flagellation
Goodell's sign
gravida
Hegar's sign
implantation
intrapartal
lanugo
mesoderm
morula
para
perinatal
postpartal
prenatal
teratogenic agent
trimester
villi
Wharton's jelly
zygote

LEARNING OBJECTIVES

After reading this chapter, the student should be able to do the following:

- Define the key terms.
- Explain the physiology of conception
- Discuss the anatomical and physiological alterations that occur during pregnancy.
- Identify the components of antepartal assessment.
- Compare the presumptive, possible, and positive signs of pregnancy.
- Discuss the common discomforts of pregnancy.
- List the danger signs that might occur during pregnancy.
- Discuss cultural practices and beliefs that may affect ongoing health care during pregnancy.
- Describe nutritional requirements during pregnancy.
- Identify nursing diagnoses relevant to care of the prenatal patient.

RELATED TOPICS OF INTEREST

- Cultural aspects of nursing care (Chapter 8)
- Signs, symptoms, and physical assessment (Chapter 9)
- Vital signs (Chapter 10)
- Basic nutrition (Chapter 18)
- Care of the patient with a reproductive disorder (Chapter 33)

Few experiences in life are as exciting and challenging as childbearing. The changes that occur in a relatively short time are profound and dramatic. Childbearing is a challenge to the new mother, to the newly developing or changing family unit, to society, and to the nurse who assists in the childbearing process. The maternity nurse is in a unique position of providing care to the unborn.

The goal of maternity care is a healthy pregnancy with a physically safe and emotionally satisfying outcome for both mother and infant. Consistent health supervision and surveillance are of utmost importance. Many maternal adaptations are unfamiliar to pregnant women and their families. The knowledgeable maternity nurse can help the pregnant woman recognize the relationship between her physical status and the plan for her care. Sharing information encourages the pregnant woman to participate in her own care, depending on her interest, need to know, and readiness to learn.

THE PHYSIOLOGY OF PREGNANCY

To comprehend the physiological changes of pregnancy, the nurse must understand the normal anatomy and physiology of the male and female reproductive systems. It is particularly important to review the menstrual cycle and related hormonal activity. It is also important to recognize that specific cells, ova in the female and sperm in the male, carry genetic messages to their offspring. These cells, when united, result in a new individual with a unique genetic makeup, parts of which come from each parent.

Fertilization

During sexual intercourse sperm carried in the ejaculatory semen of the male enters the vagina of the female. By **flagellation** (whiplike movement) the sperm travel through the mucus of the cervical canal (if the mucus is receptive), enter the uterine chamber, and move into the ampulla—the outer third of the fallopian tube. If the timing is such that an ovum has been produced and is also within the ampulla of the tube, fertilization may occur. Fertilization takes place when sperm joins or fuses with the ovum; this is also called *conception.* The fusion of the sperm into the ovum requires approximately 24 hours. Once fertilization has occurred, the new cell is referred to as a **zygote** (cell formed by the union of two reproductive cells) or fertilized ovum. This cell carries 46 chromosomes (44 autosomes and 2 sex chromosomes). At the moment of fertilization the sex of the zygote and all other genetic characteristics are determined and do not change.

Implantation

The zygote moves through the uterine tube by ciliary action and some irregular peristaltic activity. It requires 3 to 4 days to enter the uterine cavity. During this time the zygote is in a phase of rapid cell division called *mitosis.* Further changes result in formation of a structure called the **morula** (developmental stage of the fertilized ovum in which there is a solid mass of cells resembling a mulberry), which develops into the **blastocyst** (the embryonic form that is a spherical mass of cells having a central fluid-filled cavity surrounded by two layers of cells). After the blastocyst is free in the uterine cavity for 1 to 2 days, the exposed cell walls of the blastocyst (called the *trophoblast*) secrete enzymes that are able to break down protein and penetrate cell membranes. These enzymes allow the blastocyte to enter the endometrium and implant. The action of the enzymes normally stops short of the myometrium but may cause slight bleeding in some individuals. This is called *implantation bleeding.* While this bleeding is rarely more than spotting, it may confuse some women who think that they had a very light and short menstrual cycle when they are really pregnant.

The condition of the uterine lining is critical if **implantation** (embedding of the fertilized ovum in the uterine mucosa) of the zygote is to occur. The endometrium during the secretory phase of the menstrual cycle has an enriched vascular bed with enlarged blood vessels and an increased store of glycogen, which will support development of the embryo if implantation occurs. Implantation usually occurs in the fundus of the uterus on either the anterior or posterior surfaces. If uterine conditions are not suitable, it is unlikely that implantation will occur. If intrauterine vascular or hormonal conditions cannot sustain the implanted embryo, a spontaneous abortion will occur. Most spontaneous abortions occur during the first 8 weeks of pregnancy for these reasons. **Ectopic pregnancy,** where implantation occurs outside of the uterine cavity, also poses serious problems. These conditions will be discussed further in Chapter 42.

During the first few weeks after implantation, primary **villi** (short vascular processes or protrusions growing on certain membranous surfaces) appear. These villi are able to use maternal blood vessels as a source of nourishment and oxygen for the developing embryo. This occurs during the stage of development, from the time of implantation, about 2 weeks after conception, until the seventh or eighth week. It is also during these first few weeks that the first stages of the **chorionic villi** (tiny vascular protrusions on the chorionic surface that project into the maternal blood sinuses of the uterus and help to form the placenta) occur. Chorionic villi secrete human chorionic gonadotropin (HCG), a hormone that stimulates the continued production of progesterone and estrogen by the corpus luteum. This is the reason that ovulation and menstruation cease during pregnancy. Primary villi also synthesize protein and glucose for approximately 12 weeks, until the fetus is adequately developed to meet its own needs. The chorionic villi become the fetal portion of the placenta.

Embryonic/Fetal Development

Until the time of implantation, the germinal phase, the cell mass is referred to as the zygote. During this period the fertilized ovum develops from the two original cells into a many-celled organism. The zygote develops two separate and distinct cavities, the amniotic cavity and the yolk sac. The amniotic cavity has walls lined with the **ectoderm** (outer layer of embryonic tissue giving rise to skin, nails and hair) and a cavity filled with amniotic fluid. The yolk sac is lined with the **endoderm** (the innermost of the cell layers; from the endoderm arise the lining of cavities and passages of the body and the covering of most internal organs), which supplies nourishment until implantation. A third layer of primary cells, the **mesoderm** (embryonic middle layer of germ cells giving rise to all types of muscles, connective tissue, bone marrow, blood, lymphoid tissue, and all epithelial tissue) is located between the two cavities. The embryo develops at the point at which these three layers meet, called the trilaminar embryonic disk.

The embryonic stage begins with implantation and comprises approximately the first 8 weeks of pregnancy. During the embryonic stage, the three primary cell layers differentiate into tissue and layers, which form the placenta, embryonic membranes, and the embryo itself. During the embryonic stage, cell growth is rapid. A simple heart begins beating, and rudimentary (basic, initial, or primary) forms of all the major organs and systems develop. By the end of this stage, the embryo has acquired a human appearance. Starting with the ninth week the embryo is referred to as the fetus, and the fetal stage begins.

Many structures are developing simultaneously in the embryo; therefore when an infant is born with one birth defect or abnormality, the physician will check for others that are likely to be present. During the early weeks of pregnancy, often before a woman even knows that she is pregnant, **teratogenic agents** (any drug, virus, or irradiation that the exposure to can cause malformation of the fetus) can cause serious harm. Rubella, a known teratogen (a nongenetic factor that causes malformations and disease syndromes in utero), which is usually a mild childhood disease, is serious if developed at this stage of pregnancy. This virus can affect all of the germ layers and cause serious anomalies, such as cardiac defects, deafness, and mental retardation.

The prenatal calendar, Table 39-1 on pp. 1212-1220, describes fetal development and maternal changes throughout pregnancy.

Embryonic/Fetal Physiology

The Placenta. The *placenta* (Greek,"flat plate") is a disklike organ made up of about 20 sections called *cotyledons.* It is a unique structure, present only during pregnancy. From a few beginning cells this organ develops rapidly. At full term the placenta looks like a large red disk with a diameter of 15 to 20 cm (6 to 10 inches) and a thickness of 2 to 3 cm (1 inch). It normally weighs between 400 and 600 g (1 lb to 1 lb 5 oz). The bulk of the placenta is fetal in origin. It appears dark red and has a rough surface; the cotyledons are apparent as distinct lobes with clefts or divisions between each lobe. The fetal side is smooth and shiny. It consists of the membranes of the amniotic sac that encases the fetus.

As already mentioned, the placenta functions as an endocrine gland secreting HCG and the steroidal hormones estrogen and progesterone, which maintain the pregnancy. In addition, the placenta is the site of the exchange of nutrients, oxygen, and waste products between the fetus and the maternal circulation. While the placenta allows transfer of oxygen and nutrients through such processes as diffusion, active transport, and others, it also has the ability to block the transfer of certain substances. Some viruses are able to cross the placental barrier, but most bacteria are too large to cross. Some drugs do not cross the placenta, but most do cross and can cause serious harmful effects to the growing embryo/fetus. After delivery the placenta is of no further use and is expelled.

The Fetal Membranes. The amniotic sac is composed of two layers, both originating in the zygote. The outer layer, the *chorion,* attaches to the fetal portion of the placenta. The inner layer, the *amnion,* blends with the fetal umbilical cord. These membranes appear to be very fragile, but in fact are strong enough to contain the fetus and amniotic fluid even at full term.

The Umbilical Cord. The umbilical cord joins the embryo to the placenta. It originates in the fetal portion of the placenta and is normally attached near the center. The cord is normally 50 to 55 cm (20 to 22 inches) long and approximately 2 cm (less than 1 inch) in diameter at the time of delivery. Umbilical cords can vary widely in appearance. The major part of the cord is a pale white, gelatinous-mucoid substance called **Wharton's jelly** (a gelatinous tissue that remains when the embryonic body stalk blends with the yolk sac within the umbilical cord). This substance prevents compression of the blood vessels. Normally two arteries and one vein are apparent and may give a ropelike appearance to the cord. The vein carries oxygenated blood to the fetus; the arteries carry deoxygenated blood back to the placenta. The cord has no pain receptors, so cutting at the time of delivery does not cause pain.

Amniotic Fluid. Amniotic fluid acts as a cushion against mechanical injury, helps to regulate fetal temperature, and allows the developing embryo/fetus room for growth. The amount of fluid changes from about 30 ml (1 oz) at 10 weeks to as much as 1 L at delivery. This slightly alkaline fluid is changing continuously. Amniotic fluid contains albumin, urea, uric acid, creatinine, bilirubin, lecithin (phospholipids for fat metabolism), sphingomyelin (a compound consisting of lipids and sphingosine, found in high concentrations in the brain and other tissues of the nervous system), fructose, fat, leukocytes, proteins, epithelial cells, enzymes, and strands of **lanugo** (downy, fine hair characteristic of the fetus between 20 weeks gestation and birth; most noticeable over the shoulders, forehead, and cheeks but is found on nearly all parts of the body except for the palms of the hands and the soles of the feet). Amniocentesis can be done in the later stages of pregnancy. This test helps determine the development, maturity, health, and sex of the fetus. Amniocentesis is not without risks and is performed only to obtain necessary medical information.

Amniocentesis is the procedure in which a small amount of amniotic fluid is removed by passing a needle

Text continued on p. 1221.

TABLE 39-1 Fetal Development and Maternal Events During Pregnancy and Drug Substances to Avoid

	Week 1	Week 2	Week 3	Week 4	Week 5	Week 6	Week 7	Week 8
Baby's development	The ovum becomes fertilized, divides, and burrows into the uterus.	The embryonic disk (ectoderm, entoderm, mesoderm) is formed. These three primitive germ layers will generate every organ and tissue in the baby's body.	The first body segments appear, which will eventually form the primitive spine, brain, and spinal cord.	Heart, blood circulation, and digestive tract take shape. The embryo is now ⅕ inch long; the head is a third of its total length.	The heart starts to pump blood; limb buds appear. Major divisions of the brain can now be discerned.	Eyes begin to take shape; external ears develop from skin folds.	Development is proceeding rapidly. The face is now complete with eyes, nose, lips, and tongue—even primitive milk teeth. Tiny bones and muscles appear beneath the thin skin.	The embryo is now a little more than an inch long, its tiny heart beating at about 40 to 80 times a minute.
Maternal events	Ovaries increase production of "pregnancy-maintaining" hormone, progesterone.	The first period is missed.	Placenta grows to cover one fifteenth of the uterine interior. Breast may begin to feel tender. There is no weight gain.			Exchange of fetal and maternal metabolites across the placenta begins; yet the two circulations are completely separate.	No noticeable weight gain occurs.	The placenta now covers about one third of the uterine lining.

Common maternal discomforts			Morning sickness occurs because increased hormonal activity slows down the digestive system, apparently to enhance the absorption of nutrients for the baby.	Fatigue is thought to be caused by a change in ovarian hormone production (progesterone and relaxin), the purpose of which is to relax pelvic ligaments, stimulate breast growth, and soften the cervix.		Urinary frequency is caused by the uterus compressing the bladder against the pelvic bones, thus reducing its capacity, and also by hormonal changes that affect the water balance in the body.		
Remedies			Eat a few dry crackers before rising. Eat frequent, small, low-fat meals during the day to help. Drink liquids between meals.	Exercise regularly and get plenty of sleep with frequent naps during the day.		Decrease pressure on the bladder at night by sleeping on the side. Also, drink no fluids after 6 PM.		
Drug substance to avoid			Antiemetics: cyclizine (Migral, Marezine), meclizine (Antivert, Bonine), trimethobenzamide (Tigan) (Avoid throughout pregnancy.)	Stimulants: amphetamines, excessive caffeine (Avoid throughout pregnancy.)				
Acceptable alternatives	None: Avoid all drugs not prescribed by a physician for a specific condition. Avoid x-rays.							

Continued.

TABLE 39-1 Fetal Development and Maternal Events During Pregnancy and Drug Substances to Avoid—cont'd

	Week 9	Week 10	Week 11	Week 12	Week 13	Week 14	Week 15	Week 16
Baby's development	Genitalia are now well defined; the baby's sex is determined. Eyelids finish forming and seal shut. The embryo has become a fetus. 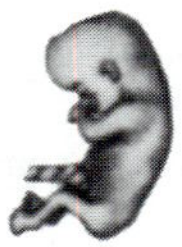	The fetus assumes a more human shape as the lower body rapidly develops. Blood and bone cells form. The first movements begin. 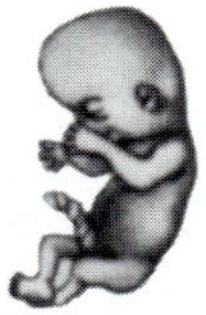	Organs begin to function. The pancreas produces insulin; the kidneys produce urine. 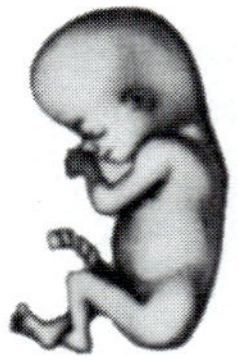	The lungs have taken shape; primitive breathing motions begin. The swallowing reflex has been mastered as the fetus sucks its thumb while floating weightlessly in the amniotic fluid. 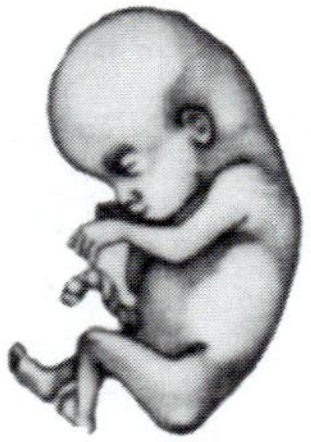	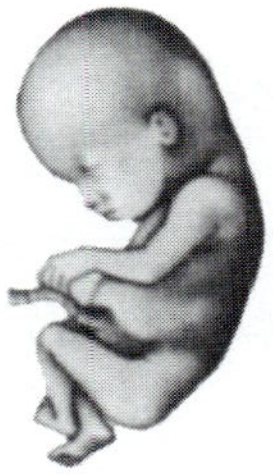	The musculoskeletal system has matured. The nervous system begins to exercise some control over the body; blood vessels rapidly develop. 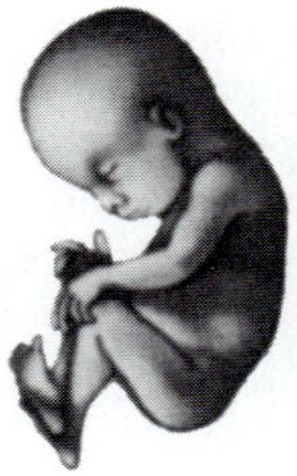	With hands ready to grasp, the fetus, now weighing about 7 ounces, kicks restlessly against the amniotic sac. 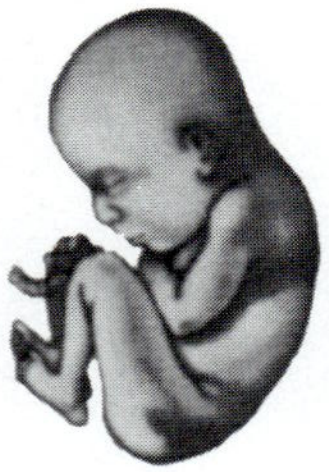	All organs and structures have been formed, and a period of simple growth begins. 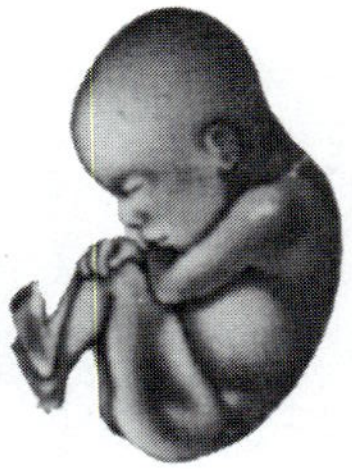
Maternal events	Maternal blood volume has increased 30% to 40%.	The sensation of these first movements has been described by some women as if something were blowing bubbles through a straw in their stomachs.	There is a 2- to 3-pound weight gain and a possible increase in perspiration.	The placenta has reached complete functional maturity, acting as the baby's lungs, kidneys, liver, and digestive and immune systems.		There is a 3- to 4-pound weight gain, and her belly begins to show.		The fetal heartbeat can now be heard with an amplified stethoscope. Placenta begins producing the estrogen hormone.

Common maternal discomforts	Sleeplessness may result from the discomfort or anxieties of pregnancy.				Vaginal secretions are the result of an increased supply of blood and glucose to the vaginal mucosa. Severe pruritus, irritation, and malodor suggest an infection.		Headaches may occur while your body becomes adjusted to changes in blood volume and vascular tone. Emotional tension may also be a factor.
Remedies	Drink a glass of warm milk before bedtime. (It is also good for the baby.)				If infection is suspected, consult a professional. Cleanse daily with warm water, keeping the area dry to prevent chafing. Apply yogurt for vulvar pruritus.		Change body positions slowly. Rest with a damp cloth on the forehead, which may help. Drink milk and/or eat a small snack to produce some relief.
Drug substances to avoid	Tranquilizers Narcotics Antihistamines Alcohol Barbiturates (Avoid throughout pregnancy.)				Vaginal anti-infectives: metronidazole (Flagyl) (Avoid throughout pregnancy.)		Analgesics: salicylates (aspirin), phenacetin/caffeine, propoxyphene (Darvon), indomethacin (Indocin) Tranquilizers (Avoid throughout pregnancy.)
Acceptable alternatives	None: Avoid all drugs not prescribed by a physician for a specific condition. Avoid x-rays.				AVC Cream Nystatin vaginal tablets (Mycostatin) Miconazole vaginal cream (Monistat)		Tylenol brand acetaminophen

Continued.

TABLE 39-1 Fetal Development and Maternal Events During Pregnancy and Drug Substances to Avoid—cont'd

	Week 17	Week 18	Week 19	Week 20	Week 21	Week 22	Week 23	Week 24
Baby's development		An oily coating protects the fetus. Fine hair covers the body and keeps the oil on the skin.	Eyebrows, eyelashes, and head hair develop.	The fetus is now following a regular schedule of sleeping, turning, sucking, and kicking and has settled on a favorite position in the uterus.		The skeleton is developing rapidly as the bone-forming cells increase their activity.	Eyelids begin to open and close.	The fetus now weighs about 27 ounces.
Maternal events		There is a 3- to 4-pound weight gain.	Breasts begin secreting colostrum in preparation for nursing.	Placenta reaches its largest size relative to the fetus, covering half the uterine lining. There are 400 ml of fluid in the amniotic sac.		There is a 3- to 4-pound weight gain.		The placenta becomes thicker rather than wider. Mother can now sense when baby is awake.
Common maternal discomforts		Faintness or dizziness when standing suddenly. This is caused by reduced blood flow to the brain as the body adjusts to new circulatory patterns. Shortness of breath may occur.	Varicose veins are often the result of rising blood pressure in the lower extremities. This is caused by the enlarged uterus cutting off blood flow back from the legs to the heart.	Allergies, such as hay fever, are a common problem for some people.		Skin changes such as darkened nipples, stretch marks, splotches on cheeks and forehead, acne, redness on palms and soles of feet are due to increased hormone levels in the blood.		Epistaxis sometimes occur because of increased blood volume and nasal congestion.

Remedies	Try to sit with your feet up when possible; rise slowly and support yourself.	When sitting, rest legs on footstool with feet elevated; avoid pressure on lower thighs. (Many women find support stockings helpful.)	Use air conditioning (with a clean filter) and wear a pollen mask to screen out allergens.		Be patient. (Virtually all of these effects will subside soon after childbirth.)		Apply a little petroleum jelly in each nostril, which should stop the bleeding. Use a humidifier. Do not irritate nasal mucosa.
Drug substances to avoid	Tranquilizers Alcohol (Avoid throughout pregnancy.)		Most antihistamines: hydroxyzine (Atarax), trimeprazine (Temaril) (Avoid throughout pregnancy.)		Tetracycline (for acne) (Avoid throughout pregnancy.)		
Acceptable alternatives (occasional use)	Smelling salts Aromatic spirits of ammonia		Chlorpheniramine for congestion; nasal spray for stuffy nose, occasionally. Calamine lotion for rashes.		If nipples or abdomen itches, a lanolin-based cream or baby oil can provide relief. A mild soap can remove the excessive facial oil produced by acne.		Pseudoephedrine or nasal spray may be used occasionally for stuffy nose, if necessary.

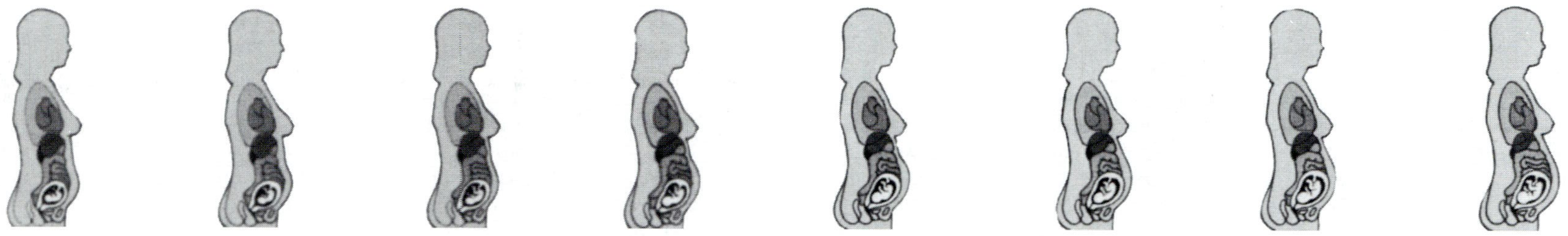

Continued.

TABLE 39-1 Fetal Development and Maternal Events During Pregnancy and Drug Substances to Avoid—cont'd

	Week 25	Week 26	Week 27	Week 28	Week 29	Week 30	Week 31	Week 32
Baby's development		To a certain extent, the baby can now breathe, swallow, and regulate its body temperature but still depends greatly on maternal support.	A substance called **surfactant** forms in the lungs, preparing them to function independently after birth.	Baby is two-thirds grown.	Fat deposits are building up beneath the skin to insulate the baby against the abrupt change in temperature at birth.	The digestive tract and the lungs are now nearly fully matured, and the skin becomes less red and wrinkled.	The baby has grown to about 14 inches.	
Maternal events		There is a 3- to 4-pound weight gain.	Respiratory movements can be detected by ultrasound. Mother sometimes feels baby's breathing as "hiccups."	The volume of amniotic fluid decreases to make room for growing fetus.		There is a 3- to 5-pound weight gain.		Mother may have trouble sleeping because of baby's activity.
Common maternal discomforts			Leg and muscle cramps may be caused by fatigue, pressure exerted on the nerves by the uterus, or too little calcium or too much phosphorus in the diet.	Pyrosis (heartburn) often occurs as the stomach emptying time is delayed, causing a burning sensation in the throat.		Edema of ankles. The pressure of the uterus on the large veins returning blood to the heart may induce water retention.	Constipation is another result of the decelerated digestive process. As food moves slowly through the intestines, more water is extracted, leaving the stool drier and harder.	Hemorrhoids may also develop.

Remedies			Exercise regularly, walking especially. Elevate legs and flex toes when resting. Increase milk consumption.	Drink milk between small, frequent meals. (This problem will disappear soon after your baby's birth.)		Elevate legs—once or twice a day for an hour or so—level with your hips. Sleep on your left side.	Eat foods containing roughage, such as raw fruits, vegetables, and cereals with bran. Drink liquids and exercise frequently.	Soak in a warm bath or sit on soft pillows to soothe the symptoms.
Drug substances to avoid			Salicylates (aspirin) Tranquilizers (Avoid throughout pregnancy.)	Antacids: calcium carbonate, magnesium trisilicate (Gaviscon), sodium bicarbonate (baking soda), cimetidine (Tagamet) (Avoid throughout pregnancy.)		Most diuretics ("water pills") (Avoid throughout pregnancy.)	Laxatives: mineral oil, castor oil (Avoid throughout pregnancy.)	
Acceptable alternatives (occasional use)			Calcium supplements with little or no phosphorus.	Maalox Mylanta (also for "gas")			For constipation: Metamucil, Senokot, teaspoon of milk of magnesia at bedtime	For hemorrhoids: Nupercainal suppositories or cream, Anusol, Medicone

Continued.

TABLE 39-1 Fetal Development and Maternal Events During Pregnancy and Drug Substances to Avoid—cont'd

	Week 33		To Term
Baby's development			
	Virtually the entire uterus is now occupied by the baby, and its activity is restricted.	Maternal antibodies against measles, mumps, rubella, whooping cough, and scarlet fever are transferred to the baby, providing protection for about 6 months until the infant's own immune system can take over.	
	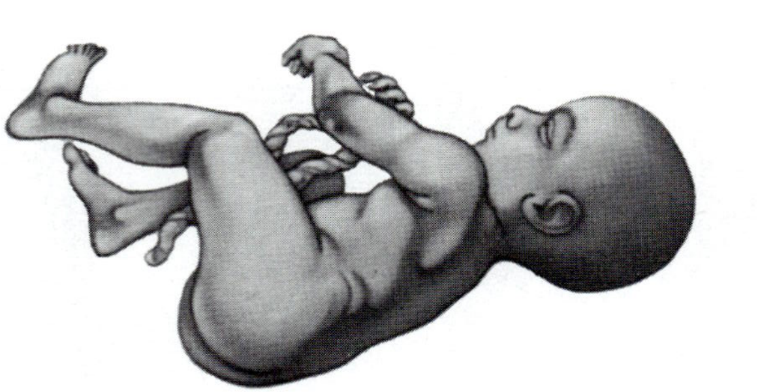		
Maternal events			
	The placenta is nearly 4 times as thick as it was 20 weeks before and weighs about 20 ounces.	Preparing for birth, the baby descends deeper into the mother's pelvis. There is a 3- to 5-pound weight gain.	In 9 short months, the miracle is complete; a single, microscopic fertilized cell has transformed into a 6 trillion-celled human being.
Common maternal discomforts			
	Backaches are often caused by muscles and ligaments relaxing in preparation for the stretching required in delivery and by the added off-center weight of the enlarged uterus.	Urinary frequency is caused—for the second time in pregnancy—by the uterus compressing the bladder against the pelvic bones, thus reducing its capacity.	Uterine contractions become perceptible as the cervix and lower uterine segment prepare for labor.
Remedies			
	Do back exercises, such as the "pelvic tilt," which can help strengthen back and abdominal muscles. Wear low-heeled shoes or flats; avoid heavy lifting.	Decrease pressure on the bladder at night by sleeping on your side. Urinate frequently.	
Drug substances to avoid		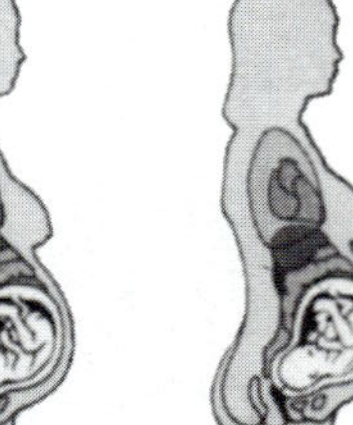 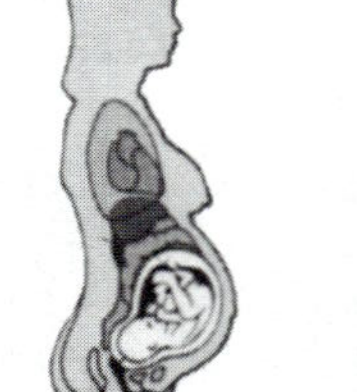	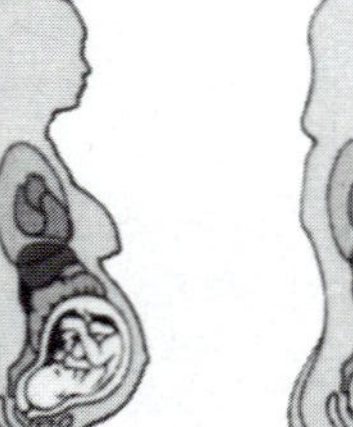 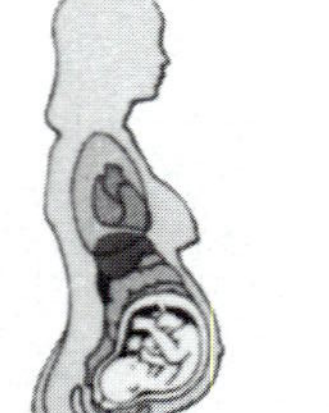
	Analgesics: salicylates (aspirin), propoxyphene (Darvon), phenacetin/caffeine, indomethacin (Indocin), codeine (Avoid throughout pregnancy.)		
Acceptable alternatives			
(occasional use)	Tylenol brand acetaminophen		

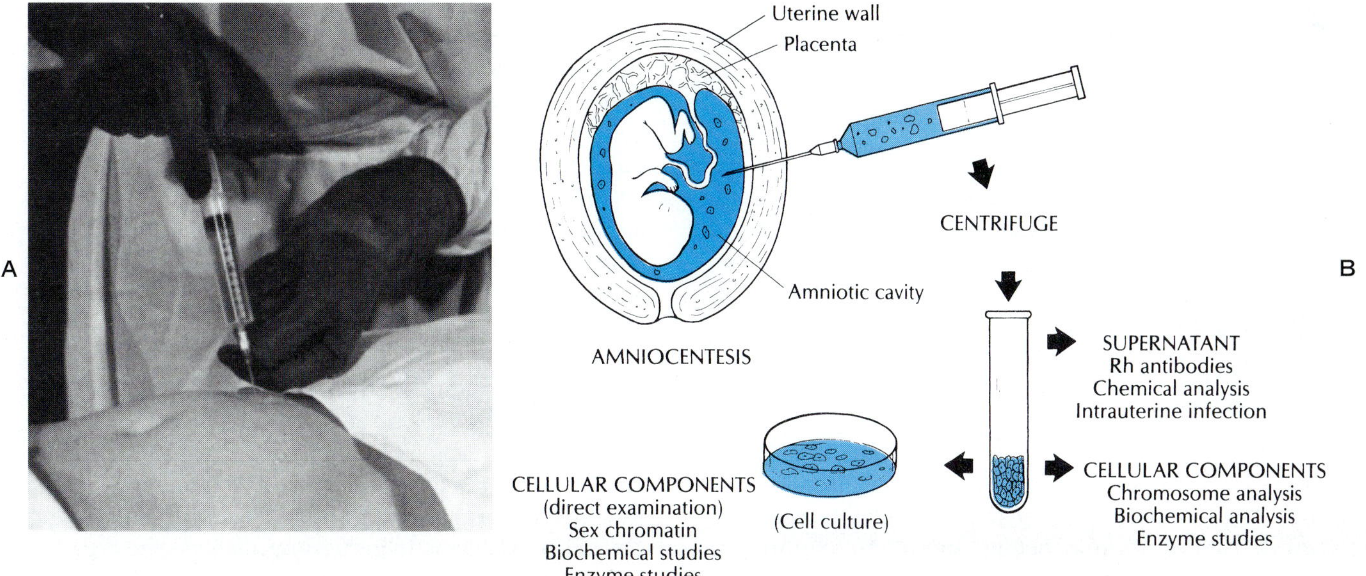

FIG. 39-1 **A,** Transabdominal amniocentesis. **B,** Amniocentesis and laboratory use of amniotic fluid aspirant. (Courtesy March of Dimes.)

though the abdominal wall (see Fig. 39-1). This procedure is usually conducted in conjunction with abdominal ultrasound, which enables the physician to visualize the location of the fetus, placenta, and pocket of amniotic fluid. Laboratory examination of the amniotic fluid can reveal valuable information regarding genetic factors such as sex and chromosomal abnormalities, health status, and maturity of the fetus.

Early amniocentesis is performed at approximately the sixteenth week of pregnancy and is used to detect the presence of biochemical or chromosomal abnormalities. Testing at this time allows the mother time to consider termination of the pregnancy before the legal point of viability (22 weeks) is reached. Later in pregnancy amniocentesis is primarily used to determine fetal lung maturity. It is sometimes performed to detect the presence of intrauterine infection or fetal distress.

Chorionic villus sampling (CVS) is a relatively new test to detect genetic disorders of the fetus. It can be performed even earlier than amniocentesis, usually at 8 to 12 weeks' gestation. During this test the physician aspirates a small amount of tissue from the chorion of the placenta through the cervix. This tissue is then analyzed for signs of chromosomal abnormality. The earliest possible detection of problems is desirable if therapeutic termination of pregnancy is being considered. First trimester abortions are generally less traumatic, physically and psychologically, than termination at a later time.

Fluorescence in situ hybridization (FISH) is a newly developed diagnostic test for fetal chromosomal abnormalities. This test is usually performed between 10 and 15 weeks' gestation and provides rapid information regarding the risk of fetal defects.

MATERNAL PHYSIOLOGY

Hormonal Changes

Estrogen and progesterone levels remain elevated for the first 8 to 10 weeks of pregnancy as a result of HCG, which supports the corpus luteum. After this time the placenta takes over production and maintains necessary levels. As long as these levels are high, follicle-stimulating hormone (FSH), luteinizing hormone (LH), and ovulation are suppressed, as is menstruation.

Uterus

The uterus enlarges during pregnancy as a result of hormonal stimulus, increased vascularity, hyperplasia (new muscle fiber and tissue), and hypertrophy (enlargement of existing fiber and tissue). The nonpregnant uterus is pear shaped and weighs approximately 50 g (2 oz). By the third trimester (the last 3 months of a 9-month pregnancy), it is egg shaped and has increased in weight to 1000 g (2.2 lb). At term it can hold a fetus, placenta, and amniotic fluid totaling more than 4000 g (8.5 lb).

The consistency of the tissue changes also. Changes in the cervix and fundus, along with an altered position in the pelvis, are early signs of pregnancy.

The uterus, which in a nonpregnant state is a pelvic organ, will rise to the base of the ribcage. The superior aspect of the uterus (the fundus) will be located at the level of the xiphoid process when the pregnancy reaches completion.

Breasts

Changes occurring in the breasts during pregnancy include hypertrophy of the mammary glandular tissue and increased vascularization, pigmentation, size, and prominence of nipples and areolae. These breast changes are all caused by hormonal stimulation.

The Maternity Cycle

The maternity cycle, which will be discussed in this and successive chapters, is divided into three distinct periods. The first portion of the cycle is called the **antepartal** (fr. Latin root *ante,* "before," and *parere,* "to bring to bear") or **prenatal** (fr. Latin root *pre,* "before," and *natal,* "birth") The antepartal period begins with conception and ends with the onset of labor.

The next portion of the cycle is referred to as the **intrapartal** period (fr. Latin *intra,* "within"). This period begins with the onset of labor and ends with delivery of the placenta. The same period is sometimes called the **perinatal** portion (fr. Latin *peri,* "around," and *natal,* "birth") because it pertains to the time and process of giving birth.

The final stage of the maternity cycle is the **postpartal** period (fr. Latin *post,* "after"). This period starts after the delivery of the placenta and lasts for approximately 6 weeks or until the reproductive organs return to the prepregnancy state.

Pregnancy spans 9 months, approximately 40 weeks. Pregnancy is also divided into 3-month periods or **trimesters.** The first trimester covers weeks 1 through 13; the second, weeks 14 through 26; and the third, weeks 27 through term gestation (38 to 40 weeks).

ANTEPARTAL ASSESSMENT

General Physical Assessment

When a woman suspects she is pregnant and visits the physician's office or clinic, assessment should begin. Ideally the woman has been receiving regular medical attention and is already known by the health care provider. Unfortunately, because of cost or frequent changes of residence, many people do not receive regular, routine health care. Many women also seek the attention of a specialist, obstetrician nurse practitioner, or midwife during pregnancy. This necessitates establishing a new primary care practitioner-patient relationship and total review of the health history.

On the first visit demographic (study of the human population) data such as age, occupation, marital status, and insurance information are obtained (see Chapter 9). This basic information helps the primary care practitioner identify potential areas of concern. For example, an adolescent who is 15, single, unemployed, and a high school dropout with no insurance presents a very different set of concerns from those of a 25-year-old, married college graduate with comprehensive insurance.

A basic family and personal medical history is obtained. To anticipate any problems, the primary care practitioner must be aware of any genetic diseases present in either the mother's or father's family. A family history that includes genetic diseases may increase the concerns of a pregnant woman until she is assured that her baby is normal. If serious genetic problems are known, many couples seek genetic counseling before they consider having children.

A personal medical history is taken and a review of systems is done. Information about such chronic diseases as cardiac problems, hypertension, diabetes mellitus, and infectious diseases (e.g., rubella, AIDS and other sexually transmitted diseases) is obtained, and any history of accidents or previous surgeries is documented. Significant findings in these areas may indicate the potential for problems and the need for early medical and nursing intervention. High-risk pregnancies will be discussed in Chapter 42.

Life-style patterns including recreational activities, nutrition, and eating habits, use of prescription medication or street drugs, alcohol, work exposure to hazardous conditions, and smoking are assessed. Early detection of problem situations and correction of these can reduce hazards to the woman and prevent detrimental effects on the growth and development of the fetus.

A basic physical examination—including measurement of height and weight and vital signs (see Chapter 10); assessment of heart, lungs, and reflexes; and a general physical inspection of skin and mobility—is normally done. Basic blood work includes (1) hemoglobin and hematocrit assessment, (2) serology tests for detection of infectious diseases such as syphilis and possibly for the human immunodeficiency virus (HIV) and hepatitis virus, (3) blood typing and Rh factor determination, and (4) rubella titer. Routine urinalysis is done to test for glucose, protein, and ketones. Pregnancy tests may be ordered if the pregnancy has not already been confirmed. All these tests increase the data available and enable the primary care practitioner to plan comprehensive care.

Obstetrical Assessment

In addition to the general health history and physical examination, information about the woman's gynecological, menstrual, and obstetrical history is obtained. This includes the use of contraceptives and the regularity of the menstrual period, including frequency, duration, amount of flow, presence of pain, and any other significant comments. Any history of gynecological surgery, vaginal discharge, or herpes infection is reviewed. The physician may ask questions also regarding exposure to DES (diethylstilbestrol), since daughters of women who took DES during pregnancy have an increased risk of spontaneous abortion caused by incompetent cervix.

The woman's number of pregnancies and their outcomes are discussed. This includes the course of the pregnancy with special attention to any complications, the type of delivery (vaginal or cesarean), the presence of any complications during delivery, the use of forceps or other medical assistance, the type of anesthetic used, the condition of the newborn, and any complications of the postpartum period.

Gynecological Examination

The gynecological examination normally includes palpation and auscultation of the abdomen, visualization of the cervix and vagina, evaluation of the bony pelvis, palpation of the uterus externally or bimanually, depending on the situation, and an examination of the vulva, perineum, anus, and rectum. If a Papanicolaou, or Pap, smear is needed, this may be obtained at the beginning of the examination. The nurse is often called on to prepare the necessary equipment and assist in this examination. The nurse should also provide explanations and emotional support to the patient (see Chapter 9).

DETERMINATION OF PREGNANCY

Many times it is a suspicion of pregnancy that brings a woman to the doctor's office. After the entire history and physical examination have been done, the physician can determine with varying degrees of certainty that this is in fact true.

Presumptive Signs

The presumptive signs given below are indicators that a woman may be pregnant, but these signs may also be indicators of other conditions not related to pregnancy. Box 39-1 lists the signs and symptoms of pregnancy.

- *Amenorrhea:* Absence of menstruation is frequently an early sign of pregnancy but can also be seen with other hormonal conditions, changes in environment, malnutrition, fatigue or stress, and menopause.
- *Nausea and vomiting:* The number of potential causes for nausea and vomiting is limitless and in and of itself is not indicative of pregnancy.
- *Frequent urination:* As the uterus enlarges, it is common for a woman to experience urinary frequency. However, many other conditions ranging from diabetes mellitus and cystitis to emotional stress can cause urinary frequency.
- *Breast changes:* Swelling, tingling, and tenderness of the breasts are common during pregnancy, along with changes in pigmentation of the areola.

Box 39-1 SIGNS AND SYMPTOMS OF PREGNANCY

PRESUMPTIVE	PROBABLE	POSITIVE
Amenorrhea Nausea and vomiting Urinary frequency Breast changes Abdominal changes Quickening Skin changes: Chadwick's sign	Changes in the reproductive organs: Hegar's sign Goodell's sign Ballottement Positive pregnancy tests	Radiographic visualization Fetal motion detected by trained observer Auscultation of fetal heart sounds

Many women experience similar changes during the normal menstrual cycle. There are several sebaceous glands (Montgomery's tubercles; Montgomery's glands) on the areolae of the breasts; these tubercles normally enlarge during pregnancy. The sebaceous material secreted from the ducts of the glands to the skin of each areola serves to lubricate and protect the breasts from infection and trauma during breast feeding.

- *Change in the shape of the abdomen:* Abdominal enlargement is typically seen in the second trimester of pregnancy but can also be caused by tumors or organomegaly (enlargement of any organ).
- *Quickening:* The subjective sensation of fetal movement first occurs at about 16 to 18 weeks' gestation. At times intestinal peristalsis or gas can be mistaken for fetal movement.
- *Skin changes:* Pigment changes, such as darkening of some areas of the body such as the areola, may occur, possibly indicating pregnancy. These changes can also be caused by endocrine disturbances. During the pelvic examination the physician may note that the vagina, cervix, and sometimes the vulva will have a violet or purplish discoloration, which appears at about 6 to 10 weeks' gestation. This is called *Chadwick's sign.* In addition to pregnancy, this sign can be caused by any condition that causes pelvic congestion.

Probable Signs

The probable signs below indicate a high likelihood that the woman is pregnant. These signs are not, however, 100% reliable indicators. Box 39-1 summarizes the signs and symptoms of pregnancy.

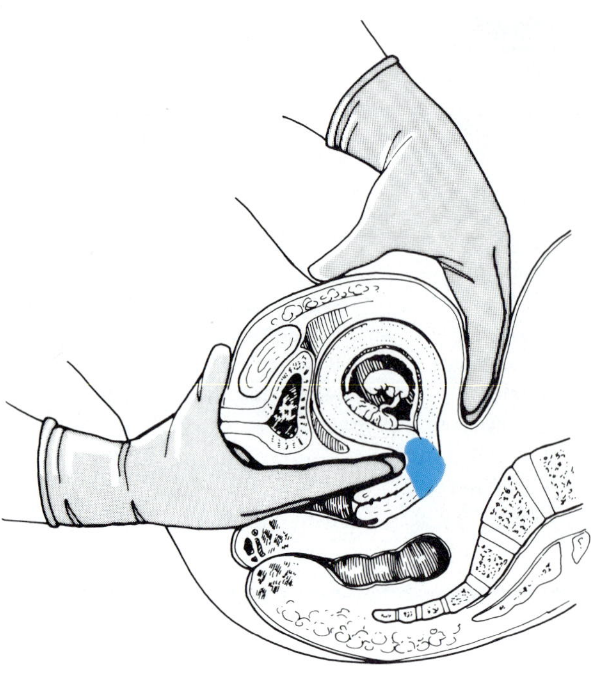

FIG. 39-2 Hegar's sign. Bimanual examination for assessing softening of isthmus while the cervix is still firm.

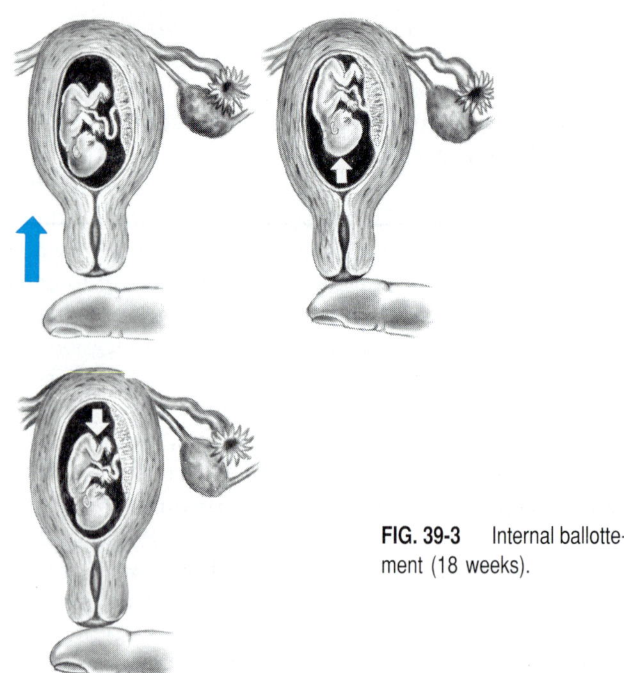

FIG. 39-3 Internal ballottement (18 weeks).

- *Changes in the reproductive organs:* Enlargement of the uterus indicates a high probability of pregnancy, particularly if accompanied by changes in the consistency of the isthmus of the uterus (the segment between the fundus and the cervix). A softening of this segment is called **Hegar's sign** (see Fig. 39-2). This change, and a softening or increased pliability of the cervix called **Goodell's sign,** are most commonly seen in pregnancy. **Ballottement,** which may be used at approximately 16 to 18 weeks' gestation, is a technique that involves palpating the uterus in such a way that the rebound of the floating fetus is felt by the examiner's finger (see Fig. 39-3).
- *Positive pregnancy tests:* Tests are administered using either blood or urine and function by measuring the level of HCG. Many of these tests are now available over the counter in drugstores; however, the reliability of these products is only as good as the technique used in collecting the urine specimen and performing the test. Tests administered by the primary care practitioner are generally between 95% and 99% accurate. Over-the-counter tests tend to yield either false positive readings, in which the woman is not pregnant but the test indicates she is, or false negative readings, in which the test indicates the woman is not pregnant when in fact she is. The greatest advantages of pregnancy tests are that they can be administered early in pregnancy and are reasonably inexpensive. If the test results are positive and other indicators such as uterine changes are abnormal, the primary care practitioner may suspect complications such as an ectopic (outside the uterus) pregnancy or hydatidiform mole (abnormal growth of a fertilized ovum in which a large vascular mass, but no fetus, develops). Hydatidiform mole frequently results in a highly reactive pregnancy test, and the test may continue to indicate positive results even after surgical removal.

Positive Signs

Positive signs are those that occur only with pregnancy and are not present at any other time. Box 39-1 summarizes the signs and symptoms of pregnancy.

- *Visualization:* The fetal skeleton seen on x-ray examination is a positive sign of pregnancy, but use of radiation is generally limited during pregnancy because of possible danger to the fetus. Ultrasonic tracing of the fetus is also a positive indication of pregnancy.
- *Fetal movement:* Fetal movement may be detected by a trained observer (the primary care practitioner).
- *Auscultation of fetal heart beat:* At 10 to 12 weeks' gestation a Doppler or ultrasonic transmitter can be used to detect the fetal heart tone. After 18 weeks, traditional equipment such as a fetoscope can be used to auscultate the fetal heart rate.

Determination of the Estimated Date of Confinement

Normal human pregnancy, counting from the first day of the last menstrual period, is about 280 days, 40 weeks, 10 lunar months (28 days each), or slightly more than 9 calendar months.

The estimated date of confinement (EDC), often known as the "due date," involves calculations based on the woman's menstrual cycle. The most common method is called *Nagele's rule*. Using this rule one would start with the *first day* of the woman's last menstrual period and add seven days, then count back 3 months. For example, if the first day of the last menstrual period was June 14, counting back three months to March 14 then adding 7 days would yield an EDC of March 21. Studies reveal that only a small percentage of infants are actually born on the date predicted; most deliveries, however, do occur within 1 to 10 days before or after the EDC.

If the woman does not keep a menstrual record, calculation of the EDC may be more difficult. The primary care practitioner must then rely on observations such as quickening, estimation of fetal size by palpation, or ultrasonic tests, all of which can be unreliable. If it is imperative that the primary care practitioner know the level of fetal maturity, specialized tests can be performed later in the pregnancy.

Obstetrical Terminology

Specific terms are used in obstetrics to describe the number of times a woman has been pregnant and has given birth. **Gravida** (fr. Latin root *gravidus,* "heavy") indicates a pregnant woman. To this term Latin numerical prefixes are added to indicate number of pregnancies, such as *primigravida* (one), *nulligravida* (none), and *multigravida* (multiple). Similarly, prefixes to the Latin root **-para** (to bring forth) denote the number of births, such as *primipara* (one), *nullipara* (none), *multipara* (multiple). A shorthand method of keeping track of a patient's obstetrical history is used in many facilities; for example, to record the gravida/para, "1/0" indicates the first pregnancy with no viable births.

A more detailed five-part description is sometimes used. The first digit represents the total number of pregnancies, including the present one; the second digit indicates the number of term deliveries; the third indicates the number of premature deliveries; and the fourth indicates the number of abortions. *Abortion* is a medical term indicating loss of a fetus before the age of viability (capable of living) (see Chapter 42). The fifth indicates the number of children living. This is sometimes confusing, because it does not indicate how a child may have died. It also does not include the outcome of an ongoing pregnancy, because this cannot be known until after the delivery. In other words, if all children died in an auto accident, the last number would be 0, even if all the pregnancies and deliveries were normal. For example, a descriptive number such as 5-3-2-0-4 indicates that a woman has been pregnant 5 times, delivered 3 full-term infants and 2 preterm infants, has had no abortions, and has 4 living children.

ANTEPARTAL CARE

Health Perception/Health Management

Most pregnant women want to learn more about pregnancy, childbirth, and motherhood (provided no serious problems in the area of role relationship, coping, or self-perception are occurring). Pregnancy is one time in life when most women see the importance of regular medical supervision and are more willing to make changes in their habits than any other time. It seems that most women are willing to think of their baby first and to do everything that is best for the infant.

A checklist for antepartal needs throughout pregnancy is a valuable tool. It provides the team of care providers with a communication tool to prevent gaps and to identify areas of repeated concerns for patients. When shared with patients, the checklist items validate their universality among gravidas and their families. Knowledge that items are common to many offers some reassurance. Reading the checklist also reminds patients of otherwise forgotten data. Boxes 39-2 through 39-4 on p. 1226 contain the checklists for the first, second, and third trimesters of pregnancy, respectively.

Once pregnancy is diagnosed, prenatal care is instituted. Nursing intervention follows the nursing process: assessment, analysis, and formulation of nursing diagnoses, planning, implementation, and evaluation.

Pregnancy is an excellent time to establish good general health practices if these have been lacking. Many women do not have regular physical examinations or Pap smears or do home screening tests such as breast self-examinations until they become pregnant. The high motivation level makes this a good time for the nurse to teach patients about health maintenance practices. (See Chapters 33 and 38 for discussions of breast self-examination.)

Early in pregnancy the woman often begins to seek information and make choices regarding how and where she wishes to give birth. The nurse can help provide information regarding the options available in a particular community. These options are discussed further in Chapter 40.

Routine care during pregnancy begins with the initial examination and history, as previously described. Appointments are recommended once a month through the seventh month, once every 2 weeks for the next month, and then once every week until delivery. If any problems occur or the primary care practitioner suspects anything

Box 39-2 FIRST TRIMESTER CHECKLIST

- Diagnosis and expected date of delivery
- Schedule and events of visits
- Counseling for self-care
  - Adaptations/discomforts
    - Breast changes
    - Urinary frequency
    - Nausea and vomiting
    - Fatigue
    - Psychosocial responses and family dynamics
- Exercise and rest
- Relaxation
- Nutrition
- Sexuality
- Danger signs
- Resources
  - Education
  - Dental evaluation
  - Medical service
  - Social service
  - Emergency room
- Diagnostic tests
  - Specify
- Other

Box 39-3 SECOND TRIMESTER CHECKLIST

- Schedule and events of visits
- Counseling for self-care
  - Adaptations/discomforts
    - Skin changes
    - Palpitations
    - Faintness
    - GI distress
    - Varicosities
    - Neuromuscular and skeletal distress
  - Safety (seat belts)
  - Exercise and rest
  - Relaxation
  - Nutrition
  - Sexuality
  - Personal hygiene
  - Danger signs
  - Preparation for childbirth and parenthood classes
- Fetal growth and development
- Diagnostic tests
  - Specify
- Other

Box 39-4 THIRD TRIMESTER CHECKLIST

- Schedule and events of visits
- Counseling for self-care
  - Adaptations/discomforts
    - Dyspnea
    - Insomnia
    - Psychosocial responses and family dynamics
    - Gingivitis and epulis
    - Urinary frequency
    - Perineal discomfort and pressure
    - Braxton Hicks contractions
    - Leg cramps
    - Ankle edema
  - Safety (balance)
  - Exercise and rest
  - Relaxation
  - Nutrition
  - Sexuality
  - Danger signs—general
  - Danger signs—preterm labor
- Fetal growth and development
- Preparation for baby
  - Feeding method
  - Nipple preparation
- Preparation for labor
- Recognition: false versus true
  - Prenatal classes
  - Control of discomfort
  - Hospital tour
  - Provision for other family members
  - Preparation for homecoming
- Diagnostic tests
  - Specify
- Other

unusual, such as a multiple pregnancy, the schedule of visits may be altered. Dental care should continue during pregnancy. Any major dental work, such as oral surgery or extractions, is usually delayed until after delivery.

Smoking during pregnancy can be dangerous to the developing fetus. Oxygen deprivation can lead to decreased intrauterine growth and low birth weight.

Drinking alcoholic beverages during pregnancy is also contraindicated, particularly during the first trimester. Fetal alcohol syndrome will be discussed in Chapter 42.

Taking any medication or drugs during pregnancy, including over-the-counter drugs, should be avoided (Box 39-5). As mentioned, most drugs are able to cross the placenta and are transmitted to the fetus. Only medications prescribed by the primary care practitioner should be taken. Street drugs such as marijuana and cocaine are very dangerous to both mother and fetus and must be avoided.

Box 39-5

FDA PREGNANCY CATEGORIES

The rational use of any medication requires a risk versus benefit assessment. Among the myriad of risk factors which complicate assessment, pregnancy is one of the most perplexing.

The FDA has established five categories to indicate the potential of a systemically absorbed drug for causing birth defects. The key differentiation among the categories rests upon the degree (reliability) of documentation and the risk: benefit ratio. Pregnancy Category X is particularly notable in that if any data exist that may implicate a drug as a teratogen and the risk: benefit ratio does not support use of the drug, the drug is contraindicated during pregnancy. These categories are summarized below:

PREGNANCY CATEGORY AND DEFINITION

A: Adequate studies in pregnant women have not demonstrated a risk to the fetus in the first trimester of pregnancy, and there is no evidence of risk in later trimesters.

B: Animal studies have not demonstrated a risk to the fetus, but there are no adequate studies in pregnant women . . . or . . . Animal studies have shown an adverse effect, but adequate studies in pregnant women have not demonstrated a risk to the fetus during the first trimester of pregnancy, and there is no evidence of risk in later trimesters.

C: Animal studies have shown an adverse effect on the fetus, but there are no adequate studies in humans; the benefits from the use of the drug in pregnant women may be acceptable despite its potential risks . . . or . . . There are no animal reproduction studies and no adequate studies in humans.

D: There is evidence of human fetal risk, but the potential benefits from the use of the drug in pregnant women may be acceptable despite its potential risks.

X: Studies in animals or humans demonstrate fetal abnormalities or adverse reaction reports indicate evidence of fetal risk. The risk of use in a pregnant woman clearly outweighs any possible benefit.

Regardless of the designated Pregnancy Category or presumed safety, no drug should be administered during pregnancy unless it is clearly needed and potential benefits outweigh potential risks.

From Facts and Comparisons, Division of JB Lippincott, St Louis, January 1994.

Today many women continue to work throughout pregnancy. It is important that the work environment be checked for chemicals and other hazards.

Danger Signs During Pregnancy

Although there are many changes and normal discomforts during pregnancy, certain signals indicate the need for immediate medical attention. These danger signs are listed in Box 39-6. The pregnant woman should be taught these danger signs. The nurse must stress the importance of contacting the primary care practitioner promptly if any of these signs are present.

Box 39-6

DANGER SIGNS AND SYMPTOMS DURING PREGNANCY

Visual disturbances—diplopia (double vision), blurring, or spots

Headaches—severe, sudden, or continuous

Edema—swelling of the face, presacral area, or fingers

Rapid weight gain—in excess of normal gain for gestation

Pain—severe abdominal or epigastric pain

Signs of infection—fever, chills, diarrhea, changes in vaginal drainage, pain or burning with urination

Vaginal bleeding—no matter how slight

Vaginal drainage—anything other than normal mucus

Persistent vomiting

Muscular irritability or convulsions

Absence or decrease in fetal movement once felt

Nutritional/Metabolic Health Pattern

Weight Gain. Nutritional needs change substantially during pregnancy, since the mother must meet not only her own nutritional needs but also those of the developing fetus. This does not mean that the woman must "eat for two" by doubling her food intake; this will only lead to extra body weight, which adds to discomfort and increases the stress on all body systems. Weight gain is no longer tightly controlled, but most primary care practitioners recommend weight gain in the 21- to 35-pound range as most desirable. Only 2 to 4 pounds should be gained during the entire first trimester; a gain of about 1 pound per week for the remainder of the pregnancy is normal. Inadequate weight gain or sudden excessive weight gain may indicate problems with nutrition or complications.

Nutritional Requirements.

Caloric intake. Pregnancy places additional demands on the mother's metabolism. To meet her needs and those of the fetus, caloric needs increase about 300 calories per day on average—slightly less early in pregnancy, slightly more later. The woman's activity level must also be taken into account when determining desirable caloric intake. If problems are encountered in determining caloric needs, a dietician should be consulted.

TABLE 39-2 Nutrient Needs of Pregnancy

Nutrient	Amount (RDA 1989) Nonpregnant Adult Need	Pregnancy Need	Reasons for Increased Nutrient Need in Pregnancy	Food Sources
Protein				
	46-50 g	60 g	Rapid fetal tissue growth Amniotic fluid Placenta growth and development Maternal tissue growth: uterus, breasts Increased maternal circulating blood volume: ■ Hemoglobin increase ■ Plasma protein increase Maternal storage reserves for labor, delivery, and lactation	Milk Cheese Egg Meat Grains Legumes Nuts
Calories				
	2200	2500	Increased basal metabolic rate, energy needs Protein sparing	See individual foods
Minerals				
Calcium	800 mg	1200 mg	Fetal skeleton formation Fetal tooth bud formation Increased maternal calcium metabolism	Milk Cheese Whole grains Leafy vegetables Egg yolks
Phosphorus	800 mg	1200 mg	Fetal skeleton formation Fetal tooth bud formation Increased maternal phosphorus metabolism	Milk Cheese Lean meats
Iron	15 mg	30 mg	Increased maternal circulating blood volume, increased hemoglobin Fetal liver iron storage High iron cost of pregnancy	Liver Meats Egg Whole or enriched grain Leafy vegetables Nuts Legumes Dried fruits
Iodine	150 μg	175 μg	Increased basal metabolic rate—increased thyroxine production	Iodized salt
Magnesium	280 mg	320 mg	Coenzyme in energy and protein metabolism Enzyme activator Tissue growth, cell metabolism Muscle action	Nuts Soybeans Cocoa Seafood Whole grains Dried beans and peas
Vitamins				
Thiamine	1.1 mg	1.5 mg	Coenzyme for energy metabolism	Pork, beef Liver Whole or enriched grains Legumes
B_6 (pyridoxine)	1.6 mg	2.2 mg	Coenzyme in protein metabolism Increased fetal growth requirement	Wheat, corn Liver Meat
B_{12}	2.0 μg	2.2 μg	Coenzyme in protein metabolism, especially vital cell proteins such as nucleic acid Formation of red blood cells	Milk Egg Meat Liver Cheese

From Food and Nutrition Board: *RDAs,* ed 10, Research Council, National Academy Press, 1989.

*Basal metabolic rate.

†Provision of adequate nonprotein calories so that protein can be utilized for tissue synthesis and maintenance rather than energy needs.

‡Iron needs during lactation are not substantially different from those of nonpregnant women, but continued supplementation of the mother for 2 to 3 months after parturition is advisable to replenish stores depleted by pregnancy.

TABLE 39-3 Sample Menus for Diet During Pregnancy

Menu 1		Menu 2
Breakfast		
1 c ready-to-eat cereal		1 c oatmeal with
1 slice wheat toast		2 tbsp raisins
1 tsp margarine		2 tsp cinnamon & sugar
1 c orange juice		1 c 1% milk
1 c 1% milk		
Snack		
1 apple		1 c strawberries
2 tbsp peanut butter		1 English muffin with
		2 tsp margarine
Lunch		
2 oz turkey on		2 slices ham and cheese pizza
2 slices wheat bread		1 slice french bread
1 tsp mayonnaise		2 c iceberg lettuce with shredded carrots
1 c spinach salad		2 tbsp low-calorie ranch dressing
6 crackers		Water
1 c 1% milk		
Snack		
½ cantaloupe with		1 c tomato soup
½ c low-fat cottage cheese		6 crackers
Supper		
3 oz lean pork chop		4 oz roast chicken
½ sweet potato with		½ c rice pilaf
1 tsp margarine		½ c asparagus
1 c steamed broccoli		1 c 1% milk
1 dinner roll with		
1 tsp jelly		
Water		
Snack		
2 oatmeal cookies		½ c ice-milk
1 c 1% milk		½ c fruit cocktail
Total number of servings provided:		
Bread group	8	9
Fruit group	3	3
Vegetable group	4	4
Milk group	3½	3½
Meat group	6 oz	6 oz
Fats, oils, and sweets	5	5

The pregnancy diet is a modification of a normal diet based on the Food Guide Pyramid, with increases in those nutrients needed for fetal development. Protein, which supplies amino acids for tissue and blood production, is very important. Two or three servings of the meat group should be included. Milk, which is rich in calcium, is an important nutrient for pregnant women. At least three servings of the milk group is recommended. Fats are important as an energy source and carbohydrates are needed to meet total caloric needs. Two to four servings of the fruit group, three to five servings from the vegetable group, and six to eleven servings from the grain group are advocated. Inadequate carbohydrate intake can lead to abnormal metabolism of protein, decreasing the amount available for growth (see Chapter 18). Dietary recommendations are summarized in Tables 39-2 and 39-3.

Minerals and vitamins. Calcium and phosphorus are necessary for bone and tooth mineralization in the fetus. They also affect the acid-base balance of the body. Iron is essential to prevent anemia, which would decrease the oxygen-carrying ability of the blood. Oxygen transport is very important during pregnancy, because the mother must not only meet her own needs but also meet the needs of the developing fetus. A normal hematocrit level in nonpregnant women is 37% to 47%. During pregnancy this may drop as low as 34% as a result of a condition called *physiological anemia of pregnancy.* The total red blood cell volume normally increases during pregnancy; however, there is an even greater increase in plasma volume. This results in a decreased hematocrit level, even if nutrition and iron intake are adequate. If iron intake is inadequate, serious anemia may result. Supplementation with 30 mg of iron daily is recommended.

Vitamin intake should follow the recommended daily allowance for both water- and fat-soluble forms. Some that are of particular importance are vitamins C and D and folic acid. With the recent information on folic acid and birth defects, it would seem prudent to recommend 400 mcg (0.4 mg) supplement of folic acid per day. Vitamin C requirements are increased in pregnancy to aid in tissue formation; vitamin D is necessary for absorption and utilization of calcium. Folic acid is necessary for fetal growth and prevention of anemia. Vitamin and mineral supplements are frequently prescribed by the physician and should be taken as directed.

Pica. Pica is the craving and eating of substances that are not normally considered edible. The reason for this condition is not known, but it is more common in certain cultural groups and regions of the country. It may be seen in children and occasionally during pregnancy. Substances such as clay or laundry starch are commonly ingested. Although not toxic, both of these may interfere with iron absorption, resulting in anemia. Large amounts of clay may also result in fecal impaction.

Common Discomforts. Many pregnant women experience some discomforts of the GI tract during pregnancy. Excessive salivation (ptyalism) is mentioned by some women; it is thought that this occurs in response to the high levels of estrogen during pregnancy. While it may be uncomfortable and awkward at times, it causes no serious problems and disappears late in pregnancy or after delivery. Use of astringent mouthwash or chewing gum or sucking on hard candy may provide relief.

Nausea in the early stages of pregnancy is a common complaint. This most typically occurs when the woman awakens in the morning; hence the name "morning sickness." It can, however, occur at any time of the day. This is thought to be caused by increased HCG levels and changes in carbohydrate metabolism. If the nausea is mild, it can usually be controlled by slowly eating a few soda crackers or dry toast before rising from bed. Smaller, more frequent meals are also suggested. Avoidance of spicy or greasy food helps in some cases. Morning sickness rarely lasts beyond the fourth month. If it lasts longer, is more severe, and particularly if it involves vomiting, the primary care practitioner should be contacted. The most severe form is called *hyperemesis gravidarum.* The cause of this is not clear, but untreated, it can lead to dehydration, fluid and electrolyte imbalance, acid-base imbalance, and altered kidney and cardiac function. Fetal death may also result. Hospitalization with close medical supervision, including administration of IV feeding, may be required (see Chapter 42).

Pyrosis (heartburn) from gastric reflux into the esophagus can be caused by the increasing size of the fetus in the abdominal cavity, which displaces the stomach. Increased progesterone level, which causes relaxation of the cardiac sphincter, and decreased gastric mobility, which delays the emptying time of the stomach, can also contribute to the problem. Smaller meals taken more often, decreased fat intake, low-sodium antacids, and avoiding lying down after meals often give relief.

Skin Changes. Changes in pigmentation are often seen during pregnancy as a result of increased amounts of melanocyte-stimulating hormone. The changes occur primarily in areas that already have greater pigmentation, such as the areolas, nipples, vulva, perianal area, and linea alba (midline of the abdomen from pubis to umbilicus), which darkens and is called the *linea nigra.*

Chloasma, the mask of pregnancy, is an irregular darkening of the pigment of the cheeks, forehead, and nose. These changes are frequently more obvious in women with darker hair and skin and may be worsened by sun exposure. This generally disappears or fades significantly soon after delivery.

Striae gravidarum, or stretch marks, are reddish, wavy streaks that can appear on the thighs, abdomen, and breasts. These are more common with distention but may occur even in relatively thin women. They usually fade after delivery.

Spider nevi (a branched growth of dialated capillaries on the skin) and *palmar erythema* (reddened palms) are sometimes seen. These are caused by increased blood flow resulting from high estrogen levels. Both usually disappear when the pregnancy ends.

Changes in hair growth and consistency, even significant loss of scalp hair, are noted by some women. This is usually temporary unless other physiological problems are active.

Occasionally, decreased emptying of the gallbladder may result in subclinical jaundice, which causes generalized pruritus (itching). See Table 39-4 for discomfort/concerns related to maternal adaptations during the third trimester.

Hygiene Practices. Bathing or showering during pregnancy should continue as part of routine hygiene. Increased perspiration is common, and good personal hygiene is important to prevent body odor. Tub bathing may become difficult in the later months of pregnancy because of changes in mobility and balance. Some primary care practitioners restrict tub baths in the last month, since the cervix may have begun to dilate.

Most primary care practitioners recommend that women avoid using hot tubs, sauna baths, and spas during pregnancy since central nervous system defects may be a result of maternal hyperthermia during the first trimester. Since early in the first trimester a woman may not be aware she is pregnant, it is probably wise for those not taking measures to prevent pregnancy to also avoid these hyperthermic baths. Douching is not recommended, even though the woman may have increased vaginal discharge. If the vaginal drainage causes pruritus or other symptoms, this should be reported to the primary care practitioner.

It is not essential for a woman to buy special clothing, but whatever garments are chosen should be comfortable and should not restrict movement. It is important to avoid circulation-restricting clothing such as garters. Larger bras may be necessary as breasts enlarge; too snug a bra may interfere with breathing.

Elimination

Gastrointestinal System. Slowing of intestinal peristalsis can result in abdominal distention, flatulence, and constipation. Constipation can also be related to the iron supplements that are being taken.

Hemorrhoids can result from straining as a result of constipation. They can also be caused by the enlarged uterus putting pressure on the pelvic blood vessels, slowing venous return from the lower extremities. Women with a history of cholelithiasis may experience problems with this as a result of an increased cholesterol level, which is common during pregnancy. Adequate fluid intake, dietary roughage, and exercise may help reduce problems related to constipation.

Urinary System. Frequency of urination is a common complaint of pregnancy. During pregnancy the mother must excrete not only her own waste products but also those of the fetus. Urinary output increases during pregnancy and the specific gravity decreases. Early in pregnancy the enlarging uterus irritates the bladder by putting pressure on it. This continues until the uterus rises into the abdominal cavity. Later in pregnancy, when the presenting part descends into the pelvis, the pressure and symptoms return. Kegel's exercises can be taught to

TABLE 39-4 Discomforts/Concerns Related to Maternal Adaptations During the Third Trimester

Discomfort	Physiology	Teaching for Self-Care
Shortness of breath and dyspnea occur in 60% of pregnant women	Expansion of diaphragm limited by enlarging uterus; diaphragm is elevated about 4 cm (1½ in); some relief after *lightening* (when the fetus settles lower in the true pelvis, leaving more space in the upper abdomen)	Good posture; flying exercise; sleep with extra pillows; avoid overloading stomach; stop smoking; refer to physician if symptoms worsen to rule out anemia, emphysema, and asthma
Insomnia (later weeks of pregnancy)	Fetal movements, muscular cramping, urinary frequency, shortness of breath, or other discomforts	Reassurance; conscious relaxation; back massage or effleurage (deep or gentle stroking); support of body parts with pillows; warm milk or shower before retiring
Psychosocial responses—mood swings, mixed feelings, increased anxiety	Hormonal and metabolic adaptations; feelings about impending labor, delivery, and parenthood	Reassurance and support from significant other and nurse; improved communication with partner, family, and others
Return of urinary frequency and urgency	Vascular engorgement and altered bladder function caused by hormones; bladder capacity reduced by enlarging uterus and fetal presenting part; lightening	Kegel's exercises; limit fluid intake before bedtime; reassurance; wear perineal pad; refer to physician for pain or burning sensation
Perineal discomfort and pressure	Pressure from enlarging uterus, especially when standing or walking; multifetal gestation	Rest, conscious relaxation, and good posture; maternity girdle; refer to physician for assessment and treatment if pain is present; rule out labor
Braxton Hicks contractions	Intensification of uterine contractions in preparation for work of labor	Reassurance; rest; change of position; practice breathing techniques when contractions are bothersome; effleurage; rule out labor
Leg cramps (gastrocnemius spasm), especially when reclining	Compression of nerves supplying lower extremities because of enlarging uterus; reduced level of diffusible serum calcium or elevation of serum phosphorus; aggravating factors: fatigue, poor peripheral circulation, pointing toes when stretching legs or when walking, drinking more than 1 L (1 qt) of milk per day; cause unclear	Rule out blood clot by checking for Homans' sign; use massage and heat over affected muscle; stretch affected muscle until spasm relaxes. Physician-prescribed oral supplementation with calcium carbonate or calcium lactate tablets; aluminum hydroxide gel, 1 oz, with each meal removes phosphorus by absorbing it.
Ankle edema (nonpitting) to lower extremities	Edema aggravated by prolonged standing, sitting, poor posture, lack of exercise, constrictive clothing (e.g., garters), or hot weather	Ample fluid intake for "natural" diuretic effect; put on support stockings before rising; rest periodically with legs and hips elevated, exercise moderately; refer to physician if generalized edema develops (diuretics are contraindicated)

help tone the muscles of the perineum and help prevent stress incontinency (see Chapter 33).

Dilation of the ureter and kidneys may occur, particularly on the right side, as a result of placental progesterone and pressure from the enlarging uterus. Restricted circulation in the pelvis as the uterus enlarges increases the risk of bladder trauma and urinary tract infection.

Activity/Exercise

Normal activity should continue throughout an uncomplicated pregnancy. If a woman regularly participates in a fitness program or sport, she probably can continue with most activities. This should be discussed with the primary care practitioner if there are any doubts. High-risk activities or those that require a great deal of balance and coordination are discouraged. Common sense is the best guide.

Fatigue is a common complaint during pregnancy. The woman must pace herself and not overdo tiring activities.

Changes in balance and posture occur as the fetus increases in size. To compensate for the shifting center of gravity, the lumbodorsal curve increases (lordosis). This may result in low backaches. Hormonal influence on pelvic bones, resulting in joint relaxation, can lead to a waddling gait. Footwear with low heels and the use of good body mechanics will help reduce discomfort.

Leg cramps are a common occurrence. These may relate to pressure on the pelvic blood vessels and nerves or altered calcium and phosphorus balance. Dorsiflexion of the foot may help reduce these cramps. Dependent edema and varicose veins can also result from increasing intraabdominal pressure. Many women wear support hose to reduce edema; resting with legs elevated is also helpful.

Round ligament pain or tenderness in the lower abdomen is a result of stretching of the ligaments by the enlarging uterus. There is no way to prevent this, but good body mechanics helps minimize discomfort.

Dyspnea (shortness of breath) may be experienced as the uterus enlarges and pushes the diaphragm upward, reducing the size of the chest cavity. Avoiding large meals, which distend the stomach, and maintaining good posture will help reduce this problem. Exercises are often recommended to help reduce discomfort and to prepare for childbirth. See Box 39-7 for exercise guidelines during pregnancy.

Rest/Sleep

Early in pregnancy few changes in sleep patterns are experienced. However, as the size of the abdomen increases it may become increasingly difficult for the woman to find a position of comfort, particularly for those women who prefer to sleep in the prone position. The supine position is not recommended as a woman approaches her due date, because this may cause excessive pressure on the aorta and vena cava as a result of the increased size of the uterus. The woman may experience syncope and vertigo. The supine position also may result in decreased circulation for the fetus. A side-lying position is recommended.

Placing pillows under the legs and abdomen will promote good body alignment and rest. Naps at intervals during the day can be helpful, but these are not always possible with busy life-styles.

Sexuality/Reproductive

Breast Changes. Breast changes begin early in pregnancy. Many women complain of tingling and a feeling of fullness. Increased sensitivity is also common. Generally the breasts increase in size preparatory to lactation.

Sexual Activity. Sexual desire and activity may change during pregnancy. Unless there are complications in the pregnancy or the bag of waters has ruptured, there is no physiological reason to limit sexual activity during pregnancy. Many factors will have a strong influence on the frequency and type of sexual activity. Both the woman and her partner may experience fears or concerns related to sexual activity during pregnancy. There are many cultural, religious, and psychological influences, and it is important for the partners to communicate their fears, concerns, and needs to each other. Many women experience a decrease in desire as a result of hormonal changes and the multiple discomforts that may be occurring. Change in body shape and body image may also cause concern. Discussion of various coital positions and sexual activity that does not include intercourse is appropriate. The primary care practitioner may promote this discussion by introducing the topic during routine prenatal care.

Increased vaginal secretions are common during pregnancy. Leukorrhea, an increase in vaginal mucus, results from hormonal changes. If the discharge changes in color or odor, the physician should be informed.

Vaginal Bleeding. Vaginal bleeding at any time during pregnancy should be reported to the physician. Sexual activity should cease until the cause of the bleeding is determined and should be resumed only when the physician determines that no danger exists.

Coping/Stress Tolerance

Pregnancy is a developmental landmark. Physiologically it marks the onset of adulthood, no matter what the actual age of the woman. As with other significant developmental changes, anxiety is normal. All the physical and hormonal changes of pregnancy place additional stress on the woman. Fears are plentiful. Will the labor and delivery be painful? Will the baby be normal? Will she be able to provide proper care? Will there be enough money? Mood swings and ambivalence (conflicting emotions) are common as the woman works through her fears and comes to grips with the reality of pregnancy and how this pregnancy will affect her life.

Problem-solving skills and methods of coping that worked in the past are used in an attempt to adjust to this new situation. It is important to provide support as this problem solving occurs and to help the woman work through her unique situation. Explanation of the normal physiological changes and discomforts is important. Listening and allowing the woman adequate time to verbalize her fears can also help reduce anxieties.

Role/Relationship

The expectant woman has generally held several roles in her life, such as child, student, employee, and wife. Pregnancy introduces a totally new role, that of mother.

Box 39-7 EXERCISE TIPS FOR PREGNANT WOMEN

- **Consult your health-care provider** when you know or suspect you are pregnant. Discuss your medical and obsetrical history, your current regimen, and the exercises you would like to continue throughout pregnancy.
- **Seek help** in determining an exercise routine that is well within your limit of tolerance, especially if you have not been exercising regularly.
- **Consider decreasing weight-bearing exercises** (jogging, running), and concentrate on non-weight-bearing activities such as swimming, cycling, or stretching. If you are a runner, you may wish to walk instead, starting in your seventh month.

  Because strenuous exercise during the last few weeks of pregnancy increases the risk of low birthweight, stillbirth, and infant death, reduce exercise sharply 4 weeks before your due date.
- **Avoid risky activities** such as surfing, mountain-climbing, sky-diving, and racquetball. Activities requiring precise balance and coordination may be dangerous.
- **Exercise regularly** at least three times a week, as long as you are healthy, to improve muscle tone and increase or maintain your stamina. Sporadic exercises may put undue strain on your muscles.
- **Limit activity to shorter intervals.** Exercise for 10 to 15 minutes, rest for 2 to 3 minutes, then exercise for another 10 to 15 minutes.
- **Decrease your exercise level** as your pregnancy progresses. The normal alterations of advancing pregnancy, such as decreased cardiac reserve and increased respiratory effort, may produce physiologic stress if you exercise strenuously for a long time.
- **Take your pulse** every 10 to 15 minutes while you are exercising. If it's more than 140 beats per minute, slow down until it returns to a maximum of 90.
- **Avoid becoming overheated** for extended periods. It's best not to exercise for more than 35 minutes, especially in hot, humid weather. As your body temperature rises, the heat is transmitted to your fetus. Prolonged or repeated fetal temperature elevation may result in birth defects, especially during the first 3 months.
- **Warm-up and stretching exercises** prepare your joints for more strenuous exercise and lessen the likelihood of strain or injury to your joints.
- **A cool-down period** of mild activity after exercising will help bring your respiration, heart, and metabolic rates back to normal and avoid pooling of blood in the exercise muscles.
- **Rest for 10 minutes after exercising,** lying on your left side. As the uterus grows, it puts pressure on a major vein carrying blood to your heart on the right side of your abdomen. Lying on your left side takes the pressure off and promotes return circulation from your extremities and muscles to your heart, increasing blood flow to your placenta and fetus.
- **Drink two or three 8-ounce glasses of water** after you exercise, to replace the body fluids you lost through perspiration. While exercising, drink water whenever you feel the need.
- **Increase your caloric intake** to replace the calories burned during exercise. Choose such high-protein foods as fish, cheese, eggs, or meat.
- **Take your time.** This is not the time to be competitive or train for activities requiring long endurance.
- **Wear a supportive bra.** Your increased breast weight may cause changes in posture and put pressure on the ulnar nerve.
- **Wear supportive shoes.** As your uterus grows, your center of gravity shifts and you compensate by arching your back. These natural changes may make you feel off balance and more likely to fall.
- **Stop exercising immediately** if you experience shortness of breath, dizziness, numbness, tingling, abdominal pain, or vaginal bleeding, and consult your health care provider.

Modified from Paglone A, Worthington S: Cautions and advice on exercise during pregnancy, *Contemp OB/GYN* 25:160, 1985 (special issue).

The woman often looks to her own life for persons to model and tends to seek guidance from family and friends. Culture will have much to do with how she will define her role.

There are also changes in the dynamics between the woman and the baby's father, particularly with the first pregnancy. The mother is no longer just a wife or girlfriend; she is also a mother. While she is coping with the role change to mother, he is coping with the role change to father.

Self-Perception/Self-Concept

The rapid changes in body shape and size can lead to changes in self-image. Many women feel that they are not attractive when they are pregnant. They may also feel a loss of control related to the changes taking place. They are no longer free to do as they please, since anything that they do may affect the growing fetus.

Cognitive/Perceptual

Although sensory changes are uncommon with pregnancy, blurring or diplopia (double vision) may indicate problems with pregnancy-induced hypertension. See Chapter 42 for further discussion.

Prenatal education is important. Most primary care practitioners give explanations during routine visits, but the time available is too brief to meet all of the average woman's needs. The nurse should play an important role in prenatal education. Many low-cost pamphlets are available and should be provided whenever possible. Libraries and bookstores also have many good books on prenatal care. Classes are held in many hospitals, clinics, public health agencies, and schools.

PREPARATION FOR CHILDBIRTH

Special classes are offered by hospitals, public health agencies, private organizations, and the Red Cross to help the childbearing family understand and prepare for the demands of pregnancy, labor, the newborn, and parenthood.

There are often a variety of courses available within a community that complement one another and meet the differing needs of specific segments of the population (Fig. 39-4). Some classes are general in nature while others are targeted toward specific groups such as adolescents, those having cesarean or VBAC (vaginal birth after cesarean) delivery, siblings, or grandparents (Box 39-8).

Common methods of prepared childbirth take their names from the physician who proposed specific methods and techniques.

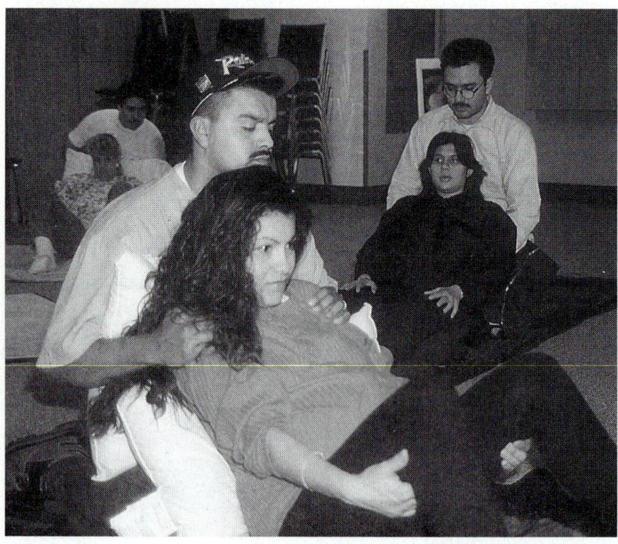

FIG. 39-4 The mother and the father during participation in a childbirth preparation course.

Dick-Read Method

Named after Dr. Grantly Dick-Read, who wrote the book *Childbirth Without Fear*, this childbirth method includes pregnancy education with the teaching of progressive relaxation techniques by the woman in labor. His teachings stress the importance of close attendance to the needs of the mother during labor and the avoidance of any unnecessary or excessive analgesics.

Lamaze Method

Named after Dr. Fernand Lamaze, who studied and adopted the techniques of psychoprophylaxis, or the mental control of pain, Lamaze techniques are based on the repetition of specific muscle control, breathing, and distraction or attention-focusing techniques. These childbirth techniques must be practiced frequently enough to become a reflex response during the patient's labor. Lamaze classes typically start early in pregnancy and are held more frequently than other types of childbirth classes.

Bradley Method

Named after Dr. Robert Bradley this method focuses on control of environmental factors such as lighting, temperature, and noise to provide a natural, calm, supportive environment for childbirth. In this method the husband plays an integral role as the coach and the comfort giver.

Box 39-8

AREAS TYPICALLY DISCUSSED IN CHILDBIRTH PREPARATION CLASSES

- A review of reproductive anatomy and physiology
- Discussion of physical and emotional changes commonly observed during pregnancy
- Fetal growth and development
- Nutrition
- Routine aspects of prenatal hygiene and exercise
- Danger signs during pregnancy
- Explanation of the birth process, both vaginal and cesarean
- Discussion of analgesia and anesthesia during labor and delivery
- Care of the newborn infant
- Breast feeding
- Sibling preparation
- Changing family dynamics
- Postpartum exercises

Cultural Variation in Prenatal Care

There are many cultural and religious influences on the pregnant woman. It is important not to generalize when giving care; not all members of a cultural group will behave in exactly the same way. It is always wise to discuss beliefs with each individual to determine her unique cultural practices, and if the practices do not cause harm, they should be included in planning care.

Because of cultural and other factors, such as lack of money, lack of transportation, and poor communication on the part of health care providers, many women do not participate in the prenatal care system. Their behavior must not be misinterpreted as uncaring, lazy, or ignorant.

A concern for modesty is also a deterrent for prenatal care for many persons. Exposing one's body parts, especially to a male practitioner, is a major violation of modesty. Thus many women may prefer a midwife over the male practitioner. Too often health care providers assume women lose this modesty during pregnancy and labor. Most women value and appreciate efforts to maintain modesty.

Virtually all cultures emphasize the importance of a socially harmonious and agreeable environment. Absence of stressful relationships is important for a successful outcome for mother and baby.

Harmony with other persons must be fostered. Visits from extended family members may be required to demonstrate continued pleasant and noncontroversial relationships. If dissonance (discord) exists in any relationship with others, it is usually dealt with in culturally prescribed ways.

In other belief systems, "magic" establishes taboos. Some Hispanics advise against pregnant women witnessing an eclipse of the moon because they believe it may cause a cleft palate in the infant. Exposure to an earthquake may result in preterm delivery or miscarriage (lay term for a spontaneous abortion). A breech presentation may occur if the earthquake was exceptionally strong. Some members of the African-American culture believe a pregnant woman must not ridicule someone with an affliction for fear her child may be born with the same handicap. There is a widely held folk belief that raising one's arm above one's head or tying knots may cause the umbilical cord to wrap around the baby's neck and become knotted.

Some cultures of the Southwest may wear amulets (charm, talisman, fetish, lucky piece), spirit medals, and beads to ward off evil spirits. Other cultural beliefs include:

Filipino's are cautioned that any activity is dangerous, and others willingly take over their work. Inactivity constitutes a protection for mother and child. The mother is encouraged to simply produce the succeeding generation. This behavior should not be misinterpreted as laziness or noncompliance.

Some food taboos of various cultural groups are as follows:

- Vietnamese women are to avoid "unclean" foods such as beef, dog, rat, and snake meat.
- Japanese women are cautioned against hot, spicy, and salty food.
- Some African-Americans in the southern United States, Guatemalans, and Hispanics may not eat acid foods or fresh vegetables and fruits.

It is imperative are the practitioner determine and explore cultural practices and beliefs with the cross cultural patient (see Chapter 8 for further discussion of the cultural aspects of nursing).

NURSING PROCESS SUMMARY

When performing a nursing assessment on a pregnant woman the various health patterns listed in Table 39-5 on pp. 1236-1238 should be reviewed to help focus observations. The nurse is not limited to the questions indicated but may use these as a starting point. Any significant observations or responses will indicate the need for a more in-depth assessment. It is important to consult with a more experienced primary care practitioner if the significance of any data is in question.

Table 39-5 also suggests possible nursing diagnoses and nursing interventions that may be helpful in planning nursing care.

TABLE 39-5 Nursing Process and the Prenatal Patient

Data Collection	Possible Nursing Diagnoses	Patient Goals/Expected Outcomes	Nursing Interventions
Health management			
Does the patient keep appointments? Are medications taken as prescribed? Does the patient avoid alcohol, cigarettes, and other drugs? Does patient perform breast self-exam? Is patient aware of danger signs?	Health maintenance, altered, related to cultural beliefs, lack of resources, lack of knowledge	The patient will use self-care behaviors to maintain an optimum level of wellness for herself and the fetus.	Identify factors that interfere with health maintenance; provide explanations and printed materials to clarify health maintenance behaviors such as BSE (breast self-exam) and danger signals; provide encouragement with health seeking behaviors
Nutritional/metabolic			
Is diet adequate per recommended daily allowance? Is fluid intake adequate? How much weight has been gained/lost? How rapidly is the weight changing? Has she noticed any edema of feet or ankles?	Nutrition, altered: less than body requirements, related to inadequate intake of nutrients to meet increased metabolic demands (nausea/vomiting, inadequate financial/nutritional knowledge) Nutrition altered: more than body requirements, related to excessive caloric intake	Patient will know that good nutrition leads to suggested weight gain in pregnancy. Patient will know additional nutrients necessary during pregnancy and how to fulfill this need. Patient will meet nutritional needs and maintain weight gain within recommended weight gain pattern.	Assess weight gain or loss at regular intervals; initiate dietary consultation; review Food Guide Pyramid; provide information regarding nutritional and fluid needs during pregnancy; assess for unique cultural practices and determine harmful effects, if any, and counsel accordingly. Explain that suggested weight gain pattern is about 4.1 kg (3 lb) in first trimester, 4.5 kg (10 lb) in second, and 4.5 kg (10 lb) in third; review Food Guide Pyramid; sources of energy—rich but nutritionally poor food should be identified and eliminated; moderate exercise should be encouraged if there is no contraindication; teach the patient that weight reduction in pregnancy by dietary manipulation is contraindicated because of potentially adverse and possibly toxic effects on fetal nutrition.
Activity/exercise			
What type of exercise is practiced? Does the woman complain of backache? Has the physician placed any limits on activity?	Injury, high risk for, related to altered balance Activity intolerance related to fatigue	Patient will be free of injury from falling. Patient (couple) will learn ways of conserving her energy.	Stress importance of wearing proper footwear; teach avoidance of hazardous activities. Teach importance of pacing activities and planning adequate rest; encourage patient to be active, to walk, and to engage in normal although not strenuous activities.

TABLE 39-5 Nursing Process and the Prenatal Patient—cont'd

Data Collection	Possible Nursing Diagnoses	Patient Goals/Expected Outcomes	Nursing Interventions
Elimination			
Has pattern of urine elimination changed? Has bowel elimination pattern changed? Is there any burning with urination? Pain with defecation? Constipation? Diarrhea?	Infection, high risk for urinary tract infection, related to physiological changes of pregnancy Incontinence, stress, related to increased intraabdominal pressure secondary to uterine enlargement Constipation, related to decreased rate of peristalsis	Patient understands information, and infection does not occur. Patient will understand and know means of coping with urinary incontinence. Patient will have usual healthy bowel habits and remain free from constipation.	Review signs and symptoms of urinary tract infections; encourage patient to drink 200 ml of fluid per day (8 to 10 oz of cranberry juice may be included because it is acidic and can lower the pH of the urinary tract, making it less hospitable to developing bacteria); teach patient correct cleansing after voiding or bowel movement (cleansing anterior to posterior to prevent contamination of bladder with fecal material, which contains *E. coli*); teach patient to wear underpants and pantyhose with cotton crotch; teach patient to urinate frequently (holding urine increases the time bacteria are in the bladder and allows them to multiply). Teach Kegel's exercises; encourage voiding at regular intervals. Teach patient the importance of eating fresh fruits, vegetables, and whole grain products and drinking 6 to 8 glasses of water daily to aid in bowel regularity.
Rest/sleep			
Has sleep pattern changed? Increased fatigue noticed? Does patient take naps or rest periods? Do any positions cause discomfort?	Sleep pattern disturbance, high risk for, related to altered body shape Fatigue, related to increased metabolic demands of pregnancy	Patient will learn ways to adjust sleep schedule and positions to aid in sleeping. Patient will schedule frequent rest period during the day to conserve energy. Patient will be able to increase activity level and resume ADLs without undue fatigue.	Teach support of body parts with pillows. The side-lying position is recommended to promote uterine perfusion and fetoplacental oxygenation by eliminating pressure on the ascending vena cava and descending aorta (supine hypotension); encourage patient to have warm milk or shower before retiring; teach avoidance of caffeine-containing fluids/food late in day; reassure patient that insomnia is a common occurrence during late pregnancy. Discuss positioning to promote comfort; assist in planning activities to promote rest periods.

Continued.

TABLE 39-5 Nursing Process and the Prenatal Patient—cont'd

Data Collection	Possible Nursing Diagnoses	Patient Goals/Expected Outcomes	Nursing Interventions
Cognitive/perceptual			
Has the patient noticed any vision changes? Blurring? Headaches? Has she enrolled in any prenatal classes? Does she attend them?	Knowledge deficit, related to lack of experience with needs of pregnancy	Patient will become knowledgeable about the needs of pregnancy, trimester by trimester.	Provide information regarding prenatal classes, prepared childbirth, and danger signs during pregnancy.
Role/relationship			
Does she feel confused regarding her changing role? Has interpersonal dynamics with husband, boyfriend, mother, friends changed?	Role performance, altered, related to expectations for pregnancy Family processes, altered, related to expectations for pregnancy	Patient (couple) will learn and demonstrate positive coping techniques.	Spend time listening to concerns; involve family members and significant others in teaching; contact social services if serious problems with dynamics are suspected.
Coping/stress tolerance			
What fears or anxieties are verbalized? How has her self-image changed?	Fear, related to real or imagined threat to self or fetus Coping, ineffective family, related to role changes, economic stressor related to childbearing	Patient will be able to verbalize fears and identify coping mechanisms. Patient (couple) will learn and demonstrate positive coping techniques.	Encourage verbalization of fears and concerns; provide explanations at patient's level of understanding. Assist family members in adjusting to new roles; explore support services; establish trusting relationship.
Value/belief			
What is the patient's cultural background? What are her religious practices?	Spiritual distress, related to separation from spiritual or cultural beliefs or practices	Patient will verbalize importance of proper care practices within the limits of her belief system to maintain adequate optimum health of her and her baby.	Incorporate cultural practices into care whenever possible; consult spiritual advisor for specific information if necessary (the nurse cannot give culturally appropriate nursing interventions without knowing the cultural and racial factors that affect the patient and family).

REFERENCES AND SUGGESTED READINGS

1. Ahumada LS: Multicultural perinatal health care, *Matern Child Health Educ Res* 6(2), 1991.
2. Bernhardt JH: Potential workplace hazards to reproductive health, *J Obstet Gynecol Neonatal Nurs* 19:53, 1990.
3. Bobak IM, Jensen MD: *Essentials of maternity nursing,* ed 3, St Louis, 1991, Mosby.
4. Bobak IM, Jensen MD: *Maternity and gynecologic care: the nurse and family,* ed 5, St Louis, 1993, Mosby.
5. Burgess MA: Rubella vaccination just before or during pregnancy, *Med J Aust* 152:507, 1990.
6. Burroughs A: *Maternity nursing,* ed 6, Philadelphia, 1992, Saunders.
7. Chez RA: Advising pregnant women about nutrition, *Contemp Obstet/Gynecol* 36(1):80, 1991.
8. Cook PS, Peterson RC, Moore DT: *Alcohol, tobacco, and other drugs may harm the unborn,* U.S. Department of Health and Human Services, DHHS Pub No (ADM) 90-1711, Rockville, Md, 1990, Office for Substance Abuse Prevention.
9. Corinne L et al: The unheard voices of women: spiritual interventions in maternal-child health, *MCN Am J Matern Child Nurs* 17:3, 1992.
10. Culpepper L: *Exercise during pregnancy*. In Merkatz IR, Thompson JE, editors: *New perspectives on prenatal care,* New York, 1990, Elsevier Science.
11. Doenges M, Moorhouse M: *Nurse's pocket guide to nursing diagnosis with interventions,* ed 3, Philadelphia, 1991, FA Davis.

12. Fischbach F: *A manual of laboratory diagnostic tests,* ed 4, Philadelphia, 1992, Lippincott.
13. Fishbein EG, Phillips M: How safe is exercise during pregnancy? *J Obstet Gynecol Neonatal Nurs* 19:45, 1990.
14. Giger J, Davidhizar R: *Transcultural nursing: assessment and intervention,* ed 2, St Louis, 1995, Mosby.
15. Haire D: Patient education in childbirth: a long way in forty years, *Int J Childbirth Educ* 6:7, 1991.
16. Hammond TL et al: The use of automobile safety restraint systems during pregnancy, *J Obstet Gynecol Neonatal Nurs* 19:339, 1990.
17. Ingalls AJ, Salerno MC: *Maternal and child health nursing,* ed 7, St Louis, 1990, Mosby.
18. Kenner CA, MacLaren A: *Essentials of maternal and neonatal nursing,* Springhouse, Penn, 1993, Springhouse.
19. Ladewig PW, London MI, Olds SB: *Essentials of maternal-newborn nursing,* ed 2, Redwood City, Calif, 1990, Addison-Wesley.
20. Lederer JR et al: *Care planning pocket guide: a nursing diagnosis approach,* Redwood City, Calif, 1993, Addison-Wesley.
21. Martin LL, Reeder SJ: *Essentials of maternity nursing: family centered care,* Philadelphia, 1991, Lippincott.
22. McDonald AD et al: Cigarette, alcohol and coffee consumption and congenital defects, *Am J Public Health* 82:1, 1992.
23. *Mosby's medical, nursing, and allied health dictionary,* ed 4, 1994, Mosby.
24. *NAACOG Standards for the Nursing Care Women and Newborns,* ed 4, Washington, DC, 1991, NAACOG.
25. Olds SB, London ML, Ladewig PW: *Maternal newborn nursing: a family centered approach,* ed 4, Menlo Park, Calif, 1992, Addison-Wesley.
26. Redman BK: *The process of patient education,* ed 7, St Louis, 1992, Mosby.
27. Reeves N et al: Fatigue in early pregnancy: an exploratory study, *J Nurse Midwife* 36:5, 1991.
28. Richardson P: Women's experiences of body change during normal pregnancy, *Matern Child Nurs J* 19:2, 1990.
29. Seidel HM et al: *Mosby's guide to physical examination,* ed 3, St Louis, 1995, Mosby.
30. Starn JR: Cultural childbearing: beliefs and practices, *Int J Childbirth Educ* 6:38, 1991.
31. Thomas CL: *Taber's cyclopedic medical dictionary,* ed 17, Philadelphia, 1993, FA Davis.
32. Thurman SK et al: Cocaine use: implications for interventions with childbearing women and their infants, *Child Health Care* 21:1, 1992.
33. Tucker SM et al: *Patient care standards,* ed 5, St Louis, 1992, Mosby.
34. Watson WJ et al: Fetal responses to maximal swimming and cycling exercise during pregnancy, *Obstet Gynecol* 77:382, 1991.
35. Wilson JR et al: *Obstetrics and gynecology,* ed 9, St Louis, 1991, Mosby.
36. Zerwekh JR: At the expense of their souls, *Nurs Outlook* 39:58, 1991.

CHAPTER CHALLENGE

KEY POINTS

- Pregnancy is a normal process that involves many complex physiological changes in the mother.
- During a period of 280 days, two initial cells join and develop into a unique, viable human being.
- Unique structures such as the placenta, membranes, umbilical cord, and amniotic fluid protect and support the developing fetus. These structures are discarded when the pregnancy is completed and they are no longer necessary.
- All aspects of the mother's life-style can potentially affect her developing fetus.
- Many drugs and viruses can cross the placenta and present serious hazards to the developing embryo, particularly during the first trimester of pregnancy.
- Sophisticated diagnostic tests are often performed to identify genetic or developmental problems during pregnancy. Early identification of problems may influence a woman's decisions regarding a pregnancy.
- Although pregnancy is a normal process, regular and ongoing health care is important throughout pregnancy.
- Many signs and symptoms of pregnancy are similar to those manifested by other medical conditions. The positive signs of pregnancy are visualization of the fetus, fetal motion detected by a trained observer, and auscultation of fetal heart sounds.
- Every pregnant woman should be aware of the danger signs during pregnancy and contact her physician if any of these are present.
- Nutritional needs change during pregnancy. To support normal growth and development of the fetus, caloric needs increase, as well as mineral and vitamin requirements.
- Many discomforts may occur during pregnancy. The nurse should be aware of measures that can reduce these discomforts without causing harm to the mother or fetus.
- Pregnancy is a time of role adjustment for both the prospective mother and father. All family members are affected by the addition of a new member.
- Adequate preparation for childbirth will enable the woman to become a knowledgeable participant in the entire childbearing process. The nurse should be aware of classes available in the community and the materials covered in these classes.
- The nurse and the patient are influenced by cultural and personal values and beliefs during the patient's pregnancy. Careful assessment is imperative.

STUDY QUESTIONS

1. Ms. Foster, age 22, is sexually active and does not use any form of birth control. She has never missed a menstrual period until now. In addition she has recently begun to experience breast tenderness and episodes of nausea. These symptoms are:
   1. Early signs of hormonal problems
   2. Presumptive signs of pregnancy
   3. Probable signs of pregnancy
   4. Positive signs of pregnancy
2. Mrs. Easterday, age 36, has come to the clinic for fertility studies. She has never been pregnant. She would be considered a:
   1. Nulligravida
   2. Nullipara
   3. Primigravida
   4. Primapara
3. Ms. Potter, states that her last menstrual period began October 30 and ended November 5. She came to the clinic on December 18 because she has not had another menstrual period. Using Nagele's rule Ms. Potter's EDC (estimated date of confinement) would be:
   1. July 23
   2. July 29
   3. August 2
   4. August 6
4. Ms. Jorgensen has many questions regarding fetal growth and development and pregnancy. She asks the nurse how the fetus obtains the necessary nutrients from her during pregnancy. The nurse would explain that these are provided by the:
   1. Amniotic fluid
   2. Chorionic membrane
   3. Placenta
   4. Uterus
5. Ms. Johnson does not smoke, but occasionally likes to have a few alcoholic drinks with friends. The nurse recognizes that Ms. Johnson understands her prenatal teaching when she states:
   1. "I'll only have one drink when we go out now."
   2. "I'll only drink wine and beer, not any hard liquor while I'm pregnant."
   3. "I'll try not to drink as often now."
   4. "I'll drink soft drinks until after I deliver."
6. Mrs. Drinen is slightly overweight and is worried about gaining too much weight during her pregnancy. The nurse would explain that during pregnancy weight gain:
   1. Should be watched carefully and not exceed 22 lb
   2. Is less important than proper nutrition
   3. Occurs more rapidly because of changes in metabolism
   4. Is not a concern because she can lose any excess weight after delivery
7. The nurse explains to Ms. Dormar that she should contact the primary care practitioner if she experiences any of the danger signs during pregnancy. The nurse determines that Ms. Dormar understands the teaching when she states that she will call if she experiences:
   1. Severe headaches
   2. Urinary frequency
   3. Backaches
   4. Mild edema of the ankles
8. As Mrs. Shaff's pregnancy progresses, she complains of episodes of heartburn. The nurse would explain that this is possibly a result of:
   1. Increased dietary intake of calcium
   2. Decreased fluid intake
   3. Increased progesterone levels
   4. Decreased estrogen levels
9. During her regular prenatal visit Mrs. Formann complains that she often forgets to take the prescribed vitamin and mineral supplements. In light of this information it is most appropriate for the nurse to ask if she has experienced any:
   1. Episodes of constipation
   2. Muscle cramps
   3. Excessive skin dryness
   4. Dental problems
10. In preparation for childbirth Ms. Smythe has started to read books on labor and delivery. She states that she doesn't think that she'll go to the classes because she's afraid. The nurse's best response is:
    1. "You should really go to classes because you'll learn a lot of important things."
    2. "You'll have the chance to meet many other pregnant women at the classes and share information with them."
    3. "Let us discuss whether there is something special that you are concerned about or afraid of?"
    4. "If you've read all the books, you probably don't need to go to the classes."

40

NORMAL LABOR AND DELIVERY

Gloria E. Wold

KEY TERMS

amniotomy
attitude
Braxton Hicks contractions
descent
effacement
engagement
episiotomy
expulsion
extension
external rotation
fetal lie
fetal position
fetal presentation
fetopelvic disproportion
flexion
internal rotation
lightening
meconium
oligohydramnios
oxytocin
restitution
surfactant
uterine inertia

LEARNING OBJECTIVES

After reading this chapter, the student should be able to do the following:

- Define the key terms.
- Discuss the signs and symptoms of impending labor.
- Discuss true and false labor.
- Describe fetopelvic disproportion.
- Discuss the "powers" involved in labor and delivery.
- Identify the mechanisms of labor.
- Describe the stages of labor.
- Explain the components of assessment during labor and delivery.
- Explain breathing techniques beneficial for the patient in labor.
- Identify nursing diagnoses relevant to the woman in labor.
- Discuss medical interventions related to labor and delivery.
- Discuss nursing interventions related to labor and delivery.

RELATED TOPICS OF INTEREST

- Cultural aspects of nursing care (Chapter 8)
- Sign, symptoms, and physical assessment (Chapter 9)
- Vital signs (Chapter 10)
- Care of the patient with a reproductive disorder (Chapter 33)
- Care of the mother and newborn at risk (Chapter 42)

NORMAL LABOR

Onset of Labor

In most pregnancies the fetus reaches maturity and the uterus begins the process of labor at exactly the right time. Although this process has been occurring throughout human history, researchers are still trying to discover the exact cause for the onset, or beginning, of labor.

Theories of Labor

Although there is no known cause for the onset of labor, there are several theories. These fall into two main categories—those based on mechanical changes and those based on hormonal changes.

One mechanical theory involves uterine stretching. It is based on the principle that once a hollow body organ reaches a certain state of distention, it will spontaneously contract and empty. For example, a full bladder will empty by incontinence and a distended stomach will empty by vomiting. It is hypothesized that when the uterus stretches to a certain size it will empty spontaneously. However, the wide variation of uterine size between different pregnancies in the same woman makes this a weak theory. For example, a woman may have one pregnancy in which she delivers a 6-pound baby at term. In her next pregnancy she may again reach term but delivers twins each weighing 6 pounds.

There are several hormonal theories for the onset of labor based on either an increase or decrease in hormones. In some of the theories, the source of the hormones is the mother; in other theories, it is the fetus. Some suggest the production of increased amounts of hormones acts as a trigger to start labor; others hypothesize a decrease in hormone levels is the trigger. Some of the more common theories relating to hormones are (1) oxytocin stimulation, (2) progesterone withdrawal, (3) estrogen stimulation, and (4) fetal cortisol. These and others are possible but not proven.

Signs of Impending Labor

Although we do not know what causes labor, we can recognize when labor is about to begin by watching for certain signs.

As early as 2 weeks before the onset of labor the woman may notice that the fetus seems to have settled or "dropped" into the pelvis. This is called **lightening** and is seen most often in nulliparas. Once lightening has occurred, the woman often notices that urinary frequency returns. She may be able to breathe more normally, since there is more space in the abdominal cavity. Multiparas may not experience this change until they are in active labor.

Occasionally a woman may experience a seepage or sudden outflow of fluid from the vagina. This may be urine, or it may be amniotic fluid, indicating a rupture of the amniotic sac. A simple test with nitrazine paper can distinguish between these. Without washing the area, the paper is moistened with the discharge. If the paper reacts (turns blue), the discharge is probably amniotic fluid. If the test is nonreactive, the membranes are probably intact. The amniotic sac generally ruptures after labor has begun. If it ruptures before labor starts, medical attention is essential. Rupture of the bag of waters (BOW) leads to increased risk of infection. If labor does not occur within 24 hours after rupture of the membranes, the physician will usually attempt to start labor by administering medication.

The amount of vaginal drainage typically increases as term approaches, and a blood-tinged mucus called the *bloody show* may be observed. This "show" is the mucus that occluded the opening of the cervix during pregnancy (mucus plug). Vaginal examination may reveal that the cervix has begun to change consistency. The cervix begins to soften, and in true labor it also begins to thin (efface) and open (dilate).

Backache and contractions of the uterus, called **Braxton Hicks contractions** (irregular tightening of the pregnant uterus that begins in the first trimester and increases in frequency, duration, and intensity as pregnancy progresses), are common as the pregnancy approaches term. These contractions vary from mild to

TABLE 40-1 Comparison of True and False Labor

True Labor	False Labor
Contractions follow a regular pattern.	Contractions rarely follow a pattern.
Contractions come closer together, are stronger, and tend to last longer.	Contractions vary in length and intensity.
Contractions get stronger with ambulation.	Contractions frequently stop with ambulation or position change.
Contractions seem to start in the lower back and then travel to the lower abdomen.	Contractions may be felt in the back, but are most often noticed in the fundus.
Contractions are usually not stopped by controlled breathing, sedation, or other relaxation interventions.	Contractions eventually stop with relaxation interventions.
The cervix softens, effaces, and dilates.	The cervix may soften, but there is little or no change in effacement or dilation.
The fetus continues descent into the pelvis.	There is no significant change in the fetal position.

moderate in severity. They remain irregular and do not dilate the cervix.

Some women notice a slight loss of weight (1 to 3 pounds) a few days before labor, and others report a last-minute burst of energy.

True labor is marked by the onset of regular, rhythmic contractions that cause progressive dilation and **effacement** (thinning and shortening or obliteration of the cervix that occurs during late pregnancy or labor or both) of the cervix.

False Labor Versus True Labor

Because many women fear that they will go to the hospital at the wrong time, nurses should explain how true labor differs from false labor. These differences are described in Table 40-1. It is also important to stress that when there is any doubt, medical attention should be obtained. At times even experienced professionals find it difficult to differentiate the early stages of true labor from false labor.

LABOR AND DELIVERY

Alternative Labor and Delivery Sites

When the woman suspects that the onset of true labor has begun, she typically notifies her primary care practitioner and her significant others. A plan for delivery should have been established during the pregnancy. Delivery can be planned in a traditional hospital setting, a birthing room, or at home. A traditional labor and delivery setting tends to be very medically oriented and may seem physically and emotionally "sterile and cold" to many women. In this traditional method visitors to the woman in labor are strictly limited. Only the spouse or one significant other is allowed to be present during labor and delivery. Typically, many room changes occur: the mother is admitted to a labor room, then transferred to a delivery room, after delivery is moved to a recovery room, and finally to a postpartum room. Many women dislike this and find the restriction of visits with loved ones and the frequent moves disturbing. Despite these considerations, the traditional hospital is a safe setting. All the personnel and equipment needed in case of emergency are readily available.

To avoid the negative aspects of the traditional system, some women want to give birth at home. This plan must be agreed on by the physician or nurse midwife. Home delivery is permitted only when an uncomplicated delivery is expected and the primary care practitioner has reasonable confidence that no harm will come to either the mother or infant. An unplanned delivery at home could lead to serious problems. If an emergency occurs, precious time is lost transporting the mother or infant to the hospital where support is available.

Birthing centers are a fairly recent development. These centers are generally located within the hospital but are structured to be more homelike. The attitude of the staff is more open and welcoming to the spouse and significant others. The entire birthing process and often the entire stay at the facility will take place in one room. This eliminates many of the negative factors of the traditional hospital setting but provides the safety of having all necessary personnel and equipment available. For these reasons, alternative birthing centers are becoming increasingly popular.

Process of Labor and Delivery

To understand the complex process of labor and delivery it is important to examine each of the factors involved. These factors are frequently called the five *P*s:

passageway	The pelvis and soft tissues
passengers	The fetus and placenta
powers	Contractions and voluntary effort
position of mother	Standing, walking, side lying, squatting, on hands and knees
process	All parts working together

Passageway

The Pelvis. The superior portion of the pelvis (iliac segment of the innominate bones) functions as a support for the uterus and fetus during the late months of pregnancy. These bones aid in directing the fetus into the inferior (lower) portion of the pelvis, which is called the *true pelvis.* The two sections are divided by an imaginary line called the *linea terminalis* or pelvic inlet.

The size and shape of the true pelvis are of more importance than those of the false pelvis, because the fetal head must be able to pass through this section of the pelvis for vaginal delivery to occur. Four different types of pelves are recognized. Each of these has a unique shape and characteristics, as shown in Table 40-2 on p. 1244.

The true pelvis is further divided into three segments, the inlet, the cavity or midpelvis, and the outlet (Fig. 40-1 on p. 1244). Several methods are available to the primary care practitioner for evaluating the size of the true pelvis:

1. *Palpation:* Externally, the primary care practitioner can use a pelvimeter to determine the distance between the ischial tuberosities. This helps the primary care practitioner estimate the distance between the ischial spines, which can otherwise be obtained only by pelvic x-ray examination. Internally, the primary care practitioner can palpate additional bony prominences to determine pelvic adequacy.

TABLE 40-2 Comparison of Pelvic Types

	Gynecoid (50% of Women)	Android (23% of Women)	Anthropoid (24% of Women)	Platypelloid (3% of Women)
Brim	Slightly ovoid or transversely rounded Round	Heart shaped, angulated Heart	Oval, wider anteroposteriorly Oval	Flattened anteroposteriorly, wide transversely Flat
Depth	Moderate	Deep	Deep	Shallow
Side walls	Straight	Convergent	Straight	Straight
Ischial spines	Blunt, somewhat widely separated	Prominent, narrow interspinous diameter	Prominent, often with narrow interspinous diameter	Blunted, widely separated
Sacrum	Deep, curved	Slightly curved, terminal portion often beaked	Slightly curved	Slightly curved
Subpubic arch	Wide	Narrow	Narrow	Wide
Usual mode of delivery	Vaginal Spontaneous Occiput anterior position	Cesarean Vaginal Difficult with forceps	Vaginal Forceps/spontaneous occiput posterior or occiput anterior position	Vaginal Spontaneous

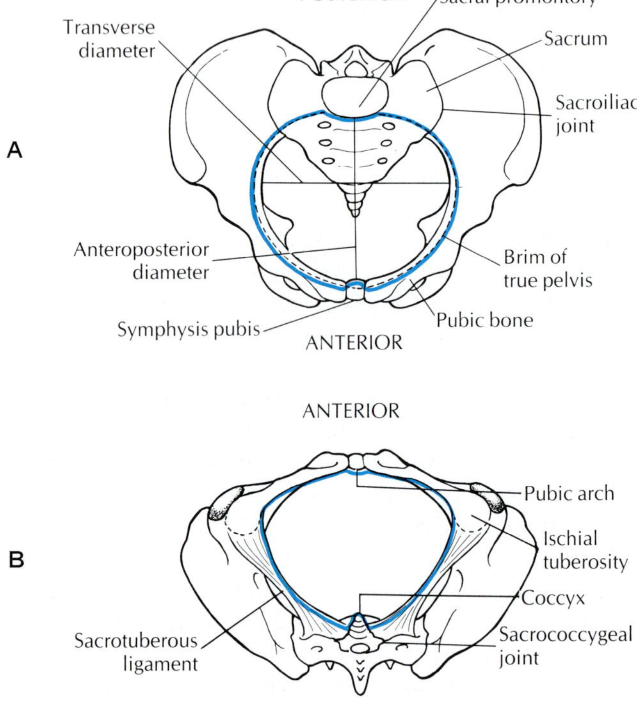

FIG. 40-1 Female pelvis. **A,** Pelvic brim (inlet, linea terminalis, or ileopectineal line) from above. **B,** Pelvic outlet from below.

2. *Pelvimetry:* With x-ray films from different views the primary care practitioner can accurately measure the bony prominences. However, this measurement is usually done at a time other than pregnancy if there has been an injury or known developmental problem, such as rickets. Pelvimetry is not routinely done during pregnancy, because the radiation may be harmful to the fetus.
3. *Ultrasonography:* Sound waves above the range of human hearing can also be used to estimate pelvic adequacy. Because ultrasound does not involve the use of radiation, it is generally regarded as safe for the fetus. In more than 20 years of obstetrical use, no detrimental effects have been observed. Because ultrasound can visualize soft tissue, it is also helpful in gathering information regarding fetal growth, multiple pregnancy, placental location, and abnormal presentation that may complicate delivery.

It is important to understand that adequacy of the pelvis is relative. At the time of each delivery the primary care practitioner must determine whether the pelvis is adequate to allow passage of the fetus. Although certain measurements are considered "normal," the size and position of the fetus make each situation unique.

Soft Tissues. During labor the uterus, cervix, vagina, and muscles of the perineum change in consistency and shape to allow passage of the fetus in the following ways.

Uterine tissues. During labor the walls of the upper section of the uterus have a thickened musculature that provides the force during contractions. The muscle walls of the lower section become thinner and act as a passive tube. Located between the two sections is a band of tissue, the physiological retraction ring (Fig. 40-2).

Cervical tissues. As contractions of the muscular upper segment apply downward pressure, the uterine

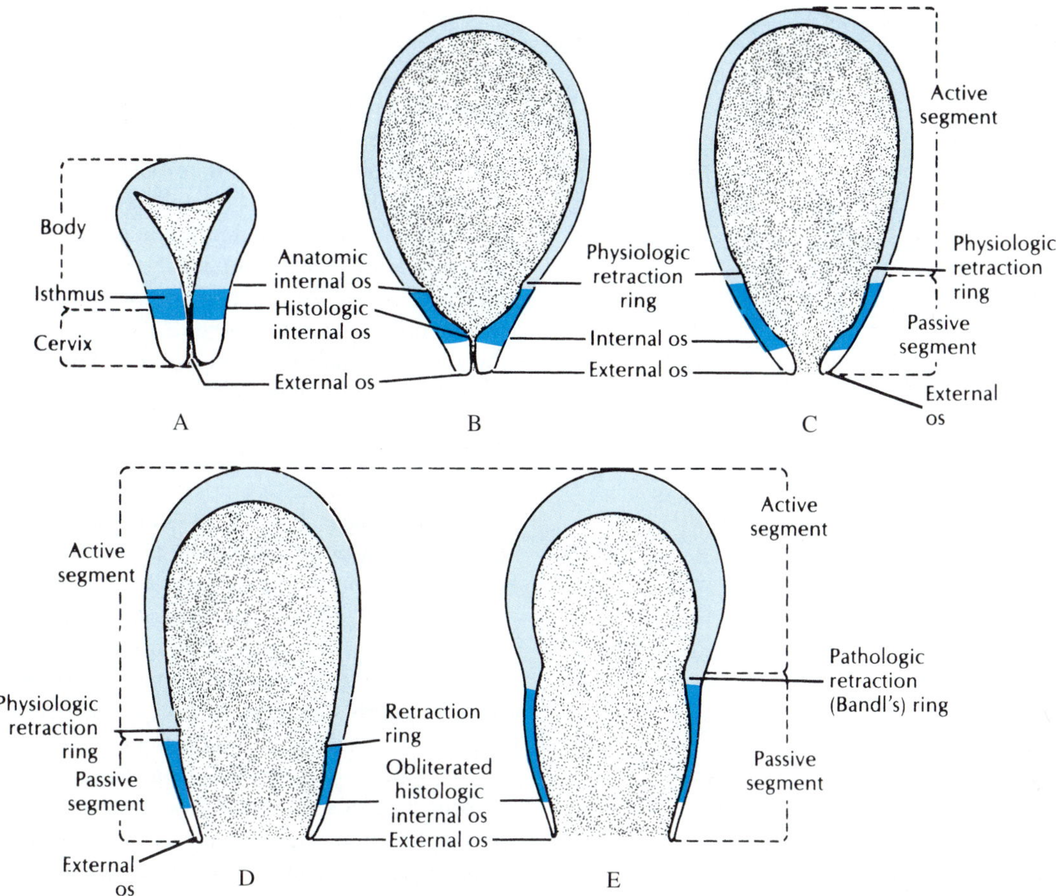

FIG. 40-2 Progressive development of segments and rings of uterus at term. Note comparison between: **A,** Nonpregnant uterus. **B,** Uterus at term. **C,** Uterus in normal labor in early first stage. **D,** Second stage. Passive segment is derived from lower uterine segment (isthmus) and cervix, and physiological retraction ring is derived from anatomical internal os. **E,** Uterus in abnormal labor in second-stage dystocia. Pathological retraction (Bandl's) ring that forms under abnormal conditions develops from physiological ring.

contents (fetal presenting part) efface and dilate the cervix.

Vagina. In response to hormonal changes during pregnancy, the vagina undergoes many changes. Increased blood supply (vascularity), increased thickness of the mucosa, loosening of the connective tissue, and enlargement (hypertrophy) of smooth muscle cells all make the vagina capable of stretching (dilating) to allow passage of the fetus.

Perineum. The muscles of the pelvic floor are stretched and thinned by the pressure of the presenting part. The anus may appear dilated and bulging.

Passengers

The Fetus. To be born, the fetus must be able to exit through the bony passageway just described. This is a major challenge, since at term the fetus often weighs 7 pounds or more and is 20 to 21 inches long.

Fetal skull. Because the fetal skull is usually the largest part of the body, the delivery of the head poses the greatest concern. The shoulders and pelvis, which are more mobile, do not often cause problems.

The bones of the fetal skull are not rigidly joined (fused). This allows the bony plates to move and overlap as they progress through the maternal pelvis. This reshaping of the skull bones in response to pressure against the maternal pelvis is called *molding.* The major bones of the skull are the two frontal bones, two parietal bones, two temporal bones, and the occiput.

These are joined by membranous spaces called the *sutures.* Where sutures meet, there are larger membranous areas called the *fontanelles* (Fig. 40-3 on p. 1246). The anterior fontanelle (bregma) tends to be larger and diamond shaped, since it is formed by four bones. The posterior fontanelle is smaller and triangular, since only three bones adjoin. Palpation of the sutures and fontanelles through the cervix permits the primary care practitioner to determine the presentation of the fetus during labor. The largest transverse diameter of the skull is the biparietal measurement. If this is too large, the skull may not be able to enter the mother's pelvis.

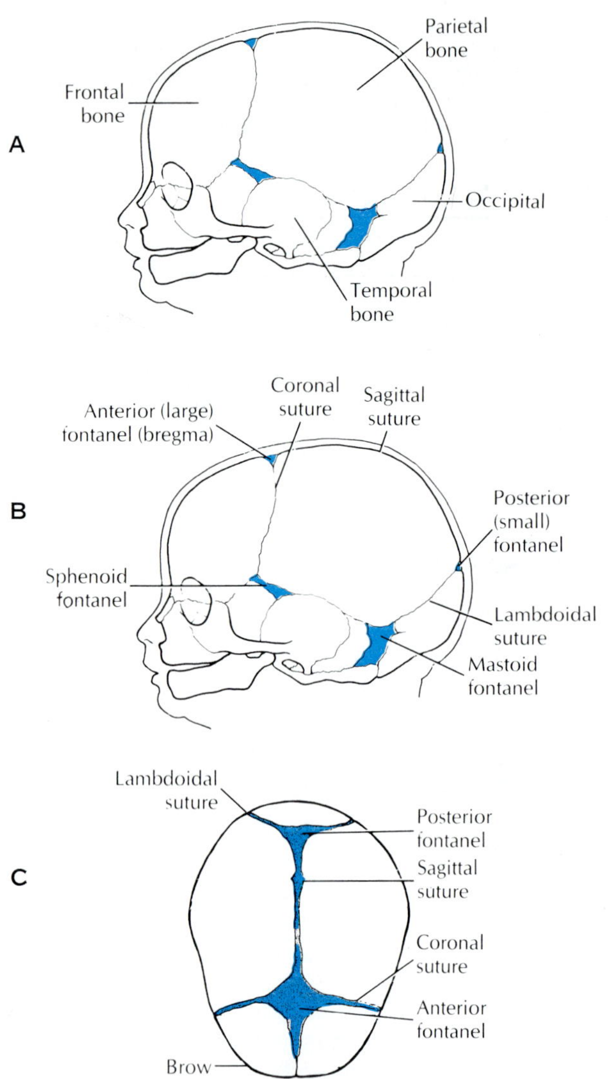

FIG. 40-3 Fetal head at term. **A,** Bones. **B,** Fontanelles. **C,** Sutures.

Fetal attitude. The relationship of fetal body parts to one another is called **attitude.** At term, the ideal attitude for the fetal body is flexion. The back is bowed outward, the chin is touching the sternum, the arms are crossed on the chest, and the thighs are flexed on the abdomen. This is called the **fetal position** (the relationship of the occiput, sacrum, chin, or scapula of the fetus to the front, back, or sides of the mother's pelvis). This attitude is ideal, because it takes up minimal space and allows the best angle of approach to the pelvis. If there is insufficient room because of too little amniotic fluid **(oligohydramnios;** abnormally small amount or absence of amniotic fluid; often indicative of fetal urinary tract defect), multiple pregnancies, or anatomical variations in the mother, the attitude may be altered, leading to complications of labor or delivery.

Fetal lie. **Fetal lie** is the relationship of the cephalocaudal (head-to-buttocks) axis of the fetus to the cephalocaudal axis of the mother. If the spine of the fetus is parallel to the spine of the mother, the lie is called *longitudinal.* This could be cephalic presentation (head down) or breech presentation (buttocks down). The lie is longitudinal in 99% of deliveries. If the spine of the fetus is perpendicular to that of the mother, it is called *transverse* lie. Only 1% of deliveries involve a transverse lie. This is most common in women who have had many pregnancies (resulting in weakened abdominal walls), maternal pelvic contracture, or placenta previa, which will be discussed in Chapter 42. During pregnancy, while the fetus is small it changes lie frequently. By term the fetal lie seldom changes because the space available is limited.

Fetal presentation. **Fetal presentation** (that part of the fetus that first enters the pelvis and lies over the inlet [head, face, breech, or shoulders]) describes the part that will be in contact with the cervix. This is determined by both attitude and lie.

In about 96% of deliveries the presentation is cephalic. In cephalic presentation some part of the fetal head is in contact with the cervix. There are four types of cephalic presentation: vertex (region between the fontanelles), brow, face, and mentum (chin).

In about 3% of deliveries the presentation is breech. In breech presentations either the buttocks or legs are in contact with the cervix. There are three types of breech presentation: complete breech, in which the buttocks present and the thighs are well flexed on the abdomen; frank breech, in which the buttocks present and the thighs are extended across the abdomen and chest; and footling breech, in which there is no flexion and one foot or two feet are present. Breech presentations are more difficult to deliver vaginally. To decrease risks to the fetus, the majority of breech births are delivered surgically. These surgical deliveries, called *cesarean births,* will be discussed later.

In about 1% of deliveries some other body part presents. These occur when the fetus has been in a transverse lie. The shoulder, hand, elbow, and iliac crest are possible presenting parts. In these cases a cesarean birth is also required.

Fetal position. Position is the relationship of the presenting fetal part to a quadrant of the maternal pelvis. Fetal position can be determined by abdominal inspection and palpation (Leopold's maneuvers, Fig. 40-4 on p. 1247), vaginal or rectal examination, auscultation of fetal heart tones, or ultrasound or x-ray examination. Once the position is determined, it is expressed in abbreviated form. For example, the most common position for delivery is LOA, left occiput anterior, in which the occiput of the fetus points toward the left anterior segment of the maternal pelvis. The ROA, right occiput anterior, position is the next most common position. Many combinations are possible, as shown on p. 1248 and in Fig. 40-5 on p. 1247 and Fig. 40-6 on p. 1248.

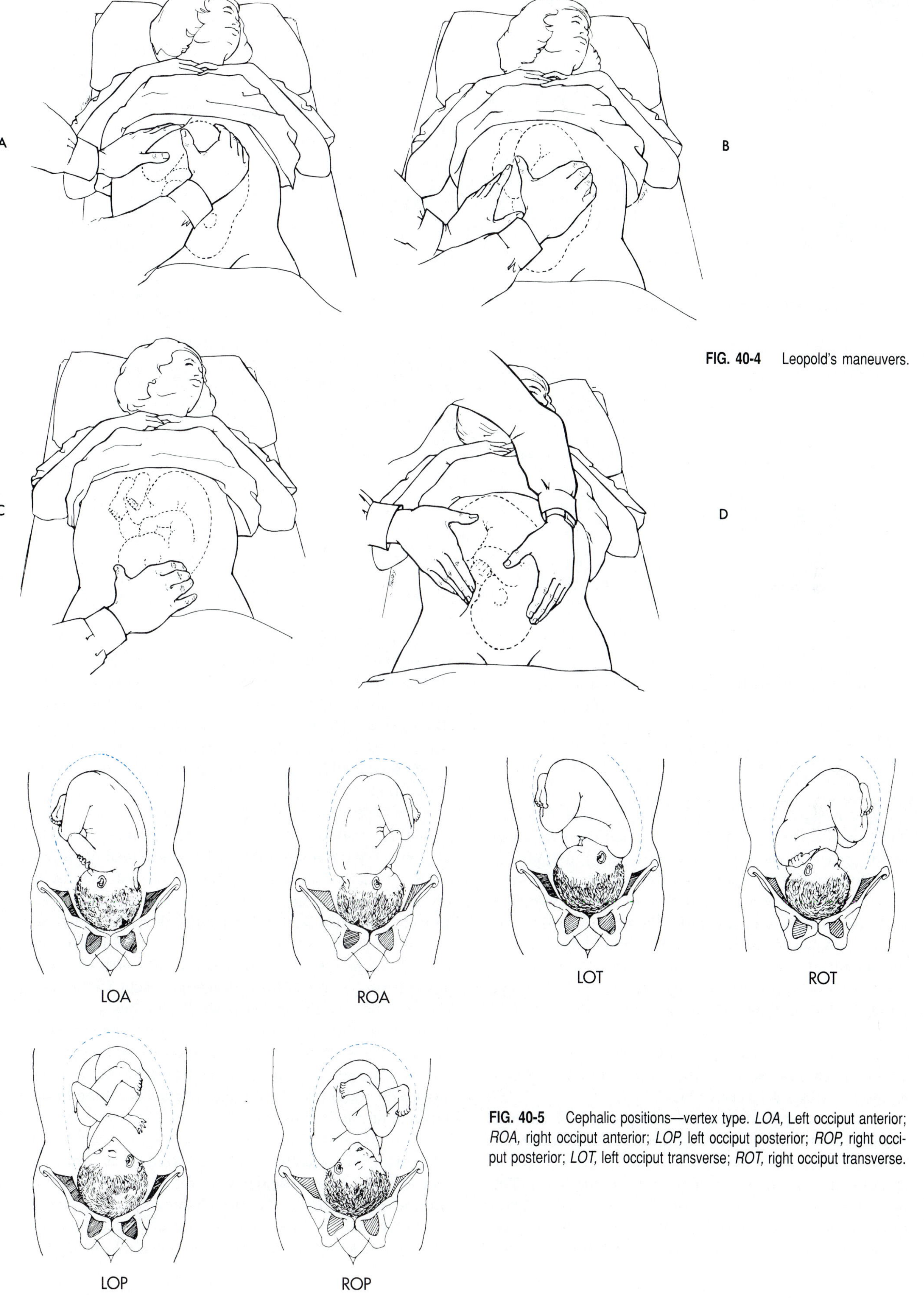

FIG. 40-4 Leopold's maneuvers.

FIG. 40-5 Cephalic positions—vertex type. *LOA,* Left occiput anterior; *ROA,* right occiput anterior; *LOP,* left occiput posterior; *ROP,* right occiput posterior; *LOT,* left occiput transverse; *ROT,* right occiput transverse.

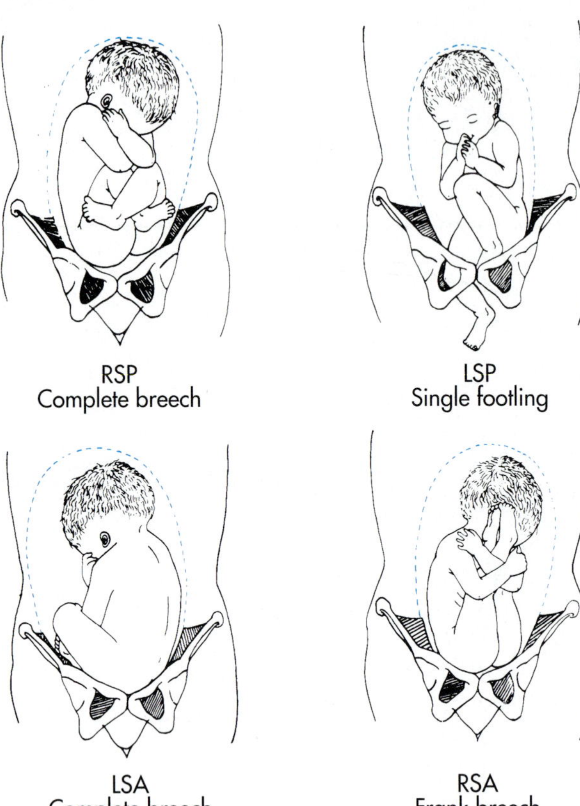

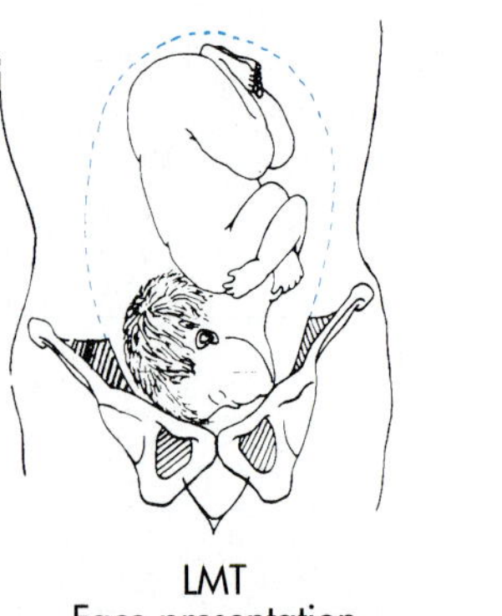

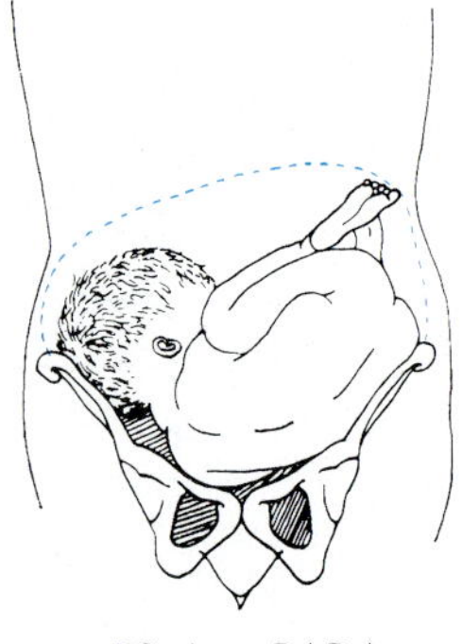

FIG. 40-6 Various presentations and positions. *RSP,* Right sacroposterior; *LSP,* left sacroposterior; *LSA,* left sacroanterior; *RSA,* right sacroanterior; *LMT,* left mentotransverse; *RScA,* right scapuloanterior; *RADA,* right acromiodorsoanterior.

Maternal pelvis side		Presenting part		Maternal quadrant	
R	Right	O	Occiput	A	Anterior
L	Left	B	Brow	P	Posterior
		M	Mentum (chin)	T	Transverse
		S	Sacrum		
		SC	Scapula		

Effect of fetal position on labor. A longitudinal lie, well-flexed attitude, with vertex presentation is the ideal. In this position the fetal skull bones are most able to mold to progress through the maternal pelvis. The fetal skull also provides a smooth, round surface, which is most effective in effacing and dilating the cervix. The smooth, regular shape also fills the cervix and prevents the umbilical cord from prolapsing, or coming before, the fetus. Cord prolapse is dangerous, because pressure on the vessels in the cord can restrict the blood flow to the fetus.

If a part other than the vertex presents, labor is generally longer, more tiring to the mother, and more likely to require surgical intervention.

Monitoring fetal status. The process of labor is stressful to the fetus, and it is important to monitor the fetus continuously during this time. Fetal heart rate (FHR) is a good indicator of the fetus's condition. The FHR is auscultated using a fetoscope or a Doppler instrument. This should be done every 15 to 30 minutes during the first stage of labor and every 5 minutes during the second stage. The FHR should also be taken immediately after rupture of the membranes, particularly if the head is not engaged (i.e., firmly settled into the pelvis). The normal FHR range is 120 to 160 beats per minute. An increase or decrease of 30 beats per minute may indicate fetal distress and should be reported immediately (Box 40-1).

Frequently electronic monitors, either internal or external, are applied. These monitors continuously track maternal contractions and the changes in fetal heart rate (Figs. 40-7 and 40-8 and Fig. 40-9 on p. 1250). Monitors are more accurate in detecting subtle changes of condition before they can be recognized by auscultation. Greenish discoloration of the amniotic fluid often indicates fetal distress. The color is a result of stool called **meconium** (first stools of the infant: viscid, sticky; dark greenish brown, almost black; sterile, odorless) being released from the fetal rectum in response to oxygen deprivation. This color is often referred to as *meconium staining.* In response to hypoxia, fetal intestinal activity increases, and the anal sphincter relaxes, resulting in the passage of meconium.

Placenta. The placenta is also referred to as a passenger. After the fetus is delivered in the presence of strong uterine contractions, the placental attachment site is markedly reduced in size. This reduced size causes the placenta to separate from its attachment. Normally, the

Box 40-1

INTERPRETING CHANGES IN FETAL HEART RATE

NORMAL BASELINE RATE

120 to 160 bpm.

TACHYCARDIA

Moderate increase to 160 to 180 bpm.

Marked increase above 180 bpm. Significant if variability is absent and late or variable decelerations (a decrease in the speed or velocity of an object or reaction) are present.

BRADYCARDIA

Moderate decrease to 100 to 120 bpm.

Marked decrease to below 100 bpm. Significant if variability decreased/absent or if late or variable decelerations are present.

VARIABILITY

Measures the normal fluctuation of the FHR from the baseline. Absent or minimal variability can be indicative of fetal distress. Variability is classified as long term (LTV) or short term (STV).

DECELERATIONS

Periodic decrease in the FHR in response to contractions. Classified as early, late, or variable.

- *Early decelerations:* due to pressure on fetal skull; tend to be uniform; onset, shape, and recovery correspond to contractions.
- *Late decelerations:* due to decreased oxygen and blood flow to fetus through the placenta; usually noted at or after the peak of the contraction; may indicate fetal distress, particularly if associated with changes in baseline FHR and absence of variability.
- *Variable decelerations:* due to compression on the umbilical cord; occur randomly and onset may be sudden; FHR decreases below normal range.

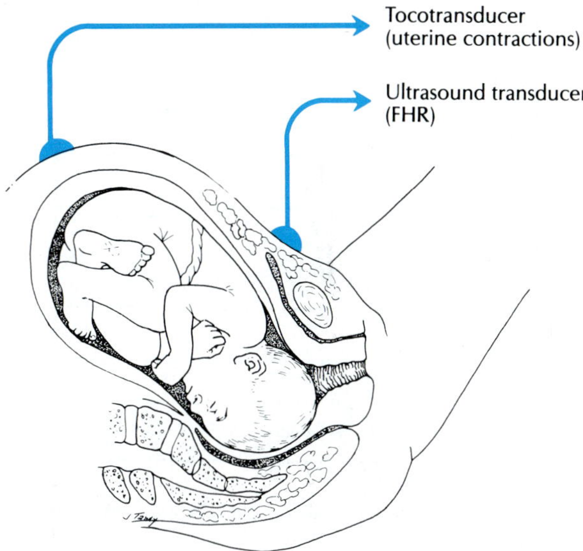

FIG. 40-7 Diagrammatic representation of external noninvasive fetal monitoring with tocotransducer and ultrasound transducer, with ultrasound transducer placed below umbilicus and tocotransducer placed on uterine fundus position.

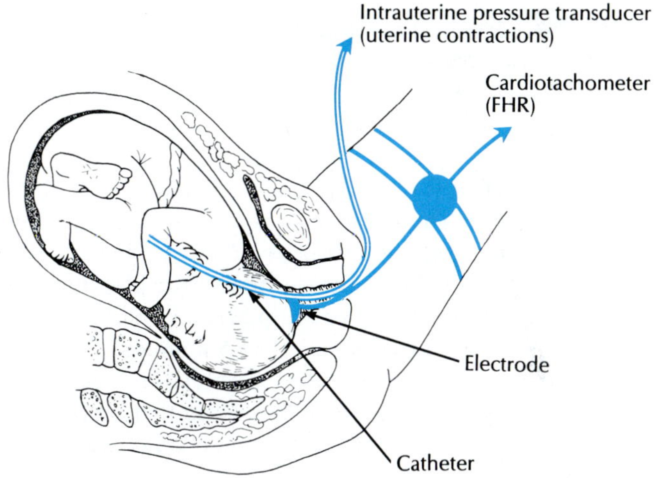

FIG. 40-8 Diagrammatic representation of internal invasive fetal monitoring with intrauterine catheter and spiral electrode in place (membranes ruptured and cervix dilated).

first few strong contractions 5 to 7 minutes after the birth of the baby shear the placenta from its base. A placenta will not easily be freed from a flaccid (relaxed) uterus because the placental attachment site is not reduced in size.

Placental separation is indicated by the following signs:

- A firmly contracting fundus
- A change in the uterus from a discoid (disklike) to a globular ovoid (egg shape), as the placenta moves to the lower segment
- A sudden gush of dark blood from the introitus (the entrance into the vagina)
- Apparent lengthening of the umbilical cord as the placenta gets closer to the introitus
- A vaginal fullness (the placenta) noted on vaginal or rectal examination or fetal membranes seen at the introitus

Whether the placenta shows its shiny fetal surface (Shiny Schultze) or its dark roughened maternal surface (Dirty Duncan) is of no clinical significance.

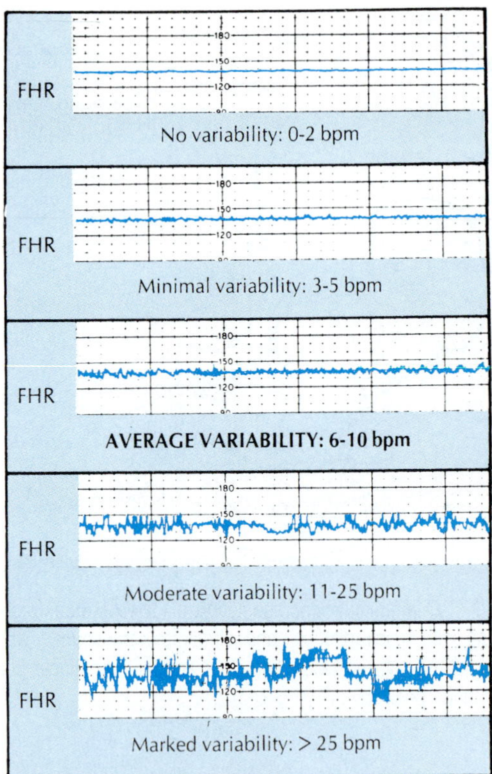

FIG. 40-9 Fetal heart rate variability. Short- and long-term variability tend to increase and decrease together.

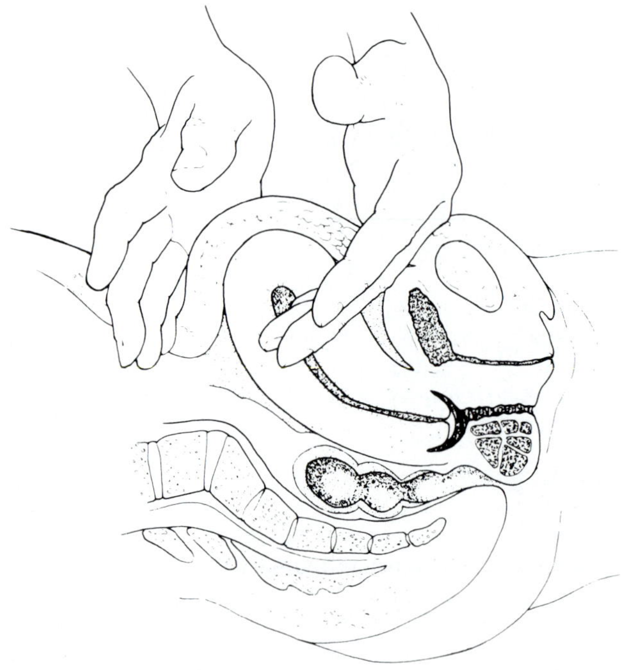

FIG. 40-10 Palpating fundus of uterus during first hour after delivery.

The delivery of the placenta completes the third stage of labor. The duration of this third stage of labor will be 15 to 30 minutes or longer if the health care practitioner waits for the mother to express the placenta herself. When the delivery of the placenta is managed actively, its duration can be less than 5 minutes.

After the placenta (with its membranes) emerges, it is examined for intactness to be certain that no portion of it remains in the uterine cavity (no retained fragments of the placenta or membranes).

The goal of this stage of labor is the prompt separation and expulsion of the placenta, achieved in the easiest and safest manner.

If the fundus is not firm, the nurse must stimulate the uterine muscle to regain tone and to expel any clots before measuring the distance from the umbilicus. The uterus is massaged gently only until it is firm; overstimulation causes uterine muscle fatigue and results in atonia (relaxation).

The uterus can contract only if it is free of intrauterine clots. Care must be taken to avoid inversion of the uterus during expulsion of clots. To expel clots the nurse keeps the hands placed as in Fig. 40-10 to support the uterus from below with one hand. With the upper hand the nurse applies firm pressure downward toward the vagina while observing the perineum for the number and size of expelled clots. As the nurse performs these assessments, the patient is taught the rationale for the assessment and how to maintain uterine tone by self-massage.

Powers

The forces that move the passengers through the passage include involuntary uterine contraction and voluntary maternal pushing.

Uterine Contractions. As already mentioned, during labor the muscles in the upper uterine segment, the fundus, thicken and contract at intervals. The intervals may be as much as 15 or 30 minutes apart in early labor and as frequent as every 2 or 3 minutes at the most active stage. Early contractions last 20 to 35 seconds; at the later stages they typically last 60 to 80 seconds. Each contraction has three parts: the increment, during which the muscles contract and the force increases in strength; the apex, during which the optimal force is exerted; and the decrement, during which the muscles relax.

These contractions are involuntary and originate at pacemaker points near the uterotubal junction. When a contraction occurs, the uterine cavity becomes smaller, and this forces the presenting fetal part or the bag of waters against the cervix. In addition, the thickening of the upper segment retracts, pulling the lower segment upward around the presenting part. In combination these actions efface and dilate the cervix. Before labor

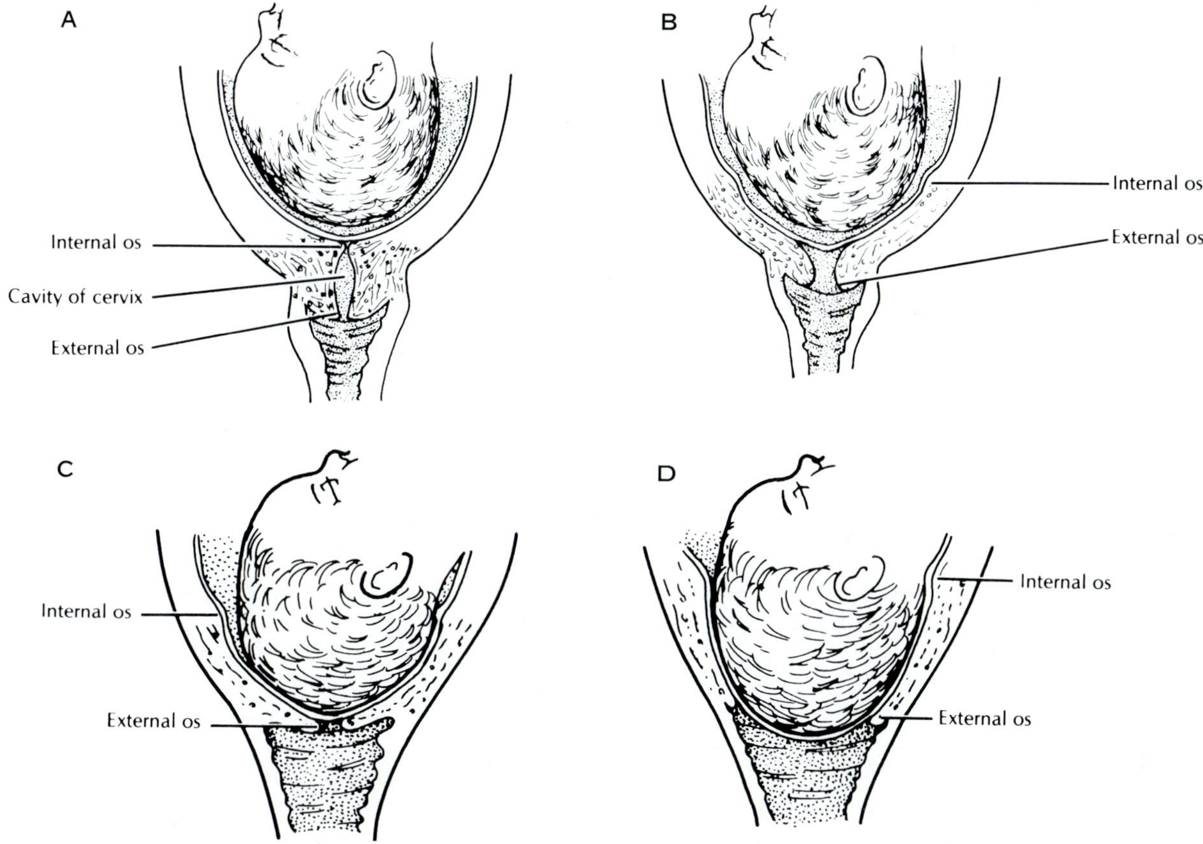

FIG. 40-11 Cervical effacement and dilation. Note how cervix is drawn up around presenting part (internal os). Membranes are intact, and head is not well applied to cervix. **A,** Before labor. **B,** Early effacement. **C,** Complete effacement (100%). Head is well applied to cervix. **D,** Complete dilation (10 cm). Some overlapping of cranial bones. Membranes still intact.

the nulliparous cervix is 2 to 3 cm long and 1 cm thick. The *os* (mouth or opening) is generally closed or open less than 1 cm. In a multiparous woman, the cervix may begin to efface and dilate before labor starts.

Labor progresses differently in nulliparas than in multiparas. In nulliparas, effacement usually precedes dilation. In multiparas, effacement and dilation usually progress simultaneously.

Effacement is described in percentages; total effacement is reached when no thickness of the cervix can be distinguished. Dilation is measured in centimeters; complete dilation is accomplished when a measurement of 10 cm is reached. This is the point at which the fetus is able to leave the uterus (Fig. 40-11).

Monitoring Contractions. Contractions can be monitored by placing a hand on the fundus of the uterus and using palpation to detect the contraction. Contractions are timed from the beginning of one contraction to the beginning of the next. Electronic monitors measure and time contractions and correlate fetal heart rate to maternal contractions (Fig. 40-12).

Voluntary Pushing. When the presenting part reaches the pelvic floor, the woman typically experiences an urge to bear down or push. Many women describe this as an urge to defecate. Pushing before the cervix is completely effaced and dilated will exhaust the woman and may actually slow the progress of labor. Once the cervix is fully effaced and dilated, the woman can assist in the progress of labor. To assist effectively, the woman must hold her breath and use her diaphragm and abdominal muscles to increase intraabdominal pressure. Such pushing assists in forcing the fetus through the birth canal.

Position of the Mother

Positioning the woman in a manner that allows gravity to assist her efforts is helpful. Squatting or using a semiseated position is more effective than a supine position. Special birthing chairs, which provide support and facilitate voluntary pushing, are available in many birthing centers. In a sitting position, such as squatting, abdominal muscles work in greater synchrony with uterine contractions during bearing-down efforts.

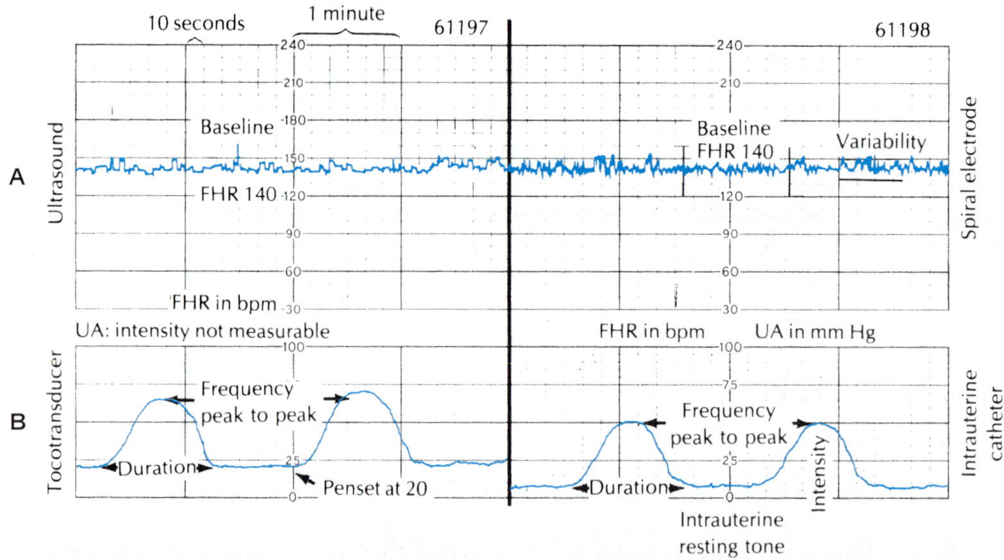

FIG. 40-12 Display of FHR and uterine activity on chart paper. **A,** External mode with ultrasound tocotransducer as signal source. **B,** Internal mode with spiral electrode and intrauterine catheter as signal source.

Process

Mechanisms of Labor. For the fetus to move through the maternal pelvis, several maneuvers are required. These turns and adjustments are called the *mechanisms of labor.* The mechanisms of labor in the vertex position are as follows:

Engagement
Descent
Flexion
Internal rotation
Extension
External rotation and restitution
Expulsion

Engagement occurs when the biparietal diameter of the fetal head crosses the inlet of the pelvis. When this occurs, the head is said to be fixed or engaged in the pelvis. This tends to occur early in nulliparous women, often several days or weeks before labor begins. Multiparous women may not experience engagement until labor has started.

Descent is the downward progress of the presenting part. The amount of progress is measured by comparing the lowest point of the presenting part to the ischial spines. This is measured in centimeters above or below the level of the spines and is referred to by *station.* For example, if the presenting part is even with the ischial spines, the station is 0; if the presenting part is 2 cm above the spines, the station is −2; if the presenting part is 2 cm below the ischial spines, the station is +2 (Fig. 40-13).

Flexion, which is the normal attitude, increases as a result of resistance from the cervix or pelvic floor.

Internal rotation enables the fetal head to progress through the maternal pelvis. The largest diameter of the fetal head aligns with the largest diameter of the pelvis.

Extension occurs when the occiput passes under the symphysis pubis. This bony structure acts as a stable point and provides leverage, enabling the head to leave the pelvis. The actual delivery of the head is done by extension. As soon as the head is delivered, it moves to realign with the body and shoulders. This is referred to as **restitution** (Fig. 40-14).

External rotation occurs as the shoulders and body move through the birth canal, using the same maneuvers as the head. The shoulders are delivered similarly to the head, with the anterior shoulder pressing under the symphysis pubis, which again acts as a leverage point, and assists in delivery of the posterior shoulder. After the shoulders are delivered the delivery ends with **expulsion** in which the body of the infant leaves the pelvis. Delivery of the body occurs rapidly once the shoulders have been delivered (Fig. 40-14 and Fig. 40-15 on p. 1254).

Stages of Labor and Delivery.

First stage: dilation. The first stage begins with the onset of regular contractions and ends with complete dilation of the cervix. This is generally the longest stage of labor. In nulliparas this stage averages 10 to 12 hours; in multiparas the average is 6 to 8 hours. This stage is often divided into the following three phases:

1. *Early latent phase,* 0 to 3 cm dilation; contractions occur 5 to 8 minutes apart and last 20 to 35 seconds. During this stage the woman gener-

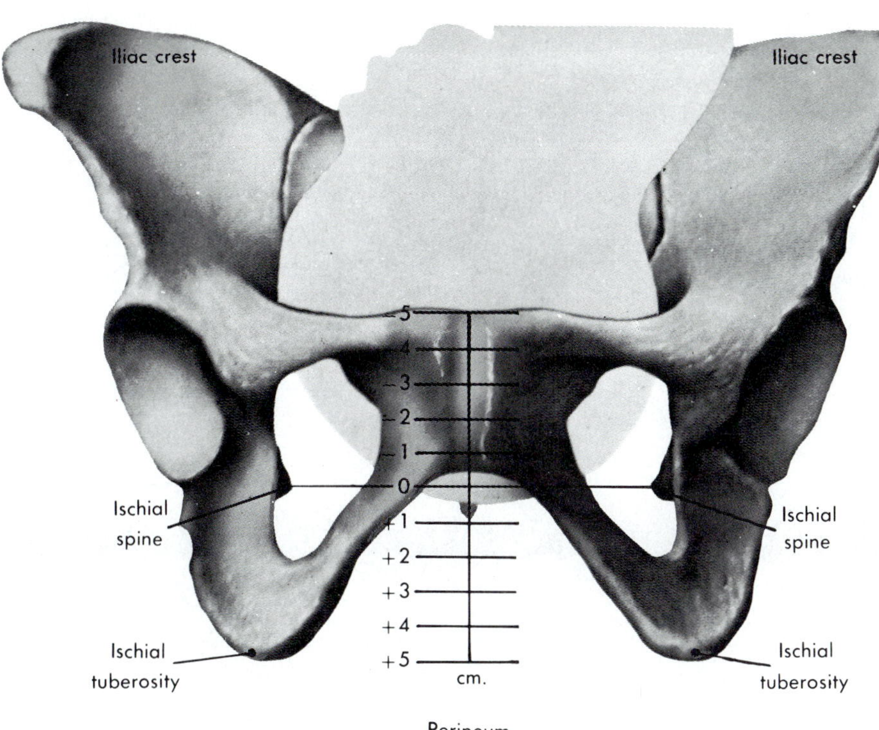

FIG. 40-13 Stations of presenting part, or degree of engagement. Location of the presenting part in relation to the level of ischial spines is designated station and indicates degree of advancement of the presenting part through pelvis. Stations are expressed in centimeters above (minus) and below (plus) the level of the ischial spines. (From *Phenomena of normal labor,* Columbus, Ohio, 1964, Ross Laboratories.)

A

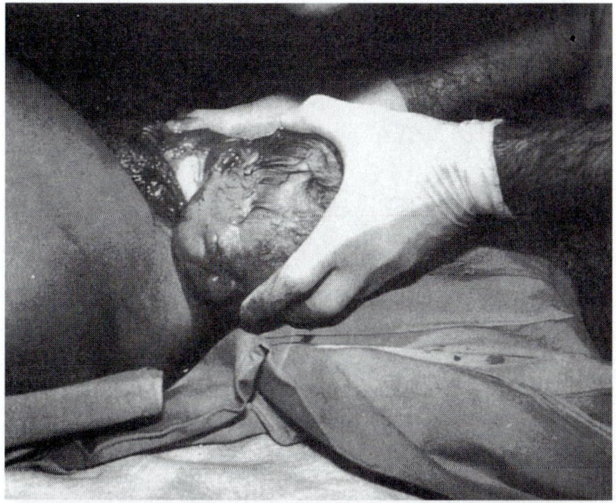

FIG. 40-14 Mechanism of labor. **A,** Restitution. **B,** External rotation. **C,** Slow expulsion of fetus/newborn. Note bulb syringe in hand in **B.**

B

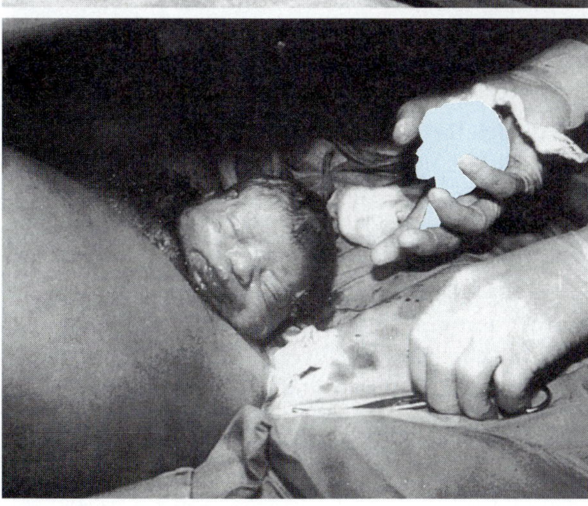

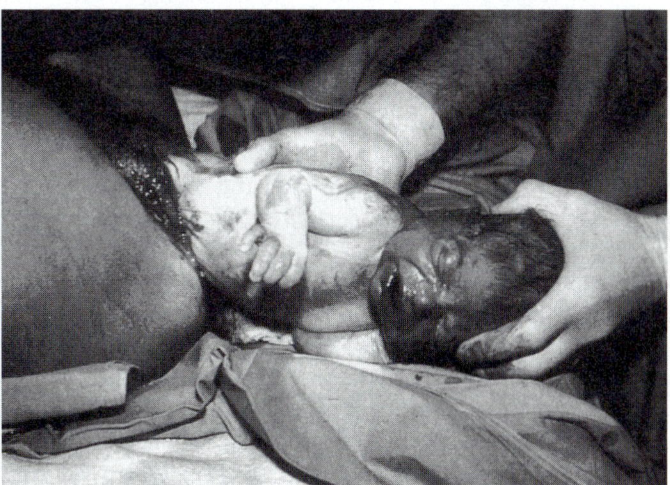

C

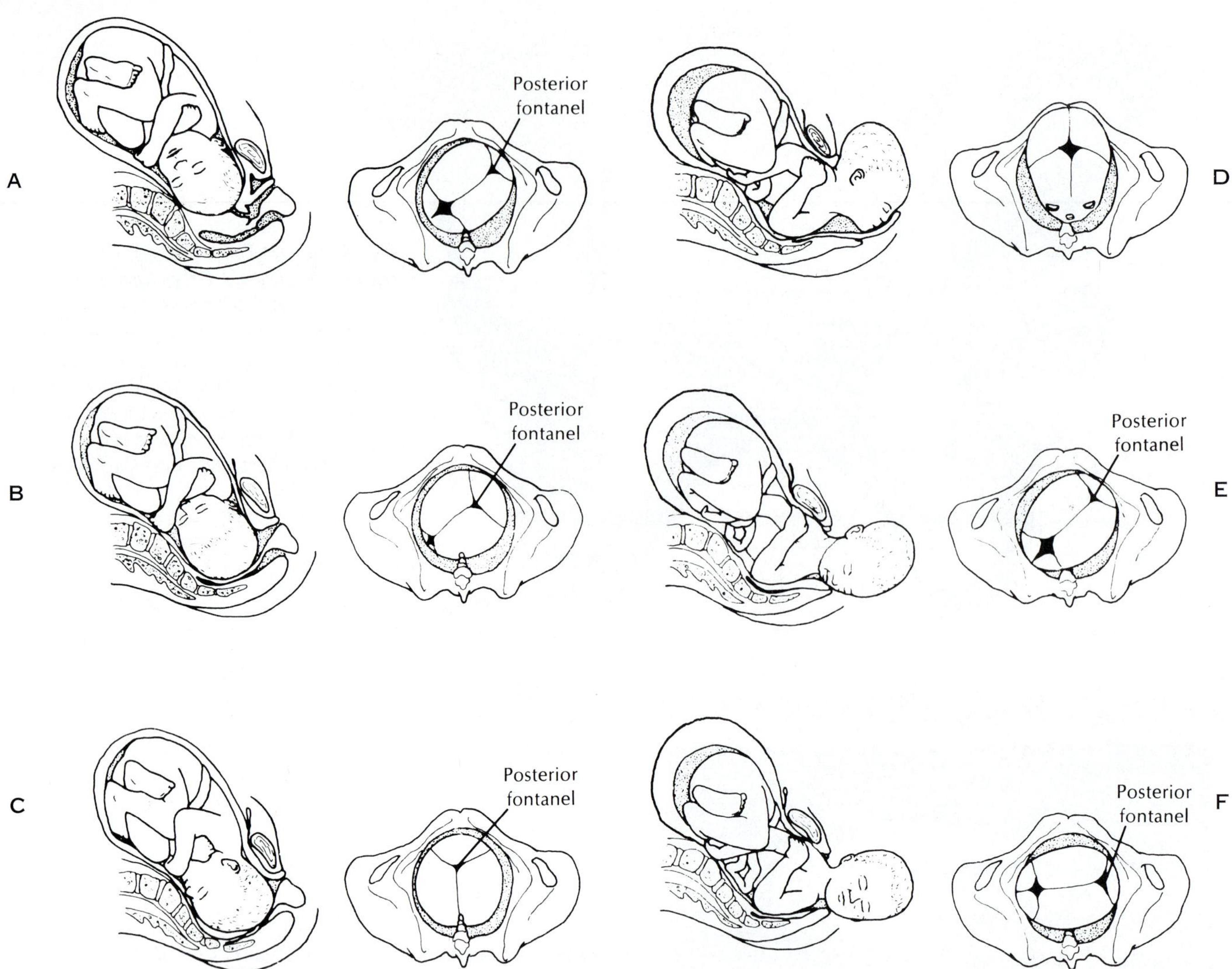

FIG. 40-15 Mechanism of labor in left occipitoanterior (LOA) presentation. **A,** Engagement and descent. **B,** Flexion. **C,** Internal rotation to OA. **D,** Extension. **E,** Restitution. **F,** External rotation.

ally is alert, frequently is talkative, and tends to be receptive to coaching on breathing techniques. This coaching may be provided by the nurse or significant other and reviews techniques learned in the prenatal classes. Pain tends to be mild and easily controlled. Backache is a common complaint. Many women, particularly multiparas, prefer to remain home during this stage. If the bag of waters has not ruptured, many women walk during this stage. The nulliparous woman may express anxiety about her ability to cope with childbirth.

2. *Mid/active phase,* 4 to 7 cm dilation; contractions occur at 3- to 5-minute intervals and last 40 to 60 seconds. During this stage the woman becomes less talkative and focuses on breathing techniques. The intensity of the pain increases but still may be manageable without medication (Box 40-2).
4. *Transitional phase,* 7 to 10 cm dilation; contractions occur at 2- to 3-minute intervals and last up to 80 seconds. This is a time of deep focus in which the woman may not wish to communicate with the nurse or significant other. If the woman has not requested pain medication earlier, she may desire it at this time. Many women experience nausea.

Second stage: delivery. The second stage of labor begins with complete dilation at 10 cm and ends with the birth of the baby. The average length of this stage is 30 minutes to 2 hours in nulliparas and 20 minutes to 90 minutes in multiparas. Contractions continue to last 80 to 90 seconds, but they may be slightly less frequent.

Box 40-2

BREATHING TECHNIQUES DURING LABOR

- Breathing techniques should be used only during contractions. Normal breathing patterns should be encouraged between contractions.
- A deep breath called a cleansing breath should be taken before and after each contraction to help the woman relax and to increase oxygen intake.
- Inspirations and expirations should be of equal duration.
- Hyperventilation, excessively rapid deep breathing, should be avoided since this can result in maternal symptoms (tingling of the fingers, hands, and mouth or vertigo) and may result in decreased oxygenation of the fetus.
- Specific breathing patterns are used during various phases of labor and delivery. If a woman has been trained in Lamaze or other methods, provide support and reminders. If a woman has not learned a specific method, the following pattern can generally be encouraged without advanced training:
  Early/latent phase: slow, deep chest or abdominal breathing at 6 to 9 breaths per minute; inhale through nose and out through pursed lips.
  Mid/active phase: Slow acceleration then deceleration of breaths through contraction; breaths shallow; approximately 16 to 20 breaths per minute.
  Transitional phase: 4-6 pants followed by a blow for duration of contraction.

Once the cervix is completely dilated, the woman is able to use the voluntary forces previously described. Generally, the woman feels the urge to push and is anxious to do so. Pushing is hard work, and the woman requires ongoing encouragement from the coach and nurse. Resting between contractions, if possible, is important to conserve energy.

During this stage the primary care practitioner may provide anesthesia and perform an episiotomy. The **episiotomy** (surgical incision of the perineum at the end of the second stage of labor to facilitate delivery and to avoid laceration of the perineum) (Fig. 40-16) is a surgical incision of the perineum that allows easier delivery. The most common type of episiotomy is a midline, or median, incision in which the tissues of the perineum are separated at an anatomical junction. If the perineum is too small, the primary care practitioner may perform a mediolateral incision in which muscle must be cut. This is generally more uncomfortable and is only done when necessary.

Immediately after delivery the baby's airway is established and the umbilical cord is clamped with two clamps and then severed between the clamps. If every-

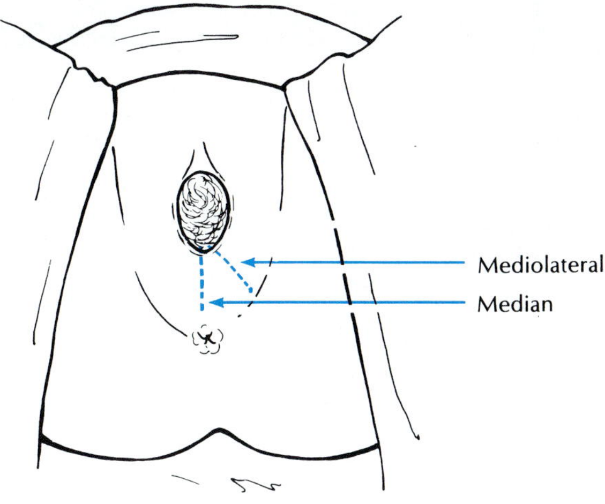

FIG. 40-16 Types of episiotomies.

thing is normal, the baby is shown to the parents. The infant then either may be given to the mother to hold or may be positioned in a special warming unit that allows for close observation and care. If any problems occur with the infant, care is administered immediately. This emergency care may, of necessity, be performed in the delivery area. The nurse should remain calm and supportive to the parents. The nurse should be aware that the parents may be alarmed and require support and explanations to allay their fears for the newborn.

Third stage: delivery of the placenta. The third stage begins with the delivery of the infant and ends with the delivery of the placenta. The average for both primiparas and multiparas is 5 to 20 minutes.

Generally speaking, the mother is less interested in the third stage. Focus and attention are usually directed to the newborn. Many women wish to inspect and possibly breastfeed the infant. When the placenta detaches from the uterine wall, a sudden outpouring of blood appears from the vagina. The cord protruding from the vagina lengthens, and the shape of the uterus becomes more rounded and firm. The woman may again experience contractions. The size and consistency of the placenta usually permit delivery with one or two pushes. Some women are curious to see the placenta; if so, it should be shown to them. During this time the primary care practitioner repairs the episiotomy if one was performed. Total blood loss is normally from 200 to 300 ml; it is considered excessive if more than 500 ml of blood is lost during delivery. It is common for an **oxytocic** (drugs that stimulate uterine contractions, thus accelerating childbirth and preventing postdelivery hemorrhage) medication, such as Pitocin or Methergine, to be administered during this stage. These medications will cause the uterus to contract firmly. This causes compression of blood vessels inside the uterus and minimizes blood loss (see the medications table on p. 1256).

MEDICATIONS FOR NORMAL LABOR AND DELIVERY

Medication	Trade Name	Action	Side Effects	Nursing Implications
Magnesium sulfate		Decreases acetylcholine in motor nerve terminals, which is responsible for seizure prevention in preeclampsia and eclampsia	Diarrhea, side effects are related to magnesium levels. Greater than 3 mg/dl: depressed CNS, blocked neuromuscular transmission leading to anticonvulsant effects. Greater than 5 mg/dl: depressed deep tendon reflexes. Greater than 12.5 mg/dl: respiratory paralysis	Obtain vital signs every 15 min after IV dose; do not exceed 150 mg/min; monitor cardiac function; time contractions and monitor fetal heart rate; monitor I&O (should remain 30 ml/hr or more).
Methylergonovine maleate	Methergine	Stimulates uterine contraction, decreases bleeding	Headache, dizziness, nausea, vomiting, chest pain, palpitation, hypertension, tinnitus, sweating, rash	Monitor blood pressure, pulse, character, and amount of vaginal bleed; monitor respiratory rate; give intramuscularly in deep muscle mass and intravenously only in emergency.
Oxytocin	Pitocin, Syntocinon	Acts directly on myofibrils producing uterine contractions, stimulates milk ejection by breasts	Fetal: bradycardia, dysrhythmias, jaundice, hypoxia, intracranial hemorrhage; maternal: anaphylaxis reactions, postpartum hemorrhage, cardiac dysrhythmias, nausea, vomiting, premature ventricular contractions, hypertension, convulsions	Monitor I&O ratio, contractions, fetal heart rate, blood pressure, pulse, and respirations.
Prostaglandin PGE (dinoprostone)	Prepidil	Stimulates uterine contraction like that seen in normal labor	Maternal: uterine contractile abnormalities, nausea, vomiting, diarrhea, back pain, warm feeling in vagina, fever; fetal: heart rate abnormalities, bradycardia	Use caution to prevent contact with skin; wash thoroughly after administration; bring to room temperature before administering; do not force warming process; have patient remain supine for 15 to 30 min after insertion.
Ritodrine hydrochloride	Yutopar	Uterine $beta_2$-adrenergic receptor stimulating effects, which reduces uterine contractions.	Erythema, rash, dyspnea, hyperglycemia, headache, restlessness, anxiety, chills, tremor, nausea, vomiting, diarrhea, constipation, altered maternal and fetal heart rate	Monitor maternal and fetal heart tones during infusion; watch intensity and length of uterine contractions; monitor fluid intake to prevent overload; monitor blood glucose level in diabetic patients.

Fourth stage: stabilization. The time immediately after delivery is critical as the mother's body attempts to recover from the efforts of labor. Usually the mother is monitored closely for 2 to 4 hours after delivery in the birthing room or in a recovery room. Some women, particularly those who had a long or difficult labor and delivery, are exhausted and wish only to rest. Others appear to be euphoric and wish to talk about the experience or spend more time with the baby and their significant other.

It is important to monitor physiological changes closely during the fourth stage. Vital signs, uterine tone, vaginal drainage, and the perineal tissue are assessed. During the first hour assessments are done every 15 minutes. If observations are within normal limits, assessments are done every 30 minutes for the next hour. If all observations remain normal, the woman is transferred to a patient room for the remainder of her hospitalization.

Response of the Newborn to Birth. The process of delivery is stressful to the newborn. Rapid adaptation from the intrauterine climate to that of extrauterine life is essential if the newborn is to survive.

The physical condition of newborn infants is evaluated at birth. An evaluation guide called the Apgar score is used in most facilities (Table 40-3). This scoring is done at 1 and 5 minutes of age. The score can range from 0 to 10. The criteria used include heart rate, respiratory effort, muscle tone, reflex irritability, and skin color. A low score indicates serious problems that may require resuscitation. A high score indicates good condition, requiring only routine care.

Breathing must be established. In utero, the fetus's need for oxygen was met by the mother. Once the umbilical cord is severed, the newborn must breathe to obtain oxygen. Fetal lungs must be adequately mature so the alveoli can expand adequately. A substance called **surfactant** is produced; it decreases surface tension within the alveoli and permits inflation. At the time of delivery a combination of chemical, thermal, tactile, and mechanical changes initiates the first breath.

The airway must be cleared of fluids that are present in the lungs. Some fluids are forced from the lungs as the thorax passes through the pelvis during delivery. A bulb syringe is used to remove excess fluid from the mouth and nasopharynx (Figs. 40-17 and 40-18).

Warmth is necessary to prevent a rapid drop in body temperature. The environment in utero was approximately 99° F (37.2° C); the external environment in the delivery room is usually about 70° F (21.1° C). To prevent hypothermia the infant should be dried immediately to help reduce heat loss from evaporation. The baby then may be placed in contact with the mother's skin if she wishes to breastfeed, or the baby may be transferred to a radiant warming unit.

If there are no complications, the infant remains in view of the mother until her care is completed. Identification bracelets are placed on both mother and baby before they leave the delivery room. These will be used to verify infant identification and match it with that of the mother until discharge. Footprinting of the infant is an-

TABLE 40-3 Apgar Scoring Chart

Sign	0	1	2
Heart rate	Absent	Slow—below 100	Above 100
Respiratory effort	Absent	Slow—irregular	Good crying
Muscle tone	Flaccid	Some flexion of extremities	Active motion
Reflex irritability	None	Grimace	Vigorous cry
Color	Pale blue	Body pink, extremities blue	Completely pink

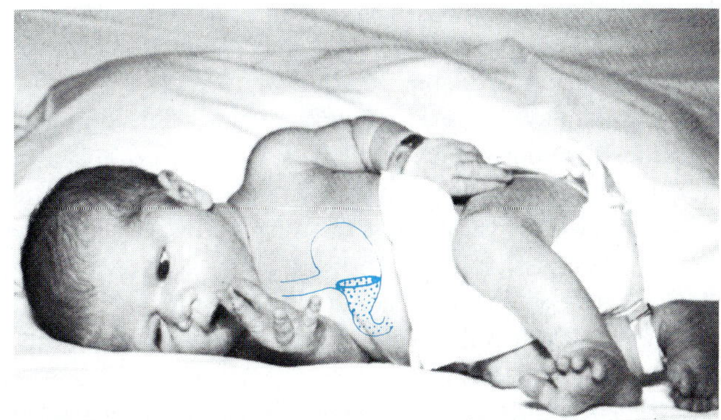

FIG. 40-17 Infant is turned to right side and supported in this position to facilitate drainage from mouth and to promote emptying of stomach contents into the small intestine.

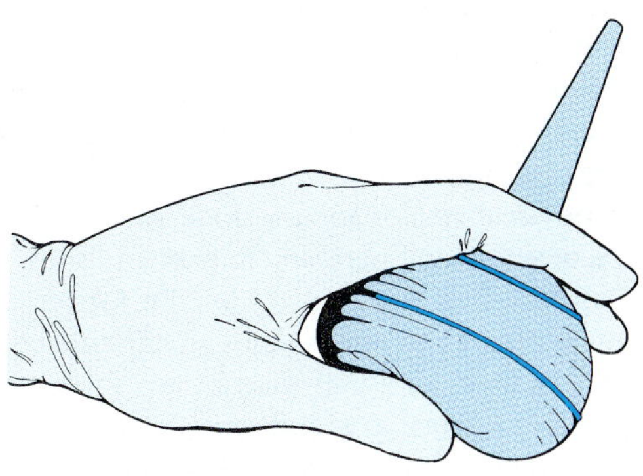

FIG. 40-18 Bulb syringe. Bulb must be compressed before insertion.

other method of identification; this may be done in the delivery area or in the nursery.

NURSING ASSESSMENT AND INTERVENTIONS

Health Perception and Health Management

It is important to know how well prepared for childbirth the woman is; the woman who has attended classes and practiced breathing techniques will require a different level of explanation and support than one who has had no preparation.

If a hospital delivery is planned, admission is generally prearranged and much of the paperwork completed ahead of time to minimize delays. If home delivery is anticipated, the family should follow whatever directions the primary care practitioner has given them.

When hospitalization is anticipated, it is a good idea for the prospective parents to prepare a suitcase with necessary items well in advance of the date of delivery. Making a "trial run" to the hospital also provides reassurance. This can reduce fears of not getting to the hospital on time. If there are children at home, plans should be made for their care. It is advisable that the parents-to-be anticipate as many problems as possible and make several alternative plans.

On admission an assessment begins. This typically includes the following:

1. Review of the prenatal record, including general medical history, past obstetrical history, and the history of this current pregnancy. This should include information about allergies and any current health problems, such as respiratory or other types of infection.
2. The mother is interviewed to gather information about signs and symptoms of the onset of labor, such as the nature and frequency of contractions; level of discomfort; and the presence of vaginal discharge such as bloody show or loss of amniotic fluid. If these data indicate that the woman is in labor, information regarding the type of preparation for childbirth, support person present, special cultural practices or expectations, type of anesthesia planned, method of infant feeding desired, and name of pediatrician are also obtained.
3. A physical examination is done, including a complete set of vital signs and fetal heart tones. These data will function as a baseline for further assessment. Heart and lung sounds are auscultated. The face, hands, legs, and sacrum are inspected for signs of edema. The abdomen is palpated to determine the fetal lie and presentation. The status of the membranes is assessed. If there is any question regarding ruptured membranes, a nitrazine test should be performed before the vaginal examination, since solutions used may make the test results unreliable. Contractions are timed to determine frequency, regularity, duration, and intensity. A vaginal examination is performed to determine the progress of labor, including position, dilation, effacement, and station.
4. Diagnostic tests include a urinalysis to check for the presence of glucose, protein, or ketones, which may indicate potential complications. If blood analyses were not performed during pregnancy, they should be done at this time. Information about hemoglobin and hematocrit levels, blood type and Rh factor, antibody titer, and screening for sexually transmitted diseases helps in assessment of actual or potential problems.

Nutritional and Metabolic Pattern

Gastrointestinal (GI) motility and absorption decrease during labor and delivery. Food eaten before labor may remain in the digestive tract and lead to complaints of nausea and vomiting. Once active labor begins, solid foods are generally withheld. It is important to know when food was last consumed in case administration of a general anesthetic becomes necessary. In addition, fluid intake should be assessed. Increased physical exertion and mouth breathing are common during labor. When these factors are combined with restricted oral intake, a fluid deficit may result. Some primary care practitioners allow small amounts of ice chips or clear beverages during labor. Orders for intravenous fluids, such as a 5% dextrose solution, to prevent fluid imbalance are very common.

Elimination

Depending on the amount of fluid intake, urine output may be normal or decreased. Voiding every 2 hours is desirable. A full bladder can interfere with the progress of labor. When membranes are intact, use of the toilet is permitted. Once membranes are ruptured, use of the bedpan is preferred. If the presenting part is compressing the urethra, catheterization may be ordered.

Bowel elimination is assessed. Some women experience diarrhea with the onset of labor. Careful hygiene technique is important to reduce the possibility of contamination. Enemas were once routinely administered to empty the colon and maximize space in the pelvic cavity; today they are given only when specifically ordered. Large-volume enemas are sometimes used to stimulate or strengthen labor. Enemas *should not be given* if there is vaginal bleeding or premature labor, if the presenting part is not engaged, or if there is other than a vertex presentation. If membranes are ruptured, the enema should be expelled into a bedpan.

The urge to defecate during labor may indicate the start of the second stage. Before allowing a woman to attempt to have a bowel movement, it is wise to inspect the perineum and assess dilation for progress of labor.

Activity and Exercise

Ambulation is generally encouraged so long as the membranes are not ruptured. Ambulation may also be permitted if the membranes have ruptured and the presenting part is fully engaged. Walking provides distraction and tends to strengthen the effectiveness of labor. When ambulation becomes too uncomfortable, or if the mother has been given analgesics, she usually is encouraged to rest. Positioning becomes important; the woman should be encouraged to assume the position most comfortable for her. Sitting or semiseated positions are preferred by some women. Low back pain is common. A side-lying position is frequently more comfortable than supine. Changing position may help reduce discomfort. If the patient is allowed to be up, a warm shower provides much relief for low back pain during labor. Side-lying positions reduce pressure on the vena cava. The left side is recommended if the FHR shows late deceleration or if the woman experiences hypotension. The Trendelenburg position is used if prolapse of the cord is suspected.

Sexuality and Reproductive Issues

Assessment of vaginal drainage continues through labor. If not observed sooner, bloody show may be seen. Moderate amounts of discharge are common, and linens should be changed to provide comfort. Any bright red bleeding should be reported immediately.

Vaginal examination to assess the progress of labor continues through the first stage of labor. Contractions are monitored for frequency, duration, and intensity.

Coping and Stress Tolerance

Fears become apparent during labor and delivery, particularly in the primigravida. Many women have unrealistic expectations for themselves and feel that they should be able to be in control of labor. Controlled breathing techniques help, but the involuntary nature of labor troubles many women. Encouragement and support in breathing exercises, along with explanations regarding the progress of labor, are helpful. Fatigue and pain lower the woman's ability to cope. It is important to understand the cultural and religious background of each woman, since these factors may strongly influence her behavior.

The nurse should pay attention to the reaction of the support person. It is important to recognize that many times the woman's significant other will experience fears and anxieties. The father particularly may exhibit concerns about the process of labor and the pain the mother is experiencing. At times fathers will express guilt about their role, either in not being able to help enough or in being responsible for the pregnancy. It is important to tell the father that he is an important participant, not an unwanted guest in the process of childbirth. He should be encouraged to help make the woman comfortable and provide the companionship and caring needed.

Role and Relationship

Many women wish their spouse or a significant other to be with them during labor and delivery. Most childbirth education programs include this individual in the preparation. Often this person works as the "coach" to remind the woman of breathing techniques and provide encouragement.

In some situations this is not the case, and the woman faces labor and delivery alone. This may be at her request, or it may be a matter of circumstances. If she is alone, the nursing staff must provide extra support. Many other individuals, such as grandparents, siblings, and extended family, may be interested in the progress of labor. Depending on the situation, the nurse should try to pay attention to the needs of these family members.

Father or Partner During Labor

The father of the baby usually is the partner who supports the woman in labor. He often is able to provide comfort measures and touch that the laboring woman needs. When the woman becomes focused on her pain, sometimes the father can persuade her to try nonpharmacological variations of comfort measures. He usually is able to interpret the woman's needs and desires to staff members. He may be totally focused and involved with the woman, or he may be more passive because of cultural norms or fear. The nurse should assess his level of comfort in asking questions and in being present and involved during the second-stage labor and birth. In this way the nurse can determine what level of support to provide to the couple during this time.

The father will be exposed to many sights and smells he may never before have experienced. It is important to tell him what to expect and to make him comfortable about leaving the room to gather his composure should something shock him. First, of course, provision should be made for someone else to support his partner during his absence. Staff members need to verbalize that the father's presence is helpful and to encourage his involvement in the care of his partner to the extent of his comfort level. This is especially true when his partner has become angry and told him to go away. The nurse must reassure the father that this is normal behavior for a woman in transition and that if he reenters after a few minutes, the woman will ask him why he was gone so long.

Participation in the birth is ego building. The father can be of assistance during the labor process; his presence is important. For example, recently a 16-year-old unwed mother in labor with her first child thrashed about, moaning and screaming with each contraction. A nurse remained at her bedside, coaching and comforting to no avail. The adolescent father arrived and was escorted into her room. The young woman continued her labor calmly and without medication through delivery.

When the father is active and supportive, the mother turns to him. The primary care practitioner remains the medical-surgical expert, without taking on the significant-other surrogate role as well. The couple's future relationship and their relationship with the child may be positively influenced. Mutuality is fostered when the mother can turn to the father and say, "I could never have done it without you. You were my pillar of strength."

Supporting the father as well as the mother during labor elevates the nurse's role. It is another step forward from merely providing custodial care to enacting a therapeutic role. Support of the father reflects the nurse's orientation and commitment to the person, the family, and the community. Therapeutic nursing actions convey to the father several important concepts.

First, he is of value as a person. He is not inept and bungling or idle, nervous, and inconsequential. Second, he can learn to be a partner in the mother's care. Finally, childbearing is a partnership.

The nurse can support the father/partner in the following ways:

1. Regardless of the degree of involvement desired, orient him to the maternity unit, including the woman's labor room, cafeteria, waiting room, nursery, and names and functions of personnel present.
2. Respect his or their decisions as to his degree of involvement, whether the decision is active participation in the delivery room or just being kept informed. When appropriate, provide data on which he or they can base decisions; offer freedom of choice as opposed to coercion. This is their experience and their baby.
3. Indicate to him when his presence has been helpful, and continue to reinforce this throughout labor.
4. Offer to teach him comfort measures to the degree he wants to know them. Reassure him that he is not assuming the responsibility for observation and management of his partner's labor, but supporting her as she progresses.
5. Communicate with him frequently regarding her progress, procedures to be performed, what to expect from procedures, and what is expected of him.
6. Prepare him for changes in her behavior and physical appearance.
7. Remind him to eat; offer snacks and fluids if possible.
8. Relieve him as necessary; offer blankets and a pillow if he is to sleep in a chair by the bedside. Acknowledge the stress of the situation on each partner and identify normal responses. The nonjudgmental attitude of staff members helps the father and mother accept their own and the other person's behavior.
9. Attempt to modify or eliminate unsettling stimuli (such as extra noise, extra light, chatter).

A well-informed father/partner can make a significant contribution to the health and well-being of the mother and child, their family interrelationship, and his self-esteem.

It has been found that a significantly lower percentage of women suffered postdelivery emotional upsets when their partners received support and assistance from parent education classes, physicians, midwives, and nurses throughout the childbearing cycle.

Self-Perception

The prepared mother generally feels more able to deal with labor and delivery than the unprepared one. Multigravidas generally have more confidence, since they have previous experience to draw on. Women who have experienced problems during pregnancy or in past labors and deliveries may need reassurance that they can be successful. The nurse should continue to be supportive. Even an unprepared woman can participate in simple breathing exercises with coaching from the nurse.

Cognitive and Perceptual Issues

Pain is a major concern during labor and delivery. Breathing exercises help reduce discomfort, but as the intensity of labor increases, most women require some form of analgesia and/or anesthesia. The physician will prescribe these medications with caution, because they pass through the placenta and affect the fetus. Timing is critical to prevent diminished or depressed respiratory effort at the time of birth. The condition of the mother and fetus must be carefully assessed before and after medication administration.

The most commonly used analgesics are meperidine HCl (Demerol) and butorphanol tartrate (Stadol), which may be given intramuscularly or intravenously. Antianxiety medications such as hydroxyzine HCl (Vistaril) and diazepam (Valium) may be administered to reduce ap-

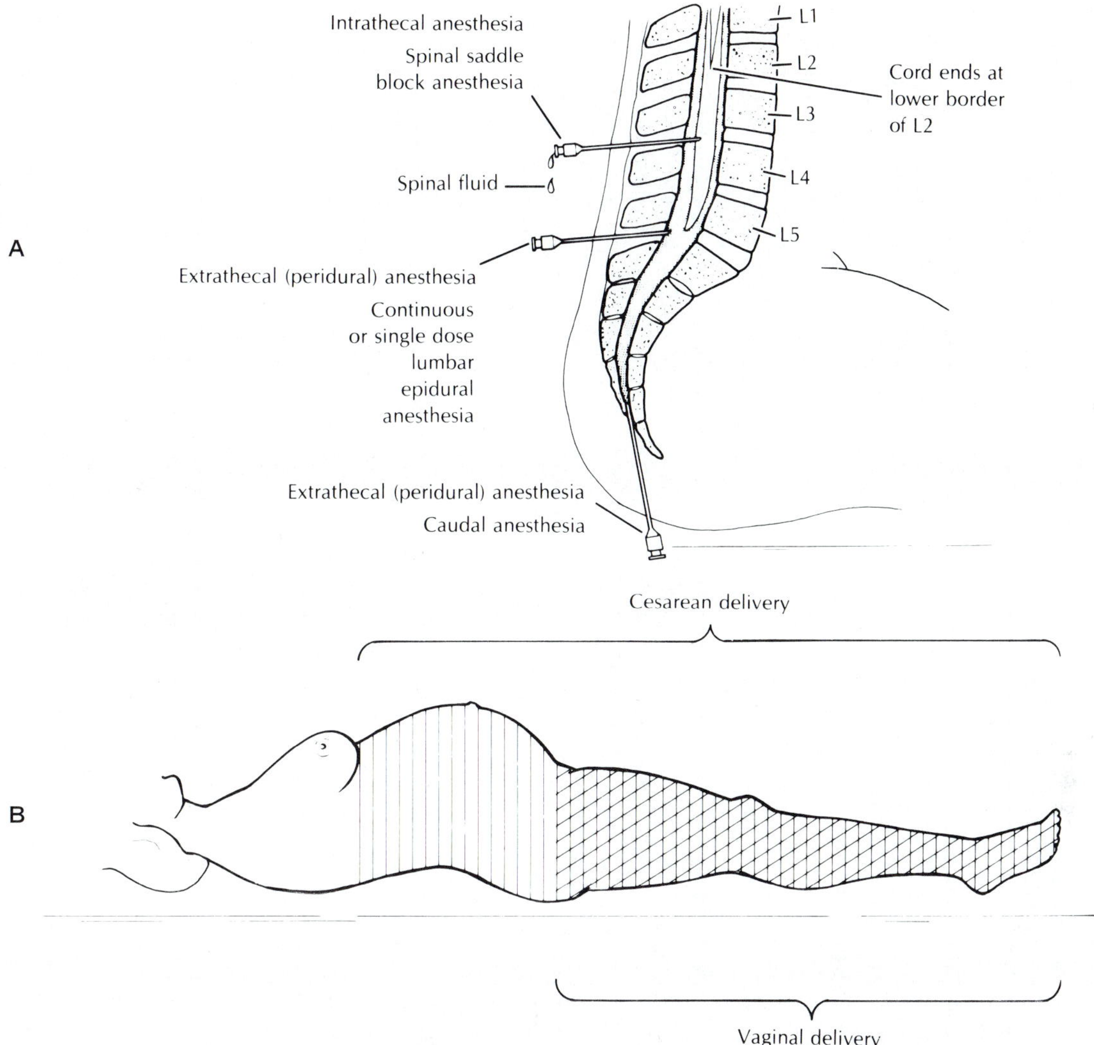

FIG. 40-19 **A,** Regional anesthesia in obstetrics. **B,** Level of anesthesia necessary for cesarean delivery and for vaginal delivery. (Courtesy Ross Laboratories, Columbus, Ohio.)

prehension and anxiety. These medications also potentiate the effects of narcotics. Occasionally, sedative/hypnotics such as pentobarbital (Nembutal) and secobarbital (Seconal) are given in early labor to promote relaxation and rest.

The form of anesthesia used will depend on the patient's wishes and the primary care practitioner's assessment of maternal and fetal need. Anesthetics are classified as general, regional, and local. Most vaginal deliveries today include a form of regional anesthetic (Fig. 40-19). Regional anesthetics include paracervical, epidural, spinal, and pudendal blocks (Table 40-4 on p. 1262).

Values and Beliefs

Cultural beliefs and practices have implications for labor and delivery, as they do in all aspects of life. The values and beliefs of women in labor should be respected. The nurse should seek information about specific cultural practices, values, and beliefs and incorporate these in the plan of care.

MEDICAL INTERVENTIONS

Although labor and delivery are essentially normal processes, sometimes complications arise. At times it becomes necessary for the physician to intervene to protect the mother or fetus.

Induction

As already discussed, the exact cause of labor is unknown. Induction is an attempt to start labor at a time other than when it begins spontaneously. This intervention may be necessary when membranes have been rup-

TABLE 40-4 Anesthesia for Labor and Delivery

Type of Anesthesia	Usual Dosage	Administration	Area Anesthetized or Effects	Possible Side Effects		Nursing Interventions After Administration
				Mother	Fetus	
Regional						
Paracervical block	5-10 ml of 1% solution of a "caine" drug	Injection, either side of cervix at 4 cm dilation	Cervix and uterus	Can slow labor	30% incidence of temporary slowing of fetal heart	Close monitoring of fetal heart tones and maternal vital signs and contractions
Pudendal block	5-10 ml of 1% solution of a "caine" drug	Injection into area of pudendal nerves for birth	Perineum	None unless allergic to drug	None	Reassurance and explanation; monitor fetal heart tones and maternal vital signs closely
Caudal and lumbar epidural	5-15 ml of 1%, 1.5%, or 2% solution of a "caine" drug	Caudal canal Epidural space at 4 cm dilation	Pelvic region	Hypotension; cannot "push" for delivery May slow labor if started too early	Slowing of fetal heart and fetal heart decelerates	Monitor fetal heart tones and maternal vital signs closely; use excellent aseptic techniques
Saddle block (low spinal)	1-1.5 ml of solution concentration, depending on "caine" drug used	Injection under dura of spinal cord for birth	Pelvic region	Postspinal headache Hypotension	None	Intravenous and O_2 usually used
General inhalation						
Nitrous oxide Ethylene Cyclopropane Ether Other similar agents		Inhaled through mask	Complete body	Could aspirate if vomits	Respiratory depression; hypoxia	Be alert and prepared for vomiting (with aspiration of food) and excessive uterine bleeding owing to uterine relaxation
Inhalant analgesia						
Methoxyflurane (Penthrane)	0.3% to 0.5% in first stage or at time of delivery	Volatile inhalant	Relieves pain	Hypotension; slow shallow respirations	Hypoxia and central nervous system depression	Inform woman of what she will experience. Allow her to administer as needed.
Trichloroethylene (Trilene)	0.5% in first stage or at time of delivery			Irregular pulse; rapid respiration		Do not hold mask for her. Check vital signs frequently.

tured longer than 24 hours, in cases of severe pregnancy-induced hypertension, or in a postterm pregnancy. Occasionally an elective induction is performed when the woman has a history of precipitous (lasting under 3 hours) labors. This is done to prevent an emergency out-of-hospital delivery.

The primary care practitioner assesses each woman carefully to determine that she is a good candidate for induction and that no harm will come to either mother or fetus.

The medically approved methods of inducing labor include the following:

1. *Amniotomy:* If the amniotic membranes have not ruptured, the primary care practitioner may use a sterile instrument (hook shaped) to open the sac and allow drainage of the fluid; this procedure is called an **amniotomy** (AROM: artificial rupture of the fetal membrane). FHR is measured immediately before and after this procedure. The amount and color of amniotic fluid are assessed. If all criteria for induction were met, labor typically starts within 6 to 8 hours.
2. *Prostaglandin (PGE) gel application:* After assessment of the mother and fetus, the primary care practitioner applies PGE gel intracervically using a plastic catheter. Contractions normally begin within an hour of instillation of the gel. Vital signs, FHR, and contractions are monitored carefully. It is common for an amniotomy to be performed in conjunction with the gel application. An internal fetal monitor is also routinely applied when PGE gel is used. In most regions the LPN/LVN does not apply this gel but the LPN/LVN does have the responsibility of monitoring/assessing labor progress.
3. *Oxytocin stimulation:* Use of oxytocin is indicated to induce labor or to stimulate a labor that is not making adequate progress because of generalized inactivity, which is known as **uterine inertia** (absence or weakness of uterine contractions). A dilute form of the medication is administered intravenously. Pitocin is most commonly used, although Syntocinon, a synthetic form of oxytocin, is occasionally used. These medications are very powerful and are started by the primary care practitioner or a specially trained nurse, if hospital policies permit. The nurse may then monitor the progress of labor. Since the contractions that result from oxytocin can be very strong, it is essential to monitor the FHR and contractions carefully and document care. The infusion is stopped and the primary care practitioner contacted if there are signs or symptoms of complications, such as changes in FHR, bradycardia, tachycardia, dysrhythmias, excessive frequency, duration, or pressure of contractions.

Forceps Delivery

Forceps are a pair of spoonlike devices that fit around the fetal head to aid in expulsion of the fetus (Fig. 40-20). As with induction, there are certain criteria that must be met before the primary care practitioner uses forceps. The nurse assisting in the delivery is responsible for providing the type of forceps requested by the primary care practitioner. Close monitoring of the FHR before and during the forceps maneuvers is essential. It is also important to explain to the mother that these actions will help the baby.

Cesarean Delivery

Cesarean birth, also referred to as a *c-section,* is delivery through an abdominal and uterine incision. This type of delivery may be anticipated in advance or may be performed in cases of emergency. The number of cesarean deliveries has increased greatly during the last 20 years. Although there is concern in the medical community and the media about this trend, approximately 20% of deliveries continue to take place by the cesarean route.

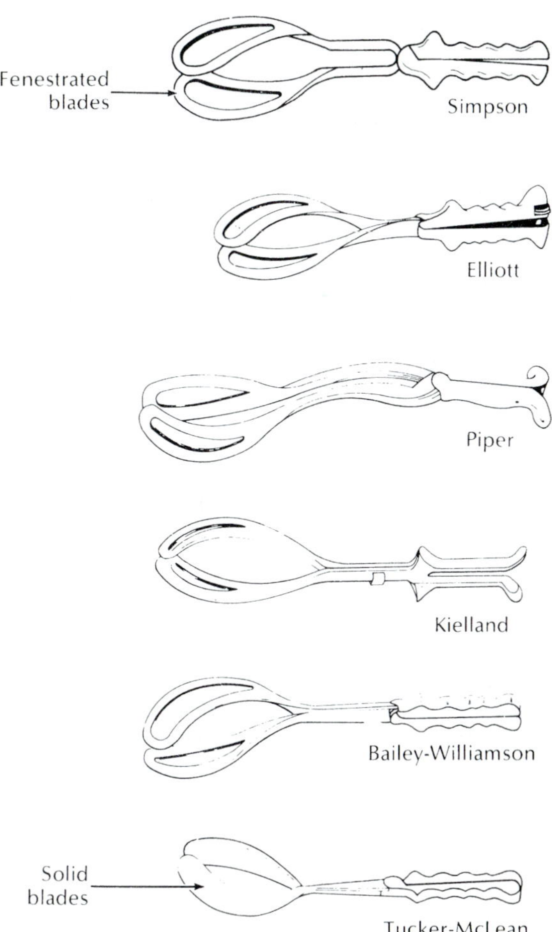

FIG. 40-20 Types of forceps.

TABLE 40-5 Nursing Process and the Patient in Labor

Data Collection	Possible Nursing Diagnoses	Patient Outcomes	Interventions
Health management			
Does the woman appear prepared for labor and delivery? Has she taken prenatal classes? Has she received routine prenatal care? What if any unusual/untoward symptoms does she present? What is the status of fetal membranes?	Health maintenance, altered, related to lack of resources and lack of knowledge	Patient will use self-care behaviors to maintain an optimum level of wellness for herself and her baby.	Identify factors that are likely to interfere with labor. Provide explanations regarding labor.
Nutritional and metabolic issues			
When was her last meal? What was consumed? Any nausea or vomiting? Any edema noted?	Nutrition, altered: less than body requirements, related to inadequate intake of nutrients	Excess glucose intake will be avoided.	Provide frequent oral hygiene. Withhold food during active labor. Monitor the administration of an electrolyte solution without glucose to avoid excess glucose in the bloodstream (excessive maternal glucose results in fetal hyperglycemia and fetal hyperinsulinism; after birth the neonate's high levels of insulin will deplete the glucose stored, and hypoglycemia will result). Per primary care provider's orders, offer clear fluids, small amounts of ice chips, hard candy.
	Fluid volume deficit, related to inadequate fluid intake	Patient's fluid balance will be maintained.	Monitor IV fluid replacement therapy. Monitor urine output. Monitor temperature. Offer clear liquids during the active phase of labor and small amounts of ice chips thereafter. Instruct patient to take small sips of clear liquids or water to prevent vomiting and its potential for aspiration of fluids into the lungs.
Activity and exercise			
What is the status of fetal membranes? What is fetal heart rate? Fetal movement? Vital signs?	Activity intolerance, high risk for, related to fatigue and effort to labor	Patient (couple) will learn ways of conserving her energy.	Encourage activity if membranes are intact. Institute safety precautions if patient is medicated for pain. Monitor maternal vital signs and FHR. Promote rest between contractions. Provide a restful environment.

TABLE 40-5 Nursing Process and the Patient in Labor—cont'd

Data Collection	Possible Nursing Diagnoses	Patient Outcomes	Interventions
Elimination			
When was last bowel movement? Amount and consistency? What is pattern of urine elimination?	Urinary retention, high risk for, related to pressure of presenting part on urethra	Patient will be able to empty her bladder.	Monitor voiding; check bladder for signs of distention or retention. Encourage voiding every 2 hours. Catheterize per primary care provider's orders.
Rest and sleep			
How long has she been in labor? How well has she slept recently?	Sleep pattern disturbance, related to labor	Patient will be able to rest between contractions.	Position patient to promote comfort. Encourage periods of rest between contractions. Encourage participation from significant other in patient comfort measures such as backrubs.
	Fatigue, related to increased physical demands of labor	Patient's fatigue will be kept to a minimum.	Maintain a comfortable, supportive atmosphere. Provide nonpharmacological management of discomfort to decrease fatigue. Encourage rest or sleep, if possible, during first stage of labor.
Cognitive and perceptual issues			
Is she knowledgeable of breathing techniques? What is level of pain? Duration? Location? How frequent are contractions?	Knowledge deficit, related to lack of experience with labor	Patient will begin self-care activities.	Review breathing techniques; explain and coach in breathing if untrained.
	Pain, related to labor contractions	Patient will report increased comfort.	Provide emotional support; maintain supportive environment. Encourage nonpharmacological methods for relief of pain and discomfort, such as focusing and feedback; reinforce relaxation breathing techniques. Provide effleurage (a light stroking of the abdomen in rhythm with breathing during contractions), sacral pressure or massage, and transcutaneous electrical nerve stimulation as ordered. Administer analgesics as ordered.

Continued.

TABLE 40-5 Nursing Process and the Patient in Labor—cont'd

Data Collection	Possible Nursing Diagnoses	Patient Outcomes	Interventions
Role and relationship			
Who has accompanied patient to hospital? How interested/involved is this person?	Role performance, altered, related to expectations for labor Family processes altered, related to expectations for labor	Patient (couple) will become knowledgeable of and demonstrate positive coping techniques.	Spend time listening to concerns; involve family members and significant other in teaching. Verbalize that the father's presence is helpful and encourage his involvement in the care of his partner to the extent of his comfort level.
Coping and stress			
What fears or anxieties are verbalized?	Anxiety, related to change in role or perceived threat to self	Patient will be able to verbalize fears and identify coping mechanisms.	Encourage verbalization of fears and concerns. Provide explanations at patient's level of understanding.
Values and beliefs			
What is the patient's cultural background? What are her religious practices?	Spiritual distress, related to separation from spiritual or cultural beliefs or practices	Patient will practice proper health care techniques within the limits of her belief system to maintain the health and safety of herself and her baby.	Incorporate cultural practices into care whenever possible. Consult a spiritual advisor for specific information if necessary.

Indications for cesarean birth can be maternal or fetal. The major maternal indications for cesarean delivery are (1) **fetopelvic disproportion** (also called *cephalopelvic;* the head of the fetus is larger than the pelvic outlet), in which the fetus is unable to pass through the maternal pelvis; (2) previous cesarean delivery; (3) breech presentation; (4) medical conditions that would endanger the mother's health, such as cardiac complications; (5) abnormal conditions of the placenta, such as placenta previa; (6) infections of the vaginal canal; and (7) pelvic abnormalities. The major fetal indicators are (1) fetal oxygen deprivation (hypoxia); (2) prolapse of the umbilical cord; (3) breech presentation; (4) malpresentations, such as transverse; and (5) congenital anomalies. These conditions will be discussed in greater depth in Chapter 42.

Current medical practice is rethinking at least one of these criteria. The old rule was "once a cesarean, always a cesarean." Today many women who have previously delivered by cesarean are candidates for vaginal birth after cesarean (VBAC). Depending on the woman's medical history, the nature of this pregnancy, and the reason for the earlier cesarean, the primary care practitioner may permit a trial labor. In these cases the woman must be very carefully monitored, and the facility must be prepared to perform an emergency cesarean if complications arise.

When a cesarean delivery is performed, the incisions are made both in the abdominal wall and in the uterine wall. Depending on the technique used by the primary care practitioner, several different incisions may be employed.

Postpartum care of the woman experiencing cesarean delivery will be discussed in Chapter 41.

NURSING PROCESS SUMMARY

Table 40-5 offers guidelines for reviewing all health patterns to help the nurse focus observations when performing an assessment on a woman in labor. Significant observations or responses will indicate the need for further questioning. If the nurse is unsure of the significance of data, it is important to consult with a more experienced nurse.

Table 40-5 also suggests possible nursing diagnoses with interventions.

REFERENCES AND SUGGESTED READINGS

1. Andrews CM, Chrzanowski M: Maternal position, labor and comfort, *Appl Nurs Res* 3:7, 1990.
2. Biancuzzo M: How to recognize and rotate an occiput posterior fetus, *MCN* 93(3):38, 1993.
3. Bobak IM, Jensen MD: *Essentials of maternity nursing,* ed 3, St Louis, 1991, Mosby.
4. Bobak IM, Jensen MD: *Maternity and gynecologic care: the nurse and the family,* ed 5, St Louis, 1993, Mosby.
5. Burroughs A: *Maternity nursing,* ed 6, Philadelphia, 1992, Saunders.
6. Cosner KR, DeJong E: Physiologic second-stage labor, *MCN* 18(1):38, 1993.
7. Doenges M, Moorhouse M: *Nurse's pocket guide to nursing diagnosis with interventions,* ed 3, Philadelphia, 1991, FA Davis.
8. Eganhouse DJ: Fetal monitoring of twins, *J Obstet Gynecol Neonatal Nurs* 21:17, 1992.
9. Fischbach F: *A manual of laboratory diagnostic tests,* ed 4, Philadelphia, 1992, Lippincott.
10. Freeman RK, Farite TJ, Nageatte MP: *Fetal heart rate monitoring,* Baltimore, 1991, Williams & Wilkins.
11. Hankins GDV: Apgar scores: are they enough? *Contemp OB/GYN* (special issue) 36:13, 1991.
12. Ingalls AJ, Salerno MC: *Maternal and child health nursing,* ed 7, St Louis, 1991, Mosby.
13. Jepson HA et al: The Apgar score: evolution, limitations, and scoring guidelines, *Birth* 18:2, 1991.
14. Kenner CA, MacLaren A: *Essentials of maternal and neonatal nursing,* Springhouse, Penn, 1993, Springhouse.
15. Ladewig PW, London MI, Olds SB: *Essentials of maternal-newborn nursing,* ed 2, Redwood City, Calif, 1990, Addison-Wesley.
16. Lederer JR et al: *Care planning pocket guide: a nursing diagnosis approach,* Redwood City, Calif, 1993, Addison-Wesley.
17. Litwack K: Managing postanesthetic emergencies, *Nurs '91* 21:49, 1991.
18. Malestic SL: Fathers need help during labor, too, *RN* 53(7):23, 1990.
19. Martin LL, Reeder SJ: *Essentials of maternity nursing: family centered care,* Philadelphia, 1991, Lippincott.
20. Miller AM, Lorkovic M: Prostaglandin E_2 for cervical ripening, *MCN* 18(1):23, 1993.
21. *Mosby's medical, nursing, and allied health dictionary,* ed 4, St Louis, 1994, Mosby.
22. Olds SB, London ML, Ladewig PW: *Maternal newborn nursing: a family-centered approach,* ed 4, Menlo Park, Calif, Addison-Wesley.
23. Pagana KD, Pagana TJ: *Mosby's diagnostic and laboratory test reference,* St Louis, 1992, Mosby.
24. Pirez-Woods MR et al: Panic control after cesarean birth: efficacy of patient-controlled anesthesia vs. traditional therapy IM morphine, *J Perinatol* 11:174, 1991.
25. Smith DP et al: *Comprehensive child and family nursing skills,* St Louis, 1991, Mosby.
26. Stroud R, Cochrane S: Midwives managing without drugs, *Nurs Times* 86:70, 1990.
27. Swinnerton T: Alternative remedies during labor, *Nurs Times* 87:64, 1991.
28. Thomas CL: *Taber's cyclopedic medical dictionary,* ed 17, Philadelphia, 1993, FA Davis.
29. Tucker SM: *Pocket guide for fetal monitoring,* ed 2, St Louis, 1992, Mosby.
30. Tucker SM et al: *Patient care standards,* ed 5, St Louis, 1992, Mosby.
31. Willson JR et al: *Obstetrics and gynecology,* ed 9, St Louis, 1991, Mosby.
32. Wright WC: Continuous epidural block for OB anesthesia, *Contemp OB/GYN* 36:89, 1991.

CHAPTER CHALLENGE

KEY POINTS

- Although various theories are proposed, the process that starts labor has not been determined.
- True labor and false labor can be confusing to the patient and health care personnel; even knowledgeable individuals can be mistaken.
- The birth process can occur in a variety of settings. The most important concern is protecting the welfare of both the mother and newborn.
- Vaginal delivery involves a complex interrelationship of the passageway, the passengers, and the powers.
- The first stage of labor is usually the longest stage. There are significant risks to both mother and fetus during this time; therefore both the mother and fetus must be carefully and continuously assessed.
- Fetal monitoring, using internal or external sensors, enhances the nurse's ability to monitor labor and recognize signs of fetal distress.
- Many women are trained in specific breathing techniques designed to reduce pain and facilitate control of the birthing process. The nurse should be prepared to assist with these.
- The fourth stage of labor, the time of stabilization, requires careful nursing assessment of the mother. Assessment of vital signs and fundal checks are essential to detect excessive blood loss.
- The process of delivery is stressful to the newborn. The Apgar scoring system is used 1 and 5 minutes after birth to assess the newborn's condition.
- Modification of functional health patterns occurs during labor and delivery. The nurse should assess all areas to detect problems quickly and report these promptly.
- In some cases the primary care practitioner may have to intervene in the process of labor and delivery and use forceps or surgical means to deliver a healthy newborn.
- The nurse can facilitate mother-infant attachment by meeting the new mother's physical, support, and teaching needs.
- Episiotomy and lacerations may be seen even with "normal" childbirth, and their appropriate and prompt repair is essential.

STUDY QUESTIONS

1. Mrs. Brown, a 27-year-old multipara, is afraid that she will go to the hospital in false labor and be sent home. The nurse would explain that it is most appropriate to go to the hospital when the contractions:
   1. Vary in length and intensity
   2. Start in the back and travel to the abdomen
   3. Are felt in the abdomen
   4. Stop or decrease with ambulation
2. Ms. O'Meara, age 19, asks if there are any signs other than contractions that will indicate the onset of labor. The nurse would explain that a normal sign of impending labor is:
   1. Increased frequency of urination
   2. Sudden, sharp pain in the lower abdomen
   3. Production of colostrum from the breasts
   4. Discharge of pink-tinged vaginal mucus
3. Mrs. Arco, age 36, has been admitted to the hospital in early labor. She calls the nurse to report a gush of warm fluid. To determine if this means the bag of waters has ruptured, the nurse would:
   1. Send a sample to the laboratory for analysis
   2. Check the fluid with nitrazine paper
   3. Test the fluid for the presence of glucose and acetone
   4. Perform a pelvic examination
4. Ms. Quick, age 25, is in active labor when her bag of waters ruptures. The first appropriate nursing action is to:
   1. Position her on her right side
   2. Assist her to the Fowler's position
   3. Offer her the bedpan
   4. Assess the fetal heart rate
5. Mrs. Brooks, age 31, has been in labor for 10 hours. Her lips are dry, and she complains of being thirsty. The most appropriate nursing intervention would be to:
   1. Offer her small amounts of ice chips
   2. Request a clear liquid diet from dietary
   3. Call the physician for an intravenous order
   4. Explain that she cannot have fluids during labor
6. Ms. Davis, age 39, has progressed in labor, and assessment reveals that the cervix is completely dilated and effaced. She has the urge to bear down. It is most appropriate to assist her into:
   1. The lateral position
   2. The supine position
   3. The squatting position
   4. The knee-to-chest position
7. Ms. Thibodeau, age 30, has been in labor for several hours. She calls for the nurse and states that she "has to move her bowels" and wants to bear down. The nurse realizes that this probably indicates that she is in the:
   1. First stage of labor
   2. Transition stage
   3. Second stage of labor
   4. Third stage of labor
8. Mrs. Brown, age 29, is a primipara in the second stage of labor and is actively bearing down. Her husband questions how long it will take for her to deliver. You would explain that stage two in a primipara usually takes:
   1. 5 to 15 minutes
   2. 15 to 30 minutes
   3. 30 minutes to 2 hours
   4. 2 to 3 hours
9. Mrs. Quincy, age 24, has delivered, and the nurse is assessing her for signs of placental separation, such as:
   1. A change in the shape of the uterus
   2. A decrease in uterine muscle tone
   3. A shortening in the length of the protruding cord
   4. Complaints of rectal pain
10. Mrs. Clinton, age 42, delivers spontaneously. The nurse is prepared to calculate the Apgar score to assess the:
    1. Status of the newborn
    2. Condition of the mother
    3. Amount of blood loss
    4. Maturity of the newborn

41

CARE OF THE MOTHER AND NEWBORN

Gloria E. Wold

KEY TERMS

acrocyanosis
autolysis
circumcision
colostrum
cryptorchidism
engorgement
fontanelle
gynecomastia
harlequin sign
Homans' sign
involution
lactation
lanugo
lochia
meconium
mummification
parent-child attachment (bonding)
physiological jaundice
polydactyly
prolactin
puerperium
pseudomenstruation
syndactyly
vernix caseosa

LEARNING OBJECTIVES

After reading this chapter, the student should be able to do the following:

- Define the key terms.
- Describe postpartum assessment of the mother.
- Identify the physiological changes that occur in the postpartum period.
- Discuss the nursing responsibilities during the postpartum period.
- Explain the importance of teaching personal and infant care.
- Discuss the psychosocial adaptations that occur postpartum.
- Describe the assessment of the normal newborn.
- Identify the physical characteristics of the normal newborn.
- Identify normal reflexes observed in the newborn.
- Describe common variations that may be observed in the newborn.
- Describe the behavioral characteristics of the newborn.
- Discuss nursing interventions for the circumcised newborn.
- Discuss parent-infant attachment (bonding)
- Discuss nutritional needs and feeding of the newborn.

RELATED TOPICS OF INTEREST

- Life span development (Chapter 7)
- Cultural aspects of nursing care (Chapter 8)
- Diet therapy (Chapter 19)
- Care of the patient with a cardiovascular disorder (Chapter 28)
- Care of the patient with a urinary disorder (Chapter 30)
- Care of the patient with a reproductive disorder (Chapter 33)

The postpartum period, also called the **puerperium,** lasts from the time the woman delivers until the reproductive organs return to approximately the nonpregnant size and position, usually in 3 to 6 weeks. This period consist oftwo stages. The immediate postpartum period, lasting up to 6 hours after delivery, is sometimes called the *fourth stage of labor* or the recovery stage. During thistime the newly delivered mother requires special care and attention after the rigors of delivery. This is a time for close observation and assessment to ensure that no problems occur. The later postpartum stage follows the stage of recovery and lasts until about 6 weeks after delivery.

During the postpartum period the mother's body makes rapid physiological adaptations. The anatomical and physiological changes that took place over 9 months reverse within just 6 weeks. Many psychological changes also occur as the woman and her family adjust to the new family member or members.

ANATOMICAL AND PHYSIOLOGICAL CHANGES

Uterus

After the birth of the baby and delivery of the placenta, the uterus contracts in response to oxytocin (hormone produced by the posterior pituitary gland that stimulates uterine contractions and release of milk in the mammary gland [let-down reflex]). This contraction compresses blood vessels at the site where the placenta separated from the uterine wall. This site, an area 8 to 10 cm (3 to 4 inches) in diameter, has open venous sinuses. If the uterus does not contract adequately, blood loss can be excessive. The placental site will heal by the process of exfoliation, in which necrotic tissue is sloughed from the uterine lining, leaving a fresh layer of endometrial tissue free from scars. This process is necessary if successive pregnancies are to occur.

Immediately after delivery the uterus can be felt at about the level of the umbilicus. It is the size of a small melon and weighs approximately 1000 g (2 lb). Within a week if will be barely palpable at the level of the symphysis pubis and will have decreased in size to about 500 g (1 lb). Within 6 weeks the uterus will again be a pelvic organ approximately the nonpregnant size of 50 g (2 oz). This decrease in size is called **involution** (Fig. 41-1).

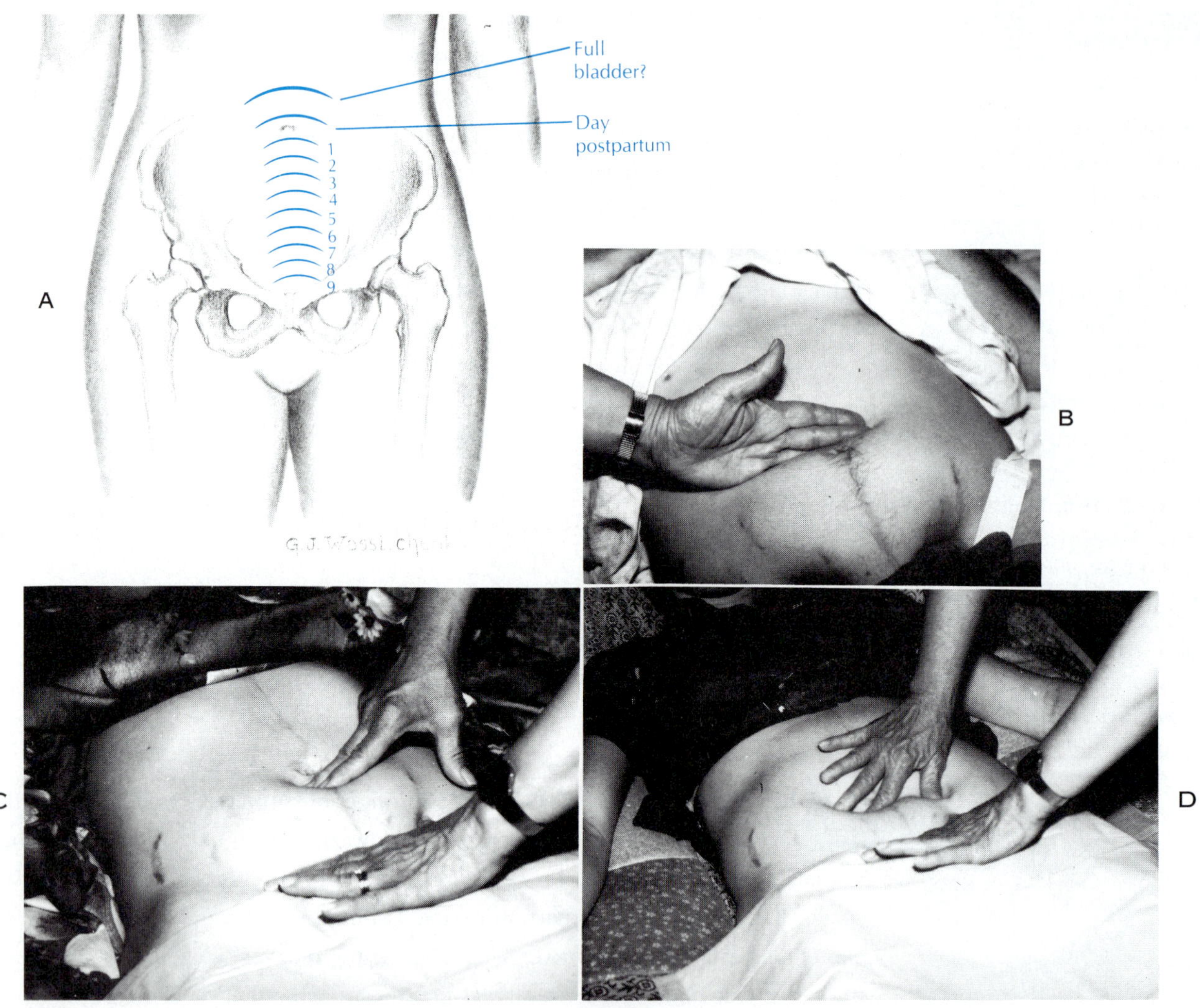

FIG. 41-1 Assessment of involution of uterus after delivery. **A,** Normal progress, days 1 through 9. **B,** Size and position of uterus 2 hours after delivery. **C,** 2 days after delivery. **D,** 4 days after delivery. (**B, C,** and **D,** courtesy Marjorie Pyle, RNC, Lifecircle, Costa Mesa, Calif.)

After contracting, the muscle fiber does not return to its original length, but remains slightly shortened, which is a unique attribute of uterine muscle that aids in preventing postdelivery hemorrhage and results in involution.

Involution is carried out by a process called autolysis. **Autolysis** (the self-dissolution or self-digestion that occurs in tissues or cells by ezymes in the cells themselves) is a result of sudden withdrawal of estrogen and progesterone. This sudden drop in hormone levels releases proteolytic enzymes into the endometrium; these enzymes cause the cells to lose protein materials and thereby shrink in size. The number of muscle cells remains the same, but the size of each cell changes dramatically.

The fluid waste discharged after delivery is called **lochia** (vaginal discharge during puerperium consisting of blood, tissue, and mucus). As the uterine lining is being shed, the necrotic tissue, blood, and mucus leave the body through the vagina. Lochia has a fleshy odor similar to menstrual discharge.

Initially, the amount of blood content is greatest, resulting in a bright red drainage called *lochia rubra.* This is generally seen the first day or two after delivery. As healing of the placental site occurs, the discharge becomes a pink-to-brown color called *lochia serosa.* This generally occurs until the seventh day. After that the drainage is slightly yellow to white and is called *lochia alba.* This continues for another 10 days to 2 weeks. If fragments of the placenta remain in the uterus, the uterus will not be able to contract and seal blood vessels adequately. This can result in excessive blood loss and may require surgical intervention (Table 41-1).

TABLE 41-1 Lochia and Nonlochia Bleeding

Lochia	Nonlochia Bleeding
Lochia usually trickles from the vaginal opening. The steady flow is greater as the uterus contracts.	If the blood discharge spurts from the vagina, there may be cervical or vaginal tears in addition to the normal lochia.
A gush of lochia may result as the uterus is massaged. If it is dark in color, it has been pooled in the relaxed vagina, and the amount soon lessens to a trickle of bright red lochia (in the early puerperium).	If the amount of bleeding continues to be excessive and bright red, a tear may be the source.

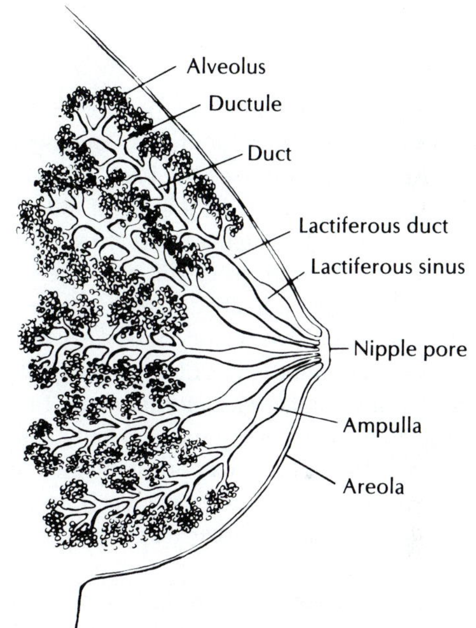

FIG. 41-2 Detailed structural features of human mammary gland.

Breasts

Breast changes begin early in pregnancy. Increased amounts of estrogen stimulate enlargement of breast size as a result of increased adipose and fluid retention. Estrogen also stimulates the growth of the milk ducts to prepare for **lactation** (function of secreting milk or period during which milk is secreted). Milk production is necessary if a woman plans to breastfeed her infant. This is a very basic yet complex process.

The first secretion produced by the breast is **colostrum.** This precursor to milk is thin, watery, and slightly yellow. It is rich in protein and calories in addition to antibodies and lymphocytes. Colostrum may be produced as early as the second trimester of pregnancy, particularly in multigravidas. Its production continues for about 2 days after delivery, when true milk production begins.

Lactation is a combination of hormonal, neurological, and psychological responses. After delivery estrogen and progesterone levels drop rapidly. While the levels of estrogen and progesterone are diminishing, the level of prolactin is increasing. **Prolactin,** a hormone secreted by the anterior pituitary gland, is responsible for stimulating milk production in the mammary alveolar cells (Fig. 41-2 and Fig. 41-3, *A*, on p. 1272). Stimulation of the nipples, particularly by the infant's sucking, causes the release of oxytocin from the posterior pituitary gland. Oxytocin stimulates contraction of the mammary ducts and causes the milk to be ejected from the breast. This cycle is called the *let-down reflex* (Fig. 41-3, *B*).

Embarrassment, fear of pain during breastfeeding, or lack of self-confidence in the ability to breastfeed may result in difficulty establishing the let-down reflex. In many women "let-down" also occurs during sexual orgasm. This may be troublesome if it is not expected.

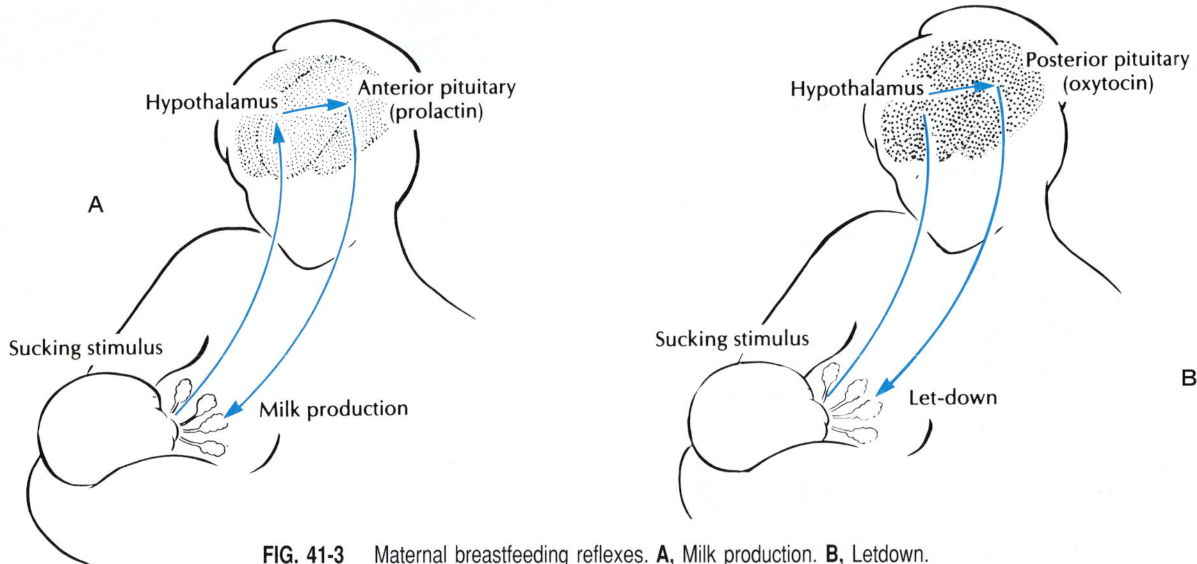

FIG. 41-3 Maternal breastfeeding reflexes. **A,** Milk production. **B,** Letdown.

Once lactation is established, the mother may feel a tingling or prickling sensation when feeding time approaches. If the mother nurses the baby at regular intervals and empties the breast, the supply of milk increases in response to the baby's demands. It is not uncommon for the breasts to become very full and uncomfortable when the milk supply initially comes in, since a combination of venous and lymphatic stasis also occurs during lactation. This fullness is called **engorgement.** Application of warm, moist washcloths to the breasts and nursing the baby more frequently usually resolve the problem. Once the milk supply is established, prolactin production decreases, and it is primarily oxytocin, released as the baby suckles, that maintains the supply of milk.

If the breast is not adequately stimulated, the lactation response may not be established. This can happen when the baby has a weak suck or is not put to breast often enough. If the breast is not emptied adequately, the pressure of the milk in the alveoli can also suppress milk production. Incorrect placement at breast may also lead to problems. If the baby's mouth grasps only the nipple and does not apply pressure on the lactiferous glands (mammary glands/Montgomery's glands, consisting of 20 to 24 glands in the areolas of the nipples) in the areola, milk will not be released and the needed stimulation will not occur. This also may lead to nipple trauma and soreness. The nurse should explain this to the new mother. Massé cream may be ordered by the primary care practitioner to soothe and soften tender nipples.

Two of the main causes for unsuccessful breastfeeding are lack of knowledge and poor self-confidence. Nurses can play an important role in supporting and encouraging the woman who wishes to breastfeed. To do this the nurse must be knowledgeable in correct techniques of breastfeeding. There are many good books available that can be useful when instructing a new mother; also many support groups such as the LaLeche league provide information and encouragement (Figs. 41-4 and 41-5).

Breastfeeding has many benefits for the mother. One benefit is a more rapid involution of the uterus as a result of the release of oxytocin during breastfeeding, which stimulates contraction of the uterus. Another benefit is a lower incidence of breast cancer in women who have nursed for at least 3 months; several studies have validated this benefit. Also, many women who breastfeed report a special closeness to their infants, because they are providing a special and important nourishment.

Bottle-feeding is the choice of many other women. If the woman chooses not to breastfeed, lactation must be suppressed. This can be accomplished by use of medication or by mechanical means. The most commonly administered antilactogenic medication is bromocriptine mesylate (Parlodel), which suppresses prolactin secretion. This medication is started promptly after delivery, when the new mother's blood pressure has stabilized. It is taken twice daily for 14 to 21 days. Regular blood pressure patient assessments should be made during the hospitalization. If mechanical suppression is to be used, it must be started before milk production begins. This is accomplished by applying a supportive bra within 4 to 6 hours after delivery. Ice to the breasts will also decrease the discomfort that may result from engorgement. Any form of breast stimulation, such as pumping the breasts, should be avoided, and application of heat to the breasts should also be minimized, even when bathing. Maternal fluid intake should not be restricted.

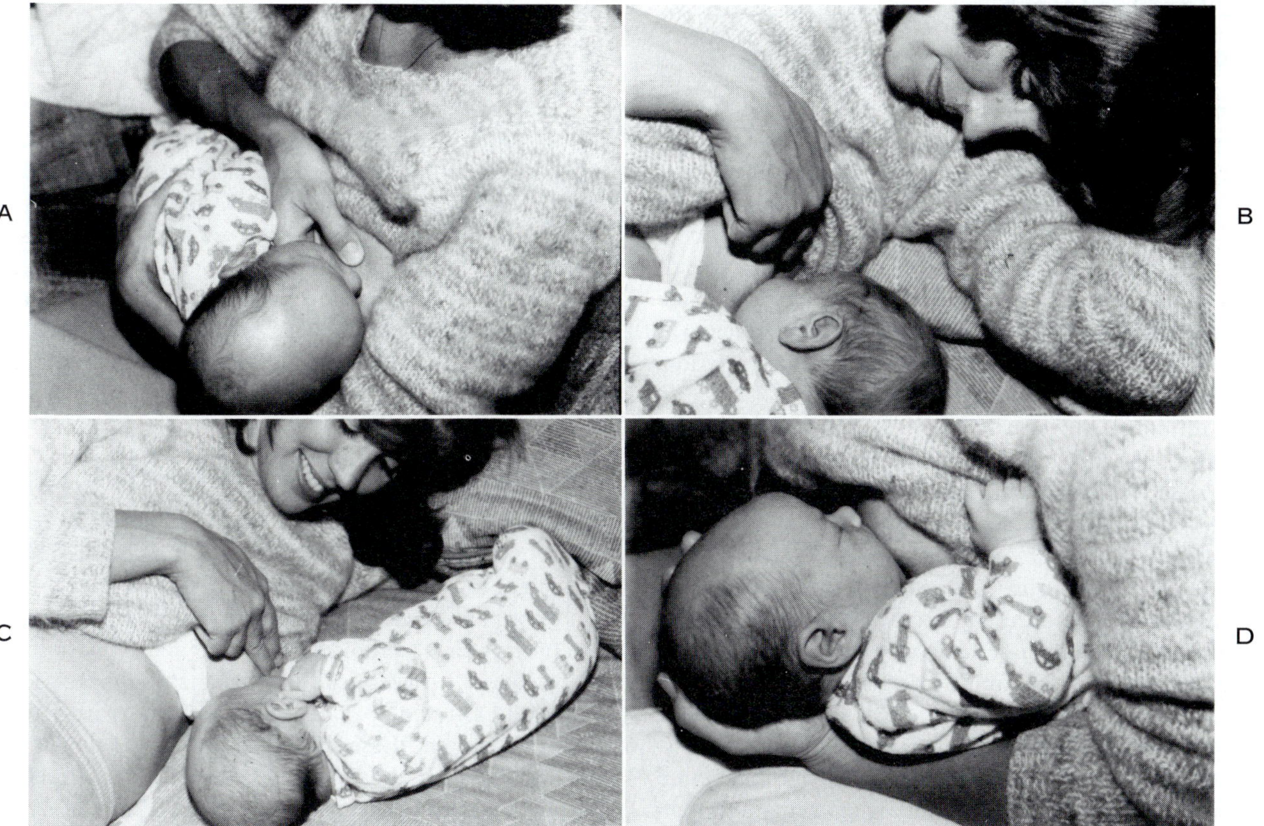

FIG. 41-4 Positioning the baby. **A,** Cradle hold. One arm and hand support baby. Other hand supports breast (thumb above and fingers below). Breast is guided into baby's mouth. **B,** Side-lying position. Pillows support mother's head. Baby is turned toward mother. Mother depresses breast to facilitate baby's breathing. **C,** Variation on side-lying position. **D,** Football hold. Baby is held in one arm with hand supporting head. (Courtesy Marjorie Pyle, RNC, Lifecircle, Costa Mesa, Calif.)

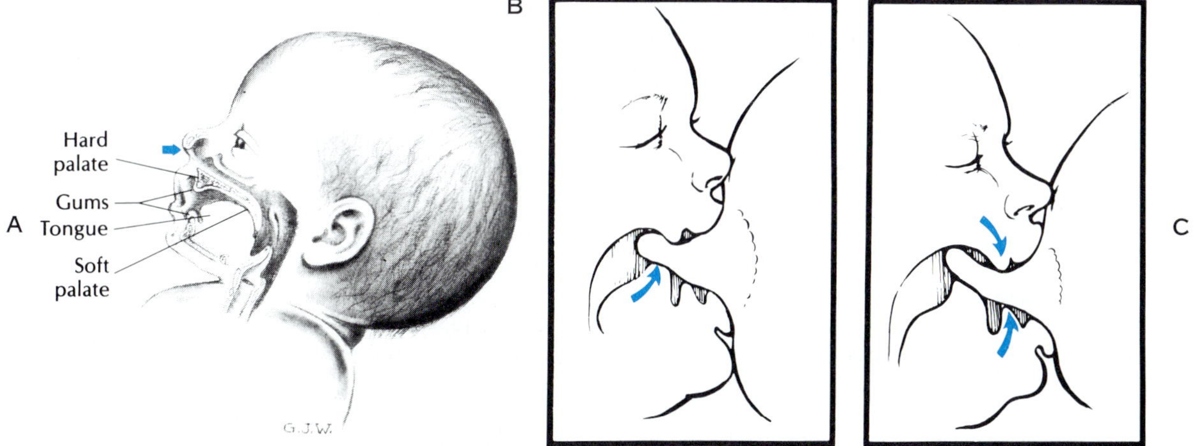

FIG. 41-5 Suckling process. **A,** Infant breathes through nose *(arrow)*. Tongue and palate meet closing esophagus. **B,** Tongue thrusts up and forward to grasp nipple. **C,** Gums compress areola and tongue moves backward, creating negative pressure for suction.

NURSING ASSESSMENT AND INTERVENTIONS

Health Perception/Health Management

Women with uncomplicated deliveries remain in the hospital a short time after giving birth. It may be only hours, or it may be 1 or 2 days after delivery. Even women who delivered by cesarean are rarely kept more than 5 to 7 days. This may be a result of financial concerns, type of insurance coverage, or personal preference. Since early discharge is increasingly common, it is important to assess the woman's ability to meet her own needs and those of her infant. Parent-newborn relationship assessments are vital.

The home situation should be discussed. If any information obtained about the home situation appears unsafe or questionable, an appointment with a social worker is necessary before discharge. It is also important to review self-care concerns before discharge. This should include information about postpartum danger signs (Box 41-1) and the importance of medical follow-up. It should also include review of infant and self-care activities and family planning information.

Parent-Newborn Relationships. The mother's reaction to the sight of her newborn may range from excited outbursts of laughing, talking, and even crying to apparent apathy. A polite smile and nod may acknowledge the comments of nurses and primary care practitioners. Occasionally the reaction is one of anger or indifference; the mother turns away from the baby, concentrates on her own pain, and sometimes makes hostile comments. These varying reactions can arise from pleasure, exhaustion, or deep disappointment. Whatever the reaction and cause may be, the mother needs continuing acceptance and support from all the staff. A written form accompanying the baby's chart should record the parents' reaction at birth. How did the parents look? What did they say? What did they do?

Some warning signs of possible difficulties in parent-child relationships, apparent immediately following delivery, are listed in Box 41-2.

Siblings should be encouraged to get acquainted with the new family member (Fig. 41-6).

Parents are responsive to praise of their newborn. Many require reassurance that the blue appearance of the baby after delivery is normal until respirations are well established. The reason for the molding of the baby's head must be reviewed with parents. Information about hospital routine as to future parent-child contacts can be repeated. The hospital staff, by their interest and their concern, can do much to make this experience a satisfying one for parents, family, and significant others.

Nutritional and Metabolic Issues

Recovery Stage. The length of time spent in labor, and the physical exertion, often result in hunger. Most physicians allow a meal after delivery if the woman is alert and not nauseated. Fluids are very important during the recovery phase to replace the fluids and blood lost during delivery; a variety of fluids such as water and juices should be offered. If intravenous (IV) fluids are ordered by the physician, these should be administered promptly. When a general anesthetic has been used, such as during a cesarean delivery, the presence of bowel sounds should be verified before solid food is given.

If the woman has been using mouth-breathing techniques during labor, the mucous membranes and lips may be dry and cracked, and breath odor may be noticeable. Good oral hygiene will relieve these symptoms and reduce discomfort. A complete sponge bath enhances well-being and provides comfort by removing perspiration and other waste products from the skin.

Box 41-1 POSTPARTUM DANGER SIGNS

- Fever with or without chills
- Malodorous vaginal discharge
- Excessive amount of vaginal discharge
- Bright red vaginal bleeding after it has changed to pink or rust color
- Edema, erythematous or painful area on the legs
- Pain or burning sensation with urination or an inability to void
- Breast changes such as localized pain, heat, edema, or malodorous drainage
- Pain in the perineal or pelvic area

Box 41-2 WARNING SIGNS: PARENT-NEWBORN RELATIONSHIPS IMMEDIATELY AFTER DELIVERY

- Passive reaction, either verbal or nonverbal (parents do not touch, hold, or examine baby or talk in affectionate terms or tones about baby)
- Hostile reaction, either verbal or nonverbal (parents make inappropriate verbalization, glances, or disparaging remarks about physical characteristics of child)
- Disappointment over sex of baby
- No eye contact
- Nonsupportive interaction between parents (if interaction seems dubious, talk to nurse and physician involved with delivery for further information)

From Gray JD et al: *Semin Perinatol* 3:95, 1979.

Later Postpartum Stage. Diet remains an important concern during the postpartum stage. Many women are very aware of the weight gained during pregnancy, and wish to lose the excess as soon as possible. It is important that dieting not deprive the woman of necessary nutrition. If the woman has not gained excessive weight during pregnancy, the prepregnant weight is normally achieved in 6 to 8 weeks without dieting. Most physicians do not recommend any weight-loss diets until after this time. The nonlactating mother should continue to eat a well-balanced diet that follows the Food Guide Pyramid. Caloric intake should be the same as before pregnancy, provided it was not excessive. Lactating mothers generally continue with the diet recommended during pregnancy; the extra calories, vitamins, and minerals are required by the body for lactation. A breastfeeding mother can consume 300 more calories daily than the bottle-feeding mother and lose weight at the same time (see Chapter 18).

Hygiene

Good personal hygiene continues to be important during the late postpartum stage. Excessive perspiration and a slight odor from drainage are common; regular bathing should be encouraged to minimize odors and promote comfort. After the first day, most women are permitted to be up ad lib and prefer to shower and shampoo by themselves. Vertigo may occur as a result of vascular shifts related to the heat of the shower. If this occurs while standing in the shower, the woman may experience syncope and injury may result. The first time the newly delivered woman takes a shower, the nurse should be particularly careful to provide for safety. This includes instruction on use of the emergency call signal and the length of time recommended and providing a chair in the shower room. The nurse should also check the patient frequently during her first shower to verify that safety is maintained. Tub baths are not recommended until after the postpartum examination at 6 weeks, so that no water that has been contaminated with body wastes enters the vaginal canal or uterus until healing is completed.

Sitz baths are sometimes ordered by the physician to reduce discomfort and to promote healing of the perineum. Vasodilation from the warm water helps reduce edema and speed tissue repair. If sitz baths are ordered, the patient should be instructed about water temperature and length of time. As with a shower, vascular changes may occur, and the nurse should check on the patient regularly to promote safety. It is important that proper cleaning of equipment take place between patients if community facilities are used (Fig. 41-7). Today some facilities use a personal, portable sitz bath that the patient can take home at discharge (see Chapter 16).

If the woman has delivered by cesarean birth, an abdominal incision is present, with sutures or staples that close the incision. This incision should be assessed in the same manner as any other surgical incision. It should remain approximated with no erythema, and there should be very little exudate and no malodorousness (foul odor). The incision may be left open to the air or a surgical dressing may be applied, depending on the physician's orders. Some physicians apply Steri-Strips

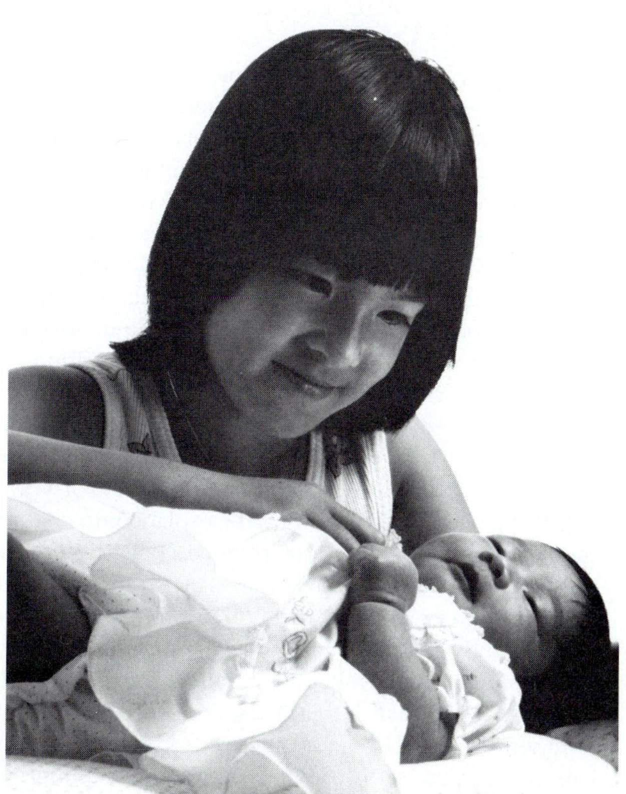

FIG. 41-6 Sibling involvement.

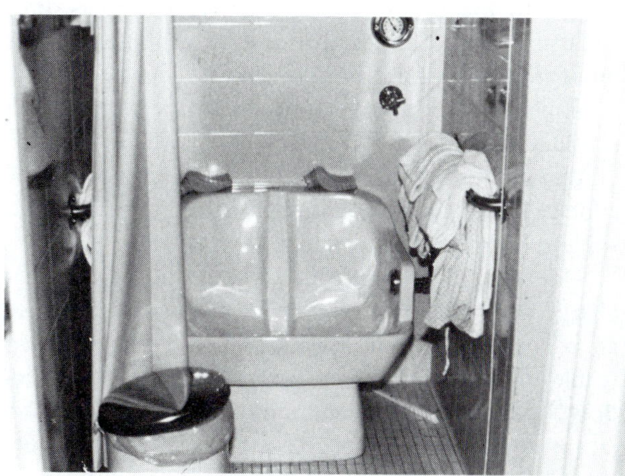

FIG. 41-7 Sitz bath. (Courtesy Marjorie Pyle, RNC, Lifecircle, Costa Mesa, Calif.)

rather than a dressing over the incision. If no dressing is used to protect the wound, care should be used so clothing does not irritate the incision.

Elimination

Recovery Stage. Diuresis and diaphoresis are common immediately after delivery. If, in addition, the woman received IV fluids, urinary output may be increased. The bladder should be supported above the symphysis pubis and palpated to check for fullness. Voiding is encouraged, because a full bladder may interfere with complete contraction of the uterus.

Many times the tissue edema from the delivery makes voiding difficult. The initial voiding should be within 4 to 6 hours after delivery. Some agencies have a policy to assess voidings three times in measurable amounts of 300 ml or more postdelivery to determine urinary elimination. Measures to stimulate voiding should be tried. If these are unsuccessful, catheterization may be required. An indwelling catheter is routinely inserted before cesarean delivery and may remain in place for 1 or 2 days after delivery.

Later Postpartum Stage. Because most women are fatigued and the perineum is still painful, the nurse must encourage the woman to void at regular intervals of every 2 to 4 hours. If the woman is voiding frequently, and in small amounts (less than 100 ml), the nurse should suspect retention with overflow. The nurse should also question the patient about any symptoms of urgency, frequency, or dysuria. If any of these are noted, they should be reported promptly. Incomplete emptying of the bladder will prevent the uterus from contracting normally; it also predisposes the patient to urinary tract infections.

It is particularly important to review proper cleansing technique after delivery. The woman should be instructed to gently cleanse and wipe from the anterior to posterior of the perineum. This method of cleaning prevents microorganisms from the rectal area being transported to the cleaner urinary or vaginal areas. Proper cleansing should be done after each urination or bowel movement. This form of perineal care can be readily accomplished using a plastic squeeze bottle with a pointed tip filled with warm (100° F [37.7° C]) water to which a certain amount of disinfectant such as Septisol has been added. The suggested formula is 1 to 3 (30 ml of Septisol and 90 ml of warm water).

Ideally, bowel elimination should occur before discharge from the hospital. Fear of discomfort because of an edematous, painful episiotomy or hemorrhoids may result in the woman's resisting the urge to defecate. Bowel peristalsis may continue to be slowed. When this fact is combined with decreased activity and loss of abdominal tone, constipation may result. To prevent this, many physicians order bulk enhancers or stool softeners. Occasionally, suppositories are administered to promote bowel evacuation. The nurse should inspect the perineum to be aware of problems and assure the patient that no harm will come from normal elimination. The importance of adequate bulk in the diet and adequate fluid intake should be stressed. Sitz baths after defecation provide cleansing and can soothe the perineum.

Cesarean birth patients, particularly those who received general anesthesia, are likely to develop problems with bowel function. The combination of general anesthesia and lost abdominal tone increases the risk of ileus, so the nurse must pay close attention to bowel function and report any abnormal observations promptly. Ambulation aids in promoting bowel function. The nurse should assist with and encourage the patient to ambulate periodically throughout the day.

Perineal pads, worn to absorb vaginal drainage, should be changed after each urination or defecation. It is essential to teach the woman about the importance of correct application and changing of the pad. Pads should be put in place from anterior to posterior and secured so as not to move about. If they are not correctly worn, contaminated areas could touch cleaner areas of the perineum and increase the risk of infection. Correct and scrupulous hand washing should be stressed to the new mother to prevent cross-contamination.

MAINTENANCE OF SAFETY

Activity/Exercise

Recovery Stage. Vital signs should be monitored every 15 minutes during the recovery stage (Table 41-2).

The mother is settled comfortably in bed. A patient who has just given birth may need to remain in bed for a period of time to allow her body systems to adjust to fluid volume changes. The nurse will decide the appropriate time for the first ambulation. The nurse takes several things into consideration when making this decision: baseline blood pressures, the amount of blood loss, type and amount of analgesic or anesthetic medications administered during labor and birth, the level of pain evident in the woman's movements, and the patient's desire to ambulate. The rapid decrease in intraabdominal pressure after birth results in a dilation of the blood vessels supplying the intestines (known as splanchnic engorgement), causing blood to pool in the viscera. This contributes to orthostatic hypotension, which tends to occur when a woman who has recently given birth stands up; consequently, she may faint or feel lightheaded.

It is imperative to keep aromatic ammonia ampules available. These can be easily broken to revive the patient who is ambulating for the first time. The nurse must caution the patient to use her call bell to summon help before she attempts to get out of bed. The nurse will

TABLE 41-2 Vital Signs and Blood Pressure After Delivery

Normal Findings	Deviations from Normal Findings and Probable Causes
Temperature	
During first 24 hours, may rise to 100.4° F (38° C) as a result of dehydrating effects of labor. After 24 hours the woman should be afebrile.	A diagnosis of puerperal sepsis is suggested if a rise in maternal temperature of 100.4° F (38° C) is noted after the first 24 hours after delivery and recurs or persists for 2 days. Other possibilities are mastitis, endometritis, urinary tract infections, and other systemic infections.
Pulse	
Bradycardia is a common finding for the first 6 to 8 days after delivery. Bradycardia is a consequence of increased cardiac output and stroke volume. The pulse returns to nonpregnant levels by 3 months after delivery. A pulse rate of between 50 and 70 beats per minute (bpm) may be considered normal.	A rapid pulse rate or one that is increasing may indicate hypovolemia as a result of hemorrhage.
Respirations	
Respirations should fall to within the woman's normal predelivery range.	Hypoventilation may follow an unusually high subarachnoid (spinal) block.
Blood pressure	
Blood pressure is altered slightly if at all. Orthostatic hypotension, as indicated by feelings of vertigo or syncope immediately after standing up, can develop in the first 48 hours as a result of the splanchnic engorgement that may occur after delivery.	A low or falling blood pressure may reflect hypovolemia secondary to hemorrhage. However, it is a late sign, and other symptoms of hemorrhage usually alert the staff. An increased reading may result from excessive use of vasopressor or oxytocic medications. Since pregnancy-induced hypertension (PIH) can persist into or occur first in the postpartum period, routine evaluation of blood pressure is needed. If a woman complains of headache, hypertension must be ruled out as a cause before analgesics are administered. If the blood pressure is elevated, the woman is confined to bed and the physician notified. (See Chapter 42.)

assess her color, pulse, and level of consciousness (LOC) in response to conversation and then assist her in ambulating to the bathroom. Once the woman has reached the bathroom, the nurse should remain outside the door and inquire as to her well-being every minute or so. If there is no answer, the nurse enters the bathroom to assess the women's condition. A wheelchair should be available in the room or just outside in the case the woman feels too weak to walk back to bed. She is encouraged to rest after the ambulation, so that she can regain her strength.

The patient who has received conduction anesthesia (epidural block) is kept in bed until she is able to fully move and feel sensation in her legs and her blood pressure and pulse are within normal limits. Ambulation can occur within the first 2 hours, depending on whether the last dose was administered intravenously or intramuscularly shortly before birth. The nurse will need to assess her ability to communicate, her LOC, and her vital signs for stability (within normal limits) before allowing the woman to get out of bed. The nurse will check that the patient is wearing slippers before she ambulates to prevent slipping or sliding.

The patient who has received analgesics needs to be watched until she is fully recovered from the medication (i.e., vital signs are stable within her normal range, and she is fully awake).

The woman's temperature may be slightly elevated if the woman is dehydrated. A temperature higher than 100.4° F (38° C) is significant and should be reported. Many women feel chilled after giving birth and appreciate an extra blanket or one that has been warmed. Sometimes offering a beverage such as hot tea or warm milk provides comfort.

Slight bradycardia, 50 to 70 beats per minute, is sometimes observed and is not considered abnormal if the other vital signs are within normal limits. Tachycardia may also occur as a response to increased blood loss or physical exertion.

Blood pressure may be slightly elevated from exertion, excitement, and possibly from the oxytocic medications. If the blood pressure is consistently elevated, or if the patient also complains of headache or visual disturbances, complications related to hypertensive disease of pregnancy could be occurring. These often persist even after delivery. The physician should be notified immediately. Decrease in blood pressure could be caused by altered intraabdominal pressure or hemorrhage. Changes should be watched closely and reported.

Little activity is observed during this stage. Most women wish to rest, hold the baby, or visit with their significant others.

Later Postpartum Stage. Vital signs normally stabilize within the first 2 hours after delivery; any abnormality persisting longer than this should be reported immediately. If vital signs have not stabilized within this time, the nurse should continue to monitor them and report significant changes.

A temperature of 100.4° F (38° C) or more on 2 successive days during the first 10 days after delivery, not including the first 24 hours after delivery, is considered indicative of puerperal infection. Any signs and symptoms of infection occurring during the postpartum stage should be monitored closely. Good aseptic technique should be used when caring for the postpartum patient. Signs and symptoms of infection should be reviewed with the new mother before discharge. The nurse should stress the importance of contacting the physician promptly if any of these should occur.

Pulse and blood pressure are also assessed. Bradycardia may persist up to 10 days after delivery. Elevated blood pressure readings or a continued decrease in blood pressure may be significant and should be reported promptly.

Most women try to get as much rest as possible while in the hospital. This is important, but activity is also needed to prevent complications such as thrombophlebitis of the lower extremities. New mothers should be encouraged to be out of bed and move about in the room. If the baby is kept in a nursery away from the mother's room, this is a good target for ambulation. If the perineum is uncomfortable, the woman should be taught to stand using the muscles of the legs while squeezing the buttocks together. This technique also helps when she attempts to sit. If unsteadiness is observed, the woman should be accompanied when she ambulates. Ambulation is very important for women who delivered by cesarean birth; they should be thought of as surgical patients and ambulated as soon as possible. It is important to remember that inactivity predisposes the woman to development of thrombophlebitis.

The flow of lochia may increase suddenly when the patient gets out of bed; secretions that pooled in the vagina drain out of the body when she stands. Once the lochia has changed to serosa or alba, excessive exercise or activity may result in the lochia's changing back to rubra. This is a good indicator to slow down and increase activity more slowly.

Postpartum exercises suitable for the new mother should begin when the physician identifies an appropriate time. These exercises are for the mother who has delivered from vaginal birth as well as the mother who had cesarean birth. The woman should begin gradually. Vigorous exercise is to be avoided until after the 6 weeks' examination, when the physician releases the new mother to do so.

The nurse may teach isometric exercises that help toning without causing undue exertion.

Rest and Sleep

Rest and sleep are important through the postpartum period. After the difficulties most women encounter at the end of pregnancy, it is a pleasure to sleep in any position desired. Many women report that the night after delivery, they get the best sleep they have experienced in weeks.

Hospital noises interrupt the sleep of many new mothers; environmental noise should be kept to a minimum to promote rest and sleep. Sleep should not be disturbed unless it is necessary to protect the patient's well-being.

If she is breastfeeding, the new mother may choose to feed the infant at intervals through the night. This results in an interrupted night's sleep. This interrupted pattern may persist for weeks until the infant is capable of sleeping for 5 or 6 hours without a feeding. The nurse should instruct the patient on the importance of naps and rest periods during the day to compensate for lost sleep. If sleep deprivation is prolonged, it may interfere with milk production and the let-down reflex.

Sexuality and Reproductive Issues

Recovery Stage. The fundus and lochia are checked every 15 minutes for the first 1 or 2 hours after delivery. The fundus should remain contracted, firm, and midline. This is critical, since severe bleeding may result if the uterus does not tightly constrict the placental site. As discussed earlier, a full bladder can displace the uterus and prevent contraction of the uterus. The patient should be encouraged to empty her bladder before the nurse checks the fundus. The uterus is palpated by placing one hand over the lower segment of the uterus near the pubic bone. The side of the other hand is used to feel the location and consistency of the uterus (Figs. 41-1 and 40-8).

If the fundus is not firm, it will be difficult to locate. An atonic uterus, one that has lost muscle tone, feels soft or "boggy." The nurse may gently massage the fundus to increase contractility. Frequently small clots will be expressed during this maneuver, and the uterus will regain good contracted tone. If this does not result in contraction, the physician may order oxytocic medication. The most commonly ordered medications are Pitocin and methylergonovine maleate (Methergine). These are usu-

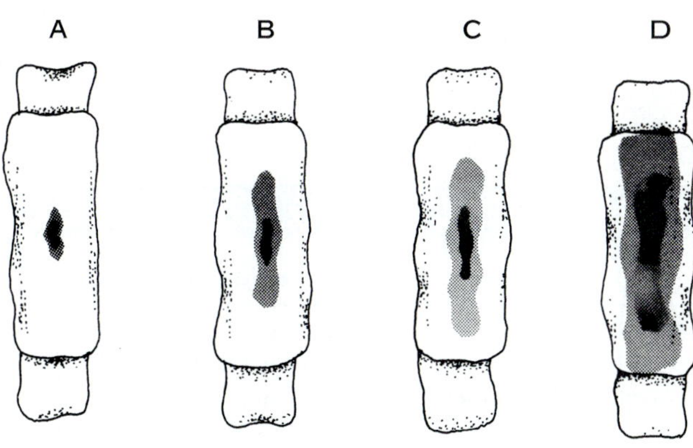

FIG. 41-8 Suggested guidelines for assessing lochia volume. The pad may also be weighed and compared with the weight of a clean, dry pad (1 g of weight equals 1 ml). **A,** Scant, less than 25 cm (1 in); **B,** light, less than 10 cm (4 in); **C,** moderate, less than 15 cm (6 in); **D,** heavy, saturated pad within 1 hour.

ally administered intravenously to obtain prompt response. Methergine may also be administered intramuscularly or orally. Vital signs must be monitored closely if these medications are being given, because they may cause alterations in blood pressure, bradycardia, nausea, headache, vertigo, and other side effects (see the medications table on p. 1280).

While the uterus is being palpated, the amount of lochia should be observed. If the uterus is contracting well, small to moderate amounts of drainage will be observed. If tone is poor, the amount of lochia will be increased. It is important to learn what is considered scant, light, moderate, and heavy amounts. This is usually determined by number of absorptive pads saturated in a period of time, such as pads per hour (Fig. 41-8). The time factor is of utmost importance when assessing lochia. One pad saturated in ½ hour is of a more serious nature than one pad saturated in 4 hours. The nurse should pay particular attention to the patient who has a small but steady trickle of lochia. Many times the blood loss in these patients is significantly greater than the loss in those who seem to bleed larger amounts (see Table 41-1). The nurse must also be sure to check under the buttocks of the patient who remains in the supine position; many times gravity causes drainage to miss the pad and pool under the patient.

Later Postpartum Stage

Daily assessments of the breasts, fundus, lochia, perineum, rectum, and the vascular condition of the legs are performed. These are often called the *postpartum checks.*

It is recommended that all new mothers wear a bra, even if the breasts are not overly large. The bra should be comfortable and fitted to provide support. Breastfeeding mothers should be encouraged to use bras large enough to accommodate the enlargement that occurs with lactation. Nonnursing mothers will need a bra that provides adequate compression to inhibit lactation without being uncomfortable.

With the bra removed, the breasts should be inspected and palpated. The nurse should observe for erythema, heat, edema, and engorgement. Filling of the breast usually occurs first near the axillary region. Engorgement is usually not observed until the third postpartum day. Because most women have been discharged from the hospital before this occurs, it is important to teach methods of obtaining relief from engorgement before sending the patient home. If the patient is breastfeeding, interventions such as manual expression of milk and application of warm, moist heat are most useful. If the patient is not breastfeeding, compression of the breasts with a firm bra, wrapped ice packs, and analgesics are most often recommended.

The nipples should be inspected for inflammation, fissures, or tenderness. The nipples generally do not cause problems for nonlactating mothers; however, if the patient is breastfeeding, the nipples should be kept soft and supple. Most physicians recommend avoiding excessive use of soap or other chemicals because they dry the skin and may be ingested by the infant. Plain water and air drying may prevent problems. Some physicians recommend allowing the nipples to dry after feeding without removal of the milk residue. If additional moisturizer is needed, small amounts of unscented lanolin are used. If the patient is allergic to wool, lanolin should be avoided, because it is obtained from the wool of sheep. Modifications in the nursing schedule and positioning of the baby may be needed if tender or cracked nipples continue to be a problem. Many references include more information on breast care.

The fundus is checked for the normal signs of involution. As in the recovery stage, the location and consistency of the uterine fundus are checked. It is normally located at the level of the umbilicus on the day of delivery. The first day postpartum it may be one fingerbreadth above or at the level of the umbilicus; after that it normally descends at the rate of one fingerbreadth per day (Fig. 41-1, *A*). When assessing the fundus of a woman delivered by cesarean birth, it is possible to carefully palpate on the sides of the incision to determine uterine tone and position.

As during the early recovery stage, the fundus should remain firmly contracted. Any atony should be handled as described. If massage does not result in adequate contraction, the physician should be notified. Lochia may begin to change within the first 2 days from the rubra to the serosa form. The amount of drainage is assessed. There is frequently less lochia observed after cesarean deliveries, because the uterine cavity is suctioned as part of the surgical procedure. The odor of the lochia should remain fleshy. If there is a fetid odor, infection may be present, and this should be reported promptly.

The perineum and rectum are inspected by having the woman assume a lateral position with the upper leg

MEDICATIONS FOR THE MOTHER AND NEWBORN

Medication	Trade Name	Action	Side Effects	Nursing Implications
Bromocriptine	Parlodel	Inhibits prolactin secretion, prevents postpartum lactation	Nausea, headache, dizziness, abdominal cramping, orthostatic hypotension	Give with meals to minimize GI effects; warn change position carefully to minimize orhtostatic hypotension; know that it is contraindicated in patients sensitive to ergot derivatives.
Codeine (with acetaminophen)	Tylenol No. 3, others	Pain reliever, narcotic	Drowsiness, sedation, nausea, vomiting, constipation, respiratory depression, urinary retention, allergic reactions, rash, urticaria	Avoid concomitant use of alcohol or other CNS depressant drugs; tell patient to avoid driving or other hazardous tasks while on this medication; warn patient that extended use may result in dependency.
Dibucaine ointment	Nupercainal	Topical anesthetic	Allergic reactions, burning, stinging	Know that it is for external use only (application to severely denuded tissue may result in systemic absorption).
Erythromycin ophthalmic ointment	Ilotycin	Ophthalmic antibiotic agent	Irritation of eye	Apply to conjunctival sacs immediately after delivery of baby.
Methylergonovine	Methergine	Oxytocic agent, stimulates uterine contraction, used to control postpartum bleeding	Headache, dizziness, nausea, chest pain, tachycardia, hypertension	Know that it is contraindicated in patients sensitive to ergot derivatives.
Oxytocin	Pitocin	Oxytocic agent, stimulates uterine contractions	Mother—nausea, vomiting, uterine spasm or rupture, water intoxication, seizures, cardiac dysrhythmias, hypotension fetus—cardiac dysrhythmias, CNS or brain damage	Carefully monitor intake and output, fetal heart tones, and length, duration, and force of uterine contractions.
Vitamin, prenatal	Materna, others	Vitamin supplement	Nausea, vomiting	Tell patient it is important that pregnant women take prenatal vitamins and not regular vitamin supplements and that prenatal vitamins contain extra folic acid, whick is needed for normal fetal growth.
Witch hazel	Tucks pads, cream	Astringent	Local irritation	Know that it is for external use only.

drawn toward the chest. The perineum should be approximated. If an episiotomy was performed, the tissue may appear edematous and erythema is common. Ecchymosis is also common, particularly after a difficult delivery. Many physicians order some form of topical anesthetic, such as Tucks or Nupercainal ointment, to soothe the perineum. This should be applied to the perineum by means of a clean, lint-free tissue, not the fingers.

If localized edema, discoloration, and intense pain are observed in the perineal area, a hematoma may be present. This hematoma is caused by excessive bleeding into the tissue. A hematoma is most common after deliveries in which forceps were used. Hematomas may be obvious, or may be concealed in the vaginal canal. If the woman complains of persistent perineal pain or fullness in the vagina, the physician should be notified. This problem requires medical attention, perhaps surgical intervention.

Although the rectum and legs are not part of the reproductive system, these areas are typically included in postpartum checks.

Hemorrhoids (varicosities of the rectum) usually disappear quickly after delivery if there is no long-standing history of this problem. Topical anesthetics are used to relieve pain if ordered by the physician. Sitz baths also provide relief and should be offered if the physician has ordered them.

The patient's legs should be examined by stretching and straightening each leg. The foot is then dorsiflexed. If pain occurs the patient is said to have a positive **Homans' sign,** which indicates inflammation of the blood vessels of the leg and possible thrombophlebitis. If Homans' sign is positive, the physician should be notified promptly.

The postpartum assessment may be completed quite readily by using eight letters that help the nurse organize a head-to-toe assessment. Those eight letters spell BUBBLE-HE, are indicated by the following:

B = *Breast:* To assess the breast, have the patient lie down and remove her bra. Palpate both breasts for engorgement or nodules. Inspect nipples for pressure, soreness, cracks, or fissures.

U = *Uterus:* The top of the uterus, the fundus, should remain very firm. If it becomes soft, the uterine muscles probably aren't contracting properly or the uterus has retained placental fragments. Both conditions predispose the patient to hemorrhage. Gently massage the uterus to help the muscles contract and expel placental fragments.

B = *Bladder:* The new mother may urinate frequently the first few days after giving birth. Be alert for signs and symptoms of infection. Also note any dysuria or urinary retention.

B = *Bowels:* Because of early discharge from the hospital many women leave without having had a bowel movement. Assess for bowel sounds, encourage activity with rest periods, and encourage adequate fluid intake.

L = *Lochia:* Lochia has a definite fleshy scent, but if it has a fetid odor, it may indicate infection. Assess carefully.

E = *Episiotomy:* Most new mothers have an episiotomy and in some cases even a laceration. Position the patient on her affected side. Instruct her to flex her top leg at the knee and draw it up toward her waist. Use a flashlight and wear gloves. Stand behind the patient and gently lift her top buttock to expose the perineum. Also assess for hemorrhoids.

H = *Homans' sign:* To assess the patient, position the legs flat on the bed while she reclines in the supine position. Dorsiflex her foot toward the ankle. Assess both extremities. If she complains of pain, Homans' sign is positive and further assessment is needed.

E = *Emotional status:* Consider the three phases most new mothers pass through:

- The first is "taking in"—the time immediately following birth (she will sleep, depend on others for nurturing and food, and relive the events surrounding the birth).
- Over the next few days she will be "taking hold." She will be preoccupied with the present, very concerned about her health and her baby's condition. She cares for herself and wants to learn to care for her newborn.
- The next phase comes later in the postpartum period, "letting go." She will reestablish relationships with other people.

Finally monitor the patient's emotional status, noting how she interacts with her family, her level of independence, sleep and rest patterns, mood swings, irritability, or crying.*

Coping and Stress Tolerance

Many new mothers feel overwhelmed by the responsibility of motherhood. New mothers feel intimidated by the nurses' capability and skill with the newborn. They often feel inept and may not wish to ask questions that might be viewed as unintelligent. Establishing a rapport is essential; listening for and anticipating fears and anxieties are important nursing measures. False reassurances are not helpful; thorough teaching and encouragement are far more beneficial.

Often women experience a period of depression after delivery that is triggered by rapid hormonal shifts. This so-called postpartum depression may be mild or rather severe. It often appears between 2 and 7 days postpartum. Preparing the woman for the possibility of this and planning a course of action if it does occur are nursing responsibilities.

Signs of Potential Problems

No assessment of psychosocial needs is complete without assessing for signs of potential problems. Not all po-

*Adapted from Fergusen H: Planning letter perfect postpartum care, *Nurs 87,* May 1987, pp 50-51.

Box 41-3
SIGNS OF POTENTIAL PROBLEMS: PSYCHOSOCIAL NEEDS

- Inability or refusal to discuss labor and birth experience
- Refusal to interact with or care for baby (e.g., does not name baby, does not want to hold or feed baby)
- Refusal to attend infant care (including breastfeeding) classes
- Refusal to discuss contraception
- Refers to self as ugly and useless
- Excessive preoccupation with self (body image)
- Marked depression
- Lack of support system

tential psychosocial problems are easily identified. However, there are some signs that may indicate a need for further evaluation by a care giver skilled in that area. Nor does the presence of one or more of these signs provide absolute proof that a problem actually exists. Box 41-3 presents some signs that may indicate a need for further assessment.

Role and Relationship

Roles and relationships are affected by the addition of a new family member. These changes are most obvious when the first child is born, but adjustments take place any time an additional child joins a family. Time, money, and emotional resources must be divided to include the new member.

The mother faces the greatest number of changes. In our society the mother still fills the role of primary caregiver to the child. The total responsibility of this role 24 hours a day, 7 days a week, is overwhelming to many women. Today, because many women are independent wage earners, the loss of freedom to come and go as they please is also difficult adjustment. Even if the woman has made plans to return to work and makes arrangements for excellent child care, role conflict can lead to guilt and confusion. The nurse should be sensitive to the mother's concerns.

The responsibilities of fatherhood often become a reality when the father actually sees his child. The realization that a totally dependent individual needs him can be frightening to many men. The financial concerns of feeding, clothing, and sheltering his family take on new significance.

A two-income family may have only his wages, at least temporarily. Even if the mother returns to work, there are new expenses for child care. The wife is now also a mother, and many times the needs of the child will supersede the husband's needs or wishes. Freedom and spontaneity give way to a life circumscribed by feeding schedules, diaper bags, and baby-sitters.

Because many men have little knowledge or experience in caring for infants, simple things, such as feeding, changing diapers, or even carrying a baby, may be intimidating. The nurse can help alleviate these fears by including the father in teaching whenever possible and by allowing him to verbalize his fears and concerns.

Additional role adjustments relate to friends and the extended family. Friendships and socialization may require adjustment. Parents now become grandparents and in-laws share grandchildren. These are all dynamic situations, and each family will make a variety of accommodations in the process of incorporating their new roles.

Self-Perception

It is common for the new mother to wish to discuss her perception of the labor and delivery. Time should be allowed for her to verbalize and work through her experiences. The reality may have differed greatly from her expectations, and explanations are needed to clarify things in her mind. The new mother may spend considerable time with friends or in telephone conversation relating her experiences through labor and delivery.

It is not uncommon for the new mother to be rather passive for the first day or two. This is what is often called the "taking in" stage. During this time the mother needs supportive care. Her primary focus may be on herself and on personal needs such as sleep, food, and attention. She may defer to the nurses and let others provide total care for the baby. This is followed by what is referred to as the "taking hold" stage. In this phase the woman is ready to assume greater authority and responsibility for herself and her baby.

Mood swings are common early in the postpartum period, related to recent stresses, fatigue, and rapid hormonal changes. This should be explained to the new mother so she does not become unduly concerned.

It is common for new mothers, particularly primiparas, to expect that they will regain their prepregnancy figure quickly after delivery. Many bring clothes that they hoped to wear home, only to be sadly disappointed. The nurse should be supportive and explain that time is required for the body to regain the prepregnancy tone and shape.

Cognitive and Perceptual Issues

Control of the discomforts during the postpartum period is important. If the woman is to resume a normal level of activity and get adequate rest, pain cannot be allowed to interfere.

The most common discomforts experienced are perineal pain from the episiotomy and the so-called *afterbirth pains.* Afterbirth pains are cramping sensations, resulting from the contraction of the uterus. Any new mother may experience afterbirth pains, but they are more common and may be more severe in multiparas.

Most physicians prescribe analgesics for these discomforts. Acetaminophen is commonly used, with or without codeine. Codeine is generally effective but is a controlled substance and also has side effects, such as constipation and vertigo, that may be undesirable in the postpartum patient. Salicylates, such as aspirin, are usually avoided, because they may interfere with clotting mechanisms. Recently ibuprofen (Motrin) has been popular. Ibuprofen is an analgesic, antiinflammatory, and prostaglandin inhibitor. It is often effective in reducing the severity of the cramping without altering the contraction of the uterine muscle. A cautionary note in using ibuprofen: ibuprofen is to be used with caution for persons with kidney or heart disease, or those taking diuretics.

Another major challenge of the postpartum period involves learning. The new mother needs to know how to care for herself and how to care for the newborn. This can be overwhelming for the first-time mother. The nurse has limited time to teach all the necessary information. Most hospitals have teaching lists and printed handouts or booklets that include all of the key areas (Box 41-4 on p. 1284). To prevent the woman from becoming overwhelmed, teaching should be paced throughout the hospital stay, not left until discharge. The nurse should also document newborn teaching (Box 41-5 on p. 1285-1286).

Values and Beliefs

Culture may prescribe activities or rituals for both mother and baby; these may include specific behaviors related to diet, hygiene, or activity. Each culture is unique as to what behaviors should occur or be avoided. Many books describe a variety of cultural practices related to childbearing. It is wise to have the patient verbalize her unique cultural practices; the nurse should listen nonjudgmentally. If any of the practices should be harmful to either mother or baby, it is important to explain the reasons the behavior should not be practiced. The ideal is finding a way to blend the cultural practice with safe health teaching.

The behavior patterns for many cultures include a period of seclusion for new mothers that lasts 7 to 40 days, with a minimum of activity allowed. These practices are based on two beliefs: that delivery has upset the balance of mother's body and that the mother, infant, and those caring for them are in a pollution state.

NORMAL NEWBORN

Immediate Assessment

In addition to the Apgar scoring, which was done immediately after the delivery, the nurse performs other assessments to establish the gestational age of the newborn. Gestational age is the actual number of weeks since conception. This is important, because many problems observed in newborns are age related. Since many women are unsure of the exact date of conception, calendar-based gestational age is unreliable. Physical and neurological assessment based on established criteria is more reliable. Physical characteristics are evaluated within the first few hours of life. Neurological assessment is done 24 hours later, after the nervous system has had the opportunity to stabilize from the trauma of delivery.

Characteristics

Body Size and Shape. The head of the newborn is disproportionately large for its body. The abdomen is prominent, with a smaller chest and narrow hips. The body is usually held in a moderately flexed position. There is a wide variation of size in normal newborns. The average newborn weighs 3400 g (7 lb 8 oz) and is approximately 50 cm (20 inches) in length. Charts are available for plotting height and weight. The head circumference averages 33 to 33.5 cm (13 to 14 inches) and is generally about 2 cm (1 inch) larger than that of the chest, which averages 30 to 33 cm (12 to 13 inches).

Skin. The skin of the infant can exhibit a wide range of rashes and color changes. Most are not significant and disappear within a few days. However, parents may be concerned by these until the changes are explained.

Skin color. The skin color is normally pink to slightly reddish in appearance. The ruddiness results from normally elevated red blood cell concentration. The hands and feet may appear slightly blue; this is called **acrocyanosis** and is caused by poor peripheral circulation. Acrocyanosis can persist for 7 to 10 days. It is most commonly observed when the infant becomes cold. Mottling, a lacy pattern with dilated vessels on pale skin, is also commonly seen. Another normal variation is called the **harlequin sign;** half of the newborn's body appears deep red and the other side of the body appears pale as a result of vasomotor disturbance, with some vessels constricting while others dilate.

When infant is placed on one side, the dependent half is noticeably pinker than the superior half. This may last for up to 20 minutes, and while disturbing to view, it is not harmful.

Jaundice, a yellow discoloration caused by deposits of bile pigments, also known as *icterus neonatarum,* is first detected over bony prominences on the face and on the mucous membranes. This is abnormal during the first 24 hours of life. After 24 hours it is not necessarily abnormal. The hemoglobin and hematocrit levels of the newborn are frequently elevated; hemoglobin may range from 14 to 24 g/dl and hematocrit from 44% to 64%. After 24 hours **physiological jaundice** (jaundice occur-

Box 41-4

POSTPARTUM TEACHING SUMMARY

MATERNAL POSTPARTUM DISMISSAL

1. *Fundus* (height, massage)
   - 1 fingerbreadth down a day
   - Back into pelvis in 10 days
   - Feels firm like a softball
   - Report bogginess to primary care practitioner immediately
   - May have cramping with nursing
2. *Lochia* (amount, changes, warning signs)
   - First 3 days, will be dark red color, like menstrual flow; 2-3 days after this, will be pinkish brown in color
   - Moderate flow: 4-8 lightly saturated pads a day
   - Flow will continue for 3-4 weeks
   - The last couple of weeks will be a yellowish color with a musty, stale odor
   - Report any foul-smelling or bright red discharge, or large clots
   - If overactive, flow may increase; rest. If flow does not subside, notify primary care practitioner
3. *Perineum* (episiotomy care, cleansing, healing, douching, tampons)
   - Sitz baths 2-3 times daily with vaginal delivery
   - Cleanse from front to back
   - Use perineal spray H_2O bottle after voiding
   - Change pad frequently; after each voiding and when soiled
   - Do not douche or use tampons until after first office visit when primary care practitioner says it is okay
   - Continue using Tucks for discomfort and to aid in healing
   - Episiotomy will heal in approximately 3 weeks (when the lochia has stopped)
4. *Breasts*
   A. Breastfeeding (nipple care, engorgement, feeding techniques, breast pump)
      - Air dry; use proper breaking technique; Massé cream if ordered; wear a good supportive bra
      - Can become pregnant while nursing; use a contraceptive
      - Engorgement—apply heat, warm shower; may pump to enable baby to latch on
      - Feeding techniques—demonstrate proper use; advise where to purchase materials; demonstrate manual expression; expressed milk may be frozen in plastic bottles for bags or up to 6 months
      - May take a mild analgesic 1 hour before nursing

   B. Dry Breasts (engorgement, fluid intake)
      - Wear supportive, well-fitting bra
      - Continue to take Parlodel if ordered
      - Avoid breast stimulation (warm showers)
      - Apply ice bags for 20 minutes four times a day
      - It takes about 5 days for lactation to be suppressed
      - Don't drink excessive amounts of fluids (normal: six to eight 8-oz glasses)
5. *Nutrition* (nursing, dieting)
   - Continue prenatal vitamins until gone
   - Nursing: need 500 kcal over prepregnant diet; need increased protein; 400 mg calcium each day; 8-10 glasses of fluid each day. Avoid onions, cabbage, chocolate, spices, and foods that may distress infant. No dieting during breast feeding
6. *Sexuality* (sexual activity)
   - 45% of nonnursing mothers resume menses by sixth week
   - Breastfeeding does not provide protection against pregnancy
   - Avoid sexual activity until after first postbirth office visit and primary care practitioner advises
   - If episiotomy is not healed and sexual activity is resumed, there is increased discomfort and chance of infection
7. *Exercise* (when, how much)
   - Increased lochia or pain means patient needs to reevaluate activity
   - Don't resume strenuous exercises until primary care practitioner advises
   - Gradually increase activity
8. *Emotions* (bonding, "baby blues")
   - Parent-child attachment—bonding: schedule time to enjoy baby. Use eye contact, cuddling and caressing. Enjoy infant feedings

   Postpartum blues:
   - May be tearful or anorexic and have difficulty sleeping
   - Hormonal factors and fatigue are often responsible
   - Notify primary care practitioner if prolonged, increased, or unmanageable
9. *Cesarean Birth* (incision, activity)
   - Notify primary care practitioner of any redness, drainage, separation of incision, temperature above 101° F (38.3° C)
   - Associated with anything heavier than baby, gradually increase activity
   - Take pain meds as ordered and needed
10. *Report to Primary Care Giver* (fever, chills, heavy flow, foul odor of vaginal flow)
    - Temperature above 101° F (38.3° C)
    - Chills
    - Change in lochia—foul smell, return to bright red, excessive amount
    - Calf pain, tenderness, or swelling
    - Evidence of mastitis: breast tenderness, cracking, redness, or a feeling of discomfort or uneasiness
    - Urinary urgency, burning, or frequency
    - Severe or incapacitating depression
11. *Safety* (car seat safety film, car seat demonstration)
    - Review infant safety from baby discharge sheet
    - Review car seat safety film
    - Volunteers have car seats to rent
    - Demonstrate proper use of car seat

The nurse should document postpartum teaching.

Box 41-5

NEWBORN TEACHING SUMMARY

1. Security
   - Know care giver. Check references. Ask others who are trusted.
   - Baby should not be left alone on flat surface because he could roll over and off of the surface.
   - Do not lay baby on abdomen; place on the side or back to prevent suffocation.
   - Car seat safety/law:
     —Use until age 4 years or 40 pounds.
     —Infant in car seat should be secured in back seat facing the rear of the car.
     —This is the law in 33 states; if you are stopped, you could be fined.
2. Bath Demonstration/Normal Skin Conditions
   - Skin should be soft, pink, and dry.
   - Clean perineum from front to back to prevent urinary tract infections.
   - Use hypoallergenic soap. Most babies need bathing only every other day.
   - Keep diaper area as clean as possible. (Use little or no powder.)
   - Keep head clean, rinsing well after each shampoo to prevent cradle cap.
3. Umbilical Cord Care
   - Use alcohol on cord stump. (Be careful to prevent alcohol from dripping down to perineal area.)
   - Keep area dry; fold diaper down with plastic side on outside to prevent moisture retention.
     —Sponge bathe for 7 to 10 days until umbilical cord comes off. (Do not soak in bath water.)
   - Report any redness, drainage, or foul odor coming from umbilical area.
4. Circumcision Care
   - If a Gamco Clamp was used, apply petroleum jelly-covered gauze to penis after every diaper change. Keep area clean to prevent infection; cleanse penis carefully with warm water at least every 4 hours.
   - If a Plastibell is used, the plastic rim remains in place for about a week while healing takes place, after which the Plastibell will fall off.
   - Petroleum gauze is not necessary.
   - Do not allow pressure on circumcised area.
   - Do not be alarmed when a yellowish crust forms; this is part of the normal healing process. Do not attempt to remove this crust; it will only last 2 to 3 days. Fanfold the diaper so that it does not press on the area.
5. Eye Care
   - Wash with water from inner to outer corner with a different area of the wash cloth for each eye.
   - Note that a special treatment was administered to baby's eyes on delivery. This may cause some swelling and redness. Do not be alarmed; this is normal.
6. Diaper Area Care
   - Change diaper as soon as possible.
     —Wash from front to back, especially on girls, to prevent urinary tract infection.
   - Cleanse with warm water and mild soap; dry well
   - If rash persists, call the physician.
     —Use very little powder. If possible, have diaper area open to the air.
7. Feeding Method
   - Breast
   - Position: entire body of infant should face the breast.
     —Direct the nipple into infant's mouth with as much of the areola tissue into the baby's mouth and over the tongue.
     —Lightly brush the infant's lips with the nipple to start the rooting reflex.
     Feed baby before baby gets frantic and very hungry.
     —Alternate breasts with each feeding.
     —Gently hold breast away from baby's nostrils; babies are nose breathers.
     —To break suction, place finger under nipple; do not pull breast away from baby.
   - Burping baby:
     —Burp between breasts, over the shoulder, sitting up supported by your hands, or lying across your lap.
   - Length of time to nurse:
     —Feed for 10 to 15 minutes from each breast.
     —Mothers who have cesarean births need to support infant so that he does not rest on the abdomen for long periods.
     —It is important to empty both breasts because an empty breast signals the woman's body to produce more milk.
   - Supplement: you may pump your breast while away from baby; keep breast milk cold during transport.
     —Breast milk can be safely stored in a refrigerator for 24 to 48 hours.
     —If breast milk will not be used within 48 hours, it should be frozen immediately after being expressed. Breast milk may be frozen for 2 weeks. To thaw, gently shake container under warm tap water. Thawed breast milk should be used immediately. It should not be refrozen. Do not use a microwave to thaw or heat breast milk. Place breast milk in container of warm water.
     —After the milk supply is established, an occasional bottle will not affect lactation or breast feeding.
   - Stooling pattern: stools of breast-fed babies are loose. Some infants have a stool with each feeding.
   - Bottle
   - Positions:
     —The bottle should never be propped.
     —The bottle should be held so that fluids fill the nipple and none of the air in the bottle is allowed to enter the nipple.
     —Avoid overfeeding; be alert to infant cues that enough formula has been taken (e.g., falls to sleep, turns head to side, or ceases to suck).
   - Burping baby:
     —Burp baby every ½ to 1 oz of milk.
     —Position baby over the shoulder, sitting up supported by your hands, or lying across your lap.
   - Preparation of bottles:
     —Formula may be purchased in powder ready-to-use, or liquid form to be mixed with water.

The nurse should document newborn teaching.

Continued.

Box 41-5 NEWBORN TEACHING SUMMARY—cont'd

—Formulas should be prepared with scrupulous cleanliness unless home conditions or the water supply is unsafe (such as from a private well); then water should be boiled 15 minutes.
—Many helpful pamphlets on formula preparations are available.
—Formula may be given at room temperature; test formula temperature on inner wrist or back of hand.

- Storing formula:
  —Opened container of ready-to-feed or concentrated formula should be discarded after 24 hours; date the opened container.

8. Clothing
   - Dress infant for the season.
   - Dress infant in soft, comfortable clothing.
   - Dress infant as you are dressed.
9. Vaginal and Breast Secretions
   - As the maternal hormones clear the infant's bloodstream, the infant may have a mucuslike, bloody vaginal discharge.
   - Both girl and boy babies may have a swelling of the breast tissue, and sometimes a thin discharge may be seen; this will subside as the mother's hormones are eliminated from infant's body.
10. When to Call Physician
    - If baby develops sudden fever, rash, excessive vomiting, diarrhea, distended abdomen, or bleeding from circumcision, call the physician.
11. Bulb Syringe
    - Correct use:
      —Squeeze out air to establish suction by compressing bulb and holding it in. Gently insert tip of syringe into the side of infant's mouth and release; then suction the nares.
      Clean well after each use.
12. Infant CPR
    - Film: be sure to see film before dismissal.
    - Teaching:
      —Give fingertip compressions (5 to 1).
      —Give puffs for breaths (1 to 5).
      —Cover baby's nose with cheek as you cover mouth.
      —Avoid stretching back too far in the head-chin lift.
13. PKU, Biotenidase, and thyroid testing should be performed on all newborns. Undetected abnormalities could lead to brain damage or death. With early detection and proper treatment, these are preventable.
14. Pamphlet Information
    - Be encouraged to keep, read, and refer to pamphlets if you have any questions. The number of the formula company is on the pamphlet.
15. Equipment Use and Medication Instruction
    - Use medication prescribed only by a physician. (Do not use nose drops because aspiration may result in lung complications.)
    - Know about the correct use of a breast pump and bulb syringe.

ring 48 hours or later after birth, gradually disappearing by the seventh to tenth day, and caused by the normal reduction in the number of red blood cells) may appear, because the excessive levels of hemoglobins are no longer required for oxygen transport. When jaundice is observed, further assessment is required to determine the cause. The physician may order laboratory and diagnostic tests to determine the nature of the problem and begin treatment to prevent complications. Causes of jaundice will be discussed further in Chapter 42.

Skin appearance. At birth the skin is covered with a yellowish-white cream cheese–like substance called **vernix caseosa.** This substance protects the infant's skin from the amniotic fluid. When the vernix caseosa is removed, the skin may appear dry and may crack, flake, and peel. A layer of soft hair called **lanugo** (downy, fine hair characteristic of the fetus, between 20 weeks' gestation and birth; lanugo is most noticeable over the shoulders, forehead, and cheeks but it is found on nearly all parts of the body except the palms of the hands and soles of the feet and the scalp) is commonly noted.

Good turgor and tissue elasticity are normally observed. Desquamation of the skin of the term infant does not occur until a few days following birth. Its presence at birth is an indication of postmaturity.

A variety of observations may be made when assessing the skin. The most commonly observed are noted in Box 41-6.

Head. The **fontanelles** (broad area or soft spot consisting of a strong band of connective tissue contiguous [touching] with cranial bones and located at the junction of the bones) should be palpable. The *anterior fontanelle* is normally large and diamond shaped and closes at approximately 18 months of age. The posterior fontanelle is smaller and triangular in shape and normally closes at 2 months of age. The sagittal suture may be felt by running the fingers between the two fontanelles.

The head of the newborn may also manifest many variations. Most of these are a result of the birth process and disappear without treatment shortly after the delivery:

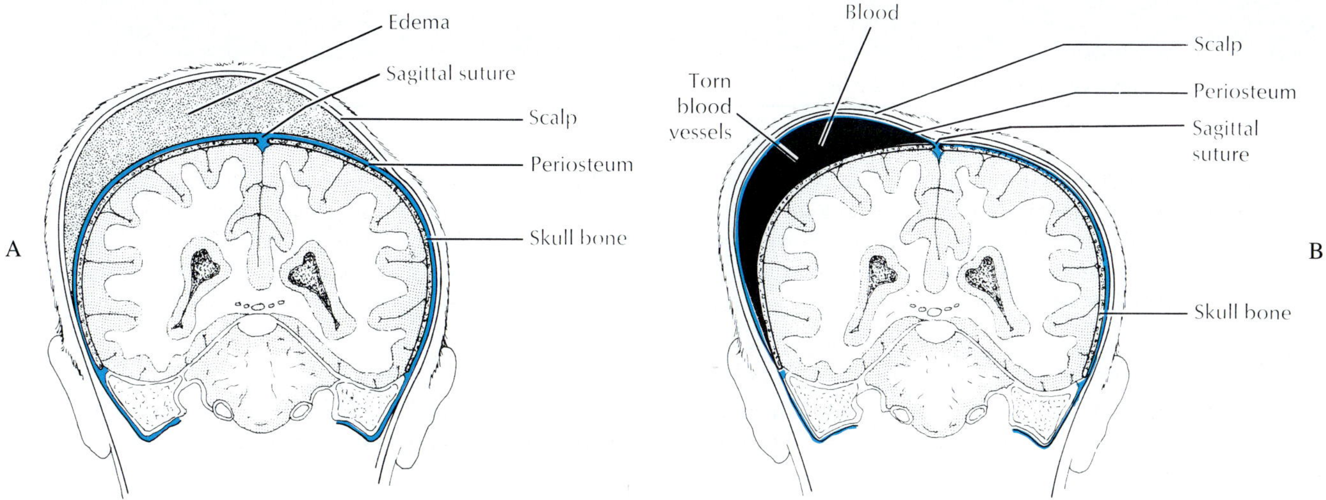

FIG. 41-9 Differences between caput succedaneum and cephalhematoma. **A,** Caput succedaneum: edema of scalp noted at birth; crosses suture line. **B,** Cephalhematoma: bleeding between periosteum and skull bone appearing within first 2 days; does not cross suture lines.

1. *Molding* is overlapping of the bones of the skull. The head may appear elongated and misshapen; this is a result of compression during delivery and normally disappears within a day or two.
2. *Caput succedaneum* is commonly seen with molding. It is the result of edema in the soft tissue of the scalp. The tissue feels spongy and may be felt over suture lines. This also disappears without treatment (Fig. 41-9 *A*).
3. *Cephalhematoma* is caused by bleeding within the periosteum of a cranial bone. It is confined to a particular bone and does not cross suture lines. This is usually a result of difficult labor. Cephalhematomas may not be apparent immediately after delivery; they generally appear 1 to 2 days after birth. These normally absorb without treatment. Large hematomas may lead to anemia and jaundice, which require medical intervention (see Fig. 41-9, *B*).

Face. The newborn's chin is receding and the nose relatively flat. Fat pads make the cheeks appear full and round. Movements of the face should be symmetrical. The mouth should open freely, and the oral cavity should be intact with a closed palate. Small white nodules called *Epstein's pearls* may be observed on the hard palate. These are a result of epithelial cells and will disappear spontaneously within a few weeks. Occasionally an infant is born with teeth. This is rare but should be watched closely, because they may become loose and be aspirated. The oral cavity should be clean and free from lesions. A fungal infection may be acquired during passage through the birth canal if the mother is infected with *Candida albicans.* This results in thrush, a white,

Box 41-6

COMMON SKIN OBSERVATIONS IN THE NEWBORN

- *Milia* are small white spots usually seen in the nose and chin. They are a result of occluded sebaceous glands and disappear spontaneously within a few weeks.
- Newborn rash, technically called *erythema toxicum neonatorum,* is an elevated, hivelike rash that may result in small white vesicles. It is not contagious, and like milia disappears without treatment.
- *Telangiectatic nevi,* "stork-bites," are flat, pink or red marks often seen on the eyelids, nose, or nape of the neck. These are dilated capillaries that become more vivid when the infant cries. They are not significant to the health of the infant and disappear at 1 to 2 years of age.
- *Mongolian spots* are areas of increased pigmentation. The lumbar dorsal area is the most common location. The area may appear bluish-black. These are most often seen in darker-skinned races.
- *Nevus flammeus,* "port-wine stain," is a reddish-purple discoloration often seen on the face. This is a capillary angioma below the epidermis. Unfortunately, these will not disappear spontaneously. Recently medical techniques have been developed that reduce or remove port-wine birthmarks.
- "Strawberry birthmarks," *nevus vasculosus,* are capillary hemangiomas. These may continue to increase in size for several months. They normally then begin to shrink spontaneously and usually disappear early in childhood.

TABLE 41-3 Assessment of Reflexes in the Normal Newborn

Expected Behavioral Response	Comments
Moro (startle)	
Sudden jarring or change in equilibrium causes extension and abduction of extremities and fanning of fingers, with index finger and thumb forming a C shape, followed by flexion and adduction of extremities; legs may weakly flex; infant may cry (see Fig. 41-10)	Elicit by holding the infant above the examining table in a supine position with one hand beneath the sacrum and the other supporting the upper back and head; the infant's head is then suddenly allowed to fall about 30 degrees. Disappears after 3-4 months, usually strongest during first 2 months.
Tonic neck	
When infant's head is quickly turned to one side, arm and leg will extend on that side, and opposite arm and leg will flex; posture resembles a fencing position (Fig. 41-11).	Disappears by 3-4 months of age, to be replaced by symmetrical positioning of both sides of body.
Crawling	
When placed on abdomen, infant will make crawling movements with the arms and legs (Fig. 41-12).	Disappears at about 6 weeks of age.
Dance or step	
If infant is held so that sole of foot touches a hard surface, there will be a reciprocal flexion and extension of the leg, simulating walking (Fig. 41-13).	Disappears after 3-4 weeks, to be replaced by deliberate movement.

patchy coating of the mucous membranes that cannot be wiped off. Treatment with antifungal medications such as nystatin or gentian violet is required.

Eyes. The eyelids may appear edematous because of prophylactic antibiotic medication that was applied to the eyes after birth to prevent *ophthalmia neonatorum* (infection in the neonate's eyes, usually resulting from gonorrheal or other infection contracted when the fetus passes through the birth canal [vagina]). The eyes appear wide-set. Strabismus (crossed eyes) and nystagmus (abnormal motion of the eyes) are commonly seen as a result of the newborn's immature nervous system. Most Caucasian infants have slate-gray to blue irises at birth; in darker-skinned races the irises may appear darker. The newborn does not produce tears, because the lacrimal structures have not fully matured. Vision has been found to be more acute than previously believed. Newborns are nearsighted and can see objects best at 8 to 10 inches; most prefer simple patterns in black and white and human faces. It is important that the parents know this, because eye contact with the baby is an important part of bonding.

Ears. The ears are normally positioned with the upper insertion of the pinna located even with the outer canthus of the eye. Low-set ears may indicate a chromosomal disorder. High-pitched sounds and the mother's voice generate the greatest attention. It is believed that the fetus becomes familiar with the mother's voice while still in utero.

Reflexes. A wide variety of reflexes are seen in the normal newborn. Some are protective reflexes, such as the rooting, sucking, gag, swallow, and sneeze reflex. Other reflexes such as the Babinski, Moro, tonic neck, and stepping are related to the immature nature of the newborn's nervous system. Many are present for a limited time and then disappear. Table 41-3 identifies the nature and significance of the most commonly observed reflexes.

Genitals. The genitals in female newborns may be edematous. Discharge of blood-tinged mucus from the vagina, called **pseudomenstruation,** may occur in response to maternal hormones. The breasts may be enlarged in either sex. This is called **gynecomastia** and is also a result of maternal hormones. The labia majora cover the minora in term infants. The scrotum in the male may be enlarged and edematous, indicating a hydrocele. The testicles are normally descended in term infants; in preterm infants they may not be descended **(cryptorchidism).** The penis should be inspected for position of the urethral meatus. Abnormal placement may result in problems with voiding. Circumcision is not normally done if there is any malplacement, since the foreskin may be used as part of the surgical correction.

Spine. The spine should be straight without curves. The normal cervical and lumbar curves will develop once the infant begins to stand. The spine should also be examined for dimples, tufts of hair, and masses that may indicate abnormalities of spinal column development.

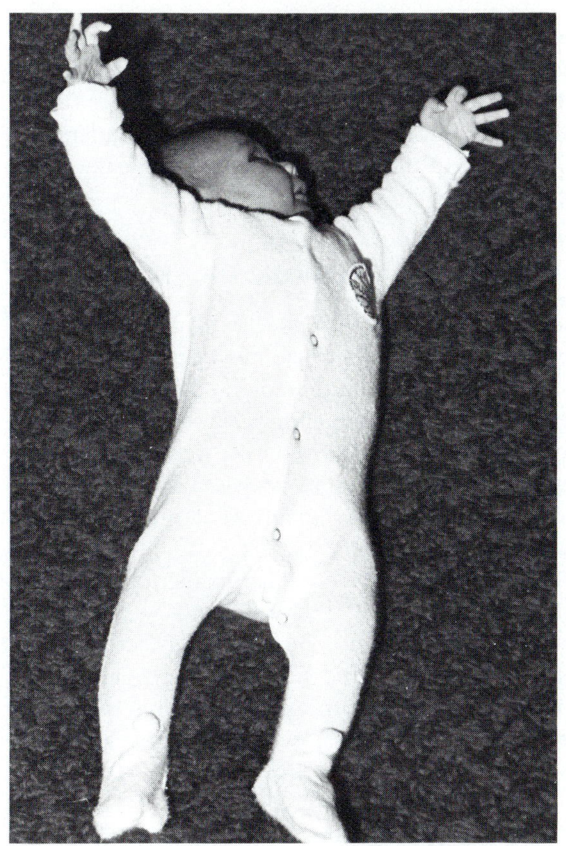

FIG. 41-10 Moro reflex (startle reflex).

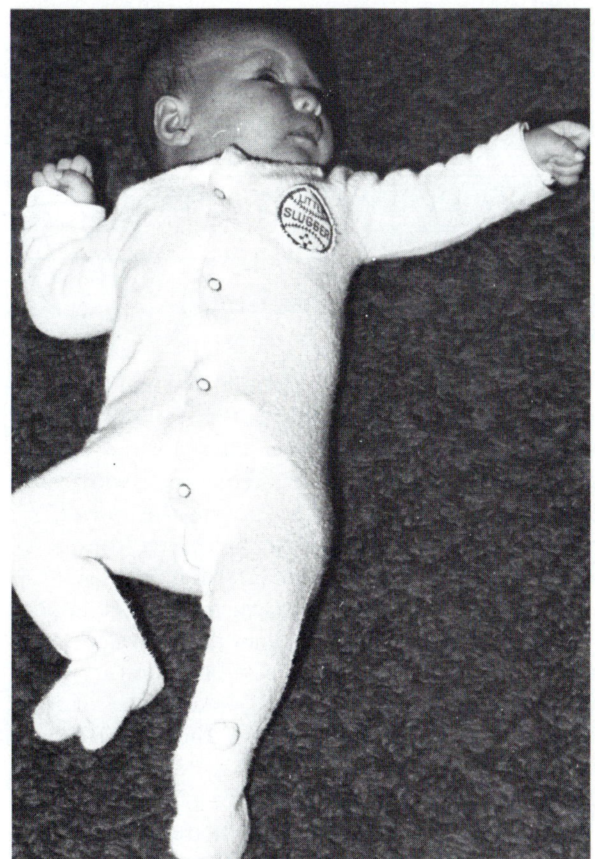

FIG. 41-11 Tonic neck reflex.

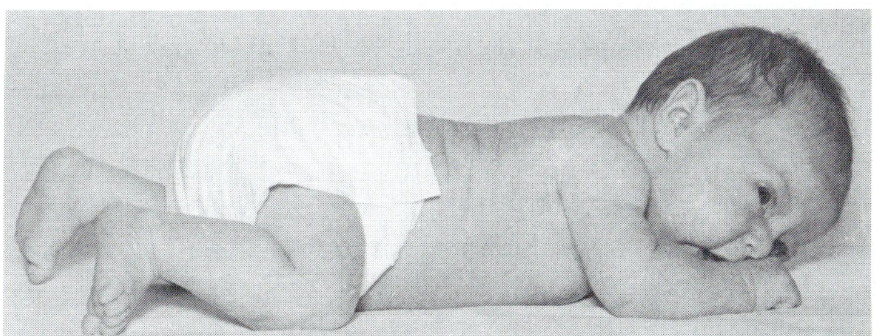

FIG. 41-12 Crawl reflex.

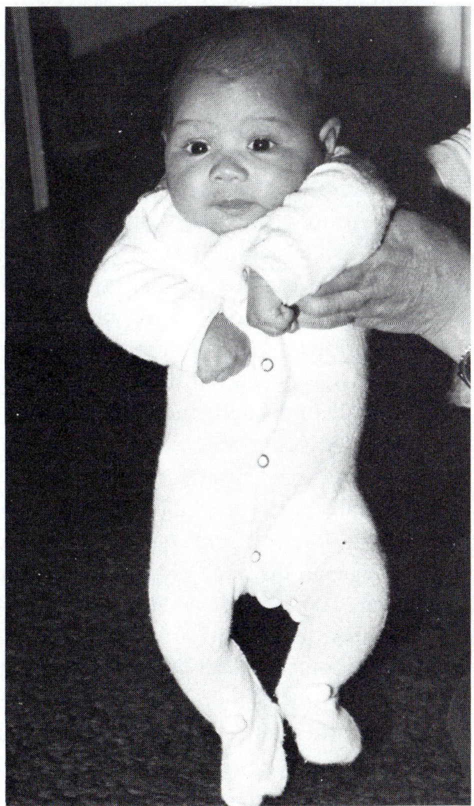

FIG. 41-13 Dance reflex.

Extremities. The arms and hands are generally flexed against the body. Both arms should move evenly. Trauma during delivery may result in fracture of the clavicle or in brachial palsy. Both hands should be free from webbing (**syndactyly;** malformation of digits, commonly seen as fusion of two or more toes to from one structure) or extra digits (**polydactyly;** excessive number of digits [fingers or toes]). A single crease in the palm of the hand, a simian line, may indicate chromosomal disorders such as Down syndrome (mongolism or trisomy 21 [three of chromosome number 21]). Nails often extend beyond the fingertips. Legs should be equal in length. If one leg appears longer or if the gluteal or popliteal folds are asymmetrical, a congenital hip dysplasia may be suspected. The hips should move freely. The feet may appear to be turned abnormally; this is often the result of the newborn's position in utero.

NURSING ASSESSMENT AND INTERVENTIONS

Health Management and Health Perception

Before giving the newborn to the mother, identification bracelets should be checked to prevent the possibility of giving the baby to the wrong mother.

The mother should be instructed about handwashing when caring for the baby to prevent the spread of microorganisms; this is important when going from performing personal hygiene to caring for the infant.

The new mother should be instructed in safety practices to reduce the likelihood of injury to the infant. Positions that provide head support while carrying and burping should be demonstrated. The large size of the head requires care when handling the infant. The mother should also be taught never to leave the baby unattended in an unsafe location, such as on a table or bed. The environment should be kept free of hazards, such as pins or other sharp objects. Bathing techniques and temperature taking should be demonstrated. The mother should be taught proper positioning of the infant. It is recommended that an infant be placed on its side after feeding to reduce the possibility of aspiration if the baby regurgitates. Bottles should never be propped for feeding, because this may lead to choking or aspiration. The use of infant car seats is now mandatory in most states.

State laws will require that certain diagnostic tests be performed on the newborn. The nurse must know the laws of the particular state. These tests are done to detect conditions that result in serious complications, such as neurological disorders and cognitive impairment. If any of these metabolic conditions are detected early in life and if proper treatment is started promptly, many of the complications may be eliminated or reduced. Most of the diseases tested for involve inborn errors of metabolism in which the newborn is unable to metabolize various nutrients. Some of the more common tests include those done to detect phenylketonuria (PKU), maple sugar urine disease (MSUD), galactosemia, and hypothyroidism. These tests involve either blood or urine samples. For most test results to be meaningful, the newborn must have consumed an adequate amount of either human milk or cow's milk formula. Because of early discharge of mothers and newborns this may not occur before the newborn goes home. If the tests are to be performed before the neonate is discharged from the hospital, completion of the necessary blood work should be verified and noted on the chart before the newborn is allowed to leave. If the tests are to be done later, usually at 2 to 5 days of age, the newborn will have to return to the hospital or physician's office. In these situations the nurse must be sure that the parents understand the importance of the tests and know specifically when the newborn is to be tested.

Nutritional and Metabolic Issues

Newborns have low prothrombin levels at birth and are at risk for hemorrhage. Because newborns are not able to synthesize vitamin K in the colon until they have adequate intestinal flora, a vitamin K (Aquamephyton) injection is routinely administered to newborns. Injections are best administered in the vastus lateralis muscle as this muscle is more developed than other muscles of the newborn's structure.

Weight is monitored daily. It is considered normal for a newborn to lose up to 10% of its body weight in the first week of life, from a combination of factors. More weight is lost through the passing of meconium and urine than is taken in by the newborn. This is particularly true in breastfed babies. Most newborns regain their birth weight within the first week.

Nutritional Requirements. The normal newborn requires approximately 120 calories per kilogram of body weight each day. This includes proteins, carbohydrates, fats, vitamins, and minerals. Breast milk and prepared formulas are balanced to meet the needs of the newborn. Since newborns cannot concentrate urine efficiently, fluid intake needs are high; 140 to 160 ml/kg/day is necessary (1 kg = 2.2 lb).

With the improved formulas available today, the fluid and nutritional needs of infants can be met by either breast feeding or bottle-feeding. The mother can choose which method she prefers. The nurse should provide support and teaching appropriate to the parent's chosen method.

Breast milk is produced in three stages. *Colostrum,* the first substance produced, is creamy and yellow-white in appearance. It contains more protein, minerals, and fat-soluble vitamins than mature breast milk. It also contains high levels of immunoglobulins, which may transfer some immunity to the newborn. Production of colostrum usually begins in the last trimester of pregnancy and continues for 2 to 4 days after delivery. Transitional milk is produced for about 1 week. This may appear thinner and more watery. This milk is high in fats, lactose, and water-soluble vitamins and contains more calories than colostrum. Mature milk is generally established by 2 weeks after delivery. This may appear very thin and watery. It provides 20 kcal/oz and contains lactose, proteins, minerals, and vitamins. If the mother is eating properly, only vitamin D may need to be supplemented.

Formulas are prepared by modifying cow's milk to make it more similar to human milk. It appears thicker and more rich, but also contains 20 kcal/oz. Formulas are available in ready-to-feed and concentrated forms. The mother must be instructed in proper preparation and storage to prevent nutritional or digestive problems in her infant.

The first feeding is normally 15 to 30 ml of sterile water. This must be given with caution to verify that the infant is able to swallow normally and that no anomalies of the digestive tract are present. If this is taken without difficulty, either breast feeding or bottle-feeding is begun. It is normal for infants to regurgitate mucus after the first few feedings. Food intake is necessary to prevent hypoglycemia, which is stressful to the newborn. Some facilities have a policy that requires that a blood glucose determination test be performed. Excessive maternal glucose results in fetal hyperglycemia and fetal hyperinsulinism. After birth, the neonate's high levels of insulin will deplete the glucose stores, and hypoglycemia will result. If the result is 40 or below, sterile glucose water is given. This is done in the very first hours after birth.

The frequency of feeding will depend on the type of feeding. Breastfed babies tend to do best on an "on demand" schedule. Most breastfed babies will nurse at 1- to 3-hour intervals. Bottle-fed babies tend to eat less frequently, usually every 2 to 4 hours, because formula is digested more slowly. Each baby will establish a pattern over a period of time. It is important not to overfeed, particularly with bottle-fed babies, since this can lead to regurgitation. Breastfed infants may receive supplements of glucose water if this is ordered by the physician. However, this may interfere with the process of establishing lactation, since the neonate may not be adequately hungry when put to breast.

It is important to burp the baby at intervals. This should be done for both bottle-fed and breastfed babies. While sucking the baby normally swallows air; if this air is not cleared from the stomach, the infant may feel satisfied and stop eating. When the air clears the stomach, the infant may again appear hungry.

Before starting, a feeding position that is comfortable for the mother should be chosen. The baby should be in a position that facilitates the flow of milk into the stomach. Many different positions are suitable for breast feeding or bottle-feeding (see Fig. 41-4).

Hypothermia. Maintenance of body temperature is a major concern when caring for the newborn. Prolonged exposure to a cold environment can result in increased oxygen consumption and depleted glycogen reserves. The newborn has a large surface area and a limited amount of protective adipose tissue. Heat is lost through radiation, evaporation, conduction, and convection. The nurse must be aware of ways heat is being lost and take precautions to minimize these when meeting the hygiene needs of the newborn (Table 41-4).

Temperature may be monitored with a skin sensor or thermometer. Before inserting a rectal thermometer it is important to verify that the anus is patent. The rectal method of temperature assessment is being used less and less. It is not considered safe. The chance of rectal irritation or perforation is great. Most facilities use the axillary route because it is considered safe. The normal axillary temperature is 97.7° to 98.6° F (36.6° to 37° C).

Skin care. Inspection and bathing of the neonate take place after the body temperature has stabilized. The frequency and type of baths will depend on the policies of the facility.

Bathing serves a number of purposes. It provides opportunities for complete cleansing of the infant, observation of the infant's condition, promotion of comfort, and parent-child family socialization. All bathing articles and the infant's change of clothing should be gathered before bathing.

The temperature of the room should be 75° F (24° C), and the bathing area should be free of drafts to prevent heat loss. The bath water should be approximately 100° F (38.7° C) to prevent chilling. Heat loss in the infant is greater than heat loss in the adult because of the relatively large ratio of the skin surface to body mass in the newborn. Heat loss must be controlled during the bath period to conserve the infant's energy. Bathing the infant quickly, padding cold surfaces, exposing only a portion of the body at a time, and thorough drying are therefore part of the bathing technique. Until the initial bath is completed, personnel must wear gloves when handling the newborn.

TABLE 41-4 Precautions to Minimize Heat Loss in Infants

Heat Loss in Infants	Nursing Interventions to Prevent Heat Loss
Radiation: loss that occurs when heat transfers from the body to cooler surfaces and objects not in contact with the body	Keep body well wrapped to prevent radiant loss. Work quickly to avoid excessive time with skin exposed. Use radiant warmer to minimize loss. Locate crib away from outside wall.
Evaporation: loss when water is converted into a vapor	Dry infant thoroughly after delivery and promptly when bathing.
Conduction: loss of heat to a cooler surface by direct skin contact	Pad surfaces under infant, including tables and scales. Warm other equipment, such as stethoscopes, before use.
Convection: loss of heat to cooler air currents	Reduce drafts from open doors, windows, or air conditioning.

Recent Centers for Disease Control and Prevention regulations related to universal precautions for HIV have increased the use of soap solutions for bathing newborn infants. A nonmedicated mild soap may be used for the initial bath. The hair is shampooed, and a brush or comb may be used to remove dried blood and vernix caseosa. Cotton balls, not gauze, are used to cleanse the nostrils and ears. Careful drying may decrease the risk of infection. The temperature is reassessed 30 minutes after completion of the bath. The order of the bath is essentially the same as for an adult, beginning with the eyes, face, and head and ending with the anal region.

After the initial bath, washing with warm water is sufficient for the first week. However, the perineal area should be carefully washed with nonmedicated mild soap and warm water and carefully dried with each diaper change.

The infant's fragile skin can be injured by too vigorous cleansing. Vernix caseosa, the white material that looks like cold cream, is not removed vigorously because it is attached to the upper layer of the skin. Too vigorous washing results in removal of the protective skin layer. Vernix caseosa may be left on for 45 hours; if it persists beyond that time, it may be washed off gently. Some nurses advocate massaging the vernix caseosa gently into the skin. To date, no studies have confirmed the benefits or disadvantages of this technique.

Questions have arisen about some routine practices: use of soap, oils, powder, lotion, and sponging. According to Whaley and Wong[39]:

> One of the most important considerations in skin cleansing is preservation of the skin's pH, which is about 5 soon after birth. The slightly acidic skin surface has bacteriostatic effects. Consequently, only warm water with a mild soap should be used for the bath. Alkaline soaps such as Ivory, oils, powder, and lotions are not used because they alter the pH, thus providing a better environment for bacterial growth. Talcum has the added risk of aspiration if applied too close to the infant's face.

The nurse should discuss the choice of cloth or disposable diapers with parents. Using disposable diapers exclusively is the most expensive method, costing several times more than cloth diapers laundered at home. Diaper service costs vary but may be more than twice as much as the self-laundry method. Over 1 or 2 years, the cost or savings can be considerable, particularly if more than one child is wearing diapers. However, some disposable diapers may help prevent diaper dermatitis.

Special attention should be given to care of the umbilical area. At delivery the cord is moist. Over the next few days a drying process called **mummification** (mortification, producing a dry hard mass) begins. It is important to avoid getting the cord wet during bathing. Most facilities have a routine to promote drying by use of alcohol or other substances (Triple Dye) that inhibit microbial growth. Odor or exudate from the cord is abnormal and should be reported promptly. Tub bathing is delayed until the fully dried cord drops off at about 10 days of age.

The mother should be given a demonstration of temperature-taking and bathing the newborn. If possible she should be encouraged to bathe the infant with a nurse observing. This will help her gain confidence and provides an opportunity to answer questions about care. It is also a good time to demonstrate safe methods of holding and positioning the infant (Fig. 41-14).

Circumcision, surgical removal of the foreskin, may be performed if the parents consent. There is little agreement among authorities about the necessity or desirability of circumcision. Because this is a surgical procedure, consent forms must be signed.

If circumcision is performed, the area should be kept clean and assessed for bleeding every hour for the first 12 hours postoperatively. Apply gentle pressure to the bleeding area with a folded gauze pad. Sterile petroleum gauze is usually applied to the penis after circumcision and is left in place for 24 hours; it is replaced if it becomes dislodged prematurely. Wash penis gently at diaper change to remove urine and feces and reapply fresh sterile petroleum gauze. Do not attempt to remove the dried yellow exudate that forms in 24 hours and persists for 2 to 3 days; this is part of the normal healing process. Cloth diapers may be recommended during the healing period (about 1 week). A plastic bell may be used to cover the glans and prevent hemorrhage and contamination, negating the need for petroleum gauze dressing. Avoid positioning the infant on the abdomen for the first few hours postprocedure. If bleeding is not controlled, continue application of intermittent pressure, notify physician, and prepare for blood vessel ligation. If the infant has undergone this procedure without anesthesia, he should be comforted until he is quieted and then returned to his crib. These infants usually are fussy for about 2 to 3 hours and may refuse a feeding.

It is vitally important for the nurse to teach the parents appropriate home care prior to the discharge of the newborn. Teaching should include measures to promote hygiene, thus reducing the risks of infection. The parents should be educated to report immediately any unusual signs and symptoms such as edema or purulent, malodorous discharge, as well as elevated temperature and delayed healing.

Elimination

The newborn should void within 24 hours of delivery. If this does not occur, the physician should be notified. The average newborn voids small amounts of poorly concentrated urine; it is normally clear and odorless. Occasionally a small pink or brownish discharge may be observed as a result of uric acid crystals that were formed in the bladder in utero. As the fluid intake increases and kidney function improves, urination becomes more frequent and assumes the normal color.

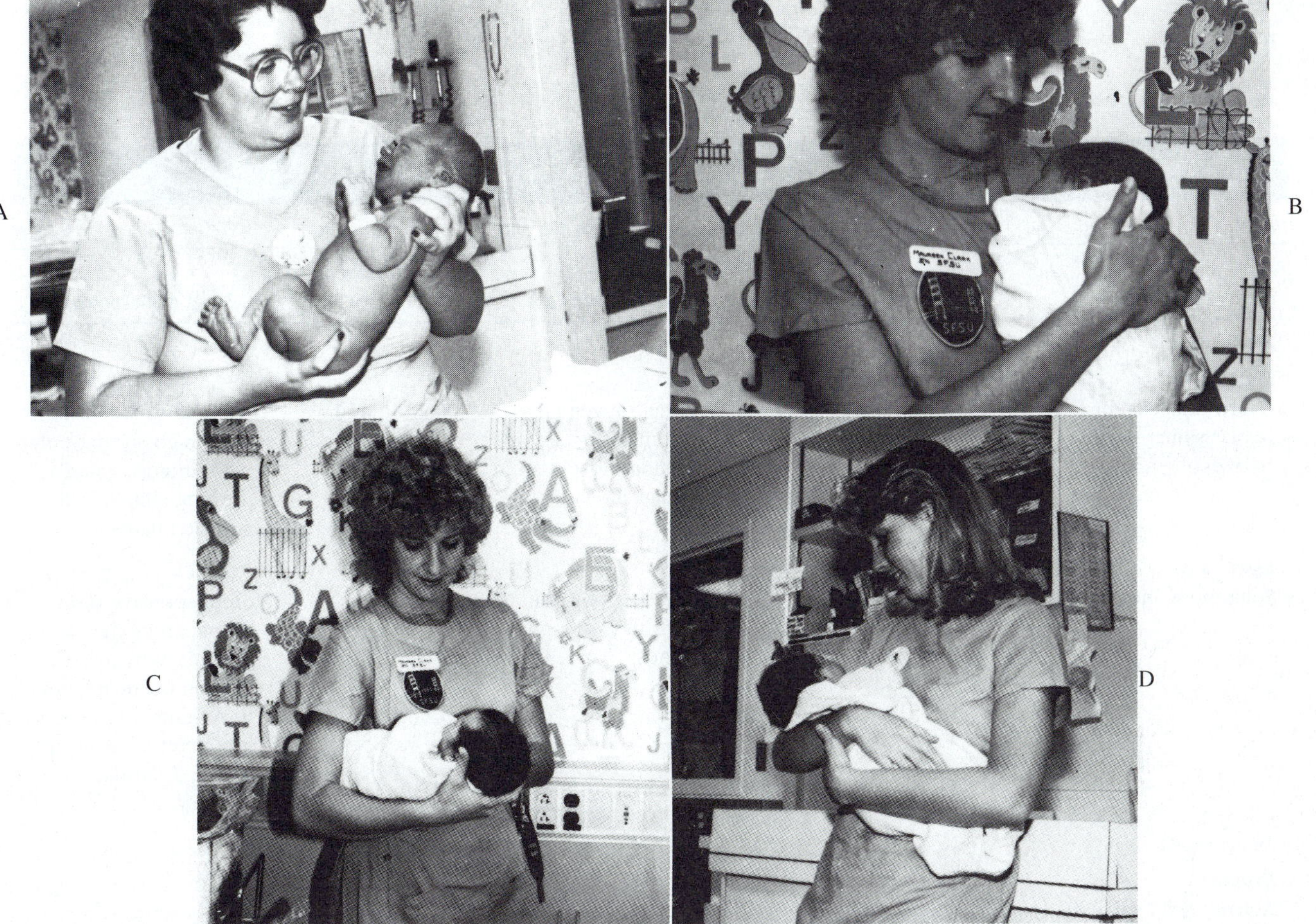

FIG. 41-14 Holding baby securely with support for head. **A,** Holding newborn while moving from one place to another. Baby is undressed to show posture. **B,** Holding newborn upright in "burping" position. **C,** "Football" hold. **D,** Cradle hold.

Bowel elimination should occur within 24 hours of birth. The initial stools of the newborn are odorless, black-green in color, and sticky in consistency. This is called **meconium** and is made up of vernix, strands of lanugo, mucus, and other substances from the amniotic fluid. Occasionally the first stool is encased in mucus and called a *meconium plug*. If no stool is observed, the physician should be notified so an examination can be performed to determine the nature of the problem. Once the infant begins to take nourishment, the nature of the stool changes. Transitional stools, which occur on about the second day, tend to be greenish and loose. These are seen until about the fourth day, when the milk stool is seen. Breastfed babies tend to pass stool frequently, sometimes with every feeding. The stool is pale yellow and sweet smelling. Small curds may be observed. Babies who are bottle-fed tend to have fewer stools, usually two or three per day. These are bright yellow in color and pasty in consistency; the odor may be slightly stronger than that of breastfed babies. This type of stool will continue until solid food is introduced. Very watery stool, green stools (after the transition), or stools expelled with a great deal of force may indicate gastrointestinal irritation or infection and should be reported promptly. Newborns can lose a great deal of fluid rapidly and become dehydrated. (It should be noted, however, that newborns normally give the impression of straining with a stool because their muscles are underdeveloped. This can cause parents undue concern if left unadvised. This will subside as growth and maturity continue.)

The skin of the perineum and buttocks can become irritated if waste products are left in contact for too long. The parents should be taught to wash the skin, wiping from anterior to posterior, after each voiding or stool. Diapers should be changed promptly. Minimal use of powders and creams, which can irritate the skin, is recommended. Disposable or cloth diapers may be chosen.

Rest and Sleep

Most newborns spend 16 to 20 hours per day sleeping. They may be observed to startle and make sucking mo-

TABLE 41-5 Behavior Summary of Sleep-Wake States in Newborn

	Characteristics of State			
Body Activity	**Eye Movements**	**Facial Movements**	**Respiratory Pattern**	**Level of Response**
Sleep states				
Deep sleep				
Nearly still, except for occasional startle or twitch	None	No facial movements, except for occasional sucking movement at regular intervals	Smooth and regular	Threshold to stimuli is very high so that only very intense and disturbing stimuli will arouse infants.
Light sleep				
Some body movements	Rapid eye movements (REM), fluttering of eyes beneath closed eyelids	May smile and make brief fussy or crying sounds	Irregular	More responsive to internal and external stimuli. When these stimuli occur, infants may remain in light sleep, return to deep sleep, or arouse to drowsy.
Awake states				
Drowsy				
Activity level variable, with mild startles interspersed from time to time; movements usually smooth	Eyes open and close occasionally, are heavy-lidded with dull, glazed appearance	May have some facial movements; often there are none, and face appears still	Irregular	Infants react to sensory stimuli although responses are delayed. State change after stimulation frequently noted.
Quiet alert				
Minimal	Brightening and widening of eyes	Face has bright, shining, sparkling looks	Regular	Infants attend most to environment, focusing attention on any stimuli that are present. Optimum state of arousal.
Active alert				
Much body activity; may have periods of fussiness	Eyes open with less brightening	Much facial movement; face not as bright as in quiet alert state	Irregular	Increasingly sensitive to disturbing stimuli (hunger, fatigue, noise, excessive handling).
Crying				
Increased motor activity, with color changes	Eyes may be tightly closed or open	Grimaces	More irregular	Extreme response to unpleasant external or internal stimuli.

tions during sleep. Breathing may be regular and even or irregular, depending on the sleep state. The time awake is spent crying, eating, or in quiet alertness. Each infant establishes a unique pattern. The pattern established by the newborn may be erratic and stabilizes over time as the nervous and digestive systems mature. Most infants do not exceed 5 continuous hours of sleep for some months, and this can be very disruptive to the mother's need for sleep (Table 41-5).

Vital Signs, Activity, and Exercise

Maintenance of a clear airway is critical. Many infants require suctioning to remove mucus from the nose and mouth. Newborns are obligate nose breathers; they must be able to breathe through their nose while suckling. Therefore the nasal passageway must be kept open and free from mucus. A small bulb syringe is most commonly used. It must be decompressed before insertion and then gently released to suction secretions. Parents should have uses of the bulb syringe explained before the first feeding. For the first few days a bulb syringe should always be kept with the newborn, particularly during feeding.

Crying is the newborn's only means of communication. The cry can be used to indicate hunger, pain, or simply the need for attention. The cry of the newborn should be strong, vigorous, and of medium pitch.

Crying in an infant may signal hunger, pain, desire for attention, or fussiness. As mother and infant become more adept at interpreting each other's behavior, some mothers state they are able to distinguish the reason for crying. The following actual report indicates that mother and baby are communicating effectively.

> I can tell when she's hungry. Crying starts in a plaintive (sorrowful, sad) way and then becomes more and more demanding. When she is hurt she lets out a startled yell as though she couldn't believe it was happening to her. Sometimes when she is put down to sleep, she starts a kind of talking cry, jerky and demanding: it gets louder, and if nothing happens, fades away in little spurts. The fussy cry is the hardest to take—nothing seems to work; like a complaining that goes on and on.

A high-pitched cry may indicate neurological problems.

The respiratory movements of a newborn are diaphragmatic and are best measured by counting the rise and fall of the abdomen. The normal respiratory rate is between 30 and 60 respirations per minute. Flaring of the nostrils, sternal retraction, or tachypnea may indicate distress and should be reported immediately.

The normal range for the newborn heart rate is between 120 and 150 beats per minute. Rates as low as 100 beats per minute when sleeping, and as high as 180 beats per minute when crying, are not unusual. The heart beat should have a regular rate and rhythm. The apical beat can be auscultated between the fourth and fifth intercostal spaces. This is best done when the infant is asleep. Murmurs are rather common in the newborn. The physician will determine whether they are significant.

Blood pressure is approximately 80/40 in a healthy newborn. The normal range is systolic: 60 to 80 mm Hg; diastolic: 40 to 50 mm Hg. Electronic equipment with a specialized sensor is required to obtain accurate readings. Blood pressure readings are taken infrequently, unless complications occur. Upon the newborn's admission to the nursery, blood pressure is assessed on all four extremities. A difference between the upper and lower extremities' pressure could denote abnormalities such as coarctation of aorta.

Parent-Child Attachment

The human infant is born quite defenseless. Without a caregiver, the infant could not survive. The parents are responsible for the infant's physical and psychological development.

Parenting is not instinctive; a new parent must bond with the baby first. **Bonding, parent-child attachment,** is defined as the initial phase in a relationship characterized by strong attraction and a desire to interact (Fig. 41-15). Without bonding it would be difficult to maintain the energy required to meet the newborn's needs. The nurse cannot make bonding occur but can facilitate its development.

Early contact with the infant is important to establish bonding. A new mother normally wishes to touch and explore her baby. Holding the infant close and looking eye to eye (the en face position) (Fig. 41-16 on p. 1296) help bonding to occur. It is normal for new mothers to talk in high-pitched tones to the baby. The nurse should encourage early and frequent interaction between the newborn and the parents. Attachment should increase when the infant begins to respond.

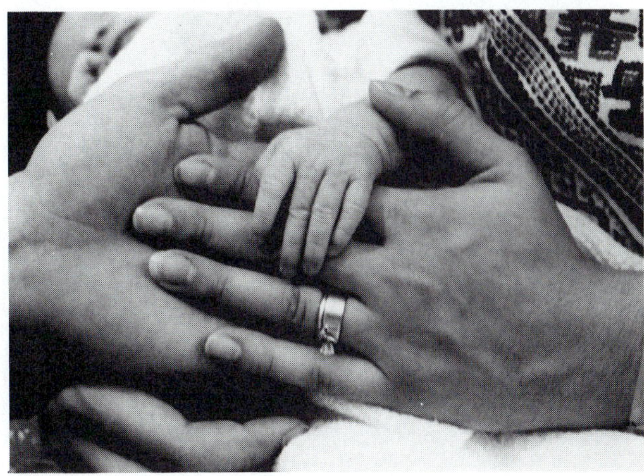

FIG. 41-15 Hands. (Courtesy St. Luke's Hospital, Kansas City, Mo.)

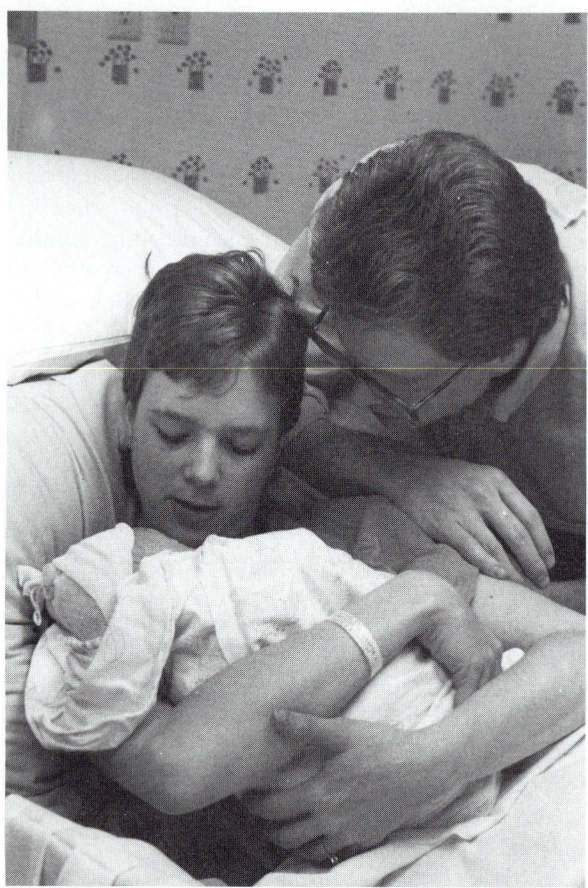

FIG. 41-16 Eye-to-eye contact. (Courtesy the Birthplace, Riverside Medical Center, Minneapolis.)

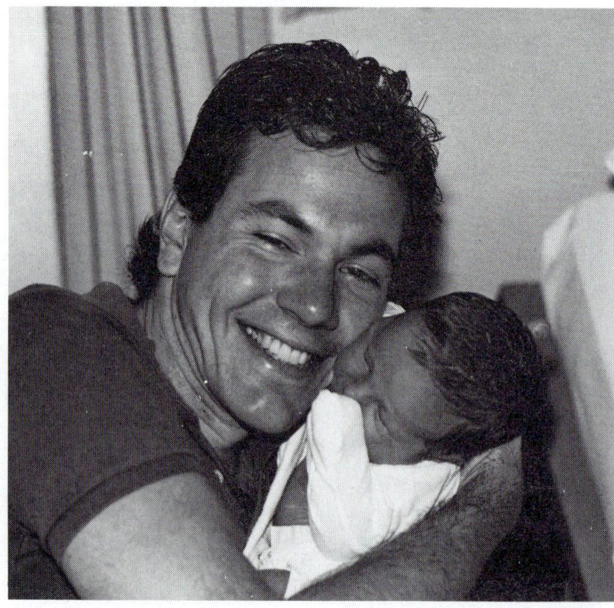

FIG. 41-17 Father and newborn son.

The newborn has amazing capabilities. The infant is a socially responsive human being who can probably learn better on the first day of life than ever again. A baby, immediately after birth, will stare intently at the parents' faces and see them. In fact, newborns prefer looking at the mother's face, especially the eyes, rather than at other objects. Other capabilities of the newborn include the ability to recognize an approaching object as a threat and to turn away to avoid it and the ability to reach for an object and usually come close to touching it. The newborn will imitate another person's facial expressions such as sticking out the tongue, opening the mouth, and pursing the lips. Newborn babies are active stimulus seekers where repetition and the level of stimulation are important. The baby is actually capable of shutting out stimuli and can even learn to respond by turning its head at the sound of the mother's voice.

Indeed, babies are not passive and unresponsive creatures to be hurried off to the hospital nursery after birth. The affectionate bond between mother and child and between father and child begins at the moment of birth (Figs. 41-16 and 41-17). As long as the newborn is responding normally, immediate skin-to-skin contact with the parents is very important in bonding. The newborn will have difficulty opening the eyes under bright spotlights but will look around if the lights are dimmed. (It is possible to dim the main lights in the delivery area and still have light focused over the perineum for episiotomy repair or other necessary procedures.) Also, shielding the infant's face with one's hands or a blanket will provide enough protection from the light to encourage the baby to open the eyes. Objects are in clearest range for the newborn at about 8 to 12 inches. Newborns prefer faces over other patterns. Refraining from using prophylactic eye drops and weighing and measuring the baby for 30 minutes to 1 hour after birth will allow the parents time alone with their baby so that the attachment process can proceed without interruption.

The mother may wish to breastfeed in the first hour after birth; the nurse or the father can assist her.

Periods of quiet alertness are best for interaction. The nurse should explain the different levels of alertness to the parents so they can recognize them (see Table 41-5). Care should be timed so that the mother is available to enjoy quiet moments with her newborn.

NURSING PROCESS SUMMARY

Tables 41-6 and 41-7 will assist the nurse in reviewing all health patterns of the mother and newborn. These guidelines will help focus observations; significant observations or responses will indicate the need for further questioning. If the nurse is unsure of the significance of data, it is important to consult with another nurse.

In addition, possible diagnoses with patient outcomes and interventions are suggested.

TABLE 41-6 Nursing Process and the Postpartum Patient

Data Collection	Possible Nursing Diagnoses	Patient Goals/Expected Outcomes	Nursing Interventions
Health management			
Is the patient interested in learning about personal care and that of the infant? Does she follow through on teaching? Did she follow through with prenatal care, and does she have a physician to care for the baby? Has she made appointments for follow-up?	Health maintenance, altered, related to lack of resources and lack of knowledge	Patient verbalizes willingness to follow nursing/medical regimen.	Provide explanations regarding postpartum care. Provide literature regarding postpartum care. Provide educational videos.
Nutritional and metabolic issues			
Is diet adequate per recommended daily allowance? Is fluid intake adequate? How much weight has been gained/lost?	Nutrition, altered: less than body requirements, related to inadequate intake of nutrients	Patient verbalizes willingness to follow diet.	Initiate dietary consultation; review Food Guide Pyramid and recommendations if breastfeeding. Discuss importance of avoiding dieting in early postpartum period.
Does she have an episiotomy? What is the condition of breasts and nipples? Is she breastfeeding?	Fluid volume deficit, related to inadequate fluid intake for process of lactation	Patient will verbalize importance of taking in an increased amount of fluids.	Monitor fluid intake; discuss importance of adequate fluid intake, particularly if breastfeeding or living in warm climate. Stress importance of taking in liquids without caffeine
	Tissue integrity, impaired, related to perineal incision or laceration	Patient will be free of perineal infection.	Review importance of correct perineal care. Assess perineum at least once a shift. Instruct in sitz bath procedures if ordered. Provide comfort measures such as use of Tucks if ordered.
Activity and exercise			
What does she know about postpartum exercise? Who is available to help with care at home? How many other children are at home? Vital signs?	Activity intolerance, related to fatigue	Patient will verbalize the importance of rest periods during the postpartum recovery period. Patient verbalizes activities that increase fatigue.	Stress the importance of pacing activities while meeting personal needs and those of newborn. Explore options for help at home.

Continued.

TABLE 41-6 Nursing Process and the Postpartum Patient—cont'd

Data Collection	Possible Nursing Diagnoses	Patient Goals/Expected Outcomes	Nursing Interventions
Elimination			
Has pattern of urine elimination changed? Has bowel elimination pattern changed? Is there any burning with urination? Pain with defecation? Constipation? Diarrhea?	Incontinence, stress, high risk for, related to changes in pelvic musculature	Patient describes plan for improved urinary elimination pattern.	Monitor voiding: Assess bladder for signs of distention or retention. Encourage regular voiding. Catheterize per physician orders. Teach Kegel exercises.
	Constipation, related to decreased abdominal muscle tone	Patient verbalizes presence of optimal bowel pattern.	Stress importance of foods high in fiber and fluid. Encourage adequate activity. Stress importance of not ignoring urge to defecate. Discuss use of stool softeners if ordered.
Rest and sleep			
Has sleep pattern changed? Increased fatigue noticed? Does patient take naps or rest periods?	Sleep pattern disturbance related to child care demands Fatigue related to increased physical demands of child care	Patient identifies measures that will increase rest/sleep.	Assist in planning day to maximize rest periods. Suggest uninterrupted nap while baby sleeps.
Cognitive and perceptual issues			
Is there any pain? Nature? Duration? Location? Is she knowledgeable about newborn care? Growth and development and safety needs of newborns?	Knowledge deficit, related to lack of experience with care of newborn	Patient verbalizes understanding of instructions/information.	Provide information regarding infant and child care. Provide materials regarding growth and development. Stress safety teaching.
Role and relationship			
Does she feel confused about her changing role? Have interpersonal dynamics with husband, boyfriend, parents, friends changed?	Role performance, altered, related to expectations for parenting Family processes, altered, related to expectations for parenting	Patient identifies personal strengths. Family members participate in decision-making processes regarding posthospital care.	Spend time listening to concerns. Involve family members and significant others in teaching. Consult social services if serious problems with dynamics are observed.
Coping and stress			
What fears or anxieties are verbalized? How has her self-image changed?	Anxiety Coping, ineffective individual Fear	Patient identifies available resources/support systems and initiates alternative coping strategies.	Identify cultural or other factors that are likely to interfere with postpartum care.
Values and beliefs			
What is the patient's cultural background? Religious practices?	Spiritual distress, related separation from spiritual or cultural beliefs or practices	Patient expresses acceptance of limited religious/cultural practices.	Incorporate cultural practices into care whenever possible. Consult a spiritual advisor for specific information if necessary.

TABLE 41-7 Nursing Process and the Newborn

Data Collection	Possible Nursing Diagnoses	Patient Goals/Expected Outcomes	Nursing Interventions
Health management			
Are the parents aware of the need for regular physical examination and the need for immunizations? Are the parents aware of normal growth and development during the first year of life?	Health maintenance, altered, related to cultural beliefs, lack of resources, lack of maternal knowledge regarding newborn care	Patient and/or significant other demonstrates adequate caretaking of infant.	Identify cultural or other factors likely to interfere with newborn care. Provide explanations regarding newborn care. Provide literature regarding newborn care.
Nutritional and metabolic issues			
What type of feeding is the infant receiving? Breastfed? Formula? What type? How much consumed at each feeding? Any breaks in skin? How much weight has been lost? More than 10% of body weight? Body temperature?	Breastfeeding, ineffective, related to maternal anxiety	Patient verbalizes what triggers her anxieties. Patient verbalizes her specific anxieties.	
	Breastfeeding, interrupted, related to illness, maternal obligations, and breast tenderness.	Patient demonstrates appropriate breastfeeding skills with minimum of discomfort.	Provide information regarding breastfeeding. Provide encouragement and restful environment. Refer to breastfeeding support groups.
	Nutrition, altered: less than body requirements, related to inadequate sucking, inability to obtain food for self	Newborn will receive adequate nutrition as evidenced by appropriate weight gain.	Assess suck, monitor changes in weight, provide mother with materials regarding infant nutrition including breastfeeding and bottle-feeding. Assess positioning of infant at breast.
	Fluid volume deficit, related to inadequate fluid intake or excessive fluid loss	Infant maintains adequate fluid volume and electrolytes for growth and weight gain as evidenced by normal skin turgor, weight, intake, and urine specific gravity.	Teach mother how to monitor fluid intake, particularly if breastfeeding or living in warm climates. Teach mother how to assess infant for dehydration. Stress importance of contacting physician if infant develops diarrhea or fever.
	Feeding pattern, ineffective infant, related to prematurity, anatomical abnormalities	Infant will receive adequate nutrition to grow within the normal limits for age	Assess suck and swallow, try alternate nipples and feeding systems. Reassure mother. Burp frequently. Instruct mother to listen for click, swallow during nursing.
	Hypothermia, related to immature thermoregulatory system, exposure to cool or cold environment, low birth weight	Infant maintains normal axillary temperature of 97.7° to 98.6° F (36.5° to 37° C).	Provide adequate warmth with clothing or radiant warmer. Bath quickly and dry thoroughly to reduce heat loss through evaporation. Maintain safe environmental temperature.
	Tissue integrity, impaired, related to healing umbilicus, circumcision	Infant will remain free of signs and symptoms of infection.	Review importance of observation of area. Teach proper cord care, circumcision care, and diapering techniques.

Continued.

TABLE 41-7 Nursing Process and the Newborn—cont'd

Data Collection	Possible Nursing Diagnoses	Patient Outcomes	Nursing Interventions
Activity and exercise			
Is the airway clear of secretions? Can infant move freely? Symmetrically? Are gluteal folds equal? Can infant lift the head? Muscle tone?	Airway clearance, ineffective, related to excessive secretions	Infant remains free of respiratory distress.	Teach proper positioning to facilitate respiratory drainage. Instruct mother in use of bulb syringe.
	Injury, high risk for, related to inability to protect self	Infant remains free of harm/injury.	Teach mother how to safety check home. Instruct in safety measures when carrying infant. Stress importance of proper child restraint in cars and use of safety seats.
Elimination			
How often does the infant void? What is the frequency, color, and consistency of stool? Are there any unusual observations about urine or stool?	Constipation, related to immature muscle development and inadequate fluid/nutritional intake	Infant will have the normal amount of stools per day for the bottle-fed baby or for the breastfed baby. Infant will have the normal number of voidings per day as evidenced by unstained, odorless, wet diapers.	Urinary elimination, altered patterns, related to newborn status and inadequate fluid intake. Teach mother normal changes in bowel and bladder elimination. Teach proper cleansing of the perineal area. Teach mother to observe stools and voidings for unusual findings—frequency, color, and consistency.
Rest and sleep			
What sleep pattern is observed? Does the infant wake readily for feeding? How many hours are spent asleep?	Sleep pattern disturbances, related to developmental stage	Infant will receive adequate sleep for normal growth.	Explain normal newborn sleep cycle to mother. Help structure environment and schedule to promote normal sleep patterns.
Cognitive and perceptual issues			
Does the infant respond to loud noises? Is eye-to-eye contact made? Does the infant appear to be in pain? Is crying continuous or intermittent?	Pain, acute, related to circumcision, gastrointestinal distress	Infant will be free of discomfort as evidenced by quiet sleep.	Assess nature and frequency of crying episodes. Change diapers, feed, burp; reposition, swaddle, rock, or use other soothing techniques.

REFERENCES AND SUGGESTED READINGS

1. Abriola DV: Mothers' perceptions of a postpartum support group, *Matern Child Nurs J* 19(2):112, 1990.
2. Barnes JE et al: Breastfeeders versus bottle feeders: differences in feminity perceptions, *MCH* 21(1):15, 1993.
3. Bobak IM, Jensen MD: *Essentials of maternity nursing,* ed 3, St Louis, 1991, Mosby.
4. Bobak M, Jensen MD: *Maternity and gynecologic care: the nurse and the family,* ed 5, St Louis, 1993, Mosby.
5. Burrough A: *Maternity nursing,* ed 6, Philadelphia, 1992, Saunders.
6. Campinba-Bacote J, Bragg EJ: Clinical assessment in maternity care, *MCH* 18(1):24, 1993.
7. Cosner KR, DeJoung E: Physiologic second-stage labor, *MCH* 18(1):38, 1993.
8. Doenges M, Moorhouse M: *Nurse's pocket guide to nursing diagnosis with interventions,* ed 3, Philadelphia, 1991, FA Davis.
9. Easterlong WE, Herbert WNP: *The puerperium.* In Scott JR et al: *Danforth's obstetrics and gynecology,* ed 6, Philadelphia, 1990, Lippincott.
10. Evans CJ: Description of a home follow-up program for childbearing families, *J Obstet Gynecol Neonatal Nurs* 20:113, 1991.
11. Fischbach F: *A manual of laboratory diagnostic tests,* ed 4, Philadelphia, 1992, Lippincott.
12. Fishbein EG, Phillips M: How safe is exercise during pregnancy? *J Obstet Gynecol Neonatal Nurs* 19:45, 1990.
13. Frantz K: Keep breastfeeding simple, keep it easy, keep it fun, *Birth* 18(4):228, 1991.
14. Giger JN, Davidhizar E: *Transcultural nursing: assessment and intervention,* ed 2, St Louis, 1995, Mosby.
15. Hall LA et al: Psychosocial predictors of maternal depressive symptoms, parenting attitudes and child behaviors in single parent families, *Nurs Res* 40:214, 1991.
16. Ingalls AJ, Salerno MC: *Maternal and child health nursing,* ed 7, St Louis, 1991, Mosby.
17. Johnstone HA, Marcinak JF: Candidiasis in the breastfeeding mother and infant, *J Obstet Gynecol Neonatal Nurs* 19(2):171, 1990.
18. Kenner CA, MacLaren A: *Essentials of maternal and neonatal nursing,* Springhouse, Penn, 1993, Springhouse.
19. Ladewig PW, London MI, Old SB: *Essentials of maternal-newborn nursing,* ed 2, Redwood City, Calif, 1990, Addison-Wesley.
20. Lederer JR et al: *Care planning pocket guide: a nursing diagnosis approach,* Redwood City, Calif, 1991, Addison-Wesley.
21. Luegenbrehl DL et al: Standardized assessment of blood loss, *MCH* 15(4):241, 1990.
22. Lukacs A: Issues surrounding early postpartum discharge: effects on the caregiver, *J Perinat Neonatol Nurs* 5(1):33, 1991.
23. Martell LK: Postpartum depression as a family problem, *MCH* 15(2):90, 1990.
24. Martin LL, Reeder SJ: *Essentials of maternity nursing-family centered care,* Philadelphia, 1991, Lippincott.
25. Matthews MK: Mother's satisfaction with neonate's breastfeeding behaviors, *J Obstet Gynecol Neonatal Nurs* 20:49, 1991.
26. McDonald AD et al: Cigarette, alcohol and coffee consumption and congenital defects, *Am J Public Health* 82(1):91, 1992.
27. Mead-Bennett E: The relationship of primigravida sleep experience and select moods on the first postpartum day, *J Obstet Gynecol Neonatal Nurs* 19(2):146, 1990.
28. *Mosby's medical, nursing, and allied health dictionary,* ed 4, St Louis 1994, Mosby.
29. Olds SB, London ML, Ladewig PW: *Maternal-newborn nursing: a family centered approach,* ed 4, Menlo Park, Calif, 1992, Addison-Wesley.
30. Pagana KD, Pagana TJ: *Mosby's diagnostic and laboratory test reference,* St Louis, 1992, Mosby.
31. Parham ES: The association of pregnancy weight gain with the mother's postpartum weight, *J Am Diet Assoc* 90:550, 1990.
32. Phillips CR: *Family-centered maternity/newborn care,* ed 3, St Louis, 1992, Mosby.
33. Reid L: Teaching what comes naturally: helping first-time mothers to breastfeed, *Nurs Times* 88(3):45, 1991.
34. Scott JR et al: *Dansforth's obstetrics and gynecology,* ed 6, Philadelphia, 1990, Lippincott.
35. Seidel HM et al: *Mosby's guide to physical examination,* ed 3, St Louis, 1995, Mosby.
36. Thomas CL: *Taber's cyclopedic medical dictionary,* ed 17, Philadelphia, 1993, FA Davis.
37. Tucker SM et al: *Patient care standards: nursing process, diagnosis, and outcome,* ed 5, St Louis, 1992, Mosby.
38. Talman L et al: Changes in functional status after childbirth, *Nurs Res* 39(2):70, 1990.
39. Wong DL: *Nursing care of infants and children,* ed 5, St Louis, 1995, Mosby.

CHAPTER CHALLENGE

KEY POINTS

- During the 6 weeks after delivery, the reproductive organs return to approximately the prepregnant size and location.
- The new mother should avoid dieting and excessive activity during the early postpartum period.
- Postpartum fatigue and depression are common as a result of hormonal and physiological changes.
- Complications can occur during the postpartum period. It is essential that the nurse assess each woman carefully.
- Before discharge the nurse should provide instruction concerning the danger signs of the postpartum period and verify that the woman knows when and how to contact her physician.
- Hormonal changes enable the woman to produce enough milk to meet the nutritional needs of the growing infant. Nutritional needs of the lactating woman are similar to those during pregnancy.
- Motherhood is a learned skill. The new mother will require extensive teaching and encouragement about parenting skills.

- Early discharge requires that the nurse provide essential teaching in a brief period. The nurse should be careful to document teaching.
- The nurse should supplement teaching with written materials so the new mother has something to refer to when at home.
- There is a wide range of normal variation among newborns. The nurse should verify any questionable observations with another nurse or physician.
- Hypothermia and infection are two major areas of concern when providing care to the newborn.
- Circumcision is an elective surgical procedure.
- The newborn has social as well as physical needs.
- The nurse should provide demonstration and teaching to educate the mother about the hygiene needs of the newborn.
- Whether or not this is the couple's first baby, parents appreciate anticipatory guidance in the care of their child.
- Parent-child attachment (bonding) is the process by which parent and child come to love and accept each other.

STUDY QUESTIONS

1. Mrs. Kidd, age 35, gravida 4 para 3, is in her first postpartum day. She had an uncomplicated pregnancy and delivery. When assessing her vital signs, the nurse obtains the following readings. It is essential that the nurse promptly report findings of:
   1. T 99° F, P 58, BP 110/70
   2. T 100.8° F, P 92, BP 116/84
   3. T 98.6° F, P 86, BP 140/92
   4. T 98.2° F, P 100, BP 100/54
2. Mrs. Langley, age 27, is breastfeeding. On the first day postpartum, the nurse would expect to find her breasts to be:
   1. Soft, free from secretions
   2. Soft, producing colostrum
   3. Firm at outer margins, producing milk
   4. Engorged, producing milk
3. On the first day postpartum the nurse examines 31-year-old Mrs. Webster's fundus and find that it is displaced to the side. The most appropriate nursing action is to:
   1. Have her turn onto her side before measuring the height
   2. Escort her to the bathroom to empty her bladder
   3. Report this immediately to the physician
   4. Document the fact that the fundus is displaced
4. When the nurse assesses Ms. Stabler, age 35, on the second postpartum day for vaginal drainage, the nurse would report immediately:
   1. Large amount of lochia rubra with fleshy odor
   2. Moderate amount of lochia rubra with a few small clots
   3. Moderate amount of lochia rubra with a foul odor
   4. Small amount of lochia rubra
5. Mrs. Sbonik, age 30, is a multipara who delivered a 7-lb, 6-oz infant. During breastfeeding she complains of strong afterbirth pains. She asks why these are occurring. The nurse explains that the pains occur because she:
   1. Delivered a large infant
   2. Is a multipara
   3. Is breastfeeding
   4. Is a multipara and is breastfeeding
6. Mrs. Peterson is 26 years old. Her physician has written orders for several PRN medications. To reduce the afterbirth pains she is experiencing, the most appropriate medication would be:
   1. Ibuprofen
   2. Aspirin
   3. Tylenol with codeine
   4. Meperidine hydrochloride
7. Mrs. Burke, age 19, a primipara, comments on the presence of several milia on the baby's nose and chin. The nurse would explain that these are a result of:
   1. An increased amount of pigmentation
   2. A cluster of capillaries located close to the skin surface
   3. A minor skin infection
   4. Clogged sebaceous glands
8. Mrs. Peek, age 41, a multipara, is scheduled for discharge tomorrow morning. Before discharge the nurse would explain that she should make an appointment with her physician for:
   1. 1 to 2 weeks after delivery
   2. 2 to 3 weeks after delivery
   3. 3 to 4 weeks after delivery
   4. 4 to 6 weeks after delivery
9. The physician has ordered an injection of vitamin K for Baby Crisp. The nurse is aware that this medication is given to:
   1. Promote healthy tissue development
   2. Supplement vitamins missing in breast milk
   3. Enhance the absorption of calcium
   4. Reduce the risk of hemorrhage
10. Baby Girl Sanders has orders for eye prophylaxis to prevent ophthalmia neonatorum. This typically involves:
    1. Patching the eyes to prevent excessive exposure to light
    2. Instillation of antibiotic drops into the conjunctival sac
    3. Application of warm moist compresses to reduce edema of the lids
    4. Careful washing of the eyes with sterile water from inner to outer canthus

42

CARE OF THE MOTHER AND NEWBORN AT RISK

Gloria E. Wold

KEY TERMS

anasarca
atony
brown fat
cotyledons
direct Coombs' test
dizygotic
eclampsia
erythroblastosis fetalis
gestational diabetes mellitus
glycosylated hemoglobin
high-risk pregnancy
hydramnios
indirect Coombs' test
kernicterus
kick count
monozygotic
morbidity
mortality
phototherapy
placental barrier
preeclampsia
pregnancy-induced hypertension (PIH)
TORCH

LEARNING OBJECTIVES

After reading this chapter, the student should be able to do the following:

- Define the key terms.
- List those conditions that increase maternal and fetal risk.
- Discuss bleeding disorders that can occur during pregnancy.
- Identify diagnostic tests used to determine high-risk situations.
- Describe the HELP syndrome.
- Discuss pregnancy induced hypertension.
- Discuss preexisting maternal health conditions that influence pregnancy.
- List the infectious diseases most likely to cause serious complications.
- Discuss the care of the pregnant adolescent.
- Discuss the problems created by alcohol and drug abuse.
- Identify concerns related to preterm infants.
- Explain the hemolytic diseases of the newborn.
- Discuss nursing diagnoses related to high-risk conditions of the mother and newborn.

RELATED TOPICS OF INTEREST

- Life span development (Chapter 7)
- Diet therapy (Chapter 19)
- Care of the patient with a cardiovascular disorder (Chapter 28)
- Care of the patient with an endocrine disorder (Chapter 32)
- Care of the patient with a reproductive disorder (Chapter 33)
- Care of the HIV-positive or AIDS patient (Chapter 37)
- The patient with an addictive personality (Chapter 47)

Although most pregnancies proceed normally, complications and high-risk situations can occur at any stage of the childbearing process, and the nurse must be aware of these so that appropriate, timely actions can be taken. Two lives are involved, and the nurse must provide care that protects the welfare of both.

Of the approximately 6 million births that occur in the United States each year, 500,000 will be categorized as high risk because of maternal or fetal complications. The united efforts of all members of the obstetrical team and close collaboration with the other medical personnel are required to adequately care for the high-risk patient.

Box 42-1 FACTORS THAT PLACE THE POSTPARTUM PATIENT AND NEWBORN AT HIGH RISK

MOTHER

Hemorrhage
Infection
Abnormal vital signs
Traumatic labor or birth
Psychosocial factors

INFANT (FACTORS FOR ADMISSION TO NICU*)

High-Risk Category

Continuing or developing signs of respiratory distress syndrome
Asphyxiation (Apgar score <6 at 5 min); resuscitation required at birth
Preterm; dysmaturity†
Cyanosis or suspected cardiovascular disease; persistent cyanosis
Major congenital malformations requiring surgery; chromosomal anomalies
Convulsions, sepsis, hemorrhagic diathesis,‡ or shock
Meconium aspiration syndrome
Central nervous system depression for >24 hr
Hypoglycemia
Hypocalcemia
Hyperbilirubinemia

Moderate-Risk Category

Dysmaturity
Prematurity (weight between 2000 and 2500 g)
Apgar score of <5 at 1 min
Feeding problems
Multifetal birth
Transient tachypnea
Hypomagnesemia or hypermagnesemia
Hypoparathyroidism
Failure to gain weight
Jitteriness or hyperactivity
Cardiac anomalies not requiring immediate catheterization
Heart murmur
Anemia
Central nervous system depression for <24 hr

*NICU; neonatal intensive care unit.
†Dysmaturity: weight less than would be expected for the known length of the gestational period.
‡Diathesis: constitutional predisposition to certain disease conditions.

A **high-risk pregnancy** is one in which the life or health of the mother or infant is jeopardized by a disorder coincidental with or unique to pregnancy. For the mother the high-risk status extends (arbitrarily based on medical judgment) through the puerperium, that is, 29 days after delivery. Postdelivery maternal complications are usually resolved within a month, but perinatal **morbidity** (state of being diseased) may continue for months or years.

A better understanding of human reproduction has greatly reduced morbidity and **mortality** (quality or state of being subject to death). Knowledge of the fetus and neonatal disorders has increased dramatically in the last 10 to 15 years. This has led to a gratifying drop in perinatal morbidity and mortality during this period. Since 1969, when the perinatal death rate in the United States dropped below 30 per 1000 live births for the first time, the rate has steadily declined. In 1985, the death rate was estimated to be 14.7 per 1000 live births. In 1988, African-American women were 3.3 times more likely than Caucasian women to die of causes associated with pregnancy, childbirth, and the perperium. Further, African-American women have 40% more hospitalizations during pregnancy than do Caucasian women (National Center for Health Statistics, 1990). This decline of the perinatal death rate in the United States is attributed to changes in social and economic factors and to availability of health care.

Understanding of the high-risk patient will allow the nurse to provide individualized therapeutic nursing interventions. Nurses can be instrumental in educating the public about the importance of obtaining early and regular care during pregnancy. See Box 42-1 for factors that place the postpartum woman and neonate at high risk.

HYPEREMESIS GRAVIDARUM

Etiology. When vomiting during pregnancy becomes excessive enough to cause electrolyte, metabolic, and nutritional imbalances, the condition is termed *hyperemesis gravidarum*. Although mild morning sickness is common, hyperemesis gravidarum, also called *pernicious vomiting*, is a serious complication.

The exact cause of this condition is not known. Hormones, particularly human chorionic gonadotropin (HCG), are suspected: hyperemesis is more common with conditions in which there are high levels of HCG involved, such as hydatidiform mole. Psychogenic factors may also be involved. Hyperemesis gravidarum is one of the most common nutrition-related discomforts of pregnancy.

Clinical Manifestations. The mother experiences vomiting and retching that far exceeds those seen with the usual morning sickness. Women with hyperemesis gravidarum may border on starvation and become severely dehydrated. Many serious complications that endanger both the mother and fetus can result. Acid-base imbalance related to the loss of excessive amounts of hydrochloric acid or intestinal juices may occur, resulting in alkalosis or acidosis. Potassium may become depleted, leading to cardiac dysrhythmias. Vitamin deficiencies can lead to jaundice and hemorrhage.

Assessment. The frequency, amount, and character of emesis should be assessed, recorded, and reported. Fluid intake and output (I&O) are measured carefully. Assessment of the fetal status is also important. The nurse must monitor fetal heart rate regularly and immediately report any significant changes (see Chapter 40).

Medical Management. Medical treatment is directed at meeting nutritional needs, thereby maintaining acid-base and electrolyte balance. Intravenous (IV) feeding must be monitored closely. Solid intake is restricted until vomiting stops and the woman feels capable of trying solid food. Bland solids, such as toast and crackers, or liquids are introduced slowly, and the woman's ability to tolerate these foods must be carefully assessed. The nurse observes the patient for any signs of complications such as metabolic acidosis, jaundice, or hemorrhage and alerts the physician should these occur.

Nursing Interventions. Typically this patient is hospitalized and given parenteral fluids. Oral hygiene is essential, because the mouth may be irritated by the vomitus. Care is needed to reduce the mother's emotional distress; fear for herself and her fetus are commonly observed. The nurse should provide emotional support and explanations. The family is included in the plan of care whenever possible. Encouraging their participation may help to alleviate some of the emotional stress associated with hospitalization.

Nursing diagnoses and interventions for the patient with hyperemesis gravidarum include but are not limited to the following:

NURSING DIAGNOSES	NURSING INTERVENTIONS
Nutrition, altered: less than body requirements, related to nausea and persistent vomiting secondary to pregnancy	Monitor food intake; caloric record may be desirable. Offer dry crackers and bland food as tolerated. Provide a pleasant atmosphere at meals. Administer antiemetics as ordered.
Fluid volume deficit, related to decreased fluid intake and excessive fluid loss	Measure and record I&O. Administer fluids as ordered. Assess skin turgor and mucous membranes. Weigh daily at same time. Monitor laboratory values and report abnormalities. Encourage oral fluids, slowly increasing amount as tolerated. Monitor IV fluids if ordered.
Oral mucous membranes altered, high risk for, related to dehydration and frequent emesis	Inspect oral cavity daily. Provide oral hygiene before meals and after each emesis, using soft bristle brush and oral swabs. Lubricate lips.
Fear, related to possibility of harm to fetus or self	Convey acceptance of patient's perception of fear. Help patient to identify personal strengths and previous coping mechanisms. Help patient identify sources of support. Provide opportunities to verbalize fears. Provide continuity of care.

Patient teaching.

- Arrange for dietary consult.
- Discuss importance of adequate nutrition during pregnancy.
- Assess the woman's willingness to follow prescribed diet plan.
- Encourage patient compliance.
- Provide patient with information related to potential risks to fetus.

Prognosis. In most instances, hyperemesis gravidarum will respond to therapy and the prognosis is good. If untreated, hyperemesis gravidarum can result in maternal and fetal death.

MULTIPLE PREGNANCY

Etiology. Pregnancy involving twins occurs in approximately 1 of 90 births in the United States. Triplets occur in approximately 1 in 7600 births. Pregnancies involving more than three fetuses are even more rare. Pregnancies involving five or more embryos are often a result of fertility drugs.

Twins are classified as monozygotic or dizygotic. **Monozygotic** twins originate with one fertilized ovum; the embryonic disk divides, causing "identical twins." Because the genetic message is identical, the twins must be of the same sex and carry an identical genetic code. They share a placenta, but each has a separate umbilical cord. **Dizygotic** twins are the result of two separate ova being fertilized at the same time. These twins, have separate placentas. The sex and genetic makeup can vary; they are no more closely related than siblings born at different times (Fig. 42-1 on p. 1306).

Pathophysiology. Maternal and fetal risks are increased during multiple pregnancy. Spontaneous abortions, maternal anemia, pregnancy-induced hypertension, hydramnios, and bleeding from placenta previa or abruptio placentae are more common in women with twins. Congenital anomalies, problems with entangled cords, and

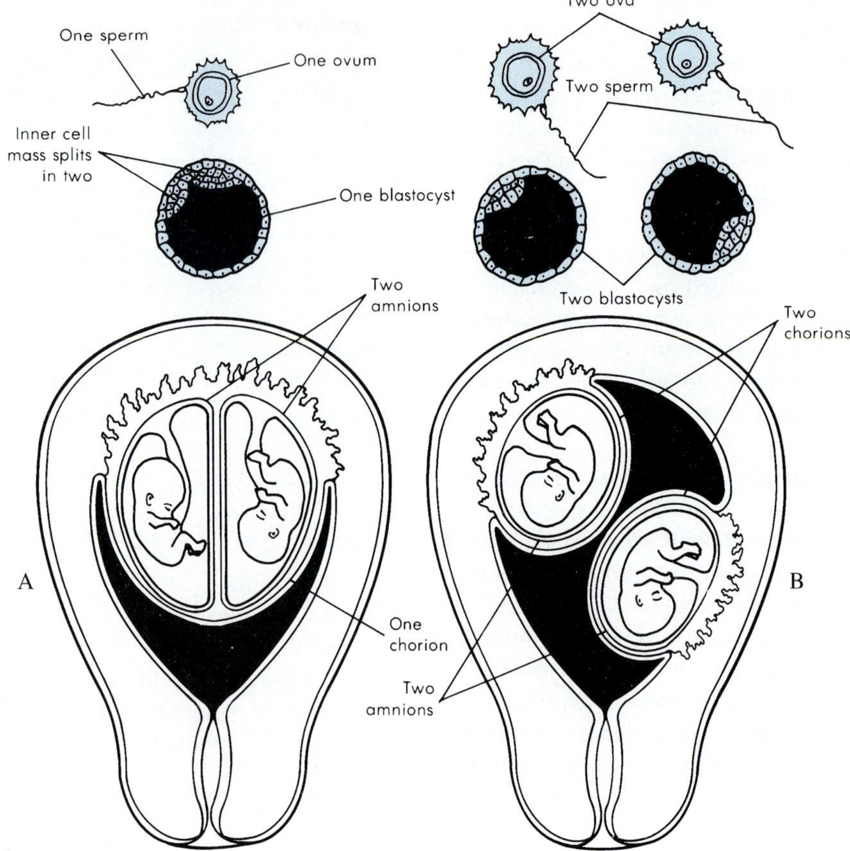

FIG. 42-1 Multiple pregnancies. **A,** Identical twins develop from one ovum and one sperm. **B,** Fraternal twins develop from two ova and two sperm.

growth problems are common in the fetuses. An incomplete separation of the embryonic disk can result in conjoined ("Siamese") twins.

Labor may be complicated by the loss of uterine tone that results from overstretching of the musculature, abnormal presentations, and preterm labor. Many twin pregnancies and almost all pregnancies with more than two fetuses result in the need for a cesarean delivery.

Because of overdistention of the uterus, twins usually deliver before term and have extended hospital stays. Twins may be double joy, but are also double the responsibility and more expensive than one baby. The parents need a great deal of support both before and after the twins arrive. It is possible to breastfeed twins. However, the woman who plans to do this needs help with her many other responsibilities because breastfeeding will consume a great deal of her time.

Clinical Manifestations. Multiple pregnancy is suspected when uterine enlargement exceeds the norm. Abdominal palpation using Leopold's maneuvers, auscultation of two distinct heart tones, and ultrasonography will reveal the presence of multiple fetuses.

BLEEDING DISORDERS

Vaginal bleeding during pregnancy is an indication that problems exist; women should be instructed to contact their physician if any bleeding occurs. Depending on the stage of pregnancy, several different conditions may cause the bleeding. Assessment, diagnostic tests, and nursing interventions for bleeding disorder will be addressed later in the chapter.

ECTOPIC PREGNANCY

Etiology. In ectopic pregnancy implantation occurs somewhere other than within the uterus. The most common site of ectopic implantation is within the fallopian tube. Other possible sites include the abdominal cavity, ovary, ligaments, or cervix (Fig. 42-2).

Ectopic pregnancy occurs when for some reason the progress of the fertilized ovum through the fallopian tube is slowed or obstructed. Pelvic inflammatory disease, resulting in tubal obstruction, is commonly a cause.

Pathophysiology. When the fertilized ovum implants and begins to develop in the fallopian tube, it soon grows

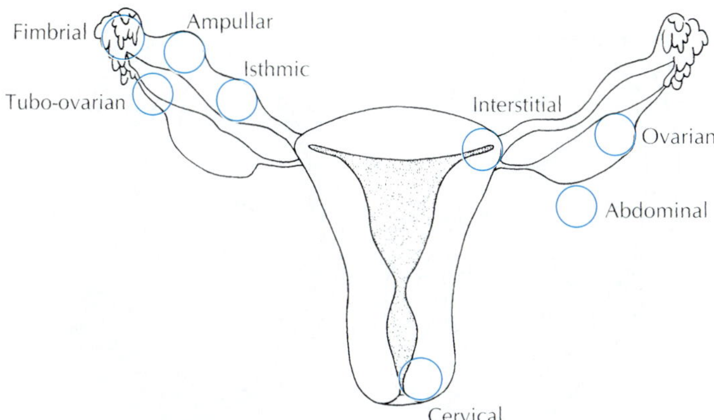

FIG. 42-2 Sites of implantation of ectopic pregnancies in order of frequency of occurrence: ampulla, isthmus, interstitium, fimbria, tuboovarian ligament, ovary, abdominal cavity, and cervix (external os).

to a size too large to be contained. This results in rupture of the tube and bleeding into the abdominal cavity. Approximately 1 out of every 200 pregnancies is ectopic and at least three fourths of those become symptomatic and are diagnosed during the first trimester. Ectopic pregnancy is a significant cause of maternal morbidity and mortality even in developed countries.

Clinical Manifestations. Vaginal bleeding may be observed and hypovolemic shock may be present. Signs of peritoneal irritation include sharp, localized, one-sided pain or pain referred to the shoulder. The abdomen may become rigid and tender.

Medical Management. In the presence of ectopic pregnancy, rapid surgical treatment and blood replacement therapy are almost always indicated.

Prognosis. The prognosis varies. Maternal death from ectopic pregnancy is about 1 in 800 in North America. Maternal morbidity and secondary surgery are high, however, principally because of inaccurate or delayed diagnosis. The physician must rule out uterine abortion, ruptured corpus luteum cyst, appendicitis, salpingitis, ovarian cysts, torsion of the ovary, and urinary tract infection. The perinatal mortality in ectopic pregnancy is virtually 100%. Ectopic pregnancy recurs in approximately 10% of women, but more than 50% of women who have had an ectopic pregnancy achieve at least one normal pregnancy thereafter. The diagnosis and management are rapidly changing as technology improves.

SPONTANEOUS ABORTION

Etiology. Abortion is the termination of pregnancy before the age of viability. Most abortions occur during the first trimester of pregnancy. It is estimated that as many as 20% of all pregnancies end in first-trimester spontaneous abortion. Many of these go unrecognized, with the woman merely thinking that her menstrual period was delayed. There are three types of abortion. Spontaneous abortion results from natural causes; therapeutic abortion is interruption of the pregnancy for medical reasons; and elective abortion is performed for social reasons.

More than half of all spontaneous abortions are caused by abnormal embryonic development, chromosomal defects, and inheritable disorders. Most of the other spontaneous abortions result from maternal causes such as advancing maternal age and parity, chronic infections, chronic debilitating diseases, poor nutrition, and recreational drug use; the reasons for the remainder are speculation. Many early pregnancies abort for unknown reasons before the diagnosis of pregnancy has ever been made.

Pathophysiology. The pathophysiology depends on the specific cause.

Clinical Manifestations. The main presenting symptom is bleeding, which may or may not be accompanied by cramps or backache. Spontaneous abortions are classified as follows:

- *Threatened:* Unexplained bleeding and cramping occur. The fetus may or may not be alive. Membranes remain intact, and the cervical os remains closed.
- *Inevitable:* Bleeding increases and the cervical os begins to dilate. Membranes may rupture.
- *Complete:* All products of conception are expelled from the uterus.
- *Incomplete:* Some, but not all, of the products of conception are expelled.
- *Missed:* The fetus dies and growth ceases, but the fetus remains in utero. Amenorrhea continues, but no uterine growth is measurable. In fact, the uterus may decrease in size.
- *Septic:* Malodorous bleeding, elevated temperature, and cramping may be present; cervical os is opened; and abdominal tenderness may be typical.

Medical Management. IV fluids may be administered, and blood loss may be replaced with transfusions when a spontaneous abortion occurs. A dilation and curettage (D&C) may be indicated to remove retained placental tissue (Box 42-2 on p. 1308).

Patient teaching. Patient teaching should include the need for rest. If significant blood loss occurred, iron supplementation may be ordered (see patient teaching box on p. 1308).

Prognosis. Prognosis is good.

Box 42-2

TYPES OF SPONTANEOUS ABORTION AND THERAPEUTIC MANAGEMENT

Threatened: Bed rest, sedation, and avoidance of stress and orgasm are recommended. Further treatment will depend on patient's course.

Inevitable, Incomplete: Prompt termination of pregnancy is accomplished, usually by D&C.

Complete: No further intervention may be needed if uterine contractions are adequate to prevent hemorrhage and if there is no infection.

Missed: If spontaneous evacuation of the uterus does not occur within 1 month, pregnancy is terminated by method appropriate to duration of pregnancy. Blood clotting factors are monitored until uterus is empty. DIC and incoagulability of blood with uncontrolled hemorrhage may develop in cases of fetal death after twelfth week if products of conception are retained for longer than 5 weeks (see pp. 1310-1311 for discussion of DIC).

Septic: Immediate termination of pregnancy by method appropriate to duration of pregnancy (see Chapter 42). Cervical culture and sensitivity (C&S) studies are done, and broad-spectrum antibiotic therapy (e.g., ampicillin) is started. Treatment for septic shock is initiated if necessary.

PATIENT TEACHING AFTER SPONTANEOUS ABORTION

- Refer to appropriate support groups, clergy, or professional counseling.
- Advise patient to report any heavy, profuse, or bright red bleeding to physician.
- Reassure patient that a scant, dark discharge may persist for 1 to 2 weeks.
- To reduce the risk of infection, remind patient not to introduce anything into the vagina until bleeding has stopped.
- Acknowledge that patient has experienced a loss and that time is required for recovery. She may experience mood swings and depression.

PLACENTA PREVIA

Etiology. Placenta previa occurs when the placenta implants in the lower uterine segment. This may be covering the cervical os completely or marginally (Fig. 42-3, *A*).

Placenta previa is described by the degree to which the placenta covers the internal cervical os: complete or total; partial with incomplete coverage; and marginal, which indicates only an edge of the placenta approaches the internal os. The term *low implantation* is used when the placenta is situated in the lower uterine segment, but away from the internal os.

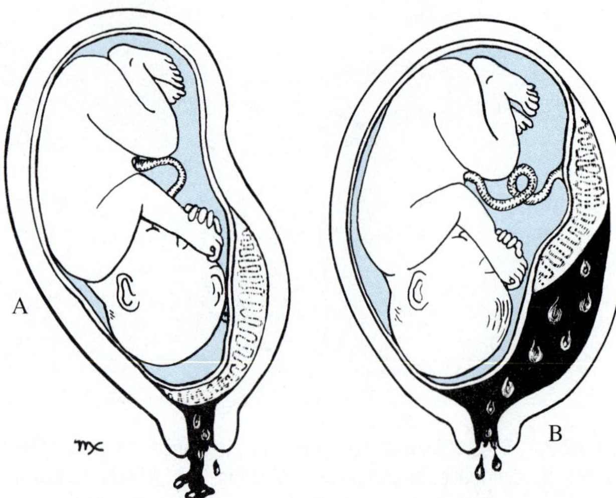

FIG. 42-3 **A,** A type of total placenta previa. **B,** Abruptio placentae, or separation of normally inserted placenta.

In the second trimester approximately 45% of all placentas are implanted in the lower uterine segment. As the lower uterine segment lengthens (stretches), the placenta seems to move upward. By term only 1 placenta in 200 is still a previa. Placentas most likely to remain unchanged are classified as complete.

The cause of placenta previa is unknown. It is more common in multiparas and seems to recur in the same woman. Some sources claim that multifetal pregnancies and uterine scarring from previous surgery are possible factors.

Pathophysiology. In the last trimester of pregnancy, uterine size increases and the cervix begins to dilate. As the placenta separates from the uterus at the internal os of the cervix, sinuses at the site begin to bleed. The amount of bleeding depends on the amount of separation that occurs.

Clinical Manifestations. The main presenting symptom of placenta previa is painless, bright red, vaginal bleeding occurring after 20 weeks' gestation.

The bright red bleeding may be intermittent, may occur in gushes, or more rarely may be continuous. It may start while the patient is resting or in the midst of any activity. Severe hemorrhage almost never occurs unless vaginal or rectal examination initiates violent bleeding before or during early labor.

The detachment of placenta previa is painless. If the first bleeding coincides with the onset of labor, the patient may experience discomfort because of uterine contractions.

Abdominal examination usually will reveal a soft (relaxed), nontender uterus of normal tone.

Obstetrical ultrasound is the diagnostic method of choice. The vaginal examination, known as the *double setup procedure,* is a serious undertaking; it is attempted only if the physician is prepared for the birth. In a double setup procedure, a sterile vaginal examination is performed in an operating room, with personnel and equipment ready to effect an immediate vaginal or cesarean birth. Since manipulation of the lower uterine segment or cervix may result in profound hemorrhage, preparation for immediate delivery is necessary.

Medical Management. Because of the relative safety of cesarean birth today, this is usually the treatment of choice for placenta previa. Some obstetricians may adopt a "wait and see" attitude and eventually deliver the baby vaginally.

Following the diagnosis of placenta previa, the patient should remain in the hospital under close supervision. Blood, typed and cross-matched, is usually available for emergency use. Delivery is delayed, if possible, until after the thirty-sixth week.

Blood loss may cease with delivery of the infant. The interlacing muscle bundles contracting around open vessels so characteristic of the upper part of the uterus are absent in the lower part of the uterus. Therefore postpartum hemorrhage may occur even if the fundus is contracted firmly.

Hemorrhage and the possible results of anemia increase the risk of infection—both placentitis and puerperal (postpartum) infection. If bleeding cannot be controlled, a hysterectomy may be necessary.

Prognosis. Maternal mortality in placenta previa has dropped almost 50%, to about 0.6%, during the past decade in most areas in North America because of conservative therapy. The perinatal mortality (resulting primarily from preterm birth) still approaches 20% in most hospitals.

ABRUPTIO PLACENTAE

Etiology. Abruptio placentae is premature separation of the normally implanted placenta from the uterine wall. This generally occurs late in pregnancy, frequently during labor (Fig. 42-3, *B*).

The cause is unknown. Some predisposing factors include trauma, chronic hypertension, and pregnancy-induced hypertension. Abruptio placentae is three times greater in women with gravidity of more than five. Women who use cocaine during pregnancy have a significant incidence of premature separation of the placenta.

Premature separation of the placenta is a serious disorder and accounts for about 15% of all perinatal deaths. Approximately one third of infants of women with premature separation of the placenta die. More than 50% of these die as a result of preterm delivery, and many others die due to intrauterine hypoxia.

Abruptio placentae occurs in about 1% of all pregnancies.

Pathophysiology. When the placenta separates from the uterine wall, bleeding from uterine sinuses occurs, as in placenta previa. Three major forms of abruptio placentae have been identified.

1. *Central:* Bleeding occurs in the center of the placenta; because the margins of the placenta remain attached, the bleeding is not visible, resulting in a concealed hemorrhage.
2. *Marginal:* Bleeding occurs when an edge of the placenta separates from the uterus; vaginal bleeding is apparent.
3. *Complete:* The entire placenta separates from the uterine wall; vaginal bleeding is profuse.

Clinical Manifestations. The major symptoms of abruptio placentae are sudden, severe pain accompanied by uterine rigidity. The uterus may also increase in size as a result of the hemorrhage. The first sign during labor may be very strong and constant contractions. Symptoms vary with the degree of separation.

Assessment. When any vaginal bleeding occurs during pregnancy, the nurse should assess the following:

1. *The duration, amount, color, and characteristics of the bleeding.* This includes assessing (a) the time since the onset of bleeding; (b) what, if any, activity preceded the bleeding episode; (c) the number of pads saturated per hour; and (d) the color of the bleeding (bright red, dark red, or brown). If any clots or tissue is passed, it should be saved for examination by the physician.
2. *The vital signs.* Depending on the origin and severity of the bleeding, signs of shock may be present. In addition to pulse and blood pressure, it is important to observe for pallor, diaphoresis, cool, clammy skin, or dyspnea. These physical signs will seem out of proportion to the amount of bleeding if the hemorrhage is concealed, as in central abruptio placentae.
3. *Pain.* The nurse should note the location, nature, and duration of pain and whether bleeding is painless. This will help the physician determine the cause of the bleeding.
4. *Fetal heart rate.* Depending on the stage of pregnancy, this may be done with fetoscope or Doppler amplifier. If pregnancy is in the early stages, fetal heart sounds may not be heard. In labor when there is utero placental insufficiency, the fe-

tus, in its struggle to obtain more oxygen, may be very restless and active. The fetal heart rate (FHR) either greatly accelerates or slows.

5. *Emotional response.* The mother's fear for her own life and the life of the fetus is common. Guilt that she did something that caused the bleeding is also common.

Medical Management. Abruptio placentae in its more severe form is an obstetrical emergency. The treatment often, but not always, includes delivery by cesarean birth and blood replacement.

A side-lying position with a wedge placed under the supine patient's right hip facilitates uterine-placental perfusion. Blood loss is restored. Blood and fluid replacement therapy is monitored carefully. A retention catheter is inserted to monitor urine output accurately. The fetus is monitored and delivered when indicated. Hysterectomy may be necessary to control bleeding. Provide emotional support to the patient and family.

Diagnostic Tests. The most common laboratory tests include determination of hemoglobin and hematocrit levels. These tests determine the amount of blood loss. Blood typing and cross-matching of blood for transfusion are ordered in case blood replacement is necessary. Hormone studies may be ordered to determine fetal death. Ultrasound scans may be done to determine placental location. Vaginal and rectal examinations are avoided, because they may cause increased bleeding.

Nursing Interventions. Nursing measures are structured to support and promote optimal physical and psychological functioning.

Oxygen should be available. If blood loss is significant, oxygen-carrying capability is decreased; oxygen may be ordered to prevent maternal or fetal hypoxia.

IV or blood replacement therapy may be required, and the nurse should be prepared for this.

Possible loss of the pregnancy is a crisis. It is important for the nurse to be supportive of the patient's and family's emotional needs. The nurse should remain with the woman as much as possible, listen to her concerns, give clear explanations about medical treatment, and prepare her for the possible loss.

Nursing diagnoses and interventions for the patient with abruptio placentae include but are not limited to the following:

NURSING DIAGNOSES	NURSING INTERVENTIONS
Cardiac output, decreased, related to excessive bleeding secondary to placenta previa	Monitor and record vital signs q 15 min until stable, then q 1 hr as indicated. Measure and record I&O. Weigh daily. Assess skin turgor and mucous membranes. Assist patient to ambulate.
Anticipatory grieving, related to possible loss of pregnancy	Allow time for patient to verbalize concerns about loss. Assist with grieving processes. Encourage contact with support system. Encourage session with spiritual advisor if the patient so desires.
Fear, related to unknown outcome	Allow time to verbalize fears. Maintain continuity of care whenever possible. Involve active participation of significant other.

Prognosis. Maternal mortality approaches 1% in abruptio placentae; this condition remains a leading cause of maternal death. The mother's prognosis depends on the extent of placental detachment, overall blood loss, degree of DIC, and time between the placental separation and delivery.

Fortunately, 80% to 90% of all abruptio placentae involves only two or three placental segments (a normal placenta has 15 to 28 visible segments called **cotyledons:** these segments—each made up of fetal vessels, chorionic villi, and an intervillous space—appear on the maternal surface of the placenta); therefore the prognosis is generally not grave.

Fetal prognosis is poor. At least one third of the babies of mothers with abruptio placentae die before, during, or soon after birth. Some of those who survive are neurologically impaired.

DISSEMINATED INTRAVASCULAR COAGULATION

Etiology. Disseminated intravascular coagulation (DIC) is a potentially life-threatening disorder that results from alterations in the normal clotting mechanism. It may be seen with abruptio placentae, incomplete abortion, hypertensive disease, or infectious process.

Pathophysiology. As a result of stressing the coagulation processes in an attempt to prevent excessive blood loss, the body produces excessive amounts of thrombin, stimulating the conversion of fibrinogen to fibrin. Elevated fibrin levels result in multiple small clots forming in small blood vessels, which may lead to obstruction of vessels, ischemia, and damage to vital organs. This clot formation also traps platelets and can result in generalized hemorrhage.

Clinical Manifestations. The onset of symptoms is sudden. The patient may complain of chest pain or dyspnea and become extremely restless and cyanotic, occasionally expectorating frothy, blood-tinged mucus. Profound circulatory shock from hemorrhage may occur rapidly. Fetal and maternal death may occur.

Assessment. All women with complications that may result in DIC should be observed closely for signs of bleeding such as epistaxis (nosebleeds), bleeding gums, or petechiae, particularly around the blood-pressure cuff on the patient's arm. The maternal and fetal conditions should continue to be monitored by assessment of vital signs, FHR, and I&O and by general careful assessment.

Diagnostic Tests. Blood testing includes determination of hemoglobin and hematocrit. Clotting factor studies, such as fibrinogen levels, platelet counts, prothrombin time (PT), and partial thromboplastin time (PTT), are typically ordered for the patient. Laboratory tests may reveal various degrees of anemia and decreased fibrinogen and platelet counts. Prolonged PT and PTT are also typical.

Medical Management. Emergency care for DIC includes IV administration of fibrinogen, blood, and other substances that will help restore normal clotting mechanisms. Paradoxically, DIC therapy may include heparin by continuous infusion pump and oxygen therapy by a tight-fitting mask at 10 to 12 L per minute. If the fetus is not yet born, delivery should occur as soon as possible. Urinary output is monitored carefully (urinary output must be maintained at more than 30 ml per hour) since renal failure is one consequence of DIC.

Nursing Interventions. Nursing interventions are directed at supporting medical treatment. Signs and symptoms must be reported promptly and completely. Caution should be used when providing care to minimize the risk of additional trauma to tissue, which may lead to further bleeding. The emotional needs of the patient and the family are recognized and supported by the nurse.

A nursing diagnosis and interventions for the patient with DIC include but are not limited to the following:

NURSING DIAGNOSIS	NURSING INTERVENTIONS
Gas exchange, impaired, high risk for, related to impaired oxygen-carrying capacity of the blood resulting from hemorrhage.	Move patient slowly to prevent orthostatic hypotension. Avoid trauma during care. Check entire body for signs of bleeding. Monitor vital signs and laboratory values; report deviations from normal promptly. Monitor urinary output closely. Monitor fluid and blood replacement therapy as ordered. Administer anticoagulants per protocol.

Prognosis. Prognosis depends on the degree and extent of the underlying disorder as well as the response of the woman to prompt and proper treatment.

POSTBIRTH HEMORRHAGE

Etiology. Postbirth hemorrhage occurs in two stages. Early postpartum hemorrhage is blood loss greater than 500 ml in the first 24 hours after delivery; late postpartum hemorrhage occurs after the first 24 hours. At least 5% of women suffer postbirth hemorrhage.

The most common causes of early hemorrhage are (1) uterine **atony** (lack of normal tone or strength), often related to excessive distention of the uterus from multiple pregnancy, hydramnios (excessive amount of amniotic fluid), or a very large infant. Atony is also more common in grand multiparas or in cases in which labor has been prolonged or traumatic; (2) retained placenta or fragments of the placenta; and (3) lacerations of the perineum. The most common cause of late postpartum hemorrhage is retained fragments of the placenta. See Box 42-3 for more risk factors of postbirth hemorrhage.

Pathophysiology. The major action that prevents hemorrhage is contraction of the uterus, which seals off the uterine sinuses. Hemorrhage results when loss of tone or tissue remaining in the cavity prevents adequate contraction of the uterus.

Assessment. Nursing assessment of uterine contraction and lochia is part of routine postpartum assessment. If the uterus is found to be boggy or if the flow of lochia is heavy, hemorrhage should be suspected. Vital signs may also change if blood loss is substantial. Any alteration noted should be reported promptly.

Postbirth hemorrhage can progress rapidly to shock; therefore, the nurse must assess the patient carefully and

Box 42-3 RISK FACTORS FOR POSTBIRTH HEMORRHAGE

Cesarean birth
Birth of a large infant
Birth assisted by forceps or vacuum extractor
Overdistended uterus from hydramnios, multifetal gestations, large fetus
Intrauterine manipulation/manual removal of the placenta
Lacerations of the birth canal
Magnesium sulfate administration during labor or postpartum
Multiparity
Previous postbirth hemorrhage
Placental abruption, retained placental fragments
Pitocin-induced/augmented labor
Uterine atony
Uterine inversion
Uterine subinvolution

thoroughly. The history should be reviewed for factors that predispose to postbirth hemorrhage (see Box 42-3).

The bleeding color, amount, and if possible, source should be assessed. Vital signs may not be reliable indicators of shock in the immediate postpartum period because of physiological adaptations of this stage. Data should include assessment for bladder distention, because a distended bladder prevents uterine contractions.

Medical Management. The medical treatment for retained placental fragments is D&C, whereby the retained tissue is surgically removed. Blood transfusions are administered if hemorrhage is severe.

Nursing Interventions. Nursing interventions are directed at reducing blood loss. Initial care includes fundal massage; normally this increases the uterine tone and decreases bleeding. If the uterus remains atonic, the physician typically prescribes an oxytocin. Vital signs should be monitored carefully when oxytocin is administered. If bleeding continues, one may suspect that placental fragments have been retained. If a D&C is required, the nurse prepares the patient for surgery. Explanations of the necessity of surgery should be given to reduce apprehension. Consent forms must be signed and all other surgical preparations completed. (See Chapter 22 for presurgical and postsurgical interventions.)

Nursing diagnoses and interventions for the patient with postbirth hemorrhage include but are not limited to the following:

NURSING DIAGNOSES	NURSING INTERVENTIONS
Cardiac output decreased, related to postpartum blood loss	Monitor vital signs until stable, and vaginal flow has diminished. Measure and record I&O. Increase activity level slowly to avoid fatigue. Administer oxygen as needed. Encourage fluids po unless contraindicated.
Fear, related to possible surgical intervention	Allow opportunities to verbalize fears. Explain all treatments and procedures. Maintain continuity of care. Include significant others.
Knowledge deficit, related to signs of hemorrhage	Select teaching strategies appropriate to patient's need and willingness to learn. Demonstrate postpartum checks of fundus and lochia. Observe patient performing self-check. Review importance of contacting the physician if signs are abnormal or questionable.
Fluid volume deficit, related to hypovolemia secondary to excessive blood loss	Perform fundal massage until firm. Monitor vital signs and I&O closely. Assess blood loss by pad saturation. Monitor for signs and symptoms of infection. Monitor IV therapy as ordered. Teach patient fundal massage.

Patient Teaching. Because today's patients leave the hospital in a relatively short time, it is important to teach the patient how to perform the postpartum checks of the fundus and lochia. They should be aware that it is important to call the physician if bleeding is excessive or persists longer than expected.

Prognosis. Although all possible medical, surgical, and nursing interventions are attempted, there still may be maternal or neonatal mortality.

PREGNANCY-INDUCED HYPERTENSION

Etiology. **Pregnancy-induced hypertension (PIH)** (disease encountered during pregnancy or early in the puerperium, characterized by increasing hypertension, albuminuria, and generalized edema; also classified as preeclampsia, and if untreated may progress to eclampsia), is a serious complication of pregnancy and places both the mother and fetus at risk.

The cause of PIH is unknown. Many theories have been proposed, but to date none have been proven. This condition was formerly called *toxemia,* because it was once thought that a toxin caused the symptoms. This condition is seen most often in primigravidas, particularly those under 20 or over 35 years of age. It is also more common in women from lower socioeconomic groups or individuals with poor nutritional status. A woman with a multiple pregnancy, diabetes mellitus, or family history of PIH is also at increased risk. PIH is a disease process unique to pregnancy. The only known "cure" is termination of the pregnancy.

Pathophysiology. Complex hormonal and vascular changes occur with PIH; these lead to increased blood pressure, decreased placental perfusion, decreased renal perfusion, altered glomerular filtration rate, and fluid and electrolyte imbalance.

Clinical Manifestations. The classic signs of PIH, in order of appearance, are (1) edema, (2) hypertension, and (3) proteinuria. These signs generally appear after the twentieth week of pregnancy (Box 42-4). PIH is a progressive disease. Depending on the severity of the symptoms, PIH is classified as preeclampsia (which is further subdivided into mild or severe forms) and eclampsia.

Mild preeclampsia. There are few clinical symptoms in early **preeclampsia.** Change in the blood pressure readings—an increase of 30 mm Hg systolic and 15 mm Hg diastolic or a reading of 140/90 in a woman who has had normal blood pressure readings—indicates a problem. This is the reason it is important to establish baseline readings early in pregnancy. Generalized edema may be evident in the face, hands, and ankles. Weight may increase as much as 3 lb (1.5 kg) per month in the

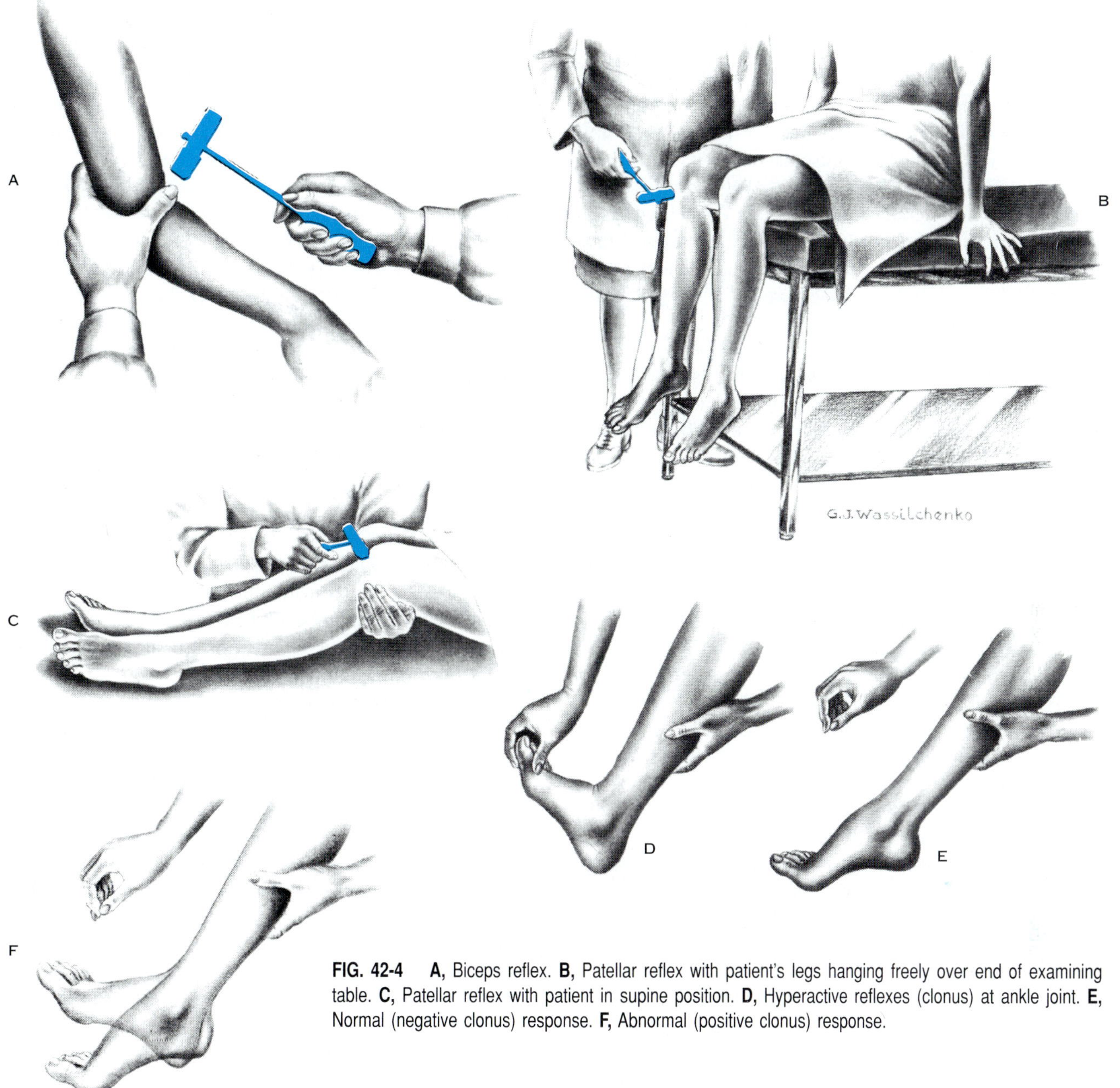

FIG. 42-4 **A,** Biceps reflex. **B,** Patellar reflex with patient's legs hanging freely over end of examining table. **C,** Patellar reflex with patient in supine position. **D,** Hyperactive reflexes (clonus) at ankle joint. **E,** Normal (negative clonus) response. **F,** Abnormal (positive clonus) response.

second trimester and 1 lb (0.5 kg) per week in the third trimester. Urine testing frequently shows 1+ to 2+ albumin readings. The urine output is not less than 500 ml/24 hours.

Severe preeclampsia. The symptoms of severe preeclampsia may appear suddenly. Blood pressure readings increase, and readings of 160/110 or higher on two separate occasions 6 hours apart with the pregnant woman on bed rest are common. Edema becomes increasingly obvious and may be observed in the face, hands, sacral area, abdomen, and throughout the lower extremities. Weight increases dramatically. As much as 2

Box 42-4 WARNING SIGNS OF PREECLAMPSIA

- Rapid rise in blood pressure
- Rapid gain in weight
- Generalized edema
- Increase in proteinuria
- Epigastric pain
- Marked hyperreflexia (Fig. 42-4, *D* through *F*), especially transient or sustained ankle clonus
- Severe headaches
- Visual disturbance
- Oliguria with urinary output of <120 ml in 4 hours
- Irritability, transient mental changes
- Nausea and vomiting, severe

lb (1 kg) can be gained in a matter of a few days or a week. Urine testing for albumin shows 3+ to 4+ readings. The urine output is less than 500 ml/24 hours.

Eclampsia. **Eclampsia** is the most severe form of pregnancy-induced hypertension. The most dramatic characteristic is grand mal seizures, with *tonic* (pertaining to or characterized by muscular tension) and *clonic* (spasmodic alternation of muscular contractions) phases. This is generally followed by a coma that lasts from minutes to hours. It is also characterized by elevated blood pressure, albuminuria, and oliguria. If untreated, this sequence of seizure-coma may repeat, and death may follow.

Assessment. Blood pressure should be assessed routinely throughout pregnancy, labor, delivery, and the postpartum period. It is important to remember that PIH can occur anytime after the twentieth week and persist until 2 days after delivery. Weight should be recorded at each prenatal visit and compared with norms. Excessive or rapid weight gain, particularly when accompanied by edema, should be reported promptly. Assessment for edema should be done at each visit. Edema is typically described using a scale of 1+ to 4+:

- 1+ Minimal edema on pedal and pretibial area
- 2+ Obvious edema of lower extremities
- 3+ Edema of face, hands, sacrum, and abdomen observed (see Chapter 28, Fig. 28-22)
- 4+ Indicates massive, generalized edema **(anasarca)**

Urine is typically tested for albumin using dipstick reagents. This should be done at each visit and on admission for labor. (If the bag of waters is ruptured, these dipstick readings may be inaccurate.) Questions about the occurrence of headaches, visual disturbance, or epigastric pain should be routinely asked, because these may also indicate problems with PIH.

If the patient is hospitalized for PIH, deep tendon reflexes (Table 42-1 and Fig. 42-4, *A* through *C*) and urinary output are monitored, as well as electronic monitoring of FHR.

Diagnostic Tests. Typical tests include hematocrit, BUN, and urine tests for specific gravity and protein. Often a 24-hour urine collection is obtained to measure creatinine and protein clearance. Electrolyte panels are commonly drawn. If symptoms indicate severe preeclampsia or eclampsia, liver function and platelet count evaluations are also done. If the physician determines that early induction of labor is required, tests for fetal maturity including estriol levels, amniocentesis, ultrasonography, and stress tests may be done.

Medical Management. The woman may or may not need to be hospitalized depending on the severity of symptoms. Very mild preeclampsia may be managed at home, but more severe symptoms require that the woman be hospitalized. Typically bed rest is ordered, preferably in the left lateral recumbent position, which will reduce pressure on the inferior vena cava and promote venous return. A well-balanced diet with adequate protein is important. Moderate sodium intake is allowed, but high-sodium foods should be avoided. Meals are allowed as long as the woman is alert and there are no signs of impending convulsions. IV therapy may be initiated to keep a line open for emergency medications. IV electrolytes may also be administered. In cases of severe preeclampsia or eclampsia, medications may be prescribed. Magnesium sulfate ($MgSO_4$) may be prescribed parenterally to prevent seizures in preeclampsia. Sedatives and antihypertensives may also be ordered (see medication table for drugs for the mother and newborn at risk).

Nursing Interventions. The goal of nursing interventions is to be alert for signs and symptoms of preeclampsia, such as complaints of headache, edema, and blurred vision.

In mild cases routine I&O is monitored; in severe cases it may be necessary to insert an indwelling catheter and record hourly urine output. Fetal condition must be monitored carefully. In mild cases routine auscultation of FHR is adequate; in severe cases fetal monitors will give more accurate information.

It is important to monitor I&O levels carefully to avoid fluid overload from IV infusions as well as magnesium sulfate toxicity (Box 42-5 on p. 1316).

Some practitioners request a **kick count,** a daily counting of fetal movements felt in 1 hour while the mother is resting. Fetal activity under three counts per hour is considered serious and needs to be reported. Fetal activity decreases if hypoxia develops.

Daily weight is recorded to determine the amount of fluids eliminated from the body. I&O should be recorded. Blood pressure is monitored every 4 hours or more frequently if condition indicates. The nurse who is alert to encouraging compliance of treatment can be instrumental in preventing the patient from convulsing. Since stress may exacerbate this condition, it is important to keep the environment quiet and nonstressful. Maintaining a stress-free environment is difficult, however, because enforced bed rest may last for several

TABLE 42-1 Assessing Deep Tendon Reflexes

Degree	Grading
Brisk with sustained clonus	5+
Hyperactive response (brisk with transient clonus)	4+
More than normal (brisk)	3+
Normal, active	2+
Low response (sluggish or dull)	1+
No response	0

MEDICATIONS FOR THE MOTHER AND NEWBORN AT RISK

Medication	Trade Name	Action	Side Effects	Nursing Implication
Acyclovir	Zovirax	Antiviral	Topical—stinging, burning, rash, pruritus; systemic—headache, seizures, renal toxicity, phlebitis at IV site	Topical—use glove to apply, cover lesion completely; systemic—ensure adequate hydration to prevent crystallization in kidneys, give IV dose for 1 hr.
Hepatitis B immune globulin (HBIG)	H-BIG, HyperHep, others	Immune globulin that provides passive immunity to hepatitis B virus	Tenderness, pain, and muscle stiffness at injection site; fever; chills; nausea; vomiting; myalgias; hypersensitivity reactions; anaphylaxis	Administer intramuscularly only (severe systemic reactions may occur if given intravenously); do not mix product with any other medications.
Lung surfactant	Exosurf—synthetic (colfosceril palmitate) Survanta—natural lung surfactant (beractant)	Replaces natural lung surfactant that maintains lung inflation and prevents lung collapse, used to treat and prevent respiratory distress syndrome in premature neonates	Synthetic—apnea, pulmonary hemorrhage, pulmonary air leak; natural—transient bradycardia, oxygen desaturation, hypotension, apnea	Administer endotracheally only; suction before administration (drug may reflux into endotracheal tube during administration); slow or stop administration until tube is clear.
Magnesium sulfate	Many	Seizure prevention in preeclampsia or eclampsia, also used to prevent premature labor, serum magnesium replacement	Flushing, bradycardia, sweating, depressed reflexes, muscle flaccidity progressing to paralysis	Monitor serum magnesium concentrations and clinical status to minimize toxicity; use caution when giving to patients with renal impairment.
Oxytocin	Pitocin	Oxytocic, stimulates uterine contraction	Mother—nausea, vomiting, uterine spasm or rupture, water intoxication, seizures, cardiac dysrhythmias, hypotension; fetus—cardiac dysrhythmias, CNS or brain damage.	Monitor intake and output carefully; monitor fetal heart tones and length, and duration; monitor force of uterine contractions carefully.
RH_O (D) Immune globulin	RhoGAM, others	Suppresses immune response of RH-antigen negative mothers exposed to Rh-positive blood	Local reaction at the injection site, myalgias, fatigue, lethargy, rare allergic reactions	Give within 72 hr of exposure; confirm that the mother is Rh-negative; give intramuscularly only.
Ritodrine	Yutopar	Tocolytic agent used for preterm labor, causes uterine relaxation	Tachycardia, hyperglycemia, anxiety, nervousness, tremor, nausea, vomiting, hypotension, cardiac dysrhythmias, hypokalemia	Monitor maternal and fetal heart tones; monitor uterine contractions during administration.
Rubella vaccine	Meruvax II	Live virus vaccine that provides active immunity to rubella	Local burning, stinging, and pain; induration; fever; influenza-like syndrome; rare hypersensitivity	Administer subcutaneously, not intravenously; do not give to patients who are immunosuppressed, pregnant, or have ongoing infectious process.

Box 42-5 DANGER SIGNS OF MAGNESIUM SULFATE TOXICITY

- Sudden hypotension
- Urinary output less than 30 ml/hr
- Respiration less than 12/min
- Hyporeflexia, absence of reflexes
- Toxic serum levels
- Sudden decrease in FHR

Box 42-6 HOSPITAL PRECAUTIONARY MEASURES

- Environment: quiet, nonstimulating, lighting subdued
- Seizure precautions: padded side rails, suction and oxygen administration equipment ready to use
- Call button within easy reach
- Emergency medication tray immediately accessible
  - Hydralazine (antihypertensive vasodilator) and magnesium sulfate in or adjacent to woman's room
  - Calcium gluconate immediately available in a well-labeled syringe at the bedside as an antidote to $MgSO_4$ toxicity
- Emergency delivery pack accessible

weeks. Enforced bed rest or hospitalization can be very disruptive for the patient and her family; there are financial implications, and the woman's condition can seriously affect family dynamics. Explanations of the necessity of treatment and clarification of care and treatment are essential. See Box 42-6 for hospital precautionary measures.

Nursing diagnoses and interventions for the patient with PIH include but are not limited to the following:

NURSING DIAGNOSES	NURSING INTERVENTIONS
Family processes, altered, related to protracted physical illness	Involve patient in family decision making whenever possible. Encourage family members to verbalize feelings about inability of wife/mother to participate in family activities.
Diversional activity deficit, related to environmental lack of stimulation	Elicit hobbies or interests that can be performed while at rest. Involve patient in conversation while performing care. Encourage family to visit and bring books or other recreational items. Provide change of scenery if possible. Encourage relaxation techniques. Encourage listening to music.
Knowledge deficit, related to treatment	Emphasize positive aspects of compliance. Explain importance of compliance to positive resolution of problem. Give positive reinforcement for compliant behavior. Determine values that lead to noncompliance. Keep couple informed about the management and progress of patient's condition.

Patient teaching. All pregnant women must be taught the danger signs of pregnancy and the importance of regular medical supervision. Many of the symptoms of PIH, particularly the mild, early symptoms, will only be detected by maintaining regular physician contact. If PIH is diagnosed, it is important to explain the consequences of failure to comply.

High-quality protein, vitamin, and mineral intake should be encouraged. Salt restriction below the normal dietary levels (4 to 6 g/24 hr) is usually not recommended.

It is important that the patient understand that bed rest is vital because it slows metabolism of the body and relieves edema.

Prognosis. Immediate and continuous care by the obstetrical team is mandatory to prevent maternal and fetal morbidity and mortality.

HELLP Syndrome. The HELLP syndrome (H, hemolysis; EL, elevated liver enzymes; LP, low platelet count) represents an extension of the pathology of severe preeclampsia and eclampsia. The initial symptoms of the HELLP syndrome usually appear early in the third trimester.

For a woman to be diagnosed as having the HELLP syndrome, her platelet count must be $<100,000/mm^3$, her liver enzyme levels must be elevated (AST and ALT), and some evidence for intravascular hemolysis must be present. The hemolysis accounts for the large drop in hematocrit, out of proportion to blood loss, that occurs in most new mothers with HELLP syndrome during the postpartum period. A unique form of coagulopathy (not DIC) occurs with the HELLP syndrome.

Recognition of the clinical and laboratory findings of the HELLP syndrome is important if early, aggressive therapy is to be initiated to prevent maternal and neonatal mortality.

An unfavorable (uneffaced and undilated) cervix and the aggressive nature of this disorder support cesarean birth. Prolonged induction of labor could increase maternal morbidity. Fresh-frozen plasma may be needed if bleeding occurs and persists. The major laboratory manifestations of the disease, however, may not appear until the early postpartum period (48 to 72 hours). Delayed transfusion of packed red blood cells (RBCs) often is necessary because of the continued hemolysis. It is important to attempt to lower the blood pressure if the diastolic pressure is consistently greater than 110 mm Hg. However, blood pressure may be normal or slightly elevated; thus it is not an adequate indicator of the severity of the disease. Hypoglycemia may be present in the woman with HELLP syndrome and, when the blood sugar is less than 40 mg/dl, is associated with a high maternal mortality.

COMPLICATIONS RELATED TO INFECTIOUS PROCESSES

Both mother and fetus must be considered in the assessment of maternal infection. In some diseases, such as tuberculosis, the fetus almost always is spared, even though the mother may be dying. With other infections, such as rubella, the fetus may be critically compromised, whereas the mother may be only slightly ill.

Pregnancy is generally regarded as an immunosuppressed condition. That a fetus is not rejected during pregnancy still remains an immunological mystery. Altered immune responses during pregnancy may decrease maternal ability to fight infection. In addition, genital tract changes may affect susceptibility. As pregnancy advances, vaginal walls engorge and the cervix enlarges. These intravaginal changes, accompanied by decreasing vaginal pH, may contribute to susceptibility.

Some consequences of maternal infection—such as infertility and sterility—last a lifetime. Psychosocial problems as a result of maternal infections may include altered interpersonal relationships and lowered self-esteem. Other conditions, such as a congenitally acquired infection, often affect a child's length and quality of life.

Education and counseling are important aspects of care for the prevention of maternal infections. Adolescent mothers are at risk because of earlier onset of intercourse and increased likelihood of multiple partners. The recent trend of exchanging sex for drugs is contributing to a rise in infection rates, especially among urban, poor, and minority women.

The prevention of disease and reduction of maternal and neonatal complications continue to be enormous challenges. Many microorganisms can increase maternal and fetal risk. Many studies show an increase in mortality and morbidity when infection is present; thus it is important to prevent infection. If not prevented, infections should be recognized and treated promptly.

*T*oxoplasmosis, *o*ther infections such as hepatitis, *r*ubella virus, *c*ytomegalovirus, and *h*erpes simplex viruses, known collectively as **TORCH** infections, comprise a group of organisms capable of crossing the placenta and adversely affecting the development of the fetus (Box 42-7 on p. 1318).

Transmission of human immunodeficiency virus (HIV), a retrovirus, occurs primarily through the exchange of body fluids. Severe depression of the cellular immune system characterizes acquired immunodeficiency syndrome (AIDS) (see Chapter 37). Although the populations at high risk have been well documented, all women should be assessed for the possibility of HIV exposure. HIV infection in women is commonly reported at a later stage in the disease, and they usually enter the hospital for initiation of treatment when the illness is more severe. The delay may be due in part to the fact that the symptoms are different from those in men. Chronic vaginitis and candidiasis are common presenting problems (Box 42-8 on p. 1319).

Etiology. The infectious diseases that may cause complications are numerous. While some are airborne or ingested, most are spread by direct contact, usually through sexual transmission (see Chapter 33 for further discussion of sexually transmitted diseases). Others are contracted by use of contaminated needles or blood transfusions.

Nursing Interventions. The presence of infection is not always evident. Because of the increased incidence of serious infectious diseases, the Centers for Disease Control and Prevention (CDC) recommends that universal precautions be taken for all patients. These precautions are most important when dealing with blood and body fluids. When providing care to mothers and newborns the nurse is frequently exposed to blood and body fluids and must be particularly alert. Use of gloves, masks, gowns, and glasses is necessary when procedures that involve splashing of body fluids, such as amniotomy, are performed. Gloves should be used when cleaning or assessing the breasts or perineal area. Gloves should also be used when bathing the newborn. Thorough hand washing, as always, is essential. Suctioning or resuscitation of the infant should be done using mechanical barriers or equipment such as mouth shields, suction devices, and ventilators. Care should be used when handling needles and syringes; these should be disposed of in special containers without breaking or recapping.

Psychological support is important to the patient with an infectious disease. Because many of these diseases are life threatening to the mother, fetus, or newborn, fear and anxiety are common. If the infection results in fetal mortality or defects, guilt may be expressed by the mother. The nurse must also cope with her own feelings about these serious infectious diseases. Caring for mothers and newborns with AIDS and other such diseases can create many moral and ethical problems that must be resolved if the nurse is to function therapeutically.

A nursing diagnosis and interventions for the patient with an infectious disease include but are not limited to the following:

Box 42-7 TORCH INFECTIONS

T—Toxoplasmosis is caused by a protozoan, *Toxoplasma gondii,* which can be contracted by eating raw, contaminated meats or having contact with the feces of infected cats. Toxoplasmosis is one of the common accompanying opportunistic infections of AIDS. The mother may be free of symptoms or may develop myalgia, enlarged posterior cervical lymph nodes, malaise, and rash that disappear in a matter of days. Diagnosis is confirmed by blood studies, and women in at-risk groups should have toxoplasmosis titer evaluated. The effects on the fetus can be profound: spontaneous abortion, stillbirth, neonatal death, blindness, retardation, and a wide range of congenital anomalies that are associated with the disease. It is important to teach all pregnant women to avoid undercooked meats. If cats are present in the environment, the woman should wear gloves whenever chance of contact with feces exists. Acute infection in pregnancy produces flulike symptoms and lymphadenopathy. The medication of choice is sulfa, or clindamycin in sulfa-allergic patients.

O—Other: The primary infection included in this category is hepatitis. Hepatitis A is a virus spread by droplets or hands and is associated with poor hand washing after defecation. Pregnancy effects include spontaneous abortion and influenza-like signs and symptoms: fever, malaise, and nausea. If exposure to the fetus occurs in the first trimester and is untreated, possible effects include fetal anomalies, preterm birth, fetal or neonatal hepatitis, and intrauterine death. Gamma globulin vaccination is given to mothers and newborns for prophylaxis.

Hepatitis B is a virus transmitted in a manner similar to that of HIV. Routes of transmission include contaminated needles, syringes, or blood products; sexual intercourse; and body fluid exchange (see Chapter 27 for further discussion).

During pregnancy, common signs and symptoms include fever, rash, anorexia, malaise, myalgias, and jaundice if the liver is acutely affected. Fetal and newborn effects are the same as listed for hepatitis A. Populations at risk should be given the hepatitis B vaccine. Vaccination during pregnancy is not thought to pose risk to the fetus by some sources. Many factors need to be taken into consideration when making the decision to administer the vaccine to the pregnant patient. Neonates exposed in utero should be given the vaccine following birth.

This group also includes the miscellaneous infections that may affect the mother and/or fetus. Urinary tract and vaginal infections can cause fever, chills, dysuria, pain, malaise, and changes in vaginal drainage. Any of these symptoms should be reported promptly to the physician. Culture and sensitivity tests will usually reveal the specific organism. The physician will base treatment on the causative organism and the severity of the problem. Treatment must be done cautiously because of the possibility of teratogenic effects from the antibiotics. Sexually transmitted diseases (STDs) are also a serious concern. Syphilis can also cross the placental barrier and infect the fetus. Chlamydia may cause pneumonia or eye infections in the newborn. Gonorrhea can cause pelvic inflammatory disease (PID) in the mother and eye infections in the newborn.

R—Rubella, German measles, or 3-day measles. A viral infection transmitted by droplets. Fever, rash, and mild lymphedema usually are seen in the affected mother. If contracted during the first trimester, rubella can have profound effects on the fetus. A wide range of congenital defects, including congenital heart disease, mental retardation, and cataracts, may result. Diagnosis is made by serological tests for rubella titer. Immunization should ideally be given before a woman reaches childbearing age. If a pregnant woman does not have immunity, she should be cautioned to avoid risk of exposure to the disease. Because this immunization involves administration of an attenuated (diluted to reduce virulence of pathogenic microorganism) virus, it is given after delivery, frequently just before discharge. This is one time the physician can be certain that the woman is not pregnant. The woman should be further cautioned to avoid becoming pregnant for 2 to 3 months after vaccination, since the attenuated virus used for immunization may still be present in the mother.

C—Cytomegalovirus (CMV) is viral and belongs to the herpesvirus group. It is a very common infection that can be spread by close contact, breastfeeding, sexual relations, and kissing. More than half of all adults have antibodies to the virus. This virus is capable of crossing the placental barrier and causing serious damage to the fetus, including cognitive impairment, hearing problems, and congenital anomalies. It is unusual in that the mother may be totally asymptomatic and that it does not always cause fetal complications. Pregnant health care providers should carefully observe universal precautions to avoid exposure to droplets of infected secretions such as saliva, urine, and respiratory discharges.

H—Herpes genitalis, also called herpesvirus type 2, causes painful lesions on the external genitals and can also involve the cervix. Intrauterine infection of the fetus can occur if the membranes rupture or vaginal delivery takes place when active lesions are present. If the virus is not treated, the neonatal mortality rate is extremely high. Diagnosis is made on the basis of maternal symptoms and a culture of the lesions. Women with active herpes infection should be delivered by cesarean birth. The pregnancy effects of primary genital herpes infection include spontaneous abortion, preterm labor, and intrauterine growth retardation. Health care providers with herpes simplex virus (HSV) infections should take precautions. Anyone with oral HSV lesions should wear a mask if in close contact with newborns, and anyone with skin lesions should not give direct care until lesions are dried and crusted. Scrupulous hand washing is essential.

Box 42-8 AIDS

Acquired immunodeficiency syndrome is a major health concern today. It has had a significant impact on all areas of health care, including maternal nursing. The causative organism is the human immunodeficiency virus (HIV) which enters the body through blood, blood products, or sexual contact. It is capable of crossing the placental barrier and infecting the fetus in utero, causing congenital defects such as microcephaly (abnormal smallness of the head) and facial deformities. Because of the long incubation period, infants born to HIV seropositive mothers may show no indication at birth but develop signs of the infection later. These include failure to thrive, recurrent infection, interstitial pneumonia, neurological abnormalities, and others. Studies place the risk of perinatal transmission at 20% to 50%. Most children diagnosed with AIDS die within the first few years of life.

NURSING DIAGNOSIS	NURSING INTERVENTIONS
Infection, high risk for, related to external factors	Practice good hand washing technique and correct use of protective gloving. Monitor vital signs, particularly temperature, every 4 hr. Observe for any drainage or discharge. Teach patient signs and symptoms of infection. Teach patient to apply clean pad and to remove soiled pad from front to back. Assess for adequate nutritional intake. Encourage fluid intake. Teach patient correct technique for perineal care following each voiding or bowel movement.

Patient teaching. Education on prevention of infection should start long before pregnancy. Infections acquired by a woman before she becomes pregnant can seriously affect the outcome of pregnancy. Immunization for rubella before childbearing years is essential, and the importance of having children routinely immunized should be stressed to all new mothers. Such hygiene practices as careful handwashing and proper storage and preparation of meats should be reviewed. Safe sex practices, including use of condoms, should be discussed with at-risk individuals, and the importance of regular medical care and treatment should be stressed.

Counseling the pregnant woman with a vaginal infection should also include measures to deal with the discomfort, such as:

- Pouring warm water over the urethra and vulva
- Urinating through an empty toilet paper tube
- Warm sitz baths for 15 minutes three to five times daily
- Avoiding strong deodorant soaps, creams, and ointments
- Drying the genital area with a blow dryer
- Using 100% cotton underwear
- Avoid tight fitting jeans
- Avoiding panties or panty hose with nylon inserts
- Obtaining early and regular Papanicolaou (Pap) smears
- Avoiding any sexual contact during outbreaks

Prognosis. The success of the prevention measures depends on the conscious effort of the health care worker in carrying out all recommended procedures carefully.

COMPLICATIONS RELATED TO EXISTING MEDICAL CONDITIONS

Diabetes Mellitus

Etiology. Diabetes mellitus is an endocrine disorder that affects metabolism and the utilization of glucose (see Chapter 32). This disease is not curable and is often difficult to control in the nonpregnant patient. In pregnancy, hormonal changes and stresses placed on all the maternal body systems result in even more complex medical and nursing management. According to recent studies, diabetes is a risk factor in approximately 1% to 2% of pregnancies.

Pathophysiology. In diabetes mellitus the pancreas does not produce adequate amounts of insulin to metabolize glucose normally. Because glucose does not enter the cells without adequate insulin, blood glucose levels remain high. The cells release stored fat and protein for energy, leading to ketosis and a negative nitrogen balance.

Various forms of this disease have been classified. Type I, insulin-dependent diabetes mellitus (IDDM), requires regular administration of insulin for control. Type II, non-insulin-dependent diabetes mellitus (NIDDM), is most often controlled by diet or oral hypoglycemics. **Gestational diabetes mellitus** (GDM) is characterized by abnormal glucose metabolism, which is manifested only during pregnancy. A significant number of women who fall into this category will later manifest NIDDM (see Chapter 32).

Clinical Manifestations. Alteration in blood glucose levels is the major manifestation of the disease. Blood glucose levels above 120 mg/dl significantly increase the risk of complications. When blood glucose levels are elevated, the classic symptoms of diabetes may be observed: polyuria, polydipsia, and polyphagia.

Effects on pregnancy. Improved control of this disease process has reduced the risk to both mother and fetus; however, the incidence of complications is still significant. Maternal complications include infections (urinary tract and vaginal), difficult labor related to increased fetal size (which frequently results in cesarean birth), vascular complications (including retinopathy), azotemia, ketoacidosis, and increased incidence of hypertensive disorders. Fetal complications include spontaneous abortion, **hydramnios** (excessive amniotic fluid), large placenta, alteration in size for gestational age, congenital anomalies, increased incidence of respiratory distress syndrome, and fetal or neonatal death.

Assessment. Urine testing should be performed at all prenatal visits. If these indicate the presence of glucose, additional testing is required. For the known diabetic, assessment of diet, activity, and medication compliance is essential. The vascular system should be assessed regularly for possible complications, and the patient should be watched closely for signs of infection. The condition of the fetus is also assessed closely by serial ultrasonography and other medical measures.

Diagnostic Tests. A 1-hour diabetes screening test or glucose tolerance tests may be ordered. If the woman is known to have diabetes mellitus, careful monitoring of blood glucose levels is important throughout the pregnancy. **Glycosylated hemoglobin** (a combination of hemoglobin and blood glucose, making up about 4% to 8% of the total hemoglobin; that is, the hemoglobin chains have glucose attached to them) tests are used to monitor glucose control during the 1 to 3 months before the test. Fingerstick blood testing is also useful.

Fetal surveillance. Diagnostic techniques for fetal surveillance often are performed during pregnancy complicated by diabetes mellitus to assess fetal growth and well-being. Efforts are made to determine the estimated date of delivery (EDD) or estimated date of confinement (EDC). A baseline ultrasound scan is done to assess gestational age of the fetus. Follow-up ultrasound examinations are performed during the pregnancy, as often as every 4 to 6 weeks, to monitor fetal growth and development and to assess for congenital abnormalities.

Biochemical analysis of amniotic fluid is performed to ascertain fetal lung maturity, typically in the third trimester. Amniocentesis earlier in gestation may be used to diagnose congenital anomalies.

Nursing Interventions. Nursing care is directed at maintaining the patient in a euglycemic (normal blood glucose) status. The patient's insulin requirements will change significantly throughout pregnancy, labor, and delivery. The nurse must assess the patient carefully at each visit, complete all blood glucose level evaluations as ordered, and report any abnormalities to the physician promptly. Because of possible teratogenic effects, oral hypoglycemics are usually discontinued. Insulin may be required by both NIDDM and GDM patients to control blood glucose levels.

A nursing diagnosis and interventions for the patient with diabetes mellitus include but are not limited to the following:

NURSING DIAGNOSIS	NURSING INTERVENTIONS
Knowledge deficit, related to diabetes mellitus, its management and potential effects on the pregnant woman and fetus	Review pathophysiology of the disease. Assist the patient in formulating questions for the physician. Clarify misconceptions. Teach home monitoring of blood glucose levels. Review effects of diabetes on the pregnant patient and fetus. Teach danger signs of diabetes and whom to notify (written as well as oral). Stress importance of weekly prenatal visits during second half of pregnancy. Refer patient to community diabetic support groups.

Patient teaching. The need for teaching will differ with the classification of the disease and the assessment of patient willingness to learn. A woman who has been diagnosed before pregnancy will need reinforcement of diet, medication, and health practices. The nurse will also need to explain the effects pregnancy has on diabetes throughout the course of pregnancy, labor, delivery, and the postpartum period. For the gestational diabetic, teaching should stress the necessity of good control of the disease, including all the teaching normally given to a new diabetic.

Prognosis. Blood glucose control is essential in pregnancy. Insulin will not cross the placental barrier; consequently, the control of the mother's blood sugar is vital to the health of the fetus.

Cardiac Complications

Pregnancy increases the demands on the cardiovascular system. This is not a problem for the normal, healthy heart, which is able to adapt to the increased demands. However, women who have preexisting cardiac disease face increased risk when cardiac function is challenged by pregnancy. The incidence of peripartum cardiomyopathies has been reported as 1 in 3000 to 4000 pregnancies. It occurs more often in multiparous women.

Etiology. The most common cardiac problems of maternity patients result from rheumatic heart disease, congenital heart defects, or mitral valve prolapse. Occasionally a condition called *peripartum cardiomyopathy* (disease of the myocardium, especially due to primary diseases of the heart muscle; in maternity patients it is *peripartum* cardiomyopathy), is observed in patients who have no history of cardiac problems. This may be seen in the last month of pregnancy or during the postpartum period. The symptoms are similar to those of congestive heart failure.

Pathophysiology. During pregnancy increased blood volume, heart rate, and cardiac output are normal. In the woman with existing cardiac problems, the muscle, valves, or vessels are overly stressed by these changes and symptoms of the underlying pathological condition are exacerbated, resulting in cardiac decompensation, congestive failure, and other medical problems.

Clinical Manifestations. The symptoms will depend on the underlying pathology. Edema, cyanosis, tachycardia, palpitations, dysrhythmias, chest pain, dyspnea, and fatigue may occur. Physical exertion may increase the symptoms. Clinical findings are those of congestive heart failure (left ventricular failure) (see Chapter 28).

Assessment. At each prenatal visit the patient's vital signs should be measured and her ability to participate in activity evaluated. Unusual fatigue with activity may reveal problems. Assessment should include monitoring for edema, weight gain, murmurs, cough, dyspnea, or abnormal lung sounds. It is important to compare these data with normal changes during pregnancy.

Diagnostic Tests. Chest x-ray evaluation, electrocardiograms, echocardiograms, and auscultation are used to determine the type and severity of the cardiac problem. Blood gas analysis may be required if severe decompensation is observed.

Nursing Interventions. Nursing care is directed at helping the woman to maintain normal physical and psychosocial function. During pregnancy the nurse should teach the importance of diet, medications, pacing activity, and adequate rest. This includes education about the specific disease and its management. Iron intake must be adequate to prevent anemia, which will further stress the heart. Sodium may be restricted to control the fluid volume and decrease cardiac stress. Stool softeners may be prescribed to decrease use of the Valsalva maneuver (holding the breath while bearing down) when defecating. The level of activity will be dictated by the severity of the cardiac problem. The nurse should be aware of the medical recommendations and help the woman incorporate these into her daily life. Patients with more severe cardiac problems will require the greatest adjustments, and the nurse must be highly sensitive to personal and family needs.

During labor, the semi-Fowler's or side-lying position with the head elevated will enhance respiratory effort and improve circulation. The efforts of labor may require oxygen administration, and the need for this should be explained. Administration of medications such as cardiotonics (digitalis), diuretics, prophylactic antibiotics, sedatives, and analgesics may be required as directed by the physician. The nurse should try to minimize unnecessary activity by the patient during labor and calmly explain everything to decrease anxiety. Fetal condition should be closely monitored for any signs of distress. A fetal monitor should be used for continuous assessment.

During delivery conservation of energy is important. Resting between contractions and using shorter, open-glottis pushing are recommended. The fetal status must be monitored very closely during this time.

Postpartum care will vary according to the severity of the cardiac problem. Methods of incorporating care of the infant into the mother's level of activity should be explored. Because extravascular fluid returns to the bloodstream following delivery, the mother is at risk for developing cardiac decompression during the 48 hours after the birth.

To promote normal parent-child attachment contact should be established as early as possible. Breastfeeding should be discussed with the physician, because the physical effort may be excessive for the mother and the transfer of medications in the breast milk may be harmful to the infant. As in all other areas of nursing, it is important to continue to assess the patient's status and give explanations for all care.

A nursing diagnosis and interventions for the patient with cardiac complications include but are not limited to the following:

NURSING DIAGNOSIS	NURSING INTERVENTIONS
Activity intolerance, related to insufficient oxygenation resulting from decreased cardiac output	Plan nursing strategies to optimize rest. Teach methods that help conserve energy. Monitor vital signs and response to activity. Identify stressors. Discuss methods of stress reduction. Encourage patient to report activities that increase fatigue Assist with activity as needed. Keep frequently used items of patient within easy reach. Minimize anxiety and stress. Administer medication as ordered. Maintain and increase strength with active and passive range-of-motion (ROM) exercises. Involve family/significant other in supporting and participating with patient in daily activities.

Prognosis. In cardiac complications the maternal mortality rate has been estimated in the range of 30% to 60%; the infant mortality rate is approximately 10%. The prognosis is good if cardiomegaly is not persistent after 6 months. The prognosis for women whose hearts remain enlarged is not as favorable. Future pregnancies usually result in some cardiac failure (50% to 88%). Mortality may be as high as 60%. Oral contraceptives are contraindicated because of the risk of thromboembolism.

AGE-RELATED COMPLICATIONS

Adolescent Pregnancy

Adolescent patients present the nurse with a unique challenge. A significant number are sexually active and in need of contraceptive counseling; many become pregnant. The pregnant adolescent, her family, and her partner require sensitive, competent nursing interventions. The young woman may choose to terminate the pregnancy or carry it to term. She may place the infant up for adoption or elect to keep the baby. The nurse plays a vital role in assisting the patient to make informed decisions and in supporting her, both physically and emotionally, in carrying out her chosen option. The nurse should never recommend a preferable choice.

Developmental tasks of adolescence must be accomplished before the child can become a mature adult. These tasks vary from culture to culture and with individual adolescents and their goals.

Adolescent female development is characterized by physical development, behaviors, and concerns approximating chronological age. The period of adolescence may be divided into three stages: early, middle, and late. The higher the developmental level, the greater the readiness to accept responsibility for self and others (Box 42-9).

Pregnancy interrupts work on identity formation and developmental tasks. Attempting to accomplish developmental tasks of pregnancy and the developmental tasks of normal adolescence simultaneously may be overwhelming. The psychological burden may lead to depression and to postponement in attaining an adult identity (see Box 42-9).

The pregnant adolescent faces further developmental tasks of parenthood. These tasks will be as important to the new adolescent parents' plan for organizing ways to behave in their environment as they are for the adult (see Box 42-9).

The number of adolescent pregnancies is increasing in most areas of the country. This trend is attributed to many sociological factors; breakdown of the traditional family and changes in social mores have resulted in earlier sexual activity. Teenagers account for an increasingly large percentage of births and abortions. Physiological immaturity, incomplete education, and unresolved developmental tasks are complicating factors. Most pregnant teenagers are unmarried. The psychological and economic support provided by a stable family is often missing. When combined with fear or denial of the pregnancy, the pregnant teenager often goes without medical attention until late in pregnancy. Lack of prenatal care increases the risk to the pregnant teenager and her infant. Teenagers under 15 years of age present the greatest risks. Older adolescents need not have increased risk if early prenatal care is obtained.

Assessment. Assessment of all health patterns for each adolescent is essential.

Nursing Interventions. Nursing diagnoses and interventions for the pregnant adolescent patient include but are not limited to the following:

NURSING DIAGNOSES	NURSING INTERVENTIONS
Coping, ineffective individual, related to depression secondary to unplanned pregnancy	Assess stressors. Assess patient's anxiety level. Allow time for expressing fears. Provide a nonthreatening atmosphere to allow for questions and expression of feelings. Assess relationship with sexual partner, and explore possible consequences of contacting him. Demonstrate interest in the patient and willingness to help. Assist the patient to develop problem-solving strategies. Find methods of fostering feeling of achievement and self-esteem. Assist in developing or strengthening support systems.
Knowledge deficit, related to choices regarding pregnancy, childbirth experiences, and parenthood	Examine own views regarding sexuality to be able to maintain nonjudgmental approach. Listen and give honest answers. Accept and expect repeated testing from the adolescent. Create a safe and stable environment that engenders trust. Evaluate which stage of development adolescent is experiencing. Teach the adolescent about pregnancy choices, childbirth, and parenthood. Encourage questions and verbalization of fears and concerns. Compliment teen on questions and references to learn issues. Encourage support persons to attend and participate in prenatal care. Refer to childbirth and parenthood class, community support and information groups.
Body image disturbance, related to the physical changes of pregnancy	Show interest in patient, her thoughts and feelings. Provide private place to discuss patient concerns in an unhurried manner. Encourage verbalization. Identify support system with teen. Evaluate teen's adolescent stage to counsel and support her in achieving her developmental task. Compliment teen on her appearance, verbalization of feelings and learning, when appropriate. Refer to outside resources, guidance counselor, tutor.

Box 42-9

TASKS OF THE PREGNANT ADOLESCENT

DEVELOPMENT TASKS OF PREGNANCY

- *Accepting the Biological Reality of Pregnancy:* Most adolescents do not expect to become pregnant. Many deny it until the signs are too obvious to be ignored. Teenagers commonly diet and wear constricting clothes to hide the pregnancy; some succeed until the birth. The level of denial in both teenagers and their families can be quite high. Some sources state that concealment of the pregnancy was the primary reason younger adolescents failed to seek prenatal care before the third trimester; whereas poor motivation frequently was the reason given by the older adolescents (18 to 19 years).
- *Accepting the Reality of the Unborn Child:* The adolescent may accept only the fantasy of having a cute, happy, healthy baby to dress up and play with like a doll. The idea of the infant's growth and development into an older child is not a reality to the adolescent.
- *Accepting the Reality of Parenthood:* Being a parent implies being loving, concerned, and capable of providing the nurturing care an infant needs. Although there usually is a desire to be a good parent, young adolescents (mother and father) have limited life experiences, their own need to grow and develop, and little ability to cope with abstractions and to problem solve. The amount and type of support available to adolescents can significantly influence the accomplishment of these tasks.

DEVELOPMENTAL TASKS OF PARENTHOOD

- *Reconciling the Imagined with the Actual:* Although it is biologically possible for the young female teen to become a parent, her egocentricity (regarding the self as the center, and having little regard for others) and concrete (logical and coherent) thinking interfere with her ability to parent.
- *Becoming Adept in Care Giving Activities:* The very young adolescent is inexperienced and unprepared to recognize early signs of illness, risks of danger, or household hazards. Children may be inadvertently neglected
- *Being Aware of the Infant's Needs:* Some sources say infants of adolescents are nine times more likely to die as a result of accidents and violence than are infants of older mothers. The higher rates of infant mortality are attributed to the inexperience, lack of knowledge, and immaturity of the adolescent mother, resulting in the inability to recognize a problem and obtain necessary resources. Nonetheless, in most instances, with adequate support and developmentally appropriate teaching, effective parenting can be learned by adolescents.
- *Establishing Oneself and One's Infant as a Family:* Maintaining a relationship with the baby's father is beneficial for the mother and the child. Involvement of the father is related to appropriate maternal behaviors and the mother's increased sense of confidence and security, as well as a healthy sense of trust, self-esteem, and social skills in the adolescent.

Labor and Birth. The very young adolescent may be frightened of needles, pelvic examinations, noises from other women in labor or from equipment, and birth rooms. Single, private rooms should be provided when possible. The adolescent in labor should have the support of a knowledgeable coach, whether husband, friend, parent, or nurse. Many teenagers come to labor lacking preparation; they are fearful and often alone. If they are admitted early in the first stage, teaching about relaxation with contractions, ambulation, side-lying positions, and comfort measures can be accomplished. The adolescent is more concerned with how the baby will get out than with fetal well-being. Even though she may show an intense response to the contractions, the adolescent is trusting and will follow suggestions. Labor often progresses quickly. Anticipatory guidance and explanation of procedures should always be a component of care. Many adolescents keep their infants and are responsive to staff members' sharing their delight. For these young parents, efforts to promote parent-child attachment are particularly important.

Postpartum Care. Physically, the adolescent mother requires the same care as any woman who has given birth. Explicit directions for self-care and infant care are required. Most adolescents view the care of the infant as their primary area of concern. The need for continued assessment of the new mother's parenting abilities during the postbirth period is essential. In addition, continued support should be provided by involving grandparents or other family members, through home visits, and group sessions for discussion of infant care and parenting problems. Outreach programs concerned with self-care, parent-child interactions, child injuries, and failure to thrive, as well as those that provide prompt and effective intervention, prevent more serious problems.

Postpartum contraception is a high priority for every young adolescent. The risk of repeat pregnancy in adolescence is very high, and all the accompanying risks of adolescent pregnancy increase with each subsequent pregnancy. Almost universally, postpartum adolescents will say they will never have sex again and therefore, "need no birth control." Nonetheless adolescents need to leave the hospital with barrier methods (foam and condoms) and the knowledge of how and when to use them. Very young adolescents may be shy or embarrassed about touching their genitals to use the barrier method. In addition, they will not likely anticipate intercourse. For these reasons, some health care providers send adolescents home on a regimen of oral contraceptives. This practice is controversial because of the increased risk of thromboembolic disease in the immediate postpartum period (first 4 weeks). Thus the decision must be based on the individual adolescent and her life situation. Adolescent males need to be considered and included in any interventions in sexuality education, family planning, and parent education.

The adolescent will need support if she is contemplating the option of adoption for her child. Health professionals need to avoid using phrases that give negative connotations to the adoption process. Phrases such as "put up for adoption" and "give up for adoption" imply a callous, uncaring, insensitive biological parent. Neither should the terms "real or natural parents" be used exclusively for genetic parents. The adoptive parents are the "real parents" because they care for the child. Neutral language, such as "arranging for an adoption," "biological parent" or "birth mother," and "adoptive parent," is preferred. The mother is given the option of either remaining on the postpartum floor or transferring to another unit. She is assured that she will have as much access to the baby as she desires.

Grief results from actual or perceived loss. The adolescent may experience grief brought on by the contemplation of adoption, giving birth to a preterm infant who may be in the intensive care unit, or the death of the infant. The nurse can help the birth mother move through the grieving process. The adolescent who gives birth to a preterm infant or one who is small for gestational age may find it extremely difficult to reconcile this tiny, scrawny infant with her fantasized "Gerber" baby. She may experience fear over the thought of caring for the child introduced to her in the intensive care unit. The confidence and trust in her abilities gained during the prenatal period may be replaced with feelings of being overwhelmed and incompetent. The consequent alienation of mother and infant may never be overcome. Intensive teaching and continuous support programs are essential if both the young mother and her vulnerable infant are not to be estranged.

Many young mothers pattern their parenting on what they themselves experienced. It is vital, therefore, to determine the kind of support that those close to young mothers are able or prepared to give and the kinds of community aid that can supplement this support. The adolescent may have conflict with dependency versus independency issues as she performs her mothering role within the framework of her family of origin. The adolescent's family of origin also may need assistance in adapting to their new roles.

The Adolescent Father. The adolescent father is also faced with immediate developmental crises: completing the developmental tasks of adolescence and making a transition to parenthood and, sometimes, to marriage. These transitions can be stressful. The nurse can initiate interaction with the adolescent father by asking his pregnant partner to bring the father to the clinic with her so that he may participate in the birth. With the pregnant teen's agreement, the father also may be contacted directly. Data needed for inclusion of the young father in all aspects of the care are based on assessment of four areas: the couple's relationship; levels of stress, concern, and coping; educational and vocational goals; and the level of health education knowledge. As do all fathers, adolescent fathers need support to discuss their emotional responses to the pregnancy. The nurse's nonjudgmental attitude is essential for open communication. The father's feelings of guilt, powerlessness, or bravado should be recognized because of their negative consequences for both parents and child. Counseling needs to be reality oriented. Topics such as finances, child care, parenting skills, and the father's role in the birth experience need to be discussed. Teenage fathers also need knowledge of reproductive physiology and birth control options.

The adolescent mother's partner, as well as her family, affects how she will deal with her pregnancy, labor and birth, and subsequent parenthood. The adolescent father may continue to be involved in an ongoing relationship with the young mother. In many instances he plays an important role in the decisions she faces in pregnancy. He may influence her decision to continue the pregnancy, to have an abortion, to keep the child, or to place the child for adoption.

The nurse supports the young father by helping him develop realistic perceptions of his role as "father to a child." The nurse encourages his use of coping mechanisms that are not detrimental to his, his partner's, or his child's well-being. The nurse enlists support systems, parents, and professional agencies on his behalf. Encouraging mutual responsibility for birth control is a constant necessity.

Patient teaching. Education of the pregnant adolescent is essential. To work effectively with adolescents the nurse must be sensitive and nonjudgmental and knowledgeable about the stages of adolescence. Because no two adolescents are alike, a wide range of skills must be used to reach each individual (see patient teaching box and Fig. 42-5).

Older Pregnant Woman

At the other end of the reproductive cycle are women who have their first child after they are 35 years of age. These women have a somewhat increased risk of maternal and fetal complications. Issues and concerns related to the over-35 age group have become increasingly prominent in the last decade. There have always been women over 35 who have continued their childbearing either by choice or because of lack or failure of contraception during the perimenopausal years. Today this

PATIENT TEACHING FOR ADOLESCENT PARENTS

- Nutrition is a major area of concern for the teenager. The young teen is often still growing herself, and her nutritional intake must meet her own needs and those of the fetus. Fad diets and food idiosyncrasies are common in teenagers; this must be taken into account when teaching nutrition. Body image disturbance is a problem for even a mature woman. The teenager, particularly one who has not yet accepted the fact of pregnancy, may limit food intake to avoid gaining weight. This can be exceedingly dangerous to both mother and infant.
- Preparation for labor and delivery is also essential. Many adolescents have little knowledge of human anatomy and have many fears and misconceptions about the process of childbirth. Many may have heard stories from friends that only increase their anxiety. The nurse should be factual without being harsh when describing the birth process.
- Many adolescents plan to raise their infants; therefore instruction should also include child care and growth and development. Referral to community agencies that will provide ongoing support is important.
- The adolescent father should not be ignored. It is important to consider the effect of pregnancy on him, particularly if he remains meaningfully involved with the teenage mother. Counseling is important for both, because the physical, financial, and emotional consequences of the pregnancy will affect both of them for the rest of their lives.

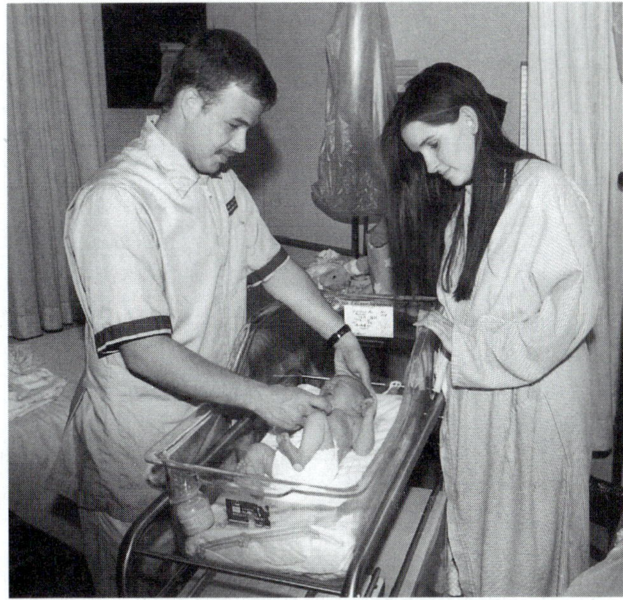

FIG. 42-5 Demonstrating infant care.

group also includes women who have postponed pregnancy because of careers or other reasons, as well as women with infertility problems who have become pregnant because of technological advances that have expanded alternatives for couples desiring children.

Changes in society, particularly the increased number of women with careers, have resulted in many women delaying pregnancy until later in life. Many women become aware of the "biological clock" as menopause approaches and wish to have a child while they are still able to do so. The potential for infertility increases with age. Although most women who wait until later in life are well educated and have consciously decided to become pregnant, conception and pregnancy are not always easy. The likelihood of ectopic pregnancy and placenta previa and the incidence of various medical conditions, such as diabetes or hypertension, increase with age.

If the woman does become pregnant, studies show that each year after age 35 increases the risk of conceiving a child with Down's syndrome or other chromosomal anomalies. Amniocentesis is commonly done to detect genetic problems. Detection of genetic disorders can raise ethical dilemmas regarding abortion or raising a disabled child.

As women maintain better overall health and fitness, increased age appears to be less of an impediment to a normal pregnancy.

Psychosocial adjustment to parenthood at this time of life depends greatly on the individual and her particular situation. Changes in income, life-style, and work routines can present challenges that are stressful, even if the pregnancy is desired.

Studies have identified certain factors that can influence parental responses in this older group. Fatigue and the need for more rest seem to be the major concerns of older parents with newborns. Many of these mothers, being less resilient than younger women, may need to stay in the hospital longer, rather than be forced to an early discharge as some third-party payers request.

Measures designed to assist the mother in regaining strength and muscle tone (e.g., prenatal and postnatal exercises) are emphasized. Some older mothers may find that the care of the newborn infant exhausts their physical capabilities. Many women might benefit from referral to supportive resources in the community.

COMPLICATIONS RELATED TO THE NEWBORN

Newborns at Risk

Many maternal conditions can place the newborn in increased danger of illness or death. It is important to iden-

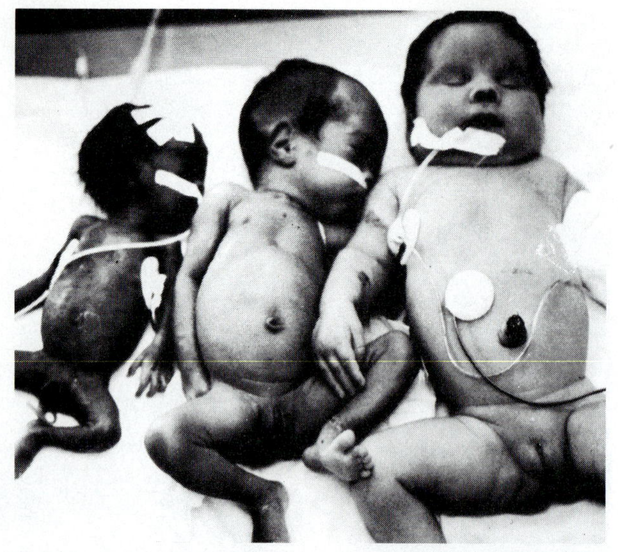

FIG. 42-6 Three babies of same gestational age, with weights of 600, 1400, and 2750 g, respectively, from left to right. Their weights are plotted in Fig. 42-6.

tify any maternal risk factors as soon as possible to decrease the risk to the fetus/newborn. Once these risks are identified, all medical and nursing measures possible should be undertaken to minimize the consequences to both the mother and newborn.

When risk factors are identified early, it is possible to be prepared to meet the needs of the newborn at risk. New equipment, such as fetal monitors and more sensitive diagnostic tests, has made recognition of problems occurring during labor and delivery easier. Despite all our progress, however, many infants still are born in need of special attention.

At the time of delivery the newborn is assessed. The Apgar gives important information about the newborn's status at 1 and 5 minutes after delivery (see Chapter 41). This is followed by a more detailed assessment of size related to gestational age. It is important to distinguish between infants who are preterm and those who are small for gestational age. While both groups are at risk, the problems they present will be different.

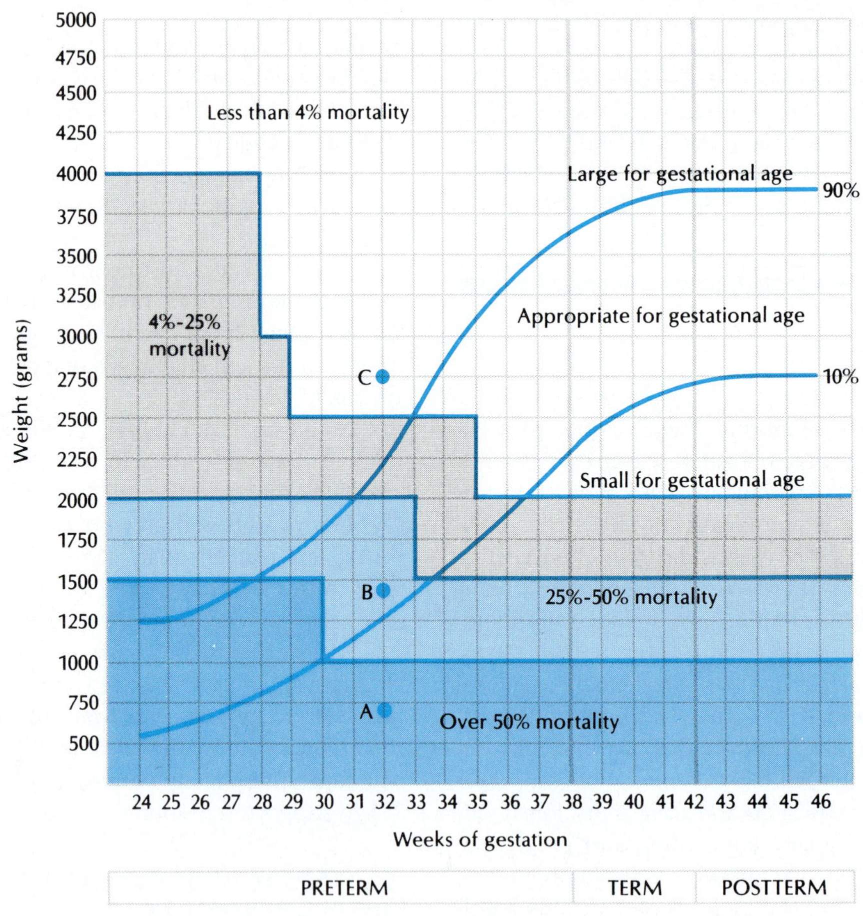

FIG. 42-7 Intrauterine growth status for gestational age and according to appropriateness of growth. Weights of infants as shown in Fig. 42-5 are plotted at points *A, B,* and *C.* (Courtesy Mead Johnson & Co, Evansville, Ind. Modified from Battaglia FC, Lubchenco LO: *J Pediatr* 71:59, 1967.)

Gestational age is significant with regard to neonatal mortality and morbidity (Figs. 42-6 and 42-7). Both preterm and postterm infants are at risk. Gestational age is classified as follows:

Preterm	0 to 37 complete weeks of pregnancy
Term	38 to 41 complete weeks of pregnancy
Postterm	42 or more weeks of pregnancy

Gestational Age

Physical assessment procedures to determine gestational age are based on the method devised by Dubowitz et al. Ideally the tests are performed between 2 and 8 hours of age. For the first hour the infant is recovering from the stress of birth, and this is reflected in muscle movements; for example, the arm recoil is slower in a fatigued infant. After 48 hours some responses change significantly. The plantar creases on the soles of the feet appear to increase in number and become visible as the skin loses fluid and dries. See Figs. 42-8 to 42-12 and Tables 42-2 and 42-3 on p. 1329-1331 for the estimation of gestational age. Fig. 42-13 on p. 1332 shows newborn maturity rating and classification.

Preterm Infant.

Etiology. The exact causes of preterm labor are unknown. In some cases it is related to maternal or placental problems, but in other cases the cause cannot be determined. The end result is delivery of an infant 37 weeks or less in age.

A

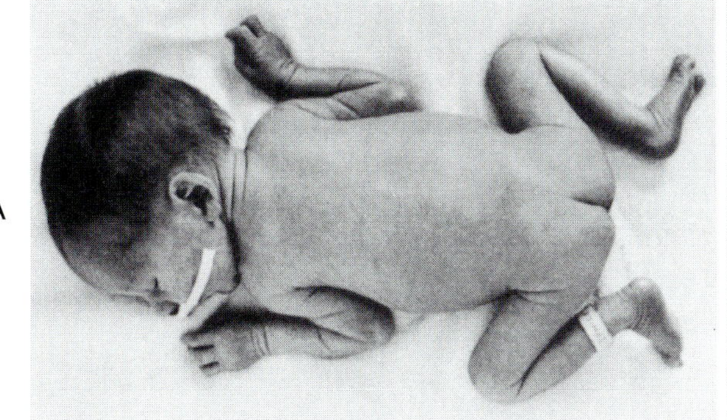

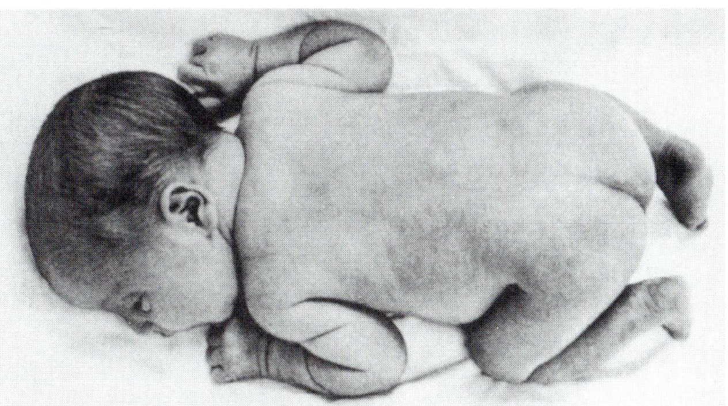

B

FIG. 42-8 Infant lie postbirth. **A,** In prone position, preterm infant lies with pelvis flat and legs splayed like a frog's. **B,** Normal full-term infant lies with limbs flexed, pelvis raised, and knees usually drawn under abdomen. (Courtesy Mead Johnson & Co, Evansville, Ind.)

A

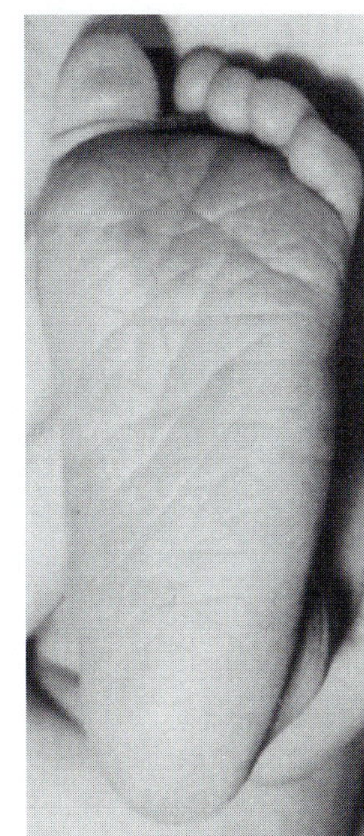

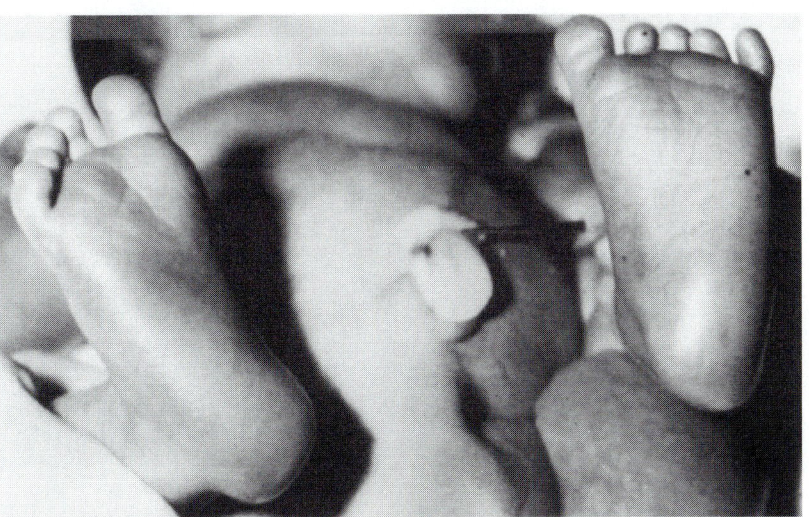

B

FIG. 42-9 **A,** Normal sole creases of full-term newborn. **B,** Sole of foot of preterm infant. As infant loses interstitital fluid after birth, creases become apparent even in preterm infants. Therefore assessment should be performed in first 2 hours after birth.

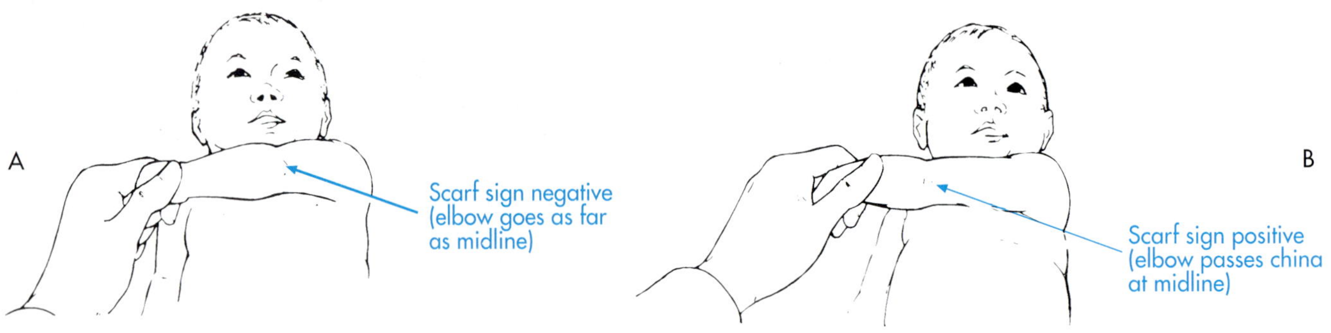

FIG. 42-10 Assessment of gestational age in term newborn **A,** and preterm newborn, **B.**

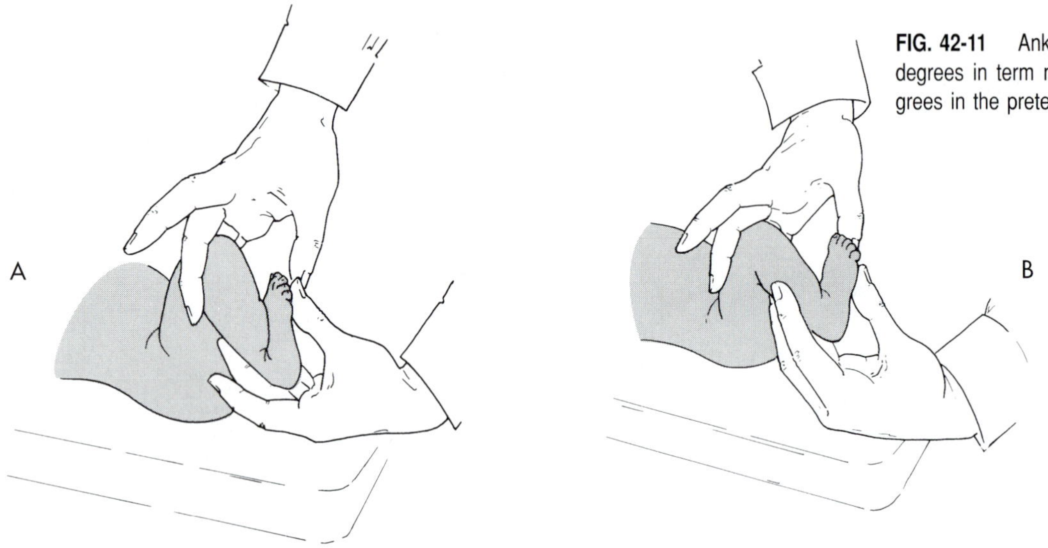

FIG. 42-11 Ankle dorsiflexion. **A,** Angle of 0 degrees in term newborn. **B,** Angle of 20 degrees in the preterm newborn.

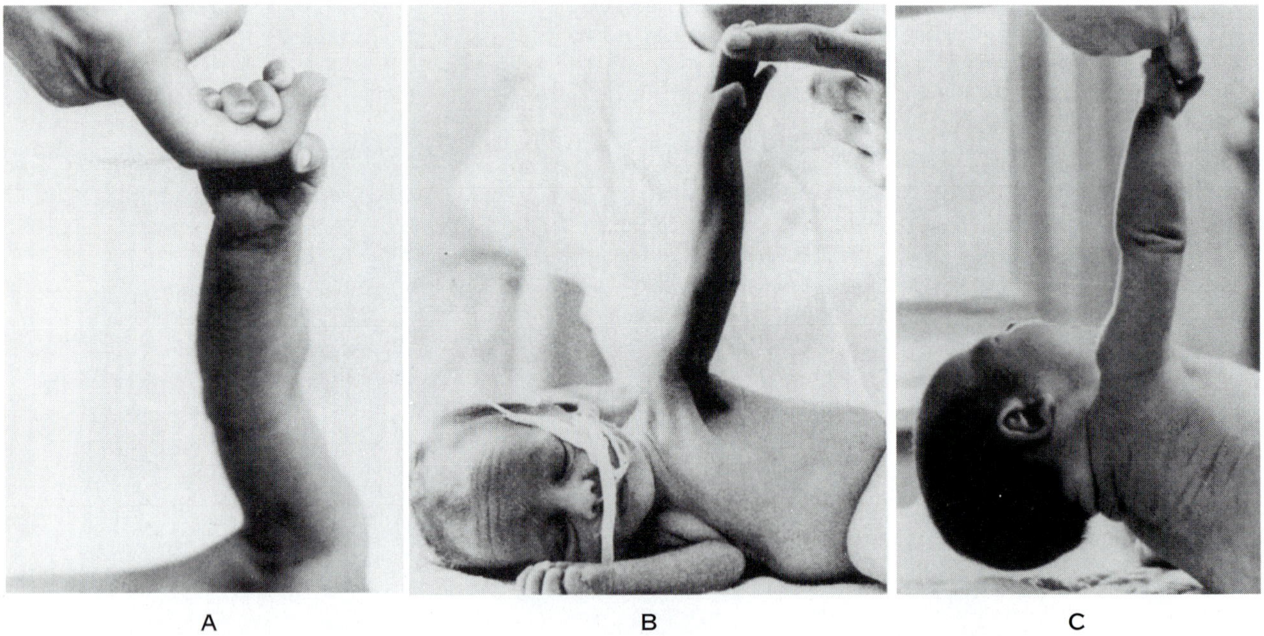

A B C

FIG. 42-12 **A,** Primitive grasp reflex present in all normal newborns usually weakens and disappears after 3 months. When palm is stimulated by finger, infant will grasp it. Full-term infant reinforces grip as finger is drawn upward. Dorsum of hand should not be touched because this excites the opposite reflex, and hand opens. **B,** Grasp reflex present in preterm infant is distinct from that noted in term infant. Grip can be obtained and arm drawn upward, but when traction is applied, grip opens and there is much less muscle tension. **C,** Once grasp is obtained in term infant, grip is reinforced when the arm is drawn upward. There is progressive tensing of muscles until baby hangs momentarily.

TABLE 42-2 Elaboration of Physical Maturity Scales

Criterion	Findings and Assigned Scores: 0	1	2	3	4	Infant Score*
Skin						
Edema	Edema evident over hands and feet; pitting seen over tibia	Pitting edema over tibia	No edema obvious	—	—	———
Texture and opacity	Gelatinous, transparent; veins seen especially over abdomen	Visible veins; thin, smooth	Few larger veins seen, especially over abdomen; medium-thick smooth skin	Veins rarely seen; some thickening, superficial cracking	No vessels; parchment-like, thick, cracking; if leathery, very cracked, and wrinkled, give score of 5	
Color	Dark red (infant is quiet for evaluation)	Pink	Pale pink	Pale; pink mainly over palms, soles, lips, and ears		
Lanugo	None	Abundant over body; long; thick	Thinning, especially over lumbosacral area	Bald areas; thinning over other areas	Mostly bald of lanugo; at least half of back bald	———
Plantar creases	No creases seen	Faint red marks on upper half of sole	Red marks obvious over more than upper half; deeper lines over less than one third	Indentations noticeable over more than one third; lines seen over two thirds	Creases cover entire sole (Fig. 42-8)	———
Breast	Nipple barely perceptible; no palpable breast tissue	Flat, smooth areola present around well-defined nipple; some breast tissue	Stippled areola but edge flat; 1-2 mm breast bud	Stippled areola with edges raised; 3-4 mm breast bud	Full areola; 5-10 mm breast bud; may have breast milk	———
Ear form						
Cartilage	Pinna flat, soft, easily folded	Slight incurving of pinna; soft, easily folded; slow recoil	Well-incurved pinna; soft; ready recoil	Upper pinna well curved; formed and firm to edge; instant recoil	Thick cartilage; ear stiff	———
Genitals						
Male	No testes in scrotum and no rugae over scrotum	—	Testes descending; few rugations	Testes within scrotum, good rugae	Scrotum pendulous with rugae covering scrotum	———
Female	Prominent clitoris and labia minora; labia majora do not cover labia minora	—	Labia majora and labia minora equally prominent	Labia majora appear large; labia minora, small	Labia majora completely cover clitoris and labia minora	
					TOTAL	———

*Highest score possible = 25.

TABLE 42-3 Elaboration of Neuromuscular Maturity Scales*

Criterion	Method of Assessment	— 0
Posture (Fig. 42-7)	Position: supine Activity: quiet Assessment: extension and flexion of arms, hips, legs	Complete extension
Square window (wrist)†	Position: supine Method: with thumb supporting back of arm below wrist, apply gentle pressure with index and third fingers on dorsum of hand; do not rotate infant's wrist Assessment: angle formed between hypothenar eminence and forearm	Very premature (<30 wk) 90 degrees
Arm recoil	Position: supine Method; flex forearms on upper arms for 5 sec; pull on hands to full extension and release Assessment: degree of flexion	No recoil; arms remain extended 180 degrees
Popliteal angle (Fig.42-10)	Position: supine; pelvic on flat, firm surface Method: flex leg on thigh; then flex high on abdomen; holding knee with thumb and index finger, extend leg with index finger of other hand behind ankle Assessment: degree of angle behind knee	Complete extension; very premature 180 degrees
Scarf sign (Fig. 42-9)	Position: supine Method: support head in midline with one hand; pull hand to opposite shoulder Assessment: position of elbow in relation to midline	Elbow to opposite arm like scarf around neck
Heel to ear	Position: supine, pelvic is kept flat on surface Method: pull foot up toward ear on same side; do not hold knee Assessment: distance of foot from ear and degree of extension of knee	Toes touch ear; leg completely extended (180 degress)

X, First examination; O, second examination.
*Compare combined scores for physical and neuromuscular maturity to the "maturity rating" scores and read estimated weeks of gestational age. Estimate of gestational age obtained is accurate only to plus or minus 2 weeks. After gestational age is estimated, infant's length, weight, and head

Pathophysiology. The preterm infant is developmentally immature. The lungs are not producing sufficient amounts of surfactant to allow adequate oxygenation. Structures within the heart may not have adapted, as they normally do in a term infant, leading to oxygenation problems. Lack of subcutaneous fat, large surface area relative to body weight, and poor reserves of glucose and **brown fat** (source of heat unique to neonates that is capable of greater thermogenic [producing heat] activity than ordinary fat; deposits are found around the adrenals, kidneys, and neck; between scapulas, and behind the sternum for several weeks after birth) all contribute to problems with heat conservation. The digestive system is formed, but problems with absorption of nutrients are common. The renal system is immature and ineffective. Fluid and acid-base imbalance is frequently observed. The infant is also neurologically immature; the gag, suck, and swallow reflexes may be

Finding and Assigned Scores					Infant Score	
1	2	3	4	5	X	0
Extension of arms; slight flexion of hips, legs	Extension of arms	Slight flexion of arms; full flexion of legs	Complete flexion	—	——	——
Premature (30-35 wk) 60 degrees	Premature (30-35 wk) 45 degrees	Maturing (35-38 wk) 30 degrees	Term: hand lies flat on ventral surface of forearm 0 degrees	—	——	——
—	Some recoil sluggish response 100 to 180 degrees	Maturing (35-38 wk) 90 to 100 degrees	Brisk recoil to complete flexion <90 degrees	—	——	——
Premature (30-35 wk) 160 degrees	Premature (30-35 wk) 130 degrees	Maturing (35-38 wk) 110 degrees	Maturing (35-38 wk) 90 degrees	Extension is resisted <90 degrees	——	——
Elbow beyond midline of thorax	Elbow just beyond midline	Elbow at midline	Elbow does not reach midline	—	——	——
Toes almost reach face (130°)	Knees flexed (110°)	Knees flexed (90°)	Knees flexed; popliteal angle is less than 90°	—	——	——
				NEUROMUSCULAR MATURITY TOTALS	——	——
				PHYSICAL MATURITY TOTALS (see Fig. 42-13)	——	——
				COMBINED SCORE	——	——

circumference are entered on appropriate graphs. All three measurements should fall within same approximate range, for example, all within SGA, LGA, or AGA. If one measurement is excessively large (falling into LGA range) and other two fall into SGA range, growth deviation should be assessed.

weak or absent, and other normal reflexes may be absent or atypical.

Clinical manifestations. The premature newborn's posture is froglike or flaccid. The color is usually ruddy, and cyanosis is common. The head appears very large in proportion to the body, and the bones of the skull are pliable with large, flat fontanelles. The skin is very thin and translucent with obvious blood vessels and little subcutaneous fat. There may be a layer of fine hair (lanugo) coating large areas of the body. Cartilage in the ears is pliable, and the ears can be easily folded. The genitals in males are small, and frequently the testes are undescended. In females the labia majora are small. The cry is weak, and reflexes are immature or absent.

Assessment. All systems of the premature newborn must be assessed carefully and continuously—changes occur rapidly and require continuous monitoring. Preterm infants are typically placed in an intensive care

ESTIMATION OF GESTATIONAL AGE BY MATURITY RATING

Symbols: X - 1st Exam O - 2nd Exam

NEUROMUSCULAR MATURITY

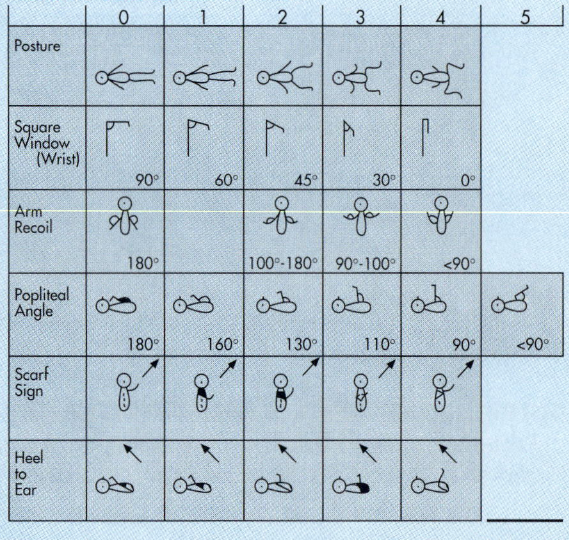

	0	1	2	3	4	5
Posture						
Square Window (Wrist)	90°	60°	45°	30°	0°	
Arm Recoil	180°		100°-180°	90°-100°	<90°	
Popliteal Angle	180°	160°	130°	110°	90°	<90°
Scarf Sign						
Heel to Ear						

Gestation by Dates ______________ wks

Birth Date ______________ Hour ______________ am pm

APGAR ______________ 1 min ______________ 5 min

PHYSICAL MATURITY

	0	1	2	3	4	5
SKIN	gelatinous red, trans-parent	smooth pink, visible veins	superficial peeling &/or rash few veins	cracking pale area, rare veins	parchment, deep cracking no vessels	leathery, cracked, wrinkled
LANUGO	none	abundant	thinning	bald areas	mostly bald	
PLANTAR CREASES	no crease	faint red marks	anterior transverse crease only	creases ant. 2/3	creases cover entire sole	
BREAST	barely percept.	flat areola, no bud	stippled areola, 1—2 mm bud	raised areola, 3—4 mm bud	full areola, 5—10 mm bud	
EAR	pinna flat, stays folded	sl. curved pinna, soft with slow recoil	well-curv. pinna, soft but ready recoil	formed & firm with instant recoil	thick cartilage, ear stiff	
GENITALS Male	scrotum empty, no rugae		testes descend-ing, few rugae	testes down, good rugae	testes pendulous, deep rugae	
GENITALS Female	prominent clitoris & labia minora		majora & minora equally prominent	majora large, minora small	clitoris & minora completely covered	

MATURITY RATING

Score	Wks
5	26
10	28
15	30
20	32
25	34
30	36
35	38
40	40
45	42
50	44

SCORING SECTION

	1st Exam X	2nd Exam O
Estimating Gest Age by Maturity Rating	______ Weeks	______ Weeks
Time of Exam	Date ______ Hour ______ am pm	Date ______ Hour ______ am pm
Age of Exam	______ Hours	______ Hours
Signature of Examiner	______ M.D.	______ M.D.

FIG. 42-13 Newborn maturity rating and classification. (Courtesy of Mead Johnson & Co, Evansville, Ind. Scoring section adapted from Ballard JL et al: *Pediatr Res* 11:374, 1977. Figures modified from Sweet AY: Classification of the low-birth-weight infant. In Klaus MH, Fanroff AA: *Care of the high-risk infant,* Philadelphia, 1977, Saunders.)

nursery and receive care from nurses specially trained to meet their needs.

The preterm infant is at risk because of immaturity of organ systems and lack of reserves. The morbidity and mortality rate for preterm infants is higher by three to four times than that of older infants of comparable weight. The potential problems and care needs of the preterm infant of 2000 g differ from those of the term, postterm, or postmature infant of equal weight.

Preterm infants are at a distinct disadvantage when they face the transition from intrauterine to extrauterine life. The degree of disadvantage depends primarily on their level of maturity. Physiological disorders and anomalous malformations affect their response to treatment as well. In general, the closer they are to the normal term infant in gestational age and birth weight, the easier will be their adjustment to the external environment.

An accurate assessment of gestational age is a good indicator of the problems a preterm newborn is likely to experience. In assessing the preterm infant, the health care provider follows a systematic approach. The response of the preterm infant to extrauterine life is different from that of the term infant. Knowing the physiological basis of these differences helps the nurse assess these infants, understand the response of the preterm infant, and determine which potential problems are most likely to occur.

Diagnostic tests. A wide range of diagnostic tests may be performed, based on the specific needs of the newborn.

Nursing interventions. The specifics of the care of the preterm newborn are too extensive for the scope of this text. The major goals include maintaining and stabilizing preterm newborns until they mature adequately. Respiratory regulation, thermal regulation, fluid and electrolytes, sensory stimulation, and promotion of bonding with the parents are all major areas of concern for the nurse.

Nursing diagnoses and interventions for the preterm child include but are not limited to the following:

NURSING DIAGNOSES	NURSING INTERVENTIONS
Thermoregulation, ineffective, high risk for, related to immature temperature regulation center, large body surface in relation to body weight, and minimal brown fat stores	Use skin probe to maintain skin temperature at 36.1° to 36.7° C (97 to 98° F). Monitor heart rate and rhythm. Keep well covered and wrapped in blankets. Pad cold surfaces. Use radiant warmer if uncovered for extended periods of time. Keep skin dry. Avoid drafts. Keep crib, warmer, or Isolette away from windows and cold external walls. Monitor for signs and symptoms of cold stress: decreased temperature, lethargy, and pallor (cold stress increases oxygen requirements). Avoid taking rectal temperature. Obtain axillary temperatures and compare to registered skin probe temperature every 30 min for 2 hr and until stable.
Anxiety (parental), high risk for, related to preterm birth, separation, and breastfeeding	Encourage parents to stay with baby in the NICU. Encourage parents to actively participate in all aspects of care as is possible. Encourage parents to hold baby and examine baby en face. Encourage mother to breastfeed. Explain the use of all equipment being used. Discuss baby's behavioral cues and physical characteristics.

NURSING DIAGNOSES	NURSING INTERVENTIONS
Anxiety (parental), high risk for, related to preterm birth, separation, and breastfeeding—cont'd	Encourage parents to express their feelings about the pregnancy, labor, and birth. Discuss parents' feeding decisions. Facilitate milk expression and storage by providing equipment and/or referral for lactation consultation.

Hemolytic Diseases.

Etiology. Hemolysis may result from basic incompatibility of blood groups, such as ABO incompatibility, or from a transfer of antibodies through the placenta.

Pathophysiology. Understanding Rh incompatibility requires an understanding of basic genetics. Rh incompatibility occurs only when the mother is Rh negative and the fetus is Rh positive. For this to occur the father of the fetus must be Rh positive (Fig. 42-14 on p. 1334).

The term *Rh negative* indicates that the woman does not possess a specific blood antigen. If the woman is sensitized (i.e., exposed to the antigen), antibodies are produced. Exposure can occur through blood transfusion of incompatible blood or during pregnancy, when some fetal blood cells can enter the maternal circulation. This transfer of antigen may occur in cases of abortion or abruption, or at the time of delivery. Once Rh antibodies are developed by the mother, they remain in her blood, as do other antibodies.

When the woman becomes pregnant, antibodies may cross the **placental barrier** (obstruction, boundary, or separation provided by the placental tissue between the fetal and maternal circulation; substances of small size, excluding blood cells, may cross this barrier). If the fetal RBCs contain the Rh antigen, the antibodies cause hemolysis (destruction). The higher the level of maternal antibodies, the greater the destruction of fetal RBCs.

Because sensitization most often occurs at delivery, the firstborn fetus generally has no signs of hemolysis; it is successive fetuses who are most likely to be affected. Today serious problems related to Rh incompatibility, such as **erythroblastosis fetalis** (a type of hemolytic anemia that occurs in newborns as a result of maternal-fetal blood group incompatibility, especially involving the Rh factor and ABO blood groups), are usually prevented by administration of a special gamma globulin.

ABO incompatibility is also an antigen-antibody process. Type O blood naturally contains anti-A and anti-B antibodies. These antibodies cross the placenta and cause hemolysis in the fetus if the fetus has blood types A or B. Incompatibility is also possible if the mother is A and the infant B or if the mother is B and the infant A. No sensitization is required, and it may affect the first and all successive pregnancies (see Chapter 29).

Clinical manifestations. The mother shows no clinical symptoms. Hemolysis may occur in utero, and de-

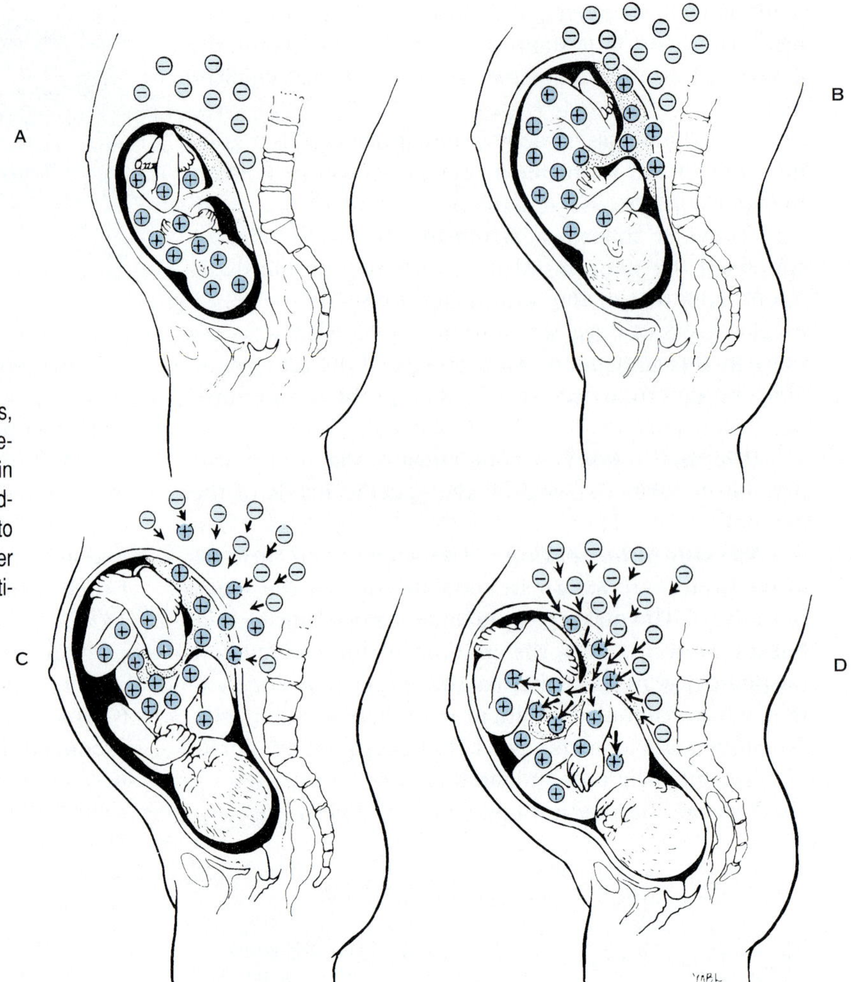

FIG. 42-14 Mechanisms of erythroblastosis fetalis, which is caused by Rh incompatibility. **A,** Rh-positive fetus is carried by Rh-negative mother. **B,** Rh protein crosses placental barrier and invades mother's bloodstream. **C,** Mother's system manufactures antibodies to destroy foreign Rh protein. **D,** Antibodies cross back over placenta and destroy fetus's blood cells, which are intimately associated with Rh protein.

tection must be made by diagnostic tests on amniotic fluid or suspected by changes in fetal condition or maternal diagnostic tests. Jaundice present at birth or observed during the first 24 hours of life is considered an indicator of a pathological condition. **Kernicterus** (an abnormal toxic accumulation of bilirubin in central nervous system tissues caused by hyperbilirubinemia (an excess of bilirubin in the blood of the newborn) may result in neurologic damage. Anemia resulting from RBC destruction is also possible.

Assessment. The maternal blood type and Rh factor are determined during pregnancy. If the mother is Rh negative, it is necessary to know the blood type of the father. If he is also Rh negative, no Rh-based problem will probably occur. However, because the negative factor is recessive and the positive factor is dominant, it is possible for two Rh-negative parents to produce a newborn with Rh-positive blood type.

If the father is Rh positive, the possibility of problems occurring is greater. It is also important to assess the woman's history for any occurrences that may have caused sensitization.

Diagnostic tests. Blood typing will reveal situations that require follow-up. **Indirect Coombs' tests** on maternal blood samples measure the number of maternal antibodies. Antibody titer tests determine the level of maternal antibodies. If the titer exceeds 1:16, amniocentesis may be performed to obtain fluid for further testing. Optical density studies, which measure bilirubin level, can be done on this fluid to assess fetal condition. (If the fetus is determined to be in grave danger, intrauterine transfusion may be necessary.) After delivery, **direct Coombs' tests** are done on infant blood to determine the presence of antibody-coated RBCs. Bilirubin levels of infant blood will measure the extent of RBC destruction.

Nursing interventions.

Maternal. If the results of an Rh-negative mother's indirect Coombs' test are negative, the mother is given an intramuscular injection of anti-Rh gamma globulin (RhoGAM). This is currently recommended at 28 weeks of pregnancy and again within 72 hours of delivery. RhoGAM provides passive antibodies and prevents development of naturally occurring maternal antibodies. RhoGAM should also be given to an Rh-negative mother in cases of abortion, ectopic pregnancy, and amniocentesis. The mother is given an identification card completed with vital information including date of last injection of RhoGAM. She should carry this card with her at all times.

Newborn. The newborn affected by a hemolytic process must be observed carefully; jaundice and anemia may become severe and lead to other complications. The nurse should monitor the bilirubin, hemoglobin, and hematocrit levels and notify the physician of any abnormal laboratory results. The infant suffering from severe jaundice may be treated with phototherapy or may require transfusions. If the infant requires phototherapy, several precautions must be taken. **Phototherapy** involves exposing the skin to fluorescent lights, which converts the bilirubin to a water-soluble form that can be excreted in the urine. It is important to maintain body temperature and protect the infant's eyes during this treatment. Stools may be loose and the urine contains excessive waste products, so it is important to maintain skin integrity by careful cleansing and frequent diaper changes. Because fluid loss is increased, adequate fluids are important to maintain necessary hydration.

Nursing diagnoses and interventions for the patient with hemolytic disease include but are not limited to the following:

NURSING DIAGNOSES	NURSING INTERVENTIONS
Fluid volume deficit, high risk for, related to insensible weight loss and dehydration from phototherapy	Do not clothe infant; to diaper is questionable. Maintain neutral thermal environment. Maintain axillary temperature at 97.7° F (36.5° C). Assess axillary temperature at least q 2 hr and prn. Avoid exposure of skin temperature probe to phototherapy lights. Weight infant daily unclothed at the same time on the same scale before feeding. Offer pacifier prn. Measure accurate I&O. Check urine specific gravity every shift. Test strength of bililight according to hospital's and manufacturer's policy. Note neurological signs of kernicterus and report immediately.
Parenting, altered, high risk for, related to disruption of parent-infant interaction secondary to phototherapy	Explain need to provide adequate fluid intake. Explain need to offer water between feedings. Discuss signs and symptoms to report to physician, such as recurrence of jaundice, persistent diarrhea. Emphasize importance of having laboratory tests done as ordered.
Parenting, altered, high risk for, related to disruption of parent-infant interaction secondary to phototherapy—cont'd	Emphasize importance of follow-up care. Encourage parent participation in infant care activities such as feeding, bathing, and cuddling. Review care of infant with hyperbilirubinemia as necessary with parents. Permit siblings to visit according to hospital policy. Turn off lights, and remove eye shields when parents visit according to time period ordered by physician. Reinforce explanation of phototherapy, reasons for particular interventions, and plan of care. Designate duties with which parents can assist.

PATIENT TEACHING. Rh-negative women should be aware of the process involved in Rh sensitization. The nurse should answer all questions that the woman or her spouse or significant other may have.

Phototherapy is likely to be disturbing to the parents and can interfere with parent-child attachment of mother and newborn. The nurse must explain the reasons for treatment and provide opportunities for maternal-infant interaction. Today many newborns are sent home receiving this form of therapy. Insurance companies are recognizing the therapeutic value of phototherapy at home. Many are now endorsing this trend by including phototherapy in their insurance policies.

The nurse must be responsible for teaching the parents correct use of the equipment and the special care required by the infant.

Drug and Alcohol Syndromes

Etiology. The pregnant woman who takes drugs or drinks alcohol not only places herself at risk but also endangers her fetus. Most drugs, including common substances such as alcohol and nicotine, are able to cross the placental barrier and affect the fetus. Depending on when in the pregnancy a drug was taken, the amount taken, and the chemical properties of the drug, a wide range of fetal and maternal complications may occur.

Pathophysiology. The exact pathophysiology varies with the drug involved.

Clinical Manifestations and Assessment.

Alcohol dependency. Use of alcohol may result in multiple anomalies called *fetal alcohol syndrome* (FAS). Characteristics of FAS are as follows:

1. Abnormalities of the CNS, including cognitive impairment, hyperactivity, and microcephaly. Withdrawal symptoms often occur within the first day of life. These include tremors, seizures, abnormal

reflexes, inconsolable crying, sleeplessness, and inattention to stimuli.
2. Facial abnormalities, such as abnormal eyelid structure, and incomplete development of the facial bones, particularly underdevelopment of the jaw and upper lip.
3. Growth retardation and failure to thrive are commonly seen and may persist long after delivery. Most affected infants are small for gestational age at birth and exhibit feeding disorders and vomiting for months afterward.
4. Miscellaneous cardiac, renal, and skeletal abnormalities may occur.

Drug dependency also manifests a wide range of problems. The symptoms depend on the particular drug used but commonly include the following:

1. Congenital anomalies, particularly of the cardiac, genitourinary, and nervous systems
2. Abnormal behavior, with difficulty responding to the environment
3. Respiratory distress related to narcotic depression or aspiration of meconium
4. Growth retardation often related to poor nutritional status of the mother during pregnancy
5. Withdrawal symptoms, including disturbed CNS function such as exaggerated reflexes, hyperirritability, sneezing, yawning, sleeplessness, tremors, and seizures. Diarrhea, stuffy nose, perspiration, flushing, and other symptoms may occur.

Diagnostic Tests. Drug screening panels may be used to detect the presence of these substances in the mother's urine or blood. These tests may be unreliable, depending on the time interval since the mother last used the drug. (See Chapter 47 for further discussion of drug screening testing.)

Nursing Interventions. Nursing care for the infant is directed at preventing further injury, particularly during the withdrawal phase. Observation of the newborn is essential to detect increasing instability. Infants of known drug and alcohol users are generally placed in a neonatal intensive care unit. Physical care includes careful temperature regulation and monitoring of vital signs. Small feedings are given, and the infant is observed for diarrhea, regurgitation, and vomiting. Positioning on the right side is helpful in preventing aspiration. IV therapy may be required. Medications may be administered as ordered to prevent the most serious withdrawal symptoms. Stimuli that may aggravate seizures are minimized. The inconsolable behavior of these infants makes providing care to them exceedingly difficult and stressful.

The parents of the newborn should be included in care whenever possible. Depending on the severity of the problems encountered, the infant may remain in the hospital, be discharged to the parent, or be placed in the custody of social services. It is a major challenge to establish a therapeutic relationship with the chemically dependent parent. Nurses should consult with social welfare or other departments that are best able to protect the newborn and also help the parent obtain the treatment needed to overcome the addiction.

A nursing diagnosis and interventions for parents of a child with a drug or alcohol syndrome include but are not limited to the following:

NURSING DIAGNOSIS	NURSING INTERVENTIONS
Coping, ineffective individual, related to lack of support system	Establish trusting relationship. Use nonjudgmental approaches. Allow patient to verbalize. Instill a sense of hope. Assist in developing improved self-esteem. Observe for medical signs of withdrawal. Provide supportive care during detoxification. Assess potential for violent or suicidal behavior. Discuss coping strategies. Initiate referrals. Encourage recognition of personal strengths. Assist in helping to develop problem-solving strategies. Explore resources for decreasing use of substances.

Other nursing diagnoses appropriate for the new mother who is also chemically dependent could be: Injury to fetus, high risk for, related to preterm labor and Nutrition, altered: less than body requirements, related to drug use/lack of knowledge.

Nursing diagnoses and interventions for the infant with a drug or alcohol syndrome include but are not limited to the following:

NURSING DIAGNOSES	NURSING INTERVENTIONS
Breathing pattern, ineffective, related to fetal alcohol syndrome (FAS)	Arrange for resuscitation equipment to be easily accessible. Place infant on cardiopulmonary monitor (set close alarm limits). Place infant in position of least distress (prone or side-lying). Suction mouth and nose as necessary. Implement seizure precautions.
Nutrition, altered: less than body requirements, related to irritability and poor sucking reflex	Elevate infant's head during and after feedings. Feed in small, frequent amounts. Evaluate different nipples for feeding. Burp well after feedings. Feed by oral gavage as necessary. Obtain daily weights. Maintain strict I&O. Keep suction easily accessible; aspirate nares as circumstance requires.

REFERENCES AND SUGGESTED READINGS

1. Acosta YM et al: HIV disease and pregnancy: antepartum and intrapartum care, *J Obstet Gynecol Neonatal Nurs* 21:2, 1992.
2. Anderson A, Anderson B: Towards a substantive theory of mother-twin attachment, *MCH* 15(6):373, 1990.
3. Arnold LS et al: Low birth weight and infant mortality: a health policy perspective, *NAACOGS Clin Issues Perinat Womens Health Nurs* 3:1, 1992.
4. Barnes LP: Pregnancy over 35: special needs, *MCN* 16:5, 1991.
5. Bastin N et al: HIV disease and pregnancy: postpartum care of the HIV positive woman and her newborn, *J Obstet Gynecol Neonatal Nurs* 21:2, 1992.
6. Bobak IM, Jensen MD: *Essentials of maternity nursing,* ed 4, St Louis, 1994, Mosby.
7. Bobak IM, Jensen MD: *Maternity and gynecologic care,* ed 5, St Louis, 1993, Mosby.
8. Burroughs A: *Maternity nursing,* ed 6, Philadelphia, 1992, Saunders.
9. Charsha DS: Effects of maternal bleeding problems on the fetus and neonate, *NAACOGS Clin Issues Perinat Womens Health Nurs* 2:3, 1991.
10. Costa T, Job Spira N, Fernandez H: Increased risk of ectopic pregnancy with maternal cigarette smoking, *Am J Public Health* 81:199, 1991.
11. Dorris M: Fetal alcohol syndrome, *Parents* 65(11):243, 1990.
12. Drug for respiratory distress syndrome: beractant—more help for premies' tiny lungs, *Nursing* 22(5):60, 1992.
13. Drummond SB: Disseminated intravascular coagulation, *NAACOGS Clin Issues Perinat Womens Health Nurs* 3:3, 1992.
14. Dubowitz LMS et al: Gestational age of the newborn, *J Pediatr* 17:1, 1970.
15. Eganhouse DJ: Fetal monitoring of twins, *J Obstet Gynecol Neonatal Nurs* 21(1):17, 1992.
16. Eganhouse DJ et al: Nursing assessment and responsibilities in monitoring the preterm pregnancy, *J Obstet Gynecol Neonatal Nurs* 21:5, 1992.
17. Fanaroff AA, Martin RJ: *Neonatal perinatal medicine: diseases of the fetus and infant,* ed 5, St Louis, 1992, Mosby.
18. Fleming BW et al: Assessing and promoting positive parenting in adolescent mothers, *MCN* 18(1):32, 1993.
19. Frager B: Teenage childbearing: the problem has not gone away, *J Pediatr Nurs* 6:2, 1991.
20. Gable SG: Diabetes mellitus: ways of individualizing care, *Contemp OB/GYN* 36(1):68, 1990.
21. Gilbert ES, Harmon JS: *High-risk pregnancy and delivery: nursing perspective,* ed 2, St Louis, 1992, Mosby.
22. Harker L et al: The last egg in the basket? Elderly primiparity: a review of the findings, *Birth* 19:1, 1992.
23. Harvey MG: Diabetic ketoacidosis during pregnancy, *J Perinat Neonat Nurs* 6:1, 1992.
24. Ingalls AJ, Salerno MC: *Maternal and child health nursing,* ed 7, St Louis, 1991, Mosby.
25. Iole J, Richardson M: Giving surfactant to premature infants, *Am J Nurs* 90(3):59, 1990.
26. Kenner CA, MacLaren A: *Essentials of maternal and neonatal nursing,* Springhouse, Penn, 1993, Springhouse.
27. Ladewig PW, Longon MI, Olds SB: *Essentials of maternal-newborn nursing,* ed 2, Redwood City, Calif, 1994, Addison-Wesley.
28. Lagrew DC: Strategies for managing embolism pregnancy, *Contemp OB/GYN* 35(1):113, 1990.
29. Laxery JP: Ultrasound in the multifetal pregnancy, *Female Patient* 17(5):116, 1992.
30. Lederer JR et al: *Care planning pocket guide: a nursing diagnosis approach,* Redwood City, Calif, 1993, Addison-Wesley.
31. Levine CD: Premature rupture of the membranes and sepsis in preterm neonates, *Nurs Res* 40:36, 1991.
32. Lindenberg CS et al: A review of the literature on cocaine abuse in pregnancy, *Nurs Res* 40:69, 1991.
33. Martin LL, Reeder SJ: *Essentials of maternity nursing: family centered care,* Philadelphia, 1991, Lippincott.
34. McDonald AD et al: Cigarette, alcohol and coffee consumption and congenital defects, *Am J Public Health* 82:1, 1992.
35. *Mosby's medical, nursing, and allied health dictionary,* ed 4, St Louis, 1994, Mosby.
36. Nager CW, Murphy AA: Ectopic pregnancy, *Clin Obstet Gynecol* 33:403, 1991.
37. National Center for Health Statistics: Advance report of mortality statistics, 1988, *Mortality Vital Statistics Report* 39(7)(suppl), 1990.
38. O'Brien WF: Predicting preeclampsia, *Obstet Gynecol* 75(3):445, 1990.
39. Olds SB, London ML, Ladwig PW: *Maternal newborn nursing: a family centered approach,* ed 4, Menlo Park, Calif, 1992, Addison-Wesley.
40. Pagana KD, Pagana TJ: *Mosby's diagnostic and laboratory reference,* St Louis, 1992, Mosby.
41. Phipps WJ, Long BC, Woods NF: *Medical-surgical nursing: concepts and clinical practice,* ed 4, St Louis, 1991, Mosby.
42. Thomas CL: *Taber's cyclopedic medical dictionary,* ed 17, Philadelphia, 1993, FA Davis.
43. Trustum A: When to expect ectopic pregnancy, *RN* 54:22, 1991.
44. Tucker SM et al: *Patient care standards: nursing process, diagnosis and outcomes,* ed 5, St Louis, 1992, Mosby.
45. Urrutia NL: Sorting the complexities of respiratory distress syndrome, *MCN* 16:308, 1991.
46. Whaley LF, Wong DL: *Nursing of infants and children,* ed 4, St Louis, 1991, Mosby.
47. Williamson WD et al: Congenital infections, clinical outcome and educational implications, *Infants Young Child* 4:4, 1992.

CHAPTER CHALLENGE

KEY POINTS

- Complications can occur during any stage of the childbearing process.
- The nurse must continually assess pregnant women and newborns for any signs of complications.
- The nurse must educate all pregnant women about danger signs that indicate complications, stressing the importance of prompt medical attention.
- Hemorrhage is a danger sign both during pregnancy and after delivery.
- Bleeding disorders of pregnancy are medical emergencies that demand expert teamwork on the part of the health care team.
- The type of spontaneous abortion determines the management.

- The cause of PIH is unknown, and there are no known reliable tests for predicting women at risk for preeclampsia.
- Magnesium sulfate, the anticonvulsive agent of choice for preventing eclampsia, requires careful monitoring of reflexes, respirations, and urinary output; its antidote, calcium gluconate, should be at the bedside.
- A wide range of infectious diseases present a threat to the mother and newborn.
- The Rh-negative mother may require special interventions to prevent sensitization, which may have an effect on future pregnancies.
- Preexisting health conditions, such as cardiac problems or diabetes mellitus, increase the risks of childbearing.
- The age of the mother is significant in childbearing. Both the very young and the older mother are at increased risk.
- Adolescents can develop trusting relationships with helping professionals whom they respect.
- Drug and alcohol use have a serious impact on the developing fetus.
- Newborns born to drug- or alcohol-abusing mothers may manifest a variety of anatomical and neurological defects.

STUDY QUESTIONS

1. Ms. Brooks, a 32-year-old multipara, is hospitalized for observation of hyperemesis gravidarum. The nurse should be particularly watchful for signs of:
   1. Abnormal bleeding
   2. Jaundice
   3. Acid-base imbalance
   4. Fluid imbalance
2. Mrs. Quinn, age 29, who delivered twin boys, asks the nurse if they are identical twins. The nurse checks the delivery record because she is knowledgeable that identical twins:
   1. Share the same placenta and umbilical cord
   2. Share the same placenta with separate umbilical cords
   3. Have separate placentae and membranes
   4. Have separate placentae and umbilical cords
3. Ms. Burns, age 26, is admitted to the hospital because of suspected ectopic pregnancy. She is at increased risk because her health history reveals:
   1. This is her first pregnancy
   2. She has used oral contraceptives for 3 years
   3. Previous treatment for pelvic inflammatory disease
   4. Multiple sex partners
4. Ms. Jones, age 16, 34 weeks' gestation, comes to the physician's office for her routine visit. In the past week she has gained 2 lb and complains of vision problems. The nurse suspects that she is experiencing problems related to:
   1. Diabetes mellitus
   2. Pregnancy-induced hypertension
   3. Hypoglycemia
   4. Impaired cardiac function
5. Baby Best, age 1 day, is noticeably jaundiced. His blood is type A, Rh negative. This is most likely to be a result of the mother having blood that is:
   1. Type A
   2. Type O
   3. Rh positive
   4. Rh negative
6. Mrs. Quinn, age 35 and a multipara, is hospitalized with severe pregnancy-induced hypertension. To provide safe care the nurse would need to be aware of the effects of the medication:
   1. Magnesium sulfate
   2. Tegretol
   3. RhoGAM
   4. Meperidine hydrochloride
7. The nurse is aware that seizures can occur with severe pregnancy-induced hypertension:
   1. Only during pregnancy
   2. During pregnancy or labor
   3. During pregnancy, labor, or delivery
   4. During pregnancy, labor, delivery, or early postpartum period
8. Mrs. Scott, age 23, is 39 weeks' pregnant when she experiences painless, bright red bleeding. The nurse suspects she has a/an:
   1. Hydatidiform mole
   2. Abruptio placentae
   3. Placenta previa
   4. Ruptured ectopic pregnancy
9. Ms. Post, age 19, a poorly controlled type I diabetic, delivered a male infant at 37 weeks. An important part of nursing interventions involves monitoring his:
   1. Blood calcium level
   2. Arterial blood gases
   3. Bilirubin levels
   4. Blood glucose levels
10. Baby Todd, born of a mother with a history of alcohol abuse, must be observed carefully for signs of withdrawal including:
    1. Respiratory distress
    2. Tremors
    3. Sneezing
    4. Excessive sleepiness

11

PEDIATRIC NURSING

I want to give service to people who need care, teaching to those who lack knowledge, comfort to those who fear. The idea of sharing a profession with intelligent colleagues who are dedicated to the same task is very appealing. The fact that the work is dynamic inspires enthusiasm. It's one of the few occupations left where high standards, honesty, and strong moral character are looked upon favorably. The woman or man in that white uniform inspires confidence because of the profession's good name. A goal to keep ever before me.

Debra D. Ledford
Student Nurse

43

BASIC PEDIATRIC NURSING CARE

Judy Holt Rollins

KEY TERMS

anticipatory guidance
birth defect (congenital anomaly)
body surface area (BSA)
burping
children with special needs
deciduous/primary teeth
en face position
family-centered care
fontanelle
morbidity
mortality
weaning

LEARNING OBJECTIVES

After reading this chapter, the student should be able to do the following:

- Define the key terms.
- Identify three events that had a significant impact on the health care of children in the United States in the twentieth century.
- Describe the purposes and outcomes of the White House Conferences.
- Describe five areas in which growth and development principles are used by a pediatric nurse.
- Outline several approaches for making the hospitalization of children a positive experience for them and their families.
- List general strategies to consider when talking with children.
- Discuss pain management in infants and children.
- Explain the needs of parents during their child's hospitalization.
- List 10 methods of preventing injuries in 1- and 2-year-old children.
- Discuss key elements of family-centered care in the pediatric patient.
- Discuss how age and developmental level influence the ways children perceive and understand experiences such as illness or disability.
- Describe alternative methods of feeding infants with health problems.
- Identify three methods of applying safety reminder devices for infants and children for safety and/or procedures.
- Describe the differences in collecting urine and blood specimens from young children.

RELATED TOPICS OF INTEREST

- Communication (Chapter 4)
- Life span development (Chapter 7)
- Vital signs (Chapter 10)
- Admission, transfer, and discharge (Chapter 11)
- Safety (Chapter 13)
- Specimen collection and diagnostic examination (Chapter 17)
- Basic nutrition (Chapter 18)
- Mathematics review (Chapter 20)
- Principles and practice of medication administration (Chapter 21)
- The surgical patient (Chapter 22)
- Care of the mother and newborn (Chapter 41)

HISTORY OF CHILD CARE IN AMERICA

For centuries children were considered miniature adults. In looking at medieval art, one observes that the bodies of children were painted with the proportions and musculature of adults rather than the physical characteristics of infants and children. Childhood was considered an unimportant stage of life.

In colonial America children were expected to assume adult responsibilities as soon as they could. The value of children was related directly to the work they could perform. Infant **mortality** (the condition of being subject to death) was high. Epidemics were common, and there were no controls or treatment plans for diseases such as smallpox, diphtheria, measles, or dysentery. Farm accidents and burns from open fireplaces or from gun powder also contributed to high mortality.

With industrialization there was a population shift from rural to urban settings and families moved into cities, where they lived in overcrowded and unsanitary conditions. Young children worked in factories 12 to 14 hours a day. The economy was poor, and survival was a real issue as family life was sacrificed. Children had no legal rights, and there were no work laws.

These conditions continued until 1860 when Dr. Abraham Jacobi, a New York physician, first lectured to medical students on the special diseases and health problems of children. Until then no effort was made to provide health care to children and their needs were not considered to be different from those of adults.

Some physicians, nurses, and social workers became interested in working with children. Pioneering efforts in the investigation of childhood diseases resulted in the establishment of "milk stations." Until then milk was not refrigerated and contained hundreds of millions of bacteria, which contributed to the development of diarrhea and tuberculosis. At milk stations, infants were weighed and mothers were taught how to prepare milk before giving it to their babies. Mothers also had access to nurses who taught them the benefits of fresh air, clean water, adequate clothing, and the recreational needs of children. This crusade for pure milk resulted in improved sanitation, the pasteurization of milk, and increased interest in infant care.

In spite of this effort, as late as 1890 about 20% of the children died before their second birthday and about 50% did not live to the age of 21 years. Families were large during this period, perhaps in an effort to compensate for these losses.

At the turn of the twentieth century deplorable social conditions continued. Children were being exploited in the work place. Many were homeless. Those in orphanages and foundling homes were subjected to cruel and inhumane treatment by caretakers. In 1909, with pressures to correct what was happening to children, President Theodore Roosevelt convened the first White House Conference on Children. It focused on such issues as child labor, dependent children, and infant care. In 1912 the U.S. Children's Bureau was established as a direct result of that conference. It was charged with investigating all aspects of child care, including infant mortality, child labor laws, conditions of social agencies, and the country's birthrate. This federal agency also published *Infant Care,* the most extensive collection of information on child care ever compiled.

With the end of World War I the second White House Conference on children was convened in 1919. It addressed the socioeconomic situation of mothers and children. The first federally supported health programs for mothers and children were established. The depression of 1929 paralyzed the United States and resulted in devastating social and economic conditions, which had their greatest effect on children. A White House Conference on Children was called in 1930 to study the economic effects of the depression on the health and well-being of children. Thereafter, a conference was held every 10 years, at the beginning of each decade, until the 1980s. In 1987, the National Commission on Children was formed on behalf of children.

These conferences have been responsible for many changes in child health and welfare, including funding for essential programs, legislation, and a shift from treating diseases to preventive health care. Those who attended were professionals who worked with children, representatives of federal and state agencies and volunteer organizations, and members of various citizens' groups. Although these people could not legislate, they raised the consciousness of public officials and private citizens regarding the status of children and families.

The United States did not recover from the 1929 depression for many years. In the interim the Children's Bureau was able to propose legislation that affected children. The most remarkable pieces of legislation were those authorized by the Social Security Act of 1937, which was signed by President Franklin D. Roosevelt. The health care needs of children were incorporated in Title V, and for the first time there was recognition of the needs of crippled children. The Women, Infants, and Children (WIC) program is one example of the benefits of this legislation.

Established in 1967, the Office of Child Development houses the Children's Bureau and the Bureau of Child Development Services, which operates such programs as Head Start. The Secretary of Health and Human Services is the cabinet officer responsible for all their activities.

In December 1987, Congress and President Ronald Reagan created the National Commission on Children to serve as a forum on behalf of the children of the nation. In May 1991, after 2½ years of intensive investigation and deliberation, the 34-member commission concluded that the United States is failing many of its children. For example, the proportion of children who are not adequately immunized for preventable childhood diseases has increased dramatically since the early 1980s. Lack of immunization resulted in 26,500 measles cases and 60 measles deaths in 1990.[6] The commission's final report listed numerous recommendations for addressing pressing children's issues such as the need to ensure income security, improve health, increase educational achievement, prepare adolescents for adulthood, strengthen and support families, and protect vulnerable children and their families.

An analysis of the progress made in child health and child care shows an increase in access to and a more equitable distribution of services in the 1960s. In the late 1970s and the 1980s the emphasis was on cost containment. Cost containment and access to care are major issues for health care reform in the 1990s.

Children are the focus of many reform initiatives in the 1990s, and solutions will emphasize collaboration between various disciplines. For example, violence, once considered solely a criminal justice problem, is now acknowledged as a preventable public health problem. The most effective solutions for this and other multifaceted problems will require the expertise of health care professionals as well as law enforcement and criminal justice officials, social workers, economists, and educators.

PEDIATRIC NURSING

The purpose of pediatric nursing is to promote the highest possible state of health in each child by (1) preventing disease or injury; (2) assisting children, including those with a permanent disability or health problem, to achieve and maintain an optimum level of health and development; and (3) treating or rehabilitating children who have health deviations.

Characteristics of a Pediatric Nurse

Pediatric nursing is different from other clinical specialties in nursing. First, the nurse must enjoy working with children of all ages. A great deal of time is spent with an individual child. Second, when a child has a health problem, the child, family, and disease become a nursing concern; one cannot be separated from the other two. Pediatric nursing is family-centered nursing in its truest sense.

The pediatric nurse must have keen observation skills, especially when caring for infants and toddlers or children who are critically ill or cannot communicate in the traditional sense. Some children have minimal communication abilities, and pain, thirst, and other discomforts must be interpreted. Also, the nurse can assess the developmental ages of children by watching them play or perform certain tasks. In addition, not all **birth defects (congenital anomalies)** (any abnormality present at birth, particularly a structural one, which may be inherited genetically, acquired during gestation, or inflicted during parturition [process of giving birth]) are diagnosed in the newborn period, and the nurse may identify a problem as a result of a physical assessment. When children are very ill, minor changes in their physical status can result in a variety of complications, and therefore any changes must be noted as early as possible. These examples typify the role observation plays in clinical practice.

Supporting a child through a difficult procedure or serious illness is an activity in which a pediatric nurse commonly becomes involved. Such an endeavor not only includes preparation for the event, it requires establishing a level of trust, which permits children to express their fear, apprehension, and anxiety. To establish a trusting relationship, a nurse must convey respect to children, talk with them at a level they can understand, and, most important, be honest.

Teaching is ongoing in pediatrics. It can range from explaining the effects of a medication to an 8-year-old to helping parents learn how to give a subcutaneous injection to their child. There also are innumerable opportunities to help children and parents adapt to a chronic illness or disorder, which requires a nurse's knowledge of community resources or volunteer agencies available for equipment or support.

Nurses also need to be aware of the indirect teaching that occurs through example. A pediatric nurse can serve as a role model for children, by demonstrating appropriate health promotion and prevention behaviors, such as maintaining good nutrition, a healthy life-style, and personal hygiene, or for parents, by exhibiting age-appropriate responses to children.

A pediatric nurse also functions as a child and family advocate, whether those activities involve an ethical decision or the quality of care given. This may involve a nurse coordinating the activities of a health team and collaborating with members of different disciplines to provide a child with the expert care that is required.

Being able to communicate effectively with a child is essential. However, to enjoy and continue working in pediatrics, a nurse must recognize and appreciate the uniqueness that each child or adolescent brings to a nurse-patient relationship. It is that special quality—uniqueness—that should be understood, respected, and practiced by anyone who provides care for children.

Children with Special Needs

Medical advances over the past two decades have resulted in significant changes in the pediatric population. Fragile or premature infants and children with severe injuries or disabilities who never would have survived in the past are now being saved. Progress has not been won without cost; many of these children are left with chronic or disabling conditions, some with very severe and involved implications. The definition of **children with special needs** includes infants and children with congenital abnormalities, malignancies, gastrointestinal

(GI) diseases, and central nervous system (CNS) anomalies. Many of these children remain dependent on technology.

Children with special needs comprise approximately 35% of the youngsters hospitalized today. However, many forms of technology previously found only in hospital settings have now been adapted for home use. With appropriate services and support, even children with very severe disabilities are living at home with their families and attending school with their peers.

Family-Centered Care

The term *family-centered care,* although part of nursing literature for many years, has only been redefined and clarified in recent years (Box 43-1). **Family-centered care** is a philosophy of care that recognizes the family as the constant in the child's life and holds that systems and personnel must support, respect, encourage, and enhance the strengths and competence of the family. Nurses and others in the community support families in their natural care-giving and decision-making roles by building on the family and individual members' unique strengths.

Box 43-1 KEY ELEMENTS OF FAMILY-CENTERED CARE

- Recognizing that the family is the constant in a child's life, while the service systems and personnel within those systems fluctuate
- Facilitating parent/professional collaboration at all levels of health care:
  - Care of an individual child
  - Program development, implementation, and evaluation
  - Policy formation
- Honoring the racial, ethnic, cultural, and socioeconomic diversity of families
- Recognizing family strengths and individuality, and respecting different methods of coping
- Sharing with parents, on a continuing basis and in a supportive manner, complete and unbiased information
- Encouraging and facilitating family-to-family support and networking
- Understanding and incorporating the developmental needs of infants, children, and adolescents and their families into health care systems
- Implementing comprehensive policies and programs that provide emotional and financial support to meet the needs of families
- Designing accessible health care systems that are flexible, culturally competent, and responsive to family-identified needs.

From Shelton TL, Stepanek JS: *Family-centered care for children needing specialized health and developmental services,* Bethesda, Md, 1994, Association for the Care of Children's Health.

To better understand family-centered care, it helps to compare how a particular situation was often handled in the past with how it is handled with a family-centered approach to care. In the past, parents were usually denied access to their child's medical records or hospital chart. With a family-centered care approach, parents have the same access to information about their child as all other members of the child's health care team. In some cases, parents actually record information on their child's chart. Other changes, such as hospitals welcoming parents 24 hours a day, reflect increased acknowledgment of the importance of family.

A family-centered approach to care is an important concept in the nursing care of all children. However, it is crucial for optimum care for children with special needs, who will likely experience repeated contact with the health care system throughout their lives.

Partnerships with Parents

Related to family-centered care is the concept of partnerships with parents. Parental involvement in their children's care has evolved from that of relinquishing their role to institutions to today's role of planners as well as recipients of services.

This role is best promoted by a partnership between parents and nurses, other care givers, and service providers. In a true partnership, parents are respected as equals and have the rightful role in deciding what is important for themselves and their family. The nurse's role is to support and strengthen the family's ability to nurture and promote its members' development.

Mutual respect is the foundation for effective partnerships with parents. Parents know their child better than anyone else and can provide the nurse with important information unobtainable from other sources. Parents of children with special needs also often become experts on their child's condition. The authoritarian tradition of the nurse of the past has been replaced by nurses who are consultants to their parents, sharing their unique knowledge and decision-making responsibility.

NURSING IMPLICATIONS OF GROWTH AND DEVELOPMENT

It is important for a nurse to know the basic principles of normal growth and development to understand what infants and children are like, what can be expected from them, what their needs are, and why they behave as they do. Although each child is unique, groups of children of the same age are more alike than they are different. For example, a number of general statements can be made about the babies in a newborn nursery and yet there are significant differences among them. In knowing their similarities, a nurse is better able to perform assessments, develop interventions, identify problems, and promote normal development (see Chapter 7).

The stages of growth and development are complex processes that occur as the body grows and the mind and personality unfold. As the newborn moves through infancy, toddlerhood, preschool age, school age, and adolescence, each stage consists of predictable, orderly events that are accomplished sequentially. When a nurse knows the normal milestones accomplished by a 6-year-old, for example, it is easier to identify a delay in the 6-year-old who has not mastered the developmental milestones expected. It is important to realize that there are differences in the rate at which a particular task is accomplished. One infant may sit up at 5 months of age and another at 7 months. However, *most* infants do so at 6 months of age. As one might expect, illness or a lack of stimulation interferes with normal development. Other variables that affect development include a baby's genetic makeup and a host of environmental factors, such as ethnic background, religion, family size, socioeconomic bracket, and education.

A student in pediatric nursing may ask why growth and development are important aspects of studying children. One of the nurse's primary responsibilities is to identify an infant or child who is demonstrating cognitive impairment (preferred term for mental retardation). The earlier intervention takes place, the greater the likelihood that improvement or remediation will be achieved. The nurse may also play a significant role in other types of interventions (Table 43-1). For example, nurses can caution expectant mothers on the hazards of consuming alcohol or smoking while pregnant, refer children with suspected delays to early interventionists, teach parents therapeutic activities and exercises to use with their children, and become knowledgeable about resources in the community that serve children and their families.

Knowledge of child development allows the nurse to use a developmental rather than a chronological approach to pediatric nursing care. A developmental approach emphasizes the child's abilities and strengths rather than disabilities and weaknesses. It considers children's individuality and personalities, and builds on

TABLE 43-1 Nurses Role in Preventing and Treating Cognitive Impairment

Characteristics	Examples
Prevention	
Directing efforts to prevention; occurs before the child is conceived or born	Genetic counseling Prenatal care Informing expectant mother about toxic substances, such as alcohol, smoking, and using drugs, and positive health practices
Diagnostic procedures	
Determining whether a disability exists, and if so, what the appropriate treatment should be	Denver Developmental Screening Test Hearing testing Early Language Milestone Scale
Corrective procedures	
Using a prosthetic device to improve the child's functioning	Hearing aid
Compensation	
Providing an enriched environment, and possibly stimulating the child's other senses to assist in functioning in an effort to offset a weakness	Infant stimulation Therapeutic play
Circumvention	
Finding a means of providing alternative sensory input	Early rich touching experiences for the visually impaired child
Remediation	
Attempting to prevent the occurrence of secondary deficits and to fill gaps in development	Physical therapy to prevent contracture deformity

Adapted in part from Anastasiow N: The effects of early intervention. In Anastasiow N, Harel S, editors: *At-risk infants,* Baltimore, 1993, Paul H Brookes.

what they *can* do rather than concentrating on what they *cannot* do.

Understanding normal growth and development enables a nurse to select age-appropriate toys for the infant or young toddler and devise activities that appeal to the school-age child or adolescent. Play is the work of childhood. It should be done in a safe environment, using toys that are safe. Children learn through every opportunity that is made available to them. One should observe a 2-year-old playing with a large, four-sided box to appreciate a child's curiosity or creativity. The child can do more things with that box than any adult could ever imagine.

Age and developmental level influence the ways in which children perceive and understand experiences such as illness or disability and, therefore, their ability to cope. Nurses with this knowledge are better prepared to develop appropriate nursing care plans. The following generalizations can be made regarding children's concept of illness at different stages of development:

- *Infants:* perceive illness as generalized discomfort and pain
- *Preschoolers:* conceive of illness as a punishment for bad behavior; believe that adults could magically cure the illness if they wanted to
- *School-age children:* may perceive illness as a result of bad or indiscreet behavior; can have an accurate awareness of the location of body parts and a beginning understanding of body processes and functions
- *Adolescents:* focus on discrete symptoms rather than overall impact of illness; can intellectually question and deal with information about illness; may use denial of illness or overcompensate in areas not affected

The nurse should keep in mind that children, particularly very young ones, can change physically and developmentally very rapidly. Therefore, continual reassessment is needed to modify nursing care plans to reflect these changes.

For a pediatric nurse a knowledge of growth and development also is the basis for anticipatory guidance with parents. **Anticipatory guidance** (psychological preparation of a patient for an event expected to be stressful, as in the preparation of a child for surgery by explaining what will happen and what it will feel like. It is also used to prepare parents for normal growth and development of their children) means to teach parents (and children when they are old enough to understand) what is likely to occur in the coming weeks and months so that the child's well-being will be protected and promoted at that time. For example, parents will know that their 9- or 10-month-old will begin to crawl from one place to another. It is normal, it is expected, and it should be allowed. However, parents must remove any harmful objects from the child's reach. Once a child becomes mobile, it is important to "child-proof" the environment, making it a safe one for the "curious crawler." Nurses play an important role in assisting parents to understand the physical and behavioral changes that occur rapidly in the developing infant or toddler. These principles also are useful in working with school-age children, who will be exposed to many new experiences once they start school, or preadolescents, who should be prepared for hormonal and growth changes they will experience.

DIFFERENCES BETWEEN ADULTS AND CHILDREN

The differences between adults and children are significant, including rate of growth, level of understanding, and means of communicating. Each stage of childhood is unique, with its own set of characteristics (see Chapter 7). A nurse must use different skills with children of different age groups. The challenges that children present to a nurse are constant, exciting, and satisfying.

At birth, all body systems are not functioning at full capacity, affecting, for example, how newborns and young children respond to medications: they are more susceptible than adults to the toxic effects of certain medications because of their limited ability to detoxify or eliminate drugs.

As the newborn grows, different systems of the body mature, teeth erupt, vision improves, nutritional patterns change, and speech develops. Gradually and through a series of complex processes, a totally dependent human being becomes a thinking, feeling, self-sufficient individual. Some of those processes are discussed here to explain the growth and development changes from childhood to adulthood.

Metabolism

The most obvious difference between an adult and an infant is size. The rate of metabolism is highest in the newborn infant because the ratio of total body surface area to body weight is much greater in the infant than it is in the adult. This proportion decreases as the child grows and matures. The basal metabolic rate (BMR) is a measure of metabolism when the body is at rest, and it changes dramatically as the body increases in size. When considering that newborns double their birth weight at 5 to 6 months and triple it at about 1 year of age, the nurse better appreciates the rapid rate at which metabolism occurs in very young children.

The body uses energy provided by foods. Whereas the energy requirements for an infant are highest during the first 6 months of life, they are fairly constant from 4 to 10 years and vary in adolescence, depending on the teen's physical development (Table 43-2 on p.1346).

Because metabolism is so high in infants and children, their ability to recover from surgery or a fractured

TABLE 43-2 Daily Caloric Needs of Infants, Children, and Adolescents

Age Group	Caloric Needs (kcal/kg)	Age Group	Caloric Needs (kcal/kg)
Infants		Adolescents	
Birth-6 mo	108	Males	
6-12 mo	98	11-14 yr	55
Children		15-18 yr	45
1-3 yr	102	Females	
4-6 yr	90	11-14 yr	47
7-10 yr	70	15-18 yr	40

Adapted from Food and Nutrition Board: *Recommended daily allowances,* ed 10, Washington, DC, 1989, National Academy Press.

TABLE 43-3 Vital Signs (Averages)

Age	Heart Rate/Min	Respirations/Min	Blood Pressure
Newborn	120	35	70/50
1-11 months	120	30	90/60
2 years	110	25	96/68
4 years	100	23	100/70
6 years	100	21	105/70
10 years	90	20	108/70
12 years	88	20	110/70
16 years	70	20	120/70

bone is swift in comparison with that of an adult. With all bodily functions accelerated, healing occurs quickly. For example, a fractured femur at birth is united in 3 weeks, but an 8-year-old with the same type of fracture requires 8 weeks for union and a 20-year-old takes 20 weeks to heal.

Vital Signs

Body temperature, which also reflects metabolism, is fairly stable from infancy through adulthood. The one exception is the newborn infant, whose temperature can be affected by the environment. An air-conditioned delivery room may result in the newborn's temperature dropping to 97° F (36.1° C) or lower, which accounts for the use of radiant warmers for newborns after delivery. Newborns also can have difficulty dissipating heat in an overheated environment, which increases the risk of hyperthermia.

Despite the ability to regulate their temperatures, infants and toddlers are prone to wide variations, especially after crying for extended periods or after active play. Temperature elevations also occur rapidly in young children when infections are present.

Although a temperature is taken rectally initially in the newborn to assess a patent anus, tympanic/axillary temperatures usually are done on infants and young children. Unless contraindicated, oral temperatures may be taken on children 6 years and older. However, many facilities are now using tympanic temperatures for all ages.

There also are great variations in the heart rates of children. Although the apical beat of a newborn may be 152 per minute, very gradually the heart slows to 72 to 75 beats per minute by adolescence (Table 43-3). The presence of infection increases the heart rate, as does physical activity. During sleep a child's pulse is at its slowest rate. Any irregularities in volume, rate, and rhythm should be noted. Whereas an apical pulse is taken on infants and young children, a radial pulse is often used instead on children over 2 years of age and adolescents. Pulse rate should be counted for a full minute. Some pediatricians request that their patients have an apical pulse taken. The respiratory rate also slows as a child progresses from infancy to adolescence. Newborns are obligatory nasal breathers, which means they breathe only through their noses, and will not breathe through the mouth until 3 or 4 weeks old. A newborn's respiratory rate is extremely erratic, which requires counting it for 1 full minute to be accurate. The rate, depth, and quality of respirations should be assessed. The rate may be as rapid as 40 or 50 breaths a minute, gradually slowing to 32 to 35 a minute by 36 hours of age. In infants both abdominal and chest movements are observed when measuring respirations. The presence of a developing pulmonary disorder is suspected when the respiratory rate increases.

The blood pressure is low in a newborn. Gradually it rises, so that by the end of adolescence it is about 120/78. When doing a blood pressure reading, it is important to use the correct cuff size to ensure accuracy. The cuff should cover two-thirds the length of the upper arm or leg. The crying of an infant or toddler can result in a falsely elevated reading.

Urine Output

A nursing responsibility is the monitoring, measuring, and/or collection of urine. Output varies and depends on the size of the infant or child. Table 43-4 identifies average volumes excreted at given ages.

At birth the renal system, like many other systems of the body, is immature. Many tests done in adults are not done in young children because of this. For example, urea clearance is impaired in young children, so it is not measured in infants or toddlers younger than 2 years.

Teeth

The **primary** (**deciduous,** baby) **teeth** (any one of the set of 20 teeth that appear normally during infancy) be-

TABLE 43-4 Urine Output

Age	Volume	Age	Volume
Preterm newborn	1-3 ml/kg/hr	1 year	22 ml/hr
Full-term newborn	3-4 ml/kg/hr	5 years	28 ml/hr
6 months	12 ml/hr	12 years	33-35 ml/hr

gin to descend between the sixth and ninth months of life. The central incisors are the first teeth to appear. By a child's third birthday, all 20 primary teeth are present. Permanent teeth begin to appear at about 6 years, and most are present by 12 years.

The eruption of teeth is distressing to the baby, whose gums are erythematous and edematous. The fussiness demonstrated may result in refusal to eat. A cold teething ring and numbing (locally anesthetizing) agents provide some relief to painful gums.

Eating Patterns

Infants begin life outside the womb nursing at the breast or ingesting formula or breast milk by bottle or tube. Whole cow's milk is not used until after 12 months of age because it can cause occult GI bleeding and iron deficiency anemia in young infants. Therefore, infants under 12 months should be given only breast milk or formula; after 12 months whole milk can be used. Skim or low-fat milk is not recommended because the essential fatty acids are inadequate and the solute concentration of protein and electrolytes, such as sodium, is too high.

Most infants are given solid foods at 4 to 6 months of age when they begin to need more iron in the diet and their teeth begin to erupt. Iron-fortified cereal is the first solid food given to a baby. Rice is easily digested and has low allergic potential, so it is commonly selected. However, oatmeal and barley are high-protein cereals that can be given also. After several months of breast milk or formula, the addition of solid foods to an infant's diet is a significant developmental step (see Chapter 18).

Although the order of introduction of foods other than cereal is arbitrary, the usual sequence is strained fruits, fruit juices, strained vegetables, and, finally, strained meats. As more teeth erupt, a finger-feeding food, such as zwieback, is offered. This helps infants develop a hand-to-mouth cycle, which is basic to feeding themselves.

It is important for each new food to be introduced at weekly intervals, so that food allergies can be identified (the presence of an allergy may take several days to appear). Development of a rash, wheezing, or diarrhea may signify the baby's allergic response to a food.

By 9 months, several teeth have erupted and junior foods, which are of much coarser texture, can be offered. These fruits, vegetables, and meats taste different and encourage the infant to chew, as a result of the different texture. Finger foods given at this time include pieces of fruit (excluding grapes, which could choke the infant) and cooked vegetables.

The cost of baby foods is significant; therefore as the infant acquires more teeth and does not experience difficulty eating solids, parents are encouraged to prepare these foods at home. Cooking fresh or frozen foods and using a blender or food processor is encouraged. By 12 to 15 months toddlers should be eating table foods prepared for the family. Although using a spoon is messy, typical toddlers become angry and frustrated when they are "ready" to feed themselves and parents continue to feed them. **Weaning** (gradually eliminating breastfeeding or bottle-feeding and instituting cup and table feedings) from the bottle or the breast is a major accomplishment of toddlerhood. That method of feeding has provided the child with a great deal of pleasure and satisfaction. However, solid foods also are pleasing to the taste buds, but when toddlers feed themselves with a spoon, turning it upside down as they navigate the utensil toward their mouth, they lose much of the food; the same situation occurs with a cup. A plastic cup with a spout decreases the amount of milk or juice that is spilled. Most 9- or 10-month-old infants, who can sit in their high chairs, begin to demonstrate a readiness to wean. They are becoming much more active and squirm when they are held for feedings. In addition, they observe siblings and adults drinking from cups or glasses and desire to do the same. Gradually, bottle-feedings or breastfeedings are replaced by the cup. Usually the bedtime feeding is the last one to be discontinued.

Sleeping Patterns

Children spend less total time sleeping as they mature. The newborn sleeps much of the time that is not occupied with feeding and other aspects of care. Most babies are sleeping through the night by the latter part of their first year and take one or two naps a day. Most 12 to 18-month-olds usually nap one time a day. The 3-year-old child has usually given up all daytime naps.

Vision

The eyes of a newborn undergo many changes before vision is comparable with that of an adult. At birth, visual acuity is 20/300, which makes it important for the adult holding a baby to assume an **"en face" position** (position in which the adult's face and the infant's face are approximately 8 inches apart and on the same plane, as when the mother holds the infant up in front of her face or when she nurses the infant) (Fig. 43-1 on p. 1348). Clear vision by the baby is achieved only at very close range. The baby should be held comfortably, so that eye contact can be made and the newborn can gaze on the

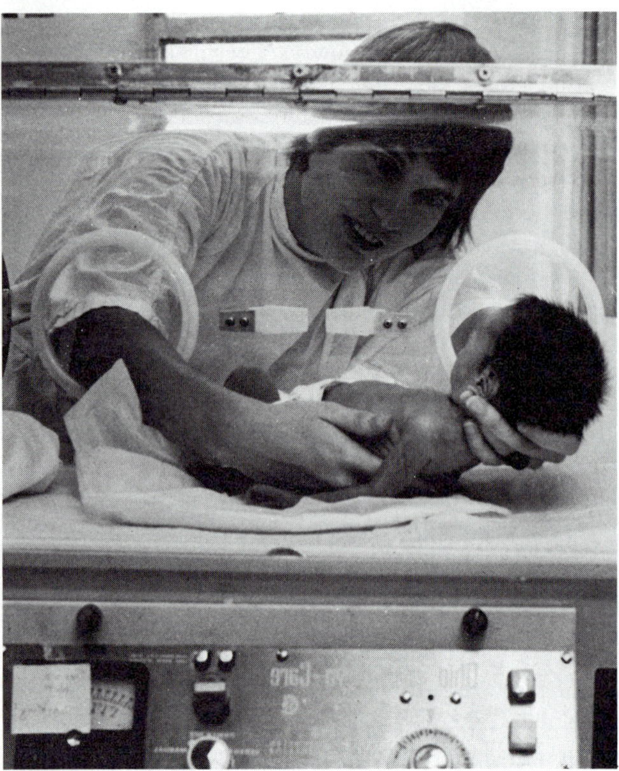

FIG. 43-1 Sometimes a mother must overcome a physical barrier to achieve the en face position.

face of the holder. Although tears are absent immediately after birth, by the second week of life, tear glands begin to function. Newborns can follow bright, colorful objects by the second or third week of life.

Although visual acuity is 20/200 by the fourth or fifth month, depth perception does not develop before the ninth or tenth month. One-year-olds, who enjoy playing with large objects (blocks, toys, and boxes), often bump into obstacles because their vision is only 20/100. By the fourth birthday, a child's vision is 20/20. When a child starts school, accommodation (changes in ciliary muscle and the lens in bringing light rays from various distances to focus on the retina) and refraction (the normal eye produces the proper image of the object on the retina) also are present. It takes almost 6 years of continual development for the parts of the eyes to function as they do in an adult.

Speech and Communication

Crying at birth is the earliest evidence of speech. Infants use this method of communicating when they are hungry, in pain, or need to be changed. Crying is gradually followed by other sounds, such as cooing, laughing, or babbling. By 9 months infants practice and painstakingly repeat the noises they can make. While they begin to express themselves, they also begin to imitate the vocal sounds of an adult. It is possible to have an actual conversation with the infant. Although no formal words are exchanged, it is a pleasant experience. The adult speaks, the infant responds, the adult answers, and so on. While each takes a turn at contributing to this verbal exchange, the "conversation" usually ends with laughter. As the infant begins to enjoy experimenting with these sounds, it is important to encourage these vocalizations; it is positive reinforcement for oral communication.

A 1-year-old has a three- or four-word vocabulary. It usually includes *mama* and *dada*. In toddlerhood more words are understood than expressed. Children usually know 25 to 50 words by 18 months, but by 2 years, they may know more than 250 words. Speech develops rapidly at this stage, as children practice and learn new words and their meanings. Soon they can say a two- or three-word sentence. Preschoolers have a fairly extensive vocabulary to convey their wants, needs, and desires (see Chapter 7).

An adult uses words confidently in speaking with others, but the same cannot be said for all children. That ability is determined by the child's stage of development, the amount of stimulation or encouragement received from adults, the child's health status, and many other factors. In addition, the development of language does not occur in isolation. It is related to the physiological, neurological, and psychosocial progress that occurs simultaneously.

A nurse should know what typifies speech at certain stages of childhood. That knowledge helps to identify a problem. For example, the lack of babbling or the inability of a 9-month-old to imitate sounds may indicate the presence of deafness or impairment of hearing. A baby who is deaf makes verbal sounds until 6 or 7 months of age, but without being able to hear, the child's verbalizations decrease and gesturing or some expression of body language (or nonverbal communication) increases.

A nurse uses verbal communication in a variety of ways. Talking softly to infants while cuddling them is an important part of establishing a relationship with babies. Although the toddler is leery of strangers, if the nurse talks with a parent first, the 2-year-old senses the trusting attitude of the adult and begins to participate in the conversation. As a result of improving verbal skills, preschoolers and school-age children understand more and share their concerns more easily. Teaching 8- and 10-year-olds is particularly satisfying because they are eager to learn. On the other hand, adolescents who have refined their verbal abilities communicate a significant amount of information nonverbally through body language, gestures, or facial expressions. General strategies to consider when talking with children include the following:

1. Use a calm, unhurried, and confident voice.
2. Speak clearly, be specific, and use as few words as possible. As a general guide, use sentences

whose sum of words is equal to the child's age in years plus one.

3. State directions and suggestions in a positive way, for example, say, "You need to stay very still" rather than, "Don't move."
4. Since children see things only in relation to themselves and from their viewpoint, focus communication on them.
5. After greeting the child, continue to talk to both the child and parent while pursuing activities that do not involve the child directly.
6. Use play as a strategy for getting to know the child. For example, if the child has a doll or stuffed animal, begin by speaking to the toy. Then initiate conversation with the child by asking simple questions about the toy.
7. Listen and observe the child at play. Often children will express important information, such as complicated and/or difficult feelings, through this familiar medium.
8. Look for opportunities to offer the child choices, but offer them only when they exist. It is confusing to children to have a choice offered when there actually is none. For example, when a child must change into a gown, a statement such as, "I need your dress off so I can listen to your chest. Shall I help you take it off?" gives the child an explanation, a choice, and some control.

Box 43-2

DEVELOPMENTAL CONSIDERATIONS WHEN COMMUNICATING WITH CHILDREN

INFANTS

- Consider body language, such as gestures and posture, as well as pitch, intonation, and intensity of voice.
- Nonverbal behaviors work especially well for infants, with cuddling, patting, or some other form of gentle physical contact often quieting them.
- Maintain a calm voice and avoid sudden, loud noises. The actual words spoken are not as important as the way they are spoken.
- Because infants can begin fearing strangers as early as 6 months, holding out the hands and asking the older infant to "come over" is seldom successful. If handling is necessary, the best approach is to pick up the infant firmly without using gestures.
- Infants are usually more at ease when upright and in visual contact with and close proximity to their parents.

PRESCHOOL AND YOUNG SCHOOL-AGE CHILDREN

- Avoid quick approaches with preschool and young school-age children. Let them make the first move whenever possible.
- Broad smiles and other facial contortions may appear threatening.
- Avoid extended eye contact until after the child is comfortable.
- Position yourself at the child's eye level. You will appear less threatening to the child, and the child's smallness will be deemphasized.
- Children may be more responsive when remaining close to the parent, such as sitting on the parent's lap.
- New or intimidating situations, such as hospitalization, are potentially stressful and may make it difficult for children to understand words with many syllables or even simple words that express unfamiliar ideas. Avoid expressions with dual meanings, such as "put to sleep."

PRESCHOOL AND YOUNG SCHOOL-AGE CHILDREN—cont'd

- Substitute words that may be interpreted as threatening with words that are less emotionally charged, such as replacing *stick* with *gently slide,* or *hurt* with *feel uncomfortable.*

OLDER SCHOOL-AGE CHILDREN

- Give children an opportunity to express their thoughts, concerns, and feelings. Listen and respond to underlying messages rather than just verbal content. Be attentive, try not to interrupt, and avoid comments that convey disapproval or surprise.
- Avoid prying, asking embarrassing questions, and lecturing when giving advice.

ADOLESCENTS

- Be prepared to deal with a wide range of emotions and behaviors with adolescents. Give concrete explanations that focus on the teenager's concerns, even though the adolescent's capacity to think in abstract terms increases with age.
- Although it is not necessary to be fluent in teen jargon, ask for clarification when necessary.
- To enhance communication, exchange information without using coercive questions. Initially confine discussions to less threatening topics to allow time for trust to develop.
- Ask broad, open-ended questions before specific questions, such as "How's school?" before asking, "What is the best/worst thing about school?"

Adapted from Clutter L et al: Communicating effectively with young children, *Children's Nurse* 5(4):1, 1987.

9. Be honest with children. Instead of saying "This will hurt" prior to a procedure it is better to prepare the child with a statement such as "Children tell me different things about how this feels. Some say it feels like a chicken pecking or a cat scratching. Afterward, will you tell me what it felt like for you?"
10. Use direct and concrete communication with young children because they are unable to work with abstractions or to separate fact from fantasy. For example, they attach literal meanings to such common phrases as "a frog in the throat" or "hold your horses."
11. Avoid using a phrase that might be misinterpreted by a young child. For example, the statement, "Let's see how warm your body is," is preferred to, "Let's take your temperature," since young children may wonder what you are going to do with their temperature and if you are planning to give it back. Words such as "shot" can be frightening if a child envisions a shot from a gun. Instead substitute, "putting some medicine under the skin."
12. Children between 5 and 8 years want concrete explanations and reasons for everything, for they rely more on what they know than what they see when faced with new problems. Continue to use relatively simple explanations, remembering that their expanding vocabulary can facilitate communication.

One of the most important points a nurse should remember is to speak with a child at the child's stage of development (Box 43-2 on p.1349). How a nurse talks with a 2-year-old differs greatly from conversation with a 12-year-old. To be successful in establishing relationships with children and to be effective in teaching or sharing information, a nurse must communicate with them at the appropriate level.

HOSPITALIZATION OF A CHILD

Hospitalization is an anxiety-producing experience for children and their families, primarily because of a basic fear of not knowing what will occur. It is an interruption in the child's normal development and routine, and it also results in separation from friends. Every member of the family is affected by the hospitalization because of its disruption in routines. Such an experience can be made less traumatic by anticipatory guidance, explanations, and preparation to help relieve fear and anxiety. However, infants and toddlers cannot understand. Therefore separation is especially painful for them. Preparation can be done for a scheduled admission; however, emergencies arise, and unplanned hospitalizations occur. In those instances, explanations should be given whenever possible and as soon as feasible to avoid traumatic situations.

Adequate preparation makes the transition from the security of a home to the unfamiliar atmosphere of a hospital less difficult. When preparation should begin and how much information should be given will vary. The age of the child influences preparation. A physician provides a family with details about a treatment plan, length of stay, and expected results or outcomes. Parents can then reinforce the information by explanations to the child, using simple, age-appropriate terms. Usually there is time before the actual admission to provide opportunities for the child to talk about what is going to occur.

Preadmission Programs

Many hospitals have orientation programs for children who are to be admitted. In some hospitals nurses conduct preadmission programs; other hospitals use child life specialists (health care professionals with extensive knowledge of child growth and development and the special emotional needs of children who are hospitalized).

The programs are based on the child's level of understanding and stage of development, with the purpose of familiarizing the child with hospital surroundings. These programs should dismiss the child's fantasies and correct misconceptions. The programs include tours and audiovisual aids, such as movies, slides, and puppet shows. The child is given simple explanations of equipment used during surgery and/or hospitalization.

It is helpful for children to handle some of the items they will see while hospitalized, such as masks and gowns, stethoscopes, anesthesia masks, and syringes. There should be time for questions. The nurse should encourage children to talk about what they have seen or heard. By doing so, problem areas or areas of concern can be identified. Some hospitals distribute coloring books or story books that focus on the information contained in the orientation program. This material reinforces information and also helps parents answer their children's questions. Brochures may be distributed at this time that describe hospital routines and list items children can bring with them to the hospital. Information is written simply, clearly, and at understandable levels.

Timing is important. Attendance at such a program should be enough in advance for the child to assimilate the information, but not so far in advance that the information is forgotten. Generally, the younger the child, the shorter the period between the time the child is told about pending hospitalization and the actual admission date. A toddler usually is told only days before. However, school-age children have a better understanding of time and the future; therefore they can be told that they are going to the hospital "in 2 weeks." Adolescents should be told as far in advance as possible to allow them time to inform peers and solicit their support.

Children should be allowed to prepare for this new experience in their own way. This preparation involves telling friends and selecting pictures of family members, toys, or clothes they wish to take, if they are permitted. Packing a bag with these items reinforces the eventuality.

Parents can benefit from such orientation programs too. They are provided with information that is helpful in answering a child's questions at home. Printed materials provide parents a reference guide for reviewing what the child has been told.

An emergency admission thrusts the child into an unknown environment surrounded by strange equipment, frightening sounds, and many unfamiliar adults. The incident that results in the hospitalization usually is sudden, serious, and possibly painful. The speed with which a health team responds to the emergency is critical, and there is little time for explanations. Whenever possible, a nurse must explain to the child and family what is happening. This can avoid an escalating crisis situation. When the child is stable and awake, a nurse can assess the child's perception of what happened, correct any misconceptions, and provide information not given initially.

Admission

In large hospitals children may be assigned to a nursing unit according to their age group. For example, a 2-year-old will be admitted to the toddler unit and a teenager to the adolescent unit. Smaller, community hospitals attempt to assign children of similar ages in rooms large enough to accommodate two to four children.

Pediatric units are usually bright, colorful, and cheery areas with cartoon figures on the walls (or ceilings of treatment rooms), many pictures, and large photographs of sports figures and popular singers. The unit or room may be decorated to reflect the age group admitted there. For example, an infant/toddler unit may have many age-appropriate toys, high chairs, playpens, and strollers. An adolescent area may have a lounge with a television, a stereo, records, tapes, and VCR. The pediatric environment is different from adult units to decrease anxiety by including many items that are found in the child's normal home or school environment.

First impressions are important and may influence the child's entire hospital stay. Therefore when children arrive on the unit, they should be greeted warmly and welcomed by name. After they are shown to their room and introduced to roommate(s), they should be given a tour of the unit. Two important locations to be pointed out are the area in which snacks or liquid refreshments are available and the playroom (or "activity" room when speaking to adolescents) where they will spend time when allowed out of bed. The play area is a safe, secure place for children. It contains an assortment of toys, games, and crafts for diversional activities. Newly admitted children also need explanations about when meals are served, how to operate their beds, and how to communicate with nurses by using a call bell or intercommunication system. Most hospitals welcome parents 24 hours a day, but others may only allow visiting at designated times, such as 10 AM to 6 PM or 2 PM to 8 PM.

Hospital Policies

There are times when anxiety levels about the admission are high. Perhaps heart surgery is to occur or a brain tumor is suspected. In those instances, a nurse may elect to postpone a tour or an in-depth orientation. The development of a therapeutic relationship with the family may be more important, because it can affect the entire course of a hospitalization. The nurse should inform parents that a tour and further orientation are available and that the timing of such events is the parent's choice. Some hospitals have facilities that allow one parent to "live-in" or "room-in," which means a parent can stay 24 hours a day. Beds, meals, and shower facilities are made available to them. Parents should be made aware that these accommodations are available. Hospitalization is especially traumatic to very young children, and having supportive parents stay increases their security.

Parents who are involved in care have a sense of contributing to the child's recovery, which is an important consideration. Having a parent present increases the teaching opportunities of a nurse. It also enables a nurse to assess a family's strengths, needs, and potential problem areas. However, parents need time to relax and to get away from the child's bedside periodically. Hospitals with a family-centered philosophy set aside a room or other specified area on the nursing unit for parents. There they can socialize, support each other, and share their thoughts. The presence of parents does not mean that nurses give up their responsibilities in caring for these children. Rooming-in can be an exhausting experience. Parents need breaks and relief to remain effective in supporting the child.

Certain hospitals allow children to wear their own clothes; this is especially important for a hospitalized adolescent. However, if a child is scheduled for surgery or an IV line is started, hospital gowns are required because of the possibility of loss or damage.

After a child is admitted, a nursing history is obtained. An identification bracelet, usually worn on the wrist, is important to verify identity when medications are given or procedures are done. These bands may be placed on the ankles of infants and toddlers because they are curiosity items on their wrists. When the band is applied, the nurse should allow space for one finger to fit between the band and the skin. The band should not be constrictive, and the skin underneath should be checked for its integrity.

Vital signs, including blood pressure, are assessed. The height (or length for infants) and weight also are measured and recorded. They are important baseline data. Height and weight may be used in calculating a

TABLE 43-5 Age-Related Concerns and Needs of Children Who Are Hospitalized

Concerns	Possible Responses	Positive Parent/Nurse Responses
Infancy		
The infant needs to have parents close by; parents are seen as powerful. Parents' presence and reactions provide best support in handling fear, pain, and separation.	Inappropriate bonding; development of distrust; anxiety due to separation and new environment; delayed skills development.	Close proximity to child (rooming in); frequent contact with child; stroking, cuddling, rocking, talking and singing, reading; communicating love for child.
Toddler		
Separation from parents is a major issue. Loss of control is viewed in terms of physical restriction, loss of routine and rituals, and dependency. The toddler fears bodily injury and pain.	Regression; lack of cooperation; not eating; no interaction with others; protest (e.g., verbal cries for parent; verbal attack on others; kicking, biting, hitting, pinching; may try to escape to find parent; clings to parent); depair (e.g., passive, depressed, disinterested in environment; uncommunicative; loss of newly learned skills); negativism; temper tantrums; resistance.	Praise for appropriate behavior (e.g., putting on slippers without help); restate reasons for hospitalization; rooming-in; continue with usual home routine (e.g., read a bedtime story); communicate love for child.
Preschool		
The presence of parents continues to be of primary importance. Hospitalization is perceived as rejection or punishment. There may be fears of mutilation. Treatment may be seen as hostile or punishment. Child is concerned with bodily penetration by surgery or injections.	Anger toward primary caretaker (parent); acting out (e.g., throwing toys, inappropriate verbalizations); refusal to listen to or look at or speak to parent; refusal to participate in hygiene and play activities; protest (e.g., less direct and aggressive than toddler, may displace feelings on others); despair and detachment; physical and verbal aggression; dependency; withdrawal; feelings of fear, anxiety, guilt, shame; physiologic responses; immature behavior.	Accept and provide outlets for child's anger; communicate love for child; maintain behavior limits (appropriate discipline); restate reasons for hospitalization; use play conversation to continue hospital experience explanation. Reassure child that hospitalization is not a punishment.
School-age		
The school-age child is primarily concerned with lack of body control and mastery. There may be feelings of inadequacy. The child may become demanding and rebellious to maintain semblance of control. Knowledge about illness is effective in handling anxiety.	Regression; inability to complete some tasks; anger related to confinement, inability to be mobile, lack of contact with friends; refusal to ambulate; loneliness; boredom; isolation; withdrawal; depression; displaced anger; hostility; frustration; excessive sleeping or TV watching; seek information.	Establish consistent visiting pattern; implement plan for continued education and teacher visit; set limits for self-care tasks that are attainable; praise for appropriate behavior (e.g., completing homework); arrange peer visit.
Adolescence		
Hospitalization may be viewed as a threat to independence. Conflicts over control issues become a focal concern. Separation from family and peers may interfere with developmental task mastery and can be interpreted as abandonment and substantiate a sense of worthlessness. There is concern about status in peer group after hospitalization.	Rejection; uncooperativeness; withdrawal; self-assertion; self-control; cooperativeness; fear; anxiety; overconfidence; may capitalize on gains from pain; depression; loneliness; withdrawal; boredom.	Support the adolescent's need for independence, confidentiality, and decision-making. Encourage opportunities to meet normal developmental tasks while in the hospital (e.g., schoolwork, visits with peers).

Adapted from Association for the Care of Children's Health: *Guidelines for adolescent units,* Washington, DC, 1980, Association for the Care of Children's Health; Magrab P: *Psychosocial development of chronically ill children.* In Hobbs N, Perrin JM, editors: *Issues in the care of children with chronic illness,* San Francisco, 1985, Jossey-Bass; Pass M, Pass C: Anticipatory guidance for parents of hospitalized children, *J Pediatr Nurs* 2(4):250-258, 1987; Whaley L, Wong D: *Nursing care of infants and children,* ed 4, St Louis, 1991, Mosby.

child's body surface area, which is important information when treating a child with burns or in calculating fluid and electrolyte requirements. Most medical centers use body weight in kilograms to compute drug dosages. An important nursing responsibility is identifying the scale used to weigh a child, if more than one is available, so that the same scale is used for subsequent weighings.

All newly admitted infants and children have routine blood samples drawn by a laboratory technician. Some hospitals make efforts to reduce the number of "sticks" a child receives by coordinating various physician requests whenever possible. Urine specimens are collected. The laboratory values provide a physician with baseline information, and they may be diagnostic. Additional x-ray examinations or procedures will be ordered as appropriate to the child's specific health problem.

Developmental Support for the Child

Hospitalization not only interrupts children's normal routines, it also threatens their normal developmental process. It is not unusual for children to regress when hospitalized. For instance, a young school-age child may resume the practice of thumbsucking. Often regression persists for several months after a child is discharged.

There are several steps nurses can take to minimize or even eliminate some of the traumatic effects of hospitalization on a child's normal development. Children's developmental level influences their understanding and response to hospitalization. Strategies for supporting the child are likely to be more effective when developmental concerns and needs are considered (Table 43-5).

Nurses should be especially concerned with meeting the psychosocial needs of children with special needs who are hospitalized. Because of the nature of their conditions, the likelihood increases that these children will experience invasive and traumatic procedures and frequent and lengthy hospital stays. These factors result in a group of children more vulnerable to the emotional and developmental consequences of hospitalization.

Pain Management

Health care professionals, including nurses, tend to underestimate pain in children. One reason is that some people falsely believe that infants or young children cannot feel pain. Another explanation is that children cannot possibly be experiencing pain if they are playing, reading, or engaging in other activity. We now know that anything that is painful to adults should be assumed to be painful to infants and children. We also know that children, like adults, may engage in activities for distraction, as a method of coping with pain.

Knowing when a child is in pain and how intense the pain is can sometimes be difficult. Infants cannot tell the nurse that they are in pain, or the pain's location. The nurse must rely on physiological variables and behavioral variables such as vocalization, facial expressions, and body movements, and keep in mind that whatever is painful for an adult will likely be painful for a person of any age. Nurses can assess pain in children with pain assessment tools such as the Wong-Baker Faces Scale (Fig. 43-2). Children may be reluctant to let the nurse know they are experiencing pain for fear of getting pain medication by injection. The nurse can advocate for IV pain medication administration, particularly when IV lines are already in place, and promote oral pain medication administration as soon as possible.

Children are often undertreated for pain for reasons other than inaccurate pain assessment. Fear of respiratory depression or addiction may mean that a child does not receive an adequate amount of pain medication, does not receive it often enough, or is not considered a candidate for certain narcotics. Although respiratory depression can be a side effect with opioids, evidence suggests that in children over 3 months of age (and possibly younger) opioids cause no greater respiratory depression than in adults. As for addiction, there is no indication that children are at any increased risk of physiological or psychological dependence from the use of opioids for pain management.

In addition to learning to accurately assess pain in children and advocating for and administering adequate

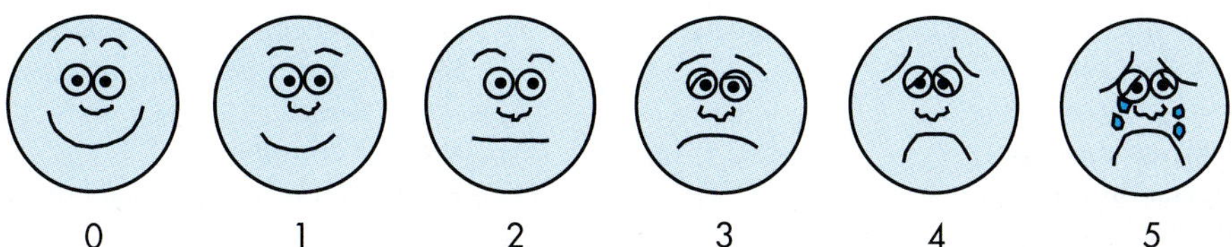

FIG. 43-2 Wong-Baker Faces pain-rating scale. Explain to the person that each face is for a person who feels happy because he has no pain (hurt) or sad because he has some or a lot of pain. *Face 0* is very happy because he doesn't hurt at all. *Face 1* hurts just a little bit. *Face 2* hurts a little more. *Face 3* hurts even more. *Face 4* hurts a whole lot. *Face 5* hurts as much as you can imagine, although you don't have to be crying to feel this bad. Ask the person to choose the face that best describes how he is feeling. Recommended for persons age 3 years and older. (From Wong DL, Baker C: Pain in children: comparison of assessment scales, *Pediatr Nurs* 14[1]:9, 1988.)

pain medication, the nurse can encourage parental presence and use sensitive care practices to lessen children's pain. Soothing talk or musical tapes can be integrated into care practices. Infants may benefit from pacifiers, swaddling, rocking, or simply being held. Care should be taken to let the child's needs determine timing of care routines, procedures, and tests whenever possible. The nurse can also take appropriate action to reduce noise and other disturbing sensations to create a soothing and calming environment for the child in pain.

Surgery

Undergoing a surgical procedure can be an especially stressful event for children and their families. Children facing surgery without information and preparation often develop misconceptions about the surgical event or any of the series of events leading up to or after surgery. Fantasies built on misconceptions may lead to fears, which in turn can lead to negative reactions and long-term consequences, such as behavioral problems or an inability to trust others.

Preparing a child for surgery entails providing information about what will happen and what the child will experience. Addressing the events surrounding surgery that are most difficult for children is a good place to begin. Six common stress points have been identified for children undergoing surgery: (1) admission, (2) blood tests, (3) the afternoon of the day before surgery, (4) injection of preoperative medication, (5) before and during transport to the operating room, and (6) return from the recovery room. The nurse can think through each stress point from the child's perspective to develop an individualized preparation plan.

Age influences the types of fears and concerns a child may experience regarding surgery. Table 43-6 lists common age-related fears and effective interventions. Nurses using children's ages as a guide increase the likelihood that children will be adequately prepared for surgery and all the surrounding events.

Parent Participation

It is essential to establish an effective, working relationship with parents as soon as possible. Parents are the most significant individuals to a child. Also, they know their child better than anyone else and may play an important role in assessing the child's responses. Therefore a nurse should project a positive attitude toward parents. It can be done by giving them a warm greeting, a smile, and establishing eye contact.

In obtaining a nursing history, it is important for the nurse to select a quiet place on the unit to listen to parents' responses and to provide them with opportunities to ask questions. The reason for hospitalization may be minor according to a physician, but a parent may perceive it as very serious. Parents may be fearful and anxious because of the seriousness of the illness, the procedures involved, or the pain a child will experience. Their apprehension then is transmitted to the child. Therefore

TABLE 43-6 Age-Related Fears Associated with Surgery

Age	Primary Concerns	Intervention
Under 5 years	What will happen when they wake up Where they will be Who will be with them	Show recovery room, if possible Tell when their parents will visit them after surgery Encourage parents to be with them as soon as possible
School-age		
Younger	Anesthesia That they might wake up during surgery How doctor knows when or if doctor knows how to awaken them	Show mask Explain "gas" or "medicine" and how it works Stress concept of "special sleep" Explain that it is a special person's job to control the sleep
Older	Same as above plus Operation itself Mutilation Possible death	Same as above Provide knowledge about procedure
Adolescents	Same as above plus Special anxiety for change in body image Loss of control while under anesthesia (in terms of behavior and for body integrity) Peer reaction to scars Impact on sexuality Impact on adolescent mode of dress	Same as above Reassure that only what is supposed to be done will be performed Introduce to peer with similar surgery

it is important to convey interest and concern and try to decrease their anxieties.

Parents experience a series of reactions when a child is hospitalized. They too are in an unfamiliar environment, meeting different groups of people who ask many questions and give them much information. Perhaps the tests or procedures mentioned are unknown to them, and they may become frustrated because they do not understand much of what is being told to them. Parents often do not know hospital rules and regulations and what is expected of them. They lose control in this setting and feel powerless. To this point, they alone have cared for their son or daughter. Now a nurse assumes control over the child's care. If an accident is the cause for hospitalization, parents may blame themselves and feel guilty. When a nurse meets the emotional needs of a parent, that mother or father is better able to support the child.

On admission parents need specific information on routines, hospital policies that affect them, any limitations that exist, and what is expected of them. When parents are given information that they can apply immediately, their anxiety levels decrease and they feel more comfortable.

Later, diagnostic tests, medications, or procedures that are planned by the physician should be explained to the parents. Anxiety and the sheer volume of information parents must absorb may result in confusion or forgetfulness about what they have been told. Any change in plans may generate anxiety and result in a parent being unable to process the information. Therefore the nurse should thoroughly explain the tests and treatments.

As the parents' comfort increases, they become more involved in meeting their child's physical needs. Mothers tend to spend more time with their hospitalized children and participate early in providing care. Fathers are often more reluctant, and they should be encouraged to become involved. When parents participate, they are contributing to the child's recovery. Another strategy is for the nurse to ask for parents' assistance in establishing goals or revising a care plan.

The equipment that surrounds a child can be overwhelming, with the strange-sounding alarms or with electrodes placed on different parts of the child's body (Fig. 43-3). When a nurse explains the function of a monitor or some other device, it often becomes less threatening. However, it is important to use terms a parent can understand.

Initially a parent may watch the nurse suction the child, perform chest physical therapy, or change a dressing. If a nurse uses these opportunities to describe what is done and why, parents become more interested. Eventually a nurse may hear, "Do you think I can suction Billy today?" The information that has been exchanged between a parent and a nurse, the demonstrations that have occurred, and the teaching that has been done have motivated this parent to perform a procedure he or she has not done before. Parents can become skillful in performing a variety of technical skills if they are taught in a patient, nonthreatening manner and if questions are encouraged. Some activities in which parents become involved include gastrostomy tube feedings, tracheostomy suctioning, and intramuscular or subcutaneous injections.

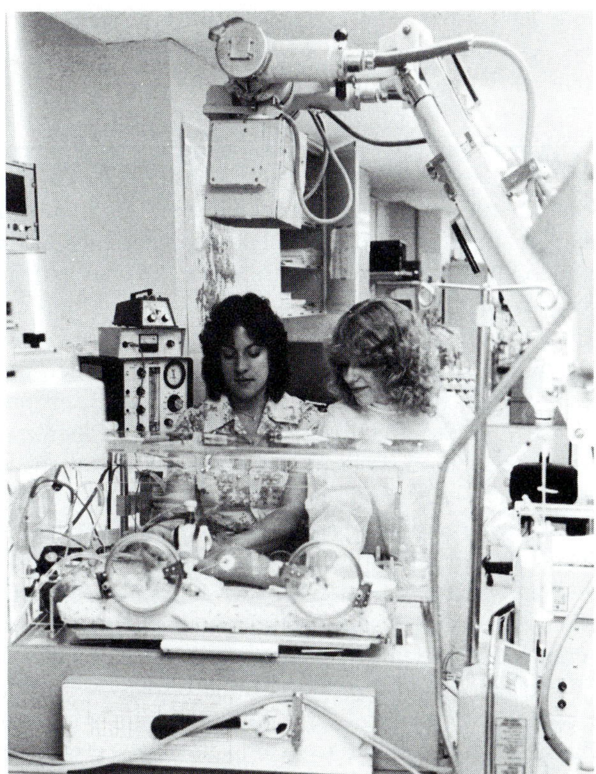

FIG. 43-3 A parent can be overwhelmed by the equipment that surrounds an infant.

Parents must be confident in their ability to perform given tasks in their child's care and should be encouraged to participate *only* in as many activities as they feel comfortable performing. Generally, the extent of parental involvement also is a good measure of a nurse's effectiveness as a teacher.

The last phase of adaptation for parents of a child who is hospitalized relates to discharge. Teaching is an ongoing process throughout the hospitalization and should not be postponed until the time of discharge. Although there may be some activity restrictions for the child, any nursing intervention measures that are required can usually be done at home. After adequate instruction and supervision by a nurse, parents usually can provide care as competently as the nurse.

The pediatric nurse must gain the trust of the parents by (1) reviewing and interpreting information from the physician as needed, (2) asking the parents if they have any questions, (3) conveying concern for the parents' well-being, (4) listening and being available, and (5) respecting them as experts on their child and soliciting their input. These activities are time consuming, and yet for a nurse who works with families, they are some of the most satisfying.

COMMON PEDIATRIC PROCEDURES

Some of the following procedures are general care of children, procedures healthy children experience in the home. Others take place primarily in health care settings. Many events that are common in health care settings can be frightening for children. Depending upon the child's age, the nurse should prepare children and/or their parents for even what may be considered insignificant procedures. Preparing children for procedures increases their cooperation, helps them cope, and promotes a sense of self-esteem and mastery.

Using a sensations-based approach is believed to be the most effective method of preparation. The nurse provides information about what the child might feel, see, smell, hear, or taste, along with emotions commonly experienced. For example, children scheduled for x-rays or CT scans might feel frightened, anxious, guilty ("Am I being punished for being bad?"), powerless, and/or curious. The sights they would see could include a "big machine" or "camera" over them and a lead shield or apron on themselves, the x-ray technician, and a parent if present. They would hear noises of the machine "buzzing" and the sliding of x-ray plates. The room and the table might feel cold, and the lead shield would feel kind of heavy on them.

Timing of preparation is important. It is usually best to prepare young children closer to the time of the procedure. Older children can be prepared further in advance. Children of all ages may be prepared just before less complicated procedures, such as injections, finger sticks, or taking vital signs.

Bathing

Bathing the child provides a nurse with the opportunity to do a complete skin assessment. When giving a bath, the nurse should protect the infant from drafts and chilling. Bathing is usually done before a feeding to prevent regurgitating or vomiting. The water temperature is checked. If the umbilical cord is still attached, a sponge bath is given. The cord and the area around it should be cleaned with alcohol, which helps drying.

Water only is used to clean areas around the eyes. A mild soap is used on the rest of the body, which is bathed from the face and down the trunk. One section of the body should be exposed, washed, rinsed, and dried thoroughly before bathing another anatomical part. A baby's creases need special attention. Babies have very short necks, and if not cleaned and dried thoroughly, the skin may become impaired.

If a sponge bath is given at the bedside, the infant should be placed across the width of the bed facing the nurse. This practice allows greater control of any movement by the baby and decreases the likelihood of the baby rolling out of the crib. Cotton-tipped applicators are *never* used to clean the ear canal, because injuries can occur with any sudden movement. A wash cloth is adequate. Special care needs to be given to the genitalia. In females, the labia are separated and washed, from anterior to posterior. The penis and scrotum of a circumcised male are washed. In an uncircumcised male, external washing and rinsing on a daily basis are all that is required. The foreskin should not be retracted because it is almost always attached to the glans. Forcing the foreskin back may harm the penis, causing pain, bleeding, and possibly adhesions. Ointments and powders usually are not recommended.

Infants enjoy being placed in basins for baths. After washing the baby's face, the nurse lathers the trunk and extremities. Using dry hands, which enables the nurse to pick up the infant more securely, the infant is placed in the basin. The head needs the support of one hand; the other hand is used to rinse the infant, who should be allowed to play and splash the water, which encourages development. After being removed from the basin, the infant is dried thoroughly.

The nurse holds the infant football-style when washing the infant's head. In this position, an infant's hip rests on a nurse's hip. While one hand of the nurse supports the baby's head, the baby's back rests on the nurse's forearm. This position allows the infant to look at the nurse's face while the hair is washed. After the hair is lathered well, the head can be rinsed over the basin at the bedside. Some nurses prefer to wash an infant's hair at a sink under running water. Parents raise questions about the baby's soft spot (anterior **fontanelle;** a space, roughly diamond-shaped, covered by tough membranes between the bones of an infant's cranium; the posterior fontanelle is triangular in shape). They should be assured that the area cannot be injured by shampooing.

Most toddlers love to be placed in a tub for their baths. Toys should be provided. They are used in splashing, water play, and bathing. It is important to remember that water is fascinating to a toddler because it has no shape or form. Safety is an issue, and a child should *never* be left in a tub without supervision. Most young children should be allowed to enjoy themselves in a tub for 15 to 30 minutes.

The school-age child may be reluctant to bathe, and many are not accustomed to a daily bath. Usually with encouragement from the nurse, children who are feeling fairly well will participate in their daily care. Nurses must use their judgment of the child's physical and mental condition and advice from the child's parents to determine how much supervision a particular child requires.

Most adolescents gradually become accustomed to bathing or showering as part of their daily routine. The need for an underarm deodorant usually becomes evident during puberty. Privacy when bathing and dressing is of paramount importance during the teenage years.

Feedings

Breastfeeding. Many mothers wish to continue breastfeeding their baby who is ill or hospitalized. The nurse can assist the mother by providing a quiet environment and a comfortable chair for her to sit in when nursing her baby. Some mothers are unable to be present for every feeding, or the baby is unable to take milk directly from the breast. The nurse can encourage the mother to use a breast pump and provide a private place for this activity. Bottles of breast milk can be frozen to be given up to 1 week later by bottle or tube feeding.

Formula. The position one assumes for feeding an infant should be comfortable for the adult and infant. The infant should be held securely in one's arms. A table or stand should be within arm's reach so the bottle can be set aside while the baby is **burped** (belching or eructation).

Formula or juice should fill the nipple entirely to decrease the amount of air swallowed in the course of the feeding. Infants cannot voluntarily push the bottle away when finished. Therefore they should be fed only as much as they voluntarily consume to prevent overfeeding. During the feeding the bottle is removed and the infant is burped. Newborns need burping more often than older babies. With experience, the nurse learns to recognize the infant's "cues," such as squirming, that signal when burping is needed.

There are three common methods of burping an infant (see Chapter 41). The infant can be placed in a sitting position on one's lap. With one hand over the infant's chin and chest supporting the body as the infant leans forward, the other hand gently pats or rubs the infant's back from the waist to the shoulders. The infant also can be placed flat across an adult's lap, using one hand to rub or pat the back and the other hand to secure the body. The third position is placing the baby upright, looking over a shoulder. One arm holds the baby and the other hand is free to rub the infant's back from the waist to the shoulders. Once air has been released, the feeding can be resumed. This process is repeated until the desired amount has been consumed by the infant.

After feeding, the infant is positioned on the right side. This permits the feeding to flow toward the lower end of the stomach and allows any swallowed air to rise above the fluid and through the esophagus.

Solids. When solid foods are started, the infant should be fed in an infant seat. The safety strap should always be in place securely. In an infant seat, the baby's eyes can focus on the adult, while both hands of an adult are free to introduce solids to the infant. Once an infant achieves control, the baby can be held in the arms of an adult. Older infants (8 or 9 months old) can be placed in a high chair with a safety strap in place. It may be necessary to provide additional support. Baby blankets rolled up and placed on either side of the infant's trunk provide effective support.

> It is important to wait to start solid foods until your baby is ready. Children do better with feeding if they have some control over the process. *The semireclining baby will have very little control over the spoon-feeding process.* The sitting baby can look at the spoon, feel the food with his fingers, get his fingers to his mouth. . . . He can open his mouth and lean forward if he wants to eat; he can close his mouth and turn his head away if he is not interested. It is easy for a parent to pick up and understand feeding cues from a sitting up baby who is eating solid food. It is much harder if you are starting out with one who is really too little, lying back in his infant seat.*

Once a toddler has begun walking, placement in a high chair is a confinement that might be vigorously resisted. In climbing out of a high chair, a toddler may fall and sustain a significant injury, despite the fact that a safety strap was used. There are two points to remember when dealing with a toddler. First, the toddler's appetite decreases at this age and this is normal. Second, resistance to the high chair may be intense, and an injury can occur. It may be advantageous to try an alternative. While they take in less solid food, toddlers continue to drink liquids freely.

> Not all walking babies vigorously resist high chairs. There are individual children who do, but this does not include all older babies. Eventually all babies/toddlers will resist a high chair, but base the timing on when to quit using the high chair on each individual baby. There are alternatives such as a booster seat, or pushing the high chair up to the table, or stools with backs/arm rests. Make sure the toddler's feet are supported—not dangling. Make sure he is at a height where he does not have to reach "up" to get his food and make sure he is close enough to the table to be somewhat confined so his attention is on eating. *Ideally* the family eats at the same time as the toddler; therefore, there is less risk for injury because parents can prevent the child from climbing all over his chair. (Sometimes *ideal* doesn't always occur.)
>
> It is usually not a good idea to put food on a chair and let the child "stroll by" and eat! First of all, the parent better know a good carpet and upholstery cleaner—the child is going to have food all over the house. Also—more seriously—children, even babies, need limits. They should learn that you eat *at the table,* you eat *at regular times,* and you eat *with the family* (ideally), you learn behavior standards at the table (manners)—toddlers learn these gradually.
>
> Parents should have three regular meals and *planned* snacks each day so the child eats about every 2-3 hours.
>
> Also, children should sit down to eat. Choking is more likely if children eat on the run.*

*Kristen Naughan, RD; educator; mother of four.

Gavage. Some infants and children need gavage feedings. This involves passing a feeding tube through the nose or mouth, down the esophagus, and into the stomach. Although in many health care settings nurses must have additional training before performing this function, they usually assist with the tube placement and are permitted to perform the actual tube feedings.

Commonly used methods to determine the length to insert the tube in children are (1) measuring from the nose to the bottom of the earlobe and then to the end of the xiphoid process or (2) measuring from the nose to the earlobe and then to a point midway between the xiphoid process and the umbilicus. However, the accuracy of these traditional methods has been questioned in recent years. Recent research indicates that using a child's height may be the more valid measurement method to predict gastric tube insertion distance.

Some restraint of infant activity may be necessary when passing the tube. Pulling up the bottom of the shirt over both arms is often all that is needed to restrain the newborn. Some infants may need to be wrapped in a mummy safety reminder device before proceeding. The mummy safety reminder device is described in a later section. A small towel folded across the chest and secured beneath the shoulders, taking care that breathing is not compromised, is usually sufficient in the unlikely event that a premature infant requires restraint.

Because infants are nose breathers, the mouth is the preferred route for tube insertion. The tube may be passed through the nose for older infants and children. Children who are able are asked to swallow while the tube is being inserted. A tube that will be indwelling is almost always inserted through the nose; alternate nares are used for reinsertion to prevent irritation. Once inserted, the tube is taped in place. If inserted through a naris, the tube is taped to the cheek, not to the forehead, to prevent possible damage to the nostril.

Before feedings, tube placement should be checked by *both* (1) aspirating for stomach contents and (2) injecting a small amount of air (0.5 to 1 ml in premature or very small infants to 5 ml in larger children) through the syringe into the tube while simultaneously listening with a stethoscope over the stomach area for sounds of gurgling or growling. If there is any doubt about tube placement, feeding should not proceed, and the practitioner should be consulted. Radiography may be necessary to confirm proper tube placement.

Whenever possible, the nurse should hold the infant during the feeding. If this is impossible, the infant or child should be positioned on the back or toward the right side with the head and chest elevated. Infants are given a pacifier during feedings to encourage sucking and help them associate sucking with satisfying hunger. The formula should be warmed to room temperature, and, after a gentle push with the plunger, allowed to flow into the stomach by gravity. Rates of no more than 5 ml every 5 to 10 minutes in premature and very small infants and 10 ml/minute in older infants and children should be followed to prevent nausea and regurgitation. At the completion of the feeding the nurse flushes the tube with sterile water (1 or 2 ml for small tubes to 5 ml or more for large ones). Indwelling tubes are clamped or capped after feeding. If the tube is to be removed, it is pinched firmly to prevent escape of fluid and withdrawn quickly. The child is positioned on the right side for at least 1 hour to minimize the possibility of regurgitation and aspiration. The infant is burped if condition permits. The nurse records the type and amount of feeding given and the child's response.

Gastrostomy. A gastrostomy tube is often used in children when passing a gastric tube is contraindicated or in children who require tube feeding over an extended period. The tube is placed when the child is under general anesthesia or percutaneously using an endoscope with the child under local anesthesia. A tube is inserted through the abdominal wall into the stomach, secured by a purse-string suture, and the stomach is anchored to the peritoneum at the operative site. Feeding is carried out is the same manner and rate as in gavage feeding. After feedings, the nurse places the child on the right side or in Fowler's position. The tube may be left open and suspended or clamped between feedings, depending on the child's condition.

Total Parenteral Nutrition (TPN). When feeding by way of the GI tract is impossible, inadequate, or hazardous, TPN (also called IV alimentation or hyperalimentation) may be used. A highly concentrated solution of protein, glucose, and other nutrients is infused intravenously through conventional tubing with a special filter attached to remove particulate matter or microorganisms. Wide-diameter vessels, such as the superior vena cava or subclavian veins, are the usual sites of infusion. In most health care settings the nurse must have additional training before assisting with TPN. Nursing responsibilities include control of sepsis, monitoring of the infusion rate, and continuous observations.

Safety Reminder Devices

There are times when, for safety, children should be restrained after surgery or during a procedure or examination. Safety reminder devices (SRDs) are used only as a last resort. They should be applied correctly, and circulation and skin integrity are monitored closely. Any SRD should be removed every 2 hours so that the body area can be exercised. If extremities are restrained, they should be released one at a time so that the child cannot pull out an IV or a nasogastric (NG) tube. The ties of all SRDs are attached to bedframes *only,* not to side rails.

Elbow SRD. Elbow SRDs prevent flexion or bending of elbows. They allow an infant or toddler to move the upper extremities, but they protect the newly repaired cleft lip/palate or scalp vein infusion site. Clean tongue blades are slipped into the parallel pockets of a wraparound SRD (see Chapter 13). The shirt or pajama sleeve is pulled down to the wrist, and the elbow is placed in the center of this SRD. The SRD is wrapped around the arm and tied securely. The sleeve is cuffed over the bottom of the SRD to protect the skin. Both the axilla and the wrist should be checked for skin impairment.

Mummy SRD. A mummy SRD is used when the trunk and upper and lower extremities should be immobilized. A jugular venipuncture or the insertion of a NG tube may require this type of SRD.

A square baby blanket is placed on a crib, and one corner is folded over. The infant is placed on the back on the blanket so the shoulders are at the level of the fold and arms are at the sides. One corner of the blanket is wrapped over the right arm and tucked under the infant's left side. The opposite corner is placed over the left arm and placed securely under the right side of the body (Fig. 43-4). A commercially prepared mummy SRD is also available.

A modified version may be necessary to expose the chest. While one corner of the blanket is placed around the right arm and tucked under the baby's body, the opposite corner encircles the left arm and it too is secured. The corner beneath the feet is brought up to the abdomen and pinned, thereby leaving the chest exposed.

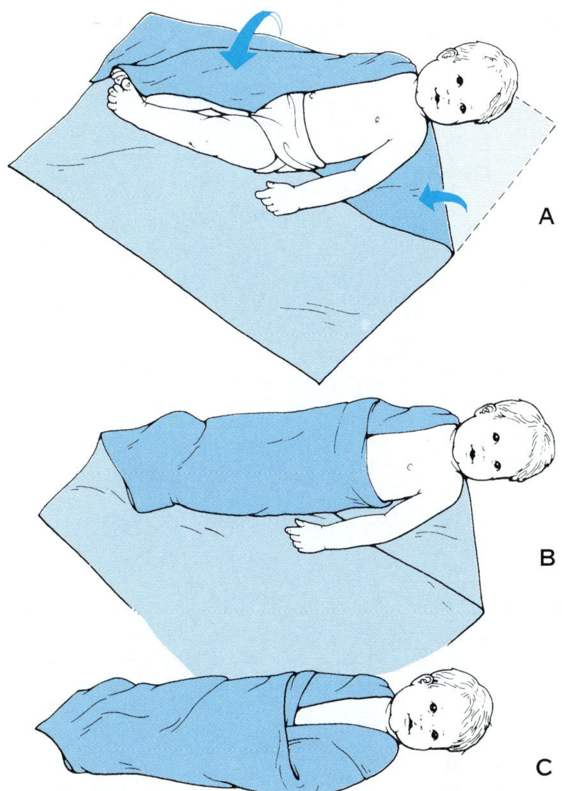

FIG. 43-4 **A** and **B,** Mummy restraint. Material is first folded over the right arm, and then corner is tucked under the left side. **C,** The opposite corner is then folded over the infant's left arm and tucked under the right side to secure.

Clove-Hitch SRD. This type of four-point SRD is used on all extremities of a child. Rolls of Kerlix, roller bandage, or strips of muslin can be used. The wrists and ankles are padded with gauze squares or other soft material. A clove hitch is *not* a square knot. A figure 8 is made with the material, slipped over the padded wrist or ankle, and tightened gently (see Chapter 13). Each SRD should be checked frequently so that circulation is not affected or there is no excessive pressure. A slip knot is used to tie the ends of these SRDs to the bed frame.

Jacket SRD. A jacket SRD is sometimes used to keep an extremely active older infant or toddler safely in bed or in a high chair. It resembles a vest and has ties in the back. The child's arms are pulled through the jacket, and the jacket is tied in the back. The long ties are attached to a bed frame or under the seat of a high chair. While children can move all body parts, they cannot climb out of beds or high chairs.

Urine Collection

Collecting a urine specimen can be a major problem in pediatrics when the child is not toilet trained. It is often a routine admission procedure that provides important information. In addition, kidney infections are common, and so urine should be collected and examined often.

A suprapubic bladder tap is sometimes done on newborns and infants (Fig. 43-5 on p.1360). Contamination is a minimal concern using this method. An infant is placed in a froglike position, similar to the position described later for femoral venipunctures. A physician prepares the skin above the bladder and inserts a 20- or 21-gauge needle into the bladder and removes several milliliters of urine. The nurse gently prevents the legs from excessive movement, which could cause injury at the insertion site, by holding the infant's legs in a froglike position. It is usually done 30 to 60 minutes after voiding.

Plastic urine collecting bags also are used. It is important to apply them correctly. Applying tincture of benzoin to the area increases the adhesiveness of these bags (Fig. 43-6 on p.1360). In girls special attention should be given to the narrow area between the vagina and the rectum. If the adhesive backing is not attached securely to this area, the anus is covered. As a result, a stool may contaminate the specimen.

When the bag is in place, a slit should be cut into the disposable diaper before it is placed on the child. By doing so the urine bag can be pulled through to the outside so it can be observed. As soon as the child voids,

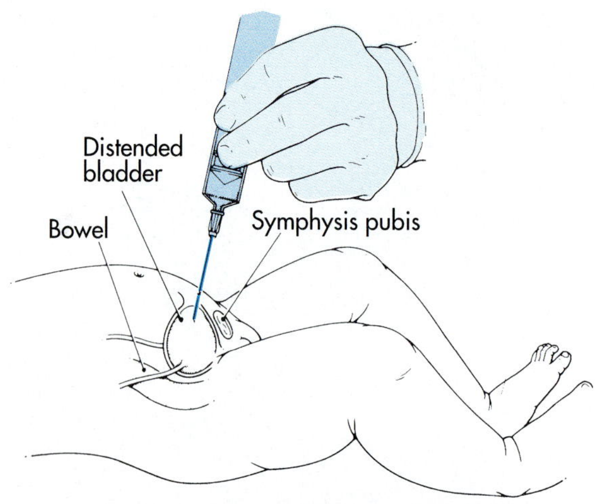

FIG. 43-5 Suprapubic bladder aspiration.

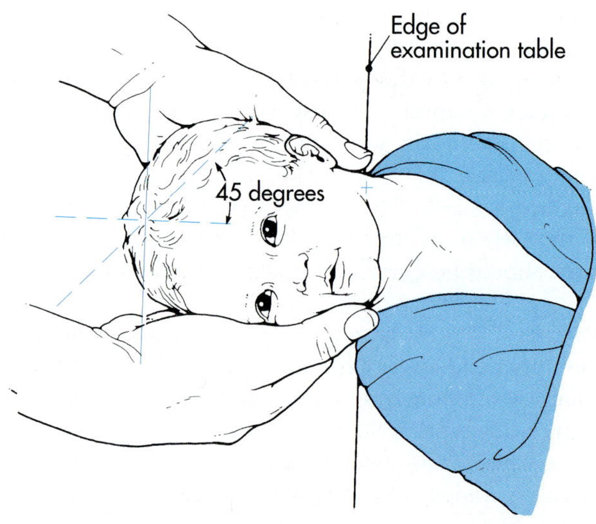

FIG. 43-7 Correct position for jugular venipuncture procedure. The puncture site is indicated by *x*. The mummy SRD is used.

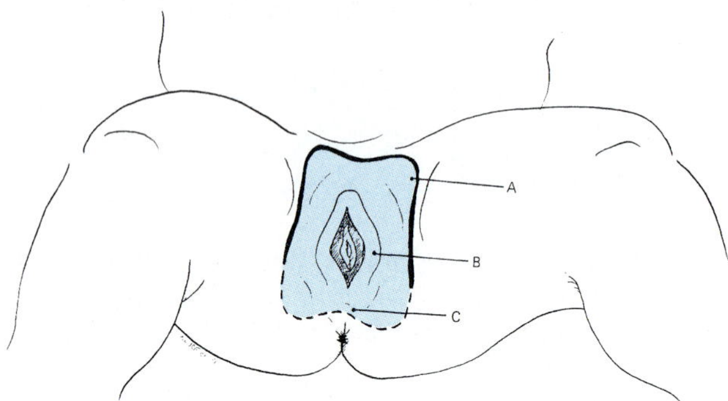

FIG. 43-6 Application of a pediatric urine bag for female infants. *A,* Pediatric urine bag. *B,* Labia majora. *C,* Pelvic floor (in female infants it is important to attach the bag securely at this point).

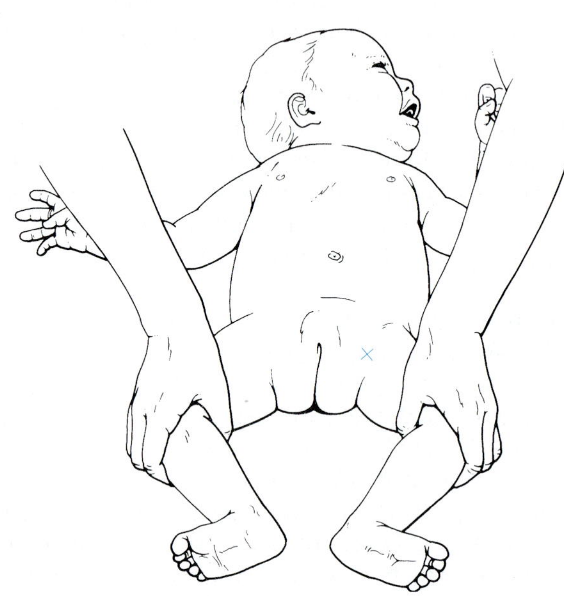

FIG. 43-8 Position for femoral venipuncture procedure. The *x* indicates the puncture site.

the bag is removed, decreasing the possibility of losing the urine specimen.

Catheterizations are done occasionally. The high possibility of contamination, especially in regard to introducing organisms into the urinary system, has resulted in avoiding this procedure as much as possible.

Venipunctures

In infants and young children, a jugular or femoral vein may be used to obtain a blood specimen. It is the nurse's responsibility to prepare, position, and restrain the child. Holding the head or lower extremities absolutely immobile is critical.

When a jugular vein is used, the child is placed in a mummy SRD beforehand. The child's body is placed on the examining table so that the shoulders are at the edge of the table (Fig. 43-7). Turning the infant's head 45 degrees provides the best angle for successful entry.

For a femoral venipuncture, the infant is placed on the back with both legs in a froglike position (Fig. 43-8). It is necessary to apply gentle pressure to both knees to restrict movement. Once the needle has been removed from the vein, pressure should be applied to the site to prevent the formation of a hematoma.

Sometimes the veins of the extremities, especially the arm and the hand, are used. Older children, with appropriate explanation, preparation, and support, will usually require only minimal if any restraint. Younger children can be restrained by having the technician on one side of the child's bed and the nurse on the other. The nurse can lean across the child's upper body to prevent movement and immobilize the venipuncture site with an arm.

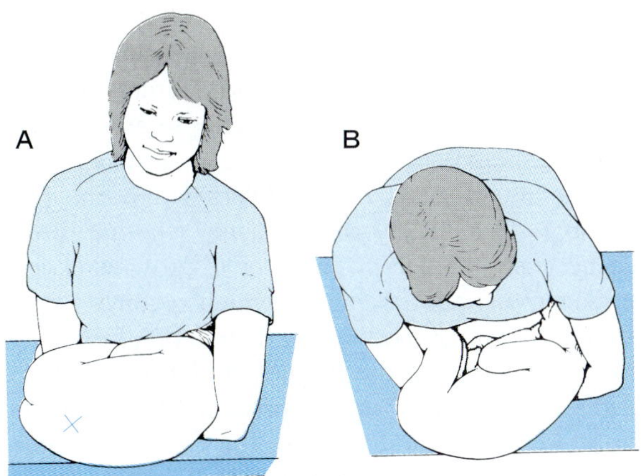

FIG. 43-9 **A,** Correct position for lumbar puncture procedure with infant at or over table edge; the *x* indicates the puncture site. **B,** View of lumbar puncture restraint from above.

Lumbar Puncture

This procedure requires positioning the child at the edge of the examining table or bed, on the side, facing the nurse. Infants are often placed in a sitting position. The neck and legs are gently flexed, as demonstrated in Fig. 43-9. This angle increases the spinal curvature and helps the physician to gain entry into the subarachnoid space of the spinal canal. It is important to observe the child for any sign of difficulty. A toddler's legs may need to be wrapped in a blanket to decrease activity. The child should be held securely in that position until the spinal tap has been completed.

Oxygen Therapy

Oxygen is used to improve a child's respiratory status. It is also used in children who have cardiac or neurological disorders. When a nurse administers oxygen to a newborn or infant, it is important to remember the harmful effects of oxygen on the developing pulmonary system. Oxygen is forced through sterile water to humidify it to counteract its drying effect. Oxygen levels must be checked frequently (q2hr).

Infants and young children receiving oxygen are monitored on an oximeter, a flexible photoelectric device with adhesive backing placed on the foot or hand of an infant or finger of an adolescent. The monitoring screen gives an instant reading of the oxygen saturation of blood. There is a high correlation between this measurement and the arterial oxygenation.

Hood and Incubator. Oxygen often is delivered to small infants through a plastic hood that fits over the baby's head (Fig. 43-10). It is an efficient method of providing oxygen at levels that can be controlled. More important, the body is accessible for starting an IV line or performing a procedure.

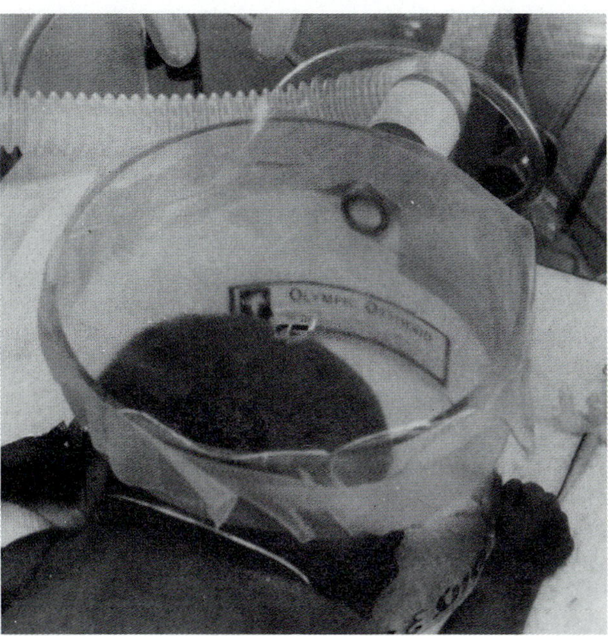

FIG. 43-10 A preterm neonate whose head is enclosed within a plastic circular hood that maintains a constant humidified and oxygenated environment.

A less efficient method of delivering oxygen to an infant is with the use of a closed incubator. Imperfectly fitted lids, uncovered vents, and portholes that must be opened often to perform an activity on the infant all contribute to fluctuations in oxygen levels. Maintaining a constant temperature within the incubator is a problem too. As an infant's metabolism increases in an effort to maintain body temperature, larger amounts of oxygen are required.

Mist Tents. The purpose of using a mist tent is to improve a child's respiratory status by liquefying pulmonary secretions. It allows a nurse to observe a child easily through the plastic canopy. All of its working parts are outside of the tent, which is a distinct advantage when a toddler needs this form of therapy. Compressed air or oxygen runs through sterile water to form the therapeutic mist. A disadvantage is that the canopy must be opened for treatments and procedures, which lowers the concentration of the mist.

A nurse must organize all activities (to limit the number of times the tent is opened) so that the desired concentrations can be maintained and the child will have longer rest periods. The tent should be tucked under the mattress of a crib to maintain humidity levels. If the tent is functioning efficiently, dampness within it is significant and frequent (q3-4hr) linen and clothing changes may be necessary.

Nasal Cannula. Delivering oxygen to newborns and all ages of children can be done using a nasal cannula. It is a mode of delivery commonly used with infants suffering from bronchopulmonary dysplasia (abnormal development of the bronchi and the lungs). Maintaining the cannula's placement can be problematic in the infant, whose random head and hand movements disturb its position. Placing clear plastic tape around the oxygen tubing and over the nose/cheek prevents its disturbance. Adjusting the device at the back of an infant's head allows a nurse to fit the tubing to the child, and hooking it over the pinnae helps in stabilizing it. In older children the nasal cannula is held in place by adjustable elastic straps on the head.

Suctioning

Maintaining a patent airway may require suctioning. Air passages are more easily occluded in children because of the small size of their respiratory tract structures. Signs that a child may need suctioning include pallor; restlessness or anxiety; increased pulse, respiration, and temperature; dyspnea; bubbling (copious amounts of thin secretions); rattling (thick, tenacious secretions); drooling; mouth breathing; nasal flaring; grunting; gasping; retractions; cyanosis; and erythema (flushed face). Infants may have an anxious look in their eyes or constantly fidget. An older child may constantly seek attention with no explanation, toss and turn in bed, or finger the edge of a blanket.

Suctioning should be used when secretions are audible in the airway or when signs of airway obstruction or oxygen deficit are present. Various devices are used to suction children, such as a bulb syringe or a straight suction catheter of the proper size for the child. In nonemergency situations the nurse should demonstrate how the suction machine operates by suctioning some water from a cup. The small child should be reassured that the machine is only suctioning excess fluid from the mouth or nose, not body contents. Recommended pressures for airway suctioning using wall suction range from 50 to 95 mm Hg for infants to 95 to 110 mm Hg for children.

The use of artificial airways has become a routine life-sustaining measure in the pediatric and neonatal population. Depth, timing, and frequency are important considerations when suctioning a tracheostomy or endotracheal tube.

- *Depth:* Approximately ¼ to ½ inch beyond the tip of the artificial airway; determine placement by placing an appropriately sized suction catheter into an artificial airway of the same size, insert the catheter to the appropriate depth, mark with tape, and keep at the bedside as a reference.
- *Timing:* Limit suctioning to not more than 5 seconds.
- *Frequency:* Allow 30 seconds between suctioning attempts.

Intake and Output

There are many health disorders that require the accurate monitoring of the amount of solids and liquids taken in and the amount excreted. For example, measuring and recording intake and output (I&O) is extremely important in infants with diarrhea, toddlers with burns, or adolescents with renal disorders. Infants who are hospitalized because they fail to thrive or to grow as expected are placed on "calorie counts," which requires the careful recording of all food ingested and liquids given. This intake is recorded at the bedside, and a nutritionist calculates the calories actually consumed by a child. It is helpful in determining whether the cause is organic or the result of an inadequate intake. These causes are ruled out before a maternal-infant problem is considered.

All fluids given to a child are documented on a record kept at the bedside. Adolescents can usually assume this responsibility after an explanation. All urine voided is measured before discarding. Older children may need to be reminded to save all urine. However, they are usually cooperative.

Measuring urine output in the infant or toddler who is not toilet trained can be a challenge. Most hospitals require routine weighing of diapers (before and after voiding) of all children who are not toilet trained. The weight of a dry disposable diaper is subtracted from the weight of a wet diaper. The difference in the weight in grams equals the milliliters voided; 1 g equals 1 ml of urine.

Weight

Fluid loss is reflected in a child's weight, especially that of infants and toddlers. The same scale should be used and the child should be weighed at the same time every day. Any error then becomes a constant one. What children wear and what is attached to them is important and affects weight. For example, the weight of a naked infant with an NG tube, electrodes, and an IV armboard differs significantly from that of the infant without these attachments. If this equipment has been added or removed, it should be noted on the graphic sheet.

Medication Administration

A critical responsibility of a pediatric nurse is the administration of medications. A nurse *must* know the drug's side effects and toxic signs and symptoms, as well as how to compute the dose correctly and administer it properly. The right amount of the right medication must be given to the right child at the appropriate time and by the correct route. Nurses also must observe and document a child's response to the drug.

There are no unit dosages in pediatrics because children are of various ages and weights. Methods of calculating dosages for children consider age, body weight, and **body surface area (BSA)** (total area exposed to the outside environment).

Calculating the proportional amount of BSA to body weight is the most reliable method for determining children's dosages. The height and weight of the child is used to estimate the BSA. This information is then applied to a formula for dosage, such as

$$\frac{\text{Body surface area of child}}{\text{Body surface area of adult}} \times \text{Adult dose} = \text{Estimated child's dose}$$

Oral Medications. Oral administration of medications is usually the preferred route whenever possible. Most oral medications for children are available in liquid form for ease of administration. It is important for the nurse to remember that household teaspoons vary greatly in capacity. Therefore, a drug ordered in teaspoons should be measured in milliliters, with 5 ml = 1 teaspoon. Several devices, such as hollow-handled medicine spoons, are available to ensure accurate measurement and administration. Some, but not all, solid drugs can be crushed and mixed with food. An unpleasant taste in a drug can often be masked in a small amount of pleasant-tasting food, or the tongue can be numbed slightly beforehand with an ice cube or frozen flavored ice treat.

Intradermal, Subcutaneous, and Intramuscular Medications. Injections are a source of pain and fear for children, so drugs are usually given by injection only when other routes cannot be used. Recommendations for injections are listed in Table 43-7. The primary site for intramuscular injections is shown in Fig. 43-11.

Intravenous Medications. The IV route of administering a medication is often selected for the following reasons:

- Medication is almost immediately distributed to tissues and prompt physiological action occurs.
- With consecutive doses, predictable drug levels can be achieved to maintain therapeutic effects.
- After initial insertion, IV administration is more comfortable for the child than other types of parenteral injections.

The IV sites in children differ from those of adults. A superficial scalp vein is commonly used in infants under 9 months of age because these veins have no valves, so a needle can be inserted in either direction. In addition, the head can be moved from side to side without dislodging the needle. Any accessible vein may be used in older children.

Converting an infusion line to an intermittent peripheral infusion device (IPID) is done when a child does not require additional IV fluids but still needs additional medications, such as antibiotics or pain medication. With an IPID, a child can move about except for those brief periods when drugs are infused. The tube is irrigated regularly to keep the line open as per agency policy.

TABLE 43-7 Needle and Site Recommendations for Selected Injections

Needle	Sites
Intradermal (ID)	
3/8-1/2 inch 25-27 gauge Short bevel	*Primary:* ventral forearm *Secondary:* scapular area; upper chest; medial aspect of thigh
Subcutaneous (SC)	
3/8-5/8 inch 23-26 gauge Medium bevel	*Primary:* upper arm; lower abdomen; anterior thigh *Secondary:* scapular area; upper buttocks (above the iliac crest)
Intramuscular (IM)	
5/8-1 1/2 inch 20-25 gauge Medium bevel	*Primary:* 0-2 years—vastus lateralis 2-12 years—vastus lateralis; ventrogluteal *Secondary:* 0-2 years—ventrogluteal 2-12 years—deltoid for small volume; dorsal gluteal

Adapted from Elliott M: Administering intradermal, subcutaneous, and intramuscular injections. In Smith D, editor: *Comprehensive child and family nursing skills,* St Louis, 1991, Mosby.

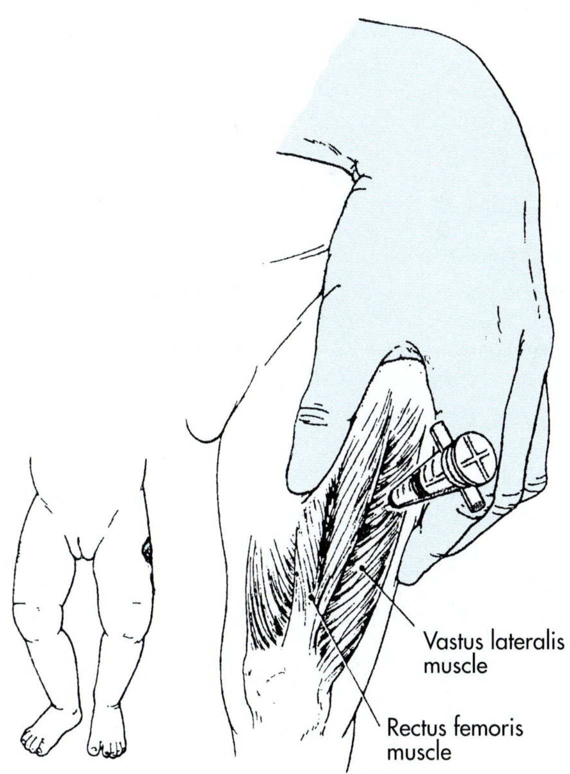

FIG. 43-11 The vastus lateralis muscle is the primary site for intramuscular injections in the thigh. The needle penetrates the midlateral thigh on a front-to-back course.

TABLE 43-8 Preventing Accidents

Behavior	Accident/Hazard	Prevention
Newborn		
Sleeping; poor head control; some body movement	Suffocation	Do not tuck blankets in. Do not use pillows. Do not use plastic bags in crib. Avoid soft, moldable mattresses. Place healthy infants in supine or side-lying positions for sleep.
	Accidents	Use an approved car seat and follow manufacturer's instructions. Check crib slats—they should be no more than 2⅜″ apart.
	Burns	Test bath water temperature. Never smoke or drink hot liquids while holding baby.
	Falls	Never leave baby alone or unattended on bed, sofa, or counter. Always have one hand on baby. Carry newborn with two hands.
	Lead poisoning	Eliminate or reduce the child's exposure to any surfaces or substances containing lead.*
1-6 Months		
Head control improving	Suffocation	Keep crib free of plastic bags. Do not use pillows.
Placing objects in mouth	Foreign body aspiration Injury from toys: loose parts or sharp edges	Inspect all toys; remove button eyes or detach small wheels. Do not offer foods on which the baby can choke, such as grapes, nuts, potato chips, and raisins. Remove open safety pins, needles, and nails from baby's reach.
Moving body from one place to another	Falls	Do not leave baby unattended on bed, sofa, or counter.
Beginning to pull self to sitting position	Burns	Test bath water; hold infant securely. Keep hot liquids in cups away from child's grasp.
7-12 Months		
Sitting up	Falls/drownings	Never leave infant unattended in high chair, on bed, or in tub.
Crawling	Accidents	Use gates at bottom and top of stairs. Place guards around fireplaces; never leave infant alone near space heater.
	Suffocation	Do not leave plastic bags or balloons in crib or playpen or within infant's reach.
Feeding self	Aspiration/ingestion	Do not offer foods on which child can choke, such as popcorn, small, hard candies, gum, or hot dogs. Lock up all medications and poisonous household substances. Purchase medicines and household cleaners in childproof containers. Keep number of the local poison control center by telephone. Keep ipecac syrup on hand, and know how to give it. Childproof the entire house, including placement of poisonous houseplants out of reach.

*This precaution should continue throughout childhood.

TABLE 43-8 Preventing Accidents—cont'd

Behavior	Accident/Hazard	Prevention
1-2 Years		
Holding on or walking	Falls, lacerations, and abrasions	Keep furniture with sharp edges and glass table tops out of child's way or protect with special corner protectors.
		Keep sharp kitchen utensils and garden equipment out of reach or locked up.
Exploring environment		Always know where the toddler is playing.
		Supervise all outdoor play activities.
Running		Do not allow child to run with objects in mouth.
		Begin teaching safety outdoors, including dangers of traffic, climbing, and walking in front of swings at playground.
	Motor vehicle accidents	Always use an approved car seat and follow manufacturer's instructions.
		Keep toddler in fenced area.
		Install childproof locks on car doors.
		Teach child to cross street holding an adult's hand.
		Keep car doors locked in garage or driveway.
		Do not allow play in driver's seat without adult present.
	Ingestion/inhalation	Keep insecticides, medications, and all harmful cleaners locked up.
	Suffocation	Supervise play with balloons.
		Do not allow plastic bags in play.
		Remove doors of refrigerators or chain shut before discarding.
	Drowning	Keep bath water level low in tub.
		Never leave child alone in tub or wading pool; empty wading pool after use.
		Supervise child closely at beach.
		Never allow child near water without an adult.
		Fence around swimming pool.
		Enroll toddler in swimming class.
	Burns	Remove matches/lighters from reach.
		Teach fire safety.
		Keep handles of pots toward center of stove when cooking.
		Keep child away from stove while preparing meals.
		Keep child away from charcoal fires.
3-5 Years		
Climbing; running Exploring environment outside the home Improving motor skills	Falls, lacerations, and abrasions	Check yard, playground, and daycare center for potential hazards.
		Begin teaching: safety in using playground equipment; dangers of pushing/shoving playmates; and avoiding strangers.
		Supervise child using scissors.
		Discourage approaching animals without an adult.
		Supervise action-related activities, such as tricycles and Big Wheels.
		Teach child name, address, and telephone number.
	Motor vehicle accidents	Use car seat/safety belts in car according to DOT (Department of Transportation) standards.
		Review acceptable behavior in a moving car.
		Review crossing street at corner, watching lights and flow of traffic.
		Teach child to keep parent informed of whereabouts.
		Confine play to yard; do not allow to play in street.
	Burns	Practice fire drills in the home.
		Implement other practices similar to those for 1- to 2-year-olds.
	Firearms	Never keep loaded guns/rifles in house or garage.
		Keep service guns locked.
		Instruct child never to touch gun or bullets.

Continued.

TABLE 43-8 Preventing Accidents—cont'd

Behavior	Accident/Hazard	Prevention
6-11 Years		
Motor skills continuing to improve; enjoying large muscle activities; becoming increasingly independent; engaging in competitive sports; unsupervised activities	Motor vehicle accidents, injuries, and fractures	Review traffic safety.
		Use safety belts.
		Teach skate board safety—control speed, refrain from jumping, use helmet, knee, and elbow pads.
		Teach bicycle safety—rules of the road, use of reflectors, proper signaling, use of helmets.
		Review safety regarding use of lawn mowers, farm equipment, and tools.
		Teach child not to hide in or play near cars.
		Caution child about playing in vacant buildings, quarries, or sand pits.
		Teach proper use of protective gear in competitive sports.
		Teach child not to throw objects at people or moving vehicles.
		Teach child how to call fire department, police, and emergency medical assistance.
	Drownings	Review swimming and boating safety.
		Do not allow ice skating on pond unless its safety has been determined.
		Never allow the child to swim or skate alone.
	Inhalation/ingestions	Evaluate health education programs at school.
		Emphasize the hazards of glue sniffing and drug or alcohol use.
		Encourage family discussions about substance abuse.
12-18 Years		
Rapid growth spurt; demonstrating risk-taking behaviors; demonstrating increased independence; engaging in extracurricular activities; reacting to peer group influence; driving a car	Motor vehicle, motorcycle, and bicycle injuries and fractures	Evaluate the high school's safety and health education programs.
		Review bicycle/motorcycle safety, including use of helmets.
		Enroll child in driver education classes.
		Establish limits regarding care, use, and consequences of drinking and driving.
		Encourage group participation in outdoor activities, such as running or jogging.
		Supervise competitive sports activities.
		Encourage enrolling in first aid classes.
		Maintain a physical conditioning program.
		Review water safety in seasonal activities.
	Drownings	Discourage risk-taking behaviors at pool or beach.
		Discuss dangers of swimming and skating alone.
		Keep guns empty and locked up.
		Teach proper care of firearms.
	Firearms	Supervise target practice in isolated areas.

Although administering medications intravenously has many advantages, the route is also the most hazardous for children. Extreme caution must be used. Most health care settings require nurses to complete extensive training before permitting them to perform this function.

Eye and Ear Drops. Administering eye and ear drops may require the assistance of a second nurse. Positioning is critical to administering them successfully. The child's head must be kept as immobile as possible and the eye should be opened for proper administration of eye drops. Likewise, after ear drops are given, the head should be kept still for the medication to run down the canal. For proper instillation of ear drops to children under 3 years, the pinna should be pulled *down and back*. For children older than 3 years, ear drops are given as to an adult—by pulling the pinna up and back.

SAFETY

Protecting a child from harm is a major issue in pediatrics. Anticipatory guidance for parents of infants and toddlers and health teaching for school-age children and adolescents are two methods of preventing accidents. However, hazards and dangers are everywhere—in the home, at the playground, at school, and in the hospital.

Injuries cause more deaths and disabilities in children than do all causes of disease combined. The risk-taking activities of adolescents also contribute to the **morbidity** (an illness or an abnormal condition or quality) and mortality of adolescence. Table 43-8 on pp.1364-1366 identifies common developmental characteristics, potential hazards, and preventive measures that can decrease the incidence of accidents and injuries.

Parents and children should talk and listen to each other to prevent many accidents. Maintaining open communication between and among all members of a family is one method of prevention. The adult who is a role model, who thinks about safety, and who identifies potential dangers in the environment or a particular activity can influence a child immensely.

REFERENCES AND SELECTED REFERENCES

1. Acute Pain Management Guideline Panel: *Acute pain management in infants, children, and adolescents: operative and medical procedures,* AHCPR Pub No 92-0020, Rockville, Md, 1992, Agency for Health Care Policy and Research, Public Health Service, US Department of Health and Human Services.
2. American Academy of Pediatrics, Committee on Nutrition: Use of whole cow's milk in infancy, *Pediatrics* 89(6):1105, 1992.
3. Anastasiow N: *The effects of early intervention.* In Anastasiow N, Harel S, editors: *At-risk infants,* Baltimore, 1993, Paul H Brookes.
4. Beck LE: *Child development,* ed 2, Needham Heights, Md, 1991, Allyn & Bacon.
5. Brantly D, Rollins J: *Preparing the child psychologically for surgery.* In Smith D, editor: *Comprehensive child and family nursing skills,* St Louis, 1991, Mosby.
6. Children's Defense Fund (CDC): *The state of America's children,* Washington, DC, 1991, The Fund.
7. Coffman, SP: Patient education for drowning prevention, *J Pediatr Health Care* 5(3):141, 1991.
8. Ellet M et al: Predicting the distance for gavage tube placement in children, *Pediatr Nurs* 18(2):119, 1992.
9. Grogan LB: Grief of an adolescent when a sibling dies, *MCN* 15(1):21, 1990.
10. Hamilton PM: *Basic pediatric nursing,* ed 6, St Louis, 1991, Mosby.
11. Jones NE: Childhood residential injuries, *MCH* 18(3):168, 1993.
12. Leff P, Walizer E: Building the healing partnership, Cambridge, Mass, 1992, Brookline.
13. Martin B: *Administering IV medications.* In Smith D, editor: *Comprehensive child and family nursing skills,* St Louis, 1991, Mosby.
14. National Association of Children's Hospitals and Related Institutions (NACHRI): *Profile of child health in the United States,* Alexandria, Va, 1988, The Association.
15. National Commission on Children: *Beyond rhetoric: a new American agenda for children and families,* Washington, DC, 1991, The Commission.
16. National Safety Council: *Accident facts,* Chicago, 1990, Council.
17. Oberc M: *Clearing an oral or nasal airway.* In Smith D, editor: *Comprehensive child and family nursing skills,* St Louis, 1991, Mosby.
18. Pazela KJ, Gerberg AK: Privileged communication: talking with a dying adolescent, *MCN* 15(1):16, 1990.
19. Rollins J, Brantly D: *Preparing the child for procedures.* In Smith D, editor: *Comprehensive child and family nursing skills,* St Louis, 1991, Mosby.
20. Runton N: Suctioning artifical airways in children: appropriate technique, *Pediatr Nurs* 18(2):115, 1992.
21. Savedra MC et al: Assessment of post-operation pain in children and adolescents using the adolescent pediatric pain tool, *Nurs Res* 42(1):5, 1988.
22. Siederman JR: Pain relief during routine procedures for children with leukemia, *MCH* 15(3):163, 1990.
23. Skale N: *Manual of pediatric nursing procedures,* 1992, Philadelphia, 1992, Lippincott.
24. Smith D, editor: *Comprehensive child and family nursing skills,* St Louis, 1991, Mosby.
25. Wong D: *Essentials of pediatric nursing,* ed 4, St Louis, 1993, Mosby.
26. US Dept. of Health & Human Services: *Quick reference guide for clinicians: acute pain management in infants, children, and adolescents: operative and medical procedures,* Washington, DC, 1992, The Department.

CHAPTER CHALLENGE

KEY POINTS

- The medical and psychosocial needs of children were considered unimportant until the twentieth century.
- The differences between adults and children are immense and demonstrate the challenges a pediatric nurse encounters daily in clinical practice.
- Knowledge of child development allows the nurse to use a developmental rather than a chronological approach to pediatric nursing care. A developmental approach emphasizes the child's abilities and strengths rather than disabilities and weaknesses.
- The traumatic effects of a child's hospitalization can be decreased by children and their parents attending a preadmission orientation program.
- Rooming-in facilities allow a parent to become as involved as desired and provide the child with the security of an adult who is known, trusted, and loved.

- Family-centered care is a philosophy of care that recognizes that the family is the constant in the child's life and that systems and personnel must support, respect, encourage, and enhance the strengths and competence of the family.
- In understanding parental responses to the hospitalization of a child, the nurse is better able to address the parents' needs.
- Health care professionals, including nurses, tend to underestimate pain in children. One reason is that some people believe that young infants or young children cannot feel pain. Nurses can assess pain in children with pain assessment tools, such as the Wong-Baker Faces Scale.
- Accidents are a leading cause of death in children and adolescents, and potential hazards should be identified so they can be avoided.
- The preparation of medications for infants and children requires precise computations of dosages.
- The urine of an infant can be obtained by using a plastic collecting bag or by the physician's doing a suprapubic tap.
- Explanations that are provided to children always should be given at age-appropriate levels so they can be understood. Age and developmental level influence the ways in which children perceive and understand experiences such as illness or disability, and therefore, their ability to cope.

STUDY QUESTIONS

1. The president responsible for the first White House conference was:
   1. F.D. Roosevelt
   2. R.B. Hayes
   3. G. Cleveland
   4. T. Roosevelt
2. A family-centered approach to care is important when caring for any children but is crucial for optimum care for:
   1. School-age children
   2. Children having minor surgery
   3. Children with special needs
   4. Children receiving routine immunizations
3. Eight-year-old Jason has had asthma since birth. He was admitted to the emergency room last night after experiencing a severe attack. The nurse's role in a partnership with his parents would include:
   1. Deciding what is best for Jason and his family
   2. Withholding information about Jason's condition from his parents so that they will not worry
   3. Ignoring what his parents have to say about the way they give Jason his medications at home
   4. Providing information about a parent-to-parent support group for parents of children with asthma
4. Tanya is 8 months old. Which of the following play activities would she most likely enjoy:
   1. A game of pat-a-cake
   2. Playing with puppets
   3. Working a puzzle
   4. Hearing a story
5. Bobby is 4 years old and has just been told that he has leukemia. What might his concept of illness be:
   1. With proper explanations, he is able to accurately understand how leukemia affects his body
   2. He believes that his parents could make the leukemia go away if they really wanted to
   3. He can have a beginning understanding of body processes and functions
   4. He will focus on discrete symptoms rather than the overall impact of his leukemia
6. The rate of metabolism is highest in the:
   1. Infant
   2. Preschooler
   3. School-age child
   4. Adolescent
7. Seven-year-old Betsy is about to have a fingerstick. The best thing the nurse could tell her to prepare her for the event is:
   1. "It will hurt but you are a big girl, so you can just grin and bear it."
   2. "It will hurt a lot, and you can cry if you want to."
   3. "Some children tell me it feels like a chicken pecking or a cat scratching."
   4. "Close your eyes, don't look, and it will be over in a minute."
8. Hannah is 18 months old and is hospitalized for surgery in the morning. Of the following interventions, the one that would be *most* helpful in relieving her stress associated with hospitalization is:
   1. Maintaining a normal routine
   2. Providing opportunities for play
   3. Encouraging parental presence and rooming-in
   4. Encouraging self-care activities
9. Roger, 10 years old, had abdominal surgery yesterday. He is quietly working a puzzle and is offering no complaints. The nurse can assume which of the following about Roger's pain status:
   1. Roger could not possibly be in pain or he would not be able to play
   2. Because Roger is a child, he cannot experience as much pain as an adult
   3. Roger may be distracting himself from the pain through play
   4. Roger should not be feeling any pain on the first postoperative day
10. Which of the following statements regarding injury prevention is true:
    1. Injuries are the leading cause of deaths and disabilities in children
    2. Child safety is not a responsibility of the pediatric nurse
    3. A child's age has no relationship to the type of accident that might occur
    4. Concern with lead poisoning ends when a child reaches 7 years of age

44

CARE OF CHILDREN WITH PHYSICAL AND EMOTIONAL PROBLEMS

Marie Ann Marino
Susan De Rienzo Vivio

KEY TERMS

acquired heart disease
alpha-fetoprotein (AFP)
amblyopia
chelation therapy
child maltreatment
cognitive impairment
congenital heart defect
"currant jelly" stools
glomerulonephritis
Gowers' sign
intelligence quotient (IQ)
Legg-Calvé-Perthes disease
lichenification
neural tube
Nissen fundoplication
nuchal rigidity
pica
pneumothorax
priapism
sickled cell
subluxation

LEARNING OBJECTIVES

After reading this chapter, the student should be able to do the following:

- Define the key terms.
- Describe the clinical manifestations of common skin disorders in infants and children.
- Demonstrate an understanding of the nursing interventions for the patient with congenital hip dysplasia.
- Describe the clinical manifestations and medical management of children with gastrointestinal system dysfunction.
- Discuss the nursing interventions for an infant or child with a congenital heart defect.
- Identify major alterations in respiratory function and specific nursing interventions for children with pneumonia.
- Identify methods of nursing assessment used to detect alterations in sensory organs.
- List five clinical manifestations of meningitis.
- Describe five nursing interventions for the child in a corrective device or cast.
- State five physical and behavioral indicators that should arouse suspicion of child abuse.

RELATED TOPICS OF INTEREST

- Basic nutrition (Chapter 18)
- Care of the patient with an integumentary disorder (Chapter 25)
- Care of the patient with a musculoskeletal disorder (Chapter 26)
- Care of the patient with a gastrointestinal or accessory organ disorder (Chapter 27)
- Care of the patient with a cardiovascular disorder (Chapter 28)
- Care of the patient with a blood or lymphatic disorder (Chapter 29)
- Care of the patient with a urinary disorder (Chapter 30)
- Care of the patient with a respiratory disorder (Chapter 31)
- Care of the patient with an endocrine disorder (Chapter 32)
- Care of the patient with an eye or ear disorder (Chapter 34)
- Care of the patient with a neurological disorder (Chapter 35)
- Care of the patient with an immune disorder (Chapter 36)

- Care of the HIV-positive or AIDS patient (Chapter 37)
- Care of the patient with cancer (Chapter 38)
- Basic pediatric nursing care (Chapter 43)
- Loss, grief, dying, and death (Chapter 52)

It is problematic to refer to the child as a "miniature adult." Many of the health problems that affect children differ from those of adults. Management of these problems may also be quite different. Nurses need to be aware of the unique way they provide care to children and their families. The care of children must be focused on the child as part of the family. In providing nursing interventions to children it is important to include parents as much as possible, delegating to them any interventions that are appropriate. Allowing parents to assist the nurse in their child's care will provide an opportunity for the nurse to teach and answer questions. Parents should be encouraged to express any fears and concerns they may have about their child's condition or care. It is also necessary to provide them with resources within their community so they may provide for the continued health of their child after discharge.

This chapter was designed to provide the reader with a thorough understanding of the unique physical and emotional problems affecting children. Although this chapter is dedicated to the understanding of the most prevalent health issues affecting children, it is beyond the scope of this chapter to address all the disorders that may affect children. Readers may also refer to other chapters within this comprehensive text that address specific systems disorders, many of which relate specific pediatric implications.

DISORDERS OF CARDIOVASCULAR FUNCTION

Many of the cardiovascular disorders in children are the result of a **congenital heart defect** (an abnormality or anomaly of the heart, present at birth). Consequences of many of these defects include congestive heart failure, predisposition to infection, hypoxia, and alterations in growth. Another group of cardiovascular disorders, *acquired heart disorders,* consist of abnormalities that compromise the heart's function and occur after birth.

Any type of cardiovascular disorder may be frightening to the child and parents. It is important for the nurse to educate and prepare them regarding the disorder and its management.

Congenital Heart Defects (CHD)

It is estimated that 5% to 10% of term newborns have a congenital heart defect (CHD). This rate is higher in infants born prematurely.

Etiology/Pathophysiology. Several environmental and genetic risk factors have been implicated in the incidence of various types of defects. Environmental factors include intrauterine rubella exposure, maternal alcoholism, diabetes mellitus, advanced maternal age, and maternal drug ingestion (e.g., lithium, thalidomide, or Dilantin). Genetic risk factors include a sibling or parent with a CHD, chromosomal anomalies (Down syndrome, trisomy 13-15, and Turner syndrome), and presence of other noncardiac congenital anomalies.

Principles of fetal and postnatal circulation. During fetal development the placenta is the source of oxygen and nutrients. Oxygenated blood is brought to the fetus by the umbilical vein and enters the fetal heart via the inferior vena cava. The fetal lungs, which are collapsed and full of fluid, pose a strong resistance to the right side of the heart, increasing the pressures in the right atrium and right ventricle. Because of the increased pressure in the right side of the heart, blood entering the heart from the inferior vena cava is directed across the right atrium through the *foramen ovale* to the left atrium. This blood is then ejected from the left ventricle into the aorta. As a result the blood richest in oxygen is pumped through the aorta to the coronary arteries, brain, and upper extremities. Venous blood returning from this region returns to the right atrium through the superior vena cava and is directed downward through the tricuspid valve into the right ventricle. From there it is pumped into the pulmonary artery, where the majority of the blood is shunted to the descending aorta through the *ductus arteriosus* and perfuses the lower body (Fig. 44-1). Only a small amount enters the fetal lungs due to high pulmonary resistance (Fig. 44-2, *A*).

At delivery, with the first breath, the newborn's lungs expand and the fluid within them is absorbed into the pulmonary circulation. As a result, pulmonary and right heart pressures fall and, with the removal of the placenta, systemic pressures rise. The foramen ovale closes as the pressure in the left atrium exceeds the pressure in the right atrium. The ductus arteriosus closes with the increased oxygen content of the newborn's blood (Fig. 44-2, *B*).

Types of defects. In the heart, blood flows from an area of high pressure to an area of low pressure (Fig. 44-3, *A,* on p.1372). Congenital heart defects are classified according to the direction blood flows across the associated defect. A *left-to-right shunt* results when there is an abnormal connection between the heart chambers and blood flows from an area of higher pressure (left side of heart) to an area of lower pressure (right side of the heart). As a result, oxygenated blood returns to the right side of the heart and reenters the pulmonary circulation; hence the term *acyanotic defect* (Fig. 44-3, *B*). These defects result in extra blood flowing into the pulmonary circulation, increased pulmonary workload, and congestive heart failure (CHF). Manifestations of CHF are summarized in Chapter 28.

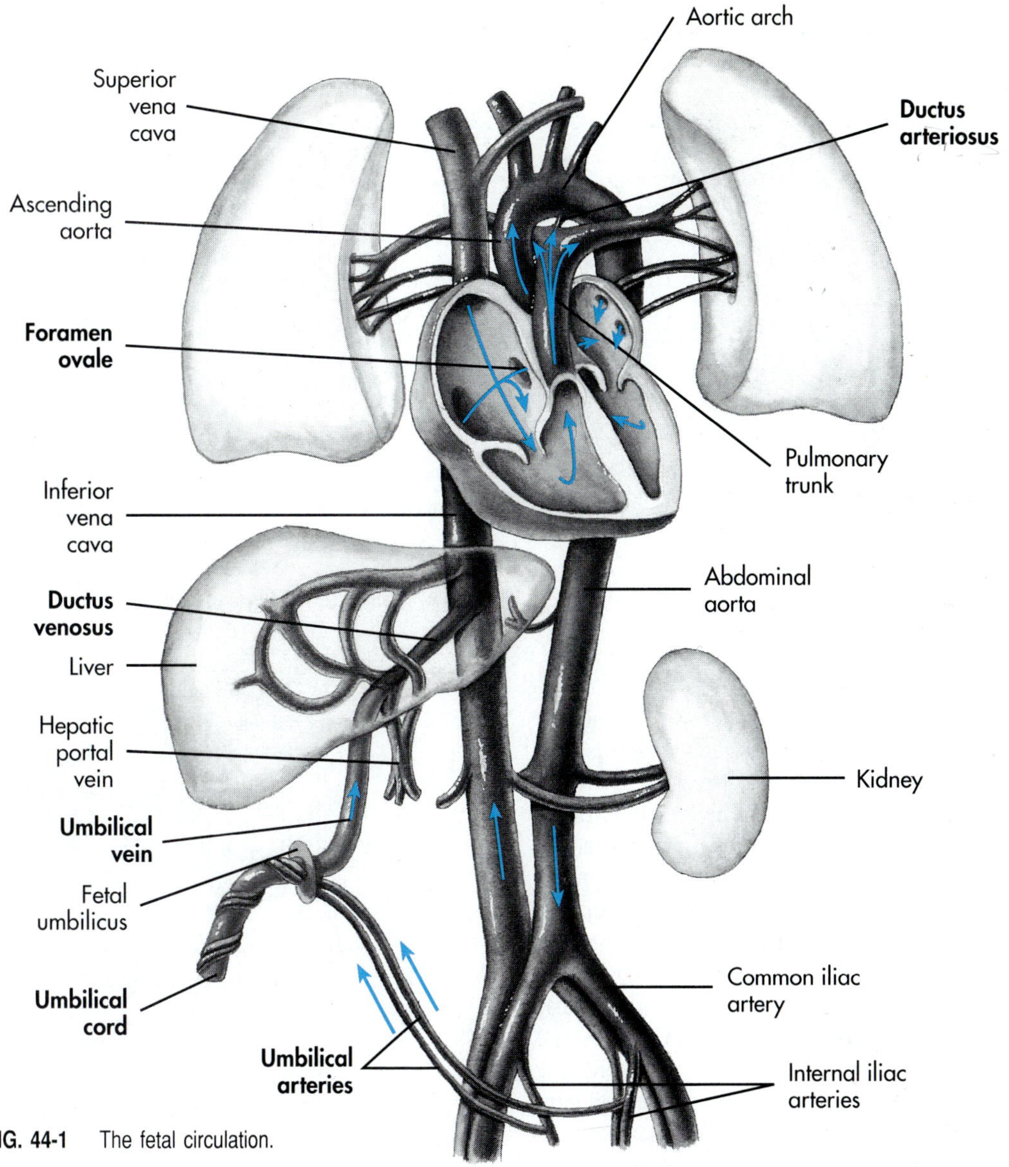

Aortic arch
Superior vena cava
Ductus arteriosus
Ascending aorta
Foramen ovale
Pulmonary trunk
Inferior vena cava
Abdominal aorta
Ductus venosus
Liver
Hepatic portal vein
Kidney
Umbilical vein
Fetal umbilicus
Common iliac artery
Umbilical cord
Umbilical arteries
Internal iliac arteries

FIG. 44-1 The fetal circulation.

Superior vena cava
Ligamentum arteriosus
Pulmonary artery
Pulmonary vein
LA
Foramen ovale
A
Descending aorta
Aortic valve
B
RA
Mitral valve
LV
Pulmonic valve
Ductus venosus
RV
Ligamentum teres
Tricuspid valve
Inferior vena cava
Saturated
Mixed
Desaturated

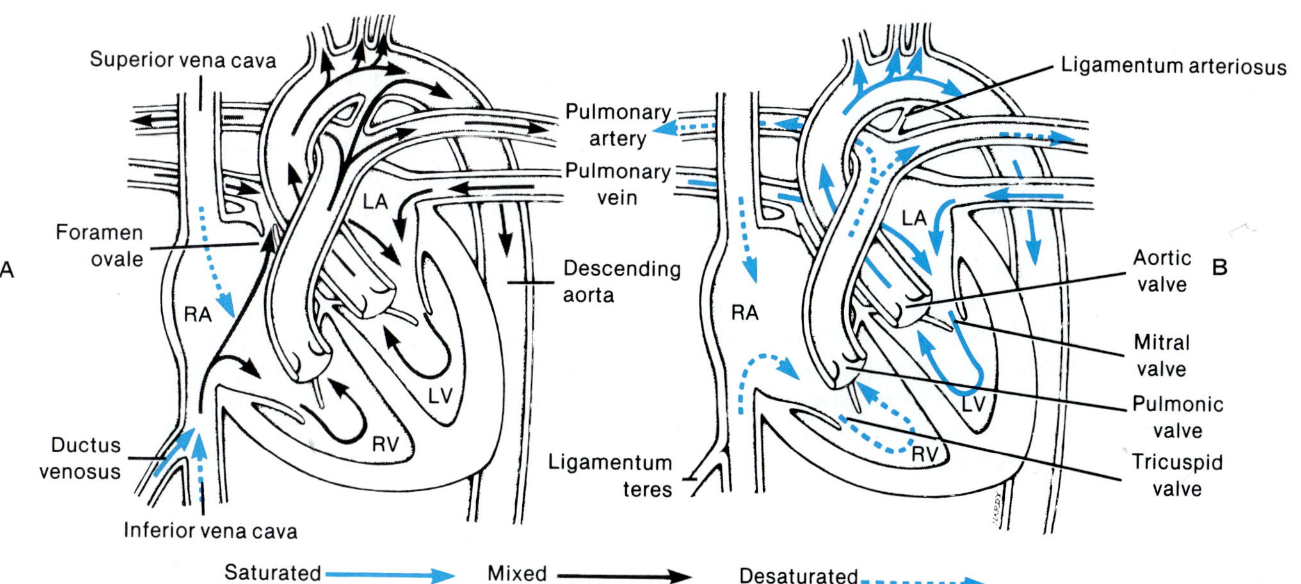

FIG. 44-2 Changes in circulation at birth. **A,** Prenatal circulation. **B,** Postnatal circulation. *Arrows* indicate direction of blood flow. *RA,* Right atrium; *LA,* left atrium; *RV,* right ventricle; *LV,* left ventricle. Although four pulmonary veins enter the LA, for simplicity this diagram shows only two.

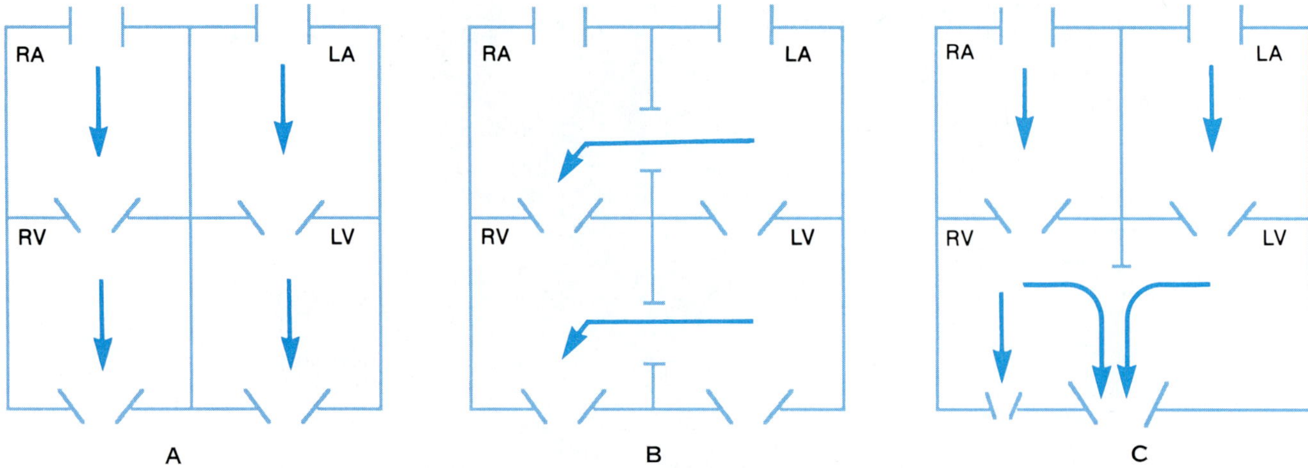

FIG. 44-3 Shunting of blood in congenital heart disease. **A,** Normal. **B,** Acyanotic defect. **C,** Cyanotic defect.

A *right-to-left shunt* results when there is an anomaly in the heart that causes the pressures on the right side of the heart to be abnormally higher than those on the left. As a result, blood is shunted from the right to the left side of the heart. Deoxygenated blood enters the left side of the heart and is pumped to the rest of the body causing *hypoxemia* (decreased oxygen content in the blood), *hypoxia* (decreased oxygen delivery to the tissues), and *cyanosis* (bluish discoloration of the skin); hence the term *cyanotic defect* (Fig. 44-3, *C*).

Clinical Manifestations. The child with suspected cardiac dysfunction may exhibit cyanosis, pallor, cardiomegaly, pericardial rubs, murmurs, additional heart sounds (S_3 and/or S_4), discrepancies between apical and radial pulses, tachypnea, dyspnea, grunting, digital clubbing, hepatomegaly, splenomegaly, discrepancies between upper and lower extremity blood pressures, crackles, and wheezing. (Specific clinical manifestations of common heart defects will be discussed later in this chapter.)

Diagnostic Tests. There are many invasive and noninvasive tests available to diagnose cardiovascular disorders. The studies performed will vary according to the nature of the suspected disorder. The more frequently conducted tests include: laboratory evaluation, such as a complete blood count (CBC), serum chemistries, urinalysis, urine culture, and arterial blood gases (ABGs); electrocardiogram; echocardiogram; fluoroscopy; angiography; and cardiac catheterization.

Major Acyanotic Defects

Acyanotic defects involve primarily left-to-right shunts. Although many children are asymptomatic, CHF is a common clinical manifestation in children with acyanotic defects. Common acyanotic defects, their specific manifestations, and medical management are presented in the next section. Nursing interventions for the child with a congenital heart defect are presented in the care plan.

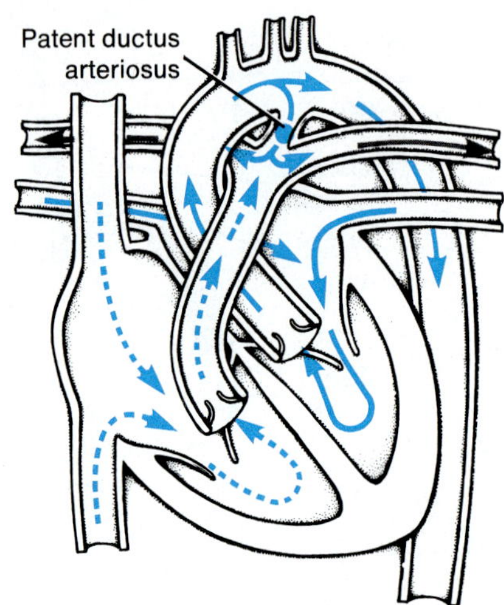

FIG. 44-4 Patent ductus arteriosus (PDA).

Patent Ductus Arteriosus (PDA). The ductus arteriosus is a fetal artery that connects the pulmonary artery to the aorta (see Fig. 44-1). Failure of the ductus arteriosus to close within the first weeks of life allows blood to shunt from the high-pressure aorta (oxygenated blood) to the low-pressure pulmonary artery (unoxygenated blood) (Fig. 44-4).

Clinical manifestations. Children may be asymptomatic or may exhibit signs and symptoms of CHF. Other clinical manifestations may include a typical "ma-

NURSING CARE PLAN THE CHILD WITH A HEART DEFECT

Debbie Bornea is a 9-month-old infant with a ventricular septal defect. She has a loud, harsh systolic murmur. She weighs 15 lb (her birth weight was 7 lb). The family has been told the septal defect will require open heart surgery when she is 18 to 24 months of age.

Nursing diagnoses	Patient goals/expected outcomes	Nursing interventions
Cardiac output, decreased, related to structural defect	Patient will exhibit improved cardiac output; heartbeat will be strong, regular, and within normal limits for age.	Administer digoxin (Lanoxin) as ordered, using established precautions to prevent toxicity; check dosage with another nurse for safety. Count apical pulse for 1 full minute before giving drug. Withhold medication and notify practitioner if pulse rate is less than 90 to 110 bpm (infants) or 75 to 85 (older children), depending on previous pulse readings. Monitor serum potassium levels (decrease in levels enhances digoxin toxicity).
Infection, high risk for, related to debilitated physical status	Patient will exhibit no evidence of infection.	Use meticulous hand washing. Avoid contact with infected persons. Monitor for signs of infection, including elevated temperature and elevated white blood count, which may indicate infection. Provide frequent rest periods. Provide adequate nutrition; assess nutritional status, including daily weight. Be alert for signs of complications: ■ CHF ■ digitalis toxicity ■ increased respiratory effort ■ hypoxemia ■ cerebral thrombosis ■ cardiovascular collapse
Activity intolerance, high risk for, related to imbalance between oxygen supply and demand	Patient will maintain adequate energy levels.	Allow for frequent rest periods. Encourage quiet games and activities for age. Help child select activities appropriate to age, condition, and capabilities. Avoid extremes of environmental temperatures.

Continued.

Growth and development, altered, related to inadequate oxygen and nutrients to tissues; social isolation	Patient will achieve normal growth and development.	Provide a diet high in nutrition. Provide pleasant environment for eating. Encourage small, frequent feedings. Provide snacks several times a day. Provide frequent rest periods between feedings and activities. Encourage activities appropriate to the child's age and developmental level. Monitor for signs of CHF and decreased cardiac output during activities. Arrange for continued family involvement during the child's hospitalization.
Injury, high risk for (complications), related to cardiac condition and therapies	Parents will recognize early signs of complications and institute appropriate action.	Teach family to recognize signs of complications: ■ CHF ■ Digoxin toxicity ■ Vomiting (earliest sign) ■ bradycardia ■ dysrhythmias ■ increased respiratory effort—tachycardia, retention, grunting, cough, cyanosis ■ hypoxemia—cyanosis, restlessness, tachycardia ■ cerebral thrombosis—compensatory polycythemia (in cyanotic heart disease) is particularly hazardous when child is dehydrated ■ cardiovascular collapse—pallor, cyanosis Teach family to intervene during hypercyanotic spells: ■ place child in knee-chest position with head and chest elevated ■ remain calm ■ call practitioner
Knowledge deficit, related to the disorder and methods of treatment	Family will demonstrate an understanding of the disorder and its treatments.	Assess the family's understanding of the diagnosis. Reinforce the physician's explanation of the child's disorder and its treatments. Provide written instructions regarding medication schedules and treatment protocols. Encourage the family to verbalize questions, fears, and concerns. Allow the family to participate in the child's care when appropriate. Provide emotional support to the child and the family.

CRITICAL THINKING QUESTIONS

1. You enter Debbie's room and notice the mother sitting at her bedside crying. She states, "I don't know how I will deal with her having heart surgery." An appropriate initial response to Mrs. Bornea would be:
2. Mrs. Bornea states Debbie has a very poor appetite. In educating the mother, two helpful suggestions could be:
3. Mrs. Bornea mentions that she is concerned Debbie will get an infection and become acutely ill. Two therapeutic nursing interventions for patient teaching would be:

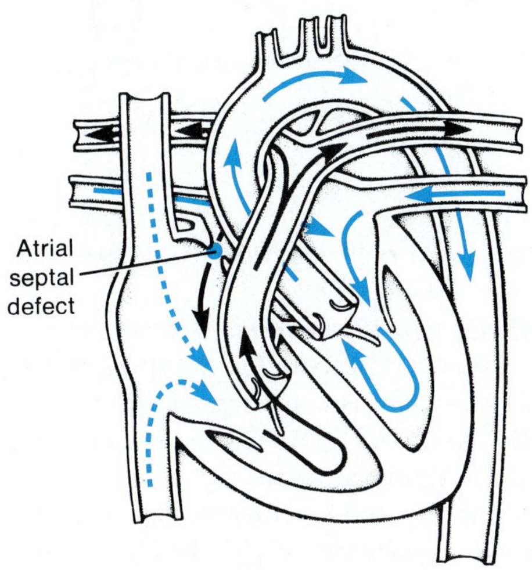

FIG. 44-5 Atrial septal defect.

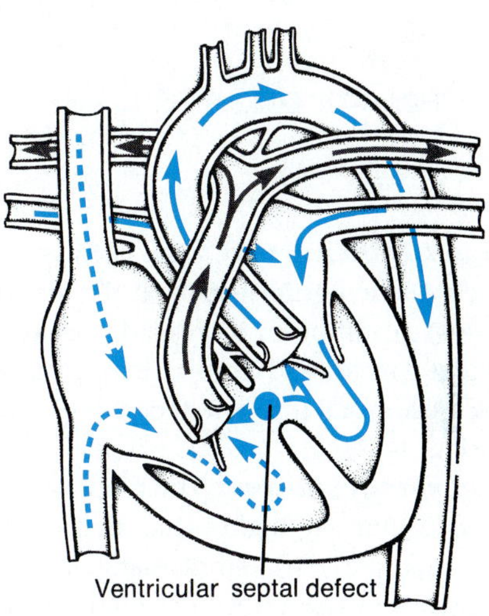

FIG. 44-6 Ventricular septal defect.

chinelike" murmur audible at the upper left sternal border, widened pulse pressure, and bounding pulses.

Medical management. Administration of indomethacin (a prostaglandin inhibitor) has been effective in closing the ductus arteriosus in newborns. Surgical correction involves ligating the ductus arteriosus through a thoracotomy incision.

Atrial Septal Defect (ASD). An ASD is an abnormal opening in the atrial septum, which enables blood to flow from the higher-pressure left atrium (oxygenated blood) to the lower-pressure right atrium (unoxygenated blood) (Fig. 44-5).

Clinical manifestations. Although some children may be asymptomatic, others may have manifestations of CHF. A characteristic harsh systolic murmur may be auscultated over the third intercostal space.

Medical management. Surgical correction is accomplished through open heart surgery with cardiopulmonary bypass. Small defects are repaired with purse-string sutures, and moderate to large defects are repaired with a patch.

Ventricular Septal Defect (VSD). A VSD is an abnormal opening in the interventricular septum, resulting in the flow of blood from the higher-pressure left ventricle (oxygenated blood) to the lower-pressure right ventricle (unoxygenated blood). The size of the defect can range in size from a pinhole to absence of the entire septum (single ventricle) (Fig. 44-6).

Clinical manifestations. Initially children may be asymptomatic, but signs of CHF eventually manifest. Other clinical manifestations include a loud, harsh systolic murmur and a palpable thrill.

Medical management. Approximately 50% of ventricular septal defects close spontaneously; the remainder require open heart surgery. A palliative procedure, known as a pulmonary artery banding, may be performed in symptomatic infants. This procedure involves impeding the flow of blood from the right ventricle to the pulmonary circulation, thus reducing pulmonary congestion. Complete surgical repair involves open heart surgery with the use of cardiopulmonary bypass. The defect is usually repaired with a patch; smaller defects may be closed with sutures.

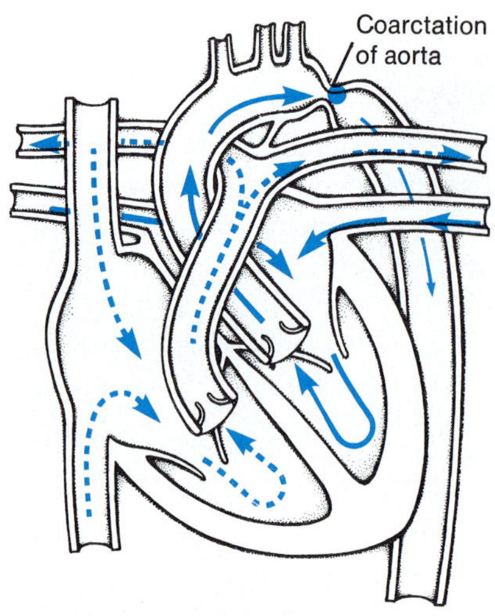

FIG. 44-7 Coarctation of the aorta.

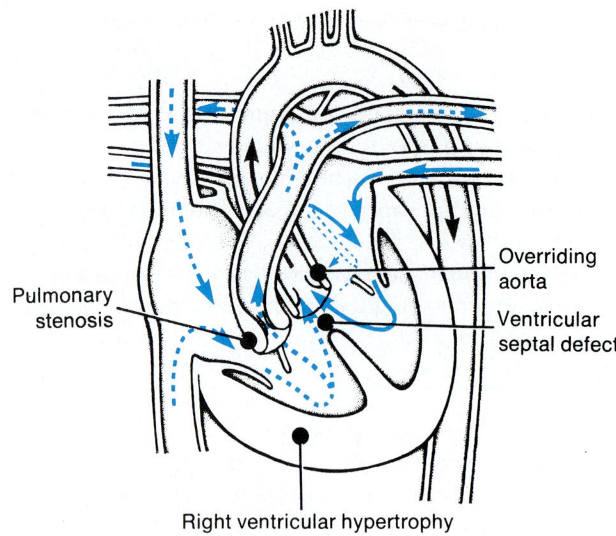

FIG. 44-8 Tetralogy of Fallot.

Coarctation of the Aorta (COA). COA is a narrowing of the lumen of the aorta (usually at the site of the ductus arteriosus), resulting in increased pressure proximal to the defect (head and upper extremities) and decreased pressure distal to the defect (body and lower extremities) (Fig. 44-7).

Clinical manifestations. The blood pressure in the arms will be 20 mm Hg higher than that in the legs (reversal of normal pattern). Other manifestations include bounding pulses in the upper extremities and weak or absent pulses in the lower extremities, signs of CHF, leg cramping on exertion in older children, and epistaxis.

Medical management. Surgical correction involves removal of the narrowed portion of the aorta with an end-to-end anastomosis or graft replacement if the narrowing is extensive.

Major Cyanotic Defects

Cyanotic defects result from the shunting of venous blood (unoxygenated) into the arterial system (oxygenated) as a result of an abnormal communication between the two systems (right-to-left shunt). Cyanosis is a primary clinical manifestation of cyanotic defects. Infants born with severe cyanosis may require a palliative surgical intervention before complete surgical correction can be performed. The purpose of the palliative procedure is to increase blood flow to the lungs to promote oxygenation. The more common cyanotic defects, their specific manifestations, and medical management will be presented in the next section. Nursing interventions for the child with a congenital heart defect will be presented in the nursing care plan.

Tetralogy of Fallot (TOF). TOF involves a combination of four defects: (1) pulmonary stenosis, (2) ventricular septal defect, (3) right ventricular hypertrophy, and (4) overriding aorta (Fig. 44-8).

Clinical manifestations. Infants may be profoundly cyanotic at birth and may experience acute episodes of severe cyanosis and hypoxia (TET spells or blue spells). Children with TOF may experience clubbing of the nailbeds, dyspnea, squatting, poor growth, mental slowness, fainting, and cerebrovascular disease.

Medical management. A palliative procedure is performed in infants with profound cyanosis and hypoxia. This temporary procedure, most commonly a *Blalock-Taussig shunt,* is designed to redirect blood flow back to the lungs to allow for oxygenation. This is accomplished by creating an artificial connection between the pulmonary artery and the aorta. Complete surgical correction involves closure of the ventricular septal defect, a pulmonic valvotomy, and repair of the overriding aorta.

Transposition of the Great Vessels (TGV). In TGV the pulmonary artery arises from the left ventricle and the aorta arises from the right ventricle. Therefore venous blood returning to the right side of the heart exits through the aorta without being oxygenated, and oxygenated blood returning from the pulmonary system is returned via the pulmonary artery to the lungs (Fig. 44-9). Some infants are born with associated defects that allow for communication between the two circulations.

Clinical manifestations. Infants born with minimal communication between the two circulations have profound cyanosis. Those who are born with an associated defect such as patent ductus arteriosus, atrial septal defect, or ventricular septal defect may have less cyanosis and experience manifestations of CHF. Cardiomegaly is usually apparent on x-ray.

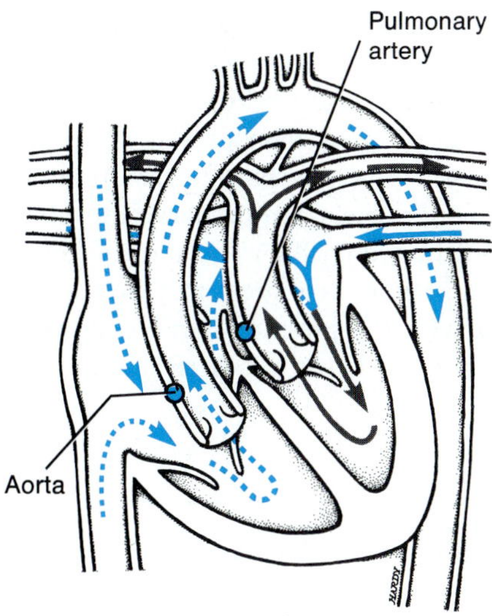

FIG. 44-9 Transposition of the great vessels.

Medical management. Initially, palliative procedures are performed to provide mixing. This is accomplished by enlarging an already present atrial septal defect or creating one by pulling a balloon catheter through the atrial septum. Complete correction of TGV is accomplished through open heart surgery and involves switching the great vessels to their proper positions.

Acquired Heart Disease

Acquired heart disease refers to those disorders that occur after birth. They result from a variety of reasons, including autoimmune processes, infection, familial tendencies, and environmental factors. One disease that has experienced a resurgence in recent years and has caused concern to health professionals is rheumatic fever. For a complete discussion of rheumatic fever, refer to Chapter 28.

DISORDERS OF HEMATOLOGICAL FUNCTION

Childhood blood disorders encompass wide ranges of etiology, severity, treatment, and prognosis; however, the majority of hematological disorders seen in infants and children stem from chronic systemic illness, nutritional deficits, and inherited blood disorders.

Anemias

Iron Deficiency Anemia. Iron deficiency anemia is the most prevalent blood disorder in infancy and early childhood, with peak incidence occurring between 6 and 24 months. The most common cause of iron deficiency anemia in this age group is an inadequate intake of dietary iron, which is essential for hemoglobin synthesis. Other causes include acute or chronic blood loss as well as malabsorption of dietary iron secondary to chronic diarrhea or malabsorption syndromes.

Etiology/pathophysiology. Anemia is defined as a decrease in red blood cell (RBC) volume, a decrease in hemoglobin, or both. Anemia reduces the oxygen-carrying capacity of the blood and can result in tissue hypoxia. Anemia can be classified as either hypoproliferative (defective erythrocyte production) or hemolytic (premature destruction of erythrocytes). Iron deficiency anemia becomes apparent at about 6 months of age in the full-term infant and about 3 months of age in the premature infant, when their maternal stores of iron become depleted and the infant becomes dependent on dietary sources of iron.

Clinical manifestations. The clinical signs and symptoms of mild to moderate anemia (hemoglobin: 6-10 g/dl) can be vague and nonspecific and include irritability, weakness, decreased play activity, and fatigue. When hemoglobin falls below 5 g/dl, the child will have anorexia, skin pallor, pale mucous membranes, inability to concentrate, tachycardia, and systolic murmurs. Children with chronic, long-term anemia may exhibit growth retardation and developmental delays.

Diagnostic tests. The diagnostic evaluation begins with an accurate history, including the child's diet, appetite, activity, weight and rate of growth, and any recent blood loss. Initial laboratory tests include a CBC, reticulocyte count, and serum ferritin (a major iron-storage protein).

Medical management. Therapeutic management involves iron replacement therapy, nutritional counseling, and treatment of any underlying conditions (hemorrhage or malabsorption). Oral iron supplementation of Fer-In-Sol (ferrous sulfate) is usually prescribed until the hemoglobin level returns to normal. Citrus fruits or juices may be given with iron supplements as ascorbic acid enhances iron absorption. Permanent dietary changes are essential to prevent recurrence. Breastfeeding, iron-fortified formulas, and iron-rich solid foods are encouraged.

Nursing interventions. Dietary counseling is of primary importance, and the nurse can assist the family in choosing iron-rich foods. Oral preparations of iron should be given three times daily between meals with citrus fruits or juices to enhance iron absorption. Parents should also be informed that their child will have dark, tarry green stools while on oral iron therapy. To avoid staining of the teeth with liquid preparations of iron, teach the family to administer the medication with a syringe placed toward the back of the mouth for infants; older children can take the preparation through straws.

Patient/family teaching. A primary nursing objective is to educate the family in how to prevent nutritional anemia. The nurse discusses with parents the importance of using iron-fortified formula and the introduction of solid foods at the appropriate age. The best solid food source of iron is commercial infant cereals.

A difficulty encountered in discouraging the parents from feeding milk to the exclusion of other foods is dispelling the popular myth that milk is a "perfect food." Many parents believe that milk is best for the infant and equate the weight gain with a "healthy child" and "good mothering." They may not be concerned about providing other foods as long as the child continues to take milk. The nurse can also stress that overweight is not synonymous with good health.

Diet education of teenagers is especially difficult since teenage girls are particularly prone to follow weight-reduction diets. Emphasizing the effects of anemia on appearance (pallor) and energy level (difficulty maintaining popular activities) may be useful.

Prognosis. The prognosis for a child with this condition is very good. However, there is some evidence that

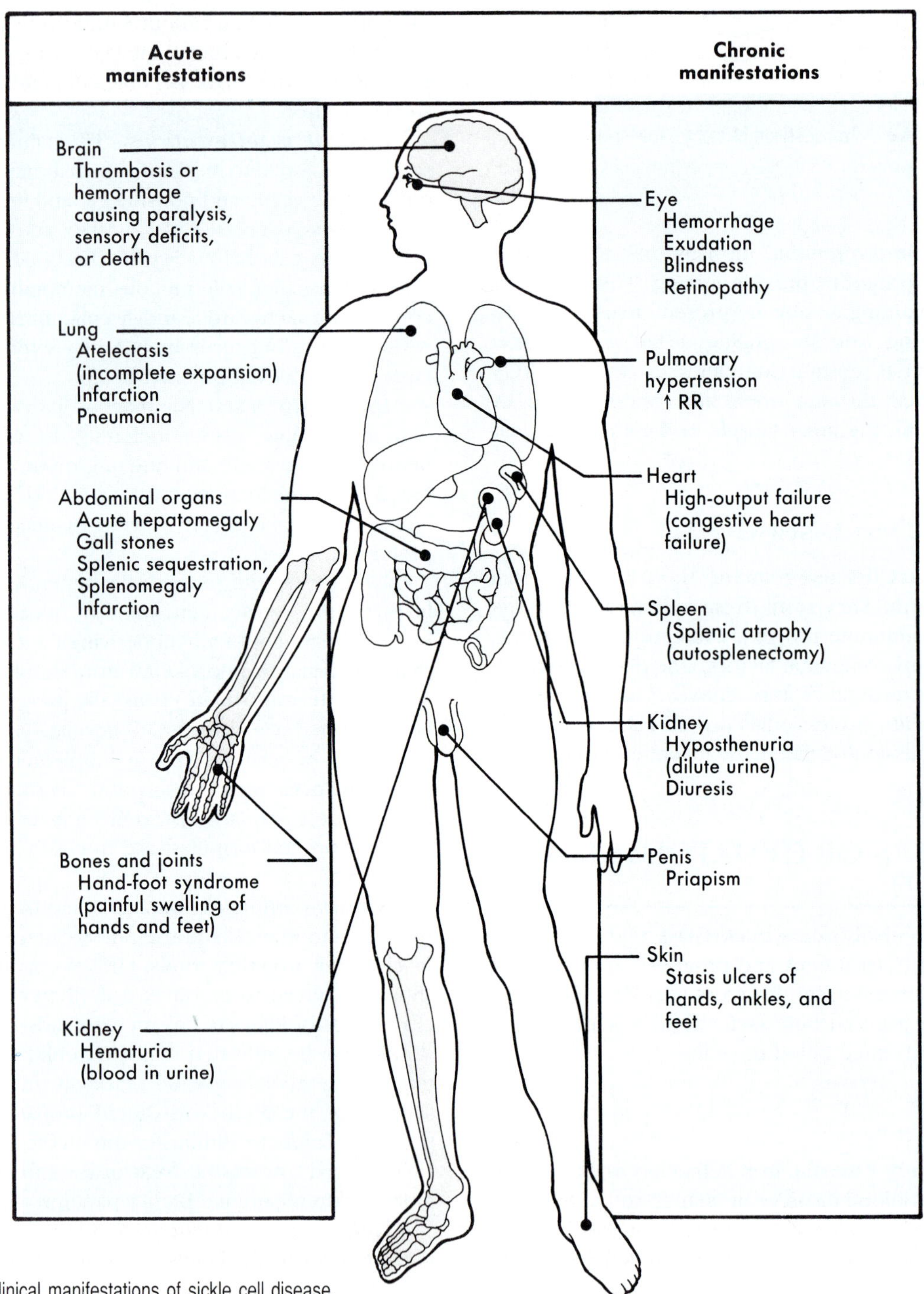

FIG. 44-10 Clinical manifestations of sickle cell disease.

if the iron deficiency anemia is long standing, mild cognitive impairment may result.

Sickle Cell Anemia. Sickle cell anemia is a genetic disorder characterized by an abnormal form of hemoglobin within the erythrocyte. In the United States, the disease is most common in the black population, with an incidence of 1:400 to 1:500 live births. Sickle cell anemia is classified as either sickle cell trait or active sickle cell disease. Sickle cell trait rarely results in clinical manifestations; however, children with sickle cell trait are carriers of sickle cell anemia. The rest of this discussion will focus on active sickle cell disease, which is the most severe and potentially fatal form of the disorder.

Etiology/pathophysiology. When oxygen is released into the tissues, the abnormal hemoglobin becomes more viscous and crystallizes, causing the erythrocyte to change from its characteristic round shape to an elongated, crescent shape **(sickled cell).** As sickled cells clump, circulation slows, resulting in obstructions with severe tissue hypoxia and necrosis. Sickling is an intermittent phenomenon that can be precipitated by infection, fever, hypoxemia, dehydration, high altitudes, cold, or emotional stress.

Clinical manifestations. Children with sickle cell disease may first present with pallor, irritability, fatigue, and jaundice. Growth impairment becomes apparent as the child's height and weight fall below average. Cardiomegaly and CHF develop in response to hypoxia and decreased cardiac output. In the older child, the joints and surrounding tissue can become edematous and painful. Strokes can occur if sickling causes cerebral occlusion, resulting in sensory deficits, paralysis, and/or death. Persistent penile erection **(priapism)** can occur in response to occluded penile veins. Severe sickling can lead to sickle cell crisis, an acutely painful period that occurs intermittently throughout the life of a child with sickle cell anemia (Fig. 44-10). Crises can be classified as one of three types: vasoocclusive, sequestration, or aplastic (Box 44-1).

Diagnostic tests. The sickle-turbidity test (Sickledex) is frequently used for screening purposes. If the test is positive, hemoglobin electrophoresis is performed to determine sickle cell trait or sickle cell disease.

Medical management. The treatment is primarily palliative, and is outlined in Box 44-1.

Nursing interventions. Nursing interventions for the child in sickle cell crisis include maintaining adequate hydration to prevent further sickling, administering analgesics as ordered, and promoting comfort measures such as warm baths and local heat.

Patient/family teaching. Families of children with sickle cell anemia should be taught to avoid situations that lead to hypoxia and sickling: infection, dehydration, emotional stress, and strenuous physical activity.

Prognosis. The prognosis varies. The greatest risk is usually in children under 5 years of age, and the majority of deaths in these children are caused by overwhelming infection. However, as the child grows older, the crises usually become less severe and less frequent, although death in early adulthood is not uncommon. Consequently, sickle cell anemia is a chronic illness with a potentially terminal outcome.

Box 44-1 TYPES AND MEDICAL MANAGEMENT OF SICKLE CELL CRISES

Vasoocclusive crisis: Obstruction of the small blood vessels of the hands and feet, resulting in edema, impaired range of motion, and pain. *Medical management:* palliative—analgesics, hydration, oxygen.

Sequestration crisis: Blood pools in the spleen and liver, resulting in hepatosplenomegaly; can progress to cardiovascular collapse and death. *Medical management:* analgesics, volume expanders, transfusions; recurrent episodes treated by splenectomy.

Aplastic crisis: Caused by premature destruction of erythrocytes, resulting in profound anemia. *Medical management:* transfusion of packed RBCs.

Aplastic Anemia. Aplastic anemia is due to the failure of bone marrow; all formed elements of the blood are defective, underdeveloped, or absent, resulting in severe anemia, leukopenia, and thrombocytopenia (pancytopenia) (for a more detailed discussion, see Chapter 29).

Coagulation Disorders

Coagulation disorders in children are characterized by abnormal bleeding either into the skin or from internal organs, secondary to clotting factor defects, platelet dysfunction, or vascular compromise.

Hemophilia.

Etiology/pathophysiology. Hemophilia is a serious, lifelong bleeding disorder inherited as an X-linked recessive disorder. Hemophilia is transmitted by female carriers and affects male offspring in 1:10,000 male births. Classic hemophilia (type A) is caused by a deficiency in factor VIII, which is a necessary component of blood coagulation.

Clinical manifestations. Diagnosis is usually made after infancy. In toddlerhood, when children typically become more active, hemophilic boys tend to have more episodes of oral bleeding and bruising. However, by age 4, 90% of these children have demonstrated persistent bleeding from minor lesions. The most frequent types of internal bleeding occur within the joints (hemarthrosis) and muscles. Pain intensifies as the bleeding continues to fill the joint cavity, limiting movement to the point where the child refuses to use the affected joint. Recurrent episodes of hemarthrosis lead to bone deformities with resulting contractures and crippling. Intracranial hemorrhage, either spontaneous or secondary to head trauma, is life-threatening and accounts for more hemophilic deaths than any other bleeding.

Diagnostic tests. Laboratory findings include a normal prothrombin time (PT), a normal bleeding time and platelet count, and a prolonged partial thromboplastin time (PTT). Factors VIII and IX are deficient or absent.

Medical management. For minor, external bleeding, pressure and cold packs may be all that is necessary. Immediate replacement of factor VIII to control more serious bleeding can minimize tissue, nerve, and joint damage. Nonnarcotic or narcotic analgesics may be prescribed. Because blood products are often used to control bleeding, the child should be protected from contracting hepatitis by receiving hepatitis B vaccine.

Nursing interventions. Nursing interventions focus on teaching the child and family to avoid injury and control bleeding. Age-appropriate toys should not have rough or sharp edges; removal of throw rugs and placement of barriers to stairs are encouraged. Playtime should be supervised to minimize hazards and injuries. Physical activity such as swimming, softball, bicycling, hiking, bowling, golf, and running is encouraged for muscle development or psychological well-being. Contact sports, such as football, hockey, or soccer, should be avoided because of their potential for injury. Early dental visits with a dentist knowledgeable in hemophilia can be beneficial in minimizing the risks of a potential bleeding source. Additionally, children with hemophilia should wear medical identification bracelets. The nurse should also inform the family about the National Hemophilia Foundation,* which can provide financial, medical, and psychological assistance.

Patient/family teaching. Parents are taught to protect the child without being overprotective. When external bleeding occurs, parents are taught to apply pressure and cold. Nurses also instruct and encourage the child and family in safely administering factor products at home. Parents are instructed to seek emergency medical care if the child has signs of increased intracranial pressure, which may indicate an intracranial bleed—severe headache, vomiting, and disorientation.

Prognosis. The progress made in hemophilia care over the past two decades has been striking. The advent of home infusion therapy, coupled with recent advances in producing safer and more effective factor concentrates, has revolutionized the treatment and management of hemophilia. Early treatment has significantly reduced the morbidity formerly associated with hemophilia.

Although there is no cure for hemophilia, its signs and symptoms can be controlled and its potentially crippling deformities markedly reduced or avoided. Children with hemophilia have a normal life expectancy in every aspect but one: they have a tendency to bleed, which is a significant inconvenience but not necessarily a life-threatening event.

Unfortunately, those individuals with hemophilia who were treated before the current purification techniques for factor VIII concentrate were established may have been exposed to human immunodeficiency virus (HIV). One estimate is that 60% of these patients under 21 years of age have seroconverted to HIV positive and a significant number have AIDS. Individuals with hemophilia who were diagnosed and treated with factor concentrates since 1989 are at virtually no risk for developing HIV infection.

Idiopathic Thrombocytopenia Purpura.

Etiology/pathophysiology. Idiopathic (cause unknown) thrombocytopenia purpura (ITP) is characterized by a marked decrease in the amount of circulating platelets with resultant bleeding beneath the skin. ITP is the most common thrombocytopenia of childhood, occurring most frequently in the 2- to 5-year age group. As its name implies, the cause of ITP is unknown, and ITP can be either acute or chronic. The acute form of ITP usually follows a viral infection (such as a respiratory infection, rubella, rubeola, mumps, or chickenpox) and is self-limiting; the chronic form has periods of remission.

Clinical manifestations. Other than bleeding, the child appears well. The platelet count drops to <20,000, ensuring impairment in clotting. Platelet counts <10,000 can be life-threatening. Ecchymoses and a pinpoint petechial rash are usually the first signs of ITP, and the areas most commonly involved are over bony prominences. Other manifestations include bleeding gums, bleeding lips, and epistaxis (nose bleeds). The most serious complication of ITP is intracranial hemorrhage, bleeding into the subdural, subarachnoid, and/or intracerebellar space, and is characterized by hematuria (blood in urine); hemarthrosis; melena (black, tarry stools); hematemesis (blood in emesis); and menorrhagia (abnormally heavy menstrual periods).

Diagnostic tests. Microscopic examination reveals not only a decreased number of platelets but platelets that are large in size. Bleeding time and clot reaction time are prolonged, and the tourniquet test for capillary fragility, where a blood pressure cuff is inflated to 100 mm Hg and left in place for 5 minutes, will be positive (that is, more than 15 petechiae present).

Medical management. ITP is a self-limiting illness in the majority of cases, and about three fourths of children recover without complications within 3 months. In most cases, ITP is allowed to run its course with supportive management. A short course of corticosteroids may be used to suppress the immune attack on platelets, thereby reducing the severity of the disease. Transfusions of packed RBCs may be necessary in treating severe, life-threatening hemorrhage. Immunosuppressive

*110 Green St., Room 303, New York, NY 10012; (212) 219-8180; (800) 42HANDI.

therapy (vincristine) and intravenous gamma globulin (IVGG) therapy have also been used with some success in treating chronic cases of ITP. Symptomatic children with recurrent or chronic ITP that fails to respond to treatment usually undergo splenectomy, which eliminates the site of antiplatelet antibody production.

Nursing interventions. Nursing interventions are largely supportive. Preventing bruising and controlling bleeding are of primary importance in managing ITP. The nurse offers education and emotional support since the majority of these children will receive no treatment other than supportive therapy.

Patient family/teaching. Families should be taught to protect the child with low platelets to restrict activity and avoid injury. Additionally, the nurse counsels the family that salicylate drugs (such as aspirin) are never used for pain because salicylates inhibit platelet function. Parents are also instructed to immediately notify their physician if the child experiences acute head trauma and especially if the child exhibits symptoms of intracranial hemorrhage: headaches, visual disturbances, lethargy, vomiting, or disorientation.

Prognosis. The majority of children have a self-limited course without major complications. Some children will develop chronic ITP and require ongoing therapy. A splenectomy may modify the disease process, and the child will be asymptomatic.

Neoplastic Disorders

Neoplastic disorders are the leading cause of death from disease in children past infancy. Although therapeutic advances in drug treatment (chemotherapy), radiation therapy, and surgical techniques have increased the potential for a normal lifespan, the diagnosis of cancer remains a catastrophic, emotionally devastating occurrence for the child and family.

Leukemia. Leukemia is the name given to a group of malignant diseases of the bone marrow and lymphatic system. Leukemia is the most common malignancy of childhood, is more common in males than in females, and has a peak incidence occurring in children between 3 and 5 years of age.

Etiology/pathophysiology. The most common leukemia seen in children is acute lymphoblastic leukemia (ALL). Although the etiology is unknown, the pathological characteristic is the uncontrollable proliferation of blast cells (immature white blood cells [WBCs]) which accumulate in the marrow, causing crowding and depression of other healthy cells (mature WBCs, RBCs, and platelets). As nonfunctional blast cells infiltrate the lymph nodes, the liver, the kidney, and the spleen, they cause these organs to enlarge, producing the clinical manifestations seen in acute leukemia.

Clinical manifestations. Anemia with pallor and fatigue is often severe and may be the first presenting sign. Other signs are leukopenia with fever and infection and thrombocytopenia with bleeding and petechiae. Blast cells can also invade bones, causing bone pain, limping, and joint pain with swelling. Hepatosplenomegaly and enlarged lymph nodes may be present at diagnosis.

Diagnostic tests. A CBC may indicate pancytopenia (decreased RBCs, WBCs, and platelets). The diagnosis is made on examination of bone marrow aspirate that essentially shows immature blast cells. A lumbar puncture may be performed to determine if infiltration of the central nervous system (CNS) has occurred.

Medical management. Highly individualized treatment protocols are instituted by the physician immediately following diagnosis. Since many of the drugs used to bring about a remission can cause a serious depletion of blood elements, the period immediately following remission can leave the child vulnerable to serious infection and hemorrhage. Supportive therapy is instituted until the bone marrow recovers.

To prevent the development of leukemia within the central nervous system (CNS leukemia), prophylactic treatment has become a standard protocol. Since the blood-brain barrier frequently prohibits most systemic drugs from penetrating the CNS, the drugs used in CNS prophylaxis are given intrathecally, that is, injected directly into the cerebrospinal fluid via lumbar puncture. The drug of choice is methotrexate, given both intrathecally and intravenously, but other chemotherapeutic agents may be used. Once remission has occurred, maintenance therapy is begun in an effort to maintain remission and further reduce leukemic cells. The protocol includes daily doses of 6-mercaptopurine (6-MP), weekly doses of methotrexate, and monthly doses of prednisone and vincristine for 2 to 3 years (see Chapter 29).

Nursing interventions. An important nursing intervention in dealing with children with any type of childhood cancer is to be available for family, especially in the early phases of diagnosis and treatment.

Nursing diagnoses and interventions for the child with cancer include but are not limited to the following:

NURSING DIAGNOSES	NURSING INTERVENTIONS
Infection, high risk for, related to impaired immune system	Provide private room; use reverse isolation if necessary. Use strict hand washing technique. Monitor temperature. Use aseptic technique for all skin punctures. Screen all visitors and staff for signs of infection.
Skin integrity, impaired, high risk for, related to treatment-induced changes	Use sheepskin, waffle pads, flotation devices to prevent pressure areas. Clean mouth with soft sponge toothbrush or cotton applicator to prevent mucosal bleeding. Give frequent mouth rinses.

NURSING DIAGNOSES	NURSING INTERVENTIONS
Nutrition, altered: Less than body requirements, high risk for, related to nausea, vomiting, and anorexia	Encourage frequent, small meals of any food tolerated; plan to improve quality of food selections when appetite increases. Take advantage of hungry period; serve small "snacks." Fortify foods with nutritious supplements, such as powdered milk or commercial supplements. Allow child to be involved in food preparation and selection when appropriate.
Anxiety, fear, related to unknown outcome	Instruct patient/family on symptoms, treatments. Promote atmosphere of open communication. Encourage patient and family to ventilate feelings. Recognize developmental fears associated with illness and procedures.

Patient/family teaching. Nurses working with families of children with cancer have a significant supportive role in helping them understand the therapies, preventing or managing expected side effects or toxicities, observing for late effects of treatment, and helping the child and family live as normal a life as possible and cope with the emotional aspects of the disease. Education is a constant feature of the nursing role, especially in terms of new treatments, clinical trials, and home care.

Prognosis. Children diagnosed between 2 and 9 years of age have consistently demonstrated a better outlook than those diagnosed before 2 or after 10 years of age, and females appear to have a more favorable prognosis than males. About 95% of children with ALL achieve initial remission through a number of chemotherapeutic agents and irradiation.

Hodgkin's Disease. Hodgkin's disease is a malignant lymphoma distinguished by painless, progressive enlargement of lymphoid tissue. Although the exact etiology of Hodgkin's disease is still unknown, it is believed to occur in one specific site with spread to nearby lymph nodes through lymphatic routes. Hodgkin's disease is more common in males and is rare in children under 5 years of age; however, the incidence increases throughout childhood and peaks between 15 and 19 years of age. Treatment protocols for children follow the same protocols established for adults. For a complete discussion of Hodgkin's disease, see Chapter 29.

Prognosis. More than 90% of those with early-stage Hodgkin's disease and up to 75% of those with advanced disease can expect long-term survival.

DISORDERS OF IMMUNE FUNCTION

Immunodeficiency disorders are the result of impaired immune function with alteration of the immune (self-defense) response. Immunodeficiency disorders are classified as primary or secondary. Primary immunodeficiency disorders result from genetic or congenital abnormalities and include X-linked agammaglobulinemia (defect in B cell development), DiGeorge syndrome (congenital absence of thymus and parathyroids), and severe combined immune deficiency (absence of both B and T lymphocytes and phagocytic cells). Secondary immunodeficiency disorders, the most common form of immunodeficiency, are acquired disorders associated with certain drug therapies such as corticosteroids, cancer chemotherapy, and antibiotics; radiation therapy; splenectomy; and viral infections. The common indicator in all immunodeficiency disorders is the development of unusual or recurrent, severe infections.

Acquired Immunodeficiency Syndrome (AIDS)

Etiology/Pathophysiology. AIDS is a chronic and usually fatal disease caused by an acquired dysfunction of the immune system. AIDS is caused by the human immunodeficiency virus (HIV), which has been found in blood and in varying amounts in body fluids (semen, vaginal secretions, breast milk, tears, saliva, and urine). The majority of children with AIDS in the United States are under 2 years of age and most have been infected perinatally by an HIV-infected mother while in utero, during parturition, or through breastfeeding. Less common, children have also become infected through the use of blood or blood product transfusions before 1985 and during sexual contact in child abuse. Although the exact mechanism of transmission is unknown, an HIV-infected mother has a 30% to 50% chance of passing the virus to her child, and the risk can increase with subsequent pregnancies.

Clinical Manifestations. Symptoms of HIV infection in children range from no symptoms to severe, life-threatening illnesses. Signs and symptoms commonly associated with AIDS include failure to thrive, progressive neurological disease, and frequent viral and bacterial infections (cytomegalovirus, herpes simplex virus, otitis media, sinusitis, enterocolitis, recurrent pneumonia, and septicemia). In contrast to adult HIV infection, most children rarely contract *Pneumocystis carinii* pneumonia (PCP) or Kaposi's sarcoma. Instead, lymphocytic interstitial pneumonitis (LIP) and malignant lymphomas are more common. Additionally, hepatosplenomegaly, lymphadenopathy, and candidiasis are common to infected adults and children.

Diagnostic Tests. In the child over 15 months of age, the diagnosis of HIV infection is made by the same serological enzyme-linked immunosorbent assay (ELISA) and Western Blot testing for the presence of serum HIV antibodies used in adults. But the diagnosis of the child less than 15 months of age is complicated by the fact that in the seropositive mother, maternal HIV antibodies cross the placenta to the fetus. Most exposed infants 0 to 15 months of age will test positive for HIV antibodies, but it is unclear whose antibodies are being detected during this time. A positive diagnosis in this age group can be supported by the presence of opportunistic infections associated with AIDS, falling CD4 counts (T cells), and abnormal serum immunoglobulins. HIV culture is also available but has limited use as a diagnostic test for HIV.

Medical Management. The medical management of pediatric HIV infection follows the same protocols used in the management of adult HIV infection with dosages adapted for the pediatric population (see Chapter 37).

Nursing Interventions. The nursing interventions are basically the same for the adult and pediatric populations. However, the HIV-infected child must be monitored closely for signs of abnormal growth and development, which are common in this group.

If there is family involvement, nursing interventions are directed at supporting the family. Whenever possible, social services and home health and nutritional services, such as Women, Infants, and Children (WIC), are made available.

Nursing diagnoses and interventions for the child with HIV include but are not limited to the following:

NURSING DIAGNOSES	NURSING INTERVENTIONS
Infection, high risk for, related to impaired body defenses, presence of infective organisms	Restrict contact with persons who have infections, including family, other children, friends, and members of staff. Observe thorough hand washing. Place child in room with noninfectious children; restrict visitors with active illnesses. Advise visitors (and hospital personnel) to practice thorough hand washing. Promote body's remaining natural defenses (e.g., good nutrition). Administer medication, as prescribed.
Social interaction, impaired, related to physical limitations, hospitalizations, social stigma toward AIDS	Assist child in identifying personal strengths. Educate school personnel and classmates about AIDS. Encourage child to participate in activities with other children.
Grieving, anticipatory, related to having a child with a potentially fatal illness	Identify stage of grieving process family is experiencing. Provide opportunities for family to express emotions. Help parents deal with their feelings, allowing them more emotional reserve to meet the needs of their children. Encourage parents to share their moments of sorrow with their children. Facilitate family's assistance with child's care.

Patient/family teaching. The adolecent population is increasingly contracting AIDS. Changing moral standards, increased sexual freedom, increased IV drug use, and misinformation about the disease in this age group render adolescents at high risk for exposure to the disease. As patient advocates, nurses become involved in educating these youngsters directly by counseling them on matters such as avoiding casual sex and using a condom during intercourse. Nurses also can help promote educational messages in the media (Fig. 44-11) (e.g., radio and Music Television [MTV]) and in places that youths frequent.

Prognosis. Early recognition and improved medical care have changed HIV disease from a rapidly fatal to a chronic, but terminal disease of childhood. The ultimate prognosis for perinatal HIV infection depends on the age of the child at diagnosis and the type of secondary diseases. Children diagnosed with AIDS in early infancy are more likely to die at an earlier age.

Juvenile Rheumatoid Arthritis (JRA)

Etiology/Pathophysiology. JRA is a chronic inflammatory, autoimmune disease of connective tissue. Peak on-

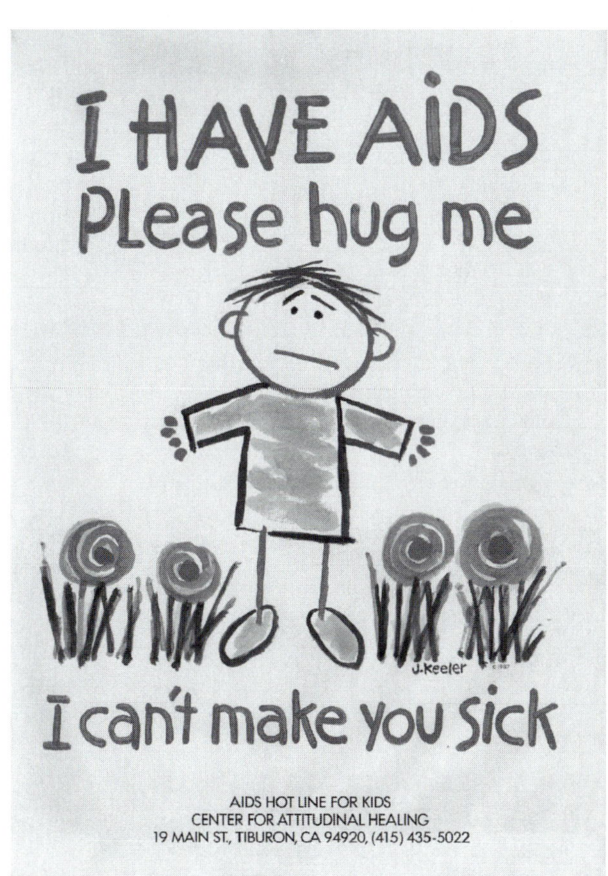
I HAVE AIDS
Please hug me
J.Keeler
I can't make you sick
AIDS HOT LINE FOR KIDS
CENTER FOR ATTITUDINAL HEALING
19 MAIN ST., TIBURON, CA 94920, (415) 435-5022

FIG. 44-11 Using one medium to promote educational messages about AIDS.

MEDICATIONS FOR CHILDREN WITH PHYSICAL AND EMOTIONAL PROBLEMS

Medication	Trade Name	Action	Side Effects	Nursing Implications
Intravenous immune globulin	Gammar-IV, Gamimune-N, Gammagard, Sandoglobulin	Replacement therapy for primary and secondary immunodeficiencies, inteferences with Fc receptors on cells of reticuloendothelial system for autoimmune cytopenias and ITP	Flushing of face and chest tightness, chills, fever, dizziness, nausea, diaphoresis, headache, hypotension, hypersensitivity reactions, pain at injection site, abdominal pain	Follow proper IV protocol for each product; be prepared for possible hypersensitivity reaction; do not admix product with any other IV product.
Chemotherapy agents—asparaginase	Elspar	Inhibits protein synthesis by deaminating asparagine and depriving tumor cells of this essential amino acid	Hypotension, chills, fever, rash, pruritus, anaphylaxis, coughing, vomiting, hyperglycemia, hepatotoxicity, pancreatitis, leukopenia, malaise, drowsiness, coma, seizures	Use two injection sites for IM doses greater than 2 ml; monitor for severe allergic reactions and onset of abdominal pain and mental status change; check CBC, differential and platelet count weekly; check liver and renal Fx tests and serum and glucose tests; watch temperature.
Chemotherapy agents—cytosine arabinoside (cytarabine)	Cytosar-U	Inhibits DNA synthesis, thus interfering with cell replication in S phase of cell cycle before mitosis	Hepatic dysfunction, fever, rash, thrombophlebitis, bleeding, nausea, vomiting, anorexia, diarrhea, alopecia, bone marrow suppression	Monitor liver function test, CBC with differential and platelet count, serum creatinine level, BUN level, serum uric acid level.
Chemotherapy agents—doxorubicin HCl	Adriamycin	Inhibits DNA synthesis by decreasing replication and free radical production	Alopecia, nausea, vomiting, bone marrow suppression, stomatitis, fever	Watch for tissue damage secondary to drug extravasation; monitor liver function test; know that urine and other bodily fluids may be red-orange for 48 hrs.
Chemotherapy agents—6-mercaptopurine (6-MP)	Purinethol	Purine antagonist that inhibits DNA and RNA synthesis	Hepatotoxicity, anorexia, nausea, vomiting, stomatitis, bone marrow suppression	Do not give with meals; monitor temperature, CBC with differential, and renal function tests.
Chemotherapy agents—methotrexate sodium	Folex	Inhibits enzyme that reduces folic acid, which is needed for nucleic acid synthesis in all cells	Alopecia, uticaria, photosensitivity, acne, bone marrow suppression, nausea, vomiting, gingivitis, pharyngitis, stomatitis, diarrhea	Monitor CBC with differential; liver function tests; renal function tests; and temperature.

MEDICATIONS FOR CHILDREN WITH PHYSICAL AND EMOTIONAL PROBLEMS—cont'd

Medication	Trade Name	Action	Side Effects	Nursing Implications
Chemotherapy agents—vincristine sulfate	Oncovin	Binds mitotic spindle, stopping cell reproduction in M and S phases	Alopecia, skin rash, weight loss, orthostatic hypotension, neurotoxicity, nausea, vomiting, anorexia	Watch for tissue damage secondary to drug extravasation; monitor serum electrolyte level, hepatic function test, and neurological examination.
Exogenous surfactant (colfosceril palmitate-exosurf) (beractant-survanta)	Exosurf, Survanta	Replaces deficient or ineffective endogenous lung surfactant in neonates with respiratory distress syndrome, reduces surface tension and stabilizes alveoli from collapsing	Pulmonary hemorrhage, apnea, mucous plugging, decrease in transcutaneous oxygen of greater than 20%, congenital pneumonia	Assess respiratory rate, rhythm, character, chest expansion, color, ABG and transcutaneous saturation; give only by endotracheal tube; suction before treatment and then do not suction for 2 hours after treatment; stop drug if there is reflux during treatment.
Ribavirin	Virazole	Selective inhibitory activity against respiratory syncytial virus	Pulmonary: worsening of respiratory status, bronchospasm, pulmonary edema, hypoventilation, ventilator dependence; cardiovascular: cardiac arrest, hypotension, bradycardia. Anemia, rash, conjuctivitis	Monitor respiratory function and I&O ratio; discard solution in SPAG (2 units every 24 hr).
Cromolyn sodium	Gastrocrom, Intal, Nasalcrom	Prevents mast cell release of histamine, leukotrienes, and slow-reacting substance of anaphylaxis by inhibiting degranulation after contact with antigen	Throat irritation, cough, nasal congestion, headache, dizziness, nausea, vomiting, bitter taste, rash, joint pain or swelling, dry mouth	Monitor eosinophil count during treatment; clear out as much mucus as possible before treatment; have patient gargle or take sip of water to decrease throat irritaion.
Nystatin suspension	Mycostatin, Nilstat	Interferes with fungal DNA replication, binds sterols in fungal cell membrane	Rash, nausea, vomiting, anorexia, diarrhea, cramps	Watch for hypersensitivity reactions; Place half dose on each cheek; try to retain in mouth as long as possible or may swab mouth.

set of JRA is between 2 and 5 years of age and 9 and 12 years of age. In JRA, there is chronic inflammation of the synovium with joint effusion. This inflammatory process leads to erosion, destruction, and fibrosis of the articular cartilage. The exact etiology of the inflammatory process is not known, but the tissue injury is thought to occur from a previous infectious process.

Clinical Manifestations. The signs and symptoms seen in acute systemic onset include daily afternoon temperature spikes, macular rash on the trunk and extremities, and joint involvement. Other systemic conditions include pericarditis, lymphadenopathy, hepatosplenomegaly, iridocyclitis, and anemia.

Diagnostic Tests. There are no specific tests for diagnosing JRA. The latex fixation test, which identifies rheumatoid arthritis in the adult, is negative in 90% of juvenile cases. Depending upon the degree of inflammation, the erythrocyte sedimentation rate (ESR) may be elevated. In some types of JRA, antinuclear antibodies (ANAs) may be present. Radiographic findings in early-onset JRA may show the widening of joint spaces and, later, fusion and articular destruction.

Medical Management. The goals of management include the prevention of joint contractures, preservation of joint function, and relief of signs and symptoms. Nonsteroidal antiinflammatory drugs (NSAIDs) are prescribed. These include tolmetin (Tolectin), naproxen (Naprosyn), indomethacin (Indocin), ibuprofen (Motrin), and aspirin. Slower-acting antirheumatic drugs (SAARDs) are usually added to the drug therapy when one or two of the NSAIDs cannot effectively control signs and symptoms. The SAARDs include gold, D-penicillamine, and hydroxychloroquine. Symptomatic treatment of JRA includes the application of moist heat to facilitate movement and physical therapy. Surgical intervention may be necessary for some children unresponsive to therapy. See the medications table on pp.1384-1385 for drugs for children with physical and emotional problems.

Nursing Interventions. The nurse discusses potential problems in the school environment such as stairs and strenuous activities and facilitates planning with the school nurse to arrange for medication administration and rest periods. JRA strongly affects the normal activities of daily living (ADLs) of children afflicted with the disorder. The nurse supports the family in expressing their fears and concerns and guides them in a daily program of rest, exercise, medication administration, and pain management. The child is encouraged to perform ADLs (bathing, dressing, grooming) with little or no help from the family to enhance self-esteem. The nurse also suggests support groups for the child and parents that provide education and resources necessary to effectively cope with a chronic, debilitating illness. Referrals to the Arthritis Foundation* and the American Juvenile Arthritis Foundation* can provide this assistance.

Nursing diagnoses and interventions for the child with JRA include but are not limited to the following:

NURSING DIAGNOSES	NURSING INTERVENTIONS
Pain, chronic, related to joint inflammation	Provide as much relief as possible with antiinflammatory medication and other therapies to help child tolerate the pain and cope as effectively as possible (although desirable, complete pain relief is probably unattainable). Apply moist heat to relieve pain and stiffness (the most efficient and practical method is tub baths).
Physical mobility, impaired, related to joint discomfort and stiffness	Promote ADLs to provide satisfactory exercise and increase mobility. Encourage lying in the prone position to straighten hips and knees. Instruct patient and family in the purpose and correct use of any splints and appliances. Instruct in use of raised toilet seat for independent toileting.

Patient/family teaching. Nursing interventions consist of educating the child and family in the disease process and management. Parents are taught to perform gentle range of motion (ROM) exercises to promote joint mobility, administer medications, apply heat (warm baths can be very effective) to relieve pain, and encourage normal play activity to promote exercise and increase joint mobility.

Prognosis. The course of JRA is highly variable. Some 30% to 40% of patients have active disease 10 years after diagnosis, have substantial disability as adults, and require long-term drug therapy.

DISORDERS OF RESPIRATORY FUNCTION

Acute respiratory infections are extremely common in infants and children. They can range from minor to life-threatening illnesses. Most respiratory illnesses involve viral pathogens. Bacterial infections most commonly involve group A β-hemolytic streptococcus, *Staphylococcus aureus,* and *Haemophilus influenzae.*

Respiratory Distress Syndrome (RDS)

Etiology/Pathophysiology. RDS, idiopathic respiratory distress syndrome (IRDS), and hyaline membrane disease (HMD) are terms that refer to the severe lung

*1314 Spring St. N.W., Atlanta, GA 30309; (404) 872-7100 or (800) 283-7800.

disorder that is the major cause of morbidity and mortality in the neonatal period. RDS is caused by a deficiency of surfactant and occurs almost exclusively in the preterm, low-birth-weight infant. RDS is seen more often in males and in infants delivered by cesarean section. Other predisposing factors include infants of diabetic mothers, asphyxia, maternal hemorrhage, and shock. Surfactant reduces the surface tension of fluids that line the avleoli, thereby permitting expansion of the lungs and alveolar inflation. Without sufficient production of surfactant, the infant is unable to keep the lungs inflated and the alveoli collapse at the end of expiration resulting in hypoxia, atelectasis, and respiratory acidosis.

Clinical Manifestations. Respiratory signs and symptoms become apparent immediately after birth. Signs and symptoms include nasal flaring; expiratory grunting; intercostal, subcostal, or substernal retractions; dusky color; tachypnea; and low body temperature. In severe cases, infants may die within hours of the onset of signs and symptoms; those who survive gradually show improvement by the fourth day.

Diagnostic Tests. The diagnosis of RDS is based on the clinical presentation and radiographic examination. Blood gas analysis indicates the degree of respiratory and metabolic acidosis.

Medical Management. The treatment of RDS is entirely supportive and directed toward correction of imbalances. Supportive measures include maintaining a neutral thermal environment, adequate oxygenation either by increasing ambient (pertaining to the surrounding area) oxygen concentration or by ventilatory assistance, and correction of respiratory and metabolic acidosis. Oxygen therapy is continually evaluated by measuring arterial oxygen to prevent hypoxia and the toxic effects of high concentrations of oxygen. Nutritional support is provided by parenteral therapy during the early acute stage to prevent aspiration.

Prevention of RDS. The administration of exogenous (originating outside the body) pulmonary surfactant to infants at high risk of developing or who have developed RDS has greatly reduced the morbidity and mortality associated with the disorder. Exogenous surfactant is administered directly into the lungs shortly after birth and a second dose is administered 12 hours later.

Nursing Interventions. The primary nursing consideration in caring for the infant with RDS is observing and assessing the infant's response to therapy. Continuous monitoring and assessment are essential so that oxygen concentrations and ventilator settings can be adjusted in response to the infant's blood gas measurements and pulse oximetry readings. The nurse performs frequent respiratory assessments, observes the infant's behavior, and observes for signs of respiratory complications and sepsis. Suctioning is performed as needed and based upon individual assessment of the neonate (auscultation, increased infant irritability, excessive moisture in the endotracheal tube). Suctioning is never carried out on a routine basis. Frequent vigorous suctioning can lead to bronchospasm, airway damage, infection, **pneumothorax** (collapse of the lung), hypoxia, and increased intracranial pressure that can lead to intraventricular hemorrhage in the neonate. Nurses can help the infant maintain an open airway by positioning the infant on the side with the head supported in alignment. The nurse assesses the infant's skin frequently and protects the skin from impairment by frequent repositioning and the use of water mattresses or pillows and sheepskin. A water-soluble ointment can be used to reduce irritation to the nares or around the mouth, and frequent oral hygiene with water can relieve dryness caused by oxygen therapy.

Family teaching. Parents will need emotional support and should be encouraged to discuss their anxieties and concerns so that the nurse can clarify information. Parents are also encouraged to touch, hold, and talk to the infant and participate in the care whenever possible to promote bonding.

Prognosis. RDS is a self-limiting disease. Infants with RDS who survive the first 96 hours have a reasonable chance of recovery. Surfactant replacement therapy may improve the survival rate and reduce the severity of RDS.

Bronchopulmonary Dysplasia (BPD)

Etiology/Pathophysiology. BPD is a chronic pulmonary disorder that develops in premature infants. BPD is associated with meconium aspiration, RDS, high concentrations of oxygen, positive pressure ventilation, and endotracheal intubation. Chronic lung changes include thickening and necrosis of alveolar walls with impairment of oxygen diffusion from the alveoli to the capillaries. Edema and inflammation of the capillary bed can cause some alveoli to collapse, some to hyperinflate, and others to rupture. The disorder is characterized by diffuse infiltrates, hyperinflation, and chronic pulmonary insufficiency.

Clinical Manifestations. The clinical signs and symptoms of BPD vary widely. Most infants show evidence of respiratory distress (wheezing, retracting, nasal flaring, irritability, abundant secretions, and cyanosis when stressed). These children are vulnerable to upper respiratory infections and frequently require hospitalization due to poor respiratory status.

Diagnostic Tests. There are no specific signs or symptoms or laboratory data to confirm a diagnosis of BPD. Radiographic examination and ABG determinations may be helpful in contributing to the diagnosis. Pulmonary function tests may also be helpful in determining the degree of lung dysfunction.

Medical Management. Precautions are taken to prevent RDS and reduce ventilation and oxygen requirements. When ventilation and oxygen are necessary, they are managed meticulously by using the lowest concentration of oxygen and ventilatory pressures to maintain adequate gas exchange to avoid further damage of lung tissue. During weaning, bronchodilators may be used to decrease airway resistance and increase lung compliance. Nutritional support is provided initially by total parenteral nutrition (TPN) and replaced by nasogastric, gavage, or breastfeeding or bottle feeding.

Nursing Interventions. Rest periods are planned to decrease respiratory effort and conserve energy. When oral feedings are begun, small, frequent feedings are provided to prevent overdistension of the stomach, which can interfere with respiratory effort. The nurse is instrumental in supporting parents and encourages them to participate in their infant's care.

Patient/family teaching. Parents are also counseled in ways to reduce the risk of respiratory infections and to notify their physician at the fist sign of a respiratory infection in their child. Parents are taught cardiopulmonary resuscitation and how to manage any other emergency that might be anticipated for their infant.

Prognosis. There is a high mortality rate in the first year. Infants who survive are at risk for chronic lung disease.

Pneumonia

Etiology/Pathophysiology. Pneumonia is an acute inflammation of the pulmonary parenchyma (tissue), small airways, and alveoli. Pneumonias are classified by etiological agent: bacterial, viral, mycoplasmal, or foreign body aspiration. Pneumonia is common throughout childhood, occurs more frequently in infants and young children, and is usually associated with an upper respiratory infection. Pneumonias are primarily seen in the winter months from November through March. Viral pneumonias are more common than bacterial pneumonias, with respiratory syncytial virus (RSV) accounting for the largest percentage of infections in children. Bacterial pneumonias most common in infants and children are caused by streptococcal, staphylococcal, pneumococcal, or *Haemophilus influenzae* organisms.

Clinical Manifestations. The clinical manifestations of viral and bacterial pneumonias are given in Box 44-2.

Diagnostic Tests. Radiographic examination establishes the location and extent of infection. Peripheral blood tests may reveal an elevated WBC, with bacterial infection showing a greater elevation in WBC than viral infection. Identification of the causative organism includes culture and Gram stain of respiratory secretions and the blood, and diagnostic thoracentesis if fluid is suspected in the pleural cavity. If no bacterial microorganism is identified, the pneumonia is considered to be viral.

Box 44-2 CLINICAL MANIFESTATIONS OF PNEUMONIA IN CHILDREN

Cough	Lethargy
Wheezes or crackles	Headache
Respiratory distress	Fever
Chest pain	Myalgia
Anorexia	Abdominal pain
Irritability	Nasal discharge
Malaise	

Medical Management. The goal of therapy in the management of pneumonia is directed toward improving oxygenation and preventing dehydration. Treatment includes antibiotic therapy, oxygen therapy, chest physiotherapy, suctioning, fluid administration, and bronchodilators. Antipyretics may be ordered to control fever. For RSV pneumonia, Ribavirin (an antiviral) treatment is started within 3 days of onset of infection. Ribavirin is delivered by a SPAG (small-particle aerosol generator) nebulizer (or Collison nebulizer) through an oxyhood or mist tent over 12 to 18 hours per day for 3 to 7 days.

Nursing Interventions. Observation of respiratory status, including skin color and respiratory effort, and monitoring of cardiovascular status are two important nursing measures. Infection control measures are instituted according to hospital protocol. Supportive nursing management includes providing for adequate rest periods to conserve energy, maintaining hydration by monitoring prescribed IV fluids, and gentle suctioning with a bulb syringe when necessary.

Patient/family teaching. Nurses encourage parents to participate in their child's care, guiding them in feeding and holding while their child is in the mist tent to prevent dislodgement of IV catheters.

Prognosis. Prognosis for pneumococcal and streptococcal pneumonias is generally good, with rapid resolution when detected and treated early. Staphylococcal pneumonias typically run a longer course, but early detection and treatment are usually effective.

Sudden Infant Death Syndrome (SIDS)

The sudden, unexpected, and unexplained death of a healthy infant evokes a variety of familial responses ranging from hysteria and denial to stoicism (impassive, indifferent to joy or pain). Nurses assume an important role in assisting the family through the death and grieving process.

Etiology/Pathophysiology. SIDS is the sudden, unexpected death of a healthy, normal infant under 1 year of age where a postmortem examination fails to establish a cause of death. The incidence is 2 to 3 per 1000 live births, with peak incidence occurring between 2 and 4 months of age. SIDS always occurs during sleep and is the leading cause of death in infants between 1 month and 1 year of age. SIDS occurs more often in males and in siblings of SIDS victims. There is an increased incidence in winter months, with peak incidence occurring in January. Native Americans and African-Americans are most often affected, and there is an increased occurrence in lower socioeconomic classes. SIDS is often associated with premature birth and low birth weight, low Apgar scores, multiple births, and with CNS and respiratory dysfunctions. SIDS is also associated with maternal smoking, drug addiction, and maternal age of less than 20 years. Breastfed infants have a lower incidence of SIDS. The cause of SIDS is unknown, and numerous theories have been proposed. Some studies show evidence of abnormalities of cardiorespiratory regulation: prolonged sleep apnea, depressed ventilatory response to increased carbon dioxide or decreased oxygen, increased frequency of short apneic episodes, and excessive periodic breathing. Other studies show a relationship between sleep position and SIDS. Sleeping in a prone position may predispose the infant to oropharyngeal obstruction or affect ventilatory arousal. Soft, polystyrene-filled mattresses or pillows may cause suffocation in the infant sleeping in a prone position.

Clinical Manifestations. Death occurs during sleep, and there is no audible outcry or sign of distress.

Diagnostic Tests. Diagnosis is confirmed at postmortem examination, which reveals pulmonary edema and intrathoracic hemorrhages.

Medical Management. Therapeutic management is directed toward assisting the family that has just lost an infant to SIDS (see Chapter 52).

Nursing Interventions. The death of an infant from SIDS propels the family into a crisis situation. The initial response is one of extreme shock and disbelief. As parents try to cope, they may experience feelings of guilt and blame. Typically, it is the mother who finds her infant dead in the crib. The appearance of the dead infant indicates that some activity has taken place prior to death. The infant is most often found with the blankets over the head and huddled in a corner of the crib. The infant's hands may be clutching the sheets or blanket. Frothy, blood-tinged secretions are noted in the mouth and the nostrils. The infant's appearance and the shock of an unexpected death lead many parents to believe that their infant has suffocated, and they become filled with self-blame. Nurses need to be aware of these circumstances so that they can effectively assist and support the family in this time of crisis. The first persons to respond to a SIDS event are the police and ambulance personnel, who are generally educated in SIDS. When talking with the parent, they should be nonjudgmental, ask few questions, and provide support to the family. Upon the family's arrival in the emergency room, the nurse is most likely the first person to interact with them. The nurse stays with the parent, listening to and supporting the family. Emergency room personnel ask only factual information about the event. If resuscitation was attempted at home, the child may have bruises and broken ribs, which may be confused with physical abuse. The physician examines the infant and pronounces death. At this time, hospital personnel will discuss autopsy so that the cause of death can be established; otherwise the circumstances surrounding the death cannot be laid to rest. The emergency room nurse becomes instrumental in assisting families with grief and mourning. The nurse cleans the infant, wraps the child in a sheet or blanket, and tidies the room where the family can spend time with their dead infant. In coming to terms with the death, the parents' last moments with their infant should be quiet, peaceful, and as meaningful as possible. The nurse offers to stay with the family or allow them private time if they wish. The baby's belongings are bagged and given to the family upon leaving.

Family teaching. The nurse arranges for a public health nurse to visit the family as soon as possible after the death to decrease feelings of isolation, help them in understanding the SIDS phenomenon, and assist with siblings' feelings. A referral to the National SIDS Foundation* is always helpful.

Upper Respiratory Tract Infections

Acute Pharyngitis (Sore Throat).

Etiology/pathophysiology. Acute pharyngitis is an inflammation of the pharynx. Approximately 80% of acute pharyngitis cases are viral in origin, while 20% are bacterial (group A β-hemolytic streptococcus). Acute pharyngitis occurs frequently between 4 to 12 years of age, when children are increasingly exposed to infections outside the home. Children less than 3 years of age with pharyngitis are usually infected with *Haemophilus influenzae.* These children should be watched for neurological signs and symptoms indicating possible menin-

*P.O. Box 2753, Landover Hills, MD 20784; (301) 459-3388. Also, Sudden Infant Death Syndrome Alliance, 10500 Little Patuxent Parkway, Suite 420, Columbia, MD 21044; (301) 964-8000 or (800) 221-SIDS.

gitis; however, with the use of Hib vaccine, infections involving this organism are beginning to decline. Acute pharyngitis is more commonly seen in later winter and early spring.

Clinical manifestations. Viral pharyngitis presents with low-grade fever, malaise, anorexia, erythema, and throat soreness. The child may also complain of headache, cough, hoarseness, rhinitis, and conjunctivitis. Streptococcal pharyngitis presents with high fever, throat soreness, white exudates on the posterior pharynx and tonsillar region, vomiting, and abdominal pain.

Diagnostic tests. A throat culture is performed to detect streptococcal pharyngitis.

Medical management. Viral pharyngitis is treated symptomatically with lozenges, gargles, and acetaminophen. Streptococcal pharyngitis must be treated with a 10-day course of antimicrobial therapy to prevent complications (rheumatic fever and glomerulonephritis). Penicillin is the drug of choice for streptococcal pharyngitis. Erythromycin is used for those with penicillin allergy.

Nursing interventions. Throat discomfort in both viral and bacterial infections is relieved with saline gargles, lozenges, warm compresses to the neck, and acetaminophen. Cool liquids (nonacid) are encouraged until the throat feels better, then soft, bland foods are introduced. Follow-up care of streptococcal pharyngitis is emphasized to ensure eradication of the causative organism.

Patient/family teaching. The nurse instructs the family in antimicrobial therapy, emphasizing the need to completely finish the medication even though the child feels better.

Prognosis. The prognosis of acute pharyngitis is usually excellent. Inadequately treated streptococcal infections sometimes trigger a response in the heart (rheumatic fever) or kidneys (acute glomerulonephritis).

Tonsillitis.

Etiology/pathophysiology. The tonsils are masses of lymphoid tissue believed to protect the respiratory and alimentary tracts from invasion by pathogenic microorganisms. They are also thought to play a role in antibody formation. Tonsillitis usually occurs as a result of pharyngitis and can be viral or bacterial (streptococcal) in origin.

Clinical manifestations. The signs and symptoms of viral and bacterial tonsillitis are similar and include sore throat, headache, edematous and tender cervical lymph glands, fever, hoarseness, and cough. Additionally, in streptococcal tonsillitis, the child may exhibit vomiting, complain of muscle aches, and have difficulty swallowing or breathing.

Diagnostic tests. A CBC may indicate a significantly elevated WBC. A throat culture is performed to detect streptococcal tonsillitis.

Medical management. The treatment for bacterial and nonbacterial tonsillitis includes the comfort measures described in acute pharyngitis. Additionally, bacterial tonsillitis is treated with a 10-day course of penicillin (or erythromycin) to prevent complications. Surgical removal of the tonsils for chronic tonsillitis is controversial. Tonsillectomy is recommended for children with hypertrophied tonsils that interfere with eating or breathing.

Nursing interventions. The nursing interventions for children with tonsillitis is the same as described in acute pharyngitis. If surgery is indicated, the nurse psychologically prepares the child preoperatively as well as assesses the child for signs of infection and loose teeth and checks the child's laboratory data, including the bleeding and clotting studies. Postoperatively, the child is kept in a semiprone position to facilitate drainage; monitored frequently for excessive bleeding, which will cause frequent swallowing even while asleep; given analgesics as prescribed; and when recovered from analgesia, provided with fluids (with the exception of acidic, grape, red, or chocolate drinks in order to distinguish fresh or old blood in emesis from ingested liquid). A soft diet follows. The use of straws has been advised against because sucking may precipitate bleeding; however, this intervention is not universally accepted.

Patient/family teaching. Discharge instructions include:

- Avoiding foods that are irritating or highly seasoned
- Avoiding the use of gargles or vigorous toothbrushing
- Discouraging the child from coughing or clearing the throat
- Using mild analgesics or an ice collar for pain
- Alerting parents that hemorrhaging may occur 5 to 10 days after surgery as a result of tissue sloughing from the healing process. Any signs of bleeding require immediate physician notification

Prognosis. The prognosis is generally excellent. Improperly treated streptococcal infections may result in rheumatic fever or glomerulonephritis.

Croup Syndromes.

Laryngotracheobronchitis (LTB)/viral group and acute epiglottitis.

Etiology/pathophysiology. LTB is the most common form of the croup syndromes affecting children 3 months to 3 years of age and is usually viral in origin. LTB usually follows an upper respiratory infection that descends to the lower respiratory tract and has a gradual, progressive onset.

Acute epiglottitis is a severe, potentially life-threatening bacterial infection of the epiglottis in older children and is usually caused by *Haemophilus influenzae,* type B. The inflamed epiglottis becomes cherry-red and edematous, which can lead to total airway obstruction.

Clinical manifestations. The child with LTB initially demonstrates hoarseness, inspiratory stridor, tachypnea, nasal flaring, suprasternal retractions, and barking cough. Body temperature may be normal or mildly elevated.

However, the child with epiglottitis is acutely ill with high fever, muffled voice, drooling, progressive respiratory distress, anxiety, and fear.

Diagnostic tests. The diagnosis of LTB is based on a history of a preceding upper respiratory infection, CBC with differential, the clinical signs and symptoms, and physical examination.

A tentative diagnosis of acute epiglottitis is established by clinical signs and symptoms and is considered a medical emergency. The child is taken to the operating or ambulatory surgery room where emergency equipment is available for immediate intubation or tracheostomy in the event of further obstruction during examination of the pharynx. Lateral neck radiographs may be done in the operating room to observe for soft tissue edema and area of obstruction. Skilled personnel with the equipment necessary to perform immediate intubation or tracheostomy never leave the child's side. Visual examination of the pharynx and invasive procedures such as blood collection and insertion of IV lines are done with the child under anesthesia. Tracheal secretions at the time of intubation are collected for culture and sensitivity.

Medical management. Management of both LTB and epiglottitis is focused on maintaining an open airway. For the child with LTB, high cool-mist humidity with low-concentration oxygen (<30%) is provided by mist tent. Epinephrine by aerosol is administered to decrease airway edema by vasoconstriction and improve oxygenation by bronchodilation. The effects of epinephrine are short-lived, and the child will most likely need repeated doses as the airway edema returns a few hours after epinephrine administration. Therefore, children receiving epinephrine are monitored very closely. During the acute phase, the child is kept NPO because rapid respirations predispose to aspiration. Adequate hydration is accomplished by IV administration of fluids. Sedatives are never used because they mask restlessness, which is a clinical indication of hypoxia and a deteriorating condition.

Immediate treatment of the child with acute epiglottitis includes an artificial airway. Respiratory care includes humidification, gentle oral suctioning, and constant observation of respiratory status. Oxygen may be ordered for moderate respiratory distress, and aerosolized epinephrine is administered to decrease airway edema by local vasoconstriction. Again, the child receiving epinephrine is closely monitored as the effects of epinephrine are short-lived and airway edema may return a few hours after administration. IV antibiotics and fluids are started. Epiglottal edema usually decreases after 24 hours of antibiotic therapy. By the third day, the epiglottis is nearly normal in size and the child can be safely extubated at this time.

Nursing interventions. LTB or acute epiglottitis can be a frightening experience for the child and the family. The nurse should respond quickly in a calm manner, supporting and reassuring parents that everything possible is being done for their child. The nurse continually assesses the child for signs of response to therapy or increasing obstruction. Treatment changes are frequently based on the nurse's observations. The child is maintained in Fowler's position, and respirations are monitored for rate, depth, retractions, and nasal flaring. The child's cardiac status is also monitored because restlessness and tachycardia are signs of increasing hypoxia. Vital signs are monitored frequently. Intubation and tracheostomy sets are kept at bedside for possible respiratory failure. Nursing interventions are carefully planned to provide for frequent rest periods to conserve energy.

Family teaching. Parents are kept informed of their child's progress and encouraged to participate in care.

Prognosis for laryngotracheobronchitis. In most children, the disease is relatively mild. Gradual improvement to recovery occurs in 3 to 7 days. The most serious complication and the one responsible for most deaths from croup is laryngeal obstruction.

Prognosis for epiglottitis. Without prompt diagnosis and treatment, the rapid course of epiglottitis can cause death within a few hours.

Lower Respiratory Tract Infections

Bronchitis (Tracheobronchitis).

Etiology/pathophysiology. Bronchitis is an inflammation of the large airways, the trachea, and the bronchi. It usually follows an upper respiratory infection and is almost always viral in origin. The most common cause is rhinovirus; although parainfluenza, adenovirus, and RSV have also been identified as causes. *Mycoplasma pneumoniae* is a common cause of bronchitis in children more than 6 years of age. Bronchitis occurs mainly in the winter months and is primarily seen in children under 4 years of age (although it can affect any age group).

Clinical manifestations. The onset is gradual with signs and symptoms of an upper respiratory tract infection (cough, coryza, little or no fever). After 2 to 3 days, the nonproductive, hacking cough becomes productive and worsens at night.

Diagnostic tests. Radiographic examination of the chest is indicated for the child with severe signs and symptoms. For the majority of children, chest radiographs are normal.

Medical management. Treatment is basically palliative. If the cough interferes with resting or eating, cough drops, lollipops, and pediatric cough preparations are usually effective. Cough suppressants are contraindicated in bronchitis unless sleep is significantly affected. Acetaminophen may be prescribed for fever. Antibiotics are not necessary in viral bronchitis. If the cough lasts beyond 10 days, a secondary bacterial infection should be suspected.

Nursing interventions/patient and family teaching. The nurse suggests the use of a cool mist humidifier to relieve the child's cough and help liquefy secretions. Fluids to decrease viscosity of secretions and prevent dehydration are encouraged.

Prognosis. Acute bronchitis is self-limiting.

Acute Bronchiolitis.

Etiology/pathophysiology. Bronchiolitis is a viral inflammation of the smaller airway passages, the bronchioles, which become inflamed causing edema. The accumulation of mucus and exudate can partially or completely obstruct the lumen. RSV is the organism responsible for the vast majority of cases. Bronchiolitis occurs in children under 2 years of age, with a peak incidence at 6 months of age.

Clinical manifestations. Upper respiratory infection signs and symptoms predominate during the first few days, followed by worsening signs and symptoms of respiratory distress. The infant exhibits retractions, tachypnea, nasal flaring, paroxysmal nonproductive coughing, and wheezing. The infant may have low-grade or very high fever; be irritable, fussy, and anxious; and have difficulty eating. Respiratory distress becomes progressively more severe during the first 72 hours.

Diagnostic tests. The diagnosis is based on the age of the child and the clinical signs and symptoms. Radiographic examination of the chest shows areas of atelectasis and hyperinflation. Nasal smears for RSV are also obtained.

Medical management. High humidity via mist tent to loosen secretions is used. If hypoxemia is present, oxygen therapy is administered with mist therapy. IV fluids are indicated if the infant is unable to tolerate oral feedings. If RSV is suspected, Ribavirin therapy is begun (see discussion under Pneumonia). Bronchodilators may be used in severe cases of bronchiolitis.

Nursing interventions. The infant is placed on respiratory isolation precautions. Thorough hand washing is encouraged to prevent cross-contamination. Acute nursing interventions focus on promoting adequate oxygenation, frequent monitoring of respiratory status, and maintaining hydration. As with any respiratory condition, parents will need reassurance and support during this stressful period.

Prognosis. The disease lasts 3 to 10 days, and the prognosis is generally good.

Pulmonary Tuberculosis.

Etiology/pathophysiology. Pulmonary tuberculosis (TB) is a chronic bacterial lung infection caused by the bacillus *Mycobacterium tuberculosis.* TB remains a leading cause of death in many underdeveloped countries. It continues to be a public health problem in the United States primarily due to immigration of foreign-born persons, the AIDS epidemic, and multiresistant strains of TB. The most important risk factor in TB infection progressing into active disease is an inadequate immune response due to age or an impaired immune system, such as is seen in young infants, the elderly, or those infected with HIV. Immunocompromised children and children less than 3 years of age are at greatest risk for TB, with the risk again increasing during the postpubertal adolescent years. The primary source of TB infection in children is exposure to an infected adult, usually a family member, babysitter, or frequent visitor.

Clinical manifestations. Most children do not exhibit any clinical signs and symptoms when first infected. Signs and symptoms are extremely variable and develop so gradually that they may go unnoticed until the disease has significantly progressed.

Diagnostic tests. Although not diagnostic, tuberculin skin testing is the most important screening measure in identifying infected children at risk for disease. To confirm the diagnosis, positive bacteriological sputum cultures for *M. tuberculosis* are essential. Infants and young children do not cough and expectorate sputum. Instead, mucus from the respiratory tract is usually swallowed. Therefore, the best way to obtain sputum samples from infants and children is by gastric aspiration. Chest radiographs are also important in determining the presence and extent of active lesions. The medical management and nursing interventions are basically the same as in the adult with active tuberculosis. Please refer to Chapter 31 for continued discussion.

Patient teaching and prognosis. Because the success of therapy depends on compliance with the drug regimen, parents are instructed regarding the importance of giving medications as often and for as long as ordered. The optimum duration of therapy is unknown, but the usual course of treatment is no less than 12 months for an initial treatment or 18 to 24 months for more serious forms of the disease.

Foreign Body Aspiration.

Etiology/pathophysiology. Foreign body aspiration is the passage of any foreign material into the lung. It can occur at any age but is most common in children under 3 years of age owing to the normal hand-mouth activity of this age group. Commonly aspirated items include pieces of food (hot dogs; small, round candies; nuts; popcorn; peanut butter), marbles, pieces of small toys (car wheels, beads, balloons), safety pins, buttons, and coins. The degree of obstruction (partial or complete) is dependent upon the item aspirated and its anatomical location. Most aspirated items become wedged in the right main bronchus because its diameter is larger than the left bronchus and it originates from the trachea at a wider angle, allowing a straight line of entry.

Clinical manifestations. Initially, aspiration of a foreign body in the bronchus produces coughing, gagging, choking, or wheezing, which subsides for a period of hours or even weeks without signs or symptoms. Secondary signs such as a chronic cough, wheeze, or dyspnea develop in response to a persistent respiratory infection distal to the obstruction. Laryngotracheal (upper airway) foreign body can cause an acute obstruction with the potential for a life-threatening crisis. Signs include hoarseness, stridor, cyanosis, or loss of consciousness.

Diagnostic tests. Foreign body aspiration is diagnosed by history, clinical signs, and thorough physical examination of the chest for evidence of uneven breath sounds. Radiographic examination may reveal the location of opaque items such as coins but are less helpful in identifying food items. In many cases, the aspiration event may not have been witnessed; therefore, the practitioner must be acutely aware of its potential in this age group.

Medical management. Clinical intervention of upper airway obstruction includes the Heimlich maneuver for children over 1 year of age, and combination back blows and chest thrusts for the child under 1 year of age. Laryngoscopy may also be necessary. Lower airway obstruction is managed by bronchoscopy to locate and extract the aspirated object. Following removal, the child is placed in a high-humidity environment, and any secondary bacterial infection is treated with antimicrobial therapy.

Nursing interventions. Nurses who work with children can encounter foreign body aspirations at any time and should be prepared to quickly identify, assess, and aid the choking child to prevent cardiorespiratory arrest. Following removal of the object, chest physiotherapy and postural drainage are carried out as well as frequent assessment of respiratory status and vital signs.

Patient/family teaching. Nurses should teach parents the correct techniques for performing back blows and the Heimlich maneuver. Nurses can also educate parents about the hazards of aspiration and encourage them to teach their children safety.

Prognosis. With immediate removal of the foreign body by back blows, the Heimlich maneuver, or direct laryngoscopy or bronchoscopy, the prognosis is generally excellent.

Cystic Fibrosis (CF).

Etiology/pathophysiology. CF is an inherited disorder of the exocrine (mucus-producing) glands, characterized by excessive thick mucus that obstructs the lungs and the gastrointestinal (GI) system. CF is a multiorgan disease, but death is usually caused by pulmonary failure. It is the most common fatal genetic disorder, occurring in about 1 out of every 1800 births. CF affects both sexes equally and is more common in Caucasian populations. The abnormally thick mucus that collects in the lung airways and organ ducts causes obstruction. Bronchiolar obstruction predisposes the lung to infection, bronchiectasis, and cystic dilations. Complications include bronchial and bronchiolar obstruction, pulmonary hypertension, and cor pulmonale. Obstruction of the pancreatic ducts leads to dilation and fibrosis and a decrease in pancreatic enzymes (lipase, amylase, and trypsin), which results in malabsorption. Obstruction in the hepatic system leads to biliary cirrhosis, portal hypertension, and splenomegaly. Elevated sodium chloride concentrations in the sweat and the saliva occur as a result of the abnormal reabsorption of chloride by epithelial cells.

Clinical manifestations. Pancreatic insufficiency and malabsorption result in *steatorrhea* (bulky, foul-smelling, fatty stools), growth failure, protruding abdomen, and thin, wasted extremities. Rectal prolapse is a common GI manifestation of CF. Appetite is often increased early in the illness in response to poor absorption. Malabsorption can also lead to a vitamin K deficiency, resulting in bleeding disorders, esophageal varicies, and ecchymoses. Diminished subcutaneous fat results in sallow, transparent skin. Pulmonary involvement is manifested by chronic cough, wheezing, sputum production, and dyspnea resulting in hypoxia, clubbing of the fingers and toes, and cyanosis. Hyperinflation of the lungs can produce a barrel chest.

Diagnostic tests. The diagnosis of CF is based on a family history of the disorder, absence of pancreatic enzymes, pulmonary involvement, and a positive sweat test. A sweat test over 60 mEq/L of chloride is diagnostic for CF.

Medical management. The goals of therapy include good nutrition, prevention and control of respiratory infections, and providing as normal a life-style as possible for the child. Pulmonary toileting is the single most important aspect of treatment. Chest physiotherapy (CPT) and postural drainage are performed several times a day to loosen and remove pulmonary secretions. Breathing exercises are encouraged to improve aeration. Inhalation therapy with bronchodilators prior to CPT facilitate secretion removal. Expectorants, mucolytic agents, and antibiotics are used to relieve obstruction and resolve infections. Digestive and nutritional therapy includes pancreatic enzyme replacement and a diet high in calories, protein, and salt.

Nursing interventions. Nursing interventions for the child with CF are highly complex and a challenge for the nurse. Management focuses on improving pulmonary function and facilitating lung clearance, preventing

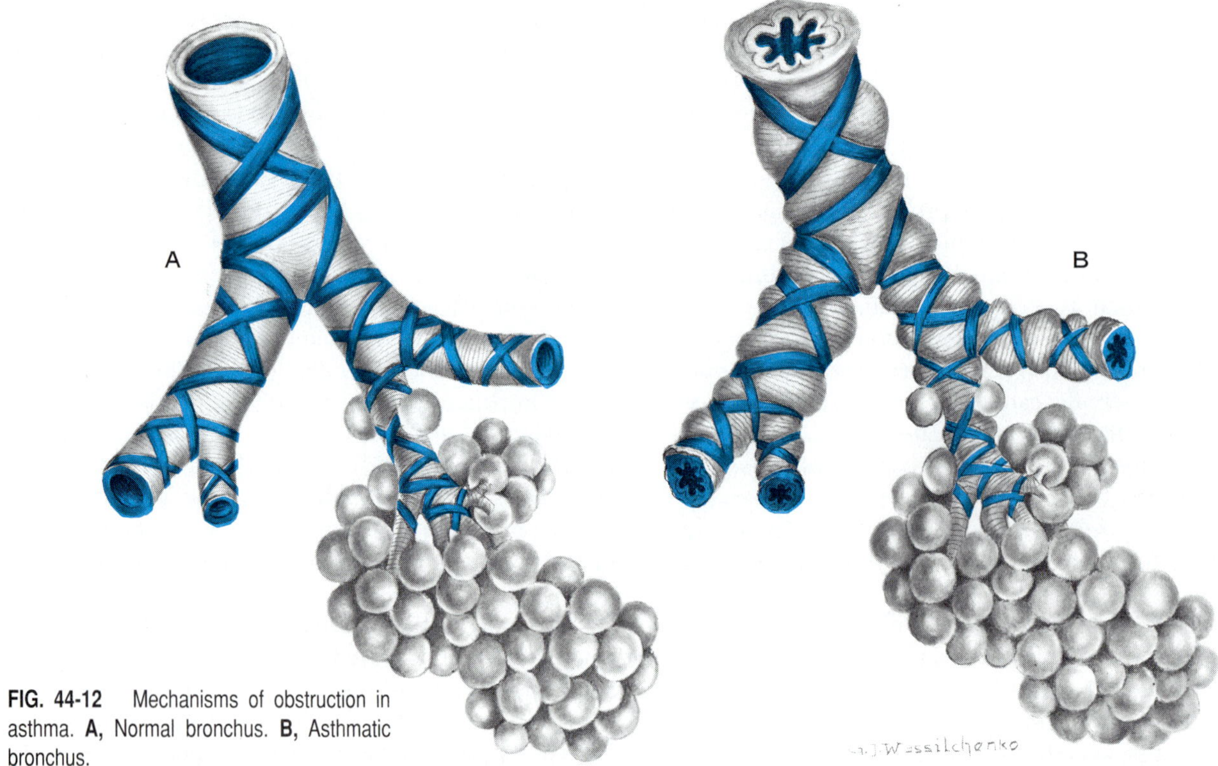

FIG. 44-12 Mechanisms of obstruction in asthma. **A,** Normal bronchus. **B,** Asthmatic bronchus.

and/or managing respiratory infections, promoting normal growth and development, optimizing nutritional status, educating about the illness and its management, planning for home care and community support, referring for counseling when needed, providing long-term support and follow-up, and encouraging medication compliance. Improving pulmonary function involves CPT, breathing exercises, and inhalation treatment. CPT is performed several times daily to loosen secretions in the lung, and postural drainage is done to facilitate the removal of these thick secretions. To encourage breathing exercises, the nurse can suggest blowing bubbles or pinwheels to help prevent tracheobronchial obstruction. Nebulizer treatments may be carried out by the respiratory therapist or the nurse. The nurse assesses the child's tolerance to therapy and monitors its effectiveness. Infection control measures are instituted to prevent cross-contamination, and the family is taught to protect the child from exposure to persons with respiratory infections. Yearly influenza immunizations are strongly recommended. Early in the course of the illness, the child may exhibit excessive appetite; as the disease progresses, the appetite decreases and the child will usually experience anorexia. Pancreatic enzymes, needed to digest proteins, fats, and carbohydrates, are mixed with a carbohydrate and administered before meals and snacks. Children with CF will have frequent hospitalizations, which can interfere with normal development and impair socialization; the nurse addresses these issues with psychological support and appropriate activities. One of the most critical aspects in providing care to the CF child and family is assisting them with positive coping strategies and providing emotional support. Support groups can be a source of great comfort and assistance to newly diagnosed children and their families. The Cystic Fibrosis Foundation* provides education and services to families and professionals.

Patient/family teaching. The nurse instructs the family in improving the nutritional status of their child to ensure adequate growth and development. Nurses are responsible for coordinating counseling, referrals to community support, and home care services, as well as for educating the child and the family in the disease process and its management.

Prognosis. No exact figures are available regarding the life expectancy of a child with CF. Many still die in infancy and early childhood, but increasing numbers are living into their third and fourth decades and even beyond. More than 50% of patients now live into adulthood.

Bronchial Asthma.

Etiology/pathophysiology. Bronchial asthma is a reversible obstructive respiratory disorder. It is a common chronic illness in children of all ages and accounts

*6931 Arlington Road, Bethesda, MD 20814-3205; (800) FIGHTCF or (301) 951-4422.

for the majority of school absences, pediatric visits to the emergency room, and admissions to the hospital. Bronchial asthma has a familial tendency and is frequently associated with allergic rhinitis and atopic dermatitis. The frequent cause of bronchial asthma is an allergic hypersensitivity to environmental factors. The common factors associated with bronchial asthma include bronchospasm, mucosal edema, and increased mucosal secretions (Fig. 44-12). Bronchospasm of the bronchial smooth muscle causes bronchial edema with a decrease in the diameter of the bronchi and bronchioles; edematous mucous membranes produce thick, tenacious secretions, which causes a further narrowing of the air passages. Mucous plugs that occlude the smaller air passages cause obstruction and air trapping distal to the obstruction, resulting in hypoxemia and increased respiratory effort.

Clinical manifestations. Initially, the child may complain of a tightness in the chest, and an audible expiratory wheeze may be heard. As the attack progresses, these signs and symptoms may be accompanied by shortness of breath, inspiratory and expiratory wheezing, tachypnea, dyspnea, coarse breath sounds, prolonged expiration, restlessness, anxiety, deep dark-red color to lips, cyanosis, paroxysmal cough progressing from dry and hacking to productive, fatigue, and diaphoresis.

Diagnostic tests. The diagnosis is determined by clinical signs and symptoms, history, physical examination, pulmonary function tests, and serum laboratory tests such as blood gases, and CBC. Radiographic examination of the chest is usually performed to rule out other pathology.

Medical management. The child is placed on oxygen therapy and subcutaneous injections of epinephrine or nebulizer treatments with Isuprel (isoproterenol), Bronkosol (isoetharine), or Nalcrom (cromolyn) are followed with CPT. An IV infusion is maintained to promote hydration and infuse medications. In severe attacks, IV aminophylline is administered to control bronchospasm. Theophylline blood levels are obtained frequently to ensure that therapeutic levels are being maintained. IV corticosteroid therapy may also be initiated to decrease inflammation.

Nursing interventions. Nursing interventions include frequent monitoring of vital signs because aminophylline infusion can induce tachycardia and dysrhythmias. Adequate hydration is maintained to replace insensible loss through diaphoresis and hyperventilation. To facilitate optimal ventilation, the nurse maintains the child in high Fowler's position, provides for rest periods, and teaches breathing exercises. It is extremely important that nurses provide a calm atmosphere and reassurance for the anxious child and family. Parents and children need to understand the illness and how to avert or prevent attacks at home. Allergens can be identified by skin testing, and measures to eliminate or avoid them can then be instituted.

Nursing diagnoses and interventions for the child with brochial asthma include but are not limited to the following:

NURSING DIAGNOSES	NURSING INTERVENTIONS
Suffocation, high risk for, related to interaction between individual and allergen(s)	Teach patient/family correct use of bronchodilators, corticosteroids. Teach patient/family how to avoid conditions or circumstances that precipitate asthmatic attack. Teach family meal planning to eliminate allergenic foods. Encourage removal of furry pets. Instruct family in modification of environment; "allergy proofing" home, especially no smoking in home. Teach patient/family to avoid extremes of environmental temperature. Encourage avoidance of undue excitement and/or physical exertion. Assist parents in obtaining assistance in installing device to control environment (humidifier, air conditioner, electronic air filter).
Breathing patterns, ineffective, related to allergenic response in bronchial tree	Teach and/or supervise breathing exercises and controlled breathing. Teach correct use of prescribed medications. Assist patient/family in selecting activities appropriate to child's capabilities and preferences. Encourage regular exercise. Encourage good posture. Encourage physical exercise involving stop-and-start activity that does not overtax the respiratory mechanism. Discourage physical inactivity.

Patient/family teaching. Parents need to know the nature of the disease and, when the allergens are determined, how they can avoid and/or relieve asthmatic attacks. Teach parents and the older child how to use the medications prescribed to relieve bronchospasms (Fig. 44-13 on p. 1396). Teach early signs and symptoms of an impending attack so it can be controlled before symptoms become distressful. Older children who use a nebulizer or aerosol device to deliver adrenergic drugs need to be taught how to use a metered-dose inhaler. The parents should be taught to avoid exposing the child to excessive cold, wind, or other extremes of weather and to smoke, sprays, or other irritants. Self-care is a hallmark of effective asthma management, and self-management programs are important in helping the child and family cope with the disease.

Prognosis. The outlook for children with asthma varies widely. Many children lose their signs and symptoms at puberty, but there is no factor that can predict which children will "outgrow" their asthma. Some develop other forms of allergy in adulthood, most fre-

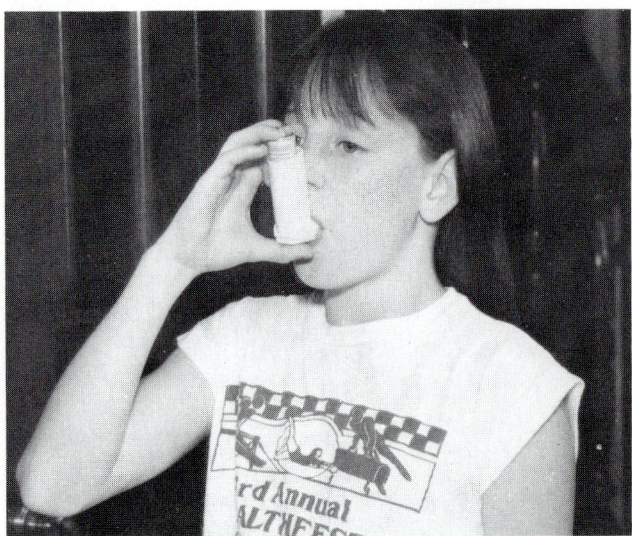

FIG. 44-13 Child using metered-dose inhaler.

quently involving the nose. Although death from asthma is rare, the death rate has been rising steadily during the last decade despite improvements in treatment.

DISORDERS OF GASTROINTESTINAL FUNCTION

The primary function of the gastrointestinal (GI) tract is the absorption and metabolism of nutrients necessary to support and promote optimal growth and development. Because the GI tract is responsible for processing nutrients for all parts of the body, an alteration in GI function can affect other body systems. If a GI problem is undiagnosed and/or untreated, the overall health of the child may be affected. However, any disease process, although it may not directly affect the GI tract, may result in manifestations of GI disturbance.

Cleft Lip and/or Cleft Palate

Clefts of the lip and palate are facial malformations that occur during embryological development. A combination of cleft lip and palate is more commonly seen than is an isolated occurrence of either.

Etiology/Pathophysiology. Cleft of the lip is due to a failure of the medial nasal and maxillary processes to join. The cleft may be unilateral or bilateral and is often associated with abnormal development of the external nose, nasal cartilages, and nasal septum (Fig. 44-14). Cleft of the palate is due to a failure of the palatal shelves to fuse. Cleft palates may involve only the soft palate or may extend into the hard palate.

Clinical Manifestations. Feeding from the breast or bottle may not be difficult in infants with less severe cleft lip and intact palate. More extensive cleft lips and clefts of the palate are associated with feeding difficulties; infants may have an ineffective suck, and saliva and feedings may leak into the nasal cavity, causing gagging and choking as the infant breathes.

Speech may also be delayed and, after development, may be hypernasal with poor articulation. Children with cleft palate may also be predisposed to recurrent otitis media or persistent otitis media with effusion due to eustachian tube dysfunction. The older child with cleft lip and palate may experience psychological difficulties because of the cosmetic appearance of the defect and problems with impaired speech.

Diagnostic Tests. Cleft lip and most cases of cleft palate are apparent at birth, and the facial appearance of the infant is of immediate concern to the parents.

Medical Management. Surgical closure of the cleft lip, whether isolated or associated with cleft palate, is usually performed at 1 to 2 months of age, when the infant has shown satisfactory weight gain and is free of any oral, respiratory, or systemic infections. The surgical technique used is Z-plasty. This method involves the use of a staggered suture line to minimize notching of the lip from retracted scar tissue. A Logan bow (a thin, arched metal bar that is taped to the cheeks) is applied immediately after the surgery to prevent tension on the suture line from crying, and the arms are restrained to prevent the infant from rubbing the incision.

Clefts of the palate are usually repaired when the child is 12 to 18 months of age. Surgical repair during this period allows for palatal changes associated with normal growth to occur without the development of faulty speech patterns.

Nursing Interventions. Nursing interventions for the child with cleft lip and palate are initially related to ensuring adequate nutritional support for the infant and assisting the parents in dealing with the diagnosis. Before surgical correction of cleft lip and palate, feeding may be a considerable problem. The primary goals for nursing are to ensure an adequate intake of food and to prevent aspiration. The best method for feeding is to support the infant's head in an upright position and to use care and patience during each feeding. Because infants with cleft lip and palate cannot generate the suction required to feed through a normal nipple or breast, special feeding devices are used (Fig. 44-15). Breastfeeding may be possible if a breast shield with a special cleft-lip nipple is used. During feedings, these infants require frequent burping because they tend to swallow large amounts of air. Another important goal is to assist the parents in dealing with the diagnosis of cleft lip and palate and to promote bonding between the parents and the infant. To accomplish this goal the nurse may emphasize positive aspects of the infant's appearance and

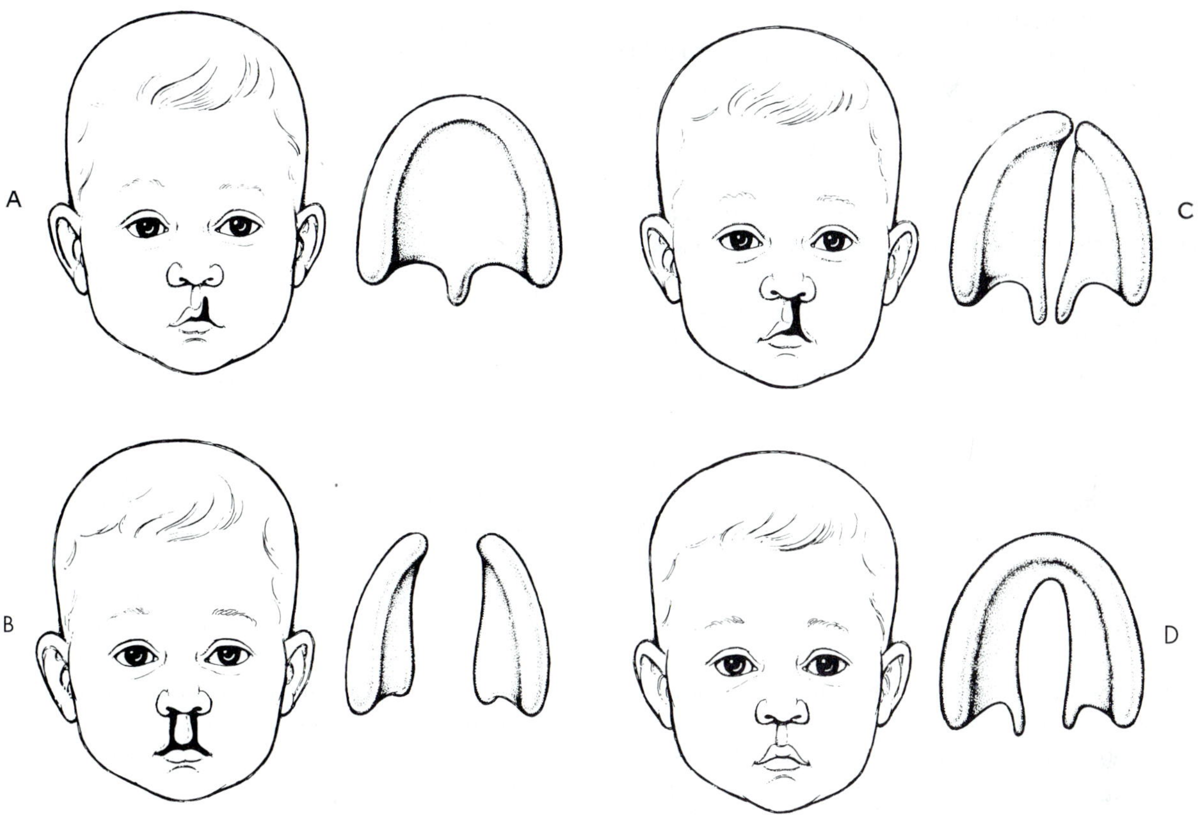

FIG. 44-14 Variations in clefts of lip and palate at birth. **A,** Notch in vermilion border. **B,** Unilateral cleft lip and palate. **C,** Bilateral cleft lip and cleft palate. **D,** Cleft palate.

behavior. The nurse may also show the parents photographs of children whose cleft lip and palate have been repaired to illustrate the positive results of surgical intervention.

Postoperative nursing interventions include protecting the integrity of the suture line, promoting optimal nutrition, and continuing support of the child and parents. Infants should be positioned only on their sides or back; positioning on the abdomen allows them to rub the face on the sheets. Safety reminder devices are placed on the child's elbows to prevent touching or rubbing of the suture line. These safety devices are removed periodically to enable movement of the arms and to provide an opportunity to observe the skin under the safety reminder device for signs of impairment or pressure.

Immediately following surgery, the infant with cleft lip may be kept NPO until the effects of the anesthesia have disappeared. Then, the infant is gradually introduced to liquids, beginning with clear liquids (water and dextrose water) and gradually progressing to formula. The use of the Breck feeder is generally preferred. The rubber tip of the feeder is slipped into the side of the infant's mouth carefully, avoiding contact with the suture line. Breastfeeding is usually contraindicated. The mother may be encouraged to pump her breasts to promote the continued production of milk until the infant

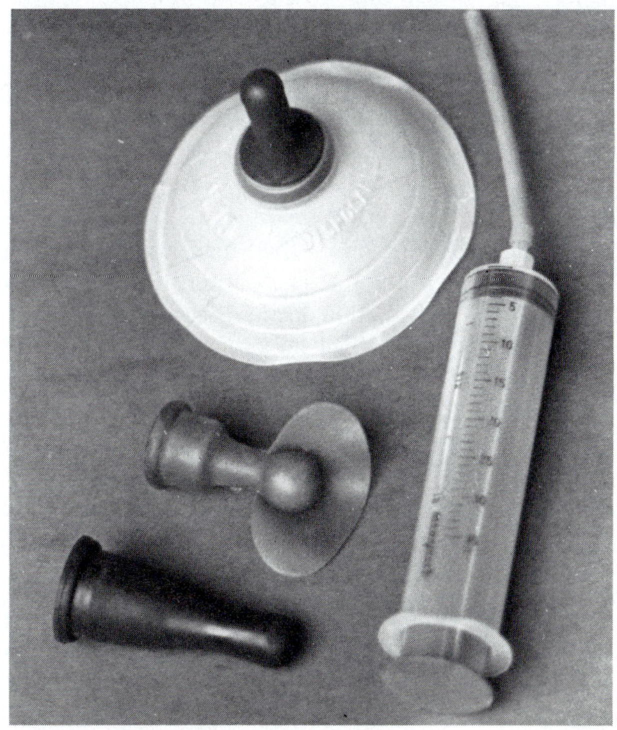

FIG. 44-15 Some devices used to feed an infant with a cleft lip and palate. *Clockwise:* Lamb's nipple, flange nipple, special nurser, and syringe with rubber tubing (Breck feeder).

is able to feed directly from the breast. After feedings, the suture line is gently cleansed with a saline-soaked cotton-tipped swab. The infant is then placed in an infant chair or on the right side to promote digestion and prevent aspiration of regurgitated formula. In addition, careful aspiration of the oral and nasopharyngeal cavities may be necessary to remove collections of mucus, blood, and saliva and to prevent aspiration. Analgesics are administered as ordered.

Postoperative care after surgical repair of cleft palate is similar to that of cleft lip repair. The child with cleft palate repair is allowed to lie on the abdomen as this will facilitate drainage of mucus and serosanguinous exudate from the oral cavity. Analgesics are administered as ordered. Liquid nourishments are usually provided by cups. Straws, pacifiers, and eating utensils are avoided as they may injure the suture line. The child is gradually advanced from a liquid diet to a blenderized diet, and parents are instructed to continue this diet after discharge until they are otherwise instructed by the surgeon.

Patient/family teaching. The nurse may assist the family by providing them with information on agencies that provide services, information, and support to families with a child who has cleft lip and palate. These agencies include the Cleft Palate Foundation and the March of Dimes–Birth Defects Foundation.

Prognosis. Even with good anatomical closure, the majority of children with cleft lip–cleft palate have some degree of speech impairment that requires speech therapy. Improper drainage of the middle ear contributes to recurrent otitis media with scarring of the tympanic membrane, which leads to hearing impairment in a large number of children with cleft palate.

Dehydration

When the body loses more fluid than it absorbs, as in diarrhea, or when it absorbs less water than it excretes, as in vomiting, dehydration occurs. Basically, dehydration occurs whenever the total fluid intake is less than the total fluid output.

Etiology/Pathophysiology. Dehydration may be the result of a number of disease processes that cause abnormal losses through the skin, respiratory, renal, and most commonly, the GI systems.

Clinical Manifestations. The physical signs of dehydration are primarily the result of a deficit in fluid volume. Table 44-1 summarizes the clinical manifestations of dehydration.

Diagnostic Tests. Diagnosis of dehydration is made on the basis of observed clinical manifestations (Table 44-1).

TABLE 44-1 Clinical Manifestations of Dehydration

Assessment	Signs and Symptoms
Skin	Cold, dry, gray
Mucous membranes	Dry
Eyes	Sunken
Fontanelle	Sunken
Behavior	Lethargic
Pulse	Rapid
Blood pressure	Low
Respirations	Rapid

Medical Management. Refer to the discussion on medical management of diarrhea, p. 1399.

Nursing Interventions. Careful nursing assessment and intervention are important in the clinical detection and management of dehydration. It is an essential nursing function to assess for any clinical manifestations of dehydration. This assessment should begin with a general survey of the child and continue with specific observations.

Observations should include the measurement of intake and output (I&O). This measurement includes oral and parenteral intake and losses from sweat, wound drainage, urine, stools, vomiting, nasogastric (NG) drainage, and fistulas. For children who are not toilet trained, wet diapers can be weighed to assess the amount of output. By subtracting the weight of a dry diaper in grams from the weight of the wet diaper, the actual fluid content of the diaper can be calculated The volume of fluid in milliliters is equal to the weight of the fluid measured in grams. Other observations that assist in the assessment of dehydration include vital signs, body weight, skin color, temperature and turgor, capillary refill, presence or absence of edema, moisture and color of mucous membranes, sensation of thirst, and, in infants, assessment of the fontanelles.

Family teaching. The parents should be taught that infants and young children have a greater need for water than adults and are more vulnerable to alterations in fluid and electrolyte balance.

Prognosis. Shock is common in severe depletion of extracellular fluid. With effective medical management and nursing interventions, the prognosis is favorable.

Diarrhea and Gastroenteritis

Diarrhea is one of the most common disorders affecting children; it can quickly render the child vulnerable to fluid deficits and electrolyte imbalances. Diarrhea is a disturbance in intestinal motility, characterized by an increase in frequency, fluid content, and volume of stools.

Box 44-3 CLINICAL MANIFESTATIONS OF DIARRHEA

- Cool, pale skin
- Lethargy
- Sunken eyes
- Sunken fontanelles
- Poor skin turgor
- Rapid pulse and respirations
- Low blood pressure
- Normal or elevated temperature
- Irritability progressing to lethargy
- Weight loss
- Vomiting

The diarrhea may be acute or chronic and infectious or noninfectious. Diarrhea caused by an inflammatory process, such as infection, is called *gastroenteritis.*

Etiology/Pathophysiology. Although diarrhea may result from a variety of causes, the most common is bacterial or viral invasion of the intestinal mucosa. The most prevalent bacterial pathogens are *Salmonella, Shigella, Campylobacter jejuni,* and *Giardia lamblia.* Infections caused by *Salmonella* or *Shigella* must be reported to the state health department. Many factors can predispose a child to diarrhea. Infants have a greater susceptibility to diarrhea, and the results are more serious because infants have a small extracellular fluid reserve. When this reserve is suddenly and quickly depleted, dehydration rapidly ensues. Children who are malnourished, debilitated, or immunocompromised are more prone to diarrhea. Poor hygiene, contaminated food and/or water, warm weather, and crowded and substandard living conditions can also predispose children to diarrhea. Other common causes of diarrhea are the ingestion of large quantities of fruit juice, such as apple juice, food sensitivities, antibiotics, and formula intolerance.

When a pathogen invades the intestinal mucosa, the resulting enterotoxins stimulate an inflammatory reaction. As a result, water and electrolytes are secreted and there is invasion and destruction of the epithelial cells of the GI mucosa. Serious disturbances, such as renal failure, dehydration, acid-base imbalances, shock, and circulatory collapse, may follow.

Clinical Manifestations. In addition to the increased number of stools and the increased fluid content of stools, other clinical manifestations of diarrhea are summarized in Box 44-3. In addition to these manifestations, the nurse should also assess the child for any signs of dehydration, which is a common complication of diarrhea (see Table 44-1).

Diagnostic Tests. A carefully obtained history should include information regarding recent travel, exposure to infected agents, personal contact, allergies, food or formula sensitivities, living conditions, and contact with contaminated water and/or food. Laboratory evaluation may include a stool culture and examination of the stool for ova and parasites, WBC, and *Clostridium difficile* toxin.

Medical Management. The goals of management are to restore fluid and electrolyte imbalances and to treat the underlying cause. Management in cases of mild to moderate diarrhea may involve resting the bowel for a short time by maintaining NPO status. After approximately 1 hour, an oral rehydration solution (ORS), such as Pedialyte or Ricelyte, may be offered in small amounts. If the infant is breastfeeding, this should continue as a supplement to the ORS. When the number and fluid content of stools have decreased, the infant can gradually be advanced to full-strength formula. In older children, solid foods can be offered when rehydration is complete. Initially, foods that are nonirritating to the bowel should be offered. These may include bananas, rice, applesauce, and toast (BRAT diet). Gradually, a regular diet may be resumed.

In cases of severe diarrhea, hospitalization and IV therapy are required. Rehydration is accomplished through IV administration of a saline solution containing 5% dextrose. This solution provides the child with fluid, sodium, and calories. Once kidney function has been verified, potassium may be added to the IV solution to correct any potassium depletion. IV rehydration should continue until the diarrhea improves. Once rehydration has begun and the severe effects of the diarrhea and dehydration have improved, measures to detect and treat the underlying cause are employed. This includes antimicrobial therapy where indicated.

Nursing Interventions. Nursing interventions for the infant or child with diarrhea are focused on assessment, including the careful recording of I&O; promotion of rehydration; correction of electrolyte imbalances; provision of age-appropriate nutrition; prevention of the spread of the diarrhea; prevention of complications; and support of the child and family.

Nursing diagnoses and interventions for the child with diarrhea and gastroenteritis include but are not limited to the following:

NURSING DIAGNOSES	NURSING INTERVENTIONS
Fluid volume deficit, related to excessive GI losses in stool	Offer oral fluids as indicated and as tolerated. Monitor IV fluids as prescribed. Maintain strict record of I&O (urine and stool); monitor urine specific gravity. Weigh child daily.

NURSING DIAGNOSES	NURSING INTERVENTIONS
Fluid volume deficit, related to excessive GI losses in stool—cont'd	Assess vital signs, skin turgor, mucous membranes, and mental status q 4 hr or as indicated.
Skin integrity, impaired, related to irritation caused by frequent, loose stools	Change diaper frequently. Cleanse buttocks gently with bland, nonalkaline soap and water or immerse child in a bath for gentle cleansing. Apply protective ointment (type of ointment may vary for each child and may require a trial period). Expose slightly erythematous intact skin to air whenever possible; apply protective ointment to very irritated or excoriated skin. Observe buttocks and perineum for infection, such as *Candida.*
Anxiety/fear, related to separation from parents, unfamiliar environment, distressing procedures	Provide mouth care and pacifier for infants who are NPO. Encourage family visitation and appropriate participation in care. Touch, hold, and talk to child as much as possible. Provide sensory stimulation and diversion appropriate for child's developmental level.

Patient/family teaching. Parents should be instructed to avoid the use of antidiarrheals such as diphenoxylate (Lomotil) or kaolin and pectin (Kaopectate). They should also be cautioned to wash their hands thoroughly after changing diapers to prevent the spread of infection. Soiled diapers, bed linens, and clothes should be properly disposed of or thoroughly cleaned.

Prognosis. Mild or moderate diarrhea is managed at home by simple methods. Severe diarrhea requires hospitalization with fluid therapy per IV route. With treatment, prognosis is usually excellent.

Constipation

Constipation is best defined as the passage of hardened stools, and may be associated with failure of complete evacuation of the colon with defecation. Constipation may present as a primary disorder or may occur in association with a wide variety of GI tract or systemic disorders.

Etiology/Pathophysiology. Constipation may occur in children of any age. In the newborn period, the infant normally passes a first meconium stool within 24 to 36 hours. Failure to do this may indicate intestinal atresia (congenital closure of any part of the intestine) or stenosis (constriction or narrowing of a passage or orifice), Hirschsprung's disease (see p. 1403), meconium ileus (ileus of the newborn due to obstruction of the bowel with meconium), or a meconium plug. In formula-fed infants, constipation may result from a high fat or protein content or inadequate fluid in the formula. In children, constipation may be associated with environmental factors such as medications (i.e., iron supplements, anticonvulsant therapy, low-fiber diet, or antacids) or may result from a learned repression of the urge to defecate. In children who have constipation, passage of hardened stools is painful. As a result, the child may repress the urge to defecate. Continuous repression results in dilation of the rectum, reduced sensation of the need to defecate, and decreased muscle tone in the lower rectum. This cycle results in chronic, incomplete evacuation of the colon, and the child becomes severely constipated. Episodes of diarrhea or encopresis (leakage around the firm stool in the rectum) may lead to "accidents" or soiling.

Clinical Manifestations. In infancy, constipation may be associated with hard stools or evidence of fresh blood in the stools. Children with "functional" constipation may experience cramping abdominal pain, anal fissures, pain on defecation, loss of appetite, and irritability.

Diagnostic Tests. Diagnosis of constipation is dependent on a careful history. Parents should be asked to describe the infant's or child's bowel patterns. Physical examination of the anus and rectum should be performed by the physician.

Medical Management. In the newborn, simple measures may effectively alleviate the problem. Modifying the formula with addition of more fluid or carbohydrates may correct the situation. For older infants, beyond 5 to 6 months, adding foods with bulk (fruits and vegetables) and increasing fluid intake may correct the problem. If the constipation is due to a tightened anal sphincter, parents may be instructed to manually dilate the sphincter two or three times daily until sufficient dilation is attained. The management of simple constipation in children is focused on emptying the rectum completely of stool with the use of mild laxatives and/or enemas and instituting dietary modifications, such as increased fluid intake and addition of high-fiber foods, to prevent further constipation. The treatment of chronic constipation in children is aimed at complete evacuation of the rectum and toileting retraining therapy. Complete evacuation of the rectum is usually achieved by using enemas and stool softeners. After complete evacuation is attained, bowel retraining therapy to sustain evacuation is instituted. This generally consists of behavioral modification, using positive reinforcement for toilet sitting and defecation, and emotional support.

Nursing Interventions. Nursing interventions begin with a careful history of bowel patterns, including stool characteristics (color, consistency, frequency, and associated pain), diet, and concomitant medications. If dietary modifications are to be instituted, the nurse will need to educate the parents regarding these and ensure their understanding. Parents may also need to be instructed about normal stool patterns and what constitutes constipation. It may be important to discuss with parents their expectations and attitudes regarding toileting, and emotional reassurance of the parents and child may be needed.

Patient/family teaching. Parents should be instructed to avoid the use of honey and corn syrup (Karo syrup) as a home remedy for constipation in young infants. Use of these products may be associated with the development of infant botulism.

Prognosis. Simple measures ordinarily correct constipation, but successful resolution depends upon the age of the child and the underlying cause. In the more complex situations, counseling and bowel retraining may be necessary.

Gastroesophageal Reflux (GER)

GER can best be defined as the regurgitation of the gastric contents into the esophagus. GER usually begins within 1 week of birth, and regurgitation occurs immediately after a feeding or when the infant is laid down after a feeding.

Etiology/Pathophysiology. GER is primarily due to an incompetent lower esophageal (or cardiac) sphincter. As a result, gastric contents are allowed to regurgitate into the esophagus.

Clinical Manifestations. Vomiting or spitting up is the primary manifestation in the first week of life. Aspiration of the gastric contents may lead to respiratory signs such as apnea, choking or gagging after feedings, and aspiration pneumonia. In young children a chronic cough, wheezing, and recurrent pneumonia are common. Growth and weight gain are a problem with a majority of children. Continuous irritation of the esophageal lining with gastric acid may lead to esophageal ulceration and bleeding. This may manifest as anemia, hematemesis, or blood in the stools.

Diagnostic Tests. A carefully obtained history may be sufficient for diagnosis in mild cases. In more severe or complex cases, diagnosis can be made by observation of reflux during barium esophagography, monitoring esophageal pH with an esophageal probe, upper endoscopy, or esophageal scintigraphy (detects radioactive substances in the esophagus after a feeding of the compound and assesses gastric emptying).

Medical Management. Treatment of GER in infants usually involves feeding them a formula that has been thickened with infant cereal. If the infant is breastfeeding, milk should be manually expressed and mixed with cereal for feedings.

Several studies have examined the effectiveness of positioning therapy for infants with GER. These studies have yielded different results. Traditionally, the upright position in an infant seat was recommended for infants with GER. Later, a head-elevated prone position maintained by use of an upper-body harness was found to be superior. A recent study found no significant difference between the flat prone and head-elevated prone positions and concluded that the head-elevated prone position is probably not worth the extra effort required to maintain this position.[20] At this time, the available information suggests that either position following feeding and at night is a reasonable measure for treating infants with GER.

Pharmacological intervention involves the administration of antacids qid to reduce the irritating effects of the gastric acid. Metoclopramide (Reglan) may also be given before meals and at bedtime to accelerate gastric emptying. Surgical management of GER may be indicated in severe cases. A **Nissen fundoplication,** which involves wrapping the fundus of the stomach around the distal esophagus to prevent reflux of the stomach contents into the esophagus, is the most commonly performed surgical procedure (see Chapter 27).

Nursing Interventions/Family Teaching. The goals of nursing include assisting in the recognition of infants with signs that may indicate GER; providing care for the child undergoing a surgical procedure, if applicable; and providing emotional reassurance that GER is a disorder and not the result of faulty feeding practices.

Patient teaching. An important aspect of teaching is educating parents about formula or breast milk thickening and proper positioning after feedings.

Prognosis. The majority of infants affected have mild GER and achieve normal function by 6 to 7 weeks of age. Generally 90% improve by about 1 year of age; they require only medical therapy. If GER is severe and remains unsuccessfully treated, multiple complications such as esophageal strictures and recurrent respiratory distress with aspiration pneumonia can occur.

Hypertrophic Pyloric Stenosis (HPS)

HPS is an obstructive disorder in which the gastric outlet is mechanically obstructed by a congenitally hypertrophied pyloric muscle. It is also the most common reason for an abdominal operation during the first 6 months of life. HPS is present in approximately 1 in 250 live births. Males are three to four times more likely to be affected than females.

Etiology/Pathophysiology. The cause of HPS is not known. There is an increased incidence in siblings and offspring of affected persons. The circular muscle that surrounds the valve between the stomach and the duodenum becomes diffusely enlarged as the result of hypertrophy and hyperplasia (Fig 44-16). As a result, it is difficult for the stomach to empty. At approximately 4 to 6 weeks of age, infants with HPS begin to vomit almost immediately after feedings. As the condition progresses, the vomiting grows more forceful and becomes projectile, the hallmark sign of HPS.

Clinical Manifestations. Initially, the signs begin as regurgitation that progresses to projectile vomiting. Lethargy, weight loss, poor skin turgor, sunken fontanelles, and loss of subcutaneous tissue may become apparent as dehydration ensues (Box 44-4).

Diagnostic Tests. Examination of the abdomen may assist in the diagnosis and reveal key signs of HPS. Visible peristaltic waves that move from left to right across the epigastric region may be evident, and palpation may reveal an olive-shaped mass in this area to the right of the midline. If the diagnosis cannot be established after history and physical examination, upper GI radiographic studies or an ultrasonic examination may be indicated.

Medical Management. Surgical relief of the pyloric obstruction as soon as the diagnosis is established is the standard treatment for HPS. The surgical correction of HPS is accomplished by performing a *Fredet-Ramstedt procedure.* This operation (a pyloromyotomy) involves surgically splitting the pylorus muscle down to the submucosa, allowing for a larger lumen.

Nursing Interventions. Nursing interventions of the infant with HPS primarily involve assisting with the establishment of a diagnosis, providing adequate nutrition, managing preoperative and postoperative care, and supporting the family. A carefully obtained history with assessment for signs and symptoms of HPS is essential for the prompt diagnosis. Correction of any metabolic disturbances and dehydration prior to surgery is essential. These are generally corrected by IV administration of fluid and electrolytes. The infant is NPO to eliminate vomiting. Careful assessment of I&O is necessary to monitor fluid replacement and rehydration. Postoperative nursing interventions are focused on preventing complications by monitoring I&O, observation of physical signs, and instituting oral feedings. Feedings of glucose water are begun 6 hours postoperatively, and if feedings are retained for 24 hours, full feedings are then started. Parents should be encouraged to express their concerns and visit their infant frequently, participating in the care when appropriate. Barring complications, infants are usually discharged within 1 to 2 days after surgery.

Patient/family teaching. Most parents need support and reassurance that the condition is caused by a structural problem and is in no way a reflection of their parenting skills and capacities.

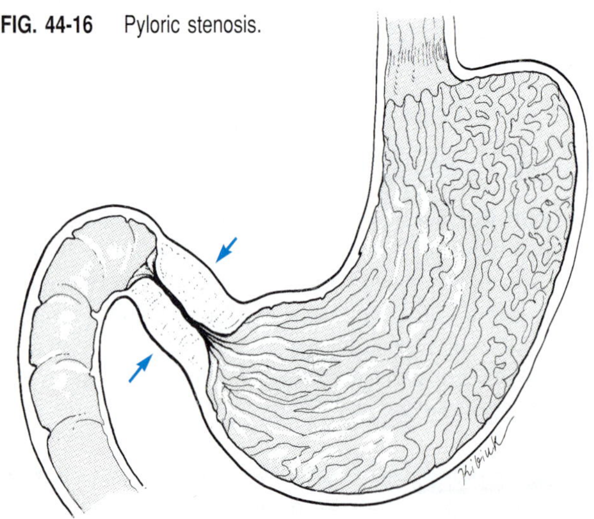

FIG. 44-16 Pyloric stenosis.

Prognosis. Most infants recover completely and rapidly following pyloromyotomy. Postoperative complications include persistent pyloric obstruction and wound dehiscence. Approximately 15% of infants with HPS also have gastroesophageal reflux.

Intussusception

Intussusception is the most common cause of intestinal obstruction in children between 3 months and 6 years of age. It is twice as common in male children. Generally, the cause of intussusception is not known.

Box 44-4 CLINICAL MANIFESTATIONS OF HYPERTROPHIC PYLORIC STENOSIS

- Projectile vomiting:
  May be ejected 3 to 4 feet from the child when in a side-lying position, 1 foot or more when in a back-lying position
  Usually occurs shortly after feeding (may not occur for several hours)
  May follow each feeding or appear intermittently
  Nonbilious (no bile) vomitus; may be blood-tinged
- Infant hungry, avid nurser; eagerly accepts a second feeding after vomiting episode
- No evidence of pain or discomfort except that of chronic hunger
- Weight loss
- Signs of dehydration
- Distended upper abdomen
- Readily palpable olive-shaped mass in the epigastrium just to the right of the umbilicus
- Visible gastric peristalsis waves that move from left to right across the epigastrium

Etiology/Pathophysiology. Intussusception is the result of the telescoping of one portion of the intestine into another (Fig. 44-17). The site most commonly affected is the ileocecal valve, at the juncture of the distal ileum and the proximal colon. As the ileum telescopes into the colon, the passage of intestinal contents distal to the defect becomes obstructed. Subsequently, as the mucosa of the intestinal walls rub against each other, blood and mucus from the mucosa leak into the intestinal lumen and form **"currant jelly" stools** (feces that is mixed with blood and mucus from the intestinal mucosa), a hallmark sign of intussusception. Serious complications include peritonitis, intestinal ischemia, and infarction, perforation, and shock. If the condition is untreated, death of the child can occur within 2 to 5 days.

Clinical Manifestations. In most cases there is a sudden onset of severe abdominal pain in a previously well child. Vomiting and lethargy usually occur. Within 12 hours of the onset of abdominal pain, the child usually passes the characteristic "currant jelly" stool.

Diagnostic Tests. The history and physical signs are usually diagnostic. Definitive diagnosis is made by barium enema, which will reveal an obstruction to the flow of barium through the intestine. A digital rectal examination reveals blood and mucus.

Medical Management. Intussusception can often be relieved by hydrostatic reduction using barium at the time of diagnostic evaluation. The force exerted by the flowing barium from the enema may successfully force the telescoped portion of the bowel into its correct position. Surgical treatment of intussusception involves manual reduction of the invagination (the process of becoming enclosed in a sheath) and, if necessary, resection of nonviable bowel with end-to-end anastomosis.

FIG. 44-17 Intussusception.

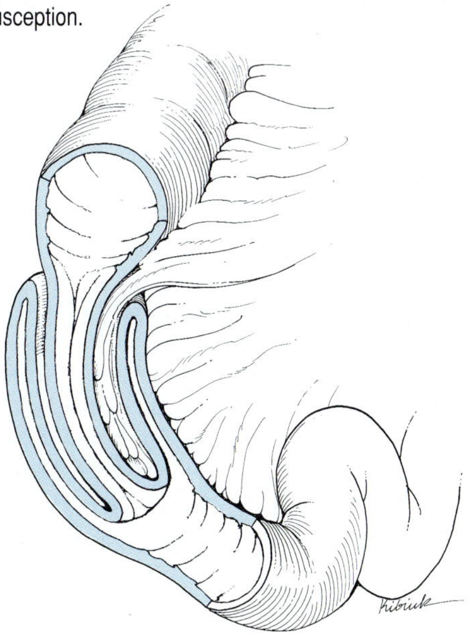

Nursing Interventions. Nursing interventions for the child with intussusception involve obtaining a thorough history from the parents and observing for physical signs that will help establish a prompt and accurate diagnosis. As soon as a diagnosis has been established, the nurse should begin to prepare the parents for the diagnostic barium enema. Parents should be informed that in many cases this procedure may be corrective, but if it is unsuccessful, surgery may be required. After the hydrostatic reduction, the nurse observes for the passage of barium and the return of normal bowel movements. Children are observed for at least 24 hours following the procedure to assess for the possibility of recurrence. If surgery is indicated, the child is kept NPO, and an IV infusion is begun to supply adequate hydration and electrolytes. Postoperative care of the child involves obtaining vital signs, monitoring the operative site, and assessing for the return of bowel sounds. When peristaltic function has returned, oral feedings may be gradually introduced.

Prognosis. Many patients with intussusception can be successfully treated by hydrostatic reduction. Surgery is required for patients in whom the barium enema was unsuccessful. If untreated, 90% of patients will worsen or die of complications such as perforation, peritonitis, and sepsis. With early diagnosis and treatment, serious complications and death are rare.

Hirschsprung's Disease

Hirschsprung's disease, also known as *megacolon,* is a functional intestinal obstruction caused by the absence of parasympathetic ganglion cells in a portion of the colon. The incidence is 1 in 5000 live births, with a predominance in males. It is more common in children with trisomy 21 (a congenital condition characterized by varying degrees of cognitive impairment and multiple defects [Down syndrome]), and a small number of cases follow a familial pattern.

Etiology/Pathophysiology. In Hirschsprung's disease there is an absence of innervation to a segment of the bowel. In most cases, the lower portion of the sigmoid colon just above the anus is affected. As a result, there are no peristaltic waves in the affected portion of the colon to propel the fecal contents, causing an intestinal obstruction and distention of the bowel proximal to the defect (Fig. 44-18 on p. 1404).

Clinical Manifestations. Clinical manifestations can vary according to age. Neonates may be diagnosed early, failuring to pass meconium within 48 hours or 1 week and having signs of partial or complete intestinal ob-

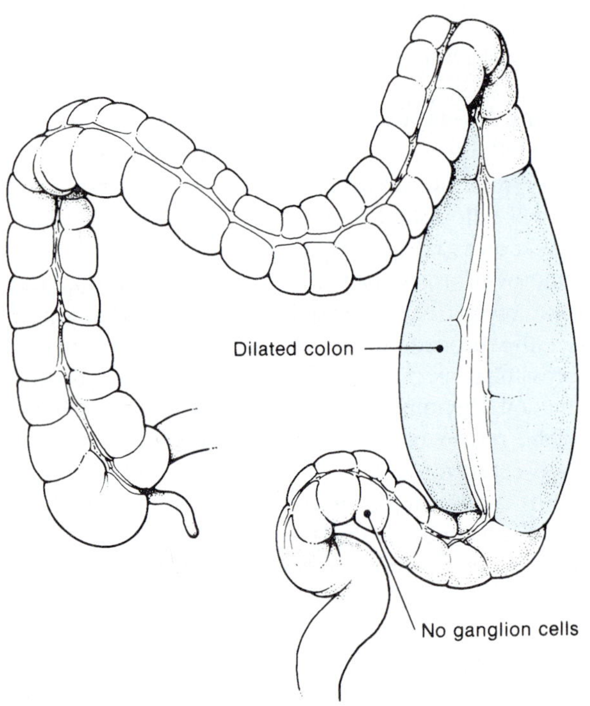

FIG. 44-18 The affected bowel in Hirschsprung's disease.

struction, such as abdominal distention, vomiting, poor feeding, and failure to pass stools. Infants may have a history of constipation or intermittent constipation and diarrhea. Dehydration, failure to thrive, abdominal distention, and fever may also be manifested. Hirschsprung's disease in the older child is associated with chronic constipation; abdominal distention; ribbonlike, foul-smelling stools; poor weight gain; malnourishment; anemia; palpable fecal mass; and visible peristalsis.

Diagnostic Tests. A carefully obtained history, associated clinical manifestations, and a barium enema assist in making a diagnosis of Hirschsprung's disease.

Medical Management. Immediate treatment involves surgical removal of the affected portion of the bowel. The surgery is performed in two stages. The first stage involves placement of a temporary colostomy in the portion of normal, innervated colon just proximal to the defect. This will allow for a period of rest during which the normal bowel will regain its tone. The second stage involves excising the affected segment and pulling the normal, innervated segment down through the anus, anastomosing it to the anal canal. This procedure, known as the *Soave endorectal pull-through,* is usually performed when the child reaches a weight of 20 pounds.

Nursing Interventions. Nursing interventions for the infant or child with Hirschsprung's disease is focused on assisting the parents with adjusting to the diagnosis, promoting parent-infant bonding, preparing the parents for surgery, and educating them regarding colostomy care. Preoperative nursing interventions are directed toward restoring the child's nutritional status by providing a low-fiber, high-protein, high-calorie diet or, in severe cases, TPN. The bowel may need to be evacuated with daily enemas and stool softeners. Oral antibiotics may be prescribed to decrease intestinal flora. Abdominal girths are measured daily. It is important to prepare the parents and child, when developmentally appropriate, for the colostomy. It should be stressed that this is a temporary procedure unless a large portion of the bowel is involved, necessitating a permanent ileostomy. Postoperative care includes assessing vital signs and bowel sounds, observing for the passage of flatus and stools, and monitoring the operative site. An NG tube is generally placed during the surgery and is removed as soon as peristalsis has returned, usually within 24 hours, and a regular diet for age in introduced.

Patient/family teaching. Before discharge parents need instruction regarding colostomy care and may be referred to a visiting nurse for assistance in caring for the colostomy.

Prognosis. Most children with Hirschsprung's disease require surgery rather than medical therapy. Once the patient is stabilized with fluid and electrolyte replacement, if needed, the temporary colostomy is performed with a high rate of success. After closure of the colostomy, most children are able to attain satisfactory defecatory function.

Hernias

A hernia is defined as the protrusion of organs or portions of an organ through a structural defect or weakened muscle wall. A complication of herniation arises when the circulation to the protruding organ is impaired (known as a strangulated hernia) or when the pressure of protruding organs impairs the function of other organs. Incarceration of a hernia occurs when the hernia cannot be manually reduced. Hernias affecting the diaphragm and the abdominal wall are outlined in Table 44-2.

DISORDERS OF GENITOURINARY FUNCTION

Disorders of the genitourinary (GU) tract are very common in children and may be caused by a variety of etiological factors. The GU system is responsible for maintaining fluid and electrolyte balance within the body. Disorders of the GU system alter the delicate balance of fluid and electrolytes within the body and may be potentially life threatening.

TABLE 44-2 Hernias

Type	Clinical Manifestations/Diagnostic Tests	Interventions
Diaphragmatic		
Protrusion of a portion of the abdominal organs through the foramen of Bochdalek (an opening in the diaphragm)	Respiratory distress within hours of delivery; cyanosis, tachypnea, retractions, dyspnea, respiratory acidosis, and absent breath sounds on the affected side (bowel sounds may be present) Abdominal pain, vomiting Diagnosis made by radiography	*Medical:* Immediate surgical repair of the diaphragm with replacement of the herniation; placement of chest tubes *Nursing:* Preoperative: Support respiratory function; provide comfort; place in semi-Fowler's position; suction, give oxygen, and monitor IV fluids. Postoperative: Maintain routine postoperative care and monitoring, place in semi-Fowler's position; do chest physiotherapy and positive pressure ventilation; monitor oxygenation; provide comfort; support parents.
Hiatal		
Intermittent protrusion of the stomach through the esophageal opening in the diaphragm	Vomiting, dysphagia, dyspnea, GE reflux, respiratory distress, bleeding Diagnosis made by history and radiography	*Medical:* Surgical repair of the esophageal opening *Nursing:* Routine preoperative and postoperative care, as above
Inguinal (Fig. 44-19 on p. 1406)		
Loop of intestine prolapses through the inguinal ring above the scrotal sac because of muscle weakness; can be unilateral or bilateral.	Hydrocele or undescended testes may be present also. Inguinal hernias are usually asymptomatic and are found only in the course of routine examination. However, a hernia can become strangulated or incarcerated (i.e., a portion of the intestine becomes tightly caught in the hernia sac, restricting blood supply)	*Medical:* Hernia can usually be reduced by gently manipulating the strapped intestine; when surgery is done (herniorrhaphy), overnight hospital stay is not necessary. *Nursing:* Apply ice to the scrotum to reduce edema; comfort and quiet the child with an incarcerated (trapped) inguinal hernia so the surgeon can reduce the incarceration; do not use diapers postoperatively even if the child is not toilet-trained; instruct parents not to give tub baths until healing is completed.
Umbilical (see Fig 44-19)		
Protrusion of the intestine through a weakness in the abdominal wall around the umbilicus	Inspection and palpation of abdomen High incidence in African-American infants Spontaneous closure at 1 to 2 years of age	*Medical:* Spontaneous closure by 2 yr of age in small defects (<2 cm); surgical closure if condition persists after ages 2 to 5 or for defects >2 cm *Nursing:* Discourage use of home remedies (i.e., coins, belly bands, abdominal taping); reassure parents

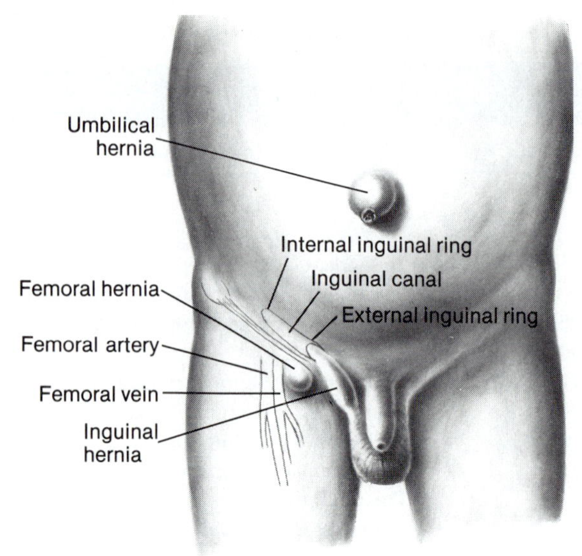

FIG. 44-19 Location of hernias.

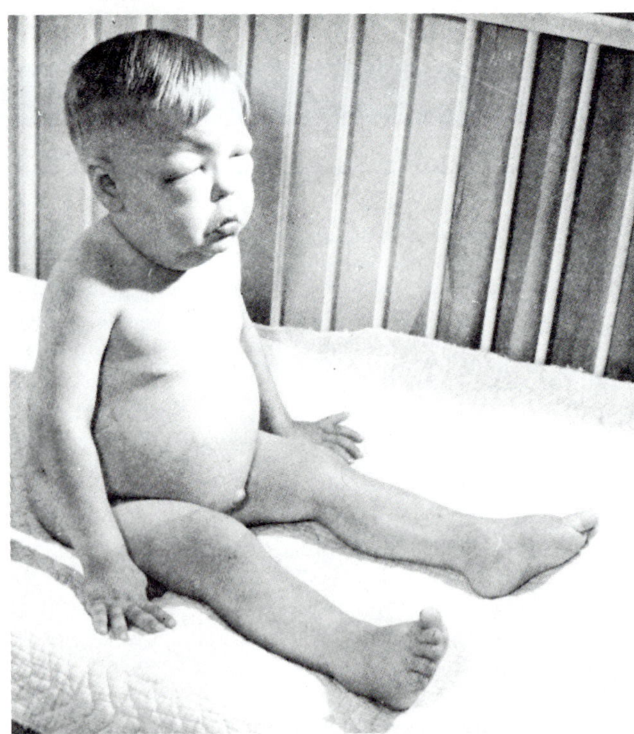

FIG. 44-20 Child with nephrotic syndrome.

Urinary Tract Infection (UTI)

UTIs may affect the upper urinary tract (kidneys and ureters) and/or the lower urinary tract (bladder and urethra). They are more prevalent in females, uncircumcised males, and sexually active adolescents. UTIs are primarily caused by bacteria, most frequently gram-negative organisms. A shorter urethra in females (2 cm in young girls and 4 cm in mature women) provides a short access route to the bladder for organisms that are common to the perineal and perianal regions. Another factor that may lead to UTIs is urinary stasis. Normally, the urine is sterile, but the warm climate within the bladder provides an excellent growth medium for bacteria. Children may also have a congenital anomaly such as urethral stenosis or vesicoureteral reflux (backward flow of urine from the bladder to the ureters) that may lead to urinary stasis and cause a UTI. Signs and symptoms of UTIs may be subtle, and parents may not realize anything is wrong with the child. Initially, the manifestations may be subtle or not present at all. In infants, fever, weight loss, failure to thrive, feeding difficulties, vomiting, and diarrhea are common. In children, urinary frequency, pain during urination, foul-smelling urine, incontinence in a toilet-trained child, abdominal and/or flank pain, hematuria, and vomiting are common signs and symptoms. For a complete discussion of UTIs, refer to Chapter 30.

Nephrotic Syndrome (Nephrosis)

Nephrotic syndrome is a clinical state characterized by proteinuria, edema, hyperlipidemia, and hypoproteinemia. Nephrotic syndrome can occur in three forms: (1) idiopathic or primary; (2) secondary (occurring as a result of glomerular damage caused by a known etiology); or (3) congenitally acquired. In children, the idiopathic form is seen most commonly.

Etiology/Pathophysiology. For most children (90%), the cause of the syndrome is unknown. Autoimmune processes and a hypersensitivity to an antigen-antibody reaction have been implicated as possible causes. The underlying pathological abnormality is proteinuria that results from glomerular damage that renders the glomerulus permeable to protein (proteinuria). This leads to low levels of protein in the blood (hypoproteinemia), decreasing colloidal osmotic pressure in the capillaries. As a result, the relative increase of hydrostatic pressure within the capillaries causes fluid to leak into the interstitial spaces (edema). This shift of fluid into the interstitial spaces causes a decrease in blood volume (hypovolemia). In compensation, the kidneys retain sodium and water, leading to an increase in the potential for edema. The mechanism by which the level of lipids in the blood is increased is poorly understood.

Clinical Manifestations. The development of manifestations is subtle. Initially, children may develop periorbital edema, which is primarily noticed upon waking from sleep. Abdominal distention may be apparent as fluid accumulates in the abdominal cavity (ascites). As the syndrome progresses, the edema becomes generalized and severe (anasarca) (Fig. 44-20). Vomiting, anorexia, diarrhea, and irritability are common. Increased body weight, decreased urine output, and marked edema are hallmark signs.

Diagnostic Tests. The diagnosis of nephrotic syndrome is made on the basis of clinical manifestations and urine studies. Analysis of the urine will reveal marked proteinuria with a high specific gravity. The urine may be dark and frothy. RBCs, hyaline casts, and fat bodies may also be present. Serum protein levels are reduced, and serum lipid levels are elevated. A renal biopsy may be performed to determine the extent of glomerular damage and evaluate the response to therapy.

Medical Management. The principal goal of management of nephrotic syndrome is to reduce the edema. This is primarily accomplished with steroid therapy. Adrenocortical steroids (prednisone) are administered to reduce the proteinuria and subsequently the edema. This response usually occurs within 7 to 21 days of initiation of the therapy; the steroids are slowly tapered over a period of several weeks and are discontinued when the child is asymptomatic. Bed rest is usually encouraged in the acute phase of the illness, with progression to ambulation as the edema subsides. Children are also placed on a low-sodium diet during the period of severe edema. Diuretics are not administered to the child with nephrotic syndrome because they will decrease the circulating blood volume, which is already a concern for these children. Relapses are an issue for a majority of children for many years.

Nursing Interventions. Nursing interventions are focused on clinical observation of the child in the acute phase and monitoring the effects of therapeutic interventions. Careful monitoring of I&O, body weight, and abdominal girth is essential in assessing the status of fluid retention or excretion. Meticulous skin care should be provided to avoid impairment of edematous skin and prevent secondary infections. Frequent monitoring of vital signs is necessary to detect early signs of complications such as infection or shock. Because the child with nephrotic syndrome has a poor appetite, eating may be a challenge. It is essential that the child have a good protein intake to offset the loss of protein through the urine. Preferred foods should be offered frequently in small amounts and served in an attractive manner. Because increased susceptibility to infection is a common side effect of steroid therapy, the child should be kept free of exposure to communicable diseases and sources of infection. As the edema decreases, the child's activity may be increased. Continuous support of the family should be provided during the acute phase of the illness and while the child recovers.

Patient/family teaching. Parents are instructed in testing urine for albumin, administration of medications, diet restrictions (if any), and the common effects of steroid therapy. Parents are also instructed regarding avoiding contact with infected playmates, but the child is permitted to attend school. Parents should be instructed how to assess for signs of relapse and told to seek immediate medical attention if this should occur.

Prognosis. A satisfactory response is more likely when relapses are detected and therapy is instituted early. Remissions are prolonged when instructions are carried out faithfully. The prognosis for ultimate recovery in most cases is good.

Acute Glomerulonephritis (AGN)

Glomerulonephritis is defined as an inflammation of the glomeruli of the kidney. Most commonly, it occurs as a postinfection phenomenon and is associated with pneumococcal, streptococcal, and viral infections. *Acute poststreptococcal glomerulonephritis (APSGN)* is the most common of the postinfection forms. APSGN primarily affects early school-age children and has a 2 : 1 predominance in males.

Etiology/Pathophysiology. APSGN follows a streptococcal infection of the throat or skin. Immune complexes that develop as a result of infection with certain strains of group A β-hemolytic streptococcus become fixed to the basement membrane of glomeruli. The glomeruli become edematous and infiltrated with WBCs. As a result, the glomerular filtration rate decreases, causing an accumulation of sodium and water in the blood, which leads to circulatory congestion and edema. Inflammation and damage to the glomeruli result in increased permeability, allowing protein molecules to escape into the urine (proteinuria).

Clinical Manifestations. Manifestations of APSGN usually appear 10 to 14 days after the streptococcal infection. Onset is characterized by a sudden onset of hematuria, proteinuria, and oliguria. Edema, abdominal pain, low-grade fever, anorexia, vomiting, and headache may be present. Hypertension and heart failure may occur as a result of hypervolemia.

Diagnostic Tests. Urinalysis reveals proteinuria, hematuria, and elevated specific gravity. Bacteria are usually not seen, and urine culture is negative. Cultures of the throat or skin are positive for the streptococcal organism. The *antistreptolysin O titer* (antibodies formed against streptococcus) is elevated, indicating that there has been a recent infection with streptococcus.

Medical Management. The acute phase of glomerulonephritis generally lasts 1 to 2 weeks. During this time bed rest is usually recommended, although many children will set their own limits based on their tolerance

TABLE 44-3 Defects of the External Genitourinary Tract

Defect	Medical Management
Hypospadias (Fig. 44-21)	
Urethral opening located along the ventral (anterior) surface of the penile shaft	Surgical correction involves extending the urethra to a normal position. After repair, the child is expected to have both normal reproductive and urinary function.
Epispadias	
Urethral opening located along the dorsal (posterior) surface of the penile shaft	Surgical correction involves penile and urethral lengthening, and, possibly, bladder neck reconstruction.
Phimosis	
Narrowing or stenosis of the opening of the foreskin	Mild cases are treated with manual retraction. Severe cases are treated with circumcision.
Hydrocele	
Fluid in scrotal sac	Surgical correction indicated if spontaneous resolution has not occurred in 1 yr.
Cryptorchidism	
Failure of one or both of the testes to descend into the scrotum	Medical management involves administration of human chorionic gonadotropin. Surgical correction: orchiopexy, which is surgical fixation of a testes. Treatment is aimed at preventing testicular damage and malignancies.
Inguinal Hernia	
Protrusion of the abdominal organs through the inguinal canal and into the scrotal sac	Surgical correction involves closure of the inguinal canal.

to activity. Moderate sodium restriction is recommended while the child is hypertensive and edematous. Regular measurement of vital signs, body weight, and I&O is necessary to monitor the progression of the disease and detect any complications. Antihypertensive medications and diuretics may be administered to control hypertension. Antibiotic therapy is indicated for children who have a persistent infection.

Nursing Interventions. Nursing interventions are focused on promoting rest and adequate nutrition, preventing and detecting complications, and supporting the child and family. During the acute phase of the illness the child may be placed on bed rest. The nurse can provide activities that require minimal energy expenditure and will keep the child's interest. Meals should reflect the child's preferences while adhering to any dietary restrictions that have been ordered. Measurement of vital signs, body weight, and I&O will provide information about the disease's progression and detect the presence of complications.

Patient/family teaching. The parents should be educated about the disease and its therapy and allowed to express their feelings and concerns.

Prognosis. Most children with APSGN recover completely, with few or no complications.

Wilms' Tumor

Wilms' tumor is the most common malignant tumor of childhood, accounting for 20% of solid tumors in children. The peak age of incidence of these tumors is 3 to 4 years.

Etiology/Pathophysiology. Wilms' tumor most commonly affects the left kidney. Both kidneys are affected in 10% of the cases. Wilms' tumor has both hereditary and nonhereditary origins. The most common sites for metastasis are the lungs, lymph nodes, liver, brain, and bone.

Clinical Manifestations. Most Wilms' tumors manifest as enlarging, asymptomatic, and firm abdominal masses. Other manifestations of the tumor include abdominal pain, hematuria, fever, hypertension, weight loss, and fatigue. If there has been metastasis of the Wilms' tumor, dyspnea, cough, and chest pain may be present.

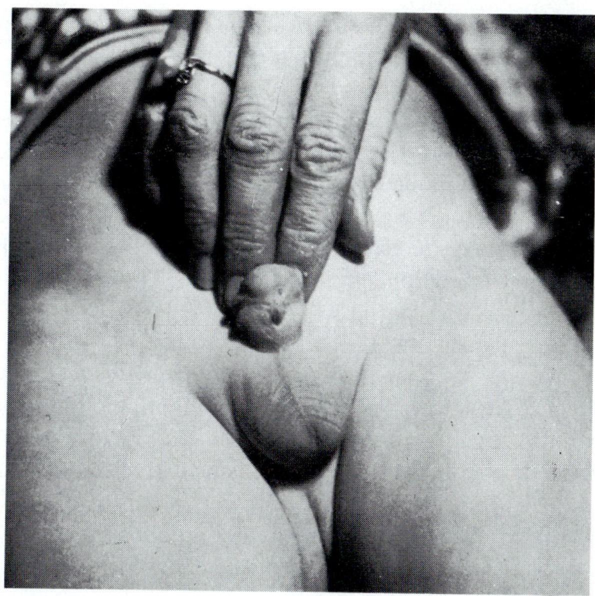

FIG. 44-21 Hypospadias.

Diagnostic Tests. Many tumors are detected by parents as they feel an enlarged abdominal mass during bathing, dressing, or carrying the child. In addition to a thorough history and physical examination, diagnostic studies include radiographic studies, computerized tomography, and hematological and chemistry studies. Definitive (final) diagnosis is based upon surgical biopsy. Because the tumor is encapsulated, the child's abdomen should not be palpated more than is necessary for diagnosis. This will decrease the possibility of rupture of the capsule and spillage of the malignant cells into the abdominal cavity.

Medical Management. Treatment of Wilms' tumor involves surgical resection as soon as possible after diagnosis. During surgery the abdomen is explored to determine the extent of the disease and if there has been metastasis of the tumor. If one kidney is affected, the tumor, kidney, and adrenal gland are removed. Meticulous care is employed during resection to avoid rupture of the capsule and spread of cancer cells throughout the abdomen. The other kidney is examined for evidence of disease. If both kidneys are involved, part of the kidney is removed on the less affected side with removal of the total kidney on the opposite side. Most children will receive radiotherapy following surgery. Chemotherapy is indicated for all children. The usual course of treatment ranges from 6 to 15 months.

Nursing Interventions. Preoperative nursing interventions involve preparing the child and family for surgery. This is a challenging responsibility for the nurse because most surgeries are performed within 24 hours of diagnosis. Postoperative nursing interventions are similar to those provided to the child undergoing abdominal surgery. Special attention is directed toward monitoring bowel sounds and assessing renal function. The nurse should be sensitive to the parents' feelings about their child's diagnosis; it is common for parents to feel that they should have identified the mass earlier.

Patient/family teaching. The overall objective in discharge planning is to return the child to a normal preoperative life-style. The nurse emphasizes the usual needs for discipline and moderate protection from infection. Treatment schedules are planned to allow uninterrupted school attendance.

Prognosis. It should be reinforced to parents that prognosis is excellent and survival rates have improved with the development of new treatment protocols. Children with localized tumor (stages I and II) have a 90% chance of cure with appropriate therapy.

Structural Defects of the Genitourinary Tract

Structural defects of the GU tract have serious implications for the psychological well-being of the child. Prompt correction is necessary to avoid a negative psychological impact on the child as well as to prevent physical complications. The major structural defects and their medical management are presented in Table 44-3.

Nursing Interventions. Nursing interventions for the child with a defect of the GU tract are focused on assisting with diagnosis and preparing the child and family for procedures and corrective surgeries. The nurse should provide the child and parents with emotional support and opportunities to express their concerns, questions, and fears.

Prognosis. Satisfactory surgical repair is successful for the more common disorders and is carried out or initiated as early as possible.

DISORDERS OF ENDOCRINE FUNCTION

The endocrine system is responsible for the production and secretion of the major chemical regulators of the body, namely the hormones. Disorders are caused primarily by an undersecretion or oversecretion of these hormones. Endocrine system dysfunctions affect all aspects of body function, including appearance, growth, and physical and psychological well-being.

Hypothyroidism

Hypothyroidism results from a deficient production of thyroid hormone (TH) by the thyroid gland. The main function of the thyroid gland is to regulate metabolism by the production of thyroxine (T_4), triiodothyronine (T_3), and calcitonin. The secretion of these hormones is controlled by thyroid-stimulating hormone (TSH) from the anterior pituitary.

Etiology/Pathophysiology. Hypothyroidism may be primary or acquired. Primary causes include (1) congenital defects or (2) defective synthesis resulting from an autoimmune process. Acquired causes of hypothyroidism include (1) insufficient stimulation of the gland by the pituitary or the hypothalamus or (2) systemic resistance to TH.

Clinical Manifestations. The clinical manifestations of hypothyroidism are described in Box 44-5.

Diagnostic Tests. Hypothyroidism may also be detected by a decrease in serum levels of TH (T_4 and T_3) and an increase in serum TSH levels (if the defect is in the thyroid) or a decrease in serum TSH levels (if the defect is in the pituitary).

Medical Management. The treatment of choice for congenital and acquired hypothyroidism is oral thyroid hormone replacement therapy. Prompt treatment is especially critical in the infant with congenital hypothyroidism to avoid permanent cognitive (the process of knowing) impairment.

Nursing Interventions. In addition to assisting in detection of the condition and implementing of TH replacement therapy, nursing interventions focus on assisting the child and family with compliance to the medical regimen and periodic monitoring of its effects. As soon as the child grows and matures, responsibility for the disorder and its treatment should be placed with the child.

Patient/family teaching. Following diagnosis and implementation of thyroid hormone therapy, the importance of compliance and periodic monitoring of the response to therapy should be stressed to the parents and to the child, when old enough.

Prognosis. If congenital hypothyroidism is present, treatment must be started shortly after birth for normal physical and intellectual growth to occur. The most significant factor adversely affecting eventual intelligence appears to be inadequate treatment, which may be related to noncompliance.

Hyperthyroidism

Hyperthyroidism is generally rare in young children, primarily affecting young adolescents. The most common form of childhood hyperthyroidism is Graves' disease.

Etiology/Pathophysiology. Although the exact causal mechanism is unknown, the most accepted theory is an autoimmune process resulting in the production of immunoglobulins that have thyroid-stimulating properties.

Clinical Manifestations. The clinical manifestations of hyperthyroidism are described in Box 44-6.

Diagnostic Tests. In addition to clinical manifestations, the diagnosis of hyperthyroidism is made on the basis of increased serum levels of T_4, T_3, and radioactive iodine uptake (RAIU).

Medical Management. The management of hyperthyroidism is directed toward decreasing the rate of TH secretion. This is usually accomplished through the administration of antithyroid medications including propylthiouracil (PTU) and methimazole (Tapazole), subtotal thyroidectomy, or iodine administration (^{131}I [iodine-131]).

Box 44-5 CLINICAL MANIFESTATIONS OF HYPOTHYROIDISM

CONGENITAL	ACQUIRED
Prolonged jaundice	Growth delay
Lethargy	Dry skin
Poor appetite	Puffy eyes
Poor sucking reflex	Constipation
Dyspnea	Lethargy
Hypothermia	Mental slowness
Cool, mottled skin	

Box 44-6 CLINICAL MANIFESTATIONS OF HYPERTHYROIDISM

- Nervousness
- Irritability
- Hyperactivity
- Tremors
- Excessive appetite
- Weight loss
- Exophthalmos (protruding eyeballs)
- Palpable thyroid gland
- Advanced bone age
- Tachycardia
- Tachypnea
- Hypertension
- Warm skin
- Accelerated growth
- Heat intolerance
- Thyroid storm
    - *Rapid onset:*
        - Severe hyperthermia
        - Vomiting
        - Diarrhea
        - Severe tachycardia
    - *May advance to:*
        - Delirium
        - Coma
        - Death

Nursing Interventions. Nursing interventions for the child with hyperthyroidism are focused on intervening with the physical manifestations of the disease. Emotional lability is often manifested by sudden episodes of crying or elation. Rest is promoted, and a quiet, nonstimulating environment is provided in the initial phase of treatment. Heat intolerance may be alleviated by dressing the child in lightweight clothing, altering the room temperature, and offering lightweight blankets for sleeping comfort. Dietary modifications include increased calories and daily vitamin supplementation. If surgery is recommended, the child and family should be provided with explanations about the nature of the surgery, where the incision will be located, and what to expect postoperatively. Postoperative care includes strict observation of bleeding and complications. The neck should be kept slightly flexed and supported to avoid strain on the suture line (see Chapter 32).

Patient/family teaching. Upon discharge a referral to a public health, school, or a home health nurse will enable continuity of care and increase compliance with the medical regimen.

Prognosis. Generally, after drug treatment, some improvement is noted within the first 2 weeks. In many children an initial treatment course of 1 to 2 years will be followed by a complete remission of the disorder. Those who relapse may benefit from a second course of medication therapy, but may be candidates for surgical intervention.

Diabetes Mellitus (DM)

DM is a syndrome characterized by a deficiency of insulin resulting in alterations in protein, carbohydrate, and fat metabolism. Insulin-dependent diabetes mellitus (IDDM) is the most frequently seen endocrine disorder in children. The etiology/pathophysiology, clinical manifestations, and diagnostic tests for DM are discussed in Chapter 32.

Medical Management. The management of DM involves a multidisciplinary approach and focuses on the child and family as a whole. Insulin replacement is the definitive treatment for DM. There are three types of insulin: rapid-, intermediate-, and long-acting. All insulins are prepared in 100 units/ml strength. The dosage of insulin for each child is dependent on levels of glucose in the blood. The serum glucose is measured by putting a drop of the child's blood on a test strip and reading the color change by comparing it with a color chart or by inserting the strip into a glucose monitor. The daily insulin dosage is also dependent on food intake and activity and exercise levels. Most children are managed with a twice-daily insulin protocol that is a combination of rapid-acting (regular) and intermediate-acting (NPH or Lente) insulins. The injections of insulin are given before breakfast and before dinner. Adjustments in the insulin dosage are needed during growth spurts, increased exercise, illnesses, infections, and surgery.

An insulin pump is also available to children with DM and is designed to deliver predetermined amounts of regular insulin continuously The device consists of a syringe that contains the supply of insulin, a plunger, and a pump that pushes the plunger to deliver the desired dosage. The insulin flows from the syringe into a needle inserted into the subcutaneous tissue. The needle is aseptically changed every 48 hours. Although the insulin pump has advantages over daily insulin injections, there is one major disadvantage. It cannot be removed for more than 2 hours under any circumstance.

The management of DM in children also centers on nutrition. A nutritionist should be available to discuss nutritional needs and restrictions with the child and family. Children with DM do not require special foods or supplements; they essentially have the same nutritional needs as other children, except for the deletion of concentrated sugars from the diet. Generally, children and their families are taught to follow the American Diabetes Association (ADA) food plan, which is based on an exchange system. This plan is based on a balanced diet that incorporates the Food Guide Pyramid Recommendations. The Pyramid's intent is to illustrate which foods should be included in a healthful diet and in what proportion (see Figs. 18-1 and 18-2).

Exercise is encouraged as it can lower blood glucose levels. Food intake and insulin requirements must be adjusted to the child's activity level.

Nursing Interventions. Nursing interventions for the child with DM is focused on educating the child and family about the disease, treatment, and complications, and providing support and reassurance. Because the treatment of DM relies upon principles of self-management, it is essential that the child and family understand the disease and its treatment. The parents and child should be encouraged to express their questions, fears, and concerns about the disease and its management. The nurse should support the child and family in their adjustment to the disease and provide them with concrete suggestions about managing the disease that will have a positive affect on their attitudes about DM and its management.

Patient/family teaching. It is important that the child and family be instructed about meal planning by a nutritionist and these instructions should be reinforced by the nurse. The child and family need to be educated about the action of insulin, including the onset, peak, and duration of action, as well as manifestations of hyperglycemia and hypoglycemia. They should also be aware of how to recognize manifestations of diabetic ketoacidosis. Both the child and family should be instructed in the proper techniques of insulin injections. The parents and child are taught to develop a rotation pattern so that injections are not given repeatedly in the same sites. Nurses should also teach the parents and child the principles and techniques of home glucose monitoring.

Prognosis. DM is a chronic metabolic disease. Compliance to treatment improves quality of life. Long-term complications involve the small, as well as larger, blood vessels. The principal microvascular complications are nephropathy and retinopathy. With poor control, vascular changes appear as early as 2½ to 3 years after diagnosis; with good control, changes have been postponed for 20 or more years.

DISORDERS OF MUSCULOSKELETAL FUNCTION

Musculoskeletal problems in childhood are common and are a result of genetics, rapid growth, or the child's natural tendency toward active mobility. Many musculoskeletal conditions are temporary, and ultimately normal function returns.

Congenital Hip Dysplasia (CHD)

Etiology/Pathophysiology. CHD or congenital dislocation of the hip is a developmental abnormality of the femoral head, the acetabulum, or both. CHD is associated with such conditions as first pregnancy, spina bifida, and breech presentation. **Subluxation** of the hip, or partial dislocation, is characterized by incorrect position of the femoral head in the acetabulum. Subluxation is the degree of CHD most commonly seen in infants. Dislocation occurs when the femoral head has no contact with the acetabulum.

Clinical Manifestations. In the infant, shortening of the femur on the affected side is present; thigh and gluteal folds are uneven (or increased on the affected side) when the infant is placed in the prone position, and there is limited abduction of the hip on the affected side (Fig. 44-22). The older, weight-bearing infant may have the affected leg shorter than the other, a waddling gait, or limping.

Diagnostic Tests. Early diagnosis of CHD in the newborn is associated with more successful and less complicated treatment. Nursing assessment of the manifestations listed above alerts the physician to the possibility of CHD. In addition, sonography or radiographic examination may be helpful in establishing the diagnosis.

Medical Management. Once diagnosed, treatment is begun immediately. Any delay in treatment can result in a worsening deformity and poorer prognosis. Treatment

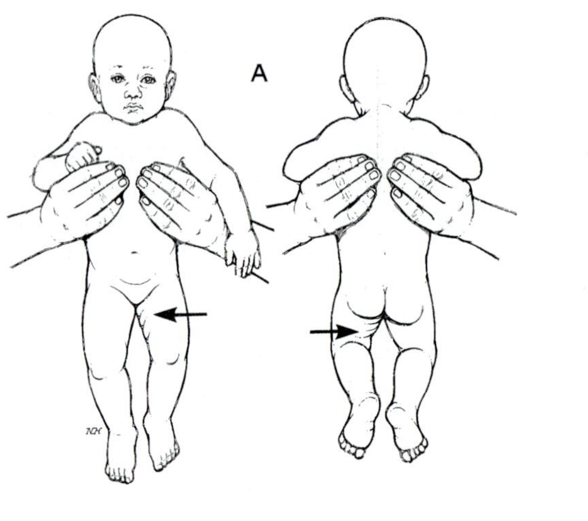

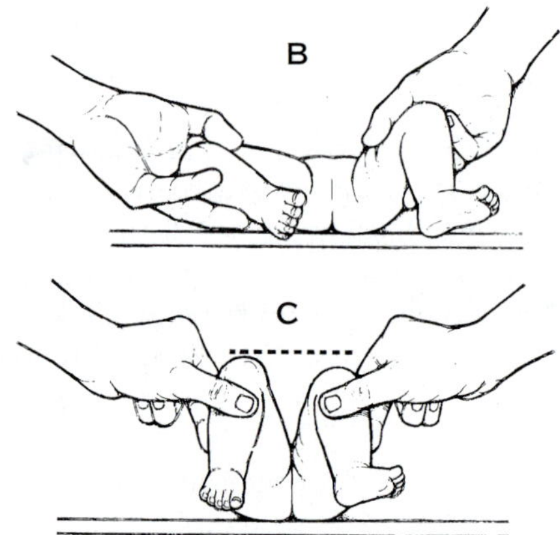

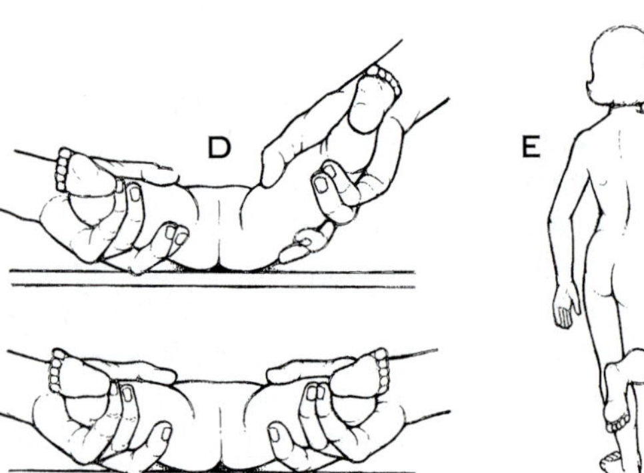

FIG. 44-22 Signs of congenital dislocation of hip. **A,** Asymmetry of gluteal and thigh folds. **B,** Limited hip abduction, as seen in flexion. **C,** Apparent shortening of femur, as indicated by level of knees in flexion. **D,** Ortolani click (if infant is under 4 weeks of age). **E,** Positive Trendelenburg sign or gait (if child is weight bearing).

will depend upon the severity of the dysplasia and the age of the infant. Treatment for infants under 6 months of age consists of positioning the head of the femur within the acetabulum and maintaining the hip in abduction for 4 to 6 months with the use of a Pavlik harness (Fig. 44-23). Once abduction is achieved, positioning is maintained in a hip spica cast for several months until the hip is stable. Infants diagnosed between the ages of 6 and 18 months will require skin traction reduction and casting until the hip is stable. Surgical open reduction may be needed if soft tissue obstructs the head of the femur from entering the acetabulum. Immobilization in a hip spica cast follows open reduction. The management of children diagnosed after 18 months is more extensive because adaptive changes have taken place. Open surgical reduction, osteotomy, and arthroplasty may be necessary.

Nursing Interventions. Nurses are in a unique position to observe newborns for evidence of CHD and other congenital defects. The earlier the defect is identified and treated, the better the chance for a favorable outcome. The primary goals in caring for a child in a corrective device or cast are to maintain the position of the hip joint, prevent complications, and provide stimulation necessary for the developing infant or child. As early as possible, parents should be involved in caring for their baby to build confidence in providing care at home. Box 44-7 provides general guidelines for the nursing interventions for a child in a corrective device or cast.

Patient/family teaching. Parents as well as all other care givers need to understand that children in corrective devices should be involved in all the activities of any child in the same age group. Confinement should not exclude children from family activities.

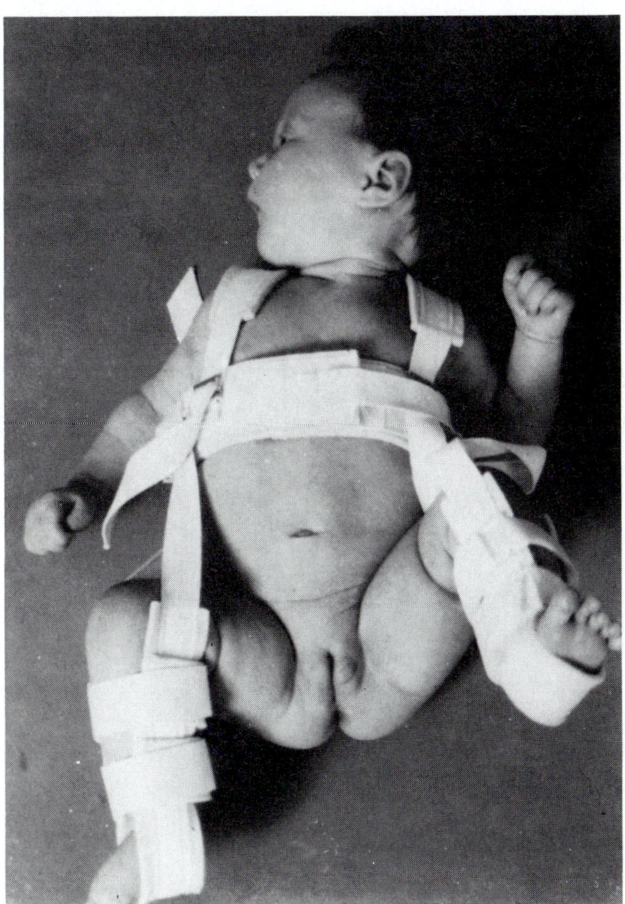

FIG. 44-23 Child in Pavlik harness.

Prognosis. With early treatment the prognosis is more favorable to the restoration of normal body function.

Legg-Calvé-Perthes Disease

Etiology/Pathophysiology. **Legg-Calvé-Perthes disease** is a disorder caused by decreased blood supply to the femoral head, which results in necrosis and regeneration of the femoral head. It occurs four times more often in boys and affects children from 3 to 12 years of age. The cause of the disorder is unknown, and the disease process itself is self-limited.

Clinical Manifestations. Signs and symptoms are usually insidious. The child may complain of pain, exhibit a limp on the affected side, and have limited ROM. The condition is aggravated by activity and decreases with rest.

Diagnostic Tests. Legg-Calvé-Perthes disease is suspected when the above signs and symptoms are present. The diagnosis is confirmed by radiographic examination.

Box 44-7 CARE OF THE CHILD IN A CAST OR CORRECTIVE DEVICE

- Do neurovascular assessment of the 5 Ps (impairments to be reported immediately): Pain, pallor or cyanosis, paresthesia (numbing/tingling, decrease in sensation), pulselessness, puffiness
- Skin monitored frequently for erythema or tenderness.
- Wash and dry skin at least daily.
- Smooth or pad sharp cast or brace edges with gauze or adhesive tape.
- Teach cast or brace maintenance and cleaning.
- Assess circular dressings for excessive tightness.
- Stimulate circulation with gentle massage over pressure areas.

Medical Management. Treatment of Legg-Calvé-Perthes disease is accomplished with bed rest, traction, casts, braces, or harnesses. The goal of therapy is to maintain the head of the femur within the acetabulum so that the femoral head will preserve its normal shape as it regenerates. If this is accomplished, full ROM can be maintained.

Nursing Interventions. While the child is in traction or in casts, braces, or harnesses, skin care and neurovascular assessment are essential. Please refer to Box 44-9 for care of the child in a cast or corrective device.

Patient/family teaching. Because most of the child's care is conducted on an outpatient basis, the major emphasis of nursing intervention is teaching the family the care and management of the corrective appliances elected for therapy. The family needs to learn the purpose, function, application, and care of the corrective device and the importance of compliance in order to achieve the desired outcome. Suitable activities must be devised to assist the child in developing a sense of initiative or industry. This is an opportune time to encourage the child to begin a hobby, such as collections, model building, or crafts.

Prognosis. Legg-Calvé-Perthes disease is self-limiting, but the ultimate outcome of therapy depends on early and efficient treatment and the age of onset of the disorder. Younger children, whose epiphyses are more cartilaginous, have the brightest prognosis for complete recovery. The later the diagnosis is made, the more damage has occurred before treatment is implemented. In most cases, with good patient compliance, the prognosis is excellent.

Scoliosis

Etiology/Pathophysiology. The most common skeletal deformity of adolescence is scoliosis. The condition is a lateral curvature of the spine that causes changes in the spine, chest, and hips. Severe curvature can affect cardiopulmonary and neurological function and result in a negative self-image. Scoliosis can occur at any age but is more often seen in adolescent females.

Clinical Manifestations. The child with idiopathic scoliosis will present with unequal hip height and shoulder height, scapular and rib prominence, and a posterior rib hump that is visible when the child bends forward at the waist (Fig. 44-24).

Diagnostic Tests. Early identification and treatment of scoliosis are vitally important for a good prognosis. Routine screening of children from 10 to 15 years of age involves posterior observation of the undressed child (bending forward at the waist with arms and head hanging downward) for curvature, asymmetry, and rib hump. Radiographs confirm the diagnosis.

Medical Management. Curvatures of less than 20 degrees require no treatment. Bracing is used for moderate curvatures, and it can slow the progression of scoliosis

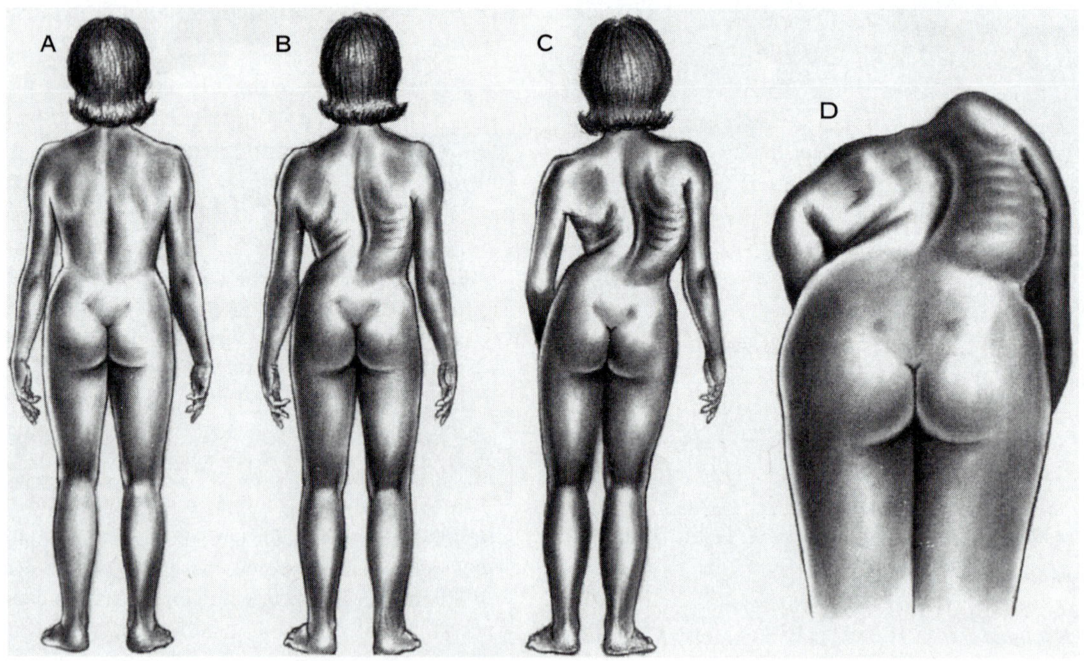

FIG. 44-24 Scoliosis in children. Normal spinal alignment and abnormal spinal curvatures associated with scoliosis. **A,** Normal. **B,** Mild. **C,** Severe. **D,** Rotation and curvature.

until the spine is mature. The most common brace available is the *Milwaukee brace*, which extends from the chin to the pelvis (Fig. 44-25). The brace is worn for 23 hours a day and may be necessary for years until spinal maturity occurs. Frequent follow-up is necessary for brace adjustment. Surgical intervention is indicated in severe scoliosis or scoliosis that does not respond to bracing. Surgery consists of spinal fusion and the insertion of a stabilizing rod such as the Harrington rod.

Nursing Interventions. The adolescent who must wear a brace may have difficulty complying with the treatment plan. Developmentally, the adolescent is trying to fit in with peers by conforming to peer norms and will need plenty of reassurance to feel attractive and worthwhile during treatment. Instruction on maintaining skin integrity is essential for the adolescent in a brace or cast. Box 44-7 outlines care for the child in a corrective device or cast.

Patient/family teaching. When a child first faces the prospect of a prolonged period in a brace, cast, or other device, the therapy program and the nature of the device must be explained thoroughly to both the child and the parents so that they will have an understanding of the anticipated results, how the appliance corrects the defect, the freedoms and constraints imposed by the device, and what to do to help achieve the desired goal.

Prognosis. Treatment for scoliosis extends over a significant portion of the child's period of growth. Prognosis is dependent upon severity of the condition and compliance with treatment.

Osteomyelitis

Osteomyelitis is an infection within the bone. In children, the metaphysis of the femur, the tibia, and the humerus are the areas most commonly affected. Although osteomyelitis can occur at any age, the peak incidence in children occurs between the ages of 3 and 15 years, and boys are affected twice as often as girls. For a more detailed discussion of osteomyelitis, see Chapter 26.

Talipes (Clubfoot)

Etiology/Pathophysiology. Talipes is a congenital deformity of the foot and ankle, of which there are many types. *Talipes equinovarus* (foot adducted and twisted inward) is the type of clubfoot deformity seen most often. The incidence is 1 in every 1000 live births and is twice as high in males as in females. Talipes can be unilateral or bilateral. The cause of talipes is unknown, but theories point to an inherited or environmental disorder. The incidence of talipes is also increased in families where there is already a child with the defect. The more

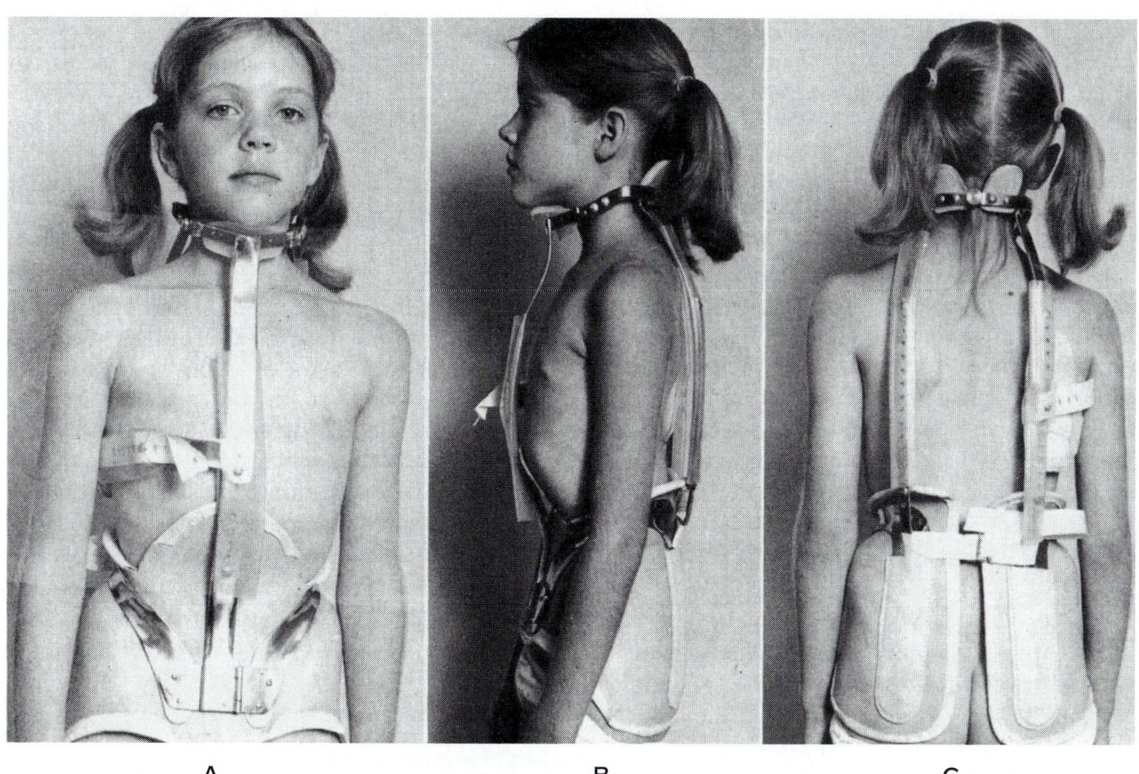

FIG. 44-25 Milwaukee brace. **A,** Front view. **B,** Side view. **C,** Rear view. (From Blount WP, Mueller KH: *Praxis* 8:139, 1972.)

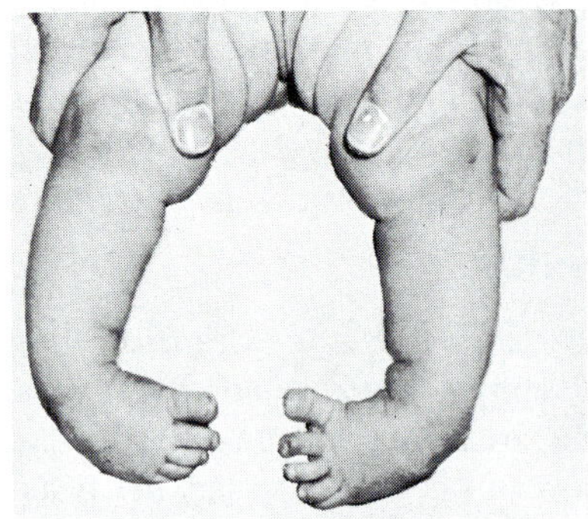

FIG. 44-26 Bilateral congenital talipes equinovarus (congenital clubfoot) in 2-month-old infant.

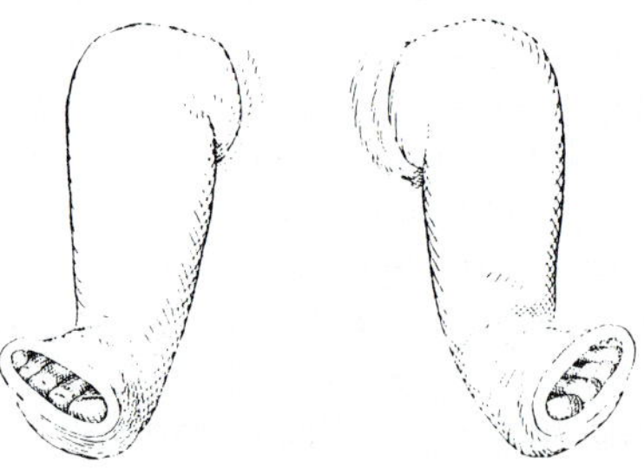

FIG. 44-27 Feet casted for correction of bilateral congenital talipes equinovarus.

flexible talipes deformities are thought to develop from environmental conditions, such as intrauterine positioning and restricted movement within the uterus, although the evidence is not conclusive.

Clinical Manifestations. Talipes varies in severity. Clubfoot may involve one foot (more common) or both feet. The most common type of clubfoot is when the foot is pointed downward and inward (Fig. 44-26).

Diagnostic Tests. Talipes is evident at birth, and diagnosis is made by examination, manipulation, and radiographs.

Medical Management. The earlier the treatment is begun, the more favorable the outcome. Treatment of talipes consists of manipulation and the application of a series of short leg casts (Fig. 44-27). The foot is gently manipulated into a more normal position and then casted to maintain the correction. Casts are changed weekly to allow for further manipulation and to accommodate the rapidly growing infant. Once the casting series is completed and the deformity is corrected, the foot (or feet) will require a combination of passive stretching exercises and corrective splints or shoes to prevent the deformity from recurring. The Denis Browne splint is the device most commonly used to maintain correction. Corrective shoes are adjusted to a prescribed angle onto a Denis Browne bar and worn continuously until the child is ready for walking, at which time corrective walking shoes are used.

Nursing Interventions. Once the neonate or infant has been diagnosed with talipes, parents will need support and education. Very often, parents will need time to adjust to the distressing fact that their child has a deformity. Nurses should take every opportunity to educate parents while encouraging them to express their feelings and concerns. Nursing care of the infant with casts is the same for any child in a cast (see Box 44-9). Often, neonates are casted before discharge from the hospital. Keeping casts clean and dry is relatively easy with a small infant. Cast edges are inspected carefully for rough edges, which can irritate newborn skin. The toes are observed frequently for coldness, pain, blueness, or edema and, if present, are reported to the physician immediately. Casts are cumbersome and heavy. Parents are assisted in finding comfortable positions for feeding, playing, and cuddling. Sponge baths are given until the infant no longer needs casting. Casts can also hinder the infant's ability to kick, move the legs, or roll over. During this time of limited activity, parents can provide audio, visual, and tactile stimulation to encourage normal development. Treatment and follow-up care are usually provided on an outpatient basis.

Patient/family teaching. Nursing responsibilities include the teaching of passive stretching exercises with a return demonstration by the parent, if this is part of the treatment plan. Parents are taught cast care and how to handle the infant. The nurse teaches the parents how to hold the heel firmly and to stretch only the forefoot; otherwise, undue force on the heel may produce a valgus deformity (twisted outward, away from midline). Stretching exercises are performed several times a day, and the parent may find it easier to remember to do the exercises if they are associated with a regular activity like diaper changing or after feedings.

Prognosis. Some feet respond to treatment rapidly; some respond only to prolonged, vigorous, and sustained efforts; and the improvement in others remains disappointing even with maximum effort on the part of all concerned. Correction of talipes equinovarus is most reliably accomplished by manipulation and the application of a series of casts begun immediately or shortly after birth and continued until marked overcorrection is reached.

Duchenne's Muscular Dystrophy

Etiology/Pathophysiology. Duchenne's muscular dystrophy (DMD) is a genetically acquired disorder characterized by gradually progressive skeletal muscle wasting and weakness. DMD is the most severe and most common form of all dystrophies. The onset of signs and symptoms occurs between the ages of 2 and 4.

Clinical Manifestations. Initial signs and symptoms, which are mild and progress gradually, can easily be overlooked. Parents may be the first to notice that the child is clumsy, frequently falls, has a waddling gait, and experiences difficulty running, climbing, and riding a bicycle. The muscles of the pelvic girdle are frequently involved, and the child shows evidence of this weakness by rising from the floor in a classic manner. The child lies on the side and flexes the knees (or gets on all fours), then extends the knees and uses the hands to "walk up" the thighs **(Gowers' sign).** As the disorder progresses, there is severe muscle wasting, resulting in contractures and deformities. By 12 years of age, ambulation is no longer possible. Respiratory tract infection usually occurs when the diaphragm and accessory muscles used in respiration become affected in the final stages.

Diagnostic Tests. DMD is considered based upon the clinical signs and symptoms described above and family history. The diagnosis is confirmed by electromyogram (EMG); elevated serum creatine phosphokinase (CPK); elevated aspartate aminotransferase (AST); and muscle biopsy that reveals fibrous and fatty tissue.

Medical Management. There is no effective treatment to arrest DMD. The goals, therefore, are to maintain ambulation and independence for as long as possible. Physical therapy is begun to optimize ROM and delay muscle atrophy; braces may be used to provide additional support; and contractures are released through surgical intervention.

Nursing Interventions. The most important nursing consideration in the care of a child with DMD is to assist the child and the family in developing positive coping strategies to deal with the progressively debilitating aspects of the illness. The goal is to maintain independence for as long as possible. Because of the progressive nature of the illness, the nurse will need to assess the child's capabilities frequently. The care of a child with DMD, or any child with a chronic, debilitating terminal illness, is extremely demanding and stressful for the family. The nurse can help the family lessen their anxiety and fears through teaching and active listening. A referral to the Muscular Dystrophy Association of America, Inc.* can provide a number of supplementary services to patients and their families.

Patient/family teaching. The nurse helps the family plan an exercise program to encourage muscle strength and delay the onset of some of the physical disabilities. The nurse counsels the family in good nutrition to prevent obesity that can cause the child to become prematurely wheelchair bound.

Prognosis. Children rarely live past age 20, with death resulting from respiratory or cardiac complications.

Septic Arthritis (Septic Joint, Suppurative Arthritis)

Etiology/Pathophysiology. Septic arthritis is an infection of a joint, which can occur from bacteria in the blood or as a direct extension of an existing infection such as osteomyelitis. Bites (human, cat, dog, rat, or tick) are a frequent cause of septic arthritis. The infection causes joint irritation and damage to the synovial membrane; synovial fluid increases and causes distention within the joint. As the infection progresses, pus accumulates and breaks down the articulating cartilage (which cannot regenerate) and leads to permanent damage. In infancy the incidence of septic arthritis occurs equally among boys and girls; in the adolescent age group, it occurs predominantly in males. The joints most commonly affected are the hip, knee, shoulder, wrist, and ankle. In the neonatal group, the causative organisms include group B *Streptococcus* and gram-negative enterics (pertaining to the intestine); in the 6 months to 5 years age group, *Haemophilus influenzae* (this may change as more children are immunized against *H. influenzae*); over 5 years of age, *Staphylococcus aureus;* and in adolescents, *Neisseria gonorrhoeae.*

Clinical Manifestations. The affected joint is erythematous, edematous, warm, and exquisitely painful. There is usually limited ROM. The extremities are maintained in a flexed position by the child. If the lower extremities are involved, the child may limp or refuse to walk. Except in infants, fever is usually present. Septic arthritis occurs very rapidly and is considered a medical emergency.

Diagnostic Tests. Radiographic examination may reveal joint edema. The joint is aspirated, and purulent matter is Gram stained and cultured. A blood culture is taken. A peripheral blood smear will show leukocytosis and elevated erythrocyte sedimentation rate (ESR) in children, which may not be demonstrated in infants.

Medical Management. Joint aspiration and surgical irrigation are essential to managing the condition. Surgical drainage and irrigation ensure that the joint will be decompressed, safeguarding the vasculature, and will clear the joint of destructive purulent matter, eradicate the infection, and prevent secondary blood-borne spread of infection. Broad-spectrum IV antibiotic therapy is initiated and switched to more specific antibiotics once the organism is identified. IV therapy will continue for 10 to

*810 Seventh Avenue, New York, NY 10019; (212) 586-0808.

14 days and be changed to oral antibiotics once there is a good IV response. Oral therapy will continue to complete a 4-week course.

Nursing Interventions. The nursing care is the same as for the child with osteomyelitis (see Chapter 26).

Prognosis. If the hip joint is involved where avascular necrosis can develop and cause deformity, long-term disability can result.

Fractures

Although any bone can be fractured, the most common fracture sites in children include the long bones of the extremities, the clavicles, the wrists, fingers, and skull. Fractures can be complete (bone and periosteum separate completely) or incomplete or greenstick (bone splits but does not completely break). Spiral fractures affect the length rather than the width of the bone and are frequently the result of child abuse. For a complete discussion of these fractures, see Chapter 26. The remainder of this section will specifically address the nursing interventions for the child with a fracture.

Nursing Interventions. Assessing the child with a possible traumatic injury involves assessment of the injury and soft tissue damage. The first priority is to calm and reassure the child and the parents so that the assessment can take place. Once the child has calmed down, the nurse assesses for pain and point of tenderness, color, sensation, motion, and pulses distal to the injury. If the injury requires casting, specific nursing measures are instituted (see Chapter 26). Pain also needs to be addressed and can be alleviated with the use of comfort measures and analgesics ordered by the physician. If the injury requires correction by traction, nursing interventions will include maintaining skin integrity and monitoring skeletal traction sites for infection. The nurse also observes for complications of immobility, especially circulatory compromise and muscle spasms. Deep-breathing exercises are encouraged; blowing bubbles or balloons (under supervision) can make this activity fun for the child.

DISORDERS OF NEUROLOGICAL FUNCTION

Disorders that affect neurological function can be classified into three major categories: (1) increased intracranial pressure, (2) hypoxia, and (3) seizure activity. The residual effects of neurological disorders can have profound effects on the child's function and future performance. It is essential to identify neurological impairments at an early stage so that they can be properly diagnosed and interventions can be instituted.

Meningitis

Meningitis is a significant cause of illness in the pediatric age group. Meningitis is defined as an infection of the meninges. Most cases affect children younger than 5 years of age. Its importance lies primarily in the frequency with which it occurs in infancy and childhood and the unnecessarily high death rates and residual damage caused by undiagnosed and untreated or inadequately treated cases.

Etiology/Pathophysiology. Although meningitis can be caused by a number of bacterial, viral, and fungal organisms, bacterial meningitis is the most common. Organisms generally spread to the meninges following an upper respiratory infection, by lymphatic drainage, or by direct deposit through a lumbar puncture or skull fracture. Following invasion of the meninges by an organism, it enters the cerebrospinal fluid (CSF) and travels throughout the subarachnoid space, spreading the infection. As the meninges become infected, an inflammatory process ensues, causing a thick exudate and WBC accumulation. With continued inflammation, CSF flow becomes occluded and the brain becomes hyperemic (increased blood to a part) and edematous.

Clinical Manifestations. The manifestations of meningitis may occur insidiously or suddenly, beginning with fever, vomiting, headache, irritability, photophobia, and **nuchal rigidity** (pain and stiffness in the neck when flexed) and may progress to decreased level of consciousness and seizures. Infants may exhibit a bulging fontanelle. Classic signs of meningeal irritation include: positive *Kernig sign* (resistance to knee extension in the supine position with the hips and knees flexed against the torso) and positive *Brudzinski sign* (flexion of the knees and hips when the neck is flexed rapidly onto the chest). Meningococcal meningitis, the most readily transmissible type of meningitis, may also produce petechiae and may rapidly progress to death without prompt initiation of proper treatment.

Diagnostic Tests. Meningitis is diagnosed by a carefully obtained history and physical and by analysis of CSF obtained by a lumbar puncture. A CSF sample is obtained for culture and sensitivity. Findings that indicate a bacterial infection include presence of a bacterial organism, elevated WBC count, elevated protein level, and decreased glucose level.

Medical Management. The management of bacterial meningitis involves immediate IV administration of appropriate antibiotic therapy. Therapy is usually continued for at least 10 days or until the CSF culture is negative. The child is usually isolated from other children, family, and staff until appropriate antibiotic therapy has been administered for at least 24 hours. Appropriate hydration, antipyretics, and comfort measures are instituted. The child is closely observed for complications of meningitis, including seizures, disseminated intravascular coagulation syndrome, and shock. Safety measures should be instituted because the child may develop seizures. After discharge the child is closely followed to assess for any sequelae of the disease, such as hearing impairments and cognitive, perceptual, language, and behavioral problems.

Prevention. The spread of bacterial meningitis can be avoided in the exposed siblings by prescribing prophylactic rifampin. Primary prevention strategies are focused on the administration of vaccines.

Nursing Interventions. Initial nursing interventions focused on rapid identification of the child with meningitis and prompt institution of appropriate antibiotic therapy. Nurses should take all necessary precautions to prevent the spread of the disease to themselves and others. Rest should be promoted for the child in the initial phase of the disease and environmental stimuli (especially noise and bright lights) should be kept to a minimum. The child may be most comfortable without a pillow and with the head of the bed elevated. Observations of vital signs, level of consciousness, I&O, and neurological signs should be made at frequent intervals. Families should be supported throughout the course of the disease; they are usually unprepared for the sudden acuteness of the disease and may feel guilty for not recognizing it earlier.

Patient/family teaching. With immunization schedules now calling for administration of Hib vaccine to infants at 2 months of age, parents should be encouraged to bring their child to a health facility so that the full series of inoculations is completed. With the high mortality associated with bacterial meningitis, early immunization can prevent families from experiencing the tragic death of a child. Nurses play a significant role in educating families regarding preventive measures such as early Hib vaccinations.

Prognosis. Although antimicrobial therapy has had a significant effect on the course of meningitis, it remains a potentially life-threatening disease. The age of the child, the type of organism, the severity of the infection, the duration of the illness before the onset of therapy, and the sensitivity of the organism to antimicrobial drugs are important factors in the prognosis. Possible residual deficits such as communicating hydrocephalus and possible hearing loss, blindness, seizures, learning disorders, and attention deficit disorder can occur.

Encephalitis

Encephalitis is defined as an inflammation of the CNS, namely, the brain tissue and spinal cord. The course of the disease closely resembles that of meningitis, and the care for each is similar.

Etiology/Pathophysiology. Encephalitis can be caused by a variety of organisms, such as bacteria, spirochetes, fungi, protozoa, and viruses. Most cases of encephalitis occur as a result of direct invasion of the CNS by a virus or from postinfectious involvement after a viral illness, such as measles, mumps, or varicella.

Clinical Manifestations. The manifestations of encephalitis can begin gradually or suddenly and may include malaise, fever, headache, dizziness, nuchal rigidity, nausea, vomiting, ataxia, tremors, seizures, and coma, and may proceed to death.

Diagnostic Tests. Diagnosis of encephalitis is based on clinical manifestations associated with the disease and, if possible, identification of the virus. Laboratory detection of the virus can be made through serological tests or CSF cultures.

Medical Management. Children suspected of having encephalitis are promptly hospitalized for strict observation and supportive care. Treatment is primarily supportive. Management is focused on controlling fever, suring adequate hydration and nutrition, monitoring vital signs, and observing for complications.

Nursing Interventions. Nursing interventions for the child with encephalitis are the same as for the child with meningitis (refer to Nursing Interventions section under meningitis). The major focus of care involves administering medication, controlling fever, monitoring neurological status and vital signs, and providing emotional support to the child and family.

Patient/family teaching. Follow-up care with periodic re-evaluation and rehabilitation are important for survivors with residual effects of the disease. The parents should be encouraged to keep appointments for follow-up examinations.

Prognosis. The prognosis depends on the child's age, the type of organism, and residual neurological damage. Children younger than 2 years of age may exhibit increased neurological disability, including learning disabilities and seizure disorders.

Hydrocephalus

Hydrocephalus is a condition characterized by an excess of fluid within the cranial vault, subarachnoid space, or both. It is caused by an imbalance between the production and absorption of CSF within the ventricular system. Hydrocephalus may develop from infancy (as a congenital lesion) and through adulthood.

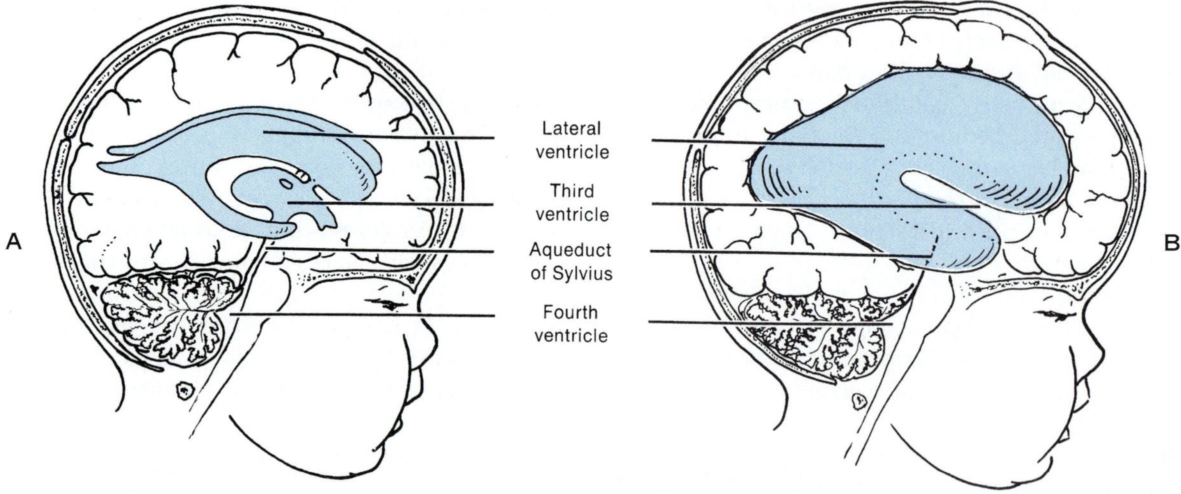

FIG. 44-28 Hydrocephalus; a block in the flow of CSF. **A,** Patent CSF circulation. **B,** Enlarged lateral and third ventricle caused by obstruction of circulation—stenosis of the aqueduct of Sylvius.

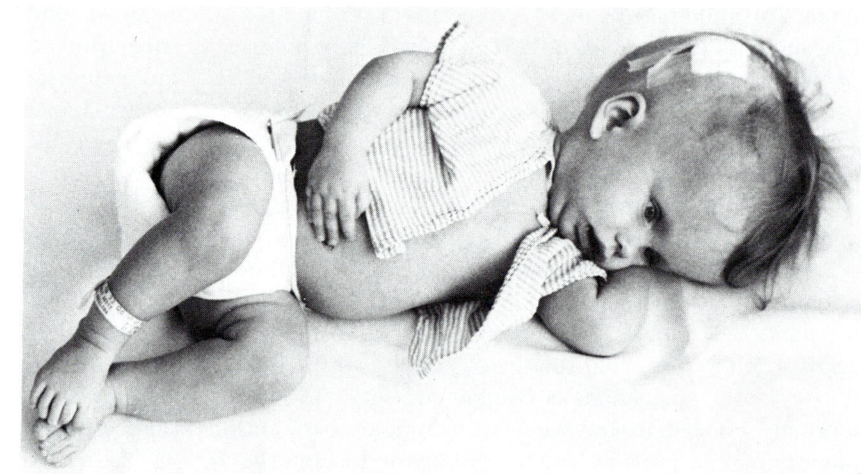

FIG. 44-29 Child with enlarged head caused by hydrocephalus.

Etiology/Pathophysiology. Hydrocephalus is caused by increased production of CSF, by obstruction within the ventricular system (noncommunicating hydrocephalus; no passage of fluid between the ventricles), or by defective reabsorption of the CSF (communicating hydrocephalus; passage of CSF between the ventricles). Overproduction of CSF is most commonly caused by a tumor in the choroid plexus. Obstruction within the ventricular system is most frequently caused by a congenital atresia, most commonly along the aqueduct of Sylvius (see Fig. 35-9). Other causes of obstruction include a hemorrhage, a growing tumor, or an infection. Defects in the body's reabsorptive process can be caused by an extensive hemorrhage within the subarachnoid space, which obscures the absorption surface of the membrane.

As CSF accumulates within the cranium, the brain is compressed against the skull and the ventricular system becomes dilated, increasing intracranial pressure (Fig. 44-28). If hydrocephalus occurs before the fusion of the cranial sutures, the skull becomes markedly enlarged (Fig. 44-29).

Clinical Manifestations. In early infancy, manifestations of hydrocephalus include widening and bulging of the fontanelles, separation of the cranial sutures, dilation of scalp veins, thin and shiny scalp, and rapidly increasing head circumference. As CSF accumulation continues, frontal "bossing" (prominence of the forehead) becomes apparent. Other manifestations are depressed eyes with "setting sun" sign (sclera is seen above the iris), slow pupil response to light, irritability, high-pitched cry, diffi-

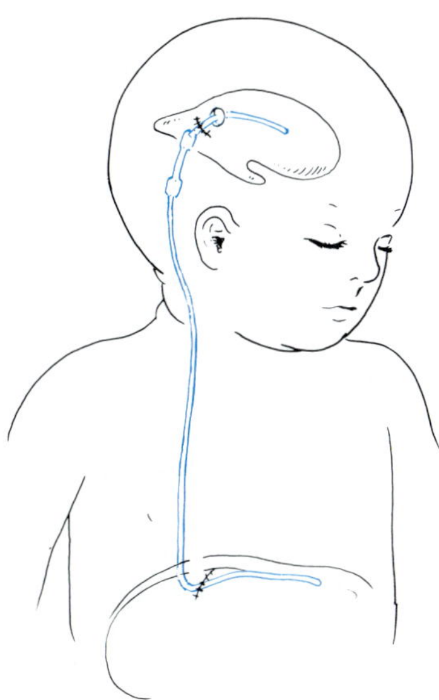

FIG. 44-30 Ventricular peritoneal shunt. Catheter is threaded subcutaneously from small incisions at the sites of ventricular and peritoneal insertions.

culty in being consoled, lethargy, altered level of consciousness, and difficulty in sucking and feeding. In children, manifestations may include headache upon awakening, hyperactive reflexes, strabismus, unsteady gait, irritability, papilledema (edema of the optic disc), lethargy, disorientation, and progression to stupor.

Diagnostic Tests. In infants, measurement of the head circumference is the most important diagnostic technique. All infants should have the head circumference measured routinely. Any measurement that crosses one or more grid lines within a 2- to 4-week period is suggestive of hydrocephalus. Other diagnostic assessments include observation of neurological signs that may indicate increased intracranial pressure, CT scan, and MRI.

Medical Management. If a tumor is the cause of hydrocephalus, it is surgically removed. If the cause of the hydrocephalus is obstruction, then the treatment involves surgical shunting of excess CSF from the ventricles to the peritoneum with a ventricular peritoneal shunt (V-P shunt) (Fig. 44-30). Revisions in the V-P shunt are needed when the shunt malfunctions, becomes infected, or when it becomes too short as the child grows.

Nursing Interventions. Nursing interventions for the child with hydrocephalus involve assisting with prompt diagnosis, observing for complications of the disease and shunt placement, and providing support and education to the family. Nutrition may be affected if intracranial pressure increases. Handling the child before, during, and after feedings should be avoided as it may lead to vomiting. Small, frequent feedings may be better tolerated, and infants should be placed on their sides after feedings to avoid aspiration. Postoperatively, the child is observed for signs of increasing intracranial pressure, vital signs are assessed, and I&O are closely monitored. The child is usually placed on the nonoperative side to avoid pressure on the shunt site. Skin care, especially to the scalp, should be meticulously performed both preoperatively and postoperatively. A sheepskin should be placed under the child's head, and position should be changed every 2 hours. The family should be supported during the hospitalization and prepared for discharge.

Nursing diagnoses and interventions for the child with hydrocephalus include but are not limited to the following:

NURSING DIAGNOSES	NURSING INTERVENTIONS
Infection, high risk for, related to presence of mechanical drainage system	Wash hands before contact with patient. Limit visitors to reduce the number of organisms in patient's environment, and restrict visitation by individuals with any type of infection. Encourage adequate diet to maintain optimal nutritional status. Maintain asepsis for dressing changes/ wound care.
Family processes, altered, related to situational crisis (child with a physical defect)	Facilitate family's acceptance of infant: ■ Allow expression of feelings ■ Convey attitude of acceptance of infant and family ■ Indicate by behavior that infant is a valuable human being

Patient/family teaching To prepare for the child's discharge and home care, the parents are instructed on how to recognize signs that indicate shunt malfunction or infection and how to pump if necessary. Safe transportation is an essential issue to discuss with parents. Small infants can be restrained reclining in an approved car bed. It is important to emphasize that hydrocephalus is a lifelong problem and that the child will require evaluation on a regular basis. The overall aim is to establish realistic goals and an appropriate educational program that will assist the child to achieve optimal potential.

Prognosis. The prognosis of children with treated hydrocephalus depends largely on the rate at which hydrocephalus develops, the duration of raised intracranial pressure (ICP), the frequency of complications, and the cause of hydrocephalus. With prompt diagnosis and proper shunt functioning, the survival rate for children with hydrocephalus is 80%.

Cerebral Palsy (CP)

CP is the most common permanent physical disability of childhood, affecting 1.2 to 2 in every 1000 live births.

CP is a general term given to a group of nonprogressive disorders of motor neuron impairment that result in motor dysfunction. In addition, the child may also exhibit intellectual, visual, language, and neurological impairments. The primary manifestations of CP involve abnormal muscle tone and poor coordination.

Etiology/Pathophysiology. Many antenatal, perinatal, and postnatal factors have been implicated in the etiology of CP. Antenatal factors include maternal nutritional deficiencies, infections, maternal drug ingestion, maternal metabolic disturbances, maternal hemorrhage, toxemia, and blood incompatibilities. Perinatal factors include cerebral trauma and anoxia during birth. Anoxia plays the most significant role in the pathology of brain damage. Anesthesia or analgesia during labor and delivery, prematurity, and metabolic or electrolyte disturbances are also factors. Postnatal factors include infection, head trauma, cerebrovascular accident, and poisoning.

Clinical Manifestations. The clinical manifestations of CP can range from moderate to severe and are described in Box 44-8.

Diagnostic Tests. The diagnosis of CP is based on history and physical examination. A careful antenatal and birth history should be obtained from the mother and documented. A thorough neurological examination is an essential component in the physical examination process and may aid in establishing a diagnosis of CP. Additional tests may include CT scan, cranial sonogram, electroencephalogram (EEG), and a serum metabolic screening.

Medical Management. There is no specific treatment for CP. Children with CP benefit from the integrated efforts of occupational, physical, and speech and hearing therapists. Care for the child is provided in the home and at an early-intervention center where children can benefit from specialized services and parents can support each other. Some orthopedic abnormalities may require corrective surgery, casting, or bracing.

Box 44-8 CLINICAL MANIFESTATIONS OF CP

- Delayed gross motor development
- Involuntary movements
- Hypertonic muscles
- Poor sucking
- Feeding difficulties
- Persistence of primitive reflexes
- Exaggerated deep tendon reflexes
- Arching of back
- Vision and hearing impairments
- Extension and scissoring of lower extremities
- Developmental disabilities

Nursing Interventions. Nursing interventions for the child with CP is focused on early recognition and prompt institution of interventions aimed at providing optimum development. Eating can be facilitated with the use of adaptive eating utensils. Self-feeding and a high-calorie diet should be encouraged. It is important to encourage mobilization. Devices such as braces, wheeled scooters, and walkers are available to assist with mobility. Protective head gear should be encouraged when a child is first learning to walk. It is important to praise children when goals are attained and encourage them to be as independent as possible within their limitations.

Nursing diagnoses and nursing interventions for the child with CP include but are not limited to the following:

NURSING DIAGNOSES	NURSING INTERVENTIONS
Physical mobility, impaired, related to neuromuscular impairment	Encourage sitting, crawling, and walking at appropriate ages. Carry out therapies that strengthen and improve control. Assist child in using appropriate leg motions when learning to walk. Provide incentives to locomote. Ensure the child is rested before attempting locomotion activities. Incorporate play that encourages desired behavior. Employ aids that facilitate locomotion such as parallel bars, crutches.
Self-care deficits, bathing/hygiene, dressing/grooming, feeding, toileting, related to physical disability	Encourage child to assist with care as age and capabilities permit. Select toys and activities that allow maximum participation by child and that improve motor function and sensory input. Avoid undue persistence by health care provider to accomplish a goal. Assist with jaw control during feeding. Adapt utensils, foods, and clothing to facilitate self-help (e.g., large-bowled spoon with padded handle; finger foods and foods that adhere to, rather than slip from, utensil; and clothing that opens in front with self-adhering closings rather than buttons). Assist parents in toilet training child.

Patient/family teaching. Parents should be taught proper handling of their children and how to assist them with ADLs. The family is taught to perform stretching and passive ROM exercises and to select play activities that provide for maximum stimulation and participation. Parents should also be educated about the disorder and the resources available to them so they may ensure optimal development for their child.

Prognosis. CP is a chronic neurological disability. There is no cure, but promotion of an optimal developmental course is vital so the child may realize full potential within the limits of the brain dysfunction.

Seizure Disorders

Etiology/Pathophysiology. The term *seizure* refers to a sudden, excessive, disorderly discharge of abnormal electrical impulses by the brain's neurons, causing a temporary alteration in CNS function. Most seizures are idiopathic, with no identifiable cause. Some seizures are acquired and result from such conditions as tumors, trauma, hypoxia, infections, poisons, fever, and metabolic disturbances. Children are most prone to seizures during the period between birth and 2 years of age. Approximately 5% of children will experience at least one seizure before they are adolescents. Epilepsy or recurrent seizures affect 1% to 2% of all children. For a complete discussion of seizure disorders, see Chapter 35.

Medical Management. The treatment of seizure disorders primarily involves drug therapy. Anticonvulsants that are most valuable in controlling partial and/or generalized seizures include carbamazepine (Tegretol) and phenytoin (Dilantin). The initial treatment of status epilepticus is focused on supporting and maintaining vital functions, including securing a patent airway, administering oxygen, establishing venous access, providing hydration, and administering lorazepam (Ativan), diazepam (Valium), or phenobarbital, as ordered. After the continuous seizure is stopped, the child may be given a loading dose of phenytoin to assure sustained control of seizures.

Anticonvulsant therapy is continued for a prolonged period. Dosage modifications are made as the child grows. There is recent evidence to support the theory that, in children with a normal EEG who have been seizure-free for at least 2 years, anticonvulsant medications can be successfully discontinued without increasing the risk of seizure recurrence. Discontinuance of the medication should be done gradually over 1 to 2 weeks. Abrupt withdrawal of anticonvulsants may result in an increase in the number and severity of seizures and can precipitate an episode of status epilepticus.

Nursing Interventions. Nursing interventions for the child with a seizure disorder involve assisting with the diagnosis, providing acute care during a seizure, providing for long-term management of the seizure disorder, and supporting and assisting the child and family. To assist with the diagnosis of a seizure disorder it is essential to observe the child during a seizure and carefully document events, including any precipitating factors, if known or suspected; behavior before the seizure; time seizure began and ended; clinical manifestations of the seizure; and postseizure behavior and signs and symptoms. It is important to recognize precipitating factors and prevent or minimize the child's exposure to them. It is important to protect the child from injury during a seizure. Measures to prevent injuries during a seizure include padding the bed siderails and keeping them upright, easing the child to the floor from a sitting or standing position, moving furniture out of the way, loosening restrictive clothing, and turning the child's head to the side to prevent aspiration of secretions. It is important not to force an object (e.g., tongue blade, airway) between the child's teeth during a seizure because it may cause oral trauma. Staying with the child during and after a seizure and providing reassurance, emotional support, and explanations will minimize the child's anxiety. A significant nursing goal is to promote a positive self-image in the child through encouragement and identification of the child's strengths and assets. Providing emotional support to the family is also essential. Encourage parents to express their fears and concerns and assist them to understand their child's condition. The family needs education regarding the nature of the disorder and possible precipitating factors, seizure precaution measures, dosage and side effects of medications, and the importance of maintaining as normal a life-style as possible.

Patient/family teaching. It is important to impress on the family the need to continue the medication regularly, without interruption, for as long as required. The nurse can help the parents plan the administration of the medication at convenient times to minimize disruption of family routine. Although anticonvulsant drugs are available in liquid extracts or emulsions, the tablet form is preferred by neurologists. The unequal distribution of the drug in the solute and the increased likelihood of inaccurate measurements make liquid medication less desirable.

Prognosis. Seizures can be controlled or greatly reduced in the majority of children, and new studies hold the promise of progress in future treatment. Seizures will not shorten the life of the child, and the child can attend school, marry, and elect to have children.

Spina Bifida (Myelomeningocele)

Spina bifida is a term used to describe a variety of congenital defects of **neural tube** (tube formed from the fusion of the neural folds from which the brain and spinal cord arise) closure. When the neural tube fails to close during embryological development, a defect is produced that may involve a small area of the neural tube or its entire length. On examination the infant may have a tuft of hair, cleft, or small, fatty mass over the defect. *Myelomeningocele* is one form of spina bifida whereby portions of the spinal cord, the meninges, spinal fluid, and nerves protrude through the neural tube defect.

Etiology/Pathophysiology. The etiology of neural tube defects is generally unknown. Poor nutrition and advanced maternal age have been implicated as contributing factors. Recent evidence supports the theory that neural tube defects may be caused by the interaction of a genetic predisposition with an essential nutrient deficiency (folic acid), and that multivitamins containing folic acid taken during the first 6 weeks of pregnancy will prevent (by more than 50%) their occurrence.[18]

Clinical Manifestations. Because the spinal cord most commonly ends at the defect, all motor and sensory function beyond the defect is absent. Most myelomeningoceles involve the lumbar and lumbosacral areas. Depending on the level of the defect, the infant may have flaccid paralysis and sensory deficits of the lower extremities, bowel and bladder incontinence, clubfoot defects, and a subluxated hip (a partial or incomplete dislocation of the hip). Hydrocephalus is present in 80% of affected infants.

Diagnostic Tests. It may be possible to detect a neural tube defect prenatally. Uterine ultrasound and elevated maternal **alpha-fetoprotein (AFP)** (antigen present in the human fetus that can be used to evaluate fetal development) level can indicate the presence of a myelomeningocele. After birth the diagnosis is made on the basis of clinical manifestations. A CT scan may be performed to assess for the presence of hydrocephalus.

Medical Management. Treatment for the infant with myelomeningocele involves surgery to replace the neural contents within the sac to eliminate the possibility of infection. A V-P shunt may have to be inserted to provide relief from hydrocephalus (for a discussion of hydrocephalus, see pp. 1419-1421). Corrective surgeries may be required for hip and lower extremity deformities. Additional measures include continuous neurological assessments and assisting the family to deal with the diagnosis and surgery.

Nursing Interventions. Nursing interventions for the child with myelomeningocele are focused on preventing infection and complications, providing postoperative care, and supporting and educating the family. Nursing interventions for the child with myelomeningocele are described in Box 44-9.

Parents will need explanations regarding their child's condition and the surgery it requires. Family members should be encouraged to express their fears and concerns and advised of resources within their community that provide support and services for families of children with spinal defects.

Patient/family teaching. Because the care that has been instituted in the hospital will be continued at home, parents will need to be instructed on positioning, feeding, bowel training, bladder catheterization, and physical exercises.

Box 44-9 NURSING INTERVENTIONS FOR THE CHILD WITH MYELOMENINGOCELE

PREOPERATIVE

- Position child on abdomen.
- Cover sac with sterile, saline-soaked guaze.
- Protect sac from contact with feces and urine.

POSTOPERATIVE

- Position child on abdomen for 10-14 days (until incision is healed).
- Monitor vital signs.
- Observe for signs of bleeding and infection.

Prognosis. The early prognosis for the child with myelomeningocele depends on the neurological deficits present at birth, including motor ability and bladder innervation and the presence of associated cerebral anomalies. Improved surgical techniques do not alter the major physical disability and deformity or chronic urinary tract and pulmonary infections that affect the quality of life for these children.

Narcotic Abstinence Syndrome

Because narcotics readily cross the placental membrane, women who use drugs while they are pregnant cause a passive addiction in their unborn children. Narcotics commonly abused by women during pregnancy include cocaine, "crack," heroin, and methadone. Shortly after birth the infant exhibits signs and symptoms of drug withdrawal, including irritability, disturbed sleeping and feeding patterns, tremors, seizures, hyperreflexia (increased reflex reaction), clonus (abnormal neuromuscular activity characterized by rapidly alternating involuntary contraction and relaxation of skeletal muscles), high-pitched cry, hypertonic muscles, tachypnea, frantic sucking of hands, vomiting, diarrhea, and inability to maintain body temperature. Signs and symptoms of narcotic withdrawal may persist for 3 to 4 months. Infants suspected of having narcotic abstinence syndrome can have their urine analyzed for metabolites of the drug. It is essential to obtain a urine sample from the infant immediately after birth because the byproducts of the drugs are quickly cleared from the body.

Infants who are suffering from narcotic abstinence syndrome are most comfortable in a nonstimulating environment that is free from bright lights and loud noises. They may prefer to be tightly swaddled in a blanket with a pacifier to satisfy their vigorous sucking needs. It is essential for the nurse to monitor the infant's I&O and vital signs. Nursing interventions should be organized in a manner that reduces the amount of disturbance to the infant.

Patient/Family Teaching. Upon discharge the infant will need to be referred to an early intervention program because they are at risk for neurological problems; parent-infant bonding difficulties; and developmental, behavioral, and learning disabilities. Mothers will need to be referred for parental education and drug treatment programs to enable an optimal outcome for both the child and family.

Neuroblastoma

Neuroblastoma is a malignant hemorrhagic tumor composed principally of cells resembling neuroblasts that give rise to cells of the sympathetic system. After brain tumors, neuroblastomas are the most common solid tumors in childhood, with an incidence of approximately 10 per million white children and 7 per million black children per year. More than 50% of the cases occur in children less than 2 years of age, and 75% are encountered during the first 4 years of life. Neuroblastoma is a malignant tumor that has a high rate of dissemination, with 70% of patients having metastasis at the time of presentation.

Etiology/Pathophysiology. These tumors originate from embryonic neural crest cells that normally give rise to the adrenal medulla and the sympathetic ganglia. Consequently, the majority of tumors develop in the adrenal gland or the retroperitoneal sympathetic chain. Other sites include the head, neck, chest, or pelvis. The most common sites for metastatic disease include the liver, skin, lymph nodes, bone, and bone marrow.

Clinical Manifestations. The clinical manifestations of neuroblastoma depend on the location of the tumor. The most common location is the abdomen, and manifestations may include a palpable, firm, irregular mass that crosses the midline; anorexia; bowel and bladder alterations related to compression by the tumor; and spinal cord compression. If the tumor is located in the upper chest, manifestations include dyspnea, difficulty swallowing, and neck and facial edema. Many of the manifestations at the time of diagnosis are the result of metastatic disease. Manifestations of metastasis are hepatomegaly, splenomegaly, anemia, bone and joint pain, skin nodules (especially in infants), periorbital edema, weight loss, pallor, and weakness.

Diagnostic Tests. Initial diagnostic studies are focused on locating the primary tumor site and areas of metastasis. In addition to a complete history and physical, other studies include skeletal survey, bone scan, CT scan, abdominal ultrasound, bone marrow aspiration and biopsy, and urine collection for catecholamine (biologically active amines, epinephrine, and norepinephrine) metabolites (adrenal tumors will stimulate the production of catecholamines). A biopsy of the tumor provides a definitive (final) diagnosis and staging information.

Medical Management. The management of neuroblastoma involves a combination of surgery, radiation therapy, and chemotherapy. If the tumor is localized, surgical removal of the tumor followed by radiation therapy will be done. If there is widely disseminated disease, as much of the tumor as possible is removed and the child will receive follow-up chemotherapy and radiation therapy.

Nursing Interventions. Initial nursing interventions are focused on preparing the child for diagnostic and operative procedures. Postoperative care is similar to that for any child undergoing abdominal surgery, including observation of any postoperative complications. Psychological support of the family is essential and involves helping them to prepare for the diagnostic and operative procedures and postoperative complications. Parents will need an opportunity to express their fears and concerns. Because of the high incidence of metastasis at diagnosis, parents may feel guilty that they did not seek medical attention sooner.

Patient/family teaching. Parents will need to be educated about any chemotherapy or radiation therapy that is needed.

Prognosis. Because of the frequency of invasiveness, the prognosis for neuroblastoma is poor. Generally the younger the child at diagnosis (especially under 1 year of age), the better the survival rates. Also, neuroblastoma is one of the few tumors that demonstrates spontaneous regression, possibly as a result of maturity of the embryonic cell or the development of an active immune system.

DISORDERS OF COGNITIVE FUNCTION

A child's mental health is an integral part of the total well-being of the child. A variety of factors influence the personality and developmental capabilities of a child, including genetic composition, environment, social support, and culture. Children should be assessed for emotional as well as physical problems during all visits with a health care provider. Children who have been diagnosed with a cognitive impairment and their families require prompt intervention by specialists in the field of mental health. The nurse is instrumental in providing appropriate referrals and offering support to the child and family.

Cognitive Impairment

Cognitive impairment (formerly referred to as mental retardation) is the most common developmental disability, affecting up to 3% of the population. It is defined as significantly subaverage general intellectual functioning existing concurrently with deficits in adaptive behavior and manifested during the developmental period.[6] Cognitive impairment is classified into four general categories on the basis of an **intelligence quotient (IQ)** (an index of relative intelligence determined through the subject's answers to arbitrarily chosen questions): (1) mild (educable cognitive impaired): IQ of 50-55 to approximately 70; (2) moderate (trainable cognitive impaired): IQ of 35-40 to 50-55; (3) severe: IQ of 20-25 to 35-40; (4) profound: IQ below 20-25.

Etiology/Pathophysiology. The causes of cognitive impairment are varied, including biochemical, infectious, genetic, endocrine, and idiopathic. Specific causes include chromosomal abnormalities such as Down syndrome, perinatal infections (e.g., cytomegalovirus, rubella, syphilis, toxoplasmosis), perinatal anoxia, maternal drug or alcohol abuse, metabolic disorders such as phenylketonuria, lead poisoning, hypothyroidism, and prematurity.

Clinical Manifestations. Manifestations vary according to the child's age and degree of impairment. Children may fail to achieve developmental milestones at appropriate ages. Generally, they may manifest delays in motor, social, cognitive, and language skills.

Diagnostic Tests. Assessment of the child suspected of having cognitive impairment should begin as soon as the parents or health care provider realizes the child is not developing normally. Diagnostic studies include neurological examination, CT scan, serum metabolic screening, developmental screening tests (e.g., Denver Developmental Screening Test), standardized intellectual tests (e.g., Stanford-Binet Intelligence Scale, Wechsler Intelligence Scale for Children), and chromosomal analysis and genetic screening.

Nursing Interventions. The nursing interventions for a child with a cognitive impairment is focused on promoting optimum development and providing the family with support, education, and referrals. The family needs to be supported at the time of initial diagnosis and encouraged to verbalize their fears and concerns. Parents should be encouraged to enroll the child in an early intervention program that can facilitate the child's self-care abilities and assist the family with future needs. Each task taught should be broken into small, specific steps because the child may not be able to understand the task as a whole. Parents should be encouraged to emphasize the normal needs of all children regardless of cognitive ability, including love, social interaction, and play.

Patient/family teaching. It is essential to provide parents with information on normal developmental milestones, stimulation techniques, safety, normal speech development, sexual development, and the role of positive self-esteem in motivating children to accomplish goals within their limitations.

Prognosis. Cognitive impairment is a chronic condition. In recent years major changes have occurred in the philosophy of care toward people with cognitive impairment. Children with cognitive impairment are no longer automatically admitted into institutional settings but often remain at home.

Down Syndrome

Down syndrome is the most common chromosomal abnormality, affecting 1 in 800 live births. It was once referred to as mongolism because affected children have a slant to their eyes that makes them appear Oriental.

Etiology/Pathophysiology. The majority of cases of Down syndrome (95%) are attributable to an extra chromosome on the 21st pair, hence the term *trisomy 21.* The risk of having a child with Down syndrome increases with increasing maternal age, especially those over 35 years of age.

Clinical Manifestations. Children with Down syndrome have a characteristic facial appearance (Fig. 44-31). Most frequently, manifestations in the infant include a small, rounded skull with a flat occiput; upward-slanting eyes; broad, flat nose; protruding tongue; short, thick neck; hypotonic extremities; mottled skin; low-set ears; and a simian crease on the palmar side of the hand. All children with Down syndrome have some degree of intellectual impairment, ranging from low normal intelligence to severe cognitive impairment. Children with Down syndrome are prone to upper respiratory infections, and many children have congenital heart defects. Other associated health problems include hypothyroidism and increased incidence of leukemia.

Diagnostic Tests. In addition to the characteristic manifestations as an adjunct to the diagnosis of Down syndrome, a chromosomal analysis should be performed to confirm the chromosomal abnormality.

Medical Management. In addition to routine medical care, corrective surgery may be indicated for congenital heart defects. Auditory and vision screening should be conducted to assess for any sensory impairments. Thyroid function tests are also recommended.

Nursing Interventions. Care for the child with Down syndrome is similar to that for the child with a cognitive impairment (refer to Nursing Intervention section under

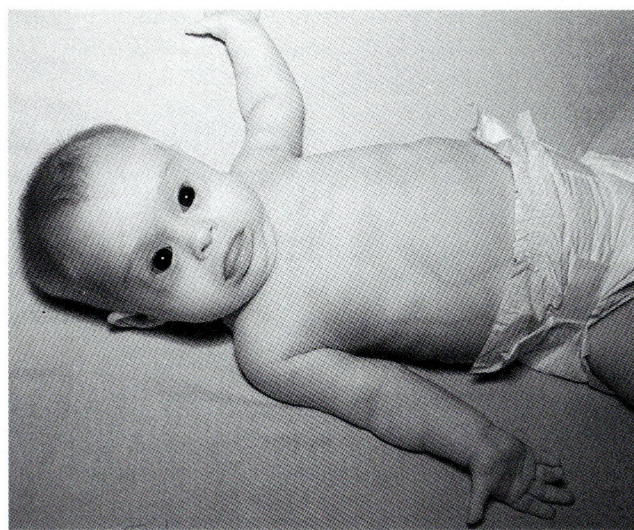

FIG. 44-31 Down syndrome in infant. Note small, square head; upward slant to the eyes; flat nasal bridge; protruding tongue; mottled skin; and hypotonia.

cognitive impairment). Primary nursing goals include supporting the family at the time of diagnosis and referring the child and family to agencies that provide support and services.

Patient/family teaching. The family will need education regarding their child's condition.

Prognosis. The life expectancy for people with Down syndrome has improved in recent years but remains lower than that for the general population. Over 80% of those afflicted survive to age 30 years and beyond. Down syndrome is associated with earlier aging, and virtually all deceased individuals have neurological changes associated with Alzheimer's disease.[3]

Lead Poisoning

Lead poisoning is one of the most common, preventable, serious health care problems affecting children in the United States today. Lead levels small enough to be asymptomatic may insidiously cause neurological deficits in exposed children. Lead levels as low as 10 micrograms per deciliter (μg/dl) have been shown to cause significant health concerns in children.

Etiology/Pathophysiology. Lead in the environment that is either ingested or inhaled continues to be the most important contributing factor in lead poisoning. The primary sources of lead exposure are lead-based paint or caulking chips, lead-contaminated soil and dust, and drinking water that has traveled through lead or lead-soldered pipes. Ingested lead is slowly excreted from the body through the GI and GU tracts. Lead that is retained is stored in the bone where it remains inactive. When the level of ingested lead exceeds the amount that can be absorbed by the bone, lead travels through the body in the circulatory system and leads to anemia. Lead poisoning may also cause serious, irreversible damage to the CNS. Low lead levels can also be detrimental to the CNS, resulting in behavioral, cognitive, intellectual, and sensory deficits.

Clinical Manifestations. Manifestations of lead poisoning include anemia, anorexia, abdominal pain, lethargy, impulsiveness, irritability, learning difficulties, decreased attention span, decreased curiosity, hearing deficits, growth and developmental failure, and **pica** (craving to eat nonfood substances).

Diagnostic Tests. Direct measurement of blood levels remains the primary diagnostic technique in the assessment of lead poisoning. Additionally, a complete history and physical examination and an environmental assessment provide valuable information that will identify exposed children and environments at highest risk. Supplemental diagnostic studies include an x-ray of the abdomen, which may show recently ingested pain chips in the intestinal tract; long-bone x-rays, which may reveal "lead lines" (areas of increased density) near the epiphyseal lines; and urine studies to detect proteinuria, ketonuria, and glycosuria, which may result from lead-induced kidney damage.

Medical Management. The management of lead poisoning is determined by the child's blood level. The primary objective of treatment is to remove lead from the body and prevent further exposure to lead. Pharmacological treatment, such as **chelation therapy** (in toxicology, to use a compound to grasp a toxic substance and make it nonactive and thus nontoxic) is utilized with children who have excessive lead levels. The precise course of therapy and chelating agent depend on the preference of the practitioner and the severity of the child's condition. Emphasis is also placed on improving nutritional deficiencies and preventing infection.

Nursing Interventions. The challenges of lead poisoning provide a unique opportunity to pediatric nurses. With a shift toward primary prevention, nurses can be instrumental in the quest to end childhood lead poisoning. Prevention strategies are directed toward identifying and responding to lead sources for the population of children at risk and the communities in which they live. This can be accomplished by completing a thorough environmental and health questionnaire at each routine health visit to assess a child's potential risk for lead exposure. Since lead is everywhere in the environment, essentially all children are at risk for lead poisoning. Therefore, the Centers for Disease Control and Prevention recommends that all children between the ages of 6 months and 6 years of age be screened for lead poisoning, except in communities where large numbers of screened children indicate there is not an excessive lead burden (lead levels less than 10 μg/dl). Parents also require support and understanding and should be provided with resources and referrals so that they may access assistance to help them with this problem.

Box 44-10 PARENT GUIDELINES FOR REDUCING BLOOD LEAD LEVELS

- Make sure child does not have access to peeling paint or chewable surfaces painted with lead-based paint, especially window sills and wells.
- If house was built before 1960 and has hard-surfaced floors, wet mop them at least once a week with a high-phosphate solution (e.g., trisodium phosphate (available in hardware stores). Wipe other hard surfaces (such as window sills and baseboards) with a similar solution. Do not vacuum hard-surfaced floors or window sills or wells, since this spreads dust. Use vacuum cleaners with agitators to remove dust from rugs rather than vacuum cleaners with suction only.
- Wash child's hands and face before eating.
- Wash toys and pacifiers frequently.
- If soil around home is likely to be contaminated with lead (e.g., if home was built before 1960 or is near a major highway), plant grass or other ground cover; plant bushes around outside of house so that child cannot play there.
- During remodeling of older homes, be sure to follow correct procedures. Be certain children and pregnant women are not in the home, day or night, until process is completed. Following deleading, thoroughly clean house using wet mopping before inhabitants return.
- In areas where lead content of water exceeds the drinking water standard, run water for at least 2 minutes from *cold-water* tap for drinking, cooking, and making formula; may use first-flush water for other purposes.
- Do not store food in open cans, particularly if cans are imported.
- Do not use pottery or ceramic ware that was inadequately fired or is meant for decorative use for food storage or service.
- Avoid folk remedies that contain lead.
- Make sure that home exposure is not occurring from parental occupations or hobbies. Household members employed in occupations such as lead smelting should shower and change into clean clothing before leaving work.
- Make sure child eats regular meals, since more lead is absorbed on an empty stomach.
- Make sure child's diet contains plenty of iron, calcium, protein, and zinc.

Modified from Centers for Disease Control: *Preventing lead poisoning in young children,* Atlanta, 1991, The Centers.

Patient/family teaching. Parent guidelines for reducing lead in the child's environment are described in Box 44-10.

Prognosis. Although most of the pathophysiological effects of lead are reversible, the most serious consequences of both high- and low-level lead exposure are the effects on the CNS. In children with lead encephalopathy, permanent brain damage results in cognitive impairment, behavior changes, possible paralysis, and seizures. However, low-dose exposure may also cause permanent neurological deficits.

DISORDERS OF INTEGUMENTARY FUNCTION

Skin function is affected by genetic factors, cleanliness, hydration, and nutrition. Dermatological disorders in children comprise a significant proportion of children's visits to physician's offices and clinics. Many of these disorders can be painful for the child as well as distressing for the family.

Noninfectious Disorders of the Skin

Contact Dermatitis.

Etiology/pathophysiology. Contact dermatitis is an inflammatory, delayed immune response of the skin resulting from contact with environmental antigens to which a person is hypersensitive. Contact dermatitis occurs more frequently in infants and toddlers, and frequently there is a family history of allergy. The most commonly affected areas include the face, neck, hands, feet, and legs. The allergens most common in children include soaps, detergents, bubble baths, shoe components, metals, chemicals, cosmetics, and plants such as poison ivy, oak, and sumac.

Clinical manifestations. The contact area becomes erythematous, edematous, and pruritic. Papules (solid, red, raised areas less than 0.5 cm in diameter) and vesicles (circumscribed raised areas filled with serous fluid and less than 0.5 cm in diameter) form and can weep and ooze if scratching breaks open the area.

Diagnostic tests. Diagnosis is made by observation of the pattern and location of the rash and by an accurate history to identify the causative agent. Skin testing may also be helpful in the identification of suspected plants, foods, or animals.

Medical management. Since the hypersensitive reaction is usually self-limiting, treatment is directed toward identifying and eliminating the cause and relieving signs and symptoms. Cool, wet dressings dipped in Burow's solution (solution of aluminum acetate, used as a drying agent for weeping skin lesions) or alkaline applications such as baking soda baths help soothe the affected area, as do topical antipruritics such as Caladryl lotion. These are all available without prescription. Topical, over-the-counter steroid creams may be applied to mild contact dermatitis. In more severe cases, systemic corticosteroids may be prescribed. Antihistamines such as Benadryl are helpful in controlling pruritus.

Nursing interventions. Advise the family to keep the child's fingernails clipped short to prevent a secondary bacterial infection from scratching. Loose, lightweight clothing during the healing phase is also comforting and decreases irritation.

Patient/family teaching. Parents are taught to keep an accurate history of possible causative agents. Once the primary irritant has been identified, it should be avoided. If the skin does come in contact with the causative agent, the affected area should be washed with a mild soap and water and dried thoroughly. Talcum powder, overheating, and hot baths should be avoided. Topical medications should be applied only as directed by a physician.

Prognosis. The reaction is usually self-limiting and should resolve within 2 weeks.

Diaper Dermatitis.

Etiology/pathophysiology. Diaper dermatitis is one of the most common skin disorders in infancy and the cause of great concern for many parents. Diaper dermatitis is a form of contact dermatitis and usually caused by an external irritant. The most common irritating agents include prolonged exposure to urine and/or feces; inadequate cleaning of the diaper area; soaps, detergents, or fabric softeners used to wash diapers; excessive use of powders or ointments; and the use of plastic pants. Fair-complexioned infants tend to have more sensitive skin and are more vulnerable to diaper rash than darker-complexioned infants. The peak age of occurrence is 9 to 12 months of age, and the incidence is higher in bottle-fed than in breastfed infants.

Clinical manifestations. The rash appears as erythematous papular lesions (similar in appearance to a scald) on the buttocks, labia or scrotum, inner thighs, and mons pubis—areas that come into direct contact with the diaper. Frequently, skin folds are spared. An excoriated perianal area may be due to frequent diarrhea. The inflammation does not take on a specific configuration; rather, it can appear in a variety of patterns. The moist, warm, dark environment created by the diaper can also promote the growth of secondary bacterial or fungal infections. The infant with diaper dermatitis is usually uncomfortable and may be fussy, irritable, and restless.

Diagnostic tests. The diagnosis of diaper dermatitis is usually made by clinical observation of the characteristics and location of the rash and an assessment of possible irritants. Bacterial or fungal cultures may be indicated for persistent secondary infections.

Medical management. Keeping the diaper area *clean and dry* is of primary importance. Measures to promote healing and prevent diaper dermatitis from recurring include changing diapers as soon as they become soiled, thorough cleansing of the diaper area with a mild soap and water and gentle drying at each diaper change, exposing the affected area to the air several times a day, avoidance of occlusive plastic pants, and the application of a small amount of a medicated powder or cornstarch to promote dryness. For more severe cases, a topical glucocorticoid may be required.

Nursing interventions. Protective ointments such as Desitin, A&D ointment, or zinc oxide may be used prophylactically. Keep diaper area clean. If powder is desired, a thin application of cornstarch or a cornstarch-based powder is preferred. Excessive amounts of powder in the presence of moisture will cake and excoriate the skin (Box 44-11).

Patient/family teaching. Parents should be taught the basics of diaper and skin care as outlined above. To prevent the infant's inhalation of powder dust, instruct parents to put a small amount in their hand and apply it to the baby's diaper area (Box 44-11).

Prognosis. Quick recognition with prompt therapy leads to a good prognosis.

Box 44-11 PARENT GUIDELINES FOR CONTROLLING DIAPER RASH

- Keep skin dry
  Use superabsorbent disposable diapers to reduce skin wetness.
  If using cloth diapers, use only overwraps that allow air to circulate; avoid rubber pants.
  Change diapers as soon as soiled, especially with stool, whenever possible, preferably once during the night.
  Expose healthy or only slightly irritated skin to air, not heat, to dry completely.
- Apply ointment, such as zinc oxide or petrolatum, to protect skin, especially if skin is very erythematous or has moist, open areas.
  When soiled, wipe off top layer of ointment and reapply.
  To completely remove ointment, especially zinc oxide, use mineral oil; do not wash vigorously.
- Avoid overwashing the skin, especially with perfumed soaps or commercial wipes that may be irritating.
  May use a moisturizer or nonsoap cleanser, such as cold cream or Cetaphil, to wipe urine from skin.
  Gently wipe stool from skin using water and mild soap, such as Dove.

NOTE: Powder helps keep the skin dry, but talc is very dangerous if breathed into the lungs. Plain cornstarch or cornstarch-based powder is safer. When using any powder product, shake it first into your hand, then apply it to the diaper area. Store the container away from the infant's reach; keep container closed when not in use.

Atopic Dermatitis (Eczema).

Etiology/pathophysiology. Atopic dermatitis is a pruritic, allergic response commonly seen in infancy and childhood. Atopy refers to an allergy for which there is a genetic or inherited predisposition. A familial history of asthma, allergic rhinitis, or dry skin is often present. The disease is also associated with hypersensitivity to histamine. The exact cause is unknown but is thought to be associated with food allergies and abnormal skin function. Infantile atopic dermatitis can occur between 2 and 5 months of age and can be problematic to age 2 or 3 years, when many children seem to "outgrow" the illness. Childhood atopic dermatitis usually occurs at age 2 or 3 years and may persist to 5 years of age. Adolescent atopic dermatitis is usually seen at 12 years of age and can last indefinitely.

Clinical manifestations. In infantile eczema the primary lesions consist of erythema, vesicles, and papules, which can ooze and crust. They appear most often on the cheeks, scalp, trunk, and extensor surfaces of the extremities. In childhood eczema the lesions appear as erythematous, scaly patches on the trunk, elbows, knees, ankles, hands, and feet and behind the ears. The skin becomes thick and leatherlike **(lichenification).** In adolescent eczema, the lesions are the same as in childhood but the distribution affects mainly the hands, feet, neck, and face. At any age, the unaffected skin is usually very dry, and the pruritus can be extremely intense. The child will often be uncomfortable and restless. Infants unable to scratch may rub their faces on linens or clothing in an effort to relieve the itch. Scratching or rubbing can also lead to secondary infections, and children with atopic dermatitis have been noted to have an increased susceptibility to bacterial *(Staphylococcus aureus),* viral (herpes simplex), and fungal skin infections. The signs and symptoms are better in humid climates and worse in fall and winter, when homes are heated and environmental humidity is lower.

Diagnostic tests. The diagnosis is made from clinical observation of the type and distribution of the lesions, a positive family history of allergy, and severity of pruritus. Skin testing to determine specific allergens is usually done in more severe cases.

Medical management. The therapeutic management includes hydration of the skin, controlling pruritus, decreasing inflammation, and preventing secondary infections. Skin hydration can be accomplished in a variety of ways. Tepid baths followed by the administration of a cream or lotion help trap moisture in the skin. The application of occlusive creams or ointments helps relieve dry skin. To decrease inflammation, thin applications of topical steroid creams or lotions are used. The strength and type of topical steroid used are determined by the degree of inflammation and the age of the child. Oral antihistamines such as diphenhydramine (Benadryl) or hydroxyzine (Atarax) are useful in controlling pruritus. Appropriate systemic antibiotics are used in secondary bacterial infections.

Nursing interventions. The nurse's role in caring for the child with atopic dermatitis involves measures to control pruritus, promote skin integrity, and provide support to the child and family. Compresses with Burow's solution soothe itching and moisten skin. Hot baths or showers are discouraged because of their drying effect on the skin. Cornstarch added to tepid bath water can provide some relief from itching as well as hydrate skin. If soap is to be used, it should be a mild, nonfragrant soap such as Dove or Neutrogena. To prevent new lesions or secondary infection, scratching must be kept to a minimum. For the infant, covering the hands with mittens or socks can reduce scratching. For the older child, gloves allow for more dexterity. At times, it may be necessary to use safety reminder devices to discourage scratching; however, it is important that the infant or child be free from these restrictions periodically.

Patient/family teaching. Overheating can intensify itching; therefore parents need to understand that dressing their child in lightweight, loose clothing made from cotton or cotton blends is preferable. Clothing, linens, and blankets should be washed and double rinsed to ensure removal of all soap residue. It is important for parents to understand that lubricants need to be applied frequently, especially after bathing while the skin is still damp to seal in moisture. Fingernails and toenails should be clipped short and kept clean to minimize the risk of infection. At any age, keeping hands busy with play activities provides the distraction needed to discourage scratching. The appearance, discomfort, and irritability displayed by children with atopic dermatitis can be very upsetting for family members. Encourage parents to verbalize their feelings and provide reassurance. Teaching stress-reduction techniques can be helpful to both the child and the parents because stress can trigger exacerbations of the illness.

Prognosis. Atopic dermatitis can be controlled but not cured. The majority of affected children (90%) "outgrow" atopic dermatitis by adolescence. Some may continue to have atopic dermatitis into adulthood.

Seborrheic Dermatitis.

Etiology/pathophysiology. Seborrheic dermatitis, or cradle cap, is a chronic inflammatory reaction of the skin commonly seen in infancy. Although the cause of the illness is unknown, it is thought to be related to sebaceous gland activity. Often, there is no family history of allergy.

Clinical manifestations. Seborrheic dermatitis most commonly affects the scalp and appears as thick, white or yellowish, crusty or scaly patches. Mild pruritus may accompany the disorder. Other areas commonly affected include the eyebrows or eyelids (blepharitis), the postauricular (behind the ear) area, the external ear (otitis externa), the nasolabial (nose and lip) folds, and the inguinal region (seborrheic diaper dermatitis).

Diagnostic tests. Diagnosis is made by clinical observation of the characteristics and location of crusty patches.

Medical management. Seborrheic dermatitis is managed by treating the signs and symptoms and simple preventive measures. Crusty, scaly patches can be removed by the application of mineral oil to the affected areas (except the eyelids) to help loosen crusts followed by shampooing with a mild, tearfree shampoo and thorough rinse. The hair is then brushed with a soft baby brush or a soft toothbrush to remove flakes from the hair. A fine-tooth comb also works well. Preventive measures include daily shampooing with an antiseborrheic shampoo. Topical corticosteroids are rarely needed.

Nursing interventions. Crusts should be soaked with warm water and cotton (or clean washcloth) compresses until loosened. The eye area is then cleansed with clean cotton (or a clean washcloth) and warm water, starting at the inner canthus and continuing to the outer canthus. For each stroke, a clean piece of cotton (or clean area on the washcloth) should be used (Table 44-4 on p. 1432).

Patient/family teaching. Often parents need reassurance that shampooing their infant's hair will not cause harm to the fontanelles. A demonstration on how to shampoo the hair may be necessary. If cradle cap is extensive, nurses should inform parents that several treatments may be necessary to loosen and remove all crusts. If the eyelids are involved, the parents should be taught how to safely clean these areas.

Prognosis. Lesions can appear shortly after birth to old age, with periods of remissions and exacerbations.

Acne Vulgaris. Acne is an inflammatory process of the skin commonly seen in adolescence. It is slightly more common in males. Peak incidence occurs between 16 and 17 years of age in females and 17 and 18 years in males, although lesions may be seen as early as age 9 or 10 years. Acne is a disease that involves the philosebaceous follicles (the hair follicles and sebaceous gland complex) of the face, neck, shoulders, back, and upper chest.

Nursing interventions. The adolescent should be informed that benzoyl peroxide and retinoic acid are incompatible together and, thus either they are prescribed for use on alternate days or one is designated for use in the morning and the other at night. The nurse should also inform the adolescent of the side effects of topical medications, especially the reddened skin that can result from compliance with the regimen prescribed by the dermatologist. The nurse should assess the psychosocial impact of acne on the adolescent's self-image. Depression, anxiety, and low self-esteem may occur during the adolescent's developmental task of developing identity. The adolescent with acne will need a great deal of emotional support in dealing with feelings of self-consciousness and frustration, especially during periods of exacerbations. For adolescents who insist on wearing make-up, water-based preparations are preferred. Meticulous skin care is emphasized, including removal of cosmetics at night. Involving the adolescent in developing the plan of care may ensure successful compliance with the measures prescribed for resolution.

Although the disease is self-limited and not life-threatening, its significance to the adolescent is great, and it is a mistake to underestimate the impact it can have on young persons. For a complete discussion of acne, please see Chapter 25. See Table 44-4 for nursing diagnoses with nursing interventions for a child with a disorder of integumentary function.

Prognosis. Acne will resolve spontaneously over a variable period, depending on the individual.

Psoriasis. Psoriasis is a chronic, proliferative skin disorder characterized by thick, scaly patches and inflammation. Psoriasis is not usually seen in children younger than 6 years of age. The disorder is characterized by remissions and exacerbations. Persons are otherwise healthy. Humidifiers may help in winter. For a complete discussion of psoriasis, see Chapter 25.

Traumatic Injuries. Animal, insect, and human bites in children account for a considerable number of visits to clinics and physicians' offices. Most bites from dogs or cats are from pets belonging to the family or neighbors. Dog bites involve lacerations or tissue avulsion injuries, while cats inflict more puncturelike wounds. Boys are bitten more often by dogs; girls are bitten more often by cats. Animal bites most often occur on the child's face, scalp, and upper extremities because children tend to keep their heads close to the animal during play. Human bites occur in young children during rough or aggressive play or when they become frustrated; bites can also be the result of child abuse. The most common traumatic injuries in children, their manifestations, management, and nursing interventions are outlined in Table 44-5 on p. 1433.

Infectious Disorders of the Skin

Bacterial Infections. Impetigo, folliculitis, and cellulitis are common bacterial infections in childhood. The assessment of systemic signs and symptoms, areas involved, and appearance of lesions are helpful in establishing the type of infection. Table 44-6 on p. 1434 reviews the etiology, clinical manifestations, management, and nursing interventions for these infections.

Prognosis. Prognosis for bacterial infections of the skin is good but becomes guarded in the more complex and puzzling cases.

TABLE 44-4 Nursing Diagnoses and Nursing Interventions for the Child with a Disorder of Integumentany Function

Nursing Diagnoses	Nursing Interventions
Skin integrity, impaired, related to irritation	Assess for signs of scratching. Advise parents to keep the child's fingernails short or cover hands with mittens or socks. Keep affected areas clean and dry. Apply medications as directed.
Pain, related to pruritus	Encourage rest. Encourage well-balanced diet. Protect skinfolds and surfaces that rub together. Keep clothing and linen clean and dry. Remove adhesives and occlusive dressings carefully. Maintain careful hand washing. Wear gloves when indicated. Assess degree of discomfort. Administer antihistamine and glucocorticoid as directed to reduce pruritus and inflammation. Advise loose, lightweight clothing to promote comfort. Apply cool compresses to soothe skin. Reduce external stimuli that aggravate discomfort, such as clothing or bed linen. Teach child to recognize agents or circumstances that produce reaction.
Infection, high risk for, related to scratching and skin impairment	Assess for signs of infection. Change diapers as soon as soiled. Administer appropriate antibiotics as directed. Implement universal precautions (see Chapter 12). Maintain careful hand washing. Teach and reinforce positive habits of hygienic care.
Body image disturbance, related to perception of appearance	Encourage child to express feelings about personal appearance and perceived reactions of others. Hold child (remember that there is no substitute for the stimulation and comfort of human contact). Touch and caress unaffected area. Teach self-care where appropriate. Involve child in planning treatment schedules. Support and encourage child in efforts to deal with multiple problems that may be associated with disorder, including discomfort, rejection, discouragement, and feelings of self-revulsion. Encourage child to maintain usual activities.
Family processes, altered, related to having a child with a severe skin condition (e.g., eczema, psoriasis)	Teach family skills needed to carry out therapeutic program. Provide written instructions. Inform family of expected and unexpected results of therapy and a course of action to follow. Help devise special techniques to carry out therapy. Be aware of overprotectiveness and restrictiveness, which can stifle child's emotional growth. Allow and encourage family members, particularly the one who cares for the child most of the time, to express negative feelings, such as anger, frustration, and perhaps guilt. Stress that negative feelings are normal, acceptable, and expected, but that they must have an outlet if family members are to remain healthy. Encourage family in efforts to carry out plan of care. Provide assistance when appropriate. Refer to agencies and services that assist with social, financial, and medical problems.

TABLE 44-5 Traumatic Injuries

Clinical Manifestation	Management	Prevention
Animal bites (dogs/cats)		
Lacerations, punctures, tissue avulsion	Wound care Avulsed tissue—put on ice, rush child to physician for possible reattachment	Supervise children during play with pets. Educate children in appropriate ways to handle pets. Teach understanding of animal behavior and respect for animals. Never leave infants alone with pet.
Human bites		
Lacerations	Wound care	Supervise young children at play.
Insect bites (fleas, mosquitoes, flies, gnats)		
Hypersensitive reactions; papular urticaria; firm papules	Cool compresses, topical antihistamines, Caladryl lotion	Use insect repellents (should not contain >10% DEET). Remove source by treating furniture, mattresses, carpets, and pets.
Insect stings (hornets, wasps, bees)		
Nonhypersensitive: local erythema, edema, tenderness, pruritus	Carefully scrape off stinger, if present; cleanse with soap and water; use cool compresses, antipruritic agents	Avoid insect breeding/nesting areas. Wear clothes that cover the extremities and feet.
Hypersensitive: systemic reactions and anaphylaxis	Intramuscular epinephrine and immediate medical attention; epinephrine kits available for home/school to prevent anaphylactic shock/death	
Sunburn		
Mild: erythema, tenderness, mild edema Severe: severe erythema, pain, edema, vesicular formation	Cool compresses, moisturizers Immediate medical attention	Use topical sunscreens containing *p*-aminobenzoic acid (PABA) and sun-protection factors (SPF) 15-30 Limit time spent in sun during period of maximum exposure (11 AM to 3 PM); also at higher altitudes, limit time on fresh snow and water, especially when sun is directly overhead.

Viral Infections.

Herpes Simplex Virus, Type 1. Herpes simplex virus is a fairly common infection, as evidenced by the presence of HSV-1 antibodies in 30% to 60% of the young adult population. HSV-1 is transmitted by direct contact of infected body fluids with nonintact skin or mucous membranes. The children most susceptible to HSV are immunosuppressed children (steroid therapy, chemotherapy, leukemia, or HIV-positive), children with burns, and infants with diaper rash or eczema. For a more complete discussion of HSV, see Chapter 25.

Prognosis. Prognosis for viral infections of the skin is usually good; however, the infection may be fatal in children with depressed immunity. Healing will occur without scarring unless secondary infection develops.

Tinea Capitis, Tinea Corporis, Tinea Cruris, and Tinea Pedis (Ringworm). Tinea infections are common fungal infections of the skin in children. The infections are classified according to the area of the body that is involved. Tinea capitis is a common infection of the scalp among school-age children. Tinea corporis can be found on the trunk and on the extremities in young children; tinea cruris ("jock itch") is found in the inguinal area of pubescent males; and tinea pedis ("athlete's foot") is found between the patient's toes. The tinea infections are discussed in greater detail in Chapter 25.

Prognosis. Prognosis for fungal infections of the skin, with treatment, is good.

TABLE 44-6 Bacterial Infections of the Skin

Etiology	Clinical Manifestations	Management
Impetigo		
Staphylcoccus aureus; group A streptococcus, or both	Erythematous papules progress to vesicles with exudative and honey-colored crusting stages; involves the face, buttocks, and extremities; pruritus is common	Mupirocin topical or systemic treatment with penicillin, erythromycin, or cloxacillin. *Nursing Interventions:* Teach family measures to control spread of infection; instruct in careful hand washing.
Folliculitis		
Staphylococcus aureus	Pustule with surrounding erythema of the hair follicle of the scalp or extremities; can progress to a furuncle (a boil from the primary folliculitis), with extension into the surrounding dermis *Systemic effects:* Malaise, if severe	Topical antibiotics and local, warm, moist compresses; more severe cases may require incision and drainage, followed by antibiotic therapy. *Nursing Interventions:* Teach family measures to control spread of infection; hygiene measures, such as careful hand washing.
Cellulitis		
Staphylococcus aureus; group A streptococcus, *Haemophilus influenzae,* type b	Can occur anywhere on the body; area is erythematous, edematous, warm, and painful; adjacent tender lymph node enlargement; may progress to abscess formation *Systemic effects:* Fever, malaise	Antibiotic therapy, rest, and warm, moist compresses. Neonates with HSV-1 are hospitalized; children under 3 years of age with facial cellulitis are usually hospitalized. *Nursing Interventions:* Gently cleanse area with saline; observe for complications; administer antibiotics and analgesics as prescribed; institute wound drainage precautions if drainage develops; teach family measures to control spread of infection, such as careful hand washing.

Candidiasis (Thrush).

Etiology/pathophysiology. Candidiasis is caused by the fungus *Candida albicans.* The infection is a common disorder in infants under 6 months of age and transmitted by contaminated hands, nipples, and pacifiers. In the neonate, candidal infection may result from passage through an infected vagina. The candidal lesion begins as a pustule on an inflammatory base. As inflammatory cells accumulate, whitish-yellow or whitish-gray curdlike patches appear over the infected area. The incidence of candidiasis is higher in immunocompromised children, infants of diabetic mothers, and children with oronasal malformations (cleft lip and/or palate).

Clinical manifestations. The white patches of *Candida* are frequently found on moist tissues, as it cannot grow on dry skin. Common areas affected include the tongue, buccal cavity, GI tract, and vagina. Often, parents mistake thrush for a formula coating on the tongue. Generally, the condition is asymptomatic and easily treated. However, severe cases can result in pain and refusal to eat or drink, causing risk of dehydration.

Diagnostic tests. Diagnosis is made by careful history and clinical observation of the plaques. Attempts to distinguish thrush from formula can be determined by rinsing the area with water or gently wiping the area with a wet washcloth. If the white coating remains, thrush is present. Scraping lesions is contraindicated because the lesions bleed easily.

Medical management. Nystatin suspension is the most common antifungal agent used in oral *Candida* infections. Nystatin suspension is administered after feedings and applied directly onto the lesions and to each side of the mouth before swallowing. Treating infections early can prevent more serious complications such as candidal infections of the upper airway and GI tract. When oral candidiasis is diagnosed, the diaper area is also inspected for signs of infection. Nystatin cream is prescribed for diaper candidiasis.

Nursing interventions/patient teaching. Nurses inform parents that the full 7-day course of nystatin suspension is to be completed even though candidal lesions may no longer be present. Prevention of reinfection includes teaching parents to sterilize bottles, nipples, pacifiers, and teethers. Hand washing is emphasized. Parents are instructed to report any oral discomfort that results in poor fluid intake. Signs of dehydration are reviewed with the family. If the mother is breastfeeding, she should be advised to wash her nipples with soap and water before and after feedings. The application of nystatin cream may also be recommended.

Prognosis. Prognosis for candidiasis (thrush) is good with prescribed therapy.

Parasitic Infections.

Scabies and Pediculosis. Scabies is an infectious parasitic disorder caused by a mite. Scabies is most commonly seen in school-age children. The scabies mite burrows under the skin, leaving behind debris, feces, and eggs. The condition causes a papular rash and intense pruritus. Transmission occurs by direct contact with an infected person, bed linen, or clothing.

Pediculosis capitis (head lice) is a scalp infection that causes intense pruritus. It is common among preschool and school-age children. The adult louse attaches to the skin and feeds by sucking blood. On the hair shaft, the mature female louse lays her eggs (nits), which hatch in 7 to 10 days. The louse does not jump or fly and is not carried or transmitted by pets. Infestations usually occur as a result of sharing contaminated combs, brushes, hats, or clothing that comes in contact with the head. Medical management and nursing interventions of scabies and pediculosis are outlined in Box 44-12.

Box 44-12 MEDICAL MANAGEMENT AND NURSING INTERVENTIONS FOR PARASITIC INFECTIONS

- Lindane (Kwell) 1% lotion, cream, or shampoo
- Simultaneous treatment of family members
- Atarax or Benadryl for pruritus
- Hot-water cleansing of contaminated clothing and linens
- Examiners should wear gloves when assessing for head lice
- Teach parents to:
  Carefully inspect the head of a child who scratches the head more than usual for bite marks, erythema, and nits
  Read directions carefully before beginning therapy
  Be aware of psychological effects, which can be highly stressful to children

Patient/family teaching.

- Dead lice and remaining nits are removed with a very fine-tooth comb. Tweezers may be necessary to remove the nits if the comb is ineffective.
- Machine wash all washable clothing, towels, and bed linens in hot water and dry in a hot dryer for at least 20 minutes. Dry-clean nonwashable items.
- Thoroughly vacuum carpets, car seats, pillows, stuffed animals, rugs, mattresses, and upholstered furniture.
- Seal nonwashable items in plastic bags for 14 days if unable to dry-clean or vacuum.
- Soak combs, brushes, and hair accessories in lice-killing products for 1 hour or in boiling water for 10 minutes.*

Prognosis. Prognosis is good with treatment.

Communicable Diseases and Immunizations. The incidence of many communicable diseases and the serious complications associated with them has been significantly reduced through the development and use of vaccines. However, health professionals will occasionally encounter children with a preventable communicable disease. The nurse is usually the first person to observe signs of illness, such as a rash, that may be related to a communicable disease. The nurse should be able to identify potentially infectious cases so that measures can be instituted to prevent exposure and transmission to others. In assessing the child with suspicious signs and symptoms, the nurse should determine whether the child has had any recent exposure to a known case and whether or not the child is experiencing any prodromal symptoms. The immunization status of the child and determining whether the child has had a prior history of the illness can help to rule out certain communicable diseases. The goals of nursing interventions for the child with a communicable disease are directed toward preventing transmission of disease to others, preventing complications, and promoting supportive management. Table 44-7 on pp.1436-1440 describes the common communicable diseases seen in childhood, their medical management, and specific nursing interventions.

The development of immunizations against communicable diseases has significantly reduced the morbidity and mortality associated with these diseases. Most children in the United States are adequately immunized against these diseases; however, a number of children remain underimmunized or unimmunized due to financial hardship, religious beliefs, diminished access to health services, or lack of education regarding the prevention of these illnesses. For recommendations for immunization administration in normally healthy infants and chil-

Text continued on p. 1440.

*From Clore ER: Dispelling the common myths about pediculosis, *J Pediatr Health Care* 3:28, 1989.

TABLE 44-7 Childhood Communicable Diseases

Disease	Clinical Manifestations	Medical Management	Nursing Interventions
Rubeola (measles)			
Etiology: Paramyxovirus Transmission: direct contact from respiratory tract secretions, blood, or urine of infected person Incubation: 7-12 days Communicable period: 4 days before to 5 days after rash appears	Prodrome: fever, malaise, cough, coryza, conjunctivitis; Koplik spots (pinpoint red spots with central white speck in buccal cavity opposite lower molars) 3-4 days before rash Acute phase: rash appears as irregular macular erythema; begins on face and behind ears and spreads to feet; rash lasts up to 7 days; child may exhibit vomiting, diarrhea, anorexia, lymphadenopathy Complications: otitis media, pneumonia, laryngotracheitis, encephalitis	Supportive management: acetaminophen, fluids, and bed rest until fever subsides: dim lights or sunglasses if photophobic	Institute seizure precautions (fever can be high [104° F (40° C)]). Cleanse eyes to remove crusting and decrease rubbing. Use a cool mist humidifier for cough. Offer small, frequent meals of bland foods Keep skin clean and dry; use tepid baths. Restrict to quiet activities until child feels better, usually by day 6 of rash. Use isolation to protect unimmunized children or the immunocompromised from exposure. Teach and encourage good hand washing technique Notify physician of ear pain, chest pain, difficulty breathing, headaches.
Rubella (German measles)			
Etiology: Rubivirus Transmission: direct contact with nasopharyngeal secretions of infected person; indirect contact with contaminated articles (fomites); transplacental transmission Incubation: 14-21 days Communicable period: 7 days before to 5 days after rash appears	Prodrome: young children—possible lymphadenopathy; adolescents/adults—low-grade fever, headache, sore throat, anorexia, clear nasal discharge, cough, lymphadenopathy 1-5 days Acute phase: pinkish-red maculopapular rash beginning on face; spreads to trunk, then extremities—3 days Complications: usually none; rare—arthritis, encephalitis; birth defects as virus crosses placenta (teratogenic)	Supportive management: acetaminophen for fever or discomfort	Provide respiratory isolation to protect unimmunized children, pregnant women. Teach and encourage good hand washing technique. Institute comfort measures as needed. Isolate child from pregnant women. Reassure parents of benign nature of illness in affected child.

TABLE 44-7 Childhood Communicable Diseases—cont'd

Disease	Clinical Manifestations	Medical Management	Nursing Interventions
Varicella (chicken pox)			
Etiology: Varicella zoster virus (herpesvirus) Transmission: direct contact with respiratory tract secretions; indirect contact with contaminated articles; airborne droplets Incubation: 10-21 days (usually 13-17 days) Communicable period: 1 day before eruption until all lesions crusted (1 week after onset)	Prodrome: low-grade fever, malaise, anorexia—24 hours Acute phase: pruritic rash 3-5 days, begins as macule, progresses to papule then vesicle on erythematous base; vesicles rupture causing oozing and crusting; all three stages present in various intensities; rash appears on trunk, face, proximal extremities, mucous membranes Complications: children—secondary bacterial skin infections possible; adults—pneumonia, encephalitis, laryngeal edema, hemorrhagic varicella, thrombocytopenia	Supportive management: acetaminophen for fever; systemic or topical antipruritics or systemic antihistamines; skin kept clean and dry; antiviral treatment—acyclovir (Zovirax); varicella zoster immune globulin within 3 days of exposure in high-risk children (immunocompromised; leukemia; newborns)	Keep nails short and smooth; give daily baths without soap; use lightweight, loose clothing; administer antipruritics or antihistamines as ordered; teach child to apply pressure on itch rather than scratching; use mittens on young children. Use strict isolation in hospital. If child is at home, instruct parents to isolate ill child from siblings and high-risk children and adults until lesions dry. Teach and encourage good hand washing technique. Administer acetaminophen as ordered. Encourage fluids.
Roseola infantum (exanthema subitum)			
Etiology: Human herpesvirus, type 6 Transmission: unknown; occurs in children age 6-24 months Incubation: unknown Communicable period: unknown	Sudden-onset, persistent high fever, lasts up to 4 days; child appears well otherwise; fever rapidly falls to normal followed by rose-pink macular/maculopapular rash on trunk and spreads to rest of body; rash lasts 1-2 days and is nonpruritic Complications: febrile seizures	Supportive management: acetaminophen for fever; seizure precautions for the child prone to febrile seizures; encourage fluids	Teach parents how to lower fever safely. Reassure parents as to benign nature of illness. If child is prone to seizures, discuss appropriate precautions.

Continued.

TABLE 44-7 Childhood Communicable Diseases—cont'd

Disease	Clinical Manifestation	Medical Management	Nursing Interventions
Erythema infectiosum (fifth disease)			
Etiology: human parvovirus B19 Transmission: respiratory tract secretions and blood Incubation: 4-14 days but up to 20 days Communicable period: unknown—most likely before signs and symptoms develop; communicability unlikely once rash develops; children with aplastic crisis contagious until 1 week after onset of signs and symptoms	Prodrome: in children with aplastic crisis—fever, malaise, myalgia; rash usually absent Acute phase: rash appears in 3 stages: 1st stage—red rash on face, "slapped cheek" appearance (fades in 1-4 days), circumoral pallor; 2nd stage—maculopapular, lacelike rash on upper extremities spreading to trunk and thighs, lasts 1 or more weeks; 3rd stage—rash can recur periodically for weeks in response to heat, sunlight, cold Complications: arthralgia, arthritis infrequently in children but common in adults. Encephalitis, myocarditis (rare); maternal infection—low risk for fetal hydrops	Supportive management: acetaminophen for fever; analgesics or antiinflammatories	For hospitalized child, use respiratory isolation/ precautions for 7 days after onset: no isolation is necessary at home. Teach and encourage good hand washing technique. Institute comfort measures as necessary.
Scarlet fever			
Etiology: group A β-hemolytic streptococcus Transmission: direct contact with respiratory tract secretions of infected person Incubation: 2-5 days (average 3 days) Communicable period: during incubation and acute illness phase	Prodrome: sudden-onset high fever, vomiting, headache, chills, malaise Acute phase: tonsillitis, pharyngitis; white strawberry tongue (tongue has white coating and papillae become red and edematous) by day 1 or 2; by day 4, white coating sloughs leaving red strawberry tongue; sandpaper-like red rash appears about 12 hours after prodrome and is intense in skin folds; cheeks are flushed and circumoral pallor present; desquamation begins by end of 1st week and continues for 3 or more weeks Complications: otitis media, pneumonia, sinusitis, glomerulonephritis, carditis, peritonsillar abscess	Antimicrobial treatment—full course of penicillin or erythromycin for those allergic to penicillin Supportive management: bed rest, analgesics, fluids	Institute respiratory isolation precautions until completion of first 24 hours of antimicrobial treatment. Teach and encourage good hand washing technique. Offer soft diet if child is able to chew; encourage fluids. Restrict to quiet activities until child feels better. Offer lozenges, gargles, cool mist humidifier for throat Maintain good oral hygiene. Advise parents to consult practitioner if fever persists after beginning therapy. Discuss procedures for preventing spread of infection.

TABLE 44-7 Childhood Communicable Diseases—cont'd

Disease	Clinical Manifestation	Medical Management	Nursing Interventions
Mumps (parotitis)			
Etiology: paramyxovirus Transmission: direct contact with respiratory tract secretions of infected person Incubation: 16-18 days Communicable period: 1-2 days and up to 7 days before parotid edema to 5-9 days after onset of signs and symptoms	Prodrome: fever, malaise, headache Acute phase: unilateral or bilateral edema and tenderness of parotid glands by day 3; chewing aggravates "earlike" pain Complications: meningoencephalitis, epididymoorchiditis, arthritis, sensorineural deafness, myocarditis; sterility in males is rare	Supportive management: acetaminophen for fever, analgesics for pain; IV fluids may be necessary for the child who refuses to eat or drink	Institute respiratory isolation/precautions for 9 days after onset of edema or until edema has subsided. Teach and encourage good hand washing technique. Offer soft, bland diet; encourage fluids. Use warm or cool compresses for edema. Dress child in tightly fitting underpants or scrotal support for orchitis.
Diphtheria			
Etiology: *Corynebacterium diphtheriae* Transmission: direct contact with nose, eye, throat discharges or skin lesions of infected person; rarely: fomite transmission or food-borne outbreaks Incubation: 2-5 days Communicable period: untreated person—2 weeks to several months	Clinical manifestations vary according to diphtheritic membrane affected: *nasal:* nasal discharge—serosanguineous and mucopurulent, can progress to epistaxis; white membrane on nasal septum *tonsillar/pharyngeal:* pharyngitis; malaise; anorexia; fever (low grade); membrane over tonsils, pharynx; lymphadenitis *laryngeal:* cough, fever, hoarseness Complications: airway obstruction, thrombocytopenia, myocarditis, vocal cord paralysis	Antimicrobial treatment—penicillin or erythromycin; antitoxin, usually IV, preceded by skin testing for horse serum sensitivity; possible tracheostomy for respiratory obstruction	Institute strict respiratory isolation/precautions. Maintain bed rest. Offer liquid or soft diet. Suction gently, as necessary. Observe for signs of respiratory distress/obstruction: dyspnea, apprehensiveness, cyanosis; and report such findings to physician. Keep tracheostomy set at bedside. Regulate humidity for optimum liquefaction of secretions.

Continued.

TABLE 44-7 Childhood Communicable Diseases—cont'd

Disease	Clinical Manifestation	Medical Management	Nursing Interventions
Pertussis (whooping cough)			
Etiology: *Bordetella pertussis* Transmission: direct contact or droplet spread of respiratory tract secretions of infected person Incubation: 7-20 days Communicable period: from prodromal stage through 4th week	Prodrome: URI signs and symptoms 1-2 weeks; cough, sneezing, little or no fever, headache, anorexia Acute phase: paroxysmal stage—dry, hacking cough followed by prolonged inspiration ("whoop" sound) most often at night; paroxysms usually followed by vomiting of thick, stringy mucus; lasts 4-6 weeks; convalescent stage—decrease in coughing and whooping and lasts 1-2 weeks Complications: pneumonia, hypoxia, atelectasis, otitis media, seizures, dehydration, weight loss, prolapsed rectum, hernia, hemorrhage (epistaxis, subconjunctival, cerebral edema, and CNS disturbances)	Antimicrobial treatment—erythromycin or sulfamethoxazole-trimethoprim (Bactrim, Septra) for 7-10 days Antiseizure treatment—for those experiencing seizures; phenytoin; supportive management—hospitalization required for infants or children with underlying pulmonary or cardiac disease, dehydration, or severe signs and symptoms; gentle suctioning to prevent choking, high humidified oxygen therapy; IV fluids; intubation set at bedside for emergency	Institute respiratory isolation precautions. Enforce strict hand washing. Maintain bed rest if child is febrile; offer quiet activities Offer liquids—small amounts frequently; if child vomits, refeed. Monitor cardiac and respiratory status. Observe for signs of airway obstruction: dyspnea, restlessness, cyanosis, and report such findings to physician. Provide high humidity and gently suction frequently to prevent choking. Reassure parents during paroxysms. Teach parents in the use of a cool mist humidifier to avoid triggers of paroxysms (dust, smoke, chilling, sudden change in temperature, excitement) Teach parents how to recognize signs of respiratory distress, and arrange for a public health nurse to visit after discharge from hospital.

dren, see Table 7-4. The information has been modified from the American Academy of Pediatrics: *Report of the Committee on Infectious Diseases,* ed 22, Elk Grove Village, Ill, 1991. These recommendations should not be interpreted to be absolute. The manufacturer's packaged insert should be consulted for handling, storage, dosage, and administration. Parents should be informed of the risks and benefits before the administration of each vaccine.

Prognosis. See Table 44-7 for possible complications of communicable diseases. With accurate diagnosis, prompt treatment, and prevention of complications, prognosis is usually good.

DISORDERS OF SENSORY ORGAN FUNCTION

Sensory impairment in young children can lead to serious adverse outcomes in growth and development. Prevention, early detection, and management are essential for favorable outcomes.

Hearing

Otitis Media (OM).

Etiology/pathophysiology. OM, an infection of the middle ear, is a common infection in children from 6 months to 2 years of age and often follows an upper respiratory infection. A significant cause of otitis media is the accumulation of bacteria in the nasopharynx. In young children, the eustachian tube, which connects the nasopharynx and the middle ear, is shorter, more horizontal, and wider, allowing nasopharyngeal flora to pass and become trapped in the middle ear. Feeding practices have also been implicated in the incidence of OM. Bottle-fed babies may have a higher incidence of OM compared with that of breastfed babies because of the more supine position assumed during bottle feeding. Toddlers and young children should always be evaluated for foreign bodies (pieces of toys, beads, pebbles, vegetables, etc.) in the ear canal, which can lead to hearing loss and local infection.

Clinical manifestations. The infant or young child with acute otitis media (AOM) may experience otalgia (earache), fever, rhinitis, fussiness, irritability, and decreased appetite. Pulling, tugging, or rubbing the affected ear or rolling the head from side to side may indicate AOM. Older children will usually complain of ear pain. Occasionally, there may be purulent discharge in the ear canal, which is indicative of a ruptured tympanic membrane (TM). When this occurs, there is a sudden cessation of ear pain.

Diagnostic tests. Visualization of the tympanic membrane by otoscopic examination, along with clinical signs and symptoms, usually confirms the diagnosis. If there is drainage in the ear canal, the material can be cultured.

Medical management. The management of AOM includes administration of antibiotics for 10 days and acetaminophen for fever and discomfort. Upon completion of antibiotic therapy, the child is seen by the practitioner to determine the effectiveness of treatment and observe for complications. If fluid accumulates and remains in the middle ear space, the surgical insertions of tympanostomy tubes may be indicated to drain the fluid and relieve the pressure. Tympanostomy tubes may also be indicated in chronic OM. Tympanostomy tubes remain in the ear an average of 6 months before being spontaneously rejected.

Nursing interventions. Children usually begin to feel better after 48 to 72 hours of antibiotic therapy. The application of heat or cold (whichever provides the greatest comfort) over the affected ear with the child lying on the affected side can also help alleviate pain. This position also facilitates drainage of the exudate if the eardrum has ruptured or if a myringotomy was performed. If the ear is draining, the external canal may be cleaned with sterile cotton swabs or pledgets soaked in hydrogen peroxide. If ear wicks or lightly rolled sterile gauze packs are placed in the ear after surgical treatment, they should be loose enough to allow accumulated drainage to flow out of the ear; otherwise the infection may be transferred to the mastoid process. The wicks need to stay dry during shampoos or baths.

Patient/family teaching. The nurse emphasizes that the medication should be taken for the fully prescribed course to ensure eradication of the infection. Nurses can educate parents in the prevention of otitis media by teaching them to hold their infants in an upright position when feeding. If tympanostomy tubes have been inserted, parents are taught postoperative care. The ear should be protected during bathing, shampooing, and swimming because bacteria in the water can be introduced into the ear.

Prognosis. With appropriate therapy, most children improve within 48 to 72 hours. The most common complication of otitis media is mild to moderate hearing loss due to chronic or recurrent effusion. The episodic (temporary) hearing loss that may occur during occasional bouts of OM is usually reversible; however, conductive hearing loss associated with chronic OM may be permanent and may interfere with language and cognitive development.

Vision

Refractive Errors (Myopia and Hyperopia). Refractive errors occur when light rays entering the lens are bent and fall in front of or behind the retina, preventing the image from falling on a single point on the retina as it should. Two of the most common refractive errors in childhood are myopia (nearsightedness) and hyperopia (farsightedness), which results in loss of visual acuity. Screening tests that measure visual acuity can assist in identifying refractive errors. Treatment consists of corrective lenses and periodic reevaluation. Nurses can play a vital role in ensuring vision screening, especially in the preschool years, to avoid school problems later on. See Chapter 34 for information on diagnostic eye tests.

Strabismus. In strabismus, there is a lack of coordination in the extraocular musculature, resulting in a crossed-eye appearance. Strabismus is caused by muscle imbalance, results from paralysis, or may be congenitally acquired. The condition can affect one or both eyes and results in two images (instead of one) received by the brain. Common clinical manifestations include squinting, closing one eye, tilting the head (to block out one image), and difficulty focusing or picking up objects. Medical management varies according to the cause of the strabismus. Occlusion therapy may be used where the good eye is patched for a period of 6 to 8 weeks in order to stimulate and strengthen the affected eye, corrective lenses or eye exercises may be prescribed, or surgical correction may be indicated. Nursing intervention includes adequate explanation of the treatment plan, care of corrective lenses, instruction in eye exercises, and reinforcement of occlusive patches if they should become loose.

Prognosis. Left untreated, the child is at risk for **amblyopia** (lazy eye; reduction or dimness of vision, especially in which there is no apparent pathological condition of the eye) in which there is a loss in visual acuity. This complication can be prevented if the underlying problem is corrected before the child is 6 years of age.

Periorbital Cellulitis.

Etiology/pathophysiology. Periorbital cellulitis is a serious inflammation of the eyelid and periorbital area. The condition is usually unilateral and has the potential to affect the eye and the CNS. Periorbital cellulitis can result from conjunctivitis, impetigo, insect bites, or trauma. Common causative organisms include *Haemophilus influenzae, Staphylococcus aureus,* and group A β-hemolytic streptococcus.

Clinical manifestations. Children with periorbital cellulitis usually experience pain, tenderness, fever, erythema (of distinctive magenta color), and edema of the eyelids and periorbital area. Headache and purulent nasal discharge may also be present.

Diagnostic tests. Cultures of the eye, the nose, and the blood are performed to identify the causative agent. Ultrasound and CT scan of the orbit may be useful to rule out abscess.

Medical management. Because of the emergent nature of the illness, the child is admitted for aggressive IV antibiotic administration. Analgesics and antipyretics may be prescribed for pain and fever. Warm compresses may also relieve discomfort.

Nursing interventions. As the edema decreases, the skin around the eye becomes dry and begins to peel. Preserving skin integrity involves the application of a thin layer of petrolatum to the area.

Patient/family teaching. Reassure parents that eye discoloration may persist for several days and that most children recover completely without complication.

Prognosis. The edema usually subsides within 36 hours of antibiotic therapy, and with appropriate treatment, the prognosis is usually excellent.

Nasal Cavity

Allergic Rhinitis.

Etiology/pathophysiology. Allergic rhinitis occurs in about 10% of the pediatric population, most commonly in children over the age of 5. Allergic rhinitis may be seasonal or perennial, and there is a familial predisposition to allergy in these children. Exposure to an inhaled allergen sets off the allergic response.

Clinical manifestations. The signs and symptoms seen in the pediatric population include congestion, sniffling, mouth breathing, itchy nose, and postnasal drip. Often there is a line across the nose from nasal rubbing (allergic salute). The medical management and nursing interventions for the child with allergic rhinitis are the same as those for the adult; see Chapter 36 for details.

CHILD MALTREATMENT

The maltreatment of children is an obscure, complicated, and prevalent problem in today's society. The problem of maltreatment is not confined to one specific race, religion, or socioeconomic level. Although certain groups have higher reported rates of abuse, this problem occurs in every level of society. **Child maltreatment** is a broad term used to describe physical and emotional neglect and physical, emotional, and sexual abuse of children. In recent years, the number of reported cases of child maltreatment has increased dramatically. In 1991 in the United States, there were nearly 3 million cases of child maltreatment reported to social service agencies. Unfortunately, many cases of child maltreatment are insidious and go undetected and unreported.

Child Neglect

Neglect can be broadly divided into two categories: physical neglect and emotional neglect. *Physical neglect* can be defined as failure of a parent or caretaker to supply a child with adequate food, clothing, shelter, education, or health care although financially able to do so or offered financial or other means to do so. *Emotional neglect* can be defined as the failure by a parent or caretaker to meet a child's needs for emotional nurturance, affection, and attention.

Child Abuse

Child abuse can be divided into three broad categories: physical abuse, emotional abuse, and sexual abuse. *Physical abuse* is defined as the intentional, nonaccidental infliction of physical injury upon a child by a parent or guardian. *Emotional abuse* can be defined as the intentional attempt by a parent or caretaker to impair or destroy the mental or emotional state of a child. *Sexual abuse* is defined as commission of a sexual offense by an older person against a child who is dependent or developmentally immature for the purpose of the perpetrator's own sexual stimulation or gratification.

Etiology. There are many factors that contribute to the etiology of child maltreatment, including parental, child, and situational factors. Parental factors include the parent's own socialization history and history of having been an abused child, the parent's age and developmental level, attitudes toward the child and childrearing, knowledge of normal child behavior and development, and the parent's psychological state. Characteristics of the child may place them at risk for maltreatment. Many factors, including temperament, age, exceptional physical needs, disabilities, and health or behavior problems may increase the potential for maltreatment by a parent or caretaker. Situational factors include sources of stress

TABLE 44-8 Clinical Manifestations of Possible Child Maltreatment

Behavioral Indicators	Physical Indicators
Physical neglect	
Begging or stealing food	Failure to thrive
Extended stays at school	Lag in growth and development
Fatigue or listlessness at school	Consistent hunger
Delinquency	Poor personal hygiene
Alcohol and/or drug abuse	Inappropriate dress for season
	Unattended medical needs
	Abandonment
Physical abuse	
Wary of contacts with parents or other adults	Bruises, welts, and bite marks
Apprehension when other children cry	Bruises reflecting the shape of object used to inflict injury (electrical cord, belt buckle, iron, radiator)
Fear of parents or going home	Bruises in various stages of healing
Wears concealing clothing to hide injuries	"Grab marks" on arms or shoulders
Low self-esteem	Evidence of human bites
Suicide attempts	Lacerations or abrasions
	Burns that are symmetrical and have no "splash marks"
	Cigar or cigarette burns on soles, palms, back, or buttocks
	Fractures:
	To skull, nose, face
	Multiple or spiral
	Various stages of healing
	Discovered in the course of examination, not reported by caretaker
Sexual abuse	
Promiscuous behavior	Difficulty in walking or sitting
Unwillingness to change for gym	Torn, stained, or bloody underclothing
Withdrawal, fantasy, or infantile behavior	Pain or pruritus in genital area
Age-inappropriate sexual knowledge	Bruises or bleeding in external genitalia, vaginal, or anal areas
Poor peer relationships	Bruises to the hard or soft palate
Delinquency	Sexually transmitted diseases in preteens
Prostitution	Adolescent pregnancy
Forcing sexual acts on other children	Enuresis/encopresis
Fear of being touched	Vaginal or penile discharge
Suicide attempts	Foreign bodies in vagina or rectum
Low self-esteem	Presence of sperm
Excessive or public masturbation	Recurrent urinary tract infections
Declining school performance	
Emotional neglect and abuse	
Stranger anxiety	Failure to thrive
Emotional withdrawal	Feeding difficulties
Inappropriate fearfulness	Enuresis/encopresis
Delinquency	Sleep disturbances
Lag in emotional and intellectual development	
Language difficulties	
Suicide attempts	

and support within the family's environment. There may be marital problems, financial difficulties, drug and/or alcohol abuse, lack of social support or the inability of the parent or caretaker to ask for support, poor social network, and poor relationships with extended families. These factors may increase the potential for an abusive reaction by adding stress to an environment in which a parent or caretaker is already lacking resources.

Clinical Manifestations. Children who have been abused or neglected may manifest certain physical and/or behavioral indicators that suggest maltreatment. These manifestations are summarized in Table 44-8 on p. 1443.

Nursing Interventions. The most important role for any health care provider, especially nurses, is the identification of a child who is being maltreated. Often, the nurse may be the first person to see the child and parent. A thorough history and physical examination are the most effective diagnostic tools in recognizing a child who has been abused or neglected. The presence of a behavioral or physical indicator of maltreatment should serve to prompt further investigation because these indicators rarely appear as single factors. Any manifestations of abuse should be carefully documented in the medical record, as should the caretakers' explanation for these findings. Special attention should be paid to injuries that are unexplained or inconsistent with the parent or caretaker's explanation of how the injury was incurred.

If abuse is suspected, it is important to question the child and parent separately. It is rare for a child to betray a parent and admit the abuse. Even the most battered of children remain loyal to the perpetrators (those guilty of committing the act). The use of drawings, play, diagrams, and anatomically correct dolls may help a child to express what has happened.

All states have regulations for the mandatory reporting of child maltreatment when a health professional has reason to suspect that a child has been abused or neglected. It is not necessary for the professional to be certain or "prove" that a child has been maltreated; it is enough for the reporter to distrust or doubt what has been observed in the child. Many states have a toll-free number where reports are taken by a state central registry and then referred to the local Department of Social Services office where the child resides.

If the child requires hospitalization as a result of the abuse, it is important for the nurse to maintain a nonjudgmental attitude toward the parents or caretakers. Establishing a rapport with the family will promote a trusting and open relationship between the nurse and parents. The hospitalization provides a unique opportunity for the nurse to demonstrate positive caretaking activities and offer education through role modeling. It is important to provide consistency in the care givers assigned to the child. All procedures and treatment should be explained to the child so that invasive or painful events are not misinterpreted. If the child is to return to the parents' care, their participation should be integrated into the daily routine. In this situation it is essential for the nurse to document interactions between the child and parents in an objective and factual manner.

Preventing child maltreatment is an area where nurses can play an active role. During the prenatal period, families at risk for abuse can be identified and referred for intervention. During the child's health care visits, the nurse can identify families at risk by observing behaviors that indicate a lack of understanding of the child's care requirements or by assessing the support systems available to the family in stress. Nurses can encourage parents to search for and access resources that will provide supportive services. Reinforcement of positive caretaking behaviors is an effective way of affirming positive parenting practices.

REFERENCES AND SUGGESTED READINGS

1. Centers for Disease Control: *Preventing lead poisoning in young children: a statement by the Centers for Disease Control,* Atlanta, 1991, The Centers.
2. Congeni BL: The resurgence of acute rheumatic fever in the United States, *Pediatr Ann* 21(12):816, 1992.
3. Cooley SC, Graham JM: Down syndrome: an update and review for the primary pediatrician, *Clin Pediatr* 30(4): 233, 1991.
4. De Rienzo-De Vivio S: Childhood lead poisoning: shifting to primary prevention, *Pediatr Nurs* 18(6):565, 1992.
5. Giordano BP et al: The challenge of transferring responsibility for diabetes management from parent to child, *J Pediatr Health Care* 6(5):235, 1992.
6. Grossman HJ, editor: Manual on terminology and classification in mental retardation, American Association on Mental Deficiency, Baltimore, 1983, Garamond Pridemark Press.
7. Farrington E: Diaper dermatitis, *Pediatr Nurs* 18(1):81, 1992.
8. Finer NN et al: Obstructive, mixed, and central apnea in the neonate: physiologic correlates, *J Pediatr* 121(6):943, 1993.
9. FitzSimmons SC: The changing epidemiology of cystic fibrosis, *J Pediatr* 122(1):1, 1993.
10. Granoff DM et al: Differences in the immunogenicity of three *Haemophilus influenzae* type b conjugate vaccines in infants, *J Pediatr* 121(2):187, 1992.
11. Halsey NA: Discussion of immunologic practices: advisory committee/American Academy of Pediatrics recommendations for universal infant hepatitis B vaccination, *Pediatr Infect Dis J* 12(5):446, 1993.
12. Himelstein BP et al: T-cell depleted bone marrow transplantation for siblings with X-linked severe combined immunodeficiency, *J Pediatr* 122(2):289, 1993.
13. Hurwitz A: Helping the Down syndrome child to reach new heights: the role of the pediatric nurse, *Pediatr Nurs* 18(5):485, 1992.
14. Leventhal JM et al: Maltreatment of children born to teenage mothers: a comparison between the 1960s and 1980s, *J Pediatr* 122(2):314, 1993.
15. Long CA, Barron D: Sudden infant death syndrome and infant positioning: implications for critical care, *Pediatr Nurs* 18(5):524, 1992.

16. Martin MB, Butler RM: Understanding the basics of beta thalassemia major, *Pediatr Nurs* 19(2):143, 1993.
17. Michaels RH, Ali O: A decline in *Haemophilus influenzae* type b meningitis, *J Pediatr* 122(3):407, 1993.
18. Milunsky A et al: Multivitamin/folic acid supplementation in early pregnancy reduces the prevalence of neural tube defects, *JAMA* 262:284, 1989.
19. Molinari F: Update on the treatment of pediculosis and scabies, *Pediatr Nurs* 18(6):600, 1992.
20. Orenstein S: Prone positioning in infant gastroesophageal reflux: is elevation of the ghead worth the trouble? *J Pediatr* 117(2):184, 1990.
21. Sanchez I et al: Effects of racemic epinephrine and salbutamol on clinical score and pulmonary mechanics in infants with bronchiolitis, *J Pediatr* 122(1):145, 1993.
22. Shannon R: Gastroesophageal reflux in infancy: review and update, *J Pediatr Health Care* 7(2):71, 1993.
23. Speers AT, Speers M: Care of the infant in a Pavlik harness, *Pediatr Nurs* 18(3):229, 1992.
24. Spitzer A et al: Complications of immunosuppression, *J Pediatr* 121(1):145, 1992.
25. Warrier RP, Regueria O: Wilms' tumor, *Pediatr Nephrol* 6:358, 1992.
26. Weingarten CT, Gomberg SM: Measles: again an epidemic, *Pediatr Nurs* 18(4):369, 1992.
27. Wong DL: *Whaley's and Wong's essentials of pediatric nursing,* ed 4, St Louis, 1993, Mosby.

CHAPTER CHALLENGE

KEY POINTS

- The most common skin disorders of infancy and childhood include diaper dermatitis, atopic dermatitis, and seborrheic dermatitis.
- Treatment initiated immediately upon diagnosis can result in a better prognosis for many of the musculoskeletal disorders seen in infancy.
- Cleft lip and palate, the most common facial malformation, usually involves nutritional, dental, and speech alterations and requires a multidisciplinary approach to treatment.
- Congenital heart defects are classified as either acyanotic or cyanotic.
- Nursing interventions in the care of a child with CHF are to assist in improving cardiac function, decreasing cardiac demands, reducing respiratory distress, maintaining nutritional status, promoting fluid loss, and providing family support.
- The most common form of neoplasm in childhood is acute lymphoblastic leukemia.
- Nursing interventions for the child with hemophilia involve preventing bleeding by decreasing the risk of injury, recognizing and managing bleeding with factor replacement, preventing the crippling effects of joint degeneration, and preparing and supporting the child and family for home care.
- Oral preparations of iron given to the child with iron deficiency anemia should be given between meals with citrus fruits or juices to enhance absorption.
- Croup is a term describing a group of signs and symptoms of varied origin. It is characterized by obstruction or edema in the region of the larynx, producing inspiratory stridor, hoarseness, and a cough described as "barking."
- Most children do not exhibit any clinical signs or symptoms when first infected with *M. tuberculosis;* therefore routine skin screening is an important measure in diagnosis.
- Hypertrophic pyloric stenosis is recognized by characteristic projectile vomiting, malnutrition, dehydration, and a palpable mass in the epigastrium, and is relieved by pyloromyotomy.
- Diabetes mellitus is a syndrome characterized by a deficiency of insulin, resulting in alterations in protein, carbohydrate, and fat metabolism.
- Early recognition of hearing, vision, and speech deficits in infants and children can be accomplished through periodic screening and assessment.
- Although meningitis can be caused by a number of bacterial, viral, and fungal organisms, bacterial meningitis is the most common.
- Lead in the environment that is either ingested or inhaled continues to be the most important contributing factor in lead poisoning.
- Acquired immunodeficiency syndromes are associated with certain drug therapies, radiation, splenectomy, and viral infections.
- The reversed ratio of helper to suppressor T cells in HIV disease results in an inadequate or absent immune response.
- The maltreatment of children is an obscure, complicated, and prevalent problem in today's society. The problem of maltreatment is not confined to one specific race, religion, or socioeconomic level.

STUDY QUESTIONS

1. Michael, 12 months old, is diagnosed with iron deficiency anemia. The most likely cause is:
   1. Hemolysis
   2. Inadequate dietary intake of iron
   3. Abnormal hemoglobin structure
   4. Lack of vitamin C
2. Sally is a 3-year-old girl who was sexually abused by her uncle. During her evaluation at the emergency room, which of the following is an appropriate nursing intervention:
   1. Avoid touching the child without the parent's permission
   2. Get the child to talk about what happened
   3. Ask the child direct questions about the incident to gather factual information
   4. Document any manifestations of abuse carefully in the medical record
3. When providing care for the child who is cognitively impaired, an important nursing goal is:
   1. Teaching self-care skills
   2. Promoting optimal development
   3. Encourage parents to verbalize their concerns
   4. All the above
4. Steven is a 6-week-old infant who has been diagnosed as having pyloric stenosis. His parents ask the nurse to explain this condition to them. The nurse's best response would be to explain that pyloric stenosis is a condition characterized by:
   1. Tightening of the pyloric muscle
   2. Weakness of the pyloric muscle
   3. Enlargement of the pyloric muscle
   4. Dilation of the pylorus
5. Brian is an 8-month-old infant with infantile eczema. Which of the following indicates the most common surfaces where the lesions of infantile eczema are found:
   1. Behind the ears and on the elbows, knees, and ankles
   2. Behind the knees and on the trunk, knees, and elbows
   3. On the cheeks, scalp, trunk, and extensor surfaces of extremities
   4. Behind the ears and on the dorsum of the hands and feet
6. Four-day-old Sarah is diagnosed as having congenital hip dysplasia. An early clinical manifestation the nurse can observe for would be:
   1. Limited adduction of the hip
   2. Shortening of the leg on the affected side
   3. Depressed dance reflex
   4. Uneven thigh and gluteal folds
7. Which of the following anatomical defects constitute a tetralogy of Fallot:
   1. Aortic stenosis, atrial septal defect, overriding aorta, hypertrophy of the left ventricle
   2. Pulmonary stenosis, ventricular septal defect, overriding aorta, hypertrophy of the right ventricle
   3. Aortic stenosis, ventricular septal defect, overriding aorta, hypertrophy of the right ventricle
   4. Pulmonary stenosis, atrial septal defect, overriding aorta, hypertrophy of the left ventricle
8. Gina's mother is HIV positive. By age 2 years, it is determined that Gina too has HIV infection. Which of the following statements is true:
   1. *Pneumocystis carinii* pneumonia (PCP) is common in HIV-infected children
   2. The majority of children with HIV infection in the United States acquired the infection perinatally from their HIV-infected mothers
   3. Most HIV-infected children die from Kaposi's sarcoma
   4. Failure to thrive is rare in HIV-infected children
9. Sarah, 2 years of age, has been hospitalized with viral pneumonia. Which of the following best describes the characteristic clinical manifestations of viral pneumonia:
   1. Cough, chest pain, nasal discharge
   2. Cough, wheeze, fever
   3. Cough, respiratory distress, irritability
   4. Cough, anorexia, abdominal pain
10. Craig, a 3-year-old boy, was just brought into the emergency room with suspected epiglottitis. Which of the following nursing interventions would be of highest priority for initial contact with a child with suspected epiglottitis:
    1. Perform a detailed nursing assessment of the child, including rectal temperature
    2. Examine the child's throat with a tongue depressor and flashlight to check for erythema and edema
    3. Maintain the child in the most comfortable position for breathing
    4. Prepare to administer a sedative so the child can relax

12

GERONTOLOGICAL NURSING

Is it the thrill of the newborn's cry, the older person's eyes that sparkle and say, "Thank you for your concern," or waving goodbye to the patient who was critically ill but now going home? These are just a few reasons why I want to be a nurse. Nursing is a wonderful array of joys, opportunities, challenges, and rewards. I enjoy being a part of nursing because it gives me the opportunity to help others. The challenges that nursing provides continually add to my knowledge and press me to work harder. Each day brings new experiences filled with blessings.

April Ottum
Student Nurse

45

CARE OF THE OLDER ADULT

Gloria E. Wold

KEY TERMS

akinesia
aphasia
ataxia
chronological age
claudication
collagen
dementia
disoriented
dysarthria
dysphagia
hemianopia
hemiplegia
kyphosis
lentigo
nocturia
orthostatic hypotension
presbycusis
presbyopia
pruritus
pyrosis
senility
shearing forces

LEARNING OBJECTIVES

After reading this chapter the student should be able to do the following:

- Define the key terms.
- Identify demographic information about the older population in the United States.
- Identify some of the common myths concerning the older adult.
- Describe biological and psychosocial theories of aging.
- Describe changes associated with aging for each of the body systems.
- Discuss methods of assessment used for each body system.
- Identify nursing diagnoses appropriate to the older adult.
- Describe appropriate nursing interventions for common health concerns of the older adult.
- Describe how older adults differ from younger individuals in their response to illness, medications, and hospitalization.
- Describe why finances and housing are major concerns for the older adult.
- Identify changes that occur with aging in intelligence, learning, and memory.
- Describe common psychosocial events that occur to the older adult.
- Describe ways to preserve dignity and to increase self-esteem of the older adult.

RELATED TOPICS OF INTEREST

- Life span development (Chapter 7)
- Signs, symptoms, and physical assessment (Chapter 9)
- Care of the patient with a cardiovascular disorder (Chapter 28)
- Care of the patient with a blood or lymphatic disorder (Chapter 29)
- Care of the patient with a respiratory disorder (Chapter 31)
- Care of the patient with an endocrine disorder (Chapter 32)
- Care of the patient with a neurological disorder (Chapter 35)
- Loss, grief, dying, and death (Chapter 52)

OVERVIEW OF THE AGING ADULT

Description

Late adulthood is recognized as beginning about age 65 and covering the remaining years until death, which could represent a span of 40 years or more. It may be more appropriate to think of late adulthood as encompassing several groups: the young older adults, who are in their late sixties and early seventies; the middle older adults, who are in their late seventies and early eighties; the older elder adults, who are older than 85; and the centenarians, who are older than 100 years of age.

Although late adulthood is tied to chronological age, it is important to note that **chronological age** (the age of an individual expressed as a period of time that has elapsed since birth) is a very poor indicator of old age. Some individuals are "old" in their fifties, and others in their nineties are physically and mentally active, involved contributors to society. Generally, people do not see themselves or others as being "old" if they are active and healthy (Fig. 45-1).

Demographics

Currently there are approximately 30 million individuals over 65 years of age (Fig. 45-2). This represents 12% of the United States population. Approximately 60% are women and 40% are men. The majority are Caucasian (90.5%). African-Americans and other races represent 9.5% of older adults. It is projected that by the year 2020, 17% to 18% of the population will be over the age of 65.

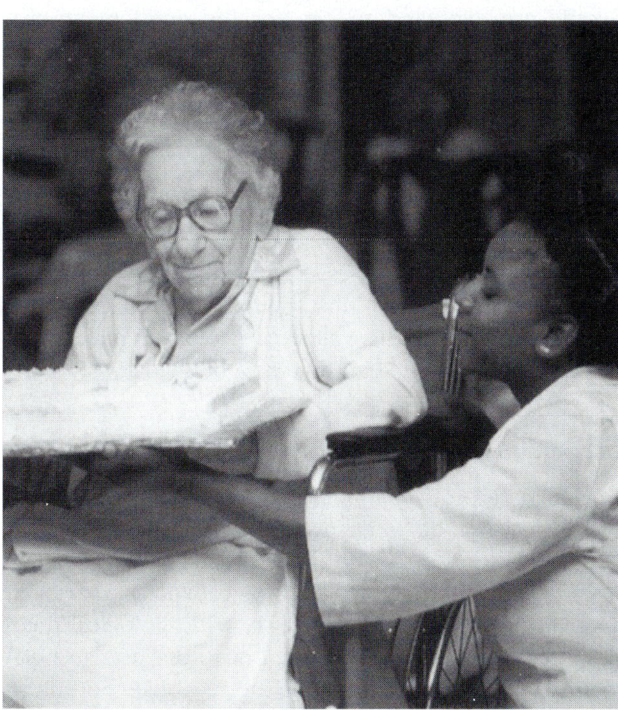

FIG. 45-1 Self-esteem is vital for successful aging.

Legislation Affecting Older Adults

The first major legislation that attempted to provide financial security for older adults was the Social Security Act of 1935. At the time this law was passed, few people lived long enough to collect significant benefits. Over time, increasing numbers of politically active older adults sought and achieved major new legislation designed to benefit themselves (Table 45-1 on p. 1450). Although this legislation has helped many older adults, the continu-

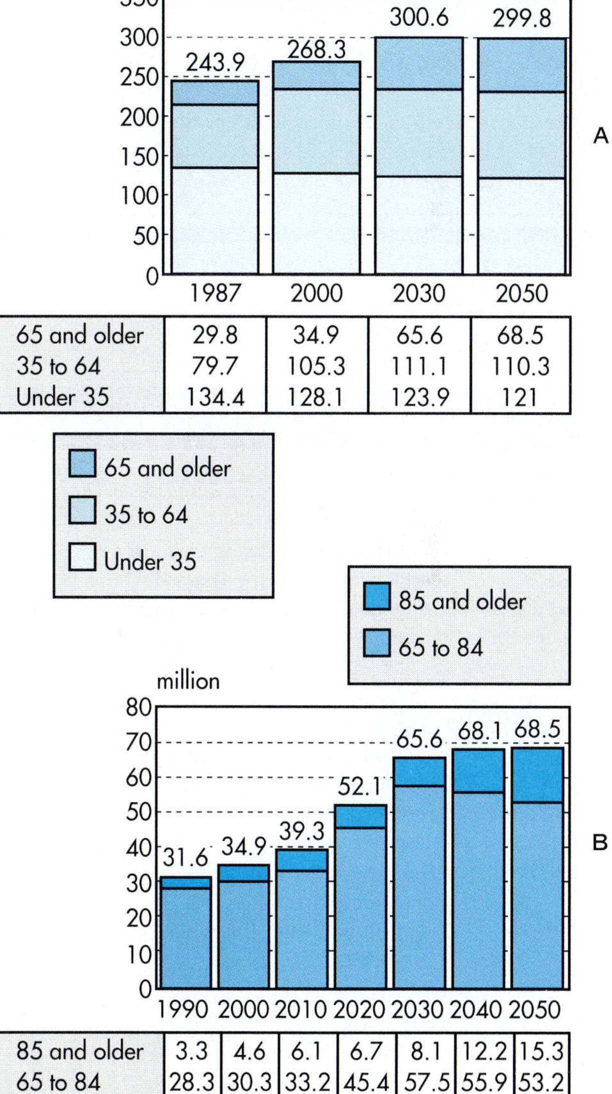

FIG. 45-2 National population projections. **A,** All ages, 1987 to 2050. **B,** Older adults, 1990 to 2050. (Data published by the U.S. Bureau of the Census, 1989.)

Box 45-1

COMMON MYTHS ASSOCIATED WITH AGING

Myth: All people become senile when they become old.
Reality: Studies and evidence indicate that decline is not inevitable. Creativity and intelligence do not appear to change. Memory and learning ability may show slight decline, since they are functions of the nervous system, which does experience some age-related changes. Serious decline in mental capabilities is generally a result of disease process—not age.

Myth: Older adults are isolated and alone.
Reality: Studies have shown that the majority of older adults have at least weekly contact with family. Many live within a half-hour's drive of at least one family member. Although it is assumed that the family is the main support and source of social activity, many older people have also developed a network of friends who provide support and relationships.

Myth: Most older adults are in nursing homes or care facilities.
Reality: Only 10% of older adults persons reside in hospitals or nursing homes. The majority of older adults own and live in their own homes.

Myth: Older adults are poor.
Reality: Although the poverty rate for people over 65 (12%) is above that of the rest of the population (10.5%), it is interesting to note that the median net worth of older households was over $60,000, compared with the U.S. average for other households of $32,000. The net worth for 16% of older households was below $5,000 and for 7% was above $250,000.

Myth: Older adults are ill and disabled.
Reality: Most older people have at least one chronic condition, but these conditions generally do not limit their ability to manage their household and activities of daily living. In a study of noninstitutionalized older adults, approximately 7 of 10 individuals reported their health as "good" or "excellent" as compared with that of others their own age.

TABLE 45-1 Legislation That Has Helped Older Adults

Year	Legislation
1965	Medicare and Medicaid established.
	Administration on Aging established.
1967	Age Discrimination Act passed.
1972	Supplemental Security Income Program instituted.
	Social Security indexed to reflect inflation, COLA.
	Nutrition Act passed, which allows for provision of nutrition programs for older adults.
1973	Council on Aging established.
1978	Mandatory retirement age was changed to age 70.
1986	Mandatory retirement age was eliminated for most employees.
1988	Catastrophic health insurance became part of Medicare.

ously increasing cost of these programs is leading to intergenerational conflict. Proportionately fewer working people are expected to pay for the entitlement programs, and resentment among the young is growing. How the opposing needs of the generations will ultimately be resolved is a major problem facing our society.

Myths and Realities

The myths and stereotypes of aging and older adults are numerous (Box 45-1). Most myths are generalizations that focus on the negative aspects of aging. In many cases research has proved such myths to be inaccurate.

Theories of Aging

Our current knowledge about aging and the aging process is very limited. In an attempt to explain aging and a person's response to aging, a number of theories have been proposed. Some of the biological and psychosocial theories of aging are listed in Box 45-2. Biological theories attempt to explain why the body ages; psychosocial theories try to give reasons for the responses and inter-

Box 45-2 COMMON THEORIES OF AGING

BIOLOGICAL

Programmed Aging

Cells in the body can reproduce only 40 to 60 times. Aging takes place when more and more cells can no longer regenerate themselves.

Error

An error in protein synthesis causes successive errors in cells of the body, resulting in decline in biological functions.

Immunological

Through the immune system becoming less effective and/or less able to distinguish between foreign and host cells, aging occurs as a result of less protection from infection or disease and the immune system destroying body cells that it misreads as defective or foreign.

Free Radical

In the metabolism of the body to produce energy, extra electrons are released that build up in the body and combine chemically, damaging cells and interfering with normal body function, resulting in aging.

Wear and Tear

Cells of the body wear out from internal and external stress, which can include chemical damage, trauma, or dysfunction of body systems and buildup of waste products.

PSYCHOSOCIAL

Erikson's Developmental Stages

In the last stage of life the task is acceptance of life and one's own life-style, which can result in ego integrity. Inability to achieve a level of acceptance results in anger and despair.

Disengagement Theory

Aging is the process in which the older adults and society mutually withdraw from one another.

Exchange Theory

Aging is reduced interaction between older adults and society as a result of the decreasing value that interaction has for both.

Activity Theory

Aging is a result of decreasing involvement of older adults in the activities and events of the world.

actions older adults have with society during late adulthood.

BODY SYSTEMS, AGING, AND RELATED NURSING INTERVENTIONS

All systems of the body experience age-related changes. The degree and rate at which changes occur vary among individuals, systems, and organs, as does a person's ability to compensate. For each body system there are changes and conditions that are more commonly found in older adults, and these changes produce needs and interventions that may be unique to the older individual. In this chapter the most common nursing diagnoses are identified and interventions given that focus on the older individual, but in all cases additional nursing diagnoses and interventions may be appropriate to meet the individual needs of the older adult, or there may be interventions that would be appropriate regardless of age and that are discussed in other chapters.

Integumentary System

Age-Related Changes. The majority of age-related changes in the integumentary system are apparent to most people: the lack of pigment in the hair (graying); thinning hair and baldness; less **collagen** (a fibrous, insoluble protein found in connective tissue, including skin, bone, and ligaments) and elasticity in the skin, with less fat under the skin (wrinkles); age spots (**lentigo** [a tan or brown macule on the skin brought on by sun exposure, usually in middle-aged or older persons]); thinning of the epidermis and reduced numbers of oil and

TABLE 45-2 Integumentary Changes With Aging

Physiological Change	Results
Decreased vascularity of dermis and decreased amount of melanin	Increased pallor in white skin Decreased hair color (graying)
Decreased sebaceous gland function	Increased dry skin
Decreased sweat gland function	Decreased perspiration
Decreased subcutaneous fat	Increased wrinkling
Decreased thickness of epidermis	Increased susceptibility to trauma
Increased localized pigmentation	Increased incidence of brown spots (senile lentigo)
Increased capillary fragility	Increased purple patches (senile purpura)
Decreased density of hair growth	Decreased amount and thickness of hair on head and body
Decreased hormone production	Decreased vaginal secretions and breast tissue mass as well as decreased speed of erection Increased brittleness of nails
Decreased peripheral circulation	Increased thickening and yellowing of nails
Decreased rate of nail growth	Increased longitudinal ridges on nails
Increased androgen to estrogen ratio	Increased facial hair in women

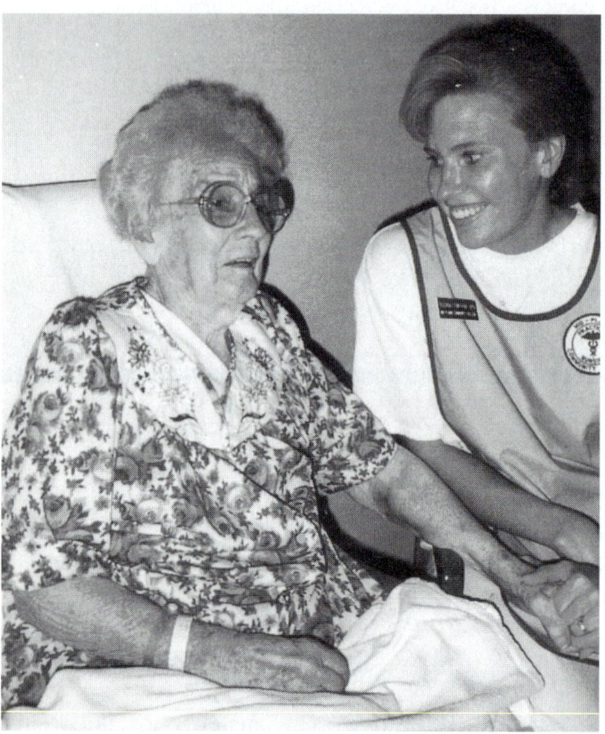

FIG. 45-3 Age-related changes in the integumentary system.

sweat glands (dry skin); and increased fragility of blood vessels, resulting in ecchymosis (bruising). See Table 45-2 and Fig. 45-3 for integumentary changes with aging.

Assessment of the Integumentary System.

- Observe skin for signs of excessive dryness, or impairment. Note presence, location, and amount of exudate.
- Observe hair for excessive loss, dryness, or oiliness.
- Observe the nails for excessive length, sharp edges, brittleness, increased thickening, and yellowing.

Common Concerns and Nursing Interventions.

Pruritus. Older persons may complain of dryness and itching **(pruritus)** of the skin, especially in cold dry weather, because of reduced glandular secretions and moisture. Soap can be drying to the skin; this is true even of soaps designed for dry skin and of the residue left after incomplete rinsing. Older individuals should use soap sparingly. For sedentary older adults, bathing once or twice a week with partial baths may be sufficient, because the normal body oils and perspiration are reduced. Water-based or light oil-based substances should replace alcohol rubs and alcohol-based substances for skin care. Application of water-based lotions to dry areas and after bathing can improve most individuals' comfort and avoid the feeling of oil residue that some persons find uncomfortable.

Decubitus ulcers. Thin skin and lack of subcutaneous fat predispose the older adults to decubitus ulcers when fragile skin is compressed between bony prominences of the body and other objects. The fragile skin also bruises and tears easily. The nurse should institute measures that will prevent pressure, friction, **shearing forces** (forces tending to produce injury by a shearing strain), and moisture (most commonly associated with incontinence). Pressure points can best be prevented by frequent repositioning. There are many types of pads and aids available that are said to prevent pressure, but it is important to use aids that will minimize pressure without restricting circulation or creating pressure on surrounding areas.

The most common situation resulting in friction occurs when fragile skin rubs against the sheets of the bed. Besides the normal safety precautions taken to prevent injury to any patient, gentle handling during turning and transfers is required. It may be necessary to use additional assistance or equipment to adequately lift and move a patient rather than risk friction "burns" and tearing of the skin while trying to reposition a patient in bed. The use of tape on the skin of older adults should be minimized, because the fragile skin can easily be torn in the process of removing tape. Urine, drainage, or fecal material left in contact with the skin even for a short period of time can cause it to become impaired. This can accelerate the formation of decubitus ulcers when it occurs at a pressure point such as the coccyx or hip. Urine, drainage, or fecal material should be removed and the skin washed, rinsed with clear water, and patted dry.

Prevention and healing of any decubiti depend on good nutritional status. A well-balanced diet with attention to protein, vitamins, and minerals plays an important role in maintaining skin integrity in the older adult.

Nursing diagnoses and interventions for the patient with decubitus ulcers include but are not limited to the following:

NURSING DIAGNOSES	NURSING INTERVENTIONS
Skin integrity, impaired, high risk for, related to physiological changes of aging	Perform daily skin inspection. Reduce frequency of bathing. Use mild, nondetergent soaps, and rinse thoroughly. Use emollients and lotions to maintain skin moisture. Turn and reposition frequently. Move and transfer carefully. Reduce sources of pressure. Keep linens clean, dry, and free from foreign objects.
Skin integrity, impaired, related to inadequate nutritional intake	Assess nutritional intake. Explain importance of nutrition. Provide adequate nutrients and fluids. Assess wounds daily including size, location, and depth. Obtain wound cultures if appropriate. Follow strict aseptic technique when performing wound care per physician orders.

Gastrointestinal System

Age-Related Changes. Older persons experience a decreased secretion of saliva and enzymes in the intestinal tract, atrophy and decreased tone of the intestine, and decreased peristalsis. The normal changes of aging may be intensified by medications commonly prescribed for other conditions, lack of fluids, and lack of exercise. Older persons also have a less active gag response, which increases the chances of choking and aspiration (Table 45-3).

TABLE 45-3 Gastrointestinal Changes With Aging

Physiological Change	Results
Increased dental caries and tooth loss	Decreased ability to chew normally Decreased nutritional status
Decreased gag reflex	Increased incidence of choking and aspiration
Decreased muscle tone at sphincters	Increased incidence of pyrosis (heartburn); esophageal reflux
Decreased gastric secretions	Decreased digestion
Decreased peristalsis	Increased constipation and bowel impaction

Assessment of the Gastrointestinal System.

- Assess oral cavity for presence of lesions, dental caries, loose teeth, and halitosis.
- Assess ability to chew and swallow. Assess for complaints of **pyrosis** (heartburn).
- Assess for complaints of intestinal cramping.
- Assess dietary intake, especially of high-fiber foods, fat, and sodium. Note amount and type of food and fluid intake.
- Assess weight. Compare with norms and note significant changes.
- Assess for signs of abdominal distention.
- Assess frequency, amount, and consistency of bowel elimination.
- Assess individual's ability to control defecation.
- Assess bowel elimination routines and use of laxatives.

Common Concerns and Nursing Interventions.

Nutrition and obesity. *Obesity* is defined as weighing 20% over ideal body weight and is commonplace in the older adult. It would be prudent and perfectly normal for older adults to consume less food than they did in their earlier, more physically active years. The general nursing diagnosis would be *nutrition, altered: more than body requirements.* The interventions would focus on reducing calories while providing the necessary nutrients in a diet acceptable to the older adult. Adults 75 to 90 years of age need approximately 30 calories per kilogram of body weight (14 cal/lb), compared with 40 calories per kilogram (18 cal/lb) for persons 20 to 37 years of age. This normally represents a diet of 1800 to 2400 calories daily, depending on gender and ideal weight. With the reduction in calories, older adults need to consume "quality foods" such as grains, vegetables, and fruits, which contain vitamins and minerals to meet their daily needs without large amounts of sugars and fats. They also need foods that provide protein and are good sources of calcium. In assisting an older adult with a reduced-calorie diet, the nurse should keep in mind foods that may be poorly tolerated as a result of changes in the digestive tract, the inability to eat certain foods because of dentures, difficulty in chewing and swallowing, and what the older adult defines as acceptable to eat or individual food preferences.

Unless there is a medical condition requiring supplementation, a well-balanced diet precludes the need for daily vitamin supplements.

Weight loss. A very gradual weight loss over the later years is a normal response to loss of body mass associated with changes of body composition of fat, muscle, and fluid. A rapid weight loss may indicate illness and should be reported to the older person's physician.

Fluids/dehydration. Fluids are necessary for the body to function and remove waste products of metabolism. It is important for an elderly person to have a minimum of 1500 ml of fluids daily. Frequently older adult individuals decrease fluid intake as a means of controlling incontinence when they have difficulty with mobility, which affects their ability to get to the bathroom, undress, and dress. Others have difficulty with hand grasp, so that pouring and drinking from a cup are difficult.

The general nursing diagnosis would be *fluid volume deficit,* and the interventions would depend on the cause of the deficit. If the deficit is caused by the older adult trying to control occurrences of incontinence resulting from an inability to get to the bathroom in time, the most appropriate interventions would be to make arrangements to have fluids available *and* toilet facilities easily accessible. This can be done by arranging the room so that access to the bathroom is unobstructed, the older adult is assisted to the bathroom on a scheduled basis, or a commode or urinal is kept where the older adult can easily use it. Older adults who have a fluid deficit because of difficulty picking up a cup or drinking may find one of the specially adapted cups with a double handle (Fig. 45-4) or a cutout for the nose to be a wonderful solution for a person who has difficulty bending the neck. Older adults who are disoriented may need to be prompted to drink, and those with severe impairments may need to be assisted to drink fluids on a scheduled basis.

Oral hygiene and dentures. Because many older people have dentures, people assume that it is normal to lose one's teeth during old age. However, it is not part of the normal aging process to lose teeth. Poor oral hygiene, untreated periodontal disease, and the fact that today's older population matured before the introduction of many modern methods of dental prophylaxis are factors in the current older population having dentures. In the future, with good oral hygiene practices throughout life, many people will maintain their natural teeth for life.

The need for mouth care is generally related to the nursing diagnosis of *self-care deficit* or *knowledge deficit.* Recommended mouth care for older adults consists of a thorough cleansing of the entire mouth structure with a soft-bristled toothbrush or foam-stick applicators in the early morning and at bedtime. Mouth care is also

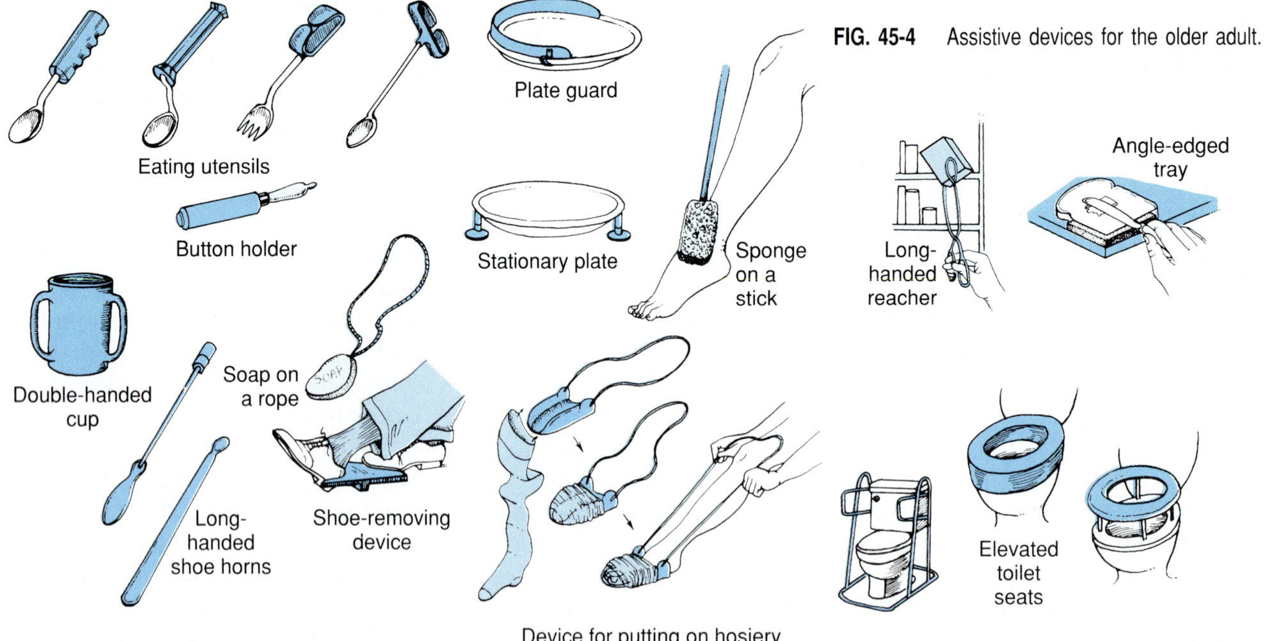

FIG. 45-4 Assistive devices for the older adult.

important when an older adult has dentures. In addition to cleaning the dentures, the gums and tongue should be brushed and the mouth rinsed.

Loss of appetite. Older adults may also experience or complain of a loss of appetite. Changes in taste resulting from decreased numbers of taste buds and saliva may make food taste different and less appealing. Missing teeth make chewing difficult and tiring. Loose-fitting dentures makes chewing difficult and can allow food under the denture resulting in lesions—both of which will decrease a person's desire to eat. Interventions begin with oral hygiene to eliminate debris that can interfere with taste or cause lesions. If dentures are in poor condition and fit poorly, interventions may include referral for dental services.

Interventions that may be appropriate when an older adult is not eating adequately because of less taste or interest in food might include preparing the food using color and garnishes, using attractive dishes and table settings with good lighting and bright colors, and providing foods that have more seasoning if there are no restrictions. Homemade frozen dinners prepared from extra portions of a favorite meal can be an easy and effective way to provide an interesting meal.

For individuals who have *impaired mobility* or *activity intolerance* that interferes with their ability to prepare food, community-based programs such as Meals-on-Wheels or home-delivered meals from a senior nutrition site can be a source of prepared meals. Also, a wide variety of fresh, canned, and frozen foods in small or single servings are available in stores. It is important to note the sodium content in canned foods.

For most individuals eating is also associated with a social setting, and food may be less appealing when an individual eats alone. Older individuals may have lost their spouses, or they may be unable to leave their home. Common nursing diagnoses involve emotional reactions or altered relationships and might be expressed as *hopelessness, grieving, or social isolation.* Appropriate interventions would depend on the nursing diagnosis. For some individuals, listening to the radio or watching television at meal time or having a pet nearby to talk to during the meal can help to relieve some of the loneliness. Another option may be for the older adult to participate in a congregate meal program in the community. This senior citizen program provides transportation, meals, and an opportunity to socialize.

Pyrosis (heartburn) and food intolerance. It is not unusual for older adults to complain of "heartburn," "sour stomach," and "gas." The nursing diagnosis may be *pain* after eating; this pain is frequently the result of a food intolerance or reflux of food into the esophagus. Reflux occurs when the sphincter at the proximal end of the stomach becomes less efficient, allowing food and digestive enzymes to flow back into the esophagus and cause irritation. Reflux can be controlled by eating small meals, avoiding eating before bedtime, and elevating the head of the bed by placing 4-inch blocks under its legs.

Lactose, which is the most common food substance to which individuals develop an intolerance, is primarily found in milk. Normally, the solution would be to avoid milk in the diet, but milk is a major source of calcium. A better answer would be to substitute other milk products, such as cheese and yogurt, that have been processed in such a way that they are better digested by lactose-intolerant individuals.

Dysphagia. Difficulty in swallowing **(dysphagia)** can be caused by neurological or vascular conditions that interfere with the coordination of swallowing and lead to nursing diagnoses of *swallowing, impaired,* and *aspiration, high risk for.* The major nursing intervention would be planning an appropriate diet, because it is usually more difficult for the older adult to swallow fluids or foods such as soup, which contain firm foods in liquid, than semisolid or solid food.

A technique to assist swallowing involves sitting the individual up straight or slightly forward, chin down, and placing small amounts of moderately textured food in the mouth. This technique can help prevent aspiration and reduces swallowing difficulty.

Constipation. Older adults are prone to constipation as a result of the decreases in intestinal secretions and mobility, but fiber in the diet, fluids, and exercise are generally adequate measures for normal function. The general nursing diagnosis would be *constipation.* Nursing interventions would be to ensure adequate fluids, exercise, and a diet that contains fiber. If dietary fiber needs to be increased and the older adult is unable to eat enough vegetables and fruits, a good source of fiber is bran. Depending on the normal diet of the older adult, up to 10 g of bran per day should be included in cereals, muffins, or breads or sprinkled over other foods. This can be achieved if the daily meals include 2 slices of whole-grain bread, 2 bran muffins or biscuits, and 2 spoonfuls of bran added to or sprinkled over other foods.

Nursing diagnoses and interventions for the older adult with gastrointestinal system changes include but are not limited to the following:

NURSING DIAGNOSES	NURSING INTERVENTIONS
Swallowing, impaired, related to altered level of awareness	Assess individual's unique needs and problems. Verify condition of teeth and/or fit of dentures. Assist to sitting position with chin flexed toward chest. Allow adequate time for meals. Feed slowly. Give frequent verbal cues to swallow. Reduce distractions during meals. Keep suction equipment available in case of problems.

NURSING DIAGNOSES	NURSING INTERVENTIONS
Nutrition, altered: less than body requirements, related to lack of interest in food	Assess reasons for loss of interest such as depression or grief. Monitor daily intake. Weigh weekly. Determine individual food preferences. Provide oral hygiene before meals. Serve meals in attractive manner; assist as needed. Supplement meals with nutritious snacks if permitted. Consult with dietitian. Provide for social interaction during meals.
Constipation, related to inadequate intake of fiber and fluids	Assess frequency and consistency of bowel movements. Increase dietary fiber by encouraging cereals such as bran and fruits such as prunes. Determine fluid preferences. Keep fluids at bedside, and offer these at frequent intervals.

TABLE 45-4 Urinary Changes With Aging

Physiological Change	Results
Decreased number of functional nephrons	Decreased filtration rate
Decreased blood supply	Decreased removal of body wastes
	Increased concentration of urine
Decreased muscle tone	Increased volume of residual urine
	Increased volume of residual urine, stress incontinence, nocturia
Decreased tissue elasticity	Decreased bladder capacity
Increased size of prostate	Increased risk of infection
	Decreased stream of urine
	Increased hesitancy, frequency, nocturia

Urinary System

Age-Related Changes. Overall kidney function decreases with age. The number of functioning glomeruli is decreased approximately 50%. Even with this decrease the body has considerable reserve to support normal body functions unless kidney disease is present. Bladder capacity decreases approximately 50%, so that it may only hold 150 ml. The bladder and sphincters lose elasticity and are less responsive to the stimulus to urinate. Men commonly experience enlargement of the prostate gland (Table 45-4).

Assessment of the Urinary System.

- Assess frequency, amount, odor, color, and consistency of urine.
- Assess individual's ability to control urination.

Common Concerns and Nursing Interventions.

Nocturia. At least 50% of older men and 70% of older women have to get up two or more times during the night to empty their bladders, a condition known as **nocturia** (excessive urination at night). This can be caused by age-related changes or medical conditions. The most significant age-related change is the decrease in bladder capacity. A decrease of bladder tone may also cause urine to remain in the bladder on emptying, causing a person to experience the sensation of a full bladder (frequency) within a brief period. Incomplete emptying of the bladder can also occur if a male has benign hypertrophy of the prostate gland, which causes the gland to enlarge, constricting the urethra and flow of urine. Although nocturia does not jeopardize an individual's physical health, it is inconvenient, interferes with sleep, and can contribute to fatigue. Significant interruptions of sleep may generate the nursing diagnosis of *sleep pattern disturbance.* In such situations, nursing interventions would focus on decreasing or controlling nocturia by limiting fluids in the evening, taking diuretic medications in the morning, and minimizing the hazards for falls when an individual has to get up to urinate. A history of nocturia or an increase in the number of episodes would require medical evaluation, because it may indicate infection and the need for medical treatment.

Incontinence. Another related problem for many older individuals is incontinence. Some older adults will not leave their home for fear they will have an "accident" in public.

Having given birth, age-related changes in muscles and ligaments, and increased abdominal pressure can cause older women to experience incontinence when they laugh, cough, or sneeze. A common age-related problem is a decrease in the time between when an individual perceives the urge to urinate and the actual relaxation of the sphincters; therefore older men and women who have problems with mobility may experience incontinence when it takes them longer to get to the bathroom.

Nursing interventions for the nursing diagnosis of *stress incontinence* begin with an understanding that an older adult is not trying to get attention by requesting to go to the bathroom frequently or is not incontinent by choice. At no time should an older adult be reprimanded or humiliated for having to urinate or having "accidents." It is more appropriate to make certain that an older adult has frequent and easy access to a bathroom or a urinal or commode. Active, ambulatory older adults may feel comfortable going out in public if fitted with external collection devices, panty liners, or absorbent briefs.

A nursing diagnosis and interventions for the older adult with urinary system changes include but are not limited to the following:

NURSING DIAGNOSIS	NURSING INTERVENTIONS
Incontinence, stress, related to age-related changes in the bladder.	Assess intake and urination patterns. Modify clothing to facilitate toileting. Answer call signals promptly. Develop a toileting schedule. Provide incontinence pads or garments when appropriate. Initiate measures to maintain skin integrity. Catheterize as prescribed by physician.

TABLE 45-5 Cardiovascular Changes With Aging

Physiological Change	Results
Decreased heart size	Decreased oxygenation
Decreased cardiac output	Increased incidence of heart failure Decreased peripheral circulation
Decreased elasticity of heart muscle and blood vessels	Decreased venous return Increased dependent edema Increased incidence of orthostatic hypotension Increased varicosities and hemorrhoids
Increased atherosclerosis	Increased blood pressure Increased myocardial infarction

Cardiovascular System

Age-Related Changes. The heart's muscle tissue loses fibers and strength with age. The valves of the heart become thick and more rigid. Nerve conduction and coordination are less efficient in the pacemaker of the heart. Cardiac output decreases approximately 1% each year after the age of 25 as heart contractions become weaker. It takes longer for the heart to contract and longer for the atria to fill. The heart is also less capable of dealing with stress; typically it takes longer for the pulse to return to normal after exercise. The vessels of the heart and body become less elastic and show calcification (arteriosclerosis) with advancing age. Systolic blood pressure generally rises to compensate for the increased resistance and loss of elasticity of vessels (Table 45-5).

Assessment of the Cardiovascular System.

- Assess for signs of pallor, rubor, or cyanosis.
- Assess apical and peripheral pulses. Compare both extremities when assessing characteristics of peripheral pulses.
- Assess capillary refill time.
- Assess for presence of vertigo or syncope.
- Assess blood pressure in lying, sitting, and standing positions. Note any significant change between positions (orthostatic hypotension).
- Assess for edema. Note location and severity.

Common Concerns and Nursing Interventions.

Dysrhythmias. Changes in the structure of and blood supply to the heart and the pacemaker system may make the heart more susceptible to irregular heart rhythms (dysrhythmias). The dysrhythmias will cause the heart to be less effective in supplying blood to the body and can lead to heart failure. Although the dysrhythmias and heart failure can be treated by the physician, the nursing diagnosis of *cardiac output, decreased,* will require nursing interventions such as observing the response to treatment by checking vital signs frequently, noting the characteristics of the pulse, accurately monitoring fluid I&O, and observing and reporting the older adult's response to medications. Other nursing interventions include minimizing stress on the heart by monitoring the response to activity and providing appropriate rest periods before and after activity. (See Chapter 28 for more specific information regarding nursing interventions for cardiac conditions.)

Peripheral vascular disease. Vascular changes affect the arteries or veins of the older adult. Arterial conditions can be caused by spasms or atherosclerosis, which causes insufficient amounts of blood to tissues in the legs and feet. The older adult may complain of cold feet, cramping (intermittent **claudication,** which is weakness of the legs accompanied by cramplike pain in the calves caused by poor circulation of the blood to the leg muscles), and numbness. Weakening of muscles and loss of elasticity in the veins are responsible for the most common venous condition in the older adult—varicose veins. The most common nursing diagnosis for peripheral vascular conditions would be *tissue perfusion, altered (peripheral).* Nursing interventions would include techniques to promote circulation, including walking to stimulate venous return, not standing in one place for long periods, and avoiding constriction of leg vessels, which can be caused by crossing the legs or knotting stockings to hold them up. For varicose veins, elastic stockings are often used to give veins needed support.

Other nursing diagnoses for peripheral vascular disease may be *infection, high risk for,* and *skin integrity, impaired, high risk for.* Nursing interventions would include cleanliness of the feet and legs; adequate shoes that will give protection, but not bind or rub; and teaching the older adult to be aware of situations that may cause injury, because sensation for hot and cold is decreased.

A nursing diagnosis and interventions for the older adult with peripheral vascular disease include but are not limited to the following:

NURSING DIAGNOSIS	NURSING INTERVENTIONS
Tissue perfusion, altered, peripheral, related to circulatory changes with aging	Assess peripheral tissue for color, temperature, sensation, movement, and the presence of pain. Assess rate, rhythm, and volume of peripheral pulses. Assess for the presence of edema. Apply antiembolism garments as ordered. Administer vasodilating medications as ordered. Handle tissue gently. Avoid temperature extremes. Discourage smoking.

Respiratory System

Age-Related Changes. The tissues of the lungs and bronchi become less elastic and more rigid with age. The chest wall is less able to expand because of changes in the skeletal system, such as **kyphosis** (an abnormal condition of the vertebral column characterized by increased convexity in the curvature of the thoracic spine) and calcification. Muscles associated with respiration are weakened, so that lung expansion and vital capacity are decreased. Overall, the older person's air exchange is reduced, and secretions and residual air remain in the lungs (Table 45-6).

TABLE 45-6 Respiratory Changes With Aging

Physiological Change	Results
Decreased body fluids	Decreased ability to humidify air
Decreased number of cilia	Decreased ability to trap debris
Decreased tissue elasticity	Decreased gas exchange Increased pooling of secretions in lower lobes
Decreased number of capillaries	Decreased gas exchange
Increased calcification of cartilage	Increased rigidity of ribcage Decreased lung capacity

Assessment of the Respiratory System.

- Assess depth, rhythm, and rate of respiration at rest and with activity.
- Assess the amount of activity the individual is able to tolerate. Note activities that result in excess respiratory effort.
- Assess for the presence of cough. Note whether productive or nonproductive.

Common Concerns and Nursing Interventions.

Chronic obstructive pulmonary disease (COPD). A common respiratory condition of older adults, COPD is not a single disease but commonly a combination of chronic bronchitis, chronic asthma, and emphysema in varying degrees that results in progressive changes that are seen as individuals become older. By age 90 nearly everyone has some degree of emphysema; therefore the disease and the age-related changes cause most older adults to experience some degree of COPD.

Nursing diagnoses would be airway clearance, ineffective, and gas exchange, impaired, and might also include ineffective breathing pattern. Nursing interventions for older adults with mild to moderate COPD include measures to liquefy secretions through adequate intake of fluids and removal of secretions by teaching proper coughing technique to improve airway clearance. Interventions for *gas exchange, impaired*, would be teaching the avoidance of smoking and areas of heavy air pollution, proper administration of prescribed medication, prevention of respiratory infections, and encouraging low-stress exercise such as walking for physical conditioning and breathing. Patient education in breathing techniques may help improve ineffective breathing patterns.

Since respiratory function affects many other systems and the functional ability of the individual, other nursing diagnoses and interventions may be appropriate for a patient with COPD (see Chapter 31).

Pneumonia. Age-related changes and decreased resistance to respiratory infections cause more older individuals to contract pneumonia and die from pneumonia than persons of younger age groups. Even with modern antibiotics and sophisticated medical treatment, pneumonia can be life threatening for the older adult. This is especially true if an older adult is hospitalized and has other chronic illnesses.

The nurse should recognize that older individuals do not always exhibit the usual signs and symptoms of pneumonia, such as high fever, cough, pain, and headache. Older individuals may show signs and symptoms only of lethargy, disorientation, anorexia, and low or mild fever. Older adults showing such signs and symptoms should be seen by a physician for appropriate treatment.

As with other respiratory conditions, nursing diagnoses would be airway clearance, ineffective, and gas exchange, impaired. Interventions would be to liquefy secretions through adequate intake of fluids and prescribed medications, assisting removal of secretions by teaching proper coughing technique to improve airway clearance, and turning and deep breathing to improve gas exchange and prevent stasis of secretions.

Nursing diagnoses and interventions for the older adult with respiratory changes include but are not limited to the following:

NURSING DIAGNOSES	NURSING INTERVENTIONS
Airway clearance, ineffective, related to obstructive pulmonary diseases	Assess respiratory patterns and effort. Observe for signs of cyanosis. Teach effective breathing and coughing techniques. Promote adequate hydration. Suction secretions if necessary. Administer supplemental oxygen as ordered. Encourage use of spirometry as ordered.
Gas exchange, impaired, related to pulmonary changes of aging	Assess respiratory patterns and effort. Observe for signs of cyanosis. Position patient to maximize chest expansion. Maintain calm, restful environment. Administer sedatives or analgesics with caution.

Musculoskeletal System

Age-Related Changes. Some of the most obvious changes associated with aging occur in the musculoskeletal system. There is a reduction in the number and size of active muscle fibers with decreased muscle strength. The joints become less elastic and flexible with the loss and calcification of cartilage. There is demineralization and loss of supporting bone matrix in the patient's skeleton, which leads to osteoporosis. In the spine, changes in the bone structure and compression of intravertebral disks result in postural changes such as kyphosis (Table 45-7).

Assessment of the Musculoskeletal System.

- Assess ability to stand, move, and perform ADLs.
- Assess gait pattern.
- Assess for muscle weakness, paralysis, joint edema, pain, or limitations in joint mobility.

Common Concerns and Nursing Interventions.

Arthritis. Two forms of arthritis may be found in the older adult. Rheumatoid arthritis, a systemic disease thought to be of immune factor origin, can affect persons of any age but is most common after the age of 60. Osteoarthritis, or degenerative joint disease, is a noninflammatory disorder in which the cartilage in the joints deteriorates and new bone forms on the surface. It is thought to be a normal response to aging. It is estimated that more than 90% of the population 40 years of age or older are affected, although a person may not experience symptoms for many years.

TABLE 45-7 Musculoskeletal Changes With Aging

Physiological Change	Results
Decreased bone calcium	Increased osteoporosis Increased curvature of the spine (kyphosis)
Decreased fluid in intervertebral discs	Decreased height
Decreased blood supply to muscles	Decreased muscle strength
Decreased tissue elasticity	Decreased mobility and flexibility
Decreased muscle mass	Decreased strength Increased risk of falls

The primary nursing diagnoses will be *physical mobility, impaired,* and *pain*. Other nursing diagnoses may be *self-care deficits, bathing/hygiene, feeding, dressing/grooming; home maintenance management, impaired; social interaction, impaired;* or *individual coping, ineffective,* since the chronic nature of arthritis affects the individual's functional ability and life-style. Interventions for older individuals with arthritis involve relieving stress on the affected joints through the use of rest and assistive devices such as splints, walkers, adapted utensils, and clothes with Velcro fasteners (see Fig. 45-4). Range-of-motion and other forms of mild exercise are recommended to maintain muscle strength and joint motion. Heat and gentle massage can help to control pain and muscle spasms, and analgesic medications may be administered.

Osteoporosis. Generally considered a normal aging process because it is so common in older adult, osteoporosis is a disease in which the bones become more porous and easily fractured. The cause is unknown, but it appears strongly related to estrogen deficiencies and low calcium levels in the blood. Most common signs and symptoms are skeletal deformities from vertebral fractures and pain in the back or extremities from compression of nerves. Hip and wrist fractures are also common with falls.

Prevention in earlier years by eating a healthy diet, maintaining the recommended calcium intake, and engaging in weight-bearing activities is recognized as much more effective for retaining bone than any treatment later in life to replace bone once it has been lost.

A nursing diagnosis for an older person with osteoporosis might be *health-seeking behaviors.* The goal would be to improve health status. Interventions would include exercise in the form of walking or swimming to stimulate the formation of bone and avoidance of heavy lifting and bending to prevent vertebral fractures. Increasing the calcium intake to 1200 to 1500 mg per day would help to reduce bone loss.

Nursing diagnoses and interventions for the older adult with musculoskeletal system changes include but are not limited to the following:

NURSING DIAGNOSES	NURSING INTERVENTIONS
Self-care deficit, bathing/hygiene, dressing/grooming, feeding, toileting, related to weakness	Assess ability to dress, feed, bathe, and toilet self. Develop plan to enhance highest level of function. Allow adequate time to perform activities. Provide assistive devices. Consult with physical and occupation therapists. Modify environment to facilitate self-care.
Mobility, impaired physical, related to musculoskeletal changes of aging	Assess strength and joint mobility. Teach maintenance of good body alignment. Have patient change position frequently. Consult with physical therapist. Provide assistive devices such as canes and walkers. Teach safe use of assistive devices.
Pain, chronic, related to joint changes	Assess nature and severity of pain. Avoid activities that increase pain. Teach maintenance of good body alignment. Teach nonpharmacological approaches to pain control. Administer analgesics as prescribed.

Falls. Falls are the leading cause of accidental death in individuals over the age of 65. The consequences of falls are much more serious for older adults than for younger people, because older adults are more likely to be injured in the fall. Because of age-related changes in the musculoskeletal system, fractures are frequently the outcome of a fall.

Falls can result from disease processes and age-related changes with advanced age. Decreased circulation to the brain; diminished coordination, space, and position perception; decreased ability to balance; decreased muscle strength; changes in gait; and slowed nervous system response are some of the major factors contributing to falls in older adults. Other factors include limited activity, side effects of medications, disorientation, and environmental hazards such as low-light situations and objects obstructing the pathway.

Injury, high risk for, is the nursing diagnosis. Appropriate interventions are to provide an environment that is free of hazards, increased lighting for decreased vision, and assistive devices such as walkers and canes to aid balance. Other adaptations would be raised toilet seats, handrails on stairs, and grab bars in the bathroom to prevent falls (see Fig. 45-4). Older adults should also be taught to sit on the side of the bed when they arise and to stand for several minutes before walking as a technique to cope with **orthostatic hypotension** (abnormally low blood pressure occurring when an individual assumes the standing posture) that may be caused by poor vascular perfusion or medications.

Endocrine System

Age-Related Changes. The levels of hormones secreted and the response of body tissue to hormones change with age. A decrease in thyroid activity causes a lower basal metabolism rate. A reduction in pituitary hormone (ACTH) levels causes a decrease of adrenal gland function and reduced levels of steroids, progesterone, androgen, and estrogen. There is a gradual decrease in the release of testosterone, estrogen, and progesterone from the gonads. The beta cells in the pancreas produce a slow and insufficient release of insulin (Table 45-8).

Assessment of the Endocrine System.

- Assess laboratory tests for abnormal calcium, glucose, or thyroid hormone levels.

Common Concerns and Nursing Intervention.

Non-insulin-dependent diabetes mellitus. Two general types of diabetes are recognized: Type I or insulin-dependent diabetes mellitus (IDDM), in which the body fails to produce insulin, and Type II or non-insulin-dependent diabetes mellitus (NIDDM), considered to be the body's inability to produce and utilize insulin appropriately. Of adult diabetics 85% to 90% have NIDDM, which often begins in middle age and does not always exhibit the usual symptoms of thirst, increased appetite, and large amounts of urine, as seen in IDDM. In older adults, repeated infections, slow healing, and sensory and nervous system dysfunctions may be the more common signs.

TABLE 45-8 Endocrine Changes With Aging

Physiological Change	Results
Decreased pituitary excretions	Decreased muscle mass
Decreased production of thyroid stimulating hormone	Decreased basal metabolic rate
Decreased production of parathyroid hormone (seen with osteoporosis)	Increased blood calcium levels
Decreased production and utilization of insulin	Increased blood glucose levels

The goal for interventions in NIDDM is to achieve and maintain a normal metabolic state through diet management, weight control, and exercise. Specific nursing diagnoses and interventions for diabetes are discussed in Chapter 32. In working with the older adult, the nurse should assist in adapting the diet, with as little change as possible to encourage compliance. Intake should be balanced, with recommended amounts of protein, carbohydrates, fats, vitamins, and minerals. Refined sugar is avoided, and a high-fiber diet is encouraged. The other aspects of care especially important include preventing complications through blood testing to monitor glucose levels, good foot care, and instituting safety precautions to prevent injury and infections.

Reproductive System

Age-Related Changes. The major changes in the reproductive system related to aging are the diminished levels of male and female hormones—estrogen and progesterone in women and androgen and testosterone in men. The process of aging diminishes sexual function but does not preclude it (Fig. 45-5). Although it takes longer for a man to be sexually aroused and achieve erection and ejaculation, men maintain the ability for sexual function into their eighties and nineties. For women, menopause is marked by a decrease in hormones, with tissue atrophy of the ovaries, fallopian tubes, cervix, and vulva. There is a decrease in the amount of vaginal secretions and the pH becomes more alkaline. Although age-related changes occur, they do not diminish the older woman's capacity to achieve orgasm and enjoy sexual relations (Table 45-9).

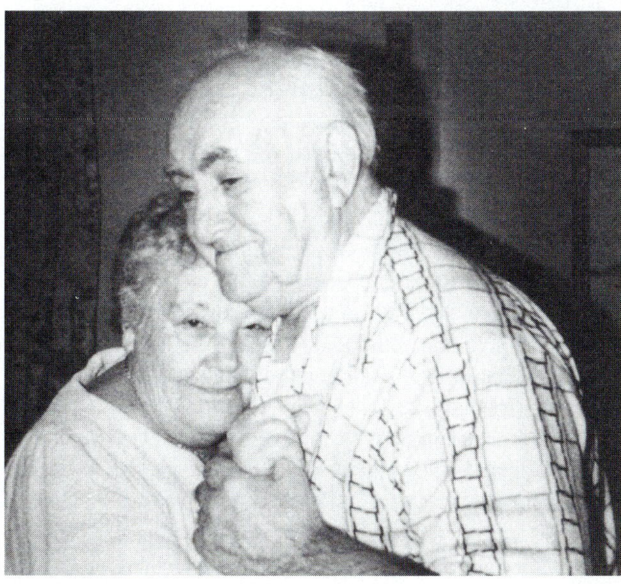

FIG. 45-5 Love, warmth, sharing. (Photo by Arthur P. Stanley. Courtesy of American Society on Aging.)

Assessment of the Reproductive System.

- Assess for signs of vaginal or penile ulceration, edema, or discharge.
- Assess for presence of dimpling or drainage from the breast.

Common Concerns and Nursing Interventions.

Sexual function. The misconceptions that older adults are impotent and asexual or that they are perverse if they are sexually active are probably the most common reasons for sexual dysfunction in older adults. If individuals continue to be sexually active on a regular basis, they retain the capability to respond sexually. In situations in which an older adult indicates that sexual intercourse is difficult or uncomfortable because of vaginal dryness, the use of estrogen creams or water-soluble lubricants can relieve the discomfort.

Research and information from a variety of sources indicate that aging individuals have the potential to be sexual, continue to have interest in sex, and are indeed sexual beings. For many older adults, the lack of a sexual partner is the main factor for decreased sexual activity.

Sexuality also encompasses sexual identity as a man or woman, intimacy (emotional closeness to others), and

TABLE 45-9 Reproductive Changes With Aging

Physiological Change	Results
Female	
Decreased estrogen levels	Decreased vaginal secretions
Decreased tissue elasticity	Decreased pubic hair
	Increased vaginal tissue fragility
	Increased tissue irritation
	Decreased size of uterus
	Decreased vaginal length and width
	Decreased size of vaginal opening
	Increased pain with intercourse (dyspareunia)
	Decreased breast tissue mass
Increased vaginal alkalinity	Increased risk of infection
Male	
Decreased testosterone	Decreased amount of facial and pubic hair
Decreased circulation	Decreased rate of ejaculation
	Decreased force of ejaculation
	Decreased speed gaining erection

touch. Regardless of age, it is important to feel good about oneself as a male or female and to have close relationships with other people.

The nurse must examine personal feelings about sexuality and aging and must become informed about age-related changes in sexual function to dispel misinformation. Sexuality of older adults can also be supported by encouraging and helping them to look their best, complimenting them when they look nice, respecting and allowing them to have privacy, not ridiculing them if they show affection for one another, and using touch to communicate acceptance. A pat on the arm or a hug can be a way of communicating concern and caring to almost anyone.

A nursing diagnosis and interventions for the older adult with sexual dysfunction include but are not limited to the following:

NURSING DIAGNOSIS	NURSING INTERVENTIONS
Sexuality patterns, altered, related to lack of privacy	Allow verbalization of concerns regarding sexual needs. Provide privacy for interaction between alert, consenting individuals. Assist individual to maintain good physical hygiene and meet cosmetic needs. Provide distraction and alternative activities for disoriented individual who masturbates; if unsuccessful, provide privacy.

Special Senses

Age-Related Changes. Age-related changes in vision include **presbyopia** (farsightedness resulting from a loss of elasticity of the lens of the eye), or narrowing of the peripheral field of vision, decreased accommodation to near objects, and a decrease in visual acuity as the pupil becomes smaller and less responsive to light. Depth perception is distorted and vision in dim light becomes difficult. There is some clouding of the lens of the eye. Yellowing of the lens and changes in color perception cause older adults to have difficulty differentiating shades of the same color and colors such as green, blue, and violet. Although the age-related changes decrease visual capability, blindness is not a normal result of aging.

Age-related changes in hearing include **presbycusis,** which is the normal loss of hearing acuity, speech intelligibility, auditory threshold, and pitch associated with aging. Hearing sensitivity decreases with age. The eardrum loses elasticity, the ossicles of the middle ear become more rigid, and there is atrophy of auditory nerve and end-organs in the inner ear. Because of exposure to a variety of loud noises throughout life and age-related changes, older individuals may have hearing losses of different tones, causing some sounds to be distorted and others to be absent.

Age-related changes affecting the sense of touch and position include a decrease in the number of receptor cells throughout the skin and joints. Older adults have increasing difficulty sensing temperature and maintaining balance, which places them at risk for burns and falls.

The effects of aging on smell and taste are relatively minor. Olfactory receptors decline in number, which may reduce or alter a person's ability to smell. There is also a decrease in the number of taste buds, although it has not been proved to what degree taste is actually affected (Table 45-10).

Assessment of the Special Senses.

- Assess eyes for dryness, tearing, or signs of irritation.
- Assess ability of individual to see both close up and at a distance. Ask about problems with or recent changes in vision.
- Assess hearing. Note use of hearing aids and effectiveness.
- Assess for reported changes in taste or smell.

THERAPEUTIC DIALOGUE

Nurse: Good morning, Mrs. Quinn. I'm Sue Gordon. I'll be taking care of you today. Mrs. Quinn? Mrs. Quinn?

Patient: I can't hear you; you have to come closer where I can see you.

Nurse: Let me help you with your hearing aid and glasses. Is that better?

Patient: Much better! I feel lost at night without them. Who did you say you were?

Nurse: I'm Sue Gordon, your nurse today. I wanted to say good morning and see if you were having any special concerns.

Patient: Nothing out of the ordinary. My joints hurt, and I didn't have a bowel movement yesterday. Will you be giving me something to help my bowels?

Nurse: I'll check what is ordered, but first let me help you with your breakfast tray. I see that you have both bran cereal and prunes. Maybe those will be enough to help your bowels.

Patient: I hope so. After breakfast I want to get dressed right away so I can go to chapel services.

Nurse: I'll make sure that we get you ready in time.

Patient: Be sure that you do. My husband died 7 years ago today, and I really want to go to the chapel.

Nurse: It's still hard, isn't it?

Patient: Yes. I still miss him; we had 52 good years together. I get lonely for him and all of the friends I've lost, but praying helps me.

Nurse: I'll let you eat so you can be ready in time. Maybe later you'd like to talk some more.

Patient: Yes, I think I'd like that. Come back later.

Common Concerns and Nursing Interventions.

Decreased vision. With increasing age comes decreasing visual capability as a result of the age-related changes previously described. The general nursing diagnosis for decreased vision would be *sensory-perceptual alteration, visual.* A number of interventions can be used to compensate for age-related changes in vision; the nurse should make sure the patient's eyeglasses are clean and are available, increase the amount of light in the environment, reduce glare by use of shades on windows and lights, and use night lights to avoid abrupt light-to-dark changes. The use of low-vision aids such as large print, strongly contrasting colors (black on a white background), and magnifying glasses can compensate for the decrease in visual acuity.

Decreased hearing. The decreased ability to hear is frequently a frustration to both older adults and individuals who are trying to talk to them. Hearing aids may help in situations in which amplification can improve hearing, but hearing aids cannot compensate for nerve damage or effectively screen out other distracting noises. To communicate with an individual with a hearing loss the nurse should speak at a normal or slightly slower pace without exaggerating or shouting, lower the tone of voice since hearing loss is frequently in the higher tones, and eliminate background noise whenever possible. Another effective communication technique is using nonverbal communication such as gestures, smiles, and nodding the head with the verbal message. The nurse should never project annoyance or impatience to the patient who has a hearing loss. Patience and acceptance are necessary in a therapeutic approach.

A nursing diagnosis and interventions for the older adult with altered senses include but are not limited to the following:

NURSING DIAGNOSIS	NURSING INTERVENTIONS
Sensory/perceptual alterations (specify), related to physiological changes of aging	Assess for sensory changes. Alert all care givers to sensory problems of individual. Determine most effective methods of communicating with sensorily impaired individual. Modify environment to remove hazards and reduce risks. Verify that assistive devices such as hearing aids or glasses are clean and functional.

TABLE 45-10 Special Sense Changes With Aging

Physiological Change	Results
Vision	
Decreased number of eyelashes	Increased risk of eye injury
Decreased tear production	Increased risk of eye irritation
Increased discoloration of lens	Decreased color perception
Decreased tissue elasticity	Increased blurring
Decreased muscle tone	Decreased diameter of pupil
	Increased refractive errors
	Decreased night vision
	Increased sensitivity to glare
Hearing	
Decreased tissue elasticity	Decreased ability to distinguish high-frequency sounds
Decreased joint mobility	Decreased high-frequency sounds
	Decreased hearing ability
Decreased number of hair cells in inner ear	Increased problems with balance
Taste and smell	
Decreased number of papillae on tongue	Decreased ability to taste
Decreased number of nasal sensory receptors	Decreased ability to detect smells

Nervous System

Age-Related Changes. With age there is a decline in the number of peripheral nerve cells and fibers, as well as brain cells. Physiologically, there is a slowing of nerve impulse transmission in the nervous system, resulting in a longer reaction time for older adults. Autonomic nervous system changes include decreased efficiency in maintaining normal body temperature and in the pulse returning to normal after exercise or stress (Table 45-11).

Assessment of the Nervous System.

- Assess alertness level.
- Assess appropriateness of behavior and responses.
- Assess changes in memory.

TABLE 45-11 Neurological Changes With Aging

Physiological Change	Results
Decreased number of brain cells	Decreased reflexes
Decreased number of nerve fibers	Decreased coordination
Decreased number of neuroreceptors	Decreased perception of stimuli
	Decreased motor responses

- Assess for the presence of pain. Note severity, location, quality, duration, and precipitating events.
- Assess sleep patterns. Note onset, duration, and quality of sleep as well as of any daytime napping.

Common Concerns and Nursing Interventions.

Insomnia. It is not unusual for older adults to state that they are not able to sleep. Studies of sleep patterns in various age-groups show that the sleep pattern changes with age. With aging there are fewer periods of deep sleep and frequent periods of wakefulness, giving the impression of sleeplessness even though the total sleep time is the same or only slightly reduced from that of young adulthood.

Many older people resort to sleeping pills in an attempt to treat their insomnia. Sleeping medications may help a person get to sleep, but they change the normal sleep patterns and may cause a person to wake up more during the night or feel drowsy and lethargic the next day.

Complaints of insomnia represent a nursing diagnosis of *sleep pattern disturbance.* Nursing interventions to help an older person sleep begin with encouraging a bedtime ritual. For most people this might include brushing the teeth, reading a book or the paper, using a favorite pillow, or listening to the radio. Exercise and activity during the day increase the likelihood of falling asleep at night. Research has also shown that the time it takes to fall asleep is related to the length of time from the last sleep period; therefore older adults may find that they can fall asleep at night if they nap in the morning rather than taking an afternoon nap.

Disorientation. **Disoriented** (to lose awareness or perception of space, time, or personal identity and relationships) is a word frequently used to describe behavior by older adults. To many people, disorientation is the same as **senility** (pertaining to, or characteristic of old age or the process of aging, especially the physical or mental deterioration accompanying aging) or dementia—conditions that are not reversible. However, the majority of causes of disorientation are reversible and should more properly be called *delirium.* Among the many causes of reversible disorientation can be anemias, electrolyte imbalances, hypoxia, drugs, sensory deficits, pain, fatigue, crisis, and sensory overload.

If an older adult suddenly becomes disoriented, it is important to look for a cause and have the older person seen by a physician for treatment. When an older adult is experiencing delirium, the nursing diagnosis will be *thought processes, altered.* Reality orientation is a useful intervention for delirium. Guidelines for reality orientation include the following:

Call patients by their correct names or as they wish to be called
Make eye contact
Converse about familiar subjects
Provide familiar objects in the older adult's environment
Explain events and procedures in concise, simple language
Be honest
Set a routine and be consistent
Engage the older adult in familiar and simple activities that have purpose, such as washing the face or brushing the teeth

Dementia/Alzheimer's disease. There are several causes of disorientation that are irreversible and are considered to be true **dementia** (a progressive impairment of intellectual [cognitive] function that interferes with normal social and occupational activities). Almost all cases of dementia are a result of either arteriosclerosis combined with small CVAs or Alzheimer's disease.

Normally seen in individuals over 60 years of age, Alzheimer's disease is a progressive condition in which there is atrophy of the brain. There is loss of cortical neurons, the ventricles are enlarged, and senile plaques and neurofibrillary tangles are found in the cortex of the brain. The onset is gradual, usually beginning with memory failure and difficulty in focusing attention. Although the older person may become anxious about the inability to remember, it may be some time before family members become aware of the decline in mental function. As the disease progresses, memory becomes worse, and the older adult has difficulty with abstract reasoning and judgment. As mental capabilities decline, behavior deteriorates. The individual becomes less sociable and alert, has less tolerance for change, and may become agitated and untidy. In the late stage of the disease, the individual becomes disoriented as to time, place, and person. Deterioration in both mental and motor function results in incoherent speech and communication difficulties. Loss of motor function creates problems with eating, dressing, and toileting. In the terminal stage, the individual is unable to communicate. There is little or no response to surroundings or recognition of family members. Physically, the patient is unable to walk or control movement, becomes incontinent of urine and feces, and is susceptible to infections.

In dementia, regardless of the cause, the main nursing diagnosis is *thought processes, altered.* Depending on the individual and the stage of the disease, other nursing diagnoses would include *self-care deficit; injury, high risk for; communication, impaired verbal;* and *anxiety.*

Interventions related to the nursing diagnoses attempt to maintain the ability of the individual to function. ADLs such as dressing may need to be divided into small steps and explained as they are done in very specific and simple terms. The individual may need to be coached as to what to do when eating and given finger foods or only one item at a time. The environment should be calm, and distracting stimuli should be eliminated. Large groups or complex activities should be avoided, because they may cause the individual to become agitated or have a catastrophic reaction (angry and aggressive behavior, which is an overreaction to a situation with which he cannot cope).

When understanding and communication become impaired, nonverbal communication becomes more important. A calm, pleasant tone of voice, gestures that correspond to the verbal message, and maintaining contact through touch and listening skills should be used. Safety measures to prevent falls must be instituted.

Wandering is a behavior frequently associated with dementia. In some situations it may be an attempt to find the bathroom or familiar surroundings; it may be the individual's way of coping with anxiety. For individuals unable to locate the bathroom or their own rooms, easily read signs with universally accepted symbols and familiar objects can help them find the way.

Restraining demented individuals can be detrimental and increase agitation. As long as there are safe areas, walking is a good activity for promoting sleep and reducing some of the anxiety and restlessness commonly found in dementia.

Care of an older adult with dementia or Alzheimer's disease requires patience and calmness. Routine is very important, and changes should be introduced very slowly. It is important to remember that the individual no longer thinks logically or understands the surroundings.

Parkinson's disease. Parkinson's disease is second only to cerebral vascular accident as the most common disorder affecting the nervous system in the older adult. It is a progressive, degenerative disease characterized by muscle rigidity, tremors, and **akinesia** (an abnormal state of motor and psychic hypoactivity). The individual has a masklike appearance, drooling, and shuffling gait and may experience emotional instability. In most cases, stress and frustration increase signs and symptoms.

Medication therapy with levodopa, amantadine HCl (Symmetrel), and anticholinergic drugs such as benztropine mesylate (Cogentin) and trihexyphenidyl HCl (Artane) may help to slow the process of the disease or may temporarily improve a patient's condition, but side effects from the drugs can also cause disorientation, blurred vision, delirium, and drowsiness.

Nursing diagnoses associated with Parkinson's disease include *mobility, impaired physical; injury, high risk for;* and *communication, impaired verbal.* Nursing interventions for an older adult with Parkinson's disease include observing the response to medication therapy and maintaining mobility through exercise and activity. Range-of-motion exercises and massage help to relieve muscle spasms and maintain joint mobility. Interventions for a safe environment such as removing throw rugs and furniture from walkways, having hand rails or objects that will not tip over if the older person uses them for support, and good lighting are important, because the lack of balance and other characteristics of the disease can contribute to falls and injuries. The use of mobility aids such as canes and walkers as well as adaptive aids for ADLs can prolong the independence of an individual with Parkinson's disease.

Intellectual function is not impaired, but the tremors and akinesia cause difficulty in communication and much frustration for both the individual and others with whom he is trying to communicate. Giving the individual time to respond, encouraging efforts to communicate, and showing acceptance of the individual through actions and nonverbal communication can help to alleviate some of the feelings of frustration.

Transient ischemic attacks. The changes in the vascular system seen in the older adult include thickening of the vessel walls and the presence to some degree of atherosclerosis and arteriosclerosis. Specific medical diagnoses related to arterial conditions in the older adult are transient ischemic attack (TIA) and CVA (stroke).

TIAs are small spasms or occlusions in the vessels of the brain. Signs and symptoms of TIA vary, depending on the vessel's location in the brain. The most common signs and symptoms are changes in vision, headache, disorientation, **ataxia** (an abnormal condition characterized by impaired ability to coordinate movement), and drop attacks (falling without losing consciousness). If the older adult has not been seen by a physician for diagnosis of the signs, a referral to a physician for medical evaluation is appropriate.

The nursing diagnosis appropriate for an individual experiencing TIAs is *injury, high risk for.* Interventions would be providing a safe environment by removing hazards, use of safety devices and mobility aids to prevent falls and assist balance, and use of memory aids such as written instructions, schedules, and lists to assist the older adult in coping with the disorientation.

Cerebrovascular accident. CVAs are the third leading cause of death in the United States and increase in likelihood after 55 years of age. Symptoms of a CVA can include **hemiplegia** (paralysis of one side of the body), **dysarthria** (difficult, poorly articulated speech, resulting from interference in the control over the muscles of speech), dysphagia (difficulty in swallowing), sensory changes such as **hemianopia** (defective vision or blindness in one half of the visual field), **aphasia** (an abnormal neurological condition in which language function is defective or absent because of an injury to certain areas of the cerebral cortex), and intellectual and emotional changes. Nursing interventions immediately after the CVA involve support of life functions and are described in Chapter 35.

Although some of the initial neurological involvement may disappear in 3 to 6 months, most individuals will have some residual dysfunction. The most common nursing diagnoses are *mobility, impaired physical; self-care deficit, bathing/hygiene;* and *communication, impaired verbal.* Interventions will focus on the rehabilitation to maximize the ability to accomplish ADLs and to be as independent as possible. Older adults may need to learn to use the nondominant hand because of hemiplegia and may require adaptive and assistive devices for ADLs, such as adapted utensils, reaching devices, and pull-on or easily secured clothing (see Fig. 45-4). Wheelchairs and canes may be necessary for the weakness, loss of balance, and loss of control of the legs. The nurse encourages or assists the patient to do exercises and activities prescribed by therapists as well as to follow the therapist's suggestions about actions that will be most beneficial for progress. Communication techniques for older adults having aphasia include listening carefully, turning down or decreasing competing stimuli such as the radio or TV, and using pictures and appropriate gestures, speaking slowly, using direct short statements, and not interrupting. With all interventions, the nurse should make sure that the older adult is not rushed and is given encouragement and praise for effort as well as success in performing tasks.

Nursing diagnoses and interventions for the older adult with neurological disorders include but are not limited to the following:

NURSING DIAGNOSES	NURSING INTERVENTIONS
Injury, high risk for, related to altered neurological or sensory function	Assess strength, joint mobility, and sensory function. Assess changes in mental status. Provide assistance during ambulation or potentially hazardous activities. Keep environment free from hazards. Answer call signal promptly. Discourage smoking and other high-risk activities. Document and report changes in behavior or physical function.
Communication, impaired verbal, related to neurological condition in which injury has occurred to certain areas of cerebral cortex	Assess communication problems and abilities. Pace communication to avoid frustration or fatigue. Use techniques determined to be most effective for individual. Keep messages simple. Repeat, rephrase, and restate messages. Use therapeutic touch. Consult with speech therapist.
Sleep pattern disturbance, related to physiological changes of aging	Assess sleep and nap patterns. Identify factors that contribute to sleep disturbance. Schedule nursing interventions to reduce interruption of sleep. Plan bedtime to meet individual's needs and preferences. Include personal sleep rituals. Modify environment to promote sleep. Provide comfort measures to promote sleep.

NURSING DIAGNOSES	NURSING INTERVENTIONS
Pain, chronic, related to joint changes	Assess nature and severity of pain. Avoid activities that increase pain. Teach maintenance of good body alignment. Teach nonpharmacological approaches to pain control. Administer analgesics as prescribed.

HEALTH CARE AND THE AGING ADULT

Signs and Symptoms and Illness

Normally we rely on a pattern of signs and symptoms to tell us when we are sick. When we assess an individual, we expect certain subjective and objective data to indicate illness. Older individuals do not always respond to illness in the same way as younger individuals. Older adults frequently respond to illness and infections by exhibiting disorientation or delirium, falling or postural instability, immobility, and incontinence. A change in behavior of an older person, especially involving the signs and symptoms listed, should be documented and reported. The change may indicate infection or illness long before any of the usual signs and symptoms appear.

Medications

Some older adults do not take any medication, but others may be taking five or more medications per day (Table 45-12). Approximately 30% of the prescriptions for medication are given to 12% of the population (people over 65). Older persons also use a high percentage of the over-the-counter (OTC) medications sold, such as antacids, laxatives, and analgesics; thus they are at risk for adverse side effects and interactions of drugs.

Age-related changes in body function can also contribute to adverse reactions. Research indicates that the body's ability to absorb, transport, and eliminate medications is decreased with age because of impaired circulation, changes in vessel walls, and a decrease in the number and efficiency of the glomeruli in the kidneys. Metabolism of medications is also decreased as a result of decreased blood flow in the liver, fewer functioning liver cells, and a decrease in the liver enzymes that function to break down and transform medications. As a result of all the changes, many medications remain in the body longer than in a younger person. Dosages may need to be reduced to prevent toxicity, since the normal adult dosage is for a 150-pound, 20-year-old individual. Many elders also have conditions such as congestive heart failure or kidney disease that further impair the body's ability to metabolize and excrete medications.

TABLE 45-12 Common Groups of Medications Used by the Older Adult

Medication Group	Nursing Interventions
Antacids	Observe for signs and symptoms of diarrhea, constipation. Teach older adult to check sodium and sugar content on the label. Encourage older adult to take antacid 1 hour after meals and not with other medications. Caution use with history of cardiac or renal conditions.
Antibiotics	Observe for disorientation, changes in hearing. Encourage fluid intake. Monitor weight, I&O, specific gravity of urine. Observe for GI disturbances, diarrhea. Observe for secondary yeast or fungal infections of mouth, vagina.
Antidepressants/antipsychotics	Observe for tremor, spasms. Teach techniques to use with vertigo when changing positions, and methods to counteract dry mouth. Caution use with glaucoma, prostate, or cardiac conditions. Observe for urinary retention.
Antihistamines	Observe for changes in blood pressure. Observe for anticholinergic effects—restlessness, delirium. Caution use with glaucoma, prostate, or cardiac conditions.
Antihypertensives	Observe for depression, anxiety, disorientation. Monitor for bradycardia, angina, hypotension.
Antiinflammatory agents	Teach importance of taking with food. Explain need for avoidance if there is a history of peptic ulcer. Observe for nausea, vomiting, GI bleeding. Observe for psychological disturbances.
Cardiovascular agents	Explain importance of keeping appointments for laboratory examinations. Observe for orthostatic hypotension. Monitor heart rate and rhythm. Observe for adverse reactions—disorientation, depression, vertigo, lethargy.
Diuretics	Observe for orthostatic hypotension, delirium, changes in mental function. Explain reasons for taking in the morning. Observe for hypokalemia. Weigh daily. Record I&O.
Narcotics	Observe for hypotension. Observe for adverse or idiosyncratic reactions—hallucinations, agitation, disorientation. Monitor respiratory function.
Oral anticoagulants	Monitor prothrombin times. Observe for bleeding. Explain importance of keeping appointments for laboratory examinations. Explain need for avoidance of aspirin-containing products. Institute safety measures to prevent injury.
Oral hypoglycemic agents	Observe for signs of hypoglycemia—weakness, headache, malaise. Monitor blood glucose levels.
Tranquilizers and sedatives	Observe for signs of oversedation—lethargy, disorientation, agitation. Explain the need to avoid other depressants and alcohol. Observe for adverse and idiosyncratic reactions—delirium, orthostatic hypotension, cardiac dysrhythmia.

Nursing interventions begin with assisting older persons to take their medications properly. Most older adults are interested in learning about the medications they are taking and appreciate techniques that will help them take the correct dose at the correct time, such as a chart or pill box with compartments labeled with the time and where the pills can be placed for each time they are to be taken. Nurses must also be alert to the possibility of medication interactions and signs and symptoms of toxicities, which can easily be misinterpreted as "signs of old age." Disorientation, fatigue, anorexia, falls, and vertigo are frequently indications of a medication reaction and should be reported to the physician for evaluation.

Hospitalization, Surgery, and Rehabilitation

Illness leading to hospitalization and surgical intervention requires the nurse to have knowledge of the aging process and the effects of anesthesia and immobility. Although responses are very individual, older adults have less reserve to cope physically and emotionally with the effects of hospitalization and surgical intervention. They require longer postoperative recovery and convalescent periods, yet during these periods it is very important to minimize the normal effects of immobility on body systems, which can include stasis of secretions, orthostatic hypotension, and digestive and perceptual disorders. This is not to say that people in their eighties and nineties should not undergo surgery, but their rehabilitation should begin as soon as they are stabilized after surgical intervention. Especially important are measures to prevent complications of immobility and techniques to support coping skills and independence. Turning, deep breathing, coughing or other techniques for ventilation, and removal of respiratory secretions are important with older adults because of the age-related changes in the respiratory tract that increase the risk of atelectasis and pneumonia. Depending on the type of surgery, older individuals should be ambulated within 8 to 24 hours to decrease the risks of stasis in the circulation, kidneys and bladder, and respiratory tract. Getting up, even to stand or take a few steps, can help to stimulate muscle activity, expand the lungs, and improve mental outlook. Older individuals should be encouraged to perform self-care activities but at their own level of tolerance and with rest periods. It is also important to remember that the hospitalization and surgical intervention may increase signs and symptoms of other chronic conditions, such as arthritis, which may be cause for complaints of discomfort or difficulty in doing ADLs.

SECURITY AND SAFETY CONCERNS FOR THE OLDER ADULT

Finances

When asked what concerns them the most in their later years, older adults will usually answer "health" and "finances." The two are frequently related. For older persons, health care can become a major expense and devastate their financial security. Because of chronic health problems in addition to acute episodes, older adults spend a greater percentage of their income on health care than younger individuals do. Many have a fixed income from retirement pensions and only limited savings to pay for the rising costs of housing, food, and health care.

For individuals in lower socioeconomic groups, pensions may not be available, and low salaries and seasonal work prevent the accumulation of finances for later in life or can be insufficient to provide basic needs. A woman who did not work outside the home may not have acquired any financial resources of her own and may become indigent when her husband dies.

Financial problems can arise when people have not planned carefully for retirement. Many people assume that adequate pensions will be available if they have to retire or if their spouses die and that Social Security pensions are available to everyone. Unfortunately, this is not true. Retirement planning, including financial planning, needs to begin early in life for both men and women. As people live longer, the retirement period could be as long as 40 years. Much of the planning involves education about the possible problems and options for retirement and financial security in the later years.

There are a number of agencies and senior programs in the community that can help older adults who have limited resources. Such programs can include homemaking assistance, legal services, low-cost housing or housing improvement, multiservice senior programs, recreation programs, and information and referral services.

Housing

Housing represents a certain amount of self-concept and status. It is also the largest expenditure in most persons' budgets; therefore it is a concern to many older adults.

The majority of older adults prefer to remain independent and have their own housing. Approximately 74% own the home in which they live, and 12% rent their house or apartment. Even when older adults own their home, the cost and difficulty of maintaining it often become a problem. Most are on fixed incomes, which do not allow for rising costs of taxes and repairs, or mobility and medical problems make it difficult or impossible to keep a home in good condition.

If an older adult chooses to have a smaller living space, it is frequently a mobile home or apartment. Other options for living arrangements might include retirement villages or senior housing apartments or single-family homes. Other innovative arrangements include group living and sharing a home.

PSYCHOSOCIAL CARE OF THE OLDER ADULT

Intelligence, Learning, and Memory

Knowledge of the psychological aspects of aging begins with the understanding that aging has little influence on intelligence, ability to learn, and memory. "Intelligence" is very hard to define and measure. Although many older adults may have had little formal education, they may be self-taught or know many things from experience. Research indicates that most older people retain their intelligence and are capable of learning throughout their lives, although it may require more time because of age-related changes in the senses and nervous system.

Loss, Grief, and Depression

Significant age-related changes experienced by the older adults in the psychosocial domain can include personal, social, and economic losses. There are changes in roles and retirement, and the loss of significant others—parents, siblings, children, spouses, and friends. Physical changes can result in losses of independence and space. For some older adults, losses occur suddenly, concurrently, or within a short period. How well a person copes with grief related to loss and how long it takes for grief to be resolved depends on many factors. For some individuals, avoiding isolation and self-pity, helping others, joining groups, adopting a pet, setting goals, maintaining independence, and retaining a sense of humor are successful coping strategies for grief or isolation.

For others, the stress and grief related to real and perceived losses lead to either short- or long-term depression. Fatigue, sadness, insomnia, anorexia, helplessness, and hypochondria are frequent symptoms of depression in older adults. These symptoms are commonly mistaken as changes that normally occur with aging. It is unfortunate that few older adults receive treatment for depression, although depression is more common in this age group than any other. Current research indicates that older persons who receive psychotherapy for depression show improvement (see Chapter 52).

Nursing diagnoses and interventions for the patient with loss, grieving, or depression include but are not limited to the following:

NURSING DIAGNOSES	NURSING INTERVENTIONS
Grieving, dysfunctional, related to losses common with aging	Encourage verbalization of feelings regarding losses. Acknowledge reality of grief. Plan care to promote consistency and reduce stress. Encourage participation in activities to provide distraction. Refer to spiritual counselor or other sources of support.
Social interaction, impaired, related to loss of significant others, illness	Assess reasons for decreased social interaction. Encourage participation in group activities. Spend time with isolated individual.
Powerlessness, related to personal, social, and economic losses	Allow older person to make choices whenever possible. Encourage person to do as much for self as possible. Adapt environment to support independence. Explain reasons for changes in plan of care.

PROMOTING HEALTHY AGING

Successful aging requires self-esteem; it is the foundation of psychosocial health. Without self-esteem a person will lack the courage to interact or cope with new situations. Although it may not be possible to alter low self-esteem created and maintained throughout life, it may be possible to improve the self-esteem of an individual when it is related to the losses common to the older adult. Programs to increase self-esteem may include reality orientation, reminiscence, and pet therapy, all of which also encourage social interaction and positive reinforcement (Fig. 45-6 on p. 1470).

Being valued by others and treated with respect builds self-esteem. Addressing an older individual as "Gramps" or "Grandma," unless the person is one's grandparent, is inappropriate. It is important to address older adults by name or what they choose to be called; it indicates respect for the individual. It is inappropriate to use an older adult's first name unless the person so specifies.

Giving an older person time to respond in a situation, respecting wishes or preferences, and listening to what an older person has to say are ways the nurse can communicate to the person that he is valued. (See Therapeutic Dialogue.)

Supporting independence of older adults and providing ways for them to control their lives contribute to self-esteem. Allowing older persons to make decisions that affect their care or to be a part of the decision-making process seems only natural but is frequently ignored. Another important nursing behavior is showing respect for privacy, space, and possessions in the home and in the hospital.

Besides the importance that independence has in maintaining self-esteem, the independence to live in their own way is necessary for many older adults to exist; this independence needs to be preserved. Ebersole speaks of the "least restrictive environment" for the frail older person. Even if their ways of coping are not the most effective or acceptable to the nurse, intervention or change that is too aggressive can exceed an older person's ability to cope. The result may be mental deterioration, physical illness, and death.

• • •

To help older adults, the nurse has a role as advocate to dispel the myths associated with aging and to educate people to the realities of aging and options that are available. Excellent sources of information and resources for older adults, their families, and care providers are the American Association of Retired Persons (AARP) and local Area Agency on Aging offices. See Box 45-3 on p. 1470 for a list of politically active senior citizen groups.

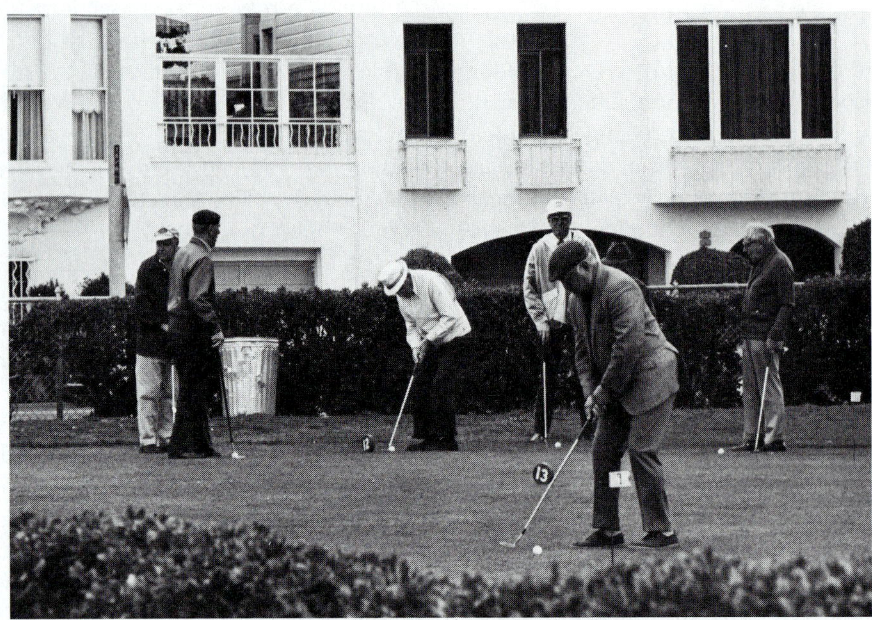

FIG. 45-6 Group activities and exercise promote healthy aging.

Box 45-3 POLITICALLY ACTIVE SENIOR CITIZEN GROUPS

AARP

American Association of Retired Persons
Consists of members who are at least age 50
Currently has 30 million members
In the future, could have 76 million members when Baby Boomers reach age 50
Uses volunteers, and employs lobbyists to advance the political and economic interest of older adults
Provides wide variety of membership benefits, including insurance programs and discounts

NCSC

National Council of Senior Citizens
Has 4.5 million members
Focuses on political and legislative issues

NASC

National Alliance of Senior Citizens
Has 2 million members
Focus on a variety of issues of concern to older adults

OWL

Older Women's League
Has 20,000 members
Focuses on needs of older women

GRAY PANTHERS

Has 75,000 members
Consists of local groups and a national organization
Attempts to increase public awareness of the needs of older adults by means of demonstrations, door-to-door canvassing, and other attention-getting methods

REFERENCES AND SUGGESTED READINGS

1. Aaronson L et al: Pressure that falls on rising, *Geriatr Nurs* 12(2):67, 1991.
2. Beare PG, Myers JL: *Principles and practice of adult health nursing,* ed 2, St Louis, 1994, Mosby.
3. Bender P: Deceptive distress in the elderly, *Am J Nurs* 92(10):29, 1992.
4. Bodey E, Robins M, Foresties M: Diversional therapy: residents in a long term care facility, *Can Nurse* 86(2):33, 1990.
5. Boondas J: Nursing home resident assessment classification and focused care, *Nurs Health Care* 12:308, 1991.
6. Burke MM, Walsh MB: *Nursing care of the frail elderly,* St Louis, 1992, Mosby.
7. Chappell ML: Living arrangements and sources of caregiving, *J Gerontol* 46(1):51, 1991.
8. Chenitz WC, Stone J, Salisbury S: *Clinical gerontological nursing,* Philadelphia, 1990, Saunders.
9. Ebersole P, Hess P: *Toward healthy aging,* ed 4, St Louis, 1994, Mosby.
10. Eliopoulos C, editor: *Caring for the elderly in diverse settings,* Philadelphia, 1990, Lippincott.
11. Eliopoulos C: *Gerontologic nursing,* ed 3, Philadelphia, 1993, Lippincott.
12. Farrell J: *Nursing care of the older person,* Philadelphia, 1990, Lippincott.
13. Fensek NA et al: Tips for treating aging skin, *Patient Care* 26(6):61, 1992.
14. Gehlsen GM, Whaley MH: Falls in the elderly. II. Balance, strength and flexibility, *Arch Phys Med Rehabil* 71:739, 1990.
15. Gray MW: Polypharmacy in the elderly: implications for nursing, *Orthop Nurse* 9(6):49, 1990.
16. Havis KA: Common dementia problems, *Geriatr Nurs* 11(2):76, 1990.
17. Herbert R: The normal aging process reviewed, *Nurs Stand* 5(51):36, 1991.
18. Hogstel MO: *Clinical manual of gerontological nursing,* St Louis, 1992, Mosby.
19. Jones PL, Millman A: Wound healing and the aged patient, *Nurs Clin North Am* 25(1):263, 1990.
20. Kain CD et al: The older adult: a comparative assessment, *Nurs Clin North Am* 25(4):833, 1990.
21. Kart CS: *The realities of aging: an introduction to gerontology,* ed 3, Boston, 1990, Allyn & Bacon.
22. Kee CC: Sensory impairment: factor X in providing nursing care to the older adult, *J Community Health Nurs* 7(1):45, 1990.
23. Kim MJ, McFarland GK, McLane AM: *Pocket guide to nursing diagnosis,* ed 5, St Louis, 1993, Mosby.
24. Kolanowski AM: The clinical importance of environmental lighting to the elderly, *J Gerontol Nurs* 18(1):10, 1992.
25. Lederer JR et al: *Care planning pocket guide: a nursing diagnosis approach,* ed 3, Redwood City, Calif, 1990, Addison-Wesley.
26. Leuckenotte AG: *Pocket guide to gerontologic assessment,* St Louis, 1990, Mosby.
27. Maas M, Buckwalter K, Hardy MA: *Nursing diagnosis and interventions for the elderly,* Redwood City, Calif, 1991, Addison-Wesley.
28. Malasanos L et al: *Health assessment,* ed 4, St Louis, 1990, Mosby.
29. Miller CA: *Nursing care of older adults: theory and practice,* Glenview, Ill, 1990, Scott Foresman/Little, Brown.
30. *Mosby's medical, nursing, and allied health dictionary,* ed 4, St Louis, 1994, Mosby.
31. Norrie JM, McHutchin E: Releasing restraints: providing safe care for the elderly, *Red Nurs Health* 14:187, 1991.
32. North American Nursing Diagnoses Association: *Ballot,* St Louis, March 1992, The Association.
33. Potter PA, Perry AG: *Fundamentals of nursing: concepts, process and practice,* ed 3, St Louis, 1993, Mosby.
34. Rantz M: *Diversional activity deficit.* In Mass M, Buckwalters KC, Hardy M, editors: *Nursing diagnosis and interventions for the elderly,* Redwood City, Calif, 1991, Addison-Wesley.
35. Ringsven MK, Bond D: *Gerontology and leadership skills for nurses,* Albany, NY, 1991, Delmar.
36. Rogers FF, editor: *Geriatric nursing care plans,* St Louis, 1991, Mosby.
37. Rubenstein LZ et al: The value of assessing falls in an elderly population, *Am J Intern Med* 113(4):308, 1990.
38. Selby TL: RNs work to keep America healthy, *Am Nurse* 22(2):3, 1990.
39. Thomas CL: *Taber's cyclopedic medical dictionary,* ed 17, Philadelphia, 1993, FA Davis.
40. Urton MM: A community home inspection approach to preventing falls among the elderly, *Public Health Rep* 106(2):192, 1991.
41. Williams SG, Dipalma JA: Constipation in the long-term care facility, *Gastroenterol Nurs* 12(3):179, 1990.
42. Wold G: *Basic geriatric nursing,* St Louis, 1993, Mosby.

CHAPTER CHALLENGE

KEY POINTS

- Although the efficiency of body systems declines with age, the body has reserves and compensatory mechanisms that normally allow an individual to function well in late adulthood in the absence of disease.
- Regardless of age, individuals have the same basic needs for physiological function, safety, security, belonging, and self-esteem.
- Although older adults are experiencing age-related changes, the rate and response to such changes are individual and require individualized care.
- In the absence of disease that affects brain tissue or thought processes, individuals retain their intelligence, ability to learn, and memory throughout their lives.
- The majority of older adults have one or more chronic conditions that may have acute episodes or affect the care necessary when treatment is occurring for other, nonrelated medical-surgical events.
- With advancing age, more coordinated and active interventions are required to support the physiological and psychological equilibrium of the individual.
- Regardless of the normal age-related changes or disease processes that occur, supportive and restorative interventions are appropriate to maintain or improve the quality of life for an older adult.

STUDY QUESTIONS

1. Mrs. Jones, a 72-year-old Caucasian, lives alone. She is physically active and provides for her own needs. She is:
   1. Typical of the older person today
   2. Not typical because she is does not live in an institutional setting
   3. Not typical because members of minority groups tend to live longer
   4. Not typical because men tend to live longer
2. Mrs. Quincy, age 81, has noticed that her skin is increasingly dry and itchy. It would be most appropriate for the nurse to encourage her to:
   1. Discuss this with her physician
   2. Bathe more frequently
   3. Use a minimal amount of soap
   4. Apply petrolatum generously to her skin
3. Mr. Borth eats many of his meals at home but frequently likes to eat out with friends. He states that his food intake has not changed over the years but his weight has steadily increased. It is most appropriate to recommend that he:
   1. Join an exercise club
   2. Go on a strict diet and take multivitamins
   3. Stop going out to eat
   4. Decrease his calorie intake by about 20%
4. After meals Mrs. Hansen complains of "heartburn." To reduce the amount of heartburn, it is *most appropriate* to recommend that she:
   1. Eat smaller, more frequent meals
   2. Take antacid medication after each meal
   3. Ingest a small glass of bicarbonate of soda
   4. Drink milk after each meal to decrease stomach acidity
5. Mr. Todd, age 78, complains of constipation. The most appropriate plan of care for this would include:
   1. Serving fresh fruits and vegetables at each meal
   2. Serving bran cereal and whole grain toast at breakfast
   3. Administration of milk of magnesia daily
   4. Use of laxative suppositories every other day
6. Mr. Jamison, an alert, ambulatory 81-year-old, is reluctant to go to physical therapy because he fears he will be incontinent. It is *most appropriate* to:
   1. Schedule therapy sessions in his room
   2. Apply a condom catheter
   3. Assist him to the bathroom before each therapy session
   4. Restrict his fluid intake on the days he has therapy
7. Mrs. Berg suffers from Parkinson's disease, for which she takes levodopa. She often experiences difficulty in stating her wishes. The nurse can best help her communicate by:
   1. Providing her with paper and pencil
   2. Anticipating her requests so she doesn't have to talk
   3. Asking her many questions
   4. Using nonverbal methods of communication
8. Mrs. Sally Cooper, age 83, is a quiet lady who prefers to spend time in her room looking through old picture albums and talking to the staff about her family. The nurse recognizes that this:
   1. Is a form of life review and reminiscence that should be encouraged
   2. Is unhealthy since she does not spend enough time with other people her own age
   3. Is a sign of avoidance or denial that should be discouraged
   4. Is not providing her with enough physical activity and should be restricted
9. The new staff nurse isn't sure how to address the residents on her unit. It is most appropriate for the nurse to:
   1. Address everyone as "Grandma" or "Grandpa" until she learns their names
   2. Ask each of the residents how he or she prefers to be addressed
   3. Ask experienced staff members what they call the person
   4. Call them by their first name to make them feel more at ease

13

MENTAL HEALTH NURSING

To be a nurse, hey! That's for me. Nursing is a never-ending road for further education. There will always be something new to learn. A schoolbook with no last chapters. The sacrifices, anguish, frustration to become a nurse are forgotten and worthwhile. Forgotten, when you know you're needed, helping, and being there as a friend to someone during his time of need. The rewards can seem so simple, yet overwhelming!

Robin E. Smith
Student Nurse

46

MENTAL HEALTH CONCEPTS

Mary Miller Werlinger

KEY TERMS

adaptation
affect
affective disorder
anxiety
behavior
compulsion
conflict
defense mechanisms
depression
mania
mental illness
motivation
multiaxial system
obsession
personality
phobia
psychosis
self-concept
somatization
stress
stressor

LEARNING OBJECTIVES

After reading this chapter, the student should be able to do the following:

- Define the key terms.
- Describe the mental health continuum.
- Identify defining characteristics of people who are mentally healthy and those who are mentally ill.
- Describe the parts of the personality.
- Describe the factors that influence an individual's response to change.
- List the five axes of DSM-IV used to examine and treat mental health–illness.
- Identify barriers to healthy adaptation.
- Identify sources of stress.
- Describe factors that contribute to the development of emotional problems or mental illness.
- Identify the major components of a nursing assessment that focuses on mental status.
- Identify and describe the major mental disorders.
- List five warning signs of suicide.
- Identify basic nursing interventions for patients experiencing various mental health problems.
- Describe the general care and treatment methods for patients experiencing mental health problems.
- Identify key elements that constitute therapeutic communication.

RELATED TOPICS OF INTEREST

- Communication (Chapter 4)
- The nursing process (Chapter 5)
- Life span development (Chapter 7)
- Cultural aspects of nursing care (Chapter 8)
- Diet therapy (Chapter 19)
- Care of the patient with a gastrointestinal or accessory organ disorder (Chapter 27)
- Care of the patient with a neurological disorder (Chapter 35)
- Care of the older adult (Chapter 45)
- The patient with an addictive personality (Chapter 47)

The LPN/LVN can expect to use knowledge of mental health nursing principles in a variety of practice settings. Basic mental health concepts will be useful in understanding a patient's behavioral responses to disease and dysfunction. Each person responds differently to change, such as the change created by illness and hospitalization. Response and **behavior** (the manner in which a person acts or performs; any or all of the activities of a person, including physical actions, which are observed directly, and mental activity, which is inferred and interpreted) will vary in accordance with a person's basic personality and past experiences. All individuals have unique personalities and resources to deal with changing situations and the changing environment. An individual's mental health status may vary depending on the situation and the available support systems.

Mental health can be defined as one's ability to manage life's problems and to derive satisfaction from living throughout the various stages of life. No clear set of characteristics can be identified as specific to mental health. Mentally healthy individuals are characterized by (1) the development of mature patterns of problem solving, (2) an ability to cope with crisis beyond the assistance of family and friends, (3) a value system characterized by respect and trust for self and others, (4) having fulfilling interpersonal relationships, and (5) having satisfying work and work relationships.

Mental illness may be evidenced by behavior that is conspicuous, threatening, and disruptive of relationships or that deviates significantly from behavior that is considered socially acceptable.

Changes in society and in the economy have altered the status and situation of many individuals. It is estimated that one of every eight people in the United States is in need of mental health services. It is also estimated that one of every three people will develop a mental health problem at some point. In part these statistics may reflect our changing societal environment. Nurses may find themselves in daily contact with battered spouses, abused children, homeless people, persons who are single parents, or substance abusers. Regardless of the practice setting, the nurse will frequently find a patient in need of emotional support.

Nurses are in a position to be a source of help to the patient. Nursing care is usually rendered in an interpersonal situation. Patients will express their feelings in a variety of ways. The nurse has the responsibility of assessing and intervening while maintaining a caring relationship of trust with the patient.

The emphasis of the mental health aspect of nursing is to assist the patient and family to achieve satisfying and productive ways of dealing with both the positive and negative aspects of daily living and to cope with situations that require a change in life-style.

This chapter is not intended to be a comprehensive course in psychiatric nursing. The focus of content will be on developing an awareness and understanding that regardless of the setting or the situation, the need for emotional well-being is a common thread among all patients.

HISTORICAL OVERVIEW OF MENTAL HEALTH

The history of mental health dates to primitive times. During early history, a mentally ill person was thought to be possessed by supernatural spirits or forces. The person was often ostracized, mistreated, and banished from the community. Historical records show that there was an interest in mental health and illness and its treatment during the Greco-Roman era. History has recorded the various directions that care and treatment of mental illness have taken. The history of psychiatric nursing is relatively brief, spanning little more than a century. However, psychiatric nursing has been affected by events in the history of psychiatry, dating back to 1793 when Pinel unchained insane men and secured a safe environment for them, thus initiating the asylum movement. Linda Richards, who practiced in the 1880s, has been credited as being the first American psychiatric nurse.

The 1970s brought about changes in mental health treatment at the community level. A goal of community treatment is to return the individual to the home environment as soon as possible and to provide a support system within the community to facilitate treatment and return to as near normal functioning as possible.

Mental health concepts and principles are practiced in a variety of settings, including public health and home health care facilities and acute care hospitals. Psychiatric units and mental health centers are not the only settings in which mental health care is practiced; the patient in need of emotional support can be found in any health care setting. The community-based mental health movement and the holistic health movement brought about an awareness that all individuals, sick or well, have emotional needs.

BASIC CONCEPTS RELATED TO MENTAL HEALTH

Nursing is a people-oriented profession. Every interaction that a nurse engages in with the patient affords an opportunity for assessment of the patient's emotional state. The nurse can create an environment that allows the patient to have as positive an experience as possible.

Mental Health Continuum

Mental health and mental illness can be viewed as being on opposite ends on a *mental health continuum.* On the illness end, the person is rarely in touch with reality. On the healthy side of the continuum, the person demonstrates high-level wellness. This form of wellness includes an assertive communication style, acceptance of strengths and weaknesses, and available energy to deal with life situations. The midpoint on the continuum can be regarded as normal mental health. Although some lack of insight may be evidenced, this level is characterized by adequate coping skills, satisfactory responses, and adjustments to life changes with some growth or possibly some mild regression.

Although many individuals function in a relatively "healthy" manner, periods of crisis or biochemical imbalances can decrease their functional capacity, placing them toward the lower end of the continuum, or "illness."

To determine placement on the continuum, several components of mental health must be assessed. These components include positive self-concept, awareness of responsibility for one's behavior and its consequences, maintenance of satisfying interpersonal relationships, adaptability to change, effective communication, awareness and acceptance of emotions and their expression, and recognition and use of supportive systems.

Mental health	**Mental illness**
Adaptive (constructive)	Maladaptive (destructive)

The point at which a person is deemed to be mentally ill is determined by the behavior exhibited as well as the context in which the behavior is observed. Mental illness results from an inability to cope with a situation that the individual finds overwhelming. Often the maladaptive behavior is in response to acute anxiety.

Personality and Self-Concept

Personality refers to the relatively consistent set of attitudes and behaviors particular to an individual; it consists of unique patterns of mental, emotional, and behavioral traits of a person. Thoughts, feelings, values, and beliefs evolve into a consistent set of traits that characterize the person. Personality development is influenced by genetics and interactions with the environment. From infancy and throughout life a person has interactions that affect personal security, values, personal identity, and relationships with others.

Many theories exist about the growth process and the development of the personality. All are attempts to explain why people behave as they do as well as how the individual evolves emotionally and physically.

Erik Erikson* provided a framework for understanding personality development in terms of task mastery (see Chapter 7). If a given task is not mastered, then a set of behaviors can be predicated.[8] Sigmund Freud† described personality development as having three parts: id, ego, and superego (Box 46-1). The id functions on a primitive level and is aimed primarily at experiencing pleasure and avoiding pain. The ego functions to integrate and mediate between self and the rest of the environment. It is the ego that experiences anxiety. The superego is the moralistic censoring force. It develops from the ego in response to reward or punishment from others. When all three substructures function in harmony, the individual experiences emotional stability, and would be considered to have a healthy self-concept. A mature, well-adjusted personality is "under the leadership" of the ego.

Freud delineated the levels of awareness: conscious, preconscious, and unconscious. At the conscious level experiences are within the person's awareness; the person is aware of and can control thoughts. Preconsciousness refers to thoughts of which the person is not aware but that can be recalled to consciousness. The preconscious state helps to screen certain thoughts and repress unpleasant thoughts and desires. The unconscious level holds memories, feelings, and thoughts that are not available to the conscious mind.

Self is a complex concept that has four distinct parts that influence behavior. The four areas of self are (1) personal identity, (2) body image, (3) role, and (4) self-esteem. Personal identity is the organizing principle of the self; it is the "I." A person with a strong identity knows who he is and is not. Body image is the picture of and the feelings toward one's body. Body image includes feelings about the way one looks, the way one's body functions, sex, size, and whether one's body image can help realize personal gains. Manifestations of body image include stance, posture, clothing, and jewelry. *Role performance* is the expected behavior of an individual in a social position. Roles are ascribed or assumed. An ascribed role involves no personal choice, such as being female or male. An assumed role is selected by the individual, such as occupation. In a lifetime an individual fills many overlapping roles and must combine these roles to achieve an integrated pattern of functioning. *Self-esteem* is the assessment one makes about personal worth. Self-esteem is the thoughts and feelings a person holds about self. **Self-concept** (how an individual views himself, which pertains to personal identity, body image, role, and self-esteem) is more than the total of the four parts—it is the frame of reference the individual uses for all he knows and experiences. Self-concept includes all perceptions and values held by the individual and the individual's behaviors and interactions.

Through the process of growth and development, the individual accumulates and processes information

*One of the most widely read and influential theorists whose concepts of identity and identity crisis have had major professional influence throughout the social sciences.

†Known as the "father of psychiatry" who proposed a new understanding of personality that profoundly affected Western culture.

Box 46-1 PARTS OF THE PERSONALITY

ID

The basic innate drive for survival and pleasure.

Demands constant gratification.

Composes the individual's entire personality at birth.

The id is not changed by experience because it is not in contact with the external world. Its goals are to reduce tension, to increase pleasure, and to minimize discomfort.

EGO

The reality factor.

Helps the individual perceive conditions accurately.

Decides how to act and when to act.

The ego is that portion of the psyche that is in contact with external reality—we might say the ego stands for reason and good sense, whereas the id stands for untamed passion.[9]

SUPEREGO

The parental/societal value system.

Strives for perfection and morality.

The superego develops from the ego. It serves as a judge or censor over the thoughts and activities of the ego. Freud describes three functions of the superego: conscience, self-observation, and the formation of ideals.

that helps form a basic perception of who he is, how he looks, and how others react to him. How a person sees himself determines behavior and interactions with others. Disturbances in self-concept are commonly seen in individuals with mental illness or emotional problems.

Stress

Every individual is continually exposed to a variety of situations that produce stress. A person's mental health fluctuates according to ability to adapt and deal with life situations. Any situation or event that requires change leads to stress. The situation or event may be either pleasant or unpleasant. **Stress** is the nonspecific response of the body to any demand made on it. By contrast, a **stressor** is a situation, activity, or event that produces stress. The meaning an individual gives to the stress determines whether the person feels distress. Stress is highly subjective, uniquely perceived by the person experiencing it. Stress in itself is neither good nor bad; however, its effect may be either positive or negative. Stress that facilitates individual growth and development and promotes change and adaptation brings positive results. Some stressors can be overwhelming for patients, yielding negative results seen in ineffective coping.

Mental health nursing concerns itself with behavior, particularly a person's response to stressors. Health factors affect this response. The stress of being ill greatly influences a person's emotional well-being. How stress is perceived by the person determines whether the stress produces anxiety in the individual. The nurse can be a resource in helping a patient develop adaptive patterns of behavior.

Anxiety

Anxiety (condition in which an individual experiences a vague feeling of apprehension resulting from a real or perceived threat to self) is said to be a universal emotion and is a response to a stressful situation. It is a state of apprehension, a vague feeling whose source is often unknown. Anxiety is an internal process experienced when there is a real or perceived threat to the physical body or self-concept. *Anxiety is a major component of all mental health disturbances.* In mild forms, anxiety readies the body for action and reaction to danger. Mild levels of anxiety enable the body to meet stressful demands, by promoting problem solving and constructive action. Higher levels of anxiety immobilize the individual's coping skills and result in emotional chaos. In severe forms, anxiety interferes with activities.

Anxiety is usually described in terms of levels, and each level is associated with certain behaviors (Box 46-2 on p.1478). Signs of higher levels of anxiety include vocal changes; rapid speech; increased pulse, respirations, and blood pressure; tremors; restlessness; increased perspiration; nausea; frequent urination; diarrhea; and occasionally vomiting.

Anxiety is created within the individual as the result of inner conflict, and subsequently behavior stems from the anxiety. Maladaptive behavior is often a defense against anxiety. A person learns a variety of ways to respond to anxiety as the individual moves through the various stages of growth and development. Behavior exhibited in response to stress and anxiety is the result of a combination of factors. The degree of anxiety experienced is influenced by the following:

- How the person views the stressor (nature of the event)
- The number of stressors (life situations) being handled at any one time
- Previous experience with similar situations
- The magnitude of change the event represents for the individual

Box 46-2 LEVELS OF ANXIETY

An individual's response depends on the level of anxiety.

MILD

Slight increase in vital signs and an awareness of danger
Able to think and make connections; heightened awareness
Is ready for action
Motivation is increased

MODERATE

Feels tension
Perception has decreased
Remains alert but only to specific information
May be prone to arguing, teasing, or complaining
Physical signs and symptoms may appear: headache, diarrhea, nausea, vomiting, low back pain

SEVERE

Experiences a feeling of impending danger
Perceptual field significantly narrows and becomes distorted
Communication may be distorted and difficult to understand
Feels fatigued
Changes in vital signs may be evident on assessment

PANIC

Feeling of extreme terror
May become immobilized
Reality is distorted
Personality may disintegrate further
Could cause harm to self and others

AGORAPHOBIA

Anxiety about or avoidance of places or situations from which escape might be difficult (or embarrassing) or in which help may not be available in the event of panic attack or panic-like symptoms.

Events that may precipitate feelings of anxiety include:

1. *Threats to physical integrity*: Decreased ability to perform activities of daily living; impending physiological disability: surgery, diagnosis of a life-threatening disorder; pain; infection; trauma
2. *Threats to self-esteem and insults to the identity*: Loss of significant relationships, loss of spouse, difficulty at work, loss of job, change in jobs, relocation to a new home

Anxiety is relieved through various coping and mental mechanisms that will be discussed later in this chapter. These mechanisms are partly conscious and partly unconscious. They serve to protect the individual from situations perceived as dangerous. Anxiety is an inevitable part of life; part of the emotional growth process is to learn to deal with stress and anxiety in an adaptive or corrective manner.

Motivation

Motivation is the gathering of personal resources or the inner drive to complete a task or reach a goal. This inner drive may be generated by the perceived reward of having performed the task or from the perceived threat of punishment. Motivation is an important aspect in treating emotional problems.

Frustration

Frustration refers to anything that interferes with goal-directed activity. Interference with goal-directed activity results in frustration. This concept is important in understanding the individual's response to frustration. Some people are more flexible and adaptable than others. When adaptive behavior fails, anxiety increases.

Conflict

Conflict (a mental struggle, either conscious or unconscious, resulting from the simultaneous presence of opposing or incompatible thoughts, ideas, goals, or emotional forces, such as impulses, denials, or drives) refers to the presence of two drives. Some conflicts are easily resolved, whereas others are more complicated and lead to increased anxiety. If the conflict is of a serious nature, maladaptive patterns of resolving the situation may become evident. An example of conflict can be seen when a person is ill and needs to see a physician but does not because all work-related sick time has been used.

Adaptation and Coping

Adaptation refers to an individual's ability to adjust to changing life situations using various strategies. Any kind of change in routines or patterns of living causes varying degrees of stress. Illness, family problems, lack of money, or inadequate transportation may all be viewed as stressful to the individual. An inability to meet basic needs or role expectations can precipitate emotional upheaval. Feelings and emotions are part of an individual's affect. The **affect** is the external manifestation of inner feelings or emotions. An emotionally healthy person finds ways of dealing with the stress and resolving it (problem solving); hence, adaptation occurs. Adaptation may be viewed as positive or negative, depending on the

TABLE 46-1 Commonly Used Defense Mechanisms

Mode	Description
Compensation	An individual makes up for a "deficiency" in one area by excelling in or emphasizing another area. *Example:* A boy who is small in stature places his emphasis on academics rather than attempting sports.
Conversion	Emotional conflicts are turned into a physical symptom, which provides the individual with some sort of benefit (secondary gain). *Example:* The individual who witnesses a murder, then experiences sudden blindness with no organic cause.
Denial	Reality is denied; it does not exist. *Example:* The patient who has suffered a severe myocardial infarction is told that he will have to severely restrict his physical activity. The evening nurse finds him on the floor of his room, doing sit-ups and push-ups.
Displacement	Emotions are expressed toward someone or something other than the source of the emotion. Unconsciously, the individual does not feel safe expressing the feelings directly. *Example:* The person has an argument with his employer and comes home and yells at the family.
Dissociation	Separation and detachment of emotional significance and affect from an idea or situation. *Example:* The person who has been traumatically victimized retells his situation, while smiling and joking about it.
Identification	Individual incorporates a characteristic (thought or behavior) of another individual or group. The individual does not give up personal identity. *Example:* A teenager who dresses like a favorite rock singer.
Introjection	A quality or attribute of another is internalized and becomes part of the individual. *Example:* The child who follows her parents' instructions when the parents are not present (e.g., carefully crossing the street).
Projection	Attributing to others characteristics that the person does not want to admit possessing. Blaming personal shortcomings on someone else. *Example:* A student who does poorly on an examination and states, "That test was unfair. The teacher did not present the material correctly."
Rationalization	A process of constructing plausible reasons to explain and justify one's behavior. The person denies actual thoughts and justifies actions by giving untrue, but seemingly more acceptable, reasons for the behavior. *Example:* The young boy who was instructed to make up his bed and clean his room before leaving for school chooses to play instead. In the afternoon, when he and his mother arrive home and she becomes angry at noticing his disregard of her instructions, states, "But Mom, Dad was in a hurry this morning and told me that if I wanted a ride to school, I'd better get in the car."
Reaction formation	The conscious behavior is completely opposite to the unconscious process. *Example:* A person who is excessively polite to an individual who is disliked.
Regression	Behavior, thought, or feelings used at an earlier stage of development are exhibited. *Example:* An 8-year-old who reverts to bed-wetting and thumb-sucking while hospitalized.
Repression	The barring from conscious thought of painful, disagreeable thoughts, experiences, and/or impulses. Energy is expended so that the individual has less available energy. *Example:* A patient who was incontinent after surgery represses the embarrassment and totally suppresses the event.
Sublimation	Sexual or aggressive energy/impulses are discharged in a socially acceptable way. *Example:* The teenager who engages in many competitive sports.
Suppression	An intentional exclusion of painful thoughts, experiences, or impulses. (This is not considered a defense mechanism by some.) *Example:* A student who fails to keep an appointment for academic counseling.

alternative that the individual selected. A person can grow or regress as the result of an experience.

Individuals may respond to anxiety through the use of coping responses. *Coping responses* are used to reduce anxiety brought on by stress. Common coping responses include overeating, drinking, smoking, withdrawal, seeking out someone to talk to, yelling, exercising, fighting, pacing, listening to music, and engaging in physical activity. Coping mechanisms are used consciously, and the individual chooses the behavior.

Defense Mechanisms. Another way of coping with anxiety is through defense mechanisms. **Defense mechanisms** (unconscious, intrapsychic reactions that offer protection to the self from a stressful situation) are used to block conscious awareness of the threatening feelings. Usually these mechanisms operate at the unconscious level. Defense mechanisms are behavior patterns that protect the individual against a real or perceived threat. This type of coping behavior develops when an individual experiences (perceives) an unconscious conflict or a threat to personal integrity (physical or self-concept). This threat or conflict results in the creation of a state of anxiety within the individual, which is then relieved or diminished in some manner. Every individual uses defense mechanisms to maintain biological integrity and protect the self. If defense mechanisms are used inappropriately or are overused, this behavior is deemed to be a maladaptive pattern of coping. Table 46-1 on p.1479 shows commonly used defense mechanisms.

COMMON HUMAN RESPONSES ASSOCIATED WITH MENTAL ILLNESS

The nurse should have a basic understanding of the classifications (human responses) and treatment methods for mental illness. The patient on a medical unit may have a physiological disorder but may also have a history of emotional problems. A more common situation is the patient who is ill and is experiencing emotional disturbance as a result of the illness or the impact of the illness. It is important for nurses to be able to deal with both the physical and emotional aspects of patient care.

The Diagnostic and Statistical Manual IV (DSM-IV), published by the American Psychiatric Association, is a **multiaxial system** (system used for organizing information in a psychiatric diagnosis) that classifies mental disorders and is used by most hospitals and health care professionals in the United States. Various disorders and descriptive references are outlined. DSM-IV, as it is commonly called, is the current tool used to facilitate medical diagnosis and to provide a guide to clinical practice and is also used by nursing.

This manual uses a multiaxial system to examine mental health–illness according to five categories called axes:

- *Axis I* Clinical disorders and other conditions that may be a focus of clinical attention
- *Axis II* Personality and developmental disorders
- *Axis III* General medical conditions
- *Axis IV* Psychosocial and environmental problems
- *Axis V* Global assessment of functioning

The psychiatrist or physician makes a diagnosis based on stated criteria for each psychiatric disorders. Nursing interventions as well as appropriate medications may be prescribed for conditions under Axis I, II, or III. Axis IV is used to assess present stressors that may or may not be symptoms identified as requiring additional nursing interventions. All five axes, when used together, facilitate a holistic assessment useful for comprehensive care. This classification system is an excellent resource and a valuable tool for psychiatric nurses and physicians.

Mental disorders that will be discussed in this chapter include the following:

- Organic mental disorders—delirium and dementia
- Thought process disorders—schizophrenia
- Affective disorders—depression
- Anxiety disorders—phobias, general anxiety
- Personality disorder
- Psychophysiological disorder
- Substance abuse and dependence
- Eating disorders

A basic description of each of the major disorders (organic, thought process, affective, and anxiety) and a summary of treatment, prognosis, and related nursing diagnoses can be found in Table 46-2.

Organic Mental Disorders: Delirium and Dementia

Organic disorders differ from other mental health disorders in that there is an identifiable brain disease or dysfunction that is the basis for the behavior. Organic disorders may result from an underlying vascular disorder, brain infection, trauma, metabolic disturbance, or poisoning (see Table 46-2; see also Chapters 35 and 45 for a discussion of Alzheimer's disease). A predominant characteristic of this type of disorder is disorientation. Some individuals will interact appropriately during the day while environmental stimulation exists. When environmental cues are reduced during the late evening and night, some individuals will become disoriented. Teaching reality orientation techniques and providing a safe environment are two key aspects of nursing care.

Thought Process Disorders: Schizophrenia

Thought process disorders are characterized by bizarre, non-reality-based thinking. Persons with thought disorders represent the largest number of mentally ill patients. The personality in these patients is disorganized and disintegrates, and there is a distortion of reality (see Table 46-2). There are five subtypes of this category of illness:

1. *Disorganized:* Flat or inappropriate affect, incoherence
2. *Paranoid:* Delusions; auditory hallucinations
3. *Catatonic:* Features stupor, negativism, rigidity, excitement, posturing
4. *Undifferentiated:* Delusions, hallucinations, incoherence, gross disorganization (does not fit criteria of other types)
5. *Residual:* Demonstrates the typical signs and symptoms associated with schizophrenia without displaying evidence of gross disorganization, incoherence, delusions, and hallucinations

TABLE 46-2 Human Responses Associated with Mental Illness

Characteristics	Treatment and Prognosis	Associated Nursing Diagnoses
Organic mental disorders		
Dementia		
Slow and progressive worsening of symptoms: poor memory, impaired judgment, personality changes, decreased cognitive function	Treatment is determined by cause Prognosis is poor; essential feature of condition is its insidious onset and deteriorating course with loss of intellectual abilities and personality changes	Thought processes, altered, related to cerebral deterioration Fear, related to sensory impairment Injury, high risk for, related to paranoia Anxiety (specify level), related to poor memory Self-care deficit, bathing/hygiene, related to decreased cognitive function
Delirium		
Acute onset of symptoms: disorientation, incoherent thought content, impaired cognitive function, symptoms worsen at night, illusions, hallucinations	Treatment is determined by cause Prognosis is guarded	Injury, high risk for, related to disorientation Violence, high risk for, directed at others, related to hallucination Thought processes, altered, related to alterations in mental status Self-care deficit, bathing/hygiene, related to impaired cognitive function
Nursing interventions for patients with organic disorders		
Reality orientation techniques: Tell the patient who he is, who the nurse is, where he is, orient to day and time, and tell the patient what is expected of him at that time. Place large clock and calendar in strategic locations to serve as memory cues. Decrease sensory stimuli; do not expose to crowds of people. Provide for safety: Bed in lowest position to the floor, side rails elevated, call light within reach, personal articles within reach on the bedside stand, sufficient night lighting from the bed to the bathroom. Provide for adequate nutrition. Assist with hygiene and toileting/grooming. Encourage and assist with mobility.		
Thought process disorders		
Schizophrenia		
Inappropriate emotional responses, incoherence, bizarre behavior, hallucinations and delusions, trouble relating to others Patient with paranoia may view the environment as threatening; symptoms present at least 6 months; inappropriate or absent affect; ideas of reference, magical thinking	Antipsychotic medication therapy Long-term social support Prognosis is variable and depends on the extent of the symptoms and responses to treatment Paranoid type may be reluctant to seek treatment	Thought processes, altered, related to presence of psychological conflict Sensory/perceptional alterations: visual, auditory, olfactory, related to slow and progressive worsening of symptoms Anxiety, related to inability to relate to others Self-care deficit, bathing/hygiene, related to side effect of psychotropic medications Social interaction, impaired, related to unacceptable social behaviors Role performance, altered, related to inadequate coping methods Family processes, altered, related to difficulty of family members in coping effectively with patient's maladaptive behaviors
Nursing interventions for patients with thought process disorders		
Use simple statements in communication. Use reality orientation techniques. Be alert to the presence of hallucinations: do not argue with the patient or enter into the hallucination. Provide for adequate nutrition. Approach the patient in an honest manner. Provide for safety. Encourage participation in self-care; assist with self-care as indicated.		

Continued.

TABLE 46-2 Human Responses Associated with Mental Illness—cont'd

Characteristics	Treatment and Prognosis	Associated Nursing Diagnoses
Affective disorders		
Bipolar affective disorder		
Mood swings with manic episodes, alternating with or without episodes of depression; symptoms of mania: grand or self-confident mood, overresponse to stimuli, irritability, decreased need for and ability to sleep, increased physical activity, flight of ideas, rapid speech, "too busy" to eat or pay attention to self-care wears bright, garish clothes	Antimanic medications (Lithium) Family and individual support with education regarding symptoms and appropriate use of medication Prognosis depends on response to medication and treatment	Injury, high risk for, related to impulsive behavior Activity intolerance, high risk for, related to manic episodes Violence, high risk for: directed at others, related to irritability and delusional thinking Thought processes, altered, related to psychological stress Social interaction, impaired, related to inadequate personal resources Nutrition, altered: less than body requirements, related to inadequate intake in relation to metabolic expenditures
Major depression		
Prolonged, intense unhappiness; symptoms include lack of ambition, pessimism, multiple physical complaints, guilt feelings, isolation, anxiety, suicidal ideation, appetite disturbances, sleep disturbance, fatigue, constipation, limited attention span	Antidepressant medication therapy Electroconvulsive therapy (when medications are contraindicated or are ineffective) An estimated 50% of individuals have at least one additional episode of depression	Violence, high risk for: self-directed, related to feelings of worthlessness Hopelessness, related to unmet expectations Coping, ineffective individual, related to inadequate support system Sleep pattern disturbance, related to fears and anxieties Powerlessness, related to multiple life changes Nutrition, altered: less than body requirements, related to reduced intake secondary to appetite disturbance Communication, impaired verbal, related to withdrawal into self Self-care deficit, dressing/grooming, related to fatigue secondary to sleep deprivation

Nursing interventions for patients with affective disorders

- Planned activity (may have to remove patient from group activity).
- Reduce environmental stimuli.
- Use a kind but firm manner in addressing the patient.
- Assist with grooming, hygiene, and selection of clothing.
- Provide nutritional foods and snacks.
- Provide for safety.
- Be alert to changes in mood or behavior.
- Administer prescribed medication.
- Do not argue with patient.
- Be consistent in assigning care givers to the patient.
- Assign patient to private (single) room.
- Consider providing activities for the patient in room.
- Avoid placing the patient in competitive activities.
- Weigh patient weekly.
- Offer fluids frequently and monitor for dehydration.
- Allow time for patient to respond to questions.
- Present information to patient in simple terms.
- Allow for rest periods.
- Sit with patient if he does not wish to initiate conversation.
- Be alert for cues that indicate a potential for self-harm: check for hazards, remove glass and sharp objects, check for clothing that might be used in suicide attempt, move patient closer to nursing area, monitor patient frequently.

Characteristics	Treatment and Prognosis	Associated Nursing Diagnoses
Anxiety disorders		
Generalized anxiety		
Characterized by a steady, pervasive level of anxiety Can occur at any age; common around age 20-30 Lasts 6 months or longer Symptoms: apprehension, irritability, insomnia, poor concentration, fear of unknown, conversation dominated by physical complaints, preoccupied or neglectful self-care	Occasionally, antianxiety medication therapy (therapy is effective in either diminishing anxiety or helping individual learn to cope with anxiety) Relaxation techniques Prognosis is variable; condition can last 6 months or longer	Anxiety, related to unmet needs Coping, ineffective individual, related to unrealistic perceptions Fear, related to phobia stimulus

TABLE 46-2 Human Responses Associated with Mental Illness—cont'd

Characteristics	Treatment and Prognosis	Associated Nursing Diagnoses
Panic disorders		
Severe anxiety Exhibits physical manifestations suddenly and without apparent reason Onset is frequently in the late twenties	Occasionally, antianxiety medication therapy Relaxation techniques Attacks last minutes to hours and may recur several times a week	Anxiety, related to actual or perceived threats Coping, ineffective individual, related to inadequate coping methods Fear, related to separation from support systems
Phobias		
Characterized by a persistent and irrational fear of a specific object, situation, or activity Leads to a life-style of self-protective avoidance Social phobias are more common in women	With desensitization, patient is taught to relax while reentering phobic situation in imagination and then in real life. Anxiety and fear are kept to minimum. Prognosis is variable and depends on response to treatment	Anxiety, related to inability to trust Coping, ineffective individual, related to personal vulnerability Fear, related to actual or imagined threat to self
Obsessive-compulsive disorders (OCDs)		
Neurotic condition characterized by inability to stop persistent, irrational, and uncontrollable acts (compulsions) or thoughts (obsessions) contrary to person's standards or judgment. Usually appears after adolescence, resulting from fear, guilt, and anticipation of punishment. Person is usually orderly, meticulous, punctual, dependable, and scrupulous, although with tendency to be rigid and stubborn. Mild forms are common Equally distributed between men and women Increase during stress	Treatment may consist of psychotherapy, to uncover the basic fears and to help the person distinguish objective dangers from imagined dangers. The antidepressant clomipramine (Anafranil) has been of great benefit in treating this condition. Prognosis is more severe than with other neurotic disorders; complete recovery is rare; however, complete disability is seen only in minority of cases	Anxiety, related to threat to self-concept Coping, ineffective individual, related to inadequate handling of stressors Thought processes, altered, related to increasing anxiety ***Nursing interventions for patients with anxiety disorders*** Encourage the patient to share thoughts and feelings. Be supportive and provide assistance. Encourage self-care and simple decision making. Avoid reinforcing concerns over physical complaints. Explain all procedures and treatments. Be on time with treatments and medications.
Personality disorders		
May exhibit a range of behaviors, depending on the type of disorder present Common characteristics poor impulse control (drinking, overeating, substance abuse, assaultive behavior), self-destructive acts such as self-mutilation, manipulation of others or dependency on others, inappropriate behavior for situation, disregard for rules	Medication therapy Support groups helpful (rehabilitative) Family counseling Prognosis is guarded; antisocial personality disorder is more socially malignant of disorders and appears to have most severe consequences	Social interaction, impaired, related to low self-esteem Coping, ineffective individual, related to lack of control of impulsive actions Family processes, altered, related to change in roles secondary to illness Violence, high risk for: self-directed or directed at others, related to response to therapy ***Nursing interventions for patients with personality disorders*** Be firm and consistent and set limits on behavior. Establish consequences for violating limits. Provide positive feedback when appropriate behavior is exhibited; encourage ventilation. Encourage decision making and patient participation. Discuss incidents with patient. Approach in a calm, confident manner. Know where the patient is at all times.

Major Affective Disorders: Bipolar Personality and Major Depression

Affective disorders are any of a group of psychotic disorders characterized by severe and inappropriate emotional responses, by prolonged and persistent disturbances of mood and related thought distortions, and by other symptoms associated with either depressed states or manic states (see Table 46-2). *Mood,* as defined by DSM-IV, is a prolonged emotion (depression or elation) that affects a person's psyche. Extremes in mood range from depression to mania. Research indicates that hereditary factors account for 60% to 80% of affective disorders.

Depression (a mood disturbance characterized by exaggerated feelings of sadness, despair, discouragement, dejection, worthlessness, and hopelessness that are inappropriate and out of proportion to reality) is a reaction to a real or perceived loss of a valued object. Depression may be prolonged and increasingly incapacitating for the patient.

Depression can be so severe that the person may contemplate or actually succeed at committing suicide. Many people find life so precious that they cannot understand why anyone would voluntarily end it. Yet the US Department of Health and Human Services in 1990 revealed that in 1987 more than 30,000 people committed suicide (the intentional taking of one's own life) in the United States. Suicide is increasing among young people and males and decreasing among females. Caucasians are almost twice as likely to kill themselves as African-Americans. Older adults have especially high rates of suicide.

Statistics probably understate the number of suicides since many go unreported and some "accidental" deaths may actually be self-inflicted. Also, the figures do not include suicide attempts. For example, there are about 6000 documented suicides a year among young people. Some mental health professionals estimate that each year as many as 400,000 children and teenagers try to kill themselves and fail (National Committee for Citizens in Education, 1986).

Some people believe that ending one's life is a rational decision, given certain circumstances, such as terminal illness; and suicide is considered a right to be defended. There is growing support for "right to die" legislation, which removes the criminal connotations from suicide and gives mature people the right to end their lives when they see fit. See Box 46-3. To help prevent suicide, the nurse needs to recognize its warning signals and learn the kinds of actions that can often avert it.

Box 46-3 WARNING SIGNS OF SUICIDE

- Withdrawal from family or friends
- Talking about death, the hereafter, or suicide
- Giving away prized possessions
- Drug or alcohol abuse
- Personality changes, such as unusual anger, boredom, or apathy
- Signs of depression, such as unusual neglect of appearance; difficulty concentrating on work or school; staying away from usual activities; complaints of physical problems when nothing is organically wrong; sleeping or eating much more or much less than usual; loss of self-esteem; feelings of helplessness, hopelessness, extreme anxiety, or panic

Mania (a mood disorder characterized by an expansive emotional state, extreme excitement, excessive elation, hyperactivity, agitation, overtalkativeness, flight of ideas, increased psychomotor activity, fleeting attention, and sometimes violent, destructive, or self-destructive behavior) is characterized by overactivity and a euphoric state.

Anxiety Disorders: Generalized Anxiety and Panic Disorders

Anxiety disorders are characterized by a high degree of anxiety and/or avoidance behavior. Table 46-2 describes generalized anxiety disorders and panic disorders. Two other disorders classified as anxiety related are phobic disorders and obsessive-compulsive disorders.

A phobic disorder is characterized by a persistent dread or fear of an object or situation. A **phobia** (an anxiety disorder characterized by an obsessive, irrational, and intense fear of a specific object, such as an animal or dirt; of an activity, such as meeting strangers or leaving the familiar setting of the home; or of a physical situation, such as heights and open or closed spaces) transfers anxiety to some object in the environment.

Obsessive-compulsive disorders frequently involve an undesirable but persistent thought about such things as violent behaviors, fear of contamination, or doubts about a situation (e.g., having turned off the burner of the stove). **Obsession** refers to the persistent thought or idea with which the mind is continually and involuntarily preoccupied and which suggests an irrational act. **Compulsion** (an irresistible, repetitive, irrational impulse to perform an act that is usually contrary to one's ordinary judgments or standards yet results in overt anxiety if it is not completed) involves carrying out the obsession. Obsessive-compulsive disorders may be expressed in the form of constant handwashing, being obsessed with the cleanliness of one's house, checking the gas jets on the stove numerous times before leaving the house, or committing a violent act.

Personality Disorders

Personality disorders are inflexible and maladaptive patterns of behavior or thinking that are associated with significant impairment of functioning. Box 46-4 outlines and describes the common personality disorders. The disorder usually surfaces during adolescence or earlier and continues through adulthood. The associated behaviors are generally more troubling to others than to the individual. The disorders are characterized by impaired relationships, lack of insight, and difficulty handling change (see Table 46-2).

Psychophysiological Disorders

Some physical disorders are thought to have a psychological basis. **Somatization** (a disorder characterized by recurrent, multiple, physical complaints and symptoms for which there is no organic cause) is the process whereby an individual's feelings, needs, and conflicts are manifested physiologically. Psychophysiological disorders are thought to have an emotional basis, manifested as a physical illness. Usually the individual has little or no awareness of the conflict underlying the illness and may even resent such an implication. Disorders thought to have emotional undertones include peptic ulcers, hypertension, asthma, certain skin disorders, arthritis, ulcerative colitis, coronary artery disease, painful or irregular menstruation, sexual indifference, and migraine headaches. Somatization is also referred to as *Briquet's syndrome.*

Substance Abuse and Dependence

Dependence on a substance may be defined as a disorder in which a person is psychologically or physically dependent, as on drugs or alcohol. Alcohol, the most abused drug in the United States, is a central nervous system (CNS) depressant. Drugs that are abused usually alter the mood, giving the individual a euphoric feeling. Drugs that are abused include illicit drugs and certain prescription drugs such as diazepam (Valium) and chlordiazepoxide (Librium) (Table 46-3; also see Chapter 47).

Eating Disorders

Certain individuals develop nutritional problems known as eating disorders. Two common eating disorders are anorexia nervosa and bulimia. See Chapter 19 for a discussion of eating disorders.

Box 46-4 PERSONALITY DISORDERS

Abusive personality: Individual who uses violent or abusive behavior to cope with anxiety (tension conflict)

Paranoid personality: Characterized by suspicion, secretiveness, distortion of reality, and oversensitivity; thinks that others are out "to get" him

Borderline personality: Has not established self-identity; fears being alone; experiences mood swings over a short period

Antisocial personality: Has a history of difficulties with personal relationships; does not profit from experience or punishment; has no real loyalties to any person, group, or code; and has a tendency to rationalize behavior

TABLE 46-3 Frequently Abused Substances

Substance	Related Effects
Opiates Meperidine Morphine Codeine Methadone	Euphoria, relaxation, constricted pupils, slurred speech, impaired judgment
Barbiturates Amytal Nembutal Seconal	Euphoria, decreased inhibition, impaired judgment, slurred speech, incoordination
Amphetamines	Euphoria, hyperactivity, irritability, anorexia, weight loss, tachycardia, hypertension
Cocaine/crack	Euphoria, agitation, grandiose thinking, anorexia, weight loss, diaphoresis, insomnia
Hallucinogens	Perceptual distortion, heightened awareness, hallucinations, illusions, dilated pupils
Phencyclidine (PCP)	Euphoria, perceptual distortion, agitation, delusions, violence
Marijuana	Mild euphoria, loss of inhibition, relaxation, decreased motivation
Antianxiety drugs	Relaxation, feeling of confidence, relief of anxiety, drowsiness, hypotension

OVERVIEW OF TREATMENT METHODS

Communication and the Therapeutic Relationship

The key component to psychiatric–mental health treatment is the development of a helping-trust relationship. The relationship maximizes the patient's strengths, maintains self-esteem, and assists the patient to develop and utilize coping skills. The helping-trust relationship is a therapeutic professional relationship; it is not social in nature. In a therapeutic relationship the nurse assists the patient in learning new ways of responding to people and situations.

Therapeutic communication is a dynamic process in which both participants (the nurse and the patient) share meaning. To be therapeutic, communication must assist with the corrective experiences that help the patient in meeting predetermined goals.

There are different types of relationships. Most relationships are social; that is, the participants are equally involved in exchanging information and meeting individual needs. In a therapeutic relationship both participants work toward goals that have been agreed on. The nurse assists the individual to learn new ways of interacting to function more effectively. The nurse attempts to establish a rapport with the patient and gain trust to facilitate positive interactions that will lead to corrective behavior. In day-to-day interactions with a patient the nurse will find that the individual will be more responsive and amenable to instruction if the nurse is trusted and seen as a competent professional.

Therapeutic communication is a dynamic process by which individuals share meaning. To be therapeutic, communication must assist with the corrective experiences that help the individual to meet predetermined goals. Therapeutic techniques for communication are included in Chapter 4. These techniques of communication can be used in every nursing situation. The therapeutic dialogues on pp.1486 and 1489 demonstrate therapeutic nurse-patient interactions.

Psychopharmacology

Psychotropic (psychoactive) medications are drugs used in conjunction with other therapies to help modify an individual's behavior. Medication is used to control symptoms. Monitoring for signs of effectiveness and evidence of side effects is an important nursing responsibility. It is clearly the role of the nurse administering these medications to understand their use. Commonly prescribed drugs are presented in Table 46-4.

Antidepressants. There are many antidepressant medications; the types that are currently in use include tricyclics, monoamine oxidase inhibitors (MAOIs), and a newer group (similar to the tricyclics) of which trazodone is a member. The newest class of antidepressants are the selective serotonin reuptake inhibitors (SSRIs). Prozac (fluoxetine), Zoloft (sertraline), and Paxil (paroxetine HCl) belong to this new class and assist in alleviating signs and symptoms of depression. Wellbutrin (bupropion) is of the aminoketone class and is another new antidepressant.

The medications work in different ways in the brain and assist in alleviating signs and symptoms of depression such as decreased appetite or sleep, lack of alertness, and prolonged sadness. These medications do not take effect immediately; it is generally 2 to 4 weeks before improvement is noted. Antidepressants should be continued for several months to prevent recurrence of symptoms. The nurse should be familiar with each drug before administration.

Antimanics. The chief drug used to stabilize the mood and behavior of a patient with mania is lithium carbonate. A therapeutic blood level is required and may take 7 to 10 days to achieve. During the interim, antipsychotic medications are frequently used for control of behavior. Toxicity is a problem encountered with this drug, and the nurse should be aware of the signs. Patient education is an important factor in lithium administration.

Antipsychotics. Antipsychotic medications are for acute and chronic management of (1) schizophrenia, (2) organic mental disorders with **psychosis** (major disorder of organic or emotional origin, characterized by impairment of thought, communication, and memory and distortion of reality), and (3) the manic phase of a bipolar affective personality disorder. These drugs provide some symptomatic control, but are not a cure. There are a number of side effects associated with these drugs.

THERAPEUTIC DIALOGUE

EXAMPLE: Starting a conversation with a patient may include several approaches:

What circumstances brought you to the hospital?
Tell me a little about what has been going on with you.
Mrs. Jones, I am Larry Smith. I'll be your nurse today.
Tell me how you are feeling today.

- Mrs. Jung underwent a hysterectomy 2 days ago for severe fibroid tumors. She is 32 years old and has a 3-year-old child. She has been married 5 years. The nurse who admitted her after surgery enters the room and finds her crying.

Nurse: (*Walks over to Mrs. Jung and touches her arm and stands there quietly.*)

Patient: (*Continues to cry but looks up at the nurse and starts to quiet.*)

Nurse: You look upset; would you like to talk? (*Pulls up a chair and sits at eye level.*)

Patient: My whole life is ruined.

TABLE 46-4 Psychoactive Medications

Generic Name	Trade Name	Side Effects	Nursing Implications
Antidepressants			
Tricyclics			
Amitriptyline Amoxapine Desipramine hydrochloride Imipramine hydrochloride Nortriptyline hydrochloride	Elavil Asendin Norpramin Tofranil Aventyl, Pamelor	Anticholinergic effects, including dry mouth, blurred vision, constipation, urinary retention, and tachycardia Other precautions: not used in patients with severe liver disease or immediately after a myocardial infarction; given with caution for persons with cardiac disease; abrupt withdrawal may cause sleep disturbance	Monitor BP for hypotension Observe for urinary retention and constipation Suggest sugarless gum or candy for dry mouth Explain that patient may experience increased appetite Caution patient against strenuous exercise and high temperature, because perspiration may be blocked by anticholinergic effects
Monoamine oxidase inhibitors			
Phenelzine sulfate Tranylcypromine sulfate	Nardil Parnate	Orthostatic hypotension, headache, abnormal heart rate and/or rhythm, blurred vision, dry mouth, fatigue, nausea and vomiting, constipation Other precautions: hypertensive crisis can result, especially if tyramine-containing foods are not restricted (e.g., red wine, beer, aged cheese, chocolate, licorice, yogurt, caffeine-rich foods, liver, and broad beans)	Monitor BP; have patient stand up slowly and move legs before rising Teach patient that foods high in tyramine must be restricted Consult physician before taking over-the-counter cough/cold products Know that it is contraindicated during therapy with other MAOIs or within 7 days of such therapy or elective surgery requiring general anesthesia Know drug interactions for parnate; all medications should be assessed by physician and pharmacist before being added to drug regimen
Other antidepressants			
Trazodone hydrochloride Fluoxetine hydrochloride	Desyrel Prozac	See tricyclics Appetite loss, insomnia, anxiety, tremors, fatigue, weight loss, hyponatremia, diarrhea, frequent urination, painful menses Any psychoactive drug may impair judgment, thinking or mental skills	Teach patient to take with food to decrease vertigo Teach patient to be alert for appetite loss Teach patient not to drink alcohol or take other antidepressant medications Because Prozac commonly causes nervousness and insomnia, tell patient to avoid taking it in afternoon to prevent sleep disturbances
Bupropion	Wellbutrin	Appetite increase, hypertension, hypotension, impotence, seizures	Advise patient to take drug as scheduled and to take each day's dosage in three doses to minimize risk of seizures
Sertaline	Zoloft	Insomnolence, ataxia, chest pain, tachycardia, dry mouth, increased appetite, sexual dysfunction	Administer once daily in morning or evening Use cautiously in patient with hepatic impairment, seizure disorders, or suicide ideation
Paroxetine hydrochloride	Paxil	Blurred vision, postural hypotension, ejaculatory disturbances, somnolence	Use cautiously in patient with history of seizure disorders or mania or hepatic or renal impairment

Continued.

TABLE 46-4 **Psychoactive Medications—cont'd**

Generic Name	Trade Name	Side Effects	Nursing Implications
Antimanic			
Lithium carbonate	Eskalith Lithobid	Possible toxicity at serum levels above 1.5 mEq/L Symptoms include nausea, vomiting, abdominal cramps, diarrhea, polyuria, polydipsia, coarse muscle tremor, ataxia, slurred speech, disorientation, and seizures Long-term effects: possible kidney damage	Teach patient signs and symptoms of toxicity and to maintain high fluid intake and stable salt use Blood tests to assess level will be needed periodically
Antipsychotics			
Chlorpromazine Thioridazine hydrochloride Trifluoperazine hydrochloride Fluphenazine hydrochloride Perphenazine Thiothixene Haloperidol	Thorazine Mellaril-S Stelazine Prolixin Permitil Trilafon Navane Haldol	Anticholinergic side effects: dry mouth, blurred vision, constipation, urinary retention, postural hypotension, confusion Extrapyramidal side effects (EPS): akathesia (severe restlessness—"I can't stand still") Parkinsonian effects: rigidity, resting tremor, shuffling gait Dystonias: bizarre movements of the face and neck, torticollis, oculogyric crisis Other precautions: lowered seizure threshold, tardive dyskinesia (characterized by involuntary movements of lip, tongue, and jaw after medications are stopped or decreased) Rare side effects: neuroleptic malignant syndrome (hyperthermia, muscle rigidity, labile BP, confusion, cardiovascular collapse)	Suggest sugarless candy or gum for dry mouth Teach patient the importance of taking medications and not stopping medications abruptly Patient should wear sunscreen product Baseline vital signs and blood counts Have patient move before rising Watch for EPS and use anticholinergic medications as ordered prn (Cogentin, Benadryl) Watch for neuroleptic malignant syndrome
Antianxiety agents			
Alprazolam Busipirone Chlordiazepoxide hydrochloride Clorazepate dipotassium Lorazepam Oxazepam	Xanax Buspar Librium Tranxene Ativan Serax	Drowsiness, ataxia, muscle weakness, occasionally disinhibition Patient may complain of "morning hangover" and transient hypotension on arising Other precautions: must be used with caution in patients with depression, psychosis, or history of drug abuse	Watch for increased side effects in older adults Explain to the patient the need to arise first to a sitting position, to equilibrate, before standing Teach patient not to operate machines while taking these medications, to avoid alcohol use, and not to stop medication abruptly

Nurse: Your life is ruined?

Patient: I wanted other children; we were going to have a large family.

Nurse: Tell me what a large family means to you.

Patients experiencing loss often need to cry. Crying begins to release emotion and should be accepted by the nurse. The close physical presence and touch communicate acceptance. Acknowledgment of feelings encourages further expression, and then the patient's sense of loss can be explored.

- Mr. Hill is a 65-year-old diagnosed with cancer of the lung. The day nurse is making initial patient rounds and enters the room. The nurse notices that Mr. Hill looks uncomfortable.

Nurse: (*Walks over to the bed.*) Good morning, Mr. Hill. You look uncomfortable.

Patient: I'm tired; I stayed awake all night.

Nurse: You had difficulty sleeping?

Patient: I have a lot on my mind. I couldn't sleep.

Nurse: (*Sits down next to the patient and pats his hand.*) Tell me what has been worrying you.

Patients should be encouraged to talk (ventilate). The nurse must be observant for nonverbal communication and for underlying meanings in the stated words. Talking brings emotions to the surface where they can be identified and dealt with.

It cannot be emphasized enough that the patient and the nurse bring their physiological, psychological, developmental, and spiritual components into the therapeutic relationship. Also brought into the relationship are previous life experiences, needs, aspirations, and frustrations. The nurse has an opportunity to help the patient explore a life event and the meaning that it has for the individual.

- Mrs. Haines, who has been pacing the halls, is now staring out the window. She is toying with a ring on her finger. The nurse notices that Mrs. Haines is vigorously tapping one foot on the floor.

Nurse: (Walks over to patient and sits beside her.) Mrs. Haines, I have noticed that you seem a little restless. Is something troubling you?

Patient: No, not really. Well, maybe I am a little upset.

Nurse: Is there something in particular that is upsetting you?

Patient: I don't know. I'm just anxious.

Nurse: Tell me how you feel.

Patient: I feel jittery and nervous.

Nurse: Is there something specific that is worrying you right now?

Patient: My husband is going to lose his job in another month, and here I am in the hospital. I just don't know how we'll pay the bills. It scares me.

Nurse: Have you and your husband discussed this situation?

Patient: (Patient continues to share her feelings with the nurse.)

Anxiety is an unpleasant feeling of tension and apprehension. A person experiencing anxiety may be unaware of the exact source of the tension. Anxiety is accompanied by an array of physical and psychological symptoms. Resolution of the anxiety begins with awareness of the source of the anxiety. An individual seeks ways to resolve the tension (problem solving) in order to be rid of the tension.

Antianxiety Agents. Antianxiety agents are used to help individuals experiencing moderate to severe anxiety. These agents reduce anxiety, but just enough so that tension is reduced and the patient remains motivated. Drugs in this category are commonly abused.

Other Forms of Treatment. Other treatment modalities are frequently used in addition to therapeutic communication and psychopharmacology. *Psychotherapy* is a process in which feelings and thoughts are explored, new ways of perceiving the environment are taught, and interventions are reinforced. Psychotherapy includes psychoanalysis, family therapy, behavior modification, and group therapy. The group therapy format serves many purposes, including the provision of an interpersonal testing ground in which feedback is given and received by multiple sources.

Electroconvulsive therapy (ECT, shock treatments) involves the passing of an electrical current through electrodes to the brain, resulting in a seizure. ECT is used to treat severe depression and compulsive suicidal tendencies. It is especially helpful in patients who are resistant to psychoactive drug therapy. In ECT, the patient loses consciousness and undergoes tonic contractions for approximately 10 seconds, followed by a somewhat longer period of clonic convulsions. On awakening, the individual has no memory of the shock. ECT is usually administered three times a week for 2 months and is used primarily for the treatment of acute depression.

Adjunctive therapies include occupational therapy, recreational therapy, music therapy, and art therapy. These types of therapy allow the expression of feelings, help increase self-esteem, and promote positive interactions and reality orientation. Such forms of adjunctive therapy may be used in a group setting or individually.

Ongoing maintenance for patients with a severe and persistent (chronic) mental illness can be very challenging, for the individual and the family. Rehospitalizations may remind them that the disorder has not been cured and must be closely monitored, even when the patient is relatively symptom-free. Special needs of the long-term mentally ill may be addressed by community mental health care and support, partial hospital programs, and assisted living environments.

HOW ILLNESS AFFECTS MENTAL HEALTH

There is a misconception that mental health principles are applicable only in a mental health facility or center. The goal of mental health nursing is to assist the individual to have a realistic and accepting view of self and to establish and maintain effective interpersonal relationships. The stress of being ill greatly influences an individual's mental state and level of functioning.

Ordinarily individuals feel "in control" of their lives. Illness reduces that control and may create instability and cause anxiety. When hospitalized, a person leaves behind the familiarity of home and work for the unfamiliar hospital setting. Activities may be limited, family visits may be restricted, possessions are locked up or returned home, and someone else is in control of the decision making. Most people do not expect to become ill or to have life-style alterations resulting from illness or accidents. Serious injury or illness may dramatically alter an individual's role performance (family, income, work), body image, life-style, and self-concept. Regardless of whether the situation is temporary or permanent, the individual's emotional state is disturbed.

Some patients will have difficulty with an illness or crisis. The "difficult" patient may cope by displaying denial, hostility, vulgarity, noncompliance, aggression, manipulation, apathy, or depression.

Behavior is learned, and patients bring their learned behavior patterns into the health care setting. All behavior has meaning; humans behave to meet needs and to communicate. The behavior the individual uses is based on past experiences and is the best available to the individual at the time. The interventions for nursing are to notice and respond therapeutically to all behavior. By understanding the relationship between stressors, anxiety, and behavior, the nurse can facilitate healthy adaptation. Special considerations regarding older adults are highlighted in the gerontological box.

GERONTOLOGICAL CONSIDERATIONS

- Older persons experiencing significant sensory changes in hearing or vision may experience behavioral changes that are mistaken for disorientation.
- Social isolation among older adults is frequently caused by physical or financial limitations.
- The behavioral characteristics and personality of older persons are often an exaggeration of their behavior at a younger age.
- Many losses, including loss of loved ones, home, job, and independence, occur with aging. These losses result in varying amount of grief. The number of losses and the rapidity with which they occur may affect the coping ability of the older person and result in anxiety, fear, or depression.
- Relocation from home to hospital or even from room to room can cause stress in the older person that may be manifested by behavioral changes.
- Hopelessness and helplessness are commonly seen in older adults. These feelings can lead older persons to lose the will to live and even to commit suicide.
- Reminiscence and life review are effective techniques to help the older adult cope with changing life circumstances.
- Alcoholism, often hidden or denied, is common among the older population. Alcohol may be used as a means of coping with grief, depression, loneliness, or boredom. If unrecognized, it can exacerbate medical conditions and lead to serious drug reactions.

Applying the Nursing Process

In every setting the nurse uses the nursing process to meet the many needs of the patient. The LPN/LVN participates in the nursing process by observing patient behavior and assisting in establishing the nursing diagnosis. Together with the RN, appropriate nursing interventions are outlined for the individual patient. The LPN/LVN and RN implement the plan and continue to observe and report behavior. It is from these observations that adjustments are made in the plans of care.

Box 46-5 outlines basic nursing assessments of emotional status. Other assessments include observation for high risk for violence, level of anxiety, use of defense mechanisms, and use of coping methods.

The role of the LPN/LVN in the planning process is to offer suggestions for intervention believed to be helpful to the patient. RN and LPN/LVN work as a team to implement the plan of care.

Box 46-5 ASSESSMENT OF EMOTIONAL STATUS

General appearance: Describe dress, makeup, and hygiene

General behavior: Describe general activity level, posture, gait, and response to examination

Speech pattern: Describe rate, tone, loudness, and quantity content of speech (descriptions include too detailed in response to questions, extreme distractibility, unable to complete an answer, uses rhyming)

Content of thought: Describe thinking being reality oriented, delusional, evidence of hallucinations, evidence of ideas of reference or other non-reality-based thinking

Mood and affect: Describe the general feeling state and affect

Sensorial function: Describe orientation, memory, attention, ability to think abstractly

Insight and judgment: Does the individual understand the present situation? What is the individual willing to do about it?

Potential for danger: Assess the individual's potential for violence or self-harm, degree of impulse control, previous history of violence or aggression toward others

NURSING CARE PLAN THE PATIENT WITH DEPRESSION

Mr. Cullin is a 68-year-old widower whose wife died 18 months ago. He was admitted to the open psychiatric unit for the diagnosis of major depression. Mr. Cullin has two grown children who live out of state. He has severe hypertension and beginning COPD. On admission Mr. Cullin states, "I just can't go on all alone like this. . . . I have so little energy." Mr. Cullin has lost 20 pounds in 6 months; he weighs 160 pounds and is 5 feet 11 inches tall. Mr. Cullin rarely leaves home, although friends ask him out frequently. He complains of difficulty sleeping and reports 2 to 3 hours of sleep per night. When asked, he admits to thinking of killing himself; he states he attempted to do so with a mild overdose of his hypertension medication before this admission.

Nursing diagnoses	Patient goals/expected outcomes	Nursing interventions
Violence, high risk for, self-directed, related to suicidal thoughts, feelings of hopelessness, and inability to cope as manifested by stating, "I can't go on alone," and overdose 2 days ago	Patient will not attempt suicide throughout hospitalization. Patient will express feelings when asked. Patient will verbalize one future-oriented goal not related to suicide.	Establish a relationship; keep staff assignment as consistent as possible. Provide a safe environment: no sharps, check to ensure patient swallowed medications. Use a kind, firm manner; tell patient that you can see that he is sad and that he still needs to do . . . At least two times per shift, while patient is awake, observe his suicide potential; ask "Are you thinking of hurting yourself now?" If yes, ask "How are you going to hurt yourself?" (Decide whether method is available.) "Can you agree not to hurt yourself for ______ *(specify time period)* without talking with me first?" If patient cannot commit to not acting, stay with him while appropriate alternative care is sought. Check on patient frequently q 30-45 min at varied intervals, such as 7:00, 7:25, 8:10, 8:35 . . . As patient begins to verbalize feelings, attempt to focus on anything that has gone right that he can feel good about. Ask what/how he can change to decrease feelings of loneliness. Assist patient to identify past meaningful activities (e.g., card game); attempt to have patient engage in these again. Have patient explore ways to cope: problem solving, physical activity, social activities, communication, etc.
Sleep pattern disturbance related to lack of activity and feelings of hopelessness, manifested by sleeping only 2 to 3 hr/night	Patient will sleep 5-6 hr/night before discharge. Patient will verbalize ability to use relaxation techniques when awake at night.	Encourage planned naps only. Help patient to establish consistent sleep time. Teach progressive relaxation exercises. Plan a physical activity while patient is awake.

Continued.

Social isolation, related to fatigue and hopelessness, manifested by failure to interact with other patients and inability to make a decision, such as choosing clothing to wear	Patient will participate in unit activities when asked by day 3. Patient will remain out of bed and room by day 3. Patient will talk about one activity that he can do after discharge from hospital.	Encourage interaction with others (e.g., at mealtimes). Get patient out of bed and room. Have patient do short, focused activities (e.g., deliver flowers to a peer, call a family member). Plan for activities after discharge.
Nutrition, altered: less than body requirements, related to grief, manifested by eating only about 40% of meals, weight loss of 20 lb in past 6 mo	Patient will eat 60% of all food offered. Patient will have adequate fluid intake. Patient will weigh 180 pounds.	Monitor eating. Encourage fluids. Try six small feedings. Present attractively prepared foods, foods patient likes.

CRITICAL THINKING QUESTIONS

1. Mr. Cullin is admitted to the psychiatric unit and placed on suicidal precautions. Mr. Cullin sits stoically staring out the window, and does not respond to the nurse's greeting. To prevent Mr. Cullin from self-destruction, the safety interventions that should be incorporated into his care are:
2. Mr. Cullin sleeps poorly, approximately 2 to 3 hours a night. To correct his sleep pattern disturbance, therapeutic interventions would include:
3. A weight loss of 20 lb is reported by Mr. Cullin's children. To help Mr. Cullin meet adequate nutritional requirements, the staff could:

Evaluation is ongoing. At intervals or when the patient's response dictates, the care plan is updated. Examination of the documentation and personal observations are considerations when evaluating the plan of care (see nursing care plan, pp.1491-1492).

All phases of the nursing process should be clearly documented. Most documentation is on an ongoing basis and should include the assessment criteria found in Table 46-4. All facilities use various forms and methods in documentation. Information should be accurate and descriptive. Documentation of the patient's actual conversation is very valuable.

In summary, humans are complex in nature and possess both physical and psychological components. The individual is affected in various ways by any change that creates stress and anxiety. Nurses in any setting must consider the emotional aspect of the individual. The nurse can be a valuable resource in helping a patient develop adaptive patterns. To accomplish this, the nurse needs a basic knowledge of human behavior, basic mental health principles, and assessment.

REFERENCES AND SUGGESTED READINGS

1. Aguilera DC, Messick JM: *Crisis intervention theory and methodology,* ed 7, St Louis, 1994, Mosby.
2. Andreason NC: Assessment issue and cost of schizophrenia, *Schizophr Bull* 17:475, 1991.
3. American Psychiatric Association: *Diagnostic and statistical manual of mental discorders (DSM-IV),* 1992, The Association.
4. Buchanan DM: Suicide: a conceptual model for an avoidable death, *Arch Psychiatr Nurs* 5:341, 1991.
5. Coffey C, Weiner R: Electroconvulsive therapy: an update, *Hosp Community Psychiatry* 41(5):515, 1990.
6. Danielson R: Counseling for young men: what does it do? *Reprod Health* 22(3):115, 1990.
7. Dzurec L: How do they see themselves? Self-perception and functioning for people with chronic schizophrenia, *J Psychosoc Nurs Ment Health Serv* 28(8):10, 1990.
8. Erikson EH: *Identity, youth and crisis,* New York, 1968, Norton.
9. Freud S: *The ego and the id*; New York, 1962, Norton (edited by J Strackey).
10. Glod C: Psychopharmacology and clinical practice, *Nurs Clin North Am* 26:375, 1991.
11. Gordon M: *Manual of nursing diagnosis: 1995-1996,* St Louis, 1995, Mosby.
12. Grainger R: Conquering fears and phobias, *Am J Nurs* 91:15, 1991.
13. Grainger R: Dealing with feelings, *Am J Nurs* 90(2):14, 1990.

14. Green A, Salzman C: Clozapine: benefits and risks, *Hosp Community Psychiatry* 41(4):379, 1990.
15. Haber J et al: *Comprehensive psychiatric nursing,* ed 4, St Louis, 1992, Mosby.
16. Hamachek D: Evaluating connectedness in the psychiatric nurse-patient relationship, *Arch Psychiatr Nurs* 1:11, 1993.
17. Heifner C: Positive connectedness in the psychiatric nurse-patient relationship, *Arch Psychiatr Nurs* 1:11, 1993.
18. Keltner N, Folk D: *Psychotropic drugs,* St Louis, 1993, Mosby.
19. Keltner N, Schwecke L, Bostrom C: *Psychiatric nursing: a psychotherapeutic management approach,* St Louis, 1991, Mosby.
20. Kemper B: Therapeutic listening: developing the concept, *J Psychosoc Nurs Ment Health Serv* 39(7):21-23, 1992.
21. Klose P, Tinius T: Confidence builders: a self-esteem group at an inpatient psychiatric hospital, *J Psychosoc Nurs Ment Health Serv* 30(7):5, 1992.
22. Knesel C: Combating anxiety, *RN* 8:50, 1990.
23. Malone J: Schizophrenia research update: implications for nursing, *J Psychosoc Nurs Ment Health Serv* 28(8):4, 1990.
24. McBride A: Mental health effects of women's multiple roles, *Am Psychol* 45(3):381, 1990.
25. McBride A: Psychiatric nursing in the 1990s, *Arch Psych* 4:21, 1990.
26. McConnel J: *Fear.* In McFarland G, Thomas M: *Psychiatric mental health nursing: application to the nursing process,* Philadelphia, 1991, Lippincott.
27. McConnell E: Do you really know what's troubling your patient? *Nursing '90* 29(2):43, 1990.
28. McFarland GK, Wasli E, Girity E: *Nursing diagnosis and process in psychiatric mental health nursing,* ed 2, Philadelphia, 1991, Lippincott.
29. Medried R: Strategies for handling angry patients and their families, *Nursing '90* 20(4):66, 1990.
30. Moorhouse MF, Doenges MS: *Nurse's clinical pocket manual: nursing diagnoses, care planning, and documentation,* Philadelphia, 1990, FA Davis.
31. Perko J, Kriegh H: *Psychiatric and mental health nursing,* East Norwalk, Conn, 1990, Appleton & Lange.
32. Rawlins R, Williams S, Beck C: *Mental health-psychiatric nursing: a holistic life-cycle approach,* ed 3, St Louis, 1993, Mosby.
33. Ricci M: The new after-care clinic: treating individuals rather than masses, *J Psychosoc Nurs Ment Health Serv* 28(8):18, 1990.
34. Robinson L: Stress and anxiety, *Nurs Clin North Am* 25:935, 1990.
35. Sadow D, Ryder M: Anxiety reduction: lessons that benefit students and patients, *J Psychosoc Nurs* 28(9):29, 1990.
36. Skidmore-Roth L: *Mosby's 1995 nursing drug reference*, St Louis, 1995, Mosby.
37. Simoni PS: Obsession: compulsive disorder, *J Psychosoc Nurs Ment Health Serv* 29(4):19, 1991.
38. Strong G: Eating disorders: to eat or not to eat? *Nurs Times* 21(86):44, 1990.
39. Stuart G, Sundeen S: *Principles and practice of psychiatric nursing,* ed 4, St Louis, 1991, Mosby.
40. Taylor CM: *Essentials of psychiatric nursing,* ed 14, St Louis, 1994, Mosby.
41. Tesson B: Who are they? Identifying and treating adult children of alcoholics, *J Psychosoc Nurs Ment Health Serv* 28(9):16, 1990.
42. Warner SL: Humor: a coping response for student nurses, *Arch Psych Nurs* 5(1):10, 1990.
43. Weiss F: The right to refuse: informed consent and the psychosocial nurse, *J Psychosoc Nurs Ment Health Serv* 28(8):25, 1990.
44. Whitley G: *Anxiety.* In McFarland G, Thomas MD: *Psychiatric mental health nursing: application to the nursing process,* Philadelphia, 1991, Lippincott.
45. Wilson H, Kneisel C: *Psychiatric nursing,* ed 4, Menlo Park, Calif, 1992, Addison-Wesley.

CHAPTER CHALLENGE

KEY POINTS

- Individuals have unique personalities. The personality consists of the id, the ego, and the superego.
- All behavior has meaning. An individual's behavior is the best that person is capable of, given the present environment.
- Corrective emotional experiences assist the individual to change. The nurse uses therapeutic communication to facilitate this.
- Personality refers to the relatively consistent set of attitudes and behaviors particular to an individual.
- Self is an important part of personality; self consists of identity, body image, role, and esteem.
- Anxiety is a universal response to a real or imagined threat to self.
- Defense mechanisms are automatic behaviors used to protect the ego in times of anxiety.
- Coping mechanisms are usually adaptive methods used to deal with feelings or stressors.
- Stress is the nonspecific response of the body to demands. Stressors are any factors causing stress.
- Mental health and illness can be viewed on a continuum.
- DSM-IV is a multiaxial system used in the diagnosis of psychiatric disorders. It consists of the physical, psychiatric, and social factors affecting the individual.
- Psychiatric nursing is a science and an art. Each individual has unique value and potential for growth. The nurse uses self in the context of a therapeutic relationship; to accomplish this, the nurse must have self-knowledge.
- The nursing process is used in psychiatry and includes assessment, nursing diagnoses formulation, planning, intervention, and evaluation. The care plan documents this process.
- To help prevent suicide the nurse needs to recognize its warning signals and learn the kinds of actions that can avert it.
- Therapeutic communication is a dynamic method of interacting with patients for problem solving and growth.
- In psychiatry, medications are used to assist individuals with feelings and behaviors.
- Behavior is observed and evaluated to determine a patient's progress and the effectiveness of the care plan.

STUDY QUESTIONS

1. The nurse is caring for a female patient who is unable to walk. There is no physiological cause for the paralysis. In talking with this patient the nurse learns that the patient suspects her husband of having an affair. He has been staying out late and attending many out-of-town meetings. Now that she has been ill, he has seldom left her side. The nurse is aware that this patient may be unconsciously using which one of the following mechanisms:
   1. Regression
   2. Suppression
   3. Introjection
   4. Conversion reaction
2. Johnny, age 10, is dressed in attire resembling that of his idol, a teenage rock star. This mechanism is an example of:
   1. Introjection
   2. Projection
   3. Identification
   4. Suppression
3. Mr. Nall, age 82, is experiencing extreme disorientation. The nurse's priority intervention is:
   1. Allowing the patient to make decisions
   2. Keeping the patient in the company of other patients for stimulation
   3. Using occupational therapy to keep his mind occupied and stimulated
   4. Limiting the staff who will be caring for him to help build a trusting relationship
4. Mr. Hernandez, age 82, is wakeful through the night. In planning nursing interventions, the staff is aware of the importance of:
   1. Nutrition
   2. Safety
   3. Elimination
   4. Family support
5. Mrs. Jean, age 32, has a history of bipolar personality. Which of the following nursing diagnoses is commonly associated with the manic phase of bipolar affective disorder:
   1. Tissue perfusion, impaired
   2. Hopelessness
   3. Social interaction, impaired
   4. Pain
6. The nurse is a member of the health care team. The entire team is involved in planning care. Which of the following is included in the role of the LPN/LVN in the planning phase of the nursing process in the mental health area:
   1. Complete responsibility for formulating and documenting the plan
   2. Setting patient goals
   3. Telling the physician the plan
   4. Offering suggestions for intervention and assisting in the implementation of the plan with the patient
7. The nurse is preparing to care for a patient known to be delusional. In responding to a delusional person the nurse must keep in mind that:
   1. Most patients require the administration of sedation
   2. The nurse in charge is the most appropriate team member to care for this patient
   3. The patient's feelings must be responded to, whatever they may be, and that outbursts are not to be allowed
   4. A factual explanation for the event the patient is perceiving as threatening should be given
8. Mr. Jerome looks at the nurse who is examining him and says, "You are one of the guards here in this prison. Leave me alone!" The nurse is aware that this statement may indicate disorientation. The most appropriate action by the nurse in this situation would be to:
   1. State factually that the patient is disoriented
   2. Ignore the remark and continue the examination
   3. Ask a family member to be present in the room
   4. Orient the patient to time, place, person, and circumstances
9. Mr. Todd, 63 years of age, has been living at home alone since the death of his wife. Mr. Todd is brought in by his son for evaluation of increasing disorientation and weakness. In performing a mental status assessment of this patient, the nurse is aware that the examination assesses mental health functioning in the area of cognition, affect, and which of the following:
   1. Intelligence
   2. Behavior
   3. Relationships
   4. Cause/effect
10. Five-year-old Brent is admitted for treatment of pneumonia. Brent clings to his mother and starts to suck his thumb. This is an example of the defense mechanism known as:
    1. Repression
    2. Suppression
    3. Regression
    4. Projection

47

THE PATIENT WITH AN ADDICTIVE PERSONALITY

Elizabeth Schenk

KEY TERMS

abstinence
addiction
addictive personality
Al-Anon
alcohol withdrawal syndrome
Alcoholics Anonymous
alcoholism
anorexia nervosa
bulimia
cannabis (marijuana)
chemical dependency
delirium tremens
detoxification
drug abuse
fetal alcohol syndrome
habituation
hallucinogen
Korsakoff's psychosis
tolerance
Wernicke's encephalopathy

LEARNING OBJECTIVES

After reading this chapter, the student should be able to do the following:

- Define the key terms.
- Name three types of addictions, and explain each one.
- Define the terms *dependence* and *tolerance* as they relate to drug and alcohol use.
- Describe one educational effort and one legal effort that have been used to decrease the incidence of chemical dependency.
- Explain the concept of intervention as it relates to alcoholism.
- Describe what is meant by enabling behavior.
- Explain two reasons that have been proposed to explain the development of chemical dependency.
- Describe three disorders associated with alcoholism and two disorders/diseases associated with drug addiction.
- Identify the six types of drugs of abuse.
- Discuss why nurses are at increased risk to develop chemical dependency.

RELATED TOPICS OF INTEREST

- Basic nutrition (Chapter 18)
- Diet therapy (Chapter 19)
- Care of the patient with a gastrointestinal or accessory organ disorder (Chapter 27)
- Mental health concepts (Chapter 46)

The treatment of patients with addictive behaviors is an important concern for nurses. Treatment centers are located in many areas, and more nurses are becoming involved in this specialty. Many patients in general hospitals also suffer from some type of addictive behavior. Persons may suffer from more than one addiction at the same time. An **addiction** has been defined as a compulsive, uncontrollable dependence on a substance, habit, practice to such a degree that cessation causes severe emotional, mental, or physiological reactions.[26] An example of this is the alcoholic person who is also a drug addict and a compulsive gambler.

Alcoholism and drug addiction are commonly referred to as **chemical dependencies.** This dependence refers to the total psychophysical state of the individual addicted to drugs or alcohol who must receive an increasing amount of the substance to prevent the onset of symptoms of abstinence and withdrawal.[26]

Alcohol is a drug, and the person addicted to alcohol may be at greater risk for drug addiction. Other addictions include compulsive gambling, compulsive shopping, compulsive working, eating disorders, and sexual addictions. Co-dependency is also a problem requiring treatment. This chapter will deal mainly with alcoholism and drug addiction but will briefly cover co-dependency and eating disorders.

Most modern definitions of dependence concerning drug addiction and alcoholism consist of two parts—physical and psychological dependence. Physical dependence refers to a physiological state where the continuous and prolonged consumption of a drug or alcohol leads to the user adapting to its presence. **Tolerance** then develops. This is the ability to endure ordinarily injurious substances, such as drugs or alcohol, without apparent physiological or psychological injury. If the use of alcohol or drugs stops, withdrawal signs and symptoms occur. Psychological dependence refers to the craving for a drug or alcohol. Another term that is frequently used is **habituation,** which is psychological and emotional dependence on a drug, tobacco, or alcohol resulting from the repeated use of the substance but without the addictive, physiological need to increase the dosage.[26]

DUAL DIAGNOSIS

Chemical dependence is a primary illness; however, chemically dependent people often have other psychological effects, such as depression or anxiety. Many problems disappear when drinking and drug use cease; it is essential to diagnose and treat chemical dependence before other psychological problems are investigated.

Psychiatric and psychological symptoms may, however, make recognition of an addiction more difficult. Determining the correct diagnosis is a task for an expert in chemical dependence and in psychiatry or psychology. Persons with a dual diagnosis may be more difficult to treat and may require treatment with medication.

PREVENTION

Prevention of chemical dependence is a complex issue. Legal efforts have been made, by restricting the sale of alcohol to minors and by instituting heavier penalties for driving while intoxicated or drug trafficking. Unfortunately, many of these efforts have not been successful.

The key to prevention is, in part, education. This includes teaching fairly young children about the dangers of drug and alcohol use and *abuse.* Many elementary schools now start these programs as early as the first or second grades. In addition, work may be done with children to increase their self-esteem so that they may be better able to resist peer pressure to drink or use drugs as they become older.[9,20]

Also, families and employers of alcoholics or drug abusers are being educated about these problems. They are taught that alcoholism is a disease that needs treatment. The alcoholic is usually surrounded by persons who enable the use and abuse. An example of this is the spouse who calls the employer on behalf of the drunk or hungover mate to report an illness, such as the flu. Without this enabling behavior, which includes making many excuses for the behavior of the alcoholic, the alcoholic might seek help sooner.

Prompt diagnosis and treatment can be important in assisting alcoholics to once again become productive members of society. It is often difficult to make the diagnosis of chemical dependence. Some indications of the problem include frequent illnesses or related illnesses, undue preoccupation with the use of chemicals, and mood swings. Other indications include violent or acting-out behavior, denial about the use of substances, and financial difficulties. The person tends to use the substance as an answer to all problems, loses control over the use, and loses the ability to express any feelings. The use of defense mechanisms, especially denial, is very common.

Prevention of complications must be considered. These complications occur not only because of effects of the substance, but also because of nutritional problems or infections. Complications for drug addicts often occur because of acquired disease from dirty needles or equipment and may prove fatal, such as with AIDS.

ALCOHOLISM

Etiology

Alcoholism is a common health problem and may add to the problems of persons with other health disorders. **Alcoholism** has been defined as the extreme dependence on excessive amounts of alcohol, associated with a cumulative pattern of deviant behaviors.[26] Excessive drinking of alcohol may lead to coma or death from acute alcohol poisoning or to numerous health problems if the drinking continues over a long period. The alcoholic begins to develop an increasing tolerance of and physical dependence on alcohol. Blackouts from episodes of drinking may start to occur. Guilt, shame, and remorse are common; the alcoholic then drinks more to relieve these feelings. As the drinking increases, problems increase and relationships with others deteriorate. The person reaches a point where "he drinks to live and lives to drink."

Estimates are that about 90 million Americans use alcohol and at least 9 to 10 million are alcoholics or problem drinkers.[23] Between 3% and 10% of Americans will be problem drinkers at some time in their lives. Although the percentage of male alcoholics is still much larger than that for female alcoholics, the margin is narrowing. Women are more likely to hide their problems and are not as likely to be detected.[23] Another group that is showing increasing numbers of alcoholics is the older adult.[19,27] In addition, alcoholism affects the functioning of another 30 million friends and relatives of alcohol abusers. Industries lose billions of dollars annually because of alcoholism. This includes medical expenses, lost wages, decreased production, motor vehicle accidents, and crime.[23,30] Alcohol is involved in nearly half of all deaths caused by motor vehicle accidents and fatal intentional injuries such as suicides and homicides. Victims are intoxicated in about one third of all homicides, drownings, and boating deaths.[23,25]

The use of alcohol predates recorded history. Cultures from many parts of the world have developed alcoholic beverages that have been used to celebrate important events. Alcohol has been used as medicine, as a form of magic, and as a part of worship services. In the United States, legal positions on the use of alcohol have varied. In 1642 drunkenness was punishable by a fine. In 1790 a law was passed that gave every soldier a daily portion of liquor. Prohibition, which forbade the production and sale of alcohol beverages, was passed in 1919 and repealed in 1933.

The average consumption of alcohol by Americans aged 14 and older in 1990 was calculated as 2.54 gallons, down from a peak of 2.76 gallons per person over the age of 14 in 1981. It is believed that this decrease can be attributed to the awareness of the dangers of alcoholism as well as to the fact that all 50 states have now raised the legal drinking age to 21.[33]

Theories of the Cause of Alcoholism

No one theory explains the cause of alcoholism. Some believe that persons are more likely to develop alcoholism because of some physical reason, such as an inner urge controlled by the nervous system or a dysfunction of the endocrine system. It has been found that alcoholism is in part genetically determined. The incidence of alcoholism is high in families, and the risk of sons of alcoholic men developing alcoholism over their lifetime is 30% to 50%. Studies of twins have shown that the identical twin of an alcoholic will be an alcoholic in 60% of the cases, whereas only 30% of the fraternal twins of alcoholics will be alcoholics.

Other theories are based on the belief that some part of the personality leads to the development of alcoholism. Certain common personality traits have been identified in addicted persons. These traits have often been grouped under the term **addictive personality** (a personality marked by traits of compulsive and habitual use of a substance or practice to cope with psychic pain engendered by conflict and anxiety).[26]

The traits include low stress tolerance, dependency, negative self-image, and feelings of insecurity and depression. It is not clear whether these traits are present before the development of alcoholism or are a result of it.

A relationship has been found between various groups in society and alcohol use. For instance, Jews, Mormons, and Moslems have a very low rate of alcoholism, whereas the French have a high rate.

Some people still believe that alcoholism develops as a result of either a moral fault or a sin of the alcoholic. Much of the early treatment of alcoholics was based on this theory. Today, alcoholism is generally accepted as a disease that is treatable.

Pathophysiology

Alcohol is a central nervous system (CNS) depressant. The so-called stimulating effect of alcohol occurs because the first areas affected are the higher centers of the brain that govern self-control and judgment. As alcohol continues to be ingested, other areas of the brain are affected. Unconsciousness may occur, respirations may be affected, and death may result.

Alcohol does not require digestion and is absorbed in the stomach and intestine. An empty stomach increases absorption. After ingestion, small amounts are lost through breathing and in the urine, but 90% is broken down by the liver. The active ingredient in alcoholic beverages is ethyl alcohol, or ethanol. A total of 12 ounces of beer, 4 ounces of wine, and 1½ ounces of "hard" liquor contain a similar amount of alcohol.

Alcohol has a diuretic effect. Increased amounts of electrolytes, especially potassium, magnesium, and zinc, may be excreted in the urine of a heavy drinker. Prolonged use of alcohol has a toxic effect on the intestinal mucosa that results in decreased absorption of thiamine, folic acid, and vitamin B_{12}.

Alcohol is not converted to glycogen; it provides the body with calories but no minerals or vitamins. One ounce of alcohol provides 200 kcal, but these are "empty calories" (calories with no nutritional value). Blood alcohol levels depend on the amount of alcohol ingested and the size of the individual. Most states designate blood alcohol serum levels of 100 mg/dl (0.10%) as the legal limit for driving a motor vehicle. Increasing blood alcohol levels have increasingly serious side effects (Table 47-1 on p. 1498).

Assessment

It is important to collect both subjective and objective data about the patient suffering from substance abuse.

TABLE 47-1 Blood Alcohol Levels and Related Side Effects

Level	Side Effects
50-75 mg/dl (0.05%-0.075%)	Pleasant, relaxed state, mild sedation, loosening of inhibitions
100-200 mg/dl (0.1%-0.2%)	Overt signs of intoxication: loosening of tongue, clumsiness, beginning emotional changes
200-400 mg/dl (0.2%-0.4%)	Severe intoxication: difficulty speaking, stumbling, emotional lability
400-500 mg/dl (0.4%-0.5%)	Stupor, coma
Over 500 mg/dl (0.5%)	Usually fatal

Collection of *subjective data* includes the person's normal using or drinking pattern, as well as the date and time of the last drink or use of drugs. The specific drink or drug used and the quantity used are important, as is the assessment of normal dietary patterns, the presence of diseases associated with alcoholism, and the use of prescribed medications. This information should be obtained in as much detail as possible. (See Therapeutic Dialogue and see latter part of chapter for specific information of drugs mentioned.)

Any history of tremors, hallucinations, delusions, seizures, or DTs should be assessed. Past periods of abstinence, normal diet patterns, the presence of problems (legal, occupational, family), and any family history of chemical dependency are assessed. It is important to remember that the defense mechanism of denial will usually be present in untreated chemical dependence. The information gained from the person may not always be accurate, and it is helpful to validate it with families or significant others.

Collection of *objective data* includes abnormal responses to preoperative medication, anesthetics, or sedatives. The presence of tremor, morning nausea, or skin conditions should be assessed, as well as mental functioning, general behavior, and the relationship of weight to height. The presence of tachycardia, hypertension, neuropathies, and petechiae is significant. The presence of ascites and a blood or urine specimen positive for alcohol or drugs should alert the nurse to take further history.

Diagnostic Tests

Routine blood tests will often reveal abnormalities that are directly related to alcoholism. These include liver enzymes, hypoglycemia, and abnormal blood protein levels. Magnesium levels may be decreased. It is not uncommon to find anemia and other evidence of poor nutrition in alcoholic patients.

Disorders Associated with Alcoholism

Fetal Alcohol Syndrome. **Fetal alcohol syndrome** is a congenital abnormality or anomaly resulting from a daily maternal intake of alcohol equivalent to 3 ounces or more of absolute alcohol per day.[26] Fetal alcohol problems occur frequently in newborns whose mothers drank heavily during pregnancy. These women have a higher incidence of delivering infants with birth defects such as mental retardation, growth disorders, and malformed body parts, as well as a high incidence of spontaneous abortions, stillbirths, and infant deaths. Even moderate drinking can result in infants with birth defects. As few as two drinks per day throughout pregnancy may cause adverse effects in an infant.[15]

Alcohol Withdrawal. When alcohol is not available to a person who has developed a physiological dependence, withdrawal signs and symptoms occur. These signs and symptoms range from mild tremors to severe agitation and hallucinations. The type and seriousness of the signs and symptoms depend on several factors. Alcoholics at high risk include older persons, persons who have had a previous history of delirium tremens, persons with nutritional problems, and persons with other illnesses. Signs and symptoms of alcohol withdrawal include diaphoresis, tachycardia, elevated blood pressure, tremors, nausea and/or vomiting, anorexia, restlessness, hallucinations, and convulsions.[26] These clinical signs and symptoms associated with cessation of alcohol consumption are called **alcohol withdrawal syndrome.**

The tremors associated with alcohol withdrawal usually are seen 6 to 48 hours after the last drink. They may persist from 3 to 5 days. The hands are involved first, but the tremors may become generalized with involvement of the feet, tongue, and trunk. Seizures may occur from 12 to 24 hours after the last drink. Usually these are grand mal seizures and are not preceded by an aura.

Delirium tremens, or DTs, is an acute complication of alcohol withdrawal that interferes with brain metabolism. This sometimes fatal psychotic reaction is caused by excessive intake of alcoholic beverages over a long period of time.[26] The rate of death can be as high as 15%, even with treatment. Signs that indicate DTs include tremors, increased activity, disorientation, fear, and an elevated temperature. DTs often occurs suddenly, 3 to 4 days after the last drink. The condition lasts from 2 days to a week, but at times can last as long as 4 weeks.

Other disorders that occur with alcoholism include those found in Table 47-2.

Two other conditions often seen in chronic alcoholics are Korsakoff's psychosis and Wernicke's encephalopathy. **Korsakoff's psychosis** is a form of amnesia and is characterized by a loss of short-term memory and an inability to learn new skills. **Wernicke's encephalopathy** is an inflammatory, hemorrhagic, and degenerative condition of the brain. It is characterized by lesions

TABLE 47-2 Disorders That May Occur With Alcoholism

System	Disorders
Hepatic	Hepatitis, cirrhosis, fatty liver (see Chapter 27)
Gastrointestinal	Cancer of the mouth and esophagus, esophageal varices, irritation of the stomach or pancreas, difficulty in absorbing food (see Chapter 27)
Neurological	Organic brain disease with confusion, Wernicke's encephalopathy (pathological condition of brain caused by thiamine deficiency), disorders of peripheral nerves (neuropathies) (see Chapter 35)
Cardiovascular blood disorders	Enlarged heart, high blood pressure, increased cholesterol levels, low blood sugar, anemia, coronary artery disease, congestive heart failure (see Chapters 28 and 29)
Musculoskeletal	Disorders of muscles (myopathies) (see Chapter 26)
Immunological	Increased susceptibility to infection (see Chapter 36)

in several parts of the brain. It is believed to be caused by a thiamine deficiency, which often accompanies the malnutrition found in chronic alcoholics.[26]

Nursing Interventions

Care for the alcoholic patient in the acute phase usually involves detoxification efforts to prevent acute withdrawal. **Detoxification** (the removal of a poison or its effects from a patient)[26] is undertaken in a controlled setting where the patient can be closely watched and treated for complications as needed.

The safety of the patient is of prime concern. If the patient is intoxicated, careful attention is given to maintaining a patent airway. Because of the high risk of aspiration, the head of the bed should be elevated at least 30 degrees, and a suction machine should be readily available. IV fluids may be necessary to maintain hydration.

In the initial withdrawal period, the alcoholic may be at risk for seizure activity. In addition to the use of anticonvulsants, side rails should be kept up and the patient observed carefully for signs of impending problems. The nurse should also be aware that the person experiencing delirium tremens may become violent and inflict injury on others. If the person becomes so agitated as to pose a risk of harm to self or others, it may be necessary to obtain a physician's order to place the person in leather safety reminder devices.

Nursing Diagnoses

Nursing diagnoses and interventions for the patient with alcoholism and/or drug addiction include but are not limited to the following:

NURSING DIAGNOSES	NURSING INTERVENTIONS
Airway clearance, ineffective, related to possible aspiration	Keep head of the bed elevated as long as intoxication continues. Give fluids with care if patient is intoxicated. Have suction machine readily available. If patient is vomiting, assign staff member to stay with patient.
Activity intolerance, related to lack of conditioning and illness	Encourage patient's participation in exercise sessions. Encourage adequate diet. Encourage patient to build up amount of exercise gradually. Encourage patient to refrain from overexertion. Administer vitamins as ordered.
Adjustment, impaired, related to use of drugs or alcohol	Explain to patient importance of stopping the use of drugs and alcohol. Explore with patient alternative ways of aiding adjustment. Assist patient in developing an aftercare plan. Link patient with AA or NA contact. Allow patient to honestly vent feelings and concerns.
Anxiety, related to uncertainty about the future	Encourage use of relaxation exercises. Encourage patient to participate in physical exercise. Refer patient to social worker or counselor to assist in sorting out concerns. Educate patient and family in finding nonpharmacological means to handle anxiety. Suggest referral to psychiatrist if needed. Refer to community resource agencies as necessary.
Coping, ineffective individual, related to abnormal use of alcohol or drugs	Plan time for patient's verbalizations. Listen carefully to patient. Encourage family participation in planning for sobriety. Reinforce teaching about disease concept of alcoholism/drug addiction. Assess present coping patterns, and identify strengths and weaknesses. Refer to community resource agencies as necessary.
Denial, related to inability to admit to being an alcoholic or drug addict	Confront the denial of the patient by relating incidents and problems to its use. Assist family in preparing for an intervention if needed. Confront denial in nonjudgmental way. Encourage patient to work on Step 1 of the 12-step program. Encourage patient to attend lectures concerning alcoholism and drug abuse. Encourage patient to attend group therapy.

NURSING DIAGNOSES	NURSING INTERVENTIONS
Family processes, altered, related to family system dysfunction	Encourage family to participate in family component part of treatment program. Encourage family to attend Al-Anon. Refer for family or marital counseling as appropriate. Answer questions of family members in honest way.
Grieving, anticipatory, related to inability to drink or use drugs	Allow time for grieving. Assist patient in accepting diagnosis. Reassure patient that grieving for not being able to use or drink is expected. Have patient talk with other recovering people.
Hopelessness, related to inability to stop drinking or using	Encourage patient to have a sense of hope, one day at a time. Encourage patient to attend and lead AA meetings. Reinforce patient gains made in treatment. Provide spiritual support if asked. Encourage patient to verbalize fears and lack of hope.
Infection, high risk for, related to poor hygiene and nutritional status	Inspect sites where drugs may have been injected for infection. Encourage good hygiene. Encourage good nutrition. Observe for signs and symptoms of infection. Medicate with antibiotics as ordered.
Injury, high risk for, related to intoxication	Use side rails in up position. Medicate as ordered to prevent or decrease symptoms of alcohol withdrawal. Explain all procedures before doing them. Use safety reminder devices as ordered, for patients in DTs, for example. Make sure call light is within reach.
Knowledge deficit, related to lack of information about alcoholism	Provide information about the disease concept and medical aspects of chemical dependency. Discuss with patient need for continued abstinence. Provide patient with information about the importance of verbalizing feelings. Give patient needed information about aftercare, AA, and NA. Discuss with patient the drugs to avoid and the importance of being honest with physician and dentist. Provide information about defense. mechanisms and signs and symptoms of impending relapse.
Noncompliance, related to past life-style	Help patient identify incidents where past life-style or health practices have negatively impacted on life. Share treatment plan with the patient. Encourage patient to be part of planning. Assist patient in making amends to those harmed in past (Steps 6 and 7) (see Box 47-1). Assist patient in identifying need to be more compliant in future.
Nutrition, altered: less than body requirements, related to anorexia and GI complications	Monitor intake. Provide well-balanced diet with adequate snacks. Medicate for GI complications as ordered. Monitor laboratory work. Assess for any GI bleeding. Encourage socialization during meals.
Powerlessness, related to inability to limit drinking or use	Involve the patient in decision making where possible. Discuss with patient meaning of powerlessness. Encourage patient to work on Steps 2 and 3 of AA or NA. Give positive reinforcement for periods of sobriety. Offer spiritual assistance as requested.
Self-esteem disturbance, related to troubled life	Encourage patient to participate fully in group therapy. Assist patient to identify issues of low self-esteem. Teach patient disease concept of alcoholism/drug addiction. Recommend individual counseling as needed. Listen carefully to patient. Give patient adequate time for verbalization.
Sleep pattern disturbance, related to alcohol use	Encourage use of relaxation tapes to help with sleep. Assist patient in setting schedule for going to bed. Encourage patient to become involved in exercise program. Prepare warm milk for the patient to drink before bedtime. Assist patient in seeing insomnia as tolerable. Reassure patient that insomnia will improve with a longer period of sobriety.
Social isolation, related to loss of friends and family due to use	Assist patient in meeting other recovering persons. Assist patient in planning for making new sober social contacts. Encourage patient to find a home AA group and a sponsor.
Spiritual distress, related to lack of concept of a loving God	Discuss with patient the difference between the spiritual and the religious. Encourage patient to participate in attending church or speaking to clergy if desired. Accept any difficulty the patient has with the concept of God. Accept patient's concept of a higher power.
Thought process, altered, related to acute intoxication or brain damage from alcohol	Administer vitamin therapy as indicated. Encourage adequate nutrition. Discuss with physician referral for psychological testing. Provide environmental cues as needed. Prepare patient for diagnostic testing as appropriate.

Rehabilitation

The object of treatment for alcoholism is to assist patients to completely stop drinking alcohol. They need to understand that they can never take one drink or mood-altering drug without the danger of relapse. Alcoholics who are not currently drinking are not considered cured—only recovering.

Group therapy is often used. The goal of this is to enable the person to see the relationship between alcohol and the negative consequences that have been suffered. Positive reinforcement, caring, emotional support, and encouragement are also important. The group can point out negative behaviors and defense mechanisms and offer possible solutions to its members.

One of the main goals of a treatment program is to decrease the denial of the alcoholism. The person usually is not aware of the damage that has been done in all areas of life. The patient is assisted to understand the concept of powerlessness. In addition, the alcoholic is given a sense of hope about stopping the use of drugs and alcohol, primarily through contact with other recovering persons. As a result, self-esteem also increases.

Many recovering alcoholics attend Alcoholics Anonymous (AA). **Alcoholics Anonymous** (AA) is an international nonprofit organization, founded in 1935, consisting of abstinent alcoholics whose purpose is to help other alcoholics stop drinking and maintain sobriety through group support, shared experiences, and faith in a power greater than themselves. The AA program emphasizes medical and religious resources for help in overcoming alcoholism. It consists of attending meetings and coping with abstinence "one day at a time." Meetings are held regularly in most communities at convenient times in factories, schools, churches, hospitals, and many other institutions and community buildings.[26]

AA is a group of self-acknowledged alcoholics whose goal is to stay sober and to help other alcoholics gain sobriety. Local AA groups are sometimes listed in the telephone book or in a local directory of meetings. A phone call to AA will bring help in the form of a telephone call or a visit by an AA member to the alcoholic desiring help.

The foundation of AA is a 12-step program that assists the alcoholic in admitting powerlessness over alcohol and other drugs. The success of AA has led to the formation of other groups that share the same 12-step approach. These groups include Al-Anon, Families Anonymous, and Overeaters Anonymous. See Box 47-1 for a listing of the 12 steps.

In addition to the alcoholic, family members also need education and, at times, counseling. This assists the patient and family to grow together and not apart. In spite of this, the divorce rate among couples where one member is an alcoholic is high.[4]

Planned Confrontations. Some still believe that it is only when the alcoholic desires and seeks help that treatment can be effective. Unfortunately, often by the time an alcoholic realizes the need for help, much has been lost. Recently a process called *intervention* has been used to assist the alcoholic in asking for help. Interventions are planned confrontations by individuals who care about the person.[16] They present facts or data about specific and descriptive events. The tone of the intervention should be nonjudgmental. The goal of the intervention is to have the alcoholic see and accept reality so that the need for help is realized. It is best to have immediate help ready.[16] See care plan on pp. 1502-1503.

Activity and Mobility. The person entering treatment may be weak because of poor nutrition as well as complications of the alcoholism. As the withdrawal from alcohol occurs, strength improves. Many alcoholics need to develop a pattern of regular exercise; for this reason, most treatment centers include a period of regular physical conditioning. This also helps the alcoholic to establish a regular pattern of sleep. Patients recovering from alcoholism are urged to maintain a regular exercise program after discharge.

Box 47-1

TWELVE STEPS OF ALCOHOLICS ANONYMOUS

1. We admitted we were powerless over alcohol—that our lives had become unmanageable.
2. Came to believe that a power greater than ourselves could restore us to sanity.
3. Made a decision to turn our will and our lives over to the care of God as we understood him.
4. Made a searching and fearless moral inventory of ourselves.
5. Admitted to God, to ourselves, and to another human being the exact nature of our wrongs.
6. Were entirely ready to have God remove all these defects of character.
7. Humbly asked Him to remove our shortcomings.
8. Made a list of all persons we had harmed, and became willing to make amends to them all.
9. Made direct amends to such people whenever possible, except when to do so would injure them or others.
10. Continued to take personal inventory and when we were wrong promptly admitted it.
11. Sought through prayer and meditation to improve our conscious contact with God as we understood Him, praying only for knowledge of His will for us and the power to carry it out.
12. Having had a spiritual awakening as a result of these steps, we tried to carry this message to alcoholics, and to practice these principles in all our affairs.

From Alcoholics Anonymous, New York, 1976, Alcoholics World Service, Inc.

NURSING CARE PLAN: THE PATIENT WITH ALCOHOLISM

Mr. Smith is a 54-year-old certified public accountant who is admitted to a treatment facility. He gives a history of drinking as much as a fifth of whiskey a day. Presently, he is slightly intoxicated, and his blood alcohol level is 0.12%. His admission liver function studies are abnormal, and his urine drug screen is negative for any other drugs. He is separated from his wife of 30 years. However, she drove him to the facility and admitted that she still cared for him, but that his drinking was the cause for her leaving him. Mr. Smith has never been treated for alcoholism before. Except for hypertension, his health is good. He has been drinking heavily, according to his wife, for about 5 years, since their son was killed in an automobile accident. On admission, he has a slight tremor and is cooperative, but tearful.

Nursing diagnoses	Patient goals/expected outcomes	Nursing interventions
Coping, ineffective individual, related to uncontrolled use of alcohol	Patient will learn to cope in healthier fashion.	Teach patient alternative ways to relax, such as biofeedback and relaxation techniques. Reinforce positive actions of patient. Encourage patient to share with other patients.
Denial, ineffective, related to inability to admit that he is an alcoholic	Patient will recognize effects of alcohol on life.	Assist patient to complete drug and alcohol history. Encourage patient to participate in group therapy. Confront inconsistencies in drug history or story. Share abnormal laboratory values and implications with patient
Injury, high risk for, related to alcohol withdrawal signs and symptoms	Patient will remain free of injury.	Observe closely for signs of alcohol withdrawal. Medicate as ordered.
Knowledge deficit, related to physical, emotional, and mental effects of alcohol	Patient will verbalize knowledge of: disease concept, medical aspects, need for abstinence, importance of expressing feelings, drugs to avoid, importance of honesty to physician, defense mechanisms, aftercare, and AA.	Teach patient after withdrawal and when ready to listen.
Powerlessness, related to alcoholism	Patient will verbalize knowledge of powerlessness.	Assist patient to learn about and taking first step of AA.
Self-esteem disturbance, related to unhealthy coping mechanisms	Patient will verbalize positive self-concept.	Give patient positive reinforcement of work. Demonstrate to patient that he is not unique. Help patient to process past events.

CRITICAL THINKING QUESTIONS

1. During Mr. Smith's assessment, the nurse notes that he has tremors, is agitated, and verbalizes visual hallucinations. To prevent injury to Mr. Smith, the nurse would perform which therapeutic interventions?
2. As Mr. Smith's physical condition improves, he discloses his hopelessness and lack of desire to continue living. An appropriate response by the nurse would be:
3. During group therapy, Mr. Smith states, "Now that I am physically better, I know I will be able to stop drinking. I don't need any help. There really isn't anything wrong with me at this time." The staff intervention at this time would be:

Patient Education. Educating the alcoholic about the disease is important. This should include information about the disease concept and medical aspects of the disease, including complications and signs and symptoms of relapse. The need for **abstinence,** defined as the voluntary avoidance of substances or the performance of an act for which the person has an appetite, is stressed.[26] The importance of aftercare, including Alcoholics Anonymous (AA), the importance of being honest with a physician, and the importance of expressing feelings are also stressed. The patient should be advised about what drugs to avoid and about products that contain alcohol, such as mouthwash and after-shave.

Education of the alcoholic should also include the family and significant other. These persons need understanding and education to help themselves and the alcoholic to recover. Al-Anon may help. **Al-Anon** is an international organization that offers guidance and counseling for relatives, friends, and associates of alcoholics.[26]

Medications. Medications used in the initial period of detoxification include chlordiazepoxide (Librium) or a similar drug. The drug is used in decreasing doses for its sedating and anticonvulsant effect during detoxification. The dosage can be as great as 50 mg every 3 hours during the first 24 hours. Anticonvulsant therapy may include phenytoin (Dilantin) and magnesium sulfate. The anticonvulsant may be continued for a longer period if the person has a history of seizures. Because nutritional problems are common with alcoholism, multivitamin supplements including thiamine and vitamin B_{12} are usually prescribed.

The drug atenolol may be used to reduce tremors and lessen the danger of cardiovascular symptoms by lowering heart rate, blood pressure, and body temperature during alcoholic withdrawal. Antipsychotic drugs are used to prevent hallucinations. Antidepressants may be used if the person is found to be depressed.

Specific medications may differ from setting to setting. In some, alcohol or paraldehyde will be used in the detoxification process. Whatever the medication used, it is important to realize that alcoholics may require large doses of medication to safely withdraw from alcohol. If medication does not control the withdrawal, safety reminder devices may be needed for safety of both the patient and the staff.

Another medication that may be used is disulfiram (Antabuse), which blocks the enzymatic action needed to metabolize alcohol. If the person drinks, the drug will cause nausea, vomiting, palpitations, and general ill feelings. Antabuse is used voluntarily by the patient to help maintain sobriety. The patient should know what effects will occur if he drinks while taking this drug. It is usually continued for some time after treatment.

Nutrition Therapy. Many alcoholics enter treatment in a poor nutritional state. They may have received most of their calories from alcohol or had no appetite for food. As the condition of the alcoholic improves, the appetite usually improves also. The emphasis is on three well-balanced meals a day, with free access to snacks. Many patients crave sugar in this period. If the alcoholic has developed cirrhosis of the liver, dietary modifications may be needed. In cases of DTs, intravenous feedings or feedings through a nasogastric tube may be necessary (see Chapter 19).

THERAPEUTIC DIALOGUE

Nurse: Welcome to our unit, Mr. Smith. My name is Sue Jones, and I am the nurse on duty tonight. Can you tell me why you are here?

Patient: They made me come.

Nurse: Can you tell me more about what you mean?

Patient: My family ganged up on me and had this meeting. They called it an intervention. They set it up for me to come here.

Nurse: That must be hard for you. Why did they have the meeting?

Patient: I only drink on the weekends, and then not that much.

Nurse: How much is not much?

Patient: About 10 beers, more or less.

Nurse: What is the most you've ever had on the weekend?

Patient: About a case and a half. But that's unusual.

Nurse: Mr. Smith, I know that it is sometimes hard to get really honest about drinking. But I want to assure you that information you share with me will be shared only with the treatment team. Also, we're not here to judge you. It's important for you to tell me as honestly as you can what and how much you've been drinking, as well as the time of your last drink. This is important so that we can help prevent withdrawal symptoms and complications that could happen. I'm not sure you've told me the whole story.

Patient: You don't think I'm terrible?

Nurse: No, I don't. I think that you're sick and need help, but I don't think you're terrible.

Patient: I guess I drink about a case a day, every day. I also use cocaine several times a week.

(Interview continues.)

Prognosis

Alcoholism is a disease that includes frequent relapses. No figure can be given for the percentage of persons treated for the disease who subsequently relapse; however, without adequate support and aftercare, many alcoholics do relapse. A high level of involvement in Alcoholics Anonymous or another support group is linked to a greater chance that recovery continues.

DRUG ABUSE

Because alcohol is in itself a drug, alcoholism and drug abuse are considered part of the disease of chemical dependence. **Drug abuse** has been defined as the use of a drug for nontherapeutic effect, especially one for which it was not prescribed or intended.[26] Much of the information covered in the section on alcoholism also pertains to the use of drugs.

The history of nonmedical drug use is thousands of years old. As early as 5000 BC, the Sumerians referred to a "joy plant" (thought to be the opium poppy plant). Since then, drugs have played a significant role in almost every culture. In recent years the incidence of drug abuse has risen. Drugs are often readily available.

The terms *habituation* and *addiction* have been used to define the nature and extent of drug use (see p. 1496 for a definition of habituation). Drug addiction is a condition characterized by an overwhelming desire to continue taking a drug to which one has become habituated through repeated consumption because it produces a particular effect. This effect is usually an alteration of mental activity, attitude, or outlook.[26] *Drug dependence* or *chemical dependence* are other terms that may be used.

The drug types discussed in this chapter will include stimulants, depressants, hallucinogens, narcotics, cannabis, and deliriants.[17]

Stimulants

Stimulants are natural or synthetic drugs that have a strong stimulating effect on the central nervous system that is accompanied by a feeling of alertness and self-confidence. Other results include dilation of the pupils, increase in pulse and blood pressure, reduction of fatigue, reduction of appetite, and an increase in concentration. However, when the feeling of alertness wears off, the person experiences fatigue and depression. Drugs included in this category are amphetamines, cocaine, caffeine, and nicotine.

Stimulants have the potential to produce tolerance, but usually not physical withdrawal. Psychological dependence is common. Side effects of stimulant use include restlessness, dizziness, insomnia, headaches, diarrhea, constipation, and lack of appetite. Persons who ingest a large amount of stimulants over a period of time may experience extreme agitation and anxiety. Death may occur as a result of a cerebral hemorrhage or myocardial infarction. Persons can collapse from exhaustion while using stimulants. Withdrawal can lead to profound depression and may lead to suicide.

Amphetamines. Amphetamines are synthetic psychoactive drugs that are available in capsule or tablet form. Medical uses of amphetamines include the treatment of narcolepsy, obesity, fatigue, and depression. Ritalin, an amphetamine-like drug, is used to treat children who are hyperactive. Common amphetamines include dextroamphetamine (Dexedrine), methamphetamine (Methedrine), and amphetamine (Benzedrine). Street names include pep pills, dexies, bennies, ups, speed, crystal, meth, and whites.

Cocaine Hydrochloride. Cocaine is a white crystalline powder used as a local anesthetic. This psychoactive drug comes from the leaves of the South American coca bush.[26] It was first used by early South American tribes. Its use was encouraged by the Spaniards, who found that the natives worked longer and harder and needed less food when they used cocaine.

At one time cocaine was used as an ingredient in many products, including syrups, nasal sprays, cigarettes, liquors, and Coca-Cola. It was also recommended as a treatment for alcoholism. In 1914 the nonmedical use of cocaine was prohibited. Medical uses now include (1) an anesthetic of choice for some procedures of the nose and throat and (2) as an ingredient of Brompton's cocktail, used for pain control in patients with cancer.

Cocaine is used by sniffing, smoking, or injecting. Cocaine may also be free-based (a process of heating the drug to separate it from impurities). When free-base cocaine is injected, it produces a "high" that is more intense and short-lived than when cocaine is smoked.

A newer form of cocaine that is increasingly available is called *crack*. It is less expensive than other forms and highly addicting. Other street names for cocaine include blow, coke, dust, flake, nose candy, rock, snow, superblow, toot, and white.[14]

Chronic sniffing of cocaine can destroy the nasal tissues. Smoking it can cause lesions in the lungs. Tolerance and psychological dependence can develop, and an overdose can cause convulsions, respiratory paralysis, and death.[7] A cocaine psychosis has been reported, which is characterized by a loss of pleasure and orientation, hallucinations, and insomnia. Abrupt withdrawal from cocaine does not lead to physical withdrawal.[28]

Because of the stimulation of the brain by cocaine, there is a surge in the systolic blood pressure with its use. This increase in blood pressure has been linked with subarachnoid hemorrhage. Cocaine use in high doses has also been found to cause seizures as well as fatal ventricular dysrhythmias.[2]

The use of cocaine during pregnancy causes constriction of the uterine blood vessels, leading to fetal distress because of oxygen deprivation. This increases the risk of spontaneous abortion in the first trimester of pregnancy. It can also cause slowed fetal growth and congenital abnormalities as well as in utero brain hemorrhage and stroke.

Caffeine. Caffeine is the most accepted and used psychoactive substance in the United States. Many beverages, medications, and other products contain caffeine. It has been used as an additive in carbonated beverages since the early 1900s. Because of its availability and widespread use, most persons do not view caffeine as a drug.

In its pure state, caffeine is a white powder or white needle-shaped crystals. It stimulates the central nervous system (CNS) and digestive system and the kidneys. Body metabolism is increased, and blood pressure is raised. Large doses of caffeine cause tachycardia, headaches, nervousness, insomnia, and stomach distress. Physical dependence occurs with a regular intake of 350 mg for an adult (a cup of brewed coffee contains 75 to 155 mg). Withdrawal symptoms include severe headache, irritability, and fatigue.

Nicotine. It is far easier to become addicted to cigarettes than to alcohol or other drugs. Smoking is also physically damaging. It has been linked to heart and blood vessel disease, chronic bronchitis, emphysema, and cancer.

The tobacco plant belongs to the genus *Nicotiana*, a member of the nightshade family. There is evidence that tobacco was used as long ago as AD 200. Tobacco is chewed or inhaled. The nicotine in tobacco stimulates the CNS and suppresses the appetite. Withdrawal signs and symptoms include decreased heart rate, weight gain, impaired psychomotor performance, nervousness and anxiety, headaches, fatigue, and insomnia.

Depressants

Depressants are synthetic drugs that have a depressant action on the CNS. Drugs included in this category are barbiturates and tranquilizers. Methaqualone is a nonbarbiturate sedative-hypnotic that is also a depressant. Commonly called Quaalude, the drug is no longer available as a legal prescription drug, but is available on the streets. Other specific examples of depressants include Valium, Seconal, Librium, and Ativan. These will be discussed further later in the chapter.

Barbiturates. Barbiturates are synthetic drugs that are classified as *sedative-hypnotics.* They arise from barbituric acid and are used medically to treat high blood pressure, epilepsy, and insomnia, and to sedate patients before and during surgery.

Barbiturates are swallowed (capsule or elixir), used as a suppository, or injected. The drugs were first synthesized in the early 1900s. Street names of barbiturates include yellow jacket (pentobarbital), red devil (secobarbital), phennie (phenobarbital), blue heaven or blue devil (amobarbital), barbs, downs or downers, rainbows, blues, or goof balls.

Barbiturates cause depression of the CNS, including slowing of physical and mental reflexes. Continued use can cause physical and psychological dependence, as well as tolerance. Barbiturates produce a feeling of well-being and relief from anxiety. Side effects include difficulty in breathing, lethargy, nausea, and dizziness. Alcohol and other CNS depressants potentiate the effects of barbiturates. Withdrawal symptoms include irritability, restlessness, anxiety, and sleep disturbances. In severe forms, withdrawal causes convulsions and delirium.

Tranquilizers. Minor tranquilizers are psychoactive drugs that are taken to reduce anxiety. First developed in 1950, they are commonly prescribed and are available in capsules, tablets, and liquid. Common types are found in the benzodiazepine family and include chlordiazepoxide (Librium), diazepam (Valium), oxazepam (Serax), lorazepam (Ativan), and clorazepate (Tranxene).

Minor tranquilizers slow the activities of the CNS. They also have anticonvulsant and muscle-relaxant properties and produce a sense of well-being. When the effects of the drug wear off, users frequently feel increased anxiety. Tranquilizers can cause physical and psychological dependence, and tolerance to them can develop.

Other CNS-depressing drugs potentiate the action of tranquilizers. Signs of an overdose include sleepiness, disorientation, loss of consciousness, and decreased reflexes. Withdrawal signs and symptoms include anxiety, diaphoresis, insomnia, vomiting, tremors, delirium, and seizures. Because of the dangers of seizures, detoxification should be medically supervised.

Hallucinogens

Hallucinogens are natural and synthetic drugs that affect the mind by causing excitation of the CNS. They produce changes in perception and thinking. Included in this category are phencyclidine (PCP), lysergic acid diethylamide (LSD), mescaline, psilocybin, and 3,4-methylenedioxyamphetamine (MDA). They are found in the streets in a wide range of forms, including powder, peyote buttons, mushrooms, capsules, and tablets. LSD may be found on blotter paper, chips, and sheets of paper containing tattoos or stamplike pictures of cartoon figures. Hallucinogens are usually taken orally, although MDA can be sniffed and injected. They may be put on sugar cubes or mixed in other food. PCP may be sprinkled on tobacco or marijuana and smoked. When it is combined with marijuana, it is called sheba. PCP may be injected or snorted. Common street names include those found in Table 47-3.

Most of the effects of hallucinogens are psychological, although nausea and vomiting are not uncommon reactions. These drugs act as stimulants at first and produce depressed appetite, dilated pupils, and increases in body temperature, heart rate, and respirations. Hallucinogens have a profound psychological effect on people, often described as a process of amplification, with the drug acting as a catalyst. This effect is called a *trip.* A person's attempts to resist the effects of the drug seem to increase the chances of a negative experience, or a bad trip, which is characterized by tremendous disorientation, unpleasant sensory images, and extreme panic. With large doses of PCP, there may be respiratory or cardiac arrest. Flashbacks may occur with the use of hallucinogens: the user reexperiences the effects of a drug without having taken it again.

Narcotics

Narcotics are drugs that are derived from the opium poppy or are produced synthetically. In general, narcotics lower the perception of pain. Narcotics include heroin, morphine, opium, codeine, meperidine, and methadone. Narcotics are injected, sniffed, smoked, or taken by mouth. Street names for heroin include H, horse, junk, hard stuff, smack, or scag.

TABLE 47-3 Common Street Names of Hallucinogens

Hallucinogen	Street Name
LSD	Acid, barrels, blotter, domes, microdots, purple haze, windowpane
Mescaline	Buttons, cactus, mesc, mescal buttons
MDA	Love drug, mellow drug of America
Psilocybin	Magic mushroom, shroom
PCP	Angel dust, animal tranquilizer, crystal, dust, hog, embalming fluid, KJ killer, peace pill, synthetic marijuana

Effects of narcotics include (1) shallow breathing; (2) reduced hunger, thirst, and sexual drive; (3) drowsiness; and (4) pinpoint pupils. The person may experience euphoria, lethargy, heaviness of limbs, and apathy. Overdoses of narcotics can cause coma, convulsions, respiratory arrest, and death. If narcotics are injected, there is risk of hepatitis B, AIDS, or other infections, such as septicemia. With narcotics, tolerance and physical and psychological addiction develop. Withdrawal may be painful and should be medically supervised. Clonidine (Catapres) is often used for detoxification. Signs and symptoms of withdrawal include nausea, cramps, chills, sweating, restlessness, and increased nasal secretions.

Cannabis

Cannabis, or **marijuana,** is a psychoactive drug derived from the flowering tops of the hemp plant. It can grow wild or is fairly easily cultivated. It is usually smoked as a cigarette (joint or reefer) or in a pipe or bong. Slang terms for marijuana include dope, grass, herb, joint, pot, reefer, roach, smoke, snuff, and weed. Marijuana has been used for medical and nonmedical purposes for more than 3000 years. Its popularity as a street drug began in the nineteenth century. It is commonly abused today. Hashish, or hash, is more concentrated than marijuana and produces more intense symptoms.

Marijuana's role in reducing eye pressure in glaucoma and in controlling side effects of chemotherapy is being evaluated. Physical effects of marijuana include drying of the eyes and mouth, increase in appetite, reddening of the eyes, and impairment of short-term memory. It raises the heart rate and blood pressure while lowering the body temperature and producing loss of coordination and possible confusion. Research shows that marijuana may affect chromosome division and cause birth defects. Marijuana is fat soluble and may be stored in the body for as long as several months.

Psychological effects of marijuana include an altering of perception of the senses. The user has a sense of well-being and intoxication, although depression and panic may occur. Psychological addiction occurs, and anxiety reactions may occur.

Deliriants

Deliriants are any chemicals that produce fumes or vapors that, when inhaled, cause signs similar to intoxication. They may be called inhalants. The fumes or vapors from inhalants are sniffed through the nose, or the vapors are put into a bag or captured in a balloon to increase the concentration of the inhaled fumes.

The use of inhalants is traced back to ancient Greece. Sniffing of commercial products and solvents was first documented in the 1950s. The deliriants or inhalants have a psychoactive or mood-altering effect when the vapors are inhaled or sniffed. Most fall into one of three categories: solvents, aerosol sprays, or anesthetics. Solvents include commercial products such as glue, gasoline, kerosene, lighter fluid, Wite-Out (correction fluid), and nail polish remover. Products such as hair sprays, deodorant, insecticides, and cookware sprays are examples of aerosols. Anesthetics that are used recreationally include ether, chloroform, and nitrous oxide. Amyl nitrate and butyl nitrate, drugs used for cardiac disease, are also abused. These may be called *whippets*.

Almost all inhalants are CNS depressants that slow the user's heart rate, brain activity, and breathing. Other effects include slurred speech, blurred vision, inflamed mucous membranes, light-headedness, ringing in the ears, watering eyes, loss of coordination, and excessive nasal secretions. With high doses, the user may lose consciousness or have seizures. The effects are immediate and usually last 20 to 45 minutes.

The prolonged use of inhalants may lead to liver, kidney, blood, and bone marrow damage. The sniffing of toluene, found in gasoline and commercial cleaners, has been linked to irreversible brain damage. This can be manifested as forgetfulness, inability to think clearly, depression, irritability, hostility, and paranoia. Use of large amounts of aerosols or solvents can cause death as a result of cardiac arrest after dysrhythmias. Death from inhalants is usually caused by suffocation because of the displacement of oxygen in the lungs. Sniffing inhalants from a bag or balloon increases the risk of suffocation.

Some inhalants cause tolerance or dependence. Signs and symptoms of withdrawal include chills, hallucinations, headaches, stomach pains, cramps, and delirium tremens. The psychological effects of deliriants include a feeling of stimulation and energy. At higher doses, the user may feel intoxicated.

Assessment

Subjective factors to assess include those found in the section on alcoholism. The objective factors found in the discussion of alcoholism also are pertinent, with the addition of the presence of "track marks"—if the person has been mainlining (injecting the drug directly into a vein), needle marks, scars, or small scabs can be seen on the hands, forearms, or insteps. However, many other veins are used as points of entry to conceal addiction, including the dorsal vein of the penis or the conjunctival artery of the eyelid. Other objective and subjective signs include those discussed in Table 47-4 on p. 1508.

Diagnostic Tests. Diagnostic testing for drug abuse can be done on urine or blood samples. The amount of time after use that drugs can be detected in the urine varies from a very short time for alcohol and cocaine to a long time for benzodiazepines and cannabis. It is possible to have a minimally positive drug test for cannabis because of a long period of "passive inhalation" (close contact with someone smoking and exhaling marijuana fumes). Urine testing is not commonly done to detect alcohol because alcohol is metabolized very rapidly; alcohol blood levels are much more accurate. A breath test is used by law enforcement agencies to determine alcohol levels in the blood. Although some persons are concerned that routine testing violates civil liberties, efforts will continue to develop an accurate, objective method for determining whether a person is under the influence of drugs or alcohol.

Other diagnostic tests that may be used include testing for hepatitis and HIV. Blood cultures may show the presence of septicemia.

Nursing Diagnoses

The reader is referred to pp. 1499-1500 in the section on alcoholism.

Nursing Interventions

Rehabilitation of the drug-dependent person follows the guidelines discussed for the treatment of the alcoholic. Also see Table 47-1 for other methods of treatment. One difference between drug and alcohol abuse is that, in most cases, the possession and use of drugs are illegal. In the United States, the illicit use of narcotics has been a crime since the 1914 Harrison Narcotic Act was passed.

Methadone Maintenance. One approach to the treatment of narcotic addiction is the methadone maintenance program. Methadone is a synthetic drug, and the average daily dose costs much less than heroin or morphine. The drug is given legally as a part of a rehabilitation program. Methadone itself is addictive. Because methadone is easily available through legal channels, some experts believe that it is essentially the same as taking maintenance doses of other drugs, such as insulin. Other persons disagree, however, because they believe that the use of methadone encourages addiction and replaces one drug with another.

Cocaine Withdrawal. Although cocaine does not produce physical tolerance, the psychological tolerance is very strong. Research has shown that long-term cocaine use has yielded symptoms similar to those of Parkinson's disease. It depletes dopamine in the brain. Because of this, bromocriptine (Parlodel) has been used to assist in controlling the symptoms of withdrawal from cocaine and to prevent relapse.

Patient Education. The reader is referred to the discussion of this topic in the section on alcoholism (p. 1503).

TABLE 47-4 Acute Intoxication and Withdrawal of Mind-Altering Drugs

Acute Intoxication		
Signs and Symptoms	**Treatment**	**Withdrawal Signs and Symptoms**
Narcotics		
Respiratory depression, depressed respirations (12 or below), bradycardia, hypotension, cold clammy skin, decreased body temperature; deep sleep, stupor, or coma; pinpoint pupils	Maintain ventilation; provide oxygen. Give narcotic antagonist: naloxone (Narcan) 0.4 mg IV. Monitor vital signs every 15 to 30 min until patient is conscious. Treat for shock.	*Not life threatening* Early: restlessness, irritability, drug craving, yawning, lacrimation, diaphoresis, rhinorrhea; followed by "yen" sleep (intense desire to sleep; sleeps restlessly) Later: awakens with more severe signs and symptoms, nausea, vomiting, anorexia, abdominal cramps, bone and muscle pain, tremors, piloerection ("gooseflesh")
Other CNS depressants		
Same as narcotics (above)	Lavage if recent oral ingestion. Maintain ventilation; provide oxygen. Monitor vital signs every 15 to 30 min until patient is conscious. Position patient side-lying or prone, not supine. Treat for shock. Hemodialysis for renal shutdown.	*May be life threatening* Insomnia, restlessness, tremors, anorexia, followed by convulsions, and signs and symptoms similar to delirium tremens (disorientation, visual and auditory hallucinations), fever, dehydration
CNS stimulants		
Labile cardiovascular signs and symptoms (flushing or pallor, pulse and blood pressure changes, dysrhythmias), hyperpyrexia, mental disturbances (agitation, paranoia, hallucinations), convulsions, circulatory collapse	Give chlorpromazine, 25 to 50 mg IM. Provide a quiet environment. Orient patient to reality. Monitor vital signs until stable.	*Withdrawal is not severe* Somnolence, apathy, irritability, depression, fatigue
Hallucinogens		
Physiological toxicity low at doses that produce strong psychological effects Acute panic reaction ("bad trip") may lead to suicide "Flashback" episodes Prolonged psychotic disorders (paranoia, depression) Phencyclidine: CNS depression or stimulation may lead to death	Provide quiet, supportive environment and constant attention. Give diazepam (Valium), 2 to 10 mg IM for severe anxiety.	*No evidence of withdrawal symptoms*
Cannabis		
Adverse reactions infrequent Simple depression, paranoid ideation, disorientation, hallucinations	Provide support and reassurance. Give tranquilizer for agitation.	*Withdrawal symptoms rare* Insomnia, anorexia

Risk of disease. Addicts who inject drugs are at risk for diseases such as hepatitis and AIDS. Often addicts share needles and equipment or reuse them without sterilization between use. Addicts may also demonstrate resistance to more responsible use because of blackouts or the character traits that accompany the disease. Many intravenous drug users test positive for the AIDS virus. Although supplying clean needles to drug users has been advocated by some, this is controversial. Those who oppose this recommendation feel that it would encourage IV drug use.

Prognosis. The prognosis for the person suffering from drug abuse is the same as that for the person with a diagnosis of alcoholism. The importance of adequate support after treatment is recognized.

CO-DEPENDENCY

Co-dependency has been defined as the set of maladaptive and/or immature responses, behaviors, and feelings experienced by someone closely associated with an actively chemically dependent person. The co-dependent person responds to life in dysfunctional ways. Commonly reported symptoms of co-dependency include the following[31,35]:

1. Self-esteem that relies heavily on feeling needed by others
2. Need to control others even when it is unrealistic to do so
3. Tendency to develop complicated relationships with chemically dependent people

Co-dependency becomes significant because persons in recovery often find that they need to address their co-dependency to gain complete peace of mind. Without this they are at increased risk of relapse and problems with relationships. Also, research has found that nursing as a profession tends to attract those who are from alcoholic homes and those who are co-dependent in nature. These nurses may have increased risk of "burnout" from nursing.[5] Al-Anon or Adult Children of Alcoholics groups may provide treatment for the person who is troubled because of co-dependency.

EATING DISORDERS

An eating disorder has been described as an obsession with weight and an addiction to food. It is also, however, a way of coping with feelings and an attempt for the persons to feel better about themselves. It is an addiction, and much of the discussion concerning alcoholism and drug addiction applies here.

Anorexia nervosa and bulimia are two common eating disorders.[10] **Anorexia nervosa** is a psychoneurotic disorder characterized by a prolonged refusal to eat, resulting in emaciation, amenorrhea, emotional disturbance concerning body image, and an abnormal fear of becoming obese.[26] **Bulimia** is an insatiable craving for food, often resulting in episodes of continuous eating followed by periods of depression and self-deprivation.[26] Regular, self-induced vomiting or the use of laxatives to purge is common. Other signs of eating disorders may include restrictive dieting, fasting, or vigorous exercise to prevent weight gain. There is also an excessive concern with body shape and weight.

Eating disorders are a way to "anesthetize" intense negative feelings and to cope with stress and relieve tension. Most of the time activities relative to eating and exercise become a part of a ritual. Most persons with eating disorders fear losing control.

Both anorexia nervosa and bulimia are common in young women. Treatment for these is important—without treatment, these conditions can be fatal. Treatment includes helping the person learn to trust others and to exercise her rights in a relationship. Patients are assisted in expressing their feelings, and individual patient education and nutritional counseling are crucial. While this treatment is carried out, the patient may require nutrition intravenously or by nasogastric tube to sustain life (see Chapter 19).

IMPAIRED NURSES

Over the past several years, many states have developed programs to assist nurses who are impaired by either alcohol or drugs. Part of the reason for this is that the rate of chemical dependence among nurses and other health providers is greater than that of the general public. Before the start of peer assistance programs, through either state boards or state nursing associations, often nurses would be fired or be free to move to other facilities, where the abuse could continue.

In 1980 two states, Maryland and Ohio, had peer assistance programs in place. By fall 1983, 25 states either had programs in place or were planning to start them. At present only a few states do not have programs. These programs work closely with state boards of nursing.

Peer assistance programs have several goals: (1) to assist the nurse who is impaired to receive treatment; (2) to protect the public from the untreated nurse; (3) to help the recovering nurse reenter nursing in a systematic, planned, and safe way; and (4) to assist in monitoring the continued recovery of the nurse for a period of time.

The reentry of the nurse may include a restriction on access to narcotics for a period of time.

The basis of these programs is one nurse helping another nurse. Most volunteers in these programs are recovering nurses or nurses who work in the area of chemical dependence or psychiatric nursing.

If a colleague is suspected, it is important to notify the supervisor, who will often notify the state nursing association or state board of nursing.[24] The best way to help a colleague who is abusing drugs or alcohol is to not cover up the use and to report it to persons who can help arrange for appropriate help.[22,32]

REFERENCES AND SELECTED READINGS

1. Alcoholics Anonymous: New York, 1976, Alcoholic World Services, Inc.
2. Amin M et al: Cocaine induced myocardial infarction: a growing threat to men in their 30's, *Postgrad Med* 90(4):50, 1991.
3. Bell K: Identifying the substance abuser in clinical practice, *Orthop Nurs* 11(2):29, 1992.
4. Captain C: Family recovery from alcoholism: mediating family factors, *Nurs Clin North Am* 24(1):55, 1989.
5. Covello B: Codependency taints nursing's goals, *RN* 54(4):132, 1991.
6. Cusack J et al: Alcoholism: uncovering the hidden diagnosis, *Emerg Med* 24(7):71, 1992.
7. Dubiel S: Action stat! Cocaine overdose, *Nurs 90* 20(3):33, 1990.
8. Dubiel S: Drug abuse: designer drugs, *Adv Clin Care* 6(5):22, 1991.
9. Eels M: Strategies for promotion of avoiding harmful substances, *Nurs Clin North Am* 26(4):915, 1991.
10. Flood M: Addictive eating disorders, *Nurs Clin North Am* 24(1):45, 1989.
11. Frances R: Substance abuse, *JAMA* 265(23):3171, 1991.
12. Grinspoon L, Bakalar J: Alcohol abuse and dependence, *The Harvard Medical School Mental Health Review*, 1990.
13. Hall S, Wray L: Codependency: nurses who give too much, *Am J Nurs* 89(11):1456, 1989.
14. House M: Cocaine, *Am J Nurs* 90(4):40, 1990.
15. Jacques J, Snyder M: Newborn victims of addiction, *RN* 54(4):47, 1991.
16. Johnson V: *Intervention,* Minneapolis, 1987, Hazeldon Foundation.
17. Kinney J: *Clinical management of substance abuse,* St Louis, 1991, Mosby.
18. Klebanoff N: Caring and nursing: explorations in feminist perspectives. Codependency: caring or suicide for nurses and nursing (pamphlet), *NLN Publ Center Hum Caring* 14-2369: 151, 1991.
19. Krach P: Discovering the secret: nursing assessment of elderly alcoholics in the home, *J Gerontol Nurs* 16(11):32, 1990.
20. Levy G, Hickey J: Fighting the battle against drugs, *RN* 54(4):44, 1991.
21. Linn L, Gelberg L, Leabe B: Substance abuse and mental health status of homeless and domiciled low-income users of a medical clinic, *Hosp Community Psychiatr* 41(3):306, 1990.
22. Lippman H: Addicted nurses: tolerated, tormented, or treated? *RN* 55(4):36, 1992.
23. Long B, Phipps W, Cassmeyer V: *Medical-surgical nursing: a nursing process approach,* St Louis, 1993, Mosby.
24. Miller H: Addiction in a coworker: getting past the denial, *Am J Nurs* 90(5):72, 1990.
25. Mitiguy J: Alcohol and head trauma, *Addict Nurs Netw* 3(2):52, 1991.
26. *Mosby's medical, nursing, and allied health dictionary,* ed 4, St Louis, 1994, Mosby.
27. Parette H: Nursing attitudes toward the geriatric alcoholic, *J Gerontol Nurs* 16(1):26. 1990.
28. Povenmire K: Recognizing the cocaine addict, *Nurs 90* 20(5):46, 1990.
29. Public Health Service: *Health United States 1989 and prevention profile,* Washington DC, 1990, US Department of Health and Human Services.
30. Rice D et al: *The economic costs of alcohol and drug abuse and mental illness,* San Francisco, 1990, Institute for Health and Aging.
31. Ryan J: Codependency in nursing: healing wounds and changing patterns, *J Christ Nurs* 8(2):10, 1991.
32. Sullivan E: *Nursing and health care: chemical dependency in the nursing profession* (pamphlet), NLN Pub No 41-2365, 1990.
33. US Department of Health and Human Services: *Healthy people 2000: national health promotion and disease prevention objectives,* Washington, DC, 1990, US Government Printing Office.
34. Williams E: Strategies for intervention, *Nurs Clin North Am* 24(1):95, 1989.
35. Zerwekh J, Michaels B: Co-dependency: assessment and recovery, *Nurs Clin North Am* 24(1):109, 1989.

CHAPTER CHALLENGE

KEY POINTS

- Examples of compulsive addictions include alcoholism, drug addiction, compulsive overeating, compulsive gambling, and compulsive working.
- Alcoholism and drug addiction are commonly referred to as chemical dependence.
- Dependence may be psychological and physical and is defined as the need to continue the use of drugs and/or alcohol to prevent withdrawal.
- Persons with chemical dependence may also suffer from a psychiatric diagnosis (called dual diagnosis).
- There is a genetic component to the development of chemical dependence.
- Alcohol provides the body with "empty calories," and heavy drinking can cause damage to many body systems, especially the liver.
- Denial and delusion are commonly found in persons with untreated chemical dependence.
- Alcoholics may require large doses of medication to safely withdraw from alcohol.
- Many of the problems found in alcoholism may be the result of nutritional problems.
- Alcoholics Anonymous or related 12-step groups have been effective in treating the addicted person, because the program helps the person accept the powerlessness over drugs or alcohol.
- The basic types of drugs that are abused are stimulants, depressants, hallucinogens, narcotics, cannabis, and deliriants.
- Drug addiction includes craving, psychological dependence, and physical dependence.
- Nurses are at increased risk of the development of alcoholism and chemical dependence.
- Disorders that occur frequently with alcoholism include hepatitis, cirrhosis of the liver, cancer of the

mouth and esophagus, high blood pressure, myopathies, increased susceptibility to infection, and organic brain disease with disorientation.

- Disorders that occur with drug addiction include cellulitis, HIV, abscesses, and hepatitis.
- Two reasons that have been proposed to identify chemical dependence include a genetic predisposition and environmental influences.
- An educational effort used to decrease the incidence of chemical dependency is the teaching of young elementary school students the hazards of taking drugs.
- One legal effort that has been used to decrease drug addiction is the raising of the legal drinking age.
- Nurses are at increased risk of alcoholism and chemical dependence because of their often co-dependent personalities and the easy access to drugs.
- The intervention consists of concerned persons presenting information to the alcoholic or drug addict in a loving and nonjudgmental way in order to make the person realize the seriousness of the problem.
- Enabling behavior helps the alcoholic maintain denial by often covering up problem areas.

STUDY QUESTIONS

1. Which of the following statements is true concerning chemical dependence:
   1. Chemically dependent persons rarely have other psychological or psychiatric problems.
   2. It is important to treat any psychiatric disorder before treating chemical dependence.
   3. Psychiatric and psychological problems make the diagnosis of chemical dependence easier.
   4. Persons with a dual diagnosis disorder are often more difficult to treat.
2. Which of the following statements is true for a person who is an alcoholic:
   1. The person's drinking is a moral problem.
   2. The person is at increased risk of becoming a drug addict.
   3. The person will be cared for only in a treatment center.
   4. The person will be able to resume social drinking.
3. Withdrawal from which type of mind altering drugs may be life-threatening:
   1. Hallucinogens
   2. CNS stimulants
   3. Narcotics
   4. CNS depressants
4. Mrs. Blum, a 35-year-old, is in her first trimester of pregnancy. During her first prenatal visit to her obstetrician, she asks, "It's all right if I drink, isn't it?" The most appropriate response for the nurse is:
   1. A few drinks never hurt anyone. It will be fine.
   2. You can drink as long as you limit it to three drinks.
   3. It is best to avoid drinking totally during pregnancy.
   4. Drinking by the mother can't influence the baby.
5. Ms. True is being discharged from a drug and alcohol treatment center after detoxification from alcoholism. In preparing the patient for discharge, what advice is important to give the patient about over-the-counter medications:
   1. All medications bought in a drugstore are considered safe for the alcoholic.
   2. The recovering alcoholic should never take over-the-counter medication.
   3. The patient's physician does not need to know about over-the-counter medications.
   4. Some medications, especially cough syrups, contain large amounts of alcohol.
6. A nurse is teaching a class of alcoholics and their families about sobriety. As part of this, the concept of abstinence is discussed. A family member asks the nurse what this term means. The best response is:
   1. Avoidance of all hard liquor and street drugs
   2. Avoidance of all mood-altering drugs and alcohol
   3. Avoidance of all alcohol products
   4. Avoidance of all street drugs and inhalants
7. Susan Block, a nursing student, is preparing to take part in an intervention concerning her father and his use of alcohol. The goal of an intervention is:
   1. To have the alcoholic see the reality of his drinking and accept help
   2. To educate the person about the dangers of drinking large amounts
   3. To discuss ways to help the alcoholic become a social drinker
   4. To present damaging evidence about the person in a judgmental way
8. During the hospitalization of Mrs. Blue, a 35-year-old patient with cirrhosis of the liver, the nurse attempts to obtain a history of alcohol use. Mrs. Blue denies drinking large amounts, even though the nurse has been told by her husband that she drinks up to a quart of whiskey each night. Which statement would best account for this denial:
   1. Mrs. Blue is a pathological liar and cannot tell the truth.
   2. Mrs. Blue knows that the nurse would not want to know the truth.
   3. Mrs. Blue's denial is a common manifestation of chemical dependency.
   4. Mrs. Blue never remembers what she does in the evening or night.
9. Mr. Smith is a 25-year-old admitted to the medical-surgical unit with acute intoxication that led to a seizure. He needs to be observed closely for what problem that may be life threatening:
   1. Delirium tremens
   2. Wernicke's encephalopathy
   3. Peripheral neuropathy
   4. Tardive dyskinesia

14

COMMUNITY HEALTH

Having been a full-time homemaker and mother for 30-some years, I evaluated my acquired skills as a caretaker and caregiver. After searching my heart, observing nurses at work, seeking inner direction and guidance, my goal was to become a nurse. Why? To provide a genuine, wholesome, love-filled, caring interest for the sick, especially older adults, who deserve and sincerely yearn for dignity and respect. To have helped even one person regain, maintain, or initiate trust and respect for the nursing profession will be an added bonus.

Helen Bieker
Student Nurse

48

HOME HEALTH NURSING

Sandra Klocke

KEY TERMS

accreditation
certification
DRG
home health care
Medicaid
Medicare

LEARNING OBJECTIVES

After reading this chapter, the student should be able to do the following:

- Define the key terms.
- Describe how home health care differs from community and public health care services.
- List at least three types of home health agencies.
- List at least four services that may be provided by home health care.
- Describe two major ways home care differs from hospital care.
- Define skilled nursing services.
- Describe the role of the LPN/LVN in the delivery of skilled nursing care.
- Relate the nursing process to home health care practice.
- List two sources of reimbursement for home care services.

RELATED TOPICS OF INTEREST

- The evolution of nursing (Chapter 1)
- Legal aspects of nursing (Chapter 2)
- Ethical aspects of nursing (Chapter 3)
- The nursing process (Chapter 5)
- Documentation (Chapter 6)
- Life span development (Chapter 7)
- Admission, transfer, and discharge (Chapter 11)
- Hospice care (Chapter 53)

Home health care services enable individuals of all ages to remain in the comfort and security of their homes while receiving health care. Family support, familiar surroundings, and participation in the care process contribute to feelings of worth and dignity. Services may include skilled nursing, physical therapy, speech language pathology, occupational therapy, medical social services, homemaker-home health aide (also referred to as home health aide), nutritional support, respiratory therapy, acquisition of medical supplies and equipment, and homemaker and companion care.

The approach to patient care is one of teamwork and blending of disciplines. Historically and currently professional nurses are primarily involved in the administration and management of agencies and the supervision of nursing interventions. The LPN/LVN is a valuable team member of this very important health care service. Although home care has traditionally been a part of public and community health services, the focus is much narrower.

DEFINITIONS

Home health care preserves individual independence and integrity and keeps families together.

The following are definitions of home health care as viewed from four different perspectives:

Official: A component of comprehensive health care in which services are provided to individuals and their families in their place of residence for the purpose of promoting, maintaining, or restoring health, or of minimizing the effects of illness and disability.

Patient: Skilled and compassionate care provided on a one-to-one basis in the comforting and familiar surroundings of the home. It is based on individual needs and personalized schedules and is provided over a period of time so that adjustment, change, and learning can most effectively take place.

Family: A means to keep the family together as a functioning, integrated unit. The goals are learning to adapt to change, preventing dysfunctional patterns, and attaining family wellness within the confines of an individual member's illness or disability. It provides needed emotional support and linkage with the larger community support systems.

Provider: Challenges all disciplines involved to provide excellent care in often less than excellent conditions and surroundings. Independence, creativity, communication, and excellent clinical skills are integral parts of daily practice. It is an opportunity for nurses to demonstrate the best of their profession and themselves in cooperation with the health care team to patients and families with physical and psychological needs.

Home care was formerly simply defined as providing physical care to the sick in their homes, but the scope and complexity of the concept and practice have grown.

HISTORICAL OVERVIEW

Roots of the concept can be traced to the New Testament, when visiting the sick was a form of charity. Sixth-century monks practiced home care as an important aspect of their work in the community. One of the earliest organized systems for home care was developed in 1617 by St. Vincent de Paul, who organized the Sisterhood of the Dames de Charite to meet social welfare and visiting nursing needs.

In the 1700s families were primary care givers. The poor were hospitalized, whereas those with financial means were cared for in their homes by the visiting physician.

The first home care program in the United States was organized in 1796 as the Boston Dispensary. In 1859 William Rathbone of Liverpool, England, established the Metropolitan Nursing Association, the first organized district nursing service, because of the outstanding home care his dying wife received. He believed that many people with long-term illnesses could be better cared for in their own homes than in a hospital—a belief central to home care today.

The first visiting nurse service in the United States was formed in Philadelphia in 1886. It was directed by nurses who provided care to all ages of persons with both acute and chronic care needs.

Lillian Wald and Mary Brewster developed a visiting nurse service for the poor in New York City in 1893 at the Nurses' Settlement House on Henry Street. In the late 1800s and early 1900s visiting nurse associations were formalized, and public health departments became widespread.

Metropolitan Life Insurance had a major impact on the growth and nature of home services when in 1909 it began offering nursing services to its millions of industrial policy holders. This initiated third-party payment for services. Payment until then had been provided primarily on a charitable or patient-paid basis.

The Social Security Act of 1935 first provided governmental rather than local charitable funding for selected services, such as maternal health, communicable disease, and the training of public health professionals. It subsidized assistance for the poor and aged. Amendments to the Act in 1950 further defined services and opened the door to direct payment for providers.

A revolution, however, occurred in 1965 when Title XVIII (known as Medicare) and Title XIX (known as Medicaid) amendments to the Social Security Act were enacted. **Medicare** provided direct federal monies for the health care of all citizens 65 and older (or disabled), regardless of socioeconomic status. The companion **Medicaid** bill covered the care needs of the poor and indigent of all ages. When Medicare became effective in 1966, it revolutionized home care by (1) changing it to a medical rather than nursing model of practice, (2) defining and limiting services it would reimburse, and (3) changing the payment source and even changing the reason home care was provided. For considerations concerning the older adult patient, see the gerontological box.

The next major influence on home care came in 1983. Congress enacted the prospective payment system as a part of the Tax Equity and Fiscal Responsibility Act for hospitals receiving Medicare reimbursement. This

GERONTOLOGICAL CONSIDERATIONS

- The growing number of older adults has resulted in an increased need for home health care services.
- Early discharge policies have resulted in very ill older adults leaving the hospital. This increases the importance of patient teaching, early discharge planning, and appropriate referral to home health agencies by hospital staff nurses
- Many older adults do not require total care but do require a limited amount of assistance. Home care reduces disruption of life-style and is more cost effective than institutional placement.
- Transfer to a hospital or nursing home even on a temporary basis increases the stress level of older persons. Stress is decreased if they receive care in a familiar environment.
- A number of service agencies exists that can assist older adult in their communities. These include Meals on Wheels, home health aide, homemaker, and home-based physical therapy services. Nurses should be familiar with home health services in their area and help older persons make arrangement for the appropriate services.

system, based on major diagnostic categories and diagnosis-related groups (**DRGs**), paid a set rate (according to diagnosis) for the hospitalized patient's care rather than the "cost" or charges traditionally billed by institutions. The net effect of the change was a major shift of patients out of the hospital into their homes, extended-care facilities, or skilled nursing facilities. Such patients were discharged earlier in their convalescence and thus required more nursing care. This created a challenge to home care in terms of volume of patients seen, necessity of more skilled nursing care over intensive times, and the evolution of highly technical procedures in the home. Existing agencies expanded, and new ones developed to meet the demand.

TYPES OF AGENCIES

In the broadest terms home care services can be delivered by any individual, service group, organization, or agency with the desire to provide services to the elderly, disabled, or ill of any age. The type and qualifications of personnel used, quality of services delivered, and standards of care can vary widely and often depend on funding sources.

The agency may have to comply with federal, state, and local laws and regulations via the following:

Licensure by the state: This gives legal permission to operate within that state only. Regulations vary widely. Not all states have such laws.

Certification by state certifying body designated by the federal government: Rules governing **certification** (a process in which an individual, institution, or educational program is evaluated and recognized as meeting certain predetermined standards) are federally mandated. Only certified agencies may receive Medicare payment. Many states piggyback Medicaid reimbursement to certification, as do some insurers.

Certificate of need granted by some states according to rules and formulas devised by state regulators: Cost of starting and running the agency, availability of personnel, and need for their services are generally considered in this process.

Accreditation by an outside agency that evaluates and judges how well the agency meets certain standards set by the accrediting organization: This **accreditation** (a process whereby a professional association or nongovernmental agency grants recognition to a school or institution for demonstrated ability in a special area of practice or training) may be granted by the National League for Nursing Community Health Accreditation Program, the Joint Commission for Accreditation of Healthcare Organizations, or the National Homecaring Council. Other groups may accredit special programs or specialized agencies. Some of these national accrediting agencies are seeking "deemed status" from federal regulators, which will allow their accreditation to also serve as the required certification. This will eliminate the need for separate surveys for some agencies.

It is still possible for some agencies to operate under no specific rules or regulations.

Before Medicare, home health care was provided primarily by visiting nurse associations, nursing divisions of state or local health departments, and hospitals. Now agencies are classified according to (1) tax status—for profit or not for profit; (2) location—freestanding or institution based; and (3) governance—private or public. Table 48-1 on p. 1516 summarizes and describes the six generally accepted types of home health agencies. The structure of some of these agencies is subject to change and variation. For example, some visiting nurse associations have reorganized and placed their home health agencies into private, nonprofit structures to ensure reimbursement that will cover the cost of providing services. Similarly, it is possible to have an official or voluntary hospital-based agency.

Growth in number of agencies has mirrored the growth of home care. In 1966 there were approximately 2000 agencies. Medicare-certified agencies numbered 2864 in 1980, 6007 in 1986, 5787 in 1988, and 9285 in 1991.

Although the late 1980s saw a decrease in agencies, the numbers have rebounded, largely because of increases in hospital-based agencies and specialized agencies providing highly technical types of care. Such high-technology care may include intravenous services, ventilator-dependent care services, and management of

TABLE 48-1 Home Health Agencies

Status	Governed By	Supported By	Services Offered	Staffed By	Time of Service	Example
Voluntary						
Public; nonprofit; freestanding	Community-based board of directors	Tax deductible contributions; grants; fees from all sources	Community health; public health; home health	RN; LPN/LVN; aide; homemaker; social worker; therapists	Generally ½-8 hr	Visiting nurse association
Official						
Public; nonprofit; freestanding	State, county, city, or other local unit of government and volunteer board representatives of the area	State, local, or county revenues; grants; fees from limited sources; charitable contributions	Community health; public health; home health	RN; LPN/LVN; aide; homemaker; may have social workers; therapists	Generally ½-4 hr	State health departments; county health departments; city health departments
Combination						
Public; nonprofit; freestanding	Jointly operated by the two types of agencies above under a combined board of directors	State, local, or county revenues; grants; fees from limited sources; charitable contributions	Community health; public health; home health	RN; LPN/LVN; aide; homemaker; may have social workers; therapists	Generally ½-4 hr	County-based visiting nurse association
Hospital						
Private; nonprofit or for profit; institution-based; hospital	Hospital board of directors	Fees from all sources	Home health; community health (limited)	RN; LPN/LVN; aide; social workers; therapists	Generally ½-4 hr	XYZ hospital home health agency
Proprietary						
Private; for profit; freestanding	Governed and owned by individual corporation, or other organization; many paid boards of directors appointed by owner	Fees from most sources; may or may not participate in Medicare/Medicaid	May have limited home health; private duty; homemaker	RN; LPN/LVN; aides	1-24 hr	Home health care of XYZ
Private not for profit						
Private; nonprofit; freestanding	Governed and owned by individual, corporation, or other organizational structure; board appointed by owner	Fees from most sources; may or may not participate in Medicare/Medicaid	May have limited home health services; private duty; homemaker	RN; LPN/LVN; aides	½-24 hr	ABC home health agency
Other						
Private; for profit or nonprofit; institution based	Based within formalized institution; governed by that board or designated board	Fees from all sources	Home health services; limited homemaker	RN; LPN/LVN; aide; therapists; may have homemaker; social worker	½-4-8 hr	ABC nursing home—home health agency; ABC rehabilitation facility home care

human immunodeficiency virus (HIV) patients in the home. The demand for this type of care is expected to increase at double-digit percentage levels into the twenty-first century.

Home care visits and Medicare expenditures for home care have quadrupled between 1980 and 1991. This can be directly attributed to shorter hospitalizations, more seriously ill patients being discharged home, and increased acceptance of higher technology care being delivered in the home.

SERVICE COMPONENTS

Most home health agencies follow the basic Medicare model of services offered. Functions and scopes of practice are dictated by state licensing boards and professional organizations. Primary services include the following:

- Skilled nursing
- Physical therapy
- Speech-language pathology
- Occupational therapy
- Medical social services
- Home health aide

Other therapy services, such as respiratory, or professional services such as nutritional counseling, pharmacy, podiatry, dentistry, and psychiatric or mental health, may be offered. Support services, such as homemaker, companion, and respite, may be provided but are not directly reimbursed by Medicare. The service mix depends on patient diagnosis, patient/family needs, and availability of resources. Medical supplies are commonly provided. Home medical equipment ranging from the traditional hospital bed to highly sophisticated items such as respirators and apnea monitors may be provided by companies specializing in equipment provision.

Medicare and Medicaid home care services are based on the medical model of treatment and depend on the physician for entry into the formalized system. Medicare requires a plan of treatment signed by the physician, outlining all disciplines, treatment, frequency, and duration. These orders must be recertified every 62 days. Third-party payers may or may not have similar requirements. Only the primary services will be explained in this chapter.

Skilled Nursing

Skilled nursing services are provided and directed by currently licensed registered nurses. Some agencies require that nurses have a bachelor's degrees in nursing, whereas others hire graduates of all types of RN programs and teach them agency policies and specific procedures. Not all nurses can be effective home health nurses. Basic nursing services may be provided by the LPN/LVN under the supervision of the RN.

Service Goals. Skilled nursing services revolve around the following four major goals:

Restorative: The return to a previous level of functioning as appropriate and realistic

Improvement: Achieving better health and a higher level of functioning than when admitted

Maintenance: Preservation of functional capacities and independence by maintaining current level of health

Promotion: Teaching health life-styles that minimize the effect of illness or disability and prevent the recurrence of illness

Provider Attributes. Nurses practicing in the home setting are care givers, teachers, counselors, case managers, and advocates. They must be technically proficient, self-motivated, innovative, and independent decision makers. Common sense, flexibility, compassion, empathy, patience, honesty, and dependability are essential. Nurses who depend on the security of the institutional setting, immediate medical direction, and frequent peer support find the independence of home care practice difficult.

Home health nursing requires that nurses and other providers adapt to the patient, family, and home environment. Staff are visitors in the patient's home. Strong communication skills are essential for teaching, counseling, interviewing, and listening. High energy level, cheerfulness, and a positive attitude are valuable attributes as nurses often work with patients and families who are under stress. Respect of the patient's dignity, privacy, and needs of autonomy is an integral part of providing effective nursing services.

Services are generally provided in the patient's home; hence nurses must feel comfortable with the unknown, as well as accept differences in ethnic cultures, mores, and value systems. Commitment to professional standards of practice, ongoing continuing education, and skills updates are important.

Nursing Process. Home health nursing uses the basic nursing process to assess the needs, establish a patient-centered plan of care, implement nursing actions, evaluate the effectiveness of actions, and plan for modification or resolution of identified problems. Interventions may range from wound care to intravenous chemotherapy. Teaching could involve diabetes instruction or the management of complex support equipment in the home. Teaching is always patient centered, with the primary goals being self-care and independent functioning within the confines of the illness or disability (Fig. 48-1 on p. 1518). In the counseling role a nurse may provide emotional support to the dying patient and the family or provide skilled psychiatric interventions (if properly qualified). Case management may include only supervision of the home health aide or involve the coordination of complex care plans with services, supplies, and

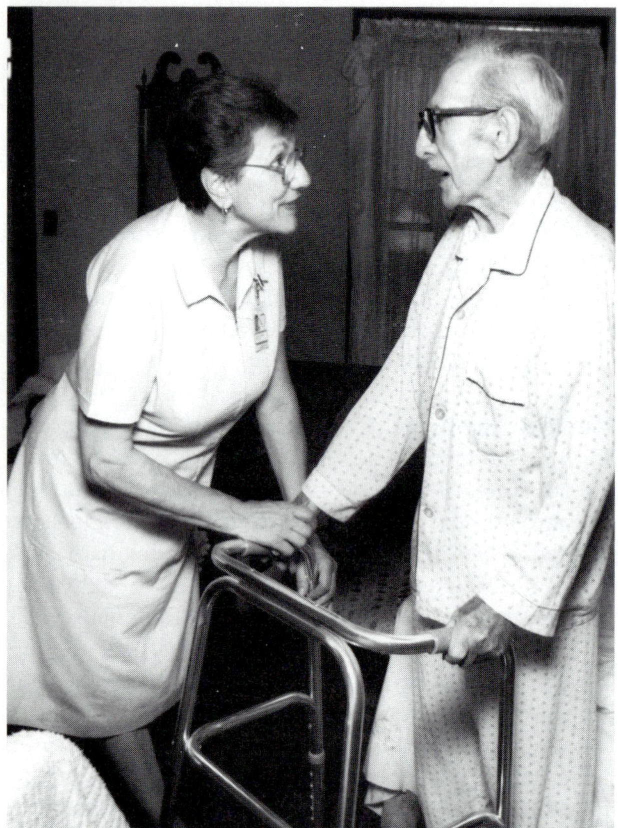

FIG. 48-1 The nurse assists an older patient to ambulate. (Photo by Marilu Halamandaris, *CARING Magazine.*)

equipment provided by many different disciplines.

RNs have been the primary providers of skilled service by both tradition and regulation. Skilled service has become, however, a growing field of practice for the LPN/LVN as agencies cope with increased staffing needs, nursing shortages, and recognition of the contributions the LPN/LVN can make to home care.

LPNs/LVNs now represent 10% to 20% of the home care work force of the major providers in urban areas. Medicare-certified agencies currently employ LPNs or LVNs as 6% of their work force.

Licensed Practical/Vocational Nurse Role

LPNs/LVNs must be supervised by the RN. Although LPNs/LVNs cannot make detailed patient assessments or clinical judgments, their observations, reporting, documentation, teaching, and technical care capabilities are important to home care.

Provider Attributes. Personal and professional attributes described for RNs also apply to the LPN/LVN. Independent practice is not allowed, but self-direction, motivation, creativity, clinical proficiency, flexibility, compassion, empathy, and patience are all essential attributes. Good communication skills, both written and verbal, are necessary. The ability to work alone, follow directions, recognize important changes in condition, and assist in patient teaching is needed. Evaluation of care interventions and recommendations for alteration of the plan of care are a part of the role. The concept of teamwork must be understood and practiced.

Functions. Depending on the agency, agency policies, and state practice acts, the LPN/LVN may provide the following services in the home as directed and supervised by the RN:

1. Catheter care and teaching
2. Ostomy care and teaching
3. Wound care and sterile dressing changes
4. Obtaining specimens for cultures
5. Injection administration
6. Prefilling of insulin syringes
7. Fingersticks for blood glucose readings
8. Monitoring of physical status (such as lung sounds, bowel sounds, pulses, edema, and weights)
9. Teaching, monitoring, or setting up medications
10. Enteral feedings
11. Specimen collection
12. Therapeutic diet teaching or reinforcement
13. Tracheostomy care including suctioning
14. Enemas for special conditions
15. Emotional support
16. Preventive health measures
17. Patient and family teaching

Assistance with highly technical procedures, such as intravenous therapies, home dialysis, and respirator management, may be allowed in some states.

Home health care offers a new and challenging area of practice for the LPN/LVN who enjoys practicing nursing in a less restrictive environment. LPNs/LVNs employed in home health agencies cite satisfaction in terms of flexibility, pay, and one-on-one relationships with patients. The need for this level of nursing practice will continue to grow. Commitment to quality of care is a common thread through skilled nursing services: hence the LPN/LVN must also pursue frequent inservice updates and continuing education to ensure current practice.

PHYSICAL THERAPY SERVICES

Services must be provided by a qualified and licensed physical therapist. A physical therapy assistant under the supervision of the licensed therapist may deliver limited services. The goals of treatment must be restorative for Medicare reimbursement but may be maintenance or preventive for other payer sources. The therapist completes a detailed assessment of the patient and then determines treatment, education, and assistive devices needed for rehabilitation. These are included as a part of the physician-approved plan of treatment. Treatments range from muscle strengthening to transcutaneous nerve stimulation and ultrasound treatments. The therapist actively teaches the patient and family the rehabilitation plan to promote self-care and independence. Communication with the physician and RN promotes continuity of care.

SPEECH LANGUAGE PATHOLOGY SERVICES

To be Medicare reimbursed, speech services must be provided by a master's-prepared clinician who has been certified by the American Speech and Hearing Association. Other insurers may accept a practitioner prepared at the bachelor's level. Therapy goals include minimizing communication disorders and their physical, emotional, and social impact. Independent functioning and maximum rehabilitation of speech and language abilities are primary treatment goals. Services may be provided after stroke or after surgery. Therapies may range from language relearning to working with eating or swallowing disorders or teaching lipreading to those with hearing disorders. Pathologists work closely with the patient and family for rehabilitation or adjustment to a new disability.

OCCUPATIONAL THERAPY

Occupational therapy services deal with life's practical tasks. Therapists are prepared at the bachelor's level and may earn the occupational therapist registered (OTR) designation if they meet the registration requirements of the National Occupational Therapy Association. Some services may be provided by the certified occupational therapy assistant under the supervision of the OTR. Based on a complete evaluation of functional level, the therapist will choose and teach therapeutic activities designed to restore functional levels. Services include (1) techniques to increase independence, (2) design, fabrication, and fitting of orthotic or self-help devices, and (3) assessment for vocational training. Patient-centered education is an integral part of attaining independence in self-care.

MEDICAL SOCIAL SERVICES

Medical social services are provided by social workers prepared at the master's level. Bachelor's-prepared workers may provide services under mastered social worker (MSW) supervision. Their focus is on the emotional and social aspects of illness. The patient, family, or other support systems are evaluated for social, emotional, and environmental factors. The care plan includes education, counseling, payment source identification, and referrals. Coping with stress and crisis intervention are also part of social worker services. Social services in home health are generally short term.

HOMEMAKER–HOME HEALTH AIDE SERVICES

Medicare refers to the homemaker–home health aide (HM-HHA) as a home health aide (HHA). These workers are an integral part of the home health care team. They provide the basic support services that can enable an elderly individual, disabled adult, or dependent child to remain at home. Medicare requires that a primary skilled or therapy service (speech or physical) be necessary before HHA services can be provided. Medicaid and some insurers have less stringent requirements. Many insurers do not reimburse this care. Family members and individuals are often willing to pay privately to prevent institutionalization.

Most aide services fall into one of three categories: (1) personal care: assistance with bathing, oral hygiene, eating, dressing, or toileting; (2) physical assistance: with transfers, medications, ambulation; or (3) household chores: cooking, light housekeeping, shopping, laundry. Medicare will not cover visits made solely for the third reason.

Although "training" of aides has long been required by Medicare, rules governing type, length, and content of preparation have been nonexistent; hence, skills and standards were not uniform. As a part of the Omnibus Budget Reconciliation Act of 1987, new standards for training and competency evaluation have been formulated and are now effective.

Medicare and Medicaid require on-site supervision of the aide every 2 weeks, principally by an RN. A licensed physical therapist may provide the supervision if skilled nursing is not involved. Private payers, however, often do not have such requirements. Aide services are sometimes provided in blocks of time ranging from 1 to 2 hours for Medicare to 8 to 24 hours for private or other payment sources.

THE TYPICAL HOME HEALTH PROCESS

Referral

The entry point to the home health care system is by referral. This can come from the patient, family, social service agency, hospital, physician, or another agency. Agencies have a variety of methods of intake for referrals ranging from a formalized hospital discharge planning process with a central agency intake coordinator to a direct call from the patient's physician to the agency staff.

Admission

The initial evaluation and admission visit are made by an RN within 24 to 48 hours of the referral. This may be completed by an RN in a formal role as admission nurse or by a staff nurse who will serve as the primary nurse on the case. The physician often is contacted for general orders before this visit, but agencies may make an evaluation visit without orders if allowed to do so by agency policy. The evaluation and admission process generally includes as a minimum:

1. Complete patient evaluation including physical and psychosocial factors
2. Environmental assessment relating specifically to safety and ability to provide services effectively in the home
3. Identification of primary functional impairments
4. Identification of the impact of the disease or disability on the patient and family
5. Assessment of the family or significant other support system
6. Determination of knowledge, and adherence to treatments and medications
7. Determination of the desire for care and services
8. Involvement of the patient and family in the development of the plan of care and goals
9. Notification to the patient of rights as a patient, along with information on costs, payment sources, and billing practices
10. Explanation of the patient's right to self-determination, including information and implementation policies for advanced directives
11. Provision of initial nursing interventions

The admission process typically takes a minimum of 1 hour. It will take longer if the patient is disoriented or in need of nursing interventions. In some hospital-based agencies an abbreviated evaluation visit may be made while the patient is still in the hospital.

Care Plan

If the patient is to be admitted, the physician must be contacted for specific orders before delivery of care. A treatment plan is drafted cooperatively with the physician. This plan describes the current physical status of the patient, medications, treatments, the disciplines needed to provide care, the frequency and duration of services, and the goals/outcomes, and the time frame for implementation. A plan of treatment must be signed by the physician and serves as the traditional physician orders. Although the treatment plan can be altered at any time, based on patient needs, through additional written, signed orders, it *must* be reviewed and renewed on a regular schedule for Medicare and Medicaid patients. Separate care plans may be written that are discipline specific, such as nursing and physical therapy. A separate detailed home health aide care plan is always required.

Visits

Visits for interventions by ordered disciplines are made to meet the patient-centered goals and progress toward identified outcomes. Skilled nursing visits typically take 30 to 45 minutes but could increase to several hours for complex procedures. Therapy visits range from 30 minutes to 1 hour. Aide visits average 1 to 2 hours but could be longer, depending on needs and payment source. Revisions to the plan of care and referrals to other agencies occur during this period. Patients may be visited as infrequently as one time a month for diabetic monitoring to several times a day over a short period to provide complex care. Several visits per week are typical. Patients may receive only skilled nursing services or may be visited by all disciplines. They may remain on the caseload a week or years, but 60 to 90 days is common.

Documentation

Throughout the care process concise and complete documentation is essential. This documentation may be handwritten, dictated, or entered into a computer. A number of agencies use the problem-oriented record system—many in combination with the nursing diagnosis system.

Many agencies are beginning to use various problem classification schemes linked with nursing diagnoses (Box 48-1), specific interventions, and defined patient outcomes. Documentation that follows the nursing process model provides an accurate picture of the type and quality of care. It reflects the effectiveness of the plan of care and progress toward goals and outcomes, or it reflects the nature and reasons for lack of progress or deterioration and includes alternative interventions. Communications with the home care team and referral sources must also be documented.

Documentation is influenced by other factors. Staff must recognize the record as a legal document subject to close scrutiny at any time. Professional standards, accountability, and quality of car are closely linked to legal implications, as well as to internal evaluation purposes.

Reimbursement sources have a major influence on documentation requirements by setting forth specific forms and formats that must be followed. Medicare requires extensive paperwork. Private insurer requirements are generally less cumbersome.

Discharge Planning

Discharge planning for home care, as in hospitals, begins with admission. When patient goals or other specific criteria are met, the discharge occurs. Patient and family

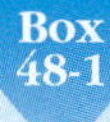

Box 48-1 EXAMPLES OF NANDA-APPROVED NURSING DIAGNOSES ROUTINELY IDENTIFIED AS REQUIRING HOME HEALTH CARE

Infection, high risk for, related to:
- Inadequate primary or secondary defenses
- Inadequate acquired immunity
- Malnutrition

Knowledge deficit, related to:
- Lack of experience
- Cognition limitation

Nutrition, altered: less than body requirements, related to:
- Inability to ingest or digest food
- Inability to absorb nutrients
- Economic deprivation

Self-care deficit, bathing/hygiene, related to:
- Pain
- Musculoskeletal impairment
- Decreased endurance
- Neurological impairment

Skin integrity impaired, related to:
- Physical immobility
- Radiation
- Impaired circulation (pressure)
- Inadequate nutrition

Pain, related to:
- Chronic illness (e.g., rheumatoid arthritis)
- Terminal cancer

participation in discharge planning is encouraged. The physician is consulted regarding the discharge and issues the final order. Many agencies follow up on a postdischarge basis to track patient progress and elicit patient satisfaction information. The purpose of discharge planning is to promote continuity of care in the patient's home.

QUALITY ASSURANCE/ ASSESSMENT/IMPROVEMENT

Quality assessment programs provide documentation for outside organizations and for internal measures for improvements and refinements of policies and procedures. Assessing quality involves evaluating all aspects of the agency operation. Three major elements are included:

1. *Structural criteria:* The agency's overall organization, philosophy, policies, procedures, bylaws, personnel practices, supervision, orientation, contracts, and physical facilities.
2. *Process criteria:* evaluation of care delivery. The activities of the health professionals and paraprofessionals and support in the management of patient care, documentation, and patient care conferences are scrutinized.
3. *Outcome criteria:* measurement of change in patient behavior, the results of patient care in terms of changes, health indicators, and satisfaction. Care standards and expected outcomes are an integral part of this area.

Specific criteria and measures are developed in each area and evaluated for compliance and effectiveness. Evaluation may be accomplished in some areas by management, by a multidisciplinary committee, or by groups of outside professionals and consumers.

In the past, measures of quality of the agency, care delivered, and staff were subjective, with little standardization and agreement. Quality assessment plans now reflect standards, objectives, and measurable outcomes and include plans for remediation or improvement as an integral part of the process.

There is currently a move by a national accreditation body (Joint Commission on Accreditation of Healthcare Organizations) and many businesses to redefine quality assessment activities in terms of quality improvement. Terms such as *total quality management, continuous quality improvement,* and *quality improvement* (for home care) relate to an agency-wide commitment to excellence that covers clinical and nonclinical functions. The following major principles are involved:

1. Quality of patient care and desired outcomes can be improved by assessing and improving governance, management, and clinical and support processes that affect patient outcomes.
2. Processes are carried out by individuals (managers, clinicians, support) and jointly by these groups.
3. Processes must be coordinated and integrated.
4. Employees of an organization arc motivated and competent to carry out processes and should be given opportunities to continuously improve.

Continued movement toward this philosophy of management is likely in home care as the twenty-first century approaches. It will have a direct impact on all staff and provide a different emphasis on how many agencies will operate.

REIMBURSEMENT SOURCES

Reimbursement for home health services comes from a variety of sources, and covered services and disciplines vary. Medicare and Medicaid are major sources of income for the majority of agencies, but reliance on these sources for reimbursement has decreased in recent years.

Medicare

Medicare is a federal program that requires agencies to be certified as meeting the federal conditions of participation, which set forth specific requirements for organization, staffing, training, types of services covered, and agency evaluation. Regulations further mandate eligibility requirements. Beneficiaries of services must be 65 or older, disabled, or have end-stage renal disease. In addition, they must be (1) under the care of a licensed physician, (2) homebound, and (3) in need of skilled nursing or therapy services on an intermittent basis.

Types of services covered and length of coverage are further delineated in guidelines developed by the Health Care Financing Administration (HCFA). Ten regional fiscal intermediaries, who act on behalf of HCFA, receive claims for payment, process reimbursement, and determine coverage.

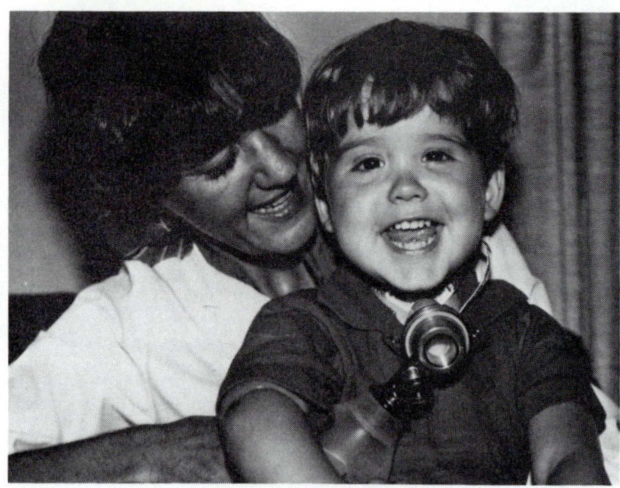

FIG. 48-2 Child with Ondine's disease, chronic obstructive pulmonary disease, and collapsible airway syndrome. With the services of home health care, he has been able to recover at home. (Photo by Marilu Halamandaris, *CARING Magazine*.)

Medicaid

The Medicaid program pays for home care services to indigent and low-income persons of all ages. It is administered by the state but is both state and federally subsidized. Many states require Medicare certification for participation in the Medicaid program. Services covered vary from state to state, but most include the basic services covered by Medicare plus expansion of aide and personal care services. This program has recently been allowed, through a waiver process, to pay for around-the-clock services to children who require high-technology care and equipment. Children who have lived in an institution can go home and be a part of the family unit (Fig. 48-2).

Third Party

Third-party insurers pay for limited home care services. Coverage, requirements, and payment rates vary. Reimbursement often is tied to posthospitalization recoveries. A few progressive companies are paying for nursing and aide services for new mothers who return home within 24 hours of delivery.

Case management by or on behalf of insurance companies and workman compensation plans is being widely practiced. A case manager (commonly a nurse or social worker) will determine and arrange for a mix of home care, therapy services, counseling, supplies, and equipment for a patient. The availability of these combined, paid-for services often allows earlier discharges and provides a planned approach to rehabilitation.

A similar approach to case management for the elderly is commonly provided by Area Agencies on Aging, social service departments, community or public health agencies, independent case managers, or contracts with groups or companies providing such services. Costs may be fully paid, depending on how the service is provided.

Private Pay

Individuals may also pay directly for home health services. Charges may be the standard full charge or may be scaled down based on the ability of the patient to pay.

Other Sources

Health maintenance organizations (HMOs) and preferred provider organizations (PPOs) have negotiated contracts with home health agencies to provide services to their patients. Both organizations are prepaid health plans operated independently or through employer groups. Again, requirements and coverage differ.

SUMMARY

Current trends support the growth of home care as an economical, humane, preferred health delivery system for certain types of care. Advances in medical knowledge coupled with high-technology health care have increased the number of individuals surviving birth traumas, prematurity, infectious diseases, acute illnesses, accidents, and other maladies that formerly were fatal.

Many illnesses are medically managed and controlled rather than cured. This has increased the number of potentially debilitating chronic illnesses. Dependency and disability are more prevalent in all age groups. One in seven persons now needs help with basic activities of daily living. Home care provides needed assessment and evaluation of chronic illnesses to prevent acute episodes. Aides and homemakers can provide necessary support in activities of daily living to enable the patient to remain in the home.

The birth rate has declined, resulting in an aging population. In the 1900s only 2% of the population was 65 or older. That figure was 12.3% in 1989 and is projected to reach 20% by the 2030. Nearly 20% of this group are considered poor or near poor. It is estimated that 80% of this group has at least one chronic disability. The age group older than 85 years is the fastest growing group today. It is estimated that by the year 2000 there will be a tenfold increase in persons older than 100 years. About 40% of those 85 and older need help with physical activities. Assistance in daily living is essential to this group. Skilled nursing and therapy offer rehabilitation and prevention of deterioration, as well as methods to cope with physical changes.

Federal and private insurers are trying to cap the rapidly rising cost of health care by shortening hospital stays and controlling admissions. Home care agencies are filling the gap for patients who are released early but who still require complex care or rehabilitation. In many cases, home care services can prevent hospitalization by offering enteral, parenteral, intravenous, and blood transfusion services.

The movement toward deinstitutionalization of technology-dependent children and adults is now possible as Medicaid and third-party payers change reimbursement criteria. Home care support makes "family life" a reality for people who once thought of hospital personnel as parents.

An emphasis on healthy living and illness prevention is supported by home health providers as part of the plan of care. This one-on-one education teaches specific techniques to avoid recurrences of illness or deterioration of condition.

Finally, individuals want to be at home as long as possible. Care provided by home health agencies and support from social service agencies and others are now making this possible throughout the life span.

REFERENCES AND SUGGESTED READINGS

1. Aitken MJ: Matching models to environments: a planning guide to the solution of pediatric home care models, *Home Healthc Nurse* 7(2):13, 1989.
2. American Nurses Association: *Standards of clinical nursing practice,* Kansas City, Mo, 1991, The Association.
3. American Nurses Association: *Standards of home health nursing practice,* Kansas City, Mo, 1986, The Association.
4. Bulau JM: *Administrative policies and procedures for home health care,* ed 2, Rockville, Md, 1991, Aspen.
5. Department of Health and Human Services: *Code of Federal Regulations (Title 42),* Washington, DC, 1989, The Department.
6. de Savorgnani A, Haring R, Galloway S: Caught in the middle: a profile of licensed practical nurses in home care, *Caring* 11(8):12, 1992.
7. Dombi WA: The patient's right to self-determination, *Caring* 10(5):78, 1991.
8. Fischbach FT: *Documenting care: communication, the nursing process and documentation standards,* Philadelphia, 1991, FA Davis.
9. Haddad A, Kapp M: *Ethical and legal issues in home care: case studies and analysis,* New York, 1990, Appleton & Lange.
10. Harris MD: *Home health administration,* Owings Mills, Md, 1988, National Health Publishing.
11. Health Care Financing Administration: *HCFA statistics,* Bureau of Data Management and Strategy, Pub No 03229, Washington, DC, 1986, US Government Printing Office.
12. *Home health and hospice manual: regulations and guidelines,* Subscriber Digest, Bulletin No 17, Owings Mills, Md, 1989, National Health Publishing.
13. Humphrey CJ, Milone-Nuzzo P: *Home care nursing: an orientation to practice,* New York, 1991, Appleton & Lange.
14. Iyer PW, Camp NH: *Nursing documentation: a nursing process approach,* St Louis, 1991, Mosby.
15. Joint Commission on Accreditation of Healthcare Organizations, *Accreditation manual for homecare: standards,* vol 1, Oak Brook, Ill, 1992, The Commission.
16. Kaye LW: *Home health care,* Newbury Park, Calif, 1992, Sage.
17. Kirsch A, Donovan S: The journey to quality improvement in home care, *Caring* 11(8):46, 1992.
18. *Managed care digest: long term care edition,* Kansas City, Mo, 1992, Marion Merrell Dow.
19. Martin KS, Scheet NJ: *The Omaha system: applications for community health nursing,* Philadelphia, 1992, Saunders.
20. Mesenheimer CG: *Quality assurance for homecare,* Rockville, Md, 1989, Aspen.
21. Rice R: *Home health nursing practice: concepts and application,* St Louis, 1992, Mosby.
22. Saba VK, Zuckerman AE: A new home health classification method, *Caring* 11(10):27, 1992.
23. Shaughnessy P, Bauman M, Kraner A: Measuring the quality of home health care: some important considerations, *Caring* 9(2):4, 1990.
24. Staebler R: Providing mental health services for the elderly, *Caring* 10(5):52, 1991.
25. Stanhope M, Lancaster J: *Community health nursing: process and practice for promoting health,* ed 3, St Louis, 1992, Mosby.
26. Twardon CA, Gartner MB: Empowering nurses: patient satisfaction with primary nursing in home health, *J Nurs Adm* 21(11):39, 1991.
27. US General Accounting Office, Report to the Chairman, Select Committee on Aging, House of Representatives: Elderly Americans: health, housing, and nutrition gaps between the poor and nonpoor, GAO/PEMD-92-29, Washington, DC, June 1992.
28. Vance M: Management by values, *Caring* 12(1):60, 1993.
29. Weaver K: Nutritional concerns of the home care patient, *Home Healthc Nurse* 9(2):36, 1991.
30. Wood JB, Estes CL: The impact of DRGs on community-based service providers: implications for the elderly, *Am J Public Health* 80(7):840, 1990.

CHAPTER CHALLENGE

KEY POINTS

- Home health care allows individuals to maintain personal control and to participate in the direction of their own care.
- Families are an important part of the success of home care services as health care workers provide care, supervision, assistance, and support in attaining the care plan goals.
- Home health care is not a new concept; however, legislative, regulatory, and current health care trends have changed the way it is provided.
- A number of different professional and paraprofessional disciplines provide home care services based on a coordinated plan of care approved by a physician. Teamwork is an essential component of the concept.
- Home health agencies are organized groups that employ or contract with professionals and paraprofessionals to provide services. Different types of agencies may be subject to varying federal, state, and local laws and regulations.
- Skilled nursing care is the most frequently provided serivce. RNs and LPNs/LVNs under the supervision of RNs provide direct care of different levels of complexity.
- Providers of care in the home must possess special qualities to effectively practice in this nontraditional environment.
- Home health care agencies strive to provide the highest quality of services in an economical manner. Success is evaluated through quality assurance plans.
- Home health services are reimbursed by federal, state, local, group, and private sources.
- Quality assessment of safe and effective care in the home is of great significance.
- Although some aspects of nursing interventions in the home are the same as practiced in other health care settings, home health care nurses pay particular attention to interaction and cooperation among family members, the patient, and other members of the health care team.
- The acuity levels of patients requiring care in their homes continues to rise, and the technological aspects of care, including use of mechanical equipment and invasive procedures such as intravenous therapies, are increasing in home care. These factors, when combined with shorter hospital stays, require extensive discharge planning to prepare patients and family for home health care.

STUDY QUESTIONS

1. Mrs. Christofer is a 79-year-old widow. She recently fractured her hip and had a bipolar hip replacement. Her daughter works during the day, but provides care in the evening. The most appropriate service agency to provide for Mrs. Christofer's daily care is a/an:
   1. private duty agency
   2. home health care agency
   3. nursing home facility
   4. outpatient rehabilitation agency
2. A student nurse asks her nurse educator why there is an increased demand for home health care. The most accurate response by the educator would be that:
   1. more family members want to care for their ill members at home
   2. there is a shortage of nurses who want to work in acute hospital care settings
   3. there is an increase in the number of older patients with chronic illnesses
   4. there is increased technology in hospitals, which is anxiety provoking to many patients
3. The nurse is assigned to home health care for Mr. Hernandez, an 83-year-old patient with a CVA with right-sided hemiplegia, difficulty swallowing, and speech impairment. He is cared for in his home by his elderly wife and retired daughter. The nurse involved in administering care in their home must provide a:
   1. strict regimen and care plan
   2. holistic, nonjudgmental philosophy
   3. teaching plan for all family members
   4. means of transporting Mr. Hernandez to his physician
4. Nurses are knowledgeable that evolving future health care trends point to:
   1. decreased reimbursement for home health care services
   2. keeping patients in the hospital longer because of the severity of their illnesses
   3. increased high-technology procedures in the home setting
   4. slowed growth in number of agencies involved in home care

5. Ms. Peterson is a 68-year-old patient recovering from an abdominoperineal resection with a permanent colostomy. Her physician has ordered home health care nursing upon her discharge. A *primary goal* for home health care nursing for Ms. Peterson would be to:
   1. return the patient to previous life-style
   2. avoid dependency on medication therapy
   3. establish self-care and independence
   4. maintain a friendly relationship with family members
6. A nursing supervisor for home health care must always be concerned with patient care and:
   1. location of the home
   2. quality assurance
   3. method of payment
   4. number of children in the home
7. When the home health care nurse makes arrangements for the patient to receive home care, data are collected from the:
   1. home care agency
   2. patient and family members
   3. insurance company
   4. community volunteer agencies
8. Upon beginning home health care visitation, Mr. Somas, a terminal cancer patient tells the nurse he has a living will. The nurse is knowledgeable that this document functions to state Mr. Soma's desire to:
   1. have all means of technical assistance and equipment utilized to prolong his life
   2. have his family members make decisions regarding his care
   3. be allowed to die without life-prolonging techniques
   4. have a lethal injection administered to relieve his suffering
9. Which of the following services is not generally provided by a home health agency:
   1. skilled nursing
   2. nutritional support
   3. home health aide
   4. recreational therapy
10. A major influence on home health care began in 1983. This system, based on major diagnostic categories and diagnosis-related groups, paid a set rate for the hospitalized patient's care rather than the "cost" or charges traditionally billed by institutions. Such patients were discharged earlier in their convalescence and thus required more home nursing care. This system is called:
    1. DRGs
    2. Medicaid
    3. Medicare
    4. Older American Act

49

REHABILITATION NURSING

Sally L. Persons Beck

KEY TERMS

autonomy
cervical cord injury
comprehensive rehabilitation plan
flaccid
functional assessment
holistic approach
lumbar cord injury
rehabilitation
spastic
spondylolisthesis
thoracic cord injury
traumatic brain injury (TBI)

LEARNING OBJECTIVES

After reading this chapter, the student should be able to do the following:

- Define the key terms.
- Define the philosophy of rehabilitation nursing.
- Discuss four members of the rehabilitation team and the functions of each member.
- Discuss the role of the LPN/LVN in the rehabilitation team.
- Discuss the four stages of disability adjustment.
- Discuss three major disabling conditions.
- Provide the nursing diagnosis, goals, and interventions for three major disabling conditions.

RELATED TOPICS OF INTEREST

- Care of the patient with a musculoskeletal disorder (Chapter 26)
- Care of the patient with a neurological disorder (Chapter 35)
- Home health nursing (Chapter 48)

Rehabilitation is the process of maximizing an individual's abilities and resources to promote optimum growth and function by focusing on the individual's decision-making ability. This begins with preventive care in the initial stage of the accident or disease, it continues through the restorative phase, and it involves adaptation to a new life.

Rehabilitation is reaching maximum achievable independence. It is restoration to the fullest physical, mental, social, vocational, and economic capacity possible for a given individual. When individuals no longer regard themselves as disabled, they become more responsive and participative members of their families and communities.

The focus in rehabilitation should be on *ability,* not *disability.* This usually requires training, education, and strengthening. Comprehensive rehabilitation helps each person as an individual see more reasons to pursue successes than to give up. For those who have the courage to try, the reward is newfound achievement and independence.

Rehabilitation nursing is an "attitude" along with knowledge and skills that must be basic to all phases of patient care. The concept of rehabilitation should be infused into general care, and the maintenance and preventive aspects should be ongoing throughout the individual's life. *Rehabilitation nursing is a vital part of health care, not just a phase of it.*

REHABILITATION PROFESSIONALS: REHABILITATION TEAM

Rehabilitation is a creative process. It requires a team to work together and contribute specialized services for a common goal (Table 49-1). The team members represent a variety of disciplines. A multidisciplinary team concept is used at a rehabilitation center. Professional staff members use their knowledge and skills to develop and implement a care plan—a plan designed to help the patient reach a maximum level of independence. This requires a holistic approach. **Holistic approach** is a system of comprehensive or total patient care that considers the physical, emotional, social, economic, and spiritual needs of the person. It is also called *comprehensive care*.

REHABILITATION NURSING

Disease and injuries can occur slowly or suddenly and result in devastating disabilities. Life-styles are dramatically altered, and families may be torn apart. Rehabilitation can make a difference. It can turn tragedy to triumph.

The rehabilitation nurse must focus on creative problem-solving techniques. The goal is to provide a supportive environment that encourages independence while helping the patient to adapt to a different life-style. The major emphasis is on "how to" and "why" and involves active patient participation. Quality rehabilitation must be consistent.

The rehabilitation nurse assists the individual to return to optimal functioning through teaching and helping the individual to cope with changes associated with illness or disability. The nurse explains concepts and facts about rehabilitation to the individual, reinforces learning, and evaluates progress. Teaching is individualized and informal.

The nurse's role in the rehabilitation program is to prevent complications, limit deficit as much as possible, and assist in planning and implementing the rehabilitation program. The nurse assists in increasing independence by planning with individuals those functions they can accomplish by themselves and those with which they need assistance. It is important to convey hope and support.

In a holistic approach to the rehabilitation process, attention must be given to all component parts of human existence. Treatment plans provide, maintain, and coordinate services in the physical, psychological, and spiritual aspects. The goals of a comprehensive rehabilitation plan are as follows:

TABLE 49-1 Rehabilitation Team

Member	Role	Goal
Patient	Key member	Participates in goal setting; takes control of own life
Physiatrist	Rehabilitation physician	Team leader; coordinator of program
Rehabilitation RN	Coordinator; educator	Provides support; promotes independence
Rehabilitation LPN/LVN	Care provider; advocate	Assists in treatment plan and implementation
Physical therapist	Designs exercise program	Provides therapy; assesses needs; provides training
Occupational therapist	Assesses independent living needs	Recommends equipment modifications; adapts equipment
Speech pathologist	Designs rehabilitation communication program	Assists in regaining communication skills; educator
Therapeutic recreation therapist	Recreation planner	Activates leisure time; promotes interest in activities
Clinical psychologist	Emotional evaluator	Assists patient in developing realistic positive attitudes
Chaplain	Consultant	Provides support and guidance
Vocational rehabilitation counselor	Vocational planner	Helps obtain training and employment

The *physical* goal involves focus on potential strengths, enhancement of body awareness, and assisting the patient in making meaning out of disorder. Patients are usually discharged from rehabilitation centers or the hospital when they master certain physical tasks. The role of the LPN/LVN may take a role similar to that of the community health nurse, who is responsible for monitoring treatment plans in terms of physical achievements.

In attaining the *emotional* goal, the nurse needs to become an ally and advocate. The nurse identifies and enhances primary support systems, identifies and understands defense mechanisms, and teaches progressive relaxation or other methods of reducing anxiety and tension.

For the *mental* goal, the nurse needs to provide diversional activities, identify previous coping patterns and survival strategies, access and provide reality orientation, provide opportunities for choice, and enhance **autonomy** (the ability or tendency to function independently). The nurse must try to provide the individual with consistent understanding, strength, friendliness, and positively oriented realism.

The goal of *psychosocial restoration* is also a part of the broad perspective of rehabilitation. The achievement of self-care and mobility does not guarantee reintegration of social functioning. The nurse must be innovative and treat each case on an individual basis to promote psychosocial restoration. Encouraging self-transcendence helps individuals to focus on others. For example, a patient who has been in a diving accident and has a spinal cord injury that requires use of a wheelchair finds meaning in volunteering in the recreational program in a nursing home. While meeting the needs of others, this person has fulfilled his own psychosocial needs.

All individuals have a spiritual (not to be confused with religious) dimension. The nurse's assistance with the *spiritual* goal may consist of discussing the meaning of disorder from a spiritual perspective, reflecting with and discussing the life history of the patient, and assessing spiritual resources.

A rehabiliation nurse must focus on the means to enable the patient to move from a totally dependent state to a level of independence. Each patient should receive individual treatment by specific nurses and therapists so that bonds of trust and friendship can develop through the difficult rehabilitation process. Extensive family and patient education, modern adaptive equipment, numerous community integration activities, specialized programs, and professional effective team therapies all combine to help the patients learn to maximize their lives.

Basic rehabilitation can be used whether the patient is suffering from arthritis, multiple sclerosis, mental illness, cerebral vascular accident (CVA, or stroke), spinal cord injury, burn, or traumatic brain injury (TBI). It is the nurse's responsibility to apply appropriate concepts and techniques.

Basic nursing measures, such as position changes, are essential to maintain body alignment. This prevents skeletal and muscular deformities (contractures) and decubitus ulcers.

Rehabilitation nursing is a challenge that requires knowledge, teamwork, coordination, planning, and patience. Rehabilitation professionals must learn to care for disabled persons and must stay informed regarding current knowledge and techniques.

A COMPREHENSIVE REHABILITATION PLAN

The more comprehensive the rehabilitation program, the better the chance for achieving substantial results. All major services that are needed to treat a patient's disability should be provided. The goal of rehabilitation specialists should be to help individuals return to home, work, or school.

There is a newly developed problem-oriented format used for medical evaluations that lists patient problems rather than a single diagnosis. The list includes the disease or injury, significant consequences and complications, physical function limitations that reflect the extent of the physical disability, and psychological, social, and vocational data. With this new approach, specific therapeutic techniques and interventions can be directed toward each of the limitations.

Initially, medical services are primary and vocational services are minimal. Gradually, medical services decrease and vocational services increase. Part of the medical **comprehensive rehabilitation plan** (planned, orderly sequence of services for a disabled individual; designed to help the patient realize maximum potential) involves team consultations, which include functional assessment, evaluation conference, and family conference. **Functional assessment** is completed on patient admission (at least within 24 hours of admission) and examines the patient's functional abilities. This assessment should include the patient's (1) level of response; (2) attitude, cooperation, and motivation; (3) bladder program; (4) bowel program; (5) skin condition; (6) sleep/activity tolerance; (7) diet and nutrition; and (8) activities of daily living (ADLs), such as bed/car transfer, toilet transfer, light hygiene, bath, and positioning. At the evaluation conference, the patient is thoroughly evaluated. A complete medical team reviews the available data and sets realistic goals. At a family conference the patient's functional status, goals, and future plans are discussed. This conference is usually arranged by the rehabilitation social worker.

Box 49-1 REHABILITATION

To understand what rehabilitation means, one must first understand what it means to become disabled.

Disability is an abrupt, apprehensible, unexpected, unrequested, unpredictable, startling, and stunning thrust into change. Feelings, emotions, health, and even the future change. Many relationships change. To become disabled is to become changed.

To become disabled means that fear, pity, discrimination, and frustration are increased. Respect, equality, security, and commitments are decreased. Some relationships become decreased.

Rehabilitation is a light, a beacon, a pathway, a new direction. It is learning and understanding. It is a bridge to a different world that holds many unknowns and uncertainties.

Rehabilitation is a challenge to the basic essence of the human being. It is a challenge to end desperation and an opportunity to cease self-pity. It is a directive to accept yourself for what you are today, and then to begin working towards a new future that contains all you could be.

Rehabilitation is a new beginning. It is a chance to regroup, an opportunity to design your own future and set your own goals. It is guidance, help, and caring from knowledgeable people. Rehabilitation is a pathway out of the pit of disability and desperation.

Rehabilitation is hope. Rehabilitation is life.

Dave Greimann,
Rehabilitation Counselor

DISABILITY ADJUSTMENT

A disability may cause behavioral and emotional changes. Roles, body image, self-concept, and family dynamics change. Adjustment to a disability is always influenced by various factors in the patient's sociocultural background and personal psychology. Major tasks in the rehabilitation process include the redefining of body image, sexuality, life goals, and career plans.

In today's society employment fulfills many basic human needs. It provides a sense of identity and independence, a feeling of accomplishment and status, and an opportunity to use skills to be responsible. It is a source of earnings and security. When introduced, individuals usually share information about occupation immediately after exchanging names. Because jobs correlate to personal identity, loss of a job affects one's identity and can create considerable anxiety and depression. Jobs provide not only personal satisfaction and socialization benefits, but a reason to get out of bed in the morning. The workplace is where an individual is expected to be, a place to come home from, and a reason to be tired.

TABLE 49-2 Stages of Adjustment

Stage	Definition	Characteristics
Reaction stage	Shock	Withdrawal; anxiety; blunted emotions; depression; anger
Adjustment stage	Defensive retreat	Persistent or reoccurring denial; refusal to accept limitations
Understanding stage	Acknowledgment	Realistic attitude; depression; goal setting
Acceptance stage	Adaptation	Utilization of assets; independence; development of self-image

After acute medical treatment, often the first barrier identified is the person's change in social status. Disabled persons are classified as some type of minority, and at times people tend to attribute negative characteristics to them. Others may see disabled persons as less attractive, less desirable, or less capable. As a result of their disability, these persons may lose their social status and suffer serious economic consequences. The disability may be so great that the cost of medical care depletes the family's resources. The tendency to stereotype and discriminate against the "disabled" can be reversed if employers and other members of society will consider them to be what they are—people with physical and/or mental limitations. The key word in disability is *ability* (Box 49-1).

Stages of Adjustment

Numerous experts have proposed various stages of adjustment. Generally it is felt that each phase is accompanied by a characteristic emotional experience, and a predominant emotional reaction changes as the person progresses through the phases of adjustment. A summary of the various stages of adjustment is provided in Table 49-2. The duration and individual reactions vary in time, intensity, and order. A person may skip a phase altogether.

OVERVIEW OF MAJOR DISABLING CONDITIONS

Rehabilitation is a bridge for the patient, spanning the gap between uselessness and usefulness, between hopelessness and hopefulness, between despair and happiness (see Box 49-1). Following are a few of the major conditions for which dedicated rehabilitative efforts are required.

Multiple Sclerosis

Multiple sclerosis (MS) is one of the most common neurological diseases. The cause is unknown. It is defined as a chronic, progressive disease characterized by scattering of demyelinating lesions in the central nervous system (CNS), which affects the white matter of the brain and spinal cord. Assessment involves observations/findings, such as fatigue, sensory impairment (numbness and tingling), dizziness, weakness of extremities, visual disturbance, speech impairment, difficulty in chewing and swallowing, staggering gait, bladder or bowel dysfunction, mood swings, depression, irritability, apathy, inattention, lack of judgment, and weeping.

Nursing diagnoses, goals/expected outcomes, and interventions for MS include but are not limited to the following:

NURSING DIAGNOSES	GOALS/EXPECTED OUTCOMES	NURSING INTERVENTIONS
Self-care deficit, hygiene, feeding, and/or toileting, related to limitations in physical mobility imposed by disease process	Patient's self-care needs will be met	Maintain quiet and relaxing environment Encourage self-care Avoid use of heating pads (heat diminishes muscle strength and increases potential for burns) Plan all activities to avoid fatigue Plan bladder and bowel dysfunction program, if appropriate Encourage fluids
Body image disturbance, related to altered perception of self	Patient will accept changes in body image and self-esteem	Establish means of communication Acknowledge concerns about body image Be supportive of emotional changes, and encourage verbalization of feelings
Airway clearance, ineffective, high risk for, related to motor weakness and/or immobility	Patient will maintain a patent airway	Suction as needed Assist and teach patient to cough and deep breathe Maintain patent airway
Knowledge deficit, related to disease process	Patient and/or significant other will demonstrate understanding of home care and follow-up instructions through interactive discussion and actual return demonstration	Explain nature of disease Explain that warm weather and hot baths may increase weakness Explain importance of avoiding fatigue Explain importance of regular exercise and rest Discuss signs and symptoms of disease progression Discuss signs and symptoms of cold and influenza and report to physician Encourage socialization Encourage independence

Cerebral Vascular Accident

A cerebral vascular accident (CVA) can be defined as a sudden onset of neurological symptoms as a result of an abnormal condition of the blood vessels of the brain, characterized by occlusion by an embolus or cerebrovascular hemorrhage, resulting in ischemia of the brain tissues normally perfused by the damaged vessels. CVA is often accompanied by other medical problems associated with the diseases of the blood vessels, such as hypertension, heart disease, or peripheral vascular disease. Nursing concerns include depression, contractures, bowel and bladder dysfunction, urinary tract infections, pneumonia, or seizures. Rehabilitation potential is directly related to the duration and depth of coma. The earlier the return of extremity function, the better the prognosis. Other rehabilitation professionals usually involved are the speech pathologist, occupational therapist, physical therapist, clinical psychologist, and vocational rehabilitation counselor if appropriate. (See Chapter 35 for nursing interventions for CVA.) For data about older adults, see the gerontological box.

Low Back Pain

Back disorders constitute a substantial percentage of all disabilities. Usually the pain is in the lower lumbosacral region. Various back disorders are diagnosed as acute sprain, chronic strain, degenerative disk disease, and **spondylolisthesis** (a partial forward dislocation of a vertebra over the one below it, most commonly the fifth lumbar vertebra over the first sacral vertebra). The range of medical intervention may include total bed rest, medications to ensure relaxation and to relieve inflammation and pain, and home exercise programs. Surgery is sometimes required. Vocation implications include careful analysis of sitting, standing, moving, lifting, pulling, pushing, and climbing requirements of the job. It is also important to identify potential sources of stress in the job. The individual with chronic back pain poses a definite challenge to achieve vocational success.

Low back pain is defined as pain in the lower back that may be caused by a variety of diseases that affect bone, but is generally the result of (1) stress on the vertebral process or (2) herniated disk. Assessment and observations include back pain (low and intense), radiating leg pain, muscle spasm, muscular weakness, obesity, and faulty posture.

Nursing diagnoses, goals/expected outcomes, and interventions for the patient with low back pain include but are not limited to the following:

NURSING DIAGNOSIS	GOALS/EXPECTED OUTCOMES	NURSING INTERVENTIONS
Pain, chronic, related to the disease process	Patient will express minimal discomfort or absence of pain	Maintain bed rest with firm mattress Administer medications as ordered: analgesics, muscle relaxants, antiinflammatory agents Application of hot or cold compresses as ordered Physical therapy as ordered Increase activity as allowed
Knowledge deficit, related to home care management	Patient and/or significant other will demonstrate understanding of home care and follow-up instructions through interactive discussion and actual return demonstration	Stress importance of prescribed rehabilitation plan Demonstrate use of transcutaneous electrical nerve stimulation (TENS) Provide diet instructions Discuss medication: name, schedule, purpose, dosage, and possible side effects Promote follow-up visits with physician

Emotional Disabilities

A disability may cause behavioral, emotional, role, body image, and self-concept changes and alterations in family dynamics. Emotional disabilities are generally grouped into diagnostic categories defined by the American Psychiatric Association, such as organic, mental, and personality disorders. The more seriously disabled individuals are usually socially isolated and vocationally inadequate and possess strong dependency needs. Additionally, they lack self-confidence and social skills necessary to effectively communicate with others. It should be emphasized that even severely disabled psychiatric patients can be helped to improve their lives through work. Work is therapeutic. Emotional disability requires close vocational counselor involvement and support.

GERONTOLOGICAL CONSIDERATIONS

- A large percentage of the individuals requiring rehabilitative nursing services are older adults. Although complete recovery may not be possible, the nurse should not underestimate the older person's potential for substantial progress.
- The rehabilitation potential of the older person will frequently be influenced by more than one health problem.
- Rehabilitation for a cerebrovascular accident (stroke), fractured hip, arthritis, or joint replacement may need to be modified because of heart disease, diabetes, or other chronic conditions that are commonly seen in the older population. Healing also takes somewhat longer. For these reasons older adults typically make slower progress in rehabilitation.
- Older persons may need more encouragement and modified procedures to motivate them to participate in rehabilitation. This is particularly true if the older persons have lost confidence in themselves or have lost hope for improvement.
- Older persons who feel that they have little to live for need a highly supportive environment and reinforcement of even small amounts of progress from caregivers.

Spinal Cord Injuries

Spinal cord injuries have increased mainly because of an increase in motor vehicle accidents. The majority of individuals paralyzed are young. Because of improved medical care, they now survive the injury, and because of their youth, they have vocational potential. Functional disabilities are related to injury level. After acute nursing intervention, other concerns involve bowel and bladder functional impairment, ambulation functions, dressing, personal hygiene, exercise, and communication (speech and writing). Rehabilitation potential is directly related to nursing concerns. It is important for the reha-

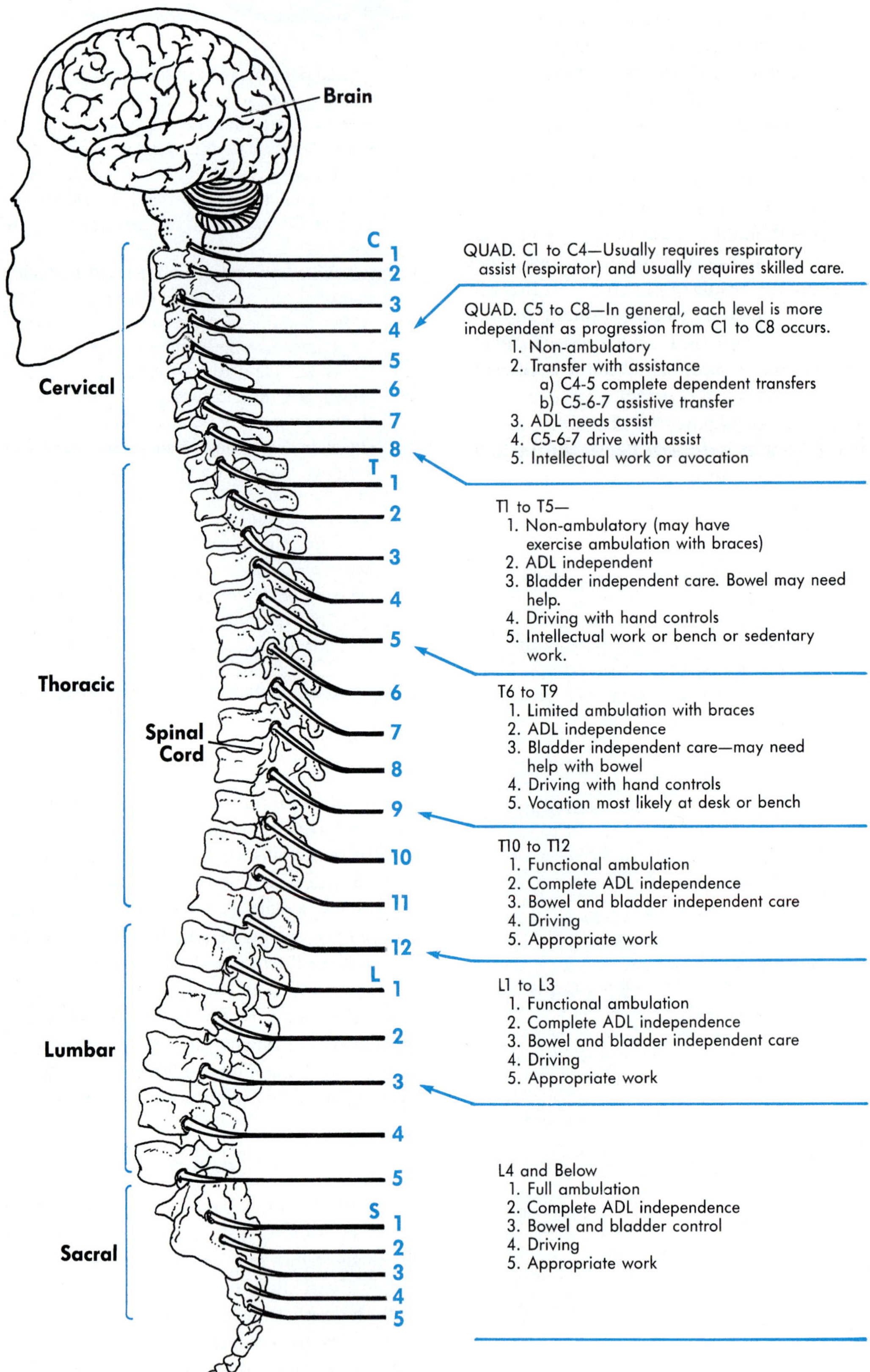

FIG. 49-1 The level of injury on the spinal cord can help to predict what a patient will be able to do. The severity of the injury also affects the abilities. Each patient must be treated individually; these are general guidelines.

bilitation professional to carefully consider education, interests, aptitudes, and physical requirements when assessing rehabilitation potential.

A spinal cord injury is any injury in which the spinal cord is compressed by fracture or displaced vertebrae, bleeding, or edema. Spinal cord injuries can be divided into the following:

1. **Cervical cord injury:** Level of injury is at cervical spine C2 to C7 and involves paralysis of all extremities and trunk, respiratory failure, bladder and bowel disturbance, bradycardia, perspiring, elevated temperature, and headache.
2. **Thoracic cord injury:** Level of injury is at thoracic spine T1 to T12 and involves paralysis of lower extremities. Initially muscles are **flaccid** (weak, soft, flabby; lacking normal muscle tone) and later become **spastic** (spasms or other uncontrolled contractions of the skeletal muscles). Paralysis of bladder, bowel, and sphincters; pain in chest or back; abdominal distention; and loss of sexual function are other potential symptoms.
3. **Lumbar cord injury:** Level of injury is at lumbar spine L1 to L2 with paralysis of lower extremities, bladder, and rectum and loss of sexual function (Fig. 49-1).

Nursing diagnoses, goals/expected outcomes, and interventions for the patient with a spinal cord injury include but are not limited to the following:

NURSING DIAGNOSES	GOALS/EXPECTED OUTCOMES	NURSING INTERVENTIONS
Breathing pattern, ineffective, related to neurogenic or traumatic injury	Patient will have a patent airway	Maintain patent airway Administer assisted ventilation Closely monitor for signs of respiratory failure, and be prepared to assist with tracheotomy if needed. Monitor vital signs and consciousness every 1 to 2 hours Assess motor/sensory function to ensure adequate rhythm and pattern of respiration
Self-care deficit, hygiene, feeding, and toileting, related to neurophysiological impairment	Patient's self-care needs will be met	Maintain IV fluids as ordered Maintain NPO until chewing, swallowing, and gastrointestinal (GI) function is established

NURSING DIAGNOSES	GOALS/EXPECTED OUTCOMES	NURSING INTERVENTIONS
Self-care deficit, hygiene, feeding, and toileting, related to neurophysiological impairment—cont'd	Patient's self-care needs will be met—cont'd	Provide nutritional support as ordered Connect indwelling catheter to closed gravity drainage Teach self-catheterization to thoracic- and lumbar-injured patients Administer catheter care Administer oral hygiene every 2 to 4 hours Administer skin care every 2 to 4 hours Explain importance of skin care Teach muscle-building exercises
Knowledge deficit, related to diagnosis and home management	Patient and significant other will demonstrate understanding of home care and follow-up instructions	Ensure patient and significant other are informed about disease prognosis Prepare for chronicity and duration of rehabilitation process Discuss medications: name, dosage, routine, possible side effects, and purpose
Skin integrity, impaired, actual or high risk for, related to immobility	Patient's skin integrity maintained, clean, dry, and intact	Bathe daily using warm water and mild soap Massage the skin with mild lanolin-based lotions to increase circulation and maintain integrity Dry skin thoroughly Assess perineal and perianal areas to observe for excoriation, vaginal discharge, and pain Apply lotions or cornstarch to areas as needed Assess feet and hands for signs of rash, dryness, or skin impairment Change position every 1 to 2 hours Maintain adequate nutrition

Traumatic Brain Injury

Although there are numerous disabilities, each with its own nursing and vocational implications, few present the challenges of the patient with **traumatic brain injury** (TBI). In spite of mandatory seat belt laws and drinking/driving reforms, the number of head injuries resulting from motor vehicle accidents continues to rise. Again, as a result of medical advances, there are an increasing number of survivors.

Head injuries can be classified as either penetrating or closed head injuries. In penetrating injuries, an object lacerates the scalp, fractures the skull, and injures the soft tissue in its path, thus destroying nerve cells. In a closed head injury, the brain collides with an inner surface of the skull. This results in widespread damage called *shearing* (when the brain mass is rotated in the cranial vault). Thus there is violent twisting action, which causes the upper section of the brain to rotate with the lower end anchored securely in a stationary position.

There appears to be direct correlation between the amount of disability resulting from a TBI and the degree of expertise and aggressiveness of those providing medical care during the acute period. Successful vocational outcome correlates with duration and depth of coma, duration of posttraumatic amnesia, preinjury level of functioning (positive achievement), rate of improvement in the 1-year postinjury stage, age of onset (the younger the age of the patient, the better the prognosis), and the presence of realistic vocational goals.

Head injuries can be classified as mild, moderate, severe, or catastrophic. Mild head injury is characterized by brief or no loss of consciousness, which constitutes the majority of head injuries. Neurological examinations are often normal. Postconcussive syndrome can persist for months, years, or indefinitely. Signs and symptoms include fatigue, headache, dizziness, lethargy, irritability, personality changes, cognitive deficits, decreased information-processing speed, and memory, understanding, learning, and perceptual difficulties. These symptoms lead to feelings of incompetence, guilt, and frustration. Family members may become impatient and frustrated.

In the moderate head injury there is a characteristic period of unconsciousness from 1 to 24 hours. There are usually cognitive impairments, which include planning, sequencing, judgment, reasoning, and computation skills. Generally there are some psychosocial problems, which include self-centeredness, denial, mood swings, agitation, depression, lethargy, sexual dysfunction, emotional lability, low frustration tolerance, poor judgment, or behavioral outbursts.

Patients with severe head injuries experience unconsciousness or posttrauma amnesia in excess of 8 days. There are cognitive, psychosocial, and behavioral disabilities.

Catastrophic head injury is characterized by a coma lasting several months or longer. These individuals may appear to be awake. However, they generally never regain significant meaningful communication with their environment.

In rehabilitative assessment of the patient with TBI, inconsistent performance, anger, and frustration should be expected, and ineffective behavior will be changeable (unless it is neurogenic in origin). Cognitive barriers to rehabilitative recovery include problems in thinking and reasoning (impaired memory), impaired concentration and attention, and impaired informational processing speed. Psychosocially, there appears to be a lack of initiative. However, this is a normal consequence of a head injury. Egocentric (self-centered) behavior is 100% normal in a head-injured individual, as is depression. Generally, the more the memory improves, the more the patient becomes depressed. Abstinence from alcohol should be considered primary with any patient with a head injury. Alcohol increases the chance of impulse and seizure activity.

Continuous and honest involvement of the family, as both a victim of the injury and an equal participant in the rehabilitation process, is critical to the successful rehabilitation of the head-injured patient. It should be remembered that the entire family is a victim of the TBI. Often the head-injured person's awareness and acceptance of the disability are determined by the flexibility of the family system itself.

The rehabilitation professionals must be available and be honest in reporting to families, including "I don't know," when appropriate. Equal communication with all family members is important, as is encouraging the family to become involved in counseling and education. The family should be encouraged to be aware of each others' needs and interests. They should be assisted in becoming involved in a support group, and technical terminology should be avoided by the nurse. It is important that the family understand that rehabilitation is not a birthright.

Nursing assessments involve observing altered levels of consciousness, including headaches, dizziness, mental changes (irritability, restlessness, disorientation, stupor, coma), pupillary response (size, equality, response to light), airway patency, seizure activity, projectile vomiting, drainage from ears and nose, elevated temperature, and elevated or decreased blood pressure.

Nursing diagnoses, goals/expected outcomes, and interventions for the patient with traumatic brain injury include but are not limited to the following:

NURSING DIAGNOSES	GOALS/EXPECTED OUTCOMES	NURSING INTERVENTIONS
Airway clearance, ineffective, related to impaired neurological function	Patent airway will be maintained	Maintain patent airway, endotracheal tube, or tracheostomy, as ordered, with suctioning prn Administer oxygen, humidification, or mechanical ventilation as ordered Assist patient in coughing and deep breathing Check blood pressure, pulse, and respiration every 15 to 30 minutes; report any pupillary or mental changes immediately, since changes signal respiratory embarrassment
Self-care deficit, bathing, feeding, and toileting, related to neurological impairment	Patient's self-care needs will be met	Administer oral hygiene every 2 to 4 hours Administer skin care every 2 hours prn Provide for all hygiene needs as indicated Provide for patient's elimination needs Initiate voiding measures as indicated Encourage early ambulation as ordered Perform active or passive range-of-motion (ROM) exercises to all extremities
Body image disturbance, high risk for, related to actual/perceived changes in physical and personal self-image	Patient will accept changes in body image and self-esteem	Provide emotional support Encourage verbalization of feelings about body image Provide for alternative communication methods if vocalization is impaired, such as Magic Slate or pencil and paper
Knowledge deficit, related to disease process and home management	Patient and/or significant other will demonstrate understanding of home care and follow-up instructions through interactive discussion and actual return demonstration	Discuss nature of disorder, treatment, and procedures Explain to family the need to encourage verbalization about body image changes or limitations Explain need for ambulation and planned rest periods Discuss possible residual effects, such as dizziness, headache, and memory loss, which may persist for 3 or 4 months after trauma Discuss medications Explain need to avoid taking over-the-counter medications Discuss signs and symptoms of progression of condition to report to physician Explain importance of ongoing outpatient care

Begin as soon as possible with vocational planning. As soon as the patient can participate, include him or her. Early intervention is necessary.

Use calm, controlled, and consistent manner.
Use short-term, goal-directed techniques.
Accentuate the positive.
Coordinate vocational and psychosocial adjustment.
Expect the unexpected.
Use group methods and videotaping.
Use positive reinforcement.
Be redundant.
Assume nothing: *review, review, review.*

Specific considerations for return-to-work evaluations include the following:

1. Initiate evaluation early.
2. Evaluate all areas of work repertoire (obtain detailed preinjury work information).
3. Identify compensatory mechanisms.
4. Seek a broad range of input from family, team, and other patients.
5. Above all, determine whether the patient's work and jobs were the central life focus.

Regardless of personality types, any disability, particularly a TBI, is a crisis that threatens many aspects of the patient's and family's life: job income, pleasures, family, community ties, health, and life itself. The fears are very real.

• • •

Rehabilitation nurses must take their responsibility seriously as professionals who can significantly affect the future of those with disabilities. Nurses must facilitate changing restraint to openness, turning inertia into action. Focus must be on the assets and successes of people who have disabilities.

Emerson summed it up succinctly when he wrote:

> It is one of the most beautiful compensations of this life that no man can sincerely try to help another without helping himself.

REFERENCES AND SELECTED READINGS

1. Beare PG, Myers JL: *Principles and practices of adult health nursing,* St Louis, 1994, Mosby.
2. Dittmar SS: *Rehabilitation nursing: process and practice,* St Louis, 1989, Mosby.
3. Gender AR et al: Rehabilitation: mending body and spirit, *Healthcare Trends and Transition* 4(1):68, 1992.
4. Harris HC: Kurt battled us before confronting the real enemy: sudden disability, *Nursing* '90 20(4):52, 1990.
5. Hood GH, Dincher JR: *Total patient care,* ed 8, St Louis, 1993, Mosby.
6. Hochuler SH et al: *Rehabilitation of the spine: science and practice,* St Louis, 1993, Mosby.
7. Long BC, Phipps WJ, Cassmeyer VL: *Medical-surgical nursing,* ed 3, St Louis, 1993, Mosby.
8. Miller M: Learning to cope with disability, *Nursing* 21(8):96, 1991.
9. *Mosby's medical, nursing, and allied health dictionary,* ed 4, St Louis, 1994, Mosby.
10. National Institute on Disability and Rehabilitation Research: *Stroke, rehab brief, XI (11),* Washington, DC, 1989, Office of Special Education and Rehabilitation Services, The Institute.
11. Phipps WJ, Long BC, Woods NF: *Medical-surgical nursing: concepts and clinical practice,* St Louis, 1991, Mosby.
12. Potter P, Perry A: *Basic nursing: theory and practice,* St Louis, ed 3, 1995, Mosby.
13. Potter PA, Perry AG: *Fundamentals of nursing: concepts, process, and practice,* ed 3, St Louis, 1993, Mosby.
14. Tucker SM et al: *Patient care standards: nursing process, diagnosis and outcomes,* St Louis, 1992, Mosby.

CHAPTER CHALLENGE

KEY POINTS

- Rehabilitation is defined as the process of maximizing an individual's capabilities or resources to foster optimal growth and functioning.
- The patient is the most important team member and must be involved in planning the programs and learning in detail about the disabilities, the ways of accomplishing the goals, and the options available.
- Rehabilitation nursing is directed toward the prevention of complications of disease or trauma and the maintenance and/or restoration of function.
- Basic rehabilitation can be used regardless of cause of disability. The nurse must individualize care by developing goal-directed actions for each patient.
- A disability can have a number of effects on both the patient and the family, including behavioral and emotional changes and changes in roles, body image, self-concept, and family dynamics.
- Holistic nursing interventions should be used to assist the patient in attaining a maximal state of functioning and well-being.
- A comprehensive rehabilitation plan is multifaceted and may involve a functional assessment, evaluation conference, and family conference.
- Stages of adjustment include shock, denial or defensive retreat, acknowledgment or constructive response, and adaptation. Individual reactions vary in time, intensity, and order.
- A decubitus ulcer is one of the most common severe skin problems faced in the health care setting.
- The number of spinal cord injuries and traumatic brain injuries has increased because of an increase in motor vehicle accidents. Medical advancements have resulted in an increasing number of survivors.

STUDY QUESTIONS

1. Amy, 19 years old, is brought to the emergency room after a diving accident. She is noted to have a spinal cord injury at the cervical level (C3). Which of the following nursing diagnoses would be correct:
   1. Breathing patterns ineffective, related to neurogenic injury
   2. Fluid volume deficit, related to osmotic diuresis
   3. Pain, acute, related to disease process
   4. Knowledge deficit, related to disease process
2. Dave, age 11, had a head injury from being struck in the skull by a baseball bat. He awoke in a hospital 3 weeks later. His head injury would be classified as:
   1. Mild head injury
   2. Moderate head injury
   3. Catastrophic head injury
   4. Severe head injury
3. Ms. Corona, age 39, has been diagnosed with multiple sclerosis (MS). Signs and symptoms for MS may include:
   1. Ataxia, paresthesia, blurred vision, dysphasia, or slurred speech
   2. Tremors, impaired chewing, increased salivation, excessive sweating, ataxia
   3. Seizures, loss of consciousness, absent gag reflex, ataxia, dysphasia
   4. Disorientation, polyuria, coma, Kussmaul's respirations, hot, flushed skin
4. Mr. Lordon, a railroad worker, is diagnosed as having degenerative disk disease. Nursing interventions may include:
   1. Observation for dyspnea and hypertension and assessment of neurovascular status
   2. Physical therapy, bed rest, or hot or cold compresses as ordered
   3. Bed rest, change postsurgical dressing, and assist with prosthesis measurement
   4. Assess location and type of pain and assist patient with use of crutches
5. Mrs. Jacobs was admitted to the hospital with a diagnosis of cerebral vascular accident (CVA). A CVA can be described as:
   1. A chronic, progressive disease characterized by scattering of demyelinating lesions in the central nervous system
   2. A progressive, degenerative disease causing destruction of nerve cells in the basal ganglia of the brain
   3. A thrombus or other foreign matter lodged in a pulmonary arterial vessel that usually arises from a peripheral vein
   4. A sudden onset of neurological symptoms as a result of an abnormal condition of blood vessels of the brain
6. Mr. Morris is admitted to the rehabilitation unit with a cervical cord injury. The nurse will anticipate that Mr. Morris may have:
   1. Lower extremity paralysis, weak trunk control, and decreased endurance
   2. Partial trunk paralysis with total lower extremity paralysis
   3. Paralysis of arms, trunk, and lower extremities, and difficulty breathing
   4. Only lower extremity paralysis with loss of sexual function
7. Working in a rehabilitation unit, the nurse is assigned to Max, age 19. Max has a spinal cord injury at T6. The nurse would expect that Max:
   1. Could not complete a transfer independently, dress or perform personal hygiene, or drive a car even with adaptations.
   2. Could complete independent self-care, would be able to drive and to utilize a standard wheelchair.
   3. Would have weak shoulder movements, low endurance, and low respiratory reserve.
   4. Could use an adapted wheelchair with hand controls, would have difficulty breathing, and could not complete self-care.
8. Ms. Sonna, a 22-year-old, was admitted with a spinal cord injury. Dr. Gillan, a physiatrist, is part of Ms. Sonna's rehabilitation team. Ms. Sonna asks the nurse why she has a physiatrist for a doctor. The nurse explains that a physiatrist is a medical specialist in:
   1. Recreational planning
   2. Pediatrics
   3. Rehabilitation
   4. Psychiatric problems
9. Mrs. Zeda, age 35, has just been diagnosed with MS. The process of assisting an individual after a disabling event has occurred is the definition of:
   1. Identification
   2. Compensation
   3. Repression
   4. Rehabilitation
10. Miss Defur, a 28-year-old, is a patient with a traumatic brain injury (TBI). When working with Miss Defur, the nurse should remember to:
    1. Be redundant and consistent
    2. Use long-term, goal-directed techniques
    3. Avoid group methods or videotaping
    4. Use a calm and inconsistent manner

15

EMERGENCY NURSING

I don't really know when I decided to become a nurse, but after my children were in school and more self-sufficient, I began attending college for the first time. Nursing was the career choice for me. It is an ever-changing field, and I have met some of the nicest people during my time as a student nurse. I know I've made the right choice.

Pam Warner
Student Nurse

50

CARDIOPULMONARY RESUSCITATION

Gloria DePole Coschigano

KEY TERMS

ABCs
biological death
BLS
brain death
cardiac arrest
clinical death
CPR
EMS
Heimlich maneuver
stridor

LEARNING OBJECTIVES

After reading this chapter, the student should be able to do the following:

- Define the key terms.
- List the reasons CPR should be performed.
- Discuss the legal implications of CPR.
- Name six causes of sudden death.
- List the steps in performing one-rescuer CPR on the adult victim.
- Name the steps in performing two-rescuer CPR on the adult victim.
- List the steps in performing CPR on the child and the infant.
- Recognize the causes of airway obstruction.
- Name the steps in performing the Heimlich maneuver on the conscious choking victim.
- Describe the steps in performing the Heimlich maneuver on the unconscious victim.
- Discuss management of airway obstruction in the child and the infant.

RELATED TOPICS OF INTEREST

- Legal aspects of nursing (Chapter 2)
- Ethical aspects of nursing (Chapter 3)
- Vital signs (Chapter 10)
- Care of the patient with a cardiovascular disorder (Chapter 28)
- Care of the patient with a respiratory disorder (Chapter 31)
- First aid (Chapter 51)

Cardiovascular disease remains the number one killer in the United States. However, communities with large numbers of people trained in cardiopulmonary resuscitation **(CPR;** a basic emergency procedure for life support, consisting of artificial respiration and manual external cardiac massage) and a rapid response emergency medical services **(EMS;** a national network of services coordinated to provide aid and medical assistance from primary response to definitive rescue, stabilization, transportation, and medical emergencies) system can successfully resuscitate victims of "sudden death," especially those "deaths" caused by cardiovascular disorders. It is important for the licensed practical/vocational nurse to be able to perform CPR, both as a responsible member of the community and as a member of the health care team.

LEGAL IMPLICATIONS

The Good Samaritan Act protects the CPR rescuer just as it protects the provider of first aid (see Chapter 2). However, it is important that the rescuer be thoroughly familiar with the CPR technique. Certification in basic life support (**BLS;** the phase of cardiopulmonary resuscitation [CPR] and emergency cardiac care [ECC] that either [1] prevents circulatory or respiratory arrest or insufficiency by prompt recognition and early intervention, by early entry into the emergency care system [ECS] or both or [2] externally supports the circulation and respirations of a victim of cardiac arrest through CPR basic life support) may be obtained through local chapters of the American Heart Association or the local American Red Cross Association. The rescuer must perform CPR according to the standards designated by the certifying agency.

ETHICAL IMPLICATIONS

Reasons why individuals choose not to become involved in performing CPR include (1) lack of motivation, (2) fear of doing harm, (3) lack of knowledge, and (4) fear of contracting communicable diseases. However, once CPR is started, it may not be discontinued except for the following reasons:

- The victim recovers.
- The rescuer is exhausted and cannot continue CPR.
- Trained medical personnel arrive on the scene and take over CPR.
- A licensed physician arrives on the scene, pronounces the victim dead, and orders CPR to be discontinued.

EVENTS REQUIRING CPR

There are many situations that require resuscitation efforts (Box 50-1). CPR is indicated in any syndrome where respiration or respiration and circulation are absent. The two purposes of CPR are:

- To keep the lungs supplied with oxygen when breathing has stopped
- To keep the blood circulating and carrying oxygen to the brain, heart, and other parts of the body

Clinical death means that heartbeat and respiration have ceased. **Biological death** results from permanent cellular damage caused by lack of oxygen. The brain is the first organ to suffer from this lack of oxygen. In many cases CPR can reverse clinical death if initiated before 4 minutes of cardiopulmonary arrest. After 10 minutes without CPR, brain death is certain. Therefore it is extremely important that CPR is begun as quickly as possible. **Brain death** is an irreversible form of unconsciousness characterized by a complete loss of brain function while the heart continues to beat. The legal definition of this condition varies from state to state. The

Box 50-1 EVENTS REQUIRING CPR

Cardiac arrest. The most common cause of cardiac arrest is myocardial infarction (MI). In addition, shock from hemorrhage, trauma to the heart, respiratory arrest, and drugs may precipitate a cardiac arrest.

Drowning. Children are common victims of drowning and boating accidents. Persons using alcohol and/or drugs near bodies of water are often victims of drowning. It is important to note that near-drowning victims may recover completely after long periods of submersion. The low water temperature that produces hypothermia reduces the metabolic rate and decreases oxygen demands. Because of this, CPR must be initiated even after 4 to 6 minutes are known to have elapsed.

Electrical shock. Persons exposed to high-voltage electricity may be subject to accidental electrocution. Electrical shock may paralyze the breathing muscles and cause cardiac arrest by interfering with the normal rhythm of the heart. The rescuer who is initiating CPR must be careful not to be exposed inadvertently to the electrical current. The rescuer must ensure that the current is deenergized before beginning CPR.

Anaphylactic reaction. Exposure to a known allergen (food, poisons, drugs) or an insect bite may produce a severe allergic reaction known as anaphylaxis. This reaction may cause spasms or edema of the upper airway and could progress to cardiovascular collapse. CPR must be initiated immediately, as with any other emergency situation.

Asphyxiation. Asphyxiation or suffocation may be caused by inhaling a gas other than oxygen, resulting from fires, chemical spills, or gas leaks. In addition, children and adults may suffer respiratory arrest and ultimately cardiac arrest from choking on food or small objects that are placed in the mouth. The Heimlich maneuver and CPR are performed in this instance.

Drug overdose. Intentional or accidental abuse of alcohol and drugs may cause respiratory and cardiac arrest. Besides treating this as a poisoning emergency, CPR should be performed as necessary.

Sudden infant death syndrome (SIDS). The unexpected and sudden death of an apparently normal and healthy infant that occurs during sleep and with no physical or autopsic evidence of disease. Home monitoring systems to detect prolonged *apnea* and early CPR are part of a prevention program.

usual clinical criteria for brain death include the absence of reflex activity, movements, and respiration. The pupils are dilated and fixed. Because hypothermia, anesthesia, poisoning, or drug intoxication may cause deep physiological depression that resembles brain death, a diagnosis of brain death requires that the electric activity of the brain be evaluated and shown to be absent on two electroencephalograms performed 12 to 24 hours apart. Brain death is also called irreversible coma.

ADULT ONE-RESCUER CPR

To remember the steps of one-rescuer or two-rescuer CPR, remember the **ABCs** (a mnemonic for assessing status emergency patients—Airway, Breathing, Circulation).

A: Airway

The initial assessment in determining the need for CPR is to determine responsiveness. This is done by gently shaking the victim and shouting, "Are you OK?" This precaution will prevent the rescuer from injuring a person who is alert, but sleeping. OK is a word that is understandable in any language.

Call for help. It is important to access the EMS System as quickly as possible. Shouting for help immediately, directing another person to make a telephone call, or the rescuer making the call is recommended (see Chapter 51).

If there is no evidence of head or neck trauma, the rescuer should use the head-tilt/chin-lift maneuver to open the airway. This method consists of placing one hand on the victim's forehead and applying firm backward pressure to tilt the head back. The fingers of the other hand are placed under the jaw (avoiding the soft tissue under the chin) to lift the chin forward (Fig. 50-1). *A word of caution:* If a neck injury is suspected, establish the airway using the jaw-thrust (or chin-lift) without the head-tilt. Jaw-thrust can be accomplished by grasping the angle of the victim's lower jaw with the rescuer's hands on both sides of the jaw and bringing the mandible forward, keeping the neck in straight alignment and *not* tilting the head back.

To determine breathlessness the rescuer should:

- Look for the rise and fall of the chest
- Listen for sounds of breathing
- Feel for the warmth of the victim's mouth against the cheek (see Fig. 50-1)

B: Breathing

Mouth-to-mouth ventilation is the quickest method of supplying oxygen to the victim's lungs. The rescuer's exhaled air has enough oxygen to supply the victim's needs until life support systems take over. The head-tilt/chin-lift position and an airtight seal must be maintained throughout rescue breathing.

To preserve the open airway, the rescuer should be at the victim's shoulders and the thumb and index finger of the hand that is maintaining the head-tilt should be used to gently pinch the nostrils closed. The rescuer should then take a deep breath, seal the lips around the outside of the victim's mouth (creating an airtight seal), and give *two* full breaths lasting 1½ to 2 seconds each (Fig. 50-2). This minimizes gastric distention and decreases the potential of the victim vomiting, which can result from rapid breaths and excessive air volume being given. Allow the victim to exhale passively.

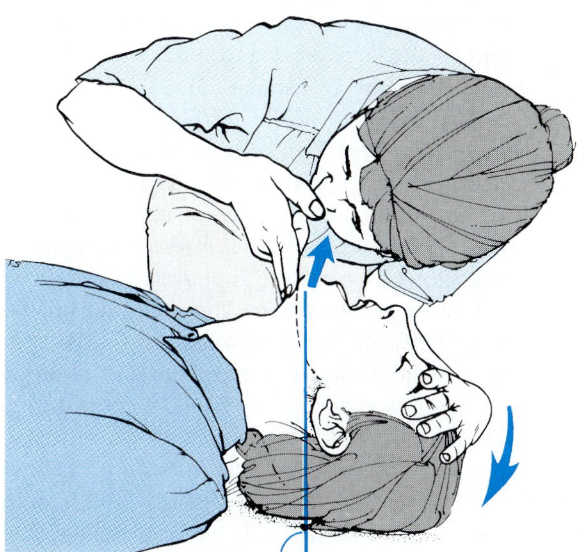

FIG. 50-1 (American Heart Association: *Textbook of basic life support for healthcare providers,* 1994.)

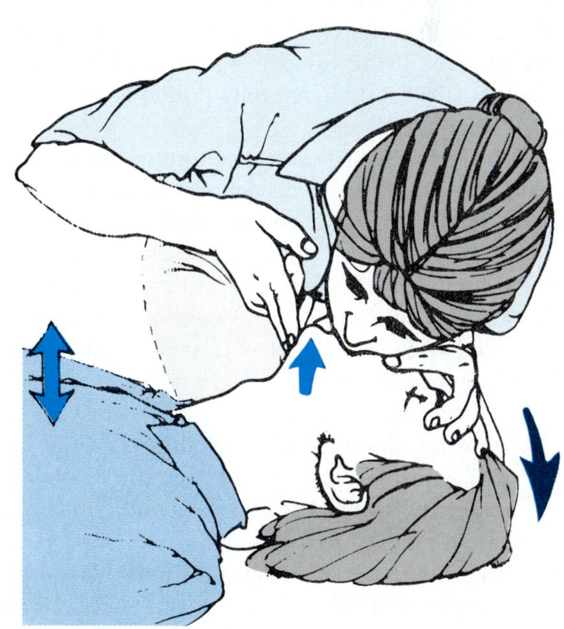

FIG. 50-2 (American Heart Association: *Textbook of basic life support for healthcare providers,* 1994.)

If the initial attempt to ventilate the victim is unsuccessful, the rescuer should reposition the head and attempt to ventilate again. Improper chin and head position is the most common reason for difficulty with ventilation. If the second attempt at ventilation is also unsuccessful, the rescuer should proceed with foreign body airway obstruction management procedures (see pp. 1545-1546).

C: Circulation

Once the ventilations have been performed, it is important to assess for the presence of the pulse. Pulselessness (cardiac arrest) indicates the need for external cardiac compressions. Respiratory arrest may occur without cardiac arrest. Performing external cardiac compressions on a victim with a pulse may result in severe physical damage. If the victim has a pulse, rescue breathing should be initiated at one breath every 5 seconds, or 12 times per minute for the adult. Cardiac arrest will follow if respiratory arrest continues.

To determine pulselessness, the carotid pulse is the most reliable and accessible for the CPR rescuer. While the head-tilt is maintained with one hand on the forehead, the rescuer should locate the victim's thyroid cartilage (Adam's apple) with two or three fingers of the other hand. The rescuer should then gently slide these fingers into the groove between the trachea and the muscles on the side of the neck until the carotid pulse is felt. The pulse must be palpated gently on one side to avoid obliteration of the artery.

If there is no pulse, the diagnosis of **cardiac arrest** (sudden cessation of functional circulation) is confirmed. At this point it is important to have someone activate the EMS system (if not already done). If another person is present, he should call the local emergency phone number. If the rescuer is alone and not able to activate the EMS system, the only option is to continue CPR.

Performing external cardiac compressions will circulate blood to the heart, lungs, brain, and the rest of the body. If external cardiac compressions are performed properly, 20% to 50% of the normal output of the heart can be maintained. This will bring enough oxygen to the body to sustain life. Proper hand position will enable as much blood to be circulated as possible. Hands should be positioned as follows:

1. With the middle and index fingers of the hand that is nearest the victim's legs, the rescuer palpates the lower edge of the victim's rib cage on the side next to the rescuer.
2. The fingers are then run up the rib cage to the xiphoid process (where the ribs meet the sternum on the lower part of the chest).
3. Keeping the middle finger on the xiphoid process, the rescuer places the index finger next to the middle finger on the lower end of the sternum.
4. The heel of the hand nearest the head is placed on the lower half of the sternum, as close as possible to the index and middle fingers (Fig. 50-3).
5. The fingers may be extended or interlaced, but must be kept off the chest.

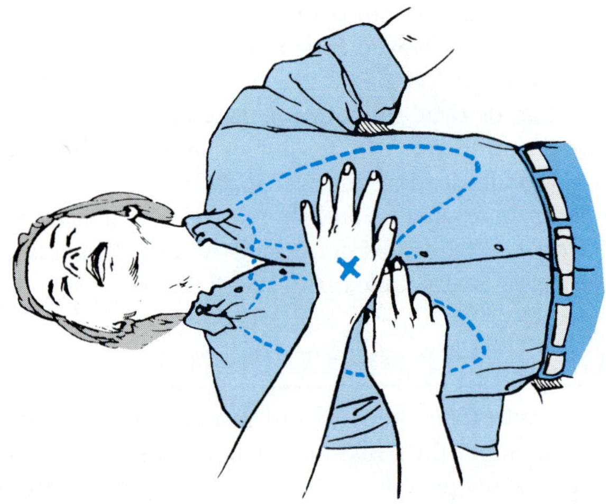

FIG. 50-3 (American Heart Association: *Textbook of basic life support for healthcare providers,* 1994.)

Proper compression techniques are important to deliver the appropriate amount of force to simulate the pumping action of the heart. Compression techniques are as follows:

1. The elbows are locked in place, with the arms straight and the shoulders positioned over the hands so that the thrusts of external cardiac compressions are in a downward motion. Some of the force of the compressions will be lost if there is a rolling or rocking motion.
2. The rescuer leans forward, creating pressure to depress the sternum 1½ to 2 inches in the adult. This is difficult to estimate, but the rescuer will feel the pliability of the sternum. The motion is smooth, never rolling or jerking (Fig. 50-4).
3. External chest compression pressure is released completely to allow the chest to return to position. This allows blood to flow into the heart. The time allowed for release should equal the time required for compression. There should not be a pause between compressions.
4. Hand positions must be maintained at all times—the hands should not be lifted or moved in any way. Hands should stay in contact with the chest.
5. Complications of external chest compressions include lacerated liver, fractured ribs, and fractured sternum, as well as bruising or bleeding of the liver, lung, and spleen. Concern for possible injuries from CPR should not interfere with prompt and energetic application.

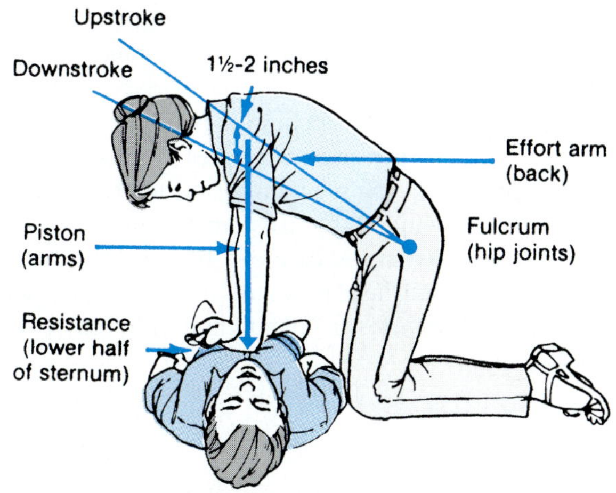

FIG. 50-4 (American Heart Association: *Textbook of basic life support for healthcare providers,* 1994.)

The sequencing of breathing to external compressions in one-rescuer and two-rescuer CPR will be discussed in the following paragraphs:

Steps to Adult One-Rescuer CPR
A: Airway

- Determine unresponsiveness.
- Call for help. Activate the EMS system.
- Position the victim (and rescuer).
- Open the airway.

B: Breathing

- Determine breathlessness.
- If victim is not breathing, give 2 breaths.
- If unable to give 2 breaths, reposition the head and reattempt to ventilate.
- If still unable, proceed with foreign body airway obstruction management procedures.

C: Circulation

- Determine pulselessness.
- If pulse is present, continue rescue breathing at 12 times per minute, or one breath every 5 seconds. Activate the EMS system.
- If pulse is not present, have someone activate the EMS system (if not done previously). Perform 15 chest compressions at a rate of 80 to 100 per minute. Count "1 and, 2 and, 3 and, 4 and, 5 and, 6 and, 7 and, 8 and, 9 and, 10 and, 11 and, 12 and, 13 and, 14 and, 15."
- Continue with 2 breaths and 15 compressions for 4 cycles.
- Reassessment: After 4 cycles of 2 breaths and 15 compressions, reevaluate the victim for the following:
  1. Return of the pulse (5 seconds). If absent, continue CPR with 2 ventilations followed by compressions.
  2. Return of breathing (3 to 5 seconds). If present, monitor breathing and pulse closely. Keep the patient in recovery position—side lying.

If the victim has spontaneous return of breathing and heart function and if *no* trauma is present, the victim should be placed in side "recovery position" to protect the airway. If not, continue CPR, checking for return of pulse and breathing every few minutes.

ADULT TWO-RESCUER CPR

Because artificial ventilation must be combined with external cardiac compressions, it is less fatiguing to perform CPR with two rescuers. The American Heart Association and American Red Cross now teach two-rescuer CPR only to professionals and paraprofessionals.

When One-Rescuer CPR Is in Progress

If CPR has been started with one rescuer, the most logical time for entrance of the second rescuer is after a completed cycle of 15 compressions and 2 breaths. If the EMS system has not been alerted, the first rescuer directs the second rescuer to do so before two-person CPR begins.

The second rescuer identifies himself by saying, "I know two-person CPR," moves to the head, opens the airway, and checks the carotid pulse. The other rescuer positions himself at the chest and finds the proper hand placement for chest compressions. This should take no longer than 5 seconds.

The compression-ventilation ratio for two-person CPR is 5 chest compressions for every 1 breath. There should be a pause of 1½ to 2 seconds to allow for ventilation (inspiration). Exhalation occurs during chest compressions. The compression rate of 2-person CPR is 80 to 100 per minute. The rescuer performing chest compressions will more likely become fatigued. He will initiate the switching procedure (see p. 1544.)

When No CPR Is in Progress

If both rescuers arrive at the scene at the same time and both acknowledge that they know two-person CPR, it is important to establish priorities. One rescuer should activate the EMS system while the other initiates one-rescuer CPR. If the EMS system can be activated by another person, the two rescuers should proceed as follows:

One rescuer goes to the victim's head and does the following:

1. Determines unresponsiveness
2. Positions the victim
3. Opens the airway

4. Checks for breathing
5. If breathing is absent, says "no breathing" and gives 2 ventilations
6. Checks for pulse; if pulse is absent, says "no pulse"

The second rescuer, at the same time, does the following:

1. Finds the location for external cardiac compressions
2. Assumes proper hand position
3. Begins external cardiac compressions after the "no pulse" statement is made by the first rescuer; the sequencing remains 5 compressions for every 1 breath

It is the responsibility of the ventilator (rescuer performing rescue breathing) to evaluate the effectiveness of chest compressions by checking the carotid pulse during chest compressions (a pulse should be felt upon each compression) and monitoring for the spontaneous return of circulation and breathing.

Switching Procedures

Switching the positions of the ventilator and the compressor prevents fatigue of either rescuer and allows time for the ventilator to evaluate the effectiveness of CPR. The switch is initiated by the rescuer performing chest compressions at the end of the 5:1 sequence. After giving a breath, the ventilator moves to the chest and gets into position to give compressions. The compressor moves to the victim's head and checks the pulse for 5 seconds. If no pulse is felt, she gives a breath and states the command to "resume CPR."

PEDIATRIC CPR—CHILD/INFANT

The basic steps of CPR and foreign body airway obstruction management are the same whether the victim is an infant, child, or adult. For the purpose of BLS, an infant may be defined as anyone younger than 1 year. A child may be defined as anyone between the ages of 1 and 8 years.

A: Airway

Unresponsiveness should be determined. The child should be gently shaken. The heels of the feet of an infant may be tapped.

Help should be called for. If the rescuer cannot immediately activate the EMS system, the new guideline is to perform BLS for 1 minute before activating the EMS system. To estimate what 1 minute would be like, do 20 breaths—one every 3 seconds and 20 cycles of CPR. Pediatric arrests are, for the majority, respiratory in nature.

The victim should be positioned on a firm, flat surface for effectiveness of CPR. Performing CPR while carrying an infant may be advantageous if help could be obtained more quickly. However, this technique is not as effective.

The head-tilt/chin-lift technique is used to open the airway of a child. However, care must be taken not to hyperextend the neck in infants. The shorter trachea may become occluded by this maneuver. The head should not be tilted in the case of a head injury: the jaw thrust may be used instead. Caution is necessary with suspected neck injuries in infants and children, as it is in adult cases.

B: Breathing

After the airway is open, the rescuer looks for movement of the chest, listens for breath sounds, and feels for exhaled airflow. If there is no breathing, the rescuer inhales and seals the mouth and nose of the infant. The rescuer pinches the nostrils closed and seals the mouth.

Two breaths (1 to 1½ seconds per breath) are given, with a pause between breaths. The volume of air in an infant's lungs is smaller than an adult's; thus the rescuer's breaths should be adjusted to allow for appropriate rise and fall of the chest. Usually the amount of air for the infant is said to be what an adult can hold in the cheeks. Gastric distention is very common in infants and children during CPR as a result of overinflation of the lungs.

C: Circulation

Assessment of the pulse should be made on the carotid artery of the child and the brachial artery of the infant. If there is a pulse, rescue breathing should be continued at a rate of 1 breath every 4 seconds for a child and 1 breath every 3 seconds for an infant. It there is no pulse, external cardiac compressions must be performed also.

When performing external cardiac compressions in the infant, the rescuer must do the following:

1. Visualize an imaginary line between the nipples.
2. Place the index finger of the hand farthest from the infant's head on this line as it intersects the sternum (breastbone). Lay the middle and ring fingers next to the index finger.
3. Then lift the index finger, and using the middle and ring fingers, compress the breastbone on this area (one finger's width below the line between the nipples). Because of the variations in sizes of infants, this measurement should be used only as a guide (Fig. 50-5).
4. The breastbone is compressed to a depth of ½ to 1 inch at a rate of at least 100 times per minute. Count aloud very quickly "one, two, three, four, five." Compression and release action should be done smoothly. It has been recommended to "think" the count rather than counting aloud, as one can easily lose count because the rate is so fast.

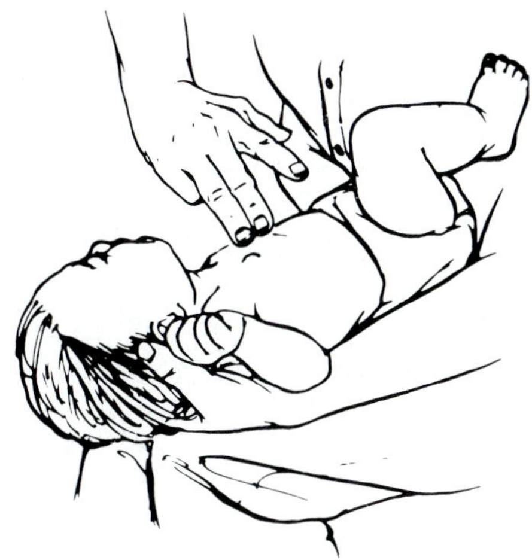

FIG. 50-5 (American Heart Association: *Textbook of basic life support for healthcare providers,* 1994.)

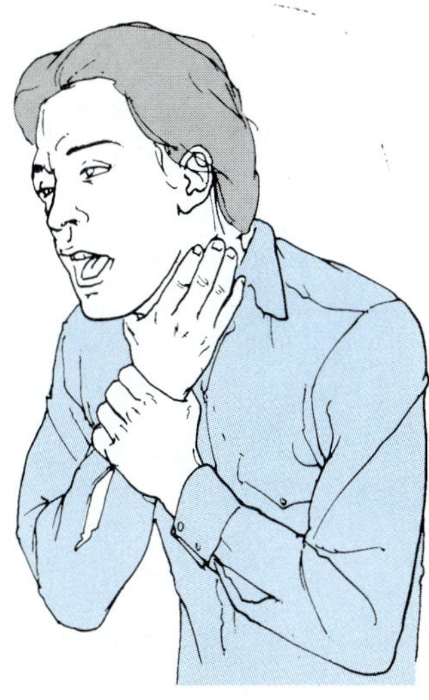

FIG. 50-6 (American Heart Association: *Textbook of basic life support for healthcare providers,* 1994.)

5. At the end of each compression, pressure is released and the sternum is allowed to return to normal position without removal of the fingers from their placement. The movements should be smooth, not jerky.
6. The sequence of compressions to ventilation is 5:1 (5 compressions to 1 breath).

When performing cardiac compressions in the child, the following must be done:

1. The lower margin of the child's rib cage is palpated with the middle and index fingers, while the head tilt is maintained by the other hand.
2. The xiphoid process (where the ribs and breastbone meet) is located.
3. With the middle finger on this notch, the index finger is placed next to the middle finger.
4. Looking at the landmark, place the heel of the hand next to where the index finger was.
5. The chest is compressed with the heel of one hand at a depth of 1 to 1½ inches 100 times per minute. The fingers should not touch the ribs.
6. The compressions should be smooth, allowing the chest to return to the natural position after each compression.
7. The sequence is 5 compressions to 1 breath.
8. If the child is older or large, the adult method of CPR should be used.

FOREIGN BODY AIRWAY OBSTRUCTION MANAGEMENT

Food, particularly meat, is the most common cause of choking or airway obstruction in the adult. Factors that contribute to this are large or poorly chewed pieces of food, the ingestion of alcohol, and loose-fitting dentures. Foreign objects (for example, marbles, beads, buttons, and food) are the most common cause of airway obstruction in children. This maneuver is the most effective method of removing foreign body airway obstructions.

If the air exchange is good, the victim is able to cough forcibly, although there may be wheezing between coughs. *Do not interfere* with the victim at this point. However, the victim should be monitored closely, because he may regress to a state of poor air exchange.

If the victim is experiencing poor air exchange, he may have a weak, ineffective cough, make a high-pitched, "crowing" noise while inhaling, have increased respiratory difficulty, and develop cyanosis. With complete airway obstruction, the victim cannot speak, breathe, or cough, and may clutch the neck (Fig. 50-6). This sign is the universal distress signal. To assess the inability to speak, ask the victim, "Are you choking?" Complete airway obstruction will prevent oxygen from entering the lungs and being circulated to the brain and vital organs. Unless prompt action is initiated, the victim will become unconscious and death will result.

Conscious Victim

Abdominal thrusts given below the diaphragm (the **Heimlich maneuver**) are recommended for relieving foreign body airway obstruction. These thrusts put pressure on the diaphragm, forcing air from the lungs to move and expel the foreign object. The victim may be in a sitting position. Standing behind the victim, the rescuer wraps her arms around the victim's waist. She should then make a fist with one hand and place the thumb of the fist against the middle of the victim's abdomen slightly above the navel and well below the tip of the xiphoid process. The other hand is wrapped over the fist to provide added force. She then presses the fist into the victim's abdomen with a quick upward thrust (Fig. 50-7 on p. 1546). The rescuer repeats each thrust

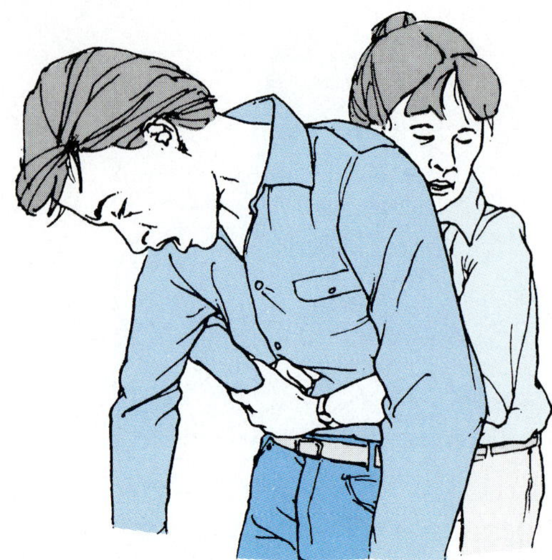

FIG. 50-7 (American Heart Association: *Textbook of basic life support for healthcare providers,* 1994.)

until the foreign body is expelled or the victim becomes unconscious. It may be necessary to repeat 6 to 10 times. If the victim is pregnant or obese, chest thrusts may be used instead of abdominal thrusts. The hands are in the same position as chest compressions in CPR.

Unconscious Victim

If the conscious victim becomes unconscious, he should be placed in a supine position with the face up. Because regurgitation is a common occurrence in an unconscious victim, a finger sweep should be performed. In performing the finger sweep, the rescuer opens the victim's mouth by grasping both the tongue and the lower jaw between the thumb and fingers and lifting upward. This draws the tongue from the back of the throat and away from the foreign body. The index finger of the rescuer's available hand is inserted along the side of the cheek and deeply into the throat to the base of the tongue. A hooking motion is used to dislodge the object and bring it into the mouth, where it can be grasped and removed. Care should be taken not to push the foreign body farther down into the throat with this maneuver.

The rescuer should then open the airway and attempt to ventilate (if the foreign body has been dislodged, the victim will need artificial respirations and possibly external cardiac compressions). If ventilation is unsuccessful, 6 to 10 abdominal thrusts should be performed. To perform abdominal thrusts on an unconscious victim, the rescuer should kneel astride the victim's thighs and place the heel of one hand against the victim's abdomen, in the midline slightly above the navel but well below the tip of the xiphoid process. The second hand remains on top of the first hand for additional force. The rescuer should press into the abdomen with a quick, upward thrust. The mouth should be opened again and a finger sweep performed. All the above steps should be repeated until the foreign body is dislodged and spontaneous breathing is restored. If spontaneous breathing is not restored, CPR must be initiated.

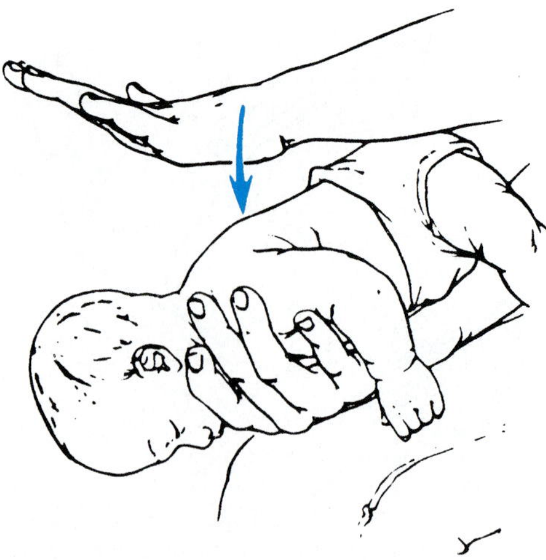

FIG. 50-8 (American Heart Association: *Textbook of basic life support for healthcare providers,* 1994.)

Infant. Of all deaths from foreign body aspiration, 65% are in the infant age group. Aspirated materials include food, such as candies and nuts, and small objects. Infants and children experience acute respiratory distress with coughing, gagging, and **stridor** (harsh sound during respirations, high-pitched and resembling the blowing of wind, due to obstruction of the air passage). The victim may become unconscious.

The child is treated like the adult with performance of the Heimlich maneuver. However, there is a potential for injury in using this maneuver in the infant. Infants should have a combination of back blows and chest thrusts, as follows:

- The infant is straddled over the rescuer's arm with head lower than the trunk, with the face down, and supported firmly at the jaw.
- With this arm resting on the rescuer's thigh, the other arm delivers four back blows between the shoulder with the heel of the hand (Fig. 50-8).
- The rescuer places her free hand on the infant's back so that the victim is sandwiched between the two hands, one supporting the neck, jaw, and chest, while the other supports the back.
- While continuing to support the head and neck, the rescuer turns the infant and places him on the thigh with the head lower than the trunk.
- Four chest thrusts are performed with the hands in the same position as when performing external cardiac compressions (see Fig. 50-5).
- The blind finger sweep technique is never used, because the foreign body could become lodged farther because of the shortened trachea of the infant. However, if the object is visualized when the mouth is open, it may be removed.

REFERENCES AND SUGGESTED READINGS

1. American Heart Association: *Healthcare provider's manual for basic life support,* Dallas, 1988, The Association.
2. American Red Cross: *Community CPR,* St Louis, 1993, Mosby.
3. Britt J: What to do when your patient codes, *Nurs '90* 20(1):42, 1990.
4. Carroll PF, Maher VF: Quick review of a code's legal aspects, *Nurs '90* 20(5):38, 1990.
5. Cummins RO et al: Improving survival from sudden cardiac arrest, *Circulation* 83:1832, 1991.
6. Ellstrom K, Bella LD: Understanding your role during a code, *Nurs '90* 20(5):36, 1990.
7. Emergency Cardiac Care Committee and Subcommittee, American Heart Association: Guidelines for cardiopulmonary resuscitation and emergency cardiac care, *JAMA* 268(16):2171, 1992.
8. Heimlich HJ: The Heimlich maneuver: best technique for saving any choking victim's life, *Postgrad Med* 87(6):38, 1990.
9. Hudak C et al: *Critical care nursing: a holistic approach,* ed 5, Philadelphia, 1990, Lippincott.
10. *Illustrated manual of nursing practice,* Springhouse, Penn, 1991, Springhouse.
11. Kinkade SL, Lohrman J: *Critical care nursing procedures: a team approach,* Philadelphia, 1990, BC Decker.
12. Martin JS et al: Early triage and treatment of the acute myocardial infarction patient: how fast is fast? *J Emerg Nurs* 16(3):195, 1990.
13. *Mosby's medical, nursing, and allied health dictionary,* ed 4, St Louis, 1994, Mosby.
14. National Safety Council: *First aid and CPR,* Boston, 1991, Jones & Bartlett.
15. Nelson NP: Near drowning, *J Emerg Nurs* 16(2):119, 1990.
16. Perry AG, Potter PA: *Clinical nursing skills and techniques,* ed 3, St Louis, 1994, Mosby.
17. Phipps WJ et al: *Medical-surgical nursing: concepts and clinical practice,* ed 4, St Louis, 1991, Mosby.
18. Potter PA, Perry AG: *Basic nursing: theory and practice,* ed 3, St Louis, 1995, Mosby.
19. Potter PA, Perry AG: *Fundamentals of nursing: concepts, process, and practice,* ed 3, St Louis, 1993, Mosby.
20. Shieby SB: *Mosby's manual of emergency care,* ed 3, St Louis, 1990, Mosby.
21. Somers MS: The shattering consequences of CPR: how to assess and prevent complications, *Nursing* 26(7):34, 1992.
22. Soud T: Airway breathing circulation and disability: what is different about kids? *J Emerg Nurs* 18(2):107, 1992.
23. Thomas CL: *Taber's cyclopedic medical dictionary,* ed 17, Philadelphia, 1993, FA Davis.
24. Timby BK, Lewis LW: *Fundamental skills and concepts in patient care,* ed 5, Philadelphia, 1992, Lippincott.
25. Wong DL: *Nursing care of infants and children,* ed 5, St Louis, 1995, Mosby.

CHAPTER CHALLENGE

KEY POINTS

- Personnel trained in CPR and a rapid response EMS system can be successful in resuscitation of victims of cardiac arrest or apparent sudden death.
- The rescuer must perform CPR according to the standards designated by the American Heart Association or the American Red Cross.
- There is a moral obligation to continue CPR once it has been initiated unless the rescuer is exhausted, the rescuer cannot continue, trained medical personnel take over CPR, or a licensed physician pronounces the victim dead.
- The best recovery from cardiopulmonary arrest occurs when CPR is begun within 4 minutes from cardiopulmonary arrest. After 10 minutes without CPR, brain death is certain.
- **A**irway, **B**reathing, and **C**irculation are the three steps to remember in one- or two-rescuer CPR.
- Rescue breathing can supply enough oxygen to meet the victim's needs until the EMS takes over.
- A tight seal of the nose and mouth during rescue breathing will help prevent gastric distention.
- If external cardiac compressions are performed accurately, enough oxygen can be supplied to the heart, lungs, brain, and the rest of the body to sustain life.
- The chest must be compressed to a depth of 1½ to 2 inches in the average-sized adult.
- The sequencing for adult one-rescuer CPR is 2 breaths for every 15 compressions.
- CPR should not be interrupted for more than 5 seconds, except for special circumstances.
- The sequencing for two-rescuer CPR is 1 breath for every 5 compressions.
- The responsibility of the ventilator in two-rescuer CPR is to evaluate the effectiveness of CPR by monitoring the carotid pulse and observing for the spontaneous return of circulation and breathing.
- According to basic child life support standards, an infant is defined as anyone younger than 1 year of age. A child is defined as anyone between the ages of 1 and 8 years.
- Two fingers are used during chest compressions in the infant.
- The heel of one hand is used during chest compressions of the child.
- If a victim is choking but has good air exchange (is coughing forcibly), do not interfere.
- The Heimlich maneuver is the most effective method of removing foreign body airway obstruction.
- The finger sweep technique must be avoided when managing foreign body airway obstruction in the infant.

STUDY QUESTIONS

1. A child, age 8, needs CPR. The ratio of chest compressions to ventilations are:
   1. 15 compressions to 2 breaths
   2. 5 compressions to 1 breath
   3. 8 compressions to 1 breath
   4. 10 compressions to 2 breaths
2. One of the few reasons to stop CPR once it has begun is that:
   1. Another rescuer pronounces the victim dead.
   2. The rescuer determines the efforts are useless
   3. The victim becomes cyanotic
   4. Another CPR-trained rescuer takes over
3. A choking victim needs the Heimlich maneuver. Chest thrusts would be used during the technique if:
   1. The victim is pregnant
   2. The victim loses consciousness
   3. The victim is age 10
   4. The victim is coughing
4. When compressing the chest of the infant, the depth of compressions should be:
   1. 1½ to 2 inches
   2. 1 to 1½ inches
   3. ½ to 1 inch
   4. 1 to 2 inches
5. The first assessment to make on a possibly unconscious victim is to:
   1. Establish unresponsiveness
   2. Check the carotid pulse
   3. Assess for breathing
   4. Monitor vital signs
6. When performing 2-person CPR on an adult, the rate of compressions to ventilations is:
   1. 5 compressions to 1 breath
   2. 10 compressions to 2 breaths
   3. 12 compressions to 1 breath
   4. 5 compressions to 2 breaths
7. Once the airway is open on an unconscious victim, the next step in one-person CPR is to:
   1. Call for help
   2. Assess for the presence of breathing
   3. Give 2 quick breaths
   4. Assess the carotid pulse
8. When compressing the chest of the adult, the depth of compression is:
   1. ½ to 1 inch
   2. 1 to 1½ inches
   3. 2 to 3 inches
   4. 1½ to 2 inches
9. If an infant is choking on a particle of food, and he is coughing vigorously:
   1. Do nothing immediately; continue to observe
   2. Perform a finger sweep to remove the food
   3. Turn him over and give 4 back blows
   4. Perform 6 to 8 abdominal thrusts
10. When performing one-person CPR, the rescuer should be positioned:
    1. At the head of the victim
    2. Astride the victim's legs
    3. Kneeling at the victim's shoulders
    4. At the foot of the victim

51

FIRST AID

Gloria DePole Coschigano

KEY TERMS

crepitus
cyanosis
embolism
epistaxis
epistaxis digitorum
Good Samaritan laws
hematemesis
hematuria
hemoptysis
melena
oliguria
pleural space
shock
tachycardia
tetanus toxoid
vesicle

LEARNING OBJECTIVES

After reading this chapter, the student should be able to do the following:

- Define the key terms.
- List priorities of assessment to be performed when arriving at a situation requiring first aid.
- Discuss moral, legal, and physical interventions of performing first aid.
- List five causes of shock.
- Discuss the signs and symptoms of shock.
- List nursing interventions to treat shock.
- Discuss three methods of controlling hemorrhage.
- Define four types of wounds.
- Discuss types of treatment including bandaging of wounds.
- Discuss methods of treating three common types of poisonings.
- List the characteristics of assessment of bone, joint, and muscle injuries.
- Discuss emergency care for suspected injuries.
- Define three types of burns.
- Discuss the nursing interventions in the first aid treatment of burns.
- Describe the nursing interventions of heat and cold emergencies.

RELATED TOPICS OF INTEREST

- Communication (Chapter 4)
- Signs, symptoms, and physical assessment (Chapter 9)
- Vital signs (Chapter 10)
- The surgical patient (Chapter 22)
- Care of the patient with an integumentary disorder (Chapter 25)
- Care of the patient with a musculoskeletal disorder (Chapter 26)
- Care of the patient with a cardiovascular disorder (Chapter 28)
- Care of the patient with a respiratory disorder (Chapter 31)
- The patient with an addictive personality (Chapter 47)
- Cardiopulmonary resuscitation (Chapter 50)

First aid is the immediate, *temporary* assistance given to a person who is injured or has become ill. First aid includes assessing the victim for life-threatening conditions, performing appropriate interventions to sustain life, and keeping the person in the best possible physical and mental condition until emergency medical services (EMS) can be obtained. It is important to remember that first aid *does not replace* medical care but is used to preserve life until medical help is obtained. Because minutes are precious in preventing permanent disability and injury, the nurse must be prepared to handle emergency conditions and administer first aid.

OBTAINING MEDICAL EMERGENCY AID

The nurse's ability to recognize the need for medical assistance and knowledge of how to obtain medical emergency aid can mean the difference between life and death to an injured or ill person. It is important to know the right phone number to call (both in the community and in the institutional setting). In most communities the emergency medical number is 911; however, the fire department, police department, or local hospital may be the correct number to call for assistance in some localities. Box 51-1 provides information to convey when calling in a medical emergency from the community.

MORAL AND LEGAL RESPONSIBILITIES OF THE NURSE

Good Samaritan laws (legal stipulation for protection of those who give first aid in an emergency situation) have been enacted in most states to protect health professionals from legal liability when providing emergency first aid. If the nurse follows a reasonable and prudent course of action, the chances of legal problems are very small. Before the nurse administers first aid, she must have verbal permission from the victim; the victim also has the right to refuse first aid. The law assumes that an unconscious person would give consent if he were able. After the nurse has initiated first aid, she has a moral and legal obligation to continue the aid until the victim can be cared for by someone with comparable or better training; for example, an EMT or a physician can arrive at the scene and assume first aid care of the victim.

Box 51-1 INFORMATION TO CONVEY IN A MEDICAL EMERGENCY

1. Name of person making the phone call
2. Location of the emergency
3. What has happened (either by direct observation or by gathering data from others)
4. Numbers of people that need assistance
5. The victim's name
6. Obvious injuries and the victim's apparent condition
7. First-aid measures that have already been administered
8. Presence of medical alert bracelet or any known history
9. The physical characteristics of the rescue (stairs, elevators)
10. Always hang up last

ASSESSMENT OF THE EMERGENCY SITUATION

Assessment of life-threatening problems is the first priority in an emergency situation. Assistance may be required to care for victims of some injuries or illnesses or to call EMS. In these cases the nurse may need to shout several times to get someone's attention. While seeking help the nurse should continue the primary survey by checking for (1) an open airway, (2) breathing, and (3) circulation (pulse and severe bleeding). This is known as checking the ABCs. An immediate life-threatening situation of highest priority is arrested or abnormal breathing. To assess whether the victim is breathing properly, the airway must be opened with a chin-lift/head-tilt maneuver unless neck injury is suspected. If neck injury is suspected, a face thrust with head-tilt should be used. Never use hyperextension of the head and neck to establish an airway because of the potential for a cervical spine injury.

The nurse determines whether the chest is rising, listens for breath sounds, and places the cheek near the victim's mouth to feel the passage of air from the victim's breathing (Chapter 50). Rhythm, depth, and rate of respirations should be assessed. The following are signs that the victim is having problems breathing: cyanosis, wheezing, stridor, and snoring.

An arrested or an abnormal pulse is also a life-threatening situation. The rate, rhythm, and strength of the carotid pulse are assessed. It is important to observe for signs of external bleeding and internal bleeding, which may result in shock. The person's skin color, temperature, pupil reaction, pulse, and respiration must be monitored. Poisonings are also life threatening. The nurse should observe for burns or stains in and around the person's mouth or hands. Depressed respirations and circulatory collapse may also result from poisonings.

After the initial assessment for life-threatening problems, the victim must be observed for indications of skull injury and brain or spinal cord damage, which require attention as soon as possible. Decreasing level of consciousness, abnormal pupil reaction, and lack of movement in the arms or legs may indicate injury to the head or spinal cord. Fractures, dislocations, and superficial ecchymosis or wounds require attention after the more serious conditions are treated.

SHOCK

Shock (an abnormal condition of inadequate blood flow to the body's peripheral tissues, with life-threatening cellular dysfunction, hypotension, and oliguria) results from the failure of the cardiovascular system to provide sufficient blood circulation (oxygen, nutrients, hormones, and electrolytes) to the body's tissues and a decreased removal of metabolic wastes. To maintain circulatory homeostasis, the following mechanisms must be present: a functioning heart to circulate blood and a sufficient amount of blood volume. The capability of the vascular system, accommodating blood flow to the capillaries and cells for perfusion and thus providing O_2, glucose, and returning carbon dioxide to the right side of the heart, is also necessary to maintain adequate circulation. Inability of the body to compensate for failure of one or more of these mechanisms results in shock.

Classification of Shock

Shock is classified according to the cause. The most common causes of shock are severe loss of blood, intense pain, extensive trauma, burns, poisons, emotional stress or intense emotions, extremes of heat and cold, electrical shock, allergic reactions, and a sudden or severe illness. Box 51-2 provides several examples of types of shock.

Box 51-2 TYPES OF SHOCK

Hypovolemic shock (also known as hemorrhagic shock): caused by a decrease in fluid volume from bleeding, prolonged vomiting, or diarrhea or loss of fluid from surgery, trauma, or burns.

Cardiogenic shock: results from poor heart function caused by various cardiovascular abnormalities. The heart is unable to maintain sufficient blood pressure to all body parts.

Neurogenic shock: caused by failure of the nervous system to maintain the normal contraction of the blood vessels. Common causes are spinal anesthesia, quadriplegia, or medications that cause vasodilation, in which the blood pressure is lower because there is not enough blood to fill the dilated blood vessels.

Septic shock: results from severe infection. Toxins from the microorganisms cause loss of fluid through the blood vessel walls; often seen in persons receiving chemotherapy or in conditions that result in an immunocompromised functioning, such as in persons with AIDS.

Psychogenic shock syncope: caused by the nervous system's reaction to an emotional stimulus. The blood vessels dilate temporarily, decreasing blood flow to the brain, which results in unconsciousness or syncope.

Anaphylactic shock: anaphylaxis (an exaggerated hypersensitivity reaction to a previously encountered antigen) results from a sudden, severe, allergic body reaction to a foreign substance. The allergen or foreign protein causes the sudden release of histamine, which decreases the amount of blood for circulation because of the release of plasma through the capillary walls as a result of capillary hyperpermeability.

Assessment

The signs and symptoms of shock can be disguised by other signs of injury; some may appear in only the late stages of shock. The nurse must be aware of the following when assessing the victim for shock:

Level of consciousness. The victim may experience changes in behavior, restlessness, anxiety, disorientation, syncope, and agitation. As the condition worsens, the victim becomes more lethargic. Coma and death can result.

Skin changes. The skin becomes cool, clammy, pale, and ashen-looking. As shock progresses, **cyanosis** (slightly bluish, grayish, slatelike, or dark purple discoloration of the skin, especially of the lips and nail beds, due to the presence of abnormally reduced hemoglobin in the blood) develops and the victim may appear dehydrated.

Cardiovascular blood pressure. Initially the blood pressure may be normal, but as shock progresses, there is steady decrease in blood pressure and capillary refill time is delayed.

Pulse. The pulse rate usually increases (**tachycardia;** abnormal rapidity of heart action, usually defined as a heart rate of over 100 beats per minute in an adult) in all types of shock. It also becomes weak and thready in character.

Respirations. The respiratory rate increases. Respirations may also be shallow, rapid, labored, or irregular as a result of vasoconstriction in the lungs, causing fluid to accumulate.

Urinary output. With decreased circulation of fluid volume, the amount of urinary output is decreased (**oliguria;** diminished amount of urine formation, less than 500 ml in every 24 hours).

Neuromuscular changes. Decreased oxygen to the tissues results in weakness and/or tremors of the arms and legs. Eyelids close and the pupils dilate.

Gastrointestinal effects. Because of loss of fluids and fluid shifts, the victim will complain of thirst. Nausea, vomiting, and dry mucous membranes may also be present.

Nursing Interventions

The nurse must *immediately treat* the cause of shock. Priority interventions are to establish an airway (Chapter 50), control bleeding, and reduce pain. Appropriate positioning of the victim in shock is determined by the type and extent of injuries; the following general guidelines are recommended. The victim should lie flat with the head slightly lower than the rest of the body (now called a *modified Trendelenburg*) unless the victim has sustained head and/or chest injuries (Fig. 51-1, *A*). If head, neck, or spinal injuries are suspected, the victim must be kept flat and not be moved, unless it is absolutely necessary, to prevent further injury (Fig. 51-1, *B*). If the victim is unconscious or is vomiting or bleeding around the nose and mouth, he should be positioned on the side to allow the airway to clear and to encourage drainage. The head and shoulders should be elevated if the victim is having problems breathing (Fig. 51-1, *C*).

The nurse must maintain the shock victim's body temperature, keeping the victim warm and dry by placing blankets or other coverings under the victim to prevent heat loss from underneath. The victim should be covered with any available material, such as a blanket or clothing; however, overheating should be avoided. The victim should never be given anything to eat or drink because internal injuries may be present, surgery may be needed immediately, and the patient may aspirate the fluid. A moistened cloth will relieve dry mouth or mucous membranes. In a clinical setting, fluids will be replaced by IV therapy.

The nurse must take measures to relieve pain in the shock victim. Nursing interventions include supporting the injury, avoiding rough handling, and adjusting tight or uncomfortable clothing or bandages. It is important not to give analgesics or drugs unless directed by a physician. Nurses should not allow others to attempt to give alcoholic substances to a victim. Because the victim may be very frightened, it is essential to give emotional support and reassurance.

BLEEDING/HEMORRHAGE

An average adult male has approximately 12 pints of blood circulating in his bloodstream. Blood is necessary to transport oxygen and nutrients to all parts of the body.

Effects of Blood Loss

The loss of blood (hemorrhage) from internal or external bleeding causes a decrease in oxygen supply to the body. Decreased blood volume also causes the blood pressure to fall; thus the heart must pump faster to com-

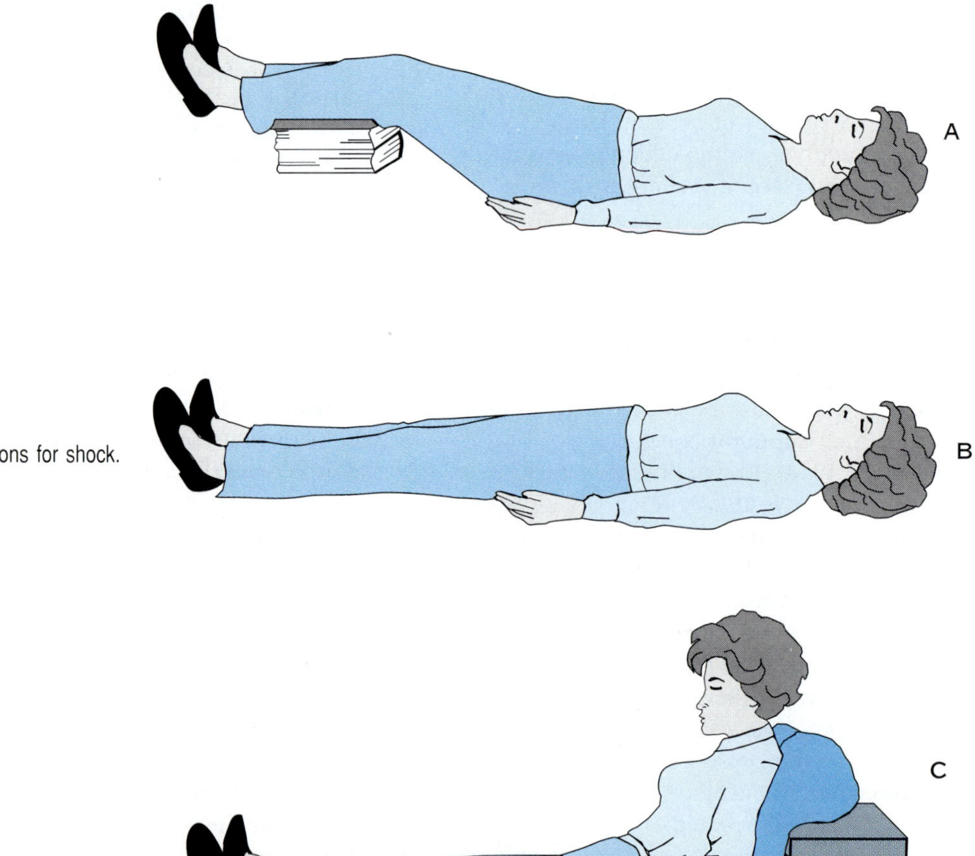

FIG. 51-1 Body positions for shock.

pensate for the decrease in blood volume and blood pressure. The body will attempt to clot the blood to halt bleeding. Clotting usually requires 6 to 7 minutes. If uncontrolled, bleeding can result in shock and death.

Types of Bleeding

Depending on the depth of the wound, bleeding may come from one or all of three sources—capillaries, veins, and arteries. Capillary bleeding, the most common type of external hemorrhage, results from damaged or broken capillaries and is characterized by the oozing of minor cuts, scratches, and abrasions.

Venous bleeding occurs when a vein is severed or punctured. The result is a slow, even flow of dark red blood. Besides shock from blood volume loss, a danger of venous bleeding is the entrance of air into the severed vein, which could result in an **embolism** (an abnormal circulatory condition in which an embolus travels through the bloodstream and becomes lodged in a blood vessel) traveling to the vital organs—heart, lung, and brain.

Arterial bleeding is the least common type of injury, because arteries are located deep in the body and are usually protected by bones, fat, and other structures. When an artery is severed or punctured, the bleeding is characterized by the heavy spurting of bright red blood in the rhythm of the heart beat. The most common arteries that can be affected are:

- Femorals (in the upper thigh and groin)
- Radials (in the lateral aspect of the lower arms)
- Brachials (in the medial aspect of the upper arm)
- Carotids (on either side of the neck)

Nursing Interventions

Direct Pressure. The most effective general treatment of bleeding is to apply direct pressure over the bleeding site. This can be accomplished by placing a dressing or the cleanest material possible over the wound and applying firm pressure with the gloved hand (Fig. 51-2). Then a bandage should be applied with the knot tied snugly over the wound to exert direct pressure. If bleeding continues after the bandage is applied, pressure should be resumed with the hand as well as the bandage. Bleeding should be controlled in 10 to 30 minutes. The bandage supplying direct pressure should not be removed except by a physician, even if it becomes saturated with blood. Another layer of dressing may be placed on top and firm pressure continued.

Raising the bleeding part of the body above the level of the heart will decrease the amount of blood flow and increase the body's ability to clot at this site. This technique should be used with direct pressure *only* if there are no suspected or known fractures or conditions that may be exacerbated by this maneuver. A splinted fracture, however, may be elevated if no other contraindications are present.

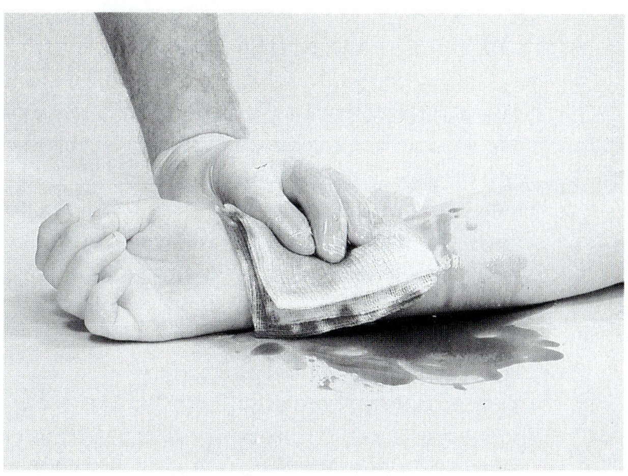

FIG. 51-2 Applying pressure to wound site.

Indirect Pressure. If direct pressure and elevation do not control bleeding, indirect pressure may be applied to any of the 26 pressure points situated along main arteries. To apply indirect pressure the fingers or the heel of the hand is used to compress the artery against the underlying bone located between the heart and the wound. This can be done only if there are no suspected fractures beneath the area where pressure must be applied. The most common pressure points are over carotid, subclavian, brachial, and femoral arteries.

Application of a tourniquet. Bleeding can almost always be controlled by the three-step measure of direct pressure, elevation, and indirect pressure. A tourniquet must be used *only* when these methods have failed and the victim's life is in danger. Extensive damage to the part may occur because of the cessation of blood flow to the area; there is a risk of sacrificing a limb to save a life. A tourniquet may also damage nerves and vessels directly below/under the tourniquet. An improperly, loosely applied tourniquet will not stop arterial flow but will hinder venous flow. Thus bleeding may be increased instead of controlled. Skill 51-1 on p. 1554 provides techniques to follow when applying a tourniquet.

Epistaxis

Epistaxis (nosebleed) is very common but is seldom a serious emergency. However, profuse bleeding from the nose can lead to shock. There are several causes of epistaxis. Trauma (especially a direct blow to the nose); **epistaxis digitorum** (self-inflicted local digital trauma from nasal picking); infections, including the common cold; high blood pressure; strenuous activity; and low humidity in winter months may precipitate epistaxis.

SKILL 51-1

APPLYING A TOURNIQUET

1. Use a strong wide, flat piece of material, if possible (e.g., towel, necktie, wide belt). Never use rope or wire, which could cut the skin.
2. Place pressure on the nearest pressure point to control bleeding while applying the tourniquet.
3. Apply a pad (piece of cloth, handkerchief, dressing) over the artery to be compressed to prevent damage to the skin.
4. Place the tourniquet between the wound and the heart; allow some uninjured skin between the wound and the tourniquet. Wrap the material around the limb twice and tie a half-knot on the upper surface of the limb.
5. Place a stick or rod (approximately 6 inches long) over the knot and secure it in place.
6. Twist the stick enough times to stop the bleeding.
7. Secure the stick firmly with the free ends of the tourniquet. Do not cover the tourniquet (see illustration).
8. Write "T" or "TK" (meaning tourniquet) on the victim's forehead and the time it was applied. Attach a note to the victim's clothing describing the time and location of the tourniquet.
9. Treat for shock and transport to the nearest medical facility.
10. Never loosen a tourniquet once it has been applied. *Always* seek medical attention once a tourniquet has been applied.

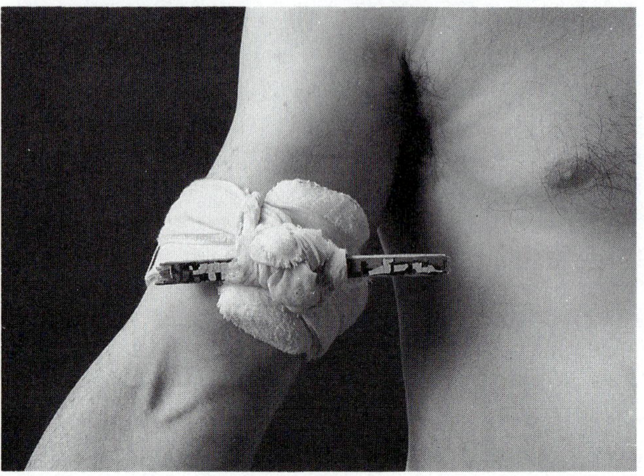

STEP 7

Nursing Interventions. The person with epistaxis must be kept quiet in a sitting position, leaning forward. If the victim is unable to sit up, he should remain supine with the head and shoulders raised (if this position is not contraindicated by other injuries).

Other interventions include:

- Asking the victim to blow all clots out of the nose
- Keeping the victim's head tilted slightly forward so that blood will not run down the back of the throat and cause choking or vomiting
- With the thumb and forefinger applying steady pressure to both nostrils for 10 to 15 minutes before releasing.
- Reminding the victim to breathe through the mouth and to expectorate any accumulated blood
- Applying ice compresses over the nose at the same time may help control bleeding

If bleeding continues despite interventions, medical assistance should be sought because the victim possibly is bleeding from a posterior site and fluid replacement as well as possible surgery may be necessary.

Internal Bleeding

Internal bleeding is a potentially life-threatening situation. It is difficult to diagnose and can progress rapidly. Common causes of internal bleeding include fractures, knife or bullet wounds, crushing injuries, organ injuries, and medical conditions such as ruptured aneurysms.

Assessment. All the signs and symptoms of shock may prevail, as discussed on p. 1551. Initially the victim may experience only vertigo or dizziness. The victim may also expectorate blood **(hemoptysis)** or vomit blood **(hematemesis).** Dark, tarry stool **(melena)** or blood in urine **(hematuria)** may also be present. Pain, tenderness, or a dislocation where injury is suspected could indicate internal bleeding, as would obvious bleeding from the mouth, rectum, or any other body opening.

Nursing Interventions. Internal bleeding is a priority medical emergency, and every effort should be made to obtain medical care immediately. Victims on anticoagulant therapy can have significant blood loss from minor injury. So too may the victim with a history of ETOH abuse as well as those victims with blood dyscrasias.

The victim should be placed on a flat surface with legs slightly elevated if this is not contraindicated by other injuries. An airway is established, and treatment for shock is instituted. A cold compress or ice is positioned on the area of the suspected injury. Ice is never applied directly to the skin as it can "burn" the tissue. Body temperature is maintained with blankets and vital signs are assessed every 5 minutes. The victim should not be given anything to eat or drink. Oxygen may be administered as ordered by the physician. The nurse decreases the victim's fear and anxiety by giving support and reassurance.

WOUNDS AND TRAUMA

A wound is an injury to the internal or external soft tissues of the body. The basic rules for the first aid treatment of all wounds include these:

1. Stop bleeding.
2. Treat for shock.
3. Prevent infection.

Closed Wounds

Closed wounds involve the underlying tissues of the body; the top layer of skin is not broken. Examples of closed wounds are ecchymoses, contusions, strains, and sprains. They most commonly occur during injury from falls, automobile accidents, or contact sports.

The following signs and symptoms are most likely to occur with a closed wound: (1) *edema* may appear within 24 to 48 hours; (2) *discoloration* is likely to occur as a result of the formation of a hematoma (swelling containing blood)—initially the discoloration is blackish-blue and then turns to green or yellow within a few days; (3) *deformity* of the limbs is caused by fractures and dislocations; (4) *shock* may follow from the force of the trauma; (5) there may be *pain and tenderness* at the site; and (6) signs of *internal bleeding* may be present.

Nursing Interventions. If the wound is small, ice packs may be applied, and padding and a soft roller bandage may be used for pressure. If the wound is large, the patient should be treated for shock; cold compresses and a pressure bandage are applied. Medical assistance should be obtained immediately. (See pp. 1562-1563 for nursing interventions in the treatment of dislocations and fractures.)

Open Wounds

Open wounds are openings or breaks in the mucous membrane or skin. Regardless of the type, there is always danger of bleeding or infection. Infection is more common in wounds that do not bleed freely, because active bleeding tends to flush bacteria from the wound. Following are five general types of open wounds—abrasions, incisions, lacerations, punctures, avulsions—and their nursing interventions.

A **tetanus toxoid** (an active immunizing agent prepared from detoxified tetanus toxin that produces an antigenic response in the body, conferring permanent immunity to tetanus infection) injection is necessary as a general treatment for all open wounds. The victim should be pretested for toxoid reaction. The decision of the attending physician should prevail at all times, especially for those wounds that have occurred as a result of a soiled object or are themselves dirty.

Abrasions. Abrasions are caused by a rubbing or scraping of the outer layers of the skin. Bleeding is limited to oozing of blood: there is danger of infection from contamination with dirt and bacteria. Examples of abrasions include rope and road burns, scratches, and abrasions of the knees and elbows.

Nursing interventions. All dirt should be removed if possible. Strong antiseptics should not be used, because they may irritate the skin. Many references point out there is no one solution to use in cleaning wounds. The solution is not as important as the technique used. The wound should be cleansed from the inside out. Many sources say normal saline is safe, is effective, and with copious irrigation will remove debris. Some sources say povidone-iodine unless properly diluted may actually cause tissue necrosis because it is too harsh. The abrasion is covered with a sterile dressing.

The victim should be advised as to the signs and symptoms of infection such as edema, erythema, pain, and purulent exudate. The victim should also be instructed to seek medical attention should these signs and symptoms occur.

Incisions. Incisions are smoothly divided wounds made by sharp instruments. Infection is not as likely to occur, because blood flows freely from the wound. However, bleeding may be extensive and muscles, tendons, and nerves may be damaged. Common examples of incisional wounds include cuts from knives, broken glass, razors, or edges of paper.

Nursing interventions. The incision is carefully cleaned and covered with a sterile dressing; an antiseptic is used only at a physician's recommendation. A "butterfly" bandage or Steri-Strips may be used to hold the edges of the wound together. Bleeding is controlled by applying pressure. Medical attention should be sought if the incision is deep, bleeding is profuse, and function is limited.

Lacerations. Lacerations are wounds that are torn with jagged, irregular edges. Bleeding may be profuse, and tissue destruction and infection may occur. Auto accidents, blunt objects, and heavy machinery accidents are common causes of lacerations.

Nursing interventions. The laceration should be carefully cleaned. Bleeding is controlled by applying pressure (see Fig. 51-2). Adhesive strips, Steri-Strips, or a "butterfly" bandage are used to close the edges of the laceration. The wound should be covered with a sterile dressing, and the victim should be taken to a physician for treatment.

Puncture Wounds. Puncture wounds are caused by the penetration of sharp objects into body tissues. The surface opening may be small; however, the object may penetrate deeply, causing severe damage to tissues and organs. Infection is common, since bleeding is minimal. Tetanus bacteria, in particular, may multiply rapidly after a puncture wound.

It is essential that health care providers determine if the victim's tetanus vaccine is current. Nails, needles, bullets, knives, animal bites, broken glass, and insect stings are common causes of puncture wounds.

Nursing interventions. If the wound is deep or if the object is protruberant, it should be stabilized before immobilizing the part. The object should not be removed (it may have to be cut from the tissues). The wound site should be immobilized and the patient taken to the physician immediately.

Avulsions. An avulsion is the forcible tearing of tissue from the body. The force of industrial or automobile accidents may amputate fingers, toes, or whole limbs of the body. Bleeding is usually extensive, and shock usually results. In some cases, a detached body part may be reattached by a surgeon if it is sent to the hospital with the victim.

Nursing interventions. The ABCs of emergency care should be followed (see Chapter 50), with airway being the first priority. Hemorrhage must be controlled by direct pressure; a tourniquet should be used as a last resort (see Skill 51-1). Because of this trauma and subsequent loss of blood, the nurse must monitor and treat for shock. If the severed part is found, it should be separated from as much dirt and debris as possible with gloved hands and covered with sterile gauze, a towel, or clean cloth. It should be put in a plastic bag, sealed shut, and the bag placed in ice or cold water. The part is transported with the victim. The severed part *must not* be frozen, immersed in a solution or water, treated with antiseptic, or thrown away.

Special Types of Wounds

Eye Injuries. Foreign bodies such as dirt, sand, cinders, or pieces of metal or chemical spills are the most common causes of eye injury. They not only cause discomfort, but if not removed, may cause inflammation or infection. The natural flow of tears when a foreign substance is present very often leads to the flushing out of a foreign object. The victim should not rub the eye, since this can scratch the tissues of the eye and further embed the object.

Assessment. The victim should be observed for edema or lacerated eyelids and/or erythema on the surface of the eye. Sometimes the nurse may see a visible scratch on the surface of the eye. Excessive tearing of the eye may also be noted, and the victim may complain of discomfort. Changes in vision or visual acuity may occur.

Nursing interventions. To remove a foreign body from the eye, the eyelids should initially be flushed gently with clean water, if available, especially if the injury is a chemical splash, holding the eyelids open and flushing from the inner canthus to the outer canthus of the eye. Gloves should be worn. If the foreign object is under the upper eyelid, it may be removed by bringing the upper lid over the lower lid. As the upper lid returns to its normal position, the undersurface will be wiped by the action of the eyelashes. A foreign body of the upper lid may also be removed by grasping the eyelashes of the upper lid and inverting it over a cotton swab or similar object. The foreign object may then be removed with the corners of a piece of sterile gauze.

Particles under the lower lid may be removed by pulling down the lower lid, exposing the inner surface. The corner of a piece of sterile gauze can be used to remove the foreign body. If the foreign body cannot be removed by these measures, if the eye is scratched, or if the object is embedded in the eye, no attempt should be made to disturb it, because this could cause further damage. A cup or cone can be positioned over the area of injury, and then a bandage can be loosely applied to *both* eyes. The head is stabilized with sandbags or pillows and the victim is transported in a supine position to the physician as quickly as possible.

Chest Injuries. Chest wounds are extremely dangerous and need immediate medical attention. In most wounds of the chest, air escapes into the chest (**pleural space;** the potential space between the visceral and parietal layers of the pleurae). Normally this space is a vacuum; therefore air entering this space may cause an increase in pressure, which will result in a pneumothorax (collapse of the lung).

Assessment. The nurse should assess the following factors:

- Sharp pain at the site of the injury
- Pain associated with breathing
- Difficult and labored breathing
- Failure of one or both sides of the chest to expand normally with inspiration
- Expectorating bright red or frothy blood (hemoptysis)
- Signs and symptoms of shock: rapid, weak, thready pulse, vertigo, and hypotension
- Cyanosis of the skin and mucous membranes
- A sucking or hissing sound as air flows in and out of the chest
- Distention or edema of the neck and arm veins
- Anxiety
- Tracheal deviation

Nursing interventions. For the first aid treatment of penetrating chest wounds, if the chest wall has been penetrated by a sharp object, the object should not be removed; this could result in further bleeding and the entrance of air into the chest wound. The object is immobilized with dressings and tape. The ABCs of treatment should be employed (see Chapter 50). The victim should be treated for shock; however, the victim's head may need to be elevated slightly to facilitate the person's breathing.

If there is a sucking chest wound (without the penetrating object in place), an airtight dressing must be applied. Any available material may be used—gauze, plastic wrap, clothing, or even the nurse's hand if that is the only thing available. This dressing must be large enough so that it is not sucked into the hole in the victim's chest, and it should be as airtight as possible. The victim should be monitored for any signs and symptoms of developing pneumothorax. If the victim shows any signs of increased respiratory distress, the nurse lifts a corner of the dressing over the wound and allows air to escape.* Liquids should be withheld, since aspiration could result.

Nursing interventions. For the first aid treatment of crushing chest wounds, it is important to know that the most common injury to the chest is fractured ribs. Simple fractures (one or two ribs) may not need to be bound, strapped, or taped. If the injury to the chest is extensive, the fractured ribs should be immobilized with gauze or clothing. Dressings should be applied carefully to open wounds to avoid pressure on the chest. The victim's head and shoulders should be elevated slightly to facilitate breathing.

Dressings and Bandages

General Principles of Bandaging. Bleeding should be controlled before the bandage is applied. The dressing is opened carefully, using sterile materials if possible. If sterile equipment is not available, the cleanest material possible should be used. The dressing should cover the entire wound. Wounds should be bandaged firmly but not too tightly; tight bandages can interfere with circulation to the tissue. Loose ends may be caught on objects. The part should always be bandaged in the alignment that is desired; a joint should never be bent after it is bandaged. The tips of the fingers and toes should remain exposed if possible, to check for circulation. The nurse should assess for edema and circulation frequently. Knots should be tied over the top of open wounds to control bleeding unless this is contraindicated.

*American Academy of Orthopaedic Surgeons: *Emergency care and transportation of the sick and injured,* ed 5, 1992.

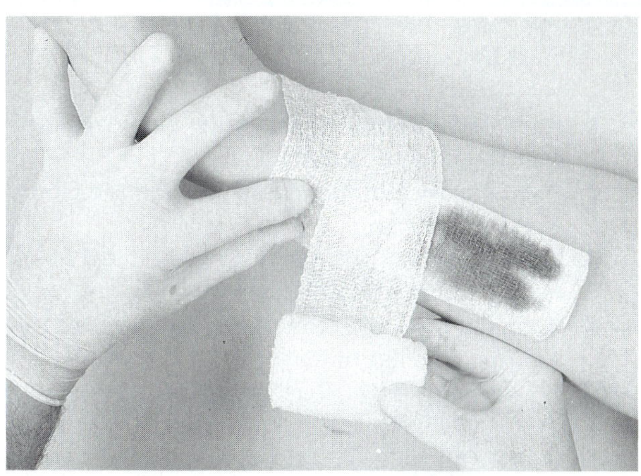

FIG. 51-3 Use of roller bandage.

Application of Common Types of Bandages.

The bandage compress. The bandage compress is the most common type of dressing. It consists of several thicknesses of gauze, covered with tape or gauze.

The triangular bandage. The triangular bandage is made of a piece of cloth that is folded diagonally and cut along the fold. This is used most commonly as a sling to support injured bones. Skill 51-2 describes the application of an arm splint using a triangular bandage.

The roller bandage. The roller bandage is used to support an injured part, apply pressure to a dressing for control of bleeding, or secure a splint to immobilize a part (Fig. 51-3). Roller bandages should be applied uniformly to ensure even pressure. The skin should be covered completely; it is safer to use a greater number of evenly spaced overlapping turns than fewer, tighter turns of the bandage. The roller bandage is started at the point of dressing or at the part of the limb with the smallest circumference (e.g., the wrist or ankle). The roller bandage is fastened with either tape or a square knot. Circular or spiral roller bandages are used to cover a cylindrical part. A figure-eight bandage may also be used, especially if splints must be used.

POISONS

Each year thousands of people die from self-inflicted or accidental poisonings. Of these people, the majority are children. A poison is any substance (solid, liquid, or gas) that even in small amounts causes damage to the body or interferes with the function of its systems. There are poison control centers throughout the country that are equipped to give information about poisons and methods of treatment on a 24-hour-a-day, 7-day-a-week basis. Most poisons act rapidly and thus require immediate first aid.

SKILL 51-2

APPLYING AN ARM SPLINT USING A TRIANGULAR BANDAGE

1. Place one end of the base of the open triangle over the uninjured shoulder.
2. Place the apex of the triangle behind the elbow of the injured arm.
3. Bend the arm at the elbow with the hand elevated slightly (4 to 5 inches).
4. Bring the forearm across the chest and over the bandage (see illustration).
5. Take the lower end of the triangle and bring it over the shoulder of the injured side. Tie the bandage on the neck at the uninjured side, so that the knot is on the side of the neck.
6. Twist the remaining end of the bandage and tuck it in at the elbow (see illustration).
7. Remember to keep fingertips exposed to assess circulation.

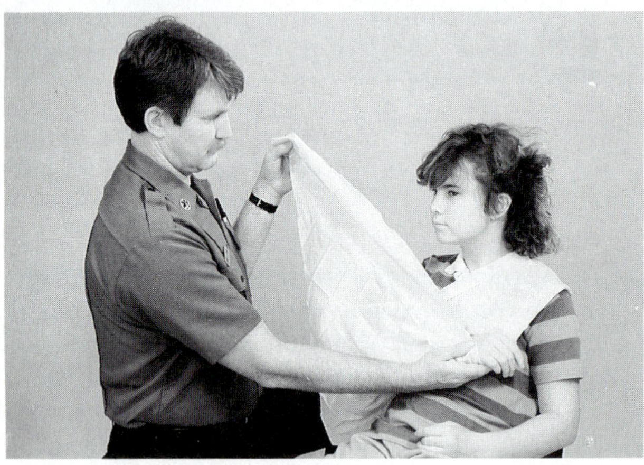

STEP 4

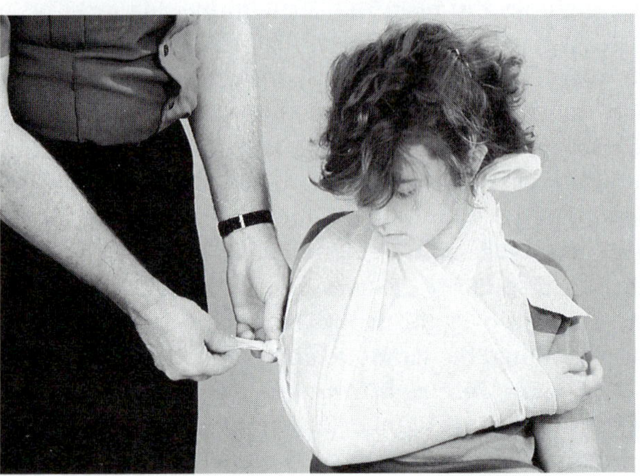

STEP 6

Poison control centers need the following information:

- Weight of patient
- Age of patient
- Substance ingested, inhaled, or injected
  How much
  When taken
- If other drugs are taken and the routes
- Status of patient at present time

General Assessment of Poisonings

Acute signs and symptoms of poisonings may be delayed for hours. The following may be indications of poisonings: respiratory distress; pulmonary edema; bronchospasm; severe nausea, vomiting, or diarrhea; seizures, twitching, or paralysis; decreased level of consciousness or unconsciousness; restlessness, delirium, agitation, or panic; color changes; pale, flushed, or cyanotic skin; signs of burns, edema around the mouth or other areas of the body; pain on swallowing, tenderness, cramps; characteristic odor on the breath; unusual urine color (red, green, bright yellow, black, bronze); slow, labored breathing or wheezing; abnormal constriction or dilation of pupils; abnormal eye movements, such as nystagmus (constant, involuntary, cyclical movement of the eyeball); skin irritation, erythema, and/or edema; and shock or cardiac arrest.

Ingested Poisons

Poisoning by mouth is the most common type of poisoning, especially in children. Common substances include household cleaning products, garden and garage supplies (e.g., insecticides, gasoline), drugs, medications, food, and plants.

Nursing Interventions. The nurse should waste no time in calling the poison control center to describe the poison ingested and receive instructions. An airway must be maintained. If the victim is an adult and is conscious, the poison control center may instruct the nurse to dilute the poison by giving 1 to 2 glasses (8 to 16 ounces) of water (for a child, 1 glass [8 ounces]). If the cause of the poison is a drug, this may be contraindicated, since water would increase the rate of absorption. If the victim is conscious and the poison is *not* a corrosive, and only when the nurse is directed to do so by the poison control center or other medical facility, vomiting should be induced. The following methods may be used.

One tablespoon of syrup of ipecac with 6 to 8 ounces of water should be given to a child, and 2 tablespoons of ipecac with 1 to 2 glasses (8 to 16 ounces) of water to an adult. Milk or carbonated beverages should never be given with syrup of ipecac. If vomiting does not occur within 20 to 30 minutes, the dose is repeated once only.

Vomiting should not be induced if the victim is having a seizure or is semiconscious or unconscious, or if the nurse suspects the victim has swallowed any caustic or corrosive substance, such as a strong acid, lye, gasoline, or rat poison. The nurse should not induce vomiting if the victim has a serious heart condition or is in the later stages of pregnancy. If the poison is corrosive, it should be diluted with water and medical help sought immediately. The nurse should treat for shock and administer CPR if needed. The substance's container and any vomitus should be brought to the medical facility to help identify and treat the poison. An antidote should never be given until the poison control center has been consulted.

Inhaled Poisons

Because inhaled poisons can be present without warning and are absorbed very rapidly, prompt first aid measures are important. Common sources of inhaled poisons include carbon monoxide (from autos, fires, heating systems, propane engines, and paint remover), carbon dioxide (from sewers or industry), and refrigeration gases. Chlorine (used in cleaning and industry) and fumes from sprays and other liquid chemicals may also give off poisonous fumes. This is seen when cleaning chemicals are mixed together, causing poisonous fumes to be released.

Nursing Interventions. The nurse must first assess the danger. The victim should be removed from the dangerous area only if there is no danger to the rescuer. Clothing should be loosened from the victim's throat and chest. An airway must be maintained, and CPR may have to be started. The victim should remain quiet and inactive while being transported to the nearest medical facility.

Absorbed Poisons

Poisons, caustic chemicals, and poisonous plants that come in contact with the skin can be rapidly absorbed, causing burning, skin irritation, allergic responses, or severe systemic reactions. Most signs and symptoms occur within 1 to 2 hours after absorption. Signs and symptoms include nausea, vomiting, diarrhea, flushed skin, dilated pupils, cardiovascular abnormalities, and CNS and respiratory reactions. Poison ivy, poison oak, and poison sumac are the most common plants that can elicit a poison response.

Nursing Interventions in the First Aid Treatment of Poisoning by Absorption. The first action must be to quickly remove the source of the irritation and then to wash the contacted area with soap and water. Skin preparations that are effective in the treatment of contact poisonings include baking soda, Burow's solution, or oatmeal to dry **vesicles** (small thin-walled, raised skin lesions containing clear fluid). Calamine lotion and hydrocortisone cream (5%) are effective to relieve pruritus.

Injected Poisons

Injections of drugs to which an individual is allergic and the venom from insects, reptiles, and animals can cause allergic reactions that can range from mild to severe. Emergency care involves minimizing the travel of the poison to the heart. The reaction to an insect bite may be mild or severe.

Minor Reactions to Insect Bites. If the individual has been stung by a bee, the stinger should be removed with the *side* of a tweezer or knife in a scraping motion. If the nurse attempts to grasp the barbed stinger with tweezers, venom may be forced further into the skin. Nursing interventions include washing the bite with soap and water and applying cold packs to relieve pain and slow the absorption of the poison. A paste of baking soda and water may relieve pruritus at the site.

Severe Reactions to Insect Bites. Within as little as 60 minutes or up to several hours, a victim of a bite or sting may experience a severe allergic reaction. Urticaria, wheezing, edema of the lips and tongue, generalized pruritus, and respiratory arrest are the most common signs and symptoms of anaphylactic shock (severe allergic reaction) (see Chapter 36).

Nursing Interventions. The victim should lie down, and the nurse should immobilize the area of the bite. Remove rings and jewelry.

A wide (4- to 5-inch) constricting band is then applied proximal to the wound. Do not release the constricting band once applied because that would bolus the patient with the toxin. The band should stop only venous blood flow, not arterial; therefore, a pulse should be present below the constriction. The affected part should be kept in a dependent position, below the level of the heart. The victim should be transported to the hospital immediately, and if possible the type of animal or insect that caused the bite should be identified. Keep the patient NPO (nothing by mouth). Ice packs are no longer recommended. Some people who know that they are allergic wear medical alert tags and carry medication (antihistamines) to take after a bite. This can be self-administered. The nurse should give this medication only if directed to do so by the physician.

DRUG AND ALCOHOL EMERGENCIES

Drugs (including alcohol) are chemical substances that can affect body functioning and can be subject to abuse and overdose.

Alcohol

Alcohol is the most commonly abused drug in the world. It is a CNS depressant that can cause many signs and symptoms, even death.

Assessment. Signs and symptoms of *mild* intoxication include nausea, vomiting, diarrhea, lack of coordination, and poor muscle control. Flushing, erythema of the face and eyes, visual disturbances, and rapid mood swings may be present. Slurred or inappropriate speech, inappropriate behavior, and lethargy (sleepiness) may also occur.

Serious alcohol intoxication is usually caused by consuming a large quantity of alcohol over a short period of time. Signs and symptoms include drowsiness that progresses to coma; rapid, weak pulse; and depressed, labored breathing or respiratory arrest. Loss of control of urinary and bowel functions and disorientation, restlessness, and hallucinations may occur. Tremors that may progress to grand mal seizures, nausea, vomiting, expectorating blood from the respiratory tract, and diarrhea may be present. This person may also experience loss of memory, visual disturbances, lack of muscle coordination, and depressed reflexes (see Chapter 47).

Drugs

Abuse of drugs is a major problem in the world today. Not only are illegal drugs abused, but also prescription and over-the-counter medications. In assessing the drug abuser the nurse observes for signs and symptoms of loss of reality orientation, hallucinations, and varying degrees of consciousness; coma could be a result. Slurred speech, extremes in mood swings, inappropriate behavior, and anxiety may also be present. The victim may have a fever and flushed skin and be experiencing diaphoresis (sweating). Lack of coordination and impaired judgment may make safety a real problem. Depending on the drug, the pulse and blood pressure may increase or decrease, the pupils may constrict or dilate, and the appetite may increase or decrease. Obvious hypodermic needle marks on the arms, legs, and neck may be present. The victim may complain of diarrhea or pain in the abdomen, legs, or joints, and may also experience tremors or seizures.

Nursing Interventions. Because an accurate nursing history is important, the nurse must obtain as much information as possible about the substance ingested and keep the containers if possible. The life-threatening situations are handled first and an airway is established. If the victim is unconscious, he should be turned to the side. Clothing is loosened to assist ventilation. If the victim is having muscle twitching and is drowsy, the nurse should not attempt to arouse him, because this may precipitate a seizure. If a fever is present, it can be reduced by applying cool, wet compresses. The nurse should protect the victim from self-injury during a seizure or hallucination by removing harmful objects. The nurse should not attempt to restrain a victim during seizure activity.

The nurse may induce vomiting if directed by the physician or poison control center; particularly if the drug was taken within 30 minutes. Vomiting should never be induced if the victim is stuporous because of the danger of aspiration. The nurse must be calm, supportive, and nonjudgmental, especially if the patient is very agitated or excited. The intoxicated person should never be left alone. Careful assessment of mental status and vital signs must be performed frequently. A substance abuse victim can go into respiratory arrest very quickly. The victim must be transported to a medical facility promptly.

THERMAL AND COLD EMERGENCIES

Heat Injuries

Excessive heat affects the body in several ways. In a hot environment, heat builds up in the body. The body automatically attempts to get rid of the excessive heat by increasing the amount of perspiration produced and slowing down muscular activity. If this mechanism fails for an external (environmental) or internal reason, heatstroke or heat exhaustion could result. Heatstroke and heat exhaustion represent different reactions to excessive heat; for this reason signs, symptoms, and treatment are also different.

Heat Exhaustion. Heat exhaustion is the most common type of heat injury and is the result of prolonged perspiration and the loss of large quantities of salt and water. It occurs most often in hot humid weather, when adequate fluids are not replaced (common in older adults who have a diminished thirst mechanism despite dehydration).

Nursing assessment of the victim of heat exhaustion would include observing for signs and symptoms such as headache, dizziness, nausea, weakness, and diaphoresis.

Mental disorientation and brief loss of consciousness may occur. The victim has a normal body temperature with pale, cold, clammy skin. The victim may complain of abdominal cramps and loss of appetite. Breathing may be rapid and shallow and the pulse may be weak and rapid; blood pressure may drop but usually returns to normal when the person is placed in a recumbent position.

Nursing interventions. The victim must be cooled off as quickly as possible; move the victim to a cool area, but avoid chilling. As much clothing as possible should be removed and constrictive clothing loosened to allow the circulation of air to cool the body. The victim should lie down with feet 8 to 12 inches higher than the head. The victim may be cooled with cold, wet compresses, and a fan or air conditioner should be used if available.

If the victim is completely conscious and alert, give ½ glass of water every 15 minutes for 1 hour. The use of salted water is controversial in the treatment of heat emergencies. The nurse must follow the advice of the physician when administering salted water. If the victim is drowsy or vomiting, fluids should not be given by mouth. In the clinical setting IV fluids are given. The victim should be transported to a medical facility as soon as possible.

Heatstroke. Heatstroke is the more serious heat injury; death can result if heatstroke is untreated. The most common cause of heatstroke is vigorous physical activity in a hot, humid environment. The body becomes overheated, but the cooling mechanism of perspiration does not operate. Deprived of this mechanism, the body stores excessive heat. (Body temperature may rise to 106° F [41° C].) Brain and CNS damage can result.

Assessment. The signs and symptoms of heatstroke include rapidly rising body temperature; hot, dry, reddened skin; and no visible perspiration. The pulse is rapid initially, then slows and weakens as the blood pressure falls. Breathing becomes deep and rapid. The victim complains of headache, dry mouth, nausea, and vomiting; the victim may experience vertigo and decreased level of consciousness and may collapse. Muscle twitching and convulsions may occur.

Nursing interventions. It is important to cool the victim as quickly as possible, moving him to a cool area. Establishing and maintaining an airway are priority nursing interventions. The victim should be undressed (retaining undergarments only). The victim's bare skin should be cooled as quickly as possible with cold water or ice compresses. Cold packs can be placed around the victim's neck, under the arms, and around the ankles to cool the blood in the main arteries. A fan or air conditioner should be used if available. Treatment continues until the victim's temperature falls below 100° F (32.2° C). The victim should be monitored for chilling (control shivering as this will only increase temperature) as the body temperature falls, and the temperature should be checked every 10 to 15 minutes to ensure that it does not rise again. Cooling efforts are continued until the victim is able to obtain medical assistance.

Exposure to Excessive Cold

When the body is exposed to severe cold, blood vessels constrict, body heat is lost, and destruction of tissue may result. Cold, moist air, fatigue, smoking, drugs, alcohol, dehydration, and age and some disease entities such as diabetes mellitus accelerate the potential for injury. Persons with darker skin are more prone to frostbite.

Frostbite. Frostbite is the most common and dangerous local cold injury involving freezing and damaging of body cells. Ice crystals actually form in the body fluid and underlying tissues. These crystals draw water from the cells, causing destruction of tissue integrity. Common areas affected by frostbite are the ears, nose, fingers, and toes.

Assessment. Initially the frostbitten skin takes on a red flush, and the victim may complain of numbness, tingling, and/or pain. Progressively the part becomes hard and loses all sensation. The color of the part changes to a grayish white color as circulation diminishes further. If thawing occurs, the color may change to blue-purple or black, indicating severe damage to or death of tissues. Vesicles and edema may develop. If frostbite is very severe, complete loss of function of the part may result from the damage.

Nursing interventions. If there is a possibility that the part will become refrozen after it has been thawed, it is better to leave it frozen until the victim arrives at a medical facility. Severe tissue damage can result from thawing and refreezing a frozen part. The victim should be treated for shock, and an airway should be established and maintained. Any constricting clothing should be removed to encourage circulation.

If there is no risk of the part being refrozen, it should be warmed in this manner. The frozen part is immersed in warm water (preferably a bathtub) at 102° to 105° F (38.8° to 40.5° C) for 20 to 45 minutes. Water temperature should be checked frequently, not allowing it to cool. If a tub is not available, a hot, moist towel may be used. The nurse must be very careful *not to rub the part;* underlying tissue may become bruised and damaged by friction. If water is not available, the part may be warmed by placing it against a warm part of the body—the axilla, abdomen, or between the legs. The frozen part should never be placed near an open flame or oven. Gentle warming must be performed to avoid burns and damage.

Once the part is warmed, the victim is encouraged to gently move the part. If the legs or feet are involved, however, the victim should not be allowed to walk. The thawed part is wrapped in clean towels or bulky dressings and elevated. The entire body should be kept warm, and warm fluids should be offered to drink. Alcohol should never be given, and the victim should not smoke, because this will cause further vasoconstriction. Ice, snow, or cold should never be placed on a frostbitten area. All frostbite injuries, no matter how minor, should be seen by a physician.

Hypothermia. Hypothermia is the lowering of the body temperature below the normal level (95° F [35° C] or below). The brain, heart, lungs, and other vital organs are affected by this drop in temperature. Hypothermia occurs most frequently when the air is windy, cold, and moist, or precipitation is present. The victim may be exhausted or intoxicated; older persons or those living in a poorly heated environment are subject to hypothermia.

Assessment. Initially, the victim may shiver uncontrollably; shivering ceases when the body temperature is below 90° F (32.2° C). Speech becomes slow, slurred, and incoherent, and the victim demonstrates memory lapses, disorientation, and poor judgment. Safety is a problem, because the gait becomes uncoordinated, and muscle activity may decrease or cease. The skin appears mottled and edematous, and the patient complains of generalized numbness. A weak, irregular pulse develops, with a depressed respiratory rate. The victim becomes lethargic, with decreasing levels of consciousness. Finally, there is a loss of all of the reflexes, and the victim appears to be dead.

Nursing interventions. Although a person in the final stages of hypothermia may appear to be dead because of the effects of the lowered metabolic rate, many such victims can be revived. First aid is always instituted in an attempt to treat hypothermia. CPR should always be initiated if necessary (see Chapter 50), even though the victim may appear dead. The victim should be placed in a supine position with the head lower than the feet. The victim is rewarmed slowly; rapid exposure to warmth can precipitate shock. The victim is moved to a warm area, and all wet clothing is removed and replaced with dry ones. The nurse should cover the victim with warm blankets.

If the victim is completely conscious, warm fluids can be given to drink. Alcohol should never be given because of its vasodilatory effect on the peripheral vessels, which causes the central temperature core to drop further. Medical help must be obtained as soon as possible for the patient.

BONE, JOINT, AND MUSCLE INJURIES

The four major types of injuries that occur to bones, tendons, ligaments, and muscles are fractures, dislocations, sprains, and strains.

Fractures

A fracture is a break in the continuity of a bone. Fractured bones seldom are an immediate threat to life, although they can cause serious complications. In administering first aid to an injured victim, establishing an airway and treating hemorrhage are considered priority situations. Considerable blood loss can be caused by fractures (750 to 3000 ml from a fractured pelvis and 500 to 3000 ml from a fractured femur).

There are several types of common fractures:

Open or compound fractures: an open wound exists over the fracture site. Very often the affected bone may be seen protruding through the skin.

Closed fractures: the skin overlying the injury is intact.

Comminuted fractures: the bone is shattered into two or more fragments or pieces.

Greenstick fractures: an incomplete break occurring most commonly in children because their bones are pliable.

Assessment. The physician, using x-ray diagnostic procedures, can determine whether a bone is definitely fractured. Fracture is suspected if there are pain and tenderness in the area of the fracture; pain also develops during movement, and the victim complains of an inability to move the affected part. A deformity of the limb may be obvious with edema and discoloration (cyanosis, erythema) of the area. Fragments of bone may be protruding through the skin. If the affected part is moved, a grating sound is heard. This is called **crepitus** and is caused by the broken bones scraping against each other. The victim may state that he heard or felt the bone snap.

Nursing Interventions. The victim should not be moved unless he is in danger. The ABCs of first aid take priority. Next the nurse must control bleeding in open fractures by cutting away the clothing around the wound and covering with a large sterile pressure dressing. The nurse should not attempt to reduce the fracture; this could cause further damage to the bone and tissue. The victim is treated for shock.

The fracture should be immobilized, but no attempt to realign the bone should be made. The rule is: "Splint the part where it lies." A fracture can be changed from a simple break to comminuted or splintered by moving it improperly. The splint should be lightweight but rigid. It must be long enough to extend past the joints above and beyond the fracture. It should be wider than the thickest part of the injury. The splint must be padded on the inner surface to avoid contact with the skin. The fracture is supported while gently sliding the splint under the limb. A roller bandage or similar material is used to secure the limb in place (Fig. 51-4). Circulation in the limb is monitored by assessing color, temperature, pulses

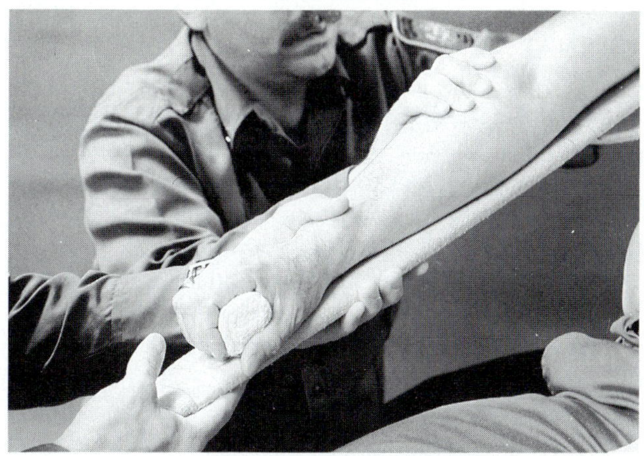

FIG. 51-4 Immobilization of fractured arm.

below the injury, complaints of numbness and tingling, and evidence of edema.

Dislocations

Dislocations occur in joints. They usually result from a blow or fall. Common areas are the jaw, shoulder, elbow, wrist, finger, hip, and ankle.

General Assessment. The victim may complain of pain and edema in the area of the dislocation. A deformity of the part may be observed. The part may be rigid and the victim is unable to move it. A common observation in the dislocated joint of an extremity is shortening of the affected part.

General Nursing Interventions. The nurse should never attempt to reduce a dislocation or push the joint back into place; this will further damage delicate ligaments, tendons, nerves (especially the olecranon elbow), and the bone. The joint must be splinted in the same manner as a fracture. The nurse should be sure the splint is large enough to support the limb in the line of the deformity. The limb is bound to the body or supported in a sling. This is useful in dislocations of the shoulder and elbow.

Strains and Sprains

Strains are injuries to muscle tissue that result from stretching and tearing from overexertion. Sprains are injuries to joints resulting from stretched and/or torn ligaments. This may be caused by twisting it beyond the normal range of motion. The most commonly affected joints are the knee and ankle. Permanent damage can occur to the tissue and joint if sprains are left untreated.

Assessment. Injuries to muscle or ligaments result in the following signs and symptoms:

Strains: spasms, or "knotting" of the muscles, acute pain, stiffness, and weakness on movement; back pain radiating down the leg; discoloration

Sprains: pain and/or tenderness around a joint; immobility of the joint; rapid and marked edema; discoloration around the joint

Nursing Interventions. A suspected musculoskeletal injury should be treated as a fracture, until fracture is definitely ruled out. In the treatment of sprains and strains, the nurse should remember the word *RICE,* which stands for:

R *Rest* the affected extremity.

I *Ice* applications to the part but not directly to the skin until the edema and pain subside (24 to 72 hours is most common). This may be followed by warm compresses to encourage healing by increasing the blood flow. The victim's skin is assessed frequently for any evidence of burns.

C *Compression:* an Ace bandage or compression bandage should be used to support the injured part.

E *Elevation:* the part is elevated above the level of the heart to promote venous flow and therefore reduce edema.

Spinal Cord Injuries

Assessment. To assess for paralysis, the nurse asks the victim if he can move his hands and/or feet and asks the victim if he feels pain or sensation. The nurse may test for sensation by touching or pinching the skin. Abrasions and ecchymosis, especially on the shoulders, back, and abdomen, may indicate injury to the victim's spinal cord.

Nursing Interventions. Spinal cord precautions are taken in all cases of head trauma and multiple traumas. There is a high correlation between neck and spinal cord injuries in patients with facial lacerations. An airway is established, keeping the head in a neutral position (never hyperextending the neck). If the victim vomits, he should be moved (by several people as one unit) on the side to allow drainage.

CPR is administered if necessary. Hemorrhage and shock must be treated. The head and neck must be kept in line with the body when moving the victim. Even a slight movement of the individual's head can cause spinal damage. The nurse should not attempt to move the victim without at least three assistants (Skill 51-3). The assistants must be trained in emergency medical care (EMTs).

SKILL 51-3

MOVING THE VICTIM WITH A SUSPECTED SPINAL CORD INJURY

1. Carefully roll the victim, supporting the entire length of the body, just enough to slip a solid board underneath the victim for support. This board must extend beyond the victim's head and feet (see illustration).
2. While another person steadies the victim's head, place a towel or padding in the space underneath the victim's neck (never put the head on a pillow).
3. Place additional padding (rolled up blankets, towels, sandbags, etc.) around the head and neck to hold the head in place, keeping the neck in line with the body. A cervical collar may be used.
4. Secure the victim to the backboard with bandages or improvise these so that the entire body is immobilized. Tape the head in place.
5. In the event of an emergency situation in which the victim is wearing a helmet, the nurse should immobilize the victim with the helmet left in place.

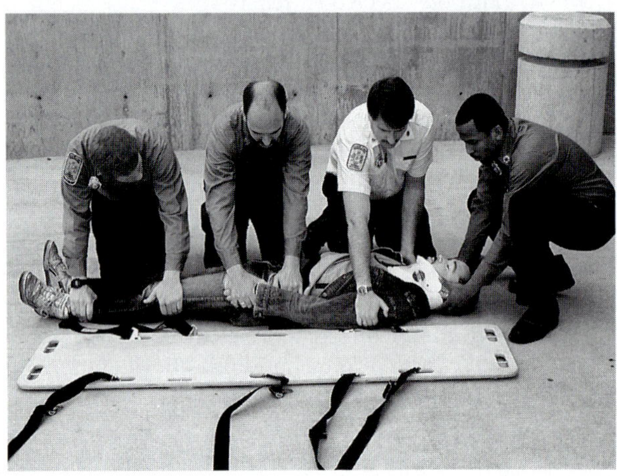

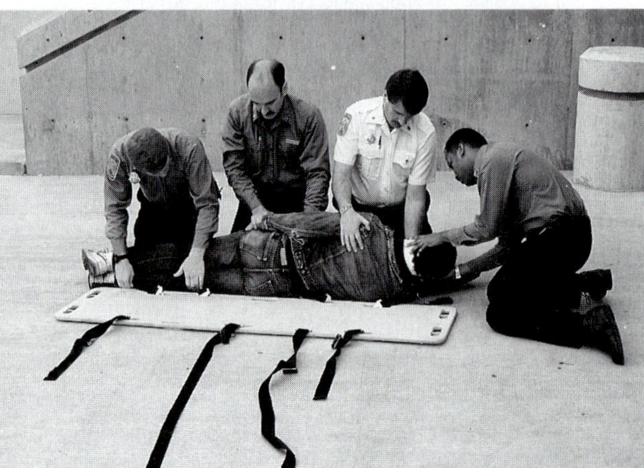

STEP 1

BURN INJURIES

Burns are a leading cause of accidental injuries, especially among children. Burns may be caused by heat from fire or steam, electricity from faulty wiring, chemicals such as lye, strong cleaning products, acids, solar radiation, and radioactive materials.

Burns may be classified according to the depth or the extent of the body surface area burned. The principal complications of all burns are shock from loss of fluids and electrolytes and trauma and infection because of the loss of skin as a barrier (see Chapter 25).

Shallow Partial-Thickness Burns

Shallow partial-thickness burns (previously classified as first-degree burns) are the least serious of all burns, involving only the outer layer of the skin. The most common first-degree burns are simple sunburn or from contact with hot objects. Healing is usually spontaneous and uncomplicated. Signs and symptoms include erythema of the skin and pain.

Nursing Interventions. The burn should be cooled immediately by soaking in cold (not ice) water or applying cold compresses to the area for as long as it takes to decrease pain (up to 30 minutes). The nurse should never put grease, butter, salt water, or topical burn ointments or sprays on the burn. A sterile dressing should be placed over the burn site to ease pain.

Deep Partial-Thickness Burns

Deep partial-thickness burns (previously classified as second-degree burns) involve the entire first layer of skin (epidermis) as well as some of the underlying tissue; scarring from vesicles and infection may occur. Common causes of second-degree burns are severe sunburn, scalding liquids, direct flame, and chemical substances.

Assessment. Signs and symptoms include the following. Deep erythema of the skin, or mottled skin with vesicular formation, may be seen. Considerable edema may result, lasting over several days. There may be a weeping of fluid through the skin surface (loss of plasma), and the person complains of intense pain.

Full-Thickness Burns

Full-thickness burns (previously classified as third-degree burns) involve destruction of the skin and underlying tissue, including fat, muscle, and bone. The area is usually charred and healing is difficult. The skin may be thick and leathery, with black or dark brown, cherry red, or dry and milky white colors. The victim may not complain of pain, since nerve endings may be severed by the burn. There is a hyperpermeability of capillaries, with plasma seeping into the interstitial spaces—thus fluid loss; the wounds weep a great deal of fluid and blood. Thus a fluid and electrolyte imbalance occurs. Hypovolemic shock and infection are common complications. Medical attention is urgent. Common causes of full-thickness burns are direct flame (ignited clothing), explosions, and gasoline or oil fires.

Nursing Interventions for Moderate to Severe Burns (Deep Partial-Thickness and Full-Thickness). An airway must be established before edema occurs. Respiratory and cardiac function is assessed. The nurse should remove all the victim's clothing, shoes, and jewelry, which may be constricting and even smoldering. Leaving clothing on can cause more severe burns. CPR is administered if necessary. The victim is treated for shock. The victim should be kept warm, with the burned area elevated. The nurse should inspect for burns around the mouth and nose, which could affect respiratory status. Chemical burns should be immediately flushed with copious amounts of water.

If medical help will be arriving within 15 to 30 minutes, the nurse should withhold oral fluids. If medical help is delayed, ½ glass of water mixed with ½ teaspoon of salt plus ½ teaspoon baking soda may be given to replace electrolytes. If vomiting occurs, fluids should not be given.

The burn should be cooled immediately, using cool compresses. This should be used only for partial-thickness burns. Cool compresses could cause hypothermia in more extensive burns. Clothing is removed from the burned area. The victim's shoes should always be removed; often heavy boots may be smoldering and can cause a more severe burn. Vesicles should not be broken, and the nurse should not touch a burn with anything except sterile dressings. Antiseptics, ointments, sprays, or creams should not be applied on a burn; this could interfere with medical treatment and cause further complications. Loose sterile dressings should be applied over the burn. The victim should be checked frequently to be sure that edema has not caused further constriction of the area near the burn.

REFERENCES AND SUGGESTED READINGS

1. *Emergency care update 93* from these reference sources: *Am Nurse* 25(6):12, 1993; *Ann Emerg Med,* 22(3):89, 1993; *J Emerg Nurs* 19(2):102, 1993; *Patient Care* 9:11, 1993; *J Emerg Nurs* 19(1):34, 1993; *J Emerg Nurs* 19(1):45, 1993; *Curr Emerg Cardiac Care* 4(1):1, 1993; now appearing in *Nursing 1993 23(9):62, 1993.*
2. American Red Cross: *Community first aid and safety,* St Louis 1993, Mosby.
3. Bailey M, Michalski J: Radial head fracture, *Nursing* 23(9):43, 1993.
4. Bergeron DJ: *Brady first responder,* Englewood Cliffs, NJ, 1991, Prentice-Hall.
5. Boyd-Monk H: Eye trauma in the workplace, *AAOHN J* 38(10):487, 1990.
6. Brown L: Emergency procedures: life savers, *Am Health* 11(2):70, 1992.
7. Dire DJ, Welsh AP: A comparison of wound irrigation solutions used in the emergency department, *Ann Emerg Med* 19:704, 1990.
8. Fontanarosa PB et al: Emergency management of epistaxis: achieving hemostasis safely and effectively, *Emerg Med Rep* 12(26), 1991.
9. Joyce SM: *Epistaxis.* In Hamilton G, Trott A, Strange G, editors: *Emergency medicine: an approach to clinical problem solving,* Philadelphia, 1991, Saunders.
10. Lammers RL et al: Effect of povidone-iodine and saline soaking on bacterial counts in acute, traumatic, contaminated wounds, *Ann Emerg Med* 19:709, 1990.
11. Long BC, Phipps WJ, Cassmeyer VL: *Medical-surgical nursing: a nursing process approach,* ed 3, St Louis, 1993, Mosby.
12. Moore EE et al: *Early care of injured patient,* ed 4, Philadelphia, 1990, BC Decker.
13. *Mosby's medical, nursing, and allied health dictionary,* ed 4, St Louis, 1994, Mosby.
14. National Safety Council: *First aid and CPR,* Boston, 1991, Jones & Bartlett.
15. Phipps W, Long B, Woods N: *Medical-surgical nursing: concepts and clinical practice,* St Louis, 1991, Mosby.
16. Potter PA, Perry AG: *Basic nursing: theory and practice,* ed 3, St Louis, 1995, Mosby.
17. Potter PA, Perry AG: *Fundamentals of nursing: concepts, process and practice,* ed 3, St Louis, 1993, Mosby.
18. Rich J: Penetrating chest injury, *Nursing* 23(3):33, 1993.
19. Shingleton JF: Eye injuries, *N Engl J Med* 325(6):403, 1991.
20. The Staff: *Nursing procedures,* Springhouse, Penn, 1992, Springhouse.

CHAPTER CHALLENGE

KEY POINTS

- First aid is used to preserve life until medical help arrives, not to replace medical care.
- Airway problems, circulatory problems, profuse bleeding, and poisonings are life-threatening situations that require priority emergency care.
- Shock should be suspected in all traumatic injuries, diseases, and physical and emotional stress situations.
- Shock can be prevented and kept from worsening by administering prompt, effective treatment.
- Steps for controlling bleeding include direct pressure, elevation, and indirect pressure. A tourniquet is seldom used, and only as a last resort.
- The chief responsibilities of the nurse caring for an open wound are to stop bleeding and prevent infection.
- The major concerns in a chest wound are to control bleeding and maintain breathing and oxygenation.
- When bandaging a part it is important to assess frequently for evidence of impaired circulation: edema, pain, change of color, coolness, and decreased capillary refill.
- Any substance, if abused or misused, may be considered a poison and needs medical assistance immediately.
- The nurse should never induce vomiting in a poisoned victim unless directed to by the poison control center or medical facility.
- Reactions to a poisonous bite may take a few minutes to several hours to appear. First aid measures should be taken immediately.
- The main objectives in administering first aid to a victim with a fracture are to immobilize the area, treat for shock, and prevent further injury.
- The nurse should always splint a fractured part in the position it is in and should never attempt to realign it.
- A splint must extend past the joint above and below the fracture.
- First aid treatment must always be given for a musculoskeletal injury as if it is a fracture.
- The spinal cord can be damaged by edema, resulting from internal hemorrhage or external pressure from fractured vertebra. Every precaution must be taken to immobilize the victim to prevent a spinal injury from resulting in cord damage.
- The dangers from burn injuries are shock, loss of fluids, and infection.
- In heat emergencies, it is important to cool the victim as soon as possible.
- The greatest danger in the treatment of frostbite is that the part becomes thawed and then refrozen. Severe tissue damage may result.
- Although a victim of hypothermia may appear dead because of low metabolic levels, many victims have been revived.

STUDY QUESTIONS

1. The priority assessment to make of the accident victim at the scene of a car accident would be whether:
   1. The victim is actively bleeding
   2. The victim has a patent airway
   3. There is an apical pulse
   4. There are signs of head trauma
2. When caring for a victim who has a head injury and is developing shock:
   1. Elevate the victim's head
   2. Lower the victim's feet
   3. Elevate the upper body
   4. Leave in a flat position
3. You find an unconscious woman in a car that is on fire. She is breathing. Her arm is fractured. She has several lacerations that are bleeding profusely. What do you do first:
   1. Splint the fractured arm
   2. Get her out of the car
   3. Give mouth-to-mouth resuscitation
   4. Stop the bleeding
4. You find a child with an open bottle of aspirin. What do you do:
   1. Wait for signs and symptoms
   2. Search the label
   3. Call the poison control center
   4. Give large quantities of milk to drink
5. The priority goal for the first aid treatment for all wounds is that:
   1. Infection will be prevented
   2. Wound healing will be promoted
   3. Bleeding will be controlled
   4. Deformities will be prevented
6. The first intervention when treating a victim with a penetrating chest wound is:
   1. Treat for shock
   2. Cover the wound with airtight dressings
   3. Monitor vital signs
   4. Irrigate the wound with normal saline solution
7. In caring for an injured victim, your first consideration should be to:
   1. Care for the burns
   2. Treat for shock
   3. Care for possible fractures
   4. Establish an airway

16

DYING AND DEATH

The nursing field can be very enriching and rewarding. I have chosen to become an LPN because I enjoy working with people, the pay is good, and I feel that this a good way of contributing to my community. Becoming a nurse can sometimes be a struggle. The classes are hard, and you spend a lot time studying. But, in the end, the benefits are worth it all. The day you graduate is worth it all; you stand there proud of all your accomplishments. Whether it is working in a hospital on the floor or caring for the elderly in a nursing home or working in the health department, nursing is a very, very rewarding career. Giving care and understanding to someone that is ill or relies on you is the greatest joy of all.

Kimberly Sue Langford
Student Nurse

52

LOSS, GRIEF, DYING, AND DEATH

Elaine Kockrow
Barbara Christensen

KEY TERMS

advanced directives
anticipatory grief
autopsy
bereavement
death
DNR
durable power of attorney
dysfunctional grieving
euthanasia
grief
grief therapy
grief work
living will
loss
maturational loss
morbidity
mortality
mortician
mourning
postmortem care
situational loss
thanatologist
thanatology

LEARNING OBJECTIVES

After reading this chapter, the student should be able to do the following:

- Define the key terms.
- Explain how the concept of loss impacts on the grief reaction.
- Identify how the changes in the health care system affect nursing interventions for the dying patient.
- Describe the stages of dying.
- Identify needs of the grieving patient and family.
- Recognize the five aspects of human functioning and how each interacts with the others during the grieving/dying process.
- Identify unique physical signs and symptoms of the near-death patient.
- Discuss nursing interventions for the dying patient.
- Describe techniques in assisting the dying patient to say "good-bye."
- Describe nursing interventions that may facilitate death in special circumstances (perinatal, pediatric, geriatric, and suicide).
- Describe nursing responsibilities in care of the body after death.
- Describe approaches to facilitate the grieving process.
- Explain concepts of euthanasia, DNR, organ donations, fraudulent methods of treatment, and the Dying Person's Bill of Rights.
- Discuss support for the grieving family.
- Discuss advanced directives, which include the living will and durable power of attorney.

RELATED TOPICS OF INTEREST

- Legal aspects of nursing (Chapter 2)
- Ethical aspects of nursing (Chapter 3)
- Communication (Chapter 4)
- Cultural aspects of nursing care (Chapter 8)
- Comfort, rest, and sleep (Chapter 15)
- Hygiene and care of the patient's environment (Chapter 16)
- Home health nursing (Chapter 48)
- Hospice care (Chapter 53)

Life is a series of losses and gains. Illness and hospitalization frequently may cause a loss. When any aspect of self is no longer available to a person, that person suffers a **loss.** Nurses work with many patients who experience different types of loss. Loss and **death** (cessation of life) are universal, yet individually unique events of the human experience. Coping mechanisms determine people's ability to face and accept loss. **Grief** (a pattern of physical and emotional responses to bereavement, separation, or loss) is a natural response to loss. Nurses assist patients in understanding and accepting loss so that life can continue. When patients do not do **grief work** (adaptation process of mourning a loss) after a loss, serious emotional, mental, and social problems may occur.

Humans can anticipate death. This causes anxiety, planning, denial, love, loneliness, achievement, and lack of achievement. Death can be an overwhelming experience that affects dying persons and their families, significant others, friends, and care givers. The style of dying reflects a person's style of living, and attitudes about death depend on a person's beliefs and emotional strengths.

Care of dying patients and their families can be one of the most challenging aspects of nursing care. Because dying is the final stage of human growth and development, it is essential that nurses be as knowledgeable about the process of dying as they are about the process of birth. Because health care usually emphasizes the cure of disease and the promotion of health, the death of a patient may represent a form of failure to health care providers. Research in the United States has shown that health care personnel caring for dying patients may withdraw from the patients socially while providing adequate physical care.

When nurses deal with grieving families and dying patients, they are confronted with their own **mortality** (the condition of being subject to death) and other discomforting issues that accompany loss. Such factors can influence quality of care. All losses have the possibility of triggering the grief process. The severity of the loss may vary, but the stages of grief that accompany the loss are still present. Understanding loss, the grief process, and the task of dying can assist the nurse in delivering quality care to those patients and families experiencing death.

CHANGES IN HEALTH CARE RELATED TO DYING AND DEATH

Before the 1950s it was common for patients to die at home in their own beds with assistance only from their family. From the 1950s to the 1980s the health care system became very mechanized and dying occurred mostly in institutions and often with very sophisticated machinery attached to the dying individual to prolong life. As recently as 1983 when diagnosis-related groups (DRGs) came into play, this trend again changed. Generally, only those persons considered medically at risk for complications or who need immediate hospital recovery time after surgery or special procedures are placed in hospital beds. Currently, the recuperating or terminally ill patient is often discharged to home, convalescent center, or nursing home. Nurses practicing in home health care settings have felt this impact as they provide care to the terminally ill patient. At home these patients are now receiving IV infusions, including blood products, and other technical and mechanical assistance. Nurses in health care facilities and homes are the health care providers most often available to the grieving family during the crisis of death. These nurses are often licensed practical/vocational nurses.

HISTORICAL OVERVIEW

Opportunities to learn the dynamics surrounding grief, dying, and death are relatively new. It was in the 1960s that pioneers in death and dying theory, such as Kübler-Ross and Glasser and Strauss, produced works that stimulated the health care industry. Dying and death became topics of research and seminars. In the 1970s hospices in the United States became recognized as health care delivery systems (see Chapter 53). **Grief therapy** (mental treatment aimed at helping a patient deal with the pain of loss; a program in assisting the bereaved to cope with their loss) was introduced in the 1980s when Benoliel and Martocchio added new insights into the needs and care of the dying patient. Care providers are assisting patients and families to become involved in determining treatment options and to choose the setting, circumstances, and management of the dying process.

The future will offer opportunities for individuals to exercise more control over their care as living wills are upheld in courts of law as legal documents and terminal health care shifts away from hospital settings. This shift will continue to provide a primary role for nurses in the care of the dying person at home and the family experiencing loss.

LOSS

Not all losses are obvious or immediate. Obvious losses are such events as the death of a loved one, divorce, breakup of a relationship, or loss of a job. Not so obvious are the losses precipitated by illness, aging, and changing schools, jobs, or neighborhoods.

Individuals experience many losses throughout life, and these losses often are **maturational loss** (a loss resulting from normal life transitions). They can occur as one experiences the loss of childhood dreams, the loss as an adolescent when a romance fails, and the loss felt when leaving the family home for college or marriage

TABLE 52-1 Losses

Types	Example
Physiological	Loss of body function, body structure, valued physical attribute
	Loss of body image through loss of extremity or breast
Psychological	Loss of self-esteem, self-concept, self-identity
	Loss of a job
Sociocultural	Loss of social identity, social role, or family constellation or cultural heritage
	Loss through divorce
	Loss of a loved one or significant other caused by death
Material	Loss of possessions, such as money, home, pet, car
	Loss of home by fire
	Loss of belongings through theft

Box 52-1 FACTORS INFLUENCING LOSS EXPERIENCES

- Childhood experiences
- Significance assigned to the loss
- Physical and emotional state
- Accumulated loss experience
- View of loss as crisis
- Visibility
- Duration and timing
- Abruptness or suddenness
- Financial impact
- Availability of resources
- Cultural factors
- Personal attributes
- Relationship with the lost person

and establishing a home of one's own. Later as one ages, the individual experiences menopause, and loss of hair, teeth, hearing, sight, and "youth." *Loss* may also be defined as a **situational loss** (loss occurring suddenly in response to a specific external event), such as the sudden death of a loved one or the unemployed person who suffers the loss of self-esteem. All these changes give the individual experience with loss and promote emotional growth and the activation of coping skills. These skills can later be used to cope with even more significant losses. Early experiences with loss can prepare individuals to deal with loss throughout the life cycle. Loss may be further described as shown in Table 52-1.

When death occurs after a long illness, each family member is affected psychologically, socioculturally, and materially. The person experiencing the death is affected in all of these areas, as well as physiologically.

Each person experiences loss as it individually affects him or her. Each loss is followed by a time of grief and grieving.

Personal loss is any significant loss that requires adaptation through the grieving process. Loss occurs when something or someone can no longer be seen, felt, heard, known, or experienced. The type of loss influences the degree of stress. For example, the loss of an object might not generate the same stress as the loss of a significant other. However, individuals respond to loss differently. The death of a family member would be expected to cause more stress than the loss of a pet, but for an older person living alone, the death of a pet that has been a constant companion would possibly cause more emotional stress than that of a cousin who had not been seen in years. The type of loss is significant to the grieving process; yet, the nurse must recognize that each person's interpretation of a loss is highly individualized.

Loss threatens self-concept, self-esteem, security, and sense of worth. The nurse must recognize the meaning of each loss to a patient and its impact on physical and psychological functioning.

Loss is a complex phenomenon influenced by many factors. See Box 52-1 for factors influencing loss experiences. A review of these factors is helpful in understanding what a specific loss means to an individual. Generalizations about personal experiences and behavior are useful only when one is committed to understanding and accepting individual variations.

GRIEF AND GRIEVING

Grief is the subjective response of emotional pain to actual or anticipated loss. Grief is a natural part of human experience. **Bereavement** is defined as a common depressed reaction to the death of a loved one. **Mourning** (reaction activated by a person to assist in overcoming a great personal loss) refers to culturally defined patterns for expressions of grief. Mourning patterns include funerals, wakes, memorials, black dress, and defined time of social withdrawal.

Nurses who work with the terminally ill and bereaved persons often develop a heightened empathy and identification with their patients. This occurs because the loss experience is so universal that everyone has experienced its impact. These losses can prepare persons for the ultimate loss in death. Grief is a normal and universal response to loss.

A review of the literature reveals many examples of increased **morbidity** (an illness or an abnormal condition or quality), both physical and mental, after significant losses. There is an increase in the breakup of marriages and other significant relationships after the loss of a child or when one partner suffers a loss of a body part or function.

Grief involves thought, feelings, and behaviors. Its purpose is to achieve more effective functioning, which takes time. The grieving person will try a variety of strategies in order to cope. The following tasks of grief facilitate healthy adjustment to loss:

1. Accepting the reality of the loss
2. Experiencing the pain of grief
3. Adjusting to an environment that no longer includes the lost person, the object, or the aspect of self
4. Reinvesting emotional energy into new relationships

These tasks are not sequential. In fact, grieving people may work on all four tasks simultaneously, or only one or two may be priorities. Nurses can assist patients and families in working through these tasks.

In the past, society discouraged openness during grief. Unhappy children were told not to cry when playmates moved away, awkward adolescents were told not to be embarrassed about sudden growth spurts, and dying persons were told to remain calm and dignified. Changes in attitudes, beliefs, and values have promoted more open expressions of grief. For example, nurses learn to seek support from peers in expressing their concerns about dealing with terminally ill patients. Similarly, family members seek support from care givers to express anger over loss. Grieving can lead to new understandings that promote growth. A person can grow from experiences of loss through openness, encouragement of others, and adequate support.

Behaviors and feelings associated with the grieving process occur in individuals suffering losses such as physical deformities or deaths of close friends. These behaviors and feelings also occur when individuals face their own deaths. The patient is also undergoing loss and the family's experience of grief.

There is no right way to grieve. The concept and theories of grief are only tools that can be used to anticipate the emotional needs of patients and families and plan interventions to help them understand their grief and deal with it.

A nurse should not classify the patient's grief; that is, the nurse should not identify a patient as experiencing a certain phase of grief or working on a certain grief-related task. The nurse's role is to assess grieving behaviors, recognize the influence of grief on behavior, and provide empathetic support.

Loss, through death or otherwise, is somewhat easier to cope with if it is expected. Sometimes the diagnosis of terminal illness allows a period of **anticipatory grief** (to expect, await, or prepare oneself for the loss of a family member or significant others) when both the dying person and the mourners can cry together and can share their affection for each other. Having time for anticipation does not necessarily ease the pain of loss, since attachment is often strengthened during the period of anticipatory grief. However, the emotions expressed at this time can make the loss less conflicted than when such exchanges never occur. When individuals achieve the maturity to realize that death is final and universal, this awareness of mortality often leads them to anticipate eventual grief and make a special effort to express affection and appreciation of their elderly relatives, even when there is no evidence of impending death.

The sudden death of someone who is not "supposed to" die (sometimes referred to as "out of sequence" death) is the most difficult grief to bear. The clearest example is the death of a child, especially one who has lived long enough to have a distinct personality and position in the family. If the death is a violent and sudden one, as most young people's deaths are, the loss is particularly devastating. Parents and siblings are often wracked by powerful and personal emotions of guilt, denial, and anger, as well as sorrow. One protective impulse is to blame someone—perhaps oneself for not having been more careful or more loving, perhaps a spouse, and perhaps even the dead child.

Blame and guilt, however, can destroy a family, just when family members need each other most. The Compassionate Friends, a self-help group for parents of dead children, finds that many married couples are driven apart by their separate reactions to the death. One parent might need to talk about the death while the other cannot bear to hear the child's name. Brothers and sisters of a dead child suffer too—partly because parents are so involved in their own grief that the surviving children are deprived of attention and partly because a child's grief may follow a different course from that of adults. Denial and regression are common at first, with sorrow and acceptance coming much later than for adults. Each family member should make an effort to understand and accept the many possible individual forms and paces of mourning that may be exhibited by others. Children in particular need to know that all questions and feelings are acceptable.

The nurse gathers data to make nursing diagnoses regarding grief or a patient's reaction to it. Clustering of patient or family behaviors, characteristics, and data involving the loss leads to an individualized nursing diagnosis. Identification of defining characteristics provides the basis for developing nursing interventions in the care plan (Box 52-2 on p. **1572**).

Nurse's Grief

Nurses may also experience grief when working with patients, especially with dying patients; as a result, their roles in supporting grieving patients and family can become complicated. However, they should never allow their grief to influence patients and families. Nurses who

Box 52-2 NANDA-APPROVED NURSING DIAGNOSES RELATED TO GRIEVING

Grieving, anticipatory, related to:
- Perceived potential loss of significant other
- Perceived potential loss of physiopsychosocial well-being
- Perceived potential loss of personal possessions

Grieving, dysfunctional, related to:
- Actual or potential object loss
- Thwarted grieving response
- Chronic fatal illness
- Lack of resolution of previous grieving response
- Loss of significant other
- Loss of physiopsychosocial well-being
- Loss of personal possessions

Adjustment, impaired, related to:
- Incomplete grieving

Nutrition, altered: less than body requirements, related to:
- Depressed grief response

Coping, ineffective family: compromised, related to:
- Temporary preoccupation by a significant person who is trying to manage emotional conflicts and personal suffering (anticipatory grieving) and is unable to perceive or act effectively in regard to patient's needs

Family processes, altered, related to:
- Situational transition or crisis

Hopelessness, related to:
- Failing or deteriorating physiological condition
- Long-term stress
- Abandonment
- Loss of belief in transcendent values or supreme being

Social isolation, related to:
- Inadequate personal resources

Spiritual distress (distress of the human spirit), related to:
- Separation from religious and cultural ties

Sleep pattern disturbance, related to:
- Stress of grief response

are not aware of their own grief issues have more difficulty in relating to patients as unique individuals; for example, a dying patient may remind the nurse of a beloved grandparent, so the nurse may become too emotionally involved. Other requisites for working with dying patients include coming to grips with understanding the grief process, appreciating the experience of the dying patient, using effective listening skills, acknowledging personal limits, and knowing when there is a need to get away and take care of the self.

Box 52-3 STRATEGIES TOWARD SURVIVAL FOR NURSES

- Take regular breaks or time-outs from the patient care area, and consider rotating out of high-stress areas.
- Identify specific patients who are the most stressful so that they can be anticipated.
- Trade off patients or ask for special assistance in working in these specific situations.
- Acknowledge physical needs as key factors in stress reduction.
- Integrate decompression routines into daily life. (Before leaving the work area take a moment to review the day and set it aside before going home.)
- Engage in life-affirming activities (for example, spend time with lively, healthy children).
- View losses as an opportunity to reevaluate and grow.
- Avoid the "rescuer" or "savior" complex; recognize limits.
- Recognize the need for support and do not hesitate to ask for it.
- Say "I choose" rather than "I should."
- Develop the skills of setting limits and feeling okay about saying "no."
- Laugh and play in the face of tragedy without guilt.
- Seek consultation on a regular basis.

When nurses experience multiple losses and fail to adequately process them, they can experience bereavement overload (the initial loss was compounded with an additional loss before resolution of the initial loss). They experience frustration, anger, guilt, sadness, helplessness, anxiety, depression, and feelings of being overwhelmed. Self-care is critical to survival. Nurses need to do for themselves what they do for their patients and families. They need to mourn their losses. This is done on an individual basis and as part of a larger group caring for the patient. Nurses need to develop personal support systems that allow time away from the care-giving setting, opportunities to share feelings in nonjudgmental, open relationships, and use of stress-management techniques that restore energy. Sometimes institutions provide opportunities for their staff to get together for mutual support and for closure and grieving over the loss of a patient. Nurses' roles in the care of the dying and bereaved are filled with experiences that bring grief and stress. They must attend to their need for relief from these demands. See Box 52-3 for strategies toward survival for nurses. Unrelieved grief and stress can lead to diminished well-being and inability to care for others.

Stages of Grief and Dying

The purpose of knowing about the stages of grief and dying is to recognize what emotions and behavior can

TABLE 52-2 Reactions to the Dying Process

Stage	Reaction	Description
Patient Reactions: Kübler-Ross*		
Stages of grieving/dying		
Denial and isolation	"No—not me." "There must be a mistake."	Serves as a buffer to the patient to shield oneself until the individual is able to mobilize alternate defenses.
Anger	"Why me?"	Hostility may be directed toward care givers or loved ones.
Bargaining	"Yes, but"	Bargaining is often made with God. It is an attempt to postpone death and is a positive way to maintain hope.
Depression	"Yes, me"	Sadness and grief. Time of introspection. Usually request only significant others to be with them. The patient struggles with painful realities of life and preparing for death.
Acceptance	"I am ready."	Resolved to the fact that death is imminent. Peaceful acceptance and positive feelings are often present.
Survivors Reaction: Martocchio†		
Manifestations of grief and bereavement		
Shock and disbelief	"Maybe this is not happening." "This is just a dream/nightmare."	Survivors feel a sense of unreality. Often reject offers of comfort and support. Disbelief may remain even though death is comprehended intellectually.
Yearning and protest	"Why do I feel this way?"	Survivors may express anger toward the deceased for leaving them.
Anguish, disorganization, and despair	"Living is a chore." "All the joy is gone out of life."	Reality and permanency of the loss are recognized.
Identification in bereavement	"I am just like him (dying or dead person)." "I will carry on her (dying person's) goals."	Bereaved may adopt behavior, ideals, mannerisms, or goals of the deceased.
Reorganization and restitution	"Life goes on." "The sun has risen on a new day."	Life stabilizes but some of the pain of loss may last for a lifetime.

*From Rawlins R, Williams S, Beck CK: *Mental health-psychiatric nursing* ed 3, St Louis, 1993, Mosby.
†From Martocchio B: Grief and bereavement healing through hurt, *Nurs Clin North Am* 20(2):327, 1985.

occur and to plan interventions accordingly as they appear.

Thanatology (the study of dying and death) sparked much interest, beginning in the 1970s. Two important works from **thanatologists** (one who studies dying and death) are Kübler-Ross' stages of dying and Martocchio's manifestations of grief. Both of these theories are essential for the nurse's understanding of the human reactions to the dying process (Table 52-2). Grief theory models demonstrate that in the normal grief process, there is an onset, active grief work, and a resolution or reorganization of the survivors' lives after their loss.

Unresolved Grief

Bereavement is a state of great risk physically, as well as emotionally and socially. For this reason, the importance of grief work cannot be stressed too much.

Various theorists have described behaviors indicative of unresolved grief. It is termed *unresolved grief* because there has been some disturbance of the normal progress toward resolution. See Box 52-4 on p. **000** for signs and symptoms of and behaviors reflecting unresolved grief. These individual signs, symptoms, and behaviors may be unremarkable during the acute stage of grief. However, they are major signs of incomplete grief work when they are manifested beyond the expected time for resolution (the power to make choices and set goals and to act on them firmly in spite of difficulty) of grief. The more signs, symptoms, and behaviors the mourner has, the stronger the likelihood of unresolved grief.

It is important for the nurse to recognize these individuals and refer them for appropriate counseling and/or treatment. See the nursing care plan on p. **000** for the patient experiencing **dysfunctional grieving,** unresolved grief, or complicated mourning (a severe

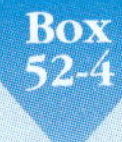

SIGNS, SYMPTOMS AND BEHAVIORS OF UNRESOLVED GRIEF (DYSFUNCTIONAL GRIEVING)

- Acquisition of symptoms belonging to the last illness of the deceased.
- Alteration in relationships with friends and relatives.
- Furious hostility against specific persons somehow connected with the death (physicians, nurses).
- Lasting loss of patterns of social interaction.
- Actions detrimental to one's social and economic well-being, for example, giving away belongings.
- Agitated depression with tension, insomnia, feelings of worthlessness, bitter self-accusation, obvious need for punishment, and even suicidal tendencies.
- History of delayed or prolonged grief.
- A feeling that the death occurred yesterday, even though the loss took place months or years ago.
- Unwillingness to move the possessions of the deceased after a reasonable amount of time.
- Inability to discuss the deceased without crying, particularly over a year after the loss.
- Major grief reactions triggered by a relatively minor event.
- Overidentification with the deceased.
- Phobias about illness or death.
- Diminished participation in religious and ritual activities that are part of the mourner's culture including avoidance of visiting the grave.
- Radical changes in life-style.
- Exclusion of friends, family members, or activities associated with the deceased.

chronic grief reaction in which the person does not complete the resolution stage of the grieving process within a reasonable time).

Supportive Care During the Dying and Grieving Process

To give compassionate nursing care and support to the family and patient during both the grieving and dying process, the nurse should consider the five aspects of human functioning. By using the nursing process, the nurse does an assessment in each aspect: physical, emotional, intellectual, sociocultural, and spiritual, to fully understand and adequately provide interventions in these areas.

Physical. While interviewing and observing the patient, the nurse should assess such areas as sleeping patterns, body image, activities of daily living (ADLs), mobility, general health, medications, and pain. The nurse also should address the basic needs of nutrition, elimination, oxygenation, activity, rest, sleep, and safety.

Goals for interventions should be (1) energy conservation, (2) pain reduction techniques, (3) comfort measures, (4) promotion of sleep and rest, and (5) increasing self-esteem through body image acceptance.

Emotional. Preparing for one's death is a personal endeavor filled with anxiety and fear. Assessing the patient and family's anxiety level, guilt, anger, level of acceptance, and identification is important. Major fears of the dying patient include fears of abandonment, loss of control, pain and discomfort, and the unknown.

The nurses intervene appropriately when they are able to accept the patient's and family's individual feelings, offer encouragement and support, and give the patient "permission to die" by assisting the patient in saying "good-bye."

Intellectual. Intellectual assessment includes an evaluation of the patient and family's educational level, their knowledge and abilities, and expectations they have in regard to how and when death will occur. Some aspects of the intellectual dimension can be altered during the dying process because of physiological changes, medications, the patient's emotional state, or the disease process. Being alert to these changes will avert problems if the patient's memory or sensations are decreased.

Intervention is directed toward patient/family education and support. Keeping all informed of procedures, changes in condition of the patient, and hospital policies contributes to well-informed decisions being made when necessary.

Social. Assessing the patient's and family's support systems is valuable. Ascertaining if family members desire to assist in the patient's daily care not only will lessen the family's sense of loss of control but also will clarify what tasks the family will do and what will be done by nursing staff. Not making these needs and desires clear can result in distrust and hostility between family and nursing staff. Each family and each individual member in that family are unique in what they wish to do. The nurse should never assume that families *want* to deliver daily care. Many do, but others do not, and they need the opportunity to make that choice (Box 52-5 on p. **1576**).

Family members must be supported through the dying and death of their loved one and, at the same time, be encouraged to provide support. In an institution, families often have greater difficulty giving support. The nurse must recognize the value of family members as resources and assist them in working with the dying person.

In the home the family becomes closely involved in the patient's care (see Chapters 48 and 53). A terminal illness places heavy demands on social and financial resources. The emotional strain often disrupts normal communication channels. The family may become afraid to interact with the patient.

NURSING CARE PLAN: PERSON EXPERIENCING DYSFUNCTIONAL GRIEVING (UNRESOLVED GRIEF)

Mrs. Swanson is 78 years old. She is being admitted for weakness, complaints of chronic fatigue, anorexia, and weight loss.

Her nursing history reveals she refuses to care for herself, has ceased participating in her church activities, and is unable to discuss the deceased without crying.

Her social history reveals her only child, a daughter, died unexpectedly at the age of 47. Her husband of 50 years died 1 year later. She is accompanied by her grandchildren who offer support and concern.

The nursing assessment reveals she lacks resolution of previous grieving response and is experiencing bereavement overload.

Nursing Goal/Expected Outcome: To promote resolution of the grieving process.

Nursing diagnosis	Patient goals/expected outcomes	Nursing interventions
Grieving, dysfunctional, related to bereavement overload secondary to death of daughter and husband manifested by refusing to care for self, abstaining from participation in church activities, the inability to discuss the deceased without crying, alterations in eating habits, and interference with performance of ADLs	1. Patient will establish new and meaningful relationships and interest. 2. Patient will engage in constructive, meaningful life-style (precrisis level of functioning). 3. Patient will relate realistically to both the pleasures and the disappointments of the loss relationships. 4. Patient will participate in decision making and cooperate with recommended treatment within 2 weeks.	Identify significance of multiple losses Discuss ambivalence Assess stage of grief and support patient's expressions of grief Use active listening Facilitate discussion of positive and negative aspects of loss Facilitate exploration of support groups Provide opportunities for social interaction, especially with those who coped with similar losses Teach patient and significant others about the grieving process Assure patient that feelings are normal Expect patient to meet responsibilities and give positive reinforcement Help patient identify ways to adapt life-style to accommodate loss Explore ways to assist patient to make new emotional investments If, you become uncomfortable with your unresolved feelings of loss, contact another nurse to counsel the patient

CRITICAL THINKING QUESTIONS

1. Mrs Swanson is admitted to the medical unit for severe weakness, weight loss, and chronic depression. She is reluctant to get out of bed to dress and have meals. To facilitate progression through the grieving process, the nurse would:
2. Mrs. Swanson appears thin, with poor tissue turgor. To encourage improvement of her nutritional status, the nurse and dietician would:
3. The nursing assessment for Mrs. Swanson revealed a flat affect, very little verbalization, and an unkempt body. To achieve patient goals/expected outcomes, the therapeutic nursing interventions would include:

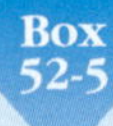

SUGGESTIONS FOR INVOLVING THE FAMILY IN THE CARE OF THE DYING PATIENT

- Assist in planning a visitation schedule for family members to prevent patient and family from becoming fatigued.
- Allow young children to visit a dying patient when the patient is able to communicate.
- Be willing to listen to family complaints about the patient's care and feelings about the patient.
- Help family members learn to interact with the dying person (e.g., using attentive listening, avoiding false reassurances, conducting conversations about normal family activities or problems).
- Allow family members to help with simple care measures such as feeding, bathing, and straightening bed linen. (Recognize that family members are often more successful than nursing staff in persuading the patient to eat.)
- When the family becomes fatigued with care activities, relieve them from their duties so that they can acquire needed rest and support. Refer them to resources for meals and lodging.
- Support the act of grieving between patient and family. Provide privacy when preferred. Do not discourage open expression of grief between family and patient.
- Provide information daily with regard to the patient's situation. Prepare the family for sudden changes in the patient's appearance and behavior.
- Communicate news of impending death when the family is together, if possible. Remember that members can provide support for one another.
- Convey the news in a private area and be willing to stay with the family.
- As death nears, help the family stay in communication with the dying person through short visits, caring silence, touch, and telling the patient of their love.
- After death, assist the family with decision making, such as selection of a mortician, transportation of family members, and collection of the patient's belongings.

When families choose to take the patient home for care, be sure that they are well prepared before discharge for what they need to know (see patient teaching box). Arrange for hospice services to assist the family, if they are receptive; emphasize continuity of care and 24-hour availability for when the patient is experiencing an emotional or physical crisis and needs ongoing support.

During the social assessment, it is necessary to learn whom the patient considers significant others. Although families are considered important, it is crucial to learn whom the patient considers the most supportive person in his or her life. It may be a friend, coworker, or church member. This person should become a part of the patient's supportive network and be included in planning the patient's care. The nurse encourages these social support persons to become involved and at the same time maintains and promotes the patient's independence whenever possible. By completing assessment, diagnosis, planning, implementation, and evaluation, the nurse can develop a nursing care plan.

PATIENT TEACHING: DYING PATIENT'S FAMILY

Goals/Expected Outcomes

- The family will be able to demonstrate basic patient care measures.
- Family will perform patient care independently as desired and appropriate.

Teaching Strategies

- Describe and demonstrate feeding techniques and selection of foods to facilitate ease of chewing and swallowing.
- Demonstrate bathing, mouth care, and other hygiene measures and allow family to perform return demonstration.
- Show video on simple transfer techniques to prevent injury to themselves and the patient; help family to practice.
- Instruct family on need to enforce rest periods.
- Teach family to recognize signs and symptoms to expect as the patient's condition worsens and information on whom to call in an emergency.
- Discuss ways to support the dying person and listen to needs and fears.
- Solicit questions from family and provide information as needed.
- Provide teaching, information, and encouragement in the use of creative outlets for expressing feelings and communicating with others. Encourage the use of tape-recorded messages, drawings, writings, imagery, music, and poetry. (This also assists patients and families in creating memories that can be very comforting later.)
- Inform patient and family of relaxation techniques.
- Observe the family and patient interacting using effective communication skills.

Spiritual. The nurse assesses the spiritual dimension by gaining insight into the patient's philosophy of life, religious resources, and how the rituals of the particular faith group have significance in dealing with his or her death.

NURSING CARE PLAN: PERSON FACING DEATH

Mrs. Borno is 68 years old and has been admitted to the hospital for weakness and debilitation caused by widespread metastatic cancer of the colon. She complains of pain and is anxious to return home. Both she and her family are aware of her terminal state.

The nursing history identified that (1) she is unable to care for herself because of severe weakness; (2) she has chronic pain; (3) she has a decreased appetite; (4) she appears anxious and wants to be home with her family; and (5) she is grieving the loss of her health and expresses fears regarding her death.

Nursing Goals: Control pain; prevent injury; ensure safety; provide for activities of daily living, including adequate nutrition, hydration, and elimination; relieve anxiety; and facilitate the normal grieving process.

Nursing diagnoses	Patient goals/expected outcomes	Nursing intervention
Pain, related to disease progression	Patient will be comfortable and without pain.	Position patient comfortably; change position gradually and unhurriedly. Provide pain-relief measures patient prefers (e.g., relaxation therapy, diversion, and distraction). Give analgesics as ordered. Evaluate pain for intensity and quality. Know that pain is what patient says it is.
Anxiety, severe, related to impending death	Patient will verbalize statements that reflect anxiety.	Allow patient to verbalize feelings and concerns. Explore how patient sees dying. Teach family members how to offer support effectively.
Self-care deficit, bathing/hygiene, dressing, toileting, related to advanced disease	Patient will carry out ADLs at highest ability.	Assist with ADLs but allow patient/family to assist when able. Provide sufficient time for ADLs.
Fear, related to evidence of metastasis	Patient will express fear of disease progression and prognosis. Patient will be able to deal with fears in a realistic way.	Encourage patient to discuss fears.Provide information as requested. Validate source of fear with patient; help identify effective coping skills. Encourage participation in support group or in one-to-one relationships.
Fatigue, related to anemia secondary to metastasis	The patient will have the energy she needs to assist with ADLs and to have short visits with significant others.	Help patient and family understand physiological basis for fatigue. Encourage patient to discuss feelings related to fatigue. Help patient plan rest and activity.
Nutrition, altered: less than body requirements, related to disease progression	The patient will be able to consume 40% of her meals.	Provide small feedings of high-calorie, high-protein foods and fluids. Assist with oral hygiene. Assist with environmental control (temperature, appearance, odors). Identify food preference and provide the preferences as often as possible.

Continued.

Nursing diagnoses	Patient goals/expected outcomes	Nursing intervention
Role performance, altered, related to inability to carry out normal functions of wife, mother, grandmother	Patient will interact with family as strength will allow.	Encourage patient to verbalize feelings and anxieties over altered role performance to facilitate normal grieving process.
Social isolation, related to hospitalization	Patient will be reunited with family.	Allow family to visit as much as possible. Involve patient in group activities.
Grieving, related to deteriorating health	Patient will be able to verbalize feelings of loss.	Allow patient to express feelings, including anger. Assist patient in identifying positive aspects of her life that can be used now.

CRITICAL THINKING QUESTIONS

1. Mrs. Borno complains of severe bone pain and nausea. She appears cachexic and extremely weak. To decrease Mrs. Borno's symptoms, the nursing interventions would include:
2. "I want to go home to die. I don't want to stay in the hospital. All I want to do is go home and be with my family," says Mrs. Borno. The hospice team could most benefically assist Mrs. Borno by:
3. When the nurse enters Mrs. Borno's room to begin ADLs, she notes extreme fatigue and lethargy. To conserve Mrs. Borno's strength, the nursing interventions would include:

Interventions in this area can come from clergy, friends, family, health care providers, and significant others. Supporting the patient and family's belief system and values is important (Chapter 8).

One aspect of this belief system is hope. Hope can take many forms; the challenge for the nurse is to help the patient and family identify those hopes that are most important to them and that will help them to cope.

Hope is multidimensional (taking many forms) and a changing life force. It is characterized by a confident, yet uncertain expectation of achieving a goal. Hope is not a single act but a complex series of thoughts, feelings, and actions that change often. Research studies have shown a significant relationship between the level of hope and the level of coping. The studies have also revealed that strength in religious connections and performance of family role responsibilities were significantly related to the variables of hope and coping.

The maintenance of hope can be difficult during the dying process. As the patient's condition deteriorates, the challenge becomes one of assisting the patient and family in translating their hope for a cure into realistic hopes that are focused on short-term, achievable goals. This may be the hope for a comfortable and pain-free life or the desire to live long enough to participate in some important family event, like the wedding of a child. A total lack of hope leads to distress of the human spirit. The relinquishment of hope is rapidly followed by death.

Special Supportive Care. Often death occurs outside the realm of serious illness, injury, or aging. Perinatal, pediatric, suicidal, and geriatric deaths are some examples that warrant special consideration.

Perinatal death. The death of a child is often viewed as one of the most devastating losses that can occur in a family. If the death of the child occurs before, during, or shortly after birth, it is called perinatal death.

Special considerations by health care providers should be addressed so that the parents and family can grieve adequately. Because there are no or few memories that loved ones can share about the child, "acting as though it never happened" places parents in jeopardy of living with unresolved grief. When possible, the parents should see, touch, and hold the infant, so that the reality of the situation can be faced and resolution of the grief can occur. Listening attentively and allowing the parents

TABLE 52-3 Children's Beliefs About Death

Age (Years)	Belief System
3	See death as a separation. Unable to comprehend permanency.
3 to 5	Fear death but see it as reversible. View death as a loss of an object.
6 to 10	Generally see death as permanent. Often have morbid feelings about death. Fear pain and mutilation.
11 to 18	Recognize death as permanent and irreversible. Attitudes and beliefs greatly influenced by parents. Often act as if they are invincible.

to express their feelings over their loss is beneficial. Referring to the baby as "your baby," "your son," or "your daughter," or using the given name can reinforce that the baby was indeed a unique individual who was loved and will be missed. The usual cultural rituals after death should take place for the baby, such as a funeral or memorial service.

Pediatric death. Children faced with death present a need for special nursing skills. Nurses should be aware of how children view or understand death, both for themselves and for others[33] (Table 52-3).

These children are usually aware that they are going to die. They often try to protect their parents. They need to be told the truth in language they can understand and be allowed to share fears, feelings, and opinions.

Parents and loved ones have much difficulty in accepting the reality of a child's impending death. Death of a child is an "out of sequence" death and therefore is often more difficult to accept. Parents often harbor extreme guilt. They may express hostility and anger toward health care providers, God, or the world in general. When a grandchild is dying, the grandparents suffer a double grief—for themselves and for their son or daughter. Siblings also are extremely affected and need much support at this time. Supportive group therapy is often beneficial for the survivors after a child's death, as well as during the dying process.

Suicide. Survivors of a person who has committed suicide suffer all the emotions of grief, in addition to profound guilt or shame (see Chapter 46). Because of this, they are at high risk for suicide themselves, and a grief counselor may be very helpful. Because suicide is usually not considered acceptable, many families of suicide victims are not given the same support from the church, community, or workplace as those whose loved ones have died from other causes. Because of the family's anger, fear, and shame, others do not reach out to help.

GERONTOLOGICAL CONSIDERATIONS

- Many older adults have long-standing religious beliefs that are likely to influence their response to death and dying. Spiritual counselors should be available if one is desired.
- Many older adults have come to acceptance of death; others remain in earlier stages. Verbalization of the "wish to die" may indicate acceptance or depression.
- Some older adults feel free to discuss death; others avoid this topic. The nurse's personal views regarding aging and death will have an impact on the older person's ability to provide appropriate emotional support.
- The older person may experience many losses that result in a grief response. These include loss of job, possessions, home, friends, spouse, and autonomy. The older adult often needs emotional support to cope with grief.
- Loss of a spouse in older adulthood is highly likely to result in a relocation. This increases the stress level of an already grieving older person and the risk of new health problems or an exacerbation of existing illness.
- Many older adults have initiated advanced directives regarding their wishes in case of terminal illness.
- Older adults have the right to a dignified death.

Gerontological death. It is often assumed that older adults will display some understanding and acceptance toward the death process. This is not always true. The older patient must be treated as an individual, and the nurse should assess the patient's needs in the same way as for any patient facing a terminal illness (see gerontological box). It is important to include the older person in self-care and in decisions to undergo or refuse extensive therapeutic or resuscitative measures. Even when aggressive technological options are rejected, patients still need to have intensive nursing interventions and pain control. Families who suffer the loss of an older person may accept the death but nonetheless must experience the grieving process.

Other considerations in caring for dying patients include such issues as euthanasia, DNR, organ donations, fraudulent treatment methods, and the Dying Person's Bill of Rights.

ISSUES RELATED TO DYING AND DEATH

Euthanasia

Euthanasia may be active euthanasia (Greek for "easy death"), an action deliberately taken with the purpose of shortening life to end suffering or to carry out the wishes of a terminally ill patient. There is also passive euthanasia, which is permitting the death of a patient that takes the form of withholding treatment that might extend life, such as medication, life-support systems, or feeding tubes.

Although active euthanasia is highly controversial, most people are not in favor of preserving life in all cases. In a New York Times–CBS Poll taken in 1990, 53% of the respondents said that physicians should be allowed to assist an ill person in taking his or her own life.[25] These changing attitudes over the past 25 years can be attributed to technologies that can keep patients alive indefinitely after the brain has, for all practical purposes, stopped functioning. These are thorny ethical questions for society and for patients and their families. There is a pressing need to define and monitor a problem that one physician has called "so fundamental that it has moved beyond the boundaries of medicine."[6]

Do Not Resuscitate

Patients and families should control any decisions relative to any conditions that withhold or withdraw treatment. Death with dignity remains a concern for all. A do not resuscitate (DNR) decision should be a joint decision of the patient, family, and health care providers. All facts regarding the patient's condition should be explained to the patient and family, as well as all treatment options. **DNR** means *only* not to resuscitate. It does not mean to withhold any other care, such as hygiene, nutrition, fluids, or medications. All DNR orders and the discussion with the patient and family should be thoroughly documented in the patient's chart (Box 52-6).

Advanced Directives

The issue of advanced directives has come to the forefront of many states within the last few years. **Advanced directives** are signed and witnessed documents providing specific instructions for health care treatment in the event that a person is unable to make those decisions personally at the time they are needed. Documents may take the form of a **living will** (a legal document drawn up by the person who is not yet near death, detailing how much medical care he or she wants to receive if terminally ill), which describes wishes regarding medical care. This document can assist the family and health care providers in carrying out an individual's wishes. In some states the living will is legally binding. Courts in some states where living wills are not recognized as legal documents have upheld treatment decisions that a competent, rational adult has personally made.

Advanced directives are based on the right to self-determination. Every adult has the freedom to accept or refuse recommended medical treatment. Every person who completes an advanced directive should give a copy to his or her regular physician and to family or friends to ensure that it is available if necessary.

Box 52-6 CHARACTERISTICS OF ACCEPTABLE DO NOT RESUSCITATE (DNR) ORDERS

A medical order *not* to resuscitate a patient is an acceptable order when:

- The order is documented in the written medical record
- The order specifies the exact nature of the treatment to be withheld
- Patients, when they are able, and families participate in the decision
- The decision not to resuscitate is discussed with care givers, including the nurses
- The order is periodically reviewed
- Staff realize the order is not equivalent to medical or psychological abandonment of patients

Do not resuscitate (DNR) orders are commonly understood to mean the withholding of CPR, which is used to treat cardiac arrest. It involves external chest compression and some form of artificial respiration. Because of potential misunderstanding of what the DNR order specifically means, it is advisable that the DNR order be written identifying the exact condition not to be treated and the specific intervention to be withheld. The practice of not writing the DNR order is unacceptable. In fact, the medical record, read as a whole, should reveal the clear responsibility for the DNR order, the rationale for it, and the process used in its formulation. Some hospitals and nursing homes may have more specific requirements in their policies that the medical/surgical nurse should follow.

Every competent adult has the right to refuse treatment, even life-sustaining procedures, such as CPR. The patient's informed consent should be obtained by the physician who will write the order, and should be documented in the medical record. Or, if the patient is unable to consent, the patient's family participation should be sought and documented. The patient's incapacity to participate must also be documented to reflect the rationale for involving the family. In some states the law may be that when it is two physicians' opinion that a patient lacks capacity to consent, a surrogate is sought from a list provided in the law. That surrogate must consent to the DNR order.

DNR orders must be reviewed periodically, because the patient's status may change or new knowledge may come to light about the patient's condition. Continual review of the DNR order helps reassure staff that they are not abandoning the patient; it will also ensure that the "hopeless" patient is still cared for.

A person may revoke the advanced directive at any time in any manner in which the person is able to communicate that intent (Box 52-7).

Organ Donations

Legally competent persons are free to donate their bodies or organs for medical use. Consent forms are available for this purpose. In many states adults may request organ donation by signing the back of their driver's licenses. A nurse may serve as a witness when individuals wish to give consent for the donations of organs, tissue, or the body.

In most states, required request laws stipulate that at the time of a person's death, a qualified health care giver must ask family members to consider organ or tissue donation. In the past this option has not been offered. Required request laws came about because of the shortage of suitable organs for transplantation.

The Uniform Anatomical Gifts Act addresses many problems of organ donation and stipulates that the physician who certifies death shall not be involved in removal or transplantation of the organs. The National Organ Transplantation Act prohibits selling or purchasing organs and facilitates this area of medical and nursing practice. Organ and tissue donations remain voluntary.

These donations can include the following:

Body organs	Body tissue
Kidney	Cornea
Heart	Bone
Lung	Skin
Heart-lung	Heart valve
Liver	
Pancreas	

Box 52-7 THE LIVING WILL AND DURABLE POWER OF ATTORNEY

People who receive extraordinary measures to prolong life are often unconscious or mentally incompetent by the time these measures are put into effect. Therefore by deciding ahead of time what kind of care you want and communicating these decisions to others, you can do much to ensure that you receive the extent of care that you want. This can be done through such documents as a living will and a medical durable power of attorney. If your state has adopted legislation for either or both documents, you should use the legally approved wording.

A living will should be addressed, and copies of it should be given to your family doctor, your attorney, and close family members. It specifies that if the time comes when you can no longer take part in decisions for your own future, this statement will stand as an expression of your wishes and directions while you are still of sound mind.

You may, for example, direct that if a situation should arise in which there is no reasonable expectation of recovery from extreme physical or mental disability, you be allowed to die and not be kept alive by medications, artificial means, or "heroic measures." You may also, of course, use a living will to request such measures to keep you alive as long as possible. You may request pain-relieving medication, even though it may shorten your life. You may spell out specific provisions with regard to, for example, cardiac resuscitation, mechanical respiration, antibiotics, tube feeding, and permission to offer your organs as transplants to other people.

Some "living will" legislation applies only to terminally ill patients—not to patients who are incapacitated by illness or injury but may live many years in severe pain, who are in a coma, or who are in some other greatly disabled state. Therefore it is advisable to draw up a **durable power of attorney,** an instrument that appoints another person to make decisions in the event of your incompetence. A number of states have enacted statutes expressly for decisions about health care, known as a "medical durable power of attorney." In these states, filling out a form is all that is required; you do not have to consult an attorney.

Depending on the statute, the agent you appoint (someone you trust and have confidence in) may give, withdraw, or withhold consent to specific medical or surgical measures; hire and fire medical personnel; gain access to your medical records; go to court to carry out your wishes; spend or withhold funds for treatment; and interpret your living will.

REMEMBER:

- Both documents need to be signed and dated before two witnesses who are not blood relatives and to whom you are not leaving property.
- For the durable power of attorney, you must have your signature notarized. If you choose more than one proxy for decision making on your behalf (a good idea in case your first choice is not available), give an order of priority (1, 2, 3).
- Give a copy to your physician to keep in your medical file, and be sure that the physician agrees with your wishes.
- Give copies to close relatives, friends, or both.
- Tell the above people about your intentions now.
- Look over your living will once a year. Redate it and initial the new date to make it clear that your wishes are unchanged.[32]

Box 52-8

THE DYING PERSON'S BILL OF RIGHTS

I have the right to be treated as a living human being until I die.

I have the right to maintain a sense of hopefulness however changing its focus may be.

I have the right to be cared for by those who can maintain a sense of hopefulness, however changing this might be.

I have the right to express my feelings and emotions about my approaching death in my own way.

I have the right to participate in decisions concerning my care.

I have the right to expect continuing medical and nursing attention even though "cure" goals must be changed to "comfort" goals.

I have the right not to die alone.

I have the right to be free from pain.

I have the right to have my questions answered honestly.

I have the right not to be deceived.

I have the right to have help from and for my family in accepting my death.

I have the right to die in peace and dignity.

I have the right to retain my individuality and not be judged for my decisions which may be contrary to beliefs of others.

I have the right to discuss and enlarge my religious and/or spiritual experiences, whatever these may mean to others.

I have the right to expect that the sanctity of the human body will be respected after death.

I have the right to be cared for by caring, sensitive, knowledgeable people who will attempt to understand my needs and will be able to gain some satisfaction in helping me face my death.

From Barbus A: The dying patient's bill of rights, *Am J Nurs* p 99, Jan 1975.

Fraudulent Methods of Treatment

Often patient and family seek unconventional methods of treatment to prolong the patient's life. Such treatments may include special diets, enemas, unproven drugs, and machines or devices. Nurses may assist patients and families in sorting out which treatments are real and which are fraudulent. Fraudulent treatments are those that are misrepresented, whether by concealment or nondisclosure of facts, for the purpose of inducing another to use the product. Any treatment that does not offer the patient informed consent with information regarding options, results, and approvals from federal agencies should be suspect.

Rights of Dying Patients

Death with dignity is the goal in caring for the dying patient. Box 52-8 shows the Dying Person's Bill of Rights.

THE DYING PATIENT

Guidelines for Communicating With the Dying Patient

Therapeutic communication expresses respect for the patient, maintains realistic hope, and offers appropriate reassurance and support. Supportive words without an accompanying supportive attitude will ring hollow and fail to provide comfort; reassurance that is unrealistic or given merely to calm a patient will not work. Stating that, "Everything will be just fine," when this is untrue, will only increase the patient's anxiety and violate the trust in the care giver. It is far better to give reassurance in a limited way that is consistent with the facts.

Therapeutic communication will also require careful attention to what the patient expresses verbally and nonverbally. Interpretations or summaries of the patient's thoughts and feelings should always be checked out with the patient for their accuracy and effect.

If patients do not wish to communicate at a particular time, they need to know that this is acceptable and will be respected. Care givers should indicate a willingness to return at another time, when the patient will feel more comfortable. The most important way in which to help is to be available to actively listen, nonjudgmentally, and with acceptance, allowing the patient to express emotions and feelings without fear.

Behavior that indicates we are listening to the patient is "attending behavior." It includes appropriate eye contact, attentive body language, and verbal following. Eye contact is especially important for dying patients, since they may receive numerous messages of rejection from other members of society.

A unique problem in communicating with physically ill patients is that the care giver is usually standing up while the patient is typically lying down in bed. This increases the patient's feelings of regression and being out of control, dependent, and helpless. Nurses should show their attentiveness in nonverbal as well as verbal ways. For instance, the nurse can choose to sit in a chair close to the patient's bed to minimize the physical distance and the emotional distance it implies. When appropriately used, touching is a very effective means of communication. Later in the illness, when strength for or interest in verbal communication has dwindled, touching is particularly important. The hand that is held, the arm that is patted, the tear that is gently wiped all indicate attending behavior as well as concern and care.

It is vitally important to remember that there is no way for a patient to "solve" the problem of dying. However, there are ways nurses can share the attendant feelings and fears of the patient. Through open and sensitive communication with the dying patient, nurses not only facilitate the expression of emotion, but also affirm that the patient is a living human being who is being supported and cared about.

Assisting the Patient in Saying Good-bye

Many terminally ill patients are fully aware that they are dying. One of their most difficult tasks is in the "saying of good-byes" to their loved ones. Saying good-bye acknowledges leaving and may be expressed in verbal, nonverbal, concrete, and symbolic ways. By working through these tasks, the family members are moving toward the completion of unfinished business with the patient. Unfinished business will compound the transition through the grieving process. This is an area where nurses can assist the dying person and the family (see therapeutic dialogue).

THERAPEUTIC DIALOGUE

Family Support

Family member: I can't go back in that room. He just lies there and stares. I don't know what to do or say.

Nurse: Being near someone who is dying can be uncomfortable.

Family member: It makes me so sad to see him like that. Do you think he knows I'm there?

Nurse: It's very possible that he does. Would you like me to go in with you?

Family member: Yes, please. I wonder if he can hear me?

Nurse: It must be very difficult for you not to be certain that he is hearing you. If there is something you want to say to him, get close, take his hand, and speak directly to him. Most people in his condition can hear but are very weak and may not have the strength to respond.

Family member: I just feel like I am not able to do anything for him anymore.

Nurse: Just being there is letting him know that you care. That's something very important to any person.

Family member: I suppose you're right. I guess I'm ready to go in now.

Nurse: I'll be right here next to you.

First, the nurse can provide a private, comfortable environment. The patient may request that the nurse or another health care provider be present or very nearby to be of assistance if emotional expression becomes overwhelming. Patients can be assisted in saying their good-byes through role playing, letter writing, or audio or video recording. Helping patients focus on what they want to say can be facilitated by asking them to talk to their loved ones as if they were going to be separated for a long time. They should be encouraged to express those feelings and thoughts they would most want their loved ones to know in their absence. Asking a dying person what he would want to say to his 6-year-old when the child is 12 can help the patient formulate appropriate letters or tape recordings. Often dying patients become depressed because they do not have a purpose in life. Working on tasks, such as poems, letters, and recordings, affords patients feelings of control and productivity in their last days.

Physical Care

The nurse has an important responsibility in assisting patients to meet their physical needs. Providing adequate nutrition and maintaining elimination patterns are priorities in providing for the dying patient's physical needs (see Chapter 53). Keeping the patient clean, dry, well groomed, odor free, and comfortable decreases the chances of skin impairment and also provides the patient with feelings of self-esteem and self-worth (see Chapter 16).

Adjusting the environment to increase comfort and safety is paramount. Side rails should be used for both safety and assisting weak patients to adjust their own positions when possible.

Assessments and Interventions for the Dying Patient

Care of the dying patient has many facets. Of all the needs of the dying patient, the three most crucial are the needs for control of pain, preservation of dignity and self-worth, and love and affection.

One of the nurse's ideal goals should be not only to allay the physical suffering of patients as best possible, but also to help them prepare for recognition and acceptance of this reality of life (death) so that they can undertake their last task in life with credit and dignity. There is a clear mandate for family, friends, and care givers to make sure that the abandonment that is so frequently a part of the dying patient's experience does not occur. It must be repeated—one of the worst fears of any individual is to be left to die alone.

The patient near death continues to need meticulous nursing interventions. Because of the increased weakness and deterioration of the body, the patient's physical needs are important. Although patients may appear comatose, unconscious, or unresponsive, this appearance is often a result of extreme fatigue, and the nurse will find that patients are aware of those activities occurring around them. Table 52-4 on p. **1584** shows signs of approaching death as expressed in physical needs and the appropriate interventions.

Changes in vital signs include (1) slow, weak, and thready pulse; (2) lowered blood pressure; and (3) rapid, shallow, irregular, or abnormally slow respirations. Mouth breathing occurs, which leads to dry oral mucous membranes. The patient often has a detached look in the

TABLE 52-4 Nursing Interventions for the Patient Near Death

Physical Needs	Nursing Interventions
1. Decreased sensations and reflexes	1. Suctioning of respiratory tract as needed.
2. Decreased circulation	2. Careful skin care and range-of-motion exercises
3. Decreased sphincter control (urinary and bowel incontinence)	3. Frequent change of position, at least q2h
4. Decreased hearing and sight	4. Meticulous hygiene, including oral care
5. Decreased need for pain medication	5. Clear and slow verbal communication; stand or sit within patient's vision
6. Increased need for touch	6. Evaluate and differentiate between pain and anxiety and treat accordingly
7. Usually conscious	7. Touch gently
	8. Involve patient in care; explain all actions
	9. Perform all nursing interventions with compassion and preservation of the patient's dignity

eyes. There is a diminished sensory and motor function in the lower extremities, progressing to the upper extremities. There is diminished touch sensation; pressure and pain sensations remain intact. As death becomes imminent, the pupils will become dilated and fixed, Cheyne-Stokes respirations will occur, the pulse will become increasingly weaker and more rapid, and the blood pressure will continue to fall. There is diminished peripheral circulation. The skin is cool and clammy; profuse diaphoresis may occur. If collection of mucus occurs in the throat, noisy respirations will be heard. This sound is referred to as the *death rattle.* A period of peace may immediately precede the moment of death. The clinical signs of death are the following:

1. Unreceptivity and unresponsiveness
2. No movement or breathing
3. No reflexes
4. Flat encephalogram
5. Absence of apical pulse
6. Cessation of respirations

Postmortem Care

In most states the physician is responsible for certifying a death in the medical record. The time of death and a description of therapies or actions taken are described in the medical record. The physician may request permission from the family for the **autopsy** (examination performed after a person's death to confirm or determine the cause of death). Autopsies are required in circumstances of unusual death (for example, violent trauma or unexpected death in the home).

The nurse may be the best person to care for the patient's body after death **(postmortem care)** because of the therapeutic nurse-patient relationship; thus, the nurse may be more sensitive to the need for caring for the patient's body with dignity and sensitivity. The body should be cared for as soon as possible after death to prevent tissue damage or disfigurement. If the family has requested organ donation, appropriate measures must be taken immediately.

The nurse offers the family the opportunity to view the body. It may help to suggest that this is an opportunity to say "good-bye" to their loved one, especially if they were not present at the time of death. If the family hesitates to view the body, the nurse lets them think about it. If they decide not to view the body, the nurse accepts their decision without judgment. If the family decides to view the body, they are assured that they will not be alone and that the nurse will be glad to accompany them or will request whomever they would like to be present. The nurse spends as much time as possible assisting the grieving family and offers to contact other support services, such as social services and the spiritual adviser. (Many health care facilities now employ a full-time chaplain who may be summoned in the event of death.) The family now becomes the patient.

After the patient has been pronounced dead by a physician or professional nurse and before the family views the body, the nurse prepares it and the room to minimize the stress of the experience. The nurse removes supplies and equipment from sight. Tubes remaining in the body are removed, clamped, or cut to within 1 inch (2.5 cm) of the skin and taped in place. Care of tubes and specimens depends on agency policy, as well as whether an autopsy will be performed. Soiled linen and other clutter should be removed. A spray deodorizer may eliminate unpleasant odors.

The nurse prepares the body by making it look as natural and comfortable as possible. If the body is placed in the supine position with arms at the sides, palms down or across the abdomen, a **mortician** (person trained in the care of the dead) can better prepare it for interment. The nurse places a small pillow or folded towel under the head to prevent discoloration from blood pooling. The eyelids usually remain closed if gently held down for a few seconds. If this does not occur, a moistened cotton ball will hold them in place.

The nurse inserts the patient's dentures to maintain normal facial features. A rolled-up towel under the chin keeps the mouth closed (Skill 52-1).

CARE OF THE BODY AFTER DEATH

Nursing action/Rationale

1. Gather equipment *to organize procedure.*
2. Wash hands *to reduce spread of organisms.*
3. Don clean gloves *to protect nurse from contamination.*
4. Close patient's eyes and mouth if needed *to provide a more normal appearance.*
5. Remove all tubings and other devices from patient's body *to make patient look more peaceful.*
6. Place patient in supine position *for access for procedures.* Elevate the head *to prevent discoloration.*
7. Replace soiled dressings with clean ones *to avoid odor.*
8. Bath patient as necessary *to reduce odor.*
9. Brush or comb hair *for more normal appearance.*
10. Apply clean gown *for appearance.*
11. Care for valuables and personal belongings *for legal considerations.*
12. Allow family to view body and remain in room *to provide emotional support if family wishes.*
13. After the family has left the room, attach special label if patient had a contagious disease *to protect those who handle the body.*
14. Close door to room *to prevent exposure to patients and visitors.*
15. Await arrival of ambulance or transfer to morgue *out of respect for patient.* Some agencies use a shroud to enclose the body before transfer to the morgue.
16. Document procedure and disposition of patient's body as well as belongings and valuables *for legal purposes.*

At the time of death, the nurse must also make notation of any valuables, such as watch, rings, or money, and secure these articles so that they may be delivered to the family according to agency policy.

Documentation

Documentation of the care given to the dying patient must be objective, complete, legible, and accurate. As death approaches, documentation should be frequent and include the signs of impending death as they occur. Recording who was present at the time of the patient's death is important. The nurse should continue to chart until the last entry states where and to whom the body was transferred.

SUPPORT OF THE GRIEVING FAMILY

The grieving family and significant others' needs should be met by a caring, compassionate health care provider. If an individual is alone at the time of the loved one's death, it is essential that all attempts be made to contact someone—family, clergy, or friends—to be with the grieving individual. Words that convey sympathy should be expressed, and if appropriate, a spontaneous touch, such as a hand on the arm or embrace, can be used as a comforting gesture. Any questions should be answered, and the family should be encouraged to view, touch, and talk to the dead family member. Be nonjudgmental as the individual expresses anger, guilt, or unfairness. Assist in notifying the mortician and any individuals involved in the procurement of donated organs.

Informing others can be a major emotional step for family members. Being present and offering assistance in this area can be very supportive. Directing family members to support groups and other referral agencies (churches, therapists, social workers) will facilitate the expansion of the family's social network, as well as foster relatedness and decrease isolation.

Grief work as described by Martocchio is as follows.

1. Emancipation of the bereaved from bondage to the deceased
2. Readjustment to an altered environment
3. Development of any new or renewed relationships
4. Learning to live in a comfortable fashion with memories of hurt, happiness, suffering, and joys associated with the deceased

EVALUATION CRITERIA FOR THE GRIEVING FAMILY

Resolution of grief has begun when, after the loss, the grieving person and/or family can complete the following tasks:

1. Have positive interactions with others
2. Participate in support groups with others similarly bereaved to share expressions of loss and offer companionship

3. Establish goals, and work to achieve them
4. Discuss the meaning of the loss and its effect on the person's life

Dealing with the grief that comes with the loss of a loved one requires support and understanding. Six months to 2 years may elapse before an individual can complete grief work and begin the full process of resolution. Many believe that four seasons must pass before the bereaved can begin to think of the deceased without feeling intense emotional pain.[15]

REFERENCES AND SUGGESTED READINGS

1. Antomacci M: Sudden death: helping bereaved parents in the PICU, *Crit Care Nurse* 10(4):65, 1990.
2. Arnold J: Grieving, *Imprint* 37(1):53, 1990.
3. Badzek LA: What you need to know about advanced directives, *Nursing* 22(6):58, 1992.
4. Beare P, Myers J: *Principles and practice of adult health nursing,* St Louis, 1990, Mosby.
5. Benner KL, Terminal weaning: a loved one's vigil, *Am J Nurs* 93(5):22, 1993.
6. Carton RW: The road to euthanasia, *JAMA* 263(16):2221, 1990.
7. Colt GH: *The enigma of suicide,* New York, 1991, Summit Books.
8. Coyle N: The last four weeks of life, *Am J Nurs* 90(12):75, 1990.
9. Coyle N et al: Character of terminal illness in the advanced cancer patient: pain and other symptoms during the last four weeks of life, *J Pain Symptoms Manage* 5:8393, 1990.
10. Devich L et al: Supportive care for the hopelessly ill, *Nurs Outlook* 38(3):140, 1990.
11. Dufault K, Martocchio BC: Hope: Its spheres and dimensions, *Nurs Clin North Am* 20:379, 1985.
12. Ebersole P, Herr P: *Towards healthy aging: human needs and nursing responses,* ed 3, St Louis, 1990, Mosby.
13. Editors of Nursing 91: Meeting the challenge of a dying patient, *Nursing* 21(2):42, 1991.
14. Freiberg KL: *Human development: a life span approach,* ed 4, Boston, 1992, Jones & Bartlett.
15. Gifford BJ, Cleary BB: Supporting the bereaved, *Am J Nurs* 90(2):48, 1990.
16. Grassman D: Turning personal grief into personal growth, *Nursing* 22(4):43, 1992.
17. Hecks B: The gift of courage, *Nursing* 22(12):88, 1992.
18. Hogan NS, Balk DE: Adolescent reaction to sibling death: perceptions of mothers, fathers, and teenagers, *Nurs Res* 39(2):103, 1990.
19. Kim MJ, McFarland GK, McLane A: *Pocket guide to nursing diagnoses,* St Louis, 1991, Mosby.
20. Kübler-Ross E: A letter to a nurse about death and dying, *Nursing* 21(11):78, 1991.
21. Kübler-Ross E: *On death and dying,* New York, 1969, Macmillan.
22. Kübler-Ross E: *To live until we say good-bye,* Englewood Cliffs, NJ, 1978, Prentice-Hall.
23. Kuntz BB: Grief has no color, *Am J Hospice Palliative Care,* 8(1): 35, 1991.
24. Long BC, Phipps WJ, Cassmyer V: *Medical-surgical nursing: a nursing process approach,* ed 3, St Louis, 1993, Mosby.
25. Malcolm AH: Giving death a hand: rending issue, *The New York Times,* June 9, 1990.
26. Martocchio B: Authenticity, belonging, emotional closeness and self-representation, *Oncol Nurs Forum* 14(4):23, 1987.
27. Martocchia B: Grief and bereavement healing through hurt, *Nurs Clin North Am* 20(2):327, 1985.
28. McIntosh JL et al: *Suicide and its aftermath: understanding and counseling the survivors,* New York, 1987, WW Norton.
29. Moses M, Perry P: *Closer to the light: learning from children's near-death experiences,* New York, 1990, Random House.
30. Mulhern RM: When there's no treatment left but the truth, *RN* 49:26, 1986.
31. O'Connor AP: Understanding the cancer patient's search for meaning, *Cancer Nurs* 13:167, 1990.
32. Paplia DE, Olds-Wendbos S: *Human development,* 5th ed, New York, 1992, McGraw-Hill.
33. Potter PA, Perry AG: *Fundamentals of nursing: concepts, process, and practice,* ed 3, St Louis, 1993, Mosby.
34. Rawlins RP, Williams SR, Beck CK: *Mental health-psychiatric nursing,* ed 3, St Louis, 1993, Mosby.
35. Rosen SL: Stillbirth: what nurses should and should not do, *Imprint* 37(1):68, 1990.
36. Salloday SA, McDonnel MM: Facing ethical conflicts, *Nursing* 22(2):43, 1992.
37. Schoenbeck SB: Exploring the mystery of near-death experiences, *Am J Nurs* 93(5):42, 1993.
38. Snyder R et al: Should nurses pronounce death? *Nurs* 90(60):41, 1990.
39. Steinman FJ: When mommy dies, *Am J Hospice Palliative Care 8(1):42, 1991.*
40. Ufema J: Helping loved ones say good-bye, *Nursing* 21(12):42, 1991.
41. Ufema J: Insights on death and dying, *Nursing* 22(8):87, 1992.
42. Wallace B: The right to die rightly—right ignored, *Hospice,* 3(3):10, 1992.
43. Waltman RE: When a spouse dies, *Nursing* 22(7):48, 1992.
44. Walfelt AD: Toward an understanding of complicated grief: a comprehensive overview, *Am J Hospice Palliative Care* 8(2):28, 1991.

CHAPTER CHALLENGE

KEY POINTS

- Care of the dying patient has moved from the home to hospitals and back again over the past 50 years.
- In 1969, Kübler-Ross was instrumental in identifying the five stages of death and dying: denial, anger, bargaining, depression, and acceptance.
- Losses occur throughout the life cycle and provide the individual experience with loss and promote emotional growth and development of coping skills.
- The effect a loss will have on a person is individualized and may be determined by duration, abruptness, extent, time required for treatment or replacement, or financial impact of the loss.
- Grief is an active not a passive process; it takes work and emotional energy.
- When people do not do "grief work" following any significant loss, they are at risk for emotional, mental, and social problems.
- The grief theory demonstrates that in the normal grief process, there is an onset, active grief work, and a resolution or reorganization of the survivors' lives after the loss.
- Nurses experience all the emotions of grief not only in response to their own loss, but also in response to the death of their patients.
- A nurse must assess whether family members are willing to be involved in a dying patient's care before using them as resources.
- The major concerns of the dying patient are (1) fear of abandonment, (2) fear of loss of control, (3) fear of pain and discomfort, and (4) fear of the unknown.
- Euthanasia is an ethical and legal issue faced by nurses. Active euthanasia is illegal in the United States.
- A do not resuscitate (DNR) order means only that. It does not mean to withhold hygiene, hydration, nutrition, or medications.
- Patients who decide ahead of time what kind of care they want and communicate these decisions to others can do much to ensure that they receive the extent of care that they want. This is called advanced directives and may involve the living will and/or durable power of attorney.
- The Dying Person's Bill of Rights speaks to the elements that may characterize dying with dignity.
- Assisting a dying patient in saying "good-byes" is an intervention nurses can initiate.
- The physical care requirements of the dying patient are primarily nursing interventions. Providing adequate nutrition, elimination, hygiene, safety, and comfort are nursing priorities.
- Continuing to speak to and include the patient in his or her care is essential, since as death approaches, the dying patient becomes weaker. Patients may appear comatose and yet be aware of activities around them.
- Signs of impending death are (1) slow, thready, and weaker pulse, (2) lowered blood pressure, (3) rapid shallow, irregular, or abnormally slow respirations, and (4) mottling of lower extremities.
- Postmortem care is the care administered to the body after death. Procedures including cleansing, positioning, and labeling the body, should be followed.

STUDY QUESTIONS

1. During end-of-shift report it is stated that Mrs. Brown, 86 years old, is dying as a result of end stage renal disease. As her nurse you recall dying is considered:
   1. undesirable at any time
   2. a failure for the nurse
   3. impossible with modern medical devices
   4. the final stage of human growth and development
2. A nurse on your unit attempts to avoid caring for Mrs. Seachord, 92 years old, who is dying of congestive heart failure. If the nurse cannot avoid caring for this patient, she provides care, but in a detached manner. This nurse is demonstrating:
   1. poor nursing care
   2. grief reaction
   3. withdrawal
   4. bereavement
3. Mrs. Burke, 65 years old, has been admitted with various physical complaints due to unresolved grief. During her morning care she says, "It's been 6 months since Harry died. When is it going to get easier?" An appropriate answer by the nurse concerning grief work completion would be that grief work is completed:
   1. when the family returns to work, school, and social activities
   2. after the funeral, wake, or memorial services
   3. as soon as the bereaved can talk freely
   4. on an individualized basis
4. Mrs. Burke, 77 years old, has been admitted with pneumonia. Her husband asks the nurse about the living will. As a licensed nurse you remember that living wills:

1. allow the courts to decide when care can be given
2. allow the individual to express his or her wishes regarding care
3. are legally binding in all states
4. allow health care workers to withhold fluids and medications

5. Mr. Lewis, 36 years old, is in the terminal stages of leukemia and has been admitted to the hospital, because it has become too difficult for his family to care for him at home. As the nurse admitting him, you recall that Mr. Lewis would experience which type of loss?
   1. aspect of self
   2. significant others
   3. known environment
   4. external objects

6. Mrs. Shank, age 35, has just died as the result of multiple injuries caused by a motor vehicle accident. To provide therapeutic support to her family, the nurse is knowledgeable that grieving:
   1. helps to promote good mental and physical health after a loss
   2. should be carried out in solitude
   3. is socially unacceptable in society today
   4. increases emotional bondage to the deceased

7. Mrs. Thomas has remained at the bedside of her dying mother throughout the night. When her mother died the following morning, Mrs. Thomas cried out angrily at the nurse and physician. As the nurse, the most appropriate action would be:
   1. explain that everything possible was done for her mother
   2. remain with Mrs. Thomas and listen to what she is saying
   3. leave Mrs. Thomas in privacy and allow her to work through her grief
   4. notify a clergyman and call other family members

8. Dale Conley, a newly licensed nurse, is assigned to his first dying patient. Nurse Conley would be best prepared to care for this patient if he:
   1. had completed a course dealing with death and dying
   2. is able to control his own emotions about death
   3. had experienced the death of a loved one
   4. has resolved the matter of his own mortality

9. The nurse is assigned to Mrs. Clark, who was recently diagnosed with a terminal illness. While the nurse was assisting her with morning care, Mrs. Clark asked about organ donations. The most appropriate action would be to:
   1. assist her in obtaining the necessary information to make this decision
   2. have the patient first discuss the subject with her family
   3. suggest she delay making a decision at this time
   4. contact the physician so consent can be obtained from the family

10. Ms. Longos, a licensed nurse, is assigned to complete postmortem care for Mrs. Jones, age 69. Ms. Longos is knowledgeable that postmortem care is:
    1. death occurring at home
    2. care of the body after death
    3. care given to family members
    4. pronouncing the patient dead

53

HOSPICE CARE

Josephine M. Estrada
Elaine Kockrow
Barbara Christensen

KEY TERMS

bereavement
cachexia
curative
holistic care
hospice
interdisciplinary hospice team
palliative
primary care giver
psychosocial
respite
spiritual
stomatitis
TENS

LEARNING OBJECTIVES

After reading this chapter, the student should be able to do the following:

- Define the key terms.
- Differentiate between curative and palliative care.
- Discuss the philosophy of hospice care.
- Discuss three requirements for hospice admission.
- Explain the roles of the interdisciplinary team.
- List three common signs or symptoms related to the terminally ill.
- Develop a care plan with patient goals related to these signs or symptoms.
- Discuss two ethical issues in hospice care.
- Explain three common hospice settings.
- Discuss the role of hospice in the family's bereavement period.

RELATED TOPICS OF INTEREST

- Ethical aspects of nursing (Chapter 3)
- Comfort, rest, and sleep (Chapter 15)
- Hygiene and care of the patient's environment (Chapter 16)
- Diet therapy (Chapter 19)
- Principles and practices of medication administration (Chapter 21)
- Care of the patient with cancer (Chapter 38)
- Home health nursing (Chapter 48)
- Loss, grief, dying, and death (Chapter 52)

Hospice is a philosophy of care that has been revived during the past decade. The concept originated in Europe and now has spread throughout the world. **Hospice** is from the Latin word *hospitium,* meaning "hospitality, lodging." It is a resting place for travelers on a difficult journey. A hospice program is family-centered care designed to help the terminally ill patient be more comfortable and maintain a satisfactory life-style through the process of dying.

In the middle ages, hospices were places of refuge for the poor and the sick and for travelers on religious journeys. Hospices emerged because the religious orders of monks and nuns believed that service to one's neighbor was a sign of

love and dedication to God. A typical medieval hospice was a combination guest house and infirmary, providing food, shelter, and illness care to the guests until they were refreshed and renewed for their journey or until they died. One of the earliest hospices was founded around AD 450 in Syria. Many hospices were established across Europe and in the Mediterranean region. In the late nineteenth and early twentieth centuries, religious groups started hospices in Dublin and London to care for the poor. As centuries passed, these hospices grew into hospitals as the religious concept gradually became dissociated from medical care.

The concept was renewed in the 1960s in London by Cicely Saunders, a nurse who later became a physician. Because of her interest in persons who were terminally ill with cancer, she became intensely involved in improving methods of pain control. She began her work at St. Joseph's Hospice, operated by the Irish Sisters of Charity. In 1968 she opened St. Christopher's Hospice of London, which has become a model for modern hospice care. This hospice offers in-patient care, home care, and bereavement services. It also serves as a national and international education, training, and research center for professionals involved in the hospice approach to terminal care.

Hospice migrated to the United States in the early 1970s. Since then, physicians, nurses, clergy, social workers, and many nonprofessional volunteers have worked together to develop more than 1800 hospice programs in the United States.

Hospices may vary greatly in structure and organization. A hospice may be affiliated with a hospital or home health agency or may be a separate organization (free-standing or community based). All types can offer inpatient as well as home care. Many hospices began as volunteer groups concentrating their efforts on psychosocial issues and family care and later developed into community-based or hospital affiliates. Some volunteer hospices continue to provide services.

In many cases, the person's home can become the hospice. Skilled doctors and nurses visit often, to give comfort as well as medication and therapy and to instruct family members in how to provide daily care. Expert help and guidance are available, by phone or in person, 24 hours a day.

If the hospice is a separate facility, the atmosphere is more like that of a friendly dormitory than that of a hospital. The patients usually wear their own clothes, move about the hospice as they choose, and socialize with each other and with the staff. The kitchen is always open for individually prepared food as well as for conversation around the coffee pot.

Today, hospice services are reimbursable through Medicare, Medicaid, and most private insurance companies. Medicare certification or state licensure ensures quality hospice services.

ISSUES AND RESPONSES OF THE TERMINALLY ILL

When a patient with a life-threatening illness has exhausted all treatment and the disease has not been arrested or cured, he must decide whether continued active therapy is feasible or beneficial. By this time, he may have already experienced many debilitating physical and emotional symptoms caused by the treatments or the progressive disease itself. Not all terminally ill patients experience all symptoms, but all have experienced at least some symptoms at one time or another.

At this point, when decisions for the appropriate type of care must be made, it is important to establish an honest and open communication among the patient, family, and physician. The patient's total physical, psychosocial, and spiritual needs are evaluated and openly discussed by those involved in the care. Dying and death are now realities affecting family roles, life-style patterns, and future goals. This total situation leads to deciding between palliative care and further **curative** (active treatment designed to cure) measures. **Palliative** (designed to relieve pain and distress, to control the signs and symptoms of disease but not to produce a cure) care is alleviating or controlling those symptoms that create physical, psychosocial, or spiritual distress. It stresses quality of life and is directed toward living life to the fullest until death occurs naturally.

HOSPICE APPROACH

Hospice care becomes appropriate when active treatment is no longer effective and supportive measures are needed to assist the terminally ill patient through the dying process. It offers the dying person a safe passage from life to death in a way that preserves dignity and important relationships. Not every terminally ill patient is suited to this type of care, because there are families and patients who choose to fight for life until the end. Hospice is appropriate mainly for those individuals who feel that the quality of life is more important and vital than the length of life. A significant number of individuals who recieve hospice care today are older adults with terminal diseases (see gerontological box).

To provide effective hospice care, an understanding of the philosophy and its relationship with the patient's responses and points of view is needed. The basic goals of hospice address the following:

1. Controlling or alleviating the patient's signs and symptoms
2. Allowing the patient and family to be involved in decision making to maintain dignity
3. Encouraging both the patient and family to live life as fully as possible
4. Providing continuous support to maintain patient and family confidence and reassurance to achieve these goals

GERONTOLOGICAL CONSIDERATIONS

- Families who are caring for terminally ill older adults may seek hospice care services as a respite.
- Medicare funding covers hospice care.
- The hospice often provides the dying older person with a higher level of control and dignity than other types of health care facilities.

This approach is defined as **holistic** (the philosophy that holds that in nature entities such as individuals and other complete organisms function as complete units that cannot be reduced to the sum of their parts) **care** because it focuses on physical, psychosocial, and spiritual issues, using an interdisciplinary team to provide this care. Specific standards of practice have been adopted by the National Hospice Organization as official guidelines in hospice care (Box 53-1).

To assist the dying patient, the team considers not only the patient but also the family regarding decisions affecting care. Hospice considers the patient and family as a unit, because families experience the stresses of dying as much as the patient. Stress extends into the **bereavement** (the expected and common depressed reaction to the loss of a loved one) period after the patient dies. For a patient to be admitted into the program for care, established criteria are considered:

1. There must be medical direction, and the physician of the patient must approve and willingly participate in the plan of care. The physician must also certify that the patient's disease is life threatening and that curative measures are no longer feasible.
2. The patient and family must agree to participate in this type of service.
3. The patient and family must understand and agree that care will be planned according to comfort and that life support measures may not necessarily be performed.

Also important is the availability of a **primary care giver** (one who assumes ongoing responsibility for health maintenance and therapy for illness). This person is usually a member of the immediate family or can be a significant other. This person becomes vital when the patient can no longer care for himself safely. A primary care giver is essential if hospice services are provided in the patient's home, but if the services are provided in a free-standing nursing home or inpatient facility, the primary care givers are the staff working in the facility. Once these criteria for admission are considered and agreed upon, the interdisciplinary team focuses on the appropriate plan of care.

Box 53-1 NATIONAL HOSPICE ORGANIZATION STANDARDS

1. Appropriate therapy is the goal of Hospice care.
2. Palliative care is the most appropriate form of care when cure is no longer possible.
3. The goal of palliative care is the prevention of distress from chronic signs and symptoms.
4. Admission to a Hospice program of care is dependent on patient and family needs and their expressed request for care.
5. Hospice care consists of a blending of professional and non-professional services.
6. Hospice care considers all aspects of the lives of patients and their families as valid areas of therapeutic concern.
7. Hospice care is respectful of all patient and family belief systems, and will employ resources to meet the personal philosophic, moral, and religious needs of patients and their families.
8. Hospice care provides continuity of care.
9. A Hospice care program considers the patient and the family together as the unit of care.
10. The patient's family is considered to be a central part of the Hospice care team.
11. Hospice care programs seek to identify, coordinate, and supervise persons who can give care to patients who do not have a family member available to take on the responsibility of giving care.
12. Hospice care for the family continues into the bereavement period.
13. Hospice care is available 24 hours a day, 7 days a week.
14. Hospice care is provided by an interdisciplinary team.
15. Hospice programs will have structured and informal means of providing support to staff.
16. Hospice programs will be in compliance with the standards of the NHO and the applicable laws and regulations governing the organization and delivery of care to patients and families.
17. The services of the Hospice program are coordinated under a central administration.
18. The optimal control of distressful symptoms is an essential part of a Hospice care program requiring medical, nursing and other services of the interdisciplinary team.
19. The Hospice care team will have a medical director on staff, physicians on staff, and a working relationship with the patient's physician.
20. Based on patients' needs and preferences as determining factors in the setting and location for care, a Hospice program provides in-patient care and care in the home setting.
21. Education, training, and evaluation of Hospice services are ongoing activities of Hospice care programs.
22. Accurate and current records are kept on all patients.

TABLE 53-1 Interdisciplinary Hospice Team

Team Member	Background	Function/Responsibility
Medical director	Licensed physician	Is a mediator between the hospice team and primary physician Provides consultation relative to medical aspect of care
Hospice coordinator	Licensed registered nurse	Manages the hospice program Explains the service, admits the patients, and then assigns the primary team Facilitates team meetings
Social worker	Certified as a social worker with a bachelor's or master's degree	Evaluates the psychosocial needs Is a resource for potential community services Assists with obtaining equipment and supplies Counsels when there are communication difficulties
Chaplain coordinator	Seminary degree; Clinical Pastoral Education (CPE) experience	Is the link between hospice team and pastoral community Coordinates pastoral support for the patient/family
Volunteer coordinator	Experience in volunteer work	Recruits and trains the volunteers Coordinates assignment of the volunteers
Bereavement coordinator	Background in bereavement counseling	Assesses the bereaved family after the death of the patient Coordinates and facilitates bereavement support group Provides bereavement counseling
Pharmacist	Licensed registered pharmacist	Provides drug consultation
Dietician	Licensed dietician	Provides diet counseling
Physical therapist	Registered physical therapist	Recommends appropriate safety devices Performs and instructs patient and family in passive exercises and transfer training

TABLE 53-2 Primary Hospice Team

Team Member	Background	Function/Responsibility
Primary physician	Licensed physician	Responsible for the medical aspect of symptom control for patient
Primary nurse	Licensed registered nurse	Is an advocate between patient, family, physician, and interdisciplinary team Evaluates patient's response to treatment Instructs the patient and family in management and effects of medication, illness, basic nursing, etc.
Secondary nurse	Licensed practical/vocational nurse	Works under supervision of physician and registered nurse to provide bedside nursing interventions appropriate to the terminally ill patient Assists in the physical, emotional, and spiritual support of the patient and family
Primary pastor	As required by church affiliation	Supports patient and family to cope with fears and uncertainty Provides opportunities for reconciliation, prayer, and **spiritual** (that aspect of life involving religious beliefs or value systems) healing. Responsible for funeral planning and performing burial services Continues to support the family during bereavement period
Hospice volunteer	Completion of volunteer training of at least 24 hr	Provides companionship for patient/family Available for family relief for respite care and emotional support Continues to be supportive throughout the bereavement period
Nurse's aide	Certified as a nurse's aide	Administers personal care and assistance with activities of daily living (ADLs)

Most hospice programs use a core of professionals who are responsible for coordinating the overall program and are referred to as the **interdisciplinary hospice team** (multiprofessional health team, such as physicians, nurses, social workers, and pastors working together in caring for the terminally ill patient) (Table 53-1). These professionals may have various educational backgrounds. The team consists of a medical director who is a licensed physician, a hospice coordinator who is a registered nurse, a social worker, a chaplain, and a volunteer coordinator. Each of these professionals has a responsibility to establish the care that will be delivered. The medical director is a liaison (link) between the hospice team and primary physician and provides consultation relating to the medical aspects of care. The hospice coordinator manages the program by explaining the services to potential patients, admitting them into the program, assigning the primary team, and facilitating the team meetings. The social worker evaluates the psychosocial needs of the patient and family, is a resource for potential community services if financial matters are a concern, counsels when communication difficulties are present, and obtains any necessary equipment and/or supplies needed for the safety and comfort of the patient. The chaplain coordinator contacts the patient's own pastor in the community to be part of the team for spiritual support. The pastor's role is vital to assist the patient and family to cope with fears and uncertainty. Support can include dealing with unfinished business and regrets and providing opportunities for reconciliation, prayer, and spiritual healing. Funeral planning and performing the burial services are included in this role also, along with continued support for the family throughout the bereavement period.

The patient's primary physician provides medical support, focusing on symptom control. The primary physician's involvement is essential to the success of the team care plan. The nurse becomes a liaison between the patient, family, physician, and interdisciplinary team regarding information about the status of the patient and effectiveness of symptom control. The nurse (1) evaluates the patient's response to treatment, (2) instructs the patient and family in management and effects of medications, illness, and basic nursing care, and (3) provides emotional support as possible.

The volunteer coordinator is responsible for training and assigning volunteers who will provide added support. When families are responsible for the total care of the patient in the home, "burnout" of the care giver becomes a concern. This is when the services of volunteers become vital. They provide companionship, family relief through **respite** (period of relief from responsibilities for the care of a patient) care and emotional support. With use of the volunteer, family can grocery shop, run errands, and participate in other activities, knowing their loved one is not alone. Volunteers become dependable friends, whose services the family can request and accept without guilt or feeling that they are imposing.

Other team members may include a pharmacist, for drug consultation; a dietician, for diet counseling and meal planning; a physical therapist, to provide safety devices, passive exercises, or transfer training; an occupational therapist, to assist in activities of daily living; and a music therapist, to provide diversional therapy to assist with pain management.

Each hospice patient and family is assigned a specific primary team who will be responsible for delivering the care (Table 53-2). A team care plan is developed by the total interdisciplinary team. Regular team conferences are held to discuss effectiveness of care (Fig. 53-1 on p. 1594). Observations by all members are reported and evaluated, and changes regarding care are made accordingly. The team must function as a cohesive unit to use all expertise and resources to provide quality patient care.

SYMPTOM CONTROL AND NURSING INTERVENTIONS

Pain

Of all the symptoms a dying patient experiences, pain is the most dreaded. To the healthy person, pain is usually temporary, but to the dying it can be constant and terrifying. Pain takes on many forms, such as physical, **psychosocial** (intellectual, emotional, and social components of the individual) and spiritual, and becomes a major factor that should be addressed and alleviated. According to Munley, although 50% of those dying with a malignancy usually do not have physical pain, and 10% may have mild pain, 40% suffer severe pain. The stress related to suffering and trying to control or alleviate it causes anxiety, anger, depression, restlessness, and isolation. The family caring for persons in this situation become frustrated and helpless as they try to control the pain, creating further feelings of guilt and inadequacy. Another issue that contributes to pain and emotional stress is the financial burden of high medical bills, inadequate funds, and unemployment. Spiritual pain may also surface, especially if there has not been any form of religious support or practices within the family unit. The patient and the family may develop a sense of hopelessness regarding the patient's impending fate, and fears related to the dying process, such as lingering, suffering, and isolation, may come into focus.

Initially, the physician may order diagnostic tests to determine if the cause of pain is related to tumor invasion or other pathological factors. Removing the cause may be impossible; therefore controlling the pain becomes vital in successful management of the person who is terminally ill. Many studies have been done regarding effective pain control (see Chapter 15), and the consen-

HOSPICE WEEKLY UPDATE

PATIENT NAME: Aletha Lindsley

DATE: 10-15-94

PRIMARY NURSE: Julie Thelen

PRIMARY PHYSICIANS: Dr. N Mack Dr. E. Schwartzkopf Dr. R. Asher Dr. M Nielson

PRIMARY CAREGIVER: Vern Lindlsey

PASTOR: G Timmons

SOCIAL WORKER: Mary Pendleton

CHURCH: Baptist

VOLUNTEER: Vesta Oerter

DIAGNOSIS: Cancer of breast with metastasis

MEDS AND FREQUENCY: phenergan 50 mgm
® q̄ 6 hrs.
Morphine rectal Supp. 20 mgm
q̄ 6 hrs.
Hydrochlorothiazide 25 mgm
tab T q̄ AM
Roximal 20 mgm '0' q̄ 4-6 hrs PRN
O_2 2L per nasal cannula
Colace tabs ῑῑ q̄ HS
tagamet 800 mgm '0' q HS

ALLERGIES: NKA

NURSING/MEDICAL UPDATE:

WEIGHT: 110 DATE: 10-15-94

VITAL SIGNS: 96-114-14 104/54

MENTAL ACUITY: occasionally disoriented to time

NEURO: unsteady gait

CARDIAC: tachycardia

RESPIRATORY: fine crackles in right apex

BOWELS: obstinate constipation

INTAKE/OUTPUT: 1000ml in/425ml out per 24 hrs

APPETITE: anorexic/eats 25% of meals

ACTIVITY LEVEL: activity intolerance

SKIN INTEGRITY: no impairment noted

PAIN SITES:	INTENSITY	CONTROL
Lower Lumbar	on a scale of 1-10 an '8'	good
spine		

PROGRESS NOTES: patient over the weekend became very nauseated and vomited approximately 300 ml of bile colored emesis. Afraid that her oral medications are causing this and is reluctant to take them Counseled, probably not the medication specifically causing the problem. Had dyspnea over weekend, O_2 was ordered and patient obtained notable relief. Husband states great concern over her increasing weakness and deteriorating mental clarity.

PLAN:
Could increase phenergan suppository q 3-4 hrs PRN
social worker will call husband to offer assistance and support.

[X] Check – Reported to primary nurse

Hospice Team Signatures: Julie Thelen
Janelle Hawks
Mary Pendleton
Gary Timmons
Vesta Oerter

FIG. 53-1 Hospice weekly update.

sus is that a pain assessment must be done to effectively control pain. Many programs use a pain assessment form to determine what mode of therapy will be effective. The following questions used for evaluation are directed to the patient:

1. Where is your pain? (The use of a body chart can be helpful so that the patient can identify the location.)
2. What kind of pain do you have? (Is it sharp, dull, continuous; a pain scale [where 0 is no pain, and 10 is severe] is useful.)
3. How long have you had pain?
4. When does your pain occur, and how often?
5. How long does your pain last?
6. What other problems add to your pain?
7. What relieves your pain? (Position of comfort, medications used, and environment can be addressed here.)

Answers to these questions are important in determining appropriate therapy. Even if the cause of pain is not apparent, the need for control is imperative.

Oral administration of medications is preferred, so that patients and families can independently manage the schedule and administration. Mild to moderate pain is controlled effectively in many cases with nonsteroidal antiinflammatory drugs. These drugs are also beneficial to use with narcotic analgesics, decreasing the required dose of narcotic. Narcotic analgesics, such as the opiates, are commonly used when severe pain cannot be controlled with nonsteroidal antiinflammatory drugs. When oral administration is not feasible because of nausea or vomiting, many of these drugs can be given rectally, topically, and parenterally (not in or through the digestive system—as a drug given by injection). Morphine sulfate has become the drug of choice in hospice care, because it can be administered orally, sublingually, rectally, and parenterally. Sustained release forms are also available. Some of the common forms of morphine used are Duramorph PF, MS Contin, Roxanol, and Roxanol SR.

Ineffective pain management is usually associated with undermedication or overmedication. Some causes of undermedication are (1) fear that the patient will become addicted; (2) fear that the patient will become dependent too soon and a stronger drug will be needed; (3) not taking the medication until the pain is intense, making it difficult to control; and (4) attempting to relieve pain with ineffective medication, holding in reserve for later the stronger ones, such as morphine. Overmedication may occur when several different narcotic analgesics are taken at the same time or close together because relief is not obtained soon enough. The goal is to prescribe a sufficient dose of an effective drug to alleviate pain and at the same time allow the patient to remain alert enough to participate in ADLs. Medication should be administered on a regular basis so that the pain does not return.

Another effective method of pain control is the use of heat or cold packs at the site of discomfort. Acupuncture and transcutaneous electrical nerve stimulation **(TENS)** (method of pain control by the application of electric impulses to the nerve endings; it causes interference with transmission of painful stimuli [see Chapter 22]) units have been used also. Some behavior techniques that can be beneficial are relaxation, hypnosis, and biofeedback.

Nursing Interventions. The nurse's role focuses on teaching the patient and family the effects and schedule of the medications so they can control the patient's pain. The patient and family should understand that pain can be controlled and that using large doses of narcotics is common and necessary to achieve that control. The nurse can assist the family in setting a schedule for administering the medications and then can monitor the patient's response to and compliance with the established treatment. Patient education regarding other techniques, such as massage, positioning for comfort, and heat or cold packs, is also the nurse's responsibility. It is important to give positive feedback to the patient and family when management of the pain is successful.

Nausea and Vomiting

Nausea is usually worse than vomiting because often it is obvious only to the patient, and so it tends to be ignored. Sometimes the drugs used for pain control cause nausea, and therefore it is recommended to give antiemetics with the narcotic analgesic. Anxiety has also been known to cause nausea, which then leads to vomiting. Patients who vomit are anxious about why they are vomiting, and this worsens the symptom. Constipation also can cause nausea. If nausea and vomiting occur because of obstruction from tumor invasion, it will be necessary to seek medical intervention. Evaluating the cause may not be easy, but once corrected it can often be prevented.

Nursing Interventions. Educating the patient and family regarding the problems that could cause or prevent nausea and vomiting is necessary. The patient should be encouraged to take the ordered antiemetics 30 minutes before meals and at bedtime on a regular basis. If vomiting occurs, eating should be discouraged for a period until peristalsis is stabilized. Relaxation and rest periods should be encouraged to avoid unusual stimulation. When the nausea and vomiting have subsided, the patient should begin drinking liquids or eating soft, bland foods. Small light meals should be served initially, with the diet as bland as possible, avoiding sweet, greasy, spicy, or strong-smelling foods (see Chapter 19). Fluids are important to prevent dehydration. The patient should eat slowly and in a pleasant atmosphere. If anxiety is causing nausea and vomiting, the patient should be encouraged to verbalize his fears.

Constipation

Constipation is one of the most common problems for the terminally ill patient. Sometimes this problem causes more anxiety and discomfort than pain itself. Because constipation can cause other symptoms, such as abdominal pain, nausea, or vomiting, prevention of the problem is important. Factors that contribute to constipation are poor dietary intake, the use of narcotics for pain control, and inactivity. When a patient begins to take medication for pain control, the use of a stool softener and stimulant laxative is necessary. Suppositories and enemas may be needed if oral laxatives produce no results. A rectal examination performed by the nurse may be necessary to check for an impaction. If an impaction is present, manual removal is necessary for relief. See Skill 27-8.)

Nursing Interventions. The following points are important for the nurse to educate the patient and family in prevention of constipation:

1. Narcotics may cause constipation, so laxatives must be given with the narcotic.
2. Patients who are not eating continue to produce waste in the bowel and can get impacted with feces.
3. High fluid intake should be maintained.
4. The patient should have a bowel movement at least every 3 days.
5. If possible, eating foods high in fiber is helpful.

Anorexia and Malnutrition

Anorexia may be caused by nausea, vomiting, constipation, dysphagia, **stomatitis** (any inflammatory condition of the mouth; may result from drugs used for cancer), and infections. These complications lead to difficulty in eating, which in turn causes loss of appetite. Odors of food cooking, inability to tolerate sweet foods, or a bitter taste in the mouth also contributes to the problem. This makes food less enjoyable, so the patient does not eat. Poor intake lowers the body's metabolism, which decreases the need for nourishment. Thus hunger is not realized. This cycle leads to **cachexia** (a state of malnutrition and wasting), resulting in muscle weakness and weight loss.

Nursing Interventions. If anorexia is related to stomatitis or infections, good oral hygiene is important. A technique to alleviate discomfort is using swabs or toothettes soaked in flavored mouthwash to cleanse the mouth. Small, frequent drinks; crushed ice; or artificial saliva can be useful to relieve dry mouth. If the odor of food causes anorexia, the patient should not be in the kitchen during meal preparation. The meals should be as attractive as possible, using foods chosen by the patient. High-protein supplements are helpful when eating is impossible. Weighing the patient should be avoided because the patient may be depressed and discouraged by attention to weight loss.

Dyspnea or Air Hunger

Breathing effectively may be difficult for many patients, especially during the very end stages of the illness. Air hunger may be caused by tumor pressure, fluid and electrolyte imbalance, or anemia. Anxiety resulting from fear or panic may accompany the problem.

Nursing Interventions. The patient may be more comfortable in an upright or orthopneic position. Oxygen therapy is of questionable value in this situation. Oral hygiene needs to be maintained for comfort. The use of a fan in the room is sometimes comforting to the patient. Mild tranquilizers may be used to decrease the patient's awareness of air hunger. The patient and family need a great deal of reassurance and support during this time.

Other Common Signs and Symptoms

Weight loss and dehydration can lead to a decrease of soft tissue, especially on the bony areas of knees, hips,

Box 53-2 NANDA-APPROVED NURSING DIAGNOSES FOR THE PATIENT RECEIVING HOSPICE CARE

Airway clearance, ineffective

Constipation

Family processes, altered

Fatigue

Fear (specify)

Grieving: anticipatory, dysfunctional

Care giver role strain, high risk for

Ineffective management of therapeutic regimen (individual)

Nutrition, altered: less than body requirements

Oral mucous membrane, altered

Pain

Powerlessness

Self-care deficit, bathing/hygiene

Skin integrity, impaired, high risk for

Social isolation

elbows, and buttocks. Increased weakness is also noted in the last stages of a terminal illness. With increased weakness, activity intolerance increases and the patient spends most of the time reclining. This leads to high risk for skin impairment and the formation of decubiti.

Nursing Interventions. It is important at this time to teach the patient and family the basics of good skin care. Cleanliness promoted by bathing can be refreshing, as well as therapeutic, in promoting comfort and the feeling of self-worth. The skin should be inspected frequently and kept as dry and clean as possible. Avoiding harsh soaps, strong detergents, or irritations from buttons, snaps, or food crumbs should be stressed. An Egg-crate mattress, sheepskin, or air-flotation mattress and heel and elbow protectors can cushion the bony areas. If decubiti occur, cleaning with normal saline, drying well, and applying a skin protector are helpful measures (see Chapter 16). Common nursing diagnoses for the patient receiving hospice care are listed in Box 53-2.

BEREAVEMENT PERIOD

The family, especially the care giver, continues to need support during the bereavement period after the patient dies. Even though the family feel they have prepared for the death, facing the future without the person who died is difficult. Hospice care does not conclude once the patient dies, but continues for at least 1 year. Many believe that four full seasons must pass before the bereaved can begin to think of the deceased without feeling intense emotional pain. The death of a loved one is a devastating agony that takes a long time to subside. Depending on the size of the program, special bereavement teams with counselors are available for the family. The team may facilitate a bereavement support group, which meets on a regular basis, providing these families the opportunity to communicate and share their feelings. Volunteers and pastors keep in touch by phone calls, cards, and remembering the bereaved person on holidays and anniversaries (see Chapter 52).

ETHICAL ISSUES IN HOSPICE

Some ethical issues when dealing with hospice patients include withholding or withdrawing nutritional support, right to refuse treatment, or "do not resuscitate" (DNR). Families find it difficult to discontinue nourishment, even when death is clearly approaching. If the patient is unconscious, decisions regarding these issues may fall on one family member. This may create guilt if other family members disagree. There are no simple answers to any of these concerns. It is hoped that the patient's wishes are made known in advance, such as in a living will, or that a power of attorney has been appointed.

An advanced directive is a document prepared while an individual is alive and competent. It provides guidance to the health care team in the event the person is no longer capable of making decisions. The directive states the individual's preferences concerning life-support measures and organ donations, and may give authority to another person to make decisions for the terminally ill patient who may be in a coma.

Death is a lonely experience, and can be done only alone, but the period leading to that point should not be lonely. It is important for the hospice team to be sensitive to the patient's and family's needs and maintain honesty at all times. The patient and the family should be included in all aspects of care and decision making. Opportunities for expression of concerns and fears should be provided, because this will make the process less fearful and threatening. Allowing the patient and family to live fully and comfortably so that dying can be truly dignified until death occurs naturally is the main goal of hospice care.

REFERENCES AND SUGGESTED READINGS

1. Bayer DL: Women approach death, *Am J Hospice Palliative Care* 10(3):28, 1993.
2. Beiter K: Lessons from the hearts of others, *Am J Hospice Palliative Care* 10(3):21, 1993.
3. Bruera E: Issues of symptom control in patients with advanced cancer, *Am J Hospice Palliative Care* 10(2):12, 1993.
4. Cooke MA: Living each moment, *Am J Hospice Palliative Care* 10(3):33, 1993.
5. Corr CA: Support for grieving children, *Am J Hospice Palliative Care* 8(4):23, 1991.
6. Coyle N et al: Character of terminal illness in the advanced cancer patient: pain and other symptoms during the last four weeks of life, *J Pain Symptoms Manage* 5:8393, 1990.
7. Coyle N et al: The last four weeks of life, *Am J Nurs* 90(12):75, 1990.
8. Eaks GG: Grief resolution in hospice nurses: an exploration of effective methods, *Nurs Health Care* 11(5):242, 1990.
9. Giffard BJ, Cleary BB: Supporting the bereaved, *Am J Nurs* 90(2): 1990.
10. Keenan M: Family forever, *Hospice,* 4(1):15, 1992.
11. Leppanen MC: Curing vs. caring, *Hospice,* 3(3):20, 1993.
12. Long B, Phipps W, Cassmeyer V: *A nursing approach,* ed 3, St Louis, 1993, Mosby.
13. Lubieniecki K: Cooperation improves patient access to hospice, *Hospice* 4(2):5, 1993.
14. McCaffery M: Nurses lead the way to new priorities, *Am J Nurs* 90(10):45, 1990.
15. *Mosby's medical, nursing, and allied health dictionary,* ed 4, St Louis, 1994, Mosby.
16. Moses M, Perry P: *Closer to the light: learning from children's near death experiences,* New York, 1990, Random House.
17. Mount B: Whole person care: beyond psychosocial and physical need, *Am J Hospice Palliative Care* 19(1):28, 1993.
18. Paice JA: Unraveling the mystery of pain, *Oncol Nurs Forum* 18(5):843, 1991.
19. Papalia DE, Olds WS: *Human development,* ed 5, New York, 1992, McGraw-Hill.
20. Potter PA, Perry AG: *Fundamentals of nursing: concepts, process, and practice,* ed 3, St Louis, 1993, Mosby.
21. *Taber's cyclopedic medical dictionary,* ed 17, Philadelphia, 1993, FA Davis.
22. Watt-Watson N, Donavan MI: *Pain management: nursing perspective,* St Louis, 1992, Mosby.

CHAPTER CHALLENGE

KEY POINTS

- Palliative care is appropriate when cure is not possible but care is still needed. This becomes the goal of hospice care.
- The goal of palliative care is to control pain and other symptoms for the prevention of distress.
- Admission to a hospice program is the decision of a patient and family, because not all persons need or desire hospice care.
- Hospice care consists of a blending of professionals and nonprofessionals to meet the total needs of the patient and family.
- Hospice care is delivered by an interdisciplinary team, because no individual or profession can meet all the needs of terminally ill patients and families all the time.
- Hospice care considers all aspects of the lives of patients and their families. Stresses and concerns may arise in many ways when families are faced with a terminal illness.
- A hospice care program considers the patient and family together as the unit of care, because families experience much stress and pain during the terminal illness of one of their members.
- Family participation in care giving is an important part of palliative care.
- Hospice care is available 24 hours a day, 7 days a week, because needs may arise at any time.
- Hospice care is respectful of all patient and family belief systems, seeking resources to meet the physical, psychosocial, and spiritual needs of the family unit.
- Hospice care for the family continues into the bereavement period. Needs of the family continue after the patient dies.
- Hospice services are reimbursable through Medicare, Medicaid, and most private insurance companies.
- Hospices allow the patient and family to live fully and comfortably so that dying can be dignified.

STUDY QUESTIONS

1. Nurse Jones has just begun working for hospice. He will become a vital member of the interdisciplinary team. This team consists of a:
   1. nurse, physician, social worker, pastor, and volunteer
   2. physician, pastor, volunteer, and nurse
   3. social worker, volunteer, pastor, and dietician
   4. physician, social worker, volunteer, and physical therapist
2. Mr. Reid, who is 89 years old, is terminally ill with cancer of the liver and has been discharged home under hospice care. Mrs. Reid asks the nurse if their Blue Cross/Blue Shield policy will cover their expenses. The nurse's correct response is that hospice care is reimbursed by:
   1. very few insurance companies
   2. Medicare and many insurance companies
   3. Medicaid and Medicare
   4. Medicaid, Medicare, and most insurance companies
3. The medication of choice for pain control in the hospice setting is:
   1. Ibuprofen
   2. Morphine
   3. Meperidine (Demerol)
   4. Codeine
4. Many hospice patients have persistent nausea and vomiting. The measure that can alleviate or reduce these signs and symptoms is:
   1. taking analgesics on a regular basis
   2. a diet high in fat and fiber with between meal snacks
   3. taking antiemetic medication on a regular basis
   4. participating in active and passive exercises
5. Mrs. Babcock, who is 40 years old, is a hospice patient. She has been taking morphine sulfate by PCA pump. Her nurse assesses her for the most common side effect of narcotic analgesics, which is:
   1. nausea and vomiting
   2. constipation
   3. anorexia
   4. muscle weakness
6. Hospice is concerned with the patient and family during the dying process as well as what length of time after death:
   1. 1 year
   2. 2 years
   3. 6 months
   4. 1 month
7. For a hospice nurse the goal of palliative care is:
   1. To provide an atmosphere in which the patient and family may socialize
   2. To cure the patient of distressing signs and symptoms commonly experienced by the terminally ill
   3. To administer primary care that involves the family in the patient's treatment
   4. To control pain and other signs and symptoms for the prevention of distress

17

THE WORLD OF THE GRADUATE

Nursing requires a commitment to be the best you can be, and then you have to be a little better than best. As students we put in long hours of study; then we are told we will earn the privilege of working long hours, probably midnight hours. As a graduated practical nurse, when you look at the above description, you think, "Why do I want to become a nurse? I must be crazy, or I must love what I am doing." When all the requirements to become licensed are accomplished and the working aspect lies ahead, I will become a part of helping to shape the world. We can either be present at life, or we can choose another profession. I choose to be a nurse.

Donna Baker
Student Nurse

54

THE WORLD OF THE GRADUATE

Carolyn Dean

KEY TERMS

advancement
contract
endorsement
interview
negligence
Nurse Practice Act
reciprocity
resignation
résumé
role
transcribe

LEARNING OBJECTIVES

After reading this chapter, the student should be able to do the following:

- Define the key terms.
- Discuss the three methods of applying for a job.
- Describe what can be expected from an interview for a new job.
- Discuss confidentiality.
- List the advantages of membership in professional organizations.
- Discuss career opportunities for the LPN/LVN.
- Explain the structure and role of the charge nurse.
- Discuss the guidelines for being an effective leader.
- Identify two reasons why an evaluation is important.
- Discuss telephone manners in professionalism.
- List the three types of physician's orders, and discuss the legal aspects of each.
- List three ways you can ensure accuracy when transcribing physicians' orders.
- List the pertinent data necessary to compile an effective end-of-shift report.
- Describe the Nurse Practice Act.
- Identify three important functions of a State Board of Nursing.
- List four reasons a State Board of Nursing could revoke a nursing license.
- Discuss the Computerized Adaptive Testing (CAT) for the National Council Licensure Examination (NCLEX) for the LPN/LVN candidate.

RELATED TOPICS OF INTEREST

- Legal aspects of nursing (Chapter 2)
- Ethical aspects of nursing (Chapter 3)
- Communication (Chapter 4)
- Principles and practice of medication administration (Chapter 21)
- Home health nursing (Chapter 48)
- Rehabilitation nursing (Chapter 49)
- Hospice care (Chapter 53)

FUNCTIONING AS A GRADUATE

The **role** (a socially expected behavior pattern associated with an individual's function in social groups) of a graduate nurse will be exciting and challenging. The LPN/LVN is a valuable member of the health care team and functions in many settings. This chapter provides some guidelines for being a conscientious nurse while assuming this new role. There are many nursing opportunities from which to choose. Methods to obtain a job are letter of application, résumé, and interview.

Letter of Application

The letter of application should always be brief, neatly typed, and correctly spelled. A sample letter of application is found in Fig. 54-1. The letter should state the exact position for which you are applying and any information about yourself and your qualifications. Box 54-1 provides guidelines for writing the letter of application.

The Résumé

The **résumé** (a summary of educational and professional experiences, including activities and honors) is a one- or two-page written document that contains certain information about you, your education, and your experience. It is a brief outline of your personal and professional life. It also describes your skills and interests. Future employers will be impressed with a well-prepared résumé; therefore you should take the preparation of your résumé very seriously. It should be well organized, neat, and accurate. You should prepare a résumé that is basic, properly arranged, and contains the most recent information. Be sure to use a variety of action words and self-descriptive words. There are several types of résumés—keep yours brief and informative. The employer is seeking the employee with the most potential for the job. The résumé may be the first means by which the employer gains an impression of you. A sample résumé is presented in Fig. 54-2 on p.1602.

(return address) 1314 East 17th Street
Sedalia, MO 65301
(date) Sept. 3, 1995

Mr. Greg Derk *(inside address)*
Personnel Manager
North Central Hospital
615 South Tryon Street
Kansas City, MO
64156
Dear Mr. Derk: *(salutation)*

I am interested in the position of LPN on a surgical unit for which you advertised an opening in the Kansas City Star on Sunday, Sept. 2.

I will graduate on Sept. 23 from North Central Missouri College and will take the LPN licensure examination in October. Throughout my education, I have maintained a keen interest in medical-surgical nursing. In addition, I worked part-time as a nurse assistant on a surgical floor at St. Francis Hospital in Marceline for a year while I was in nursing school. My résumé is enclosed for further information about my background and experience.

I am a highly motivated individual and perform well in stressful situations. I am energetic, systematic, organized, and efficient and provide quality nursing care to patients. I am enthusiastic about my career in nursing and look forward to reviewing my qualifications with you.

I will be in Kansas City on Friday, Sept. 7, and if it is convenient for you, I would like to talk with you then about this position. You can reach me by phone at (816) 827-1032. I look forward to hearing from you.

(complimentary close) Sincerely yours,

(provide signature)
Sue Renfro

Enclosure

FIG. 54-1 Sample letter of application.

Box 54-1

GUIDELINES FOR WRITING LETTERS OF APPLICATION

1. Include your full address above the date of your letter.
2. Address the letter appropriately. If you are responding to a classified advertisement that provides a return box only, use the address given and the salutation *Ladies and Gentlemen.* If you have learned about a position through your school office or through a friend, you should have the name of the person in charge of employment. In this case, include the name in the inside address as follows:

   Mr. Thomas L. Leeper
   Personnel Manager
   The Azzaro Corporation
   3689 Wilson Street
   Atlanta, GA 30315

   The proper salutation is *Dear Mr. Leeper:*
3. In the first paragraph, state your interest:

   The nursing position that you advertised in the *Atlanta Times* on Monday, June 2, is of interest to me.

   or

   Miss Cathie Royer, the placement counselor at Greenville College, has suggested that I apply for the nursing position that is available in your facility.
4. In the second paragraph refer to your résumé, which you will enclose. This paragraph should highlight the main points of your education and experience.
5. In the final paragraph of your application, indicate your interest in a personal interview and the times you are available.
6. The complimentary close may be a simple *Sincerely yours.* Include your signature above your typewritten name, and indicate the enclosure.

LINDA PATTERSON
2777 EAST EIGHTH
TRENTON, MO 64683

PHONE: (816) 359-8888

JOB OBJECTIVES: Staff LPN leaning toward inservice or home health care.

EDUCATION:

North Central Missouri College, Trenton, MO 64683
Licensed Practical Nurse: Graduation, Sept. 1995; License, 1995

Kirksville Health Center, Kirksville, MO 63501
Advanced Cardiac Life Support, 1994
Advanced Fluid and Electrolyte Course, 1994

EXPERIENCE:

St. Francis Hospital, Marceline, MO 64668, August 1993 to July 1994, Nurse Assistant

Brookfield Nursing Center, Brookfield, Mo 64628, January 1992 to July 1993, Nurse Assistant

Grim-Smith Hospital, Kirksville, MO 63501, June 1991 to December 1991 Nursing Assistant

HONORS AND ACTIVITIES:

North Central Missouri College: Dean's Honor Roll; Class Secretary; Intramural sports

High School: Member, National Honor Society; Class President; Who's Who Among American High School Students; Girls' State delegate; Member, concert and marching band; Softball; Basketball.

Community: Girl Scout; Community Betterment; Youth Leadership Award from the governor—1990; Extension Club president.

REFERENCES:

Mrs. Lynn Myers	Ms. Cherie Urton	Mrs. Carol Jacobs
Health Occupations Division	Instructor	Director of Nursing
North Central Missouri	North Central Missouri	St. Francis Hospital
Trenton, MO 64683	1301 Main Street	Marceline, MO 64668
(816) 359-3948	Trenton, MO 64683	(816) 359-3939
	(816) 359-4562	

FIG. 54-2 Sample résumé.

The Personal Interview

The **interview** (a meeting of people face to face, as for evaluating or questioning a job applicant) is important, and every effort should be made to make it a success. First impressions are sometimes incorrect, and whether they are positive or negative, they have a lasting effect. Prepare carefully for the interview, and make a good impression. Box 54-2 provides steps to a successful interview.

Box 54-2 STEPS TO A SUCCESSFUL INTERVIEW

1. Be well groomed.
2. Arrive at the interview a few minutes earlier than the appointment; if there is a receptionist or secretary, identify yourself, and give the name of the person you are to see.
3. Be cheerful and polite.
4. Be knowledgeable about the position for which you are applying.
5. Be patient while waiting for an interview.
6. Smile, and give name distinctly when greeting the interviewer.
7. Use a firm handshake.
8. Address interviewer by name, using Mr., Mrs., or Ms.
9. Use appropriate body language (refer to Chapter 4).
10. Maintain eye contact with the interviewer.
11. Allow the interviewer to take the initiative.
12. Answer questions concisely. Try to make the interview interesting and informative. Use the time effectively.
13. Articulate (to present yourself clearly).
14. Be factual.
15. Avoid being critical.
16. Convey genuine interest and enthusiasm.
17. Avoid discussing personal problems, unless applicable to job.
18. Be prepared to relate qualifications and experiences.
19. Inquire as to job description, work schedule, and fringe benefits.
20. If requested, state salary desired; if salary offered is unacceptable, do not mislead the interviewer.
21. Inquire about starting salary, pay increases, and maximum salary allowed.
22. If asked, indicate preference of position desired.
23. Look for clues when the interview is over. Usually an employer will ask, "Do you have any more questions?" This is probably a good time to say, "No thank you, but I enjoyed our interview and hope that you will consider me for the position with your company."
24. Express appreciation for the interview.
25. Suggest when and where you might be contacted, if necessary.
26. Send additional information promptly, upon request.

For a good working relationship, your skills and nursing care values should be in harmony with the objectives of the job description.

Contracts

A **contract** is a promise or a set of promises between two or more persons that creates a legal relationship between them and a legal obligation that one or more of them must fulfill. The usual contract the LPN/LVN will encounter is the employment contract. Although it is desirable to have a written employment contract, an oral employment contract may be binding on the nurse and the employer. Under the employment contract it is the nurse's obligation to perform nursing functions with the skill and knowledge of a LPN in accordance with the standards of the profession and any additional qualifications the nurse claimed to possess. The employer is responsible for providing a safe working environment, sufficient and competent fellow workers, and safe equipment. Failure on the part of the nurse or the employer to perform these duties is a breach of contract. Breach of contract can result in a lawsuit seeking a court to order the breaching party to perform the obligations of the contract or to pay money to the party who was damaged by the breach. However, because the contract is one for personal services, a nurse will usually not be forced to work for the employer. Rather, the nurse might be liable for money damages to an employer for breach of contract.

The employment contract should specify the length of the contract period; hours the nurse is to work; salary; vacation; sick leave pay; medical, maternal, disability, and liability insurance coverage; educational benefits; and any other benefits or working conditions that the nurse and employer agree on. The employment contract can be terminated legally, without a breach, by completion of all obligations under the terms of the contract or by consent of all parties to the termination.

Retaining Your Position

To retain your position you must accept its imposed responsibilities. This includes reporting on and off duty, notifying the proper person if ill, and giving your employer sufficient time to secure a replacement. You should understand your duties and show interest in their performance. Be willing to give the best of your abilities and show their worth to others. Above all, try to find happiness and success in your job. All jobs have desirable and undesirable elements, but usually the desirable elements outweigh the undesirable. Do not change jobs too frequently. Recommendations are better the longer you retain a certain position. Never walk away from your duties or responsibilities. Remember that in return for your services the employer has contracted to pay you a definite salary with certain fringe benefits. Employers have the right to demand a good day's work in return for a just salary. If you take a strong character and a good personality to a new position, you will advance both personally and professionally. Joy in what you are doing, together with sufficient preparation and knowledge, will help you to give quality nursing care to the patient and be a pleasant co-worker.

Advancement

Advancement (a rise in rank or importance, a promotion, progress, improvement) may result from additional preparation or additional experience. It may be gained by learning the position more thoroughly and by assuming new and greater responsibilities. Advancements, together with the difficulties and obstacles that they bring, stimulate interest and enthusiasm. They are usually based on a person's qualifications, behavior, performance, and preparation.

Terminating Employment

Resigning from a position properly is another skill that you should have. Employers will sometimes question a résumé that reflects frequent job changes; therefore it is in your best interest to remain at the first place of employment at least 1 year. If this is impossible, the proper **resignation** (the act of resigning to give up a position of employment) procedure should be followed. A verbal statement and a letter of resignation, if given, may be beneficial in obtaining your next position. If the facility has a formal resignation form, it should be completed neatly and legibly. If a letter of resignation is expected, it should be brief and courteous. In concise terms, state your reason for leaving. Address the letter to your immediate supervisor or employer. It is delivered in a sealed envelope. A sample letter of resignation is in Fig. 54-3.

THE GAP BETWEEN STUDENT AND GRADUATE

Know Who You Are

Sometimes it is difficult to clearly understand the exact responsibilities of each health team member. Job descriptions to fit some of the new roles have not been written. The LPN/LVN is responsible to an RN or to the physician. The role of the LPN/LVN, like the roles of others

406 Martin Lane
Edinburg, MO 64683
May 6, 1995

Ms. Nel Pitts, RN
Director of Nurses
Memorial Hospital
Edinburg, MO 64683

Dear Ms. Pitts:

Because of unforeseen circumstances, I must resign my position as staff LPN on 1-E. My husband has been transferred to another city, and I must seek employment there.

I would like my resignation to be effective as of May 29, 1995.

I would appreciate it if I could have my accrued benefits added to my terminal salary check.

I thank you for all the courtesies extended to me during my employment. The staff has been helpful, and I have enjoyed my 4 years of employment at Memorial Hospital. I hope that in the future I can seek employment again at this facility.

Sincerely yours,

(provide signature)
(Mrs.) Kelly Anderson, LPN

FIG. 54-3 Sample letter of resignation.

associated with health care, is constantly changing. As the services of health care facilities are extended to meet the increasing demand of the population, the role of the LPN/LVN does not remain static. Many technical and scientific changes in the health care system have resulted in a multiplicity and complexity of functions placed on nurses. As a result, those who work with patients must be extremely careful not to lose sight of their principal concern, the human being. Patients quickly recognize nurses who have a genuine concern for their individual needs. Your enthusiasm and zest for nursing are clearly evident in the personalized quality of care given. Stay focused on the patient and the patient's needs.

Confidentiality

Consider as confidential all information the patient gives. The information may be exchanged with other members of the health care team only in the performance of your duties. Release of information to anyone other than the health care team without the consent of the patient is a violation of the right to privacy. Important reminders concerning confidentiality are listed in Box 54-3.

Box 54-3 CONFIDENTIALITY REMINDERS

1. Discuss patient information only in conferences or reports. Be mindful of conversations in the cafeteria and at the nurses' station.
2. Keep confidential all information gathered from medical records, reports, or conferences.
3. Be nonjudgmental in observations of patients, hospital staff, family members, or other personnel.
4. Do not store patient statistics on any retrievable or permanent computer system unless authorized.
5. Do not keep or copy any patient information except when necessary for required report. All notes should be destroyed after submitting required report.
6. Never copy any original medical records for any reason unless ordered by a physician.
7. Do not leave patient chart where unauthorized persons can access it.
8. It is generally not the nurse's responsibility to release patient information to the police, media, relatives, or visitors.
9. Familiarize yourself with how patient information is to be handled within the facility.
10. You are ethically obligated to treat information about your patient as confidential.

Remember:

WHAT YOU SEE HERE,
WHAT YOU HEAR HERE,
WHILE YOU ARE HERE,
LET IT STAY HERE,
WHEN YOU LEAVE HERE.

Expectations of an LPN/LVN in the Community

The LPN/LVN participates in activities that promote the community's attitude toward positive health care. The nurse uses community resources to promote a better understanding of the health services available to the general public and promotes and participates in community health projects and other health-oriented activities such as maternal and child health clinics, disabled children clinics, mental health clinics, blood pressure clinics, and community health fairs.

Professional Organizations

If you want a voice in your vocation, it will be a benefit to join that vocation's organizations. No organization can be any more active or effective than its members. Some professional organizations provide opportunities for continuing education to their members and associated allied health staff.

Two national organizations are designed to support and meet the needs of the LPN/LVN: the National Association for Practical Nurse Education and Service (NAPNES) and the National Federation of Licensed Practical Nurses (NFLPN).

NAPNES was founded in 1941 to promote an understanding of practical nursing schools and continuing education for the LPN/LVN. The organization also developed a position on the education of the practical nurse and defines ethical conduct and publishes standards of practical/vocational nursing practice. The *Journal of Practical Nursing* is the official publication, and *NAPNES Forum* is the newsletter that informs members of activities. Membership is open to students, graduates, faculty, and others who are interested in the practical/vocational nurse. For more information, write to: NAPNES, 1400 Spring Street, Suite 310, Silver Spring, MD 20910.

NFLPN was founded in 1949 to promote the licensed practical nurse. The membership is limited to practical/vocational nursing students and graduates. It informs members of the most current issues of interest and makes available to its members malpractice, personal liability, health, and accident insurance. The NFLPN also lobbies on both the state and national levels for issues that are of interest and concern to its members. The *Licensed Practical Nurse* is the official publication. For further information write to: NFLPN, 214 South Drive, PO Box 11038, Durham, NC 27703.

Members who constitute these two organizations all share the common goals of the LPN/LVN.

The National League for Nursing (NLN) was founded in 1952 and is involved with all types and levels of nursing. The NLN is a large organization that has divisions called *councils.* The Councils of Practical Nursing Program (CPNP) is the division of the NLN that accredits education programs and provides continuing education for faculty. The official publication is *Nursing and Health Care.* Professional testing services, studies, and surveys on nursing education are provided by the NLN organization. Membership is open to all nurses and others interested in health care.

Updating and Continuing Education

The health care system is changing daily as a result of rapidly developing technology, and it is critical to keep current on nursing trends and issues. More excellent opportunities to learn new nursing skills are available to the nurse today than ever. Facilities are offering employees continuing education through seminars or workshops using current videos, journals, textbooks, and computers.

To renew nursing licenses, some states require a given number of hours per year in continuing education units (CEUs). This is to improve the quality of patient care by educating nurses on the most recent trends in nursing interventions.

LPNs/LVNs who wish to pursue further education may receive credit for education. Progressive LPN/LVN to RN programs have been developed throughout the nation, making it possible for an LPN/LVN to become an RN in a shorter period of study. There are various names for these programs, such as *career ladder, upper mobility, level I and level II, 1 + 1,* and *accelerated/associate degree nursing program.* Programs vary, and each should be investigated thoroughly.

CAREER OPPORTUNITIES

Never before has nursing been so exciting; today the new graduate has a variety of job opportunities available. The options will require considerable thought to make the correct decision. The job opportunities for the LPN/LVN have expanded and now extend beyond those in the nursing home and hospital.

Hospital Nursing

In hospital nursing, the responsibilities of the LPN/LVN will depend on the policies and philosophy of the facilities. Hospital schedules may be of three shifts: 7 AM to 3 PM, 3 PM to 11 PM, and 11 PM to 7 AM. Some schedule two 12-hour shifts: 7 AM to 7 PM and 7 PM to 7 AM. Most offer different options to meet the personal needs of the employee (Fig. 54-4). In the hospital, the LPN/LVN is usually the bedside nurse, and the RN is usually the charge nurse. In many hospitals total patient care is given. Total patient care can best be described as follows: the nurse assigned to the patient gives the bath, makes the bed, gives the medications, performs various procedures necessary, and charts; each care giver has fewer patients but gives total care to those patients for the entire shift.

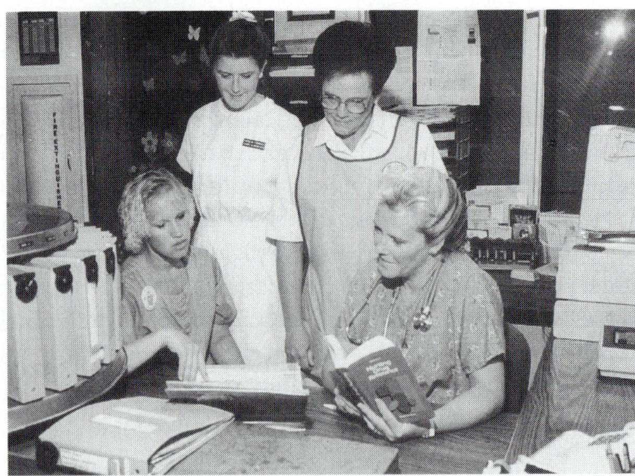

FIG. 54-4 Various positions are available in the hospital setting.

In some hospitals other work experiences may be available for the LPN/LVN. Such areas are intensive care units, renal dialysis, pediatrics, surgery, and emergency room. These areas usually require specialized education beyond the LPN/LVN education. Many hospitals offer further education to the LPN/LVN who is interested in one of these specialties.

Same-day surgery units within the hospital setting are becoming more common. In this type of unit, patients are admitted, undergo surgery, and are discharged in the same day. The LPN/LVN must be skilled in preoperative, postoperative, and recovery care.

Private Duty Nursing

The private duty nurse gives total care to one patient. The setting for the private duty nurse may change from patient to patient, but basically the job description is the same. This type of nursing is totally independent nursing care service. Private duty nursing may take place in the hospital, home, other facility, and while traveling aboard or in the United States. You not only accept the patient when doing private duty nursing but the family as well. The nurse is paid directly by the patient or responsible person. When the setting for private duty nursing is in a health care facility, the nurse is expected to follow the policies and procedures of that facility.

When doing private duty nursing, you are legally responsible for your own actions. If you should experience any doubt about an order or procedure, obtain clarification from the physician before carrying out the order or procedure. Charts must be kept carefully. In the home, set up a type of record in which you can list necessary items, such as medications given, vital signs, and the condition of the patient. This home record may be requested by and released to the physician. Narcotics not used are returned to the physician before you leave the case.

The major problems of private duty nursing are the irregular assignments and the economic aspects. In private duty nursing there is no certainty of work or payment. However, because today there are so many unfilled demands for private duty nurses, the availability of cases presents fewer problems for the LPN.

If you should choose this field of nursing, it is advisable to remember that you will be responsible for the payment of your Social Security, as well as your federal, state, and city taxes. This means that you must keep continuous, accurate records of your days worked and payments received.

An advantage of private duty nursing is that you may work as many days as you like, or you may accept a case for as long a period of time as you desire. You have more freedom and fewer restrictions in your workday.

Home Health Nursing

Home health care is expanding rapidly. The hours of employment with this type of nursing may fit into your lifestyle. Some facilities prefer you to have some experience in hospital nursing first, for you to function with a broader knowledge base. An established health care program that is funded and operated by local, state, or federal government agencies provides the nursing care. The LPN/LVN will work under the supervision of an RN or physician. The nursing care may be given in the home or in a community health center. The nurse may have an opportunity to do patient teaching in public or community health. This may range from prenatal classes to teaching patients to give their insulin injections. The nurse is allowed to be flexible and works autonomously. Therefore skillful time management and an interest in working independently are helpful in this area. Advantages to home health nursing are steady employment, less formal environment, and opportunities to assess and provide for patients' needs.

Armed Services Nursing

There are various branches of services that offer educational benefits to nurses. The United States Army offers the LPN/LVN financial assistance with education. This area offers a wide range of experience, including traveling and working in Veterans Administration hospitals. If you are interested in the armed services, it is advisable to contact the recruiter in your area.

Armed Services (Army). The Army requires the LPN/LVN to be between 17 and 34 years of age and a United States citizen of high moral standards and personal qualifications. The nurse must be a graduate of a 1-year practical nursing program and currently licensed.

Advantages are patriotic service to country, travel, the opportunity for different experiences, special rank and pay, allowance given for clothing and quarters, and benefits of education, training, medical and dental care, and survivors' insurance. Disadvantages are varied shifts, often rotating divisions, and a regimented life-style.

Government Nursing

Civil Service. The LPN/LVN may work in a Veterans Administration hospital or other government hospitals. Advantages are good salary, fringe benefits, and good insurance and retirement plans. The disadvantage is that the ratio of nurses to patients is sometimes low.

Industrial Nursing

The focus in industrial nursing is on promoting wellness and preventing accidents. Safety is emphasized, and usually the nurse is first-aid oriented. The industrial nurse may do physical assessment, health surveys, insurance forms preparation, and health education, as well as nursing intervention for patients injured in industrial accidents. The LPN/LVN will work under the supervision of an RN or physician. Depending on the size of the industrial site, this type of nursing may offer shifts and benefits different from those of other career opportunities.

In this field of nursing you must have patience, understanding, observational skills, and current first-aid techniques and principles. You must possess organizational skills and neatness in keeping records. You must be able to adjust to all types of situations and people.

Office Nursing

The LPN/LVN may work in a physician's office, clinic, or other health practice. In these settings, the nurse may be responsible for various duties other than nursing skills, such as receptionist, bookkeeper, and laboratory assistant, and may be responsible for ordering supplies. The LPN/LVN who makes this choice must be flexible and be able to adjust easily to various roles. Advantages to working in this field are Social Security coverage; Sundays and most evenings free; and holiday, vacations, and salaries determined by the physician.

Rehabilitation Nursing

This field requires responsibility for guiding the patient toward health and independence. Advantages are steady employment, a less formal environment, and an opportunity to provide good care.

Psychiatric Nursing

Psychiatric nursing requires a mature person (not in years) to handle the responsibilities of the job. This type of nursing may be done in an open ward in a general hospital, outpatient clinic, mental health agency, psychiatric hospital, or institution. Advantages are a good salary and advancement in leadership areas.

Nursing Home and Extended-Care Facilities

The job opportunities in the field of geriatrics are increasing daily. In the nursing home or extended-care facilities, a large number of LPN/LVNs are needed, and in many instances they function as charge nurses. The amount of responsibility for the LPN/LVN depends on the facility and the level of care given. Working at this type of setting requires many special qualities, such as patience, interest in working with the same people over a long period, good communications, and leadership skills. Advantages to working in these settings are steady employment, less formal environment, hours usually more stable, and greater opportunity for advancement.

Hospice Nursing

Hospice nursing offers care to terminally ill patients in either an institution or home setting, usually under the auspices of home health nursing. The qualifications for a hospice nurse are to have a clear understanding of his or her own feelings concerning death and to understand the philosophy of the hospice setting. The nurse closely supports the patient and family without interfering with family interpersonal relationships. Advantages of hospice nursing are steady employment, less formal environment, and opportunities to provide good bedside care that is concerned with pain relief and comfort measures. Disadvantages are always caring for dying patients and the possibility of having to travel to more than one home each shift (see Chapter 53).

Leadership

No single management style is always appropriate. The most effective leaders (ones who have the ability to influence others to the attainment of a goal) select aspects from several styles as the situation requires. The eclectic leader realizes that both the tasks and the people involved are important. In situations involving nursing interventions, the supervising nurse must keep complete control. If something must be done, or must be done in a particular way, it is the leader's responsibility to see that it is done promptly and correctly. Nurses reporting to the supervisor must recognize her authority and responsibility. In cases of emergency the supervisor must know that an order will be followed.

In other areas, however, the nurse in charge may use a more democratic style. Making daily assignments, assigning miscellaneous tasks, and scheduling breaks and lunch are simple examples of where the employees could and should have input. These areas affect the employee directly and can greatly affect job satisfaction.

When you are the charge nurse in a nursing home or extended-care facility, it will be you from whom others will be seeking advice and guidance. You are expected to make the correct decisions effectively for the shift. Every nurse needs a basic set of guidelines to assist in functioning efficiently as a charge nurse. Box 54-4 provides guidelines to assist in more effective leadership.

Time Management

Using time to good advantage will be of great value. Learn good time management skills, and practice them frequently until they become fully developed. These

Box 54-4 GUIDELINES FOR EFFECTIVE LEADERSHIP

1. Orient the team you will be working with. They deserve to hear what is expected of them by you. Each one should be aware of his or her job description. The workplace will be less stressful if everyone is familiar with any uniqueness you or others may have concerning the nursing care given.
2. Keep notepad and pencil with you (document on notepad pertinent information that may be needed later). Also have available a pocket calculations guide on drug doses and IV drop rate.
3. Develop your own system of abbreviations for your information—use only standard abbreviations on legal documents.
4. Make patient rounds as soon as report is over. If you are to be responsible for the direct care of a certain number of patient, make certain you can document accurate information concerning their conditions. Note on your "pocket notes" date and time, and briefly state what you observe or hear. This is helpful if the patient's condition changes.
5. Check all equipment and supplies that you will be responsible for during your shift. You may assign these duties to another responsible person if available. These checks can become part of the routine and will assist in the proficiency of the staff.
6. Everyone performs best when the team works together and each receives recognition for individual performance.
7. Keep informed of the events within the facility.
   a. Attend necessary meetings.
   b. Become familiar with rules and regulations of the facility in which you are employed.
   c. Learn what surveys or inspections will be conducted.
   d. Learn where the policy and procedure documents are kept; also ensure that they are updated and located in a central area.

skills will help you manage not only at work but also in daily living. See Box 54-5 for 10 steps to effective time management.

Manage your time so you can accomplish both what you must do and what you *want* to do.

Transcribing Physicians' Orders

Physicians' orders are written, telephoned, or verbal. The written orders are recorded on the chart by physicians. Some facilities employ ward clerks, ward secretaries, or unit secretaries to transcribe the physician's orders. But in long-term care facilities, there usually are no unit secretaries. In facilities that do employ unit secretaries, the secretaries usually do not work at night. Therefore in many facilities, the nurse is expected to transcribe the order from the chart. There will be times when the order will be difficult to read—NEVER GUESS. If in doubt, get a second opinion. Also if the written order does not read like a "routine order" or if it is a little different from usual, check with the physician or other responsible person. It is imperative to check on the written order before carrying out the order. If in doubt about the physician's order, always recheck for clarity (Fig. 54-5).

The policy for verbal or telephone orders varies in different facilities. Be certain to check the policy of the facility for the LPN/LVN regarding accepting verbal or telephone orders. The orders given by telephone or verbal communication are more subject to error. If you are responsible for accepting this type of order, be certain of the accuracy. Clarify the order by repeating it to the person giving it. This gives both people a chance to hear the order. Always write a telephone or verbal order immediately. If it is given too rapidly, ask that it be repeated more slowly. When the correct spelling of a medication is questionable, refer to a list of commonly ordered medications or to the *Physicians' Desk Reference* (PDR). Be cautious when medications look alike when written, have similar spelling, or sound alike. There are several drugs that sound alike but have very different actions (for example, Xanax and Zantac). Xanax is an antianxiety agent, and Zantac is a histamine antagonist for the treatment of ulcers.

When **transcribing** (to write or type a copy of) from physicians' orders, the precautions in Box 54-6 on p.1610 will assist in avoiding errors.

When there is an order for a medication to be discontinued or changed, the steps in Box 54-7 on p.1610 should be followed (again, this procedure will vary in different facilities).

Orders to be transcribed are diet, preoperative and postoperative instructions, all medical treatments, activity, procedures, medications, diagnostic imaging and other diagnostic studies, and laboratory tests. When a patient undergoes surgery, all preoperative orders are automatically canceled. The physician must rewrite the orders postoperatively if the orders are to be continued.

Box 54-5 10 STEPS TO EFFECTIVE TIME MANAGEMENT

1. Set goals, plan, and evaluate feedback relative to your goals.
2. Set priorities—know what you want, how you want it, and when you want it.
3. Use "do" lists daily, weekly, monthly. Mark off tasks as completed.
4. Do not procrastinate. Identify and confront underlying problems that lead to procrastination, and resolve them.
5. Be organized. Avoid time wasters and learn to delegate.
6. Stay focused.
7. Be self-disciplined—it generates pride and satisfaction.
8. Do one of four things with paperwork: complete it, act on it, save it (if valid reason), or destroy it (if it is of no value).
9. Keep motivated—think in a positive manner.
10. Learn to use computers efficiently—thoroughly learn a computer program.
11. Learn your peak time when energy and attention levels are optimal; match your energy level with complexity of task to be completed.

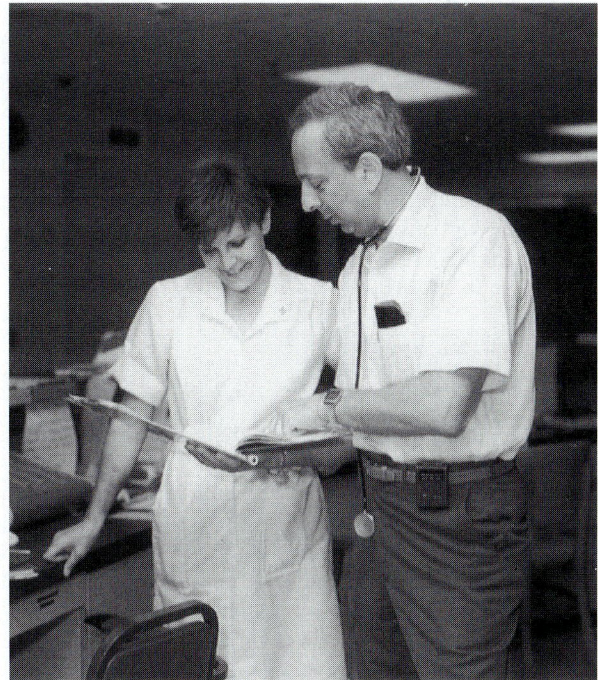

FIG. 54-5 Clarifying the physician's order.

Many physicians have routine postoperative orders, which have been prepared beforehand. This sheet is placed in the patient's chart, and the orders are transcribed as discussed. There will be a procedure for each order according to policy of the facility. When transcribing any order, follow completely through all steps one order at a time, and then check it off on the order sheet. The nurse transcribing orders should record the time and sign full name on each order. When appropriate, complete the proper requisition slip. As a charge nurse, report any new orders or changes to other staff members so that optimum care will be provided to the patient.

Box 54-6 PRECAUTIONS FOR TRANSCRIBING ORDERS

The information that follows applies to all physicians' orders.

1. Check that orders are written on the correct chart.
2. If there is more than one order, read through *all* orders before beginning.
3. Process stat orders first. (A stat order signifies that a single dose of medication is to be given immediately and only once.)
4. If there is some confusion during a telephone order, have another nurse listen in on the line for clarification.

The items below are basic guidelines and may vary from one facility to another. Check the agency's policy.

5. The medication needed should be ordered from the pharmacy: include the date, patient's name, room number, time, medication, route of administration, dosage, and frequency.
6. Record the orders in the required areas, such as Kardex, Medex, or medication card. Be certain to include the date.
7. A stat medication may need to be written on a card of a different color. Write STAT on the card, and also write the room number, patient's name, drug dose, route, and time. Pay special attention to STAT orders—the card should be destroyed after the order is given and recorded. STAT orders are to be carried out *immediately,* not at the next routine time for medication administration or procedure performance.
8. Make very certain that all orders have been carried out and recorded in the proper record. (Have a second nurse verify for accuracy until you gain experience.)
9. Each order should be checked off on the physicians' order sheet and signed with your name or initials.
10. Those nurses responsible for administering medications should be notified of any new order.
11. Most facilities use a sign that indicates a new order. A red flag may be placed on each chart, or perhaps the physician places the chart in a specific place, such as on the unit secretary's desk.
12. Preferably the charge nurse should be assigned to examine all patients' charts for new orders. This should happen during each shift.

End-of-Shift Report

As an LPN/LVN, you are often responsible for giving an end-of-shift report. See Box 54-8 for an example. The following material will assist you in organization of data for a more efficient and accurate report.

The purpose of the shift report is to provide the next shift with pertinent information about the patient. The quality of nursing care the patient receives is contingent on how well each shift communicates with the other.

Before beginning the report, plan your communication. Be cognizant of what you want to express. Consider your choice of words. Be precise. Use accepted medical/nursing terminology. Practice pronouncing difficult vocabulary to enhance pronunciation.

Before starting the report, write down all necessary information, such as vital signs, type of intravenous (IV) fluids, rate of infusion, and credit left in IV bottles and continuous bladder irrigations. Report the condition of the IV site. Record the patient's appetite, intakes, and output for feces, urine, and gastric secretion. Report output from drainage tubes, such as Davols, Hemovacs, T-tubes, Malecot drains, Solcotrans, and closed chest tubes. Report color of all body excretions. Have information of analgesics given, the time administered, and effect. Record the amount of patient-controlled analgesia (PCA) used. Write down narcotic credits from the PCA. Write down the assessment results of your patient's lung sounds, bowel sounds, abdomen (soft or distended), and condition of the skin—report abnormal color and turgor for dehydration or edema. Note circulatory checks if pertinent, as well as presence or absence of pedal pulses. If the patient has a bruit, report it. Note dressing changes, amount and color of exudate, and the condition of the

Box 54-7 PROCEDURE FOR DISCONTINUING OR CHANGING A MEDICATION

1. Mark old medication order off the Kardex or Medex by crossing through with a highlighter marking pen. If it is an order change, write new order.
2. Notify the nurse responsible for carrying out new orders about discontinued and newly ordered medications.
3. See that the old medication card is destroyed, if medication card issued.
4. Check off on the physicians' order sheet.

incision. Note any abnormal signs and symptoms, such as dyspnea, tachycardia, or abnormal mental status or level of consciousness. Note neurological deficits, such as flaccid extremity, drooping side of face, hemianopia, or difficulty swallowing (dysphagia).

Once all the above data are compiled, use Kardex and begin the report. Be systematic and report the following:

1. State patient's room and bed number, name, age, physician, all diagnoses, and date of surgery if patient is postoperative.
2. Summarize patient's day/evening/night.
3. Report all pertinent nursing care.
4. Describe change in patient's condition. Usually most facilities report only abnormal vital signs except first postoperative day, and then last set of vital signs are given.
5. Report special medications, intravenous solutions, infusion rate, IV credits. State time, method, and dosage of analgesics given and the effect.
6. Report all intakes and outputs.
7. Report status of lungs and bowel sounds.
8. Report mental status and level of consciousness.
9. Report circulatory checks, pedal pulses, and skin abnormalities in turgor or color.
10. State diagnostic procedure, such as CT scans, x-ray studies, MRI, endoscopy, proctoscopy, thoracentesis, and surgery. Report diet changes, special permits, preoperative procedures, daily weights, activity status, Accuchecks, Hematest for stools, clean catch urine for analysis and/or C&S, sputum specimen for C&S, respiratory therapy, and physical therapy orders. Report all nursing interventions, such as dressings, packs, ostomy care, and oxygen.
11. Discuss patient and family education.
12. Note other services, such as social services, pastoral care, and discharge planning.
13. State any pertinent information helpful in patient care.
14. Report "no code" status.
15. Present the report in an unbiased, nonjudgmental manner.

Box 54-8 SAMPLE OF A SHIFT REPORT

348A Mabel Lauritsen, age 87, patient of Dr. Hartman, in with congestive heart failure and stasis ulcer of the right leg. She is alert and cheerful, has had a comfortable day. She has a slight decrease of the edema in her lower extremities. Received an additional 40 mg of Lasix orally at 10 AM; weight is 165 lb, down 10 lb since admission 2 days ago. Vital signs unremarkable except BP 168/100. Has an IV of D_5W with 20 mEq of KCl infusing at 60 ml per hr with a credit of 600 ml. IV site is without edema or erythema. Has been up about 1 hour today. Appetite has been good. Received Bancap tablets two at 1400 for pain in right leg. Intake 480 ml IV, 350 ml oral; voided 650 ml of clear, amber urine. Lung sounds clear except for fine crackles in base of right lung. She is expectorating a small amount of clear mucus. No dyspnea noted. Bowel sounds present; abdomen soft. Had moderate amount soft brown stool. Pedal pulses 2+ bilaterally. Has a 2 by 3 cm stasis ulcer of right leg treated with whirlpool and Betadine dressing. The dressings are to be changed qid; TED hose are on. There is an order for Hematest of stools × 3, clean catch urine for C&S, and a chest x-ray. She is to be NPO after midnight for surgery at 9 AM for débridement of the ulcer of her right leg. A preoperative consent form is needed. Social services will be seeing the patient and her daughter Ann Zahrt for discharge planning a few days after surgery.

LICENSURE EXAMINATION

There are review courses available to assist the graduate nurse in preparing for the National Council Licensure Examination for Practical Nurses (NCLEX-PN). Before you sign up, evaluate which course will be most beneficial to you. In considering a review course, remember the objective is to review, not primary learning.

- Plan ahead, and make an intelligent decision regarding a review course.
- Carefully evaluate your need for a review course.
- Look for a course that utilizes faculty from areas outside your school.
- Know how the course is taught. Some are taught via video.
- Consider the cost; most review courses cost about $200 to $250.
- Know the following: How long the course will last; where the course is held; the size of the class; when the course is offered.

There are review books available to aid the new graduate in preparing for the NCLEX-PN. It is important to select a review book that meets your study needs. Nursing faculty, friends with review books, the school library, and the bookstore are all sources of information regarding review books. Plan on purchasing a review book while you are still in school. Review books are revised about every 3 years.

The National Council of State Boards of Nursing, Inc., has adopted computerized adaptive testing (CAT) for the NCLEX for RN and LPN/LVN candidates, beginning in 1994. Traditional paper and pencil testing is a thing of the past. The NCLEX/CAT exam takes a maximum of 5 hours; some candidates will be able to complete the exam in less time. There will be approximately 1200 computer testing stations nationwide, distributed among a minimum of 200 centers in 150 geographical markets. The test center will be quiet and comfortable with specially designed work stations to enhance security while providing a personal testing environment.

The examinee takes a CAT exam by sitting at an individual computer or terminal and answering questions on the screen. As the examinee answers each question, the computer recalculates the examinee's estimated ability level. Using that estimate, the next question is chosen by the computer. The test is thus adapted to each examinee, depending on how each question is answered. No two persons receive the same test questions in the same order. Everyone takes a different test.

The first question for the examinee is of low to moderate difficulty. If the question is answered correctly, the following question will be more difficult. If the question is answered incorrectly, the following question will be easier.

The test stops when the examinee's ability level can be estimated at a predetermined degree of accuracy. To meet these stopping criteria, the examinee will be required to answer a specified minimum number of questions. As long as the examinee's ability level cannot be accurately determined, the test will continue until a specified maximum number of questions are presented or until the time allotted (e.g., 5 hours) has elapsed. Ability is calculated independently, in other words, it does not depend on how the examinee compares in the group (norms group).

Security is maintained by direct staff observation of the testing session, in addition to continuous monitoring by video camera and audio taping. The proctor is able to observe all candidates simultaneously and continuously during testing without entering the room, which eliminates the noise and movement of persons moving about the room.

The candidate's application is approved by the board of nursing in the jurisdiction where the NCLEX is to be taken. The candidate receives a ticket of admission from the Educational Testing Service (ETS) Data Center, which has been selected as the CAT service vendor. The candidate also receives information that describes the test, the protocol for making an appointment for the exam, and a list of available centers and their toll-free numbers. Testing is offered 15 hours a day, 6 days a week. The center schedules an appointment for a 5-hour time slot within 30 days of the call. Score reports are printed and sent to the board of nursing in each jurisdiction within 24 hours. Each board of nursing schedules its own notification timetable; thus, a candidate no longer need wait 6 to 8 weeks for the results of the examination. Most test results are received in about 1 week.

On successful completion of the examination, you can practice as an LPN/LVN. The scores are on a pass/fail basis. At the present, if the test is failed, it may be taken as many times as necessary to pass. The state board of nursing has the authority to refuse any graduate the right to take the examination. Sometimes graduates do not understand that completing the required hours of theory and clinical practice does not automatically make them eligible to take the examination. If there is a question as to the moral character of the applicant, an individual state board hearing may occur. A recommendation as to the applicant's moral character may be written by a person who is knowledgeable about the applicant. Often a nurse educator will be asked to submit such a letter to the state board of nursing. The state board has the authority to accept or reject an applicant to sit for the national licensure. The director of the school of nursing must recommend the graduate to sit for the national licensure. After receiving the license, the LPN/LVN is responsible for renewing it and keeping the state board informed of any changes of address, name, and employment (i.e., active or inactive) status. The nurse cannot legally practice nursing without a license. Licensure permits persons to offer special skills to the public, but it also provides legal guidelines for protection of the public.

The NCLEX-PN makes it possible to practice nursing in other states if one has successfully passed the examination and if the nurse's education fulfills the issuing state's requirements. After a move to another state, the nurse must apply for a license or temporary practice permit before practicing nursing. This licensure from one state to another is called **endorsement** (a statement of recognition of the license of a health practitioner in one state by another state; the applicant would need to meet the current state's licensing requirements). Some states called this licensure **reciprocity.** This is a mutual agreement to exchange privileges, dependence, or relationships as, for example, an agreement between two governing bodies to accept credential of care givers licensed in the other's state. True reciprocity means that an individual licensed in one state can automatically receive licensure in the other, even if the licensing requirements of the states differ. If the nurse travels with a patient from one state to the other or to Canada, the license the nurse has in her possession is valid for the length of the stay in the other state or Canada.

NURSE PRACTICE ACT

The Nurse Practice Act is a statute enacted by the legislature of any of the states or by appropriate officers of the districts or possessions.

The **Nurse Practice Act** is the licensing law. It defines the title and regulations governing the practice of nursing. The act delineates the legal scope of the practice of nursing within the geographical boundaries. Its provisions assist the nurse in staying within the legal scope of nursing practice in each state. Some states have separate governing boards for professional and practical/vocational nursing. The Nurse Practice Act defines the regulations for practical nursing and includes requirements for an approved school of nursing. It also states the requirements for licensure and conditions for which a license may be revoked or suspended (see Chapter 2).

STATE BOARD OF NURSING

The state board of nursing consists of members who represent the different levels of nursing and who are appointed by the governor. The purpose of the board is to protect the public by administering the Nurse Practice Act. The board is responsible for approving schools of nursing and renewing and issuing licenses. The board has the authority to suspend or revoke a license. Some of the conditions under which a nurse license may be suspended or revoked because of inability to perform competently are drug addiction, alcohol abuse, and lack of mental or physical well-being. A nursing license can be revoked also for **negligence** (the commission of an act that a prudent person would not have done or the omission of a duty that a prudent person would have fulfilled, resulting in injury or harm to another person; it must be proved that other prudent members of the same profession would ordinarily have acted differently under the same circumstances) in patient care, endangering a patient's life, or failing to comply to the standard and requirements of the Nurse Practice Act of the state in which the nurse is practicing (see Chapter 2).

REFERENCES AND SUGGESTED READINGS

1. Adams-Ender CL: Mentoring: nurses helping nurses, *RN* 91(4):21, 1991.
2. Aiserstein TJ: Taking charge: how to land the job you want, *RN* 53(2):15, 1990.
3. American Nurse's Association: *Standards of nursing practice,* Kansas City, Mo, 1991, The Association.
4. Becker BG, Finder DT: *Vocational and personal adjustments in practical nursing,* ed 7, St Louis, 1994, Mosby.
5. Begany T: Put these on your bookshelf, *RN* 56(11):49, 1993.
6. Beninger CJ et al: Preparing for state boards, *Nurs '90* 29(2):1990.
7. Bersky A: Computerized adaptive testing, National Council of State Board of Nursing, Inc, NCLEX; Third Regional Invitational, New Orleans, April 22-23, 1992.
8. Bostwick B: *Résumé writing,* ed 4, New York, 1990, Wiley.
9. Calfee B: 7 things you should never chart, *Nurs* 24(3):43, 1994.
10. Chenevert M: *Mosby's tour guide to nursing school,* ed 2, St Louis, 1992, Mosby.
11. Chin PL, Kramer MK: *Theory and nursing: a systematic approach,* ed 3, St Louis, 1991, Mosby.
12. Chitty KK: *Professional nursing: concepts and challenges,* Philadelphia, 1993, Saunders.
13. Cohen MR: Better ways to transcribe orders, *Nurs* 20(1):9, 1990.
14. Council of Practical Nursing Programs: *Practical nursing care 1989-1990* (pub no 38-1328), New York, 1990, National League for Nursing.
15. Cox SS: Taping report tips to record by, *Nursing* 24(3):64, 1994.
16. Deloughery G: *Issues and trends in nursing,* St Louis, 1991, Mosby.
17. Douglass LM: *The effective nurse: leader and manager,* St Louis, 1992, Mosby.
18. Ellie JR, Hartley CL: *Nursing in today's world: challenges issues, and trends,* ed 4, Philadelphia, 1992, Lippincott.
19. Engram B: Yes, you can —: the job you really want, *Nurs '91* 21(2):116, 1991.
20. Flores DW: Marketing yourself in an interview, *Nursing* 22(8):100, 1992.
21. Grensing L: A formula to avoid miscommunicating, *Nurs '90* 10(9):122, 1990.
22. Hall J, Stevens P: Nursing shortage, *Nurs Outlook* 39:2, 1991.
23. Hanger TI: Presenting yourself successfully, *Nurs '91* 21(6):87, 1991.
24. Hart PD: What the public thinks, *J Pract Nurs* p 29, March 1991.
25. Hill SS, Howlett HA: *Success in practical nursing: personal and vocational issues,* ed 2, Philadelphia, 1993, Saunders.
26. Hurley ML: What do the new JCAHO standards mean for you? *RN* 54(6):42, 1991.
27. Kurzen CR: *Contemporary practical/vocational nursing,* ed 2, Philadelphia, 1993, Lippincott.
28. Lloyd A: Stop, look and listen, *Nurs Times* 87(12):30, 1991.
29. Mattera MD, editor: *RN presents: nursing opportunities 1992,* ed 23, Montvale, NJ, Medical Economics.
30. Merker L: *Meet the challenge: health care in the 1990s,* p 32, Sept 1991.
31. *Mosby's medical, nursing, and allied health dictionary,* ed 4, St Louis, 1994, Mosby.
32. Moss J: *Membership services,* Raleigh, NC, 1992, NFLPN.
33. Murphy T: Improving nurse/doctor communications, *Nurs '90* 19(8):114, 1990.
34. National Council adapts CAT for NCLEX administration, *Nurs Health Care* 12(8):440, 1991.
35. *Nursing data source,* vol 2, New York, 1991, National League for Nursing.
36. Potter PA, Perry AG: *Basic nursing: theory and practice,* ed 3, St Louis, 1995, Mosby.
37. Potter PA, Perry AG: *Fundamentals of nursing: concepts, process and practice,* ed 3, St Louis, 1993, Mosby.
38. Raudsepp E: Seven ways to cure communication breakdowns, *Nurs '90* 10(4):132, 1990.
39. Ringsven MK, Bond D: *Gerontology and leadership skills for nurses,* Albany, NY, 1991, Delmar.
40. Smith CE: Changing jobs: making the right move, *Nurs '90* 20(9):107, 1990.
41. Yannes-Eyles M: *Mosby's comprehensive review of practical nursing for NCLEX-PN,* ed 11, St Louis, 1994, Mosby.
42. Yates MJ: *Resumes that knock 'em dead,* Boston, 1992, Bob Adams.
43. Zwewekh J, Claborn JC: *Nursing today,* Philadelphia, 1994, Saunders.

CHAPTER CHALLENGE

KEY POINTS

- A well-prepared résumé broadens interview opportunities.
- An interview is important, and every effort should be made to guarantee a successful one.
- The release of information to anyone other than the health care team is a violation of the patient's right to privacy.
- The nurse may be found guilty of invasion of privacy, slander, or libel if the patient's health care information is not kept confidential.
- Learning does not cease upon graduation.
- The new graduate has a variety of job opportunities available. Options will require considerable thought to make the correct decision.
- The nurse should follow the correct procedure for transcribing physician's orders.
- The purpose of the end-of-shift report is to accurately communicate pertinent patient information from one shift to another.
- LPNs/LVNs are legally liable for their actions; therefore, they should understand the legal framework within which they are practicing.
- Endorsement/reciprocity enables a nurse to practice in another state without retaking the NCLEX-PN.
- The National Council of State Boards of Nursing, Inc., has adopted the CAT for the NCLEX-PN.
- The Nurse Practice Act is the licensing law.
- The main function of a state board of nursing is to ensure safety for the consumer of nursing services.
- Licensure permits persons to offer special skills to the public, but it also provides legal guidelines for protection of the public.

STUDY QUESTIONS

1. A group of new LPNs/LVNs are discussing the function of the state board of nursing, which is to:
   1. Establish certain nursing procedures in the hospital
   2. Renew and issue licenses as well as suspend or revoke a license
   3. Separate schools of nursing in the state
   4. Establish inservice programs in the hospital
2. The following organizations are totally committed to practical/vocational nursing and its continuing education:
   1. NAPNES and NFLPN
   2. NPANES and NLN
   3. NLN and ANA
   4. ANA and NFLPN
3. The LPN license permits:
   1. Giving first aid
   2. Recommending a particular physician
   3. Supervising care in a long-term care facility
   4. Rendering safe nursing service to the public
4. The primary purpose of states' requiring nurses to be licensed to practice nursing is to:
   1. Protect the LPN/LVN employer and the nurse
   2. Provide legal guidelines to protect the public
   3. Protect the patient and employer
   4. Protect the LPN/LVN from malpractice
5. Ms. Brown will join a professional organization. The national organization for LPNs/LVNs is:
   1. ANA
   2. NLN
   3. NAPNES
   4. NRN
6. In a long-term care facility, the LVN knows that the following physician orders take priority:
   1. PRN orders
   2. One-time-only orders
   3. Routine orders
   4. Stat orders
7. The physician's order that is the least subject to error is:
   1. Written
   2. Telephone
   3. Verbal
   4. Transcribed
8. Mr. Limus, LVN, is contemplating which field of nursing he will seek employment. Several options are available to him. He is aware that in private duty nursing:
   1. He must always work fixed hours and days
   2. He will care for three or four patients
   3. The pay is the same as for an RN
   4. He is directly responsible to the individual employer for salary and schedule
9. A statute enacted by the legislature of any of the states to delineate the legal scope of the practice of nursing within the geographical boundaries of the jurisdiction is called the:
   1. NLN Act
   2. Nurse Practice Act
   3. NCLEX Act
   4. JCOAH Act
10. It is 14:30, time for the end-of-shift report. During a change-of-shift report, the nurse:
    1. Repeats gossip about specific patients
    2. Drinks coffee and visits with colleagues
    3. Identifies nursing diagnoses
    4. Gives her impression of the patient
11. Every nurse giving an end-of-shift report must realize it is important to:
    1. Evaluate results of nursing interventions
    2. Discuss various opinions about the patient
    3. Criticize the patient's behavior
    4. Discuss the patient's finances

CREDITS

We thank Mosby for the use of its extensive art library during the preparation of this text. We also acknowledge the following Mosby authors and their books from whom we have borrowed select illustrations and display material.

Anderson KN, Anderson I, Glanze WD: *Mosby's medical, nursing, and allied health dictionary,* ed 4, 1994.

Barkauskas VH et al: *Health and physical assessment,* 1994.

Beare PG, Myers JL: *Principles and practice of adult health nursing,* ed 2, 1994.

Belcher AE: *Cancer nursing: Mosby's clinical nursing series,* 1992.

Bobak I: *Maternity and gynecologic care: the nurse and the family,* ed 5, 1993.

Brundage D: *Renal disorders: Mosby's clinical nursing series,* 1992.

Clayton BD, Stock YN: *Basic pharmacology for nurses,* ed 10, 1993.

Dison N: *Simplified drugs and solutions for nurses,* ed 10, 1992.

doCarmo PB: *Basic EMT skills and equipment: techniques and pitfalls,* 1988.

Ebersole P, Hess P: *Toward healthy aging: human needs and nursing response,* ed 4, 1994.

Hamilton PM: *Basic maternity nursing,* ed 6, 1989.

Harkness Hood G, Dincher JR: *Total patient care: foundations and practice of adult health nursing,* ed 8, 1992.

Ingalls AJ, Salerno MC: *Maternal and child health nursing,* ed 7, 1991.

Korones SB: *High-risk newborn infants: the basis for intensive nursing care,* ed 4, 1986.

LaRocca J, Otto S: *Pocket guide to intravenous therapy,* ed 2, 1993.

Long BC, Phipps WJ: *Medical-surgical nursing: a nursing-process approach,* ed 3, 1993.

Malasanos L et al: *Health assessment,* ed 4, 1990.

McCance KL, Huether SE: *Pathophysiology: the biological basis for disease in adults and children,* ed 2, 1994.

Meeker MH, Rothrock J: *Alexander's care of the patient in surgery,* ed 9, 1991.

Mudge-Grout C: *Immunologic disorders: Mosby's clinical nursing series,* 1993.

Nolte J: *The human brain: an introduction to its functional anatomy,* ed 3, 1993.

Pagana KD, Pagana TJ: *Mosby's diagnostic and laboratory test reference,* 1992.

Perry AG, Potter PA: *Clinical nursing skills and techniques,* ed 3, 1994.

Perry AG, Potter PA: *Pocket guide to basic skills and procedures,* ed 3, 1994.

Phillips C: *Family-centered maternity/newborn care,* ed 3, 1992.

Phipps WJ et al: *Medical-surgical nursing: concepts and clinical practice,* ed 4, 1991.

Potter PA, Perry AG: *Basic nursing: theory and practice,* ed 3, 1995.

Potter PA, Perry AG: *Fundamentals of nursing: concepts, process, and practice,* ed 3, 1993.

Prior JA, Silberstein JS, Stand JM: *Physical diagnosis: the history and examination of the patient,* ed 6, 1981.

Schneeburg NG: *Essentials of clinical endocrinology,* 1979.

Seeley RR, Stephens TD, Tate P: *Anatomy and physiology,* ed 2, 1992.

Seidel HM et al: *Mosby's guide to physical examination,* ed 3, 1995.

Smith S: *Communications in nursing: communicating assertively and responsibly in nursing—a guidebook,* ed 2, 1992.

Sorentino SA: *Mosby's textbook for nursing assistants,* ed 3, 1992.

Thibodeau G: *Anthony's textbook of anatomy and physiology,* ed 13, 1990.

Thibodeau G: *Structure and function of the body,* ed 9, 1992.

Thompson JM et al: *Mosby's clinical nursing,* ed 3, 1993.

Tucker SM: *Fetal monitoring and fetal assessment in high-risk pregnancy,* 1978.

Whaley LF, Wong DL: *Nursing care of infants and children,* ed 4, 1991.

Williams SR: *Essentials of nutrition and diet therapy,* ed 6, 1994.

Wilson SF, Thompson JM: *Respiratory disorders: Mosby's clinical nursing series, 1990.*

Wong DL: *Whaley and Wong's Essentials of pediatric nursing,* ed 4, 1993.

Worthington-Roberts B, Williams SR: *Nutrition in pregnancy and lactation,* ed 5, 1993.

ANSWER KEY

Chapter 1

1. 1
2. 4
3. 3
4. 4
5. 1
6. 3

Chapter 2

1. 2
2. 3
3. 1
4. 3
5. 4
6. 4
7. 2

Chapter 3

1. 1
2. 4
3. 2
4. 4
5. 3
6. 2
7. 1

Chapter 4

1. 3
2. 1
3. 3
4. 1
5. 2
6. 2
7. 2
8. 2

Chapter 5

1. 1
2. 2
3. 1
4. 1
5. 4
6. 4
7. 4
8. 3

Chapter 6

1. 3
2. 1
3. 4
4. 2
5. 3
6. 2
7. 1
8. 3
9. 1

Chapter 7

1. 2
2. 3
3. 3
4. 2
5. 2
6. 1
7. 2
8. 3
9. 3
10. 3

Chapter 8

1. 2
2. 3
3. 4
4. 2
5. 4
6. 3
7. 1

Chapter 9

1. 4
2. 2
3. 2
4. 1
5. 2
6. 2
7. 1

Chapter 10

1. 1
2. 2
3. 3
4. 2
5. 2
6. 4
7. 2
8. 3

Chapter 11

1. 2
2. 1
3. 4
4. 4
5. 1
6. 4
7. 2
8. 4

Chapter 12

1. 1
2. 3
3. 4
4. 1
5. 4
6. 2
7. 1
8. 2
9. 4
10. 2

Chapter 13

1. 3
2. 4
3. 1
4. 4
5. 1
6. 4
7. 4
8. 3
9. 4
10. 2

Chapter 14

1. 3
2. 1
3. 2
4. 1
5. 3
6. 2
7. 1
8. 4
9. 3
10. 1

Chapter 15

1. 3
2. 1
3. 3
4. 1
5. 3
6. 4
7. 2
8. 4
9. 4
10. 1
11. 1
12. 2
13. 2
14. 2

Chapter 16

1. 3
2. 4
3. 2
4. 4
5. 4
6. 2
7. 4
8. 1
9. 1
12. 4
13. 3
14. 3
15. 4
16. 1
17. 4
18. 3
19. 4

Chapter 17

1. 1
2. 3
3. 2
4. 4
5. 1
6. 2
7. 4
8. 3
9. 2
10. 1

Chapter 18

1. 4
2. 4
3. 1
4. 2
5. 3
6. 4
7. 1
8. 2
9. 3
10. 2

Chapter 19

1. 2
2. 2
3. 2
4. 3
5. 2
6. 2
7. 1
8. 4
9. 2
10. 3

Chapter 20

Section I

1. 1
2. 2
3. 1
4. 3

Section II

1. 2
2. 2
3. 1

Section III

1. 3
2. 4
3. 3
4. 1
5. 2

Section IV

1. 3
2. 3
3. 4
4. 1

Chapter 21

1. 1
2. 4
3. 2
4. 1
5. 2
6. 3
7. 1
8. 4
9. 1
10. 4

Chapter 22

1. 4
2. 4
3. 2
4. 3
5. 1
6. 2
7. 2
8. 3
9. 2
10. 3
11. 1
12. 4

Chapter 23

1. 2
2. 3
3. 1
4. 4
5. 1
6. 2
7. 4
8. 1
9. 3
10. 2

Chapter 24

1. 1
2. 1
3. 1
4. 1
5. 3
6. 3
7. 4
8. 1
9. 2
10. 3

Chapter 25

1. 2
2. 1
3. 2
4. 3
5. 1
6. 2
7. 3
8. 4
9. 1
10. 2
11. 3
12. 1
13. 2
14. 3
15. 4
16. 4
17. 1

Chapter 26

1. 3
2. 2
3. 4
4. 1
5. 1
6. 2
7. 1
8. 2
9. 4
10. 2
11. 1
12. 2
13. 2
14. 4
15. 1
16. 2
17. 3
18. 2
19. 4
20. 1

Chapter 27

1. 2
2. 3
3. 2
4. 2
5. 2
6. 2
7. 1
8. 2
9. 3
10. 4
11. 1
12. 2
13. 2
14. 1
15. 1
16. 4
17. 1
18. 2
19. 3

Chapter 28

1. 1
2. 2
3. 1
4. 3
5. 2
6. 3
7. 2
8. 4
9. 4
10. 3
13. 4
14. 1
15. 4
16. 4
17. 2
18. 2
19. 4
20. 2
21. 3
22. 1

Chapter 29

1. 3
2. 1
3. 2
4. 3
5. 1
6. 3
7. 4
8. 2
9. 4
10. 2
11. 3
12. 2
13. 4
14. 3
15. 1
16. 4
17. 3
18. 2
19. 3

Chapter 30

1. 1
2. 3
3. 2
4. 3
5. 3
6. 4
7. 2
8. 1
9. 4
10. 3
11. 2
12. 2

Chapter 31

1. 2
2. 4
3. 3
4. 2
5. 3
6. 4
7. 3
8. 2
9. 4
10. 4
11. 1
12. 2
13. 3
14. 4
15. 2
16. 3
17. 3
18. 2
19. 1
20. 2
21. 4

Chapter 32

1. 3
2. 1
3. 4
4. 3
5. 3
6. 3
7. 4
8. 1
9. 4
10. 4
11. 1
12. 1
13. 4
14. 3
15. 4

Chapter 33

1. 1
2. 2
3. 3
4. 4
5. 1
6. 3
7. 4
8. 2
9. 1
10. 2
11. 3
12. 1
~~13. 1~~

Chapter 34

1. 2
2. 2
3. 3
4. 2
5. 1
6. 2
7. 2
8. 1
9. 2
10. 3
11. 3
12. 2
13. 1
14. 4
15. 3
16. 4
17. 1

Chapter 35

1. 1
2. 3
3. 2
4. 1
5. 3
6. 2
7. 1
8. 3
9. 1
10. 3
11. 1
12. 2
13. 2
14. 1
15. 4
16. 4
17. 4
18. 2
19. 4
20. 4

Chapter 36

1. 3
2. 2
3. 1
4. 2
5. 2
6. 1
7. 3
8. 3
9. 4
10. 2
11. 2

Chapter 37

1. 2
2. 1
3. 1
4. 3
5. 2
6. 2
7. 2
8. 2
9. 3
10. 4

Chapter 38

1. 1
2. 1
3. 3
4. 1
5. 1
6. 4
7. 3
8. 1
9. 2
10. 3

Chapter 39

1. 2
2. 1
3. 4
4. 3
5. 4
6. 2
7. 1
8. 3
9. 2
10. 3

Chapter 40

1. 2
2. 4
3. 2
4. 4
5. 1
6. 3
7. 3
8. 3
9. 1
10. 1

Chapter 41

1. 2
2. 2
3. 2
4. 3
5. 4
6. 1
7. 4
8. 4
9. 4
10. 2

Chapter 42

1. 3
2. 2
3. 3
4. 2
5. 3
6. 1
7. 4
8. 3
9. 4
10. 2

Chapter 43

1. 4
2. 3
3. 4
4. 1
5. 2
6. 1
7. 3
8. 3
9. 3
10. 1

Chapter 44

1. 2
2. 4
3. 4
4. 3
5. 3
6. 4
7. 2
8. 2
9. 2
10. 3

Chapter 45

1. 1
2. 3
3. 4
4. 1
5. 2
6. 3
7. 4
8. 1
9. 2

Chapter 46

1. 4
2. 3
3. 4
4. 4
5. 2
6. 3
7. 4
8. 4
9. 4
10. 2
11. 3

Chapter 47

1. 4
2. 2
3. 4
4. 3
5. 4
6. 2
7. 1
8. 3
9. 1

Chapter 48

1. 2
2. 3
3. 3
4. 3
5. 3
6. 2
7. 2
8. 3
9. 4
10. 1

Chapter 49

1. 1
2. 4
3. 1
4. 2
5. 4
6. 3
7. 2
8. 3
9. 4
10. 1

Chapter 50

1. 2
2. 4
3. 1
4. 3
5. 1
6. 1
7. 2
8. 4
9. 1
10. 3

Chapter 51

1. 2
2. 4
3. 2
4. 3
5. 3
6. 2
7. 4
8. 2
9. 1
10. 4

Chapter 52

1. 4
2. 3
3. 4
4. 2
5. 3
6. 1
7. 2
8. 4
9. 1
10. 2

Chapter 53

1. 1
2. 4
3. 2
4. 3
5. 2
6. 1
7. 4

Chapter 54

1. 2
2. 1
3. 4
4. 2
5. 1
6. 3
7. 4
8. 1
9. 4
10. 2
11. 3
12. 1

GLOSSARY

ABC Mnemonic for assessing status of emergency patients: **A**irway, **B**reathing, **C**irculation; utilized in one- or two-rescuer CPR.

abduct To draw away (as a limb) from the axis of the body.

abduction Movement of an extremity away from the midline of the body.

ablation Amputation or excision of any part of the body; removal of a growth or harmful substance.

abrasion Scraping or rubbing away of a surface, such as the skin, by friction.

abstinence Voluntary avoidance of substances; refraining from the performance of an act.

accommodation Adjustment of the eye for various distances whereby it is able to focus the image of an object on the retina by changing the curvature of the lens.

accountability Being answerable for one's own actions.

accreditation Process whereby a professional association or nongovernmental agency grants recognition to an institution or agency for demonstrated ability in a special area of practice.

accrue To bring together so as to increase in number or mass.

acetabulum *L. "vinegar cup"* Large, cup-shaped articular cavity at the junction of the ilium, the ischium, and the pubis, containing the ball-shaped head of the femur.

acetone Colorless, aromatic ketone found in small amounts in normal urine and in larger quantities in the urine of patients with diabetes mellitus.

acetylcholine Neurotransmitter substance widely distributed in body tissues, with a primary function of mediating synaptic activity of the nervous system.

achalasia Abnormal condition characterized by the inability of a muscle to relax, particularly the cardiac sphincter of the stomach.

Achilles tendon Common tendon of the soleus and gastrocnemius muscles; begins near the middle of the posterior part of the leg.

achlorhydria Abnormal condition characterized by the absence of hydrochloric acid in the gastric secretions.

ACLS (advanced cardiac life support) Provision of basic life support plus use of adjunctive equipment for establishing an intravenous line, administering fluid and drugs, monitoring the heart, performing defibrillation, controlling dysrhythmias, and providing postresuscitation care.

acquired heart disorder Cardiovascular disorder that consists of postnatal abnormalities that compromise the heart's function.

acquired immunodeficiency syndrome (AIDS) Acquired condition that impairs the body's ability to fight infection; the end stage of continuum of HIV infection in which the infected person has a CD_4 count (lymphocytes) of 200 cells/mm^3 or less.

acrocyanosis Peripheral cyanosis; the blue discoloration of the hands and feet in most infants at birth that may persist for 7 to 10 days.

acromion process Slightly flaring projection at the lateral end of the scapula; it forms the highest point of the shoulder.

action potential (or **action current**) Electrical impulse consisting of a self-propagating series of polarizations and depolarizations transmitted across the cell membranes of a nerve fiber during the transmission of a nerve impulse and across the cell membranes of a muscle cell during contraction or other activity of the cell.

active transport Force that moves molecules into cells without regard for the positive or negative charge by osmosis.

actual nursing diagnosis Statement of a health problem that a nurse is licensed and competent to treat.

acuity Sharpness or acuteness of hearing or sight.

acute Having a short and relatively severe course; a disease process characterized by a relatively short duration of signs and symptoms that are usually severe and begin abruptly.

acute pain Intense, unpleasant sensation of short duration, lasting less than 6 months.

adaptation Adjustment to changing life situations by using various strategies.

adaptive immunity Protection that provides a specific reaction to each invading antigen and has the unique ability to remember the antigen that caused the attack.

addiction Compulsive, uncontrollable dependence on a substance, habit, or practice to such a degree that cessation causes severe emotional, mental, or physiological reactions.

addictive personality Personality marked by traits of compulsive and habitual use of a substance or practice to cope with psychic pain engendered by conflict and anxiety.

adduction Movement of an extremity toward the axis of the body.

adenosine triphosphate (ATP) Enzyme involved in obtaining energy for cellular energy metabolism.

adhesion Band of scar tissue that binds together two anatomical surfaces that are normally separate.

adipose tissue Type of body tissue composed of cells containing stored fat.

adjunct Additive substance or treatment to increase the effectiveness of a primary procedure or to facilitate its performance.

ADL Activity of daily living.

admission Entry of a patient into a health care facility.

adolescence Period that begins with puberty and extends for 8 years or longer, until the person is physically and psychologically mature and ready for adult responsibilities.

adoptive family Family unit with adoptive children, children chosen and taken into the family by legal process and raised as one's own.

adrenal glands (suprarenal glands) Small, yellow endocrine glands that lie directly atop the kidneys; they contain an outer section, the adrenal cortex, and a small inner section, the adrenal medulla.

adrenocorticotropic hormone (ACTH) Peptide hormone secreted by the anterior pituitary gland; stimulates the endocrine activity of the cortex portion of the adrenal glands.

advanced directives Signed and witnessed document providing specific instructions for health care treatment in the event that a person is unable to make those decisions at the time they are needed.

advancement Rise in rank or importance; a promotion, progress, improvement.

adventitious Abnormal sounds superimposed on breath sounds.

adverse drug reaction Harmful, unintended reaction to a drug administered at the normal dosage.

advocate Person who works on behalf of another person who is in a vulnerable or underprivileged position.

afebrile Without fever.

affect External manifestation of inner feelings or emotions.

afferent Proceeding toward a center, as applied to arteries, veins, lymphatics, and nerves.

against medical advice (AMA) Charting notation when a patient leaves a health care facility without a physician's order for discharge.

ageism Discrimination against older persons.

aggression Interpersonal behavior that dominates, humiliates, or violates the rights of others.

aggressive communication Overpowering, bold, forceful way of expressing one's opinions.

agility Ability to move with quick, easy grace.

aging Process of growing old, which begins at conception and ends at death.

agnosia Total or partial loss of the ability to recognize familiar objects or persons through sensory stimuli as a result of organic brain damage.

agonist Drug that produces a predictable response at the intended site of action.

AHA American Heart Association.

AIDS Acquired immunodeficiency syndrome.

akinesia Abnormal state of motor and psychic hypoactivity.

Al-Anon International organization offering guidance and counseling for relatives, friends, and associates of alcoholics.

albuminuria Presence of albumin in the urine.

alcohol sponge Sponge bath with alcohol and water to reduce body temperature.

alcohol withdrawal syndrome Clinical signs and symptoms associated with cessation of alcohol consumption, including tremors, hallucinations, autonomic nervous system dysfunction, and seizures.

Alcoholics Anonymous (AA) International nonprofit organization, founded in 1935, of abstinent alcoholics whose purpose is to help other alcoholics stop drinking and maintain sobriety through group support, shared experiences, and faith in a power greater than themselves. The AA program, which emphasizes both medical and religious resources for help in overcoming alcoholism, focuses on attending meetings and coping with abstinence "one day at a time." Meetings are held at convenient times in factories, schools, churches, hospitals, and many other institutions and community buildings.

alcoholism Extreme dependence on excessive amounts of alcohol, associated with a cumulative pattern of deviant behaviors.

alignment Relationship of various body parts to each other.

alimentary canal Musculomembraneous tube extending from the mouth to the anus.

allergen Substance that can produce a hypersensitive reaction in the body but that is not necessarily inherently harmful.

alopecia Loss of hair resulting from destruction of hair follicles.

alpha-fetoprotein (AFP) Antigen present in the human fetus; can be used to evaluate fetal development.

alveoli Small, saclike structures through which gas exchange takes place in the lungs.

alveolus Combining form meaning "trough, channel, cavity"; a small grapelike structure.

amblyopia Reduction or dimness of vision, especially when there is no apparent pathological condition of the eye.

amenorrhea Absence of menstrual flow.

amino acids Building blocks of which proteins are constructed and are the end products of protein digestion.

amniocentesis Obstetrical procedure in which a small amount of amniotic fluid is removed for laboratory analysis; usually performed between the sixteenth and twentieth weeks of gestation to aid in the diagnosis of fetal abnormalities.

amniotomy Artificial rupture of the fetal membranes (AROM).

ANA Standards of Nursing Practice Evaluation that serves as a basis for comparison of similar occurrences, set forth by the American Nurses' Association.

anabolism The building aspect in which the energy released from catabolism allows the cells to build more complex, usable forms of nutrients; the building and repairing phase of metabolism.

analysis Separation of substances into their constituent parts.

anaphylactic shock Severe, life-threatening hypersensitivity reaction that may cause spasms or edema of the upper airway and could progress to cardiovascular collapse.

anaphylaxis An exaggerated, life-threatening hypersensitivity reaction to a previously encountered antigen.

anaplasia Change in the structure of cells; a loss of differentiation characteristic of a malignancy.

anasarca Severe generalized edema.

anastomosis Surgical joining of two ducts or blood vessels to allow flow from one to the other.

anatomy Study, classification, and description of structures and organs of the body.

androgen Male sex hormones.

anemia Blood disorder characterized by RBC, hemoglobin, and hematocrit levels below normal range.

anesthesia absence of sensation (*an* meaning "without" and *esthesia* meaning "awareness or feeling").

aneurysm An enlarged, dilated portion of an artery.

angina pectoris Paroxysmal thoracic pain and choking feeling caused by anoxia of the myocardium.

animism Attribution of human characteristics to nonhuman or inanimate objects.

anion Negatively charged ion that when in solution is attracted to the positive electrode.

ankylosis Fixation of a joint, often in an abnormal position, usually resulting from destruction of articular cartilage and subchrondral bone.

anomalies Congenital malformations, such as the absence of a limb or the presence of an extra finger.

anorexia Lack or loss of appetite, resulting in the inability to eat.

anorexia nervosa A psychoneurotic disorder characterized by a prolonged refusal to eat: self-imposed starvation.

anoxia Abnormal lack of oxygen.

answer Response of a defendant to the complaint of a plaintiff.

antagonist Drug that will block the action of another drug.

antepartal First stage of the maternity cycle; also known as the *prenatal* or the *antenatal period*.

anterior Front of a structure.

anterior fontanelle Diamond-shaped area at the superior, anterior area of the head.

antibody Protein molecule essential to the immune system, produced by lymphoid tissue in response to bacteria, viruses, or other antigenic substances; an antibody is specific to an antigen.

anticipatory grief Expectation of or preparation for the loss of one or more valued or significant objects; accomplishment of part of the grief work before the actual loss.

anticipatory guidance Psychological preparation of a patient for an event expected to be stressful, as in the preparation of a child for surgery by explaining what will happen and what it will feel like. It is also used to prepare parents for normal growth and development of their children.

antidiuretic hormone (ADH) Hormone that decreases the production of urine by increasing the reabsorption of water by the renal tubules.

antigen Substance recognized by the body as foreign that can trigger an immune response.

antioxidant Chemical or other agent that delays or prevents the breakdown of a substance by oxygen.

anuria Urinary output of less than 100 to 250 ml/day.

anxiety Condition in which an individual experiences a vague feeling of apprehension resulting from a real or perceived threat to self.

aorta Largest artery of the body; the main track of the systemic arterial circulation, comprised of four parts: the ascending aorta, the arch, the thoracic portion of the descending aorta, and the abdominal portion of the descending aorta.

apex Pertaining to the top, the end, or the tip of a structure—as the apex of the heart.

aphasia Abnormal neurological condition in which language function is defective or absent because of an injury to certain areas of the cerebral cortex.

apical pulse Heart beat as measured with the bell or disk of the stethoscope placed over the apex of the heart.

aplasia In hematology, a failure of the normal process of cell generation and development.

apnea Absence of spontaneous respirations.

appeal Request for review and/or retrial of legal issues.

approved program Program that meets minimum standards established by the state agency responsible for overseeing educational programs.

apraxia Impairment of the ability to perform purposeful acts.

aqueous humor A clear, watery fluid similar to blood plasma circulating in the anterior chamber of the eye; it is constantly being formed, drained, and replaced in the anterior chamber.

arachnoid membrane Thin, delicate membrane enclosing the brain and the spinal cord, interposed between the pia mater and the dura mater. The subarachnoid space lies between the arachnoid membrane and the pia; the subdural space lies between the arachnoid membrane and the dura.

areola Darker tissue surrounding the nipple.

areolar gland One of the large sebaceous glands in the areolae encircling the nipples on women's breasts.

arrhythmia See *dysrhythmia.*

arteries Large vessels carrying blood in a direction away from the heart.

arteriole Smallest vascular branch of the arterial circulation.

arteriosclerosis Common arterial disorder characterized by thickening, loss of elasticity, and calcification of arterial walls resulting in a decreased blood supply, especially to the cerebrum and lower extremities.

arthrocentesis Puncture of a joint with a needle to withdraw fluid performed to obtain synovial fluid for diagnostic purposes.

arthrodesis Surgical fusion of a joint.

arthroplasty Surgical repair or refashioning of one or both sides, parts, or specific tissues within a joint.

arthroscopy Examination of the interior of a joint performed by inserting a specially designed endoscope through a small incision.

articulation Gliding, rotation, and angular movement of a joint.

ascites Accumulation of fluid and albumin in the peritoneal cavity.

asepsis Absence of infection.

asphyxia Severe lack of oxygen to the blood, leading to hypercapnia, loss of consciousness, and, if not corrected, death.

assertive communication Communication that considers the feelings and requests of patients yet honors nurses' rights in the relationship.

assertiveness Nurses' ability to confidently and comfortably express thoughts and feelings while still respecting the legitimate rights of others.

assessment Evaluation or appraisal of a condition; includes observing, gathering, verifying and communicating pertinent data, usually information pertaining to the patient.

asterexis Hand-flapping tremor usually induced by extending the arm and dorsiflexing the wrist; frequently seen in hepatic coma.

asthenia General feeling of tiredness and listlessness.

asthma Respiratory disorder characterized by recurring episodes of paroxysmal dyspnea, wheezing on expiration due to constriction of the bronchi, coughing, and viscous mucoid bronchial secretions.

astigmatism Defect in the curvature of the eyeball surface.

asymptomatic Without indication of disease; without subjective or objective signs and symptoms.

ataxia Abnormal condition characterized by impaired ability to coordinate movement.

atelectasis Collapse of lung tissues, preventing the respiratory exchange of carbon dioxide and oxygen.

atheroma Abnormal mass of fat or lipids deposited on the arterial wall.

atherosclerosis A common arterial disorder characterized by yellowish plaques of cholesterol, lipids, and cellular debris in the inner layer of the walls of large and medium-sized arteries.

atony Lack of normal tone or strength.

atrioventricular valve Valve in the heart through which blood flows from the atria to the ventricles.

atrium (atria) Chamber or cavity, such as the upper chamber of the heart.

atrophy Decrease in size or physiological activity of a part of the body because of disease or lack of use.

attachment Close, mutual relationship between two people that involves contact and proximity and endures through time.

attenuation Weakening the virulence of a disease organism.

attitude Relationship of fetal body parts to each other.

audiometry Testing of hearing acuity.

auditors Person appointed to examine a patient's charts and health records to assess the quality of care.

auditory hallucination Perception of sound without an external stimulus.

aura Sensation, as of light or warmth that may precede an attack of migraine or an epileptic seizure.

auscultate To listen for sounds within the body to evaluate the condition of the heart, lungs, pleura, intestines, or other organs or to detect fetal heart sounds.

autistic behavior Self-absorbed, isolated, repetitive behavior and lack of communication with others.

autocratic family Family unit with unequal relationships; parents attempt to control with strict rigid rules and expectations.

autograft Surgical transplantation of any tissues from one part of the body to another location in the same individual.

autoimmunity Immune response (autoantibodies or cellular immune response) to one's own tissues.

autologous Originating within the self.

autolysis Self-dissolution or self-digestion in tissues or cells by enzymes in the cells.

autonomy Ability or tendency to function independently.

autopsy Examination performed after death to confirm or determine the cause of death.

axilla Underarm area or armpit.

axis Line that passes through the center of the body or through a part of the body.

axon Cylindric extension of a nerve cell that conducts impulses away from the neuron cell body.

azotemia Retention in the blood of excessive amounts of nitrogenous compounds.

B cell Type of lymphocyte that responds to stimulation of antigens entering the body, causing an immunological response.

babbling Incoherent sounds made by an infant while vocally playing with sounds.

back rub (massage) Manipulation of the soft tissue by rubbing and kneading to increase circulation, improve muscle tone, and promote relaxation in the patient.

bacteriuria Presence of bacteria in the urine.

Ballottement Technique of palpating an organ or floating structure by bouncing it gently and feeling it rebound. Ballottement of a fetus within the uterus is a probable objective sign of pregnancy.

Bartholin's gland One of the two small, mucus-secreting glands bilateral to the vaginal opening.

basal metabolic rate (BMR) Amount of energy used by the body at rest to maintain vital functions such as respiration, circulation, temperature, peristalsis, and muscle tone.

base of support Area on which an object rests.

basophils Granulocytic leukocytes essential to the nonspecific immune response to inflammation because of their important role in releasing histamine during tissue damage or invasion.

bath basin Small plastic pan used to hold water for bathing a patient.

bath mitt Wash cloth folded over the hand to form a mitt; prevents wet ends of cloth from touching the patient.

battered woman syndrome Repeated episodes of physical assault on a woman by a man with whom she has a close relationship.

bedpan Device for receiving feces or urine from patients confined to bed; may be used for specimen collection.

bedside commode Chair with a hole in the seat containing a vessel for urination and defecation.

behavior Manner in which a person acts or performs; any or all of the activities of a person, including physical actions that are observed directly, and mental activity, which is inferred (to conclude from certain premises as evidence) and interpreted.

beneficence Bringing about of good.

benign Not recurrent or progressive; opposite of *malignant.*

benign neoplasm Localized tumor that has a fibrous capsule, limited potential for growth, and cells that are well differentiated.

bereavement Common depressed reaction to the death of a loved one.

beriberi Disease of the peripheral nerves caused by a deficiency of or an inability to assimilate thiamin.

bicarbonate Main anion of the extracellular fluid.

biographical Relating to the facts and events of a person's life.

biological age Person's present position with respect to potential life span, which may be younger or older than chronological age and encompasses measures of vital organ functions.

biological death Results from permanent cellular damage caused by a lack of oxygen. The brain is the first organ to suffer from this lack of oxygen.

biopsy Removal of a small piece of living tissue from an organ or another part of the body for microscopic examination to confirm or establish a diagnosis, estimate prognosis, or follow the course of a disease.

bipolar hip replacement Prosthetic implant used to replace the femoral head and neck in fractures when the vascular supply to the femoral head is or may eventually be compromised; also called *hemiarthroplasty.*

birth defect (congenital anomaly) Abnormality present at birth, particularly a structural abnormality that may be inherited genetically, acquired during gestation or inflicted during the parturition process of giving birth.

blanching Causing to become pale by applying digital pressure.

blastocyst Embryonic form that is a spheric mass of cells having a central, fluid-filled cavity (blastocell) surrounded by two layers of cells; the outer layer forms the placenta, and the inner layer later forms the embryo.

blended/reconstructed family (step family) Family unit formed by parents who bring unrelated children from prior marriages into a new, joint-living situation.

blood pressure Pressure exerted by the circulatory volume of blood on the arterial walls, veins, and chambers of the heart.

BLS (basic life support) Phase of cardiopulmonary resuscitation (CPR) and emergency cardiac care (ECC) that prevents circulatory or respiratory arrest or insufficiency by prompt recognition and early intervention or by early entry into the emergency care system (ECS) or both or externally supports the circulation and respirations of a victim of cardiac arrest through CPR.

Bobath technique Treatment designed to normalize muscle tone by providing as many sensations of normal muscle tone, posture, and movement as possible.

body mechanics Physiological study of the muscular actions and the functions of muscles in maintaining the posture of the body.

body substance isolation (BSI) Isolation system that emphasizes the potential infectiousness of all moist body substances; effective for all patients except for those with diseases spread by the respiratory tract, such as tuberculosis.

body surface area (BSA) Total area exposed to the outside environment.

bolus Food broken down and mixed with saliva and ready to be swallowed; concentrated mass of pharmaceutical preparations given intravenously.

bonding Initial phase in a relationship characterized by strong attraction and a desire to interact.

bony prominence Area of the body where bones can be easily palpated. Bony areas have greater potential for impaired skin integrity than other areas of the body.

Bowman's capsule Cup-shaped end of a renal tubule containing a glomerulus.

bradycardia Slow rhythm characterized by a pulse of less than 60 beats per minute.

bradykinesia Abnormal condition characterized by slowness of all voluntary movement and speech, as caused by Parkinsonism and certain tranquilizers.

bradypnea Abnormally slow rate of breathing.

brain death Irreversible form of unconsciousness characterized by a complete loss of brain function while the heart continues to beat. The legal definition of this condition varies from state to state.

brain stem Portion of the brain comprising the medulla oblongata, the pons, and the mesencephalon. It performs motor, sensory, and reflex functions. The 12 pairs of cranial nerves are attached to the base of the brain.

Braxton Hicks contractions Irregular tightening of the pregnant uterus that begins in the first trimester and increases in frequency, duration, and intensity as pregnancy progresses. Near term, strong Braxton Hicks contractions are often difficult to distinguish from true labor.

bronchiole Small airway of the respiratory system extending from the bronchi into the lobes of the lung.

bronchitis Acute or chronic inflammation of mucous membranes of the tracheobronchial tree.

bronchopulmonary Of or pertaining to the bronchi and the lungs of the respiratory system.

bronchopulmonary dysplasia Abnormal development of the bronchi and lungs.
bronchoscopy Visual examination of the tracheobronchial tree using the standard rigid, tubular metal bronchoscope or the narrower, flexible fibertropic bronchoscope.
bronchus Large passage into the lungs through which pass inspired air and exhaled waste gases.
brown fat Source of heat unique to the neonate that is capable of greater thermogenic (heat-producing) activity than ordinary fat. Deposits are formed around the adrenals, kidneys, and neck; between scapulas; and behind the sternum and remain for several weeks after birth.
bruit Abnormal swishing sound heard over organs, glands, and arteries.
buccal In or directed toward the cheek.
buffer Chemical system that circulates through the body in pairs neutralizing excess acids or alkalines by contributing or accepting hydrogen ions; can be considered chemical sponges.
bulimia (also called *bulimia nervosa*) an eating disorder involving an insatiable craving for food, often resulting in episodes of continuous eating followed by periods of depression, self-deprivation, and/or purging.
burnout Mental or physical energy loss related to a job, accompanied by feelings of hopelessness or loss of creativity.
burping Belching or eructation.
bursa Fibrous sac between certain tendons and the bones beneath them. Lined with a synovial membrane that secretes synovial fluid, the bursa acts as a small cushion that allows the tendon, as it contracts and relaxes, to move over the bone.

cachexia General ill health and malnutrition marked by weakness and emaciation and usually associated with a serious disease such as cancer.
calcaneus Heel bone.
calcitonin Polypeptide hormone released by the thyroid gland; works as an antagonist to parathyroid hormone to decrease blood calcium levels by causing calcium to be stored in bones.
calcium Silvery yellow metal; the most abdundant mineral in the body; a positively charged ion known as a *cation.*
callus Bony deposits formed between and around the broken ends of a fractured bone during healing.
calyx Cup-shaped organ or cavity.
canal of Schlemm Tiny venous sinus located at the border or junction of the sclera and corner; drains the aqueous humor and funnels it into the bloodstream.
candidiasis Mild fungal infection that appears in men and women; usually caused by *Candida albicans* and *Candida tropicalis.*
cannabis (marijuana) Psychoactive drug derived from the flowering tops of hemp plants.
canthus Angle at the medial and lateral margins of the eyelid (corners of the eye).
capillaries Tiny blood vessels joining arterioles and venules.
carbohydrate Any of a group of organic compounds, the most important being sugar, starch, cellulose, and gum.
carcinoembryonic antigen (CEA) Oncofetal glycoprotein antigen found in colonic adenocarcinoma and other cancers and in nonmalignant conditions.
carcinogen Substance known to increase the risk for the development of cancer.
carcinoma Malignant tumor composed of epithelial cells, with a tendency to metastasize.
carcinoma in situ Preinvasive, asymptomatic carcinoma that can be diagnosed only be microscopic examination of cervical cells.
cardiac arrest Sudden cessation of functional circulation.
cardiac output Volume of blood expelled by the ventricles of the heart.
cardiovascular Of or pertaining to the heart and blood vessels.
cardioversion Restoration of the heart's normal sinus rhythm by delivery of a synchronized electric shock through two metal paddles placed on the patient's chest.
care giver role Function of giving care to others.
carotid pulse Pulse of the carotid artery, felt by gently pressing a finger into the groove between the larynx and the sternocleidomastoid muscle in the neck.
carrier Person or animal that harbors and spreads an organism causing disease in others but who does not become ill.
catabolism Break down or destructive phase of metabolism. Catabolism occurs when complex body substances are broken down to simpler ones; opposite of *anabolism.*
cataract Opacity or clouding of the lens.
catatonic state Extreme immobility and muscular rigidity, usually associated with panic or schizophrenia.
cation Positively charged ion that when in solution is attracted to the negatively charged electrode.
CDC See Centers for Disease Control and Prevention.
cell Fundamental unit of all living tissue.
cellular immunity Acquired immunity characterized by the dominant role of small T lymphocytes.
center of gravity Midpoint or center of weight of a body or object. In the standing adult human the center of gravity is in the midpelvic cavity, between the symphysis pubis and the umbilicus.
Centers for Disease Control and Prevention (CDC) Federal agency that provides facilities and services for investigation, identification, prevention, and control of disease; headquartered in Atlanta, Georgia.
central nervous system One of the two main divisions of the nervous system, consisting of the brain and the spinal cord.
centrifuge Equipment that spins test tubes at high speeds.
centriole Intracellular organelle, associated with cell division.
cerebellum Part of the brain located in the posterior cranial fossa behind the brain stem. It consists of two lateral cerebellar hemispheres, or lobes, and a middle section called the *vermis.* Its functions are concerned with coordinating voluntary muscular activity.
cerebral dominance Specialization of each of the two cerebral hemisphers in the integration and control of different functions.
cerebrospinal fluid Fluid that flows through and protects the four ventricles of the brain, the subarachnoid space, and the spinal canal.
cerebrovascular accident (CVA) Abnormal condition of the blood vessels of the brain characterized by occlusion by an embolus or cerebrovascular hemorrhage, resulting in ischemia of the brain tissues normally perfused by the damaged vessels. The sequelae depend on the location and extent of ischemia.
cerebrum Largest and uppermost section of the brain, divided by a central sulcus into the left and the right cerebral hemispheres.
certification Process in which an individual, an institution, agency, or educational program is evaluated and recognized as meeting certain predetermined standards.
cerumen Yellowish or brownish waxy secretion produced by vestigial apocrine sweat glands in the external ear canal; earwax.
ceruminous gland One of a number of tiny structures in the external ear canal, believed to be modified sweat glands.
cervical cord injury Injury to the spinal column at the cervical spine C2 to C7 and involves paralysis of all extremities and trunk, respiratory failure, bladder and bowel disturbance, bradycardia, perspiring, elevated temperature, and headache.
cervix Smaller, narrower, lower portion of the uterus.
chancre Painless erosion or papule that ulcerates superficially with a scooped-out appearance.
chart (health care record) Legal record that is used to meet many demands of the health accreditation, medical insurance, and legal systems.
charting by exception Recording only new data or changes in patient status or care; charting the exceptions to the previously recorded data.
charting, documenting, or *recording* Process of noting data in a patient record, usually at prescribed intervals.
chelation therapy In toxicology, use of a compound to group a toxic substance and make it nonactive and thus nonotoxic.
chemical dependence Total psychophysical state of one addicted to drugs or alcohol who must receive an increasing amount of the substance to prevent abstinence signs and symptoms.
chemoreceptors Sensory nerve cell activated by chemical stimuli.
Cheyne-Stokes respiration Abnormal respiratory pattern characterized by periods of apnea altering with deep, rapid respirations.
child maltreatment Emotional, physical, or sexual abuse of a child.
children with special needs Infants and children with congenital abnormalities, malignancies, gastrointestinal diseases, and central nervous system anomalies.
Chlamydia trachomatis Gram-negative, intracellular bacterium that causes several common sexually transmitted diseases.
chloride Negatively charged extracellular anion; a salt of hydrochloric acid.
cholesterol (dietary) Fat-soluble sterol found in animal fats and oils, organ meats, and egg yolk.
cholesterol (serum) Fat-soluble sterol that circulates in the bloodstream. It is continuously synthesized in the body, primarily in the liver.
chorionic villi Tiny vascular protrusions of the chorionic surface that project into the maternal blood sinuses of the uterus and help to form the placenta.
choroid Posterior portion of the middle layer of the vascular tunic of the eye. It is highly vascular and supplies nutrients to the retina.

chromatin Material within the cell nucleus from which the chromosomes are formed. It consists of fine, threadlike strands.

chromosomes Threadlike structure in the nucleus of a cell that functions in the transmission of genetic information.

chronic Developing slowly and persisting for a long period, often for the remainder of the life of the individual.

chronic obstructive pulmonary disease (COPD) Progressive and irreversible condition characterized by diminished inspiratory and expiratory capacity of the lungs.

chronic pain Pain lasting longer than 6 months; can be as intense as acute pain, can be continuous or intermittent.

chronological age Age of an individual expressed as time elapsed since birth.

Chux Waterproof, disposable underpad.

Chvostek's sign Abnormal spasm of the facial muscles elicited by light taps on the facial nerve in patients who are hypocalcemic; seen in tetany.

chyme Viscous, semifluid contents of the stomach present during digestion of a meal.

cilia Small, hairlike processes on the outer surfaces of some cells, aiding metabolism by producing motion, eddies, or current in a fluid, most often associated with the respiratory passageway.

circumcision Surgical procedure in which a part of the foreskin is removed, leaving the glans penis uncovered.

circumorbital around an orbit, often referring to the eye.

cisterna chyli Enlarged pouchlike structure in the abdominal thoracic duct that serves as a storage area for lymph moving toward its point of entry into the venous system.

classification Sorting of objectives into groups according to certain attributes, such as color, size, or shape.

claudication Weakness of the legs accompanied by cramplike pain in the calves caused by poor circulation of the blood to the leg muscles.

cleft lip Congenital anomaly consisting of one or more clefts in the upper lip, resulting from failure of the maxillary and median nasal processes to close.

cleft palate Congenital defect characterized by a fissure in the midline of the palate, resulting from failure of the two sides to fuse during embryonic development.

climacteric Phase of the aging process marking the transition from the reproductive phase to a nonreproductive stage of life.

clinical death Cessation of heartbeat and respirations. In many cases CPR can reverse clinical death if initiated within 4 minutes of cardiopulmonary arrest.

clonus(ic) Abnormal pattern of neuromuscular activity, characterized by rapidly alternating involuntary contraction and relaxation of skeletal muscle.

closed bed Hospital bed made with all linens pulled toward the head of the bed.

CMV See *cytomegalovirus.*

cocaine hydrochloride White crystalline powder used as a local anesthetic. It was originally derived from coca leaves, but can also be prepared synthetically.

cochlea Part of the inner ear, it resembles a snail's shell and contains the organ of Corti, the organ of hearing.

code System of notification that allows information to be transmitted rapidly.

co-dependency Situation in which a person is overly affected by and concerned with controlling other people's behaviors.

coffee ground vomitus/emesis Dark brown vomitus the color and consistency of coffee grounds, composed of gastric juices and old blood; indicative of slow upper gastrointestinal bleeding.

cognitive behavior Mental processes characterized by knowing, thinking, learning, and judging.

cognitive impairment Significantly subaverage general intellectual functioning; formally referred to as *mental retardation.*

cognitive learning Learning concerned with problem-solving abilities, intelligence, and conscious thought.

cohabitation Two people living together in a sexual relationship without marriage.

coitus Sexual union of two people of the opposite sex.

collaborative problem Actual or potential health problem (complication) that focuses on the pathophysiological response of the body that nurses are responsible and accountable for identification and treatment in collaboration with the physician.

collagen Fibrous insoluble protein found in connective tissue, including skin, bone, and ligaments.

Colles' fracture A fracture of the distal portion of the radium within 1 inch of the joint of the wrist.

collodion Clear or slightly opaque, highly inflammable liquid composed of pyroxylin, ether, and alcohol. It dries to a strong, transparents film that is used as a surgical dressing.

color blindness Inability to distinguish colors of the spectrum.

colostrum Breast fluid that may be excreted from the second trimester of pregnancy onward but is most evident in the first 2 to 3 days after birth and before the onset of true lactation. This thin, yellowish fluid is rich in proteins and calories in addition to antibodies and lymphocytes.

colporrhaphy Surgical correction of cystocele and rectocele by shortening the muscles that support the bladder and repair the rectocele.

colposcopy Examination of the cervix and vagina using a colposcope.

comfort To give strength and hope, to cheer and to ease the grief or trouble of another.

command hallucination Imaginary voice commanding the individual to do something.

commiseration Sharing of mutual predicaments when nurses have experienced patients' circumstances.

communication Vehicle for establishing a therapeutic relationship, since it involves conveying information and exchanging thoughts and feelings.

community health nursing Blend of nursing and public health, promoting prevention, education, and maintenance.

compartment syndrome Pathological condition caused by progressive development of arterial compression and reduced blood supply to an extremity.

compassion Strong emotion or sentiment stimulated by the presence of suffering that evokes recognition and mutual sharing of the despair or pain of the sufferer.

compatibility Quality or state or existing together in harmony.

complaint Pleading by a plaintiff made under oath to initiate a lawsuit.

comprehensive rehabilitation plan Planned, orderly sequence of services designed to help a disabled individual realize maximum potential.

compressor Individual in two-rescuer cardiopulmonary resuscitation (CPR) who performs external cardiac compressions.

compulsion Irresistible, repetitive, irrational impulse to perform an act that is usually contrary to one's ordinary judgments or standards yet results in overt anxiety if it is not completed.

computed tomography Painless x-ray technique that films a cross section of tissue (CT scan); also called *computerized axial tomography.*

computer terminal On-line terminal at a nursing work station used to access a larger mainframe computer for data processing.

conception/fertilization Beginning of pregnancy.

concrete operational stage Phase of Piagetian theory in which thoughts become increasingly logical and coherent so that the child is able to classify, sort, and organize facts while still being incapable of generalizing or dealing with abstractions; occurs between 7 to 11 years of age.

condyle Rounded projection at the end of a bone that anchors muscle ligaments and articulates with adjacent bones.

confidentiality Nondisclosure of certain information except to another authorized person; process of keeping information and records private or secret.

conflict Mental struggle, either conscious or unconscious, resulting from the simultaneous presence of opposing or incompatible thoughts, ideas, goals, or emotional forces, such as impulses, desires, or drives.

confront To challenge.

confrontation Communication skill of informing patients how their behavior is destructive to themselves or others and asking patients to change this behavior.

congenital heart defect Abnormality of the heart present at birth.

congestive heart failure (CHF) Abnormal condition characterized by circulatory congestion resulting from the heart's inability to act as an effective pump.

congruent In agreement or harmony.

conjunctiva Thin mucous membrane lining the inner aspect of the eyelids and the anterior surface of the eyeball to the edges of the cornea.

conjunctivitis Inflammation of the conjunctiva.

connective tissue Tissue that supports and binds other body structures. The types are bone, cartilage, and fibrous tissue.

conservation Mental process of understanding the sameness of a situation or object in spite of a change in some aspect (e.g., that the mass or quantity of an object is the same even if it changes shape or position).

consolation Soothing and encouraging expressions used to ease discomfort or pain.

consumer One who uses goods or services.

contact lens Small, curved glass or plastic lens shaped to fit the eye and to correct refraction or inability of the lens of the eye to focus accurately.

contamination Condition of being soiled, stained, touched, or otherwise exposed to harmful agents by the entry of infectious or toxic material into a previously clean or sterile environment, making an object potentially unsafe for use as intended.

context Meaning of language within a particular setting.

continuity of care Continuing of established patient care from one setting to another.

contract Promise or a set of promises between two or more persons that creates a legal relationship between them and a legal obligation that one or more of them must fulfill.

contracture Abnormal, usually permanent condition of a joint characterized by flexion and fixation and caused by atrophy and shortening of muscle fibers.

convalescence Period of recovery after an illness, injury, or surgery.

conversion Unconscious defense mechanism in which repressed emotions are transformed into physical signs and symptoms; also called *conversion hysteria* or *conversion reaction.*

cooing Hum of contentment made by an infant.

coping Voluntary pattern of behavior used to relieve stress or anxiety.

cordotomy Operation in which an incision is made high in the thoracic area and two laminae are removed; then the pain pathways in the spinothalamic tract (anterior and lateral aspect of the cord) on the side opposite the pain are severed.

corium/dermis True skin; the layer of skin just below the epidermis, consisting of papillary and reticular layers and containing blood and lymphatic vessels, nerves and nerve endings, glands, and hair follicles.

cornea Transparent central anterior portion of the sclera; allows light rays to enter the inner portion of the eye.

coronary In anatomy, of or pertaining to encircling structures, as the coronary arteries of the heart.

coronary artery disease (CAD) Variety of conditions that obstruct blood flow in the coronary arteries.

cor pulmonale Abnormal cardiac condition characterized by hypertrophy of the right ventricle of the heart as a result of hypertension of the pulmonary circulation.

corpuscle Any cell of the body; a red or white blood cell.

cortex Outer part; from the Latin word for "bark" or "rind", so the cortex of an organ is its outer layer.

corticosteroid Any one of the natural or synthetic hormones associated with the adrenal cortex, which influences or controls by process of the body.

cortisol Steroid hormone occurring naturally in the body.

coryza (acute rhinitis) Acute inflammation of the mucous membranes of the nose, usually accompanied by edema of the mucosa and nasal discharge.

costovertebral angle Pertaining to a rib and a vertebrae; one of two angles that outline a space over the kidneys.

cotyledon One of the 15 to 28 visible segments of the placenta on the maternal surface, each made up of fetal vessels, chorionic villi, and an intervillous space.

countertraction Force that counteracts the pull of traction.

Couvade syndrome Man's physical and emotional reaction to his partner's pregnancy.

Cowper's gland Either of two pear-shaped glands beneath the bulb of the male urethra; they correspond to the Bartholin's glands in the female.

coxsackievirus Any of 30 serologically different enteroviruses associated with a variety of signs and symptoms and primarily affecting children during warm weather.

CPR (cardiopulmonary resuscitation) Basic emergency procedure for life support, consisting of artificial respiration and manual external cardiac massage.

craniotomy Any surgical opening into the skull, performed to relieve pressure, to control bleeding, or to remove a tumor.

crackles Abnormal sound heard on auscultation of the chest and produced by passage of air through the bronchi that contain secretions or exudate or that are constricted by spasms or a thickening; may be heard on inspiration and expiration. Formerly called *rales.*

creatinine Nitrogenous compound produced by metabolic processes in the body.

crepitus Sound that resembles the crackling noise heard when rubbing hair between the fingers or throwing salt on an open fire. It is associated with gas gangrene, the rubbing of bone fragments, or the crackles of a consolidated area of the lung in pneumonia.

crisis Time of change or turning point in life when patterns of living must be modified to prevent disorganization of the person or family.

cryosurgery Procedure to "freeze" the border of a retinal hole with a frozen-tipped probe.

cryptorchidism Failure of testes to descend into the scrotum.

crystalline lens Transparent colorless structure of the eye, biconvex in shape, enclosed in a capsule and held in place just behind the pupil by the suspensory ligament. Its function is to focus light rays so that they form a perfect image on the retina.

cue Word, phrase, or symptom that indicates the nature of something perceived. Cues are grouped to assist the nurse in interpretations of data.

culdoscopy Diagnostic procedure that provides visualization of the uterus and adnexa (uterine appendages), ovaries, fallopian tubes, and small intestine.

cultural healing beliefs Beliefs that reflect a specific culture's orientation to health and illness.

culture Nonphysical traits such as values, beliefs, attitudes, and customs shared by a group and passed from one generation to the next.

culture Procedure for laboratory test involving cultivation of microorganisms or cells in a special growth medium.

cumulative Type of drug build up in the body that can lead to a toxic or even lethal (deadly) effect.

cumulative action Increased activity demonstrated by a drug when repeated doses accumulate in the body.

curative Active approach to treatment, designed to cure.

curettage Scrapping of material from the wall of a cavity or other surface performed to remove tumors or other abnormal tissue for microscopic study.

Curling's ulcer Duodenal ulcer that develops 8 to 14 days after severe burns on the surface of the body.

currant jelly stools Feces mixed with blood and mucus from the intestinal mucosa.

cushingoid Having the habitus and facies characteristic of Cushing's disease: fat pads on the upper back and face, striae on the limbs and trunk, and excess hair on the face.

custom Habitual practice; the usual way of acting under given circumstances.

cyanosis Slightly bluish, gray, slatelike, or dark purple discoloration of the skin resulting from the presence of abnormally reduced amounts of hemoglobin in the blood.

cytological valuation Study of cells.

cytology Study of cells: their formation, origin, structure, biochemical activities, and pathology.

cytomegalovirus (CMV) Member of a group of large, species-specific, herpes-type viruses with a wide variety of disease effects.

cytoplasm "Living matter"; the protoplasm of a cell outside the nucleus.

damages Monies asked for by the plaintiff or compensation for any loss, detriment, or injury to the plaintiff's person, property, or rights caused by the wrong doing or negligence of the defendant.

dander Dry scales shed from the skin or hair of animals or feathers of birds that may cause an allergic reaction in some individuals.

data base Large store or bank of information.

death Cessation of life.

debridement Removal of damaged cellular tissue from a wound or burn to prevent infection and to promote healing.

decentering Coordination mentally of two or more ideas or characteristics, such as space and length.

deciduous/primary teeth Set of 20 teeth that appear normally during infancy.

decorticate rigidity Abnormal postural reflex characterized by flexion of the arms, wrists, and fingers. The legs may also be flexed.

decubitus ulcer Inflammation or sore in the skin over a bony prominence. It results from ischemic hypoxia of the tissue because of prolonged pressure on the part.

defendant Person to whom the complaint is directed.

defense mechanism Unconscious, intrapsychic reaction that offers protection to the self from a stressful situation.

defibrillation Termination of ventricular fibrillation by delivering a direct electrical countershock to the pericardium.

defining characteristics Clinical signs and symptoms that furnish evidence that the problem exists.

dehiscence Partial or complete separation of the wound edges.

delirium tremens (DTs) Acute, sometimes fatal psychotic reaction caused by excessive intake of alcoholic beverages over a long period.

delusion Persistent, afferent (deviating from the normal) belief or perception held inviolable by a person even though it is illogical, unique, and probably wrong.

dementia Progressive impairment of intellectual (cognitive) function that interferes with normal social and occupational activities.

democratic family pattern Family style in which the adult members are considered equal and children are treated with respect and recognized as individuals.

demographics Statistical study of human populations, especially with reference to size and density, distribution and vital statistics, and typical characteristics.

dendrite Branching process that extends from the cell body of a neuron and receives impulses.

denial Unconscious defense mechanism in which emotional conflict and anxiety are avoided by refusing to acknowledge those thoughts, feelings, desires, impulses, or external facts that are consciously intolerable.

denominator Bottom number of a fraction.

dentin Calcified tissue that gives shape and structure to the tooth.

denture Artificial teeth not permanently fixed or implanted.

deposition Out-of-court, under-oath statement of a witness.

depression Mood disturbance characterized by exaggerated feelings of sadness, despair, discouragement, dejection, worthlessness, and hopelessness that are inappropriate and out of proportion to reality.

despair Second response to separation from attachment figure, involving quiet hopelessness, sadness, and mourning.

detoxification Removal or reduction of a poison or its effects.

development Gradual process or change and differentiation from a simple to a more advanced level of complexity.

developmental delay Mental retardation.

diabetic retinopathy Disorder of retinal blood vessels characterized by capillary microaneurysms, hemorrhage, and formation of new vessels; appears approximately 10 years after onset of diabetes mellitus.

diagnose To identify a disease or condition by a scientific evaluation of physical signs, symptoms, history, laboratory tests, and procedures.

diagnosis-related group (DRG) System that classifies patients by age, diagnoses, and surgical categories; used to predict the use of hospital resources, including the length of stay.

dialysis Medical procedure for the removal of certain elements from the blood or lymph by virtue of the difference in their rates or diffusion through an external semipermeable membrane or, in the case of peritoneal dialysis, through the peritoneum.

diaphragm Domelike muscular partition between the thoracic and abdominal cavities.

diaphysis Shaft of a long bone, composed of a compact bone, yet shaped like a long, hollow tube.

diarthrosis Freely movable joint in which contiguous bony surfaces are covered by articular cartilage and connected by ligaments lined with synovial membrane.

diastole Period between contractions of the atria or the ventricles during which blood enters the relaxed chambers from the systemic circulation and the lungs.

diastolic Minimum level of blood pressure measured between contractions of the heart; recorded as the lower blood pressure measurement.

diencephalon Division of the brain between the telencephalon and the mesencephalon. It consists of the hypothalamus, thalamus, metathalamus, and the epithelamus and includes most of the third ventricle.

diet therapy Treatment of disease through diet.

dietary fiber Generic term for nondigestible chemical substances in plants.

differential white blood cell count Laboratory examination in which the different kinds of white blood cells are counted and reported as percentages of the total examined or absolute (actual) number.

differentiation Process of cellular development in which unspecialized cells or tissues are systemically modified to achieve specific and characteristic physical forms, physiological functions, and chemical properties.

diffusion Process in which solid particles in a fluid move from an area of higher concentration to an area of lower concentration, resulting in an even distribution of the particles in the fluid.

digestion (chemical) Series of reactions that break the proteins, fats, and carbohydrates into molecules that the cells can readily use.

digestion (mechanical) Breakup of food into smaller particles and propelling of the particles through the gastrointestinal system to become mixed with various enzymes.

dilemma Situation requiring a choice between two equally desirable or undesirable alternatives.

diplopia Double vision.

direct Coombs (direct antiglobulin) test Laboratory blood test to detect autoantibodies against red blood cells, which can cause cellular damage. These antibodies result in hemolytic anemia. Normal findings: negative, no agglutination.

disaster manual Written agency instructions specifying departmental responsibilities, chain of command, call-back procedures, assignment procedures, patient evacuation procedures and routes, procedures for the receipt and management of casualties, and policies related to the overall management of supplies and equipment.

disaster-preparedness plan Formal plan of action, usually prepared in written form, for coordinating the response of the hospital staff in the event of a disaster within the hospital or the surrounding community.

disaster situation Uncontrollable, unexpected, psychologically shocking event.

discharge Release of a patient from a health care facility.

discharge planning Schedule of events often planned by a multidisciplinary team leading to the return of a patient from hospital confinement to life at home or another health care setting.

discovery Pretrial procedures allowing one party to examine vital witnesses and/or documents held exclusively by the adverse party.

disengagement stage Period of family life when the grown children depart from the home. In some family units it is very brief because the adult children return to live in the family home.

disinfection Process by which pathogens, but not necessarily their spores, are destroyed.

disorientation Mental confusion characterized by inadequate or incorrect perceptions of place, time, and identity.

disoriented To lose awareness or perception of space, time, or personal identity and relationships.

disseminated intravascular coagulation (DIC) Acquired hemorrhage syndrome of clotting, cascade overstimulation, and anticlotting processes.

diuresis Secretion and passage of large amounts of urine.

diverticulitis Inflammation of one or more diverticula (pouchlike herniations through the colon).

diverticulosis Presence of pouchlike herniations through the muscular layer of the colon.

dizygotic Related to or proceeding from two zygotes (fertilized ova).

DNR Do not resuscitate.

documenting Process of adding written information to the chart, usually at prescribed intervals.

dominant group Group of persons exercising authority or influence; ruling or prevailing group.

dorsal Toward the back.

dorsiflexion Bending or flexing backward, as in upward bending of the fingers, wrist, foot, or toes.

double bagging Infection control practice of placing a bag of contaminated items into another bag that is clean and is held outside the isolation room.

drainage Free flow or withdrawal of fluids from a wound or cavity by some sort of system (e.g., a catheter or T-tube).

dramatic play Play that acts out adult roles.

drawsheet Sheet smaller than a bed sheet, usually placed across the middle of the bottom sheet to keep the mattress and bottom linens dry; can also help turn or move a patient in bed.

drip factor Apparatus that is used to deliver measured amounts of IV solutions at specific flow rates based on the size of drops of the solution.

DRG See *diagnosis-related groups.*

drug abuse Use of a drug for a nontherapeutic effect, especially one for which it was not prescribed or intended.

drug addiction Condition characterized by an overwhelming desire to continue taking a drug to which one has become habituated through repeated consumption because it produces a particular effect, usually an alteration of mental activity, attitude, or outlook.

drug interaction Modification of the effect of a drug when administered with another drug.

Duchenne's muscular dystrophy Abnormal congenital condition characterized by progressive symmetric wasting of the leg and pelvic muscles. It is an X-linked recessive disease that appears insidiously between 3 and 5 years of age and spreads from the leg and pelvic muscles to the involuntary muscles. It usually results in death within 10 to 15 years of the onset of symptoms; also called *pseudohypertrophic muscular dystrophy.*

dullness Low-pitched, thudlike sound produced by performing percussion over a dense organ such as the liver.

dumping syndrome Combination of profuse perspiration, nausea, vertigo, and weakness experienced by patients who have had a subtotal gastrectomy; symptoms are felt soon after eating, when the contents of the stomach empty too rapidly into the duodenum.

dura mater Outermost and most fibrous of the three membranes surrounding the brain and spinal cord.

durable power of attorney Instrument that appoints one person to make decisions in the event of another person's incompetence.

dysarthria Difficult, poorly articulated speech, resulting from interference in the control over the muscles of speech.

dysfunctional grieving State in which actual or perceived object loss exists; objects include people, possessions, job status, home, ideals, and parts and processes of the body.

dysmenorrhea Painful menstruation.

dyspnea Shortness of breath or a difficulty in breathing that may be caused by certain heart conditions, strenuous exercise, or anxiety.

dysphagia Difficulty in swallowing.

dysplasia Abnormal development of tissue.

dysrhythmia Any cardiac rhythm that deviates from normal sinus rhythm, also called *arrhythmia.*

dysuria Painful or difficult urination.

eclampsia Most severe form of pregnancy-induced hypertension characterized by toxic and clonic convulsions, coma, elevated blood pressure, albuminuria, and oliguria occurring during pregnancy or shortly after delivery.

ectoderm Outer layer of embryonic tissue giving rise to skin, nails, and hair.

ectopic Of an object or organ, situated in an unusual place, away from its normal location.

ectopic pregnancy Implantation of the fertilized ovum outside the uterine cavity in, for example, the abdomen, fallopian tubes, or ovaries.

edema Abnormal accumulation of fluids in interstitial spaces of tissue; a combining form meaning "swelling."

effacement Thinning and shortening or obliteration or the cervix that occurs during late pregnancy, labor, or both.

efferent nerve Nerve that transmits impulses away or outward from a nerve center, such as the brain or spine.

ego integrity Feelings of acceptance of life for what it has been, with no wish to relive it.

egocentric Self-centered; unable to consider another's viewpoint.

electromyogram (EMG) Record of the intrinsic electric activity in a skeletal muscle.

ELISA (enzyme-linked immunosorbent assay) Antibody test that detects the presence of HIV antibodies; used in diagnosing HIV-positive persons.

embolism Obstruction of a blood vessel by a foreign substance or blood clot.

embolus Foreign object, a quantity of air or gas, a bit of tissue or tumor, or a piece of thrombus that circulates in the blood stream until it becomes lodged in a vessel.

emesis basin Small, kidney-shaped basin used to collect vomitus.

empathy Ability to recognize and to some extent share the emotions and states of mind of another and to understand the meaning and significance of that person's behavior.

emphysema Overinflation and other destructive changes of alveolar walls, resulting in loss of lung elasticity and decreased gas exchange.

empyema Accumulation of pus in a body cavity, especially the pleural space, as a result of infection.

EMS (emergency medical services) National network of services coordinated to provide aid and medical assistance from primary response to definitive care, involving personnel trained in the rescue, stabilization, transportation, and advanced treatment of traumatic or medical emergencies.

electrolytes Substances that are sometimes called *minerals* or *salts;* develop tiny electrical charges when dissolved in water and break up into particles known as *ions.*

en face Position in which the mother's face and the infant's face are approximately 8 inches apart and on the same plane, as when the mother holds the infant up in front of her face or when she nurses the child.

enamel Hard, white, dense substance forming a covering for the crown of the teeth; the hardest substance in the body.

endarterectomy Surgical removal of the intimal lining of an artery.

endocrine glands Ductless glands; that is, they release their secretions directly into the blood stream.

endocrinologist Physician who specializes in endocrinology.

endoderm Innermost cell layer; from the endoderm arises the lining of cavities and passages of the body and covering for most of the internal organs.

endogenous Growing within the body; originating from within the body or produced from internal causes, such as a disease caused by the structural or functional failure of an organ or system.

endogenous infection Infection caused by nonpathogenic bacteria.

endometriosis Condition in which endometrial tissue appears outside the uterus.

endorphin Any one of the neuropeptides composed of many amino acids, elaborated by the pituitary gland and acting on the central and the peripheral nervous system to reduce pain.

endorsement Statement of recognition of the license of a health practitioner in one state by another state.

engagement Fixation of the presenting part of the fetus in the maternal pelvis. The lowest part of the presenting part is at or below the level of the ischial spines.

engagement/commitment stage Period when the couple prepares for marriage and becomes free of parental domination.

engorgement Process of swelling of the breast tissue brought about by an increase in blood and lymph supply to the breast, occurs around 48 hours postpartum and usually reaches a peak between the third and fifth day.

engrossment Father's initial response to newborn.

enteral Pertaining to the intestines.

enteral nutrition Administration of nutrients into the GI tract; usually refers to tube feeding.

enteric Pertaining to the intestines.

enteric coated Encasement of tablet in candylike coated shell to prevent medications from being absorbed in the stomach; absorption takes place in the intestine.

enucleation Removal of the eyeball.

environment All the factors that influence the life and survival of a person.

enzyme Complex proteins produced by living cells capable of inducing chemical changes in other substances without being changed themselves.

enzyme-linked immunosorbent assay (ELISA) Antibody test that detects HIV antibodies.

eosinophils Granulocytic leukocytes that play a role in allergic reactions and are effective against certain parasitic worms.

epidermis Superficial layers of the skin, made up of an outer, dead portion and a deeper, living cellular portion.

epididymis Tightly coiled tube structure that lies superior to the testes and extends posteriorly.

epididymitis Infection of the cordlike excretory duct of the testicles.

epiphysis End of the long bones; composed of spongy bone and contains the red bone marrow.

episiotomy Surgical incision of the perineum at the end of the second stage of labor to facilitate delivery and to avoid laceration of the perineum.

epistaxis Hemorrhage from the nose; nosebleed.

epistaxis digitorum Self-inflicted local digital trauma (i.e., from nasal picking).

epithelium Covering of the external and internal organs of the body, including the lining of the vessels.

erythema Redness or inflammation of the skin or mucous membrane resulting from dilation and congestion of superficial capillaries. Examples are mild sunburn or nervous blushes.

erythroblastosis fetalis Hemolytic anemia in newborns, resulting from maternal-fetal blood group incompatibility, especially involving the Rh factor and ABO blood groups.

erthrocytes Mature red blood cells.

erythrocytosis Abnormal increase in the number of circulating red cells.

eschar Black, leathery crust; a slough that the body forms over burned tissue.

esophageal varices Complex of longitudinal, tortuous veins at the lower end of the esophagus.

essential nutrients Carbohydrates, proteins, fats, minerals, vitamins, and water necessary for growth, normal function, and body maintenance. These substances must be supplied by food—they are not synthesized by the body in the quantities required for normal health.

establishment stage Period between the wedding and the birth of the first child.

estrogens Hormones that produce female physical charcteristics.

ethnic stereotype A fixed concept of how all members of an ethnic group act or think; may not bear any relationship to reality.

ethnicity A group's affiliation as a result of shared linguistic, racial, religious and/or cultural background.

ethnocentrism Tendency to view members from one cultural or ethnic group in terms of the standards of behavior, values, and customs of a person's own group.

etiology The study of all factors that may be involved in the development of a disease; the cause of disease.

eustachian tube Tube lined with mucous membrane that joins the nasopharynx and the middle ear cavity; this tube equalizes the air pressure on either side of the tympanic membrane.

euthanasia Deliberately bringing about the death of a person who is suffering from an incurable disease or condition; actively or passively.

evaluation The determination made about the extent to which the established outcomes have been achieved in the nursing care plan.

evaluation conference A complete medical team thoroughly evaluates the patient; this team reviews available data and sets realistic goals.

evisceration When the patient's viscera protrude through the disrupted wound.

exacerbation An increase in the seriousness of a disease or disorder as marked by greater intensity in the signs or symptoms of the patient being treated.

excoriation Injury to the surface layer of skin caused by scratching or abrasion.

exocrine Of or pertaining to the process of secreting outwardly through a duct to the surface of an organ or tissue or into a vessel, as a gland that secretes through a duct.

exocrine glands Glands that secrete through a series of ducts; examples are the sebaceous and sudoriferous of the skin.

exogenous Outside the body; originating outside of the body or produced from external causes, such as a disease caused by a bacterial or viral agent foreign to the body.

exogenous infection Infection caused by microorganisms not present in the human body.

exophthalmos An abnormal condition characterized by a marked protrusion of the eyeballs.

expectant stage The period of family life which begins when conception occurs and continues through the pregnancy.

expectoration Ejection of mucus, sputum, or fluids from the trachea and lungs by coughing or spitting.

expiration Breathing out, normally a passive process, depending on the elastic qualities of lung tissue and the thorax; also known as *exhalation.*

expressing opinions Nurses' disclosing what they think or feel about health care situations or health care options affecting their patients.

expulsion Having the tendency to drive out or expel.

extended family A family group consisting of the biologic parents, their children, the grandparents and other family members.

extension Movement allowed by certain joints of the skeleton that increases the angle between two adjoining boxes.

external genitalia Reproductive structures located outside the body; also called *vulva* in the female.

extracellular Fluid outside the cells of the body; lost from the body more rapidly than intracellular fluid.

extravasation The escape of fluids into surrounding tissue.

extremes Outer terms of the proportion.

extrinsic Caused by external factors.

extubation Removal of an endotracheal tube from an airway.

exudate Fluid, cells, or other substances that have been slowly exuded.

fallopian tubes Pair of ducts opening at one end into the upper portion (fundus) of the uterus and the other end into the peritoneal cavity, over the ovaries.

family Two or more persons who are related by blood, marriage, or adoption, and who live together.

family conference Consultation between the rehabilitation team and the family to discuss the patient's functional status, goals, and future.

family interaction Total of all roles and behaviors shown in a family at a given time.

family-centered care Philosophy of care that recognizes the family as the constant in the child's life and that personnel must support, respect, encourage, and enhance the strengths and competence of the family.

fanfold Folded like a fan lengthwise, such as the top linen on a hospital bed.

fasciculation Localized, uncoordinated, uncontrollable twitching of a single motor muscle group innervated by a single motor nerve.

fat Substance composed of lipids or fatty acids, ranging from oil to tallow.

fatigue State of exhaustion or a loss of strength or endurance.

febrile Pertaining to or characterized by an elevated body temperature.

feces Waste from the intestine; BM (bowel movement).

feedback Nurses' reactions (thoughts or feelings) about patients' behavior.

feelings All emotional and physical responses and sensations. Feelings are indicators of well-being.

fetal alcohol syndrome Congenital abnormality or anomaly resulting from a daily maternal intake of alcohol equivalent to 3 ounces or more of absolute alcohol.

fetal lie Relationship existing between the long axis of the fetus and the long axis of the mother.

fetal position The relationship of the occiput, sacrum, chin, or scapula on the presenting part of the fetus to its location in the front, back, or sides of the maternal pelvis.

fetal presentation That part of the fetus which first enters the pelvis and lies over the inlet; may be head, face, feet, or shoulders.

fetal pelvic disproportion Also referred to as *cephalopelvic*—the head of the fetus is larger than the pelvic outlet.

fibrin Stringy, insoluble protein; a product of the action of thrombin on fibrinogen in the clotting process.

fibroblast Flat, elongated, undifferentiated cell in connective tissue that forms fibrous, binding, and supporting tissue.

fibromyositis Any one of a large number of disorders in which the common element is stiffness and joint or muscle pain.

fibula One of the two bones of the lower leg, lateral to and smaller than the tibia.

filtration Movement of water and particles through a membrane by a force from either pressure or gravity; this membrane contains spaces through which the liquid may pass but that are too small to permit the solid particles to pass.

filtration The transfer of water and dissolved substances from an area of higher pressure to an area of lower pressure.

first intention healing Primary union of the edges of the wound, progressing to complete healing without scar formation or granulation.

first-level patient-focused response Reflexive, spontaneous identifications that nurses make with patients' suffering.

fistula Abnormal opening between two organs.

fixative Any substance used to preserve gross or histological specimens of tissue for examination.

flaccid Weak, soft, and flabby; lacking normal muscle tone.

flagella Hairlike projections that extend from some unicellular organisms and aid in their movement.

flagellation Whiplike movement.

flatness High-pitched flat sound produced by performing percussion over tissue such as muscle tissue.

flatulence Excess formation of gases in the stomach or intestine.

flatus Air or gas in the intestine that is passed through the rectum.

flossing Mechanical cleansing of tooth surfaces with stringlike waxed or unwaxed dental floss.

fluid Body fluid, either intracellular or extracellular, that is involved in the transport of electrolytes and other vital chemicals to, through, and from tissue cells.

fluoroscopy Technique in radiology for visually examining a part of the body or the function of an organ using a fluoroscope.

focus charting Expansion of the *data* and *need* columns in nurses' notes to include topics concerning the whole patient, such as behavior or treatment and response. The charting format is DAR (data, action, response).

focused assessment Concentration of attention on that part of the body where signs and symptoms are localized or most active in order to determine their significance.

follicle stimulating hormone (FSH) Secreted by the anterior pituitary gland—FSH stimulates the growth of the graffian follicle that leads to ovulation in the female; in the male it leads to the production of sperm cells.

fomite Nonliving material, such as bed linens, that may convey pathogenic microorganisms.

fontanelle A space roughly diamond-shaped covered by tough membranes between the bones of an infant's cranium. The posterior fontanelle is triangular shaped.

footboard Board placed at the foot of the patient's bed so that the feet rest firmly against the board at right angles to prevent footdrop.

foramen Round openings through a bone.

foramen magnum Opening located at the base of the occipital bone, which allows the spinal cord to communicate with the brain.

formal operational thought phase Piagetian phase that begins during adolescence, permitting abstract reasoning and systematic scientific problem solving.

fossa A shallow depression in a bone.

foster family Family unit who cares for, supervises, and nurtures children whose parents are unable to care for them.

fracture pan Small bedpan often used for patients with fractures to help prevent pain by reducing the amount of movement required for its placement.

frustration Feeling experienced when there is interference with goal-directed activity.

functional assessment Is completed upon admission and examines the patients functional abilities.

fundus Larger part, base, or body of a hollow organ.

gait Manner or style of walking.

gang Group whose membership is formed on the basis of skilled performance of some activity; a group of persons having informal and unusually close social relations.

ganglion One of the nerve cells, chiefly collected in groups outside the central nervous system.

gate control theory Suggests that pain impulses can be regulated or even blocked by gating mechanisms located along the central nervous system.

gauge A standard or scale of measurement.

generation gap Conflict between parents and offspring.

generativity Concern about providing for others that is equal to the concern of providing for the self.

genuineness Congruent (harmonious) verbal and nonverbal communication demonstrating nurses' trustworthiness.

geriatrics Medical and nursing specialty concerned with the physiological and pathological changes of later maturity, including study and treatment of health problems.

gerontology Study of the individual in later maturity and the aging process from physiological, pathological, psychological, sociological, and economic points of view.

gestational diabetes mellitus (GDM) Disorder characterized by an impaired ability to metabolize carbohydrates, usually caused by a deficiency of insulin;

occurs in pregnancy and disappears after delivery, but in some cases returns years later.

gingivae Gums.

Glasgow coma scale A quick, practical, and standardized system for assessing the degree of conscious impairment in the critically ill and for predicting the duration and ultimate outcome of coma, primarily in patients with head injuries.

glaucoma An abnormal condition of elevated pressure within an eye because of obstruction of the outflow of aqueous humor.

glioma Malignant tumor of the brain.

global cognitive dysfunction Generalized impairment of intellect, awareness, and judgment.

glomerulonephritis Inflammation of the glomeruli of the kidney.

glomerulus Tightly bound network of capillaries in a cluster and enveloped in a thin wall located in the kidneys.

glucagon Hormone produced by the alpha cells in the islets of Langerhans in the pancreas that stimulates the conversion of glycogen to glucose in the liver.

gluten Insoluble protein constituent of wheat and other grains.

glycogen Polysaccharide that is the major carbohydrate stored in animal cells.

glycosuria Presence of albumin in the urine.

glycosylated hemoglobin This test produces an accurate long-term index of the patient's average blood glucose level by measuring the patient's glycohemoglobin or GHB. Glycohemoglobin is a minor hemoglobin that makes up 4% to 8% of the total hemoglobin. It is a combination of hemoglobin and blood glucose. This test can have a blood sample drawn at any time because it is not affected by short-term variations. This test reflects the average blood sugar level for the 100-120 day period before the test.

goal The purpose to which an effort is directed.

Golgi apparatus One of many small membranous structures found in most cells, composed of various elements associated with formation of carbohydrate and protein compounds.

Good Samaritan law Legal stipulation for protection of those who give first aid in an emergency situation.

Goodell's sign Softening of the uterine cervix; a probable sign of pregnancy.

Gower's sign Classic sign of Duchenne's muscular dystrophy; the child positions on all fours and uses the hands to "walk up" the thighs.

graafian follicle Mature ovarian vesicle that ruptures during ovulation to release the ovum.

graduated Container that has markings indicating marked intervals.

granulation Any soft-pink fleshy projection that forms during the healing process in a wound not healing by first intention.

gravida A pregnant woman.

gray matter Gray tissue that makes up the inner core of the spinal column, arranged in two large lateral masses connected across the midline by a narrow commissure; also, gray tissue on the surface of the cerebral hemisphere comprising the cerebral cortex.

greater trochanter Large protuberance located at the top of the shaft of the femur, on the lateral side.

grief A pattern of physical and emotional responses to bereavement, separation, or loss.

grief therapy Mental treatment aimed at helping a patient deal with the pain of loss.

grief work Adaptation process of mourning a loss.

growth Increase in the size of an organism or any of its parts.

growth hormone Hormone released by the anterior pituitary gland that produces normal growth of the body.

gynecomastia Development of abnormally large mammary glands in the male that sometimes may secrete milk. When observed in the newborn, it is in response to maternal hormones; may be noted in either sex of the newborn.

gyrus One of the tortuous convolutions of the surface of the brain caused by infolding of the cortex.

habituation Psychological and emotional dependence on a drug, tobacco, or alcohol, resulting from the repeated use of the substance but without the addictive, physiological need to increase dosage.

hallucination Sensory perception that does not result from an external stimulus; it can occur in any of the senses and is classified accordingly as auditory, gustatory (taste), olfactory (smell), tactile (touch), or visual.

hallucinogen A substance that causes excitation of the central nervous system.

handroll Device, usually a washcloth rolled and placed in the patient's hand, to support the hand while squeezing.

harlequin sign Rare color change of no pathological significance occurring between the longitudinal halves of the newborn's body; when the infant is placed on one side, the dependent half is noticeably pinker than the superior half.

Hazardous Communication Act Requires hospitals to inform employers about the presence of or potential for harmful exposures and how to reduce the risk of exposures.

head injury Any traumatic damage to the head resulting from penetration of the skull or from too rapid acceleration or deceleration of the brain within the skull.

health Physical, mental, and social well-being and the absence of disease or other abnormal conditions.

health care facility Agency or institution that provides health care.

health care system Complete network of agencies, facilities, and all providers of health care in a specified geographical area.

health history (in medicine) A collection of information obtained from the patient and from other sources concerning the patient's physical status and psychologic, social and sexual functions.

Hegar's sign Softening of the isthmus of the uterine cervix early in gestation; a probable sign of pregnancy.

height The vertical measurement of a structure, organ, or other object from bottom to top, when it is placed or projected in an upright position.

hemarthrosis Bleeding into a joint space.

hematemesis Vomiting blood.

hematocrit Measure of the packed cell volume of red cells, expressed as a percentage of total blood volume.

hematoma Escaped blood trapped in tissues of the skin or in an organ as a result of trauma.

hematopoiesis The normal formation and development of blood cells in the bone marrow.

hematuria Presence of blood in the urine.

hemianopsia Blindness in one half of the visual field.

hemiplegia Paralysis of one side of the body.

hemocult test Detects occult (hidden) blood in feces.

hemoglobin Complex, protein-iron compound in the blood that carries oxygen to the cells from the lungs and carbon dioxide away from the cells to the lungs.

hemophilia A Hereditary coagulation disorder due to lack of antihemophiliac factor VIII, which is needed to convert prothrombin to thrombin.

hemophiliac Person with an inherited disorder characterized by excessive bleeding caused by a clotting defect.

hemoptysis Expectorating blood from the respiratory tract.

hemostasis Body process that arrests the flow of blood and prevents hemorrhage.

heparin lock Device used with an Angiocath or butterfly needle allowing maintenance of an IV route without continuous administration of IV fluid.

heterograft (xenograft) Tissue from another species, used as a temporary graft.

heterozygous Having two different genes.

high-risk nursing diagnosis A clinical judgment that an individual, family or community is more vulnerable to develop the problem than others in same or similar situation.

high-risk pregnancy Condition in which the life or health of the mother or infant is jeopardized by a disorder coincidental with or unique to pregnancy.

hilus Notch or indentation

hirsutism Excessive body hair in a masculine distribution.

HIV See *human immunodeficiency virus.*

HIV disease Symptomatic HIV infection that is not severe enough for a diagnosis of AIDS; symptoms of HIV disease are persistent unexplained fever, night sweats, diarrhea, weight loss, and fatigue.

HIV infection State in which HIV enters the body and under favorable conditions multiplies, producing injurious effects to the body.

holistic Of or pertaining to the whole; considering all factors, as holistic medicine.

holistic care The philosophy which holds that, in nature, entities such as individuals and other complete organisms function as complete units that cannot be reduced to the sum of their parts.

holistic health care A system of comprehensive or total patient care that considers the physical, emotional, social, economic, and spiritual needs of a person.

Homan's sign Early sign of thrombophlebitis of the deep veins of the calf in which there are complaints of pain when the leg is in extension and the foot is dorsiflexed.

home health agency An organization that provides health care in the home.

home health care Services that enable individuals of all ages to remain in the comfort and security of their homes while receiving health care.

homeostasis Relative constancy in the internal environment of the body, naturally maintained by adaptive resources that promote healthy survival.

homograft (allograft) The transfer of tissue between two genetically dissimilar individuals of the same species, such as a skin transplant between two humans who are not identical twins.

homosexual family Family group made up of same-sex adults who share bonds of emotional commitment and roles of childbearing.

homozygous Having two identical genes for a particular characteristic inherited from each parent.

hormones Chemical messengers that travel through the blood stream to their target organ; when the hormone reaches it target, a metabolic change occurs.

hospice From the Latin word *hospitum,* meaning "hospitality"; a resting place for travelers on a difficult journey.

host A person or group who because of risk factors, may be susceptible to disease or illness.

human immunodeficiency virus (HIV) Retrovirus that causes AIDS.

humanistic nursing approach Nursing perspective that considers the nurse-patient relationship as a human-to-human event.

humoral immunity One of the two forms of immunity that respond to antigen such as bacteria and foreign tissue. It is mediated by the B cells.

hydramanos Abnormal condition of pregnancy characterized by an excess of amniotic fluid.

hydrocephaly Pathological condition characterized by an abnormal accumulation of cerebrospinal fluid, usually under increased pressure, within the cranial vault and subsequent dilation of the ventricles. In infants the head grows at an abnormal rate, with separation of the structures, bulging fontanelles, and dilated scalp veins. Typical behavior includes irritability with lethargy and vomiting.

hydronephrosis The dilation of the renal pelvis and calyces.

hydrostatic pressure Pressure exerted by a liquid.

hygiene The science of health.

hymen Fold of mucous membrane, skin, and fibrous tissue covering the external opening of the vagina.

hypercalcemia A condition in which there is too much calcium in the blood.

hypercapnia Greater than normal amounts of carbon dioxide in the blood.

hyperextension Position of maximum extension.

hyperglycemia A greater than normal amount of glucose in the blood.

hyperkalemia Abnormally high levels of potassium in the blood.

hyperlipidemia Excess of lipids in the blood.

hypermenorrhea Excessive bleeding at the time of regular menstrual flow.

hyperopia Farsightedness; inability to see objects at close range.

hyperplasia Increase in the number of cells of a body part.

hyperreflexia Neurological condition characterized by increased reflex reactions.

hypersensitivity An abnormal condition characterized by an excessive reaction to a particular stimulus.

hypertension A common, often asymptomatic disorder characterized by elevated blood pressure persistently exceeding 140/90 mm Hg.

hyperthermic Much higher than normal body temperature.

hypertonic A solution of higher osmotic pressure.

hypertrophy Increase in the size of an organ caused by an increase in the size of the cells rather than the number of cells.

hyperventilation The rate of ventilation exceeds normal metabolic requirements for exchange of respiratory gases.

hyphema Hemorrhage into the anterior chamber of the eye, usually caused by a blunt or percusive injury; also called *hyphemia.*

hypocalcemia A deficiency of calcium in the serum.

hypoglycemia A less than normal amount of glucose in the blood, usually caused by administration of too much insulin, excessive secretion of insulin by the islet cells of the pancreas, or dietary deficiency.

hypokalemia A condition in which an inadequate amount of potassium, the major intracellular cation, is found in the circulatory blood stream.

hypotension An abnormal condition in which the blood pressure is not adequate for normal perfusion and oxygenation of the tissues.

hypothermia An abnormal and dangerous condition in which the temperature of the body is below 95° F (35° C), usually caused by prolonged exposure to cold.

hypotonic A solution of lower osmotic pressure.

hypoventilation An abnormal condition of the respiratory system that occurs when the volume of air is not adequate for the metabolic needs of the body.

hypoxia An inadequate, reduced tension of cellular oxygen.

hysterosalpingooophrectomy Removal of the entire uterus plus one or both fallopian tubes, and ovaries.

icterus Yellow color of the skin, mucous membranes, and sclera of the eyes (jaundice).

ileal conduit Ureters are implanted into a loop of the ileum that is isolated and brought to the surface of the abdominal wall.

ideas of reference Obsessive delusion that statements or actions of others refer to oneself, seen in paranoid disorders.

identity Sense of uniqueness as a person; of internal stability, sameness, and continuity, which resist extreme change.

idiopathic Cause unknown.

idiopathic hyperplasia Increase in number of cells without a known cause.

idiosyncratic Individual's unique hypersensitivity to a particular drug; it is an unexpected response to a medicine.

illness An abnormal process in which aspects of the social, emotional, or intellectual condition and function of a person are diminished or impaired.

illusion False perception or experience occurring in response to an environmental stimulus.

immune response Reaction of the body to foreign substances.

immune serum Serum of an animal or human containing antibodies against a specific disease; used to confer passive immunity to that disease.

immunity Quality of being insusceptible to or unaffected by a particular disease condition.

immunization A process by which resistance to an infectious disease is induced or increased.

immunocompetent The ability of an immune system to mobilize and deploy its antibodies and other responses to stimulization by an antigen.

immunodeficiency Abnormal condition of the immune system in which cellular or humoral immunity is inadequate and resistance to infection is increased.

immunogen Any agent or substance capable of provoking an immune response or producing immunity.

immunoglobulins Proteins capable of acting as antibodies; present in serum, body fluid, and body secretions.

immunology Study of the immune system; the reaction of tissues of the immune system of the body to antigenic stimulation.

immunosuppressed Administration of agents that significantly interfere with the ability of the immune system to respond to antigenic stimulation by inhibiting cellular and humoral immunity.

immunosurveillance The immune system's recognition and destruction of newly developed abnormal cells.

immunotherapy Special treatment of allergic responses: administering increasingly large doses of the offending allergens to gradually develop immunity.

immunotropic Tendency to have an influence on or be influenced by the immune system.

impaction Condition of being tightly wedged into a part such, as eruption of a tooth blocked by other teeth; the presence of a large or hard fecal mass in the rectum or colon.

implantation Embedding of the fertilized ovum in the uterine mucosa.

implementation The phase of nursing process that includes ongoing activities of data collection, prioritization, and performance of nursing intervention, and documentation.

incision Cut produced surgically by a sharp instrument to create an opening into an organ or space in the body.

incus One of the three ossicles in the middle ear; resembling an anvil.

indirect Coombs (blood antibody screening test) Laboratory blood test that detects circulating antibodies against RBCs. The major function of this test is to determine if the patient has serum antibodies (other than the major ABO system) to specific RBCs. Normal findings: negative; no agglutination.

induration Hardening of a tissue, particularly the skin, because of edema, inflammation, or infiltration by neoplasm.

industry Interest in doing work of the world, formation of responsible work habits and attitudes, and mastery of age-appropriate tasks.

infancy First 12 to 24 months of life.

infant mortality Statistic rate of infant death during the first year after live birth, expressed as the number of such births per 1000 live births in a specific geographical area of institution in a given period.

infarct Localized area of necrosis in tissue, a vessel, or an organ resulting from tissue anoxia; caused by an interruption in the blood supply to an area.

infection process cycle Five-point cycle that enables microorganisms to move from place to place and cause infection. If the cycle is broken, the microorganisms cannot grow, spread, or cause disease.

inferiority Feeding inadequate, defeated, lazy, unable to learn or do tasks, and unable to compete, compromise, or cooperate, regardless of actual competence.

inflammation Protective response of body tissues to irritation or injury, such as pain, swelling, redness, heat, and lack of function.

inflammatory bowel disease Refers to both Crohn's disease and ulcerative colitis, involving inflammation and tissue changes in intestinal walls.

inhibit To stop or slow a process.

initial/establishing stage Period when a couple establishes a home.

injecting drug user (IDU) One involved in nonprescribed drug use by needles, including street drugs and steroids.

innate immunity The body's first line of defense, providing physical and chemical barriers to invading pathogens and protect locally against the external environment.

inner canthus of the eye Inner angle at the medial margins of the eyelid.

innominate Without a name. The term is traditionally applied to certain anatomical structures, often identified by their descriptive names, such as hipbone, brachiocephalic artery, and brachiocephalic vein.

insertion The more moveable end of a muscle attachment.

inspection Visual examination of the external surface of the body as well as of its movements and posture.

inspiration Exchange oxygen for carbon dioxide. Also known as *inhalation.*

institutionalize To place a person in an institution for psychological or physical treatment or for the protection of the person or society.

insulin Naturally occurring hormone, secreted by the beta cells of the islets of Langerhans in the pancreas as a response to increased levels of glucose in the blood.

insulin lipodystrophy Loss of local fat deposits in diabetic patients as a complication of repeated insulin injections.

insulin reaction Adverse effects caused by excessive levels of circulating insulin.

integument Covering or skin.

intelligence Ability to learn from experience, to acquire and retain knowledge, to solve problems, and to respond to a new situation.

intelligence quotient (IQ) Index of relative intelligence determined through the subject's answers to arbitrarily chosen questions.

interagency Between two health care facilities.

interdisciplinary hospice team Multiple professional health team, such as physicians, nurses, social workers, and pastors, working together in caring for the terminally ill patient.

intermittent claudication A weakness of the legs accompanied by cramplike pains in the calves caused by poor circulation of the blood to the leg muscles.

intermittent peripheral intravenous device (formally called *heparin lock* An IV infusion device with a male adaptor covered by a rubber diaphragm that is filled with anticoagulant or saline.

interrogatories Written questions of witnesses taken from witnesses before the scheduled trial.

interstitial Fluid between the cells or in the tissues of the body.

intervention Specific therapeutic techniques directed toward each of the limitations.

interview Meeting of people face to face, as for evaluating or questioning a job applicant.

intimacy Reaching out and using the self to form a commitment to and an intense, lasting relationship with another person, or even a cause, an institution, or a creative effort.

intraagency Within a health care facility.

intracellular Fluid inside the cells of the body.

intraoperative Pertaining to a period of time during a surgical procedure.

intrapartal Period that begins with the onset of labor and ends with the delivery of the placenta, also called *perinatal.*

intrathecal Of or pertaining to a structure, process, or substance within a sheath, as the cerebrospinal fluid within the theca of the spinal canal.

intravascular Fluid or plasma within the vessels of the body.

intrinsic Originating from or situated within an organ or tissue: from internal causes.

intussusception Infolding of one segment of the intestine into the lumen of another segment in children.

involuntary Occurring without conscious control or direction.

involution Reduction in size of the uterus after delivery and its return to its normal size.

ion Electrically charged particle resulting from the breakdown of an electrolyte; will be negatively or positively charged.

iridectomy Surgical removal of part of the iris.

iris Circular, contractile disc suspended in aqueous humor between the cornea and the crystalline lens of the eye and perforated by a circular pupil.

iron deficiency anemia A microcytic, hypochromic anemia caused by inadequate supplies of iron needed to synthesize hemoglobin, characterized by pallor, fatigue, and weakness.

irradiation Exposure to x-rays.

ischemia Decreased blood supply to a body organ or part often marked by pain and organ dysfunction.

ischium Lower portion of the innominate or hip bone.

isolation Separation of a seriously ill patient from others.

isolation and self-absorption Inability to be intimate, spontaneous, or close with another.

isolation precautions Practices of infection control to reduce or eliminate the transmission of pathogens; precautions include wearing protective apparel such as gowns, gloves, and masks and following the procedure for double bagging.

isotonic A solution of the same osmotic pressure.

jaundice Yellowish discoloration of the skin, mucous membranes, and sclerae of the eyes, caused by greater than normal amounts of bilirubin in the blood.

joint Any one of the connections between bones.

judgment The decision of the law given by a court as a result of court proceedings.

jurisdiction Power and authority of a constitution of the state and/or local system to pronounce the sentence of the law.

JVD Jugular vein distention, which reflects increased right arterial pressure.

Kaposi's sarcoma (KS) A rare cancer of the skin or mucous membrane characterized by blue, red, or purple raised lesions.

Kardex A card system used to consolidate patient orders and care needs in a centralized, concise way.

Kegel's exercises A regimen of isometric exercises in which a woman executes a series of voluntary contractions of the muscles of her pelvic diaphragm and perineum to increase the contractility of her vaginal muscles or improve the retention of urine; also called *pubococcygeus exercises.*

keloid Overgrowth of collagenous scar tissue at the site of a skin wound.

keratoplasty excision of the corneal tissue, followed by surgical implantation of a cornea from another human donor.

kernicterus Abnormal toxic accumulation of bilirubin in central nervous system tissue caused by hyperbilirubinemia (an excess of bilirubin in the blood of the newborn).

ketoacidosis Acidoses accompanied by an accumulation of ketones, in the blood, resulting from faulty carbohydrate metabolism.

ketoaciduria Presence in the urine of excessive amounts of ketone bodies, occurring as a result of uncontrolled diabetes mellitus, starvation, or any other metabolic condition in which fats are rapidly catabolized.

ketone bodies Normal metabolic products, β-hydroxybutyric and aminoacetic acid, from which acetone may arise spontaneously.

kick-count Daily counting of fetal movements felt in 1 hour while the mother is resting.

kilocalorie Unit that denotes the heat expenditure of an organism and the fuel or energy value of food, often abbreviated kcalorie or kcal.

Korotkoff's sounds Sounds heard during the taking of blood pressure using a sphygmomanometer and stethoscope.

Korsakoff's psychosis Form of amnesia often seen in chronic alcoholics, characterized by a loss of short-term memory and an inability to learn new skills.

Kussmaul's respirations Abnormally deep, very rapid, sighing respirations characteristic of diabetic acidosis.

kwashiorkor A malnutrition disease, primarily of children, caused by severe protein deficiency, usually occurring when the child is weaned from the breast.

kyphosis An abnormal condition of the vertebral column characterized by increased convexity in the curvature of the thoracic spine.

labia majora Two large folds of tissue extending from the mons pubis to the perineal floor.

labia minora Two smaller folds of skin between the labia majora.

labile Unstable; characterized by a tendency to change or to be altered.

labyrinthitis Inflammation of the labyrinthine canals of the inner ear.

lactation Function of secreting milk from the breasts in the nourishment of an infant or breastfeeding child.

lacteals Lymphatic capillaries in the villi of the small intestine that transport fats obtained from food to the blood stream.

lalling Infant's movement of tongue with crying and vocalization.

laminectomy Surgical chipping away of the bony arches of one or more vertebrae.

language Combination of sounds into a meaningful whole to communicate thoughts and feelings.

lanugo Downy, fine hair characteristic of the fetus between 20 weeks gestation and birth that is most noticeable over the shoulders, forehead, and cheeks, but is found on nearly all parts of the body except for the palms of the hands and the soles of the feet.

lanula Half-moon structure, such as the crescent-shaped, pale area at the base of the nail of a finger or toe.

laparoscopy This examination provides direct visualization of the uterus and adnexa.

larynx The organ of voice that is part of the air passage, is supported by nine areas of cartilage, and connects the pharynx with the trachea.

law The reference to a rule, principle, or regulation established and made known by a government to protect or to restrict the people affected.

leadership Ability to influence others to the attainment of goals.

Legge-Calvé-Perthes disease A disorder caused by decreased blood supply to the femoral head which results in necrosis and regeneration of the femoral head.

leisure Freedom from obligations and formal duties of paid work, and opportunity to puruse, at one's own pace, mental nourishment, enlivenment, pleasure, and relief from fatigue of work.

lens Crystalline lens of the eye; a curved transparent disc that is capable of refracting light.

lentigo A tan or brown macule on the skin brought on by sun exposure, usually in middle-aged or older person.

leukemia Malignant disorder of the hematopoietic system, in which an excess of leukocytes accumulates in the bone marrow and lymph nodes.

leukocytes White blood cells.

leukopenia Reduction in the number of circulating white blood cells due to depression of the bone marrow.

leukoplakia mucosa A white patch on the mouth or tongue.

leukorrhea Normal white vaginal discharge.

liability Legal concept that one is responsible and will be held accountable for one's actions (personal liability); that a corporation is responsible and answerable for its own decisions (corporate liability); or that an employer is responsible for an employee's acts done within the scope of employment.

license The granting of permission by a competent authority (usually a government agency) to an organization or individual to engage in a practice or activity that would otherwise be illegal.

lichenification Hypertrophy of the epidermis, resulting in rough, thickened, leatherlike skin.

lie Relationship between the long axis of the fetus and the long axis of the mother.

ligament Bonds of connective tissue binding joints together and connecting various bones and cartilages.

lightening Sensation of decreased abdominal distention produced by uterine descent into pelvic cavity as the fetal presenting part settles into the pelvis. It usually occurs 2 weeks before the onset of labor in nulliparous.

lipids Group name for organic substances of a fatty nature, including fats, oils, sterols (such as cholesterol), phospholipids, waxes, and related compounds.

lipodystrophy Abnormality in the metabolism or deposition of fats. Insulin lipodystrophy is the loss of local fat deposits in diabetic patients as a complication of repeated insulin injections.

lipoprotein A protein and lipid molecule that facilitates transport of lipids in the blood stream.

lithotomy Incision of a duct or organ, especially the bladder, for removal of stone.

lithotomy position Position assumed by the patient lying supine with the hips and knees flexed and the thighs abducted and rotated externally.

litigate To carry out a lawsuit or to contest one.

litigation A lawsuit.

living will A legal document (a form of advanced directives) drawn up by a person who is not yet near death, detailing how much medical care they want to receive if they become terminally ill.

LOC Level of consciousness.

lochia Vaginal discharge during the puerperium consisting of blood, tissue, and mucus.

lordosis An increase in the curve at the lumbar space region that throws the shoulder back, making the appearance "lordly or kingly."

loss Any aspect of one's self that is no longer available to that person.

lumbar cord injury Trauma to the spinal column at the lumbar spine, L1 and L2, with paralysis of lower extremities, bladder, and rectum, and loss of sexual function.

lumen Space within an artery, vein, intestine, or tube such as a needle or catheter.

luteinizing hormone (LH) Secreted by the anterior pituitary gland; initiates ovulation and release of the egg, followed by the formation of the corpus luteum, which in turn produces the hormone estrogen and progesterone.

lymphadenopathy Disease of the lymph nodes, including hypertrophy and proliferation of lymphoid tissue.

lymphangitis Inflammation of one or more lymphatic vessels, usually resulting from an acute streptococcal or staphylococcal infection in an extremity.

lymphedema Primary or secondary disorder characterized by edema and the accumulation of lymph in soft tissue.

lymphocytes White blood cells that occur in two forms, B cells and T cells.

lymphokine One of the chemical factors produced and released by T-lymphocytes that attract macrophages to the site of infection or inflammation and prepare them for attack.

lysosome Cytoplasmic, membrane-bound particle containing hydrolytic enzymes that function in intracellular digestive processes.

macrophage Cell that "eats" pathogenic microorganisms.

macule Small, flat blemish or discoloration that is flush with the skin surface.

magical thinking Belief that merely thinking about an event in the external world can cause it to occur.

magnesium The second most abundant cation in the intracellular fluid of the body.

magnetic resonance imaging (MRI) Medical imaging that uses nuclear magnetic resonance as its source of energy.

major affective disorder Any of a group of psychotic disorders characterized by severe and inappropriate emotional responses, prolonged and persistent disturbances of mood and related thought distortions, and other symptoms associated with either depressed or manic states.

malignant Growing worse, resisting treatment; said of cancerous growths, tending or threatening to produce death, harmful.

malignant neoplasm Tumor that progressively spreads to other areas of the body.

malleolus Rounded, bony process on each side of the ankle.

malleus One of the three ossicles in the middle ear; resembles a hammer.

malpractice (in law) Professional negligence that is the proximate cause of injury or harm to a patient resulting from a lack of professional knowledge, experience, or skill that can be expected in others in the profession or from a failure to exercise reasonable care or judgment in the application of professional knowledge, experience, or skill. Malpractice is the failure to meet a professional standard of care.

mammogram X-ray of the breast; use of radiography of the breast to diagnose breast cancer.

mammography Radiography of the soft tissue of the breast to allow identification of various benign and neoplastic processes.

management The act, art, or manner of managing or handling; controlling, directing, to have charge of.

mandatory Required by a command, order, or law.

mania Mood disorder characterized by an expansive emotional state, extreme excitement, excessive elation, hyperactivity, agitation, overtalkativeness, flights of ideas, increased psychomotor activity, fleeting attention, and sometimes violent, destructive, or self-destructive behavior.

manubrium One of the three bones of the sternum, presenting a broad, quadrangular shape that narrows where it unites with the superior end of the sternum.

marasmus A condition of extreme malnutrition and emaciation, occurring chiefly in young children, that is characterized by progressive wasting of subcutaneous tissue and muscle. It results from a lack of adequate calories and proteins.

masticate To crush and grind food.

mastoiditis Infection of one of the mastoid bones.

matriarchal family patterns, also known as *matrifocal* A style in which the female assumes primary dominance in areas of child care and homemaker.

matrix Basic substance from which a specific type of tissue develops.

mattress pad (cover) Material that fits over a mattress to protect it from soiling.

maturational loss A loss resulting from normal life transition (such as a child going off to school for the first time).

means Inner terms of the proportion.

meconium First stools of the infant: viscid, dark greenish brown, almost black; sterile; odorless.

mediastinum The mass of organs and tissues separating the lungs; it contains the heart, and its large vessels, trachea and esophagus.

edicaid A federally funded, state-operated program of medical assistance to people with low incomes, authorized by Title XIX of the social security act.

medical asepsis A group of techniques that inhibit the growth and spread of pathogenic microorganisms. Sometimes referred to as *clean technique*.

medical diagnosis The identification of a disease or condition by scientific evaluation of physical signs, symptoms, history, laboratory tests, and procedures.

Medicare A federally funded national health insurance for certain persons over 65 years of age.

medicated tub bath Therapeutic bath in which medication is dispersed in water, usually in treating a dermatological disorder.

medicine Art and science of diagnosis, treatment, and prevention of disease and the maintenance of good health.

medulla The most internal part of a structure or organ, as the renal medulla.

medulla oblongata Most vital part of the brain; continuing as the bulbous portion of the spinal cord just above the foramen magnum and separated from the pons by a horizontal groove.

melana Abnormal, black tarry stool containing digested blood.

melanin Black or dark brown pigment that occurs naturally in the hair and skin and in the iris and choroid of the eye.

melanoma Malignant neoplasm, primarily of the skin.
membrane Thin layer of tissue that covers a surface, lines a cavity, or divides a space, such as the membrane that lines the abdominal wall.
menarch The first menstrual cycle.
meninges Any of the three membranes that enclose the brain and spinal cord, comprising the dura mater, the pia mater, and the arachnoid.
meningomyelocele Developmental defect of the central nervous system in which a hernial sac containing a portion of the spinal cord, its meninges, and cerebrospinal fluid protrudes through a congenital cleft in the vertebral column; also called *myelomeningocele.*
meniscus Curved formed by liquid's upper surface.
menometrorrhagia Excessive spotting between cycles.
menopause Permanent ceasing of ovulation and menstruation, which causes loss of reproductive ability (female climacteric).
menorrhagia Excessively heavy or long menstral periods.
menstruation Periodical discharge through the vagina of a bloody secretion from the shedding of the endometrium.
mental health continuum Mental health and mental illness can be viewed as opposite ends on a continuum. The point at which the person is deemed mentally ill is determined by behavior, as well as by the circumstances in which the behavior is seen.
mental illness May be evidenced by behavior that is conspicuous, threatening, and disruptive of relationships or that deviates significantly from behavior that is considered socially acceptable.
mesentery A peritoneal fold shaped like a giant, pleatal fan encircling the greater part of the small intestine and connecting the intestine to the posterior abdominal wall.
mesoderm Embryonic middle layer of germ cells giving rise to all types of muscles, connective tissue, bone marrow, blood lymphoid tissue, and all epithealial tissue.
metabolism The aggregate of all chemical processes that take place in living organisms.
metabolites Substances produced by metabolic action.
metastasis Process by which tumor cells spread to distant parts of the body.
microorganism Any tiny, usually microscopic entity capable of carrying on living processes. Kinds of microorganisms include bacteria, fungi, protozoa, and viruses; seen only by a microscope.
micturition Urination.
middle age Period of life from mid-40s to mid-60s or 70.
midlife crisis Major turning point in one's life related to identity crisis and self-absorption; involves changes in commitments to career and/or spouse and children, as well as emotional turmoil for the individual and others.
midstream urine specimen Urine collected after voiding is initiated and terminated before voiding is completed—midstream.
milliequivalent (mEq) Number of grams of solule dissolved in 1 ml of normal solution.
mineral An inorganic substance ingested as a compound (such as sodium chloride) rather than a free element. Minerals play a vital role in regulating many bodily functions.
minority group A racial religious, ethnic or political group smaller than and differing from the larger, controlling group in a community or nation.
miotic Causing constriction of the pupil of the eye.
miter Fold and tuck made on the corner of a sheet; gives the hospital bed a finished appearance.
mitochondria Powerhouses of the cell. They are bean shaped and convert food to an energy form (ATP) for the cell.
mitosis Type of cell division of somatic (pertaining to nonreproductive cells) cells in which each daughter cell contains the same number of chromosome as the parent cell.
monocytes Agranulocytic, phagocytic leukocytes that circulate in the blood stream and move into tissue where they engulf foreign antigens and cell debris.
monozygotic Originating or coming from a single fertilized ovum, such as identical twins.
mood Particular state of mind or feeling, such as humor or temper.
morals Generally accepted customs of conduct and right living in a society.
morbidity An illness or an abnormal condition or quality; the rate at which an illness occurs in a particular area of population.
mores Folkways of central importance, accepted without question and embodying the fundamental moral views of a group.
morphology Study of physical shape and size.
mortality The condition of being subject to death; number of deaths in a specific population, usually expressed as deaths per 1000, 10,000, or 100,000.
mortician Person certified in the care of the dead.
morula Developmental stage of the fertilized ovum in which there is a solid mass of cells resembling a mulberry.
motivation The gathering of personal resources or the inner drive to complete a task or reach a goal.
motor Pertaining to motion, the body apparatus involved in movement, or the brain functions that direct purposeful activities.
motor neuron One of various efferent nerve cells that transmit nerve impulses from the brain or from the spinal cord to muscular or glandular tissue.
mourning Reaction activated by a person to assist in overcoming a great personal loss.
multiaxial system System used for organizing information in a psychiatric diagnosis.
multigravida Woman who has been pregant more than once.
multipara Woman who has been delivered of more than one viable infant.
multiple myeloma Malignant neoplasm of the bone marrow.
mummification Mortification producing a dry, hard mass.
muscle tone Muscle strength; the normal state of balanced tension in muscles.
myalgia Diffuse muscle pain, usually accompanied by malaise, occurring in many infectious diseases.
mydriatic Causing pupillary dilatation.
myelin Fatty sheath covering neurons.
myelogram X-ray film taken after injection of a radiopaque medium into the subarachnoid space; demonstrates any distortions of the spinal cord, spinal nerve roots, and subarachnoid space.
myeloproliferative Producing excessive bone marrow.
myelosuppression Inhibition of the production of blood cells and platelets in the bone marrow.
myocardial infarction An occlusion of a major coronary artery or one of its branches caused by atherosclerosis or an embolus resulting in necrosis of a portion of cardiac muscle.
myocardium Thick, contractile, middle layer of uniquely constructed and arranged muscle cells that form the bulk of the heart wall.
myopia Condition of nearsightedness; inability to see objects at a distance.
myositis Inflammation of muscle tissue.
myringotomy A surgical incision of the tympanic membrane to relieve pressure and release purulent exudate from the middle ear.

NANDA North American Nursing Diagnosis Association.
narcotic abstinence syndrome (NAS) Condition affecting babies born to narcotic-addicted mothers whose addiction is passed on to the child. The baby will demonstrate signs of hyperreflexia, hypertonia, a high-pitched cry, tremors, sneezing, and yawning.
narrative charting Traditional style of charting in which the nurse documents in story form all pertinent patient observations, care, and responses in the *nurse's notes* section of the patient's record.
negative feedback In physiology, a decrease in function in response to a stimulus.
neglect Failure of care givers to provide a child with basic necessities of life.
negligence The commission of an act that a prudent person would not have done or the omission of a duty that a prudent person would have fulfilled, resulting in injury or harm to another person. It must be proved that other prudent members of the same profession would ordinarily have acted differently under the same circumstances.
neonatal period First 4 weeks of life.
neonate Infant during first 4 weeks of life.
neoplasia New and abnormal growth of cells, which may be benign or malignant.
neoplasm Any abnormal growth of new tissue, which may be benign or malignant.
neoplastic Any abnormal growth of new tissue benign or malignant also called *tumor.*
nephron Structural and functional unit of the kidney, resembling a microscopic funnel with a long stem and two convoluted sections.
nephrotoxin Substances with specific destructive properties for the kidneys such as certain antibiotics, heavy metals, solvents, and chemicals.
neural tube Tube formed from the fusion of the neural folds from which the brain and spinal cord arise.
neurilemma Layer of cells composed of one or more Schwann cells, which enclose the segmented myelin sheaths of peripheral nerve fibers. The nerve fibers of the brain and the spinal cord are not enclosed by neurilemma.
neuromuscular junction Area of contact between the ends of a large myelinated nerve fiber and a skeletal muscle fiber.
neuron Basic nerve cell of the nervous system, containing a nucleus within a cell body and extending one or more processes.
neuropathy Any abnormal condition characterized by inflammation and degeneration of the peripheral nerves.
neurotransmitter Any one of numerous chemicals that modify or result in the transmission of nerve impulses between synapses.

neurotropic Having a tendency to influence or be influenced by the nervous system.

neutrophil Granular circulating leukocyte essential for phagocytosis (process by which bacteria, cellular debris, and solid particles are destroyed and removed).

nevus Pigmented, congenital skin blemish that is usually benign but may become cancerous.

Nissen fundoplication Surgical procedure to wrap the fundus of the stomach around the distal esophagus to prevent reflux of the stomach contents into the esophagus.

nitrogen balance Difference between intake and output of nitrogen in the body. If intake is greater, a positive nitrogen balance exists and anabolism occurs. If output is greater, a negative nitrogen balance exists and catabolism occurs. When nitrogen intake equals output, the body is in zero nitrogen balance.

nocturia Excessive urination at night.

nocturnal emissions Ejaculation of semen during sleep; physiological marker of puberty in male.

nodule A firm, fixed mass, small and rounded.

nonrapid eye movement (NREM) One of two highly individualized sleeping states divided into four stages through which a sleeper progresses during a typical sleeping cycle; represent three fourths of a period of typical sleep.

nonspecific immunity Passive immunity; acquired immunity transmitted naturally through the placenta to a fetus, through the colostrum to an infant, or artificially by injection.

nonverbal communication Messages conveyed by eye movements, facial expression, and body posturing.

normotensive Having normal blood pressure.

nosocomial infection A hospital (or any other health care facility) acquired infection; an infection acquired at least 72 hours after admission.

noxious A stimulation of the sensory nerve endings that is harmful, injurious, or detrimental to physical health.

nuchal rigidity Pain and stiffness of the neck when flexed.

nuclear family A family unit consisting of the biologic parents and their offspring.

nullipara Woman who has not been delivered of a viable infant.

numerator Top number of a fraction.

Nurse Practice Act A statute enacted by the legislature of any of the states or by the appropriate officers of the districts or possessions. The act delineates the legal scope of the practice of nursing within the geographic boundaries of the jursidiction.

nurse's notes Nurse's written documentation of patient observations, care, and responses.

nursing Practice in which a nurse assists the individual, sick or well, in the performance of those activities contributing to health or its recovery (or to a peaceful death) that he would perform unaided if he had the necessary strength, will, or knowledge.

nursing assessment Identification by a nurse of the needs, preferences, and abilities of a patient. Assessment provides the scientific basis for a complete nursing care plan.

nursing care plan Plan of care based on a nursing assessment and a nursing diagnosis; lists nursing actions necessary to meet a patient's needs.

nursing diagnosis A clinical judgment about individual, family, or community responses to actual or high risk (potential) health problems/life processes.

nursing health history Data collected about the patient's level of wellness, changes in life patterns, sociocultural role, and mental and emotional reactions to illness.

nursing intervention Activity performed by nurses that should promote the achievement of the desired patient outcome.

nursing notes See *nurse's notes.*

nutrient Chemical compound or element found in food that is necessary for good health. Nutrients perform any or all of these basic functions: providing energy, building and repairing tissues, and/or regulating body processes.

nutrient density Nutrients relative to calories. Food providing a high quantity of one or more nutrients in a small number of calories is nutrient dense.

nutrition All the processes involved in taking in nutrients and in their assimilation and use for proper body functioning and maintenance of health.

nystagmus Involuntary, rhythmic movement of the eyes. Oscillations maybe horizontal, vertical, rotary, or mixed.

obesity Abnormal increase in the proportion of fat cells, mainly in the viscera and subcutaneous tissues of the body; overfatness.

objective data Of or pertaining to a clinical finding that is observed, palpated, or auscultated. Laboratory findings as well as radiologic and other studies are included; observable and measurable signs.

objective data collection Process in which data relating to the patient's problems are obtained through direct physical examination, laboratory analysis, and radiological studies.

OBRA (Omnibus Budget Reconciliation Act) Federal legislation that mandates specific guidelines and prohibits routine use of safety reminder devices in nursing homes.

obsession Refers to the persistent thought or idea with which the mind is continually and involuntarily preoccupied and which suggests an irrational act.

occiput Back of the head; of or pertaining to the occipital region.

occlusion A blockage in a canal, vessel, or passage of the body.

occult Hidden.

occult blood Blood that is obscure or hidden from view.

occupied bed Hospital bed that must be made up while it is occupied by a patient.

Oddi's sphincter A circular muscle located at the opening of the common bile duct into the duodenum at the papilla of Vater.

olecranon The upper end of the ulna, which forms the point of the elbow.

oligohydramnios Abnormally small amount of absence of amniotic fluid; often indicative of fetal urinary tract defect.

oliguria A diminished capacity to form and pass urine, less than 500 ml in 24 hours, so the end products of metabolism cannot be excreted efficiently.

oncology The sum of knowledge regarding tumors; it is the branch of medicine that deals with the study of tumors.

open bed Fanfolded top linens on a hospital bed, for easy access for patient.

ophthalmoscope Device used to examine the interior of the eye.

opportunistic Disease characteristic caused by normally nonpathogenic organisms in a host whose resistance has been decreased by such disorder as AIDS.

opportunistic infection Infection in a person whose resistance to disease has been decreased by other disorders, such as diabetes mellitus, cancer, or AIDS or by a procedure, such as surgery or catheterization.

oral hygiene Care of the oral cavity; mouth.

oral swabs Swabs impregnated or soaked with various solutions for oral hygiene, such as glycerin and lemon juice.

ordinariness Nurses' sharing of sense of common humanity, creating a bond of humaness with patients.

organ Structure made up of two or more kinds of tissues organized in such a way that the tissues can together perform a more complex function than can any tissue alone.

orientation Awareness of one's physical environment with regard to time, place, and the identity of other persons.

ORIF Open Reduction Internal Fixation is a surgical procedure allowing fracture alignment under direct visualization while using various internal fixation devices applied to the bone.

orifice Entrance to or outlet of any cavity in the body.

origin Less moveable or fixed end of a muscle attachment.

orthopedic bed Bed designed to accommodate a patient with fractures.

orthopnea An abnormal condition in which a person must sit or stand in order to breathe deeply or comfortably.

orthopneic Pertaining to posture assumed by the patient sitting up in bed at a 90-degree angle; patient may also lean forward supported by a pillow on over bed table.

orthostatic hypotension A drop of 25 mm Hg in systolic pressure and a drop of 10 mm Hg in diasystolic pressure when moving from a lying to sitting or sitting to standing position.

Ortolani's test Procedure used to evaluate the stability of the hip joints in newborns and infants. A click or a popping sensation (Ortolani's sign) may be felt if the joint is unstable, because the head of the femur moves out of the acetabulum under pressure from the examiner's hands during rotation and abduction.

OSHA Occupational Safety and Health Administration.

osmosis The passage of water across a semipermeable membrane. The water moves from an area of lower concentration to an area of higher concentration.

osseous Pertaining to bone.

ossicle Small bone, such as the malleus, the incus, or stapes of the middle ear.

osteoclasia Destruction and absorption of bony tissue by osteoclasts, such as during growth or the healing of fractures.

osteoclast Large type of multinucleated bone cell that functions in periods of growth or repair, such as the breakdown and resorption of osseous tissue.

otitis Inflammation or infection of the ear.

outcome Description of the specific measurable behavior (outcome criteria) that the patient will be able to exhibit after the nursing interventions.

outer canthus of the eye Outer angle at the lateral margins of the eyelid.

ovulation Release of a mature ovum (egg) from the ovary.

oxidation Process in which the oxygen content of a compound is increased.

oxytocin Hormone produced in the hypothalamus, stored in the posterior pituitary; when needed, promotes the release of breast milk and stimulates uterine contractions during labor.

oxytocins Drugs that stimulate uterine contractions thus accelerating childbirth and preventing post delivery hemorrhage. They may be used to increase the letdown reflex during lactation.

pacemaker Battery-operated generator that initiates and controls the heart rate by delivering an electrical impulse via an electrode to the myocardium.

pain Unpleasant sensation caused by noxious stimulation of the sensory nerve endings.

palliation Therapy to relieve or reduce uncomfortable symptoms but not to cure.

palliative Designed to relieve pain and distress, control the signs and symptoms of disease but not to produce a cure.

palpation A technique used in physical examination in which the examiner feels the texture, size, consistency, and location of certain parts of the body with the hands.

pancytopenia Condition of all three major blood elements (red cells, white cells, and platelets) from the bone marrow being reduced or absent.

Papanicolaou test A simple smear method of examining stained exfoliative cells; used most commonly to detect cancers of the cervix.

papule Palpable, circumscribed, solid elevation in skin, smaller than 0.5 cm

para To bring forth.

paracentesis Procedure in which fluid is withdrawn from the abdominal cavity.

parallel play Playing alongside a peer or same-aged child.

paralysis Abnormal condition characterized by loss of muscle function or loss of sensation.

paralytic ileus Most common type of intestinal obstruction; a decrease in or absence of intestinal peristalsis that may occur after abdominal surgery.

paranoia Transitory mental state characterized by illogical thought processes and generalized suspicion and distrust.

parasite Plant or animal that lives upon or within another living organism at whose expense it obtains some advantage.

parasympathetic Of or pertaining to the craniosacral division of the autonomic nervous system, consisting of the oculomotor, facial, glossopharyngeal, vagus, and pelvic nerves. The parasympathetic slows heart rate, increases intestinal peristalsis and gland activity, and relaxes sphincters.

parathyroid glands Hormone glands located on the posterior surface of the thyroid gland; these gland secrete parathyroid hormone.

parathyroid hormone (parathormone) Produced by the parathyroid glands and working as an antagonist to calcitonin, this hormone tends to increase the concentration of calcium in the blood.

parenchyma Tissue of an organ, as distinguished from supporting or connective tissue.

parenteral Not in or through the digestive system.

parenteral nutrition Administrative of nutrients by a route other than the alimentary canal, such as intravenously.

parenthood stage Begins at the birth or adoption of the first child.

paresthesia Any subjective sensation such as a pricking pins and needles, or numbness.

partial bath Patient's incomplete bath. A nurse usually must bathe the back, legs, and feet.

passive transport The movement of small molecules across the membrane of a cell with no cellular energy required.

patella Knee cap.

patent Condition of being open and unblocked, such as a patent airway.

pathogen Any microorganism capable of producing disease.

pathogenic Capable of causing disease.

pathognomonic Sign or symptom specific to a disease condition.

patient Recipient of a health care service.

patient-controlled analgesia A drug delivery system that allows patients to administer pain medications when they need them.

patients' rights Legal and regulatory rights to participate in the planning of care, be informed of services, know by whom and how payment will be made, have privacy and grievance procedures, and be shown respect for personal possessions.

patriarchal family pattern A family style in which the male assumes the dominant role.

PCP *Pneumocystic carinii* pneumonia.

pectoris major Large fan-shaped muscle that covers the anterior chest from the sternum to the proximal end of the humerus.

pediculosis Lice infestation.

peer Person deemed an equal for the purpose at hand. A peer is usually about the same age and mental level.

peer review An appraisal by professional co-workers (of equal status) or the way an individual nurse conducts practice, education, or research.

pellagra Disease resulting from deficiency of the vitamin niacin.

pepsin The chief enzyme of gastric juices that converts proteins into proteoses and peptones.

peptic ulcer Loss of the mucous membrane of the stomach, duodenum, or any part of the gastrointestinal system exposed to gastric juices.

percent Hundredth; symbolized as %.

perception Understanding based on impressions and feelings.

percussion Technique used to evaluate size, border, and consistency of some organs and to discover the presence and evaluate the amount of fluid in a body cavity.

perennial Present at all seasons of the year, permanent, consistent.

perinatal Period during pregnancy that begins with the onset of labor and ends with delivery of the placenta; sometimes called *intrapartal.*

perinatal death Death of an infant before, during, or shortly after birth.

perineal care Care given the genitalia.

periodontal disease Disease of the tissues around the teeth.

perioperative period Entire surgical inpatient period, from admission to date of discharge.

periorbital edema Swelling around the eyes, which may indicate a pathological condition of the kidney.

periosteum A protective fibrous vascular membrane that covers the diaphysis of the bone.

peripheral Pertaining to the outside, surface, or surrounding area.

peripheral nervous system The motor and sensory nerves and ganglia outside the brain and spinal cord, consisting of 12 pairs of cranial nerves, 31 pairs of spinal nerves, and their various branches in body organs.

peripheral parenteral nutrition (PPN) Administration of a nutritionally adequate solution into a peripheral vein.

peristalsis Coordinated, rhythmic, serial contraction of smooth muscle that forces food through the digestive tract, bile through the bile duct, and urine through the ureters.

pernicious Capable of causing great injury or destruction; deadly, fatal.

pernicious anemia A progressive megaloblastic, macrocytic anemia, affecting mainly older people, that results from a lack of intrinsic factor essential for the absorption of vitamin B_{12}.

personality Refers to the relative consistent set of attitudes and behaviors particular to an individual; it consists of patterns of mental, emotional, and behavioral tracts of a person.

PGL Persistent generalized lymphedema.

phagocytes White blood cells that are able to surround, engulf, and digest microorganisms and cellular debris.

phagocytosis The process by which certain cells engulf and digest microorganisms and cellular debris.

phalanges Any one of 14 tapering bones composing the fingers of each hand and the toes of each foot.

pharmacology Study of drugs and their action on the living body.

pharynx Throat; a tubular structure about 6 inches long that extends from the base of the skull to the esophagus and is situated just anterior to the cervical vertebrae. It is the passageway for both air and food.

phimosis A condition in which the prepuce is too small to allow retraction of the foreskin over the glans penis.

phlebothrombosis Abnormal condition in which a clot forms within a vein.

phobia An anxiety disorder characterized by an obsessive, irrational, and intense fear of a specific object, such as an animal or dirt, of an activity, such as meeting strangers or leaving the familiar setting of the home; or of a physical situation, such as heights and open or closed spaces.

phosphorus Chiefly, an intracellular anion in fluid of the body.

phototherapy Treatment for hyperbilirubinemia and jaundice in the newborn that involves the exposure of an infant's bare skin to intense fluorescent light. The blue range of the light accelerates the excretion of bilirubin in the skin, decomposing it by photooxidation.

physiatrist Physician who specializes in the field of rehabilitation.

physician's orders Specific orders by a physician for a patient's medical care.

physiological jaundice Jaundice usually occuring 48 hours or later after birth, gradually disappearing by the seventh to tenth day; caused by the normal reduction in the number of red blood cells. The infant is otherwise well.

physiology Study of functions of the various organs and tissues of the body.

pia mater Innermost of the three meninges covering the brain and the spinal cord. It is closely applied to both structures and carries a rich supply of blood vessels, which nourish the nervous tissue.

pica Craving to eat non food substances.

PIH Pregnancy-induced hypertension.

pinna Outer flap of external ear composed of tissue and cartilage.

pinocytosis The process by which extracellular fluid is taken into the cell.

pituitary gland Small gland attached to the hypothalamus and couched in the sphenoid bone, supplying numerous hormones that govern many vital processes.

pity Expression of regret or sorrow for patients who are suffering, distressed, or unhappy.

placebo An inactive substance or procedure that is given to a patient for it's suggestive effect.

placental barrier Barrier (obstruction, boundary, or separation) produced by the placental tissue, between the fetal and maternal circulation. Substances of small size, excluding blood cells, may traverse (to go across) this barrier.

plaintiff Person who files a lawsuit initiating a legal action.

planning The phase of the nursing process in which the nurse establishes priorities of care, writes desired patient outcomes, selects and converts nursing interventions into nursing orders, and communicates the plan of care.

pleural effusion An abnormal accumulation of fluid in the interpleural spaces of the lungs, characterized by fever, chest pain, dyspnea, and a nonproductive cough.

pleural friction rub Low-pitched, grating or creaking lung sounds that occur when inflamed pleural surfaces rub together during respiration.

pleural space Potential space between the visceral and parietal layers of the pleurae.

pleurisy Inflammation of the parietal pleura of the lungs, characterized by dyspnea and stabbing pain, leading to restriction of ordinary breathing with spasm of the chest on the affected side.

pluralistic society Society in which numerous distinct ethnic, religious, or cultural groups coexist within one nation.

***Pneumocystis carinii* pneumonia (PCP)** Unusual pulmonary disease caused by a parasite; usually seen in patients with AIDS, infants, or debilitated or immunosuppressed people.

pneumonia Acute inflammation of the lungs, often caused by inhaled pneumococci.

pneumothorax Collection of air or gas in the pleural cavity causing the lung to collapse.

poisoning The condition or physical state produced by the ingestion, injection, inhalation, or exposure of a poisonous (toxic) substance.

polycythemia Abnormal increase in the number of red blood cells in the blood.

polydactyly Excessive number of digits (fingers or toes).

polydipsia Excessive thirst.

polyphagia Eating to the point of gluttony.

polyuria Excretion of an abnormally large quantity of urine.

pons Prominence on the ventral surface of the brainstem, between the medulla oblongata and the cerebral peduncles of the midbrain. The pons consists of white matter and a few nuclei and is divided into a ventral portion and a dorsal portion.

portal of entry Route by which microorganisms enter the human body.

position Relationship of a fetal reference point with respect to its location in the maternal pelvis.

possible nursing diagnosis A problem that is considered feasible.

postmortem care Care of the body after death.

posterior Back part of a structure; toward the back.

posterior fontanelle Triangular-shaped area at center back of head.

postictal period The time pertaining to the period after a convulsion.

postpartal Final stage of the maternity cycle; begins after the delivery of the placenta and lasts for approximately 6 weeks.

postprandial After a meal.

posture Position of the body with respect to the surrounding space; the sense of balance.

potassium The dominant intracellular cation in fluid of the body.

potentiation Synergistic action in which the effect of two drugs given at the same time is greater than the effect of the drugs given separately.

PQRST Method used when gathering information during a patient interview; P—provocative, palliative; Q—quality, quantity; R—region, radiation; S—severity scale; T—timing.

preadolescence (prepubescence) Period from about age 9 or 10 until onset of puberty, characterized by an increase in hormone production.

preeclampsia Abnormal condition of pregnancy characterized by the onset of acute hypertension after the twenty-fourth week of gestation.

pregnancy-induced hypertension (PIH) Disease encountered during pregnancy or early in the puerperium characterized by increasing hypertension, albuminuria, and generalized edema; further classified as *preeclampsia* or *eclampsia.*

premenstrual syndrome Group of signs and symptoms occurring about a week before menstruation, associated with fluid retention.

prenatal Occurring or existing before birth, referring both to the care of the patient during pregnancy and the growth and development of the fetus; also known as *antepartal.*

preoperational thought stage Piagetian phase of child development during the period of 2 to 7 years of age, when the child focuses on the use of language as a tool. The child has the emerging ability to reason.

prepuce Fold of skin that forms a retractable cover, such as the foreskin of the penis or the fold around the clitoris.

presbycusis Impairment of hearing in old age.

presbycusis A normal loss of hearing acuity, speech intelligibility, auditory threshold, and pitch associated with aging.

presbyopia Defect in vision in advancing age involving loss of accommodation or recession of near vision; due to loss of elasticity of crystalline lens.

preschooler Child aged 3 to 5½ years.

presentation Part of the fetus that first appears in the pelvis.

priapism Persistent penile erection.

primary caregiver One who assumes ongoing responsibility for health maintenance and therapy for illness.

primipara Woman who has given birth to one viable infant.

prn *(pro re nata)* When required.

problem Any health care condition that requires diagnostic, therapeutic, or educational action.

problem list for POMR Prioritized master list of the patient's active, inactive, temporary, and potential medical and other problems; serves as an index to the rest of the record.

problem-oriented medical record (POMR) Method of recording data about the health status of a patient in a problem-solving system. Parts included are the data base, problem list, initial plan, and progress notes.

procidentia Uterine prolapse or herniation of the uterus into the vagina and at times beyond the vulva.

progesterone Female hormone that prepare the uterus to accept a fetus and maintain the pregnancy.

progress notes Notes made by a nurse, physician, or another team member that describe the patient's condition and the treatments given and planned.

prolactin A hormone secreted by the anterior pituitary gland. It is responsible for stimulating milk production in the mammary alveolar cells.

proliferation Reproduction, or multiplication of similar forms.

pronate Ventral surface of the body faces downward.

prone The body in horizontal position when lying face downward.

proportion Relationship between two ratios.

proprioception Sensation pertaining to stimuli originating from within the body regarding spatial position and muscular activity or to the sensory receptors that they activate. This sensation gives one the ability to know the position of the body without looking at it and the ability to "know objectively the sense of touch."

proprioceptor Any sensory nerve ending, such as those located in muscles, tendons, and joints, that responds to stimuli originating from within the body regarding movement and spatial position.

prostatodynia Pain in prostate gland.

prosthesis Artificial replacement for a missing body part.

protein (dietary) Any large group of naturally occurring, complex, organic nitrogenous compounds necessary for proper growth, development, and maintenance of health.

protest Initial grief response in separation from attachment figure.

pruritus The symptom of itching. An uncomfortable sensation leading to the urge to scratch. Scratching often results in secondary infection. Some causes of pruritus are allergy, infection, jaundice, and skin irritation.

pseudomenstruation Bleeding from the uterus, not accompanied by the usual changes in the endometrium. May be observed with the newborn in response to maternal hormones.

PSRO (Professional Standards Review Organization) Physicians review the services provided under Medicare, Medicaid, and Maternal-Child Health programs to ensure standards are being met and to ascertain the need for the program.

psychoactive material Substance that affects mental activity.

psychological age Behavioral capacity of the person to adapt to changing environmental demands; includes capacities of memory, learning, intelligence, skills, feelings, and motivations for exercising behavioral control or self-regulation.

psychosis Major disorder of organic or emotional origin, characterized by impairment of thought, communication, and memory and distortion of reality.

psychosocial Intellectual, emotional, and social components of the individual.

psychotic State characterized by gross distortion of reality and impaired social functioning.

ptosis Drooping of the eyelids.

pubarche Beginning development of certain secondary sex characteristics preceding physiological puberty.

puberty State of physical development when sexual reproduction first becomes possible, with menstruation and spermatogenesis (10 to 14 years for females; 12 to 16 years for males).

public health nursing Nursing assessment, identification of high-risk groups, intervention directed at disease prevention, and health education and promotion for all ages, groups, and individuals.

puerperium Period of time after the third stage of labor and lasting until involution of the uterus takes place, usually about 3-6 weeks.

pulmonary edema Accumulation of extravascular fluid in lung tissues and alveoli, caused most commonly by congestive heart failure.

pulmonary embolus (PE) Occlusion of a pulmonary artery by foreign matter, such as fat, air, tumor tissue, or a thrombus, that usually arises from a peripheral vein.

pulse A rhythmic beating or vibrating movement regular, recurrent expansion and contraction of an artery produced by waves of pressure caused by the ejection of blood from the left ventricle of the heart as it contracts.

pulse deficit A condition that exists when the radial pulse is less than the ventricular rate as auscultated at the apex.

pulse pressure Difference between systolic and diastolic pressure, usually 30 to 40 mm Hg.

pulverized Crushed to a powder.

punctum Tiny opening in the margin of each eyelid that opens into the tear duct.

pupil A circular opening in the iris or the eye, located slightly to the nasal side of the center of the iris.

pupillary reflex Adjustment of the eyes for near vision, consisting of pupillary constriction.

purulent Producing or containing pus.

pustulant vesicles Small, circumscribed pus-containing elevations of the skin.

pustule Small elevation of the skin containing fluid that is usually purulent.

pyrexia Fever or febrile condition in which the body's temperature is above 98.6° F (37° C).

pyrosis A burning sensation in the epigastric and sternal region, with raising of acid liquid from stomach; heartburn.

pyuria Pus in the urine.

quadrantectomy Another form of segmental mastectomy in which the quadrant of the breast in which the tumor is located is removed.

quality assurance/assessment/improvement In health care, any evaluation of services provided and the results achieved as compared to accepted standards.

RACE A formula to enable nurses to be prepared when safety is threatened by fire; *R*escue the patient, sound the *A*larm, *C*onfine the fire, *E*xtinguish or *E*vacuate.

racism Any ethnocentric activity—cultural, individual, or institutional, deliberate or note—that is based on a belief in the superiority of one racial group over other racial groups, thus maintaining the oppression and control of these groups.

radial pulse Pulse felt over the radial artery.

range of motion (ROM) Normal movement that any given joint is capable of making.

rapid eye movement One of the two highly individualized sleeping states that follow NREM state. May last from a few minutes to a half an hour and alternate with NREM periods; dreaming occurs during this time.

ratio Relationship of one number or quantity to another number or quantity.

reagent Substance producing a chemical reaction.

receptors Molecules that recognize or respond to specific invaders.

reciprocity Mutual agreement to exchange privilege, dependence, or relationships as an agreement between two governing bodies to accept the credit of care givers licensed in each state. True reciprocity means: Individuals licensed in one state can automatically receive licensure in the next, even if the licensing requirements of the states differ.

reconstituted/blended family Divorced or widowed adult and a new spouse, with each adult's own child(ren) plus the child(ren) of the new partnership, if any, who live together.

recording Process of adding written information to the chart, usually at prescribed intervals.

recumbent Lying down or leaning backwards.

Reed-Sternberg cells Atypical histiocytes; large, abnormal, multinucleated cells in the lymphatic system, found in Hodgkin's disease.

referred pain Pain that is felt at a site other than the injured or diseased organ or part of the body.

reflection Therapist's repetition of statements made by the patient; helps to clarify information.

reflex Reflected action, particularly an involuntary action or movement.

refraction Bending of light rays.

regurgitation Backward flowing, as the casting up of undigested food.

rehabilitation The process of maximizing an individual's abilities and resources to promote optimum growth and function by focusing on the individual's decision-making ability.

remission A decrease in the severity of the disease of any of its symptoms.

request for action Patient's request for physical activities or treatment nurses carry out, such as providing physical comfort measures or ensuring a safe and convenient environment.

request for comfort Patients' request to nurse for strength, cheer, or the easing of grief or trouble.

request for information Factual knowledge that the patient requires in order to understand and make decisions about health care.

request for understanding Patient's need to have the nurse demonstrate comprehension of what the patient is feeling or experiencing and the patient's reactions.

reservoir Any natural habitat of a microorganism that promotes growth and reproduction.

residual urine Urine remaining in the urinary tract after voiding.

residue Bulk in the colon that includes undigested food, fiber, bacteria, body secretions, and cells.

resignation Act of resigning; giving up a position of employment.

respiration The process of molecular exchange of oxygen and carbon dioxide within the body's tissue from the lungs to cellular oxidation processes.

respite Period of relief from responsibilities for the care of a patient.

responsibility Condition, quality, fact, or instance of being responsible. *Responsible* means expected or obliged to account for something to someone. It also means being able to distinguish between right and wrong and to think and act rationally and hence be accountable for one's behavior.

restitution In obstetrics, the turning of the fetal head to the left or right after it has completely emerged from the introitus as it assumes a normal alignment with the infant's shoulders.

restraint Any one of numerous devices used in aiding the immobilization of patients; the preferred term is now safety reminder device (SRD).

resumé A summary of educational and professional experiences, including activities and honors, to be used in seeking employment for biological citations on professional meeting programs or related purposes; curriculum vitae.

retention The inability to void even in the presence of an urge to void.

retina Ten-layered, delicate nervous tissue membrane of the eye, continuous with the optic nerve, that receives images of external objects and transmits impulses through the optic nerve to the brain.

retinal detachment Separation of the retina from the choroid in the posterior area of the eye.

retraction Visible sinking in of soft tissue of the chest between and around the firmer tissue of the ribs as occurs with increased respiratory effort.

retrovirus Composed of a genetic material called *RNA* instead of the more common DNA found in most living cells, retroviruses carry their genetic code in RNA rather than DNA material.

reversibility Performance of opposite mental actions with the same problem or situation, such as addition and subtraction or multiplication and division.

review of system (ROS) System-by-system review of the body functions. ROS is begun during the initial interview.

rhizotomy Resection of a posterior nerve root just before it enters the spinal cord, usually performed to control severe pain in the upper trunk or to relieve severe spasms.

ribosome Cytoplasmic organelle composed of ribonucleic acid and protein that functions in the synthesis of protein.

role A socially expected behavior pattern associated with an individual's function in various social groups.

ROM Range of motion.

rubor Redness, especially when accompanying inflammation.

rugae Fold or crease, especially one of the folds of the mucous membrane on the internal surface of the stomach.

rule of nines Divides the body into multiples of nine; is used to determine the total body surface area (BSA) involved in burn trauma.

safety reminder device Any one of numerous devices used to immobilize a patient; formerly referred as *restraint.*

sanguineous Pertaining to blood.

sarcoma Malignant tumor of connective tissues such as muscle or bone.

satiety Feeling of fullness and satisfaction from food.

scale Small, thin flake of keratinized (dried-out) epithelium.

scar Connective tissue that is avascular, pale, contracted, and firm after the earlier phase of healing.

schema Innate knowledge structure that allows a child to organize its mind.

school age Period from about 6 to 16 years of age.

sclera Outermost tunic of the eyebulb composed of thick, white connective tissue that gives shape and protection to the eyeball.

scoliosis Curvature of the spine usually consisting of two curves: the original abnormal curve and a compensatory curve in the opposite direction.

scurvy Condition resulting from lack of ascorbic acid (small sacs)(vitamin C) in the diet.

sebaceous gland One of the many small sacculated organs in the dermis that secrete oil.

sebum Oily secretion from the sebaceous glands.

second intention Wound closure in which the edges are separated, granulation tissue develops to fill in the gap, and epithelium grows in over the granulation producing a scar.

secondary gain Material, emotional, or social advantage acquired as a result of a symptom or an illness.

second-level patient-focused responses Learned professional communication responses controlling the amount of nurses' personal investment in patients' suffering.

self-bath Bath done by the patient in bed or at the bedside.

self-concept How an individual views the self; pertains to personal identity, body image, role, and self-esteem.

self-despair Feeling that life has not been satisfactory and having a desire to relive it.

self-disclosure Nurses' revelations about self to a patient for the purpose of communicating understanding.

semicircular canals Any of three bony, fluid-filled loops in the osseous labyrinth of the internal ear, associated with the sense of balance.

semi-Fowler's position Position the patient assumes while lying in bed; the head of bed is raised to about 30 degrees, and the foot of bed is raised slightly.

semilunar valve Valve with half-moon-shaped cusps, such as the aortic valve and the pulmonary valve.

seminal vesicles Paired structures that lie at the base of the bladder and produce 60% of the volume of semen.

senescence phase The last stage of the life cycle which requires the older adult to cope with a long range of changes.

senility Pertaining to or characteristic of old age or the process of aging, especially the physical or mental disorientation accompanying aging.

sensitivity A laboratory method of determining the effectiveness of antibiotics. A report of resistance means the antibiotic is not affective in inhibiting the growth of a pathogen, whereas use of an effective antibiotic results in a "sensitive" report.

sensorimotor The developmental phase of childhood, encompassing the period from birth to 2 years of age, according to Piaget's psychology. In this stage, an infant's knowledge of the work comes about primarily through sensory impressions and motor activities.

sensory (afferent) neurons Cell of the nervous system consisting of afferent fibers that conduct sensory impulses from the periphery of the body to the brain or spinal cord via the dorsal spinal roots.

separation anxiety Fear and apprehension caused by separation from familiar surroundings and significant persons.

septum The muscular partition that separates the right and left heart.

sequela Any abnormal condition that occurs after a disease, treatment, or injury.

sequestrum A fragment of necrotic bone that is partially or entirely detached from the surrounding or adjacent healthy bone.

seriation Mental ordering of objects according to height, weight, or strength.

seroconversion The development of detectable levels of antibodies; a change in serologic tests from negative to positive as antibodies develop in reaction to an infection.

seronegative Lacking HIV antibodies; confirmed by blood tests.

serosanguineous Thin and red fluid composed of serum and blood.

serous Pertaining to, resembling, or producing serum; the clear watery portion of the blood.

sex education Factual teaching about anatomy and physiology related to the sex act and reproduction.

sex hormones Biochemical agents that influence structure and function of sex organs and appearance of sexual characteristics.

sexuality education Learning about self as a sexual being.

shearing Applied force or pressure exerted against the surface and layers of the skin as tissue slides in opposite but parallel planes.

shock Abnormal condition of inadequate blood flow to the peripheral tissues, with life-threatening cellular dysfunction, hypotension, and oliguria.

sibling Brother or sister.

sickled cell Erythrocyte whose characteristic round shape has altered to an elongated crescent shape.

sigh A periodic deep inspiration.

sign An objective finding as perceived by the examiner.

Sims position Lying on the left side with the right knee and thigh drawn upward toward the chest; the chest and abdomen are allowed to fall forward.

single parent One parent who lives with the child(ren).

single parent family Family group occurs when one parent leaves the nuclear family because of divorce, separation, desertion, or death. May also be the result of unwed parents living alone or the decision of a single person to adopt a child.

singultus Hiccups.

situational loss Loss occurring suddenly in response to a specific external event such as the sudden death of a loved one or the unemployed person who suffers the loss of self-esteem.

sitz bath Bath in which only the hips and buttocks are immersed in water or saline solution; the time allotted is 20 to 30 minutes.

skin graft Portion of skin implanted to cover areas where skin has been lost by burns or injury.

skin impairment Disruption of the surface skin that breaks open and becomes a decubitus ulcer that can penetrate to the bone.

smear Material placed on a glass slide or culture medium for microscopic examination.

Snellen Eye chart test for visual acuity; letters, number, or symbols are arranged on the chart in decreasing size from top to bottom.

SOAPE charting Charting format used in POMR. Components include subjective data (S) reported by the patient; objective data (O) acquired by inspection, percussion, auscultation, and palpation and by tests, usually measurable findings; assessment (A) of the problem; plan (P) of care; and evaluation (E) of patient's response to the treatment plan.

SOAPIER charting Same as SOAPE charting except that intervention (I) and revision (R) are added. Interventions are specific actions carried out, and revisions are the changes to be made to the original plan.

social age Roles and habits of a person with respect to other members of society, resulting from the person's life course through various social institutions.

social contract family/cohabitation Unmarried couple living together and sharing roles and responsibilities similar to the nuclear family structure.

social network Interconnected group of cooperating significant others, related or not, with whom a person interacts.

sodium The most abundant electrolyte in the body; the major extracellular electrolyte.

somatization A disorder characterized by recurrent, multiple, physical complaints and symptoms for which there is no organic cause.

somatotropin Human growth hormone (HGH) secreted by the anterior pituitary gland; speeds up the cells' anabolism of amino acids, stimulating the anabolism of amino acids which in turn stimulate the systemic growth of the body.

sonorous wheezes Low-pitched, loud, course, snoring lung sounds.

souffle cup Ungraduated disposable paper cup.

spastic Spasms or other uncontrolled contractions of the skeletal muscles.

specific immunity (or **active acquired immunity**) Form of acquired immunity that results from production of antibodies in the cells.

specimen A small sample of something, intended to show the nature of the whole, such as a urine specimen.

speech Uttering of vocal sounds that form words and express thoughts.

spermatogenesis The process of development of spermatozoa.

sphenoid Central part of floor of cranium; large bone at base of the skull between the occipital and ethmoid in front, and the parietal and temporal bones at the side.

sphygmomanometer Device for measuring arterial blood pressure.

spiritual life That aspect of life involving religious beliefs or value systems.

spondylolisthesis Partial forward dislocation of a vertebra over the one below it, most commonly the fifth lumbar vertebra over the first sacral vertebra.

spores The reproductive cell of some genera of fungi or protozoa. These cells are highly resistant to heat and chemicals. Under proper environmental conditions they may revert to the actively multiplying form of bacterium (e.g., gas gangrene or tetanus).

stagnation or self-absorption Regression into adolescent or younger behavior, characterized by physical and psychological invalidism.

standards of care Those acts that are permitted to be performed or prohibited from being performed by a prudent person working within the parameters of training, license, and experience and the conditions existing at the time; the nurse's duty to a patient with whom there is an established nurse-patient relationship to provide reasonable, prudent care required by the circumstances.

standard operating procedure Written documents that contain rules, policies, procedures, regulations, and orders for the conduct of patient care in various stipulated circumstances that are unique to the agency.

stapedectomy The removal of the stapes of the middle ear and insertion of a graft and prosthesis.

stapes One of three tiny ossicles in the middle ear, resembling a stirrup.

stasis Disorder in which the normal flow of a fluid through a vessel of the body is slowed or halted.

statute Legislative act declaring, commanding, or prohibiting something.

steatorrhea Excessive fat in the feces.

sterile Free of germs.

sterilization A process by which all microorganisms, including their spores, are destroyed.

stertorous Pertaining to a respiratory effort that is strenuous and struggling; having a snoring sound.

stethoscope. An instrument used in mediate auscultation, consisting of two ear pieces connected by means of flexible tubing to a diaphragm, which is placed against the patient's chest or back to hear heart and lung sounds.

stoma Combining form meaning a mouth or opening.

stomatitis Inflammation of the mouth due to destruction of normal cells of the oral cavity that may result from infection by bacteria, viruses, or fungi from exposure to certain chemicals or drugs, vitamin deficiency, or systemic inflammatory disease.

strabismus Eyes unable to focus in the same direction, commonly called *cross-eyed.*

stress The nonspecific response of the body to any demand made on it.

stressor A situation, activity, or event that produces stress.

stridor Harsh sound during respirations high pitched and resembling the blowing of wind, due to obstruction of air passages.

subcultures An ethnic, regional, economic or social group with characteristic patterns of behavior and ideals that distinguish it from the rest of a culture or society.

subjective data Symptoms, verbal statements provided by the patient. That which arises from within or is perceived by the individual and related to the examiner.

subjective data collection Process in which data relating to the patient's problems are elicited from the patient.

sublingual Under the tongue.

subluxation Partial dislocation.

sudoriferous gland One of about 3 million tiny structures within the dermis that produce sweat.

suicide The intentional taking of one's own life.

sulfate (SO_4) Salt of sulfuric acid, which is plentiful in the body.

summons A court order advising the defendant that a lawsuit against him is pending.

supination One of the kinds of rotation allowed by certain skeletal joints that allows the palm of the hand to turn upward.

supine Being in the horizontal position, lying face upward.

support Anything nurses communicate or provide patients that helps them function more effectively or makes them feel better about how they are functioning.

suppression Cessation of urine production (anuria).

suppuration To produce purulent matter.

surface tension The tendency of the surface of a liquid to minimize the area of its surface by contracting; this property affects the exchange of gases in the pulmonary alveoli.

surfactant Lipoprotein necessary for normal respiratory function that prevents alveolar collapse (atelectasis).

surgery Branch of medicine concerned with diseases and trauma requiring operative procedures.

surgical asepsis A group of techniques that destroy all microorganisms and their spores (sterile technique).

surveillance Exercise of continuous scrutiny of and watchfulness over the distribution and spread of infections and factors related thereto, of sufficient accuracy and completeness to be effective control.

suture Surgical stitch taken to repair a tear, incision, or wound.

sweat test Method for evaluating sodium and chloride excretion from the sweat glands; often the first test performed in the diagnosis of cystic fibrosis.

sympathetic nervous system Part of the nervous system that accelerates heart rate, constricts blood vessels, and raises blood pressure.

sympathy Expressions of nurses' own sorrow or regret at patients' plight.

symptom Subjective indication of a disease or a change in condition as perceived by the patient.

synapse Region surrounding the point of contact between two neurons or between a neuron and an effector organ, across which nerve impulses are transmitted through the action of a neurotransmitter such as acetylcholine or norepinephrine.

synarthrosis Any one of many immovable joints, such as those of the skull segments, in which a fibrous tissue or a hyaline cartilage connects the bones.

syncope A transient loss of consciousness due to inadequate blood flow to the brain (fainting).

syndactyly Malformation of digits, commonly seen as a fusion of two or more toes to form one structure.

syndrome Complex of signs and symptoms.

synergistic Action of two or more substances or organs to achieve an effect of which each is incapable.

synovectomy Excision of a synovial membrane of a joint.

syntaxis (consensual) communication Communication in which two people can understand the meaning of their dialogue together, explore and agree on meanings of words used, and speak in cause-effect relationships.

system A group of organs arranged in such a way that they can together perform a more complex function than can any organ alone.

systole The contraction of the heart, driving blood into the aorta and pulmonary arteries.

systolic Maximum blood pressure; occurs during contractions of the blood vessels, recorded as the upper blood pressure measurement.

T cell A small, circulating lymphocyte that participates in cellular immune responses, such as graft rejection and delayed hypersensitivity.

tachycardia An abnormal condition in which the myocardium contracts regularly but at a rate greater than 100 beats per minute.

tachypnea An abnormally rapid rate of breathing.

tactile fremitus Tremulous vibration of the chest wall felt on palpation.

TBI Traumatic brain injury.

temperature Relative measure of sensible heat or cold.

tendons White glistening, fibrous bonds of tissue that attach muscle to bone.

tenesmus Ineffective and painful straining with defecation.

TENS See *transcutaneous electrical nerve stimulation.*

tepid Moderately warm to the touch.

teratogenic agent Any drug, virus, or irradiation, the exposure to which can cause malformation of the fetus.

tertiary intention (or third intention) Wound closure in which granulation tissues fill the gap between the edges of the wound with epithelium growing over the granulation at a slower rate and producing a larger scar than results from healing from second intention. Suppuration is also usually found.

testosterone Male hormone that contributes to development of male characteristics.

tetanus toxoid Active agent prepared from detoxified tetanus toxin that produces an antigenic response in the body, conferring permanent immunity to tetanus infection.

tetany Condition characterized by cramps, muscle twitching, and possible convulsions as a result of low blood calcium.

thanatologist One who studies dying and death.

thanatology The study of dying and death.

therapeutic Beneficial.

therapeutic communication Process in which a nurse helps the patient to a better understanding through verbal or nonverbal communication.

therapeutic diet A diet used as a medical treatment.

third party payers Entities (persons or elements) other than the giver or receiver of service responsible for payment (e.g., medicare or insurance company.)

thoracentesis The surgical perforation of the chest wall and pleural space with a needle for the aspiration of fluid for diagnostic or therapeutic purposes or for the removal of a specimen for biopsy.

thoracic cord injury Injury to the spinal column at the thoracic spine T1 and T12 and involves paralysis of lower extremities.

thrill Fine vibration felt by the examiner, indicating an organic murmur.

thrombocytes The smallest cells in the blood that are essential for the coagulation of blood and to maintain hemostasis.

thrombocytopenia Reduction in the number of circulating platelets, due to depression of the bone marrow.

thrombophlebitis Inflammation of a vein in conjunction with the formation of a thrombus.

thrombus Of or pertaining to a clot.

thymus gland It lies in the upper thorax, posterior to the sternum; it produces the hormone thymosin, which plays an active role in the immune system.

thyroid gland Butterfly-shaped endocrine gland with one lobe lying on either side of the trachea; it secretes thyroxine (T_4); triiodothyronine (T_3) and calcitonin.

thyroid-stimulating hormone (TSH) Secreted by the anterior pituitary gland; acts on the thyroid gland to increase thyroid hormone secretion.

tibia Lower leg bone, it articulates with the femur, lies medially, and bears the major portion of the body weight.

tinnitus A subjective noise sensation in one or both ears; ringing or tinkling sound in the ear.

tissue Collection of similar cells that act together in the performance of a particular function.

TMJ Temporomandibular joint.

toddler Child between the ages of 1 and 3 years.

tolerance A reduced response to a drug.

tolerance The ability to endure hardship, pain, or ordinarily injurious substances, such as drugs, without apparent physiological or psychological injury.

tongue depressor Wooden blade used to facilitate examination of the throat.

tonus(ic) Normal state of balanced tension in the tissues of the body, especially the muscles.

tophi Calculi containing sodium urate deposits that develop in periarticular fibrous tissue; typically found in patients with gout.

topical Applied to the skin.

TORCH (toxoplasmosis, other, rubella virus, cytomegalovirus, and herpes simplex viruses) Group of agents that can infect the fetus or the newborn infant, causing a constellation of morbid effects called *TORCH syndrome.*

tort The category of law involving civil wrongs against another's person or property. Torts include neglience, false imprisonment, assault, and battery.

total parenteral nutrition (TPN) Administration of a nutritionally complete solution through a central vein.

toxicity A condition that results from exposure to excess amounts of a substance that does not cause adverse effects in smaller amounts.

toxicological analysis Scientific study of poisons, their detection, and their effect.

trachea Windpipe; a tubelike structure that extends from the larynx approximately 5 inches to the midchest, where it divides into the right and left bronchi.

tracheostomy A surgical opening into the trachea through which an indwelling tube may be inserted.

tracheotomy Incision made into the trachea through the neck below the larynx, performed to gain access to the airway below blockage with a foreign body, tumor, or edema of the glottis.

tract In neurology, the neuronal axons grouped together to form a pathway.

traction Having a limb, bone, or group of muscles under tension with weights and pulleys; aligns or immobilizes the part and relieves pressure on it.

traditional or block chart Conventional patient chart broken down into sections or blocks; included are admission data, physicians' orders, history and physical, nursing care plan, nurses' notes and graphics, progress notes, and test data.

transcribe To write or type a copy of.

transcutaneous electrical nerve stimulation (TENS) A unit of pain control that is a pocket-sized, battery-operated device that provides a continuous, mild electrical current to the skin via electrodes.

transfer Moving a patient from one unit to another (intraagency transfer) or moving a patient from one health care facility to another (interagency transfer).

transformation Shift from one state to another, such as water to ice to vapor.

transient ischemic attack (TIA) Episode of cerebrovascular insufficiency, usually owing to partial occlusion of an artery by an atherosclerotic plaque or embolism.

trauma Physical injury caused by violent/disruptive action or psychic injury resulting from a severe emotional shock.

traumatic brain injury head injury, classifed as either penetrating or closed; may also be classified as mild, moderate, severe, or catastrophic.

Trendelenburg A position in which the patient is lying supine with his head lower than the body with body and legs elevated and on an incline.

trichomoniasis A sexually transmitted disease caused by protozoan *Trichomonas vaginalis.*

trigone Region between the two openings of the two ureters and the urethra.

trimester Three months.

trophic Having to do with nutritional status.

Trousseau's sign A test for latent tetany in which carpal spasms are induced by inflating a sphygmomanometer cuff on the upper arm; seen in hypocalcemia and hypomagnesemia.

trust Risk-taking process whereby an individual's situation depends on the future behavior of another person.

tube feeding Administration of nutritionally balanced, liquified foods or formula into the stomach, duodenum, or jejunum by way of a nasoenteric tube or a feeding ostomy.

turgor The normal resiliency of the skin caused by the outward pressure of the cells and interstitial fluid. May be assessed as increased or decreased skin turgor.

tylectomy The removal of a circumscribed area that includes the tumor; also called a *lumpectomy.*

tympanic Pertaining to the membranous eardrum.

tympanic membrane A thin, semi transparent membrane in the middle ear that transmits sound vibrations to the internal ear by means of the auditory ossicles (eardrums).

tympanoplasty One of several operative procedures on the ear drum or ossicles of the middle ear designed to restore or improve hearing in patients with conductive hearing loss.

tympanostomy tube Tubes inserted under general anesthesia to drain accumulated fluid from the middle ear space; also called *pressure equalizer (PE) tubes.*

tympany A high-pitched, drumlike sound produced by peforming percussion over a hollow organ such as the stomach.

type I diabetes mellitus Condition in which impaired glucose tolerance results because of destruction of beta cells in the pancreatic islets, resulting in deficient insulin production, but the patient retains normal sensitivity to insulin action; insulin-dependent diabetes mellitus.

type II diabetes mellitus Condition in which impaired glucose tolerance results from an abnormal resistance to insulin action; non-insulin-dependent diabetes mellitus.

umbilical cord Bluish-white, gelatinous structure that transports maternal blood from the placenta to the fetus.

umbilicus Point on the abdomen at which the umbilical cord joined the fetus. In most adults it is marked by a depression.

unassertive communications Nurses' failure to stand up for legitimate rights.

unilateral neglect Condition in which an individual is perceptually unaware of and inattentive to one side of the body.

universal donor Person with type O, Rh factor–negative blood. Such blood may be used for emergency transfusion with minimal risk of incompatibility.

universal precautions An approach to infection control designed to prevent transmission of blood-borne diseases such as AIDS and hepatitis B in health care settings.

urate Any salt of uric acid, as sodium urate.

ureters Extension of the kidney pelvis that extends 10 to 12 inches to the lower part of the urinary bladder.

urinal A device for receiving urine; may be male or female; may be used for specimen collection

urolithiasis Formation of urinary calculi.

urticaria Itching skin eruption characterized by welts of varying sizes with well-defined, inflamed margins and pale centers (also called *hives*).

uterine inertia Absence or weakness of uterine contractions during labor.

vagina Thin-walled, muscular, tubelike structure of the female genitalia, approximately 3 inches (7.5 cm) long.

value system The accepted mode of conduct and set of norms, goals, and values that the person has developed over many years, beginning in childhood.

values Intrinsic beliefs about the worth of an entity or concept that provide a basis for attitudes and behaviors and help persons to establish a hierarchy of needs and goals.

valve Combining form meaning "a thing that regulates the flow of."

varicose veins Tortuous, dilated vein with incompetent valves.

vegan Vegetarian whose diet excludes all foods of animal origin.

vehicle The means by which organisms are carried about.

veins Vessels that convey blood from the capillaries to the heart.

vena cava One of the two large veins returning blood from peripheral circulation to the right atrium of the heart.

venous stasis Disorder in which the normal flow of blood through a vein is slowed or halted.

ventilator Person in two-rescuer CPR who performs rescue breathing technique.

ventral Anterior, to face forward; the front of the body.

ventricles A small cavity, either of two lower chambers of the heart that when filled with blood contracts to propel it into the arteries.

venule Any of the small blood vessels that gather blood from the capillary plexuses and anastomose to form the veins.

verbal communications Messages nurses send through words, voice inflection, and rate of speech.

vernix caseosa Protective, gray-white fatty substance of cheesey consistency covering the fetal skin at birth.

verruca Benign, viral, warty skin lesion with a rough, papillomatous (nipple-like) growth).

vertigo The sensation that the outer world is revolving about oneself or that one is moving in space.

vesicle Circumscribed elevation of skin filled with serous fluid, smaller than 0.5 cm.

viable Capable of living, such as a normal human fetus that has reached a stage of development, usually 24 weeks, which will permit life outside the uterus.
villi Short vascular processes or protrusions clustered over the entire mucous surface of the small intestine.
virulence Power of a microorganism to produce disease; of or pertaining to a very pathogenic or rapidly progressive condition.
viscus Any large inferior organ in any of the great body cavities.
visual analog scale An objective means of assessing pain severity; it consists of a straight line, representing a continuum of intensity and has visual descriptors at each end.
vital signs Measurements of temperature, pulse, respiration, and blood pressure.
vitamin Organic compound essential in small quantities for normal physiological and metabolic functioning of the body.
vitreous humor A transparent jellylike substance filling the cavity behind the crystalline lens of the eye.
Volkmann's contracture A permanent contracture with clawhand, flexion of wrist and finger, and atrophy of the forearm that can occur as a result of compartment syndrome.
volvulus Twisting of the bowel on itself, causing intestinal obstruction.
vomer Bone forming the posterior and inferior part of the nasal septum, having two surfaces and four borders.

weaning Gradually eliminating breast or bottle feedings, replaced by cup and table feeding.
weight The force exerted on a body by the gravity of the earth. Normal weight depends upon the frame of the individual.
wellness Dynamic state of health in which an individual progresses toward a higher level of functioning, achieving an optimum balance between internal and external environments.
wellness nursing diagnosis A clinical judgment about an individual, group, or community in transition from a specific level of wellness to a higher level of wellness.
Wernicke's encephalopathy Inflammatory, hemorrhagic, degenerative condition of the brain caused by thiamine deficiency, seen in association with chronic alcoholism.
Western blot A laboratory blood test to detect the presence of antibodies to a specific antigen; used in diagnosing HIV.
Wharton's jelly Gelatinous tissue that remains when the embryonic body stalk blends with the yolk sac within the umbilical cord.
wheal Irregularly shaped, elevated area or superficial localized edema, varies in size (e.g., hive, mosquito bite).
wheeze A whistling or sighing sound resulting from narrowing the lumen of a respiratory passageway. May be heard both on inspiration and expiration. Wheezes characteristically clear on coughing; crackles do not.
whirlpool bath Immersion of the body or part of the body in a tank of hot water agitated by a jet of equally hot water and air.
white matter Tissue surrounding the gray matter of the spinal cord, consisting mainly of myelinated nerve fibers but with some unmyelinated nerve fibers embedded in a spongy network of neuroglia.
widow(er)hood Status of the surviving spouse after the death of husband or wife.
Wilms' tumor Malignant neoplasm of the kidney, occuring in young children. The tumor, an embryonial adenomyosarcoma, is well encapsulated in the early stage but may later extend into the lymph nodes and the renal vein or vena cava and metastasize to the lungs or other sites.
withdrawal symptoms Unpleasant, sometimes life-threatening, physiological changes that occur when certain drugs are withdrawn after prolonged, regular use.
wound Any physical injury involving a break in the skin; caused by an act or accident rather than by a disease.

xerostomia Dryness of the mouth caused by cessation of normal salivation.
xiphoid Distal portion of the sternum.

young adulthood Chronologically, a period of life from the mid-20s to the mid-40s.

zygot Cell formed by the union of two reproductive cells; the fertilized ovum resulting from the union of a sperm and ovum; developing ovum from the time it is fertilized until, as a blastocyst, it is implanted in the uterus.

INDEX

Q

R

W

X

Y

Z

COMMON ABBREVIATIONS

° C	degrees Centigrade
° F	degrees Fahrenheit
ʒ	dram
@	at
♀	female
♂	male
>	greater than
<	less than
↑	increase
↓	decrease
1°	primary
2°	secondary
△	change
$\overline{aa}$	indicating equal amounts of each
ABG	arterial blood gas
ac	before meals
ad lib	freely as desired
ADL	activities of daily living
a.m.a.	against medical advice
BE	barium enema
bid	two times a day
BP	blood pressure
BRP	bathroom privileges
BUN	blood urea nitrogen
$\bar{c}$	with
c/o	complains of
cap	capsule
CBC	complete blood count
cc	cubic centimeter
CDC	Centers for Disease Control
cm	centimeter
CO	carbon monoxide
CO_2	carbon dioxide
CPR	cardiopulmonary resuscitation
CT	computed tomography
D_5W	5% dextrose in water
dl	deciliter
DNR	do not resuscitate
dx, Dx	diagnosis
ECG, EKG	electrocardiogram
EEG	electroencephalogram
elix	elixir
ER	emergency room
ESR	erythrocyte sedimentation rate
ETOH	ethyl alcohol
f ℥	fluid ounce
FUO	fever of unknown origin
Fx, fx	fracture, fractional urine test
g, gm, Gm	gram
GI	gastrointestinal
gr	grain
gt, gtt	drop, drops
GTT	glucose tolerance test
h/hr	hour
H&P	history and physical examination
Hct, HCT	hematocrit
Hgb	hemoglobin
HIV	human immunodeficiency virus (AIDS)
hs	at bedtime
I&O	intake and output
IDDM	insulin-dependent diabetes mellitus
IM	intramuscular
IV	intravenous
IVP	intravenous push; intravenous pyelogram
IVU	intravenous urogram
K	potassium
kg	kilogram
KUB	kidney, ureters, and bladder (radiograph)
KVO	keep vein open
L	liter
m	meter
m, min, ♍	minim
mcg	microgram
mg	milligram
ml	milliliter
mm	millimeter
mm Hg	millimeters of mercury
MRI	magnetic resonance imaging
O_2	oxygen
OD	right eye; optical density; overdose
OS	left eye
OZ, ℥	ounce
pc	after meals
PERRLA	pupils equal, round, and reactive to light and accommodation
pH	hydrogen ion concentration (acidity and alkalinity)
PO, po	orally
prn	when required, as often as necessary
q	every
qd	every day
qh	every hour
qid	four times a day
qod	every other day
ROM	range of motion
Rx	take; treatment
$\bar{s}$	without
sos	if necessary
SQ, subq, SC	subcutaneous
ss	half
SSE	soapsuds enema
stat	immediately
tid	three times a day
TLC	tender loving care
TKO	to keep open
TPR	temperature, pulse, and respirations
WBC	white blood cell, white blood count

NURSING CARE PLANS